Revised and Edited by

CLAYTON L. THOMAS, M.D., M.P.H

Consultant in Human Reproduction
Department of Population Sciences
Harvard School of Public Health

Vice President Medical Affairs
Tampax Incorporated

Taber's
CYCLOPEDIC
MEDICAL
DICTIONARY

EDITION **12** ILLUSTRATED

Taber's
CYCLOPEDIC
MEDICAL
DICTIONARY

F. A. DAVIS COMPANY PHILADELPHIA

United States of America
F. A. DAVIS COMPANY
1915 Arch Street, Philadelphia, Pa., 19103
Great Britain, Europe, and British Commonwealth
(Except as noted)
BLACKWELL SCIENTIFIC PUBLICATIONS LTD.
Osney Mead, Oxford, OX2 0EL, England
Canada
McGRAW-HILL RYERSON LIMITED
330 Progress Ave., Scarborough, 707, Ontario
India, Burma and Ceylon
THE KOTHARI BOOK DEPOT
King Edward Road, Parel, Bombay 12, India

INTRODUCTION TO EDITION 12

To have the privilege and responsibility of continuing the work of the accomplished medical lexicographer, the late Mr. Clarence Wilbur Taber, is awesome in view of the tradition of excellence he established for this Dictionary. Nevertheless, speaking for myself and the F. A. Davis Company, we can assure you, the reader, the high quality has been maintained so that this volume will be one of the most useful books you will ever own.

This Dictionary is intended for all concerned with promotion of health, care of the sick, and prevention of disease. Evidence of its usefulness to those persons is indicated by the fact that three million copies have been sold throughout most of the world.

The new and improved look of this edition is due in part to the fact that for the first time the Dictionary type has been set by computer. The Videocomp system provided easy retrieval of entries for editorial review and correction and permitted additions up to the setting of final pages.

For this reason we have been able to add terms not found in other medical dictionaries. Examples are blastokinin, careinoembryonic antigens, cup arthroplasty of the hip, donor card, endometrial jet washing, isotope cisternography, ketamine hydrochloride, laminar air flow, Lassa fever, liquid crystals, marantology, opportunistic infections, Optacon, organ perfusion system, primary physician, umbrella filter, umbrella pack, and zero population growth.

Obsolete tables and terms have been deleted. Important new tables have been added. The Medical Emergencies section of the Appendix has been carefully reviewed and revised where indicated. This includes a list of Poison Control Centers in the United States and Canada. A table for Radiological Emergencies has been added to the text. Fifty illustrations are either new or revised.

Because the metric system will become the accepted international standard for weights and measures, all values for weight, measure, or volume have been provided in both the metric and English system units.

As in previous editions we note our considerable debt to the many persons who have taken the time to provide us with their constructive criticism and suggestions. These are most welcome and are given careful consideration in preparing each new edition.

On a very personal note I would like to thank the staff of the F. A. Davis Company, particularly the President Mr. Robert H. Craven, and Mrs. Miriam Maritato and Mrs. Eleanor Mora.

The assistance and understanding of a loving spouse permits many men and women the great luxury of doing the work which they find satisfying. Thus, to my wife Peggy I say thank you for being all things to me.

It has been my good fortune to be associated with a variety of persons who excel in their fields of endeavor. Two of these to whom I shall always be grateful are Hilton A. Salhanick, M.D., Professor in and Chairman of the department in which I am a consultant at the Harvard School of Public Health; and my employer Mr. Thomas F. Casey, President of Tampax Incorporated. The model of intellect and industry provided by both of these gentlemen is a continuing source of inspiration.

Clayton Lay Thomas, M.D., M.P.H.

SOURCES CONSULTED

This volume represents the labor of a great number of persons. Originally the scholarly endeavors of the late Clarence Wilbur Taber and the editorial staff of the F. A. Davis Company combined to produce a volume of such excellence as to stimulate attempts at imitation. The sources consulted by Mr. Taber included books, periodicals, other scholars, and practitioners in all areas of nursing and medicine. They would, if listed, fill a great number of pages.

There is no reason to alter this formula. We would, however, be negligent if we failed to express our debt to the world of learning as represented by the work of physicians, scientists, and nurses in all branches of human biology and medicine. Their work product available in texts and journals are the life blood of all of us who strive to produce and maintain the quality of this Dictionary.

The gratitude of us all to libraries and their staffs must be acknowledged as the *sine qua non* for the production of a dictionary.

Clayton Lay Thomas, M.D., M.P.H.

FEATURES AND THEIR USE

ONLY a thoroughly trained mechanic would pretend to understand the workings of a complicated piece of machinery with its thousands of parts. Almost anyone, however, feels competent to use and understand a dictionary that in reality represents hundreds of highly specialized subjects. To most persons, a dictionary is a dictionary. Nevertheless, *Taber's Cyclopedic Medical Dictionary* contains many subjects and features never before incorporated in such a reference work.

This work is a medical dictionary, but it is more than that. It is as much a dictionary of medical subject matter as it is a dictionary of medical terms. It is a source book of medical knowledge that will save much time in consulting a great many other works. A few of its more outstanding features are the following:

Pronunciations: At least 90% of all main entries are respelled for pronunciation. Long and short vowels are marked diacritically, and primary and secondary accents are shown. Latin rules cannot be depended upon for the pronunciation of medical words, and authorities do not agree upon standardized pronunciations. Common usage, however, seems to prevail, and this has been followed as much as feasible in this book. Respellings for pronunciation are accurate and do not distort the actual spelling of the word any more than is necessary to indicate the proper phonetic sound.

Spellings: Diphthongs are eliminated where possible. In most cases the letter "k" is substituted for "c" in such words as leukocytes. Words formerly hyphenated are now indicated as one word, i.e. gastrointestinal. Only proper nouns are capitalized, but proper nouns used as adjectives do not take a capital initial.

Vocabulary: This glossary is sufficiently extensive to meet the daily needs of the practicing physician, medical student, nurse, and others concerned with all aspects of medicine. Obsolete words and highly specialized topics which belong in separate lexicons have been eliminated. Hundreds of drugs which have not been in general use for many years, have been eliminated to make room for new drugs. Medical literature is constantly searched in order to provide the latest terms in good medical standing.

Definitions: These stand out in a paragraph separate and apart from all collateral terms and apart from additional supplementary matter, thus making it easy to read the definitions. The majority of synonyms have their own complete definitions, even at the risk of duplication.

There probably is no profession in which there is less agreement regarding certain subjects than Medicine. The prevailing opinion of the profession, however, has been given in this dictionary, in so far as this has been available. Unfortunately this may result in an adverse opinion in some instances, especially if the consultant is not familiar with opposing views or unduly favorable to a definition other than the one expressed.

Subtopics: Many related words are listed and defined in most dictionaries in the same paragraph, such as the many acids, or different forms of the same disease. In this dictionary each of these words has its own vocabulary entrance with its definition separate and apart from other material. These topics are listed in alphabetical order, making access to them easy and quick.

Etymologies: This is the only abridged medical dictionary containing the derivations of words indicating their Latin, Greek, and other sources with their meanings. These are not merely reproductions from other works, but the result of research which has made possible a great degree of accuracy. Prefixes and Suffixes also appear in alphabetical order.

Medical Synonyms: Medical synonyms are incorporated with the definition of a word. This is a great aid to medical writers and speakers.

Words Pertaining To: In many cases a list of other words pertaining to the one defined follows important main entries. Therefore a complete study of a given term may be made by reading the definitions of words on the list. In some instances a short list of related subjects will follow the word defined.

First Aid: Practically every form of accident is listed with first aid treatment. Included among these are poisons and their antidotes, bites and stings of all kinds, fractures, and other accidents, including different forms of unconsciousness. Tables concerning these emergencies are located in the Appendix.

Diseases: The principal diseases with their various forms are given together with diagnosis, symptoms, prognosis, treatment, and nursing procedures, including diet.

Dietetics: A great number of foods are listed along with nutritional data including caloric, fat, protein, carbohydrate, vitamin, and mineral content.

Drugs: Many of the terms for drugs are given their trade-mark names, even though no references to the trade-mark or proprietary nature of the drug may be given in the individual listing. These names are in common use by physicians and nurses who may be more familiar with them than with their scientific names.

Nursing Procedures: More of these are given than are usually found in the handbooks of nursing on the market.

Tabulations: Many important tabulations are found in the text, but long tables which interfere with finding words in the dictionary are grouped in the Appendix.

The Interpreter: This contains the questions and statements which are most often used during examination and in taking the patient's history to aid in establishing diagnoses. To aid the physician in finding specific questions and possible answers, the phrases are grouped in distinct categories in the Table of Contents to The Interpreter. Each item is in five languages: English, Spanish, Italian, French, and German.

Continual use of this dictionary reveals its value and usefulness to those who are concerned with preventing illness and caring for the sick.

FACT FINDING INDEX

The user of reference works seldom is aware of the many subjects they contain. The following index lists a few of the entries in this Dictionary covering such important subjects as Diagnosis, First Aid, Nursing Procedures and Poisoning. Many other subjects could be listed in the same manner; however, they will be found in regular alphabetical order.

PRONUNCIATION

Diacritics: These are marks over or under vowels to indicate pronunciation. It is impractical in a specialized abridged dictionary to mark all the vowel sound variances as used in dictionaries of the English language. Therefore only two diacritics are used in this dictionary: the macron ‾ showing the name sound or long sound of vowels, as the *a* in rāte, *e* in rēbirth, *i* in īsle, *o* in ōver, and *u* in ūnite; and the breve ˘ showing the short sound of vowels, as the *a* in ăpple, *e* in ĕver, *i* in ĭt, *o* in nŏt, *u* in cŭt. Occasionally, vowels of a foreign language are indicated.

Accents: These are marks used to indicate stress upon certain syllables. A single accent ′ is called a primary accent. A double accent ″ is called a secondary accent; it indicates less stress upon a syllable than that given by a primary accent. Examples are *ŏb′jĕct* and *ŏb-jĕk″tĭ-fĭ-kā′shŭn.*

ABBREVIATIONS
USED IN THE TEXT

ABBR.	abbreviation	I.V.	intravenous(ly)
AmerInd.	American Indian	K	potassium, kalium
approx.	approximately	kcal.	kilocalorie, Calorie
AS.	Anglo-Saxon	kg.	kilogram
at. no.	atomic number	L.	Latin
at. wt.	atomic weight	LL.	Late Latin
C.	Centigrade	ME.	Middle English
C	carbon	Mg	magnesium
Ca	Calcium	mg.	milligram
Cal.	large Calorie (i.e. kilocalorie)	ml.	milliliter
		N	nitrogen
cal.	small calorie	NA	Nomina Anatomica (Parisiensia)
cc.	cubic centimeter		
Cl	chlorine	Na	sodium, natrium
CNS.	central nervous system	NP.	nursing procedure
CONTRA.	contraindication	O	oxygen
Cu	copper, cuprum	OB.	obstetrics
D.	Dutch	O.Fr.	Old French
E.	English	ONP.	operating nursing procedure
e.g.	for example		
esp.	especially	P	phosphorus
ETIOL.	etiology	pert.	pertaining
Ex.	example	pl.	plural
F.	Fahrenheit	PROG.	prognosis
F.A.	first aid	q.v.	which see
Fe	iron, ferrum	rel.	relating, related
Fr.	French	RS.	related subjects
FUNCT.	function	S	sulfur
Ger.	German	sing.	singular
gm.	gram(s)	Sp.	Spanish
Gr.	Greek	sp. gr.	specific gravity
gr.	grain(s)	SYM.	symptoms
H	hydrogen	SYMB.	symbol
I	iodine	SYN	synonym
i.e.	that is	USP.	United States Pharmacopoeia
I.M.	intramuscular(ly)		
I.U.	International Unit	viz.	namely

A

Å. Abbr. for *Angstrom unit.*

A₂. Abbr. for *aortic second sound.*

A.A. Abbr. for *achievement age; Alcoholics Anonymous.*

a. Abbr. for *accommodation; ampere; anode; anterior; area; artery.*

āā. Abbr. Gr. *ana,* of each. Prescription sign meaning the *stated amount of each of the substances is to be taken.*

a-, an-. Prefix meaning *without, away from, not.*

A.A.A.S. Abbr. for *American Association for the Advancement of Science.*

A.A.F.P. Abbr. for *American Academy of Family Practice.*

A.A.G.P. Abbr. for *American Academy of General Practice,* former name of the American Academy of Family Practice.

A.A.M.R.L. Abbr. for *American Association of Medical Record Librarians.*

A.A.P. Abbr. for *American Academy of Pediatrics.*

Aaron's sign (ār'ŏn). [Charles D. Aaron, Amer. physician, 1866-1951] Distress in region of heart or stomach upon pressure over McBurney's point, q.v., in appendicitis.

ab- [L.]. Prefix meaning *from, away from, negative, absent.*

abactus venter [L. *abactus,* driven away, + L. *venter,* belly]. Induced abortion, q.v.

Abadie's sign (ă-bă-dēz'). 1. [Charles A. Abadie, Fr. ophthalmologist, 1842-1932]. In exophthalmic goiter, spasm of the levator palpebrae superioris. 2. [Jean Abadie, Fr. neurologist, 1873-1946]. In tabes dorsalis, insensibility to pressure over the Achilles tendon.

abaissement (ă-bās'mon) [Fr., a lowering]. 1. Depression. 2. In ophthalmology, a synonym for lenticular displacement (couching). 3. Falling.

abalienated (ăb-āl'yĕn-ă-tĕd) [L. *abalienare,* to separate from]. Insane.

abalienatio mentis (ăb-āl''yĕn-ā'shī-ō mĕn'tĭs). Insanity.

abalienation (ab-āl-yen-ā'shun) [L. *abalien-āre,* to separate from]. Physical or mental decay; lunacy or derangement.

abaptiston (ă''bap-tis'ton) [Gr. *abaptistos, a-,* not + *baptistos,* dipped]. Trephine that cannot slip and injure the brain.

abarognosis (ăb''ăr-ŏg-nō'sĭs) [Gr. *a-,* not, + *baros,* weight, + *gnosis,* knowledge]. Loss of sense of weight. SYN: *baragnosis.*

abarthrosis (ab-ar-thrō'sis) [L. *ab,* from, + Gr. *arthron,* joint]. A movable joint or point

upon which bones move freely upon each other. SYN: *diarthrosis.*

abartic'ular ["+ *articulus,* joint]. At a distance from a joint.

abarticula'tion. 1. Dislocation of a joint. 2. Diarthrosis.

abasia (ă-bā'zī-ă) [Gr. *a-,* not, + *basis,* step]. Motor incoordination in walking. Inability to walk due to impairment of coordination.

    a. **-astasia.** Lack of motor coordination with inability to stand or walk. SYN: *astasia-abasia.*

    a., **atactic.** Uncertain movements in walking. SYN: *ataxic abasia.*

    a., **choreic.** Associated with chorea of the legs.

    a., **paralytic.** That in which the leg muscles are paralyzed.

    a., **paroxysmal trepidant.** That caused by trembling and sudden stiffening of legs on standing, making walking impossible.

    a., **spastic.** Paroxysmal trepidant abasia.

    a., **trembling, a. trepidans.** That due to trembling of the legs.

abasic (ă-bā'sik). Pert. to abasia. SYN: *abatic.*

abate (ă-bāt') [L. *ab,* from, + *battere,* to beat]. 1. To lessen or decrease. 2. To cease or cause to cease.

abatement (ă-bāt'mĕnt). Decrease in severity of pain or symptoms.

abatic (ă-băt'ĭk). Pert. to abasia. SYN: *abasic.*

abaxial, abaxile (ab-ak'sī-al, ab-ak'sĭl) [L. *ab,* from + *axis*]. 1. Not in line of axis of the body or a part. 2. At opposite end of the axis of a part.

Abbe's condenser (ab'bā). [Ernst Abbe, Ger. physicist, 1840-1905] Several achromatic lenses attached to a microscope to increase illumination.

Abbe's operation. [Robert Abbe, Amer. surgeon, 1851-1928] 1. Resection of fifth nerve for tic douloureux. 2. Lateral anastomosis of the intestine.

Abbe-Zeiss apparatus. [E. A.; Carl Zeiss, Ger. optician, 1816-1888] A device for counting blood cells in a specific quantity of blood. SYN: *Thoma-Zeiss counting cell hemocytometer.*

Abbott's method. [Edville G. Abbott, Amer. orthopedic surgeon, 1870-1938] Treatment of scoliosis by a series of plaster jackets.

Abbott-Miller tube. [W. Osler Abbott, Amer. physician, 1902-1943; T. Grier Miller,

Amer. physician, 1866 -] A double channel intestinal tube used to relieve intestinal distention. Commonly called Miller-Abbott tube.

Abbott-Rawson tube. [W. O. A.; Arthur J. Rawson, Amer. scientist, 1896-] Double barrelled gastroenterostomy tube.

abdomen (ab-do'men, ab'do-men) [L., *belly*]. [NA] That portion of the trunk located between the chest and the pelvis; the upper portion of the abdomino-pelvic cavity.

Contains the stomach with lower part of esophagus, small and large intestines, liver, gallbladder, spleen, pancreas, and bladder. A serous membrane, the peritoneum, lines this cavity. SEE: *abdominal cavity; a. regions.*

a., accordion. Swelling of the abdomen which comes and goes rapidly. Due to nervousness. SYN: *abdominal pseudotympany.*

a., acute. Medical jargon used to denote any acute abdominal condition demanding prompt operation.

a., boat-shaped. A., scaphoid, q.v.

a., carinate. A., scaphoid, q.v.

a., navicular. A., scaphoid, q.v.

a. obstipum. Congenital shortness of the rectus abdominis muscle.

a., pendulous. Condition in which the excessively relaxed anterior wall of the abdomen hangs down over the pubis.

a., scaphoid. One in which the anterior wall is hollowed, presenting a sunken appearance as in emaciation and some cerebral diseases.

a., surgical. A., acute, q.v.

abdominal (ab-dom'i-nal). Pert. to the abdomen, its function and disorders.

a. cavity. The cavity within the abdomen. It is lined with a serous membrane, the peritoneum, and contains the following organs: stomach with lower portion of esophagus, small and large intestines (except sigmoid colon and rectum), liver, gallbladder, spleen, pancreas, kidney and ureter. It is continuous with the pelvic cavity, the two comprising the abdomino-pelvic cavity.

a. crisis. Severe pain in the abdominal area. Usually refers to the pain which occurs during sickle cell anemia crisis or that due to syphilis.

a. decompression. Technique used in obstetrics to facilitate childbirth. The abdominal area is surrounded by an airtight chamber in which pressure may be intermittently decreased below atmospheric. During labor pains, the pressure is decreased and the uterus is permitted to work more efficiently because the abdominal muscles are elevated away from the uterus.

a. examination. AUSCULTATION: Listening to sounds produced in the abdomen. Useful in diagnosing aneurysm of abdominal aorta, fetal heart sounds and vascular sounds from placenta. Intestinal sounds may be absent in paralytic ileus, q.v.

INSPECTION: Most satisfactorily performed with patient on back with thighs slightly flexed. In health, abdomen is of an oval form, marked by elevations and depressions corresponding to abdominal muscles, umbilicus, and in some degree by form of adjacent viscera. Is larger relative to size of chest in children than in adults; more rotund and broader inferiorly in females than in males.

Alterations in shape due to disease are *first,* enlargement, which may be general and symmetrical, as in ascites; or partial and irregular, from tumors, hypertrophy of organs, as the liver and spleen, or from distention of portions of intestines by gas, as the colon in typhoid fever; *second,* retraction, as in extreme emaciation, and in several forms of cerebral disease, esp. noticeable in tuberculous meningitis of children.

The respiratory movements of abdominal walls bear a certain relation to movements of the thorax; are often increased when the latter are arrested and vice versa; thus abdominal movements are increased in pluerisy, pneumonia, pericarditis, etc., but decreased or wholly suspended when disease causes abdominal pain, or in peritonitis.

The superficial abdominal veins are also at times visibly enlarged, indicating an obstruction to the flow of blood, either in the portal system as in cirrhosis, or in the inferior vena cava.

PALPATION: May be performed with tips of fingers, whole hand, or both hands; pressure may be slight or forcible, continuous or intermittent. To obtain greatest amount of information, patient should be placed in horizontal position with head slightly raised and thighs flexed. Sometimes necessary to place in standing position or leaning forward.

Findings Detectable by Palpation: Size and position of viscera; existence of tumors and swellings, whether superficial or deep, large or small, hard or soft, smooth or nodulated, movable or fixed, solid or liquid, and whether they change position with respiration. Also ascertain whether tenderness exists in any portion of the abdominal cavity, and if pain is increased or relieved by firm pressure.

Impulse, if one exists, is systolic and expansive, though when situated high up there also may be a slight diastolic movement. A thrill is rarely perceptible. Surface of tumor, when not ruptured is rounded and smooth. Effusion of blood into surrounding tissues may produce lobulations.

PERCUSSION: Patient should be placed in same position as for palpation, and percussion should be for most part mediate. In exploring abdomen by means of percussion, finger should first be placed immediately below the xiphoid cartilage, pressed firmly down, and carried along the median line toward the pubes, striking it all the way, now forcibly, now gently. The different tones of stomach, colon, and small intestines will be distinctly heard. Percussion should then be made laterally, alternately to one side, then the other, till whole surface is percussed. Abdominal aneurysm gives dullness or flatness over it unless a distended intestine lies above it.

a. gestation. Abdominal pregnancy. Extrauterine pregnancy in belly cavity.

a. inguinal ring. The internal opening of the inguinal canal, bounded inferiorly by the inguinal ligament, medially by the inferior epigastric vessels, and above and laterally by the lower free border of the transversus abdominis muscle. SYN: *deep inguinal ring; interior abdominal ring.* SEE: *inguinal canal; inguinal ring.*

a. quadrants. Four parts or divisions of the abdomen determined by drawing a vertical and a horizontal line through the umbilicus. The quadrants and their contents are:

Right upper q.: Right lobe of liver, gallbladder, part of transverse colon, part of pylorus, hepatic flexure, right kidney, and duodenum. *Right lower q.:* Cecum, ascending colon, small intestine, appendix, bladder if distended, right ureter, right spermatic duct in male, right ovary and right tube, uterus if enlarged in female.

Left upper q.: Left lobe of liver, stomach, transverse colon, splenic flexure, pancreas, left kidney, and spleen. *Left lower q.:* Small intestine, left ureter, sigmoid flexure, descending colon, bladder if distended, left spermatic duct in male, left ovary and left tube, uterus if enlarged in female.

a. reflexes. Contraction of the muscles of the abdominal wall upon stimulation of the overlying skin. Absence of these reflexes indicates damage to the pyramidal tract.

a. regions. The abdomen and its external surface are divided into nine regions by four imaginary planes: two horizontal, one at the level of the ninth costal cartilage (or the lowest point of the costal arch), and the other at the level of the highest point of the iliac crest; two vertical, through the centers of the inguinal ligaments (or through the nipples, or through the centers of the clavicles), or curved and coinciding with the lateral borders of the two abdominal rectus muscles.

a. rings. The apertures in the abdominal wall. *a.r., external:* An interval in aponeurosis of external oblique muscle, just above and to outer side of crest of the pubic bone. *a.r., triangular:* About one inch from base to apex, and half an inch transversely; gives passage to spermatic cord in male, round ligament in female. *a.r., internal or deep:* Situated in the transversalis fascia, midway between the anterior superior spine of ilium and symphysis pubis, half inch above Poupart's ligament; oval form, larger in male. Transmits spermatic cord in male, round ligament in female.

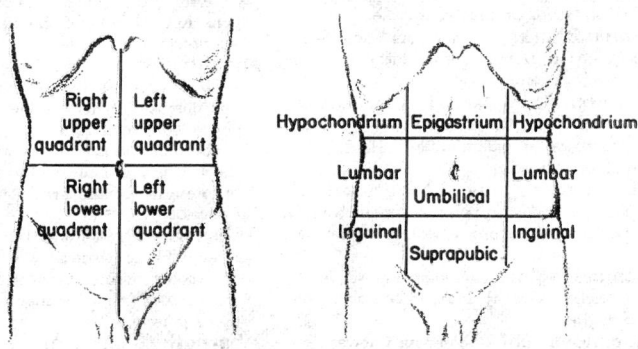

ABDOMINAL REGIONS

a. section. Abdominal incision for any operation on abdominal organs. SEE: *laparotomy.*

abdominalgia (ab-dom-ĭ-nal'jĭ-ă) [L. *abdomen,* + Gr. *algos,* pain]. Pain in the abdomen.

abdomino- (ab-dom'ĭ-nō). Combining form; relating to the stomach.

abdominoanterior (ab-dom''ĭ-nō-an-tē'rĭ-or). Position of fetus in uterus with belly facing anterior abdominal wall of mother.

abdom"inocar'diac re'flex. A change in heart rate, usually a slowing, resulting from mechanical stimulation of abdominal viscera.

abdominocentesis (ab-dom''ĭ-nō-sen-tē'sis) [L. *abdomen,* + Gr. *kentēsis,* puncture]. Puncture of the abdomen with an instrument for withdrawal of fluid from the abdominal cavity. SYN: *paracentesis abdominis.*

abdom"inocys'tic ["+ Gr. *kystis,* bladder]. Pertaining to abdomen and bladder.

abdominogenital (ăb-dŏm''ĭ-nō-jĕn'ĭ-tal) ["+ *genitalis*]. Pertaining to the abdomen and genital organs.

abdom"inohysterec'tomy ["+ Gr. *hystera,* uterus, + *ektomē,* excision]. Removal of uterus through abdominal incision.

abdominohysterotomy (ăb-dŏm''ĭ-nō-hĭstĕr-ŏt'ŏ-mĭ) ["+ "+ *tomē,* a cutting]. Incision of the uterus through a surgical opening in the abdomen.

abdom"inoposte'rior. Position of fetus in uterus with abdomen toward mother's back.

abdominoscopy (ăb-dom''ĭ-nŏs'kŏ-pĭ) [L. *abdomen,* belly, + Gr. *skopein,* to view]. Examination, especially by instrument, of abdomen or its viscera.

abdom"inoscro'tal ["+ *scrotum,* bag]. Pertaining to the abdomen and scrotum.

a. muscle. Cremaster muscle.

abdominothoracic (ab-dom''ĭ-nō-tho-ras'ĭk) ["+ Gr. *thōrax,* breastplate]. Pert. to the abdomen and thorax.

a. arch. The costal arch, a line dividing the thorax from the abdomen.

abdominous (ăb-dŏm'ĭ-nŭs). Having a prominent abdomen.

abdominouterotomy (ab-dom''ĭ-nō-ū-tĕr-ŏt'ŏ-mĭ) [L. *abdomen,* belly, + *uterus,* womb, + Gr. *tomē,* incision]. Abdominohysterotomy.

abdominovaginal (ăb-dŏm''ĭ-nō-văj'ĭ-năl) ["+ *vagina,* sheath]. Pert. to the abdomen and vagina.

abdominovesical (ăb-dŏm''ĭ-nō-vĕs'ĭ-kl) ["+ *vesica,* bladder]. Pert. to the abdomen and the urinary bladder.

a. pouch. Peritoneal fold which includes urachal folds.

abducens (ab-dū'senz) [L. drawing away from]. 1. Abducent nerve, q.v. 2. The rectus lateralis muscle of the eye, which moves the eyeball outward. 3. Pert. to drawing away from the median line of the body.

a. labiorum. Elevates angle of mouth. SYN: *caninus muscle; levator anguli oris muscle.* SEE: *Table of Muscles* in *Appendix.*

a. oculi. Rectus lateralis muscle of eye. SEE: *Table of Muscles* in *Appendix.*

a. oris. Elevates angle of mouth. SYN: *caninus muscle; levator anguli oris muscle.* SEE: *Table of Muscles* in *Appendix.*

abducent (ăb-dū'sĕnt) [L. *abducens,* drawing away]. 1. Abducting, leading away from. 2. Abducens.

a. nerve. Innervates rectus lateralis muscle of eye which rotates the eyeball outward. SYN: *6th cranial nerve.* SEE: *cranial nerves.*

abduct (ăb-dŭkt') [L. *abductus,* led away]. To draw away from the median plane of the body or one of its parts.

abduction (ăb-dŭk'shŭn). 1. The lateral movement of the limbs away from the median plane of the body, or the lateral bending of the head or trunk. 2. The movement of the digits away from the axial line of a limb. 3. In ophthalmology, outward rotation of the eyes.

abductor (ăb-dŭk'tŏr). A muscle which upon contraction draws a part away from median plane of body or axial line of an extremity. Opposed to adductor. SEE: *Table of Muscles* in *Appendix.*

Abel's bacillus. [Rudolf Abel, Ger. bacteriologist, 1868-1942]. Klebsiella ozaenae; found in ozena.

abenteric (ab-en-ter'ik) [L. *ab,* from, + Gr. *enteron,* intestine]. Rel. to or involving organs located outside the intestines. SYN: *apenteric.*

abepithymia (ab-ep-ĭ-thĭ'mĭ-ă) ["+ Gr. *epithymia,* desire]. 1. Paralysis of the celiac (solar) plexus. 2. This word is related to the Greek word thymos, meaning soul. The seat of the soul and desire was thought to be in the diaphragm. Thus the term has been used to describe unnatural or pathological desires.

Abernethy's fascia (ăb'ĕr-nē''thē). [John Abernethy, Br. surgeon, 1764-1831]. A layer of areolar tissue separating the external iliac artery from the iliac fascia over the psoas muscle.

Abernethy's sarcoma. A circumscribed, usually malignant, fatty tumor occurring principally on the trunk.

aberrant (ăb-ĕr′ănt) [L. *ab*, from, + *errare*, to wander]. Wandering from the normal or usual course.

a. pyramidal tract. Several groups of fibers from the midbrain to the cranial nerve motor nuclei and separating from the main fibers of the cortex.

aberratio (ăb-ĕr-ā′shĭ-ō). Aberration.

a. lactis. Secretion of milk from a site other than the breast.

a. mensium. Vicarious menstruation.

a. testis. Location of a testis in a position away from the path of normal descent.

aberration (ăb-ĕr-ā′shŭn) [L. *ab*, from, + *errare*, to wander]. 1. Deviation from a normal course. 2. Mental unsoundness, but not insanity. 3. Imperfect refraction.

a., chromatic. Unequal refraction of different wave lengths of light through a lens, producing a colored image.

a., chromosomal. Variations in chromosomes as to number (aneuploidy, polyploidy) or those involving alterations in chromosomal material (translocation, deletion, duplication).

a., diopteric. Spherical a.

a., distantial. Blurring of a distant object.

a., lateral. Deviation of a ray from the focus measured on a line perpendicular to the axis.

a., longitudinal. Deviation of a ray from the focus measured along the axis.

a., mental. Any deviation from normal mental functions.

a., spherical. Unequal refraction of different wave lengths of light through a lens, producing a blurred image.

aberrometer (ăb″ĕr-ŏm′ĕ-tĕr) [L. *ab-*, from, + *errare*, to wander, + Gr. *metron*, measure]. An instrument for measuring errors in delicate observations or instruments.

abevacuation (ăb-ē-văk″ū-ā′shŭn) [″+ *eva-cuare*, to empty]. 1. Abnormal evacuation either in excess or in deficiency. 2. Metastases.

abeyance (a-bā′ăns) [O. Fr.]. A temporary suspension of activity, sensation, or pain.

abient (ăb′ē-ĕnt). Tending to move away from the source of a stimulus. Opposed to adient.

abiogenesis (ăb-ĭ-ō-jĕn′ĕ-sĭs) [Gr. *a-*, not, + *bios*, life, + *genesis*, production]. Spontaneous generation of life; theoretical production of living from nonliving matter.

abiogenetic, abiogenous (ăb-ē-ō-jĕ-nĕt′ĭk, ăb-ē-ŏj′ĭ-nŭs). Pert. to spontaneous generation.

abiologic, abiological (ă-bī-ō-loj′ĭk, -al). Not related to biology or the science of life.

abionarce (ăb″ĭ-ō-năr′sē) [Gr. *a-*, not, + *bios*, life, + *narke*, stupor]. Infirmity, especially of the aged, due to weakness of mind and body.

abionergy (ăb″ĭ-ŏn′ŭr-jĭ) [Gr. *a-*, not, + *bios*, life, + *energeia*, action, energy]. Premature degeneration. SYN: *abiotrophy*.

abiosis (ăb-ĭ-ō′sĭs) [Gr. *a-*, not, + *bios*, life]. Absence of life.

abiotic (ab-ĭ-ŏt′ĭk). Incompatible with life; not viable.

abiotrophia (ăb″ĭ-ō-trō′fĭ-ă) [Gr. *a-*, not, + *bios*, life, + *trophē*, nutrition]. Abiotrophy.

abiotrophy (ăb-ĭ-ŏt′rō-fĭ). Premature loss of vitality or degeneration of tissues and cells with consequent loss of endurance and resistance.

abirritant (ăb-ĭr′ĭ-tănt) [L. *ab-*, from, + *irritare*, to irritate]. Relieving irritation; soothing.

abirrita′tion. 1. Asthenia, or atony. 2. Decreased response to stimuli.

ablactation (ăb-lăk-tā′shŭn) [L. *ab-*, from, + *lac*, milk]. Free of, or cessation of, milk secretion; weaning.

ablastemic (ă-blăs-tĕm′ĭk) [Gr. *a-*, not, + *blastos*, germ, seed]. Not germinal.

ablate (ăb-lāt′) [L. *ablatus*, taken away]. To remove, especially by excision.

ablatio (ăb-lā′shĭ-ō) [L. *ablatio*, carrying away]. Ablation, removal, detachment.

a. placentae. Premature detachment of a normally situated placenta; apoplexy of placenta; abruptio placentae, q.v. SEE: *placenta*.

a. retinae. Detachment of retina. SEE: *retina*.

ablation (ăb-lā′shŭn) [L. *ab*, from, + *latus*, carried]. Removal of a part, as by cutting.

ablepharia (ăb-lĕ-fā′rĭ-ă) [Gr. *a-*, not, + *blepharon*, eyelid]. Congenital reduction in size or absence of the eyelids.

ablepharon (ă-blĕf′ă-ron). Ablepharia.

ablepharous (ă-blĕf′ă-rŭs). Without eyelids.

ablephary (ă-blĕf′ă-rĭ). Ablepharia.

ablepsia (ă-blĕp′sĭ-ă) [Gr. *a-*, + *blepein*, to see]. Lack of or loss of sight. Blindness.

abluent (ăb′lū-ĕnt) [L. *ab*, from, + *luens*, washing]. An agent possessing cleansing qualities, as a detergent.

ablution (ăb-lū′shŭn). A cleansing or washing.

ablutomania (ă-blū″tō-mā′nĭ-ă) [L. *ablutio*, a washing, + Gr. *mania*, frenzy]. Compulsion to wash or clean oneself.

abmor′tal [L. *ab*, from, + *mors*, death]. The electrical current produced by dying tissue. It passes to the surrounding living tissue.

abner′val [L. *ab*, from, + *nervus*, nerve]. Away from a nerve, esp. with reference to the passage of an electric current through a muscle away from point where nerve enters the muscle. Opposed to adnerval.

abneural (ab-nū'ral) [L. *ab*, from, + Gr. *neuron*, nerve]. 1. Ventral. Remote from neural or dorsal aspect. 2. Abnerval.

abnormal (ăb-nōr'măl) ["+ *norma*, rule]. Deviating from normal. Contrary to the usual size, location, condition or system.

abnormality (ăb"nōr-măl'ĭ-tĭ). That which is not normal.

abnormity (ăb-nōr'mĭ-tĭ). 1. Deformity; abnormality. 2. A monstrosity.

abocclusion (ăb"ŏ-klū'zhŭn). Dentition in which the teeth of the mandible and the maxilla are not in contact.

aborad (ăb-ō'răd) [L. *ab*, from, + *oris*, mouth]. Away from the mouth.

aboral (ăb-ō'răl). Opposite to, or away from, the mouth.

abort (ă-bōrt') [L. *abortare*, to miscarry]. 1. To cause expulsion of an embryo or of the fetus before time of viability. 2. To arrest progress of disease. 3. To arrest growth or development.

aborticide (ă-bōr'tĭ-sĭd) ["+ *caedere*, to kill]. Destruction of the fetus in the uterus.

abortient (ă-bōr'shĕnt) [L. *abortio*, abortion]. 1. Producing abortion. 2. Abortifacient.

abortifacient (ă-bor-tĭ-fā'shent) [L. *abortus*, abortion, + *facere*, to make]. Anything used to cause or induce an abortion.

abortion (ă-bōr'shŭn) [L. *abortio*]. 1. The arrest of any physical action or disease. 2. The termination of pregnancy before the stage of viability, i.e., sometime between the twentieth and twenty-eighth week of gestation, the fetus measuring less than 14 inches (20 cm.) and weighing less than 500 gm. Because laymen interpret the word abortion to mean criminal interruption of pregnancy, it is advisable to use the word miscarriage when discussing spontaneous abortion with a patient or her family. 3. The immature product of conception which has been expelled prematurely.

ETIOL: Among most common causes are faulty development of embryo, abnormalities of the placenta, endocrine disturbances, acute infectious diseases, severe trauma or shock.

SYM: Abdominal cramps and bleeding from vagina.

NP: Send for doctor. Keep patient quiet. Care as for uterine hemorrhage. Save discharges for doctor's inspection. Watch for shock and symptoms of sepsis.

a., accidental. That which occurs spontaneously and accidentally without criminal intent.

a., ampullar. Tubal abortion occurring from the ampulla of the oviduct.

a., artificial. When induced or performed purposely, as by a surgeon.

a., cervical. One in which the ovum is retained in the cervical canal.

a., complete. Abortion in which the complete product of conception has been expelled.

a., criminal. A. which is deliberately produced for other than medical purposes.

a., embryonic. One that occurs before the fifth month of pregnancy.

a., fetal. One that occurs after the fifth month of pregnancy.

a., habitual. A. in the course of three or more pregnancies, with no apparent cause.

a., imminent. That characterized by bleeding and colicky pains which progressively increase. Cervix usually effaced and patulous.

a., incomplete. Abortion in which part of the product of conception has been retained in the uterus.

a., induced. One brought on intentionally, as a criminal or therapeutic a. Abortions may be induced by use of drugs, instruments, or exposure to radiation. SEE: *curettage.*

a., inevitable. That which cannot be halted.

a., infected. When accompanied by infection of retained material with resultant febrile reaction.

a., justifiable. A. performed to save the mother's life. SEE: *a., therapeutic.*

a., missed. That in which a dead nonviable fetus and other products of conception are retained in the uterus for two months or longer.

a., ovular. That which occurs within first three weeks after conception.

a., partial. In multiple pregnancy, aborting of only one fetus, or less than the entire number.

a., septic. That in which there is an infection of the product of conception and the endometrial lining of uterus usually resulting from attempted interference during early pregnancy.

a., spontaneous. Occurring without having been induced.

a., therapeutic. A. performed legally before viability under certain conditions, as when the mental or physical health of the mother is endangered by continuation of the pregnancy.

a., threatened. The appearance of signs and symptoms of possible loss of embryo. Vaginal bleeding with or without intermittent pain is usually the first sign. If embryo is still alive and attachment to uterus has not been interrupted, pregnancy may continue. Absolute bed rest essential with avoidance of coitus, douches, and strong cathartics.

   a., tubal. 1. A tubal pregnancy in which the fetus has been expelled through the distal end of a uterine tube. 2. The escape of the product of conception into the peritoneal cavity by way of the uterine tube.

abortionist (ă-bŏr′shŭn-ĭst). One who performs abortion.

abortive (ă-bor′tiv) [L. *abortivus*]. 1. Preventing the completion of. 2. Abortifacient; that which prevents the normal continuation of pregnancy. 3. Rudimentary.

abortus (ă-bŏr′tŭs) [L.]. An aborted fetus weighing less than 500 gm.

abouchement (ă-būsh-mŏn′) [Fr.]. The ending of a small vessel in a large one.

aboulia (ă-bū′lĭ-ă) [Gr. *a-*, not, + *boulē*, will]. Inability to exercise will power. SYN: *abulia,* q.v.

aboulomania (ă-bū″lō-mā′nĭ-ă) [Gr. *a-*, not, + *boulē*, will, + *mania*, frenzy]. Mental disorder with loss of will power. SYN: *abulomania.*

abrachia (ă-brā′kĭ-ă) ["+ *brachiōn,* arm]. The congenital anomaly of armlessness.

abrachiocephalia (ă-brā″kē-ō-sĕ-fā′lĭ-ă) ["+ "+ *kephalē*, head]. Congenital anomaly consisting of absence of arms and head.

abrachiocephalus (ă-brā″kĭ-ō-sĕf′ă-lŭs). A fetal anomaly without head or arms.

abrachius (ă-brā′kĭ-ŭs) [Gr. *a-*, not, + *brachiōn,* arm]. An individual without arms.

abradant (ă-brād′ĕnt). Abrasive.

abrade (ă-brād′) [L. *ab,* from, + *radere,* to scrape]. 1. To chafe. 2. To roughen or remove by friction.

abra′sio cor′neae [L., abrasion of cornea]. Removal of corneal excrescences by scraping.

abrasion (ă-brā′zhŭn) [L. *ab,* from, + *radere,* to scrape]. 1. A scraping away of a portion of skin or of a mucous membrane as a result of injury or mechanical means, as in dermabrasion for cosmetic purposes. A brush burn. 2. The wearing away of the substance of a tooth. Normally occurs from mastication; may be accomplished by mechanical or chemical means. SEE: *avulsion; bruise.*

abra′sive. 1. Producing abrasion. 2. That which abrades.

abreaction (ăb″rē-ăk′shŭn) [L. *ab,* from, + *rē,* again, + *actus,* acting]. In psychoanalysis, release of, or discharge of, emotional tension by consciously recalling or acting out a painful experience which had been ei-

ther forgotten or repressed. Abreaction may allow this painful or consciously intolerable experience to become bearable because of the insight gained during the process.

abrosia (ă-brō′zĭ-ă) ["+ *erodere,* to gnaw away]. 1. Fasting; abstaining from food. 2. A wasting away.

abruptio (ă-brŭp′shĭ-ō) ["+ *abruptus,* broken off]. A tearing away from.

   a. placentae. Premature detachment of normally situated placenta; ablatio placenta. SEE: *placenta.*

   ETIOL: Unknown, but is associated with hypertension or preeclampsia in many cases.

   PATH: Extravasation of blood between placenta and uterine wall, occasionally between muscle fibers of the uterus.

   SYM: Hemorrhage, concealed or evident, or a combination of both. Pain, constant at point of separation of placenta due to blood extruding between muscle fibers. Uterine contraction constant; occasionally tetanic in nature. Evidences of fetal asphyxia and death, increased fetal movements, and changes in heart rate until final cessation of both. Albumin in urine. Anemia.

   TREATMENT: In mild cases, rest in bed. In severe cases, shock must first be combated. A soft and partially dilated cervix is an indication for immediate artificial rupture of membranes followed by natural or artificial induction of labor. If the fetus is viable and alive, and if the mother's cervix is firm and not dilated, a cesarean section is the treatment of choice. If the uterus fails to contract after cesarean section, a rapid hysterectomy usually is necessary.

abscess (ăb′sĕs) [L. *abscessus,* a going away]. A localized collection of pus in any part of the body. The result of disintegration or displacement of tissue. SEE: *inflammation; pus.*

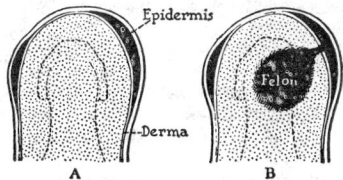

SUBEPITHELIAL ABSCESS
A, Abscess located at tip of finger lies between dense epidermis and derma. B, Subepithelial abscess developed from felon which perforated derma, spread out beneath epidermis, and lifted up in a manner similar to a blister.

a., acute, or warm. A. with local symptoms of inflammation, with fluctuation, and pointing; also pressure and constitutional symptoms. Inflammation becomes intensified with increased heat, redness, swelling, and edema. Pain becomes throbbing and greater, with impaired loss of function of the part. An elevation appears with fluctuation and softening as it reaches the surface, becoming necrotic and yellow, giving way with evacuation of pus. Pressure symptoms, according to size and depth. In floor of mouth or neck, swelling may cause dyspnea and dysphagia. Constitutional symptoms vary, from slight temperature (fever may be absent in a well walled-off abscess) to high temperature, with rigors and sweats if associated with pyemia and septicemia. Any or all general symptoms may be absent in deep-seated abscesses except loss of weight and strength.

TERMINATION: This may be by pointing, evacuation, and discharge of the pus; or it may become inspissated, encapsulated, and at times absorbed.

a., alveolar. Abscess about root of a tooth in alveolar cavity. Usually the result of necrosis and infection of dental pulp following dental caries.

a., amebic, of liver. Abscess occurring in the liver developing as a complication of amebic dysentery. Caused by Entamoeba histolytica.

a., anorectal. One in the tissue near the rectum. SYN: *ischiorectal a.; perirectal a.*

a., apical. One at the apex of lung or at extremity of root of a tooth.

a., appendiceal, appendicular. Pus formation around an inflamed vermiform appendix.

a., arthrifluent. A wandering abscess having origin in a diseased joint.

a., atheromatous. Softening in the wall of a blood vessel as the result of atherosclerosis.

a., axillary. One or multiple abscesses in axilla.

a., bartholin. A. of Bartholin's gland.

a., bicameral. One with two pockets.

a., bile duct. A. of the bile duct. SYN: *cholangitic a.*

a., bilharziasis. One in an intestinal wall caused by Schistosoma.

a., blind. An abscess with no external opening such as a dental granuloma.

a., bone. Brodie's abscess, q.v.

a., brain. An intracranial abscess; one involving the brain or its membranes. They are seldom primary, usually occurring secondary to infections of middle ear, nasal sinuses, face, or skull, or from contamination from penetrating wounds or skull fractures. They may also have a metastatic origin arising from septic foci in the lungs (bronchiectasis, empyema, lung abscess), in bone (osteomyelitis), or in the heart (endocarditis). Infection of nervous tissue by the invading organism results in necrosis and liquefaction and edema of surrounding tissues.

Brain abscesses may be acute, subacute, or chronic. Their clinical manifestations depend on part of brain involved, size, virulence of infecting organisms, and other factors.

SYM: Severe and persistent headache usually localized over infected area; fever, vomiting, vertigo, malaise, sometimes irritability and other mental symptoms.

TREATMENT: Chemotherapy and antibiotic agents; sometimes puncture and aspiration or surgical extirpation is necessary.

a., breast. A. of breast marked by acute inflammation. SYN: *mammary a.*

a., Brodie's. Tuberculosis with suppuration of articular end of a bone, especially the tibia. SYN: *bone a.*

a., bursal. One in a bursa.

a., canalicular. An abscess of breast discharging into the milk ducts.

a., caseous. One in which the pus has a cheesy appearance.

a., cerebral. A brain abscess. SYN: *intracranial a.*

a., cheesy. Caseous abscess.

a., cholangitic. One of the bile duct.

a., chronic. One with pus but without signs of inflammation; usually of slow development. Formed by liquefaction of tuberculous tissue. May occur anywhere on the body but more frequently in the spine, hips, genitourinary tract, and lymph glands. Symptoms may be very mild, pain when present being due to pressure upon surrounding parts. Tenderness often absent. Chronic septic intoxication with hectic fever occurs when there is mixed infection. Amyloid disease may develop if the abscess persists for a prolonged period. SYN: *cold a.*

a., circumscribed. An abscess limited or confined by surrounding tissue.

a., circumtonsillar. An abscess around the tonsil. SYN: *quinsy; peritonsillar abscess.*

a., cold. Chronic abscess, q.v.

a., collar-button. Two cavities, one larger than the other, containing pus and connected by a narrow channel. SYN: *shirt-stud abscess.*

a., congestive. One that shows pus at a point distant from where formed.

a., deep. One arising from below the deep fascia.

a., dental. An abscess beside a tooth, usually near the root.

a., dentoalveolar. One in the alveolar process surrounding the root of a tooth.

a., diffuse. A collection of pus not circumscribed by a well-defined capsule.

a., dry. One that disappears without pointing or breaking.

a., embolic. One due to a septic embolus.

a., emphysematous. Tympanitic a., q.v.

a., encysted. One with pus circumscribed in a serous cavity.

a., endamebic; a., entamebic. Amebic a., q.v.

a., epidural. Extradural a., q.v.

a., epiploic. One in the omentum.

a., extradural. A. on the dura mater.

a., fecal. An abscess containing feces.

a., filarial. One caused by filaria.

a., follicular. One forming in a follicle.

a., frontal. Abscess in the frontal lobe of the brain.

a., fungal. Abscess caused by a fungus.

a., gangrenous. One attended with gangrene of surrounding parts.

a., gas. A typanitic abscess; one containing gas due to presence of gas-forming organisms such as Clostridium perfringens.

a., gingival. An abscess of the gum.

a., glandular. One around a lymph node.

a., gravitation. An abscess in which the pus migrates, sinking to a lower part of the body.

a.'s, heart. In interstitial myocarditis, multiple small abscesses.

a., helminthic. One due to the presence of a parasitic worm.

a., hematic. One due to an extravasated blood clot.

a., hemorrhagic. One containing blood.

a., hepatic. Abscess of the liver, esp. an amebic a.

a., hot. An acute abscess, q.v.

a., hypostatic. A wandering abscess, q.v.

a., idiopathic. One due to unknown causes.

a., iliac. One in the iliac region.

a., intracranial. A. of brain. SYN: *cerebral a.*

a., intradural. A. within the layers of the dura mater.

a., intramammary. An abscess of the mammary gland. SYN: *mammary a.; breast a.*

a., intramastoid. A mastoid process abscess of the temporal bone.

a., ischiorectal. One in the ischiorectal fossa.

a., kidney. One or multiple abscesses of renal cortex. SYN: *renal a.*

a., lacrimal. Suppuration of a lacrimal gland.

a., lacunar. One in the urethral lacunae.

a., lateral; a., lateral alveolar. A periodontal abscess.

a., lumbar. Abscess in the lumbar region.

a., lung. A. occurring in the lung.

a., lymphatic. An abscess of a lymph node.

a., mammary. One in the female breast, esp. an abscess involving the glandular tissue. Usually seen during lactation or at time of weaning. SYN: *breast a.; intramammmary a.*

a., marginal. One near the orifice of the anus.

a., mastoid. Suppuration of the mastoid portion of the temporal bone.

a., mediastinal. Suppuration in the mediastinum.

a., metastatic. A secondary one at a distance from focus of infection.

a., migrating. A wandering abscess, q.v.

a., miliary. A small embolic abscess. One discharging numerous small collections of pus.

a., milk. A mammary abscess during lactation.

a., mother. A primary abscess giving rise to other abscesses.

a., multiple. A group of abscesses accompanying pyemia.

a., mural. One in tissues of the abdominal wall.

a., nocardial. One caused by Nocardia.

a., orbital. Suppuration in the orbit.

a., ossifluent. One dependent on degeneration of bone tissue.

a., palatal. One in an upper lateral incisor, erupting toward the palate.

a., palmar. A purulent effusion into the tissues of the palm of the hand.

a., parafrenal. Abscess on the side of the frenulum of the penis. Usually involves Tyson's gland.

a., parametric; a., parametritic. One between the folds of the broad ligaments of the uterus.

a., paranephric; a., paranephritic. One in the tissues around the kidney.

a., parapancreatic. One in the tissues next to the pancreas.

a., parietal. A periodontal abscess arising in the periodontal tissue other than the orifice through which the vascular supply enters the dental pulp.

a., pelvic. Abscess of the pelvic peritoneum, especially Douglas' pouch.

a., pelvirectal. A deep rectal abscess.

a., periapical. A periodontal abscess at the root apex of a tooth.

a., pericemental. An alveolar abscess not involving the apex of a tooth.

a., pericoronal. One around the crown of an unerupted molar tooth.

a., peridental. Periodontal abscess.

a., perinephric. One in tissue about the kidney. SYN: *perirenal a.*

a., periodontal. An abscess arising in the periodontal tissue (structures of support for teeth).

a., peripleuritic. In the tissue surrounding the parietal pleura.

a., periproctic. One in the areolar tissue about the anus. SYN: *perirectal a.*

a., perirenal. An a. in the tissue surrounding the kidney. SYN: *perinephric a.*

a., peritoneal. An abscess within the peritoneal cavity usually following peritonitis.

a., peritonsillar. Quinsy.

a., periurethral. One formed in tissue surrounding the urethra.

a., perivesical. One in the tissues around the urinary bladder.

a., phlegmonous. An acute abscess in the connective tissue.

a., pneumococcic. One due to infection with pneumococci.

a., postcecal. One sometimes occurring in appendicitis.

a., postmammary. Retromammary abscess, q.v.

a., post-typhoid. A chronic abscess occurring as a complication of typhoid fever.

a., prelacrimal. One of the lacrimal bone producing a swelling at inner canthus.

a., premammary. A subcutaneous or subareolar abscess of the mammary gland.

a., primary. One originating at point of infection.

a., prostatic. A. within the prostate gland.

a., protozoal. One caused by a protozoan.

a., psoas. One with pus descending in sheath of psoas muscle due to vertebral disease, usually tuberculous in origin.

a., pulmonary. A. of the lungs. Nontuberculous suppuration of lung tissue with one or more localized areas of necrosis resulting in pulmonary cavitation.

a., pulp. 1. A cavity discharging pus formed in the pulp of a tooth. 2. An a. of the tissues of the pulp of a finger.

a., pyemic. A metastatic one, usually multiple, due to pyogenic organisms.

a., rectal. One in the rectum.

a., renal. One or multiple abscesses of the renal cortex. SYN: *kidney a.*

a., residual. One occurring from old inflammatory products at the site of an earlier abscess.

a., retrocecal. Abscess situated behind the cecum.

a., retromammary. One between the mammary gland and the chest wall.

a., retroperitoneal. One located between the peritoneum and the posterior abdominal wall.

a., retropharyngeal. An a. of the lymph nodes in the walls of the pharynx. I sometimes simulates diphtheritic pharyngitis.

a., retrovesical. One behind the bladder.

a., root. An abscess of the root of a tooth. SYN: *apical a.*

a., sacrococcygeal. An a. over the sacrum and coccyx.

a., satellite. A secondary one arising from and located near the primary abscess.

a., scrofulous. One due to tuberculous degeneration of bone or lymph nodes.

a., secondary. Embolic abscess.

a., septicemic. An a. resulting from septicemia.

a.'s, shirt-stud. Two cavities, one larger than the other, containing pus and connected by a narrow channel. SYN *collar-button abscess.*

a., spermatic. An a. of the seminiferous tubules.

a., spinal. One due to necrosis of a vertebra.

a., spirillary. One containing Spirilla.

a., splenic. One of the spleen.

a., stercoral; a., stercoralaceous. An abscess containing feces. SYN: *fecal abscess.*

a., stitch. One formed about a stitch of suture.

a., streptococcal. An abscess caused by streptococci.

a., subaponeurotic. One beneath an aponeurosis or fascia.

a., subarachnoid. A. of the midlayer of the covering of the brain and spinal cord *a., subareolar.* One underneath the areola of the mammary gland, sometimes draining through the nipple.

a., subdiaphragmatic. An a. beneath the diaphragm. SYN: *subphrenic a.*

a., subdural. One beneath the dura of brain or spinal cord.

a., subepidermal. One beneath the epidermis.

a., subfascial. One beneath a fascia.

a., submammary. An a. beneath the mammary gland.

a., subpectoral. One beneath the pectoral muscles.

a., subperiosteal. Bone abscess below the periosteum.

a., subperitoneal. One between the parietal peritoneum and the abdominal wall.

a., subphrenic. An a. beneath the diaphragm. SYN: *subdiaphragmatic a.*

a., subscapular. One between the serratus anterior and the posterior thoracic wall.

a., subungual. One beneath the distal portion of a fingernail. May follow injuries with pins, needles, or splinters.

a., sudoriparous. An a. of a sweat gland.

a., superficial. One occurring above the deep fascia.

a., suprahepatic. One in the suspensory ligament between the liver and the diaphragm.

a., sympathetic. One arising some distance from the primary cause.

a., syphilitic. One occurring in the tertiary stage of syphilis.

a., thecal. One in a tendon sheath.

a., thymus. An a. of the thymus. SYN: *Dubois' a.*

a., tonsillar. Acute suppurative tonsillitis, or quinsy.

a., tooth. An alveolar abscess.

a., traumatic. One caused by injury.

a., tropical. Amebic a. of the liver.

a., tuberculous. Same as chronic a.

a., tympanitic. An abscess that contains air or gas.

a., tympanocervical. One arising in the tympanum and extending to the neck.

a., tympanomastoid. A combined abscess of the tympanum and mastoid.

a., urethral. One of the urethra.

a., urinary. One caused by escape of urine into the tissues.

a., urinous. One which contains pus with urine.

a., verminous. One which is caused by or contains insect larvae or other animal parasites.

a., wandering. One at a distance from focus of disease with pus along fascial sheaths of muscles. SYN: *migrating abscess.*

a., warm. An acute abscess, q.v.

a., worm. One caused by or containing worms.

abscission (ăb-sĭ'zhŭn) [L. *abscindere,* to cut off]. The removal of a part by excision.

absence (ăb-sĕnz). Temporary mental inattention.

absentia epileptica (ăb-sĕn'shĭ-ă ĕp-ĭ-lĕp'-tĭk-ă) [L.]. The loss of consciousness in the mild form of epilepsy.

abs. feb. Abbr. for *absente febre,* in the absence of fever.

Absidia (ăb-sĭd'ĭ-ă). Genus of pathogenic fungi of the order Phycomycetes and the family Mucoraceae.

absinthe, absinth (ăb'sĭnth) [L. *absinthium,* wormwood]. A liquor containing oil of wormwood, anise, and other herbs. It is highly toxic, adversely affecting the nervous system.

absinthism (ăb'sĭnth-ĭ"zm). Deterioration of the nerve centers following excessive use of absinthe.

absolute alcohol. Alcohol with not more than 1% of water.

absolute temperature. Temperature reckoned from absolute zero.

absolute zero. –273.15° C or –459.67° F. The lowest possible temperature.

absorb [L. *absorbere,* to suck in]. To take in, suck up, or imbibe. SEE: *absorption.*

absorbefacient (ăb-sŏr"bē-fā'shĕnt) ["+ *facere,* to make]. Causing or that which causes absorption.

absorbent (ăb-sŏr'bĕnt). 1. A substance which absorbs, esp. a substance which brings about the absorption of diseased tissue. 2. Having the power to absorb.

absorptiometer (ăb-sŏrp'shĭ-ŏm'ē-tĕr) [L. *absorptio,* absorption, + Gr. *metron,* measure]. 1. An instrument for measuring thickness of liquid, drawn by capillary attraction, between glass plates. 2. Instrument for measuring the absorption of gas by a liquid.

absorption (ăb-sŏrp'shŭn) [L. *absorptio,* to suck in]. 1. The taking up of liquids by solids, or of gases by solids or liquids. 2. The taking up of light or of its rays by black or colored rays. 3. The taking up by the body of radiant heat, causing a rise in body temperature. 4. PHYS: The passage of a substance through some surface of the body into body fluids and tissues, as the passage of ether through the respiratory epithelium of lungs into the blood during anesthesia, or passage of oil of wintergreen through the skin, the result of several processes: diffusion, q.v., filtration, q.v., osmosis, q.v.

RS: chondrolysis; imbibition; osmosis; resorption.

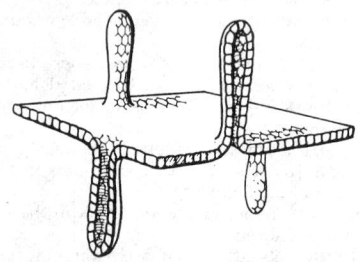

ABSORPTION—INTESTINAL SURFACE
Showing villi and crypts, which greatly increase the number of cells that have access to an epithelial surface and the contents of the lumen.

a., colon. Water (important in the conservation of body fluids) and products of bacterial action are normally absorbed esp. in the ascending colon. Some nutrients and drugs are absorbed by the lower bowel. Cellulose is not digested but passes from the body as residue.

a., cutaneous. A. through the skin.

a., disjunctive. Separation of a slough by absorption of a layer of adjacent healthy tissue.

a., external. Taking up of material by the skin and mucous membrane.

a., internal. Normal digestion.

a., interstitial. Removal of wastes by absorbent system.

a. lines. Dark lines of solar spectrum. SYN: *Fraunhofer's lines,* q.v.

a., mouth. Some substances, but no food nutrients, can be absorbed from the mouth; some drugs, esp. alkaloids, can be absorbed through the oral mucosa.

a. of radiation. Grotthuss' law states that only rays which are absorbed are physiologically active. Sometimes called Draper's law.

a., pathologic. Absorption into the blood or lymph of substances normally excreted or of a product of disease processes, e.g., pus.

a., protein. In the form of amino acids, produced by digestive hydrolysis, proteins enter the portal vein from the intestinal walls, and through the liver into the general circulation whence they are absorbed by the tissues. Each tissue synthesizes its own form of protein from the amino acids received from the blood.

a., small intestine. The most important absorption of products of digestion occurs in the small intestines, esp. the ileum. Products of digestion absorbed from the gastrointestinal tract pass into either blood or lymph. The mesenteric veins unite to form the portal vein and carry such blood to the liver; the mesenteric lymphatics are called lacteals because during absorption of a fatty meal the lymph which they contain looks milky and is called chyle. The lacteals empty into the cisterna chyli and are joined by lymphatics from other parts of the body; the mixed lymph travels, via the thoracic duct, to the subclavian vein where it empties into the blood stream.

a. spectrum. A spectrum showing absorption lines.

a., stomach. Water, alcohol, and some salts can be absorbed through the gastric mucosa.

absorptive (ăb-sörp'tĭv). Absorbent.

abstergent (ăb-stěr'jĕnt) [L. *abstergere,* to cleanse.]. Cleansing, purifying.

abstinence (ăb'stĭ-nĕns) [L. *abstinere,* to abstain]. Going without voluntarily, esp. refraining from indulgence in food, alcoholic beverages, or sexual intercourse.

a. symptoms. Partial collapse resulting from withdrawal of alcohol, stimulants, and some opiates.

abstract (ăb'străkt, ăb-străkt') [L. *abstrahere,* to draw away]. 1. A preparation containing the soluble principles of a drug concentrated and mixed with lactose. 2. A summary or abridgment of an article, book, address, etc.

abstraction (ăb-străk'shŭn). 1. Removal or separation of a constituent from a mixture or compound. 2. Removal of blood; bloodletting. 3. Absorption of the mind; inattention or absent-mindedness.

abterminal (ăb-tĕr'mĭ-năl) [L. *ab,* from, + *terminus,* end]. Away from an end and toward the center, said of electric currents in muscles.

abulia (ă-bū'lĭ-ă) [Gr. *a-,* not, + *boulē,* will]. Absence of or inability to exercise will power; hesitation; indecision. Seen in schizophrenic reactions. SYN: *aboulia.*

abuse (ă-būs'). Misuse; excessive or improper use.

abutment (ăb-bŭt'mĕnt) [Fr. *abouter,* to place end to end]. The tooth to which a partial denture is anchored.

A.C. Abbr. for *anodal closure; adrenal cortex; air conduction; alternating current; antiphlogistic corticoid; atriocarotid; auriculocarotid; axiocervical.*

a.c. Abbr. for L. *ante cibum,* before meals.

Ac. Chem. symbol for actinium.

acacia (ă-kā′shĭ-a). USP. Gum arabic. A dried, gummy exudation from the tree Acacia senegal. Used as a suspending agent or vehicle in pharmaceutical or other industrial products.

acalcicosis (ă-kăl″sĭ-kō′sĭs). Condition resulting from deficiency of calcium in diet. SYN: *acalcerosis.*

acalculia (ă-kăl-kū′lĭ-ă) [Gr. *a-,* not, + L. *calculare,* to reckon]. Inability to solve simple or complex mathematical problems.

acampsia (ă-kămp′sĭ-ă) [" + *kamptein,* to bend]. Inflexibility of a limb; rigidity, ankylosis.

acan′tha [Gr. *akantha,* thorn]. 1. The spine. 2. A vertebral spinous process.

acanthesthesia (ă-kăn″thĕs-thē′zĭ-ă) [Gr. *akantha,* thorn, + *disthésis,* sensation]. A sensation as of a pinprick; a form of paresthesia, q.v.

Acanthia lectularia (ă-căn′thĭ-ă lĕc-tū-lā′rĭ-ă). The bedbug. SYN: *Cimex lectularis.*

acan′thion [Gr. *akanthion,* a thorn]. Tip of anterior nasal spine.

acantho-. Combining form meaning thorn, spine.

Acanthocephala (ă-kăn″thō-sĕf′ă-lă) [Gr. *akantha,* thorn, + *kephalē,* head]. A class of wormlike entozoa related to the Platyhelminthes, including a few species parasitic in man.

acanthocephaliasis (ă-kăn″thō-sĕf-ă-lĭ′ă-sĭs). Infestation with Acanthocephala.

acan′thoid [Gr. *akantha,* thorn, + *eidos,* form]. Thorny; spiny; of a spinous nature.

acanthokeratodermia (ă-kăn″thō-kĕr″ă-tō-dĕr′mĭ-ă) [" + *keras,* horn, + *derma,* skin]. Hypertrophy of the horny portion of the skin of the palms of hands and soles of feet, and thickening of the nails.

acantholysis (ă-kăn-thŏl′ĭ-sĭs) [" + *lysis,* solution]. Any disease of the skin accompanied by degeneration of the cohesive elements of the cells of the outer or horny layer of the skin.

   a. bullosa. A skin condition of large bullae produced by irritation or trauma. SYN: *Epidermolysis bullosa,* q.v.

acanthoma (ăk″ăn-thō′mă) [" + *-ōma,* tumor]. Previously used to denote cancer of skin. Benign tumor of the skin.

   a. adenoides cysticum. A cystic tumor, often familial, occurring on chest, face and in axillary regions. Tumors contain tissues resembling sweat glands and hair follicles. SYN: *epithelioma adenoides cysticum.*

acanthopel′vis (ă-kăn″thō-pĕl′vĭs) [Gr. *akantha,* a thorn, + *pelyx,* pelvis]. A prominent and sharp pubic spine on a rachitic pelvis.

acanthosis (ăk″ăn-thō′sĭs) [Gr. *akantha,* a thorn, + *-ōsis,* condition]. Increased thickness of prickle cell layer of skin.

   a. nigricans. Rare chronic inflammatory disease of skin in adult life sometimes associated with cancer of some internal organ. Characterized by symmetrically distributed hard and soft papillary growths accompanied by hyperpigmentation and hyperkeratosis. SYN: *keratosis nigricans.*

acanthotic (ăk″ăn-thŏt′ĭk). Pert. to acanthosis.

acap′nia [Gr. *akapnos,* smokeless]. The presence of less than normal amount of carbon dioxide in blood and tissues, e.g., after voluntary overbreathing. SEE: *hyperventilation.*

   SYM: Depressed respiration, giddiness, paresthesia, cramps, occasionally convulsions.

acapnial (ă-căp′nĭ-ăl). Showing or pert. to acapnia.

acarbia (ă-kăr′bĭ-ă) [Gr. *a-,* not, + L. *carbo,* coal]. Diminution of bicarbonate in the blood.

acardia (ă-kăr′dĭ-ă) [" + Gr. *kardia,* heart]. Congenital absence of the heart.

acardiac (ă-kăr′dĭ-ăk). Having no heart.

acardiacus (ă-kăr-dĭ′ă-kŭs). A parasitic twin without a heart, therefore utilizing the circulation of its twin. SYN: *acardius.*

acardiohemia (ă-kăr″dĭ-ō-hē′mĭ-ă) [Gr. *a-,* not, + *kardia,* heart, + *haima,* blood]. Lack of blood in the heart.

acardionervia (ă-kăr″dĭ-ō-nĕr′vĭ-ă) [" + " + *neuron,* sinew]. Lack of nerve stimulus to the heart.

acardiotrophia (ă-kăr″dĭ-ō-trō′fĭ-ă) [" + " + *trophē,* nutrition]. Atrophy of the heart.

acar′dius. Acardiacus, q.v.

acariasis (ăk″ă-rĭ′ă-sĭs) [L. *acarus,* mite, + Gr. *-iasis,* condition]. Any disease caused by a mite or acarid. SYN: *acarinosis.*

acaricide (ă-kăr′ĭ-sīd) [" + *caedere,* to kill]. 1. An agent that destroys acarids. 2. Destroying a member of order Acarina.

acarid, acaridan (ăk′ă-rĭd, ă-kăr′ĭ-dăn) [L. *acarus,* mite]. A tick or mite; member of the order Acarina.

acaridi′asis (ă-kăr″ĭ-dĭ′ăs-ĭs) [" + Gr. *-iasis,* condition]. Disease caused by a mite. SYN: *acariasis.*

Acarina (ăk″ă-rĭ′nă). An order of the class Arachnida which includes a large number of species of minute animals known as mites or ticks. Most are ectoparasites, infestation causing local dermatitis with pruritus and sometimes systemic reactions. They also are vectors of a number of diseases. SEE: *Ixodidae; Sarcoptidea; scabies; tick.*

acarinosis (ă-kăr″ĭ-nō′sĭs) [L. *acarus*, mite, + Gr. *-ōsis*, condition]. Disease caused by a mite. SYN: *acariasis.*

acarodermatitis (ak-ă-ă-rō-der-mă-tī′tis) ["+ Gr. *derma*, skin, + *-itis*, inflammation]. The itch. Inflammation of skin caused by a mite.

acaroid (ăk-ă-royd) ["+ *eidos*, resemblance]. A mite, or resembling one.

acarophobia (a-kar-ō-fō′bĭ-ă) [L. *acarus*, mite, + *phobos*, fear]. Delusion that the skin is infested with mites or worms.

acarpia (ă-kărp′ĭ-ă) [Gr. *a-*, not, + *karpos*, fruit]. Barrenness; sterility.

Acarus (ăk′ăr-ŭs) [L., mite]. A genus of mites.

acarus [L.]. Any mite or tick.

acaryote (ă-kăr′ĭ-ōt) [Gr. *a-*, not, + *karyon*, nucleus]. Without a nucleus.

acatalepsia, acatalepsy (ă-kăt″ă-lep′sĭ-ă, -sĭ) ["+ *katalambanein*, to comprehend]. 1. Mental deficiency; inability to understand. 2. Diagnostic uncertainty.

acatalep′tic (ă-kăt″ă-lĕp′tĭk). 1. Deficient mentally. 2. Uncertain or doubtful.

acatamathesia (ă-kăt″ă-mă-thē′zĭ-ă) [Gr. *a-*, not, + *katamathēsis*, understanding]. 1. Loss of ability to understand spoken words. 2. Inability to comprehend as a result of a brain lesion.

acataphasia (ă-kăt″ă-fā′zĭ-ă) ["+ *kataphasis*, affirmation]. Inability to coherently express thoughts verbally. This condition is due to a cerebral lesion.

acataposis (ă-kăt″ă-pō′sĭs) ["+ *kataposis*, gulping down]. Dysphagia. Difficulty in swallowing.

acatastasia (ă-kăt-ăstă′zĭ-ă) [Gr. *akatastasis*, disorder]. Irregularity; deviation from normal.

acatharsia (ak″ă-thăr′zĭ-ă) [Gr. *akatharsis*, uncleanness]. Foulness; impurity; lack of purging.

acathexia (ă″kă-thĕks′ĭ-ă) [Gr. *a-*, not, + *kathexis*, retention]. An inability to retain normal secretions.

acathexis (ă″kă-thĕks′ĭs). In psychoanalysis, lack of emotion toward a thing or idea which is unconsciously important to the individual.

acathisia (ă″kă-thĭz′ĭ-ă) [Gr. *a-*, not, + *kathisis*, sitting]. Inability to sit down because the thought of doing so causes severe anxiety. Patient has a feeling of restlessness and an urgent need of movement and complains of a feeling of muscular quivering. This symptom may appear as a complication of thera-

py with antipsychotic tranquilizers such as phenothiazines or reserpine. Also spelled akathisia or akatizia.

acaudal, acaudate (ă-kŏ′dăl, -dăt) ["+ L. *cauda*, tail]. Having no tail.

ACC. Abbr. for *anodal closure contraction.*

acc. Abbr. for *accommodation.*

acceleration (ăk-sĕl″ĕr-ā′shŭn) [L. *acceleratus*]. Increasing the speed of motion or rate, as pulse or respiration.

    a., angular. A change in direction of motion, as when the body rotates about its own axis.

    a., central. A., centripetal, q.v.

    a., centripetal. Movement of the body in a circular or curved course. SYN: *central acceleration.*

    a., linear. A change in velocity either forward or backward.

    a., negative. Acceleration which produces a force acting on the body in the long axis from seat to head, as when a pilot goes into a dive. SYMB: –G.

    a., positive. Acceleration which produces a force acting on the body in the long axis from head to seat, as when a pilot pulls out of a dive. SYMB: +G.

accelerator (ăk-sĕl′ĕr-ā″tŏr). Anything which increases action or function. In chemistry, a catalyst.

    a. nerves. Sympathetic nerves which contain fibers whose impulses increase rate and force of heart beat. Postganglionic fibers arise principally in cervical and thoracic ganglia.

    a. reflexes. Statokinetic reflexes, q.v.

    a. urinae. Obsolete term for bulbocavernosus muscle. SEE: *Table of Muscles* in *Appendix.*

accentuation (ăk-sĕn″chū-ā′shŭn) [L. *accentus*, accent]. Marked with a special stress; emphasis.

accept′or (ăk-sĕp′tŏr) [L. *accipere*, to accept.]. A substance absorbing nascent hydrogen or oxygen freed by a reducing enzyme.

    a., hydrogen. Substance which receives hydrogen from a hydrogen donator.

accessorius (ăk″sĕs-ō′rĭ-ŭs) [L., supplementary]. Accessory, supplementary, as certain muscles, glands, nerves.

accessory (ăk-sĕs′ō-rĭ). Auxiliary; assisting. Term applied to a lesser structure which resembles in structure and function a similar organ, as the accessory pancreatic duct (of Santorini) or accessory suprarenal glands. An organ or structure which assists other organs in performing their functions as accessory reproductive organs.

    a. food substances. Substances necessary to maintain normal health but which are not sources of energy. Include water, inorganic salts, and vitamins.

a. nerve. 11th cranial nerve; spinal accessory nerve. Motor nerve made up of a cranial and a spinal part which supplies the trapezius and sternomastoid muscles and pharynx. Accessory portion joins the vagus, to which it supplies its motor and some of its cardio-inhibitory fibers.

a. sign. A nonpathognomonic sign.

accident (ăk'sĭ-dĕnt) [L. *accidens,* happening]. 1. An unexpected event. 2. An unforeseen occurrence of an unfortunate nature; a mishap. 3. An unexpected complicating event in the course of a disease, or following surgery.

a., cerebrovascular. A sudden, unexpected interference in brain function resulting from a vascular disturbance such as cerebral hemorrhage, occlusion of a vessel by a thrombus or embolus, vasospasm, or vasodilation. ABBR: CVA. SYN: *apoplexy.*

a., serum. An allergic reaction following the therapeutic introduction of a foreign serum into a hypersensitive individual. SEE: *anaphylaxis.*

accidental (ăk"sĭ-dĕn'tăl). Occurring suddenly, unexpectedly, inadvertently; under unforeseen circumstances.

accident-prone. Said of persons having an unusually high rate of accidents.

accipiter (ăk-sĭp'ĭ-tĕr) [L., a hawk]. A nose bandage with clawlike ends which spread over the face.

ACCl. Abbr. for *anodal closure clonus.*

acclimation, acclimatization (ăk-lĭ-mā'shŭn, a-klī-mă-tĭ-zā'shun) [Fr. *acclimater,* acclimate]. The act of becoming accustomed to a new climate.

acclimatize (ăk-klī'mă-tīz). To become accustomed to a different environment and climate.

accommodation [L. *accomodare,* to suit]. 1. Adjustment or adaptation, esp. adjustment of the eye for seeing at different distance. ABBR: a.; acc. SEE: *adaptation.* 2. In opthalmology, the term is applied to a phenomenon noted in receptors in which continued stimulation fails to elicit a sensation or response.

The adjustment of the eye whereby it is able to focus the image of the object on the retina. In accommodation for near vision, the following changes occur: contraction of ciliary muscle causes relaxation of the zonule which is attached to the lens. This reduces tension on the lens allowing it to assume the shape of a sphere. This in turn allows the visual image of near objects to be focused on the retina. In addition, the pupil

contracts and the optic axes converge. These three actions, all reflex in nature, comprise the accommodation reflex. In accommodation for far vision, the reverse changes occur. The ability of the eye to accommodate decreases with age.

a., absolute. The amount of accommodation of one eye separately.

a., amplitude of. The difference between refracting power of the eye when accommodating for near and far vision. It is measured in diopters (D) and normally diminishes progressively from childhood to old age. It is approximately 16 D at age 12, 6.5 D at age 30, and 1 D at age 50.

a., binocular. Meeting of both eyes at a point in order to carry the object's image to the retina of both.

a., excessive. Greater-than-needed accommodation of the eye.

a., histologic. Change in cell form and function due to change in surrounding conditions.

a., mechanism. Method by which curvature of eye lens is changed in order to focus close objects on the retina.

a., negative. Relaxation by the eye to adjust itself for long distances.

a., positive. Contraction by the eye to adjust itself for short distances.

a., range of. Space of vision between its closest and most remote points.

a. reflex. A group of three reflexes closely associated with each other which facilitate the production of sharp images on corresponding points of the retinae. They are contraction of ciliary muscle resulting in rounding of lens, contraction of pupil, and convergence of eyes. SYN: *near reflex.*

a., relative. The extent to which accommodation is possible for any specific state of convergence of eyes.

a., spasm of. A spasm of the ciliary muscle usually resulting from excessive strain from over-use. Common in myopia in which accommodation is continually used in order to see anything, even distant objects, clearly.

a., subnormal. Insufficient accommodation of the eye.

a., synaptic. Condition in which nerve cells at synapses become less excitable to presynaptic impulses.

accommodative iridoplegia (ă-kŏm'ō-dā"tĭv ĭr"ĭ-dō-plē'jĭ-ă). Noncontraction of pupils during accommodation.

accouchement (ă-kūsh-mon'). The act of delivery in childbirth; parturition.

a. forcé. Forced delivery, especially by version, forceps or other means. Formerly denoted forcible hand delivery.

accoucheur (ă-kū-shŭr′) [Fr.]. An obstetrician.

accoucheuse (ă-kū-shūz′) [Fr.]. A midwife.

accrementition (ăk″rĕ-mĕn-tĭsh′ŭn) [L. *accrescere,* to increase]. Growth of tissues by addition of similar tissue.

accretio (ă-krē′shĭ-ō) [L.]. Adhesion of parts normally separate from each other.

a. cordis. Condition in which fibrous bands extend from external pericardium to surrounding structures resulting in angulation and torsion of heart.

accretion (ă-krē′shŭn) [L. *accrēscere,* accrue]. 1. Increase by external addition; accumulation 2. The growing together of parts naturally separate. 3. Accumulation of foreign matter in a cavity.

acculturation. The process in which a member of one culture assumes the values, attitudes, and behavior of a second culture in order to become an accepted member of that culture.

ACD. Abbr. for *absolute cardiac dullness.*

ACD sol. Citric acid, trisodium citrate, dextrose solution. The anticoagulant used when collecting blood for transfusions.

ACE. Abbr. for *adrenal cortical extract.*

acedia (ă-sē′dĭ-ă) [Gr. *a-,* not, + *kedos,* care]. Mental state of indifference, insensibility, lack of emotion. SYN: *apathy.*

acenesthesia (ă-sĕn″ĕs-thē′zĭ-ă) [″+ *koinos,* common, + *aisthēsis,* sensation]. Absence of a feeling of well-being, present in such disorders as hypochondriasis and neurasthenia.

acentric (ă-sĕn′trĭk) [Gr. *a-,* not, + L. *centrum,* center]. Not central; peripheral.

A.C.E.P. Abbr. for *American College of Emergency Physicians.*

acephalia, acephalism (ă-sĕ-fā′lĭ-ă, ă-sĕf′ă-lĭzm) [″+ *kephalē,* head]. A developmental disorder in which the head is absent.

acephalo- (ă-sĕf′ă-lō-) [Gr. *a-,* not, + *kephalē,* head]. Combining form meaning without a head.

acephalobrachia (ă-sĕf′ă-lō-brā′kĭ-ă) [″+ ″+ *brachion,* arm]. A developmental anomaly in which head and arms are absent.

acephalus (ă-sĕf′ă-lŭs). A malformed fetus.

acerate (ăs′ĕr-āt) [L. *ācer*]. Sharp, pointed.

acerbity (ă-sĕrb′ĭ-tĭ) [L. *acerbus,* sharp]. Astringency combined with acidity.

acervuline (ă-sĕr′vū-lĭn) [L. *acervulus,* a little heap]. Aggregated, occurring in clusters.

acervuloma (ă-sĕr″vū-lō′mă) [″+ *-ōma,* tumor]. Intracranial tumor containing psammoma bodies.

acer′vulus (ă-sĕr′vū-lŭs) [L.]. Sandy, gritty, sabulous.

a. cer′ebri. Gritty matter filling the follicle of the pineal gland. SYN: *brain sand.*

acescence (ă-sĕs′ĕns) [L. *acescere,* to become sour]. 1. Slight acidity. 2. Process of souring.

acescent (ă-sĕs′ĕnt). Slightly acid.

acesodyne (ă-sĕs′ō-dĭn) [Gr. *akesis,* cure, + *odynē,* pain]. An agent for relieving pain. SYN: *anodyne.*

acestoma (ă-sĕs-tō′mă) [Gr. *akestos,* curable, + *-ōma,* tumor]. The fresh granulations which later form a cicatrix.

acetabular (ăs′ĕ-tăb′ū-lăr). Pert. to the acetabulum.

acetabulum (ăs′ĕ-tăb′ū-lŭm) [L., a little saucer for vinegar]. 1. The rounded (cotyloid) cavity on the external surface of the innominate bone (os coxae or os innominatum) which receives head of femur. 2. The ventral sucker of the fluke.

acetanilid (ăs″ē-tăn′ĭ-lĭd). A white powder or crystalline substance obtained by interaction of glacial acetic acid and aniline. Originally introduced as antifebrin.

ACTION AND USES: Analgesic, antipyretic, and anti-inflammatory. Acute or chronic poisoning may develop following prolonged administration or drug idiosyncrasy. Because of its toxicity, it is rarely used.

POISONING SYM: Cyanosis due to formation of methemoglobin, cold sweat, irregular pulse, dyspnea, and unconsciousness. Sudden cardiac failure may occur.

F.A. TREATMENT: In acute poisoning, analeptics such as caffeine, external heat, inhalation of oxygen, gastric lavage or emetics, artificial respiration, blood transfusion. In chronic poisoning, stop use of drug; iron preparations for secondary anemia.

acetarsone (ăs″ē-tăr′sōn). An arsenical compound, acetylamino-hydroxy-phenyl-arsonic acid, contains 27% arsenic. Used in amebiasis and trichomonas vaginalis infections.

acetate (ăs′ē-tāt). A salt of acetic acid.

acetazolamide (ăs″ĕt-ăz″ōl-ăm′ĭd). USP. A fine white powder, slightly soluble in alcohol or water. It is a sulfonamide compound used as a diuretic. It has been used also in glaucoma and in epilepsy.

acetic (ă-sē′tĭk) [L. *acetum,* vinegar]. Pert. to vinegar; sour.

a. acid. CH_3COOH. The acid in vinegar. An aqueous solution containing not less than 36% or more than 37% by weight of CH_3COOH. Used as a reagent, a caustic; sometimes taken internally. SYN: *ethanoic acid.*

a. acid glacial. USP. A solution containing not less than 99.5% by weight of $C_2H_4O_2$.

acetify (ă-sĕt'ĭ-fī) [L. *acetum,* vinegar, + *fieri,* to become]. To produce acetic fermentation or vinegar.

acetimeter (ă-sĕ-tim'ĕ-tĕr) ["+ Gr. *metron,* measure]. An apparatus which determines the acetic acid in fluid.

acetoacetic acid (ăs"ĭ-tō-ă-sē'tĭk). A ketone body formed when fats are incompletely oxidized as in diabetes. Appears in the urine in abnormal amounts in starvation or diabetes. SYN: *diacetic acid.*

Acetobacter (as-ē-tō-bak'tĕr) [L. *acetum,* vinegar, + Gr. *bacterion,* little rod]. A genus of non-pathogenic bacteria of the family Pseudomonadeceae.

A. aceti. Produces vinegar from wine or cider. This produces a stringy substance in the liquid called mother of vinegar.

acetolase (a-set'o-lās). An enzyme which catalyzes conversion of alcohol into acetic acid.

acetonasthma (as"ē-tōn-as'ma). A form of asthma associated with acetonuria. SYN: *uremic asthma.*

acetone (ăs'ē-tōn). Dimethyl ketone $(CH_3)_2$-CO, a colorless, volatile, inflammable liquid, miscible with water, useful as a solvent, and having a characteristic sweet, fruity, ethereal odor. Found in the blood and urine in diabetes, faulty metabolism, and after lengthy fasting, produced when the fats are not properly oxidized, due to inability to oxidize glucose in the blood. SEE: *acetonuria, acidosis, ketone, ketosis, tests.*

a. bodies. Certain substances related to acetone. An example is acetoacetic acid, q.v. SYN: *ketone bodies,* q.v.

a. in urine, test for. Take five cc. of urine; add a few crystals of ammonium sulfate and dissolve; add a small crystal of sodium nitroprusside, and shake a little. Cover with a layer (about two cc.) of strong ammonia. The presence of acetone is indicated by the formation of a purple ring between the layers of liquid.

Test may also be done by wetting a specially treated paper with urine. If acetone is present, the paper will turn a certain color. These test papers or "sticks" are commercially available.

acetonemia (ăs"ē-tō-nē'mĭ-ă). Large amounts of acetone in blood.

SYM: Abnormal excitement, gradual depression, acidosis.

acetonitrile (ăs"ē-tō-ni'trĭl). CH_3CN. Methyl cyanide. A substance which is found in an increased amount in the urine of persons

who smoke three or more cigarettes a day.

acetonuria (ăs"ē-tō-nū'rĭ-ă). The occurrence of acetone and diacetic bodies in the urine, as in the ketosis of diabetes, starvation, etc., which may be due to incomplete oxidation of fats. SEE: *acetone; acidosis; tests.*

acetophenetidin (as"ē-tō-fē-nĕt'ĭ-dĭn). An odorless, white, crystalline substance derived from coal tar. An antipyretic and analgesic. Must be used cautiously as it is toxic and may cause hemolysis of red blood cells. Prolonged use causes serious damage to the kidneys. SYN: *phenacetin.*

acetous (ăs'ē-tŭs) [L. *acetum,* vinegar]. 1. Pert. to vinegar. 2. Sour in taste.

acetum (ă-sē'tŭm) [L.]. (pl. *aceta*) 1. Vinegar. 2. A drug dissolved in a weak vinegar solution.

acetyl (ăs'ē-tĭl) [L. *acetum,* vinegar, + Gr. *hylē,* matter]. The univalent radical, CH_3-CO.

acetylation (ă-sĕt'ĭ-lā'shŭn). The introduction of one or more acetyl groups into an organic compound.

acetylbetamethylcholine (ăs"ē-tĭl-bā"tă-mĕth"ĭl-kō'lĭn). A derivative of acetylcholine which is a strong stimulus to the parasympathetic nervous system.

ACTION: Lowers blood pressure, vasodilation, stimulates peristalsis, and increases sweating. Used in tachycardia.

acetylcholine (ă"sĕt-ĭl-kō'lēn). An ester of choline occurring in various organs and tissues of the body. It is thought to play an important role in the transmission of nerve impulses at synapses and myoneural junctions. It is quickly destroyed by an enzyme, cholinesterase. Either excessive or deficient action of acetylcholine at the motor endplates may result in neuromuscular block. ABBR: ACh. SEE: *cholinergic fibers.*

a. chloride. A salt of acetylcholine injected intramuscularly or subcutaneously as a parasympathetic stimulant. It lowers blood pressure by dilating peripheral vessels and relaxes smooth muscle spasms.

acetylene (a-sĕt'ĭ-lēn). C_2H_2. A colorless explosive gas with a garlic-like odor.

acetylsalicylic acid (ăs"ĕt-ĭl-săl"ĭ-sĭl'ĭk). USP. A white crystalline solid formed by the action of acetic anhydride on salicylic acid. It is one of the most widely used analgesics and antipyretics. Also, because it is widely available, it is often misused, and is one of the most frequent causes of accidental poisoning in children. SYN: *aspirin.*

POISONING: In acute, signs vary with increasing doses from mild lethargy and hyperpnea to coma and convulsions. Sweating, dehydration, and restlessness may be present with moderate doses. In chronic poisoning, tinnitus, skin rash, bleeding tendency, weight loss, and mental symptoms may be present.

TREATMENT: In acute, gastric lavage or emetics. Give sodium sulfate by mouth to remove remaining salicylate. Artificial respiration with administration of oxygen may be required.

For a child if blood pressure is low, give whole blood transfusion at the rate of 10-15 ml./kg. for one hour. Glucose by mouth or intravenously is indicated if hypoglycemia is present. For convulsions not due to hypoglycemia give succinylcholine intravenously and at the same time give artificial respiration. Be certain to maintain the airway. In very severe cases, exchange transfusion or dialysis of the blood by using an artificial kidney.

ACH. 1. Abbr. for *adrenal cortical hormone.* 2. An index of nutrition based on *a* rm girth, *c* hest depth, and *h* ip width.

ACh. Abbr. for *acetylcholine.*

achalasia (ăk″ă-lā′zĭ-ă) [Gr. *a-*, not, + *chalasis*, relaxation]. Failure to relax; said of muscles, such as sphincters, the normal function of which is a persistent contraction with periods of relaxation.

　　a. of the cardia. Failure of relaxation of lower segment of esophagus resulting in difficulty in passage of foods to the stomach. In advanced cases, dysphagia is marked and dilatation of the esophagus may occur. SYN: *cardiospasm.*

　　a., pelvirectal. Congenital dilatation of the colon.

　　a., sphincteral. Failure of intestinal sphincters to relax.

AChE. Abbr. for *acetylcholinesterase.*

ache (āk) [AS. *ācan*]. 1. A continued pain as distinguished from a sudden or spasmodic pain. May be dull or severe. 2. To suffer continued pain.

acheilia (ă-kī′lĭ-ă) [Gr. *a-*, not, + *cheilos*, lip]. Developmental anomaly in which there is an absence of one or both lips.

acheiria (ă-kī′rĭ-ă) [″+ *cheir*, hand]. 1. Congenital absence of one or both hands. 2. Loss of sensation in, with accompanying sense of loss of, one or both hands. May result from temporary or permanent injury or malfunction of sensory mechanism, or may occur in hysteria. 3. Inability to determine to which side of the body a stimulus has been applied. SYN: *achiria.*

acheiropodia (ă-kī″rō-pō′dĭ-ă) [″+ ″+ *pous*, foot]. Developmental anomaly in which there is an absence of hands and feet.

achievement age. Determined by test for proficiency in a subject. The result is compared with the score obtained by average children of that age group. ABBR: A. A. SEE: *age.*

　　a. a. quotient. A state of progress in learning ascertained by dividing the achievement age by the mental age. ABBR: A. Q.

Achilles jerk. [Achilles, hero of the *Iliad*, whose vulnerable spot was his heel because it was the place where his mother held him when she immersed him in the river Styx.] The Achilles tendon reflex.

Achilles tendon (ă-kĭl′ēz tĕn′dŏn). The tendon of the gastrocnemius and soleus muscles of the leg. SYN: *tendo calcaneus.*

　　A. t. reflex. Plantar flexion extension of foot resulting from contraction of calf muscles following a sharp blow to the Achilles tendon. The variations and their significance correspond closely to those of the knee jerk. It is exaggerated in upper motor neuron disease and diminished or absent in lower motor neuron disease. The character of the response is influenced by the metabolic rate. Thus attempts have been made to use this reflex as an index of thyroid function. The value of such use is questionable.

achillobursitis (ă-kĭl″ō-bŭr-sī′tĭs) [″+ L. *bursa*, a pouch, + Gr. *-itis*, inflammation]. Inflammation of the bursa lying over the tendo calcaneus.

achillodynia (ă-kĭl″ō-dĭn′ĭ-ă) [″+ *odyne*, pain]. Pain caused by inflammation between the tendo calcaneus and the bursa.

achillorrhaphy (ă-kĭl-ŏr′ă-fĭ) [″+ Gr. *raphē*, sewing]. Suture of tendo calcaneus.

achillotomy (ă-kĭl-ŏt′ō-mĭ) [″+ *tomē*, incision]. A division of tendo calcaneus. SYN: *achillotenotomy.*

achiria (ă-kī′rĭ-ă) [Gr. *a-*, not, + *cheir*, hand]. 1. Congenital lack of hands. 2. Loss of sense of possession of one or both hands. 3. Inability to tell on which side of body a stimulus is applied. SYN: *acheiria.*

achlorhydria (ā″klōr-hī′drĭ-ă) [″+ *chlōros*, green, + *hydōr*, water]. Absence of free hydrochloric acid in the stomach.

　　ETIOL: May be due to gastric carcinoma, gastric ulcer, pernicious anemia, adrenal insufficiency, chronic gastritis. SEE: *achylia.*

　　a., histamine proved. Absence of free acid in gastric secretion even after subcutaneous injection of histamine hydrochloride.

achloride (ă-klō′rĭd). A salt other than a chloride; nonchloride.

achloropsia (ă-klō-rop′sĭ-ă) [Gr. *a-*, not, + *chloros*, green, + *opsis*, vision]. Color blindness in which green cannot be distinguished. SEE: *deuteranopsia.*

acholia (ă-kō'lĭ-ă) ["+ *cholē,* bile]. An absence or want of bile or a condition which prevents bile from entering the duodenum.

    a., pigmentary. Bile deficiency indicated by clay-colored feces in the absence of jaundice.

acholic (ă-kō'lĭk). Pert. to acholia.

acholuria (ă-kō-lū'rĭ-ă) [Gr. *a-,* not, + *cholē,* bile, + *ouron,* urine]. In some forms of jaundice, absence of bile pigments in the urine.

achondroplasia (ă-kŏn"drō-plā'sĭ-ă) ["+ *chondros,* cartilage, + *plasis,* a moulding]. Defect in the formation of cartilage at the epiphyses of long bones, producing a form of dwarfism; sometimes seen in rickets. SYN: *chondrodystrophy.*

achoresis (ă-kō-rē'sĭs) [Gr. *a-,* not, + *chōrein,* to make room]. A permanent reduction in size of the bladder, stomach, or other hollow viscus thus reducing its capacity.

achreocythemia (ă-krē"ō-sī-thē'mĭ-ă) [Gr. *achroios,* colorless, + *kytos,* cell, + *haima,* blood]. Absence of coloring in the red blood cells as a result of deficiency or lack of hemoglobin. SYN: *achroiocythemia.*

achroacyte (ă-krō'ă-sīt). A lymphocyte; a colorless cell.

achroacytosis (ă-krō"ă-sī-tō'sis) [Gr. *achroios,* colorless, + *kytos,* cell, + *-ōsis,* condition]. Many lymphocytes in the peripheral circulation.

achroiocythemia (ă-kroy"ō-sī-thē'mĭ-ă) ["+ "+ *haima,* blood]. *Achreocythemia,* q.v.

achroma (ă-krō'mă) [Gr. *a-,* not, + *chrōma,* color]. An absence of color or normal pigmentation as in leukoderma, albinism, etc. Hereditary, circumscribed skin areas deficient in pigmentation.

achromacyte (ă-krō'mă-sīt) ["+ "+ *kytos,* cell]. A decolorized erythrocyte; one in which hemoglobin is lacking or has been lost. SYN: *achromatocyte; ghost corpuscle; phantom corpuscle; Ponfick's shadow.*

achromasia (ăk"rō-mā'zĭ-ă) [Gr. *achromatos,* without color]. 1. Absence of normal pigmentation of the skin as in albinism, vitiligo, leukoderma. 2. Pallor. 3. The lack of the ability to be stained, said of cells or tissues.

achromate (ă-krō'māt) [Gr. *a-,* not, + *chrōma,* color]. A person who is color blind.

achromatic (ak"rō-măt'ĭk) [Gr. *achrōmatos,* without color]. 1. Lacking in color. 2. Not dispersing light into its constituent components. 3. Not containing or composed of chromatin. 4. Staining with difficulty, with reference to cells and tissues.

    a. lens. One which transmits light without separating the spectral colors.

achromatin (ă-krō'mă-tĭn). The weakly staining substance of a cell nucleus.

achro'matism. Colorlessness.

achromatocyte (ăk"rō-măt'ō-sīt) [Gr. *a-,* not, + *chrōma,* color, + *kytos,* cell]. A decolorized red blood cell. SYN: *achromacyte; ghost corpuscle; phantom corpuscle.*

achromatolysis (ă-krō"mă-tŏl'ĭ-sĭs) ["+ "+ *lysis,* loosing]. Dissolution of cell achromatin. SYN: *plasmolysis.*

achromatophil (ā"krō-mat'ō-fĭl) ["+ "+ *philos,* love]. A cell or tissue that is not stainable in the usual manner.

achromatopsia (ă-krō"mă-top'sĭ-ă) [Gr. *achrōmatos,* without color, + *opsis,* vision]. Color blindness.

achromatosis (ă-krō"mă-tō'sĭs) ["+ *ōsis,* condition]. Condition of being without natural pigmentation. SEE: *achroma.*

achromatous (ă-krō'mă-tŭs). Without color.

achromaturia (ă-krō"mă-tū'rĭ-ă) [Gr. *achrōmatos,* without color, + *-ouron,* urine]. Colorless or nearly colorless urine.

achromia (ă-krō'mĭ-ă) [Gr. *a-,* not, + *chroma,* color]. 1. Absence of color; pallor. 2. Achromatosis. 3. Condition in which erythrocytes are pale and have large central pale areas; hypochromia.

    a., congenital. Albinism, q.v.

achromic (ă-krō'mĭk). Lacking color.

achromoderma (ă-krō"mō-dĕr'mă) [Gr. *a-,* not, + *chroma,* color, + *derma,* skin]. Lack of color in skin. Leukoderma.

achromophil (ă-krō'mō-fĭl) ["+ "+ *philos,* fond]. Achromatophil, q.v.

achromotrichia (ă-krō"mō-trĭk'ĭ-ă) ["+ "+ *trichia,* condition of the hair]. Lack of color or graying of the hair. SYN: *canities.*

    a., nutritional. Grayness of hair due to dietary deficiency.

achromycin (ăk"rō-mī'sĭn). Proprietary name for tetracycline, an antibiotic effective in treatment of many bacterial infections.

achroodextrin (ak"rō-ō-dĕks'trĭn) [Gr. *achroos,* colorless, + dextrin]. One of the varieties of dextrin resulting from hydrolysis of starch.

achylia (ă-kī'lĭ-ă) [Gr. *a-,* not, + *chylos,* chyle]. Absence of chyle or other digestive ferments.

    a. gastrica. Complete absence or marked diminution in amount of gastric juice. SEE: *achlorhydria.*

    a. pancreat'ica. Absence or deficiency of pancreatic secretion. Usually a manifestation of chronic pancreatitis.

achylosis (ā"kī-lō'sis). Achylia, q.v.

achylous (ă-kī'lŭs) [Gr. *achylos,* without chyle]. 1. Lacking in any kind of digestive secretion. 2. Without chyle.

achymia, achymosis (ă-kī'mĭ-ă, ak-ĭ-mō'-sis) [Gr. *a-,* not, + *chymos,* juice]. Deficiency or absence of chyme.

acicular (ă-sĭk'ū-lăr) [L. *aciculus,* little needle]. Needle-shaped.

acid [L. *acidus,* sour]. 1. Any substance of a group which characteristically is sour in taste, neutralizes basic substances, makes litmus paper red, and produces hydrogen ions (protons) when reacting with certain metals. SEE: *indicator.* 2. A sour substance.

a., acetic. USP. $C_2H_4O_2$. Gives sour taste to vinegar. Also used as a reagent, a caustic; sometimes taken internally. SYN: *ethanoic acid.*

a., acetic dilute. Containing 6% pure acetic acid.

a., acetic glacial. USP. Contains not less than 99.5% of acetic acid ($C_2 H_4O_2$) by weight.

a., acetoacetic. CH_3COCH_2COOH. A ketone body formed when fats are incompletely oxidized. Appears in urine in abnormal amounts in starvation or diabetes. SYN: *acetylacetic acid; diacetic acid; 3-oxobutanoic acid.*

a., acetylsalicylic. USP. CH_3COOC_6-H_4COOH. Derivative of salicylic acid. It occurs as white crystals or powder and is odorless. Used extensively for analgesic and antipyretic actions. Poisoning may occur from an overdose. SYN: *Aspirin.*

TREATMENT: SEE: *acetylsalicylic acid.*

a., adenylic. A nucleotide; it occurs in muscle, blood corpuscles and yeast as well as other nuclear material. SYN: *adenosine monophosphate.*

a., amino. An organic acid containing one or more NH_2 (amino) groups and a COOH (carboxyl) group; these compounds are the basic building blocks for all of the body's protein elements. The end-products of digestion of proteins which are absorbed finally into the tissues. Certain of these acids are essential in the human body for growth and repair of tissues. Oral preparations of essential amino acids may be used as dietary supplements when necessary. SEE: *amino acid.*

a., aminoacetic. NH_2CH_2COOH. One of the simplest examples of an amino acid. Same as glycine.

a., aminosalicylic. Para-aminosalicylic acid, q.v.

a., ascorbic. USP. $C_6H_8O_6$. A vitamin which occurs naturally in fresh fruits, esp. citrus fruits, and in fresh vegetables. Essential in maintenance of collagen formation, osteoid tissue of bones, and formation and maintenance of dentin. This essential vitamin is used as a dietary supplement and in the prevention and treatment of scurvy. It requires about three months of lack of ascorbic acid in the diet for scurvy to develop. The usefulness of large daily doses (1-5 gm. a day) of this vitamin in preventing or treating the common cold in otherwise healthy persons has not been established. Continuous treatment with large doses may cause kidney stones to form. SYN: *vitamin C; antiscorbutic vitamin.*

a., aspartic. $COOHCHNH_2CH_2COOH$. An amino acid; one of the products of pancreatic digestion.

a., barbituric. $C_4H_4O_3N_2$. A crystalline compound from which phenobarbital and other barbiturates are derived. SYN: *malonylurea.*

a., benzoic. USP. $C_7H_6O_2$. A white crystalline material having a slight odor. Used in keratolytic ointments, and as a food preservative. Saccharin is a derivative of this acid.

a., bile. Any substance occurring in the form of salt in the bile; glycocholic acid and taurocholic acid. On combination with a base they give rise to bile salts. They are formed by the reaction of glycocoll (glycine) or taurin with cholic acid.

a., boracic. A., boric, q.v.

a., boric. H_3BO_3. A white crystalline substance giving very weak acid solutions, poisonous to plants and animals. Soluble in water, alcohol, or glycerin.

CAUTION: Because of its toxicity, the use of boric acid should be quite limited. It is particularly dangerous in areas where it could be accidentally swallowed by children or used in food because of its physical resemblance to sugar. SEE: *boric acid.*

a., butyric. C_3H_7COOH. A liquid having a rancid odor; found in rancid butter, in cheese, perspiration, and cod liver oil.

a., carbolic. Obsolescent name for phenol.

a., carbonic. H_2CO_3. An acid formed from carbon dioxide dissolved in water.

a., carboxylic. Any one containing the group COOH. The simplest examples are formic and acetic.

a., chaulmoogric. A cyclic unsaturated fatty acid in chaulmoogra oil, formerly used in treatment of leprosy (Hansen's disease).

a., chromic. CrO_3. Escharotic sometimes used to remove warts. SYN: *chromic anhydride; chromium trioxide.*

a., citric. USP. $C_6H_8O_7$. Prepared synthetically or from lemon or lime juice in form of colorless crystals or white crystalline powder. Soluble in water, ether or alcohol. Used as a preventive of scurvy. Hydrous form is used as a flavoring agent or vehicle.

a., deoxyribonucleic. The material of which chromosomes are primarily composed. It is believed to be the entire inheritable substance in living tissue. Sugar, phosphoric acid and a nitrogenous base are the essential components of this acid. ABBR: DNA.

a., desoxyribonucleic. A., deoxyribonucleic, q.v.

a., diacetic. A., acetoacetic, q.v.

a., ethanoic. A., acetic, q.v.

a., ethylenediaminetetracetic. A compound which, in the form of its calcium or sodium salts, is useful in removing certain substances such as lead and digitalis from the body. This is done by chelation, q.v. ABBR: EDTA.

a., fatty. One of a series of carboxylic acids, with a general formula of RCOOH or $C_nH_{2n}O_2$, which can be combined with *glycerol* to form fats; the simplest members of the series are formic and acetic; most typical, stearic and palmitic. A fatty acid which contains carbon atoms with double bonds between them, i.e. $C=C-C=C$ etc. instead of $C-C-C-C$ etc. The former is called an unsaturated fatty acid. In human nutrition the diet should contain unsaturated rather than saturated fatty acids because of the importance of the latter in cholesterol metabolism.

a., folic. USP. A member of the vitamin B complex. Used in treatment of sprue. Found naturally in green plant tissue, liver and yeast. Produced synthetically, its formula is $C_{19}H_{19}N_7O_6$ and is identical with pteroylglutamic acid.

CAUTION: Folic acid should not be used in the treatment of pernicious anemia because it does not protect patients against the development of changes in the central nervous system which accompany this type of anemia.

a., formic. HCOOH. The first member of the monobasic fatty acid series, but is a much stronger acid than the others in the series. It occurs naturally in animal secretions and in muscle, but it may also be prepared synthetically. It is one of the irritants present in the sting of insects such as bees and ants. SYN: *methanoic acid.*

a., formiminoglutamic. $C_6N_2O_4H_{10}$. An intermediate product in the metabolism of histidine. Its increase in the urine after administration of histroline in patients with folic acid deficiency is the basis for the Figlu excretion test. ABBR: Figlu.

a., gallic. $C_6H_2(OH)_3COOH$. A colorless crystalline acid. It occurs naturally in plants such as nut galls and tea. It is used as a skin astringent, and in the manufacture of writing inks and dyes. SYN: *3,4,5-trihydroxybenzoic acid.*

a., glucuronic. $CHO(CHOH)_4COOH$. An oxidation product of glucose. Found in the urine. Toxic products (such as salicylic acid, menthol, and phenol) that have entered the body through the intestinal system are detoxified in the liver by conjugation with glucuronic acid. SYN: *glycuronic acid.*

a., glutamic. $COOH(CH_2)_2CH(NH_2)$-COOH. A non-essential amino acid formed during protein metabolism. Is used orally as an anticonvulsant. SYN: *aminoglutaric acid; glutaminic acid.*

a., glyceric. $CH_2OHCHOHCOOH$. An intermediate product of oxidation of fats. SYN: *2,3-dihydroxypropanoic acid.*

a., glycocholic. $C_{24}H_{39}O_4NHCH_2$-COOH. A conjugate with glycine in the bile.

a., homogentisic. An acid found in the urine in alkaptonuria. SYN: *alkapton.*

a., hydriodic. HI. In solution, it is used in various forms of chemical analyses (quantitative, qualitative, etc.). A well-diluted solution is used orally in iodide treatment of thyroid gland disease. SYN: *hydrogen iodide.*

a., hydrochloric. USP. HCl. An inorganic acid. Occurs naturally in the gastric juice. Presence of this acid is essential to digestion. It also destroys fermenting bacteria which might cause intestinal tract disturbances. A further-diluted solution of 25% hydrochloric acid is used in hypoacidity or achlorhydria.

Caution: When so used, it must be diluted accurately and swallowed by using a drinking straw. This will prevent the acid from damaging the teeth. SYN: *muriatic acid.*

a., hydrocyanic. HCN. A colorless, extremely poisonous, highly volatile liquid. Occurs naturally in plants. It is obtained synthetically by several methods. Has many industrial uses: electroplating, fumigation, and production of dyes, pigments, synthetic fibers, and plastic. Exposure of man to 200-500 parts of acid per 1,000,000 parts of air for 30 minutes is fatal. It acts by preventing cellular respiration. SYN: *prussic acid; hydrogen cyanide.*

TREATMENT: SEE: *cyanide* in *Table of Poisons and Poisoning* in *Appendix.*

a., hydroxytoluic. A., mandelic, q.v.

a., imino. An acid formed as a result of oxidation of amino acids in the body.

a., lactic. USP. $C_3H_6O_3$. Occurs in sour milk from fermentation of lactose present and is formed in muscles during the metabolic changes which occur during strenuous exercise. Lactic acid milk (buttermilk or acidophilus milk) is administered to help prevent growth of putrefactive bacteria in the large intestine. SYN: *2-hydroxypropanoic acid; 2-hydroxypropionic acid.*

a., linoleic. $C_{18}H_{32}O_2$. An unsaturated fatty acid, a dietary essential. First isolated from linseed oil but is also found in corn oil. SYN: *linolic acid; 9,12-octadecadienoic acid.*

a., linolenic. $C_{18}H_{30}O_2$. An unsaturated fatty acid, a dietary essential.

a., linolic. A., linoleic, q.v.

a., lysergic. A crystalline substance, $C_{16}H_{16}N_2O_2$ derived from ergot. Its derivative, lysergic acid diethylamide, LSD, is a potent hallucinogen. SEE: *LSD.*

a., malic. $C_4H_6O_5$. Found in certain sour fruits as apples and apricots. Active in aerobic metabolism of carbohydrate.

a., malonic. $C_3H_4O_4$. A dibasic acid formed by oxidation of malic acid. Occurs in beets. Active in the tricarboxylic acid cycle in carbohydrate metabolism. Its inhibition of succinic dehydrogenase is the classic example of competitive inhibition.

a., mandelic. $C_8H_8O_3$. A colorless hydroxy acid. Its salt is used in urinary tract infections.

a., methanoic. A., formic, q.v.

a., mineral. Acids prepared from inorganic materials, as sulfuric, hydrochloric, nitric, and phosphoric acids.

a., muriatic. A., hydrochloric, q.v.

a., nicotinic. $C_6H_5NO_2$. A member of the vitamin B complex. Occurs naturally in liver, yeast, milk, cheese, and cereals. Used for prevention and specific treatment of pellagra. SYN: *niacin.*

a., nitric. HNO_3. A strong corrosive acid prepared from sulfuric acid and a nitrate. It is used in manufacture of explosives and dyes, and as a coagulant in testing urine for albumin (Heller's ring test).

a., nucleic. Combines with protein to form nucleoprotein, a substance in the nuclei of cells of all living things. SEE: *deoxyribonucleic a.*

a., oleic. $C_{18}H_{34}O_2$. An unsaturated fatty acid that can be prepared from various fats and oils. SYN: *9-octadecenoic acid.*

a., organic. An acid containing the carboxyl radical COOH.

a., oxalic. $H_2C_2O_4$, or $(COOH)_2$. The simplest dibasic organic acid occurring as colorless monoclinic crystals. It occurs naturally in rhubarb, wood sorrel and many other plants. It is the strongest organic acid and is poisonous. It is effective in removing ink or rust stains from cloth. It is used also as a reagent. SYN: *ethanedioic acid.*

a., palmitic. $C_{15}H_{31}COOH$. A saturated fatty acid occurring as esters in most natural fats and oils. SYN: *hexadecanoic acid.*

a., pantothenic. $C_9H_{17}NO_5$. A member of the vitamin B complex.

a., para-aminobenzoic. $NH_2C_6H_4$-COOH. A member of the vitamin B complex. It is used as a dietary supplement and as an antirickettsial drug. It is also used as a reagent. Also known as p-aminobenzoic acid. ABBR: PABA.

a., para-aminosalicylic. USP. C_7H_7-NO_3. It is a white or nearly white and practically odorless powder that darkens when exposed to air or light. It is an antituberculosis drug, but its effectiveness is greatly enhanced when used in combination with streptomycin and isoniazid; it is believed to delay development of bacterial resistance. SYN: *aminosalicylic acid.*

a., pectic. An acid derived from pectin.

a., perchloric. $HClO_4$. A colorless unstable liquid; the highest oxygen acid of chlorine.

a., phenylglycolic. A., mandelic, q.v.

a., phosphoric. An oxygen acid of phosphorus, used as an alkaloidal reagent. The phosphoric acids are: orthophosphoric acid, H_3PO_4; pyrophosphoric, $H_4P_2O_7$; metaphosphoric, HPO_3; and hypophosphoric, $H_4P_2O_6$. The salts of these acids are phosphates.

a., phosphorous. An oxygen acid of phosphorus. The phosphorous acids are: ortho-, $H_2(HPO_3)$; pyro-, $H_4P_2O_5$; meta-, HPO_2; and hypo-, $H(H_2PO_2)$. The salts of these acids are phosphites.

a., phosphotungstic. $H_3PW_{12}O_{40}$-$.24H_2O$. A trigonal crystalline organic acid, the water content of which may vary. Used in the form of its sodium salt in testing for alkaloids.

a., picric. $C_6H_2(NO_2)_3OH$. A yellow crystalline substance which precipitates proteins.

a., prussic. A., hydrocyanic, q.v.

a., pteroylglutamic. A., folic, q.v.

a., pyruvic. $CH_3CO.COOH$. An intermediate product of glycolysis in muscle tissues.

a., ribonucleic. A substance found in cytoplasm and chromosomes. It assists in selection and synthesis of proteins from the amino acid sequences. ABBR: RNA.

a., salicylic. USP. $C_7H_6O_3$. Occurs as white needle-shaped crystals or as white crystalline powder. It is used as a local antiseptic or keratolytic.

a., saturated fatty. Fatty acid in which the carbon atoms are linked to other carbon atoms by single bonds. SEE: *fatty acids; unsaturated fatty acids.*

a., silicic. Any one of a group of substances containing silica. May be H_2SiO_3, H_2SiO_4, or H_2SiO_6. When precipitated, silica gel is obtained.

a., stearic. USP. $C_{18}H_{36}O_2$. A monobasic fatty acid occurring naturally in plants and animals. Used in manufacture of soap and pharmaceutical products such as glycerin suppositories.

a., succinic. $COOH(CH_2)_2COOH$. An intermediate in carbohydrate metabolism.

a., sulfonic. Any organic compound of the general formula SO_2OH derived from sulfuric acid by replacement of a hydrogen atom.

a., sulfosalicylic. A crystalline acid, soluble in water or alcohol. Used as a reagent for precipitating proteins, as in testing for albumin in urine.

a., sulfuric. H_2SO_4. A colorless, corrosive, heavy liquid prepared from sulfur and indispensable in the industries, being used in the production of nearly all industrial products. It is rarely used in medicine. SYN: *oil of vitriol.*

a., sulfurous. H_2SO_3. An inorganic acid. It is a powerful chemical reducing agent and is used commercially especially for its bleaching properties.

a., tannic. A glucoside prepared from oak galls and sumac and yielding gallic acid and glucose on hydrolysis. SYN: *tannin,* q.v.

a., tartaric. $C_4H_6O_6$. Obtained from by-products of wine fermentation. Widely used in industry in manufacture of carbonated drinks, flavored gelatins, dyes, metals, etc. Also used as a reagent.

a., taurocholic. A substance occurring in bile and yielding cholic acid and taurine on hydrolysis.

a., trichloroacetic. $C_2HCl_3O_2$. A caustic crystalline substance.

a., unsaturated. Organic acid in which some of the carbon atoms are linked to other carbon atoms by double bonds, thus containing less than the maximum possible number of hydrogen atoms. For example, compare unsaturated oleic and linoleic acids with the saturated stearic acid. SEE: *fatty acid; saturated fatty acid.*

a., uric. $C_5H_4N_4O_3$. An important organic constituent of normal urine. Usually occurs in form of salts (urates).

a., valeric. $C_5H_{10}O_2$. An oily liquid of the fatty acid series, existing in four isomeric forms and having a distinctly disagreeable odor. SYN: *pentanoic acid.*

acidaminuria (ăs''ĭd-ăm''ĭ-nū'rĭ-ă) [L. *acidum,* acid, + amine + Gr. *ouron,* urine]. Excess of amino acids in urine.

acid-base balance. The mechanisms by which the acids and alkalies are kept in a state of equilibrium so that the hydrogen ion concentration of the arterial blood is maintained between pH 7.35 and 7.45. This is accomplished by action of buffer systems of the blood, and the regulatory (homeostatic) functions of the respiratory and urinary systems. Disturbances in acid-base balance result in acidosis or alkalosis, q.v.

acidemia (as-ĭ-dē'mĭ-ă) [L. *acidum,* acid, + Gr. *haima,* blood]. A condition in which uncompensated reduction in alkaline substances or uncompensated increase in circulating acid substances results in increased acidity of the blood, so that the pH drops from a normal range of 7.35 to 7.45 to more acid values, e.g., 7.0 to 7.3. SEE: *acid-base balance; acidity; acidosis.*

acid-fast. Not decolorized easily when stained by acids. Pertaining to bacteria which after staining are decolorized by a mixture of acid and alcohol. The acid-fast bacteria retain the red dyes, but the surrounding tissues are decolorized. In clinical medicine an example of this type of organism is Mycobacterium tuberculosis.

acid foods. The effect of foods once they have been digested cannot be determined by their taste. In general, fruits and vegetables are alkali-producing foods. There is no reason for the normal individual to avoid eating acid foods such as those containing a large amount of protein.

acidifiable (ă-sĭd'ĭ-fī''ă-bl) [L. *acidum,* acid, + *fieri,* to be made, + *habilis,* able]. Capable of being transformed to produce an acid reaction.

acidification (ă-sĭd'ĭ-fĭ-kā'shŭn) ["+ *factus,* made]. Becoming sour; conversion into an acid.

acidimeter (ăs''ĭ-dĭm'ě-těr) [L. *acidum,* acid, + Gr. *metron,* measure]. Instrument for testing purity of acids.

acidimetry (ăs''ĭ-dĭm'ĭ-trĭ). Determination of an acid's strength, or of the acidity of a fluid.

ac'idism, acidis'mus [L. *acidus,* sour]. Poisoning due to acids introduced from outside the body.

acidity (ă-sĭd'ĭ-tĭ). Quality of being acid; having an excess of acid; sourness.

In chemistry denoting: (1) the quality of possessing the characteristics of any acid and so, in acids or acid salts, equivalent to basicity; (2) the capacity for saturating an acid evinced by a base; (3) the intensity of an acid reaction, expressed usually in terms of the hydrogen-ion concentration. SEE: *hydrogen ion*.

a. of stomach. Sourness due to fermentation of food in the stomach, or oversecretion of acid.

acidocyte (ăs'ĭ-dō-sīt'') [L. *acidum,* acid, + Gr. *kytos,* cell]. An eosinophil; eosinophilic leukocyte.

acidocytopenia (ăs'ĭ-dō-sī''tō-pē'nĭ-ă) ["+ "+ *penia,* poverty]. Abnormal reduction of number of eosinophils in the blood.

acidocytosis (ăs'ĭ-dō-sī-tō'sĭs) ["+ "+ *-osis,* condition]. Abnormal increase in number of eosinophilic leukocytes in the blood.

acidophil(e (ă-sĭd'ō-fĭl, -fĭl) [L. *acidum,* acid, + Gr. *philos,* love]. 1. Capable of being stained by acid stains such as eosin. Said of cells or parts of cells prepared for microscopic study. SYN: *acidophilic; acidophilous.* 2. An acid-staining cell of the anterior pituitary. 3. A bacterial organism which grows well in an acid medium.

acidophilic (ă-sĭd''ō-fĭl'ĭk). 1. Having affinity for acid or pert. to certain tissues and cell granules. 2. A cell capable of being stained by acid stains; eosinophil. SYN: *acidophilous.*

acidophilus milk (ăs'ĭ-dŏf'ĭ-lŭs). Milk fermented by Lactobacillus acidophilus cultures. Used to change intestinal flora. SEE: *milk.*

acidoresistant (ăs'ĭ-dō-rē-zĭs'tănt). Acid-resisting; said about bacteria.

acidosic (ăs'ĭ-dō'sĭk). Having acidosis.

acidosis (ăs'ĭ-dō'sĭs) [L. *acidum,* acid, + Gr. *-ōsis,* condition]. A disturbance in the acid-base balance of the body in which there is an accumulation of acids (as in diabetic a. or renal disease) or an excessive loss of bicarbonate (as in renal disease). SEE: *acid-base balance; acidemia; buffer.*

a., carbon dioxide. That resulting from CO_2 retention as in drowning or decreased respiration. SYN: *gaseous a.*

a., compensated. Condition in which the ratio of bicarbonate to carbonic acid in blood plasma remains constant even though the blood bicarbonate may be decreased. Normally the ratio is approximately 20 to 1.

a., diabetic. A. occurring in advanced stages of diabetes mellitus due to loss of sodium and potassium along with ketone bodies in the urine. Serum carbon dioxide is decreased as base is lost, fixed acids increase. SEE: *diabetic coma.*

a., gaseous. A., carbon dioxide, q.v.

a., metabolic. A. resulting from increase in acids other than carbonic acid. Possible causes are excessive ingestion of acids or acid salts, ketosis, severe dehydration, diarrhea, vomiting, renal disease, impaired liver function.

a., renal. A. due to impaired kidney function. The a. is induced by loss of excessive amounts of base or inability to excrete phosphoric and sulfuric acids.

a., respiratory. A. secondary to pulmonary insufficiency resulting in retention of carbon dioxide.

acidotic (ă''sĭd-ŏt'ĭk). Pert. to acidosis.

acid poisoning. Acids have a sour taste and many of them are corrosive or poisonous. SEE: *Acids* in *Table of Poisons and Poisoning* in *Appendix.*

F. A. TREATMENT: Dilute and wash with large volumes of water. Give orally milk, egg white, magnesium oxide, milk of magnesium, lime water, or aluminum hydroxide gel. Avoid carbonates as neutralizers because in the presence of strong acids they will react to produce carbon dioxide gas. This may cause distention and rupture of the stomach. Give demulcents and morphine for pain. The use of emetics and stomach tubes is dangerous.

acid-proof. Acid-fast.

acid salt. A compound formed when only a part of the hydrogen of an acid is replaced by a metal.

acid'ulate [L. *acidulus,* slightly acid]. To make somewhat sour or acid.

acidulous (ă-sĭd'ū-lŭs). Slightly sour or acid.

acidum (ăs'ĭ-dŭm) [L.]. Acid.

aciduria (as-ĭd-ū'rĭ-ă) ["+ Gr. *ouron,* urine]. The condition of acid in the urine.

acidu'ric [L. *acidus,* sour, + *durare,* to endure]. Capable of growing in an acid medium, but preferring a slightly alkaline medium, as certain bacteria.

acies (ā'sē-ēz) [L. edge]. Margin or border.

acinar (ăs'ĭ-năr) [L. *acinus,* grape]. Rel. to or affecting an acinus.

acinesia (ăs'ĭ-nē'sī-ă). Akinesia, q.v.

acinesic, acinetic (ăs-ĭ-nē'sĭk, -nĕt'ĭk). Akinetic, q.v.

acini (ăs'ĭ-nī). Pl. of acinus.

aciniform (ă-sĭn'ĭ-form) [L. *acinus,* grape, + *forma,* shape]. Resembling grapes. SYN: *acinous.*

acinitis (ăs'ĭ-nī'tĭs) ["+ Gr. *itis,* inflammation]. Inflammation of glandular acini.

acinous (ăs'ĭ-nŭs). Pert. to glands resembling a bunch of grapes; resembling as acini and alveolar glands. SYN: *aciniform.*

acinus (ăs'ĭ-nŭs) [L., grape]. (pl. *ac'ini*) [NA] Smallest division of a gland; a group of secretory cells surrounding a cavity.

acladiosis (ăk-lăd'ĭ-ō'sĭs). An ulcerative skin disease believed to be due to the genus Acladium.

aclasis (ăk'lă-sĭs) [Gr. *a-*, not, + *klasis,* a breaking away]. Abnormal tissue arising from and continuous with a normal structure, as in chondrodysplasia. SYN: *aclasia.*

    a., diaphyseal. Imperfect formation of cancellous bone in cartilage between diaphysis and epiphysis.

aclastic (ă-klăs'tĭk) ["+ Gr. *klan,* to break]. Not refracting light rays.

acleistocardia (ă-klīs"tō-kăr'dĭ-ă) [Gr. *akleistos,* not closed, + *kardia,* heart]. Patent foramen ovale.

aclu'sion [Gr. *a-*, not, + L. *claudere,* to close]. Imperfect adjustment of opposing tooth surfaces when jaws are closed.

acmastic (ăk-măs'tĭk) [Gr. *akmē,* prime]. Pert. to disease with regular increase of symptoms to a peak level (epacmastic) and decrease (paracmastic), or period of decline.

acme (ăk'mē) [Gr. *akmē,* point]. 1. The highest point, peak. 2. The time of greatest intensity of a symptom or disease process.

acne (ăk'nē) [Gr. *akmē,* point]. This is a general term but is often used alone to indicate acne vulgaris, q.v. A chronic inflammatory disease of the sebaceous glands and hair follicles of the skin characterized by comedones, papules, pustules. Cysts and nodules may develop and scarring is common. Usually associated with seborrhea.

    a. artificialis. A. caused by external disturbance or irritation.

    a. atrophica. A. with residual pitting and scarring.

    a. cachecticorum. A type of acne seen in debilitated patients.

    a. ciliaris. That which affects the edges of the eyelids.

    a. conglobata. Acne vulgaris with abscesses, cysts, and sinuses that leave scars.

    a. decalvans. Quinquad's disease; a purulent folliculitis of the scalp resulting in irregular bald patches. SYN: *folliculitis decalvans.*

    a. indurata. Form of a. vulgaris with chronic discolored indurated surfaces.

    a. keloid. Infection about the hair follicles at back of neck causing scars and thickening of skin.

    a. urticaria. A form with itching patches.

    a. varioliformis. Vesiculopustular folliculitis which occurs most commonly on temples and frontal margins of the scalp but may be seen on chest, back or nose.

    a. vulgaris. Common acne.

    ETIOL: Unknown. Predisposing causes include hereditary or familial tendencies and disturbances in androgen-estrogen balance affecting activity of sebaceous glands. Specific exciting factors may include excess carbohydrates and fats, food allergies, foods rich in iodine, gastrointestinal disturbances, endocrine disorders, psychogenic factors. Vitamin deficiencies, ingestion of halogens, and contact with chemicals such as tar and chlorinated hydrocarbons may be specific causative factors. That bacteria are important once the disease is present is indicated by the successful results following antibiotic therapy.

    For unexplained reasons the lesions may become worse during the premenstruum.

    SYM: There may be either papules about comedones with black centers, or pustules, or hypertrophied nodules caused by overgrowth of connective tissue. In the indurative type the lesions are deep-seated and cause scarring. Face, neck, shoulders are common sites.

    PROG: Obstinate and recurrent.

    TREATMENT: Local in all; systemic when indicated. Topical cleansing and peeling agents. Extraction of comedones and incision and drainage of cysts and pustules. Avoidance of foods which are known to cause exacerbations, and bromides and iodides. Vitamin A therapy and antibacterial therapy have been successful in some patients.

acnegenic (ăk"nē-jĕn'ĭk) [Gr. *akmē,* point, + *gennan,* to produce]. That which causes or produces acne.

acneiform (ăk-nē'ĭ-form) ["+ L. *forma,* shape]. Resembling acne. Also spelled acneform.

acnemia (ăk-nē'mĭ-ă) [Gr. *a-*, not, + *knēmē,* lower leg]. Wasting of the calves of the legs.

acni'tis [Gr. *akmē,* point, + *-itis,* inflammation]. A papular eruption which becomes pustular, leaving slight scars.

acoin (ăk'ō-ĭn). A white crystalline powder; guanidine derivative. Used as a local anesthetic.

acomia (ă-kō'mĭ-ă) [Gr. *a-*, not, + *komē,* hair]. Baldness. SYN: *alopecia.*

aconite (ăk'ō-nīt) [Gr. *akoniton*]. A poisonous and very powerful alkaloid. The dried tuberous root of Aconitum, esp. A. napellus (monkshood) and A. lycoctonum (wolfsbane). Its action, which is due to the presence of two very potent alkaloids, was well known to the ancients, and believed to have been used as an arrow poison early in Chinese history, and perhaps also by the inhabitants of ancient Gaul.

Aconite is no longer in general use but is of historical interest.

aconuresis (ă-kŏn″ū-rē′sĭs) [Gr. *akōn*, involuntary, + *ourēsis*, urination]. An involuntary voiding of urine.

acoprosis (ă″kō-prō′sĭs) [Gr. *a-*, not, + *kopros*, feces]. Marked reduction or absence of feces in the intestine.

acoprous (ă-kŏp′rŭs). Pert. to lack of feces in the intestine.

acor (ā′kōr) [L., a sour taste]. Acidity. SEE: *acid.*

acorea (ă-kō-rē′ă) [Gr. *a-*, not, + *korē*, pupil]. Absence of the pupil of the eye.

acoria (ă-kō′rĭ-ă) ["+ *koros*, satiety]. 1. Lacking in satisfaction after eating but not from hunger. 2. Gluttony.

RS: bulimia; hyperorexia; polyphagia.

acormus (ă-kōr′mŭs) ["+ *kŏrmŏs*, trunk]. 1. Lack of a trunk. 2. A fetal abnormality consisting of a head and extremities without a trunk.

acouesthesia (ă-kū″ĕs-thē′zĭ-ă) [Gr. *akouein*, to hear, + *aisthēsis*, sensation]. Sense of hearing.

acoumeter (ă-kū′mĕ-ter) ["+ *metron*, measure]. An instrument for determining acuteness of hearing.

acouophonia (ă-kū″ō-fō′nĭ-ă) ["+ *phonē*, sound]. Auscultatory percussion.

acousia (ă-kū′zĭ-ă) [Gr. *akousis*, hearing]. The hearing faculty.

acousma (ă-kūz′mă) [Gr. *akousma*, a thing heard]. Nonverbal auditory hallucination.

acousmatagnosia (ă-kūs″măt-ăg-nō′sĭ-ă) ["+ *agnosia*, ignorance]. Inability to understand what is said due to mental disorder.

acousmatamnesia (ă-kūs″măt-ăm-nē′zĭ-ă) ["+ *amnēsia*, forgetfulness]. Loss of memory for sounds.

acoustic (ă-kū′stĭk) [Gr. *akoustikŏs*]. Pert. to sound or to the sense of hearing.

    a. center. In the temporal lobe of the cerebrum.

    a. meatus. The external or internal auditory canal.

    a. nerve. Consists of two separate parts, vestibular and cochlear nerve with superficial origin at junction of pons and medulla. SYN: *auditory n.; 8th cranial n.; statoacoustic n.; nervus vestibulocochlearis* [NA].

    FUNCT: Special senses of hearing and equilibrium. Vestibular and cochlear nerves consist of special somatic afferent fibers. Cells of origin of vestibular nerve are bipolar

and lie in the vestibular ganglion, peripheral branches terminating in receptors of semicircular ducts, saccule, and utricle. Cells of origin of cochlear nerve are bipolar and lie in spiral ganglion, peripheral branches terminating in spiral organ of Corti. The two nerves become joined, enter the internal acoustic meatus with the facial nerve, and then separate.

acoustics (ă-kū′stĭks). The science of sounds and their perception.

ACP. Abbr. for *American College of Physicians; anodal closing picture.*

acquired [L. *acquirere*, to get]. Not hereditary or innate.

    a. characteristic. One resulting from the effects of the environment and not inherited.

acral (ă′krăl) [Gr. *akron*, extremity]. Pert. to extremities.

acrania (ă-krā′nĭ-ă) [Gr. *a-*, not, + *kranion*, skull]. Congenital absence of the cranium, either partial or complete.

acrasia (ă-krā′zĭ-ă) [Gr. *akrasia*, bad mixture]. Without self-control; intemperate.

acratia (ă-krā′shĭ-ă) [Gr. *akrateia*, want of power]. 1. Loss of strength; impotence. 2. Incontinence, or loss of control.

acraturesis (ă-krăt″ū-rē′sis) [Gr. *akratēs*, powerless, + *ouresis*, urination]. Inability to urinate, or difficulty in urination, due to bladder atony or weakness.

acremoniosis (ăk″rē-mō-nĭ-ō′sĭs). A condition marked by fever and development of swellings, due to infection with the fungus Acremonium.

Acremonium (ăk″rē-mō′nĭ-ŭm). A pathogenic fungus.

acribometer (ăk″rĭ-bŏm′ĕ-tĕr) [Gr. *acribēs*, exact, + *metron*, measure]. Instrument which measures minute objects.

acrid (ăk′rĭd) [L. *acer, acris,* sharp]. Burning, bitter, irritating.

acriflavine (ăk-rĭ-flā′vĭn). A dye; a derivative of acridine which is obtained from coal tar. Has been used as a germicide and in urinary tract infections.

acrimony (ăk′rĭ-mō″nĭ) [L. *acrimonia*, pungency]. Quality of being pungent, acrid, irritating.

acrinia (ă-krĭn′ĭ-ă) [Gr. *a-*, not, + *krinein*, to separate]. Decreased or absent secretion.

acrisia (ă-krĭs′ĭ-ă) [Gr. *akrisia*, want of judgment]. Condition of uncertainty in diagnosis and prognosis.

acritical (ă-krĭt′ĭ-kăl) [Gr. *a-*, not, + *kritikos*, critical]. Not marked by a crisis.

acritochromacy (ă-krĭt″ō-krō′mă-sĭ) [Gr. *akritos*, not distinguishing, + *chrōma*, color]. Color blindness.

acro- (ăk′rō) [Gr. akron, extremity]. A combining form meaning extremity, top, extreme point.

acroagnosis (ăk″rō-ăg-nō′sĭs) ["+ gnōsis, knowledge]. Absence of feeling that one has a limb.

acroanesthesia (ăk″rō-ăn-ĕs-thē′zĭ-ă) [Gr. akron, extremity, + an-, not, + aisthesis, sensation]. Lack of sensation in one or more of the extremities.

acroarthritis (ak-rō-ar-thrī′tis) ["+ arthron, joint, + -ītis, inflammation]. Arthritis of the hands or feet.

acroasphyxia (ăk″rō-ăs-fĭks′ĭ-ă) ["+ asphyxia, pulse stoppage]. Cold, pale condition of hands and feet; symptom of Raynaud's disease.

acroataxia (ăk″rō-ă-tăks′ĭ-ă) [Gr. akron, extremity, + ataktos, out of order]. Ataxia involving, or limited to, the fingers and toes.

acrobystiolith (ăk″rō-bĭs′tĭ-ō-lĭth) [Gr. akrobystia, prepuce, + lithos, stone]. A calculus of the prepuce.

acrobystitis (ăk″rō-bĭs-tī′tis) ["+ -ītis, inflammation]. Preputial inflammation.

acrocentric (ăk″rō-cĕn′trĭk). Type of chromosome in which the centromere is located near one end. At metaphase it has the appearance of a wishbone. SYN: subterminal.

acrocephalia (ăk″rō-sĕf-ă′lĭ-ă) [Gr. akron, extremity, + kephalē, head]. Pointed condition of the top of the cranium. SYN: acrocephaly.

acrocephalic (ăk″rō-sĕ-fāl′ĭk). A skull with a vertical index above 77; pert. to one with a peaked head.

acrocephalosyndactylia (ăk″rō-sĕf″ă-lō-sĭn″dăk-tĭl′ĭ-ă) [Gr. akron, extremity, + kephalē, head, + syn, without, + daktylos, a finger]. A congenital condition marked by a peaked head and webbed fingers and toes. SYN: Apert's syndrome.

acrocephaly (ăk″rō-sĕf′ă-lĭ). A malformed cranial vault having a high or peaked appearance due to premature closure of the coronal, sagittal, and lambdoidal sutures. SYN: acrocephalia.

acrochordon (ăk″rō-kŏr′dŏn) [Gr. akron, extremity, + chordē, cord]. A soft pedunculated growth.

acrocinesia, acrocinesis (ăk″rō-sĭn-ē′sĭ-ă, -sis) ["+ kinesis, movement]. Excessive motility or freedom of movement.

acrocinetic (ăk″rō-sĭn-ĕt′ĭk). Showing excessive motion.

acrocontracture (ak″rō-kŏn-trăkt′ūr) [Gr. akron, extremity, + L. contrahere, to draw together]. Contracture of the hands or feet.

acrocyanosis (ăk″rō-sī-ă-nō′sĭs) ["+ kyanosis, dark blue color]. Cyanosis of finger tips, and other extremities.
   ETIOL: Due to vasomotor disturbances. Seen in catatonia, hysteria, etc.

acrodermatitis (ăk″rō-dĕr-mă-tī′tis) [Gr. akron, extremity, + derma, skin, + -ītis, inflammation]. Dermatitis of the extremities.
   a. chronica atrophicans. Progressive dermatitis of hands and feet that moves slowly upward on the affected limbs.
   a., continuous. An obstinate eczematous eruption confined to the extremities.
   a. hiemalis. A form occurring in winter, affecting the extremities and tending to disappear spontaneously.

acrodynia (ăk″rō-dĭn′ĭ-ă) ["+ odynē, pain]. 1. Disorder of skin and limbs in children. 2. Multiple neuritis of digits.

acroedema (ăk″rō-ē-dē′mă) ["+ edema]. Chronic edema of the hands or feet.

acroesthesia (ăk″rō-ĕs-thē′zĭ-ă) [Gr. akron, extremity, + aisthēsis, sensation]. 1. Marked hyperesthesia. 2. Pain in the extremities.

acrogeria (ăk″rō-jēr′ĭ-ă) ["+ geron, old man]. A condition wherein the skin of the hands and feet shows signs of premature aging.

acrognosis (ăk″rŏg-nō′sĭs) ["+ gnōsis, knowledge]. Sensory perception of limbs.

acrohyperhidrosis (ăk″rō-hī″pĕr-hĭ-drō′sĭs) [Gr. akron, extremity, + hyper, above, + hidrōsis, sweating]. Excessive perspiration of hands and feet.

acrohypothermy (ăk″rō-hī″pō-thĕr′mĭ) ["+ hypo, under, + thermē, heat]. Abnormal coldness of extremities.

acrokinesia (ăk″rō-kĭn-ē′sĭ-ă) ["+ kinesis, movement]. Excessive motion. SYN: acrocinesia.

acrolein (ăk-rō′lē-ĭn) [L. acer, acrid, + oleum, oil]. A volatile liquid produced by dry distillation of glycerin. Irritating to the eyes. Used in chemical warfare. SYN: acrylaldehyde.

acromacria (ăk″rō-măk′rĭ-ă) [Gr. akron, extremity, + makros, long]. Spider-fingers. SYN: arachnodactyly.

acromastitis (ăk″rō-măs-tī′tĭs) ["+ mastōs, breast, + -ītis, inflammation]. Inflammation of the nipple; thelitis.

acromegalia, acromegaly (ăk″rō-mĕ-gā′lĭ-ă, -mĕg′ă-lĭ) ["+ megas, megal-, big]. A chronic disease of middle-aged persons characterized by elongation and enlargement of bones of the extremities and certain head bones, esp. frontal bone and jaws, accompanied by enlargement of nose and lips and thickening of soft tissues of the face.

ETIOL: Hyperfunction of the eosinophilic cells of the anterior lobe of the pituitary resulting in excess production of growth hormone.

SYM: Onset of the disease is so gradual that neither the patient nor his associates notice it. Facial features are enlarged, mandible and malar bones becoming prominent with protrusion of orbital ridge. Teeth become widely separated. Hands and feet become gradually enlarged. About one third of patients will develop diabetes. Early complaints include muscular pains, headache, sweating. As the disease progresses, muscular weakness is a serious feature and visual impairment may go to the point of blindness.

TREATMENT: X-ray therapy or surgery of pituitary gland.

acromelalgia (ăk″rō-mĕl-ăl′jĭ-ă) [Gr. *akron*, extremity, + *melos*, limb, + *algos*, pain]. Bilateral vasodilation of the vessels of the hands and feet. The skin is reddened, warm, and painful. Cause is unknown. Treatment is symptomatic.

acromelic (ăk″rō-mĕl′ĭk) ["+ *melos*, limb]. Referring to or affecting the end of the extremities.

acrometagenesis (ăk″rō-mĕt″ă-jĕn′ĕ-sĭs) ["+ *meta*, beyond, + *genesis*, origin]. Abnormal growth of extremities.

acromial (ăk-rō′mĭ-al) [Gr. *akron*, extremity, + *ōmos*, shoulder]. Rel. to the acromion.

a. angle. The angle at edge of spine of the scapula where it ascends to become the acromion.

a. process. The acromion, q.v.

a. reflex. Flexion of forearm with internal rotation of hand resulting from quick blow upon acromion. Elicited in hyperkinetic states.

acromicria (ăk″rō-mĭk′rĭ-ă) ["+ *mikros*, small]. Congenital shortness or smallness of the extremities.

acromioclavicular joint (ă-krō″mĭ-ō-klă-vik′ū-lar) [Gr. *akron*, extremity, + *ōmos*, shoulder, + L. *clavicula*, small key]. An arthrodial joint between the acromion and the acromial end of the clavicle.

acromiocoracoid (ă-krō″mĭ-ō-kōr′ă-koyd) ["+ "+ *korax*, crow, + *eidos*, resemblance]. Pert. to the acromion and coracoid process.

acromiohumeral (ăk-rō′mĭ-ō-hū′mĕr-ăl) ["+ L. *humerus*, shoulder]. Pert. to acromion and humerus.

acromion (ă-krō′mĭ-ŏn) [Gr. *akron*, extremity, + *ōmos*, shoulder]. [NA] The lateral, triangular projection of spine of scapula, forming point of the shoulder, and articulating with the clavicle. SYN: *acromial process*. SEE: *acromioclavicular*.

acromiothoracic (ă-krō″mĭ-ō-thō-răs′ĭk) ["+ "+ *thorax*, breastplate]. Pert. to acromion and thorax.

a. artery. A branch of the axillary artery.

acromphalus (ăk-rŏm′făl-ŭs) ["+ *omphalos*, umbilicus]. 1. Center of navel. 2. Beginning of umbilical hernia, marked by abnormal projection of umbilicus.

acromyotonia (ăk″rō-mī-ō-tō′nĭ-ă) ["+ *mys*, muscle, + *tonōs*, tension]. Myotonia of extremities causing spasmodic deformity.

acronarcotic (ăk″rō-năr-kŏt′ĭk) [L. *acer, acris,* sharp, + Gr. *narcosis,* a benumbing]. Having the property of a narcotic and yet irritant in local effects.

acroneurosis (ăk″rō-nū-rō′sĭs) [Gr. *akron,* extremity, + *neuron,* nerve]. Any neurosis, usually vasomotor, in extremities.

acronym (ăk′rō-nĭm) ["+ *onym,* name]. Word formed by combining the first letter or letters of a name or a phrase. EX: MASH for Mobile Army Surgical Hospital.

acronyx (ăk′rō-nĭks″) [L. *acer, acris,* sharp, + Gr. *onyx,* claw]. A nail edge growing into the lateral tissue of a finger or toe.

acroosteolysis (ăk″rō-ŏs″tĭ-ō-lĭ′sĭs) [Gr. *akron,* extremity, + *osteon,* bone, + *lysis,* dissolution]. 1. A familial disease in which dissolution of the tips of the extremities of young children occur. There is no history of trauma and spontaneous amputation does not occur. Etiology unknown. 2. An occupational disease seen in workers who come in contact with vinyl chloride polymerization processes. Characterized by Raynaud's phenomenon. Scleroderma-like skin changes and x-ray evidence of bone destruction of the distal phalanges of the hands. Recovery follows after removal from exposure. SEE: *Raynaud's disease.*

acropachy (ăk′rō-păk″ĭ) [Gr. *akron,* extremity, + *pachys,* thick]. Thickening of fingers or toes.

acroparalysis (ăk″rō-pă-răl′ĭ-sĭs) ["+ *paralyein,* to disable at the side]. Paralysis of one or more extremities.

acroparesthesia (ăk″rō-păr-es-thē′zĭ-ă) [Gr. *akron,* extremity, + *para,* beside, + *aisthesis,* sensation]. Paresthesia (intense prickling, tingling or numbness) of fingers and hands occurring usually following sleep, more often in women than men. May be severe in some instances.

acropathology (ăk″rō-pă-thŏl′ō-jĭ) ["+ *pathos,* suffering, + *logos,* science]. Pathology of disease of extremities.

acropathy (ăk-rŏp′ă-thĭ) Any disease of extremities.

acrophobia (ăk-rō-fō'bǐ-a) [Gr. *akron*, extremity, + *phobos*, fear]. Morbid fear of high places.

acroposthitis (ăk"rō-pŏs-thī'tis) [Gr. *akroposthis*, prepuce, + *-itis*, inflammation]. Inflammation of prepuce.

acroscleroderma (ăk"rō-sklĕr-ō-dĕr'mă) [Gr. *akron*, extremity, + *scleros*, hard, + *derma*, skin]. Hard, thickened skin condition of toes and fingers. SYN: *sclerodactylia.*

acrosclerosis (ăk"rō-sklĕr-ō'sǐs) ["+ "+ *-osis*, condition]. A scleroderma of the upper extremities, sometimes extending to neck and face. Usually follows Raynaud's disease.

acrose (ăk'rōz). A sugar prepared synthetically by formaldehyde or glucose condensation.

acrosome (ăk'rō-sōm) [Gr. *akron*, extremity, + *sōma*, body]. The anterior end of head of the spermatozoon.

acrosphacelus (ăk"rō-sfās'ĕ-lŭs) ["+ *sphakelos*, gangrene]. Gangrene of digits. May be symptom of Raynaud's disease.

acroteric (ăk"rō-tĕr'ĭk) [Gr. *akrōtērion*, summit]. Pertaining to the outermost parts of the extremities, as the tips of the fingers.

acrotic (ă-krŏt'ĭk). 1. [Gr. *a-*, not, + *krotos*, striking]. Pert. to failure of or defective beating of the pulse. 2. [Gr. *akrotēs*, an extreme]. Pert. to the surface or glands of the skin.

acrotism (ăk'rō-tizm) [Gr. *a-*, not, + *krotos*, a striking.]. Apparent absence of the pulse.

acrotrophoneurosis (ăk-rō-trō"fō-nū-rō'sis) [Gr. *akron*, extremity, + *trophē*, nourishment, + *neuron*, nerve, + *-osis*, condition]. Trophoneurosis of extremities with trophic, neuritic, and vascular changes. Usually caused by prolonged immersion in water.

acrylaldehyde (ăk"rĭl-ăl'dĕ-hĭd). A volatile liquid from glycerin. SYN: *acrolein.*

acrylate (ăk'rĭ-lāt). A salt or ester of acrylic acid.

acrylic acid (ă-krĭl'ĭk). A colorless corrosive liquid, $H_2C=CHCOOH$. Used in making acrylic polymers and resins.

ACS. Abbr. for *American Cancer Society; American Chemical Society; American College of Surgeons; anodal closing sound; antireticular cytotoxic serum* (Bogumolets serum).

A.C.S.M. Abbr. for *American College of Sports Medicine.*

ACTH. Abbr. for *adrenocorticotropic hormone,* a pituitary hormone that stimulates the cortex of the adrenal glands. SEE: *cortisone.*

actin (ăk'tĭn). One of the proteins in muscle fiber, the other being myosin.

actinic (ăk-tĭn'ĭk) [Gr. *aktis*, ray]. 1. Pert. to radiant energy such as X rays, ultraviolet light, sunlight, particularly the photochemical effects. 2. In physical therapy, pert. to actinism, q.v. Capable of producing chemical changes as applied to radiant energy.

a. burns. Those caused by ultraviolet or sun rays.

F. A. TREATMENT: As for dry heat burns. SEE: *burns.*

a. dermatitis. Inflammation and erythema of the skin due to exposure to actinic rays such as are present in X rays, sunlight, ultraviolet light.

actinism (ăk'tĭn-ĭzm). That property of radiant energy which produces chemical changes, as in photography or heliotherapy.

actinium (ak-tĭn'ē-ŭm) [Gr. *aktis*, ray or beam]. SYMB: Ac. At. wt. of the longest lived isotope, 227; at. no. 89. A radioactive element.

actinochemistry (ăk"tĭ-nō-kĕm'ĭs-trī) [Gr. *aktis*, ray, + *chēmeia*, chemistry]. Branch of chemistry concerned with the effect of light on substances and systems.

actinodermatitis (ăk"tĭn-ō-dĕr-mă-tī'tis) ["+ *derma*, skin, + *-itis*, inflammation]. Dermatitis caused by exposure to actinic rays.

actinogen (ăk-tĭn'ō-jĕn) ["+ *genesis*, production.]. Any radioactive element.

actinogenesis (ăk"tĭn-ō-jĕn'ē-sĭs). The source or production of actinic rays.

actinogenic (ăk"tĭn-ō-jĕn'ĭk) [Gr. *aktis*, *aktin*, ray, + *gennan*, to produce]. Producing rays; radiogenic.

Actinomyces (ăk"tĭn-ō-mī'sēz) [Gr. *aktis*, ray, + *mykes*, fungus]. A vegetable parasite (Actinomycetaceae) causing actinomycosis.

A. antibioticus. A species of fungus from which the antibiotic Actinomycin is obtained.

A. bovis. The fungus causing actinomycosis (lumpy jaw).

A. israelii. The species isolated from human actinomycosis. Pathogenic for man.

actinomycetic (ăk"tĭ-nō-mī-sĕt'ĭk). Pert. to Actinomyces.

actinomycetin (ăk"tĭn-ō-mī-sĕt'ĭn). A substance that is antibacterial from Actinomyces, effective against some gram-positive and gram-negative organisms.

actinomycin A (ăk"tĭn-ō-mī'sĭn). An antibacterial substance from Actinomyces antibioticus, heat-stable and highly toxic, effective against gram-positive organisms. It is orange-colored, soluble in alcohol and ether.

actinomycin B. Similar to actinomycin A but not soluble in alcohol. Not used clinically because of its toxicity.

actinomycoma (ăk″tĭ-nō-my-kō′mă) [Gr. *aktis*, ray, + *mykēs*, fungus, + *-ōma*, tumor]. A tumor produced by actinomycosis.

actinomycosis (ăk″tĭn-ō-mĭ-kō′sĭs) ["+ *osis*, condition]. A noncontagious ray fungus disease in animals, sometimes communicated to man, invading the brain, lungs, gastrointestinal tract, or, most often, the jaw (lumpy jaw).

ETIOL: Actinomyces bovis in cattle; A. israelii in man. This organism is normally present in the mouth.

SYM: Formation of slow growing granulomata, which later break down, discharging viscid pus containing minute yellowish ("sulfur") granules.

TREATMENT: Prolonged administration of penicillin is usually effective. Tetracyclines are the second choice. Surgical incision and drainage of accessible lesions is helpful when combined with chemotherapy.

actinomycotic (ăk″tĭn-ō-mĭ-kŏt′ĭk). Pert. to actinomycosis.

actinon (ăk′tĭn-ŏn) [Gr. *aktis, aktin*, ray]. Emanation from actinium, which is one of the radium, actinium, and thorium series. SYN: *radon^{219}*.

actinoneuritis (ăk″tĭn-ō-nū-rī′tĭs) ["+ *neuron*, nerve, + *-itis*, inflammation]. Neuritis due to exposure to radium or X rays.

actinopraxis (ăk″tĭn-ō-prăk′sĭs) ["+ *praxis*, a doing]. Employment of light or radioactive rays in diagnosis and treatment.

actinotherapy (ăk″tĭn-ō-thĕr′ă-pī) [Gr. *aktis*, ray, + *therapeia*, healing]. Treatment of disease by rays of light, esp. actinic or photochemically active rays, or by X rays or radium.

actinotoxemia (ăk″tĭn-ō-tŏks-ē′mĭ-ă) ["+ *toxikon*, poison, + *haima*, blood]. A toxic reaction produced by an excessive dose of radiation.

action (ăk′shŭn) [L. *actio*]. Performance of a function, or process; in pathology, a morbid process.

    a., antagonistic. The ability of a drug or a muscle to oppose or resist the action or effect of another drug or muscle. Opposed to synergistic a.

    a. of arrest. Inhibition.

    a., astringent. One in which the tissue cells are contracted by a chemical combination of drug and tissues, forming an albuminate. If this is not dissolved in fluids surrounding tissues, they are not acted upon further by the drug.

    a., bacteriocidal. The lethal effect on bacteria.

    a., bacteriostatic. The effect of stopping or preventing growth of bacteria without killing them.

    a., ball-valve. Intermittent obstruction of a passageway or opening so that the flow of fluid or air is prevented from moving in the normal direction and at the usual rate.

    a., cumulative. Sudden increased action of a drug after several doses have been given.

    a. current. Used in physical therapy. SEE: *a. potential.*

    a., drug. SEE: *drug action.*

    a. potential. The momentary difference in electrical potential between active and resting parts of a nerve fiber found when the two parts are connected with a sensitive galvanometer.

    a., reflex. Involuntary movement produced by a sensory nerve and carried to a center and returned by an efferent nerve to its origin or source of stimulus.

    a., specific dynamic. Stimulation of metabolic rate by ingestion of certain foods, esp. proteins.

    a., synergistic. The ability of a drug or muscle to aid or enhance the effect of another drug or muscle. Opposed to antagonistic a.

activate (ăk′tĭ-vāt). 1. To make active. 2. To make radioactive.

activator (ăk′tĭ-vā″tŏr). 1. A substance in the body which converts an inactive substance into an active agent, as the action of hydrogen ions on pepsinogen converting it to pepsin. 2. Any substance which specifically induces an activity such as an inductor or organizer in embryonic development, or a trophic hormone.

active principle. The chemical substance in a pharmacological preparation which is responsible for the effects of the medicine. SEE: *drug action.*

actomyosin (ăk″tō-mĭ′ō-sĭn). The combination of actin and myosin in a muscle. Upon muscle stimulation these substances shorten without changing their volume and thus cause contraction of the muscle.

actual (ăk′chū-ăl) [L. *actus*, doing]. Real, existent.

    a. cautery. Cautery acting by virtue of its heat and not chemically.

acufilopressure (ăk″ū-fĭ′lō-prĕsh″ūr) [L. *acus*, needle, + *filum*, thread, + *pressura*, pressure]. Acupressure increased by a ligature.

acuity (ă-kū′ĭ-tĭ) [L. *acuere*, to sharpen]. Clearness, sharpness.

a., visual. Acuteness or sharpness of vision.

acuminate (ă-kū′mĭn-āt) [L. *acuminatus,* sharpened]. Conical or pointed.

acupressure (ăk′ū-prĕsh″ŭr) [L. *acus,* needle, + *pressura,* pressure]. Compression of blood vessels by means of needles in surrounding tissues.

   a. forceps. Spring-handled forceps for compressing blood vessels.

   a. needles. Elastic needles for compressing blood vessels.

acupuncture (ăk″ū-pŭngk′tūr) [″+ *punctura,* puncture]. Puncture with needles for diagnostic and therapeutic (counterirritation) purposes.

acus (ā′kŭs) [L., needle]. A surgical needle.

acusection (ăk″ū-sĕk′shŭn) [″+ *secare,* to cut]. Section by an electrosurgical needle.

acusticus (ă-kū′stĭ-kŭs) [Gr. *akoustikos,* hearing]. The acoustic nerve, q.v.

acute (ă-cūte′) [L. *acutus,* sharp]. 1. Sharp, severe. 2. Having rapid onset, severe symptoms and a short course; not chronic.

acutenaculum (ăk″ū-tĕn-ăk′ū-lŭm) [L. *acus,* needle, + *tenaculum,* holder]. A needle holder.

acutorsion (ăk″ū-tŏr′shŭn) [″+ *torsio,* twisting]. Twisting of an artery with a needle to control hemorrhage.

acyanoblepsia (a-sī″ă-nō-blĕp′sĭ-ă) [Gr. *a-,* not, + *kyanos,* blue, + *blepsis,* vision]. Inability to discern blue colors. SYN: *acyanopsia.*

acyanopsia (ă-sī″ă-nŏp′sĭ-ă). Acyanoblepsia, q.v.

acyanotic (ă-sī″ă-nŏt′ĭk) [Gr. *a-,* not, + *kyanos,* blue]. Pert. to the absence of cyanosis.

acyclic (ă-sī′klĭk). 1. In chemistry, aliphatic; open chain compounds. 2. Without a cycle.

acyesis (ā″sī-ē′sĭs) [Gr. *a-,* not, + *kyēsis,* pregnancy]. 1. Absence of pregnancy. 2. Sterility of the female.

acystia (ă-sĭs′tĭ-ă) [″+ *kystis,* bladder]. Congenital absence of bladder.

acystinervia, acysteneuria (ă-sĭs″tĭ-nĕr′vĭ-ă, -nū′rĭ-ă) [″+ *kystis,* bladder, + *neuron,* nerve]. Defective nerve supply to or paralysis of the bladder.

AD. Abbr. for *anodal duration; average deviation; diphenylchlorarsine.*

ad- [L.]. Prefix indicating adherence, increase, toward, as adduct.

-ad. [L.]. Suffix meaning toward; in direction of, as cephalad.

a.d. Abbr. for L. *auris dextra,* right ear.

A.D.A. Abbr. for *American Dental Association; American Dietetic Association.*

adactylia (ā″dăk-tĭl′ĭ-ă) [Gr. *a-,* not, + *daktylos,* finger]. A congenital anomaly consisting of absence of digits of hand or foot.

adamantine (ăd″ă-măn′tĭn) [Gr. *adamantinos,* very hard]. Very hard, said of enamel of teeth.

adamantinoma (ăd″ă-măn″tĭ-nō′mă) [″+ -*ōma,* tumor]. A tumor of the jaw, esp. the lower one, arising from the enamel organ. May be partly cystic, partly solid, and may reach a large size; of low-grade malignancy. SYN: *ameloblastoma.*

adamantoblast (ăd″ă-măn′tō-blăst) [Gr. *adamas,* hard surface, + *blastos,* germ]. An enamel cell from which tooth enamel is formed.

adamantoblastoma (ăd″ă-măn″tō-blăs-tōmă) [″+ ″+ -*ōma,* tumor]. Overgrowth of an adamantoblast.

adamantoma (ăd″ă-măn-tō′mă) [Gr. *adamas,* hard surface, + -*ōma,* tumor]. Adamantinoma, q.v.

Adam's apple. The laryngeal prominence formed by the two laminae of the thyroid cartilage. SYN: *pomum Adami, prominentia laryngea* [NA].

Adams-Stokes syndrome. [Robert Adams, Irish physician, 1791-1875; William Stokes, Irish physician, 1804-1878]. Altered state of consciousness due to decreased flow of blood to the brain. Caused by any transient interference with cardiac output such as incomplete or complete heart block. The patient may be light-headed or become completely unconscious and have convulsions.

adaptation (ăd″ăp tā′shŭn) [L. *adaptare,* to adjust]. 1. In biology, the ability of an organism to adjust to a change in environment. 2. In ophthalmology, the ability of the eye to adjust to light of various intensities, accomplished by changing size of pupil accompanied by chemical changes occurring in the rods. 3. In psychology, a change in quality, intensity, or disturbance of a sensation which occurs after continuous stimulation of constant intensity. 4. In dentistry, the proper fitting of dentures, bands, etc. to the teeth, or closeness of a filling to walls of a cavity.

   a., chromatic. A change in hue or saturation or both resulting from pre-exposure to light of other wave lengths.

   a., dark. The adjustment of the eyes for vision in dim light. SYN: *scotopia.*

   a., light. Adjustment of the eyes for vision in bright light. SYN: *photopia.*

adapter (ă-dăp′tĕr). A device for joining one part of an apparatus to another part.

adaxial (ăd-ăks'ĭ-ăl) [L. *ad*, toward, + *axis*, axis]. Toward the main axis. Opposed to abaxial.

ADC. Abbr. for *anodal duration contraction; axiodistocervical.*

add. In prescription writing, abbr. for L. *adde*, let there be added.

addict (ăd'ĭkt) [L. *addictus*, given over]. One habituated to the use of alcohol or a drug.

addiction (ă-dĭk'shŭn). Enslavement to some habit, esp. the drug habit.

Addis count method (ăd'ĭs). [Thomas Addis, Amer. physician, 1881-1949]. Method for counting the sediment (casts and cells) in a 12-hour sample of urine.

addisonism (ăd'ĭ-sŭn-ĭzm″). Symptom complex not due to disease of suprarenal glands but resembling Addison's disease. The presence of abnormal skin pigmentation with debility. Seen in pulmonary tuberculosis.

Addison's disease. [Thomas Addison, Eng. physician, 1793-1860]. Disease resulting from deficiency in the secretion of adrenocortical hormones. SYN: *adrenal cortical hypofunction; chronic hypoadrenocorticism.*

ETIOL: Progressive destruction of the adrenal cortex which is often invaded by chronic infectious diseases as tuberculosis, histoplasmosis, cryptococcosis and other fungus diseases. Commonly, idiopathic atrophy of the adrenal is the cause.

SYM AND SIGNS: Increased pigmentation of skin and mucous membranes, irregular milk-white patches (vitiligo) on skin, black freckles over head and neck, weakness, fatigability, hypotension, nausea, vomiting, anorexia, weight loss, and occasional hypoglycemia.

PROG: If untreated, the disease will continue a chronic course with progressive but relatively slow deterioration; in some patients the progression may be a rapid one of deterioration. Patients treated properly have an excellent prognosis.

NP: Freedom from anxiety, the prevention of fatigue. If confined to bed, as during an adrenal crisis, the patient should be kept warm and bedsores must be guarded against. Watch the pulse for sudden changes, as fainting and syncope may occur, and patient may die in such an attack. He never should be left alone if confined to the bed. Keep the patient as cheerful as possible.

TREATMENT: Adrenocortical hormone therapy is dramatic in its effect and in adrenal crisis must be given promptly in order to prevent death. SEE: *adrenal; adrenalin.*

addition (ă-dĭ'shŭn). In chemistry, a reaction in which two substances unite without loss of atoms or valence.

adduct (ă'dŭkt) [L. *adductus*, brought toward]. 1. To draw towards the main axis of body or a limb. 2. In optics, to turn eye inwardly.

adduction (ă-dŭk'shŭn). 1. Movement of a limb, or bending of trunk or head toward median plane of body or in case of digits, toward axial line of a limb. 2. In optics, turning the eyes toward the midline.

   a., convergent-stimulus. Convergence of eyes upon fixation of gaze on an object at the near point of vision.

adductor (ă-dŭk'tŏr) [L. a bringer toward]. A muscle which draws toward the medial line of the body or to a common center.

   a. reflex. Contraction of adductors of the thigh upon applying pressure to, or tapping, medial surface of thigh or knee.

adelomorphous (ăd″ĕl-ō-mŏr'fŭs) [Gr. *adelōs*, not seen, + *morphē*, shape]. Having undefined form. Word is applied to the central cells of the gastric glands.

adelphotaxis (ă-dĕl'fō-tăk″sis) [Gr. *adelphos*, brother, + *taxis*, arrangement]. Grouping of cells in mutual relationships. SYN: *adelphotaxy.*

adenalgia (ăd″ĕn-ăl'jĭ-ă) [Gr. *adēn*, gland, + *algos*, pain]. Pain in a gland. SYN: *adenodynia.*

adenase (ăd'ĕ-nāz) ["+ *ase*, enzyme]. Enzyme secreted by the pancreas, spleen, and liver and which converts adenine, q.v., into hypoxanthine, q.v. SEE: *enzyme.*

adenasthenia (ăd″ĕn-ăs-thē'nĭ-ă) ["+ *astheneia*, weakness]. Deficient glandular functional activity.

adendritic (ă″dĕn-drĭt'ĭk) [Gr. *a-*, not, + *dendritēs*, rel. to a tree]. Without dendrites, as certain cells in spinal ganglia. SYN: *adendric.*

adenectomy (ăd″ĕn-ĕk'tō-mĭ) [Gr. *adēn*, gland, + *ek*, out, + *temnein*, to cut]. Excision of a gland.

adenectopia (ăd″ĕ-nĕk-tō'pĭ-ă) ["+ "+ *topos*, place]. A gland out of its normal place.

adenemphraxis (ăd″ĕ-nĕm-frăk'sĭs) ["+ *emphraxis*, stoppage]. Obstruction to discharge from a gland.

adenia (ă-dē'nĭ-ă). Chronic inflammation of a lymph gland with resulting enlargement.

adeniform (ă-dĕn'ĭ-fŏrm) [Gr. *adēn*, gland, + L. *forma*, shape]. Like a gland in form.

adenine (ăd'ĕ-nin). 6-aminopurine, $C_5H_5N_5$, a solid substance of the uric acid group, and derivable from the nucleic acids.

adenitis (ăd″ĕ-nī′tĭs) [Gr. *adēn,* gland, + *-ītis,* inflammation]. Inflammation of lymph nodes or a gland.

adenization (ăd″ĕ-nĭ-zā′shŭn). Abnormal change into a glandlike structure.

adeno- [Gr. *adēn,* gland]. A prefix denoting a gland.

adenoacanthoma (ăd″ĕ-nō-ăk″ăn-thō′mă) ["+ *akantha,* thorn, + *-ōma,* tumor]. Adenocarcinoma in which some cells have undergone squamous metaplasia.

adenocarcinoma (ăd″ĕ-nō-kăr″sĭn-ō′mă) ["+ *karkinos,* cancer]. A malignant adenoma arising from epithelium of a glandular organ.

adenocele (ăd′ĕ-nō-sēl″) [Gr. *adēn,* gland, + *kēlē,* tumor]. A cystic tumor arising from a gland. A tumor of glandular structure.

adenocellulitis (ăd″ĕ-nō-sĕl-ū-lī′tĭs) ["+ L. *cella,* small chamber, + Gr. *-ītis,* inflammation]. Inflammation of a gland and adjacent cellular tissue.

adenochondroma (ăd″ĕ-nō-kŏn-drō′ma) ["+ *chondros,* cartilage, + *-ōma,* tumor]. Adenoma with added characteristics of chondroma.

adenocyst (ăd′ĕ-nō-sĭst″) ["+ *kystis,* sac]. A cystic tumor arising from a gland.

adenocystoma (ăd″ĕ-nō-sĭs-tō′mă) [Gr. *adēn,* gland, + *kystis,* sac, + *-ōma,* tumor]. Cystic adenoma.

adenodynia (ăd″ĕ-nō-dĭn′ĭ-ă) ["+ *odynē,* pain]. Pain in a gland. SYN: *adenalgia.*

adenoepithelioma (ăd″ĕ-nō-ĕp″ĭ-thĕl-ĭ-ō′ma) ["+ *epi,* on, + *thēlē,* nipple, + *-ōma,* tumor]. Tumor consisting of glandular and epithelial elements.

adenofibroma (ăd″ĕ-nō-fī-brō′mă) [Gr. *adēn,* gland, + L. *fibra,* fiber, + Gr. *-ōma,* tumor]. Fibrous and glandular tissue tumor frequently in uterus.

adenogenous (ăd″ĕ-nŏj′ĕ-nŭs) ["+ *gennan,* to produce]. Having origin in glandular tissue.

adenohypersthenia (ăd″ĕ-nō-hī″pĕr-sthē′nĭ-ă) [Gr. *adēn,* gland, + *hyper,* excess, + *sthenos,* strength]. Excessive glandular activity.

adenohypophysis (ăd″ĕ-nō-hī-pŏf′ĭ-sĭs) ["+ *hypo,* under, + *phyein,* to grow]. The anterior lobe or glandular portion of the hypophysis cerebri.

adenoid (ăd′ĕ-noyd) [Gr. *adēnoeides,* glandular]. Lymphoid; having the appearance of a gland.

   a. hypertrophy. Enlargement of the pharyngeal tonsil occurring commonly in children. May result from infection of Waldeyer's ring or may be congenital.

   a. tissue. The pharyngeal tonsil; adenoids, q.v.

adenoidectomy (ăd″ĕ-noyd-ĕk′tō-mĭ) ["+ *ektomē,* excision]. Excision of adenoids. SEE: *tonsillectomy.*

   NP: Watch color and pulse for signs of excessive bleeding; children often swallow blood; and signs are only as above.

adenoids (ăd′ĕ-noyds). Lymphatic tissue forming a prominence on the wall of the pharyngeal recess of the nasopharynx. SYN: *pharyngeal tonsil.*

adenolipoma (ăd″ĕ-nō-lĭp-ō′mă) [Gr. *adēn,* gland, + *lipos,* fat, + *-ōma,* tumor]. A benign tumor having glandular characteristics but composed of fat.

adenolymphitis (ăd″ĕ-nō-lĭm-fī′tĭs) ["+ L. *lympha,* lymph, + Gr. *-ītis,* inflammation]. Inflammation of a lymph gland. SYN: *lymphadenitis.*

adenolymphocele (ăd″ĕ-nō-lĭm′fō-sēl) ["+ "+ Gr. *kēlē,* tumor]. Cystic dilatation of a lymph node from obstruction.

adenolymphoma (ăd″ĕ-nō-lĭm-fō′mă) ["+ "+ *-ōma,* tumor]. A lymph gland adenoma.

adenoma (ăd-ĕ-nō′mă) [Gr. *adēn,* gland, + *-ōma,* tumor]. (pl. *adenomata*) A neoplasm of glandular epithelium.

   a., acidophil(ic. A tumor of the pituitary gland whose cells stain with acid dyes. Cause of acromegaly and gigantism. SYN: *eosinophil a.*

   a., basophil(ic. A tumor of the pituitary gland whose cells stain with basic dyes. Cause of Cushing's syndrome.

   a., chromophobe. Tumor of pituitary gland composed of cells that do not stain readily. May cause pituitary deficiency or diabetes insipidus.

   a., eosinophil(ic. Same as acidophil(ic a., q.v.

   a., fibroid. Fibroadenoma. SYN: *a. fibrosum.*

   a., islet. Nonmalignant neoplasm of the pancreas sometimes containing beta cells. May be cause of hypoglycemia. SYN: *insuloma; langerhansian a.*

   a., langerhansian. Islet a., q.v.

   a., malignant. Adenocarcinoma, q.v.

   a. sebaceum. Benign tumorlike growths on face developing from epithelium of sebaceous glands which undergo fatty but never colloid metamorphosis. Sometimes associated with mental deficiency.

   a., tubular. An adenoma of the form of a tubular gland.

adenomalacia (ăd″ĕ-nō-mă-lā′shĭ-ă) [Gr. *adēn,* gland, + *malakia,* softening]. Glandular softening.

adenomatome (ăd″ĕ-nō′mă-tōm) ["+ *tomē*, a cutting down]. Instrument for removing adenoids.

adenomatosis (ăd″ĕ-nō-mă-tō′sĭs) [Gr. *adēn*, gland, + *-ōma*, tumor, + *-osis*, increase]. The condition of multiple glandular tissue overgrowths.

adenomatous (ăd″ĕ-nō′mă-tŭs). Pert. to adenomas.

adenomere (ăd′ĕ-nō-mēr″) [Gr. *aden*, gland, + *mēros*, part]. The functional part of a gland.

adenomyoma (ăd″ĕ-nō-mī-ō′mă) ["+ *mys*, muscle, + *-ōma*, tumor]. A tumor containing glandular and smooth muscular tissue.

adenomyometritis (ăd″ĕ-nō-mī″ō-mĕ-trī′-tĭs) ["+ "+ *metra*, womb, + *-ĭtis*, inflammation]. A hyperplastic condition of the uterus which is the result of pelvic inflammation and grossly resembles an adenomyoma.

adenomyosis (ăd″ĕ-nō-mī-ō′sĭs) [Gr. *adēn*, gland, + *mys*, muscle, + *-ōsis*, increase]. Benign invasive growth of the endometrium into the muscular layer of the uterus.

adenomyxoma (ăd″ĕ-nō-mĭk-sō′mă) ["+ *myxa*, mucus, + *-ōma*, tumor]. A benign tumor with adenoma and myxoma characteristics.

adenomyxosarcoma (ăd″ĕ-nō-mĭk″sō-săr-kō′mă) ["+ "+ *sarx*, flesh, + *-ōma*, tumor]. A malignant tumor with adenoma, myxoma, and sarcoma characteristics.

adenoncus (ăd″ĕ-nŏn′kŭs) [Gr. *adēn*, gland, + *onkos*, tumor]. A tumor of a gland or its enlargement.

adenopathy (ăd-ĕ-nŏp′ă-thĭ) ["+ *pathos*, suffering]. Swelling and morbid change in lymph nodes; glandular disease.

adenopharyngitis (ăd″ĕ-nō-făr″ĭn-jī′tĭs) ["+ *pharynx*, throat, + *-ĭtis*, inflammation]. Inflammation of tonsils and pharyngeal mucous membrane.

adenophthalmia (ăd″ĕ-nŏf-thăl′mĭ-ă) [Gr. *adēn*, gland, + *ophthalmos*, eye]. Inflammation of the meibomian glands.

adenosarcoma (ăd″ĕ-nō-săr-kō′mă) ["+ *sarx*, flesh, + *-ōma*, tumor]. A tumor with characteristics of adenoma and sarcoma.

adenosclerosis (ăd″ĕ-nō-sklĕ-rō′sĭs) ["+ *sclērōsis*, hardening]. Glandular hardening.

adenose (ăd′ĕ-nōs). Glandlike.

adenosine (ăd′ĕ-nō-sīn). A nucleotide containing adenine and ribose.

    a. diphosphate. A compound of adenosine containing two phosphoric acid groups. This enzyme is produced during muscle contraction. It is reformed when the muscle relaxes. ABBR: ADP.

    a. triphosphate. A compound of adenosine containing three phosphoric acid

groups. An enzyme found in all cells but particularly muscle cells. When this substance is split by enzyme action, energy is produced. The energy of the muscle is stored in this compound. ABBR: ATP.

adenosis (ăd″ĕ-nō′sĭs) [Gr. *adēn*, gland, + *-ōsis*, increase]. Any disease of a gland, esp. of a lymphatic gland.

adenovirus (ăd″ĕ-nō-vī′rŭs). One of a group of closely related viruses which can cause infections of the upper respiratory tract. A large number have been isolated.

adeps (ăd′ĕps) [L.]. Lard; omental hog-fat.

    a. benzoina′tus. Benzoinated lard.

    a. la′nae. Wool fat. Purified anhydrous lanolin from sheep wool. Used as an ointment base.

    a. lanae hydrosus. Hydrous wool fat; lanolin.

adequacy. In nutrition, the relationship between intake of nutrients and individual requirements.

ader′mia [Gr. *a-*, not, + *derma*, skin]. Defect of or lack of skin, congenital or acquired.

ader″mogen′esis ["+ "+ *genesis*, production]. Imperfect growth or repair of skin.

ADH. Abbr. for *antidiuretic hormone* (vasopressin).

adherent (ad-hē′rent) [L. *ad*, to, + *haerēre*, to stick]. Attached to, as of two surfaces.

adhe′sion. 1. A holding together by new tissue, produced by inflammation or injury, of two structures which are normally separate. 2. A fibrous band which holds parts together which are normally separated. 3. An attraction to another substance; thus molecules or blood platelets adhere to each other or to dissimilar materials.

    a., abdominal. Adhesion in the abdominal cavity, usually involving the intestines. Caused by inflammation or trauma. They are treated surgically if causing great pain or intestinal obstruction.

    a., pericardial. Adhesion of the pericardial sac. If extensive enough may lead to restriction of the normal movement of the heart. SEE: *pericarditis.*

adhesiotomy (ad-hē″zĭ-ŏt′ō-mĭ) [L. *ad*, to, + *haerere*, to stick, + Gr. *ektomē*, excision]. Surgical division of adhesions.

adhesive (ăd-hē′sĭv) [Fr. *adhésion*]. 1. Causing adhesion. 2. Sticky; adhering. 3. That which causes two bodies to adhere.

    a. inflammation. A serous membrane inflammation exudating fibrinous matter making adhesions possible.

    a. plaster, a. tape. USP. A fabric or film, one side of which is coated with an adhesive substance, that remains in place after application to the skin.

adiadochokinesis (ă-dī''ă-dō-kō-kĭn-ē'sis) [Gr. *a-*, + *diadochas*, successive, + *kinēsis*, movement]. 1. Inability to make rapid alternating movements. 2. In neurology, rapid antagonistic movements which cannot be carried out with accuracy. Seen in cerebellar disease. SYN: *adiadochokinesia*. RS: asynergia; dysmetria; gait.

adiaphoresis (ă-dī''ă-fō-rē'sĭs) [Gr. *a-*, not, + *diaphorein*, to perspire]. Deficiency or absence of sweat.

adiaphorous (ă''dĭ-ăf'ō-rŭs) ["+ *diaphoros*, different]. Neither harmful nor beneficial. Neutral.

adiapneustia (ă''dĭ-ăp-nū'stĭ-ă) [Gr. *a-*, not, + *diapnein*, to breathe through]. Anhidrous. Failure to, or lack of sweat.

adiastole (ă''dĭ-ăs'tō-lē) ["+ *diastolē*, dilatation]. Imperceptibility of diastole.

adiathermancy (ă-dī''ă-thur'măn-sī) ["+ *dia*, through, + *thermē*, heat]. State of being impervious to heat.

adient (ăd'ī-ĕnt) [L. *adeo*, to go toward]. Tending to move toward a stimulus. Opposed to abient.

adipectomy (ad''ĭ-pek'tō-mĭ) [L. *adeps*, fat, + Gr. *ektomē*, a cutting out]. Excision of fat or adipose tissue, usually a large quantity.

adipic (ă-dīp'ĭk). Rel. to adipose tissues.

adipocele (ad'ĭ-pō-sēl) [L. *adeps*, fat, + Gr. *kēlē*, tumor]. A hernia which contains fat or fatty tissue. Lipocele.

adipocere (ad'ĭ-po-sēr) ["+ *cera*, wax]. A brown waxlike substance composed of fatty acids and calcium soaps. It is formed in animal tissues which have been buried in a moist place. SYN: *grave wax*.

ad''ipofibro'ma ["+ *fibra*, fiber, + Gr. *-ōma*, tumor]. A fibroma and adipoma.

adipogenous (ad''ĭ-pŏj'ĭn-ŭs) ["+ Gr. *gennan*, to produce]. Inducing the formation of fat.

adipoid (ad'ĭ-poyd) [L. *adeps*, fat, + Gr. *eidos*, form]. Fatlike; lipoid.

adipolysis (ad''ĭ-pŏl'ĭ-sĭs) ["+ Gr. *lysis*, setting free]. The hydrolysis or digestion of fat.

adipoma (ad''ĭ-pō'mă) ["+ Gr. *-ōma*, tumor]. Fatty tissue tumor. SYN: *lipoma*.

adipometer (ad-ĭ-pŏm'ĕ-ter) ["+ Gr. *metron*, measure]. Instrument for measuring thickness of the skin. Useful in determining thickness of subcutaneous fat layer and is therefore used to judge degree of obesity.

adiponecrosis (ad''ĭ-po-nĕ-krō'sĭs) [L. *adeps*, fat, + Gr. *nekrōsis*, deadness]. Necrosis affecting fatty tissue.

ad''ipopex'ia ["+ Gr. *pēxis*, fixation]. The storing of fat. SYN: *lipopexia*.

ad'ipose [L. *adiposus*, fatty]. Fatty; pertaining to fat.

a. capsule. Renal fat.

a. fossae. Fatty accumulations on outer mammary surface.

a. tissue. Connective or areolar tissue containing masses of fat cells.

adiposis (ad''ĭ-pō'sĭs) [L. *adeps*, fat, + Gr. *-ōsis*, condition]. Abnormal accumulation of fat in the body. SYN: *corpulence; liposis.*

a. cerebralis. Obesity due to intracranial disease esp. of the hypophysis or pituitary.

a. doloro'sa. A disease the symptoms of which are fatty painful formations, and nerve lesions.

a. hepat'ica. Fatty degeneration or infiltration of the liver.

adipositis (ad''ĭ-pō-sī'tĭs) [L. *adiposus*, fatty, + Gr. *-itis*, inflammation]. Infiltration of an inflammatory nature in and beneath subcutaneous adipose tissue.

adipos'ity. Excessive fat in the body. SYN: *adiposis; obesity.*

adiposogenital dystrophy (ad''ĭ-pō''sō-gen'ĭ-tal dĭs'trō-fĭ) [L. *adiposus*, fatty, + *genitalis*, belonging to birth, Gr. *dys-*, bad, disordered, + *trophē*, nutrition]. Combination of adiposity, impaired development of genital organs, and change in secondary sex characteristics. SYN: *Fröhlich's syndrome; sexual infantilism.*

ETIOL: A disturbance or tumor of the hypothalamus and pituitary gland.

adiposuria (ad''ĭ-pō-sū'rĭ-ă) ["+ Gr. *ouron*, urine]. Fat in the urine. SYN: *lipuria.*

adip'sia, ad'ipsy [Gr. *a-*, not, + *dipsa*, thirst]. Absence of thirst.

ad'itus [L.]. An approach; an entrance.

a. ad antrum. The recess of the tympanic cavity which leads from epitympanic recess to the tympanic antrum.

a. ad aquaeductum cerebri. The entrance to the sylvian aqueduct, situated at lower posterior angle of third ventricle of brain.

a. ad infundibulum. A small canal leading from the third ventricle into the infundibulum.

a. glottidis inferior. Inferior entrance to the glottis.

a. glottidis superior. Superior entrance to the glottis.

a. laryngis. [NA] Upper aperture of larynx.

adjuster (ad-jus'ter). Device for holding together the ends of the wire forming a suture.

adjustment (ad-just'ment) [L. *adjuxtāre*, to bring together]. 1. Biological adaptation to an altered or changing condition, particularly in the environment. 2. Mechanical change in a microscope so that the tube containing the lenses is moved up or down in order to bring the object into focus.

ad'juvant [L. *adjuvans*, aiding]. That which assists, esp. a drug added to a prescription to hasten or increase the action of a principal ingredient; synergist.

ad lib. Abbr. for L. *ad lib'itum*, at pleasure or as much as is wanted.

ad nauseum (ad-naw'sē-ăm) [L.]. Of such degree or extent as to produce nausea.

adner'val [L. *ad*, to, + *nervus*, nerve]. Near or toward a nerve.

adneural (ad-nū'răl) ["+ Gr. *neuron*, nerve]. Adnerval.

adnex'a [L.]. Accessory parts of a structure.

    a. oculi. Lacrimal glands.

    a. uteri. Ovaries and oviducts.

adnex'al. Adjacent or appending.

adnexi'tis [L. *adnexa*, appendages, + Gr. *-itis,* inflammation]. Inflammation of the adnexa uteri.

adnexopexy (ăd-nĕks'ō-pĕks'ī) ["+ Gr. *pēxis,* a putting together]. Fixing the fallopian tube and ovary to the abdominal wall.

adolescence (ăd"ō-lĕs'ĕns) [L. *adolēscēns*, from *adolēscere*, to grow up]. The period from the beginning of puberty until maturity. The onset of puberty and maturity is a gradual process and variable among individuals. Thus it is not practical to set exact age or chronological limits in defining the adolescent period.

ad"oles'cent. 1. Pert. to adolescence. 2. Young man or woman not fully grown.

adoral (ăd-ō'răl) [L. *ad*, to, + *os, oris,* mouth]. Toward or near the mouth.

A.D.P. Abbr. for *Adenosine diphosphate.*

adrenal (ăd-rē'năl) [L. *ad*, to, + *ren*, kidney]. Originally used to indicate nearness to the kidney. Now used in reference to the a. gland or its secretions.

    a. gland. A triangular-shaped body adjacent to and covering the superior surface of each kidney. It is a gland of internal secretion. SYN: *suprarenal gland.*

EMBRYOLOGY: The adrenal gland is essentially a double organ composed of an outer cortex and an inner medulla. The cortex arises in the embryo from a region of the mesoderm which also gives rise to the gonads or sex organs. The medulla arises from ectoderm which also gives rise to the sympathetic nervous system.

ANAT: The entire gland is enclosed in a tough connective tissue capsule from which trabeculae extend into the cortex. The cortex consists of cells arranged into three zones: the outer zona glomerulosa, the middle zona fasciculata, and the inner zona

reticularis. The cells are arranged in a cordlike fashion. The medulla consists of chromaffin cells arranged in groups or anastomosing cords. The two adrenal glands are situated retroperitoneally, each embedded in perirenal fat above its respective kidney. In the adult the average weight is 5 gm., and the range is 4-14 gm. The gland usually is heavier in males than in females.

PHYS: Synthesizes and stores three catecholamines: dopamine, norepinephrine, and epinephrine. Dopamine's chief effects are dilation of systemic arteries, increased cardiac output, and increased flow of blood to the kidneys. The primary action of norepinephrine is to constrict the arterioles and venules with resulting increased resistance to blood flow, elevated blood pressure, and slowing of the heart. Epinephrine dilates arteries, increases heart activity, dilates the bronchi by relaxing bronchial musculature, increases level of glucose in the blood by stimulating the production of glucose from glycogen in the liver, increases the amount of fatty acid in the blood, and diminishes activity of the gastrointestinal system. The three catecholamines are also produced in other parts of the body.

The a. medulla is under the control of the sympathetic nervous system and functions in conjunction with it. It is intimately related to adjustments of the body in response to emotional states. Anticipatory reactions tend to bring about the release of norepinephrine. More intense emotional reactions, esp. those in response to extreme stress, tend to increase the secretion of both; epinephrine induces reactions which adapt the organism to meet emergency situations.

Cortex: Secretes a group of hormones which vary in quantity and quality. They are all synthesized from cholesterol and contain the basic steroid nucleus perhydrocyclopentanophenanthrene, q.v. These compounds are grouped according to their chemical structure and biological activity as follows: glucocorticoids (cortisol, corticosterone) which act principally on carbohydrate metabolism; mineralocorticoids (aldosterone, dehydroepiandrosterone) which affect metabolism of the electrolytes sodium and potassium; androgens (17-ketosteroids), estrogens (estradiol), and progestins (progesterone), all three of which are important in the physiology of reproduction. It is important to realize that there is considerable overlap in the biological activity of many of these compounds.

There is hardly a body system which is not influenced by the action of adrenal cortical hormones. Cortisol and cortisone are important in carbohydrate, water, muscle, bone, central nervous system, gastrointestinal, cardiovascular, and hematological metabolism. They are also important anti-inflammatory agents. The principal long-term effect of cortisone and cortisol is catabolic.

The 17-ketosteroids act principally as androgenic and anabolic agents. Aldosterone's principal action is to control sodium and potassium levels in the blood.

PATHOLOGY: *Medulla:* Increased secretion of catecholamines occurs when a pheochromocytoma develops. In this condition the patient develops hypertension, excessive sweating, paroxysmal attacks of blanching or flushing of the skin, tachycardia, headache, anorexia, weight loss, altered personality changes, signs of increased metabolism, constipation, and postural hypotension. Diagnosis may be confirmed by determining the level of catecholamines or their metabolic end-products in the urine.

Cortex: When excess secretion of cortical hormones occurs one of a variety of syndromes may result, depending upon which hormones or group of hormones are increased. If cortisol is increased, the signs of Cushing's syndrome result: obesity with striae and redistribution of fat to produce a "buffalo hump" and "moon face," muscle wasting, osteoporosis, decreased glucose tolerance, atherosclerosis, and systolic hypertension. If the androgens are increased male sex characteristics are accentuated in the female with voice change, hirsutism, clitoral enlargement, and pronounced muscular development. Baldness and acne will develop in either sex with this condition. It is termed adrenogenital syndrome.

When aldosterone is elevated hypertension, low serum potassium, elevated serum sodium, increased urine volume, and rarely edema will be present. This is called primary aldosteronism.

Adrenal cortical deficiency may be acute or chronic. The chronic form is called Addison's disease and is characterized by anemia, sluggishness, weakness, weight loss, hypotension, hypoglycemia, nausea, vomiting, diarrhea, abnormal skin pigmentation, and mental changes.

In acute adrenocortical insufficiency (adrenal crisis) death due to circulatory collapse will result unless the disease is treated promptly and vigorously. The cause may be a hemorrhage into the adrenal cortex due to infection or it may occur at birth due to trauma. In the adult, headache, lassitude, confu-

sion, restlessness, vomiting, and shock progressing to death if the cortex is destoyed. A less acute form of adrenal crisis may develop in a person who has recently discontinued taking cortisone and is suddenly subjected to severe stress. Adrenal crisis due to hemorrhage into the adrenal caused by meningococcal infection is called the Waterhouse-Friderichsen syndrome.

adrenalectomy (ăd-rē″năl-ĕk′tō-mĭ) [L. *ad*, to, + *ren*, kidney, + Gr. *ektomē*, excision]. Excision of an adrenal gland.

adrenalin (ă-dren′ă-lĭn). Proprietary name for epinephrine, q.v.

adrenaline (ă-drĕn′ă-lēn). British designation for epinephrine, q.v.

adrenaline′mia [L. *ad*, to, + *rēn*, kidney, + Gr. *haima*, blood]. Epinephrine in the blood.

adrenalinu′ria ["+ Gr. *ouron*, urine]. Epinephrine in the urine.

adren′alism. Illness caused by abnormal function of adrenal glands.

adrenalitis (ad-rē″năl-i′tĭs) [L. *ad*, to, + *ren*, kidney, + *-itis*, inflammation]. Inflammation of the adrenal glands; adrenitis.

adrenergic (ăd-rĕn-ĕr′jĭk) ["+ "+ Gr. *ergon*, work]. Term applied to nerve fibers which when stimulated release epinephrine (adrenaline) at their endings. Includes nearly all sympathetic post-ganglionic fibers except those innervating sweat glands.

adreni′tis. Adrenalitis, q.v.

adrenochrome (ăd″rē′nō-krōm) [L. *ad*, to, + *rēn*, kidney, + Gr. *chrōma*, color]. A red pigment obtained by oxidation of epinephrine.

adrenocorticotropic (ăd-rē″nō-kōr″tĭ-kō-trōp′ĭk) ["+ "+ *cortex*, bark, + Gr. *tropos*, a turning]. Having a stimulating effect on the adrenal cortex.

a. hormone. A hormone secreted by anterior lobe of hypophysis which is essential to the growth, development, and continued function of the adrenal cortex. In some animals this hormone has a melanaphore-stimulating-hormone action as well as the effect of liberating free fatty acids from fat tissue. The possibility that these effects also occur in man is good but unproven. ABBR: ACTH. SYN: *corticotropin.*

adrenogenital ["+ "+ *genitalis,* genital]. Pert. to the adrenal glands and the genitalia.

adrenogenous (ăd″rē-nŏj′ĭ-nŭs) ["+ "+ Gr. *gennan,* to produce]. Originating in or produced by the adrenal gland.

adrenolytic (ăd″rĕn-ō-lĭt′ĭk) [L. *ad*, to, + *rēn,* kidney, + Gr. *lysis,* a loosening]. Pervading or inhibiting the activity of adrenergic nerves. Interfering with the response to epinephrine.

adrenopathy (ăd″rĕn-ŏp′ă-thĭ) ["+ "+ Gr. *pathos*, disease]. Any disease of the adrenal glands.

adrenoprival (ăd-rĕn′ō-prī′văl) ["+ "+ *privāre*, to deprive]. Pert. to or characterized by deprivation of the function of the adrenal glands.

adrenosterone (ăd″rĕn-ŏs′tē-rōn). An androgenic hormone secreted by the adrenal cortex.

adrenotoxin (ăd-rē″nō-tŏks′ĭn) [L. *ad*, to, + *rēn*, kidney, + *toxicum*, poison]. A substance toxic to the adrenal glands.

adrenotropic (ad-rē″nō-trōp′ĭk) ["+ "+ Gr. *tropos*, a turning]. Nourishing or stimulating to the adrenal glands with reference especially to hormones which stimulate function of the adrenal glands.

ADS. Abbr. for *antidiuretic substance.* SEE: *antidiuretic hormone (ADH).*

adsorb′ent. A substance which leads readily to adsorption, such as activated charcoal or magnesia.

adsorption (ăd-sŏrp′shŭn) [L. *ad*, to, + *sorbere*, to suck in]. Adhesion by a gas or liquid to the surface of a solid.

adsternal (ăd-stĕr′năl) [L. *ad*, toward, + Gr. *sternon*, chest]. Near or toward the sternum.

ADT. 1. Abbr. for *adenosine triphosphate.* 2. Abbr. placed on a placebo prescription, indicating A (any) D (what you desire) T (thing). 3. Obsolete abbr. for *agar-gel diffusion test.*

adter′minal [L. *ad*, to, + *terminus*, boundary]. Toward extremity of any structure, as end of nerve or muscle.

adtorsion (ăd-tŏr′shŭn) [L. *ad*, to, + L. *torsiō*, twisted]. Convergent squint; inward rotation of both eyes.

adultera′tion [L. *adulterāre*, to pollute]. The addition of an impure or weaker, and usually cheaper, substance to another.

advancement (ăd-văns′mĕnt) [Fr. *avancer*, to set forth]. Operation to remedy strabismus, by which the ocular muscle is severed and then attached at a point further removed from its origin.

    a., capsular. Attachment of capsule of Tenon in front of its normal position.

adventitia (ăd″vĕn-tish′ē-ă) [L. *adventicius*, coming from abroad]. The outermost covering of a structure or organ, such as the tunica adventitia, or outer coat of an artery.

adventitious (ăd″vĕn-tish′ŭs). 1. Acquired; accidental. 2. Arising sporadically. 3. Pert. to adventitia.

adverse reactions. In pharmacology and therapeutics, the development of undesired side effects or toxicity due to the administration of drugs. Onset of such reactions may be

sudden or take days to develop. Early detection by use of laboratory tests is sometimes possible in the case of drugs which might adversely affect the blood-forming organs, the liver or kidneys. It is important that all persons who care for sick persons be alert to the possibility of a patient's developing an adverse reaction to the drug or drugs administered. SYN: *adverse effects.*

adynamia (ăd″ĭ-nā′mĭ-ă) [Gr. *a-*, not, + *dynamis*, strength]. Weakness or loss of strength; asthenia, q.v.

adynamic (ăd″ĭ-năm′ĭk, ā-dī-năm′ĭk). Pert. to adynamia.

    a. ileus. Intestinal obstruction due to lack of intestinal motility. This causes abdominal distention and interferes with postsurgical recovery, particularly from abdominal surgery.

Aedes (ā-ē′dēs) [Gr. *aēdēs*, unpleasant]. A genus of mosquitoes belonging to the family Culicidae. Many species are troublesome pests and some are transmitters of disease.

    A. aegypti. A species of A. which transmits yellow fever and dengue.

aeluropsis (ē″lū-rōp′sĭs) [Gr. *ailouros*, cat, + *opsis*, vision]. Condition in which the eye or palpebral fissure is slanting and narrow.

aer- (air, ā′ĕr) [Gr. *aer*, air]. Combining form meaning relationship to gas or air.

aerated (air′, ā′ĕr-ā-tĕd) [Gr. *aer*, air]. Containing air or gas.

aeration (air-, ā″ĕr-ā′shŭn). 1. Act of airing. 2. Change of venous into arterial blood in the lungs. 3. Saturation or charging of a fluid with gases.

aerendocardia (air-ĕn″dō-kăr′dĭ-ă) [Gr. *aer*, air, + *endon*, in, + *kardia*, heart]. Bubble of air in the blood within the heart.

aerenterectasia (air″ĕn-tĕr-ĕk-tā′zĭ-ă) ["+ *enteron*, intestine, + *ektasis*, stretching out]. Distention of intestine with gas.

aeriform (air′, ā-ĕr′ĭ-form) ["+ L. *forma*, shape]. Airlike; gaseous.

aero- (air′o, ā-ĕr′ō). Combining form indicating relationship to air or gas.

Aerobacter (ā″ĕr-ō-băk′tĕr) [Gr. *aēr*, air, + *baktērion*, little rod]. A genus of aerobic, nonspore-bearing, gram-negative bacilli of the family Enterobacteriaceae.

    A. aerogenes. A species of A. It occurs normally in the intestine of man and other animals and is found in decayed matter, on grains and plants.

aerobe (air′ōb) ["+ *bios*, life]. (pl. *aerobes*) A microorganism which requires free oxygen in order to be able to live and grow. SYN: *aerobion.*

    a., facultative. A microorganism which prefers an environment that is devoid of free oxygen but which has adapted so that it can live and reproduce in the presence of free oxygen.

    a., obligate. A microorganism which grows and reproduces only when free oxygen is present.

aerobic (ă-rō'bĭk). 1. Living only in presence of oxygen. 2. Concerning an organism living only in oxygen.

    a. exercise. Exercise during which the energy needed is supplied by the oxygen inspired. A. exercise is required for sustained periods of hard work and vigorous athletic ability. Opposed to anaerobic exercise, q.v.

aero'bion. Aerobe, q.v.

aerobiosis (air''ō-bī-ō'sĭs) [Gr. *aēr*, air, + *biōsis*, mode of living]. Living in an atmosphere containing oxygen.

aerocele (air'ō-sēl) ["+ *kēlē*, tumor]. Gas within and distending a cavity.

aerocolpos (air-ō-kŏl'pŏs) ["+ *kolpos*, vagina]. Distention of the vagina with air.

aerocoly (air-ŏk'ō-lĭ) [Gr. *aēr*, air, + *kōlon*, colon]. Distention of colon with gas.

aerocystoscopy (air''ō-sis-tos'kō-pī) ["+ *kystis*, bladder, + *skopein*, to view]. Examination of the bladder, when distended by air, with a cystoscope.

aerodermectasia   (air-ō-der''mek-tā'zĭ-ă) ["+ *derma*, skin, + *ektasis*, stretching out]. Subcutaneous emphysema.

aerodontalgia (air''ō-dŏnt-ăl'gĭ-ă) [Gr. *aēr*, air, + *odous*, tooth, + *algos*, pain, + *-ia*, condition]. Pain in the teeth resulting from reduction in atmospheric pressure, as at high altitudes.

aerodontia (air-ō-dŏn'shĭ-ă). A branch of dentistry concerned with the effect of flying on the teeth.

aerodynam'ics [Gr. *aēr*, air, + *dynamis*, force]. Science of air or gases in motion.

aeroembolism (air''ō-em'bō-lizm) ["+ *embolos*, plug]. A condition in which nitrogen bubbles form in fluids and tissues of body during rapid ascent to high altitudes.

    SYM: Boring, gnawing pain in joints; itching of skin and eyelids; unconsciousness; convulsions; and paralysis. Symptoms are relieved by recompression, i.e., return to lower altitudes. Even though oxygen by mask may be available, ascents above 25,000 feet should be avoided except in planes with pressurized cabins. SEE: *bends; caisson disease*.

aeroemphysema (air''ō-ĕm-fĭ-zē'ma) ["+ *emphysēma*, an inflation]. Aeroembolism, q.v.

aerogen (air'ō-jĕn'') [Gr. *aēr*, air, + *gennan*, to produce]. A gas-forming microorganism.

aerogenesis (air-ō-jĕn'ē-sis) ["+ *genesis*, production]. Formation of gas.

aerogenic (air-ō-jen'ik). Gas-forming.

aerogenous (air-, ā''er-ŏj'en-us). Gas-forming.

aerogram (air'ō-grăm) [Gr. *aēr*, air, + *gramma*, mark]. Roentgenogram of an organ after it has been inflated or filled with air or gas.

aerohydrother'apy ["+ *hydrō*, water, + *therapeia*, treatment]. Treatment by application of air and water. SYN: *aerohydropathy*.

aeromed'icine. Aviation medicine.

aerometer (ă-rŏm'ē-tĕr) [Gr. *aēr*, air, + *metron*, measure]. Device for measuring density of gases.

aeroneurosis (air''ō-nū-rō'sĭs) ["+ *neuron*, nerve, + *-ōsis*, condition]. A chronic functional nervous disorder affecting aviators.

aeropathy (air-ŏp'ă-thī) ["+ *pathos*, suffering]. Morbid condition caused by a marked change in atmospheric pressure, such as mountain sickness or caisson disease.

aeroperitoneum (air''ō-pĕr''ĭ-tō-nē'ŭm) [Gr. *aēr*, air, + *per*, around, + *teinein*, to stretch]. Distention of peritoneal cavity with gas. SYN: *aeroperitonia*.

aerophagia (air''ō-fā'jĭ-ă) ["+ *phagein*, to eat]. Swallowing of air. SYN: *aerophagy*.

aerophilous (air-, ā''ēr-ŏf'ĭ-lŭs) ["+ *philein*, to love]. Requiring air for growth and development. SYN: *aerobic*.

aerophobia (air-ō-fō'bĭ-ă) [Gr. *aēr*, air, + *phobos*, fear]. Morbid fear of a draft or of fresh air.

aerophore (air'ō-for) ["+ *phoros*, bearing]. A portable apparatus for inflating the lungs of stillborn or asphyxiated infants.

aerophyte (air'ō-fīt) ["+ *phyton*, plant]. A plant or vegetative organism which derives its sustenance from air.

aeropiesotherapy (air''ō-pī-ē''sō-thĕr'ă-pī) [Gr. *aēr*, air, + *piesis*, pressure, + *therapeia*, service for the sick]. Therapeutic use of air at either increased or decreased barometric pressure. SEE: *decompression chamber; hyperbaric oxygen*.

aeroplethysmograph (air''ō-plē-thiz'mō-graf) ["+ *plēthysmos*, enlargement, + *graphein*, to write]. Instrument for recording air respired.

aeropleura (air''ō-plū'rā) ["+ *pleura*, side]. Pneumothorax; air in pleural cavity.

aeroporotomy (air''ō-pō-rot'ō-mĭ) [Gr. *aēr*, air, + *poros*, passage, + *tomē*, cutting]. Operation, such as a tracheotomy, for admitting air into the air passages.

aeroscope (air″ō-skōp″) ["+ *skopein*, to view]. Device for examining visible particles in the air.

aerosinusitis (air″ō-sī″nus-ī′tĭs) ["+ L. *sinus*, a hollow, + Gr. *-itis*, inflammation]. Chronic inflammation of nasal sinuses due to changes in atmospheric pressure.

aerosis (air-, ā″er-ō′sĭs) ["+ *-osis*, condition]. Accumulation of gas in any of the tissues.

aerosol (air′ō-sōl, sōl) [Gr. *aër*, air, + L. *solutio*, solution]. 1. Atomized particles of a substance suspended in air. 2. A solution of a bactericidal substance which can be atomized for sterilizing the air of a room. 3. A colloidal mixture in which gas is the continuous phase (dispersion medium).

 a. therapy. The use of aerosolized medicines in the treatment of disease, especially pulmonary conditions such as asthma, bronchitis, and emphysema.

aerosolization. Producing an aerosol.

aerospace medicine. The branch of medicine which is concerned with the physiologic, pathologic, and psychologic problems man encounters in the environment of space.

aerosporin (air-, ā″ĕr-ŏs′-pō-rĭn). One of a group of antibiotics known as polymyxins and derived from Bacillus polymyxa (aerosporus), a soil organism. SEE: *polymyxin.*

aerotaxis (air″ō-tăk′sĭs) [Gr. *aër*, air, + *taxis*, arrangement]. Movement of organisms away from or toward air, said of aerobic and anaerobic bacteria.

aerotherapy (air′ō-ther″ă-pĭ) ["+ *therapeia*, treatment]. The use of air in the treatment of disease, utilizing changes in composition and density. SEE: *aeropiesotherapy; decompression chamber; hyperbaric oxygen.*

aerothermotherapy (air-ō-ther″mō-ther′ă-pĭ) ["+ *thermos*, heat, + *therapeia*, treatment]. Therapeutic use of hot air.

aerothorax (air″ō-thō′raks) ["+ *thōrax*, chest]. Presence of air in the intrapleural space. SYN: *pneumothorax.*

aerotitis (air-ō-tī′tĭs) [Gr. *aër*, air, + *ot-*, ear, + *-itis*, inflammation]. Inflammation of the ear, esp. the middle ear, due to failure of the eustachian tube to remain open while the patient experiences alteration in barometric pressure. This may occur while flying, diving, or working in a pressure chamber. SYN: *barotitis.*

aerotonometer (air″ō-tō-nom′ē-ter) ["+ *tonos*, tension, + *metron*, measure]. Apparatus for measuring tension of gases of the blood.

aerotropism (air-ŏt′rō-pĭsm) ["+ *tropē*, a turn]. The tendency of organisms, esp. bacteria and protozoa, to move toward (positive)

a region where air is available as toward the surface of water or toward an air bubble, or to move away (negative) from the air supply.

aerourethroscope (air″ō-ū″rē′thrō-skōp″) ["+ *ourēthra*, urethra, + *skopein*, to view]. An apparatus for examination of the urethra after dilatation by air.

aerourethroscopy (air″ō-ū″rē-thros′kō-pī). Examination of the urethra when distended with air.

Aesculapius (es″kū-lā′pē-us). The Latin name for the Greek god of medicine; son of Apollo and the nymph Coronis.

 A., staff of. A staff or crude stick with a snake wound around it so that its head is at the top of the stick. This symbol is used to signify the art of healing and is used by many medical organizations.

aet. Abbr. for L. *aetas*, at the age of, aged.

afebrile (ă-fĕb′rĭl) [Gr. *a-*, not, + L. *febris*, fever]. Without fever.

af′fect [L. *affectus*, exerting influence on]. In psychology, the emotional reactions associated with an experience.

affec′tion. 1. Love, feeling. 2. Disease, physical or mental.

affec′tive. Pert. to an emotion or mental state.

 a. insanity. Impulsive or emotional insanity.

 a. memory. Memory of a psychic trauma causing recurrence of emotion.

 a. psychosis. A psychotic reaction characterized by serious disorder of mood or emotional feeling. SYN: *manic-depressive reaction.*

 a. spasms. Attacks of laughing, screaming or weeping in hysteria.

af′ferent [L. *ad*, to, + *ferre*, to bear]. Carrying impulses toward a center, as when a sensory nerve carries a message toward the brain; also said of certain veins and lymphatics. Opposed to efferent, q.v.

affiliation (ă-fil-ĭ-ā′shŭn) [L. *affiliāre*, to take to oneself as a son]. In nursing education, the administrative association of two hospitals or schools of nursing. This enables nurses to obtain specialized training and experience which might not otherwise be available to them.

affinity (ă-fĭn′ĭ-tĭ) [L. *affinis*, neighboring]. 1. Common relationship; attraction. 2. Chemical attraction between two substances, i.e., oxygen and hemoglobin. SEE: *chemoreceptor.*

 a., chemical. Force combining atoms of various substances.

 a., elective. Force causing a substance to elect one substance rather than another with which to unite.

a., selective. A., elective, q.v.

af'flux [L. *ad*, to, + *fluere*, to flow]. Rush of blood to a part.

affu'sion [L. *affūsus*, pour upon]. The pouring of water upon, as on the body, for cooling, cleansing, or therapeutic purposes. Used in fever or agitation. Contraindicated in typhoid accompanied by complications, or decompensating heart, or hemorrhagic cases.

NP: Patient may lie on a rubber sheet arranged to direct the water into a pail at bedside. A thin sheet may cover patient. Water can be poured on body through a watering can.

afibrinogenemia (ă-fī''brin-ō-jĕ-nē'mĭ-ă) [Gr. *a-*, not, + L. *fibra*, fiber, + Gr. *gennan*, to produce, + *haima*, blood]. A rare blood disease characterized by the absence or decrease of fibrinogen in the blood plasma so that the blood is incoagulable; may be congenital or acquired. (The term "hypofibrinogenemia" more accurately describes the disease process.) The acquired type is due to one of several causes which can reduce the plasma concentration of fibrinogen. This has been observed in severe trauma and burns; following extensive surgery; obstetric complications of abruptio placentae or retention of a dead fetus; neoplastic disease; hepatic cirrhosis; leukemia; sarcoidosis; and polycythemia vera.

TREATMENT: The clinical picture may develop suddenly. Administration of whole fresh blood and fibrinogen may prevent death from hemorrhage.

afteraction. Continued reaction for some time after the stimulus ceases, particularly in nerve centers. In the sensory centers this action gives rise to aftersensations.

afterbirth. Placenta and membranes expelled after birth of child.

aftercare. Care of a convalescent after conclusion of treatment in a hospital or mental institution.

aftercataract. 1. Secondary cataract. 2. Development of an opacity of the lens capsule after cataract removal.

afterdischarge. The discharge of impulses from a reflex center after stimulation of the receptor has ceased. Results in prolongation of response.

aftereffect. A response occurring some time after the original stimulus or condition has produced its primary effect.

afterhearing. Persistence of sensation of sound after the stimulus causing the sound has ceased.

afterimage. Image which persists subjectively after the cessation of stimulus.

If colors are same as object it is called positive; negative if complementary colors are seen. In the former case, the image is seen in its natural bright colors without any alteration; in the latter, the bright parts become dark, while dark parts are light.

afterimpression. An aftersensation, q.v.

afterpains. Uterine cramps due to contraction of uterus, occurring during first few days after childbirth (puerperium); commonly seen in multiparae. Pains more severe during nursing. The pain rarely lasts for longer than 48 hours postpartum.

TREATMENT: Codeine, aspirin. The earlier given, the less needed.

afterperception. Perception of a sensation after cessation of stimulus.

aftersensation. Sensation persisting after stimulus causing it has ceased.

aftertaste. Persistence of gustatory sensations after cessation of stimulus.

aftertreatment. Secondary treatment; that following a primary treatment regimen. SEE: *aftercare.*

aftervision. SEE: *afterimage.*

Ag [L. *argentum*]. Chem. symb. for silver.

agalactia (ag''ă-lak'shĭ-ă) [Gr. *a-*, not, + *gala*, milk, + *-ia*, condition]. Absence of milk secretion after childbirth.

agalorrhea (ă-gal''ō-rē'ă) ["+ "+ *rhoia*, flow]. Arrest of milk flow.

agamic (ă-gam'ik) [Gr. *a-*, not, + *gamos*, marriage]. 1. Reproducing asexually. 2. Asexual.

agammaglobulinemia (ă-găm''ă-glŏb''ū-lĭn-ē'mĭ-ă) ["+ *gamma globulin*, + *haima*, blood]. A rare disease characterized by the virtual absence of gamma globulin from the blood plasma with resulting loss of the ability to produce immune antibodies, and the absence of natural blood group isoantibodies from the serum; may be congenital or acquired. The sex-linked congenital form is inherited like hemophilia as a sex-linked recessive characteristic, and occurs only in male children. The nonsex-linked form occurs as an autosomal dominant characteristic. This latter form is quite rare.

agamogen'esis ["+ *gamos*, marriage, + *genesis*, development]. 1. Asexual reproduction. 2 Parthenogenesis.

agar (ā'gĕr, ăg'ĕr) [Malay, gelatin]. 1. Sea weed (alga) belonging to the genus Gelideum. The source of agar-agar. 2. A dried mucilaginous product obtained from certain species of algae, especially Gelideum. It is unaffected by bacterial enzymes, hence widely used as a solidifying agent for bacterial culture media; also used as a laxative because of its great increase in bulk upon absorption of water. 3. A culture medium containing agar.

agar-agar. Agar, q.v.

agastria (ă-gas'trĭ-ă) [Gr. *a-*, not, + *gastēr*, stomach]. Absence of the stomach.

agastric (ă-gast'rĭk). Lacking an alimentary canal as in certain animals such as tapeworms.

AgCl. Chem. symb. for silver chloride.

age [Fr. *áge*, L. *aetās*]. 1. The time from birth to the present for a living individual as measured in units of time. 2. A particular period of life, as middle age or old age. 3. To grow old. 4. In psychology, the degree of development of an individual expressed in terms of the age of an average individual of comparable development or accomplishment.

a., achievement. One determined by a proficiency test, the results of which are measured with the mental ability of the average child of the same chronological age. ABBR: A.A.

a., bone. X-ray studies of the stage of development of ossification centers of the extremities can be utilized to estimate the age of children. The estimate obtained is called bone age. SEE: *epiphysis.*

a., chronological. Age as determined by years of existence. ABBR: C.A.

a. of consent. In legal terms, the age at which one is capable of giving deliberate and voluntary agreement, esp. to marriage or to unlawful sexual intercourse. It implies physical and mental power and free action. The age of consent to unlawful sexual intercourse in general is 13-18 years.

a., menarcheal. Elapsed time expressed in years from menarche.

a., mental. The age of a person with regard to his mental development; this is determined by a series of mental tests as devised by Binet. Thus, if a woman of 30 can pass only the tests of a child of 12, she is said to have a mental age of 12. ABBR: M.A.

a., physiological. Age as determined by functional activity.

age, words pert. to: adolescence; climacteric; geriatrics; maturation; puberty; senility.

agenesia, agenesis (ă"jen-ē'sĭ-ă, ă-jen'ē-sĭs) [Gr. *a-*, not, + *genesis*, production]. 1. Failure of an organ or part to develop or grow. 2. Lack of potency.

agenitalism (ă-jĕn'ĭ-tăl-ĭsm) ["+ L. *genitālis*, belonging to birth]. Symptoms resulting from absence of the testicles or ovaries.

agenosomia (ă-jen"ō-sō'mĭ-ă) ["+ *gennan*, to beget, + *sōma*, body]. Condition of fetus in which the genitals are absent or poorly de-

veloped and the intestines protrude from an incompletely developed abdominal wall.

agent (ā'jent) [L. *agere*, to do]. Something which causes an effect. Thus bacteria which cause disease are said to be agents of the specific diseases they cause. A medicine would be classed as a therapeutic agent.

agerasia (ă-jĕr-ā'sĭ-ă). Healthy, vigorous old age; youthful appearance of an old person.

ageusia (ă-gū'sĭ-ă) [Gr. *a-*, not, + *geusis*, taste]. Absence, a partial loss, or an impairment of the sense of taste.

ETIOL: May be due to disease of the chorda tympani on one side or of the gustatory fibers; excessive use of condiments; effect of certain drugs; or lesions involving sensory pathways or taste centers in the brain.

a., central. That due to a cerebral lesion.

a., conduction. That due to a lesion involving sensory nerves of taste.

a., peripheral. That due to a disorder of taste buds of mucous membrane of tongue.

agger (aj'ĕr) [L.]. A small elevation or eminence; a mound.

a. nasi. [NA]. A small elevation, the anterior part of the ethmoidal crest on medial surface of the frontal process of the upper jaw (maxilla), forming part of the nasal cavity.

agglomerate (ă-glom'ĕ-rāt) [L. *ad-*, to, + *glomerāre*, to wind into a ball]. To congregate; to form a mass.

agglu'tinable [L. *agglutinans*, gluing]. Capable of agglutination.

agglutinant (ă-glū'tĭ-nant). 1. Anything causing adhesion. 2. Causing to unite or adhere, as healing of a wound. 3. An antibody produced in the body in response to stimulation by an antigen (agglutinogen). SYN: *agglutinin.*

agglutination (ă-glū"tĭ-nā'shun). 1. Clumping of microorganisms when a specific immune serum is added to a bacterial culture. 2. Clumping of blood corpuscles when incompatible bloods are mixed. 3. Adhesion of surfaces of a wound.

agglu'tina"tive. Causing or capable of causing agglutination.

agglutinin (ă-glū'tĭ-nĭn) [L. *agglutinans*, gluing]. An antibody which causes agglutination; more specifically a substance present in normal or immune serum capable of causing agglutination or clumping of specific antigens (bacteria or cells). SEE: *agglutinogen; blood groups; blood typing; isoagglutinin.*

a., anti-Rh. A factor normally absent in human plasma but sometimes occurring in Rh-negative mothers bearing an Rh-positive fetus or in Rh-negative individuals who have

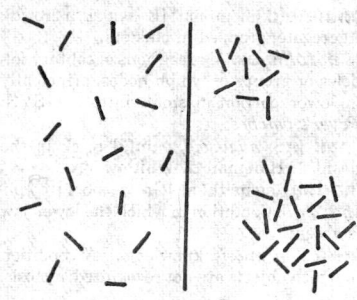

AGGLUTINATION REACTION

Left, negative, with uniform distribution of bacilli; Right, positive, with the formation of clumps.

received multiple transfusions of Rh-positive blood.

    a., chief. A specific one in the blood of a person who has been immunized against a specific disease or microorganism. It is active in higher dilutions than are the other agglutinins present.

    a., cold. Agglutinins which act only at low temperatures. They are present in the serum of patients with atypical pneumonia and in certain blood diseases.

    a., flagellar. One which agglutinates only the flagella of an organism.

    a., group. A. acting as a specific on one species, but which will act on others.

    a., haupt. A., chief, q.v.

    a., immune. A. causing immunity, found in the blood either because of recovery from the disease or of having been inoculated with the microorganism.

    a., major. A., chief, q.v.

    a., minor. One acting on an organism related to the one utilized for immunization but in lower dilutions.

    a., nonspecific. One found in individuals who have had a certain disease and which agglutinates organisms having no relation to the disease. Utilized in certain diagnostic tests.

    a., O. One acting on the bodies of organisms, in contrast to flagellar or motile agglutinins. SYN: *somatic a.*

    a., partial. Minor agglutinin, q.v.

    a., somatic. O agglutinin, q.v.

agglutinogen (ă-glū-tin′ō-jĕn) [Gr. *agglutinans,* gluing, + Gr. *gennan,* to produce]. 1. A substance which stimulates the development of a specific agglutinin, thereby acting as an antigen. 2. A specific antigen used in agglutination tests. SEE: *blood groups.*

    a.'s, A and B. Discovered by Karl Landsteiner in 1901. These two antigenic substances are found in the red blood cells of human beings and react with the alpha (anti-A) and beta (anti-B) isoagglutinins in the blood. The red corpuscles may contain A, B, or a combination of A and B agglutinogens, or may not contain either A or B; the four resulting blood groups are A, B, AB and O. Blood groups are inherited according to Mendel's law.

    a.'s, M and N. These two antigenic substances are found in the red corpuscles of human beings. Anti-M and anti-N agglutinins are rarely found in normal serum. The red blood cells may contain M, N, or M and N agglutinogens, resulting in blood types M, N, or MN, respectively.

    a., Rh. A specific substance called the Rh factor, present in red cells. It was discovered in 1940 by Landsteiner and Wiener who prepared anti-Rh serum by injecting red cells from Rhesus monkeys into rabbits or other animals. They found that the red cells of 85% of Caucasians will be agglutinated when in contact with anti-Rh. These persons are termed Rh-positive. The remaining 15% whose red cells are not agglutinated by anti-Rh are termed Rh-negative. More than 25 blood factors are known to belong to the Rh-Hr system. Their importance in blood typing and blood type incompatibility between mother and fetus makes this blood group system second in importance only to the ABO group.

agglutinoid (ă-glū′tin-oid) ["+ "+ Gr. *eidos,* resemblance]. An agglutinin that has lost its zymophore group as a result of the effect of heat, age, chemicals, etc., and, consequently, its ability to agglutinate its specific antigen although its ability to combine with its antigen remains.

agglutinophilic (ă-glū″tin-ō-fil′ik) ["+ "+ Gr. *philos,* fond]. Contributing to agglutination.

agglu′tinophore ["+ "+ Gr. *pherein,* to bear]. The active agent producing agglutination.

agglutogenic (ă-glū″tō-jen′ik) [L. *agglutinans,* gluing, + Gr. *gennan,* to produce]. 1. Pert. to substances from which agglutinins originate. 2. Producing agglutinins.

agglutom′eter ["+ "+ Gr. *metron,* measure]. Device to simplify the agglutination or Widal test without the use of an ordinary microscope.

ag′gregate [L. *aggregātus,* collect]. 1. Total substances making up a mass. 2. To cluster or come together.

aggression (ă-grĕsh'ŭn) [L. *aggredi,* to approach with hostility]. In psychology, a forceful attacking action, physical, verbal, or symbolic. May be justified and real or unrealistic and the result of disordered mental processes. In some forms of mental illness aggression may be directed toward the self, and physical damage including suicide may result.

aging (āj'ing). Growing old, maturing. Progressive changes related to the passage of time. There is no precise method for determining the rate or degree of aging.

agitated depression. A psychiatric depression characterized by continuous restlessness.

SYM: Patients are restless, depressed, and agitated, pacing up and down, wringing hands, crying, picking and rubbing. They have feelings of guilt, unworthiness, and ideas of persecution, phobias, and obsessions.

NP: Similar to manic-depressive cases. Prevent patient from hurting self, as from pulling out hairs and tearing skin, etc. Divert patient but do not argue with him. Hydrotherapy may be indicated.

agitation (ăj'ĭ-tā'shun) [L. *agitāre,* to drive]. 1. Excessive restlessness and increased mental and especially physical activity. 2. Tremor. 3. Shaking of a container so that the contents are rapidly moved and mixed.

agitographia (ăj''ĭ-tō-grăf'ĭ-ă) ["+ Gr. *graphein,* to write]. Writing with excessive rapidity, with unconscious omission of words, syllables, etc.

agitophasia (ăj'ĭ-tō-fā'zĭ-ă) ["+ Gr. *phasis,* speech, + *-ia,* condition]. Excessive rapidity of speech, with slurring, omission, and distortion of sounds. SYN: *agitolalia.*

aglaukopsia (ă''glaw-kŏp'sĭ-ă) [Gr. *a-,* not, + *glaukos,* green, + *opsis,* vision]. Green blindness.

aglossia (ă-glos'ĭ-ă) ["+ *glōssa,* tongue, + *-ia,* condition]. 1. Congenital absence of tongue. 2. Lack of ability to speak.

aglossostomia (ă''glos-ō-sto'mĭ-ah) ["+ "+ *stoma,* mouth, + *-ia,* condition]. Congenital absence of tongue and mouth opening.

aglutition (ag-lū-tish'un) ["+ L. *glutire,* to swallow]. Difficulty in swallowing or inability to swallow.

aglycemia (ă''glī-sē'mĭ-ă) [Gr. *a-,* not, + *glykys,* sweet, + *haima,* blood]. Lack of sugar in the blood.

aglycosu'ric ["+ "+ *ouron,* urine]. Free from glycosuria.

agmatology (ăg''mă-tol'ō-jĭ) [Gr. *agma,* fragment, + *logos,* study of]. The study of fractures.

agminate(d (ăg'mĭ-nāt) [L. *agmen,* a crowd]. Aggregate; grouped in clusters.

　　a. follicles. Aggregations of solitary follicles or groups of lymph nodes, principally in lower portion of small intestine. SYN: *Peyer's patches.*

ag'nail [AS. *angnaegl,* painful prick in the flesh]. 1. Hangnail. 2. Whitlow, q.v.

agnathia (ag-nā'thĭ-a) [Gr. *a-,* not, + *gnathos,* jaw]. Condition in which the lower jaw is absent.

agne'a ["+ *gnōsis,* knowledge]. A condition in which objects are not recognized; agnosis, q.v.

AgNO₃. Chem. symb. for silver nitrate.

agnogenic (ag-nō-jen'ik) [Gr. *a-,* not, + *gnōsis,* knowledge, + *gennan,* to produce]. Of unknown origin or etiology.

agno'sia. Loss of comprehension of auditory, visual, or other sensations although the sensory sphere is intact; inability to recognize an object. SYN: *mind blindness.*

　　a., auditory. Mental inability to interpret sounds.

　　a., optic. Mental inability to interpret images that are seen.

　　a., tactile. Inability to distinguish objects by sense of touch.

-agogue (ă-gog) [Gr. *agōgos,* leading, inducing]. Suffix meaning a producer or leader.

agomphiasis (ag''ŏm-fĭ'ă-sĭs) [Gr. *a-,* not, + *gromphios,* molar, + *iasis,* state]. 1. Looseness of the teeth. 2. Without teeth.

agonad (ă-gō'năd) ["+ *gonē,* seed]. A person without gonads.

agon'adal. Having no gonads.

ag'onal [Gr. *agōn,* a contest]. Rel. to death, or to agony.

ag'onist. The muscle directly engaged in contraction as distinguished from muscles which have to relax at the same time.

Thus in bending the elbow, the m. biceps brachii is the agonist and the triceps the antagonist.

agony (ăg'ō-nĭ). 1. Extreme suffering, mental or physical. 2. Death struggle.

agoraphobia (ăg''ō-ră-fō'bĭ-ă) [Gr. *agora,* market place, + *phobos,* fear]. Morbid dread of open spaces.

-agra [Gr. *agra,* a seizure]. Suffix indicating relationship to a severe pain; seizure.

agraffe (ă-grăf') [O.F. *agrafer,* to hook, fasten]. An appliance for clamping together edges of a wound.

agrammatism (ă-gram'ă-tizm'') [Gr. *agrammatos,* unlettered]. Inability to form a grammatical or intelligible sentence or to arrange words in grammatical sequence.

ETIOL: Cerebral disease.

agranulocyte (ă-grăn'ū-lō-sīt) [Gr. *a-*, not, + L. *granulum,* granule, + Gr. *kytos,* cell]. A nongranular leukocyte.

agranulocytic (ă-grăn-ū-lō-sĭt'ĭk). Pert. to agranulocytosis.

agranulocytosis (ā″grăn″ū-lō-sī-tō'sĭs). An acute disease in which the white blood cell count drops to extremely low levels and neutropenia becomes pronounced. Characterized by high fever, prostration, necrotic ulcerations of the mouth, rectum, and vagina. Some cases idiopathic; others resulting from drugs or radiation. SYN: *granulocytopenia.*

agranuloplas'tic [Gr. *a-*, not, + L. *granulum,* granule, + Gr. *plastikos,* formative]. Inability to form granular cells.

agranulo'sis. Same as agranulocytosis.

agraphia (ā-grăf'ĭ-ă) [Gr. *a-*, not, + *graphein,* to write, + *-ia,* condition]. A loss of ability to express oneself in writing due to a central lesion, or to muscular incoordination.

Copying or writing from dictation may still be possible. It is analogous to or associated with motor aphasia. SYN: *logographia.* SEE: *anorthography; aphasia, motor.*

  a., absolute. Complete inability to write.

  a., acoustic. Inability to write words heard.

  a., amnemonic. Inability to write a connected sentence expressing an idea, but letters or words may be written.

  a., atactic. Absolute agraphia, q.v.

  a., cerebral. Inability to express thoughts in writing.

  a., mental. Cerebral a.

  a., motor. A. due to inability to coordinate muscle movements.

  a., optic. Inability to copy words.

  a., verbal. Inability to write words although letters can be written.

agria (āg'rĭ-ă) [Gr. *agrios,* wild]. Malignant pustules; severe pustular eruption.

agroma'nia [Gr. *agros,* field, + *mania,* frenzy]. Unreasonable desire for solitude or solitudinous wandering. Morbid desire to live in solitude or in the country.

agrypnia (ă-grĭp'nĭ-ă) [Gr. *agrypnos,* sleepless]. Inability to sleep. SYN: *ahypnia; ahypnosis; insomnia.*

agrypnot'ic. 1. Afflicted with insomnia. 2. That which causes wakefulness.

ague (ā'gū) [Fr. *aigu,* sharp, acute]. Originally used to indicate a chill or fever, esp. if due to malaria. Rarely used except colloquially.

ah. Abbr. for *hypermetropic astigmatism.*

Ahlfeld's sign (ahl'felts). [Friedrich Ahlfeld, Ger. obstetrician, 1843-1929]. Uterine irregular contractions after the 3rd month of pregnancy.

ahypnia (ă-hĭp'nĭ-ă) [Gr. *a-*, not, + *hypnos,* sleep]. Insomnia or sleeplessness. SYN: *agrypnia; ahypnosis.*

A.I. Abbr. for *aortic insufficiency; artificial insemination; axioincisal.*

aichmophobia (āk″mō-fō'bĭ-ă) [Gr. *aichmē,* point, + *phobos,* fear]. Morbid fear of pointed instruments or of being touched by them or with a finger.

AID. Abbr. for *artificial insemination by donor* (heterologous insemination).

AIH. Abbr. for *artificial insemination by husband* (homologous insemination).

ailment. A physical or mental illness, esp. one which is mild.

ailurophobia (ă-lū″rō-fō'bĭ-ă) [Gr. *ailouros,* cat, + *phobos,* fear]. Morbid fear of cats. A symbolism of psychoneurotic origin.

ainhum (ān'hŭm) [African]. A fissured constriction of unknown origin causing eventual amputation of the digit. Affects usually the fourth or fifth toes and less commonly other digits of the feet or hands. It is predominately a disease of members of dark-skinned races; it apparently does not occur in Caucasians. There is no specific treatment.

air (ār) [Gr. *aēr,* air]. The invisible, tasteless, odorless mixture of gases surrounding the earth.

The air, so-called "breath of life," is made up of approximately 21% oxygen, 0.8% argon, 78% nitrogen, aqueous vapor, carbon dioxide, and traces of ammonia, helium, neon, krypton, xenon, and other rare gases. However, in mines and industrial communities and their environs it is polluted. The proportions, esp. of water vapor, are variable.

  a., alveolar. Air in the alveoli; that involved in the pulmonary exchange of gases between air and the blood. Its content is determined by sampling the last portion of a maximal expiration.

  a., complemental. The amount that may be breathed in over and above the tidal air, by deepest possible inspiration. SYN: *inspiratory reserve volume.*

  a., dead space. The volume of air that fills the respiratory passageways and not available for exchange of gases with the blood.

  a., functional residual. The volume of air left in the lungs at the end of a natural unforced expiration. It is the sum of expiratory reserve volume (supplemental air) and residual air.

a., liquid. Air liquified by great pressure. It produces intense cold on evaporation.

a., minimal. The small amount of air left in the alveoli by collapse of small bronchi when the supplemental and residual air is driven out when the lungs collapse with the thorax open. This makes it possible for the excised lungs of animals to float, hence the term "lights."

a., reserve. A., supplemental, q.v.

a., residual. The amount remaining in the lungs after the fullest possible expiration. About 1500 cc.

a., supplemental. Amount that may be forcibly expired after a quiet expiration. About 1600 cc. SYN: *expiratory reserve volume.*

a., tidal. The amount that flows in and out of the lungs with each quiet respiration; average of adult male about one pint (500 cc.).

air, words pert. to: "aer-" words; aspiration; atelectasis; expiration; inspiration; respiration; ventilation.

air bed. 1. Large inflated air cushion used as a mattress. SEE: *air cushion.* 2. A special bed which permits the patient actually to float on a cushion of air. The air which comes from the surface of the bed prevents the body from coming in contact with the surface. Esp. useful in treating patients with burns or patients with bedsores.

air cell. An air vesicle, q.v.

air conditioning. Providing, usually by use of special equipment, for control of temperature and humidity of the air while insuring adequate ventilation.

air curtain. Method of directing an air current around a patient so that air which would normally circulate around and contaminate the patient is prevented by the curtain of air. Used in isolating patients from bacteria or dust-borne allergens.

air cushion. An airtight inflatable cushion. To inflate, a pump, as a bicycle pump may be used.

NP: When inflating orally, place layer of gauze over opening and between lips.

air em′bolism [L. *embolismus,* from Gr. *en,* in, + *ballein,* to throw]. Obstruction of a blood vessel brought about by entrance of air into the blood stream.

ETIOL: A postoperative possibility, or air may enter during hypodermic injection if syringe is not properly filled. Air should be excluded when giving an intravenous injection.

air flow, laminar. SEE: *laminar air flow.*

air-fluidized bed. A special bed consisting of a mattress filled with approx. 100 billion ceramic spheres which are suspended by a continual flow of warm air at the rate of approx. 40 cubic feet (1.13 cubic meters)/minute. This creates a surface that feels like a liquid, having a specific gravity of 1.3.

The patient "floats" on the mattress with only minimal penetration. Because of the even distribution of weight the bed is particularly useful in treating burn patients and decubitus ulcers. Nursing care of the patient is greatly simplified because the patient can be moved by finger-tip pressure.

air hun′ger. Shortness of breath marked by rapid, labored breathing. SEE: *dyspnea.*

air sac. An air vesicle, q.v.

airsickness. Condition similar to seasickness occurring during aircraft flight.

air swal′lowing. Oral intake of air either voluntarily or involuntarily. Involuntarily, this condition mainly occurs in infants as a result of improper feeding; in adults it occurs in neurasthenia or hysteria or when on a fluid diet. SYN: *aerophagia.*

air vesicle. Pulmonary tissue saccule filling with air during breathing.

airway. 1. Any natural passageway for air in the body. 2. A device used to prevent or correct obstructed respiratory passage, especially during anesthesia.

akaryocyte (ă-kar′ē-ō-sīt′) [Gr. *a-,* not, + *karyon,* kernel, + *kytos,* hollow vessel]. Erythrocyte; red blood cell; a nonnucleated cell.

akatamathesia (ă-kăt″ă-mă-thē′zĭ-ă) ["+ *katamathēsis,* understanding]. The mental condition of being unable to understand.

akathisia (ăk″ă-thĭ′zĭ-ă). SEE: *acathisia.*

akinesia (ā″kĭ-nē′zĭ-ă) [Gr. *a-,* not, + *kinēsis,* movement]. Complete or partial loss of muscle movement. SEE: *acinesia.*

a. algera. Form with intense pain caused by any movement.

a. amnestica. Form marked by failure of muscular power due to lack of use.

akinet′ic. 1. Pert. to akinesia. 2. Rel. to or characterized by amitosis.

Al. Chem. symb. for aluminum. (British: aluminium.)

-al [L.]. 1. Suffix indicating connection with, as in abdominal, marginal. 2. In chemistry indicates an aldehyde.

ala (ā′lă) [L. *ala,* wing]. (pl. *alae*) 1. An expanded or winglike structure or appendage. 2. Axilla, q.v.

a. auris. The pinna of the ear.

a. cerebelli. [NA] A. of central lobule. SYN: *a. lobuli centralis.* .

a. cinerea. Dark triangular area on the floor of the fourth ventricle. The autonomic fibers of the vagus nerve arise from the cells of the nucleus of this area. SYN: *triangle of the vagus nerve; trigonum nervi vagi.*

a. of ethmoid. Small projection on each side of the ethmoid bone.

a. of ilium. Broad, thin upper portion of the os ilium or iliac bone.

a. major ossis sphenoidalis. [NA]. Greater wing of the sphenoid bone.

a. minor ossis sphenoidalis. [NA]. Lesser wing of the sphenoid bone.

a. nasi. [NA]. Lower extended portion of lateral wall of nose.

a. of nose. A. nasi, q.v.

a. of sacrum. Large triangular surface on either side of the base of the sacrum.

a. vomeris. [NA]. One of the two lateral extensions of bone on the superior border of the vomer.

alae (ā'lē). Plural of ala, q.v.

a. lateralis. 1. Greater wing of sphenoid bone. 2. Extended processes on each side of frontal bone.

ala'lia [Gr. *a-*, not, + *lalein*, to talk]. Loss of ability to speak due to defect or paralysis of the vocal organs. Aphasia.

ETIOL: Psychic or due to lesion.

alar (ā'lăr) [L. *ala*, wing]. 1. Pert. to or like a wing. 2. Axillary.

a. artery. Supplies tissues of ala of nose.

a. cartilage. One on each side of nose forming the tip.

alastrim (ă-lăs'trĭm) [Portuguese, *alastrar*, to spread]. A modified smallpox with sparse rash and low-grade fever. SYN: *variola minor.*

alate (ā'lāt) [L. *ala*, wing]. Winged.

al'ba [L. *albus*, white]. 1. White. 2. White substance of the brain.

albedo (ăl-bē'dō) [L.]. Whiteness. Reflection of light from a surface.

a. ret'inae. Retinal edema.

a. unguium. White semilunar area at nail root. SYN: *lunula.*

Albers-Schönberg disease (ăl-bărs-shĕn'bärg). [Heinrich Ernst Albers-Schönberg, Ger. roentgenologist, 1865-1921] Abnormal bone calcification giving bones spotted, marblelike appearance and causing them to fracture spontaneously. SYN: *marble bones; osteopetrosis.*

Al'bert's disease. [Eduard Albert, Austrian surgeon, 1841-1900]. Inflammation of the bursae lying over the Achilles tendon. SYN: *achillobursitis.*

al'bicans [L.]. (pl. *albicantia*) 1. White or whitish. 2. One of the corpora albicantia.

a., corpus. Whitish body in ovarian cortex.

albidum (ăl'bĭ-dum) [L.]. White.

albidu'ria [L. *albidus*, whitish, + Gr. *ouron*, urine]. 1. Passing of white or colorless urine of low specific gravity. SYN: *albinuria.* 2. Chyluria, q.v.

albidus (ăl'bĭ-dŭs) [L.]. Whitish.

albinism (ăl'bĭn-ĭsm) [L. *albus*, white]. Abnormal, nonpathological absence of pigment in skin, hair, and eyes, partial or total, frequently accompanied by astigmatism, photophobia, and nystagmus, because the choroid is not sufficiently protected from light because of lack of pigment.

Albini's nodules (ăl-bē'nē). [Giuseppe Albini, It. physiologist, 1830-1911]. Minute nodules on margins of mitral and tricuspid valves of the heart; sometimes seen in newly born.

albino (ăl-bī'nō). A person deficient in pigment; one afflicted with albinism.

albinu'ria [L. *albus*, white, + Gr. *ouron*, urine]. Passing of white or colorless urine of low specific gravity. SYN: *albiduria.*

albocinereous (ăl''bō-sĭn-ē'rē-ŭs) ["+ *cinereus*, gray]. Pert. to both white and gray matter of brain and spinal cord.

Albright's disease. [Fuller Albright, Amer. physician, 1900 —]. Same as Recklinghausen's disease and osteitis fibrosa cystica, q.v.

albuginea (ăl-bū-jĭn'ĭ-ă) [L. from *albus*, white]. A layer of firm, white, fibrous tissue forming the investment of an organ or part, as of the eye, testicle, ovary or spleen. SYN: *tunica albuginea.*

a. corporum cavernosorum. A strong, very elastic white fibrous coat, forming a sheath common to both corpora cavernosa of the penis.

a. oc'uli. Sclera, or tough white supporting covering of the eyeball.

a. ovarii. The layer of firm fibrous tissue lying beneath the epithelial ovarian covering.

a. testis. The thick, unyielding layer of white fibrous tissue lying under the tunica vaginalis.

albugineotomy (ăl''bū-jĭn''ē-ŏt'ō-mĭ) [L. *albugenea*, + Gr. *tomē*, cutting]. Incision of tunica albuginea of the testis.

albuginitis (ăl''bū-jĭn-ī'tĭs) ["+ Gr. *-itis*, inflammation]. Inflammation of any tunica albuginea.

albu'go [L.]. White opacity of the cornea.

albu'men. 1. White of an egg. 2. Former spelling for albumin, q.v.

albu'min [L. *albumen*, egg white]. One of a group of simple proteins.

It is found in the blood as serum albumin; in milk as lactalbumin; and in the white of egg as albumen. It is soluble in cold water;

coagulated on heating, then no longer dissolved by cold or hot water. In the stomach coagulated albumins are made soluble by peptase, being changed at the same time into albumoses and peptones.

In general, albumins from animal sources are of higher quality than those from vegetable sources, because animal proteins contain greater quantities of essential amino acids. SEE: *albumoses; amino acids; peptones.*

a. test. The commonest type of albumin found in urine is serum albumin. Before testing, certain precautions must be observed: The specimen of urine must be fresh. The specimen must also be clear; the safest way to ensure this is to filter it through special filter paper (blotting paper makes a good substitute). The urine must be acid.

There are many tests for albumin, but the usual ones follow.

Acetic acid test: Over a Bunsen burner, heat the top inch (1.3 cm.) or so of a test tube filled three parts full of urine. A cloudiness will occur, which may be due to phosphate or albumin. Add 2-3 drops of acetic acid. If the cloud disappears it is due to phosphates; if it becomes intensified, albumin is present.

Heller's cold test: Pour about 1/2 in. (1.3 cm.) of concentrated nitric acid in a test tube, and overlay it carefully with the urine, using a pipette. An opaque line appears at the junction of the fluids. This may take a few minutes to develop.

Paper strip or tablet tests: There are several forms of tests available which are based on the principle that certain chemicals impregnated in paper or in tablet form will change color when exposed to protein-containing urine. Within certain limits, these tests are reliable and have the advantage of providing a result in a few seconds.

Sulfosalicylic acid test: Add 10-20 drops of sulfosalicylic acid to urine in a test tube. Albumin is shown as a white, cloudy precipitate. This may be carried out as a ring test, as in Heller's test.

Since albuminuria can be caused by many different conditions, the results require careful interpretation.

Quantitative methods are available. SEE: *Esbach's method.*

a., acid. Compound resulting from action of acid on a.

a., alkali. Compound resulting from action of weak alkalies on a.

a., blood. Serum a., q.v.

a., circulating. A. present in body fluids.

a., derived. A. changed by chemical action; albuminate.

a., egg. White of an egg; albumen; ovalbumin.

a., muscle. Form found in muscular tissue.

a., native. Any a. present in an organism normally, as serum a.

a., normal human serum. USP. Sterile solution of serum albumin from healthy donors. Administered intravenously to restore blood volume.

a., serum. The main proteins found in the blood. SYN: *blood a.*

a., urinary. Serum albumin, serum globulin, and any other proteins in urine.

a., vegetable. Any albumin in, or derived from, plant tissue.

albu'minate. The compound formed when albumin combines with an acid or alkali (base).

albuminatu'ria [L. *albūmen,* white of egg, + Gr. *ouron,* urine]. Albuminates in voided urine.

albuminiferous (ăl-bū″mĭn-ĭf'ĕ-rŭs) ["+ *ferre,* to bear]. Producing albumin.

albuminimeter (ăl-bū″mĭn-ĭm'ĕ-ter) ["+ Gr. *metron,* measure]. Instrument for measuring amount of albumin in urine.

albuminiparous (al-bū″mĭn-ĭp'ă-rŭs) ["+ *parere,* to bear]. Yielding albumin.

albuminogenous (al-bū″mĭn-oj'ĕ-nus) [L. *albumen,* white of egg, + Gr. *gennan,* to produce]. Producing albumin.

albu'minoid ["+ Gr. *eidos,* form]. 1. Resembling albumin. 2. A protein. 3. Scleroprotein.

albuminolysis (ăl-bū″mĭn-ōl'ĭ-sĭs) ["+ Gr. *lysis,* dissolution]. Proteolysis; decomposition of protein.

albuminone (al-bū″mĭ-nōn). Noncoagulable protein in blood serum. SYN: *albumone.*

albuminoptysis (al″bū-mĭn-ŏp'tĭ-sĭs) [L. *albumen,* white of egg, + Gr. *ptyein,* to spit]. Albumin in sputum.

albuminoreac'tion ["+ *rē,* again, + *agere,* to act]. The presence or absence of albumin in the sputum. Positive reaction indicates inflammatory condition of lungs.

albuminorrhe'a ["+ Gr. *rhoia,* flow]. Albumin in urine. SYN: *albuminuria,* q.v.

albuminose (al-bū'min-ōs). 1. Albumose. 2. Albuminous.

albumino'sis [L. *albumen,* white of egg, + Gr. *-osis,* condition]. Abnormal increase of albuminous constituents in blood plasma.

albu'minous. Having the nature of or containing albumin.

albu"minuret'ic ["+ Gr. *ourētikos,* causing urine to flow]. Pert. to albuminuria.

albuminuria (al-bū-min-ū'rĭ-ă) ["+ Gr. *ouron,* urine]. Presence of readily detectable amounts of serum protein, especially serum albumin but also serum globulin and others, in the urine. It is usually a sign of renal impairment; its presence, however, is not always a sign of disease because it may be found in normal persons following vigorous exercise. SYN: *proteinuria.*

It occurs in febrile states, malignant hypertension, congestive heart failure, nephrotic syndrome and other kidney disorders. SEE: *nephritis; nephrosis.*

  a., cardiac. Caused by disease of the heart valves.

  a., cyclic. Finding at regular diurnal intervals of small amounts of albumin in the urine, esp. in childhood and adolescence.

  a., digestive. A. that occurs following the eating of certain foods. SYN: *dietetic a.*

  a., extrarenal or accidental. Due to contamination of urine with pus, chyle, or blood.

  a., functional or transient. One in which the only finding is occasional presence of albuminuria; not usually associated with kidney disease. Occurs in some after taking certain foods.

  a., intrinsic. A. excreted in urine as a result of intrinsic renal disease. SYN: *true a.*

  a., orthostatic. Postural albuminuria, q.v.

  a., pathological. A. caused by a disease.

  a., physiological. A., in a temporary form, existing without evidence of pathology.

  a., postural. Albuminuria in normal individuals who have remained in an erect position for a considerable length of time. SYN: *orthostatic a.*

  a., renal. Due to changes in epithelial cells of kidneys, making them pervious to proteins of the blood, as in all forms of nephritis.

  a., toxic. Due to toxins generated within the body or by poison from outside source.

albuminu′ric retini′tis. Inflammation of retina characterized by hazy retina, blurred disk margin, distention of retinal arteries, retinal hemorrhages, and white patches in the fundus, esp. the stellate figure at the macula. SEE: *retinitis.*

albumone (al-bū′mōn, al′bū-mōn″). A noncoagulable protein in blood serum. SYN: *albuminone.*

albu′moscope [L. *albumen,* white of egg, + Gr. *skopein,* to view]. An instrument for determining the presence of albumin in the urine.

al′bumose. The intermediate product produced by enzymes in the splitting of proteins which, in the course of digestion, become peptones.

albumosemia (al″bū-mō-sē′mĭ-ă) [L. *albumen,* white of egg, + Gr. *haima,* blood]. Albumose in the blood.

albumosuria (ăl″bū-mō-sū′rĭ-ă) ["+ Gr. *ouron,* urine]. The presence of albumose in urine. There is considerable doubt that protein in this form is execreted in the urine.

Alcaligenes (al″kă-lĭj′ĭ-nēz). Rod-shaped, gram-negative, or gram-variable bacteria found in the intestinal tract of man, soil, and dairy utensils and products.

  a. faecalis. Found normally in the intestinal tract of man. Rarely becomes pathogenic.

Alcock's canal. [Benjamin Alcock, Irish anatomist, 1801 —]. A space in the external fascia of the ischiorectal fossa, above the tuberosity of the ischium. It contains the internal pudendal artery, veins, and nerve.

al′cohol [Arabic *al-koh′l,* something subtle]. 1. A class of organic compounds formed from hydrocarbons by substituting one or more hydroxyl (OH) group for a similar number of hydrogen atoms. 2. Ethyl alcohol, a colorless, volatile, flammable liquid of the formula C_2H_5OH. Its molecular weight is 46.07; boiling point 78.5° C. It is a product of fermented or distilled liquors, and is obtained, in its pure form, from grain by fermentation and fractionation distillation. The USP standard is a liquid that contains not less than 92.3% by weight of C_2H_5OH. SYN: *ethanol; ethyl alcohol; grain alcohol; spirit of wine.*

ACTION AND USES: Used in preparing essences, tinctures, extracts; manufacturing of ether, ethylene and other industrial products; as a rubbing compound; as an antiseptic when in 70% solution. Arrests growth of putrefactive bacteria and is, therefore, used as a preservative of biological specimens and in certain patent medicines. Used in antifreeze products because of its low freezing point. Instruments may be sterilized by placing them in a 70% solution of alcohol for 30 minutes. Acts as a depressant to the nervous system when taken in excessive amounts.

  a., absolute. Contains 99% alcohol and not more than 1% by weight of water.

  a., dehydrated. Absolute a., q.v.

  a., denatured. Alcohol rendered unfit for use as a beverage or medicine by adding toxic ingredients. Used commercially as a solvent.

  a., diluted. USP. Alcohol containing not less than 41% and not more than 42% by weight of ethyl alcohol. Used as a solvent. SYN: *diluted ethanol; proof spirit.*

a., ethyl. Ordinary or grain alcohol. SEE: *alcohol* (def. 2).

a., grain. SEE: *ethyl a.*

a., methyl. CH_3OH. A colorless, volatile, flammable liquid obtained from distillation of wood. Even though its physical properties are similar to those of ethyl alcohol, it is not fit for human consumption. Poisoning with methyl alcohol can lead to blindness and death. It is used as a solvent, for fuel, as an additive for denaturing ethyl alcohol, and in the preparation of formaldehyde. SYN: *carbanol; methanol; wood alcohol.*

a., wood. Same as methyl a., q.v.

alcoholase (al'ko-hŏl-ās). A ferment converting lactic acid into alcohol.

alcohol'ic [L. *alcoholicus*]. 1. Pertaining to alcohol. 2. One afflicted with alcoholism.

a. fermentation. That in which carbohydrates are converted to alcohol through action of yeast.

Alcoholics Anonymous. An altruistic organization whose members are former chronic alcoholics who are interested both in overcoming their own difficulties and in helping others with similar problems. The organization has groups in most cities in the U.S.A. and can be contacted through its listing in telephone books. ABBR: A.A.

alcoholism (ăl'kŏ-hŏl-ĭzm) [Arabic *al-koh'l*, something subtle]. A disorder manifested by complete absorption with and loss of control over consumption of alcohol and characterized by chronicity, intoxication, and tendency toward relapse. Excessive drinking causes physical disability leading to impaired emotional, occupational, and social adjustments.

ETIOL: Unknown. Psychological, physiological, and sociological factors play an important part. A deep-seated neurosis, subconscious feelings of insecurity and inadequacy, conflicts and frustrations are factors. The exhilaration factor is often the cause of intoxication in normal persons. Alcoholism is an illness and should be so treated.

a., acute. Acute intoxication with temporary mental disturbances and muscular incoordination.

CAUTION: When stupor or coma is observed in a patient who is suspected of being intoxicated by alcohol, other causes such as intracranial disease, insulin shock, etc., should also be considered. Acute alcoholism can cause death.

SYM AND SIGNS: There may be motor instability (staggered gait, blurred or double vision, impaired reflex action); reduced mental function; increased pulse rate; decreased blood pressure; dilated pupils; flushing of skin; drowsiness or stupor.

TREATMENT: When enough alcohol has been consumed to cause coma, vigorous therapeutic measures are indicated; thus insulin, dextrose, thiamine, chlorpromazine, and oxygen are used.

a., chronic. Pathological state from habitual use of alcohol in toxic amounts.

SYM AND SIGNS: Malnutrition; vitamin deficiency; alcoholic cirrhosis of liver; gastritis; pancreatitis; and neurological disorders such as tremulousness, hallucinosis, seizures, delirium tremens.

TREATMENT: Psychotherapy, tranquilizing drugs, withdrawal of alcohol, correction of vitamin deficiency. SEE: *delirium tremens; intoxication.*

a. psychoses. These conditions include pathological intoxication, delirium tremens, Korsakoff's psychosis, acute hallucinosis. SEE: *delirium tremens; hallucinosis, acute; intoxication; Korsakoff's syndrome.*

alcoholomania (al'kō-hol''ō-mā'nĭ-ă) [Arabic *al-koh'l*, something subtle, + Gr. *mania,* frenzy]. Abnormal craving for intoxicants.

alcoholometer (al'kō-hol-om'ĕ-ter) ["+ Gr. *metron,* measure]. An instrument for measuring quantity of alcohol in a fluid.

alcoholophilia (al'kō-hŏl-ō-fil'ĭ-ă) ["+ Gr. *philein,* to love]. Morbid craving for alcohol.

alcoholu'ria ["+ Gr. *ouron,* urine]. Alcohol in the urine.

aldehyde (al'dĕ-hīd). [*alcohol dehydrogenatum,* q.v.] 1. Oxidation product of a primary alcohol; has the characteristic group —CHO. 2. Acetaldehyde. CH_3CHO. A colorless, fuming, flammable liquid. SYN: *acetic aldehyde; ethanol.*

aldolase (ăl'dō-lās). An enzyme present in skeletal and heart muscle and the liver; important in converting glycogen into lactic acid. Its serum level is increased in certain muscle diseases and in viral hepatitis.

al'dose. A carbohydrate of the aldehyde group (—CHO).

aldosterone (ăl-dŏs'tĕr-ōn, al''dō-stēr'ōn). The most biologically active mineralocorticoid hormone secreted by the adrenal cortex. Functions in regulation of metabolism of sodium, chloride and potassium. SEE: *adrenal gland.*

aldos'teronism, aldoster'onism. A condition in which the blood contains abnormally high levels of aldosterone. This causes retention of sodium; urinary loss of potassium; and alkalosis. The patient develops episodes of tetany; weakness; paralysis; hypertension; cardiac irregularity; polyuria; and polydipsia. SYN: *Conn's syndrome.*

alemmal (ă-lĕm'al) [Gr. *a-*, not, + *lemma*, husk]. Without a neurilemma, as a nerve fiber.

Alep'po boil, button, evil, sore. Cutaneous leishmaniasis, caused by infection with the parasite Leishmania tropica. Characterized by one or multiple ulcerations of the skin. SYN: *Delhi boil; Oriental sore.*

alethia (ă-lē'thĭ-ă) [Gr. *a-*, not, + *lēthē*, forgetfulness]. Inability to forget.

aleukemia (ă-lū-kē'mĭ-ă) ["+ *leukos*, white, + *haima*, blood]. 1. Deficiency of white blood corpuscles. The existence of leukopenia or aleukocytosis. 2. Aleukemic leukemia. A form of leukemia in which the leukocytes in the blood are not greatly increased. SEE: *leukemia.*

aleukemic (a''lū-kē'mik). Marked by aleukemia. SEE: *leukemia.*

aleukia (ă-lū'kĭ-ă). 1. Absence or abnormal decrease in number of white blood cells. 2. Absence or abnormal decrease in number of blood platelets.

aleukocytosis (ă-lū-kō-sī-tō'sĭs) [Gr. *a-*, not, + *leukos*, white, + *kytos*, cell + *-osis*, process]. A diminished production of white corpuscles in the blood.

aleuron, aleurone (al-ū'rŏn) [Gr. *aleuron*, flour]. The protein granules present in the outer layer of the endosperm of cereal grain.

Alexand'er-Adams operation. [William Alexander, Brit. surgeon, 1844-1919; James A. Adams, Scottish gynecologist, 1857-1930]. Shortening the round ligaments of the uterus and suturing their ends to the exterior or abdominal ring. Used in treating uterine displacement.

alexeteric (ă-lĕk''sē-tĕr'ik) [Gr. *alexētērios*, fit to keep off]. Protective against infection, venom, and poison.

alex'ia [Gr. *a-*, not, + *lexis*, speech]. Inability to read, due to a central lesion; word blindness. A form of sensory, optic, or visual aphasia.

    a., cortical. That due to lesions involving the left angular gyrus.

    a., motor. That in which printed or written words cannot be read aloud but are understood.

    a., musical. Inability to read music. It may be sensory, optical or visual, but not motor. SEE: *anarthria; aphemia.*

alexic (ă-lĕks'ĭk). 1. Defensive, as an alexin. 2. Pert. to alexia.

alexin (ă-lĕks'ĭn) [Gr. *alexein*, to ward off]. Defensive substance in normal serum which, in presence of a sensitizer, destroys bacteria and exerts a lytic action on cells. SYN: *complement, q.v.* RS: *immunity.*

alexin'ic un'it. The lowest amount of alexinic serum required to dissolve a measured quantity of red blood corpuscles in the presence of an excessive amount of hemolytic serum.

alexipharmac (ă-lĕks''ĭ-far'măk) [Gr. *alexein*, to ward off,\ + *pharmakon*, poison]. 1. An antidote. 2. Antidotal. Warding off the ill effects of a poison.

alexipyretic (ă-lĕk''sĭ-pī-ret'ĭk) ["+ *pyretos*, fever]. That which lessens fever. SYN: *febrifuge.*

alexocyte (ă-lĕks'ō-sīt) ["+ *kytos*, cell]. A leukocyte supposed to secrete alexin.

a-Leydigism (ă-lī'dĭg-ĭzm). Absence of Leydig cell function resulting in hypogonadism.

algae (al'jē) [L. *alga*, seaweeds]. Plants belonging to the subphylum Algae of the phylum Thallophyta, the lowest division of the plant kingdom. They are independent plants without roots, stems or leaves but which contain chlorophyll, have a simple life history, and vary in size from microscopic forms to massive seaweeds. They live in fresh or salt water or in moist places. Some serve as food or as sources of medicinal products. Ex: rockweed, kelp, and Irish moss.

algefacient (ăl''jē-fā'shent) [L. *algere*, to be cold, + *faciens*, making]. Cooling, or refrigerant.

algesia (al-jē'zĭ-ă) [Gr. *algēsis*, sense of pain]. Supersensitiveness to pain; hyperesthesia.

algesic (ăl-jē'sik). Hyperesthesic; painful.

algesichronometer (ăl-jē''zē-krō-nom'ē-tĕr) [Gr. *algēsis*, sense of pain, + *chronos*, time, + *metron*, measure]. An instrument for measuring time taken to feel pain.

algesimeter (ăl''jē-sĭm'ē-tĕr) [Gr. *algēsis*, sense of pain, + *metron*, measure]. An instrument for measuring skin sensitivity to pain. SYN: *algometer.*

algesthesia (ăl''jes-thē'zē-ă) [Gr. *algos*, pain, + *aisthēsis*, sensation]. Unusual sensitivity to sensory stimuli, as pain or touch. SYN: *hyperesthesia.*

algetic (ăl-jĕt'ĭk). Painful.

-algia [Gr.]. Suffix signifying pain, as in neuralgia.

algicide (al'jĭ-sīd) [L. *alga*, seaweeds, + *caedere*, to kill]. That which destroys algae.

algid (ăl'jĭd) [L. *algidus*, cold]. Cold; chilly.

    a. pernicious fever. A form of malaria with symptoms of collapse.

    a. stage. Cold and cyanotic skin occurring in cholera and some other diseases.

algiomotor (ăl''jē-ō-mō'tor) [Gr. *algos.*, pain, + L. *motor*, a mover]. Causing painful contraction of muscles, particularly pain during peristalsis.

algiomus'cular ["+ L. *musculus*, muscle]. Algiomotor, q.v.

algogenic (al-gō-jen'ik) [Gr. *algos*, pain, + *genesis*, production]. 1. Causing neuralgic pain. 2. [L. *algor*, cold + Gr. *gennan* to produce]. Lowering body temperature below normal.

algolagnia (al"gō-lag'nĭ-ă) [Gr. *algos*, pain, + *lagneia*, lust]. A perversion whereby sexual satisfaction is derived by experiencing pain or by inflicting pain on others. SEE: *masochism; sadism.*

algolagnist (al-gō-lag'nist). One who practices algolagnia.

algomenorrhea (al"go-men"o-rē'ă) [Gr. *algos*, pain, + *mēn*, month, + *rhoia*, flow]. Painful menstruation. SYN: *dysmenorrhea.*

algom'eter ("+ *metron*, measure). Instrument for testing the sensitiveness to pain, as pinching the skin. SYN: *algesimeter.*

algophily (al-gŏf'ĭ-lĭ) ["+ *philein*, to love]. Morbid love of pain. Algolagnia, q.v.

algophobia (al"gō-fō'bĭ-ă) ["+ *phobos*, fear]. Morbid aversion to witnessing or experiencing pain.

algopsychalia (al"gō-sī-kā'lĭ-ă) ["+ *psychē*, mind]. Mental distress of hysterical origin. SYN: *psychalgia.*

al'gor [L. cold]. 1. A chill. 2. The sensation of cold; cold.

    a. mortis. The chill of death.

algos (al'gos) [Gr.]. Pain.

algospasm (ăl'gō-spăzm) [Gr. *algos*, pain, + *spasmos*, spasm.]. A painful cramp or spasm.

alible (al'ĭ-ble) [L. *alibilis*, nutritive]. Absorbable; nutritive; assimilable.

alices (ăl'ĭ-sēz) [L.]. The red spots appearing before pustulation in smallpox. q.v.

alicyclic (ăl-ĭ-sī'klik). Having properties of both aliphatic (open-chain) and cyclic (closed-chain) compounds.

alienation (āl"yen-ā'shun) [L. *aliēnāre*, to make strange]. 1. Mental disorder; insanity. 2. Hostility or withdrawl.

a'lienism. Science of mental diseases.

a'lienist. Obsolete term for psychiatrist.

aliform (al'ĭ-form) [L. *ala*, wing, + *forma*, shape]. Having form of a wing.

    a. process. Wing of the sphenoid.

alignment (ă-līn'ment) [Fr. *aligner*, to put in a straight line]. 1. Arranged in a straight line. 2. In orthopedics, the placing of portions of a fractured bone into correct anatomical position. SEE: *alinement.*

al'iment [L. *alere*, to nourish]. Nutriment, food.

alimen'tary [L. *alimentum*, nourishment]. Of or pertaining to nutrition.

    a. canal or tract. The digestive tube from the mouth to anus, including mouth or buccal cavity, pharynx, esophagus, stomach, small amd large intestine and rectum. Drugs administered orally (by mouth) are absorbed in the stomach or intestine by the portal vein and pass through the liver before entering the general circulation, or they may be absorbed into the lacteals and enter the blood stream by way of the thoracic duct.

    a. duct. The thoracic duct.

alimenta'tion. The general process of nourishing the body; it includes mastication; swallowing; digestion; absorption; and assimilation.

    RS: absorption; anabolism; catabolism; digestion; foods; metabolism.

    a., artificial. Feeding, usually intravenous, of patient unable to take nourishment normally.

    a., forced. 1. Feeding of a patient unwilling to eat. 2. Therapeutic feeding of more nourishment than necessary.

    a., rectal. Injection, by enema, of food through the rectum.

alimentotherapy (al"ĭ-men"tō-ther'ă-pī) [L. *alimentum*, nourishment, + Gr. *therapeia*, healing]. Treatment employing dietetics. SYN: *dietotherapy.*

alina'sal [L. *ala*, wing, + *nasus*, nose]. Pert. to the alae nasi or wings of the nose.

alinement (ă-līn'ment) [Fr. *aligner*, to put in a straight line]. 1. Arranging in a line. 2. In dentistry, bringing artificial or natural teeth into normal articulation.

aliphatic (al'ĭ-fat'ik) [Gr. *aleiphar*, *aleiphatos*, fat, oil]. Belonging to that series of compounds characterized by open chains of carbon atoms rather than by rings.

aliquot (al'ĭ-kwŏt) [L. *alius*, other, + *quot*, how many]. A fractional part divisible into the whole without a remainder. A portion of a liquid or solid substance which represents a known quantitative relationship to the original amount.

alisphenoid (al-ĭ-sfē'noyd) [L. *ala*, wing, + Gr. *sphēn*, wedge, + *eidos*, resemblance]. Pert. to the greater wing of the sphenoid bone.

alizarin (ă-lĭz'ă-rĭn) [Arabic *ala sara*, extract]. A red dye obtained from coal tar or madder.

alkalemia (ăl"kă-lē'mĭ-ă) [Arabic *al-qalīy*, ashes of salt wort, + Gr. *haima*, blood]. An excessive alkalinity of the blood due to a decrease in the hydrogen ion concentration or an increase in hydroxyl ions. The blood is normally slightly alkaline (pH 7.35 to 7.45).

alkales'cence. 1. Slight alkalinity. 2. Process of becoming alkaline.

alkales'cent. Alkaline or becoming alkaline.

al′kali [Arabic *al-qaliy,* ashes of salt wort]. 1. A metallic hydroxide (except ammonia) that has the property of combining with an acid to form a salt, or with fatty acids to form soap. 2. Any substance that can neutralize acids and affect indicators in certain ways. Alkalis form an excess of OH⁻ ions over H⁺ ions in an aqueous solution. Ex: sodium hydroxide which turns red litmus paper blue.

SEE: *"alkal-" words; corrosive alkali.*

a. poisoning. Poisonings by lye, sodium, potassium hydroxide, etc.

F.A. TREATMENT: Large amounts of water by mouth; diluted vinegar or lemon juice. Then olive oil or milk and egg whites by mouth. Mild stimulants to prevent shock. Tracheotomy if necessary. If esophagus is known to be injured it is imperative to use corticosteroid therapy beginning as soon as possible. It is advisable to use a broad-spectrum antibiotic if corticosteroids are used.

FOLLOW-UP TREATMENT: Morphine is useful to allay pain. Rest, heat, quiet, and adequate fluid intake are imperative. *Caution:* Avoid emetics, strong acids, or lavage.

alkalimeter (al″kă-lĭm′ĕ-ter) ["+ Gr. *metron,* measure]. Device for measuring strength of alkalies alone or in a mixture.

alkalim′etry. Measurement of degree of alkalinity in a mixture.

al′kaline. Pert. to an alkali or having the reactions of one.

al′kaline-ash diet. One consisting chiefly of milk, fruits and vegetables with very small amounts of protein foods such as meat, fish, cheese, poultry.

al′kaline effects of foods. Fruits and vegetables contain salts of alkaline metals, such as calcium, magnesium, potassium, and sodium and they exert an alkaline effect in the body. Original acid parts of the salts, and the free acids, such as citric, malic, tartaric, and lactic, are burned in the body to carbonic acid, eliminated by the breath. This makes possible the neutralization of the acidic products from proteins by the alkaline metals. The blood stream and tissues are protected against sudden changes in normal faintly alkaline reaction by the bicarbonates, phosphates, and proteins serving as buffer agents. The body never becomes actually acid in reaction although the alkaline reserve may become depleted.

al′kaline reserve. The amount of base in the blood, principally bicarbonates, available for neutralization of fixed acids (hydrochloric, lactic, etc.). A fall in a. reserve is called acidosis; a rise, alkalosis.

Normally, the carbon dioxide-combining power of the serum is 24-35 mEq./L. and the carbon dioxide content is 24-33 mEq./L.

al′kaline tide. The increase in alkaline reserve and occasional occurrence of alkaline urine during gastric digestion.

alkalin′ity. State of being alkaline. SEE: *hydrogen ion.*

al′kalinize. To make alkaline; alkalize.

alkalinu′ria [*alkali* + Gr. *ouron,* urine]. An alkaline urine.

alkalipe′nia ("+ Gr. *penia,* poverty). Low alkali reserve of the body.

alkalither′apy. Therapeutic use of alkalies.

alkaliza′tion. Process of making alkaline.

al′kalize. To make alkaline.

al′kaloid [*alkali* + Gr. *eidos,* resemblance]. 1. An active bitter principle obtained from plants that reacts with an acid to form a salt, the latter being used because of its solubility, rather than the alkaloid. 2. An alkaline principle of organic origin; any nitrogenous base, esp. one of vegetable origin having a toxic effect. Ex: Morphine, nicotine, quinine, strychnine.

INCOMPATIBILITIES: Coffee (caffeine), tea (tannin).

alkalom′etry ["+ Gr. *metron,* measure]. Dosimetry. A system of dosage in administration of alkaloids.

alkalo′sis ["+ Gr. *-ōsis,* condition of]. A condition in which the alkalinity of the body tends to increase beyond normal due to excess of alkalies or withdrawal of acid or chlorides from the blood.

a., altitude. A condition due to exposure to high altitudes. This causes respiratory alkalosis, q.v.

a., metabolic. A condition characterized by a pH of blood and other body fluids that is higher than normal and a carbon dioxide content of the serum that is greater than 70 volumes per cent (30 mEq./L.). Commonly a result of loss of acid from excessive vomiting, but also of loss of potassium or ingestion of excessive amounts of sodium bicarbonate. Symptoms and signs are apathy; irritability; delirium; dehydration and occasionally tetany.

TREATMENT: Correct primary disorder; administer sodium or potassium chloride, nonalkalinizing gels.

a., respiratory. A condition characterized by a pH of blood and other body fluids that is greater than normal but with a carbon dioxide content of the serum that is less than 21 mEq./L. Caused by hyperventilation of a neurotic or systemic source, as hysteria; salicylate poisoning; lesion of central nervous system; or decreased oxygen content of the air. Symptoms and signs are lightheadedness, fainting, tetany.

TREATMENT: Discontinue use of salicylates (in salicylate poisoning); inhalation of expired CO_2 from paper bag (in neurosis); correction or alleviation of central nervous system disorder or lesion. SEE: *hyperventilation.*

alkalother'apy. Therapeutic use of alkalies.

alkalot'ic. Pert. to alkalosis.

alkaluria (al″kă-lū′rĭ-ă) [*alkali* + Gr. *ouron,* urine, + *-ia,* condition]. The condition of alkali in the urine.

alkap'ton(e (al-kap′tōn) [″+ Gr. *hapto,* to bind to]. A yellowish-red substance sometimes occurring in urine, the result of incomplete oxidation of tyrosine and phenylalanine.

alkaptonuria (al″kap-tō-nū′rĭ-ă) [*alkapton* + Gr. *ouron,* urine]. A rare inherited disorder characterized by the excretion of large amounts of homogentisic acid in the urine, a result of incomplete metabolism of the amino acids tyrosine and phenylalanine. Presence of the acid is indicated by the darkening of urine when alkalinated and the dark staining of diapers or other linen.

alkene (al′kēn). A bivalent aliphatic compound formed by removal of two hydrogen atoms. Thus when the ethane molecule,

$$\begin{array}{cc} H & H \\ | & | \\ HC\!-\!CH \\ | & | \\ H & H \end{array}$$

loses two hydrogen atoms it becomes ethylene,

$$\begin{array}{cc} H & H \\ | & | \\ HC\!=\!CH \end{array}$$

with a double bond between two carbons. These are also called unsaturated hydrocarbons.

alkyl (ăl′kĭl) [Ger. *alkohol,* alcohol, + Fr. *-yle,* a radical]. A hydrocarbon molecule from which one atom of hydrogen is absent. The resulting substances are called alkyl groups or alkyl radicals. Thus the methane hydrocarbon molecule,

$$\begin{array}{c} H \\ | \\ H\!-\!C\!-\!H \\ | \\ H \end{array}$$

becomes an alkyl radical when it loses one hydrogen molecule to become the methyl radical,

$$\begin{array}{c} H \\ | \\ H\!-\!C \\ | \\ H \end{array}$$

In chemical formulae hydrocarbon radicals are abbreviated **R.**

alkylating agent (al′kĭ-lāt-ing). 1. A substance which introduces an alkyl radical into a compound in place of a hydrogen atom. 2. One which adds a side chain to an aromatic compound.

alkylation (al″kĭ-lā′shun). A chemical process in which an alkyl group (or radical) becomes part of a compound by taking the place of a hydrogen atom.

allachesthesia (al″ă-kes-thē′zĭ-ă) [Gr. *allachē,* elsewhere, + *aisthēsis,* sensation]. Tactile sensation perceived as being remote from the actual point of stimulation.

allantiasis (al-an-ti′ă-sis) [Gr. *allantos,* sausage]. 1. Sausage poisoning. 2. Any poisoning caused by Clostridium botulinum. SEE: *botulism.*

allantochorion (al-lăn″tō-ko′rĭ-ŏn). Fusion of the allantois and chorion into one structure.

allanto'ic. Pert. to the allantois.

allan'toid [Gr. *allantos,* sausage, + *eidos,* resemblance]. 1. Sausage-shaped. 2. Pert. to the allantois.

allan'toin (ă-lan′tō-in). A white crystalline substance derived from purine metabolism and also produced synthetically. Occurs in allantoic and amniotic fluids. At one time was used to promote wound healing.

allantoinu'ria [*allantoin* + Gr. *ouron,* urine]. Allantoin in the urine.

allantois (ă-lan′tō-ĭs) [Gr. *allantos,* sausage, + *eidos,* resemblance]. A kind of elongated bladder, between the chorion and amnion of the fetus which grows out from the caudal extremity of the embryo and communicates with the bladder of the urachus. It is very apparent in quadrupeds, but not in the human species. In primates, including man, the allantois has no function but its blood vessels develop, becoming the umbilical vein and paired umbilical arteries. SEE: *chorion.*

alleles (ă-lēl′, ă-lēl′) [Gr. allēlōn, of one another]. A pair of genes, situated on the same site on paired chromosomes, containing specific inheritable characteristics. A pair of alleles is usually indicated by the alphabetical letter with a capital used for the dominant and a lower case letter for the recessive. An individual possessing a pair of identical alleles, either two dominant or two recessive, is said to be "pure" for the characteristic controlled by the gene and is therefore homozygous for this gene. The union of a dominant gene and its recessive allele produces an heterozygous individual for that characteristic. More than one inheritable characteristic may be present on the same pair of genes (alleles). For example the genes for blood type A, B, and O are at the same position on alleles.

allelic genes (ă-lěl′ĭk). Genes which occupy the same locus on a specific pair of chromosomes and control the heredity of a particular characteristic. The heredity of eye color appears to depend on a series of allelic genes; the A-B-O blood groups are determined by allelic genes; the standard Rh-Hr types are transmitted by allelic genes. SYN: *allele; allelomorph,* q.v.

allelocatal′ysis [Gr. *allēlōn,* reciprocally, + *katalysis,* dissolution]. Stimulation of a bacterial culture by the addition of cells of same type.

allelomorph (ă-lē′lō-morph, ă-lĕl′ō-morph) [″+ *morphē,* form]. Alleles, q.v.

allelotaxis (a-lē″lō-tăk′sĭs) [″+ *taxis,* order]. Development of a part from different embryonic structures.

Allen-Doisy unit (al′ĕn doy′sĭ). [Edgar V. Allen, Amer. anatomist, 1892-1943; Edward A. Doisy, Amer. biochemist and physiologist, 1893 —]. Injection in a spayed mouse of the smallest amount of estrus-producing hormone secreted during pregnancy, producing desquamation of vaginal epithelium in the mouse.

allen′thesis [Gr. *allos,* other, + *en,* in, + *thesis,* a placing]. Introduction of a foreign substance into the body.

allergen (al′er-jen) [Gr. *allos,* other, + *ergon,* work, + *gennan,* to produce]. Any substance which indicates a state of, or brings on manifestations of, allergy. It may or may not be a protein or an antigen. Among common allergens are *inhalants:* dusts, pollens, fungi, smoke, perfumes, odors of plastics; *foods:* wheat, eggs, milk, chocolate, strawberries; *drugs:* aspirin, antibiotics, serums; *infectious agents:* bacteria, viruses, fungi, animal parasites; *contactants:* chemicals, animals, plants, metals; *physical agents:* heat, cold, light, pressure, radiations.

allergenic (ăl″er-jĕn′ĭk). Producing or causing allergy.

aller′gic. Pert. to, sensitive to, or caused by an allergen.

allergization (ăl″er-jĭ-zā′shŭn). Introduction of a foreign substance into the body in order to bring about a state of sensitivity.

al′lergy [Gr. *allos,* other, + *ergon,* work]. An altered reaction of body tissues to a specific substance (allergen) which in nonsensitive persons will, in similar amounts, produce no effect.

It is essentially an antibody-antigen reaction but in some cases the antibody cannot be demonstrated. The reaction may be due to the release of histamine, or histamine-like substances from injured cells.

Ex: An infection of a common cold may render a patient more susceptible to future infection, while an attack of mumps or measles renders the patient less liable; hypersensitiveness of body cells due to proteins such as ferment in the protein molecules, and which causes hay fever or asthma through inhalation, resulting in lesions, or skin eruptions.

Allergic conditions include eczema; allergic rhinitis, or coryza; hay fever; bronchial asthma, and urticaria or hives. Gastrointestinal allergy may appear in children.

NP: *In children:* Avoid extremes of temperature and humidity. Skin must not be chilled and sweating must be kept to a minimum. Soap and water must not be used on eczematous parts of the skin. An ointment may be ordered which should be applied many times during the day in a thin layer, and as often as the child rubs it off.

Woolen clothing and blankets should not be used, or feather-stuffed pillows or mattresses. To prevent scratching, cuffs should be used so the child cannot bend the arm at the elbow. Other restraints of arms and legs may be necessary. Elimination diets are indicated.

ETIOL: Heredity; pollen, dust, hair, fur, feathers, scales, or dandruff; also specific foods, such as eggs, chocolate, milk, wheat, tomatoes, citrus fruits, oatmeal, potatoes.

SYM: Eosinophilia frequently present; urticaria, eczema, rash, asthma, hay fever, migraine, or gastrointestinal disturbances.

RS: anaphylaxis; atopy; hay fever; hypersensitiveness; immunity.

a., food. Find the offending food by placing the patient on a diet consisting of commonly nonallergenic foods and suspected foods. Then add foods suspected to be allergenic to the diet one at a time. Skin tests are sometimes useful. Offending food should be eliminated. SEE: *anaphylaxis.*

a., heat and cold. Changes of temperature may cause cutaneous reactions such as urticaria; and also internal reactions with sensitive persons. Itching, redness of skin, headache, asthmatic symptoms, dyspnea, and shock can follow exposure to cold water. Heat may produce same symptoms.

allesthesia (al″ĕs-the′sĭ-ă) [″+ *aisthēsis*, sensation]. A sensation in one limb which is referred to the other one; allochiria.

alliaceous (al″ĭ-ā′shus) [L. *allium*, garlic, + *-āceus*, of a specific kind]. Tasting like garlic or onions.

alliesthesia (ăl″ĭ-ĕs-the′sĭ-ă) [Gr. *allios*, changed, + *aisthesis*, sensation]. The perception of an external stimulus as pleasant or unpleasant depending upon stimuli coming from inside the body. A particular stimulus may be perceived as pleasant at one time and unpleasant at another.

allitera′tion [L. *ad*, to, + *litera*, letter]. A form of dysphasia in which many of the spoken words have the same sound or begin with the same consonant as other words used. For example: The red rooster reluctantly rested.

allo- [Gr. *allos*, other]. 1. A prefix indicating divergence, difference from or opposition to the normal. 2. Indicating a body made stable by heat. 3. In chemistry, an isomer, close relative or variety of a compound. Isomerism when there is relative asymmetry.

allobiosis (ăl″ō-bĭ-ō′sĭs) [″+ *bios*, life]. The altered responses produced in organisms exposed to environmental or physiological changes.

allochesthesia (al″ō-kĕs-the′zĭ-ă) [Gr. *allache̅*, elsewhere, + *aisthēsis*, sensation]. Tactile sensation remote from point of stimulation. SYN: *allesthesia; allochiria.*

allochezia, allochetia (ăl″ō-ke̅′zĭ-ă, ăl″ō-ke̅′shĭ-ă) [Gr. *allos*, other, + *chezein*, to defecate]. 1. Excretion of nonfecal matter from the bowels. 2. Excretion of feces through an abnormal opening.

allochiria, allocheiria (ăl″ō-kī′rĭ-ă) [″+ *cheir*, hand + *-ia*, condition]. Sensation referred to side of body opposite its origin; allesthesia. Observed in locomotor ataxia and in hysteria.

allochroism (ăl-ŏk′rō-ĭzm, ăl″ō-krō′ĭzm) [″+ *chroa*, color + *-ism*]. Change in color.

allochromasia (al″ō-krō-mā′sĭ-ă). Change in color of hair or skin.

allocinesia (ăl″ō-sĭn-e̅′sĭ-ă) [Gr. *allos*, other, + *kine̅sis*, movement]. Movement on side of body opposite to the one the patient has been requested to move. SEE: *allokinesis.*

alloerot′icism. Alloerotism, q.v.

alloerotism (ăl″ō-ĕr′ō-tĭsm) [Gr. *allos*, other, + *Eros*, god of love]. Sexual urges stimulated by and directed toward another person. Opposed to autoerotism. SEE: *heterosexual.*

allogeneic. Arising from or obtained from another individual. Ex: tissue obtained for grafting is of different genetic constitution than the host tissue.

allokinesis (ăl″ō-kĭ-ne̅′sĭs) [Gr. *allos*, other, + *kinesis*, movement]. Movement on side of body opposite to the one the patient has been requested to move.

allokinetic (ăl″ō-kĭ-nĕt′ĭk). Movement caused by external forces, i.e., passive not active motion.

allola′lia [Gr. *allos*, other, + *lalia*, talk]. 1. Speech defect or impairment due to a brain lesion. 2. A type of dysphasia in which words are spoken unintentionally, or inappropriate words are substituted for appropriate ones.

allomorphic (al″lō-morph′ĭk) [″+ *morphe̅*, form]. Assuming a different form but remaining unchanged in character.

al′lopath. A practitioner of medicine who utilizes allopathy, q.v.

allopathy (ăl-ŏp′ă-thĭ) [Gr. *allos*, other, + *pathos*, disease]. A system of medicinal practice involving use of medicines which produce effects different from those of the disease treated; in principle, the opposite of homeopathy. A term erroneously used for the regular practice of medicine by physicians.

allophasis (ăl-of′ă-sĭs) [″+ *phasis*, speech]. Incoherency, delirium.

alloplasia (ăl″ō-plā′zĭ-ă) [″+ *plasis*, a molding]. Replacement of normal cell forms by other cell forms in the tissue. SEE: *heteroplasia.*

al′loplasty. Plastic surgery with non-human tissue.

allopolyploidy (al″ō-pŏl′e̅-ploy-de̅). Having more than two sets of chromosomes derived from different ancestral species.

allopsychic (al-ō-sī′kĭk) [Gr. *allos*, other, + *psyche̅*, mind]. Ideas not related to the patient's personality, but to the external environment.

allopsycho′sis [″+ ″+ *-osis*, condition]. Derangement of perceptive powers.

allorhythmia (ăl″ō-rĭth′mĭ-ă) [″+ *rythmos*, rhythm]. Irregular cardiac rhythm.

all-or-none law. That a stimulus to a nerve or muscle causes it to respond to its greatest extent or not at all. Applied specifically to a single striated muscle fiber, a single nerve fiber, or the heart as a whole.

allotherm (ăl′ō-thĕrm) [Gr. *allos*, other, + *therme̅*, heat]. An organism whose temperature is directly dependent on its environment. SEE: *homothermal; poikilotherm.*

allotox′in (″+ *toxikon*, poison). A substance within the body which protects by destroying toxins inimical to it.

allotransplantation (al″lo-trans-plan-tā′-shun) [″+ L. *trans*, through + *plantāre*, to plant]. Grafting or transplanting tissue from one individual into another.

allotriogeustia (ă-lot″rĭ-ō-jŭst′ĭ-ă, -gŭ′stĭ-a) [Gr. *allotrios*, strange, + *geusis*, taste]. Perverted appetite or sense of taste.

allotriophagy (ă-lot″rĭ-ofʹă-jĭ) [″ + *phagein*, to eat]. A perverted appetite for injurious, unusual, and nonedible substances. SEE: *pica*.

allotriuria (a-lot″rĭ-ū′rĭ-ă) [″ + *ouron*, urine]. Abnormal urine.

allotropic (ăl″ō-trŏp′ĭk) [Gr. *allos*, other, + *tropos*, direction]. 1. In chemistry, pert. to different forms of the same element without change of chemical composition. 2. Altered by digestion so as to be changed in its nutritive value. 3. Indicating one who is concerned with the welfare and interests of others, i.e. not self-centered.

allot′ropism, allot′ropy. Presence of an element in two or more distinct forms with unlike properties.

allowance. General term for the amount of food or nutrients recommended per person each day.

allox′an [*allantoin* + *oxalic*]. $C_4H_2N_2O_4$. A substance obtained as an oxidation product of uric acid. In experimental medicine, has caused diabetes in animals. It gives a red color to the skin, and has been used as a basis of cosmetic preparations.

allox′in. Any one of a series of xanthin bases derived from the splitting of chromatin which, on oxidation, produces uric acid.

allox′ur bases or bodies [*alloxan* + *urea*]. Xanthine bases. Nitrogenous substances formed by splitting of nucleins.

alloxuremia (al-oks-ū-rē′mĭ-ă) [*alloxur* + Gr. *haima*, blood]. Xanthine bases in the blood.

alloxu′ria [″ + Gr. *ouron*, urine]. Xanthine bases in the urine.

alloy (al′oy, ă-loy′) [Fr. *aloyer*, to combine]. A metallic substance (e.g., brass) resulting from the fusion, mixture or combination of two or more metals. Also, a substance (e.g., steel) formed from the fusion of a metal and a nonmetal.

al′lyl [L. *allium*, garlic + Gr. *hylē*, matter]. C_3H_5. A univalent unsaturated radical. It is present in garlic and mustard.

almond (ă′mund) [Gr. *amugdalē*]. Fruit of the almond tree. Highly nutritive and rich in protein. High fat content. Source of thiamine, riboflavin and niacin.

Food value of 100 gm. (roasted and salted): Cal. 627; protein 18.6 gm.; fat 57.7 gm.; sodium 198 mgm.

alochia (ă-lō′kĭ-ă) [Gr. *a-*, not, + *lokhos*, pert. to childbirth]. Absence of puerperal, q.v., vaginal discharge following childbirth.

aloe (al′ō). USP. The dried juice of several species of aloe. It is a necessary ingredient for compound benzoin tincture.

alo′gia [Gr. *a-*, not, + *logos*, speech]. Inability to express oneself through speech. SYN: *aphasia*.

alopecia (al″ō-pē′shĭ-ă) [Gr. *alōpekia*, fox mange]. Natural or abnormal baldness or deficiency of hair, partial or complete, localized or generalized.

ETIOL: May result from: 1. Physiologic changes as a part of the aging process. 2. Effects of serious illness, e.g., typhoid fever. 3. Drugs, e.g., arsenic, thallium. 4. Endocrine disorders, e.g., hypothyroidism. 5. Certain forms of dermatitis. 6. Hereditary factors.

TREATMENT: Treatment of seborrheic dermatitis if present. Scalp baldness may be treated by surgical transplantation of hair follicles from another part of the body to the scalp.

a. adnata. Congenital baldness.

a. areata. Baldness is sharply defined; circumscribed patches which leave the scalp smooth and white.

a., congenital. Form with absence of hair bulbs at birth.

a. follicularis. Inflammation of the hair follicles of the scalp causing loss of hair from affected areas.

a. furfuracea. Chronic in course and marked by dandruff and itching, and falling out of hair (exfoliation of scales). SYN: *a. pityroides.*

a. neurotica. Baldness following a nervous disease or injury to nervous system, and occurring at site of injury.

a. pityroides. Falling of both scalp and body hair, together with abundant branlike desquamation.

a. prematura. Premature baldness.

a. senilis. Baldness of old age.

a. simplex. Baldness prematurely.

a. symptomatica. Loss of hair after prolonged fevers or during course of some disease; also may result from changes in internal secretions.

a. totalis. Complete loss of hair from the entire body.

a. toxica. Loss of hair thought to be due to toxins of infectious disease.

a. universalis. General loss of hair from all parts of body.

al′pha. First letter A, or α of Greek alphabet. In chemistry, denotes first in a series of isomeric compounds.

a. rhythm. In electroencephalography, rhythmical oscillations in electric potential occurring at a rate of 8 to 13 per second. They are best recorded when the eyes are positioned in a particular way.

a. tocopherol. One of a group of substances with vitamin E activity.

a. wave. Alpha rhythm, q.v.

alphelasma (al''fel-as'ma). Leukoplakia.

alternans (awl-tĕr'nanz) [L. *alternāre,* to alternate]. Alternation.

a., pulsus. Regular heart rhythm in which strong beats alternate with weak ones.

al'ternating cur'rent. An electrical current the direction of which reverses at regular intervals.

al'ternator. So-called sinusoidal alternator; an electromagnetic device consisting of a revolving armature which cuts the lines of force in a magnetic field and which delivers a sinusoidal current from secondary coil of the apparatus.

al'therm, altherm pad. A device containing heat-producing chemicals for applying heat to the eye or a sinus.

Alt. hor. Abbr. for *alternis horis,* every other hour.

altricious (al-trish'us) [L. *altrix,* nourisher]. Slow in developing; requiring long nursing.

al'um (L. *alumen).* (ammonium alum, or aluminum ammonium, sulfate). Large, colorless crystals, or white powder, with sweetish, strongly astringent taste. Used locally, in solution, as a mild astringent for mucous membranes.

Its manufacture (which is of great antiquity) is by subjecting alum stone to a roasting process, and treating with sulfuric acid.

alu'men (L.). Alum.

a. exsiccatum. Alum that has been dried or burnt; used as a dusting powder.

aluminosis (al-ū''min-ō'sis) ["+ Gr. *-ōsis,* condition of]. Chronic catarrhal inflammation of the lungs in alum workers.

alu'minum. SYMB: Al. At. wt. 26.9815; at. no. 13. sp. gr. 2.699. A silver-whitish metal.

a. acetate. A salt formed by the reaction between aluminum sulfate and lead acetate. Its aqueous solution, containing 4 to 5%, is known as Burow's solution.

USES: Regarded as a valuable local astringent.

a. hydroxide gel. USP. A white viscous suspension containing aluminum hydroxide and hydrated aluminum oxide; an antacid especially useful in treatment of peptic ulcer.

alveobronchioli'tis, alveobronchi'tis [L. *alveolus,* little tub, + Gr. *bronchos,* windpipe, + *-ītis,* inflammation]. Inflammation of the bronchioles, and pulmonary alveoli; bronchopneumonia, q.v.

alve'olar. Pert. to an alveolus, q.v.

a. air. That determined by sampling the last portion of a maximal expiration. SEE: *air; spirometry.*

a. bone. Bone of the alveolar processes of mandible and maxilla.

a. periosteum. The periodontal membrane.

a. process. One of four processes which make up each maxillary bone.

alveolar-capillary block. Impaired ability of gases to pass through the pulmonary alveolar-capillary membrane.

alve'olate. Honeycombed: pitted.

alveoli (al-vē'ō-li) [L.]. Pl. of alveolus, q.v.

a. dentales. [NA]. Tooth sockets.

a. pulmonis. [NA]. Air cells of the lungs.

alveoli'tis [L. *alveolus,* + Gr. *-ītis,* inflammation]. Inflammation of the alveolar processes; pyorrhea, q.v.

alveoloclasia (al-vē''o-lo-klā'zī-ă) ["+ Gr. *klasis,* fracture]. Absorption of any part of the alveolar process.

alveolus (al-vē'ō-lus) [L. small hollow or cavity]. (pl. *alve'olī)* 1. A little hollow. 2. The socket of a tooth. 3. Air cell of the lungs. 4. A small depression such as those contained in the honeycomb cells of the gastric mucous membrane. 5. A follicle of a racemose gland.

a., mucous, of the salivary glands Those that secrete the ropy material of the saliva, containing mucin.

a., parietal. An air space in the wall of an alveolar passage in the lung.

a. pulmoneus. A pulmonary air space.

a., serous, of the salivary glands. Those that secrete the serous albumin of the saliva, coagulating when heated.

a., terminal. An air space connected with a pulmonary infundibulum.

alveus (al've-us) [L.]. A channel or groove.

a. hippocampi. [NA]. A layer of white fibers covering ventricular surface of the hippocampal formation of the rhinencephalon.

alvine (al'vin) [L. *alvus,* belly]. Pert. to the intestines or abdomen.

a. concretion. Intestinal stone.

a. discharge. Stools.

a. flux. Watery feces.

alvi'nolith ["+ Gr. *lithos,* stone]. An intestinal mass formed from calcareous salts and other matter. SEE: *bezoar.*

al'vus [L.]. Abdomen and viscera.

alymphopotent (a-lĭm″fō-pō′tĕnt) [Gr. *a-*, not, + L. *lympha*, water, + *potens*, able]. Unable to develop lymphocytes or lymphoid cells.

Alzheimer's disease (ahlts′hī-merz). [Alois Alzheimer, Ger. neurologist, 1864-1915]. Presenile dementia, which is similar to senile dementia but occurs in the 40-60-year age group. The disease has a relentless and irreversible course but may take from a few months to four or five years to go to the stage of complete helplessness.

Am. Chem. symbol for americium. Abbr. for *mixed astigmatism; ametropia*.

ama (ā′mä) [L. *vessel*]. Enlargement of a bony canal of labyrinth of the internal ear at the end opposite the ampulla.

A.M.A. Abbr. for *American Medical Association.*

amaas (ä′mäl ɔ̃). A mild form of smallpox; alastrim.

am′acrine cell [Gr. *a-*, not, + *makros*, long, + *is, inos*, fiber]. Cell in inner nuclear layer of retina possessing only one branching process.

amah, ama [Portuguese *ama*, wet nurse]. In the Orient a household maid who cares for children.

   a., diving. In the Orient, esp. Japan and Korea, a woman who earns her living diving for marine life.

amal′gam [Gr. *malagma*, soft mass]. Any alloy containing mercury.

amal′gamate. To make an amalgam.

Amantadine hydrochloride (ă-man′tă-dĕn hi″dro-klor′īd). An antiviral agent originally used for prophylaxis against certain strains of the influenza virus.

amara (am-ā′rä) [L. *amarus*, bitter]. Bitters, an alcoholic concoction made with herbs or roots. Used to flavor alcoholic drinks.

amarthritis (am″ar-thri′tis) [Gr. *hama*, at same time, + *arthron*, joint, + *-itis*, inflammation]. Polyarthritis. Inflammation of more than one joint at the same time.

amasesis (ā-mas-ē′sis) [Gr. *a-*, not, + *masēsis*, chewing]. Inability to masticate food.

amas′tia ["+ *mastos*, breast]. Lack of breast development. SYN: *amazia.*

am′ativeness [L. *amare*, to love]. 1. Sexual desire. 2. Propensity to love.

amaurosis (am″aw-rō′sus) [Gr. *amaurōsis*, darkening]. Complete loss of vision, esp. that in which there is no evidence of pathologic condition of the eye.

   a., albuminuric. A. caused by kidney affection.

   a., amaurotic. A. caused by the atrophying of optic nerve or vision centers.

   a., cerebral. A. caused by brain malady.

   a., congenital. A. from birth on.

   a., diabetic. A. in connection with diabetes.

   a., epileptoid. Sudden blindness following an epileptic seizure and lasting up to two weeks.

   a. fugax. Temporary loss of vision in one eye due to insufficient flow of blood to the eye. May last for up to 10 minutes.

   a., lead. A. caused by lead poisoning.

   a. partialis fugax. Sudden transitory blindness with symptoms similar to migraine: nausea; vomiting; dizziness; and disturbances of vision.

   a., reflex. A. due to reflex action caused by irritation of a remote part.

   a., saburral. A. in conjunction with acute gastritis.

   a., toxic. Blindness from optic neuritis caused by toxins which may be endogenous such as diabetes or exogenous such as alcohol or tobacco.

   a., uremic. A. caused by uremic condition.

amaurotic (am-aw-rot′ik). Pert. to one afflicted with amaurosis.

   a. familial idiocy. Term for a group of related familial diseases marked by dementia, impaired vision, and lipid defect.

   a. familial idiocy, infantile. That occuring in infants between the ages of one and 12 months. Generally, the patients are members of Jewish families. It is marked by degeneration of the retina (cherry-red spot); progressive blindness; mental deterioration; loss of motor control; and death by age three years. SYN: *Tay-Sachs disease.*

   a. familial idiocy, juvenile. That form occurring between ages six and 14 years. Marked by deposits of pigment around macula of eye; progressive blindness; progressive loss of motor control; mental deterioration; and death. SYN: *Batten-Mayou disease; Spielmeyer-Vogt disease.*

   a. familial idiocy, late infantile. That type occurring usually at the age of three or four years. Marked by optic atrophy; progressive blindness; spasticity and tremor; seizures; and death. SYN: *Jansky-Bielschowsky disease; late infantile cerebral lipoidosis.*

   a. familial idiocy, late juvenile. Similar to the juvenile form except for loss of vision which rarely occurs in the late juvenile type. Onset usually takes place between the ages of 15 and 25 years. Marked by tremors; muscle rigidity; dementia; convulsions; and death. SYN: *adult a. familial idiocy; Kufs's disease.*

amaxophobia (ă-maks″ō-fō′bĭ-ă) [Gr. *hamaxa,* carriage, + *phobos,* fear]. Morbid dread of vehicles or of riding in them.

amazia (ă-mā′zĭ-ă) [Gr. *a-,* not, + *mazos,* breast]. Lack of development of the breasts. SYN: *amastia.*

ambi- [LL. *ambi-,* on both sides]. Prefix indicating both or both sides; around; about, as ambidextrous.

ambidex′trous ["+ L. *dexter,* right]. Ability to work effectively with either hand.

ambilat′eral ["+ L. *latus,* side]. Pert. to both sides.

ambilevous (am-bĭ-lē′vus) ["+ L. *laevus,* left-handed]. Awkward in use of either hand.

ambio′pia ["+ Gr. *ōps,* eye]. Double vision. SYN: *diplopia,* q.v.

ambisin′ister ["+ L. *sinister,* left]. Awkward in use of either hand. SYN: *ambilevous.*

ambiten′dency ["+ L. *tendere,* to stretch]. Ambivalence of the will. SEE: *Ambivalence.*

ambivalence (am-biv′ă-lens) ["+ L. *valentia,* strength]. Simultaneous concurrent contradictory feelings and/or actions about the same object, person or idea. Ambivalence is present to some degree throughout life but is reduced in late childhood from its peak in the 2-to-5-year period. May be of minor diagnostic significance in schizophrenia, the neuroses, and manic-depressive psychosis.

ambiv′alency. The condition of being ambivalent.

ambiv′alent. Have equal power of value in both directions.

    a. feelings. Two opposite emotions, such as love and hate, for the same person at same time. SEE: *ambivalence.*

ambivert (ăm′bĭ-vĕrt) [L. *ambio-,* + L. *vertere,* to turn]. One intermediate between an extrovert and an introvert.

amblyacousia (am″blĭ-ă-koo′sĭ-ă) [Gr. *amblys,* dull, + *akousis,* hearing]. Dullness of hearing.

amblyaphia (am-blĭ-af′ĭ-ă) ["+ *haphe,* touch]. Dull sense of touch.

amblychromasia (am″blĭ-krō-mā′sĭ-ă) ["+ *chrōma,* color]. The state in which the cell nucleus stains faintly.

amblychromat′ic. Staining faintly.

amblygeustia (am″blĭ-jūs′tĭ-ă, am″blĭ-gūs′tĭ-ă) [Gr. *amblys,* dull, + *geusis,* taste]. Defective or blunted taste.

amblyopia (ăm″blĭ-ō′pĭ-ă) ["+ *ōps,* eye]. Reduced or dimness of vision, not dependent upon visible changes in the eye and not a refractive error. Causes may be alcoholic, astigmatic, diabetic, malaria, drugs or tobacco, toxic, or uremic.

    a., crossed. That of one eye with hemianesthesia of the opposite side of the face. SYN: *a. cruciata.*

    a. ex anopsia. Dimness of vision resulting from disuse of the eyes. Usually in one eye and associated with convergent squint or very poor visual acuity.

    a., reflex. A. due to irritation of peripheral area.

    a., toxic. That due to effect of toxic substances such as alcohol or tobacco.

amblyoscope (am′blī-ō-skōp″) ["+ "+ *skopein,* to view]. Instrument for training an amblyopic eye for better vision.

am′bo, ambon [Gr. *ambon,* edge of a dish]. Annular fibrocartilage producing an elevation about a joint cavity; also the elevation itself.

amboceptor (am-bō-sep′tor). A term now obsolete. Used by Ehrlich to explain basic immune mechanisms.

am′bos [Ger.]. Incus or anvil bone of the middle ear.

am′bulance [L. *ambulāre,* to move about]. A vehicle for transportation of the sick and wounded.

am′bulant, ambulatory. Able to walk, not confined to bed.

    a. typhoid fever. A mild attack of typhoid fever, in which the patient is not confined to bed. SEE: *typhoid.*

Ameba. A genus of protozoa, class Sarcodina.

    A. proteus. The common, large, freshwater species.

ame′ba, amoeba [Gr. *amoibē,* change]. (pl. *amebae, amoebae; amebas, amoebas*) A one-celled protozoan minute animal form of life that constantly changes its shape by sending out processes of its protoplasm, by which it moves about and obtains its nourishment.

    It is found in a variety of pools, and in the green slime on the top of the water. It is also found in the mud at the bottom. It possesses an outer translucent substance called the ectoplasm; but the inner substance, endoplasm, is denser and contains a nucleus. It feeds by surrounding its victim and enclosing it in the so-called food vacuole. Oxygen is absorbed from the surrounding water, and CO_2 is eliminated through the plasma membrane. The organism moves by extending fingerlike protrusions of the protoplasm called pseudopodia. Reproduction is by binary fission in which the nucleus is divided by mitosis. One of the species found in the human colon, Entamoeba histolytica, may be pathogenic to man, causing amebic dysentery. In parasitic forms, encystment may occur.

amebiasis (am″ē-bī′ă-sĭs). An infectious disease due to Ameba, esp. Entamoeba hystolytica.

ETIOL: Entamoeba histolytica; acquired by ingesting food or drink containing encysted forms.

PATH: Small abscesses and, later, ulcers of mucous membrane of colon, sometimes resulting in perforation. Liver abscesses may result from amebas being carried to liver via portal vein.

SYM: Many patients are asymptomatic. Disease is generally characterized by dysentery with diarrhea, weakness, and prostration. Nausea, vomiting and pain may be present and stools frequent. Complications may result in amebic hepatitis.

DIAG: Cysts or trophozoites of E. histolytica in stools.

TREATMENT: In acute amebiasis, metronidazole (Flagyl), tetracycline or emetine hydrochloride. Chloroquine, metronidazole or emetine is useful in liver abscess. Repeated treatment at intervals for up to three months are necessary to assure the amebae have been eliminated.

a., hepatic. Infection of the liver by amebas, usually with abscess formation.

ame′bic. Pert. to or caused by amebas.

a. carrier state. That in which an individual harbors a form of pathogenic ameba but has no clinical signs of the disease.

a. dysentery. That caused by Entamoeba histolytica. SEE: *amebiasis.*

a. hepatitis. Amebic abscess of the liver.

ame′bicide, amebacide [Gr. *amoibē,* change, + L. *caedere,* to kill]. Destructive to or any agent that kills amebas.

ame′biform [″+ L. *forma,* shape]. Formed like an ameba.

amebocyte (ă-mē′bō-sīt) [″+ Gr. *kytos,* hollow vessel]. A cell showing ameboid movements.

ame′boid [″+ Gr. *eidos,* resemblance]. Having the appearance and characteristics of an ameba.

a. movements. Those possessed by leukocytes which "wander" through capillary walls into surrounding tissues; a process known as diapedesis.

ame′boidism. Ameba-like movements, noting a condition shown by certain nerve cells.

amebula (a-mē′bū-lă) [L. *ameba,* little spore]. A spore which moves by means of pseudopodia, esp. the spore of a protozoan.

amebu′ria [Gr. *amoibē,* change, + *ouron,* urine]. Amebas in the urine.

amelanotic (ā″mĕl-ă-not′ĭc). Without melanin; unpigmented.

amelia (ă-mē′lĭ-ă) [Gr. *a-,* not, + *melos,* limb, + *-ia,* condition]. A congenital anomaly characterized by the absence of one or more limbs.

amelioration (ă-mē″lĭ-or-ā′shun) [L. *ad,* to, + *melior,* better]. Improvement; moderation of a condition.

ameloblast (ă-mĕl′ō-blast) [O. Fr. *amel,* enamel, + Gr. *blastos,* germ]. A cell from which tooth enamel is formed.

ameloblastoma (ă-mĕl″ō-blas-tō′mă). Highly destructive tumor of the jaw. SYN: *adamantinoma.*

ameloden′tinal [O.Fr. *amel,* enamel, + L. *dens, dent-,* tooth]. Pert. to both enamel and dentine.

ame′nia [Gr. *a-,* not, + *mēn,* month]. Absence of the menses; amenorrhea, q.v.

amenomania (ă-mē-nō-mā′nĭ-ă) [L. *amoenus,* pleasant, + Gr. *mania,* frenzy]. Manic phase of manic-depressive psychosis marked by excessive gaiety, lightheartedness, and morbidly cheerful disposition.

amenorrhea (ă-men″ō-rē′ă) [Gr. *a-,* not, + *mēn,* month, + *rhoia,* flow]. Absence or suppression of menstruation; normal before puberty, after the menopause, during pregnancy and lactation.

ETIOL: Congenital abnormalities of the reproductive tract; metabolic disorders (obesity, malnutrition, diabetes); systemic diseases (syphilis, tuberculosis, nephritis); emotional disorders (excitement, anorexia nervosa); endocrine disorders, esp. those involving the ovaries, pituitary, thyroid, and adrenal glands; hormonal imbalance (excesses or inadequacies) of estrogen or progesterone, or of follicle-stimulating hormones. These are common causes.

TREATMENT: Underlying cause should be determined and corrected. If hormone deficiencies exist, substitutional therapy is recommended.

a., emotional. That resulting from shock, fright, hysteria, etc.

a., functional. Condition with varying intervals of amenorrhea interspersed with normal menstrual periods.

a., partial. Appearing occasionally and at irregular intervals.

a., pathologic. That before the menarche, after menopause, and during pregnancy and lactation.

a., physiological. Periods when normally free from menstruation: prepuberty, pregnancy, lactation, postmenopause periods.

a., primary. Emansio mensium. That in which menses have never made their appearance.

a., secondary. Suppressio mensium. That in which, having appeared, the menses subsequently cease.

amenorrhe'ic. Pert. to amenorrhea.

ament (ā'ment) [L. *ab*, from, + *mens*, mind]. An idiot; one without evidence of mind.

amentia (a-men'shĭ-a). 1. Congenital mental deficiency; feeblemindedness. 2. In psychology, condition marked by subnormal intelligence; on the basis of intelligence tests, an I.Q. of 70 or below. SEE: *dementia.*

RS: idiot; imbecile; intelligence test; moron.

a., nevoid. Amentia with a nevoid condition, calcification of parts of the brain, glaucoma and epilepsy.

a., phenylpyruvic. A. with secretion of phenylpyruvic acid in urine.

americium (ăm-ĕr-ĭs'ĭ-ŭm) [L., the Americas]. A metallic element. SYMB: Am. The mass number of the longest-lived isotope is 243; at. no. 95.

Amerind. [*Ameri*can *Ind*ian] General term for an American Indian or an Eskimo.

ameristic (ā''mer-is'tik) [Gr. *a*, not, + *meristos*, divided]. Undifferentiated, not split into fragments.

ametria (ă-mē'trĭ-ă) ["+ *mētra*, uterus]. Congenital absence of the uterus.

ametrohemia (ah-mĕt''rō-hē'mĭ-ă) ["+ "+ *haima*, blood]. Lack of uterine blood supply.

ametrom'eter [*ametropia*, + Gr. *metron*, measure]. Instrument for measuring ametropia.

ametropia (ă''mĕ-trō'pĭ-ă) [Gr. *ametros*, disproportionate, + *ōps*, eye, + *-ia*, condition]. Imperfect refractive powers of eye (hyperopia, myopia, astigmatism), in which the principal focus does not lie on the retina.

amicro'bic [Gr. *a-*, not, + *mikros*, small, + *bios*, life]. Lacking in microbes or microorganisms. Not due to microbes.

am'icron(e. A colloid particle unrecognizable through the ultramicroscope. Thus particles smaller than 10^{-8} mm.

amicroscop'ic. Too small to be detected through the ultramicroscope.

am'idase. A deamidizing enzyme, one that catalyzes the hydrolysis of urea.

amide (am'ĭd). A chemical compound produced by the substitution of an acid radical for one of the hydrogen atoms of ammonia.

amidin [Fr. *amidon,* starch]. The part of starch soluble in water.

amido-. A prefix signifying the presence of the radical $CO.NH_2$.

amid'ulin [Fr. *amidon,* starch]. Soluble starch.

amimia (a-mim'ĭ-ă) [Gr. *a-*, not, + *mimos*, mimic]. Loss of power to express ideas by signs or gestures.

a., amnesic. That in which signs and gestures can be made but their meaning is not remembered.

a., ataxic. That in which signs and gestures cannot be made because of nervous or muscular disorders.

amine (ă-mēn', am'ĭn). One of a group of nitrogen-containing organic compounds formed when one or more of the hydrogens of ammonia have been replaced by one or more hydrocarbon radicals.

amino- (ă-mē'nō, am'in-ō). Prefix denoting presence of the amino (NH_2) group combined with a radical, other than an acid radical.

aminoacetic acid (ăm''ĭn-ō-ă-sē'tĭk). One of the simplest examples of an amino acid, $NH_2 CH_2COOH$. It is synthesized in the body. SYN: *glycine.*

aminoacetic acidemia. Amino acids in the blood.

amino acid. One of a large group of organic compounds marked by presence of both an amino (NH_2) and a carboxyl (COOH) radical. Their basic formula is NH_2-R-COOH in which R stands for any aliphatic or aromatic radical. They are amphoteric and exhibit properties marked by both the amino and carboxyl groups. They are the building blocks of which proteins are constructed, and they are the end-products of protein digestion or hydrolysis.

There are twenty or more amino acids. All of these are necessary for metabolism or growth but because some are supplied by food and the others can be produced by the body, the ones provided by food are called "essential." These are: histidine (may be essential for children but not for adults); isoleucine; leucine; lysine; methionine; phenylalanine; threonine; tryptophan; and valine. The "nonessential" amino acids are: alanine; aspartic acid; arginine; citrulline; cystine; glutamic acid; glycine; hydroxyglutamic acid; hydroxyproline; norleucine; proline; serine; and tyrosine.

Arginine, while "non-essential" for the adult, cannot be formed quickly enough to supply the demand in infants and thus is classed as "essential" in early life. Also tyrosine may be formed from phenylalanine or it would be classed as "essential." SEE: *deaminization; digestion; protein.*

Not all proteins contain all the essential amino acids as is the case with milk, cheese, eggs, and meat. Unused amino acids are converted into urea. They pass unchanged through the intestinal wall and portal vein into the blood, then through the liver into the general circulation from which they are absorbed by the tissues according to the specific protein for a specific tissue, each tissue making its own protein from the amino acid, and each deaminizing that which remains unused.

a. compound. Substance containing the group NH$_2$; same as amine, q.v.

a. group. The NH$_2$ group which characterizes the amines.

aminoacidop'athies. Various disorders of amino acid metabolism of which there are nearly 100 including cystinuria, alcaptonuria and albinism.

aminophylline (ăm-ĭ-nŏf'ĭ-lĭn, ăm''ĭ-nō-fĭl'-in). USP. C$_{16}$H$_{24}$N$_{10}$O$_4$·2H$_2$O. A mixture of theophylline and ethylenediamine. Used esp. in acute asthma that has not responded to epinephrine. Used also as a stimulant to the respiratory center and heart muscle, and as a diuretic. SYN: *theophylline ethylenediamine.*

aminopterin (ăm-ĭ-nŏp'tĕr-ĭn). A proprietary name for 4-aminopteroylglutamic acid, a folic acid antagonist used in treatment of acute leukemia.

aminopyrine (ăm''ĭn-ō-pī'rēn, -rĭn). An antipyretic and analgesic. Because this drug is considerably more toxic than acetylsalicylic acid (aspirin), it should not be used routinely.

aminosis (am''ĭ-nō'sĭs) [*amino-,* + Gr. *-ōsis,* state]. Excessive production of amino acids in the body.

aminuria (am-ĭ-nū'rē-ă) ["+ Gr. *ouron,* urine]. Amines in voided urine.

amitosis (am''ĭ-tō'sĭs) [Gr. *a-,* not, + *mitos,* a thread]. Simple or direct cell division without change in the nucleus.

amitotic (am''ĭ-tŏt'ĭk). Characterized by amitosis.

am'meter [*ampere,* + Gr. *metron,* measure]. In physical therapy, an instrument calibrated to measure in amperes the strength of a current flowing in a circuit. SEE: *milliammeter.*

ammone'mia [*ammonia,* + Gr. *haima,* blood]. Ammonia in the blood. Normally only faint traces of ammonia are found in the blood. Increased amounts of ammonia in the blood are due to a pathological condition such as impaired liver function. SYN: *ammoniemia.*

ammonia (ă-mō'nĭ-ă) [*Amūn,* Egyptian deity]. A gas formed by decomposition of nitrogen-containing substances such as proteins and amino acids. Ammonia is

converted into urea in the liver. Its formula, NH$_3$, relates it to many poisonous substances but also to the proteins and to many useful chemicals. Dissolved in water, it neutralizes acids and turns litmus blue.

a., aromatic spirit of. A flavored solution of ammonia and ammonium carbonate in water and alcohol.

a., blood. Ammonia in the blood. Increased values are found in liver failure.

a. toxicity. Ammonia is produced in the intestinal tract by bacterial action. After absorption it is transported to the liver where it is metabolized. In diseases such as cirrhosis of the liver the ammonia absorbed may be shunted past the liver. This results in an accumulation of ammonia in the blood. The resulting alteration in consciousness; neurologic changes; abnormal electroencephalogram; and a "flapping tremor" (asterixis) are due at least in part to ammonia toxicity.

TREATMENT: Directed to the prevention of production and absorption of ammonia in the intestinal tract by giving enemas and antibiotics such as neomycin to prevent growth of the bacteria which produce ammonia. Limit protein in diet.

a. water. A strong ammonia solution. It has a very pungent odor. A necessary agent for aromatic ammonia spirit. SYN: *ammonia solution.*

a. water, stronger. A 28% solution of ammonia in water. SYN: *strong ammonia solution.*

ammoni'acal. Having the characteristics of or pert. to ammonia.

ammo'niated. Containing ammonia.

ammoniemia (a-mō''nĭ-ē'mĭ-ă) [*ammonia* + Gr. *haima,* blood]. Ammonia in the blood. SEE: *ammonemia.*

ammonium car'bonate. Occurs as hard masses with strong odor of ammonia. On exposure to air, loses CO$_2$ and ammonia. It is a necessary agent in preparation of aromatic ammonia spirit.

ammonium chlor'ide. USP. White crystalline powder without odor. It is used as an expectorant, a diuretic, and as an aid in restoring acid-base balance.

ammonium hydrox'ide. This is a solution of ammonia gas in water, used about the house for cleaning purposes and as a refrigerant.

POISONING: SEE: *Ammonia* in *Table of Poisons and Poisoning* in *Appendix.*

ammoniuria (ă-mō''nĭ-ū'rĭ-ă) [*ammonia* + Gr. *ouron,* urine]. An excessive amount of ammonia in the urine.

amnesia (ăm-nē'zĭ-ă) [Gr.]. A loss of memory.

This may be for recent experiences, those subsequent to the disease, and is then termed anterograde. When it involves more remote memory stores it is called retrograde. Amnesia is often applied to episodes during which the patient forgets his identity, though he may conduct himself properly enough, and following which no memory of the period persists. Such episodes are often hysterical, sometimes epileptic; while trauma, senility, alcoholism, and other organic reaction types account for a smaller number.

In psychoanalysis, partial a. is seen in confusional insanity; lack of retention in senility; and in hysteria there may be lack of recall.

    a., auditory. Loss of memory for word meanings.

    a., lacunar. Loss of memory for isolated events.

    a., periodic. A. occurring in a period of double consciousness.

    a., retroanterograde. A memory disorder in which present-day events are referred to the past and vice versa.

    a., tactile. Inability to distinguish objects by sense of touch. SYN: *astereognosis.*

    a., transient global. Transient amnesia which occurs in otherwise healthy persons. Onset is usually sudden and may last for a few hours. Remote memory is retained even though memory for recent events is absent. Recovery is usually rapid.

    a. traumatica. A. caused by injuries.

    a., visual. Inability to remember the appearance of objects that have been seen or to be cognizant of printed words.

amnesic (am-nē'sik). Pert. to amnesia.

    a. aphasia. Loss of memory. SYN: *amnesia.*

amnestic (am-nes'tik). Amnesic, or causing amnesia.

amniocentesis (am"nĭ-ō-sen-tē-sis) [Gr. *amnion,* lamb, + *kentēsis,* puncture]. Puncturing the amniotic sac, usually by using a needle and syringe, in order to remove amniotic fluid. The material obtained may be studied chemically or cytologically. Technique may be used to decompress an overdistended uterus.

amniochorial, amniochorionic (am"nĭ-ō-kō'rĭ-ăl, -kō-rĭ-on'ik). Relating to both amnion and chorion.

am"nioclep'sis [Gr. *amnion,* lamb, + *kleptein,* to steal]. Gradual unperceived loss of amniotic fluid.

amniog'raphy ["+ *graphein,* to write]. Radiography of amniotic sac.

am'nion [Gr. *amnion,* lamb]. The inner of the fetal membranes, a thin, transparent sac which holds the fetus suspended in the liquor amnii or amniotic fluid, q.v. The amnion grows rapidly at the expense of the extra-embryonic coelom, and by the end of the second month it fuses with the chorion forming the amniochorionic sac. Commonly called the bag of waters or caul. SEE: *"amnio-" words; oligohydramnios.*

amniorrhea (am"nĭ-or-rē'ă) ["+ *rhoia,* flow]. Escape of the amniotic fluid, liquor amnii.

amniorrhexis (ăm"nĭ-ō-rĕk'sĭs) ["+ *rhēxis,* rupture]. Rupture of the bag of waters, or amnion.

amnios (am'nĭ-os). The amnion, or the liquor amnii.

amnioscope (ăm'nĭ-ō-skōp) [Gr. *amnion,* + *skapein,* to examine]. Apparatus for looking inside the amniotic cavity.

    a., suction. One designed to allow suction to be applied so that it is held in place against the fetal scalp. This permits evacuation of the amniotic fluid from the area pressing against the scalp, thus leaving a clear field for sampling blood from that site.

amniotic (am-nĭ-ot'ik). Pert. to the amnion.

    a. cavity. 1. One that appears in the embryonic mass of the ovum. It is lined with a layer of cells called the embryonic ectoderm. The cavity enlarges rapidly as the embryo develops. 2. The fluid-filled cavity of the amnion.

    a. fluid. Liquor amnii. The liquid or albuminous fluid contained in the amniotic sac, q.v. This fluid is transparent and almost colorless. The liquid protects the fetus from injury; helps maintain an even temperature; prevents formation of adhesions between the amnion and the skin of the fetus; and prevents conformity of the sac to the fetus (the last being an important consideration during labor). Premature rupture of the amniotic sac results in a so-called "dry labor." The amniotic fluid is continually being absorbed and renewed at a rapid rate. About one-third of the water in the amniotic fluid is replaced each hour.

    a. sac. The bag or sac formed by the amnion, q.v.

amniotitis (ăm-nĭ-ō-tī'tĭs) [Gr. *amnion,* lamb, + *-itis,* inflammation]. Inflammation of the amnion.

amniotome (am'nĭ-ō-tōm) ["+ Gr. *tomē,* cutting]. Instrument for puncturing fetal membranes.

amnitis (am-nī'tis). Inflammation of the amnion. SYN: *amniotitis.*

amobarbital (ăm"ō-bar'bĭ-tăl). USP. $C_{11}H_{18}$ N_2O_3. An odorless, white, crystalline powder. Used as a sedative of intermediate action.

 a. sodium. $C_{11}H_{17}N_2NaO_3$. An odorless, white, granular powder. Following administration, it is absorbed rapidly, and is inactivated rapidly in the liver. Used as a sedative.

amoeba (ă-mē′ba) [Gr. *amiobē,* change]. A one-celled protozoan animal form. SEE: *ameba.*

amok, amuck (ă-mŏk′, ă-mŭk′) [Malay]. A state of murderous frenzy.

amor (a′mor) [L]. Love, esp. sexual love.

 a. insanus. Unrestrained libido in the insane. SYN: *erotomania,* q.v.

 a. lesbicus. Lesbianism, q.v.

 a. sui. Vanity; love of self.

amoralia (ă″mō-rā′lĭ-ă) [Gr. *a-,* not, + L. *mōrālis,* moral]. Moral imbecility.

amoralis (a″mō-rā′lis). A moral imbecile.

amorphia, amorphism (ă-mor′fĭ-ă, ă-mor′-fĭzm) [Gr. *a-,* not, + *morphē,* form]. State of being without definite form.

amorphous (a-mor′fus). Without definite structure.

amotio (a-mō′shĭ-ō) [L. *amovere,* to move from]. A detachment.

 a. retinae. Detached retina.

am″pelother′apy [Gr. *ampelos,* grape vine, + *therapeia,* treatment]. Grape cure; therapeutic use of grapes.

amperage (ăm-pĕr′ĭj). Strength of the electrical current expressed in amperes or milliamperes.

ampere (ăm′pēr). Practical unit of intensity of electric current, which is produced by 1 volt acting through resistance of 1 ohm. ABBR: amp.

 a. meter. Instrument denoting in amperes the strength of a current. SEE: *ammeter.*

amphetamine (am-fĕt′ă-mēn, -mĭn). A colorless liquid which volatilizes slowly at room temperature. It is a central nervous system stimulant. The preparation most commonly used is the sulfate, marketed in tablet or capsule form.

 a. sulfate. $(C_9H_{13}N)_2H_2SO_4$. A synthetic, white, crystalline substance which acts as a stimulant of the central nervous system. Used in treatment of narcolepsy and certain types of mental depression. Use of amphetamines to control appetite in treating obesity has not proven to be effective. Large doses are toxic, and prolonged use may cause drug dependence.

amphi- [Gr. *amphi,* on both sides]. Prefix indicating on both sides, at both ends, on all sides or around. In chemistry, it denotes certain positions or configurations.

amphiarthrosis (ăm″fĭ-ăr-thrō′sĭs) [Gr. *amphi,* on both sides, + Gr. *arthrosis,* joint]. A form of articulation intermediate between diarthrosis and synarthrosis, in which the articulating bony surfaces are connected by an elastic cartilaginous substance; the mobility is slight, but may be exerted in all directions. The articulations of the bodies of the vertebrae are examples.

amphiaster (ăm″fĭ-ăs′tĕr) ["+ *astēr,* star]. Double star formed during mitosis, q.v.

Amphibia (ăm-fĭb′ĭ-ă) [Gr. *amphibios,* double life]. A class of animals which live on land and in water, as salamanders, frogs, etc.

amphibious (ăm-fĭb′ĭ-ŭs). Able to live both on land and in water.

amphiblas′tula [Gr. *amphi,* on both sides, + *blastula,* little sprout]. A form of blastula in which the blastomeres are of unequal size. Seen in sponges.

amphiblestri′tis ["+ *blēstron,* fish net, + *-itis,* inflammation]. Inflammation of retina. SYN: *retinitis.*

amphicelous (ăm-fĭ-sē′lŭs) ["+ *koilos,* hollow]. Concave on each end, as a vertebrae.

amphicentric (ăm-fĭ-sĕn′trĭk) [Gr. *amphi,* on both sides, + *kentron,* center]. Centering or converging at both ends.

amphichroic, amphichromatic (ăm-fĭ-krō′ik, -krō-mat′ik) ["+ *chroma,* color]. 1. Turning red litmus paper blue, and blue, red. 2. Reacting both as an acid and an alkali.

amphicra′nia ["+ *kranion,* skull]. Pain on both sides of head.

amphicreatine, amphicreatinine (ăm″-fĭ-krē′ă-tĭn, -krē-ăt′ĭ-nĭn) [Gr. *amphi,* on both sides, + *kreas,* flesh]. A leukomaine formed in muscles.

amphicyte (ăm′fĭ-sīt) ["+ *kytos,* cell]. One of the capsule cells enveloping the bodies of cerebrospinal ganglionic neurons.

amphicyt′ula ["+ L. *cytula,* little cell]. In mammals, the impregnated ovum.

amphidiarthrosis (ăm-fĭ-dī-ăr-thrō′sĭs) [Gr. *amphi,* on both sides, + *diarthrosis,* articulation]. An articulation with amphiarthrosis and diarthrosis, such as that of the lower jaw.

amphigas′trula ["+ L. *gastrula,* little stomach]. The human ovum in advanced gastrula stage.

amphigony (ăm-fĭg′ō-nĭ) ["+ *gonos,* begetting]. Sexual reproduction.

amphimixis (ăm-fĭ-mĭks′ĭs) [Gr. *amphi,* on both sides, + *mixis,* mingling]. Mixing of maternal and paternal germ cells in reproduction, thus giving hereditary characteristics from both parents.

amphimorula (ăm″fĭ-mŏr′ū-lă) ["+ L. *morula*, little mulberry]. The morula in ovum with unequal composing cells.

amphipyrenin (ăm″fĭ-pī′rĕn-ĭn) ["+ *pyrenōs*, stone of a fruit]. The basophile substance of the nuclear membrane of a cell.

amphithe′ater [Gr. *amphi*, on both sides, + *theatron*, theater]. An operating room with rising tiers of seats arranged around it for students and other observers.

amphitrichate, amphitrichous (ăm-fĭt′-rĭ-kāt, -kŭs) ["+ *thrichos*, hair]. Pert. to certain organisms having flagella or a flagellum at both ends.

ampho- [Gr. *amphō*, both]. Prefix meaning both.

amphodiplopia (ăm-fō-dĭ-plō′pī-ă) [Gr. *amphō*, both, + *diploos*, double, + *ōps*, vision]. Double vision in each eye.

amphojel (ăm′fō-jĕl). A proprietary name for a suspension of aluminum hydroxide.

am″phopep′tone. First peptone formed by tryptic digestion of protein.

amphophil, amphophilous (ăm′fō-fĭl, ăm-fŏf′ĭ-lŭs) [Gr. *amphō*, both, + *philos*, fond]. Having affinity for acid and/or basic dyes.

amphor′ic [L. *amphoricus*]. Pert. to a sound as that caused by blowing across the mouth of a bottle; a resonance; a cavernous sound on percussion of a pulmonary cavity.

amphoricity (ăm″fōr-ĭs′ĭ-tĭ). Producing amphoric sounds.

amphoriloquy (ăm″fōr-ĭl′ō-kwē) [L. *amphora*, jar, + *loqui*, to speak]. The presence of amphoric sounds in speaking.

amphorophony (ăm″fōr-ŏf′ō-nĭ) [Gr. *amphoreus*, jar, + *phōnē*, voice]. Amphoric voice sound.

amphoter′ic, amphot′erous [Gr. *amphoteros*, both]. Having properties of both an acid and a base.

    a. compounds. Those which may act as a base or an acid, i.e., protein.

    a. reaction. A double reaction of certain liquids which turn red litmus paper blue, and blue, red.

amphotericin B (ăm″fō-tĕr′ĭ-sĭn). USP. An antibiotic agent obtained from a strain of Streptomyces nodosus. It is used in treatment of deep-seated mycotic infections. The drug usually is administered parenterally.

amphoterism (am-fō′ter-izm). Having both acid and basic properties.

amphoterodiplopia (ăm-fōt″ĕr-ō-dĭ-plō′pī-ă) [Gr. *amphoteros*, both, + *diploos*, double, + *ops*, vision]. Double vision in each eye. SYN: *amphodiplopia*.

amphoton′ic [Gr. *amphō*, both, + *tonos*, tone]. Pert. to both vagotony and sympathicotony.

amphotony (ăm-fŏt′ō-nĭ) ["+ *tonos*, tone]. Tonicity of the sympathetic and parasympathetic nervous systems.

ampliation (ăm-plĭ-ā′shŭn) [L. *ampliare*, to make wider]. Distention of a part or cavity.

am′plifier. Something which enlarges, extends, or increases the strength of an effect. In electronics, this would be a device for increasing the electrical current or signal.

amplification (ăm″plĭ-fĭ-kā′shŭn) [L. *amplificatio*, making larger]. 1. Enlargement of visual area in microscopy. 2. Magnification of sound in telephony.

amplitude (ăm′plĭ-tūd) [L. *amplitudo*]. 1. Amount, extent, size, abundance or fullness. 2. In physics, the extent of movement, as of a pendulum or sound wave. The maximum displacement of a particle, as that of a string vibrating as measured from the mean to the extreme.

ampule (ăm′pūl) [L. *ampulla*]. A small glass that can be sealed and its contents sterilized. This is a French invention for containing hypodermic solutions. SYN: *ampoule; ampul.*

ampulla (ăm-pŭl′lă) [L., little jar]. (pl. *ampul′lae*) [NA] 1. Sac-like dilatation of a canal or duct, as the semicircular canals or ductus deferens, q.v. 2. A small, hermetically sealed flask containing a solution for parenteral use; an ampule.

    a. ductus deferens. An irregular and nodular dilatation of the vas deferens just before its junction with the excretory duct of the seminal vesicle.

    a. of lacrimal duct. The slight dilatation of the lacrimal duct medial to the punctum.

    a. of rectum. Slight dilatation of rectum proper just before continuing as anal canal. Also called infraperitoneal portion of rectum proper.

    a. of semicircular canal. A dilatation at end of semicircular canal which houses an ampulla of a semicircular duct.

    a. of semicircular ducts. Dilatation of semicircular ducts near their junction with the utricle. In their walls are the crista ampullares.

    a. of uterine tube. The dilated distal end of a uterine tube terminating in a funnel-like infundibulum.

    a. of vas deferens. A. ductus deferens, a dilatation at the base of the bladder near the end of the vas deferens.

    a. of Vater. The duodenal end of the drainage systems of the pancreatic and common bile ducts. Although in common usage, the name is being discarded in favor of the more accurate papilla of Vater.

ampulli'tis [L. *ampulla,* little jar, + Gr. *-itis,* inflammation]. Inflammation of any ampulla, esp. of ductus deferens.

amputation (ăm″pū-tā′shŭn) [L. *amputāre,* to cut around]. Surgical removal of a diseased limb, part, or organ.

   a., congenital. A. of parts of the fetus in utero, believed formerly to be caused by constricting bands but now believed to be a developmental defect.

   a. in contiquity. A. at a joint.

   a. in continuity. A. elsewhere than at a joint.

   a., double-flap. A. in which two flaps of soft tissue are formed.

   a., primary. A. performed before inflammation sets in.

   a., secondary. A. performed during period of suppuration.

   a., spontaneous. Nonsurgical separation of an extremity or digit. SEE: *ainhum.*

   a., tertiary. A. performed following abatement of inflammatory reaction.

amuck (ă-mŭk′) [Malay *amok,* furious attack]. State of murderous frenzy. Syn: *amok.*

amusia (ă-mū′sĭ-ă) [Gr. *amousos,* unmusical]. Music-deafness; inability to produce or comprehend music, as loss of the ability to play a musical instrument.

   ETIOL: Brain lesion, but cause not clearly understood.

   a., motor. Condition in which music is understood, but without ability to produce by singing, humming, or playing.

   a., sensory. Music deafness. Inability to understand the sounds of music.

Amussat's operation (ăm′ū-sŏ). [Jean Z. Amussat, Fr. surgeon, 1796-1856] Surgical formation of an artificial anus, by lumbar colotomy in ascending colon.

amychophobia (ă-mī″kŏ-fō′bĭ-ă) [Gr. *amyche,* scratch, + *phobos,* fear]. Morbid fear of being scratched; fear of the claws of any animal.

amyctic (ă-mĭk′tĭk) [Gr. *amyktikos,* mangling]. 1. Irritating, caustic. 2. A Caustic or corrosive agent.

amyelencephalia (ă-mī″ĕl-ĕn-sĕf-ā′lĭ-ă) [Gr. *a-,* not, + *myelos,* marrow, + *enkephalos,* brain]. Congenital malformation consisting of absence of brain and spinal cord.

amyelia (ă-mī-ē′lĭ-ă). Absence of spinal cord.

amyeloneuria (ă-mī″ĕl-ō-nū′rĭ-ă) [Gr. *a-,* not, + *myelos,* marrow, + *neuron,* nerve]. Incomplete paralysis or impaired function of the spinal cord.

amyelotrophy (ă-mī″ĕl-ŏt′rō-fī) [″+ ″+ *atrophia,* atrophy]. Spinal cord atrophy.

amygdala (ă-mĭg′dă-lă) [L., almond]. (pl. *amygdalae*) 1. A mass of gray matter in the anterior portion of the temporal lobe. 2. Obsolete term for the tonsil.

amygdalin (ă-mĭg′dă-lĭn). A bitter tasting glucoside in bitter almonds and cherry laurel leaves. Used as a flavoring agent.

amygdaline (ă-mĭg′dă-lĭn, -līn) [L. amygdalinus]. 1. Pert. to a tonsil. 2. Pert. to or shaped like an almond. SYN: *amygdaloid.*

amygdaloid (ă-mĭg′dă-loyd) [Gr. *amygdalē,* almond, + *eidos,* resemblance]. Resembling a tonsil or an almond.

   a. fossa. A depression for the tonsil.

   a. tubercle. A projection from the middle cornu of the lateral ventricle, marking area of the amygdaloid nucleus.

amygdalolith (ă-mĭg′dă-lō-lĭth″) [″+ *lithos,* stone]. Stone in a distended crypt of a tonsil.

amygdalopathy (ă-mĭg″dă-lŏp′ă-thī) [″+ *pathos,* suffering]. Any disease of a tonsil.

amygdalothrypsis (ă-mĭg″dă-lō-thrĭp′sĭs) [Gr. *amydalē,* almond, "+ *thrypsis,* a crushing]. Crushing of a tonsil followed by excision.

amygdalotome (ă-mĭg′dă-lō-tōm″) ["+ *tome,* a cutting]. Instrument for excision of a tonsil.

amyl (ăm′ĭl) [L. *amylum,* starch, + Gr. *ylē,* material]. A hypothetical univalent radical, C_5H_{11}, nonexistent in a free state.

   a. nitrite. USP. $C_5H_{11}NO_2$, a volatile and highly flammable clear liquid. Used as a vasodilator, esp. for anginal pain.

amylaceous (ăm′ĭ-lā′shē-ŭs). Starchy.

amylase (ăm′ĭ-lās) [L. *amylum,* starch, + Gr. *-asis,* colloid enzyme]. A ferment or amylolytic enzyme of the saliva, pancreatic juice, and intestinal juice that hydrolyzes starch, producing achroödextrin and maltose. These products are later acted upon by the maltase of the intestines and converted into dextrose before absorption. A. is more powerful than ptyalin and it acts on uncooked as well as cooked starch. SEE: *antiamylase; enzymes.*

   a., pancreatic. Amylopsin, q.v.

   a., salivary. Ptyalin, q.v.

   a., vegetable. Diastase, q.v.

amylemia (ăm′ĭ-lē′mĭ-ă) ["+ Gr. *haima,* blood]. Presence of starch in the blood.

amylin (ăm′ĭ-lĭn). 1. Part of starch soluble in water. 2. A monacid base. The group $C.NH.NH_2$. SYN: *amidin.*

amylodextrin [L. *amylum,* starch, + *dexter,* right]. Soluble substance produced during the change of starch into sugar.

amylodyspepsia (ăm′ĭ-lō-dĭs-pĕp′sĭ-ă) ["+ Gr. *dys,* bad, + *pepsis,* digestion]. Inability to digest starchy foods.

amylogen (ăm-ĭl′ō-jen) ["+ Gr. *gennan,* to produce]. Soluble starch.

amylogenesis (ăm″ĭ-lō-jĕn′ĕ-sĭs) [L. *amylum*, starch, + Gr. *genesis*, production]. The production of starch.

amylogenic (ăm″ĭ-lō-jĕn′ĭk) ["+ Gr. *gennan*, to produce]. Starch-producing

amyloid (ăm′ĭ-loyd) ["+ Gr. *eidos*, resemblance]. 1. Resembling starch; starchlike. 2. A protein complex having starchlike characteristics produced and deposited in tissues during certain pathological states. It is a homogeneous, highly refractile substance staining readily with Congo red.

Amyloid is a protein-polysaccharide complex of varying composition. It is associated with a variety of chronic disease, particularly tuberculosis, osteomyelitis, leprosy, Hodgkin's disease, and carcinoma.

   a. degeneration. Degeneration of organs or tissues from deposition of amyloid. Structures are waxy and translucent, having hyaline appearance. Liver, spleen, and kidneys most involved but any tissue may be infiltrated.

   a. disease. Amyloidosis.

   a. kidney. Enlarged, firm, smooth kidney usually associated with amyloid diseases of spleen or liver. Sym: Face pale, waxy skin which may be edematous. Liver and spleen may also be enlarged; not tender under pressure. Diarrhea if intestines are involved. Albumin, hyaline, and waxy casts in urine.

   a. nephrosis. A nephrotic syndrome from myeloid degeneration of kidney.

amyloido′sis [L. *amylum*, starch, + Gr. *eidos*, resemblance, + *-ōsis*, condition]. A metabolic disorder marked by deposition of amyloid in organs and tissue. Thought to be the result of disordered function of the reticuloendothelial system and abnormal immunoglobulin synthesis. There is no known method of preventing amyloid deposits from forming except to control the primary disease with which it is associated.

   a., lichen. A form limited to the skin.

   a., localized. A. in which isolated amyloid tumors are formed.

   a., secondary. A. associated with chronic suppuration and tissue necrosis, as in tuberculosis, syphilis, Hodgkin's disease, rheumatoid arthritis, and in extensive tissue destruction. Spleen, liver, kidneys, and adrenal cortex most frequently involved.

amylolysis (ăm″ĭl-ŏl′ĭ-sĭs) [L. *amylum*, starch, + Gr. *lysis*, solution]. Changing of starch into sugar in the process of digestion.

amylolytic (ăm″ĭl-ō-lĭt′ĭk). Pert. to the digestion of starches or their conversion into simple sugars (amylolysis, q.v.).

   a. enzyme. A ferment that hydrolyzes starch, producing achroodextrin and maltose. SYN: *amylase.*

amylophagia (ăm-ĭ-lō-fā′jĭ-ă) [L. *amylum*, starch, + Gr. *phagein*, to eat]. Abnormal craving for starch.

amylopsin (ăm″ĭ-lŏp′sĭn) ["+ Gr. *opsis*, appearance]. Diastatic enzyme in pancreatic juice which changes starch into achroodextrin and maltose. SEE: *digestion; duodenum; enzymes.*

amylose (ăm′ĭ-lōs). A group of carbohydrates containing starch, cellulose, and dextrin. SEE: *saccharose.*

amylosis (ăm″ĭ-lō′sĭs) [Gr. *amylon*, starch, + *-ōsis*, condition]. Albuminoid degeneration of the cells.

amylosuria (ăm″ĭ-lō-sū′rĭ-ă) ["+ *ouron*, urine]. Amylose in the urine.

amylum (ăm′ĭ-lŭm) [L.]. Starch; corn starch. Used as dusting powder.

amylu′ria [L. *amylum*, starch, + Gr. *ouron*, urine]. Starch in the urine.

amyocardia (ă-mī″ō-kăr′dĭ-ă) [Gr. *a-*, not, + *mys*, muscle, + *kardia*, heart]. Weakness of the heart muscle. SYN: myasthenia cordis.

amyostasia (ă-mī″ō-stā′sĭ-ă) ["+ "+ *stasis*, standing]. Difficulty in standing because of lack of coordination or because of muscular tremors. SEE: *tremor.*

amyosthenia (ă-mī″os-thē′nĭ-ă) ["+ "+ *sthenos*, strength]. Lack of muscular tone or power.

amyosthen′ic. Pert. to muscular weakness.

amyotaxy (ă-mī″ō-tăks′ĭ) [Gr. *a-*, not, + *mys*, muscle, + *taxis*, order]. Muscular ataxia.

amyotonia (ă-mī″ō-tō′nĭ-ă) ["+ "+ *tonos*, tone]. Deficiency or lack of muscular tone.

   a. congenita. A non-inherited but sometimes familial disease characterized by absence of muscular development, with the lower extremities being the first involved. It is first seen at, or shortly after, birth. SYN: *myatonia congenita, Oppenheim's disease.*

amyotrophia (ă-mī″ō-trō′fĭ-ă) ["+ "+ *trophē*, nourishment]. Muscular wasting.

   a., progressive spinal. Progressive muscular atrophy.

amyotrophic (ă-mī″ō-trŏf′ĭk). Pert. to atrophy.

   a. lateral sclerosis. A syndrome marked by muscular weakness and atrophy with spasticity and hyperreflexia due to degeneration of motor neurons of spinal cord, medulla, and cortex. Prognosis is very poor. If only cells of motor cranial nuclei in the medulla are involved, condition is called progressive bulbar palsy.

amyotrophy (ăm-ĭ-ŏt′rō-fĭ). Muscular wasting. SYN: amyotrophia.

amyous (ăm'ĭ-ŭs) [Gr. *a-*, not, + *mys*, muscle]. 1. Weak; deficient in muscular strength. 2. Without muscle.

amyxia (ă-mĭks'ĭ-ă) ["+ *myxa*, mucus]. Deficient mucous secretion.

amyxorrhea (ă-mĭks-ō-rĭ'ă) ["+ "+ *rhoia*, flow]. Lack of normal secretion of mucus.

An. 1. Chem. symb. for actinon. 2. Abbr. for *anisometropia; anode.*

an- [Gr.]. A negative prefix indicating without or not.

A.N.A. Abbr. for *American Nurses' Association.*

ana (ăn'ă) [Gr.]. Meaning "one of each"; used in writing prescriptions as āā. SEE: *prescription.*

anabasis (ă-năb'ă-sĭs) [Gr. *ascend*]. Period of increased severity in a disease.

anabatic (ăn''ă-băt'ĭk). 1. Increased severity. 2. Pert. to anabasis.

anabiosis (ăn''ă-bĭ-ō'sĭs) [Gr. *anabiōsis*, revive]. Revival of a body which seemed lifeless. SYN: *resuscitation.*

anabiotic (ăn-ă-bĭ-ŏt'ĭk). 1. Restorative. 2. Any agent that resuscitates or restores.

anabol'ic [Gr. *anabolikos*]. Promoting or pert. to anabolism.

   a. agents. Testosterone, or a steroid hormone resembling testosterone, which stimulates anabolism (rather than catabolism) in the body as a whole. *CAUTION:* Indiscriminate use of anabolic agents is inadvisable because of the undesired side effects they may produce.

anabolin (ă-năb'ō-lĭn). A product of anabolism. SYN: *anabolite.*

anabolism (ă-năb'ō-lĭzm) [Gr. *anabolē*, a building up]. The building up of the body substance; the constructive or synthetic chemical reactions included in metabolism; a process by which a cell takes from the blood the substance required for repair and growth, building it into a cytoplasm, thus converting a nonliving material into the living cytoplasm of the cell.

   RS: assimilation; catabolism; metabolism; nutrition; synthesis.

anab'olite. Any product of anabolism. SYN: *anabolin.*

anabrosis (ăn''ă-brō'sĭs) [Gr.]. Superficial ulceration of soft tissue.

anacamptics (ăn''ă-kămp'tĭk) [Gr. *anakamptein,* to bend back]. Study of reflection of light or sound.

anacamptometer (ăn''ă-kămp-tŏm'ē-ter) ["+ *metron,* measure]. Device for measuring intensity of deep reflexes.

anacatharsis (ăn''ă-kă-thăr'sĭs) [Gr. *anakatharsis,* upward cleansing]. Severe prolonged vomiting; expectoration.

anacathar'tic. That which causes vomiting.

anachlorhydria (ăn''ă-klōr-hĭd'rĭ-ă). Decreased amount of free hydrochloric acid in the gastric juice.

anacidity (ăn''ă-sĭd'ĭ-tĭ) [Gr. *an-,* not, + L. *aciditas,* acid]. Abnormal deficiency of acidity.

anaclisis (ă-năk'lĭ-sĭs) [Gr. *anaklisis,* a leaning back]. 1. Reclining. 2. State of being emotionally dependent upon another.

anaclit'ic choice. An early expression of psychosexual development in which the object of one's love is influenced by dependence upon the mother or whoever is responsible for the child's early care, more or less inhibiting other expression of the sex instinct. Opposed to narcissism, q.v.

anacroasia (ăn''ă-krō-ā'zĭ-ă) [Gr. *an-,* not, + *akroasis,* hearing]. Inability to understand spoken words.

anacrotic (ăn''ă-krŏt'ĭk) [Gr. *ana,* up, + *krotos,* stroke]. 1. Pert. to a pulse with more than one expansion of the artery. 2. Pert. to two heartbeats traced on the ascending line of a sphygmogram. SYN: *anadicrotic.* SEE: *pulse.*

   a. limb. Ascending or vertical upstroke of a sphygmogram.

   a. pulse. Pulse in which one or more small waves occur on ascending limb of tracing of pulse wave, as in aortic stenosis.

anac'rotism. Existence of a double beat on ascending line of sphygmogram. SYN: *anadicrotism.*

anacusia, anacusis (ăn-ă-kū'sĭ-ă, -sĭs) [Gr. *an-,* not, + *akouein,* to hear]. Complete deafness.

anadenia (ăn-ă-dē'nĭ-ă) ["+ *adēn,* gland]. 1. Absence of glands. 2. Reduced glandular function.

anadicrotic (ăn''ă-dĭ-krŏt'ĭk) [Gr. *ana,* up, + *dikrotos,* double beating]. 1. Pert. to a pulse with more than one artery expansion. 2. Pert. to two heartbeats traced on the ascending line of a sphygmogram. SYN: *anacrotic.*

anadicrotism (an-ă-dĭk'rō-tizm). Existence of a double beat on ascending line of the sphygmogram. SYN: *anacrotism.*

anadidymus (ăn''ă-dĭd'ĭ-mŭs) ["+ *didymos,* twin]. A developmental abnormality in which the lower extremities of two fetuses are joined together.

anadipsia (ăn''ă-dĭp'sĭ-ă) ["+ *dipsa,* thirst]. Intense thirst.

anaerobe (ăn-ā'ĕr-ōb) [Gr. *an,* + *aer,* air, + *bios,* life]. A microorganism which thrives best or lives only without oxygen.

   a., facultative. An organism showing preference for free oxygen, yet capable of growing in its absence.

a., obligatory. Organism growing only in absence of free oxygen.

anaerobic (ăn″ā-ĕr-ō′bĭk). Having the power to use oxygen for metabolism from oxygen compounds; having the ability to live without air as some microbes.

a. exercise. Exercise during which the energy needed is provided without utilization of inspired oxygen. This type of exercise is limited to short bursts of vigorous activity. SEE: *aerobic exercise.*

anaerobiosis (ăn-ā″ĕr-ō-bī-ō′sĭs) [Gr. *an-*, not, + *aēr*, air, + *bios*, life, + *-ōsis*, condition]. 1. Life in an oxygen-free atmosphere. 2. Functioning of an organ or tissue in absence of free oxygen.

anaerobiotic (ăn-ā″ĕr-ō-bī-ŏt′ĭk). Able to exist without free oxygen.

anagnosasthenia (ăn″ăg-nōs-ăs-thē′nĭ-ā) [Gr. *anagnōsis*, reading, + *astheneia*, weakness]. 1. Distressing symptoms when trying to read, caused by neurosis rather than organic disease of the eye. 2. Inability to read even though the words can be seen.

anagoge, anagogy (ăn″ā-gō′jĭ) [Gr. *anagōgē*, a leading up]. In psychology, spiritual, moral, or idealistic phases of thought.

anakatadidymus (ăn″ā-kăt″ā-dĭd′ĭ-mŭs) [Gr. *ana*, up, + *kata*, down, + *didymos*, twin]. A congenital anomaly wherein twins are divided above and below but joined in the middle.

anakatesthesia (ăn″ā-kăt″ĕs-thē′zĭ-ā) ["+ "+ *aisthēsis*, sensation]. A sensation as of hovering or bearing down upon one.

anakusis (ăn″ā-kū′sĭs) [Gr. *an-*, not, + *akouein*, to hear]. Complete deafness. SYN: *anacusia.*

anal (ā′năl) [L. *analis*]. Rel. to the anus or outer rectal opening.

a. canal. The terminal portion of the large intestine, its external aperture being the anus. This is protected by an internal and external sphincter muscle, and remains closed except during defecation. It is about 1 1/2 inches (2.5–4 cm.) long.

a. character. In psychology, a pattern of adult behavior characterized by excessive orderliness, stinginess, and obstinacy. If carried to an extreme, these qualities lead to the development of obsessive-compulsive type of behavior.

a. erotism. Stage in pregenital libido in which pleasurable sensations are experienced in the anal region.

a. reflex. Contraction of anal sphincter following irritation of skin about anus. Reflex is lost in lesions of posterior columns of cord and is exaggerated in anal fissures.

analepsis (ăn″ā-lĕp′sĭs) [Gr. *analēpsis*, a taking up]. Gaining strength after an illness. Restoration to health.

analeptic (ăn″ā-lĕp′tĭk) [Gr. *analēptikos*, restorative]. 1. A drug used to stimulate the central nervous system. Used esp. in treatment of poisoning by drugs which depress the central nervous system, such as the barbiturates. 2. A restorative agent.

analgesia (ăn-ăl-jē′zĭ-ā) [Gr. *an-*, not, + *algos*, pain]. Absence of normal sense of pain.

a. algera, a. dolorosa. Severe pain with loss of sensitivity in a part.

a., paretic. Complete a. of upper limb in conjunction with partial paralysis.

analgesic (ăn″ăl-jē′sĭk). A medicine which relieves pain.

analgetic (ăn″ăl-jĕt′ĭk). Analgesic; producing freedom from pain, or an agent that lessens pain.

analgia (ăn-ăl′jĭ-ā) [Gr. *an-*, not, + *algos*, pain]. State of being without pain.

analgic (ăn-ăl′jĭk). Without pain.

analogue, analog (ăn′ā-lŏg) [Gr. *analogōs*, proportionate]. An organ or part similar in function, but differing in structure. In chemistry, a compound which is structurally similar to another but differs in that one molecule or radical has been replaced by one of the same valence.

analogy (ăn-ăl′ō-jĭ) [L. *analogia*, analogous]. 1. Likeness or similarity between two things which otherwise are unlike. 2. In biology, similarity in function, but difference in structure or embryonic origin. Opposed to homology.

analysand (ăn-ăl′ĭ-zănd). A patient who is being psychoanalyzed.

analysis (ă-năl′ĭ-sĭs) [Gr. a dissolving]. (pl. *analyses*) 1. Separation of anything into its constituent parts. 2. In chemistry, determination, or separation into, its constituent parts of a substance or compound. 3. Treatment by a physician trained as a psychoanalyst.

a., chromatographic. Separation of substances on the basis of color reaction of the constituents as they are differentially absorbed on one of a variety of materials such as filter paper.

a., colorimetric. The separation, by adsorption, of a compound and the identification of its elements by color.

a., densimetric. A. by determination of the specific gravity (density) of a solution, and then estimation of the amount of solids.

a., gastric. A. of the stomach contents to determine the concentration of free hydrochloric acid and combined (total) acid, presence or absence of lactic acid, presence or absence of occult blood, presence of pus and excessive mucus, and amount and types of bacteria.

a., qual'itative. Determining the nature of the elements in a substance.

a., quantita'tive. Determining the nature and the quantity of elements in a substance.

a., spectrophotometric. Determination of the presence of materials in a compound by measuring amount of light they absorb in the infrared, visible, or ultraviolet regions of the spectrum.

a., spectrum. A. of substances by use of a spectroscope.

a., volumetric. Quantitative a. performed by the measurement of the volume of solutions or liquids.

analyst (ăn'ă-lĭst) [Fr. *analyse*, analysis]. 1. One who analyzes. 2. A licensed practitioner of psychoanalysis. SYN: *psychoanalyst.*

analytic (ăn-ă-lĭt'ĭk) [Gr. *analytikos*]. Pert. to any analysis.

analytical balance. A balance for chemical analysis.

analyze (ăn'ă-līz) [Fr. *analyse*, analysis]. To separate into parts or principles in order to determine the nature of the whole; methodical examination.

anamnesis (ăn"ăm-nē'sĭs) [Gr. *anamnēsis*, recalling]. 1. Recollection; faculty of remembering. 2. That which is remembered. 3. The personal and case history of a patient and his family history. SEE: *catamnesis.*

anamnestic (ăn"ăm-nĕs'tĭk). 1. Pert. to previous medical history of patient. 2. Assisting the memory.

anamniot'ic [Gr. *an-*, not, + Gr. *amnion*, amnion]. Without an amnion.

ananabasia (ăn-ăn"ă-bā'sĭ-ă) ["+ *anabasis*, an ascending]. An abulia (loss of will) in which the person seems unable to ascend heights.

ananaphylaxis (ăn-ăn"ă-fĭ-lăk'sĭs) ["+ *an-*, not + *phylaxis*, protection]. That which neutralizes anaphylaxis, q.v.

ananastasia (ăn-ăn"ă-stā'sĭ-ă) [Gr. *an-*, not, + *anastasis*, a rising up]. Loss of will power (abulia) in which the person is unable to rise from a sitting position.

anandria (ăn-ăn'drĭ-ă) [Gr. *anandros*, without a man]. Impotence; lack of virility.

anangioplasia (ăn-ăn"jĭ-ō-plā'sĭ-ă) [Gr. *an-*, not, + *angeion*, vessel, + *plassein*, to form]. Imperfect vascularization of a part.

anangioplas'tic. Pert. to imperfect development of the vascular system.

anapeiratic (ăn"ă-pī-răt'ĭk) [Gr. *anapeirasthai*, to try again]. Pert. to a condition arising from excessive muscular activity.

a. cramp. Cramp arising from excessive muscular activity.

a. cramp, cyclist's. Pain in scrotum, perineum, and thighs from excessive bicycling.

a. cramp, occupational. Writer's cramp.

a. cramp, professional. Spasmodic disorder affecting groups of muscles used in special work or movements.

anaphalantiasis (ăn-ăf'ă-lăn-ti'ă-sĭs) [Gr. *ana*, up, + *phalanthos*, front baldness]. Loss of hair of the eyebrow.

anaphase (ăn'ă-fāz) ["+ *phainein*, to appear]. Stage in mitosis between metaphase and telophase in which longitudinal halves of chromosomes (the chromatids) separate and move toward their respective poles.

anaphia (ăn-ā'fĭ-ă, ăn-ăf'ĭ-ă) [Gr. *an-*, not, + *aphē*, touch]. 1. Abnormal sensitiveness to touch. 2. Loss or diminished sense of touch.

anaphoresis (ăn"ă-fō-rē'sĭs) [Gr. *an-*, not, + *phoresis*, sweating]. 1. Insufficient activity of the sweat glands. 2. Transmission of electropositive bodies into tissues by passage of electric current, the flow toward the positive pole.

anaphoria (ăn"ă-fōr'ĭ-ă) [Gr. *ana*, up, + *phorein*, to carry]. Tendency of eyeballs to turn upward. SYN: *anatropia.*

anaphrodisia (ăn-ăf'rō-dĭz'ĭ-ă) [Gr. *an-*, not, + *aphrodisia*, sexual desire]. Diminished or absent sex desire.

anaphrodisiac (ăn"ăf-ro-dĭz'ĭ-ăk). An agent that will depress the sexual desire or function.

anaphrodite (ăn-ăf'rō-dĭt). One with an impairment of sexual desire or with an absence of it.

anaphylactia (an-ă-fĭ-lak-shĭ-ă) [Gr. *ana*, again, + *phylaxis*, protection]. Any anaphylactic condition.

anaphylactic (ăn-ă-fĭ-lăk'tĭk). 1. Pert. or rel. to anaphylaxis. 2. Denoting increased activity to agents which are innocuous to others.

a. shock. State of collapse resulting from injection of a substance to which an animal has become sensitized. SEE: *anaphylaxis.*

anaphylactin (ăn"ă-fĭ-lăk'tĭn). The substances supposed to produce hypersusceptibility following injection of a foreign protein.

anaphylac'togen [Gr. *ana*, again + *phylaxis*, protection, + *gennan*, to produce]. That which produces anaphylaxis or anaphylactin. SYN: *allergen.*

anaphylactogen'esis. The process of producing anaphylaxis.

anaphylactogenic

anaphylactogenic

anaphylactogenic (ăn″ă-fĭ-lăk-tō-jĕn′ĭk). 1. Producing anaphylaxis. 2. The agent producing anaphylactic reactions.

anaphylaxis (ăn″ă-fĭ-lăks′ĭs) [Gr. *ana*, again, + *phylaxis*, protection]. A hypersensitive state of the body to a foreign protein or drug, induced by a preliminary injection; a condition produced artificially and experimentally in lower animals and dependent upon well-defined antigen-antibody reaction. Hypersensitivity so that the injection of a second dose in 10-12 days brings about an acute reaction, known also as protein sensitization and serum sickness, q.v. The term implies symptoms severe enough to produce serious shock.

Reactions which constitute anaphylactic shock occur suddenly. They include increased irritability, dyspnea, cyanosis, sometimes convulsions, unconsciousness, and death. Reactions primarily due to contraction of smooth muscle fibers and increased permeability of capillary endothelium. Death usually results from spasm of muscles of bronchioles.

Such diseases as asthma, hay fever, and urticaria (hives) are thought to be of an anaphylactic nature, being caused by the irritation of a food or by the pollen of some plants and flowers, to which the individual may have become sensitized. Sometimes marked a. follows a blood transfusion. Serum sickness is an anaphylactic reaction which occasionally follows injection of foreign serums, esp. horse serum.

SYM: *Mild a.*: Fever (slight), redness of skin, itching, urticaria *Severe a.*: Dyspnea, violent cough, chest constriction, cyanosis, fever, skin eruption, pulse variations, convulsions, collapse.

PROG: In mild cases, favorable; symptoms are self-limited. In severe cases, death may occur if emergency treatment is not given.

TREATMENT: Vasopressor agents, esp. epinephrine; corticosteroids; oxygen, artificial respiration.

NP: Oxygen inhalations, treatment for shock.

a., active. A. resulting from injection of an antigen.

a., heterologous. Passive a. by transfer of serum from an animal of a different species.

a., homologous. Passive a. by transfer of serum from an animal of the same species.

a., local. Local inflammatory reaction following repeated injections of antigenic material. SYN: *Arthus phenomenon.*

a., passive. A. induced by injection of serum from a sensitized animal into a normal one. After a few hours the latter becomes sensitized.

anaplasia (ăn-ă-plā′zĭ-ă) [Gr. *ana*, backward + *plasis*, a molding]. 1. Reversion of cells to a more embryonic type. 2. Alteration in cells which is believed, by some authorities, to produce malignancy.

anaplas′tic [Gr. *ana*, again, + *plassein*, to form]. Pert. to anaplasia or restoration of lost part.

anaplasty (ăn′ă-plăs″tĭ). Grafting or restoring lost parts.

anaplerosis (ăn″ă-plē-rō′sĭs) [Gr. *anaplērōsis*, a filling up]. Surgical transplantation of tissue to fill a defect.

anapnea (ăn″ăp-nē′ă) [Gr. *anapnein*, to breathe again]. 1. Respiration. 2. Regaining the breath.

anapneic (ăn″ăp-nē′ĭk). Pert. to anapnea or relieving dyspnea.

anapophysis (ăn″ă-pŏf′ĭ-sĭs) [Gr. *ana*, back + *apophysis*, offshoot]. An accessory spinal process of a vertebra.

anap′tic [Gr. *an-*, not, + *aptein*, to touch] Pert. to anaphia or diminished or lost tactile sense.

anarithmia (ăn″ă-rĭth′mĭ-ă) ["+ *arithmos* enumeration]. Inability to count or to use numbers.

ETIOL: Brain lesion.

anarthria (ăn-ăr′thrĭ-ă) ["+ *arthron*, joint] Loss of motor power to speak distinctly. May be a result of a neural lesion or a muscular apparatus defect.

a. centralis. Partial aphasia caused by a lesion of the central nervous system.

a. literalis. Stammering.

anasarca (ăn″ă-săr′kă) [Gr. *ana*, again, + *sarkos*, flesh]. Severe generalized edema. SEE: *edema.*

anasarcous (ăn″ă-săr′kŭs). Dropsical; edematous.

anaspadias (ăn″ă-spā′dĭ-ăs) [Gr. *ana*, up, + *spadon*, a rent]. Epispadias, q.v.

anastaltic (ăn″ă-stăl′tĭk) [Gr. *anastaltikos* checking]. 1. Very astringent. 2. Afferent.

anastasis (ă-năs′tă-sĭs) [Gr., a rising up]. 1. Return to health. 2. Resuscitation.

anastate (ăn′ă-stāt) [Gr. *anastatos*, raised up]. Any substance formed by, or condition characteristic of, an anabolic process.

anastole (ăn-ăs′tō-lĭ) [Gr. *anastolē*]. Shrinking away or retraction of the lips of a wound

anastomose (ă-năs′tō-mōs) [Gr. *anastomōsis*, opening]. 1. Opening of one vessel into another, or the union of one nerve with another. 2. To make such a connection surgically.

anastomosis (ă-năs″tō-mō′sĭs) [Gr., opening]. (pl. *anastomo′ses*) 1. A communication between two vessels. 2. The surgical or pathological formation of a passage between any two normally distinct spaces or organs. 3. An end-to-end union, joining together, or intercommunication of parts of any network or set of fibers such as nerves, or connective tissue fibers.

a., antiperistaltic. Enterostomy in which the two parts are so joined that the peristaltic wave in one part proceeds in a direction opposite to the other.

a., arteriovenous. A. between an artery and a vein.

a., collateral. A natural a., as that of the arteries at knee joint.

a., crucial. An arterial a. on the back of the thigh, formed by the medial femoral circumflex, inferior gluteal, lateral femoral circumflex, and first perforating arteries.

a., Galen's. The a. between the superior and inferior laryngeal nerves.

a., heterocladic. A. between branches of different arteries.

a., homocladic. A. between branches of the same artery.

a., Hyrtl's. An occasional looplike anastomosis between right and left hypoglossal nerves in geniohyoid muscle.

a., intestinal. The establishment of a communication between two portions of the intestines. SYN: *enterostomy.*

a., isoperistaltic. Intestinal a. in which the two parts are so joined that the peristaltic wave in each part is in the same direction.

a., Jacobson's. The union of a nerve from the petrous ganglion with the Vidian nerve, or with the tympanic branch of the glossopharyngeal.

a., precapillary. A. between small arteries just before they become capillaries.

a., Schmidel's. Abnormal communications between the vena cava and the portal system.

a., side-to-side. A. between two structures lying side by side or which are in that position after the procedure.

a., terminoterminal. A. between the peripheral end of an artery and the central end of the corresponding vein, and between the central end of the artery and peripheral end of vein.

a., ureterotubal. An a. between the ureter and the fallopian tube.

anastomot′ic. Pert. to, or marked by, anastomosis.

anatherapeusis (ăn″ă-thĕr″ă-pū′sĭs) [Gr. *ana*, up, + *therapeia*, treatment]. Treatment by steadily increasing doses.

anatomic (ăn″ă-tŏm′ĭk) [Gr. *anatomē*, dissection]. Of or rel. to the anatomy or structure of an organism.

anatomist (ăn-ăt′ō-mĭst). An individual skilled in anatomy.

anatomy (ăn-ăt′ō-mī) [Gr. *anatomē*, dissection]. 1. The structure or study of structure of organisms, or a treatise on same. 2. Dissection or cutting apart.

a., applied. Study applied to diagnosis and treatment, esp. surgical treatment.

a., comparative. Comparison of structure of different animals.

a., descriptive. Study of individual parts of physical structure.

a., gross. Study of structures seen with the naked eye. SYN: *macroscopic anatomy.*

a., microscopic. Study of structure by use of a microscope. SYN: *histology.*

a., morbid or pathological. Study of abnormal structure.

a., surface. Study of form and markings of the structure of the body, esp. as they relate to underlying tissues and organs.

anatopism (ă-năt′ō-pĭzm) [Gr. *ana*, without, + *topos*, place, + *-ismos*, condition]. Inability to conform to social customs of the group to which an individual belongs.

anatoxic (ăn″ă-tŏks′ĭk) ["+ *toxikon*, poison]. 1. Pert. to anatoxin. 2. Anaphylactic.

anatoxin (ăn″ă-tŏks′ĭn). A modified toxin retaining the antigenic properties with lessened toxic properties.

anatricrotic pulse (ăn″ă-trī-krŏt′ĭk) ["+ *treis*, three, + *krotos*, stroke]. Three beats on the ascending curve of a pulse wave.

anatripsis (ăn″ă-trĭp′sĭs) [Gr., friction]. 1. A centripetal or upward movement in massage. 2. Inunction. Rubbing or removing by scraping. 3. Crushing as of a stone.

anatriptic (ăn-ă-trĭp′tĭk) [Gr. *anatriptos*]. An agent to be rubbed in.

anatro′pia [Gr. *ana*, up, + *tropē*, a turning]. Tendency of eyeballs to turn upward; anaphoria.

anaxon)e (ăn-ăk′son) [Gr. *an-*, not, + *axon*, axis]. A nerve cell, as of the retina, having no neuraxon.

anazoturia (ăn″ă-zō-tū′rĭ-ă) ["+ *a-*, not, + *zōē*, life, + *ouron*, urine]. Without urea or nitrogenous substances in the urine.

ANC. Abbr. for *Army Nurse Corps.*

AnCC. Abbr. for *anodal closure contraction.*

anchone (ang-kō′nē) [Gr. *anchein*, to strangle]. Spasm of the throat in hysteria.

anchorage (ăng′kĕr-āj) [Gr. *ankura*, anchor]. 1. Operative fixation of displaced viscus. 2. The part to which anything is fixed, as a tooth to which a bridge is fastened.

anconad (ăn′kō-năd) [Gr. *ankōn*, elbow, + L. *ad*, to]. Toward the elbow.

anconagra (ăn″kŏn-ăg′rä) [″+ *agra*, a seizure]. Gout of the elbow.

anconal, anconeal (ăn′kō-năl, an-kō′nī-ăl). Pert. to the elbow.

    a. fossa. Fossa olecrani.

anconeus (ăn-kō′nē-ŭs) [Gr. *ankōn*, elbow]. Short extensor muscle of forearm located on the back of the elbow. It arises from the back portion of the lateral epicondyle of the humerus, and its fibers insert on side of the olecranon and upper fourth of shaft of ulna. Assists in extension of the elbow.

anconitis (ăn″kō-nī′tĭs) [″+ *-itis,* inflammation]. Inflammation of the elbow joint.

Ancylostoma (ăn″sĭl-ŏs′tō-mä) [Gr. *ankylos,* crooked, + *stoma,* mouth]. A genus of nematodes of the family Ancylostomatidae including the hookworms. SEE: *Necator americanus.*

    A. braziliense. Species of hookworm infesting dogs and cats, larvae of which may cause creeping eruption in man.

    A. caninum. Species of hookworm infesting dogs and cats. Its larvae may cause creeping eruption in man.

    A. duodenale. The hookworm found in Mediterranean countries and the Nile Valley. Also found along with Necator Americanus in Asia, Central and South America, and West Indies. Commonly infests man causing ancylostomiasis, q.v. Adult male hookworms average 8-11 mm. in length and females 10-13 mm. Buccal capsule of the worm contains two pairs of teeth.

Ancylostomatidae (ăn″sĭ-lŏs″tō-măt′ĭ-dē). A family of nematodes belonging to the suborder Strongylata. It includes the genera Ancylostoma and Necator, common hookworms of man.

ancylostomiasis (ăn″sĭ-lŏs-tō-mī′ä-sĭs) [Gr. *ankylos,* crooked, + *stoma,* mouth, + *-iasis,* condition]. Infestation by either hookworm, Ancylostoma duodenale or Necator americanus, in the preintestinal phase. Infecting larvae enter through the skin of the bare foot of a person and cause ground itch or water sore characterized by inflammation, itching and sometimes allergic reactions. Passing from the skin through the lungs, larvae may predispose to pulmonary infections, or if larvae are numerous, pneumonia or pneumonia-like symptoms may occur. In intestines, may cause nausea, colicky pains, and diarrhea. Loss of blood leads to anemia; and, in children, normal mental and physical growth is retarded.

Ancyclostomiasis, known as hookworm disease, is common in tropical and semitropical areas where the climate, plus poor sanitation and damp earth, brings the larvae in contact with bare skin, usually of the foot.

TREATMENT: Tetrachlorethylene for Necator americanus infestation. Thiabendazole is effective as is Bephenium hydroxynaphthoate which is the drug of choice for Anclystoma duodenale. Anemia and malnutrition should be treated simultaneously.

ancyroid (ăn′sī-royd) [Gr. *ankyra,* anchor, + *eidos,* resemblance]. Shaped like fluke of an anchor.

Andernach's ossicles (ŏn′dĕr-nŏk). [Johann Winther von Andernach, Ger. physician, 1487-1574]. Small bones found in cranial sutures. SYN: *Wormian bones.*

Andral's decu′bitus (ăn′drăl). [Gabriel Andral, Fr. physician, 1797-1876] Lying on sound side during beginning of pleurisy.

andriatrics (ăn″drī-ăt′rĭks) [Gr. *anēr,* man, + *iatreia,* medical treatment]. Study of diseases of male genitals.

andro- [Gr. *andros,* man]. A prefix signifying man, male, or masculine.

androgalactozemia (ăn″drō-găl-ăk″tō-zē′mī-ä) [″+ *gala,* milk, + *zemia,* loss]. Oozing of milk from male breast.

androgen (ăn′drō-jĕn) [″+ *gennan,* to produce]. Substance producing or stimulating male characteristics as the male sex hormone, testosterone.

androgyne (ăn′drō-jĭn) [Gr. *andros,* man, + *gynē,* woman]. Androgynus.

androgynoid (ăn-drōj′ī-noyd) [″+ ″+ *eidos,* resemblance]. A person possessing female gonads (ovaries) but secondary sex characteristics of a male; a female pseudohermaphrodite. Term is less commonly used for a person possessing male gonads (testes) but secondary sex characteristics of a female; a male pseudohermaphrodite.

androgynus (ăn-drōj′ī-nŭs) [Gr. *andros,* man, + *gynē,* woman]. 1. Resembling or pert. to an androgynoid, q.v. 2. Without definite sexual characteristics.

androg′ynus. A female pseudohermaphrodite.

android (ăn′droyd) [Gr. *andros,* man, + *eidos,* resemblance]. Resembling a male; manlike.

andrology (ăn-drŏl′ō-jī) [″+ *logos,* study]. Study of diseases of the male, esp. the male sex organs.

andromania (ăn″drō-mā′nī-ä) [″+ *mania,* frenzy]. Abnormally increased sexual desire in the female. SYN: *nymphomania,* q.v.

andromimetic (ăn″drō-mĭm-ĕt′ĭk) [Gr. *andros,* man, + *mimētikos,* imitative]. Simulating human processes, as certain types of protozoa.

androp'athy ("+ *pathos*, suffering). Any disease peculiar to the male.

androphile (ăn'drō-fīl) ["+ *philos*, fond of]. Preferring man; said of certain parasitic organisms.

androphobia (ăn"drō-fō'bǐ-ă) [Gr. *andros*, man, + *phobos*, fear]. Abnormal fear of the male sex.

androstane (ăn'drō-stān). A steroid hydrocarbon $C_{19}H_{32}$ which is the precursor of androgenic hormones.

androsterone (ăn"drō-stēr'ōn, ăn-drŏs'tēr-ōn). $C_{19}H_{30}O_2$, an androgenic steroid found in the urine and considered to be a metabolite of testosterone. It has been synthesized. As one of the androgens (male sex hormones), androsterone contributes to the characteristic changes of growth and development of the genitals and axillary and pubic hair, deepening of the voice, and development of the sweat glands in the male.

-ane. In chemistry, indicates a saturated hydrocarbon.

anebous (ăn-ē'bŭs) [Gr. *anebos*, immature]. Immature; below the age of puberty.

anedeous (ăn-ē'dǐ-ŭs) [Gr. *an-*, not, + *aidoia*, genitals]. Not possessing genitals.

anelectrotonus (ăn"ĕl-ĕk-trŏt'ō-nŭs) [Gr. *ana*, up, + *elektrōn*, electric, + *tōnōs*, tension]. The state of diminished irritability of a nerve or muscle produced in region near the anode during the passage of an electric current.

Anel's operation (ă-nĕl'). [Dominique Anel, Fr. surgeon, 1679-1730]. Ligation of an artery immediately above and on proximal side of an aneurysm.

Anel's probe. A probe for the lacrimal and nasal ducts.

anemia (ă-nē'mǐ-ă) [Gr. *an-*, not, + *haima*, blood]. A condition in which there is a reduction in number of circulating red blood cells or in hemoglobin, or in the volume of packed red cells per 100 ml. of blood, or a combination of two or more of these factors. It exists when hemoglobin content is less than 13-14 gm./100 ml. for males or 11-12 gm./100 ml. for females.

If the onset of a. is slow the body may adjust so well that there will be no functional impairment, even though the hemoglobin may be less than 6 gm./100 ml. of blood.

Anemias are classified on basis of morphological differentiation and mean corpuscular volume (MCV) as normocytic, macrocytic and microcytic; mean corpuscular hemoglobin concentration (MCHC) as

normochromic, hypochromic, and hyperchromic; and etiology.

ETIOL: A. may result from excessive blood loss or destruction or from decreased blood cell formation. A. may follow acute or chronic hemorrhage or excessive blood cell destruction, as occurs in hemolytic diseases or hypersplenism. Anemias due to decreased blood formation may result from defective nucleoprotein synthesis (as in pernicious and other macrocytic anemias), iron deficiency, inhibition of bone marrow as occurs in certain toxic states, loss of bone marrow, or bone marrow failure.

SYM: Pallor of skin, fingernail beds, and mucous membranes; weakness; vertigo; headache; sore tongue; drowsiness; general malaise; dyspnea; tachycardia; palpitation; angina pectoris; gastrointestinal disturbances; amenorrhea; loss of libido; slight fever. In severe cases BMR may be increased.

NP: The nursing care of patients with anemia provides adequate rest; proper care of the skin, mouth, and teeth; proper elimination; a regulated diet; and antianemic medication prescribed by the physician.

Rest: Usually patients with mild and moderately severe anemias are ambulatory, but patients with very severe anemias must be kept in bed and spared all possible exertion. In acute a. due to blood loss absolute rest is essential; the foot of the bed should be elevated, the patient kept comfortably warm but not hot. Warm, stimulating drinks may be given if the hemorrhage is not from gastrointestinal tract.

Care of the skin: Daily warm baths and light massage are beneficial. In very severe anemias, special care of the buttocks and heels may be necessary to prevent the formation of pressure sores. Fresh air and sunshine are indicated, but chilling should be avoided.

Care of the mouth and teeth: Besides ordinary oral hygiene, special care of the mouth is indicated in anemic patients who have soreness of the tongue, mouth and pharynx. Alkaline mouthwashes are beneficial; if the gums are very sore, pledgets of cotton or gauze may be substituted for a toothbrush for cleaning the teeth.

Diet: The nurse's principal function in this regard is to see that the patient takes the diet which has been prescribed for him. This may be a difficult task since he often has a poor appetite and his mouth and tongue may be sore. Tact and gentle persuasion often necessary. severe anemias the function of the kidneys may be impaired; for this reason, fluids should be given freely to insure an adequate output of urine.

Medicines: If the patient is taking iron or liver, it is most important that he does not miss a single dose. If he is given a transfusion the nurse must watch carefully for reaction, and notify the doctor immediately if the patient complains of chilliness, pain in the chest or back, or shortness of breath, or if his temperature rises. Also if tenderness or swelling appears at the site of injection of liver extract.

Teaching the patient: Throughout the patient's illness the nurse should never lose the opportunity to impress the patient with the importance of his continuing proper treatment after he leaves the hospital. He should be made to understand that in order to get well and stay well he must continue to follow his diet and to take his medicine. He must also understand that he must revisit his doctor at frequent intervals for checkups and blood counts so that relapse may be prevented.

RS: antianemic; ischemia.

a., achlorhydric. A. in which there is an absence of free hydrochloric acid in gastric juice.

a., achrestic. A rare hyperchromic, macrocytic a. resembling pernicious a. yet gastric secretion is normal. Probably due to inability of bone marrow to utilize antianemic principle.

a., Addisonian. A., pernicious, q.v.

a., aplastic. A. caused by aplasia of bone marrow and destruction of same by chemical agents (benzene, arsenic, nitrogen mustards) or physical factors (X rays and other sources of ionizing radiation). An idiopathic form may occur.

a., blind loop. Megaloblastic a. due to a blind loop or multiple diverticulosis of the jejunum which becomes infected with bacteria. These organisms destroy vitamin B_{12}, thus causing a. May be treated by removing blind loops or administering vitamin B_{12} and antibiotics. SEE: *a., megaloblastic.*

a., chlorotic. Form of a. in adolescent girls and young women thought to be due to faulty diet. SYN: *chloranemia; chlorosis; green sickness; iron-deficiency a.,* q.v.

a., congenital hemolytic. Inherited, chronic disease characterized by hemolysis of blood cells, jaundice, and splenomegaly. SYN: *congenital hemolytic icterus; jaundice.*

a., Cooley's. A. resulting from inheritance of a recessive trait responsible for interference with hemoglobin synthesis. SEE: *thalassemia.*

a., crescent cell. A., sickle cell, q.v.

a., deficiency. Condition resulting from lack of an essential ingredient such as iron or vitamins in the diet, or the inability of the intestine to absorb such. SYN: *nutritional a.*

a., drepanocytic. A., sickle cell, q.v.

a., erythroblastic. Thalassemia, q.v.

a., essential. Idiopathic a.; pernicious a.

a., hemolytic. A. resulting from hemolysis of red blood cells. Is either acquired as from the effects of toxic agents, or congenital (familial).

a., hyperchromic. A. in which mean corpuscular hemoglobin concentration (MCHC) and color index (C.I.) are greater than normal (30% and 1.1 respectively). Term is actually a misnomer as red cells cannot contain an excess of hemoglobin.

a., hypersplenic. Condition resulting from excessive destruction of red blood cells in the spleen.

a., hypochromic. A. in which there is a hemoglobin deficiency, and mean corpuscular hemoglobin concentration is below 30%.

a., idiopathic. A. in which there is a lesion of the blood-forming tissue of unidentified cause.

a., iron-deficiency. A. resulting from a greater demand on the stored iron than can be supplied. Most commonly caused by a chronic loss of blood. Usually successfully treated with oral ferrous sulfate or ferrous gluconate and a well-balanced diet.

a., Jaksch's. Infantile pseudoleukemia; a painless, progressive enlargement of the lymphoid tissues, often beginning in the neck.

a., lymphatic. A. associated with tumors of the lymph nodes. SEE: *Hodgkin's disease.*

a., macrocytic. A. marked by abnormally large erythrocytes.

a., megaloblastic. A. in which megaloblasts are found in the blood.

a., microcytic. A. with abnormally small erythrocytes.

a., myelopathic, myelophthisic a. A. caused by disruption, usually by metastasis, in bone marrow function.

a., normocytic. A. in which size and hemoglobin content of red blood cells remain normal.

a., nutritional. A., deficiency, q.v.

a., pernicious. A chronic, macrocytic a. characterized by achlorhydria. Occurs most commonly in the white race after 4th decade of life; occurs rarely before the age of 35. SYN: *Addisonian pernicious a.; Biermer's a.*

ETIOL: Failure of the stomach to secrete enough intrinsic factor to insure intestinal absorption of vitamin B_{12}, the extrinsic factor. This is due to atrophy of the glandular mucosa of the fundus of the stomach and is associated with absence of hydrochloric acid.

SYM: Weakness, sore tongue, paresthesias (tingling and numbness) of extremities, and gastrointestinal symptoms as diarrhea, nausea, vomiting, pain; signs of cardiac failure may be present in severe anemia.

TREATMENT: Intramuscular injection of vitamin B_{12}.

a., primary. A., pernicious, q.v.

a., secondary. A. which occurs as the result of a severe disease such as cancer, tuberculosis, infection, or hemorrhage.

a., septic. A. due to severe infection.

a., sickle cell. A hereditary, chronic, hemolytic a. characterized by presence of large numbers of crescent or sickle-shaped red blood cells in the blood. Occurs almost exclusively in Negroes. Due to an abnormality in the hemoglobin molecule.

a., splenic. Condition characterized by enlargement of the spleen (with accompanying a., leukopenia and sometimes thrombocytopenia), gastric hemorrhage, and usually cirrhosis of the liver. SYN: *Banti's syndrome; chronic congestive splenomegaly.*

anemic (ă-nē'mĭk). Pert. to anemia; deficient in red blood cells, in hemoglobin, or in volume of blood.

a. hypoxia. Reduction in amount or capability of hemoglobin to transport oxygen.

anemophobia (ăn"ē-mō-fō'bĭ-ă) [Gr. *anemos*, wind, + *phobos*, fear]. Abnormal fear of drafts or of the wind.

anemot'rophy [Gr. *an-*, not, + *haima*, blood, + *trophē*, nourishment]. Anemia from deficient formation of blood.

anempeiria (ăn"em-pī'rĭ-ă) ["+ *empeiria*, experience]. Deficiency in practical knowledge or experience.

anencephalus (ăn"ĕn-sĕf'ă-lŭs) ["+ *engkephalos*, the brain]. A congenital deformity characterized by absence of brain and spinal cord, the cranium being open throughout its whole extent and the vertebral canal converted into a groove.

anephrogenesis (ă-nĕf'rō-jĕn'ĕ-sĭs) [Gr. *a-*, not, + *nephros*, kidney, + *genesis*, beginning]. Congenital anomaly consisting of lack of kidney tissue.

anepia (ăn-ē'pĭ-ă) [Gr. *an-*, not, + *epos*, word]. Inability to speak.

anergasia (ăn"ĕr-gā'sĭ-ă) ["+ *ergon*, work]. Anergia; functional inactivity resulting from a structural lesion of the central nervous system.

anergastic reaction (ăn"ĕr-găs'tĭk). Disorder involving cerebral lesions or organic psychoses. Loss of memory, impairment of mental activity, function, or judgment.

anergia (ăn-ĕr'jĭ-ă) [Gr. *an-*, not, + *ergon*, work]. Inactivity; sluggishness.

anergic (ăn-ĕr'jĭk). Sluggish; inactive. Deficient in energy; listless.

a. stupor. Acute phase of dementia.

anergy (ăn'ĕr-jĭ). 1. Asthenia. 2. Impaired or absent ability to react to specific antigens.

aneroid (ăn'ĕr-oyd) [Gr. *a-*, not, + *nēron*, water, + *eidos*, form]. Operating without a fluid as an aneroid barometer which utilizes atmospheric pressure instead of a liquid such as mercury.

anerythrocyte (ăn"ē-rĭth'rō-sīt) [Gr. *an-*, not, + *erythros*, red, + *kytos*, cell]. A red blood cell without hemoglobin.

anerythroplasia (ăn"ē-rĭth"rō-plā'zĭ-ă) ["+ "+ *plasis*, a molding]. Without formation of red blood cells.

anerythroplastic (ăn"ē-rĭth"rō-plăs'tĭk). Marked by anerythroplasia.

anerythropsia (ăn"ē-rĭ-thrŏp'sĭ-ă) [Gr. *an-*, not, + *erythros*, red, + *opsis*, vision]. Inability to distinguish red clearly.

anesthecinesia, anesthekinesia (ăn-ĕs-thē"sĭn-ē'sĭ-ă, -kĭ-nē'sĭ-ă) ["+ *aisthesis*, sensation, + *kinesis*, movement]. Combined sensory and motor paralysis.

anesthesia (ăn"ĕs-thē'zĭ-ă) [Gr. *an-*, not, + *aisthesis*, sensation]. Partial or complete loss of sensation with or without loss of consciousness as result of disease, injury, or administration of a drug or gas.

STAGES OF PHARMACOLOGICALLY-INDUCED GENERAL ANESTHESIA: First stage includes preliminary excitement until voluntary control is lost. Hearing is last sense to be lost. Avoid talking in presence of patient.

Second stage consists of loss of voluntary control with corneal reflex still present.

In the third stage there is entire relaxation, no rigidity, deep regular breathing, sluggish corneal reflex, and loss of conjunctival reflex.

TESTS FOR ANESTHESIA: *Reaction to light:* Exclude light by holding hand over eyes; withdraw hand quickly. Pupil will reduce in size if anesthesia is complete.

Conjunctival reflex: Place soft clean object at corner of eye on conjunctiva. The eyelid will attempt to close. This reflex is lost during third stage.

Corneal reflex: If cornea is lightly touched with soft clean object the eyelid attempts to close. Reflex is brisk during first and second stages, sluggish during third stage, and lost only in deep anesthesia.

Danger signals: If too deep due to overdose corneal reflex is lost, pupils widely dilate and cease to react to light. Cardiac and respiratory centers fail, patient ceases to breathe, and heart action stops.

EMERGENCY MEASURES: Artificial respiration by anesthetist; injection of cardiac stimulant, inhalation of oxygen, several seconds of brisk slapping over heart, injection of epinephrine into heart muscle. SEE: *resuscitation, heart-lung.*

a., audio. A. produced by sound; used by dentists to kill pain.

a., block. A. resulting from nerve blocking by injection of alcohol or other substance into or very near a nerve trunk. SYN: *conduction a.; nerve block a.*

a., bulbar. Pons lesion causing central a.

a., caudal. A form of a. in which needle is inserted into sacrococcygeal notch and local anesthetic injected into the epidural space.

a., dissociative. A type of anesthesia characterized by catalepsy, amnesia, and marked analgesia. Agents which produce this type of anesthesia have been used experimentally.

a., dolorosa. Painfulness of a part with a. of that part, as in thalamic lesions.

a., general. One that is complete and affecting the entire body with loss of consciousness when the anesthetic acts upon the brain. This type of a. is usually accomplished following administration of inhalation or intravenous anesthetic. Commonly used for surgical procedures.

a., Gwathmey's. A. induced by injecting an olive oil and ether solution into the rectum.

a., hysterical. Bodily a. occurring in hysteria.

a., infiltration. Local a. achieved by injecting the local anesthetic solution directly into the tissues, such as injection of procaine solution into the gums for dental procedures.

a., inhalation. General a. achieved by inhaling vapor or gas anesthetics such as ether, nitrous oxide, methoxyflurane.

a., local. A. affecting a local area only, the anesthetic acting upon nerves or nerve tracts. SEE: *a., block; a., infiltration.*

a., mixed. Production of general a. by more than one drug, as nitrous oxide gas for

induction followed by ether for maintenance of a.

a., neural. Injection of an anesthetic into a nerve or immediately around it (intraneural and paraneural). SYN: *block a.*

a., primary. First stage of a. q.v., before unconsciousness.

a., rectal. General a. produced by introduction of anesthetic agent into rectum.

a., refrigeration. A. induced by lowering temperature of a part to near freezing by topical ethyl chloride spray or by immersion of the body or a part in a container of finely cracked ice.

a., regional. Nerve or field blocking, causing insensibility over a particular area.

a., sexualis. Anaphrodisia or absence of sexual desire.

a., spinal. 1. A. resulting from injury to conduction pathways of the spinal cord. 2. A. produced by injection of anesthetic into subarachnoid space of spinal cord.

a., surgical. When depth of a. produces relaxation of muscles and loss of sensation and/or consciousness.

a., tactile. Loss of sense of touch.

a., topical. Local a. induced by application of an anesthetic directly to surface of body.

a., traumatic. Loss of sensation resulting from injury to nerve.

a., twilight. State of light a. SEE: *twilight sleep.*

anesthesia, words pert. to: words beginning "anesthe-"; carbon dioxide; chloroform; cocaine; cyclopropane; ether; ethyl chloride; ethylene; labor; nitrous oxide; para-anesthesia; paraldehyde; procaine.

anesthesimeter (ăn″ĕs-thĕ-sĭm′ĕ-tĕr) [Gr. *an-*, not, + *aisthesis*, sensation, + *metron*, measure]. A device for measuring the amount of inhalation anesthetic administered.

anesthesiology (ăn″ĕs-thē-zĭ-ŏl′ō-jĭ) ["+ "+ *logos*, science]. Science of anesthesia.

anesthetic (ăn″ĕs-thĕt′ĭk). 1. Causing or pert. to anesthesia. 2. An agent that produces insensibility to pain or touch. According to action, they are subdivided into general and local. SEE: *anesthesia.*

anesthetist (ăn-ĕs′thĕ-tĭst). One who administers anesthetics, esp. for general anesthesia.

a., nurse. A registered nurse who has had special training in anesthesia so that she is capable of administering anesthetic agents.

an″esthetiza′tion. Induction of anesthesia.

anesthetize (ăn-ĕs′thĕ-tīz). To induce anesthesia, either local or general.

anetic (ă-nĕt'ĭk) [Gr. *anetikos*]. Relaxing, soothing.

anetiologic (ăn-ē"tĭ-ō-lōj'ĭk). Not etiologic; not according to the principles of etiology.

anetoderma (ăn-ĕt-ō-dĕr'mă) [Gr. *anetos*, relaxed, + *derma*, skin]. 1. Atrophy of the skin. 2. Soft fibromata of the skin, forming large, pendulous masses.

anetus (ăn'ē-tŭs). Any intermittent fever.

aneuploidy (ăn'ū-ploy'dĭ) [Gr. *an-*, not, + *eu*, well, + *ploos*, fold, + *eidos*, form]. Having an abnormal number of chromosomes for the species indicated.

aneurysm (ăn'ū-rĭzm) [Gr. *aneurysma*, a widening]. Localized abnormal dilatation of a blood vessel. Due to congenital defect or weakness of the wall of the vessel.

ETIOL: In the aorta usually occurs secondary to syphilitic aortitis. Arteriosclerosis and atherosclerosis accompanied by hypertension are contributing causes. Bacterial or mycotic infection or trauma are common causes of aneurysms in peripheral arteries.

NP: No exertion permitted. Absolute rest in bed. Later, patient may get up, but warn against vigorous effort. General care in heart conditions should be observed.

Observe circulation of the affected part. Keep limb warm with an electric pad or blanket, but, as sensation is impaired, apply heat with great care. Inspect affected part every 15 minutes, and adjust limb to aid circulation.

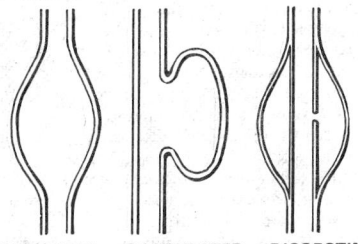

FUSIFORM   SACCULATED   DISSECTING
ANEURYSM   ANEURYSM   ANEURYSM

a., aortic. A. affecting any part of the aorta, usually resulting from syphilitic infection, but may result also from necrosis of the structure of the aorta or from atherosclerosis. SEE: *a., dissecting*.

PATH: Pressure on trachea, esophagus, veins, or nerves.

SYM: Dyspnea, cough, sputum, dysphagia, congestion of head and neck. Inequality in the two radial pulses.

TREATMENT: Surgery.

a., arteriovenous. A. in which artery and vein become connected by a saccule.

ETIOL: Trauma. Weak point, in walls of an artery, due to syphilis, sudden strain, or injury.

SYM: Pain, expansile pulsation, bruit.

NP: Avoid increasing heart action or raising blood pressure.

a., cirsoid. A dilatation of a network of vessels commonly occurring on the scalp. The mass may form a pulsating subcutaneous tumor. SYN: *racemose a.*

a., dissecting. A. in which the blood makes its way between the layers of a blood vessel wall, separating them; a result of necrosis of the medial portion of the arterial wall.

a., fusiform. All the walls of the blood vessels dilate more or less equally, creating a tubular swelling.

a., mycotic. A. due to bacterial infection.

a., racemose. SYN: *cirsoid a.*, q.v.

a., sacculated. A. due to the yielding of a weak patch on one side of the vessel and not involving the entire circumference; usually due to an injury.

a., varicose. A. forming a blood-filled sac between an artery and a vein.

a., venous. Aneurysm of a vein.

aneurysmal (ăn"ū-rĭz'măl) [Gr. *aneurysma*, a widening]. Pert. to aneurysm.

aneurysmectomy (ăn"ū-rĭz-mĕk'tō-mĭ) ["+ *ektomē*, excision]. Extirpation of an aneurysm by removal of its sac.

aneurysmorrhaphy (ăn"ū-rĭz-mŏr'ă-fĭ) ["+ *rhaphe*, suture]. Surgical repair of an aneurysm.

aneurysmotomy (ăn"ū-rĭz-mŏt'ō-mĭ) [Gr. *aneurysma*, a widening, + *tomē*, cut]. Incision of the sac of an aneurysm, allowing it to heal by granulation.

anfractuosity (ăn-frăk"tū-ŏs'ĭ-tĭ) [L. *anfractus*, a winding]. A cerebral sulcus or fissure.

anfractuous (ăn-frăk'tū-ŭs). Bending; sinuous.

angel's wing. A condition usually caused by paralysis of the serratus anterior muscle and characterized by scapula projecting posteriorly. SYN: *winged scapula.*

Angelucci's syndrome (ăn"jĕ-lū'chē). [Arnaldo Angelucci, It. opthalmologist, 1854-1934]. Great excitability, palpitation, and vasomotor disturbance associated with vernal conjunctivitis.

angi-, angio- (ăn'jĭ, ăn'jĭ-ō) [Gr. *angeion*, vessel]. Prefix meaning a blood or lymph vessel.

angiasthenia (ăn"jĭ-as-thē'nĭ-ă) ["+ *a-*, not, + *sthenos*, strength]. Loss of vascular tone.

angiectasia, -sis (ăn"jĭ-ĕk-tā'zĭ-ă, -ĕk'tă-sĭs) ["+ *ektasis*, stretching]. Enlarged capillaries or abnormal dilation of a vessel.

angiectomy (ăn″gī-ĕk′tō-mĭ) [Gr. *angeion*, vessel, + *ektomē*, excision]. Excision or resection of a blood vessel.

angiectopia (ăn″jī-ĕk-tō′pī-ă) [Gr. *angeion*, vessel, + *ektopos*, out of place]. Displacement of a vessel.

angiemphraxis (ăn″jī-em-fraks′is) [″+ *emphraxis*, stoppage]. Obstruction of any vessel.

angiitis (ăn″jī-ī′tĭs) [Gr. *angeion*, vessel, + *-itis*, inflammation]. Inflammation of a blood or lymphatic vessel.

angina (ăn-jī′nă, L. ăn′jī-nă) [L. quinsy, from *angere*, to choke]. 1. A sense of suffocation. 2. Disease of the pharynx or fauces. 3. Any disease characterized by attacks of choking or suffocation.

a. abdominis. Severe abdominal pain resulting from sclerosis of abdominal blood vessels.

a., acute. Simple sore throat.

a. cruris. A. due to obstruction of an artery, causing pain and cyanosis of the affected part, with periodic lameness.

a. decubitus. Attacks of a. pectoris occurring during rest or sleep.

a., follicular. A. of the larynx and pharynx from public speaking, excessive drinking of alcoholic liquors.

a. laryngea. Inflammation of the larynx.

a. ludovici, a. ludwigii. A., Ludwig's, q.v.

a., Ludwig's. Submaxillary cellulitis; a deep infection of tissues of the floor of the mouth.

a. maligna. Gangrenous inflammation of the throat; septic sore throat.

a., necrotic. Form with gangrenous patches in the mucosa of the air passages, seen in scarlet fever and occasionally in diptheria.

a. parotidea. Inflammation of the parotid glands. SYN: *mumps.*

a. pectoris. Pain and oppression about the heart; a paroxysmal affection characterized by severe pain radiating from the heart to the shoulder, thence down the left arm, or, rarely, from the heart to the abdomen; apparently dependent upon some lesion of the coronary arteries of the heart, its walls, or valves.

SYM: Severe, steady pain and feeling of pressure in region of the heart; great anxiety, fear of approaching death (angor animi), and fixation of the body; face pale, ashen, or livid; brow bathed in sweat. Dyspnea often noted; pulse variable, usually tense and quick. Blood pressure is raised during an attack. Attack lasts from a few seconds to several minutes.

PROG: May be grave. Attacks may be intermittent, and with proper rest and care recovery is possible.

TREATMENT: During attack, inhalation of amyl nitrite or nitroglycerin sublingually. Avoidance of excitement; physical rest.

a. pectoris vasomotoria. Angina pectoris in which symptoms are relatively mild. Pallor, cyanosis, and coldness and numbness of the extremities are characteristic. Also called mock, spurious, or false angina.

a., phlegmonous. Inflammation of the deep tissues of the throat with edema and usually suppuration.

a. simplex. Sore throat. SEE: a., acute.

a. streptococcus. A. caused by the streptococcus.

a. tonsillaris. Quinsy.

a. trachealis. Croup.

a., Vincent's. A pseudomembranous affection of the mouth involving gingivae, oral mucosa, and sometimes pharynx and tonsils. Fusiform bacilli and a spirochete, Borrelia vincenti, are invariably associated with the disease but their relationship to it is not definitely established. SYN: *trench mouth.* SEE: *Vincent's a.*

anginal (ăn′jī-nal). Pert. to angina.

anginoid (ăn′jī-noyd) [L. *angina*, choking, + Gr. *eidos*, resemblance]. Resembling angina pectoris, or any angina.

anginophobia (ăn″jī-nō-fō′bī-ă) [″+ Gr. *phobos*, fear]. Intense fear of an attack of angina pectoris.

anginose (ăn′jī-nōs) [L. *angina*, choking]. Pert. to or resembling angina.

anginous (ăn′jī-nŭs). Resembling angina. SYN: *anginose.*

angio- (ăn′jī-ō) [Gr. *angeion*, vessel]. A combining form denoting a seed, vessel, or something contained within a vessel.

angioataxia (ăn″gī-ō-ă-tăk′sē-ă) [″+ *ataktos*, out of order]. Variability in arterial tonus.

angioblast (ăn′jī-ō-blast) [″+ *blastos*, germ]. 1. The earliest tissue arising from mesenchyme cells of the embryo from which blood vessels develop. 2. A cell which participates in vessel formation.

angiocardiography (ăn″jī-ō-kar″dī-og′ră-phē) [Gr. *angeion*, vessel, + *kardia*, heart, + *graphein*, to write]. Roentgenography of the heart and great vessels after intravenous injection of a radiopaque diagnostic solution.

angiocardiokinetic (ăn″jī-ō-kar″dī-ō-kĭ-nĕt′ĭk) [″+ ″+ *kinesis*, movement]. Stimulating or that which affects movements of heart and blood vessels.

angiocarditis (ăn″jĭ-ō-kăr-dī'tis) ["+ "+ -*itis*, inflammation]. Inflammation of the heart and large blood vessels.

angiocavernous (ăn″jĭ-ō-kăv'er-nŭs) [Gr. *angeion*, vessel, + L. *caverna*, cavern]. Rel. to angioma cavernosum.

angiocholecystitis (ăn″jĭ-ō-kō″lĕ-sĭs-tī'tĭs) ["+ *cholē*, bile, + *kystis*, bladder, + -*itis*, inflammation]. Inflammation of gallbladder and bile vessels.

angiocholitis (ăn″jĭ-ō-kō-lī'tis) ["+ "+ -*itis*, inflammation]. Inflammation of biliary vessels; cholangitis.

angiocrine (ăn'jĭ-ō-krĭn) [Gr. *angeion*, vessel, + endocrine]. Marked by vasomotor disorders resulting from disturbances of the endocrine glands.

angiodermatitis (ăn″jĭ-ō-der-mă-tĭ'tĭs) ["+ *derma*, skin, + -*itis*, inflammation]. Inflammation of cutaneous vessels.

angiodystrophia (ăn″jĭ-ō-dĭs-trō'fĭ-ă) ["+ *dys*, bad, + *trophē*, nourishment]. Faulty nutrition of vessels.

angioedema (ăn″jĭ-ō-ĕ-dē'mă). Angioneurotic edema, q.v.

angioendothelioma (ăn″jĭ-ō-en″dō-thē″lĭ-ō'mă) [Gr. *angeion*, vessel, + *endotheli*, + -*ōma*, a tumor]. (pl. -*mata* or -*mas*) A tumor consisting of endothelial cells, commonly occurring as single or multiple tumors of bone.

angiofibroma (ăn″jĭ-ō-fĭ-brō'mă) ["+ L. *fibra*, fiber, + Gr. -*ōma*, tumor]. (pl. -*mas* or -*mata*) An angioma having connective tissue overgrowth.

angiogenesis (ăn″jĭ-ō-jen'ĕ-sis) ["+ *genesis*, origin]. Development of blood vessels.

angiogenic (ăn″jĭ-ō-jĕn'ĭk). Pert. to angiogenesis; of vascular origin.

angioglioma (ăn″jĭ-ō-gli-ō'mă) [Gr. *angeion*, vessel, + *glia*, glue, + -*ōma*, tumor]. A mixed angioma and glioma.

angiogram ["+ *gramma*, mark]. A series of x-ray film of a blood vessel taken in rapid sequence following the injection of a radiopaque substance into the vessel. This technique has been used to define the size and shape of various veins and arteries of organs and tissues.

    a., cerebral. A. of blood vessels, esp. the arterial system, of the brain.

angiograph (an'jĭ-ō-grăf') ["+ *graphein*, to write]. A variety of sphygmograph.

angiography (an″jĭ-ŏg'ră-fĭ). 1. A description of blood vessels and lymphatics. 2. Examination of blood vessels by roentgen rays. Vessels are made visible by injection of radiopaque substance. 3. Recording the movements of the arterial pulse by use of a sphygmograph.

    a., cerebral. An x-ray of the vascular system.

angiohyallnosis (ăn″jĭ-ō-hī″ă-lin-ō'sis) [Gr. *angeion*, vessel, + *yalos*, glass, + -*ōsis*, production]. Hyaline or glassy degeneration of the muscular coat of blood vessels.

angiohypertonia (ăn″gĭ-ō-hī″pĕr-tō'ni-ă) ["+ *hyper*, over, + *tonos*, tension]. Condition marked by spasm of blood vessels, esp. arteries. SYN: *vasospasm*. SEE: *hypertension*.

angiohypotonia (ăn″jĭ-ō-hī″po-tō'ni-ă) ["+ *hypo*, under, + *tonos*, tension]. Angioparalysis; angioparesis; vascular dilatation. SEE: *hypotension*.

angioid (ăn'jĭ-oyd) [Gr. *angeion*, vessel, + *eidos*, resemblance]. Resembling a blood vessel.

    a. streaks. Dark, wavy, anastomosing striae lying beneath retinal vessels.

angiokeratoma (ăn″jĭ-ō-ker″ă-tō'mă) ["+ *keras*, horn, + -*ōma*, tumor]. A skin disorder occurring chiefly on feet and legs, and characterized by formation of telangiectases or warty growths (in groups), accompanied by thickening of the epidermis along the course of dilated capillaries.

angiokinetic (ăn″jĭ-ō-kĭ-nĕt'ĭk) ["+ *kinesis*, movement]. Pert. to action of blood vessels.

angioleukasia (ăn″gĭ-ō-lū-kā'sĭ-ă) [Gr. *angeion*, vessel, + *leukos*, white, + *asia*, condition]. Dilatation of lymphatics.

angioleukitis (ăn″jĭ-ō-lū-ki'tis) ["+ "+ -*itis*, inflammation]. Inflammation of lymphatics.

angiolipoma (ăn'jĭ-ō-lip-ō'-mă) ["+ *lipos*, fat, + -*ōma*, tumor]. A mixed angioma and lipoma.

angiolith (ăn'jĭ-ō-lĭth) [Gr. *angeion*, vessel, + *lithos*, stone]. Calcareous deposit in wall of a blood vessel.

angiology (ăn″jĭ-ŏl'ō-jĭ) ["+ *logos*, science]. The science of the blood vessels and lymphatics.

angiolupoid (ăn″jĭ-ō-lu'poyd). A tuberculous skin lesion consisting of small, oval, red plaques.

angiolymphitis (an″jĭ-ō-lim-fī'tĭs) [Gr. *angeion*, vessel, + L. *lympha*, lymph, + -*itis*, inflammation]. Inflammation of the lymphatics. SYN: *lymphangitis*.

angiolymphoma (ăn″jĭ-ō-lim-fō'mă) ["+ "+ -*ōma*, tumor]. Tumor formed principally of dilated lymphatics.

angiolysis (ăn″jĭ-ŏl'ĭ-sis) ["+ *lysis*, destruction]. Obliteration of blood vessels as in the umbilical cord when it is tied just after birth.

angioma (ăn″jĭ-ō'mă) [Gr. *angeion*, vessel, + -*ōma*, tumor]. A form of tumor, usually benign, consisting principally of blood or lymph vessels. Considered to be remnants of fetal tissue misplaced or undergoing disordered development. SYN: *hemangioma; lymphangioma*. SEE: *choristoma; epithelioma; hamartoma; nevus*.

a. cavernosum. A. that is congenital; appears as an elevated dark red tumor, ranging in size from a pea to that of the hand. It may pulsate; commonly involves the subcutaneous or submucous tissue. It is nonmaligant and small ones may disappear without therapy. SYN: *strawberry mark*.

a., flat. A superficial a. which may occur at any part of the body. SYN: *nevus flammeus; port-wine stain*.

a., senile. An a. common in elderly persons and consisting of a compressible mass of blood vessels. SYN: *ruby spot*.

a., serpiginous. A skin disorder characterized by appearance of small, red vascular dots arranged in rings on the skin.

a. simplex. One that is congenital, made up of capillaries, nonelevated, bright red or purple-red in color; may cover a large surface; usually found on the face, commonly called "Mother's mark." No satisfactory treatment. Cosmetic creams are usually sufficient. SYN: *nevus flammeus; port-wine stain*.

a., stellate. An a. in which numerous telangiectatic vessels radiate from a central point. They usually occur on the face and are commonly associated with hepatic disease, hypertension, and pregnancy. SYN: *spider hemangioma; spider nevus*.

a. venosum racemosum. Swelling associated with greatly enlarged superficial varicose veins.

angiomalacia (an″jĭ-ō-mă-lā′sĭ-ă) ["+ *malakia*, softness]. Softening of blood vessel walls.

angiomatosis (an″jĭ-ō-mă-tō′sis) ["+ *-ōma*, tumor, + *-ōsis*, condition]. Condition of multiple angiomata.

a. retinae. Primary angioma of retina.

angiomatous (an″jĭ-ō′mă-tus). Resembling an angioma.

angiomegaly (ăn″jĭ-ō-mĕg′ă-lĭ) [Gr. *angeion*, vessel, + *megas*, large]. Enlargement of blood vessels, esp. in the eyelid.

angiometer (an″jĭ-ŏm′ĕ-ter) ["+ *metron*, measure]. Instrument for measuring tension and diameter of vessels.

angiomyocardiac (ăn″jĭ-ō-mĭ″ō-kar′dĭ-ak) ["+ *mys*, muscle, + *kardia*, heart]. Pert. to blood vessels and cardiac muscle.

angiomyoma (ăn″jĭ-ō-mĭ-ō′mă) [Gr. *angeion*, vessel, + *mys*, muscle, + *-ōma*, tumor]. An angioma mixed with a myoma.

angiomyosarcoma (ăn″jĭ-ō-mĭ″ō-sar-kō′mă) ["+ "+ *sarx*, flesh, + *-ōma*, tumor]. Tumor containing elements of angioma, myoma, and sarcoma.

angioneurectomy (ăn″jĭ-ō-nū-rĕk′tō-mĭ) [Gr. *angeion*, vessel, + *neuron*, nerve, + *ektomē*, excision]. Excision of vessels and nerves.

angioneurosis (ăn″jĭ-ō-nū-rō′sis) ["+ "+ *-ōsis*, condition]. Spasm or paralysis of blood vessels, resulting from a disturbance of vasomotor system.

angioneurotic (ăn″jĭ-ō-nū-rot′ik). Pert. to angioneurosis.

a. edema. A condition characterized by development of local allergic wheals accompanied by swelling of subcutaneous or submucous tissues. It is benign and thought to be an allergic disorder, usually a food allergy. SYN: *angioedema; hives; giant urticaria; Quincke's disease; urticaria.*

angioneurotomy (ăn″jĭ-ō-nū-rŏt′ō-mĭ) [Gr. *angeion*, vessel, + *neuron*, nerve, + *tomē*, cutting]. Cutting of vessels and nerves.

angionoma (ăn″jĭ-ō-nō′mă) ["+ *nomē*, ulcer]. Ulceration of a vessel.

angioparalysis (ăn″jĭ-ō-pă-ral′ĭ-sĭs) ["+ *paralyein*, loosen, dissolve]. Vasomotor relaxation of blood vessel tone.

angioparesis (ăn″jĭ-ō-pă-rē′sis) [Gr. *angeion*, vessel, + *paresis*, weakness]. Partial paralysis of the vasomotor system.

angiopathology (ăn″jĭ-ō-pă-thŏl′ō-jĭ) ["+ *pathos*, suffering, + *logos*, science]. Morbid changes of the blood vessels.

angiopathy (ăn-jĭ-ŏp′ă-thĭ). Any disease of blood vessels or lymphatics.

angioplany (ăn′jĭ-ō-plan′ĭ) [Gr. *angeion*, vessel, + *planē*, wandering]. Abnormal location, course, or structure of a blood vessel.

angioplasty (ăn′jĭ-ō-plas″tĭ) ["+ *plassein*, to form]. Plastic surgery upon blood vessels.

angiopoietic (ăn″jĭ-ō-poy-ĕt′ĭk) ["+ *poiein*, to make]. Pertaining to or causing the formation of blood vessels.

angiopressure (ăn′jĭ-ō-prĕsh″ŭr) [Gr. *angeion*, vessel, + *pressure*]. Control of hemorrhage by pressure.

angiopsathyrosis (ăn″jĭ-ō-sath″ĭ-rō′sĭs) ["+ *psathyrousthai*, to crumble away]. Fragility of blood vessels.

angiorhigosis (ăn″jĭ-ō-rĭ-go′sĭs) ["+ *rhigos*, cold]. Rigidity of vessels.

angiorrhaphy (ăn″jĭ-or′a-fĭ) [Gr. *angeion*, vessel, + *rhaphē*, seam]. Suture of a vessel or vessels.

angiorrhea (ăn″jĭ-ō-rē′ă) ["+ *rhoia*, flow]. Oozing of blood from vessels.

angiorrhexis (ăn″jĭ-or-eks′is) ["+ *rhēxis*, rupture]. Rupture of a blood vessel.

angiosarcoma (ăn″jĭ-ō-sar-kō′mă) [Gr. *angeion*, vessel, + *sarx*, flesh, + *-ōma*, tumor]. Mixed sarcoma and angioma.

angiosclerosis (ăn″jĭ-ō-sklĕ-rō′sĭs) [″+ *sklērōsis*, hardening]. Hardening of the walls of the vascular system.

angioscope (ăn′jĭ-ō-skōp) [″+ *skopein*, to view]. A microscope for studying capillary vessels.

angiosialitis (ăn″jĭ-ō-sī-ă-lī′tĭs) [Gr. *angeion*, vessel, + *sialon*, saliva, + *-itis*, inflammation]. Inflammation of a salivary duct.

angiosis (ăn″jĭ-ō′sĭs) [″+ *-ōsis*, condition]. Any disease of the lymphatics or blood vessels.

angiospasm (ăn′jĭ-ō-spazm) [″+ *spasmos*, tension, spasm]. Spasmodic contraction of blood vessels. May cause cramping of muscles or intermittent claudication.

angiospastic (ăn″jĭ-ō-spăs′tĭk). Pert. to angiospasm.

angiostenosis (ăn″jĭ-ō-stĕ-nō′sĭs) [″+ *stenoein*, to make narrow, + *-ōsis*, condition]. Narrowing of a tube or passage, especially a blood vessel.

angiosteosis (ăn″jĭ-os″tē-ō′sĭs) [″+ *osteon*, bone]. Calcareous degeneration of walls of blood or lymph vessels.

angiostomy (ăn″jĭ-ŏs′to-mĭ) [Gr. *angeion*, vessel, + *stoma*, mouth]. Operation making artificial fistulous opening into a blood vessel.

angiostrophy (ăn″jĭ-os′trō-fĭ) [″+ *strophē*, twist]. Twisting cut end of a vessel.

angiosynizesis (ăn″jĭ-ō-sĭn″ĭ-zē′sĭs) [″+ *synizesis*, contraction]. Collapse of walls of a vessel and their subsequent adhesion.

angiotaxis (ăn″jĭ-ō-tăk′sĭs) [Gr. *angeion*, vessel, + *staxis*, trickling]. 1. Hemophilia or hemorrhagic diathesis. 2. Oozing of blood.

angiotelectasis (ăn″jĭ-ō-tĕl-ek′tă-sĭs) [Gr. *angeion*, vessel, + *telos*, end, + *ektasis*, stretching out]. Dilatation of terminal arterioles.

angiotenic (ăn″jĭ-ō-ten′ĭk) [″+ *teinen*, to stretch]. Characterized by or caused by distention of blood vessels.

angiotensin (ăn″jĭ-ō-ten′sin). A pressor substance that is formed in the body by interaction of renin and a serum globulin fraction. It increases arterial muscle tone. Formerly called angiotonin or hypertensin.

angiotitis (ăn″jĭ-ō-tī′tĭs) [Gr. *angeion*, vessel, + *ous*, *ōt-*, ear, + *-itis*, inflammation]. Inflammation of blood vessels of the ear.

angiotome (ăn′jĭ-ō-tōm″) [″+ *tomē*, cutting]. One of the segments of the vascular tissues of the embryo.

angiotomy (ăn″jĭ-ŏt′ō-mĭ). Dissection of blood vessels.

angiotonic (ăn″jĭ-ō-ton′ĭk) [Gr. *angeion*, vessel, + *tonos*, tension]. Pert. to increase of arterial tension.

angiotonin (ăn″jĭ-ō-tōn′in). Former name for angiotensin, q.v.

angiotribe (ăn′jĭ-ō-trīb″) [Gr. *angeion*, vessel, + *tribein*, to crush]. Instrument for crushing the end of an artery to check hemorrhage. SYN: *vasotribe*.

angiotripsy (ăn′jĭ-ō-trip″sĭ) [″+ *tripsis*, friction]. The use of an angiotribe to check hemorrhage.

angiotrophic (ăn″jĭ-ō-trof′ik) [″+ *trophē*, nourishment]. Pert. to nutrition of blood vessels.

angitis (ăn-jī′tĭs) [″+ *-itis*, inflammation]. Inflammation of the blood vessels or lymphatics. SYN: *angiitis*.

angle (ăng′gl) [L. *angulus*]. 1. The space or area enclosed near the point or line where two lines or planes meet. 2. A projecting or sharp corner.

a., acromial. Point of junction of lateral and posterior borders of the acromion.

a., acute. An a. less than 90°.

a., alpha. One found by intersection of visual line with optic axis.

a., alveolar. Meeting point of the base of the nasal spine and the middle point of the alveolus of the upper jaw.

a., basilar. Formed by the intersection of a projection line from the nasal point to a line drawn at the base of the nasal spine.

a., biorbital. Formed by the meeting of the axes of the orbits.

a., carrying. A. made at the elbow by extending the long axis of the forearm and the upper arm. This obtuse angle is more pronounced in the female than in the male.

a., cerebellopontile, a., cerebellopontine. Junction of the cerebellum and pons.

a. of convergence. A. between the visual axis and the median line when an object is looked at.

a., costal. Meeting point of the lower border of the false ribs with the axis of the sternum.

a., craniofacial. A. formed at the point where the basifacial and basicranial axes join at the midpoint of the sphenoethmoidal sutures.

a., facial. A. made by lines from the nasal spine and external auditory meatus meeting between the upper middle incisor teeth.

a., gamma. A. formed by line of fixation with optic axis.

a. of incidence. A. between a ray incident on a surface and a line drawn perpendicular to the surface at the point of incidence.

a. of iris. A. between the cornea and iris at the periphery of the anterior chamber of the eye.

a. of jaw. A. at the point where the posterior edge of the ramus of the mandible and the lower surface of the body of the mandible join.

a. of mandible. A. of the jaw.

a., metafacial. A. between the base of the skull and the pterygoid process.

a., obtuse. An a. greater than 90°.

a., occipital. Formed by the intersection of lines from the basion and from the lower border of the orbit at the opisthion.

a., ophryospinal. A. formed by the joining of lines drawn from the auricular point and the glabella at the anterior nasal spine.

a., optic. SEE: *visual angle.*

a., parietal. Formed by the meeting of the prolongation of the two lines tangent to the prominent portion of the zygomatic arch and the parietofrontal suture.

a., pontine. Same as cerebellopontine a., q.v.

a., pubic. Junction of the rami of the pubes.

a., sphenoid. Formed by the intersection of lines coming from the nasal point and the tip of the rostrum of the sphenoid, at top of the sella turcica.

a., sternal. A. between the manubrium and the body of the sternum.

a., venous. A. of the internal jugular and subclavian vein.

a., visual. The a. formed by drawing lines from the nodal point of the eye to the extreme edges of the visual object.

angophrasia (an″gō-frā′zǐ-ā) [Gr. *anchein,* to choke, + *phrasis,* utterance]. Drawling, choking speech in paralytic dementia.

angor (ang′gor) [L., strangling]. Violent distress as in angina pectoris.

angor animi (ang′ōr ăn′ĭ-mī) [″ + soul]. Overwhelming feeling of impending death or disaster.

angstrom unit (ōng′strŭm). [Anders J. Ångström, Swedish physicist, 1814-1874]. An internationally adopted unit of measurement of wave length: one ten-millionth of a millimeter, or one two hundred and fifty-four millionth of an inch. Used especially to specify radiation wavelengths. Also called angstrom. SYMB: Å.

Anguillula (ang-gwil′ū-lā) [L., eel]. Genus of nematode worms.

A. aceti. Vinegar eel.

A. intestinalis. Parasitic form of nematode infesting intestine in tropics and near-tropics. SYN: *Strongyloides intestinalis.*

A. stercoralis. Free stage of A. intestinalis. SYN: *Strongyloides stercoralis,* q.v.

anguilluliasis (ang-gwil-ū-lī′ā-sĭs). Infestation with anguillula.

angular [L.]. Having corners or angles.

a. artery. The artery at the inner canthus of the eye; facial artery.

angulation (ăng″ū-lā′shŭn). Formation of angular loops in the intestine, a blood vessel, or ureter.

anhaphia (ăn-hā′fĭ-ā) [Gr. *an-,* not, + *aphē,* touch]. Abnormal or defective sense of touch. SYN: *anaphia.*

anhedonia (ăn″hē-dō′nĭ-ā) [″ + *ēdonē,* pleasure]. Lacking in interest or pleasure in acts which are normally pleasurable. May be an early sign of schizophrenia.

anhedonic (ăn″hē-don′ik). Pert. to anhedonia.

anhelation (ăn-hĕl-ā′shŭn) [L. *anhelare,* to pant]. Dyspnea, shortness of breath.

anhematopoiesis (ăn-hē-mă-tō-poi-ē′sĭs) [Gr. *an,* not, + *haima,* blood, + *poiein,* to make]. Defective blood formation. SYN: *anhematosis.*

anhematosis (ăn″hēm-ă-tō′sĭs) [″ + *haimatoein,* to change into blood]. Defective or insufficient blood formation.

anhemolytic (ăn-hē-mō-lĭt′ĭk) [″ + *haima,* blood, + *lytikos,* dissolving]. Not destructive to the blood cells.

anhepatia (ăn-hē-pā′shĭ-ā) [Gr. *an-,* not, + *ēpar,* liver]. Failure or deficiency of liver function.

anhepatic (an-he-păt′ĭk). Not produced by the liver.

anhepatogenic (an-hep-ă-tō-jen′ĭk) [Gr. *an-,* not, + *hēpar,* liver, + *gennan,* to produce]. Not produced by or arising in the liver. SYN: *anhepatic.*

anhidrosis (ăn″hĭ-drō′sis) [Gr. *an-,* not, + *hidros,* sweat]. Diminished or complete absence of secretion of sweat. May be generalized or localized, temporary or permanent, accompanying disease conditions or may be a congenital anomaly. SYN: *anidrosis.*

TREATMENT: Treatment of cause or accompanying conditions. Soft, nonirritating clothing; bland, soothing ointments and lubricants for skin. Air conditioning provides comfort in most instances.

anhidrotic (ăn″hĭ-drot′ik). Inhibiting or preventing, or anything that inhibits or prevents perspiration. SYN: *anidrotic.*

anhistic, anhistous (ăn-hĭs′tĭk, -hĭs′tŭs) [Gr. *an-*, not, + *histos*, tissue]. Seemingly without structure.

anhydration (an-hī-drā′shŭn) ["+ *hydōr*, water]. The state of not being hydrated; dehydration.

anhydremia (an-hī-drē′mĭ-ä) ["+ "+ *haima*, blood]. A lessening of the normal quantity of fluids in the blood.

anhydride (an-hī′drĭd) [Gr. *an-*, not, + *hydōr*, water]. A substance from which the hydrogen and oxygen, in the ratio in which they exist in water, have been removed.

anhydrochloric (an-hī-drō-klō′rĭk) ["+ "+ *chlōros*, green]. Lacking in hydrochloric acid.

anhydromyelia (an-hī-drō-mī-e′lĭ-ä) ["+ "+ *myelos*, marrow]. Deficiency in spinal fluid.

anhydrous (an-hī′drŭs) [Gr. *an-*, not, + *hydōr*, water]. Containing no water.

anhypnia (an-hip′nĭ-ä) [Gr. *an-*, not, + *hypnos*, sleep]. Insomnia; sleeplessness; anhypnosis.

anhypnosis (an-hĭp-nō′sĭs). Insomnia.

anianthinopsy (an-ī-an′thin-op″sī) [Gr. *an-*, not, + *ianthinos*, violet, + *opsis*, vision]. Inability to recognize violet tints.

anidrosis (an-ĭ-drō′sĭs) [Gr. *an-*, not, + *hidrōs*, sweat]. Abnormal deficiency of sweat. SYN: *anhidrosis.* q.v.

anidrotic (an-ĭ-drot′ĭk). Pert. to anidrosis. SYN: *anhidrotic.*

anile (ăn′ĭl, ā′nĭl) [L. *anus*, an old woman]. 1. Infirm; as an old woman. 2. Senile.

aniline (an′ĭ-lĭn) [Ar. *an-nil*, the indigo plant]. The simplest aromatic amine, $C_6H_5NH_2$, an oily liquid derived from benzene. Used in manufacture of dyes for medical and industrial purposes. SYN: *aminobenzene; phenylamine.*

anilinophil, anilinophilous (an″ĭ-lin′ō-fĭl, -lin-of′ĭ-lus) ["+ Gr. *philos*, fond]. A structure staining readily with aniline dyes.

anilism (ăn′ĭl-ĭzm) ["+ *-ismos*, condition]. Chronic aniline poisoning. SYN: *anilinism.*
SYM: Cardiac block, weakness, intermittent pulse, vertigo, muscular depression, cyanosis. SEE: *aniline* in *Table of Poisons and Poisoning* in *Appendix.*

anility (ă-nĭl′ĭ-tĭ) [L. *anus*, an old woman]. Old age in females.

anima (an′ĭ-mä) [L. soul]. 1. Soul. 2. According to Jung, an individual's true inner self as distinguished from the "image" or appearance or external character *(persona)* presented to the observer. Anima refers to the feminine inner personality, esp. as present in men, as compared to animus, which refers to the masculine personality, esp. as present in women.

a. mundi. Paracelsus' term for the vital force essential to the continuity of life.

animal (ăn′ĭ-mäl) [L. *animālis, living*]. 1. A living organism, not a plant, which has certain features: mobility; a nervous system; nutritional requirements involving changing complex substances into simpler ones and then resynthesizing them. Animals usually do not store or manufacture chlorophyll. In some acellular organisms the distinction between plant and animal cannot be made. 2. Any animal, especially a four-footed one, other than man. 3. Pert. to or from an animal. 4. A subhuman or inhuman person, one who is beastlike.

animalcule (ăn″ĭ-mal′kūl) [L. *animalculum*, little animal]. Any microscopic animal organism. A protozoan.

animation (ăn-ĭ-mā″shŭn) [L. *animus*, soul]. State of being alive, or active.

a., suspended. Temporary cessation of vital activities such as respiration with loss of consciousness; state of apparent death.

animi agitatio ["+ *agitore*, to turn over in the mind]. Mental agitation.

anincretinosis (an-in″krē-tĭ-nō′sis) [Gr. *an-*, not, + *incrētus*, sifted in, + *-ōsis*, condition]. A disorder due to failure of an endocrine gland or system to produce a hormone.

anion (an′ĭ-on) [Gr. *ana*, up, + *iōn*, going]. An ion carrying a negative charge. Since unlike forms of electricity attract each other, this ion is attracted by, and travels to, the positive anode. Examples are acid radicals and corresponding radicals of their salts. SEE: *ion.*

anionic (an″ĭ-on′ĭk). Containing or pert. to anions.

a. detergent. A chemical substance with disinfectant properties due to the presence of an active negatively-charged chemical group. May be natural or synthetic.

anirid′ia [Gr. *an-*, not, + *iris*, rainbow, iris]. Congenital absence, complete or partial, of iris. SYN: *irideremia.*

anischuria (an″ĭs-kū′rĭ-ä) ["+ *ischouria*, retention of urine]. Incontinence of urine; enuresis.

aniseikonia (ăn-īs-ĭ-kō′nĭ-ä) [Gr. *anisos*, unequal, + *eikōn*, image]. A condition in which the size and shape of the ocular image of one eye differs from that of the other.

anisergy (ăn-is′ĕr-jĭ) ["+ *ergon*, work]. Varying degrees of blood pressure in different parts of the system.

aniso- (an-is-o). Prefix denoting unequal, unsymmetrical in combination.

anisochromatic (an-ī″sō-krō-mat′ĭk) [Gr. *anisos*, unequal, + *chrōma*, color]. Not of uniform color.

anisocoria (an-ĭ″sō-kō′rĭ-ă) ["+ *korē*, pupil]. Inequality of the diameter of the pupils; may be normal or congenital.

Often seen in early stages of insanity, each pupil alternating in contraction and dilation. Found in aneurysms, head trauma, diseases of the nervous system, brain lesion, paresis, and locomotor ataxia.

anisocytosis (an-ĭ″sō-sī-tō′sis) ["+ *kytos*, cell, + *-ōsis*, condition]. Inequality in size of cells, esp. erythrocytes. An abnormal condition.

anisogamy (an″ĭ-sog′ă-mĭ) [Gr. *anisos*, unequal, + *gamos*, marriage]. Sexual fusion of two gametes of different form and size.

anisognathous (an″ĭ-sog′nă-thus) ["+ *gnathos*, jaw]. Having upper jaw wider than lower one.

anisohypercytosis (an-ĭ″sō-hī″per-sī-tō′sis) ["+ *hyper*, above, + *kytos*, cell]. Increase in number of leukocytes with altered proportion of the different varieties. Opposed to anisohypocytosis.

anisohypocytosis (ăn-ĭ″sō-hī″pō-sī-tō′sĭs) ["+ *hypo*, below, + "]. Decrease in number of leukocytes with altered proportion of different varieties. Opposed to anisohypercytosis.

anisoiconia (ăn-ĭ″sō-ĭ-kō′nĭ-ă) [Gr. *anisos*, unequal, + *eikōn*, image]. Condition in which ocular image in one eye is different in size and shape from that of other. SYN: *aniseikonia*, q.v.

anisomastia (ăn-ĭ-so-măs′tĭ-ă) ["+ *mastos*, breast]. Breasts unequal in size.

anisomelia (ăn-ĭ″so-me′lĭ-ă) ["+ *melos*, limb]. Inequality between two paired limbs.

anisometrope (ăn-ĭ″sō-mĕt′rōp) [Gr. *anisos*, unequal, + *metron*, measure, + *ops*, vision]. One afflicted with anisometropia.

anisometropia (ăn-ĭ″sō-me-trō′pĭ-ă). Inequality in refractive power of the two eyes.

anisometropic (an-ĭ″sō-mĕ-trŏp′ĭk). Having unequal refractive power.

anisonormocyto′sis (ăn-ĭ″so-nŏr″mo-sī-tō′sĭs) [Gr. *anisos*, unequal, + L. *norma*, rule, + Gr. *kytos*, cell]. Abnormal relation in numbers of different forms of leukocytes but with normal number of total leukocytes.

anisopia (ăn″ĭ-so′pĭ-ă) ["+ *ops*, vision]. Inequality of visual power of both eyes.

anisopiesis (an-ĭ″sō-pī-ē′sis) ["+ *piesis*, blood pressure]. Apparent inequality of blood pressure in different parts of the body.

anisorhythmia (ăn-ĭ″so-rith′mĭ-ă) [Gr. *anisos*, unequal, + *rythmos*, rhythm]. Absence of synchronism in rate of the atria and ventricles or irregular heart action.

anisospore (an′ĭ-sō-spōr) ["+ *sporos*, seed]. A sexual cell. Opposed to isospore.

anisosthen′ic (ăn-ĭ″sos-then′ĭk) ["+ *sthenos*, strength]. Not of equal muscle strength.

anisotropal (ăn″is-ot′rō-pal) [Gr. *anisos*, unequal, + *tropos*, a turning]. 1. Not equal in every direction. 2. Unequal in power of refraction. SYN: *anisotropous*.

anisotrop′ic (ăn-ĭ″so-trŏp′ĭk). Having different optical properties in different directions, as have certain crystals; double polarizing.

anisotropous (ăn-ĭ-sot′ro-pus). 1. Not equal in every direction. 2. Unequal in refractive power. SYN: *anisotropal*.

anisuria (an″is-ū′rĭ-ă) [Gr. *anisos*, unequal, + *ouron*, urine]. Alternate polyuria and oliguria, q.v.

ankle (ăng′kl) [AS. *ancléow*]. 1. The joint between the foot and lower end of leg. 2. In popular usage the region of this joint, including the tarsus and lower end of leg.

   a. bone. The talus.

   a. clonus. Repetitive extension-flexion movement of muscles of ankle, associated with increased muscle tonus. Commonly a symptom of corticospinal disease.

   NP: Keep patient's feet at right angles on a rectangular foot splint. When splint is removed for examination, etc., avoid dorsiflexion of foot to prevent movement of ankle, clonus or spasm.

   a. clonus reflex. Elicited by quick, vigorous dorsiflexion of the foot while the knee is held in a flexed position, resulting in repeated clonic movement of the foot so long as the foot is maintained in dorsiflexion.

   a. jerk. Contraction of calf muscles resulting in extension of the foot following a blow upon the Achilles tendon.

   a. joint. A hinge joint. Lower part of tibia, its medial malleolus and lateral malleolus of fibula, forming socket for the talus.

   a., tailor's. An abnormal bursa over the head of the fibula in tailors from pressure caused by sitting cross-legged on the floor.

ankylo- (ăng′kĭ-lō) [Gr. *ankylē*, a stiff joint, from *ankulos*, bent]. Combining form meaning crooked, bent, a fusion or growing together of parts.

ankyloblepharon (ăng″kĭ-lo-blef′ar-on) ["+ *blepharon*, eyelid]. Adhesion of ciliary edges of lids to each other.

ankylochilia (ăng″kĭ-lo-ki′lĭ-ă) ["+ *cheilos*, lip]. Adhesion of lips to each other.

ankylocolpos (ăng-kĭ-lo-kol′pos) [Gr. *ankylē*, a stiff joint, + *kolpos*, vagina]. Imperforation or atresia of the vagina.

ankylodactylia (ăng-kĭ-lo-dak-til′e-ah) ["+ *daktylos*, finger]. Adhesion of two or more fingers or toes to one another.

ankyloglossia (ăng″kĭ-lo-glos′sĭ-ă) ["+ *glōssa*, tongue]. Abnormal shortness of frenum of tongue; tongue-tie.

ankyloproctia (ăng″kĭ-lo-prok′shĭ-ă) [Gr. *ankylē*, a stiff joint, + *prōktos*, anus]. Stricture or imperforation of the anus.

ankylosed (ăng′kĭ-lōst). Denoting fixation of a joint. Stiffened; held by adhesions; affected with ankylosis, q.v.

ankylosis (ăng″kyl-o′sis) [Gr. *ankylē*, stiff joint]. Abnormal immobility and fixation of a joint due to pathological changes in the joint or its surrounding tissue.

ETIOL: May be congenital, sometimes hereditary, or it may be result of disease. Seen in many joint conditions. May be performed surgically.

NP: If done surgically, maintain complete immobility of joint until bone has firmly united, which may be from six to 12 weeks. Keep joint in perfect position.

　　a., artificial. The surgical fixation of a joint.

　　a., bony. The abnormal union of the bones of a joint, also called true ankylosis.

　　a., extracapsular. That caused by rigidity of parts outside a joint.

　　a., false. Spurious a.; that due to rigidity of the surrounding parts.

　　a., fibrous. That due to the formation of fibrous bands within a joint only.

　　a., intracapsular. That due to the undue rigidity of structure within a joint.

　　a., ligamentous. A. by ligaments or fibrous structures.

　　a., true. Same as a., bony, q.v.

Ankylostoma (ăng″kĭ-los′to-mă) ["+ *stoma*, stomach]. Genus of nematode parasites; Ancylostoma, q.v.

ankylostoma (ăng″kĭ-los′to-mă). Trismus, lockjaw.

ankylostomiasis (ăng″kĭ-lo-sto-mi′ă-sĭs). Hookworm disease; ancylostomiasis, q.v.

ankylotia (ăng″kĭ-lō′shĭ-ă) [Gr. *ankylos*, crooked, + *ot-*, ear]. Closure or imperforation of external auditory meatus of ear.

ankylotome (ăng″kil-ō-tōm, ăng-kil′o-tōm) ["+ *tomē*, a cutting]. An instrument for cutting the frenulum of the tongue in tongue-tie.

ankylurethria (ăng″kĭl-ū-rē′thrĭ-ă) ["+ *ourethra*, urethra]. Stricture or imperforation of the urethra.

ankyroid (ang′kĭ-royd) [Gr. *ankyra*, hook, + *eidos*, form]. Hook-shaped.

　　a. cavity. The posterior or descending cornu of lateral ventricle of the brain.

anlage (än′lă-gē) [Ger., a laying on]. Primordium; the first accumulation of cells in an embryo which constitutes the beginning of a future tissue, organ, or part.

annatto (ă-nŏ′tŏ) [Cariban]. Reddish coloring matter obtained from the pulp of Bixa orellana, a tropical tree. Also spelled anatto, arnato.

annectent (ă-nek′tent) [L. *annectens*, tying or binding to]. Linking together.

Annelida (ă-nel′ĭ-dă). The phylum which includes the segmented worms. Ex: earthworm. The only annelids of medical significance are leeches, belonging to the class Hirudinea, q.v. Some annelids serve as intermediate hosts for parasitic worms.

annexa (ă-nĕks′ă) [L. *annectere*, to tie or bind to]. Accessory parts. SYN: *adnexa.*

annexitis (ă-nĕks-ī′tĭs) ["+ Gr. *-itis*, inflammation]. Inflammation of adnexa uteri. SYN: *adnexitis.*

annexopexy (ă-nĕks′ō-pĕks-ē) ["+ Gr. *pexis*, putting together]. Fixation of fallopian tubes and ovary to abdominal wall. SYN: *adnexopexy.*

annular (ăn′ū-lăr) [L. *annulus*, ring]. Circular; ring-shaped.

annulorrhaphy (an″ū-lor′ă-fĭ) ["+ Gr. *rhaphē*, seam]. Closure of a hernial ring by suture.

annulus (ăn′ū-lŭs) [L.]. (pl. *annuli*) A ring-shaped structure; a ring. SYN: *annulus.* [NA].

　　a. abdominalis. The internal or deep inguinal ring.

　　a. ciliaris. Boundary between choroid and iris.

　　a. femoralis. The femoral ring.

　　a. inguinalis profundus. The abdominal inguinal ring.

　　a. inguinalis superficialis. Subcutaneous inguinal ring; superficial or external inguinal ring.

　　a. migrans. A disease of the tongue characterized by appearance of yellow-bordered red patches on dorsum and sides of tongue.

　　a. tympanicus. The tympanic ring.

　　a. umbilicalis. Fibrous ring which, in late fetal life, surrounds opening through which umbilical vessels enter and leave cord.

　　a. urethralis. Circular elevated ring in bladder surrounding internal orifice of urethra.

anoci-association (ă-nŏ″sĭ-ă-sō″sĭ-ā′shŭn) [Gr. *a*, not, + L. *nocere*, to injure + association]. An anesthetic technique for helping to prevent shock from continuous preoperative apprehension. This is done by careful, prolonged use of preoperative sedation and narcotics, also local anesthesia used in conjunction with general anesthesia. This complex procedure is little used now.

anococcygeal (ā"nō-kok-sī'je-al) [L. *anus*, + Gr. *kokkyx*]. Rel. to both anus and coccyx.

a. body. The muscle and fibrous tissue lying between the coccyx and anus.

a. ligament. A band of fibrous tissue joining the tip of the coccyx with the external sphincter ani.

anodal (ăn-ō'dăl) [Gr. *ana*, up, + *hodos*, way]. Pert. to the anode.

a. closure contraction. Contraction of muscles at anode on closure of circuit. ABBR: ACC.

anode (ăn'ōd). The positive pole of an electrical source. SEE: *cathode.*

anodinia (ăn"ō-din'ī-ă) [Gr. *an-*, not, + *ōdis*, pain of childbirth]. Absence of childbirth pains.

anodmia (an-od'mī-ă) ["+ *odmē*, stench]. The want or absence of the sense of smell; anosmia, q.v.

anodontia (an"o-don'shī-ă) ["+ *odous*, tooth]. Absence of teeth. SYN: *edentia.*

anodyne (ăn'ō-din) [Gr. *an-*, not, + *odynē*, pain]. An agent that will relieve pain. Ex: acetylsalicylic acid; codeine; morphine.

anodynia (an"ō-din'ī-ă). 1. Cessation or absence of pain. 2. Loss of sensation.

anoesia (ăn"ō-ē'zī-ă) [Gr. *anoēsia*, want of understanding]. Without power of comprehension; anoia; imbecility; idiocy.

anoetic (an"ō-et'ik) [Gr. *anoētos*, unthinkable]. Rel. to the borderline of consciousness; not fully conscious.

anoia (ă-noy'ă) [Gr. *a-*, not, + *noos*, understanding]. Anoesia, q.v.

anomalous (ă-nom'ă-lŭs) [Gr. *anōmalos*, uneven]. Irregular; contrary to the normal.

anomaly (ă-nŏm'ă-lī) [Gr. *anomalia*, irregularity]. 1. Anything contrary to general rule. 2. An organ or structure which is abnormal with reference to form, structure, or position; a malformation. SEE: *monster; teras; teratology.*

anomia (a-nō'mī-ă) [Gr. *a-*, not, + *onoma*, name]. Inability to remember names of persons and objects.

anonychia (an-ō-nik'ī-ă) [Gr. *an-*, not, + *onyx*, nail]. Absence of the nails.

anoopsia (an"ō-op'sī-ă) [Gr. *anō*, upward, + *opsis*, vision]. Tendency of one eye to turn upward. SYN: *hyperphoria.*

anoperineal (a"no-per-ī-ne'al). Concerning the anus and perineum.

Anopheles (ă-nŏf'ē-lēz) [Gr. *anōphelēs*, harmful, useless]. A genus of mosquitoes belonging to the family Culicidae, order Diptera. It is a vector of Plasmodium, the causative agent of malaria, and may be involved in the transmission of causative agent of dengue, filariasis, and possibly other diseases.

anophoria (ăn-ō-fo'rī-ă) [Gr. *ana*, up, + *pherein*, to bear]. Tendency of one eye to turn upward. SYN: *hyperphoria.*

anophthalmia (an-of-thal'mī-ă) [Gr. *an-*, not, + *ophthalmos*, eye]. Congenital absence of eyes.

anopia (an-ō'pī-ă) ["+ *ops*, eye]. Anophthalmos; lack of one eye or both.

Anoplura (an-o-plu'ră) [Gr. *anoplos*, unarmed, + *owia*, tail]. An order of the class insects which includes the sucking lice. SEE: *louse; pediculosis.*

anopsia (an-op'sī-ă) [Gr. *an-*, not, + *opsis*, sight]. 1. Hyperphoria. 2. Inability to use the vision as in those confined in the dark, or from disuse of an eye in strabismus, or resulting from cataract, or in refractive errors.

anorchism (an-or'kizm) ["+ *orchis*, testicle]. Congenital absence of one or both testes.

anorectal (an-ō-rek'tal) [L. *anus* + *rectum*]. Pert. to the anus and rectum.

anorectic, anorectous (an-ō-rek'tic, -tus) [Gr. *anorektos*, without appetite for]. Having no appetite.

anorexia (an-ō-reks'ī-ă) [Gr. *an-*, not, + *orexis*, appetite]. Loss of appetite. Seen in malaise, commencement of all fevers and illnesses, also in disorders of alimentary tract, esp. of stomach, and as a result of alcoholic excesses and drug addiction, esp. cocaine. Also result of food fads and faulty feeding.

RS: acoria, ageusia, bulimia, hyperorexia, nausea, parageusia, parorexia, pica, polyphagia, pyrosis, taste.

a. nervo'sa. Loss of appetite for food not explainable by local disease. It is the symptom of a mental illness. Occurs most commonly in females between the ages of 12 and 21 but may occur in older women and men. This symptom is not associated with a specific neurosis or psychosis. There is loss of weight, and amenorrhea in women and impotence in men. In young children it is one of the few psychiatric disorders which may lead to death. Psychiatric therapy in a hospital is usually required if patient refuses to eat anything.

anorexigenic (an"o-reks'ī-jen'ik) ["+ "+ *gennan*, to produce]. 1. A substance which produces loss of appetite. 2. Causing loss of appetite.

anorganic. Same as inorganic, q.v.

anormal [Gr. *a-*, not, + L. *normalis*, according to pattern]. Abnormal.

anorrhorrhea (an-or-or-ē'ă) [Gr. *an-*, not, + *orros*, serum, + *roia*, a flow]. Diminished or imperfect secretion of serous fluid.

anorthography (an-or-thog′rä-fĭ) ["+ *orthos*, straight, + *graphein*, to write]. Agraphia, esp. motor agraphia; loss of power to express oneself in writing. SEE: *agraphia.*

anorthopia (an-or-thō′pĭ-ă) ["+ "+ *ops*, eye]. 1. Vision in which straight lines do not appear straight; symmetry and parallelism not properly perceived. 2. Strabismus.

anorthosis (an-or-thō′sis) ["+ "+ *ōsis*, condition]. Absence of, or diminished, erectility.

anoscope (a′no-skōp) [L. *anus*, + *skopein*, to view]. Speculum for examining the anus and lower rectum.

anosmatic (an-oz-mat′ĭk) [Gr. *an-*, not, + *osmē*, smell]. Deficient sense of smell.

anosmia (an-oz′mĭ-ă). Absence of the sense of smell. Frequent in neurasthenia, hysteria, and sometimes in ataxia. SYN: *anodmia; anosphrasia.*

anosmic (an-oz′mik). Lacking in sense of smell.

anosmous (an-oz′mus). Anosmic. Pert. to anosmia.

anosodiaphoria (an-ō-sō-dĭ-ă-for′ĭ-ă) [Gr. *a-*, not, + *nosos*, disease, + *diaphoria*, difference]. Real or pretended indifference to presence of disease, esp. paralysis.

anosognosia (an-ō-sog-nō′zĭ-ă) ["+ "+ *gnosis*, knowledge]. Real or pretended ignorance of the presence of disease, esp. paralysis. Opposed to pathodixia, q.v.

anosphrasia (an-os-frā′zĭ-ă) [Gr. *an-*, not, + *osphrēsis*, smell]. Absence or imperfect sense of smell.

anospinal (a″no-spī′năl) [L. *anus* + *spina*, thorn]. Pert. to the anus and spinal cord, the center in the spinal cord which controls the contraction of the anal sphincter.

anostosis (an-os-tō′sis) [Gr. *an-*, not, + *osteon*, bone]. A defective formation or development of bone; failure to ossify.

anotia (an-ō′shē-ă) ["+ *ous, ōt-*, ear]. Congenital malformation with absence of the ears.

anotropia (an″o-tro′pĭ-ă) [Gr. *ana*, up, + *tropē*, a turning]. Tendency of the eyes to turn upward and away from the visual axis.

ANOVA. *An*alysis *o*f *va*riance.

anovaginal (a″no-vaj′ĭ-năl). Pertaining to the anus and vagina.

anovarism (an-ō′var-ĭzm) [Gr. *an-*, not, + L. *ovarium*, ovary]. Absence of ovaries.

anovesical (a″no-ves′ĭ-kal) [L. *anus* + *vesica*, bladder]. Rel. in any way to both anus and urinary bladder.

anovular, anovulatory (an-ov′u-lar, an-ov′u-la-tō″rĭ) [Gr. *an-*, not, + L. *ovarium*, ovary]. Not accompanied by production of and discharge of an ovum.

    a. cycle. Menstrual cycle wherein the menstrual flow was not preceded by ovulation.

anoxemia (an-oks-ē′mĭ-ă) ["+ oxygen + *haima*, blood]. A diminution in the amount of oxygen in the blood. SEE: *hypoxia.*

anoxia (an-oks′ĭ-ă) [Gr. *an-*, not, + oxygen]. Deficiency of oxygen. SEE: *hypoxia.*

    a., anemic. Deficiency in the oxygen-carrying power of the blood.

    a., anoxic. Diminished oxygen in the arterial blood despite normal ability of the blood to contain and carry oxygen (oxygen capacity). May be due to reduced oxygen supply, respiratory obstruction, reduced surface area in lungs for exchange of gases (as in pneumonia) or inadequate respiratory movements.

    a., hypokinetic. A., stagnant, q.v.

    a., stagnant. Generalized or localized oxygen lack due to deficiency in volume of blood as occurs in cardiac failure. shock, arterial spasm, thrombosis or other conditions which result in reduced circulation of blood.

anoxic (an-oks′ĭc). Pert. to or caused by a general lack of oxygen, and characterized by a generally subnormal oxygen tension of the blood.

ansa (an′să) [L. a handle]. (pl. *ansae*) [NA] Any anatomical structure in the form of a loop or arc.

    a. capitis. The zygomatic arch.

    a. cervicalis. [NA]. Formerly called a. hypoglossi. A loop in the middle of the neck formed by the descending hypoglossal nerve and the descending cervical nerve.

    a. hypoglos′si. [NA]. A. cervicalis, q.v.

    a. lenticula′ris. [NA]. Fibers entering the lenticular nucleus from the thalamus by way of the thalamic radiation.

    a. nervorum spinalium. [NA]. A. of spinal nerves. Connecting loops of fibers between the anterior spinal nerves.

    a. peduncularis. [NA]. Fibers passing from the thalamus through the thalamic radiation, under the lenticular nucleus to the cortex of the temporal lobe and insula.

    a. sacralis. Nerve cord connecting the sympathetic trunk with the ganglion impar.

    a. subclavia. [NA]. Loop of nerve fibers winding around the anterior aspect of the subclavian artery.

anselaphesia (ăn″sĕl-ă-fē′zĭ-ă). Absence of sense of touch or feeling or sensation, esp. of tactile sensibility.

anserine (ăn′sĕr-ĭn) [L. *anser*, goose]. 1. Pert. to a goose. 2. A specific substance first found in goose muscle and later in many animals but not man, dog, cattle or horse.

ansiform (ăn′sĭ-form) [L. *ansa*, a handle]. Shaped like a loop.

ant-, anti- [Gr.]. Prefix denoting opposed to, counteracting, against.

antabuse (ăn′tă-būs″). Proprietary name for disulfiram. Administered orally in alcoholism. Ingestion of alcohol following taking of drug causes unpleasant reaction including nausea and vomiting.

antacid (ant-as′ĭd) [Gr. *anti*, against, + L. *acidum*, acid]. An agent that will neutralize acidity, esp. in digestive tract. Ex: aluminum hydroxide; magnesium oxide.

antagonism (ăn-tăg′ō-nĭzm″) [Gr. *antagōnizesthai*, to struggle against]. Opposition or contrary action, as between muscles or medicines.

    a., bacterial. The inhibition of or killing of one bacterial organism by another.

antagonist (an-tag′o-nist). That which counteracts the action of anything, as a muscle or drug.

antalgesic (ant-al-jē′sĭk) [Gr. *anti*, against, + *algos*, pain]. Pain-relieving agent. SYN: *anodyne*.

antalgic (ant-al′jĭk). An anodyne or analgesic.

antalkaline (ant-al′ka-lin, -lĭn) [Gr. *anti*, against, + alkaline]. Neutralizing or reducing alkalinity.

antaphrodisiac (ant″af-ro-diz′ĭ-ak) [″+ *aphrodisiakos*, sexual]. Lessening sexual desire.

antarthritic (ănt″ăr-thrĭt′ĭk) [″+ *arthritikos*, gouty]. Remedy for gout.

antasthenic (ănt″ăs-thĕn′ĭk) [Gr. *anti*, against, + *astheneia*, weakness]. 1. Strengthening, invigorating. 2. Agent which invigorates.

antasthmatic (ant″az-mat′ĭk) [″+ *asthma*]. 1. An agent that prevents an asthmatic attack. 2. Relieving asthma.

antatrophic (ant″ă-trō′fĭk) [″+ *atrophia*, atrophy]. Preventing or curing atrophy.

ante- [L.]. Prefix meaning before.

antebrachium (an″tē-bra′kē-um) [L. *ante*, before, + *brachium*, arm]. [NA]. The forearm.

ante cibum (an′te si′bum) [L.]. Before meals.

antecornu (an″te-kor′nu) [L. *ante*, before, + *cornu*, horn]. Anterior cornu or horn of the lateral ventricle of the brain.

antecubital (an″te-ku′bĭ-tal) [″+ *cubitum*, elbow]. In front of the elbow; at the bend of the elbow.

    a. fossa. Triangular area at the bend of the elbow. It contains several veins, cephalic and basilic, which are frequently used for diagnostic venapuncture or for administering solutions intravenously.

antecurvature (an″tē-ker′va-tūr″) [″+ *curvatura*, bend]. Bending forward abnormally. SYN: *anteflexion*.

antefebrile (an″tē-fē′brĭl, -fē′bril, -fēb′rĭl) [L. *ante*, before, + *febris*, fever]. Pert. to the period before a fever.

anteflect (an′te-flekt) [″+ *flectere*, to bend]. To bend or cause to bend forward.

anteflexion (an″te-flek′shun). Abnormal bending forward, esp. bending forward of the uterus at its body and neck.

antelocation (an″te-lo-kā′shun) [L. *ante*, before, + *locare*, to place]. Forward displacement of an organ or part of the human body.

antemetic (ant″ē-mĕt′ĭk) [Gr. *anti*, against, + *emetikos*, emetic]. 1. Arresting vomiting. 2. Remedy that controls vomiting and nausea. SEE: *antiemetic*.

ante mortem (an′te mor′tem) [L.]. Before death.

    a.-m. statement. One made immediately preceding death. If made with belief that death is approaching, it is held in law as equally binding with a statement made on oath. SYN: *deathbed statement*.

antenatal (ăn″tē-nā′tal) [L. *ante*, before, + *natus*, born]. Occurring before birth.

ante partum (an′te par′tum) [L.]. The time before the onset of labor.

antephialtic (ant″ē-fĭ-al′tik) [Gr. *anti*, against, + *ephialtēs*, nightmare]. A medicine effective in preventing nightmare.

anteposition (an″te-po-zish′un) [L. *ante*, before, + position]. Anterior displacement of the uterus.

anteprostate (an″tē-pros′tāt) [″+ prostate]. One of the bulbo-urethral glands; Cowper's gland.

anteprostatitis (an″te-pros-tă-ti′tĭs) [″+ ″+ Gr. *-itis*, inflammation]. Inflammation of glands of Cowper.

antepyret′ic [L. *ante*, before, + Gr. *pyretos*, fever]. Before the development of fever; antefebrile. SEE: *antipyretic*.

anterior (an-te′rĭ-or) [L.]. Before, or in front of.

    a. chamber. Aqueous chamber of eye. Bounded in front by cornea, behind by iris and lens.

antero- [L.]. Prefix denoting anterior, front, before.

anterograde (an′ter-o-grād″) [L. *antero*, anterior, + *gradior*, to step]. Extending frontward.

antero-inferior (an″ter-o-in-fe′rĭ-or) [″+ *inferior*, below]. In front and below.

anterolateral (an″ter-o-lat′er-al) [″+ *latus*, side]. In front and to one side.

anteromedian (an″ter-o-mē′dĭ-ăn) [L. *antero,* anterior, + *medius,* middle]. In front and toward the central line.

anteroposterior (an″ter-o-pos-tē′rĭ-or) ["+ *posterior,* rear]. Passing from front to rear.

anterosuperior (an″ter-o-su-pē′rĭ-or) ["+ *superior,* above]. In front and above.

anteversion (an″te-vĕr′zhŭn) [L. *ante,* before, + *vertere,* to turn]. 1. A tipping or bending forward of an organ. 2. A forward placement of the uterus.

  a. uteri. A forward tipping of the uterus.

anteverted (an″te-vĕrt′ĕd). Inclined or bent forward; said of uterus.

anthelix (ant′hē-lĭks, an′thē-lĭks) [Gr. *anti,* against, + *helix,* coil]. Curved prominence of the external ear parallel to and in front of the helix. SYN: *antihelix.*

anthelmintic (ant″hel-min′tik) [Gr. *anti,* against, + *helmins,* worm]. An agent useful in treating parasitic intestinal worms.

Anthemis (ăn′thĕm-ĭs). Genus of plant, the flowers of which are used medicinally.

anthemis (ăn′thĕm-ĭs). Camomile; chamomile; dried blossoms of A. nobilis. A bitter tonic; an antispasmodic.

anthemorrhagic (ant″hĕm-ō-raj′ik) [Gr. *anti,* against, + *haima,* blood, + *rēgnunai,* to discharge]. Agent for preventing or arresting hemorrhage.

anthocyanin (an″thō-sī′ă-nĭn) [Gr. *anthos,* flower, + *kyanos,* a blue substance]. Any one of a group of pigments that cause flowers and plants to be reddish purple in color.

anthocyaninemia (an″thō-sī″ă-nĭn-e′mĭ-ă) ["+ "+ *haima,* blood]. Anthocyanin in the blood.

anthocyaninuria (an″thō-sī″ă-nĭn-ū′rĭ-ă) ["+ "+ Gr. *ouron,* urine]. Anthocyanin in urine.

Anthomyia (an″thō-mī′yă) [Gr. *anthos,* flower, + *myia,* fly]. A genus of fly of the order Diptera, related to the housefly. Larvae sometimes infest man.

  A. canalicularis. A small black horse fly, whose larvae may infest the human intestine, often resulting in alarming gastrointestinal symptoms.

anthophobia (ăn″thō-fō′bĭ-ă) ["+ *phobos,* fear]. Morbid dislike of flowers.

anthracemia (an″thra-sē′mĭ-ă) [Gr. *anthrax,* coal, + *haima,* blood]. Presence in the blood of B. anthracis.

anthracia (an-thrā′sĭ-ă) [Gr. *anthrax,* coal, carbuncle]. Presence of carbuncles.

anthracoid (an′thra-koid) ["+ *eidos,* form]. Resembling or pert. to anthrax.

anthracometer (an″thrä-kom′ĕ-ter) ["+ *metron,* measure]. An instrument for measuring the carbon dioxide in the air.

anthraconecrosis (an″thrä-ko-nĕ-krō′sĭs) [Gr. *anthrax,* coal, carbuncle, + *nekrōsis,* deadness]. Necrosis of tissue into dry, black gangrene.

anthracosilicosis (an″thrä-ko-sĭl′ĭ-kō′sĭs) ["+ L. *silex,* flint, + Gr. *-ōsis,* condition]. A form of pneumoconiosis due to breathing coal dust. SYN: *coal miner's pneumoconiosis.*

anthracosis (an-thrä-kō′sĭs) ["+ *-ōsis,* condition]. Black discoloration of the lungs seen in those who work in coal mines or are exposed to coal soot or smoke; a pneumoconiosis caused by breathing coal dust and silica. SYN: *Black lung.*

anthrax (ăn′thrăks) [Gr. coal, carbuncle]. Acute, infectious disease caused by Bacillus anthracis, usually attacking cattle, sheep, horses and goats. Man contracts it from contact with animal hair, hides, or waste.

  ETIOL: B. anthracis. Workers in wools, hides, and brushes are commonly affected.

  SYM: Disease may attack lungs (woolsorter's disease) or the loose cellular tissue, giving rise to malignant edema; more commonly it occurs in form of a pustule called anthrax boil or malignant pustule. Rarely, the disease may occur in intestinal tract. Anthrax often proves fatal if untreated.

  TREATMENT: Penicillin or tetracyclines.

  NP: Isolation and complete bed rest of patient until lesions are free of anthrax bacilli. Strict isolation for inhalation type of anthrax. Daily cleansing baths and daily mouth and nose care. Diet—fluids when temperature is elevated, followed by progressive return to regular diet. Alcohol or tepid sponges for elevated temperature.

  Medical aseptic technique. Dressings burned. Bed linen, gowns, instruments and gloves autoclaved. Fluid body wastes and bath water placed in cresol or solution of chloride of lime. Terminal disinfection of room and its contents after patient is discharged.

anthropo- (ăn″thrō-pō, -pŏ) [Gr. *anthrōpos,* man]. Prefix denoting relation to man or human life.

anthropogeny (an″thrō-poj′ĕ-nĭ) [Gr. *anthrōpos,* man, + *gennan,* to produce]. Origin and development of man.

anthropoid (an′thrō-poid) ["+ *eidos,* form]. 1. Resembling a man. 2. An ape.

anthropology (an″thro-pol′o-jĭ) ["+ *-logy,* study of]. The science which treats of man in all aspects, social, cultural, behavioral and biological.

anthropometry (an-thro-pom′et-rĭ) [Gr. *anthrōpos,* man, + *metron,* measure].

Science of measuring the human body and its parts.

anthropophagy (an''thrō-pof'ă-jĭ) [" + *phagein*, to eat]. The eating of human flesh; cannibalism.

anthropophile (an-thro'po-phĭl) [" + *philein*, to love]. One with a preference for man, esp. an insect which chooses the blood of man rather than that of other mammals.

anthropophobia (an''thro-po-fō'bĭ-ă) [Gr. *anthrōpos*, man, + *phobos*, fear]. A morbid fear of society or of a particular person. An early symptom of mental disorder.

anthroposomatology (an''thrō-pō-sō-mă-tol'ō-jĭ) [" + *sōma*, body, + *logy*, study of]. Branch of anthropology dealing with human body.

anthropotomy (an''thrō-pot'ō-mĭ) [" + *tomē*, cut]. Human anatomy.

anthypnotic (ant''hip-not'ik) [Gr. *anti*, against, + *hypnos*, sleep]. 1. Preventing sleep. 2. Agent hindering sleep.

anthysteric (ant''his-ter'ik) [" + *hystera*, womb]. 1. Relieving hysteria. 2. Agent soothing hysteria.

anti- [Gr.]. Prefix meaning against.

antiagglutinin (an''tĭ-ă-glŭ'tĭ-nin). A specific antibody opposing action of agglutinin.

antialbumate, antialbuminate (an''tĭ-al'bū-māt, -al-bū'mĭn-āt) [Gr. *anti*, against, + *albumin*]. A product resulting from incomplete proteolysis or digestion of albumin; parapeptone.

antiamylase (an''tĭ-am'ĭ-lās). Substance neutralizing action of amylase.

antianaphylactin (an''tĭ-an-ă-fĭ-lak'tĭn). An antibody specific to anaphylactin.

antianaphylaxis (ăn''tĭ-ăn-ă-fĭ-lăks'ĭs) [Gr. *anti*, against + *anaphylaxis*]. Prevention of anaphylaxis. Usually attained by administering repeated doses of the sensitizing substance too small to cause an anaphylactic reaction.

antianemic (an''tĭ-ă-nē'mĭk). Curing or preventing anemia.

antiantibody (an''tĭ-an'tĭ-bod-ĭ) [Gr. *anti*, against, + antibody]. An antibody counteracting effect of antitoxin which produced it.

antiapoplectic (an''tĭ-ăp''ō-plek'tĭk). Relieving or preventing apoplexy.

antiarthritic (ăn''tĭ-ar-thrĭt'ĭk) [Gr. *anti*, against, + *arthritikos*, gouty]. Medicine given to relieve arthritis.

antibacterial (an''tĭ-băk-tē'rĭ-ăl). Destroying or stopping the growth of bacteria.

antibechic (an''tĭ-bek'ik) [Gr. *anti*, against, + *bex*, cough]. 1. Relieving cough. 2. A cough remedy.

antibiosis (an''tĭ-bĭ-ō'sĭs) [" + *bios*, life]. The association or relationship between two organisms wherein one is harmful to the other.

antibiotic (ăn''-tĭ-bī-ŏt'ĭk). Any of a variety of substances both natural and synthetic which inhibit growth of or destroy microorganisms. Used extensively in treatment of infectious diseases in plants, animals and man.

 a., bacteriocidal or bactericidal. One which kills microorganisms.

 a., bacteriostatic. One which prevents growth of microorganisms.

 a., broad-spectrum. One which is effective against a variety of microorganisms.

antibody (ăn'tĭ-bŏd''ē). Protein substances developed by the body, usually in response to the presence of an antigen which has been administered parenterally or has otherwise gained access to the body. Normal antibodies are also present in the circulation, and may be transferred from the mother to the infant in utero or may be developed during life by subclinical contact with the disease-producing agent, thereby providing immunity to diseases.

 a., fluorescent. An a. reaction made visible by incorporating a fluorescent dye into the antigen-antibody reaction. The dye fluoresces under the fluorescent light. Its presence is detected by examining the specimen, so treated, with a microscope equipped for fluorescent microscopy.

 a., hepatitis associated. A. used in testing for presence of human Australian antigen. This antigen is present in the blood of persons who have had viral hepatitis. SYN: *human anti-Australian antigen.*

antibrachium (an-tĭ-brā'kĭ-um) [Gr. *anti*, against, + *brachion*, arm]. The forearm.

antibromic (ăn''tĭ-brō'mĭk) [" + *brōmos*, smell]. 1. Deodorizing. 2. A deodorant.

anticanitic (ăn''tĭ-kă-nĭt'ĭk) [Gr. *anti*, against, + L. *canities*, gray hair]. A word indicating something which prevents or counteracts graying of hair. No substance other than a hair dye has this ability.

anticardium (ăn''tĭ-kăr'dĭ-ŭm) [" + *kardia*, heart]. Precordium.

anticarious (ăn''tĭ-kā'rĭ-ŭs) [Gr. *anti*, against, + *caries*, decay]. Preventing decay of teeth.

anticatarrhal (ăn''tĭ-kă-tăr'ăl) [" + L. *catarrhus*, catarrhal]. Relieving catarrh.

anticathode (ăn-tĭ-kăth'ōd) [" + *kata*, down, + *hodos*, way]. Portion of vacuum tube opposite cathode. SYN: *target.*

anticheirotonus (ăn''tĭ-kĭ-rŏt'ō-nŭs) [Gr. *anticheir*, thumb, + *tonos*, tension]. Spas-

Antibiotics

This list of antibiotics (some of which are of historic interest and are not used clinically) can only be considered as being representative.

Substance	Source
p-aminosalicylic acid	synthetic
amphotericin B	*Streptomyces nodosus*
ampicillin	semisynthetic penicillin
bacitracin	*Bacillus subtilis*
cephalothin	*Cephalosporium species*
chloramphenicol	*Streptomyces venezuelae*
chlortetracycline	*Streptomyces aureofaciens*
cloxacillin	semisynthetic penicillin
colistin	*Bacillus colistinus*
cycloserine	*Streptomyces orchidaceus*
dapsone	synthetic
erythromycin	*Streptomyces erythreus*
ethionamide	synthetic
glucosulfone	synthetic
griseofulvin	*Penicillium griseofulvin*
isoniazid	synthetic
kanamycin	*Streptomyces kanamyceticus*
lincomycin	*Streptomyces lincolnensis*
methenamine mandelate	synthetic
methicillin	synthetic penicillin
metronidazole	synthetic
nafcillin	synthetic penicillin
nalidixic acid	synthetic
neomycin	*Streptomyces fradiae*
nitrofurantoin	synthetic
novobiocin	*Streptomyces niveus* or *S. spheroides*
nystatin	*Streptomyces noursei*
oleandomycin	*Streptomyces antibioticus*
oxacillin	synthetic penicillin
oxytetracycline	*Streptomyces rimosus*
paromomycin	*Streptomyces rimosus*
penicillin	*Penicillium notatum* or *P. chrysogenum*
phenethicillin	semisynthetic penicillin
phenoxymethyl penicillin	semisynthetic penicillin
polymyxin B	*Bacillus polymyxa*
pyrazinamide	synthetic
rifampin	semisynthetic
ristocetin	*Nocardia lurida*
streptomycin	*Streptomyces griseus*
sulfonamides	synthetic
tetracycline	*Streptomyces species*
tyrothricin	*Bacillus brevis*
vancomycin	*Streptomyces orientalis*
viomycin	*Streptomyces floridae*

modic bending inward of thumb in epilepsy or before attack.

anticholagogue (ăn"tĭ-kō'lă-gŏg) [Gr. *anti*, against, + *cholē*, bile, + *agōgos*, drawing forth]. Depressing hepatic function.

anticholinergic (ăn"tĭ-kō"lĭn-ĕr'jĭk). 1. Impeding the impulses or action of the fibers of the parasympathetic nerves. 2. An agent that provides a cholinergic blocking action. SYN: *parasympatholytic*.

anticlinal (ăn"tĭ-klī'nal) [Gr. *anti*, against, + *klinein*, to incline]. Leaning in opposite directions.

a. vertebra. Tenth thoracic vertebra.

anticoagulant (ăn"tĭ-kō-ăg'ū-lănt) ["+ L. *coagulans*, forming clots]. 1. Delaying or preventing blood coagulation. 2. An agent which prevents or delays blood coagulation.

anticonvul'sive ["+ L. *convulsio*, pulling together]. 1. Relieving convulsions. 2. Agent preventing convulsions.

anticritical (ăn"tĭ-krĭt'ĭ-kăl). Preventing the crisis of a disease.

anticus (ăn-tī'kŭs) [L., foremost]. Anterior. That part nearest the ventral or front surface.

anticytolysin (ăn"tĭ-sītōl'ĭ-sĭn) [Gr. *anti*, against, + *kytos*, cell, + *lysis*, dissolution]. Something which interferes with or prevents cytolysis.

anticytotoxin (ăn"tĭ-sī"tŏ-tŏks'ĭn) ["+ "+ *toxikon*, poison]. An antibody specifically inhibiting cytotoxin.

antidiabetic (ăn"tĭ-dī"ă-bĕt'ĭk). 1. Preventing or alleviating diabetes. 2. Something which is useful in treating diabetes.

antidinic (ăn"tĭ-dĭn'ĭk) [Gr. *anti*, against, + *dinos*, dizziness]. 1. Relieving vertigo. 2. Agent preventing vertigo.

antidiuretic (ăn"tĭ-dī-ū-rĕt'ĭk) ["+ *dia*, intensive, + *ourēsis*, urination]. 1. Lessening urine secretion. 2. A drug having such an action.

antidotal (ăn"tĭ-dō'tal). Acting as or pert. to an antidote.

antidote (ăn'tĭ-dōt) [Gr. *antidoton*, given against]. A substance which neutralizes poisons or their effects.

a., chemical. These act chemically by reacting with the poison to produce an insoluble compound which is inert or less toxic. For example, table salt precipitates silver nitrate and forms an insoluble, harmless silver chloride. Chemical antidotes should be used sparingly and should be removed, as they may produce serious results if allowed to remain in the stomach.

a., mechanical. Those that envelop the poison inside the stomach or coat the mucous membrane of the stomach. These are fats, oils, milk (casein coagulum), whites of eggs, finely divided charcoal, fuller's earth, or mineral oil. (Fats and oils are not desirable in phosphorus, camphor, aspidium, and cantharides poisonings.)

a., physiologic. These produce physiological effects opposite to the effects of the poison, e.g., sedatives are given for convulsives and hypnotics. These should not be given without physician's definite instructions.

a., universal. Two parts activated charcoal, one part tannic acid, and one part magnesium oxide. (The charcoal absorbs; the tannic acid precipitates metals, alkaloids, and some glucosides; and the magnesium oxide neutralizes acids). Give orally by dissolving five teaspoonsful of the mixture in 1/2 glass of warm water. After the patient has swallowed the antidote, the stomach contents should then be removed by gastric lavage.

antidromic (ăn"tĭ-drŏm'ĭk) [Gr. *anti*, against, + *dromos*, running]. Running in a direction opposite the usual stream, as when a nervous impulse runs along a sensory fiber in the direction of the sense organ.

antidysenteric (ăn"tĭ-dĭs"ĕn-tĕr'ĭk). 1. Relieving or preventing dysentery. 2. An agent curing dysentery.

antidysuric (ăn"tĭ-dĭs-ū'rĭk) [Gr. *anti*, against, + *dys*, painful, + *ouron*, urine]. 1. Relieving or preventing dysuria. 2. A medicine that relieves or prevents dysuria.

antiemetic (ăn"tĭ-ē-mĕt'ĭk) ["+ *emetikos*, inclined to vomit]. An agent that will prevent or arrest vomiting.

antienzyme (ăn"tĭ-ĕn'zīm). Something which interferes with the action of an enzyme.

antiepileptic (ăn"tĭ-ĕp'ĭ-lĕp'tĭk). 1. A medicine, procedure, or diet which combats epilepsy. 2. Opposing epilepsy.

antifebrile (ăn"tĭ-fē'brĭl, -fē'brĭl, -fĕb'rĭl) [Gr. *anti*, against, + L. *febris*, fever]. 1. A physical agent, such as ice water or cool air, or a medicine, which abolishes or relieves fever. 2. Reducing or relieving fever.

antifermentative (ăn"tĭ-fĕr-mĕn'tă-tĭv). Preventing the fermentation process.

antifungal (ăn"tĭ-fŭng'găl). Destroying or preventing the growth of fungi.

antigalactagogue (ăn"tĭ-gă-lăk'tă-gŏg) [Gr. *anti*, against, + *gala*, milk, + *agogos*, drawing forth]. Something which prevents or decreases the secretion of milk.

antigalactic (ăn"tĭ-gă-lăk'tĭk). Diminishing or preventing the secretion of milk.

antigen (ăn'tĭ-jĕn) [Gr. *anti*, against, + *gennan*, to produce]. A substance which induces the formation of antibodies. An antigen may be introduced into the body or it may be formed within the body. Examples are bacteria, bacterial toxins, foreign blood cells.

antigenic (ăn-tĭ-jĕn'ĭk). Capable of causing the production of an antibody.

antigenotherapy (ăn"tĭ-jĕn"ō-thĕr'ă-pĭ). Utilization of an antigen in treatment of a disease. SYN: *antigentotherapy.*

antiglobulin (ăn"tĭ-glŏb'ū-lĭn). A precipitin which precipitates globulin.

antigoitrogenic (ăn"tĭ-goy"trō-jĕn'ĭk) [Gr. *anti,* against, + goiter, + *gennan,* to produce]. Preventing the formation of a goiter.

antigonorrheic (ăn"tĭ-gŏn"ō-rē'ĭk). 1. Curing gonorrhea. 2. An agent relieving gonorrhea.

anti-G suit. Garment designed to produce uniform pressure on the lower extremities and abdomen. This is accomplished by having inflatable compartments in the garment.

Normally the suit is used by aviators to help prevent pooling of blood in the lower half of the body when the pilot is subjected to centrifugal force greater than gravity. The garment has also been used in treating certain forms of internal bleeding.

antihelix [Gr. *anti,* against, + *helix,* coil]. Inner curved ridge of external ear parallel to the helix.

antihemolysin (ăn"tĭ-hē-mŏl'ĭsĭn). A substance which neutralizes hemolysin.

antihemorrhagic (ăn"tĭ-hĕm-ō-răj'ĭk). Something which prevents hemorrhage or bleeding.

antihidrot'ic (ăn"tĭ-hĭ-drŏt'ĭk) [Gr. *anti,* against, + *hidrotikos,* sweating]. Preventing or decreasing perspiration. SYN: *anhidrotic.*

antihistamine (ăn"tĭ-hĭs'tă-mēn, -mĭn). Any medicine which counteracts the effect of histamine.

antihistaminic (ăn"tĭ-hĭs"tă-mĭn'ĭk). 1. Inhibiting the production of or neutralizing the effect of histamine. 2. An agent used to counteract histamine.

antihormone (ăn"tĭ-hor'mōn). That which antagonizes or interferes with the action of a hormone.

antihydropic (ăn"tĭ-hĭ-drŏp'ĭk) [Gr. *anti,* against, + Gr. *hydrōpikos,* dropsical]. 1. Relieving generalized edema. 2. Agent used to treat edema.

anti-icteric (ăn"tĭ-ĭk-tĕr'ĭk) ["+ *ikteros,* jaundice]. 1. Relieving icterus. 2. Agent for treating jaundice.

anti-immune (ăn"tĭ-ĭ-mūn'). Preventing immunity.

anti-infectious (ăn"tĭ-ĭn-fĕk'shŭs). Counteracting infection.

anti-inflammatory (ăn"tĭ-ĭn-flăm'ă-tō-rĭ). Counteracting or diminishing inflammation or its effects.

anti-isolysin (ăn"tĭ-ĭ-sŏl'ĭ-sĭn). A substance inhibiting action of an isolysin.

antiketogenesis (ăn"tĭ-kē-tō-jĕn'ē-sis) [Gr. *anti,* against, + *ketone* + *gennan,* to produce]. The prevention or inhibition of ketone formation. During starvation, diabetes, and certain other conditions, the metabolism of the ketone bodies, B-hydroxybutyric acid, acetoacetate and acetone is decreased, thus they accumulate in the blood. Providing increased carbohydrates in the diet or intravenously will help to prevent or treat this. Carbohydrates are therefore antiketogenic. In ketonemia due to diabetes, both insulin and carbohydrates are required in order to permit the metabolism of carbohydrate to proceed at a rate which would control ketone formation.

antiketogenetic, antiketogenic (ăn"tĭ-kē"tō-jĕn-ĕt'ik, -jĕn'ik). Pert. to antiketogenesis.

antilactase (ăn"tĭ-lăk'tās) [Gr. *anti,* against, + *lac,* milk]. A substance counteracts lactase.

antilemic (ăn"tĭ-lē'mĭk) ["+ *loimos,* plague]. 1. Preventing plague. 2. An agent curing the plague.

antilepsis (ăn"tĭ-lĕp'sĭs) ["+ *lepsis,* a receiving in return]. 1. Application of a remedy to a healthy part; treatment by removing something, such as a body fluid, (derivation), or shifting blood from the site of pathology to a healthy part of the body, (revulsion), or in counterirritation. 2. Support, as of a bandage.

antileptic (ăn"tĭ-lĕp'tĭk) [Gr. *antileptikos,* able to check]. Pertaining to antilepsis.

antilethargic (ăn"tĭ-lĕ-thăr'jĭk) [Gr. *anti,* against, + *lethargia,* drowsiness]. Preventing sleep.

antilithic (ăn"tĭ-lĭth'ĭk) ["+ *lithos,* stone]. An agent that prevents the formation of, or favors the removal of stones or calculi in the urinary or biliary tracts.

antilobium (ăn"tĭ-lō'bĭ-ŭm) ["+ *lobos,* ear lobe]. The tragus of the ear.

antilogia (ăn-tĭ-lō'jĭ-ă) [Gr. *anti-,* against, + *logos,* science]. Contradictory symptoms which render diagnosis uncertain.

antiluetic (ăn"tĭ-lū-ĕt'ĭk) ["+ L. *lues,* pestilence]. Antisyphilitic.

antilymphocytic serum (ăn"tĭ-lĭm"fō-sĭt'-ĭk). A substance used experimentally to reduce host rejection response to transplanted tissues. Produced by inoculating animals with certain tissues from other animals. ABBR: ALS.

antilysin (ăn-tī-lī'sĭn). A substance neutralizing the lysins of a disease against which an animal has been immunized, thus preventing the lysis of cells.

antilysis (ăn-tĭl'ĭ-sĭs). The result of the action of antilysin.

antilyssic (ăn-tĭ-lĭs'ĭk) [Gr. *anti,* against, + *lyssa,* frenzy]. Preventing or inhibiting rabies. SYN: *antirabic.*

antimalarial (ăn''tĭ-mă-lā'rĭ-ăl). An agent, such as quinine, that will prevent or relieve malaria.

antimere (ăn'tĭ-mēr) ["+ *meros,* a part]. Any body segment bounded by planes at right angles to the long axis of the body.

antimetabolite (ăn''tĭ-mĕ-tăb'ō-līt). A substance which, due to its similarity of structure, is utilized by an organism as if it were a preferred metabolic substance. The antimetabolite, once ingested, does not benefit the organism. It is believed that certain antibiotics are effective because they act as antimetabolites.

antimetropia (ăn''tĭ-mĕ-trō'pĭ-ă) [Gr. *anti,* against, + *metron,* measure, + *ops,* eye]. An ocular disorder in which the eyes have different powers of refraction. Ex: one eye may be hypertropic; the other, myopic.

antimiasmatic (ăn''tĭ-mī''ăz-măt'ĭk) ["+ *miasma,* pollution]. Antimalarial.

antimicrobic (ăn''tĭ-mī-krō'bĭk) ["+ *mikros,* small, + *bios,* life]. 1. Not believing in the pathogenicity of microorganisms. 2. Preventing the development or pathogenic action of microbes.

antimonial (ăn''tĭ-mō'nĭ-ăl). Pert. to or containing antimony.

antimony (ăn'tĭ-mō''nĭ). SYMB: Sb. At. wt. 121.75, at. no. 51. An element of metallic appearance and crystalline structure. Its compounds are used in alloys and medicines, and may form poisons.

     a. poisoning. SYM: Acrid metallic taste. Cardiac and arterial depressants with additional properties of inducing sweating and vomiting about 30 minutes after injection. In large doses they irritate lining of alimentary tract, resembling arsenic.

     F. A. TREATMENT: Vomiting caused by the poison may be sufficient. Wash stomach with strong tea or dilute tannic acid. BAL (British antilewisite) is effective especially if the poisoning is due to a trivalent form such as tartar emetic. Otherwise treat symptomatically.

antimycotic (ăn''tĭ-mī-kŏt'ĭk) [Gr. *anti,* against, + *mykēs,* fungus]. Inhibiting or preventing the growth of fungi. SYN: *antibacterial.*

antinarcotic (ăn''tĭ-năr-kŏt'ĭk) ["+ *narkōtikos,* benumbing]. Counteracting the action of a narcotic either by alleviating the symptoms produced or by preventing the drug from exerting its pharmacological effect.

antinatriuresis (ăn''tĭ-nā''trī-ū-rē'sĭs) ["+ L. *natrium,* sodium, + Gr. *ourēsis,* making water.]. Decreasing the excretion of sodium in the urine.

antinausea (ăn''tĭ-nŏ'sĭ-ă). Preventing or decreasing nausea.

antinephritic (ăn''tĭ-nĕ-frĭt'ĭk). Effective in treating nephritis.

antineuralgic (ăn''tĭ-nū-răl'jĭk) [Gr. *anti,* against, + *neuron,* nerve, + *algos,* pain]. 1. Relieving neuralgic pain. 2. Agent curing neuralgia.

antineuritic (ăn''tĭ-nū-rĭt'ĭk). 1. Counteracting nerve inflammation. 2. An agent which relieves neuritis.

antinion (ăn-tĭn'ĭ-ŏn) [Gr. *anti,* against, + *inion,* nape of the neck]. Frontal pole of the skull.

antinuclear antibodies. Antibodies found in patients with various connective tissue diseases.

antioxidation (ăn''tĭ-ŏks'ĭ-dā'shŭn). Prevention of oxidation.

antioxygen (ăn-tĭ-ok'sĭ-jĕn). A substance hindering oxidation.

antipaludian (ăn''tĭ-pă-lū'dĭ-ăn). Preventing malaria fever.

antiparalytic (ăn''tĭ-păr-ă-lĭt'ĭk). Reputedly relieving paralysis.

antiparasitic (ăn''tĭ-păr-ă-sĭt'ĭk). 1. Destructive to parasites. 2. Insecticide.

antiparastatitis (ăn''tĭ-păr''ăs-tă-tī'tĭs) [Gr. *anti,* against, + *parastates,* testicle, + *-itis,* inflammation]. Inflammation of Cowper's glands.

antipathic (ăn''tĭ-păth'ĭk) ["+ *pathein,* to feel]. Opposite; unlike.

antipathy (ăn-tĭp'ă-thē). 1. Aversion; disgust; or that which excites repugnance. 2. Chemical incompatibility.

antipepsin (ăn''tĭ-pĕp'sĭn). An antienzyme counteracting pepsin.

antipeptone (ăn''tĭ-pĕp'tōn). Peptone derived from antialbumose through hydrolysis.

antiperiodic (ăn''tĭ-pē-rĕ-ŏd'ĭk) [Gr. *anti,* against, + *periodos,* a circle]. Antimalarial; preventing regular recurrences.

antiperistal'sis ["+ *peri,* around, + *stalsis,* constriction]. A wave of contraction in the gastrointestinal tract moving towards the oral end. In the duodenum it is associated with vomiting; in the ascending colon it occurs normally. SEE: *peristalsis.*

antiperistaltic (ăn″tĭ-pĕr′ĭ-stăl′tĭk). 1. Pert. to antiperistalsis. 2. Impeding peristalsis.

antiperspirant (ăn″tĭ-pĕr′spĭ-rant). Inhibiting, or a substance which inhibits, perspiration.

antiphlogistic (ăn″tĭ-flō-jĭs′tĭk) [Gr. *anti,* against, + *phlogistos,* on fire]. An agent that tends to relieve inflammation. Ex: kaolin, ichthyol.

antiplas′tic (ăn″tĭ-plăs′tĭk). 1. An agent which interferes with or prevents healing by preventing formation of granulation tissue. 2. One which thins the blood.

antipodal (ăn-tĭp′ō-dăl) [Gr. *antipous,* with feet opposite]. Located at the opposite end or side.

    a. cell. One of two nuclear cells at the base of embryo sac in a seed.

antipraxia (ăn″tĭ-prăks′ĭ-ă). Functions or symptoms antagonistic to each other.

antiprostate (ăn″tĭ-prŏs′tāt). Anteprostate; Cowper's gland.

antiprostatitis (ăn″tĭ-prŏs″tă-tĭ′tĭs). Inflammation of Cowper's gland.

antiprothrombin (ăn″tĭ-prō-thrŏm′bĭn) [Gr. *anti,* against, + *prō,* before, + *thrombos,* clot]. Agent preventing formation of thrombin; anticoagulant. SEE: *clotting.*

antiprotozoal (ăn″tĭ-prō″tō-zō′ăl). Destructive to protozoa.

antipruritic (ăn″tĭ-prū-rĭt′ĭk). That which relieves itching.

antipsoric (ăn″tĭ-sō′rĭk) [Gr. *anti,* against, + *psōra,* itch]. An agent used to prevent or arrest itching.

antiputrefactive (ăn″tĭ-pū″trē-făk′tĭv). Preventing putrefaction.

antipyic (ăn-tĭ-pī′ĭk) [Gr. *anti,* against, + *pyon,* pus]. Preventing or inhibiting suppuration; antipyogenic.

antipyogenic (ăn″tĭ-pī-ō-jĕn′ĭk) [" + " + *gennan,* to produce]. Preventing or inhibiting pus formation.

antipyresis (ăn″tĭ-pī-rē′sĭs) [Gr. *anti,* against, + *pyretos,* fever]. Use of antipyretics in fever.

antipyretic (ăn-tĭ-pī-rĕt′ĭk). An agent that reduces febrile temperatures. Ex: acetylsalicylic acid.

antipyrine (ăn″tĭ-pī′rēn) [" + *pyr,* fire]. White crystalline powder, odorless and having a slightly bitter taste. An analgesic and antipyretic. Its toxicity is similar to acetanilid. It should not be used when a less toxic analgesic, such as aspirin, is available.

antipyrotic (ăn″tĭ-pī-rŏt′ĭk) [Gr. *anti,* against, + *pyrōtikos,* burning]. Substance or technique used to treat, or effective in the treatment of, burns.

antirabic (ăn″tĭ-rā′bĭk). Preventive of, or curing rabies; antilyssic.

antirachitic (ăn″tĭ-ră-kĭt′ĭk) [Gr. *anti,* against, + *rachitis,* rickets.]. 1. Helping to cure rickets. 2. Agent for treating rickets.

    a. vitamin. Vitamin D, q.v.

antireticular cytotoxic serum. A serum obtained from horses which have been inoculated with certain human tissues. Believed, by some investigators, to stimulate the reticuloendothelial system when serum is given in small doses but to destroy the reticuloendothelial cells when given in large doses.

    The developer of this serum, Alexander A. Bogomolets, a Russian biologist, allegedly believed that humans treated with it would live longer than their normal life spans. There is no evidence to support this. The serum is not available commercially. ABBR: ACS.

antirheumatic (ăn″tĭ-rū-măt′ĭk). An agent that will combat rheumatism.

antiricin (ăn″tĭ-rī′sĭn). An antibody to ricin.

antiscabious (ăn″tĭ-skā′bĭ-ŭs) [Gr. *anti,* against, + L. *scabies,* itch]. Preventing or relieving scabies.

antiscorbutic (ăn″tĭ-skŏr-bū′tĭk) [" + L. *scorbutus,* scurvy]. An agent effective against or a remedy for scurvy. Vitamin C is antiscorbutic.

antisepsis (ăn″tĭ-sĕp′sĭs) [" + *sepsis,* putrefaction]. The prevention of sepsis by the exclusion, destruction, or inhibition of multiplication of microorganisms including viruses within body tissues.

antiseptic (ăn″tĭ-sĕp′tĭk). 1. Preventing decay, putrefaction, or sepsis. 2. An agent that will prevent the growth or arrest the development of microorganisms.

    Chemically, antiseptics may be inorganic, such as the mercury preparations, or organic, such as carbolic acid (phenol). Oxidizing disinfectants liberate oxygen when in contact with pus or organic substances. When in use they should be washed away and replaced frequently to help remove pus, blood, and other substances. Different types of bacteria are sensitive to different antiseptics. SEE: *disinfectant* for table.

    RS: asepsis; disinfectant; deodorant; germicide; sterilization.

antisepticism (ăn″tĭ-sĕp′tĭ-sĭzm). Therapeutic employment of antiseptic measures.

antiserum (ăn″tĭ-sē′rŭm). A serum obtained from human donors (or an experimental animal, usually a goat or horse) who have been immunized against a specific bacterium or other antigenic agent. The serum contains antibodies specific for the antigen. SYN: *immune serum.*

antisialagogue (ăn″tĭ-sĭ-ăl′ă-gŏg) [Gr. *anti,* against, + *sialon,* saliva, + *agogos,* drawing forth]. An agent, as atropine, that lessens or prevents the flow of saliva.

antisialic (ăn″tĭ-sĭ-ăl′ĭk). Checking or that which checks the secretion of saliva.

antisocial (ăn″tĭ-sō′shăl). Pert. to a person whose outlook or actions are socially negative, or to one who fails to obey the rules of society. SEE: *asocial.*

antispasmod′ic [Gr. *anti,* against, + *spasmos,* convulsion]. 1. Relieving or preventing spasm. 2. An agent that will relieve spasm. SEE: *spasm.*

antispastic (ăn″tĭ-spăs′tĭk). Agent relieving muscular spasm. SYN: *antispasmodic.*

anti-stain formulary. An anti-stain formulary for removing stains from bed linens and other cotton fabrics is as follows:

Balsam of Peru: Use waste ether to dissolve it before laundering. Caution: Ether is explosive and toxic. It should not be used in closed areas. Use in open air or under a properly ventilated hood. Never use in presence of a flame or lighted cigarette.

Blood: Soak in cold water, then wash in lukewarm soap solution. For old stains, soak in 1% ammonia solution and then launder.

Chocolate or cocoa: Allow hot water to run through stained fabric; then wash in hot soap solution. Javelle water to bleach if necessary. Carbona for remaining grease stain.

Cod liver oil: Soak stained fabric in kerosene oil for one hour, rubbing lightly occasionally. Then boil for 10 minutes in water to which a naphtha soap product has been added. Rinse in clear water. Caution: Kerosene is inflammable. Do not use in a closed area or near a flame.

Cosmetics: Nail polish, lipstick, or rouge —ordinary washing; stubborn stains remaining can be removed by acetone, followed by warm chlorine bleach.

Feces: Soak in cold water, rinse, then wash with soap and hot water. Use a brush to scrub.

Fruit stains: Stretch stained article over a basin, pour boiling water directly over the spot until it disappears. If this fails, use Javelle water (a preparation of washing soda and chloride of lime), rinsing between each application.

Grass stains: Use alcohol, then wash with household baking soda and hot water. Put in the sun to bleach.

Ink (ordinary): If fresh, immerse in cold or tepid water or skimmed milk. Old ink stains respond well to lemon juice, salt, and sunlight. Whatever is used, the material should be rinsed thoroughly after using to remove all of the solution.

Iodine: Soapy water, ammonia solution, and hot water rinse.

Iron rust: Use lemon juice and salt; expose to the sunlight. For firm fabrics, use strong solution of oxalic acid. Rinse very thoroughly.

Meat juices: Same as for blood.

Mercurochrome: Pour hot water through the material. Acid alcohol does very well, or Dakin's solution and 5% acetic acid (vinegar), equal parts of each. Then wash thoroughly.

Mildew: If fresh, use strong soapsuds and hang in the sunlight. If an old stain, use Javelle water, rinse thoroughly, and repeat the washing if indicated.

Paints, varnishes: Turpentine or benzol (use only in a well ventilated area). If old stain, soak well in grease to soften, then apply turpentine or the other solutions. Chloroform dissolves lacquer paint stains. Acetone sponged on fabric removes varnish. Shellac is soluble in 50% solution of alcohol. Caution: Chloroform is toxic and should be used only in a very well ventilated area.

Perspiration: Wash in strong soap solution and dry in sunlight.

Picric acid: Boil fabric in dilute sodium hydroxide solution for one-half hour and bleach in Javelle water.

Scorch: Hydrogen peroxide applied to the area; then rub well while the material is soaked in strong soap solution. Dry in sunlight.

Silver salts: If not too old, silver stains can be removed by sodium thiosulfate (photographer's hypo).

Tea or coffee: If fresh, pour boiling water through it. If old, soak in borax before pouring boiling water over it.

Urine: Soak in boiling water, then pour 5% Lysol solution over it.

antistalsis (ăn″tĭ-stăl′sĭs) [Gr. *anti,* against, + *stalsia,* contraction]. Reverse movement of bowel contents. Opposed to peristalsis, q.v.

antistaphylococcic (ăn″tĭ-stăf′ĭ-lō-kŏk′sĭk) ["+ *staphylē,* bunch of grapes, + *cocci,* bacteria.]. Destructive to staphylococcus.

antistaphylolysin (ăn″tĭ-stăf′ĭ-lŏl′ĭ-sĭn) ["+ "+ *lysis,* dissolution]. Blood serum substance counteracting staphylolysin.

antistreptococcic (ăn″tĭ-strĕp″tō-kŏk′sĭk). Destructive to streptococcus.

antistreptococcin (ăn″tĭ-strĕp″tō-kŏk′sĭn). The antitoxin of any type streptococcus.

antistreptolysin-O (ăn″tĭ-strĕp-tŏl′ĭ-sĭn). An antibody stimulated by infection with various streptococcus organisms and present in the serum of patients who have the infection. ABBR: ASLO.

antisudoral (ăn″tĭ-sū′dŏr-ăl) [Gr. *anti,* against, + L. *sudor,* sweat]. Inhibiting or preventing perspiration. SYN: *anhidrotic; antihidrotic.*

antisudorific (ăn″tĭ-sū″dŏr-ĭf′ĭk). 1. Inhibiting or preventing perspiration. 2. An agent that reduces the secretion of sweat.

antisyphilitic(ăn″tĭ-sĭf′ĭ-lĭt′ĭk) ["+ L. *syphiliticus,* pert. to syphilis]. An agent that will cure or relieve syphilis.

antitabetic (ăn″tĭ-tă-bĕt′ĭk) ["+ L. *tabes,* wasting away]. 1. Preventing tabes dorsalis. 2. Agent that mitigates tabetic symptoms.

antithenar (ăn-tĭth′ĕn-ăr) [Gr. *anti,* against, + *thenar,* palm, sole]. Placed opposite to the palm of hand or sole of foot.

antither′mic ["+ *thermē,* heat]. 1. Reducing temperature. 2. Agent lowering temperature. SEE: *antipyretic; febrile.*

antithrombin (ăn″tĭ-thrŏm′bĭn). A substance which inhibits coagulation of blood by preventing reaction between thrombin and fibrinogen.

antithromboplastin (ăn″tĭ-thrŏm′bō-plăs-tĭn). Substance which counteracts thromboplastin, thus interfering with normal blood coagulation.

antithy′roid [Gr. *anti,* against, + *thyreoeides,* thyroid]. That which interferes with the action of the thyroid gland or its hormones.

antithyroidin (ăn″tĭ-thī-roy′dĭn). A serum from sheep's blood after thyroid has been removed from animal.

    USES: Exophthalmic goiter and other diseases due to hypersecretion of thyroid gland.

antitonic (ăn″tĭ-tŏn′ĭk) [Gr. *anti,* against, + *tonos,* tone]. Diminishing tone or tonicity.

antitoxic (ăn″tĭ-tŏk′sĭk) ["+ *toxikon,* poison]. Neutralizing a poison, esp. a toxin such as bacterial toxin.

antitoxigen (ăn″tĭ-tŏks′ĭ-gĕn) ["+ "+ *gennan,* to produce]. An antigen stimulating antitoxin production in the blood. SYN: *antitoxinogen.*

antitox′in. An antibody capable of neutralizing a specific toxin. It is produced by the body cells in response to the presence of a toxin. Examples are diphtheria a., gas-gangrene a., and tetanus a. which counteract the toxins produced by the diphtheria, gas-gangrene, and tetanus bacteria. Antitoxins are used for prophylactic and therapeutic purposes. SEE: *antivenin.*

a. serum. A serum that contains the antitoxin of a disease organism. The serum is obtained from the blood of an animal. It is given in toxic diseases, either subcutaneously, intramuscularly, intravenously.

antitoxinogen (ăn″tĭ-tŏks-ĭn′ō-jĕn) [Gr. *anti,* against, + *toxikon,* poison, + *gennan,* to produce]. An antigen promoting production of antitoxin in the blood. SYN: *antitoxigen.*

antitragicus (ăn″tĭ-trăj′ĭ-kŭs). A small muscle in the pinna of the ear.

antitragus (ăn″tĭ-trā′gŭs) [Gr. *anti,* against, + L. *tragus,* goat]. [NA] A projection on the ear of the cartilage of the auricle in front of the tail of the helix, posterior to the tragus.

antitrismus (ăn″tĭ-trĭs′mŭs) ["+ Gr. *trismos,* grinding]. A condition in which the mouth cannot close because of tonic spasm.

antitrope (ăn′tĭ-trōp) ["+ *tropē,* a turn]. 1. A symmetrical pair of organs. 2. Antibody.

antitro′pin. An antibody, q.v.

antitrypsin (ăn″tĭ-trĭp′sĭn). A substance that inhibits the action of trypsin.

antitryptic (ăn″tĭ-trĭp′tĭk). Inhibiting the action of trypsin.

antituberculotic (ăn″tĭ-tū-bĕr′kū-lŏt-ĭk). Inhibiting the spread or progress of tuberculosis in the body.

antitussive (ăn″tĭ-tŭs′ĭv) [Gr. *anti,* against, + L. *tussis,* cough]. 1. Relieving or preventing coughing. 2. An agent that prevents or inhibits coughing.

a., centrally acting. An agent that depresses medullary centers, thus suppressing the cough reflex.

antiuratic (ăn″tĭ-ū-răt′ĭk) ["+ L. *uras,* urate]. 1. Preventing the precipitation of urates. 2. Substances that inhibit or prevent formation of urates.

antivaccina′tion. Opposition to vaccination.

antivaccina′tionist. One who is opposed to vaccination.

antivenene (ăn″tĭ-vĕn′ēn). Antivenin, q.v.

antivenereal (ăn″tĭ-vĕ-nē′rĭ-ăl). Preventing or curing venereal diseases.

antivenin (ăn″tĭ-vĕn′ĭn). An antigenic substance prepared from immunized animal sera.

a., black widow spider. An antitoxic serum obtained from horses immunized against venom of the black widow spider (Latrodectus mactans). Specific in treatment of bites of black widow spider.

a., crotaline, polyvalent. USP. Antisnakebite serum obtained from serum of horses immunized against venom of four types of pit vipers: Crotolus atrox, C. adamanteus, C. terrificus, and Bothrops atrox

(Fam. Crotalidae). Specific in treatment of snakebites of these pit vipers.

antiven'om. A snake venom antitoxin.

antiven'omous. Inhibiting venom.

antiviral (ăn″tĭ-vī′răl). Inhibiting a virus.

antivitamin. A vitamin antagonist; one of a group of substances, natural or synthetic, which inhibits the normal functioning of certain vitamins.

antivivisection (ăn″tĭ-vĭv′ĭ-sĕk′shŭn). Opposition to the use of animals in experimentation.

antixenic (ăn″tĭ-zē′nĭk) [Gr. *anti*, against, + *xenos*, strange]. Pert. to living tissue reaction to any foreign substance.

antizymot'ic ["+ *zymōsis*, fermentation]. An agent that will prevent or arrest fermentation. Ex: alcohol; salicylic acid.

antodontalgic (ăn″tō-dŏn-tăl′jĭk) ["+ *odont*, tooth, + *algos*, pain]. 1. Relieving toothache. 2. Remedy for toothache.

an'tra [L.]. Pl. of antrum.

antracele (ăn′tră-sēl) [L. *antrum*, cavity, + Gr. *kēlē*, tumor]. Accumulation of fluid in Highmore's antrum, i.e., the maxillary sinus. SYN: *antrocele*.

antral (ăn′trăl). Pert. to an antrum.

antrec'tomy [L. *antrum*, cavity, + Gr. *ektomē*, excision]. Excision of the walls of an antrum.

antritis (ăn″trī′tĭs) ["+ Gr. *-itis*, inflammation]. Inflammation of an antrum, esp. that of the maxillary sinus.

antroatticotomy (ăn″trō-ăt″ĭ-kŏt′ō-mī) ["+ *atticus*, attic, + Gr. *tomē*, cutting]. Operation to open and remove contents of the antrum and the attic of the tympanum.

antrocele (ăn′trō-sēl) [L. *antrum*, cavity, + Gr. *kēlē*, tumor]. Fluid accumulation in the maxillary sinus. Syn: *antracele*.

antrona'sal ["+ *nasalis*, nasal]. Rel. to the maxillary sinus and nasal fossa.

antrophore (ăn′trō-fōr) ["+ Gr. *phorein*, to carry]. A medicated bougie for local treatment of any accessible cavity or canal.

antroscope (ăn′trō-skōp) [L. *antrum*, cavity, + Gr. *skopein*, to view). An instrument for examining the maxillary sinus.

antros'copy. Examination of any cavity by the antroscope.

antrostomy (ăn-trŏs′tō-mī) ["+ Gr. *stoma*, mouth]. Operation to open an antrum for drainage.

antrotome (ăn′trō-tōm) ["+ Gr. *tomē*, incision]. An instrument for cutting open a cavity, esp. in bone.

antrotomy (ăn″trŏt′ō-mē). Opening an antral wall.

antrotympanic (ăn″tro-tĭm-păn′ĭk) [L. *antrum*, cavity, + Gr. *tympanon*, drum]. Rel.

to the mastoid antrum and the tympanic cavity.

antrotympanitis (ăn″trō-tĭm″păn-i′tĭs). Chronic inflammation of tympanic cavity and mastoid antrum.

an'trum [L. cavity]. (pl. *an'tra*) [NA]. Any nearly closed cavity or chamber, esp. in a bone.

   a. auris. External acoustic meatus.

   a. cariacum. The thoracic portion of the esophagus, functionally the superior portion of the stomach.

   a., duodenal. The duodenal cap, a dilatation of duodenum near pylorus and seen during digestion.

   a. mastoideum. [NA]. Tympanic antrum.

   a., maxillary. The maxillary sinus. SEE: *sinus.*

   a. of Highmore. The air sinus in the maxillary bone. Maxillary sinus.

   a. puncture. Puncture made in maxillary sinus by placing trocar through sinus wall. Instrument enters from near floor of nose 1 1/2 inches (3.7 cm.) from external opening. Pus is then drained.

   NP: Irrigate antrum 24 hours after puncture. May be necessary for first few days to cocainize nose before passing cannula. Attach syringe to cannula when placed. Teach patient to hold it and to treat self at home.

   a. pyloricum. [NA]. Bulge in the pyloric portion of the stomach along the greater curvature on distention.

   a. tympanicum. The mastoid antrum.

ANTU. Alpha-naphthylthiourea, a powerful rat poison.

anuclear (ā-nū′klē-ĕr). Without a nucleus, said of erythrocytes.

anulus (ăn′ū-lŭs) [L., a little ring]. (pl. *an'uli*) [NA] SEE: *annulus.*

anuresis (ăn-ū-rē′sĭs) [Gr. *an-*, not, + *ouresis*, urination]. Failure of kidney to secrete sufficient urine, or suppression or failure to reach bladder if secreted. Found in acute nephritis, congestion, renal abscess, and last stages of chronic nephritis. SEE: *anuria.*

   ETIOL: Inhalation of ether; lead, phosphorus, cantharides, or turpentine poisoning; Asiatic cholera; gastrointestinal perforation; shock; collapse; reaction to having been transfused with the incorrect type of blood; typhoid fever; yellow fever; pernicious anemia; hysteria; acute yellow atrophy of the liver. Obstructive suppression is the result of occlusion of one or both ureters.

   NP: Aid action of skin and bowels. Care as in nephritis. Wash skin with hot water, 116° - 120°F., twice a day. Hot drinks. Cover patient well. Prevent chilling and keep out of drafts.

anuretic (ăn-ū-rĕt′ĭk). Pert. to anuresis, q.v.

anuria (ăn-ū′rĭ-ă) [Gr. *an-*, not, + *ouron*, urine]. Complete urinary suppression or failure of kidney function. SYN: *anuresis*.

ETIOL: Severe dehydration, shock, transfusion reactions, poisoning by metallic or industrial poisons, sulfonamide nephrosis, kidney disease, obstruction of ureters or renal pelves, obstruction of or reduction in blood flow to kidneys, severe hypotension.

    a., postrenal. A. due to obstruction of renal flow in renal pelvis or ureter. May result from stone, sulfonamide crystals, tumor, or spasm of ureter.

    a., prerenal. Condition resulting from inadequate blood flow to kidney. May result from low blood pressure or low blood volume or both.

    a., reflex. A. which may follow trauma, stone, or instrumentation of the urinary tract.

    a., renal. A. due to lesions involving kidney itself.

anus (ā′nŭs) [L.]. [NA] The outlet of the rectum lying in the fold between the nates or buttocks. The end of the anal canal (2.5-3 cm.). Fissures of anus in newly born indicative of congenital syphilis.

    a., artificial. Opening of the bowel formed usually by colostomy.

    a., fissure in. A crack in mucosa of rectum.

    a., fistula in. A fistulous connection between lumen of rectum and perianal skin. SYN: *fistula in ano.*

    a., imperforated. Condition in which the natural opening is closed.

    a., vulvovaginal. An opening into the vulva from the anus.

anvil (ăn′vĭl) [AS. *anfilt*]. Middle ossicle of ear. SYN: *incus.*

anxietas (ăng-zī′ĕ-tăs) [L.]. Anxiety, apprehension, restlessness.

    a. tibia′rum. Tiredness, twitching, and unrest in legs when in bed.

anxiety (ăng-zī′ĕ-tĭ). A troubled feeling; experiencing a sense of dread or fear, esp. of the future, or distress over a real or imagined threat to one's mental or physical well-being.

Everyone has been anxious at some time. A. is the normal reaction to that which is threatening to one's body, life style, values, or loved ones. A certain amount of a. is normal and stimulates the individual to purposeful action. Excess a. interferes with efficient functioning of the individual. SEE: *a. neurosis.*

    a. neurosis. A functional disease in which fear (or the somatic evidences of fear) out of proportion to any apparent external cause is the essential characteristic.

A symptomatic fear state can be differentiated by recognizing a justifiable organic cause such as thyrotoxicosis. Fear may exist consciously or present a group of somatic symptoms not recognized for what they are; in fact, even denied as representing anxiety. Ordinarily, fear as a response to an environmental threat is quite conscious; it may be equally conscious without the patient having the slightest insight as to its causation.

Anxiety neurosis is manifested when an intact personality without organic disease, during clear consciousness, complains of palpitation; heart pain; dyspepsia; cold, sweaty, tremulous extremities; constriction of the throat; bandlike pressure about head, among other symptoms. Often these are interpreted as meaning regional disease.

The real significance is a feeling of inadequacy in meeting some situation, e.g., a tempting situation which is so completely repressed as to be totally unacceptable to the patient as of significance. Homosexuality is such a frustrated impulse that may lead not only to an anxiety state but to the much more intense picture of panic—psychotic terror. It is always very important not to rationalize the symptoms as being due to some physical disease. SYN: *a. reaction.*

TREATMENT: The anxious patient needs therapy as much as if the disease were due to an organic illness. Comprehensive and understanding counseling may be provided by the family physician or by a psychiatrist. It is essential that the time required be made available if it is done by the family physician. The use of drugs may be indicated; this decision must be made for each patient individually.

anxious agitated depression. Depression accompanied by worry, uneasiness, and agitation, esp. rel. to poverty, want, or ruin.

    SYM: Hallucinations may be present but generally they are absent. Other symptoms are delusions that a well-known phenomenon of nature has ceased to exist, such as the day or the night, the sun or the moon; aversion to eating; or the hearing of voices accusing the subject.

A. O. A. 1. Abbr. for *Alpha Omega Alpha,* an honorary medical fraternity in the U. S.; *American Osteopathic Association.*

A. O. C. Abbr. for *anodal opening contraction.*

aochlesia (ă-ŏk-lē'zĭ-ă) [Gr. *a-*, not, + *ochlesis*, disturbance]. Tranquillity; rest; catalepsy.

aorta (ā-ŏr'tă) [L.]. (pl. *aortas, -tae*) [NA]. The main trunk of the arterial system of the body. It is about 3 cm. in diameter at its origin. It arises from the upper surface of the left ventricle, passes upward as the ascending aorta, turns backward and to the left (arch of the aorta) at about the level of the fourth thoracic vertebra and then passes downward as the descending aorta, which is divided into the thoracic and abdominal aorta. The latter terminates at its division into the two common iliac arteries. At its exit from the ventricle, the aortic orifice is guarded by three semilunar valves.

The three divisions of the aorta are as follows: 1. Aortic arch (5 branches): *Two coronary arteries* (right and left) provide blood supply to myocardium. The *innominate artery* divides into right subclavian artery, which provides blood for the right arm and other areas, and right common carotid artery which supplies the right side of the head and neck. The *left common carotid artery* supplies the left side of the head and neck. The *left subclavian artery* provides blood for the left arm and portion of the thoracic area.

2. Thoracic aorta: Two or more *bronchial arteries* provide blood for bronchi. Four or five *esophageal arteries* provide blood to esophagus. *Pericardial arteries* supply pericardium. Nine pairs of *intercostal arteries* supply blood for intercostal areas. *Mediastinal branches* supply lymph glands and posterior mediastinum. *Superior phrenic arteries supply diaphragm.*

3. Abdominal aorta: *Celiac artery* supplies stomach, liver and spleen. *Superior mesenteric artery* supplies all of small intestine except superior portion of duodenum. *Inferior mesenteric artery* supplies all of colon and rectum except right half of the transverse colon. *Middle suprarenal branches* supply adrenal (suprarenal) glands. *Renal arteries* supply kidneys, ureters, and adrenals. *Testicular arteries* supply testicles and ureter. *Ovarian arteries* (correspond to *internal spermatic arteries* of the male) supply the ovaries, part of ureters, and uterine tubes. *Inferior phrenic arteries* supply diaphragm and esophagus. *Lumbar arteries* supply lumbar and psoas muscles and part of abdominal wall musculature. *Middle sacral artery* supplies sacrum, coccyx. *Right and left common iliac arteries* supply lower pelvic and abdominal areas and the lower extremities.

aortal (ā-ŏr'tăl). Pert. to the aorta.

aortalgia (ā"or-tăl'jĭ-ă) [Gr. *aortē*, aorta, + *algos*, pain]. Pain in the aortic area.

aortarctia (ā"or-tărk'shĭ-ă) ["+ L. *arctare*, to narrow]. Aortic narrowing.

aortectasia (ā"ŏr-tĕk-tā'zĭ-ă) ["+ *ek*, out, + *tasis*, a stretching]. Dilatation of the aorta.

aor'tic. Pert. to aorta or its orifice in the left ventricle of the heart.

　　a. murmur. Symptom of a. valvular disease.

　　a. opening. 1. Path through diaphragm for aorta. 2. Posterior opening in the diaphragm.

　　a. regurgitation. Leakage of the blood from the aorta back into the left ventricle at the recoil of the aorta's elastic walls.

　　ETIOL: Diseases of the heart or aortic valves with defects or weakness of heart muscle. SYN: *a. insufficiency.*

　　a. stenosis. Narrowing of aorta or its orifice due to lesions of the wall with scar formation, infection as in rheumatic fever, or embryonic anomalies. Hypertrophy of the heart is a common result.

　　a. valves. Three valves in left ventricle at the a. opening.

aortitis (ā-ŏr-tī'tĭs) [Gr. *aortē*, aorta, + *-itis*, inflammation]. Inflammation of the aorta. Associated with syphilis in which vascular changes have taken place. A common cause of aortic aneurysm.

　　SYM: Possible cough, cyanosis, dyspnea, cardiac asthmatic attacks, hemoptysis.

aortoclasia (ā"ŏr-tō-klā'zĭ-ă) ["+ *klasis*, a breaking]. Aortic rupture.

aortog'raphy ["+ *graphein*, to write]. Examination of aorta by x-ray pictures after injection of contrast fluid.

aortolith (ā-ŏr'tō-lĭth) [Gr. *aortē*, aorta, + *lithos*, stone]. Calcareous deposit in the aortic wall.

aortomalacia (ā-ŏr"tō-mă-lā'shĭ-ă) ["+ *malakia*, softness]. Softening of the aorta's walls.

aortopathy (ā"ŏr-tŏp'ă-thĭ) ["+ *pathos*, disease]. Any aortic disease.

aortoptosia, aortoptosis (ā"ŏr-tŏp-tō'zĭ-ă, -sĭs) [Gr. *aortē*, aorta, + *ptosis*, a falling]. Downward displacement of abdominal aorta.

aortorrhaphy (ā"ŏr-tor'ă-fĭ) ["+ *rhaphē*, suture]. Suture of the aorta.

aortosclerosis (ā-ŏr"tō-sklĕr-ō'sĭs) ["+ *skleros*, hard]. Aortic sclerosis.

aortostenosis (ā-ŏr"tō-stĕn-ō'sĭs) [Gr. *aortē*, aorta, *stenosis*, a narrowing]. Narrowing of the aorta.

aortotomy (ā"ŏr-tŏt'ō-mĭ) ["+ *tomē*, a cutting]. Incision of the aorta.

AOS. Abbr. for *anodal opening sound.*

aosmic (ā-ŏz'mĭk) [Gr. *a-*, not, + *osmē*, smell]. Without odor.

A.O.T.A. Abbr. for *American Occupational Therapy Association.*

A.P.A. Abbr. for *American Pharmaceutical Association; American Physiotherapy Association; American Psychiatric Association.*

apallesthesia (ă-păl "ĕs-thē'zĭ-ă) [Gr. *a-*, not, + *pallein*, to tremble, + *aisthēsis*, feeling]. Inability to detect vibrations of a tuning fork placed against the body.

apandria (ăp-ăn'drĭ-ă) [Gr. *apo*, from, + *andros*, man]. Aversion to males.

apanthropia, apanthropy (ăp"ăn-thrō'pĭ-ă, ăp-ăn'thrŏ-pĭ) ["+ *anthrōpos*, man]. 1. Morbid aversion to society or fear of human companionship. 2. Apandria, q.v.

aparalytic (ă-păr"ă-lĭt'ĭk) [Gr. *a-*, not, + *paralyein*, to loosen]. Marked by lack of paralysis.

aparathyrosis (ă-păr"ă-thī-rō'sĭs) ["+ *para*, near, + *thyreos*, an oblong shield, + *ōsis*, condition]. Parathyroid deficiency.

apareunia (ā"păr-ū'nĭ-ă) ["+ *pareunos*, lying with]. Inability to accomplish sexual intercourse. Usually due to mechanical obstruction of the entrance to the vagina. SEE: *dyspareunia.*

aparthrosis (ăp"ăr-thrō'sĭs) [Gr. *apo*, from, + *arthron*, joint, + *-osis*, condition]. 1. A joint, such as the shoulder joint, which moves freely in any direction. SYN: *diarthrosis.* 2. Dislocation of a joint.

apastia (ă-păs'tĭ-ă) [Gr., fasting]. Abnormal refusal to eat.

apathetic (ăp"ă-thĕt'ĭk) [Gr. *a-*, not, + *pathos*, disease]. Indifferent; without interest. SYN: *apathic.*

apathic (ă-păth'ĭk). Indifferent. SYN: *apathetic.*

apathism (ăp'ă-thĭzm) [Gr. *a-*, not, + *pathos*, disease, + *ismos*, condition]. Slow to react to stimuli. Opposed to erethism, q.v.

ap'athy [Gr. *apatheia*]. Indifference; insensibility; without emotion, sluggish. Opposed to erethism, q.v.

A.P.C. Abbr. for *acetylsalicylic acid, phenacetin,* and *caffeine,* common ingredients in various headache and cold tablets.

apectomy (ă-pĕk'tō-mĭ) [L. *apex*, tip, + Gr. *ektomē*, incision]. Eradication of apex of a tooth root. SYN: *apicoectomy.*

ape hand. Nerve lesion in which the thumb remains extended at right angle from hand.

apeidosis (ăp"ī-dō'sĭs) [Gr. *apo*, away + *eidos*, form]. Slow modification or disappearance of the clinical and histological characteristics of a disease.

apellous (ă-pĕl'ŭs) [Gr. *a-*, not, + L. *pellis*, skin]. 1. Without skin or lack of formation of scar tissue in wounds. 2. Having a short prepuce, or circumcised.

apenteric (ăp"ĕn-tĕr'ĭk) [Gr. *apo*, from, + *enteron*, intestine]. Outside the intestine. SYN: *abenteric.*

apep'sia [Gr. *a-*, not, + *pepsis*, digesting]. 1. Absence of pepsin in the gastric juice. 2. Imperfect digestion or its cessation.

apepsin'ia. Absence of pepsin in the gastric juice.

aperient (ă-pĕr'ĭ-ĕnt) [L. *aperiens*, opening]. A very mild laxative. Ex: magnesium oxide.

    NP: Usually given at night on an empty stomach if the drug acts slowly (10-12 hours). Saline a. and those having rapid action are given first thing in morning on an empty stomach, half-hour before first fluids are ingested.

    Aperients should not be given in suspected appendicitis, in colic as a rule, in enteritis if diarrhea and vomiting are present.

aperistal'sis [Gr. *a-*, not, + *peri*, around, + *stalsis*, constriction]. Absence of peristalsis.

apéritif (ă-pĕr"ĭ-tēf') [L. *aperīre*, to open]. An alcoholic beverage such as wine taken before a meal to stimulate the appetite.

aperitive (ă-pĕr'ĭ-tĭv). 1. An appetizer. 2. Mild purgative. SYN: *aperient,* q.v.

apertura (ăp"ĕr-tū'ră) [L.]. (pl. *aperturae*) [NA] An opening.

aperture (ăp'ĕr-chūr"). An orifice or opening.

apex (ā'pĕks) [L. tip]. (pl. *ap'ices*) [NA]. The summit or extremity of anything.

    a. beat. The point of maximum impulse of the heart against the chest wall felt in the 5th left intercostal space, approx. 3 1/2 inches from middle of sternum, about an inch within a line drawn from middle of clavicle parallel with sternum (the mammary line).

    Generally may be detected by inspection or palpation; when these fail, may be localized by auscultation. In recumbent position apex beat may be elevated an inch or more. When body is inclined to left, beat may be detected in or outside the mammary line. During forced inspiration, may become imperceptible or be found below its usual place. During forced expiration, beat becomes more forcible and position elevated. Patient as a rule should be examined in erect or sitting posture, while breathing quietly.

    A weak apex beat may be noted in healthy persons at rest, heart failure, pericardial effusion, emphysema, shock or collapse.

    Deformity of chest may cause displacement in any direction.

    Changes in force and extent: May be increased by hypertrophy of heart; excited action of heart from exercise, drugs, reflex irritation, excitement; or disease (as exophthalmic goiter).

Displacement to the left: May result from hypertrophy and dilatation of the heart (down and to the left); pneumothorax on the right; pericardial effusion (up and to left); chronic diseases of left lung and pleura, associated with retraction--as fibroid phthisis and pleural adhesions; abdominal tumors and effusions (up and to left); pressure of a pleural effusion on the right side (up and to left).

Displacement to right: May be caused by chronic disease of the right lung or pleura, associated with retraction; pneumothorax on the left; pressure of a pleural effusion on left side.

Displacement downward: May result from hypertrophy and dilatation of heart, chiefly the left ventricle; pressure of solid growths in upper mediastinum; aneurysm of aortic arch; enlargement of liver, causing traction through central tendon of diaphragm.

Precordial prominence: May result from deformity, enlargement of heart, pericardial effusions.

a. murmur. Murmur over the apex of the heart.

a. root. The end of the root of a tooth.

apex'igraph, apex'ograph [L. *apex*, tip, + Gr. *graphein*, to write]. An instrument for determining location and size of apex of a tooth root.

Apgar score. System of scoring infant's condition one minute after birth. The heart rate, respiration, muscle tone, color, and response to stimuli are scored 0, 1, or 2. The maximum score for a normal baby is 10. Those with low scores require immediate attention if they are to survive.

A.P.H.A. Abbr. for *American Public Health Association.*

aphacia (ă-fā'sĭ-ă). Aphakia, q.v.

aphacic (ă-fā'sĭk). Aphakic.

aphagia (a-fā'jĭ-ă) [Gr. *a-*, not, + *phagein*, eat]. Inability to swallow.

aphakia (ă-fā'kĭ-ă) ["+ *phakos*, lentil]. Absence of eye's crystalline lens.

aphakic (ă-fā'kĭk). Pert. to aphakia.

aphalangia (a"fā-lan'jĭ-ă) [Gr. *a-*, not, + *phalanx*, row]. Absence of fingers or toes.

aphanisis (ă-făn'ĭ-sĭs) [Gr. *aphaneia*, disappearance.]. Fear or apprehension that sexual potency will be lost.

aphasia (ă-fā'zĭ-ă) [Gr. *a-*, not, + *phasis*, speaking]. Inability to express oneself properly through speech, or loss of verbal comprehension.

It is considered to be complete or total when both sensory and motor areas are involved.

RS: agraphia; alalia; anarthria; aphemia; atactic; paraphasia; word blindness.

a., amnesic. Loss of memory for words.

a., ataxic. Inability to articulate. Similar to motor a., q.v.

a., auditory. Inability to understand meaning of spoken words; word deafness.

a., Broca's. A., motor, q.v.

a., conduction. A. due to lesion of conduction path between motor and speech centers.

a., gibberish. Utterance of meaningless phrases.

a., motor. Patient knows what he wants to say but cannot say it. Unable to coordinate muscles controlling speech. May be complete or partial. Broca's area is disordered or deseased.

a., nominal. Inability to name objects.

a., optic. Inability to call name of an object recognized by sight without the aid of sound, taste, or touch; a form of agnosia, q.v.

a., semantic. Inability to understand meaning of words.

a., sensory. Inability to understand spoken words if word center is involved (auditory a.) or the written word if visual

Apgar Score

Sign	Score		
	0	1	2
Heart rate	Absent	Slow or less than 100	Greater than 100
Respiratory effort	Absent	Slow, irregular	Good; crying
Muscle tone	Limp	Some flexion of extremities	Active motion
Reflex irritability	No response	Grimace	Cough or sneeze
Color	Blue, pale	Body pink; extremities blue	Completely pink

word center is affected (visual a.). If both centers are involved, will not understand spoken or written word.

    a., syntactic. Loss of proper grammatical construction.

    a., traumatic. A. caused by head injury.

    a., Wernicke's. A., sensory, q.v.

aphasic, aphasiac. Pert. to aphasia.

aphelotic (ăf-ĕl-ŏt'ĭk) [Gr. *aphelkein,* to draw away]. Absent minded; given to reverie.

aphemesthesia (ă-fem″es-thē'zĭ-ă) [Gr. *a-,* not, + *phēmē,* speech, + *aisthēsis,* sensation]. Word deafness, or word blindness.

aphemia (ă-fē'mĭ-ă). Loss of speech due to impairment of the word memory center; ataxic aphasia.

aphephobia (af″ĕ-fō'bĭ-ă) [Gr. *haphē,* touch, + *phobos,* fear]. Abnormal aversion to being touched by anyone.

aphilopony (ă″fĭl-op'ŏ-nĭ) [Gr. *a-,* not, + *philein,* to love, + *ponos,* bodily exertion]. An abnormal dread of or dislike for work.

aphlogistic (ă″flō-jĭs'tĭk, af″lō-jĭs'tĭk) [″+ *phlogistos,* inflammable]. 1. Not inflammable. 2. Burning without flame.

aphonia (ă-fō'nĭ-ă) [″+ *phōnē,* voice]. Inability to produce speech sounds from larynx. Not due to a brain lesion. May occur in chronic laryngitis.

    ETIOL: Disease of vocal cords, paralysis of laryngeal nerves, pressure on recurrent laryngeal nerve, or it may be functional due to hysteria or psychiatric causes.

    a. clericorum. Clergyman's sore throat.

    a., paralytic. A. resulting from paralysis of speech muscles.

    a. paranoica. The silence of the mentally ill.

    a., spastic. A. resulting from spasm of vocal muscles, esp. that initiated by efforts to speak.

aphonogelia (ă-fo″no-je'lĭ-ă) [″+ ″+ *gelōs,* laughter]. Inability to laugh out loud.

aphoresis (ăf″ō-rē'sĭs) [Gr. *a-,* not, + *phorēsis,* being transmitted]. 1. Lack of endurance, especially of pain. 2. Any separation or removal of a part.

aphose (af'ōz) [″+ *phōs,* light]. A subjective visual perception of darkness, or of a shadow.

aphrasia (ă-frā'zĭ-ă) [″+ *phrasis,* speech]. Inability to use connected phrases when speaking.

    a., paralytic. Due to paralysis of the faculty of ideation.

    a., superstitious. Avoidance of certain words because of scruples or aversion to their use.

aphrenia (a-frē'nĭ-ă) [Gr. *a-,* not, + *phrēn,* mind]. An apparent lack of intellect seen in some forms of dementia.

aphrenic, aphrenous (ă-frĕn'ĭk, -ŭs). Pert. to dementia.

aphrodisia (af″rō-dīz'ĭ-ă) [Gr. *aphrodisios,* rel. to *Aphroditē,* goddess of love]. Sexual passion, esp. when extreme or violent.

aphrodisiac (af″rō-diz'ĭ-ak). An agent which stimulates sexual desire.

aphronesia (ă-fro-ne'sĭ-ă) [Gr. *a-,* not, + *phronēsis,* common sense]. 1. Silliness. 2. Dementia.

aphronia (ă-frō'nĭ-ă) [″+ *phronein,* to understand]. Mental deficiency; defective functional activity of cerebrum.

aphtha (af'thă) [Gr. small ulcer]. (pl. *aph-thae*) 1. Small ulcer on a mucous membrane of the mouth. 2. Thrush.

    a., Bednar's. Whitish ulceration of hard palate in young children.

    a., cachectic. Lesions formed beneath the tongue; accompanied by severe constitutional symptoms.

aphthenxia (af-thenks'ĭ-ă) [Gr. *a-,* not, + *phthegxis,* utterance]. Aphasia characterized by inability to enunciate.

aphthongia (af-thon'jĭ-ă) [Gr. *a-,* not, + *phthongos,* voice]. Aphasia due to spasm of muscles controlling speech.

aphthous (af'thus) [Gr. *aphtha,* small ulcer]. Pert. to, or characterized by, ulcers.

aphylactic (a″fi-lak'tik) [Gr. *a-,* not, + *phylaxis,* a protecting]. Absence of immunity to a disease.

aphylaxis (ă-fi-laks'is). Without immunity against disease.

apical (ăp'ĭ-kal, ā'pĭ-kal) [L. *apex,* tip]. Pert. to the apex.

apicectomy (ap″is-ĕk'tō-mĭ) [L. *apex,* tip, + Gr. *ektomē,* excision]. Resection of apex of a tooth root. SYN: *apicoectomy; apicotomy.*

apices (ā'pĭ-sēz, ăp'ĭ-sēz) [L.]. Pl. of apex.

apicitis (ap-ĭ-sī'tis) [″+ Gr. *-itis,* inflammation]. Inflammation of any apical structure, esp. apex of lung or tooth root.

apicoectomy (ap-ĭ-kō-ĕk'tō-mĭ) [L. *apex,* tip, + Gr. *ektomē,* excision]. Amputation of apex of a tooth root. SYN: *apicectomy; apicotomy.*

apicolocator (a″pĭ-ko-lō'kā-tor) [″+ *locare,* to place]. Instrument for locating apex of a tooth root.

apicolysis (ap″i-kol'ĭ-sĭs) [″+ Gr. *lysis,* dissolution]. Artificial collapse of the apex of a lung by making an opening through the anterior chest wall.

    NP: Keep patient on affected side and watch for shock and hemorrhage.

apicotomy (ap″ĭ-kot′ō-mĭ) [L. *apex.*, tip, + Gr. *tomē*, incision]. Removal of apex of a tooth root. SYN: *apicoectomy.*

apinealism (ă-pin′ĕ-al-izm) [Gr. *a-*, not, + L. *pīnea*, pine cone, + Gr. *ismos*, condition]. Syndrome due to absence of pineal gland.

apinoid (ap′ĭ-noyd) ["+ *pinos*, filth, + *eidos*, form]. Free from dirt; clean.

apiphobia (ă″pĭ-fō′bĭ-ă) [L. *apis*, bee, + Gr. *phobos*, fear]. Abnormal fear of bees or of insects which buzz like a bee.

apituitarism (ă″pĭ-tū′ĭ-tar-izm) [Gr. *a-*, not, + L. *pituita*, phlegm, + *ismōs*, condition]. Condition due to loss of function or removal of pituitary body. Leads to dwarfism or pituitary cachexia. SEE: *Simmond's disease.*

APL. 1. Abbr. for *anterior pituitary-like* (hormone), a substance with activity similar to chorionic gonadotropin. 2. Proprietary name for a preparation of chorionic gonadotropin.

aplanatic lens (ă″plă-nŏt′ĭk lĕnz) [Gr. *a-*, not, + *planētos*, wandering]. Free from spherical or chromatic aberration.

aplasia (ă-plā′zĭ-ă) ["+ *plasis*, a developing]. Failure of an organ or part of the body to develop naturally.

    a. axialis extracorticalis congenita. Congenital defect of the axon formation on the surface of the cerebral cortex.

aplastic (ă-plăs′tĭk) ["+ *plastikos*, shaped]. Pert. to aplasia; having deficient or arrested development.

apnea (ăp-nē′ă) [Gr. *a-*, not, + *pnoē*, breathing]. Cessation of breathing, usually of a temporary nature. May result from reduction in stimuli to the respiratory center as in overbreathing in which carbon dioxide content of the blood is reduced; from failure of respiratory center to discharge impulses as occurs when the breath is held voluntarily; or during Cheyne-Stokes respiration, q.v.

    It is a serious symptom, esp. in such conditions as arteriosclerosis, meningitis, coma, heart and kidney diseases, and also following an injury to the brain where concussion results. Sometimes this type of breathing is noticed in perfectly healthy children and in the aged during profound sleep.

    SYM: It is characterized by a gradual increase in the rate until it ends in a gasp followed by a gradual decrease until the respiration ceases, then it begins again. Another form is sometimes noticed when the respirations gradually increase in force and frequency and then suddenly cease.

    a. alarm mattress. A mattress which is designed to sound an alarm when the infant lying on it ceases to breathe.

apneumatosis (ap″nū-mă-tō′sĭs). Noninflation of air cells of lung; congenital atelectasis.

apneusis (ăp-nū′sĭs). A sustained respiratory inspiratory effort. Due to surgical removal of the upper portion of the pons.

apo-, ap- (ap′o) [Gr. *apo*, from]. Prefix denoting from, away, separation, as apophysis.

apobiosis (ap″o-bi-ō′sis) ["+ *bios*, life]. In physiology, death of a part.

apocamnosis (ap″ō-kam-nō′sĭs) [Gr. *apokamnein*, to grow weary]. Weariness, easily induced fatigue.

apochromatic (ăp″ō-krō-măt′ĭk) [Gr. *apokenoein*, to drain, + *chrōmatikos*, colored]. Free from spherical and chromatic aberration, said of lenses.

apocope (ă-pok′ō-pē) [Gr. *apokopē*, a cutting off]. Amputation.

apocoptic (ap-ō-kop′tik) [Gr. *apo*, off, + *koptein*, to cut]. The effect resulting from the removal of a part.

apocrine (ap′ō-krēn, -krĭn, -krīn) [Gr. *apo*, from, + *krinein*, to separate]. 1. Pert. to cells which lose part of their cytoplasm while functioning, esp. gland cells such as those of the mammary glands and certain sweat glands. 2. Describes sweat glands which differ from the usual (eccrine) in that they appear only in hairy areas such as axillae, groin, and mammary. They appear after puberty, are better developed in women than in men and in Negroes than in Caucasians. The characteristic odor of perspiration is produced by the action of bacteria on the material secreted by the apocrine sweat glands. SEE: *eccrine; holocrine; merocrine.*

apocrustic (ap″ō-krus′tĭk) [Gr. *apokroustikos*, able to ward off]. 1. Astringent. 2. Repellent.

apodal (ă-pō′dal) [Gr. *a-*, not, + *pous*, pod- foot]. Having no feet.

apodemialgia (ăp″ō-dē″mĭ-ăl″gĭ-ă) [Gr. *apodēmia*, away from home, + *algos*, pain]. An abnormal desire to wander from one's abode or environment; wanderlust. Opposed to nostalgia.

apodia (ă-pō′dĭ-ă) [Gr. *a-*, not, + *pous, pod-*, foot]. Developmental defect with absence of one or both feet.

apogee (ap′ō-jē) [Gr. *apo*, from, + *gē*, earth]. Most critical stage of a disease.

apokamnosis (ap″ō-kam-nō′sis) [Gr. *apokamnein*, to grow weary, + *-ōsis*, denoting increase]. Abnormal tendency to fatigue, as in neurasthenia.

apolepsis (ap″ō-lep′sis) [Gr. *apolepsis*, a leaving off]. 1. Cessation of a function. 2. Retention or suppression of an excretion or secretion.

apomorphine (ap″ō-mor′fēn) [Gr. *apo-*, change from, + morphine]. A morphine derivative prepared from the alkaloid by removal of one molecule of water.

    a. hydrochloride. A grayish white powder which becomes green in color on exposure to water or air.

    As an emetic, it is sometimes valuable in cases of poisoning when stomach pump cannot be employed. In small doses may be used as an expectorant.

apomyttosis (ap″o-mĭt-to′sis) [Gr. *apomysein*, to blow the nose]. Any disease in which stertorous breathing or sneezing is a characteristic sign.

aponeurol′ogy (ap″o-nū-rŏl′o-jĭ) [Gr. *apo*, from, + *neuron*, tendon, nerve, + *-logy*, study of, from *logos*, word]. The science of aponeuroses.

aponeurorrhaphy (ap″o-nū-ror′ă-fĭ) [″ + ″ + *rhaphē*, seam]. Aponeurotic suture.

aponeurosis (ăp″ō-nū-rō′sĭs) [Gr. *apo*, from, + *neuron*, nerve, tendon]. (pl. *aponeuroses*) A flat fibrous sheet of connective tissue which serves to attach muscle to bone or other tissues at their origin or insertion.

    a., epicranial. The galea aponeurotica. A fibrous membrane extending from occipital muscles anteriorly to frontal muscles.

    a., lumbar. Superficial sheet of the a. of origin of the transversus abdominis muscle. With the lumbocostal a., encloses the sacrospinalis muscle.

    a., lumbocostal. Deep sheet of the a. of origin of the transversus abdominis muscle. With the lumbar a., encloses the sacrospinalis muscle.

    a., pharyngeal. Sheet of connective tissue lying just under the mucosa of pharynx.

aponeurositis (ăp″o-nū-rō-sī′tĭs) [″ + ″ + *-itis*, inflammation]. Aponeurotic inflammation.

aponeurotic (ap″o-nū-rot′ĭk) [Gr. *apo*, from, + *neuron*, nerve, tendon]. Pert. or rel. to an aponeurosis.

aponeurotome (ap″ō-nū′rō-tōm) [″ + ″ + *tomē*, cutting]. Knife for dividing an aponeurosis.

aponeurotomy (ap″ō-nū-rot′ō-mĭ). Surgical cutting of an aponeurosis.

aponia (ă-pon′ĭ-ă) [Gr. *a-*, not, + *ponos*, toil, pain]. 1. Abstaining from exertion. 2. Absence of pain.

aponic (a-pon′ik). Rel. to aponia. Relieving pain or fatigue.

aponoia, aponoea (ap″ō-noy′ă, ap″ō-nē′ă) [Gr. *apo*, from, + *nous*, mind]. Amentia.

apophlegmatic (ap″ō-fleg-mat′ĭk) [″ + *phlegmatikos*, abounding in mucus]. Producing a mucous discharge; expectorant.

apophyseal (ap″ō-fiz′ē-al) [″ + *physis*, growth]. Rel. or pert. to an apophysis.

apophysis (ă-pŏf′ĭ-sĭs) [Gr. *apophysis*, offshoot]. (pl. *apophyses*) [NA] A projection esp. from a bone, an outgrowth without an independent center of ossification. Ex: a tubercle or tuberosity.

    a. cerebri. The pineal body.

    a. of Ingrassia. Smaller wing of sphenoid bone.

    a. lenticularis. Temporal bone's orbicular process.

    a. of Rau, a. raviana. Long process of malleus.

apophysitis (ă-pŏf″ĭ-sī′tis) [Gr. *apo*, from, + *physis*, growth, + *-itis*, inflammation]. Inflammation of an apophysis.

apoplectic (ap″ō-plĕk′tĭk) [Gr. *apoplēktikos*, crippled by stroke]. Pert. to apoplexy.

apoplectiform (ăp″ō-plĕk′tĭ-form) [Gr. *apoplexia*, stroke, + L. *forma*, appearance]. Like apoplexy. SYN: *apoplectoid*.

apoplectigenous (ăp″ō-plĕk-tĭj′ĭ-nŭs) [″ + *genos*, origin]. Causing apoplexy.

apoplectoid (ap″o-plĕk′toyd) [″ + *eidos*, form]. Like apoplexy. SYN: *apoplectiform*.

apoplexia (ap″o-plex′ĭ-ă) [LL. from Gr. *apoplēssein*, to cripple by a stroke]. Apoplexy, q.v.

    a. uteri. Sudden hemorrhage from the uterus due to arterial degeneration or infarct.

apoplexy (ăp′ō-plĕk″sĭ) [Gr. *apoplēssein*, to cripple by a stroke]. 1. Sudden loss of consciousness followed by paralysis due to hemorrhage into brain, or formation of an embolus or thrombus, which occludes an artery. May also be caused by rupture of an extracerebral artery causing subarachnoid hemorrhage. SYN: *shock; stroke*, q.v. 2. Condition of an organ marked by a hemorrhage into its substance, as apoplexy of the lung.

    SYM: Onset acute. Unconsciousness. Stertorous breathing due to paralysis of portion of the soft palate; expiration puffs out the cheeks and mouth. Pupils sometimes unequal, the larger one being on the side of the hemorrhage. Paralysis usually involves one side of the face, arm and leg of one side, with eyeballs turned away from the side of the body-paralysis, skin covered with clammy sweat, the surface temperature of which is often subnormal; speech disturbances. Onset more gradual if caused by a thrombosis, q.v.

    F.A. TREATMENT: Keep patient quiet and sitting up or lying down with head and shoulders elevated. Do not give stimulants. Apply cooling applications to head and neck.

Do not transport unless absolutely imperative, and then very carefully.

PROG: Depends upon symptoms. Often
grave.

NP: As patient recovering from unconsciousness may hear all that is said in the
room, care should be exercised about talking
in presence of patient. Complete quiet except to reassure patient in a calm gentle
voice. Guard against self-inflicted injuries to
nonparalyzed side from movements due to
irritation. Supine position: Head and body
on same plane. Avoid pressure sores by moving patient frequently. Ease breathing by
change of position once an hour, turning
from paralyzed side to back and reverse. To
lie on paralyzed side may require much effort to breathe. Turn body as a whole, not in
part, flexing a paralyzed arm across chest,
lower extremities flexed. Frequent cleansing of oropharyngeal passages.

Maintain body heat, but care must be exercised lest the unconscious patient be
burned by using heating pad or hot water
bottle at incorrect temperature. Guard
against sacral bed sores (not due to pressure;
a cutaneous indication of lowered vitality).
This is indicated by redness of skin which
may be followed by superficial blisters, resulting in a gangrenous ulcer. Constant
asepsis and antisepsis if break occurs in
skin. Binders to hold dressings; no adhesive
plasters.

A retention catheter may be used to avoid
a wet bed. Use of a closed urinary drainage
system is essential to prevent infection.
Enemas instead of purgatives. Avoid pressure of bed clothes by using a bed cradle.
Watch for contractures of muscles and avoid
these by change of position and passive exercise.

Convalescence: Liquid or soft foods; solid
ones as patient begins to masticate. Slight
elevation of head when feeding which
should be done from the paralyzed side unless patient exhibits imperfect sight, when
position should be reversed to accommodate.

Feed slowly to avoid aspiration of food.
Loss of muscular power of pharynx, tongue
and cheeks must be considered. Frequent bathing; emollients or cocoa butter
applied afterward. Watch for danger from
heat or cold if loss of sensation is manifested
in any part. Systematic massage. No strenuous rubbing. Passive exercises until active
movements are possible.

Hemiplegic or chronic state: Careful
training of muscles and organs of speech is
necessary. Physical therapy, later followed
perhaps by occupational therapy. Confi-
dence must be inspired, memory trained,
and emotions controlled by patient. Nurse
should teach patient how to sit and how to
stand and walk.

RS: Aaron's sign; coma; hemiplegia.

aporrhipsis (ap-ō-rip'sis) [Gr. *apo,* away, +
riptein, to throw]. Removal of clothing or
bed clothes; seen in some psychotic conditions or in delirium.

aposia (ă-pō'zĭ-ă) [Gr. *a-,* not, + *posis,* drink].
Absence of thirst.

apositia (ăp"ō-sĭt'ĭ-ă, -sĭsh'ĭ-ă) [Gr. *apo,* away,
+ *sitos,* food]. Anorexia associated with disgust for food.

apospory (ă-pos'pō-rĭ) ["+ *sporos,* seed]. In
botany, absence of spore-producing ability.

apostasis (ă-pos'tă-sĭs) [Gr. *apostasis,* departure from]. 1. The crisis or end of a disease.
2. An abscess.

apostem, apostema (ap'ō-stem, -stē'mă)
[Gr. *apostēma,* abscess]. An abscess.

aposthia (ă-pos'thĭ-ă) [Gr. *a-,* not, + *posthē,*
foreskin]. Congenital absence of the prepuce.

apothanasia (ap"ō-thă-nā'zĭ-ă) [Gr. *apo,*
away, + *thanatos,* death]. Prolongation of
life.

apothecaries' weights and measures
An outdated and obsolete system of
weights and measures used by physicians
and pharmacists. Has been replaced by the
metric system, q.v.

The scruple and the pound are now seldom used. A portion of a grain is expressed
fractionally, as gr. 1/2, not decimally. The
quantity is written in Roman numerals, q.v.,
with the symbol before it, as gr. v to indicate
five grains,

$$\mathfrak{Z} \underset{xv}{\overline{}} \text{ for 15 ounces.}$$

Some points to remember: The character $\mathfrak{Z}$
represents 60 grains, while f $\mathfrak{Z}$ represents 60
minims. $\mathfrak{Z}$ represents 480 grains only, while
f $\mathfrak{Z}$ is necessary to express 480 minims. A
minim is not the equivalent of a grain. 480
minims (1 f $\mathfrak{Z}$) of water weighed at standard
temperature weigh 456.37 grains. This
should be remembered for percentage solutions. SEE: *weights and measures* in *Appendix.*

apothecary (ă-poth'ē-kā-rĭ) [Gr. *apothēkē,*
storing place]. A druggist or pharmacist. In
England and Ireland one licensed by the Society of Apothecaries as an authorized physician and dispenser of drugs.

apothem, apotheme (ap'ō-thĕm, -thĕm)
[Gr. *apo,* away, + *thema,* deposit]. The
brown precipitate which appears when vege-

table decoctions or infusions are exposed to the air or are boiled a long time.

apothesis (ă-pŏth'ĕ-sĭs) [Gr. *apothesis*, a placing back]. Reduction of a fracture or dislocation.

apotheter (ă-poth'ĕ-ter) [Gr. *apothēni*, to put away]. An instrument used during delivery to push up a prolapsed umbilical cord.

apotripsis (ap"o-trip'sis) [Gr. *apotribein*, to abrade]. Removal of opacity in cornea.

apparatus (ap"ă-rā'tŭs, -răt-ŭs) [L. *apparāre*, to prepare]. 1. A number of parts acting together in the performance of some special function. 2. In anatomy, a group of structures or organs which work together to perform a common function. 3. A mechanical appliance or appliances, used in operations and experiments.

  a., acoustic. Auditory apparatus, the assemblage of parts essential for hearing.

  a., biliary. The structures concerned with secretion and excretion of bile. Includes liver, gallbladder, and hepatic, cystic and common bile ducts.

  a., Clover's. A device used in administering ether or chloroform.

  a., Fell-O'Dwyer's. An instrument for performing artificial respiration, and for preventing collapse of the lung in chest operations.

  a., Golgi. See: *a., internal reticular.*

  a., internal reticular. A cell organoid of variable shape—sometimes granular, reticular, or canalicular—present in most cells, esp. nerve and gland cells. It is rich in lipid materials and varies in size with functional activity of the cell. Its exact function is unknown but it is thought to be involved in secretory activity. SYN: *Golgi a.; Golgi complex; lipochondria; canalicular a.*

  a., juxtaglomerular. Thickened portion of an afferent arteriole in the cortex of a kidney. Consists of modified smooth muscles which acquire a clear swollen appearance. Considered to be the possible source of renin.

  a., lacrimal. The tear-secreting gland and various structures by which tears are conveyed to the nasal cavity.

  a. ligamentosus colli. The occipitoaxial ligament.

  a., respiratory. The entire respiratory system.

  a., sound conducting. Those parts of the acoustic apparatus that transmit sound.

  a., sound perceiving. Those central parts of the acoustic apparatus that are essential for the perception of sounds.

  a., vocal. The various organs collectively that subserve phonation.

appendage (ă-pĕn'dĭj). Anything attached or appended to a larger or major part, as a tail or a limb. SEE: *appendix*.

  a., atrial. A small muscular pouch attached to each atrium of the heart.

  a., auricular. Atrial a.

  a., cutaneous. A.'s of the skin, as the nails, hair, sebaceous and sweat glands.

appendalgia (ap"en-dal'jĭ-ă) [L. *appendere*, hang to, + Gr. *algos*, pain]. Pain in lower right quadrant in region of vermiform appendix.

appendectomy (ap"en-dek'tō-mĭ) [L. *ad*, to, + *pendere*, hang, + Gr. *ektomē*, cut out]. Surgical removal of the vermiform appendix.

appendical, appendiceal (ă-pĕn'dĭ-kal, ap-ĕn-dĭs'ĕ-al). Pert. to an appendix.

  a. reflex. Tenderness at McBurney's point accompanied by rigidity considered a reflex expression by way of sympathetic cerebrospinal arc.

appendicectasis (a-pen-dis-ek'tă-sis) [L. *appendere*, hang to, + Gr. *ektasis*, a stretching]. Dilatation of the vermiform appendix.

appendicectomy (a-pen"dis-ek'tō-mĭ) ["+ Gr. *ektomē*, excision]. Surgical removal of the appendix.

appendices (a-pen'dĭ-sēz). Pl. of appendix.

  a. epiploicae. Pouches of peritoneum, filled with fat and attached to the colon.

appendicitis (a-pen"dĭ-si'tis) [L. *appendere*, hang to, + Gr. *-itis*, inflammation]. Inflammation of the vermiform appendix.

It generally occurs in the young, very rarely before the fifth year or after the fiftieth. It is more common in male adults than in female adults. The disease may be acute, subacute, or chronic.

When this diagnosis is considered in the adult female, it must be differentiated from pain associated with ovulation (mittelschmerz, q.v.), ruptured ectopic pregnancy and pelvic inflammatory disease.

  a., acute. SYM: Abdominal pain, usually severe and generally throughout the abdomen, followed by nausea and vomiting; localization of pain in the right lower quadrant of abdomen with tenderness and rigidity over right rectus muscle or McBurney's point; fever usually rising within several hours, 99°-101° F.; pulse increasing with temperature; patient lying on back with right lower extremity frequently flexed to relieve muscle tension; leukocytosis present shortly after onset. In mild cases symptoms begin to subside on the second day, but in more severe cases there may be a cessation of pain indicating that the appendix has ruptured. After a few hours a well-defined abscess may be felt in the right iliocecal region showing that nature has walled off the area.

TREATMENT: Notify physician as soon as possible. Refrain from giving foods, liquids, cathartics, enemas, and from applying heat. Surgery as soon as the diagnosis is made is the safest procedure.

a., chronic. May follow an acute attack leaving a cicatricial narrowing of the lumen of the appendix, or adhesions. SYM: Gastric indigestion, frequently simulating a gastric ulcer, duodenal ulcer, or gallbladder disease. Tenderness manifested in the right lower abdomen. TREATMENT: Surgical.

a. obliterans, a., protective. A. with adhesions closing the appendiceal cavity.

appendicoenterostomy (a-pen″dik-o-enter-os′to-mĭ) [″+ Gr. *enteron,* intestine, + *stoma,* mouth]. 1. Appendicostomy. 2. The establishment of an anastomosis between appendix and intestine.

appendicolithiasis (ă-pĕn″dĭ-kō″lĭ-thĭ′ă-sĭs) [″+ Gr. *lithos,* stone]. Formation of calculi in the vermiform appendix.

appendicolysis (a-pen″dĭ-kol′ĭ-sis) [L. *appendere,* to hang to, + Gr. *lysis,* a loosening]. Operation which frees appendix from adhesions by a slit in the serosa at its base.

appendicopathy (a-pen″dĭ-kop′ath-ĭ) [″+ Gr. *pathos,* disease]. Any disease of the vermiform appendix.

a. oxyurica. Lesion of the appendical mucosa supposedly due to oxyurids (intestinal parasitic worms).

appendicostomy (a-pen″dĭ-kos′tō-mĭ) [″+ Gr. *stoma,* mouth]. Operation for irrigating cecum and colon.

appendicular (ap″ĕn-dĭk′ū-lăr) [L. *appendere,* to hang to]. 1. Appendical. 2. Pert. to limbs or that appended to another part.

appendix (ă-pĕn′dĭks) [L.]. (pl. *appendixes, appendices*) [NA] An appendage, esp. the vermiform appendix.

a., atrial. A small muscular pouch attached to each atrium of the heart.

a., auricular. Atrial a.

a., ensiform. The third or lowest portion of the sternum.

a. epididymidis. [NA] A cystic structure attached to epididymis, a vestigial remnant of cranial tip of mesonephric duct.

a., gangrenous. When inflammation is extreme, blood vessels are blocked in the mesentery, circulation to appendix cut off, and diffuse peritonitis ensues.

a. testis. [NA] A vestigial remnant of cranial portion of Müllerian duct forming a small bladderlike structure at cranial end of testis.

a. vermiformis. [NA] A worm-shaped process projecting from the cecum, whose mucous membrane also lines the appendix, which contains many solitary glands. Its average length is 8.3 cm. SYN: *processus vermiformis; vermiformis a.*

a., vesicular. A cystic structure found in the broad ligament near the ovary attached to epoöphoron. It is a vestigial structure representing remains of cranial portion of mesonephric duct.

a., xiphoid. The xiphoid process, small terminal portion of sternum.

appendotome (ă-pĕn′do-tōm) [L. *appendere,* hang to, + Gr. *tomē,* a cutting]. An instrument for excision of appendix.

apperception (ăp″ĕr-sĕp′shŭn) [L. *ad,* to, + *percipere,* to perceive]. 1. The process of receiving (perceiving) and interpreting sensory stimuli. 2. Mental perception, consciousness, recognition.

apperceptive (ap″ĕr-sĕp′tĭv). Pert. to apperception.

appestat (ap′ĕ-stat) [L. *appetītus,* longing for, + Gr. *statēs,* stand, from *histanai,* to make stand]. An area of the hypothalamus which is supposed to control appetite for food.

appetence, appetency (ăp′ĕ-tĕns, -tĕn-sĭ) [L. *appetere,* to strive for]. A strong appetite or desire.

appetite (ăp′ĕ-tĭt) [L. *appetītus,* longing for]. Desire, esp. for food; not necessarily hunger.

a. juice. Gastric secretion brought about by psychic causes such as sight or odor of food, and by tasting and chewing. It ceases 15 to 20 minutes after mastication is completed.

a., perverted. Desire to eat unnatural and indigestible substances such as paint or laundry starch.

appetite, words pert. to: acoria; anorexia; apositia; bulimia; dysorexia; hyperorexia; malacia; parageusia; pica; polyphagia; taste.

appetition (ăp″ĕ-tĭsh′ŭn) [L. *ad,* toward, + *petere,* to seek]. Desire for some object.

appetizer (ăp′ĕ-tī″zĕr). That which promotes appetite.

applanation (ap″lă-nā′shŭn) [L. *ad,* to, + *planare,* to flatten]. Abnormal flattening, as of the corneal surface.

apple (ăp′l) [AS. *aeppel*]. Most widely used of fleshy, many-celled fruits having a core. Fruit of tree of the genus Malus.

Food value of 100 gm. (raw, not pared): Cal. 58; trace of protein and fat; carbohydrate 14.5 gm.; vitamin A, 90 I.U.; ascorbic acid 4 mg.

a., Adam's. The laryngeal prominence formed by the two laminae of the thyroid cartilage.

a. packer's diseases. Those which can afflict persons whose work involves the picking, sorting, or packing of apples.

a. packer's epistaxis. Nosebleed due to handling packing trays containing certain dyes.

a. picker's disease. Bronchitis due to a fungicide used on apples.

a. sorter's disease. Contact dermatitis due to chemicals used in washing apples.

a. thinner's disease. Mild intoxication due to pesticide residues on apples.

pplehead. Broad, thick skull of a dwarf.

pplicator (ăp′lĭkā″tĕr) [L. *applicāre*, to attach]. Device, usually a slender rod of glass or wood, used with a pledget of cotton on the end, to apply medicine to the nose, throat, uterus, or any other body cavity.

pposition (ap″ō-zĭ′shŭn) [L. *ad*, to, + *pōnere*, to place]. 1. Development by accretion. 2. Addition of parts. 3. Fitting together, as the edges of two surfaces.

pproximal (ă-proks′ĭ-mal) [″+ *proximus*, nearest]. Contiguous; next to.

pproximate (ă-prŏks′ĭ-māt) [″+ *proximāre*, to come near]. To bring a part toward another, as when bringing the fingers together or an arm toward the body.

praxia (ō-prăks′ĭ-ă) [Gr. *a-*, not, + *praxis*, action]. 1. Inability to perform certain purposive movements without loss of motor power, sensation, or coordination. 2. Ridiculous and out of the ordinary acts performed by the insane. 3. Inability to understand the meaning of things.

a., akinetic. Inability to carry out spontaneous movements.

a., amnesic. Condition resulting from inability to remember orders or instructions.

a., ideational. Misuse of objects due to failure to identify them.

a., motor. Inability to willfully perform acts.

prication (ap-rĭ-kā′shun) [L. *apricare*, expose to sun]. 1. Sunstroke. 2. Sun-bathe. Basking in the sun.

pricot (ā′prĭ-kŏt, ăp′rĭ-kŏt) [L. *praecoquum*, early-ripening plum]. Fruit resembling small peach in appearance.

Food value of 100 gm. (raw): Cal. 51; protein 1.0 gm.; negligible amount of fat; calcium 17 mg.; phosphorus 23 mg.; vitamin A, 2700 I.U.; ascorbic acid 10 mg.

Food value of 100 gm. (dried uncooked): Cal. 260; protein 5.0 gm.; trace of fat; carbohydrate 66.5 gm.; calcium 67 mg.; phos-

phorus 108 mg.; iron 5.5 mg.; sodium 26 mg.; potassium 979 mg.; vitamin A, 10900 I.U.; ascorbic acid 12 mg.

aproctia (ā-prŏk′shĭ-ă) [Gr. *a-*, not, + *prōktos*, anus]. Imperforation or absence of anus.

apron (ā′prŏn) [O.Fr. *naperon*, cloth]. Garment to cover front of the body, for protection of clothing during surgical operations, during certain nursing procedures, while working with plaster of Paris, etc.

a., Hottentot. Abnormally long labia minora. SYN: *velamen vulvae.*

aprosexia (ap″ro-sĕk′sĭ-ă) [Gr. *a-*, not, + *prosechein*, to heed]. Unintentional inattention, esp. from defective hearing, sight, or mental weakness. Inability to concentrate on anything.

aprosopia (ap″rō-sō′pĭ-ă) [″+ *prosōpon*, face]. Congenital defect in which part or all of the face is absent.

apselaphesia (ap″sel-ă-fē′zĭ-ă) [″+ *psēlaphēsis*, feeling]. Absence of tactile sense.

apsithyria (ap″sĭ-thī′rĭ-ă) [Gr. *a-*, not, + *psīthyrizein*, to whisper]. Hysterical loss of voice including inability to whisper.

apsychia (ap-sĭk′ĭ-ă, -sī′kĭ-ă) [″+ *psychē*, mind]. Unconsciousness; a faint.

apsychosis (ap-sī-kō′sĭs, ā″sī-ko′sĭs) [″+ ″+ *-ōsis*, increased]. Inability to think.

A.P.T. Abbr. for *alum-precipitated toxoid.*

aptyalia, aptyalism (ap″tī-ā′lĭ-ă, ăp-tī′ă-lĭzm, ă-tī′a-lĭzm) [Gr. *a-*, not, + *ptyalon*, saliva]. Lack of, or deficiency in, secretion of saliva. SYN: *dry mouth; oligosialia; xerostomia.*

ETIOL: Disease (mumps, typhoid fever); dehydration; effect of drugs; x-ray irradiation; old age; obstruction of salivary ducts. Sjogren's syndrome in which there is deficient secretion of lacrimal, salivary, and other glands.

apulmonism (ă-pul′mon-ĭzm) [″+ L. *pulmo*, lung]. Defect in which a part of or the entire lung is absent.

apulosis (ăp″ū-lō′sĭs) [Gr. *oulein*, to cicatrize]. A cicatrix.

apus (ā′pŭs) [Gr. *a-*, not, + *pous*, foot]. A malformed fetus without feet.

apyetous (ă-pī′ĕ-tus) [″+ *pyēsis*, suppuration]. Nonsuppurative; nonpurulent.

apyknomorphous (ă-pik″nō-mor′fus) [″+ *pyknos*, thick, + *morphē*, form]. Not pyknomorphous; pert. to a cell which does not stain deeply because its stainable material is scattered.

apyogenous (ā-pi-oj′en-us) [Gr. *a-*, not, + *pyon*, pus, + *genos*, origin]. Not due to pus.

apyous (ā-pī′us). Without pus.

apyretic (ă-pī-ret'ik) [Gr. *a-*, not, + *pyretos*, fever]. Without fever. SYN: *afebrile.*

apyrexia (ā-pī-reks'ĭ-ă) ["+ *pyrexis*, feverishness]. 1. Absence of or intermission of fever. 2. Nonfebrile period of an intermittent fever.

apyrogenetic, apyrogenic (ā-pī-rō-jĕ-net'-ik, -jen'ĭk) ["+ "+ *genos*, origin]. Not causing fever.

A.Q. Abbr. for *achievement quotient.*

aq. Abbr. for L. *aqua*, water.

aqua (ak'wă) [L. *aqua*]. (pl. *aquae*) Water. ABBR: a.; aq.

    a. ammoniae. Water charged with ammonia and stimulants.

    a. calcariae. Lime water.

    a. camphorae. Camphor water.

    a. chlori. Water charged with chlorine for antisepsis and cleaning.

    a. destillata. A water obtained by distillation.

    a. ferveṇt. Hot water.

    a. fontana. Spring water.

    a. fortis. Weak nitric acid.

    a. labyrinthi. The fluid in the labyrinth of the ear.

    a., medicated. An aqueous solution of a volatile substance. Usually contains only a comparatively small percentage of the active drug. Many of them are merely water saturated with a volatile oil. They are used more as vehicles and to give odor and taste to solutions.

    a. oculi. The fluid (aqueous humor) of the eye.

    a. pura. Purified water.

    a. purificata. Purified water.

    a. re'gia. Nitrohydrochloric acid water (20% nitric acid and 80% hydrochloric acid).

    a. tepida. Lukewarm water.

aquacapsulitis (ak"wa-kap"su-li'tis) ["+ *capsula*, a small box, + Gr. *-itis*, inflammation]. Serous iritis. SYN: *aquocapsulitis.*

aquapuncture (ăk"wă-pŭngk'chūr) [L. *aqua*, water, + *punctura*, puncture]. 1. Injection of water hypodermically as a placebo. 2. A fine jet of water sprayed on the skin as a counterirritant.

aqueduct (ak"we-dukt") ["+ *ductus*, duct]. Canal or passage. SYN: *aqueductus.*

    a., cerebral. Canal in midbrain connecting third and fourth ventricles. SYN: *aqueductus cerebri.*

    a., vestibular. Small passage reaching from the vestibule to the posterior surface of the temporal bone's petrous section. SYN: *aqueductus vestibuli.*

aqueductus (ăk"wŭ-dŭk'tŭs). [NA] A channel or canal to convey fluids.

    a. cerebri. [NA] Canal lined with ciliated epithelium and going from the posterior end of the third ventricle through the mesencephalon to the fourth ventricle. SYN: *aqueduct of Sylvius.*

    a. cochleae. Canal connecting subarachnoid space and the perilymphatic space of the cochlea.

    a. Fallopii. Canal for facial nerve in petrous part of temporal bone.

    a. Sylvii. Aqueductus cerebri.

    a. vestibuli. [NA] Canal from vestibule of ear extending into temporal bone.

aqueous (ā'kwē-ŭs) [L. *aqua*, water]. Of the nature of water; watery.

    a. chamber. Anterior chamber of the eye.

    a. humor. Watery transparent liquid containing trace of albumin and small amount of salts. Produced by the iris, ciliary body, and cornea. It circulates through the anterior and posterior chambers of the eye and leaves the eye through one of three routes: the posterior route through the zonula, the iris, and the canal of Schlemm. To enter the latter, it passes through the spaces of Fontana to the pectinate villi through which it is filtered.

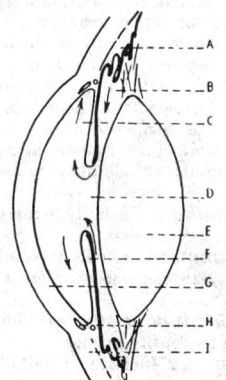

MOVEMENT OF AQUEOUS HUMOR IN THE EYE

Formed by the ciliary body in the posterior chamber, the aqueous humor streams out through the pupil into the anterior chamber and disappears into the sinus venosus sclerae (Schematic). A, Ciliary body with ciliary glands. B, Posterior chamber. C, Anterior chamber. D, Pupil. E, Lens. F, Iris. G, Cornea. H, Sinus venosus sclerae (Schlemm's canal). I, Sclera.

aquiferous (ak-wif'er-us) [L. *aqua*, water, + *ferre*, to bear]. Carrying water or lymph.

aquiparous (ak-wǐp'ǎ-rus) ["+ L. *parere*, to produce]. Producing water.

aquocapsuli'tis. Serous iritis.

AR. Abbr. for *achievement ratio; alarm reaction.*

Ar. Chem. symb. for argon.

arabinose (ǎ-rab'ǐ-nōs). Gum sugar, a pentose, obtained from boiling gum arabic and 0.5% sulfuric acid. Sometimes found in urine. SYN: *l-arabinose; pectinose.*

arabinosuria (ǎ-rǎb''ǐ-no-su'rǐ-ǎ) [arabinose + Gr. *ouron*, urine]. Arabinose in the urine.

arachnid (a-rak'nǐd). A member of the class Arachnida.

Arachnida (ǎ-rak'nǐ-dǎ) [Gr. *arachnē*, spider]. A class of the Arthropoda, including the spiders, ticks, and mites.

arachnidism (ǎ-rak'nǐd-izm) ["+ *eidos*, form, + *ismos*, condition of]. Systemic poisoning from spider bite. SYN: *arachnism.*

arachnitis (ǎ-rak-nǐ'tis) ["+ *-itis*, inflammation]. Inflammation of the arachnoid membrane. SYN: *arachnoiditis.*

arachnodactyly (ǎ-rak''nō-dak'tǐl-ǐ) [Gr. *arachnē*, spider, + *dactylos*, finger]. Spider fingers; a state in which fingers and sometimes toes are abnormally long, slender, and curved. SYN: *Marfan's syndrome.*

arachnoid (ǎ-rak'noyd) ["+ *eidos*, form]. 1. Resembling a web. 2. Arachnoid membrane; arachnoidea, q.v.

    a. cavity. (a) The space between the arachnoid membrane and the dura mater (cavum subdurale); (b) the space between the arachnoid membrane and the pia mater (cavum subarachnoidale or subarachnoid space). The latter contains the cerebrospinal fluid.

    a., cranial. SEE: *arachnoidea encephali.*

    a. membrane. One (the middle) of the three membranes which cover the brain and spinal cord. SEE: *arachnoidea.*

    a., spinal. SEE: *arachnoidea spinalis.*

arachnoidea (ǎ-rǎk-noyd'ē-ǎ). [NA]. A thin, delicate membrane, being the intermediate membrane which encloses the brain and spinal cord. It is located between the pia mater and dura mater, being separated from the pia by the subarachnoid space and from the dura by the subdural space.

    a. encephali. The arachnoidea, the outer surface of which is separated from the dura over the brain by the subdural space. SYN: *cranial arachnoid.*

    a. spinalis. The arachnoidea, the inner surface of which is separated from the pia mater by the subarachnoid space over the spinal cord. It is continuous with a. encephalis. SYN: *spinal arachnoid.*

arachnoidism (ǎ-rǎk'noyd-ǐzm) [Gr. *arachnē*, spider]. The result produced by the bite of poisonous spiders.

arachnoiditis (ǎ-rǎk''noyd-ǐ'tis) ["+ *eidos*, form, + *itis*, inflammation]. Arachnitis; inflammation of the arachnoid membrane.

arachnolysin (ǎ-rǎk-nōl'ǐ-sǐn) ["+ *lysin*]. The hemolysin present in spider venom.

arachnopia (ǎr''ǎk-nō'pǐ-ǎ) [Gr. *arachnē*, spider, + L. *pia*, protective membrane]. Pia and arachnoid considered as one membrane.

Aran-Duchenne disease (ǎr-ŏn' dū-shěn'). [François Amilcar Aran, Fr. physician, 1817-1861; Guillaume Duchenne, Fr. neurologist, 1806-1875] Muscular atrophy beginning in the extremities and progressing to other parts of the body. SYN: *progressive muscular atrophy.*

araneous (ǎ-rā'nē-us) [L. *aranea*, cobweb]. Arachnoid; resembling a cobweb.

Arantius' body, nodule (ǎr-ǎn'shǐ-ǔs). (pl. *Arantii*) [Julius Caesar Arantius, It. anatomist and physician, 1530-1589] Small nodule at center of each of the aortic valve cusps. SYN: *noduli valvularum aortae.*

arborescent (ǎr''bor-es'ent) [L. *arborescere*, to become a tree]. Branching; tree-like.

arborization (ǎr''bor-ǐ-zā'shun) [L. *arbor*, a tree]. 1. Interlacing; ramification; applied to nerve processes, terminations, fibers and arterioles. 2. A structure having the conformation of a tree. SEE: *nerve.*

    a., terminal. The treelike termination of a nerve cell process, esp. the axis cylinder; the telodendria.

arbor vitae (ǎr'bor vī'tī) [L. *arbor*, tree, + *vita*, life]. In anatomy, 1. A tree-like structure; a tree-like outline seen in a section of the cerebellum. 2. A series of branching ridges within the cervix of the uterus. SYN: *plica palmatae.*

arc (ǎrk) [L. *arcus*, bow]. A curved line; portion of the circumference of a circle.

    a., reflex. The path followed by a nerve impulse in a reflex action. The impulse originates in a receptor at the point of stimulation, passes through an afferent neuron or neurons to a reflex center in the brain or spinal cord, and from the center out through efferent neurons to the effector organ, a muscle, or gland where the response occurs.

arcade (ǎr-kād'). Any anatomic structure composed of a series of arches.

    a., Flint's. The arteriovenous anastomosis at the base of the pyramid of the kidney.

arcanum (ar-kā'num) [L. *arcānum*, a secret]. (pl. *arcana*) Secret remedy or nostrum; an elixir.

arcate (ar'kāt) [L. *arcatus*, bow shaped]. Arched, bow-shaped.

arch-, arche-, archi- [Gr. *archē,* beginning]. Prefix meaning first, principal, chief, beginning, ultimate of a kind, as in archetype.

arch [L. *arcus,* a bow]. Any structure of a curved or bow-like outline.

a., abdominothoracic. The lower boundary of the front of the thorax.

a., alveolar. A. of the alveolar process of either jaw.

a., aortic; a. of the aorta. Proximal curved part of the aorta, extending downward to the lower border of the fourth thoracic vertebra. The innominate, left common carotid, and left subclavian arteries arise from the aortic a.

a.'s, aortic. A series of six pairs of vessels which develop in the embryo and connect the aortic sac with the dorsal aortas. During the fifth to seventh weeks, the a.'s undergo transformation, some persisting as functional vessels, others persisting as rudimentary structures, and some disappearing entirely.

a.'s, branchial. A series of a.'s which support the gills of fishes. They occur in the human embryo and play an important role in the development of the head and neck. First is the mandibular, second, the hyoid. The third, fourth and fifth are transitory. SYN: *gill a.'s; visceral a.'s.*

a., carotid. The third aortic a. which provides the common carotid artery.

a.'s of Corti. A series of a.'s made up of the rods of Corti.

a., costal. A. formed by the ribs.

a., crural. Femoral a.; Poupart's ligament.

a., deep crural. A band of fibers arching in front of sheath of femoral vessels; the downward extension of the transversalis fascia.

a., dental. An a. formed by the alveolar process on either jaw, containing teeth and covered by the gums.

a.'s, embryonic. Fetal a.'s, the aortic, branchial, mandibular, hyoid, pulmonary, and thyrohyoid a.'s.

a., femoral. Poupart's ligament.

a.'s of foot. The instep of the foot formed by longitudinal a. and transverse a.

a., glossopalatine. The anterior pillar of the fauces, q.v.

a., hemal. A. formed by the body and processes of a vertebra, a pair of ribs and the sternum, or other like parts; also the sum of all such a.'s.

a., hyoid. The second branchial a. which persists in the styloid process, the stylohyoid ligament, and lesser cornu of the hyoid bone.

a., Langer's axillary. A thickened border of fascia forming a bridge across the occipital groove.

a., longitudinal. One of the two anteroposterior a.'s of the foot; the medial formed by calcaneus, talus, navicular, cuneiforms, and first three metatarsals; the lateral by the calcaneus, cuboid, and fourth and fifth metatarsals.

a., mandibular. The first branchial a. from which the upper and lower jawbones and associated structures develop. It also gives rise to the malleus and incus.

a., nasal. The a. formed by the nasal bones and by the nasal processes of the superior maxilla.

a., neural. The a. of a vertebra formed by its pedicles and laminae; also the sum of all such a.'s. SYN: *vertebral a.*

a., palmar. *Deep,* an a. formed in the palm by the communicating branch of the ulnar and the radial artery. *Superficial,* an a. in the palm forming the termination of the ulnar artery.

a.'s, pharyngeal. The branchial a.'s of the fetus.

a., pharyngopalatine. The posterior pillar of the fauces, q.v.

a., plantar. The a. formed by the external plantar artery and deep branch of the dorsalis pedis artery.

a.'s, postaural. The branchial a.'s.

a., pubic. The portion of the pelvis formed by the rami of the ischia and the ossa pubis on either side.

a., pulmonary. The fifth of the aortic a.'s on the left side. It becomes the pulmonary artery.

a., stylohyoid. One of the embryonic a.'s made up of four segments, viz: the pharyngobranchial, which develops into the styloid process, the epibranchial, developing into the stylohyoid ligament, the ceratobranchial and hypobranchial which together develop into the lesser cornu of the hyoid bone.

a., superciliary. A curved process of the frontal bone lying just above the orbit and subjacent to the eyebrow.

a., supraorbital. A bony a. formed by the upper margin of the orbit.

a., tarsal. One of two branches, superior and inferior, of the median palpebral artery which supply the upper and lower eyelids, respectively.

a., thyroid. The third fetal a.; its cartilage is represented by the greater cornu of the hyoid bone.

a., transverse. An a. of the foot formed by the proximal portions of the metatarsal bones and anterior bones of the tarsus.

a., vertebral. The arched dorsal portion of a vertebra which, with the body, encloses the vertebral canal. SYN: *neural arch.*

a.'s, visceral. Branchial a.'s, q.v.

a., zygomatic. The a. formed by the malar and temporal bones.

archaic type of reaction. An inadequate immature reaction to reality; a reversion to a type once acceptable as normal (e.g., in infancy).

archamphiaster (ärk-ăm'fĭ-ăs''tĕr) [Gr. *archē,* origin, + *amphi,* around, + *astēr,* star]. Amphiaster formed when polar globules are extruded during the process of mitosis, or division, of a cell.

archegenesis (är''kē-jĕn'ē-sĭs) ["+ *genesis,* origin]. Generation spontaneously. SYN: *abiogenesis; archebiosis.*

archenteron (ärk-ĕn'tĕr-ŏn) ["+ *enteron,* intestine]. The primitive digestive cavity of the gastrula which is lined with entoderm. Its opening to the outside is the blastopore. SYN: *gastrocoele; primary gut.*

archeocyte (ar'kē-ō-sīt) [Gr. *archaios,* ancient, + *kytos,* a cell]. A wandering cell.

archeokinetic (ar''kē-o-kĭ-nĕt'ĭk) ["+ *kinētikos,* concerning movement]. Pert. to a low and primitive type of motor nerve mechanism as found in the peripheral and ganglionic nervous systems. SEE: *neokinetic; paleokinetic.*

archepyon (ar-kep'ĭ-on) [Gr. *archē,* a beginning, + *pyon,* pus]. Unusually thick pus.

archespore, archesporium (ar'kē-spor, ar''ke-spō'rĭ-ŭm) ["+ *spora,* a seed]. Cells giving rise to mother cells of spores.

archetype (ar'kē-tīp) ["+ *typos,* model]. 1. Primitive type, from which other forms have developed by differentiation. 2. An ideal or perfect anatomical type. Used as a standard in judging other individuals.

archiblast (ar'kĭ-blast) [Gr. *archi,* first, + *blastos,* a germ, bud]. The outer layer which surrounds the germinal vesicle.

archiblastic (ar''kĭ-blas'tĭk). Derived from, or pert. to, the archiblast.

archiblastoma (ar''kĭ-blas-tō'mă) [Gr. *archē,* origin, + *blastos,* germ, + *-ōma,* tumor]. Tumor of archiblastic tissue.

archigaster (ar'kĭ-gas''ter) ["+ *gastēr,* belly]. The primitive embryonic alimentary canal.

archinephron (ar''kĭ-nef'ron) ["+ *nephros,* kidney]. Primordial kidney, an organ of the embryo. SYN: *mesonephros; wolffian body.*

archineuron (ar-kĭ-nū'ron) [Gr. *archē,* origin, + *neuron,* nerve, tendon]. The central cell of the cerebral cortex, and all its processes. The nervous impulse which is transmitted to initiate physiological function originates in the archineuron.

archipallium (ar''kĭ-pal'ĭ-um) ["+ L. *pallium,* a cloak]. Olfactory cortex, older than neopallium.

archiplasm (ar'kĭ-plăzm) ["+ *plasma,* a mold]. 1. The most primitive living substance. 2. The substance of the fertilized ovum.

archistome (ar'kĭ-stōm) [Gr. *archē,* origin, + *stoma,* mouth]. Invagination of blastula making little opening into archenteron. SYN: *blastopore.*

architis (ar-kī'tis) [Gr. *archos,* anus, + *-itis,* inflammation]. Inflammation of the anus; proctitis.

arch-, archo [Gr. *archos,* rectum, from *archē,* beginning]. Prefix denoting relationship to the rectum or anus.

archocele (ar'kō-sēl) ["+ *kēlē,* tumor]. Hernia of the rectum.

archocolposyrinx (ar''kō-sĭs''tō-kol''pō-sir'inks) ["+ *kystis,* bladder, + *kolpos,* vagina, + *syrinx,* tube, fistula]. Fistula of rectum, vagina, and bladder.

archocystosyrinx (ar''kō-sĭs''tō-sir'inks) ["+ "+ *syrinx,* tube, fistula]. Anovesical fistula.

archoptoma (ar''kop-tō'mă, ar''ko-tō'mă) [Gr. *archos,* anus, + *ptōma,* a fall]. Prolapse of the rectum.

archoptosia, archoptosis (ar''kop-tō'sĭ-ă, -sĭs; ar''ko-tō'sĭ-ă, sĭs) ["+ *ptōsis,* a falling]. Prolapse of rectum.

archorrhagia (ar''kō-ra'jĭ-ă) ["+ *rhēgnunai,* to break out]. Hemorrhage from the rectum; archorrhea.

archorrhea (ar-kō-rē'ă) [Gr. *archos,* anus, + *rhein,* to flow]. Rectal hemorrhage. SYN: *archorrhagia.*

archostenosis (ar''kō-stĕ-nō'sis) ["+ *stenōsis,* a narrowing]. Stricture of the rectum.

arciform (ar'sĭ-form) [L. *arcus,* bow, + *forma,* shape]. Bow-shaped; shaped like an arc. SYN: *arcuate.*

arctation (ark-tā'shun) [L. *arctatus,* from *arctare,* to press together]. Stricture of any canal opening.

arcuate (ar'kū-āt) [L. *arcuatus,* bowed]. Bowed, shaped like an arc. SYN: *arciform.*

arcuation (ar-kū-ā'shun). A bending, curvature.

arculus (ar'kū-lŭs) [L. *arculus,* a small arch]. Support, in the form of an arch for bedclothes, to protect a part. SYN: *cradle.*

arcus (ar'kŭs) [L. *arcus,* a bow]. (pl. *arcus*) An arc or arch.

a. alveolaris maxillae. [NA] Formerly called limbus alveolaris. The arch of the alveolar process of either jaw.

a. dentalis. Dental arch.

a. juvenilis. Opaque ring about the corneal periphery similar to a. senilis; occurs in young individuals.

a. plantaris. [NA] The plantar arch.

a. senilis. Opaque white ring about corneal periphery, seen in aged persons. Due to deposit of fat granules in cornea or to hyaline degeneration.

ARD. Abbr. for *acute* (undifferentiated) *respiratory disease.*

ardanesthesia (ar″dan-es-the′zĭ-ă) [L. *ardor,* heat, + Gr. *an-,* not, + *aisthēsis,* feeling]. Inability to feel heat. SYN: *thermanesthesia.*

ardent (ar′dent) [L. *ardens,* burning]. Burning; feverish.

ardor (ar′dor) [L., heat]. Burning; great heat.

a. urinae. A burning sensation during urination.

a. veneris. Sexual desire.

a. ventriculi. Heart burn; pyrosis.

area (a′rē-ă, ăr′ē-ă) [L. *area,* an open space]. (pl. *areas, areae*) 1. A circumscribed space; one having definite boundaries. 2. A region of the cerebral cortex which differs in structure and function from other regions.

a. acustica. A. vestibularis, q.v.

a., association. A. of the cerebral cortex connected with other cortical a.'s through association and commissural fibers. Thought to be a region in which higher mental processes are mediated.

a., auditory. The hearing center of cerebral cortex located in floor of lateral fissure and coming to surface on dorsal surface of superior temporal gyrus. It receives auditory fibers from medial geniculate body.

a., Broca's. A. in the left hemisphere in posterior portion of inferior frontal convolution. Controls speech. In left-handed persons it is in the right hemisphere. SYN: *motor speech a.*

a.'s Brodmann's. Specific a.'s of the cerebral cortex, considered to be the seat of specific functions of the brain.

a. germinativa. A. of germination of the ovum.

a., Kiesselbach's. A. of anterior portion of nasal septum. Because of its abundant supply of capillaries it is a common site of nosebleed.

a., occipital. Portion of brain below the occipital bone.

a. pellucida. Clear central portion of a. germinativa of the earliest stages of the embryo.

a., rolandic. A. situated in anterior central convolution in front of fissure of Rolando in each hemisphere. Governs motor acts of the body.

a. vestibularis. A rounded elevation in lateral portion of fourth ventricle above the vestibular nucleus. SYN: *a. acustica.*

areatus (a″re-a′tus). Occurring in circumscribed areas or patches.

areflexia (ă″rĕ-flek′sĭ-ŏ) [Gr. *a-,* not, + L. *reflectere,* to bend back]. State without reflexes.

arenaceous (ar″ĕ-na′se-us) [L. *arenaceus,* sandy]. Resembling sand or gravel.

arenation (ar″ĕ-na′shun) [L. *arena,* sand]. A sand bath or application of hot sand.

arenoid (ar′e-noyd) [″ + Gr. *eidos,* form]. Like sand.

areola (ă-rē′ō-lă) [L. *areola,* a small space]. (pl. *areolae*) 1. A small space or cavity in a tissue. 2. A form of macula, q.v., showing a hyperemic area about a skin lesion such as that about a boil. 3. A ringlike discoloration as that about the nipple. 4. The part of the iris enclosing the pupil.

a. mammae. [NA]. The dark pigmented portion of the mammary gland which surrounds the nipple.

a. papilla'ris. A. mammae, q.v.

a., primary. A space appearing in calcified cartilage which is undergoing degeneration in formation of endochondral bone.

a., secondary. An additional ring which during pregnancy is added around the areola mammae.

areolar (ă-rē′o-lar). Rel. to the areola.

a. glands. Large modified sweat glands lying beneath areola of the breast with ducts opening on its surface. They secrete a lipoid material which lubricates the breast and protects nipple during nursing. SYN: *glands of Montgomery.*

a. tissue. Connective tissue which occupies the interspaces of the body.

areolitis (ar″e-o-li′tĭs) [L. *areola,* a small space, + Gr. *-itis,* inflammation]. Inflammation of mammary areola.

areometer (a-re-om′ē-ter) [Gr. *araios,* thin, + *metron,* a measure]. Hydrometer; instrument for measuring specific gravity of fluids.

areosis (ar-e-o′sis) [L. *area,* open place, + Gr. *ōsis,* increased]. Dilution; less compact.

arevareva (ăr-ē″vă-rā′vă) [Tahitian, skin rash]. Severe skin disease accompanied by general debility.

ETIOL: Thought to be due to excess use of kava, an intoxicating beverage.

argamblyopia (ar″gam-bli-o′pĭ-ă) [Gr. *argos*, idle, + *amblus*, dulled, + *ops*, eye]. Amblyopia due to not using the eye.

Argasidae (ar-gas′ĭ-di) [Gr. *argēēis*, shining]. Family of ticks usually infecting birds, but may attack man, causing severe pain, also fever.

argema (ăr-jē′mă) [Gr. *argema*, ulcer]. White corneal ulcer.

argentaffin, argentaffine (ar-jent′ă-fĭn) [L. *argentum*, silver, + *affinis*, associated with]. Taking a silver stain. SYN: *argyrophil.*

argentaffinoma (ar″jen-taf′ĭ-no′mă) ["+ "+ Gr. *ōma*, tumor]. Growth containing argentaffin elastic fibers. May be located in several body sites but usually in the ileum.

May be benign or malignant. When malignant will produce the carcinoid syndrome, q.v.

argentum (ar-jĕn′tŭm) [L.]. SYMB: Ag. At. wt. 107.868; at. no. 47. Silver.

argilla (ar-jĭl′ă) [Gr. *argillos*, white clay]. Clay or kaolin.

argillaceous (ar″jĭl-a′shus). Resembling or composed of clay.

arginase (ar′jĭ-nās). Enzyme of the liver that splits up arginine in hydrolysis, forming urea and ornithine.

arginine (ar′jĭ-nēn, -nĭn) [L. *argentum*, silver]. Crystalline basic amino acid. $C_6H_{14}N_4$-O_2. Obtained from decomposition of vegetable tissues, protamines, proteins and, also prepared synthetically.

It is a guanidine derivative, yielding urea and ornithine on hydrolysis. It is a hexone base. SEE: *amino acid.*

argol, argal (ar′gol, ar′gal). Impure cream of tartar formed in wine casks.

argon (ar′gon) [Gr. *argos*, inactive]. SYMB: Ar. At. wt. 39.948; at. no. 18. An inert gas in the atmosphere.

Argyll Robertson pupil (ar-gĭl′ rob′ert-son). [Douglas Argyll Robertson, Scottish ophthalmologist, 1837-1909] More properly the name of a symptom often present in paralysis and locomotor ataxia (due to syphilis), in which the light reflex is absent but there is no change in the power of contraction during accommodation. Usually bilateral.

argyria (ar-jir′ĭ-ă) [Gr. *argyros*, silver]. Bluish discoloration of skin and mucous membranes as a result of the administration of silver.

argyriasis (ar″jĭ-rī′ă-sĭs). Bluish discoloration of skin due to use of silver. SYN: *argyria.*

argyric (ar-jir′ik). Pert. to silver.

argyrism (ar′jĭr-izm) [Gr. *argyros*, silver]. Bluish discoloration of skin due to use of silver. SYN: *argyria.*

Argyrol (ar′jĭ-rol). Silver vitellin. Proprietary name for a dark-brown, crystalline, protein substance containing 20% silver.

Used as an antiseptic in infections of the eye, nose and throat, and for urethral irrigations.

argyrophil (ar-jĭ′ro-fĭl) [Gr. *argyros*, silver, + *philos*, fond]. Staining readily or easily impregnated with silver. SYN: *argentaffin.*

argyrosis (ar″jĭ-ro′sĭs) ["+ *ōsis*, increased]. Bluish discoloration of skin due to use of silver. SYN: *argyria.*

arhyth′mia. Arrhythmia, q.v.

Arias-Stella reaction. An endometrial gland cell abnormality which may be present in normal or ectopic pregnancy. It is not a sign of endometrial adenocarcinoma.

ariboflavinosis (ă-rī″bō-flā″vĭn-ō′sĭs) [Gr. *a-*, not, + *riboflavin*, + Gr. *-osis*, disease]. Condition arising from a deficiency of riboflavin in the diet.

SYM: Lesions on the lips; stomatitis and, later, fissures in the angles of the mouth; seborrhea around the nose; vascularization of cornea.

TREATMENT: Riboflavin, given orally.

aridura (ar-ĭd-ū′ra) [L. *aridus*, parched]. Dryness, wasting, withering.

aristocardia (ă-ris″to-car′dĭ-ă) [Gr. *aristos*, best, + *kardia*, heart]. Cardiac deviation to the right.

aristogenics (ă-ris″to-jen′ĭks) ["+ *genesis*, generation]. Attempt to control and improve the genetic end-product by encouraging the mating of those with particularly desirable physical and mental characteristics. SYN: *eugenics.*

arithmomania (a-rĭth″mō-mā′nĭ-ă) [Gr. *arithmos*, a number, + *mania*, madness]. Repetition of consecutive numbers, unnecessary counting, and morbid interest in numbers.

arkyochrome (ar′kĭ-ō-krōm) [Gr. *arkys*, net, + *chrōma*, color]. A nerve cell in which the stainable substance is arranged in a network.

arkyostichochrome (ar″kĭ-ō-stik′ō-krōm) ["+ *stichos*, row, + *chrōma*, color]. A nerve cell in which the stainable material is arranged both as a network and in parallel lines.

arm [AS.]. 1. In anatomy, the upper extremity from shoulder to elbow. 2. In popular usage, the upper extremity from shoulder to hand or the entire upper extremity.

 a., bird. Atrophy of forearm muscles.

 a. bone. The humerus.

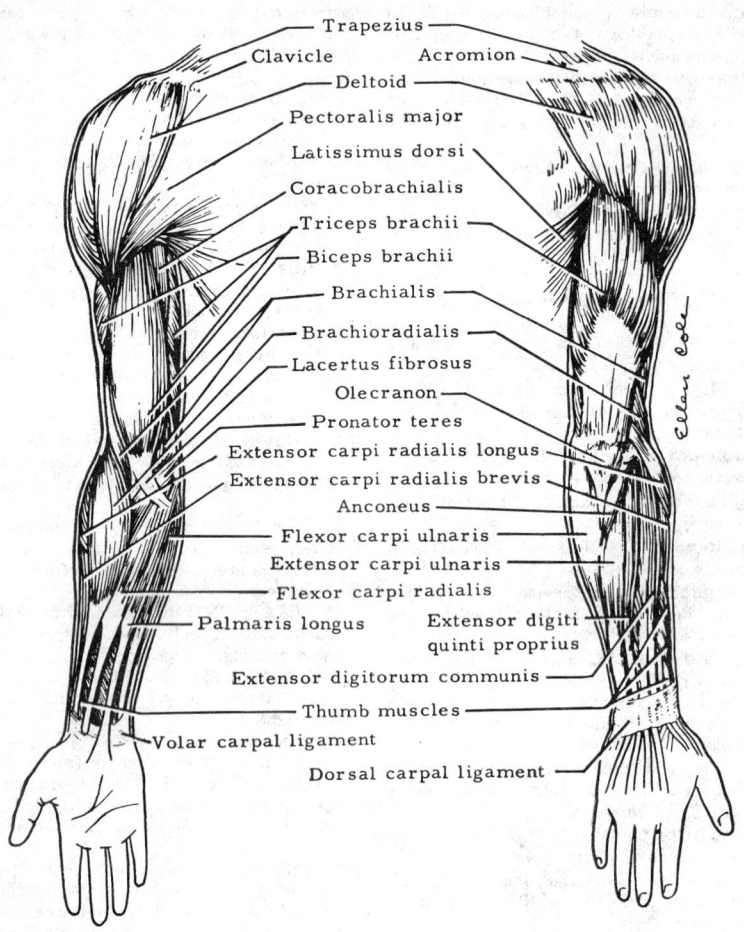

Trapezius
Clavicle   Acromion
Deltoid
Pectoralis major
Latissimus dorsi
Coracobrachialis
Triceps brachii
Biceps brachii
Brachialis
Brachioradialis
Lacertus fibrosus
Olecranon
Pronator teres
Extensor carpi radialis longus
Extensor carpi radialis brevis
Anconeus
Flexor carpi ulnaris
Extensor carpi ulnaris
Flexor carpi radialis
Palmaris longus   Extensor digiti quinti proprius
Extensor digitorum communis
Thumb muscles
Volar carpal ligament
Dorsal carpal ligament

ANTERIOR MUSCLES OF ARM   **POSTERIOR MUSCLES OF ARM**

a., brawny. Hard, swollen arm after removal of a breast, due to lymphedema.

a. center. Center in rolandic area controlling arm motion.

a., Saturday-night. A form of paralysis of the brachial plexus, sometimes seen in intoxicated persons. ETIOL: Sleeping in a chair, with the arm hanging over the back of the chair while the head rests on the shoulder or arm.

arm, words pert. to: axilla; "brachio-" words; brachium; forearm; humerus; radius; ulna.

armamentarium (ar"mă-men-tā'rĭ-um) [L. *armamentum,* implement]. All that a physician or surgeon uses in his practice such as instruments, drugs, books.

armature (ar'mă-tūr) [L. *armatūra,* equipment]. A part of an electrical generator, consisting of a coil of insulated wire mounted around a soft iron core.

armilla [L. *armilla,* bracelet]. (pl. *armillae)* The annular ligament of the wrist.

armpit. Axilla.

arm-to-arm vaccination. Transferring vaccine virus from one patient to another.

army itch. Chronic itch prevalent during U. S. Civil War. SYN: *camp itch.*

Arneth's classification of neutrophils (ar'nāt). [Joseph Arneth, Ger. physician, 1873-1955] Based on the number of nuclear lobes which polynuclear neutrophils contain. The normal are

Lobes	1	2	3	4	5
%	5	35	41	17	2

Arneth's formula. Method of procedure for elaborate differential blood count to estimate number of immature leukocytes.

Arnold-Chiari deformity, malformation. [Julius Arnold, Ger. pathologist, 1835-1915; Hans Chiari, Ger. pathologist, 1851-1916] A condition in which the inferior poles of the cerebellar hemispheres and the medulla protrude and may herniate through the foramen magnum. It is one of the causes of hydrocephalus and is usually accompanied by spina bifida and meningomyelocele.

Arnold's canal. [Friedrich Arnold, Ger. anatomist, 1803-1890] Passage in the temporal bone for small superficial petrosal nerve.

Arnold's ganglion. Otic ganglion.

Arnold's nerve. Auricular branch of vagus nerve. Stimulation of this nerve causes coughing.

aroma (ă-rō'mă) [Gr. *arōma,* spice]. An agreeable odor.

aromatic. 1. Having an agreeable odor. 2. Belonging to that series of carbon compounds in which the carbon atoms form closed rings (as in benzene) as distinguished from the aliphatic series in which the atoms form straight or branched chains.

  a. ammonia spirit. Contains 34 grams of ammonium carbonate in 1000 ml. of a solution containing diluted ammonia solution, fragrant oils, alcohol, and purified water.

  Used as antacid and carminative. Reflex stimulant when vapor is inhaled.

  a. compounds. Ring or cyclic compounds related to benzene, many having a fragrant odor.

arrachment (ă-răsh-mon') [Fr. extraction]. Pulling out the capsule in a membranous cataract through a corneal incision.

arrectores pilorum (ă"rek-tō-rĕz pĭl-ō'rum) [L. *arrectores,* raisers, + *pilus,* hair]. (sing. *arrector pili)* Involuntary muscle fibers arising in the skin and extending down to connect with the hair follicles on the side toward which the hair slopes. Under the influence of cold or fright they contract, straighten the follicles, and raise the hairs, resulting in "gooseflesh" or cutis anserina.

arrest (ă-rĕst'). Stoppage, particularly the cessation of motion of a part which is normally in motion.

  a., cardiac. Cessation of the heart.

  a., epiphysial. Arrest of longitudinal growth of bone.

  a., pelvic. In obstetrics, condition in which presenting part of fetus becomes fixed in maternal pelvis.

  a., sinus. Condition in which sinus node does not initiate impulses for heart beat.

arrhenoblastoma (ă-rē"nō-blas-tō'mă) [Gr. *arrēn,* male, + *blastos,* germ, + *-ōma,* tumor]. An ovarian tumor which secretes male sex hormone and thus causes secondary male sex characteristics (virilization) in the female.

arrhythmia (ă-rith'mī-ă) [Gr. *a-,* not, + *rythmos,* rhythm]. Absence of rhythm; irregularity.

  a., cardiac. Irregular heart action caused by disturbances, either physiological or pathological, in discharge of cardiac impulses from SA node or their transmission through conductile tissue of the heart. See: *bradycardia; tachycardia.*

  a., sinus. Irregular heart beat occurring commonly in children or in the aged in which the rate alternately increases and decreases.

arrhythmic (ă-rith'mĭk). Signifying loss of rhythm.

arrosion (ă-rō'zhŭn) [L. *ab,* away, + *rodere,* to gnaw]. Ulcerous destruction of vessel walls.

arsenfast (ar'sen-fast). Resistant to the poisonous action of arsenic, esp. spirochetes which acquire immunity after repeated arsenic administration.

arseniasis (ar"se-ni'ă-sĭs) [L. *arsenium,* arsenic]. Chronic arsenical poisoning.

arsenic (ar'sĕ-nĭk). SYMB: As. At. wt. 74.922; at. no. 33; sp. gr. 5.73. A metallic element of grayish white color, very poisonous, used in the manufacture of dyes and medicines.

  Minute traces of arsenic are found in vegetables and animal forms of life. It is a constant element of cell life and is present in eggs.

  Many household and garden pesticides contain various forms of arsenic. All of these are toxic if ingested or inhaled in sufficient quantity.

  CUMULATIVE EFFECT: Disorders of alimentary tract, nausea, vomiting, diarrhea, dehydration, neuritis, paralysis of wrist and ankle muscles.

  a. triox'ide. As_2O_3. A white powder. Used internally in form of Fowler's solution (solution of potassium arsenite) 1%. Previously used for a variety of conditions but is little used now. More than a few grains may be fatal. SYN: *arsenous powder; white a.*

POISONING SYM: In acute poisoning, may appear in a few minutes or, when taken with solid food, may not appear for many hours. Metallic taste and odor of garlic on breath, burning pain throughout gastrointestinal tract, vomiting and purging, dehydration, shock syndrome, coma, convulsions, paralysis, death.

F.A.: Lavage stomach with copious amounts of water. If this cannot be done, induce vomiting. Administer dimercaprol (British antilewisite).

TREATMENT: After first aid, maintain fluid and electrolyte balance. Morphine for pain. Treat for shock and pulmonary edema. Blood transfusion may be required to treat blood hemolysis.

SEE: *Table of Poisons and Poisoning* in *Appendix.*

arsenic, words pert. to: acetarsone; arsephenamine; tryparsamide.

arsenical (ăr-sĕn'ĭ-kăl). 1. Pertaining to or containing arsenic. 2. A drug containing arsenic.

arsenic-fast (ar'sĕn-ĭk-fast). Resistant to toxic action of arsenic. SYN: *arsenfast.*

arsenicism (ar-sen'ĭ-sĭzm) [L. *arsenicum,* arsenic, + Gr. *ismos,* condition of]. Chronic arsenic poisoning. SYN: *arseniasis.*

arsenicophagy (ar″sen-ĭ-kof'ă-jĭ) ["+ *phagein,* to eat]. Habitual eating of arsenic. SYN: *arsenophagy.*

arsenionization (ar″sen-ĭ″on-ī-zā'shŭn). Electrolytic diffusion of arsenic ions in tissues.

arsenium (ar-se'nĭ-um) [L]. Arsenic.

arsenoblast (ar-sen'o-blast) [Gr. *arsĕn,* male, + *blastos,* germ]. Male element in nucleus of impregnated ovum; a male pronucleus.

arsenophagy (ar″se-nof'a-jĭ) [L. *arsenium,* arsenic, + Gr. *phagein,* to eat]. Habitual eating of arsenic. SYN: *arsenicophagy.*

arsenoresistant (ar-sen″o-re-zis'tant) ["+ *resistāre,* to withstand]. Resistant to arsenic compounds.

arsenotherapy (ar″sĕ-no-thĕr'ă-pĭ) ["+ Gr. *therapeia,* treatment]. Treatment with arsenic and its compounds.

arsenous (ar'sĕ-nŭs) [L. *arsenium,* arsenic]. Of the nature of, or pert. to, arsenic or its compounds, esp. those containing arsenic in its lower valency. SYN: *arsenical.*

arsine (ar'sĕn). A very poisonous gas used in chemical warfare. SYN: *arsenous hydride.*

arsphenamine (ars-fĕn'ă-mēn). A light yellow powder containing about 30 % arsenic.

Formerly used in treatment of syphilis. SYN: *salvarsan; 606.*

artefact (ar'tĕ-fakt) [L. *ars,* art, + *factus,* made]. Artifact, q.v.

arterectomy (ar″tĕ-rĕk'tō-mĭ) [Gr. *artēria,* artery, + *ektomē,* excision]. Excision of an artery or arteries.

arteria (ar″tĕ'rĭ-ă). (pl. *arteriae)* Artery, q.v.

arteriagra (ar″tĕ-rĭ-og'ră) [Gr. *artēria,* artery, + *agra,* a seizure]. Pain in an artery.

arterial (ar-tē'rĭ-ăl). Pert. to one or more arteries.

    a. bleeding. Blood is bright red and comes in spurts. Arrest by pressure on proximal side of vessel (nearest heart).

    a. circulation. It is maintained by the pumping of the heart, elasticity and extensibility of arterial walls, peripheral resistance in the areas of small arteries, and by the quantity of blood in the body. SEE: *circulation.*

    a. varix. An enlarged and tortuous artery.

arterialization (ar-tē″rĭ-al-ĭ-zā'shŭn). Aeration of the blood, changing it from venous to arterial.

arteriarctia (ar″tĕ-rĭ-ark'shĭ-ă) [Gr. *artēria,* artery, + L. *arctus,* bound]. Stenosis or constriction of an artery.

arteriasis (ăr″tĕ-rĭ'ă-sĭs) ["+ *iasis,* condition]. Degeneration of an artery.

arteriectasis, arteriectasia (ar″tĕ-rĭek'tă-sis, -ek-tā'zĭ-ă) ["+ *ektasis,* a stretching out]. Arterial dilatation.

arterio- [Gr. *artēria,* artery]. Combining form indicating artery or arterial.

arterioatony (ar-tē″rĭ-ō-at'ō-nĭ) ["+ *atonia,* languor]. Lack of tone in arterial walls.

arteriocapillary (ar-tē″rĭ-o-kap'ĭ-la″rĭ) ["+ L. *capillus,* like hair]. Pert. to arteries and capillaries.

    a. fibrosis. Sclerosis of capillaries and arterioles.

arteriofibrosis (ar-tē″rĭ-o-fi-bro'sĭs) [Gr. *artēria,* artery, + L. *fibra,* fiber, + *ōsis,* increased]. Arteriocapillary fibrosis.

arteriogram (ar-tē'rĭ-o-gram) ["+ *gramma,* inscription]. 1. Recording of arterial pulse. SYN: *sphygmogram.* 2. X-ray picture of an artery which contains a radiopaque dye.

arteriography (ar″te-rĭ-og'ră-fĭ) ["+ *graphein,* to write]. 1. Description of arteries. 2. Sphygmography. 3. Roentgenography of arteries.

arteriola (ar-tē″rĭ-o'lă) [L. *arteriola,* small artery]. (pl. *arteriolae)* [NA]. Small artery; an arteriole.

    a. rec'ta. [NA]. One of the small renal arteries going to the medullary pyramids.

arteriole (ar-tē'rĭ-ōl). (pl. *arterioles*) A minute artery, especially one which, at its distal end, leads into a capillary. Arteriola.

arteriolith (ar-tē'rē-o-lith) [Gr. *artēria*, artery, + *lithos*, stone]. An arterial calculus.

arteriology (ar-tē''rĭ-ol'o-jĭ) ["+ -logy, study]. Science of arteries, usually combined with study of other vessels, as in angiology, q.v.

arteriolosclerosis (ar-tē''rĭ-o'lo-sklĕ-rō'sĭs) [L. *arteriola*, small artery, + Gr. *sklērōsis*, hardening]. Thickening of the walls of the arterioles with loss of elasticity and contractility. A type of arteriosclerosis.

arteriolosclerotic (ar-tē''rĭ-ō'lo-sklĕ-rot'ĭk). Rel. to arteriolosclerosis.

arteriomalacia (ar-tē''rĭ-o-mă-la'shĭ-ă) [Gr. *artēria*, artery, + *malakia*, softening]. Softening of the arteries.

arteriometer (ar''te-rĭ-om'ĕ-tĕr) ["+ *metron*, measure]. Instrument measuring variations in the size of an artery as blood pulses through it.

arteriomotor (ar-tē''rĭ-o-mō'tor) ["+ L. *movere*, to move]. Causing changes in size of arteries by dilatation and constriction.

arteriomyomatosis (ar-tē''rĭ-ō-mĭ-ō-mă-tō'-sĭs) [Gr. *artēria*, artery, + *mys*, muscle, + *ōma*, tumor, + *-ōsis*, increased]. Thickening of arterial walls due to overgrowth of muscle fibers.

arterionecrosis (ar-tē''rĭ-o-ne-kro'sĭs) ["+ *nekros*, dead, + *ōsis*, condition]. Arterial necrosis.

arteriopalmus (ar-tēr'ĭ-o-palm'us) ["+ *palmus*, palpitation]. Pulsation of an artery or arteries.

arteriopathy (ar''tē-rĭ-op'ă-thĭ) [Gr. *artēria*, artery, + *pathos*, disease]. Any disease of the arteries.

arterioplania (ar-tē''rĭ-o-pla'nĭ-ă) ["+ *planasthai*, to wander]. The presence of an anomalous course of an artery.

arterioplasty (ar-tē''rĭ-ō-plăs'tĭ) ["+ *plassein*, to form]. Repair or reconstruction of an artery.

arteriopressor (ar-tē''rĭ-o-pres'or) [Gr. *artēria*, artery, + L. *pressura*, force]. Causing increased arterial blood pressure.

arteriorrhaphy (ar-tē''rĭ-or'ă-fĭ) ["+ *raphē*, suture]. Arterial suture.

arteriorrhexis (ar-tē''rĭ-ō-reks'ĭs) ["+ *rhēxis*, rupture]. Rupture of an artery.

arteriosclerosis, arteriolosclerosis (ăr-tē''rĭ-o-, ăr-tē''rĭ-ō-lō-sklē-ro'sĭs) [L. *arteriola*, small artery, + Gr. *sklērōsis*, hardening]. Term applied to a number of pathological conditions in which there is thickening, hardening, and loss of elasticity of the walls of blood vessels, esp. arteries. This results in altered function of tissues and organs.

Changes may occur either in the intima or media.

ETIOL: Cause is unknown. Involutional changes associated with aging, altered lipoid metabolism and other factors are possibly involved.

TREATMENT: Moderate and regular exercise as walking; diet low in animal or hydrogenated vegetable fats; minimal use of tobacco; general moderation in all things to reduce or avoid stress; drugs for hypertension if present.

NP: Avoid all conditions which induce increase of blood pressure. Avoid either cooling or overheating of extremities. It is dangerous to apply intense local heat (hot water bottle or heating pad) to the arms or legs of an individual with inadequate blood supply due to arteriosclerosis. Massage of limbs to avoid cramps and start circulation.

Moderation in food, drink, and exercise. Avoid indigestion. It is not necessary to remain in bed unless heart is affected by strain, but rest is imperative. Anxiety should be eliminated. Avoid all strain upon the heart. Watch for signs of cerebral hemorrhage and guard against cerebral thrombosis by prevention of sudden or continued exertion by the patient.

a. **of legs.** A form due to failure of circulation in the legs.

a., **medial.** Arteriosclerosis involving the muscular arteries in which changes occur primarily in the media. SYN: *Monckeberg's a.*

a., **Monckeberg's.** Medial a., q.v.

arteriosclerotic (ar-tē''rĭ-o-skle-rot'ik). Pert. to arteriosclerosis.

arteriospasm (ar-tē''rĭ-o-spazm'') [Gr. *artēria*, artery, + *spasmos*, pain]. Arterial spasm.

arteriostenosis (ar-tē''rĭ-o-ste-no'sĭs) ["+ *stenōsis*, a narrowing]. Narrowing of the lumen of an artery, either temporary or permanent.

arteriostosis (ar-tē''rĭ-os-tō'sĭs) ["+ *osteon*, bone, + *ōsis*, increased]. Calcification of an artery.

arteriostrepsis (ar-tē''rĭ-ō-strep'sĭs) [Gr. *artēria*, artery, + *strepsis*, a twisting]. Twisting of divided end of an artery to arrest hemorrhage.

arteriosympathectomy (ar-tē''rĭ-s-sĭm''pă-thĕk'tō-mĭ) ["+ *sympatheia*, suffer with, + *ektomē*, excision]. Removal of arterial sheath containing fibers of sympathetic nerve.

arteriotome (ar-tē''rĭ-ō-tōm) ["+ *tomē*, incision]. Knife for opening an artery.

arteriotomy (ar''tē-rī-ot'ō-mĭ). Surgical division or opening of an artery.

arteriotony (ar-tē''rī-ot'ō-nĭ) [Gr. *artēria*, artery, + *tonos*, tension]. Blood pressure; intra-arterial blood tension.

arteriovenous (ar-tē''rī-ō-vē'nŭs) ["+ L. *vena*, a vein]. Rel. to both arteries and veins.

arterioversion (ar-tē''rī-o-vĕr'shŭn) ["+ L. *versiō*, a twining]. Everting wall of artery to arrest hemorrhage from open end.

arterioverter (ar-tē''rī-ō-ver'ter). An instrument for everting cut end of an artery for arresting hemorrhage.

arteritis (ar''tē-rī'tis) [Gr. *artēria*, artery, + *-ítis*, inflammation]. Inflammation of an artery. SEE: *polyarteritis*.

   a. **defor'mans.** Inflammation of inner coat of an artery. SYN: *chronic endarteritis.*

   a. **oblit'erans.** Inflammation of intima of artery causing closure of vessel's lumen. SYN: *endarteritis obliterans.*

artery (ar'ter-ĭ) [Gr. *artēria*, windpipe]. (pl. *arteries*) One of the vessels carrying blood from the heart to the tissues.

   Frequently is nearly empty after death. The ancients supposed that air circulated through them; from which supposition the name, artery, was derived.

   The arteries carry the blood from the right and left ventricles of the heart to all parts of the body. There are two sets, the pulmonary and the systemic. The pulmonary artery carries the venous blood from the right ventricle to the lungs. The systemic system begins as the aorta from the left ventricle.

   ANAT: They have three coats: The inner, tunica intima, or serous; the outer, tunica adventitia, or white fibrous; and the middle, tunica media, or yellow fibrous. The blood they carry is, normally, red. SEE: *Tables* in Appendix.

   a. **coiled.** A., spiral, q.v.

   a. **elastic.** An a. in which elastic tissue is predominant in the tunica intima and tunica media. They include the aorta and its larger branches (innominate, common carotid, subclavian, and common iliac)—vessels which conduct blood to the muscular arteries.

   a. **end.** An artery whose branches do not anastomose with those of other arteries, e.g., arteries to brain and spinal cord.

   a. **muscular.** An artery with smooth muscle tissue in its wall, esp. the tunica media, by means of which the flow of blood to tissues can be regulated through contraction and relaxation. These arteries also contract spastically when injured thus preventing excessive loss of blood.

   a., **sheathed.** The terminal portion of a pulp artery in the spleen which has a peculiar thickened wall.

   a., **spiral.** The coiled terminal branch of a uterine artery. It supplies the superficial two-thirds of the endometrium and, in a pregnant uterus, it empties into intervillous spaces supplying blood which bathes the chorionic villi.

   a., **terminal.** A., end, q.v.

artery, words pert. to: adventitia, aneurysm, angina pectoris, circulation, endarteritis, hypertonia, hypotonia, lumen, media, mesarteritis, periarteritis, sclerosis.

arthragra (ăr-thrăg'ră) [Gr. *arthron*, joint, + *agra*, seizure]. An attack of acute pain in the joints. SYN: *gout.*

ar'thral. Pert. to a joint.

arthralgia (ar-thral'jĭ-ă) [Gr. *arthron*, joint, + *algos*, pain]. Pain in a joint.

   a. **saturnina.** Joint pain resulting from lead poisoning.

arthrectomy (ar-threk'tō-mĭ) ["+ *ektomē*, excision]. Excision of a joint.

arthredema (ar-thrĕ-dē'mă) ["+ *oidēma*, a swelling]. Edema of a joint.

arthrempyesis (ar''threm-pī-ē'sis) ["+ *empyēsis*, suppuration]. Suppuration in a joint.

arthresthesia (ar''thres-thē'zĭ-ă) ["+ *aisthēsis*, sensation]. Joint sensibility; the perception of articular motions.

arthric (ar'thrik). Pert. to a joint.

arthritic (ar-thrĭt'ik). 1. Pert. to a joint. 2. Pert. to arthritis. 3. A person afflicted with arthritis.

arthritides (ar-thrĭt'ĭ-dēz). 1. Collective term applied to various joint disorders. 2. Pl. of arthritis.

arthritis (ar-thrī'tis) [Gr. *arthron*, joint, + *-ítis*, inflammation]. (pl. *arthritides*). Inflammation of a joint, usually accompanied by pain and, frequently, changes in structure.

   ETIOL: Arthritis may result from or be associated with a number of conditions including: infection (gonococcal, tuberculous, pneumococcal); rheumatic fever; ulcerative colitis; trauma; neurogenic disturbances as tabes dorsalis; degenerative joint disease as osteoarthritis; metabolic disturbances as gout; neoplasms as synovioma; hydrarthrosis; para- or periarticular conditions as fibromyositis, myositis, or bursitis; various other conditions as acromegaly, Raynaud's disease, etc. SEE: *bursitis; rheumatism.*

   a., **acute secondary.** A. caused by osteitis. Severe pain, redness, and swelling.

   a., **acute suppurative.** Purulent distention of synovial sac; a serious form.

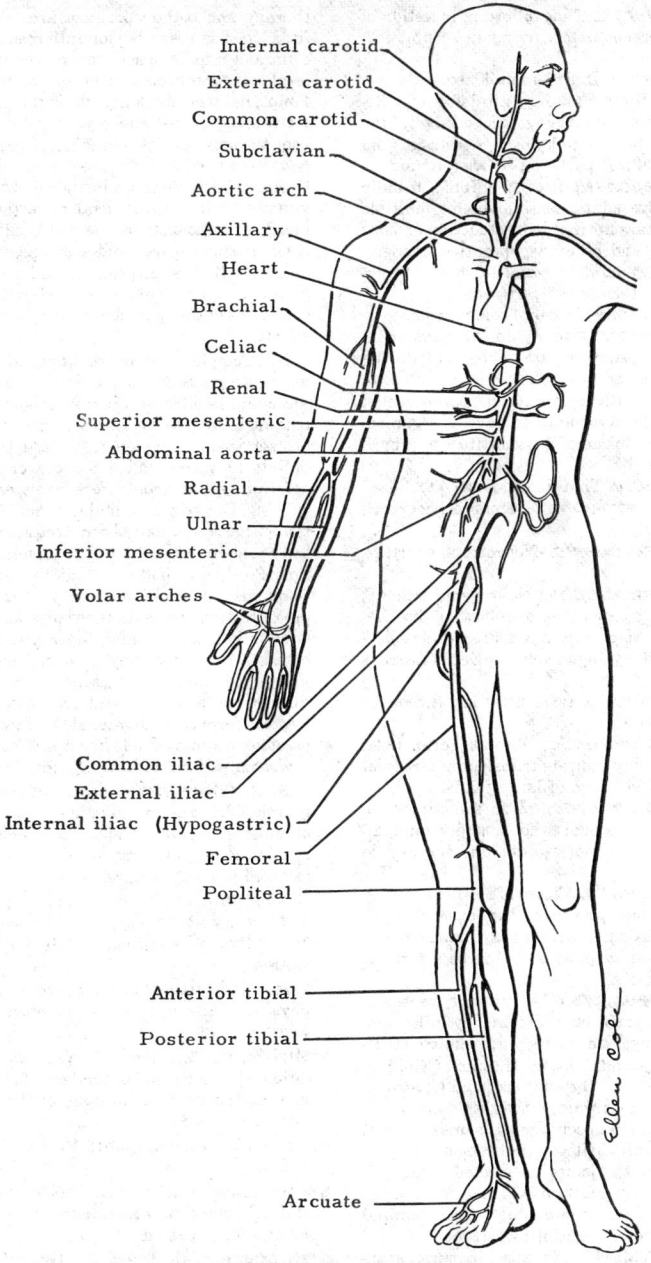

Internal carotid

External carotid

Common carotid

Subclavian

Aortic arch

Axillary

Heart

Brachial

Celiac

Renal

Superior mesenteric

Abdominal aorta

Radial

Ulnar

Inferior mesenteric

Volar arches

Common iliac

External iliac

Internal iliac (Hypogastric)

Femoral

Popliteal

Anterior tibial

Posterior tibial

Arcuate

PRINCIPAL ARTERIES OF THE BODY

a., allergic. That following ingestion of food allergens or occurring in serum sickness.

a., atrophic. Rheumatoid arthritis, q.v.

a. deformans. A. with deformity. Begins in fingers; develops progressively. Deformity due to ankylosis, exostosis, and atrophy of soft parts. SYN: *rheumatoid a.*

a., degenerative. A chronic, usually progressive joint disease involving multiple joints, characterized by destruction of joint cartilage and other degenerative changes. SYN: *degenerative joint disease; hypertrophic arthritis; osteoarthritis.*

a. fungosa. Tuberculosis of a joint.

a., gonorrheal. A. due to gonorrheal infection. Usually attacks knee joint; during acute stage several joints may be affected.

TREATMENT: Penicillin, parenterally, in large doses for 10 to 14 days. If organism is resistant to penicillin, substitute appropriate antibiotic.

a., gouty. That due to gout, q.v.

a., hypertrophic. Degenerative arthritis, q.v.

a., neurogenic. Neurotrophic arthritis, q.v.

a., neurotrophic. Neurogenic arthritis or that accompanying or following diseases of the nervous system. Occurs in tabes dorsalis and syringomyelia. SEE: *Charcot's joint.*

a., osteo-. A form affecting the bones and joints.

a., palindromic. Obsolete term. Used at one time to indicate transient arthritis, of unknown etiology, of large joints.

a., pneumococcal. A. sometimes appearing as a sequel to lobar pneumonia, affecting one or more joints, and the middle ear.

a., psoriatic. A form of a. which usually accompanies psoriasis, the exacerbations and remissions of arthritic symptoms paralleling those of psoriasis. May be a form of rheumatoid a.

a., rheumatoid. A systemic disease of unknown cause characterized by inflammatory changes in joints and related structures. It tends to be chronic. Crippling deformities are the end result. SYN: *atrophic arthritis; chronic proliferative arthritis.*

ETIOL: The specific cause is unknown but it is generally believed that the pathological changes in the joints are related to an antigen-antibody reaction which is poorly understood. Environmental and familial factors are of doubtful importance.

TREATMENT: No specific cure; spontaneous remissions often occur. Physical therapy and orthopedic measures are utilized. Rest is essential for inflamed joints. Pain and muscle spasm can be relieved by local measures such as heat (hot baths, heat lamps, hot poultices). Aspirin is the most effective and safest analgesia for long-term use. Various special methods of treatment have been tried with diverse degrees of effectiveness. These methods include dietary and vitamin regimens; artificial hyperthermia; blood transfusions; use of gold salts and BAL; hormones (adrenal cortical steroids and ACTH); foreign proteins and vaccines. Hormone treatments often relieve acute symptoms but may produce undesirable side effects.

NP: Complete rest in bed imperative during acute stage when hands and feet and joints are swollen and painful. Usually the patient is unable to use them. In order to protect them, complete rest is necessary. Splints may be applied for prevention of deformities but avoid pressure sores from rubbing. Due to poor circulation and limitation of motion, a daily bath necessary. Rub bony prominences with oily massaging solution. Position of patient should be changed frequently. A cradle may be used to avoid pressure from bedclothes. Apply heat over swollen joints. Maintain proper elimination by diet. An enema may be necessary. The mental condition needs special consideration. Strive to keep patient's mind occupied by some form of occupational therapy and if possible, a radio or television set placed in the room will aid in arousing interest.

a., suppurative. A. occurring commonly in children; due to infection by pyogenic organisms, usually Streptococcus hemolyticus and Staphylococcus aureus. Commonly referred to as a "surgical joint."

a., syphilitic. A. occurring in secondary and tertiary stages of syphilis; characterized by tenderness, swelling, and limitation of motion.

a., tuberculous. A. involving epiphyseal cartilage, synovial membrane and joint.

arthritism (ar'thrĭ-tizm) ["+ Gr. *ismos*, condition of]. A condition or tendency to inflammation and gouty conditions of the joints and their processes.

arthro- [Gr. *arthron*, joint]. Prefix: Pert. to joints.

arthrobacte′rium ["+ Gr. *baktērion*, little staff]. A bacterium which reproduces by segmentation or fission.

arthrocace (ar-throk′ă-sĭ) ["+ Gr. *kakē*, badness]. Caries of a joint.

arthrocele (ar'thrō-sēl) ["+ Gr. *kēlē*, tumor]. 1. Hernia of a synovial membrane, penetrating the capsule of a joint. 2. Any joint swelling.

arthrochondritis (ar''thrō-kon-drī'tĭs) ["+ Gr. *chondros*, cartilage, + -*itis*, inflammation]. Inflammation of an articular cartilage.

arthroclasia (ar''thrō-klā'zĭ-ă) ["+ Gr. *klasis*, a breaking]. Artificial breaking of an ankylosed joint to provide movement.

arthrodesis (ar-throd'ĕ-sis) ["+ Gr. *desis*, binding]. The surgical fixation of a joint; artificial ankylosis.

arthrodia (ar-thrō'dĭ-ă) [Gr. *arthrōdia*, a gliding joint]. Gliding joints articulating by surfaces which glide upon each other.

arthrodynia (ar''thrō-dĭn'ĭ-ă) [+ Gr. *odynē*, pain]. Pain in a joint.

arthrodysplasia (ar''thrō-dĭs-plā'zĭ-ă) [*arthro-* + Gr. *dys*, bad, + *plassein*, to form]. A familial disease characterized by deformity of various joints.

arthroempyesis (ar''thrō-em-pī-ē'sĭs) ["+ Gr. *empyēsis*, suppuration]. Suppuration in a joint. SYN: *arthrempyesis*.

arthroendoscopy (ar''thrō-ĕn-dos'kō-pī) [*arthro-*, + Gr. *endon*, within, + *skopein*, to examine]. Inspection of interior of a joint by using an endoscope.

arthrog'raphy ["+ Gr. *graphein*, to write]. 1. A description of the joints. 2. Roentgenography of a joint.

arthrogryposis (ar''thrō-grĭ-pō'sĭs) ["+ Gr. *grypos*, curved, + -*ōsis*, increased]. 1. Persistent contracture of a joint. 2. Tetany.

arthrokleisis (ar''thrō-klī'sĭs) ["+ Gr. *kleisis*, a closure]. Ankylosis, or fixation, of a joint either natural or produced surgically.

arthrolith (ar''thrō-lĭth) ["+ Gr. *lithos*, stone]. Calculous deposit in a joint.

arthrology (ar-throl'ō-jī) ["+ Gr. *logos*, study]. The science of joints.

arthrol'ysis ["+ Gr. *lysis*, a loosening]. The operation of restoring mobility to an ankylosed joint.

arthromeningi'tis ["+ Gr. *mēninx*, membrane, + -*itis*, inflammation]. Inflammation of a synovial membrane. SYN: *synovitis*.

arthrometer (ar-throm'ĕ-ter) ["+ Gr. *metron*, measure]. Instrument for measuring the degree of movement of a joint.

ar'thron. An articulation or joint.

arthroncus (ar-throng'kus) [Gr. *arthron*, joint, + *onkos*, mass]. 1. Tumor of a joint. 2. Swelling of a joint.

arthroneural'gia [*arthro-* + Gr. *neuron*, nerve, + *algos*, pain]. Pain in a joint.

arthrono'sos ["+ Gr. *nosos*, disease]. Joint disease.

a. defor'mans. Arthritis causing deformity. SYN: *arthritis deformans*, q.v.

arthropathol'ogy ["+ Gr. *pathos*, disease, + *logos*, study]. The pathology of joint disease.

arthropathy (ar-throp'ă-thĭ) ["+ Gr. *pathos*, disease]. Any joint disease.

a., Charcot's. Neurogenic arthropathy, q.v.

a., inflammatory. An inflammatory joint disease; arthritis.

a., neurogenic. A trophic joint disease with effusion of fluids into a joint, seen in locomotor ataxia due to syphilis, and in syringomyelia and sometimes in general paresis. SYN: *Charcot-Marie-Tooth disease*, q.v.; *Charcot's joint*, q.v.

a., osteopulmonary. Enlargement and swelling of the ends of the long bones following pulmonary disease.

a., static. A disturbance in a joint of a given extremity secondary to a disturbance in some other joint of the same extremity, as one in the right knee joint secondary to one in the right hip joint.

a., tabetic. A., neurogenic, q.v.

arthrophyma (ar''thrō-fī'mă) ["+ Gr. *phyma*, swelling]. An articular swelling.

ar'throphyte ["+ Gr. *phyton*, growth]. Abnormal growth in joint cavity.

arthroplasty (ar''thrō-plas'tĭ) ["+ Gr. *plassein*, to form]. Surgical formation or reformation of a joint.

arthropod (ar'thrō-pod). A member of the phylum Arthropoda.

Arthropoda (ar-throp'ō-dă) [*Arthro-* + Gr. *pous*, foot]. A phylum of invertebrate animals characterized by bilateral symmetry, esp. chitinous skeleton, segmented bodies, and jointed paired appendages. Includes the crustaceans; insects; myriapods; arachnids; and similar forms. It is the largest animal phylum, containing over 700,000 species. Many are of medical importance as causative agents of disease, as vectors, or as noxious pests.

arthropyosis (ar''thrō-pī-ō'sis) ["+ Gr. *pyōsis*, suppuration]. Suppuration of a joint.

arthrorheu'matism ["+ Gr. *rheumatismos*, flux]. Rheumatism of the joints.

arthrorrhagia (ar''thrō-rā'jĭ-ă) ["+ Gr. *rhegnynai*, to burst forth]. Hemorrhage into a joint.

arthrosclero'sis ["+ Gr. *sklērōsis*, a hardening]. Stiffening or hardening of the joints, esp. in the aged.

ar'throscope ["+ *skopein*, to examine]. An endoscope for examining interior of a joint.

arthros'copy. Direct joint visualization by means of an arthroscope.

arthro'sis [*arthro-* + Gr. *-ōsis*, increased]. 1. Joint. 2. Joint affection due to trophic degeneration.

ar'throspore ["+ Gr. *sporos*, a seed]. A bacterial spore formed by segmentation.

arthrosteitis (ar"thros-tī-i'tĭs) ["+ Gr. *osteon*, bone, + *-itis*, inflammation]. Inflammation of the bony structures of a joint.

arthros'tomy ["+ Gr. *stoma*, an opening]. The formation of a temporary opening into a joint for drainage purposes.

arthrosynovi'tis ["+ Gr. *sny*, with, + *ōon*, egg, + *-itis*, inflammation]. Inflammation of synovial membrane of a joint.

arthrotome (ar'thrō-tōm) ["+ Gr. *tomē*, cut]. Knife for making incisions into a joint.

arthrotomy (ar-throt'ō-mĭ). Cutting into a joint.

arthrous (ar'thrus) [Gr. *arthron*, joint]. Jointed or pert. to a joint.

arthroxesis (ar-thrak'sĭ-sis) [*arthro-* + Gr. *xesis*, scraping]. Scraping of diseased tissue from a joint.

Arthus's reaction (ar-toos'). [Maurice Arthus, Fr. physiologist, 1862-1945] A severe local inflammatory reaction which occurs at site of repeated injection of a nonirritating but antigenic substance such as egg albumin. SYN: *Arthus's phenomenon.*

ar'tichoke [It. *articiocco*]. Perennial plant with edible flowery head. The globe artichoke is the edible variety cultivated for market in the United States. It is also known as the common, green, Italian, French or Paris artichoke.

Usually served with a thick, high-fat sauce. Food value of 100 gm. (boiled): Cal. 8 to 44; protein 2.8 gm.; fat, a trace. The carbohydrate present is in the form of inulin which is of doubtful availability.

artic'ular [L. *articularis*]. Pert. to articulation.

artic'ulate [L. *articulatus*, jointed]. 1. To join together as a joint. 2. To adjust artificial teeth properly. 3. Clearly spoken. 4. To enunciate clearly.

artic'ulated. State of articulation or of being jointed.

articula'tion. 1. The connection of bones; a joint. It is classified as being immovable (synarthrosis), slightly movable (amphiarthrosis), or freely movable (diarthrosis). Cartilage, or fibrous or soft tissue lines the opposing surfaces of all joints. 2. The relative position of the tongue and palate necessary to produce a given sound. 3. Speech, clearly enunciated; enunciation.

    a., confluent. Speech in which syllables are not clearly enunciated.

artic'ulo mor'tis. At the time of death.

articulus (ăr-tĭk'ū-lŭs) [L.]. 1. A knuckle or a joint. 2. A segment.

ar'tifact, artefact [L. *ars*, craft, + *facere*, to make]. 1. Anything artificially produced. 2. An apparent structure produced in a cell or tissue by fixation, staining, or other manipulation.

artifi'cial. Not natural; formed in imitation of nature. SEE: *feeding.*

    a. hyperemia. Bringing blood to the superficial tissues by means of counterirritation such as may be produced by cupping or acupuncture.

    a. impregnation. Same as a. insemination, q.v.

    a. insemination. Mechanical injection of semen into the vagina.

    a. pneumothorax. Artificial introduction of air into pleural cavity. Oxygen or nitrogen, or filtered atmospheric air is used.

artifi'cial respira'tion. Maintenance of respiratory movements by artificial means.

Call a doctor at once. Laryngeal spasm often blocks air from lungs. Passage of catheter or airway tube may be necessary to convey air to lungs. Drugs may be needed to counteract spasm and promote circulation. If such a spasm exists, attempts at artificial respiration may be useless.

METHODS: *Manual methods:* In the past, several relatively ineffective manual methods involving applying pressure to the chest and releasing it have been used. The most effective method is mouth-to-mouth breathing.

Mechanical methods: These include Eve's rocking method and various pressure-cycling devices designed to alter pressure within the lungs and bring about the exchange of gases. Ex: resuscitators; respirators (iron lungs); pulmotors; and lung motors. Devices with stimulation of phrenic nerves are used also.

Choice of method depends upon individual case. If respiration needs only to be started and maintained artificially for a limited period, as in asphyxia from such causes as gases, drowning, and electric shock, the mouth-to-mouth method is effective. If resuscitation apparatus is available, the use of O_2 and CO_2 is indicated. In cases where artificial respiration must be maintained for days, as in morphine poisoning and infantile paralysis, apparatus such as a respirator is used.

IMPORTANT: Artificial respiration may be required to be continued for hours. It should not be discontinued until the patient has been declared dead by a physician.

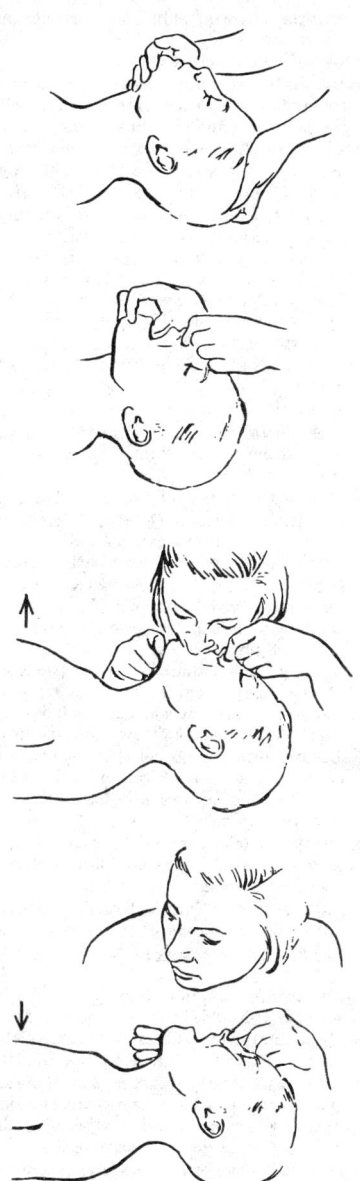

SUPPLEMENTARY TREATMENT: Keep warm with blankets; massage with friction; hot water bottles, etc. If possible, head should be directed downhill to aid circulation to brain; it is desirable to turn the mouth toward the wind. Circulation must be maintained by massaging extremities toward the heart. Stimulants such as aromatic spirits of ammonia applied to nostrils intermittently, and injections of drugs, such as epinephrine (adrenalin), and ephedrine.

RS: asphyxia; collapse; coma; drowning; Eve's method; Laborde's method; respiration; respirator; resuscitation; resuscitation, heart-lung; shock; syncope; unconsciousness.

ar'tisan's cramp. A spasmodic affection of the muscles induced by prolonged work requiring delicate coordination and occurring only in performance of that particular work.

Occupations in which most apt to occur are writing, piano playing, sewing, and telegraphing.

artus (är'tŭs) [L. *artus,* joint]. A joint or joints; a limb.

aryepiglottic (ăr''ĭ-ĕp''ĭ-glŏt'ĭk) [Gr. *arytaina,* pitcher, + *epi,* upon, + *glŏttis,* glottis]. Pert. to the arytenoid cartilage and epiglottis.

ar'yl-. A prefix denoting a radical of the aromatic series.

    a. group. In chemistry, a radical group of the aromatic or benzene series.

arylarsonate (ăr-ĭl-ăr'sō-nāt). Salt of arylarsonic acid.

arytenoid (ar''ĭ-tē'noyd) [Gr. *arytaina,* ladle, + *eidos,* form]. 1. Resembling a ladle or pitcher-mouth. 2. Relating to the a. cartilage, gland, ligament, or muscle.

arytenoidectomy (ar-ĭ-tē''noyd-ek'tō-mĭ) ["+ "+ *ektomē,* excision]. Excision of arytenoid cartilage.

arytenoiditis (ar-ĭt''ĕ-noy-dī'tis). Inflammation of arytenoid cartilage.

Arzberger's pear (ărz'bĕr-gĕr). [Friedrich Arzberger, Austrian physicist, 1833-1905] A hollow pear-shaped device used to pass cool water through after it has been inserted into the rectum. Used in treating rectal diseases such as hemorrhoids.

As. 1. Abbr. for *astigmatism.* 2. Chem. symb. for arsenic.

A.S. Abbr. for L. *auris sinistra,* left ear.

asafetida or asafoetida (as-ă-fet'id-ă) [L. *asa,* gum, + *foetida,* smelly]. A gum resinous substance with characteristic strong odor and garlic taste. Even though this substance is no longer used in medicine, it is of historical interest. In the early part of the 20th century it was used as a carminative and

ARTIFICIAL RESPIRATION
Mouth-to-mouth breathing (Rescue breathing) method.

also as an amulet, suspended in a small bag around the neck. When so used, asafetida was supposed to ward off disease.

asaphia (as-ă-fī′ă, ă-saf′ĭ-ă) [Gr. *asapheia*, obscurity]. Inability to articulate properly due to cleft palate.

asbes′tiform [*asbestos* + L. *forma*, appearance]. Having structure similar to asbestos.

asbes′tos [Gr. *asbestos*, unquenchable]. Fibrous form of magnesium and calcium silicate.

asbesto′sis [*asbestos* + Gr. *-ōsis*, increased]. Lung disease, a form of pneumonoconiosis, q.v., due to protracted inhalation of asbestos particles.

ascariasis (as″kă-rī′ă-sĭs) [Gr. *askaris*, pinworm]. Condition resulting from infestation by Ascaris lumbricoides, the large roundworm. SEE: *Ascaris.*

ascar′ides. Pl. of Ascaris, q.v.

Ascaris (as′ka-ris). (pl. *ascarides*). A genus of nematodes belonging to the superfamily Ascaridoidea. They inhabit the intestines of invertebrates.

A. lumbricoides. A species of Ascaris which lives in the human intestine. Eggs are passed with the feces and are transmitted by contaminated water, food, or hands. After being swallowed, the eggs containing embryos hatch and the larvae enter the blood stream or lymph vessels, pass through the liver and heart to the lungs from which they migrate up the respiratory passages and are swallowed. A new cycle is then started.

Aschheim-Zondek test (ăsh′hĭm-tsŏn′dĕk) [Selmar Aschheim, Ger. gynecologist, 1878 —; Bernhardt Zondek, Ger. gynecologist, 1891 —]. A test for pregnancy. SEE: *test.*

Asch′ner's phenomenon, reflex, sign [Bernhard Aschner, Austrian gynecologist, 1883-1960]. Slowing of the pulse caused by eyeball pressure. Sometimes used to slow the heart during attacks of supraventricular tachycardia. May also be used as a diagnostic test for angina pectoris. Slowing of the heart produced by this reflex may relieve anginal pain. SYN: *oculocardiac reflex.*

Aschoff's bodies (ăsh′ŏf) [Ludwig Aschoff, Ger. pathologist, 1866-1942]. Aschoff's nodules, q.v.

Aschoff's cells. Large cells with basophilic cytoplasm and a large vesicular nucleus often multinucleated. Characteristic of Aschoff's nodules.

Aschoff's nodules. Small nodules found chiefly in association with small arteries in myocardium, a pathognomonic lesion of rheumatic fever. They may also occur in adventitia or aorta, pulmonary arteries and diaphragm.

asci (ăs′ī). Pl. of ascus.

ascia (as′ī-ă, as′kī-ă) [L. *ascia*, ax]. A form of spinal bandage with each turn overlapping the previous one for a third of its width.

ascites (ă-sī′tez) [Gr. *askitēs*, from *askos*, bag]. The excessive accumulation of serous fluid in the peritoneal cavity. SEE: *edema.*

ETIOL: Interference in venous return as occurs in cardiac disease, obstruction of flow in vena cava or portal vein; obstruction in lymphatic drainage; disturbance in electrolyte balance as occurs in sodium retention or in depletion of plasma proteins.

a. chylosus. Chyle in the ascetic fluid usually resulting from rupture of thoracic duct.

ascit′ic. Pert. to ascites

a. fluid. Sp. gr. 1.005-1.015, clear and pale, straw-colored fluid occurring in ascites.

Ascoli's reaction (ahs-kō′lē) [Alberto Ascoli, It. serologist, 1877-1956] Precipitation test for anthrax. Also called Ascoli's test utilized for detection of anthrax bacilli in meat.

Ascomycetes (as″kō-mī-sē′tēz) [Gr. *askos*, a bladder, + *mykēs*, fungus]. The sac fungi; the largest class of Eumycetes, the true fungi (of the phylum Thallophyta). Organisms in this group are characterized by possession of a saclike sporangium (ascus, q.v.) in which ascospores are developed. Includes the yeasts, blue molds, mildews, and truffles.

ascorbic acid (ăs-kor′bĭk) [Gr. *a-*, not, + L. *scorbūtus*, scurvy]. Vitamin C. It occurs naturally and can be synthesized. SEE: *acid, ascorbic; vitamin C.*

ascospore (as′kō-spŏr) [Gr. *askos*, bag, + *sporos*, seed]. A spore produced within an ascus or spore sac.

ascus (as′kus). (pl. *asci*). A saclike structure within which ascospores, typically eight, are formed; characteristic of the Ascomycetes, q.v.

-ase. A suffix used in forming the name of an enzyme. It is added to the name or a part of the name of the substance upon which it acts, as lipase which acts on fats (lipids).

asemia, asemasia (ă-sē′mĭ-ă, as″ĭ-mā′zĭ-ă) [Gr. *a-*, not, + *sēmasia*, the giving of a sign]. Inability to comprehend any type of symbol; a form of aphasia. SEE: *asymbolia.*

asep′sis ["+ *sēpesthai*, to decay]. A condition free from germs; free from infection; sterile, free from any form of life. SEE: *antisepsis, sterilization.*

asep′tic. Rel. to asepsis; free from septic matter.

asep'tic-antisep'tic [Gr. *a-*, not, + *sēpsis*, decay, + *anti*, against, + *sēpsis*]. Both aseptic and antiseptic.

asep'ticize. To make sterile; to free from pathogenic matter.

asexual (ă-sek'shoo-al) [Gr. *a-*, not, + L. *sexualis*, having sex]. Without sex; nonsexual.

asexualiza'tion. Ablation of the ovaries or testes and in this manner desexing the individual.

ash (ăsh) [AS. *aesc*, ash]. Incombustible, powdery residue of a substance that has been completely incinerated.

asialia (as-ī-a'lī-ă, ā''sī-ā'lī-ă) [Gr. *a-*, not, + *sialon*, spittle]. Failure to secrete saliva or deficiency of it. SYN: *aptylism*.

Asiat'ic cholera. An epidemic, acute infectious disease. SEE: *cholera*.

asiderosis (ā''sĭd-ĕ-rō'sĭs) [Gr. *a-*, not, + *sidēros*, iron, + *-ōsis*, condition]. Deficiency of iron reserve in the body.

asitia (a-sish'ī-ă) ["+ *sitos*, food]. 1. Aversion to food. SEE: *anorexia*. 2. The want of food.

ASLO. Abbr. for *antistreptolysis-O*.

asocial (ā-sō'shĭl). 1. Withdrawn from society. 2. Inconsiderate of the needs of others.

asonia (ă-sō'nĭ-ă) [Gr. *a-*, not, + L. *sonus*, sound]. Tone deafness.

Aspar'agus [Gr. *asparagos*]. A genus of liliaceous herbs.

    A. officinalis. Plant of which the tender shoots are eaten as food, and the root is used as a diuretic.

aspar'agus. The common food asparagus; the tender shoots of A. officinalis. Eating asparagus causes the urine to have a peculiar odor.

    Food value of 100 gm. (canned, green, drained solids): Cal. 21; protein 2.4 gm.; vitamin A 800 I.U.; ascorbic acid 15 mg.; calcium 19 mg.

aspastic (ă-spas'tik) [Gr. *a-*, not, + *spastikos*, having spasms]. Nonspastic.

aspecific (ă-spē-sĭf'ĭk). Not specific.

as'pect [L. *aspectus*, a view]. 1. That part of a surface looking in any designated direction. 2. Appearance, looks.

aspergillin (as''pĕr-jĭl'ĭn). 1. A pigment produced by Aspergillus niger. 2. An inappropriate name applied to a number of antibiotic substances produced by various species of Aspergillus.

aspergillosis (ăs''pĕr-jĭl-ō'sĭs). Aspergillus in the tissues or on any mucous surface and the condition produced thereby. This condition may develop in the bronchi; lungs; mucous membranes of the eye, nose, or urethra; the aural canal, or the skin. It may even extend through the various viscera, producing my-

cotic nodules in the lungs, liver, kidney, and other organs.

    a., aural. Otomycosis.

    a., pulmonary. Disease of the lungs caused by Aspergillus.

Aspergillus (ăs''pĕr-jĭl'ŭs) [L. *asper'gere*, to sprinkle]. A genus of Ascomycetes, including several species of the molds, some of which are pathogenic. The principal pathogenic species is Aspergillus fumigatus, although others (A. flavus, A. nidulans and A. niger) may be involved. SEE: *aspergillosis*.

    A. auricula'ris. A species in the external auditory meatus.

    A. bar'bae. A species found in mycosis of the head.

    A. bouffardi. Found in black mycetoma.

    A. bronchialis. A species in the bronchi of a diabetic patient.

    A. concen'tricus. A species once thought to be the cause of Tinea imbricata ringworm.

    A. fla'vus. A mold found on corn and grain.

    A. fumiga'tus. A species that has been found in the ear, nose, and lungs.

    A. glau'cus. A bluish mold found on dried fruit, also in the human ear.

    A. mucoroid'es. A form found in the lungs.

    A. nid'ulans. A species causing one form of white mycetoma.

    A. ni'ger. A pathogenic form with black spores, frequently present in the external auditory meatus.

    A. ocra'ceus. The species which produces the characteristic and desirable odor of coffee.

    A. pic'tor. A species found in the patches of pinta.

    A. re'pens. A species found in the auditory canal.

aspermat'ic [Gr. *a-*, not, + *sperma*, seed]. Pert. to aspermatism.

aspermatism (ă-sper'mă-tizm) ["+ "+ *ismos*, condition of]. Absence or nonemission of semen. SYN: *aspermia*. SEE: *azoospermia*.

asper'mia. Lack of, or failure to ejaculate, semen.

asper'mous. Pert. to aspermia. SYN: *aspermatic*.

as'perous [L. *asper*, rough]. Uneven; having minute elevations.

asper'sion [L. *aspersio*, sprinkling]. Sprinkling an affected part with water; a form of hydrotherapy, q.v.

asphalgesia (as''fal-jē'zĭ-ă) [Gr. *asphe-*, self, + *algos*, pain]. A burning sensation sometimes felt during hypnosis on touching certain articles.

asphyctic, asphyctous (as-fik'tik, -tus) [Gr. *a-*, not, + *sphyxis*, pulse]. 1. Asphyxiated. 2. Without pulse.

asphyxia (ăs-fĭk'sĭ-ă). A decrease in the amount of oxygen and an increased amount of carbon dioxide in the body as a result of some interference with respiration.

ETIOL: *Extrinsic Causes:* Choking; gas (illuminating, sewer); exhaust gas (principally carbon monoxide); electric shock; drugs; anesthesia; traumatic asphyxia; crushing injuries of chest; compression of chest; injury of respiratory nerves or centers; diminution of oxygenation of environment; drowning. *Intrinsic Causes:* Hemorrhage into lungs or pleural cavity; foreign bodies in throat; swelling of air passages; diseases of air passages; ruptured aneurysm or abscess; edema of the lung; cardiac deficiency. Tumors, such as goiter; pharyngeal and retropharyngeal abscesses. *Other Causes:* Paralysis of the respiratory center; profound anesthesia; pneumothorax; narcotic drugs and electrocution.

SYM: In general include dyspnea; cyanosis; rapid pulse; impairment of senses; mental disturbances; and in extreme cases convulsions; unconsciousness; and death.

F.A. TREATMENT: Artificial respiration, q.v.

     a. carbonica. Suffocation from inhalation of coal or water gas.

     a., fetal. That occurring in a fetus; results from interference with placental circulation or from premature separation of placenta as in placenta praevia.

     a. livida. Asphyxia with cyanosis of the skin.

     a., local. That in which a limited portion of the body is involved as the fingers, hands, toes, or feet.

     a. neonatorum. Imperfect breathing in the newborn child.

     a. pallida. When difficulty in breathing is accompanied by weak and thready pulse, pale skin, and absence of reflexes. This is the most serious type.

asphyx'ial. Pert. to asphyxia; asphyctic.

asphyx'iant. An agent, esp. any gas, that will produce asphyxia.

asphyx'iate. To cause asphyxiation or asphyxia.

asphyx"ia'tion [Gr. *a-*, not, + *sphyxis*, pulse]. A state of asphyxia or suffocation. Act of producing asphyxia. SEE: *asphyxia.*

aspidium (as-pĭd'ĭ-um) [Gr. *aspiction*, little shield]. The root and stalk of Dryopteris flix-mas (male fern) or Dryopteris marginalis

(marginal fern). Used medicinally in form of oleoresin. SYN: *male fern.*

     a. oleoresin. Extract of male fern; male fern oleoresin.

USE: As an anthelmintic in treatment of tapeworm infestations of intestines. Care should be taken that it is not administered with an oil, since absorption may occur.

as'pirate [L. *ad,* to, + *spirāre,* to breathe]. 1. Aspiration; to remove by suction. 2. A sound like that of the letter *h.*

aspiration (ăs-pĭ-rā'shŭn). 1. To draw in or out as by suction. Foreign bodies may be aspirated into the nose, throat, or lungs on inspiration. 2. The withdrawing of a fluid from a cavity by means of suction with an instrument called an aspirator.

Cavities most commonly aspirated are: pericardial c.; pleural c.; theca (lumbar puncture); abscess c.

The object of a. is to remove fluid from an affected area such as pleural effusion; and ascites; to obtain specimens, as blood from a vein or serum from the spinal canal.

NECESSARY ARTICLES: Disinfecting solution for the skin; local anesthetic; two aspirating needles with the aspirating apparatus as indicated; utensil for receiving the fluid and a sterile receptacle for the specimen; sterile sponges, towels, basins, etc.; sterile gloves, face masks, and gowns; sterile forceps; surgical dressings as the case may require; stimulant ordered if indication arises.

NP: Place patient in a comfortable position. Drape; be sure patient is warm. Have all equipment in order and in readiness for the use of the physician. Physician and nurse should wear face masks. If aspiration site is close to patient's face, patient should also wear a face mask. SEE: *foreign bodies, lumbar puncture.*

aspirator (as'pĭ-rā-tor). 1. Apparatus for evacuating fluid contents of a cavity. Varieties are piston pump; compressible rubber tube; rubber bulb; and siphon aspirators; a trocar and cannula; and hypodermic needle and syringe.

2. Instrument used in chemical analysis of gases.

aspirin (ăs'per-ĭn). Acetylsalicylic acid, q.v.

     a. poisoning. SEE: salicylate in *Table of Poisons and Poisoning* in *Appendix.*

asplenia (ă-splē'nĭ-ă) [Gr. *a-*, not, + L. splēn, spleen]. Absence of or failure of function of the spleen.

asporogenic (as"pō-rō-jĕn'ik) ["+ *sporos* seed, + *gennan,* to produce]. Not reproducing by spores.

asporous (ă-spō'rus). Having no spores.

assanation (as″ă-nā′shun) [L. *ad*, to, + *sānitās*, health]. Improvement of sanitary conditions.

assay (ă-sā′, ăs′ā) [O. Fr. *assai*, trial]. The analysis of a substance to determine its constituents and the relative proportion of each. Physical, chemical, and biological methods are used.

assident (as′ĭ-dent) [L. *assidēre*, to sit by]. A term applied to symptoms to indicate they are usually but not invariably present with a certain disease.

assimilable (ă-sĭm′ĭ-lă-bl) [L. *ad*, to, + *similare*, to make like]. Capable of assimilation.

assim′ilate. To absorb digested food.

assimila′tion. The processes whereby the products of digestion are changed to resemble the chemical substances of the body tissues, first passing through the lacteals and blood vessels; transformation of food into living tissue. The constructive phase of metabolism, i.e., anabolism.

asso′ciated movements. Synchronous correlation of two or more muscles (or muscle groups) which, though apparently not essential for the performance of some function, normally accompany it, as the swinging of arms accompanies normal walking.

Associated movements are lost rather characteristically in cerebellar disease.

associa′tion [L. *ad*, to, + *socius*, companion]. A joining or uniting together; coordination with another idea, structure, etc.

　　a. areas. Areas of the cerebral cortex which are connected to motor and sensory areas of the same side and to similar areas on the other side and to other regions of the brain as the thalamus. They serve to integrate the simpler motor and sensory functions.

　　a. center. One controlling associated movements.

　　a., controlled. An idea suggested by a word uttered by the physician.

　　a., free. In psychoanalysis, the uninhibited and uncensored oral expression of ideas as they arise in the mind.

　　a. of ideas. The linking together in a memory chain of two or more ideas, associated by some similarity, relationship, or by both having been experienced at the same time.

　　a. neuron. A neuron which transmits impulses from afferent to efferent neurons.

　　a. test. The patient is given a word (stimulus word) and he replies immediately with another word (reaction word) suggested to him by the first. The words chosen and the time taken in responding (association time) may be indicative of the patient's mental condition.

assonance (as′ō-nans) [L. *assonāre*, to respond to]. Abnormal impulse to use alliteration.

assuetude (as′wē-tūd) [L. *ad*, to, + *suēscere*, to become accustomed]. 1. Becoming habituated to conditions. 2. Acquiring tolerance to a drug until it loses its effect.

Ast. Abbr. for *astigmatism.*

astasia (ă-stā′zĭ-ă) [Gr. *a-*, not, + *stasis*, stand]. Inability to stand or sit erect due to motor incoordination.

　　a. -abasia. 1. Combined incoordination for standing or walking. 2. In psychiatry, a mental conflict making it difficult to stand or walk without swerving or swaying.

astatine (ăs′tă-tēn, -tĭn) [Gr. *astatos*, unstable]. SYMB: *At.* At. wt., the mass number of the most stable isotope is 210; at. no. 85. An unstable element.

asteatosis (as″tĭ-ă-tō′sis) [Gr. *a-*, not, + *stear*, tallow, + *-ōsis*, condition]. Any disease condition in which there is scantiness or absence of the sebaceous secretion.

　　a. cutis. A dry, fissured condition of the skin together with deficient secretion.

　　ETIOL: Symptomatic form due to senility, constitutional or local affections which give rise to trophic changes in the nervous system. Local form may be caused by frequent contact with irritants.

　　TREATMENT: Removal of underlying cause. Local application of oils and fats.

as′ter [Gr. *astēr*, star]. The stellate rays forming round the dividing centrosome during mitosis.

astereognosis (ă-stĕr″ē-ŏg-nō′sĭs) [Gr. *a-*, not, + *stereos*, solid, + *gnōsis*, recognition]. Inability to recognize objects or forms by touch.

aste′rion [Gr. *asterion*, starlike]. A craniometric point at junction of occipital, parietal, and temporal bones.

asterixis (as″ter-ix′is) [Gr. *a-*, not, + *stērixis*, fixed position]. Involuntary abnormal jerking muscular movements induced by dorsiflexion of the wrist and extension of fingers. May also be seen in other muscle groups such as those in the tongue and the feet. May be due to one of many illnesses which interfere with metabolism of the brain. When due to liver disease asterixis is caller liver flap or liver tremor.

aster′nal [Gr. *a-*, not, + *sternon*, chest]. 1. Not connected with the sternum. 2. Having no sternum.

asternia (ă-stĕr′nĭ-ă). Congenital anomaly with absence of the sternum.

asteroid (as'ter-oyd) [Gr. *astēr*, star, + *eidos*, shape]. Star-shaped.

asthenia (as-thē'nĭ-ă) [Gr. *a-*, not, + *sthenos*, strength]. Lack or loss of strength; debility. Any weakness, but one esp. originating in muscular or cerebellar disease.

   a. neurocirculatory. A psychosomatic disorder characterized by mental and physical fatigue, dyspnea, giddiness, precordial pain and palpitation esp. on exertion. SYN: *cardiac neurosis; effort syndrome; irritable heart; soldier's heart.*

   ETIOL: Unknown but occurs in individuals who are under conditions of stress, either conscious or unconscious. It is common among soldiers.

   TREATMENT: Removal from stress situation, and psychotherapy.

asthenic (as-then'ik). Weak; pert. to asthenia.

   a. body type. In psychology, a thin, more or less tall person with flat chest, accompanied by inferior muscular development, who centers his interest in his inner self. Usually an introvert. SEE: *pyknic type.*

asthenobiosis (ăs-thē"nō-bī-ō'sĭs) [Gr. *asthenēs*, without strength, + *bios*, life, + *-ōsis*, condition]. Reduced activity of an animal, resembling hibernation but not related to either temperature or climate.

asthenocoria (as-thē"nō-cō'rĭ-ă) [*asthenia*, + Gr. *korē*, pupil]. A sluggish pupillary light reflex.

asthenometer (as"thē-nom'ē-ter) [*asthenia*, + Gr. *metron*, measure]. An instrument for determining loss of strength.

asthenope (as'thĕ-nōp) [Gr. *a-*, + *sthenos*, strength, + *opsis*, power of sight]. An individual who is affected with asthenopia, q.v.

asthenopia (as"thĕ-nō'pĭ-ă). Weakness or tiring of eyes due to fatigue of ciliary muscle or extraocular muscles. Painful vision.

   SYM: Pain in or around eyes; headache, usually aggravated by use of eyes for close work; fatigue; vertigo; reflex symptoms, as nausea, twitching of facial muscles, migraine.

   a., accommodative. Refractive errors such as hyperopia and astigmatism.

   a., muscular. A. caused by weakness of extrinsic ocular muscles.

   a., nervous. Of hysteric and/or neurasthenic origin.

   a., photogenous. Caused by excessive or improper illumination.

   a., reflex. Disease in other organs, as nose, sinuses, teeth.

asthenop'ic. Rel. to asthenopia.

asthenox'ia [Gr. *a-*, not, + *sthenos*, strength, + *oxygen*]. Deficient oxygenation of waste products. Insufficient oxidation of fatty acids giving rise to ketosis.

asthma (ăz'mă) [Gr. *asthma*, panting]. Paroxysmal dyspnea accompanied by the adventitious sounds caused by a spasm of the bronchial tubes or due to swelling of their mucous membrane.

   Status asthmaticus is a more or less continuous asthmatic state which may last for hours or days.

   In all cases of asthma, but particularly in the intrinsic group, the importance of the emotions must be considered and the patient treated accordingly.

   No age is exempt but occurs most frequently in childhood or early adulthood.

   ETIOL: *Extrinsic causes.* Allergens inhaled in the air (such as pollen, mold spores, animal dander, or dust); or infections of the respiratory tract. Occasionally foods (such as eggs, shellfish, or chocolate); or drugs (such as aspirin) may precipitate an attack. *Intrinsic causes.* In this situation asthma develops in persons who are found not to be allergic to specific antigens.

   TREATMENT: Acute attacks may be relieved by a number of drugs such as epinephrine, ephedrine, or aminophylline. For persistent asthma (status asthmaticus), the use of adrenal cortical hormones may be required; even though their use may provide dramatic relief, these hormones should be used only as long as is necessary to control the acute asthmatic attack. Prolonged use of adrenal cortical hormones will lead to the development of serious side effects. The use of sedatives and expectorants is sometimes necessary. In all cases effort should be made to control causative factors including the component of the disease due to emotional disturbance. Elimination of antigen, or counteractivities such as immunization, desensitization, or hyposensitization is desirable. For asthma due to infections of respiratory tract, antibiotics should be used to control infection or prevent recurrence.

   a., bronchial. Allergic asthma. Common form of asthma due to hypersensitivity to an allergen.

   a., cardiac. Dyspnea due to heart disease.

   TREATMENT: Upright position, morphine and venesection, if patient does not have anemia. When acute pulmonary edema sets in, strophanthin or digitalis.

   a. convulsivum. A., bronchial, q.v.

a., extrinsic. Asthma due to dusts or other allergens inhaled in air or taken in with food.

a., hay. Hay fever, q.v.

a., intrinsic. Asthma resulting from allergens arising internally, usually the result of respiratory infections.

a., nonatopic. Intrinsic asthma, q.v.

a., renal. A. occurring in Bright's disease.

a., thymic. A. caused by a sudden closure of the larynx. Occurs in children, and it is believed to result from enlargement of the thymus.

asthmat'ic [L. *asthmaticus*]. Pert. to or of the nature of asthma.

astigmatic (as"tig-mat'ik). Pert. to or afflicted with astigmatism.

astigmatism (a-stig'mă-tizm) [Gr. *a-*, not, + *stigma*, point, + *ismos*, condition of]. Form of ametropia in which refraction of several meridians of eyeball is different, usually due to change in curvature of cornea and lens. ABBR: As. or Ast. SYN: *astigma.*

ETIOL: Congenital or acquired. Images do not properly focus on retina.

a., compound. Astigmatism in which both horizontal and vertical curvatures are involved.

a., index. Astigmatism resulting from inequalities in refractive indices of different parts of the lens.

a., mixed. Astigmatism when one meridian is myopic and the other hyperopic.

a., simple. Astigmatism along one meridian only.

astigmatometer, astigmometer (ă"stig-ma-tom'ĕ-ter, ă-stig-mom'ĕ-ter) [Gr. *a-*, not, + *stigma*, point, + *metron*, measure]. An instrument for measuring astigmatism.

astigmat'oscope ["+ "+ *skopein*, to examine]. Instrument for detecting and measuring astigmatism.

astigmatos'copy. Use of the astigmatoscope.

astig'mia. Astigmatism, q.v.

astigmom'eter. Astigmatometer, q.v.

astigmoscope. Astigmatoscope, q.v.

astomatous, astomous (as-tom'ă-tŭs, as'tō-mŭs) [Gr. *a-*, not, + *stoma*, mouth]. Without mouth or oral aperture.

astomia (ă-stō'mĭ-ă). Congenital absence of the mouth.

astragalar (as-trag'ă-lar). Pert. to the astragalus or talus.

astragalectomy (as"trag-ă-lek'tō-mĭ) [*astragalus*, + Gr. *ektomē*, excision]. Excision of astragalus or talus.

astragalus (as-trag'ă-lus) [Gr. *astragalos*, ball]. Obsolete term for bone of the foot which articulates with the tibia, fibula, calcaneus and navicular bone. SYN: *ankle bone; talus.*

astraphobia (as-tra-fō'bĭ-ă) [Gr. *astrapē*, lightning, + *phobos*, fear]. Anxiety and terror of thunderstorms.

astrict' [L. *astringere*, to bind fast]. 1. To contract or constrict, as the action of an astringent. To compress, as an artery in a hemorrhage. 2. To constipate.

astriction (ă-strik'shun). 1. Action of astringent. 2. Constipation.

astringent (a-strin'jĕnt) [L. *astringere*, to bind fast]. 1. Drawing together, constricting, binding. 2. An agent that has a constricting or binding effect, e.g., one which checks hemorrhages, secretion, etc. The principal astringents are salts of metals such as lead, iron, zinc (e.g., ferric chloride, zinc oxide); permanganates; and tannic acid. SEE: *styptic.*

astro- [Gr. *astron*, star]. Prefix indicating relationship to a star, or star-shaped.

astroblast (as'trō-blast) ["+ Gr. *blastos*, germ]. A cell which gives rise to an astrocyte. It develops from spongioblasts derived from embryonic neuroepithelium.

astroblasto'ma ["+ "+ *-ōma*, tumor]. Tumor composed of astroblasts.

astrocyte (as'trō-sīt) [*astro-*, + Gr. *kytos*, hollow vessel]. A star-shaped neuroglial cell possessing many branching processes.

astrocyto'ma ["+ "+ *ōma*, tumor]. Tumor formed from astrocytes.

astrog'lia ["+ *neurologia*]. Astrocytes making up neuroglial tissue.

astrokinet'ic motions ["+ Gr. *kinēsis*, motion]. Movements of centrosome.

astropho'bia ["+ *phobos*, fear]. Morbid fear of stars and celestial space.

astrosphere (ăs'trō-sfēr) ["+ Gr. *sphaira*, sphere]. A group of fibrils or fine rays which radiate from the centrosome (microcentrum) of the cell center. SYN: *aster.*

astrostat'ic ["+ *statikos*, standing]. Pert. to astrosphere in its resting condition.

asurre'nalism [Gr. *a-*, not, + L. *super*, over, + *ren*, kidney, + Gr. *ismos*, condition]. Deficient suprarenal function.

asyllabia (ă"sil-ă'bĭ-ă) ["+ Gr. *syllabē*, syllable]. Recognition of letters but not syllables or words.

asylum (ă-sī'lum) [L. from Gr. *asulos*, safe from violence]. An institution for the care of those unable to care for themselves, as the infirm, aged, insane, blind.

asymbolia (ă-sim-bō'lĭ-ă, ă-) [Gr. *a-*, not, + *symbolon*, a sign]. Inability to comprehend words, gestures, or any type of symbol; asemia. Sensory aphasia.

asymmetry (ă-sim′ĕ-trĭ) ["+ Gr. *symmetria,* symmetry]. Lack of symmetry of parts or organs on opposite sides of body.

asymphytous (ă-sim′fĭ-tus) ["+ Gr. *symphysis,* a growing together]. Not grown together.

asymptomat′ic ["+ Gr. *sumptoma,* phenomenon]. Without symptoms.

asynchronism (ă-sĭn′krō-nizm) ["+ Gr. *syn,* together, + *chronos,* time, + *-ismos,* condition of]. 1. The failure of events to occur in time with each other as they usually do. 2. Incoordination.

asynclitism (ă-sin′klĭ-tism) ["+ Gr. *synklinein,* to lean together]. An oblique presentation of the fetal head.

   a., anterior. Anterior parietal presentation. SYN: *Naegele's a.*

   a., posterior. Posterior parietal presentation.

asynechia (a″sin-ē′kĭ-ă) [Gr. *a-,* not, + *synecheia,* continuity]. Lack of continuity of structure in an organ or tissue.

asynergia, asynergy (a-sin-er′jĭ-ă, ă-sin′er-jĭ) ["+ Gr. *synergia,* cooperation]. Lack of coordination between muscle groups. Movements are in serial order instead of being made together. Seen in cerebellar diseases.

asynesia (ă-sĭn-ē′zĭ-ă) [Gr. *asynesia,* lack of intelligence]. Stupidity or intellectual dullness.

asynovia (ă-sin-ō′vĭ-ă) [Gr. *a-,* not, + *syn,* with, + *ōon,* egg]. Lack, or insufficient secretion, of synovial fluid of a joint.

asystemat′ic ["+ LL. *systēma,* arrangement]. Diffuse; not limited to one system or set of organs.

asystole, asystolia (ă-sĭs′tō-lē, a″sis-to′lĭ-ă) [Gr. *a-,* not, + *sustellein,* to draw together]. Faulty contraction of ventricles of the heart.

At. Chem. symb. for astatine.

atabrine (ăt′ă-brĭn). Proprietary name for quinacrine hydrochloride. Used in treatment of malaria and certain connective-tissue disease.

atactic (a-tak′tik) [Gr. *ataktos,* irregular]. Incoordinate, irregular, as muscular incoordination, esp. in aphasia. SYN: *ataxic.*

atactiform (ă-tak′tĭ-form) [Gr. *a-,* not, + L. *forma,* form]. Similar to ataxia.

atactilia (ă-tak-til′ĭ-ă) ["+ L. *tactilis,* pert. to touch]. Inability to recognize tactile impressions.

ataractic (at″ă-rak′tĭk) [Gr. *ataraktos,* quiet]. 1. Of or pertaining to ataraxia. 2. A drug that produces ataraxia, q.v.

atarax′ia, at′araxy [Gr. *a-,* not, + *taraktos,* disturbed]. A state of complete mental calm and tranquility. SYN: *imperturbability.*

atavism (ăt′ă-vĭzm) [L. *atavus,* ancestor]. 1. Recurrence of characteristics of a remote ancestor after remaining latent for one or more generations. 2. Reappearance, in a descendant, of a disease or abnormality experienced by a remote ancestor. A reversion to an original type.

atavis′tic. Pert. to atavism.

ataxaphasia (ă-taks-ă-fā′zĭ-ă) [Gr. *ataxia,* lack of order, + *phasis,* speech]. Inability to arrange words in sentences.

ataxaphemia (ă-taks-ă-fē′mĭ-ă) ["+ *phēmē,* speech]. Lacking in lingual coordination. SEE: *ataxophemia.*

ataxia (ă-tăks′ĭ-ă) [Gr., lack of order]. 1. Disorder or irregularity. 2. Muscular incoordination, esp. that manifested when voluntary muscular movements are attempted. SYN: *ataxy.*

   a., alcoholic. A. seen in drinkers, and caused by peripheral neuritis.

   a., autonomic. Incoordination between sympathetic and parasympathetic nervous systems.

   a., Briquet's. Hysteria accompanied by skin and leg muscle anesthesia.

   a., Brun's frontal lobe. Condition resulting from lesions of the frontal lobes. Ability to perform skilled movements is lost but capacity for crude movements is retained.

   a., bulbar. That due to a lesion in medulla oblongata or pons.

   a., cerebellar. Muscular incoordination due to cerebellar disease.

   a., choreic. Lack of muscular coordination seen in persons with chorea.

   a., Friedreich's. A., hereditary, q.v.

   a., hereditary. Hereditary degenerative disorder in which spinal pathways are involved. A cause of paraplegia in children and young adults. SYM: Ataxia in lower, and extending to upper, extremities; paralysis and contractures follow. SYN: *Friedreich's a.*

   a., hereditary cerebellar. Disease of late adolescence. ETIOL: Atrophy of cerebellum. SYM: Ataxic gait, hesitating and explosive speech, nystagmus, and sometimes optic neuritis. SYN: *Marie's ataxia.*

   a., hysterical. Ataxia of leg muscles due to hysteria.

   a., intrapsychic. A state in which emotional expressions appear to have no logical bases or relationship, other than those found in the unconscious. Thus a patient may cry when laughter would be appropriate.

   a., locomotor. A sclerosis affecting the posterior columns of spinal cord, most commonly due to syphilis. SYN: *tabes dorsalis*

SYM: Characterized by incoordination; loss of deep reflexes; disturbances of nutrition; various ocular phenomena; sometimes loss of sexual power; paralysis of sphincters; epileptiform seizures and dementia. Inability to control gait or to touch an article with the hand. See: *gait.*

TREATMENT: Penicillin. Response to treatment is often poor.

    a., Marie's. A., hereditary cerebellar, q.v.

    a., motor. Lack of ability for proper coordination of muscles.

    a., sensory. A. resulting from interference in conduction of sensory responses, esp. proprioceptive impulses from muscles. SEE: a., spinal.

    a., spinal. Due to spinal cord disease, as in locomotor a.

    a., static. Loss of deep sensibility causing inability to preserve equilibrium in standing.

ataxiadynamia (ă-tăks″ĭ-ăd-ĭ-năm′ĭ-ă) [Gr. *ataxia,* lack of order, + *a-,* not, + *dynamis,* strength]. Muscular weakness in combination with incoordination. SYN: *ataxoadynamia.*

atax′iagram ["+ Gr. *gramma,* writing]. Ataxiagraph record or tracing.

ataxiagraph (ă-taks′ĭ-a-graf) ["+ Gr. *graphein,* to write]. Instrument measuring swaying in ataxia.

ataxiam′eter ["+ Gr. *metron,* measure]. Apparatus measuring ataxia.

ataxiamnesia (a-taks′ĭ-am-nē′zĭ-ă) ["+ *amnēsia,* forgetfulness]. Suffering from muscular ataxia and amnesia.

atax′ic, atax′ial. Pert. to, or marked by, ataxia.

ataxoadynamia. Ataxiadynamia, q.v.

ataxophe′mia [Gr. *ataxia,* lack of order, + *phēme,* speech]. Incoordination of speech muscles.

ataxopho′bia ["+ *phobia,*]. Morbid dread of disorder or untidiness.

at′axy. Ataxia.

-ate. Word ending noting a specific action of the affixed noun. Ex: activate, hemolysate, pulsate.

atelectasis (at″ĕ-lek′tă-sis) [Gr. *atelēs,* imperfect, + *ektasis,* expansion]. 1. Condition in which lungs of a fetus remain unexpanded at birth. May be partial or total. 2. A collapsed or airless condition of the lung. May be caused by obstruction by foreign bodies, mucous plugs or excessive secretions, or by compression from without as by tumors, aneurysms, or enlarged lymph nodes. It sometimes is a complication following abdominal operations. A special chronic form,

designated middle lobe syndrome, results from compression of a bronchus by surrounding lymph nodes.

atelencephalia (ăt-ĕl″ĕn-sĭ-fā′lĭ-ă) [Gr. *ateleia,* incompleteness, + *enkephalos,* brain]. Congenital anomaly with imperfect development of the brain.

atelia (a-tī′lĭ-ă) [Gr. *ateleia,* incompleteness]. The retention of childish characteristics in the adult. SYN: *ateliosis.*

ateliosis (ă-tī″lĭ-ō′sis) [Gr. *a-,* not, + *teleios,* complete, + *-ōsis,* condition]. A form of infantilism due to pituitary causes in which growth may be arrested without deformity. The voice and face may resemble those of a child.

ateliot′ic. Infantile.

atelo- (at′ĕ-lō) [Gr. *atelēs,* imperfect]. Prefix denoting developmental or structural defect.

atelocardia (ăt″ĕ-lō-kăr′dĭ-ă) ["+ *kardia,* heart]. Congenital anomaly with incomplete development of the heart.

atelocephalus (ăt-ĕ-lō-sĕf′ă-lŭs) ["+ *kephalē,* head]. Having an incomplete head.

atelocheilia (ăt″ĕ-lō-kī′lĭ-ă) ["+ *cheilos,* lip]. Incomplete development of the lip.

atelocheiria (ăt″ĕ-lō-kī′rĭ-ă) ["+ *cheir,* hand]. Incomplete development of the hand.

ateloencephalia (at″ĕ-lō-en″sĕ-fā′lĭ-ă). Atelencephalia.

ateloglossia (ăt″ĕ-lō-glŏs′ĭ-ă) [Gr. *atelēs,* imperfect, + *glōssa,* tongue]. Defective development of tongue.

atelognathia (ăt″ĕ-lŏg-nā′thĭ-ă) ["+ *gnathos,* jaw]. Incomplete development of jaw.

atelomyelia (ăt″ĕ-lō-mī-ē′lĭ-ă) ["+ *myelos,* marrow]. Incomplete development of spinal cord.

atelopodia (ăt″ĕ-lō-pō′dĭ-ă) [Gr. *atelēs,* imperfect, + *pous,* foot]. Developmental defect of foot.

ateloprosopia (ăt″ĕ-lō-prō-sō′pĭ-ă) ["+ *prōsopon,* face]. Defective development of face.

atelostomia (ăt″ĕ-lō-stō′mĭ-ă) ["+ *stoma,* mouth]. Incomplete development of mouth.

athelia (ă-thē′lĭ-ă) [Gr. *a-,* not, + *thēle,* nipple]. Absence of the nipples.

athermic, athermous (ă-ther′mĭk, -mus) ["+ *thermē,* heat]. Without fever.

athermosystaltic (ă-thĕr″mō-sĭs-tăl′tĭk) ["+ "+ *systaltikos,* drawing together]. Not contracting or expanding due to action of heat or cold, said of striated muscle.

atheroma (ath″ĕr-ō′mă) [Gr. *athērē,* porridge, + *ōma,* tumor]. 1. A sebaceous cyst. SYN: *steatoma.* 2. Fatty degeneration or thickening of the wall of the larger arteries. SEE: *arteriosclerosis; atherosclerosis.*

atheromasia (ath″er-ō-mā′zĭ-ă). Atheromatous degeneration.

atheromatosis (ath″er-ō″mă-tō′sis). Generalized atheromatous condition.

atheromatous (ath″er-ō′mă-tus). Pert. to atheroma.

atheronecrosis (ath″er-ō″nĕ-crō′sĭs) [Gr. *athērē*, porridge, + *nekros*, dead, + *-ōsis*, condition]. Necrosis or degeneration accompanying arteriosclerosis.

atherosclero′sis [″+ Gr. *sklērōsis*, hardness]. A form of arteriosclerosis in which there are localized accumulations of lipid-containing material (atheromas) within or beneath the intimal surfaces of blood vessels. It is thought to be due to a metabolic defect involving lipids and lipoproteins. It is one of the common causes of arterial occlusion.

atherosis (ath″er-ō′sis) [″+ *-ōsis*, condition]. Fatty degeneration of arterial walls. SYN: *arteriosclerosis.*

athetoid (ath′ĕ-toid) [Gr. *athetos*, not fixed, + *eidos*, resemblance]. 1. Similar to athetosis. 2. Affected with athetosis.

athetosis (ath-ĕ-tō′sis) [″+ *-ōsis*, condition]. A condition wherein there are slow, irregular, twisting, snakelike muscular movements seen mostly in the upper extremities, esp. in the hands and fingers. The symptoms may be due to one of several diseases including some in children and encephalitis and tabes dorsalis in adults.

ath′lete′s foot. A fungus infection of the foot caused by various dermatophytes, esp. Trichophyton rubrum, T. mentagrophytes, and Epidermphyton floccosum. SYN: *dermatophytosis; ringworm of the foot; tinea pedis; trichophytosis pedis.*

TREATMENT: Various antifungal preparations are available, choice depending on seriousness of infection. Ointments, when used, should be applied at night and removed in the morning. Strong irritating medicaments should not be used. Soaking feet in 1:10,000 potassium permanganate solution and application of a drying lotion, such as calamine, or powder are usually effective.

athrepsia, athrepsy (ă-threp′sĭ-ă, -ĭ) [Gr. *a-*, not, + *threpsis*, nourishment]. Malnutrition, marasmus, q.v.

athreptic (ă-thrĕp′tĭk). Marasmic; pert. to or afflicted with athrepsia.

athrom′bia [Gr. *a-*, not, + *thrombos*, a clot]. Defective blood clotting.

athymia (ă-thĭ′mĭ-ă) [″+ *thymos*, mind]. Without feeling or emotion, seen in certain mental disorders.

athymic (ă-thĭ′mĭk). Pert. to athymia.

athy′mism [Gr. *a-*, not, + *thymos*, mind, + *-ismos*, condition of]. Absence of thymus gland or its secretions. SYN: *athymia.*

athyrea (ă-thĭ′rĭ-ă). Athyreosis.

athyreo′sis [Gr. *a-*, not, + *thymos*, mind, + *-ōsis*, increased]. Hypothyroidism resulting from absence or malfunctioning of thyroid gland which may be due to maldevelopment, operative removal, or inactivation by irradiation or use of antithyroid agents. SYN: *athyrea; athyria.* SEE: *hypothyroidism.*

athyria (ă-thĭ′rĭ-ă). Athyreosis.

athy″roide′mia [″+ ″+ Gr. *eidos*, form, + *haima*, blood]. Anemia associated with deficiency of thyroid hormone.

athyroidism (ă-thĭ′roy-dĭzm) [″+ ″+ ″+ Gr. *-ismos*, condition of]. Suppression of thyroid secretions, or absence of the thyroid gland; athyrea.

athyrosis (ă-thĭ-rō′sis). Athyreosis.

atlan′tad. Toward the atlas.

atlan′tal. Pert. to the atlas.

at′las. [NA]. The first cervical vertebra by which the head articulates with the occipital bone, so called because of Atlas who was supposed to support the world on his shoulders.

atloaxoid (at″lō-aks′oyd) [Gr. *atlas*, a support, + L. *axis*, a pivot, + Gr. *eidos*, form]. Pert. to atlas and axis.

atlodidymus (ăt-lō-dĭd′ĭ-mus) [″+ Gr. *didymos*, twin]. A malformed fetus with one body and two heads.

atm. Abbr. for *atmosphere; atmospheric.*

atmiatrics, atmiatry (at-mĭ-at′riks, at-mĭ′ă-trĭ) [Gr. *atmos*, vapor, + *iatrikos*, art of healing]. Treatment of respiratory disease by medicated vapors.

atmic (at′mik). Consisting of or pert. to vapor.

atmo- [Gr. *atmos*, vapor or steam]. Prefix indicating rel. to steam or vapor.

atmocau′sis [″+ Gr. *kausis*, burning]. Application of superheated steam; substitute for uterine curettage.

atmocautery (at-mō-kaw′ter-ĭ). Device for cauterization with steam.

at′mos [Gr. *atmos*, air]. A unit of air pressure; one dyne per square centimeter.

at′mosphere [″+ Gr. *sphaira*, sphere]. 1. The gases surrounding the earth. 2. Climatic condition of a locality. 3. In physics, pressure at sea level of the atmosphere—14.7 lbs. to the sq. in. (1033 grams per sq. meter). 4. In chemistry, any gaseous medium around a body.

atmospher′ic. Pert. to the atmosphere.

atmospheriza′tion. Process of transforming venous into arterial blood.

atmother′apy [Gr. *atmos*, air, + *therapeia*, treatment]. 1. Treatment of disease by medicated vapors. SYN: *atmiatrics,* q.v. 2. Treatment involving reduction of rate of respiration.

at. no. Abbr. for *atomic number.*

atocia (at-o′sĭ-ă) [Gr. *a-*, not, + *tokos*, birth]. 1. Female sterility. 2. Nulliparity.

at′om [Gr. *atomos*, indivisible]. The smallest particle of an element that can exist and take part in a chemical change, retaining its identity, and which cannot further be divided without change of its structure.

One hundred and three elements have been identified and named, which in combination with one another or others like themselves make up all the various types of matter that we know. The elements are made up of atoms which are themselves composed of still smaller particles called electrons, protons, and neutrons. More than 30 entities in the atomic nucleus have been identified, and the search for others continues. Those identified include positrons, mesons, neutrinos, pi-zero mesons. Dimensions of atoms are of the order of 10^{-8} centimeters. SEE: *atomic theory; electron.*

    a., tagged. An atom that has been made radioactive so that its course may be followed in the body. SYN: *radioactive tracer.*

atom′ic. Pert. to an atom or atoms.

    a. number. Number of protons in the nucleus of an atom. ABBR: at. no.

    a. theory. 1. Theory that all matter is composed of atoms. 2. Theories pert. to the structure, properties, and behavior of the atom.

    a. weight. The weight of an element compared to the weight of 1/12 the weight of a carbon atom. Carbon has an atomic weight of 12; oxygen, 16; hydrogen, 1.008; and nitrogen, 14.008. ABBR: at. wt.

atomicity (at″ō-mis′-ĭ-tĭ). 1. Chemical valence or combining power. 2. Number of hydroxyl groups in an alcohol, or in a base.

atomiza′tion. Converting a fluid into spray or vapor form.

at′omize. To reduce a liquid to the form of a spray or a vapor.

atomizer (at′om-ī-zer) Apparatus for changing jet of liquid to a spray.

atonic (a-ton′ik) [Gr. *a-*, not, + *tonos*, stretching]. Without tension or tone.

atonicity (at-ŏ-nĭs′ĭ-tĭ). State of being atonic, or without tone.

atony (ăt′ō-nĭ). Debility; or lack of normal tone.

    a., gastric. Lack of muscle tone in stomach and failure to contract normally, causing slow movement of food out of stomach. Secondary to certain diseases.

DIET: Small feedings at frequent intervals; soft foods; little fat. Avoid bulky foods and those requiring much mastication.

at′open [Gr. *a-*, not, + *topos*, place]. An allergen, exciting cause of atopy, q.v.

atop′ic. 1. Pert. to atopy. 2. Displaced; misplaced.

atopognosis (ă-top″og-nō′sis) [Gr. *a-*, not, + *topos*, place, + *gnōsis*, knowledge]. An inhibited sense of touch or feeling, the victim not being able to know where his skin has been touched.

atopomenorrhea (ăt″ō-pō-měn-ō-rē′ă) ["+ "+ *mēn*, month, + *rhoia*, flow]. Periodic hemorrhage from any part of the female body other than the uterus; vicarious menstruation.

atopy (ăt′ō-pĭ). A term used clinically to apply to a group of diseases of an allergic nature. They differ from most allergies in that (1) they are inherited, (2) the antibody produced, called atopic reagin or skin-sensitizing antibody, is deposited in cutaneous tissues and may enter the blood stream, and (3) the primary reaction which appears is edema as occurs in hay fever or rhinitis. The principal atopic manifestations are bronchial asthma, vasomotor rhinitis, and chronic urticaria.

atox′ic [Gr. *a-*, not, + *toxikon*, poison]. Nonpoisonous.

ATP. Abbr. for *adenosine triphosphate.*

atremia (ă-trē′mĭ-ă) [Gr. *a-*, not, + *tremein*, to tremble]. 1. Absence of trembling or tremor. 2. Inability to walk due to hysteria.

atrepsy (ă-trĕp′sĭ) ["+ *trepsis*, nutrition]. Infantile atrophy; progressive wasting and emaciation. SYN: *marasmus.*

atre′sia ["+ *trēsis*, a perforation]. 1. Pathological closure of a normal anatomical opening, or congenital absence of the same, esp. that of the esophagus. 2. Retrogression and disappearance of follicles in the mammalian ovary.

atre′sic. Imperforate; pert. to atresia.

atreto- (ă-trē′tō) [Gr. *atrētos*, imperforate]. Prefix signifying absence of an opening.

atretogastria (ă-trēt″ō-gas′tri-a) [Gr. *atretos*, imperforate, + *gastēr*, stomach]. Absence of normal opening of the cardiac and/or pyloric orifice of the stomach.

atreturethria (ă-trēt″ū-rē′thrĭ-ă) ["+ *ourēthra*, urethra]. Imperforation of the urethra.

atria (ā′trĭ-ă). Pl. of atrium, q.v.

atrial (ā′trĭ-al). Pert. to the atrium.

    a. fibrillation. Irregular and rapid contractions of the atria working independently of the ventricles. Instead of the contraction beginning at the sinoatrial node and being conducted along the bundle of His to the ventricles, there is a rapid succession of beats at the atria. Contraction of the atrial muscle causes the waves to pass round and round the atrium. There is no atrial diastole or atrial heartbeat. SYN: *auricular fibrillation.*

ETIOL: Degeneration of cardiac muscle. Occurs in late stages of mitral disease of heart, after strain of the degenerated cardiac muscle; hyperthyroidism; infiltration of the atria by neoplastic tissue; and in acute rheumatism in children.

atrichia (ă-trik'ĭ-ă) [Gr. *a-*, not, + *thrix*, hair, + *-ia*, condition]. 1. Absence of hair. 2. Lacking cilia or flagella.

atrichosis (ă-trĭ-kō'sis) ["+ "+ *-ōsis*, increased]. Having no hair, atrichia, q.v.

atri'chous. 1. Being without flagella. 2. Without hair.

atrionector (ăt"rĭ-ō-nek'tor) [L. *atrium*, corridor, + *nector*, connector]. Sinoatrial node.

at'riotome ["+ Gr. *tomē*, cutting]. Instrument which cuts connections between the cardiac atrium and ventricle.

atrioventric'ular ["+ *ventriculus*, ventricle]. Pert. to both atrium and ventricle.

   a. bundle. A bundle of modified cardiac muscle fibers which forms a part of the impulse-conducting system of the heart. It extends from the atrioventricular (A-V) node a short distance in the intraventricular septum, then divides into two branches which supply fibers to the two ventricles. SYN: *bundle of His.*

atriplicism (ă-trip'lĭ-sizm). Poisoning due to eating one form of spinach, *Atriplex littoralis.*

atrium (ā'trĭ-um) [L. *atrium*, corridor]. (pl. *atria*). A cavity or sinus.

   a. of ear. Portion of the tympanic cavity lying below the malleus; the tympanic cavity proper.

   a. of heart. The upper chamber of each half of the heart. The right atrium receives deoxygenated, dark red blood from the entire body (except lungs) through the superior and inferior vena cavae and coronary sinus; the left atrium receives oxygenated red blood from the lungs through the pulmonary veins. Blood passes from the atria to the ventricles through the atrioventricular orifices. In the embryo the atrium is a single chamber which lies between the sinus venosus and the ventricle.

   a., infection of. Site of entrance of bacteria causing an infectious disease.

   a. of lungs. The space at the end of an alveolar duct which opens into the alveoli or air sacs of the lungs.

atro'phia [Gr.]. Wasting of a part from lack of nutrition. SYN: *atrophy.*

atrophic (ă-trō'fik). Pert. to, or marked by, atrophy.

atrophied (ăt'rō-fĭd). Wasted. Afflicted with atrophy.

atrophoderma (ăt"rō-fō-der'mă) [Gr. *a-*, not, + *trophē*, nourishment, + *derma*, skin]. Atrophy of the skin.

   a. pigmentosum. Rare skin disease characterized by ulcers, disseminated pigment discolorations, etc. SYN: *xeroderma pigmentosum*, q.v.

atrophodermato'sis ["+ "+ "+ *-ōsis*, increased]. Any skin disease which has atrophied skin as a symptom.

at'rophy. 1. A wasting due to lack of nutrition of any part. 2. The reduction in size of a structure after having come to full functional maturity, as atrophy of the ovary during menopause or atrophy of an embryonic structure after having played its role in development, as the ductus arteriosus.

ETIOL: Disuse, disease, injury to trophic nerve centers in spinal cord, or interference with nerve or blood supply.

   a., acute yellow. Extensive degeneration of liver cells with jaundice, mental disturbances, and cutaneous hemorrhages.

SYM: Early nervous symptoms before jaundice sets in; slow onset; some fever with nausea and vomiting; black vomit; malaise.

   a., compression. Compression of a part causing a.

   a., correlated. Wasting of a part following destruction of another part.

   a., Cruveilhier's. Progressive wasting of the muscles.

   a. of disuse. A. from failure to normally use a part.

   a., healed yellow. Postnecrotic cirrhosis of the liver.

   a., Hoffman's. Progressive muscular wasting, in the legs, hands and forearms.

   a., Landouzy-Dejerine. A form of progressive muscular dystrophy, q.v., in which muscles of face, shoulders, and upper arms are the first involved. Called facioscapulohumeral type.

   a., muscular. Atrophy of muscle tissue which may result from interruption in nerve supply, or from a disorder involving motor centers of the brain, motor pathways of the spinal cord, motor neurons of the cord, or their endings in muscle; disuse as may occur following immobilization of joints; or pathological conditions involving muscles directly. Some conditions are hereditary and of unknown etiology.

a., myelopathic. Muscular atrophy resulting from degeneration of motor cells in anterior horns of gray matter of spinal cord.

a., myotonic. SEE: *myotonia congenita.*

a., optic. Atrophy of the second cranial (optic) nerve.

a., pathologic. That which results from the effects of disease processes.

a., peroneal muscular. A hereditary disease of unknown etiology in which peroneal nerves are primarily involved, the atrophy of muscles occurring secondary to nerve involvement. SYN: *Charcot-Marie-Tooth disease*, q.v.

a., physiologic. That which occurs as a result of the normal developmental and physiologic processes in the body (e.g., atrophy of embryonic structures; atrophy of childhood structures upon reaching maturity, as the thymus; atrophy of structures in cyclic phases of activity, as the corpus luteum; atrophy of structures following cessation of functional activity, as the ovary and mammary glands; and, finally, atrophy of structures with aging).

a., progressive muscular. Chronic disease marked by progressive wasting of the muscles and paralysis, beginning with the extremities and ultimately causing death from paralysis of muscles of respiration. SYN: *Aran-Duchenne disease.* SEE: *dystrophy, progressive muscular; sclerosis, amyotrophic lateral.*

a., trophoneurotic. Wasting due to disease of the nerves or nerve centers.

a., unilateral facial. Progressive a. of the facial tissues on one side only.

a., white. Wasting of nerve, leaving only white connective tissue.

atropine sulfate (ăt'rō-pēn sŭl'fāt). USP. The salt of an alkaloid obtained from belladonna. It is a parasympatholytic agent; counteracts effects of parasympathetic stimulation.

ACTION AND USES: Respiratory and circulatory stimulant; also used to overcome spasm of involuntary muscles; to inhibit secretions. This property makes atropine particularly useful as a premedication for inhalation anesthesia. When applied to the eye, it causes the pupil to dilate (mydriasis) and paralyzes the ciliary muscle (cycloplegia). This allows the eye to be easily examined for refractive errors.

Atropine is used to relieve muscle spasm, and for many other systemic effects.

POISONING SYM: Dryness of mouth; thirst; burning pain in throat; skin is dry,

hot and flushed; hyperpyrexia; palpitations; restlessness; excitement; delirium.

F.A. TREATMENT: Lavage with slurry of activated charcoal or 1% tannic acid. Pilocarpine will make patient more comfortable, but barbiturates must be used for controlling excitement. SEE: *Table of Poisons and Poisoning* in *Appendix.*

at'ropinism, at'ropism. Atropine poisoning.

atropiniza'tion. Production of physiologic effect of atropine.

attack. The onset of an illness or sympton. One speaks of a heart attack or an attack of gout.

attendant. A paramedical hospital employee who assists in the care of patients.

atten'tion [L. *attendere*, wait upon]. Power to focus on some phase of consciousness including some aspect of the world of reality.

a. reflex. Change in size of pupil when attention is suddenly fixed. SYN: *Piltz's reflex.*

atten'uant [L. *attenuāre*, to thin]. 1. Diluting, making thin or weak. 2. An agent that thins the blood.

atten'uate. To render thin; or make less virulent.

atten'uated. 1. Diluted. 2. Pert. to reduced virulence of pathogenic microorganism.

a. virus. One made less virulent.

attenua'tion. 1. Dilution. 2. Lessening of virulence. This may be accomplished with bacteria and viruses by heating, drying, treating with chemicals, passing through another organism, or culturing under unfavorable conditions.

at'tic. The upper portion of the middle ear or the portion lying above the tympanic cavity proper. SYN: *epitympanic recess.* SEE: *ear; tympanum.*

a. disease. Chronic suppurative inflammation of attic.

atticitis (at''ĭ-sī'tĭs) [*attic*, + Gr. *-ītis*, inflammation]. Inflammation of the tympanic attic.

atticoantrotomy (at''ĭ-kō-an-trot'ō-mĭ) ["+ Gr. *antron*, cave, + *tomē*, cutting]. Operation to remove contents of the attic and mastoid antrum.

atticot'omy ["+ Gr. *temnein*, to cut]. Surgical opening of tympanic attic.

at'titude [LL. *aptitūdo*, fitness]. Bodily posture or position assumed, esp. with reference to position of limbs. It is often a symptom of disease or abnormal mental state, e.g., the sterotyped position assumed by catatonics or theatric expression seen in hysteria.

a. of combat. The rigid defensive position a corpse assumes with flexion of legs, arms, and fingers; due to postmortem contraction of muscles.

a., crucifixion. Body rigid with arms at right angles.

a., defense. Position automatically assumed to avert pain.

a., forced. Abnormal position due to disease or contractures.

a., frozen. Stiffness of gait, seen in amyotrophic lateral sclerosis.

a., illogical. Peculiar attitudes caused by disease, esp. hysteroepilepsy.

a., passional, a., passionate. Theatric or dramatic gestures and expressions of face and figure assumed by hysteric patients.

a., stereotyped. Position taken and held for a long period, seen frequently in mental diseases.

attollens (a-tŏl'enz) [L.]. Raising or lifting up.

attrac'tion [L. *attrahere,* to draw toward]. Tendency of particles to approach each other.

a., capillary. The force by which liquids rise in fine tubes or through pores of loose material.

a., chemical. The tendency of atoms of one element to unite with those of another to form compounds.

a., molecular. The tendency of molecules with unlike electrical charges to attract each other. SEE: *adhesion; cohesion.*

attrahens (at'rä-henz). Drawing toward, as a muscle.

attrition (ă-trish'un) [L. *attritiō,* a rubbing against]. 1. A chafing or abrasion. 2. Any friction that breaks the skin. 3. A wearing away, as of teeth in normal use.

at. wt. Abbr. for *atomic weight.*

atylosis (at-ĭ-lō'sĭs) [Gr. *a-,* not, + *tylōsis,* a callus]. Nontypical tuberculosis.

atyp'ical ["+ *tupikos,* impressionable]. Deviating from the normal.

Au. Chem. symb. for gold.

A.U. Abbr. for *Angstrom unit.*

Aub-Dubois table (ōb-dū-boy'). [Joseph C. Aub, Amer. physician, 1890—; Eugene F. Dubois, Amer. physician, 1882—]. Table of normal basal metabolic rates according to age.

audile (aw'dil). 1. Pert. to hearing. 2. Ear-minded. 3. In psychoanalysis, one whose mental images are auditory. SEE: *motile; visile.*

audio-anesthesia. Anesthesia produced by sound; used by dentists to kill pain.

audiogram (aw'dĭ-ō-gram") [L. *audīre,* to hear, + Gr. *gramma,* writing]. Record of the audiometer.

audiom'eter ["+ Gr. *metron,* measure]. A delicate instrument for testing hearing.

audiom'etry. Testing of the hearing sense.

audiosound (aw'dĭ-ō-sound). Sound waves of frequencies perceptible to the human ear (12 to 20,000 cycles per second).

audiphone (aw'dĭ-fŏn) [L. *audīre,* to hear, + Gr. *phōnē,* voice]. Instrument for conveying sound to auditory nerve through the teeth or a bone.

audi'tion [L. *auditiō,* hearing]. Hearing.

a., chromatic. Condition in which certain color sensations are aroused by sound stimuli.

a., colored. Color sensation is perceived when certain sounds reach ear.

a., gustatory. Condition in which certain taste sensations are aroused by sound stimuli.

a., mental. The recollection of a sound based on previous auditory impressions.

auditive (aw'di-tiv). One who is auditory minded, depending upon hearing in learning, or recall.

auditognosis (aw"dĭt-og-nō'sĭs) [L. *auditiō,* hearing, + Gr. *gnōsis,* knowledge]. 1. Understanding and interpretation of sounds. 2. Diagnosis by percussion and auscultation.

audito-oculogyric reflex (aw"dĭt-ō-ok"ū-lō-jĭ'rĭk). The sudden turning of the head and eyes in direction of an alarming sound.

aud'itory [L. *auditorius*]. Pert. to the sense of hearing.

a. canal. One of two canals leading to the ear. They are the external auditory meatus, leading from concha to tympanic membrane, length 2.5 cm.; and the internal auditory meatus, located on posterior surface of petrous portion of temporal bone and leading from cranial cavity to inner ear, transmitting the acoustic nerve.

a. evoked response. Response to auditory stimuli as determined by a method independent of the individual's subjective response. The electroencephalogram has been used to record response to sound. By measuring intensity of sound and presence of response it is possible to test the acuity of hearing of psychiatric patients, persons who are asleep, and children too young to cooperate in a standard hearing test. ABBR: a.e.r.

a. muscles. The tensor tympani and stapedius muscles. SEE: *Table of Muscles* in *Appendix.*

a. nerve. The 8th cranial nerve; it is a sensory nerve with two sets of fibers: cochlear n. (hearing), and vestibular n. (equilibrium), the latter having three branches, the superior, inferior, and middle branch.

SYN: *nervus acusticus; nervus vestibulocochlearis* [NA]; *vestibulocochlear nerve*.

a. ossicles. The ear bones.

a. reflex. Blinking of the eyes upon the sudden unexpected production of a sound.

a. teeth. Toothlike projections in the cochlea.

a. tube. Eustachian tube, q.v.

aud'itus. The power or the sense of hearing.

Auenbrugger's sign (ow-ĕn-brŭg'er). [Leopold Joseph Auenbrugger, Austrian physician, 1722-1809]. Epigastric prominence due to marked pericardial effusion.

Auerbach's plexus (ow'er-băk). [Leopold Auerbach, Ger. anatomist, 1828-1897]. A plexus of sympathetic nerve fibers situated between the longitudinal and circular fibers of the muscular coat of the stomach and intestines. Also called the plexus myentericus.

Auer's bodies (ow'er). [John Auer, Amer. physician, 1875-1948]. Rod-shaped structures present in the cytoplasm of the cells in myeloid types of luekemia. The bodies may be found in myeloblasts, myelocytes and monocytes, and are peroxidase-positive.

Aufrecht's sign (owf'rekht). [Emanual Aufrecht, Ger. physician, 1844-1933]. Diminished breathing sound heard above the jugular notch in tracheal stenosis.

augment (ŏg-mĕnt'). [L. *augmentum*, increase]. To add to or increase.

augmentation. The increasing stage of a fever, or of symptoms of an acute disease.

augmen'ter. Increasing.

a. nerves. Those increasing force and rapidity of the heartbeat.

augnathus (ŏg-nā'thŭs) [Gr. *au*, again, + *gnathos*, jaw]. Fetus with a double lower jaw.

aula (ŏ'lă) [Gr. *aulē*, hall]. 1. Anterior part of third ventricle. 2. Inflamed area around vaccination vesicle.

aulatela (ŏ-lă-tē'lă) ["+ *tela*, web]. Membrane covering the aula.

auliplexus (ŏ-lĭ-plĕks'ŭs) ["+ L. *plectere*, to twist]. Aulic part of choroid plexus.

aulix (ŏ'lĭks) [L. *aulix*, furrow]. Monro's sulcus or sulcus hypothalamicus.

aura (ŏ'ră) [L. *aura*, breeze]. A premonitory awareness of an approaching physical or mental disorder. In epilepsy the aura may precede the attack by several hours or only by a few seconds. Epileptic aura may be of a psychic nature or sensory with olfactory, visual, auditory or taste hallucinations.

aural (ŏ'ral) [L. *auris*, the ear]. 1. Pert. to the ear. 2. Pert. to an aura.

auranti'asis [L. *aurantium*, orange, + Gr. *-iasis*, condition]. Yellowish skin color due to eating large quantities of oranges.

auran'tium [L.]. Orange.

aureomycin. A proprietary name for chlortetracycline, q.v.

auric (ŏ'rĭk) [L. *aurum*, gold]. Pert. to gold.

auricle (ŏ'rĭ-kl). Auricula, q.v.

auricula (ŏ-rĭk'ū-lă) [L., little ear]. (pl. *auriculae*) 1. [NA] The protruding portion of the external ear which surrounds the opening of the external acoustic meatus; the pinna. 2. A small conical pouch forming a portion of the right and left atria of the heart. Each projects from the upper anterior portion of each atrium. 3. A common erroneous term for the atrium.

auric'ular. 1. Rel. to the auricle of the ear. 2. Atrial.

auriculare (ŏ-rĭk"ū-lā'rĭ). (pl. *auricula'ria*). A craniometric point at center of opening of external auditory canal.

auric"ulocer'vical nerve reflex. Congestion of ear on same side resulting from stimulation of distal end of divided auriculocervical nerve. SYN: *Snellen's reflex*.

auric"ulopal'pebral reflex. Closure of an eye resulting from stimulation by heat or some tactile irritant on the exterior auditory meatus or deeper portions of canal up to the tympanum. SYN: *Kisch's reflex*.

auriculoventric'ular. Former term for atrioventricular.

a. bundle. Former name for atrioventricular bundle, q.v.

auriform (ŏ'rĭ-form) [L. *auris*, ear, + *forma*, shape]. Ear-shaped.

auriginous (ŏ-rĭj'ĭ-nŭs) [L. *auriginosis*, jaundiced]. Pert. to jaundice.

aurilave (ŏ'rĭ-lăv) [L. *auris*, ear, + *lavāre*, to wash]. An apparatus for cleansing the ear.

auripuncture (ŏ'rĭ-pŭnk"tūr) ["+ *punctura*, puncture]. Surgical puncture of tympanic membrane.

auris (ŏ'ris) [L.]. The ear.

a. dextra. Right ear. ABBR: a.d.

a. externa. The external ear (pinna and external auditory meatus).

a. interna. The internal ear (semicircular canals, vestibule, cochlea).

a. media. The middle ear (tympanum).

a. sinistra. Left ear. ABBR: a.s.

au'riscalp, auriscal'pium [L. *auris*, ear, + *scalpere*, to scrape]. 1. Scraping instrument to remove foreign matter from ear. 2. Earpick.

auriscope (ŏ'rĭ-skōp) ["+ Gr. *skopein*, to view]. Instrument for making an aural examination.

aurist (ŏ'rist). Ear specialist. SYN: *otologist*.

auris′tics. Art of treating ear diseases.

auristil′lae [L.]. Ear drops.

aurococcus (ŏ″rō-kŏk′ŭs) [L. *aurum*, gold, + Gr. *kokkos*, berry]. Pyogenic microbe forming golden cultures found in boils, abscesses, carbuncles, pyemia, etc. SYN: *Staphylococcus pyogenes aureus.*

aurother′apy [″+ Gr. *therapeia*, treatment]. Treatment of disease by administration of gold salts; used in the treatment of rheumatoid arthritis. SYN: *chrysotherapy.*

aurum (ŏ′rŭm) [L.]. Gold.

auscult (ŏs-kult′). Auscultate, q.v.

auscultate (aws′kul-tāt) [L. *auscultāre*, listen to]. To examine by auscultation.

auscultation (ŏs-kul-tā′shun). Process of listening for sounds produced in some of the body cavities, esp. chest and abdomen, in order to detect or judge some abnormal condition.

    PROCEDURE: The chest should be draped with a loose-fitting garment which can easily be moved aside to allow the stethoscope to be placed directly against the skin. When chest is covered with hair moisten latter as otherwise it will produce friction sounds, resembling rales. Auscult all over chest anteriorly and posteriorly, on full inspiration, full expiration, and after coughing. In comparing the two sides auscult symmetrical parts. Parts should be in perfect repose. Position of examiner as unrestrained as possible, lest sounds of his own blood vessels be confused with sounds from within the subject.

    a., immediate. When ear is applied directly to bared or thinly covered surface.

    a., mediate. When sounds are conducted from the surface to ear through an instrument such as a stethoscope.

auscultation, words pert. to: abdominal a.; bruit; cat's purr; egophony; percussion; rales; souffle; vocal resonance.

auscul′tatory. Pert. to auscultation.

    a. percussion. Auscultation at the same time percussion is made.

auscultoplec′trum [L. *auscultāre*, listen to, + Gr. *plēktron*, hammer]. Instrument used for both auscultation and percussion.

Australian antigen. Antigen present in some patients who have had viral hepatitis. Test for its presence may be helpful in diagnosing hepatitis. SYN: *hepatitis-associated antigen.*

autarcesis (ŏ-tăr′sĭ-sĭs, ŏ-tăr-sē′sĭs) [Gr. *autos*, self, + *arkein*, to ward off]. Resistance to infection through natural immunity.

autarcetic (ŏ-tăr-sĕt′ĭk). Pert. to autarcesis.

autechoscope (ŏ-tĕk′ō-skōp) [Gr. *autos*, self, + *echos*, sound, + *skopein*, to inspect]. Instrument for self-auscultation.

autemesia (ŏ-tĕ-mē′zĭ-ă) [″+ Gr. *emesis*, vomiting]. Vomiting without apparent cause.

autism (ŏ′tizm) [″+ Gr. *-ismos*, condition of]. In psychiatry, mental introversion in which the attention or interest is fastened upon the victim's own ego. A self-centered mental state from which reality tends to be excluded.

autistic child. A child who has a sense of aloneness and wants to maintain that condition. He does not seek or respond to affection. Speech disturbances are frequent; movements are typically purposeless, rhythmic, and repetitious. Such children are not mentally retarded and siblings usually are normal.

    ETIOL: Unknown. TREATMENT: Symptomatic.

auto- [Gr. *autos*, self]. Prefix meaning self.

autoactiva′tion [Gr. *autos*, self, + L. *agere*, to act]. Gland activation by its own secretion.

autoagglutina′tion [″+ L. *agglutināre*, adhere to]. Blood corpuscle agglutination of an individual by his own serum.

autoanal′ysis [″+ *analuein*, break down]. Patient's own analysis of mental state underlying his mental disorder.

autoanalyzer (ŏ″tō-ăn′ă-līz-ĕr). Apparatus for performing analytic tests on a large number of laboratory specimens. The testing is done automatically with the specimens being tested sequentially.

autoan′tibody [Gr. *autos*, self, + *anti*, against, + AS. *bodig*, body]. Antibody acting against tissue products of the same organism in which it is formed.

autoantitox′in [″+ ″+ *toxikon*, poison]. Antitoxin produced by body itself.

autoau′dible [Gr. *autos*, self, + L. *audire*, to hear]. Audible to oneself; pert. to sounds produced in one's own body.

au′toblast [″+ *blastos*, germ]. Independent cell, as a bacterium.

autocatalysis (ŏ-tō-kă-tăl′ĭ-sĭs) [″+ *kataluein*, to dissolve]. Increase in the rate of a chemical reaction as result of products produced in the reaction which act as catalysts.

autocatharsis (ŏ-tō-kă-thăr′sĭs) [″+ *katharsis*, a cleansing]. A form of psychotherapy in which the patient in discussing his own problems gains an insight into his mental difficulties.

autocath′eterism [″+ *kathetēr*, catheter]. Passage of the catheter by oneself.

autochthonous (ŏ-tŏk'thō-nŭs) [Gr. *autos*, self, + *chthōn*, earth]. Found where developed, as in the case of a blood clot or a calculus. Also originating in an organ itself without a stimulus from outside the organ. Thus the heart will beat even though no nervous stimuli are present.

    a. ideas. Ideas which compel attention, which are not in harmony with one's character, and which arise spontaneously, including auditory hallucinations.

autocinesia, autocinesis (ŏ"tō-sĭ-nē'sĭ-ă, -nē'sĭs) ["+ *kinēsis*, motion]. Voluntary movement.

autoclasis (ŏ'tŏk'lă-sĭs) ["+ *klasis*, a breaking]. Destruction of a part from internal causes.

autoclave (ŏ'tō-klāv) [Gr. *autos*, self, + L. *clavis*, a key]. Apparatus for sterilization by steam pressure, usually at 250° F. (121° C.) for a specified length of time. SEE: *sterilization.*

autocys'toplasty ["+ *kystis*, bladder, + *plassein*, to mold]. Plastic repair of bladder with grafts from patient's own body.

autocytolysin (ŏ-tō-sĭ-tŏl'ĭ-sĭn) ["+ *kytos*, cell, + *lysis*, dissolution]. Agent within patient's own blood plasma which destroys erythrocytes. SYN: *autolysin.*

autocytolysis (ŏ-tō-sĭ-tŏl'ĭ-sĭs). Self-digestion or self-destruction of cells.

autoder'mic [Gr. *autos*, self, + *derma*, skin]. Pert. to one's own skin, esp. rel. to dermatoplasty with patient's own skin.

autodiagno'sis ["+ *dia*, through, + *gignō-skein*, to perceive]. Diagnosis of one's own disease.

autodiges'tion ["+ L. *dis*, apart, + *gerere*, to carry]. Digestion of tissues by their own secretion as digestion of the stomach wall by gastric juice as occurs in certain stomach disorders.

autodrain'age ["+ AS. *drēahnian*, drain]. Drainage of a cavity by sending the fluid through a channel made in patient's own tissues.

autoecholalia (ŏ"tō-ĕk-ō-lā'lĭ-ă) ["+ *ēchō*, echo, + *lalia*, babble]. Repetition of words of one's own statements.

autoecic (aw-tē'sik) [Gr. *autos*, self, + *oikos*, house]. Pert. to parasite which goes through its entire life cycle in one organism.

autoerotic (ŏ"tō-ĭ-rŏt'ĭk) ["+ *erōtikos*, rel. to love]. Being sexually aroused or stimulated by oneself as in masturbation.

autofundoscope (ŏ"tō-fŭn'dō-skōp) ["+ L. *fundus*, bottom, + Gr. *skopein*, to examine]. Apparatus for autoexamination of eye vessels about macular region.

autogenesis (ŏ-tō-jĕn'ĕ-sĭs) ["+ *genesis*, production]. Abiogenesis; self-production; spontaneous generation.

autogenetic (ŏ-tō-jĕ-nĕt'ĭk). Pert. to self-production or autogenesis.

autogenic (ŏ-tō-jĕn'ĭk). Rel. to self-production. SYN: *autogenetic.*

autogenous (ŏ-tŏj'ĕ-nŭs). 1. Self-producing. 2. Originating within the body. 3. Denoting a vaccine from a culture of bacteria from the patient who is to be inoculated with it.

    a. vaccine. A suspension of killed or attenuated bacteria prepared from bacteria obtained from the patient to whom the vaccine will be administered.

au'tograft [Gr. *autos*, self, + L. *graphium*, pencil]. A graft taken from one part of a person's body to fill in another part.

autog'raphism ["+ *graphein*, to write]. Condition in which tracings made upon the skin, with the edge of a tongue depressor or similar instrument, will be followed by appearance of wheals or elevated red areas. SYN: *dermographia.*

autohem'ic [Gr. *autos*, self, + *haima*, blood]. Done with one's own blood.

autohemol'ysin ["+ "+ *lysis*, dissolution]. Antibody acting on corpuscles of individual in whose blood it is formed.

autohemol'ysis. Hemolysis of a person's blood corpuscles by his own serum.

autohemother'apy [Gr. *autos*, self, + *haima*, blood, + *therapeia*, treatment]. Treatment by withdrawal and injection of patient's own blood.

autohypnosis. Self-induced hypnosis.

autoimmune disease [Gr. *autos*, self, + L. *immūnis*, safe]. Disease in which body produces disordered immunological response against own body.

    Normally the body's immune mechanisms are able to distinguish clearly between what is a normal substance and what is foreign. In autoimmune diseases this system becomes defective and produces antibodies against normal parts of the body to such an extent as to cause tissue injury. Certain diseases such as hemolytic anemia, some forms of glomerulonephritis, rheumatoid arthritis, myasthenia gravis, and scleroderma are considered to be autoimmune diseases.

autoimmuniza'tion. Immunization produced by an attack of the disease or by processes occurring within the body.

autoinfec'tion [Gr. *autos*, self, + L. *inficere*, to taint]. Infection by bacteria present within one's own body.

autoinfu'sion ["+ L. *in*, into, + *fundere*, to pour]. Forcing blood from extremities to body by applying Esmarch bandages.

autoinocula'tion [" + L. *inoculāre*, to in-graft]. Inoculation by use of organisms obtained from another part of the body.

au"tointoxica'tion [" + L. *in*, into, + Gr. *toxikon*, poison]. A condition caused by poisonous substances produced within the body.

autoisolysin (ŏ"tō-ĭ-sŏl'ĭ-sĭn). An antibody which causes dissolution of corpuscles of the individual from whom it was obtained. It also causes lysis of cells of other individuals of the same species.

autokeratoplasty (ŏ"tō-kĕr'ă-tō-plăs"tĭ) [Gr. *autos*, self, + *keras*, harm, + *placcein*, to form]. Corneal grafting using tissue from the patient's other eye.

autokinesis (ŏ"tō-kĭ-nē'sis) [" + *kinēsis*, motion]. Voluntary action.

autokinet'ic. Being able to move voluntarily.

autolesion (ŏ'tō-lē"shŭn) [Gr. *autos*, self, + L. *laedere*, to wound]. Injury self-inflicted.

autolysate (ŏ-tŏl'ĭ-sāt) [" + *lysis*, dissolution]. Specific product of autolysis.

autolysin (ŏ-tŏl'ĭ-sĭn). Agent in serum destroying erythrocytes.

autol'ysis. 1. The self-solution or self-digestion which occurs in tissues or cells by ferment in the cells themselves, even after death and in the absence of putrefactive bacteria. 2. Hemolysis of blood cells occurring as result of the action of an animal's own serum or plasma.

autolyt'ic. Rel. to autolysis. SEE: *enzyme.*

automat'ic [Gr. *automatos*, self-acting]. Spontaneous; involuntary.

automatism (ŏ-tŏm'ă-tĭzm) [Gr. *autos*, self, + *ismos*, condition of]. 1. Automatic actions or behavior without conscious purpose or knowledge. The subject, though amnesic, appears normal to an observer but the real personality is latent during a secondary state or period of automatism, usually a hysterical trance. The patient is not responsible for his acts and must not be left for a second. He may carry out complicated acts without any idea of them and without any after-memory. 2. The spontaneous activity of cells or tissues, as the movement of cilia or the contraction of smooth muscles in tissues or organs removed from the body.

automat'ograph [Gr. *automatismos*, self-action, + *graphein*, to write]. Instrument which records involuntary movements.

automysopho'bia [Gr. *autos*, self, + *mysos*, dirt, + *phobos*, fear]. Morbid dread of personal uncleanliness.

autonephrec'tomy [" + *nephros*, kidney, + *ektomē*, excision]. Complete atrophy of the kidney and complete obliteration of the

ureter. May be caused by one of several diseases including tuberculosis of the kidney.

autonomic (ŏ-tō-nŏm'ĭk) [" + *nomos*, law]. Spontaneous, self-controlling.

    a. nervous system. A part of the nervous system which is concerned with control of involuntary bodily functions. It controls function of glands, smooth muscle tissue and the heart. It is commonly defined so as to include the sympathetic or thoracolumbar division and the parasympathetic or craniosacral division.

The sympathetic system is made up of the paired ganglionated sympathetic trunk; its connections (rami communicantes) with the thoracic and lumbar parts of the spinal nerve; the large and small splanchnic nerves; and certain ganglia in the abdomen (e.g., the mesenteric ganglia).

The parasympathetic system consists of certain fibers of some cranial nerves such as the motor fibers of the vagus and of other fibers connected with the sacral part of the spinal cord.

It is best to use the word autonomic only in connection with efferent fibers; sensory fibers coming from the viscera and passing through the above named ganglia and trunks to reach the cord may be called visceral afferents.

GENERAL FUNCTIONS: Stimulating sympathetic fibers usually produces vasoconstriction in the part supplied; general rise in blood pressure; erection of the hairs; goose-flesh; pupillary dilation; secretion of small quantities of thick saliva; depression of gastrointestinal activity; and acceleration of the heart. In general these activities occur under emergencies such as fright and are associated or correlated with expenditure of energy. They are mediated through the release of a transmitter agent, norepinephrine.

Stimulating parasympathetic nerves generally produces vasodilation of the part supplied; general fall in the blood pressure; contraction of the pupil; copious secretion of thin saliva; increased gastrointestinal activity; and slowing of the heart. SEE: *autonomotropic; nervous system.*

auton'omin. A hormone supposed to correlate endocrine gland activity, inhibiting or stimulating secretions of each according to systemic need.

autonomotrop'ic [Gr. *autos*, self, + *nomos*, law, + *tropos*, turning]. Drawn to the autonomic nervous system.

auton'omous. Independent of external influences.

auton'omy. Functional independence.

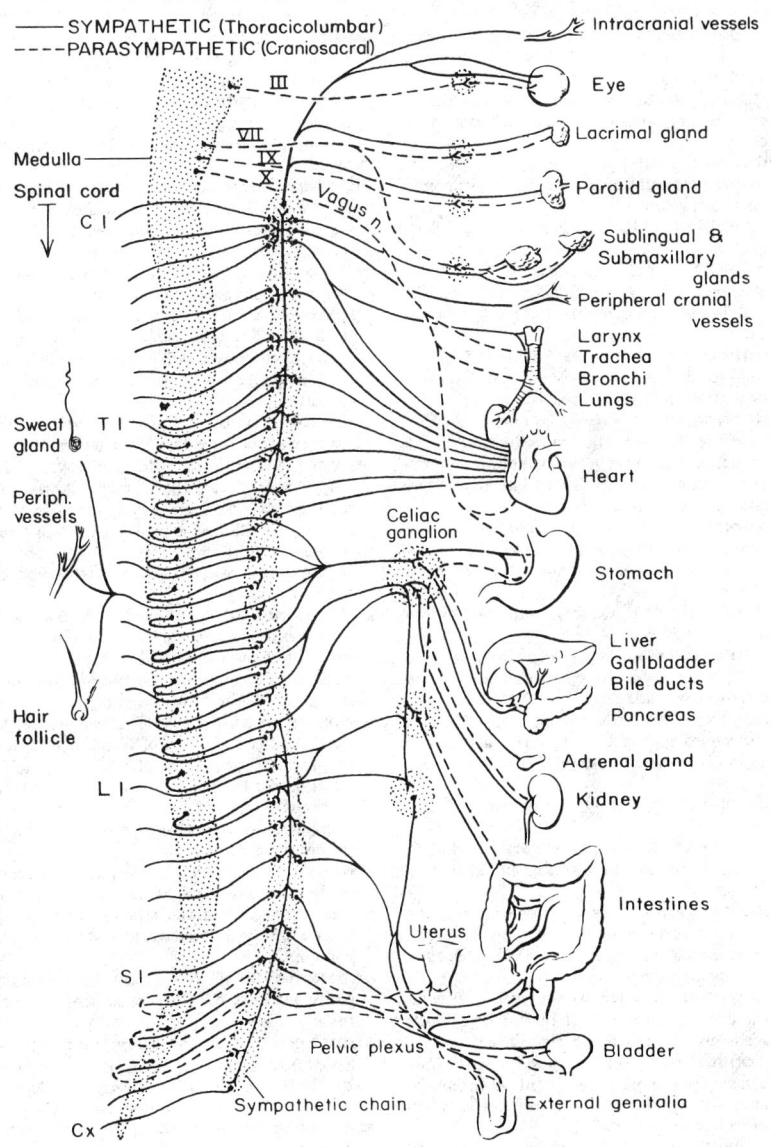

AUTONOMIC NERVOUS SYSTEM

autopathy (ŏ-tŏp′ă-thĭ) [Gr. *autos*, self, + *pathos*, disease]. A disease originating without apparent external cause. SYN: *ideopathy.*

autopep′sia ["+ *peptein*, to digest]. Digestion by self, as of gastric wall by its own secretion.

autopha′gia, autoph′agy ["+ *phagein*, to eat]. Biting oneself; self-consumption of a cell.

autophil (ŏ′tŏ-fĭl) [Gr. *autos*, self, + *philein*, to love]. Person having sensitive autonomic nervous system.

autophilia (ŏ-tŏ-fĭl′ĭ-ă). Narcissism, q.v. Self-love.

autophobia (ŏ″tŏ-fō′bĭ-ă) [Gr. *autos*, self, + *phobos*, fear]. 1. A psychoneurotic fear of being alone. 2. Abnormal fear of being egotistical.

autophonomania (ŏ″tŏ-fō″nō-mā′nĭ-ă) ["+ *phonos*, murder, + *mania*, madness]. Insanity with suicidal impulses.

autophony (ŏ-tŏf′ō-nĭ) ["+ *phône*, voice]. The vibration and echolike reproduction of the patient's own voice, breath sounds, and murmurs; usually due to diseases of middle ear and auditory tube.

autoplasmother′apy ["+ *plasma*, a thing formed, + *therapeia*, treatment]. Treatment through injecting patient's own blood plasma.

autoplas′tic ["+ *plassein*, to form]. Pert. to autoplasty, q.v.

autoplasty (ŏ′tŏ-plăs″tĭ). A grafting of fresh parts taken from the patient's body for the repair of wounds.

autoprecipitin (ŏ″tŏ-prē-sĭp′ĭ-tĭn) ["+ L. *praecipitāre*, to cast down]. Precipitin active against serum of animal in which it was formed.

autopsia (ŏ-tŏp′sĭ-ă) ["+ *opsis*, view]. Autopsy.

a. in vivo. An exploratory incision to determine cause of a disorder or nature of a disease.

autopsy (ŏ′tŏp-sĭ). Examination of the organs of a dead body to determine cause of death, or pathological conditions. SYN: *post-mortem examination.*

autopsycho′sis (Gr. *autos*, self, + *psyche*, the soul). Mental disease in which patient's ideas about himself are disordered.

autopyother′apy ("+ *pyon*, pus, + *therapeia*, treatment). Treatment of disease by administration of patient's own pathological excretions.

autoreinfu′sion ("+ L. *re*, back, + *in*, into, + *fundere*, to pour). Intravenous injection of patient's blood which has been collected from a site in which bleeding had occurred. SEE: *autotransfusion.*

autorrhaphy (ŏ-tŏr′ă-fĭ) ["+ *rhaphē*, suture]. Wound closure by using strands of tissue taken from edges of the wound.

autoseptice′mia [Gr. *autos*, self, + *septos*, rotten, + *haima*, blood]. Septicemia from poisons existing within the organism.

autoserodiagno′sis ["+ L. *serum*, whey, + Gr. *dia*, through, + *gnōsis*, knowledge]. Diagnosis through serum from patient's blood.

autoserother′apy ["+ "+ Gr. *therapeia*, treatment]. Treatment by hypodermic injection of patient's own blood serum.

autose′rous. Pert. to autoserum.

autose′rum. Serum obtained from patient's own blood or cerebrospinal fluid.

autosite (ŏ′tŏ-sīt) [Gr. *autos*, self, + *sitos*, food]. The fairly normal member of asymmetrical conjoined twins, the other twin being dependent on the autosite for its nutrition.

autosmia (ŏ-tŏz′mĭ-ă) ["+ *osmē*, smell]. Awareness of the odor of one's own body.

autosomatognosis (ŏ″tŏ-sō″mă-tog-nō′-sĭs) ["+ *sōma*, body, + *gnosis*, recognition]. The feeling that a part of the body that has been removed is still present. SEE *phantom limb.*

autosome (ŏ′tŏ-sōm). Any of the paired chromosomes other than the sex (X and Y) chromosomes.

autosplenectomy (ŏ″tŏ-splen-ĕk′tŏ-mĭ) [Gr. *autos*, self, + *splēn*, spleen, + *ektomē*, excision]. Multiple infarcts of the spleen which cause it to become fibrotic and nonfunctioning. Seen in sickle cell anemia.

autosuggestibil′ity ["+ L. *suggerēre*, to suggest]. Peculiar lack of resistance to any suggestion that may be offered by oneself.

autosugges′tion. The acceptance of an idea or thought arising from within one's own mind bringing about some physical or mental action or change.

autosynnoia (ŏ″tŏ-sĭn-noy′ă) [Gr. *autos*, self, + *synnoia*, meditation]. In psychoanalysis, intense concentration to the extent of loss of interest in the outside world; a state of introversion.

autotemnous (ŏ″tŏ-tĕm′nŭs) ["+ *temnein*, to divide]. Pert. to cells propagating by spontaneous division.

autother′apy ["+ *therapeia*, treatment]. 1. Spontaneous cure. 2. Treatment of disease by administering patient's own pathological secretions, usually as autogenous vaccine.

autotopagnosia (ŏ″tŏ-tŏp-ăg-nō′zĭ-ă) ["+ *topos*, place, + *a-*, not, + *gnōsis*, knowledge]. Inability to orient various parts of body correctly.

autotoxe′mia, autotoxico′sis ["+ *toxikon*, poison, + *haima*, blood]. Self-poisoning due to absorption of a toxic substance generated within the body.

autotox'in. Poison generated within the body upon which it acts.

autotransform'er [Gr. *autos*, self, + L. *trans*, across, + *forma*, form]. A transformer that has part of its turns common to both primary and secondary circuits. SEE: *transformer.*

autotransfusion (ŏ″tō-trăns-fū'shŭn) [″+ ″+ *fundere*, pour]. 1. Bandaging the limbs to force the blood to the vital centers. 2. A method of returning the patient's own extravasated blood to the circulation. Blood that is shed into the peritoneal cavity, particularly in a ruptured ectopic pregnancy or ruptured spleen, is collected during operation and transfused immediately into the circulation of the patient.

autotransplanta'tion [″+ ″+ *plantāre*, to plant]. Transferring a piece of tissue from one part to another in same person.

autotrophic (ŏ″tō-trō'fĭk) [″+ *trophē*, nourishment]. Self-nourishing; pert. to green plants and bacteria which form protein and carbohydrate from inorganic salts and carbon dioxide, i.e., capable of growing in absence of organic compounds.

autotuber'culin [″+ L. *tuberculum*, a small swelling]. Tuberculin prepared from cultures of patient's own sputum.

autovaccina'tion [″+ *vacca*, cow]. 1. Vaccination with autogenous vaccine or autovaccine. 2. A vaccination resulting from virus or bacteria from a sore of a previous vaccination, as may occur following scratching the sore of a smallpox vaccination and subsequent transfer of the virus to a break in the skin elsewhere.

autovac'cine. Vaccine prepared from virus developed in patient's own body.

autoxida'tion [Gr. *autos*, self, + *oxys*, acid, + *gennan*, to produce]. Spontaneous combining of a substance with oxygen.

auxanography (ŏks″ăn-ŏg'rā-fĭ) [Gr. *auxanein*, to increase, + *graphein*, to write]. Determination of most suitable medium for bacterial cultivation.

auxanology (ŏks″ăn-ŏl'ō-jĭ) [″+ *logos*, study]. Scientific study of growth.

auxesis (ŏks-ē'sĭs) [Gr. *auxēsis*, to increase]. Enlarged in bulk or size.

auxet'ic. Promoting proliferation in leukocytes and other cells.

auxilytic (ŏks-ĭ-lĭt'ĭk) [Gr. *auxanein*, to increase, + *luein*, dissolve]. Favoring lysis (2), q.v.

aux'in [Gr. *auxē*, increase]. Plant-sprout hormone promoting growth in plant cells and tissues.

auxocyte (ŏks'ō-sīt) [Gr. *auxanein*, to increase, + *kytos*, cell]. Early-growth stage of certain cells.

auxogluc (ŏks'ō-glŭk) [″+ *glykys*, sweet]. A group of tasteless atoms which combine with gluciphores to form sweet-tasting compounds.

auxol'ogy [″+ *logos*, study]. Scientific study of growth of organisms, esp. microorganisms.

auxotroph (ŏks'ō-trōf) [″+ *trophē*, nutrition]. A mutant or other organism needing a specific factor for growth different from that required by the parent organism.

A-V. Abbr. for *atrioventricular.*

availability. In nutrition, the extent to which a nutrient is present in a form that can be absorbed and utilized.

av'alanche theory [Fr. *avaler*, to descend]. Theory that nervous impulses are reinforced and thereby become more intense as they travel peripherally.

avascular (ă-văs'kū-lar) [Gr. *a-*, not, + L. *vasculum*, little vessel]. Lacking in blood vessels or having a poor blood supply, said of tissues such as cartilage.

avasculariza'tion. Expulsion of blood, as by use of Esmarch bandage.

Avel'lis's paralysis syndrome. [George Avellis, Ger. laryngologist, 1864-1916] Paralysis of one-half of soft palate, the pharynx, larynx, and loss of pain and heat and cold sensation on opposite side.

aviation medicine. The branch of medicine concerned with diseases and pathologic conditions resulting from, or incident to air travel.

aviation physiology. The branch of physiology which deals with conditions encountered by man in high altitudes as in aircraft flights, mountain climbing, or in space vehicles. The principal factors dealt with are hypoxia; physical factors such as extreme temperatures and radiation; effects of forces of acceleration and deceleration; weightlessness; enforced inactivity; and disturbance of biological rhythm.

avidin (ăv'ĭ-dĭn) [L. *avidus*, greedy]. A protein isolated from raw egg white. Said to be an inhibitor of biotin, thereby causing a deficiency in biotin. Formerly called vitamin H.

avirulent (ă-vĭr'ū-lent) [Gr. *a-*, not, + L. *virus*, poison]. Without virulence.

avitaminosis (ā-vī″tă-mĭ-nō'sĭs). Disease due to lack of vitamins in the diet; a deficiency disease. SEE: *vitamin.*

avitaminotic (ā-vī-tăm-ĭn-ŏt'ĭk). Pert. to or affected with avitaminosis.

avivement (ă-vēv-mŏn') [Fr.]. Surgical trimming of wound edges prior to suturing them together.

avocado (ăv''ō-kä'dō) [Sp. *aguacate*]. Pear-shaped, green fruit; alligator pear.

Avocados contain a sugar, mannoneptose, which is excreted in the urine. This sugar will cause a positive test for reducing substances in the urine, i.e., a false-positive reaction for excess sugar in the urine.

Food value of 100 gm. (half, peeled): Cal. 167; fat 164 gm.; carbohydrates 6.3 gm.; vitamin A, 290 I.U.; ascorbic acid 14 mg.

Avogadro's law (ŏv-ō-gŏd'rō). [Amadeo Avogadro, It. physicist, 1776-1856]. Equal volumes of gases contain equal numbers of molecules, pressure and temperature being same.

Avogadro's number. Number of molecules, 6.0225×10^{23}, in one gram-molecular weight of a compound. SYN: *Avogadro's constant*.

avoirdupois' measure (ăv''ĕr-dĕ-poyz') [Fr., to have weight]. A system of weighing or measuring all coarse and heavy articles. 7000 grains equal one pound. Some medicines are bought and sold by avoirdupois weight.

To find the capacity of a vessel or space in gallons, divide the contents in cubic inches by 231 for liquid gallons, or by 268.8 for dry gallons.

To convert gallons to cubic inches, multiply the given number of liquid gallons by 231; then change to higher denominations if required. The dry gallon (half-peck) contains 268.8 cu. in. Six dry gallons are equal to nearly seven liquid gallons.

The bushel contains 2150.42 cu. in. and is a cylindrical measure 18 1/2 in. in diameter and 8 in. deep. Measures of capacity are all cubic measures. The number of pounds in a bushel depends upon the article contained therein. SEE: *apothecaries' measure; household measures; metric system; Troy weight; Table of Weights and Measures* in *Appendix*.

avulsion (ă-vŭl'shŭn) [Gr. *a-*, not, + L. *vellere*, to pull]. A tearing away forcibly of a part or structure. If surgical repair is necessary, merely apply a sterile dressing while waiting for surgery to be done. If fingers, toes, feet, or hands are completely avulsed, they may be successfully rejoined to the body if prompt and expert care is available.

axanthopsia (aks''an-thop'sĭ-ă) ["+ *xanthos*, yellow, + *opsis*, vision]. Yellow blindness.

axenic (ăks-ĕn'ĭk) ["+ *xenos*, stranger]. Germ-free, as pertaining to animals, or pure, as pertaining to cultures or microorganisms.

axial (aks'ĭ-al) [L. *axis*, axis]. Situated in or pert. to an axis.

 a. line. A line running in the main axis of the body or part of it. The axial line of the hand runs through the middle digit; the axial line of the foot runs through the second digit.

 a. skeleton. Head and trunk.

axifugal (aks-if'ū-gal) ["+ *fugere*, to flee]. Receding from the axis. SYN: *centrifugal*.

axilem'ma [L. *axis*, axis, + Gr. *lemma*, husk]. The plasma membrane of an axon.

axil'la [L. *axilla*, armpit]. (pl. *axil'lae*) [NA]. The armpit.

axillary (ăks'ĭ-lār-ĭ). Pert. to the axilla.

ax''illofem'oral bypass graft. Surgical establishment of a connector between the axillary artery and the common femoral arteries. Synthetic artery graft is used and implanted subcutaneously. Used in treating patients with insufficient blood flow to the legs.

ax'ion [Gr. *axōn*, axle]. Brain and spinal cord. The cerebrospinal axis.

axioplasm (aks'ĭ-ō-plazm) ["+ *plasma*, a thing formed]. Neuroplasm of an axis cylinder.

axip'etal [L. *axis*, axis, + *petere*, to seek]. Directed toward the axis. SYN: *axopetal; centripetal*.

ax'is. (pl. *axes*). 1. A line, real or imaginary, which runs through the center of a body, or about which a part revolves. 2. [NA] The second cervical vertebra or epistropheus which bears the odontoid process (dens) about which the atlas rotates.

 a., basicranial. A. connecting basion and gonion.

 a., basifacial. A. from subnasal point to gonion.

 a., binauricular. A. between the two auricular points.

 a., celiac. Celiac artery from abdominal aorta.

 a., cerebrospinal. Central nervous system.

 a., cylinder. An axon (def. 2), q.v.

 a., frontal. Imaginary line running transversely through the center of the eyeball.

 a., neural. SEE: *cerebrospinal a.*

 a., optic. A line which connects the anterior and posterior poles of the eye.

 a., principal. In optics, a line which passes through the optical center or nodal point of a lens perpendicular to the surface of the lens.

a., sagittal. Imaginary line running through the eyeball anteroposteriorly.

a., visual. A line passing from object of vision directly through center of cornea and lens to the fovea.

axis traction (ăks'ĭs trăk'shŭn). Traction made on the fetus in the direction of the birth canal.

a. t. forceps. Device used to aid in traction made on the fetus.

axite (aks'īt). Any terminal filament of an axis cylinder.

axo- [Gr. *axōn*, axis]. Prefix pert. to axis or axon.

axodendrite (ăks″ō-děn'drĭt) [Gr. *axōn*, axis, + *dendron*, tree]. Process given off from a nerve cell axon (not an axis cylinder).

axofugal (ăks-ŏf'ū-găl) ["+ L. *fugere*, to flee]. Axifugal, q.v.

axolem'ma ["+ *lemma*, husk]. Axis cylinder sheath of a nerve fiber. SYN: *axilemma.*

axolysis (ăks-ŏl'ĭ-sĭs) ["+ *lysis*, dissolution]. Destruction of the axis cylinder of a nerve.

ax'on, ax'one [Gr. *axōn*, axis]. 1. A process of a neuron which conducts impulses away from the cell body. Typically one arising from a portion of the cell devoid of Nissl granules, the axon hillock. Axons may possess either or both of two sheaths (myelin sheath and neurilemma) or neither. Axons are usually long and straight, and most end in synapses in the central nervous system or ganglia or in effector organs (e.g., motor neurons). They may give off side branches or collaterals. An axon with its sheath(s) constitutes a nerve fiber. 2. A nerve cell process which resembles an axon in structure, specifically the peripheral process of a dorsal root ganglion cell (sensory neuron) which functionally and embryologically is a dendrite, but structurally is indistinguishable from an axon. SYN: *axis cylinder.* SEE: *nerve; neuron.*

axoneme (ăks'ō-nēm) ["+ *nēma*, a thread]. Axial thread of a chromosome.

axoneuron (ăks-ō-nū'rŏn) ["+ *neuron*, nerve]. A nerve cell of the cerebrospinal system.

axonometer (ăks-ō-nŏm'ĕ-ter) ["+ *metron*, a measure]. Device for determining the axis of astigmatism.

axopetal (ăks-ŏp'ĕ-tăl) ["+ L. *petere*, to seek]. Conducted along an axon toward a cell body of a neuron.

axophage (ăks'ō-fāj) [Gr. *axōn*, asix, + *phagein*, to eat]. Glia cell found in myelin excavations in myelitis.

ax'oplasm ["+ *plasma*, a thing formed]. The cytoplasm (neuroplasm) of an axon which encloses the neurofibrils.

axospongium (ăks-ō-spŏn'jĭ-ŭm) ["+ *spongos*, sponge]. The fine fibrillar network of axon of a nerve cell.

Ayerza's disease, syndrome (ŏ-yĕr'thŏ). [Abel Ayerza, Brazilian physician, 1861-1918]. One characterized by dyspnea; chronic cyanosis; erythemia; enlargement of spleen and liver; and hyperplasia of bone marrow. Polycythemia usually results from pulmonary insufficiency.

Az. Abbr. for *azote.*

aza'lein [L. *azalea*, azalea]. A red dye. SYN: *fuchsin.*

azo-. Prefix indicating the presence of —N-N— group in a chemical. This group is usually connected at either end with carbon atoms. SEE: *azo compounds.*

azoamyly (ăz-ō-ăm'ĭ-lĭ) [Gr. *a-*, not, + *zōon*, animal, + *amylon*, starch]. Diminution of amount of glycogen stored up in the liver.

azo compounds. Organic substances which contain the azo group. An example is azobenzene, $C_6H_5N:NC_6H_5$.

They are related to aniline, and include important dyes and indicators. SEE: *indicator* for table.

azoic (ă-zō'ĭk) [Gr. *a-*, not, + *zōe*, life]. Containing no living organisms.

azoospermia (ă-zō-ō-spĕr'mĭ-ă) ["+ *zōon*, animal, + *sperma*, seed]. Absence of spermatozoa from the semen.

azotation (ăz″ō-tā'shŭn) [*azote*, nitrogen]. Nitrogen absorption from the air.

az'ote [Gr. *a-*, not, + *zōe*, life]. Nitrogen.

azotemia (ăz″ō-tē'mĭ-ă) ["+ "+ *haima*, blood]. Presence of nitrogenous bodies, especially urea in increased amount, in the blood. SYN: *uremia*, q.v.

azotenesis (az-ō-tē-nē'sĭs). Disease due to excess of nitrogen in system.

azotifica'tion. Atmospheric nitrogen fixation.

azotized (az'ō-tīzd). 1. Containing nitrogen. 2. Converted into an azo compound.

Azotobacter (ă-zō″tō-bak'tĕr). Rod-shaped, gram-negative, nonpathogenic, soil and water bacteria that fix atmospheric nitrogen. The single genus of the family Azotobacteraceae.

azotom'eter [Gr. *a-*, not, + *zōē*, life, + *metron*, measure]. Instrument measuring amount of uric acid and urea in urine.

azotorrhea (az″ō-tō-rē'ă) ["+ "+ *rhoia*, flow]. Excess of nitrogenous matter in the feces or urine.

azotu'ria ["+ "+ *ouron*, urine]. An increase in nitrogenous compounds, esp. urea, in urine.

azure lunulae (az'ūrlŭ'nū-lĭ) [O.Fr. *azur*, + L. *lunula*, little moon]. Blue discoloration of the base, or lunulae, of the fingernails. May be seen in patients with hepatolenticular degeneration (Wilson's disease). Blue discoloration of the entire nail may be present in argyria and following therapy with quinacrine hydrochloride.

azurophil(e (az-ū'ro-fil) ["+ Gr. *philein,* to love]. Staining readily with azure dye.

azurophil'ia. Condition in which some blood cells have azurophil granules.

azygos (ăz'ĭ-gŏs) [Gr. *a-,* not, + *zygon,* yoke]. Occurring singly, not in pairs.

azygous (ăz'ĭ-gŭs). Single, not paired.

    a., vein. A single vein arising in the abdomen as a branch of the ascending lumbar vein. It passes upward through the aortic hiatus of the diaphragm into the thorax, then along right side of vertebral column to level of fourth thoracic vertebra where it turns and enters superior vena cava. In the thorax it receives the hemiazygous, accessory azygous and bronchial veins, as well as right intercostal and subcostal veins. In cases of obstruction to inferior vena cava, the azygous vein is the principal vein by which blood can return to the heart.

azymia (a-zī'mĭ-ä) [Gr. *a-,* not, + *zymē,* ferment]. State of being without a ferment or enzyme.

azymic, azymous (ā-zī'mĭk, -mŭs, az'ĭ-mus). 1. Unfermented or unleavened. 2. Denoting the absence of a ferment.

B

B. 1. Chem. symb. for boron. 2. Abbr. for *Bacillus, Balantidium, barometric, base, bath, behavior, buccal.*

Ba. Chem. symb. for barium.

Bab'bitt metal. [Isaac Babbitt, Amer. inventor, 1799-1862] Antifriction alloy of copper, antimony, and tin used occasionally in dentistry.

Babesia (bă-bē'zĭ-ă). [named for Victor Babes] A genus of Haemosporidia which are parasites in the blood of cattle, sheep, horses, dogs, and other vertebrate animals. They infest red blood cells bringing about their destruction with resulting hemoglobinuria. They are transmitted by ticks.

    B. bigemina. The causative organism of Texas fever in cattle.

    B. bovis. Causes hemoglobinuria and jaundice (red water fever) in cattle.

babesiasis, babesiosis (bă-be-zī'ă-sis, bă-bē"zĭ-ō'sĭs). Infection caused by a species of Babesia.

Babinski's reflex (bă-bĭn'skĭ). [Joseph Babinski, Fr. neurologist, 1857-1932] Normally, when the lateral aspect of the sole of the relaxed foot is stroked, the great toe is flexed. If the toe extends instead of flexes and the outer toes spread out, the Babinski reflex is present. This occurs in disease of the corticospinal tract. The Babinski reflex is normally present in infants under the age of six months. Also, care must be taken to avoid interpreting voluntary extension of the toe as a Babinski reflex.

Babinski's sign. Loss of or diminshed Achilles tendon reflex in sciatica.

baby. An infant.

    b., blue. Infant born with cyanosis due to a congenital anomaly of the heart which permits venous blood to travel directly from the right to the left side of the heart without going through the lungs.

bacca (bak'ă) [L. berry]. (pl. *baccae*) A berry.

bacciform (bak'sĭ-form) [L. *bacca*, berry, + *forma*, form]. Berry-shaped; coccal.

Bacillaceae (bas-ĭ-lā'sē-ē). A family (order Eubacteriales) of rod-shaped cells that can produce endospores. Usually gram-positive, commonly found in soil. Genera of family are Bacillus and Clostridium.

bacillaemia. Bacillemia, q.v.

bacillar, bacillary (bas'il-ar, bas'il-a-rĭ). 1. Pert. to or caused by bacilli. 2. Rodlike.

bacillemia (bas-ĭ-lē'mĭ-ă) [L. *bacillus*, rod, + Gr. *haima*, blood]. Presence of bacilli in the blood.

bacilli (bă-sĭl'ĭ). Pl. of bacillus.

bacillicide (ba-sil'ĭ-sīd). An agent destructive to bacilli.

bacilliculture (ba-sil'ĭ-kul-chur) [L. *bacillus*, rod, + *cultura*, cultivation]. 1. Propagation of bacilli. 2. Culture containing bacilli.

bacilliform (ba-sil'ĭ-form) ["+ *forma*, form]. Resembling a bacillus in shape.

bacilliparous (băs-ĭ-lĭp'ă-rŭs) ["+ *parere*, to produce]. Producing bacilli.

bacillogenic, bacillogenous (ba-sĭl"o-jen'-ik, ba-sĭl-oj'en-us) ["+ Gr. *gennan*, to produce]. 1. Producing bacilli. 2. Originating in bacilli.

bacillophobia (bas-ĭ-lō-fō'bĭ-ă) ["+ Gr. *phobos*, fear]. Morbid fear of bacilli.

bacillosis (bas"ĭ-lo'sis) ["+ Gr. -*ōsis*, infection]. Condition due to infection by bacilli.

bacilluria (bas-ĭ-lū'rĭ-ă) [L. *bacillus*, rod, + Gr. *ouron*, urine]. Bacilli in the urine. Most common infective organism is bacillus from the colon, usually Escherichia coli. SEE: *cystitis.*

Bacillus (bă-sĭl'ŭs). A genus of bacteria belonging to the family Bacillaceae. All species are rod-shaped, sometimes occurring in chains. They are spore-bearing, aerobic, motile or nonmotile; most are gram-positive and nonpathogenic. Only two species are pathogenic to man, the most important being B. anthracis.

    B. an'thracis. An aerobic, spore-forming bacillus pathogenic to man and domestic animals, being the causative agent of anthrax, q.v. SYN: *Davaine's bacillus.*

    B. subti'lis. The common hay bacillus but has a close resemblance to B. anthracis. It is considered to be nonpathogenic generally, but is believed by some occasionally to cause conjunctivitis in man. It is sometimes found as a contaminant of laboratory specimens. SYN: *hay bacillus.*

bacil'lus. (pl. *bacilli*) 1. Any rod-shaped microorganism. 2. A rod-shaped microorganism belonging to the class Schizomycetes. SEE: *Bacillus.*

    b., abortus. Brucella abortus. Causes infectious abortion in cattle and other domestic animals. Causative agent of brucellosis (undulant fever) in man.

    b., acid-fast. Bacillus not readily decolorized by acids or other means when stained.

    b., Bang's. Brucella abortus. SEE: *b., abortus,* q.v.

b., Bordet-Gengou. Bordetella pertussis, formerly Haemophilus pertussis. Causative agent of whooping cough.

b., Calmette-Guerin. Attenuated Mycobacterium bovis. Used in BCG vaccine as a preventive of human tuberculosis.

b., cholera. Vibrio comma. Causative agent of cholera.

b., colon. Escherichia coli. A normal inhabitant of the intestinal tract; the cause of urinary tract infections. Certain types are responsible for enteritis in infants.

b., comma. Vibrio comma. Causative agent of cholera.

b., diphtheria. Corynebacterium diphtheriae. The causative agent of diphtheria.

b., Döderlein's. A large gram-positive bacillus usually present in the vagina. Considered identical with Lactobacillus acidophilus.

b., Ducrey's. Haemophilus ducreyi. The cause of soft chancre or chancroid infection of the genitalia.

b., dysentery. A bacillus of the genus Shigella that causes bacillary dysentery.

b., Flexner's. Shigella flexneri. The most common cause of epidemic dysentery.

b., Friedländer's. Klebsiella pneumoniae. A cause of pneumonia.

b., fusiform. Fusobacterium fusiforme. The causative organism of Vincent's infection; it is found also in the normal mouth.

b., Gärtner's. Salmonella enteritidis. The cause of Salmonella gastroenteritis and Salmonella food poisoning.

b., gas. Clostridium perfringens. A cause of gas gangrene.

b., Ghon-Sachs. Clostridium septicum. A causative agent of gas gangrene.

b., Hansen's. Mycobacterium leprae. Causative organism of Hansen's disease (leprosy).

b., hay. Bacillus subtilis. Nonpathogenic bacillus, sometimes found as a contaminant of laboratory specimens.

b., Hofmann's. Corynebacterium pseudodiphtheriticum. Causative agent of a type of diptheria.

b., influenza. As Haemophilus influenzae type B, it is the cause of meningitis. Other types cause conjunctivitis, septicemia, and respiratory infections. May cause complications, as a secondary invader, in influenza, pertussis, or other diseases.

b., Klebs-Loeffler. Corynebacterium diphtheriae. The cause of diphtheria.

b., Koch-Weeks. Haemophilus aegyptius. Cause of infectious conjunctivitis.

b., leprosy. Mycobacterium leprae. Cause of leprosy (Hansen's disease).

b., Morax-Axenfeld. Moraxella lacunata, a cause of conjunctivitis in man.

b., Morgan's. Proteus morganii. May cause abscesses and urinary tract infections. Usually a secondary invader. Isolated from patients with summer diarrhea.

b., paracolon. Paracolobactrum. Found in gastroenteritis.

b., paratyphoid. Salmonella paratyphi. One of the causes of paratyphoid fever.

b., Pfeiffer's. Haemophilus influenzae. SEE: *b., influenza.*

b., plague. Pasteurella pestis. The cause of bubonic plague.

b., Shiga. Name given to a representative dysentery bacillus first described in 1898 by Kiyoshi Shiga, a Japanese bacteriologist for whom the genus Shigella was named.

b., smegma. Mycobacterium smegmatis. Found in smegma, and occasionally in feces and urine, of males and females.

b., Sonne. Shigella sonnei. A cause of bacillary dysentery in man.

b., swine plague. Pasteurella multocida. Causes plague in swine.

b., timothy. Mycobacterium phlei. An organism found in timothy grass.

b., tubercle. Mycobacterium tuberculosis. The cause of tuberculosis in human beings.

b., typhoid. Salmonella typhi. The cause of typhoid fever.

b., Vincent's. Fusobacterium fusiforme. The cause of Vincent's infection also found in the normal mouth.

b., Welch's. Clostridium perfringens. A cause of gas gangrene.

b., Whitmore. Pseudomonas pseudomallei. An infection, similar to glanders, that is pathogenic in man in India and Indochina.

bacitracin (băs-ĭ-trā′sĭn). USP. An antibiotic substance obtained from a strain of Bacillus subtilis. Its antibacterial actions are similar to those of penicillin, including gram-positive cocci and bacilli and some gram-negative organisms. Though available for intramuscular and for topical use, bacitracin is usually employed only topically in the form of ointment because of its toxicity when used parenterally.

back. 1. The dorsum or posterior surface of the body. 2. The posterior region of the body from neck to pelvis.

Misuse of the back is common among those whose duties include care of the sick. Therefore, it is important to learn basic concepts in care of the back.

backache. A common syndrome character-

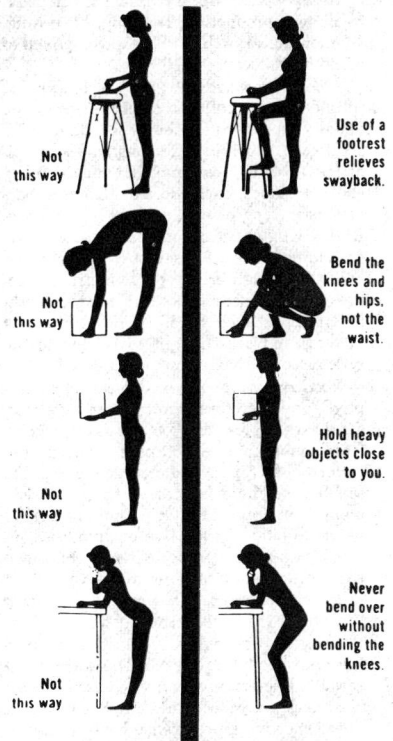

Use of a footrest relieves swayback.

Bend the knees and hips, not the waist.

Hold heavy objects close to you.

Never bend over without bending the knees.

Not this way

**HOW TO STAY ON YOUR FEET
WITHOUT TIRING YOUR BACK**

To prevent strain and pain in everyday activities, it is restful to change from one task to another before fatigue sets in. Check body position frequently, drawing in the abdomen, flattening the back, bending the knees slightly. Adapted from "Your Back and How to Care for It," Copyright 1965, Schering Corporation, Bloomfield, N.J.

ized by pain and tenderness in the muscles or their attachments in the lower lumbar, lumbosacral, or sacroiliac regions. Pain is often referred to leg following distribution of sciatic nerve.

ETIOL: 1. Infection or abnormality in another part of the body, e.g., uterine or prostatic disorders. 2. Disorders of vertebral column, such as intervertebral disk abnormality. 3. Local disturbances such as lumbar or sacral fractures, lumbosacral strain or sprain. 4. Structural inadequacies of supporting ligaments of the spinal col-

umn. 5. Muscle injury, spasm, myositis, or inflammation of fascial attachments. 6. Psychogenic factors.

TREATMENT: Treatment of specific primary cause. General treatment includes measures to allay pain and discomfort such as analgesics, preferably salicylates (codeine in severe cases), heat, and massage. Tender areas or "trigger points" may be anesthetized by local infiltration with 1% procaine or application of ethyl chloride spray. Special measures to relax tense muscles and improve blood flow are helpful. Orthopedic supports and strapping necessary in special cases. Muscle reeducation. Psychogenic treatment when necessary, esp. in excessive muscle tension resulting from emotional maladjustments.

backbone. The vertebral column; spinal column.

backflow. Abnormal backward flow of fluids.

    b., pyelovenous. Drainage from the renal pelvis into the venous system under some conditions of back pressure.

back-pressure arm-lift artificial respiration. Place the victim prone (face down) with elbows bent, one hand on the other, head to one side, cheek resting on folded hands. Kneel on one knee—or both, if you achieve better balance—at the victim's head.

Place your hands on the flat of the victim's back below the armpit with your thumbs barely touching, fingers spread outward and downward. Rock forward slowly, keeping your elbows straight, until your arms are nearly vertical, thus exerting a steady downward pressure. Now rock backward, releasing pressure. Slide your hands outward to grasp the victim's arms just above the elbows. Continue to rock backward. As you rock backward, raise and pull the victim's arms toward you until you feel tension in his shoulders. Then stop. Repeat the full cycle about 12 times a minute.

IMPORTANT: When the victim begins to breathe on his own, synchronize your efforts with his breathing until he breathes strongly. Then stop.

NOTE: The preferred method of artificial respiration is mouth-to-mouth. SEE: *resuscitation, oral.*

bacteremia (băk-tĕr-ē'mĭ-ă) [Gr. *baktērion,* rod, + *haima,* blood]. Bacteria in the blood.

bacteria (băk-tĕr'ĭ-ă) [Gr. *baktērion,* rod]. (sing. *bacterium*) Unicellular plantlike microorganisms, lacking chlorophyll.

There are three principal forms of b. *Spherical or ovoid forms:* When appearing singly, they are called micrococci; when in pairs, diplococci; when in irregular clusters, staphylococci; when in chains, streptococci; when in regular groups of eight, sarcinae. *Rod-shaped forms:* These are known as bacilli. When the rods are somewhat oval, they are called coccobacilli; when attached end to end forming a chain, streptobacilli. *Spiral forms:* When the spiral organisms are rigid they are called spirilla; when flexible, spirochetes; when forming curved rods, vibrios.

Most b. are relatively constant in form in growing cultures. But in old cultures or cultures grown under adverse environmental conditions, aberrant forms such as oversized and Y-shaped appear. These are considered by some to be involution or degenerating forms; by others to be stages in complex life cycles.

CHARACTERISTICS: *Size:* An average rod-shaped bacterium measures about 1 micron in diameter by 4 microns in length. They vary considerably in size from 0.2 x 0.5 micron (influenza bacillus) to 2 x 20 microns (some of the longer spiral cells).

Motility: Some b. are incapable of movement (all cocci) but most bacilli and spiral forms exhibit independent movement. The power of locomotion depends on the possession of one or more flagella, slender whiplike appendages. B. having no flagella are called atrichous; those having a flagellum at one end, monotrichous; those having flagella at each end, amphitrichous; those having a tuft at one end, lophotrichous; those having flagella protruding from all surfaces of the cell, peritrichous.

Capsules: Many b. possess a capsule, a layer of slimy mucoid substance which surrounds each cell. The presence of a capsule is associated with the virulence of certain pathogenic forms.

Spores: Certain species of the rod-shaped b. have the ability to develop an encysted or resting stage known as a spore or endospore. The size, shape and position of the spore within the cell are characteristic of particular species. Spores are terminal if formed at the end of a cell, central if formed at the center, subterminal if formed between the center and end. Spore formation is common among the bacilli but does not usually occur in the cocci or spiral forms. Bacterial spores are remarkably resistant to heat, drying, and the action of disinfectants. Few bacteria pathogenic to man form spores, i.e., anthrax, botulinus, gas gangrene, and tetanus bacilli. Unfavorable environmental conditions favor spore formation.

Reproduction: Binary fission is the usual mode of reproduction. Budding, branching, filamentous growth, and the development of conidia also occur.

Colony formation: A group of b. growing in one place is called a colony. A colony is usually composed of the descendants of a single cell. Colonies differ in shape, size, color, texture, type of margin, and in other characteristics. Each species of b. has a characteristic type of colony formation. Sometimes a single species may produce two types of colonies: one the smooth or S-type, the other the rough or R-type. Sometimes colonies contain clear spots and have a motheaten appearance. Such colonies are called plaques and are thought to be due to the lytic action of bacteriophage.

Food requirements: B. possess no chlorophyll, and therefore cannot carry on photosynthesis. A few can obtain their energy from inorganic substances. These are termed autotrophic and include many of the soil b. The majority derive their nourishment from organic material and are termed heterotrophic. If they live on living organisms, they are called parasites; if their food is from nonliving organic matter, they are called saprophytes. If b. produce disease in their host, they are pathogenic.

Oxygen requirements: Most b. require free or atmospheric oxygen. These are called aerobes. Bacteria living in the absence of atmospheric oxygen are called anaerobes. Those showing a preference for free oxygen and yet capable of living in its absence are called facultative anerobes; those which grow only in the absence of oxygen are called obligate anaerobes.

Temperature requirements: Most b. grow best at moderate temperatures. These are called mesophilic. Cold-loving b. which thrive in temperatures between 0° and 30° C. (32° and 86° F.) are called psychrophilic; those which thrive in high temperatures between 40° and 70° C. (104° and 158° F.) are called thermophilic. The optimum temperature for most saprophytes is around 25° C., for most pathogens, 37° C.

ACTIVITIES: *Enzyme production:* B. produce enzymes which act on complex food molecules breaking them down into simpler materials capable of assimilation. Carbohydrases act on sugars breaking them down to alcohol and carbon dioxide, a process called fermentation. Proteolytic enzymes bring about the decomposition of proteins with the formation of ill-smelling products, a process called putrefaction. Putrefaction is the decomposition of organic substances, esp. nitrogenous substances, in the absence of air and with resulting unpleasant odors. Decay is the gradual decomposition of organic matter exposed to air by b. and fungi. B. are the principal agents of decay and putrefaction.

Toxin production: Many b. produce poisonous substances called toxins. There are two types: exotoxins which diffuse from the bacterial cell into the surrounding medium and endotoxins which are liberated only when the bacterial cell dies and disintegrates. B. well known for their toxin production are the diphtheria, tetanus, and botulinus organisms.

Miscellaneous: Some b. produce pigments; some produce light, appearing luminescent at night. Many chemical substances are produced as a result of bacterial activity, among them acids, gases, alcohol, aldehydes, ammonia, indol. Pathogenic forms produce hemolysins, leukocidins, coagulases, and fibrolysins. Soil b. play an important role in various phases of the nitrogen cycle (nitrification, nitrogen fixation, and denitrification).

METHODS OF STUDYING: Principal methods used in the study of bacteria follow:

(1) Examination of unstained b. in a hanging-drop preparation. Darkfield illumination is necessary to see extremely small forms.

(2) Staining methods include general stains, differential stains, stains for special bacteria, and stains for specific parts. Of the differential stains, Gram's method and staining for acid-fast b. are the most widely used. B. fall into three groups: gram-positive b. (those which retain the stain); gram-negative b. (those which are decolorized by alcohol); acid-fast b. (those which, when stained with certain dyes, retain the stain even when treated with an acid).

(3) In cultural methods, The b. are grown on various culture media. The media may be synthetic or nonsynthetic. In the former, the exact composition of the medium is known; in the latter, the constituents are uncertain. Media, on the basis of consistency, may be liquid (nutrient broth, milk, blood serum); liquefiable solid which consist of liquid media made solid by addition of gelatin or agar-agar; nonliquefiable solid (potato, carrots, starch paste).

(4) Animal inoculation. (5) Immunological methods.

(6) Sterilization methods. Sterilization is the process of rendering any material free of living microorganisms. It may be accomplished by physical or chemical means. The use of chemical agents is usually designated disinfection. Physical agents employed are heat, light, and filtration. Sterilization may be accomplished in a flame, in a hot-air oven (150°-170° C. for one hour), in streaming steam (100° C. for 20 min. or longer), or by steam under pressure (10-15 lbs.) in an autoclave (121° C. for 20 min). Ultraviolet light is destructive to b. as are certain gases such as ethylene oxide, methyl bromide, and hydrogen cyanide. Filtration is accomplished by the use of cotton or by special filters (Berkefeld, Pasteur-Chamberland) of unglazed procelain.

Chemical agents which inhibit bacterial growth are called antiseptics and their action is described as being bacteriostatic; those which kill are called germicides or bactericides. Among disinfectants are strong acids and alkalies, metallic salts (bichloride of mercury), halogens (chlorine, iodine), oxidizing agents (hydrogen peroxide), organic compounds (phenol, formaldehyde, salicylic acid), and other substances such as boric acid. Substances used in the treatment of diseases caused by bacteria are called chemotherapeutic agents. They include the sulfonamide compounds and the antibiotics.

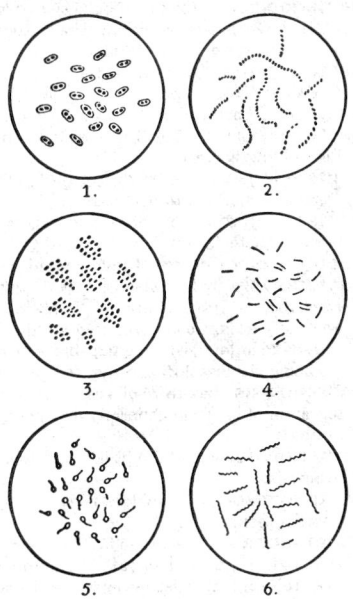

SHAPES OF BACTERIA

1, Diplococci. 2, Streptococci. 3, Staphylococci. 4, Bacilli. 5, Bacilli with spores. 6, Spirilla.

bacterial resistance. Development of resistance to a drug by an organism previously susceptible to it. Such has been manifested by pathogenic organisms (as gonococci, streptococci, staphylococci, and tubercle bacilli) to various chemotherapeutic drugs. It occurs both in vitro and in vivo. It may be due to appearance of resistant mutant strains, development of alternate metabolic pathways, decomposition of the drug, or other factors.

bactericidal (bak″ter-ĭ-sī′dal). Bacteriocidal, q.v.

bactericide (bak-ter′ĭ-sīd) [Gr. *baktērion,* rod, + L. *caedere,* to kill]. That which destroys bacteria.

bacteriemia (bak-ter-ĭ-ē′mĭ-ă). Bacteremia, q.v.

bacterio- (bak-tē′rĭ-ō). Prefix pert. to bacteria.

bacterioagglutinin (băk-tē″rĭ-ō-ă-glū′tĭ-nĭn). An agglutinin formed by the action of bacteria.

bacteriocidal (băk″tĕr-ĭ-ō-sī′dăl). Having the characteristic of destroying bacteria.

bacteriocin. A protein produced by certain gram-negative and gram-positive bacteria which kill sensitive organisms.

bacterioclasis (bak-tē″rĭ-ok′lă-sĭs) [*bacteria,* + Gr. *plasis,* breaking]. The break-up or fragmentation of bacteria.

bacteriogenic (bak-tē″-rē-ō-jen′ik) [Gr. *baktērion,* rod, + *gennan,* to produce]. 1. Caused by bacteria. 2. Producing bacteria.

bacterioid (bak-tēr′ĭ-oyd) [″+ *eidos,* form.]. Resembling bacteria.

bacteriolog′ic, bacteriolog′ical [″+ *logos,* study]. Pert. to bacteriology.

bacteriol′ogist. One whose field of competence is bacteriology.

bacteriol′ogy. Science of microorganisms.

bacteriolysin (bak-tē″rĭ-ol′ĭ-sĭn) [Gr. *baktērion,* rod, + *lysis,* solution]. A substance, especially an antibody produced within the body of an animal, which is capable of bringing about the dissolution or lysis of bacteria.

bacteriolysis (bak-tē″rē-ŏl′ĭ-sĭs). The disintegration of bacteria generally by a specific antibody.

bacteriolytic (bak-te″rĭ-ō-lit′ik). Pert. to bacteriolysis.

bacterioopsonin (bak-tē″rĭ-ō-op-sō′nĭn). Bacteriopsonin, q.v.

bacteriophage (băk-tē′rĭ-ō′fāj″) [Gr. *baktērion,* rod, + *phagein,* to eat]. Term applied to a group of transmissible agents which are capable of inducing lysis or dissolution of certain bacterial cells. They are widely distributed in nature having been isolated from feces, sewage, and polluted surface waters.

They are regarded as bacterial viruses, the phage particle consisting of a head composed of DNA and a tail by which it attaches to host cells SYN: *phage.*

bacteriophagia (băk-tē″rĭ-ō-fā′jĭ-ă). Destruction of bacteria by bacteriophage.

bacterioprecip′itin. Precipitin occurring in bacteria-treated serum.

bacteriopro′tein. One of the proteins in bacteria bodies.

bacteriopsonin (bak-tē″rĭ-op′sō-nĭn). An opsonin acting on bacteria.

bacterioscopy (bak″tē-rĭ-os′ko-pe) [Gr. *baktērion,* rod, + *skopein,* to examine]. Microscopic examination of bacteria.

bacteriostasis (băk-tē″rĭ-ōs′tă-sĭs) [″+ *stasis,* a stopping]. The arrest of bacterial growth.

bacte′riostat. An agent inhibiting bacterial growth.

bacteriostatic (bak-tē-rĭ-ō-stat′ic). Inhibiting or retarding bacterial growth.

bacteriotox′ic. 1. Toxic to bacteria. 2. Due to bacterial toxins.

bacteriotox′in. Toxin specifically destructive to bacteria.

bacteriotropin (bak-tē″rĭ-ot′rō-pĭn). An opsonin or a substance which enhances the ability of phagocytes to engulf bacteria.

bacteristatic. Inhibiting the growth of bacteria. The preferred term for bacteriostatic. SEE: *bacteriocidal.*

Bacterium (băk-tē′rĭ-ŭm). A former genus designation for rod-shaped bacteria without flagella. Term is no longer used in the taxonomic sense because of lack of an identified type species. The species formerly classified as Bacterium are now assigned to other genera such as Aerobacter, Alcaligenes, Mycobacterium, Pasteurella and Salmonella.

    B. aerogenes. Aerobacter aerogenes.

    B. aertrycke. Salmonella typhimurium.

    B. ambiguus. Shigella ambigua.

    B. cholerae suis. Salmonella cholerae-suis.

    B. coli. Escherichia coli.

    B. paratyphi (Type A). Salmonella paratyphi.

    B. paratyphi (Type B). Salmonella schottmuelleri.

    B. tularense. Pasteurella tularensis.

    B. (Eberthella) typhi. Salmonella typhosa.

    B. typhosum. Salmonella typhosa.

bacterium. Singular of bacteria, q.v.

bacteriuria (bak-tē″rĭ-ū′rĭ-ă) [Gr. *baktērion,* rod, + *ouron,* urine]. Presence of bacteria in the urine.

b., significant. Presence of more than 100,000 bacteria per ml. of urine. This is determined by culturing known dilutions of urine and counting the number of colonies.

bacteroid (băk'tĕr-oyd) ["+ *eidos*, appearance]. Resembling a bacterium.

Bacteroides (băk-ter-oyd'ēz). A genus of nonspore-forming anaerobic bacilli normally present in digestive, respiratory, and genital tracts, frequently found in abscesses, and oftentimes in the blood following infections. The species most commonly encountered is B. funduliformis.

baculiform (bak-ū'li-form) [L. *baculum*, rod, + *forma*, shape]. Rod-shaped.

bag, hydrostatic [F. *bague*, sack]. Rubber or silk bag which is inserted into the uterine cavity and then distended with fluid in order to initiate labor and aid in dilatation of cervix.

The types of bags most frequently used are Barnes and Voorhees.

b., Pol'itzer's. Soft rubber bag for middle ear inflation.

b., of waters. The amnion. The membrane enclosing the liquor amnii and the fetus. It refers sometimes to that portion of the membrane protruding into the os uteri. It is the inner embryonic membrane, the chorion being the outer envelope.

bagassosis (bag-ă-sō'sĭs). Pulmonary disorder resulting from inhalation of bagasse dust, the dusty fibrous waste of sugar cane after removal of sugar-containing sap.

baker [AS. *bacan*, cook by dry heat]. Two or more electric lamps mounted in semicircular containers, called electric light bakers. Used for applying heat to various parts of the body.

baker leg. Knock-knee; genu valgum.

Baker's cyst. [William M. Baker, Eng. surgeon, 1839-1896] One containing synovial fluid communicating with synovial fluid of a joint.

baker's dermatitis. Eczematous affection of hand caused by yeast. SYN: *baker's itch.*

baker's itch. Manual eczema from irritation of yeast.

baker's stigmata. Manual callosities from kneading dough.

BAL. Abbr. for British anti-lewisite. Proprietary name for dimercaprol, a compound used as an antidote in poisoning from heavy metals. SEE: *dimercaprol.*

balance (băl'ăns) [L. bilanx]. 1. A device for weighing. 2. A state of equilibrium; condition in which the intake and output of substances such as water and nutrients are approx. equal. SEE: *homeostasis.*

b., acid-base. Condition in which the pH of the blood is maintained at a constant level (7.35-7.45). Accomplished by the action of buffers, respiration, and work of the kidney in formation of urine of varying degrees of acidity.

b., electrolyte. Condition in which electrolytes (Na+, Ca++, Cl-, K+, Mg++, etc.) are maintained in suitable concentration for maintenance of fluid and osmotic environment proper for cellular and metabolic processes.

b., fluid. Condition in which the amount of water in the body and in various compartments (intracellular and extracellular) is maintained within certain optimal limits.

b., heat. Condition in which heat gain and heat loss are approximately equal thus maintaining a temperature of approximately 98.6° F. (37° C.).

b., nitrogen. Condition in which intake of nitrogen in protein foods is equal to nitrogen outgo, principally through loss of nitrogenous substances in the urine and feces.

balanic (ba-lan'ik) [Gr. *balanos*, glans]. Pert. to the glans clitoridis or glans penis.

balanism (bal'ă-nizm) ["+ *ismos*, condition of]. Gynecological treatment by use of pessaries or suppositories.

balanitis (bal-ă-nī'tĭs) ["+ *-itis*, inflammation]. Inflammation of the glans penis and of mucuous membrane beneath it. A purulent discharge is usually present. The prepuce is often affected.

balano- (băl-ă-nō) [Gr.]. Combining form pert. to the glans penis or the glans clitoridis.

balanoblennorrhea (băl"ă-nō-blĕn"ō-rē'-ă) [Gr. *balanos*, glans, + *blennos*, mucus, + *rhoia*, flow]. Gonorrheal inflammation of the external glans penis.

balanoplasty (bal'a-nō-plas"tĭ) ["+ *plassein*, to form]. Plastic surgery of glans penis.

balanoposthitis (bal"ă-nō-pos-thī'tis) ["+ *posthe*, prepuce, + *-itis*, inflammation]. Inflammation of the glans penis and prepuce; balanitis.

balanopreputial (bal"ă-nō-prē-pū'shĭ-al). Pert. to glans penis and prepuce.

balanorrhagia (bal"an-ō-ra'jĭ-ă) [Gr. *balanos*, glans, + *rēgnunai*, flow forth]. Hemorrhage from glans penis.

balanorrhea (băl-ăn-ō-rē'ă) ["+ *rhoia*, flow]. Balanitis with purulent discharge.

balantidial (băl-ăn-tĭd'ĭ-āl). Pert. to Balantidium, a genus of protozoans.

balantidiasis (băl"ăn-tĭ-dī'ă-sĭs). Disease caused by infestation with Balantidium coli.

SYM: Abdominal pain, diarrhea, vomiting, weakness, and loss of weight.

TREATMENT: Tetracyclines or diiodohydroxyquin.

Balantidium (băl-ăn-tĭd'ĭ-ŭm) [Gr. *balantidion,* a bag]. A genus of ciliated protozoans belonging to the order Spirotrichida. It contains a number of species parasitic in the intestines of both vertebrates and invertebrates.

B. coli. A species of Balantidium, parasitic in man. It lives in the large intestine and is the cause of balantidiasis. It is a normal parasite of hogs.

balanus (bal'ă-nus). The glans penis or glans clitoridis.

baldness [ME. *balled,* without hair]. Lack of or partial loss of hair on head. SEE: *alopecia.*

Balkan frame. A framework to fit over a bed so that weights may be suspended from it to produce the desired continuous traction and yet permit freedom of motion while maintaining desired immobilization of the part being treated.

ball. A spherically shaped object.

b. of foot. The widest part of the dorsal surface of the foot.

b., hair. Mass of hair which has accumulated in the intestine or stomach. SEE: *trichobezoar.*

b., thrombus. A round blood clot, esp. one in the heart. SEE: *thrombus.*

b. of thumb. Thenar eminence of the thumb.

ball-and-socket joint. Joint in which one rounded bone head fits into cavity of another bone. SYN: *enarthrosis.*

ballism (bal'izm) [Gr. *ballismos,* jumping about]. 1. Condition characterized by jerking, twisting movements. 2. Paralysis agitans.

ballistics (bă-lĭs'tĭks) [Gr. *ballein,* to throw]. Science of curves of projectiles.

ballistocardiograph (ba-lĭs"tō-kar'dĭ-ō-graf). Mechanism for measuring the impact by the discharge of blood from the heart at each beat and the resulting recoil.

ballistophobia (bă-lĭs"tō-fō'bĭ-ă) [Gr. *ballein,* to throw, + *phobos,* fear]. Morbid fear of missiles.

balloon [It. *ballone,* great ball]. To expand or dilate or puff out. To expand a cavity by filling it with air or water in a bag.

balloon'ing. The distention of a cavity, as vagina, by air or otherwise for examination.

ballottable (bă-lŏt'ă-bl). Capable of showing the ballottement, q.v., phenomenon.

ballottement (bal-ot-mon') [Fr. *balloter,* to toss about]. The rebound of a fetal part when lightly tapped when displaced by the examining finger either through abdominal wall or vagina. Technique may be used for examining the abdomen particularly when ascites is present.

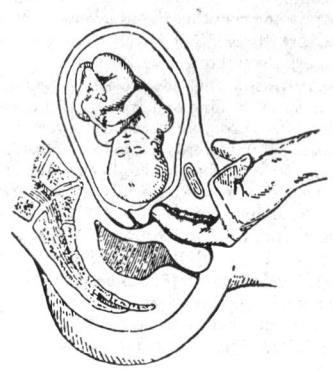

BALLOTTEMENT

ball-valve action. Action of a mass, such as a pedunculated cyst or thrombus, moving to open and close the passageway of a tube or chamber to cause intermittent obstruction. Thus a ball-valve thrombus may form in the heart and cause repeated blockage of an opening connecting two chambers of the heart.

balm [Gr. *balsamon,* balsam]. 1. A balsam. 2. A soothing or healing ointment.

b. of Gilead. 1. Mecca balsam from Commiphora opobalsamum, probably Biblical myrrh. 2. Balsam fir, source of Canadian balsam. 3. Poplar bud resin.

balneology (bal-ne-ol'o-jĭ) [L. *balneum,* bath, + Gr. *logos,* study]. The science of treating diseases by baths.

balneotherapy (bal-nē-ō-ther'ă-pĭ) [" + Gr. *therapeia,* treatment]. The treatment of disease by baths.

balneum (bal'nē-ŭm) [L. a bath]. (pl. *bal'nea*) A bath.

b. are'nae. A sand bath.

b. lu'teum. A mud bath.

balopticon (băl-ŏp'tĭ-kŏn) [Gr. *ballein,* to throw, + *optikos,* pert. to sight]. Apparatus for projecting image of an opaque object on a screen.

balsam (băwl'săm) [Gr. *balsamon,* balsam]. Oleoresin or resin containing aromatic acids or essential oils.

b. of Peru. A dark-brown, viscid, resinous liquid. ACTION AND USES: Locally for healing wounds; same as benzoin. It is used topically on the skin, usually in an alcohol solution or in ointment.

balsamic (băwl-săm′ĭk). 1. Pert. to balsam. 2. Aromatic.

b. tincture. Compound tincture of benzoin.

Balser's fatty necrosis (băl′zĕr). [W. Balser, Ger. physician 19th century] Gangrenous pancreatitis with fatty necrotic areas in interlobular tissue and sometimes in pericardial fat and bone marrow.

banana. The edible fruit of the perennial herb Musa sapientum. Food value of 100 gm. (raw): Cal. 85; protein 1.1 gm.; trace of fat; carbohydrate 22.2 gm.; calcium 8 mg.; 190 I.U. vitamin A; ascorbic acid 10 mg.; iron 0.7 mg.; 75.5 per cent water.

b. oil. Amyl acetate.

Bancroft's filariasis. [Joseph Bancroft, Eng. physician 1836-1894] A filarial infection caused by Wuchereria bancrofti. SEE: *elephantiasis.*

band. A cord or tapelike tissue which connects or holds structures together. SEE: *bundle; ligament; tract.*

bandage [ME. *bande,* a band]. Piece of gauze or other material for application to a limb or other portion of the body. Caution: When bandaging, do not allow skin of one part to be held against the skin of another part, or severe skin infection can result.

Bandages are made up of various types and materials and are used to hold dressing in place, apply pressure to a part, immobilize a part, obliterate cavities, give support to an injured area, aid in checking hemorrhages.

Types are roller; triangular; four-tailed and many-tailed (scultetus); quadrangular; elastic (elastic knit, rubber, synthetic, or combinations of these); adhesive; elastic adhesive; newer cohesive bandages under various proprietary names; impregnated bandages such as plaster of Paris, waterglass (silica), starch; stockinet. SEE: *sling.*

b., abdomen. (Triangular). A single wide cravat or several narrow ones may be used to hold dressing in place, or to exert a moderate pressure. A folded towel or handkerchief should be used to keep it from digging into the flesh.

b., amputation-stump. (Triangular). This is made in a similar way to the open-hand b., the limb being placed on the base of the b.

b., ankle. One loop is brought around the sole of foot and the other around the ankle and tied in front or side.

b., axilla. This is a spica-type turn starting under the affected axilla, crossing over the shoulder of the affected side and making the long loop under the opposite armpit.

b., back. (Triangular). Open b. to the back. This is applied the same as the chest b., the point being placed above the scapula of the injured side.

b., Barton's. For the lower jaw. A double figure-of-eight.

b., Borch's. An eye b. covering both eyes.

b., breast. (Roller). Suspensory bandages and compresses for the breasts.

b., buttocks. Use T or double-T b. or open triangle.

b., capeline. A b. applied to the head or shoulder, or to a stump, like a cap or hood.

b., chalk. A b. made of immovable stiffening with a mixture of chalk and gum.

b., chest. (Roller). Figure-of-eight (spica), many-tailed (scultetus), and triangular b. (open-chest) are used.

b., circular. A b. applied in circular turns about a part.

b., cohesive. Material which has an intense power of sticking to itself, but not to other substances. Used to make encircling applications about fingers, extremities, etc., or to build up pads.

b., cravat. Triangular b. folded to form a band around the injured part. This is done by pulling the point over towards the base, folding the base over the point, and then folding again. This makes a bandage wide enough to cover a large knee. When folded a 2nd time, it is wide enough to make the cravat bandage of the elbow. Folded a 3rd time, it could be used in making a figure-of-eight for the foot, ankle, hand, wrist, head, etc. It is an effective b. in arresting hemorrhages, retaining splints, dressings, and poultices. The center of the cravat should be laid against the affected part, the ends of the cravat carried around the limb and tied over the center of the base. When used to retain splints, it should be tied on the outer side of the limb and against the splint, thus preventing the knot from irritating the skin. When used to retain a dressing in the axilla, the center of the cravat should be placed under the arm and the ends carried upward and crossed over the shoulder and tied in the axillary space of the opposite side, thus forming a figure-of-eight. The cravat can also be used as a sling when only a simple support is needed.

In using cravats for ties or splints, care should be taken so that the knots do not pass over and press unduly on the surface of the limb. Knots should be placed where they are easily found and not subject to pressure; the ends should be neatly tucked in. All knots should be square or reef knots.

GENERAL BANDAGING TECHNIQUES

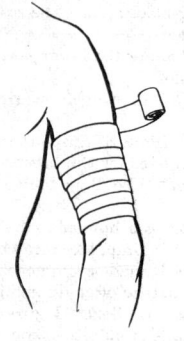 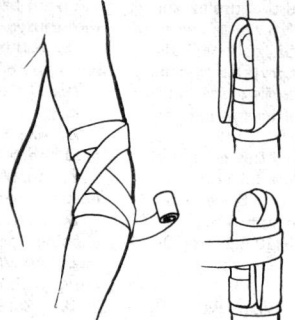 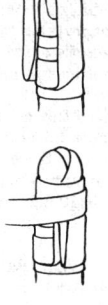 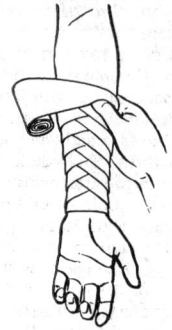

Circular   Figure-of-eight   Recurrent   Reverse spiral

SPECIAL APPLICATIONS

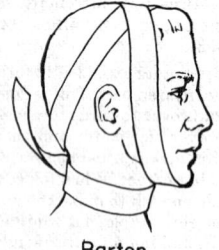

Barton

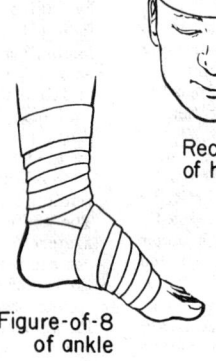

Figure-of-8
of ankle

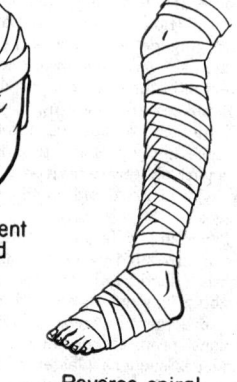

Recurrent
of head

Reverse spiral
of leg

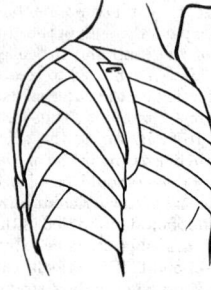

Spica of shoulder

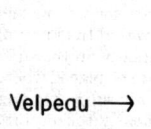

Velpeau ⟶

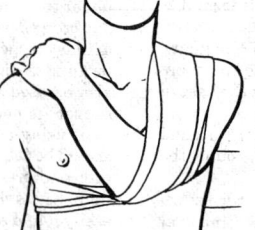 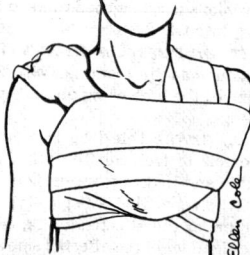

b., cravat elbow. Bend the elbow about 45 degrees. Place center of b. over point of elbow. Bring one end around forearm, and the other end around upper arm. Pull tight and tie.

b., cravat, for clenched fist. (Squire's diagonal figure-of-eight). This is a hand b. to arrest bleeding or to make pressure. The wrist is placed on the center of the cravat, one end is brought around over the fist and back to the starting point, and the same procedure is then repeated with the other end. The two ends are pulled tight, twisted, and carried around the fist again so that pressure is placed on the flexed fingers.

b., cravat, for fracture of clavicle First put a soft pad (2x4 in. or 5.1 x 10.2 cm.) in the forepart of the axilla. A sling made by placing the point of the open bandage on the affected shoulder, the hand and wrist laid on it and directed toward the opposite shoulder, the point brought over and tucked underneath the wrist and hand. The ends are then lifted and the bandage is laid flat on the chest, the covered hand is carried up on the shoulder, the ends are brought together in the back and tied, the tightness being decided by how high the shoulder should be carried. A cravat bandage is then applied horizontally above the broad part of the elbow, and tied over a pad on the opposite side of the chest. Tightening this cravat pushes out the shoulder.

b., cravat, sling. This is used for the support of the hand and in fracture of the upper arm. The wrist is laid upon the center of the cravat bandage, the forearm being held at right angle, and the two ends are carried around the neck and tied. SEE: *binder.*

b., crucial. SEE: *b., T.*

b., demigauntlet. A b. that covers the hand but leaves the fingers uncovered.

b., ear. (Roller). T b. for the ear. A piece is sewn across the right angle of the T b. large enough to suit the occasion.

b., elastic. B.'s which have the property of stretching and hence making compression when correctly applied. Usually made of special weaves or of material incorporating rubber. Applied over swollen extremities or joints, on the chest in empyema, on fractured ribs, or for supporting varicose veins, etc.

b., Esmarch's. 1. Triangular b., q.v. 2. Rubber b. wrapped about an extremity after elevation from its periphery toward the heart to force blood out of the extremity prior to operation or to increase circulating blood. On removal for surgery, a proximal band is left in place to prevent blood returning to the extremity.

b., eye. One to retain dressings. The simple roller b. for one eye or the monocle or crossed b. The binocular or crossed b. for both eyes (2 inches by 6 yards or 5.1 cm. by 5.49 meters).

b., figure-of-eight. A b. in which the turns cross each other like the figure eight. To retain dressings or to exert pressure. For joints or to leave joint uncovered; to fix splints for the foot or hand; for the great toe and for sprains or hemorrhage.

b., finger. (Roller). Oblique fixation at wrist optional at start.

b., foot. (Open triangular b. of the foot). The foot should be placed on the triangle with the base of the b. backward and behind the ankle; the apex is carried upward over the top of the foot. The ends are brought forward, folded once or twice, crossed and carried around the foot and tied on top.

b., forearm. (Triangular). Open sling b. for support of the forearm.

b., four-tailed. A strip of cloth with each end split into two. Tails used to cover prominences as elbow, chin, nose, knee, etc.

b., Fricke's. A special immobilizing b. of the male genitalia.

b., Galen's. A b. with each end split into three pieces; the middle placed on the crown of the head; the two anterior strips are fastened at the back of the neck, the posterior (two) ones on the forehead, and the two middle ones are tied under the chin.

b., Garretson's. A b. for the lower jaw, running above the forehead and back again to cross under the occiput and ending under the chin.

b., Genga's. B., Theden's, q.v.

b., Gibson's. A roller or cravat b. for fracture of the lower jaw.

b., groin. (Special). This b. is most easily applied with the patient standing or lying on a pelvic rest. A spica bandage encircles the trunk and the crossing is either placed anteriorly or laterally. To b. both groins the double spica is used. Such a double b. is used principally in applying a plaster cast.

b., hand. (Roller, 1 inch or 2.5 cm. wide). Demigauntlet b. for the hand to hold a dressing on the back of the hand. For thumb and hand, the ascending spica of the thumb, with spiral of the hand is used. A triangular b. for open b. of the hand. A descending spica is used for the thumb and figure-of-eight b. for amputation stump or clenched fist.

b., head. Single recurrent roller capeline or skull cap. *Scalp:* The double roller recurrent b. for the scalp. *Skull* (Segmental skull cap): Any of the quadrants of the skull may be bandaged. *Head* (open b. of): Use triangular or shawl b. *Tommy head b.:* Place center of narrow cravat under chin, bring ends to top of head and tie single knot. Have patient or an assistant hold ends, and separate knot which forms two loops, place one low on back of head and bring the other forward over forehead, eyes, or chin as necessary; adjust if symmetrical and tie ends on top of head.

b., heel. The triangular b. is used.

b., hip. (Triangular). Open b. of the hip: A cravat b. or other band is tied around the waist, the point of another b. is slipped under that and rolled or pinned directly above the position of the wound. The base is rolled up, the ends carried around the thigh, crossed and tied.

b., Hippocrates'. B., capeline, q.v.

b., Hueter's. A spica b. for the perineum.

b., immovable. A b. for immobilizing a part.

b., impregnated. Wide meshed b. Material impregnated with substances as plaster of Paris which have the power of solidifying after application—used to make molds or immobilize parts of the body.

b., knee. The knee cravat, the triangular, and the figure-of-eight b. are used.

b., knotted. To exert pressure on a compress or pad over a bleeding wound.

b., leg. Fix the initial end by a circular or oblique fixation at the ankle or with a figure-of-eight of the foot and ankle.

b., Maissonneuve's. A plaster of Paris b. made of folded cloth held in place by other bandages.

b., many-tailed. For trunk and limbs. A piece of roller to which slips are stitched in an imbricated fashion. One with ends split. SEE: *b., four-tailed; b., scultetus.*

b., Martin's. Roller b. of rubber used to make pressure on an extremity as for varicose veins, etc., and for exsanguination, as Esmarch's b., q.v.

b., neck. (Roller). *Spica for the neck:* B. 2 1/2 inches by 8 yards (6.4 cm. by 7.32 meters). *B. for use after operations on the thyroid gland:* Roller b. 2 1/2 inches by 9 yards (5.1 cm. by 8.23 meters). *Adhesive plaster b. for use after thyroidectomy:* Used to hold dressing on wound in place, and so far has proved more satisfactory. Apply a small dressing to center of strip, and then apply to back of neck. *Special b.:* A double loop b. of the head and neck is made by using a figure-of-eight turn.

b., oblique. A b. applied obliquely to a limb, without reverses.

b., plaster. A b. stiffened with a paste of plaster of Paris, which sets and becomes very hard.

b., postoperative. (Dressing). This is a simple divergent or convergent spica b.

b., pressure. A b. for applying pressure, usually used to stop hemorrhage.

b., protective. A b. for the purpose of covering a part or of keeping dressings in place.

b., quadrangular. A towel, large handkerchief, etc., folded variously and applied as a b. of head, chest, breast, abdomen, etc.

b., recurrent. A b. over the end of a stump.

b., reversed. One applied to a limb in such a way that the roller is inverted or half twisted at each turn so as to make it fit smoothly.

b., Ribble's. The spica of the instep.

b., Richet's. A b. of plaster of Paris to which a little gelatin has been added.

b., roller. A long strip of soft material, usually from 1/2 to 6 inches (1.3 to 15.2 cm.) wide and 2 to 5 yards (1.83 to 4.57 meters) long, rolled on its short axis. When rolled from both ends to meet at center it is called a double-headed roller.

b., rubber. A roller b. of rubber used for pressure as in swollen parts for immobilization, etc.

b., scultetus. Many-tailed b. A succession of interlocking, overlapping bands originally used to enclose a rigid support against a fractured extremity, but now used without the splint or impregnated as a supporting b. of the abdomen or lower extremity.

b., shoulder. *Open b. of the shoulder:* Spica b. *Shoulder and neck:* Shawl b. of both shoulders and neck.

b., spica. B. in which a number of figure-of-eight turns are applied, each a little higher or lower, overlapping a portion of each preceding turn so as to give an imbricated appearance. For breast, shoulder, limbs, thumb, and great toe. For support, to exert pressure, or to retain dressings. Also for hernia at the groin.

b., spiral reverse. Technique of folding a b. on itself during application to make it fit more uniformly. These reverse folds may be necessary every turn or less depending on contour of part being bandaged.

b., suspensory. A b. for supporting the scrotum.

b., T. One shaped like the letter T. For the perineum and, in certain cases, for the head.

b., tailed. One with ends split.

b., Theden's. A roller b. applied from below upward over a graduated compress to control hemorrhage.

b., toe. Small b. should be used, about 2 inches (5.1 cm.) wide.

b., triangular. A 36- to 42-inch (232 to 271 cm.) square, usually muslin cut diagonally, making two triangular b.'s. Frequently used in first aid. SYN: *Esmarch's b.*

b., Velpeau's. A special immoblizing roller b. which incorporates the shoulder, arm and forearm.

bandage roller. A device for rolling bandages.

band forms. Neutrophil granular leukocytes with band-like or horseshoe-shaped nuclei. Constitute about 4% of total leukocytes.

Bandl's ring (băn'dl). [Ludwig Bandl, Ger. obstetrician, 1842-92] Line of depression corresponding to the junction of the upper and lower uterine segments.

ban'dy leg. Bowleg. SYN: *genu varum.*

bank. A reserve stock of body fluids or parts for therapeutic use, e.g., blood bank, eye bank, kidney bank, tissue bank.

Banti's disease (băn'tē). [Guido Banti, It. physician, 1852-1925] A syndrome combining anemia, splenic enlargement, hemorrhages, and ultimately cirrhosis of liver.

baragnosis (băr-ăg-nō'sĭs) [Gr. *baros,* weight, + *a-,* not, + *gnōsis,* knowledge]. Inability to estimate weights.

barber's itch. 1. An affection of the face due to infection of hair follicles and associated glands by staphylococci. Characterized by formation of papules and pustules. SYN: *folliculitis barbae; sycosis vulgaris.* 2. A dermatomycosis caused by a fungus, Microsporum lanosum or Trichophyton mentagrophytes, T. violaceum or T. purpureum. SYN; *ringworm of the beard; tinea barbae; tinea sycosis.*

barbital (băr'bĭ-tăl). 5,5-diethylbarbituric acid. A crystalline powder, a derivative of barbituric acid. Used as a hypnotic. It is habit-forming.

POISONING: SEE: *barbiturates* in *Table of Poisons and Poisoning* in *Appendix.*

b. sodium. (soluble barbital, medicinal). Has same properties as barbital but because of greater solubility, more rapidly absorbed.

barbiturate (băr-bĭt'ū-rāt, băr-bĭ-tū'rāt). A salt of barbituric acid.

barbituric (băr-bĭ-tū'rĭk). Pert. to, or derived from, barbiturate acid.

barbiturism (băr-bĭt'ū-rĭzm, băr'bĭ-tū-rĭzm). Acute or chronic poisoning from use of any barbituric acid derivatives. Overdoses cause respiratory depression, cyanosis, circulatory collapse, stupor, coma, and possibly death. SYN: *barbituism. SEE: barbiturates* in *Table of Poisons and Poisoning* in *Appendix.*

barbotage (băr-bo-tŏzh') [Fr. *barboter,* to dabble]. Spinal anesthesia by withdrawal of spinal fluid to which the drug is added before reinjection.

baresthesia (băr-ĕs-thē'zĭ-ă) [Gr. *baros,* weight, + *aisthēsis,* perception]. Sense of weight or pressure; pressure sense.

baresthesiometer (băr''-ĕs-thē''zĭ-ŏm'ĕ-ter) ["+ "+ *metron,* measure]. Instrument for determining sensibility to pressure in different parts of body.

bariatrician (băr''ĭ-ă-trĭsh'ăn) ["+ *iatrikos,* treatment]. One who treats obesity.

bariatrics (băr''ĭ-ā'trĭks). Branch of medicine dealing with obesity.

ba'ric [Gr. *baros,* weight]. 1. Pert. to barium. 2. Pert. to weight and specific gravity.

barium (bā'rĭ-ŭm). SYMB: *Ba.* At. wt. 137.34; at. no. 56. A soft metallic element of the alkaline earth group.

b. compounds. Largely used in the paint industries to kill pests; to color fireworks, and in the form of soluble barium sulfate to visualize the hollow viscera in x-ray examinations. Poisoning occasionally comes from using the soluble salts in place of the insoluble sulfate. SEE: *Table of Poisons and Poisoning* in *Appendix.*

b. sulfate. A b. compound used in x-ray examination of the gastrointestinal tract.

bark [Old Norse *börkr*]. The outer cover of the woody parts of a plant. Ex: cascara sagrada, cinchona, wild cherry.

barley. The seed or grain of the cereal grass of the genus Hordeum.

Food value of 100 gm. (pearled, light): Cal. 349; protein 8.2 gm.; calcium 16 mg.; iron 2 mg.; niacin 3.1 mg.

Barlow's disease. [Sir Thomas Barlow, Eng. physician, 1845-1945] A deficiency disease due to lack of vitamin C (ascorbic acid). Occurs in both natural and bottle-fed babies who fail to receive adequate supplementary quantities of vitamin C. Occurs usually between 6 and 12 months of age. SYN: *infantile scurvy; Moeller-Barlow disease.*

TREATMENT: Supplemental vitamin C. Then adequate daily intake of fruit juices (orange, grapefruit, tomato).

Barnes' bag. [Robert Barnes, Eng. obstetrician, 1817-1907] Rubber bag used to induce premature labor by dilating uterine cervix. SYN: *Barnes' dilator.*

Barnes' curve. The segment of a circle whose center is the sacral promontory.

baro- [Gr. *baros*, weight]. Prefix indicating weight, heaviness.

barognosis (băr-ŏg-nō'sĭs) ["+ *gnōsis*, knowledge]. The ability to estimate weights. Opposed to baragnosis.

barograph (băr'ō-grăf) ["+ *graphein*, to write]. Recording barometer.

bar'oscope [Gr. *baros*, weight, + *skopein*, to examine]. Instrument which registers changes in the density of air.

barospirator (băr"ō-spī'rā-tor) ["+ L. *spirāre*, to breathe]. Apparatus producing artificial respiration by means of air pressure variations in a closed chamber.

barotaxis (băr"ō-tăks'ĭs) ["+ *taxis*, turning]. Stimulation of cells by altering the pressure of the atmosphere.

barotitis (băr"ō-tī'tĭs) [Gr. *baros*, weight, + *-itis*, inflammation]. Inflammation of the ear due to sudden changes in barometric pressure such as occur while flying. Closure of the eustachian tube due to upper respiratory infection prevents the middle ear from adjusting to pressure changes encountered during flight.

barotropism (băr-ŏt'rō-pĭzm) ["+ *tropē*, turning]. Barotaxis, q.v.

Barr bodies. [Murray L. Barr, Canadian anatomist, 1908 —] Sex chromatin. The deeply staining chromatin mass at the periphery of the cell nucleus. Found in normal females but not in males.

bar'rel chest. A chest that is rounded as in inspiration and has no apparent movement during respiration. Seen in emphysema.

bar'ren [O.Fr. *barhaine*, unproductive]. Sterile; incapable of producing offspring.

bar'rier [O.Fr. *barriere*]. An obstacle or impediment.

    b., blood-brain. A b. which exists between circulating blood and the brain preventing certain substances such as acid fat-soluble dyes from reaching brain tissue. It consists of either the perivascular glial membrane or the vascular endothelium or both. SYN: *hematoencephalic barrier*.

    b., hematoencephalic. B., blood-brain, q.v.

Bartholin's abscess (băr'tō-lĭn). [Casper Bartholin, Dan. anatomist, 1655-1738] An abscess which develops when Bartholin's glands become occluded in an acute inflammatory process.

Bartholin's cyst. In chronic inflammation of B.'s glands, q.v., cysts are commonly formed. Carcinoma is rare.

Bartholin's ducts. Large ducts of the sublingual salivary gland. They parallel Wharton's duct, q.v., and open with it.

Bartholin's glands. Two small compound, racemose, mucus glands, pea to bean size, situated beneath the vestibule, one on each side of the vaginal opening and at the base of the labia majora.

bartholinitis (băr"tō-lĭn-ī'tis) [Bartholin + Gr. *-itis*, inflammation]. Inflammation of Bartholin's gland.

Bartonella (băr"tō-nĕl'ă). [A. L. Barton, S. Amer. physician] A genus of bacilli of the family Bartonellaceae.

    B. bacilliformis. Motile gram-negative bacillus; the cause of bartonellosis.

bartonellosis (băr"tō-nĕl-ō'sĭs). A disease caused by infection with Bartonella bacilliformis, transmitted by female sandflies (Phlebotomus). The first clinical (noneruptive) stage is called Oroya fever, a severe anemia; the second (eruptive) stage is called verruga peruana, marked by appearance of small tumors on the skin and mucous membranes.

    TREATMENT: Disease responds to several antibiotics, but chloramphenicol has the added advantage of being effective against Salmonella which may be present as a secondary infection.

Baruch's law (băr'ūk). [Simon Baruch, Amer. physician, 1840-1921] Theory that water has a sedative effect when its temperature is the same as that of the skin, and a stimulating effect when it is below or above the skin temperature.

baruria (băr-ū'rĭ-ă) [Gr. *baros*, weight, + *ouron*, urine]. Urine having a high specific gravity.

bary- [Gr. *barys*, heavy]. Prefix indicating heavy, dull, hard.

baryecoia (băr'ĭ-ē-koy'ă) [Gr. *baryēkoia*, deafness]. Hardness of hearing; partial deafness.

baryglossia (băr-ĭ-glŏs'ĭ-ă) [Gr. *barys*, heavy, + *glōssa*, tongue]. Having a slow, thick utterance of speech.

barylalia (băr-ĭ-lā'lĭ-ă) ["+ *lalia*, speech]. Indistinct, husky speech.

baryodmia (băr-ĭ-ŏd'mĭ-ă) ["+ *odmē*, stench]. Disagreeable, heavy odor.

baryodynia (băr'ĭ-ō-dĭn'ĭ-ă) [Gr. *barys*, heavy, + *odynē*, pain]. Severe pain.

baryphonia (băr-ĭ-fō'nĭ-ă) ["+ *phōnē*, voice]. Difficulty in speaking words.

barythymia (băr-ĭ-thī'mĭ-ă) ["+ *thymos*, mind]. Sullen, gloomy, or melancholy state of mind.

basad (bā′săd) [Gr. *basis,* base, + L. *ad,* toward]. Denoting the direction toward the base of anything.

ba′sal. 1. Pert. to the base of anything; the base. 2. Of primary importance.

b. ganglia. Four masses of gray matter located deep in the cerebral hemispheres, viz., caudate, lentiform, and amygdaloid nuclei, and the claustrum. The caudate and lentiform nuclei and the fibers of the internal capsule which separate them constitute the corpus striatum.

b. lamina. SYN: *basement lamina,* q.v.; *basement membrane.*

b. metabolic rate. The metabolic rate as measured under so-called basal conditions: 12 hours after eating, after a restful sleep, no exercise or activity preceding test, elimination of emotional excitement, and in a comfortable temperature (between 62° and 87° F.).

It is usually expressed in terms of Cal. (i.e. kilocalories) per square meter of body surface per hour. ABBR.: BMR.

b. metabolism. The amount of energy needed for maintenance of life when the subject is at digestive, physical, and emotional rest.

b. temperature chart. A daily chart of temperature obtained upon awakening. Some women are able after several months to predict the time of ovulation by carefully analyzing the character and rhythm of the temperature chart. Reliability of this method to control conception is questionable, particularly in individuals with irregular menstrual cycles.

bascula′tion [Fr. *basculer,* to swing]. 1. Replacement of a retroverted uterus by swinging it into place. 2. Systolic recoil of the heart.

base [Gr. *basis,* base]. 1. The lower part of anything. 2. The principal substance in a mixture. 3. In chemistry, a compound containing a metal or the ammonium radical combined with the hydroxyl (OH) radical. In general, any substance which will neutralize an acid. Bases react with acids to form salts, turn red litmus blue, and have a bitter taste. Strong bases feel slippery and are corrosive to human tissues. Ex: sodium hydroxide (NaOH) (lye or caustic soda); potassium hydroxide (KOH) (caustic potash).

This includes compounds of metallic elements as sodium hydroxide, and various complex nonmetallic substances as ammonia, the amines, and the alkaloids. Whether an unknown chemical compound is a base or acid may be determined by the color produced when it is added to a solution containing an indicator, q.v. SYN: *alkali.* SEE: *pH.*

b. of heart. Heart surface back and upward, containing pulmonary vein and venae cavae openings.

baseball finger. Condition resulting from violent backward dislocation of the terminal phalanx onto the dorsum of the middle phalanx, as when a finger is struck on its tip when extended. SYN: *hammer finger; mallet finger.*

Basedow's disease (bāz′ē-dō). [Karl A. von Basedow, Ger. physician, 1799-1854] Graves' disease; exophthalmic goiter.

basement lam′ina [Gr. *basis,* base, + L. *lamina,* thin plate]. Preferred term for a thin layer of delicate noncellular material of a fine filamentous texture underlying the epithelium. Its principal component is collagen.

basement membrane. Basement lamina, q.v.

base′plate. Plastic material for making dental trial plates.

basi-, basio- [Gr. *basis,* base]. Prefixes denoting base or basion.

ba′sial [L. *basialis*]. Pert. to the basion.

basiarachnoiditis (bā″sĭ-ă-răk″noy-dī′tĭs) [Gr. *basis,* base, + *arachnē,* spider, + *eidos,* form, + *-itis,* inflammation]. Inflammation of the arachnoid membrane at base of brain. SYN: *basiarachnitis.*

basibregmat′ic axis ["+ *bregmata,* front of heads, + *axis,* pivot]. Vertical line from the basion to junction of coronal and sagittal sutures.

ba′sic. 1. Possessing properties opposite to those of an acid. 2. Fundamental.

b. salt. A compound formed when only part of the hydroxide radicals of a base are replaced by the acid radical of an acid.

basicra′nial axis [Gr. *basis,* base, + *kranion,* skull, + *axis,* pivot]. Straight line from the basion to point of angle of mandible.

basifa′cial axis ["+ L. *facies,* face, + Gr. *axis,* pivot]. Straight line from the point of angle of mandible to the subnasal point.

basihyal (bā″sĭ-hī′ăl) ["+ *oeidēs,* hyoid]. The body of the hyoid bone.

bas′ilar [L. *basilaris*]. Basal; pert. to a base.

basilat′eral [Gr. *basis,* base, + L. *lateralis,* pert. to the side]. Both lateral and basilar.

basil′ic [L. *basilicus*]. Prominent, important.

b. vein. Large vein on inner side of biceps. Usually chosen for intravenous injection or withdrawal of blood.

basiloma (băs-ĭ-lō′mă) [Gr. *basis,* base, + *-ōma,* tumor]. Basal cell carcinoma.

basilysis (bă-sĭl'ĭ-sĭs) ["+ *lysis,* loosening]. Crushing the fetal head in labor to aid delivery.

basilyst tractor (băs'ĭ-lĭst). Instrument devised by Sir A. R. Simpson consisting of three blades for perforating the fetal head and obtaining a substantial grasp to facilitate delivery of the child.

basio- [Gr. *basis,* base]. Prefix denoting basion.

basioccipital bone (bā"sĭ-ŏk-sĭp'ĭ-tăl) ["+ L. *occiput,* head]. Basilar process of occipital bone.

ba'sion. Point at middle border of the foramen magnum.

basiotribe (bā'sĭ-ō-trĭb) [Gr. *basis,* base, + *tribein,* to crush]. Instrument for crushing the fetal head.

basiotripsy (bā"sĭ-ō-trĭp'sĭ). Basilysis, q.v.

basiphobia (bā"sĭ-fō'bĭ-ă) [Gr. *basis,* base, + *phobos,* fear]. Fear of walking.

basirrhinal fissure (bā-sĭ-rī'năl) ["+ *rhis,* nose]. 1. Pert. to base of brain and nose. 2. A cerebral fissure at base of olfactory lobe.

basis (bā'sĭs) [L., Gr]. (pl. *bases*). Base.

   b. cranii. Base of skull.

basisphenoid (bā-sĭ-sfē'noyd) [Gr. *basis,* base, + *sphēn,* wedge, + *eidos,* form]. Lower portion of sphenoid bone.

basisyl'vian fissure. Transverse basilar portion or stem of sylvian fissure.

basket [ME.]. A netlike terminal arborization of an axon (or its collateral) of a basket cell which forms a network about the cell body of a Purkinje cell.

   b. cell. Deep stellate cells (neurons) of the molecular layer of the cerebellum whose axons or collaterals terminate in baskets.

basocyte (ba'sō-sīt) [Gr. *basis,* base, + *kytos,* cell]. A basophil cell or leukocyte.

basocytopenia (bā"so-sī"tō-pē'nĭ-ă) ["+ "+ *penia,* poverty]. Reduced number of basophil leukocytes in the blood.

basocytosis (bā"sō-sī-tō'sĭs) ["+ "+ *-ōsis,* condition]. Excess of basophilic leukocytes of the blood.

ba'sograph [Gr. *basis,* base, + *graphein,* to write]. Device for registering abnormalties of gait.

basophil(e (bā'sō-fĭl, -fīl) ["+ *philein,* to love]. In histology, (1) cells or parts of cells which are readily stained with basic dyes like methylene blue; (2) a type of white blood cell (leukocyte) characterized by possession of coarse granules which stain intensely with basic dyes; and (3) a type of cell found in the anterior lobe of the hypophysis.

   Constituting 0.5-1% of leukocytes, basophils are thought to bring anticoagulant substances to inflamed tissues. Increased numbers are found during the healing phase of inflammation and in chronic inflammation.

basophilia (bā-sō-fĭl'ĭ-ă). 1. A pathological condition of the blood in which the erythrocytes develop basophil granules. 2. A condition in which many mast cells are present.

basophilic (bā-sō-fĭl'ĭk). Pert. to the staining characteristics of various cells.

basophilism (bā-sŏf'ĭ-lĭzm). Condition characterized by excessive numbers of basophils.

   b., pituitary. A clinical syndrome (Cushing's syndrome) characterized by basophilic invasion or adenoma of the pituitary gland. SEE: *Cushing's syndrome.*

basophobia (bās-ō-fō'bĭ-ă) [Gr. *basis,* base, + *phobos,* fear]. 1. Abnormal fear of walking. 2. Emotional inability to stand or walk in the absence of muscle pathology.

bass deafness. Deafness to bass notes, the higher ones being heard.

Bassini's operation (bă-sē'nē). [Edoardo Bassini, It. surgeon, 1844-1924] Surgery for inguinal hernia.

bas'tard [O.Fr. *batard,* bastard]. 1. One born out of wedlock; illegitimate. 2. Not genuine; irregular.

bath [AS. *baeth*]. The medium and method of cleansing the body or any part of it or to treat it therapeutically as with air, light, steam, vapor, water.

   The temperature of the cleansing bath for a bed patient may be from 110°-115° F. (43.3°-46.1° C.) with a room temperature of 75°-80° F. (23.9°-26.7° C.).

   THERAPEUTIC EFFECT: Warm and hot baths and applications act to soothe both the psyche and the soma. Thus they calm and relax a nervous, agitated patient. Gradually elevated hot tub and vapor baths relax all the muscles of the body.

   Hot baths relax tissues, including the capillaries of the skin, drawing blood from the deeper tissues, and also help to relieve pain and stimulate nerves. Cold baths and applications abstract heat and stimulate reaction, esp. if followed by brisk rubbing of the skin, and contract the small blood vessels when applied locally.

   b., acid. Five oz. (150 ml.) hydrochloric acid or one gal. (3.8 liters) vinegar to 30 gal. (114 liters) water.

   b., air. Therapeutic use of air, warmed or vaporized, on the nude body.

   b., alcohol. Application of alcohol to the patient as a stimulant and defervescent, in dilute form.

   b., alkaline. Eight oz. (227 gm.) of sodium bicarbonate or washing soda to 30 gal.

Bath Temperatures

Room Temperature	Water Temperature Should Be
Below 76° F. (24.4°C.)	94–96° F. (34.4–35.6° C.)
Above 76° F. (24.4°C.)	92–94° F. (33.3–34.4° C.)
On hot summer days	90° F. (32.2° C.)

Rectal Temperature	Bath Water Should Be
103° F. (39.4° C.)	90° F. (32.2° C.)
104° F. (40° C.)	86° F. (30° C.)
104.5° F. (40.3° C.)	82° F. (27.8° C.)
105° F. (40.6° C.)	76° F. (24.4° C.)
105.5° F. (40.8° C.)	70–60° F. (21.1–15.6° C.)

Baths May Be Indicated As:

Cold	45– 65° F. (7.2–18.3° C.)
Cool	65– 75° F. (18.3–23.9° C.)
Tepid	75– 85° F. (23.9–29.1° C.)
Warm	85– 95° F. (29.1–35° C.)
Hot	95–105° F. (35–40.6° C.)
Very Hot	105–110° F. (40.6–43.3° C.)

(114 liters) of water.

b., alum. Use of alum in washing solution as an astringent.

b., antipyretic. A b. in cool water (65° to 75° F. or 18.3° to 23.9° C.).

b., aromatic. B. to which some volatile oil or perfume, or some herb, is added.

b., astringent. Bathing in liquid containing an astringent.

b., bed. For bedridden patient.

NP: Prevent an irrational or comatose patient from falling out of bed. Also replace siderails if they were in place prior to beginning the bath.

Check temperature of room; clear bedside table for bath articles. Offer bedpan or urinal. Remove top covers of bed, placing patient under cotton bath blanket; remove pillows if possible. Bring clean linens and bath basin of hot water (150° F. or 65.6° C.) to bedside.

Place towel under area to be bathed; wash carefully, rinse, dry and cover immediately with bath blanket. The usual sequence is as follows: face, neck and ears, chest, abdomen, arms and hands, back, legs and feet, and genitalia and perineum. Change bath water as often as necessary. Finish by rubbing back and buttocks with rubbing lotion. It is particularly important to use a lotion which does not dry the skin. In order to reduce friction between skin and bedclothes, dust the skin with a bland powder at the completion of the bath.

Place clean gown on patient, comb hair, and clean finger and toe nails. Remake bed with clean linen. Remove all bath articles, straighten and damp-dust room. Place call bell, drinking water, etc. within easy reach of patient. Clean up all used articles and restore to proper place. SEE: *bed.*

b., bland. A b. containing substances such as starch, bran, or oatmeal for the relief of skin irritation; an emollient bath.

b., blanket. B. in which wet pack and blankets are used.

b., borax. Glycerin and borax solution for bathing.

b., box. B. in which patient is completely enclosed in box except for his head.

b., bran. Place bran (2-3 lb. or 901 gm.-1.4 kg.) in a muslin bag and soak in hot water 15 min. Then add bag and hot water to bath water (30 gal., 95° F. or 114 liters, 35° C.), using bag as a washing-sponge.

b., brine. B., saline, q.v.

b., bubble. A b. in which the water contains many small bubbles produced mechanically as by an air pump or chemically by bubble-bath preparations.

b., cabinet. Exposure of the skin of the body except the head, to heat from electric lamps, live steam, steam radiators, or electric heaters.

b., carbon dioxide. An effervescent saline bath consisting of water, salts, and CO_2. The natural CO_2 baths are known as Nauheim baths, and approach closely CO_2 baths in their therapeutic effects.

b., cold. B. in water at a temperature below 65° F. (18.3° C.).

b., colloid. B., emollient, q.v.

b., continuous. B. that is administered for hours, days, weeks, or months. It is a continuous, flowing bath if the prescribed temperature is maintained by keeping a stream of water flowing through the tub.

b., contrasted. B. used for hands or feet. Two large basins or pails of sufficient depth, filled with water, one as hot as the patient can stand, the other as cold as he can stand. Change or add hot and cold water frequently to keep temperatures same as in beginning. Put part to be treated in hot water for one minute, then into cold for one-half minute, then again into hot water. Repeat for prescribed length of time, ending with cold water.

b., drip sheet. Modified sheet b. SEE: *b., sheet.*

b., earth. Bathing in warmed earth or sand.

b., emollient. Used for irritation and inflammation of skin, and after erysipelas. SEE: *b., glycerin; b., oatmeal; b., powdered borax; b., starch.*

b., foam. Tub b. to which has been added an extract of a saponin containing vegetable fiber, and through this mixture, oxygen, O_2, or carbon dioxide, CO_2, is driven to form foam.

b., foot. Immersion of feet and legs to a depth of 4 inches (10 cm.) above ankles in water at 98° F. (36.7° C.).

b., full. The whole body except the head is immersed in water.

b., glycerin. 10 oz. (300 ml.) of glycerin added to 30 gal. (114 liters) of water.

b., half. Tub bath with about 18 inches (46 cm.) of water; the temperature depends on the case and the desired action.

b., herb. 1-2 lb. (454-901 gm.) of herbs, such as chamomile, wild thyme, or spearmint, are tied in bag, boiled with 1 gal. (3.8 liters) of water and the decoction added to the full b.

b., hip. B., sitz, q.v.

b., hot. Tub b. with the water covering the body to a little above the nipples and temperature gradually raised from 98° F.

(36.7° C.) to desired degree, usually to 108° F. (42.2° C.).

b., hot air. Exposure of entire body except head to hot air contained in a b. cabinet.

b., hyperthermal. B. in which the body except head is immersed in water from 105°-120° F. (40.6°-48.9° C.) for one to two minutes.

b., immersion. Tub b.

b., kinetotherapeutic. B. given for underwater exercises of weak or partially paralyzed muscles.

b., lukewarm. B. in which patient's body except head is immersed in water from 94°-96° F. (34.4°-35.6° C.) for 15-60 minutes.

b., medicated. B. to which bran, oatmeal, starch, sodium bicarbonate, epsom salts, pine products, tar, sulfur, postassium permanganate, or salt is added.

b., milk. B. taken in milk for emollient or cosmetic purposes.

b., mud. Old form of applying moist heat depending on availability of certain soils heated by thermal springs or by artificial means.

b., mustard. For stimulative hot foot b., a mixture of one tablespoon of dry mustard in a quart of hot water added to a pail or large basin filled with water of 100°-104°F. (37.8°-40° C.). Used in rheumatic conditions and in sprains or other muscular foot pains caused by trauma.

b., Nauheim. A b. in which the human body is immersed in warm water through which carbon dioxide is bubbled.

b., neutral. B. in which no circulatory or thermic reaction occurs, temperature 92°-97° F. (33.3°-36.1° C.).

b., neutral sitz. Same as hot sitz b. except temperature between 92°-97° F. (33.3°-36.1° C.), for foot bath, 104°-110° F. (37.8°-40° C.), duration 15-60 minutes.

b., oatmeal. Two to three lb. (901 gm.-1.4 kg.) oatmeal to 30 gal. (114 liters) water.

b., oxygen. Given by introducing O_2 into the b. through a special device which is connected to an oxygen tank or by generating the O_2 by chemicals.

b., paraffin. Limb is immersed in warm paraffin (104°-150° F. or 37.8°-65.6° C.), quickly withdrawn, immersed again, withdrawn repeatedly until it is encased. For larger joints, may be applied with paint brush.

b., powdered borax. One-half lb. (227 gm.) to 30 gal. (114 liters) water; five oz. (150 ml.) glycerin may be added.

b., reducing. B. given to reduce patient's temperature.

b., Russian. Warm vapor b. followed by rubbing and cold plunge.

b., saline. Given in artificial sea water made by dissolving 8 lb. (3.6 kg.) of sea salt, or a mixture of 7 lb. (3.2 kg.) of sodium chloride and one-half lb. (227 gm.) of magnesium sulfate in 30 gal. (114 liters) of water.

b., sauna. A type of steam b. where the steam is produced by pouring water on heated rocks.

b., seawater or salt. B., saline, q.v.

b., sedative. A prolonged warm b. Continuous flow of water may be used. Use air cushion and back rest.

b., sheet. Given by wrapping the patient in a sheet previously dipped in water 80°-90° F. (26.7°-32.2° C.), and rubbing the whole body with vigorous strokes on the sheet, until all parts of the sheet feel warm.

b., shower. Water sprayed down upon the body from an overhead source.

b., sitz. Immersion of thighs, buttocks, and abdomen below the umbilicus in water. In a hot sitz b. the water is first 92° F. (33.3° C.) and elevated to 106° F. (41.1° C.), duration 3-10 minutes.

b., sponge. B. in which patient's body is washed by using a wash cloth and without immersing the body in a tub.

b., starch. Mix one pound (454 gm.) of starch in cold water; add boiling water to make a solution of gluelike consistency. Add this to 30 gal. (114 liters) of water.

b., steam. Given in a chamber into which steam under low pressure is allowed to escape. Best form of application is that in which subject sits in cabinet or lies in box with head outside. Caution: Temperature must be controlled carefully to avoid burning the patient.

b., stimulating. One which increases cutaneous effect; used for tonic purposes. SEE: *b., cold; b., mustard; b., saline.*

b., sulfur. A b. made by adding potassium sulfide (3 oz. or 85 gm.) or zinc sulfate (8 tsp. or 1.3 oz.), or sulfurated lime sol. N.F. (6 oz. or 180 ml.) to 30 gal. (114 liters) water. Bath should be limited to 20 min.

b., sweat. B. given to induce perspiration.

b., towel. Given by applying towels dipped in water 60°-70° F. (15.6°-21.1° C.) to arms, legs, anterior and posterior surfaces of trunk successively, removing towel, drying part.

b., vapor. Exposure of skin of body except head to vapor. Sometimes the vapor is impregnated with substances thought to possess therapeutic value, as sulfur, mercury, or camphor.

b., whirlpool. Continuous localized jets of water for the arm and leg. Water 105°-120°

F. (40.6°-48.9° C.) from a thermostatic mixer is given a swirling motion in special reservoir as it mixes with air forced through an aerator.

bath'mism [Gr. *bathmos*, threshold]. Force regulating nutrition and growth.

bathophobia [Gr. *bathos*, deep, + *phobos*, fear]. Abnormal fear of depths or of looking down from a high place.

bathyanesthesia (băth-ē-ăn″ĕs-thē′zĭ-ă) ["+ *an-*, not, + *aisthēsis*, perception]. Loss of deep sensibility.

bathycardia (băth″ĭ-kăr′dĭ-ă) ["+ *kardia*, heart]. Abnormally low position of the heart in the thorax.

bathyesthesia (băth″ĭ-ĕs-thē′zĭ-ă) ["+ *aisthēsis*, sensation]. A consciousness of muscles, joints, and organs under skin.

bathygastry (bath-ĭ-gas′trĭ) [Gr. *bathys*, deep, + *gastēr*, stomach]. Abnormally low stomach. SYN: *gastroptosis.*

bathyhyperesthesia (băth-ĭ-hī″pĕr-ĕs-thē′-zĭ-ă) ["+ *hyper*, above, + *aisthēsis*, sensation]. Excessive sensitiveness of muscular tissues and deep structures.

bathyhypesthesia (băth″ĭ-hĭp″ĕs-thē′zĭ-ă) ["+ *hypo*, under, + "]. Impairment of sensitiveness in muscular tissues and other deep structures of body.

battarism (băt′ă-rĭzm). Stuttering, battarismus.

battered child syndrome. Physical violence inflicted upon a child by adults, usually one or both of the parents or guardians, often under circumstances which make it appear that the injury was accidental.

bat'tery [Fr. *battre*, to beat]. Device for generating electrical current by chemical action.

Baudelocque's diameter (bō-dlok′). [Jean Louis Baudelocque, Sr., Fr. obstetrician, 1746-1810] Distance between the depression just beneath the spine of the last lumbar vertebra and the anterior and upper margin of the symphysis pubis. The exterior conjugate diameter of the pelvis.

Baudelocque's method. Manipulation to convert a face presentation into one of the vertex.

Baumé scales (bō-mā′). [Antoine Baumé, Fr. chemist, 1728-1805] Hydrometer scales for determination of the specific gravity of liquids, one being used for liquids heavier and one for liquids lighter than water.

bay'onet leg. Backward dislocation at knee joint of tibia and fibula.

Bazin's disease (bă-zan′). [Antoine P. E. Bazin, Fr. dermatologist, 1807-1878] Erythema induratum; tuberculosis of the skin.

BCG. Abbr. for *bacillus Calmette-Guérin.*

BCG vaccine. Tuberculosis vaccine. A freeze-dried preparation of an attenuated strain of Mycobacterium tuberculosis (bacillus Calmette-Guérin). Proposed for use in adults and children for immunization against tuberculosis. Also called bacillus Calmette-Guérin vaccine.

b.d. Abbr. for L. *bis die*, twice a day.

bdellometer (del-om'ĕ-ter) [Gr. *bdella*, leech, + *metron*, measure]. Artificial substitute for a leech.

Be. Chem. symb. for beryllium.

beaded (bēd'ĕd) [AS. *bed*, prayer]. Referring to disjointed colonies along the inoculation line in a streak or stab.

beads, rachitic (bēdz, ră-kĭ'tĭk) ["+ Gr. *rhakhitis*, disease of the spine]. Visible swelling where the ribs join their cartilages, seen in rickets. SYN: *rachitic rosary.*

beaker (bē'ker). Glass vessel with wide mouth for mixing or holding liquids.

beans [AS.]. The seeds, and sometimes immature pods containing seeds, usually of the genus Phaseolus or Vicia.

Fresh green snap beans: Food value of 100 gm. (one cup; cooked, boiled for short time in small amt. of water and drained): Cal. 25; protein 1.6 gm.; fat 0.2 gm.; carbohydrate 5.4 gm.; calcium 50 mg.; phosphorous 37 mg.; iron 0.6 mg.; sodium 4 mg.; potassium 151 mg.; vitamin A, 540 I. U.; thiamine 0.07 mg.; riboflavin 0.09 mg.; niacin 0.5 mg.; ascorbic acid 12 mg.

Fresh white beans (common varieties as navy beans): Food value of 100 gm. (one cup; cooked): Cal. 118; protein 7.8 gm.; carbohydrate 21.2 gm.; calcium 50 mg.; phosphorus 148 mg.; iron 2.7 mg.; sodium 7 mg. (if cooked in unsalted water); potassium 416 mg.; thiamine 0.14 mg.; riboflavin 0.07 mg.; niacin 0.7 mg.

bearing down. The expulsive effort of a parturient woman, in second stage of labor.

beat [AS. *bēatan*, to strike]. A pulsation or throb resulting from contraction of the heart, or the passage of blood through a vessel.

   b., apex. Impulse of the heart beat felt by the hand when held over the fifth intercostal space in left midclavicular line.

   b., ectopic. One beginning at a place other than sinoatrial node.

   b., forced. Extrasystole brought on by artificial heart stimulation.

   b., premature. An extrasystole.

Bechterew's reflex (bĕk'tĕr-ĕv). [Vladimir Mikhailovich von Bechterew, Russ. neurologist, 1857-1927] 1. Contraction of facial muscles due to irritation of nasal mucosa. 2. Dilatation of pupil on exposure to light. 3. Plantar flexion of foot. 4. Flexion of foot in dorsal direction and flexive movement of knee and hip following passive flexion of toes and plantar extension of foot. 5. Contraction of lower abdominal muscles when skin of inner surface of thigh is stroked.

bed [AS. *bedd*, bed]. A piece of furniture for resting of body.

HOW TO MAKE AN OCCUPIED BED: Caution: Special drainage and irrigation tubes must be handled carefully in order not to disturb their function or to cause the patient great pain by tugging on them.

Assemble all necessary articles; place clean linens on back of chair at bedside. Tell the patient what you are going to do; check temperature of room and adjust windows if necessary. Loosen all bedclothes; remove and fold spread and all but one blanket. Hang on back of chair. Remove top sheet from under remaining blanket. Place in laundry bag or fold and place on seat of chair to form receiver for dirty linens. Turn patient away from you if possible, and insure safety by placing chair or bedrail for security. Fold draw sheet to patient's back; straighten rubber draw sheet and fold likewise. Bottom sheet is also folded in neat, flat folds to center of bed.

Place clean bottom sheet on exposed half of mattress, folding neatly to center creases. Tuck top of sheet under head of mattress, miter corner and tuck under mattress to foot of bed. Sheet must cover mattress completely. Pull rubber draw sheet out, straighten and place clean draw sheet with center crease to patient's back. Fold top of clean draw sheet over top edge of rubber sheet and tuck both securely under mattress. Assist patient to roll toward you under blanket to clean side of bed. Again insure safety.

Proceed to other side of bed. Remove soiled draw sheet and bottom sheet and place in first piece of soiled linen on chair. Pull through clean bottom sheet, rubber sheet, and draw sheet. Proceed as for first side, tightening draw sheet to avoid any wrinkles. Ask patient to raise buttocks, if possible. Remove pillows and pillow cases; replace cases with clean ones. Pull mattress to head of bed; replace pillows and adjust to patient's comfort. Place clean top sheet, wide hem to top, over blanket; draw blanket out from under sheet and replace with top of blanket well over patient's shoulders. Put on spread and turn top hem of sheet over spread at least 8 inches. Remake foot of bed, allowing sufficient room for feet and toes of patient to move freely.

Remove soiled linens. Avoid shaking any bedclothes in order to prevent spreading dust which is a possible source of infection. Place patient's signal or call device in proper and convenient place, straighten room and evaluate comfort and appearance carefully.

b., air. B. inflatable with air. Also, a special b. which literally floats the patient on a cushion of air which comes from holes in a special mattress. Used to prevent bed sores and in burn cases.

b., air-fluidized. SEE: *air-fluidized b.*

b., anesthetic. B., recovery, q.v.

b. blocking. Placing bedblocks under bed to raise it at head or foot.

Foot of b. raised: In shock; bleeding from lower limbs; edema of lower limbs, vulva, or scrotum; some cases of hemorrhoids; to retain enema; when weight is used on lower limbs; in reduction of inguinal hernia.

Head of b. raised: To drain abdomen or pelvis; to aid respiration; in treatment for bleeding from head, neck, or upper chest.

b., capillary. A network of capillaries.

b., circular. Special b. which allows a patient to be turned end-over-end while held between two frames. This permits turning the patient without distrubing him, by turning the two frames inside a circular apparatus which holds the ends of the frames.

b., closed. B. prepared to receive a new patient; an unoccupied bed.

b., ether. B., recovery, q.v.

b., float. A b. in which the patient is supported either on a water mattress or on minute ceramic beads with air flowing through them. This type of b. is particularly useful in treating decubitus ulcers.

b., flotation. B. in which the patient reclines in a hollow, flexible, mattress-shaped device which is filled with water. This enables equal distribution of pressure on the body. Used in treating and preventing decubiti.

b., fracture. B. for patients who have fractures.

b., Gatch. An adjustable b. which provides elevation of the back and knees.

b., hydrostatic. B., water, q.v.

b., metabolic. B. arranged to facilitate collecting the feces and urine.

b., nail. The skin at tip of digit which lies beneath a nail.

b., open. B. which is assigned to a patient who is not occupying it at the time it is made.

b., recovery. B. prepared to receive patient immediately following an operative procedure requiring anesthesia. SYN: *anesthetic b.; ether b.*

b., surgical. B. equipped with a mechanism by which the head or the foot of the b. can be raised or lowered independently of each other.

b., unoccupied. B., closed, q.v.

b., water. A rubber mattress filled with water. Used for prevention of bedsores.

bedbug. An insect, Cimex lectularius, the saliva of which contains an irritating substance causing a purpuric reaction, or an urticarial wheal.

TREATMENT: Antipruritic lotions containing phenol, camphor, and menthol.

CONTROL: Largely a matter of cleanliness. In heavy infestations use appropriate insecticide, spraying furniture, mattresses, floors, baseboards, walls.

bedfast. Unable or unwilling to leave the bed; bedridden.

Bed'nar's aph'thae. [Alois Bednar, physician in Vienna, 1816-1888] Two symmetrically placed, infected, traumatic ulcers appearing on hard palate of infants.

bedpan [AS. *bedd,* bed, + *panna,* flat vessel]. A pan-shaped device which is placed under a bedridden patient for collecting and containing fecal and urinary excreta.

NOTE: In general, the use of a bedpan is uncomfortable and, because of the awkwardness of the position, requires more exertion on the patient's part than using a bedside toilet. Thus patients who are recovering from myocardial infarction and others should not be forced to use a bedpan if it is possible to move them from bed to bedside toilet.

bedrest. 1. A device for propping up patients in bed. 2. The confining of a patient continuously to his bed for rest.

bedridden. Unable or unwilling to leave the bed; bedfast.

bedsore [AS. *bedd,* bed, + *sāre,* open wound]. Pressure sore, esp. over a bony prominence.

Consists of ulceration and gangrene of a localized area, due to pressure from prolonged confinement in bed or from a cast or splint. Emaciated, weak, elderly patients and those who must remain in one position because of orthopedic or similar problems are especially likely to develop bedsores.

Located on the bony prominences thinly covered with flesh, as the end of the spine; buttocks; heels; elbows; shoulder blades; back of the head and ears in children. SYN: *decubitus; decubitus ulcer.*

PREDISPOSING CAUSES: Any factor which interferes with the circulation of the blood and mobility of the patient; prolonged fever; emaciation; obesity; paralysis; old age or senility; poorly made beds or those containing irritating bits of debris; lack of cleanliness; bruising; infrequent change of positions; cardiac diseases, nephritis, diabetes, anemia, etc.

TREATMENT: Best nursing care possible because prevention is easier than a cure; prophylactic measures in keeping the bed dry and clean; relieving the pressure as soon as the first signs of redness appear; report to the nurse in charge or attending physician at once; use the prescribed medication as directed by the physician;.

Thorough drying of skin after baths and gentle massage with alcohol to harden the skin and for stimulation of circulation; frequent change of position of patient if possible; exposure of area and protection of skin by silicone or similar preparation such as tincture of benzoin; maintenance of proper nutrition; chemical or surgical debridement of ulcers; use of sheepskin under vulnerable area; placing patient on special air bed, q.v., or flotation bed, q.v.

bed'wetting. Enuresis, q.v.

beef [Fr. *boeuf*]. Meat from cattle that are one or more years old. Nitrogen is the essential nutrient in beef, it being richer in protein than any other food excepting cheese. The leaner the beef the greater the percentage of nitrogen.

Poorer grades of beef contain fewer calories than do the choice portions.

Food value of 100 gm. (rib roast; oven-roasted; choice grade; 55% lean and 45% fat): Cal. 481; protein 18.3 gm.; fat 44.7 gm.; calcium 8 mg.; iron 2.4 mg.; vitamin A, 90 I.U.; riboflavin 0.14 mg.; niacin 3.4 mg.

beer [AS. *béor*, fermented drink]. Fermented alcoholic beverage from a malt infusion of barley, malt, or hops, with aid of brewer's yeast.

Contains about 4.5% alcohol by volume, 1% sugar, and approximately 42 calories per 100 gm. portion or 115 per 8 oz. glass.

Beer's operation. [Georg Joseph Beer, Ger. ophthalmologist, 1763-1821] Flap operation for cataract or artificial pupil.

bee sting [AS. *béo*, bee, + *stingan*, to pierce]. The stinger, which is barbed, usually remains in the wound. Pain, mottled redness and edema result.

TREATMENT: Application of fairly strong household ammonia or baking soda paste. Remove stinger if present. If pain is severe, injection of 2% procaine solution. Antihistamines help to relieve discomfort. Some individuals are hypersensitive and may suffer severe anaphylactic reactions even leading to death. In such cases subcu-

taneous or intravenous administration of epinephrine is effective.

beeswax (bēz'wax). Yellow wax obtained from honeycomb of bees. A purified form is used in ointments.

beets [L. *beta*]. A plant of the genus Beta, the common garden variety being Beta vulgaris. The root is most often eaten, but young plants (beet greens) are consumed also.

Food value of 100 gm. (one cup; red; cooked, boiled, drained): Cal. 32; carbohydrate 7.2 gm.; calcium 14 mg.; iron 0.5 mg.; vitamin A, 20 I.U.; ascorbic acid 6 mg.

beeturia (bēt-ū'rĭ-ă). Pink to deep red color of urine which sometimes follows eating of beets.

behav'iorism. A theory of conduct which regards normal and abnormal behavior as the result of conditioned reflexes quite apart from the concept of will. It does not apply to conditions resulting from structural disease.

behavior reflex. One acquired as result of training and repetition.

bel (bĕl). A unit to measure the intensity of sound. It is expressed as a logarithm.

belch [AS. *baelcan*, to eructate]. Escape of gas from the stomach through the mouth; to eructate.

belching. Raising of gas from the stomach.
ETIOL: Gastric fermentation; air swallowing; gas-containing foods.

belemnoid (bĕ-lĕm'noyd) [Gr. *belemnon*, dart, + *eidos*, shape]. Dart-shaped; styloid.

belladonna (bel"ă-dŏn'ă) [It., fair lady]. Atropa belladonna, a poisonous plant with reddish flowers and shining black berries. Active principle of atropine. SYN: *deadly nightshade.*

Used mainly for sedative and spasmolytic effects on gastrointestinal tract.

b. and atropine poisons. These include stramonium, hyoscyamus, scopolamine, belladonna, and atropine. SEE: *atropine* in *Table of Poisons and Poisoning* in *Appendix.*

b. leaf. USP. Powder from dried leaf and flowering top of Atropa belladonna Linné or A. belladonna acuminata. A parasympatholytic agent, it is used generally in tincture form though the dry extract in tablet form may be used. SYN: *deadly nightshade leaf.*

b. tincture. USP. An alcoholic extract of belladonna. Has same action as belladonna leaf, q.v.

Bellini's ducts (bĕ-lē'nē). [Lorenzo Bellini, It. anatomist, 1643-1704] Ducts in the kidney which open at tip of a renal pyramid after receiving several straight tubules. SYN: *papillary ducts.*

Bell-Magendie's law. Bell's law, q.v.

bell-metal resonance. A metallic sound heard in pneumothorax.

Bellocq's cannula (bel-ok'). An instrument for drawing in a plug through nostril and mouth to control epistaxis. SYN: *Bellocq's sound.*

Bell's law. [Sir Charles Bell, Scot. physiologist and surgeon, 1774-1842] That anterior spinal nerve roots contain only motor fibers, and posterior roots only sensory fibers. SYN: *Bell-Magendie's law; Magendie's law.*

Bell's nerve. Long thoracic nerve; nervus thoracicus longus [NA].

Bell's palsy. Acute inflammatory reaction in or around the seventh, or facial, nerve at the stylomastoid foramen. Marked by pain and paralysis of muscles controlling facial expression, causing distortion of the face.

TREATMENT: Splint for prevention of drooping of lower face, massage of affected muscles, protection of eye during sleep to prevent ulceration of cornea, analgesics for pain.

bell sound. Bell-metal resonance.

belly [AS. *baelg*, bag]. 1. The abdomen or abdominal cavity. 2. The fleshy, central portion of a muscle.

 b. ache. Colic, gastralgia.

 b. button. Umbilicus; the navel.

belonephobia (bel''ō-nĕ-phō'bĭ-ă) [Gr. *belonē*, needle, + *phobos*, fear]. Morbid fear of sharp-pointed objects.

belonoid (bel'ō-noyd) ["+ *eidos*, shape]. Needle-shaped.

belonoskiascopy (bel''ō-nō-skī-as'kō-pī) ["+ *skia*, shadow, + *skopein*, to see]. Subjective retinoscopy by means of shadows and movements to determine refraction.

benadryl (ben'ă-drĭl). Proprietary name for diphenhydramine hydrochloride, an antihistaminic agent.

Bence Jones albumose. [Henry Bence Jones, Eng. physician, 1813-1873] SEE: *protein, Bence Jones.*

bends. Painful condition caused by bubbles of nitrogen in blood and tissues as a result of too rapid decompression from greater-than-atmospheric pressure, or ascending too rapidly to a high altitude while flying. SEE: *caisson disease.*

Benedict's solution (bĕn'ĕ-dĭkt). [Stanley R. Benedict, Amer. chemist, 1884-1936] A solution used to test for presence of sugar. To 173 gm. sodium or potassium citrate and 100 gm. anhydrous sodium carbonate (dissolved in 700 ml. water) is added 17.3 gm. crystalline copper sulfate that has been dissolved in 100 ml. of water. Sufficient water is added to the mixture to make 1000 ml.

Benedict's test for sugar. Add 8 drops of clear urine (filtered if necessary) to a test tube containing 5 ml. of B's solution. Boil from 1 to 2 minutes, agitating the test tube during this time, and then allow it to cool undisturbed. Formation of red, yellow, olive green, or green precipitate indicates presence of sugar (2% or more [plus 4], 1% [plus 3], 3/4% [plus 2], 1/2% [plus 1], respectively).

Ben'edikt's syndrome. [Moritz Benedikt, Austrian physician, 1835-1920] Hemiplegia with oculomotor paralysis and clonic spasm or tremor on opposite side. It is caused by either arteriosclerosis or syphilis.

benign (bē-nīn') [L. *benignus*, mild]. 1. Not recurrent. 2. Not malignant. 3. Mild.

 b. stupor. A stupor sometimes seen in the depression of manic-depressive psychosis.

benzalkonium chloride (benz''al-kō'nĭ-um klō'rĭd). USP. A bitter, aromatic, white powder. Used as a detergent and germicide.

benzedrine (bĕn'zĕ-drēn). Proprietary name for amphetamine, q.v.

 b. sulfate. Proprietary name for amphetamine sulfate, q.v.

benzene (bĕn'zēn, bĕn-zēn') [benz(oin) + Gr. *ene*, suffix used in chemistry to denote unsaturated compound.]. C_6H_6. A volatile liquid, immiscible with water, able to dissolve fats.

Important theoretically because it is the simplest member of the aromatic series of hydrocarbons, and useful practically because, prepared in the distillation of coal tar, it serves in the synthesis of innumerable dyes, drugs, etc. The phenyl radical, C_6H_5, will be recognized in the formulae for phenol, dimethylaminoazobenzene (which see under azo compounds), and benzoic acid. SYN: *benzol.*

SEE: *benzene* and *b. hydrochlorate* in *Table of Poisons and Poisoning* in *Appendix.*

benzestrol (ben-zes'trol). A synthetic substance, which has an estrogenic effect when taken orally.

benzidine test. A test used to determine the presence of blood. Prepare benzidine solution as follows: to a saturated solution of benzidine in glacial acetic acid, add equal volume of 3% hydrogen peroxide and about one ml. of the suspected fluid. Appearance of a blue color indicates presence of blood.

benzidine test diet. This consists of milk, crackers and rice.

An iron-free diet, its purpose being to free the alimentary tract of any iron; often the stool is tested for iron. Since no iron was in the food, if any is present in the food masses, it must come from the hemoglobin of the blood. Such a result is a positive test of bleeding into the intestinal tract, and an evidence of an ulcer. Patients should be watched to be sure that they eat nothing but those foods which are served at the prescribed times.

benzoate (běn'zo-āt). Any salt of benzoic acid.

benzocaine (ben'zō-kān). Nontoxic local anesthetic.

benzo'ic acid. SEE: *acid, benzoic.*

benzoin (běn'zoyn, -zō-ĭn) [Fr. benjoin, ultimately from Arabic *luban jawi*, frankincense of Java]. USP. A balsamic resin obtained from various species of a tree, Styrax, esp. S. benzoin or S. paralleloneuris. Used as a stimulant expectorant, as an inhalant in laryngitis and bronchitis, or as a protective coating for ulcers, etc.

ben'zol. Same as benzene, q.v., but not in technical use.

benzyl benzoate (běn'zĭl ben'zō-āt). A sharp, colorless oily liquid, used externally in scabies.

beolocator. Device for locating and detecting hard metallic and nonmetallic objects in human tissues. When one end of the device comes in contact with the object being sought, the sound made is amplified. May be used in detecting a foreign body in the uterus.

Bérard's aneurysm (bā-rär'). [Auguste Bérard, Fr. surgeon, 1802-1846] An arteriovenous aneurysm in the tissues surrounding the injured vein.

Béraud's valve (bā-rō'). [Bruno J. J. Béraud, Fr. surgeon, 1823-1865] Fold of mucous membrane at junction of lacrimal sac with lacrimal duct. SYN: *Krause's valve.*

beriberi (běr'ĭ-ber'ĭ) [Singhalese *beri*, weakness]. A deficiency disease associated with malnutrition. Endemic in the Orient, Philippines and other islands of the Pacific, and formerly in rice-growing sections of the U. S.

ETIOLOGY: Deficiency of thiamine (vitamin B₁). Diet is usually a low-fat, low-protein, high-carbohydrate one, esp. in which there is a high intake of rice highly milled.

SYM: Multiple neuritis, cardiovascular changes, and edema.

TREATMENT: Oral or parenteral administration of thiamine; establishment of a properly balanced diet.

berkelium (běrk'lē-ŭm). [U. of California at Berkeley, where first produced] SYMB: Bk. At. wt. of best known istope is 247; at. no 97. A transuranium element.

Bernard's canal, duct (běr-nar'). [Claude Bernard, Fr. physiologist, 1813-1878] An accessory pancreatic duct; ductus pan-

creaticus accessorius [NA]. SYN: *Santorini's duct.*

Bernard's granular layer. Inner layer in cells lining acini of pancreas.

Bernreuter test (bern'rū-ter). A "yes" and "no" test of 125 questions used to ascertain the attitudes and interests of a person.

Bertin, columns of (ber'tan). [Exupère Joseph Bertin, Fr. anatomist, 1712-1781] Renal cortical columns supporting the blood vessels in the kidneys. The part that separates the medullary pyramids.

Bertin's ligament. Iliofemoral ligament.

beryllium (bĕ-rĭl'ĭ-um) [Gr. *béryllos*, beryl]. SYMB: Be. At. wt. 9.0122; at. no. 4; sp. gr. 1.848. A metallic element.

besoin de respirer (ba-zwan'dĕ res'pĭ-rā') [Fr. need to breathe]. Sensation inducing act of breathing.

bestiality (běs-tĭ-āl'ĭ-tĭ) [L. *bestia*, beast]. Coition with an animal.

beta (bā'tă). 1. Second letter of Greek alphabet, written β. 2. Used as a prefix to chemical words to note isomeric variety or position in compounds of subsituted groups.

b. cells. 1. Basophilic cells in the anterior lobe of hypophysis which give a positive periodic acid stain reaction. 2. Cells of the islets of Langerhans of the pancreas which secrete insulin.

b. particles, b. rays. Negatively charged particles emitted by radium; more penetrating than alpha rays. Absorbed by 1 mm. lead or 0.6 mm. platinum. SEE: *electron.*

betacism (bā'tă-sĭzm) [Gr. *bēta*, the letter b.]. Speech defect giving the *b* sound to other consonants.

betaine hydrochloride (bē'tă-ēn) [L. *beta*, beet]. A colorless crystalline substance, containing 23% hydrochloric acid, and obtained from an alkaloid found in the beet, and other plants. Used as a substitute for hydrochloric acid in hypochlorhydria.

Betz cells. [Vladimir A. Betz, Russ. anatomist, 1834-1894] A form of giant pyramidal cell in the cortical motor area of the brain. The axons of these cells are included in the pyramidal tract.

bezoar (bē'zōr) [Persian pad, protecting against, + *zahr,* poison]. A hard mass of entangled material from the stomachs and intestines of animals, and also in man as a hairball (trichobezoar), hair and vegetable fiberball (trichophytobezoar), and foodball (phytobezoar).

Bi. Chem. symb. for bismuth.

bi- (bī-) [L. *bis*, twice]. Prefix indicating two, double, twice.

biartic'ular ["+ *articulus,* joint]. Pert. to two joints; diarthric.

bibasic (bī-bā'sĭk) ["+ Gr. *basis,* foundation]. Pert. to an acid with two hydrogen atoms replaceable by bases to form salts.

bibulous (bĭb'ū-lŭs) [L. *bibulus,* drinking]. Absorbent.

bicameral (bī-kam'ĕr-ăl) [L. *bis,* twice, + *camera,* a chamber]. Having two cavities or hollows, esp. an abscess divided by a septum.

bicap'sular ["+ *capsula,* container]. Having a double capsule.

bicar'bonate. A salt resulting from the incomplete neutralization of carbonic acid, or from the passing of an excess of carbon dioxide into a solution of a base.

Sodium bicarbonate is $NaHCO_3$; calcium bicarbonate is $CaH_2(CO_3)_2$. A carbonate composed of two equivalents of carbonic acid and one of a base.

b., blood. B. in the blood. The amount present is an indicator of the alkali reserve.

b. ion. $HCO_3{}^-$.

bicellular (bī-sĕl'ū-lăr) [L. *bis,* twice, + *cellulāris,* little cell]. 1. Composed of two cells. 2. Having two chambers or compartments.

biceps (bī'sĕps) ["+ *caput,* head]. A muscle with two heads.

b. brachii. Muscle of the upper arm, having two heads. Flexes arm and forearm and supinates hand.

b. femoris. One of the hamstring muscles lying on posterior lateral side of thigh. Flexes knee and rotates it outward.

b. reflex. B. muscle contraction when tendon is percussed.

Bichat (bē-shā'). [Marie Francois X. Bichat, Fr. physiologist and anatomist, 1771-1802] Founder of scientific histology and pathological anatomy.

B.'s canal. The subarachnoid canal extending from third ventricle to middle of B.'s fissure carrying the veins of Galen.

B.'s fat ball or pad. Mass of fat behind the buccinator muscle.

B.'s fissure. The horseshoe fissure separating cerebrum from cerebellum.

B.'s foramen. SYN: B.'s canal.

B.'s ligament. Lower fasciculus of posterior sacroiliac ligament.

B.'s tunic. The tunica intima of the blood vessels.

bichloride of mercury (bī-klo'rīd). Corrosive mercuric chloride. A crystalline salt, $HgCl_2$. SEE: *mercuric chloride.*

POISONING: SEE: *mercuric chloride* in *Table of Poisons and Poisoning* in *Appendix.*

biciliate (bī-sĭl'ī-āt) [L. *bis,* twice, + Gr. *kyla,* eyelids]. Having two cilia.

bicipital (bī-sĭp'ī-tal) [L. *biceps,* two heads]. 1. Pert. to a biceps muscle. 2. Having two heads.

$Bi_2(CO_3)_3$. Bismuth carbonate.

biconcave (bī-kŏn'kāv) {L. *bis,* twice, + *concavus,* concave]. Concave on each side, as a lens.

bicon'vex ["+ *convexus,* rounded raised surface]. Convex on two sides, as a lens.

bicornuate, bicornuous (bī-kŏrn'ū-āt, ū-ŭs) ["+ *cornutus,* horned]. Having two processes or hornlike projections.

b. uterus. Anomalous uterus resulting from incomplete union of the mullerian ducts. May be double or single organ with two horns.

bicoro'nal [L. *bis,* twice, + Gr. *korōnē,* crown]. Pert. to the two coronas.

bicor'porate ["+ *corpus,* body]. Having two bodies.

bicuspid (bī-kŭs'pĭd) ["+ *cuspis,* point]. Having two cusps or projections (e.g., bicuspid tooth) or having two cusps or leaflets (e.g., bicuspid valve).

b. tooth. One of two teeth above and below on each side between the molars and canines.

b. valve. Valve between left atrium and left ventricle of the heart. SYN: *mitral valve.* SEE: *heart.*

b. i. d. Abbr. for L. *bis in die,* twice daily.

bidet (bē-dā') [Fr., a small horse]. A waist-high basin designed so that one may sit astride it. There are attachments which allow a stream of water to flow over the genital and perineal area. Thus a bidet provides an excellent means of cleaning the perineum.

biduous (bĭd'ū-ŭs) [L. *bis,* twice, + *diēs,* a day]. Continuing for two days.

Bielschowsky disease (bē''ĕl-shō'skī). [Max Bielschowsky, Ger. neuropathologist, 1869-1940] SEE: *amaurotic familial idiocy, late infantile.*

Bier's cup (bēr). [A. Karl G. Bier, Ger. surgeon, 1861-1949] A clear glass cup provided with a pump and bulb. Its use is to induce hyperemia where there is pronounced external inflammation.

Bier's spots. White spots occurring in a congested extremity when arterial supply is occluded following venous obstruction.

bifa'cial [L. *bis,* twice, + *faciēs,* face]. Having similar opposite surfaces.

bifid (bī'fĭd) ["+ *findere,* to cleave]. Cleft or split into two parts.

b. spine. Congenital fissure of vertebral column.

b. tongue. Cleft tongue.

bifo'cal ["+ *focus,* hearth]. Having two foci, as b. eyeglasses.

bifurcate (bī'fūr-kāt, bī-fūr'kāt) ["+ *furca,* fork]. Having two branches or divisions; forked.

bifurcated (bī'fūr-kāt″ĕd). Having two branches; forked.

bifurcation (bī-fūr-kā'shŭn) [L. *bis,* twice, + *furca,* fork]. A separation into two branches; the point of forking.

bigeminal (bī-jĕm'ĭ-năl) [L. *bigeminum,* twin]. Double, paired.

    b. body. One of the two anterior eminences of the corpora quadrigemina.

    b. pulse. Pulse in which beats are in groups of two with pause in between groups. SEE: *pulse, b.*

bigem'inum [L.]. (pl. *bigem'ina*) A bigeminal body.

bigeminy (bī-jĕm'ĭ-nĭ). Condition occurring in pairs, esp. pulse marked by occurrence of two beats close together followed by a pause before next pair of beats. SYN: *bigeminal pulse.*

bilat'eral [L. *bis,* twice, + *latus,* side]. Pert. to, affecting, or rel. to two sides of the body.

    b. symmetry. Symmetry of paired organs. SYN: *bilateralism.*

bilateralism (bī-lăt'ĕr-ăl-ĭzm) ["+ "+ Gr. *ismos,* condition]. Identical arrangement on two sides; symmetry.

bile (bīl) [L. *bilis,* bile]. A secretion of the liver.

It is a thick, viscid fluid with a bitter taste which passes from the bile duct of the liver into the common bile duct and then into the duodenum as needed. The bile from the liver is straw color, while that from the gallbladder varies from yellow to brown and green. There are more solids in green bile and it is mixed with mucus.

B. also is stored in the gallbladder, drawn upon as needed, and discharged into the duodenum. Contraction of the gallbladder is brought about by a hormone, cholecystokinin, produced by the duodenum, its secretion being brought about by the entrance of fatty foods (esp. egg yolk and cream) into the duodenum. Added to water, b. decreases surface tension, giving a foamy solution favoring the emulsification of fats and oils; this action is due to the b. salts, mainly sodium glycocholate and taurocholate.

COMP: The b. pigments (principally bilirubin, q.v., and biliverdin, q.v.) are responsible for the variety of the colors observed. In addition, b. contains cholesterol, lecithin, mucin, and other organic and inorganic substances.

FUNCT: Its importance as a digestive juice is due to its emulsifying action which facilitates the digestion of fats in the intestines by pancreatic steapsin, plus a further effect of the b. salts which form compounds with the fatty acids and are necessary for their absorption. B. also stimulates peristalsis.

Normally the ejection of b. only occurs during duodenal digestion. B. is both an antiseptic and a purgative. About 1800-2000 ml. are secreted/24 hr. in the normal adult. SEE: *gallbladder.*

PATH: Interference with the flow of b. produces jaundice, resulting in unabsorbed fats being found in the feces. In such instances, fats should be restricted in the diet. Gallstones also may be produced in the gallbladder when the free flow of b. from the gallbladder is impeded, or when pathological conditions interfere with b. production.

TESTS: There are several methods of testing for bile in the urine.

Gmelin's Test: 1 in. of concentrated nitric acid is carefully overlaid with the sample of urine. B. is present when there is a play of colors at the junction of the fluids. This test also can be carried out by pouring some urine onto blotting or filter paper, and then placing a drop of concentrated nitric acid on the moist paper. From the spreading edge of the drop of acid will develop a ring of various colors in which green predominates and forms the outer band.

Iodine Test: Pour urine into a test tube to a depth of 1 in. (2.5 cm.) and carefully overlay it with dilute tincture of iodine. A bright green ring will appear at the junction of the fluids if b. is present.

RS: "bili-" words, "chol-" words, stercobilin, urobilin.

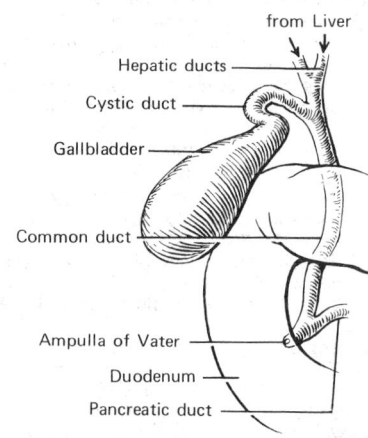

BILE AND PANCREATIC DUCTS

b. acids. Complex acids, of which cholic, glycocholic, and taurocholic acids are examples, and which occur as salts (e.g., sodium taurochlate) in b. They give b. its foamy character, are important in the digestion of fats in the intestine, and are reabsorbed from the intestine to be used again by the liver. This circulation of b. acids is called the enterohepatic circulation.

In Hay's test for b. acids, some urine is placed in a watchglass and a little powdered sulfur is sprinkled on the surface. If b. acids are present, the sulfur sinks because of the lowering of the surface tension by the b. salts.

b. ducts. Intercellular biliary passages conveying the b. from the liver to the hepatic duct which joins the duct from the gallbladder (cystic duct), to form the common b. duct (ductus choledochus), and which enters the duodenum about 3 in. (7.6 cm.) below the pylorus. SEE: *duct, common bile; duct, cystic; duct, hepatic; gallbladder.*

b. pigments. Complex, highly colored substances found in b. derived from the red pigment (hemoglobin) of the blood and imparting brown color to intestinal contents and feces. Ex: bilirubin, biliverdin.

Van den Bergh's test, q.v., is used to detect the type of bilirubin in the blood serum.

b. salts. Alkali salts of b. Sodium glycocholate and sodium taurocholate.

Bilharzia (bĭl-här'zĭ-ă). [Theodor M. Bilharz, Ger. helminthologist 1825-62] Former name for Schistosoma, the human blood fluke. SEE: *Schistosoma.*

bilharzial, bilharzic (bĭl-här'zĭ-ăl, -zĭk). Pert. to Bilharzia (Schistosoma).

bilharziasis (bĭl″här-zĭ'ă-sĭs). Schistosomiasis.

bili- [L. *bilis*]. Prefix pert. to bile.

biliary (bĭl'ĭ-ār-ĭ). Pert. to or conveying bile.

b. calculus. Cholelithiasis. Formation of stone in any of the biliary passages or in the gallbladder.

b. colic. Pain caused by the pressure or passing of gallstones.

b. ducts. Passages conveying bile from liver to hepatic duct. SEE: *bile ducts.*

bilicyanin (bĭl'ĭ-sī'ă-nĭn) [L. *bilis*, bile, + *cyaneus*, blue]. A blue or purple pigment, an oxidation product of biliverdin.

bilifaction. Bilification.

bilifica'tion [L. *bilis*, bile, + *facere*, to make]. The formation of bile.

biliflavin (bĭl'ĭ-flā'vĭn) [″ + *flavus*, yellow]. A yellow pigment derived from biliverdin.

bilifulvin (bĭl'ĭ-fŭl'vĭn) [″ + *fulvus*, tawny]. Bilirubin mixed with other substances.

bilifuscin (bĭl'ĭ-fŭs'ĭn) [L. *bilis*, bile, + *fuscus*, brown]. A dark brown pigment from bile and gallstones.

biligenesis (bĭl'ĭ-jĕn'ĕ-sĭs) [″ + Gr. *genesis*, origin]. The formation of bile.

biligenetic, biligenic (bĭl'ĭ-jĕn-ĕt'ĭk, -jĕn'ĭk) [″ + Gr. *gennan*, to produce]. Forming bile.

bilihumin (bĭl'ĭ-hū'mĭn) [L. *bilis*, bile, + *humus*, earth]. A dark insoluble residue after applying solvents to bile or gallstones.

bilineurine (bĭl'ĭ-nū'rĭn) [″ + Gr. *neuron*, nerve]. Choline, q.v.

bilious (bĭl'yŭs) [L. *bilosus*]. 1. Pert. to bile. 2. Afflicted with biliousness.

b. fever. Fever with vomiting of bile.

biliousness (bĭl'yŭs-nĕs). 1. A symptom of a disordered condition of the liver causing constipation, headache, loss of appetite, and vomiting of bile. 2. Excess of bile; bilious fever. Fever with vomiting of bile.

biliprasin (bĭl'ĭ-prā'sĭn) [L. *bilis*, bile, + Gr. *prason*, green]. Green pigment, similar to biliverdin and found in gallstones.

bilipurpin, bilipurpurin (bĭl'ĭ-pŭr'pĭn, bĭl″-ĭ-pŭr'pū-rĭn) [″ + *purpur*, purple]. A purple pigment derived from biliverdin.

bilirachia (bĭl-ĭ-rā'kĭ-ă) [″ + Gr. *rhachis*, spine]. Bile in the spinal fluid.

bilirubin (bĭl-ĭ-rū'bĭn) [″ + *ruber*, red]. ($C_{33}H_{36}O_6N_4$). The orange-colored or yellowish pigment in bile.

It is carried to the liver by the blood. It is produced from hemoglobin of red blood cells by reticuloendothelial cells in bone marrow, in the spleen, and elsewhere. It is changed chemically in the liver and excreted in the bile through the duodenum. As it passes through the intestines it is converted into urobilinogen by bacterial enzymes, most of it being excreted through the feces. If urobilinogen passes into the circulation it is excreted through the urine or reexcreted in the bile.

bilirubinate (bĭl'ĭ-rū'bĭn-āt). A salt of bilirubin.

bilirubinemia (bĭl'ĭ-rū-bĭn-ē'mĭ-ă) [L. *bilis*, bile, + *ruber*, red, + Gr. *haima*, blood]. Bilirubin in blood. Normally it is present in small amounts. However in certain pathological conditions in which excessive destruction of red blood cells occurs, or in which there is interference with bile excretion, the amount is increased.

bilirubinuria (bĭl'ĭ-rū-bĭn-ū'rĭ-ă) [″ + ″ + Gr. *ouron*, urine]. Bilirubin in urine.

biliuria (bĭl-ĭ-ū'rĭ-ă). Bile in the urine.

biliverdin (bĭl-ĭ-vĕr'dĭn) [″ + Gr. *viridis*, green]. $C_{33}H_{34}O_6N_4$. A greenish pigment in bile formed by the oxidation of bilirubin.

billion [Fr. *bi*, two, + *million*, million]. 1. In the U.S., b. is a number equal to one followed by 9 zeros (1,000,000,000 or 10^9). 2. In Europe, b. is a number equal to one followed by 12 zeros (10^{12}), i.e. bi million, or twice the number in a million (10^6). SYN: *milliard.*

bilobate (bī-lō'bāt) [L. *bis*, twice, + *lobus*, lobe]. Having two lobes.

bilobular (bī-lŏb'ū-lär). Having two lobules.

biloc'ular ["+ *loculus*, cell]. 1. Having two cells. 2. Divided into compartments.

biloc'ulate. Bilocular.

bilophodont (bī-lŏf'ō-dŏnt) [L. *bis*, twice, + Gr. *lophos*, ridge, + *odous*, odont, tooth]. Said of animals, such as the kangaroo, having teeth with two ridges.

biman'ual ["+ *manus*, hand]. With both hands; with two hands, as b. palpation.

bimax'illary ["+ *maxillaris*, pert. to the jaw]. Pert. to or afflicting both jaws.

binary (bī'nār-ī) [L. *binarius*, of two]. 1. Compounded of two elements. 2. Separating into two branches.
 b. acid. Acid containing hydrogen and one other element.
 b. digit. One of two digits, usually 0 or 1, used in a binary system of enumeration.

binaural (bĭn-ŏ'räl) [L. *bini*, two, + *auris*, ear]. Pert. to or having two ears.
 b. arc. The arc from one aural point to another across top of cranium.

binauricular (bĭn-ŏ-rĭk'ū-lär) ["+ *auricula*, little ear]. Binaural.

binder [AS. *bindan*, to tie up]. A broad bandage most commonly used as an encircling support of abdomen or chest. SEE: *bandage.*
 b., abdominal. A wide band fastened snugly about the abdomen for support.
 b., chest. A broad band used for encircling the chest to apply heat, dressings, or pressure, and supporting the breasts. Improved by using shoulder straps to keep from slipping.
 b., double-T. A horizontal band about the waist to which two vertical bands are attached in back, brought around leg and again fastened to horizontal band. Holds dressings about perineum or genitalia, esp. in males.
 b., obstetrical. A broad bandage encircling entire abdomen from ribs to pelvis, affording support.
 b., T. Two strips of material fastened together resembling a T, used as a bandage to hold a dressing on perineum of women.
 b., towel. A towel encircling abdomen or chest with ends pinned or sewed together for support.

binocular (bĭn-ŏk'ū-lär) [L. *bini*, two, + *oculus*, eye]. Pert to both eyes.

 b. vision. Normal vision involving si multaneous use of both eyes.

binotic (bĭn-ŏt'ĭk) ["+ Gr. *ous*, ear]. Pert. to o having two ears. SYN: *binaural*, q.v.

binovular (bĭn-ŏv'ū-lär) ["+ *ovum*, egg] Derived from or pert. to two ova. SYN: *b ovular.*

binuclear, binucleate (bī-nū'klē-ăr, -āt) [L *bis*, twice, + *nucleus*, kernel]. Having tw nuclei.

bio- [Gr. *bios*, life]. Prefix indicating relation ship to life.

bio-assay (bī"ō-ăs'ā) [Gr. *bios*, life, + O.Fr *asaier*, to try]. Estimation of strength of drug by noting its effect in a test animal an comparing such with effects of a standar preparation.

bioastronautics. Study of the effects o space travel on living plant and animal life

biocatalyst (bī-ō-kăt'ä-lĭst) [Gr. *bios*, life, + *katalyein*, to dissolve]. An enzyme; a bio chemical catalyzer.

biochem'istry ["+ *chēmeia*, chemistry] The chemistry of living things; the science o the chemical changes accompanying the vi tal functions of plants and animals.

biochemorphic (bī"ō-kĕm-ŏr'fĭk) ["+ "+ *morphē*, shape]. Pert. to the relationship be tween biologic action of drugs and foods and their chemical constitution.

biochemorphology (bī"ō-kĕ-mŏr-fŏl'ō-jī ["+ "+ "+ *logos*, study]. Science of chemica structure of substances as related to thei action on the body.

biocide (bī"ō-sīd) ["+ L. *-cida*, killer]. Matter esp. a pesticide or antibiotic, capable of de stroying living organisms.

bioclimatology (bī"ō-klī-mä-tŏl'ō-jī) [Gr *bios*, life, + *klima*, climate, + *logos*, study] Relationship of climate to life.

biocoenosis, biocenosis (bī"ō-sē-nō'sĭs ["+ *koinos*, common]. The relationship be tween plants and animals sharing the same area and conditions. SEE: *ecology.*

biocolloid (bī-ō-kŏl'oyd) ["+ *kollōdēs*, gluti nous]. A colloid in animal or vegetable or ganism.

biodeterioration. Any undesirable change in the properties of a material caused by the vital activities of organisms.

biodynam'ics [Gr. *bios*, life, + *dynamis* force]. The science of living force or energy biophysiology.

bioelectric impedance. The resistance o biological systems to the flow of electrica current. This resistance varies with the ions available in the tissues or fluids. Impedance can be used in determining presence of fluid in body cavities, cardiac output, and blood flow in extremities without using instruments or needles on the patient.

bioenergetics (bī″ō-ĕn″ĕr-jĕt′ĭks). Science of energy transformation taking place within living tissues.

biofeedback. A training program designed to develop the individual's ability to control his autonomic (involuntary) nervous system. After learning the technique, the patient may be able to control heart rate, blood pressure, and skin temperature or to relax certain muscles. The patient learns by using monitoring devices which indicate changes in pulse, blood pressure, brain waves, and muscle contractions; then he attempts to reproduce conditions which caused the desired changes.

biogenesis (bī″ō-jĕn′ĕ-sĭs) [Gr. *bios*, life, + *genesis*, origin]. Begetting living things from living things. Opposed to spontaneous generation.

biogenet′ic. Pert. to biogenesis.

biokinet′ics [Gr. *bios*, life, + *kinētikos*, moving]. The science of changes in developing organisms.

biolog′ic, biolog′ical [″+ *logos*, study]. Pert. to biology.

biological false positive. A serological test for syphilis which is positive in the absence of infection with Treponema.

biolog′icals. 1. Complex substances of organic origin depending for their action on the processes effecting immunity, used esp. in diagnosis and treatment of disease as vaccines, serums, or antigens. 2. Complex products of organic or synthetic origin, obtained or standardized by biological methods, as insulin.

biological warfare. The use of biological agents such as viruses, bacteria, toxins, and molds to kill or injure enemy soldiers and civilians. SEE: *chemical warfare.*

biol′ogist. A professional student of, or a specialist in, biology.

biology (bī-ŏl′ō-jī) [Gr. *bios*, life, + *logos*, study]. Science of life and living things. It includes the study of plants (botany) and animals (zoology) and all their subdivisions.

biolysis (bī-ŏl′ĭ-sĭs) [″+ *lysis*, dissolution]. Devitalization or destruction of living tissue by action of living organisms.

biolytic (bī-ō-lĭt′ĭk). Capable of destroying life.

biomet′rics. Biometry.

biometry (bī-ŏm′ĕ-trī) [Gr. *bios*, life, + *metron*, measure]. 1. Application of statistics to biological science. 2. Computation of life expectancy.

bion (bī′-ŏn) [Gr. *biōn*, living]. Any living organism.

bionergy (bī-ŏn′ĕr-jī) [Gr. *bios*, life, + *ergon*, work]. Vital energy or force.

bionics (bī-ŏn′ĭks) [*bio*-electr*onics*]. Study of how living organisms perform tasks and solve problems and the application of these findings to the design of machines, esp. computers.

bionomics (bī″ō-nŏm′ĭks) [Fr. *bionomique*, pert. to ecology]. Ecology, q.v.

bion′omy. The science pert. to life processes. SEE: *physiology; ecology.*

biono′sis [Gr. *bios*, life, + *nosos*, disease]. Any disease due to pathogenic organisms.

biophagism, biophagy (bī-ŏf′ă-jĭzm, -ă-jī) [″+ *phagein*, to eat]. Absorbing nourishment from living matter.

biophagous (bī-ŏf′ă-gŭs). Feeding on nonparasitic matter.

biophylactic (bī″ō-fī-lăk′tĭk) [Gr. *bios*, life, + *phylaktikos*, preservative]. Tending to preserve life.

biophysics (bī-ō-fĭz′ĭks) [″+ *physikos*, natural]. Application of physical laws to life processes and functions.

bioplasm (bī′ō-plazm) [″+ *plasma*, matter]. Protoplasm. Living substance.

biopsy (bī′ŏp-sī) [Gr. *bios*, life, + *opsis*, vision]. Excision of a small piece of tissue for microscopic examination.

biorhythms (bī″ō-rĭth′ŭms) [″+ *rhythmos*, rhythm]. Cyclic phenomena characteristic of life processes. Ex: menstrual cycle in women and estrus cycle in some mammals other than the human.

bios (bī′ŏs) [Gr., life]. 1. Organic life. 2. A group of substances (including esp. inositol, biotin, and thiamine) necessary for the most favorable growth of some yeasts.

bioscopy (bī-ŏs′kō-pī) [″+ *skopein*, to examine]. Examination to determine life.

biospectrometry (bī″ō-spĕk-trŏm′ĕ-trī) [″+ L. *spectrum*, image, + Gr. *metron*, measure]. Use of a spectroscope to determine the amounts and kinds of substances in tissues.

biospectroscopy (bī″ō-spĕk-trŏs′kō-pī) [″+ ″+ Gr. *skopein*, to examine]. Examination of tissue by use of a spectroscope.

biostatics (bī″ō-stăt′ĭks) [Gr. *bios*, life, + *statikos*, standing]. Science of the relationship of structure to function.

biostatis′tics. 1. Application of statistical processes and methods to the analysis of biological data. 2. Vital statistics.

biota (bī-ō′tă) [Gr. *bios*, life]. Combined and total animal and plant life in an area.

biotax′is, bi′otaxy [″+ *taxis*, arrangement]. 1. The selecting and arranging activity of living cells. 2. Systematic classification of living organisms.

biot'ics [Gr. *biōtikos*, living]. The sum of knowledge regarding life processes.

biotin (bī'ō-tĭn). A component of the vitamin B complex formerly designated as vitamin H. This water-soluble, heat-sensitive substance is essential for the activity of many enzyme systems in bacteria, animal, and presumably man. Present in many foods, but liver, kidney, milk, egg yolks, and yeast are particularly rich sources. Deficiency states have been reported in man only when the diet contains large amounts of raw egg white. This is due to b. being bound to a protein in the egg white, thus interfering with absorption. Humans with biotin deficiency develop lassitude, anorexia, depression, muscle pains, hyperesthesia of the skin, and dermatitis.

biotomy (bī-ŏt'ō-mĭ) [Gr. *bios*, life, + *tomē*, incision]. Operation on living animals for pathological or physiological study. SYN: *vivisection*.

biotoxin (bī-ō-tŏks'ĭn) ["+ *toxikon*, poison]. A toxin produced by or found in a living organism.

biotransformation. The biological process of changing the chemical characteristics of a substance so that it may be metabolized or excreted.

biotrip'sis [Gr. *bios*, life, + *tripsis*, rubbing]. A condition of the skin seen in old people in which skin wears away. May be smooth, pigmented, shiny, esp. on forehead, backs of hands, and shin.

Biot's breathing (bē-ō'). [Camille Biot, 19th century Fr. physician] Two to three short breaths with long, irregular periods of apnea. Seen in patients with increased intracranial pressure.

biotype (bī'ō-tīp) [Gr. *bios*, life, + *typos*, mark]. 1. Fundamental genetic constitution of an organism or those possessing it. Opposed to phenotype or external appearance of an organism. 2. A genotype.

biov'ular twins [L. *bis*, twice, + *ovulum*, ovum]. Twins from two separate ova.

bipara (bĭp'ă-rā) ["+ *parēre*, to give birth]. Woman who has borne two children in separate labors.

biparasitic (bī"păr-ă-sĭt'ĭk) ["+ Gr. *para*, beside, + *sitos*, food]. Pert. to parasite living upon another parasite.

biparen'tal ["+ *parēre*, to give birth]. Derived from both parents.

biparous (bĭp'ă-rŭs). Giving birth to two at a time.

bipolar (bī-pōl'ăr) [L. *bis*, twice, + *polus*, a pole]. 1. Having two poles or processes. 2. Pert. to the use of two poles in electrotherapeutic treatments. The term bitermi-

nal should be used when referring to an alternating current.

b. nerve cell. Cell with two processes.

biramous (bī-rā'mŭs) ["+ *ramus*, a branch]. Possessing two branches.

birefrac'tive, birefrin'gent ["+ *refrangere*, to break up]. Splitting a ray of light in two.

birhinia (bī-rĭn'ĭ-ā) [L. *bis*, twice, + Gr. *rhis*, nose]. A congenital deformity consisting of a double nose.

birth [Old Norse *burdhr*]. Act of being born; passage of a child from uterus.

b. canal. The uterus and vagina.

b. certificate. A legal form filled out by the physician or one in attendance at a birth and filed with the local health dept., giving pertinent information regarding the parents and child.

b., complete. The instant of complete separation of the body of the infant from that of the mother, regardless of cord or placenta detached.

b. control. Any method used to control the number of children conceived or born. This includes devices used by either the male or the female; medicines and abortion. Abstention from sexual intercourse is a form of birth control as is surgical sterilization.

b., cross. Labor with fetus lying across the uterus.

b., dry. B. following premature rupture of the fetal membranes.

b., live. An infant showing one of the three evidences of life (breathing, heart action, movements of a voluntary muscle) after complete birth.

b. mark. Nevus; mark from birth injury.

b. palsy. Paraplegia or hemiplegia caused by birth injury. Injury to shoulder muscles may cause Erb's palsy.

b., premature. B. of a fetus sometime after it is old enough to survive but before reaching 2500 gm. in weight. This weight limitation does not apply to races of small stature and weight.

b. rate. The number of live births in a given year/1000 of total population.

b., still. An infant not exhibiting evidence of life after complete b.

bisacromial (bĭs"ă-krō'mĭ-ăl) [L. *bis*, twice, + Gr. *akron*, point, + *ōmos*, shoulder]. Pert. to both acromial processes.

bisection (bī-sĕk'shŭn) ["+ *sectiō*, a cutting]. Division into two parts.

bisex'ual ["+ *sexus*, sex]. Hermaphroditic; having imperfect genitalia of both sexes in one person.

bisferious (bĭs-fēr'ĭ-ŭs) [L. *bis,* twice, + *ferire,* to beat]. Having two beats; dicrotic.

bisiliac (bĭs-ĭl'ĭ-ăk) ["+ *ilium,* ilium]. Pert. to the two most distant points of the two iliac crests.

bis in d., bis in die [L.]. Twice a day. ABBR: b.i.d.

bismuth (bĭz'mŭth) [Ger. *Wismuth,* white mass]. SYMB: *Bi.* At. wt. 208.980, at. no. 83. A silvery metallic element. Its compounds are used as a protective for inflamed surfaces, and as an opaque medium for x-ray visualization. Its salts are used as an antiseptic, astringent, sedative, and in treatment of diarrhea.

POISONING SYM: Metallic taste, foul breath, fever, gastrointestinal irritation, bluish line at gum margin, ulcerative process of gums and mouth, headache. Albuminuria; resembles lead poisoning with an absence of the blood changes and paralyses.

F.A. TREATMENT: Removal of source of bismuth; gastric lavage; high enemas; stimulants for respiration and heart if necessary; treat symptomatically.

   b. subcarbonate. USP. An odorless, tasteless powder.

USES: As an antacid, astringent, and protective.

INCOMPATIBILITIES: Sulfides, acids, acid salts.

   b. subgallate. A bright yellow powder without odor or taste.

USES: First introduced for treatment of skin diseases. General use is the same as bismuth subnitrate.

   b. subnitrate. Occurs as heavy white odorless powder.

USES: Astringent, protective antiseptic.

INCOMPATIBILITIES: Acids, tannins, and sulfides.

bistoury (bĭs'tū-rĭ) [Fr. *bistouri,* surgical knife]. Small surgical knife used in minor operations. Special varieties are tenotomes, gum lancets, hernia knives, and lithotomy bistouries.

bite (bīt) [AS. *bītan,* to bite]. 1. To cut with the teeth. 2. Puncture or tearing of the skin by the teeth as by an animal. SEE: *bites or stings.* 3. In dentistry, the angle and manner at which the upper and lower teeth meet.

   b., balanced. Balanced occlusion of the teeth.

   b., close, closed. B. in which lower incisors lie behind upper incisors.

   b., end-to-end. B. in which incisors of both jaws meet along cutting edge when jaw is closed.

   b., open. B. in which a space exists between the upper and lower incisors when the mouth is closed.

   b., over. B. in which upper incisors overlap lower ones when jaws are closed.

   b. rim. A rim of wax placed on base plate as a guide for inserting artificial teeth. SYN: *occlusion rim.*

   b., under. Condition in which lower incisors pass in front of upper incisors upon closing the mouth. SYN: *underhung b.*

bitelock. Device used in dentistry for retaining bite rims outside the mouth in the same position they were inside the mouth.

bitem'poral [L. *bis,* twice, + *temporalis,* pert. to a temple]. Pert. to both temples or temporal bones.

bites or stings. Injuries in which body surfaces are torn by insects or animals, resulting in abrasions, punctures, or lacerated wounds. SEE: *dog bite; rabies; snake bite.*

SYM: May be evidence of a wound usually surrounded by a zone of redness and swelling, often accompanied by pain, itching, or throbbing. Often become infected and may contain specific noxious materials as bacteria or venom of rabies.

F.A. TREATMENT: If suspected of poison, apply tourniquet first. Wash wound with saline solution thoroughly, apply dry sterile dressing. Administer appropriate antitetanus therapy. Treatment for shock may be needed.

Insect bites or stings contain an acid substance resembling formic acid and consequently are relieved by alkalies, as ammonia water or baking soda paste. For intense local pain injection of local anesthetic may be required. Systemic medication may be needed for generalized pain.

Others, such as the bee, wasp, and hornet, contain unknown organic substances for which there is no specific antidote. Remove the stinger if one is present. At the site of bites or stings by poisonous spiders, esp. the black widow, q.v., scorpions, tarantulas, and poisonous fish, the tourniquet should be applied promptly.

Intravenous calcium gluconate given very slowly is specific for controlling muscle pain due to black widow spider bite. It is also effective in relieving muscular cramps due to contact with jellyfish or Portugese man-of-war.

For jellyfish stings apply dilute ammonia water to area; then apply hot Epsom salt soaks. Morphine may be required for pain and supportive therapy for shock.

A sting ray injures by penetrating the skin with the barb in its tail. This causes intense pain, local swelling, nausea, vomiting, weakness, and perhaps shock. Treat symptomatically, cleanse wound thoroughly, and remove all foreign material. Soak site of wound in hot water (113°-140° F., 45°-60° C.) for 30-60 minutes; surgical debridement and closure of wound. SEE: *black widow; scorpion; tarantula.*

bite-wing x-ray. X-ray pictures taken with the film holder held between the teeth and the film parallel to the teeth. This technique permits film to be taken of several upper and lower teeth at the same time.

Bitot's spots (bē'tōz). [Pierre A. Bitot, Fr. physician, 1822-1888]. Triangular, shiny, gray spots on the conjunctiva seen in vitamin A deficiency.

bitter (bĭt'ĕr) [AS. *biter,* strong]. Having a disagreeable taste.

bituminosis (bĭ-tū″mĭ-nō'sĭs). Pneumoconiosis from dust of soft coal.

biuret (bĭ'ū-rĕt) [L. *bis,* twice, + *urea*]. A crystalline decomposition derivative of urea.

  b. reaction. Rose to violet coloring in an aqueous solution of protein when dilute solution of copper sulfate and sodium hydroxide are added to it.

  b. test. Use of above reaction to detect presence of urea or any soluble protein.

bivalent (bī-vā'lĕnt) ["+ *valens,* powerful]. 1. Having a valence of two. 2. Double, as a chromosome consisting of two joined chromosomes. 3. A bivalent chromosome.

biven'ter ["+ *venter,* belly]. A muscle with two bellies; pert. to several muscles.

biven'tral. Digastric; with two bellies.

Bjerrum's screen (byĕr'ūm). [J. Bjerrum, Dan. ophthalmologist, 1827-1892] Tangent plane for mapping field of vision, esp. central and paracentral scotomata.

Bjerrum's sign. One seen in glaucoma, an arcuate or comet-shaped blind spot usually found in central zone of the visual field.

Bk. Chem. symb. for berkelium.

B.L. Abbr. for *buccolingual.*

black (blăk) [AS. *blaec*]. 1. Devoid of color; reflecting no light. 2. Marked by dark pigmentation.

  b. bone. Animal charcoal.

  b. death. A contagious, malignant disease, as the bubonic plague.

  b. eye. Subcutaneous extravasation of blood into the eye or orbit, usually the result of injury. SYM: Pain, swelling, discoloration. TREATMENT: Cold applications with pressure for 12-24 hr. tend to prevent swelling.

  b. fever. Kala-azar, q.v.

  b. heel. Small bluish-black areas of macular pigmentation in the keratin layer of the heel. Due to small areas of spontaneously-occurring hemorrhage. Condition is harmless but may be mistaken for a plantar wart or melanoma.

  b. measles. A severe type of measles in which the eruption is very dark because of hemorrhage under the skin.

  b. vomit. The vomiting of black matter as in yellow fever. The black discoloration usually is caused by the presence of blood in the vomitus.

blackberries. The dark fruit of a plant of the genus Rubus.

  Food value of 100 gm. (canned, water packed without sugar added): Cal. 40; protein and fat less than 1%; calcium 22 mg.; iron 0.6 mg.; vitamin A, 140 I.U.; ascorbic acid 7 mg.

blackhead. A plug of dried sebum in a sebaceous gland. SYN: *comedo.*

black lung. Lay term for the chronic lung disease or pneumoconiosis found in coal miners. SYN: *coal worker's pneumoconiosis.*

blackout. 1. Temporary loss of consciousness. 2. In aviators, temporary or transient loss of vision or consciousness due to a fall of blood pressure in the head. This is caused by the centrifugal force experienced in high-speed aircraft maneuvers.

  b., alcoholic. B. which occurs in advanced, severe, chronic alcoholism.

blackwater fever. Malarial hemoglobinuria following chronic falciparum malaria.

  SYM. AND SIGNS: Sudden onset, fever, tender and enlarged liver and spleen, dark urine, epigastric pain, vomiting, jaundice, sudden shock.

black widow. A poisonous spider, Lactrodectus mactans. Its bite causes severe abdominal cramps.

  TREATMENT: Intravenous injection of calcium gluconate.

bladder [AS. *blaedre*]. 1. A membranous sac or receptacle for a secretion, as the gallbladder, q.v. 2. The vesicle which acts as a reservoir for urine. SEE: *b., urinary; genitourinary system* and *urinary tract* for illustrations.

  b., atony of. Inability to urinate due to lack of muscular tone.

  b., autonomous. One in which there is interruption in both afferent and efferent limbs of reflex arcs. Bladder sensations absent; dribbling constant; residual urine large in amount.

  b., exstrophy of. Congenital eversion of the urinary b. The abdominal wall fails to close and the inside of the b. may be seen to protrude through the abdominal wall.

b., hypertonic. 1. B. with excessive muscular tone. 2. Increased muscular activity of the b.

b., irritable. Marked by a constant desire to urinate.

b., nervous. Irritable b. with incomplete urination.

b., neurogenic. Dysfunction from lesion of central nervous system or nerves supplying the b.

b., spastic. An overactive b. with reduced capacity and incontinence.

b., stammering of. Interruption of urination.

b., urinary. The muscular, membranous, distensible reservoir for the urine which it receives from the kidneys through the ureters and which it discharges from the body through the urethra. Its function is that of a reservoir for urine. SYN: *vesica urinaria* [NA].

ANAT: The lower portion continuous with the urethra, called the neck; its upper tip, connected with the umbilicus by median umbilical ligament, called the apex. The region between the two openings of the two ureters and the urethra is the trigone. The wall of the bladder consists of an inner mucous layer of transitional epithelium, a muscular coat of smooth muscle, the outer layer comprising the detrusor urinae, and a fibrous layer. On its free superior surface is a layer of peritoneum.

The bladder is supported by numerous ligaments, supplied by the superior, middle, and inferior vesical arteries, and numerous veins and lymphatics, and innervated with nerves derived from the third and fourth sacral by way of the hypogastric plexus.

It is situated in the anterior part of the pelvic cavity, in front of the anterior wall of the vagina and the uterus, and in the male it lies in front of the rectum. It has a storage capacity in health of one-half liter (500 ml.) or more. In disease states it may be greatly distended. A frequent cause of distention of the bladder in elderly males is hypertrophy of the prostate gland which surrounds the urethra and neck of the bladder.

PHYS: An average of 40-50 oz. (about 1.2-1.5 liters) of urine are secreted within a 24-hr. period. This value is quite dependent upon amount of fluid ingested and loss of fluid through sweat and the bowels. Inability to empty the bladder is known as retention and may call for catheterization. Sphincter muscles are part of the mechanism which controls retention within the b.

The force of urination is much greater in the child than in the adult because the bladder is more nearly an abdominal than pelvic organ in the child. Thus the abdominal muscles help to expel the urine in the child.

PALPATION OF: The b. cannot be palpated when empty. When full it appears as a tumor in the hypogastric region, which, on palpation, is smooth and oval.

PERCUSSION OF: When containing urine its rounded margin is easily made out by observing the tympanic sound of the intestines on one hand, and dull sound of the bladder on the other.

b. worm. A larval form of tapeworm with a rounded cyst or b. into which a scolex is invaginated. The bladder worm of Taenia solium (pork tapeworm) encysts in muscles of pigs; that of Taenia saginata (beef tapeworm) in muscles of cattle. SYN: *cysticercus.*

bland [L. *blandus*]. Soothing, mild.

b. diet. Diet soothing in flavor and texture; all food which causes chemical, mechanical, or thermal irritation is avoided.

Blandin's glands (blŏn-dăn'). [Phillippe F. Blandin, Fr. surgeon, 1798-1849]. Glandula lingualis anterior or Nuhn's glands. Glands near tip of tongue.

blast [Gr. *blastŏs*, germ]. 1. A primitive cell of any group. The word may be used as a word termination as in erythroblast. 2. A violent movement of air such as accompanies the explosion of a shell or bomb; a violent sound as the blast of a horn.

b. injury. A clinical condition which follows severe nonpenetrating chest injuries due to explosions. Underwater explosions may cause this injury to swimmers.

blaste'ma [Gr. *blastēma*, sprout]. Immature or primitive material from which cells and tissues are formed.

blas'tid [Gr. *blastos*, germ]. The clear space marking site of the organizing nucleus in the impregnated ovum.

blasto- [Gr. *blastos*, germ]. Prefix indicating germ or bud.

blastocele (blăs'tō-sēl) ["+ *koilos*, hollow]. The cavity of the blastula, an embryonic stage of development; the segmentation cavity.

blastochyle (blăs'tō-kīl) ["+ *chylos*, juice]. Blastocelic fluid.

blastocyst (blăs'tō-sīst) [Gr. *blastos*, germ, + *kystis*, bag]. A stage in the development of a mammalian embryo which follows the morula. It consists of an outer layer or trophoblast to which is attached an inner cell mass. The enclosed cavity is the blastocele. The whole is called blastodermic vesicle or blastocyst.

blastocyte (blăs'tō-sīt) ["+ *kytos*, cell]. The morula after change into a cyst.

blastocytoma (blăs-tō-sī-tō'mă) ["+ "+ -ōma, tumor]. Blastoma, q.v.

blas'toderm ["+ derma, skin]. A disk of cells (germinal disk or blastodisk) that develops on the surface of the yolk in an avian or reptilian egg from which the embryo develops; also applied to the embryonic disk of mammalian embryos, a disk of cells lying between the yolk sac and the amniotic cavity from which the embryo develops. From the blastoderm, the three germ layers, ectoderm, mesoderm, and endoderm, arise.

blastoderm'ic vesicle. A blastocyst, q.v.

blastogenesis (blăs"tō-jĕn'ĕ-sĭs) [Gr. blastos, germ, + genesis, generation]. 1. Multiplication by budding. 2. Transmission of characteristics from parents to offspring by the germ cells.

blastokinin (blăs"tō-kī'nĭn). Protein present in the rabbit uterus at the time of implantation of the fertilized ovum. Its role in reproductive physiology is being investigated. SYN: uteroglobin.

blastol'ysis ["+ lysis, dissolution]. Lysis or destruction of a germ cell or a blastoderm.

blasto'ma ["+ -ōma, tumor]. (pl. blastomata) A granular tumor formed by a single type of tissue, including fibromas and chondromas.

blastomere (blăs'tō-mēr) [Gr. blastos, germ, + meros, a part]. One of the cells resulting from the cleavage or segmentation of a fertilized ovum.

blastomerotomy (blăs"tō-mēr-ŏt'ō-mĭ) ["+ "+ tomē, incision]. Destruction of blastomeres.

Blastomyces (blăst-ō-mī'sēz) [Gr. blastos, germ, + mykes, fungus]. (pl. Blastomycetes) A genus of pathogenic yeastlike organisms. They are dimorphic, occurring as budding yeastlike forms in tissues, but forming a mycelium in cultures.

   B. brasiliensis. Fungus causing South American blastomycosis. This organism and disease are also called coccidiodes brasiliensis and paracoccidioidomycosis, respectively.

   B. dermatitidis. The pathogen that causes North American blastomycosis, a rare fungus infection in man.

blastomycetes (blăs"tō-mī-sē'tēz). Saccharomycetes; budding fungi; yeast fungi.

blastomyco'sis [Gr. blastos, germ, + mykēs, fungus, + -ōsis, condition]. A disease caused by budding yeastlike fungi in the tissues.

   b., North American. A rare fungus infection caused by Blastomyces dermatitidis. Marked by inflammatory lesions of skin (cutaneous form) or lungs (pulmonary form), or a generalized invasion of skin, lungs,

bones, central nervous system, kidneys, liver, and spleen (systemic form).

   b., South American. A serious infection caused by Blastomyces brasiliensis. Marked by inflammatory lesions of skin, mucous membranes, and internal organs. SYN: paracoccidiodes brasiliensis.

blastophore (blăs'tō-fōr) ["+ phoros, bearing]. The part of the sperm cell which is not converted into the sperm.

blastopore (blăs'tō-pōr) [Gr. blastos, germ, + poros, passageway]. The small opening into the archenteron made by invagination of the blastula.

blas'tospore ["+ sporos, seed]. A spore formed by budding from a hypha.

blastula (blăs'tū-lă) [L.]. (pl. blastulae) An early stage in the development of an ovum, consisting of a hollow sphere of cells enclosing a cavity, the blastocele. In large-yolked eggs, the blastocele is reduced to a narrow slit. In mammalian development, the blastocyst or blastodermic vesicle corresponds to the blastula of lower forms.

blas'tular. Pert. to a blastula.

Blatta (blăt'ă) [L.]. A genus of insects of the order Orthoptera which includes the cockroaches.

   B. germanica. The German cockroach or croton bug.

   B. orientalis. The oriental cockroach, a common house pest. SYN: black beetle.

bleaching powder. Chlorinated lime or calcium hypochlorite.

blear-eye. Marginal blepharitis. Chronic inflammation of margins of eyelids.

bleb. Elevation of the epidermis, irregularly shaped. A blister or a bulla.

   May vary in size from a bean to a goose egg and contain serous, seropurulent, or bloody fluid. A primary skin lesion. May occur in dermatitis herpetiformis, pemphigus and syphilis. SEE: bulla.

bleeder [AS. blēdan, to bleed]. One whose ability to coagulate blood is either deficient or absent. Thus small cuts and injuries lead to profuse bleeding. Such a person may be treated with one of several blood fractions to assist in arresting bleeding following trauma. SEE: hemophilia.

blee'der's disease. Hemophilia; a congenital blood condition marked by inability of blood to coagulate. SEE: coagulation.

bleeding [AS. blēdan, to bleed]. 1. Emitting blood. 2. Process of emitting blood, as a hemorrhage or operation of letting blood.

   Normally when plasma of the blood is exposed to air it changes to allow fibrin to form. This entangles the corpuscles and

Bleeding: Arrest of*
For Wounds of the Face

Artery	Bone Against Which Pressure Is Applied	Course	Spot to Apply Pressure
Temporal	Temporal bone	Upwards of $\frac{1}{2}$ in. (13 mm.) in front of ear	Against bony prominence immediately in front of the ear or on temple
Facial	Low part of lower maxilla	Across the jaw diagonally upward from below	An inch (2.5 cm.) in front of angle of lower jaw on the face
Carotid	Cervical vertebrae	From outer upper edge of sternum to angle of jaw	Deeply down and backwards an inch (2.5 cm.) to the side of the prominence of the windpipe

For Wounds of the Upper Extremity

Artery	Bone Against Which Pressure Is Applied	Course	Spot to Apply Pressure
Subclavian	First rib behind clavicle	Across middle of first rib to armpit	Deeply down and backwards over center of clavicle against first rib (depress the shoulder first)
Axillary	Head of humerus	Descends across outer side of armpit to inside of humerus	High up in the armpit against upper part of humerus
Brachial	Shaft of humerus	Along inner side of humerus under edge of biceps muscle	Against shaft of humerus by pulling aside and gripping biceps, pressing deep down tips of fingers against the bone

For Wounds of the Lower Extremity

Artery	Bone Against Which Pressure Is Applied	Course	Spot to Apply Pressure
Femoral	Brim of pelvis	Down the thigh from the pelvis to the knee from a point midway between iliac spine and symphysis pubis to inner side of end of femur at knee joint	Against brim of pelvis, midway between iliac spine and symphysis pubis
Femoral	Shaft of femur		High up on the inner side of the thigh, about 3 inches (7.6 cm.) below brim of pelvis, over the line given in the direction of the knee
Posterior Tibial	Inner side of tibia, low down above ankle	Downwards to foot in hollow just behind the prominence of inner ankle	For wounds in the sole of the foot: against the tibia in center of the hollow behind the inner ankle

*Hilda M. Gration, R.N.

forms a blood clot. SEE: *blood, clotting of; hemorrhage.*

b., **arterial.** Indicated by bleeding in spurts. Color, bright red.

TREATMENT: Pressure with fingers at nearest pressure point between it and heart. Locate artery and apply digital pressure above it until bleeding stops or until the artery is ligated.

b., **breakthrough.** Intermenstrual bleeding, esp. that which occurs during use of progestational agents.

b., **occult.** Inapparent bleeding, esp. that which occurs into the intestines and can be detected only by chemical tests of the feces.

b. time. Time required for blood to stop flowing from a small wound. This test is done by using one of several techniques. Depending on the method used, the time may vary from 1-3 minutes (Duke method) to 1-9 minutes (Ivy method).

b., venous. Continuous flow of dark red blood.

TREATMENT: Patient recumbent. Pressure below wound with wound between heart and hand. Bandage over wound above and below.

blenn-, blenno- [Gr. *blennos,* mucus]. Combining form meaning mucus or pert. to it.

blennadenitis (blĕn-ăd-ĕ-nī′tĭs) [″+ *adēn,* gland, + *-itis,* inflammation]. Inflammation of mucous glands.

blennemesis (blĕn-ĕm′ĕ-sĭs) [″+ *emesis,* vomiting]. Vomiting of mucus.

blennogenic, blennogenous (blĕn-ō-jĕn′ĭk, blĕn-ŏj′ĕ-nŭs) [″+ *gennan,* to produce]. Secreting mucus.

blennoid (blĕn′oyd) [Gr. *blennos,* mucus, + *eidos,* form]. Like mucus; mucoid.

blennometritis (blĕn-ō-mĕ-trī′tĭs) [″+ *mētra,* womb, + *-itis,* inflammation]. Inflammation of the uterus.

blennophthalmia (blĕn-ŏf-thăl′mĭ-ă) [″+ *ophthalmos,* eye]. 1. Catarrhal conjunctivitis. 2. Gonorrheal ophthalmia.

blennorrhagia (blĕn-ō-rā′jĭ-ă) [″+ *rhēgnynai,* to break forth]. 1. A discharge from mucus membranes, esp. gonorrheal discharges from the genital or urinary tract. 2. Gonorrhea. SEE: *blennorrhea.*

blennorrhagic (blĕn-ō-răj′ĭk). Pert. to blennorrhea; blennorrheal.

blennorrhea (blĕn-ō-rē′ă) [Gr. *blennos,* mucus, + *rhoia,* flow]. Discharge from mucus membranes, esp. gonorrheal discharge from genital or urinary tract. SYN: *blennorrhagia.*

b., inclusion. Inflammation of conjunctiva in newborn. Caused by a filtrable virus that forms cytoplasmic inclusion bodies in the epithelial cells.

b. neonatorum. Ophthalmia neonatorum caused by gonococci.

blennorrheal (blĕn-ō-rē′ăl). Blennorrhagic; pert. to blennorrhea.

blennostasis (blĕn-ŏs′tă-sĭs) [Gr. *blennos,* mucus, + *stasis,* a halt]. The checking of any mucus discharge.

blennostat′ic. Diminishing mucus secretion.

blennothorax (blĕn″ō-thō′răks) [Gr. *blennos,* mucus, + *thōrax,* chest]. Accumulation of mucus in bronchial tubes or alveoli.

blennuria (blĕn-ū′rĭ-ă) [″+ *ouron,* urine]. Excess of mucus in the urine.

blepharadenitis (blĕf′ăr-ăd-ĕ-nī′tĭs) [Gr. *blepharon,* eyelid, + *adēn,* gland, + *-itis,* inflammation]. Inflammation of the meibomian glands. SYN: *blepharoadenitis.*

blepharal (blĕf′ăr-ăl). Pert. to an eyelid.

blepharectomy (blĕf′ă-rĕk′tō-mī) [Gr. *blepharon,* eyelid, + *ektomē,* excision]. Surgical excision of a lesion of the eyelid.

blepharedema (blĕf-ăr-ĕ-dē′mă) [″+ *oidēma,* swelling]. Swelling of the eyelids.

blepharelosis (blĕf″ăr-ĕl-ō′sĭs) [″+ *eilein,* to roll]. Ingrowing eyelashes.

bleph′arism [Gr. *blepharon,* eyelid, + *ismos,* condition]. Twitching or blinking of the eyelids.

blepharitis (blĕf′ăr-ī′tĭs) [″+ *-itis,* inflammation]. Inflammation of the edges of the eyelids involving hair follicles and glands opening on surface; ulcerative and nonulcerative.

ETIOL: In ulcerative type, bacterial infection usually by staphylococci; in nonulcerative type, cause is often unknown. May be due to allergy, exposure to dust, smoke, or irritating chemicals.

SYM: Lids red, tender, and sore with sticky exudate, ulcers on edges; lids may become inverted with lashes falling out and epiphora, q.v., occurring. Styes and meibomian cysts are associated with the condition.

NP: Bathe lids with warm saline solution to remove crusts. Ointment to edges.

b. angularis. B. in which medial angle of the eye is involved with blocking of openings of lacrimal ducts.

b. ciliaris. Inflammation affecting the ciliary margins of the eyelids.

b. marginalis. B. ciliaris, q.v.

b. parasitica. B. caused by parasites such as mites or lice.

b. squamosa. B. with scaling.

b. ulcerosa. B. with ulceration.

blepharo- [Gr. *blepharon,* eyelid]. Prefix pert. to the eyelid.

blepharoadenitis (blĕf′ăr-ō-ăd″ĕ-nī′tĭs) [″+ *adēn,* gland, + *-itis,* inflammation]. Inflammation of meibomian glands.

blepharoadenoma (blĕf′ăr-ō-ăd-ĕ-nō′mă) [″+ ″+ *-ōma,* tumor]. Adenoma or glandular tumor of eyelid.

blepharoatheroma (blĕf′ăr-ō-ăth″ĕ-rō′mă) [Gr. *blepharon,* eyelid, + *athērē,* thick fluid, + *-ōma,* tumor]. Sebaceous cyst of an eyelid.

blepharochalasis (blĕf′ăr-ō-kăl′ă-sĭs) [″+ *chalasis,* relaxation]. Relaxation of skin of eyelid due to loss of elasticity following edematous swellings such as in recurrent angioneurotic edema of lids. The redundant skin may droop over the edge of the eyelid when the eyes are open.

blepharochromidrosis (blĕf'ăr-ō-krō-mī-drō'sĭs) ["+ *chrōma,* color, + *hidrōs,* sweat]. Discolored sweat of the eyelid.

blepharoclonus (blĕf'ă-rŏk'lō-nŭs) [Gr. *blepharon,* eyelid, + *klonos,* tumult]. Clonic spasm of the muscles that close the eyelids (orbicularis oculi).

blepharoconjunctivitis (blĕf'ă-rō-cŏn-jŭnk"tĭ-vī'tĭs) ["+ L. *conjunctiva,* + Gr. *-itis,* inflammation]. Inflammation of eyelids and conjunctiva.

blepharodiastasis (blĕf-ă-rō-dī-ăs'tă-sĭs) ["+ *diastasis,* separation]. Excessive separation of eyelids, causing eye to open wide.

blepharolithiasis (blĕf'ă-rō-lĭth-ī'ă-sĭs) ["+ *lithos,* stone]. Concretions within the eyelid.

blepharon (blĕf'ă-rŏn) [Gr.]. The eyelid; palpebra.

blepharoncus (blĕf'ă-rŏn'kŭs) ["+ *onkos,* tumor]. Tumor of the eyelid.

blepharopachynsis (blĕf'ă-rō-pă-kĭn'sĭs) ["+ *pachynsis,* thickening]. Thickening of the eyelid.

blepharophimosis (blĕf-ă-rō-fī-mō'sĭs) [Gr. *blepharon,* eyelid, + *phimōsis,* narrowing]. Narrowing of slit between eyelids at external angle of eye due to angle being covered by vertical fold of skin.

blepharophryplasty (blĕf'ă-rŏf'rĭ-plăs"tĭ) ["+ *ophrys,* eyebrow, + *plassein,* to mold]. Plastic operation for restoration of eyelid and eyebrow.

bleph'aroplast. A minute mass of chromatin in a cell forming the base of a flagellum. Morphologically it is identical to a centriole. SYN: *basal body.*

blepharoplasty (blĕf'ă-rō-plăs-tĭ). Plastic operation upon the eyelid.

blepharoplegia (blĕf'ă-rō-plē'jĭ-ă) [Gr. *blepharon,* eyelid, + *plēgē,* a stroke]. Paralysis of an eyelid.

blepharoptosis (blĕf'ă-rō-tō'sĭs) ["+ *ptōsis,* a falling]. Drooping of the upper eyelid.

blepharopyorrhea (blĕf'ă-rō-pī-ō-rē'ă) ["+ *pyon,* pus, + *rhoia,* flow]. Pus flowing from the eyelid.

blepharorrhaphy (blĕf'ă-rōr'ă-fĭ) [Gr. *blepharon,* eyelid, + *rhaphē,* seam]. Reducing length of or obliterating palpebral fissure by stitching margins of eyelids. May be required to prevent damage to the cornea. SYN: *tarsorraphy.*

blepharorrhea (blĕf-ă-rō-rē'ă) ["+ *rhoia,* flow]. Discharge from the eyelid.

blepharospasm (blĕf'ă-rō-spăsm) ["+ *spasmos,* spasm]. A twitching or spasmodic contraction of the orbicularis oculi muscle due

to habit spasm, eyestrain, or nervous irritability.

blepharosphincterectomy (blĕf'ă-rō-sfĭnk-tĕr-ĕk'tō-mĭ) [Gr. *blepharon,* eyelid, + *sphinktēr,* a constrictor, + *ektomē,* excision]. Excision of part of the orbicularis palpebrarum to relieve pressure of eyelid on cornea.

blepharostat (blĕf'ă-rō-stăt) ["+ *histanai,* cause to stand]. Device for separating the eyelids during an operation.

blepharostenosis (blĕf'ă-rō-stĕn-ō'sĭs) ["+ *stenōsis,* a narrowing]. Narrowing of the palpebral slit through inability to open the eye normally.

blepharosynechia (blĕf'ă-rō-sĭ-nĕk'ĭ-ă) [Gr. *blepharon,* eyelid, + *synecheia,* a holding together]. Permanent adhesion of the eyelids.

blepharotomy (blĕf-ă-rŏt'ō-mĭ) ["+ *tomē,* a cutting]. Cutting of eyelid.

blepsopathia (blĕp"sō-păth'ĭ-ă) [Gr. *blepsis,* sight, + *pathos,* disease]. Neurasthenia caused by excessive eyestrain.

blind [AS. *blind*]. Without the sense of sight.

   b. spot. Physiological scotoma situated 15° to outside of visual fixation point; corresponds to point where optic nerve enters the eye (optic disk), a region devoid of rods and cones. SYN: *optic disk.*

blindness. Amaurosis; loss of sight.

   b., amnesic color. Inability to remember names of colors seen.

   b., color. Inability to distinguish one or more primary colors. SYN: *achromatopsia.*

   b., cortical. B. resulting from a lesion of visual area of cerebral cortex.

   b., day. Inability to see in daylight; hemeralopia.

   b., eclipse. B. due to burning the macula while viewing an eclipse without using protective lenses.

   b., hysterical. Partial or total b. associated with attacks of hysteria and occurring in absence of any organic defect.

   b., letter. Inability to understand the meaning of letters; a form of aphasia.

   b., night. Nyctalopia; inability to see at night.

   b., psychic. Sight without recognition due to brain lesion.

   b., snow. B. resulting from glare of sunlight upon the snow. May result in photophobia and conjunctivitis, the latter resulting from effects of ultraviolet rays. Usually temporary.

   b., word. Inability to understand written or printed words.

blindness, words pert. to: ablepsia; acatamathesia; achloropsia; "achro-" words;

acritochromacy; aglaukopsia; amaurosis; amaurotic; aphemesthesia; axanthopsia; blindness; blind spot; chionablepsia; hemeralopia; hemiachromatopsia; hemianopia; meropia; nyctamblyopia; nyctophobia; nyctotyphlosis; tritanopia; typhlology; xanthocyanopia.

blister [M. Dutch *bluyster,* a swelling]. 1. A bleb or vesicle containing serum, sometimes caused by a pressure. 2. A collection of fluid below the epidermis, usually the result of a burn. 3. An agent producing a bleb.

TREATMENT: Mild antiseptic, protective dressing; if extremely painful because of pressure, may be aseptically punctured and then treated as a wound.

b., blood. Small subcutaneous or intracutaneous extravasation of blood due to rupture of blood vessels.

TREATMENT: Apply antiseptic and a firm dressing with moderate pressure to aid in stopping extravasation and hasten absorption. Sometimes desirable to puncture aseptically and aspirate.

b., fever. Herpes simplex of lip.

b., fly. Produced by application of cantharides to the skin.

b., flying. A therapeutic b. used long enough to produce redness but not actual blistering.

b., water. B. containing water.

bloated (blōt'ĕd) [AS. *blouɫ*]. Swollen or distended beyond normal size as by serum, water, gas, etc.

block [M. Dutch *blok,* trunk of a tree]. 1. An obstruction or stoppage. 2. To stop the passage of sensory impulses in a nerve, nerve trunk, dorsal root of a spinal nerve, or spinal cord thus depriving a patient of sensation in the area involved. Accomplished by injection of a local anesthetic. SEE: *anesthesia.* 3. To obstruct any passageway or opening.

b., air. A leakage of air from the respiratory passageways and its accumulation in connective tissues of the lungs, there forming an obstruction to the normal flow of air.

b., atrioventricular. SYN: *A-V block.* SEE: *heart block.*

b., ear. Blockage of auditory tube to the middle ear. May result from trauma or from infection.

b., field. Regional anesthesia in which a limited operative area is walled off by an anesthetic.

b., heart. Interferences with the heart's contraction, causing dissociation of the atrial and ventricular rhythms. Due to failure of the contractile impulses to pass through the conductile tissue (atrioventricular node and bundle of His). SEE: *heart block.*

b., neuromuscular. A disturbance in transmission of impulses from motor endplate to a muscle. May be caused by an excess or deficiency of acetylcholine or by drugs which have an action simulating these effects.

b., paravertebral. Infiltration of stellate ganglion with a local anesthetic.

b., sinoatrial. SEE: *heart block, sinoatrial.*

b., spinal. Blockage in the flow of cerebrospinal fluid within spinal canal.

b., ventricular. Interference in the flow of cerebrospinal fluid between the ventricles or from the ventricles through the foramina to the subarachnoid space.

blocking. 1. Interruption in free association during psychoanalysis as a defense against unpleasant ideas. 2. A sudden, unaccountable stoppage of speech or thought. May be due to a conflict or painful thought. 3. Process of obstructing or deadening, as a nerve.

blood [AS. *blōd*]. The fluid that circulates through the heart, arteries, veins, and capillaries carrying nourishment, electrolytes, hormones, vitamins, antibodies, heat, and oxygen to the tissues and taking away waste matter and carbon dioxide. SYN: L. *sangius;* Gr. *haima.*

FUNCT: Nutrition and respiration of tissues located far from the food and air supplies; transportation of waste from the tissues to the excretory organs; chemical and thermal regulation and coordination of the body; defense against infection through the action of antibodies, q.v., and phagocytes, q.v.

COMP: Human blood is composed of a fluid part (plasma) in which are suspended red and white corpuscles, platelets, and fat globules, and a great variety of chemical substances including carbohydrates, proteins, hormones, and some oxygen. Blood consists of 22% solids and 78% water.

Expressed in metric units, an adult weighing 70 kg. has a blood volume of about 5 liters or 70 ml./kg. of body weight. The blood specific gravity varies from 1.048 to 1.066, the corpuscles being heavier and plasma lighter than this. Blood is of slightly higher specific gravity in men than in women. Specific gravity is higher after exercise and at night.

In passing through the lungs the blood gives up carbon dioxide; after leaving the heart it is carried to the tissues as arterial blood, and then returned to the heart. It moves in the aorta at an average speed of 30 cm./second and it makes the circuit of the vascular system in about 20 seconds. It constitutes approximately 7 to 8% of the body weight. SEE: *blood count; circulation; corpuscle; plasma; platelet.*

CHARACTERISTICS: It has a distinctive odor. Arterial blood is bright red or scarlet; the venous blood dark red or crimson.

b., clotting of. The process whereby blood changes into a jelly-like, nonfluid mass. Blood plasma normally contains fibrinogen, a protein. Thrombin is formed from elements present in the blood when blood is exposed to air, foreign substances, or juices from injured tissues. Thrombin converts fibrinogen into the insoluble fibrin, a stringy, elastic substance that forms a meshwork in which the corpuscles are caught. Calcium deficiency causes tendency to slow clotting. SEE: *coagulation.*

b. components. Blood may be transfused in its whole state or one of its components may be administered. The following are blood components.

Antihemophilic concentrates: Fractions of the blood rich in antihemophilic globulin. Prepared from quick-frozen plasma. *Immune and hyperimmune serum (gamma) globulin.* Protein fractions used for persons who are deficient in gamma globulin or to produce passive immunity against certain diseases such as viral hepatitis.

Packed red cells: Blood from which the plasma has been removed. Used for patients who need red blood cells but do not need plasma. Use of this component reduces over-

Blood Components

				Mean Values
Blood	Water 78%	Proteins (serum)	. . . .	14%
		Glucose	. . . .	0.80
	Solids 22%	Lipids (fats) (serum)	. . . .	0.45–0.85

Blood
- Cells
  - Red blood cells (Erythrocytes)
  - White blood cells (Leukocytes)
  - Platelets
- Plasma
  - Water
  - Gases
    - Oxygen
    - Carbon dioxide
    - Nitrogen
  - Nutrients
    - Carbohydrate (Glucose)
    - Fat (fatty acids)
    - Protein (amino acids)
  - Blood proteins
    - Serum albumin
    - Serum globulin
    - Fibrinogen
  - Salts
    - Chlorides
    - Bicarbonates
    - Sulfates
    - Phosphates
    —— of ——
    - Sodium
    - Calcium
    - Potassium
    - Magnesium
  - Protective substances
    - Antibodies
    - Opsonins
    - Agglutinin
    - Bacteriolysins
  - Hormones
  - Excretory products
    - Urea
    - Uric acid
    - Creatinine
    - Xanthine
    - Hypoxanthine
    - Guanine
    - Adenine
    - Carnine

load of the circulatory system and the risk of undesired antigenic response to the blood. *Packed frozen red cells:* Type O, Rh-negative blood cells which have been separated from the plasma and frozen in a solution of glycerol, glucose, fructose, and sodium ethylenediamine tetra-acetic acid (Na_2 EDTA). The cells are thawed just before transfusion. The advantage of this technique is that the blood may be stored in a frozen state at –80° C. for as long as a year.

Plasma: Blood from which the cellular material has been removed. Though widely used in World War II and subsequently, the use of plasma has decreased. The risk of viral hepatitis when pooled plasma is used is considerable.

b., cord. A specimen of blood obtained from the umbilical cord vein or artery of the fetus.

b., defibrinated. If whole blood is stirred in a dish (e.g., with a stick of wood) the stringy, elastic fibrin comes out on the stirrer; it can be washed until white. The remaining thick, red blood can no longer clot, and is called defibrinated blood.

If it is centrifuged, the clear liquid which now appears in the upper half of the centrifuged tube is called serum; this differs from plasma chiefly in that it does not contain fibrinogen (the parent substance of fibrin). The corpuscles are in the lower half of the tube.

b., occult. The presence of blood in such quantity that it is not apparent to the eye. Thus blood may be present in feces but of such color and consistency as to be unnoticed by the patient.

b., sludged. Blood in which red corpuscles have massed together in the smaller blood vessels, and block or slow the blood flowing through the vessels.

RS: erythrocyte; leukocyte.

blood bank. The place where whole blood and certain derived components are processed, typed, and stored until needed for transfusion. Blood is mixed with sodium citrate, physiological saline solution, and glucose (ACD solution), and is stored at 4° C. (39° F.).

Banked blood should be used as soon as possible because the longer it is stored the fewer red blood cells survive in usable form. 90% of the red cells survive up to 14 days of storage but only 70% remain after 24 days.

blood cell. Minute body in the blood of two types: erythrocytes or red blood corpuscles, and leukocytes or white blood corpuscles. SYN: *blood corpuscle.*

b.c. casts. Masses of red cells molded by

the renal tubules, the blood originating from the glomeruli. Abnormal microscopic body in the urine composed of coagulated serum covered with red blood cells.

blood clot. Coagulated mass of blood. SYN: *coagulum.* SEE: *blood, clotting of.*

blood corpuscles. The solid or cellular elements in the blood. SYN: *b. cell.* SEE: *erythrocytes; leukocytes.*

blood count. Enumeration of the red corpuscles and the leukocytes per cu. mm.

A blood count indicates the number of cells. The differential blood count tells the percentage of the various white cells in each 100 cells counted.

Normally in each cu. mm. of blood there are an average of five million erythrocytes in the male and four and a half million in the female. Prolonged exposure to altitude increases the number. The leukocytes average 5,000 to 10,000/cu. mm. Platelets average 200,000 to 300,000/cu. mm. by direct counting method.

A special chamber is filled with blood and the cells are counted using the microscope. The type of fluid used to dilute the blood depends upon whether the white or red cells are to be counted.

The differential white blood cell count is done by counting at least 200 cells in the blood which has been placed on a microscope slide in a thin layer and stained. Pathologic cells are looked for also. The platelets are either counted or estimated from the appearance of the blood on the microscope slide. Hemoglobin and hematocrit are deter-

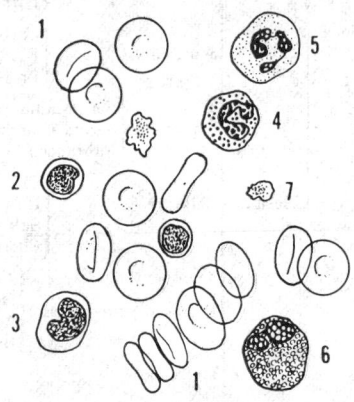

BLOOD CELLS

1, Red blood cells. 2, Immature (nucleated) red blood cells. 3, Lymphocyte. 4, Eosinophil. 5, Neutrophilic leukocyte. 6, Basophil. 7, Blood platelet.

Tabular Summary of Blood Corpuscles

Corpuscles (Cells)	Nucleus	Cytoplasm		Average diameter (Microns)	Number per cu. mm.
		Color	Granules		
Erythrocytes or red blood corpuscles	Absent	Red	None	7.2–7.8	4.2–6.2 million (lower in women than in men)
Platelets (Not true cells)	?	None	None	2–4	150,000 to 450,000
Leukocytes or white blood corpuscles	Varies with different types	None	Varies with different types	7–20	5,000 to 10,000

mined from samples of whole blood.

b.c., differential. Determined by microscopic examination of a very thin layer of blood on a glass slide after it has been suitably stained in order to demonstrate the various cells. The number of the variety of white cells in each 200 counted is obtained. Also, even though the red cells are not counted by this method, their shape, size, and color can be evaluated.

Some blood diseases and inflammatory conditions may be recognized in this way. In a differential count, the varieties of the leukocytes and their percentages normally should be: Neutrophils (segmented), 40-60%; eosinophils, 1-3%; basophils, 0-1.0%; lymphocytes, 20-40%; monocytes, 4-8%. SEE: *blood examinations.*

blood crossmatching. The process of mixing a sample of the donor's red blood cells with the recipient's serum (major crossmatching), and mixing a sample of the recipient's blood with the donor's serum (minor crossmatching). This is used before transfusion to determine compatibility of blood.

blood donor. One who gives blood to be used for transfusion.

blood dust. Minute colorless bodies in the blood, particles of the blood corpuscle. SYN: *hemoconia.*

blood examinations. Morphological, chemical, physical, bacteriological, or serological studies of blood.

Blood is difficult to study because it clots so promptly unless anticoagulants are added to it. SEE: *blood components* for table.

WHAT THE EXAMINER LOOKS FOR: The number and character of red blood cells, the percentage of hemoglobin, the coagulation time, q.v., the number and character of white blood cells, the presence of parasites; also in chemical tests the amount of sugar, urea, urea-nitrogen, nonprotein nitrogen, creatinine, and uric acid. Immunological and serological tests may determine various infections including syphilis and certain viral diseases. Culture should be made if bacteria are suspected.

CHEMICAL FINDINGS: The following ranges of values for some of the chemical constituents of blood are within so-called normal limits. Deviations from these amounts, while not necessarily a sign of disease, indicate a need for further investigation or repeat of the test to help validate the original result.

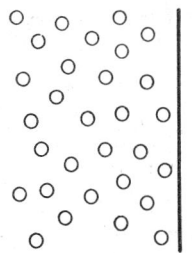 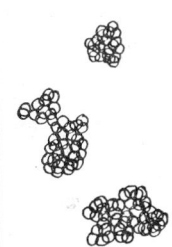

BLOOD—MAJOR CROSSMATCHING
The red blood cells of the donor are mixed with the serum of the recipient. Left, compatibility, no agglutination; Right, incompatibility with formation of clumps. This donor's blood cannot be used for this particular patient.

Calcium: 4.5-5.5 mEq./L. (9.0 to 11 mg./100 ml.) serum. Carbon dioxide combining power: 24-29 mEq./L., 53-64 vol.% (whole blood). Chloride: 100-106 mEq./L. serum. Cholesterol, total: 150-250 mg./100 ml. serum. Creatinine: 0.7-1.5 mg./100 ml. serum. Glucose (fasting): 61-100 mg./100 ml. of blood. Nonprotein nitrogen: 15-35 mg./100 ml. serum. Sodium: 136-145 mEq./L. serum. Urea nitrogen: 10-20 mg./100 ml. whole blood. Uric acid: 3.0-6.0 mg./100 ml. serum.

Whenever blood is to be collected from a vein the following points should be observed: (1) Not only should the syringe and needle be sterile, but also dry or washed out with sterile normal saline solution. In particular the syringe should contain no trace of alcohol or ether, and preferably no distilled water.

(2) The blood withdrawn is put into test tubes which are sterile and either plain dry or oxalated (i.e., containing a small quantity of sodium or potassium oxalate powder). Plain tubes are required for Wassermann reaction, Widal and other agglutination reactions, van den Bergh reaction, blood calcium. Oxalated tubes are required for blood sugar, blood urea, nonprotein nitrogen (N.P.N.), etc.

(3) Immediately after the blood has been expelled from the syringe, both the needle and syringe should be washed out with normal saline or cold water. In this way jamming of the piston is avoided. Of course this is unnecessary if disposable needles and syringes are used.

blood groups. The separation of human bloods into four groups based on the presence or absence of agglutinogens in red cells and agglutinins in the plasma. Agglutination and hemolysis may occur when incompatible bloods are mixed, followed by severe systemic reactions and possibly death. Blood groups have a hereditary basis and are dependent upon a series of alternative gene (triple alleles), a fact sometimes utilized in helping to solve problems of disputed parentage. The groups are designated by the letters O, A, B, AB. SYN: *blood types.* SEE *agglutinogen.*

bloodless. Without blood.

b. operation. Operation in which the blood is expelled by compresses from the part which is to be operated upon, or performing surgery by using electrocautery.

blood-letting. Removal of blood from the body, usually by venipuncture.

Method of Testing Blood Groups

Serum of Group	Agglutinin in Serum	Recipient Red Blood Cells of Group				Remarks
		O	A	B	AB	
O	Anti-A and Anti-B					Cells of Group O *not* agglutinated by any sera. Contains no agglutinable substances
A	Anti-B					Cells of Group A agglutinated by sera of Groups O and B
B	Anti-A					Cells of Group B agglutinated by sera of Groups O and A
AB	None					Cells of Group AB agglutinated by sera of Groups O, A, B. Serum of Group AB contains no isoagglutinins

When recipient is Group   O, select Donor from Group O
When recipient is Group   A, select Donor from Group O or A
When recipient is Group   B, select Donor from Group O or B
When recipient is Group AB, select Donor from Group O, A, B, AB

blood platelets. Small, colorless bodies in circulating blood, averaging about 3 microns in diameter, which tend to agglutinate into small clusters in shed blood. They may originate from giant bone marrow cells (megakaryocytes). They play an important role in clotting through release of thrombokinase which, in the presence of calcium, reacts with prothrombin to form thrombin.

The normal number in circulating blood is about 200,000-500,000/cu. mm. Reduction below normal is called thrombocytopenia. In certain forms of hemophilia, blood platelets are abnormally stable and fail to release thrombokinase, thus increasing coagulation time.

blood poisoning. A vague term usually used to indicate the presence of large numbers of bacteria in the circulating blood. SEE: *pyemia; septicemia; toxemia.*

blood pressure. As popularly used, the pressure, determined indirectly, existing in the large arteries at the height of the pulse wave; the systolic intra-arterial pressure.

More generally, the pressure exerted by the blood on the wall of any vessel. This pressure reaches its highest values in the left ventricle during systole. It decreases in the arterial system as the distance from the heart increases, and is lower in capillaries than in the arteries.

The systolic arterial blood pressure itself rises during activity or excitement and falls during sleep. In the normal, relaxed, sitting adult, it may be as low as 100 and as high as 140 mm. of mercury.

The following findings are considered abnormal: systolic pressure persistently above 140; diastolic pressure persistently above 100; pulse pressure constantly greater than 50.

Blood pressure varies with age, sex, altitude, muscular development, and according to states of worry and fatigue. Usually it is lower in women than in men, low in childhood and high in advancing age as a rule. SEE: *b.p., normal.*

b.p., central. B.p. in the heart chambers, in a great vein, or close to the heart. If determined in a vein it is termed central venous b.p.; if in the aorta or a similar large artery close to the heart it is designated central arterial b.p.

b.p., diastolic. That existing during relaxation phase between heart beats, normally about 80 mm. Hg. It is dependent primarily upon the elasticity of the arteries and peripheral resistance which in turn is dependent upon caliber of arterioles and capillaries.

b.p., direct measurement of. Determining the b.p. in one of several arteries. Done by placing a sterile needle or small catheter inside an artery and having the b.p. transmitted through that system to a suitable recorder. As the b.p. fluctuates the changes are recorded graphically.

b.p., indirect measurement of. A simple method for measuring b.p.

Palpatory method: The same arm, usually the right, should be used each time the pressure is measured. The arm should be at the level of the heart and the patient should be sitting or recumbent. Either a mercury-gravity or aneroid-manometer type of blood pressure apparatus may be used. The blood compression cuff should be the width and length appropriate for the size of the subject's arm: narrow (2.5-6 cm.) for infants and children and wide (13 cm.) for adults.

The deflated cuff is placed evenly and snugly around the upper arm so that its lower edge is about one inch above the point of the brachial artery where the bell of the stethoscope will be applied. While feeling the radial pulse, inflate the cuff until the pressure is about 30 mm. above the point where the radial pulse was no longer felt. Deflate the cuff slowly and record as accurately as possible the pressure at which the pulse returns to the radial artery. Systolic b.p. is determined by this method; diastolic b.p. cannot be determined by this method.

Auscultatory method: Begin as above. After inflating the cuff until the pressure is about 30 mm. above the point where the radial pulse disappears, place the bell of the stethoscope over the brachial artery just below the blood pressure cuff. Then deflate the cuff slowly, about 2-3 mm. of mercury per heart beat. The first sound heard from the artery is recorded as the systolic pressure. The point at which sounds are no longer heard is recorded as the diastolic pressure. For convenience the blood pressure is recorded as figures separated by a slant. The systolic value is recorded first. For example, 120/80 indicates systolic pressure of 120 and diastolic of 80.

Sounds heard over the brachial artery change in quality at some point prior to the point the sounds completely disappear. Some physicians consider this the diastolic pressure. This value should be noted when recording the b.p. by placing it between the systolic pressure and the pressure noted when the sound disappears. Thus 120/90/80 would indicate a systolic pressure of 120 with a first diastolic pressure of 90 and a second diastolic pressure of 80. The latter pressure would be the point of disappearance of all sounds from the artery. When the values are so recorded the physician may use either of the last two figures as the diastolic pressure. When the change in sound and the disappearance of all sound coincide, the result should be written as follows: 120/80/80.

b.p., mean. Half of the sum of systolic and diastolic values. For a normal person in good health, about 100 mm. Hg.

b.p. monitor. A device which automatically obtains and usually records the b.p. at certain intervals. The apparatus may use the direct or indirect method of determining pressure. In some models an alarm or light signal is activated if the pressure rises or falls to abnormal levels.

b.p., negative. That which is less than atmospheric pressure as in the great veins near the heart.

b.p., normal. In healthy young persons, 100-120 mm. of mercury systolic and 60-80 mm. diastolic. Upper limits of normal are 140/100, with systolic pressure greater than 140 mm. generally believed to be abnormal. Loss of resilience in the vascular tree and physiological changes of age must be considered when levels above 140 mm. are obtained in apparently healthy, older persons.

b.p., systolic. The greatest force caused by the contraction of the left ventricle of the heart.

RS: diastole; hypertension; hypotension; pulse pressure; systole.

bloodshot. Locally congested with blood.

blood shunting. A condition in which blood, by going through an abnormal pathway or bypass, does not travel its normal route. May occur when an arteriovenous fistula forms, or in congenital anomalies of the heart in which the blood passes from the right auricle or ventricle directly to the left auricle or ventricle respectively, through a defect in the wall (septum) that normally separates the auricles and ventricles.

blood smear. Drop of blood spread on a slide for purpose of examination.

PROCEDURE: Clean glass with alcohol, rinse in warm water, and wipe clean with lint-free towel or lens paper. Slide must be grease-free. Place a small drop of blood on the slide. Bring the end of another slide (spreader slide) against first slide at a 45° angle and pull it back against drop of blood so that the drop will spread between the two slides. Then push spreader slide forward against the first slide and the blood will follow forming an even smear. Smear must be thin. Dry slide by waving in air. Do not heat.

STAIN: A common method is as follows: Cover the blood smear with Wright's stain. Allow to stand 2 min. Add an equal amount of distilled water or buffer solution, mixing uniformly. Let stand 5 min. Gently wash off stain. Allow to dry. If permanent slide is desired, mount with balsam or methacrylate.

blood substitute. One of several substances used to expand the plasma volume of the blood in cases where whole blood is unavailable.

blood sugar. Sugar in the form of glucose, normally 60-100 mg./100 ml. of blood.

It rises after a meal to as much as 150 mg./100 ml. of blood but this may vary.

b.s. test. Increased glucose content of the blood or presence of glucose in the urine indicates impaired metabolism which may be due to diabetes.

blood test. A test to determine the chemical, physical, or serological characteristics of the blood or some portion of it.

blood, test for, in urine. To several ml. of urine in a test tube, add 1 or 2 drops of tincture of guaiacum. Carefully overlay this with 1/2 in. (1.2 cm.) of ether. Hold the tube in the hand to warm it for a few minutes. Blood is indicated by the appearance of a blue line at the junction of the fluids.

blood transfusion. Transfer of blood of one person into blood vessels of another. In direct or immediate transfusion, the blood is transferred via a tube directly from the donor to the recipient. In indirect or mediate transfusion, the blood is collected in a receptacle from the donor before transfusion.

blood typing. The method used to determine various factors when blood is tested according to blood group systems such as A-B-O, M-N, and Rh-Hr.

PROCEDURE: Place a drop of 2% saline suspension of patient's blood cells on each end of a slide labeling the drops A and B. Add a small drop of A typing serum to the A drop, of B typing serum to the B drop. Mix thoroughly. After 5 min. examine for agglutination. Type of blood can be determined by reactions as follows: No agglutination—Type O; Drop A only agglutinated—Type B; Drop B agglutinated only—Type A; Both drops agglutinated—Type AB. SEE: *blood groups* for table.

bloody flux. Dysentery.

bloody sweat. Excretion of blood or blood pigment through the sweat glands. SYN: *hemathidrosis.*

bloody vomit. A result of rupture of the blood vessels of the upper alimentary tract due to injury, disease, or swallowing of blood.

TREATMENT: Do not give stimulants; nothing by mouth. Keep patient quiet and lying down. Cold applications to lower chest and upper abdomen.

loody weeping. Hemorrhage from conjuctiva.

lotch. A blemish, spot, or area of discoloration on the skin.

low'fly. One of a number of genera of flies belonging to the family Calliphoridae. Most are scavengers, their larvae living in decaying flesh or meat although occasionally they may live in decaying or suppurating tissue. However, one species, the screw-worm fly, Callitroga hominivorax, attacks living tissue, laying its eggs in the nostrils or open wounds of the host domestic animals or man giving rise to myiasis.

blowpipe. A tube through which a gas is passed under pressure, the gas being directed upon a flame. It is employed to concentrate and intensify the heat of the flame.

blue [O.Fr. *bleu*]. 1. A primary color of the spectrum; sky color; azure. 2. Cyanotic.

b. baby. A child born with a very b. color due to mixture of the venous and arterial blood through a defect in the heart.

b., brilliant cresyl. A dye used in staining blood.

b. drum. Bluish appearance of tympanic membrane.

b., Evans. A dye, injected intravenously, for determining blood volume.

b. mass. A compound pill of mercury.

b., methylene. A dye used for staining tissues or as an indicator.

b. ointment. Mercurial ointment.

b. stone. Copper sulfate, q.v.

b., toluidine. A metachromatic dye used as a stain for tissues.

b. vitriol. Copper sulfate, q.v.

blueberries. The blue or blue-black fruit of several types of bush of the genus Vaccinium.

Food value of 100 gm. (raw): Cal. 62; protein 0.7 gm.; carbohydrate 15.3 gm.; calcium 15 mg.; iron 1.0 mg.; vitamin A, 100 I.U.; ascorbic acid 14 mg.

bluecomb. A disease of turkeys characterized by cyanosis. It is due to infection with Erysipelothrix rhuziopathiae.

Blumberg's sign (blum'berg). [Jacob Moritz Blumberg, Ger. surgeon and gynecologist, 1873-1955]. The occurrence of a sharp acute pain when the examiner presses his hand over McBurney's point and then releases the hand pressure suddenly. This sign is indicative of peritoneal inflammation.

Blumenbach's clivus (blu'men-bach). [Johann F. Blumenbach, Ger. physiologist and anthropologist, 1752-1840]. Sloping part of sphenoid bone behind posterior clinoid processes.

blush'ing [AS. *blyscan*, to be red]. Rush of blood to the face and neck caused by embarrassment or other emotion.

Blyth's test. [Alexander W. Blyth, Eng. physician, 1846-1921]. A test for the detection of lead in drinking water. In the presence of lead a white precipitate forms on the addition of a small amount of alcoholic tincture of cochineal to the water to be tested.

B.M.A. Abbr. for *British Medical Association.*

B.M.R. Abbr. for *basal metabolic rate.*

B.M.S. Abbr. for *Bachelor of Medical Science.*

BNA. Abbr. for *Basle Nomina Anatomica*, an anatomical nomenclature adopted by the German Anatomical Society in 1895, at Basel, Switzerland. It includes some 4500 terms.

Boas' point (bo'az). [Ismar I. Boas, Ger. physician, 1858-1938]. A tender spot left of the 12th dorsal vertebra in patients with gastric ulcer.

Boas' reagent. Formula for testing hydrochloric acid in gastric juice.

Boas' sign. The presence of lactic acid in the gastric contents.

Bochdalek's ganglion (bŏk'dăl-ĕk). [Victor Bochdalek, anatomist in Prague, 1801-1883]. Ganglion of plexus of dental nerve in the maxilla above the canine tooth.

Bodo (bo'do). A genus of the Bodonidae, flagellate protozoa often found in stale feces or urine and sometimes in the urinary bladder. Nonpathogenic.

body [AS. *bodig*, body; Gr. *sōma*; L. *corpus*]. 1. The physical man. 2. The trunk without the head and extremities. 3. The principal part of anything. 4. A small organ or a structure within an organ.

EXAMINATION: The nude body is examined and both sides compared. Physical examination is made by inspection, palpation, manipulation, mensuration, and auscultation, q.v. Physical examination should also include observation of the body as the person walks and as he goes through the various ranges of motions of the trunk, neck, and extremities. Chemical and microscopic examination may be made of the blood, sputum, feces, urine, cerebrospinal fluids, and other fluids of the body. X-ray or roentgen ray is also used and checked with clinical findings. The electrocardiograph is used for determining heart rhythms.

b., acetone. One of a number of substances which increase in the blood as the result of faulty fat metabolism. SYN: *b.'s, ketone, q.v.*

b., aortic. Two small b.'s located in the arch of the aorta which contain the endings of the aortic nerve. They respond to oxygen concentration in the blood and to changes in blood pressure.

b., Aschoff. Microscopic foci of fibrinoid degeneration and granulomatous inflammation found in various tissues in rheumatic fever.

b., Barr. Sex chromatin present at the edge of the nucleus of cells from the female.

b., basal. A basal granule or blepharoblast. A small granule usually present at the base of a flagellum or a cilium in protozoa.

b., carotid. A flat structure at the bifurcation of the common carotid artery. Contains cells which respond to changes in concentration of oxygen in the blood and to changes in blood pressure.

b., cavernous. One of three cylindrical b.'s of erectile tissue found in the penis. SEE: *corpora cavernosa penis.*

b. cavities. The thorax, abdomen, and pelvis.

b. cell. 1. The main portion of a cell, esp. a neuron; the portion that contains the nucleus. 2. Somatic cell. Any cell of the body excepting the reproductive or germinal cells.

b., chromaffin. A number of b.'s composed principally of chromaffin cells, q.v., which lie serially arranged along both sides of the dorsal aorta. Also called paraganglionic b.'s. They are ectodermal in origin, having the same origin as cells of the sympathetic ganglia.

b., chromatoid. Darkly staining b.'s found in the encysted forms of parasitic amebae. Thought to serve as reserve food. They disappear as cysts grow older.

b., chromophilic. One of the granular bodies in cytoplasm of a nerve cell which stain readily with basic dyes.

b., ciliary. A structure in the eye consisting of the ciliary muscle and ciliary processes. Functions in accommodation.

b., coccygeal. A mass of tissue consisting of one or several small nodules located at tip of coccyx. It contains an arteriovenous anastomosis. Its function is unknown.

b., Donovan's. Donovania granulomatis. Organism causing granuloma inguinale.

b., geniculate, lateral. Two b.'s forming elevations on the lateral portion of the posterior part of the thalamus. Each is the termination of afferent fibers from the retina which they receive through the optic nerves and tracts.

b., geniculate, medial. Two b.'s lying in the posterior part of the dorsal thalamus. Each receives fibers from the acoustic center of the medulla and from the inferior colliculus through the brachium.

b., Hassall's. Hassall's corpuscle, found in the medulla of the thymus.

b., Hensen's. A modified Golgi net found in the hair cells of the organ of Corti.

b., inclusion. Cell inclusions. Non-living substances in the protoplasm of a cell. Seen in virus infections.

b.'s, ketone. One of a number of substances which increase in the blood as a result of faulty fat metabolism. Among them are B-hydroxybutyric acid, acetoacetic acid and acetone. They increase in diabetes mellitus and are the primary cause of acidosis. They may also occur in other metabolic disturbances. SYN: *acetone b.'s.*

b.'s, Leishman-Donovan. Small b.'s found in the spleen and liver of victims of kala-azar or dum-dum fever. Now known to be Leishmania donovani, causative organism of the disease. They are found both within and outside of living cells and in circulating blood.

b., malpighian. (1) A renal corpuscle consisting of a glomerulus enclosed in Bowman's capsule; (2) a lymph nodule found in the spleen.

b., mammillary. A rounded b. of gray matter found in the diencephalon. It forms a rounded eminence projecting into the anterior portion of the interpeduncular fossa. Their nuclei constitute an important relay station for olfactory impulses.

b., medullary. The deeper white matter of the cerebellum enclosed within the cortex.

b., metachromatic. Metachromatic granule, q.v.

b.'s, Negri. Inclusion b.'s found in the cells of the central nervous system of animals infected with rabies. They are acidophilic masses appearing in large ganglion cells or in cells of the brain esp. those of the hippocampus and cerebellum.

b.'s, Nissl. Also called Nissl granules or chromophil substance. Conspicuous structures in nerve cells demonstrated by selective staining. They are absent in the axon and axon-hillock. They show changes under various physiological conditions and in pathological conditions may dissolve and disappear (chromatolysis). SYN: *tigroid b.*

b., pacchionian. Arachnoid granulation. Numerous small ovoid or villus-like projections of the arachnoid membrane of the brain. They may project into the superior sagittal sinus as arachnoid villi or they may press against the outer dura and grow into the inner plate of the cranium forming ovoid depressions. SYN: *arachnoid villi.*

b., perineal. The mass of tissue which separates the anus from the vestibule and the lower part of the vagina.

b., pineal. A gland-like structure in the brain which is shaped like a pine cone. It is located in a pocket near the splenium of the corpus collosum. Its exact neuroendocrine function is unknown. SYN: *pineal gland.*

b., pituitary. The hypophysis; pituitary gland, q.v.

b., polar. A small cell produced in oogenesis resulting from the divisions of the primary and secondary oocytes. It has no functional significance.

b., postbranchial. Ultimobranchial b.'s. Two b.'s which develop from the posterior wall of the 4th pharyngeal pouch. They become incorporated into the thyroid gland.

b., psammoma. Laminated calcareous b.'s seen in certain types of tumors. Term also applied to sandlike b.'s (brain sand) found in the pineal b. Also seen in prostate gland.

b., restiform. The inferior cerebellar peduncles. Two bands of fibers which connect the medulla with the cerebellum.

b., tigroid. The chromophil substance of neurons; Nissl bodies.

b., vertebral. A short column of bone forming the weight-supporting portion of a vertebra. From its dorsolateral surfaces project the roots of the arch of a vertebra.

b., vitreous. A jelly-like substance within the eye which fills the space between the lens and the retina. It is colorless, structureless, and transparent.

b., wolffian. The mesonephros or middle kidney of the embryo.

body image. The subjective image or picture an individual has of his physical appearance based on his own observations and the reaction of others.

body mechanics. Mechanical correlation of the various systems of the body.

body snatching. Robbing a grave of its body. Done in the past to obtain bodies for anatomical study in medical schools.

body type. Classification of the human body according to certain physical characteristics. SEE: *somatotype.*

Boeck's sarcoid (bĕk). [Caesar P. M. Boeck, Norwegian physician, 1845-1917]. Sarcoidosis, q.v.

boil [AS. *byl,* a swelling]. A furuncle. An acute circumscribed inflammation of the subcu-

taneous layers of the skin, gland, or hair follicle.

The deeper tissue inflammation is so severe that blood clots in the vessels and the center dies. This is the cause of the acuteness of the pain; the dead core is ultimately expelled or reabsorbed. Contrary to general opinion, boils do not arise from "bad blood," but are the result of local infection due to an invasion of staphylococci.

TREATMENT: Protect from irritation; apply moist heat intermittently. Keep skin scrupulously clean and avoid injury or trauma to involved region. Bed rest may be necessary in severe cases. After lesions are fluctuant, surgical incision and debridement may be desirable. The area around draining abscesses should be protected by an antibiotic ointment to prevent new lesions on surrounding areas. If lesions are large and located on the face, penicillin or some other antibiotic should be used systemically to prevent possible complications such as meningitis or septicemia.

b., Aleppo. SEE: *leishmaniasis, cutaneous.*

b., oriental. SEE: *leishmaniasis, cutaneous.*

boiling. Vaporization of a liquid. Boiling water destroys most microorganisms but may not kill spores and some viruses; toughens and hardens albumin in eggs; toughens fibrin and dissolves tissues in meat; bursts starch granules; softens cellulose in cereals and vegetables.

b. point. The degree of heat required to bring a liquid to a boil. It depends upon the liquid. Water boils at 212° F. (100° C.) under ordinary conditions at sea level. To kill microorganisms, water should be boiled 3-15 minutes. Aeration (pouring from one vessel to another) will overcome the flat taste of boiled water. ABBR: bp.; b.p.

bolometer (bō-lŏm'ĕ-tĕr) [Gr. *bolē,* a throw, ray, + *metron,* measure]. 1. Device for measuring the force of the heart beat apart from blood pressure. 2. An instrument for gauging minute degrees of radiant heat.

bo'lus [L. from Gr. *bōlos,* a lump]. A pill-shaped mass.

b., alimentary. A mass of masticated food ready to swallow.

bond. A force which binds ions or atoms together. It is represented by a line drawn from one molecule or atom to another as in H—O—H.

bone [AS. *bān,* bone]. 1. Osseous tissue, a specialized form of dense connective tissue consisting of bone cells (osteocytes) embedded in a matrix consisting of calcified intercellular substance. 2. An individual unit of the skeleton. SYN: *os*, q.v.

B.'s give shape to and support the body. They also serve as a storage place for mineral salts and play an important role in the formation of blood cells.

B. consists of about 50% water and 50% solid matter, the solids being chiefly cartilage hardened by impregnation with inorganic salts, esp. carbonate and phosphate of lime. The proportion of lime in b. gradually increases and in old age there is such a large proportion that the b.'s are brittle and break easily.

They surround and protect some vital organs, and give points of attachment for the muscles, serving as levers and making movement possible.

The outer surface is less porous than the inner and is called the compact tissue; the more porous portion is called cancellous tissue. The compact tissue is tunneled by a central canal containing marrow and fine branching canals. In these canals run small blood vessels and lymphatics for the maintenance and repair of b. tissue. This is known as the haversian system or canals. The exterior covering of the b., or periosteum, serves to extend the blood supply to the b. According to their shape, b.'s are classified as flat, irregular, long, and short.

For depressions, openings, and cavities in b.'s: SEE: *antrum* (nearly enclosed cavity); *canal; fissure* (slitlike opening); *foramen* (opening for blood vessels and nerves); *fossa* (concavity); *groove; meatus* (tubelike passage or opening; canal); *sinus* (air cavity within a bone; or groove lodging a blood sinus); *sulcus* (groove).

For processes (enlargements or protrusions) of b.'s: SEE: *crest* (a ridge); *condyle* (rounded process for articulation); *head* (rounded end of a bone separated from body by a constricted region, the neck); *spine* (pointed process); *trochanter* (very large process); *tubercle* (small rounded process); *tuberosity* (large rounded process).

For names of principal b.'s: SEE: *skeleton.*

b. age. Result of x-ray studies of the stage of development of ossification centers of the extremities. Can be utilized to estimate the age of children. SEE: *epiphysis.*

b., ankle. The astragalus or talus.

b. bank. Place for storage of b. to be used in b. grafts.

b., breast. The sternum.

b., brittle. Abnormal brittleness of b.'s. SYN: *osteogenesis imperfecta.*

b., cancellous. A spongy b. in which the matrix forms connecting bars and

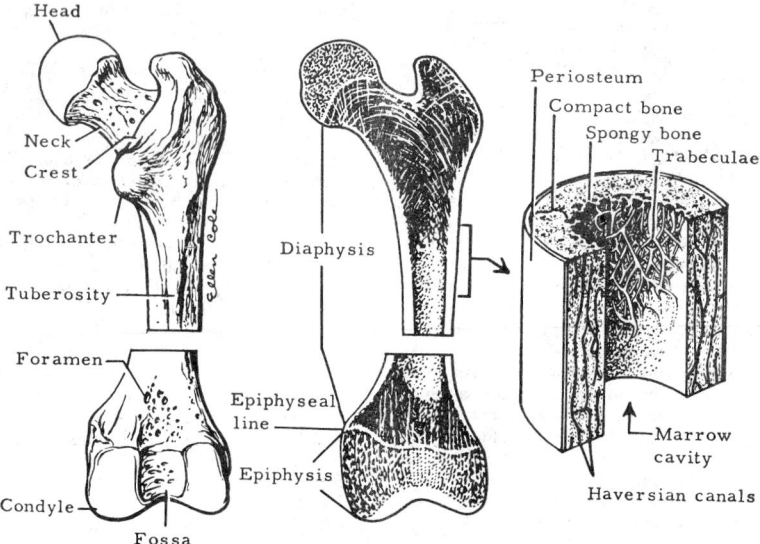

Head
Neck
Crest
Trochanter
Tuberosity
Foramen
Condyle
Fossa
Diaphysis
Epiphyseal line
Epiphysis
Periosteum
Compact bone
Spongy bone
Trabeculae
Marrow cavity
Haversian canals

BONE—Inner and outer structures

plates, partially enclosing many intercommunicating spaces filled with b. marrow.

b., cartilage. Endochondral b. which develops from cartilage.

b., cavalry. Rider's b. Bony formation in adductor magnus femoris.

b. cell. Cell in osseous tissue or b. It may be an osteoblast or bone-forming cell; an osteocyte which lies within a lacuna in bone matrix; or an osteoclast, a giant, multi-nucleated cell occupying deep groves (Howship's lacunae).

b., collar. The clavicle.

b., compact. Dense, hard b. with microscopic spaces.

b., cotyloid. One which during development forms a part of medial portion of the acetabulum. It fuses with the pubis.

b., cranial. A b. of the cranium or brain case.

b. cyst. B. tumor of cystic variety.

b., dermal. A membrane b.

b., endochondral. Cartilage b.

b. graft. A piece of b. taken either from some animal (foreign) or from the body of the patient in which it is to be used (autogenous) and positioned so as to encourage its growth and union with the bone against which it is being placed.

b. grafting. Transplanting a healthy b. to replace missing or defective b.

b., Inca. An incarial b.

b., incarial. The interparietal b., part of the occipital b.

b., incisive. Part of maxilla bearing the incisor teeth.

b., innominate. Hip b., composed of the ilium, ischium, and pubis.

b., intracartilaginous. Cartilage or endochondral b.

b., ivory. B., marble, q.v.

b., marble. Abnormally calcified b.'s with spotted appearance in a roentgenogram. SYN: *Albers-Schönberg disease; ivory b., osteopetrosis.*

b. marrow. Medulla or soft tissues in the hollow of long bones and in the extremities of long bones. SEE: *marrow.*

b. marrow aspiration. Use of a special aspirating needle to obtain a specimen of b. marrow for examination. The material usually is obtained from the upper portion of the sternum or the iliac crest. Examination of the stained marrow is helpful in diagnosing a great number of blood disorders, infections, and malignant diseases.

b., membrane. The intramembranous b.

b., perichondrial. B. formed beneath the perichondrium.

b., periosteal. B. formed by osteoblasts of the periosteum.

b., ping pong. The thin shell of osseous tissue covering a giant cell sarcoma in a b.

b. reflex. A reflex action resulting from tapping or percussion; actually a tendon or muscle reflex.

b., replacement. Cartilage b., one which replaces cartilage.

b., sesamoid. One which develops in tendon, as the patella, or in a joint capsule.

b., spongy. B., cancellous, q.v.

b., sutural. B., wormian, q.v.

b., thigh. The femur.

b., wormian. A small, irregularly shaped b. often found in the sutures of the cranium.

bone'let. A small b.; ossicle.

bonine (bo'nēn). Proprietary name for meclizine hydrochloride, an agent used for prevention and treatment of motion sickness and vomiting. Formerly marketed as bonamine.

bo'ny. Resembling or of the nature of bone. SYN: *osseous.*

boopia (bō-ōp'ī-ă) [Gr. *bous*, ox, + *ōps*, eye]. The uninterested cowlike gaze seen in hysteria.

booster (boo'stĕr). An additional dose of an immunizing agent to increase the protection afforded by the original series of injections. The booster is given some months or years after the initial immunization.

borate (bō'rāt). A basic salt of boric acid.

bo'rated. That to which borax has been added.

borax (bōr'ăks) [L. from Arabic, from Persian *būrah*]. Sodium borate. It is found in some arid regions. Its chief use is as a detergent and water softener; also a weak antiseptic.

borborygmus (bor'bō-rig'mus) [Gr. *borborygmos*, rumbling in the bowels]. (pl. borborygmi) A gurgling, splashing sound heard over the large intestine; caused by passage of flatus through the intestine.

    PATH: Its absence may denote such obstruction of the bowels as torsion, volvulus, or strangulated hernia.

border (bōr'dĕr). The outer part or edge; boundary.

b., brush. A brushlike structure found on the free surface of epithelial cells in the proximal convoluted portion of a renal tubule. It consists of nonmotile hairs.

b., striated. A modified layer of the surface protoplasm of columnar epithelial cells lining the intestine. It consists of regular, perpendicular striations consisting of minute protoplasmic processes.

Bordetella (bor″dĕ-tĕl′lă). [Jules Bordet]. A genus of Brucellaceae. Hemolytic gramnegative coccobacilli. The cause of whooping cough or an infection similar to whooping cough. SYN: *Bordet-Gengou bacillus.*

    B. pertussis. The cause of whooping cough. First isolated by Bordet and Gengou. Formerly called Hemophilus pertussis.

Bordet-Gengou bacillus (bŏr-dā′zhongoo′). [Jules Bordet, Belg. physician, bacteriologist and physiologist, 1870-1961; and Octave Gengou, Fr. bacteriologist, 1875-1957]. Bordetella pertussis, the cause of whooping cough.

boredom. Feeling of tiredness or depression because of lack of activity or challenging and meaningful stimuli. May be due to an inability to become stimulated despite the character of the stimulus. In this case boredom may be considered to be pathological. It is seen in persons who stubbornly cling to the status quo.

boric acid. H_3BO_3. USP. An odorless, white, crystalline powder obtained by condensation and evaporation from certain mineral salts.

    In solution it is used as mild antiseptic wash, esp. for the eyes, mouth, and bladder. As an ointment it is valuable in dressing burns, blisters, etc. When large doses are accidentally taken by mouth, as in children, it may be poisonous.

    POISONING: SEE: *Table of Poisons and Poisoning* in Appendix.

    SYM: Nausea, vomiting, diarrhea.

    TREATMENT: Wash out stomach. Give saline cathartic and large volumes of water. Oxygen and plasma or blood transfusions as necessary.

bo′rism. Symptoms caused by internal use of borax or boron compounds include dry skin, eruptions, gastric disturbances.

boroglycerin (bor″ō-glis′ĕr-ĭn). A compound ($C_3H_5BO_3$) formed when boric acid and glycerin are heated together.

    b. glycerite. A solution of boroglycerin (47-52%) in glycerin.

boroglycerol (bo″ro-glis′er-ŏl). Boroglycerin.

bo′ron [bor(ax) + (carb)on]. SYMB: B. At. wt. 10.81; at. no. 5. A nonmetallic element, found only as a compound such as boric acid or borax.

Borrelia (bor-rel′ĭ-ă). A genus of spirochetes including organisms responsible for relapsing fever.

    B. duttonii. Causative agent for tickborne relapsing fever.

    B. recurrentis. Causative agent of louse-borne relapsing fever.

    B. vincen′tii. A species found in Vincent's angina.

boss [O. Fr. *boce,* a swelling]. Any protuberance, esp. a round circumscribed swelling or growth such as occurs on a bone or tumor.

bosselated (bŏs′ĕ-lāt-ĕd). Marked by numerous bosses.

bossela′tion. One or more small bosses.

Bossi's dilator (bos′sē). [Luigi Maria Bossi, Swiss gynecologist, 1859-1919]. Metal instrument used to dilate the cervix by means of force.

Boston arm. A particular type of prosthesis for persons who have had an arm amputated above the elbow. The arm, which operates by means of a small battery-driven motor, obeys signals received from electric energy produced by movement of the remaining muscle groups. As these muscles move they make the arm function like a normal arm with respect to direction and strength of motion.

botfly (bŏt′flī). (pl. *botflies*) Insects belonging to the order Diptera of the family Oestridae. Parasitic on mammals, especially horses and sheep. Human infestation is rare.

botryoid (bot′rĭ-oyd) [Gr. *botrys,* bunch of grapes, + *eidos,* appearance]. Resembling a bunch of grapes.

botryomycosis (bŏt″rĭ-ō-mī-kō′sĭs) [″ + *mykēs,* fungus]. Condition characterized by chronic granulomatous lesions caused by a fungus of the family Actinomycetaceae. SYN: *staphylococcal actinophytosis.*

bot′tle nose. Acne rosacea of the nose.

botuliform (bot-u′lĭ-form) [L. *botulus,* sausage, + *forma,* shape]. Shaped like a sausage.

botulin′ic acid. A toxin found in putrid sausage.

botulism (bŏt′ū-lĭzm) [L. *botulus,* sausage, + *-ismos,* condition]. A severe form of food poisoning from food containing the botulinus toxin, produced by Clostridium botulinum. This organism is widely found in the soil and in the intestinal tract of domestic animals. Cases of human botulism are usually associated with development of the bacteria under anaerobic conditions in raw, improperly canned or otherwise preserved foods, esp. meats (as ham, sausage) and nonacid vegetables (as string beans). The toxin is a powerful exotoxin. It is very thermolabile losing its toxic properties when exposed to temperature of 80° C. for 30 min. or boiling for 10 min.

    POISONING: The toxin has a selective action on the central nervous system. In fatal cases, cardiac and respiratory paralysis occur through involvement of the medullary centers.

SYM: Fatigue, weakness, dizziness, headache, and digestive complaints as nausea, vomiting, diarrhea and abdominal pain. Progresses to paralysis in the central nervous system, and of the cardiac and respiratory systems.

TREATMENT AND PROPHYLAXIS: Bivalent antitoxin for type A and B toxin should be administered to persons with clinical symptoms and to those persons who have eaten contaminated food but do not have symptoms. Type E antitoxin, which is available only from the Communicable Disease Center, Atlanta, Ga., should also be given. Careful and continuous nursing care is necessary. SEE: *botulinum toxin* in *Table of Poisons and Poisoning* in *Appendix.*

bouba (bū′bă). Spanish-American term for yaws, q.v.

Bouchut's respiration (boo-shooz′). [Jean A. E. Bouchut, Fr. physician, 1818-1891]. Expiration longer than inspiration in children with bronchopneumonia and asthma.

Bouchut's tube. One used for intubation.

bougie (boo′zhē) [Fr. *bougie*, candle]. Instrument for exploring and dilating canals, esp. the male urethra.

    b., armed. One with caustic attached.

bouillon (boo-yawn′) [Fr. *bouillir*, to boil]. Clear broth.

    b. culture. Bouillon used as a basis for a bacteriological culture.

boulimia (boo-lim′ĭ-ă) [Gr. *bous*, ox, + *limos*, hunger]. Abnormal hunger sensation a short time after a meal. SYN: *bulimia*, q.v.

bouquet (boo-kā′) [Fr. nosegay]. 1. The aroma of a wine. 2. A cluster of anything, esp. of blood vessels or nerves.

bourdonnement (boor-dōn-mon′) [Fr. a droning]. A humming sound.

boutonnière operation (boo-tōn-yăr′) [Fr. buttonhole]. 1. Incision through perineum behind an impervious stricture. 2. A buttonhole-like opening in a membrane.

boutons terminaux (boo-tōn′ter-min-ō′) [Fr. terminal button]. Bulblike expansions at the tip of axons which come into synaptic contact with the cell bodies of other neurons.

bovine (bō′vīn) [L. *bovinus*, pert. to a cow]. Pert. to cattle.

    b. lymph. Vaccine virus from a heifer.

bovinoid (bō′vĭ-noyd) ["+ Gr. *eidos*, resemblance]. Like that of cattle; term applied to form of tubercle bacillus found in man which resembles true bovine tubercle bacilli.

bow'el [O. Fr. *boel*, intestine, from L. *botellus*, little sausage]. The intestine.

    b. movement. Evacuation of feces. Number of b. movements varies in normal individuals, some having a movement after each meal, others one in the morning and one at night, and still others only one in several days. Thus to say that the healthy person must have at least one bowel movement a day in order to maintain health is unreasonable and not based on factual evidence. Also it is completely within the range of normal variation to have two to three bowel movements each day. SYN: *defecation.*

bowleg (bō′lĕg). A bending outward of the lower limb. SYN: *bandy leg; genu varum.*

Bowman's capsule (bō′măn). [Sir William Bowman, Eng. physician, 1816-1892] The expanded end of a renal tubule or nephron which invests a glomerulus, the two constituting the renal or malpighian corpuscle. It consists of a visceral layer closely applied to the glomerulus and an outer parietal layer. It functions as a filter in the formation of urine.

Bowman's glands. Branched tubulo-alveolar glands located in the lamina propria of the olfactory membrane which serves to keep the olfactory surface moist.

Bowman's membrane. Thin homogeneous membrane separating corneal epithelium from corneal substance. SEE: *membrane.*

box-note. A hollow sound heard on percussion in emphysema.

box splint. Splint for fractures below the knee.

Boyer's bursa (bwă-yā′). [Baron Alexis de Boyer, Fr. surgeon, 1757-1833]. One anterior to the thyrohyoid membrane.

Boyer's cyst. A subhyoid cyst.

Boyle's law. [Robert Boyle, Brit. physicist, 1627-1691]. The volume of a given mass of gas, at any given temperature, varies inversely with the pressure put upon it.

Bozeman-Fritsch catheter (bōz′man-frĭtch). [Nathan Bozeman, Amer. surgeon, 1825-1905; and Heinrich Fritsch, Ger. gynecologist, 1844-1915] Double lumen uterine catheter with several openings at tip.

B. P., B. Ph. Abbr. for *British Pharmacopoeia.*

Br. Chem. symb. for bromine; abbr. for Brucella.

brachia (brā′kĭ-ă). Pl. of brachium.

brachial (brā′kĭ-ăl) [L. *brachiolis*, from *brachium*, arm]. Pert. to the arm.

    b. artery. Main artery of arm. Continuation of the axillary artery on the inside of the arm.

b. plexus. Network of lower cervical and upper dorsal spinal nerves supplying arm, forearm and hand. SEE: *nerve plexuses* in *Appendix*.

b. veins. Those accompanying the brachial artery.

brachialgia (brā″kĭ-ăl′jĭ-ă) ["+ Gr. *algos,* pain]. Intense pain in the arm.

brachialis (brā-kĭ-ăl′ĭs) [L. *brachiolis,* from *bracchium,* arm]. A muscle of the arm lying immediately under the biceps brachii.

brachio- [L. *bracchium,* arm, from Gr. *brakhiōn,* shorter, hence "upper arm" as opposed to longer forearm]. Prefix: Pert. to the brachium, arm, specifically the upper arm from shoulder to elbow.

brachiocephalic (brā″kĭ-ō-sĕ-fal′ĭk) ["+ Gr. *kephalē,* head]. Pert. to arm and head.

brachiocrural (brā″kĭ-ō-kru′ral) ["+ L. *cruralis,* pert. to the leg]. Pert. to arm and thigh.

brachiocubital (brā″kĭ-ō-kū′bĭ-tăl) ["+ L. *cubitus,* forearm]. Pert. to the arm and forearm.

brachiocyllosis (brā″kĭ-ō-sil-ō′sis) [L. *bracchium,* arm, from Gr. *brakhiōn,* shorter, hence "upper arm" as opposed to longer forearm]. Abnormal curvature of the arm.

brachiofacial (brā″kĭ-ō-fā′shăl) ["+ L. *facialis,* pert. to face]. Pert. to arm and face.

brachioncus (brā-kĭ-on′kus) ["+ Gr. *ogkos,* a swelling]. A chronic, hard swelling of the arm.

brachioradialis (brā″kĭ-ō-rā″dĭ-ā′lĭs) ["+ L. *radialis,* radius]. A muscle lying on lateral side of the forearm. SEE: *Muscles of the Body* in *Appendix*.

brachiotomy (brā″kĭ-ot′ō-mĭ) ["+ Gr. *tomē,* a cutting]. Surgical removal or cutting of an arm of the fetus to facilitate delivery.

brachium (brā′kĭ-um) [L. *bracchium,* arm, from Gr. *brakhiōn,* shorter, hence "upper arm" as opposed to longer forearm]. (pl. *brachia*) [NA]. 1. The upper arm from shoulder to elbow. 2. Anatomic structure resembling an arm.

b. conjunctivum. The superior cerebellar peduncle, q.v.

b. pontis. The middle cerebellar peduncle, q.v.

brachy- [Gr. *brachys,* short]. Prefix for short.

brachybasia (brăk-ĭ-bā′sĭ-ă) ["+ *basis,* walking]. A slow, shuffling gait seen in partial paraplegia. SEE: *gait*.

brachycardia (brăk-ĭ-kar′dĭ-ă) ["+ *kardia,* heart]. Slowness of heart action. SYN: *bradycardia,* q.v.

brachycephalic,   brachycephalous (brăk″ĭ-sĕ-fal′ĭk, -sef′ă-lus) [Gr. *brachys,* short, + *kephalē,* head]. Having a head disporportionately short.

brachycephalism,   brachycephaly (brăk″ĭ-sĕf′ă-lĭzm, -ă-lĭ). Shortness of the head.

brachycheilia (brăk″ĭ-kĭ′lĭ-ă) [Gr. *brachys* short, + *cheilos,* lip]. Condition of having abnormally short lip or lips.

brachydactylia (brăk″ĭ-dăk-tĭl′ĭ-ă) ["+ *daktylos,* finger]. Shortness of the fingers.

brachygnathia (brăk-ĭg-nā′thĭ-ă) ["+ *gnathos,* jaw]. Abnormal shortness or recession of under jaw.

brachymetropia (brăk″ĭ-mĕ-trō′pĭ-ă) [Gr. *brachys,* short, + *metron,* measure, + *opsis* sight]. Myopia; nearsightedness.

brachymetropic (brăk″ĭ-mĕ-trŏp′ĭk). Nearsighted; myopic.

brachyphalangia (brăk″ĭ-fă-lăn′jĭ-ă) [Gr. *brachys,* short, + *phalanx,* finger bone]. Shortness of phalanges.

brachypnea (brăk-ĭp-nē′ă) ["+ *pnoē,* breathing]. Shortness of breath.

brachystasis (brā-kĭs′tă-sĭs) ["+ *stasis,* standstill]. Condition in which a muscle upon contracting does not relax but maintains its shortened state.

brachyuranic (brăk″ĭ-ū-răn′ĭk) ["+ *ouranos,* roof of mouth]. Having a short palate, or a palatomaxillary index over 115.

bradesthesia (brăd-ĕs-thē′zĭ-ă) [Gr. *bradys,* slow, + *aisthēsis,* sensation]. Blunted perception. SYN: *bradyesthesia,* q.v.

Bradford frame. [Edward H. Bradford, Amer. orthopedic surgeon, 1848-1926]. An oblong frame, about 7 x 3 feet, made of 1 in. pipe, covered with canvas strips, which run from one side of the frame to the other and which are movable, thus permitting the patient to urinate and defecate without moving the spine or changing position.

brady- [Gr. *bradys,* slow]. Prefix indicating slow, as bradycardia.

bradyacusia (brad′ĭ-ă-koo′sĭ-ă)   ["+ *akouein,* to hear]. Hardness of hearing.

bradyarthria (brad′ĭ-ar′thrĭ-ă) ["+ *arthron,* articulation]. Bradylalia; unusual slowness of articulation of words.

bradyauxesis (brăd′ĭ-awks-ē′sĭs)   [Gr. *bradys,* slow, + *auxēsis,* increase]. Term applied to the type of growth in which a part grows at a slower rate than that of the organism of which it is a part.

bradycardia (brad′ĭ-kar′dĭ-ă) ["+ *kardia,* heart]. Slow heart action. SEE: *arrhythmia,* *tachycardia.*

b., sinus. A sinus rhythm with a rate below 60 in an adult, or below 70 in a child.

bradycar′dic. Pert. to bradycardia.

bradycinesia (brad′ĭ-sĭ-nē′sĭ-ă) [Gr. *bradys,* slow, + *kinēsis,* movement]. Extreme slowness of movement. SYN: *bradykinesia.*

bradycrotic (brad″ĭ-krot′ik) ["+ *krotos,* pulsation]. Pert. to slowness of pulse.

bradydiastole (brad″ĭ-dĭ-as′tō-lē) [Gr. *bradys,* slow, + *diastole,* dilatation]. Prolongation of the diastolic pause, as in myocardial lesions.

bradyecoia (brad″ĭ-ē-koy′ă) [Gr. *bradyēkoos,* hard of hearing]. Partial deafness.

bradyesthesia (brad″ĭ-ĕs-thē′zĭ-ă) [Gr. *bradys,* slow, + *aisthēsis,* perception]. Blunted perception.

bradyglossia (brad″ĭ-glos′ĭ-ă) ["+ *glōssa,* tongue]. Unusual slowness of speech. SYN: *bradyarthria; bradylalia; bradylogia; bradyphasia; bradyphemia.*

bradykinesia (brad″ĭ-kĭ-nē′sĭ-ă) ["+ *kinēsis,* motion]. Extreme slowness of movement. SYN: *bradycinesia.*

bradykinin (brăd″ĭ-kī′nĭn). A plasma kinin. SEE: *kinin.*

bradylalia (brad″ĭ-lā′lĭ-ă) [Gr. *bradys,* slow, + *lalein,* to talk]. Slowness of speech. SYN: bradylogia; bradyphasia; bradyphemia. SEE: *speech.*

bradylexia (brad″ĭleks′ĭ-ă) ["+ *lexis,* word]. Slowness of reading not attributable to lack of intelligence. SEE: *dyslexia.*

bradypepsia (brad″ĭ-pep′sĭ-ă) ["+ *pepsis,* digestion]. Slow digestion.

bradyphagia (brad″ĭ-fā′jĭ-ă) [Gr. *bradys,* slow, + *phagein,* to eat]. Slowness in eating.

bradyphrasia (brad″ĭ-frā′zĭ-ă) ["+ *phrasis,* utterance]. Slowness of speech; seen in some types of mental disease.

bradyphrenia (brad″ĭ-fre′nĭ-ă) ["+ *phrēn,* mind]. Slowness of mental activity such as may result from epidemic encephalitis.

bradypnea (brad″ip-nē′ă, brad″ĭ-nē′ă) [Gr. *bradys,* slow, + *pnoē,* breathing]. Abnormally slow breathing.

bradyrhythmia (brad″ĭ-rĭth′mĭ-ă) ["+ *rhythmos,* rhythm]. 1. Slowness of heart or pulse rate. 2. In electroencephalography, slowness of brain waves (one to six per sec.).

bradyspermatism (brad-ĭ-sper′mă-tizm) ["+ *sperma,* semen]. Abnormally slow ejaculation of semen.

bradysphygmia (brad″ĭ-sfig′mĭ-ă) [Gr. *bradys,* slow, + *sphygmos,* pulse]. Abnormally slow pulse.

bradystalsis (brad″ĭ-stal′sĭs) ["+ *stalsis,* constriction]. Slow peristalsis.

bradytocia (brad″ĭ-to′sĭ-ă) ["+ *tokos,* childbirth]. Slow parturition.

bradyuria (brad″ĭ-ū′rĭ-ă) [Gr. *bradys,* slow, + *ouron,* urine]. Slowness in passing urine.

braidism (bra′dizm). [James Braid, Eng. surgeon, 1795-1860]. Hypnotism.

braille (brāl). [Louis Braille, Fr. teacher of blind, 1809-1852]. Raised dots on paper used to communicate written language, signs, and symbols to the blind. The dots, which represent numerals and letters of the alphabet, are palpated by the fingers.

brain (brān) [AS. *braegen*]. A large, soft mass of nerve tissue contained within the cranium; the encephalon. Cranial portion of the central nervous system.

STRUCTURE: The b. is composed of neurons which are nerve cells, and neurologia or supporting cells. The brain consists of gray and white matter. Gray matter is composed principally of nerve-cell bodies and is concentrated in the cerebral cortex and the nuclei and basal ganglia. White matter is composed of nerve-cell processes which form tracts or commissures connecting various parts of the brain with each other.

The b. consists of five parts: the cerebrum; cerebellum; pons varolii; medulla oblongata; and midbrain. Of these, the cerebrum represents seven-eighths of the weight of the brain. *Lobes:* Frontal; parietal; occipital; temporal; insula. *Glands:* Pituitary; pineal. *Membranes:* Meninges, consisting of the dura mater (external), arachnoid (middle), and pia mater (internal). *Nerves:* Cranial. SEE: *Nerves, cranial,* in *Appendix.*

Subdivisions of the brain are (1) diencephalon including the epithalamus, thalamus, and hypothalamus (optic chiasma, hypophysis, tuber cinereum, and maxillary bodies); (2) myelencephalon including the corpora quadrigemina, tegmentum, crura cerebri, and the medulla oblongata; (3) metencephalon including the cerebellum and pons; (4) telencephalon including the rhinencephalon, corpora striata, and cerebrum (cerebral cortex).

Ventricles: The cavities of the brain are: the lateral ventricles (one and two) which lie in the cerebral hemispheres; the third ventricle of the diencephalon; and the fourth ventricle of the medulla. The first and second communicate with the third by the interventricular foramina; the third with the fourth by the cerebral canal (aqueduct of Sylvius); the fourth with the subarachnoid spaces by the two foramina of Luschka and the foramen of Magendie. The ventricles are filled with cerebrospinal fluid which is formed by the choroid plexuses in the walls and roofs of the ventricles.

FUNCTIONS: The brain is the primary center for regulating and coordinating body activities. Sensory impulses are received through afferent nerves; these register as sensations which are the basis for perception. It is the seat of consciousness, thought, memory, reason, judgment, and emotion.

Motor impulses are discharged through efferent nerves to muscles and glands initiating activities. Through reflex centers automatic control of body activities is maintained. The most important reflex centers are the cardiac, vasomotor, and respiratory centers which regulate circulation and respiration.

The weight of brain and cord is about 1350-1400 gm., of which total the cord represents 2%. SEE: *spinal cord.*

b. fever. Meningitis.

b. sand. Laminated bodies consisting principally of phosphates, and carbonates of

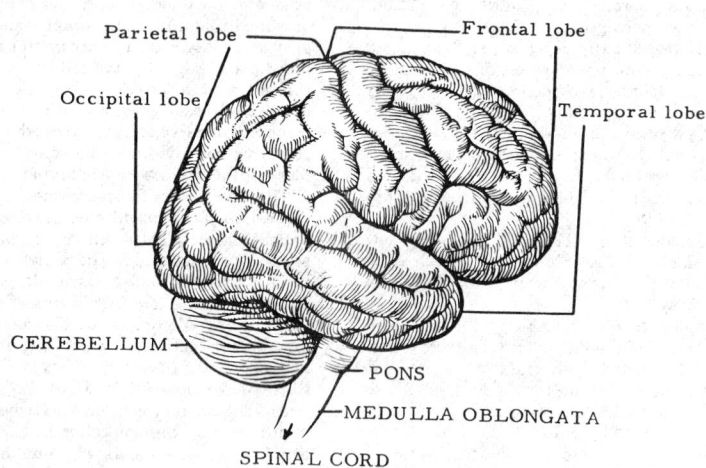

CEREBRUM

Parietal lobe — — Frontal lobe

Occipital lobe — — Temporal lobe

CEREBELLUM —

— PONS

— MEDULLA OBLONGATA

SPINAL CORD

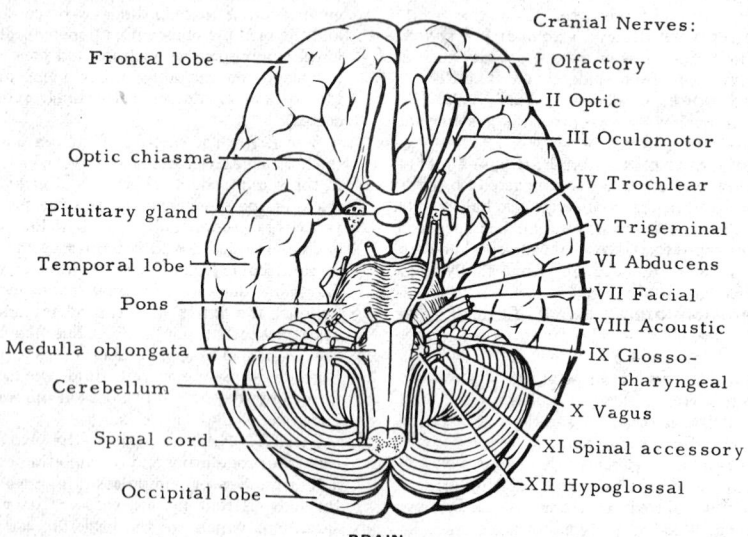

Cranial Nerves:

Frontal lobe — — I Olfactory

— II Optic

— III Oculomotor

Optic chiasma — — IV Trochlear

Pituitary gland — — V Trigeminal

— VI Abducens

Temporal lobe — — VII Facial

Pons — — VIII Acoustic

Medulla oblongata — — IX Glossopharyngeal

Cerebellum — — X Vagus

Spinal cord — — XI Spinal accessory

Occipital lobe — — XII Hypoglossal

BRAIN
Above, lateral exterior view; Below, base of brain.

calcium, and magnesium found in the pineal body called corpora arenacea.

b. stem. All the b. except the cerebellum and cerebrum.

b. storm. Temporary outburst of mental excitement; often maniacal, esp. in paranoia.

b. tumor. Usually used inexactly to describe any intracranial mass, neoplastic, cystic, inflammatory (abscess), or gummatous. Except the latter, treatment depends on surgery and thus on accurate diagnosis.

SYM: The general symptoms are those due to an increase in intracranial pressure such as headache, the change in the retina recognized by opthalmoscopic examination as choked disk, and vomiting (without nausea).

Neoplasms of the brain do not metastasize to other parts of the body.

Malignancies of perineural nerves may appear as isolated lumps. They contain almost no blood vessels. May produce pain or other sensations. The most malignant ones in childhood are gliomas, q.v.

Mental changes (esp. dullness), epileptiform convulsions, giddiness, are often general but may be localized signs. In addition, history and cranial x-ray pictures are of great value. The injection of air into the ventricles prior to x-ray examination is known as pneumoventriculography.

Brain's reflex. [W. Russell Brain, Brit. physician, 1895 —]. Extension of flexed arm on assuming quadripedal posture.

branchial (brăng'kĭ-ăl) [L. *branchia,* gills]. Pert to gills.

b. arches. Five pairs of arched structures which form the lateral and ventral walls of the pharynx of the embryo. They are partially separated from each other externally by the b. clefts; internally, by the pharyngeal pouches. The fifth arch is rudimentary. They play an important role in the formation of structures of the face and neck. The first is the mandibular arch, the second the hyoid arch. They are also called the visceral arches.

b. clefts. A series of openings between the branchial arches. They become functional gill slits in fishes.

b. grooves. A series of furrows separating the branchial arches. They are homologous to the branchial clefts of fishes and amphibians.

b. muscles. Those which develop from the mesoderm of the branchial arches. Include most of muscles of face and neck.

branchiogenic. Branchiogenous, q.v.

branchiogenous (brăng'kĭ-ŏj'ĕ-nŭs) [L. *branchia,* gills, + Gr. *gennan,* to generate]. Having origin in a branchial cleft.

branchioma (brang'kĭ-ō'mă) ["+ *-ōma,* tumor]. A tumor related to the branchial arches.

branchiomeric (brang'kĭ-ō-měr'ĭk) ["+ *meros,* part]. Of or pertaining to the branchial arches.

branchiomerism (brang'kĭ-om'er-izm). Segmental division of the entoderm.

brandy. Spiritous liquor distilled from wine and containing about 50% alcohol by volume.

brash. A burning sensation in the stomach sometimes accompanied by belching of sour fluid. SYN: *heartburn; pyrosis; water b.*

brass founders' ague (ā'gū). Tremors due to zinc poison from inhalation of toxic fumes.

brass poisoning. Due to the inhalation of fumes of zinc and zinc oxide with destruction of tissue in respiratory passage.

SYM: Dryness and burning in respiratory tract; cough; headache; chills; rarely fatal.

TREATMENT: Entirely symptomatic; inhalations of humidified air make patient more comfortable.

Braune's canal (brow'nĕ). [Christian Braune, Ger. anatomist, 1831-1892]. The parturient canal formed by the uterus, dilated cervix and vulva.

Braun's hook (brown). [Gustave von Braun, Austrian gynecologist, 1829-1911]. Instrument for fracturing clavicle or to assist in decapitation of the fetal head.

brawny induration. Pathological hardening and thickening of tissues.

Braxton Hicks sign. [John Braxton Hicks, Eng. gynecologist, 1825-1897]. Intermittent painless uterine contractions which may occur every 10 to 20 minutes. They occur more frequently as pregnancy nears completion. These contractions do not represent true labor pains but are often so interpreted.

Brazil nut. An oily, three-sided nut from the tree Bertholletia excelsa.

Food value of 100 gm. (raw): Cal. 654; protein 14 gm.; fat 67 gm.; calcium 186 mg.; iron 3.4 mg.; carbohydrate 11 gm.

bread. A food made by baking a doughy mixture of flour (wheat, corn, rye, etc.), shortening, a leavening agent, and water. The dough may or may not contain yeast, which would cause air cells due to gas generated during its growth. Food value varies with type of bread.

break. 1. In orthopedics, a fracture. 2. To interrupt continuity in a tissue or electric circuit or channel of flow or communication.

b., chromatid. Fracture of the chromatid. This causes misalignment of the parts and leads to genetic abnormalities.

breakbone fever. Acute epidemic febrile disease. SEE: *dengue.*

breast [AS. *brēost*]. 1. The upper anterior aspect of the chest. 2. Mammary gland, a compound alveolar gland consisting of 15-20 lobes of glandular tissue separated from each other by interlobular septa. Each lobe is drained by a lactiferous duct which opens on the tip of the nipple. The mammary gland secretes milk used for nourishment of young. SEE: *lactiferous glands; milk.*

DEVELOPMENT: During puberty, estrogens from the ovary stimulate growth and development of the duct system; during pregnancy progesterone secreted by the corpus luteum and placenta acts synergistically with estrogens to bring the alveoli to complete development. Following parturition, prolactin (luteotrophin) in conjunction with adrenal corticoids initiates lactation, and oxytocin from the posterior pituitary induces ejection of milk. Suckling or milking reflexly stimulates both milk secretion and discharge of milk.

CHANGES IN PREGNANCY: 6-12 1/2 weeks, fullness and tenderness, erectile tissues in nipples, nodules felt, pigment deposited around nipple (primary areola), (in blondes the areolae and nipples become pinkish, in brunettes they become dark brown and in some cases even black), and few drops of fluid may be squeezed out. 16-20 1/2 weeks (secondary areola), small, whitish spots in pigmentation. Due to hypertrophy of the sebaceous glands. These are the so-called glands of Montgomery.

NP: *Preventive Care:* Most complications of the breast during the puerperal period will not occur if proper care is given.

Use aseptic technique in breast care to avoid infection of infant's mouth as well as mother's breasts. Clean nipples with sterile water before and after each nursing.

Early treatment of soreness, cracks and fissures by the use of sterile nipple shield while the baby nurses and by taking the baby off the breast and pumping the breasts at the time the baby would be due to nurse. Pumping should be done under very low pressure and should be repeated until the nipple is well healed. This does away with the danger of infection from the infant's mouth and prevents him from making matters worse by his forceful nursing suction. Antiseptic oil, ointments, etc., may be used to favor the healing process.

Limit the nursing period during the first three days when no breast milk is available and during the engorgement period when the breasts are extremely sensitive from congestion and distention with milk. The use of the electric pump is stressed during this time.

Avoid bruising of the breasts. The use of the electric breast pump in place of excessively firm manual massage during the extreme sensitive period will prevent this.

Keep the nipples soft to avoid cracking. Applications which harden them predispose to cracking.

Avoid caking of the breasts by the use of the breast pump to remove any excess milk which may plug the ducts. In the home it

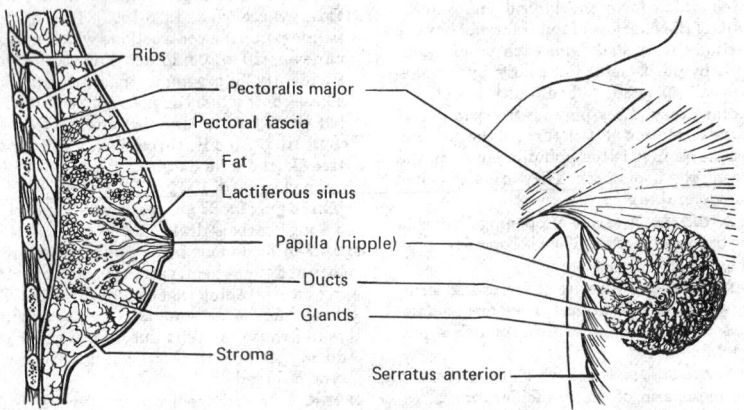

Ribs
Pectoralis major
Pectoral fascia
Fat
Lactiferous sinus
Papilla (nipple)
Ducts
Glands
Stroma
Serratus anterior

BREAST

will be necessary to resort to the hand breast pump or proper manual expression of the milk.

Proper support of the breast with a binder which pulls upward and inward. Do not bind so tightly that circulation is restricted.

Use ice bags during the engorgement period and when there is any tenderness. The ice bags are particularly soothing to cracked nipples as they relieve congestion.

When abscess occurs: When abscesses occur and drainage has been established, there is danger of carrying infection on your hands to other parts of the mother's body. The nurse must protect the mother, herself, and other patients by the use of proper technique. Gloves should be worn during the dressings. Dressings should be disposed of at once and before removing the gloves. Appropriate systemic antibiotic will be prescribed by the physician.

The infant's milk supply is endangered. The infant is taken off the affected breast, but sometimes is permitted to nurse the normal breast. At other times pumping of the good breast is ordered during the height of the infection. Nursing orders will, of course, vary with the physician, but the infant's food intake must be kept up, if necessary by artificial means.

An abscess may not only impair the function of the breast at this time, but may also affect it in subsequent pregnancies.

b., chicken; b., pigeon. Deformity in which chest is protruding, caused by rickets or obstructed respiration in infancy.

b. milk. Mother's milk. SEE: *colostrum.*

b. pump. One to draw milk from the female b. May be electric or hand-operated.

breath (brĕth) [AS. *brāēth,* odor]. The air inhaled and exhaled in act of respiration.

DIAG: *Foul odor (os fetor):* May indicate neglect of mouth or teeth; improper diet; constipation; mouth breathing; lack of exercise; use of drugs, alcohol, or tobacco. It also depends upon the food ingested and may indicate stomatitis, necrosis of jaw, caries of teeth, tonsillitis, diphtheria, gangrene and abscess of the lungs, fetid bronchitis, bronchiectasis, pyothorax, catarrh, diabetes, kidney disease, and other disorders. Mouth washes and gargles are ineffective in removing the odor if os fetor is due to systemic causes or ingestion of food such as garlic.

Urinous odor: Indicates uremia. *Sweetish odor* (that of ripe apples): Found in diabetes mellitus, esp. during coma. This sweet odor is due to the excretion of acetone in the breath. This condition develops quickly in infants and children who have gone several hours without food. *Odor of carnivorous animals:* Noted in critical illness, acidosis, and alkalosis.

Rattling and shortness of b.: Edema; presence of fluids in the air passages. *Sighing b.:* Air hunger; occurs in internal hemorrhage. Therefore be observant of this symptom following abdominal surgery and in typhoid fever.

breathing (brĕth´ĭng). Act of inhaling and exhaling air. SEE: *chest; respiration.*

b., asthmatic. Harsh b. with a prolonged wheezing expiration. Is heard all over the chest.

b., bronchial or tubular. Harsh b. with a prolonged high pitched expiration which has sometimes a tubular quality. Heard in consolidation of lung tissue.

b., cog-wheel. Respiratory murmur not continuous, but broken into waves, not indicative of any special disease, but frequently observed in bronchitis and in incipient phthisis. SYN: *jerky b.*

b., continuous positive pressure. SEE: *ventilation, continuous positive pressure.*

b. of emphysema. Weak with prolonged, low pitched or inaudible expiration.

b., exaggerated. Almost same peculiarity as puerile b. Heard over lung that is doing extra work necessitated by some impairment of its fellow.

b., intermittent positive pressure. SEE: *ventilation, intermittent positive pressure.*

b., periodic. Cheyne-Stokes respiration, q.v.

b., puerile. Type heard normally over lungs of children, loud expiration, higher pitched than in vesicular b. and almost as long as inspiration.

b., rapid. In pneumonia, high fevers, or interference with oxygenation.

b., slow. Found in narcotic poisoning, sleep, or rest, and in cases of increased intracranial pressure.

b., stertorous. Due to a relaxation of the palate and is characterized by a deep snoring sound on inspiration. It is most always present in apoplexy; the cheeks puff out with each breath on expiration. It is not regarded as a serious symptom, although it may indicate brain or nerve pressure. It is found in deep sleep and in coma.

b., weak or shallow. Noted when chest walls are thick; in the old and feeble; in emphysema; in pleural effusion; in incipient phthisis; in painful affections of the chest, like pleurodynia and beginning pleurisy; in pulmonary edema.

breatholyzer (breth'o-li-zer). Apparatus used to analyze the contents of expired air. One such device is used to test for presence of alcohol in expired air in order to determine whether or not a person is "legally" intoxicated.

bredouillement (brā-dwē-mon') [Fr.]. Pronunciation of only part of a word due to rapid utterance.

breech [AS. *brēc,* buttocks]. The nates, or buttocks.

    b. presentation. The presentation of the buttocks instead of the head in childbirth. Occurs in over 3% of all labors.

breeze. A movement of air; applied also to electricity.

bregma (brĕg'mă) [Gr. front of head]. (pl. *bregmata*) That point on the skull where the coronal and sagittal sutures join. The anterior fontanel in the fetus and young infant.

bregmat'ic. Pert. to the bregma.

bregmocardiac reflex (brĕg''mo-kard'ĭ-ăk) [Gr. *bregma,* front of head, + *kardia,* heart]. Reduced heart rate following pressure on posterior fontanel.

brei (brī) [Gr., pulp]. Tissue which has been finely divided; pulp.

Breisky's disease (bri'skē). [August Breisky, Ger. gynecologist, 1832-1889]. Atrophy of the vulva. Kraurosis vulvae.

Brenner's tumor. [Fritz Brenner, Ger. pathologist, 1877 —]. A benign fibroepithelioma of the ovary.

brevilineal (brev-ĭ-lĭn'ē-al) [L. *brevis,* short, + *linea,* line]. Shorter and broader than usual, with reference to body type. SYN: *brachymorphic.*

bridge (brĭj) [AS. *brycg*]. 1. Narrow band of tissue. 2. Dental plate fastened to a tooth at each end.

    b. of nose. The ridge formed by the nasal bones.

bridgework (brĭj'work). A partial plate held in place by permanent attachments to other teeth.

    b., fixed. Partial plates held by crowns or inlays fastened to the natural teeth.

    b., removable. Partial plates held by clasps which permit their removal.

Bright's disease. [Richard Bright, Eng. physician, 1789-1858]. A vague term for acute and chronic disease of the kidneys. It is usually associated with dropsy and albuminuria. SEE: *nephritis.*

brim. 1. An edge or margin. 2. Brim of pelvis. Superior aperture of the lesser or true pelvis; the inlet. Formed by the iliopectineal line

of the innominate bone and the sacral promontory. Oval-shaped in the female; heart-shaped in the male.

brisèment forcé (brēz-mon' fōr-sā') [Fr., crushing]. Breaking, by forcible means, of adhesions.

Brissaud's reflex (brĭs-sō'). [Edouard Brissaud, Fr. physician, 1852-1909] Contraction of tensor fascia latae muscle following stroking or tickling of sole of foot. A component of the extensor plantar response.

British anti-lewisite. Dimercaprol, q.v. ABBR: BAL.

British thermal unit. Amount of heat necessary to raise the temperature of one pound of water from 39° F. to 40° F. One BTU is equal to 0.2522 Calories (i.e. kilocalories) or 1,055 joules. ABBR: BTU.

broach (brōch) [ME. *broche,* pointed rod or pin]. A dental instrument for enlarging a tooth canal or for removing the pulp.

broad ligament of uterus. A transverse fold of peritoneum arising from floor of the pelvic cavity between the bladder and rectum, dividing the minor pelvis into anterior and posterior compartments. In its median portion lies the uterus to which it is attached on both sides. Its free superior border contains the uterine tube. A lateral portion of the upper border forms the suspensory ligament of the ovary.

Broadbent's sign. [Sir William Henry Broadbent, Eng. physician, 1835-1907]. A visible retraction of the left side and back in region of 11th and 12th ribs synchronous with the cardiac systole, in adhesive pericarditis.

Broca's area (brō'kă). [Pierre Paul Broca, Fr. surgeon, 1824-1880] On left side of brain, controlling movements of tongue, lips, vocal cords, and motor speech area. Loss of speech may follow hemorrhage into this area. Area parolfactoria. SYN: *motor speech area.* SEE: *aphasia, motor.*

broccoli (brok'ō-li). Green tops and stalks of a type of cauliflower.

    Food value of 100 gm. (cooked): Cal. 26; protein 3.1 gm.; fat 0.3 gm.; carbohydrate 4.5 gm.; calcium 88 mg.; phosphorus 62 mg.; iron 0.8 mg.; sodium 10 mg.; potassium 267 mg.; vitamin A, 2500 I.U.; riboflavin 0.2 mg.; niacin 0.8 mg.; ascorbic acid 90 mg.

Brodie's abscess. [Sir Benjamin Collins Brodie, Eng. surgeon, 1783-1862]. An abscess of the head of a bone, esp. of the head of the tibia.

    ETIOL: It is usually of tubercular origin or from subacute staphylococcal infection.

    SYM: May be aching pains in area, followed by slight swelling and tenderness on movement. Symptoms less acute but similar to osteomyelitis.

rom-, bromo- [Gr. *brōmos*, stench]. Prefixes indicating presence of bromine.

romhidrosis (brŏm″hī-drō′sis). Bromidrosis, q.v.

romide (brō′mĭd) [Gr. *brōmos*, stench]. A binary compound of bromine combined with an element or a radical. It is a central nervous system depressant.

POISONING SYM: Prompt vomiting; drowsiness; irritability; ataxia; vertigo; confusion; mania; hallucinations; coma. Also skin rashes (bromide acne) and neurological disturbances.

F.A. TREATMENT: Large doses of sodium or ammonium chloride by any route. Give saline cathartic. SEE: *Table of Poisons and Poisoning* in *Appendix.*

bromidrosiphobia (brō″mid-rō-sĭ-fō′bĭ-ă) ["+ *hidrōs,* sweat, + *phobos,* fear]. Abnormal fear of personal odors, accompanied by hallucinations.

bromidrosis (brŏm″ĭ-dro′sis) ["+ *hidrōs,* sweat]. Fetid or offensive sweat. It occurs mostly on feet, groins, and axillae.

NP: Cleanliness, use of an antiseptic, daily change of clothing, deodorant antiseptic powders.

RS: anhidrosis; chromidrosis; uridrosis.

bromine (brō′mēn, -mĭn) [Gr. *bromos,* stench]. SYMB: *Br.* At. wt. 79.904; at. no. 35. Liquid nonmetallic element. It is obtained from natural brines from wells and sea water. Its compounds are used in medicine, photography and coal tar derivatives. SEE: *bromide.*

bromism, brominism (bro′mĭzm, bro′mĭn-ĭzm) ["+ *ismos,* state of]. Poisoning resulting from prolonged use of bromides, q.v. SEE: *bromide; bromides* in *Table of Poisons and Poisoning* in *Appendix.*

bromoderma (brō″mŏ-der′mă) ["+ *derma,* skin]. Acne-like eruption due to chronic bromide poisoning.

bromohyperhidrosis (brō″mŏ-hī″pĕr-hid-rō′sĭs) [Gr. *bromos,* stench, + *hyper,* over, + *hidrōsis,* perspiration]. Fetid and excessive sweat. SEE: *bromidrosis.*

bromoiodism (brō″mŏ-ī′ŏ-dĭzm) ["+ iodine, + Gr. *ismos,* state of]. Poisoning from bromoiodides.

bromomania (brō″mŏ-mā′nĭ-ă) ["+ Gr. *mania,* insanity]. Psychosis caused by use of bromides.

bromomenorrhea (brō″mŏ-men-o-rē′ă) [Gr. *bromos,* stench, + *mēnes,* menses, + *rhoia,* flow]. Foul odor to menstrual discharge.

bromopnea (brŏm″op-ne′ă) ["+ *pnoē,* breath]. Offensive breath.

bronchadenitis (brong″kad-ĕ-nī′tis) [Gr. *bronchos,* windpipe, + *adēn,* gland, + *-itis,* inflammation]. Inflammation of bronchial glands.

bronchi (brŏng′kī). (sing. *bronchus*) [NA] The two main branches leading from the trachea. They provide the passageway for air moving to and from the lungs. The trachea divides opposite the 3rd dorsal vertebra into the right and left main bronchi. The point of division is called the carina tracheae [NA] and is the site where foreign bodies too large to enter either bronchus would rest after passing through the trachea.

The right bronchus is shorter and more vertical than the left one. They penetrate the lungs, one for the right and the other for the left lung, and terminate in the bronchioles or bronchial tubes.

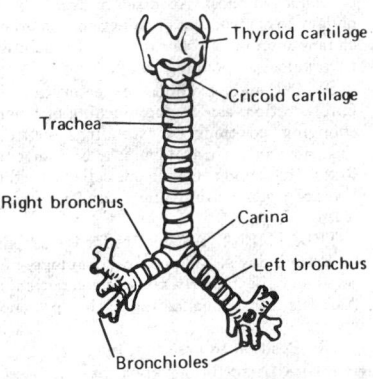

BRONCHI AND TRACHEA

    b., foreign bodies in. May cause various diseases of bronchi, large objects leading to collapse of the lung. Metal bodies, if small, may produce no symptoms. Beans, nuts, seeds, etc., may cause pneumonia, bronchitis, or lung abscess.

SYM: Choking and gagging immediately. Later, symptoms of bronchitis, atelectasis, pneumonia, or lung abscess.

PROG: Good, if removed before complications. Better in case of metallic objects than in vegetable bodies.

TREATMENT: Removal through bronchoscope.

bronchi, words pert. to: alveobronchitis, "bronch-" words; mesobronchitis; rales.

bronchial (brŏn′kĭ-ăl). Pert. to the bronchi or bronchioles.

    b. crises. Paroxysms of coughing in locomotor ataxia.

b. glands. Mucous or mixed glands in the bronchi or bronchioles.

b. tree. Bronchi and bronchial tubes.

b. tubes. The smaller divisions of the bronchi.

b. washing. Irrigation of one or both bronchi in order to collect cells for cytologic study or to help cleanse the bronchi.

bronchiarctia (brong″kĭ-ark′shĭ-ä) [Gr. *bronchos,* windpipe, + L. *arctāre,* to compress.]. Bronchial tube stenosis. SYN: *bronchiostenosis.*

bronchiectasis (brong″kĭ-ek′tă-sis) ["+ *ektasis,* dilatation]. Dilatation of a bronchus or bronchi, usually secreting large amounts of offensive pus. Dilatation may be in an isolated segment or spread throughout the bronchi.

ETIOL: Acquired or congenital, on one or both sides of chest. Acquired b. usually secondary to obstruction or infections, as bronchopneumonia, chronic bronchitis, tuberculosis, whooping cough.

SYM: Cough, dyspnea, expectoration of foul secretion, esp. in the morning or when changing position. On standing, sputum separates into three layers: a bottom one that is thick and contains pus cells; a middle layer of greenish fluid; and an upper layer of froth.

TREATMENT: Antibiotics for treatment and prophylaxis, and postural drainage. Resection of affected areas in selected patients. Aerosols for bronchodilation in bronchospasm.

NP: Position to assist drainage.

bronchiectatic (brong″kĭ-ek-tät′ĭk) ["+ *ektasis,* dilation]. Pert. to bronchiectasis.

bronchiloquy (brong-kil′ō-kwĭ) [Gr. *bronchos,* windpipe, + L. *loquī,* to speak]. Unusual vocal resonance over a bronchus covered with consolidated lung tissue.

bronchiocele (brong′kĭ-ō-sēl) ["+ *kēlē,* tumor]. Circumscribed dilatation of a bronchus.

bronchiogenic (brong″kĭ-ō-jen′ĭk) ["+ *gennan,* to originate]. Having origin in the bronchi.

bronchiole (brong′kĭ-ōl) [L. *bronchiolus,* air passage]. (pl. *bronchioles)* One of the smaller subdivisions of the bronchi. They lack cartilage.

b., respiratory. The last division of the bronchial tree. They are branches of terminal bronchioles and lead to alveolar ducts leading to the alveoli.

b., terminal. Next to the last subdivision of a bronchiole, leading to the respiratory bronchioles.

bronchiolectasis (brong″kĭ-ō-lek′tă-sis) ["+ Gr. *ektasis,* dilatation]. Dilatation of the bronchioles; capillary bronchiectasis.

bronchiolitis (brong″kĭ-ō-lī′tis) ["+ Gr. *-itis* inflammation]. Inflammation of the bronchioles.

b., exudativa. A form with fibrinous exudation.

b., vesicular. Bronchopneumonia.

bronchiolus (brong-kī′ō-lus). (pl. *bronchioli* [NA] Bronchiole, q.v.

bronchiospasm (brong′kĭ-ō-spazm) [L. *bronchiolus,* air passage, + Gr. *spasmos,* fit] Spasmodic narrowing of the lumen of the bronchial tubes.

bronchiostenosis (brong″kĭ-ō-stĕ-nō′sĭs. ["+ Gr. *stenōsis,* a narrowing]. Narrowing of the bronchial tubes. SYN: *bronchiarctia.*

bronchismus (brong-kis′mus) ["+ Gr. *ismos,* state of]. Bronchiospasm, q.v.

bronchitic (brong-kī′tĭk). Pert. to bronchitis

bronchitis (brŏng-kī′tĭs) [Gr. *bronchos,* windpipe, + *itis,* inflammation]. Inflammation of bronchial mucous membrane.

ETIOL: Infectious agents such as viruses esp. influenza virus or pyogenic organisms such as various species of Streptococcus, Pneumococcus, Staphylococcus, and Hemophilus. Infection often preceded by the common cold. Predisposing factors are exposure, chilling, fatigue and malnutrition. Acute bronchial irritation may also be caused by various physical and chemical agents such as dusts and fumes. Allergic factors may be of importance.

NOTE: Even though the pathway of air to the bronchi and lungs is capable of warming inspired cold air, there are limits beyond which this system fails. Thus it is inadvisable to let anyone sleep in an area which is extremely cold or to exercise vigorously in extremely cold air without wearing a face mask of a type which stores the heat of expired air so it will be available to warm the inspired air.

b., acute. Chilliness, malaise. Soreness and constriction behind sternum, increased by coughing; slight fever, 100°-102° F. Cough at first dry and painful, later mucopurulent expectoration which becomes free as inflammation subsides.

TREATMENT: Bed rest, increased intake of fluids, an antipyretic and analgesic, antibiotics, steam inhalations.

b., capillary. Inflammation of the secondary bronchi in children and debilitated persons.

SYM: Severe spells of coughing; rapid respiration—30 to 80 per minute; dyspnea, high fever—104°-105° F.; weak, rapid pulse. Later lips become blue, extremities cold, mind dull.

PROG: In young children very grave. May develop into bronchopneumonia.

TREATMENT: Absolute rest. Temp. of room kept uniformly at 70° or 75° F.—atmosphere kept moist by steam. Antibiotics.

b., chronic. A longstanding disease of the tracheobronchial tree characterized by chronic inflammation accompanied by fibrotic and atrophic changes in the mucous membrane.

SYM: Persistent cough, mucopurulent expectoration. Soreness behind sternum. Fever absent unless disease is severe; dyspnea on exertion.

NP: Whenever possible it is advisable for a person with chronic bronchitis to live in a mild stable climate, esp. during the winter. The ward or room in the hospital should be kept warm. General health should be maintained. Diet should be nourishing. Anti-tussive agents, antibiotics, expectorants, steam or other inhalations.

b., plastic. Fibrinous bronchitis, q.v.

b., putrid. Chronic form with foul-smelling sputum.

b., vegetal. Bronchitis resulting from the lodgement of foods of vegetable origin such as a peanut in the bronchus.

bronchium (brong'kĭ-um) [L. *bronchus*]. (pl. *bronchia*) A bronchial tube.

broncho-, bronch- [Gr. *bronchos*, windpipe]. Prefix: Rel. to the bronchi or windpipe.

bronchoadenitis (brŏng''kō-ad''e-nī'tĭs) ["+ *adēn*, gland, + *-itis*, inflammation]. Bronchadenitis, q.v.

bronchoblennorrhea (brŏng''kō-blen''o-rē'ă) ["+ *blennos*, mucus, + *rhoia*, flow]. Copious, thick sputum accompanying chronic bronchitis.

bronchocele (brŏng'kō-sēl) [Gr. *bronchos*, windpipe, + *kēlē*, tumor]. A dilatation of a bronchiole.

bronchoclysis (brŏng-kok'lĭ-sĭs) [Gr. *bronchos*, windpipe, + *klysis*, washing]. Introduction of a medicated solution into the bronchi.

bronchoconstriction (brŏng''kō-kŏn-strĭk'-shŭn) ["+ L. *constringere*, to draw together]. Constriction of the lumen of the bronchi.

bronchodilatation (brŏng''kō-dĭl-ă-tā'shun) ["+ L. *dilatāre*, to open]. Dilatation of a bronchus.

bronchoedema (brŏng''kō-ĕ-dē'mă) [Gr. *bronchos*, windpipe, + *oidēma*, tumor, from *oidein*, to swell]. Edematous swelling of the mucosa of the bronchial tubes reducing size of air passageways and inducing dyspnea.

bronchoegophony (brŏng''kō-ĕ-gof'ō-nĭ) ["+ *aig-*, goat, + *phōnē*, voice]. Egobronchophony; a goatlike sound.

bronchogenic (brŏng-kō-jĕn'ĭk) ["+ *gennan*, to originate]. Having origin in the bronchi.

bronchogram (brŏng'kō-grăm) [Gr. *bronchos*, windpipe, + *gramma*, a writing]. A roentgenogram of the lungs and bronchi.

bronchography (brŏng-kog'ră-fĭ) ["+ *graphein*, to write]. Radiography of the bronchi after a radiopaque substance has been injected into them, making a bronchogram.

broncholith (brŏng'kō-lĭth) ["+ *lithos*, stone]. Calculus in the bronchus or bronchial tube.

broncholithiasis (brŏng''kō-lĭth-ī'ă-sis) [Gr. *bronchos*, windpipe, + *lithos*, stone]. Calculi in the bronchi.

bronchomoniliasis (brŏng''kō-mon-ĭ-lī'ă-sis) ["+ L. *monile*, necklace]. Infection of the bronchial mucosa by Monilia.

bronchomo'tor ["+ L. *motus*, moving]. Causing change of caliber of the bronchi.

bronchomycosis (brŏng''kō-mī-kō'sĭs) [Gr. *bronchos*, windpipe, + *mykēs*, fungus]. A fungus infection of the bronchi or bronchial tubes, usually caused by fungi of the genus Candida.

bronchopathy (brŏng-kŏp'ăth-ĭ) ["+ *pathos*, disease]. Any pathological condition involving the bronchi or bronchioles.

bronchophony (brŏng-kof'ō-nĭ) ["+ *phōnē*, voice]. The voice as heard over a normal bronchus.

b., whispered. B. when patient whispers.

bronchoplasty (brŏng'kō-plăs''tĭ) [Gr. *bronchos*, windpipe, + *plassein*, to form]. Surgical repair of a bronchial defect.

bronchoplegia (brŏng''kō-plē'jĭ-ă) ["+ *plēgē*, stroke]. Paralysis of the bronchial tubes.

bronchopleural (brŏng''kō-plūr'ăl) ["+ *pleura*, side, rib]. Pertaining to the bronchi and the pleural cavity.

bronchopneumonia (brŏng''kō-nū-mō'nĭ-ă) [Gr. *bronchos*, windpipe, + *pneumonia*, lung inflammation]. Inflammation of the terminal bronchioles and alveoli. SEE: *pneumonia*.

ETIOL: May be caused by various types of pneumococci; Group A hemolytic streptococcus; Klebsiella pneumoniae (Friedlander's bacillus) types A & B; various staphylococci; and Pasteurella tularensis. May also be caused by other pathogenic bacteria as well as by viruses, rickettsias, and fungi.

SYM: Cough and expectoration; respiration short and shallow from 50-75/minute.

Cyanosis may ensue. Nostrils dilate with each inspiration, and in children the temperature reaches 103° or 105° F.; before death, 108° F. Pulse, 140. Duration two to three weeks. Improvement may be followed by increased severity as new patches form. In the aged many of these symptoms are absent; slight cough and little sputum; temperature, 100 to 101° F. may or may not be in evidence. Weakness, sore throat, chills, chest pain. The elderly and bedridden are susceptible.

PROG: Depends principally upon time at which treatment is initiated, recovery generally occurring quicker in those treated during the first three days. Also prognosis more favorable for those under 50; unfavorable for the very young and very old. Mortality greatly reduced by use of antibiotics.

COMPLICATIONS: Lung abscess, atelectasis, empyema, pericarditis, and paralytic ileus.

TREATMENT: Bed rest, increased intake of fluids, analgesics for pain, antibiotics, soft diet, oxygen for cyanosis, abdominal distention, and general comfort, treatment of shock if it occurs.

NP: Hygienic. Room, 65°-70° F. (18.3°-21.1° C.), humidified air. Cold sponge bath if necessary to control hyperpyrexia. Oxygen inhalations with usual precautions concerning humidification. Liquid or semiliquid food. Beware of relapse.

bronchopulmonary (brŏng″kō-pul′mo-nă-rĭ) ["+ L. *pulmonarius*, pert. to lung]. Pert. to bronchi and lungs.

bronchorrhagia (brŏng″kor-ā′jĭ-ă) [Gr. *bronchos*, windpipe, + *rhēgnunai*, to break forth]. Bronchial hemorrhage.

bronchorrhaphy (brŏng-kŏr′ă-fĭ) ["+ *rhaphē*, suture]. Suturing of a wound of the bronchus.

bronchorrhea (brŏng-kō-rē′ă) ["+ *rhoia*, flow]. Abnormal secretion from the bronchial mucous membrane, sometimes very offensive.

bronchorrhoncus (brŏng″kor-on′kus) [Gr. *bronchos*, windpipe, + *rhonchos*, snore]. A bronchial rale.

bronchoscope (brŏng′kō-skōp) ["+ *skopein*, to see]. An instrument for visual examination of the interior of a bronchus.

bronchoscopy (brŏng-kos′kō-pĭ). Examination of the bronchi through a bronchoscope.

bronchosinusitis (brŏng″kō-sī″nus-ī′tĭs) [Gr. *bronchos*, windpipe, + L. *sinus*, a hollow, + Gr. -*itis*, inflammation]. Infection of bronchi and sinuses at the same time.

bronchospasm (brŏng′kō-spăzm) ["+ *spasmos*, a spasm]. Spasm of the bronchus.

bronchospirochetosis (brŏng″kō-spī″rō-kē-tō′sis) ["+ *speira*, coil, + *chaitē*, wavy hair]. Hemorrhagic bronchitis; bronchopulmonary spirochetosis resulting from spirochetes.

bronchospirometer (brŏng″kō-spī-rom′ē-ter) [Gr. *bronchos*, windpipe, + L. *spirare*, to breathe, + Gr. *metron*, measure]. An instrument for determining the volume of air inspired from one lung and for collecting air for analysis.

bronchostaxis (brŏng″kō-stăk′sĭs) ["+ Gr. *staxis*, dripping]. Hemorrhage from the walls of a bronchus.

bronchostenosis (brŏng″kō-sten-ō′sĭs) ["+ *stenōsis*, a narrowing]. Narrowing of a bronchus.

bronchostomy (brŏng-kos′tō-mĭ) [Gr. *bronchos*, windpipe, + *stoma*, mouth]. Formation from without of an opening into a bronchus.

bronchotetany (brŏng″kō-tĕt′ă-nĭ) ["+ *tetanos*, stretched]. Extreme dyspnea due to spasm in the bronchi preventing access of air.

bronchotome (brŏng′kō-tōm) ["+ *tomē*, incision]. Instrument for making an incision of the trachea.

bronchotomy (brŏng-kot′ō-mĭ). Surgical incision of a bronchus, the larynx, or trachea.

bronchotracheal (brŏng″kō-trā′kē-ăl) [Gr. *bronchos*, windpipe, + *trachea*]. Pert. to both bronchi and trachea.

bronchotyphoid (brŏng″kō-tī′foyd) ["+ *typhos*, fever, + *eidos*, resemblance]. Typhoid fever marked by severe bronchitis in initial stage.

bronchovesicular (brŏng″kō-vē-sĭk′ū-lăr) ["+ L. *vesicula*, small bladder]. Pert. to bronchial tubes and air vesicles with special reference to sounds intermediate between bronchial or tracheal sounds and vesicular sounds.

bronchus (brŏng′kus) [Gr. *bronchos*, windpipe.]. (pl. *bronchi*) One of the two large branches of the trachea. The trachea proper terminates at the level of the 4th dorsal vetebra. SEE: *bronchi*.

brontophobia (brŏn″to-fō′bĭ-ă) [Gr. *brontē*, thunder, + *phobos*, fear]. Abnormal fear of thunder.

bronzed skin. A characteristic symptom of Addison's disease which is due to adrenal cortical insufficiency. Also seen in hemochromatosis.

brood capsule or cyst. Cystlike bodies which develop within a hydatid cyst of Echinococcus granulosus.

brossage (brō-sazh') [Fr. brushing]. Brushing the everted eyelids with stiff brush, to remove granulations, as in trachoma.

broth. 1. A nutrient drink such as bouillon usually served hot. 2. A liquid medium for culturing bacteria.

brownian movement (brow'nĭ-ăn). [Robert Brown, Eng. botanist, 1773-1858] Oscillatory movement of microscopic particles or particles of a colloidal system resulting from movement of the surrounding molecules, based on the kinetic theory of matter. This may be observed in bacteria but is distinguished from true motility resulting from activities initiated within the organism itself.

Brown-Séquard's paralysis (brown'sā-kär'). [Charles E. Brown-Séquard, Fr. physician, 1818-1894]. Reflex flaccid paraplegia occurring during some urinary tract affections.

Brown-Séquard's syndrome. Hemisection of the spinal cord with paralysis below the lesion on the affected side and with anesthesia and loss of tactile, pain, and temperature sensibility on the opposite side below the lesion.

brow presentation. When the brow or face of the infant comes first on presentation in labor; makes birth almost impossible. Cesarean section is frequently needed if the presentation cannot be altered.

Brucella (brū-sĕl'ă). [Sir David Bruce, Brit. bacteriologist, 1855-1931] A genus of bacteria, nonmotile, aerobic, gram negative, and pathogenic to man, causing undulant fever, and contagions and abortion in cattle, hogs, and goats.

brucel'lar. Pert. to Brucella.

brucellosis (brū''sĕl-ō'sĭs) [Brucella, + Gr. -ōsis, disease]. A widespread infectious, febrile disease affecting principally cattle, swine, and goats, but sometimes affecting other animals including man. It is caused by bacteria of the genus Brucella, three species being involved: B. melitensis and B. suis the cause of brucellosis in goats and swine, respectively, and B. abortus, the cause of contagious abortion in cattle and other domestic animals. In man it is called undulant fever or Malta fever and is caused by any of the three species.

Bruch's membrane (brook). [Karl. W. L. Bruch, Ger. anatomist, 1819-1884]. A glassy membrane of the uvea of the eye lying between the chorioid membrane and the pigmented epithelium of the retina.

brucine (brū'sēn, brū'sĭn). [J. Bruce, African traveler, 1730-1794]. A poisonous alkaloid from Strychnos nux vomica and other

Strychnos species. Similar to but less powerful than strychnine, q.v.

Bruck's disease (brook). [Alfred Bruck, Ger. physician, 1865 —]. A rare disease characterized by muscle atrophy and skeletal disorders such as multiple fractures and ankyloses.

bruise (brūz) [O.Fr. *bruiser,* to break]. An injury with diffuse effusion into subcutaneous tissue, and in which skin is discolored but not broken. A contusion, q.v.

b. of head, chest, and abdomen.
May be associated with internal injuries.

SYM: Pain, swelling, tenderness, discoloration. NP: Mild antiseptic if skin is scratched. Cold applications with pressure.

b. or contusion of breast. SYM: Pain, swelling, discoloration. NP: Apply cold applications and snug bandage with pressure and elevation. SEE: *contusion.*

bruissement (bru-ēs-mon') [Fr. droning noise]. A purring sound heard by auscultation.

bruit (brū'ē) [Fr. noise]. An adventitious sound of venous or arterial origin heard on auscultation.

b. de craquement. Crackling.

b. de diable. 1. The venous hum of anemia. 2. Subjective tinnitus of chlorotic patients and a humming hallucination of hearing in the insane.

b. de frottement. Friction-like sound.

b., placental. A purring or blowing noise heard in the pregnant uterus due to fetal circulation of blood, and synchronous with the maternal pulse.

b. de pot fêlé. Cracked pot sound.

b. de rape. Rasping.

b. de soufflet. Bellows sound.

Brunner's glands (brun'er). [Johann C. Brunner, Swiss anatomist, 1653-1727] Compound glands of the duodenum and upper jejunum. Also known as duodenal glands.

They are embedded in the submucous tissue and lined with columnar epithelium. They are similar to the pyloric glands of stomach, but their secretion increases in response to feeding. They secrete a clear, alkaline mucinous solution.

Brussels sprouts. The small, green, cabbage-like heads of the plant Brassica oleracea gemmiferma.

Food value of 100 gm. (cooked): Cal. 36; protein 4.2 gm.; fat 0.4 gm.; carbohydrate 6.4 gm.; calcium 32 mg.; phosphorus 72 mg.; iron 1.1 mg.; sodium 10 mg.; potassium 273 mg.; vitamin A, 520 I.U.; riboflavin 0.14 mg.; niacin 0.8 mg.; ascorbic acid 87 mg.

bruxism (brŭks'ĭzm) [Gr. *brychein,* to grind the teeth]. Grinding of the teeth, esp. during sleep.

BSR. Abbr. for *basal skin resistance.*

bubo (bū'bō) [Gr. *boubōn,* groin, swollen gland]. (pl. *buboes)* An inflamed, swollen or enlarged lymph node often exhibiting suppuration, occurring commonly after chancroid, gonorrhea, or lymphogranuloma venereum. Nodes most commonly affected are those of the groin and axilla. Buboes may also develop after other infectious diseases, esp. bubonic plague.

   b., axillary. B. in the axilla or armpit.

   b., indolent. B. in which suppuration does not occur.

   b., inguinal. B. in the region of the groin.

   b., pestilential. B. occurring in bubonic plague.

   b., venereal. B. resulting from a venereal disease.

bubonadenitis (bu-bon-ad-en-ī'tĭs) ["+ *adēn,* gland, + *-itis,* inflammation]. Inflammation of an inguinal gland.

bubonalgia (bu"bo-nal'jĭ-ä) ["+ *algos,* pain]. Pain in the groin.

bubon d'emblée (bu-bŏ"dăm-blā') [Gr. *boubōn,* groin, swollen gland, + Fr., at the first onset]. Venereal bubo appearing without previous lesion; primary bubo.

bubon'ic plague ["+ L. *plāga,* stroke, wound]. An acute, infectious disease common in the Orient, esp. India. The Black Death of the Middle Ages. Frequently it is fatal.

   ETIOL: Caused by Pasteurella pestis, usually from infected rats and ground squirrels, which is imparted to human beings by bite of the rat flea. It is characterized by enlargement of lymphatic glands, severe toxic symptoms, accompanied by intense adenitis or pneumonia. SEE: *plague.*

bubononcus (bū-bŏn-ŏn'kŭs) ["+ *onchos,* tumor]. A swelling of the inguinal region.

bucardia (bu-kär'dĭ-ä) [Gr. *bous,* ox, + *kardia,* heart]. Severe hypertrophy of the heart.

bucca (buk'ä) [L. cheek]. (pl. *buccae*) [NA] The cheek; fleshy portion of side of face.

buc'cal. Pert. to the cheek or mouth.

   b. cavity. The mouth.

   b. fat pad. The corpus adiposum or suctorial pad, an encapsulated mass of fat lying superficial to the buccinator muscle. It is well developed in infants and is thought to aid in the act of sucking.

   b. glands. Small glands situated in the mucous membranes of the mouth which secrete saliva.

buccinatolabialis (buk-sin-at-o-lä-bĭ-a'lis) [L. *buccinator,* trumpeter, + *labialis,* pert. to the lips]. The buccinator and orbicularis oris as one.

buccinator (buk'sĭn-ä-tŏr) [L. *buccinator,* trumpeter]. The muscle of the cheek. SEE: *muscle.*

buccoversion (bŭk"ō-vĕr'zhŭn) [L. *bucca,* mouth, + *versiō,* a turning]. Position of buccal part to line of occlusion; said of a tooth.

buccula (buk'ū-lä) [L. a little cheek]. A fold of redundant fatty tissue under the chin. Known as a double chin.

Buck's extension. [Gurdon Buck, Amer. surgeon, 1807-1877]. An apparatus consisting of a weight and pulley for applying extension to a limb.

bucnemia (buk-ne'mĭ-ä) [Gr. *bous,* ox, + *knēmē,* leg]. Tense inflammatory swelling of the leg; elephantiasis.

bud [ME. *budde,* to swell]. 1. In anatomy, a small structure resembling a bud of a plant, as a taste bud. 2. In embryology, a small protuberance or outgrowth which is the anlage or primordium of an organ or structure, as a limb bud.

   b., taste. An ovoid body embedded in the stratified epithelium of the tongue and also found sparingly on the epiglottis and soft palate. Buds contain the sensory receptors for taste.

bud'ding. A method of asexual reproduction in which a budlike process grows from the side or end of the parent and develops into a new organism which in some cases remains attached, in others separates and lives an independent existence. It is common in lower animals (sponges, coelenterates) and plants (yeasts, molds).

Buerger's disease (bur'ger). [Leo Buerger, Amer. physician, 1879-1943] A chronic recurring inflammatory vascular occlusive disease, chiefly of the peripheral arteries and veins of the extremities, with an extraordinary affinity for young adult Jewish males. It is fairly rare in occurrence. SYN: *thromboangiitis obliterans.*

   SYM: Paresthesia of the foot, or pain confined to one toe. Easy fatigue. Cramps in legs but not to be confused with those occurring in the aged. Legs give out, esp. when walking. Ulceration or moist gangrene may set in; amputation may be necessary.

   TREATMENT: Absolute and continued abstinence from tobacco in all forms is extremely important. Avoid excessive use of affected limb, exposure to temperature extremes, trauma, use of drugs which diminish blood supply to extremities, fungus infections. If gangrene, rest pain, or ulceration is present, complete bed rest is advised. For arterial spasm, blocking of the sympathetic nervous system by injection of various drugs or by sympathectomy may be done. SEE: *thromboangiitis obliterans.*

buffer (bŭf'ĕr) [Fr. *buffe*, blow]. 1. A substance, esp. a salt of the blood, tending to preserve original hydrogen-ion concentration of its solution, upon adding an acid or base. 2. A substance tending to offset reaction of an agent administered in conjunction with it.

b. action. Ability of chemical solutions to neutralize excess acid or base and thus prevent change in the pH of the solution.

b., blood. B. present in the blood. The principal b.'s are: carbonic acid, carbonates and bicarbonates, monobasic and dibasic phosphates, and proteins. Hemoglobin is an important protein b.

b. salts. Substances in the blood which act as a b.

buf'fy coat [Fr. *buffe*, buffalo]. Light stratum of a blood clot seen when the blood is allowed to stand in a test tube. The red blood cells settle to the bottom, then between the plasma and the red blood cells there is a light-colored layer which contains mostly white blood cells.

bug. A term applied loosely to any small insect or arthropod; more specifically a member of the order Hemiptera which includes the squash bug, chinch bug, and bedbug. They have sucking mouth parts, incomplete metamorphosis, and two pairs of wings, the fore pair being half membranous. The following bugs are of medical importance:

b., assassin. One belonging to the family Reduviidae. Many are predaceous; others are blood-sucking. Pantastrongulus, Triatoma, and Rhodnius are vectors of trypanosome diseases (Chagas' disease) in man.

b., bed. A member of the family Cimicidae, esp. of the genus Cimex. SEE: *bedbug.*

b., kissing. Several species of the family Reduviidae. Melanolestes picipes is the common kissing bug, or black corsair.

b., red. The larvae of mites of the family Trombiculidae, commonly called chiggers.

bulb (bŭlb) [L. *bulbus*, bulbous root, onion, from Gr. *bolbos*, name for bulbous plants]. 1. An expansion of a canal, vessel, or organ. 2. Obsolete term for the medulla oblongata.

b., aortic. Dilated portion of the truncus arteriosus in the embryo which gives rise to the roots of the aorta and pulmonary arteries.

b., duodenal. Upper duodenal area just beyond pylorus.

b. of the eye. The eyeball.

b., hair. The expanded portion at the lower end of the hair root.

b., olfactory. The anterior enlargement of the olfactory tract.

b., terminal, of Krause. An encapsulated sensory nerve-ending similar in structure to the corpuscles of Pacini. Also called corpuscle of Golgi-Manzoni.

b. of the urethra. The posterior portion of the spongy body.

b. of the vestibule. The vaginal b. or bulbus vestibuli, q.v.

bulbar (bŭl'băr). 1. Pert. to a bulb. 2. Shaped like a bulb. 3. Pert. to the medulla oblongata.

b. paralysis. Paralysis due to changes in motor centers of the oblongata. SEE: *paralysis.*

bul'biform [L. *bulbus*, bulbous root, + *forma*, shape]. Shaped like a bulb.

bulbitis (bŭl-bī'tĭs) ["+ Gr. *-itis*, inflammation]. Inflammation of the urethra in its bulbous portion.

bulbocavernosus (bŭl'bo-kăv''ĕr-nō'sŭs) [L. *bulbus*, bulbous root, + *cavernosus*, hollow]. A muscle ensheathing the bulb of the penis in the male or covering the bulbus vestibuli in the female. Also called in the male ejaculator urinae, accelerator urinae; in the female sphincter vaginae.

bulbocav'ernous reflex. Contraction of bulbocavernous muscle on percussing dorsum of penis.

bulbomimic reflex (bŭl'bo-mĭm'ĭk) [L. *bulbus*, bulbous root, + Gr. *mimikos*, imitator]. Contraction of facial muscles following pressure on eyeball.

bulbonuclear (bŭl''bo-nū'kle-ăr) ["+ *nucleus*, kernel]. Pert. to the nuclei in the medulla oblongata.

bulbourethral glands (bŭl''bō-ū-rē'thral) ["+ Gr. *ourēthra*, urethra]. Cowper's glands. Two small glands about the size of a pea, one on each side of the prostate gland, each with a duct about one inch (2.5 cm.) long, terminating in the wall of the urethra. They secrete a viscid fluid forming part of the seminal fluid.

RS: prostate; urethra.

bulbous (bŭl'bŭs) [L. *bulbus*, bulbous root, onion]. Bulb-shaped; swollen; terminating in an enlargement.

bul'bus [L. from Gr. *bolbos*]. Bulb, q.v.

b. corpus cavernosum. Bulb of the urethra. A bulbous swelling of the corpus cavernosum at base of the penis.

b. vestibuli. [NA]. Two oval masses of erectile tissue lying beneath the vestibule and resting on the urogenital diaphragm. They are homologous to the bulbus cavernosum urethra of the male.

bulesis (bu-lē'sis) [Gr. *boulēsis*, a willing]. An act of the will; the will.

bulimia (bu-lim'ĭ-ă) [L. from Gr. *bous*, ox, + *limos*, hunger]. Hunger experienced a short time after a meal; morbid hunger.

bulim'ic. Pert. to bulimia.

bulla (bul'lă) [L. a bubble]. (pl. *bullae*) A large blister or skin vesicle filled with fluid; a bleb, q.v. SEE: *pompholyx*.

    b. ethmoidalis. [NA]. A rounded projection into the middle meatus of the nose underneath the middle turbinated bone, formed by an anterior ethmoid cell.

    b. ossea. The dilated portion of the bony external meatus of the ear. SEE: *pompholyx*.

bullate (bul'āt). Said of a surface growth which appears blistered because of convex prominences.

bullation (bul-a'shŭn) [L. *bulla*, a bubble]. 1. Division into small compartments. 2. Inflation.

bullet wound. Puncture wound from a bullet. SEE: *wound*.

bullous (bul'us) [L. *bulla*, bubble]. Having the nature of a bulla.

BUN. Abbr. for *blood urea nitrogen*.

bun'dle. A group of fibers; a fasciculus.

    b., Arnold's. The frontopontile tract. It passes from the cerebral cortex of frontal lobe through the internal capsule and cerebral peduncle to the pons.

    b., atrioventricular. A bundle of fibers of the impulse-conducting system of the heart. From its origin in the A-V node it enters the interventricular septum where it divides into two branches whose fibers pass to the right and left ventricles respectively, the fibers of each trunk becoming continuous with the Purkinje fibers of the ventricles. SYN: *A-V bundle; bundle of His.* SEE: *heart block*.

    b. of His. B., atrioventricular, q.v.

    b., Schultze's. Comma-shaped path of fibers in middle of spinal cord's fasciculus cuneatus.

    b. of Turck. The temporopontile tract. Fibers pass from the cerebral cortex of temporal lobe and terminate in the pons.

bundle branch block. A defect in the heart's electrical conduction system wherein there is failure of conduction down one of the main branches of the bundle of His. SEE: *heart block*.

bunion (bun'yun). Inflammation and thickening of the bursa of the joint of the great toe, usually associated with marked enlargement of the joint and displacement of the toe, laterally. SEE: *hallux valgus*.

bunodont (bū'nō-dŏnt) [Gr. *bounos*, mound, + *odous*, tooth]. Having round or conical cusps, said of molar teeth, in contrast to lophodont in which crowns bear ridges or crests.

bunogaster (bu-nō-gas'ter) ["+ *gastēr*, belly]. Protrusion of the abdomen.

Bunsen burner (bŭn'sĕn). [Robert W. E. von Bunsen, Ger. chemist, 1811-1899] A gas burner with an adjustment by which the air holes at the bottom of the tube can be closed or open and the flame made either yellow or blue. If the holes are closed, the flame burns yellow, i.e., it will give light but a relatively small amount of heat. By adjusting the air intake a blue flame is produced. This is the hottest, most efficient and smokeless flame that can be produced by the burner.

buphthalmia, buphthalmos (bŭf-thal'mĭ-ă, -mos) [Gr. *bous*, ox, + *ophthalmos*, eye]. Condition of infantile glaucoma resulting in uniform enlargement of eye, particularly the cornea.

    Disease may stop spontaneously or continue until it produces blindness.

    TREATMENT: Iridectomy, sclerotomy, miotics. SEE: *hydrophthalmos*.

Burdach's tracts (bŭr'dak). [Karl F. Burdach, Ger. physiologist, 1776-1847]. Continuation of dorsolateral column of spinal cord into medulla oblongata. SYN: *cuneate fasciculus*.

buret, burette (bū-rĕt') [Fr., small holder for fluid]. A special hollow glass tube usually with a stopcock at the lower end. It is marked so that the amount of liquid released through the outlet will be known. Used in chemical analysis to measure the amount of liquid reagent used.

burn (bŭrn) [AS. *baernan*, to burn]. Tissue injury resulting from excessive exposure to thermal, chemical, electrical, or radioactive agents. The effects vary according to the type, duration, and intensity of the agent and part of body involved. The effects may be local resulting in cell injury or death, or both local and systemic involving primary shock (that occurring immediately after the injury and rarely fatal) or secondary shock (that developing insidiously following severe burns and often fatal).

    Burns are usually classified as:

    First degree burns. Superficial burns, damage being limited to outer layer of the epidermis. Characterized by erythema, hyperemia, tenderness and pain. No vesiculation.

    Second degree burns. Burns in which damage extends through the epidermis and into the dermis but not of sufficient extent to interfere with regeneration of epidermis. If secondary infection results, the damage from a second degree burn may be equivalent to that of a third degree. Vesicles usually present.

Third degree burns. Burns in which both epidermis and dermis are destroyed with damage extending into underlying tissues. Tissues may be charred or coagulated.

TREATMENT: Emergency treatment of burns which cover less than one half of the body should be cooling of the burned portion by immersion in water of approximately 50° F. temperature. This will bring about almost immediate relief of pain and will aid subsequent healing of the wound. If facilities for immersion are not available, cold compresses may be used. Treatment varies with type of burn and extent of body involved. Therapy for all burns involves asepsis and proper care of wounds, relief from pain, prevention or control of infection if it occurs, prevention or relief of shock, maintenance of water and electrolyte balance, and proper nutrition esp. to correct hypoproteinemia which usually accompanies burns. Loss of water and heat from the local burned area due to evaporation is greatly increased. Thus maintenance of water and caloric intake is essential.

In severe burns shock is always present and may cause death. Morphine is administered immediately, followed by intravenous injections of whole blood and of salt and water solutions to prevent shock. When pain has eased, charred clothing is removed and burned area is gently washed with a sterile normal saline solution.

Treatment may be by use of pressure dressings or by open technique. Experimentation with techniques such as an air bed, which keeps the body suspended on a layer of air, and use of topical silver nitrate are in progress and show promise. Also, the use of split-thickness skin grafts from the patient are being used much sooner after the burn than formerly.

The use of appropriate antibiotics, blood protein, and fluid replacement has made possible the salvage with full recovery of extensively burned patients who were formerly almost certain to die.

PRECAUTIONS: Never allow a person whose clothing is burning to run. Make him lie down and roll. Wrap him in a rug, blanket, or anything within reach and smother the flames. Be careful not to allow him to inhale the smoke. Cut away the clothing, taking care not to pull any portion of the skin away. Do not open any blisters, as this increases the chance for infections.

COMPLICATIONS (in burns and scalds): Sloughing, gangrene, erysipelas, nephritis, pneumonia, or intestinal disturbances; sudden attacks of rigor, vomiting, rise of temperature or convulsions are all suspicious symptoms. A superficial burn covering a large part of the body is more serious than a small, deep one, unless important nerves and blood vessels are involved. If two thirds of the skin is destroyed, death may be expected, even in a burn of the first degree. Shock must always be anticipated regardless of degree of burn.

b., acid. Due to exposure to corrosive acids, as sulfuric, hydrochloric, nitric, etc.

F.A. TREATMENT: Wash with large volumes of water; apply dilute alkalies, as baking soda (sodium bicarbonate) paste, soap solution dressing, chalk paste, etc. Follow with a bland oil or ointment.

b., alkali. Due to caustic alkalies, as lye, caustic potash (potassium hydroxide), caustic soda (sodium hydroxide), etc.

SYM: Painful lesion of skin often associated with gelatinization of tissue.

F.A. TREATMENT: Wash with large volumes of water. Follow by wet dressings of dilute acid, as citrus fruit juices, weak vinegar, dilute acetic acid, etc. Later dress with bland ointments or oils, or irrigate with boric acid solution. Follow by instillation of liquid paraffin or other bland oil.

b., brush. A combined burn and abrasion resulting from friction. Treatment: Like abrasion, q.v.

b., chemical. Injuries due to the action of corrosive or irritating chemicals, as acid burns, q.v., alkali burns, q.v.

Burns from chemical acids or alkalies should be treated by flushing the surface with water, thereby removing all traces of the drug. Do not delay irrigation because sterile water or saline is unavailable, even for eye burns. Use the nearest available supply of clean water. Remember that usually an acid counteracts an alkali, so that weak vinegar or weak ammonia is always safe. A carbolic acid burn is almost always counteracted by alcohol. Never use oil as it helps in the absorption of acid. If lime gets into the eye, flush the eye with water and follow with normal saline solution irrigation.

b., electric. A result of exposure to electricity. The extent of destruction is much greater than that evidenced by initial inspection. Treatment: SEE: *electric contacts and injuries.*

b. of eye. F. A. Treatment: Wash immediately with the nearest available supply of water. Do not delay because water is un-sterile or cool. Irrigation may need to be continued for hours if burn is due to lye.

b., fireworks. Fireworks injuries are usually burns, often with embedded foreign bodies and a high incidence of infection and tetanus which should be prevented by meticulous care of injury and use of antitetanus serum.

b., flash. A b. resulting from an explosive blast such as occurs from ignition of highly imflammable fluids, or in war, from a high-explosive shell or a nuclear blast.

b., gunpowder. Often followed by tetanus which should be prevented by administration of antitetanus serum and meticulous care of injury.

b., radiation. B. resulting from overexposure to radiant energy as from roentgen rays, radium emanations, sunlight, or nuclear blast.

b., respiratory. B. in which the respiratory tract is injured, as from inhalation of hot gases.

b., thermal. B. resulting from contact with fire, hot objects, or fluids.

b., x-ray. SEE: *burn, radiation.*

burning foot syndrome. A sensation of burning of the sole of the foot. Occurs in certain vitamin deficiencies. SYN: *electric foot syndrome.*

Burns' amaurosis (bŭrnz am″au-rō′sĭs) [Gr. *amaurōsis,* darkening]. [John Burns, Scottish obstetrician, 1774-1850] Dimness of sight or blindness following sexual excesses. SYN: *postmarital amblyopia.*

Note: There is no evidence that this is a disease entity. The entry is retained in this edition for historical reasons.

burrow (bŭr′ō). A tunnel made in the skin by the itch mite, Sarcoptes scabei.

bur'rowing. The formation of a subcutaneous tunnel made by a parasite, or of a fistula or sinus containing pus.

bur'sa [Gr., a leather sack]. (pl. *bursae*) 1. A padlike sac or cavity found in connecting tissue usually in the vicinity of joints. They are lined with synovial membrane and contain a fluid, synovia, which acts to reduce friction between tendon and bone, tendon and ligament, or between other structures where friction is likely to occur. 2. A blind sac or cavity.

b., Achilles. B. located between the tendon of Achilles and the calcaneus.

b., adventitious. B. not usually present but which develops in response to friction or pressure.

b., olecranon. B. at the elbow joint lying between olecranon process and the skin.

b., omental. The lesser peritoneal cavity; the cavity of the great omentum. It communicates with the greater or true peritoneal cavity via the vestibule and epiploic foramen.

b., patellar. One of several bursae located in region of the patella. Includes the suprapatellar, infrapatellar, and prepatellar bursae. Some communicate with the cavity of the knee joint.

b., pharyngeal. A small, median, blind sac found in lower portion of the pharyngeal tonsil.

b., subacromial. A large bursa lying between the acromium and coracoacromial ligament above, and the insertion of the supraspinatus below.

bursae. Pl. of bursa, q.v.

bur'sal. Pert. to a bursa.

bursa'lis [L. *bursalis,* pert. to a bursa]. Obturator internus muscle.

bursalogy (bŭr-săl′ō-jĭ) [Gr. *bursa,* leather sack, + *-logy,* study]. Anatomy, pathology, and physiology of bursae.

bursectomy (bŭr-sĕk′tō-mĭ) [″+ *ektomē,* excision]. Excision of a bursa.

bursitis (bŭr-sī′tĭs) [″+ *-itis,* inflammation]. Inflammation of a bursa, esp. those located between bony prominences and muscle or tendon, as the shoulder, knee, etc.

Common forms include painful shoulder (bursa, subacromial, q.v.) miner's or tennis elbow (bursa, olecranon, q.v.), housemaid's knee (prepatellar bursitis, q.v.), and bunion, q.v.

TREATMENT: Rest, immobilization of affected part during acute stage. Active mobilization as soon as acute symptoms subside will help to prevent adhesions. Analgesics, heat, and diathermy are helpful. Injection of local anesthetics or cortisone into bursa may be required. In chronic bursitis surgical removal of calcification may be necessary.

bursolith (bŭr′so-lĭth) [Gr. *bursa,* leather sack, + *lithos,* stone]. A calculus formed in a bursa.

bursopathy (bŭr-sop′ă-thĭ) [″+ *pathos,* disease]. Any pathological condition of a bursa.

bursula (bur′sū-lă) [L., little sack]. A small bursa.

b. testium. The scrotum.

Burton's line (bŭr′tŏn). [Henry Burton, Brit. physician, 1799-1849] A blue line along the margin of the gums visible in chronic lead poisoning.

butacaine sulfate (bū′tă-kān). A topical local anesthetic.

butane (bū′tăn). C_4H_{10}. A gaseous, inflammable hydrocarbon from petroleum.

butazolidin (bū″tă-zol′ĭ-din). Proprietary name for phenylbutazone, used in treatment of acute rheumatic disease. It has a potent anti-inflammatory action.

butisol sodium (bū′tĭ-sol sō′dĭ-ŭm). Proprietary name for butabarbital sodium, a sedative and hypnotic.

butter (bŭt′ĕr) [Gr. *bouturon,* from *bous,* cow, + *turos,* cheese]. Soft, yellowish, or whitish oily mass produced by churning cream. Consists largely of butter fat which is made up of stearin. Butyric, palmitic, and oleic acid are the acids found in butter fat.

     Food value of 100 gm. salted (approx. 10 pats or 7 tablespoons): Cal. 716; fat 81 gm.; carbohydrate 0.4 gm.; calcium 20 mg.; phosphorus 16 mg.; sodium 987 mg.; potassium 23 mg.; vitamin A, 3300 I.U. (Unsalted butter contains less than 10 mg. of sodium or potassium per 100 gm.)

buttermilk. Sour fluid obtained by separating the butterfat from cream or milk which has been churned.

     Food value of 100 gm.: Cal. 36; protein 3.6 gm.; fat 0.1 gm.; carbohydrate 5.1 gm.; calcium 121 mg.; phosphorus 95 mg.; sodium 130 mg.; potassium 140 mg.; riboflavin 0.18 mg.; niacin 0.1 mg.; ascorbic acid 1.0 mg.

buttocks (bŭt′ŭks) [AS. *buttuc,* end]. The external prominences posterior to the hips. Formed by the gluteal muscles and underlying structures. Commonly called seat.

buttonhole. A straight cut through the wall of a cavity.

     b. fracture. Perforation of a bone by a missile.

     b., mitral. Contraction of any orifice to a slit, as that of the heart.

     b. operation. Boutonnière operation. An artificial slit in a membrane.

button suture. Suture in which threads are passed through buttons on the surface and tied to prevent thread from cutting through or into underlying tissue.

butylchloral hydrate (bū″tĭl-klō′răl hī′drăt). A preparation similar in action to chloral, but said to be less depressant and more analgesic. Used for temporary relief of facial neuralgia.

butyraceous (bū″tĭ-rā′shŭs) [L. *butyrum,* butter, from Gr. *bouturon,* butter]. Containing or resembling butter.

butyrate (bū′tĭ-rāt). A salt of butyric acid.

butyric acid (bū-tĭr′ĭk) [L. *butyrum,* butter]. A fatty acid (C_3H_7COOH); derived from butter but rare in most fats. It is a viscid liquid with a rancid odor. Used in disinfectants, emulsifying agents and pharmaceuticals.

butyrin (bū′tĭr-ĭn). A soft, yellowish, semi-liquid fat which is present in butter.

butyroid (bū′tĭ-royd) [L. *butyrum,* butter, from Gr. *bouturon,* butter, + *eidos,* appearance]. Having the appearance or consistency of butter.

butyrometer (bū″tĭ-rom′ĕ-ter) ["+ *metron,* measure]. Device for estimating amt. of butter fat of milk.

butyrous (bŭt′ĭ-rŭs). Of butter-like consistency.

Byrd-Dew method. [Harvey L. Byrd, Amer. physician, 1820-1884; James H. Dew, Amer. physician, 1843-1914] Method for resuscitating newborn child suffering from asphyxia. Operator supports supine child on palms of his hands, allowing head to fall backward. By supination of forearms, operator flexes child's body and effects expiration. By pronation of arms, body is again extended, causing inspiration.

bysma (bĭs′mă) [Gr., plug]. A plug or tampon.

byssinosis (bĭs″ĭ-nō′sĭs) [Gr. *byssos,* cotton, + *-ōsis,* disease]. Pulmonary disease caused by the inhalation of cotton dust and the foreign materials contained therein, including bacteria, mold, and fungi.

byssocausis (bĭs″ō-kaw′sĭs) ["+ *kausis,* burning]. Cauterization by moxa; moxibustion.

byssoid (bĭs′oyd) ["+ *eidos,* form]. Consisting of a filamentous fringe, the filaments being of unequal length.

byssophthisis (bĭs″o-this′ĭs) [Gr. *byssos,* cotton, + *phthisis,* a wasting away]. Byssinosis, q.v.

byssus (bĭs′us). The growth of hair on the pubic region.

C

C. 1. Chem. symb. for carbon. 2. Abbr. for *Celsius* (scale or thermometer); *centigrade;* L. *centum,* one hundred; *clonus; closure; compound; congius* (gallon); L. *cum,* with.

C¹⁴. Radioactive carbon.

Ca. 1. Chem. symb. for calcium. 2. Abbr. for *cathode.*

cabbage (kăb'ij) [Fr. *cabocher,* to make a swelling]. A leafy vegetable, growing as a head on a short, thick stalk. A base-forming food.

Food value of 100 gm. (1 cup) (raw; shredded): Cal. 24; protein 1.3 gm.; carbohydrate 5.4 gm.; calcium 49 mg.; phosphorus 29 mg.; iron 0.4 mg.; sodium 20 mg.; potassium 233 mg.; vitamin A, 130 I.U.; niacin 0.3 mg.; ascorbic acid 47 mg.

Cabot's ring bodies. [Richard C. Cabot, Amer. physician, 1868-1939] Ring-shaped bodies sometimes seen in red blood cells in pernicious anemia, lymphatic leukemia, and lead poisoning.

cac-, caco- [Gr. from *kakos,* bad]. Prefix denoting bad or diseased.

CaC₂. Calcium carbide.

cacanthrax [Gr. *kakos,* bad, + *anthrax,* carbuncle]. Malignant form of anthrax.

cacao (kă-kā'ō, kă-kā'ō) [Mexican Spanish from Nahuatl *cacahuatl,* cacao beans]. 1. Seed of Theobroma cacao used to prepare cacao butter (theobroma oil), chocolate, and cocoa. 2. A reddish to brown powder prepared from the roasted ripe seeds of Theobroma cacao Linné (family Sterculiaceae) and having a chocolate odor and taste. Used in a syrup base, as a flavoring vehicle for certain medications. SEE: *cocoa.*

cacesthesia (kak″es-thē'zĭ-ă) [Gr. *kakos,* bad, + *aisthēsis,* sensation]. 1. Disorder of sensibility, morbid or otherwise. 2. Malaise.

caché (kă-shā') [Fr., covered]. A lead cone covered with paper layers, with mica bottom, used for applying radiotherapy, radium, or any radioactive substance.

cachectic (kă-kĕk'tĭk) [Gr. *kakos,* bad, + *hexis,* condition]. Pert. to cachexia.

cachet (kă-shā') [Fr., a seal]. Two concave pieces of wafer (rice paper) between which is placed medicine to be administered, the margins being pressed together so they will adhere. Used for administering medicines which have an unpleasant taste. The cachet is swallowed whole.

cachexia (kă-kĕks'ĭ-ă) [Gr. *kakos,* bad, + *hexis,* condition]. A state of ill health, malnutrition and wasting. It may occur in many chronic diseases as certain malignancies, advanced pulmonary tuberculosis, etc.

c., cancerous. C. caused by cancerous condition.

c., hypophyseal. C., pituitary, q.v.

c. hypophysiopri'va. Symptoms resulting from removal of the hypophysis cerebri.

c., lymphatic. C. caused by Hodgkin's disease of the lymph nodes.

c., malarial. C. due to chronic malaria.

c., pachydermic. C. due to myxedemic condition.

c., pituitary. Group of symptoms caused by atrophy of pituitary gland, including emaciation, premature aging, atrophy of genitals with loss of secondary sex characteristics and lowering of basal metabolic rate. SYN: *Simmond's disease.*

c. strumipri'va. Myxedema due to removal of the thyroid gland.

c., thyreopriva. C., strumipriva, q.v.

cachinnation (kak-ĭ-nā'shun) [L. *cachinnāre,* to laugh aloud]. Hysterical laughter.

CaCl₂. Calcium chloride; a bleaching powder.

Ca(ClO₃)₂. Calcium chlorate.

caco-, cac- [Gr. from *kakos,* bad]. Prefix denoting bad or diseased.

CaCO₃. Calcium carbonate; chalk.

CaC₂O₄. Calcium oxalate.

cacochylia (kăk-ō-kī'lĭ-ă) [Gr. *kakos,* bad, + *chylos,* juice, chyle]. Impaired digestion.

cacodontia (kak-o-don'shĭ-ă) [″+ *odous, odont-,* tooth]. Bad teeth.

cacodylate (kak'o-dil-āt). A salt of cacodylic acid, used in skin diseases or where arsenic is indicated.

cacoethes (kăk″ō-ē'thēz) [Gr. *kakos,* bad, + *ēthos,* character]. Any bad habit, propensity, or disorder.

cacogenesis (kăk″ō-jĕn'ē-sĭs) [Gr. *kakos,* bad, + *genesis,* development]. Any abnormal development or growth.

cacogenic. Pert. to race degeneration.

cacogenics (kăk″ō-jĕn'iks) [Gr. *kakos,* bad, + *gennan,* to produce]. Race degeneration resulting from reproduction of inferior persons.

cacogeusia (kăk″ō-gū'sĭ-ă) [″+ *geusis,* taste]. The production of an abhorrent, obnoxious taste by chewing or the introduction of food into the mouth.

cacomelia (kak″ō-me'lĭ-ă) [″+ *melos,* limb]. Congenital deformity of a limb.

cacomorphia (kak″ō-mor'fĭ-ă) [″+ *morphē,* form]. Malformation; deformity.

cacopathy (kăk-ŏp'ă-thĭ) [Gr. *kakos,* bad, + *pathos,* disease]. Malignant disease; a severe disorder.

cacoplastic ["+ *plastikos,* formed]. 1. Pert. to or causing morbid growth. 2. Incapable of normal development or formation.

cacorhythmic (kak"o-rith'mĭk) ["+ *rythmos,* rhythm]. Showing irregularity of rhythm.

cacosmia (kă-koz'mĭ-ă) [Gr. *kakos,* bad, + *osmē,* smell]. 1. An unpleasant odor. 2. Abhorrent, obnoxious smell produced by inhaling something which has an odor, but not the unpleasant one perceived.

cacothenics (kak"ō-then'ĭks) ["+ *thēnia,* state of being]. Racial degeneration from hostile environment.

cacothymia (kak"o-thi'mĭ-ă) ["+ *thymos,* spirit]. A disorder of the mind; moral depravity; insane morbidity of temper.

cacotrophy (kăk-ŏt'rō-fĭ) [Gr. *kakos,* bad, + *trophē,* nourishment]. Malnutrition.

cacumen (kak-ū'mĕn) [L. *cacūmen,* summit]. (pl. *cacumina*) 1. Part of cerebellum below the declivis. 2. The top or apex of an anatomical structure.

cadaver (kă-dav'er) [L., corpse]. (pl. *cadav'era*) A dead body; a corpse.

cadaveric (kă-dav'er-ĭk). Pert. to a dead body.

cadaverous (kă-dav'er-us). Resembling, esp. having the color or appearance of, a corpse.

cadmium (kad'mĭ-ŭm) [Gr. *cadmia,* earth]. SYMB: Cd. At. wt. 112.40; at. no. 48; sp. gr. 8.65. A metallic element occurring in zinc. It is a soft, bluish white metal and is used industrially in electroplating and in atomic fission.

caduca (kă-dū'kă) [L. *cadūcus,* falling off]. Thickened membrane of the uterus; the decidua of the uterus.

caduceus (kă-dū'sē-ŭs) [L., a herald's wand]. In mythology, the wand or staff carried by Hermes or Mercury, having two serpents entwined around it, and surmounted by two wings. Used as the medical insignia of certain groups such as the U.S. Army Medical Corps. Even though it is sometimes used to symbolize the medical profession, the staff of Aesculapius, q.v., Roman god of medicine, is usually considered to be the more appropriate symbol.

caffeine (kăf'ēn, kă-fēn'). USP. $C_8H_{10}N_4O_2$. An alkaloid of coffee and tea that is a central nervous system stimulant and a diuretic. About 100 mg. are found in a strong cup of coffee.

    Used as a diuretic, cardiac, and respiratory stimulant, and as a headache remedy. Incompatibilities are alkalies, tannic acid, quinine sulfate.

    c., citrated. A mixture of caffeine and citric acid, containing about 52% caffeine. Possesses same properties as caffeine, but more likely to disagree with the digestive functions.

    c. and sodium benzoate injection USP. A mixture of equal parts of caffeine and sodium benzoate. Action and uses same as caffeine.

    c. and sodium salicylate. A mixture of caffeine with sodium salicylate, containing about 52% caffeine. Uses same as caffeine.

caffeinism (kăf'en-ĭzm). Chronic effects of excessive use of coffee.

    SYM: Sudden flushing of the face, palpitation of the heart, trembling, general depression, anxiety, insomnia, and nervousness.

cainotophobia (ki-no"to-fo'bĭ-ă) [Gr. *kainotēs,* novelty, + *phobos,* fear]. Fear of novelty. Cenotophobia, q.v.

caisson disease (kā'sŏn) [Fr. *caisse,* a box, from L. *capsa,* box]. A condition which develops in divers subjected to too rapid reduction of air pressure after coming to the surface following exposure to compressed air. The cause is nitrogen bubbles in the tissue spaces.

    TREATMENT: Recompression and then slow decompression. This is done in a special hyperbaric chamber. SYN: *decompression sickness; bends,* q.v.

caked breast. Accumulation of milk in the secreting ducts of the breast following delivery.

Cal. Abbr. of *large Calorie.* One large Calorie is equal to 1000 calories. A large Calorie may be noted by capitalizing the initial letter of the word; or by using kilocalorie (abbr. kcal.).

cal. Abbr. of *small calorie.* When a small calorie is indicated the initial letter should not be capitalized, to differentiate from large Calorie. SEE: *Cal.*

calage (kal-ăzh') [Fr., wedging]. Fixation of body in a berth by means of pillows to prevent movement and so to relieve seasickness.

calamine (kal'ă-mīn). USP. A pink powder, containing zinc oxide with small amt. of ferric oxide.

    Used externally in various skin conditions, as a protective and astringent, as an ointment, or as a lotion.

calcaneal, calcanean (kal-kā'nē-ăl, -an) [L. *calcaneus,* heel bone]. Pert. to the calcaneus, the heel bone.

calcaneodynia (kal-kă″nē-ō-din′ĭ-ă) [″+ Gr. *odynē*, pain]. Pain in the heel.

calcaneum (kal-kā′nē-ŭm) [L. *calcaneus*, heel bone]. (pl. *calcanea*) Calcaneus, q.v.

calcaneus (kal-kā′nē-us). (pl. *calcanei*) 1. [NA] The heel bone, or os calcis. It articulates anteriorly with the cuboid bone, and with the astragalus above. 2. Talipes calcaneus, q.v.

calcanodynia (kal″kan-o-din′ĭ-ă) [L. *calcaneus*, heel bone, + *odynē*, pain]. Pain in the heel when standing or walking; calcaneodynia.

calcar (kăl′kar) [L., a spur]. A spurlike process.

    c. avis. [NA] Hippocampus minor, lower of two elevations on inner wall of posterior horn of lateral ventricle of brain.

    c. femorale. A bony spur that strengthens the femoral neck.

    c. pedis. The heel.

calcareous (kal-ka′re-us) [L. *calcarius*, pert. to lime]. Of the nature of lime; chalky.

calcarine (kal′kar-īn) [L. *calcar*, spur]. Spurshaped.

calcariuria (kal-kar′ĭ-ū′rĭ-ă) [L. *calcarius*, pert. to lime, + Gr. *ouron*, urine]. Presence of calcium lime salts in the urine.

calcaroid (kăl′kăr-oyd) [″+ Gr. *eidos*, appearance]. Calciumlike deposit in brain tissue.

calcemia (kal-sē′mĭ-ă) [″+ Gr. *haima*, blood]. Excess of calcium in the blood.

calcic (kal′sĭk) [L. *calcarius*]. Pert. to calcium or lime.

calcicosis (kăl″sĭ-ko′sis) [L. *calx*, lime, + Gr. *-ōsis*, infection]. Pneumoconiosis caused by inhaling dust from limestone, esp. by marblecutters.

calciferol (kăl-sĭf′ĕr-ol). Vitamin D₂. A synthetic vitamin D; it has the most vitamin D activity of those substances derived from ergosterol. It is used for prophylaxis and treatment of vitamin D deficiency, rickets and in hypocalcemic tetany.

calciferous (kal-sif′er-us) [L. *calx*, lime, + *ferre*, to carry]. Containing calcium, chalk, or lime.

calcific (kal-sif′ĭk) [″+ *facere*, to make]. Forming lime.

calcification (kal″sĭ-fĭ-kā′shun). Deposit of lime salts in the tissues, and commonly in bone.

    c., arterial. Deposition of calcium in walls of arteries.

    c., metastatic. That of soft tissue with transference of calcium from bone, as in osteomalacia and disease of the parathyroid glands.

calcigerous (kal-sij′er-us) [L. *calx*, lime, + *gerere*, to bear]. Containing lime or lime salts.

    c. tubes. Dentinal tubules of dentin.

calcimeter (kăl-sĭm′ĕ-ter) [″+ Gr. *metron*, measure]. Device for measuring the calcium in the blood.

calcination (kăl″sĭ-nā′shun) [L. *calcinare*, char]. Drying by roasting to produce a powder.

calcinorrhachia (kal″sin-o-ra′kĭ-ă) [L. *calx*, lime, + Gr. *rhachis*, spine]. Calcium in the spinal fluid.

calcinosis [″+ Gr. *-ōsis*, infection]. Deposit of lime salts in tissues.

calcipectic (kal″sĭ-pek′tik) [″+ Gr. *pēgnunai*, to fix]. Pert. to calcipexis, q.v.

calcipenia (kăl″sĭ-pē′nĭ-ă) [L. *calx*, lime, + Gr. *penia*, poverty]. Calcium deficiency in body tissues and fluids.

calcipexic (kal″sĭ-pĕx′ĭc) [L. *calx*, lime, + Gr. *pēgnunai*, to fix]. Pert. to calcipexis.

calcipexis, calcipexy (kăl″sĭ-pĕk′sis, -pĕks′ĭ). The fixation of calcium in body tissues.

calciphilia (kal-sĭ-fĭl′ĭ-ă) [L. *calx*, lime, + Gr. *philein*, to love]. Tendency to calcification.

calciphylaxis (kăl″sĭ-fĭ-lăks′ĭs) [″+ Gr. *phylaxis*, a guarding]. A state of induced tissue sensitivity characterized by calcification of tissue when challenged by an appropriate stimulus.

calciprivia (kal″sĭ-priv′ĭ-ă) [″+ *privus*, without]. Deficiency or absence of calcium.

calciprivic (kal″sĭ-priv′ĭk). Pert. to deficiency or absence of calcium in the body.

calcitonin. A hormone from the thyroid gland in man. It is important in bone and calcium metabolism. In other mammals it is produced by the ultimobranchial bodies which become fused with the thyroid. For that reason it formerly was designated thyrocalcitonin.

calcium (kăl′sē-um) [L. *calx*, lime]. SYMB: Ca. At. wt. 40.08; at. no. 20. Silver-white metallic element, the basis of limestone.

    Lime is its oxide. Calcium phosphate constitutes 75% of the body ash, and about 85% of mineral matter in bones.

    FUNCTION: Calcium must be carried by the blood in solution before being available for bone growth. Unless certain activating substances, such as vitamin D, are present, increased calcium intake does not affect the tissues or blood calcium. The secretions of the parathyroid glands are a factor in the utilization of calcium, making it possible for the blood to carry dissolved calcium.

    Quantities of bread, rice, oatmeal, and corn in the diet decrease absorption of calcium and phosphorus, and the alkalinity of the small intestines promotes the formation of insoluble salts.

Calcium is of great importance for coagulation of the blood; to give firmness and rigidity to bones and teeth; as a preventive of rickets; as an ion balance; as essential to lactation; for activating enzymes; for the functions of the muscles, nerves, and heart; and for maintaining the permeability of membranes.

Calcium is taken into the body as a constituent of various foods. While much of it may prove insoluble and escape absorption, some of it passes through the intestine into the blood, where it can be found by chemical tests. Its level in the serum is normally 10.5-11.0 mg./100 ml. Low blood calcium causes tetany with muscular twitching, spasms, and convulsions. Blood deprived of its calcium will not clot, and milk without calcium will not curdle.

Calcium is deposited in the bones, but can be mobilized again to keep the blood level constant when there is a period of insufficient intake. At any given time the body of an adult contains about 700 gm. of calcium phosphate; of this, 120 gm. are the element calcium. Ordinarily an adult takes in 0.8 gm. of calcium per day. During pregnancy 1.3 gm. of calcium a day will be required.

SOURCES: *Excellent:* Beans; cauliflower; chard; cheese; cream; egg yolk; kale; milk; molasses; rhubarb. *Good:* Almonds; beets; bran; cabbage; carrots; celery; chocolate; dates; figs; kohlrabi; lemons; lettuce; oatmeal; oranges; oysters; parsnips; pineapples; raspberries; rutabagas; shell fish; spinach; turnips; walnuts; watercress.

SEE: *acalcicosis; "calci-"* words.

c. carbonate, precipitated. $CaCO_3$ (precipitated chalk). USP. A fine, white, tasteless and odorless powder.

ACTION AND USES: An antacid, also antidote to corrosive acid poisoning.

c. chloride. ($CaCl_2$). USP. A very deliquescent salt occurring as translucent crystals having a sharp saline taste.

ACTION AND USES: To raise the calcium content of the blood in disorders resulting from lack of sufficient calcium, such as in hypocalcemic tetany. Used in solution and administered intravenously.

INCOMPATIBILITIES: Ephedrine.

c. deficiency. SYM: Brittle bones; poor development of bones and teeth; dental caries; rickets; tetany; heart atony; hyperirritability; excessive bleeding.

DIAGNOSIS: Normal content in blood serum is 9 to 10.5 mg. per 100 ml. of blood.

In evaluating the calcium level, laboratory error and variation may be the causes of inaccurate or inconsistent values.

c. disodium edetate. USP. A substance used to bind certain metallic ions in the body. Used in treating poisoning due to those metals.

c. gluconate. USP. A granular or white powder without odor or taste.

ACTION AND USES: Same as calcium chloride. More pleasant to taste and nonirritating when administered orally or intramuscularly in a 10% solution.

c., high, in diet. A normal adequate diet including 1 1/2 qt. milk, cheese, eggs, clams, and vegetables, esp. broccoli, cauliflower, beans, beets, and other greens.

c. hydroxide. USP. A white powder used in preparing calcium hydroxide solution, which is used as an astringent applied to the skin and mucous membranes.

c. lactate. A white, odorless and nearly tasteless powder, less irritating than the chloride.

Used orally or parenterally as an alternative to calcium gluconate.

c. levulinate. Soluble white powder used when intravenous administration of calcium is required.

c., low, in diet. Milk, cheese, and other foods high in calcium are avoided.

c. oxide. A corrosive and easily pulverized mineral occurring as a hard white or grayish-white mass. Used as germicide and disinfectant.

c. phosphate, precipitated. A white, amorphous powder used as an antacid in treatment of gastric hyperacidity.

calciuria (kal″sĭ-ū′rĭ-ă) [L. *calx*, lime, + Gr. *ouron*, urine]. Calcium in the urine.

calcopherous (kal-kof′er-us) [″+ Gr. *phoros*, bearing]. Containing or producing lime or any salts of calcium.

calcospherite (kăl″kō-sfē′rit) [″+ Gr. *sphaira*, sphere]. One of many small calcareous bodies found in tumors, nervous tissue, the thyroid and prostate.

calcreose (kal′kre-oze). A chemical combination of creosote and lime containing approximately 50% creosote.

calculary (kal′ku-la-rī) [L. *calculus*, pebble]. Pert. to calculus.

calculi (kăl′kū-lī). Pl. of calculus, q.v.

calculifragous (kăl″kū-lĭf′ră-gŭs) [L. *calculus*, pebble, + *frangere*, to break]. Breaking or reducing a stone in the bladder.

calculosis (kăl″kū-lō′sĭs) [″+ -*ōsis*, infection]. Having a calculus.

calculous (kal′kū-lŭs). Like a calculus.

calculus (kal'kū-lŭs) [L., pebble]. (pl. *calculi*) Commonly called stone; any abnormal concretion within the animal body, usually composed of mineral salts.

These pathological concretions occur in the kidneys, ureter, bladder, urethra, usually formed of crystalline, urinary salts held together by viscid organic matter. SYN: *stone.*

ETIOL: Abnormal function of the parathyroid glands; disordered uric acid metabolism as in gout; excess intake of milk and alkali. However, most kidney stones form from a cause which is unexplainable.

c., biliary. Cholelithiasis, q.v.; gallstones. SEE: *gallbladder.*

c., hemic. One formed of coagulated blood.

c., pancreatic. Calculus in the pancreas, q.v.

c., renal. Calculus in the kidney. SYN: *nephrolithiasis.*

SYM: Blockage of flow of urine from kidney if the ureter is blocked by the stone; sudden, severe, and paroxysmal renal colic; ureteral stricture; inflammation of various degrees.

PROG: Serious if allowed to continue untreated.

TREATMENT: Relief of pain, force fluids unless passage is completely blocked by the calculus. Medicines to relax smooth muscle help to allow the stone to pass and to relieve pain. If the stone is preventing urine flow or if the stone continues to grow and cause infection, surgery must be performed.

c., salivary. Calculus in salivary duct. Usually affects duct of submaxillary gland.

SYM: Obstructs flow of saliva, causing severe pain and swelling of gland, esp. when eating.

TREATMENT: Removal of stone by surgery.

c., urinary. Calculus in any part of the urinary system.

SYM: Sudden stoppage of flow of urine with sharp pain in obstruction, and, if firmly impacted, complete retention of urine.

TREATMENT: Removal of calculus by surgical means or special techniques involving the use of instruments introduced through the urethra into the bladder and ureter.

c., vesical. Calculus in the bladder.

SYM: Frequency of urination, pain, diurnal hematuria increased by exercise are suggestive.

PROG: Stone is usually small enough to pass through urethra.

TREATMENT: The use of an analgesic and an antispasmodic if necessary; adequate fluid intake. Special urological or surgical procedure if stone is large or impacted.

calculus, words pert. to: "calcu-" words; "chol-" words; gravel; "lith-" words.

calefacient (kăl''ē-fa'shĕnt) [L. *calere,* to be warm, + *facere,* to make]. Conveying or that which conveys a sense of warmth when applied to a part of the body.

calf [AS. *cealf*]. The fleshy, muscular back part of the leg below the knee formed by the gastrocnemius and soleus muscles.

caliber (kăl'ĭ-bĕr) [Fr. *calibre,* diameter of bore of gun]. The diameter of any orifice or opening.

calibration (kal-ĭ-brā'shun). Estimation of the caliber of an opening.

calibrator (kăl'ĭ-bra-tor). 1. Instrument for measuring the size of tubes or orifices. 2. Device for dilating tubes such as the esophagus or ureter.

c., anastomosis. One for determining size of opening to be anastomosis.

c., vaginal. One for determining degree of vaginal relaxation.

caliculus (kă-lik'ū-lŭs) [L. *calyculus,* small cup]. A cup-shaped structure.

c. gustato'rius. [NA]. A taste bud.

c. ophthal'micus. [NA]. The optic cup.

caliectasis (kal'ĭ-ek'tas-is) [Gr. *kalyx,* cup, + *ektasis,* dilatation]. Dilatation of the renal calyx; calicectasis.

californium (kal'ĭ-for'nĭ-ŭm). [Named for California, the state and university where it was first discovered in 1950] SYMB: Cf. At. wt. 244 to 254; at. no. 98. A chemical element prepared by bombardment of curium with alpha particles. It has properties similar to dysprosium.

caligation (kal'ĭ-gā'shŭn). Caligo, q.v.

caligo (kă-li'go) [L., darkness]. Dimness of vision. SYN: *caligation.*

caliper(s (kăl'ĭ-pĕr) [Fr. *calibre,* diameter of bore of gun]. Instrument for measuring diameters, as those of chest or pelvis.

calix (ka'liks). Calyx, q.v.

Calliphora vomitoria (kă-lĭf'ĕr-ă). Common blowfly sometimes causing myiasis disorders.

callisection [L. *callus,* hardened, insensitive, + *sectio,* a cutting]. Vivisection under anesthesia.

callomania (kal''o-mā'nĭ-ă) [Gr. *kalos,* beautiful, + *mania,* madness]. Belief in one's own beauty; a delusion of the insane.

callosal (kă-lō'sal) [L. *callus,* tough substance]. Pert. to the corpus callosum.

callosity, callositas (kă-los'ĭ-tĭ, -tas) [L. *callōsus,* thick-skinned]. Circumscribed thickening and hypertrophy of the horny layer of the skin. SYN: *callus*.

ETIOL: Friction, pressure, or other irritation, oval or elongated, on flexor surfaces of hands and feet, grayish or brownish and slightly elevated, with smooth, burnished surfaces.

TREATMENT: Temporary removal by salicylic acid or careful shaving. Permanent removal only by removal of cause. SEE: *porosis*.

callosomarginal (kă-lo″so-mar′jĭ-nal) [L. *callus*, tough, + *margo*, margin]. Pert. to the corpus callosum and marginal gyrus, marking sulcus between them.

callosum (kă-lo′sum) [L. *callōsus*, hard]. The great commissure of the brain between the cerebral hemispheres. SYN: *corpus callosum*.

callous (kăl′ŭs) [L. *callus*, hard]. Hard; like a callus.

callus (kăl′ŭs). 1. Hypertrophied thickening of circumscribed area of horny layer of skin; callosity, q.v. 2. The osseous material thrown out between ends of a fractured bone.

    c., definitive. Cartilage found between two ends of a fractured bone.

    c., provisional. Temporary deposit between ends of a fractured bone.

calmative (kăm′ă-tĭv, kăl′mă-). 1. Sedative; soothing. 2. An agent that acts as a sedative.

Calmette's reaction (kăl-mĕt′). [Leon Charles A. Calmette, Fr. bacteriologist, 1863-1933] Severe reaction of conjunctiva in one with an infective disease upon introduction of toxins of the same disease. SYN: *ophthalmoreaction*.

calomel (kăl′ŏ-mĕl) [Gr. *kalos*, beautiful, + *melas*, black]. Mercurous chloride, q.v.

calor (ka′lor) [L., heat]. 1. Heat. 2. Moderate heat of fever. Along with rubor, tumor, dolor (i.e., redness, swelling, pain), it represents the four classical signs of inflammation.

calorescence (kal″or-es′ens). Producing incandescence of a body by heating with radiation by means of a lens.

caloric (kă-lor′ĭk) [L. *calor*, heat]. Relating to heat or to a calorie.

    c. excess. Intake of calories in excess of that required for growth and metabolic processes, or for maintenance of desirable weight in the adult.

caloricity (kal″or-is′ĭ-tĭ). Heating power of the body.

calorie (kăl′ŏ-rē) [L. *calor*, heat]. A unit of heat. Also spelled *calory*.

    A calorie may be equated to work or to other units of heat measurement. The following conversion factors are commonly

used: to convert from calories to joules, multiply by 4. 1858 × 10² ; to convert from calories per minute to watts, multiply by 6. 9733 × 10⁻².

    c., gram. C., small, q.v.

    c., kilogram. C., large, q.v.

    c., large. The amount of heat needed to change temperature of one kilogram of water from 14.5° C to 15.5° C. Commonly employed in metabolic studies. When writing of human nutrition the large or kilogram calorie is used. Calorie is always capitalized in order to distinguish it from a small calorie. ABBR: Cal., or kcal. in scientific literature. SYN: *kilogram calorie*.

    c̄., small. The amount of heat needed to change temperature of one gram of water one degree centigrade. SYN: *gram calorie; microcalorie*. ABBR: cal.

calorific (kal″ō-rĭf′ĭk). Producing heat; calorifacient.

calorigenic (kă-lor′ĭ-jĕn′ĭk) [L. *calor*, heat, + Gr. *gennan*, to produce]. Pert. to heat production or its increase.

calorimeter (kal″ō-rĭm′ē-ter) [L. *calor*, heat, + Gr. *metron*, measure]. Instrument for determining heat of bodies.

    c., bomb. Apparatus for determination of potential energy of foods by measuring heat in combustion.

    c., respiratory. Apparatus for determination of heat production calculated from exchange of respiratory gases.

calorimetry (kal″ō-rĭm′ē-trĭ). Determination of heat loss or gain.

    c., indirect. Determination of heat production from amt. of oxygen used and carbon dioxide eliminated.

caloripuncture (kaľ″ō-rĭ-punk′tūr). Use of heated needles in cauterization by puncture. SYN: *ignipuncture*.

Calori's bursa (kal-ō′rē). [Luigi Calori, It. anatomist, 1807-1896] Bursa sometimes found between arch of aorta and trachea.

cal′ory. Calorie, q.v.

calvaria (kăl-va′rĭ-ă) [L., human skull]. [NA] Skull cap; cranium; skull.

calvities (kal-vish′ĭ-ēz) [L. *calvus*, bald]. Baldness; alopecia, q.v.

calx (kalks) [L., lime]. 1. Lime. 2. [NA] The heel.

    c. chlorinata. Chlorinated lime. Used as a deodorant and disinfectant.

    c. sulfurata. Sulfurated lime. Used as a depilatory.

    c. usta, c. viva. Burnt lime; quicklime.

calyciform (ka-lis′ĭ-form) [Gr. *kalix*, cup, + L. *forma*, shape]. Cup-shaped.

calyx (kā′lix) [Gr. *kalix*, cup]. (pl. *calyces*) Any

cuplike division of the kidney pelvis. The minor calyces enclose the tips of the renal pyramids, receiving the urine from the papillary ducts which open at their tips.

c. major. One of the major subdivisions of the renal pelvis, two or three in number.

c. minor. A subdivision of a major calyx, each terminating in relation to one to three papillae.

camera (kăm'ĕr-ă) [L., vault]. In anatomy, a chamber, cavity or open space.

c. anterior bulbi. The anterior chamber of the eye between the cornea and the iris.

c. posterior bulbi. Posterior chamber of the eye between the iris and the lens.

camisole (kăm'ĭ-sōl) [Fr., little shirt]. A straitjacket used for restraining violent mental patients.

cam'omile. SEE: *chamomile.*

cam'phor [Malay *kāpūr,* chalk]. USP. A gum obtained from an evergreen tree native to China and Japan.

ACTION AND USES: Topically, as 0.1% preparation, as an antipruritic.

cam'phorated. Combined with or containing camphor.

c. oil. Liniment containing camphor.

camphoromania (kam-for-ō-mā'nĭ-ă) [Malay *kāpūr,* chalk, + Gr. *mania,* madness]. Abnormal craving for camphor.

campimeter (kamp-im'ĕ-ter) [L. *campus,* field, + Gr. *metron,* measure]. Device for measuring field of vision.

campimetry (kamp-im'ĕ-trĭ). Measurement of field of vision. SYN: *perimetry.*

campospasm (kăm'pō-spăzm). Camptocormia, q.v.

camptocormia (kamp"to-kor'mĭ-ă) [Gr. *kamptos,* bent, + *kormos,* trunk]. Abnormal flexing of body.

camptodactylia (kamp"to-dak-til'ĭ-ă) ["+ *dactylos,* finger]. Permanent flexion of fingers or toes.

camptospasm (kamp'to-spăzm) ["+ *spasmos,* spasm]. Camptocormia, q.v.

canal (kă-năl') [L. *canālis,* channel]. (pl. *canals*) A narrow tube, channel, or passageway. SEE: *duct; foramen; groove; space.*

c., adductor. Hunter's c.; a triangular space lying beneath the sartorius muscle and between the adductor longus and the vastus medialis muscles. It extends from the apex of the femoral triangle to the popliteal

Recommended Daily Caloric Intake*

	Age years	kg.	Weight pounds	cm.	Height inches	Kilocalories
Children	1–2	12	26	81	32	1250
	2–3	14	31	91	36	1400
	3–4	16	35	100	39	1600
	4–6	19	42	110	43	2000
	6–8	23	51	121	48	2200
	8–10	28	62	131	52	2500
Women	10–12	35	77	142	56	2250
NOTE: During pregnancy a woman needs an	12–14	44	97	154	61	2300
	14–16	52	114	157	62	2400
additional 200 kilocalories per day; during	16–18	54	119	160	63	2300
	18–22	58	128	163	64	2000
lactation an additional 1000	22–35	58	128	163	64	2000
	35–55	58	128	160	63	1850
	55–75+	58	128	157	62	1700
Men	10–12	35	77	140	55	2500
	12–14	43	95	151	59	2700
	14–18	59	130	170	67	3000
	18–22	67	147	175	69	2800
	22–35	70	154	175	69	2800
	35–55	70	154	173	68	2600
	55–75+	70	154	171	67	2400

*Adapted from Recommended Dietary Allowances, ed. 7. Publication 1694, National Academy of Sciences, Washington, D.C., 1968.

space and transmits the femoral vessels and the saphenous nerve.

c., Alcock's. A c. on the pelvic surface of the obturator internus muscle formed by the obturator fascia. It transmits the pudendal vessels and nerve. SYN: *canalis pudendalis* [NA]; *pudendal c.*

c., alimentary. The digestive tract from mouth through the intestine.

c.'s, alveolar. C.'s in the maxilla for transmitting the posterior superior alveolar blood vessels and nerves to the upper teeth. SYN: *canales alveolares* [NA]; *dental c.'s.*

c., alveolar, inferior. C., mandibular, q.v.

c., anal. The terminal portion of the rectum opening at the anus. SYN: *canalis analis* [NA].

c., auditory, external. The external auditory meatus; transmits sound waves.

c., auditory, internal. A c. in the petrous portion of the temporal bone which transmits the acoustic and facial nerves and the acoustic artery.

c., birth. Parturient c.; passageway through which the fetus passes in parturition, specifically the uterus and vagina.

c., carotid. A c. in the petrous portion of the temporal bone which transmits interior carotid artery and the interior carotid plexus of sympathetic nerves. SYN: *canalis caroticus* [NA].

c., central. A small c. lying in the center of the spinal cord extending from the fourth ventricle to the conus medullaris. Contains cerebrospinal fluid. SYN: *.canalis centralis* [NA].

c., cervical. C. in cervix of uterus extending from internal to external os. SYN: *canalis cervicis uteri* [NA].

c., cochlear, spiral. A part of the bony labyrinth of the ear. A spiral tube about 30 mm. long making two and three-quarters turns about a central bony axis, the modiolus. Contains the scala tympani, scala vestibuli, and cochlear duct. SYN: *canalis spiralis cochleae* [NA].

c., condylar. A c. in the occipital bone which transmits emissary vein from the transverse sinus. Opens anterior to the occipital condyle. SYN: *canalis condylaris* [NA]; *condyloid c.*

c., craniopharyngeal. A c. in the sphenoid bone of a fetus which contains the stalk of Rathke's pouch.

c.'s, dental. Alveolar c.'s, q.v.

c., ethmoidal. Two grooves running transversely across the lateral mass of the ethmoid bone to the cribiform plate. Lie between ethmoid and frontal bones. The an-

terior ethmoidal c. transmits the anterior ethmoidal vessels and the nasociliary nerve; the posterior ethmoidal c. transmits the posterior ethmoidal vessels and nerve.

c., facial. A c. in the internal acoustic meatus of the temporal bone which transmits the facial nerve. SYN: *canalis facialis* [NA].

c., femoral. The medial division of the femoral sheath. It is a short compartment about 1.5 cm. long lying behind the inguinal ligament. Contains some lymphatic vessels and a lymph node. SYN: *canalis femoralis* [NA].

c., gastric. A longitudinal groove on the inner surface of the stomach following the lesser curvature. Extends from esophagus to pylorus.

c., haversian. Minute c.'s found in compact bone which contain blood and lymph vessels, nerves, and sometimes marrow. Each is surrounded by lamellae of bone comprising a haversian system. SEE: *bone.*

c., hyaloid. A c. in the vitreous body of the eye extending from the optic papilla to the posterior surface of lens. It serves as a lymph channel. In the fetus it transmits the hyaline artery to the lens. SYN: *canalis hyaloideus* [NA].

c., hypoglossal. C. in the occipital bone which transmits the hypoglossal nerve and a branch of the posterior meningeal artery. SYN: *canalis hypoglossi* [NA].

c., incisive. A short c. in the maxillary bone leading from incisive fossa in roof of mouth to the floor of nasal cavity. Transmits nasopalatine nerve and branches of the greater palatine arteries to the nasal fossa. SYN: *canalis incisivus* [NA].

c., infraorbital. C. in the maxilla lying in the floor of the orbit which transmits the infraorbital nerve and artery. It terminates anteriorly at the infraorbital foramen. SYN: *canalis infraorbitalis* [NA].

c., inguinal. A slit in the lower lateral portion of the abdominal wall, extending from the abdominal inguinal ring to the subcutaneous inguinal ring. It is an oblique passageway about 1 1/2 inches long and serves in the male to transmit the spermatic cord and the ilioinguinal nerve and in the female the round ligament of the uterus and the ilioinguinal nerve. It forms a channel through which an inguinal hernia descends. SYN: *canalis inguinalis* [NA].

c., intestinal. The alimentary c. from stomach to anus.

c., lacrimal. The lacrimal duct, q.v.

c., mandibular. C. in the mandible that transmits the inferior alveolar blood vessels and nerve to the teeth. SYN: *canalis man-dibulae* [NA].

c., maxillary. Alevolar c.'s, q.v.

c., nasolacrimal. C. lying between the lacrimal bone and the inferior nasal conchae. Contains the nasolacrimal duct.

c., Nuck's. In the female, a persistent peritoneal pouch which accompanies the round ligament of the uterus through the inguinal canal.

c., nutritive. An opening on the surface of compact bone through which blood vessels gain access to the medullary cavity of long bones. Also transmits veins.

c., obturator. An opening in the obturator membrane of the hip bone which transmits the obturator vessels and nerve.

c., pharyngeal. C. between sphenoid and palatine bones for transmission of branches of sphenopalatine vessels.

c., portal. The connective tissue (continuation of Glisson's capsule) and its contained vessels (interlobular branches of hepatic artery, portal vein, and bile duct and lymphatic vessel) located between adjoining liver lobules.

c., pterygoid. C. of the sphenoid bone transmitting pterygoid vessels, artery, and nerve. Also called canal of Vidian. SYN: *canalis pterygoideus* [NA].

c., pterygopalatine. C. lying between maxillary and palatine bones which transmits descending palatine nerves and artery. SYN: *canalis palatinus major* [NA].

c., pudendal. C., Alcock's, q.v.

c., pulp. The central cavity of a tooth filled with pulp. Contains blood vessels and sensory nerve endings.

c., sacral. Cavity within the sacrum, a continuation of the vertebral c. SYN: *canalis sacralis* [NA].

c., Schlemm's. A space or series of spaces at the junction of the sclera and the cornea of the eye into which aqueous humor is drained from the anterior chamber through the pectinate villi.

c.'s, semicircular, bony. Located in the bony labyrinth of the internal ear and enclose the three semicircular ducts: the superior, posterior, and lateral which open into the vestibule. They are enclosed within the petrous portion of the temporal bone.

c.'s, semicircular, membranous. Semicircular ducts. SEE: *duct.*

c., spinal. C., vertebral, q.v.

c., spiral, cochlear. C., cochlear, spiral.

c., spiral, of the modiolus. A series of irregular spaces which follow the course of the attached margin of the osseous spiral

lamina to the modiolus. They serve for the transmission of filaments of the cochlear nerve and blood vessels. The spiral ganglion lies in the spiral c. SYN: *canalis spiralis modioli* [NA].

c., uterine. The cavity of the uterus.

c., uterocervical. The cavity of the cervix of the uterus.

c., uterovaginal. The combined cavity of the uterus and vagina.

c., vaginal. The cavity of the vagina.

c., vertebral. The cavity formed by the foramina of the vertebral column. Also called spinal c., neural c. It contains the spinal cord and its meninges. SYN: *canalis vertebralis* [NA].

c., Volkmann's. Small c.'s found in bone through which blood vessels pass from the periosteum. They connect with the blood vessels of haversian c.'s or the marrow cavity.

canales (kă-nā'lēz). Pl. of canalis.

canalicular (kăn″ă-lĭk'ū-lar) [L. *canalicularis,* pert. to a small channel]. Pert. to a canaliculus.

canaliculi (kăn″ă-lĭk'ū-lī). Pl. of canaliculus.

canaliculus (kan″ă-lĭk'ū-lus) [L.]. (pl. *canaliculi*) A small channel or canal.

canalis (kă-nā'lĭs) [L.]. (pl. *canales*) Canal, q.v.

canalization (kă-năl″ĭ-zā'shŭn). Formation of channels in tissue.

cancellated (kăn'sĕ-lāt″ĕd) [L. *cancellus,* lattice]. Reticulated; latticelike.

cancelli (kan-sel'ī) [L. *cancellus,* lattice]. Pl. of cancellus. Reticulations forming spongy tissue of bones.

cancellous (kăn'sĕl-ŭs) [L. *cancellus,* a grating]. Having a reticular or latticework structure, as the spongy tissue of bone.

cancellus (kăn-sĕl'us). (pl. *cancelli*) An osseous plate of which cancellous bone is composed.

cancer (kan'ser) [L., a crab; ulcer]. A malignant tumor or neoplasm; a sarcoma or carcinoma.

ETIOL: Origin unknown. May be caused by various forms of chronic irritation. Some forms in animals at least are apparently caused by viruses.

SYM: The important warning signals of cancer are unusual bleeding or discharge from any internal or external body site; a lump or thickening in any area but esp. the breast; a sore that does not heal; a change in bowel or bladder habits; hoarseness or persistent cough; indigestion or difficulty in swallowing; change in size or shape or appearance of a wart or mole; unexplained loss of weight. These are the major signs of cancer and once any one of them is observed in oneself or in a patient it should be brought to a physician's attention without delay.

TREATMENT: Surgery, cytotoxic agents, radium and x-rays are recognized effective methods of treatment for cancer.

Early diagnosis and application of proper method or combination of methods are necessary for complete cure.

NP: Small pillows and sandbags to relieve strained muscles. Cradles to hold bedclothes away from painful parts. Light bedclothes; one wool blanket instead of several cotton ones. Olive oil added to rubbing alcohol prevents chafing and rawness. Bland, neutral soap should be used for bathing.

Cater to individual idiosyncrasies. Do not deny particular foods unless there is a good reason for it. Serve four to six small meals. Attractively decorated trays help to stimulate appetite in patient. Diet should contain a minimum of 2000 cal. per day.

Keep patient cheerful. Talk and soothe patient out of complaint when possible. Censor literature and talk of visitors so that cheerful attitude will be maintained.

c., black. C. with dark pigmentation.

c. cell. A cell found in neoplasm which possesses characteristics which differentiate them from normal tissue cells. Among such are degree of anaplasia, irregularity in shape, indistinctness of cell outline, nuclear size, changes in structure of nucleus and cytoplasm, increased number of mitoses and ability to metastasize.

c., hard. C. composed of fibrous tissue.

c., lip. Epithelioma, usually in men, smokers, on lower lip.

c., scirrhous. SEE: *c., hard.*

cancer, words pert. to: adenocarcinoma; carcinoma; epithelioma; sarcoma; scirrhus.

cancerogenic (kăn″sĕr-o-jĕn′ĭk) [L. *cancer,* crab, ulcer, + Gr. *genesis,* generation]. Carcinogenic.

cancerology (kan-ser-ol′o-jĭ) ["+ Gr. *logos,* study]. The science and study of cancer.

cancerophoʹbia ["+ Gr. *phobos,* fear]. Morbid fear of cancer.

canʹcerous. Pert. to malignant growth.

cancra (kang′krä). Pl. of cancrum.

cancriform (kang′krĭ-form) [L. *cancer,* crab, ulcer, + *forma,* appearance]. Having the appearance of cancer.

cancroid (kang′kroyd) ["+ Gr. *eidos,* appearance]. 1. Like a cancer. 2. A type of keloid, q.v. 3. Epithelioma, q.v.

cancrology (kang-krol′o-jĭ). Cancerology, q.v.

cancrum (kang′krum) [L. *cancer,* ulcer]. (pl. *cancra*) A rapidly spreading ulcer.

c. naʹsi. Gangrenous inflammation of nasal membranes.

c. oʹris. Gangrenous stomatitis, noma.

TREATMENT: Good oral hygiene and massive doses of appropriate antibiotic.

c. pudenʹdi. Ulceration of vulva.

candela (kă-dĕl′ä) [L. *candēla,* candle]. A unit of luminous intensity.

Candida (kăn′dĭ-dä) [L. *candidus,* glowing white]. A genus of yeastlike fungi which develop a pseudomycelium and reproduce by budding. They are the primary etiologic agents for many mycotic infections in man. Formerly called Monilia.

C. albicans. A small oval, budding fungus which is the primary etiologic organism of moniliasis (candidiasis). Formerly called Monilia albicans.

candidiasis (kan″dĭ-dĭ′ă-sĭs). Infection with any species of Candida, q.v. SEE: *moniliasis.*

candle, international. A unit of luminosity.

candlepower. Amt. of light thrown out, measured in international candles. SEE: *candela; light unit; lux; unit.*

cane. A slender stick held in the hand and used for support during walking.

canescent (kă-nĕs′ĕnt) [L. *canus,* gray]. Grayish in color.

cane sugar. Sucrose. Table sugar obtained from sugarcane. SEE: *saccharose.*

canine (kā′nīn) [L. *caninus,* pert. to a dog]. 1. Pert. to a dog. 2. Pert. to the canine teeth or the four teeth known as the eyeteeth (upper and lower) between the incisors and molars. 3. A canine tooth.

c. appetite. Abnormal hunger a short time after eating. SYN: *bulimia,* q.v.

c. eminence. Ridge on anterior surface of superior maxilla.

c. fossa. Depression on superior maxilla external to the c. eminence.

c. tooth. Tooth situated between incisors and 1st premolar tooth. SEE: *dentition; tooth.*

canities (kan-ish′ĭ-ēz) [L., gray hair]. Congenital (rare) or acquired whiteness of the hair.

Acquired form may develop rapidly or slowly, partial or complete.

c. unguium. Gray or white streaks in nails.

canker (kăng′kĕr) [L. *cancer,* ulcer]. White spots on mucous membrane of the mouth; aphtha; noma; gangrenous stomatitis; thrush.

cannabis (kăn′ă-bĭs) [Gr. *kannabis,* hemp]. Marijuana, q.v.

cannula (kăn′u-lä) [L., a small reed]. A tube or sheath enclosing a trocar, the tube allowing the escape of fluid after withdrawal of the trocar from the body.

cantaloupe, cantaloup (kăn'tă-lōp) [It. *cantalupo*, first grown at Cantalupo, papal villa near Rome]. A type of muskmelon.
Food value of 100 gm. raw: Cal. 30; protein 0.7 gm.; fat 0.1 gm.; carbohydrate 7.5 gm.; calcium 14 mg.; phosphorus 16 mg.; iron 0.4 mg.; sodium 12 mg.; potassium 251 mg.; vitamin A, 3400 I.U.; niacin 0.6 mg.; ascorbic acid 33 mg.

canthal (kăn'thăl) [Gr. *kanthos*, angle]. Pert. to a canthus.

cantharidal (kăn-thăr'ĭ-dăl) [Gr. *kantharis*, beetle, + *eidos*, form]. Pert. to or containing cantharides.

cantharides (kăn-thăr'ĭ-dēz). (sing. *cantharis*) Dried insects of the species Cantharis vesicatoria obtained from Spain or Russia. SYN: *Spanish fly.*
Formerly used externally as a counterirritant and vesicant, and internally as an aphrodisiac. Its use has been almost entirely discontinued. Poisonous if taken internally in large doses.

Cantharis (kăn'thă-rĭs). (pl. *Cantharides*) A genus of beetles, C. vesicatoria, known as Spanish fly. SEE: *cantharides.*

canthectomy (kăn-thĕk'tō-mĭ) [Gr. *kanthos*, canthus, + *ektomē*, excision]. Excision of a canthus.

canthi (kăn'thī). Pl. of canthus.

canthitis (kăn-thī'tĭs) [Gr. *kanthos*, canthus, + *-itis*, inflammation]. Inflammation of a canthus.

cantholysis (kăn-thŏl'ĭ-sĭs) ["+ *lysis*, a loosening]. Incision of a canthus to widen palpebral slit.

canthoplasty (kăn'thō-plas''tĭ) ["+ *plassein*, to form]. Plastic surgery of canthus of the eye. Enlargement of palpebral fissure by division of the external canthus.

canthorrhaphy (kăn-thor'ă-fĭ) [Gr. *kanthos*, canthus, + *rhaphē*, suture]. Suturing of a canthus.

canthotomy (kan-thot'ō-mĭ) ["+ *tomē*, a cutting]. Division of a canthus.

canthus (kăn'thŭs) [Gr. *kanthos*, corner of the eye]. (pl. *canthi*) The angle at either end of the slit between the eyelids; the external canthus or commissura palpebrarum lateralis [NA], and the internal canthus or commissura palpebrarum medialis [NA].

CaO. Calcium oxide, quicklime, calx.

CaOC. Abbr. for *cathodal* (or negative pole) *opening contracture.*

Ca(OH)$_2$. Calcium hydroxide; slaked lime.

cap (kăp) [AS. *caeppe*, from LL. *cappa*, hood]. 1. A covering. SYN: *tegmentum.* 2. First part of the duodenum. SYN: *pyloric cap.*

c., cradle. Seborrhea, oily crusts on the head, seen in infants.

c., knee-. Bone in front of the knee. SYN: *patella*, q.v.

capacitance (kă-păs'ĭ-tăns) [L. *capăcitās*, taking, from *capere*, to hold, contain]. That property of a system of conductors and dielectrics which permits the storage of electric charges. SYMB: C.

c., unit of. SEE: *farad.*

capac'ity. 1. Capability. 2. Cubic content. 3. Holding power. 4. A measure of the electric output of a generator.

c., cranial. Volume of the cranial cavity.

c., vital. Volume of air that can be forcibly exhaled after a full inspiration.

capeline (kăp'ĕ-lĭn) [Fr. a hat]. A bandage used for the head, or the stump of an amputated limb.

capiat (ka'pĭ-at) [L. "let it take"]. An instrument for removing foreign substances or bodies from a body cavity, esp. from the uterus.

capillarectasia (kap'ĭ-lăr''ĕk-tā'sĭ-ă) [L. *capillaris*, hairlike, + Gr. *ektasis*, dilatation]. Dilatation of capillary vessels.

Capillaria philippinensis (căp'ĭ-lăr'ĭ-ă fĭl-ĭ-pĭn-ĕn'sĭs). Species of roundworm discovered in the Philippines. It causes severe diarrhea, malabsorption, and enteric protein loss in man.

capillariasis, intestinal. A disease, first described in 1968, due to infestation of the small bowel with a roundworm, Capillaria philippensis. Reported from northern Luzon in the Philippine Islands. TREATMENT: Thiabendazole.

capillaries (kăp'ĭ-lă-rēz). 1. Minute blood vessels. 2. Small lymphatic ducts. Pl. of capillary, q.v.

capillaritis (kăp'ĭ-lăr-i'tĭs) [L. *capillaris*, hairlike, + Gr. *-itis*, inflammation]. Inflammation of the capillaries; telangiitis.

capillarity (kăp'ĭ-lăr'ĭ-tĭ). Process by which a liquid's surface, at the point of contact with a solid, is elevated or lowered. SYN: *capillary attraction.*

capillaropathy (kăp'ĭ-lăr-ŏp'ă-thĭ) [L. *capillaris*, hairlike, + Gr. *pathos*, disease]. Capillary disorders or disease.

capillaroscopy (kăp'ĭ-lăr-ŏs'ko-pĭ) ["+ Gr. *skopein*, to examine]. Examination of capillaries for diagnostic purposes.

capillary (kăp'ĭ-lăr'ĭ) [L. *capillaris*, hairlike]. (pl. *capillaries*) 1. Minute blood vessel, 0.008 mm. in diameter, carrying blood and forming the capillary system. Capillaries connect the smallest arteries (arterioles) with the smallest veins (venules). 2. One of the small lymphatic ducts which allow passage of nutrient matter and oxygen from the blood to the tissues, and of waste matter from the tissues into the blood. 3. Pert. to a hair; hairlike.

c.'s, arterial. The very small vessels which are the terminal branches of the arterioles or metarterioles.

c. attraction. Capillarity, q.v.

c., bile. Intercellular biliary passageways which convey bile from liver cells to the interlobular bile ducts.

c.'s, blood. Minute blood vessels which convey blood from the arterioles to the venules. They form an anastomosing network which brings the blood into intimate relationship with the tissue cells. Their wall consists of a single layer of squamous cells called endothelium through which blood and oxygen diffuse to the tissue and products of metabolic activity enter the blood stream. They average about 8 microns in diameter, but are capable of being constricted so as to have almost no lumen at all.

c.'s, lymphatic. The smallest lymphatic vessels. They are thin-walled tubes forming a dense network in most tissues of the body. They differ from blood capillaries in that they are generally slightly larger in diameter and end blindly. They collect tissue fluid from the tissues. Lymph capillaries unite to form larger lymphatic vessels.

c. permeability. The ability of substances to diffuse through capillary walls into the tissue spaces. It is influenced by anoxia, adrenal cortical hormone and the concentration of calcium ions in the blood.

c.'s, venous. The minute vessels which convey blood from a capillary network into the small veins or venules.

capillus (kă-pĭl′us) [L., a hair]. (pl. *capilli*) 1. A hair, esp. of the head. 2. A filament. 3. A hair's breadth.

cap′ital [L. *capitalis*, pert. to the head]. 1. Pert. to the head. 2. Of great importance to life.

capitate (kăp′ĭ-tāt) [L. *caput*, head]. Head-shaped; having a rounded extremity.

c. bone. Capitatum, q.v.

capitatum (kap′ĭ-tā′tum). Third bone in distal row of carpus. SYN: *capitate bone; os capitatum* [NA]; *os magnum.*

capitellum (kăp′ĭ-tel′ŭm) [L., small head]. The round eminence at lower end of the humerus articulating with radius; its radial head. SYN: *capitulum humeri* [NA].

capitular (kă-pĭt′ū-lăr). Pert. to a capitulum.

capit′ulum (kă-pĭt′ū-lum, kă-pĭch′u-lum) [L., small head]. [NA]. A small, rounded articular end of a bone.

c. fibulae. The proximal extremity or head of the fibula; articulates with tibia.

c. humeri. [NA]. Rounded prominence at distal end of humerus. Articulates with the radius. SYN: *capitellum.*

c. mallei. The head or large rounded extremity of the malleus; bears facet for the incus.

c. stapedis. The head of the stapes; articulated with lenticular process of incus.

capotement (kă-pōt-mon′) [Fr.]. A splashing sound in the stomach.

capsicum (kăp′sĭ-kŭm). Cayenne pepper; dried, ripe fruit of capsicum. Used as a carminative, stimulant and rubefacient.

capsitis (kap-sī′tis) [L. *capsa,* box]. Capsulitis of crystalline lens.

cap′sula [L., little box]. (pl. *cap′sulae*) [NA] In anatomy, a sheath or continuous enclosure around an organ or structure.

c. articula′ris. [NA] Capsule of a joint.

c. bul′bi. Tenon's capsule.

c. fibro′sa perivascularis. Glisson's capsule.

c. glomer′uli. [NA]. Bowman's capsule; malphighian capsule.

c. len′tis. [NA]. Crystalline lens capsule.

capsulae (căp′sū-lē) [L.]. Pl. of capsula, q.v.

cap′sular. Pert. to a capsule.

c. ligament. A ligament that surrounds a movable joint.

capsula′tion. Enclosure in a capsule.

cap′sule [L. *capsula,* little box]. 1. Capsula, q.v. 2. A special container made of gelatin for a single dose of a drug; the enclosure prevents the patient from tasting the drug.

c., auditory. Embryonic cartilaginous capsule enclosing the developing ear.

c., Bowman's. The glomerular capsule of the kidneys.

c., cartilage. The layer of matrix which forms the innermost portion of the wall of a lacuna enclosing a single cell or a group of cartilage cells. It is basophilic.

c., Glisson's. An outer capsule of fibrous tissue in which is invested the liver, its ducts and vessels. SYN: *capsula fibrosa perivascularis.*

c., joint. The fibrous tissues enclosing a joint.

c. of the kidney. Fat-containing connective tissue surrounding the kidney.

c., lens. A transparent structureless membrane which surrounds and encloses the lens of the eye.

c., nasal; c., optic; c., otic. Cartilaginous capsules which develop in embryonic skull enclosing each of the paired sense organs as nasal cavity, eyes, and ears, respectively.

c., suprarenal. A tough connective tissue capsule which encloses the adrenal gland. SYN: *adrenal c.*

c. of Tenon. A thin fibrous sac enveloping the eyeball, forming a socket in which it rotates. SYN: *fascia bulbi.*

capsuli'tis [L. *capsula*, little box, + Gr. *-itis*, inflammation]. Inflammation of a capsule.

cap'sulocil"iary ["+ *ciliāris*, pert. to the eyelashes]. Pert. to capsule of lens and ciliary structures.

cap'suloplas"ty ["+ Gr. *plassein*, to mold]. Plastic surgery of a capsule, esp. one of a joint.

capsulorrhaphy (kăp"sū-lōr'ă-fĭ) [L. *capsula*, little box, + Gr. *rhaphē*, suture]. Suture of a joint capsule or of a tear in a capsule.

capsulotome (kăp'sū-lō-tōm") ["+ Gr. *tomē*, incision]. Instrument for incising into capsule of crystalline lens.

capsulotomy (kăp"sū-lŏt'ō-mĭ). Cutting of capsule of crystalline lens.

captation (kăp-tā'shŭn) [L.*captātiō*, seizure]. The first stage of hypnosis.

caput (kā'pŭt, kăp'ŭt) [L.]. (pl. *cap'ita*) [NA] 1. The head. 2. The upper part of an organ.

c. gallinaginis. Round protuberance on urethral floor. SYN: *colliculus seminalis* [NA].

c. medusae. Plexus of veins about the umbilicus in one form of cirrhosis of the liver (Cruveilhier-Baumgarten syndrome) indicating portal vein obstruction.

c. obstipum. Wryneck; torticollis.

c. succedaneum. Swelling produced on the presenting part of the fetal head during labor. It may be mistaken for the bag-of-waters.

ETIOL: Effusion of serum into cellular tissue of exposed scalp through venous interference from pressure.

carbamide (kăr'bă-mīd, kăr-băm'īd). Urea, $CO(NH)_2$.

carbarsone (kăr'băr-sōn). A white, crystalline, odorless powder; contains about 28% arsenic, having a chemical structure resembling tryparsamide.

Digestion of Carbohydrates

Enzyme	Found in	Carbohydrates	End product
Sucrase (invertase)	Intestine	Sucrose	Glucose and fructose
Maltase	Intestine	Maltose	Glucose
Lactase	Intestine	Lactose	Glucose and galactose
Salivary amylase (ptyalin)	Saliva (mouth)	Starch	Dextrin to maltose
Pancreatic amylase (amylopsin)	Pancreas	Starch	Dextrin to maltose

Classification of Important Carbohydrates

Classification	Examples	Some Properties
Monosaccharides (monoses) $(C_6H_{10}O_5)_1 \cdot H_2O$ or $C_6H_{12}O_6$	Glucose Fructose	Crystalline, sweet, very soluble, readily absorbed
Disaccharides (dioses) $(C_6H_{10}O_5)_2 \cdot H_2O$ or $C_{12}H_{22}O_{11}$ hydrolyzed to simple sugars	Sucrose Lactose Maltose	Crystalline, sweet, soluble, digestible
Polysaccharides (polyoses) $(C_6H_{10}O_5)n$ composed of many molecules of simple sugars (Since the molecular weight is unknown, *n* refers to an unknown number of these groups, the exact molecular weight being undetermined.)	Starch Dextrin Cellulose Glycogen	Amorphous, little or no flavor, less soluble. Vary in solubility and digestibility. Form colloidal solutions which cannot be dialyzed.

USES: An antiamebic agent.

carbohydrase (kăr''bō-hī'drās). One of a group of enzymes (such as amylase and lactase) that hydrolyze carbohydrates.

carbohydrate foods. Foods containing only carbon combined with hydrogen and oxygen, such as sugars, starch, and cellulose. Carbohydrates, principally starches, provide a major source of calories in an average diet.

carbohy'drates [L. *carbo,* carbon, + Gr. *hydor,* water]. The monosaccharoses, disaccharoses, and polysaccharoses. A class of organic compounds so called because in them the hydrogen and oxygen are in the same ratio as they are in water, so that the group can be represented by the formula $C_x(H_2O)_y$.

Glucose, $C_6H_{12}O_6$, and sucrose, $C_{12}H_{22}O_{11}$, are typical carbohydrates, but the group also includes the noncrystalline dextrins and starches.

carbohydratu'ria [L. *carbo,* carbon, + Gr. *hydor,* water, + *ouron,* urine]. Sugar in the urine. SYN: *glycosuria.*

carbolic acid [L. *carbo,* coal, + *oleum,* oil]. Obsolete name for phenol, q.v.

carbolism (kăr'bŏl-ĭsm). Poisoning by carbolic acid SEE: *phenol.*

car'bolize. To add or mix with carbolic acid.

carbolu'ria [L. *carbo,* coal, + *oleum,* oil, + Gr. *ouron,* urine]. Phenol in the urine.

carbomycin (kăr-bō-mī'sĭn). An antibiotic obtained from Streptomyces halstedii and effective against gram-positive bacteria.

car'bon [L. *carbo,* coal]. SYMB: *C.* At. wt. 12.0111; at. no. 6. This nonmetallic element is the characteristic constituent of organic compounds.

A common form is coal. C. is found in all living things in its various forms and combinations. It is the basis of all organic matter and makes life possible through a number of combinations with hydrogen, nitrogen, and oxygen. In foods it is a fuel creating heat. The diamond is crystallized carbon.

car'bonate [L. *carbo,* carbon]. A salt of carbonic acid.

c. of soda. Sodium carbonate commercially in crude form, as washing soda. The free alkali present is irritating and in larger concentrations has the effect of sodium hydroxide, q.v.

car'bon diox'ide. CO_2. USP. A colorless gas, heavier than air, generally produced in the combustion, decomposition, or fermentation of carbon or its compounds, and found in the air and exhaled by all animals.

The final product of combustion of carbon in food. The body eliminates CO_2 through the lungs, in urine, and in perspiration.

It is also given off by decomposition of vegetable or animal matter, or formed by alcholic fermentation as in rising bread. It is necessary to all plant life and it is absorbed directly from the air.

Although a waste product, in small quantities (up to about 5%) in inspired air, it stimulates respiration; in greater quantities, it produces an uncomfortable degree of hyperpnea with mental confusion.

Although not supposed to be poisonous, it will cause death by suffocation. Over 500,000,000 tons are passed into the air per year, but as it is used by green plants, the air content is kept down to about 0.03%. One sq. yd. of leaf surface can absorb the carbon dioxide from 2500 liters of air in 1 hour. An acre of trees uses 4 1/2 tons a year.

c. d. combining power test. This test, done on blood serum, is a determination of the amount of carbon dioxide which the blood serum can hold in chemical combination.

The blood serum is saturated with CO_2 by blowing one's breath into it, removing the CO_2 by producing a vacuum, and measuring its volume directly. It is used to detect acidosis or alkalosis and to determine their degree. Carbon dioxide in solution forms a weak acid (H_2CO_3), and the amount of this acid which the blood serum can take up is a measure of its reserve power to prevent the occurrence of acidosis. The normal amount is from 50-70 ml./100 ml. of blood (usually expressed as 50-70 volumes %). Values below 50 indicate acidosis, above 70 alkalosis.

c. d. inhalation. CO_2 (5 to 7 1/2%), mixed with oxygen for inhalation stimulates breathing the same way as increased CO_2 production from exercise. Inhalation of oxygen and CO_2 is used as an accessory during artificial respiration and as a continuation of resuscitation after spontaneous breathing has returned. Also used to stimulate respiration in patients with pulmonary diseases such as pneumonia.

c. d. poisoning. CO_2 gas is most commonly used in carbonated drinks and commercially used in dry ice; of itself, it is rarely fatal unless the patient is in a closed space. It is a profound respiratory stimulant.

SYM: Violent increased breathing; sensation of pressure in the head; ringing in ears, acid taste in mouth; slight burning in nose. Within a short time, respiration almost ceases and patient becomes unconscious.

TREATMENT: Remove to fresh air, administer artificial respiration, inhalation of oxygen.

c. d. test. The alkalinity reserve in the plasma is indicated by the volume percentage of CO_2 in the blood. Acidosis shows a percentage below 50, while in coma it is as low as 20. Acidosis indicates faulty metabolism. Diacetic acid is produced as the result of accumulated fatty acids, the product of incomplete oxidation of fats.

c. d. (solid) therapy. Solid carbon dioxide (CO_2 snow) is used for therapeutic refrigeration. Solid CO_2 has a temperature of $-80°$ C. Application to skin 1-2 seconds causes superficial frostbite, 4-5 seconds a blister, 10-15 seconds superficial necrosis, 15-45 seconds ulceration. Now used mostly for certain nevi and warts, occasionally for telangiectasia.

carbonemia (kăr″bō-nē′mĭ-ă) ["+ Gr. *haima*, blood]. Excess accumulation of carbonic acid in the blood.

carbon′ic. Pert. to carbon.

c. acid. H_2CO_3. Acid resulting from mixture of carbon dioxide and water.

c. anhydrase. An enzyme which catalyzes union of H_2O and CO_2 to form carbonic acid or reverse action. Present in red blood cells.

car′bonize. To char or convert into charcoal.

car′bon monox′ide. CO. An insidious poisonous gas. It is a colorless, tasteless, odorless gas; gives no warning of its presence; and is widely distributed as the result of imperfect combustion and oxidation.

It is found in the exhaust gas from all internal combustion engines such as are used in most motor-powered vehicles. It is present in illuminating gas and results from the inefficient and incomplete combustion of coal. It is found in sewers, cellars, and mines.

POISONING: May take place from small amounts inhaled over a long period of time, or from large amounts inhaled over a short time. For example, riding in a closed automobile or parking in an automobile with motor running may cause death from the inhalation of these noxious fumes, from leaking exhausts and exhaust heaters. Another cause of death is the operation of a gasoline motor in an enclosed area such as a closed garage or basement.

Poisoning from CO is produced as a result of a chemical combination of this gas with the hemoglobin of the blood, thus preventing the blood from carrying oxygen to the tissues. Since this combination is a relatively stable one, such a patient may need oxygen administration for prolonged periods in addition to artificial respiration.

SYM: The symptoms of CO poisoning are somewhat variable. Respiration is deep and difficult. There may be reddish patches of color about the face and chest. The mucous membrane may have a brighter red hue than normal. The pulse may be slowed initially but it soon becomes increased. There may be pounding of the heart; dizziness is frequent; the muscular system often is affected so that the extremities may fail. There may be ringing in the ear; throbbing in the temples; headache; faintness and nausea; dilated pupils. If the patient is breathing when found, he usually recovers when brought into the fresh air and given stimulants.

TREATMENT: Remove patient from area containing CO. Give 100% oxygen by mouth, and artificial respiration if necessary. Keep patient warm and maintain blood pressure. Give up to 2 liters of washed red blood cells I.V. if this can be done within 30 minutes of exposure. 50% glucose or mannitol I.V. should be used for cerebral edema.

COMPLICATIONS: When such patients recover they often have some nervous system involvement including various types of paralysis, blindness, interference with sensation, muscular spasms, or twitchings for an indefinite period of time. Most of these complications disappear in time, but occasionally they remain permanently.

carbono.n′etry [L. *carbo*, carbon, + Gr. *metron*, measure]. Determination of presence and amount of carbon dioxide exhaled.

car′bon tetrachloride (tĕt″ră-klō′rĭd). CCl_4 A clear, colorless liquid with ethereal odor resembling chloroform; not inflammable.

USES: Although having narcotic and anesthetic properties resembling chloroform, it is too toxic to be suitable as an anesthetic. In general this substance is too toxic for use. Inhalation of a small quantity has been known to produce death. The mechanism of injury is acute atrophy of the liver and kidney.

POISONING: Toxic effects due to prolonged inhalation.

SYM: Irritation of eyes, nose, and throat; headache; nausea; anorexia; weakness; abdominal pain.

F. A. TREATMENT: Remove clothes contaminated with carbon tetrachloride. Oxygen inhalation and artificial respiration. Lavage with saline solution. Leave saline cathartic in stomach.

SEE: *Table of Poisons* in *Appendix.*

carbonu'ria [L. *carbo,* carbon, + Gr. *ouron,* urine]. The presence or excretion of carbon compounds in the urine.

carbonyl (kăr'bŏn-ĭl) ["+ Gr. *hylē,* matter]. The divalent radical CO, characteristic of aldehydes and ketones.

carboxyhemoglobin (kăr-băs'ĭ-hē"mōglō'-bin) [L. *carbo,* carbon, + Gr. *oxys,* acid, + *haima,* blood, + L. *globus,* sphere]. Compound formed by carbon monoxide and hemoglobin in poisoning by carbon monoxide.

carboxyl (kăr-bŏks'ĭl). The characteristic group (COOH) of organic carboxylic acids, e.g., formic acid (H-COOH), acetic acid (CH_2 COOH).

carboxylase (kăr-bŏks'ĭ-lās). An enzyme which brings about the removal of the carboxyl group (COOH) from amino acids; an enzyme found in brewer's yeast which catalyzes the decarboxylation of pyruvic acid with the production of acetaldehyde and carbon dioxide. In the body this requires the presence of vitamin B_1 (thiamine) which acts as a coenzyme.

carbuncle, carbunculus (kăr'bŭng"kl, kăr-bŭng'kū-lŭs) [L. *carbunculus,* small glowing ember]. A circumscribed inflammation of the skin and deeper tissues which terminates in a slough and suppuration and is accompanied by marked constitutional symptoms.

ETIOL: Staphylococci. Predisposing factors the same as in furuncle, q.v. Occurs more frequently in men and in adults than children. Diabetics are particularly susceptible.

SYM: It is characterized by a painful node, at first covered by tight reddened skin which later becomes thin and perforates, discharging pus through several openings. Also fever, leukocytosis, and sometimes prostration. Most commonly found on nape of neck, on upper back or on buttocks.

TREATMENT: Antibiotics given systemically are usually effective. Incision and drainage when lesion is about to point. Keep covered with warm compresses to promote blood supply to the area.

NP: Use sterile technique when dressing area. Disinfect all contaminated equipment and destroy soiled dressings.

carbun'cular. Pert. to a carbuncle.

carbunculosis (kăr-bŭng"kū-lō'sĭs) [L. *carbunculus,* small glowing ember, + Gr. *-ōsis,* condition]. Appearance of several carbuncles in succession.

carcinectomy (kăr"sĭn-ĕk'tō-mĭ) [Gr. *karkinos,* crab, + *ektomē,* excision]. The excision of a cancerous growth.

carcinelcosis (kăr"sĭ-nĕl-kō'sĭs) ["+ *helkōsis,* ulceration]. An ulcer of a cancerous nature.

carcinoembryonic antigens (kăr"sĭn-ō-ĕm'brĭ-ŏn-ĭk). Antigens present in fetal tissues and which, if found in the adult, are thought to be specific for malignant tumors. Test for presence of the antigen may facilitate diagnosing certain cancers, help to assess adequacy of surgical resection of a malignancy, and aid in detecting presence and extent of metastases. ABBR: CEA.

carcinogenesis (kăr"sĭ-nō-jĕn'ĕ-sĭs) ["+ *genesis,* production]. The production or origin of cancer.

carcinogenic (kăr"sĭ-nō-jĕn'ĭk). Causing cancer.

carcinoid (kăr'sĭ-noyd) [Gr. *karkinos,* cancer, + *eidos,* resemblance]. An argentaffin cell tumor which may arise in the intestinal tract, bile ducts, pancreas, bronchus, or ovary. These tumors secrete serotonin (5-hydroxytryptamine).

   c. syndrome. A group of symptoms which develop when a carcinoid tumor, by metastasis or on its own, produces excess amounts of serotonin.

   SYM: Include one or more of the following: brief episodes of flushing, esp. of the face and neck; tachycardia; facial and periorbital edema; hypotension; intermittent abdominal pain with diarrhea; valvular lesions of the heart; loss of weight; hypoproteinemia; signs of pellagra. The latter symptom is due to the body's available tryptophan, which is the precursor of serotonin, being used for serotonin production instead of for manufacture of niacin and protein.

   TREATMENT: Symptoms usually develop only after the tumor has metastasized; nevertheless surgical removal of accessible tumors is indicated. High protein diet with niacin supplement. Serotonin antagonist for control of diarrhea and malabsorption. Cortisone may be helpful in controlling inanition.

carcinolysis (kăr"sĭ-nŏl'ĭ-sĭs) [Gr. *karkinos,* cancer, + *lysis,* destruction]. Destruction of carcinoma cells.

carcinolytic (kăr"sĭ-nō-lĭt'ĭk). Destructive to cancer cells.

carcinoma (kăr-sĭ-nō'mă) ["+ *-ōma,* tumor]. An epithelial cell new growth or malignant tumor, enclosed in connective tissue, and tending to infiltrate and give rise to metastases.

   It may affect almost any organ or part of the body and spread through the blood stream. Etiology is unknown. SYN: *cancer.*

c., basal cell. An epidermoid c. common on face of elderly. It has a low degree of malignancy. It gives rise to the typical rodent ulcer.

c., chorionic. A tumor containing cells characteristic of the chorion of the embryo. It occurs in the testis, ovary, and other parts of the body. SYN: *choriocarcinoma.*

c., cylindrical-cell. A c. of glands usually of entodermal origin including adenocarcinoma and carcinoma simplex.

c., epidermoid. A tumor on a surface such as the skin which is covered with stratified epithelium. Usually of two types, one a wartlike growth, slow-growing, mildly malignant; the other a flat and rapidly infiltrating neoplasm.

c., glandular. C. with cells of the secreting variety. SEE: *adenocarcinoma.*

c., lipomatous. C. with fatty tissue.

c., melanotic. C. containing melanin.

c., scirrhous. A form of cylindrical-cell c. with a firm, hard structure.

c., squamous-cell. A form of epidermoid c. principally of squamous cells.

carcinomatophobia (kăr″sĭ-nō″mă-tō-fō′bĭ-ă) [Gr. *karkinos*, cancer, + *ōma*, tumor, + *phobos*, fear]. Morbid fear of carcinoma.

carcinomatosis (kăr″sĭ-nō″mă-tō′sĭs) [″+ ″+ -*ōsis*, infection]. The condition of having a carcinoma anywhere in the body. SYN: *carcinosis.*

carcinomatous (kăr″sĭ-nō′mă-tŭs). Pert. to or affected with cancer.

carcinomec′tomy [Gr. *karkinos*, cancer, + -*ōma*, tumor, + *ektomē*, excision]. Excision of a cancer.

carcinomelcosis (kăr″sĭ-nō-mĕl-kō′sĭs) [″+ ″+ *helkōsis*, ulceration]. An ulcerating cancer.

carcinopho′bia [″+ ″+ *phobos*, fear]. Morbid fear of cancer.

carcinosarco′ma [″+ ″+ *sarx*, flesh, + -*ōma*, tumor]. A mixed tumor of carcinoma and sarcoma.

carcinosectomy (kăr″sĭ-nō-sĕk′tō-mĭ) [Gr. *karkinos*, cancer, + -*ōma*, tumor, + *ektomē*, excision]. Excision of a cancer.

carcinosis (kăr″sĭ-nō′sĭs) [″+ -*ōsis*, infection]. Carcinomatosis, q.v.

car′damom, car′damon [Gr. *kardamō-mon*]. Dried ripe fruit of an herb, Elettaria repens or E. cardomomum, used as an aromatic and carminative.

Cardarelli's sign (kăr″dă-rĕl′lē). [Antonio Cardarelli, It. physician, 1831-1926]. Tracheal tugging significant of aneurysm of aorta.

cardia (kăr′dĭ-ă) [Gr. *kardia*, heart]. 1. Upper orifice (esophageal) of stomach connecting with the esophagus. 2. The heart.

cardiac (kăr′dĭ-ăk) [L. *cardiacus*]. 1. Pert. to the heart or to the cardiac orifice into the stomach. 2. Having heart disease. 3. A heart tonic.

c. arrhythmia. SEE: *arrhythmia.*

c. atrophy. Fatty degeneration of the heart.

c. compensation. The ability of the heart through its reserve power to compensate for impaired functioning of its valves.

c. cycle. The period from the beginning of one beat of the heart to the beginning of the next succeeding beat, including the *systole*, contraction of the atria and ventricles propelling the blood onward, and the *diastole*, the period during which the cavities are being refilled with blood.

The atria contract immediately before the ventricles. The ordinary cycle lasts 8/10 of a second with the heart beating approx. 60-85 times a minute in the adult at rest. The atrial systole lasts 0.1 second; the ventricular systole, 0.3 second, and the diastole, 0.4 second, thus even though the heart seems to be working continuously, it actually rests for a good portion of each cardiac cycle.

RS: circulation; diastole; heart; systole.

c. failure. Condition resulting from inability of the heart to pump sufficient blood to meet the needs of the body. SEE: *heart failure.*

c. hypertrophy. Enlargement of the heart. SEE: *heart, hypertrophy of.*

c. insufficiency. Inadequate c. output due to failure of the heart to function properly as in valvular deficiency.

c. output. The amount of blood discharged from the left (or right) ventricle per minute. For an average adult, c. output is approx. 3.0 liters per square meter of body surface area each minute. SYN: *minute volume.*

c. plexus. Plexus cardiacus [NA]. SEE: *plexuses* in *Appendix.*

c. reflex. A reflex in which the response is a change in c. rate. Stimulation of sensory nerve endings in the wall of the carotid sinus by increased arterial blood pressure reflexly slows the heart (Marey's law); stimulation of vagus fibers in the right side of the heart by increased venous return reflexly increases heart rate (Bainbridge's reflex).

c. reserve. The capacity of the heart to increase c. output and raise blood pressure above basal pressure to meet body requirements.

cardiactia (kăr-dĭ-ăk'tĭ-ă) [Gr. *kardia*, heart, + L. *actio*, function]. Cardiac stenosis.

cardiagra (kăr-dĭ-ăg'ră) ["+ *agra*, seizure]. Serious pains in the chest of a constricting nature. SEE: *angina pectoris*.

cardialgia (kăr''dĭ-al'jĭ-ă) ["+ *algos*, pain]. Pain at the pit of the stomach or region of the heart, usually occurring in paroxysms.

cardiam'eter [Gr.*kardia*, heart, + *metron*, measure]. Device for marking position of the cardia of the stomach.

cardianastrophe (kăr''dĭ-ăn-ăs'trō-fĭ) ["+ *anastrophē*, reversal of position]. Congenital transposition of the heart to the right side. SYN: *dextrocardia*.

cardianesthe'sia ["+ *anaisthēsia*, lack of sensation]. Lack of sensation in the heart.

cardiant (kăr'dĭ-ănt). 1. Affecting, or that which affects, the heart. 2. A cardiac stimulant.

cardiaortic (kăr-dĭ-ā-ōr'tĭk) [Gr. *kardia*, heart, + *aortē*, aorta]. Pert. to the heart and the aorta.

cardiasthenia (kăr''dĭ-ăs-thē'nĭ-ă) ["+ *astheneia*, weakness]. Type of neurasthenia with predominance of cardiac symptoms.

cardiasthma (kăr-dĭ-az'mă) ["+ *asthma*, panting]. Dyspnea due to heart disease.

cardiectasia, cardiectasis (kăr''dĭ-ek-ta'sĭ-ă, -ĕk'tă-sĭs) [Gr. *kardia*, heart, + *ektasis*, dilatation]. Dilatation of the heart.

cardiectomy (kăr''dĭ-ĕk'tō-mĭ) ["+ *ektomē*, excision]. Excision of the cardiac end of the stomach.

cardinal [LL. *cardinalis*, important]. Of primary importance such as the cardinal symptoms: temperature, pulse, respiration.

cardio- [Gr. *kardia*, heart]. Prefix pert. to the heart.

cardioaccel'erator ["+ L. *accelerāre*, to hasten]. That which increases the rate of the heart beat.

cardioangiology (kăr''dĭ-ō-ăn''jĭ-ōl'ō-jĭ) ["+ *angeion*, vessel, + *logos*, study]. The science of the heart and blood vessels.

cardioaortic (kăr''dĭ-ō-ā-ōr'tĭk) [Gr. *kardia*, heart, + *aortē*, aorta]. Pert. to the heart and the aortic artery.

cardiocele (kăr'dĭ-ō-sēl) ["+ *kēlē*, tumor]. Hernia of the heart.

cardiocentesis (kăr''dĭ-ō-sĕn-tē'sĭs) ["+ *kentesis*, puncture]. Surgical incision or puncture of the heart.

cardiocinetic (kăr''dĭ-ō-sĭ-nĕt'ĭk) [Gr. *kardia*, heart, + *kinesis*, motion]. Cardiokinetic, q.v.

cardiocirrhosis (kăr''dĭ-ō-sĭ-rō'sĭs). Cirrhosis of the liver associated with or occurring secondary to heart failure.

cardioclasia, cardioclasis (kăr''dĭ-ō-klā'-zĭ-ă, kăr-dĭ-ŏk'lă-sĭs) [Gr. *kardia*, heart, + *klasis*, break]. Rupture of the heart.

cardiodi'lator ["+ L. *dilatāre*, to enlarge]. Device for dilating the cardia of the esophagus.

cardiodynamics (kăr''dĭ-ō'dĭ-năm-ĭks). Science of forces involved in propulsion of blood from heart to tissues and back to heart.

cardiodynia (kăr''dĭ-ō-dĭn'ĭ-ă) [Gr. *kardia*, heart, + *odynē*, pain]. Pain in the region of the heart.

cardiogenic (kăr''dĭ-ō-jĕn'ĭk) ["+ *gennan*, to produce]. Having origin in the heart itself.

car'diogram ["+ *gramma*, mark]. A graph, on special paper, of the electrical activity of the heart muscle. Made with an electrocardiograph machine. SYN: *electrocardiograph*.

cardiograph (kăr'dĭ-ō-grăf) [Gr. *kardia*, heart, + *graphein*, to write]. A device for registering the electrical activity of the heart muscle.

cardiograph'ic. Pert. to cardiography.

cardiog'raphy. The recording and study of the electrical activity of the heart.

cardiohepat'ic [Gr. *kardia*, heart, + *hēpatos*, liver]. Pert. to heart and liver.

car''dioinhib'itory ["+ L. *inhibere*, to check]. Slowing action of the heart.

cardiokinet'ic ["+ *kinēsis*, motion]. Pert. to that which excites heart action.

car'diolith [Gr. *kardia*, heart, + *lithos*, stone]. A concretion or calculus in the heart.

cardiol'ogist ["+ *logos*, study]. A specialist in treatment of heart disease.

cardiol'ogy. The study of the heart.

cardiolysin (kăr''dĭ-ōl'ĭ-sĭn) [Gr. *kardia*, heart, + *lysis*, loosening]. A lysin acting on heart muscle.

cardiolysis (kăr-dĭ-ōl'ĭ-sĭs). Freeing pericardial adhesions to surrounding tissues, involving resection of the ribs and sternum.

cardiomalacia (kăr''dĭ-ō-mă-lā'shĭ-ă) [Gr. *kardia*, heart, + *malakia*, softening]. Softening of the heart walls.

cardiomegaly (kăr''dĭ-ō-mĕg'ă-lĭ) ["+ *megas*, large]. Hypertrophy of the heart.

cardiometer (kăr-dĭ-ŏm'ĕ-tĕr) ["+ *metron*, measure]. Device for locating impulse or apex of the heart's beat.

cardiomotil'ity [Gr. *kardia*, heart, + L. *motilis*, moving]. The ability of the heart to function.

cardiomyoliposis (kăr''dĭ-ō-mĭ''ō-lĭp-ō'sĭs) ["+ *mys*, muscle, + *lipos*, fat]. Fatty degeneration of the heart.

cardionecro'sis ["+ *nekros*, dead]. Necrosis of the heart.

cardionephric (kăr″dĭ-ō-nĕf′rĭk) [Gr. *kardia,* heart, + *nephros,* kidney]. Pert. to heart and kidney.

cardioneural (kăr″dĭ-ō-nū′răl) ["+ *neuron,* nerve]. Pert. to nervous control of the heart.

cardioneurosis (kăr″dĭ-ō-nū-rō′sĭs) ["+ "+ *-ōsis,* condition]. Functional neurosis with cardiac symptoms.

cardiopalmus (kăr″dĭ-ō-păl′mŭs) [Gr. *kardia,* heart, + *palmos,* palpitation]. Palpitation of the heart.

cardiopal′udism ["+ L. *palus,* marsh, + Gr. *ismos,* condition]. Heart disease due to growth of malarial parasites in the capillaries of the heart muscle.

car′diopath ["+ *pathos,* disease]. A person with heart disease.

cardiopathy (kăr″dĭ-ŏp′ă-thĭ). Any disease of the heart.

cardiopericarditis (kăr″dĭ-ō-pĕr″ĭ-kăr-dī′tĭs) [Gr. *kardia,* heart, + *peri,* around, + *kardia,* heart, + *-itis,* inflammation]. Inflammation of myocardium and pericardium.

cardiophobia (kăr″dĭ-ō-fō′bĭ-ă) ["+ *phobos,* fear]. Morbid fear of heart disease.

cardiophone (kăr′dĭ-ō-fōn) ["+ *phonē,* voice]. Device, esp. a stethoscope, for listening to sound of the heart.

cardioplasty (kăr″dĭ-ō-plăs′tĭ) [Gr. *kardia,* heart, + *plassein,* to form]. Operation on the cardia to relieve cardiospasm.

cardioplegia (kăr″dĭ-ō-plē′jĭ-ă) ["+ *plēgē,* stroke]. Paralysis of the heart.

cardiopneumatic (kăr″dĭ-ō-nū-măt′ĭk) ["+ *pneuma,* breath]. Pert. to the heart and the lungs.

cardiopneumograph (kăr″dĭ-ō-nū′mō-grăf) ["+ "+ *graphein,* to write]. Device for recording motion of heart and lungs.

cardioptosis (kăr-dĭ-ōp-tō′sĭs) [Gr. *kardia,* heart, + *ptōsis,* falling]. Prolapse of the heart.

cardiopul′monary ["+ L. *pulmō,* lung]. Pert. to both heart and lungs.

car′diopuncture ["+ L. *punctura,* piercing]. Surgical puncture of the heart. SYN: *cardiocentesis.*

cardiopylor′ic [Gr. *kardia,* heart, + *pyloros,* gatekeeper]. Pert. to the cardiac and pyloric ends of the stomach.

cardiore′nal ["+ L. *rēnalis,* pert. to kidney]. Pert. to both heart and kidneys.

cardiorrhaphy (kăr″dĭ-ōr′a-fĭ) ["+ *rhaphē,* a suture]. Suturing of the heart muscle.

cardiorrhexis (kăr″dĭ-ō-rĕks′ĭs) [Gr. *kardia,* heart, + *rhēxis,* rupture]. Rupture of the heart.

cardiosclerosis (kăr″dĭ-ō-sklĕ-rō′sĭs) ["+ *sklērōsis,* hardening]. Hardening of the cardiac tissues and arteries.

car′dioscope ["+ *skopein,* to examine]. Instrument for examining the interior of the heart.

cardioscopy (kăr″dĭ-ŏs′kō-pĭ). Examination of the interior of the heart without opening the chest, by using a cardioscope.

cardiospasm (kăr′dĭ-ō-spăzm) [Gr. *kardia,* heart, + *spasmos,* spasm]. Disordered motor function of the distal end of the esophagus and failure of the esophageal orifice (cardia) of the stomach to relax. Thus the word is a misnomer in that failure of relaxation (achalasia) and absence of esophageal motility (aperistalsis) are the disease processes involved.

ETIOL: Due to absence or injury of ganglion cells in Auerbach's plexus.

SYM: Substernal fullness, dysphagia, regurgitation, esp. at night.

TREATMENT: Bland semi-solid foods warmed to body temperature are of some help, but dilatation of the esophageal sphincter will allow the esophagus to drain by force of gravity. It may be possible to do this mechanically; if not, surgical myotomy may be required.

cardiosphygmograph (kăr″dĭ-ō-sfĭg′mō-grăf) ["+ *sphygmos,* throb, + *graphein,* to write]. Instrument for graphically recording movements of the heart and pulse.

cardiostenosis (kăr″dĭ-ō-stĕn-ō′sĭs) ["+ *stenōsis,* narrowing]. Heart constriction and its development.

cardiosymphysis (kăr″dĭ-ō-sĭm′fĭ-sĭs) [Gr. *kardia,* heart, + *symphysis,* growing together]. Mediastinopericarditis, q.v.

cardiotachometer (kăr″dĭ-ō-tăk-ŏm′ĕ-tĕr) ["+ *takos,* speed, + *metron,* measure]. An instrument for measuring the total number of heart beats over a long period of time.

cardiother′apy ["+ *therapeia,* treatment]. The treatment of cardiac diseases.

cardiotomy (kăr″dĭ-ŏt′ō-mĭ) [Gr. *kardia,* heart, + *tomē,* cutting]. Incision of the heart.

cardioton′ic ["+ *tonos,* tone]. Increasing tonicity of the heart.

cardiotoxic (kăr″dĭ-ō-tŏks′ĭk) ["+ *toxikon,* poisoning]. Exercising a poisonous effect upon the heart.

cardiovalvuli′tis [Gr. *kardia,* heart, + L. *valvula,* valve, + Gr. *-itis,* inflammation]. Inflammation of valves of the heart. Valvular endocarditis.

cardiovalvulotome (kăr″dĭ-ō-văl′vū-lō-tom″) ["+ "+ Gr. *tomē,* cut]. An instrument for excising part of a valve, esp. the mitral valve.

cardiovas'cular ["+ L. *vasculum*, small vessel]. Pert. to the heart and blood vessels.

c. reflex. 1. Sympathetic increase in heart rate when increased pressure in, or distention of, great veins occurs. SYN: *Bainbridge reflex.* 2. Reflex vasoconstriction resulting from reduced venous pressure.

cardiovasology (kăr″dĭ-ō-văs-ŏl′ō-jĭ) [Gr. *kardia*, heart, + L. *vas*, vessel, + Gr. *logos*, study]. Science of the heart and blood vessels. SYN: *cardioangiology.*

cardioversion. Conversion of a pathological cardiac rhythm (arrhythmia), such as ventricular fibrillation, to normal sinus rhythm. Usually accomplished by use of a device called a cardioverter which administers electrical shocks to the heart through electrodes placed on the chest wall.

CAUTION: C. should not be used in sinus tachydardia or arrhythmias (other than ventricular fibrillation) caused by digitalis toxicity. It should be used only in emergency situations when potassium administration and other measures have failed. The cardioverter may induce lethal ventricular fibrillation unresponsive to further electrical shocks.

cardioverter. Electrical device used to administer electrical shocks to the heart when electrodes are placed on the chest wall. Useful in treating (on an emergency basis) cardiac arrhythmias such as ventricular fibrillation. Changing the arrhythmia to normal sinus rhythm is called cardioversion, q.v.

carditis (kăr″dĭ′tĭs) [Gr. *kardia*, heart, + *-itis*, inflammation]. Inflammation of the heart muscles. Usually involves two of the following: pericardium, myocardium, or endocardium.

caries (kăr′ēz, kăr′ĭ-ēz) [L., rottenness]. Gradual decay and disintegration of a bone or tooth. If the decay is allowed to progress, the surrounding tissue will become inflamed and an abcess will form.

Chronic abcess, tuberculosis, and bacterial invasion of teeth are examples. In caries the bone disintegrates by pieces, while in necrosis large masses of bone are discharged. Deficiency of vitamins C and D has a direct influence upon caries of the teeth.

c., dental. Decay of the teeth. A progressive decalcification of the enamel and dentine of a tooth. The etiology is not fully known. Early detection and dental fillings offer the best form of control. Topical application of fluorine promotes resistance to dental caries if applied during the stage of tooth formation.

c. fung'sa. A type of tuberculosis of bone.

c., necrotic. C. with masses of bone in a suppurative cavity.

c., radiation. Dental caries which develop as an undesired side effect of treatment of malignancies of the oral cavity with ionizing radiation.

c. sic'ca. Dry tuberculosis of ends of bones and joints unaccompanied by fluid or swelling.

c., spinal. Pott's disease; c. of the vertebrae, usually tuberculous.

carina (kă-rī′nă) [L., keel of a boat]. (pl. *cari'-nae*) A structure with a projecting central ridge.

c. nasi. A cleftlike space between the agger nasi and roof of nasal cavity. SYN: *olfactory sulcus.*

c. tracheae. [NA]. A ridge at lower end of trachea separating openings of the two bronchi.

c. urethralis. Ridge extending posteriorly from urethral orifice and continuous with anterior column of the vagina.

carinae (kă-rī′nē) [L.]. Pl. of carina.

carinate (kăr′ĭ-nāt) [L. *carina*, keel of a boat]. Keel-shaped; possessing a conspicuous central ridge.

cariogenic (kā″rĭ-ō-jĕn′ĭk) [L. *caries*, rottenness, + Gr. *gennan*, to produce]. Conducive to caries formation.

carious (kā′rĭ-ŭs). 1. Affected with or rel. to caries. 2. Having pits or perforations. SEE: *caries.*

carmin'ative [L. *carminātivus*, cleanse]. An agent that will remove gases from the gastrointestinal tract.

carnal (kăr′năl) [L. *carnālis*, flesh]. Rel. to the flesh.

c. knowledge. A phrase used in medicolegal cases to denote sexual intercourse, esp. with a minor female child.

carneous (kăr′nē-ŭs) [L. *carneus*]. Fleshy.

carnification (kăr″nĭ-fĭ-kā′shŭn) [L. *carō*, flesh, + *facere*, to make]. Alteration of tissues, esp. the change of pulmonary tissue to a form resembling skeletal muscle.

carnitine (kăr′nĭ-tĭn). A base derived from betaine.

carnivorous (kăr-nĭv′ō-rŭs) [L. *carnivorus*]. Flesh eating.

carnopho'bia [L. *carō*, flesh + Gr. *phobos*, fear]. Abnormal aversion to meat.

carnose (kăr′nōs). Having the consistency of or resembling flesh.

carnosity (kăr-nŏs'ĭ-tĭ) [L. *carnōsitās,* fleshiness]. An excrescence resembling flesh; a fleshy growth.

carot'enase [Gr. *karōton,* carrot]. An enzyme that converts carotene into vitamin A. SYN: *carotinase.*

carotene (căr'ō-tēn) [Ger. *karotin*]. A yellow crystalline pigment present in various plant and animal tissues. It is abundant in yellow vegetables (carrots, squash, corn). C., which exists in several forms, is the precursor of vitamin A. It is stored in the liver and converted to vitamin A in the liver.

carotenemia, carotinemia (kăr''ō-tĕnē'mĭ-ă) [Ger. *Karotin,* carrot, + *haima,* blood]. Carotene in the blood characterized by yellowing of the skin (pseudojaundice). C. can be distinguished from true jaundice by the lack of yellow discoloration of the conjunctivae in carotenemia. SYN: *carotenosis.*

carotenoid (kă-rŏt'ĕ'noyd) ["+ *eidos,* form]. 1. One of a group of pigments (as carotene, q.v.) ranging in color from light yellow to purple, widely distributed in plants and animals. 2. Resembling carotene.

caroteno'sis ["+ *-ōsis,* condition]. Carotenemia, q.v.

carotic (kă-rŏt'ĭk) [Gr. *karos,* deep sleep]. 1. Carotid. 2. Resembling stupor; stupefying. 3. A sleep-producing drug.

carotid (kă-rŏt'ĭd) [Gr. *karōtides*]. 1. The right and left common carotid arteries, both of which arise from the aorta, are the principal blood supply to the head and neck. Each of these two arteries divides to form external and internal c. arteries. 2. Pert. to any c. part, as c. sinus.

   c. body. SEE: *body, carotid.*

   c. sinus. A dilated area at the bifurcation of the common carotid artery which is richly supplied with sensory nerve endings of the sinus branch of the vagus nerve. These, when stimulated by distention of the vessel wall brought about by a rise in blood pressure, bring about reflex vasodilation and a slowing of the heart rate.

carotidynia (kăr-ŏt''ĭ-dĭn'ĭ-ă) ["+ *odynē,* pain]. Pain elicited by pressure on the common carotid artery. Also spelled carotodynia.

car'otin [Gr. *karōton,* carrot]. Carotene, q.v.

car'otinase. Carotenase, q.v.

carotine'mia. Carotenemia, q.v.

car'pal [Gr. *karpalis*]. Pert. to the carpus or wrist.

   c. articulation. Wrist joint.

   c. tunnel syndrome. Pressure on the median nerve at the point at which it goes through the carpal tunnel of the wrist.

Causes soreness, tenderness, and weakness of the muscles of the thumb.

   TREATMENT: Surgical relief of tension if conservative therapy fails.

carpale (kăr-pā'lē) [Gr. *karpos*]. Any wrist bone.

carpec'tomy ["+ *ektomē,* excision]. Excision of the carpus or portion of it.

carphologia, carphology (kăr-fō-lō'jĭ-ă, -fōl'ō-ji)[Gr. *karphos,* dry twig, + *legein,* to pluck]. Involuntary picking at bed clothes, seen esp. in febrile or exhaustive delirium of the low muttering type. A grave symptom in cases of extreme exhaustion or approaching death. SYN: *floccillation.*

carpo- [Gr. *karpos*]. Prefix pert. to the carpus.

car''pometacar'pal ["+ *meta,* beyond, + *karpos,* wrist]. Pert. to both carpus and metacarpus.

carpopedal (kăr''pō-pēd'ăl) ["+ L. *ped,* foot]. Pert. to both the wrist and the foot.

   c. spasm. Spasm of the hands and feet, sometimes seen in laryngismus stridulus, q.v.

carpoptosis (kăr''pŏp-tō'sĭs) ["+ *ptōsis,* a falling]. Wrist drop.

carpus (kar'pus) [L.]. [NA]. The eight bones of the wrist joint. SEE: *wrist.*

Carrel-Dakin treatment. [Alexis Carrel, Fr.-Amer. surgeon, 1873-1944; Henry D. Dakin, Amer. chemist, 1880-1952]. Method of wound irrigation first utilized in 1915.

   Most suitable for deep septic wounds. A special apparatus is necessary—a glass receptacle for the solution constructed on the principle of a vacuum flask for maintaining a constant temperature. From this leads a rubber tube attached to a glass connection piece from which are suspended several perforated fine gauge rubber tubes. Each is tied at the lower end and perforated for about half its length. Any number of tubes can be used depending on size of wound. The flow is regulated so that there is a continual slow dropping, thus keeping the wound bathed constantly. A Dakin's special solution of sodium hypochlorite (0.45-0.50%) is used. It decomposes under light. Must be kept in dark bottle and not be older than 36-72 hours.

carrier [O.Fr. *carier,* to bear]. 1. A person who harbors a specific pathogenic organism in the absence of discernible symptoms or signs of the disease and who is potentially capable of spreading the organism to others. 2. That which carries anything as an insect such as a fly which passively carries infectious organisms; a substance which, when combined with another substance (transport substance), is capable of passing through cell

membranes as occurs in active transport mechanisms. SEE: *microorganisms; vector.*
3. An instrument or device for conveying or placing something.

CLASSIFICATION: *Infection by Animal Carriers:* Some microorganisms may be carried from animal to man by direct contact, indirect transfer, or by intermediary hosts.

Air-borne Infection: Pathogenic organisms in the respiratory tract, discharged from the mouth or nose, may be borne on the air and settle on food, clothing, walls, and floors, and if they are of the type which resists drying for a long period they may remain virulent until transmitted to another person. Coughing, sneezing, and expectorating may be responsible for droplet infection.

Contact Infection: This is the result of transmission from person to person as in kissing, coming in contact with those afflicted with communicable diseases, or with utensils handled by one with an infection.

Food-borne Infection: Bacteria may be communicated through food. Root and salad vegetables may carry bacteria from the soil or from manure. Cooking safeguards by destroying micro-organisms on food.

Human Carriers: Some parasites may live in or upon the body of those who themselves do not suffer from them, but may be carried by them to others. Carriers may be contact carriers, those who never show symptoms; incubationary carriers, those in whom the infection is starting but has not completed the incubation period; and convalescent carriers, those who have recovered but still harbor the organism causing their disease.

Insect Vectors: An insect may act as a physical carrier, as the tick which may transmit the organism causing Rocky Mountain spotted fever, or one that acts as an active intermediate host, such as the Anopheles mosquito which transmits malaria.

Prenatal Infection: This is the result of the fetus being infected from the mother's blood stream, or from contiguity with the maternal membranes.

Soil-borne Infection: Soil-borne, spore-forming organisms commonly enter the body through wounds as in tetanus and gas gangrene.

Water-borne Infection: Organisms producing typhoid, dysentery, cholera, and amebic infections may be carried through a water supply, or water in public pools used for bathing. These organisms may pass into the water from the feces of an infected person and be communicated to others.

c., active. One who harbors a pathogenic organism for a considerable period following recovery from disease due to the organism. A chronic carrier.

c., chain saw. Instrument for carrying one end of a thread around a bone to be cut.

c., chronic. C., active, q.v.

c., convalescent. One who harbors the organism during recovery from the disease caused by the organism.

c., drainage tube. Instrument for placing drainage tubes in narrow or deep seated tracts.

c., healthy. One who harbors an infectious organism but infection is inapparent throughout entire course.

c., incubatory. One who harbors and spreads an infectious organism during the incubation period of a disease.

c., intermittent. One who is capable of spreading infectious organisms at intervals.

c., ligament. Flat needlelike instrument for drawing ligament through perforations made in the fascia.

c., ligature. An instrument for carrying ligatures through tissue.

c., passive. C., healthy, q.v.

c., suppository bladder. C. for depositing suppositories, etc., in the bladder.

c., temporary. C., healthy, q.v.

c., urethral. C. for introduction into ureters. Flexible ones, about 12 in. long.

Carrion's disease (kăr-ē-ŏn'). [Daniel A. Carrion, a Peruvian student who lost his life after voluntarily taking an injection, 1850-85] Bartonellosis, q.v.

car'rots [Gr. *karōton,* carrot]. The orange root of a plant Daucus carota.

Food value of 100 gm. (raw): Cal. 42; protein 1.1 gm.; trace of fat; carbohydrate 9.7 gm.; calcium 37 mg.; vitamin A, 11,000 I.U.; ascorbic acid 8 mg.

car sickness. Sickness induced by riding in cars. A form of motion sickness, q.v.

cartilage (kăr'tĭ-lĭj) [L. *cartilago,* gristle]. A type of dense connective tissue consisting of cells embedded in a ground substance or matrix. The matrix is firm and compact, rendering it capable of withstanding considerable pressure or tension. C. has a bluish white or gray color and is semiopaque; it has no nerve or blood supply of its own. The cells lie in cavities called lacunae. They may be single or in groups of two, three, or four.

C. constitutes a part of the skeleton occurring in the costal cartilages of the ribs, the nasal septum, in the external ear and lining the eustachian tube, in the wall of the larynx, in the trachea and bronchi, between bodies of the vertebrae, and covering the articular surfaces of bones. It forms the major portion of the embryonic skeleton.

c., articular. Hyaline c. covering the articular surfaces of bones.

c., costal. C. connecting the true ribs and the sternum.

c., fibrous. C. containing visible collagenic fibers. SYN: *fibrocartilage,* q.v.

c. hyaline. A bluish-white glassy translucent cartilage. The matrix appears homogeneous although it contains collagenous fibers forming a fine network. The walls of the lacunae stain intensely with basic dyes. Hyaline c. is flexible and slightly elastic. Its surface is covered by the perichondrium except on articular surfaces. Found in articular c., in costal cartilages, in septum of nose, in larynx and trachea.

c., semilunar. One of the interarticular cartilages of the knee joint.

c., thyroid. Shield-shaped c. of the larynx, forming the prominence known as the Adam's apple.

c., yellow or elastic. A network of yellow elastic fibers, holding c. cells, and pervading intercellular substance. Found in the epiglottis, the external ear, the auditory tube, strengthening them and maintaining their shape.

cartilage, words pert. to: "cartilag-" words; "chondr-" words; cricoid.

cartilaginification (kăr″tĭ-lă-jĭn″ĭ-fĭ-kā′shun) [L. *cartilagō,* cartilage, + *facere,* to make]. Cartilage formation or chondrification; the development of cartilage from undifferentiated tissue.

cartilaginoid (kăr-tĭ-lăj′ĭ-noyd) ["+ Gr. *eidos,* form]. Resembling cartilage.

cartilaginous (kăr″tĭ-lăj′ĭ-nŭs). Pert. to or consisting of cartilage.

cartilago (kăr″tĭ-lā′gō) [L.]. (pl. *cartilag′ines*) [NA] Cartilage, q.v.

car′uncle [L. *caruncula,* small flesh]. A small fleshy growth.

c., lacrimal. C. found on the conjunctiva near the inner canthus. A small, reddish elevation of modified skin. SYN: *caruncula lacrimalis* [NA].

c., urethral. A small, red, papillary growth, highly vascular, sometimes found in the urinary meatus in females. It is characterized by pain on urination and is very sensitive to friction.

caruncula (kăr-ŭng′kū-lă) [L.]. (pl. *carun′culae*) [NA] A tiny, fleshy protuberance. SYN: *caruncle.*

c., hymenales. Small irregular nodules representing remains of the hymen. SYN: *c. myrtiformes.*

cary-, caryo- [Gr. *karyon,* nucleus]. A combining form meaning nucleus. SEE: words beginning with *kary-, karyo-.*

cascara sagrada ₍kăs-kăr′ă să-grä′dă₎. USP. The dried bark of Rhamnus purshiana, a small tree grown on western U. S. coast, and in parts of S. A. The main ingredient in aromatic cascara sagrada fluid extract, a cathartic.

case [L. *cāsus,* happening]. 1. An occurrence of disease; incorrectly used to refer to a patient. 2. An enclosing structure.

c., brain. The cranium, q.v.

c. fatality rate. Number per thousand of fatal terminations from a disease or operation.

c. history. The complete medical, family, social, and psychiatric history of a patient up to the time of admission for the present illness.

c., index. The initial patient, also called the *propositus* or *proband,* which led to the investigation of other members of a family for presence of genetic factors in the disease the original (index) case has.

caseate (kā′sē-āt) [L. *caseus,* cheese]. 1. To undergo cheesy degeneration. 2. A lactate.

caseation (kā″sē-ā′shŭn). 1. Process of conversion of necrotic tissue into a granular amorphous mass resembling cheese. 2. Precipitation of casein during coagulation of milk.

casein (kā′sē-ĭn) [L. *caseus,* cheese]. The principal protein in milk, seen in milk curds. It supplies all of the amino acids necessary for body tissue. It is a derived protein. When coagulated by rennin or acid it becomes one of the principal ingredients of cheese. SEE: *caseinogen.*

caseinogen (kā-sē-ĭn′ō-jĕn) ["+ Gr. *gennan,* to produce]. The principal protein in milk from which casein is derived. It is the substance in solution, and casein is the result of its precipitation. Its conversion into casein is the essential process in the curdling of milk.

caseous (kā′sē-ŭs). Resembling cheese; pert. to transformation of tissues into a cheesy mass.

CaSO₄. Calcium sulfate.

Casoni's reaction (kŏ-sō′nĭ). [Tomaso Casoni, It. physician, 1880-1933]. Appearance of a wheal surrounded by an erythematous zone following intradermal injection of sterile hydatid fluid. A test for presence of hydatid cysts resulting from infection with Echinococcus granulosus.

cassava (kă-sä′vă) [Sp. *casabe,* starch]. A tropical plant, the starch of which is used to make tapioca and bread. The rootstocks, from which the starch is obtained, are used also as a vegetable in tropical countries.

cassete (kă-sĕt´) [Fr., little box]. A flat, light-proof box with an intensifying screen in it, for holding x-ray film.

cast [ME. *casten*, to carry]. 1. A solid mold of a part, usually applied in situ for immobilization as in fractures, dislocations, and other severe injuries. Most often made of plaster of Paris, sodium silicate, starch, or dextrin which is rubbed into crinoline, then soaked in water, carefully applied to the immobilized part, and allowed to harden.

2. Plastic or fibrous material thrown off in various pathological conditions, the product of effusion. It is molded to the shape of the part in which it has been accumulated. According to source, casts are classified as bronchial, intestinal, nasal, esophageal, renal, tracheal, urethral, and vaginal; as to constituents, classified as bloody, fatty, fibrinous, granular, hyaline, mucous, and waxy.

HOW TO RECOGNIZE: They have a limiting membrane enclosing a matrix or substance in which are epithelial cells, pus cells, red blood cells, granules, and fat globules. From these latter characters they take their name as epithelial casts, red blood casts, etc. Casts usually have square ends, their diameter is the same throughout, and usually they do not bend or twist.

  c., blood. A c. composed principally of red blood cells.

  c., bronchial. Seen in sputum of patients with asthma and some with bronchitis.

  c., epithelial. Contain cells from inner lining of uriniferous tubules. Seen in acute nephritis.

  c., fatty. Those containing epithelium that has undergone degenerative changes, found in very advanced cases of renal degeneration.

  c., fibrinous. Yellowish-brown, sometimes with ragged fractures and highly refractile.

  c., granular. Of varying sizes and made up of albumin and white blood cells, and of serious import in nephritis in its acute and chronic forms.

  c., hyaline. Pale cylinders with rounded edges and variable size. Found in certain conditions of the kidneys.

  c., pseudo-. These are epithelial cells swollen and held in groups, resembling casts. Alkaline urine has a tendency to dissolve casts.

  c., pus. Found in urine in suppuration of kidney.

  c., urinary. Those found in the urine.

  c., uterine. Those from the uterus passed in exfoliative endometritis or membranous dysmenorrhea.

  c., waxy. Light yellowish, well defined, with tendency to split transversely, found in some cases of amyloid degeneration, and advanced nephritis.

Castellani's paint (kăs-tĕl-ăn´ĭ). [Aldo Castellani, It. physician, 1878 —] Paint used as a disinfectant for skin and in treatment of fungus infections of the skin. Composed of phenol, resorcinol, basic fuchsin, boric acid, and acetone.

Castle's intrinsic factor. [William Bosworth Castle, Amer. physician and educator, 1897 —]. A substance secreted by the stomach, essential for the absorption of cyanocobalamin (vitamin B_{12}; extrinsic factor). Absence of intrinsic factor causes pernicious anemia.

cas'tor oil. USP. A fixed oil expressed from the seed of the plant Ricinus communis.

  USES: Externally as an emollient; internally as a cathartic. In the digestive tract it is hydrolyzed to ricinoleic acid which acts as an irritant type of laxative.

cas'trate [L. *castrāre*, to prune]. 1. To remove the testicles or ovaries. SEE: *geld; spay.* 2. One who has been castrated.

cas'trated. Desexed; emasculated.

castration (kăs-trā´shŭn). 1. Emasculation; excision of the testicles or ovaries. 2. Destruction or inactivation of the gonad.

  c. complex. Morbid fear of castration.

  c., female. Removal of the ovaries. SYN: *oophorectomy; spaying.*

  c., male. Removal of the testes. SYN: *orchiectomy; orchotomy.*

  c., parasitic. Destruction of the gonads by parasitic organisms. It may result from direct infestation of the gonad or indirectly from effects of infestation in other parts of the body.

casualty (kăz´ū-ăl-tĭ) [L. *casualis,* accidental]. 1. Accident causing injury or death. 2. Person injured or killed in an accident. 3. Serviceman captured, missing, injured, or killed.

casuistics (kăz-ū-ĭs´tĭks) [L. *cāsus,* chance]. 1. Maintaining of records of clinical cases for study. 2. The determination of right and wrong in moral questions by application of ethical principles to a particular case.

cata- [Gr. *kata,* down]. Prefix indicating down or downward, against, or according to.

catabasis (kă-tăb´ă-sĭs) [Gr. *kata,* down, + *basis,* going]. The decline of a disease.

catabatic (căt-ă-băt´ĭk). Pert. to catabasis, q.v.

catabolic (kăt´´ă-bŏl´ĭk). Pert. to catabolism.

catabolin (kă-tăb'ō-lĭn). Catabolite, q.v.

catabolism (kă-tăb'ō-lĭzm) [Gr. *katabolē*, a casting down]. 1. The destructive phase of metabolism, the opposite of anabolism, the constructive phase. 2. Catabolism includes all the processes in which complex substances are converted into simpler substances, usually with the release of energy. SEE: *anabolism; metabolism.*

catabolite (kă-tăb'ō-līt). Any catabolism product. SYN: *catabolin.*

catacrotic [Gr. *kata*, down, + *krotos*, beat]. Manifesting the downstroke of a pulse tracing interrupted by an upstroke.

catacrotism (kă-tăk'rō-tĭzm) ["+ "+ *ismos*, conditon]. A pulse with one or more secondary expansions of artery following main beat.

catadicrotic (kăt-ă-dĭ-krŏt'ĭk) ["+ *dis*, twice, + *krotos*, beat]. Manifesting one or more secondary expansions of a pulse on the descending limb of the tracing.

catadi'crotism ["+ "+ "+ *ismos*, condition]. Two minor expansions following the main beat of an artery.

catadioptric (kăt"ă-dĭ-ŏp'trĭk) [Gr. *kata*, down, + *diopsesthai*, to see through]. Pert. to refraction and reflection of light simultaneously.

catagenesis (kăt-ă-jĕn'ĕ-sĭs) ["+ *genesis*, production]. Retrogression or involution.

catalase (kăt'ă-lās). An enzyme present in cells, esp. anaerobic bacteria which catalyzes the decomposition of hydrogen peroxide to water and oxygen.

catalepsy (kăt'ă-lĕp"sĭ) [Gr. *kata*, down, + *lēpsis*, seizure]. A condition seen in psychotic patients wherein there is generalized diminished responsiveness usually characterized by a trance-like state. Doctors and nurses should keep in mind that even though the patient is in a trance, conversations may be heard. Therefore one's actions toward and talk about the patient should be no different than if he were not in a cataleptic state.

catalep'tic. Pert. to catalepsy.

cataleptiform (kăt-ă-lĕp'tĭ-fŏrm) [Gr. *kata*, down, + *lēpsis*, seizure, + L. *forma*, shape]. Having the form of catalepsy.

catalep'toid ["+ "+ *eidos*, resemblance]. Resembling or simulating catalepsy.

catalysis (kă-tăl'ĭ-sĭs) [Gr. *katalysis*, dissolution]. The speeding up of the rate of a chemical reaction by a catalyst, q.v.

catalyst (kăt'ă-lĭst). An agent producing catalysis; a substance which speeds up the rate of a chemical reaction without itself being permanently altered in the reaction. Catalysts are effective in small quantities and are not used up in the reaction, i.e., they can be recovered unchanged. Ex: hydrochloric acid which catalyzes the hydrolysis of sucrose; ptyalin which catalyzes the hydrolysis of starch. SYN: *catalytic agent; catalyzer.*

catalytic (kăt-ăl-ĭt'ĭk) [Gr. *katalysis*, dissolution]. Pert. to catalysis, q.v.

   c. agent. A catalyst, q.v.

catalyzer (kăt'ă-lī-zĕr). A catalyst, q.v.

catamenia (kăt-ă-mē'nĭ-ă) [Gr. *katamēnia*]. The menses; periodic menstrual discharge of blood from the uterus.

catame'nial (kat"ă-mēn'ĭ-ăl). Pert. to the menses or catamenia.

   c. device. That which collects or absorbs the menstrual flow. SEE: *perineal pad; vaginal tampon.*

catamnesis (kăt-ăm-nē'sĭs) [Gr. *kata*, down, + *mnēmē*, memory]. A patient's history, after first being seen by physician, including all subsequent examinations. SEE: *anamnesis.*

cataphasia (kăt-ă-fā'zĭ-ă) ["+ *phasis*, speech]. A speech disorder causing an involuntary repetition of the same word.

cataphora (kă-tăf'ŏ-ră) [Gr. *kataphora*]. Lethargy with short remissions.

cataphoresis (kăt-ă-fō-rē'sĭs) [Gr. *kata*, down, + *phorēsis*, being carried]. The transmission of electronegative ions or drugs into the body tissues or through a membrane by use of an electric current.

cataphoria (kăt"-ă-fō'rĭ-ă). Tendency of visual axes to incline below the horizontal plane.

cataphor'ic. Pert. to cataphora or cataphoresis.

cataphre'nia [Gr. *kata*, down, + *phrēn*, mind]. A dementia type tending to recovery but which shows mental debility.

cataphylaxis (kăt-ă-fĭ-lăks'ĭs) ["+ *phylaxis*, guard]. 1. The process of carrying antibodies, leukocytes, etc., to the site of an infection. 2. The breaking down of the body's natural defenses against infection.

cataplasia (kăt-ă-plā'zĭ-ă) ["+ *plassein*, to form]. Degenerative change in tissues or cells. SYN: *cataplasis.*

cataplasis (kă-tăp'lă-sĭs). Cataplasia, q.v.

cat'aplasm [L. *cataplasma*]. A poultice, q.v.

cataplectic (kăt-ă-plĕk'tĭk) [Gr. *kata*, down, + *plēxis*, stroke]. Pert. to cataplexy.

cataplexy, cataplexia (kăt'ă-plĕks-ĭ, kăt-ă-plĕks'ĭ-ă). A form of sudden emotional shock, or stroke, accompanied by loss of muscular tone, without loss of consciousness, the patient falling to the floor.

   ETIOL: May be the result of intense emotion or the sudden onset of a disease or rarely a part of a narcoleptic attack.

cat'aract [L. *cataracta*]. Opacity of lens of eye or its capsule or both. Varieties are capsular, polar, lamellar, nuclear, cortical, morgagnian (fluid cataract with hard nucleus), congenital, infantile, traumatic, diabetic, and senile (occurring between 50-60 years).

STAGES: Incipient stage (spoke-shaped opacities, cloudlike opacities, opacity of cortex or nucleus). Stage of swelling or immature stage (swollen lens, shallow anterior chamber). Mature stage (lens shrinks due to loss of fluid and becomes opaque, anterior chamber regains its normal depth, no shadow thrown by iris or lens with focal illumination). Hypermature stage (lens becomes either solid and shrunken or soft and liquid).

ETIOL: Common form is result of the aging process; other forms may be congenital or caused by infection or injury.

TREATMENT: Surgical removal of lens except in presence of associated inflammation. Corrective eyeglasses.

c., capsular. C. from opacity of the capsule.

c., lenticular. Occurring in the lens.

c., morgagnian. A fluid cataract with a hard nucleus.

c., operation for. NP: *Preoperative:* Explain to patient the need for postoperative restriction of movement and covering of the eyes. Cathartic and/or enema; sedative if ordered. *Postoperative:* Avoid turning, jarring, or startling patient. Always announce your approach to the patient in a calm, unhurried tone. If medicines are to be instilled into the eyes, be certain to warn the patient several times. Sand bags at sides of head to prevent turning until permitted. Knee roll and small pillow under small of back to relieve strain. Liquid diet for first few days with gradual return to regular diet. Bowel movement not encouraged for first 48 hours to prevent straining which could exert pressure on eye. Dressing changed after first 48 hours unless otherwise ordered; patient's unoperated eye then uncovered and he is permitted to turn to that side. He is allowed up in chair by end of week. Dark glasses for patient as ordered. Use skill in feeding patient in calm, quiet atmosphere.

c., overripe. Stage following a mature c. in which lens solidifies and shrinks or becomes soft. SYN: *hypermature c.*

c., senile. C. of old persons.

cataractous (kăt″ă-răk′tŭs). Affected with or of the nature of a cataract.

catarrh (kă-tär′) [Gr. *katarrhein,* to flow down]. Term formerly applied to inflammation of mucous membranes.

c., dry. Severe spells of coughing with little or no expectoration. Generally seen in the old in association with emphysema or asthma.

SEQUELAE: Emphysema, bronchiectasis, and dilation of right ventricle.

PROG: Perfect recovery rarely attainable, but not incompatible with long life.

TREATMENT: Careful regulation of the hygiene. Constitutional.

catarrhal (kă-tär′ăl). Of the nature of or pert. to catarrh.

catastalsis (kăt-ă-stăl′sĭs) [Gr. *kata,* down, + *stalsis,* contraction]. Movement of a contraction-wave of the stomach downward, not preceded by a wave of inhibition.

catato′nia ["+ *tonos,* tension]. 1. A phase of schizophrenia in which the patient is unresponsive. The tendency to assume and remain in a fixed posture, and refusal to move or talk are characteristic of this phase. 2. Stupor.

cataton′ic. Stuporous; pert. to catatonia.

catatoxic steroids [Gr. *kata,* down, + *toxikon,* poison]. Steroids that act to increase resistance to the toxic effects of various drugs.

catatricrotic (kăt″ă-tri-krŏt′ĭk) [Gr. *kata,* down, + *treis,* three, + *krotos,* beat]. Manifesting a third impulse in the descending stroke of the sphygmogram.

catatricrotism (kăt″ă-tri′krō-tĭzm). State in which the pulse is catatricrotic.

catatropia (kăt″ă-trō′pĭ-ă) [Gr. *kata,* down, + *tropos,* turning]. Having both eyes turned downward.

cat bite. Usually a punctured or lacerated wound, potentially infected. Frequently wounds become infected later, even under careful management. If animals are rabid, may lead to rabies.

TREATMENT: Generously applied antiseptic to all parts of bite. Consider cautery and debridement. Antirabies treatment when indicated. Sterile dressings. SEE: *bites.*

catecholamines (kăt″ē-kōl-am′ēn). Biologically active amines, epinephrine and norepinephrine, derived from the amino acid tyrosine. They have marked effect on the nervous and cardiovascular systems, metabolic rate, temperature, and smooth muscle.

catelectrotonus (căt″ē-lĕk-trŏt′ō-nŭs) [Gr. *kata,* down, + *ēlektron,* amber, + *tonos,* tension]. The state of increased excitability produced in a nerve or muscle in the region near the cathode during the passage of an electric current.

catenating (kăt′ĕn-āt″ing) [L. *catena,* chain]. 1. Concerning a disease which is linked with another. 2. Formation of a series of symptoms. SEE: *concatenation.*

catenoid (kăt′ē-noyd) ["+ Gr. *eidos,* resemblance]. Chainlike; pert. to protozoan colonies whose individuals are joined end-to-end.

cat'gut. Sheep's intestine twisted for use as an absorbable ligature.

cathar'sis [Gr. *katharsis*, purification]. 1. Purgative action of the bowels. 2. The freudian method of freeing the mind by recalling the patient's memory of an event or experience that was the exciting cause of a psychoneurosis; abreaction, q.v.

cathar'tic [Gr. *kathartikos*, purging]. An active purgative, usually producing several bowel movements that may or may not be accompanied by pain or tenesmus.

Ex: cascara sagrada; castor oil. SEE: *purgative.*

catheresis (kăth-ĕ-rē'sĭs) [Gr. *kathairesis*, destruction]. 1. Weakness resulting from medication. 2. Weak action.

catheter (kăth'ĕ-tĕr) [Gr. *katheter*, something inserted]. A tube for evacuating or injecting fluids. Made of elastic, elastic web, rubber, glass, or metal.

c., cardiac. A long, fine catheter especially designed for passage through the lumen of a blood vessel into the chambers of the heart. SYN: *intracardiac c.* SEE: *cardiac; catheterization.*

c., double channel. C. providing for inflow and outflow. SYN: *two-way channel c.*

c., elbowed. C. which has an acute bend near the beak. USES: Cases of enlarged prostate. SYN: *prostatic c.*

c., eustachian. C. for injection into eustachian tube through nasal passages.

c., female. A short c., about 5 inches in length, used to pass into bladder of the female.

c. fever. Reactionary rise in temperature caused by a urinary tract infection following passage of a c. or urethral bougie.

c., Foley. A urinary tract catheter which has a balloon attachment at one end. After the catheter is inserted the balloon is filled with sterile water. Thus the catheter is prevented from leaving the bladder until the balloon is emptied.

c., indwelling. C. which is allowed to remain in place in the bladder.

c., male. C. used to pass into the bladder of the male. C. is 12-13 inches long.

c., prostatic. C., 15-16 inches long, designed to pass prostatic obstruction. SYN: *elbowed c.*

c., self-retaining. C. which can be retained at will, effecting bladder drainage.

c., vertebrated. C. in sections to be fitted together, so that it is flexible.

c., winged. C. with little flaps at each side of beak to aid in retaining it in the bladder.

catheterization (kăth"ĕ-tĕr-ĭ-zā'shŭn) [Gr. *katheterismos*, an inserting of a catheter]. Use or passage of a catheter.

c., cardiac. The passage of a catheter into the heart through an arm vein and blood vessels leading into the heart for the purpose of obtaining cardiac blood samples, detection of abnormalities, and determination of intracardiac pressure.

c., urinary bladder. Introduction of a catheter through the urethra into the bladder for withdrawal of urine.

NP: (for female patient) Treatment should be explained to patient who lies on back with knees drawn up, slightly separated; pillows under head and shoulders to relax abdominal muscles; feet flat on bed. Place screen around bed, tray at right side within reach. Arrange top covers so they may be separated with elbow. This is an aseptic procedure; scrub hands and place sterile towels, one above and one below vulva of female patient. Separate labia with first and second finger of left hand and pick up sterile cotton balls dipped in soap solution with right hand. Use downward stroke on one side of vulva, discard cotton ball, and proceed to cleanse area, swabbing orifice of meatus last.

Sterile receiver is placed between patient's legs. Nurse holds catheter about inch from open end, inspects for flaws, and inserts it into meatus of urethra, being careful not to touch any other part of vulval surface. Insert gently until urine begins to flow, holding it steadily until flow ceases. By withdrawing it slowly more urine may flow. Repeat until catheter is withdrawn.

Place finger over open end of c., invert over receiver and empty. Dry patient and cover. Report findings, condition of patient and time of c. Place urine in appropriately labelled container and send to laboratory for tests. SEE: *autocatheterism.*

catheterize (kăth'ĕ-tĕr-īz). To pass or introduce a catheter into a part, usually indicating catheterization of bladder.

cathexis (kă-thĕks'ĭs) [Gr. *kathexis*, retention]. The emotional or mental energy imparted to an idea.

cathodal (kăth'ō-dăl) [Gr. *kathodos*, downward path]. Pert. to the cathode.

cath'ode. 1. The negative pole. Opposed to the anode or positive pole. 2. In a vacuum tube, the electrode which serves as the source of the electron stream. ABBR: ca.

c. stream. Negatively charged electrons, sent out as particles from the cathode in discharges through the vacuum. SEE: *ray, cathode.*

cathodic (ka-thŏd'ĭk). 1. Pert. to a cathode. 2. Proceeding outwardly or efferently as applied to a nerve impulse.

cation (kăt'ĭ-ŏn) [Gr. *katiōn,* descending]. The element or elements of an electrolyte in electrochemical decomposition appearing as a positive ion at the negative pole or cathode.

catlin (kăt'lĭn). Surgical knife with double edges.

catoptric (kă-tŏp'trĭk) [Gr. *katoptrikos,* reflecting]. Pert. to reflected light or mirrors.

catoptrophobia (kăt''ŏp-trō-fō'bĭ-ă) [Gr. *katoptron,* mirror, + *phobos,* fear]. Morbid fear of mirrors or of breaking them.

cat scratch disease. A benign, self-limited disease lasting from two weeks to several months following a cat scratch or other skin injury. Etiology unknown but thought to be caused by a virus. There is no specific therapy. SYN: *benign inoculation lymphoreticulosis; cat scratch fever.*

cat's-eye pupil. A slitlike pupil.

cauda (kō'dä) [L.]. (pl. *cau'dae*) [NA] A tail or tail-like structure.

c. epididymidis. [NA]. The inferior portion of the epididymis which is continuous with the ductus deferens.

c. equina. [NA]. The terminal portion of the spinal cord and the roots of the spinal nerves below the first lumbar nerve. SEE: *coccyx* for illustration.

c. helicis. [NA]. A pointed process extending inferiorly from the helix of the auricular cartilage of the ear.

c. pancreatis. [NA]. The tail of the pancreas.

c. striati. Tail-like posterior extremity of the corpus striatum.

caudad (kō'dăd) ["+ *ad,* toward]. Toward the tail; in a posterior direction.

caudal (kŏd'ăl) [L. *caudalis*]. 1. Pert. to any tail-like structure. 2. Inferior in position.

caudate (kō'dāt) [L. *caudātus,* having a tail]. Possessing a tail.

caudation (ko-dā'shŭn) [L. *cauda,* tail]. 1. A lengthened or elongated clitoris. 2. Having a tail or tails.

caul (kōl) [O. Fr. *cale,* a small cap]. 1. The great omentum. 2. Membranes or portions of the amnion covering head of fetus at birth.

caul'iflower [L. *caulis,* cabbage, + *floris,* flower]. The edible thickened flower head of the plant Brassica oleracea botrytis, a member of the cabbage family.

Food value of 100 gm. (cooked, boiled, drained): Cal. 22; protein 2.3 gm.; trace of

fat; carbohydrate 4.1 gm.; calcium 21 mg.; ascorbic acid 55 mg.

cauliflower ear. Malformation of ear due to trauma, as seen in boxers.

caumesthesia (kō''mĕs-thē'zĭ-ă) [Gr. *kauma,* burn, + *aisthēsis,* sensation]. A sense of heat when surrounding temperature is normal.

causalgia (kŏ-săl'jĭ-ă) [Gr. *kausis,* heat, + *algos,* pain]. Intense burning pain.

cause [L. *causa*]. That which induces or brings about a particular condition, result, or effect.

c., constitutional. C. that is inherent within the body.

c., predisposing. C. which favors, but does not directly induce, an effect.

c., primary. The immediate or precipitating cause.

caustic (kŏ'stĭk) [Gr. *kaustikos,* capable of burning]. 1. Corrosive and burning. 2. An agent, particularly an alkali, that will destroy living tissue. Ex: silver nitrate, potassium hydroxide, nitric acid.

c. Lugol's. One part iodine, one part potassium iodide, and two parts water.

c., lunar. Toughened silver nitrate.

c. potash. Potassium hydroxide, q.v.

c. soda. Sodium hydroxide, q.v.

cauterant (kŏ'tĕr-ănt) [Gr. *kautēr,* a burner]. 1. Escharotic; caustic. 2. A caustic agent.

cauterization (kŏ''tĕr-ĭ-zā'shŭn) [Gr. *kautēriazein,* to burn]. Burning a part; cautery.

RS: chemicocautery; electrocautery; galvanocautery; moxibustion; ustion.

c., actual. C. by hot iron.

c., chemical. C. by the use of chemical agents, esp. caustic substances.

c., electrical. C. by platinum wires heated to incandescence by an electric current. SYN: *electrocautery,* q.v.; *galvanocautery.*

cauterize (kŏ'tĕr-īz). To burn with a cautery, or to apply one.

cautery (kŏ'tĕr-ĭ) [Gr. *kautēr,* a burner]. A means of destroying tissue by electricity, heat, or corrosive chemicals. Used in potentially infected wounds; to destroy exuberant granulations (proud flesh) or some neoplasms. Thermocautery consists of red hot or white hot object, usually piece of wire or pointed metallic instrument, heated in a flame or with electricity (electrocautery, galvanocautery).

caval (kā'văl). Pert. to the vena cava.

cav'alry bone. Rider's bone; bony deposit in the adductor muscles of the thigh.

cavascope (kăv'ă-skŏp) [L. *cavum,* hollow, + Gr. *skopein,* to examine]. Instrument for examining cavities.

cavernitis C-29 ceasmic

caverni'tis [L. *caverna,* hollow, + Gr. *-itis,* inflammation]. Inflammation of the corpus cavernosum penis.

caverno'ma ["+ Gr. *-ōma,* tumor]. A cavernous angioma.

cavernosi'tis [L. *cavernosus,* having hollows, + Gr. *-itis,* inflammation]. Inflammation of the corpora cavernosa.

cavernosum (kăv-ĕr-nō'sŭm). One of two erectile columns of the dorsum of the penis or clitoris. SYN: *corpus cavernosum.*

cavernous (kăv'ĕr-nŭs) [L. *caverna,* a hollow]. Containing hollow spaces.

  c. angioma. A vascular tumor with many large spaces.

  c. body. Corpus cavernosum.

  c. rale. Bubbling hollow sound.

  c. resonance. Amphoric resonance.

  c. respiration. Hollow sound heard when there is a lung cavity.

  c. rhoncus. A cavernous rale.

  c. sinus. A venous space in the dura mater on either side of the sphenoid bone.

  c. tumor. An angioma.

cavita'tion [L. *cavitas,* a cavity]. Formation of a cavity. May occur as a normal process as in the formation of the amnion in human development or pathologically as in the development of cavities in lung tissue in pulmonary tuberculosis.

cavitis (kā-vī'tĭs) [L. *cavum,* hollow, + Gr. *-itis,* inflammation]. Inflammation of a vena cava.

cavity (kăv'ĭ-tĭ) [L. *cavitas,* hollow]. A hollow space, such as a body organ or the hole in a carious tooth.

  c., abdominal. The c. of the peritoneum between the diaphragm and pelvis.

  c., alveolar. A tooth socket.

  c., amniotic. That within the amnion.

  c., articular. The synovial c. of a joint.

  c., body. In vertebrates the space between the body wall and the visceral organs; the coelom, q.v.

  c., buccal. The mouth.

  c., cotyloid. The acetabulum, q.v.

  c., cranial. The c. of the skull which contains the brain.

  c., glenoid. A shallow concavity on lateral surface of the head of the scapula which receives the head of the humerus.

  c., oral. The mouth or buccal c. Includes the vestibule and the oral cavity proper.

  c., pelvic. The c. of the pelvis. Includes the major pelvic c. which lies between the iliac fossa and above the iliopectineal lines and the minor pelvic c. which lies below the iliopectineal lines or the inlet of the pelvis.

  c., pericardial. The space between the epicardium (visceral pericardium) and the parietal pericardium.

  c., peritoneal. The potential space between the parietal peritoneum lining the body-wall and the visceral peritoneum forming surface layer of visceral organs.

  c., peritoneal, lesser. The omental bursa. SYN: *lesser peritoneal sac.*

  c., pleural. The potential space between the parietal pleura and visceral pleura.

  c., pulp. C. in a tooth containing the dental pulp and nerve termination.

  c., Rosenmüller's. C. on either side of openings of eustachian tube.

  c., serous. A space between two layers of serous membrane. Ex: pleural, pericardial, and peritoneal cavities.

  c., splanchnic. One of three, the cranial, thoracic, and abdominal, including the pelvic cavity.

  c., tympanic. The cavity of the middle ear.

cavum (kā'vŭm) [L. *cavus,* a hollow]. [NA]. A cavity or space.

  c. abdominis. [NA]. The abdominal cavity.

  c. conchae. [NA]. The inferior portion of the cavity of the auricle of the ear. It leads to the external acoustic meatus.

  c. mediastinale. The mediastinum, q.v.

  c. medullare. [NA]. The medullary cavity of a long bone.

  c. oris. [NA]. The oral cavity.

  c. pelvis. [NA]. The pelvic cavity.

  c. tympani. [NA]. Middle ear cavity.

  c. uteri. [NA] The cavity of the uterus.

cavus (kā'vŭs) [L., hollow]. Condition of exaggerated height of arch of foot. SYN: *talipes cavus.*

cayenne pepper (kī-ĕn', kā-ĕn'). Capsicum, q.v.

C.B.C. Abbr. for *complete blood count.*

C.C. Abbr. for *Commission Certified,* with reference to certification of stains by the Biological Stain Commission; *chief complaint.*

cc. Abbr. for *cubic centimeter.*

CCl₃.CHO. Chloral.

CCl₄. Carbon tetrachloride.

C.C.U. Abbr. for *coronary care unit.*

Cd. Chem. symb. for cadmium.

CDC. Abbr. for *Center for Disease Control,* q.v.

Ce. Chem. symb. for cerium.

ceasmic (sē-ăs'mĭk) [Gr. *keasma,* chip]. Pert. to an abnormal cleavage of parts or to a fissure.

cecal (sē'kăl) [L. *caecalis*, pert. to blindness]. 1. Pert. to cecum. 2. Blind, terminating in a closed extremity.

cecectomy (sē-sĕk'tō-mĭ) [L. *caecum*, blindness, cecum, + Gr. *ektomē*, excision]. Removing part of, or incision into, the cecum.
NP: Preparation for appendectomy slightly modified.

cecitis (sē-sī'tĭs) [" + Gr. *-itis*, inflammation]. Inflammation of the cecum.

cecoileostomy (sē''kō-ĭl''ē-ŏs'tō-mĭ) [" + *ileum*, ileum, + Gr. *stoma*, opening]. Making an opening through the abdominal wall into the ileum at the ileocecal valve.

cecopexy (sē'kō-pĕks'ĭ) [L. *caecum*, blindness, cecum, + Gr. *pēxis*, fixation]. Surgical fixation of the cecum to the abdominal wall.

cecoplication (sē''kō-plĭ-kā'shŭn) [" + *plica*, fold]. Reduction of a dilated cecum by making a fold in its wall.

cecoptosis (sē-kŏp-tō'sĭs) [" + Gr. *ptōsis*, a dropping]. Falling displacement of the cecum.

cecosigmoidostomy (sē''kō-sĭg''moyd-ŏs'tō-mĭ) [L. *caecum*, blindness, cecum, + Gr. *sigmoeidēs*, shaped like letter S, + *stoma*, opening]. Formation of a communication between the cecum and sigmoid.

cecostomy (sē-kŏs'tō-mĭ) [" + Gr. *stoma*, opening]. Surgical formation of a cecal fistula or artificial anus.

cecotomy (sē-cŏt'ō-mĭ) [" + Gr. *tome*, a cutting]. Cutting into the cecum.

cecum (sē'kŭm) [L. *caecum*, blindness]. A blind pouch or cul-de-sac which forms the first portion of the large intestine, located below the entrance of the ileum at the ileocecal valve. It averages about 6 cm. in length and 7.5 cm. in width and bears at its lower end the vermiform process or appendix.

-cele [Gr. *kēlē*, hernia]. Suffix indicating a swelling.

celectome (sē-lĕk'tōm) [Gr. *kēlē*, tumor, + *tomē*, a cutting]. Instrument for obtaining a piece of tissue from a tumor for examination.

celery [Gr. *selinon*]. The edible stalks and leaves of the plant Apium graveolens.
Food value of 100 gm. (raw): Cal. 17; protein 0.9 gm.; trace of fat; carbohydrate 3.9 gm.; calcium 39 mg.; ascorbic acid 9 mg.

celiac (sē'lĭ-ăk) [Gr. *koilia*, belly]. Rel. to the abdominal regions.

c. artery. The first branch of the abdominal aorta. Branches supply the stomach, liver, spleen, duodenum, and pancreas.

c. axis. C. artery, q.v.

c. disease. Intestinal malabsorption characterized by diarrhea, malnutrition, bleeding tendency, and hypocalcemia.
TREATMENT: Gluten-free diet which may have to be continued for an indefinite period.

c. plexus. Sympathetic plexus lying near the origin of c. artery. SEE: *plexus*.

celialgia (sē''lĭ-ăl'jĭ-ă) [Gr. *koila*, belly, + *algos*, pain]. Abdominal pain.

celiectasia (sē''lĭ-ĕk-tā'sĭ-ă) [" + *ektasis*, distention]. Distention of the abdomen.

celiectomy (sē''lĭ-ĕk'tō-mĭ) [" + *ektomē*, excision]. Complete or partial removal of an abdominal organ.

celiocentesis (sē''lĭ-ō-sĕn-tē'sĭs) [Gr. *koila*, belly, + *kentēsis*, puncture]. Puncture of the abdomen.

celiocolpotomy (sē''lĭ-ō-kŏl-pŏt'ō-mĭ) [" + *kolpos*, vagina, + *tome*, incision]. Surgical incision of the vagina through the abdominal wall.

celioenterotomy (sē''lĭ-ō-ĕn''tĕr-ŏt'ō-mĭ) [" + *enteron*, intestine, + *tome*, incision]. Incision in the abdominal wall to gain access to the intestines.

celiogastrostomy (sē''lĭ-ō-găs-trŏs'tō-mĭ) [Gr. *koila*, belly, + *gastēr*, stomach, + *stoma*, opening]. Incision in the abdominal wall for making a gastric fistula.

celiogastrotomy (sē''lĭ-ō-găs-trŏt'ō-mĭ) [" + " + *tome*, incision]. Incision into the stomach through the abdominal wall.

celiohysterectomy (sē''lĭ-ō-hĭs-tĕr-ĕk'tō-mĭ) [" + *hystera*, uterus, + *ektomē*, excision]. Removal of uterus through the abdomen.

celiohysterotomy (sē''lĭ-ō-hĭs''tĕr-ŏt'ō-mĭ) [" + " + *tome*, incision]. Opening into the uterus through an abdominal incision.

celioma (sē-lĭ-ō'mă) [Gr. *koila*, belly, + *-ōma*, tumor.]. An abdominal tumor.

celiomyalgia (sē''lĭ-ō-mĭ-ăl'gĭ-ă) [" + *mys*, muscle, + *algos*, pain]. Rheumatic pain in muscles of the abdomen.

celiomyomotomy (sē''lĭ-ō-mĭ''ō-mŏt'ō-mĭ) [" + " + *tome*, incision]. Incision of muscles of abdomen.

celiomyositis (sē''lĭ-ō-mĭ''ō-sī'tĭs) [" + " + *-itis*, inflammation]. Inflammation of muscles of the abdomen.

celioncus (sē''lĭ-ŏn'kŭs) [Gr. *koila*, belly, + *onkos*, tumor]. An abdominal tumor.

celioparacentesis (sē''lĭ-ō-păr''ă-sĕn-tē'sĭs) [" + *para*, beside, + *kentēsis*, puncture]. Puncture of the abdomen for purposes of tapping or drainage.

celiopathy (sē''lĭ-ŏp'ă-thĭ) [" + *pathos*, disease]. Any disease of the abdomen.

celiopyosis (sē″lĭ-ō-pī-ō′sĭs) [Gr. *koila*, belly, + *pyōsis*, suppuration]. Purulent peritonitis.

celiorrhaphy (sē″lĭ-ōr′ă-fĭ) ["+ *rhaphē*, suture]. Suture of wound in the abdominal wall.

celiosalpingectomy (sē″lĭ-ō-săl″pĭn-jĕk′tō-mĭ) ["+ *salpinx*, tube, + *ektomē*, excision]. Removal of the fallopian tubes through an abdominal incision.

celiosalpingotomy (sē″lĭ-ō-săl″pĭn-gŏt′ō-mĭ) ["+ "+ *tomē*, incision]. Opening of the fallopian tube through an abdominal incision.

celioscope (sē′lĭ-ō-skōp) [Gr. *koila*, belly, + *skopein*, to examine]. Device for visual examination of a body cavity.

celioscopy (sē″lĭ-ŏs′kō-pĭ). Use of the celioscope.

celiotomy (sē″lĭ-ŏt′ō-mĭ) [Gr. *koila*, belly, + *tomē*, incision]. Surgical incision into the abdominal cavity.

    c., vaginal. Entering the abdomen through the vagina.

celitis (sē-lī′tĭs) ["+ *-itis*, inflammation]. Peritonitis; abdominal inflammation.

cell [L. *cella*, a chamber]. 1. A small enclosed or partly enclosed cavity such as an air cell. 2. A mass of protoplasm containing a nucleus or nuclear 'material. It is the unit of structure of all animals and plants and is the physical basis of all life processes.

Cells and the products of cells comprise all the tissues of the body. All functional activities of the body are carried on by cells, and the structure and form of a cell is closely correlated with its functioning. Cells arise only from preexisting cells, new cells arising by cell division. Growth and development result from the increase in numbers of cells and the differentiation of cells into different types of tissues. Reproduction is accomplished by specialized germ cells, the spermatozoa and ova, which contain in their nuclei the genes or determiners for hereditary characteristics.

Cell inclusions or paraplastic bodies include food substances (fat droplets, glycogen and protein granules); chromophilic substance (Nissl bodies); pigment granules (melanin); crystals of various substances; and secretory granules.

Also present in the cytoplasm are submicroscopic bodies once called microsomes.

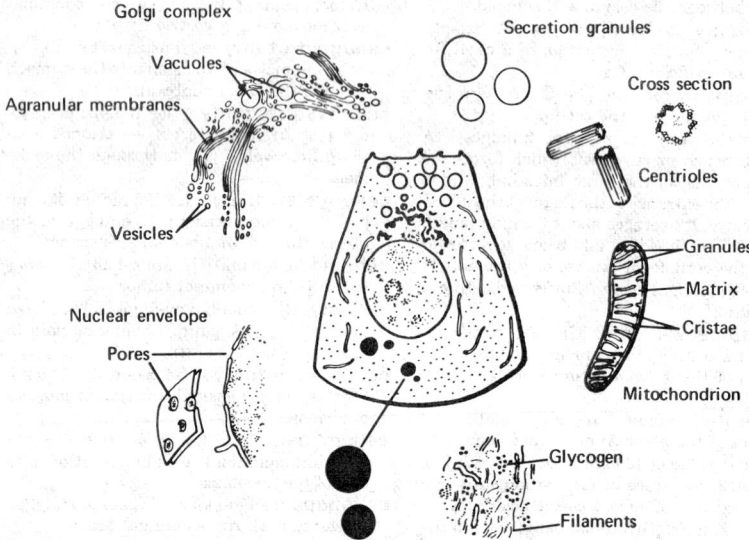

THE CELL

In the center the cell is shown as it would appear using ordinary light microscopy. The diagrams around the cell illustrate submicroscopic portions as they would be seen in a picture taken by using an electron microscope.

demonstrated by differential centrifugation. They are small fragments of the endoplasmic reticulum and contain particles of ribonucleoprotein (ribosomes). Thus microsomes should be called ribosomes. Ribosomes are important in protein synthesis within the cell.

STRUCTURE: When a typical cell is killed, fixed, and stained it exhibits a centrally located nucleus surrounded by cytoplasm.

Nucleus: The nucleus possesses a nuclear membrane which encloses a clear nuclear sap or karyoplasm. One or more densely staining bodies, the nucleoli, usually are present.

Cytoplasm: This includes the cell protoplasm lying outside the nucleus. Its outermost layer constitutes the cell membrane which forms the limiting membrane of the cell. Within the ground substance of the cytoplasm is the ergastoplasm (granular endoplasmic reticulum) which contains ribonucleoprotein, a substance which can be identified only by use of the electron microscope. Ribonucleoprotein is important in protein synthesis.

A cell may produce other cells, and it has the power of exercising the vital processes of life. Cells of one tissue differ from those of other tissues, depending upon the function they perform. Those of one tissue in man are very similar to those of corresponding tissues in other vertebrates.

c., acidophil. A c. that stains with eosin or other acid dyes.

c., acinar. A c. present in the acinus of an acinar gland, as those of the pancreas.

c.'s, adelomorphous. Transparent columnar cells lining the glands of the stomach, believed to secrete pepsinogen.

c., adipose. A fat c.

c., adventitial. A macrophage along a blood vessel, together with perivascular undifferentiated cells associated with it.

c., air. A small cavity in one of the bones of the skull containing air (e.g., mastoid air cells, air cells comprising the ethmoid sinus).

c.'s, alpha. Acidophil cells of the hypophysis (anterior lobe) and the pancreas. In the latter they are the source of glucagon.

c.'s, argentaffin. Cells found in the epithelium of the digestive tract (stomach, intestine, appendix). Cytoplasm of the c.'s contains granules which stain selectively with silver.

c., basal. 1. C., basket, q.v. 2. A type of c. in the olfactory epithelium lying between bases of the supporting cells.

c., basket. 1. A branching basal or myoepithelial c. of the salivary and other glands. 2. Certain cells of the molecular layer of the cerebellar cortex.

c.'s, beta. 1. Insulin-secreting cells of the pancreatic islets of Langerhans. 2. Basophil cells of the anterior lobe of the hypophysis.

c.'s, Betz. Large pyramidal cells of the motor area of cerebral cortex.

c., bipolar. A neuron with two processes, an axon, and dendrite. Found in retina of eye and in cochlear and vestibular ganglia of the acoustic nerve.

c., blood. Erythrocyte or leukocyte.

c. body. Part of the nerve c. or neuron which contains the c. nucleus and cytoplasm. SEE: *nerve.*

c.'s, capsule. Cells forming a single layer about the c. bodies of sensory neurons of spinal ganglia. SYN: *amphicytes; satellite cells.*

c., castration. An enlarged and vacuolated basophil c. of the hypophysis in gonadal insufficiency or following castration.

c. center. Centrosome, q.v.

c., centro-acinar. Duct cells of the pancreas more or less invaginated into the lumen of an acinus.

c., chief. 1. The cells of the parathyroid gland which secrete the hormone. 2. Zymogenic cells of gastric glands which secrete pepsin or its precursor. 3. Chromophobe cells of the hypophysis.

c., columnar. An epithelial c. with height greater than width.

c., cone. A c. in the retina whose scleral end forms a cone which serves as a light receptor. Vision in bright light, color vision, and acute vision depend upon functioning of the cones.

c., cuboidal. A c. with height about equal to width and depth.

c., daughter. C. from a mother c.

c., delomorphous. Large cells in the glands of the stomach, believed to secrete the acid of gastric juice.

c. division. Mitosis, q.v. SEE: *amitosis.*

c., endothelial. A flat c. making up the lining membranes of vessels.

c., epithelial. C. forming epithelial surfaces of membranes and skin.

c., ethmoidal. One of several cavities which honeycomb the lateral masses of the ethmoid bone, forming a part of the paranasal air sinuses. SYN: *ethmoid sinus.*

c., ganglion. 1. Any neuron whose c. body is located within a ganglion. 2. A neuron of the retina of the eye whose cell body lies in the ganglion c. layer. The axons of ganglion cells form the fibers of the optic nerve.

c., giant. Large multinucleated cells found in bone marrow; a megakaryocyte. They are thought to give rise to blood platelets.

c., glia. C., neuroglia, q.v.

c., goblet. Epithelial c. distended with mucus.

c., granule. Certain small neurons of the cerebrum and cerebellum.

c., gustatory. A neuroepithelial c. or taste c. of a taste bud.

c., horizontal. A neuron of the inner nuclear layer of the retina. The axons of these cells run horizontally and serve to connect various parts of the retina.

c., interstitial. One of the many cells found in connective tissue of the ovary and the seminiferous tubules of the testes, accounting for their internal secretion.

c., Kupffer. A fixed phagocytic c. found in the sinusoids of the liver.

c., L.E. A lupus erythematosus c.

c., Leydig's. C., interstitial, q.v.

c., littoral. A macrophage found in the sinuses of lymphatic tissue.

c., lupus erythematosus. Cells characteristic of lupus erythematosus disseminatus in which denaturation of nuclear material of leukocytes occurs. Such cells are highly chemotactic causing phagocytic leukocytes to congregate about them in a rosette fashion.

c., lutein. A c. of the corpus luteum of the ovary which contains lutein. Granulose lutein cells are hypertrophied follicle cells; these lutein (paralutein) cells develop from the theca interna.

c. mass. In embryology, a mass of cells which is the anlage or primordium of an organ or structure.

Inner c. mass is a mass of cells attached eccentrically to the inner surface of the wall of the blastocyst of mammals. From it develops the embryo proper and certain related structures as the amnion and yolk sac. The intermediate c. mass is a nephrotome, q.v.

c., mast. A c. found in connective tissue of vertebrates. Contains heparin and histamine.

c. membrane. A thin membrane (plasmalemma) which encloses a cell. It is too thin to be seen with the light microscope.

c., microglia. Neuroglial cells of mesodermal origin present in the brain and spinal cord.

c., mother. Any type of c. which divides and gives rise to two or more cells. The latter are called daughter c.'s.

c., mucous. 1. A c. which secretes mucus found in mucus-secreting glands. 2. A goblet c.

c., neuroglia. Non-nerve cells found in the central nervous system and the retina of the eye. Includes astrocytes, oligodendrocytes, and microglia.

c. organelle. A specific structure in the cytoplasm of a cell consisting of organized living substance, in contrast to inclusions which are lifeless constituents. Cell organelles include the c. membrane (plasma membrane), mitochondria, endoplasmic reticulum (ergastroplasm), Golgi complex or apparatus, ribosomes, agranular reticulum, lysosomes, c. center, and centriole.

c., parent. C., mother, q.v.

c.'s, phalangeal. Cells which support the hair cells of the organ of Corti. They form several rows of outer phalangeal cells (Deiter's cells) and a single row of inner phalangeal cells.

c., plasma. Cells derived from lymphoid elements. They are found in lymphoid tissue and the cellular connective tissue of the intestinal tract. They are important in antibody production.

c., prickle. A c. possessing spinelike protoplasmic processes that connect with similar processes of adjoining cells. Found in the stratum germinativum of the epidermis.

c., pus. A leukocyte present in pus. Cells of this type are often degenerated or necrotic.

c., pyramidal. A nerve c. of the cerebral cortex.

c., Rieder. Myeloblast which may be present in acute leukemia, possessing a lobulated or double nucleus.

c., rod. A c. in the retina of the eye whose scleral end is long and narrow, forming a rod, a sensory element of the eye. Rods are stimulated by dim light.

s., Rouget. Cells with branching processes which, in a frog, surround the walls of a capillary. They are capable of contracting upon stimulation.

c., satellite. A neuroglia c. lying adjacent to the c. body of a sensory neuron in cranial or spinal ganglia.

c., segmented. A segmented neutrophil, i.e., one with a nucleus of two or more lobes connected together by slender filaments.

c., sensory. A sensory neuron; a c. which when stimulated gives rise to nerve impulses which are conveyed to the central nervous system.

c.'s, septal. Cells attached to or in the septa of the lungs. They function in some animals as macrophages.

c., sickle. An abnormal erythrocyte shaped like a sickle. SEE: *anemia, sickle-cell.*

c., spider. An astrocyte.

c., squamous. Flat, scalelike, epithelial cell.

c., sympathicotrophic. Large epithelial cells occurring in groups in the hilus of the ovary. Thought to be chromaffin cells.

c., sympathochromaffin. Chromaffin cells of ectodermal origin present in fetal adrenal from which sympathetic and medullary cells arise.

c., target. An erythrocyte with a rounded, central area surrounded by a clear ring lightly stained, and this in turn surrounded by a dense ring of peripheral protoplasm. Present in certain blood disorders.

c., Türk's irritation. A c. resembling a plasma c., found in cases of severe anemia or chronic infection.

c., visual. A rod or cone c. of the retina.

c. wall. C. membrane, q.v. Plant cells are enclosed by a wall which contains cellulose. Some animal cells have a thin coat outside the c. membrane. It is not known whether or not this should be regarded as part of the c.

c.'s, zymogenic. Chief cells or enzyme producing cells of the gastric glands.

Cellano factor (se'lăn-ō). A hereditary factor found in most human blood; 99.8% of population have it. Named for woman who did not have this blood factor but possessed the antibody. SYN: *k factor.*

cellobiose (sĕl″ō-bī′ōs). A disaccharide resulting from the hydrolysis of cellulose.

cellophane (sĕl′ō-fān). Thin, transparent, waterproof sheet of viscose. Used as a wound dressing because it does not crack, is singularly free of infection, and wound can be seen without its removal.

cell'ula [L., little cell]. (pl. *cellulae*) [NA]. 1. A minute cell. 2. A small compartment.

cell'ular. Pert. to, composed of, or derived from cells.

c. therapy. Implantation of cells from a donor to a recipient. Ex: blood transfusions, organ transplants, skin grafting. SYN: *cell therapy.*

cell'ulase. An enzyme which converts cellulose to cellobiose. Present in some microorganisms and marine life.

c. high diet. High residue diet. SEE: *high cellulose diet.*

cellulicidal (sĕl″ū-lĭ-sī′dăl) [L. *cellula*, little cell, + *caedere*, to kill]. Destructive to cells.

cellulifugal (sĕl″ū-lĭf′ū-găl) ["+ *fugere*, to flee]. Extending or moving away from a cell.

cellulipetal (sĕl″ū-lĭp′ĭ-tăl) ["+ *petere*, to seek]. Extending or moving toward a cell.

cellulitis (sĕl-ū-lī′tĭs) [L. *cellula*, little cell, + Gr. *-itis*, inflammation]. Inflammation of cellular or connective tissue, spreading as in erysipelas.

An infection in or close to the skin is usually localized by the body defense mechanisms. If this does not happen and the inflammation spreads through the tissue, the process is called cellulitis.

c., pelvic. Parametritis; inflammation of the parametrium, q.v. May occur in puerperal fever or septic conditions of the uterus and appendages.

cellulofi'brous ["+ *fibra*, fiber]. Both cellular and fibrous.

celluloneuritis (sĕl″ū-lō-nū-rī′tĭs) ["+ Gr. *neuron*, nerve, + *-itis*, inflammation]. Inflammation of nerve cells.

c., acute anterior. Acute anterior poliomyelitis.

cellulose (sĕl′ū-lōs) [L. *cellula*, little cell]. Plant fiber; a fibrous form of carbohydrate constituting the supporting framework of plants. It is composed of a great number of glucose units.

It stimulates peristalsis and aids in intestinal elimination. Ordinarily it is not chemically changed or absorbed in digestion, remaining a polysaccharide, q.v.

c. foods. Apples, apricots, asparagus, beans, beets, bran flakes, broccoli, cabbage, celery, mushrooms, oatmeal, onions, oranges, parsnips, prunes, spinach, turnips, wheat flakes, whole grains, whole wheat bread. SYN: *fiber-containing foods.*

c. high diet. High residue diet, q.v.

c., oxidized. USP. C. which has been oxidized by nitrogen dioxide and is made in the form of cotton or gauze. Used to arrest bleeding by direct application to site of hemorrhage.

cellulotox'ic [L. *cellula*, little cell, + Gr. *toxikon*, poison]. 1. Poisonous to cells. 2. Caused by cell toxins.

celology (se-lŏl′ō-jĭ) [Gr. *kēlē*, hernia, + *logos*, study]. The surgical study of hernias.

celom, celoma (se′lŏm, se-lō′mä) [Gr. *koilōma*, a hollow]. The coelom, q.v.

celonychia (se′lō-nĭk′ĭ-ä) [Gr. *koilos*, hollow, + *onyx, onych-*, nail]. Koilonychia, q.v.

celoschisis (se-lŏs′kĭ-sĭs) [Gr. *koilia*, belly, + *schisis*, fissure]. Congenital fissure of the abdominal wall.

celoscope (se′lō-skōp) [Gr. *koilos*, hollow, + *skopein*, to examine]. Device for visual examination of a body cavity.

celosomia (sē-lō-sō'mĭ-ă) [Gr. *kēlē,* hernia, + *sōma,* body]. Herniation of fetal viscera.

celotomy (sē-lŏt'ō-mĭ) ["+ *tomē,* incision]. Kelotomy, q.v.

celozo'ic [Gr. *koilia,* belly, + *zōon,* animal]. Inhabiting any cavity of the body, such as parasitic protozoa.

Celsius scale (sĕl'sĭ-ŭs). [Anders Celsius, Swedish astronomer, 1701-44]. A temperature scale on which the boiling point of water is 100° and the melting point of ice is 0°. This is the official scientific name of the temperature scale which is also known as centigrade.

cementitis (sē"mĕn-tī'tĭs) [L. *cementum,* cement, + Gr. *-itis,* inflammation]. Inflammation of the dental cementum.

cementoblast (sē-mĕn'tō-blăst) ["+ Gr. *blastos,* germ]. A cell of the inner layer of the dental sac of a developing tooth. It deposits cementum, q.v., upon the dentine of the root.

cementocla'sia ["+ Gr. *klasis,* breaking]. Decay of the cementum of a tooth root.

cementoma (sē"mĕn-tō'mă) [L. *cementum,* cement, + Gr. *-ōma,* tumor]. A tumor having its origin in the substantia ossea.

cementum (sē-mĕn'tŭm) [L.]. [NA]. Thin layer of modified bone formed by cementoblasts and deposited upon the dentine of the root of a tooth; the substantia ossea. To it is attached the alveolar periosteum or peridental membrane which binds the tooth to its socket.

cenesthesia (sĕn-es-the'zĭ-a, sē"nĕs-) [Gr. *koinos,* common, + *aisthēsis,* feeling]. The normal feeling of being alive and aware. SYN: *coenesthesia.*

cenesthe'sic, cenesthet'ic. Pert. to cenesthesia.

cenesthopathia, cenesthopathy (sē-nĕs-, sĕn-ĕs-thō-păth'ĭ-ă, -thŏp'ă-thĭ) [Gr. *koinos,* common, + *aisthēsis,* feeling, + *pathos,* disease]. Malaise or a general feeling of lack of well-being in illness.

cenogenesis (sĕn"ō-, sē"nō-jĕn'ē-sĭs) [Gr. *kaīnos,* new, + *genesis,* production]. The development of characteristics in an individual which are absent in ancestors and which do not have a phylogenetic significance. They indicate adaptation to environment.

cenopsychic (sē"nō-, sĕn-ō-sī'kĭk) ["+ *psychē,* mind]. Only recently appearing in mental development.

cenosis (sĕn-ō', sē-nō'sĭs) [Gr. *kenos,* empty, + *-ōsis,* condition]. 1. A morbid discharge. 2. Inanition.

cenosite (sĕn'ō-, sē"nō-sīt) [Gr. *koinos,* common, + *sitos,* food]. A microorganism not depending for life upon its host, but parasitic in character. SYN: *coinosite.*

cenotic (sĕn-ŏt', sē-nŏt'ĭk) [Gr. *kenos,* empty]. 1. Purgative; drastic. 2. Pert. to cenosis.

cenotophobia (sĕn"ō-, sē"nō-tō-fō'bĭ-ă) [Gr. *kainotēs,* novelty, + *phobos,* fear]. Morbid aversion to new things and new ideas. SYN: *cainotophobia.*

cenotype (sē'nō-, sĕn'ō-tīp) [Gr. *koinos,* common, + *typos,* a type]. An original type.

censor (sĕn'sĕr) [L. *cēnsor,* judge]. In psychoanalysis, a psychic inhibition that prevents abhorrent unconscious thoughts or impulses from seeking objective expression unless in a form unrecognized by consciousness.

center (sĕn'tĕr) [L. *centrum,* center]. 1. Middle point of a body. 2. A group of nerve cells within the central nervous system which control a specific activity or function.

   c., auditory. C. for hearing in the gyri in sylvian fissure. SEE: *area, auditory.*

   c., autonomic. A c. in the brain or spinal cord which regulates any of the activities under the control of the autonomic nervous system. There are a few cortical centers but most are located in the hypothalamus, medulla oblongata, and spinal cord.

   c., Broca's. Speech c.

   c., cardioaccelerator. A c. in the medulla oblongata which gives rise to impulses which speed up the heart rate. Impulses reach the heart by way of sympathetic fibers.

   c., cardioinhibitory. A c. in the medulla oblongata containing neurons whose axons, parasympathetic fibers, pass by way of the vagus nerves to the heart. Impulses slow down heart rate.

   c., chondrification. A c. of cartilage formation.

   c., ciliospinal. A c. in the spinal cord from which arise sympathetic impulses which dilate the pupils of the eyes.

   c.'s, defecation. Two centers, a medullary c. located in the medulla oblongata and a spinal c. located in second to fourth sacral segments of the spinal cord. The anospinal centers controlling the sphincter reflexes for the process of defecation.

   c., deglutition. A c. in the medulla oblongata on the floor of the fourth ventricle which controls swallowing.

   c., epiotic. Ossification c. of mastoid process.

   c., gustatory. Little is known about it but it is thought to be in the hypothalamus. SYN: *gustatory area; taste c.*

   c.'s, heat-regulating. Two centers, a heat loss c. and a heat-production c. located in the hypothalamus. They regulate body temperature.

c., higher. 1. A c. in the cerebrum from which impulses based on conscious sensations, wishes, or desires are initiated. 2. A c. in any portion of the brain in contrast to one in the cord.

c., lower. C. in the brain stem or spinal cord.

c., micturition. C. controlling reflexes of urinary bladder. Located in second to fourth and fourth to sixth sacral segments of the cord; higher centers are present in medulla oblongata, hypothalamus and cerebrum.

c., motor cortical. The area in the frontal lobe, the origin of impulses for voluntary movements.

c., nerve. One of many in cerebrospinal or ganglionic systems originating or controlling vital function.

c., ossification. Spot where ossification begins in bones.

c., pneumotaxic. C., respiratory, q.v.

c.'s, psychocortical. Centers of cerebral cortex concerned with mental operations.

c., reflex. A region within the brain or spinal cord where connections (synapses) are made between afferent and efferent neurons of a reflex arc.

c., respiratory. A region in the medulla oblongata which controls respiratory movements. It consists of inspiratory, expiratory, and pneumotaxic centers.

c., speech. SEE: area, Broca's.

c., taste. C., gustatory, q.v.

c., temperature. C., thermoregulatory, q.v.

c., thermoregulatory. Temperature-regulating centers in the hypothalamus.

c., trophic. One of many centers located in cerebrospinal and sympathetic systems presiding over nutrition.

c., vasoconstrictor. A c. in the medulla which brings about the constriction of blood vessels.

c., vasodilator. A c. located in the medulla oblongata which brings about vasodilation of blood vessels.

c., vasomotor. A c. through which the diameter of blood vessels is controlled; the vasoconstrictor and vasodilator centers.

c., visual. C. in occipital lobe which controls sight.

c., vomiting. A c. in the medulla oblongata.

enter for Disease Control. Division of the U.S. Public Health Service in Atlanta, Georgia, for investigation and control of various diseases, esp. those which have epidemic potential.

centesis (sĕn-tē′sĭs) [Gr. *kentēsis*, puncture]. Puncture of a cavity.

centigrade (sĕn′tĭ-grād) [L. *centum*, a hundred, + *gradus*, a step]. 1. Having 100 degrees. 2. Pert. to a thermometer divided into 100°. The boiling point is 100° and the freezing point is 0°. The official scientific name for the centigrade scale is Celsius. ABBR: C. SEE: *thermometer.*

cen′tigram ["+ Gr. *gramma*, a small weight]. A measure of weight; the hundredth part of a gram; 0.15432 gr. SEE: *metric system; metric system* in *Appendix.*

centiliter (sĕn′tĭ-lē-tĕr) ["+ Gr. *litra*, measure of wt.]. One-hundredth part of a liter; 10 cc. ABBR: cl.

centimeter (sĕn′tĭ-mē-tĕr) [L. *centum*, a hundred, + Gr. *metron*, measure]. Unit of length in metric system. One-hundredth part of a meter; 2/5 of an inch (0.3937 in.). ABBR: cm.

centinormal (sĕn″tĭ-nor′măl) ["+ *norma*, rule]. One-hundredth part of the normal, as the strength of a solution.

centipede (sĕn′tĭ-pēd″) ["+ *pes, ped-*, foot]. An arthropod of the subclass Chilopoda characterized by an elongated, flattened body of many segments each with a pair of jointed legs. The first pair of appendages are hooklike claws bearing openings of ducts from poison glands. The bites of large tropical centipedes may cause severe local and sometimes general symptoms but they are rarely fatal.

centrad (sĕn′trăd) [Gr. *kentron*, center, + L. *ad*, toward]. Toward the center.

central (sĕn′trăl). Situated at, or rel. to, a center.

c. bodies. Attraction center of a cell. SYN: *centrosome*, q.v.

c. nervous system. Brain and spinal cord, including their nerves and end organs, controlling voluntary acts.

Composed of nerve tissue which forms the brain, spinal cord, and the nerves from both. Tissue is made up of gray and white matter. Gray matter is composed of cells of nervous tissue, while the white matter is composed of nerve fibers from the cells. White matter in the brain and cord carries messages or impulses from the body, or outside world, to the cells or gray matter.

C. nervous system includes parts of the brain governing consciousness and mental activities; parts of brain, spinal cord, and their sensory and motor nerve fibers controlling skeletal muscles; and end-organs of the body-wall. SYN: *cerebrospinal system;*

voluntary nervous system. SEE: *autonomic, parasympathetic,* and *sympathetic nervous systems.*

c. venous pressure. The venous blood pressure obtained by inserting a catheter, attached to a manometer, into the right atrium through the veins of the arm. Useful in

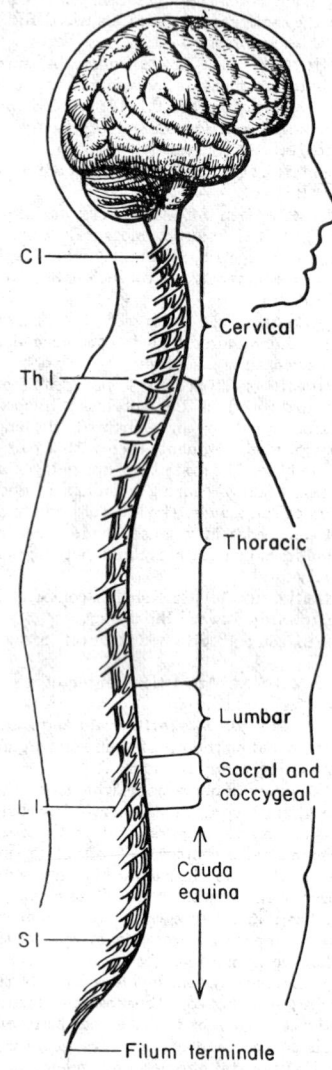

CI

Cervical

Th I

Thoracic

Lumbar

Sacral and coccygeal

L I

Cauda equina

S I

Filum terminale

THE CENTRAL NERVOUS SYSTEM

determining effective blood volume shock. When CVP exceeds 10-12 cm. of water, there is danger of overloading the circulatory system if additional fluids are given. ABBR: CVP.

centraphose (sĕn'tră-fōz) [Gr. *kentron,* center, + *a-,* not, + *phōs,* light]. A subjective sensation of darkness originating in the optic brain centers. SEE: *centrophose; chromphose.*

cen'tre. Center.

centriciput (sĕn-trĭs'ĭ-pŭt) [Gr. *kentron,* center, + L. *caput,* head]. The central part upper surface of skull between the occiput and sinciput.

centrifugal (sĕn-trĭf'ū-găl) [Gr. *kentron,* center, + L. *fugere,* to flee]. Receding from the center. SEE: *axifugal; centrifuge.*

c. force. The force which impels a thing or parts of it, outward from the center of rotation. SEE: *centrifuge.*

centrifuge (sĕn'trĭ-fūj). A device which spins or whirls test tubes at high speeds. Thus centrifugal force, q.v., causes the heavy particles in the liquid in the tubes to settle to the bottom and the lighter liquid to go to the top. When unclotted blood is centrifuged the plasma goes to the top and the heavy red cells go to the bottom of the tube. The white blood cells are heavier than the plasma but lighter than the red blood cells. Therefore they form a thin layer between the red blood cells and the plasma.

centriole (sĕn'trĭ-ōl). A minute hollow cylinder closed at one end and open at the other, found in the cell center or attraction sphere of a cell. Preceding mitosis it divides, forming two daughter centrioles (diplosome). During mitosis the centrioles migrate to opposite poles of the cell and each forms the center of the aster to which the spindle fibers are attached. SEE: *mitosis.*

centripetal (sĕn-trĭp'ĕ-tăl) [Gr. *kentron,* center, + L. *petere,* to seek]. Moving toward the center.

centrocyte (sĕn'trō-sīt) ["+ *kytos,* cell]. cell having single and double hematoxylin stainable granules of varying size in protoplasm.

centrodesmus (sĕn-trō-dĕz'mŭs) ["+ *smos,* a band]. The matter connecting the two centrosomes in a nucleus during mitosis.

centrolecithal (sĕn"trō-lĕs'ĭ-thăl) [Gr. *kentron,* center, + *lekithos,* yoke]. Pert. to egg, esp. an ova, with the yolk centrally located.

centromere (sĕn'trō-mēr) ["+ *meros,* part A clear region on a chromosome which marks the junction of its two arms.

centrophose (sĕn'trō-fōz) ["+ phōs, light]. A subjective sensation of a light spot having its origin in the optic brain centers. SEE: centraphose; chromophose.

centrosome (sĕn'trō-sōm) [Gr. kentron, center, + soma, body]. A region of the cytoplasm of a cell usually lying near the nucleus, containing in its center one or two centrioles, the diplosome. The cell spare center is active during cell division. SYN: cell center.

centrosphere (sĕn'trō-sfēr) ["+ sphaira, sphere]. The envelope encasing two centrosomes.

centrostaltic (sĕn"trō-stăl'tĭk) ["+ stellein, send forth]. Pert. to a center of motion.

centrother'apy [Gr. kentron, center, + therapeia, therapy]. Any local application that acts upon nerve centers.

centrum (sĕn'trŭm) [L.]. (pl. cen'tra) 1. Any center, esp. an anatomical one. 2. Body of a vertebra.

    c. semiova'le. A mass of white matter at center of each cerebral hemisphere.

    c. tendin'eum. Central tendon of the diaphragm.

cephalad (sĕf'ă-lad) [Gr. kephalē, head, + L. ad, toward]. Toward the head.

cephalalgia (sĕf-ă-lăl'jĭ-ă) ["+ algos, pain]. Headache, pain in the head. A symptom of numerous diseases and disorders. SEE: headache.

cephalalgic (sĕf-ăl-ăl'jĭk). Of the nature of cephalalgia.

cephalea (sĕf-ă-lē'ă) [Gr. kephalē, head]. Cephalalgia, q.v.

cephaledema (sĕf-ăl-ĕ-dē'mă) ["+ oidēma, swelling]. Edema of the head.

cephalhematocele (sĕf'ăl-hē-măt'ō-sēl) [Gr. kephalē, head, + haima, blood, + kēlē, tumor]. A bloody tumor communicating with the dural sinuses.

cephalhematoma (sĕf'ăl-hē'mă-tō'mă) ["+ "+ -ōma, tumor]. A subcutaneous swelling containing blood, often found on the head of a baby several days after birth, when delivery was accompanied by use of forceps. The swelling disappears within two to three months.

    RS: caput succedaneum.

cephal'ic [L. cephalicus]. 1. Cranial; pert. to the head. 2. Superior in position.

    c. version. Turning the fetus during labor so head will present.

cephalin (sĕf'ă-lĭn) [Gr. kephalē, head]. A phospholipid, resembling lecithin, present in the brain of mammals.

cephalitis (sĕf'ăl-ī'tĭs) ["+ -itis, inflammation]. Encephalitis, q.v.

cephalocele (sĕf'ă-lō-sēl) ["+ kēlē, hernia]. Protrusion of the brain from the cranial cavity.

cephalocentesis (sĕf'ă-lō-sĕn-tē'sĭs) [Gr. kephalē, head, + kentēsis, puncture]. Surgical puncture of cranium.

cephalodynia (sĕf'ă-lō-dĭn'ĭ-ă) ["+ odynē, pain]. Pain in the head; headache, cephalalgia.

cephalogyric (sĕf'ă-lō-jĭ'rĭk) ["+ gyros, a turn]. Of or pertaining to rotation of the head.

cephalohemometer (sĕf'ă-lō-hē-mŏm'ē-tĕr) [Gr. kephalē, head, + haima, blood, + metron, measure]. Instrument for determining changes in intracranial blood pressure.

cephalo'ma ("+ -ōma, tumor). A soft carcinoma.

cephalomenia (sĕf'ă-lō-mē'nĭ-ă) ["+ mēn, month]. Vicarious menstruation from the nose or head.

cephalomeningitis (sĕf'ă-lō-mĕn'ĭn-jī'tĭs) [Gr. kephalē, head, + meninx, membrane, + -itis, inflammation]. Inflammation of the cerebral meninges.

cephalometer (sĕf-ă-lŏm'ē-tĕr) ["+ metron, measure]. Device for measuring the head.

cephalometry (sĕf'ă-lŏm'ē-trĭ). Measurement of the head.

cephalomo'tor [Gr. kephalē, head, + L. motus, motion]. Pert. to movements of the head.

cephalone (sĕf'ă-lōn) ["+ ōn, being]. An idiot with a large head and sclerotic enlargement of the brain.

cephalonia (sĕf'ă-lo'nĭ-ă). A condition marked by idiocy, enlarged head, and sclerotic enlargement of the brain.

cephalopathy (sĕf'ă-lŏp'ă-thĭ) [Gr. kephalē, head, + pathos, disease]. Any disease of the head or brain.

cephaloplegia (sĕf'ă-lō-plē'jĭ-ă) ["+ plēgē, stroke]. Paralysis of muscles about head or, less accurately, face.

cephalorhachidian (sĕf'ă-lō-ră-kĭd'ĭ-ăn) ["+ rhachis, spine]. Pert. to the head and spine.

cephaloscope (sĕf'ă-lō-skōp) ["+ skopein, to examine]. Device for auscultation of the head.

cephalothoracopagus (sĕf'ă-lō-thō"ră-kŏp'ă-gŭs) [Gr. kephalē, head, + thōrakos, chest, + pagus, firmly set]. A double fetus joined at head and thorax.

cephalotome (sĕf'ă-lō-tōm) ["+ tomē, cutting]. Instrument for cutting the head of the fetus.

cephalotomy (sĕf-ă-lŏt'ō-mĭ). Cutting the fetal head to facilitate delivery.

cephalotractor (sĕf'ă-lō-trăk'tōr) [Gr. *kephalē*, head, + L. *tractus*, drawing along]. Obstetrical forceps.

cephalotribe (sĕf'ă-lō-trīb) ["+ *tribein*, to crush]. Instrument for crushing head of fetus.

cephalotripsy (sĕf'ă-lō-trĭp-sĭ). Crushing of fetal head in dystocia.

cephalotrypesis (sĕf'ă-lō-trĭp-ē'sĭs) [Gr. *kephalē*, head, + *trypesis*, a boring]. Removing a portion of bone from the skull. SYN: *trephination*.

cephaloxia (sĕf'ă-lōks'ĭ-ă). Torticollis or wryneck, q.v.

ceptor (sĕp'tor) [L. *receptor*, receiver]. General term for a nerve ending which, upon being stimulated, passes the stimulus on to the cell to which the ceptor is attached.

c., chemical. C. which initiates chemical reactions in the body.

c., contact. C. which apprehends stimuli contributed by direct physical contact.

c., distance. C. which perceives stimuli at a distance by aerial or ethereal forces.

cera (sē'ră) [L.]. Wax.

c. alba. White wax.

c. flava. Yellow wax.

ceram'ics, dental [Gr. *keramos*, potters' clay]. The use of porcelain or porcelain-type materials in dental work.

ceramodon'tia ["+ *odous*, tooth]. Dental ceramics.

ceramuria (sĕr"ăm-ū'rĭ-ă) ["+ *ouron*, urine]. Excessive phosphate excretion in urine. SYN: *phosphaturia.*

cerate (sē'rāt) [L. *ceratum*]. Unctuous substance containing wax and of such consistency that it may be spread easily at ordinary temperature upon muslin or similar material with a spatula, and yet not so soft as to liquefy and run when applied to the skin. Rarely prescribed.

ceratocele (sĕr'ă-tō-sēl) [Gr. *keras*, horn, + *kēlē*, hernia]. Hernia of Descemet's membrane through outer layer of the cornea. SYN: *keratocele.*

ceratotome (sē-răt'ō-tōm) ["+ *tomē*, incision]. A knife for division of the cornea.

ceratum (sē-rā'tŭm) [L., waxed]. An unctuous solid for application to the skin. SYN: *cerate*, q.v.

cercaria (sĕr-kā'rĭ-ă) [Gr. *kerkos*, tail]. (pl. *cerca'riae*) A free-swimming stage in the development of a fluke or trematode. Cercariae develop within sporocysts or redia which parasitize snails or bivalve molluscs. They emerge from the mollusc and either enter their final host directly or encyst in an intermediate host which is eaten by the final host. In the latter case, the encysted tailless form is known as a metacercaria. SEE: *fluke; trematode.*

cerclage (sār-klōzh') [Fr., hooping]. Tying parts together by encircling them with a ligature, wire, or loop.

Cercomonas (sĕr-kŏm'ō-năs) [Gr. *kerkos*, tail, + *monas*, unit]. A genus of free-living, coprozoic, flagellate protozoa. May be present in stale specimens of feces or urine. Not pathogenic.

cercomoniasis (sĕr"kō-mō-nī'ă-sĭs). Infestation with Cercomonas intestinalis.

cercus (sĕr'kŭs) [L., tail]. (pl. *cer'ci*) A hairlike structure.

cerea flexibilitas (sē'rē-ă flĕks'ĭ-bĭl'ĭ-tăs) [L. *cera*, wax, + *flexibilitas*, flexibility]. In psychoanalysis, a condition in which the limbs can be molded into any desired position.

ce'reals [L. *cereālis*, of grain]. Edible grains.

COMP: The composition of all cereals is of a similar character. The carbohydrates are the principle nutrient present and protein is next. Cereals contain 70-80% carbohydrate in the form of starch; and 8-15% protein.

Vitamin B complex abundant in wheat

Comparison of Food Value of Principal Cereals*
In Their Raw Unenriched Flour Form

	Cal. per 100 gm.	Protein gm.	Carbohydrate gm.	Fat gm.	Fiber gm.	Calcium mg.	Phosphorus mg.	Potassium mg.
Barley	349	8.2	78.8	1.0	0.5	16	2	160
Corn	368	7.8	76.8	2.6	0.8	6	164	—
Oatmeal	390	14.2	68.2	7.4	1.2	53	405	352
Rice	363	6.7	80.4	0.4	0.3	24	94	92
Rye	357	9.4	77.9	1.0	0.4	22	185	156
Wheat	365	11.8	74.5	1.2	0.4	20	97	95

* Adapted from USDA Handbook #8, 1963.

germ. Sodium chloride small, potash and phosphorus predominate. Magnesium abundant. Iron found in the germ and outer layer. Water low. Some of the cellulose is lost in milling. Whole grain contains about 1% fat.

cerebellar (sĕr-ē-bĕl'är) [L., little brain]. Pert. to the cerebellum.

cerebellifugal (sĕr"ĕ-bĕl-ĭ-fū'găl) ["+ fugere, to flee]. Extending or proceeding from the cerebellum.

cerebellipetal (ser"ĕ-bĕl-lĭp'ĭ-tăl) ["+ petere, to seek]. Extending toward the cerebellum.

cerebellitis (sĕr"ĕ-bĕl-ī'tĭs) [L. cerebellum, cerebellum, + Gr. -itis, inflammation]. Inflammation of the cerebellum.

cerebellospinal (sĕr"ĕ-bĕl-ō-spī'năl) ["+ spina, a thorn]. Pert. to cerebellum and spinal cord.

cerebellum (sĕr-ē-bĕl'ŭm) [L.]. [NA]. A portion of the brain forming the largest portion of the rhombencephalon. It lies dorsal to the pons and medulla oblongata, overhanging the latter. It consists of two lateral cerebellar hemispheres and a narrow medial portion, the vermis. It is connected to the brain stem by three pair of fiber bundles, the inferior, middle, and superior peduncles. The cerebellum is involved in synergic control of skeletal muscles and plays an important role in the coordination of voluntary muscular movements. It receives afferent impulse and discharges efferent impulse but does not serve as a reflex center in the usual sense; however it may reinforce some reflexes and inhibit others.

cerebral (sĕr'ē-brăl, sĕ-rē'brăl) [L. cerebrum, brain]. Pert. to the cerebrum.

    c. hemorrhage. The result of rupture of a sclerosed or diseased blood vessel in brain. Often associated with high blood pressure.

    RS: apoplexy; hemiplegia.

    c. infantile lipoidosis. SEE: amaurotic familial idiocy, infantile.

cerebration (sĕr"ē-brā'shŭn) [L. cerebratiō, brain activity]. Mental action of the brain.

cerebrifugal (sĕr"ē-brĭf'ū-găl) ["+ fugere, to flee]. Away from the brain; pert. to efferent nerve fibers.

cerebrip'etal [L. cerebrum, brain, + petere, to seek]. Proceeding toward the cerebrum, as nerve fibers or impulses.

cerebri'tis ["+ Gr. -itis, inflammation]. Inflammation of the brain, esp. the cerebrum.

cerebromalacia (sĕr"ē-brō"mă-lā'shĭ-ă) ["+ Gr. malakia, softening]. Softening of the brain, esp. of the cerebrum.

cerebromedullary (sĕr"ē-brō-mĕd'ū-lā-rī). Pert. to the brain and spinal cord; cerebrospinal.

cerebromeningitis (sĕr"ē-brō-mĕn"ĭn-jī'tĭs) [L. cerebrum, brain, + Gr. meninx, membrane, + -itis, inflammation]. Inflammation of the cerebrum and its membranes.

cerebropathy (sĕr-ē-brŏp'ă-thĭ) ["+ Gr. pathos, disease]. Any disease of the brain, esp. cerebrum.

cerebrophysiology (sĕr"ē-brō-fĭz-ĭ-ŏl'ō-jĭ) ["+ Gr. physis, nature, + logos, study]. Physiology of the brain.

cerebropontile (sĕr"ē-brō-pŏn'tĭl) [L. cerebrum, brain, + pons, pont-, bridge]. Pert. to the cerebrum and pons varolii.

cerebropsychosis (sĕr"ē-brō"sī-kō'sĭs) ["+ psychōsis, life]. Any mental disorder due to cerebral lesion.

cer"ebrosclero'sis ["+ Gr. sklērōsis, hardening]. Hardening of the brain, esp. of the cerebrum.

cerebroscope (sĕr-ē'brō-skōp) ["+ Gr. skopein, to examine]. An ophthalmoscope used in diagnosing diseases of the brain.

cerebroscopic (sĕr-ē"brō-skŏp'ĭk). Pert. to cerebroscopy.

cerebroscopy (sĕr-ē-brŏs'kō-pĭ) [L. cerebrum, brain, + Gr. skopein, to examine]. Diagnostic use of the ophthalmoscope in diseases of the brain.

cerebrose (sĕr'ē-brōs). $C_6H_{12}O_6$, a compound (brain sugar) derived from brain tissue.

cerebroside (sĕr'ē-brō-sīd"). One of a class of substances present in brain tissue which upon hydrolysis yield galactose, a nitrogenous base, and a fatty acid, e.g., kerasin, phrenosin, nervone. SYN: galactolipids.

cerebrosis (sĕr"ē-brō'sĭs) [L. cerebrum, brain, + Gr. -ōsis, condition]. Any brain disease.

cerebrospinal (sĕr"ē-brō-spī'năl) ["+ spina, thorn]. Referring to the brain and spinal cord, as the c. axis.

    c. axis. The central nervous system.

    c. fever. C. meningitis. Inflammation of the meninges of the brain and spinal cord; sometimes called spotted fever because of rash on the body.

    c. fluid. A water cushion protecting the brain and spinal cord from shock. Usually shrinking or expanding of the cranial contents is quickly balanced by increase or decrease of this fluid. Possibly cell nourishment and the removal of waste are minor functions.

    FORMATION OF: The fluid is formed by the choroid plexuses of the lateral and third ventricles, that of the lateral ventricles pass-

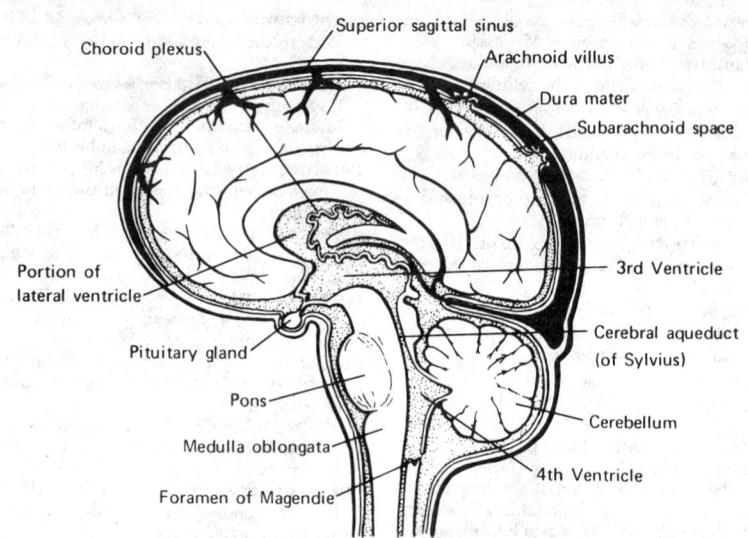

Choroid plexus
Superior sagittal sinus
Arachnoid villus
Dura mater
Subarachnoid space
Portion of lateral ventricle
3rd Ventricle
Pituitary gland
Cerebral aqueduct (of Sylvius)
Pons
Medulla oblongata
Cerebellum
Foramen of Magendie
4th Ventricle

Stippled areas contain cerebrospinal fluid.

MEDIAN SAGITTAL SECTION OF BRAIN
The foramen of Magendie connects the 4th ventricle with the subarachnoid space.

ing through the foramen of Monro to the third, and through the aqueduct of Sylvius to the fourth ventricle. Here it may escape through the central foramen of Magendie, or the lateral foramen of Luschke into the cisterna magna, and so over the brain and cord surfaces, occupying the subarachnoid spaces. It is absorbed by the arachnoid villi and through the perineural lymph spaces of both brain and cord.

CHARACTERISTICS: The fluid is watery, clear, and colorless. Normally the initial pressure of spinal fluid in a recumbent man, as determined by spinal puncture, is equivalent to 70-180 mm. of water. Amount in normal adult is 100-140 ml. Sp. gr.: 1.003-1.008.

Total cell count in adults is 0-10 cu. ml.; in children 0-20 cu. ml. (they should be counted at once and not remain in the fluid); total protein 20-45 mg./100 ml.; and glucose 50-75 mg./100 ml. Its concentration and alkaline reserve are similar to that of the blood. It does not clot on standing. Although the choroid plexuses can reflect certain blood constituents (e.g., iodides), changes in blood sugar, chloride, or urea will manifest themselves quickly in the fluid as well. Other-

wise, changes take place largely subsequent to secretion. Turbidity suggests an excessive cell count, if due to red blood cells. Centrifugalization will show a red deposit.

Formation of a web after a clear fluid has stood is characteristic of tuberculous meningitis (rarely other inflammatory reactions).

It usually shows a yellowish discoloration when containing blood from the subarachnoid spaces (in contrast to blood from trauma of puncture), although for a few days the cells may not be entirely disintegrated. A similar appearance may result from a spinal block above the point of puncture; the fluid spontaneously coagulating due to an excessive albumen content.

Total protein is increased in infections (as meningitis, brain abscess, tabes dorsalis), various types of hemorrhage or thrombosis, virus diseases (as encephalitis, anterior poliomyelitis, lymphocytic meningitis), and conditions such as chronic alcoholism.

Cell count increases especially in tuberculous meningitis, epidemic encephalitis, lymphocytic choriomeningitis, poliomyelitis several days after onset), syphilis of central nervous system, certain types of tumors of the spinal cord or brain.

c. ganglia. Sensory ganglia on the roots of cranial and spinal nerves.

c. nerves. The cranial and spinal nerves, q.v.

c. puncture. A puncture for the collection of c. fluid. It may be collected from spaces around the spinal cord (lumbar puncture), from the cisterna magna (cisternal puncture), or in infants with open fontanelles (by ventricular puncture).

cerebrosuria (sĕr″ĕ-brō-sū′rĭ-ă) [L. *cerebrum*, brain, + Gr. *ouron*, urine]. Cerebrose in the urine.

cerebrotomy (sĕr″ĕ-brŏt′ō-mĭ) ["+ Gr. *tomē*, incision]. 1. Incision of the brain to evacuate an abscess. 2. Dissection of the brain.

cerebrovascular (sĕr″ĕ-brō-văs′kū-lăr) ["+ *vasculum*, vessel]. Pert. to the blood vessels of the brain, esp. to pathological changes.

cerebrum (sĕr′ĕ-brŭm, sĕr-ē′brŭm) [L.]. The largest part of the brain consisting of two hemispheres separated by a deep longitudinal fissure. They are united by three commissures—the corpus callosum and the anterior and posterior hippocampal commissures. The surface of each hemisphere is thrown into numerous folds or convolutions called gyri separated by furrows called fissures or sulci.

c., areas of. On the basis of function, several areas have been identified and located. Among them are motor projection areas which give rise to fibers carrying efferent impulses to effector organs, the skeletal muscles; sensory projection areas which receive impulses from sense organs or sensory receptors by way of the brain stem, including the somesthetic (visual, auditory, gustatory, and olfactory) areas; association areas which are concerned with the higher mental faculties.

c., basal ganglia of. Masses of gray matter deeply embedded within each hemisphere. They are the caudate, lentiform, and amygdaloid nuclei and the claustrum.

c., embryology of. The c. develops from the telencephalon, the most anterior portion of the prosencephalon or forebrain.

c. fissures and sulci. Lateral cerebral fissure (of Sylvius), central sulcus (of Rolando), parieto-occipital fissure, calcarine fissure, cingulate sulcus, collateral fissure, sulcus circularis, longitudinal cerebral fissure.

c., functions of. The c. is concerned with sensations or the interpretation of sensory impulses, and all voluntary muscular activities; it is the seat of consciousness and is the center of the higher mental faculties such as memory, learning, reasoning, judgment, intelligence, and the emotions.

c., gyri of. Superior, middle, and inferior frontal gyri; anterior and posterior central gyri; superior, middle, and inferior temporal gyri; cingulate, lingual, fusiform, and hippocampal gyri.

c., lobes of. The principal lobes: frontal, parietal, occipital, temporal, and central (insula or island of Reil).

c., structure of. Each cerebral hemisphere consists of three primary portions—the rhinencephalon or olfactory lobe, the corpus striatum, and the pallium or cerebral cortex. The cortex is a layer of gray matter that covers the surface of each hemisphere. The part covering the rhinencephalon (phylogenetically the oldest) is called archipallium; the larger nonolfactory cortex is called neopallium. Within the c. are two cavities, the lateral ventricles (right and left) and the rostral portion of the third ventricle.

c., white matter of. The white matter or medullary substance of each hemisphere consists of three kinds of fibers: commissural fibers which pass from one hemisphere to the other, projection fibers which convey impulses to and from the cortex, and association fibers which connect various parts of the cortex within one hemisphere.

cerium (sē′rĭ-ŭm) [L.]. SYMB: *Ce*. At. wt. 140.12; at. no. 58. A metallic element obtained from the rare earths. It is used as a sulfate, in quantitative analysis.

ceroma (sē-rō′mă) [L. *cera*, wax, + Gr. *-ōma*, tumor]. A waxy tumor that has undergone amyloid degeneration.

ceroplasty (sē′rō-plăs″tĭ) ["+ *plassein*, to mold]. Manufacture of anatomical models and pathological specimens in wax.

certifiable (sĕr″tĭ-fī′ă-bl). Pert. to infectious diseases which must be reported to the health authorities.

ceruloplasmin. A glycoprotein, blue in color, to which the majority of the copper in the blood is attached. It is decreased in Wilson's disease.

cerumen (sē-rū′mĕn) [L. *cera*, wax]. The waxlike, soft brown secretion found in the external canal of the ear; inspissated, dried earwax.

ceruminal (sē-rū′mĭ-năl). Pert. to the cerumen.

ceruminosis (sē-rū″mĭ-nō′sĭs) [L. *cera*, wax, + Gr. *-ōsis*, condition]. Excessive wax formation.

ceru′minous. Pert. to cerumen.

c. glands. Modified sweat glands in the skin lining the external auditory canal, which secrete cerumen.

ceruse (sē'rūs) [L. *cerussa*]. White lead paint.

cervical (sĕr'vĭ-kăl) [L. *cervicalis*]. 1. Of, pert. to, or in the region of the neck. 2. Pert. to the cervix of an organ, as the cervix uteri.

    c. nerves. The first eight spinal nerves.

    c. plexus. That formed by loops joining the anterior rami of first four cervical nerves; it receives communicating rami from the sympathetic ganglia. SEE: *Nerve plexuses* in *Appendix.*

    c. vertebrae. First seven bones of the spinal column. SEE: *skeleton.*

cervicectomy (sĕr"vĭ-sĕk'tō-mĭ) [L. *cervix*, neck, + Gr. *ektomē*, excision]. Removal of the cervix uteri.

cervicitis (sĕr-vĭ-sī'tĭs) ["+ Gr. *-itis*, inflammation]. Inflammation of the cervix uteri.

cervico- (sĕr'vĭ-kō) [L. *cervix*]. Prefix pert. to the neck or the neck of an organ.

cervicobrachial (sĕr"vĭ-kō-brā'kĭ-ăl) ["+ Gr. *brachion*, arm]. Pert. to the neck and arm.

cervicobuccal (sĕr"vĭ-kō-bŭk'ăl) ["+ *bucca*, cheek]. Pert. to the cheek side of neck of a molar or premolar tooth.

cervicodynia (sĕr"vĭ-kō-dĭn'ĭ-ă) [L. *cervix*, neck, + Gr. *odynē*, pain]. A pain or cramp of the neck; cervical neuralgia.

cervicofa'cial ["+ *faciēs*, face]. Pert. to the neck and face.

cervicovagini'tis ["+ *vagina*, sheath, + Gr. *-itis*, inflammation]. Inflammation of the cervix of the uterus and the vagina.

cerviocovesical (sĕr"vĭ-kō-vĕs'ĭ-kăl) [L. *cervix*, neck, + *vesica*, bladder]. Pert. to the cervix uteri and bladder.

cervix (sĕr'vĭks) [L.]. (pl. *cer'vices*) [NA]. The neck or a part of an organ resembling a neck. SEE: words beginning with *cervico.*

    c. uteri. Neck of the uterus. The lower part from the internal os outward to the external os. It is rounded and conical in shape, and a portion protrudes into the vagina. It is about 1 in. (2.5 cm.) long, penetrated by the cervical canal through which the fetus and menstrual flow escape. It is apt to be torn in childbirth, in which case it must be sutured.

    c. uteri, laceration of. There may be slight tearing in most primipara. Deeper tears in manual dilatation and use of forceps; breech presentation also may be a cause. Laceration may be single, bilateral, stellate, or incomplete. Tears are repaired by suturing in order to prevent hemorrhage and later complications.

    c. vesicae, c., vesical. Neck of the bladder.

c.e.s. Abbr. for *central excitatory state.*

cesarean section (sē-sār'ĭ-ăn) [L. *caesarea*, cut]. Removal of the fetus by means of an incision into uterus, usually by way of abdominal wall. May be performed by extraperitoneal or intraperitoneal abdominal route. There are several varieties of c.s., differing mainly in the technique employed.

The most frequent cause for c.s. is dystocia due to fetopelvic (also called cephalopelvic) disproportion, i.e., for some reason the fetus is too large to be delivered through the pelvic outlet, the pelvis is abnormally small, or there is a combination of these factors.

    c.s., absolute. Where the child cannot be delivered through the natural passages under any circumstances.

    IND: Contraction of the bony pelvis with a conjugata vera diameter of less than 5.5 cm.; exostoses of the bony pelvis completely obstructing the birth canal; tumor masses of the soft parts which hinder the passage of the fetus (fibroid tumors, ovarian cysts); placenta previa and premature separation of the placenta; previous cesarian section without an absolute indication but where the postoperative course was stormy and a weakened uterine scar is suspected.

    c.s., conservative. C.s. in which the uterus is not removed. *Classical:* The incision is made across the fundus of the uterus. *Low Fundal:* The incision is made through the lower contractile portion of the uterus from a point just above the reflection of the bladder upward for a space of 2-3 inches (5-6.3 cm.). *Laparotrachelotomy:* Low cervical cesarean section. The incision is made in the noncontractile lower uterine segment after stripping back the bladder flap. After removal of the fetus and placenta the uterus is sutured and the bladder flap is sewed up over the uterine scar, thus peritonealizing the scar. *Extraperitoneal:* An abdominal incision is made parallel to Poupart's ligament. The incision in the uterus is made extraperitoneally by pushing the bladder to the side.

    c.s., radical. *Porro:* Cesarean section with removal of the uterus after the fetus has been taken out. This is a supracervical hysterectomy. *Total:* This is a total hysterectomy after the removal of the fetus, used in cases of badly lacerated cervices or in cases of early carcinoma of the cervix.

    c. s., relative. C.s. in which the child could be delivered through the natural passages but where the danger of such a delivery might be greater than through surgery.

IND: Moderate degrees of contraction of the bony pelvis with a conjugata vera diameter of about 9.5 cm.; prolapsed cord in some instances; transverse presentation of the fetus; oblique presentation of the fetus; a large baby with a moderate degree of disproportion; habitual death of the fetus during the course of labor; impacted brow or face presentation where the fetus is alive; preeclamptic toxemia in patients where a difficult labor is anticipated; carcinoma of the cervix with rigidity; in cases where hysterectomy is indicated and is to be done in conjunction with the cesarean section; in cases where oophorectomy is indicated; in cases where sterilization is desired, although to allow that patient to deliver normally and sterilize through the vaginal route at a later time is more satisfactory.

cesarotomy (sěz″ă-rŏt′ō-mĭ) [L. *caesarea*, cut, + Gr. *tomē*, incision]. Cesarean section, q.v.

cesium (sē′zĭ-ŭm) [L. *caesius*, sky blue]. SYMB: *Cs*. At. wt. 132.905; at. no. 55. A metallic element. It has a number of isotopes, radioactive isotopes Cs^{137} being used therapeutically for irradiation of cancerous tissue.

Cestoda (sěs-tŏd′ă) [Gr. *kestos*, girdle]. A subclass of the class Cestoidea, phylum Platyhelminthes, which includes the tapeworms, having a scolex and a chain of segments (proglottids). Ex: Taenia. Intestinal parasites of man and other vetebrates.

cestode (sěs′tŏd) [″+ *eidos*, form]. A tapeworm; one of the Cestoda.

cestodiasis (sěs″tŏ-dī′ă-sĭs) [″+ *-iasis*, condition]. Infestation with tapeworms. SEE: *Cestoda; tapeworm.*

ces′toid [Gr. *kestos*, girdle, + *eidos*, form]. Like a tapeworm.

Cestoidea (sěs-toy′dĭ-ă). A class of flatworms of the phylum Platyhelminthes. Includes the tapeworms.

Cetraria (sē-trā′rĭ-ă). 1. A genus of lichens, chiefly found in northern latitudes. 2. C. islandica, or Iceland moss, a lichen used in treating lung and bowel disorders.

CF. Abbr. for *citrovorum factor.*

Cf. Chem. symb. for californium.

C.F.T. Abbr. for *complement fixation test.*

C.G.S. Abbr. for *centimeter-gram-second*, a name given to a system of units for distance, weight, and time.

C$_2$H$_4$. Ethylene.

CH$_4$. Methane; marsh gas.

C$_2$H$_2$. Acetylene.

C$_6$H$_6$. Benzene.

Chaddock's reflexes (chăd′ŏk). [Charles G. Chaddock, Amer. neurologist, 1861-1936].
1. Extension of great toe resulting from irritation around external malleolus. 2. Flexion of wrist and fanning of fingers when forearm is irritated above and near wrist.

chaeromania (kē-rō-mā′nĭ-ă) [Gr. *chairein*, to rejoice, + *mania*, madness]. Mania characterized by exaltation and cheerfulness. SYN: *amenomania.*

chafe (chāf) [O.Fr. *chaufer*, to warm]. To injure by rubbing or friction.

chaf′ing. A superficial inflammation which develops when skin is subjected to friction from clothing or adjacent skin as may occur at the axilla, groin, anal region, or between digits of hands and feet or at the neck or wrists. Erythema, maceration, and sometimes fissuring occur. Bacterial or mycotic infection may result secondarily. SYN: *erythema intertrigo.*

Chagas′ disease (chăg′ăs). [Carlos Chagas, Braz. physician, 1879-1934]. S. A. trypanosomiasis. Caused by Trypanosoma cruzi and transmitted by the biting reduviid bug. SYN: *Chagas-Cruz disease.*

chain (chān) [O.F. *chaine*, chain]. 1. In bacteriology, three or more cells attached end to end. 2. In chemistry, a series of atoms held together by valence bonds.

c. reflex. One in a consecutive series.

chalarosis (kăl″ă-rō′sĭs). Infection with Chalara, a fungus producing subcutaneous nodules which break down, forming ulcers.

chalazion (kă-lā′zĭ-ŏn) [Gr. *khalaza,* hailstone]. (pl. *chala′zia, -zions*) Small, hard tumor analogous to sebaceous cyst developing on the eyelids, formed by distention of a meibomian gland with secretion. A meibomian cyst. SEE: *steatoma.*

chalcosis (kăl-kō′sĭs) [Gr. *chalkos,* copper, + *-ōsis,* condition]. 1. Chronic poisoning from copper. 2. Copper deposits in lungs and tissues.

chalice cell (chăl′ĭs) [L. *calix,* cup]. Crateriform shell remaining after mucus has been discharged from an epithelial cell. SYN: *goblet cell,* q.v.

chalicosis (kăl-ĭ-kō′sĭs) [Gr. *chalix,* limestone, + *-ōsis,* condition]. Lung disorder due to inhalation of stone particles. SYN: *pneumoconiosis,* q.v.

chalinoplasty (kăl′ĭ-nō-plăs″tĭ) [Gr. *chalinos,* corner of mouth, + *plassein,* to mold]. Plastic surgery of the mouth and lips, esp. of corners of mouth.

chalone (kăl′ōn) [Gr. *chalan,* to relax]. A poorly-defined substance which acts to regulate certain intracellular activity, including cell division.

chalybeate (kă-lĭb'ē-āt) [Gr. *chalyps,* steel].
1. Pert. to or composed of iron; ferruginous.
2. Agent containing iron.

chamber (chăm'bĕr) [Gr. *kamara,* vault].
Compartment or closed space.

c., anterior. The space between the cornea and iris.

c., aqueous. Anterior and posterior chambers of the eye, containing the aqueous humor.

c., hyperbaric. An airtight enclosure strong enough to withstand high internal pressure. Used to expose animals or an entire surgical team to increased air pressure. Used to treat gas gangrene, bends, and for certain surgical procedures.

c., low pressure. One designed to simulate high altitudes by exposing men or animals to low atmospheric pressure. Such studies are essential for simulated flights into the atmosphere and space.

c., posterior. Space behind the iris, anterior to the lens.

c., vitreous. Cavity behind the lens in the eye containing the vitreous humor.

Chamberland filter (chăm'bĕr-länd). [Charles E. Chamberland, Fr. bacteriologist, 1851-1908]. An unglazed porcelain filter through which water can be forced under pressure. Intercepts all but ultramicroscopic microorganisms.

chamomile, camomile (kăm'ē-mīl) [Gr. *khamaemēlon,* earth apple]. Flowers of the Anthemis yielding a bluish volatile oil and a bitter infusion.

chancre (shăng'kĕr) [Fr., ulcer]. A hard, syphilitic primary ulcer. The first sign of syphilis, approx. two to three weeks after infection.

Caution: During the chancre stage, the patient is highly contagious and the chancre itself contains many spirochetes. Discovery of these organisms in the chancre is the basis for the positive darkfield test for syphilis. Syphilis may occur, however, without a chancre developing. SEE: *syphilis.*

SYM: Begins as erosion or papule which ulcerates superficially. Generally single; sometimes multiple. Has a scooped out appearance due to level or sloping edges which are adherent. It has a shining red or raw floor with some deposit. Induration constant. No pain. Slightly purulent secretion. Heals without leaving scar. May appear at almost any site including mouth, penis, urethra, eyelid, conjunctiva.

c., hard; c., hunterian. Primary lesion of syphilis. SEE: *chancre.*

c., simple; c., soft. A nonsyphilitic venereal ulcer. SYN: *chancroid,* q.v.

c., true. The primary lesion of syphilis. SEE: *chancre.*

chancroid (shăng'kroyd) [Fr. *chancre,* ulcer, + Gr. *eidos,* form]. A nonsyphilitic venereal ulcer, highly infectious; a simple or soft chancre. It is caused by Hemophilus ducreyi (also called Ducrey's bacillus), a gram-negative bacillus.

INCUBATION: Approx. three to five days.

SYM: Begins with pustule or ulcer, multiple, abrupt edges, rough floor, yellow exudate, purulent secretion, sensitive and inflamed. Scar remains. Rapid progress. May affect the penis, urethra, vulva, or anus. Multiple lesions may develop by autoinoculation. Types include transient, phagedenic, giant, and serpiginous.

TREATMENT: Sulfonamides, tetracyclines, chloramphenicol.

chancrous (shăng'krŭs). Pert. to or of the nature of chancre.

change of life. The menopause, q.v.; climacteric, q.v.

chapped (chăpt) [ME. *chappen*]. Inflamed, roughened, fissured, as from exposure to cold.

charbon (shăr-bŏ') [Fr., coal]. Infection with Bacillus anthracis. SYN: *anthrax.*

charcoal (chăr'kōl) [ME. *charcole*]. Activated charcoal (USP), very fine powder prepared from soft charred wood.

ACTION AND USES: Internally for adsorption of gastrointestinal gas. Also for adsorption of poisonous alkaloids which have been swallowed.

c. fumes. SEE: *carbon monoxide.*

Charcot-Leyden crystals (shăr-kō'lī'dĕn). [Jean M. Charcot, Fr. neurologist, 1825-1893; Ernest V. von Leyden, Ger. physician, 1832-1910] Colorless, hexagonal, doublepointed and often needlelike crystals found in the sputum in asthma and bronchial bronchitis or in the feces in ulcerative cases of the intestine, esp. amebiasis.

Charcot-Marie-Tooth disease. [Charcot; Pierre Marie, Fr. neurologist, 1853-1940; Howard Tooth, Eng. physician, 1856-1926] A form of progressive neural muscular atrophy, a disease with hereditary tendencies characterized by progressive weakness of distal muscles of the arms and feet. The muscles atrophy, reflexes are lost, foot drop develops, and there is loss of cutaneous sensations. Usually develops in childhood but may occur in adults; more commonly in males. Its cause is unknown. SYN: *peroneal muscular atrophy.*

Charcot's joint (shăr-kō) (A type of joint associated with tabes dorsalis, syringomyelia, or other conditions involving disease or injury to the spinal cord, characterized by hypermobility. Decalcification of bone on joint surfaces occurs accompanied by overgrowth of bone about margins. Pain is usually absent although there are exceptions. Deformity and instability of the joint are characteristic. SYN: *neurogenic arthropathy.*

charlatan (shär'lä-tăn) [It. *ciarlatano*]. A boasting pretender to special knowledge or ability, as in medicine. SYN: *quack.*

charlatanry (shär'lä-tăn-rĭ). Undue pretension to knowledge or skill or an instance of it. SYN: *quackery.*

Charles' law (shärl). [Jacques A. C. Charles, Fr. physicist, 1746-1823]. At constant pressure a given amount of gas will expand its volume in direct proportion to the absolute temperature. SYN: *Gay-Lussac's law.*

charleyhorse. A pulled muscle, intramuscular bleeding; torn muscle fibers commonly of the quadriceps muscle or the hamstrings, associated with soreness and stiffness. Often occurs as an athletic injury.

F. A. TREATMENT: Cold applications.

charpie (shär-pē') [Fr.]. Shreds of linen for dressing wounds.

chart [L. *charta*, paper]. 1. A simple form or sheet of paper for recording the course of a patient's illness. Includes records of temperature, pulse, respiratory rate, blood pressure, urinary and fecal output, and doctors' and nurses' notes. 2. To record on a graph the sequence of events such as vital signs. SEE: *charting.*

charta (kăr'tă) [L.]. Preparation intended principally for external application, made either by saturating paper with medicinal substances or by applying the latter to the surface of the paper by the addition of some adhesive liquid.

chart'ing. The making of a tabulated record of the progress of a disease; a clinical record.

Record information about the patient and his treatment that may be gathered only by the attending nurse. The doctor needs detailed information which the nurse may contribute through her observation of and contact with the patient. These notes containing details of patient's reactions and progress, aid the doctor in making his diagnosis. The nurse's responsibility for supplying this information is very great. Verbal reports are not sufficient; they take time and make mistakes possible.

GENERAL RECORDS: *Blood Pressure:* Record under "Remarks". *Diet:* If patient is on regular diet, it is sufficient to chart breakfast, dinner, and supper, but when on any other diet, chart exactly what the patient takes. The amount of liquids taken, not "Water P.R.N." hours of giving; kind: full, light, soft, liquid, special; appetite: good, poor, special likes and dislikes. *Discharge or Death:* Discharge or death of patient with hour and date of same.

Dressings: Change of dressings on wounds and the amount and character of drainage (remark "Specimen Saved" if this has been done); hour; by whom; stitches or drains removed; patient's reaction if pained or shocked by dressing. *Drugs:* Any unfavorable reaction from drugs or treatments. Chart time when drugs or treatments are administered. All medicines, treatments, preparation, etc., are to be charted by the nurse who administers them whether she has charge of the patient or not. Confine name of medicine and dose to the prescribed column. When administering soluble salts, dispensed in solution, state dose actually administered, not the amount of solution. The administration of medicines other than by mouth should be indicated, as per hypodermic, per injection, per inunction, or per rectum. Any prominent or unusual therapeutic action or idiosyncrasy resulting from a drug should be recorded as a "Remark." A special prescription is written in full in the medication column the first time it is given. After that, chart ℞ Medicine or ℞ Capsule, as the case may be. After first charting, chart the name of principal ingredient, adding the word "Compound." Note discontinuance of medicine or treatment as a "Remark."

Fluids: Hours of giving; kind; amount. The amount should be totaled and the total charted every 12 hours. *Heat:* Chart by whose order heat is applied to an unconscious patient, and who executed the order. *Infant Feeding:* The formula should be charted the first time; afterwards, amount given, and if regurgitated, approximate the amount. *Laboratory:* Hour; kind of specimen; by whom taken; by whom ordered (not necessary in case of routine urine specimen on admission).

Medications: Hour of giving; kind (name of drug and preparation); amount; by whom given; manner of giving (mouth, hypo, rectum, intravenous); patient's reaction. *Nursing Care:* Hour; baths and shampoos; alcohol rubs and decubitus dressing; special mouth care; sitting up for first time; out of bed for first time; walking for first time; narcotics (Treatments are also charted, but as treatments). *Operations:* Name of operation; preparation; preliminary anesthetic if given by nurse or in ward; hour of going to O.R.;

hour of going to and leaving recovery room; hour of return to room; condition on return to room; hour of recovery from anesthetic; condition every half hour for next three or four hours, depending on state patient is in and severity of operation. Recovery room staff members will record treatment and condition while patient is in their care.

Personal Care: Baths, personal hygiene, and patient's reactions to these. For women, record menstruation. *Physician:* Record his visit. Doctor's orders must be recorded and time when they are carried out. *Physiotherapy:* Hour of going for treatment and hour of return; condition of patient. *Postoperative:* Changing position of postoperative patients should be recorded under "Remarks." Record passive and active exercise of patient. *Specimens:* Record the taking of specimens of blood, exudates, transudates, etc., for examination. The result will be shown by the report of the pathologist. *Surgical Preparations:* The nurse who does surgical preparations will sign her name after "Preliminary preparation of field of operation." Observe the same rule for narcotics.

Symptoms: Accurate description of all symptoms, i.e., character of pulse and respiration, psychic condition, description of pain, and nature of any discharge, etc. The remarks should be appropriate and well chosen. Subjective as well as objective symptoms should be recorded. *Time:* Everything relating to the patient's progress should be charted as it occurs. Record the hour with all statements on charts. Record on the first line of the sheet the day, date of admission, whether the patient walked in, or was admitted by ambulance, and condition of patient. Four-hour graphic charts are kept for all surgical and obstetrical cases the first three days (time 8-12-4); and for all patients whose temperature is above normal. The T.P.R. of all other patients are charted at 6 a.m. and 4 p.m.

Treatments: Hour of giving; nature of treatment; by whom given; patient's reaction. *Visits of Clergyman* (specially important in case of Roman Catholic patients): Hour; name of clergyman; rite performed. *X-ray:* Hour; to x-ray room or portable at bedside; return from x-ray room; condition of patient.

Miscellaneous: Any sudden or marked change in patient's condition; notification of patient's relatives and clergyman. Special charts are also provided for certain purposes such as the temperature, pulse and respiration chart; anesthesia chart generaly kept by the anesthetist; blood-pressure chart used in conditions apt to affect the blood pressure; intake and output charts used in all patients with fluid and electrolyte imbalance; and laboratory records usually filed with the patient's chart. If any laboratory records have been made and not filed with the chart, their existence should be noted on the clinical chart at the time made and also upon the final page of the chart.

PHYSICAL SYMPTOMS: *Appetite:* Good, poor, special likes or dislikes. *Convulsions:* Type, duration, consciousness lost; note fecal or urinary incontinence; was patient injured during convulsion or in fall which came with convulsion; aura. *Defecation:* (see Excretions; Feces; Urine in this entry.) *Diaphoresis* (perspiration): State whether slight, moderate, or profuse. *Emesis:* Amount, color, odor, consistency of the vomitus, and manner of ejecting. (See Nausea in this entry.)

Enemas: Results and unusual appearances, distention before or after; describe results fully. Note whether or not flatus was expelled with the return of the enema. Chart the solution, strength, and amount used. Also douches and irrigations.

Excretions: Time, character, and other facts. *Feces:* Enema or natural movement; amount; consistency; color; abnormal odor; abnormal constituents. Defecation accompanied by pain or tenesmus.

General Appearance: Color; posture; rash; mood; mental state. *Hemorrhages, Discharges, etc.:* Description, etc. When unusual save specimens for examination. *Nausea:* Accompanied by vomiting; following certain foods, drugs, or treatments. *Nerves:* All nervous symptoms, excitability, etc. *Pain:* Location; time of onset; character; sharp, dull, burning, grinding, throbbing; duration (constant, how long); intermittent; intervals.

Pathological Conditions: Vomiting, convulsions, etc. Record time, duration, severity, general appearance of patient before, during, and after the attack. T.P.R. immediately after, and what was done to relieve condition. Explanation as to the cause if known. *Pulse:* Rate: beats per minute. Character: full, bounding, weak, thready, faint. Rhythm: regular, irregular, intermittent. *Respiration:* Rate per minute. Character deep, shallow, difficult, easy, labored, quiet, stertorous, Cheyne-Stokes. Rhythm: regular, irregular, gasping.

Sleep: Hours of sleeping during the day as well as the night. If impossible to estimate accurately, approximate it. Time and amount. Sleepwalking, nightmares, or talking in sleep should be recorded. *Tempera-*

Charting: Abbreviations and Their Meanings

A considerable number of these abbreviations are used rarely if at all. They are recorded for historical purposes.

Abbr.	Latin Phrase	Meaning
a or āā.	ana	of each
abs. feb.	absente febre	when there is no fever
a.c.	ante cibum	before eating
ad	ad.	to, up to
ad effect.	ad effectum	until effectual
ad grat. acid.	ad gratum aciditatem	to an agreeable acidity
ad grat. gust.	ad gratum gustum	to an agreeable taste
adhib.	adhibendus	to be administered
ad lib.	ad libitum	at pleasure; as much as is needed
ad neut.	ad neutralizandum	to neutralization
ad part. dolent.	ad partes dolentes	to the painful parts
ad sat.	ad saturandum	to saturation
adst. feb.	adstante febre	when fever is present
ad us.	ad usum	according to custom
ad us. ext.	ad usum externum	for external use
aeq.	aequales	equal
ag. feb.	aggrediente febre	when the fever increases
agit. ante sum.	agita ante sumendum	shake before taking
alt. dieb.	alternis diebus	every other day
alt. hor.	alternis horis	every other hour
alt. noc.	alternis nocte	every other night
aq.	aqua	water
aq. bull.	aqua bulliens	boiling water
aq. cal.	aqua calida	warm water
aq. dest.	aqua destillata	distilled water
aq. ferv.	aqua fervens	hot water
aq. frig.	aqua frigida	cold water
aq. menth. pip.	aqua menthae piperitae	peppermint water
aq. pur.	aqua pura	pure water
arg.	argentum	silver
bal.	balneum	bath
bal. sin.	balneum sinapis	mustard bath
bib.	bibe	drink
b. i. d.	bis in die	twice daily
bis.	bis	twice
bis in 7d.	bis in septem diebus	twice a week
b.p.		blood pressure; boiling point
bull.	bulliat	let it boil
C.		Centigrade
		carbon
		Calorie (kilocalorie)
c.	cum	with
cap.	capsula	a capsule
cat.	cataplasma	a poultice
cc.		cubic centimeter
chart.	charta	paper
cito disp.	cito dispensetur	let it be dispensed quickly

Charting: Abbreviations and Their Meanings *(Continued)*

Abbr.	Latin Phrase	Meaning
c.m.	cras mane	tomorrow morning
c.m.s.	cras mane sumendus	to be taken tomorrow morning
c.n.	cras nocte	tomorrow night
cochl. amp.	cochleare amplum	heaping spoonful
cochl. mag.	cochleare magnum	a tablespoonful
cochl. med.	cochleare medium	a dessertspoonful
cochl. parv.	cochleare parvum	a teaspoonful
comp.	compositus	compounded of
cong.	congius	a gallon
contra	contra	against
cont. rem.	continuetur remedia	let the medicines be continued
c.v.	cras vespere	tomorrow night
cyath.	cyathus	glassful
cyath. vinos.	cyathus vinosus	wineglassful
D.	dosis	dose
d.	da	give
d. d. in d.	de die in diem	from day to day
decub.	decubitus	lying down
det.	detur	let it be given
dieb. alt.	diebus alternis	on alternate days
dil.	dilue	dilute
dim.	dimidius	half
div.	divide	divide
div. in p. saeq.	divide in partes aequales	divide into equal parts
don.	donec	until
emp.	emplastrum	a plaster
en., enem.		enema
exhib.	exhibeatur	let it be given
ext.	extractum	extract
ext. liq.	extractum liquidum	liquid extract
F., Fahr.		Fahrenheit (temperature scale)
Fe.	ferrum	iron
f.h.	fiat haustus	let a draught be made
f.m.	fiat mistura	let a mixture be made
f.p.	fiat potio	let a potion be made
f. pil.	fiat pilula	let a pill be made
ft.	fiat	let it be made
Gm., gm.		gram
gr.	granum	grain
gt.	gutta	a drop
gtt.	guttae	drops
h. n.	hoc noc'te	tonight
hor. som, h. s.	hora somni	at bedtime
in d.	in dies	daily
inf.	infusum	an infusion
inj.	injectio	an injection
liq.	liquor	a liquor or liquid
m.	misce	mix
mod. praesc.	modo praescripto	as prescribed

Charting: Abbreviations and Their Meanings (Continued)

Abbr.	Latin Phrase	Meaning
mor. dict.	more dicto	in the manner directed
mor. sol.	more solito	in the usual manner
n. b.	no'ta be'ne	note well
noct.	noc'te	night
non rep.	non repetatur	do not repeat
O.	octarius	a pint
o. d.	oculus dexter	right eye
ol.	oleum	oil
o.m.	omni mane	every morning
omn. bid.	omnibus bidendis	every 2 days
omn. bih.	omni bihoris	every 2 hours
omn. hor.	omni hora	every hour
omn. noct.	omni nocte	every night
o. s.	oculus sinister	left eye
p.a.a.	parti affectae applicetur	let it be applied to the affected region
part aeq.	partes aequales	equal parts
post. cib. or p. c.	post cibum	after meals
p.r.	per rectum	through the rectum
p. r. n.	pro re nata	as needed
pulv.	pulvis	a powder
p.v.	per vaginam	through the vagina
q. i. d.	qua'ter in di'e	four times a day
q.l.	quantum libet	as much as is wanted
q. p.	quantum placeat	at will
q. s.	quantum sufficiat	a sufficient quantity, as much as may be needed
℞	recipe	take (thou)
rep.	repetatur	let it be repeated
s.a.	secundum artem	by skill
sig.	signetur	let it be labeled
sing.	singulorum	of each
s. o. s.	si o'pus sit	if necessary
ss.	semis	one-half
stat.	statim	at once
sum.	sumat, sumendum	let him take, to be taken
s.v.	spiritus vini	alcoholic spirit
s. v. v.	spiritus vini vitis	brandy
T.		temperature
tab.	tabella, tabellae	a tablet, tablets
t. i. d.	ter in die	thrice daily
tinct. or tr.	tinctura	tincture
ung.	unguentum	ointment
ur.		urine

ture: If for some legitimate reason temperature is omitted, write hour in designated space and leave temperature space unmarked. When recording next temperature, bring line across this space to the adjoining space and record the next temperature. Indicate by mouth, rectum, or axilla; degree; following chill or treatment. If temperature is quite high and patient does not appear to have fever of that extent, take temperature again but remain at bedside to be sure patient is not placing thermometer against some hot object.

T. P. R.: Temperature, pulse, and respiration taken as ordered. The nurse charts the T.P.R. and general condition of the patient before going to the operating room, and the pulse and respiration with general condition upon return from the operating room. *Unconsciousness or Coma:* Time of onset; conditions associated with or which caused onset; appearance of patient while in coma; medicines or treatment given while in coma; duration. *Unusual Conditions:* Chart these such as appearance of blood, twitching, convulsions, coma, drowsiness, lethargy, unconsciousness.

Urine: State time of voiding, amount, color and appearance, whether voided or per catheter. Note time of beginning 24-hour specimen; when bladder is emptied for the purpose, this specimen is sent to laboratory for qualitative test. Remark the ending of 24-hour specimen; note amount on chart and on laboratory label. Send specimen to the laboratory for all patients remaining in the hospital over night. At 7 p.m. and 7 a.m., day and night nurses remark whether or not very ill patients voided during the day or night. Immediately upon admission begin 24-hour specimen of urine for all diabetic patients. Check may be used in the urine column: when patient uses lavatory, when he voids with defecation. At all other times the amount of urine is to be charted (totaled every 12 hours and total charted also). Accompanied by pain or burning; any abnormal appearance; specimen to laboratory.

Visitors: Reaction to visitors and mood change after visitors depart. Especially important in depressed and psychiatric patients. *Vomiting:* Cause; forcible or projectile; vomitus amount, color, odor, consistency, any unusual constituents.

MENTAL SYMPTOMS: Calmness; cheerfulness; delirium (kind); depression (degree); apparent effect of visitors, etc.; delusions and on what subjects; hallucinations; illusions and on what subjects; temper fits; willingness to cooperate; worry.

chartula (kăr'tū-lä) [L., small piece of paper]. A paper folded to form a receptacle containing a dose of medicinal substance.

chaude-pisse (shōd-pēs') [Fr.]. A burning sensation during urination, esp. in acute gonorrhea.

chauffage (shō-fōzh') [O.Fr. *chaufer,* to heat]. A heated cautery at low temperature applied over a part about 1/4 in. from it.

chaulmoogra oil, chaulmugra, chaulmaugra (chŏl-mü'grŭ, chŏl-mŏ'grŭ) [Bengali *caulmugrā*]. A vegetable oil used in treatment of leprosy and some dermatoses. Though generally replaced by sulfones in treatment of leprosy, c. is still used in endemic areas where it is readily available and has a low cost.

Chaussier's areola (shō-sē-ä'). [Francois Chaussier, Fr. physician, 1746-1828]. Indurated tissue around the lesion of a malignant pustule.

check [O. Fr. *eschec*]. 1. To slow down or arrest the course of. 2. To verify.

 c. bite. Impression of teeth on plastic material to check articulation.

 c. experiment. Control experiment, or one checked against another.

cheek [AS. *cēace*]. Side of face forming lateral wall of mouth below eye. SYN: *bucca.*

 c. bone. The malar bone; os zygomaticum [NA]; zygomatic bone.

 c. retractor. Device for enclosing cheek at the mouth's angle for properly exposing operating field.

cheese [L. *cāseus*]. The compressed casein of milk, flavored and altered by bacterial action.

 Food value of 100 gm. (pasteurized process, often called American): Cal. 370; protein 23.2 gm.; fat 30 gm.; carbohydrate 2 gm.; calcium 697 mg.; vitamin A, 1200 I.U.

cheilitis (ki-lī'tĭs) [Gr. *cheilos,* lip, + *-itis,* inflammation]. Inflammation of the lip.

 c. actinica. Irritation of lips resulting from exposure to sunlight.

 c. exfoliativa. Seborrheic dermatitis of the lips.

 c. glandularis. Disorder of the lips resulting from hypertrophy of mucous glands and their ducts.

 c. venenata. Dermatitis of the lips resulting from chemicals present in lipsticks, lip cream, and various other materials.

cheilognathopalatoschisis (kī''lō-nä''thō-păl-ä-tŏs'kĭ-sĭs) ["+ *gnathos,* jaw, + *L. palatum,* palate, + Gr. *schisis,* cleft]. Malformation in which there is a cleft in the hard and soft palate, upper jaw, and lip. SYN: *cheilognathouranoschisis.*

cheiloplasty (kī'lō-plăs''tĭ) ["+ *plassein,* to form]. Plastic operation upon the lips.

cheiloschisis (kī-lŏs'kĭ-sĭs) ["+ *schisis,* cleft]. Harelip.

cheilosis (kī-lō'sĭs) [Gr. *cheilos,* lip, + *-ōsis,* condition]. Morbid condition of lips with reddened appearance and fissures at the angles, seen frequently in deficiency of vitamin B complex, esp. riboflavin.

cheilostomatoplasty (kī''lō-stō-măt'ō-plăs''tĭ) ["+ *stoma,* mouth, + *plassein,* to form]. Plastic surgery and restoration of mouth.

cheilotomy, chilotomy (ki-lŏt'ō-mĭ) ["+ *tomē,* incision]. Excision of part of the lip.

cheirognostic (kī″rŏg-nŏs′tĭk) [Gr. *cheir,* hand, + *gnostikos,* knowing]. 1. Able to distinguish left from right side of body. 2. Able to perceive which side of the body is being stimulated.

cheiropompholyx (kī″rō-pŏm′fō-liks) [Gr. *cheir,* hand, + *pompholyx,* bubble]. A skin disease with groups of blebs or vesicles on the palms of hands, soles of feet.

cheirospasm (ki′ro-spasm) [" + Gr. *spasmos,* spasm]. Writer's cramp.

chelation (kē-lā′shun) [Gr. *chēlē,* claw]. Combining of metallic ions with certain heterocyclic-ring structures so that the ion is held by chemical bonds from each of the participating rings. When this structure is diagrammed it appears that the metallic ion is being held by a claw. Calcium disodium edetate, q.v., is a chelating agent.

cheloid (kē′loyd) [Gr. *kēlē,* tumor, + *eidos,* form]. Keloid, q.v.

chem′ical [Gr. *chēmeia,* chemistry]. Pert. to chemistry.

    c. change. A change in which a substance breaks up or combines with other substances to make new substances with new properties or characteristics. Ex: Oxygen and hydrogen combine to form water. Sodium (a metal) and chlorine (a gas) combine to form sodium chloride, or common salt. Oxygen combines with hemoglobin when the hemoglobin in the blood comes into contact with the oxygen in the air in the alveoli of the lungs to form oxyhemoglobin. The difference can be seen by comparing the bright scarlet of the arterial blood containing oxyhemoglobin with the bluish color of the venous blood containing hemoglobin.

    c. compound. 1. A substance consisting of two or more chemical elements in definite proportions and in chemical combination and for which a chemical formula can be written. Ex: water (H_2O); salt (NaCl). 2. A substance which can be separated by chemical means into simpler substances.

    c. element. 1. Element, q.v. 2. Any chemical compound or substance composed of chemical elements. SEE: *Appendix.*

Chemical Substances and Their Common Names

Chemical Names	Common Names
Nitric acid	Aqua fortis
Nitrohydrochloric acid	Aqua regia
Copper sulfate	Blue vitriol
Potassium bitartrate	Cream of tartar
Calcium carbonate	Chalk
Potassium carbonate	Salt of tartar
Potassium hydroxide	Caustic potash
Sodium chloride	Common salt
Ferrous sulfate	Copperas or Green vitriol
Aluminum and Potassium sulfate	Dry alum
Magnesium sulfate	Epsom salts
Sodium sulfate	Glauber's salts
Glucose	Grape sugar
Nitrous oxide	Laughing gas
Calcium oxide	Lime
Silver nitrate	Lunar caustic
Calcium chloride	Muriate of lime
Potassium nitrate	Niter or Saltpeter
Sulfuric acid	Oil of vitriol
Iron oxide	Rust of iron
Ammonium chloride	Sal ammoniac
Calcium hydroxide	Slaked lime
Sodium bicarbonate	Soda, baking
Ammonia	Spirits of Hartshorn
Hydrochloric acid	Spirits of salt
Calcium sulfate	Stucco or Plaster of Paris
Basic copper acetate	Verdigris
Acetic acid (diluted)	Vinegar
Hydrogen oxide	Water
Zinc sulfate	White vitriol

c. reflex. Any reflex action initiated by a chemical stimulus.

chemical and biological warfare. The tactics and technique of conducting warfare by use of toxic chemical agents and the deliberate introduction of disease-producing organisms into populations of people, animals, or plants. The chemicals include nerve gases; agents which cause temporary blindness, paralysis, hallucinations, or deafness; eye and lung irritants; mustard gas; defoliants; and herbicides. The biological warfare diseases include anthrax, brucellosis, plague, Q-fever, and tularemia. ABBR: CBW. SEE: *gases, war.*

chemicocautery (kem″ĭ-kō-kaw'ter-ĭ) ["+ *kautērion,* branding iron]. Cauterization by chemical agents.

chemiluminescence (kem″ĭ-lū″mĭ-nes'-ens). Cold light or light produced as a result of a chemical reaction and without the production of heat, e.g., the light produced by certain bacteria, fungi, or fireflies.

cheminosis (kem″in-o'sis) [Gr. *chēmeia,* chemistry, + *-ōsis,* infection]. Any disease caused by chemical agents.

chemiotaxis (kem-ĭ-o-taks'is) ["+ *taxis,* arrangement]. Chemotaxis, q.v.

chemise (shĕ-mēz') [LL. *camīsa,* linen shirt]. Surgical dressing consisting of a square bandage tied around a catheter passing through the center of the bandage.

chemist (kĕm'ĭst). One trained in chemistry.

chem'istry [Gr. *chēmeia,* chemistry]. The science that treats of the molecular and atomic structure of matter and of the composition of substances—their formation, decomposition, and the various transformations which they may undergo.

c., analytical. That concerned with the detection of the presence of chemical substances (qualitative analysis) or the determination of the amounts of substances present (quantitative analysis).

c., biological. The chemistry of living things, involving all the chemical processes which take place within an organism such as the digestion of food, anabolism, and catabolism. SEE: *biochemistry.*

c., general. The study of the entire field of chemistry with emphasis on fundamental concepts and laws.

c., inorganic. The chemistry of compounds not containing carbon.

c., nuclear. Radiochemistry or the study of changes which take place within the nucleus of an atom esp. when the nucleus is bombarded by electrons, neutrons, or other subatomic particles.

c., organic. The chemistry of carbon compounds.

c., pathological. The study of chemical changes induced by disease processes, e.g., changes in the chemistry of organs and tissues; blood; secretions; excretions, etc.

c., physical. Theoretical chemistry or that concerned with fundamental laws underlying chemical changes and the expression of these laws mathematically.

c., physiological. The study of the chemical nature of living matter and the changes occurring in the metabolic activities of plants and animals.

chemoceptor (kem'ō-sep-ter). A chemoreceptor, q.v.

chemocoagulation (chem″ō-kō-ag″ū-lā'-shun) [Gr. *chēmeia,* chemistry, + L. *coaglutio,* coagulation]. Coagulation brought about by chemical agents.

chemoreceptor (chem″ō-rē-sĕp'tor) ["+ L. *recipere,* to receive]. A sense organ or sensory nerve ending (as a taste bud) which is stimulated by a chemical substance.

chemore'flex ["+ L. *reflectere,* to bend back]. Reflex resulting from chemical stimulus.

chemosis (ke-mo'sis) [Gr. *chēmē,* cockleshell, + *-ōsis,* infection]. Swelling of conjunctiva about the cornea.

chemosurgery. Destruction of tissue by use of chemical compounds.

chemotactic (kem″o-tak'tĭk). Pert. to chemotaxis.

chemotaxis (kem″ō-tak'sis) [Gr. *chēmeia,* chemistry, + *taxis,* arrangement]. Attraction and repulsion of living protoplasm to a chemical stimulus.

chemotherapy (kem″ō-ther'a-pī) ["+ *therapeia,* treatment]. In the treatment of disease, the application of chemical reagents which are not harmful to the patient but which have a specific and toxic effect upon the disease-causing microorganism.

chemotic (kē-mŏt'ĭk). Pert. to chemosis.

chemotropism (kē-mŏt'rō-pĭzm) [Gr. *chēmeia,* chemistry, + *tropos,* a turning]. Ability or impulse to progress or turn in a certain direction due to the influence of certain chemical stimuli, as the root of a plant towards its food supply.

chenodeoxycholic acid. Oral drug used experimentally to dissolve cholesterol gallstones.

chenopodium oil (ken-o-po'dĭ-um) [Gr. *chēn,* goose, + *pous,* foot]. Oil of American wormseed. A pale-yellow, volatile oil with pungent, irritating odor.

ACTION AND USES: Antihelmintic against hookworm.

cherophobia (kē″rō-fo′bĭ-ă) [Gr. *chairein,* to rejoice, + *phobos,* fear]. Morbid fear of and aversion to gaiety.

cherries [L. *cerasus,* cherry]. The fruit of the tree of the genus Prunus, P. cerasus bearing the sour variety of cherry and P. avium bearing the sweet fruit.

    Food value of 100 gm. (raw): Cal. 58; protein 1.2 gm.; fat 0.3 gm.; carbohydrate 14.3 gm.; vitamin A, 1000 I.U.; calcium 22 mg.

chest [AS. *cest,* a box]. The thorax.

    MENSURATION: The object of measuring the c. is for ascertaining the comparative bulk of the two sides and the amt. of expansion and retraction accompanying inspiration and expiration of the two sides.

    The points of measurement are the spinous processes behind and the median line in front on the level of the 6th costosternal articulation. The right side is from half an inch to an inch (1.3-2.5 cm.) larger than the left.

    When a pleural cavity is distended with air or fluid the measurement of the affected side may exceed that of the healthy side by two or three inches; after removal of the fluid there may be an equal diminution in the measurement of the affected side, as compared with the healthy one. In emphysema the total difference between the fullest inspiration and fullest expiration on the affected side will scarcely exceed 1/16 of an inch (1.6 mm.), while on the other side there may be a difference of two or three inches (5-6.3 cm.).

    PALPATION: Serves to detect any thoracic tenderness, edema, friction fremitus, or rales, and to determine the vocal fremitus and pitting of expansion. Edema of chest walls is recognized by pitting when pressure is made with finger; it may be observed in empyema and in certain types of heart failure.

    The friction sound of pleurisy and harsh, sonorous rales can be detected sometimes by palpation. Thoracic tenderness is observed in pleurisy, pneumonia associated with pleurisy; pleurodynia, intercostal neuralgia (confined to certain spots); surgical affections like caries and fracture of the ribs; and in contusion and inflammation of the pleural surfaces.

    PERCUSSION: Place finger being used as a pleximeter firmly against chest and preferably parallel to ribs. Make finger which is used as plexor strike the one on chest perpendicularly, fix forearm, and use no more force than can be obtained from a gentle swing of the wrist. Percuss all parts of chest anteriorly and posteriorly, both inspiration and expiration. In comparing sides be sure to percuss corresponding parts.

    Normal Resonance: On the right side pulmonary resonance extends from half an inch to an inch (1.3-2.5 cm.) above the clavicle, downward to upper border of 6th rib in front, and to a line drawn through the 10th spinous process posteriorly. On left side pulmonary resonance extends from a half inch to an inch above the clavicle downward within the mammary line to the 10th rib, and posteriorly to a line drawn through the 10th spinous process.

    Cracked Pot Sound: Modified tympany can be simulated by percussing over the cheek when mouth is partially open. May be heard normally over the chest of a crying infant. In the adult it usually indicates a cavity which has a free communication with a bronchus. Best detected by keeping ear near open mouth of patient while percussing.

    Dullness or flatness: Recognized in tuberculous condition, pneumonic consolidation, pleural effusions of all kinds exept air, collapse of lung, congestion and edema of lung, enlargement of liver or spleen (at base), and morbid growths in the lung.

    It is important to determine the extent of movement of the diaphragms. To do this have the patient hold his breath in deep inspiration while in a sitting position. Then quickly percuss the chest on both sides posteriorly to find and mark the lowest point of pulmonary resonance. Repeat this while the patient holds his breath following complete expiration. On both sides of the chest the top and bottom marks should be from 2-6 cm. apart. The top line on the right is usually a cm. or two higher than the left due to the presence of the liver below the right diaphragm. Diseases which interfere with aeration of the lungs or which paralyze the diaphragms will cause the normal movement of the diaphragms to be altered.

    Hyperresonance: Observed in pneumothorax, tuberculous or bronchiectatic cavities, emphysema, lowered pulmonary tension in the initial stage of pneumonia and above a pleural effusion (Skoda's resonance), flatulent distention of the stomach or colon frequently observed over the left base.

    Tympanitic Note: A hollow drumlike sound, like that which is normally obtained by percussing the larynx or empty stomach. The above conditions are capable of producing tympany also.

    Pitch: Depends largely upon the volume of air, tension of walls of cavity, and upon size of opening that communicates with the cavity. The less the air the greater the tension, and the smaller the opening the higher will be the pitch of the note. In beginning tuberculous consolidation, the note over the affected apex is higher pitched. It must be remembered that normally the note over the right apex is higher pitched than that over the left.

Resistance: The greater the dullness the greater will be the resistance; therefore, there is always more resistance over a large pleural effusion than over a pneumonic or tuberculous consolidation

RS: breathing; fremitus; resonance; respiration; symptom, chest; "thoraco-" words.

c., emphysematous. In advanced emphysema, thorax is short and round; anterior-posterior diameter is often as long as the transverse diameter; ribs are horizontal; angle formed by divergence of the costal margin from the sternum is very obtuse or quite obliterated. Often termed barrel-shaped.

c. expansion, normal. Expansion denotes capacity of air taken into lungs. This varies with age, the young adult having a greater capacity than the aged. Those given to exercise or physical work have a greater lung capacity than others. In the male, 2 in. (5 cm.); in the female, 2 1/2 in. (6.3 cm.). Capacity: In the normal male, 22 yr. old, 69 1/2 in. (177 cm.) in height, 230-240 cu. in. (3,770-3,933 cc.); normal female, 19 yr. old, 63 in. (160 cm.), 145-150 cu. in. (2,376-2,458 cc.).

c. flail. The condition of the chest wall when, due to multiple fractures of the rib cage, it moves paradoxically in with inspiration and out during expiration.

c. prominences and depressions. An unnatural prominence or depression is often observed over the lower part of the sternum and is generally congenital. The term funnel breast or shoemaker's breast (because it may result from pressure of tools) has been applied to the sternal depression. The correct term is pectus excavatum.

A unilateral or local depression may be caused by consolidation, cavity, or pleurisy with fibrous adhesions.

A unilateral or local prominence may be due to pleurisy with effusion; pneumothorax, hydrothorax, hemothorax; aneurysm or tumor; compensatory emphysema resulting from impairment of the opposite lung; cardiac enlargements (left side); enlargments of abdominal organs, esp. liver and spleen.

c., phthinoid. Anterior posterior diameter is short, thorax long and flat, ribs oblique. Scapula prominent; spaces above

and below clavicles are depressed. Angle formed by divergence of the costal margins from the sternum is very acute.

c., rachitic. May resemble phthinoid, but usually sides are considerably flattened and sternum prominent, so term pigeon breast has been applied. The sternal ends of the ribs are enlarged or beaded and this characteristic has given rise to the term rachitic rosary. Often a circular construction of the thorax at level of the xiphoid cartilage.

c. regions. Anterior, posterior and lateral. *Anterior Divisions* (R. and L.): Clavicular, infra- and supraclavicular, mammary and inframammary, upper and lower sternal. *Posterior Divisions* (R. and L.): Scapular, infrascapular, interscapular, and suprascapular. *Lateral Divisions:* Axillary and infra-axillary.

c. thump. A sharp blow to the chest in the precordial area. Done to attempt restoration of normal heartbeat in patients with cardiac standstill or ventricular tachycardia.

Cheyne-Stokes respiration (chān′stōks). [John Cheyne, Scot. physician, 1777-1836; William Stokes, Irish physician, 1804-1878]. An irregular or cyclic type of arrhythmic breathing occurring in certain acute diseases of the central nervous system, heart, lungs, and in intoxications.

At first it is slow and shallow, then it increases in rapidity and depth until it reaches a maximum. Then it decreases gradually until it stops for 10 to 20 seconds, then repeating in the same manner. It may occur in heart failure, intracranial pressure, cerebral disease, or drug sensitivity; all of which interfere with the blood-oxygen supply to the centers in the brain which control respiration.

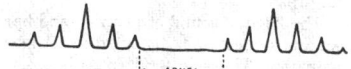

RESPIRATORY MOVEMENTS IN CHEYNE-STOKES BREATHING

Chiari's deformity (kē-ar′ēz). SEE: *Arnold-Chiari deformity.*

chiasm, chiasma (ki′azm, ki-az′ma) [Gr. *khiasma,* cross]. A crossing or decussation.

c., optic. An incomplete crossing of the optic fibers (the outer fibers not crossing each other); the point of crossing of the fibers of the optic nerves.

chicken [AS. *cicen,* chicken]. The common domestic fowl.

Food value of 100 gm. (dark meat fried without skin): Cal. 220; protein 30.4 gm.; fat 9.3 gm.; carbohydrate 1.5 gm.; vitamin A, 130 I.U.; calcium 14 mg.

Light meat fried without skin has almost the same food value as dark meat. It contains about 10% fewer Calories, 7% more protein, two-thirds as much fat and less than half as much vitamin A.

chicken breast. Abnormal prominence of the sternum. SYN: *pectus carinatum; pigeon b.*

chicken-fat clot. A yellowish blood clot formed after death.

chickenpox. Varicella; a mild, highly contagious disease, marked by an eruption of vesicles on skin and mucous membranes. SEE: *varicella.*

chig'gers. Redbugs. The six-legged larvae of mites of the family Trombiculidae, order Acarina of the class Arachnida. They are parasitic on insects, various vertebrates, and man. Eggs are laid on the ground and hatch in about 12 days, after which they attach to host at first opportunity. The redbugs attach themselves to the surface of the skin and inject a salivary secretion which dissolves the surrounding tissue. A tubular structure, a stylostome, is developed which is used in ingesting the semidigested tissue debris. The mites do not feed on blood. The most common species attacking humans in N. America is Trombicula alfreddugesi. The irritation is the result of sensitization to the injected saliva. To prevent being infested when exposed, wear clothes which are tight at the neck and arms and stuff pant legs into shoe with high tops. Certain chemical compounds such as diethyltoluamide (Off) will repel chiggers. SYN: *harvest mites; rougets; scrub mites.*

TREATMENT: Commercial preparations are available which, when applied to the affected area, asphyxiate the mite. One of these, Kwell, contains hexachlorohexane. Benzyl benzoate ointment is also effective.

chigo, chigre (chē'gō, chē'grä) [Sp.]. A jigger or sand flea.

chilblain (chil'blān) [AS. *cele,* cold, + *blēgen,* to puff]. Inflammation and swelling of the feet, toes, or fingers caused by cold, damp, atmosphere. SYN: *frostbite; pernio.*

SYM: Reddish, violaceous plaques or patches on hands and feet, occasionally the ears. Persistent, giving rise to smarting, burning, itching, esp. when parts become warm. In severe types frostbite corresponds to second degree burns, showing vesicles; bullae; ulcer; and necrosis.

NP: If circulation is not restored, warm gradually by placing parts in lukewarm water or with warm hands. Do not rub. Place patient in warm but not hot room; give warm nutritious drinks (no alcohol). Protect the part from abrasion of bed clothes by using a cradle.

TREATMENT: Analgesics; antibiotics; anticoagulants; and vasodilators are used to attempt to prevent loss of blood supply to the affected area. SEE: *windchill; windchill factor.*

child [AS. *cild,* child]. A young person of either sex, between infancy and puberty. SEE: *pediatrics.*

childbed. Puerperium. Period during and immediately subsequent to parturition.

c. fever. Puerperal sepsis, q.v.

childbirth. The process of bringing forth a child; parturition. SEE: *labor.*

c., psychophysical preparation for. Physical and mental preparation and training of the patient for labor and delivery. Patients who participate in such a program are believed to have easier and less complicated labor and delivery.

child crowing. Spasmodic closure of glottis, of brief duration, and succeeded by noisy inspiration. SYN: *laryngismus stridulus.*

chilectro'pion [Gr. *cheilos,* lip, + *ektropē,* turning out]. Eversion of the lip. Cheilectropion.

chilitis (kī-lī'tĭs) ["+ -*itis,* imflammation]. Inflammation of the lips. SEE: *cheilitis.*

chill (chĭl) [AS. *cele,* cold]. An attack of shivering accompanied by the sensation of coldness and pallor of the skin. It is due to a disturbance in the temperature-regulating centers of the hypothalamus.

Chills accompany various diseases, esp. malaria and pneumococcal pneumonia, and are coarse or fine; diffuse; trembling; etc.

ETIOL: Infections or diseases (as malaria, pneumococcal pneumonia, bacteremia); parasites in blood; bacterial vaccines; and transfusion reactions. Postoperative chills or chills in puerperium are indicative of infection.

SYM: A real chill is ushered in by extreme sensation of cold; shivering; chattering of the teeth and, in extreme cases, a marked tremor of the entire body followed by a rapidly rising temperature.

NP: Make patient comfortable by supplying external heat and extra blanket. Give hot drink when permitted or tolerated. Give patient moral support. Take temperature as soon as possible, then again about 20 minutes after chill subsides. Chart a report to attending physician noting duration and degree of severity of chills, and temperature. SEE: *ague; windchill.*

   c., nervous. Accompanied by a chilly sensation but not with fever. It may follow severe pain or extreme nervousness. It usually passes quickly and is seldom serious.

chilo-, cheilo- [Gr. *cheilos,* lip]. Prefix denoting relationship to the lip.

chiloangioscopy (kī″lō-an″jī-os′kō-pĭ) ["+ *angeion,* vessel, + *skopein,* to examine]. Microscopic examination of the circulation in the lip.

chilognathopalatoschisis (kī″lō-nā″thō-pal″ā-tos′kis-is) ["+ *gnathos,* jaw, + L. *palatum,* palate, + Gr. *schisis,* fissure]. Fissure of the lip, palate, and alveolar process.

Chilomastix mesnili (kī″lō-măs′tĭks měs-nīl′ī). A species of Mastigophora. A nonpathogenic protozoa which is parasitic in the intestines.

chiloschisis (kī-lŏs′kĭs-ĭs) [Gr. *cheilos,* lip, + *schisis,* fissure]. Harelip.

chilostomatoplasty (kī″lō-stō-mat′ō-plas″-tĭ) ["+ *stoma,* mouth, + *plassein,* to form]. Plastic operation for harelip.

chim′ney-sweeps′ cancer. Epithelioma of the scrotum. Due to chronic irritation by coal soot.

chin [AS. *cin,* chin]. Point of the lower jaw; mentum; region below lower lip.

   c. jerk. Reflex contraction of muscles of mastication on suddenly depressing the jaw.

   c. reflex. Clonic movement resulting from percussing or stroking lower jaw.

Chinese restaurant syndrome. A group of symptoms which some persons develop after eating food which contains a considerable amt. of monosodium glutamate.

   SYM: Burning sensation; headache; facial pressure; perspiration; and chest pain.

chionablepsia (kī″ō-nă-blep′sĭ-ă) [Gr. *chiōn,* snow, + *ablepsia,* blindness]. Snow blindness.

chiragra (kī-răg′ră) [Gr. *cheir,* hand, + *agra,* seizure]. Pain in the hand.

chiralgia (kī-răl′jĭ-ă). Pain in the hand of nontraumatic or neuralgic origin.

   c. paresthetica. Numbness and pain in the hand, esp. in the region supplied by the radial nerve.

chirapsia (kī-răp′sĭ-ă) [Gr. *cheirapsia,* a touching with the hands]. Friction; massage.

chirismus (kī-rĭs′mŭs). Spasm of hand muscles.

chirognostic (kī″rog-nŏs′tĭk) [Gr. *cheir,* hand, + *gnōstikos,* knowing]. Having the ability to distinguish the right from the left, or the side of body being stimulated.

chirokinesthesia (kī″rō-kin″ēs-thē′zĭ-ă) ["+ *kinēsis,* movement, + *aisthēsis,* sensation]. Subjective perception of motions of the hand.

chiromeg′aly ["+ *megas,* large]. Enlargement of the hands, wrists, or ankles.

chi′roplasty ["+ *plassein,* to form]. A plastic operation on the hand.

chiropodist (kī-rop′ō-dist, kī-) ["+ *pous,* foot]. One who practices chiropody. SYN: *podiatrist.*

chiropody (kī-rop′ō-dĭ). Treatment of minor disorders of the feet.

chiropompholyx (kī″rō-pom′fō-liks) [Gr. *cheir,* hand, + *pompholyx,* a bubble]. Inflammatory disease of skin confined to hands and feet. SYN: *pompholyx,* q.v.

chiropractic (kī″rō-prak′tik) ["+ *prattein,* to do]. A system of manipulative treatment which teaches that all diseases are caused by impingement on spinal nerves and can be corrected by spinal adjustments.

chi′roprac″tor. One who practices chiropractic methods.

chirospasm (kī′rō-spazm) [Gr. *cheir,* hand, + *spasmos,* spasm]. Spasmodic affection of muscles of hand; writers' cramp.

chirurgery (ki-rur′jer-ĭ) ["+ *ergon,* work]. Surgery.

chirurgia (ki-rur′jī-ă). Surgery.

chirurgical (ki-rur′jik-al). Surgical.

chitin (kī′tin) [Gr. *chitōn,* tunic]. A white horny substance in outer covering of body of invertebrates such as crabs. Also occurs in some fungi.

chitinous (kĭt′ĭ-nus). Pert. to or composed of chitin.

   c. degeneration. Amyloid degeneration.

Chlamydia (clă-mĭd′ĭ-ă) [Gr. *chlamys,* cloak]. A generic term for those microorganisms which cause psittacosis-ornithosis (parrot fever), lymphogranuloma venereum, trachoma, and inclusion conjunctivitis. Although these organisms were formerly considered to be viruses, the evidence indicates they resemble bacteria, esp. rickettsiae, much more than viruses. They are members of the family Chlamydozoaceae which is divided into two genera: Miyagawanella (also called Bedsonia) and Chlamydzoon (also called TRIC agents).

   C. have been divided into three groups according to their hosts: avian agents which infest birds primarily and man occassionally; human agents which are predominately infectious for man; and mammalian agents which infect various mammals (mouse, cat, cow) other than man.

chloasma (klō-az'mä) [Gr. *chloazein,* to be green]. Pigmentary skin discolorations, usually those occurring in yellowish brown patches or spots.

SYM: Areas rounded or oval with ill-defined margins; light yellow to black. In those due to external factors pigmentation develops only at site of irritation or beyond. In symptomatic forms constitutional cause underlies.

TREATMENT: Constitutional when indicated.

c. gravida'rum. Brownish pigmentation of the face, often occurring in pregnancy. It usually disappears after delivery. Also seen in some persons who take progestational agents. SYN: *mask of pregnancy.*

c. hepaticum. So-called liver spot following dyspepsia.

c., idiopathic. C. caused by external agents such as sun; heat; mechanical means; X rays, etc.

c., symptomatic. C. caused by various diseases, as syphilis or cancer.

c. traumaticum. Skin discolorations from traumatic agents.

c. uteri'num. Chloasma of pregnancy and seen in other uterine conditions.

chloral (klo'ral) [Gr. *chlōras,* green]. 1. An oily liquid having a bitter taste. 2. Chloral hydrate.

c. hydrate. USP. Colorless, transparent crystals having aromatic, slightly acrid odor, and caustic, faintly bitter taste; soluble in alcohol and water.

ACTION AND USES: As a sedative and hypnotic. When used to aid sleep it allows almost normal sleep pattern in most patients.

POISONING: Depresses and eventually paralyzes the central nervous system. Can be toxic to the liver. There may be nausea and vomiting due to gastric irritation. Pulse is feeble, respirations are shallow and irregular; lassitude; weakness; dizziness; sleep.

F. A. TREATMENT: Gastric lavage with coffee or tea. Central nervous system stimulants by mouth, injection, or rectum. Artificial respiration, Trendelenburg position, I.V. glucose. SEE: *Table of Poisons and Poisoning* in *Appendix.*

chloramines (klō'rä-mīns). Organic chlorine compounds which decompose slowly, liberating chlorine. Used extensively in dairies, food manufacturing establishments, etc., as a germicide. Ex: chloramine-T; dichloramine-T.

chloramphenicol (klor''ăm-phĕn'i-cōl). USP. An antibiotic orginally isolated from Streptomyces venezuelae. It is now made synthetically. It is a broad-spectrum agent and is especially useful in typhoid fever (in which it is the antibiotic of choice) and other infections caused by Salmonellae, and in rickettsial infections.

CAUTION: Certain blood dyscrasias may follow the use of chloramphenicol, consequently it should not be used indiscriminately or for minor infections. If used for prolonged periods, careful blood checks should be made. Be sure to read the literature which comes with each package of this medicine prior to deciding to use it rather than another antibiotic.

chloranemia (klor''a-nē'mĭ-ă) [Gr. *chlōros,* green, + *a-,* not, + *haima,* blood]. A form of iron-deficiency anemia. SEE: *anemia.*

chlorate (klō'rāt). A salt of chloric acid. SEE: *potassium chlorate.*

chlorbu'tol. Chlorobutanol, q.v.

chlorcy'clizine hydrochloride. Official name for the hydrochloride of 1-(p-Chloro-α-phenylbenzyl)-4-methylpiperazine, an antihistamine.

chloremia (klō-rē'mĭ-ă) [Gr. *chlōros,* green, + *haima,* blood]. 1. An iron-deficiency anemia. SEE: *anemia, chlorotic.* 2. Excess chloride in the blood.

chlorephidrosis (klor''ef-ĭ-drō'sis) ["+ *ephidrōsis,* perspiration]. Greenish perspiration.

chlorhydria (klor-hī'drĭ-ă) ["+ *hydōr,* water]. Excess of hydrochloric acid in stomach.

chloride (klō'rĭd) [Gr. *chlōros,* green]. A binary compound of chlorine; a salt of hydrochloric acid. Blood serum contains 100-110 mEq./L. (350-390 mg./100 ml.), principally as sodium chloride. Chlorides are increased in nephritis, eclampsia, anemia, and cardiac disease; decreased in fevers, diabetes, and pneumonia.

c., test for, in urine. To a test tube half filled with urine add a drop or two of nitric acid, which holds the phosphates in solution. Then a 3% solution of silver nitrate is added to the specimen, drop by drop, until about six drops have been added. This forms a white, curdled precipitate at once. The test should be compared with a known normal specimen of urine. Diminished chlorides are found in chronic nephritis, early stages of pneumonia; malignant disease; and in gastritis. Chlorides are increased in a diet rich in salt; in rickets; and in hepatic cirrhosis.

chloridemia (klor''ĭ-de'mĭ-ă) ["+ *haima,* blood]. Chlorides in the blood.

chloridim'eter ["+ *metron,* measure]. An instrument for estimating amt. of chlorides in a fluid. SYN: *chloridometer.*

chloridimetry (klor-ĭ-dim'ĭ-trĭ). Determination of amt. of chlorides in the body fluids.

chloridom'eter. Chloridimeter, q.v.

chloriduria (klor''ĭ-dū'rĭ-ă) [Gr. *chlōros*, green, + *ouron*, urine]. Presence of excess of chlorides in urine.

chlorinated (klor'in-ā-ted). Impregnated with chlorine.

   c. lime. Calcium hypochlorite; widely used in solution as a bleach and as an antiseptic.

chlorina'tion. Treatment of water by addition of chlorine and its compounds for the killing of bacteria. For effective disinfection, a concentration of 0.5 to 1 part of chlorine per million parts of water is necessary.

chlorine (klo'rēn) [Gr. *chlōros*, green]. SYMB: *Cl*. At. wt. 35.453; at. no. 17. A highly irritating gas and destructive to the mucous membranes of the respiratory passages. It is very poisonous and excessive inhalation may cause death. Carefully inhaling ammonia or alcohol will counteract the effects of chlorine inhalation. Chlorine is an active bleaching agent and germicide. Both of these effects are due to its oxidizing powers. It is used extensively in the disinfection of water supplies and in treatment of sewage.

   FUNCTIONS: Chlorine is found combined with sodium in the blood and exercises some influence upon metabolism; helps to maintain osmotic pressure; and aids in the regulation and stimulation of muscular action. The body fluids contain 0.85% salt solution. The inorganic salts keep in solution proteins of the blood; milk; and other secretions. Chlorine is present in the hydrochloric acid of the gastric juice. It aids digestion, activates enzymes, and is essential to normal gastric secretion.

   EXCRETION: The excretion of chlorine during a 31-day fast measured from 3.77 gm. on the first day to 0.13 gm. on the last day of the fast. It leaves the body in the form of chloride ions.

   c. preparations. Those used for disinfecting.

   Compounds (hypochlorites), as Dakin's solution or Javelle water, are very effective in their germicidal power. As a disinfecting agent in washing dishes and utensils used by infected patients, 1/10 of 1% solution should be used; the dishes should then be washed well in soap and hot water and rinsed well, or boiled and then washed well after the boiling.

   For disinfection of the stools of patients, 5% or even stronger solutions may be used for one-half hour or longer. The utensil is set aside and covered while the solution functions. Dakin's solution is nonirritating and is used as a wound disinfectant, but it must be carefully prepared daily by the laboratory and used only when fresh.

chlorite (klo'rīt). A salt of chlorous acid; used as a disinfectant and bleaching agent.

chlormerodrin (klor-mer'o-drin). Generic name, 1-[3-(Chloromercuri)-2-methoxypropyl]-urea, an orally effective mercurial diuretic.

chloroanemia (klor''o-ă-ne'mĭ-ă) [Gr. *chlōros*, green, + *a-*, not, + *haima*, blood]. A type of iron-deficiency anemia. SEE: *anemia.*

chloroazodin (klŏr-ō-ăz'ō-dĭn). α,α'-Azobis [chloroformamidine], a germicidal preparation of chlorine.

chlorobutanol (klō-ro-bū'tă-nol). USP. Colorless crystals, with camphor odor and taste. SYN: *chlorbutanol; chlorbutol.*

   USES: Antiseptic and local anesthetic, and as a preservative in many pharmaceuticals.

   INCOMPATIBILITIES: Decomposed by alkalies, and should not be mixed with borax, carbonates, etc. Soluble in ether, chloroform, and volatile oils.

chlor'oform [Gr. *chlōros*, green + L. *forma*, form]. CHCl₃. A heavy, clear, colorless liquid with strong etherlike odor, formed by the action of chlorinated lime on methyl alcohol.

   ACTION AND USES: A general anesthetic, having a small margin of safety. Locally an irritant used in liniments. Internally a carminative and sedative.

   c. anesthesia. For some time chloroform anesthesia was more popular than ether. It is six times as strong, but it was found to be more toxic.

   When employed, the chloroform is well diluted with air. It is not flammable except when mixed with alcohol, although volatile at low temperatures. It tends to decompose and to form hydrochloric acid and carbonyl chloride. Chloroform should be kept in tightly closed, dark containers, in a cool place with temperature not exceeding 85° F.

   ADVANTAGES: The period of excitement following anesthesia is relatively short. It does not irritate the mucous membranes and it produces excellent muscular relaxation. Neither does it cause excessive secretion of the respiratory mucous membrane. It has a pleasant odor and causes a minimum of side effects.

   PHYSIOLOGICAL ACTION: When inhaled it is promptly absorbed through the mucous membranes of the respiratory tract. After being eliminated by the lungs it seems to remain unchanged.

CAUTION: Dangerous symptoms may develop very suddenly. Circulatory depression may develop with cardiac arrest. It is a severe cardiac and respiratory depressant. It lowers body temperature and blood pressure. It produces toxic changes in body chemistry, and is very detrimental to the bladder and kidney functioning. It should never be given without an excess of oxygen. This form of anesthesia should not be used for a patient with disease of the heart, liver, or kidneys. Because it is not flammable it may be used when work is to be done with a cautery, diathermy, or when the X ray is used around the head or mouth. It also may be used in acute pulmonary pathology.

chloroformism (klō'rō-form''ĭzm). The habit of inhaling chloroform for pleasure.

chloroleukemia (klo''ro-lū-ke'mĭ-ă) [Gr. *chlōros*, green, + *leukos*, white, + *haima*, blood, + *ia*, condition]. Leukemia with chlorosis.

chloroma (klo-ro'mă) ["+ *-ōma*, growth]. A greenish sarcoma of the periosteum of cranial bones; green cancer.

chloromycetin (klor''ō-mī-se'tĭn). Proprietary name for chloramphenicol, q.v.

chloromyeloma (klo''ro-mī-ĕ-lō'mă) [Gr. *chlōros*, green, + *myelos*, marrow, + *-ōma*, growth]. Chloroma accompanied by multiple growths in bone marrow.

chloropenia (klo''ro-pe'nĭ-ă) ["+ *penia*, poverty]. Deficiency in chlorine; hypochloremia.

chloropenic (klo''ro-pēn'ĭk). Deficient in chlorine.

chlorophane (klo'ro-fān) [Gr. *chlōros*, green, + *phainein*, to show]. A green-yellow pigment in the retina.

chlorophenothane (klo''rō-phĕn'o-thān). USP. An insecticide, better known as DDT, which is quite effective but should not be used because of its toxicity; except in situations where no suitable substitute is available.

chlorophyll, chlorophyl (klo'ro-fĭl) [Gr. *chlōros*, green, + *phyllon*, leaf]. The green coloring matter in plants consisting of chlorophyll a and chlorophyll b. It acts as a catalytic agent in the process of photosynthesis in which carbon dioxide from the air reacts with water from the soil to form simple carbohydrates, which are used for energy or converted into more complex substances and stored.

Chemically it is quite similar to hemoglobin except the element in chlorophyll which corresponds to iron in hemoglobin is magnesium.

chloro'pia ["+ *opsis*, vision, + *ia*, condition]. Vision in which all things appear green.

chloroplast (klō'rō-plast) ["+ *plastos*, formed]. Small round green bodies found in the cells of leaves and stem of plants which are important in the process of photosynthesis. They possess a stroma and contain four pigments: chlorophyll a, chlorophyll b, carotene, and xanthophyll.

chloroplas'tid. A chloroplast, q.v.

chloroprivic (klor-o-priv'ĭk) [Gr. *chlōros*, green, + L. *privāre*, to deprive of]. Lack of, or due to loss of, chlorides.

chlorop'sia ["+ *opsis*, vision]. Vision in which all things seem green. SYN: *chloropia.*

chloroquine. USP. $C_{18}H_{26}ClN_3 \cdot 2H_3PO_4$. A white crystalline powder used for its antimicrobial action, esp. in the treatment of malaria. It is useful also in amebic dysentery complicated by liver abscess and in treating lupus erythematosus.

chlorosarco'ma [Gr. *chlōros*, green, + *sarx*, flesh, + *-ōma*, tumor]. Sarcomatous form of chloroma.

chloro'sis ["+ *-ōsis*, infection]. A form of iron-deficiency anemia, q.v. SEE: *anemia.*

chlorotic (klo-rot'ĭk). Of the nature of or afflicted with chlorosis.

chlorpromazine (klor-prō'mă-zēn). USP. A tranquilizing agent, it is used, primarily in its hydrochloride form, in major and minor psychotic states. Proprietary name is thorazine.

chlortetracycline (klor''tĕt-ră-sī'klēn). A golden colored antibiotic isolated from a strain of Streptomyces aureofaciens. It is a broad-spectrum antibiotic, inhibiting growth of or destroying some strains of streptococci, staphylococci, pneumococci, rickettsiae, and viruses. Proprietary name is Aureomycin.

Ch.M. Abbr. for *Chirur'giae magis'ter*, Master of Surgery.

choana (kō'ă-nă) [Gr. *choanē*, funnel]. (pl. *choa'nae*) A funnel-shaped opening, esp. one of the posterior nares, the communicating passageways between the nasal fossae and the pharynx.

choanoid (ko'an-oyd) ["+ *eidos*, shape]. Shaped like a funnel.

chocolate [Aztec *xococ*, bitter, + *atl*, water]. 1. Preparation made by grinding roasted cacao or theobroma seeds. 2. Beverage prepared by dissolving chocolate in water or milk. SEE: *cocoa.*

choke. 1. To strangle or suffocate. 2. To inhibit or prevent progress, growth, or an action.

choked disk. Edema of the optic disk. SEE: *papilledema.*

chokes. Respiratory symptoms, such as substernal distress, paroxysmal cough, tachypnea, or asphyxia, which may occur in decompression illness, esp. in cases of aeroembolism resulting from exposure to pressure lower than atmospheric. SEE: *caisson disease.*

choking [AS. *acēocian*, to suffocate]. Obstruction within respiratory passage or constriction about the neck, interfering with breathing and circulation of brain. May also result from spasm of the larynx induced by an irritating gas.

SYM: Face purple; eyes protrude; arms thrown about; coughing; constriction and injury about neck; cyanosis; dizziness; unconsciousness.

TREATMENT: Remove constriction. Artificial respiration. Slap violently on back. Severe blow between shoulders. With children, compress chest with the hands, squeezing suddenly and vigorously. If foreign body in throat, such as meat, insert thumb and forefinger and try to grasp it. If child, grasp by legs and hold upside down for a moment. If the article is swallowed, do not give purgative. If lodged in throat and breathing is possible, interference should be limited until professional aid is at hand. Tracheotomy may be needed.

cholago'gia [Gr. *cholē*, bile, + *agein*, to lead forth]. Excretion of bile from gallbladder.

cholagogue (kō'lă-gŏg). An agent which increases the flow of bile into the intestine, i.e., a choleretic, or cholecystagogue.

cholangiogastrostomy (ko-lan"jĭ-o-gas-tros'to-mĭ) [Gr. *cholē*, bile, + *angeion*, vessel, + *gastēr*, stomach, + *stoma*, mouth]. Formation of a communication between bile duct and the stomach.

cholangiography (ko-lan"jĭ-og'ră-fĭ) ["+ "+ *graphein*, to write]. X-ray or skiagraphic examination of the bile ducts.

cholangioma (ko-lan-jĭ-o'mă) [Gr. *cholē*, bile, + *angeion*, vessel, + *-ōma*, tumor]. A tumor of the biliary ducts.

cholangiostomy (kō'lan-jĭ-ŏs'tŏ-mĭ) ["+ "+ *stoma*, mouth]. The surgical formation of a fistula into the gallbladder.

cholangiotomy (kō'lan-jĭ-ŏt'ŏ-mĭ) ["+ "+ *tomē*, incision]. Incision of an intrahepatic bile duct for removal of gallstones.

cholangitis (kō'lăn-jī'tĭs) [Gr. *cholē*, bile, + *angeion*, vessel, + *-ītis*, inflammation]. Inflammation of the bile ducts.

cholascos (kō-lăs'kŏs) ["+ *askos*, bag]. Escape of bile into the peritoneal cavity.

cholecyst (kō'lē-sĭst) [Gr. *cholē*, bile, + *kystis*, bladder]. The gallbladder, q.v.

cholecystalgia (ko'lē-sis-tal'jĭ-ă) ["+ "+ *algos*, pain, + *-ia*, condition]. Biliary colic.

cholecystectasia (ko'lē-sis-tĕk-tā'zĭ-ă) ["+ "+ *ektasis*, dilatation]. Dilatation of the gallbladder.

cholecystectomy (ko'lē-sis-tĕk'tō-mĭ) ["+ "+ *ektomē*, excision]. Excision of a gallbladder.

cholecystendysis (ko'lē-sis-tĕn'dĭ-sis) [Gr. *cholē*, bile, + *kystis*, cyst, + *endysis*, entrance]. Removal of a gallstone by incision, suturing wound in gallbladder to the abdominal incision. The wound is then closed.

cholecystenterorrhaphy (ko'lē-sis-ten"-ter-or'ă-fĭ) ["+ "+ *enteron*, intestine, + *rhaphē*, suture]. Suture of gallbladder to intestinal wall.

cholecystenterostomy (kō-lē-sĭs-tĕn"ter-ōs'tō-mĭ) ["+ "+ *enteron*, intestine, + *stoma*, opening]. The establishment of a connection between the gallbladder and the small intestine.

cholecystic (ko'le-sis'tĭk). Pert. to the gallbladder.

cholecystitis (kō"lē-sĭs-tī'tĭs) [Gr. *cholē*, bile, + *kystis*, bladder, + *-ītis*, inflammation]. Inflammation of the gallbladder. It may be acute or chronic.

ETIOL: Acute c. nearly always caused by gallstones. Other causes may be bacteria or chemical irritants. Chronic c. may occur with or without stones. However, not all patients with gallstones experience cholecystitis.

SYM: In acute c. there is fever, gradually developing or sudden pain in upper abdomen, nausea, vomiting, visible jaundice in about 25% of patients. Frequently pain is referred to back or right shoulder. Approximately 10% of patients do not have pain. In chronic c. symptoms less severe than in acute c., but recurring. May be with or without stones.

TREATMENT: In acute c., cholecystectomy; if this is not possible, draining of gallbladder (cholecystostomy) followed by cholecystectomy at a later date.

In chronic c., cholecystectomy if stones are present. If there are no stones, antispasmodics, laxatives, rest, and sedation if necessary, and further study to determine cause.

NP: Postoperative patient in bed in semi-Fowler position to aid drainage. Inspect dressing and drainage tube for bleeding. Check to be sure tube is fastened securely to dressing. Inspect dressings and check pulse rate and blood pressure frequently during first 24 hours. Observe color of skin, sclera, urine, and stools for evidence of jaundice. Encourage patient to move from side to side and to take deep breaths; this is essential to help prevent postoperative complications. Be alert for complications as shock or hemorrhage. Maintain drainage, check for obstruction of drainage tube by patient's position, chart amount of drainage every 24 hours. Low-fat diet.

cholecystnephrostomy (ko″lē-sist′nē-fros′tō-mĭ) [Gr. *cholē*, bile, + *kystis*, cyst, + *nephros*, kidney, + *stoma*, mouth]. Making an anastomosis of gallbladder into renal pelvis.

cholecystocolostomy (kō″lē-sĭs″tō-kō-lŏs′tō-mĭ) [″+ ″+ *kolon*, colon, + *stoma*, mouth]. Making a passage from gallbladder to colon.

cholecystocolotomy (ko″lē-sis″tō-kō-lot′o-mĭ) [″+ ″+ *tome*, incision]. Incision into gallbladder and colon.

cholecystoduodenostomy (kol″e-sis″tō-dū-o-dē-nos′to-mĭ) [″+ ″+ L. *duodeni*, twelve, + Gr. *stoma*, mouth]. Surgical formation of a passage from gallbladder to duodenum.

cholecystogastrostomy (ko″lē-sĭs″tō-gas-tros′tō-mĭ) [Gr. *cholē*, bile, + *kystis*, cyst, + *gastēr*, belly, + *stoma*, mouth]. Surgical formation of a passage from the gallbladder to the stomach.

cholecys′togram (″+ ″+ *gramma*, mark). An x-ray picture of the gallbladder.

cholecystography (ko″lē-sĭs-tŏg′rä-fĭ) [″+ ″+ *graphein*, to write]. Examination of the gallbladder by x-ray study.

cholecystoileostomy (ko″lē-sĭs″tō-ĭl-e-os′to-mĭ) [Gr. *cholē*, bile, + *kystis*, bladder, + L. *ileum*, ileum, + Gr. *stoma*, mouth]. Forming a communication between the gallbladder and ileum.

cholecystojejunostomy (kō″lē-sis″to-jē-jū-nos′tō-mĭ) [″+ ″+ L. *jejunum*, empty, + Gr. *stoma*, mouth]. Forming a communication between the gallbladder and jejunum.

cholecystokinin (ko″lē-sĭs″tō-kĭ′nĭn) [″+ ″+ *kinein*, to move]. A hormone secreted by the mucosa of the duodenum which induces contraction of the gallbladder.

cholecystolithiasis (ko″lē-sĭs″tō-lĭ-thĭ′ä-sĭs) [″+ ″+ *lithos*, stone, + *iasis*, condition]. Gallstones in the gallbladder.

cholecystolithotripsy (ko″lē-sĭs″tō-lĭth′o-trĭp″sĭ) [″+ ″+ ″+ *tripsis*, a rubbing]. Crushing of a gallstone in the unopened gallbladder.

cholecys′tomy [Gr. *cholē*, bile, + *kystis*, bladder, + *tome*, incision]. Cholecystotomy, q.v.

cholecystopathy (ko″lē-sĭs-top′ä-thĭ) [″+ ″+ *pathos*, disease]. Any gallbladder affection.

cholecystopexy (kō″lē-sĭs′to-pek″sĭ) [″+ ″+ *pēxis*, fixation]. Suturing the gallbladder to the abdominal wall.

cholecystoptosis (kō″lē-sĭs-tō-to′sĭs) [″+ ″+ *ptōsis*, fall]. Displacement of the gallbladder downward.

cholecystorrhaphy (kō″lē-sĭs-tor′ä-fĭ) [Gr. *cholē*, bile, + *kystis*, bladder, + *rhaphē*, suture]. Suturing of the gallbladder.

cholecystostomy (kol″ē-sĭs-tos′tō-mĭ) [″+ ″+ *stoma*, opening]. Surgical formation of an opening into gallbladder through abdominal wall.

cholecystotomy (kō″lē-sĭs-tot′o-mĭ) [″+ ″+ *tome*, incision]. Incision of gallbladder through the abdominal wall for removal of gallstones.

choledochal (kō-lē-dŏk′äl) [Gr. *cholē*, bile, + *dochos*, receptacle]. Rel. or pert. to the common bile duct.

choledochectasia (kō-led″o-kek-ta′zĭ-ä) [″+ ″+ *ektasis*, distention]. Distention of the common bile duct.

choledochectomy (kō-led″ō-kek′tō-mĭ) [″+ ″+ *ektomē*, excision]. Excision of a portion of the common bile duct.

choledochitis (kol″ē-dō-kī′tis) [″+ ″+ *-itis*, inflammation]. Inflammation of common bile duct.

choledochoduodenostomy (kō-led″o-kō-dū-o-dē-nos′to-mĭ) [″+ L. *duodeni*, twelve, + Gr. *stoma*, opening]. Surgical communication between the common bile duct and duodenum.

choledochoenterostomy (kō-led″ō-kō-en-ter-os′to-mĭ) [″+ ″+ *enteron*, intestine, + *stoma*, opening]. Surgical passage between common bile duct and intestine.

choledochography (kō-lēd″ō-kog′räfĭ) [Gr. *cholē*, bile, + *dochos*, receptacle, + *graphein*, to write]. X-ray examination of the bile duct following administration of a radiopaque substance.

choledocholithiasis (ko-led″o-ko-lĭ-thĭ′ä-sis) [″+ ″+ *lithos*, stone]. Calculi in the common bile duct.

choledocholithotomy (ko-led″o-ko-lith-ot′-o-mĭ) [″+ ″+ ″+ *tome*, incision]. Removal of a gallstone through an incision of the bile duct.

choledocholithotripsy (ko-led′o-ko-lith″o-trĭp-sĭ) [″+ ″+ ″+ *tripsis*, a crushing]. Crushing of a gallstone in the common bile duct.

choledochoplasty (ko-led′o-ko-plas″tĭ) [Gr. *cholē*, bile, + *dochos*, receptacle, + *plassein*, to form]. Operation for repair of common bile duct.

choledochorrhaphy (ko″led-o-kor′ă-fĭ) ["+ "+ *rhaphē*, suture]. Suturing the severed ends of the common bile duct.

choledochostomy (ko-led″o-kos′to-mĭ) ["+ "+ *stoma*, mouth]. Surgical formation of an opening into common bile duct through abdominal wall.

choledochotomy (ko″led-o-kot′o-mĭ) ["+ "+ *tomē*, incision]. Surgical incision of the common bile duct.

choledochus (ko-led′o-kus) [Gr. *cholē*, bile, + *dochos*, receptacle]. The common bile duct. SYN: *ductus choledochus.*

cholehemia (ko-lē-he′mĭ-ă) ["+ *haima*, blood]. Cholemia, q.v.

choleic (ko-lē′ĭk). Cholic; pert. to the bile.

chol′elith [Gr. *cholē*, bile, + *lithos*, stone]. A biliary concretion of gallstone.

cholelithiasis (ko″lē-lĭ-thi′as-is) ["+ "+ *-iasis*, condition]. Formation or presence of calculi or bilestones in the gallbladder or common duct. The stones may remain dormant or be responsible for few symptoms.

   SYM: Digestive disturbances; heaviness in right hypochondrium; tenderness on pressure over gallbladder. Gallstone colic when passing through bile duct if obstructed. Pain may radiate to back and right shoulder. Colic usually manifest when stomach is empty. Jaundice if flow of bile is obstructed. Pain may be associated with vomiting and sweating. Gallbladder may be palpated if distended.

   TREATMENT: Cholecystectomy; in very poor-risk patients, cholecystostomy.

cholelithic (ko-lē-lith′ĭk). Pert. to or caused by biliary calculus.

cholelithotomy (ko″lē-lĭ-thot′o-mĭ) [Gr. *cholē*, bile, + *lithos*, stone, + *tomē*, incision]. Removal of gallstones through a surgical incision.

cholelithotripsy (ko″lē-lith′ō-trĭp-sĭ). Cholelithotrity, q.v.

cholelithotrity (ko″lē-lĭ-thot′rĭ-tĭ) [Gr. *cholē*, bile, + *lithos*, stone, + *tribein*, to crush]. Crushing of a biliary calculus.

cholemesis (kol-em′e-sis) ["+ *emein*, to vomit]. Bile in the vomitus.

cholemia (ko-lē′mĭ-ă) ["+ *haima*, blood]. Bile or its pigments in the blood.

cholemic state (kō-lē′mĭk). A condition of stupor and delirium which progresses into somnambulence and coma, accompanied by intense jaundice, seen in final stages of Laennec's cirrhosis or in carcinoma of the liver.

cholepathia (ko″lē-path′ĭ-ă) [Gr. *cholē*, bile, + *pathos*, disease]. Faulty contractions of bile ducts.

   c. spas′tica. Spasmodic contraction of biliary ducts.

choleperitoneum (ko″lē-per′ĭ-to-nē′um) ["+ *peri*, around, + *teinein*, to stretch]. Bile in the peritoneum.

cholepoiesis (ko″lē-poy-ē′sis) ["+ *poiein*, to make]. The formation of bile.

cholepyrrhin (ko″lē-pir′ĭn) ["+ *pyrrhos*, flame-colored]. A mixture of bile pigments. SYN: *biliphein.*

chol′era [L. *cholera*, bilious diarrhea]. An acute, specific infectious disease characterized by diarrhea with severe loss of fluids and electrolytes; painful cramps of muscles; and tendency to collapse. SYN: *algid c.; Asiatic c.; asphyctic c.; epidemic c.; Indian c.; malignant c.; pestilential c.*

   ETIOL: Causative organism, Vibrio comma (also called Vibrio cholerae; cholera bacillus; comma bacillus; Koch's bacillus) which is a short, curved, motile, gram-negative rod producing a potent endotoxin which interferes with cellular metabolism, and a mucolytic enzyme. Transmission is through water, milk, or other foods contaminated with excreta of patients or carriers.

   INCUBATION: A few hours to four to five days.

   SYM: Four stages are usually described as follows:

   Invasion: At the conclusion of the incubation period there is malaise, headache, diarrhea, and anorexia. Headache and slight fever are present. May last a few days, and then subside. Under such circumstances, may be termed cholerine. Sometimes this stage is lacking entirely.

   Evacuation: Purging, violent vomiting, and muscular cramps. Stools loose, copious, and watery, and present a typical rice-water appearance. Sometimes there are particles of blood, as well as mucus. Vomiting severe and persistent; material expelled may also resemble rice water. Muscular cramps commonly start in extremities; involve calves of legs; and later even arms, hands, feet, and trunk. Thirst unquenchable and hiccough sometimes develops. Signs of depression soon terminate in collapse. Duration of stage, two to 12 hours, seldom more.

   Stage of Collapse: Almost complete arrest of circulation; eyes sunken; cheeks hollow; nose pinched; skin dry and wrinkled; body surface cold; covered with clammy sweat; breath cool; temperature in axilla 85-95° F. (29.4-32.2° C.), while in the rectum it may be 103° F. (39.4° C.) or more. Respirations quickened, pulse weak, systolic blood pressure from 50 to 60, urine suppressed; evacuation and cramps may continue. Mind usually clear until shortly prior to death, when coma develops. Stage lasts from few hours to one or two days, and generally ends in death.

Stage of Reaction: Sometimes, even when death seems imminent, surface temperature begins to rise, vomiting ceases, bowel evacuations become less frequent, more feculent, q.v., and convalescence is established. Complete recovery may ensue in from one to two weeks. Occasionally, typhoid symptoms set in, temperature goes to 106-107° F. (41.1-41.7° C.) and outcome is fatal. Sometimes in this stage, an erythemal eruption or one of the urticarial type appears, particularly on extremities. Such eruptions have no special significance.

TREATMENT: Vigorous replacement of fluid and electrolytes by intravenous administration of saline solution. Sodium lactate or sodium bicarbonate intravenously for acidosis. Tetracycline therapy is effective in limiting the diarrhea.

PROPHYLAXIS: Proper sanitation. Cholera vaccine: Following the initial two or three injections, booster doses should be administered every six months if the person remains in an endemic area.

c. infantum. An acute disease of childhood usually occurring in summer months, accompanied by vomiting, purging, and collapse. An obsolete term.

c. morbus. Old term formerly applied to an inflammatory intestinal disease resembling cholera, characterized by intense cramps and purging.

c. sicca. A term sometimes applied to a fulminating variety of cholera which occurs without vomiting or purging.

cholerase (kol′er-ās). The special bacteriolytic enzyme of cholera vibrio.

choleresis (kol-ĕr-ē′sis, kō-ler′ĕ-sis) [Gr. *cholē*, bile, + *hairesis*, removal]. The secretion and excretion of bile by the liver.

choleretic (kol-er-et′ĭk). Pert. to choleresis, or any agent that increases excretion of bile by the liver.

choleric (kol′er-ik). Irritable; quick-tempered without apparent cause.

choleriform (kol-er′ĭ-form) [L. *cholera*, bilious diarrhea, + L. *forma*, shape]. Appearing like cholera.

cholerigenous (kol-er-ij′en-us) [″ + Gr. *gennan*, to produce]. Giving rise to cholera.

cholerine (kol′er-ĭn). A mild form or initial stages of Asiatic cholera.

choleroid (kol′ĕr-oyd) [L. *cholera*, bilious diarrhea, + Gr. *eidos*, form]. Having a resemblance to cholera.

choleromania (kol-ĕr-ō-mā′nĭ-ă) [″ + Gr. *mania*, madness]. 1. Morbid fear of contract-

ing cholera. 2. Madness occasionally seen in cholera.

cholerophobia (kol″er-o-fo′bĭ-a) [″ + *phobos*, fear]. Morbid fear of acquiring cholera.

cholerrhagia (kol-er-rā′jĭ-ă) [Gr. *cholē*, bile, + *rhēgnynai*, to burst forth]. A flow of bile.

cholesta′sia [″ + *stasis*, stoppage]. Arrest of the bile excretion.

chol″estat′ic. Pert. to or caused by cholestasia.

cholesteatoma (kō″lē-stē″ă-tō′mă) [Gr. *cholē*, bile, + *steatos*, fat, + *-ōma*, tumor]. 1. Primary. A slow growing benign tumor of the skull or brain. It has a glistening pearly appearance. Because c.'s may arise from any site no characteristic clinical picture is presented. 2. Secondary. Tumor of suppurative otitic origin in presence of marginal perforations. Fatty degeneration of epithelium containing cholesterin crystals caused by nature's effort to arrest suppuration.

cholesteremia (ko-les″tere′mĭ-ă) [″ + *stereos*, solid, + *haima*, blood]. Excess cholesterol in the blood.

cholesterin (ko-les′ter-in). Cholesterol, q.v.

cholesterinemia (ko-les″ter-in-e′mĭ-ă). Cholesteremia, q.v.

cholesterinuria (ko-les″ter-ĭn-ū′rĭ-ă) [Gr. *cholē*, bile, + *stereos*, solid, + *ouron*, urine]. Presence of cholesterin in the urine.

cholesterol (ko-les′ter-ol) [Gr. *cholē*, bile, + *steros*, solid]. A monohydric alcohol ($C_{27}H_{45}OH$). A sterol widely distributed in animal tissues and occurring in the yolk of eggs, various oils, fats, and nerve tissue (brain and spinal cord). It can be synthesized in the liver and is a normal constituent of bile. It is the principal constituent of most gallstones. It is important in metabolism serving as a precursor of various steroid hormones, e.g., sex hormones, adrenal corticoids, etc.

cholesterolemia (ko-les″ter-ol-e′mĭ-ă) [″ + ″ + *haima*, blood]. Cholesteremia, q.v.

cholesteroluria (ko-les″ter-ol-u′rĭ-ă) [″ + ″ + *ouron*, urine]. Cholesterol in voided urine.

cholesterosis (ko-les-ter-o′sis) [″ + ″ + *-ōsis*, condition]. Cholesterol deposition, esp. in excessive amounts, as in the gallbladder.

cholestyramine resin (ko″lē-stī′rā-mĭn). USP. An ion-exchange resin used to treat itching associated with jaundice. It acts by lowering the level of bile acids in the serum.

choletelin (ko-let′el-ĭn) [Gr. *cholē*, bile, + *telos*, end]. Yellow pigment derived from bilirubin.

choleuria (ko″le-u′rĭ-ă) [″ + *ouron*, urine]. Bile in urine.

choleverdin (ko″lē-ver′din) [″ + L. *viridis*, green]. Green pigment appearing in gallstones and in urine in jaundice. SYN: *biliverdin*, q.v.

choline (kō'lǐn, -lēn) [Gr. *cholē*, bile]. $C_5H_{15}NO_2$. An amine, widely distributed in plant and animal tissues, a constituent of lecithin and other phospholipids. It is essential in normal fat and carbohydrate metabolism, a deficiency resulting in lipoidosis of the liver. It is also involved in protein metabolism serving as a methylating agent, and is a precursor of acetylcholine.

cholinergic (kō''lǐn-ĕr'jĭk) [Gr. *cholē*, bile, + *ergon*, work]. Nerve endings which liberate acetylcholine.

c. fibers. They include all preganglionic fibers; all postganglionic parasympathetic fibers; postganglionic sympathetic fibers to sweat glands; efferent fibers to skeletal muscle.

cholinesterase (kō''lǐn-ĕs'ter-ās). Any enzyme which catalyzes the hydrolysis of choline esters, e.g., acetylcholinesterase which catalyzes the breakdown of acetylcholine to acetic acid and choline. Cholinesterases are inhibited by physostigmine (eserine).

cholochrome (ko'lo-krōm) [Gr. *cholē*, bile, + *chrōma*, color]. Any bile pigment.

cholohemothorax (ko''lo-hĕm''o-thō'raks) [''+ *haima*, blood, + *thōrax*, chest]. Bile and blood in the thorax.

chololith (kol'o-lith) [''+ *lithos*, stone]. A gallstone; biliary calculus.

chololithiasis (kol''o-lith-ī'ăs-is). Presence of concretions in the gallbladder. SYN: *cholelithiasis*.

cholorrhea (kol''or-rē'ă) [Gr. *cholē*, bile, + *rhoia*, flow]. Excessive secretion of bile.

choloscopy (ko-los'ko-pī) [''+ *skopein*, to examine]. Testing the biliary function.

choluria (ko-lu'rǐ-a) [''+ *ouron*, urine]. Bile salts in the urine.

chondral (kon'dral) [Gr. *chondros*, cartilage]. Pert. to cartilage.

chondralgia (kon-dral'jǐ-ă) [''+ *algos*, pain]. Pain in or around a cartilage.

chondralloplasia (kon''dral-o-plā'zǐ-ă) [''+ *allos*, other, + *plassein*, to form]. Presence of cartilage in abnormal places.

chondrectomy (kon-drek'tō-mī) [''+ *ektomē*, excision]. Surgical excision of a cartilage.

chondric (kon'drik) [Gr. *chondros*, cartilage]. Pert. to cartilage.

chondrification (kon-drĭ-fĭ-kā'shun) [''+ L. *facere*, to make]. Conversion into cartilage.

chon'drigen [''+ *gennan*, to produce]. Basal substance of cartilage, which turns into chondrin on boiling. SYN: *chondrogen*.

chondrin (kon'drǐn) [Gr. *chondros*, cartilage]. Gelatinlike matter obtained by boiling cartilage.

chondriosome (kon'drǐ-o-sōm) [''+ *sōma*, body]. Any of the organelles of a cell comprising the chondriome. Includes the mitochondria.

chondritis (kon-drī'tis) [''+ *-itis*, inflammation]. Inflammation of cartilage.

chon''droadeno'ma [''+ *adēn*, gland, + *-ōma*, tumor]. Cartilaginous tissue in an adenoma.

chon''droangio'ma [''+ *angeion*, vessel, + *-ōma*, tumor]. Cartilaginous elements in an angioma.

chondroblast (kŏn'drō-blăst) [Gr. *chondros*, cartilage, + *blastos*, germ]. A cell which forms cartilage.

chondroclast (kon'dro-klast) [''+ *klastos*, broken into bits]. A cell involved in the absorption of cartilage.

chondrocostal (kon''dro-kos'tal) [''+ L. *costa*, rib]. Pert. to costal cartilages.

chondrocranium (kon-dro-krā'nǐ-um) [''+ *kranion*, head]. The cartilaginous embryonic cranium before ossification.

chondrocyte (kon'dro-sīt) [Gr. *chondros*, cartilage, + *kytos*, hollow vessel]. A cartilage cell.

chondrodynia (kon''dro-din'ǐ-ă) [''+ *odynē*, pain]. Pain in or about a cartilage.

chondrodysplasia (kon''dro-dis-plā'zǐ-ă) [''+ *dys-*, bad, + *plassein*, to form]. Chondrodystrophy.

chondrodystrophy (kon-dro-dis'tro-fī) [''+ ''+ *trophē*, nourishment]. Defect in cartilage formation at epiphyses of long bones. SYN: *dyschondroplasia*, q.v.

c., hypoplastic. Achondroplasia, q.v.

chondrofibroma (kon''dro-fĭ-brō'mă) [Gr. *chondros*, cartilage, + L. *fibra*, fiber, + Gr. *-ōma*, tumor]. A mixed tumor with elements of chondroma and fibroma.

chondrogen (kon'dro-jen) [''+ *gennan*, to produce]. Chondrigen, q.v.

chondrogenesis (kon''dro-jen'es-is) [''+ *genesis*, production]. Formation of cartilage.

chondroid (kon'droyd) [''+ *eidos*, resemblance]. Resembling cartilage; cartilaginous.

chondroituria (kon-dro-ĭ-tū'rǐ-ă) [''+ *ouron*, urine]. Chondroitic acid in urine.

chondrolipoma (kon-dro-lip-o'mă) [Gr. *chondros*, cartilage, + *lipos*, fat, + *-ōma*, tumor]. Cartilaginous and fatty tissue tumor.

chondrology (kon-drol'o-jī) [''+ *logos*, study]. The science of cartilages.

chondrolysis (kon-drol'ĭ-sis) [Gr. *chondros*, cartilage, + *lysis*, dissolution]. The breaking down and absorption of cartilage.

chondro′ma [" + -ōma, tumor]. A cartilaginous tumor of slow growth. It may occur any place where there is cartilage. It causes no pain.

chondromalacia (kŏ-drō-măl-ā′shĭ-ă) [" + malakia, softness]. Softness of any cartilage.

chondromatous (kon-drŏm′ă-tus) [" + -ōma, tumor]. Pert. to chondroma, or tumor of a cartilage.

chondromucoid (kon″drō-mū′koyd) [Gr. chondros, cartilage, + L. mucus, mucus, + Gr. eidos, form]. A basophilic glycoprotein present in interstitial substance of cartilage.

chondromyoma (kon″dro-mī-o′mă) [" + mys, muscle, + -ōma, tumor]. Myoma and cartilaginous neoplasm combined.

chondromyxoma (kon″dro-mĭk-sō′mă) [Gr. chondros, cartilage, + myxa, mucus, + -ōma, tumor]. Chondroma with myxomatous elements.

chondromyxosarcoma (kon-dro-mĭk″sō-sar-kō′mă) [" + " + sarx, flesh, + -ōma, tumor]. A cartilaginous and sarcomatous tumor.

chondropathology (kŏn″drō-pă-thŏl′ō-jī) [" + pathos, disease, + logos, study]. Pathology of cartilages.

chondropathy (kon-drop′ath-ī). Any disease of cartilage.

chondroplast (kon′drō-plast). Chondroblast, q.v.

chondroplasty (kon′dro-plas″tī) [Gr. chondros, cartilage, + plassein, to mold]. Plastic or reparative surgery on cartilage.

chondroporosis (kon″dro-po-ro′sis) [" + poros, passage]. The porous condition of cartilage, pathological or normal, during ossification.

chondroproteins (kon-dro-pro′tī-ins) [" + prōtos, first]. A group of glucoproteins found in cartilage, tendons, and connective tissue.

chondrosarcoma (kon-dro-sar-ko′mă) [" + sarx, flesh, + -ōma, tumor]. Cartilaginous sarcoma.

chondro′sis [Gr. chondros, cartilage, + -ōsis, process]. The development of cartilage.

chon″droster′nal [" + sternon, chest]. Pert. to sternal cartilage.

chondrotome (kon′dro-tōm) [" + tomē, a cutting]. Device for cutting cartilage.

chondrotomy (kon-drot′o-mī). Dissection or surgical division of cartilage.

Chondrus [L., cartilage]. A genus of red algae which includes Chondrus crispus, the source of carrageenin, a mucilaginous substance used as an emulsifying agent. Commonly called Irish moss or carrageen.

Chopart′s amputation (shō-păr′). [François Chopart, Fr. surgeon, 1743-1795] Disarticulation at the midtarsal joint.

chorda (kor′da) [Gr. chordē, cord]. (pl. chordae) A string or tendon.

 c. dorsalis. The notochord.

 c. gubernaculi. An embryonic structure forming a part of the gubernaculum testis in the male and the round ligament in the female.

 c. obliqua. [NA]. The oblique ligament, an oblique cord which connects the shafts of the radius and ulna. Extends from lateral side of tubercle of ulna to a point just below radial tuberosity.

 c. tympani. [NA]. A branch of the facial nerve which leaves the cranium through the stylomastoid foramen, traverses the tympanic cavity and joins a branch of the lingual nerve. Efferent fibers innervate the submaxillary and sublingual glands; afferent fibers convey taste impulses from anterior two thirds of the tongue.

 c. umbilicalis. Umbilical cord connecting fetus and placenta.

 c. Willisii. One of several fibrous cords across the superior longitudinal sinus.

chordae tendineae. [NA] Small tendinous cords which connect the free edges of the atrioventricular valves to the papillary muscles.

chordal (kor′dal). Pert. to a chorda, esp. the notochord.

Chordata (kor-dā′tă) [New Latin, notochord]. A phylum of the animal kingdom which includes all vertebrates.

chordèe (kōr-dē′) [Fr., corded]. Downward, painful curvature of the penis on erection in gonorrhea caused by inflammatory infiltration of the corpus spongiosum which interferes with its distensibility.

chorditis (kor-dī′tis) [Gr. chordē, cord, + -ītis, inflammation]. Inflammation of a cord, esp. the spermatic or vocal cord.

 c. nodo′sa. Formation of small whitish nodules on one or both vocal cords.

 SYM: Hoarseness, inability of singers to register tones properly.

 TREATMENT: Voice rest. Surgical removal of nodules if they do not respond to conservative therapy.

chordot′omy [" + tomē, a cutting]. Division of any cord to relieve pain.

chorea (ko-rē′ă) [Gr. choreia, dance]. A nervous affection marked by muscular twitching. SEE: c., Sydenham's.

 c., electric. A rare form characterized by sudden involuntary contraction of a group of muscles. This causes violent movements as if the patient had been stimulated by an electric current.

 c., epidemic. Religious emotional neurosis, manifest in the 14th century in

Europe, exhibited in form of dancing mania. SYN: *dancing mania.*

c. gravidarum. A form of Sydenham's c. seen in some pregnant women, usually in those who have had chorea before, esp. in their first pregnancy.

c., Huntington's. A hereditary and chronic form manifested in adult life.

c., hyoscine. Movements simulating chorea, and sometimes accompanied by delirium, seen in acute hyoscine intoxication.

c. major. C. with violent hysterical muscular action.

c., mimetic. C. due to imitative movements.

c. minor. Sydenham's c., q.v.

c., posthemiplegic; c., postparalytic. Involuntary movements of patients subsequent to a hemiplegic attack.

c., rheumatic. Sydenham's c., q.v.

c., rhythmic. C. with movements at regulated times.

c., senile. C. developing in senility.

c., Sydenham's. A disease of childhood commonly occurring between five and 15 years of age; more females than males are affected. Usually associated with rheumatic fever. Characterized by involuntary, purposeless contractions of the muscles of the trunk and extremities; anxiety; impairment of memory and sometimes of speech.

SYN: *chorea minor; infectious chorea; rheumatic chorea; St. Vitus' dance.*

PROG: Usually recover in course of six to 10 weeks. Relapses not infrequent esp. in pregnancy. Rare complication is death from heart disease. A possible sequel is chronic chorea.

TREATMENT: Rest of body and mind, remove child from school; place under most favorable hygienic conditions. Protection against injury in severe cases. Sedation in most cases.

choreal (ko-rē'al, kō'rĭ-al). Pert. to chorea.

choreic (ko-rē'ik). Pert. to or of nature of chorea.

choreiform (kō-rē'ĭ-form) [Gr. *choreia,* dance, + L. *forma,* form]. Of the nature of chorea.

choreomania (kō''rē-ō-mā'nĭ-ă) ["+ *mania,* madness]. Epidemic chorea, as the dancing mania of the Middle Ages.

chorioadenoma (ko''rĭ-o-ad''en-ō'mă) [Gr. *chorion,* outer membrane enclosing an embryo, + *adēn,* gland, + *-ōma,* tumor]. Adenoma of the chorion.

chorioangioma (ko''rĭ-o-an-jĭ-o'mă) ["+ *angeion,* vessel, + *-ōma,* tumor]. A vascular tumor of the chorion.

choriocapillaris (ko''rĭ-o-kap-il-lā'ris) [Gr. *choroeidēs,* resembling a membrane, + L. *capillaris,* hairlike]. Capillary layer of choroid, q.v.

choriocarcinoma (kō''rĭ-ō-kăr''sĭ-nō'mă) [Gr. *chorion,* outer membrane enclosing an embryo, + *karkinōma,* cancer]. An extremely rare, very malignant neoplasm, usually of the uterus but sometimes at site of ectopic pregnancy. Though actual cause is unknown, it may occur following hydatid mole, pregnancy, abortion.

choriocele (ko'rĭ-o-sēl) [Gr. *choroeidēs,* resembling a membrane, + *kēlē,* hernia]. A protrusion of the chorioid coat of the eye through a defective sclera.

chorioepithelioma (ko''ri-o-ep''ĭ-thē''lĭ-o'mă). Choriocarcinoma, q.v.

chorioid (ko'rĭ-oyd). Choroid, q.v.

chorioma (ko''rĭ-o'mă) [Gr. *chorion,* outer membrane enclosing an embryo, + *-ōma,* tumor]. (pl. *chorio'mata*) A tumor of the chorion. There are a number of types including chorioadenoma, choriocarcinoma, and syncytioma, q.v.

choriomeningitis (ko''rĭ-o-men''in-jī'tis) ["+ *mēninx,* membrane, + *-itis,* inflammation]. Cerebral meningitis with cellular infiltration of the meninges.

c., lymphocytic. An acute central nervous system disease probably of viral origin characterized by grippelike symptoms (fever, malaise, headache, etc.) sometimes followed by acute septic meningitis.

chorion (kō'rĭ-ŏn) [Gr.]. An extraembryonic membrane which, in early development, forms the outer wall of the blastocyst. It is formed from the trophoblast and its inner lining of mesoderm. From it chorionic villi develop which establish an intimate connection with the endometrium, giving rise to the placenta. SEE: *embryo* for illustration; *trophoblast.*

chorionepithelioma. Choriocarcinoma, q.v.

chorionic (ko-rĭ-on'ik). Pert. to the chorion.

c. villi. The vascular projections from the chorion.

chorionitis (ko''rĭ-on-ī'tis) [Gr. *chorion,* skin, + *-itis,* inflammation]. 1. Inflammation of the chorion. 2. Scleroderma, q.v.

chorioretinitis (ko''rĭ-o-ret''in-ī'tis) ["+ L. *rete,* network, + Gr. *-itis,* inflammation]. Inflammation of choroid and retina.

chorista (kō-rĭs'tă) [Gr. *chōristos,* separated]. An error of development showing separation from the rudiments in a developing embryo.

choristoma (ko-ris-to'mă) ["+ *-ōma,* tumor]. A neoplasm due to overdevelopment of embryonic rudiments.

choroid (kō'royd) [Gr. *chorioeidēs*, skinlike]. Dark brown, vascular coat of eye between sclera and retina, extending from ora serrata to optic nerve.

Consists of blood vessels, united by connective tissue containing pigmented cells, and is made up of five layers: suprachoroid; layer of large vessels; layer of medium-sized vessels; layer of capillaries; lamina vitrea (homogeneous membrane placed next to pigmentary layer of retina).

It is a part of the uvea or vascular tunic of the eye.

choroideremia (ko-roy-der-ē'mĭ-ă) ["+ *erēmia*, destitution]. Absence of the choroid coat of the eye.

choroiditis (ko''royd-ī'tis) ["+ *-itis*, inflammation]. Inflammation of choroid.

   c., anterior. When outlets of exudation are at the choroidal periphery.

   c., areolar. In which inflammation spreads from around the macula lutea.

   c., central. Exudation is limited to the macula.

   c., diffuse or disseminated. When the fundus is covered with spots.

   c., exudative. When covered with patches of inflammation.

   c. guttata senilis. Tay's c., q.v.

   c., metastatic. When due to embolism.

   c., suppurative. When suppuration occurs.

   c., Tay's. A familial condition characterized by degeneration of the choroid, esp. in the region about the macula lutea. Occurs in aged persons.

choroidocycli'tis [Gr. *chorioeidēs*, skinlike, + *kyklos*, a circle, + *-itis*, inflammation]. Inflammation of the choroid coat and ciliary processes.

choroidoiritis (ko-royd''o-ī-rī'tis) ["+ *iris*, iris, + *-itis*, inflammation]. Inflammation of the choroid coat and iris.

choroidoretinitis (ko-royd''o-ret''in-ī'tis) ["+ L. *rete*, network, + Gr. *-itis*, inflammation]. Inflammation of choroid and retina.

choromania (ko''ro-mā'nĭ-ă) [Gr. *choros*, dance, + *mania*, madness]. Epidemic chorea, q.v.

Christian Science. A system of religious teaching based on Christian Scientists' interpretation of Scripture, founded in 1866 by Mary Baker Eddy. The system emphasizes full healing of disease by mental and spiritual means because a major belief is that cause and effect is mental.

Christmas disease. A form of hemophilia in males resulting from plasma thromboplastin component (PTC or Factor IX) deficiency. Named for person in whom the disease was discovered.

Christmas factor. A thromboplastin activator present in blood plasma, viz., plasma thromboplastin component (PTC).

chromaffin (krō-măf'ĭn) [Gr. *chrōma*, color, + L. *affīnis*, having affinity for]. 1. Staining readily with chromium salts. 2. Denoting pigmented cells forming medulla of the adrenal glands and the paraganglia.

   c. cells. Cells such as those of the adrenal medulla which contain granules which stain brown when cells are stained with a fluid containing potassium bichromate. SEE: *c. reaction.*

   c. reaction. The turning brown of cytoplasmic granules containing epinephrine when subjected to stains containing chromium salts. Such granules stain green with ferric chloride, yellow with iodine, and brown with osmic acid. SEE: *c. cells.*

   c. system; c. tissue. The mass of tissue forming paraganglia and medulla of suprarenal glands, which secretes adrenalin and stains readily with chromium salts. Similar tissue is found in the organs of Zuckerkandl, and in the liver, testes, ovary, and heart. SEE: *adrenal gland.*

chromaffino'ma ["+ "+ Gr. *-ōma*, tumor]. A chromaffin cell tumor. SYN: *paraganglioma.*

chromaffinopathy (kro''maf-in-op'ă-thĭ) ["+ "+ Gr. *pathos*, disease]. Any disease of chromaffin tissue.

chromaphil (kro'maf-ĭl) ["+ *philein*, to love]. Pert. to a histological element or cell which stains readily with chromium salts. SYN: *chromaffin*, q.v.

chromate (krō'māt) [Gr. *chrōmatos*, color]. A salt of chromic acid. SEE: *potassium c.*

chromatelopsia (krō''mat-ē-lop'sĭ-ă) [Gr. *chrōma*, color, + *atelēs*, imperfect, + *opsis*, sight]. Color blindness.

chromat'ic. Pert. to color.

chromatid (kro'mă-tĭd). Either of the two bodies resulting from longitudinal splitting of a chromosome.

chromatin (krō'mă-tĭn) [Gr. *chrōma*, color]. A deeply staining substance present in the nucleus of a cell, and considered to be the physical basis of heredity. In a cell in interphase, it is in the form of a fine network bearing coarse granules.

chromatinolysis (kro''mă-tin-ol'ĭ-sis) ["+ *lysis*, dissolution]. 1. Destruction of chromatin. 2. The emptying of a cell, bacterial or other, by lysis.

chromatinorrhexis (kro''mă-tin-or-rek'sis) ["+ *rhēxis*, rupture]. Splitting of chromatin.

chromatism (kro′mă-tĭzm) [Gr. *chrōma*, color, + *-ismos*, condition]. 1. Unnatural pigmentation. 2. Chromatic aberration.

chromatodysopia (kro″mă-to-dis-o′pĭ-ă) [″+ *dys*, ill, + *opsis*, sight]. Color blindness.

chromatogenous (kro″mă-toj′en-us) [″+ *gennan*, to produce]. Causing pigmentation or color.

chromatogram (krō-mat′ō-gram) [Gr. *chrōma*, color, + *graphein*, to write]. Record produced by chromatography.

chromatography (krō″mă-tog′ră-fī). Chemical analysis by which a mixture of substances is separated by fractional extraction or adsorption on a porous solid (column of aluminum oxide or filter paper) by means of flowing solvents.

    c., paper. C. in which paper strips are used as the porous solid medium.

chromatolysis (kro″mă-tol′ĭ-sis) [Gr. *chrōma*, color, + *lysis*, dissolution]. Dissolution of chromophil substance (Nissl's bodies) in neurons in certain pathological conditions, or following injury to the cell body or axon.

chromatometer (krō-mă-tom′et-er) [″+ *metron*, measure]. A scale of colors for testing color perception.

chromatopathy (kro″mă-top′ă-thī) [″+ *pathos*, disease]. Any skin disease that is marked by pigmentation.

chromat′ophil, chromatophil′ic [″+ *philein*, to love]. Staining easily.

chromatophore (kro-mat′o-fōr) [Gr. *chrōma*, color, + *phoros*, bearing]. A pigment-bearing cell.

chromatopsia (kro″mă-top′sĭ-ă) [″+ *opsis*, vision]. Abnormally colored vision.

chromatoptometry (kro″mat-op-tom′ē-trĭ) [″+ *optos*, visible, + *metron*, measure]. Measurement of color perception.

chromatosis (kro″mă-tō′sis) [″+ *-osis*, condition]. 1. Pigmentation. 2. The pathological deposition of pigment in any part of the body where it is not normally present or excessive deposition where it is present.

chromaturia (kro-mă-tu′rĭ-ă) [Gr. *chrōma*, color, + *ouron*, urine]. Abnormal color of the urine.

chromesthe′sia [″+ *aisthēsis*, perception]. The association of color sensations with words, taste, smell or sounds.

chro′micized. Mixed with a chromium salt.

chromidiosis (kro-mid-ĭ-o′sis) [Gr. *chrōma*, color, + *-osis*, condition]. Overflow of chromatin and nuclear substance into cell protoplasm.

chromid′ium [″+ *-idion*, a dim. termination]. (pl. *chromidia*) An extranuclear granule seen in the cytoplasm of a cell.

chromidrosis (kro″mid-ro′sis) [″+ *hidrōs*, sweat]. Excretion of colored sweat. It may be black. This may be present in hysteria due to indican in the sweat. Red sweat may be due to an exudation of blood into the sweat glands, or to microorganisms in those glands.

    ETIOL: May be due to ingestion or absorption of certain substances, as pigment-producing bacteria. May be caused by certain disorders of metabolism.

    SYM: Localized in eyelids, breasts, axillae, genitocrural regions; occasionally on hands and limbs. It is grayish, bluish, violaceous, brownish; it collects on skin, giving a greasy, powdery appearance to parts.

    TREATMENT: Relief of underlying nervous affection.

    RS: anhidrosis; bromidrosis; chromidrosis; hidrosis; hyperidrosis; uridrosis.

chromium (kro′mĭ-um) [Gr. *chrōma*, color] SYMB: *Cr.* At. wt. 51.996; at. no. 24. A very hard, metallic element.

    POISONING: SYM: A disagreeable taste in the mouth, pain, diarrhea, collapse and cramping. If fatal, death is due to uremia.

    TREATMENT: Chalk, magnesia, and other weak alkalies to neutralize its acid effects. Wash out stomach and give cathartics, analgesics for pain.

chro′moblast [″+ *blastos*, germ]. An embryonic cell that becomes a pigment cell.

chromoblastomycosis (kro″mo-blas″tō-mĭ-kō′sĭs) [″+ *mykēs*, fungus, + *-osis*, condition]. One of a group of diseases marked by itching and warty plaques on the skin and subcutaneous swellings of feet, legs, and other exposed areas. SYN: *verrucous dermatitis.*

    ETIOL: Several fungi including Phialophora verrucosa, P. pedrosi, P. compactum, P. dermatidis, and Cladosporium carrionii.

chromocenter [″+ *kentros*, middle]. Karyosome, q.v.

chromocholoscopy (kro″mo-ko-los′ko-pĭ) [Gr. *chrōma*, color, + *cholē*, bile, + *skopein*, to examine]. Examination of the biliary function by a pigment-excretion test.

chromocrinia (kro″mo-krin′ĭ-ă) [″+ *krinein*, to separate]. The secretion or excretion of pigmented matter.

chromocystoscopy (kro″mo-sis-tos′ko-pĭ) [″+ *kystis*, bladder, + *skopein*, to examine]. Determination of functional activity of kidneys by use of dyes.

chromocyte (kro′mo-sit) [Gr. *chrōma*, color, + *kytos*, cell]. Any colored cell.

chromocytometer (kro″mo-sī-tom′et-er) [″+ ″+ *metron*, measure]. Instrument for determining the hemoglobin in red blood corpuscles.

chromodermatosis (kro"mo-der-mă-tō'sis) ["+ *derma*, skin, + *-ōsis*, condition]. Any pigmented skin disease.

chromogen (kro'mo-jen) [Gr. *chrōma*, color, + *gennan*, to produce]. Any principle that may be changed into coloring matter.

chromogen'esis ["+ *genesis*, production]. Production of pigment.

chromogen'ic. Pigment producing.

chromolipoid (kro"mo-lip'oyd) [Gr. *chrōma*, color, + *lipos*, fat, + *eidos*, appearance]. Any lipoid, such as carotin, that is pigmented. SYN: *lipochrome*.

chromolume (kro'mo-lūm) ["+ L. *lumen*, light]. Device for producing colored light rays used for therapeutic purposes.

chromolysis (kro-mol'ĭ-sĭs) ["+ *lysis*, dissolution]. Chromatolysis, q.v.

chromomere (kro'mo-mēr) [Gr. *chrōma*, color, + *meros*, part]. 1. One of a series of chromatin granules found in a chromosome. 2. A highly refractile purple granule which forms the central portion of a blood platelet.

chromometer (kro-mom'ĕ-ter) ["+ *metron*, measure]. Device for determining the pigment in a substance. SYN: *colorimeter*.

chromometry (kro-mom'et-rĭ). The estimation of coloring matter.

chromomycosis. Chromoblastomycosis, q.v.

chromopar'ic [Gr. *chrōma*, color, + L. *parēre*, to produce]. Producing color; chromogenic. Usually refers to bacteria which color their immediate surroundings.

chromopex'ic ["+ *pēxis*, fixation]. Pert. to fixation of coloring matter, as the liver function in forming bilirubin.

chromophage (kro'mo-fāj) ["+ *phagein*, to eat]. A phagocyte that destroys pigment; believed to be present in the blanching of hair. SYN: *pigmentophage*.

chromophane (kro'mo-fān) [Gr. *chrōma*, color, + *phainein*, to show]. Retinal pigment.

chromophil(e (kro'mo-fil, -fīl) ["+ *philein*, to love]. 1. Any structure that stains easily. 2. One of two types of cells present in pars distalis of the pituitary gland. It is considered a secretory cell.

chromophilic (kro-mo-fil'ik). Staining readily; chromophilous.

chromophilous (kro-mof'il-us). Chromophilic.

chromophobe (krō'mō-fōb) [Gr. *chrōma*, color, + *phobos*, fear]. Any cell or tissue which stains either poorly or not at all. A type of cell found in pars distalis of the pituitary gland.

chromophobic (krō-mō-fō'bĭk). Resistant to staining.

chromophor'ic [Gr. *chrōma*, color, + *phere-in*, to bear]. Pert. to or bearing color.

chromophose (kro'mo-fōz) ["+ *phōs*, light]. A subjective sensation of a spot of color in the eye. SEE: *centraphose; centrophose*.

chromophytosis (kro"mo-fi-tō'sis) ["+ *phyton*, plant, + *-ōsis*, infection]. Pigmentation of skin due to a vegetable parasite. Tinea, or pityriasis versicolor.

chro'moplasm ["+ *plasma*, that which is formed]. The network of a cell nucleus.

chromoplas'tid [Gr. *chrōma*, color, + *plastos*, formed]. Colored plastids other than chloroplasts present in plant cells.

chromoprotein (kro"mo-pro'tī-in) ["+ *prōtos*, first]. One of a group of conjugated proteins consisting of a protein combined with hematin or another colored, metal-containing, prosthetic group. Ex: hemoglobin; hemocyanin; chlorophyll; flavoproteins; cytochromes.

chromop'sia ["+ *opsis*, vision]. Chromatopsia; colored vision.

chromoptometer (kro"mop-tom'ĕ-ter) [Gr. *chrōma*, color, + *opsis*, sight, + *metron*, measure]. Instrument for determining keenness of color vision.

chro"moradiom'eter ["+ L. *radius*, ray, + Gr. *metron*, measure]. An instrument for measuring penetrative power of roentgen rays.

chromoscope (krō'mō-skōp) ["+ *skopein*, to examine]. Instrument for determining color perception.

chromoscopy (krō-mos'kō-pī). Examination for color vision.

chromosome (kro'mō-sōm) [Gr. *chrōma*, color, + *sōma*, body]. 1. A microscopic rod-shaped (J- or V-shaped) body which develops from the nuclear material of a cell and is esp. conspicuous during mitosis. Chromosomes stain deeply with basic dyes. They contain the genes or hereditary determiners.

The normal number of chromosomes is constant for each species, being 46 in man (i.e., 23 pairs in all somatic cells). These constitute the diploid number. In the formation of the gametes the number is reduced to one-half (haploid number), i.e., the ovum and sperm each contain 23, or one of each of the 23 pairs. Of these, 22 are autosomes and one is the sex chromosome (X or Y).

At time of fertilization the chromosomes from the sperm unite with the chromosomes from the ovum. At that moment the sex of the embryo is determined. The female sex chromosome from the ovum may contribute only an X to the embryo. The sperm or male sex chromosome may contribute an X or a Y as its half to join with the chromosome derived from the ovum. Thus the embryo may have XX in its sex chromosome in which case a female would develop; or XY, in which case a male would develop.

2. The unit of chromatin in the nucleus of a cell.

SEE: *heredity.*

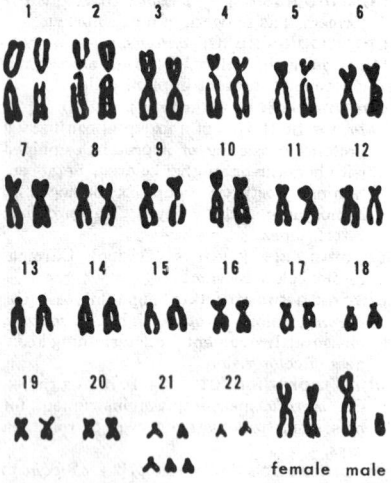

PAIRED HUMAN CHROMOSOMES

The normal number of chromosomes in a cell is 46 (23 pair). The first 22 pair are found in both men and women. The other pair is designated XX in the female and XY in the male. Occasionally, rather than the normal two chromosomes in pair 21, three chromosomes will appear as shown in the lower margin. When this occurs the patient has a mental deficiency known as trisomy-21.

   c., accessory. An unpaired monosome, a sex c., q.v.

   c., bivalent. A double chromosome resulting from the conjugation of two homologous chromosomes in synapsis which occurs during the first meiotic division.

   c.'s, giant. Extremely large chromosomes seen in the salivary glands and in other organs and tissues of insects. Also called polytenic chromosomes.

   c., sex. One of two chromosomes, the X- and Y-chromosomes, which are concerned with the determination of sex and carry the genes for sex-linked characters. In birds,

they are designated the Z- and W-chromosomes.

   c., somatic. An autosome, i.e., any chromosome except a sex chromosome.

   c., X-. One of a pair of female-determining chromosomes (XX) present in the somatic cells of all human females.

   c., Y-. The male-determining member of a pair of chromosomes (XY) present in the somatic cells of all human males. It is usually devoid of genes and in certain lower animals may be absent.

chro"mother'apy [Gr. *chrōma,* color, + *therapeia,* treatment]. The use of colored light in the treatment of disease.

chromotox'ic ["+ *toxikon,* poison]. Caused by toxic action on the hemoglobin.

chromoureteroscopy (kro"mo-ū-rē"ter-os'-ko-pĭ) ["+ *ouretēr,* ureter, + *skopein,* to examine]. Inspecting orifices of ureters after giving a substance to dye the urine.

chronaxia (kron-ak'sĭ-ă). Chronaxie, q.v.

chronaxie (krō'nak-sĭ) [Gr. *chronos,* time, + *axia,* value]. A number expressing the sensitiveness of a nerve to electrical stimulation.

It is the minimum duration, measured in seconds, during which a current of prescribed strength must pass through a motor nerve in order to cause contraction in the associated muscle; the strength of direct current (the rheobasic voltage) which will just suffice if given an indefinite time is first determined, and exactly double this strength is taken for the final determinations.

chronaximeter (kron"aks-im'et-er) ["+ "+ *metron,* measure]. Device for measuring chronaxia.

chron'ic [Gr. *chronos,* time]. Long, drawn out; applied to a disease that is not acute.

chronicity (kro-nis'it-ĭ). State of being chronic.

chronic obstructive lung disease. Disease process which causes decreased ability of the lungs to perform their function of ventilation. Diagnostic criteria include history of persistent dyspnea on exertion, with or without chronic cough, and less than one-half normal predicted maximum breathing capacity. Diseases which cause this are chronic bronchitis, pulmonary emphysema, chronic asthma, and chronic bronchiolitis.

chronobiol'ogy [Gr. *chronos,* time, + *bios,* life, + *logos,* study]. Study of the timing characteristics of life processes to attempt to describe the factors which influence biological rhythms.

chronograph (kron'o-graf) ["+ *graphein,* to write]. Device for recording short intervals of time.

chronological (krŏn″ō-lŏj′ĭ-kăl) [Gr. *chronos*, time, + *logos*, study]. Occurring in natural sequence according to time.

c. age. The number of years of one's life.

chron′oscope ["+ *skopein*, to examine]. Device for measuring extremely short intervals of time.

chronot′ropism ["+ *tropikos*, turning, + -*ismos*, condition]. Modification of periodic events such as the heart beat through external causes.

chrysarobin (kris″ă-rō′bin) [Gr. *chrysos*, gold, + Brazilian *a raraba*, bark]. A mixture of neutral principles obtained from goa powder, which is deposited in the wood of Araroba, a leguminous tree of South America. It is used topically, as an ointment, for treatment of psoriasis.

chthonophagia (thon″o-fā′jĭ-ă) [Gr. *chthōn*, earth, + *phagein*, to eat]. Eating clay or dirt; geophagy.

Chvostek's sign (vōs′tĕk). [Franz Chvostek, Austrian surgeon, 1835-1884] Local spasm following a tap on one side of face over area of facial nerve.

chylangioma (kī″lan-jĭ-o′mă) [Gr. *chylos*, juice, + *angeion*, vessel, + -*ōma*, tumor]. 1. Tumor of intestinal lymph vessels containing chyle. 2. Retention of chyle in lymphatic vessels with dilatation.

chyle (kīl) [Gr. *chylos*, juice]. The milklike contents of the lacteals and lymphatic vessels of the intestine consisting of the products of digestion and principally absorbed fats. It is carried by the lymphatic vessels to the cisterna chyli and then by way of the thoracic duct to the left subclavian vein where it enters the blood stream. A large quantity is formed in 24 hours. Reaction is alkaline.

    RS: achylia; cisterna chyli; oligochylia; receptaculum chyli; secretion.

chylemia (kī-lē′mĭ-ă) ["+ *haima*, blood]. Chyle in the peripheral circulation.

chylidrosis (kī-lĭ-drō′sis) ["+ *hidrōs*, sweat]. A milklike sweat resembling chyle.

chylifacient (kī″lĭ-fā′shent) ["+ L. *facere*, to make]. Forming chyle.

chylifaction (ki-lĭ-fak′shun). The formation of chyle. SYN: *chylification*.

chylifactive (ki-lĭ-fak′tiv). Forming chyle; chylifacient.

chyliferous (ki-lif′er-us) [Gr. *chylos*, juice, + L. *ferre*, to carry]. Carrying chyle.

chylification (ki-lĭ-fĭ-kā′shun). Chylifaction, q.v.

chylocele (ki′lo-sēl) [Gr. *chylos*, juice, + *kēlē*, tumor]. Infused chyle in tunica vaginalis testis.

chyloderma (ki″lo-der′mă) ["+ *derma*, skin]. Lymph accumulated in the enlarged lymphatic vessels and thickened skin of the scrotum; lymph scrotum; scrotal elephantiasis.

chylology (ki-lŏl′ō-jĭ) ["+ *logos*, study]. The study of chyle.

chylomediastinum (ki″lo-me″dĭ-as-ti′num) ["+ L. *mediastinum*, median]. Chyle in the mediastinum.

chylomicron (ki″lo-mi′kron) [Gr. *chylos*, juice, + *mikros*, small]. Small particle of fat in the blood after digestion and absorption of fat in the food, and perceptible under a microscope.

chylopericardium (ki″lo-per″ĭ-kar′dĭ-um) ["+ L. *peri*, around, + Gr. *kardia*, heart]. Chyle in the pericardium.

chyloperitone′um ["+ "+ *teinein*, to stretch]. Effused chyle in peritoneal cavity.

chylophoric (ki″lo-for′ĭk) ["+ *phoros*, bearing]. Conveying chyle; chyliferous.

chylopoiesis (ki″lo-poy-ē′sis) [Gr. *chylos*, juice, + *poiēsis*, production]. Formation of chyle and absorption by lacteals in the intestines. SYN: *chylification*.

chylotho′rax ["+ *thōrax*, chest]. Chyle in pleural cavities.

chylous (ki′lus). Pert. to or of the nature of chyle.

chyluria (ki-lu′rĭ-ă) [Gr. *chylos*, juice, + *ouron*, urine]. Chyle or fat globules in the urine.

chyme (kīm) [Gr. *chymos*, juice]. The mixture of partly digested food and digestive secretions found in the stomach and small intestine during digestion of a meal; it is a varicolored, thick, but nearly liquid mass. SEE: *oligochymia*.

chymosin (ki′mō-sin) [Gr. *chymos*, juice]. The enzyme in gastric juice which converts the milk protein caseinogen into casein. Calcium ions are necessary for this reaction. SYN: *rennin; chymase.*

chymosinogen (ki″mo-sin′o-jen) ["+ *gennan*, to produce]. A substance from which chymosin is formed.

chymotrypsin (ki″mo-trip′sin) ["+ *tryein*, to rub, + *pepsis*, digestion]. A proteolytic enzyme present in the intestine which, with trypsin, hydrolyzes proteins to peptones or further. It is secreted by the pancreas.

C.I. Abbr. for *color index; chemotherapeutic index* (parasitology).

cibisotome (sĭ-bis′o-tōm) [Gr. *kibisis*, pouch, + *tomē*, cut]. Instrument for incision of capsule of the lens.

cibophobia (sĭ″bō-fō′bĭ-ă) [L. *cibus*, food, + Gr. *phobos*, fear]. A morbid aversion to or fear of food.

cicatricial (sik″ă-trish'al) [L. *cicatrix,* scar]. Pert. to a cicatrix, q.v.

cicatricotomy (sik″ă-trik-ot'o-mĭ) ["+ Gr. *tomē,* incision]. Incision of a cicatrix or scar.

cicatrix (sik'ă-triks, sik-ā'triks) [L.]. A scar left by a healed wound.

Lack of color is due to absence of pigmentation. Cicatricial tissue is less elastic than normal tissue, hence it usually presents a contracted appearance. SEE: *keloid.*

cicatrizant (sĭk-at'rĭ-zant) [L. *cicatrix,* scar]. Favoring or causing, or an agent that aids in, cicatrization.

cicatrization (sik″ă-trĭ-zā'shun). Healing by scar formation. SEE: *intention.*

cicatrize (sik'ă-triz). To heal by scar tissue.

cicutism (sĭk'ū-tizm). Poisoning resulting from ingestion of Cicuta maculata or C. virosa, water hemlock.

cilia (sĭl'ĭ-ă) [L.]. (sing. *cilium*) 1. [NA] Eyelashes. 2. Hairlike processes projecting from epithelial cells, as in the bronchi, which propel mucus, pus, and dust particles. SEE: *biciliate.*

ciliariscope (sil″ĭ-ă'rĭ-skōp) [L. *ciliaris,* pert. to eyelash, + Gr. *skopein,* to examine]. Instrument for examination of the ciliary region of the eye.

ciliarotomy (sil″ĭ-ă-rot'o-mĭ) ["+ Gr. *tomē,* incision]. Surgical section of the ciliary zone in glaucoma.

cil'iary [L. *ciliaris,* pert. to eyelash]. Pert. to any hairlike processes, esp. to the eyelashes, and to eye structures such as the ciliary body.

c. arteries. Branches of the ophthalmic artery which supply the choroid layer.

c. body. Thickened part of vascular tunic of eye between base of iris and anterior part of choroid. Consists of three zones: c. disk, c. crown, and c. muscle.

c. ganglion. A ganglion lying in the posterior part of the orbit. Receives preganglionic fibers through the oculomotor nerve from the nucleus of Edinger-Westphal of the midbrain. From it six short ciliary nerves pass to the eyeball. Postganglionic fibers innervate the ciliary muscle, sphincter of the iris, and the smooth muscles of blood vessels of these structures, and also the cornea.

c. glands. Glands of Moll, a form of sweat glands of the eyelid.

c. muscle. Smooth muscle forming a part of the ciliary body of the eye. Contraction pulls the choroid forward, lessening tension on fibers of the zonula (suspensory ligament), thereby allowing the lens, which is elastic, to assume a more spherical shape; thus accomodation for near vision is accomplished.

c. nerves, long. Two or three branches of the nasal nerves supplying the c. muscle, iris, and cornea.

c. nerves, short. Several branches of the c. ganglion supplying the c. muscle, iris, and tunics of the eyeball.

c. processes. Consist of about 70 folds arranged meridionally so as to form a circle, have same structure as rest of choroid and secrete nutrient fluids which nourish neighboring parts, as cornea, lens, vitreous body. They also serve as points of attachment for the suspensory ligament of the lens. SYN: *processus ciliaris* [NA].

c. reflex. Normal contraction of pupil in accommodation of vision from distant to near.

cil'iate [L. *cilia,* eyelashes]. Ciliated.

ciliated (sil'ĭ-a-ted). Possessing cilia.

c. epithelium. Epithelium with hairlike processes on surface. They waft only in one direction and line the respiratory tract and fallopian tubes.

ciliectomy (sil″ĭ-ek'to-mĭ) [L. *cilium,* eyelash, + Gr. *ektomē,* excision]. Excision of portion of ciliary body or ciliary border of eyelid.

ciliospinal (sil″ĭ-o-spi'nal) ["+ *spinalis,* pert. to a spine]. Pert. to the ciliary body and spinal cord.

c. center. Spinal cord center which controls dilation of the pupil.

c. reflex. Dilation of pupil following stimulation of the skin of the neck by pinching or scratching the skin.

ciliostatic (sil″ĭ-o-stat'ik) ["+ *statos,* placed]. Interfering with or preventing movement of the cilia.

cilium (sĭl'ĭ-um) [L.]. [NA]. Sing. of cilia, q.v.

cillosis (sil-ō'sis) [L.]. Spasmodic twitching of the eyelid.

cimbia (sim'bĭ-ă) [L.]. Slender band of white fibers crossing the ventral surface of a cerebral peduncle.

Cimex lectularius (sī'mĕks lĕk-tū-lā'rĭ-ŭs). The bedbug. An insect belonging to the order Hemiptera.

cinchona (sĭn-kō'nă, -chō'nă) [Sp. *cinchon,* Countess of Cinchon]. The dried bark of the tree cinchona, the source of quinine. SYN: *Peruvian bark.* SEE: *quinine.*

cinchonism (sin'kon-izm) ["+ Gr. *ismos,* condition]. Poisoning from cinchona or its alkaloids.

cinchophen (sin'ko-fen). Atophan. Light yellow powder with slightly bitter taste. It frequently produces serious side effects, e.g., a fatal form of hepatitis; consequently it is seldom used in present-day medical therapy.

c. poisoning. SYM: Gastric irritation; nausea; vomiting; belching; heartburn; vertigo; weakness; diarrhea; itching; rash; jaundice; stupor. When chronic it is often associated with profound liver damage. Those with gallbladder disease; inflammation or cirrhosis of liver; the undernourished and those suffering from alcoholism are esp. susceptible.

F.A. TREATMENT: Largely symptomatic. Wash out stomach; give large quantities of fluids and saline catharsis.

cincture sensation (sĭnk'chŭr) [L. *cinctūra*, girdle]. Sensation of a tight girdle about the waist. SYN: *zonesthesia*.

cinemat'ics [Gr. *kinēma*, motion]. Science of motion; kinematics.

cinematoradiography (sin"ĭ-mat-o-rā"dĭ-og'ra-fĭ) ["+ L. *radius*, ray, + Gr. *graphein*, to write]. Radiography of an organ in motion.

cineplas'tics [Gr. *kinein*, to move, + *plassein*, to form]. Formation of muscles in a stump after amputation so that it is possible to impart motion and direction to an artificial limb.

cineraceous (sin-ē-rā'shus) [L. *cinis*, ashes]. Like ashes.

cinerea (sin-ē'rĭ-ā) [L. *cinēreus*, ashen-hued]. Gray matter of the brain or spinal cord.

    c., ala. An area at the posterior end of the fourth ventricle. Called the triangle of the vagus nerve.

cine'real. Pert. to the cinerea.

cineritious (sin"er-ish'us) [L. *cineritius*, ashen]. Ashen-gray color.

cinesi- [Gr. *kinēsis*, motion]. Prefix rel. to motion. SEE: words beginning with *kinesi-*.

cingulum (sin'gū-lum) [L. *cingulum*, girdle]. (pl. *cin'gula*) [NA] 1. A band of association fibers in the cingulate gyrus extending from anterior perforated substance posteriorly to the hippocampal gyrus. 2. An eminence on the lingual surface of the incisor teeth, esp. the upper ones. It is situated near the gum. Also called basal ridge.

cion (sī'ŏn) [Gr. *kiōn*, pillar]. The uvula, q.v.

circa (sĭr'kă) [L.]. About. Used before dates or figures which are approximate. ABBR: c.

circadian (sĭr"kă-dī'an) [L. *circa*, about, + *dies*, day]. Pert. to events which occur at approximately 24-hour intervals, such as certain biological rhythms. SEE: *clock, biological*.

circinate (sur'sĭ-nāt) [L. *circinatus*, made round]. Circular.

cir'cle [L. *circulus*, a little ring]. Any ring-shaped structure.

    c. of diffusion. One or more on projection plane of an image not in focus of the lens of the eye.

    c. of Willis. Union of the anterior and posterior cerebral arteries (branches of the carotid) forming an anastomosis at base of the brain.

cir'cuit [L. *circuire*, to go around]. 1. Course or path of an electric current. 2. The path followed by a fluid circulating in a system or tubes or cavities. 3. The path followed by nerve impulses in a reflex arc from sensory receptor to effector organ.

cir'cular [L. *circularis*]. 1. Shaped like a circle. 2. Recurrent.

    c. insanity. That in which manic and depressive attacks follow one another without intervals of lucidity.

circulation [L. *circulatio*]. Movement in a circular course.

    c. of the aqueous humor of the eye. SEE: *aqueous*.

    c. of bile salts. The sodium glycocholate and taurocholate found in hepatic bile pass with it into the duodenum and then into the intestine, where they are absorbed along with the fats.

    c. of the blood. The blood leaving the left ventricle enters the aorta, from which it escapes into the various large arteries. It thus reaches the coronary arteries of the heart itself and the arteries of the head, body wall, abdominal viscera, and extremities. Passing through the various capillary systems, it is gathered into veins, of which there are two systems: (1) Most veins empty their blood into the venae cavae superior and inferior. (2) The veins from the stomach, pancreas, spleen, and intestine unite to form the portal vein, which runs to the liver. In the latter, it breaks up into a new capillary system, which drains through the hepatic veins into the vena cava inferior. The combined blood of the venae cavae and the coronary veins enters the right atrium, passes through the right ventricle, and is forced out into the pulmonary artery. The pulmonary capillary system drains by way of the pulmonary veins into the left atrium and thence into the left ventricle.

    c. of the cerebrospinal fluid. SEE: *cerebrospinal*.

    c., collateral. Circulation which is established through an anastomosis between two vessels supplying or draining two adjacent vascular areas. This enables the blood to bypass an obstruction in the larger vessel supplying or draining the two areas, or will enable blood to flow to or from a tissue even though the principal vessel involved may be obstructed.

    c., coronary. Circulation through the

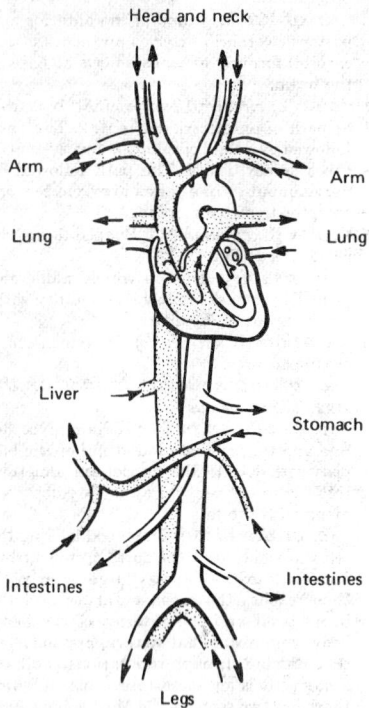

Head and neck

Arm

Arm

Lung

Lung

Liver

Stomach

Intestines

Intestines

Legs

CIRCULATION IN ADULT

muscular tissue of the heart. Blood leaves the aorta through the right and left coronary arteries which supply the myocardium. Blood passes through capillaries and is collected in veins most of which empty into the coronary sinus, which opens into the right atrium. A few of the small veins open directly into the atria and ventricles.

c., fetal. Circulation through the fetus. Blood, oxygenated in the placenta, passes through the umbilical vein and ductus venosus to the inferior vena cava and thence to the right atrium from which it may follow one of two courses—Through the foramen ovale to the left atrium and thence through the aorta to the tissues, or through the right ventricle, pulmonary artery, and ductus arteriosus to the aorta, and thence to the tissues. In either case the blood bypasses the lungs which are not functioning before birth. Blood is returned to the placenta through the umbilical arteries, which are continuations of the hypogastric arteries. At birth or shortly after, the ductus arteriosus and the foramen ovale close, establishing

normal circulation. Failure of either to occur gives rise to a "blue baby."

c. of the lymph. Lymph is formed from the tissue fluid which fills the tissue spaces of the body. It is collected into lymph capillaries which carry the lymph to the larger lymph vessels. These converge to form one of two main trunks, the right lymphatic duct and the thoracic duct. The right lymphatic duct drains the right side of the head, neck, and trunk and right upper extremity; the thoracic duct drains all the remaining portion of the body. It has its origin at the cisterna chyli, which receives the lymphatics from the abdominal organs. It courses upward through the diaphragm and thorax and empties into the left subclavian artery near its junction with the left interior jugular vein. The right lymphatic duct empties into the right subclavian vein. Along the course of lymph vessels there are lymph nodes which function as filtering structures. They filter out bacteria and particulate substances, thus preventing their entrance into the blood stream. Lymph flow is maintained by difference in pressure at the two ends of the system. Important accessory factors aiding the flow of lymph are breathing movements and muscular activities.

c., portal. Blood from the systemic arteries is supplied to the abdominal organs and is collected into the portal vein through which the blood enters the liver. It passes into sinusoids which lead to central veins of the lobules and eventually to the hepatic veins which empty into the inferior vena cava.

c., pulmonary. The venous blood which is received into the right atrium passes through the tricuspid valve into the right ventricle. From there into the pulmonary artery, which divides into two branches, one going to each lung. (This is the only instance when an artery contains venous or dark blood deficient in oxygen.) The artery branches in the lung into capillaries, and here, by means of the hemoglobin in the red corpuscles, the blood takes up oxygen from the inspired air. Red arterial blood returns to the heart by the four pulmonary veins, two from each lung, entering the left atrium. (This is the only instance where veins contain fully oxygenated blood.)

c. rate. The minute volume or output of the heart per minute. In an average size adult with a pulse rate of 70, the amount is about three liters per square meter of body surface each minute.

c., systemic. General circulation through the whole body except the lungs.

c., venous. C. of the blood via the veins.

circulation time. The time required by a particle of blood to make the complete circuit of both the systemic and pulmonary systems. C. t. is determined by injecting a substance into a vein and timing its reappearance in arteries at the point of injection. This procedure necessitates that the blood with the contained substance passes through veins to the heart and through the right atrium and ventricle, through the pulmonary circuit to the lungs, and back through the left atrium and ventricle, and then out through the aorta and arteries to the place where detected. Dyes such as florescein, methylene blue or substances such as potassium ferrocyanide or histamine have been used as tracers. Average circulation time is 18-24 seconds.

C. t. is reduced in anemia and hyperthyroidism; increased in hypertension, myxedema, and cardiac failure. C. t. may also be measured by injecting into a vein a substance which can be detected by the sense of taste when it is transported to the tongue. The normal c. t. from an arm vein to the tongue is 10-16 seconds.

c. time, pulmonary. The time required for blood to pass through the lungs. Average time 11 seconds.

cir'culatory. Pert. to circulation.

c. failure. Failure of the cardiovascular system to provide body tissues with an adequate amount of blood for proper functioning. It may be due to heart (cardiac) failure or peripheral circulatory failure, as occurs in shock, in which there is loss of blood plasma into the tissues with resulting decreased venous return.

c. system. The cardiovascular system consisting of the heart and blood vessels (arteries, arterioles, capillaries, venules, veins, and sinuses) and the lymphatic system.

c. system, inspection of. Inspection detects any abnormal centers of pulsation; the apex beat and its position, force, and extent; and any unnatural prominence over the precordial region. SEE: *abdomen; apex beat; chest; heart; lungs; pulsation.*

circum- [L.]. Prefix meaning around, as circumduction.

circumarticular (sĭr"kŭm-ar-tĭk'ū-lar) [L. *circum*, around, + *articulus*, small joint]. Surrounding a joint. SYN: *periarthric.*

circumcision (sir"kŭm-sī'shun) [L. *circumcisio*, a cutting around]. Surgical removal of the end of the prepuce of the penis. Done for hygienic reasons. Rate of occurrence of carcinoma of the penis is much less in persons who were circumcised at birth compared to those who were not.

NP: The foreskin is often tight after birth. It should be pulled back gently at birth to see that the meatus is clear, and then left alone for 8 days. After this, if still tight, it should be picked up in the thumb and finger and gently coaxed backwards twice a day. If it is inclined to bleed, smear it with an antiseptic ointment. Care must be taken not to strip it backwards too far or constriction of the glans (paraphimosis) may occur. If tightness still persists or there is any difficulty in passing urine, a doctor should be consulted. Often the gentle passage of a probe by the doctor, underneath the skin of the prepuce, will obviate any need to circumcise. Strict asepsis must be maintained in the dressing of a circumcision.

c., ritual. The religious rite performed by the Jews and Muslims at the time of removal of the prepuce.

circumclusion (sir"kŭm-klū'zhun) [L. *circumcludere*, to shut in]. Acupressure by use of a pin under an artery and a wire loop over it, attached to each end of the pin.

circumcor'neal [L. *circum*, around, + *corneus*, horny]. Around the cornea.

circumduction (sir"kŭm-duk'shun) ["+ *ducere*, to lead]. 1. The action or swing of a limb, such as the arm, in such a manner that it describes a cone-shaped figure, the apex of the cone being formed by the joint at the proximal end, while the complete circle is formed by the free distal end of the limb. 2. Circular movement of the eye.

circumflex (sir'kum-fleks) ["+ *flectere*, to bend]. Winding around, as a vessel.

c. nerve. A motor and sensory nerve. SYN: *axillary nerve; nervus axillaris* [NA]. SEE: *Table of Nerves* in *Appendix.*

circumin'sular [L. *circum*, around, + *insula*, island]. Surrounding the island of Reil in the cerebral cortex.

circumlen'tal ["+ *lens*, lens]. Situated around the lens.

circumnu'clear ["+ *nucleus*, kernel]. Surrounding the nucleus.

circumoc'ular ["+ *oculus*, eye]. Surrounding the eye.

circumor'al [L. *circum*, around, + *os, oris*, mouth]. Encircling the mouth.

c. pallor. White area around the mouth contrasting vividly with color of face, esp. seen in scarlet fever.

circumorbital (sir"kŭm-or'bĭt-ăl) ["+ *orbita*, orbit]. Around an orbit.

circumpolariza'tion ["+ *polaris*, polar]. The rotation of a ray of polarized light.

circumre'nal ["+ *renalis*, pert. to kidney]. Around or about the kidney.

cir'cumscribed ["+ *scribere*, to write]. Limited in space by that which is drawn around or confines an area.

cir"cumstantial'ity [L. *circum*, around, + *stāre*, to stand]. The mention of irrelevant facts and details in conversation. Usually a symptom of mental disorder.

circumval'late ["+ *vallāre*, to wall]. Surrounded by a wall or raised structure.

    c. papillae. V-shaped row of papillae at base of tongue.

circumvas'cular ["+ *vasculum*, vessel]. Perivascular; around a blood vessel.

cirrhosis (sĭ-rō'sĭs) [Gr. *kirrhos*, orange yellow, + *-ōsis*, infection]. A chronic disease of the liver characterized by formation of dense perilobular connective tissue; degenerative changes in parenchymal cells; alteration in structure of the cords of liver lobules; fatty and cellular infiltration; and sometimes development of areas of regeneration.

    In addition to the clinical signs and symptoms inherent in the cause of the c., those due to c. are the result of loss of functioning liver cells and increased resistance to flow of blood through the liver (portal hypertension).

    ETIOL: May be due to various factors such as nutritional deficiency (lack of proteins, choline, or methionine); or poisons (carbon tetrachloride, phosphorus); or may be due to previous inflammation caused by a virus or by bacteria.

    c., alcoholic. That occurring commonly in alcoholics. When c. occurs in persons who are chronic alcoholics, it is due to the alcohol and impaired nutrition, not to alcohol alone. SEE: *C., Laennec's.*

    c., biliary. That marked by prolonged jaundice due to chronic retention of bile and inflammation of bile ducts. SEE: *c., obstructive biliary; c., primary biliary.*

    c., cardiac. Congestive c. resulting from passive congestion of the liver due to congestive heart failure.

    c., coarse nodular. C., postnecrotic, q.v.

    c., fatty. C. with fatty infiltration of the liver cells.

    c., hypertrophic. C. in which the connective tissue hyperplasia causes the liver to be greatly enlarged.

    c., infantile. C. occurring in childhood, resulting from protein malnutrition. Also called kwashiorkor.

    c., Laennec's. The most common type of c. seen in North America. Its etiology is

unknown but is related to a combination of chronic alcoholism and impaired nutrition. In early stages the liver is enlarged, but as the disease progresses the liver becomes atrophic and nodular. Also called portal c. and alcoholic c., but these are misnomers.

    c., obstructive biliary. C. resulting from obstruction of the common duct by a stone, tumor, etc.

    c., postnecrotic. Form characterized by extensive destruction of liver cells as occurs in poisoning or following infections. Massive scarring occurs with areas of regeneration. SYN: *coarse nodular c.; healed yellow atrophy; toxic c.*

    c., primary biliary. A rare, progressive form of c. characterized by enlargement of the liver, jaundice, and pruritus. SYN: *cholangiolitic c.*

    c., syphilitic. Form occurring in tertiary syphilis in which gummas form in the liver and, on healing, cause coarse lobulation. SYN: *hepar lobatum.*

    c., toxic. That resulting from toxic substances as in poisoning by carbon tetrachloride or phosphorus. SEE: *C., postnecrotic.*

    c., zooparasitic. C. resulting from infestation with animal parasites, esp. blood flukes of the genus Schistosoma, or liver flukes, Clonorchis sinensis.

cirrhotic (sĭ-rŏt'ĭk). Pert. to or affected with cirrhosis.

cirsectomy (sir-sek'tō-mĭ) [Gr. *kirsos*, varix, + *ektomē*, excision]. Excision of a portion of a varicose vein.

cirsenchysis (sir-sen'kĭ-sis) ["+ *enchysis*, a pouring in]. Injection of varicose veins with a sclerosing substance.

cirsocele (sir'sō-sēl) ["+ *kēlē*, hernia]. Dilation of veins of spermatic cord. SYN: *varicocele*, q.v.

cirsodesis (sir-sod'ĕ-sis) [Gr. *kirsos*, varix, + *desis*, ligation]. Ligation of varicose veins as a method of treating them.

cirsoid (sir'soyd) ["+ *eidos*, resemblance]. Resembling a varix. SYN: *varicose.*

cirsomphalos (sir-som'fă-los) ["+ *omphalos*, navel]. Varicose veins around the navel.

cirsotome (sir'so-tōm) [Gr. *kirsos*, varix, + *tomē*, cut]. Instrument for cutting varicose veins.

cirsotomy (sir-sot'ō-mĭ) ["+ *tennein*, to cut]. Treatment of a varicosity by multiple incisions.

C.I.S. Abbr. for *central inhibitory state.*

cister'na [L.]. [NA] A reservoir or cavity.

    c. chy'li. [NA]. Receptaculum chyli. A dilated sac into which empties the intestinal, two lumbar, and two descending lymphatic trunks; the origin of the thoracic duct.

c., subarachnoidalis. [NA]. Wide spaces in the cranial cavity between the arachnoid and the pia mater. They contain cerebrospinal fluid.

cisternal (sĭs-ter'năl). Concerning a cavity filled with fluid.

c. puncture. A spinal puncture with a hollow needle between the cervical vertebrae, through the dura mater into the cisterna at base of brain.

PURPOSE: To inject a drug or a serum as in cerebral meningitis or cerebral syphilis, or to remove spinal fluid for diagnostic purposes or to reduce intracranial pressure. Should be used as a source of spinal fluid only if fluid cannot be obtained by lumbar puncture. SEE: *cerebrospinal fluid; spinal puncture.*

cisternography, isotope. SEE: *isotope cisternography.*

cisvestitism (sĭs-vĕs'tĭ-tĭzm) [L. *cis,* on this side of, + *vestitus,* dressed]. Wearing of clothes appropriate to one's sex but suitable for a calling or profession other than one's own. Ex: a civilian who dresses in a uniform of the armed services.

Citel'li's syndrome (che-tel'ĭ). [Salvatore Citelli, It. laryngologist, 1875-1947] Symptoms of poor memory, mental backwardness, insomnia or drowsiness, and lack of concentration in those with infected adenoids or sphenoid sinusitis.

citrate (sīt'rāt, sī'trāt). Compound of citric acid and a base.

c. solution. Solution used to prevent clotting of the blood. Its use permits whole blood to be stored in a refrigerator until it is needed for transfusion.

citric acid. $C_6H_8O_7.H_2O$. A tribasic acid present in the juice of many fruits, esp. citrus fruits. SEE: *acid.*

citric acid cycle. A complicated series of reactions in the body involving the oxidative metabolism of pyruvic acid and liberation of energy. It is the main pathway of terminal oxidation in the process of which not only carbohydrates but proteins and fats are utilized. SYN: *Kreb's cycle; tricarboxylic acid cycle.*

Cl. 1. Chem. symb. for chlorine. 2. Abbr. for *chloride; clavicle; Clostridium.*

cladosporiosis (klăd''ō-spō-rĭ-ō'sĭs) [Gr. *klados,* branch, + *sporos,* seed, + *-ōsis,* condition]. An infection, usually of the central nervous system, with a fungus, Cladosporium.

Cladosporium. A genus of fungi. Tinea nigra is caused by either C. werneckii or C. mansonii.

clam. A bivalve belonging to the phylum Mollusca.

Food value of 100 gm. (soft, raw): Cal. 82; protein 14 gm.; fat 1.9 gm.; carbohydrate 1.3 gm.

clamp (klămp) [MD. *klampe,* metal clasp]. Device used in surgery to grasp, join, compress, or support an organ, tissue, or vessel.

clang [L. *clangere,* to peal]. A loud, metallic sound.

c. tint. A delicate tone.

clap. Colloquial term for gonorrhea.

clapotage, clapotement (klă''po-tazh', klă-pot-maw') [Fr.]. Any splashing sound in succussion of a dilated stomach.

Clap'ton's lines. Green lines on dental margin of gums in copper poisoning.

clar'et stain [L. *clārāre,* to make clear]. Capillary nevus of cheek. SYN: *claret cheek; nevus flammeus.*

clarificant (klar-if'ik-ant) [L. *clarus,* clear, + *facere,* to make]. Any agent that clears the turbidity of a liquid.

Clarke's bodies. [Jacob A. L. Clarke, Eng. anatomist, 1817-1880] Alveolar sarcomatous intranuclear bodies of breast.

Clarke's column. The dorsal nucleus of the spinal cord.

clasmatoblast (klaz-mat'o-blast) [Gr. *klasma,* fragment, + *blastos,* germ]. A mast cell.

clasmatocyte (klaz-mat'o-sit) [" + *kytos,* cell]. A large, wandering, uninucleated cell with many branches.

A fixed macrophage of loose connective tissue. It is capable of ingesting particulate material and has the property of electively storing certain dyes in colloidal solution. In inflammatory conditions it becomes actively ameboid and is important in providing protection against local invasion by bacteria which it ingests. SYN: *histiocyte; tissue macrophage.*

clasmatodendro'sis [" + *dendron,* tree, + *-ōsis,* condition]. A breaking up of astrocytic protoplasmic expansions.

clasmato'sis. Crumbling into small bits; fragmentation, as of cells.

clasp-knife rigidity. Spastic action in a joint in cerebral palsies.

class [L. *classis,* division]. 1. In biology, a group of clearly defined animals or plants below a phylum and above an order. 2. In statistics, a group of variables which fall within certain value limits.

clastic (klas'tik) [Gr. *klastos,* broken]. Causing division into parts.

clastothrix (klas′tō-thriks) [″+ *thrix*, hair].
Splitting of the hair. SEE: *trichorrhexis.*

claudication (klaw-dĭ-kā′shun) [L. *claudicāre*, to limp]. Lameness; limping.

    c., intermittent. A severe pain in calf muscles occurring during walking but which subsides with rest. It results from inadequate blood supply which may be due to arterial spasm, atherosclerosis, arteriosclerosis, or an occlusion.

    c., venous. That resulting from inadequate venous drainage.

Claudius′ cells (klaw′dĭ-us). [Friedrich Claudius, Austrian anatomist, 1822-69] Large columnar cells external to the organ of Corti.

Claudius′ fossa. Small depression in posterior part of pelvis, on either side, in which lies the ovary.

claustrophilia (klaws-tro-fil′ĭ-ă) [L. *claustrum*, a barrier, + Gr. *philein*, to love]. Dread of being in an open space; a morbid desire to be shut in with doors and windows closed.

claustrophobia (klaws-tro-fō′bĭ-ă) [″+ *phobos*, fear]. Fear of being confined in any space, as in a locked room. Opposed to agoraphobia, q.v.

claustrum (klŏs′trŭm) [L.]. 1. A barrier. 2. Thin layer of gray matter separating the external capsule from the island of Reil.

clausura (klŏ-sū′ră) [L.]. Atresia of a passage, closure.

clava (kla′vă) [L., club]. (pl. *clavae*) An elevation on dorsal surface of the medulla oblongata caused by the underlying nucleus gracilis, the superior extremity of the fasciculus gracilis.

cla′vate. Club-shaped.

clav′icle [L. *clavicula*, little key]. The collarbone; a bone, curved like the letter f, that articulates with the sternum and the scapula.

    c., dislocation of. Forward, Sternal End: TREATMENT: Place knee against spine and draw shoulders back; apply c. bandage with pad on dislocated end of bone.

    Outer Extremity: Bone upon upper surface of acromion, or upon anterior part of spine of the scapula.

    SYM: Prominence upon surface of acromion which disappears when arm is raised. Shoulders flattened, arm hanging close to trunk.

    TREATMENT: Raise shoulder, draw backward; place pad in axilla, bringing elbow close to side; secure arm and forearm to chest with pad in axilla; pressure by pad and gutta percha plate on projecting clavicle strapped in place. SEE: *jugulum.*

    c., fracture of. SYM: Swelling, pain, protuberance with sharp depression over the injured bone. Patient holds the immobile arm by supporting it at the elbow.

    F.A. TREATMENT: Place ball of cloth, one or two handkerchiefs, tightly rolled, under armpit. Apply arm sling; bandage elbow to side, hand and forearm extending across the chest. Or lay patient on back on the floor with rolled-up blanket under shoulders until medical aid arrives. This position keeps shoulders back and prevents broken ends of bone from rubbing.

    TREATMENT: Have assistant draw arms and shoulders backward. Raise shoulders and support in upward, backward, and outward direction. Cover parts with adhesive plaster and bandage.

clavicular (klă-vĭk′ū-lăr). Pert. to the clavicle.

clavus (klā′vŭs) [L., nail]. 1. A corn or callosity. 2. A sharp head pain described as feeling like a nail being driven into the head.

clawfoot. A deformity of the foot characterized by excessively high longitudinal arch, usually accompanied by dorsal contracture of toes. SYN: *contracted foot; hollow foot; pes cavus.*

clawhand. A hand characterized by hyperextension of the proximal phalanges of the digits and extreme flexion of middle and distal phalanges. Usually the result of injury to ulnar and median nerves. SYN: *main en griffe.*

claw toe. A hammer toe; extreme flexion of a toe.

Clayton gas. Sulfur dioxide.

clear′ance. The elimination of a substance from the blood plasma by the kidneys. SEE: *renal clearance test.*

clear′ing agent. One that makes tissues prepared for microscopic examination more transparent.

cleavage (klē′vĕj) [AS. *cleofian*, to cleave]. 1. Splitting a complex molecule into two or more simpler ones. 2. Cell division following the fertilization of an egg. SYN: *segmentation.*

    c. cell. The blastomere.

    c., hydrolytic. Hydrolysis.

    c. lines. Lines indicating the prevailing direction of fibers in the corium of the skin. In a living subject or fresh cadaver, a puncture wound does not remain round but becomes elliptical in the direction of the fibers. Lines in general run obliquely. This is important to the surgeon because an incision parallel to these lines will heal with much less scarring than one across the lines. SYN: *Langer's lines; tension lines.*

cleft [ME. *clift*, crevice]. 1. A fissure. 2. Divided or split.

   c., **branchial.** An opening between the branchial arches of an embryo. In lower vertebrates it becomes a gill cleft.

   c. cheek. Macrostomia; transverse facial cleft.

   c., *facial.* An anomaly resulting from failure of facial processes of embryo to fuse. Common ones are oblique facial cleft, an open nasolacrimal furrow extending from eye to lower portion of nose which is sometimes continuous with a cleft in upper lip; transverse facial cleft which extends laterally from the angle of the mouth.

   c. foot. A bipartite foot resulting from failure of a digit and its corresponding metatarsal to develop.

   c. hand. A bipartite hand resulting from failure of a digit and its corresponding metacarpal to develop.

   c. palate. A congenital fissure in the palate (roof of mouth) forming a communicating passageway between mouth and nasal cavities. May be unilateral or bilateral, complete or incomplete.

   c. sternum. A congenital fissure of the breastbone.

   c. tongue. A bifid tongue; one with a separated tip.

cleido- (kli'do) [Gr. *kleis,* used for closing]. Prefix pert. to the clavicle.

cleidorrhexis (kli''dō-rek'sis) [Gr. *kleis,* used for closing, + *rhéxis,* rupture]. Fracture or bending the clavicles of the fetus for delivery.

cleidotomy (kli-dot'o-mī) ["+ *tomē,* a cutting]. Dividing a fetal clavicle to facilitate delivery.

cleptomania [Gr. *kleptein,* to steal, + *mania,* madness]. Compulsive stealing, the intrinsic value of the article not being the motive. SYN: *kleptomania,* q.v.

climacteric (kli-măk'ter-ĭk, kli-mak-ter'-ĭk) [Gr. *klimaktēr,* a rung of a ladder]. That period that marks the cessation of a woman's reproductive period (female climacteric or menopause); a corresponding period of lessening of sexual activity in the male (male climacteric).

climatology [Gr. *klima,* sloping surface of the earth, + *logos,* study]. Branch of meteorology which includes the study of climate and its relationship to disease. SEE: *bioclimatology.*

climatotherapy (kli''mat-ō-ther'ap-ĭ) ["+ *therapeia,* treatment]. Treatment of disease by having patient move to a more favorable climate.

climax [Gr. *klimax,* ladder]. 1. Period of greatest intensity. 2. The orgasm, q.v.

climograph [Gr. *klima,* sloping surface of the earth, + *graphein,* to write]. A graph of the effect of climate on health.

clinic (klĭn'ĭk) [Gr. *klinikos,* pert. to a bed]. 1. Medical instruction in which patients are observed directly, symptoms noted, treatment discussed, etc. 2. A center for physical examination and treatment of ambulant patients who are not hospitalized. 3. A place where individuals gather together with patients for the study of disease. 4. A place where preliminary diagnosis is made and treatment given, as an x-ray clinic or child-guidance clinic.

   c., *free standing.* Medical outpatient clinic which is community based and not part of a hospital.

clinical. 1. Founded on actual observation and treatment of patients as distinguished from data or facts obtained by experimentation or pathology. 2. Pert. to a clinic.

   c. analysis. The chemical analysis and study of body fluids, excreta, and tissues in the diagnosis and treatment of disease.

   c. pathology. That division of pathology which utilizes clinical analysis and other laboratory procedures in the diagnosis and treatment of disease.

   c. procedures. Procedures usually carried out by a physician or under his immediate supervision, and usually at the patient's bedside, in contrast to bedside procedures (those carried on by nurses), or office procedures. C. p. involves route of medication, local anesthesia, aspiration of fluids, administration of oxygen, etc.

   c. thermometer. Thermometer which measures body temperature. It may be disinfected by first cleansing with cotton and soap solution, using a rotary motion downward to bulb end. This removes adherent mucus which coagulates in some disinfectants, thereby retaining organisms. Rinse thoroughly in tepid, not hot, water and submerge in 70% alcohol for 10 minutes. Rinse before use. SEE: *thermometer.*

clinician (klin-ish'an) [Gr. *klinikos,* pert. to a bed]. A practicing physician.

clinodactylism (kli''no-dak'tĭ-lizm). Clinodactyly.

clinodactyly (kli''no-dak'tĭ-lĭ) [Gr. *klinein,* to bend, + *daktylos,* finger]. Permanent deflection, either medial or lateral, of one or more fingers.

clinoid (kli'noyd) [Gr. *klinē,* bed, + *eidos,* appearance]. Resembling a bed in shape.

   c. processes. Three pairs of prominences on upper surface of sphenoid bone.

clinom'eter [Gr. *klinein*, to slope, + *metron*, measure]. Instrument for estimation of torsional deviation of eyes. This is used to measure ocular muscle paralysis. SYN: *clinoscope.*

cli'noscope [" + *skopein*, to examine]. Instrument for measuring the weakness of ocular muscles.

clinostat'ic [Gr. *kline*, bed, + *stasis*, position]. Occurring when the patient is in a recumbent position.

clinostat'ism. The recumbent position.

clip. Instrument for holding tissue or other material together.

cliseometer (klis"ē-om'et-er) [Gr. *klisis*, inclination, + *metron*, measure]. Device for measuring the inclination which the female pelvis makes with the spinal column.

clithrophobia (klith"ro-fo'bĭ-ā) [Gr. *kleithria*, keyhole, + *phobos*, fear]. Morbid fear of being locked in.

clition (klit'ĭ-on) [Gr. *kleitys*, slope]. A craniometric point in center of highest part of the clivus on the sphenoid bone.

clitoridauxe (klĭ"tō-rid-awk'sĭ) [Gr. *kleitoris*, clitoris, + *auxe*, increase]. Hypertrophy of the clitoris.

clitoridectomy (klĭ"tō-rid-ek'tō-mĭ) [" + *ektomē*, excision]. Excision of clitoris.

clitoriditis (klĭ"tō-rid-i'tis) [" + *-itis*, inflammation]. Inflammation of the clitoris.

clitoridotomy (klĭ"tō-rid-ot'ō-mĭ) [" + *tomē*, cut]. Incision of the clitoris, female circumcision.

clitoris (klĭ'tō-rĭs, klit'ō-rĭs) [Gr. *kleitoris*, clitoris]. One of the structures of the female genitalia. It is an erectile part, located beneath the anterior labial commissure and partially hidden by the anterior ends of the labia minora. It is homologous to the penis of the male.

STRUCTURE: It consists of three parts: a body, two crura, and a glans. The body, about an inch (2.5 cm.) in length, consists of two fused corpora cavernosa. It extends from the pubic arch above to the glans below. The two crura are continuations of the corpora cavernosa and serve to attach them to the inferior rami of the pubic bones. They are covered by the ischiocavernosus muscles. The glans, which forms the free distal end, is a small rounded tubercle composed of erectile tissue. It is highly sensitive. The glans is usually covered by a hood-like prepuce and its ventral surface is attached to the frenulum of the labia.

c. crises. Recurring involuntary crises of excess of sexual excitement in women. Occurs in tabes dorsalis.

clitorism (klĭ'tō-rizm). 1. The counterpart of priapism. A long-continued, painful condition in the female with recurring erection of the clitoris. 2. Enlargement of the clitoris.

clitoritis (klĭ"tō-ri'tis). Inflammation of the clitoris. SYN: *clitoriditis.*

clivus (kli'vus) [L. *clivus*, a slope]. A surface that slopes, as the sphenoid bone.

c. blumenbach'ii. The slope at base of skull.

clo. A unit of thermal insulation.

cloaca (klo-ā'kă) [L. *cloaca*, a sewer]. 1. Cavity lined with endoderm at the posterior end of the body which serves as a common passageway for urinary, digestive, and reproductive ducts. Present in adults of birds, reptiles, and amphibia and in the embryos of all vertebrates. 2. An opening in the sheath covering necrosed bone.

clock [LL. *clocca*]. Device for measuring time.

c., biological. An internal mechanism which apparently regulates cyclic phenomena such as the wake-sleep cycle, menstrual cycle, and hourly variations in the level of hormones such as those from the adrenal cortex. SEE: *circadian.*

clomid. SEE: *clomiphene citrate.*

clomiphene citrate. A nonsteroidal agent used to stimulate ovulation in women who have potentially functioning pituitary and ovarian systems. Persons treated with this medicine who become pregnant have an increased incidence of multiple births. SYN: *clomid.*

clone (klōn) [Gr. *klōn*, a cutting used for propagation]. In tissue culture, a group of cells descended from a single cell.

clonic (klōn'ik) [Gr. *klonos*, turmoil]. Pert. to alternate contraction and relaxation of muscles.

c. spasm. One marked by muscular rigidity and then relaxation.

clonicity (klōn-ĭs'ĭ-tĭ). Being clonic.

clonicotonic (klōn"ĭ-kō-tŏn'ĭk) [Gr. *klonos*, turmoil, + *tonikos*, tonic]. Both clonic and tonic, as some forms of muscular spasm.

clon'ism, clonis'mus [" + *-ismos*, condition of]. Condition of being affected with clonic spasms, or a succession of them.

clon'ograph [" + *graphein*, to write]. An instrument for registering spasmodic movements.

clon'ospasm [" + *spasmos*, spasm]. Rapid alternation of muscular contraction and relaxation.

The rate is much slower than a tremor. In upper motor neuron paralysis, sharp flexion of ankle often produces ankle clonus.

clo'nus. Spasmodic alternation of contraction and relaxation; opposite of tonus.

Cloquet's canal (klō-kā'). [Jules Germain Cloquet, Fr. surgeon, 1790-1883]. An irregular passage (hyaloid) through center of the vitreous body in the fetus.

Clostrid'ium [Gr. *klōstēr,* spindle]. A genus of bacteria belonging to the family Bacillaceae. They are anaerobic, spore-forming rods and are widely distributed in nature. They are common in the soil and in the intestinal tract of man and animals and are frequently found in wound infections. Several are pathogenic in man, being the primary causative agents for gas gangrene.

Cl. botulinum. Grows in improperly processed food. Produces a powerful toxin, the cause of botulism, q.v.

Cl. chauvoei. Cause of blackleg, or symptomatic anthrax, in cattle.

Cl. histolyticum. A proteolytic organism found in gas gangrene.

Cl. novyi. Found in cases of gas gangrene. SYN: *Novy's bacillus.*

Cl. perfringens. A cause of gas gangrene. SYN: *gas bacillus; Cl. welchii.*

Cl. septicum. Found in cases of gangrene in man, cattle, hogs, and other domestic animals.

Cl. sporogenes. Frequently associated with other organisms in mixed gangrenous infections. It is non-pathogenic.

Cl. tetani. The causative organism of tetanus or lockjaw. Produces a powerful exotoxin, a portion of which affects nerve tissue, another portion is hemolytic.

Cl. welchii. Cl. perfringens, q.v.

clot (klōt) [AS. *clott,* lump]. 1. To coagulate. 2. A thrombus; a coagulum, as of blood or lymph.

SEE: *blood, clotting of; thrombosis.*

c., agony. One formed in the heart when death ensues from prolonged heart failure.

c., antemortem. One formed in the heart or its cavities before death.

c., blood. A coagulum formed of blood.

c., chicken fat. A yellow-colored blood clot appearing to contain no erythrocytes.

c., currant jelly. A clot of fibrin of reddish color and jellylike consistency.

c., distal. One formed in a vessel on distal side of a ligature.

c., external. One formed outside a blood vessel.

c., heart. A thrombus within the heart.

c., internal. One formed by coagulation of blood within a vessel.

c., laminated. One formed in a succession of layers filling an aneurysm.

c., muscle. One formed in muscle tissue.

c., passive. One formed in the sac of an aneurysm.

c., plastic. One formed from the intima of an artery at the point of ligation.

c., postmortem. One formed in the heart or blood vessel after death.

c., proximal. One formed on the proximal side of a ligature.

c., stratified. Thrombus consisting of layers of different colors.

clothes louse. Pediculus corporis; a body louse.

cloth'ing [AS. *clāth,* cloth]. Wearing apparel. Used both functionally and decoratively. From the medical standpoint clothes serve to conserve heat or to protect the body. Ex: gloves, sunhelmets, and shoes.

Air spaces in a fabric conserve heat. It is texture, not the material alone, that makes for warmth. Woolen fabrics lose in warmth when the material is matted down and the air spaces are destroyed. Wool and silk absorb more moisture than other fabrics but silk loses it more readily. Cotton and linen come next but linen loses moisture more quickly than cotton. Open mesh is necessary to prevent chill from evaporation. Knitted fabrics absorb and dry more readily than woven fabrics of the same material. Temperature inside a hat worn by a man varies from 13°-20° warmer than the outside temperature. Body heat is increased when moisture from wet garments cannot escape.

clot'ting. Coagulation, q.v.

c. time. Coagulation time, q.v.

clouding of consciousness. A state of mental confusion characterized by insufficiency of perception and impaired attention, and resulting in loss of orientation of time and place, amnesia and ill-adjusted reactions. Occurs in toxic, febrile, and other deliria as well as in cases where insufficient oxygen is being supplied to the brain. SEE: *consciousness.*

clou'dy swelling. Degeneration in which the tissues swell and become turbid.

clo'ven spine. Spina bifida. Congenital defect of spinal canal walls caused by lack of union between laminae of the vertebrae.

clove oil [L. *clavus,* a nail or spike]. USP. A volatile oil distilled from the dried flower buds of the clove tree. SYN: *Caryophyllus.*

ACTION AND USES: Antiseptic and aromatic. Useful also as an anodyne in dental practice.

clown'ism. Grotesque actions and attitudes, esp. that in certain hysterical states or in epilepsy.

clubbed fingers. Rounding of ends and swelling of fingers in children with congenital heart disease and in older children and adults with long standing pulmonary disease.

clubfoot. Nontraumatic congenital foot deformity. SEE: *talipes.*

clubhand. Deformity of the hand resembling clubfoot. SYN: *talipomanus,* q.v.

clumping [AS. *clympre,* a lump]. Thick grouping of microorganisms in a culture when specific immune serum is added. SYN: *agglutination.*

clu'nes [L. pl. of *clunis,* buttock]. [NA]. The buttocks; nates.

cluster headache. A headache similar to migraine, occurring as often as two or three times a day over a period of weeks. After this cluster of headaches, the patient may be free of symptoms for weeks or months.

SYM: The headaches come on abruptly and are characterized by intense throbbing pain behind the nostril and one eye. The eye and nose water, the skin over the throbbing area becomes red, and the pupil of the eye may become constricted. An attack rarely lasts longer than two hours.

TREATMENT: Ergotamine tartrate is useful for both treatment and prophylaxis.

cluttering. A speech defect characterized by omission of letters or syllables.

Clutton's synovitis. [Henry Hugh Clutton, Eng. surgeon, 1850-1909] Hydroarthrosis of the knee joint often associated with interstitial keratitis, seen in congenital syphilis. SYN: *Clutton's joint.*

clysis (kli'sis) [Gr. *klyzein,* to cleanse]. Injection of fluid into the body. This may be done by injecting the fluid into tissue spaces, into the rectum or the abdominal cavity.

clysma (klis'mä) [Gr. *klysma,* a drenching]. An enema, q.v.

clys'ter [Gr. *klystēr,* syringe]. An enema; a clysma.

C.M. Abbr. for *chirurgiae magister,* Master in Surgery.

C/M. Abbr. for *counts per minute.*

cm. Abbr. for *centimeter.*

CN. Abbr. for *cyanogen.*

cnemial (nē'mĭ-al). Pert. to the leg, esp. the shin.

cnemis (nē'mĭs) [Gr. *knēmis,* legging]. Shin, lower leg, tibia.

cnemitis (nē-mi'tis) ["+ *-itis,* inflammation]. Inflammation of the tibia.

CNS. Abbr. for *central nervous system.*

CO. Chem. formula for carbon monoxide.

CO₂. Chem. formula for carbon dioxide.

    CO₂ therapy. Therapeutic application of low temperatures with solid carbon dioxide. Also inhalation of carbon dioxide to stimulate breathing. SEE: *refrigeration.*

Co. Chem. symb. for cobalt.

coadunation (kō"ad-u-nā'shun) [L. *co-,* together, + *ad,* to, + *unus,* one]. Union or junction of dissimilar substances in one mass.

coagglutina'tion [L. *coāgulāre,* to curdle]. Clumping by an antigen and the homologous antibody of the corpuscles of another organism.

coag'ula [L.]. Pl. of coagulum. Blood clots or curds.

coagulable (kō-ag'u-lä-bl). Capable of clotting; apt to clot.

coagulant (ko-ag'u-lant) [L. *coagulans,* congealing]. 1. That which causes a fluid to coagulate. 2. Causing coagulation.

coagulase (ko-ag'u-lāz) [L. *coagulum,* blood clot]. Any enzyme, such as thrombin, which causes coagulation.

coagulate (ko-ăg'ū-lāt) [L. *coāgulāre,* to congeal]. To solidify or to change from a fluid state to a semisolid mass.

coag'ulated. Clotted or curdled.

    c. proteins. Derived proteins (insoluble), resulting from the action of alcohol on protein, or heat on protein solutions.

coagula'tion. The process of clotting.

Coagulation depends upon the presence of several substances. Some of the most important are prothrombin; thrombin; thromboplastin (thrombokinase); calcium in ionic form; and fibrinogen. Prothrombin is converted to thrombin by the action of thromboplastin in the presence of calcium ions. Thrombin then acts on the soluble fibrinogen of the plasma, converting it to insoluble fibrin. The fibrin forms a meshwork of fibers in which the corpuscles of the blood become entangled, thus forming a clot. Shrinkage of the fibrin causes the exudation of plasma—minus—fibrinogen, which constitutes blood serum. When blood is shed through an injured vessel, thromboplastin is liberated from the injured tissues and from degenerating blood platelets. This initiates the clotting mechanism.

In schematic (and quite simplified) form, the clotting process is as follows:

prothrombin + thromboplastin + calcium ions → thrombin

thrombin + fibrinogen → fibrin.

Clotting is retarded by cold; smooth surfaces; substances which combine with calcium, such as EDTA (ethylenediamine tetraacetic acid); neutral salts such as magnesium or sodium sulfate; certain substances of biological origin such as hirudin, heparin, snake venoms, cysteine, and dicoumarol.

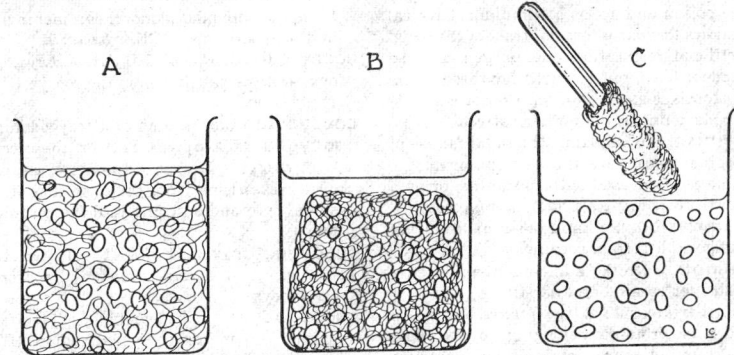

COAGULATION AND DEFIBRINATION

A, A fresh clot contains fibrin threads, corpuscles, and serum. B, On standing, the fibrin contracts, retaining most of the corpuscles but releasing some of the serum. C, If blood is stirred before and during the process of coagulation, the fibrin clings to the stirring rod and leaves the mixture of corpuscles and serum called defibrinated blood.

Clotting is hastened by warming; providing a rough surface; use of a chemical substance such as adrenalin, thrombin, thromboplastin.

   c. time. The time required for a small amount of blood to coagulate. This can be determined by collecting blood in a small test tube and noting elapsed time from moment blood is shed to time it coagulates or by collecting blood in a small capillary tube and breaking off small pieces of the tube at 30-second intervals. Coagulation is indicated by the appearance of fine threads of fibrin between the broken ends of the tube. Normal time, using the capillary tube method, is six to 17 minutes. SYN: *clotting time.*

coag'ulative. Causing coagulation.

coagulometer (ko-ag''u-lom'et-er) [L. *coāgulāre,* to congeal, + Gr. *metron,* measure]. Device for measuring the blood's coagulation time.

coag'ulum [L.]. 1. A blood clot. 2. A curd.

coalesce (ko-al-es') [L. *coalēscere,* to grow together]. To fuse; run or grow together.

coales'cence. Fusion or growing together of two or more parts of bodies.

coal tar. USP. A tar that is produced in the destructive distillation of bituminous coal. Used as an ingredient of ointments for treating eczema.

coal worker's pneumoconiosis. Chronic lung disease produced by breathing coal dust. SYN: *black lung.*

coapta'tion [L. *coaptāre,* to fit together]. The adjustment of separate parts to each other, as the edges of fractures.

coarctate (kō-ark'tāt) [L. *coarctāre,* to tight-

en]. To press or pressed together.

   c. retina. Funnel-shaped retina.

coarcta'tion. 1. Compression of the walls of a vessel. 2. Shriveling. 3. A stricture.

   c. of aorta. Narrowing of the aorta.

coarctotomy (ko''ark-tot'o-mī) [L. *coarctus,* pressed together, + Gr. *tomē,* incision]. Cutting or division of a stricture.

coat [L. *cotta,* a tunic]. A covering or a layer in the wall of a tubular structure, as the inner coat (tunica intima), middle coat (tunica media), and outer coat (tunica adventitia) of an artery.

cobalt (kō'balt). SYMB: *Co.* At. wt. 59.933; at. no. 27; sp. gr. 8.9. A chemical element, a gray, hard, ductile metal. In experimental animals it stimulates erythropoiesis.

cobra venom solution. Minute quantities of the secretion of the cobra in sterile physiological salt solution.

cocaine hydrochlor'ide (ko-kān', kō'kān). USP. The hydrochloride of an alkaloid obtained from erythroxylin cocoa.

   CHIEF USES: Local and topical anesthetic on mucous membranes. A habit-forming drug.

   POISONING SYM: Initially, a stimulation of the nervous system, with excitement, incoherent talking, restlessness, hallucinations, etc., followed by profound depression, nausea, dizziness, tingling of hands and feet, alterations of pulse, increased respiration, dilated pupils; occasionally convulsions, collapse, and death.

   TREATMENT: When taken by mouth, evacuate stomach. Administer tannic acid, strong black coffee, or strong tea to dilute the poison and act as a stimulant. Give cathartics to clear intestinal tract of the drug. Artificial respiration and oxygen may be needed. If patient survives for three hours prognosis is good. Caution: Do not administer morphine or opium derivatives.

cocainism (ko'kăn-izm). The habitual use of cocaine; more rare than morphinism. Cocaine is often used with morphine, or as a substitute. SEE: *cocaine hydrochloride.*

cocainization (ko"kăn-ĭ-za'shun). Inducing analgesia by use of cocaine.

cocainomania (ko"kăn-o-mā'nĭ-ă). Intense desire for cocaine and its effects.

Coccidia (kok-sĭd'ĭ-ă) [Gr. *kokkos,* berry]. An order of protozoa belonging to the class Sporozoa. All are intracellular parasites usually infecting epithelial cells of the intestine and associated glands. They are principally parasites of lower animals and cause great economic loss due to their toxic effect upon domestic and game animals. Only one species, Isospora hominis, infects humans. The geographic area of infestation is largely confined to the Far East.

coccidioidomycosis (kŏk-sĭd"ĭ-oyd-ō-mĭ-kō'sĭs) ["+ *eidos,* form, + *mykēs,* fungus, + *-ōsis,* condition]. A coccidioidal granuloma.

Exists in two forms: primary coccidioidomycosis, which is an acute, self-limiting disease involving only the respiratory organs; and progressive coccidioidomycosis, a chronic, diffuse, malignant disease that may involve almost any part of the body.

ETIOL: Caused by a pathogenic fungus, Coccidioides immitis.

PROG: For the primary type, favorable; for the progressive type, grave, often fatal.

SYN: *desert rheumatism; San Joaquin Valley fever; valley fever.*

coccidiosis (kok-sid-ĭ-o'sis) ["+ *-ōsis,* condition]. Pathogenic condition resulting from infestation with coccidia. SEE: *Coccidia.*

coccobacilli (kŏk"ō-bă-sĭl'ĭ). Bacilli which are short and thick and somewhat ovoid in form.

coccogenous (kok-oj'en-us) [Gr. *kokkos,* berry, + *gennan,* to produce]. Produced by cocci.

coccoid (kok'oyd) ["+ *eidos,* appearance]. Resembling a micrococcus.

coccus (kok'us) [Gr. *kokkos,* berry]. (pl. *cocci*) A type of bacteria which is spherical or ovoid in form. When cocci appear singly they are designated micrococci; in pairs, diplococci; in clusters like bunches of grapes, staphylococci; in chains, streptococci; in cubical packets of eight, sarcinae. Many are pathogenic causing such diseases as septic sore throat; erysipelas; scarlet fever; rheumatic fever; pneumonia; gonorrhea; meningitis and puerperal fever. SEE: *bacteria.*

coccyalgia (kok"sĭ-al'jĭ-ă) [Gr. *kokkyx,* coccyx, + *algos,* pain]. Pain in the coccyx. SYN *coccygodynia.*

coccydynia (kok"sĭ-din'ĭ-ă). Coccygodynia.

coccygeal (kok-sij'ĭ-al). Pert. to the coccyx.
  c. nerves. Lowest of spinal nerves; pair of nerves arising from the c. section of the spinal cord and entering into the pudendal plexus.

coccygectomy (kok"sĭ-jek'tō-mĭ) [Gr. *kok kyx,* coccyx, + *ektomē,* excision]. Excision of the coccyx.

coccygodynia (kok-sĭ-gō-din'ĭ-ă) ["+ *odynē* pain]. Pain in the coccygeal region. SYN: *coccyalgia; coccydynia; coccyodynia.*

coccyodynia (kok"sĭ-ō-din'ĭ-ă). Coccygodynia.

coccyx (kŏk'sĭks) [Gr. *kokkyx,* coccyx]. Small bone at the base of the spinal column in man, formed by four fused rudimentary vertebrae. Usually ankylosed and articulating with the sacrum above.

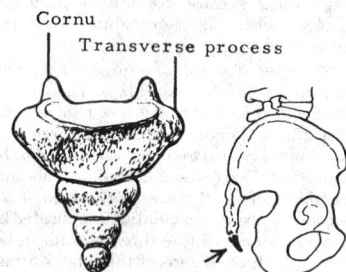

COCCYX
On left is enlarged anterior view of tip of spine seen in lateral view on right.

cochineal (koch'in-ēl) [L. *coccinus,* scarlet]. Dried female insect, used as a dye in laboratory work.

cochlea (kok'lē-ă) [Gr. *kokhlos,* land snail]. A winding cone-shaped tube forming a portion of the inner ear. It contains the organ of Corti, the receptor for hearing.

The cochlea is coiled, resembling a snail shell, winding two and three-quarters turns about a central bony axis, the modiolus. Projecting outward from the modiolus is a thin bony plate, the spinal lamina, which partially divides the cochlear canal into an upper passageway, the scala vestibuli, and a lower one, the scala tympani. Lying between the two scalae is the cochlear duct, in the floor of which lies the spiral organ (of Corti). The base of the cochlea adjoins the vestibule; at the cupola or tip, the two scalae are joined at the helicotrema.

cochlear (kok'lĭ-ar). Pert. to the cochlea.

c. nerve. The division of the stato-acoustic nerve (8th cranial nerve) which supplies the cochlea. SEE: *vestibulocochlear nerve.*

cochleare (kok"lē-ā'rĭ) [L.]. Latin word used in writing prescriptions. Indicates a spoon or spoonful.

cochleariform (kok"le-ar'ĭ-form) ["+ L. *forma*, shape]. Spoon-shaped.

cochleitis (kok"lē-ī'tis) [Gr. *kokhlos*, land snail, + *-itis*, inflammation]. Inflammation of the cochlea. SYN: *cochlitis.*

cochleo-orbicular reflex (kok"lē-ō-or-bik'-u-lar). Contraction of orbicularis palpebrarum muscle resulting from sudden noise being produced near ear. SYN: *cochleopalpebral reflex.*

cochleopalpebral reflex (kok"lē-ō-pal'pē-bral). Contraction of orbicularis palpebrarum muscle resulting from sudden noise being produced near ear. SYN: *cochleo-orbicular reflex.*

cochleovestibular (kok"lē-ō-ves-tib'ū-lar) [Gr. *kokhlos*, land snail, + L. *vestibulum*, vestibule]. Pert. to the cochlea and vestibule of the ear.

cochlitis (kok-lī'tis) ["+ *-itis*, inflammation]. Cochleitis, q.v.

cock'roach [Sp. *cucaracha*]. Blatta orientalis. A common insect belonging to the order Orthoptera, which infests homes and eating places. They are swift-running omnivorous insects averaging about two cm. in length. Through their dual contact with filth and food, they may mechnically transmit bacteria, protozoan cysts, and helminth ova. Common genera are Blatta, Blatella, and Periplaneta.

COCL. Abbr. for *cathodal opening clonus.*

co'coa [Sp. *coco*]. 1. A food substance obtained from the ripe seed of the cacao or cocoa tree. Theobroma cacao. It is prepared by pulverizing the residue after most of the fat has been removed from plain chocolate. 2. A beverage prepared from the powder.

Food value of 100 gm. (mix for hot-chocolate beverage): Cal. 392; protein 9.4 gm.; fat ~ 10.6 gm.; carbohydrate 74 gm.; calcium 2.75 mg.

cocoa butter. Theobroma oil (USP). The fat obtained from the roasted seed of Theobroma cacao.

USES: Suppositories and in toilet preparations as a lubricant.

cocon'sciousness. Conscious states of which we are unaware because they are not in the focus of attention but are at the fringe of consciousness.

cocontraction (kō"kon-trak'shun). Adjustment of two muscles during contraction, said of antagonist muscles in coordination.

co'conut. The edible fruit of the coconut palm, Cocos nucifera.

Food value of 100 gm. (dried, shredded, and sweetened): Cal. 548; protein 3.6 gm.; fat 39 gm.; carbohydrate 53 gm.; calcium 1.6 mg.; iron 2 mg.

c. water. Liquid from coconuts. Also called coconut milk.

Food value of 100 gm: Cal. 22; trace of protein and fat; carbohydrate 4.7 gm.

coctolabile (kok"tō-lā'bĭl) [L. *coctus*, cooked, + *labilis*, perishable]. Something which is altered or destroyed when heated to the temperature of boiling water.

coctoprecipitin (kok"tō-pre-sip'it-in) ["+ *praecipitāre*, to cast down]. A precipitin produced by injecting a serum that has been boiled.

coctostabile (kok"tō-stā'bĭl) ["+ *stabilis*, resisting]. Incapable of being altered or destroyed by boiling water.

codeine (ko'dēn) [Gr. *kōdeia*, poppyhead]. An alkaloid obtained from opium, or synthetically from morphine as methylmorphine.

ACTION AND USES: Analgesic, hypnotic sedative, with effects resembling morphine. Used commonly for its effectiveness in suppressing coughs.

POISONING SYM: Depression of central nervous system to the point of sleep.

TREATMENT: Similar to treatment for morphine.

INCOMPATIBILITIES: Ferrous iodide, Lugol's solution.

c. phosphate. USP. Phosphate of the alkaloid codeine, used because of its free solubility in water. Much weaker than morphine.

c. sulfate. The sulfate of the alkaloid codeine. Used the same as codeine.

Codivilla's extension (kō"dĭ-vīl'ä). [Alessandro Codivilla, It. surgeon, 1861-1912] Extension for fractures made by weight pulling on a nail passed through the lower end of the bone.

cod liver oil. A fixed oil obtained from the fresh livers of the codfish. The official oil is standardized for its vitamins A and D contents.

ACTION AND USES: Used in cases of nutritional deficiency to supply vitamins A and D. Esp. used for prophylaxis of rickets in infants.

INCOMPATIBILITIES: Light and air, both of which cause the oil to become rancid. SYN: *oleum morrhuae.*

coefficient (ko"ef-fish'ent) [L. *co-*, together, + *efficere*, to produce]. A figure put before a chemical formula or compound to indicate the number of molecules of that substance taking part in the chemical reaction.

   c. of absorption. Volume of gas absorbed by a unit volume of a liquid at 0° C. and a pressure of 760 mm.

   c., isotonic. Number indicating the amt. of salt to be added to distilled water to prevent the destruction of erythrocytes when the salt solution is added to the blood.

   c., lethal. Concentration of disinfectant that will kill bacteria in the shortest length of time at 20-25° C.

coelom (sē'lom) [Gr. *koilōma,* a cavity]. The cavity in an embryo between the split layers of lateral mesoderm. In mammals it develops into the pleural, peritoneal, and pericardial cavities.

   c. extraembryonic. In man, the cavity in the developing blastocyst which lies between the mesoderm of the chorion and the mesoderm covering the amniotic cavity and yolk sac.

coenocyte (sē'nō-sīt, sĕn'ō-sīt) [Gr. *koinos,* common, + *kytos,* hollow vessel]. A multinucleated mass of protoplasm; a mass of protoplasm in which cell membranes are lacking between the nuclei; a syncytium.

coen'zyme [L. *co-,* together, + Gr. *en,* in, + *zymē,* leaven]. Enzyme activators. A diffusible, heat-stable substance of low molecular weight which, when combined with an inactive protein called apoenzyme, forms an active compound or a complete enzyme called holoenzyme. Examples are adenylic acid, riboflavin, and coenzymes I and II.

coetaneous (ko"e-tā'nĭ-us) ["+ *aetās,* age]. Having the same age or date.

coexcitation (ko-ek-sĭ-tā'shun) ["+ *excitāre,* to arouse]. Simultaneous excitation of two parts or bodies.

coferment (ko-fer'ment) ["+ *fermentum,* leaven]. A coenzyme.

cof'fee [Turkish *kahve*]. Seed of the berry of Coffea arabica.

   COMP: Coffee has no nutritive value, but a cup of coffee, prepared by steeping the roasted, ground berries in boiling water, contains about 1% caffeine. This accounts for coffee's slight stimulant effect. SEE: *chocolate; cocoa; tea.*

   c. -ground vomitus. Vomit similar to coffee grounds in pigment and consistency, occurring as a result of blood mixed in the vomitus.

Cogan's syndrome (kō'găn). Interstitial keratitis, associated with tinnitus, vertigo, and usually deafness.

cogni'tion [L. *cognōscere,* to know]. Awareness, having perception and memory. The mental process by which knowledge is acquired.

COGTT. Abbr. for *cortisone oral glucose tolerance test.*

cog'wheel respira'tion. A sudden, brief halt in inspiration and expiration.

cohabita'tion [L. *cohabitāre,* to dwell together]. 1. Living together as man and wife without being legally married. 2. Sexual intercourse.

coherent (kō-hēr'ĕnt) [L. *cohaerēre,* to stick together]. 1. Sticking together, as parts of bodies or fluids. 2. Consistent; making a logical whole.

cohe'sion. The property of adhering.

cohe'sive. Adhesive; sticky.

Cohnheim's areas (kōn'hīm). [Julius Friedrich Cohnheim, Ger. pathologist, 1839-1884]. Irregular groups of fibrils seen in a cross section of a striated muscle fiber. SYN: *Cohnheim's fields.*

Cohnheim's theory. Theory that tumors result from embryonal cells not utilized for fetal development.

coiled posture. A natural position with some, but esp. assumed in cerebral diseases; in hepatic, intestinal, or renal colic. SEE: *posture.*

coilonychia (koy"lo-nik'ĭ-ă). Koilonychia, q.v.

coin counting. A sliding movement of tips of thumb and index finger over each other in

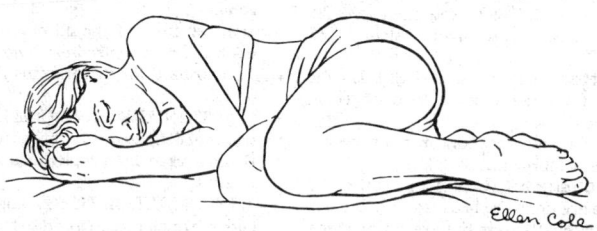

COILED POSTURE

paralysis agitans. SYN: *pill-rolling tremor.*

coin test. Test for pneumothorax. A coin placed on the chest, over the suspected area, is struck with another coin. If a cavity containing air is underneath, a metallic ringing sound is heard.

coital (ko'ĭ-tal). Pert. to sexual intercourse.

coition (ko-ish'un) [L. *coīre,* to come together]. Coitus, sexual intercourse.

coitophobia (ko"ĭ-tō-fo'bĭ-ă) ["+ Gr. *phobos,* fear]. Morbid fear of sexual intercourse.

coitus (kō'ĭ-tŭs). Coition, copulation, q.v. Sexual intercourse between man and woman.

c. à la vache. Coitus from behind with the female in the knee-chest position.

c. interrup'tus. Withdrawal of the penis from the vagina before the seminal emission occurs.

c. reserva'tus. Coitus with intentional suppression of ejaculation.

c. Saxonius. Manual pressure on the urethra at the underside of the penis or in the perineum to block the emission of semen at the time of ejaculation.

cola (kō'lă). A genus of tropical trees which produce the kola nut. An extract of the kola nut is used in pharmaceutical preparations and as a main ingredient in some carbonated beverages. SEE: *kola.*

colal'gia [Gr. *kōlon,* colon, + *algos,* pain]. Pain in the colon.

colation (ko-lā'shun) [L. *colāre,* to strain]. Straining, filtering.

colauxe (kol-awks'ĭ) [Gr. *kōlon,* colon, + *auxē,* increase]. Distention of the colon.

cold [AS. *ceald,* cold]. 1. A general term for coryza or inflammation of the respiratory mucous membranes known as the common cold. 2. The opposite of heat, q.v.

c., chest. Bronchitis, q.v. Inflammation of the bronchial mucous membranes.

c., common. Acute catarrhal inflammation of the upper respiratory tract. It is highly contagious. Incubation period is from 18 to 48 hours. Lasting immunity does not develop. SYN: *rhinitis.*

ETIOL: May be due to one of a considerable number of viruses.

SYM: Congestion of nasal mucosa with partial or complete occlusion of nostrils; continuous watery discharge with more or less continuous sniffling and blowing of nose. Headaches and dull pains in the face and head are common. Constitutional symptoms may appear, such as fever, body aches, easy fatigability and sensations of chilliness. Symptoms are usually resolved within five to 10 days.

TREATMENT: Treatment is mainly for the relief of symptoms. Spraying with ephe-

drine hydrochloride, or inhalation of benzedrine or menthol relieves nasal congestion. Analgesics are useful to relieve aching. Preparations containing codeine will usually relieve a cough but should not be used when the cough is productive. Antihistamines sometimes are effective in controlling the nasal secretions. Bed rest is recommended for febrile patients.

c. cream. USP. White perfumed ointment used mainly as a cosmetic and as an ointment base.

c., head. A common cold, q.v.

c. pack. Used to apply cold to an area, usually for pain, swelling or inflammation.

c. pressor test. Determining the rise in blood pressure after immersion of hand in cold water for one minute.

c. sore. Fever blister. Eruption of vesicles on an inflammatory base. SEE: *herpes simplex.*

colectomy (ko-lek'tō-mĭ) [Gr. *kōlon,* colon, + *ektomē,* excision]. Excision of part or of all of the colon.

coleitis (kol-ĭ-ī'tĭs) [Gr. *koleos,* sheath]. SEE: *vaginitis.*

coleocele (kō'lĭ-ō-sēl) ["+ *kēlē,* hernia]. A vaginal hernia.

coleocystitis (ko"lĭ-o-sĭs-tī'tĭs) [Gr. *koleos,* sheath, + *kystis,* bladder, + *-itis,* inflammation]. Inflammation of the vagina and bladder.

coleoptosis (kō"lē-op-tō'sĭs) ["+ *ptōsis,* falling]. Prolapse of the wall of the vagina.

coleot'omy ["+ *tomē,* incision]. Incision into the pericardium or into the vagina. SYN: *colpotomy.*

colibacellemia (ko"lĭ-bas-ĭl-le'mĭ-ă) [Gr. *kōlon,* colon, + L. *bacillus,* little rod, + Gr. *haima,* blood]. Colon bacillus in the blood.

colibacillo'sis ["+ "+ Gr. *ōsis,* condition]. Infection with the colon bacillus.

colibacilluria (ko-lĭ-bas-ĭl-u'rĭ-ă) ["+ "+ Gr. *ouron,* urine]. Colon bacillus in the urine.

colibacil'lus ["+ L. *bacillus,* little rod]. The colon bacillus, Escherichia coli.

colic (kol'ik) [Gr. *kōlikos*]. 1. Spasm in any hollow or tubular soft organ accompanied by pain. 2. Pert. to the colon. SEE: *cholecystalgia; tormina.*

c., biliary. In bile ducts usually associated with a gallstone.

c., infantile. Occurring in infants, principally during the first few months.

c., intestinal. Pain may occur throughout the abdomen.

c., lead. Associated with lead poisoning, occupations such as painting, etc. Severe abdominal c. Lead line may be found on gums and basic stippling in red blood cells. SYN: *Devonshire c.*

   c., menstrual. Abdominal pain during menses. SYN: *dysmenorrhea.*

   c., renal. In region of one of the kidneys and toward the thigh. Pain radiates from kidney region around and over abdomen into the groin. It accompanies the passage of calculus.

   c., uterine. Painful menstruation. SYN: *dysmenorrhea.*

col'ica [L.]. Colic.

colicin. A bacteriocin produced by Escherichia coli which is lethal to other E. coli.

colicoli'tis [Gr. *kōlon*, colon, + -*itis*, inflammation]. Colitis due to Escherichia coli.

colicople'gia [" + *plēgē*, stroke]. Colic and paralysis due to lead poisoning.

colicystitis (ko''lĭ-sĭs-tī'tĭs) [Gr. *kōlon*, colon, + *kystis*, bladder, + -*itis*, inflammation]. Inflammation of bladder resulting from infection with Escherichia coli.

colicystopyelitis (ko-lĭ-sĭs''tō-pī''ĕ-lī'tĭs) [" + *pyelos*, pelvis, + -*itis*, inflammation]. Inflammation of bladder and of pelvis of kidney caused by Escherichia coli.

col'iform [" + L. *forma*, form]. 1. Sieve form; cribriform. 2. Pertaining to a group of bacteria which includes Aerobacter aerogenes and Escherichia coli. Their presence in water, esp. that of E. coli, is presumptive evidence of fecal contamination.

colilysin (ko-lil'ĭ-sin) [Gr. *kōlon*, colon, + *lysis*, dissolution]. A hemolysin formed by Escherichia coli.

colinephri'tis [" + *nephros*, kidney, + -*itis*, inflammation]. Nephritis caused by the colon bacillus, Escherichia coli.

coliplication (ko''lĭ-pli-kā'shun) [Gr. *kōlon*, colon, + L. *plica*, fold]. Operation for correcting a dilated colon.

colipuncture (kō'lĭ-pŭnk''chūr) [" + L. *punctura*, a piercing]. Puncture of the colon to relieve distention. SYN: *colocentesis.*

colipyuria (ko''lĭ-pī-u'rĭ-ă) [" + *pyon*, pus, + *ouron*, urine]. Pus in urine due to Escherichia coli.

colisep'sis [" + *sēpsis*, putrefaction]. Infection caused by the colon bacillus.

coli'tis [Gr. *kōlon*, colon, + *itis*, inflammation]. Inflammation of the colon.

   c., mucous. C. accompanied by large quantities of mucus.

   SYM: Attacks occur paroxysmally and are sometimes followed by constipation. Spastic, colicky pain in midabdomen. Tenacious gelatinous mucus and shreds of mucous membrane may be passed.

   c., ulcerative. Ulceration of mucosa of colon.

   SYM: Passage of watery, offensive stools with mucus and pus. Abdominal pain, tenderness, or colic. Intermittent or irregular fever. Hemorrhage and perforation may occur.

colitoxemia (ko''lĭ-toks-ē'mĭ-ă) [" + *toxikon*, poison, + *haima*, blood]. Toxemia caused by the colon bacillus, Escherichia coli.

colitoxico'sis [" + " + -*ōsis*, condition]. Systemic poisoning caused by the colon bacillus, Escherichia coli.

colitox'in [Gr. *kōlon*, colon, + *toxikon*, poison]. A toxin produced by the colon bacillus.

coliuria (kō''lĭ-u'rĭ-ă) [" + *ouron*, urine]. Presence of the Escherichia coli in the urine. SYN: *colibaciluria.*

collagen (kol'ă-jen) [Gr. *kolla*, glue, + *gennan*, to produce]. A fibrous insoluble protein found in the connective tissue, including skin, bone, ligaments and cartilage. Collagen represents about 30% of the total body protein.

   c. diseases. A group of clinical syndromes which cause similar cellular changes. That is, they affect the body's connective tissue or soft skeleton. The joints, blood vessels, heart, skin and supporting tissue of various organs contain lesions. How these lesions are spread throughout the body determines the clinical picture in the various diseases. Collagen diseases include systemic lupus erythematosus (SLE); dermatomyositis; acute hemorrhagic glomerulonephritis; rheumatoid arthritis; rheumatic fever and scleroderma. SYN: *connective-tissue disease.*

collapse [L. *collapsus*, fallen to pieces]. 1. An abnormal retraction of the walls of an organ. 2. A sudden failure of vital power due to reflex inhibition of the heart and respiratory system, or to loss of blood, low metabolism, or undue lowering of the blood pressure.

   The term collapse designates a profound degree of shock, q.v., induced by functional inhibition of the vasomotor center, to distinguish it from the shock of exhaustion of the same center resulting from physical violence or impressions of fear. Intense fear may induce a complete collapse, as is sometimes seen in a victim about to be executed.

   SYM: Similar to those of hemorrhage. The peripheral arteries are depleted of blood, and the veins, esp. in the splanchnic region, are congested; apathy; extreme pallor; cold, clammy perspiration; thin, rapid pulse; fall of blood pressure; unconsciousness.

   NP: The head of bed, or head and shoulders of patient should be lowered. Hot blankets and hot water bottles may be placed about the patient's body. SEE: *shock.*

c. of lung. Artificially induced by pneumothorax; thoracoplasty; or avulsion of phrenic nerve. May occur spontaneously due to rupture of a bleb on the pleural surface of the lung.

collap'sing. Falling into extreme and sudden prostration resembling shock.

c. pulse. Pulse of aortic insufficiency or regurgitation; water-hammer pulse. SYN: *Corrigan's pulse.*

collapsother'apy [L. *collapsus,* fallen to pieces, + Gr. *therapeia,* treatment]. Treatment of pulmonary affections by unilateral pneumothorax and immobilization of affected lung. SYN: *collapse therapy.*

collar (kol'ar) [L. *collum,* neck]. 1. A band worn round the neck. 2. Structure or marking formed like a neckband.

c. of Venus; c., venereal. Mottled appearance of the skin of the neck occasionally seen in syphilis. SYN: *melanoleukoderma colli.*

col'larbone. The clavicle, q.v.

collat'eral [L. *con,* together, + *lateralis,* pert. to a side]. 1. Accompanying, as side by side. 2. Subordinate or secondary. 3. Not related lineally. 4. An accessory nerve or blood vessel. 5. A minute side branch of the axon or axis cylinder of a neuron which passes outward at right angles to the axon.

c. circulation. That of small anastomosing vessels, esp. when a main artery is obstructed.

c. eminence. An elevation in the floor of the lateral ventricle.

c. fissure. A fissure on the median surface of the cerebral hemisphere.

c. ganglia. Ganglia of the sympathetic division of the autonomic nervous system, located near origins of the celiac and mesenteric arteries. These include the celiac and mesenteric ganglia. SYN: *prevertebral ganglia.*

c. trigone. The angle between the diverging inferior and posterior horns of the lateral ventricle.

collat'erals. Plural of collateral.

collecting tubules. Small ducts which receive urine from several renal tubules and discharge it into papillary ducts which open into a renal calyx at the tip of a papilla.

Colles' fascia (kŏl'ēz). [Abraham Colles, Ir. surgeon, 1773-1843]. Inner layer of superficial fascia of perineum.

Colles' fracture. The transverse fracture of the distal end of radius (just above wrist) with displacement of hand backward and outward.

Colles' law. A theory, long accepted but now obsolete, that a child affected with congenital syphilis, its mother showing no signs of the disease, will not infect its mother.

colliculectomy (kol-lik″u-lek'tō-mī) [L. *colliculus,* mound, + Gr. *ektomē,* excision]. Removal of the colliculus seminalis.

colliculi'tis ["+ Gr. *-itis,* inflammation]. Inflammation of the colliculus seminalis.

collic'ulus [L.]. A little eminence.

c. bulbi; c. bulbi intermedius. Erectile tissue encircling the male urethra at the entrance to the bulb.

c. cervicalis. Urethrae muliebris. The crest on the posterior wall of the female urethra.

c. inferior. One of two elevations forming the lower portion of the corpora quadrigemina of the midbrain.

c. seminalis. An oval enlargement on the crista urethralis, an elevation in the floor of the prostatic portion of the urethra. On its sides are the openings of the ejaculatory ducts and numerous ducts of the prostate gland.

c. superior. One of two elevations forming the upper portion of the corpora quadrigemina of the midbrain.

c. urethralis. C. seminalis.

collimation (kol″ī-mā'shun) [L. *collineare,* to align]. The process of making parallel. Thus x-ray machines are fitted with a collimator to insure that the rays are parallel and not diffuse.

colliquation (kol-ī-kwā'shun) [L. *con,* together, + *liquāre,* to melt]. 1. Abnormal discharge of a body fluid. 2. Softening of tissues to liquefaction. 3. A wasting.

colliquative (kŏ-lik'wā-tiv). Pert. to a liquid and excessive discharge, as a c. diarrhea.

collodion (ko-lo'dī-on) [Gr. *kollōdēs,* resembling glue]. USP. A preparation containing pyroxylin dissolved throughly in ether and alcohol. It is a viscous liquid having an odor of ether and is highly flammable. When applied, it dries to form a strong, thin transparent film and is useful in sealing the edge of a dressing, esp. on the scalp.

c., flexible. USP. A preparation of collodion containing camphor and castor oil. It is more elastic than collodion in ether and alcohol.

c., salicylic acid. Flexible c. with salicylic acid. Used as a keratolytic agent, commonly for corns.

colloid (kol'oyd) [Gr. *kollōdēs,* glutinous]. 1. A colloidal system. A gluelike substance such as a protein or starch whose particles (molecules or aggregates of molecules) when dispersed in a solvent to the greatest possible degree remain uniformly distributed and fail to form a true solution. The size of colloid particles ranges from 1-100 millimicrons. 2. A homogeneous gelatinous substance found within the follicles of the thyroid gland and containing the thyroid secretion.

c. chemistry. This deals with such systems and substances, and with the problems of emulsions, mists, foams, and suspensions.

c. cyst. A sac containing a jellylike liquid.

c. degeneration. A mucoid degeneration seen in the protoplasm of epithelial cells.

c. suspension. A mixture holding particles in suspension, the forms of which change with the forces acting upon them, such as milk, fat, etc.

c. thyroid. Semifluid, jellylike substance filling the follicles of the thyroid gland. It contains the thyroid hormone.

colloidal (kol-loyd′ăl). Pert. to a colloid.

c. dispersion. A mixture containing colloid particles which fail to settle out and are held in suspension. They are common in animal and plant tissues, the protoplasm of cells being a colloidal mixture. Particles of colloidal dispersions are too large to pass through cell membranes and such dispersions usually appear cloudy.

colloidin (kol-loy′din). A jellylike substance seen in colloid degeneration.

colloidoclasia (kol-oyd″o-klā′sĭ-ă) [Gr. *kollōdes*, glutinous, + *klasis*, fracture]. An alteration in the equilibrium of body colloids resulting from entrance into the blood stream of unaltered colloids such as proteins with an end result of anaphylactic shock.

colloidopexy (kol-oyd′o-pek″sī) ["+ *pēxis*, fixation]. Fixation of colloids during metabolism.

collo′ma [Gr. *kolla*, glue, + *-ōma*, tumor]. A colloid degeneration of a cancer.

collonema (kol″o-nē′mă) ["+ *nēma*, yarn]. A tumor, esp. a lipoma, which has undergone mucoid degeneration.

collopexia (kol″o-peks′ĭ-ă) [L. *collum*, neck, + Gr. *pēxis*, fixation]. Fixation of the cervix uteri.

col′lum [L.]. (pl. *colla*) 1. The necklike part of an organ. 2. The neck.

collutory (kol′ū-tō″rĭ) [L. *colluere*, to rinse]. A gargle or mouth wash.

collyrium (kō-lir′ĭ-um) [Gr. *kollyrion*, eye salve]. An eyewash.

colobo′ma [Gr. *kolobōma*, a mutilation]. A lesion or defect of the eye, usually a fissure or cleft of the iris, ciliary body or choroid.

May be congenital, pathological or surgical. Sometimes the eyelid is involved.

colocentesis (kō″lō-sen-tē′sis) [Gr. *kōlon*, colon, + *kentēsis*, puncture]. Surgical puncture of the colon to relieve distention.

colocholecystostomy (ko″lo-kō″lē-sis-tos′-to-mī) ["+ *cholē*, bile, + *kystis*, bladder, + *stoma*, opening]. Surgical formation of a communication between colon and gallbladder. SYN: *cholecystocolostomy.*

colocleisis (ko-lo-klī′sis) ["+ *kleistos*, closed]. Occlusion of the colon.

coloclysis (ko-lok′lī-sis) ["+ *klysis*, washing]. A colonic enema.

coloclyster (kō″lō-klis′ter). A colonic enema.

colocolostomy (ko″lo-ko-los′to-mī) ["+ *kōlon*, colon, + *stoma*, mouth]. Formation of a connection between two portions of the colon.

colocynth (kol′o-sinth) [Gr. *kolokynthē*, fruit of Citrullus colocynthis]. Dried pulp of unripe colocynth fruit.

ACTION AND USES: A type of cathartic which has such drastic action that it should not be used.

coloenteritis (ko″lo-en″ter-ī′tis) [Gr. *kōlon*, colon, + *enteron*, intestine, + *-itis*, inflammation]. Inflammation of mucous membrane of small and large intestines.

colofixa′tion ["+ L. *figere*, to fasten]. Suspension of the colon in ptosis.

co′lon [Gr. *kōlon*]. The large intestine from the end of the ileum and beginning with the cecum to the anus, about 59 inches (1.5 meters) long, and divided into the ascending, transverse, descending, and the sigmoid or pelvic colon.

Beginning at the cecum, the first part of the large intestine, the ascending colon, passes upward to the right colic or hepatic flexure, where it turns as the transverse colon passing ventral to the liver and stomach. On reaching the spleen, it turns downward (left colic or splenic flexure) and continues as the descending colon to the brim of the pelvis where it is continuous with the sigmoid colon.

c. bacteria. Escherichia coli is the most common one found. Whatever digestion takes place in the colon is due to bacteria. A large number of fermentative bacteria are found in the middle portion of the colon. They change carbohydrates into carbon dioxide, alcohol, and lactic acid. This is the only way cellulose may be acted upon in the body. Putrefying bacteria are found in the lower part of the colon. These may produce toxic products, e.g., indol, skatol; however, if absorbed, such products undergo detoxification in the liver.

c. functions. *Mechanical:* Mixing the contents of the intestines.

Chemical: No digestive enzymes are secreted in the colon, but an alkaline fluid aids in the completion of digestion begun in the small intestines. Those products of bacterial action which are absorbed into the blood stream are carried by the portal circulation to the liver before they get into the general circulation. There is also a great deal of water absorbed in the colon rather than in the small intestines. The fluids of the body are conserved in this way, and in spite of the large volumes of secretions (saliva, etc.) added to the food during its progress through the alimentary canal, the contents of the colon are gradually dehydrated until they assume the consistency of normal feces or even become quite hard.

SEE: *absorption; defecation.*

c. syndrome, irritable. A common, benign condition of the colon appearing in two types - a form with abdominal pain, constipation, diarrhea, or one alternating with the other; and a type characterized by painless intermittent or continuous diarrhea. Heartburn, flatulence, anorexia, nausea, abdominal distention after meals, and vomiting may be present. SYN: *irritable bowel; spastic c.*

ETIOL: Unknown, but heredity, previous specific gastrointestinal disease, and emotional stress may be important.

TREATMENT: The disease is benign and the patient should be so informed after other diseases are excluded. There are no specific medicines and the patient should be taught to live with the symptoms. Bland diet, bulk laxatives, and antispasmodics may provide symptomatic relief. Sedatives, tranquilizers, and opiates should be reserved for acute attacks.

colon, words pert. to: anus; appendices; epiploicae; cecum; cholecystocolostomy; colalgia; colitis; "colo-" words; diverticulitis; jejunum; peristalsis; rectum; small intestines.

colonalgia (ko″lon-al′ji-a) [Gr. *kōlon,* colon, + *algos,* pain]. Pain in the colon.

colonic (kō-lŏn′ik). Pert. to the colon.

c. irrigation. Injection into the colon of a large amt. of fluid which is intended to fill colon and flush it.

Administered not to induce defecation but to wash out material situated above the defecation area and to wash the wall of the bowel as high as the water can be made to reach. Two primary methods: one tube, involving filling colon to capacity through a single tube and allowing liquid to run out through the same tube; and two tube method, employing separate inflow and outflow tubes.

colonitis (ko-lon-i′tis) [Gr. *kōlon,* colon, + *-itis,* inflammation]. Colitis, q.v.

colonom′eter [L. *colonia,* colony, + Gr. *metron,* measure]. Device for estimating colonies of bacteria on a culture plate.

colonopexy (ko-lon′o-pek″si) [Gr. *kōlon,* colon, + *pēxis,* fixation]. Process of attaching part of colon to abdominal wall.

colonorrhagia (ko″lon-o-rā′jī-ā) ["+ *rhēgnynai,* to burst forth]. Hemorrhage from the colon.

colonorrhea (ko″lon-o-rī′ă) ["+ *rhoia,* flow]. Mucous colitis.

colonoscope (ko-lon′o-skōp) ["+ *skopein,* to examine]. Instrument for examination of the colon. SEE: *sigmoidoscope.*

colonos′copy. Examination of upper portion of rectum with an elongated speculum.

col′ony [L. *colonia*]. A growth of microorganisms in a culture. Usually considered to have grown from a single organism.

colopexos′tomy [Gr. *kōlon,* colon, + *pēxis,* fixation, + *stoma,* mouth]. Resection of the colon and fixation to abdominal wall to establish an artificial anus.

colopexotomy (ko″lo-peks-ot′o-mī) ["+ "+ *tomē,* incision]. Incision and fixation of colon.

colopexy, colopexia (ko′lo-pek″sī, ko″lo-peks′ī-ā). Fixation of the sigmoid or cecum to the abdominal wall by suture.

coloplication (ko″lo-pli-kā′shun) [Gr. *kōlon,* colon, + L. *plica,* fold]. Making a fold in the colon to reduce its lumen.

coloprocti′tis ["+ *prōktos,* anus, + *-ītis,* inflammation]. Colonic and rectal inflammation. SYN: *colorectitis.*

coloproctostomy (ko″lo-prok-tos′to-mī) ["+ "+ *stoma,* opening]. Making a communication between a segment of colon and the rectum.

coloptosia (ko″lop-to′sī-ā) ["+ *ptōsis,* dropping]. Prolapse of the colon, esp. of the transverse colon.

coloptosis (ko-lop-to′sis). A downward displacement of the colon.

colopuncture (ko′lo-punk-chur) [Gr. *kōlon,* colon, + L. *punctura,* piercing]. Puncturing the colon.

col′or [L.]. A visible quality, distinct from form, and light and shade.

c. blindness. Inability to identify one or more of the primary colors. SYN: *daltonism.*

c. gustation. A sense of color aroused by stimulation of taste receptors.

c. hearing. A sense of color caused by a sound.

c. index. An outmoded method of expressing the amount of hemoglobin present in each red cell.

color, words pert. to: achromate; achromodermia; "acro-" words; alba; albedo; albicans; allochroism; allochromasia; anerythropsia; anisochromatic; aurantiasis; auric; canescent; carotene; "chrom-" words; flavescent; isochromatic; melanin; nigrescent; pigmentation; rubescent; rubiginous; rubor; vermilion; versicolor; xanthic.

colorectitis (ko″lo-rek-ti′tis) [G. *kōlon*, colon, + L. *rectum*, straight, + Gr. *-itis*, inflammation]. Inflammation of colon and rectum. SYN: *coloproctitis*.

colorectostomy (ko″lo-rek-tos′to-mĭ) ["+ "+ Gr. *stoma*, opening]. Formation of passage between colon and rectum.

colorim′eter [L. *color*, color, + Gr. *metron*, measure]. Instrument for measuring intensity of color in a substance or fluid, esp. one for determining the amt. of hemoglobin in the blood.

colostomy (ko-los′to-mĭ) [Gr. *kōlon*, colon, + *stoma*, mouth]. Incision of the colon for purpose of making a more or less permanent fistula between the bowel and the abdominal wall. The location is usually indicated in the description as inguinal colostomy, lumbar colostomy, etc.

    c. diet. A low residue diet.

    c., inguinal. Incision of colon to form artificial anus.

    NP: Change dressings p.r.n. Protect skin around opening from discharge by covering with sterile zinc-oxide ointment. Remove ointment by cleansing with olive oil. Chart amt. and nature of discharge. Prevent impaction, watch diet orders, irrigate through upper or lower loop as ordered. Special colostomy bags which cover the opening and greatly facilitate colostomy care are available.

colostra′tion [L. *colostrum*, colostrum]. Infant diarrhea assumed to be caused by colostrum.

colostrorrhea (ko-los″tro-rĭ′ă) ["+ Gr. *rhoia*, flow]. Abnormal secretion of colostrum.

colos′trum [L.]. Secretion from the breast before the onset of true lactation two or three days after delivery.

    The secretion contains, mainly, serum and white blood corpuscles. So-called "first milk. "

colotomy (ko-lot′o-mĭ) [Gr. *kōlon*, colon, + *tomē*, incision]. Incision of colon.

colotyphoid (kol″ō-ti′foyd) ["+ *typhos*, fever causing, + *eidos*, resemblance]. Typhoid fever with ulceration of colon.

colpalgia (kol-pal′ji-ă) [Gr. *kolpos*, vagina, + *algos*, pain]. Vaginal pain.

colpatresia (kol-pă-tre′zĭ-ă) ["+ *a-*, not, + *trēsis*, a perforation]. Occlusion or pathological closure of the vagina; vaginal atresia.

colpectasia (kol-pek-tā′sĭ-ă) ["+ *ektasis*, distention]. Dilatation of the vagina.

colpec′tomy (Gr. *kolpos*, vagina, + *ektomē*, excision). Surgical removal of the vagina.

colpeurynter (kol′pū-rin″ter) ["+ *eurynein*, to dilate]. A bag for dilatation of the vagina.

colpeurysis (kol-pū′ris-is). Dilatation of the vagina by surgery.

colpitis (kol-pi′tis) [Gr. *kolpos*, vagina, + *-itis*, inflammation]. Inflammation of the vagina. SEE: *vaginitis*.

colpocele (kol′po-sēl) ["+ *kēlē*, hernia]. Hernia into the vagina.

colpoceliotomy (kol″po-sē″lĭ-ot′o-mĭ) ["+ *koilia*, belly, + *tomē*, a cut]. Entering the abdomen surgically through the vagina.

colpocleisis (kol″po-kli′sis) ["+ *kleisis*, a closure]. Operation of occluding the vagina.

colpocystitis (kol″po-sis-ti′tis) ["+ *kystis*, bladder, + *-itis*, inflammation]. Inflammation of vagina and bladder.

colpocystocele (kol″po-sis′tō-sēl) [Gr. *kolpos*, vagina, + *kystis*, bladder, + *kēlē*, hernia]. Prolapse of the bladder into the vagina.

colpocystoplasty (kol″po-sis′tō-plas″tĭ) ["+ "+ *plassein*, to form]. Treatment of vesicovaginal fistula.

colpocystosyrinx (kol″po-sis-tō-sir′inks) ["+ "+ *syrinx*, fistula]. Fistula between bladder and vagina.

colpocystotomy (kol″po-sis-tot′o-mĭ) ["+ "+ *tomē*, incision]. Cutting into the bladder through the vagina.

    NP: Prevent bladder distention. Record intake and output. If retention catheter is present, irrigate twice daily with solution ordered and be sure catheter is kept draining. Keep patient clean and comfortable with external irrigations over the vulva. Dry skin thoroughly after each irrigation.

colpocystoureterocystotomy (kol″po-sis″tō-u-rē″ter-o-sis-tot′o-mĭ) [Gr. *kolpos*, vagina, + *kystis*, bladder, + *ourētēr*, ureter, + *kystis*, bladder, + *tomē*, incision]. Incision into the ureter through the walls of the bladder and vagina.

colpodesmorrhaphy (kol″po-des-mor′ă-fĭ) ["+ *desmos*, band, + *rhaphē*, suture]. Repair of the vaginal sphincter.

colpodynia (kol″pō-din′ĭ-ă) ["+ *odynē*, pain]. Pain in the vagina. SYN: *colpalgia*.

colpohyperplasia (kol″pō-hī-per-plā′zĭ-ă) [Gr. *kolpos*, vagina, + *hyper*, over, + *plasis*, a forming]. Excessive growth of mucous membrane of the vagina.

c. cystica. Infectious inflammation of the vaginal walls which is characterized by the production of small blebs.

colpo"hysterec'tomy [" + *hystera*, uterus, + *ektome*, excision]. Removal of the uterus through the vagina.

colpohysteropexy (kol"po-his'ter-o-pek"si) [" + " + *pexis*, fixation]. Fixation of uterus through the vagina.

colpohysterot'omy [Gr. *kolpos*, vagina, + *hystera*, uterus, + *tome*, incision]. Incision through the vagina into the uterus, as for excision of a fibroma.

colpomyomectomy (kol"po-mi"o-mek'to-mi) [" + *mys*, muscle, + *-oma*, tumor, + *ektome*, excision]. Removal of a fibroid tumor of the uterus through the vagina.

colpomyomotomy (-mot'o-mi) [" + " + " + " + *tome*, incision]. Incision of uterus through the vagina for removal of tumor.

colpopathy (kol-pop'a-thi) [Gr. *kolpos*, vagina, + *pathos*, disease]. Any pathology of the vagina.

colpoperineoplasty (kol"po-per"in-e'o-plas"ti) [" + *perinaion*, perineum, + *plassein*, to form]. Plastic operation on vagina and perineum.

colpoperineorrhaphy (kol"po-per"in-e-or'ra-fi) [" + " + *rhaphe*, suture]. Operation for mending perineal tears in vagina. SYN: *colpoperineoplasty.*

col'popexy [" + *pexis*, fixation]. Suture of a relaxed and prolapsed vagina to the abdominal wall.

colpoplasty (kol'po-plas"ti) [" + *plassein*, to form]. Plastic operation upon vagina.

colpoptosis (kol"pop-to'sis) [Gr. *kolpos*, vagina, + *ptosis*, a falling]. Prolapse of the vagina.

colporrhagia (kol"po-ra'ji-a) [" + *rhegnynai*, to burst forth]. Excessive vaginal discharge. Vaginal hemorrhage.

colporrhaphy (kol-por'a-fi) [" + *rhaphe*, suture]. Suture of vagina.

colporrhexis (kol"po-reks'is) [" + *rhexis*, rupture]. Laceration or rupture of the vaginal walls.

colposcope (kol'po-skop) [" + *skopein*, to examine]. An instrument for examining the fornices of the vagina and cervix uteri.

col'pospasm; colpospas'mus [Gr. *kolpos*, vagina, + *spasmos*, spasm]. Spasm of the vagina. SYN: *vaginismus.*

col'postat [" + L. *stare*, to stand]. Device for holding an instrument such as a radium applicator in place in the vagina.

colpostenosis (kol"po-sten-o'sis) [" + *stenosis*, narrowing]. Stenosis or narrowing of the vagina.

colpostenotomy (kol"po-sten-ot'o-mi) [" + " + *tome*, incision]. A cutting operation for dilating the lumen in stricture of the vagina.

colpotherm (kol'po-thurm) [" + *therme*, heat]. Electrical device introduced into the vagina to convey heat.

colpotomy (kol-pot'o-mi) [Gr. *kolpos*, vagina, + *tome*, incision]. Incision into the wall of the vagina.

colpoureterocystotomy (kol"po-u-re"ter-o-sis-tot'o-mi) [" + *oureter*, ureter, + *kystis*, bladder, + *tome*, incision]. Exposure of the ureteral orifices by incision through the walls of the vagina and bladder.

colpoureterot'omy [" + " + *tome*, incision]. Incision of the ureter through the vagina.

colpoxerosis (kol"po-ze-ro'sis) [" + *xerosis*, dryness]. Abnormal dryness of the vulva and vagina.

columbium. SEE: *niobium.*

columella (kol"u-mel'la) [L., small column]. 1. A little column. 2. In bacteriology, portion of the sporangiophore upon which are borne the spores.

    c. cochleae. The modiolus of the cochlea.

    c. na'si. The anterior part of the septum of nose; a turbinate bone.

column (kol'um) [L. *columna*, pillar]. A cylindrical supporting structure.

    c., anterior. The anterior portion of the gray matter on each side of the spinal cord. Also called anterior horn. With reference to white matter, the posterior funiculus.

    c. of Burdach. The fasciculus cuneatus, q.v.

    c., Clarke's. A group of large cells in medial portion of the base of the posterior gray column of the spinal cord.

    c., fornicis. A column of the fornix, two arched bands of fibers which form the anterior portion of the fornix. Fibers lead to mammillary body.

    c. of Goll. The fasciculus gracilis, q.v.

    c. of Gowers. Tract of ascending fibers anterior to the direct cerebellar column and on the lateral surface of the spinal cord.

    c., lateral. A column in lateral portion of gray matter of spinal cord. Contains cell bodies of preganglionic neurons of sympathetic nervous system. The lateral funiculus or the white matter between roots of spinal nerves.

    c. of Morgagni. One of several vertical ridges in mucous membrane at junction of anus and rectum.

c., posterior. The posterior horn of the gray matter of the spinal cord. It consists of an expanded portion or caput connected by a narrower cervix to the main portion of gray matter. The posterior funiculus of the white matter.

c., renal. A column of Bertin, cortical material of the kidney which extends centrally, separating the pyramids.

c., spinal. The line of vertebrae from the head to the pelvis, making up the bony flexible case for the spinal cord. The vertebral column, q.v.

c., vertebral. The spinal column; the portion of the axial skeleton consisting of vertebrae (7 cervical, 12 thoracic, 5 lumbar, a sacrum and coccyx) joined together by intervertebral disks. It forms the main supporting axis of the body, encloses and protects the spinal cord, and serves for attachment of the appendicular skeleton and muscles for moving the various bodily parts.

c., vesicular. Line of ganglion cells on inner side of posterior column.

columna (ko-lum'na) [L.]. (pl. *columnae*) A column or pillar.

c. bertini. Interpyramidal extension or renal column supporting renal blood vessels.

c. carnea. A muscular projection within the cardiac ventricles. SYN: *trabecula carnea.*

c. nasi. Nasal septum.

c. rugarum vaginae. Fold of mucous membrane of the vagina which is arranged in a columnar fashion.

colum'nar layer. Retinal rod-and-cone layer.

columning (kol'um-ing). Introduction of tampons in vagina to support the prolapsed uterus.

co'ma [Gr. *kōma*, a deep sleep]. An abnormal deep stupor occurring in illness, or as a result of it, or due to an injury. The patient cannot be aroused by external stimuli.

More than 50% of cases are due to trauma to the head or circulatory accidents in the brain caused by hypertension, sclerosis, thrombosis, tumor, abscess formation, or insufficient flow of blood to the brain. Other frequent causes of c. are acute infections of the brain or meninges; acute infections and bacterial intoxications as in fevers, botulism, and other diseases; effects of drugs (alcohol, atropine, barbiturates, chloral, hyoscine, paraldehyde, and phenols); trauma as in accidents, hemorrhage, and shocks; gases or fumes such as carbon dioxide or carbon monoxide; extreme temperature; neurosis such as in malingering.

GENERAL TREATMENT: First aid treatment should be strictly limited; patient should not be moved other than to slightly raise the head. Movement without aid of a physician is dangerous. The collar should be loosened. Cold compresses to head and hot ones to the spine and abdomen may be indicated. Stomach pump in case of poisoning indicated. Insulin injection for diabetic coma may be given unless the coma is due to too much insulin. *Caution:* If there is a question of whether the coma is due to an over dose of insulin or diabetic coma, it is safe to give glucose intravenously; insulin might be disastrous.

Urine should be examined for albumin and sugar.

In uremic coma, stimulate elimination. In coma due to hysteria, the patient requires careful nursing care and observation but no specific therapy is indicated.

NP: Test urine for cause, and for retention. Clean mouth. Keep water out of trachea. Keep eyes cleansed. Apply an ointment to prevent lids from sticking together. Guard against bed sores. May have to be fed artificially.

c., alcoholic. Due to alcohol.

c., apoplectic. Due to cerebral hemorrhage or apoplexy; one side of body, and/or one or more of the extremities will be paralyzed. No fever at first but one pupil may be larger than the other. Coma usually indicates increased intracranial pressure. SEE: *apoplexy.*

c., diabetic. Occurring in diabetes, due to lack of insulin which causes metabolic changes with excess production of acetone bodies, q.v., and metabolic acidosis. Paralysis not present. SYM: Sweet breath. Hyperglycemia is present, and eyeballs may be soft due to dehydration.

TREATMENT: Correct use of insulin has prevented diabetic coma to a large extent but an overdose may induce hypoglycemic coma. Thus do not give insulin until the diagnosis of diabetic coma is made. Examine urine hourly for dextrose; if urine is sugar-free, more dextrose must be given.

c., uremic. The result of disturbed kidney metabolism, causing autointoxication through the retention of metabolic end products which would normally be excreted by the kidneys. Interference with the acid-base balance develops.

SYM: In general, respiration stertorous; face livid; skin dry and may be covered with "uremic frost," which is a collection of urea excreted in the sweat; hard and rapid pulse;

Diagnosis of Diabetic and Hypoglycemic Coma*

	Diabetic Coma	Hypoglycemic Coma
Onset	Gradual	Often sudden
History	Often of acute infection in a diabetic or no previous history of diabetes	Recent insulin injection, or inadequate meal or excessive exercise after insulin
Skin	Flushed, dry	Pale, sweating
Tongue	Dry or furred	Moist
Breath	Smell of acetone	No acetone
Respiration	Deep (air hunger)	Shallow
Pulse	Rapid, feeble	Normal or bounding
Eyeball Tension	Low	Normal or raised
Urine	Sugar and acetone	None, unless bladder has not been emptied for some hours
Blood Sugar	Raised [over 200 mg. %]	Subnormal [20–50 mg. %]
Blood Pressure	Low	Normal
Abdominal Pain	Common and often acute	Sometimes sense of constriction

* Sears, W. G., Winwood, R. S.: Medicine for Nurses, ed. 11. Edward Arnold Publishers Ltd., London, 1970.

blood pressure elevated; sphincters relaxed according to cause; urinous odor on breath, urine scanty and containing many casts and albumin. Complete retention may occur.

c. vigil. Delirious lethargy with open eyes and partial consciousness.

co'matose. In a condition of coma.

comedo (kom'e-do) [L. *comedere*, to eat up]. (pl. *comedon'es, com'edos*) Blackhead. Discolored dried sebum plugging an excretory duct of the skin.

ETIOL: Either increased activity of sebaceous glands or material secreted is unable to escape through a too-narrow opening.

SYM: Commonly affects the face, back, and ears; chronic, frequently associated with seborrheic dermatitis, or acne, usually during adolescence.

PROG: Obstinate and persistent, but amenable to treatment.

TREATMENT: Aside from careful and gentle removal of plugs, treatment is essentially that of acne, q.v.

comes (ko'mēz) [L., companion]. (pl. *com'ites*) A blood vessel which accompanies a nerve or another blood vessel.

comma bacillus. Vibrio comma, the causative organism of cholera. Named for its shape.

comma tract of Schultz. The fasciculus interfascicularis, a tract of descending fibers located between the fasciculus cuneatus and fasciculus gracilis in the posterior funiculus of the spinal cord.

commen'sal [L. *com-*, together, + *mensa*, table]. One of two organisms which live in an intimate, nonparasitic relationship.

commensalism (kom-men'sal-izm"). The symbiotic relationship of two organisms of different species in which neither is harmful to the other and one gains some benefit such as protection or nourishment. Ex: nonpathogenic bacteria in human intestine.

comminute (kom'in-ūt) [L. *com-*, together, + *minuēre*, to crumble]. To break into pieces.

com'minuted fracture. A crushed bone.

comminution (kom"in-ū'shun) [L. *comminutiō*, crumbling]. Reducing a solid body to varying sizes by grating, pulverizing, slicing, granulating, and by other processes. SEE:*attenuation; dynamization.*

commissu'ra [L.]. (pl. *commissurae*) A commissure.

commissu'ral. Pert. to a commissure.

commissure (kŏm'ĭ-shūr) [L. *commissura*, a joining together]. 1. A transverse band of nerve fibers passing over the midline in the central nervous system. 2. The coming together of two structures, as the lips, eyelids, or nymphae.

c., anterior cerebral. A band of white fibers which passes through lamina terminalis connecting the two cerebral hemi-spheres.

c., anterior gray. One in spinal cord lying anterior to central canal.

c., anterior white. One in spinal cord lying anterior to central canal and anterior to the anterior gray commissure.

c. of fornix. A band of fibers connecting the two crura.

c., middle. SEE: *mass, intermediate cell.*

c., posterior, of brain. One just above the midbrain containing fibers which connect the superior colliculi.

c., posterior, of spinal cord. A gray commissure connecting two halves of spinal cord. It lies posterior to central canal.

common bile duct. Duct carrying bile to the doudenum and receiving it from the cystic and hepatic ducts. SYN: *common duct; ductus choledochus.* SEE: *bile.*

Method of Transfer of Some Common Communicable Diseases

Disease	How Agent Leaves the Bodies of the Sick	How Organisms May Be Transferred	Method of Entry Into the Body
Typhoid fever	Feces and urine	Direct contact Hands of nurse or attendant Linen and all articles used by and about patient Hands of carriers soiled by their own feces Water polluted by excreta Food grown in or washed with such water Milk diluted with contaminated water Flies	Through mouth in infected food or water and thence to intestinal tract
Diphtheria	Sputum and discharges from nose and throat Skin lesions	Direct contact Droplet infection from patient coughing Hands of nurse Articles used by and about patient	Through mouth to throat or nose to throat
Streptococcal sore throat	Discharges from nose and throat Skin lesions	Direct contact Hands of nurse Articles used by and about patient	Through mouth and nose
Pneumonia	Sputum and discharges from nose and throat	Direct contact Hands of nurse Articles used by and about patient	Through mouth and nose to lungs
Influenza	As in pneumonia	As in pneumonia	As in pneumonia

Method of Transfer of Some Common Communicable Diseases *(Continued)*

Disease	How Agent Leaves the Bodies of the Sick	How Organisms May Be Transferred	Method of Entry Into the Body
Tetanus	Excreta from infected herbivorous animals and man	Soil, especially that with manure or feces in it Dust, etc. Articles used about stables	Directly into blood stream through wounds (Is anaerobe and prefers deep, incised wound)
Tuberculosis, Human	Sputum Lesions Feces	Direct contact such as kissing Droplet infection from person coughing with mouth uncovered Sputum from mouth to fingers, thence to food and other things Soiled dressings	Through mouth to lungs and intestines From intestines via lymph channels to lymph vessels and to tissues
Tuberculosis, Bovine		Milk from infected cow	Same as Tuberculosis, Human
Cholera	Excreta from intestinal tract	As in typhoid fever	As in typhoid fever
Hookworm	Feces	Direct contact with soil polluted with feces Eggs in feces hatch in sandy soil Feces may also contaminate food	Larvae enter through breaks in skin, especially skin of feet, and after devious passage through the body settle in the intestine
Meningitis, meningococcal	Discharges from nose and throat	Direct contact Hands of nurse or attendant Articles used by and about patient Flies	Mouth and nose
Poliomyelitis	Discharges from nose and throat, and via feces	Direct contact Hands of nurse or attendant Rarely in milk	Through mouth and nose
Measles (Rubella)	As in streptococcal sore throat	As in streptococcal sore throat	As in streptococcal sore throat

Method of Transfer of Some Common Communicable Diseases (*Continued*)

Disease	How Agent Leaves the Bodies of the Sick	How Organisms May Be Transferred	Method of Entry Into the Body
Gonococcal disease	Lesions Discharges from infected mucous membranes	Direct contact as in sexual intercourse Towels, bathtubs, toilets, etc. Hands of infected persons soiled with their own discharges Hands of attendant	Directly onto mucous membrane Through breaks in membrane
Ophthalmia neonatorum (gonococcal infection of eyes of newborn)	Purulent discharges from the eye	Direct contact with infected areas as vagina of infected mother during birth Other infected babies Hands of doctor or nurse Linens, etc.	Directly on the conjunctiva
Whooping cough	Discharges from respiratory tract	Direct contact with persons affected	Mouth and nose
Mumps	Discharges from infected glands and mouth	Direct contact with persons affected	Mouth and nose
Smallpox	Discharges from nose and throat Skin lesions	Direct contact Hands of nurse Articles used by and about patient	Thought to be through mucous membrane of respiratory tract
Syphilis	Infected tissues Lesions Blood Transfer through placenta to fetus	Direct contact Kissing or sexual intercourse Needles and syringes	Directly into blood and tissues through breaks in skin or membrane Needles and syringes
Trachoma	Discharges from infected eyes	Direct contact Hands, towels, handkerchiefs, possibly clothing	Directly on conjunctiva
Leprosy	Uncertain, may be from lesions Bacilli found in nodules which may break down, forming lesions	Uncertain	Uncertain

commu'nicable disease. 1. A disease which may be transmitted directly or indirectly from one individual to another. 2. One due to an infectious agent or toxic products produced by it.

communicable disease, words pert. to carrier; contagion; endemic; epidemic; host, alternate; immunity; incubation; infection; isolation; microbe; micrococcus; microorganism; quarantine; transmissible; vector.

commu'nicans [L. *communicāre*, to connect with]. One of a number of communicating nerves or arteries.

Comolli's sign (kō-mōl'lī). A triangular swelling corresponding to the outline of the scapula when fractured.

compact' [L. *compactus*, joined together]. Dense, packed, solid.

    c. bone. Hard or dense bone which forms the superficial layer of all bones, in contrast to spongy or cancellous bone found chiefly in the ends of long bones.

compar'ative anat'omy. Human anatomy compared with that of animals.

compatibil'ity [L. *compati*, to sympathize with]. 1. State of suitability to be mixed or taken together without unfavorable results, as drugs. 2. The ability of two individuals or groups to live together without undue strife or tension.

compat'ible. Not opposed to; able to mix with another substance without destructive changes.

com'pensating. Making up for a deficiency.

    c. operation. Tenotomy of the associated antagonists in diplopia.

compensa'tion [L. *cum,* with, + *pensāre,* to weigh]. 1. Making up a defect, as cardiac circulation competent to meet demands made upon it, regardless of valvular defect. 2. In psychoanalysis, a psychic mechanism, best described by an example. The individual handicapped by a physical deformity or variation, or by a character defect, may escape the consciousness or revelation of the inferiority, by accomplishment resulting from compensatory ambition. More simply, the short man may strut or the incompetent brag.

    Sublimation, q.v., is often similar, but varies in that the substitution of a higher social goal gratifies the infrasocial drive by replacement—rather than going to the opposite extreme in a merely camouflaging manner.

    c., failure of. Inability of heart muscle to cope with cardiac output required. It indicates a diseased heart muscle.

    ETIOL: Diseased myocardium; back pressure, due to mitral regurgitation, mitral or aortic stenosis, or aortic regurgitation.

comp'lement [L. *complēre*, to complete]. A substance or body producing bacteriolysis or hemolysis which, by means of an amboceptor, is connected with a bacterial or animal cell.

    It is present in all sera. Strictly speaking, c. is not an antibody, but a natural property of blood.

    RS: albumin; Ehrlich's theory.

    c. fixation. SEE: *fixation, complement.*

complement'al, complement'ary. Supplying something that is lacking.

    c. air. Amount of air that can be inspired over and above the tidal air by the deepest inspiration. SEE: *air.*

    c. colors. Any two primary colors which, when blended, produce white light.

complemen'toid [L. *complēre*, to complete, + Gr. *eidos,* form]. A complement, the lysis-causing power of which has been destroyed.

complementophil (kom"plē-ment'o-fil) ["+ Gr. *philein,* to love]. Having the power to combine with a complement.

com'plex [L. *complexus,* woven together]. 1. All the ideas, feelings, and sensations connected with a subject. 2. Intricate. 3. An atrial or ventricular systole as it appears on an electrocardiograph tracing.

    4. A subconscious idea (or group of ideas) which has become associated with a repressed wish or emotional experience and which may influence behavior although the person may not have any appreciation of the connection between the repressed thoughts or actions.

    In Freudian psychology a grouping of ideas with an emotional background. These may be harmless, and the individual fully aware of them, e.g., an artist sees every object with a view to a possible picture and is said to have established a c. for art. Often, however, the c. is aroused by some painful emotional reaction, such as fright or excessive grief, which, instead of being allowed a natural outlet, becomes unconsciously repressed, and later manifests itself in some abnormality of mind or behavior. According to Freud, the best method of determining the c. is through the medium of psychoanalysis. SEE: *Electra c.; Oedipus c.*

    c., castration. Morbid fear of being castrated.

    c., Electra. Excessive love of the father by an adult female. SEE: *Electra complex.*

    c., inferiority. A state of mind in which one feels himself inferior to others.

c., Oedipus. Excessive love for his mother manifested by an adult male, usually accompanied by hostility toward father. SEE: *Oedipus complex.*

c., superiority. Exaggerated conviction of one's own superiority; also pretense of being superior to compensate for a supposed inferiority.

complex'us [L.]. Semispinalis capitis muscle.

complica'tion [L. *cum,* with, + *plicāre,* to fold]. An added difficulty; a complex state. A disease or accident superimposed upon another without being specifically related, yet affecting or modifying the prognosis of the original disease, e.g., pneumonia is a complication of measles, and is the cause of many deaths from that disease.

compo'nent. A constituent part.

c. blood therapy. Use of a specific blood component, such as plasma, or washed red cells, instead of an entire unit of whole blood. This practice reduces the chances for adverse reaction to whole blood transfusion while permitting the desired and essential ingredient of blood to be administered.

compos mentis (kŏm"pŭs mĕn'tĭs) [L.]. Of sound mind; sane.

com'pound [L. *componere,* to place together]. 1. A substance composed of two or more units or parts combined in definite proportions by weight and having specific properties of its own. Compounds are formed in plants and animals and are of two types, organic and inorganic. 2. Made up of more than one part.

c. astigmatism. Myopia of both vertical and horizontal meridians.

c. fracture. Fracture of bone where broken end of bone has penetrated the skin.

c., inorganic. One of many compounds which, in general, contain no carbon.

c. microscope. One consisting of two or more lenses.

c., organic. A compound containing carbon. Examples are carbohydrates, proteins, and fats.

compress [L. *compressus,* squeezed together]. 1. (kŏm'prĕs) Cloth, wet or dry, folded and applied firmly to a part. 2. (kŏm-prĕs') To press together into smaller space. 3. To close by squeezing together, as a wound.

c., chest. Application of two pieces of linen of sufficient size to fit the entire chest from the clavicles down to the umbilicus.

c., cold. Soft, absorbent cloth, several layers thick, dipped in cold water, slightly wrung out, applied to given part. To maintain constant temperature, c. is frequently renewed or ice bag or rubber coil through

which ice water is circulating is placed on it. Duration, 30-60 minutes.

c., forehead. A soft, moist towel renewed at least every two minutes.

c., hot. Soft, absorbent cloth folded into several layers, dipped in hot water (107-115° F. or 41.7-46.1° C.), barely wrung out and placed on part to be treated; covered with a piece of flannel large enough to overlap the linen slightly. Temperature is maintained at constant level by renewing c. or by rubber coil through which hot water (107-115° F. or 41.7-46.1° C.) is circulated.

c., wet. Application of two or more folds of soft cloth wrung out of water at prescribed temperatures and covered with flannel.

compression [L. *compressio,* a compression]. A squeezing together; state of being pressed together.

c. atrophy. Atrophy in a part due to steady compression.

c., cerebral. Pressure on the brain produced by increased intercranial fluids, embolism, thrombosis, tumors, and skull fractures. More serious than concussion, q.v.

SYM: Deep unconsciousness; full, bounding pulse; deep, stertorous, slow respiration; flushed face; high blood pressure; pupils varying in size. Temperature may rise and there may be retention or incontinence of urine and feces. *Danger Signals:* Coma; Cheyne-Stokes respiration; rise in temperature; quickening of pulse.

NP: Watch for change of symptoms; pulse, respiration, color, urine; and for bed sores; also convulsions, bleeding from ears and nose, and oozing at back of throat; for cerebrospinal fluid from ears, which may indicate fracture. Constant care of mouth and eyes.

c., digital. Compression of blood vessels by means of the fingers in order to stop hemorrhage.

c., myelitis. That caused by pressure on the spinal cord, often due to a tumor.

compres'sor. 1. Instrument for making pressure on a part. 2. A muscle which compresses a part as the compressor hemispherium bulbi which compresses the bulb of the urethra.

compul'sion [L. *compulsiō,* compulsion]. Repetitive stereotyped act performed to relieve fear connected with obsession; dictation by the patient's subconscious against the subject's wishes and, if denied, causing uneasiness.

c. neurosis. Obsession or psychoneurosis urging one to perform an absurd act or to say something silly.

compul'sive. Pert. to compulsion.

c. ideas. An idea that continues, against one's will, to suggest the commitment of an overt act which would normally be against one's better judgment.

compul'sory. Compelling action against one's will.

c. movements. Movements caused by injury to a nerve center.

con- [L.]. Prefix meaning together with.

conarium (ko-nā'rĭ-um) [Gr. *kōnarion,* a little cone]. Obsolete name for the pineal body. SYN: *corpus pineal* [NA].

conation (ko-nā'shun) [L. *conātio,* an attempt]. The desire or impulse, arising from inside one, to act.

concassation (kon"kas-ā'shun) [L. *con,* with, + *quatere,* to shake]. 1. Shaking of a precipitate in a bottle or pulverizing by beating. 2. Mental distress.

concatenation (kon-kat"ĭ-nā'shun) [L. *con,* together, + *catena,* chain]. A group of events or effects acting in concert or occurring at the same time.

Concato's disease (kŏn-kŏ'tō). [Luigi M. Concato, It. physician, 1825-1882]. Progressive inflammation of serous membranes in tuberculosis.

concave (kon'kāv) [L. *con,* with, + *cavus,* hollow]. Having a spherically depressed or hollow surface.

concav'ity. A surface, with curved, bowl-like sides.

conca"vocon'cave [L. *con,* with, + *cavus,* hollow, + *con,* with, + *cavus,* hollow]. Concave on opposing sides.

concavocon'vex ["+ "+ *convexus,* vaulted]. Concave on one side and convex on opposite surface. SEE: *convex.*

conceive (kŏn-sēv') [L. *concipere,* to take to oneself]. 1. To become pregnant. 2. To form a mental image or to bring into mind; to form an idea.

concentration (kon-sen-trā'shun) [L. *con,* together, + *centrum,* center]. 1. Increase in strength of a fluid by evaporation. 2. Medicine strengthened by evaporation. 3. Fixation of mind on one subject to exclusion of all other thoughts.

c., hydrogen ion. Concentration of hydrogen ions in a solution; the symbol is pH.

con'cept [L. *conceptum,* something understood]. An idea.

concep'tion. 1. The mental process of forming an idea. 2. The union of the male sperm and the ovum of the female; fertilization.

With a cycle of 28 days, menstruation normally lasts five days followed by a period of repair and proliferation of about a week. Until ovulation occurs the female is sterile. In general, ovulation occurs about 12-14 days prior to the beginning of the next menstrual period. Thus sexual intercourse during the

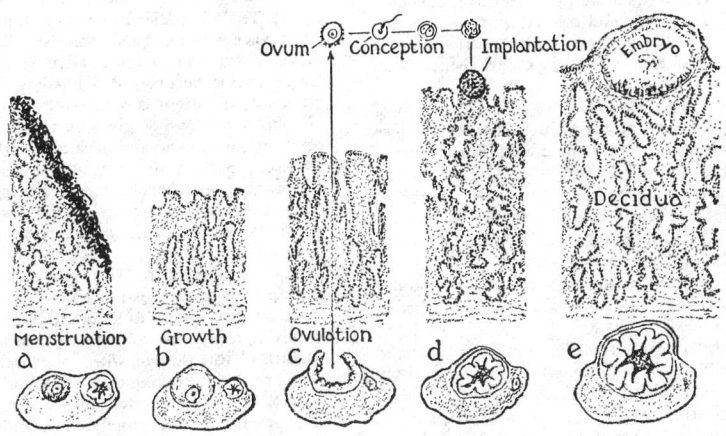

MENSTRUATION, CONCEPTION, AND IMPLANTATION
Above, Endometrium, lining of uterus; Below, graafian follicle of ovary. A, Menstruation. Lining is shed; graafian follicle begins to develop in ovary. B, Growth. Endometrium is repaired and thickens; follicle continues to grow. C, Ovulation and conception. Graafian follicle ruptures to free the ovum which becomes impregnated. D, Ovum in morula stage becomes implanted in lining of uterus. Endometrium now in pregravid stage; corpus luteum· of pregnancy developing. E, Endometrium becomes decidua and ovum is growing in it.

middle of the menstrual cycle is most likely to result in conception. During this period, the ovum is discharged from the follicle and makes its way through the fallopian tube to the uterus. If fertilization does not occur during this time the ovum disintegrates and for the remaining portion of the menstrual cycle (the 10 days preceding menstruation) conception is very unlikely to occur.

However, one of the most variable events known in human biology is the menstrual cycle. It is therefore quite difficult, and in many cases impossible, to predict optimum time of conception or the reverse by attempting to calculate ovulation time from the time the last menstrual period occurred. Also sperm survival time in the female reproductive tract is variable.

concep'tus. The products of conception.

concha (kong'kă) [Gr. *konchē,* shell]. (pl. *conchae*) 1. The outer ear or the pinna. 2. One of the three nasal conchae, q.v.

    c. auriculae. [NA] A concavity on the median surface of the auricle of the ear, divided by a ridge into the upper cymba conchae and a lower cavum conchae. The latter leads to the exterior auditory meatus.

    c. bullosa. Distention of turbinate bone due to cyst formation.

    c. nasal. One of the three scroll-like bones which project medially from the lateral wall of the nasal cavity; a turbinate bone. The superior and middle conchae are processes of lateral mass of the ethmoid bone; the inferior concha is a face bone. Each overlies a meatus.

    c. sphenoidalis. In a fetal skull, one of two curved plates located on anterior portion of body of sphenoid bone. Forms part of roof of nasal cavity.

conchitis (kong-ki'tis) ["+ *-itis,* inflammation]. Inflammation of any concha.

conchoidal (kong-koy'dal) ["+ *eidos,* shape]. Having the shape of a shell.

conchoscope (kong'ko-scōp) ["+ *skopein,* to examine]. Instrument for examination of the nasal cavity.

conchotome (kong'ko-tōm) [Gr. *konchē,* shell, + *tomē,* incision]. Device for excision of middle turbinated bone.

concoc'tion [L. *con,* with, + *coquere,* to cook]. Mixture of two medicinal substances usually done with the aid of heat.

concom'itant ["+ *comes,* companion]. Accessory; taking place at the same time.

concrement [L. *concrementum*]. A concretion as of protein and other substances. If infiltrated with calcium salts, such is termed a calculus.

concrescence (kon-kres'ens) [L. *con,* together, + *crescere,* to grow]. The union of separate parts; coalescence.

concrete (kon'krēt, kon-krēt') [L. *concretus,* solid]. Condensed, hardened, or solidified.

concre'tion [L. *con,* with, + *crescere,* to grow]. A calculus.

concub'itus [L.]. Coitus, sexual intercourse.

concus'sion [L. *concussus,* shaken violently]. 1. An injury resulting from impact with an object. 2. Loss of function either partial or complete as that resulting from a blow or fall.

    c. of the brain. Cerebral concussion. A common result of a blow to the head, or fall on the end of spine with force sufficient to be transmitted upward. This usually causes unconsciousness, either temporary or prolonged. Return of consciousness may be gradual. Patient may suddenly draw up knees and vomit. Resembles result of skull fracture.

    SYM: Vary with location and extent of injury from transient dizziness to various paralyses, or unconsciousness; unequal pupils, shock. If uncomplicated, patient regains consciousness in a short period of time. Period of reaction, accompanied by vomiting, temperature 99° or 100° F. (37.2-37.8° C.) rapid pulse, flushed face, restlessness, headache, cerebral irritation, lasts for from 12 to 24 hours.

    F.A. TREATMENT: Keep patient quietly lying down with head and shoulders slightly elevated. Do not give stimulants. Transportation should be delayed if possible. Sedatives only if patient is hyperexcited.

    CAUTION: Do not give morphine. Cool applications to head and neck are soothing. Reassure patient if conscious. Warm extremities if cold. Report any adverse symptoms, such as bleeding, at once. Darkened room best. SEE: *contusion; transportation of injured.*

    c. of labyrinth. Deafness resulting from a blow to the head or ear.

    c., spinal. Loss of function in spinal cord resulting from a blow or severe jarring.

condensa'tion [L. *con,* with, + *dēnsāre,* to make thick]. 1. Making more dense or compact. 2. Changing a liquid to a solid or a gas to a liquid. 3. In psychoanalysis, the union of ideas to form a new mental pattern. 4. In chemistry, a type of reaction in which two or more molecules of the same substance react with each other and form a new and heavier substance with different chemical properties.

conden'ser. Device for solidifying vapors and liquids. SEE: *capacitance.*

c., electrical. Device for storing of electricity by using two conducting surfaces and a nonconductor.

con'diment [L. *condire,* to pickle]. Appetizing ingredient added to food.

CLASSIFICATION: *Aromatic:* Vanilla; cinnamon; cloves; chervil; parsley; bay leaf, etc. *Acrid or Peppery:* Pepper; ginger; allspice, etc.*Alliaceous or Allylic:* Onion; mustard; horseradish. *Acid:* Vinegar; capers; gherkins; citron. *Animal Origin:* Caviar; anchovies.

In general, condiments have little nutritional value. Sugar is an exception. They are extremely useful in making food more appetizing.

ACTION: They are appetizers and stimulate the secretion of saliva and intestinal juices.

condi'tioned reflex. One acquired as result of training and repetition.

con'dom [L. *condus,* a receptacle]. A thin, flexible sheath worn over the penis. It is used during sexual intercourse to prevent sperm from entering the vagina and to help prevent venereal disease.

conduc'tance [L. *conducere,* to lead]. The conducting ability of a body or a circuit for electricity.

The best conductor is that which offers the least resistance. Examples of good conductors are gold, silver, and copper. When expressed in figures, c. is the reciprocal of resistance. The unit is the ohm.

conduc'tion. 1. The process whereby a state of excitation affects successive portions of a tissue or cell, so that the disturbance is transmitted to remote points. C. occurs not only in the fibers of the nervous system, but also in muscle fibers. 2. The transfer of electrons, ions, heat, or sound waves through a conductor or conducting medium.

c., bone. Sound conduction through cranial bones.

conductiv'ity. The specific electric conducting ability of a substance.

Numerically, c. is the reciprocal of unit resistance, or resistivity. The unit is the ohm/cm. Specific c. is sometimes expressed as a percentage. In such cases the c. is given as a percentage of the c. of pure copper under certain standard conditions.

conductor (kon-duk'tor). 1. Medium transmitting a force. 2. A guide directing a surgical knife or probe.

condylar (kon'di-lăr) [Gr. *kondylos,* knuckle]. Pert. to a condyle.

condylarthrosis (kon"dil-ar-thrō'sis) ["+ *arthrōsis,* a joint]. A form of diarthrosis, q.v.; an ovoid head in an elliptical cavity.

condyle (kon'dīl) [Gr. *kondylos,* knuckle]. (pl. *condyles*) A rounded protuberance at the end of a bone forming an articulation.

condylectomy (kon"di-lek'to-mī) ["+ *ektomē,* excision]. Excision of a condyle.

condylion (kon-dīl'ī-on) [Gr. *kondylion,* knob]. A point on either the lateral or medial surface of the mandibular condyle.

condyloid (kon'dī-loyd) [Gr. *kondylos,* knuckle, + *eidos,* appearance]. Pert. to or resembling a condyle.

c. process. Articular process on ramus of mandible consisting of a capitulum and neck. Articulates with mandibular fossa of temporal bone.

c. tubercle. A tubercle on capitulum of condyloid process of the mandible for attachment of temporomandibular ligament.

condyloma (kŏn-dī-lō'mă) [Gr. *kondylōma,* wart]. A wartlike growth of the skin, usually seen on the external genitalia or near the anus.

There are two types, a pointed variety, and a broad, flat form which is usually of syphilitic origin.

c. latum. A mucous patch on the vulva or anus, coated with gray exudate, flattened in form, with delimited area, characteristic of syphilis.

condylomatous (kon"dī-lo'mă-tus). Pert. to a condyloma.

condylotomy (kon"dī-lot'o-mī) [Gr. *kondylos,* knuckle, + *tomē,* incision]. Division without removal of a condyle.

condylus (kon'dī-lus). (pl. *condylī*) Condyle.

cone (kōn) [Gr. *kōnos,* cone]. 1. A three-dimensional figure with circular base with sides sloping to a point above. May be solid or hollow. 2. Retinal flask-shaped figure in layer of rods and cones. 3. A receptor cell of the retina concerned with color vision.

c. of light. Triangular light areas on the membrana tympani extending downward from the umbo.

c., ocular. C. of light in eye with tip on the retina.

confabula'tion [L. *confabulāri,* to talk together]. In psychoanalysis, the relating of imaginary experiences to fill in gaps in the memory.

confec'tio, confect'tion [L. *conficere,* to prepare]. Sugarlike soft solids in which one or more medicinal substances are incorporated with the object of affording an agreeable form for their administration and a convenient method for their preservation. Not often prescribed, and not official.

confinement (kon-fin'ment) [O.Fr. *confiner,* to restrain in a place]. The puerperal state or period of childbirth.

con'flict [L. *confligere*, to contend]. 1. Opposing action of incompatibles. 2. In psychiatry, the conscious or unconscious struggle between two opposing desires or courses of action. A technical term applied to a state in which social goals dictate behavior contrary to more primitive (often subconscious) desires.

confluence of sinuses. The union of the sagittal sinus with the transverse sinuses. SYN: *Confluens sinuum* [NA]; *torcular Herophili.*

con'fluent [L. *confluere*, to run together]. Running together, as when the pustules in smallpox merge.

confrontation (kon"frun-tā'shun) [L. *con*, together, + *frons*, face]. 1. The examination of two patients together, one with a disease and the other from whom the disease was supposed to be contracted. 2. A method employed in determining extent of visual fields in which that of the patient is compared with that of the examiner.

congelation (kon"jĕ-lā'shun) [L. *congelāre*, to freeze]. Freezing, or a frostbite.

congenerous (kon-jen'er-us) [L. *con*, together, + *genus*, race]. Possessing the same function, as synergistic muscles.

congen'ital [L. *congenitus*, born together]. Present at birth.

congested (kon-jes'ted) [L. *congerere*, to heap together]. Hyperemic; containing an abnormal amt. of blood.

conges'tion. The presence of an excessive amt. of blood or tissue fluid in an organ or in tissue.

    c., active. C. resulting from increased flow of blood to a part or dilatation of blood vessels.

    c., passive. Hyperemia resulting from interference with flow of blood from capillaries into venules. May also result from myocardial insufficiency.

congestive (kon-jes'tiv). Pert. to congestion.

congius (kon'jĭ-us) [L.]. (pl. *con'gii*) A gallon.

conglo'bate [L. *con*, together, + *globāre*, to make round]. In one mass, as lymph glands.

congloba'tion. Aggregation of particles in a rounded mass.

conglom'erate [L. *con*, together, + *glomerāre*, to heap]. 1. An aggregation in one mass. 2. Clustered; heaped together.

conglutin (kon-glu'tin) [L. *conglutināre*, to glue together]. A protein resembling casein found in peas, beans, and almonds.

conglu'tinant. Promoting adhesion, as of the edges of a wound.

conglu'tinate. Having the quality of adhesiveness.

conglutination (kon-glū"tin-a'shun). 1 Coalescence, adhesion. 2. Reaction, such as agglutination.

coniasis (kō-nī'ă-sis) [Gr. *konis*, dust]. Dust like calculi in gallbladder and bile ducts.

conidia (ko-nid'ĭ-ă). (pl. of *conidium*) Asexual spores of fungi.

conidiophore (kon-id'ĭ-o-for) [Gr. *konis* dust, + *phoros*, bearing]. The stalk supporting conidia.

coniol'ogy ["+ *logos*, study of]. The study of dust and its effects.

conio'sis ["+ *-ōsis*, infection]. Any condition caused by inhalation of dust.

coniza'tion [Gr. *kōnos*, cone]. Excision of a cone of tissue, as of the mucous membrane of the cervix.

conjugata (kon"ju-gā'tă) [L. *conjugatus* yoked together]. [NA] Diameter of pelvis, measured from center of the promontory of the sacrum to the back of the symphysis pubis. SYN: *conjugate.*

    c. vera. Sometimes written c.v. Same as conjugata.

conjugate (kon'jū-gāt). 1. Paired or joined 2. An important diameter of the pelvis, measured from the center of the promontory of the sacrum to the back of the symphysis pubis. In obstetrics the diagonal conjugate is measured and the true conjugate is estimated. SYN: *c. diameter.* SEE: *c., diagonal; c., external.*

    c. deviation. Deviation of both eyes to either side.

    c., diagonal. Measured from the lower edge of the symphysis to the sac and can be determined during life, whereas the true conjugate cannot be measured. The true conjugate is estimated by deducting 1.5 to 2.0 cm. from the length of the diagonal conjugate. It is about 1/2-3/4 in. (1.3-1.9 cm.) longer than the true conjugate, or about 5 in. (12.7 cm.).

    c. diameter. Conjugate, q.v.

    c., external. Measured from the spine of the last lumbar vertebra to the front of the pubes (this is done by using calipers), and is normally about 8 in. (20.3 cm.).

    c., true. Conjugate, q.v. SYN: *conjugata vera.*

conjuga'tion. A coupling together. In biology, the union of two unicellular organisms accompanied by an interchange of nuclear material as in Paramecium.

conjunctiva (con"junk-ti'vă) [L. *conjungere*, to join together]. Mucous membrane which lines eyelids and is reflected onto eyeball.

    DIVISIONS: Palpebral c. covers under-surface of lids; bulbar c. coats anterior portion of eyeball; fornix c. is the transition portion forming fold between lid and globe.

INSPECTION: Palpebral and ocular portions should be examined. Color and degree of moisture and presence of foreign bodies should be observed; also petechial hemorrhages and inflammation.

PATH. CONDITIONS: Trachoma and panus as well as discoloration. *Yellowish discoloration:* Seen in jaundice. *Pale conjunctivae:* Observed in anemias.

conjunctival reflex (kon″junk-tī′val). Closure of eyelids when conjunctiva is touched or threatened.

conjunctivitis (kon-junk″tī-vī′tis) [L. *con,* with, + *jungere,* to join, + Gr. *-itis,* inflammation]. Inflammation of conjunctiva.

TREATMENT: Directed against the specific type of infection.

c., actinic. Conjunctivitis resulting from exposure to ultraviolet (actinic) rays.

c., acute contagious. Pink eye. ETIOL: Koch-Weeks bacillus.

c., angular, of Morax-Axenfeld. That affecting the inner angle of the conjunctivae.

c., catarrhal. One due to a variety of causes such as foreign bodies, various bacteria, or irritation from heat, cold, or chemicals.

c., follicular. Type characterized by pinkish round bodies in retrotarsal fold.

c., gonorrheal. A severe, acute form of purulent conjunctivitis caused by the gonococcus, Neisseria gonorrhea. SEE: *ophthalmia neonatorum.*

c., granular. Acute, contagious, inflammatory c. with granular elevations on the lids which ulcerate and cicatrize. SYN: *trachoma.*

c., membranous. Acute conjunctivitis characterized by a false membrane; with or without infiltration.

c. of newborn. Ophthalmia neonatorum, q.v.

c., phlyctenular. An allergenic form commonly seen in children. Characterized by nodules which may ulcerate.

c., purulent. Form due to organisms producing purulence, esp. gonococcus.

c., vernal. One beginning in the spring. Most probably due to allergy.

conjunctivo′ma [" + " + Gr. *-ōma,* tumor]. A tumor of the conjunctiva.

conjunctivoplasty (kon″junk-tī′vo-plas″tī) [" + " + Gr. *plassein,* to form]. Removal of part of cornea, but replacing with flaps from the conjunctiva.

connec′tive [L. *connectere,* to bind together]. That which connects or binds together.

c. tissue. One of the four main tissues of the body. It includes an embryonic connective tissue (mesenchyme and mucous) and adult connective tissue. The latter is subdivided into four general groups: vascular tissues (blood, lymph); connective tissue proper (areolar, white fibrous, yellow fibrous, reticular, adipose); cartilage; and bone. Connective tissues are concerned primarily with supporting bodily structures and binding parts together. They also are involved in other functions such as food storage, blood formation, and defensive mechanisms of the body.

c. tissue diseases. SEE: *collagen diseases.*

co′noid [Gr. *kōnos,* cone, + *eidos,* shape]. Resembling a cone; conical.

c. ligament. Lower and inner portion of coracoclavicular ligament.

c. tubercle. Eminence on inferior surface of clavicle to which is attached the c. ligament.

consanguinity (kon″san-gwin′ĭ-tĭ) [L. *consanguinitās,* kinship]. Relationship by blood, i.e., being descended from a common ancestor.

conscious (kon′shus) [L. *conscius,* aware]. Being aware and having perception. SEE: *coma.*

con′sciousness. A state of awareness.

It implies an orientation to time, place, and person; i.e., the individual knows approximately the date, the nature of his environment, his name and other pertinent personal data.

The content of consciousness is a composite of memories and the comprehension of external reality; the emotional status and the individual's goals also enter. It is then a large part of that described as "personality" in its largest sense.

Consciousness varies its intensity and extent from minute to minute. In crises, vivid ideational association may lead to an exaggerated state of awareness. In states of relaxed contentment, it lessens, to disappear completely in sleep. This differs from the pathological condition of coma in which the patient cannot be aroused.

In so-called pathological sleep (e.g., encephalitis lethargica) and in stupor, though aroused, the patient is unable to postpone again lapsing into dullness, whereas, up to a point, normal sleep can be adequately combated by the demands of reality. Stupor is produced largely by the factors resulting in coma; the personality is relatively intact but "hazy." However, there are conditions in which a real personality change manifests itself. Clouding of consciousness may simulate the dullness but usually not the other characteristics of stupor. On the contrary, such patients may impress one as relatively alert.

Alteration of consciousness and attention; impaired orientation and recent memory are characteristic of delirium. A quiet delirium may not easily reveal itself, even in certain states of automatism in which one finds evidence of the "real personality;" there may appear on casual examination little to arouse suspicion, yet brutal acts or total absence of memory may indicate major abnormalities.

Clouding of consciousness may be diagnosed from the appearance of the patient in catatonic stupor and it may be difficult to realize the patient is quite lucid and that experiences are being registered accurately and can be later recalled. In true clouding, stimuli usually fail to register.

Again, in somnambulistic (i.e. sleepwalking) states, experiences may register but cannot be recalled after return to a normal state. During a later secondary state, it is apparent that the failure of memory is only a repression and not truly absent. Consciousness, on the other hand, may erroneously appear to be present in so-called "coma vigil" because the eyes are open and expression may be alert.

   c., clouding of. A phase of delirium in which the patient's consciousness is cloudy or not clear.

   c., cosmic. The inner reaches of consciousness in which there is recognition of knowledge or facts independent of physical influence.

   c., levels of. Altered consciousness from any cause may be classified as follows:

Somnolence. Patient may be delirious and restless, or still, and fall asleep when left alone. Even though he can answer questions he may be confused.

Stupor. Patient may be restless or combative, and may make twitching or picking motions. He should be protected from injuring himself. Responds to sensory stimuli including bright lights and loud sounds.

Semicoma. Spontaneous movement is absent unless the patient is roused. Even then, the response may be only a groan or a mutter. Withdraws from painful stimuli and is usually incontinent.

Deep coma. If patient responds at all, it is only to very painful stimuli. Spontaneous movements and resistance to passive movement are absent.

consen'sual [L. *consensus*, agreement]. Reflex stimulation of one part or side as the result of excitation of another part or opposite side.

   c. light index. When one eye is exposed to an intensity of light different from that to which the other is exposed, both pupils will react.

   c. reflex. Any reflex occurring on opposite side of body from point of stimulation.

consolidation (kon-sol-ĭ-dā'shun) [L. *consolidāre*, to make firm]. The act of becoming solid. Esp. used in connection with the solidification of the lungs due to engorgement of the lung tissues, as occurs in acute pneumonia.

constella'tion [L. *con*, together, + *stella*, star]. Ideas arising from unrepressed emotions.

constipation (kŏn"stĭ-pā'shun) [L. *constipāre*, to press together]. Difficult defecation; infrequent defecation with passage of unduly hard and dry fecal material; sluggish action of the bowels.

CAUSES: Predisposing: No regular bowel movements from childhood; worry, anxiety, fear, sedentary life. Direct: Failure to establish definite and regular times for bowel movements; improper diet; intestinal obstruction; tumors; excessive use of laxatives; weakness of intestinal musculature (atony) or excessive tonicity (spasticity); use of certain drugs; presence of anal lesions.

GENERAL CORRECTIVE MEASURES: Plenty of fresh vegetables, fruits, milk, and an abundance of water. Attempt to establish regular bowel, exercise, and eating habits.

   c., atonic. That due to weakness of muscles of colon and rectum.

   c., obstructive. Due to an obstruction in the intestines. Surgical aid may be needed. Preoperative diet should contain low residue and no gas-forming foods.

   c., spastic. That due to excessive tonicity of the intestinal wall, esp. the colon.

constitu'tion [L. *constituere*, to establish]. The physical makeup and functional habits of the body.

constitu'tional. Pert. to the body as a whole.

   c. disease. 1. One that affects the entire body rather than a specific part. 2. One that is dependent upon an individual's hereditary makeup, e.g., hemophilia.

constric'tion [L. *con*, together, + *stringere*, to draw]. 1. A binding or squeezing of a part. 2. The narrowing of a vessel or opening, as constriction of blood vessels or the pupil of the eye.

constric'tor. 1. That which binds or restricts a part. 2. A muscle which constricts a vessel, opening, or passageway, as the constrictors of the faucial isthmus and pharynx, the circular fibers of the iris, intestine, and blood vessels.

construct'ive metabolism. The binding up or anabolic process.

consult'ant [L. *consultāre*, to counsel]. A consulting physician or surgeon who acts in an advisory capacity.

consulta'tion. Diagnosis and proposed treatment by two or more physicians at one time.

consumption (kon-sump'shun) [L. *consumere*, to waste away]. 1. Tuberculosis, q.v. 2. Wasting. 3. The using up of anything.

consumption-coagulopathy. Clinical condition of altered blood coagulation wherein depletion of the clotting factors I, II, V, VIII, and platelets occurs. A pathological state secondary to a variety of diseases. SYN: *disseminated intravascular coagulation.*

consump'tive. Pert. to or afflicted with tuberculosis.

con'tact [L. *con*, with, + *tangere*, to touch]. 1. Mutual touching or apposition of two bodies. 2. One who has been recently exposed to a contagious disease.

   c., complete. When entire surface of a tooth touches entire surface of an adjoining tooth, proximally.

   c., direct. Transmission of a contagious disease by a healthy person coming in contact with a person who is a carrier of or has the disease.

   c., immediate. C., direct, q.v.

   c., indirect. The spread of a contagious disease by some medium other than directly touching an infected person.

   c. lens. A thin bowl-shaped shell of corrective glass made to fit over the cornea.

   c. lens, soft. Contact lens made of a soft hydrophilic plastic. It is softer, more comfortable to wear, and can be worn longer than conventional contact lenses made of glass. Also, because it is hydrophilic, medicine can be effectively applied to the cornea by using the soft lens as a bandage.

   c., mediate. C., indirect, q.v.

   c., proximal. Touching of teeth on their adjacent surfaces. SYN: *proximate c.*

   c. surface. Proximal surface of a tooth.

conta'gion [L. *contingere*, to touch]. 1. The process of transferring a specific disease either by direct or indirect contact. 2. A contagious disease. 3. Any virus or bacterium which causes a contagious disease. SEE: *virulent; virus.*

conta'gious. Communicable; transmitted readily from one person to another either directly or indirectly, with reference to the organism which causes a disease.

contagium (kon-tā'jĭ-um) [L.]. The agent causing infection or contagion.

containers, care and handling of. Contamination of the container in which a specimen is to be placed may render the results of the examination futile and therefore interfere with the doctor's diagnosis. The nurse must avoid contamination of any container used for the collection of specimens.

See that the containers are perfectly clean inside and outside and that the surfaces are intact. Cracked or broken containers must not be used. The containers must never be completely filled. If the presence of bacteria is suspected the container must first be sterilized, unless this has already been done by the laboratory.

Cleaning glassware: Use very little soappowder; boil glassware in water. Brush well under running water and rinse in running water. Place in potassium bichromate solution for 20 minutes. *Note:* This is a powerful chemical solution which must be kept off the skin and clothing and out of the eyes. Glasses or a protective face shield must be worn while using potassium bichromate. Rinse well in running water; rinse in distilled water; rinse again in distilled water. Invert in basket and drain dry or dry in a hot-air oven.

Sterilization of glassware: This is accomplished by hot air or dry heat, boiling water, flowing steam, steam under pressure, certain gases, and the use of germicidal chemicals.

Labels: All containers should be labeled with the name of the patient and his room number and the name of the attending physician. Request forms, sometimes used as labels, are made up to suit the individual laboratory or hospital. Provision is made for recording necessary data as indicated, including date when specimen was taken, under what circumstances, and for what substances the examination is to be done, together with other information desired.

Time: If the required specimen cannot be furnished at once, make a note of what is needed; inform the patient, the supervisor, and any other nurse who may attend the patient in your absence.

Charting: Note on the chart all specimens sent to the laboratory, when sent, and any other data that seem pertinent such as the appearance of the specimen or unusual occurrences while obtaining it.

Care of specimen: Cover immediately after depositing in the container: check label or request form. Make sure that the container is intact and that there is no danger of spilling while in transit.

contam'inate [L. *contamināre*, to render impure]. 1. To soil, stain, or pollute. 2. To render unfit for use through introduction of a substance which is harmful or injurious. 3. To make impure or unclean.

contamina'tion. 1. The act of contaminating, esp. introduction of disease germs or infectious material into or on normally sterile objects. 2. In psychiatry, the fusion and condensation of words so that they run together when spoken.

con'tent. That which is contained in something.

c., dream. What one dreams.

contiguity (kon"tĭ-gū'ĭ-tĭ) [L. *contiguus*, touching]. Contact or closely associated.

c., amputation in. Amputation through a joint.

c., law of. If two ideas occur in association they are apt to be repeated.

c., solution of. Dislocation or displacement of two normally contiguous parts.

con'tinence [L. *continēre*, to hold together]. Self-restraint, used esp. in connection with refraining from sexual indulgence. Also used in reference to the ability to control urination and defecation.

continent (kon'tĭ-nent). 1. Capable of controlling urination and defecation. 2. Not yielding to sexual desire. SEE: *continence*.

continuity (kon"tĭ-nū'ĭ-tĭ) [L. *continuus*, continued]. The state of being continuous or intimately united.

c., amputation in. Amputation through a long bone.

c., solution of. Division of normally continuous parts by fracture, rupture, laceration, incision.

contin'uous [L. *continēre*, to hold together]. Without break, cessation, or interruption.

c. spec'trum. An unbroken series of wave lengths, either visible or invisible.

Such a spectrum is produced by light from incandescent solids, liquids, or gases under high pressure, passed through a prism. Also an unbroken range of radiations of different wave lengths in any portion of the invisible spectrum.

contor'tion [L. *contorquēre*, to twist together]. A twisting into an unusual shape.

contour (kon'toor) [It. *contornare*, to go around]. Outline or surface configuration of a part.

contoured (kon'toord). Having an irregular, undulating surface resembling a relief map, said of bacterial colonies.

contra- [L.]. Prefix indicating opposite or against, as contraindication.

contra-ap'erture [L. *contra*, against, + *apertura*, opening]. A second opening made in an abscess.

contraception (kon"trä-sep'shun) ["+ *conceptiō*, a conceiving]. The prevention of conception.

contracep'tive. Any agent or device used to prevent conception.

c., oral. A medicine, usually the combination of a progestational agent and an estrogen, taken by mouth to prevent conception. Sometimes referred to as "the pill."

contract' [L. *contrahere*, to draw together]. 1. To draw together, reduce in size, or shorten. 2. To acquire through infection, as to contract a disease.

contrac'tile. Able to contract or shorten.

contractil'ity. Having the ability to contract or shorten.

contrac'tion. A shortening or tightening, as that of a muscle, or a reduction in size; a shrinking.

c., isometric. Muscular in which the muscle does not change its length.

c., isotonic. Muscular c. in which the muscle maintains constant tension by changing its length during the action.

contracture (kon-trak'chur) [L. *contractura*]. 1. Permanent contraction of a muscle due to spasm or paralysis. 2. A condition of fixed high resistance to the passive stretch of a muscle, as may result from fibrosis of tissues surrounding a joint.

c., Dupuytren's. Flexion deformity of hands and fingers due to contraction of the palmar fascia.

c., functional. Decrease of a c. during anesthesia or sleep.

c., physiological. A temporary condition in which tension and shortening of a muscle are maintained for a considerable time although there is no tetanus. May be induced by heat, action of drugs, acids, etc.

c., Volkmann's. Pronation and flexion of the hand, with shrinking and hardening of the muscles of the forearm.

contrafissura (kon"trä-fĭ-shū'rä) [L. *contra*, against, + *fissura*, fissure]. A skull fracture at a point opposite from where the blow was received.

contraindication (kŏn"trä-ĭn-dĭ-kā'shŭn) ["+ *indicāre*, to point out]. Any symptom or circumstance indicating the inappropriateness of a form of treatment otherwise advisable.

contralat′eral ["+ *latus*, side]. Originating in, or affecting, the opposite side of the body. Opposed to homolateral and ipsilateral.

    c. reflexes. 1. Passive flexion of one part following flexion of another. 2. Passive flexion of one leg causing similar movement of opposite leg.

contrast media. A radiopaque substance used to provide, during x-ray study, a contrast in density between the tissue or organ being filmed and the media. Thus barium sulfate will when swallowed help to demonstrate the outline of the intestinal tract as x-ray films are taken during the passage of that particular contrast media.

con′trast sprays. Those administered by sitting on side of bathtub, spraying feet and legs with warm water for one minute and cold water for one minute. Alternate for 10 minutes twice daily.

contravolitional (kon″trä-vō-lĭ′shun-al) [L. *contra*, against, + *velle*, to wish]. In opposition to or without the will; involuntary.

contrecoup (kontr-koo′) [Fr. *contrecoup*, counterblow]. Occurring on the opposite side.

    c. injury. An injury to parts of the brain located on the side opposite that of the primary injury, as when the frontal and temporal lobes of the brain are forced against the irregular bones of the anterior portion of the cranial vault as a result of a blow on the back of the head.

contrectation (kon″trek-tā′shun) [L. *contrectāre*, to handle]. 1. Touch with the hands. 2. Caressing or sexually fondling one of the opposite sex.

control (kon-trōl′) [L. *contra*, against, + *rotulus*, little wheel]. 1. To regulate or maintain. 2. A standard against which observations or conclusions may be checked in order to establish their validity, as a control animal, one which has not been exposed to the treatment or condition being studied in the other animals.

    c. animal. An animal subjected to the same conditions as the experimental animal except for the specific factor being tested.

    c., birth. Practice of contraception.

contrude (kon-trud′) [L. *con*, with, + *trūdere*, to thrust]. 1. Abnormal lingual curve or line of dental arch. 2. To crowd together, as the teeth.

contru′sion. Having the teeth crowded.

contuse (kon-tūz′) [L. *contundere*, to bruise]. To bruise.

contusion (kon-tu′zhun). An injury in which the skin is not broken; a bruise.

SYM: Pain, swelling, and discoloration.

    F. A. TREATMENT: Apply cold applications. Follow with firm bandage to prevent swelling. Twenty-four to 48 hours later, heat is desirable, followed by gentle massage. SEE: *concussion.*

co′nus [Gr. *kōnos*]. 1. A cone. 2. Posterior staphyloma of myopic eye.

    c. arteriosus. [NA]. Right cardiac ventricle's upper rounded anterior angle, where pulmonary artery arises.

    c. medullaris. [NA]. Conical portion of lower spinal cord.

convalescence (kon″val-es′ens) [L. *convalescere*, to become strong]. The period of recovery after the termination of a disease or an operation.

convales′cent. 1. Getting well. 2. One who is recovering from a disease or operation.

    c. diet. A diet suitable for the condition from which the patient is recovering.

convection (kon-vek′shun) [L. *convehere*, to convey]. The transference of heat by means of currents in liquids or gases.

convergence (kon-ver′jens) [L. *con*, with, + *vergere*, to incline]. 1. Visual lines directed to a nearby point. 2. The moving of two or more objects toward the same point. 3. In reflex activity, the coming together of several axons or afferent fibers upon one or a few motor neurons; the condition whereby impulses from several sensory receptors con-

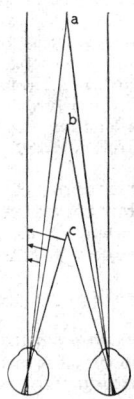

CONVERGENCE

When an object is brought from a distant position (a) to a near position (b), the eyes are rotated medially to make the lines of vision meet at the object. The closer the object, the greater the degree of convergence as measured by the angles indicated by arrows.

verge upon the same motor center, resulting in a limited and specific response.

convergent (kon-ver'jent). Tending toward a common point.

conver'sion [L. *convertere*, to turn round]. Change from one state to another. In obstetrics, the change in position of a fetus in the uterus in order to facilitate delivery. SEE: *version*.

   c. symptom. A term for a repressed emotion that becomes manifest through a physical symptom; seen in hysteria.

convex (kon'veks, kon-veks') [L. *convexus,* vaulted, arched]. Curved evenly; resembling the segment of a sphere.

convexoconcave (kon-vek"sō-kon'kāv, -kon-kāv') [" + *concavus,* vaulted hollow]. Concave on one side and convex on opposite surface. SYN: *concavoconvex.*

convexoconvex [L. *convexus,* arched]. Convex on two opposite faces.

convolute (kon'vo-lūt) [L. *convolvere,* to roll together]. Rolled, as a scroll.

con'voluted. Convolute, rolled.

   c. tubule. In the kidney the proximal c. t. lies between Bowman's capsule and the loop of Henle; the distal c. t. lies between the loop of Henle and the collecting duct.

convolution (kŏn"vō-lū'shŭn) [L. *convolvere,* to roll together]. 1. A turn, fold, or coil of anything which is convoluted. 2. In anatomy, a gyrus, one of the many folds on the surface of the cerebral hemispheres. They are separated by grooves (sulci or fissures). SEE: *gyrus.*

   c., angular. A gyrus forming posterior portion of inferior parietal lobule.

   c.'s, annectant. The four gyri connecting the c.'s on upper surface of occipital lobe with parietal and temporosphenoidal lobes.

   c., anterior central. Ascending frontal c., q.v.

   c., anterior choroid. Gyrus choroides.

   c., anterior orbital. A c. which lies in front of the orbital sulcus.

   c., anteroparietal. Ascending frontal c., q.v.

   c., Arnold's. Gyri posteriores inferiores.

   c., ascending frontal. A c. forming anterior boundary of fissure of Rolando.

   c., ascending parietal. A c. parallel to ascending frontal c., separated from it by fissure of Rolando, except at extremities, where they are generally united.

   c., Broca's. The inferior, or third, frontal c.

   c., callosal. Gyrus fornicatus. SYN: *callosomarginal c.*

   c.'s, cerebral. Those of the cerebrum.

   c. of the corpus callosum. Gyrus fornicatus.

   c., cuneate. Gyral isthmus.

   c., dentate. A small, notched gyrus, rudimentary in man, situated in dentate fissure.

   c.'s, exterior olfactory. Small projections forming outer boundary of the olfactory grooves.

   c., hippocampal. Uncinate gyrus.

   c., inferior frontal. The lower and outer part of frontal lobe.

   c., inferior occipital. A small c. lying between middle and inferior occipital fissures.

   c., inframarginal. Superior temporosphenoidal c.

   c., insular. One of a group of small c.'s forming the island of Reil, entirely concealed by the operculum.

   c. interior orbital. The gyrus next outside of the gyrus rectus.

   c.'s, intestinal. The coils of the intestines.

   c., marginal. C. beginning in front of locus perforatus anterior and bounding longitudinal fissure on mesial aspect of the hemisphere.

   c., middle frontal. C. continuous posterior with ascending frontal c. and extending forward over anterior end of hemisphere to its orbital surface.

   c., middle occipital. A c. between the first and third occipital c.'s.

   c., middle temporosphenoidal. A small gyrus continuous with the middle occipital or angular gyrus.

   c.'s, occipitotemporal. Two small c.'s on lower surface of temporosphenoidal lobe.

   c., olfactory. Olfactory lobe.

   c.'s, orbital. Small gyri on orbital surface of frontal lobe.

   c.'s, parietal. Ascending parietal c. and superior parietal c.

   c., posterior orbital. A small c. on posterior and outer side of orbital sulcus, and continuous with inferior frontal c.

   c., second frontal. A c. on the frontal lobes, lying posteriorly between the superior and inferior frontal sulci. SYN: *middle frontal c.*

   c., superior frontal. A c. which bounds great longitudinal fissure, arising posterior from upper end of ascending frontal c.

   c., superior occipital. Upper of the three c.'s on superior surface of occipital lobe.

   c., superior parietal. Portion of parietal lobe limited anteriorly by upper part of the fissure of Rolando, posteriorly by exterior parieto-occipital fissure, and inferiorly by intraparietal sulcus.

c., superior temporosphenoidal. Upper of three c.'s forming temporosphenoidal lobe. It lies just below and is parallel with sylvian fissure.

c., supramarginal. The anterior portion of interior parietal lobule behind inferior extremity of intraparietal fissure (sulcus), below which it joins the ascending parietal c.

c. of the sylvian fissure. The c. that bounds the fissure of Sylvius.

c., transverse orbital. The gyrus occupying posterior portion of inferior surface of frontal lobe, at anterior extremity of fissure of Sylvius.

c., uncinate. A c. extending from near posterior extremity of occipital lobe to apex of temporosphenoidal.

convul'sant [L. *convellere,* to pull together]. 1. An agent which produces a convulsion. 2. Causing onset of a convulsion.

c. poisons. The common ones are strychnine and other drugs of the nux vomica groups, and various infrequently used drugs, such as picrotoxin.

SYM: These produce a sense of suffocation, dyspnea, and then muscular rigidity; there are powerful tetanic contractions which may be very painful. These spasms may be brought on by trivial stimuli, such as touching the patient or they may come on at varying intervals of from three to 30 minutes and may last from one to five minutes. Trismus, cyanosis, and tachycardia are frequent accompaniments. Death results from asphyxia or exhaustion.

TREATMENT: Appropriate therapy will depend upon substance which caused the convulsion. General measures for emptying the stomach or attempting to neutralize the drug may be indicated. Sedatives may be ordered by the physician. Oxygen and artificial respiration may be indicated.

convul'sion. Paroxysms of involuntary muscular contractions and relaxations.

Convulsions due to tetanus and rabies are easily distinguished and for the most part involve a small portion of the voluntary musculature. On the contrary, in strychnine-poisoning convulsions involve the entire body. The word is accurately applied to unilateral attacks as seen in jacksonian epilepsy and, less likely, in hysteria. These attacks are usually accompanied by unconsciousness. This is not the case in strychnine poisoning, hysteria, or in jacksonian epileptic attacks until the second side is involved.

Note: It is important for the person who observes the convulsion to record on the chart the following: time of onset; duration; whether or not convulsion started in a certain area of the body or became generalized from the start; type of contractions; whether or not the patient became incontinent; was there an abnormal odor to the patient's breath; did the convulsion cause the patient to be injured or strike his head during the convulsion. This information will be quite valuable in diagnosing the patient's illness and caring for him.

ETIOL: In general: Epilepsy; eclampsia; meningitis; tetanus; uremia; poisoning from camphor, cyanides, strychnine. In children, the cause is often dietary or due to fever. Other causes: Rickets; syphilis; malnutrition; malaria; acute infectious disease; cervical disease; toxemias, or unknown. In adults, c.'s may be caused by epilepsy; heat cramps; strychnine; brain lesions; or food poisoning.

TREATMENT: If an infant, put him in a bath of 95° F. (35° C.) with cold applications to head. In adult, cause must first be found or injury may result from bath. If cause is undetermined, keep patient from injuring self. Soft pad between teeth to avoid biting tongue or cheeks. If fever is present, tepid or cool bath. Sedatives or anesthesia may be advised by physician. Aftercare: Rest in bed; absolute quiet; careful diagnosis without unduly disturbing patient.

c., clonic. One having intermittent contractions, muscles being alternately contracted and relaxed.

c., epileptiform. One accompanied by unconsciousness.

c., hysterical. C. caused by hysteria.

c., mimetic. A spasm of facial muscles.

c., oscillating. One involving separate bundles of muscle fibers which contract alternately.

c., puerperal. Eclamptic c. in pregnant or puerperal woman.

c., salaam. Nodding spasm. SEE: *eclampsia nutans.*

c., tonic. One in which the contractions are maintained for a time, as in tetany.

c., toxic. C. caused by action of a toxin on nervous system.

c., uremic. C. caused by uremic condition.

convulsion, words pert. to: anticonvulsive; athetosis; chill; chorea; epilepsy; hysteria; ictus; mimetic; paroxysm; rabies; strychnine; tetanus; tic; tremor.

convul'sive. Pert. to convulsions.

c. reflex. Incoordinate contraction of muscles in a convulsive manner.

c. tic. Spasm of face.

cook'ing [L. *coquere,* to cook]. The process of preparing foods for eating.

C. makes most foods more palatable, easier to masticate, improves their digestibility, and destroys or inactivates harmful organisms or toxins which may be present. C. releases the aromatic substances and extractives that contribute odors and taste to foods. These odors help to stimulate the appetite.

Most microorganisms and parasites are destroyed in the ordinary processes of cooking, but some require a higher degree of heat and longer cooking to effect this result. Pork has to be cooked completely throughout in order to kill the encysted larvae of Trichinella. SEE: *trichinosis.*

Action on Protein: Soluble proteins become coagulated.

Action on Soluble Substances: These are often lost in boiling, and even mineral substances and starches, though insoluble to a certain extent, suffer loss in this process.

Action on Starch: The starch granules now swell and are changed from insoluble (raw) starch to soluble starch capable of being converted into sugar in the process of digestion and of being assimilated in the system.

Cooley's anemia. [Thomas Cooley, Amer. pediatrician, 1871-1945]. Anemia resulting from inheritance of a recessive trait responsible for interference with hemoglobin synthesis. SYN: *thalassemia,* q.v.

Coo'lidge tube. An x-ray tube whose cathode consists of a spiral tungsten wire surrounded by a molybdenum tube.

Coombs' test. [R. R. A. Coombs, Brit. immunologist, 20th century]. A test for antiglobulins in the red cell; used in diagnosing various hemolytic anemias.

coordination (kō-ōr''dĭn-ā'shŭn) [L. *co-,* same, + *ordināre,* to arrange]. The working together of various muscles for the production of a certain movement.

More generally, the working together of different systems of the body in a given process, as the coordination between the system of glands and involuntary muscles in digestion.

cope (kōp). The ability to effectively deal with and handle the stresses to which one is subjected.

copiopia (ko-pī-o'pĭ-ă) [Gr. *kopos,* fatigue, + *opsis,* sight]. Eyestrain causing eye fatigue.

copodyskinesia (ko''po-dis''kin-e'sĭ-ă) [''+ *dys,* difficult, + *kinēsis,* motion]. Fatigue of or difficulty in moving a group of muscles used in working. May be out of proportion to that which would be expected from the amount of work done, in which case it is called occupational neurosis.

cop'per (cuprum) [Gr. *Kupros,* Cyprus]. SYMB: *Cu.* At. wt. 63.54; at. no. 29; sp. gr. 8.96. A metal, small quantities of which are utilized by the body. Its salts are an irritant poison.

FUNCTION AND USES: It functions with iron in its transformation into such substances as hemoglobin, and it seems to be an activating principle when used in the treatment of blood dyscrasias. It aids tissue respiration and the synthesis of cytochrome. It is present in the liver at all times and is excreted by the kidneys.

DEFICIENCY SYM: Anemia; weakness; impaired respiration and growth; and poor utilization of iron.

SOURCES: Found in many vegetable and animal tissues.

copperas (kŏp'ĕr-ăs). $FeSO_4 \cdot 7H_2O$. Pale bluish-green crystals of ferrous sulfate. Used as disinfectant and deodorizer. SYN: *green vitriol.* SEE: *ferrous sulfate.*

copperhead. A poisonous snake, Agkistrodon contortrix, common in the southern United States.

cop'per sul'fate. Blue vitriol $CuSO_4 \cdot 5H_2O$. Deep blue, shiny cyrstals or granular powder. Astringent when used in proper dilution. Also used as an algicide in reservoirs.

POISONING: SYM: A disagreeable, coppery, metallic taste, with tightness in the throat, nausea and vomiting, thirst; abdominal pains, cramps, and suppression of urine.

F. A. TREATMENT: Wash out stomach, give egg whites raw or beaten. Give demulcent drinks.

copremesis (kop-rĕm'ĕ-sĭs) [Gr. *kopros,* dung, + *emesis,* vomiting]. The vomiting of fecal material.

coprolagnia (kŏp''ro-lag'nĭ-ă) [''+ *lagneia,* lust]. An erotic satisfaction at the sight or odor of excreta.

coprolalia (kŏp''ro-la'lĭ-ă) [''+ *lalia,* babble]. A morbid desire to use sacrilegious or obscene words in ordinary conversation. Seen in obsessional neurosis or dementia precox.

coprolith (kop'ro-lith) [Gr. *kopros,* dung, + *lithos,* stone]. Hard, inspissated feces.

coprology (kŏp-rŏl'ŏ-jĭ) [''+ *logos,* study of]. Study of the feces. SYN: *scatology.*

coprophagy (kŏp-rŏf'ă-jĭ) [''+ *phagein,* to eat]. The eating of excrement.

coprophilia (kŏp''rŏ-fĭl'ĭ-ă) [Gr. *kopros,* dung, + *philein,* to love]. Abnormal interest in feces; a perversion in adults.

coprophil'ic. Term applied to organisms which normally live in fecal material.

coprophobia (kŏp″rō-fō′bĭ-ă) [Gr. *kopros*, dung, + *phobos*, fear]. A morbid disgust at defecation and feces.

coproporphyrin (kŏp″rō-por′fĭr-ĭn). A porphyrin present in feces. Coproporphyrins I and II are normally present in minute and equal amounts, but quantities are altered in certain diseases as poliomyelitis, infectious hepatitis and in lead poisoning.

coprostanol (kŏp″rō-sta′nol). A derivative of cholesterol present in feces, usually the result of bacterial action in the large intestine.

coprozoa (kŏp″rō-zō-ă) [Gr. *kopros*, dung, + *zōon*, animal]. Protozoa in fecal matter outside of the intestine.

coprozo′ic. Pert. to coprozoa; found in feces or fecal matter.

copula (kŏp′ū-lă) [L., link]. 1. Any connecting part. 2. A median elevation on floor of embryonic pharynx representing future root of the tongue; copula linguae.

copulation (kŏp″ū-lā′shŭn) [L. *copulātiō*]. Sexual intercourse. SYN: *coition; coitus; concubitus.*

cor (kor) [L.]. [NA] The heart.

    c. pulmonale. Hypertrophy or failure of right ventricle resulting from disorders of the lungs, pulmonary vessels, or chest wall.

coracoacromial (kor″ă-ko-ă-kro′mĭ-ăl) [Gr. *korax*, raven, + *akron*, point, + *ōmos*, shoulder]. Pert. to acromial and coracoid processes.

coracoid (kŏr′ă-koyd) [″+ *eidos*, appearance]. Resembling, in shape, a crow's beak.

    c. process. Process on upper anterior surface of scapula.

coramine (kō′ră-mēn). Proprietary name for nikethamide, a respiratory stimulant.

cord [Gr. *khordē*]. 1. A stringlike structure. 2. The umbilical cord.

    c. bladder. Distention of the bladder without discomfort. Tending to void frequently and dribbling after urination.

    ETIOL: Lesion affecting the posterior roots of the spinal column at the level of bladder innervation.

    c., spermatic. Cord by which the testis is connected to the abdominal inguinal ring. It consists of the ductus deferens, blood vessels, lymphatics, and nerves supplying the testis and epididymis. These are enclosed in the cremasteric fascia which forms an investing sheath. SYN: *funiculus spermaticus* [NA].

    c., spinal. That portion of the central nervous system contained in the spinal canal. The center of the cord consists of gray matter, which is composed of nerve cells, dendrites, and their processes. The white matter is arranged in tracts outside the gray

matter. It consists of medullated nerve fibers which are going to and from the brain; connecting various layers of gray matter in the cord; and leaving and entering the spinal column. The cord serves as a conducting pathway for sensory impulses to the brain and motor impulses from the brain. It also serves as a reflex center for many reflex acts. SYN: *medulla spinalis* [NA].

    c., umbilical. One which connects the umbilicus of the fetus to the placenta.

cordate (kŏr′dāt) [L. *cor*, heart]. Shaped like a heart.

cor′diform [L. ″+ *forma*, shape]. Shaped like a heart.

corditis (kŏr-dī′tĭs) [Gr. *khordē*, cord, + *-ītis*, inflammation]. Inflammation of the spermatic cord; funiculitis.

cordopexy (kŏr′do-pĕk″sĭ) [″+ *pēxis*, fixation]. Operative fixation of an anatomical cord, esp. the vocal cords.

cordotomy (kŏr-dot′ō-mĭ) [″+ *tomē*, incision]. Spinal cord section of lateral pathways to relieve pain. SYN: *chordotomy.*

core (kŏr). The center of a structure.

    c. temperature. The body's temperature in deep structures such as the liver or heart.

coreclisis (kŏr″e-kli′sis) [Gr. *korē*, pupil of the eye, + *kleisis*, closure]. Occlusion of the pupil. SYN: *iridencleisis.*

corectasia, corectasis (kŏr-ek-ta′zĭ-ă, ek′ta-sis) [″+ *ektasis*, dilatation]. Dilatation of the pupil of the eye resulting from disease.

corectome (kō-rĕk′tōm) [″+ *ektomē*, excision]. Instrument used for cutting or removing the iris. SYN: *iridectome.*

corectomedialysis (kŏr-ek″to-me-dĭ-al′ĭ-sis) [Gr. *korē*, pupil, + *ektomē*, excision, + *dialysis*, separation]. Coredialysis, q.v.

corectomy (ko-rek′tō-mĭ). Surgical removal of the iris. SYN: *iridectomy.*

corectopia (kŏr-ĕk-tō′pĭ-ă) [Gr. *korē*, pupil, + *ek*, out of, + *topos*, place]. Having the pupil to one side of center of iris.

coredialysis (ko″re-di-al′ĭ-sis) [″+ *dialysis*, separation]. Separation of iris' outer border from its ciliary attachment. SYN: *corectomedialysis.*

corediastasis (kŏr″e-dĭ-as′ta-sis) [″+ *diastasis*, a standing apart]. Dilatation of pupil.

corelysis (kor-el′ĭ-sis) [Gr. *korē*, pupil, + *lysis*, destruction]. Obliteration of pupil because of adhesions of iris to cornea.

coremorphosis (kŏr″e-mor-fo′sis) [″+ *morphē*, form, + *-ōsis*, infection]. Establishment of an artificial pupil.

corenclesis (kŏr″en-kli′sis). Iridencleisis, q.v.

coreometer (kŏ″re-ŏm′ē-tĕr) [Gr. *korē,* pupil, + *metron,* measure]. Instrument for measurement of the pupil.

coreometry (kŏ″re-ŏm′ē-trĭ). Measurement of the pupil of the eye.

coreoplasty (kŏ′re-o-plas′tĭ) ["+ *plassein,* to form]. Any operation for forming an artificial pupil.

corestenoma (kŏr″e-sten-o′mă) [Gr. *korē,* pupil, + *stenōma,* contraction]. Narrowing of pupil.

   c. congen′itum. Partial congenital obliteration of pupil by outgrowths from the iris which form a partial gridlike covering over the pupil.

coretomedialysis (kor″et-o-mē-dī-al′ĭ-sĭs) ["+ *temnein,* to cut, + *dialysis,* division]. Making of an artificial pupil through the iris. SYN: *iridodialysis.*

coretomy (kŏ-rĕt′ō-mĭ) ["+ *tomē,* incision]. Any cutting of the iris. SYN: *iridotomy,* q.v.

Cori cycle (kō′rĭ). [Carl F. Cori, Amer. pharmacologist and biochemist, 1896-; Gerty T. Cori, Amer. biochemist, 1896-1957]. In carbohydrate metabolism, the breakdown of muscle glycogen, with formation of lactic acid which enters the blood stream, is converted to liver glycogen which in turn breaks down into glucose which is carried to muscles where it is reconverted to muscle glycogen.

corium (kō′rĭ-ŭm) [L., skin]. (pl. *coria*) [NA] The layer of the skin lying immediately under the epidermis, the dermis, or true skin. Consists of two layers, papillary and reticular. It is composed of loose connective tissue in which are numerous capillaries, lymphatics, and nerve endings. In it lie hair follicles, sebaceous glands, sweat glands and their ducts and smooth muscle fibers. SYN: *cutis vera; dermis.*

corm (kŏrm) [Gr. *kormos,* a trimmed tree trunk]. A short bulb-shaped, underground stem of a plant. Ex: Colchicum.

corn [AS.]. Indian corn or maize.

   Food value of 100 gm. (fresh, cooked after kernels cut off cob): Cal. 83; protein 3.2 gm.; fat 1 gm.; carbohydrate 18.8 gm.; calcium 3 mg.; vitamin A, 400 I.U. (yellow c. only); ascorbic acid 7 mg.

corn [L. *cornu,* horn]. Horny induration and thickening of the skin, hard or soft, according to location. SYN: *clavus.*

   ETIOL: Pressure or friction or both from ill-fitting shoes.

   SYM: Hard corns on exposed surfaces have a horny core of conical shape extending down into the derma, causing pain and irritation. Soft corns occur between the toes, kept soft by moisture and maceration, and

may lead to inflammation beneath the corn. Infection with pyogenic organisms results in suppuration.

   TREATMENT: Remove cause. Properly fitting shoes of soft leather and proper shape. New materials for absorbing energy and thus preventing friction are available for lining shoes or bandaging the area of the foot being abraded. Local application of a keratolytic agent for removal of corn. Corn pads to relieve pressure. Services of a chiropodist may be necessary. Special care to patients with diabetes or a circulatory condition. Soft corns dissected similarly with cotton pad protection to prevent maceration.

cornea (kŏr′nē-ă) [L. *corneus,* horny]. [NA]. The clear, transparent anterior portion of the fibrous coat of the eye comprising about one-sixth of its surface. Its curvature being greater than that of the remainder of the bulb enables it to function as an important refractive medium. It is continuous at its periphery with the sclera.

   Composed of five layers: layer of epithelium; Bowman's membrane (anterior limiting membrane); substantia propria corneae [NA]; Descemets' membrane; and layer of endothelium.

cornea, words pert. to: abrasio corneae; albugo; anterior chamber; arcus senilis; argema; "cera-" words; chemosis; circumcorneal; "kerat-" words; leukoma; macula cornea; megalocornea; microcornea; nebula; obfuscation; pannus; peritomy; phlyctenula; rhytidosis; rutidosus; staphyloma; synechia.

cor′neal. Pert. to the cornea.

   c. reflex. Closure of eyelids resulting from direct corneal irritation.

corneitis (kŏr″nē-ĭ′tĭs) [L. *corneus,* horny, + Gr. *itis,* inflammation]. Inflammation of the cornea. SYN: *keratitis.*

corneoiritis (kŏr″nē-o-i-rī′tĭs) ["+ Gr. *iris,* iris, + *itis,* inflammation]. Inflammation of iris and cornea.

corneomandibular reflex (kŏr″nē-o-măn-dĭb′ū-lăr). Deflexion of mandible toward opposite side when cornea is irritated while mouth is open and relaxed.

corneoscloera (kŏr″nē-o-sklē′ră) [L. *corneus,* horny, + *sklēros,* hard]. The cornea and sclera considered together comprising the tunica fibrosa [NA] or fibrous coat of the eye.

corneous (kŏr′nē-ŭs) [L. *corneus*]. Horny; hornlike.

   c. layer. Horny outer layer of the epidermis. SYN: *stratum corneum* [NA].

corniculum (kŏr-nĭk′ū-lŭm) [L., little horn]. A small, hornlike process.

cornification (kŏr″nĭ-fĭ-kā'shŭn) [L. *cornu*, horn, + *facere*, to make]. The process by which squamous epithelial cells are converted into hard, horny material as in the corneum of the skin or in structures such as horns, hair, and feathers which are derived from epithelium.

cornu (kŏr'nū) [L., horn]. (pl. *cornua*) [NA] Any excrescence like a horn.

c. ammo'nis. Hippocampus major of brain.

c. anterius. [NA]. The anterior horn of the lateral ventricle.

c. coccy'geum. [NA]. Two upward projecting processes which articulate with the sacrum.

c. cuta'neum; c. huma'num. Hornlike excrescence on skin.

c. of the hyoid. The greater and lesser horns of the hyoid bones, q.v.

c. inferius. [NA]. The inferior horn of the lateral ventricle.

c. posterius. [NA]. The posterior horn of the lateral ventricle.

c. of the sacrum. Two small processes projecting inferiorly on either side of the sacral hiatus leading into the sacral canal.

cor'nua. Pl. of cornu.

cor'nual. Pert. to a cornu.

corona (kō-rō'nă) [Gr. *korōnē*, crown]. [NA]. Any structure resembling a crown.

c. capitis. Crown of head.

c. ciliaris. [NA]. Circular figure on inner surface of ciliary body.

c. dentis. [NA]. Crown of a tooth.

c. glandis. [NA]. Posterior border of glans penis.

c. radiata. 1. [NA]. Ascending and descending fibers of the internal capsule which, above the corpus callosum, extend in all directions to the cerebral cortex. Many of the fibers arise in the thalamus. 2. A thin mass of follicle cells which adhere firmly to the zona pellucida of the human ovum following ovulation.

c. veneris. Syphilitic blotches on forehead parallel to hairline.

co'ronal. Pert. to a corona.

c. suture. One which joins the parietal and frontal bones of the cranium.

coronary (kŏr'o-nă-rĭ) [L. *coronarius*, pert. to a crown or circle]. A term applied to blood vessels which supply blood to the heart muscle, i.e., myocardium. Coronary pain is usually dull and heavy; typically the patient describes the pain as being viselike or producing a feeling of compression or squeezing of the chest.

c. arteries. 1. One of a pair of arteries which supply blood to the myocardium of the heart. They arise within the right and left aortic sinuses at base of the aorta. Decreased flow of blood through these arteries induces attacks of angina pectoris. 2. The cervical branch of the uterine artery.

c. plexus. A network of autonomic nerve fibers which lies close to base of heart.

c. sinus. The vessel cavity or passage which receives the cardiac veins from the heart. It opens into right atrium.

c. thrombosis. Occlusion of one or more of the coronary arteries of the heart.

coronary care unit. A specially equipped area of a hospital for providing intensive nursing and medical care for patients who have acute coronary thrombosis.

cor'oner [L. *corona*, crown]. An official (originally, English crown officer) who investigates and holds inquests over those dead from unknown or violent causes. He may or may not be a physician, depending upon the law in each state.

cor'onoid [Gr. *korōnē*, something curved, kind of crown, + *eidos,* appearance]. Shaped like a crown.

c. fossa. An oval depression on anterior surface of distal end of humerus. Receives coronoid process of ulna.

c. process. 1. A process on proximal end of ulna. Forms anterior portion of semilunar notch. 2. A process on the ramus of the mandible which serves for attachment of the temporalis muscle.

coroparelcysis (kŏr″o-par-el'sĭ-sĭs) [Gr. *korē*, pupil, + *parelkein,* to draw aside]. Surgically bringing the pupil to one side in central corneal opacity so that it lies under a transparent area.

coroscopy (kō-ros'ko-pī) ["+ *skopein*, to examine]. Shadow test to determine refractive error of an eye. SYN: *skiascopy.*

corot'omy ["+ *tomē*, incision]. Surgical incision of the iris. Iridotomy, q.v.

cor'pora. Pl. of corpus, q.v.

c. Arantii. Tubercle found in center of semilunar valves of heart.

c. arenacea. Brain sand; psammoma bodies found in the pineal body.

c. cavernosa penis. Two columns of erectile tissue on dorsum of the penis.

c. olivaria. Two oval masses behind pyramids of the oblongata.

c. quadrigemina. The superior portion of the midbrain consisting of two pairs of rounded bodies, the superior and inferior colliculi.

corpsman (kŏr'măn). (pl. *corpsmen*) An enlisted member of a military medical service, esp. the U.S. Navy. During duty in the armed forces he receives training and experience in one or more health related fields. In wartime he may be assigned as the only medically trained person to a field unit or a small ship.

corpulence (kŏr'pū-lĕns) [L. *corpulentia*]. Fatness of the body. SYN: *obesity*.

corpulent (kŏr'pū-lĕnt). Fat; obese.

cor'pus [L., body]. (pl. *corpora*) The principal part of any organ; any mass or body.

c. albicans. [NA]. A mass of fibrous tissue which replaces the regressing corpus luteum following rupture of the graafian follicle. It forms a white scar which gradually decreases in size and eventually disappears.

c. amylaceum. A mass having an irregular, laminated structure like a starch grain, found in the prostate, meninges, lungs, and other organs in various pathological conditions.

c. annulare. Pons varolii.

c. callosum. [NA]. The great commissure of the brain between the cerebral hemispheres.

c. cavernosum. Any erectile tissue, esp. the erectile bodies of the penis, clitoris, male or female urethra, bulb of the vestibule, or the nasal conchae.

c. cerebellum. The two lateral portions of the cerebellum exclusive of the central flocculonodular node.

c. ciliare. [NA]. Ciliary body.

c. dentale; c. dentatum. Gray layer in white substance of the cerebellum.

c. fimbriatum. White layer edging the lower cornu of the lateral ventricle.

c. flavum. A waxy body seen in the central nervous system.

c. fornicis. [NA]. The body of the fornix.

c. geniculatum. The medial or lateral geniculate body, q.v.; a mass of gray matter lying in the thalamus.

c. hemorrhagicum. Blood clot formed in the cavity left by rupture of the graafian follicle.

c. highmorianum. Mediastinum testis.

c. interpedunculare. Gray matter between peduncles before the pons varolii.

c. luteum. [NA]. A small yellow body which develops within a ruptured ovarian follicle. It is an endocrine structure secreting progesterone.

c. mammillare. [NA]. A mammillary body; a rounded body in the anterior part of the interpeduncular fossa.

c. pampiniforme. Parovarium, or the remnant of the wolffian body of the female.

c. pineale. [NA]. The pineal body or pineal gland.

c. pyramidale. 1. Pyramid of the oblongata. 2. A lobe of the epididymus.

c. restiforme. The restiform body or inferior cerebellar peduncle. A band of fibers, principally ascending, in the medulla oblongata which connects the spinal cord below with the cerebellum.

c. rhomboidale. SEE: *c. dentatum.*

c. spongiosum. Erectile tissue surrounding the urethra.

c. striatum. [NA]. A structure in the cerebral hemispheres consisting of two basal ganglia (the caudate and lentiform nuclei), and the fibers of the internal capsule which separate them.

c. subthalamicum. The subthalamic nucleus (corpus Luysii), lying in the ventral thalamus.

c. trapezoideum. [NA]. The trapezoid body, q.v.

c. vitreum. [NA]. Vitreous portion of eye.

c. wolffianum. Wolffian body.

corpuscle (kŏr'pŭs-ĕl) [L. *corpusculum*, little body]. 1. Any small rounded body. 2. An encapsulated sensory nerve ending. 3. Old term for a blood cell. SEE: *erythrocyte; leukocyte.*

c., amniotic; c., amylaceous. Corpus amylaceum, q.v.

c., axile; c., axis. The center of a tactile c.

c., blood. An erythrocyte or leukocyte.

c., bone. A bone cell.

c., cancroid. Characteristic nodule in cutaneous epithelioma.

c., cartilage. A cell characteristic of cartilage.

c., chromophil. Tiny body found in cytoplasm of a nerve cell. SYN: *Nissl's body.*

c.'s, chyle. C. seen in chyle.

c., colloid. Corpus amylaceum, q.v.

c., colostrum. A cell containing phagocytosed fat globules present in milk secreted the first few days after parturition. SYN: *colostrum body.*

c.'s, corneal. Connective tissue c.'s found in fibrous tissue of cornea.

c.'s, Drysdale's. Transparent cells found in the fluid of certain ovarian cysts.

c., genital. Encapsulated sensory nerve endings resembling pacinian c.'s present in skin of external genitalia and nipple.

c., ghost. A decolorized red blood cell. SYN: *achromatocyte; phantom c.*

c.'s, Gierke's. Particles seen in the thymus gland. SYN: *Hassall's c.'s.*

c.'s, Gluge's. Particles seen in diseased nervous tissue.

c., *Golgi-Mazzoni.* Tactile corpuscles in the skin of the finger tips.

c.'s, *Hassall's.* C.'s found in the thymus gland. SYN: *Gierke's c.'s.*

c.'s, *Krause's.* Sensory encapsulated nerve endings in mucosa of genitalia, mouth, nose and eyes.

c., *lymph.* A lymphocyte, q.v.

c., *malpighian.* 1. A renal c. consisting of a glomerulus and Bowman's capsule which encloses it. 2. A malpighian body of the spleen.

c.'s, *Mazzoni's.* Nerve endings resembling Krause's c.'s.

c., *Meissner's.* A tactile c.; an encapsulated touch receptor found in connective tissue immediately underlying the epidermis of the skin, esp. on palmar and volar surfaces of hands and feet.

c., *milk.* Fat-filled globules present in milk. They represent the distal ends of mammary gland cells which are broken off in apocrine secretion.

c., *pacinian.* A large, ovoid, sensory end-organ consisting of concentric layers or lamella of connective tissue surrounding a nerve ending. They are present in tendons, intermuscular septa, connective tissue membranes, and sometimes internal organs, and function as proprioceptive receptors and as receptors of deep pressure.

c., *phantom.* Ghost c.

c., *red.* An erythrocyte, q.v.

c., *renal.* A glomerulus and the capsule (Bowman's capsule) which surrounds it. It is located at proximal end of a renal tubule. SYN: *malpighian c.*

c., *reticulated.* Erythrocytes which when properly stained show filamentous reticulations.

c., *splenic.* A nodule of lymphatic tissue present in the spleen.

c., *tactile.* A sensory end-organ which responds to touch, as Meissner's c., q.v.

c., *terminal.* A nerve ending. SEE: *nerve.*

c., *thymic.* C., Hassal's, q.v.

c., *touch.* C., tactile, q.v.

c., *Wagner's.* C., tactile, q.v.

c., *white.* A leukocyte, q.v.

corpuscular (kŏr-pŭs'kū-lăr). Pert. to corpuscles.

corpus'culum [L., little body]. (pl. *corpuscula*) [NA] Corpuscle, q.v.

c. renis. [NA] SEE: *corpuscle, renal.*

correc'tive [L. *corrigere,* to correct]. 1. A drug that modifies action of another. 2. Pert. to such a drug.

correla'tion [L. *com-,* together, + *relatio,* relation]. The processes by which the various activities of the body, especially nervous impulses, occur in proper relation to each other.

correspondence. The act or state of corresponding, i.e., occurring in proper relationship to other phenomena.

c., *retinal.* Condition occurring in normal vision in which images formed on the maculae or other points of the retinas of the two eyes are mentally blended and seen as a single image.

corresponding. Agreeing with, matching, or fitting.

c. points of retina. Identical points; points on the retinas of the two eyes which when stimulated give rise to a single image.

Corrigan's pulse (kŏr'ĭ-găn). [Sir Dominic J. Corrigan, Irish physician, 1802-1880]. A full bounding pulse, which appears to be completely empty between beats; is associated with aortic insufficiency. SYN: *water-hammer pulse.*

corro'sion [L. *corrodēre,* to corrode]. Slow disintegration or wearing away of something by a destructive agent.

corro'sive. Producing corrosion, q.v.

c. alkalies. These are corrosive hydroxides most commonly of sodium, ammonium, and potassium, as well as carbonates.

Because of their great combining power with water, and their action on the fatty tissues they cause rapid deep destruction. They have a tendency to gelatinize tissue with a somewhat grayish color forming a soapy, slippery surface, accompanied by pain and burning.

c. poisons. These include strong acids, alkalies, strong antiseptics, including bichloride of mercury, carbolic acid (phenol), lysol, cresol compounds, tincture of iodine, and arsenic compounds. They are destructive and cause disintegration similar to that caused by burns, and may result in death. If swallowed, any part of alimentary canal may be affected. Tissues involved are altered, easily perforated, or destroyed. Death comes very shortly from shock, or swelling of throat and pharynx, which causes choking; or by closure of esophagus, causing slow starvation.

SYM: Intense burning about mouth, throat, pharynx, and abdomen; abdominal cramping, retching, nausea, vomiting, and often collapse. There may be bloody vomitus (hematemesis) and diarrhea, the stools being watery, mucoid, bloody, and possibly stained with the poison or its products, resulting from its action on the contents of the alimentary tract. Stains about the lips, cheeks, tongue, mouth, or pharynx are often characteristic brown; violaceous or black stains on mucous membranes, which appear dry or parched. Carbolic acid or phenol leaves a white or gray stain resembling boiled meat; hydrochloric acid stains are grayish; nitric acid leaves a yellow stain; sulfuric acid leaves tan or dark burns.

TREATMENT: First, dilute the poison before giving any emetic and apply weak acids for prolonged periods.

Such dilution always delays absorption somewhat and makes it easier to induce vomiting. Second, remove the poison; this is best done by making the patient vomit. Emesis is more easily produced in a distended stomach. Titillate the uvula or pharynx with the finger, and again give the patient more fluid, repeating the process until the fluid returns clear. Among the most useful diluents and emetics for this purpose are tepid water; soapy water; salty water; baking soda (sodium bicarbonate) water (*do not use washing soda*); milk. A useful and widely available first aid emetic of this type is warm, soapy, greasy dish water. Any of these emetics should be used in generous amounts in all ordinary cases. (About four to seven glassfuls may be used).

Where the corrosives, such as lye or mineral acids, have been in the stomach for some time, there may be danger of perforating the stomach. In such cases there is excruciating abdominal pain, muscular rigidity, and often collapse. Following the washing of the stomach, the appropriate antidote may be administered if it is available.

In addition to the therapy directed toward removing the corrosive substance from the gastrointestinal tract, analgesic drugs and intravenous fluids may be required.

corrugator (kor'u-gā"tŏr) [L. *con*, together, + *rugāre*, to wrinkle]. A muscle which lies above the orbit arising medially from frontal bone and having its insertion on skin of medial half of the eyebrows. It draws the brow medially and inferiorly.

cortex (kŏr'tĕks) [L. rind]. (pl. *cortices*) 1. [NA] The outer layer of an organ as distinguished from the inner medulla as in the adrenal gland, kidney, ovary, lymph node, thymus, and cerebrum and cerebellum of the brain. 2. The outer layer of a structure as a hair, or the lens of the eye. 3. The outer superficial portion of the stem or root of a plant.

c., cerebellar. The surface layer of the cerebellum consisting of three layers: outer or molecular, middle, and inner or granular layer. Purkinje's cells are present in the middle layer.

c., cerebral. The thin, convoluted surface layer of gray matter of the cerebral hemispheres, consisting principally of cell bodies of neurons arranged in five layers. There are also numerous fibers.

c., interpretive. The temporal c. where memories of the past may be evoked by electric stimulation.

c., renal. SEE: *kidney*.

c., temporal. Outer layer of brain behind the temples.

Corti, canal of (kŏr'tī). [Alfonso Corti, It. anatomist, 1822-1888]. SEE: *Corti, tunnel of*.

Corti, organ of. An elongated spiral structure running the entire length of cochlea in the floor of the cochlear duct and resting on the basilar membrane. It is the end organ of hearing containing hair cells, supporting cells, and neuroepithelial receptors stimulated by sound waves. SYN: *papilla basilaris*.

Corti, tunnel of. A triangular-shaped canal extending the entire length of the organ of Corti. Its walls are formed by the external and internal pillar cells.

cortiadrenal (kor"tī-ad-rē'nal) [L. *cortex*, rind, + *ad*, toward, + *rēn*, kidney]. Pert. to cortex of adrenal gland.

cortical (kŏr'tĭ-kŏl). Pert. to a cortex.

cortices (kŏr'tĭ-sēz'). Pl. of cortex.

corticifugal (kor"tĭ-sif'u-gal) [L. *cortex*, rind, + *fugere*, to flee]. Conducting impulses arising within, and passing away from the outer surface, or cortex; denoting particularly axons of pyramidal cells of the cerebral cortex. SYN: *corticoefferent*.

corticipetal (kŏr"tĭ-sĭp'ĕ-tăl) ["+ *petere*, to seek]. Conducting impulses originating without, and passing to or toward the outer surface, or cortex; denoting particularly fibers of the thalamic radiation conveying impulses to sensory areas of cerebral cortex. SYN: *corticoafferent*.

corticoadrenal (kŏr"tĭ-ko-ăd-rē'năl) ["+ *ad*, toward, + *rēn*, kidney]. Pert. to cortex of adrenal gland.

corticoafferent (kŏr"tĭ-ko-ăf'fĕr-ĕnt) [L. *cortex*, rind, + *adferre*, to bear to]. Corticipetal, q.v.

corticobul'bar (kŏr"tĭ-ko-bŭl'băr) ["+ *bulbus*, bulb]. Pertaining to the cerebral cortex and upper portion of the brain stem, as corticobulbar tract.

corticoefferent (kŏr"tĭ-ko-ĕf'ĕr-ĕnt) ["+ *efferre*, to bring out of]. Corticifugal, q.v.

corticoid (kŏr'tĭ-koyd) [L. *cortex*, rind, + Gr. *eidos*, form]. Any of a number of steroid substances obtained from the cortex of the adrenal gland. SYN: *corticosteroid*.

corticopeduncular (kŏr″tĭ-ko-pe-dŭng′kū-lăr) [″+ *pedunculus*, little foot]. Pert. to cortex and cerebral peduncles.

corticopleuritis (kŏr″tĭ-ko-plū-rī′tĭs) [″+ Gr. *pleura*, rib, + *-itis*, inflammation]. Inflammation of the outer parts of the pleura.

corticospinal (kŏr″tĭ-ko-spī′nōl) [L. *cortex*, rind, + *spina*, thorn]. Pert. to cerebral cortex and spinal cord.

corticosteroid (kŏr″tĭ-ko-stēr′oyd). Corticoid, q.v.

corticosterone (kŏr″tĭ-kŏs′tĕ-rōn). A hormone of the adrenal cortex. Corticosterone influences carbohydrate metabolism and metabolism of potassium and sodium. It is essential for normal absorption of glucose, the formation of glycogen in the liver and tissues, and the normal utilization of carbohydrates by the tissues.

corticotrophic, corticotropic (kŏr″tĭ-ko-trof′ĭk, -trop′ĭk) [L. *cortex*, rind, + Gr. *trophē*, nourishment, *trope*, a turn]. Pert. to corticotrophin.

corticotrophin, corticotropin (kŏr″tĭ-ko-tro′fĭn, -tro′pĭn). The adrenocorticotrophic factor or principle in the anterior lobe of the pituitary gland. Stimulates adrenal cortex in secreting steroid hormones. SYN: *ACTH*, q.v.

   c. releasing factor. A substance found in the hypothalamus which controls secretion of adrenocorticotrophin.

cortin (kŏr′tĭn) [L. *cortex*, rind]. An extract of the cortex of the adrenal gland; contains the active steroid agents such as corticosterone.

cortisol (kŏr′tĭ-sol). An adrenal cortical hormone, usually referred to pharmaceutically as hydrocortisone. Closely related to cortisone, q.v., in physiological effects.

cortisone (kŏr′tĭ-sōn). A hormone isolated from the cortex of the adrenal gland and also prepared synthetically. It is closely related to cortisol. It is important for its regulatory action in metabolism of fats, carbohydrates, sodium, potassium, and proteins.

coruscation (kŏ-rŭs-kā′shun) [L. *coruscāre*, to glitter]. The subjective sensation of flashes of light.

Corynebacterium (kō-rī″nē-băk-tē′rī-ŭm) [Gr. *coryne*, a club, + *bacterium*, a small rod]. A genus of the family Corynebacteriaceae. The bacteria are rod-shaped, gram-positive, and non-motile. Though many of the species are pathogens in domestic animals, birds, reptiles, and plants, the most important is the species, C. diphtheriae, q.v., pathogenic in man.

   C. diphtheriae. The cause of diphtheria in man. SYN: *diphtheria bacillus; Klebs-Loeffler bacillus.*

coryza (kō-rī′ză) [Gr. *koryzal*, catarrh]. Cold in the head; an acute catarrhal inflammation of the nasal mucous membrane.

   c. spasmod′ica. Hay fever.

cosensitize (kō-sĕn′sĭ-tīz) [L. *con*, with, + *sensitivus*, sensitive]. To sensitize to more than one infection.

cosmesis (kŏs-mē′sĭs) [Gr. *kosmēsis*, ordering, adorning, from *kosmos*, order]. 1. Use of cosmetics. 2. In surgery, the performing of procedures intended to preserve or enhance beauty.

cosmetic (kŏz-mĕt′ĭk). 1. Preparation such as powder or cream for improving complexion. 2. Serving to preserve or promote beauty.

   c. surgery. Surgical procedures, usually plastic surgery, directed towards preserving beauty or correcting ugly scars or burns.

cos′mic [Gr. *kosmos*, order, the universe]. Pert. to the universe as a whole.

cos′ta [L.]. (pl. *costae*) [NA]. Rib.

   c. fluctuans. A floating rib.

   c. spuria. [NA]. A false rib.

   c. vera. [NA]. A true rib.

cos′tal. Pert. to a rib.

   c. cartilage. A cartilage which connects the end of a true rib with the sternum or the end of a rib with the costal cartilage above.

   c. pit. Cup-shaped depression at distal end of transverse process of a thoracic vertebra for articulation with tubercle of rib.

costalgia (kŏs-tăl′jĭ-ă) [L. *costa*, rib, + Gr. *algos*, pain]. Pain in a rib or in the intercostal spaces, e.g., intercostal neuralgia.

costectomy (kŏs-tĕk′tō-mĭ) [″+ *ektomē*, excision]. Operation of excising or resecting a rib.

cos′tive [L. *constipāre*, to press together]. Constipated.

cos′tiveness. Constipation.

costochondral (kŏs″to-kŏn′drăl) [L. *costa*, rib, + Gr. *chondros*, cartilage]. Pert. to a rib and its cartilage.

costoclavicular (kŏs″to-klă-vĭk′ū-lăr) [″+ *clavicula*, a little key]. Pert. to ribs and clavicle.

costocoracoid (kŏs″to-kor′ă-koyd) [″+ Gr. *korax*, crow, + *eidos*, form]. Pert. to ribs and coracoid process of scapula.

costopneumopexy (kŏs″to-nū′mo-pĕk-sĭ) [L. *costa*, rib, + Gr. *pneumōn*, lung, + *pēxis*, fixation]. Anchoring a lung to a rib.

costosternal (kŏs″to-stēr′năl) [″+ Gr. *sternon*, chest]. Pert. to a rib and the sternum.

costotome (kŏs′to-tōm) [″+ Gr. *tomē*, incision]. Knife or shears for cutting through a rib or cartilage.

costotomy (kŏs-tŏt′ō-mǐ). 1. Incision or division of a rib or part of one. 2. Excision of a rib; costectomy.

costotransverse (kŏs″to-trans-vĕrs′) [L. *costa*, rib, + *transvertere*, to turn across]. Pert. to the ribs and transverse processes of articulating vertebrae.

costovertebral (kŏs″to-vĕr′tĕ-brăl) ["+ *vertebra*, joint]. Pert. to a rib and a vertebra.

cot death. Sudden infant death syndrome, q.v.

cot′ton [ME. *cotoun*, from Arabic *qutn*, cotton]. A soft, white, fibrous material obtained from the fibers enclosing the seeds of various plants of the Malvaceae, esp. those of the genus Gossypium.

    c., absorbent. C. fibers from which the oil has been completely removed, enhancing ability to absorb liquids.

    c., styptic. C. impregnated with an astringent.

cotyledon (kŏt′ĭ-lē′dŏn) [Gr. *kotylēdōn*, hollow of a cup]. 1. Mass of villi on chorionic surface of the placenta. 2. Any of rounded portions into which the placenta's uterine surface is divided. 3. Seed leaf of a plant embryo.

cotyloid (kŏt′ĭ-loyd) [Gr. *kotyloeidēs*, cup shaped]. Shaped like a cup.

    c. cavity. The acetabulum or socket receiving the head of the femur.

couching (kow′ching) [Fr. *coucher*, to lay down]. Displacement of the lens downward in cataract.

cough (kŏf) [ME. *coughen*]. A forceful and sometimes violent expiratory effort preceded by a preliminary inspiration. The glottis is partially closed, the accessory muscles of expiration are brought into action, and the air is noisily expelled.

    A c. may be due to a variety of conditions, as can be seen below. There is no one course of therapy. Each disease is evaluated and treated accordingly. In c.'s due to inflammation of the respiratory tract it is usually inadvisable to completely suppress it. This is particularly true if sputum is produced as a result of coughing. SEE: *expectorant.*

    c., aneurysmal. Brassy and clanging, heard in patients suffering from aneurysm.

    c., asthmatic. More like an attack of dyspnea than a c.

    c., brassy. Heard in patients in whom there is pressure on the left recurrent laryngeal nerve, as in aortic aneurysm.

    c., bronchial. Heard in patients with bronchiectasis, q.v. May be provoked by change of posture, as in getting up in morning. Sputum: Fetid odor and copious; dirty gray. C. heard in bronchitis, q.v., in earlier stages, is hacking and irritating; in later stages, looser and easier. Sputum is thin frothy mucus.

    c., diphtherial. Heard in laryngeal diphtheria; noisy and brassy, with stridulous breathing.

    c., dry. C. unaccompanied by moisture.

    c., ear. A reflex c. induced by irritation in the ear which stimulates Arnold's nerve (ramus auricularis nervi vagi).

    c., effective. When sputum or any exudate is expectorated. SYN: *productive c.*

    c., hacking. A series of repeated efforts, as occurs in the early stages of pulmonary tuberculosis.

    c., harsh. A metallic c. occurring in laryngitis.

    c., moist. A loose c. accompanied by moisture.

    c., paroxysmal. C. occurring in whooping c. and bronchiectasis. SYN: *spasmodic.*

    c., productive. C. in which mucus or an exudate is expectorated. SYN: *effective c.*

    c., pulmonary. Hard and painful in pneumonia. Hacking and irritating in early stages of tuberculosis; in later stages, frequent and paroxysmal. SEE: *sputum.*

    c., reflex. Due to irritation from the middle ear, pharynx, stomach, or intestine. It may occur singly or coupled, or may be hacking in character.

    c., uterine. A reflex c. resulting from irritation of female organs, esp. the uterus.

    c., whooping. 1. Pertussis, q.v. 2. The paroxysmal cough ending in a whooping inspiration which occurs in pertussis.

coulomb (koo′lŏm, -lōm). [Charles A. de Coulomb, French physicist, 1736-1806] Unit of electrical quantity. It is the quantity of electricity transferred by one ampere in one second. ABBR: C.

count. The number obtained by determining the number of units of the object being counted per unit of volume, as bacteria count, red cell count, platelet count, reticulocyte count, differential count, parasite count, etc.

counteract (koun″tĕr-ăkt′). To act against or in opposition to.

counterac′tion. That action, or a drug or chemical agent having an action, opposing that of another agent.

counterextension (kown-tĕr-ĕks-tĕn′shŭn) [L. *contra*, against, + *extendere*, to extend]. Back pull or resistance to extension on a limb.

counterirritant (kown″tĕr-ĭr′ĭ-tănt) ["+ *irritāre*, to excite]. An agent that is applied locally to produce inflammatory reaction for the purpose of affecting some other part, usually adjacent to or underlying the surface irritated; e.g., mustard plaster, q.v.

There are three degrees of irritation produced by the following classes of agents: rubefacients, which redden the skin, the 1st degree; vesicants, q.v., which produce a blister or vesicle, the 2nd degree; and escharotics, which form an eschar or slough or cause death of tissue, the 3rd degree. SEE: *acupuncture; escharotic; moxibustion.*

counterirritation (kown″tĕr-ĭr′ĭ-tā′shŭn). Superficial irritation which relieves some other irritation of deeper structures.

countero′pening [L. *contra*, against, + AS. *open*, open]. A second opening, as in an abscess, not draining satisfactorily from first incision.

coun′terpressure instrument. To provide counter-retraction to offset that exerted by exit of needle.

coun′terpuncture [L. *contra*, against, + *punctura*, puncture]. Counteropening. An additional opening made to help drainage, as an abscess.

coup de soleil (kū-dă-sō-lā′) [Fr.]. Sunstroke.

coupling. In cardiology, the regular occurrence of premature systole just after a normal systolic beat. SYN: *bigeminal rhythm; coupled beats.*

courses (kōr′sĭz) [L. *cursus*, a flowing]. Menses; catamenia.

Courvoisier's law (koor-vwă′ze-ā). [Ludwig Courvoisier, Fr. surgeon, 1843-1918] Law pert. to dilatation of gallbladder. Disease processes which cause sudden blockage of the common bile duct, i.e. a stone, do not usually cause dilatation of the gallbladder. When the duct is obstructed slowly, as would be the case in infiltration of tissue around the duct (as in cancer), dilatation of the gallbladder is usually present.

couvade (koo-văd′) [Fr. to brood upon, hatch]. A custom among some primitive peoples which entails the father going to bed when his child is born. He stays there until his wife has recovered.

cov′erglass. Thin glass disk to cover a tissue or bacterial specimen to be examined microscopically.

cowperitis (kŏw″pĕr-ī′tĭs) [Cowper + Gr. -*itis*, inflammation]. Inflammation of Cowper's glands, q.v.

Cowper's glands. [William Cowper, Eng. anatomist, 1666-1709]. The bulbourethral glands. A pair of compound tubular glands about the size of a pea beneath the bulb of the male urethra, and emptying a mucous secretion into it. They are small round bodies, yellow in color. They correspond to the Bartholin glands, q.v., in the female.

cowpox (kŏw′pox). Vaccinia; pustular eruption on teats and bag of a cow in form of bluish vesicles, similar to smallpox. When given to humans, usually by vaccination, some degree of immunity against smallpox is obtained.

coxa (kŏk′să) [L., the hip, hipbone]. (pl. *coxae*) 1. The hipbone; or coxae [NA]. 2. [NA]. Hip or hip joint.

 c. valga. Deformity produced when angle of head of femur with the shaft is increased above 120°. Opposite of c. vara.

 c. vara. A deformity produced by decrease in angle made by head of femur with the shaft. Normally it should be 120°; but in c. vara it may be 80-90°. It occurs in rickets or may be due to bone injury.

coxalgia (kŏk-sŏl′jĭ-ă) [″+ Gr. *algos*, pain]. 1. Pain in the hip. SYN: *coxodynia.* 2. Hip joint disease. SYN: *coxitis.*

coxarthrosis (kŏks″ărth-rō′sĭs) [″+ Gr. *arthron*, joint, + *osis*, disease]. Term used in foreign literature to indicate arthritis of the hip.

coxitis (kŏk-sī′tĭs) [″+ Gr. -*itis*, inflammation]. Hip joint disease. SYN: *coxalgia* (def. 2).

coxodynia (kŏk″so-dīn′ĭ-ă) [L. *coxa*, hip, hipbone, + Gr. *odyne*, pain]. Pain in the hip joint. SYN: *coxalgia.*

coxofemoral (kŏk″so-fēm′ō-răl) [″+ *femur*, thigh]. Pert. to the hip and femur.

coxotuberculosis (kŏk″so-tu-bĕr″kū-lō′sĭs) [″+ *tuberculum*, a little swelling, + *osis*, diseased condition]. Tuberculous condition of the hip joint.

C.P. Abbr. for *candle power; cerebral palsy; chemically pure.*

CPK. Abbr. for *creatine phosphokinase.*

CPPV. Abbr. for *continuous positive pressure ventilation.*

Cr. Chem. symb. for chromium.

crab louse. Phthirus inguinalis and Phthirus pubis. One that infests the pubic region and other hairy areas of the body. SEE: *pediculosis.*

crachotement (kră-shŏt-mon′) [Fr.]. Inability to spit, even when the patient has a strong desire to do so; usually accompanied by syncope following utero-ovarian operation.

cracked pot sound. Percussion sound resembling that heard when striking a cracked pot, indicative of a pulmonary cavity.

cradle [AS. *cradel*]. Frame for keeping bedclothes from pressing on a wound or fractured part. SYN: *arculus.*

craigiasis (kră-gĭ′ă-sĭs). [Charles F. Craig, Amer. surgeon, 1872-1950]. Infection with

Craigia microorganism causing symptoms peculiar to dysentery.

cramp [ME. *crampe*]. A spasmodic, esp. a tonic, contraction of one or many muscles, usually painful.

In certain occupations, the attempted use of muscle groups habitually employed may lead to a so-called "professional cramp," though other motor formulae are easily executed by the affected muscles. In writer's cramp, the attempt to write induces painful spasm of the hand muscles (similarly telegrapher's, watchmaker's, seamstress' cramp, etc.).

SYM: Excruciating pain, hard and contracted lumps of muscle.

TREATMENT: Depends upon cause and location. In muscular c.'s try to extend muscle, compress it and apply heat and massage.

SEE: *heat cramp; systremma; writer's cramp.*

c., clonic. Wryneck caused by rheumatism. SYM: *rheumatic torticollis,* q.v.

c., heat. SEE: *heat cramp.*

cran'berries. A bright red, acid berry of the plant Oxycoccus.

Food value of 100 gm. (cooked sweetened sauce): Cal. 146; trace of protein; fat 0.2 gm.; carbohydrate 37.5 gm.; calcium 6 mg.

cra'nial [L. *cranialis*]. Pert. to the cranium.

c. bones. Those bones that comprise the cranium or brain case.

c. nerves. Twelve pair of nerves which have their origin in the brain. In addition to the 12 pair of c. nerves, there is a small combined efferent and afferent nerve which goes from the olfactory area of the brain to the nasal septum. This nerve, which is thought by some anatomists to be the first cranial nerve, is called terminal nerve.

DIAG: Lesions of the cranial nerves give rise to the following manifestations (lesions are described as if one of each pair of nerves were diseased): *First* (Olfactory): Loss or disturbance of the sense of smell. *Second* (Optic): Blindness of various types, depending upon the exact location of the lesion. *Third* (Oculomotor): Ptosis (drooping) of the eyelid, deviation of the eyeball outward, dilatation of the pupil, double vision.

Fourth (Trochlear): Rotation of the eyeball upward and outward, double vision. *Fifth* (Trigeminal): Sensory root: Pain or loss of sensation in face, forehead, temple, and eye. Motor root: Deviation of the jaw toward paralyzed side, difficulty in chewing. *Sixth* (Abducens): Deviation of the eye outward, double vision. *Seventh* (Facial): Paralysis of all the muscles on one side of the face; inability to wrinkle the forehead, to close the eye,

to whistle; deviation of the mouth toward the sound side.

Eighth (Vestibulocochlear): Deafness or ringing in the ears; dizziness; nausea and vomiting; reeling. *Ninth* (Glossopharyngeal): Disturbance of taste; difficulty in swallowing. *Tenth* (Vagus): Disease of the vagus nerve is usually limited to one or more of its divisions. Paralysis of the main trunk on one side causes hoarseness and difficulty in swallowing and talking. The commonest disease of the vagus is of its left recurrent branch which causes hoarseness as its principal manifestation.

Eleventh (Spinal Accessory): Drooping of the shoulder; inability to rotate the head away from affected side. *Twelfth* (Hypoglossal): Paralysis of one side of the tongue; deviation of tongue toward paralyzed side; thick speech.

craniectomy (krā-nĭ-ĕk'tō-mĭ) [Gr. *kranion,* skull, + *ektomē,* excision]. Opening of skull and removal of a portion of the skull.

NP: Take blood pressure every 15 minutes for first 12 hours, every half hour for second 12 hours, and then as ordered until discontinued. Do not leave patient alone for first 24 hours. Watch for and report at once any change in blood pressure, pulse, respiration, temperature, and any evidence of paralysis.

cranio- [Gr. *kranion,* L. *cranium,* skull]. Prefix pert. to the skull or cranium.

cranioacromial (krā″nĭ-ō-ă-krō'mĭ-al) [Gr. *kranion,* skull, + *akron,* extremity]. Rel. to the cranium and the acromion.

craniocele (krā'nĭ-ō-sēl) ["+ *kēlē,* hernia]. Protrusion of the brain from the skull. SEE: *encephalocele.*

craniocer'ebral ["+ L. *cerebrum,* brain]. Rel. to skull and brain.

cranioclast (krā'nĭ-ō-klăst) [Gr. *kranion,* skull, + *klastos,* broken]. Instrument for crushing fetal skull in delivery.

cranioclasty (krā'nĭ-ō-klăs″tĭ). Crushing of fetal head in dystocia.

craniocleidodysostosis (krā″nĭ-ō-klī″dō-dĭs-ŏs-tō'sis) [Gr. *kranion,* skull, + *kleis,* clavicle, + *dys,* bad, + *osteon,* bone, + *-ōsis,* infection]. Defective ossification of bones of head, face and clavicles; a congenital condition.

craniograph ["+ *graphein,* to write]. Device for making graphs of the skull.

craniol'ogy ["+ *logos,* study]. The study of the skull, its size, and shape, esp. in reference to different races.

craniomalacia (krā-nĭ-ō-mă-lā'shĭ-ă) [Gr. *kranion,* skull, + *malakia,* softening]. Softening of the skull bones.

craniometer (krā-nĭ-ŏm′ĕ-tĕr) ["+ *metron*, measure]. Instrument for making cranial measurements.

craniomet′ric points. Any prominences or marks on skull for defining the configuration of the cranium; for use in craniometry.

craniom′etry [Gr. *kranion*, skull, + *metron*, measure]. Study of the skull and measurement of its bones.

craniopagus (krā-nĭ-ōp′ă-gŭs) ["+ *pagos*, a fixed or solid thing]. Twins joined at the skulls.

craniopharyngeal (krā″nĭ-ō-făr-ĭn′jē-ăl) ["+ *phayrnx*, pharynx]. Pert. to cranium and pharynx.

craniopharyngioma (krā″nĭ-ō-făr-ĭn-jĭ-o′mă) ["+ "+ *-oma*, tumor]. Tumor of portion of the hypophysis cerebri.

cranioplasty (krā′nĭ-ō-plăs-tĭ) [Gr. *kranion*, skull, + *plassein*, to form]. Plastic operation on skull.

cra′niopuncture ["+ L. *punctura*, puncture]. Puncture of the skull.

craniorhachischisis (krā″nĭ-ō-ră-kĭs′kĭ-sĭs) ["+ *rhachis*, spine, + *schizein*, to split]. Congenital fissure of skull and spine.

craniostosis (krā-nĭ-ōs-tō′sĭs) [Gr. *kranion*, skull, + *osteon*, bone]. Congenital ossification of cranial sutures.

craniotabes (krā″nĭ-ō-tā′bēz) ["+ L. *tabes*, a wasting]. In infancy, abnormal softening of the skull bones. Those in the occipital region become almost paper thin.

ETIOL: Marasmus, rickets, or syphilis.

craniotome (krā′nĭ-ō-tōm) ["+ *tomē*, incision]. Device for forcibly perforating and dividing of fetal skull in labor in order to allow labor to continue. This is done in cases where the fetus has died in utero.

craniotomy (krā-nĭ-ŏt′ō-mĭ). 1. Breaking up fetal skull to facilitate delivery in difficult parturition. 2. Incision through the cranium.

craniotonos′copy [Gr. *kranion*, skull, + *tonos*, tone, + *skopein*, to examine]. Auscultatory percussion of cranium.

craniotympan′ic ["+ *tympanon*, kettledrum]. Pert. to skull and middle ear.

cra′nium [L.]. (pl. *crania*) That portion of the skull which encloses the brain; consists of single frontal, occipital, sphenoid, and ethmoid bones and the paired temporal and parietal bones. SEE: *skeleton*.

crap′ulent, crap′ulous [L. *crapula*, excessive drinking]. Rel. to, or excessive, drinking and eating. Intoxicated.

crassamen′tum [L.]. Coagulum, blood clot.

crateriform (krā-tĕr′ĭ-form) [Gr. *kratēr*, bowl, + L. *forma*, shape]. In bacteriology, indicates colonies which are saucer-shaped, craterlike, or goblet-shaped.

cravat′ ban′dage [Fr. *Cravate*, a Croatian]. Triangular bandage folded to form a band around the injured extremity. SEE: *bandage*.

crazy bone. The olecranon, q.v.

cream [L. *crāmum*]. The rich, yellowish part of milk.

Food value of 100 gm. or about 7 1/2 tablespoons (light table or coffee): Cal. 211; protein 3.0 gm.; fat 20.6 gm.; carbohydrate 4.3 gm.; calcium 102 mg.; phosphorus 80 mg.; sodium 43 mg.; potassium 122 mg.; vitamin A, 840 I.U.; riboflavin 0.15 mg.

c. substitute. Dried, containing cream, skim milk and lactose. Food value of 100 gm.: Cal. 508; protein 8.5 gm.; carbohydrate 61.3 gm.; vitamin A, 960 I.U.

creamalin (krēm′ă-lĭn). Proprietary name for an antacid preparation.

cream of tartar. Potassium bitartrate, $KHC_4H_4O_6$. Used in baking powder. SEE: *argol*.

crease (krēs) [ME. *crest*, crest]. A line produced by a fold.

c., gluteofemoral. The crease that bounds the buttocks below. SYN: *ileofemoral c.*

creatinase (krē-ăt′ĭn-ās) [Gr. *kreas*, flesh, + *ase*, enzyme]. An enzyme that decomposes creatinine.

creatine (krē′ă-tĭn) [Gr. *kreas*, flesh]. Methylglycocyamine, $NH:C(NH_2)N(CH_3)\cdot CH_2\cdot COOH + H_2O$, a colorless, crystalline substance that can be isolated from various animal organs and body fluids.

It combines readily with phosphate to form phosphocreatine (creatine phosphate) which serves as a source of high energy phosphate released in the anaerobic phase of muscle contraction.

Found esp. in muscle juice and in blood. Creatine may be present in a greater quantity in the urine of women than men. Creatine excretion is increased in pregnancy and decreased in hypothyroidism.

creatinemia (krē″ă-tĭn-ē′mĭ-ă) ["+ *haima*, blood]. Excess of creatine in circulating blood.

creatine phosphokinase. Enzyme present in skeletal and cardiac muscle and the brain. Catalyzes the reversible transfer of high energy phosphate between creatine and phosphocreatine and between adenosine diphosphate (ADP) and adenosine triphosphate (ATP).

Serum CPK is increased 10 to 25 times the normal level in the first few hours following myocardial infarction. The level returns to normal within two to four days. CPK serum levels are also increased in progressive muscular dystrophy and surgical damage to skeletal muscle. ABBR: CPK.

creatinine (krē-ăt'ĭn-ĭn) [Gr. *kreas*, flesh]. 1-methylglycocyamidine, $C_4H_7ON_3$, the end product of creatine metabolism.

It also can be isolated as colorless crystals from animal material. It is one of the nonprotein constituents of blood, and increased quantities of it are found in advanced stages of renal disease. It is a normal and an alkaline constituent of urine and blood. About 0.02 gm./kg. of body weight is excreted by the kidneys per day.

creatinuria (krē-ă'tĭn-ū'rĭ-ă) ["+ *ouron*, urine]. Creatinine in urine.

creatorrhea (krē''ă-tō-rē'ă) ["+ *rhoia*, flow]. The presence of undigested muscle fibers in the feces, seen in some cases of pancreatic disease.

crèche (krěsh) [Fr.]. A day nursery for children.

Credé's method (krā-dā'). [Karl S. F. Credé, Ger. gynecologist, 1819-1892]. 1. The means whereby the placenta is expelled by downward pressure on the uterus through the abdominal wall with the thumb on the posterior surface of the fundus uteri and the flat of the hand on the anterior surface, the pressure being applied in the direction of the birth canal. 2. For treatment of the eyes of the newborn, the use of 1% silver nitrate solution instilled into the eyes immediately after birth for the prevention of ophthalmia neonatorum (gonorrheal ophthalmia).

creek dots. Small shining dots sometimes present in the retina. Their nature or cause is unknown. Sometimes familial.

creeping eruption. Larva migrans, q.v.

cremaster (krē-măs'tĕr) [L., to suspend]. One of the fascialike muscles suspending and enveloping the testicles and spermatic cord.

cremaster'ic. Pert. to the cremaster muscle.

   c. fascia. One of the coverings of the spermatic cord.

   c. reflex. Retraction of testis when skin is stroked on front inner side of thigh.

cremate (krē'māt) [L. *crematio*, a burning]. To dispose of the body of a dead person by burning. The ashes may or may not be buried.

crematorium [L.]. A place for the burning of corpses.

crenate (krē'nāt) [L. *crenatus*]. Notched or scalloped, as crenated condition of blood corpuscles.

crenation (krē-nā'shŭn). The conversion of normally round red corpuscles into shrunken, knobbed, starry forms, as when blood is mixed with salt solution of 5% strength. SEE: *plasmolysis*.

creosote (krē'ō-sōt) [Gr. *kreas*, flesh, + *sōzein*, to preserve]. A mixture of phenols obtained from wood tar. Used as a disinfectant and as a preserver of wood.

crepitant (krěp'ĭ-tănt) [L. *crepitāre*, to crackle]. Crackling; having or making a crackling sound.

crepitation (krěp-ĭ-tā'shŭn). 1. A crackling sound heard in certain diseases, as the rale heard in pneumonia. 2. A grating sound heard on movement of ends of a broken bone.

crep'itus (krěp'ĭ-tŭs) [L.]. 1. The noise of gas discharged from the intestines. 2. Crepitation.

   c. redux. Rale indicating approaching recovery in pneumonia.

crepuscular (krē-pŭs'kū-lăr) [L. *crepusculum*, twilight]. Pert. to twilight; used to describe twilight mental state.

crescent (krěs'ěnt) [L. *crēscēns*]. Shaped like a sickle or the new moon.

   c., articular. A crescent-shaped cartilage present in certain joints as the menisci of the knee joint.

   c. of Gianuzzi. A crescent-shaped group of serous cells lying at the base of or along the side of a mucous alveolus of a salivary gland. SYN: *demilune of Heidenhein*.

   c., myopic. Grayish patch in fundus of eye due to atrophy of choroid.

crescentic (krěs-ĕn'tĭk). Sickle-shaped.

cresol (krē'sōl). Yellowish-brown liquid obtained from coal tar and containing not more than 5% of phenol.

   USE: A disinfectant in a 1-5% solution for articles or areas which do not come in direct contact with food.

cresomania; croesomania (krē''sō-mā'nĭ-ă). [Croesus, wealthy king of Lydia, 6th century B. C.] Hallucination of possessing great wealth.

crest [L. *crista*, crest]. A ridge or an elongated prominence, esp. one on a bone.

cretin (krē'tĭn) [Fr.]. One afflicted with congenital myxedema; a mentally retarded dwarf. Characterized by lack of growth and mental development; rarely if ever exceeds the mental age of 10.

The skin is rough and dry, and the hair coarse, dry, and brittle. Teeth erupt slowly and are of poor quality and irregularly placed. The tongue is large and apt to protrude from a mouth which constantly drools saliva. A cretin child is potbellied, swaybacked, and prone to umbilical hernia. Adult cretin is myxedematous. SEE: *cretinism*.

cretinism (krē'tĭn-ĭzm) ["+ Gr. *ismos*, condition]. Congenital affection, characterized by a lack of physical and mental development.

ETIOL: A congenital deficiency in secretion of the thyroid hormones.

SYM: An abnormal condition of the thyroid gland, myxedema and impaired mental ability.

TREATMENT: Dessicated thyroid orally.

c., endemic. C. resulting from iodine deficiency of mother during pregnancy or genetic factors.

c., sporadic. C. resulting from congenital absence of, or lack of normal development of, the thyroid gland.

cretinoid (crē'tĭ-noyd) ["+ Gr. *eidos*, resemblance]. Having the symptoms of cretinism, or resembling a cretin, due to a congenital condition.

cre'tinous. Pert. to a cretin or to cretinism.

crevice (krĕv'ĭs) [Fr. *crever*, to break]. A small fissure or crack.

c., gin'gival. The fissure produced by the marginal gingiva with the tooth surface.

crevicular (krĕv-ĭk'ū-lăr). Pert. to the gingival crevice.

CRF. Abbr. for *corticotrophin-releasing factor,* esp. the substance present in extract of the hypothalamus which brings about the release of ACTH from the anterior pituitary.

crib [AS. *cribbe*, manger]. 1. A framework around a denture or a natural tooth to serve as a brace or supporting structure. 2. Bassinette for newborn to lie in.

c. death. Sudden infant death syndrome, q.v.

cribbing. Aerophagia; swallowing air.

crib'rate [L. *cribratus*]. Profusely pitted or perforated like a sieve.

cribra'tion. The state of being perforated.

crib'riform [L. *cribrum*, a sieve, + *forma*, form]. Sievelike.

c. fascia. The portion of deep fascia which covers the fossa ovalis of the thigh.

c. plate. The thin, perforated, medial portion of the horizontal plate of the ethmoid bone.

cricoarytenoid (krī"kō-ă-rĭt'ĕn-oyd) [Gr. *krikos*, ring, + *arytaina*, pitcher, + *eidos*, form]. Extending between the cricoid and arytenoid cartilages.

cricoderma (krī-kō-dĕr'mă) ["+ *derma*, skin]. Ringshaped infiltrations in center of indurations on the skin.

cricoid (krī'koyd) [Gr. *krikos*, ring, + *eidos*, form]. Shaped like a signet ring.

c. cartilage. The lowermost cartilage of the larynx. It is shaped like a signet ring, the broad portion or lamina being posterior, the anterior portion forming the arch.

cricoidectomy (krī"koyd-ĕk'tō-mĭ) ["+ "+ *ektomē*, excision]. Excision of cricoid cartilage.

cricoidynia (krī-koy-dĭn'ĭ-ă) ["+ "+ *odynē*, pain]. Pain in cricoid cartilage.

cricopharyngeal (krī"kō-făr-ĭn'jĭ-ăl) [Gr. *krikos*, ring, + *pharynx*, gullet]. Pert. to the cricoid cartilage and pharynx.

cricothyreotomy (krī"kō-thī"rē-ŏt'ō-mĭ) ["+ *thyreos*, shield, + *tomē*, a cut]. Division of the cricoid and thyroid cartilage.

cricothyroid (krī-kō-thī'royd) ["+ "+ *eidos*, form]. Pert. to the thyroid and cricoid cartilages.

cricot'omy [Gr. *krikos*, ring, + *tomē*, incision]. Division of the cricoid cartilage.

cricotracheotomy (krī"kō-trā"kī-ŏt'ō-mĭ) ["+ *tracheia*, windpipe, + *tomē*, incision]. Division of the cricoid cartilage and upper trachea in closure of the glottis.

Crigler-Najjar syndrome. A rare congenital disease characterized by nonhemolytic jaundice. SYN: *congenital familial nonhemolytic jaundice.*

criminal [L. *crimen*, crime]. 1. Pertaining to crime. 2. A person who has committed or been convicted of a crime.

c. abortion. Illegal abortion.

c. neglect. In legal medicine, to fail to act in a manner which would be in the best interest of the patient.

c. responsibility. In legal medicine, being able to distinguish between right and wrong while committing a crime.

crinogenic (krĭn"ō-jĕn'ĭk) [Gr. *krinein*, to secrete, + *gennan*, to produce]. Producing or stimulating secretion.

crisis (krī'sĭs) [Gr. *krisis*, turning point). (pl. *crises*) 1. The turning point of a disease; a very critical period often marked by a long sleep and profuse perspiration. 2. The term used for the sudden descent of a high temperature to normal or below; generally occurs within 24 hours. 3. Sharp paroxysms of pain occurring over the course of a few days in certain diseases, e.g., Dietl's c.

c., abdominal. Severe abdominal pain due to one of several causes. SEE: *c., sickle cell; c., tabetic.*

c., blood. The appearance in the blood of large numbers of nucleated erythrocytes over the course of a few days.

c., Dietl's. In cases of floating kidney, the ureter becomes kinked and urine is obstructed, producing symptoms of renal colic.

c., false. Condition when temperature falls and the pulse rate remains high, suggesting that later on the temperature may rise again.

c., sickle cell. Severe abdominal pain

due to sickle cell anemia.

c., tabetic. Abdominal pain due to syphilis.

c., thyroid. Sudden increase in severity of symptoms of thyrotoxicosis; marked by fever and extreme tachycardia. Outcome occasionally fatal. SYN: *thyroid storm.*

c., true. Temperature drop accompanied by a fall in the pulse rate.

crista (kris'tä) [L.]. (pl. *cristae*) 1. [NA] A crest or ridge. 2. A projection, sometimes branched, of the inner wall of a mitochondrion into its fluid-filled cavity.

c. ampullaris. [NA]. A localized thickening of the membrane lining the ampullae of the semicircular canals; it is covered with neuroepithelium containing auditory cells.

c. galli. [NA]. A ridge on the ethmoid bone to which the falx cerebri is attached.

c. lacrimalis posterior. [NA]. A vertical ridge on the lateral surface of the lacrimal bone.

c. spiralis. A ridge on the spiral lamina of the cochlea, q.v.

criterion (kri-tē'rī-ŏn) [Gr. *kriterion,* a means for judging]. (pl. *criteria*) Standard or attribute for judging a condition or establishing a diagnosis.

critical (krĭt'ĭ-kǎl) [Gr. *kritikos,* critical]. 1. Pert. to a crisis. 2. Dangerous.

c. reflex. Abnormal tension of an area resulting from direct stimulation of that area.

crock. Medical slang for a person with a multiplicity of complaints, or repeated complaints, for which efforts to diagnose or treat are in vain. Besides the fact that the individual so labeled may have an organic ba-

sis for his complaints, the person may also be in need of sympathetic attention.

Crohn's disease (krŏn). [Burrill B. Crohn, Amer. gastroenterologist, 1884 —]. Regional ileitis; regional enteritis.

Crookes' dark space. [Sir William Crookes, Eng. physicist, 1832-1919]. Nonluminous region enveloping outline of the cathode in a discharge tube. SEE: *cathode.*

Crookes' tube. An early form of vacuum discharge tube used for the study of cathode rays.

cross [L. *crux*]. In genetics, the mating or the offspring of the mating of two individuals of different strains, races, or species.

c. fertilization. The combining of gametes of two different individuals of the same species.

cross birth. Presentation of the fetus where the long axis of the fetus is at right angles to that of the mother and requires version.

crossed. Passing from one side to the other, as crossed pyramidal tract in which nerve fibers cross from one side of the medulla to the other.

c. reflexes. 1. Passive flexion of one part following flexion of another. 2. Passive flexion of one leg causing similar movement of opposite leg.

cross-eye. Manifest inward deviation of one eye when looking at an object. SYN: *esotropia; squint; strabismus.*

crossing over. In genetics, the mutual interchange of blocks of genes between two homologous chromosomes. It occurs during synapsis in miosis.

crossmatching. Test to establish blood compatibility before transfusion. SEE: *blood crossmatching.*

crossover. An individual resulting from a new combination of linked genes.

Crotalus (krŏt'ă-lŭs) [Gr. *krotalon,* rattle]. A genus of snakes which includes most rattlesnakes. All are highly poisonous.

crotaphion (krō-tăf'ĭ-ŏn) [Gr. *krotaphos,* the temple]. Tip of greater wing of sphenoid bone.

crotchet (krŏch'ĕt) [Fr. *crochet,* small hook]. Sharp hook for extracting fetus after craniotomy.

crotonism (krō'tŏn-izm). Poisoning from croton oil.

croton oil (krō'tŏn) [Gr. *kroton,* castor oil plant seed]. Oleum tiglii; a fixed oil expressed from the seed of the croton plant, Croton tiglium.

ACTION: Drastic cathartic, externally as a rubefacient. This chemical has no place in medicine and should not be used.

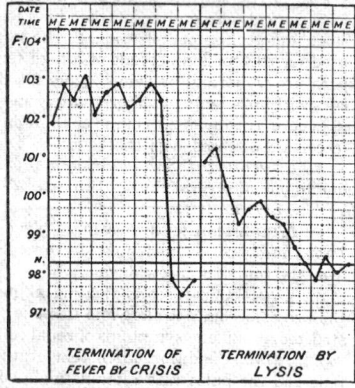

TERMINATION OF FEVER BY CRISIS   TERMINATION BY LYSIS

(After Sears, W. G., Winwood, R. S.: Medicine for Nurses, ed. 11. Edward Arnold Publishers Ltd., London, 1970.)

POISONING SYM: Severe burning pain in mouth and stomach; vomiting; marked diarrhea; and shock. Skin cold and clammy; face pinched; pulse rapid and small; collapse follows.

TREATMENT: Stomach pump or an emetic. Give soothing drinks such as milk or whites of eggs; then saline cathartic. Stimulate; apply external heat. Atropine, belladonna, or morphine to relieve cramping. Intravenous fluids may be required to maintain hydration.

crounotherapy (krū"nō-thĕr'ă-pĭ) [Gr. *krounos*, spring, + *therapeia*, treatment]. Use of mineral waters for therapeutic purposes. SYN: *crenotherapy*.

croup (krūp). Disease characterized by suffocative and difficult breathing, laryngeal spasm, and sometimes by the formation of a membrane.

    c., catarrhal. Acute catarrhal laryngitis.

    c., diphtheritic. Diphtheria of the larynx.

    c., false. C., spasmodic, q.v.

    c., membranous. Croupous laryngitis or true c. Inflammation of larynx with exudation forming in false membrane.

    SYM: Those of laryngitis; loss of voice; noisy, difficult, and stridulous breathing; weak, rapid pulse; livid surface, fever moderate.

    PROG: Grave, unless tracheostomy has been performed.

    TREATMENT: Similar to that for diphtheria, q.v. Hot fomentations to throat; emetics; and medicated steam inhalations. SEE: *carpopedal spasm; steam tent.*

    c., spasmodic. Catarrhal laryngitis without formation of false membrane, but with spasm of the glottis. Occurs in children. SYN: *false c.*

    SYM: Difficult breathing, metallic cough, swollen membrane with tenacious mucus.

    PROG: Favorable.

    TREATMENT: Hot fomentations to throat; inhalation of steam.

croupous (krū'pŭs). Pert. to croup or having a fibrinous exudation.

crown [L. *corona*, wreath]. The top or highest part of an organ or other structure. Ex: top of the head. Corona [NA], q.v.

crown'ing [L. *corōna*, wreath]. Stage in delivery when fetal head presents at the vulva.

crownwork. Artificial crown for a tooth.

crucial (krū'shăl) [L. *crucialis*]. 1. Crossshaped. 2. Decisive; of supreme importance; critical.

cruciate (krū'shĭ-āt). Cross-shaped as in the cruciate ligaments of the knee.

cru'cible [L. *crucibulum*]. A dish or container for substances which are being melted, burned, or dehydrated while exposed to high temperatures.

cruciform (krū'sĭ-form) [L. *crux,* cross, + *forma,* shape]. Shaped like a cross.

crude (krūd) [L. *crudus,* raw]. Raw, unrefined, or in a natural state. When used to describe a person, indicates one who is unrefined or uncouth.

crura (krū'ră) [L., legs]. (sing. *crus*) A pair of elongated masses or diverging bands, resembling legs.

    c. cerebel'li. Cerebellar peduncles.

    c. cer'ebri. Pair of bands joining cerebellum to medulla and pons.

    c. of diaphragm. Two pillars connecting spinal column and diaphragm.

    c. of the fornix. Arches made by division of the fornicate extremities.

crural (krū'ral) [L. *cruralis*]. Pert. to the leg or thigh; femoral.

    c. arch. Femoral arch.

    c. hernia. Femoral hernia.

    c. nerve. Femoral nerve. SEE: *nerves* in *Appendix.*

    c. palsies. Those of the nerves of the legs (e.g., 12th thoracic, 1st to 5th lumbar, and 1st to 3rd sacral spinal nerves).

crus (krŭs) [L.]. [NA]. 1. The leg. 2. Any structure resembling the leg.

    c. cerebri. [NA]. Either of the two peduncles connecting the cerebrum with the pons.

crush syndrome. Renal failure following severe local injuries, esp. those involving crushing of the lower extremities.

crust [L. *crusta*]. 1. A scab. A secondary lesion; dry serous or seropurulent, brown, yellow, red, or green exudations on a free surface. 2. An outer covering or coat.

    Seen in eczema, seborrhea, syphilis, impetigo, favus, and ringworm of the scalp.

crust'a [L.]. (pl. *crus'tae*) Crust, q.v.

    c. lactea. Seborrhea of scalp in nursing infants.

crutch [AS. *crycc*]. 1. A device for aiding a lame or weak person in walking. Usually a long staff with padded crescent-shaped portion at the top for placing under the armpit. A great variety of crutches are available: the most common, the axillary; various forms of walkers which provide a mobile stable platform which the patient holds on to while walking; forearm crutch which provides points of contact between the hand and the forearm; the shelf crutch, an adapted forearm crutch, which permits a person who can't bear weight on the hands to use a crutch; three- or four-legged cane for the person with poor balance who needs mild support.

2. In psychoanalysis, the use of some affliction which may be real or imaginary to explain personal inadequacy or failure.

Cruveilhier-Baumgarten syndrome (krū-val-yā' bŏm'gär-tĕn). [Jean Cruveilhier, Fr. pathologist, 1791-1874; P. Clemens von Baumgarten, Ger. pathologist, 1848-1928]. Thrombosis of the portal vein with cirrhosis of the liver, splenomegaly, and portal hypertension

cryalgesia (krī-ăl-jē'zĭ-ă) [Gr. *kryos*, cold, + *algos*, pain]. Pain from the cold. SYN: *crymodynia.*

cryanesthesia (krī-ăn-ĕs-thē'zĭ-ă) ["+ *an-*, not, + *aisthēsis*, sensation]. Loss of sense of cold.

cryesthesia (krī-ĕs-thē'zĭ-ă) ["+ *aisthēsis*, sensation]. Sensitiveness to the cold.

crymodynia (krī-mō-dīn'ĭ-ă) [Gr. *krymos*, frost, + *odynē*, pain]. Pain from cold, esp. rheumatic pain aggravated by cold or damp weather. SYN: *cryalgesia.*

crymophilic (krī-mō-fĭl'ĭk) ["+ *philein*, to love]. Showing preference for cold. Ex: psychrophilic bacteria. SYN: *cryophilic.*

crymophylactic (krī-mō-fĭ-lăk'tĭk) ["+ *phylaxis*, protective]. Resistant to cold.

crymother'apy ["+ *therapeia*, treatment]. The use of cold in treating disease. SYN: *cryotherapy.*

cryoaerotherapy (krī"ō-ā"ĕr-ō-thĕr'ă-pī) [Gr. *kryos*, cold, + *aēr*, air, + *therapeia*, treatment]. Cold air bath in which, by degrees, the patient is accustomed to freezing temperature.

cryobiology (krī"ō-bī-ōl'ō-jī) ["+ *bios*, life, + *logos*, study]. Study of effect of cold on biological systems.

cryocautery (krī"ō-kŏ'tĕr-ī) ["+ *kauter*, a burner]. Device for application of cold sufficient to kill tissue.

cryogen (krī'ō-jĕn) [Gr. *kyros*, cold, + *gennan*, to produce]. Substances which produce low temperatures.

cryogenic (krī"ō-jĕn'ĭk). Producing or pert. to low temperatures.

cryoglobulinemia (krī"ō-glōb"ū-lĭn-ē'mĭ-ă) [Gr. *kryos*, cold, + L. *globulus*, globule, + Gr. *haima*, blood]. Presence in the blood of an abnormal protein which forms gels at low temperatures. Found in association with pathological conditions such as multiple myeloma, leukemia, and certain forms of pneumonia.

cryom'eter ["+ *metron*, measure]. A thermometer for measuring very low temperature.

cryophilic (krī"ō-fĭl'ĭk) ["+ *philein*, to love]. Preferring low temperatures.

cryoprotectants. Drugs which permit cells to survive freezing and thawing.

cryosurgery ["+ ME. *surgerie*, surgery]. Technique of exposing tissues to extreme cold in order to produce well demarcated areas of cell injury and destruction. The tissue is usually cooled to below −20° C. Used in malignant tumors, to control pain, to produce lesions in the brain, and to control bleeding. The cold is usually produced by use of a probe containing liquid nitrogen.

cryothalamotomy (krī"ō-thăl"ă-mŏt'ō-mī) [Gr. *kryos*, cold, + L. *thalamus*, inner chamber, + Gr. *tomē*, a cutting]. Destruction of a portion of the brain by cooling the end of a slender probe placed in the thalamus. This is usually done by circulating liquid nitrogen through the hollow stylus. Used in treating parkinsonism.

cryotherapy (krī-ō-thĕr'ă-pī) ["+ *therapeia*, treatment]. The therapeutic use of cold.

cryotol'erant ["+ L. *tolerāre*, to bear]. Able to tolerate very low temperatures.

crypt (krĭpt) [Gr. *kryptos*, hidden]. 1. A small sac or cavity extending into an epithelial surface. 2. A tubular gland, esp. one of the intestine.

   c., anal. One of a number of small indentations lying immediately behind junction of anal skin and rectal mucosa.

   c. of the iris. An irregular excavation on anterior surface of the iris near pupillary and ciliary margins.

   c. of Lieberkuhn. A tubular gland of the intestine which secretes intestinal juice. Its wall is composed of columnar epithelium containing argentaffin cells and, at the base of the gland, cells of Paneth. They open between bases of the villi.

   c., synoviparous. A saclike extension of the synovial cavity into capsule of a joint. Sometimes they become blind sacs.

   c., tonsillar. A deep invagination of the surface stratified epithelium into substance of the lingual or palatine tonsils. It is surrounded by lymph nodules and may be branched.

cryptanamnesia (krĭpt"ăn-ăm-nē'zĭ-ă) [Gr. *kryptos*, hidden, + *an-*, not, + *amnēsia*, forgetfulness]. Subconscious memory.

cryptectomy (krĭp-tĕk'tō-mī) ["+ *ektomē*, excision]. Excision of a crypt.

cryptesthesia (krĭp-tĕs-thē'zĭ-ă) ["+ *aisthēsis*, sensation]. Subconscious awareness of facts or occurrences other than through the senses or through rational thinking. Ex: intuition; clairvoyance.

cryptic (krĭp'tĭk) [Gr. *kryptikos*, hidden]. 1. Having a hidden meaning; occult. 2. Tending to hide or disguise. Ex: cryptic coloring.

cryptitis (krĭp-tī'tĭs) [Gr. *kryptos*, hidden, + *-itis*, inflammation]. Inflammation of a crypt or follicle, esp. an anal crypt.

cryptococcosis (krĭp''tŏ-kŏk-ō'sĭs) ["+ *kokkos*, berry, + *-ōsis*, condition]. A systemic fungus infection which may involve any organ of the body, lungs, skin, but having a marked predilection for the brain and its meninges. SYN: *torulosis.*

ETIOL: Cryptococcus neoformans (Torula histolytica), a fungus.

SYMPTOMS: Development of single or multiple abscesses. In the cerebral type there is headache, dizziness, vertigo, stiffness of neck muscles; in final stages, coma and respiratory failure. Often mistaken for brain tumor.

PROG: Poor; in cerebral and meningeal forms usually fatal.

TREATMENT: Amphotericin B is somewhat beneficial in certain cases.

Cryptococcus (krĭp''tŏ-kŏk'ŭs). A genus of pathogenic yeastlike fungi which is the causative agent of cryptococcosis. SYN: *Torula.*

cryptodidymus (krĭp-tŏ-dĭd'ĭ-mŭs) [Gr. *kryptos*, hidden, + *didymos*, twin]. A congenital anomaly in which one fetus is concealed within another.

cryptogenetic (krĭp''tŏ-jĕn-ĕt'ĭk) ["+ *gennan*, to produce]. Of unknown or indeterminate origin.

c. infection. The invasion of bacteria without outward evidence of entry into the body. SEE: *infection.*

cryptolith (krĭp'tŏ-lĭth) ["+ *lithos*, stone]. A concretion in a glandular follicle.

cryptomenorrhea (krĭp''tŏ-mĕn''ŏ-rē'ă) [Gr. *kryptos*, hidden, + *mēn*, month, + *rhoia*, flow]. Monthly subjective symptoms of menses without flow of blood. May be due to imperforate hymen.

cryptomerorachischisis (krĭp''tŏ-mĕr''ŏ-ră-kĭs'kĭ-sĭs) ["+ *meros*, part, + *rhachis*, spine, + *schisis*, cleavage]. Spina bifida occulta without a tumor but with bony deficiency.

cryptomnesia (krĭp-tŏm-nē'zĭ-ă) ["+ *mnēsis*, memory]. Subconscious memory.

cryptophthalmus (krĭp''tŏf-thăl'mŭs) [Gr. *kryptos*, hidden, + *ophthalmos*, eye]. Complete congenital adhesion of eyelids to globe of eye.

cryptoplas'mic ["+ *plasma*, matter]. Having existence in a concealed form.

cryptopodia (krĭp''tŏ-pō'dĭ-ă) ["+ *pous*, foot]. Fibromata of feet so diffuse as to resemble pads.

cryptopyic (krĭp''tŏ-pī'ĭk) [Gr. *kryptos*, hidden, + *pyon*, pus]. Having concealed suppuration, as a pyemia without apparent etiology.

cryptorchid (krĭpt-or'kĭd) ["+ *orchis*, testis]. An individual with testicles which have not descended into the scrotum.

cryptorchidectomy (krĭpt''or-kĭ-dek'tŏ-mĭ) ["+ "+ *ektomē*, excision]. Operation for an undescended testicle.

cryptorchidism (krĭpt-or'kĭd-ĭzm) [Gr. *kryptos*, hidden, + *orchis*, testis, + *ismos*, condition of]. Failure of testicles to descend into scrotum.

cryptorchis (krĭpt-or'kĭs). Cryptorchid, q.v.

cryptorchism (krĭpt-or'kĭzm). Cryptorchidism, q.v.

cryptorrhea (krĭp-tō-rē'ă) [Gr. *kryptos*, hidden, + *rhoia*, flow]. Excessive secretion of a ductless gland.

cryptorrhetic (krĭp''tŏ-rĕt'ĭk). Pert. to the internal secretions. SYN: *cryptorrheic.*

cryptoscope (krĭp'tŏ-skōp) [Gr. *kryptos*, hidden, + *skopein*, to examine]. Fluoroscope.

cryptotoxic (krĭp''tŏ-tŏks'ĭk) ["+ *toxikon*, poison]. Having unknown toxic properties.

cry reflex. 1. Normal ability of an infant to cry. Not present in premature infants. 2. Spontaneous crying by infants during sleep. Due to some painful disease such as tuberculosis of the joints.

crystal (krĭs'tăl) [Gr. *krystallos*, ice]. A solid body in which the atoms are arranged in a definite symmetrical pattern and having faces lying at definite angles to each other as crystals formed from salts, water, etc.

c.'s, Böttcher's. C., spermin, q.v.

c.'s, Charcot-Leyden. Found in sputum from patients with asthma, leukemic blood, etc. Octahedral and composed of a phosphate.

c.'s, Charcot-Neumann. Spermin crystals found in semen and some animal tissues.

c.'s, Charcot-Robin. A type formed in blood in leukemia.

c.'s of hemin. Yellowish or brown crystals which appear when dried blood or hemoglobin is heated with a few drops of acetic acid and salt. They are crystals of hemin, the hydrochloride of heme. Their presence constitutes a delicate and reliable test for blood. SYN: *Teichmann's c.'s.*

c.'s, spermin. Crystals composed of spermine phosphate and seen in prostatic fluid on addition of a drop of ammonium phosphate solution.

crystallin (krĭs'tăl-ĭn). Globulin of the crystalline lens.

crys'talline. Resembling crystal.

   c. deposits in urine. Acid group includes the urates, oxalates, carbonates, and sulfates. The alkaline group includes the phosphates, cholesterin ammonium urate.

   c. lens. The lens of the eye in the capsule behind the pupil. It separates the aqueous from the vitreous humor. It is transparent and refracts the rays of light, impinging them upon the surface to bring them to a focus on the retina.

crystalliza'tion [Gr. *krystallos,* ice]. The formation of crystals.

crys'talloid ["+ *eidos,* form]. 1. Like a crystal. 2. A substance capable of crystallization, which in solution can be diffused through animal membranes. Opposed to colloid.

crystalloiditis (krĭs-tăl-oyd-ī'tĭs) ["+ "+ -*itis,* inflammation]. Inflammation of crystalline lens.

crystallopho'bia [Gr. *krystallos,* ice, + *phobos,* fear]. Abnormal fear of glass or objects made of glass.

crystalluria (krĭs-tă-lū'rĭ-ă) ["+ *ouron,* urine]. The appearance of crystals in the urine. May occur following the administration of sulfonamides. Their formation can be prevented by administration of adequate amounts of alkali.

crystalluridrosis (krĭs"tă-lū"rĭ-drō'sĭs) ["+ "+ *hidrōs,* sweat]. Crystallization of urinary elements on the skin.

Cs. Chem. symb. for cesium.

C.S.F. Abbr. for *cerebrospinal fluid.*

CS gas. A gas, orthochlorobenzalmalonitrile, used in riot control. Named after its two inventors, Corson and Stoughton.

Ctenocephalides (tĕn-ō-sĕf-ăl'ĭ-dēz) [Gr. *ktenodēs,* like a cockle, + *kephalē,* head]. A genus of fleas belonging to the order Siphonaptera. Common species are Ct. canis and Ct. felis, the dog flea and cat flea. The adults feed on their hosts while larvae live on dried blood and feces of adult fleas. Adults may attack man and other animals. They serve as intermediate host of the dog tapeworm, Dipylidium caninum, and may transmit other helminth and protozoan infections.

Cu. Chem. symb. for L. *cuprum,* copper.

cubic measure. SEE: *Appendix.*

cu'bital [L. *cubitum,* elbow]. Pert. to the ulna or to the forearm.

   c. fossa. Triangular area lying anterior to and below the elbow, bounded medially by the pronator teres and laterally by the brachioradialis muscle.

cu'bitus [L]. [NA] Elbow; forearm; ulna.

   c. valgus. A deformity of the arm in which the forearm deviates laterally. May be congenital or due to injury or disease. In females, slight cubitus valgus is normal and is one of the secondary sex characteristics.

   c. varus. A deformity of the arm in which the forearm deviates medially.

cu'boid [Gr. *kubos,* cube, + *eidos,* resemblance]. Like a cube.

   c. bone. Outer bone of tarsal or instep bones articulating posteriorly with the 4th and 5th metatarsus. SYN: *os cuboideum* [NA].

cucumbers [L. *cucumis*]. Fruit of Cucumis saturis vine.

   Food value of 100 gm. (raw, unpared): Cal. 15; protein 0.9 gm.; carbohydrate 3.4 gm.; calcium 25 mg.; iron 1.1 mg.; vitamin A, 250 I.U.; ascorbic acid 11 mg.

cucurbit (kū-kĕr'bĭt) [L. *cucurbita,* gourd]. Cupping glass.

cue. In psychology, a stimulus or set of stimuli to which a person has learned to respond.

cuff (kŭf) [ME. *cuffe,* glove]. Anatomical structure encircling a part.

cul-de-sac (kŭl'dī-săk') [Fr., bottom of the sack]. 1. A blind pouch or cavity. 2. The rectouterine pouch or pouch of Douglas, an extension of the peritoneal cavity which lies between rectum and posterior wall of uterus.

culdoscope (kŭl'dō-skōp). An endoscope used in performing a culdoscopic examination.

culdos'copy. Examination of the viscera of the pelvic cavity of the female after introduction of an endoscope through the wall of the posterior fornix of the vagina.

-cule, -cle [L.]. Suffix indicating little, as molecule, corpuscle.

Culex (kū'lĕks) [L., gnat]. A genus of small to medium sized mosquitoes of cosmopolitan distribution. Some species are vectors of disease organisms.

   C. pipiens. The common house mosquito. Serves as a vector of Wuchereria bancrofti, the causative agent of filariasis.

   C. quinquefasciatus. Common in the tropics and subtropics; the most important intermediate host of Wuchereria bancrofti.

Culicidae (kū-lĭs'ĭ-dē). A family of insects belonging to the order Diptera. Includes the mosquitoes.

culicifuge (kū-lĭs'ĭ-fūj) [L. *culex,* gnat, + *fugere,* to flee]. An agent to repel mosquito attacks.

cul'men [L., summit]. (pl. *cul'mina*) 1. Top or summit of a thing. 2. [NA] Most prominent part of the vermis superior near its anterior extremity. SYN: *c. cerebelli.*

cultiva'tion [L. *cultivāre*, to cultivate]. Growing microorganisms in an artificial medium.

cultural (kul'tu-ral) [L. *cultūra*, tillage]. Pert. to cultures of microorganisms.

cul'ture. 1. In psychology, the total pattern or life style of an individual or a group as judged by speech, intellectual attainment, and degree of realization of potential. 2. In bacteriology, a mass of microorganisms growing in laboratory culture media.

c., blood. Used in the diagnosis of specific infectious diseases. Test consists of withdrawing blood from a vein under sterile precautions, placing it in or upon suitable culture media, and determining whether or not bacteria grow in the media. If organisms do grow, they are identified by bacteriological methods.

c., contaminated. A c. whereupon bacteria from a foreign source have infiltrated the orginal bacteria being grown.

c., gelatin. A c. of bacteria on gelatin.

c., hanging block. A thin slice of agar seeded on its surface with bacteria, and then inverted on a cover slip and sealed in the concavity of a hollow glass slide.

c., hanging drop. A c. accomplished by inoculating the bacterium into a drop on a cover glass and mounting it in the depression on a concave slide.

c. medium. A substance on which microorganisms may grow. Those most commonly used are broths, gelatin, and agar which contain the same basic ingredients.

c., negative. A c. made from suspected matter which fails to reveal the suspected organism.

c., physical. The training of the body by means of gymnastics.

c., positive. A c. which reveals the suspected organism.

c., pure. The c. of a single form of microorganism uncontaminated by other organisms.

c., stab. A bacterial c. made by thrusting into the c. medium a point inoculated with the matter under examination.

c., stock. A permanent c. from which transfers may be made.

c., tissue. The growing of tissue cells in artifical nutrient media.

cu. mm. Abbr. for *cubic millimeter.*

cumulative (kū'mū-lā-tǐv) [L. *cumulus*, a heap]. Increasing in effect by successive additions.

c. drugs. Those which, after being received into the body in small doses, often repeated, are not immediately eliminated, but tend to accumulate in the system and eventually produce symptoms of poisoning. Carbolic acid, lead, silver, and mercurial preparations are examples of drugs which act in this way.

cu'mulus [L., a little mound]. A raised place; a heap of cells.

c. oophorus. A mass of follicle cells which surrounds the ovum. It projects into the antrum of the graafian follicle. SYN: *discus proligerus.*

cuneate (kū'nē-āt) [L. *cuneus*, wedge]. Wedge-shaped.

c. fasciculus. Continuation of posteroexternal column of cord into the medulla. SYN: *c. funiculus.*

c. nucleus. Gray matter at end of cuneate fasciculus.

cuneiform (kū-nē'ĭ-form) ["+ *forma*, shape]. Wedge-shaped.

c. bones. Those of the internal, middle, and external tarsus.

c. cartilage. One of two small pieces of yellow elastic cartilage which lies in the aryepiglottic fold of the larynx immediately anterior to the arythenoid cartilage.

cuneo- (kū'nē-ō) [L. *cuneus*, wedge]. Prefix rel. to a wedge.

cuneocuboid (kū"nē-ō-kū'boyd) [L. *cuneus*, wedge, + Gr. *kubos*, cube, + *eidos*, shape]. Pert. to cuboid and cuneiform bones.

cuneohysterectomy (kū"nē-ō-hǐs"tĕr-ĕk'tō-mǐ) ["+ *hystera*, uterus, + *ektomē*, excision]. Excision of a wedge of tissue from the posterior surface of the cervix uteri to correct abnormal anteflexion.

cu'neus [L., wedge]. (pl. *cu'nei*) Wedge-shaped lobule of brain on mesial surface of occipital lobe.

cuniculus (kū-nǐk'ū-lŭs) [L., an underground passage]. (pl. *eunic'uli*) Burrow in epidermis made by the itch mite.

cunnilinguist (kŭn-ǐ-lǐn'gwǐst) [L. *cunnus*, pudenda, + *lingua*, tongue]. One who practices cunnilingus, q.v.

cunnilingus (kŭn-ǐ-lǐn'gŭs). Sexual activity in which the mouth and tongue are used to stimulate the female genitalia.

cun'nus [L.]. The vulva, q.v.; pudenda.

cup [LL. *cuppa*, drinking vessel]. 1. Small drinking vessel. 2. A cupping glass. 3. An athletic supporter (jockey strap) reinforced with a piece of firm material to cover the genitalia. Worn to protect the penis and testicles during vigorous and contact sports. 4. Either of the two cup-shaped halves of a brassiere which fits over a breast. 5. A method of producing counterirritation. SEE: *cupping.*

Surgical technique for remodeling the femoral head and acetabulum and then covering the head with a metal cup (Vitallium). The cup prevents the raw bone surfaces from growing together. Used in treating arthritis of the hip. In older patients total hip replacement, q.v., is usually the treatment of choice.

c., favus. A cup-shaped crust which develops in certain fungus infections. SEE: *favus.*

c., glaucomatous. A depression in the optic disk occurring in late stages of glaucoma.

c., optic. In the embryo, a double layered cuplike structure connected to the diencephalon by a tubular optic stalk. It gives rise to the sensory and pigmented layers of the retina.

c., physiologic. A slight concavity in the center of the optic disk.

Cupid's bow. The normal bow-shape of the upper lip of the mouth.

cupola (kū'pō-lä) [L. *cūpula*, little tub]. 1. The little dome at apex of cochlea and of spiral canal. 2. The portion of costal pleura which extends superiorly into the root of the neck. It is dome shaped and accommodates the apex of the lung.

cupping. Application to the skin of a glass vessel, from which air has been exhausted by heat, or of a special suction apparatus in order to draw blood to the surface. This is done to produce counterirritation. SEE: *leech, moxibustion.*

cu'prum [L.]. Copper, q.v. ABBR: Cu.

curare (kyū-, kū-rä're). [Phonetic equivalent of Indian name for extracts of plants used as arrow poisons] One of several different resinous substances obtained from extracts of South American trees including species of chondrodendron. The pharmacologically-active ingredient of curare used medically is the alkaloid d-tubocurarine. This drug is used to facilitate skeletal muscle relaxation during anesthesia. SYN: *urari, woorari, woorali.* SEE: *tubocurarine chloride* (USP).

curarization (kū''rär-ĭ-zā'shŭn). Condition following introduction of a purified form of curare: eyelids heavy; nystagmus; husky voice; weak jaw and throat muscles; inability to raise head, arms, and legs.

Employed to lessen severity of convulsions produced by pentylenetetrazol and electric shock therapy and relaxation of muscles as in tetanus, etc.

cur'ative [L. *curare,* to take care of]. Having healing or remedial properties.

curd [ME.]. Milk coagulum, comprised mainly of casein.

cure [L. *cūra,* care]. 1. Course of treatment to restore health. 2. Restoration to health.

curet, curette (kū-rĕt') [Fr. *curette,* a cleanser]. A spoon-shaped scraping instrument for removing foreign matter from a cavity.

curettage (kyū''rĕ-tŏhz') [Fr.]. Scraping of a cavity.

c., uterine. Scraping with a curette to remove contents of uterus, as is done following inevitable or incomplete abortion, or to obtain specimens for use in diagnosis, and to remove growths, as polyps.

NP: It is essential that the patient's buttocks are not pulled down below edge of table. If this is done when legs are elevated in leg rests or stirrups, an undue strain is placed on the sacroiliac structures. Prolonged pressure on the leg muscles by stirrups is to be avoided, if possible, to prevent muscular soreness, paralysis of muscles, or thrombosis of a varicose vein.

The exterior surfaces are either scrubbed and irrigated with sterile water or painted using an antiseptic. The vaginal surfaces and cervix are included. The patient has already been placed on a Kelly pad, on which a sterile towel has been placed. One sterile towel is placed across the pubes and another is placed crosswise across the buttocks.

The floating nurse takes a strip of narrow adhesive plaster, about 18 in. (46 cm.) long, holding it by the ends, well away from her. The sterile nurse then throws over the middle of the tape a sterile towel so that tape holds towel in middle fold. The floating nurse places edges of tape around patient's hips so that sterile towel is stretched tightly across rectum. Sterile leggings are now pulled over patient's legs and a lithotomy sheet draped down on the perineum.

Sterile packing for the uterus should be ready. This form of packing is usually of gauze 1 1/2 in. (3.8 cm.) wide and 18 in. (46 cm.) long.

curettement (kū-rĕt'mĕnt) [Fr.]. Curettage, q.v.

Curie (kyūr'ē, kyū-rē'). 1. Marie, Polish-born Fr. chemist, 1867-1934; discovered radioactivity of thorium; discovered polonium and radium, and isolated radium from pitchblende. Awarded Nobel Prize in physics in 1903 with her husband, and in chemistry in 1911. 2. Pierre, Fr. chemist, 1859-1906; winner of Nobel Prize in 1903 with his wife.

curie. [Marie Curie] The standard unit of quantity of radon, being the amt. in equilibrium with 1 gm. of radium element. This quantity decays at the rate of 3.7×10^{10} disintegrations per second. ABBR: Ci.

cu'riegram [Curie + Gr. *gramma,* writing]. A photogram made by radium rays.

curiether'apy ["+ Gr. *therapeia*, treatment]. Radium therapy.

curium (kū'rǐ-ŭm). [Pierre and Marie Curie] SYMB: *Cm*. At. wt. of the longest-lived isotope, 247; at. no. 96. A transuranium element.

curled. In bacteriology, said of parallel chains in wavy strands, such as in anthrax colonies.

Curling's ulcer. [Thomas Curling, Brit. physician, 1811-1888]. Acute peptic ulcer which sometimes occurs following a severe burn. A form of stress ulcer, q.v.

cur'rant jelly clot. Postmortem, soft, red clot in heart and vessels.

cur'rent [L. *currere*, to run]. A flow, as of water or the transference of electrical impulses.

    c., alternating. A c. which periodically flows in opposite directions. Alternating c. waves may be either sinusoidal or nonsinusoidal. The alternating c. wave used most commonly therapeutically is the sinusoidal.

    c., direct. A c. that flows in one direction only. When used medically it is called the galvanic c.

curriculum (kǔ-rǐk'ū-lǔm) [L.]. A course of study in a special field or covering a specific time.

Curschmann's spirals (kūrsh'man). [Heinrich Curschmann, Ger. physician, 1846-1910]. Coiled spirals of mucus occasionally seen in sputum of asthma patients, etc. SEE: *sputum*.

curvature [L. *curvatura*, a slope]. A normal or abnormal bending or sloping away; a curve.

    c., angular. A sharp bending of the vertebral column. SYN: *Pott's curvature.*

    c. of the spine. One of four normal curves or flexures of the vertebral column as seen in profile, viz. cervical, thoracic, lumbar, and sacral. Abnormal curvatures may occur as a result of maldevelopment or disease processes. SEE: *kyphosis; lordosis; scoliosis.*

curve [L. *curvus*]. A bend.

    c. of Carus. An arc corresponding to the pelvic axis.

    c., temperature. Line representing changes of temperature during a given period.

curvi- [L. *curvus*, curve]. Combining form meaning curved.

Cusco's spec'ulum (kūs'kō). [Edouard Gabriel Cusco, Fr. surgeon, 1819-94]. A duckbill vaginal speculum manipulated by a screw.

Cushing's syndrome. [Harvey Cushing, Amer. surgeon, 1869-1939]. A syndrome resulting from hypersecretion of the adrenal cortex in which there is excessive production of glucocorticoids. May be due to a tumor of the adrenal gland or to excess stimulation of that gland as a result of hyperfunction of the anterior pituitary. Prolonged administration of large doses of adrenal cortical hormones will also cause this syndrome. Symptoms are protein loss, adiposity, fatigue and weakness, osteoporosis, amenorrhea, impotence, capillary fragility, edema, excess hair growth, diabetes mellitus, skin discoloration and turgidity (plethora), and purplish striae of skin.

cushion. In anatomy, a mass of connective tissue, usually adipose, which acts to prevent undue pressure upon underlying tissues or structures.

cusp (kŭsp) [L. *cuspis*, point]. 1. Point of the crown of a tooth. 2. One of the leaflike divisions or parts of the valves of the heart. SEE: *bicuspid valve; semilunar valves; tricuspid valve.*

cuspid (kŭs'pǐd). The four teeth with conic crowns (canine).

cuspidate (kŭs'pǐ-dāt) [L. *cuspidatus*]. Having cusps.

cuta'neous [L. *cutis*, skin]. Pert. to the skin.

    c. nerves. Sensory nerves of the skin of the arms and legs.

    c. respiration. The transpiration of gases through the skin.

cu'ticle [L. *cuticula*, little skin]. 1. A layer of solid or semisolid substance which covers the free surface of a layer of epithelial cells. It may be of a horny or chitinous consistency; sometimes it is calcified. Ex: enamel of a tooth, capsule of lens of eye. 2. The epidermis of the skin.

    c. of hair. A single layer of clear cells which forms the outer layer of a hair.

    c. of inner root sheath. A layer of scalelike cells which forms innermost layer of the root sheath. Lies next to the cuticle of the hair.

cuticula (kū-tǐk'u-lǎ) [L.]. Cuticle.

    c. dentis. A skinlike membrane which may cover the teeth after they have erupted. The membrane is easily removed by a dentist. SYN: *Nasmyth's membrane.*

cuticulariza'tion. Growth of skin over a sore or wound.

cutireaction. Reaction appearing on the skin; skin reaction.

    c., von Pirquet's. Reaction of skin after inoculation with tuberculosis toxins.

cutis (kū'tǐs) [L.]. [NA] The skin.

    c. anserina. Gooseflesh caused by erection of skin papillae, as from cold, shock, fright, or fear.

c., aurantiasis. Yellow discoloration of the skin resulting from ingesting excessive quantities of vegetables, such as carrots, containing carotenoid pigments.

c., hyperelastica. A congenital or familial condition characterized by excessive elasticity of the skin, loose-jointedness, easy bruisability, and development of pseudotumors at joints. SYN: *Ehlers-Danlos syndrome.*

c. laxa. Dermatolysis or hypertrophy of the skin and subcutaneous tissue.

c. marmorata. Purplish discoloration of skin on exposure to cold.

c. pendula. Condition in which the skin hangs in flabby folds or wrinkles.

c. testacea. Condition characterized by formation of plates of greasy material on trunk and extremities. SYN: *seborrhea.*

c. unctosa. Excessive secretion of sebaceous glands. SEE: *seborrhea.*

c. vera. The corium, q.v.; deep layer of skin, the dermis, q.v.

c. verticis gyrata. Looseness and hypertrophy of the scalp skin which may hang in folds.

cutitis (kū-tī′tĭs) [L. *cutis*, skin, + Gr. *-itis*, inflammation]. Inflammation of skin. SYN: *dermatitis.*

cutization (kū-tī-zā′shŭn). Skinlike condition of a mucous membrane as result of continued exposure.

cut throat. Laceration of throat. Seriousness of injury depends upon angle of thrust of cutting object and location.

F.A. TREATMENT: Send for doctor. Have subject lying down, head and shoulders raised. Press head on chest. If trachea is severed, keep open and free from clot. Compress bleeding points with clean, wet cloths. Reassure patient, keep his lips moist, do not leave him for an instant. Artificial respiration if necessary.

CVP. Abbr. for *central venous pressure,* q.v.

cyanemia (sī″an-ē′mĭ-ă) [Gr. *kyanos,* dark blue, + *haima,* blood]. Blue color of blood.

cyanephidrosis (sī″ăn-ĕf′ĭ-drō′sĭs) [″+ *ephidrōsis,* sweating]. Bluish sweat.

cyanhidrosis (sī-ăn-hī-drō′sĭs) [″+ *hidrōsis,* sweat]. Exuding bluish sweat.

cyanide (sī′ă-nīd″). A compound containing the radical —CN, as potassium cyanide (KCN), sodium cyanide (NaCN).

c. poisoning. Cyanides are among the most common and most deadly poisons known. They stop cellular respiration by inhibiting the action of cytochrome oxidase, carbonic anhydrase, and other enzyme systems. The seeds of certain stone fruits, jetberry bush and toyon, contain chemicals which upon digestion yield cyanide. This occurs only if the seeds are broken. The fatal dose for a small child varies from 5-25 seeds.

SYM: Start within a few seconds, rarely longer than two minutes. The patient utters a cry and falls insensible. Respiration is first rapid and convulsive, later slow and gasping. Death usually comes within five minutes. When smaller doses are taken, there is an acrid taste, a choking feeling, anxiety, dizziness, confusion, and headache. Convulsions with frothing of the mouth. Often incontinence. Pulse rapid, feeble, and irregular.

F.A. TREATMENT: Must be very prompt. Have victim inhale amyl nitrite immediately for 15-30 seconds. Do this every 2-3 minutes. While this is being done, give I.V. sodium nitrate 0.3 gm. in 10 ml. of water at rate of 2.5-5 ml. per minute. As soon as this is completed, administer through the same needle 25-50 ml. of 50% solution of sodium thiosulfate.

Immediate artificial respiration with 100% oxygen is required also. In one hour repeat half doses of medicines above.

External heat, epinephrine for collapse, and keep the patient in a recumbent position.

cyano- [Gr. *kyanos,* dark blue]. Combining form meaning dark blue.

cyanochroia (sī-ăn-ō-kroy′ă) [Gr. *kyanos,* dark blue, + *chroia,* color]. Cyanosis.

cyanocobalamin (sī″ăn-ō-cō-băl′ă-mĭn). USP. A component of the vitamin B complex. It is essential for blood formation. Used in treating pernicious anemia. SYN: vitamin B_{12}.

cyanoder′ma [Gr. *kyanos,* dark blue, + *derma,* skin]. Blue discoloration of skin. SYN: *cyanosis.*

cyan′ogen [″+ *gennan,* to produce]. 1. The radical CN. 2. A poisonous gas, CN-CN.

cyanomycosis (sī″ăn-ō-mī-kō′sĭs) [″+ *mykēs,* fungus, + *-ōsis,* condition]. Development of blue pus due to Micrococcus pyocyaneus.

cyanopathy (sī″ăn-ŏp′ă-thī) [″+ *pathos,* disease]. Blue discoloration of skin. SYN: *cyanosis.*

cyanophil (sī-ăn′ō-fĭl) [Gr. *kyanos,* dark blue, + *philein,* to love]. Blue staining substance of plants and animals.

cyanophilous (sī-ăn-ŏf′ĭl-ŭs). Having an affinity for a blue dye or stain.

cyanopia, cyanopsia (sī-ăn-ō′pĭ-ă, -ŏp′sī-ă) [Gr. *kyanos,* dark blue, + *opsis,* vision]. Vision in which all objects appear to be blue.

cy′anosed. Affected with cyanosis.

cyanosis (sī-ăn-ō′sĭs) [Gr. *kyanos*, dark blue, + *-ōsis*, condition]. Slightly bluish, grayish, slatelike, or dark purple discoloration of the skin due to presence of abnormal amounts of reduced hemoglobin in the blood. May not appear in patients with severe anemia even though their blood is poorly oxygenated because there is not enough reduced hemoglobin present to cause the blue color to be visible.

When entire body is affected the color is dusky leaden.

ETIOL: Deficiency of oxygen and excess of carbon dioxide in blood caused by gas or any condition interfering with entrance of air in the respiratory tract; overdoses of certain drugs; or any form of asphyxiation.

TREATMENT: Remove cause. Artificial respiration together with oxygen inhalation or oxygen plus carbon dioxide. Stimulants; heat and massage are valuable adjuncts. SEE: *asphyxia; unconsciousness.*

c., congenital. Usually associated with stenosis of the pulmonary orifice, an imperfect ventricular septum, or a patulous foramen ovale or ductus arteriosus. SEE: *tetralogy of Fallot.*

c., delayed. C., tardive, q.v.

c., enterogenous. Induced by intestinal absorption of toxins. SEE: *methemoglobinemia.*

c., hereditary methemoglobinemic. Presence of methemoglobin in the blood; present at birth, and occurring generally in males.

c. retinae. Bluish appearance of retina seen in congenital heart disease, polycythemia, and in certain poisonings as dinitrobenzol.

c., tardive. C. resulting from an interatrial or interventricular septal defect. SYN: *delayed cyanosis.*

cyanotic (sī-ăn-ŏt′ĭk). Of the nature of, affected with, or pert. to cyanosis.

cyasma (sī-ăz′mă) [Gr. *kyēsis*, pregnancy]. Freckling type of pigmentation of skin during pregnancy.

cyclamate. A non-nutritive artificial sweetener which is about 30 times as sweet as sugar. Its general use has been restricted because of the chemical's toxic effect on lower animals.

cyclarthrosis (sī-klăr-thrō′sĭs) [Gr. *kyklos*, circle, + *arthron*, join, + *-ōsis*, condition]. A lateral ginglymus or pivot joint which makes possible rotation.

cycle (sī′kl) [Gr. *kyklos*, circle]. A series of movements or events; a sequence usually recurring at regular intervals.

c., cardiac. The series of consecutive movements through which the heart passes in performing one heart beat; it includes contraction or systole, relaxation or diastole, and a short rest pause called the diastasis cordis. A complete cycle corresponds to one pulse beat, which requires a variable length of time depending upon the heart rate.

c., Cori. A series of reactions which accounts for the disposal of lactate formed during muscular activity, i.e., muscle glycogen to lactic acid to liver glycogen to blood glucose to muscle glycogen.

c., gastric. Progression of peristaltic waves over the stomach.

c., genesial. The period from puberty to menopause.

c., glycolytic. The successive steps by which glucose is broken down in living tissue.

c., Krebs′. A series of reactions occurring in muscle cells and possibly all tissues in which pyruvic acid (or two-carbon derivatives of carbohydrate, fat, or protein) formed anaerobically are converted through a series of interrelated oxidation-reduction and other reactions to carbon dioxide and water with the release of energy principally utilized in the formation of adenosinetriphosphate (ATP). It is considered to be the final common pathway for the oxidation of and interconversions between the three primary classes of foods. SYN: *citric acid c.; tricarboxylic acid c. (TCA).*

c., menstrual. A series of periodically recurring changes in endometrium of the uterus culminating in menstruation, q.v.

cyclectomy (sī-klěk′tō-mǐ) [Gr. *kyklos*, circle, + *ektomē*, excision]. 1. Excision of a portion of the ciliary body or muscle. 2. Excision of the ciliary border of the eyelids.

cy′clic. Periodic; occurring in cycles.

c. insanity. Manic-depressive psychosis; a form in which mania, melancholia, and sanity succeed each other at intervals; circular insanity.

c. vomiting. Periodic and recurring attacks of vomiting occurring in persons of a nervous temperament. The condition is usually associated with acidosis.

SYM: Dizziness, loss of appetite, headache, nausea may occur. Patient then vomits about every 1/2 hr. for 1-2 days. Great thirst, slight rise of temperature, rapid pulse, prostration.

NP: At first, glucose or another easily assimilated carbohydrate. Nothing during attacks. Keep warm in bed; mouth washes.

SEE: *nausea; vomiting.*

cyclic adenosine monophosphate. A chemical compound important to the action of many peptide hormones and important in transmission of nerve impulses. ABBR: cyclic AMP.

cyclicot'omy [Gr. *kyklikos*, circular, + *tomē*, incision]. Cutting of the ciliary muscle.

cycli'tis [Gr. *kyklos*, circle, + *-itis*, inflammation]. Inflammation of ciliary body.

SYM: Tenderness in ciliary region, swelling of upper lid, circumcorneal injection, deposits on Descemet's membrane, reduced or hazy vision, increased or decreased tension. Pain in or about the eye, worse at night and on pressure. Its course is rapid, progressively unfavorable.

COMPLICATIONS: Iritis, choroiditis, scleritis, glaucoma.

TREATMENT: Local: atropine, heat, protection from light. General: salicylates, diaphoresis, rest; treat underlying cause if possible.

c., plastic. Ciliary body inflammation accompanied by that of entire uveal tract, giving rise to a fibrinous exudate in anterior chamber and vitreous.

c., purulent. Suppurative inflammation of ciliary body and iris.

c., serous. Simple inflammation without iritis.

cyclo- [Gr. *kyklos*, circle]. 1. A combining form meaning circular or pert. to a cycle. 2. A combining form pert. to the ciliary body of the eye.

cycloceratitis (si″klo-ser″ă-ti′tis). Cyclokeratitis, q.v.

cyclochoroiditis (si″klo-ko″royd -i′tis) [Gr. *kyklos*, circle, + *chorioeidēs*, skinlike, + *-itis*, inflammation]. Inflammation of ciliary body and choroid coat of eye.

cyclodialysis (si″klo-dī-ăl′ĭ-sis) [″+ *dialysis*, dissolution]. Operation performed in certain types of glaucoma to produce communication between anterior chamber and suprachoroidal space for the escape of aqueous humor.

cycloid (si′kloyd) [″+ *eidos*, form]. 1. Resembling a circle. 2. Denoting a ring of atoms. 3. Extreme variations of mood from elation to melancholia. SEE: *cyclothymia.*

cyclokeratitis (si″klo-ker-ă-ti-tis) [Gr. *kyklos*, circle, + *keras*, cornea, + *-itis*, inflammation]. Inflammation of cornea and ciliary body.

cyclophoria (si″klo-fo′rĭ-ă) [″+ *phoros*, bearing]. Rotation of eyeball due to weakness of oblique muscles.

cycloplegia (si″klŏ-plē′jĭ-ă) [″+ *plēgē*, a stroke]. Paralysis of ciliary muscle.

cycloplegic (si-klŏ-plē′jĭk). Producing cycloplegia.

cyclopropane (si″klŏ-prō′pān). C_3H_6. A gaseous anesthetic agent, colorless, slightly heavier than air, with a not unpleasant odor. Administered with 70-95% oxygen it produces unconsciousness in 1-2 minutes. Fire and explosion must be guarded against.

cyclops (si′klŏps). A fetal malformation with one eye.

cyclosis (si-klŏ′sis) [Gr. *kyklōsis*, circulation]. A streaming movement of protoplasm such as is seen in certain plant and animal cells.

cyclothymia (si″klŏ-thi′mĭ-ă) [Gr. *kyklos*, circle, + *thymos*, mind]. In psychiatry, mild fluctuations of the manic-depressive type. They may be so mild as to be almost normal.

cyesedema (si″e-se-dē′mă) [Gr. *kyēsis*, pregnancy, + *oidēma*, swelling]. Thickening of cutis; bloating in pregnancy.

cyesiology (si-ē″sĭ-ŏl′o-jĭ) [″+ *logos*, study]. The study of pregnancy.

cyesis (si-ē′sis) [Gr. *kyēsis*]. (pl. *cyeses*) Pregnancy.

cyetic (si-et′ĭk). Pert. to pregnancy.

cylicotomy (sĭl″ĭ-kŏt′ŏ-mĭ) [Gr. *kylix*, cup, + *tomē*, incision]. Cutting of ciliary muscle. SYN: *cyclotomy.*

cylindroadenoma (si-lĭn″dro-ad″e-no′mă) [Gr. *kylindros*, cylinder, + *adēn*, gland, + *-ōma*, tumor]. An adenoma containing cylindrical masses of hyaline material.

cylindroid (sĭl-in′droyd) [″+ *eidos*, shape]. 1. Cylinder shaped. 2. A mucous, spurious cast in urine. Recognized by their twists and turns, varying markedly in diameter in different places, most frequently pointed at the ends and frequently crossing an entire field. They do not usually have cellular intrusions.

cylindroma (sĭl″ĭn-dro-ma′) [″+ *-ōma*, tumor]. Malignant tumor containing a collection of cells forming cylinders.

cylindrosarcoma (si-lĭn″dro-săr-kō′mă) [Gr. *kylindros*, cylinder, + *sarkos*, flesh, + *-ōma*, tumor]. A tumor containing properties of a cylindroma and sarcoma.

cylindruria (sĭl″ĭn-drū′rĭ-ă) [″+ *ouron*, urine]. Cylindroids in the urine.

cyllosis (sĭl-ō′sis) [Gr. *kyllōsis*]. Clubfoot.

cymbocephalic (sim″bo-sē-fāl′ĭk) [Gr. *kymbē*, boat, + *kephalē*, head]. Having a boatshaped head.

cynanthropy (sĭn-ăn′thrō-pī) [Gr. *kyon*, dog, + *anthrōpos*, man]. Insanity in which the patient behaves like a dog.

cynic spasm (sĭn′ĭk spăzm) [Gr. *kynikos*, doglike]. Spasm of face muscles causing a grin or snarl like a dog. SYN: *risus sardonicus.*

cynobex (sī'nō-bĕks) [Gr. *kyon*, dog, + *bēx*, cough]. Dry, barking cough.

cynophobia (sī''nō-fō'bĭ-ă) ["+ *phobos*, fear]. Unreasonable fear of dogs. SYN: *lyssophobia*.

cynorexia (sī''no-rek'sĭ-ă) ["+ *orexis*, appetite]. Morbid appetite, bulimia, q.v.

cyotrophy (si-ot'ro-fī) [Gr. *kyos*, fetus, + *trophē*, nutrition]. Nourishment of the fetus.

cypridopathy (sĭp''rĭ-dop'ă-thī) [Gr. *Kypris*, Venus, + *pathos*, disease]. Any venereal disease.

cypridophobia (sĭp''rī-do-fo'bĭ-ă) ["+ *phobos*, fear]. 1. Morbid fear of venereal disease. 2. Abnormal fear of the sexual act. 3. False belief of having a venereal disease.

cypriphobia (sĭp-rī-fo'bĭ-ă). Morbid aversion to and fear of coitus.

cyrtometer (sir-tom'ĕ-ter) [Gr. *kyrtos*, bent, + *metron*, measure]. Instrument for measuring circumference of chest and comparison of chest curves. Also used to measure other curved portions of the body.

cyrtosis (sir-tō'sĭs) ["+ *-ōsis*, condition]. Having any abnormal curvature of the spine. SEE: *kyphosis*.

cyst (sĭst) [Gr. *kystis*, bladder, sac]. 1. A closed sac or pouch with a definite wall which contains fluid, semifluid or solid material. It is usually an abnormal structure resulting from developmental anomalies, obstruction of ducts, or from parasitic infection. 2. In biology, a structure formed by, and enclosing, certain organisms in which they become inactive, as the cyst of certain protozoans or of the metacercariae of flukes. It may serve as a reproductive structure as in hydatid cysts.

c., **adventitious.** C. formed about a foreign body.

c., **blood.** Bloody tumor. SYN: *hematoma*.

c., **branchial.** A cervical c., q.v.

c., **cervical.** A closed epithelial sac derived from a branchial groove or its corresponding pharyngeal pouch.

c., **chocolate.** Ovarian c. with darkly pigmented gelatinous content.

c., **colloid.** C. with gelatinous contents.

c., **congenital.** C. present at birth resulting from abnormal development, as a dermoid c., imperfect closure of a structure, e.g., spina bifida; or nonclosure of embryonic clefts, ducts, or tubules, e.g., cervical c.'s, q.v.

c., **daughter.** C. growing out of the walls of another c.

c., **dentigerous.** C. containing teeth. SYN: *follicular odontoma. SEE: cyst, dermoid.*

c., **dermoid.** C. containing elements of hair, teeth, or skin. They occur commonly in the ovary and contain derivatives of all three germ layers.

c., **distention.** C. formed in a natural enclosed cavity as a follicular c. of the ovary.

c., **extravasation.** C. arising from hemorrhage into tissues.

c., **follicular.** C. arising from a follicle, as a follicular c. of the thyroid gland or ovary.

c., **Gartner's.** C. developing from a vestigial mesonephric duct (Gartner's duct) in a female.

c., **hydatid.** C. formed by the growth of the larval form of the Echinococcus granulosus, usually in the liver.

c., **implantation.** C. resulting from displacement of portions of the epidermis as may occur in injuries.

c., **intraligamentary.** Cystic formation between the layers of the broad ligament.

c., **involutional.** C. occurring in the normal involution of an organ or structure as in the mammary gland.

c., **meibomian.** Tumor or c. produced by inflammation of a meibomian gland of the eyelid. SYN: *chalazion*

c., **mucous.** Retention c. composed of mucus.

c., **nabothian.** Cystic formation caused by closure of the ducts of the nabothian glands in the cervix uteri as a result of healing of an erosion.

c., **odontogenic.** C. associated with the teeth as a dentigerous or radicular cyst, q.v.

c., **ovarian.** Cystic formation in the ovary. SEE: *ovary.*

c., **parasitic.** C. enclosing the larval form of certain parasites as the cysticercus or hydatid of tapeworms or the larva of certain nematodes, e.g., Trichinella.

c., **parovarian.** Cystic formation of the parovarium.

c., **pilonidal.** An elongated closed sac lined with stratified epithelium and usually containing hair, usually occurs in midline over sacral area of back. SYN: *pilonidal sinus.*

c., **porencephalic.** An anomalous cavity of the brain which communicates with the venticular system.

c., **proliferative.** C. lined with epithelium which proliferates, forming projections which extend into the cavity of the cyst.

c., **radicular.** A granulomatous c. located alongside the root of a tooth.

c., **retention.** C. retaining the secretion of a gland, as in a mucous or sebaceous cyst.

c., sebaceous. C. of a sebaceous gland.

c., seminal. C. of the epididymis, ductus deferens, or other sperm-carrying ducts which contains semen.

c., suprasellar. A cyst of the hypophyseal stalk just above the floor of the sella turcica. Its wall is frequently calcified or ossified.

c., tubo-ovarian. An ovarian c. which ruptures into the lumen of an adherent uterine tube.

c., unilocular. C. containing only one cavity.

c., vaginal. Cystic formation in the vagina.

cyst, words pert. to: encysted; endocyst; hydrocyst; hydroma; steatoma.

cystadenoma (sīst″ăd-ĕn-ō′mä) [Gr. *kystis*, bladder, + *adēn*, gland, + *-ōma*, tumor]. An adenoma containing cysts. Cystoma blended with adenoma.

c., pseudomucinous. C. filled with a thick, viscid fluid and lined with tall epithelial cells.

c., serous. C. filled with a clear, serous fluid and lined with cuboidal epithelial cells.

cystalgia (sīs-tăl′jĭ-ă) [″+ *algos*, pain]. Pain in the bladder.

cystauxe (sīs-tŏk′sē) [″+ *auxe*, increase]. Enlargement or thickening of the urinary bladder.

cystectasy (sīs-tĕk′tă-sē) [Gr. *kystis*, bladder, + *ektasis*, dilatation]. 1. An operation for extracting calculus from the bladder by dividing the membranous portion of the urethra, and then dilating neck of bladder. 2. Dilatation of bladder.

cystectomy (sīs-tĕk′tō-mē) [″+ *ektomē*, excision]. 1. Removal of a cyst. 2. Excision of the cystic duct and the gallbladder, or just the cystic duct. 3. Excision of the urinary bladder or a part of it.

cysteine (sīs-tē′-ĭn, sīs-tē′ĭn). A sulfur-containing amino acid, SHCH₂, CH(NH₂)- COOH, which is contained in many proteins. Is valuable as a source of sulfur in metabolism.

cystic (sīs′tĭk) [Gr. *kystis*, bladder]. 1. Of or pertaining to a cyst. 2. Pertaining to the gallbladder. 3. Pertaining to the urinary bladder.

c. duct. The duct of the gallbladder which unites with the hepatic duct from the liver to form the common bile duct.

c. fibrosis. A disease of infants, children, adolescents, and young adults involving the exocrine glands, especially those secreting mucus, and resulting in pancreatic insufficiency, chronic pulmonary disease, abnormally high sweat electrolyte levels, and, in some cases, cirrhosis of the liver. Incomplete forms lead to variations in the manifestations. It has become apparent that cystic fibrosis is a disease which affects all of the exocrine glands including in most cases the pancreas and sweat glands. The affection is believed to be genetically transmitted. Although prognosis is poor, with the advent of effective antibiotics the life span of many of these patients has been prolonged. SYN: *fibrocystic disease of the pancreas; mucoviscidosis.*

c. tumor. Tumor composed of cysts.

cysticercoid (sīs″tĭ-sĕr′koyd) [″+ *kerkos*, tail, + *eidos*, appearance]. The larval encysted form of a tapeworm. It differs from a cysticercus in having a much reduced bladder.

cysticercosis (sīs″tĭ-sĕr-kō′sĭs) [″+ ″+ *-ōsis*, condition]. Infestation with cysticerci.

cysticercus (sīs″tĭ-sĕr′kŭs). (pl. *cysticerci*) The encysted larval form of a tapeworm consisting of a rounded cyst or bladder into which the scolex is invaginated. SYN: *bladderworm.*

c. cellulosae. Infestation by bladderworms of the pork tapeworm, Taenia solium.

cysticotomy (sīs″tĭ-kot′ō-mē) [Gr. *kystis*, bladder, + *tomē*, incision]. Incision of cystic bile duct. SYN: *choledochotomy.*

cystiform (sīs′tĭ-form) [″+ L. *forma*, form]. Having the form of a cyst.

cystigerous (sīs-tĭj′er-us) [″+ L. *gerere*, to bear]. Containing cysts.

cystine (sīs′tēn) [Gr. *kystis*, bladder]. C_6H_{12}-$N_2S_2O_4$. A sulfur-containing amino acid, which is produced by the action of acids on proteins which contain this compound. It is an important source of sulfur in metabolism.

cystinemia (sīs″tĭ-nē′mĭ-ă) [cystine + Gr. *haima*, blood]. The presence of cystine in blood.

cystinuria (sīs″tĭ-nū′rĭ-ă) [″+ *ouron*, urine]. 1. The presence of cystine in urine. 2. A hereditary, metabolic disorder characterized by excretion of large amounts of cystine, lysine, arginine, and ornithine in the urine. Results in the development of recurrent urinary calculi.

cystistaxia (sīs″tĭ-stăk′sĭ-ă) [Gr. *kystis*, bladder, + *staxis*, dripping]. Blood oozing from the mucous membrane of the bladder.

cystitis (sīs-tī′tĭs) [″+ *-itis*, inflammation]. Inflammation of the bladder usually occurring secondarily to infections of associated organs (kidney, prostate, urethra). May be acute or chronic.

SYM: *Acute:* Frequent and painful urination. *Chronic:* Secondary to some other lesion with possibly pyuria as only symptom.

TREATMENT: Antibiotics are useful in treating the infection but more definitive therapy will be required if the basic cause is a renal calculus or a structural defect in the urinary tract such as obstruction.

cystitome (sĭs'tĭ-tōm) ["+ *tomē*, incision]. Instrument for incision into sac of crystalline lens.

cystitomy (sĭs-tĭt'ō-mĭ). 1. Incision of capsule of crystalline lens. 2. Incision into the gallbladder. SYN: *cholecystotomy.*

cysto-, cyst- [Gr. *kystis*, bladder]. Prefix pert. to the urinary bladder or a cyst.

cystoadenoma (sĭs"to-ad"ē-nō'mă) ["+ *adēn*, gland, + *-ōma*, tumor]. A tumor containing cystic and adenomatous elements.

cystocarcinoma (sĭs"to-kăr"sĭ-nō'mă) ["+ *karkinos*, ulcer, + *-ōma*, tumor]. Glandular tumor distended with fluid secretion of the gland.

cystocele (sĭs'to-sēl) [Gr. *kystis*, bladder, + *kēlē*, hernia]. A bladder hernia.

Injury to the vesicovaginal fascia during delivery may allow the bladder to pouch into the vagina causing a cystocele.

cystocolostomy (sĭs"to-ko-los'tō-mĭ) ["+ *kōlon*, colon, + *stoma*, mouth]. Formation of communication between the gallbladder and colon.

cystodiaphanoscopy (sĭs"to-di"ă-făn-os'ko-pĭ) ["+ *dia*, through, + *phanein*, to shine, + *skopein*, to examine]. Transillumination of abdomen by an electric light in bladder.

cystodynia (sĭs"to-din'ī-ă) [Gr. *kystis*, bladder, + *odynē*, pain]. Pain in the urinary bladder. SYN: *cystalgia.*

cystoelytroplasty (sĭs"to-el'ī-tro-plas-tĭ) ["+ *elytron*, sheath (vagina), + *plassein*, to form]. Repair of a vesicovaginal fistula.

cystoepiplocele (sĭs"to-ē-pip'lo-sēl) ["+ *epiploon*, omentum, + *kēlē*, hernia]. Herniation of a portion of the bladder and the omentum.

cystoepithelioma (sĭs"to-ĕp"ī-thē'lĭ-ō'mă) [Gr. *kystis*, bladder, + *epi*, upon, + *thēlē*, nipple, + *-ōma*, tumor]. Epithelioma in stage of cystic degeneration.

cystofibroma (sĭs"to-fi-brō'mă) ["+ L. *fibra*, fiber, + Gr. *-ōma*, tumor]. Fibrous tumor containing cysts.

cystogram (sĭs'to-gram) ["+ *gramma*, mark]. A roentgenogram of the bladder.

cystography (sĭs-tog'ră-fĭ) [Gr. *kystis*, bladder, + *graphein*, to write]. Taking roentgenograms of the bladder by using a radiopaque dye injected into the bladder.

cystoid (sĭs'toyd) ["+ *eidos*, appearance]. Bladderlike.

cystolith (sĭs'to-lĭth) ["+ *lithos*, stone]. A vesical calculus.

cystolithectomy (sĭs-to-lĭ-thĕk'tō-mĭ) [Gr. *kystis*, bladder, + *lithos*, stone, + *ektomē*, excision]. Excision of a stone from the bladder.

cystolithiasis (sĭs-to-lĭ-thi'ă-sĭs) ["+ "+ *iasis*, condition]. Calculi in the bladder.

cystolith'ic. Pert. to a vesical calculus.

cystolutein (sĭs"to-lu'te-in) [Gr. *kystis*, cyst, + L. *luteus*, yellow]. Yellow color found in some ovarian cysts.

cystoma (sĭs-tō'mă) ["+ *-ōma*, tumor]. (pl. *cysto'mata, cysto'mas*) A cystic tumor; a growth containing cysts.

cystometer (sĭs-tŏm'ē-tĕr) ["+ *metron*, measure]. Device for estimating the capacity of the bladder and its changing pressure reactions.

cystomorphous (sĭs"to-mor'fus) [Gr. *kystis*, bladder, + *morphē*, form]. Cystlike; cystoid.

cystomyxoadenoma (sĭs"to-mik"so-ad"en-ō'mă) ["+ *myxa*, mucus, + *adēn*, gland, + *-ōma*, tumor]. Myxoma and adenoma with cystic degeneration.

cystomyxoma (sĭs"to-mik-sō'mă) ["+ "+ *-ōma*, tumor]. Myxoma with cystic formation.

cystopexy (sĭs'to-pek"sĭ) [Gr. *kystis*, bladder, + *pēxis*, fixation]. Surgical fixation of bladder to wall of abdomen.

cystoplasty (sĭs'to-plas"tĭ) ["+ *plassein*, to form]. Plastic operation upon the bladder.

cystoplegia (sĭs"to-plē'jĭ-ă) ["+ *plēgē*, stroke]. Paralysis of the bladder.

cystoptosia, cystoptosis (sĭs"top-tō'sĭ-ă, -sĭs) [Gr. *kystis*, bladder, + *ptōsis*, a dropping]. Prolapse into the urethra of the vesical mucous membrane.

cystopyelitis (sĭs"to-pi-ē-li'tis) ["+ *pyelos*, pelvis, + *-itis*, inflammation]. Cystitis with pyelitis.

cystopyelonephritis (sĭs"to-pi"ē-lo-nef-ri'tĭs) ["+ "+ *nephros*, kidney, + *-itis*, inflammation]. Inflammation of urinary bladder, kidney, and pelvis of kidney.

cystoradiography (sĭs"to-rā"dĭ-ŏg'ră-fĭ) [Gr. *kystis*, bladder, + L. *radius*, ray, + Gr. *graphein*, to write]. Radiography of the gallbladder or urinary bladder.

cystorectostomy (sĭs"to-rĕk-tos'tō-mĭ) ["+ L. *rectum*, + Gr. *stoma*, mouthlike opening]. Establishment of a surgical communication between the bladder and rectum.

cystorrhagia (sĭs"to-ra'jĭ-ă) ["+ *rhēgnunai*, to burst forth]. Hemorrhage from the urinary bladder.

cystorrhaphy (sĭst-or'ă-fĭ) [Gr. *kystis*, bladder, + *rhaphē*, suture]. Suture of bladder.

cystorrhea (sĭs"to-rē'ă) ["+ *rhoia*, flow]. A discharge of mucus from the urinary bladder.

cystosarcoma (sĭs"to-sar-kō'mă) ["+ *sarx*, flesh, + *ōma*, tumor]. Sarcoma containing cysts or cystic formations.

cystoscope (sĭst'o-skōp) [Gr. *kystis*, bladder, + *skopein*, to examine]. Instrument for interior examination of bladder and ureter. It is introduced through the urethra into the bladder.

cystoscopy (sĭs-tos'ko-pĭ) ["+ *skopein*, to examine]. Examination of the bladder with the cystoscope.

cystospasm (sĭs'to-spăzm) ["+ *spasmos*, spasm]. Spasmodic contractions of the urinary bladder.

cystostomy (sĭs-tos'to-mĭ) [Gr. *kystis*, bladder, + *stoma*, mouthlike opening.]. Surgical incision into the bladder to establish a temporary opening.

cystotome (sĭs'to-tōm) ["+ *tomē*, incision]. Knife for incision of bladder.

cystotomy (sĭs-tot'o-mĭ) ["+ *tomē*, incision]. Incision of bladder.

cystotrachelotomy (sĭs"to-tra"ke-lot'ō-mĭ) [Gr. *kystis*, bladder, + *trachēlos*, neck, + *tomē*, incision]. Incision into neck of bladder.

cystoureteritis (sĭs"to-ū-rē"ter-i'tĭs) ["+ *ourētēr*, ureter, + *-itis*, inflammation]. Inflammation of ureter and urinary bladder.

cystoureterogram (sĭs"to-ū-rē'tēr-ō-grăm) ["+ "+ *gramma*, mark]. Reontgenographic study of the bladder and ureter.

cystourethroscope (sĭs"to-ū-rē'thro-skōp) [Gr. *kystis*, bladder, + *ourēthra*, urethra, + *skopein*, to examine]. Device for examining the posterior urethra and urinary bladder.

cystovesiculography (sĭs"to-vĕ-sĭk-ū-lŏg'ră-fē). Roentgenographic examination of the bladder and seminal vesicles.

cytase (sī'tās) [Gr. *kytos*, hollow vessel, cell + *-ase*, enzyme]. A ferment in phagocytes.

-cyte (sīt) [Gr. *kytos*, hollow vessel, something that contains or covers, hence cell]. Suffix denoting cell.

cyto-, cyt-. Prefix denoting the cell.

cytoarchitectonic (sī"tō-ark"ĭ-tĕk-tŏn'ĭk) [Gr. *kytos*, cell, + *architektonikē*, architecture]. Pert. to structure and arrangement of cells.

cytobiology (sī"tō-bī-ŏl'ō-jĭ) ["+ *bios*, life, + *logos*, study of]. Biology of cells.

cytobiotaxis (sī"tō-bī-ō-tak'sĭs) ["+ "+ *taxis*, arrangement]. The influence of cells upon other living cells. SYN: *cytoclasis*.

cy'toblast [Gr. *kytos*, cell, + *blastos*, germ]. A cell nucleus. SEE: *cyton*.

cytocentrum (sī"tō-sĕn'trŭm) ["+ *kentron*, center]. Minute body in cytoplasm of cell

close to nucleus. SYN: *cell center; centrosome*, q.v.; *sphere of attraction*. SEE: *sphere, attraction*.

cytocerastic (sī"to-se-ras'tĭk) ["+ *kerastos*, mixed]. Pert. to cells changing to a higher form. SYN: *cytokerastic*.

cytochemism (sī"tō-kĕm'ĭzm) [Gr. *kytos*, cell, + *chēmeia*, chemistry, + *-ismos*, condition]. Reaction of body cells to chemical agents or the injections of antitoxin.

cytochem'istry. The chemistry of the living cell.

cytochrome (sī'tō-krōm) [Gr. *kytos*, cell, + *chrōma*, color]. A pigment widely distributed in animals and plants. It plays an important role in cellular respiration. It is a mixture of three hemochromogens designated cytochromes A, B, and C.

   c. oxidase. An enzyme of importance in biological oxidations functioning in the transfer of electrons from cytochromes to oxygen, thus activating oxygen which unites with hydrogen to form water.

   c. P-450. A protein similar to hemoglobin in the microsomes of liver cells and in organs producing steroids such as the ovary, adrenal, testes, and placenta. Important in catalyzing the metabolism of steroid hormones and fatty acids and in the detoxification of a variety of chemical substances.

cytochylema (sī"to-ki-le'mă) ["+ *chylos*, juice]. The more fluid constituent of cell protoplasm. SYN: *hyaloplasm*, q.v.

cytocidal (sī"tō-sī'dăl) ["+ L. *caedere*, to kill]. Lethal to cells.

cytocide (sī'tō-sīd). An agent which causes the death of cells.

cytoclas'tic [Gr. *kytos*, cell, + *klasis*, destruction]. Destructive to cells.

cytoclesis (sī"tō-kle'sĭs) ["+ *klēsis*, a call]. The influence of living cells upon other cells. SYN: *cytobiotaxis*.

cytocyst (sī'tō-sĭst) ["+ *kystis*, a cyst]. The remains of a cell enclosing a mature schizont.

cytodendrite (sī"tō-dĕn'drĭt) [Gr. *kytos*, cell, + *dendron*, tree]. A dendrite given off from the body of a nerve cell.

cytodiagnosis (sī"tō-dī"ag-nō'sĭs) ["+ *dia*, through, + *gignōskein*, to know]. Diagnosis of pathogenic conditions by the study of cells present in exudates, fluids, etc.

cytodieresis (sī"tō-dī-ĕr'ē-sĭs) ["+ *diairesis*, division]. Cytokinesis, q.v.

cytodistal (sī"tō-dĭs'tăl) [Gr. *kytos*, cell, + *distāre*, to be distant]. Pert. to a neoplasm remote from the cell of origin.

cytogenesis (sī"tō-jĕn'ĕs-ĭs) ["+ *genesis*, origin]. Origin and development of the cell.

cytogenetics (sī″tō-jĕ-nĕt′ĭks). The study of cytology in relation to genetics, esp. the study of chromosomal behavior in mitosis and meiosis. Modern cytogenetics has led to the identification of chromosomes as bearers of the genes and deoxyribonucleic acid (DNA) as the key molecule of the gene.

cytogenous (sī-tŏj′ĕn-ŭs) [Gr. *kytos*, cell, + *gennan*, to produce]. Producing cells.

cytogeny (sī-tŏj′ĕ-nĭ) [″+ *genesis*, beginning]. The formation and development of the cell.

cytoglobin (sī″tō-glō′bĭn) [″+ L. *globus*, sphere]. A globin from lymphocytes and leukocytes. SYN: *cytoglobulin.*

cytoglycopenia (sī″tō-glī-ko-pe′nī-ă) [Gr. *kytos*, cell, + *glukos*, sweet, + *penia*, poverty]. Deficient glucose of blood cells. Also spelled *cytoglucopenia.*

cytohistogenesis (sī″to-hĭs″to-jĕn′ĕ-sĭs) [″+ *histos*, web, + *genesis*, origin]. The structural development of cells.

cytohyaloplasm (sī″to-hī′ăl-o-plăzm) [″+ *hyalos*, glass, + LL. *plasma*, a form, from Gr. *plassein*, to mold, spread out]. Fibrillary network of protoplasm.

cytoid (sī′toyd) [Gr. *kytos*, cell, + *eidos*, form]. Resembling a cell.

cytoinhibition (sī″to-ĭn″hĭ-bĭsh′ŭn) [″+ L. *inhibere*, to restrain]. Phagocytic cell action in preventing the destruction of ingested bacteria.

cytokalipenia (sī″to-kal-ĭ-pē′nī-ă) [″+ L. *kalium*, potassium, + Gr. *penia*, poverty]. A potassium deficiency in body or blood cells.

cytokerastic (sī″to-kĕ-răs′tĭk) [Gr. *kytos*, cell, + *kerastos*, mixed]. Pert. to cellular development from a lower to a higher form.

cytokinesis (sī″tō-kĭ-nē′sĭs) [″+ *kinēsis*, movement]. The separation of the cytoplasm into two parts which occurs in the latter stages of mitosis or cell division. SYN: *cytodieresis.*

cytology (sī-tŏl′ō-jĭ) [″+ *logos*, study of]. The science which deals with the formation, structure, and function of cells.

cytolymph (sī′to-lĭmf) [Gr. *kytos*, cell, + L. *lympha*, lymph]. Matrix of cytoplasm of cells. SYN: *cytochylema; cytohyaloplasm; hyalomitome; hyaloplasm,* q.v.

cytolysin (sī-tŏl′ĭ-sĭn) [″+ *lysis*, dissolution]. An antibody which causes disintegration of cells.

cytol′ysis. Dissolution or destruction of living cells. Hemolysis is the term used in case of red blood corpuscles, and bacteriolysis for bacteria.

cytomachia (sī″to-mak′ĭ-ă) [Gr. *kytos*, cell, + *machē*, fight]. Cellular activities and resistance during infection by microorganisms.

cytomegalovirus. A virus which has been included in the Herpes virus family. The virus is probably found worldwide but rarely produces clinically detectable disease except in infants up to four months of age. It is transmitted transplacentally to the fetus from a mother with a latent infection. Most infected infants are symptom-free, but when the disease does produce illness the eventual result is death. There are no effective methods of preventing or treating the illness.

cytometaplasia (sī″to-mĕt″ă-pla′zĭ-ă) [Gr. *kytos*, cell, + *metaplasis*, change]. Change of form or function of cells.

cytometer (sī-tŏm′ĕ-ter) [″+ *metron*, measure]. Instrument for counting and measuring cells.

cytom′etry. The counting and measuring of cells.

cytomicrosome (sī-to-mī′kro-sōm) [Gr. *kytos*, cell, + *mikros*, small, + *sōma*, body]. One of the minute granules in the protoplasm (cytoplasm) of the cell.

cytomitome (sī″to-mi′tōm) [″+ *mitos*, thread]. Any part of the network of the cytoplasm.

cytomorphology (sī″to-mŏr-fŏl′ō-jĭ) [″+ *morphē*, form, + *logos*, study of]. The study of the structure of cells.

cytomorphosis (sī″to-mor′fŏ-sĭs, -mor-fo′sis) [″+ ″+ -*ōsis*, formation]. The cellular transformations which a cell undergoes during its life.

cyton (sī′tŏn) [Gr. *kytos*, cell]. 1. A cell. 2. The body of a nerve cell. SYN: *perikaryon.*

cytopathogenic effect (sī″tō-păth″o-jĕn′-ĭk) [″+ *pathos*, disease, + *gennan*, to produce]. In tissue culture, the morphologic changes seen in the cultured cells due to the effect of some pathogenic agent such as a virus.

cytopathology (sī″tō-păth-ŏl′ō-jĭ) [″+ ″+ *logos*, study]. Study of the cellular changes in disease.

cytope′nia [Gr. *kytos*, cell, + *penia*, lack]. Diminution of cellular elements in blood or other tissues.

cytophagocytosis (sī″to-făg″o-sī-tō′sĭs) [″+ *phagein*, to eat, + *kytos*, cell, + -*ōsis*, condition]. Destruction of other cells by phagocytes. SYN: *cytophagy.*

cytophagous (sī-tŏf′ă-gŭs). Devouring or destructive of cells.

cytophagy (sī-tŏf′ă-jĭ). Cell destruction by phagocytes. SYN: *cytophagocytosis.*

cytophilic (sī-to-fil′ĭk) [Gr. *kytos*, cell, + *philein*, to love]. Having an affinity for or attracted by cells, e.g., antibodies.

cytophylaxis (sī″to-fĭ-lăk'sĭs) ["+ *phylaxis*, guarding against]. The protection of cells against lysis.

cytophylet'ic ["+ *phylē*, tribe]. Pert. to genealogy of cells.

cytophysics (sī″to-fĭz'ĭks) [Gr. *kytos*, cell, + *physikē*, (study of) nature]. The physics of cellular activity.

cytophysiology (sī″to-fĭz-ĭ-ŏl'ō-jĭ) ["+ *physis*, nature, + *logos*, study]. Physiology of the cell.

cytoplasm (sī'to-plăzm) ["+ LL. *plasma*, a form, from Gr. *plassein*, to mold, spread out]. The protoplasm of a cell outside the nucleus. SYN: *cytosome*.

cytoplast (sī'to-plăst). The cytoplasm of a cell body as distinguished from the contents of the nucleus.

cytoplas'tin [Gr. *kytos*, cell]. The plastin substance of the cytoplasm.

cytoproximal (sī-to-prŏks'ĭ-măl) ["+ L. *proximus*, nearest]. Pert. to the portion of an axon nearest to the cell body from which it originates.

cytoreticulum (sī″to-rĕ-tĭk'ū-lŭm) ["+ L. *reticulum*, network]. The fibrillar network supporting fluid of protoplasm.

cytoscopy (sī-tos'kō-pī) [Gr. *kytos*, cell, + *skopein*, to examine]. Microscopic examination of cells for purposes of diagnosis.

cytosome (sī'tō-sōm) ["+ *sōma*, body]. The cytoplasm or the portion of the protoplasm of a cell exclusive of the nucleus. SYN: *cytoplasm*.

cytospongium (sī″to-spun'jĭ-um) ["+ *sphongos*, sponge]. The fibrillar network of the cytoplasm of a cell. SYN: *spongioplasm*.

cytost (sī'tost) [Gr. *kytos*, cell]. A specific toxin given off by an injured or destroyed cell.

cytostasis (sī-tos'tă-sĭs) ["+ *stasis*, stoppage]. Stasis of white blood corpuscles, as in

incipient stage of inflammation.

cytostatic (sī″to-stăt'ĭk) ["+ *stasis*, standing still]. Preventing the growth and proliferation of cells.

cytotactic (sī″to-tăk'tĭk). Pert. to cytotaxia.

cytotaxia, cytotaxis (sī-to-tăk'sī-ă, -sĭs) [Gr. *kytos*, cell, + *taxis*, arrangement]. Attraction or repulsion of cells for each other.

cytother'apy ["+ *therapeia*, treatment]. 1. Treatment by use of glandular extracts; organotherapy. 2. Use of cytotoxic or cytolytic substances or serums in treating disease.

cytothesis (sī-toth'ĕ-sĭs) ["+ *thesis*, a placing]. Restoration or repair of injured cells.

cytotoxin (sī″to-toks'ĭn) [Gr. *kytos*, cell, + *toxikon*, poison]. An antibody or toxin which attacks the cells of particular organs.

SEE: *endotoxin; erythrotoxin; exotoxin; leukocidin; lysis; neurotoxin.*

cytotrophoblast (sī″to-tro'fo-blast) ["+ *trophē*, nourishment, + *blastos*, germ]. The thin inner layer of the trophoblast composed of cuboidal cells, the outer layer being the syntrophoblast. SYN: *layer of Langhans.*

cytotropic (sī″tō-trŏp'ĭk, - trōp'ĭk) ["+ *tropē*, a turn]. Having an affinity for cells.

cytozoic (sī″tō-zō'ĭk) [Gr. *kytos*, cell, + *zōon*, animal]. Living within or attached to a cell, as certain protozoa.

cytozoon (sī-tō-zō'ŏn). A protozoon which lives as an intracellular parasite.

cytula (sī'tū-lă) [L., small cell]. The impregnated ovum.

cyturia (sī-tu'rĭ-ă) [Gr. *kytos*, cell, + *ouron*, urine]. Presence of any kind of cells in the urine.

Czermak's spaces (chăr'măk). [Johann N. Czermak, Bohemian physician, 1828-1873] The interglobular spaces in dentine because of failure of calcification.

D

D. 1. Abbr. for L. *dad*, give; *date; daughter; deciduous; dermatologist;* L. *detur*, let it be given; *died; diopter; divorced; doctor.* 2. Chem. symb. for deuterium.

D-. Chemical prefix which indicates that the substance is structurally related to D-glyceraldehyde. Opposed to L-.

d. Abbr. for *density;* L. *dexter* or *dextro*, right; L. *dies*, day; *distal; dorsal; duration.*

D. and C. Abbr. for the surgical procedure of *dilatation* of the cervix and *curettage* of the uterus.

dacnomania (dăk″nō-mā′nĭ-ă) [Gr. *dæknein*, to bite + *mania*, insanity]. An irrational impulse to kill.

dacrocystitis (dăk″rō-sĭs-tī′tĭs) [Gr. *dakyron*, tear, + *kystis*, cyst, + *-itis*, inflammation]. Inflammation of the lacrimal (tear) sac. SYN: *dacryocystitis*, q.v.

dacryadenalgia (dăk″rĭ-ăd-ĕn-ăl′jĭ-ă) ["+ *adēn*, gland, + *algos*, pain]. Pain in a lacrimal gland.

dacryadeni′tis ["+ "+ *-itis*, inflammation]. Inflammation of a lacrimal gland.

dacryadenoscirrhus (dăk-rĭ-ăd-ĕn-ō-skĭr′us) ["+ "+ *skirrhos*, hardening]. Induration of a lacrimal gland.

dacryagogatresia (dăk″rĭ-ă-gŏg″ă-trē′sĭ-ă) [Gr. *dakyron*, tear, + *agōgos*, leading, + *a-*, not, + *trēsis*, perforate]. Occlusion of a tear duct.

dacryagogue (dăk′rĭ-ă-gŏg). That which stimulates the secretion of tears.

dacrycystalgia (dăk″rĭ-sĭs-tăl′jĭ-ă) [Gr. *dakyron*, tear, + *kystis*, cyst, + *algos*, pain]. Pain in a lacrimal gland; dacryocystalgia.

dacryelcosis (dăk″rĭ-ĕl-kō′sĭs) ["+ *elkōsis*, ulceration]. Ulceration of the lacrimal apparatus.

dacryoadenalgia (dăk″rĭ-ō-ăd″ĕn-ăl′jĭ-ă) [Gr. *dakyron*, tear, + *adēn*, gland, + *algos*, pain]. Dacryadenalgia; pain in a lacrimal gland.

dacryoadenitis (dăk″rĭ-ō-ăd″ĕn-i′tĭs) ["+ "+ *-itis*, inflammation]. Inflammation of lacrimal gland.

D. is rare; seen as complication in epidemic parotitis (mumps of lacrimal gland); also present in Mikulicz's disease; may be acute or chronic.

dacryoblennorrhea (dăk″rĭ-ō-blĕn″ō-rē′ă) ["+ *blenna*, mucus, + *rhoia*, flow]. Discharge of mucus from a lacrimal sac, and chronic inflammation of the sac.

dacryocele (dăk′rĭ-ō-sēl) [Gr. *dakryon*, tear, + *kēlē*, hernia]. Protrusion of a lacrimal sac.

dacryocyst (dăk′rĭ-ō-sĭst) ["+ *kystis*, cyst]. The lacrimal (tear) sac.

dacryocystalgia (dăk″rĭ-ō-sĭs-tăl′jĭ-ă) ["+ "+ *algos*, pain]. Pain in the lacrimal sac.

dacryocystectomy (dăk″rĭ-ō-sĭs-tĕk′tō-mĭ) [Gr. *dakryon*, tear, + *kystis*, cyst, + *ektomē*, excision]. The excision of membranes of lacrimal sac.

dacryocystitis (dăk-rĭ-ō-sĭs-tī′tĭs) ["+ "+ *-itis*, inflammation]. Inflammation of the tear sac involving mucus membrane of the lacrimal sac, together with submucus membrane, which later extends to connective tissue surrounding it with resulting cellulitis. Usually secondary to prolonged obstruction of the nasolacrimal duct.

SYM: Profuse tearing (epiphora), redness and swelling in area of sac which may also extend to lids and conjuctiva; pain, esp. on pressure over the lacrimal sac; overflow of tears.

TREATMENT: Hot compresses; oral and ophthalmic antibiotic preparations; incision and drainage if fluctuant; attempt to restore permeability of duct with probe when acute symptoms have subsided; in chronic cases extirpate sac or do intranasal operation (dacryocystorrhinostomy).

dacryocystoblennorrhea (dăk″rĭ-ō-sĭs″tō-blĕn-ō-rē′ă) ["+ "+ *blenna*, mucus, + *rhoia*, flow]. Chronic inflammation of and discharge from the lacrimal sac.

dacryocystocele (dăk″rĭ-ō-sĭs′tō-sēl) [Gr. *dakryon*, tear, + *kystis*, cyst, + *kēlē*, hernia]. Protrusion of lacrimal sac.

dacryocystoptosis (dăk″rĭ-ō-sĭ-tŏp-tō′sĭs) ["+ "+ *ptōsis*, a falling]. Prolapse of the lacrimal (tear) sac.

dacryocystorrhinostomy (dăk″rĭ-ō-sĭs″tō-rĭ-nŏs′tō-mĭ) ["+ "+ *rhis*, nose, + *stoma*, opening]. Surgical connecting of lumen of tear sac with nasal cavity.

dacryocystosyringotomy (dăk″rĭ-ō-sĭs″tō-sĭr″in-gŏt′ō-mĭ) [Gr. *dakryon*, tear, + *kystis*, cyst, + *syrinx*, tube, + *tomē*, incision]. Making an opening between the lacrimal sac and the nasal cavity.

dacryocystotome (dăk″rĭ-ō-sĭs′tō-tōm) ["+ *tomē*, incision]. Device for incision of lacrimal sac.

dacryocystotomy (dăk″rĭ-ō-sĭs-tŏt′ō-mĭ). Incision of the lacrimal sac.

dacryohemorrhea (dăk″rĭ-ō-hĕm″ō-rē′ă) ["+ *haima*, blood, + *rhoia*, flow]. Shedding of bloody tears.

dacryolin (dăk'rĭ-ō-lĭn) [Gr. *dakryon*, tear]. An albuminous matter in tears.

dac'ryolith ["+ *lithos*, stone]. Concretion in lacrimal passages. SYN: *dacryolite*.

dacryoma (dăk"rĭ-ō'mă) ["+ *-oma*, tumor]. 1. A lacrimal tumor. 2. Obstruction of lacrimal puncta with consequent profuse tearing (epiphora).

dacryon (dăk'rĭ-ŏn) [Gr. *dakryon*]. The lacrimal point of juncture of the lacrimal, frontal, and upper maxillary bones.

dacryops (dăk'rĭ-ŏps) ["+ *ops*, eye]. Constant flow of tears; dacryorrhea.

dacryopyorrhea (dăk"rĭ-ō-pī"ō-rē'ă) ["+ *pyon*, pus, + *rhoia*, discharge]. Discharge of pus from lacrimal duct.

dacryopyo'sis ["+ *pyōsis*, suppuration]. Suppuration in the lacrimal sac or duct.

dacryorrhea (dăk"rĭ-ō-rē'ă) [Gr. *dakryon*, tear, + *rhoia*, flow]. Excessive flow of tears.

dacryosolenitis (dăk"rĭ-ō-sō-lēn-ī'tĭs) ["+ *sōlēn*, duct, + *-itis*, inflammation]. Inflammation of a lacrimal or nasal duct.

dacryostenosis (dăk"rĭ-ō-stĕn-ō'sĭs) ["+ *stenōsis*, narrowing]. Stricture of a lacrimal or nasal duct.

dacryosyrinx (dăk"rĭ-ō-sī'rĭnks) ["+ *syrinx*, tube]. A lacrimal fistula.

dactyl (dăk'tĭl) [Gr. *daktylos*, finger]. A finger or toe; a digit of the hand or foot.

dactyl'ion. Adhesions between or union of fingers or toes.

dactyli'tis [Gr. *daktylos*, finger, + *-itis*, inflammation]. Chronic inflammation of bones of fingers and toes in very young children.

  ETIOL: Usually tuberculous or syphilitic.

  d., sickle cell. Painful swelling of the feet and hands during the first several years of life of children with sickle cell anemia, q.v.

dactylocampsodynia (dăk"tĭ-lō-kămp"sō-din'ĭ-ă) ["+ *kampsis*, bend, + *odynē*, pain]. Painful contraction of one or more fingers.

dactyl'ogram ["+ *gramma*, mark]. A fingerprint.

dactylog'raphy [Gr. *daktylos*, finger, + *graphein*, to write]. 1. The study of fingerprints. 2. The act of using a machine for blind deaf mutes to convey the signs of speech by touch.

dactylogryposis (dăk"tĭ-lō-grĭ-pō'sĭs) ["+ *grypōsis*, curve]. Permanent contraction of the fingers.

dactylology (dăk-tĭl-ŏl'ō-jĭ) ["+ *logos*, study]. Representing words by signs made with the fingers. SYN: *sign language*.

dactylomegaly (dăk"tĭ-lō-mĕg'ă-lĭ) [Gr. *daktylos*, finger, + *megas*, large]. Abnormally large size of fingers and toes.

dactyloscopy (dăk"tĭ-lŏs'kō-pĭ) ["+ *skopein*, to examine]. Examination of fingerprints for purpose of identification.

dactylospasm (dăk'tĭ-lō-spăzm) ["+ *spasmos*, spasm]. Cramp of a finger or toe.

dactylus (dak'ti-lŭs) [Gr. *daktylos*]. A toe or finger.

dairy food substitute. Foods resembling existing dairy foods but different in composition and constituents from the dairy food for which they are substituting. Ex: imitation cheese, ice cream, cream.

Dakin's solution (dā'kĭn). [Henry D. Dakin, Amer. chemist, 1880-1952] A solution for cleansing wounds, developed during World War I. A very dilute neutral solution (0.45-0.5%) of sodium hypochlorite and 0.4% boric acid.

daltonism (dŏll'tŏn-ĭzm). [John Dalton, Eng. chemist, 1766-1844] Color blindness to perception of red and green.

dam. A thin sheet of rubber used in dentistry and surgery to isolate a part from the flow of fluid. Frequently a rubber d. is used as a surgical drain.

damp. 1. Moist, humid. 2. A noxious gas.

  d., after-. Air containing large percentage of carbon dioxide.

  d., black. A gas formed by oxygen and the giving off of carbon dioxide by the coal. SYN: *choke d.*

  d., cold. Vapor charged with carbon dioxide.

  d., fire. Methane, CH_4, found in coal mines.

  d., stink. Hydrogen sulfide.

  d., white. Carbon monoxide.

damping. The steady diminution of the amplitude of successive vibrations as of an electric wave or current.

dance, St. Vitus'. A disease characterized by involuntary and irregular jerkings and movements in diverse groups of muscles. SEE: *chorea.*

Dance's sign. [Jean B. H. Dance, Fr. physician, 1797-1832] Slight retraction in the right iliac region in some cases of intussusception.

dancing disease. Epidemic dancing mania of Europe during the Middle Ages, supposed to have been caused by the bite of the tarantula. SEE: *tarantism.*

dancing mania. Epidemic chorea.

dandelion greens [L. *dēns leōnis*, lion's tooth]. Leaves of a well-known plant which grows as a weed or may be cultivated. The leaves are bitter and tonic and are eaten like spinach.

  Food value of 100 gm. (cooked): Cal. 33; protein 2 gm.; fat 0.6 gm.; carbohydrate 6.4

gm.; calcium 140 mg.; vitamin A, 11,700 I.U.; ascorbic acid 18 mg.

dan'druff. Normal exfoliation of the epidermis of the scalp in the form of dry, white scales. May be worse in diseased condition. Sometimes due to seborrhea, q.v.

dandy fever. Dengue, q.v. An acute, epidemic, febrile disease occuring in tropical areas.

danger list. List of critically ill patients in a hospital. Relatives of a patient on the list are usually notified and told of the serious nature of the illness.

dartoid (dăr'toyd) [Gr. *dartos,* skinned, + *eidos,* form]. Resembling the tunica dartos in its slow, involuntary contractions.

dar'tos [Gr.]. The muscular, contractile tissue beneath the skin of the scrotum. SYN: *tunica dartos* [NA].

    d. muscle reflex. Wormlike contraction of d. muscle following sudden cold application to perineum.

dar'trous [Gr. *dartos,* skinned]. Of the nature of herpes; herpetic.

darwin'ian ear. [Charles Robert Darwin, Eng. naturalist, 1809-1882] An exaggeration of darwinian tubercle, q.v.

darwinian tubercle. A blunt point projecting from upper part of the helix of the ear.

Darwinism (dăr″wĭ-nĭz'ĕm). The theory of biological evolution (origin of species, q.v.) through natural selection, q.v.

dasetherapy (dăs″ĕ-thĕr'ă-pĭ) [Gr. *dasos,* forest, + *therapeia,* treatment]. Treatment of disease by residency in a region of pine and spruce trees.

dasym'eter. Device for estimating density of gases.

date. The fruit of the palm; an oblong berry with a grooved seed.

    Food value of 100 gm. (natural, dry): Cal. 274; protein 2.2 gm.; fat 0.5 gm.; carbohydrate 73 gm.; calcium 59 mg.; vitamin A, 50 I.U.

daughter cell. Cell formed by the division of a mother cell.

daughter cyst. A small cyst growing out of the walls of a large cyst.

daugher nucleus. Formation of a new nucleus by a diaster.

Davidsohn's sign. [Hermann Davidsohn, Prussian physician, 1842-1911] The lessening or absence of pupillary light reflex when an electric light is held in the closed mouth. Indicates presence of a tumor or fluid in the maxillary sinus.

day blind'ness. Inability to see well in a bright light.

DDT. Abbr. for dichloro-diphenyltrichloroethane now called chlorophenothane. A powerful insecticide effective against a wide variety of insects, esp. the flea, fly, louse, mosquito, bedbug, cockroach, Japanese beetle, and European corn borer.

    Because it is so slowly excreted from the body, DDT should not be used if suitable substitutes are available.

    When ingested orally may cause acute poisoning. Symptoms are vomiting, numbness and partial paralysis of limbs, anorexia, tremors, depression, resulting in death.

de- [L. *dē,* from]. Prefix indicating down or from.

deacidifica'tion [L. *dē,* from, + *acidus,* sour, + *facere,* to make]. Neutralization of acidity.

deactivation [" + *activus,* acting]. The process of becoming inactive.

dead[AS. *dēad*]. Cessation of life or life processes.

    When death has occurred in a hospital or other institution for care of the sick, the patient's name, hour of death, and name of the ward should be written on a piece of paper and attached to the body or otherwise identified according to the custom of the institution. It is important that the "laying out" be completed before the commencement of rigor mortis. Immediate steps must be taken to inform the doctor if he is not present at time of death because no preparation of the body may be begun until the doctor has officially pronounced the patient dead. The private duty nurse may be asked to continue on duty for several hours. In any case, she should not leave until assured everything in the room is in order and that she can be of no further service. SEE: *death.*

deaf [AS. *dēaf*]. 1. Partially or completely lacking the sense of hearing. 2. Unwillingness to listen; heedless.

deaf-mute. A person who is unable to hear or speak.

deaf-mut'ism. The state of being both deaf and unable to speak.

deafness [AS.]. Complete or partial loss of ability to hear.

    ETIOL: May occur from several causes such as injury or disease of that part of the cortex controlling the center for hearing; disease of the middle ear or the eighth cranial nerve; toxic effects of certain drugs; hysteria without any abnormality of the ear or brain; injury of the ear from loud noises such as the firing of a gun at close range; an abnormal mental state producing auditory aphasia or psychic d., q.v.; congenital defects.

    Some forms of conduction d. may be remedied by a fenestration operation or stapes mobilization. SEE: *otosclerosis.*

d., aviator's. A temporary or permanent nerve d. found in a moderate percentage of aviators. This form of d. is due to prolonged exposure to loud noise levels.

d., bass. Inability to hear low tones.

d. central. D. resulting from lesions of auditory tracts of the brain or auditory centers of the cerebral cortex.

d., cerebral. D. due to brain lesion.

d., ceruminous. D. due to plugs of cerumen (ear wax).

d., conduction. D. resulting from any condition which prevents sound waves from being transmitted to the auditory receptors. May be due to wax obstructing external auditory meatus; inflammation of the middle ear; ankylosis of ear bones; fixation of footplate of stirrup. SEE: *otosclerosis.*

d., cortical. D. due to disease of the cortical centers.

d., nerve. D., perception, q.v.

d., occupational. D. caused by working in places where noise levels are quite high. Persons working in such an environment should wear devices to protect the hearing sense from the noise.

d., perceptive. D. resulting from lesions involving sensory receptors of cochlea or fibers of the acoustic nerve. SYN: *nerve d.*

d., psychic. Condition in which auditory sensations are perceived but not comprehended.

d., simulated. Malingering.

d., tone. Inability to distinguish musical sounds.

d., word. Condition in which sounds are heard but interpretation of the words is impossible.

dealbation (dē-ăl-bā'shŭn) [L. *dē*, from, + *albāre*, to whiten]. Bleaching.

deam'inase. An enzyme that causes deaminization.

deamina'tion. Deaminization, q.v.

deaminiza'tion. A chemical reaction whereby substances like the amino acids and alkaloids lose their amino groups and form ammonia.

Alanine can be deaminized to give ammonia and pyruvic acids: $CH_3CH(NH_2)COOH + O = CH_3.CO.COOH + NH_3$. Deaminization may be simple, oxidative, or hydrolytic. Oxidizing enzymes are called deaminizing enzymes when the oxidation is accompanied by splitting off of amino groups.

deanesthesiant (dē-ăn-ĕs-thē'zĭ-ănt) [L. *dē*, from, + Gr. *an-*, not, + *aisthēsis*, sensation]. Agent or action that will overcome anesthesia.

deaquation (dē''ă-kwā'shŭn) ["+ *aqua*, water]. Dehydration, q.v.

dearterialization (dē''ar'tēr''ĭ-ăl-ĭ-zā'shŭn) ["+ Gr. *artēria*, artery]. Changing character of arterial into venous blood; deoxygenation.

death [AS. *dēath*]. Permanent cessation of all vital functions.

The following definitions of death have also been considered: (1) Total irreversible cessation of cerebral function, spontaneous function of the respiratory system, spontaneous function of the circulatory system. (2) The final and irreversible cessation of perceptible heart beat and respiration. Conversely, as long as any heart beat or respiration can be perceived, either with or without mechanical or electrical aids, and regardless of how the heart beat and respiration were maintained, death has not occurred.

Defining death is complicated. Conditions such as cardiac standstill or complete lack of renal function would have meant certain death at one time. The use of cardiac pacemakers, artificial hearts and kidneys, heart transplants, and kidney transplants have made delaying death possible.

ETIOL: Gradual wearing out of tissue and loss of energy with cessation of function without disease as in old age. Result of disease represented by the culmination of its ravages in the ordinary progress of the affection or as sudden death. Injury from accidents is considered the major cause of death.

Sudden death may result from circulatory failure, cerebral causes, respiratory causes, neuroendocrinohumeral causes, shock, intoxications, obstetrical causes, infantile causes.

In some cases persons who would be expected to recover from their illness die despite extreme effort made to keep them alive. For want of a better explanation, these persons are said to have lost their will to live. They have in fact willed to die.

SIGNS: The principal sign of death is cessation of the heart's action. Other indications are opaqueness of the cornea; absence of reflexes; manifestations of rigor mortis, q.v.; and a mottled discoloration of the body, esp. over all parts where there is pressure. Many cases of death have been reported only to find after 24 hours that the person was not dead. For such reasons more or less elaborate tests have sometimes been used to determine without doubt whether life is or is not extinct. The signs mentioned usually are sufficient to confirm one's opinion that death has taken place. In all cases, however, it is advisable to call a physician to confirm that death has occurred.

In case of an emergency, the usual symptoms of death often are found to be unreliable. Attempts at resuscitation should continue to be made indefinitely. No harm can be done in attempting to resuscitate one who seems to be deceased; successes are numerous.

SEE: *d. tests.*

DETERMINING TIME LAPSE SINCE D. OCCURRED: Take the rectal temperature. In general the body loses one degree of Fahrenheit temperature each hour following death. Of course the rate of heat loss varies with temperature of the surrounding air, water, or snow.

d., black. Plague, q.v.

d., crib. Sudden infant death syndrome, q.v.

d., local. Gangrene or necrosis of a part.

d., molar. D., local, q.v.

d., molecular. D. of cell life.

d. point. A limit in environment, i.e. temperature, moisture, radiation, beyond which man cannot survive.

d. rate. Number of deaths occurring per 1000 of the population in a given area within a specified time.

d. rattle. Sound heard in the throat of the dying.

d., somatic. That of the entire organism.

d. tests. Both the electrocardiogram and electroencephalogram have been used to determine death but neither test is infallible.

d., voodoo. In primitive societies the witch doctor or shaman, q.v., may at least appear to cause death in persons whom he has caused to believe are under his spell or control.

death, words pert. to: agonal; ante mortem; autopsy; demise; euthanasia; in articulo mortis; in extremis; lethal; "necr-" words; posthumous; post mortem; putrefaction; rigor mortis; suicide.

death-bed. 1. The bed on which a person dies. 2. The final hours preceding death.

d. statement. A declaration made at the time immediately preceding death. Such a statement, if made with the consciousness and belief that death is impending, is held in law as equally binding with a statement made under oath. SYN: *ante-mortem statement.*

debil'itant [L. *debilis,* weak]. 1. A remedy used to reduce excitement. 2. That which weakens.

debil'itate. To produce weakness or debility.

debil'ity. Weakness of tonicity in functions or organs of the body.

débouchement (dā-būsh-mŏn′) [Fr.]. Opening or emptying into another part.

Debove's membrane (dē-bōv′). [George Maurice Debove, Fr. physician, 1845-1920] Layer of connective tissue cells between the epithelium and basement tissue of respiratory and intestinal epithelia.

débridement (dā-brēd-mŏn′) [Fr.]. In surgery, the removal of foreign material and dead or damaged tissue, esp. in a wound.

debris (dē-brē′) [Fr., remains]. The remains of broken down or damaged cells or tissue.

deca-, dec- [Gr. *deka*]. Prefix indicating ten.

decagram (děk′ă-grăm) [Gr. *deka,* ten, + *gramma,* weight]. A weight of 10 grams.

decalcification (dē″kăl-sĭ-fĭ-kā′shŭn) [L. *dē,* from, + *calx,* lime, + *facere,* to make]. The removal of, or the withdrawal of, lime salts from bone.

decal'cify. To soften bone by removal of calcium or its salts by acids.

decaliter (děk′ă-lē″ter) [Gr. *deka,* ten, + Fr. *litre*]. A measure of 10 liters.

decalvant (dē-kăl′vănt) [L. *dēcalvāre,* to make bald]. Destroying hair or making bald.

decameter (děk′ă-mē-ter) [Gr. *deka,* ten, + *metron,* measure]. A measure of 10 meters; 393.71 in.

decanormal (děk″ă-nor′măl) ["+ L. *norma,* rule]. Pert. to a solution 10 times as strong as a normal one. It contains 10 gm. equivalent weights of the substance per liter. SEE: normal.

decant (dē-kănt′) [L. *dē,* from, + *canthus,* rim of a vessel]. To pour off liquid so the sediment remains in the bottom of the container.

de″canta′tion. The gentle pouring off of a liquid from its sediment.

decapitation (dē-kăp″ĭ-tā′shŭn) [L. *dē,* from, + *caput,* head]. 1. The separation of the head from the body; beheading. 2. In obstetrics, the separation of the head of the fetus from the body to facilitate delivery. 3. Separating the head from the shaft of a bone. SYN: *decollation.*

decapsula′tion ["+ *capsula,* little box]. Removal of a capsule of an organ.

decarboxylation, decarboxylization (dē″kăr-bŏks-ĭ-lā′shŭn, ĭ-zā-shŭn). A chemical decomposition whereby substances like the amino acids lose their carboxyl (COOH) groups.

decay (dē-kā′) [L. *dē,* down, + *cadere,* to fall]. 1. Gradual loss of vigor with physical and mental deterioration as in aging. SEE: *senility.* 2. To waste away. 3. Decomposition of organic matter by the action of microorganisms. SEE: *cementoclasia.* 4. Disintegration of radioactive substances.

deceleration (dē-sĕl″ē-rā′shŭn). To decrease velocity.

decerebrate (dē-sĕr′ē-brāt) [L. *dē,* from, + *cerebrum,* brain]. A person or animal who has been subjected to decerebration.

decerebration (dē-sĕr-ē-brā′shŭn). Removal of the brain or cutting the spinal cord at the level of the brain stem.

dechlorina′tion [L. *dē,* from, + Gr. *chloros,* green]. Reduction in the amount of chlorides in the body by reduction of or withdrawal of salt in the diet. SYN: *dechloridation.*

deci- [L. *decimus,* tenth]. Prefix indicating one tenth.

decibel (dĕs′ĭ-bĕl) [L. *decimus,* tenth, + *bel,* unit of sound]. The unit for expressing the difference in power, usually between acoustic energy signals, i.e., sound.

decidua (dē-sĭd′ū-ă) [L. *deciduus,* falling off]. The name given to the endometrium or mucous membrane which envelops the impregnated ovum.

This may be seen in both uterine and ectopic pregnancies. The gland structures of the endometrium and the interstitial cells undergo marked hypertrophy. The decidua divides itself into an outer, or compact layer, and an inner spongy layer.

    d. basalis. [NA]. That part of the decidua which unites with the chorion to form the placenta. SYN: *d. serotina.*

    d. capsularis. [NA]. That part of the decidua which surrounds the chorionic sac. SYN: *d. reflexa.*

    d. graviditatis. The pregnancy d.

    d. menstrualis. The layer of the uterine endometrium that is shed during menstruation.

    d. parietalis. [NA]. The nonplacental lining of the uterus; the decidua. SYN: *d. vera.*

    d. reflexa. D. capsularis, q.v.

    d. serotina. D. basalis, q.v.

    d. vera. D. parietalis, q.v.

decidual (dē-sĭd′ū-ăl). Pert. to or resembling the decidua.

decidualitis (dē-sĭd″ū-ăl-ĭ′tĭs) [L. *deciduus,* falling off, + Gr. *-itis,* inflammation]. A bacterial infection of the decidua.

deciduation (dē-sĭd″ū-ā′shŭn). The loss of the decidua during menstruation.

deciduitis (dē-sĭd″ū-ī′tĭs) [L. *deciduus,* falling off, + Gr. *-itis,* inflammation]. Inflammation of the decidua.

deciduoma (dē-sĭd″ū-ō′mă) [″+ Gr. *-ōma,* tumor]. A uterine tumor containing decidual tissue. Thought to arise from portions of decidua retained within the uterus following an abortion.

    d., benign. The more or less normal invasion of the uterine musculature by the syncytium which disappears after the gestation is completed.

    d., Loeb′s. Decidual tissue produced within the uterus of experimental animals as a result of mechanical or hormonal stimulation.

    d., malignant. A tumor consisting of syncytial and Langhans cells which have a tendency to invade the general system by means of the blood stream with a high mortality rate. SYN: *choriocarcinoma; chorionepithelioma.*

    ETIOL: This tumor may arise following a full term pregnancy, an ectopic pregnancy, an abortion, a miscarriage, and particularly a vesicular mole.

    DIAG: May be made by histological study, aided by the symptoms and the Aschheim-Zondek test which remains strongly positive during the presence of this type of tumor.

    TREATMENT: Chemotherapy with the folic acid antagonist Methotrexate (USP).

deciduomatosis (dē-sĭd″ū-ō-mă-tō′sĭs) [L. *deciduus,* falling off, + *-ōma,* tumor, + *-ōsis* condition]. Excessive and irregular formation of decidual tissue in the nonpregnant state.

deciduosarco′ma [″+ Gr. *sarx,* flesh, + *-ōma,* tumor]. A tumor of the chorion. SYN: *choriocarcinoma; chorionepithelioma.*

deciduous (dē-sĭd′ū-ŭs) [L. *deciduus*]. Falling off.

    d. teeth. The milk teeth or temporary teeth, 10 in each jaw: 4 incisors, 2 canines, and 4 molars. They usually appear at 6 months and are lost by the end of 6 years. Those of the lower jaw appear before the upper ones, as follows: Lower central incisors at 5-9 months; upper incisors at 8-12 months; lower lateral incisors and first molars at 12-15 months; canines at 18-24 months; second molars at 24-30 months. SEE: dentition.

decigram (dĕs′ĭ-grăm) [L. *decimus,* tenth, + Gr. *gramma,* weight]. One tenth of a gram.

deciliter (dĕs′ĭ-lē-ter) [″+ Fr. *litre*]. One tenth of a liter.

decimeter (dĕs′ĭ-mē″tĕr) [″+ Gr. *metron,* measure]. One tenth of a meter.

decinor′mal (dĕs′ĭ-nor′măl) [″+ *norma,* rule]. Having one tenth the strength of a normal solution. SEE: *normal.*

Declaration of Geneva. A statement adopted in 1948 by the Second General Assembly of the World Medical Association. Some medical schools use it at graduation exercises.

At the time of being admitted as Member of the Medical Profession I solemnly pledge myself to consecrate my life to the service of humanity. I will give to my teachers the respect and gratitude which is their due; I will practice my profession with conscience and dignity; The health of my patient will be my first consideration; I will respect the secrets which are confided in me; I will maintain by all the means in my power, the honor and the noble traditions of the medical profession; My colleagues will be my brothers; I will not permit considerations of religion, nationality, race, party politics or social standing to intervene between my duty and my patient; I will maintain the utmost respect for human life, from the time of conception; even under threat, I will not use my medical knowledge contrary to the laws of humanity. I make these promises solemnly, freely and upon my honor. SEE: *Hippocratic oath; Prayer of Maimonides.*

declinator (dĕk'lĭn-ā''tor) [L. *declināre,* to turn aside]. Instrument used during trephining for holding apart the dura mater.

decline (dē-klīn'). 1. Progressive decrease. 2. Declining period of a disease.

declivis cerebel'li (dē-klīv'ĭs sĕr-ĕ-bĕl'ī) [L.]. Sloping posterior portion of the monticulus of the superior vermis of the cerebellum.

decoction (dē-kŏk'shŭn) [L. *dē,* down, + *coquere,* to boil]. A liquid preparation made by boiling vegetable substances with water.

When the strength and method of preparation are not otherwise specified, it is made by boiling five parts of the coarsely comminuted drug for 15 minutes with enough water to make 100 parts. There are no official decoctions.

decollation (dē''kŏl-ā'shŭn) [L. *dē,* from, + *collum,* neck]. Fetal decapitation. SYN: *detruncation.*

decollator (dē'kŏl-ā-tĕr). Device for decapitation of the fetus.

décollement (dā-kŏl-mŏn') [Fr., ungluing]. Separation of two normally adherent structures.

decompensa'tion [L. *dē,* from, + *compensāre,* to make good again]. Failure of compensation, as in circulation of the heart.

decom'plementize. To take away the complement from.

decomposition (dē-kŏm-pō-zĭsh'ŭn) [L. *dē,* from, + *componere,* to put together]. 1. The putrefactive process; decay. 2. Reducing a compound body to its simpler constituents. SEE: *fermentation, resolution.*

   d., double. A chemical change in which the molecules of two interacting compounds exchange a portion of their constituents.

   d., hydrolytic. Chemical change in substances due to addition of a molecule of water.

   d., simple. A chemical change by which a molecule of a single compound breaks into its simpler constituents or substitutes the entire molecule of another body for one of these constituents.

decompres'sion ["+ *compressio,* a squeezing together]. 1. The removal of pressure, as from gas in the intestinal tract. SEE: *Wangensteen's apparatus.* 2. The slow reduction or removal of pressure on deep-sea divers and caisson workers to prevent development of bends, q.v.

   d. chamber. A tank in which patients suffering from d. sickness are placed. After entry into the chamber, the barometric pressure is increased to that level which relieves the patient's symptoms, and then very slowly decreased until pressure is equal to outside pressure.

   d., explosive. In aviators or divers, d. resulting from an extremely rapid rate of change from one pressure to a much less pressure. This may occur if a high altitude aircraft suddenly loses its cabin pressurization or if a diver ascends quite rapidly. Causes violent expansion of body gases.

   d. illness. Caisson disease, or bends, q.v., compressed air illness. SYN: *d. sickness.*

de"contamina'tion. The process of rendering an object, person, or area free of a contaminating substance such as a bacteria, poison-gas or radioactive substance.

de"cortica'tion [L. *dē,* from, + *cortex,* bark]. The removal of the surface layer of an organ or structure, as the removal of a portion of the cortex of the brain from the underlying white portion.

   d. pulmonary. Removal of the pleura of the lung or a portion of the surface lung-tissue.

   d. renal. Removal of capsule of the kidney.

dec'rement [L. *decrementum,* decrease]. The period in the course of a febrile disease when the fever subsides.

decrep'itate [L. *decrepitāre,* to crackle]. To cause decrepitation or a crackling noise.

decrepita'tion. A crackling noise.

decrepitude (dē-krĕp'ĭ-tūd). State of general feebleness and decline which accompanies old age; weak; infirm.

decubation (dē-kū-bā'shŭn) [L. *dē,* down, + *cumbere,* to lie]. 1. The act of lying down. 2. The recovery stage of an infectious disease.

decu'bital. Pert. to a bed sore.

decubitus (dē-kū'bĭ-tŭs) [L., a lying down]. 1. A bedsore, q.v. 2. A patient's position in bed.

d., acute. A severe, sometimes fatal, bedsore which can occur on the affected side in hemiplegia.

decussate (dē-kŭs'āt) [L. decussāre, to make an X (10)]. 1. To cross, or crossed, as in the form of the letter "x." 2. Interlacing or crossing of parts.

decussa'tion. 1. A crossing of structures in form of an "x." 2. The place of crossing; chiasma.

    d. of the pyramids. Crossing of fibers of pyramids of the medulla oblongata from one pyramid to the other.

    d., optic. The crossing of the fibers of the optic nerves; the optic chiasma.

decussorium (dē-kŭs-ō'rĭ-ŭm). Instrument for depression of the dura following trephining.

dedifferentiation. In biology, development or differentiation of a tissue to a less well-developed or more primitive structure. Thus development proceeds in a reverse order.

deep [AS. deop]. 1. Below the surface. 2. Quality of the voice, such as a bass sound.

    d. reflexes. Reflexes within, or fractional stretch reflexes. Opposed to superficial or skin reflexes.

deer fly. A biting fly, Chrysops discalis, which transmits the causative organism of deerfly fever, a form of tularemia.

    d.f. fever. Tularemia, q.v.

defat'ted [L. dē, from, + AS. fāelt, to fatten]. Freed from or deprived of fat.

defecalgesiophobia (dēf'ē-kăl'jē-sĭ-ō-fō'bĭ-ā) [L. defaecāre, to remove dregs, + Gr. algēsis, pain, + phobos, fear]. Fear of defecating because of pain.

defecation (dĕf-ē-kā'shŭn) [L. defaecāre, to remove dregs]. Evacuation of the bowels.

    The bulk of the feces depends upon the amount and composition of food ingested. One does not, however, have to eat in order to have bowel movements. A large quantity of cellular material is desquamated from the epithelial lining of the intestinal tract each day.

    The food residues, reaching the rectum, cause the urge to defecate. The sensation is related to periodic increase of pressure within the rectum and contracture of its musculature.

    The expulsion of a fecal mass is accompanied by coordinated action of the following mechanisms: involuntary contraction of the circular muscle of the rectum behind the mass followed by contraction of the longitudinal muscle; relaxation of the internal (involuntary) and external (voluntary) sphincter ani; voluntary closure of the glottis, fixation of the chest, and contraction of the abdominal muscles, causing an increase in intra-abdominal pressure. SEE: constipation; feces; stool.

defect (dē'fekt, dĭ-fĕkt). A flaw or imperfection.

    d., congenital. Imperfection present at birth.

    d., filling. Interruption in the contour of the inner surface of the stomach or intestine revealed by roentgenography.

defec'tive [L. defectus, a failure]. 1. Not perfect. 2. A person deficient in one or more physical, mental, or moral powers.

defeminization. To lose or cause the loss of female sexual or social characteristics.

defense [L. defendre, to repel]. 1. Resistance to disease. 2. Acting to protect one's self from harm or injury.

    d. mechanism. 1. Any reaction, whether general or cellular, which serves to protect against something harmful. Ex: immune reactions. 2. In psychoanalysis, a method of unconscious behavior used to resolve or conceal conflicts or anxieties. Ex: compensation; denial; projection.

    d. protein. An antibody, q.v.

    d. reflex. Retraction or tension in defense against an action or threatened action.

defensive. Defending; a means of protecting from injury.

deferens (dĕf'er-enz) [L., carrying away]. Ductus or vas deferens.

deferent (dĕf'ĕr-ĕnt). Away from or downward. SEE: afferent; efferent.

    d. duct. Ductus deferens or vas deferens, q.v.

deferentectomy (dĕf-ĕr-ĕn-tĕk'tō-mĭ) [L. deferens, carrying away, + Gr. ektomē, excision]. Cutting of the ductus deferens. SYN: vasectomy.

deferential (dĕf-ĕr-ĕn'shăl) [L. deferre, to bring to]. Pert. to or accompanying the ductus deferens.

deferentitis (dĕf'ĕr-ĕn-tī'tĭs) [" + Gr. -itis, inflammation]. Inflammation of the ductus deferens.

deferred shock. Delayed onset of symptoms of shock.

deferves'cence [L. defervescere, to become calm]. The period that marks the subsidence of fever to normal temperature.

defibrillation. Stopping fibrillation of the heart through the use of drugs or by physical means. SEE: cardioversion; defibrillation, electrical.

    d., electrical. Stopping defibrillation of the heart by using an electrical device which applies shocks to the heart through electrodes placed on the chest wall. SEE: cardioversion; cardioverter.

defibrina'tion, defibriniza'tion [L. *dē*, from, + *fibra*, fiber]. Process of being deprived of fibrin. SEE: *coagulation*.

defi'ciency [L. *dēficere*, to lack]. A lack, something missing.

d. disease. One due to a deficiency of a substance essential in body metabolism.

The deficiency may be due to inadequate intake, inadequate digestion, inadequate absorption, inadequate utilization, excessive loss through excretory channels, or excessive loss to a parasite such as a hookworm or tapeworm.

Ex: Night blindness and keratomalacia due to lack of vitamin A; beriberi or polyneuritis due to lack of thiamine; pellagra due to lack of niacin; scurvy due to lack of vitamin C; rickets and osteomalacia due to lack of vitamin D; pernicious anemia due to lack of gastric intrinsic factor and vitamin B_{12}.

d., mental. Subnormal in intelligence.

definition [L. *dēfīnīre*, to limit]. The precise determination of the limits of anything, esp. a disease process.

defin'itive. Clear and final; without question.

deflagra'tion (dĕf'lă-grā'shŭn) [L. *deflagrāre*, to burn furiously]. Sudden, sharp combustion, usually with a crackling sound.

defloration (dĕf'lō-rā'shŭn) [L. *dē*, from, + *flos, flor-*, flower]. Rupture of the hymen during coitus, by accident, surgically, or through vaginal examination.

Not many females have a hymen which is of such size or consistency as to require its rupture. SEE: *hymen; virginity*.

deflores'cence. Disappearance of an eruption of the skin.

defluvium (dē-flū'vĭ-ŭm) [L.]. Falling out.

d. capillorum. Loss of hair.

defluxio (dē-flŭk'sĭ-ō) [L.]. A flowing down.

d. capillorum. A falling out of hair.

d. ciliorum. A falling out of eyelashes.

defluxion (dē-flŭk'shŭn). A flowing down; copious discharge or loss of any kind.

deforma'tion [L. *dē*, from, + *forma*, form]. The act of deforming; a disfiguration.

deform'ity. An unnatural alteration in the natural form of a part or organ. Distortion of any part or general disfigurement of the body. It may be acquired or congenital. If present after injury, usually implies presence of fracture, dislocation, or both. May be due to extensive swelling, extravasation of blood, rupture of muscles, etc.

d., anterior. Abnormal anterior convexity of the spine. SYN: *lordosis*, q.v.

d., gunstock. D. in which the forearm when extended makes an angle with the

arm because of displacement of axis of the extended arm. ETIOL: Condylar fracture at elbow.

d., Madelung's. Distortion of the radius at its lower end with ulnar displacement backward.

d., seal fin. Outward deflection of the fingers in rheumatoid arthritis.

d., silverfork. The peculiar deformity seen in Colles' fracture of the forearm. SEE: *Colles' fracture*.

d., Sprengel's. Congenital upward displacement of the scapula.

d., Velpeau's. D., silverfork, q.v.

d., Volkmann's. Congenital tibiotarsal dislocation.

defunda'tion [L. *dē*, from, + *fundus*, base]. Excision of the uterine fundus.

defurfura'tion ["+ *furfur*, bran]. Shedding of epidermis in scales; branny desquamation.

Deg. Abbr. for *degeneration; degree*.

deganglionate (dē-găn'glĭ-ŏn-āt'') [L. *dē*, from, + Gr. *ganglion*, knot]. To deprive of ganglia.

degen'erate [L. *dēgenerāre*, to fall from one's ancestral quality]. 1. A person who never had moral character, or lost it. 2. To deteriorate.

degenera'tion [L. *degeneratio*]. Deterioration or impairment of an organ or part in structure of cells and the substances of which they are a part.

ETIOL: Due to changes in size (decrease or increase) and other changes.

d., Abercrombie's. D., amyloid, q.v.

d., adipose. D., fatty, q.v.

d., albuminoid. D., amyloid, q.v.

d., amyloid. D. resulting from deposition of amyloid between cells in various organs and tissues, esp. affecting blood vessels.

d., ascending. Nerve fiber d. progressing to the center from the periphery.

d., bacony. D., amyloid, q.v.

d., calcareous. Deposits of lime salts in tissues and parts.

d., caseous. Cheesy alteration of tissues seen in tuberculosis of same.

d., cloudy swelling. A condition in which protein substances in cells become cloudy, the cells increasing in size with minute droplets of protein substances. Occurs in infectious diseases and in those of the kidneys, liver, the heart and its muscles, and in the glands.

d., colloid. Jellylike disorganization of a part.

d., cystic. Cyst formation accompanying d.

d., descending. Nerve fiber d. progressing toward the periphery from the original lesion.

d., fatty. Deposition of abnormal amounts of fat in cells, or the replacement or infiltration of tissues by fat cells.

d., fibroid. Change of membranous tissue into that of a fibrous nature.

d., gray. Gray d. in nerve tissue due to chronic inflammation.

d. hepatolenticular. D. of the liver and of the lenticular nucleus. SEE: *Wilsons's disease.*

d., hyaline. A form in which the tissues assume a homogeneous and glassy appearance. Caused by hyaline deposits replacing musculoelastic elements of blood vessels with a firm, transparent substance which causes loss of elasticity. It is responsible for hardening of the arteries and is often followed by calcification or deposit of lime salts in dead tissue. Calcification also may result in concretions.

d., lardaceous. D., amyloid, q.v.

d., mucoid. Deposition of mucus in the connective tissues.

d., myxomatous. D., mucoid, q.v.

d., Nissl. Nerve cell d. after division of the axon.

d., parenchymatous. D., cloudy swelling, q.v.

d., polypoid. Formation cf polyplike growths on mucous membrane.

d., secondary. D., wallerian, q.v.

d., senile. Bodily and mental changes of the aged.

d., vitreous. D., hyaline, q.v.

d., wallerian. Nerve fiber d. after separation from its nutritive center.

d., waxy. Amyloid or lardaceous d.

d., Zenker's. Amyloid d. in muscular tissue.

degeneration, words pert. to: amylosis; "ather-" words; athetoid; atrophic; cacogenic; caseation; catalysis; colloid; sarcomatosis; steatosis.

degen'erative. Pert. to or accompanied by degeneration.

deglutible (dē-glū'tĭ-bl) [L. *dēglūtire,* to swallow]. Capable of being swallowed.

deglutition (dē''glū-tĭsh'ŭn). The act of swallowing.

deglu'titive. Pert. to deglutition.

degradation (dĕg''rĕ-dā'shŭn) [LL. *dēgradāre,* to go down a step]. Physical, metabolic, or chemical change to a less complex form. Thus foods are physically degraded during chewing, and then chemically degraded from complete compounds, such as proteins and starches, to amino acids and sugars respectively.

degustation (dē''gŭs-tā'shŭn) [L. *degustatio*]. The sense of taste.

dehiscence (dē-hĭs'ĕns) [L. *dehiscere,* to gape]. A bursting open, as of a graafian follicle or a wound, esp. an abdominal wound.

dehy'drate [L. *dē,* from, + Gr. *hydōr,* water]. 1. In chemistry, to deprive of, lose, or become free of water. 2. The loss of or deprivation of water from the body or tissues. To become dry.

dehydration (dē''hī-drā'shŭn). The process of dehydrating. Occurs when output of water exceeds water intake. May result from deprivation of water, excessive loss of water, reduction in total quantity of elecrolytes, or injection of hypertonic solutions.

dehydroandrosterone (dē-hī''drō-an-drō-stēr'ōn, drŏs'ter-ōn). An androgenic substance $C_{19}H_{28}O_2$, present in urine with about one fifth the potency of androsterone. SYN: *dehydroisonandrosterone.*

dehydrocholesterol (dē-hī''drō-kō-lĕs'tēr-ol). A sterol found in the skin and other tissues which after activation by radiation forms vitamin D.

dehydrocorticosterone (dē-hī''drō-kor-tĭ-kōs'tēr-ōn). 11-dehydrocorticosterone (Kendall's compound A). $C_{21}H_{28}O_4$. A physiologically active steroid isolated from the adrenal cortex. It is important in water and salt metabolism.

dehydrogenase (dē-hī-drŏj'ĕ-nās). An enzyme which catalyzes the oxidation of a specific substance causing it to give up its hydrogen.

dehydrogenatum (dē-hī''drō-jĕn-ā'tŭm). Alcohol deprived of hydrogen.

dehydroisoandrosterone (dē-hī''drō-i''sō-ăn-drŏs'tēr-ōn). A 17-ketosteroid excreted in normal male urine. It possesses androgenic activity.

deionization (dē-i''ŏn-ī-zā'shŭn). Removal of ions from a substance, thus producing a substance free of minerals.

Deiters' cells (dī'tĕrz). [Otto F. C. Deiters, Ger. anatomist, 1834-1863]. 1. Supporting cells in organ of Corti. 2. Neuroglia cells.

Deiters' nucleus. Collection of cells back of the acoustic nucleus.

Deiters' process. Axis cylinder process or neuraxon.

déjà vu (da-zhŏ vū) [Fr., already seen]. The impression that something seen or some situation being experienced for the first time has been previously seen or experienced.

dejecta (dē-jĕk'tă) [L. *dejectio,* dejection]. Feces; intestinal waste.

dejection, dejecture (dē-jĕk'shŭn, -tūr). 1. A cast down feeling or mental depression. 2. Defecation or act of defecation.

Dejerine's disease (dā-zēr-ēn). [Joseph J. Dejerine, Fr. neurologist, 1849-1917]. Interstitial neuritis of infants.

Dejerine's syndrome. Condition with deep sensitivity repressed but with normal tactile sense, caused by lesion of long root fibers of posterior column.

delacrimation (dē-lăk″ri-mā'shŭn) [L. *dē*, dawn, + *lacrimā*, tear]. Excessive flow of tears. SEE: *epiphora*.

delactation (dē″lăk-tā'shŭn) [L. *dē*, from, + *lactāre, to suckle*]. Weaning or cessation of lactation.

delamina'tion [" + *lamina*, plate]. The division into laminae, esp. that of a blastoderm into two layers; epiblast and hypoblast.

delayed reflex. Any in which the response is abnormally delayed.

delayed symptoms. Delayed onset of symptoms, as of shock.

deligation (dĕl-ĭ-gā'shŭn) [L. *deligāre*, to tie up]. The application of ligatures or binder.

delimita'tion [L. *dē*, from, + *limitāre*, to limit]. Determination of limits of an area or organ in diagnosis.

deliquesce (dĕl-ĭ-kwĕs) [L. *dēliquēscere*, to melt away]. To cause liquefaction.

deliquescence (dĕl″ĭ-kwĕs'ĕns). The process of becoming liquefied as result of absorption of water from the air. Ordinary table salt has this property.

deliquescent (dĕl″ĭ-kwĕs'ĕnt). Pert. to a substance which absorbs water from the atmosphere.

delire de toucher (dā-lēr'dŭ-tū-shā'). An abnormal desire to touch or feel things.

deliriant (dē-lĭr'ĭ-ănt) [L. *dēlīrāre*, to be deranged]. An agent that will produce delirium. Ex: atropine, hyoscine.

delirifacient (dē-lĭr″ĭ-fā'shĭ-ĕnt) [" + *facere*, to make]. A drug causing delirium. SYN: *deliriant.*

delirium (dē-lĭr'ĭ-ŭm) [L.]. Disorientation for time and place, usually with illusions and hallucinations. A state of mental confusion and excitement.

The mind wanders and speech is incoherent, and the patient is in a state of continual, aimless physical activity. There are many forms of delirium, depending mainly upon the cause.

RS: alcoholism; carphologia; consciousness, clouding of; dipsomania; restraints.

    d., acute. D. developing suddenly and speedily, resulting in recovery or death.

    d., alcoholic. D. tremens, q.v.

    d., chronic. D. of chronic psychoses without febrile characteristics.

    d. constantium. D. of patients with reiteration of fixed idea.

    d. cordis. Violent heart beat; atrial fibrillation.

    d. epilepticum. D. either following an epileptic attack or appearing instead of an attack.

    d., febrile. D. occurring with fever.

    d. hystericum. D. of hysteria.

    d., lingual. Form where meaningless sounds are muttered constantly.

    d. mussitans. Excitement causing lingual d.

    d. of negation. Form in which patient thinks parts of his body are missing.

    d., partial. D. reacting on only a portion of the mental faculties, causing only some of the patient's actions to be unreasonable.

    d. of persecution. D. in which patient feels he is being persecuted by those about him.

    d., toxic. D. produced by presence of toxins in the body.

    d., traumatic. D. following injury or shock.

    d. tremens. A physic disorder involving visual and auditory hallucinations found in habitual and excessive users of alcoholic beverages.

SYM: Hallucinations as seeing snakes or monsters or hearing noises. Patient is excited and usually talking or yelling incoherently.

F.A. TREATMENT: Sedatives, esp. paraldehyde and bromides. Treat for shock if present. Glucose and fluids in large quantities. Induce free perspiration. Restraints may be necessary. Intramuscular apomorphine hydrochloride may sedate the maniacal individual, but should not be given if patient is an alcoholic with impaired liver function.

NP: The patient must never be left alone for an instant because attempts at suicide are frequent in such cases. The nursing of delirium needs endless patience, tact, and understanding. Restraint should be avoided if possible.

    d., violent. Feverish d. with exaltation and great strength.

delitescence (dĕl″ĭ-tĕs'ĕns) [L. *dēlitēscens*, hiding]. 1. An unusually complete and speedy resolution of an inflammation. 2. The latent period prior to development of symptoms following poisoning.

deliv'er [L. *dēliberāre*, to free completely]. 1. To aid in childbirth. 2. To remove or extract as a tumor from a cystic enclosure or a cataract.

deliv'ery. Expulsion of the child with placenta and membranes from the mother at birth. SEE: *labor.*

    d., abdominal. Removal of the child by Cesarean section.

    d., forceps. D. of the child by the use of instruments.

    d., postmortem. D. of the child either by the abdominal or vaginal route after death of the mother.

    d., precipitate. D. that occurs under nonaseptic conditions and when the physician is not present. In the true sense it is one which follows a rapid labor, regardless of who is present.

    NOTE: Watch the patient carefully. A multipara needs more careful watching than a primipara. However, this should not be taken as an excuse because it is possible for it to occur in a primipara.

    Do not wait for the head to be visible in a multipara if she is having frequent hard pains, particularly if they are bearing down in type. Have a physician see her immediately. In a primipara it is fairly safe to wait in the majority of cases until a small portion of the head is seen at the vaginal orifice during a pain before putting the patient up for delivery.

    Remember to watch the primipara or multipara who has received an analgesic, since precipitation can occur with little or no warning. This means watching for bulging of the perineum during the pains by viewing the vulva and not taking it for granted that because the patient is fairly quiet no progress is being made.

    d., premature. D. of a fetus after the twenty-eighth week but before full term.

    d., spontaneous. D. of the child without external aid.

delomorphous (dĕl″ō-mor'fŭs) [Gr. *dēlos,* evident, + *morphē,* form]. Having definite form and shape.

    d. cells. Granular cells which stain easily; found next to basement membrane in stomach, glands in cardiac region.

delousing (dē-lows'ing) [L. *dē,* from, + AS. *lus,* louse]. Ridding of lice by their destruction.

delta fornicis (dĕl″tă-for'nĭ-sīs) [L.]. A triangular surface on lower side of fornix; commissura hippocampi.

del'toid [Gr. *delta,* letter d, + *eidos,* resemblance]. Shaped like the Greek letter; triangular.

    d. ligament. Internal lateral ligament of ankle joint.

    d. muscle. The musculus deltoideus which covers the shoulder prominence.

    d. ridge. Ridge on humerus where deltoid muscle is attached.

de lunatico inquirendo (dē-lū-năt′ĭ-kō-in-kwī-rĕn'dō) [L.]. Legal process to determine alleged mental incompetence of a person.

delusion (dē-lū'zhŭn) [L. *dēlūdere,* to cheat]. A false belief, as the individual's believing he is Napoleon. Differs from hallucination which involves the false excitation of one or more of the senses.

    The most important delusions are those which cause the patient to harm others or himself, such as fear of being poisoned causing the patient to refuse food; those leading to suicide or inflicting injury upon self; false beliefs such as having been guilty of an unpardonable sin; those of persecution. SEE: *hallucination.*

    d., depressive. D. causing a saddened state.

    d., expansive. Conviction of one's own fineness, power, or importance.

    d., fixed. D. that remains unaltered.

    d., fleeting. A type of d. that comes and goes.

    d. of grandeur. A false sense of possessing wealth or power. SYN: *megalomania.*

    d. of negation. D., nihilistic, q.v.

    d., nihilistic. D. that causes the victim to believe that everything has ceased to exist.

    d. of persecution. D. in which patient feels everyone about him is against him.

    d., reference. D. that causes the victim to read a meaning not intended in the acts or words of others, usually an interpretation of slight or ridicule.

    d., systematized. Logical correlation with false reasoning and deduction.

    d., unsystematized. D. without any correlation between ideas and surroundings.

delu'sional. Pert. to a delusion.

dement' [L. *dēmentāre,* to make insane]. One who has lost his sanity.

demented. Of sound mind.

dementia (dē-mĕn'shĭ-ă) [L. *dēmentāre,* to make insane]. Irrecoverable deteriorative mental state, the common end result of many entities.

    d., alcoholic. D. in terminal portion of chronic alcoholic state.

    d., apathetic. D. with diminished sensitivity, occurring usually in the last stages of disease.

    d., apoplectic. Form following cerebral hemorrhage or tumors.

    d., catatonic. A form of d. praecox.

d., chronic. An incurable form occurring at any time of life.

d., epileptic. D. accompanied by mental deterioration and due to long continued epilepsy.

d. naturalis. Congenital form; idiocy.

d., organic. D. caused by lesions of nerve centers.

d. paralytica. Paresis or general paralysis of the insane. A paretic form of neurosyphilis characterized by progressive dementia and a diffuse generalized paralysis. Lasts several months to three or four years if untreated. Generally terminates in death if untreated.

ETIOL: Antecedent syphilitic infection.

d. paranoides. D. with paranoid tendencies.

d., postfebrile. D. following severe cases of infectious diseases.

d. praecox. An obsolete term. SEE: *schizophrenia.*

d., presenile. D. beginning in middle age, usually resulting from cerebral arteriosclerosis. Symptoms are apathy, loss of memory, disturbances of speech and gait.

d., primary. D. occurring by itself, without relationship to another form of psychosis.

d., secondary. D. occurring after a primary mental disease, such as mania.

d., senile. D. occurring in the aged. SYM: Progressive mental deterioration with loss of memory, esp. for recent events, with occasional intercurrent attacks of excitement.

d., syphilitic. D. caused by lesion of syphilis.

d., tabetic. D. that may occur following tabes dorsalis.

d., terminal. D. following another form of mental disease. SEE: *secondary d.*

d., toxic. D. due to excessive use of some drug.

demerol (dĕm'ĕr-ŏl). Proprietary name for meperidine hydrochloride, a white, colorless, crystalline compound, soluble in water, having a neutral reaction and an analgesic effect similar to morphine. It may be habit forming.

demi- [L. *dimidius,* half]. Prefix indicating half.

demibain (dĕm'ĭ-bān) [Fr., half bath]. Half a bath; sitz bath.

demic (dĕm'ĭk) [Gr. *demos,* people]. Concerning the living body of man.

demilune (dĕm'ĭ-lūn) [L. *dimidius,* half, + *luna,* moon]. A crescent-shaped group of serous cells which form a caplike structure over a mucous alveolus. They are present in mixed glands, esp. the submandibular gland.

demineraliza'tion [L. *dē,* from, + *minare,* to mine]. Loss of mineral salts, esp. from the bones.

demise (dē-mīz') [L. *dimittere,* to dismiss]. Death.

Dem'odex [Gr. *dēmos,* fat, + *dēx,* worm]. Genus of mites and ticks of the class Arachnida and order Acarina.

D. folliculorum. The hair follicle or face mite, an elongated wormlike organism that infests hair follicles and sebaceous glands of various mammals including man.

demography (dē-mŏg'rä-fĭ) [Gr. *demos,* people, + *graphein,* to write]. Statistical study of births, marriages, and deaths, and physical, moral, and intellectual development.

demonomania (dē"mŏn-ō-mā'nĭ-ă) [Gr. *daimon,* demon, + *mania,* madness]. Obsolete term for psychotic belief that one is possessed by demons.

Demours' membrane (dē-mūr'). [Pierre Demours, Fr. opthalmologist, 1702-95]. A fine membrane between the endothelial layer of the cornea and the substantia propria. SYN: *Descemet's membrane; lamina elastica posterior.*

demucosation (dē"mū-kō-sā'shŭn) [L. *demucosatio].* Excision of mucosa of any part of body.

demul'cent [L. *dēmulcēns,* stroking softly]. An agent that will soothe the part or soften the skin to which applied. The term is usually restricted to agents acting on mucous membrane. Ex: glycerin honey, lanolin, olive oil.

demutization (dē"mū-tĭ-zā'shŭn) [L. *dē,* from, + *mutus,* mute]. Overcoming mutism by teaching the patient to speak or to use the sign language.

demyelinate (dē-mī'ĕ-lĭn-āt) [" + Gr. *myelos,* marrow]. Destruction or removal of the myelin sheath of nerve tissue.

dena'tured [" + *natura,* nature]. Subject to having the nature of a substance changed, or to render unfit for consumption, as alcohol, q.v.

d. protein. A protein which has been treated in some manner that caused it to lose some of its physical and chemical properties. Cooking egg white denatures the albumin present.

dendraxon (dĕn-drăks'ŏn) [Gr. *dendron,* tree, + *axōn,* axle]. The terminal filaments of the neuraxon of a nerve cell.

den'dric. Pert. to or possessing a dendron.

dendriform (dĕn'drĭ-form) [Gr. *dendron,* tree, + L. *forma,* shape]. Branching, or like a tree in shape.

den'drite [Gr. *dendritēs*, pert. to a tree]. A branched protoplasmic process of a neuron which conducts impulses to the cell body. There are usually several to a cell. They form synaptic connections with other neurons.

d., extracapsular. Dendrites of neurons of autonomic ganglia which pierce the capsule surrounding the cell and extend for considerable distances from the cell body.

d., intracapsular. Dendrites of neurons of autonomic ganglia which ramify beneath the capsule forming a network about the cell body.

dendrit'ic. Treelike in form.

d. calculus. A renal stone molded in the form of the pelvis and calyces.

dendroid (dĕn'droyd) [Gr. *dendron*, tree, + *eidos*, form]. 1. Dendriform, pert. to dendrites. 2. Arborescent, treelike.

dendron (dĕn'drŏn) [Gr., tree]. A dendrite; a protoplasmic branch from a nerve cell.

dendrophagocytosis (dĕn"drō-făg-ō-sī-tō'-sis) ["+ *phagein*, to eat, + *kytos*, cell, + *-ōsis*, condition]. The absorption of portions of astrocytes by microglia cells.

dener'vated [L. *dē*, from, + Gr. *neuron*, nerve]. 1. Excision, incision, or blocking of a nerve supply. 2. A condition in which the nerve supply is blocked or cut off.

dengue (dĕng'gā, -gē) [Sp.]. Acute epidemic febrile disease lasting 5-7 days; seldom fatal. SYN: *breakbone fever; dengue fever.*

ETIOL: A virus transmitted by the mosquito, Aedes aegypti, and other species of Aedes. Incubation period is 3-15 days, usually 5-6 days.

SYM: Two fever periods with intermissions; eruptions similar to measles; severe pain in muscles and joints.

TREATMENT: No specific treatment. Analgesic and sedative agents. Mosquito control for prophylaxis.

denidation (dĕn"ī-dā'shŭn) [L. *dē*, from , + *nidus*, nest]. Removal during menstruation of the superficial mucosal surface of the lining of the uterus.

dens (dĕnz) [L.]. (pl. *dentes*) [NA]. 1. A tooth. 2. The odontoid process of the axis. A process on the body of the axis which serves as a pivot for the rotation of the atlas. SEE: *dentition* for illustration.

d. bicuspidus. D. premolaris, q.v.

d. caninus. (pl. *dentes canini*) [NA]. The canine tooth.

d. deciduus. (pl. *dentes decidui*) [NA]. Milk tooth, first tooth.

d. incisivus. (pl. *dentes incisivi*) [NA]. Incisor tooth.

d. moliris. (pl. *dentes molares*) [NA]. Molar tooth, grinder.

d. permanens. (pl. *dentes permanentes*) [NA]. One of the 32 teeth making up the so-called permanent teeth.

d. premolaris. (pl. *dentes premolares*) [NA]. One of the premolar teeth.

d. sapientiae. A wisdom tooth; late tooth; third molar; SYN: *d. serotinus.*

d. serotinus. [NA]. A wisdom tooth third molar.

densimeter (dĕn-sīm'ē-tĕr) [L. *densus*, thick + Gr. *metron*, measure]. Instrument for measuring densities.

densitometer (dĕn"sī-tŏm'ē-tĕr). A special densimeter for measuring bacterial growth and effect upon it of antiseptics and bacteriophages.

den'sity [L. *densitās*, thickness]. 1. Relative weight of a substance compared with some other substance of equal bulk. SEE: *specific gravity.* 2. The quality of being dense.

dentag'ra [L. *dens*, tooth, + Gr. *agra*, seizure]. 1. Toothache. 2. Forceps for removing teeth.

den'tal. Pert. to the teeth.

d. abscess. SEE: *abscess, dental.*

d. arch. The arch formed by the cutting and chewing surfaces of the teeth.

d. caries. Decay of the teeth. SEE: *caries.*

d. consonant. A consonant pronounced with the tongue at or near the front upper teeth. Term used in speech therapy

d. curve. The curve or bow of the line of the teeth in the jaw. The different portions of the curve are described as follows: *alignment curve,* the line passing through the center of the teeth from the middle line through the last molar; *buccal curve,* the curve extending from the cuspid to the 3rd molar; *compensating curve,* the occlusal line of bicuspids and molars; *labial curve,* the curve extending from cuspid to cuspid.

d. disk. A thin, circular piece of paper cloth, or other substance charged with abrasive powder for cutting or polishing teeth and fillings.

d. dysfunction. Malfunctioning of the parts of the dental structure.

d. engine. A machine operated with foot power or by an electric or a water motor to give a swift rotary motion to drills, burs, and burnishers.

d. engineering. Use of the principles of engineering in dentistry.

d. floss. Waxed or unwaxed thread used for cleaning between the teeth and testing for defects in the teeth.

d. formula. A method of expressing briefly the dentition of mammals in which the numbers of the teeth are given in the form of a fraction, the numbers of the upper teeth forming the numerator, those of the lower teeth the denominator.

Using *i* for incisors, *c* for canine, *b* for bicuspid, *pm* for premolar, and *m* for molar, the dental formula of man is:

$$\text{i. } \frac{2\text{-}2}{2\text{-}2} \quad \text{c. } \frac{1\text{-}1}{1\text{-}1} \quad \text{b. or pm. } \frac{2\text{-}2}{2\text{-}2} \text{ m } \frac{3\text{-}3}{3\text{-}3} \text{ 32.}$$

d. geriatrics. The scientific study and treatment of dental conditions of the aged.

d. hygienist. A trained person who professionally cleans teeth and, usually in schools or institutions, offers instruction on general care of the teeth.

d. index. A system of numbers for indicating comparative size of the teeth.

d. prosthesis. An artificial part used in the mouth to replace missing structural tissue or teeth. SYN: *denture.*

dentalgia (dĕn-tăl'jĭ-ă) [L. *dens*, tooth, + Gr. *algos*, pain]. Toothache.

dentaphone (dĕn'tă-fōn) ["+ Gr. *phōnē*, sound]. Device for conveying sound through the teeth.

dentate (dĕn'tāt) [L. *dentātus*, toothed]. Notched; having short triangular divisions of the margin; toothed.

den'tes [L.]. Teeth. Pl. of dens, q.v.

dentibuccal (dĕn-tĭ-bŭk'l) [L. *dens*, tooth, + *bucca*, cheek]. Pert. to both the cheek and teeth.

denticle (dĕn'tĭ-kl) [L. *denticulus*, little tooth]. 1. A small toothlike projection. 2. A small tooth.

dentic'ulate [L. *denticulātus*, small toothed]. Finely toothed or serrated.

d. body. Corpus dentatum of the cerebellum.

dentifica'tion [L. *dens*, tooth, + *facere*, to make]. Conversion into dental structure.

den'tiform ["+ *forma*, shape]. Toothlike.

dentifrice (dĕn'tĭ-frĭs) ["+ *fricāre*, to rub]. A powder or other substance for cleaning teeth.

dentigerous (dĕn-tĭj'ĕr-ŭs) [L. *dens*, tooth, + *gerere*, to bear]. Having or containing teeth.

dentilabial (dĕn-tĭ-lā'bĭ-ăl) ["+ *labium*, lip]. Pert. to both teeth and lips.

dentilinqual (dĕn-tĭ-lĭn'gwăl) ["+ *lingua*, tongue]. Pert. to both teeth and tongue.

dentimeter (dĕn-tĭm'ē-tĕr) ["+ Gr. *metron*, measure]. Device for measuring teeth.

dentin (dĕn'tĭn) [L. *dens*, tooth]. The main, or osseous, tissues of a tooth surrounding the pulp cavity. SYN: *dentine.*

den'tinal. Pert. to dentin.

dentinalgia (dĕn-tĭn-ăl'jĭ-ă) [L. *dens*, tooth, + Gr. *algos*, pain]. Pain in dentin, q.v.

dentine (dĕn'tēn). Dentin, q.v.

dentinifica'tion [L. *dens*, tooth, + *facere*, to make]. Formation of dentin.

dentini'tis ["+ Gr. *-itis*, inflammation]. Inflammation of dentin.

dentinoblast (dĕn'tĭn-ō-blast) ["+ Gr. *blastos*, germ]. A dentin-forming cell.

dentinogenesis (dĕn"tĭn-ō-jĕn'ē-sĭs) [L. *dens*, tooth, + *gennan*, to produce]. Formation of dentin in development of a tooth.

d. imperfecta. Aplasia or hypoplasia of the enamel and dentin of a tooth.

d. nucleus. A mass of gray matter in the medulla of each cerebellar hemisphere.

den'tinoid ["+ Gr. *eidos*, form]. 1. Resembling dentin. 2. A tumor arising from dentin; a dentinoma.

dentino'ma ["+ Gr. *ōma*, tumor]. A dentin tumor.

dentinosteoid (dĕn"tĭn-ŏs'tĭ-oyd) [L. *dens*, tooth, + Gr. *osteon*, bone, + *eidos*, form]. Dentinoid.

dentiparous (dĕn-tĭp'ă-rŭs) ["+ *parere*, to bear]. Pert. to development and formation of teeth.

den'tist [L. *dens*, tooth]. A practitioner of dentistry.

den'tistry. 1. That branch of medicine which deals with the care of the teeth and associated structures. It is concerned with the prevention, diagnosis, and treatment of diseases of the teeth and gums. 2. The art or profession of a dentist.

d., esthetic. Repair and restoration or replacement of carious or broken teeth.

d., operative. Phase of dentistry dealing with dental operations on mouth as contrasted with dental laboratory work.

d., prosthetic. Pert. to prosthodontia.

d., prosthodontic. The art of replacing defective or missing teeth through the use of artificial appliances such as bridges, crowns, artificial dentures, etc.

denti'tion [L. *dentitiō*]. 1. The type, number, and arrangement of teeth in the dental arch. 2. The cutting of teeth. SYN: *teething.* SEE: *teeth* for illustration.

d., primary. Eruption of 20 deciduous or milk teeth. The order of eruption follows: Two lower central incisors, 5-9 months; two upper central incisors, 8-12 months; two upper lateral incisors, 10-12 months; two lower lateral incisors, 12-15 months; four anterior molars, 12-15 months; four canines, 18-24 months; four posterior molars, 24-30 months.

d., secondary. (32 teeth) The eruption of the permanent teeth beginning at about

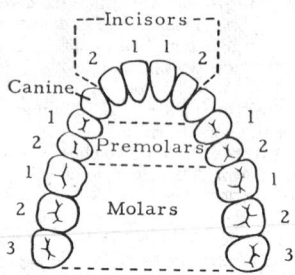

DENTITION—Teeth in situ

the age of six years. Completed by the 15th year with the exception of the wisdom teeth which appear between the 17th and 25th years. The order of eruption follows: The incisors and canines are followed by the same teeth; the frontal molars are followed by 1st bicuspids; the posterior molars are followed by 2nd bicuspids, then the 1st, 2nd, and 3rd molars follow. SEE: *teeth.*

dentoalveolar (dĕn″tō-ăl-vē′ō-lăr) [L. *dens,* tooth, + *alveolus,* small hollow]. Pert. to alveolus of a tooth.

dentoalveolitis (dĕn″to-ăl″vē-ō-lī′tĭs) ["+ "+ Gr. *-ītis,* inflammation]. A purulent inflammation of the tooth socket linings characterized by looseness of the teeth and shrinkage of the gum. SYN: *pyorrhea alveolaris.*

den′toid ["+ Gr. *eidos,* form]. Dentiform; odontoid; tooth-shaped.

dentoid′in. Organic substance of a tooth.

dentoliva (dĕn″tō-lī′vă) [L. *dens,* tooth, + *oliva,* olive]. Olivary body.

denture (dĕn′chur). A set of natural or artificial teeth, but usually artificial.

    d., artificial. A dental appliance for support of one or more artificial teeth. Used in the mouth to replace missing natural teeth. Dentures are usually made of a combination of synthetic plastic and metal.

    NP: Dentures should be cleaned after each meal. When patient's condition prevents his doing this for himself it will need to be done by the nursing staff. The simplest method of cleaning dentures is to use a soft brush and either plain soap or tooth paste, with lukewarm water (hot water may damage dentures). They should be thoroughly rinsed after each washing.

    Instruct patient to store dentures in covered opaque jar. If wrapped in tissue paper they are easily lost or thrown away.

Dentures are removed from comatose or moribund patients and prior to any surgical procedure.

    The following solutions and mixtures are accepted by the Amer. Dental Assn. for cleaning dentures: (1) Ammonia water 28% Dilute 2 ml. in 2 oz. of water. (2) Trisodium phosphate, 600 mg. in 2 oz. of water. (3) Sodium hypochlorite (bleach), 2 ml. in 4 oz. of water.

    d., full. Denture which replaces all of the teeth in both jaws.

    d., immediate. A complete set of artificial teeth to be inserted immediately after removal (extraction) of natural teeth.

    d., partial. A dental appliance replacing less than the full number of teeth in either jaw.

denucleated (dē-nū′klē-āt-ĕd) [L. *dē,* from + *nucleus,* kernel]. Deprived of a nucleus.

denuda′tion [L. *denudāre,* to lay bare]. Removal of a protecting layer or covering through surgery, pathological change, or trauma.

denutrition (dē″nū-trĭsh′ŭn) [L. *dē,* from, + *nutrīre,* to nourish]. Malnutrition.

deobstruent (dē-ŏb′strū-ĕnt) ["+ *obstruere* to block up]. Having the property of removing obstructions.

deodorant (dē-ō′dor-ănt) [L. *dē,* from, + *odorāre,* to perfume]. An agent that destroys or neutralizes foul odors. Those in common use are chlorinated lime, creolin, iodoform, permanganate of potash, chlorine, and hydrogen peroxide. SEE: *odor.*

    d., body. D. applied directly to the body to either neutralize malodor or to inhibit the growth of bacteria which produce odor.

deodorize (dē-ō′dor-īz) ["+ *odor,* odor]. To remove foul odor.

deodorizer (dē-ō′dor-īz-er). That which deodorizes.

deontology (dē″ŏn-tŏl′ō-jĭ) [Gr. *deonta,* needful, + *logos,* study]. The theory or study of professional obligations and committments; medical ethics. SEE: *ethics.*

deoppila′tion [L. *dē,* from, + *oppilatio,* obstruction]. Removal of obstructions, particularly of the bowels.

deorsum (dē-or′sŭm) [L.]. Downward or turning downward.

    d. ver′gens. Turning downward.

deorsumduction (dē-or″sŭm-dŭk′shŭn) ["+ *ducere,* to lead]. Bending downward.

deos′sification (dē-ŏs′ĭ-fĭ-kā′shŭn) [L. *dē,* from, + *os,* bone, + *facere,* to make]. Loss of or removal of mineral matter from bone or osseous tissue.

deox′idate ["+ Gr. *oxys,* sharp]. To deprive a chemical of oxygen.

deoxida'tion. Process of depriving a chemical compound of oxygen.

deoxidizer (dē-ŏk'sĭ-dī-zẽr). A deoxidizing substance.

deoxycholic acid (dē-ŏk″sĭ-kō'lĭk). $C_{24}H_{40}$ O_4, a crystalline acid found in bile.

deoxyribonuclease (dē-ŏk″sĭ-rī″bō-nū′klē-ās). An enzyme, produced by certain streptococci, which hydrolyzes deoxyribonucleoprotein of cells.

deoxyribonucleic acid (dē-ŏk″sĭ-rī″bō-nū′klē-ĭk). A complex protein of high molecular weight consisting of deoxyribose, phosphoric acid, and four bases (two purines, adenine and guanine, and two pyrimadines, thymine and cystosine). These are arranged as two long chains which twist around each other to form a double helix joined by bonds between the complementary components.

It is a nucleic acid present in chromosomes of the nuclei of cells and is considered the chemical basis of heredity and the carrier of genetic information. Formerly spelled desoxyribonucleic acid. ABBR: DNA.

deoxyribose (dē-ŏk″sĭ-rī′bōs). A phosphoric ester of a pentose present in nucleic acid.

depancreatize (dē-păn'krē-ă-tīz). To remove the pancreas surgically.

dependence (dĭ-pĕn'dĕns) [L. *dependēre*, to hang down]. In narcotic addicts, the mental and physical state of being dependent upon narcotics in order to achieve a feeling of well being. The nature of most narcotics is such that an increasingly larger dose is required to obtain that feeling. Decreasing the dose causes withdrawal signs and symptoms. SEE: *habituation; withdrawal.*

deper″sonaliza'tion [L. *dē*, from, + *persona*, person]. A sense of being someone else; a lessened sense of one's own identity.

deper'sonalize. To make impersonal; to deprive of personality or individuality.

depilate (dĕp'ĭl-āte) [L. *dēpilāre*, to deprive of hair]. To remove hair.

depilation (dĕp″ĭl-ā'shŭn). The process of hair removal. SEE: *epilation.*

depil'atory. An agent used for the removal of hair.

deplete (dĭ-plēt') [L. *dēplētus*, emptied]. To empty, as in blood letting; to produce depletion.

depletion (dĭ-plē'shŭn). Removal of substances from the body such as blood, fluids, iron, fat, protein.

deplumation (dē″plū-mā'shŭn) [L. *dē*, from, + *plūma*, feather]. Falling of eyelashes as result of disease.

depolarization (dē-pō″lăr-ĭ-zā'shŭn) [″ + *polus*, pole]. The process of reducing to a nonpolarized condition; destruction of polarity.

deposit (dĭ-pŏz'ĭt) [L. *dēpositus*, having put aside]. 1. Sediment. 2. Matter collected in any part of an organism, normal or diseased.

depravation (dĕp″ră-vā'shŭn) [L. *dēprāvāre*, completely destroyed]. 1. Pathological deterioration of function or secretion. 2. Moral or ethical perversion or corruption.

depraved (dē-prāvd'). 1. Perverted; abnormal. 2. Deteriorated.

depress'ant [L. *depressus*, pressed down]. An agent that will depress a body function or nerve activity. Ex: bromides; chloral hydrate.

    d., cardiac. D. which lessens heart action so that it beats slower and weaker.

    d., cerebral. D. lessening brain activity, making patient dull and less active. Large doses may produce sleep.

    d., motor. D. which lessens contractions of involuntary muscles.

    d., respiratory. A drug lessening frequency and depth of breathing.

    d., secretory. Agent causing decreased glandular secretions.

depressed (dē-prĕst'). 1. Below the normal level as when fragments of bone are forced below their normal level and that of surrounding portions of bone. 2. Low in spirits; dejected. 3. Decreased level of function.

depression (dē-prĕsh'ŭn) [L. *depressiō*, a pressing down]. 1. A hollow or lowered region. 2. The lowering of a part as the mandible. 3. The lowering of a vital function such as respiration. 4. A mental state characterized by dejection, lack of hope, and absence of cheerfulness. Observed in manic depressive psychoses. Depression is to be differentiated from grief which is realistic and is proportionate to that which has been lost.

    d., adverse. Melancholia.

    d., cardiac. Notch in anterior margin of left lung for the cardiac apex.

    d., pacchionian. Depression in the skull containing pacchionian bodies.

depressomotor (dē-prĕs'ō-mō'tor) [L. *depressus*, pressed down, + *motor*, mover]. A drug which diminishes muscular movements by lessening the impulses for motion sent from the brain or spinal cord.

depress'or [L.]. Instrument for depressing a part.

    d. nerve. A nerve, the stimulation of which brings about a fall in blood pressure through reflex vasodilation and slowing of heart beat.

    d. reflex. More or less transient stimulation of depressor fibers.

d., tongue. Device used to flatten tongue for throat examinations.

deprimens oculi (dĕp″rĭ-mĕns-ŏk′ū-lē) [L.]. Musculus rectus inferior oculi.

deprival (dē-prī′văl) [L. *dē,* from, + *privāre,* to remove]. Deprived of or without organs, parts, or functions.

deprivation (dĕp″rĭ-vā′shŭn). Deprival.

d., emotional. Isolation of an individual, esp. an infant, from normal emotional stimuli. In infants this produces impairment of mental and physical development. SEE: *maternal deprivation syndrome.*

d., sensory. A situation or environment wherein the usual sensory stimuli, such as noise and light, as well as human contact are absent or, in the case of noise, masked by a continuous dull noise. Persons exposed partially or completely to such an environment include astronauts, patients in artificial respirators, and patients with both eyes bandaged. Prolonged exposure to lack of sensory stimuli may cause hallucinations and other signs and symptoms of mental disorder.

deprivement (dē-prĭv′mĕnt). Being without function, parts, or organs. SYN: *deprival.*

depth [ME. *depthe*]. Richness; intensity; quality of being deep.

d. perception. Perception of spatial relationships; three dimensional perception.

d. psychology. Psychology of unconscious behavior. Opposed to psychology of conscious behavior.

depulization (dē-pūl″ĭ-zā′shŭn) [L. *dē,* from, + *pulex,* flea]. Destruction of fleas which carry the plague bacillus.

depurant (dĕp′ū-rănt) [L. *dēpūrāre,* to purify]. 1. A medicine that helps to purify by promoting the removal of waste material from the body. 2. Removal of waste material.

depura′tion. Process of freeing from impurities.

dep′urative. Cleansing.

depura′tor. 1. That which purifies. 2. An emunctory; an organ or tissue that serves to remove body wastes. Ex: bowels, kidneys, skin.

deradelphus (dĕr-ă-dĕl′fŭs) [Gr. *dere,* neck, + *adelphos,* brother]. Malformed twins, fused above the thorax and having one head, but separated below the chest as two bodies.

deradenitis (dĕr″ăd-ĕn-i′tĭs) ["+ *adēn,* gland, + *-itis,* inflammation]. Inflammation of a lymph gland of the neck.

deradenoncus (dĕr″ăd-ĕn-ŏnk′ŭs) ["+ *onkos,* tumor]. Swelling or tumor of a neck gland.

derangement (dē-rānj′mĕnt) [Fr. *dēranger,* unbalance]. Disorder of the mental functions, esp. those involving the intellect.

Dercum's disease (dĕr′kŭm). [Francis X Dercum, Amer. neurologist, 1856-1931]. A rare progressive condition with painful sub cutaneous plaques, ecchymoses, hypogona dism, and emotional instability. Seen mostly in menopausal women. The cause is un known and there is no effective treatment SYN: *adiposis dolorosa.*

dereistic (dē″rē-ĭs′tĭk) [L. *dē,* from, + *res* thing]. Pert. to overexercise of the imagina tion to the extent of ignoring reality, as seen in day dreaming. SEE: *autism.*

deric (dĕr′ĭk) [Gr. *deros,* skin]. Pert. to the skin or surface of the body. Opposed to enter ic.

derivation (dĕr″ĭ-vā′shŭn) [L. *dērivāre,* to draw off]. 1. Diversion of fluids from one part to another. 2. The formation of a substance from its source.

derivative (dē-rĭv′ă-tĭv). 1. That which is not original or fundamental. 2. Anything derived from another body or substance. 3. That which produces derivation. 4. In embryology, that which develops from a preceding structure as the derivatives of the germ layers.

derm, derma [Gr. *derma,* skin]. The cutis vera, or true skin.

dermabrasion (dĕrm′ă-brā″zhŭn) ["+ L. *abrasio,* wearing away]. A procedure for removal of acne scars or nevi on the skin by using sandpaper or another abrasive. Procedure is dangerous and should not be used indiscriminately.

Dermacentor (dĕr″mă-sĕnt′or). A genus of ticks belonging to the order Acarina, family Ixodidae.

D. andersoni. The wood tick, a species of ticks which is parasitic on man or other mammals during some part of their life cycle. May transmit causative agents of Rocky Mountain spotted fever, scrub typhus, tularemia, anaplasmosis, brucellosis, Q fever, and several forms of virus encephalomyelitis. Also causes tick paralysis.

D. variabilis. A species of ticks similar to D. andersoni. On east coast of U.S. it is the common dog tick and transmits esp. Rocky Mountain spotted fever.

der′mad [Gr. *derma,* skin, + L. *ad,* toward]. Toward the skin; externally.

dermal. Rel. to the skin or derma.

dermalaxia (dĕr″mă-lăks′ĭ-ă) [Gr. *derma,* skin, + *malaxis,* softening]. Morbid relaxation or softness of the skin.

dermalgia (dĕr-măl′jĭ-ă) ["+ *algos,* pain]. Pain in the skin.

dermametropathism (dĕr″mă-mē-trŏp′ă-thĭzm) ["+ *metron,* measure, + *pathos,* disease]. Diagnosis of skin disease by observing the markings made by drawing a blunt pencil across the skin.

dermamyiasis (dĕr-mă-mi-i'ă-sĭs) ["+ *myia,* fly, + *-iasis,* condition]. Skin disease caused by invasion of larva of dipterous insects.

dermanaplasty (dĕr-măn'ă-plăs"tĭ) [Gr. *derma,* skin, + *anaplassein,* to reform]. Skin grafting.

dermapostasis (dĕr"mă-pŏs'tă-sĭs) ["+ *apostasis,* a falling away]. Abscess formation accompanying a skin disease.

dermat-, dermato- [Gr. *dermatos*]. Prefixes indicating relationship to skin.

dermatalgia (dĕr"mă-tăl'jĭ-ă) ["+ *algos,* pain]. Paresthesia with localized pain in the skin. SYN: *dermalgia.*

dermatatrophia (dĕrm"ăt-ă-trō'fĭ-ă) ["+ *atrophia,* atrophy]. Atrophy of the skin.

dermatauxe (dĕr-mă-tŏk'sē) ["+ *auxē,* increase]. Hypertrophy of the skin.

dermatitis (dĕr"mă-ti'tis) [L. *dermatos,* skin, + *-itis,* inflammation]. Inflammation of skin evidenced by itching, redness, and various skin lesions.

ETIOL: May be due to one of several causes: skin irritants as poison ivy, corrosives, acids, and alkalies; or hypersusceptibility on part of patient to conditions which would not cause skin irritation in persons who were not hypersusceptible.

TREATMENT: Remove primary cause if due to systemic effect. If caused by local agent remove irritant by washing with soap and water. Dress with calamine lotion or bland oils or ointment.

d., actinic. Reaction of skin to sunlight or other sources of photochemical activity such as X rays or ultraviolet light.

d. aestivalis. Hot weather dermatitis.

d., allergic. Inflammation believed to be due to an allergy.

d. calorica. Inflammation due to heat or cold. Ex: sunburn.

d., cercarial. D. resulting from infestation with the cercaria of blood flukes belonging to the genus Schistosoma. SYN: *schistosome d.; swimmer's itch.*

d. congelationis. Frostbite, chilblain. SEE: *chilblain.*

d., contact. Inflammation and irritation of the skin due to contact with an irritating substance. Usually due to a combination of reduced ability of the skin to resist injury and exposure to a material in strong concentration such as soap or chemical. Some individuals are sensitive to such apparently innocuous compounds as perfumes and deodorants.

TREATMENT: Remove patient from offending material and treat skin as indicated. SYN: *d. venenata.*

d. exfoliativa. Chronic inflammation of the skin commonly involving whole surface and characterized by redness and abundant flaky desquamation.

ETIOL: Unknown.

SYM: May be primary with constitutional symptoms (fever, debility, and gastrointestinal upset), with sudden eruption, pink turning dark red, followed by thin, flaky, loosely adherent, grayish or brownish scales, tender skin, tension, and stiffness. In secondary type it follows certain scaly diseases of the skin (eczema, seborrheic d., psoriasis). Pigmentation (slate or mahogany color) is frequent.

TREATMENT: Attention to general health. Locally, soothing oily applications. Corticosteroid and antibiotic therapy.

d. gangrenosa. Skin inflammation of gangrenous form.

d. herpetiformis. Chronic inflammatory disease characterized by erythematous, papular, vesicular, bullous, or pustular lesions with tendency to grouping and with itching and burning.

ETIOL: Direct cause unknown. Occurs mostly in adult males though no age is exempt.

SYM: Slight; constitutional. Lesions develop suddenly and spread peripherally. Disease is variable and erratic and attack may be prolonged for weeks or months. Secondary infection may follow from trauma.

PROG: Amelioration of attack, but permanent relief cannot be promised.

TREATMENT: Removal of sources of reflex irritation. Soothing mixtures externally. Excoriated areas to be protected by mild antiseptics.

d. hiemalis. D. occurring in cold weather.

d. infectiosa eczematoides. Pustular eruption during or following a pyogenic disease. SYN: *Engman's disease.*

d. medicamentosa. Drug eruption.

ETIOL: Idiosyncrasy or sensitization to the drug in question. Cosmetics, arsenic (wallpaper, etc.), iodides, bromides, phenobarbital, etc., are some of the offending drugs.

SYM: With exception of bromine and iodine, the eruption is not characteristic and may resemble almost any condition or disease.

TREATMENT: Removal of cause.

d. multiformis. Form with lesions of a pustular nature.

d. papillaris capillitii. Formation on scalp and neck of surface elevations interspersed with pustules and ending in scarlike elevations resembling keloids.

d., poison ivy. D. resulting from ivy poisoning. SYN: *rhus d.* SEE: *poison ivy d.*

d., rhus. A contact dermatitis caused by substances present in certain plants. SEE: *poison ivy d.*

d. seborrheica. Acute or subacute inflammatory skin disease beginning on the scalp, characterized by rounded, irregular, or circinate lesions covered with yellowish or brownish-gray greasy scales. SYN: *alopecia furfuracea; pityriasis capitis; seborrhea corporis; seborrhea sicca.*

ETIOL: Unknown.

SYM: On the scalp it may be dry with abundant grayish branny scales, or oozing and crusted, constituting eczema capitis, and may spread to forehead and postauricular regions. On the forehead it shows scaly and infiltrated lesions with dark red bases, some itching, localized loss of hair. On eyebrows and eyelashes dry, dirty white scales, itching. On nasolabial folds or vermilion border of lips inflammation with itching. On sternal region, greasy and unctuous to the touch. May appear in interscapular, axillary, and genitocrural regions also.

TREATMENT: When limited to scalp, frequent shampooing and use of mild keratolytic agents. Selenium-containing shampoos have been helpful. Generalized seborrheic d. requires careful attention including scrupulous skin hygiene, keeping skin as dry as possible, dusting powders. Topical and systemic cortisone preparations may be required.

d. venenata. Any inflammation caused by local action of various animal, vegetable, or mineral substances on the surface of the skin. Commonly called ivy poisoning. SEE: *poison ivy d.*

ETIOL: Drugs, acids, alkalies, plants (poison ivy, oak, or sumac). Runs an acute course with recurrence on reexposure to the sensitizing agent.

SYM: Vary from simple hyperemia to gangrene and sloughing. Majority are erythematous, limited to part touched by irritant, becoming papular, vesicular, or pustular with burning or itching.

TREATMENT: Locally, apply drying solutions such as aluminum acetate. Calamine lotion is helpful in drying the lesions and for control of itching. In ivy poisoning desensitization with poison ivy extract injections may be effective. In severe cases, the use of topical and systemic cortisone may be needed.

d. verrucosa. D. characterized by the formation of wartlike nodules on the skin. These may enlarge and form papillomatous structures which sometimes ulcerate. SYN: *chromoblastomycosis,* q.v.

ETIOL: May be due to one of several fungi including Hormodendrum pedrusoi or Phialophora verrucosa.

d., x-ray. Skin inflammation due to overdose of X rays.

dermatoautoplasty   (dĕr″mă-tō-ō′tō-plăs″tĭ) [Gr. *dermatos,* skin, + *autos,* self, + *plassein,* to form]. Grafting of skin taken from some portion of the patient's own body.

Dermatobia (dĕr″mă-tō′bĭ-a) [″ + *bios,* life]. A genus of botflies belonging to the order Diptera of the family Oestridae.

D. hominis. A species of botflies, found in parts of tropical America, whose larvae infest man and cattle. The eggs are transported by mosquitoes.

dermatobiasis (dĕr″mă-tō-bī′ă-sĭs). Infestation by the larvae of Dermatobia hominis, the eggs of which are carried to the skin by mosquitoes. The larvae then hatch and bore into the skin while the mosquito feeds. Marble-like boils form at the site of infestation.

dermatocele (dĕr′mă-tō-sēl″) [Gr. *dermatos,* skin, + *kēlē,* hernia]. Tendency of hypertrophied skin and subcutaneous tissue to hang loosely in folds. SYN: *dermatolysis.*

d. lipomato′sis. A pedunculated lipoma with cystic degeneration.

dermatocelidosis (dĕr″mă-tō-sĕl″ĭ-dō′sĭs) [″ + *kēlis,* spot, + *-ōsis,* condition]. Freckles; a macular eruption. SYN: *dermatokelidosis.*

dermatocellulitis (dĕr″mă-tō-sĕl″ū-lī′tĭs) [″ + L. *cellula,* little cell, + Gr. *-itis,* inflammation]. Inflammation of subcutaneous connective tissue.

dermatoconiosis (dĕr″mă-tō-kō″nĭ-ō′sĭs) [Gr. *dermatos,* skin, + *konia,* dust]. Any irritation of the skin caused by dust, esp. one due to occupational exposure.

dermatocyst (dĕr′mă-tō-sĭst) [″ + *kystis,* cyst]. A skin cyst.

dermatodynia (dĕr″mă-tō-dīn′ĭ-ă) [″ + *odynē,* pain]. Pain in the skin; dermatalgia, q.v.

der″matofibro′ma [Gr. *dermatos,* skin, + L. *fibra,* fiber, + Gr. *-ōma,* tumor]. A skin fibroma.

dermatogen (dĕr-măt′ō-jĕn) [″ + *gennan,* to produce]. Antigen from a skin disease.

dermatogenous (dĕr″mă-tŏj′ĕn-ŭs). Producing skin or disease of skin.

dermatoglyphics (dĕr″mă-tō-glĭf′ĭks) [Gr. *dermatos,* skin, + *glyphē,* a carving]. Study of surface markings of the skin, esp. those of hands and feet. Useful in identification and genetic studies.

lermat'ograph ["+ *graphein*, to write]. 1. A device for marking the body for diagnosis. 2. A wheal made on the skin in dermatography. SYN: *dermographia*.

lermatograph'ia, dermatog'raphy. 1. A treatise on the skin. 2. A form of urticaria in which wheals are made by pressure. SYN: *dermographia*.

lermatoheteroplasty (dĕr″mă-tō-hĕt′ĕr-ō-plăs″tĭ) [Gr. *dermatos*, skin, + *heteros*, other, + *plassein*, to mold]. Skin grafting with grafts from another's skin.

lermatoid (dĕr′mă-toyd) ["+ *eidos*, form]. Resembling skin.

lermatokelidosis (dĕr″mă-tō-kĕl′ĭ-dō′sĭs) ["+ *kelidoun*, to stain]. A macular eruption; freckle.

lermatol'ogist ["+ *logos*, study]. A physician who specializes in the pathology and physiology of skin.

lermatol'ogy. The science of the skin and its diseases.

lermatolysis (dĕr″mă-tŏl′ĭ-sĭs) [Gr. *dermatos*, skin, + *lysis*, a loosening]. Tendency of hypertrophied skin and subcutaneous tissue to hang in folds. Loose skin. SYN: *cutis laxa; cutis pendula*.

lermatoma (der″mă-tō′mă) ["+ *-ōma*, tumor]. Circumscribed thickening of skin.

der'matome ["+ *tomē*, incision]. 1. Instrument for incising the skin or for cutting thin transplants of skin. 2. A segmental skin area innervated by various spinal cord segments. 3. The lateral portion of the somite of an embryo which gives rise to the dermis of the skin; the cutis plate.

dermatomere (der′mă-tō-mēr) [Gr. *dermatos*, skin, + *meros*, part]. A segment of embryonic integument.

dermatomucosomyositis (der″mă-tō-mū-ko″sō-mi-ō-si′tis) ["+ L. *mucosa*, mucus membrane, + Gr. *mys*, muscle, + *-itis*, inflammation]. Inflammation of the skin, involving mucosa and muscles.

dermatomycosis (dĕr″mă-tō-mĭ-kō′sĭs) ["+ *mykes*, fungus, + *-ōsis*, condition]. (pl. *dermatomycoses*) A skin infection caused by certain fungi of the genera Trichophyton, Epidermophyton, and Microsporum.

der″matomyo'ma [Gr. *dermatos*, skin, + *mys*, muscle, + *-ōma*, tumor]. Myoma of the skin.

dermatomyositis (dĕr″mă-tō-mĭ″ō-sĭ′tĭs) ["+ "+ *-itis*, inflammation]. A disease of connective tissue, q.v. An acute, subacute, or chronic disease of unknown etiology. Char-

acterized by edema, dermatitis, and inflammation of the muscles.

SYM: Fever, malaise, general weakness, weakness of the pelvic and shoulder girdle muscles; skin and mucosal lesions often present. About one third of patients will have esophageal weakness.

TREATMENT: Symptomatic: bed rest, physiotherapy, salicylates. Adrenal cortical steroids are helpful in most cases.

NP: Rest in bed with skillful turning is essential. Mouth lesions should be irrigated frequently with saline solution. Hot baths and heat applications help stiffness. Avoid fatigue and chilling. Massage, graduated exercise, and resistance exercises are helpful in preventing or treating muscular atrophy and contractures.

dermatoneuro'sis [Gr. *dermatos*, skin, + *neuron*, nerve. + *-ōsis*, condition]. Skin disease of nervous origin. SEE: *neurodermatitis*.

dermatopath'ia ["+ *pathos*, disease]. Any disease of the skin.

dermatopathol'ogy ["+ "+ *logos*, study]. Study of diseases of the skin.

dermatop'athy. Any skin disease. SYN: *dermatopathia*.

dermatopho'bia [Gr. *dermatos*, skin, + *phobos*, fear]. Abnormal fear of having a skin disease.

dermatophylaxis (dĕr″mă-tō-fĭ-lăks′ĭs) ["+ *phylaxis*, protection]. Protecting the skin from infection.

dermatophyte (dĕr′mă-tō-fit) ["+ *phyton*, plant]. A plant parasite which grows in or on the skin. They rarely penetrate deeper than the epidermis or its derivatives, hair, and nails. They cause such skin diseases as favus, tinea, ringworm, eczema, and erythrasma. Important dermatophytes include the genera Microsporum, Trichopyton, and Epidermophyton. All are fungi.

dermatophytid (dĕr′mă-tōf′ĭ-tĭd). A toxic rash or eruption occurring in dermatomycosis.

dermatophytosis (dĕr″mă-tō-fĭ-tō′sĭs) [Gr. *dermatos*, skin, + *phyton*, plant, + *-ōsis*, condition]. A fungus infection of the skin of the hands and feet, esp. between the toes. SYN: *athlete's foot; ringworm of feet; tinea pedis*.

dermatoplas'tic ["+ *plassein*, to form]. Pert. to skin grafting.

dermatoplasty (dĕr′mă-tō-plăs″tĭ). Transplanting living skin to cover cutaneous defects caused by injury, operation, or disease. Any restoring operation on the skin.

NP: These wounds are sometimes dressed with a light compress of sterilized gauze, saturated with a warm physiologic saline solution. Great care must be taken in adjusting bandage; if too much pressure is put on grafts they will die because of lack of vascularity.

dermatorrhagia (dĕr″mă-tō-rā′jĭ-ă) [Gr. *dermatos*, skin, + *rhegnynai*, to burst forth]. Hemorrhage into or from the skin.

dermatorrhea (dĕr″mă-tō-rē′ă) [″+ *rhoia*, flow]. Excessive secretion of sebaceous glands.

dermatosclerosis (dĕr″mă-tō-sklĕr-ō′sĭs) [″+ *sklērōsis*, hardening]. Scleroderma, q.v.

dermatoscopy (dĕr″mă-tōs′kŏ-pĭ) [Gr. *dermatos*, skin, + *skopein*, to examine]. Examination of the skin with a high powered lens or microscope.

dermatosiophobe (dĕr″mă-tō′sĭ-ō-fōb) [″+ *-ōsis*, condition, + *phobos*, fear]. One having a morbid fear of acquiring a skin disease.

dermatosiophobia (dĕr″mă-to″sĭ-ō-fō′bĭ-ă). Dread of skin disease.

dermatosis (dĕr″mă-tō′sĭs) [Gr. *derma*, skin, + *-ōsis*, condition]. (pl. *dermatoses*) Any disease of the skin in which inflammation is not necessarily a feature. Not a synonym for dermatitis.

　　d. papulosa nigra. Eruption consisting of many tiny tumors on skin of face.

　　d., progressive pigmentary. Reddish papules principally on legs; eruption is progressive. SYN: *Schamberg's disease.*

dermatosome (dĕr′mă-tō-sōm) [Gr. *dermatos*, skin, + *sōma*, body]. Section of equatorial plate in mitosis.

dermatother′apy [″+ *therapeia*, treatment]. Treatment of skin diseases.

dermatothlasia (dĕr″mă-tō thlă′zĭ-ă) [″+ *thlasis*, a bruising]. An uncontrollable tic or impetus to bruise, rub, or pinch the skin.

dermatotome (dĕr′mă-tō-tōm″) [″+ *tomē*, incision]. 1. One of the fetal skin segments. 2. A knife for incising the skin or small lesions.

dermatotropic (dĕr″mă-tō-trōp′ĭk) [Gr. *dermatos*, skin, *tropē*, a turning]. Acting esp. on the skin.

dermatoxerasia (dĕr″mă-tō zē-rā′zĭ-ă) [″+ *xērasia*, dryness]. Roughening of skin SYN: *xeroderma.*

dermatozo′on [″+ *zōon*, animal]. Animal parasite of the skin.

dermatrophia (dĕr-mă-trō′fĭ-ă) [″+ *atrophia*, atrophy]. Atrophy of the skin.

dermic (dĕr′mĭk) [Gr. *derma*, skin]. Pert. to the skin.

dermis (dĕr′mĭs) [L.]. The skin; cutis vera or true skin. SYN: *corium* [NA].

dermi′tis [″+ *-itis*, inflammation]. Inflammation of skin. SYN: *dermatitis.*

der′moblast [″+ *blastos*, germ]. Part of mesoblastic layer, developing into the corium.

dermographia, dermography (dĕr-mō-graf′ĭ-ă, -mog′ră-fĭ) [″+ *graphein*, to write] The appearance of elevated red marks on the skin as the result of pressure or stroking its surface.

dermoid (dĕr′moyd) [Gr. *derma*, skin, + *eidos*, form]. 1. Resembling the skin. 2. A dermoid cyst.

　　d. cyst. A nonmalignant cystic tumor in which are found elements derived from the ectoderm, such as hair, teeth, or skin. These tumors occur frequently in the ovary but may develop in other organs such as the lungs. 2. An ovarian teratoma.

dermoidectomy (dĕr″moyd-ĕk′tō-mĭ) [″+ *ektomē*, excision]. Excision of a dermoid cyst.

dermolysis (dĕr-mōl′ĭ-sĭs) [″+ *lysis*, loosening]. A rare destructive disease of the skin

dermomycosis (dĕr″mō-mĭ-kō′sĭs) [″+ *mykēs*, fungus, + *-ōsis*, condition]. A skin disease produced by a vegetable parasite SYN: *dermatomycosis.*

dermonosology (dĕr″mō-nō-sōl′ō-jĭ) [Gr. *derma*, skin, + *nosos*, disease, + *logos*, study]. The classification of skin affections

dermopathy (dĕr-mōp′ă-thĭ) [″+ *pathos*, disease]. Any skin disease.

dermophlebitis (dĕr″mō-flĕ-bī′tĭs) [″+ *phleps*, vein, + *-itis*, inflammation]. Inflammation of superficial veins and surrounding skin.

dermophylax′is [″+ *phylax*, protection] The protective function of the skin in warding off infections. SYN: *dermatophylaxis.*

dermophyte (dĕr′mō-fīt) [Gr. *derma*, skin, + *phyton*, plant]. A vegetable skin parasite SYN: *dermatophyte.*

dermoskel′eton (″+ *skeleton*, skeleton) The exoskeleton, q.v. The remnants in man are seen in the hair, nails, and teeth.

dermostenosis (dĕr′mō-stĕn-ō′sĭs) [″+ *stenōsis*, narrowing]. A tightening of the skin SEE: *scleroderma.*

dermosynovitis (dĕr′mō-sĭn-ō-vī′tĭs) [″+ *syn*, together, + L. *ovum*, egg, + Gr. *-itis*, inflammation]. Inflammation of the synovial sheaths and the adjacent skin.

dermosyphilopathy (dĕr″mō-sĭf′ĭ-lōp′ă-thĭ) [″+ ″+ *philein*, to love, + *pathos*, disease]. Any syphilitic disease of the skin.

dermotropic (dĕr″mō-trōp′ĭk) [Gr. *derma*, skin, + *tropē*, a turning]. Acting esp. on the skin.

dermovac′cine [″+ L. *vaccinus*, pert. to a cow]. A vaccine obtained by scraping the skin lesion produced by inoculation of the skin with a virus.

Ierodidymus (dĕr″ō-dĭd′ĭ-mŭs) [Gr. *derē*, neck, + *didymos*, double]. A malformed fetus with two necks and heads but a single body and normal limbs. SYN: *dicephalus*.

Iesalination. Partial or complete removal of salts from seawater or brackish water so that it is suitable for agriculture or household purposes.

Iesatura′tion [L. *dē*, from, + *saturāre*, to fill]. A process whereby a saturated organic compound is converted into an unsaturated one, as when stearic acid, $CH_3.(CH_2)_{16}$-.COOH, is changed into oleic acid, $C_{17}H_{33}$-.COOH. The product has different physical and chemical properties after this transformation.

Desault′s appara′tus (dĕ-sō′). [Pierre J. Desault, Fr. surgeon, 1744-95] Bandage used for fracture of clavicle. SYN: *Desault's bandage*. SEE: *bandage*.

Descemet′s membrane (dĕs-ĕ-mā′). [Jean Descemet, Fr. anatomist, 1732-1810]. A fine membrane between the endothelial layer of the cornea and the substantia propia; lamina elastica posterior.

descemetitis (dĕs″ĕ-mĕ-tī′tis). Inflammation of Descemet's membrane on the corneal posterior surface; serous cyclitis.

descemetocele (dĕs″ĕ-mĕt′ō-sēl). Protrusion of Descemet's membrane.

descendens (de-sen′dens) [L. *dē*, from, + *scandere*, to climb]. Descending; a descending structure.

    d. hypoglossi. A branch of the hypoglossal nerve given off at the point where it curves around the occipital artery, which passes down obliquely across the sheath of the carotid vessels (sometimes within it) to form a loop just below the middle of the neck with branches of the 2nd and 3rd cervical nerves. SYN: *d. noni.*

descensus (de-sen′sus) [L., a falling]. Falling, descent. SYN: *ptosis.*

    d. testis. Passage of the testicle down into the scrotum. SYN: *migration of testicle.*

    d. uteri. Defective pelvic floor allowing the uterus or part of the uterus to protrude out of the vagina. SYN: *prolapse of uterus; prolapsus uteri; procidentia.*

    VARIETIES: First Degree: Where the cervix uteri reaches down to the vaginal introitus. Second Degree: Where the cervix uteri protrudes out of the vagina. Third Degree: Where the entire uterus lies outside of the vagina. This is the condition known as procidentia uteri.

    ETIOL: This condition may be congenital or acquired, although it is most usually acquired. The etiological factors are congenital weakness of the uterine supports and injury to the pelvic floor or uterine supports during childbirth.

    SYM: The condition is most often seen following instrumental deliveries or where the patient has been allowed to bear down before the cervix is fully dilated. Frequently associated with this is a prolapsus of the anterior and posterior vaginal walls, as seen in cystocele and rectocele. In the early stages there are dragging sensations in the lower abdomen, backache while standing and on exertion, sensation of weight and bearing down in the perineum, frequency of urination and incontinence of urine in cases associated with cystocele. In the later stages a protrusion or a swelling at the vulva is noticed on standing or straining, and leukorrhea is present. In procidentia there is frequently pain on walking, inability to urinate unless the mass is reduced, and quite commonly cystitis.

    TREATMENT: The treatment depends upon the age of the patient, the degree of prolapsus, and the associated pathology. Where conservation is desired the use of the pessary is clearly indicated, or conservative surgery (round ligament shortening and pelvic floor repair) may be practiced. In the elderly patient where the uterus is pathological, a hysterectomy (abdominal or vaginal) accompanied by vaginal plastic procedure is indicated.

    d. ventriculi. Downward displacement of the stomach. SYN: *gastroptosis.*

desensitiza′tion. 1. Term applied to the condition when sensitized animals on recovering from an anaphylactic shock do not react to a subsequent injection of the antigen within a reasonable period. 2. Loss of sensitivity.

desen′sitize [L. *dē*, from, + *sentire*, to perceive]. 1. To deprive of or lessen sensitivity by nerve section or blocking. 2. To abate anaphylactic sensitiveness by administration of the specific antigen in low dosage.

desexualize (dē-seks′ū-al-īz) ["+ *sexus*, sex]. To castrate; to remove testicles or ovaries.

deshydremia (dĕs-hī-drē′mĭ-ă) ["+ Gr. *hydōr*, water, + *haima*, blood]. Diminished fluid content of the blood.

desiccant (des′ĭ-kant). Causing desiccation or dryness.

desiccate (des′ĭ-kāt) [L. *desiccāre*, to dry up]. To dry.

desiccation (des′ĭ-ka′shun). The process of drying up. SEE: *electrodesiccation.*

    d., electric. Electric therapy to cure a lesion.

desiccative (dĕs′ĭ-kā″tĭv). Causing to dry up.

desmalgia (dĕz-măl′jĭ-ă) [Gr. *desmos*, band, + *algos*, pain]. Pain in a ligament.

desmectasia, desmectasis (dĕs-mĕk-tā′zĭ-ă, -tā-sĭs) [″+ *ektasis*, dilatation]. Stretching of a ligament.

desmepithelium (dĕs-mĕp-ĭ-thē′lĭ-ŭm) [″+ *epi*, upon, + *thēlē*, nipple]. The epithelial lining of vessels and synovial cavities.

desmitis (dĕs-mī′tĭs) [″+ *-itis*, inflammation]. Inflammation of a ligament.

desmo- [Gr. *desmos*]. Prefix indicating a bond, a ligament.

desmocyte (dĕs′mō-sīt) [Gr. *desmos*, band, + *kytos*, cell]. A supporting tissue cell. SYN: *fibroblast; fibrocyte.*

desmocytoma (dĕs″mō-sī-tō′mă) [″+ ″+ *ōma*, tumor]. A tumor formed of desmocytes; a sarcoma.

desmodyn′ia [″+ *odynē*, pain]. Pain in a ligament.

desmo′enzyme. An enzyme that is bound to the protoplasm of cells and is difficult to extract, in contrast to lyoenzymes which can be extracted readily. Desmoenzymes are important in metabolic reactions involving the release of energy.

desmogenous (dĕs-mōj′ĕ-nŭs) [Gr. *desmos*, band, + *gennan*, to produce]. Of connective tissue origin.

desmography (dĕs-mŏg′ră-fĭ) [″+ *graphein*, to write]. A description of or treatise on ligaments.

desmoid (dĕs′moyd) [″+ *eidos*, form]. 1. Tendonlike; fibroid. 2. A very tough and firm fibroma.

desmology (dĕs-mŏl′ō-jĭ) [Gr. *desmos*, band, + *logos*, science]. Science of tendons and ligaments.

desmo′ma [″+ *-ōma*, tumor]. A tumor of the connective tissue.

desmoneoplasm (dĕs″mō-nē′ō-plăzm) [″+ *neos*, new, + *plasma*, matter]. A connective tissue tumor.

desmopathy (dĕs-mŏp′ă-thĭ) [Gr. *desmos*, band, + *pathos*, disease]. Any disease affecting ligaments.

desmopexia (dĕs″mō-pĕks′ĭ-ă) [″+ *pēxis*, fixation]. Fixation of round ligaments for the abdominal wall for the correction of uterine displacement.

desmoplas′tic [″+ *plassein*, to form]. Causing or forming adhesions.

desmopyknosis (dĕs″mō-pĭk-nō′sĭs) [Gr. *desmos*, band, + *pyknosis*, condensation]. Surgical procedure for shortening of round ligaments by attaching them by loops to the anterior uterine wall. SYN: *Dudley's operation.*

desmorrhexis (dĕs-mō-rĕks′ĭs) [″+ *rhēxis*, rupture]. Rupture of a ligament.

desmosis (dĕs-mō′sĭs) [″+ *-ōsis*, condition]. Any disease of the connective tissue.

desmosome (dĕs′mō-sōm) [Gr. *desmo*, band, + *sōma*, body]. A small thickening i an intercellular bridge.

desmotomy (dĕs-mŏt′ō-mĭ) [″+ *tomē*, incision]. Dissection of ligament.

desoxy-. Prefix meaning deoxidized or a reduced form of. SEE: words beginning wit *deoxy-.*

desoxycorticosterone (dĕs-ŏk″sĭ-kŏr-tĭ-kōs′tĕr-ōn). An active steroid hormone produced by the adrenal cortex. It plays an important role in the regulation of water an salt metabolism.

d. acetate. USP. An acetate ester c desoxycorticosterone and the form in which the hormone is usually administered in it therapeutic use. It may be injected in tramuscularly or used buccally.

desoxyribonucleic acid (dĕs″ŏk-sĭ-rīb″ō nū′klē-ĭk). Former spelling for deoxyribonu cleic acid, q.v.

despumation (dĕs″pū-mā′shŭn) [L. *dē*, from + *spuma*, froth]. Separation of froth or scun from a liquid.

desquamate (dĕs′kwă-māt) [L. *dēsquāmāre* to remove scales.]. To shred or scale off the surface epithelium.

desquamation (dĕs″kwă-mā′shŭn). Shed ding of the epidermis.

d., furfuraceous. Shedding of branlike scales.

desquamative (dĕs-kwŏm′ă-tĭv). Of the na ture of desquamation, or pert. to or causing it.

destructive [L. *dēstructus*, destroyed]. Caus ing ruin or destruction. Opposed to construc tive.

d. lesion. A pathological change such as an infection, tumor, or injury which causes the death of tissue or an organ.

desudation (dē-sū-dā′shŭn) [L. *dē*, from, + *sudāre*, to perspire]. Excessive sweating oft en followed by slight pustular eruption.

desynchronosis (dē-sĭn″krō-nō′sĭs) [″+ Gr *synkhronos*, same time]. The time difference between that of a person's present location and that to which he is accustomed. This causes an upset of the individual's internal biological clock. Occurs in traveling.

det. Abbr. for L. *detur*, let it be given.

detach′ment [O.Fr. *destachier*, to unfasten] To become separate.

d., retinal. The pathological condition where the retina or a part of it becomes sepa rated from the choroid.

detec'tor [L. *dētectus*, uncovered]. Device for determining the presence of something.

d., lie. A device which, by indicating changes in pulse rate and force and electrical property of the skin, may be useful in indicating when a person is telling a lie.

detelectasis (dē-těl-ěk'tǎ-sĭs) [L. *dē*, from, + *ektasis*, dilatation]. Lack of normal inflation; collapse of an organ.

deter'gent [L. *dētergēre*, to cleanse]. 1. A medicine that purges or cleanses; cleansing. 2. A cleaning or wetting agent prepared synthetically from higher alcohols, sulfuric acid, and caustic soda.

deteriora'tion [L. *dēteriōrāre*, to deteriorate]. Retrogression; said of impairment of mental or physical functions.

determina'tion [L. *determinātus*, limiting]. 1. A tendency in a definite direction, as of blood to a part. 2. A quantitative analysis.

determinism (dē-term'ĭn-ĭzm) ["+ Gr. *ismos*, condition of]. The theory that all human action is the result of predetermined and inevitable physical, psychological, or environmental conditions which are uninfluenced by the will of the individual.

deter'sive [L. *dētergēre*, to cleanse]. Detergent; cleansing or purging.

dethyroidism (dē-thī'royd-ĭzm) [L. *dē*, from, + Gr. *thyreoeides*, like a shield]. Condition resulting from removal of the thyroid.

dethyroidized (dē-thī'royd-īzd). Without a thyroid gland.

det. in dup. Abbr. for L. *detur in duplo*, let twice as much be given.

detonation (dět'n-ā'shŭn) [L. *dētonāre*, to thunder loudly]. A violent noise caused by an explosive combustion.

detoxicate (dē-tŏk'sĭ-kāt) [L. *dē*, from + Gr. *toxikon*, poison]. To remove the toxic principle of a substance. SYN: *detoxify*.

detoxification [L. *dē*, from, + Gr. *toxikon*, poison, + L. *facere*, to make]. Reduction of the toxic properties of a poisonous or toxic substance.

detoxify (dē-tŏks'ĭ-fī). To remove the toxic quality of a substance. SYN: *detoxicate*.

detrition (dē-trĭsh'ŭn) [ML. *dētritiō*]. The wearing away of a part, esp. through friction, as that of the teeth.

detritus (dē-trī'tŭs) [L., wearing away]. Any broken down or degenerative tissue or carious matter.

detruncation (dē''trŭn-kā'shŭn) [L. *dē*, from, + *truncus*, trunk]. Decapitation, esp. of a fetus. SYN: *decollation*.

detrusor urinae (dē-trū'sōr-ū-rī'nē) [L.]. External longitudinal layer of muscular coat of bladder.

detumescence (dē''tū-měs'ěns) [L. *dē*, down, + *tumescere*, to swell]. 1. Subsidence of a swelling. 2. Subsidence of erectile tissue of genital organs (penis and clitoris) following erection.

deutencephalon (dūt-ěn-sěf'ǎ-lŏn) [Gr. *deuteros*, second, + *enkephalos*, brain]. The interbrain. SYN: *diencephalon; thalamencephalon*.

deuteranopia, deuteranopsia (dū''těr-ăn-ō'pǐ-ă, -ŏp'sǐ-ă) ["+ *anopia*, blindness]. Green blindness, so named because green is the 2nd of the primary colors. SEE: *protanopia; tritanopia*.

deuterium (dū-tē'rǐ-ŭm) [Gr. *deuteros*, second]. SYMB: H²; D. Heavy hydrogen; the mass two isotope of hydrogen.

d. oxide. Heavy water. SEE: *water, heavy*.

deutero-, deuter-, deuto- [Gr. *deuteros*, second]. Prefix indicating second or secondary.

deutero-albumose (dū''těr-ō-ăl'bū'mōs) ["+ L. *albumen*, white of egg]. An albumose formed by hydrolyzing and splitting a protein molecule and precipitating it by strong salt solutions.

deuteroelastose (dū''těr-ō-ē-lăs'tōs) ["+ L. *elasticus*, elastic]. A deutero-albumose formed in the peptic digestion of elastin.

deuteromyosinose (dū''těr-ō-mī-ŏs'ĭn-ōs). A product of myosin digestion.

deuteron (dū'těr-ŏn). SYMB: d. The nucleus of deuterium or heavy hydrogen. SYN: *deuton*.

deuteropathi'a, deuterop'athy [Gr. *deuteros*, second, + *pathos*, disease]. A disease associated with or secondary to another disease.

deu'teroplasm ["+ *plasma*, matter]. The reserve food supply in the yolk or ovum. SYN: *deutoplasm*.

deutoscolex (dū''tō-skō'lěks) ["+ *skōlēx*, worm]. Secondary daughter cysts which develop on the inner wall of a hydatid cyst.

devasation (dē-văs-ā'shŭn) [L. *dē*, from, + *vasa*, vessel]. Destruction of blood vessels.

devascularization (dē-văs''kū-lăr-ĭ-zā'shŭn) ["+ *vascularis*, pert. to a vessel]. 1. Loss or draining of blood from a part. 2. To decrease the blood supply to a part of the body.

devel'opment [O.Fr. *desveloper*, to unwrap]. Growth to full size or maturity; i.e., progress of an egg to the adult state. SYN: *evolution*.

RS: aplasia; apposition; chorista; dysplasia.

devel''opmen'tal. Pert. to development.

deviate (dē'vĭ-āt") [L. *dē*, from, + *via*, way]. 1. To move steadily away from a designated norm. 2. An individual whose attitude or behavior differs from the norm. SYN: *deviant.*

deviation (dē-vĭ-ā'shŭn). Going out of the way; departure from normal.

    d., axis. A change in the direction of the major electrical axis of the heart as determined by the electrocardiogram.

    d., conjugate. D. of face and eyes to the same side in paralytics.

    d., minimum. The smallest deviation that a prism can produce.

    d., standard. In statistics, the measure of variability of any frequency curve.

deviometer (dē"vĭ-ŏm'ē-tĕr) [L. *dē*, from, + *via*, way, + Gr. *metron*, measure]. Device for estimating degree of strabismus.

devisceration (dē-vĭs"ēr-ā'shŭn) ["+ *viscus*, internal organ]. Removal of viscera. SYN: *evisceration.*

devitaliza'tion ["+ *vita*, life]. 1. Destruction or loss of vitality. 2. Anesthetizing sensitive pulp of a tooth; known as killing the nerve.

devolution (dĕv"ō-lū'shŭn) [L. *dēvolvere*, to roll down]. Catabolism, q.v.; degeneration, q.v. Opposed to evolution.

dew cure. Walking with bare feet in grass wet with dew. A form of hydrotherapy. SYN: *kneippism.*

dew point. Temperature at which dew begins to form.

dexter (dĕks'tĕr) [L.]. On the right side.

dextrad (dĕks'trăd) [L. *dexter*, right, + *ad*, toward]. Toward the right side.

dextral (dĕks'trăl). Pert. to the right side.

dextran (dĕks'trĕn) [L. *dexter*, right]. $C_6H_{10}O_5$. A monodextrin, it is used as a substitute for blood plasma in severe burns and shock.

dextrase (dĕks'trās). An enzyme that splits dextrose and converts it into lactic acid.

dextrin (dĕks'trĭn) [L. *dexter*, right]. A yellowish-white powder which forms mucilaginous solutions in water and can be prepared by the action of heat or acid on starch.

    It is a carbohydrate of the formula $(C_6H_{10}O_5)_n$. In digestion it is a soluble or gummy matter into which starch is converted by diastase; it is the result of the first chemical change in the digestion of starch.

dextrinuria (dĕks"trĭn-ū'rĭ-ă) ["+ Gr. *ouron*, urine]. Dextrin in the urine.

dextro- [L. *dexter*, right]. Prefix indicating to the right.

dextroamphetamine sulfate (dĕks"trō-ăm-fĕt'ă-mēn sul'făt). USP. A compound related to amphetamine sulfate (i.e., an isomer of amphetamine). Sometimes written d-amphetamine sulfate or dextro-amphetamine sulfate.

    Used as a central nervous system stimulant in treatment of mild depression. The long-term value of this substance to control appetite in treating obesity is questionable.

dextrocardia (dĕks"trō-kăr'dĭ-ă) [L. *dexter*, right, + Gr. *kardia*, heart]. Having the heart on the right side of the body.

dextrocar'diogram ("+ "+ *gramma*, a writing). A cardiogram representing action of the right ventricle.

dextrocular (dĕks-trŏk'ū-lăr) ["+ *oculus*, eye]. Having a stronger right eye than left.

dextrocularity (dĕks"trŏk-ū-lăr'ĭ-tĭ). The condition of having the right eye stronger than the left.

dextroduc'tion [L. *dexter*, right, + *ducere*, to lead]. The movement of visual axis to the right.

dextrogas'tria ("+ Gr. *gastēr*, belly). Having the stomach on right side of body.

dextrogyrate (dĕks"trō-jĭ'rāt) ["+ *gyrare*, to turn]. To turn to the right. Bending of light rays to the right.

dextrogyre (dĕks'trō-jīr). A substance turning to the right.

dextroman'ual [L. *dexter*, right, + *manus*, hand]. Righthanded.

dextropedal (dĕks-trŏp'ē-dăl) ["+ *pēs, ped-*, foot]. Having greater dexterity in using the right leg than the left one.

dextropho'bia ["+ Gr. *phobos*, fear]. Abnormal aversion to objects on right side of body.

dextrorotatory (dĕks"trō-rō'tă-tor-ĭ) ["+ *rotāre*, to turn]. Turning rays of light to the right.

dextrose (dĕks'trōs). A simple sugar of the monosaccharose group; also known as glucose or grape sugar. Dextrose (USP) is $C_6H_{12}O_6$, a crystalline solid which can be made by the action of acids on starches.

    It is very soluble in water, is an important constituent of corn syrup and honey, and is an example of one kind of carbohydrate, q.v. The most important of the monosaccharide group. It is usually associated with levulose. Its presence in the urine in large amounts is most probably due to diabetes. However, its presence may be indicated also in brain injuries, cirrhosis of the liver, normal pregnancies, and as a result of the administration of epinephrine or thyroxin. It is formed in the digestive tract by the action of enzymes on carbohydrates. It occurs naturally in plants and in the body fluids of animals.

    NP: A 5% solution of glucose in sterile pyrogen-free water solution is used for rectal, intravenous, or subcutaneous injection.

RS: diabetes; glycosuria; hyperglycemia; hypoglycemia; monosaccharoses.

dextrosinistral (dĕks″trō-sĭn′ĭs-trăl) [L. *dexter*, right, + *sinister*, left]. From right to left.

dextrosuria (dĕks-trō-sū′rĭ-ă). Dextrose in the urine.

dextrotropic, dextrotropous (dĕks″trō-trop′ik, -trō′pŭs) [L. *dexter*, right, + Gr. *tropos*, a turning]. Turning to the right.

dextrover′sion ["+ *vertere*, to turn]. Turned toward the right.

dezymotize (dē-zī′mō-tiz) [L. *dē*, from, + Gr. *zymē*, leaven]. To free of ferments or germs.

dg. Abbr. for *decigram*.

dhobie itch (dō′bē) [Hindi, laundryboy]. Tropical name for form of Tinea cruris which is more intense than that observed in temperate zones.

di- [Gr. *dis*, twice]. Prefix indicating twice, double, or two.

diabetes (dī″ă-be′tēz) [Gr. *diabetes*, passing through]. SEE: *d. mellitus*.

    d., brittle. Diabetic condition which is difficult to regulate. Occurs in approx. 15% of cases of d. mellitus. Many of these patients developed their condition prior to age 15. SYN: *unstable d.*

    d., bronze. Hemochromatosis. A disease of metabolism characterized by deposition of pigment in various organs of the body, cirrhosis of the liver and pancreas, and diabetes.

    d. insipidus. Polyuria and polydipsia caused by inadequate secretion of vasopressin, the antidiuretic hormone, by the neurohypophysis (main portion of the posterior lobe of the pituitary gland). More common in the young.

    SYM: Urine output of 5-10 liters/24 hours is common. Sp. gr. usually 1.001-1.005 and free of sugar and albumin. Thirst, weakness, dry skin.

    ETIOL: In almost half of all cases, the cause is unknown. Trauma to the head which causes damage to the pituitary or a tumor in that area causes the remainder of cases.

    PROG: Essentially chronic.

    TREATMENT: Eradication of causative factor if determined. When not due to specific injury of the pituitary, the disease is easily controlled by use of vasopressin replacement therapy. This may be given by injection or nasal spray.

    d., juvenile-onset. D. which has its onset prior to the age of 15 years. This form usually is quite difficult to regulate.

    d. melli′tus. A disorder of carbohydrate metabolism, characterized by hyperglycemia and glycosuria and resulting from inadequate production or utilization of insulin.

    ETIOL: Basic cause is still unknown but direct cause is failure of beta cells of the pancreas to secrete an adequate amount of insulin. In most instances d. mellitus is due to a genetic disorder, but may be due to a deficiency of beta cells caused by inflammation, malignant invasion of the pancreas, or the result of surgery. In the absence of insulin, glycogenesis and glycolysis are adversely affected. It is currently thought that insulin acts primarily at the cell membrane facilitating transport of glucose into cells.

    SYM: Principal symptoms are elevated blood sugar (hyperglycemia), sugar in urine (glycosuria), excessive urine production (polyuria), excessive thirst (polydipsia), and increase in food intake (polyphagia).

    Urine sp. gr. 1.020-40; sugar excessive; urine shows diacetic acid, betaoxybutyric acid, acetone when disease process is in advanced stage. More common in women and after the age of 40. Increased thirst; frequent urination, 3-10 qt. a day; itching, frequently about the genitals. Fasting blood sugar raised above normal range of 90-120 mg./100 cc. (ml.) of blood; boils and carbuncles. Loss of weight; emaciation; weakness; and debility. When severe diabetes is allowed to progress without proper treatment, coma ensues with weakness and sweet odor of breath; nausea, headache, vomiting, dyspnea, sense of intoxication, delirium, deep coma, resulting in death.

    COMPLICATIONS: Diabetic acidosis due to excessive production of ketone bodies; low resistance to infections, esp. those involving extemities; increase in incidence of toxemia in pregnancy and cardiovascular disorders; disturbances in electrolyte balance; eye disorders.

    PROG: Diabetes is a chronic, incurable disease but symptoms can be ameliorated and life prolonged by modern treatment. The isolation and eventual production of insulin in 1921 by Doctors Banting and Best made it possible to allow persons with this disease to lead a normal life.

    TREATMENT: Consists of diet, insulin, and exercise. At first the patient should be placed on well-balanced diet adequate in all basic essentials: carbohydrates, proteins, fats, vitamins, minerals, and fluids. In many patients this may be all that is required. It is important that obese persons with this disease be placed on a diet which will enable them to lose weight. Control of diabetes is much more difficult in an obese person. Blood sugar determinations should be made at frequent intervals. *NOTE:* Blood sugar and glucose are considered to be the same.

When a patient is given an adequate diet and the glucose still appears in the urine, insulin may be necessary. Its use is not required in every case and may be dangerous if not properly given. In the last several years certain drugs have been given by mouth for the control of mild cases of diabetes. These have been used with success mostly in middle-aged and older patients.

Diet: Standardization of patients—a balanced diet of approximately 1000-1200 cal. may be prescribed. This should be increased promptly if levels of glucose in the blood are brought within normal limits. The age, weight, and type of work or physical activity in which the patient is engaged is important in planning a diet. Standardized diets have been worked out in which the necessary proportions of carbohydrates, proteins, and fats are outlined. The diets vary from 1200-3000 cal. Frequent feedings (5-6/24 hours) rather than the standard three meals is preferred. The older the patient, as a rule, the smaller the proportion of fat in the diet.

NP: Nursing care of the patient with diabetes includes general hygienic care, giving insulin, collecting specimens, preventing and treating complications, serving the prescribed diet, and teaching the patient how to take care of himself.

General hygienic care: Care of the skin and feet. The skin must be kept scrupulously clean. Daily warm baths are essential. Irritation or bruises should be promptly attended to because any break in the skin heals with difficulty, and diabetics are susceptible to bedsores, infection, and gangrene.

Because of poor circulation, feet should have special care, being kept clean and dry, esp. between the toes. Care should be taken in trimming the toenails as the slightest abrasion of the skin may become infected. Olive oil or lanolin to keep the feet soft and smooth. Tight shoes must be avoided. Also because of poor circulation, it is dangerous to apply local heat to legs and feet; to do so could lead to gangrene.

Care of the mouth and teeth is most important. The teeth should be brushed well at least three times a day and a mouthwash should be used before and after eating. The patient should be encouraged to see his dentist regularly.

Regular bowel movements are important. Diarrhea is more frequent than constipation.

Administration of Insulin: The dosage and frequency in which insulin is given will depend on the individual patient and the physician prescribing it. In administering the drug, precautions necessary in giving hypodermic injections should be observed and care taken not to inject the drug repeatedly in the same area. Trauma should be avoided. Every diabetic patient should be taught to give himself insulin or if he is unable to give it to himself, some member of the family should be instructed.

Collecting Specimens: Both single and 24-hour urine specimens may be collected. Usually they are examined daily. It is especially important that specimens are accurately collected and labeled, and sent to the laboratory on time. Diagnosis and treatment are based mostly upon the results of urine examination. Specimens of blood may be collected by the physician for blood chemistry. The specimen is taken early in the morning before the patient has his breakfast.

Prevention of Complications: Close observation of the patient is necessary. Shock may be avoided if the patient is closely watched or if the patient has been taught that when he has the slightest symptom of insulin reaction to call the nurse. He may be instructed to eat a lump or two of sugar or to keep a piece of hard candy within his reach.

Acidosis and coma also may be prevented by the recognition of first symptoms and prompt treatment. The chief symptoms of acidosis are pain in the abdomen; nausea; vomiting; drowsiness; and difficult breathing. The doctor should be notified when the first symptoms appear. The patient kept warm with blankets but not hot water bottles or electric blankets. He should not be left alone. His pulse should be closely watched.

Teaching the Patient: Probably there is no other disease in which it is as important that the patient be taught all the factors involved in the management and treatment. The patient should understand that he will have to continue treatment all his life and that he must abide strictly by everything taught him in the hospital.

His mouth and teeth should be kept in good condition; it is necessary to pay particular attention to his feet; his diet must be followed. He should also understand the complications that may arise and the measures he may take to prevent them. He is taught to take his insulin and examine his urine. He should be taught importance of reporting to physician for frequent checkups. SEE: *coma, diabetic.*

d., pancreatic. D. associated with disease of the pancreas.

d., phlorizin. Glycosuria caused by administration of phlorizin.

d., renal. Renal glycosuria; condition characterized by a low renal threshold for sugar. Glucose tolerance is normal and diabetic symptoms are lacking.

d., true. D. mellitus, q.v.

diabetic (di-ă-bĕt′ĭk). Pert. to diabetes.

d. center. Area in the floor of the fourth ventricle.

d. coma. Loss of consiousness due to severe diabetes mellitus which has not been treated or to treatment which has not been adequately regulated.

d. ear. Otitis media diabetica.

d. neuritis. Multiple neuritis of diabetes.

d. sugar. Glucose in the sugar of the urine of diabetics.

d. tabes. Diabetes with neuritic pains in leg and loss of patellar tendon reflex.

diabetide (di-ă-bē′tid) [Fr.]. A cutaneous manifestation of diabetes.

diabetogenic (di″ă-bĕt″ō-jĕn′ĭk) [Gr. diabētēs, passing through, + gennan, to produce]. Causing diabetes.

diabetogenous (di″ă-bē-tŏj′ĕn-ŭs). Caused by diabetes.

diabetometer (di″ă-bē-tŏm′ē-ter) [Gr. diabētēs, passing through, + metron, a measure]. A device for measuring sugar in diabetic urine.

diaboleptic (di-ăb″ō-lĕp′tĭk) [Gr. diabolos, devil, + lēpsis, a seizure]. One professing to have supernatural communication, esp. with the devil.

diabrosis (di″ă-brō′sĭs) [Gr., eating through]. A corrosion causing perforation of a vessel or organ.

diabrotic (di-ă-brŏt′ĭk). 1. Corrosive. 2. An escharotic or corrosive.

diacele (di′ă-sēl) [Gr. dia, between, + koilia, a hollow]. The 3rd ventricle of the brain. SYN: diacoele.

diacetate (di-ăs′ē-tāt). A salt of diacetic acid.

diacetemia (di-ăs″ē-tē′mi-ă). Diacetic acid in the blood.

diacetic acid (di″ă-sĕt′ĭk). Acetoacetic acid, found in acidosis and in the urine of the diabetic. It is similar to acetone and is found in serious diabetes and in any condition which produces starvation, such as persistent vomiting.

d. a. test. Half fill a test tube with freshly voided urine. Then add, drop by drop, some ferric chloride solution which will cause a deposit of iron phosphate to form. Now filter the mixture and add a few more drops of ferric chloride. If diacetic acid is present a port wine color develops. The specimen is now divided into two parts, one being used as a control. One part is boiled; the color will quickly disappear if it is due to diacetic acid.

diacetonuria (di-ăs″ē-tō-nū′rĭ-ă). Diacetic acid in urine; diaceturia.

diaceturia (di-ăs″ē-tū′rĭ-ă). Diacetonuria; diacetic acid in urine.

diacid (di-ăs′ĭd) [Gr. dis, twice, + L. acidus, soured]. Having two atoms of hydrogen replaceable with a base.

diaclasia (di-ă-klā′zĭ-ă) [Gr. dia, through, + klan, to break]. A fracture, esp. breaking a bone before surgery.

diaclast (di′ă-klăst) ["+ klan, to break]. Device for perforating the fetal skull.

diacoele (di′ă-sēl). The third ventricle of brain. SYN: diacele.

diacrinous (di-ăk′rĭn-ŭs) [Gr. diakrinein, to separate]. Pert. to cells which secrete outwardly; exocrine, q.v.

diacrisis (di-ăk′rĭ-sis) [Gr. diakrisis, separation]. 1. A change in the character of a secretion. 2. Any disease having an altered secretion. 3. A critical discharge or excretion in a disease.

diacrit′ic, diacrit′ical [Gr. dia, through, + krinein, to judge]. Diagnostic; said of symptoms.

diad (di′ăd) [Gr. dis, twice]. An element or radical having an atomicity of two; a bivalent element. SEE: dyad.

di′aderm [Gr. dia, through, + derma, skin]. Blastoderm composed of ectoderm and entoderm, and containing between them the segmentation cavity.

diadochokinesia (di-ăd″ō-kō-kĭn-ē′zĭ-ă) [Gr. diadokos, succeeding, + kinēsis, motion]. Ability to make antagonistic movements, as pronation and supination, in quick succession. SEE: disdiadochokinesia.

diagnose (di′ăg-nōs) [Gr. diagignōskein, to discern]. To determine the cause and nature of a pathological condition; to recognize a disease.

diagnosis (di″ăg-nō′sĭs). (pl. diagno′ses) 1. The term denoting name of the disease a person has or is believed to have. Ex: one is found to have pneumonia; thus the diagnosis is pneumonia. 2. The use of scientific and skillful methods to establish the cause and nature of a sick person's disease. This is done by evaluating the history of the disease process; the signs and symptoms present; laboratory data; special tests such as x-ray pictures and electrocardiograms.

The value of establishing a d. is to provide a logical basis for treatment and prognosis.

d., clinical. D. determined by symptoms alone; they may be objective (visible symptoms); subjective (those of internal or mental origin); and cardinal (those pert. to respiration, pulse, and temperature). Symptoms may be local or conditions may be pathological. Most diseases have a symptom or symptoms in common with some other disease.

d., cytological. D. based on cells present in body tissues or exudates.

d., differential. Comparison of symptoms of two similar diseases to determine from which the patient is suffering.

d. by exclusion. Establishing a diagnosis by eliminating other possibilities.

d., pathological. D. based on structural lesions present.

d., physical. D. by external examination only.

d., serological. D. made by using a serological test such as that for syphilis or typhoid.

diagnosis, words pert. to: abdomen; auscultation; blood; breathing; chest; colic; coma; constipation; convulsion; cough; examination, physical; eye; face; fatigue; feces; fever; gait; gums; head, examination of; headache; infection; inflammation; inspection; nail; nausea; pain; pallor; palpation; palpitation; percussion; perspiration; position; pulse; pus; reflexes; respiration; skin; sputum; syncope; teeth; temperature; tongue; unconsciousness; urine; vertigo; vomiting.

diagnos'tic. Pert. to a diagnosis.

diagnostician (dī″ăg-nŏs-tĭsh′ŭn) [Gr. *diagignōskein*, to discern]. One skilled in diagnosis.

diagraph (dī′ă-grăf) [Gr. *dia*, through, + *graphein*, to write]. Device for recording outlines, esp. of the cranium.

dialy- [Gr. *dia*, through, + *lysis*, dissolution]. Prefix meaning to separate.

dialysate (dī-ăl′ĭ-sāt). A liquid that has been dialyzed.

dialysis (dī-ăl′ĭ-sĭs) [Gr. *dia*, through, + *lysis*, dissolution]. 1. The passage of a solute through a membrane. 2. A process in which a liquid to be purified or studied is enclosed in a thin, membranous sack and exposed to water or any other solvent which continually circulates or changes outside the sack. Diffusible substances pass through the membrane, but colloidal material does not. SEE: *absorption; diffusion; osmosis.*

d. acidosis. Metabolic acidosis due to prolonged hemodialysis wherein the pH of the dialysis bath has been inadvertently reduced by the action of contaminating bacteria.

d., renal. D. of blood in order to remove liquid and chemicals that the kidneys would normally remove if they were present and functioning.

dialyt'ic. Belonging to or resembling the process of dialysis.

dialyzable (dī-ă-lĭz′ă-bl). Capable of dialysis.

dialyze (dī′ă-līz). To make a dialysis or to have made one.

dialyzer (dī′ă-līz″er) [Gr. *dia*, through, + *lysis*, dissolution]. Membrane used in performing dialysis.

diamagnet'ic ["+ *magnēs*, magnet]. 1. Repelled by a magnet. 2. Assuming a position at right angles to the lines of force of a magnetic field.

diameter (dī-ăm′ĕ-tĕr) ["+ *metron*, a measure]. The distance from any point on the periphery of a surface, body, or space to the opposite point.

d., anterior transverse, of the fetal head. SEE: *d., temporal.*

d., anteroposterior, of the pelvic cavity. The distance between middle of symphysis pubis and upper border of 3rd sacral vertebra.

d., anteroposterior, of pelvic inlet The distance from upper part of symphysis pubis to promontory of sacrum (about 11 cm. in female). SYN: *true conjugate d. of pelvic inlet.*

d., anteroposterior, of pelvic outlet. Distance between tip of coccyx and lower edge of symphysis pubis (9-11.5 cm. in female).

d., anteroposterior, of skull. The distance in a straight line between the metopic point and the most remote point upon the external surface of the tabular portion of the occipital bone, or between the most prominent point of the glabella and the most prominent point upon the external surface of the occipital bone.

d., basilobregmatic. Distance in a straight line between basilon and bregma.

d., biauricular. 1. Distance in a straight line between two points on a line passing over the vertex and uniting the two auricular points, each immediately above the ridge which continues the zygomatic arch backward. 2. Transverse distance between the centers of external auditory meatuses, or between middle point of the upper margins of each external auditory meatus.

d., biglenoid. Distance between the center of one glenoid cavity of the temporal bone and that of the other.

d., biischial. D. between the ischial spines.

d., bijugal. Horizontal distance between two malar points.

d., bijugular. Transverse distance between two jugular points.

d., bimalar. The transverse distance between two malar points.

d., bimandibular. Transverse distance between tubercles on the inferior borders of the inferior maxilla.

d., bimastoid. Transverse distance between two mastoid processes of the temporal bone.

d., biparietal. Transverse distance between parietal eminences on each side (about 9.25 cm.).

d., bisacromial. Transverse distance between two acromial processes.

d., bisiliac. Transverse distance between most distant points of the iliac crests. SYN: *intercristal d.*

d., bisischiadic. SEE: *d., transverse, of pelvic outlet.*

d., bitemporal. Distance between the temporal bones (about 8 cm.).

d., bitrochanteric. Distance between the highest point of one of the greater trochanters and that of the other. SYN: *intertrochanteric d.*

d., bizygomatic. Greatest transverse distance between most prominent points of the zygomatic arches.

d., cervicobregmatic. Distance between anterior fontanel and junction of the neck with floor of the mouth.

d., diagonal conjugate, of the pelvis. The distance from the upper part of the symphysis pubis to the most distant part of the brim of the pelvis.

d., external biorbital. Greatest transverse distance between outer borders of external orbital apophyses of the frontal bone.

d., external conjugate, of the pelvis. Anteroposterior d. of the pelvic inlet measured externally; distance from the skin over the upper part of symphysis pubis to the skin over a point corresponding to the sacral promontory.

d. of fetal skull. Important diameters at full term are suboccipitobregmatic, 3 3/4 in. (9.5 cm.); cervicobregmatic, 3 3/4 in. (9.5 cm.); frontomental, 3 1/5 in. (8.1 cm.); occipitomental, 5 in. (12.7 cm.); supraoccipitomental, 5 1/2 in. (14 cm.); occipitofrontal, 4 1/2 in. (11.4 cm.); suboccipitofrontal, 4 in. (10.2 cm.); biparietal, 3 3/4 in. (9.5 cm.); bitemporal, 3 1/5 in. (8.1 cm.).

d., frontomental. Distance from top of forehead to point of chin.

d., inial. Distance in a straight line, in median line of skull, between most prominent points of the inion and the glabella.

d., internal biorbital. Greatest transverse distance between inner borders of the external orbital apophyses of the frontal bone.

d., interspinous. Distance between the two anterior superior spines of the ilia.

d., maximum anteroposterior, of the skull. Distance, in the median line, between the most prominent part of the glabella and the most prominent point in the middle line upon the tabular portion of the occipital bone.

d., maximum frontal. Distance between two stephanions.

d., maximum occipital. Distance in a straight line between two asterions.

d., maximum transverse, of the skull. Longest horizontal transverse line that can be drawn within the cranium.

d., mentobregmatic. Distance from chin to middle of anterior fontanel.

d., minimum frontal. Distance between two extremities of supraorbital line.

d., oblique, of pelvic inlet. Distance from iliopectineal eminence of one side to sacroiliac articulation on opposite side (about 12.5 cm. in female).

d., obstetric, of pelvic inlet. Shortest distance between sacrum and symphysis. This d. is shorter than the true conjugate.

d., occipitofrontal. Line extending from the most prominent parts of the frontal and occipital bones (about 12 cm.).

d., occipitomental. Greatest distance between occiput and point of chin (about 13 cm.).

d. of pelvis. *Anteroposterior:* the distance between the sacrovertebral angle and the symphysis pubis. *Biischial:* between the ischial spines. *Conjugata diagonalis:* between the sacrovertebral angle and the symphysis pubis. *Conjugata vera:* the true conjugate; between the sacrovertebral angle and the middle of the posterior aspect of the symphysis pubis (about 1.5 cm. less than the diagonal conjugate). *Deventer's Oblique:* between the sacroiliac synchondrosis on one side and the ileopectineal eminence on the other side. *Intercristus:* between the crests of the ilium. *Interspinous:* between the spines of the ilium. *Intertrochanteric:* between the greater trochanters when the hips are extended and the legs are held together. *Internal conjugate:* between the promontory of the sacrum and the upper edge of the symphysis pubis. *Pelvic:* any diameter of the pelvis found by measuring a straight line between any two points. *Transverse d. of the inlet:* Distance from the middle of brim across greatest width of pelvic inlet to same point of opposite side (about 13.5 cm. in female). *Transverse d. of the pelvic outlet:* between the tuberosities of the ischium. SEE: *pelvis.*

d., posterior sagittal, of midpelvis Distance between midpoint of interspinous diameter and sacrum (about 5.0 cm.).

d., sacrosubpubic. Distance between middle of promontory of sacrum and middle of lower border of the triangular ligament of pubic symphysis.

d., sagittal. SEE: *d., basilobregmatic.*

d., sternovertebral. Distance from sternum to vertebral column measured externally.

d., suboccipitobregmatic. Line extending from the bregma to the undersurface of the occiput (about 9.5 cm.).

d., suboccipitofrontal. Greatest distance between forehead and junction of occiput with the neck.

d., subtemporal. Distance between point upon sphenotemporal suture which is crossed by the ridge upon the inferior surface on the greater wing of the sphenoid bone of one side and a similar point on the other side.

d., temporal. Greatest horizontal distance between two opposite points upon the line passing over the vertex and uniting the two auricular points on surface of the temporal bones.

d., trachelobregmatic. D. between anterior fontanel and meeting point of neck with floor of mouth.

d., transverse, of pelvic inlet. Distance from middle of brim across greatest width of pelvic inlet to same point on opposite side (about 13.5 cm. in female).

d., transverse, of pelvic outlet. Distance between posterior portions of ischial tuberosities (about 11 cm. in female).

d., true conjugate, of pelvic inlet. Distance between sacrovertebral angle and symphysis pubis (about 11 cm. in female). SYN: *anteroposterior d. of pelvic inlet.*

d., vertical, of fetal head. That extending from highest point of head to anterior margin of foramen magnum.

diamid(e (dī-ăm′ĭd, -ĭd) [L. *di,* two, + *amide*]. A compound which contains two amine (CONH₂) groups. Sometimes used incorrectly to indicate a diamine or hydrozine.

diamine (dī-ăm′ĭn, ēn). A chemical compound with two NH₂ radicals.

diaminuria (dī-ăm″ĭ-nū′rĭ-ă). Diamines in the urine.

dianoetic (dī″ă-nō-ĕt′ĭk) [Gr. *dia,* through, + *nous,* mind]. Pert. to intellectual function, particularly logic and orderly analysis.

diapason (dī″ă-pā′sŭn) ["+ *pasōn,* all]. A diagnostic tuning fork used to determine the degree of deafness.

diapedesis (dī″ă-pĕd-ē′sĭs) ["+ *pēdan,* to leap]. Passage of blood cells, esp. leukocytes, by ameboid movements through the unruptured wall of a capillary vessel.

diaphane (dī′ă-fān) [Gr. *dia,* through, + *phainein,* to appear]. 1. The investing membrane of a cell. 2. A very small electric light utilized in transillumination.

diaphanometer (dī″ă-făn-ŏm′ē-tĕr) ["+ "+ *metron,* measure]. A device for estimating the amount of solids in a fluid by its transparency.

diaphanometry (dī″ă-făn-ŏm′ĕt-rĭ). Determination of translucency of a fluid, as the urine.

diaphanoscope (dī-ă-făn′ō-skōp) [Gr. *dia,* through, + *phainein,* to appear, + *skopein,* to examine]. Device for electric examination of body cavities.

diaphanoscopy (dī″ă-făn-ŏs′kō-pĭ). Examination of fluids by the diaphanoscope.

diaphemetric (dī″ă-fē-mĕt′rĭk) [Gr. *dia,* through, + *aphē,* touch, + *metron,* measure]. Pert. to degree of tactile sensibility.

diaphoresis (dī″ă-fō-rē′sĭs) ["+ *pherein,* to carry]. Profuse sweating.

diaphoretic (dī″ă-fō-rĕt′ĭk) [Gr. *dia,* through, + *pherein,* to carry]. A sudorific or an agent which increases perspiration. The term sudorific is usually confined to those active agents that cause drops of perspiration to collect on the skin. Ex: camphor, opium, pilocarpine. Heat may also be included as such an agent.

d. drugs. These produce their effects either by stimulation, general applications, or both.

d., refrigerant. One that acts on sweat centers in the spinal cord and medulla, and reduces circulation, i.e., lobelia, tobacco.

d., sedative. One, such as warm drinks or sweat baths, which dilates superficial capillaries and causes relaxation.

diaphragm (dī′ă-fram) [Gr. *diaphragma,* a partition]. 1. Thin membrane such as one used for dialysis. 2. In microscopy, an apparatus located beneath the opening in the stage by means of which the amt. of light passing through the object can be regulated. 3. A rubber or plastic cup which fits over the cervix uteri and is used for contraceptive purposes. 4. A musculomembranous wall separating the abdomen from the thoracic cavity with its convexity upward. It contracts with each inspiration, flattening out downward, permitting the descent of the bases of the lungs. It relaxes with each expiration, elevating it and restoring its inverted basin shape. The deeper the inspiration, the lower the descent of the d.; the greater the expiration, the higher does it rise.

Its origin is at a level with the 6th ribs or intercostal spaces anteriorly, and the 11th or 12th ribs posteriorly. The right half rises higher than the left. The lower surface is in relation to the suprarenal bodies of the kidney, the liver, spleen, and cardiac end of the stomach. It aids in defecation and parturition by its ability to cause an increase in intra-abdominal pressure while the person attempts to exhale with the glottis closed. It becomes spasmodic in hiccoughs and sneezing.

SEE: *midriff; phrenic; "phren-" words; straining; Valsalva maneuver.*

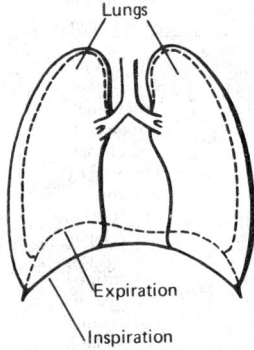

DIAPHRAGM
Movement of diaphragm and lungs in inspiration and expiration.

d., Bucky. A grid, suspended immediately beneath the x-ray table and above the film tray, so constructed that the effects of backscatter and secondary radiation are eliminated when x-ray photographs of dense structures are taken.

d., hernia of. Protrusion of abdominal contents through the d. ETIOL: Congenital or through injury.

d., pelvic. The musculofascial layer forming the lower boundary of the abdominopelvic cavity.

It is funnel-shaped, and is pierced in the midline by the urethra, vagina, and rectum. Consists of a muscular layer made up of the paired levator ani and coccygeus muscles. The fascial layer consists of two portions, the parietal and visceral layers, the former being made up of the peritoneum continuous with the connective tissue sheaths of the psoas and iliac muscles; the visceral layer is split from the parietal layer at the white line passing downward and inward to form the upper sheath of the levator ani muscles; the anterior part of this layer unites the bladder to the posterior wall of the pubes.

The middle portion splits into three parts: The vesical layer investing bladder and urethra; rectovaginal layer forming the rectovaginal septum; the rectal layer investing the rectum; the posterior part is the base of the broad ligament where it sheaths the uterine arteries and supports the cervix.

d., urogenital. Urogenital trigone, or triangular ligament. A musculofascial sheath which lies between the ischiopubic rami. It lies superficial to the pelvic diaphragm and in the male surrounds the membranous urethra; in the female it surrounds the vagina.

diaphragmalgia (di″ă-frag-mal′jĭ-ă) [Gr. *diaphragma*, barrier, + *algos*, pain]. Pain in the diaphragm.

diaphragmat′ic. Pert. to the diaphragm.

diaphragmati′tis. Diaphragmitis, q.v.

diaphragmatocele (di″ă-frag-mat′o-sēl) [Gr. *diaphragma*, partition, + *kēlē*, hernia]. Hernia of the diaphragm.

diaphragmitis (di″ă-frag-mī′tis) ["+ *-itis*, inflammation]. Inflammation of the diaphragm. SYN: *diaphragmatitis.*

di″aphragmodyn′ia ["+ *odynē*, pain]. Pain in the diaphragm.

diaphysary (di-af′ĭ-ză-rī) [Gr. *diaphysis*, a growing through]. Pert. to or affecting the shaft of a bone. SEE: *diaphysis.*

diaphysec′tomy ["+ *ektomē*, excision]. Removal of part of the shaft of a long bone.

diaphysis (di-af′ĭ-sis). The shaft or middle part of a long cylindrical bone. SEE: *apophysis; epiphysis.*

diaphysitis (di″ă-fī-zī′tis) [Gr. *diaphysis*, a growing through, + *-itis*, inflammation]. Inflammation of shaft of a long bone.

diaplasis (di-ă-plā′sis). Reduction of a fracture or dislocation. SYN: *diorthosis.*

di′aplex [Gr. *dia*, through, + L. *plexus*, a plaiting]. Choroid plexus of third ventricle.

diaplex′al. Pert. to the diaplex.

diaplex′us [Gr. *dia*, through, + L. *plexus*, braid]. Choroid plexus of third ventricle.

diapnoic (di-ăp-no′ĭk) [Gr. *diapnein*, to perspire]. 1. Pert. to or causing perspiration, esp. insensible p. 2. A mild sudorific.

diapophysis (di-ă-pŏf′ĭ-sis) [Gr. *dia*, through, + *apophysis*, outgrowth]. An upper articular surface of transverse process of a vertebra.

diapyetic (dī-ă-pī-et'ik) [Gr. *dia*, through, + *pyron*, pus]. Pert. to or causing suppuration.

diarrhea (dī-ă-rē'ä) [Gr. *dia*, through, + *rhein*, to flow]. Frequent passage of watery bowel movements. It is a frequent symptom of gastrointestinal disturbances and is primarily the result of increased peristalsis.

ETIOL: Diet; inflammation or irritation of the mucosa of the intestines; gastrointestinal infections; certain drugs; psychogenic factors.

d., acute. That characterized by sudden onset. TREATMENT: Strong tea; whey; rice milk; arrowroot; corn flour; blackberry brandy; adsorbents as aluminum hydroxide. Gradual return to ordinary diet.

The above are more or less home remedies which act as demulcents or astringents for the irritated intestinal mucosa. They are often effective but severe cases of diarrhea may require additional therapy specifically directed to the etiology of the disease. Also in severe cases fluid- and electrolyte-replacement therapy may be needed. Agents that reduce intestinal activity, such as antispasmodics and paregoric, may provide distinct relief.

d., emotional. Form caused by emotional stress.

d., epidemic, in newborn. D. in newborn caused by pathogenic strains of Escherichia coli and occurring in epidemics in hospitals.

d., fatty. D. with stools containing undigested fat particles.

d., infantile. In children under two years. Dysentery, q.v. SYM: Skin dry, temperature high; thirst, pains, increase of stools with change of color and consistency.

d., lienteric. Watery stools with undigested food particles.

d., membranous. D. with passage of pieces of intestinal mucosa.

d., mucous. D. with mucus in stools.

d., purulent. Presence of pus in stools, a result of intestinal ulceration.

d., simple. Variety in which stools contain only normal excreta.

d., summer. D. occurring in children during summer heat.

d. of travelers. That experienced by travelers. The cause is unknown; there is no effective method of prophylaxis except to attempt to avoid eating uncooked food or drinking beverages which could be contaminated. In general the disease is self-limiting. There is no specific therapy.

d., ulcerative. Severe d. with ulceration of mucosa of intestines.

diarthric (dī-ar'thrĭk) [Gr. *dis*, two, + *arthron*, joint]. Pert. to two or more joints.

diarthro'sis [Gr. *diarthrōsis*, a movable articulation]. An articulation in which opposing bones move freely; a hinge joint.

diartic'ular [Gr. *dis*, two, + L. *articulus*, joint]. Pert. to two joints.

diaschisis (dī-ăs'kī-sis) [Gr. *dia*, apart, + *schizein*, to split]. Disturbance or injury to one part of central nervous system may cause alteration in function of some distant part.

diascope (dī'ă-skōp) ["+ *skopein*, to examine]. A glass plate held against the skin for ascertaining noncongestive changes.

diastalsis (dī-ă-stal'sis) ["+ *stalsis*, contraction]. A wave of inhibition before a downward contraction in the intestine. Similar to peristalsis.

diastal'tic. 1. Pert. to diastalsis. 2. Denoting reflex action.

diastase (dī'ăs-tās) [Gr. *diastasis*, a separation]. A specific enzyme or ferment in plant cells, such as in sprouting grains and malt, and in the digestive juice which converts starch into sugar.

diastasis (dī-ăs'tă-sis) [Gr.]. 1. In surgery, injury to a bone involving separation of an epiphysis. 2. In cardiac physiology, the last part of diastole.

It follows the period of most rapid diastolic filling of the ventricles, consists of a period of retarded inflow of blood from atria into ventricles, lasts (in man under average conditions) about 0.2 seconds, and is immediately followed by atrial systole.

d. recti. A separation lateralward of the two halves of the musculus rectus dominis.

diastema (dī'ă-stē'mä) [Gr. *diastēma*, an interval or space]. (pl. *diaste'mata*) 1. A fissure. 2. A space between two teeth.

diastematocrania (dī''ă-stem''ă-tō-krā'nĭ-ă) ["+ *kranion*, cranium]. Congenital sagittal fissure of the skull.

diastematomyelia (dī''ă-stem''ă-tō-mī-ē'lĭ-ă) ["+ *myelos*, marrow]. Congenital fissure of the spinal cord.

diastematopyelia (dī''ă-stem''ă-tō-pī-ē'lĭ-ă) ["+ *pyelos*, pelvis]. Median slit of the pelvis; congenital.

dias'ter [Gr. *dis*, two, + *astēr*, star]. In mitosis the achromatic figure consisting of a double star. SYN: *amphiaster*. SEE: *mitosis*.

diastole (dī-as'tō-lī) [Gr. *diastellein*, to expand]. The normal period in the heart cycle during which the muscle fibers lengthen, the heart dilates, and the cavities fill with blood; d. of the atria occurs before that of the ventricles. Roughly, the period of relaxation alternating with systole or contraction. SEE: *heart; murmur; pulse; systole.*

diastolic (di-ăs-tol'ĭk). Pert. to diastole.

   d. pressure. This is the point of least pressure in the arterial vascular system.

   The failure of the diastolic pressure to drop in proportion to the systolic pressure is a danger sign.

   RS: blood pressure; pulse p.; systolic p.

diatax'ia [Gr. *dis*, two, + *ataxia*, lack of order]. Ataxia of both sides of body.

   d. cerebra'lis infanti'lis. Birth palsy.

diatela, diatele (di-ă-tē'lă, tēl) [Gr. *dia*, between, + L. *tela*, web]. Membranous roof of third ventricle.

diater'ma ["+ *terma*, end]. Portion of the floor of third ventricle.

diathermal (di''ă-ther'mal) ["+ *thermē*, heat]. Ability to absorb heat rays.

diather'manous. Diathermal, q.v.

diather'mia [Gr. *dia*, through, + *thermē*, heat]. Diathermy, q.v.

diather'mic. Of the nature of diathermy or of its results.

diathermy (di'ă-ther''mĭ) [Gr. *dia*, through, + *thermē*, heat]. The therapeutic use of a high frequency current to generate heat within some part of the body.

   The frequency is greater than the maximum frequency for neuromuscular response, and ranges from several hundred thousand to millions of cycles per second.

   d., medical. The generation of heat within the body by the application of high-frequency oscillatory current for warming, but not damaging, tissues.

   d., short wave. Treatment by use of wave lengths of three to 30 meters.

   d., surgical. D. of high frequency for electrocoagulation, cauterization, etc.

diathesis (di-ath'ĕ-sis) [Gr. *diatithenai*, to dispose]. Constitutional predisposition to a certain disease, condition, or group of diseases. Ex: allergic d., hemorrhagic d., or rheumatic d.

diathet'ic. Pert. to diathesis.

diatom (di'ă-tom) [Gr. *diatemnein*, to cut through]. One of a group of unicellular microscopic algae. They possess a siliceous cell wall.

diatom'ic. 1. Containing two atoms; said of molecules. 2. Bivalent.

diato'ric [Gr. *diatoros*, bored through]. Artificial teeth attached with vulcanized rubber to their bases.

diax'on, diax'one [Gr. *dis*, two, + *axōn*, axis]. A neuron having two axons.

diazo-. Prefix used in chemistry to note that a compound contains the N_2 radical.

   d. reaction. A deep red color in urine produced by the action of *p*-diazobenzenesulfonic acid and ammonia on aromatic substances found in the urine in certain conditions. SYN: *Ehrlich's diazo reaction.*

dibasic (di-bā'sik) [Gr. *dis*, two, + *basis*, base]. Containing in each molecule two atoms of hydrogen replaceable by a base; said of acids.

diblastula (di-blas'tu-lă) ["+ *blastos*, sprout]. A blastula containing the ectoderm and entoderm.

Dibothriocephalus (di-bŏth''rĭ-ō-sĕf'ăl-ŭs). Diphyllobothrium, q.v.

dibucaine hydrochloride. USP. A local anesthetic similar to cocaine in action when applied topically and similar to procaine and cocaine when injected.

dicalcic (di-kal'sik) [Gr. *dis*, two, + L. *calx*, lime]. Containing two atoms of calcium in a molecule.

   d. orthophosphate. $CaHPO_4$. A salt, often found in the urine.

dicalcium phosphate (di-kal'sī-um-fos'-făt). Dibasic calcium phosphate. Used as a source of calcium to supplement the diet.

dichloramine-T (di-klor'a-mēn). White powder containing about 28% chlorine.

   ACTION AND USES: Germicide and disinfectant.

dichotomy, dichotomization (di-kot'o-mĭ, di-kot''o-mi-za'shun) [Gr. *dicha*, twofold, + *tomē*, a cut]. 1. Bifurcation of a vein. 2. Cutting or dividing into two parts.

dichroic (di-krō'ĭk). Pert. to dichroism.

dichroism (di'kro-izm) [Gr. *dis*, two, + *chroa*, color]. Property of a substance appearing to be one color by direct light and another by transmitted light.

dichromasy (di-krō'-mă-sĭ). Able to see only two colors. Partial colorblindness. SYN: *dichromatism.*

dichromat'ic. Being able to see only two colors.

dichromatopsia (di''kro-mă-top'sĭ-ă) [Gr. *dis*, two, + *chrōma*, color, + *opsis*, sight]. Ability to distinguish only two primary colors.

dichro'mic. 1. Containing two atoms of chromium. 2. Seeing only two colors.

dichro'mophil [Gr. *dis*, two, + *chrōma*, color, + *philein*, to love]. Double staining with both acid and basic dyes.

dichromophilism (di''krō-mŏf'ĭl-ĭzm) ["+ "+ "+ *ismos*, condition of]. Having the capacity for double staining.

dick. A gas, ethyldichlorarsine, used in chemical warfare.

Dick method. [George F. and Gladys H. Dick, Amer. physicians, 1881 —] A toxin-antitoxin injection for the prevention of scarlet fever.

Dick test. In a negative reaction there may occur some slight inflammatory changes due to irritation by proteins in fluid administered.

In a manner somewhat similar to the Schick testing for diphtheria, a person's susceptibility to scarlet fever may be ascertained by the injection of a standardized toxin of the Streptococcus hemolyticus. A positive (susceptible) reaction in the shape of erythema appears in about 12 to 24 hours. Patients convalescing from scarlet fever invariably give a negative reaction. SEE: *Schick test.*

dicliditis (dĭk-lĭ-dī'tĭs) [Gr. *diklis,* double door, + *-itis,* inflammation]. Inflammation of heart valve. SYN: *valvulitis.*

diclidostosis (dĭk'lĭd-ŏs-tō'sĭs) ["+ *osteon,* bone]. Ossification of the venous valves.

diclidot'omy ["+ *tomē,* incision]. Cutting a valve, esp. a rectal or heart valve. SYN: *valvotomy.*

dicoria (dī-ko-rī'-ă) [Gr. *dis,* two, + *korē,* pupil]. Double pupil in each eye.

dicrotic (dī-krŏt'ĭk) [Gr. *dikrotos,* beating double]. Having one heartbeat for two arterial pulsations; rel. to a double pulse.

    d. notch. In a pulse tracing, a notch on the descending limb.

    d. wave. A positive wave following the dicrotic notch.

dicrotism (dī'krŏt-ĭzm) ["+ *ismos,* condition of]. The state of being dicrotic.

dictyoma (dĭk"tĭ-o'ma) [Gr. *diktyon,* net, + *-ōma,* tumor]. A retinal tumor. Also spelled diktyoma.

dicumarol (di-koo'mă-rol). Proprietary name for bishydroxycoumarin (USP), an anticoagulant that decreases activity of prothrombin in the blood plasma and hence increases prothrombin time.

Used in prophylaxis and treatment of intravascular clotting, in postoperative thrombophlebitis, pulmonary embolism, acute peripheral embolism and thrombosis, and recurrent idiopathic thrombophlebitis. Used also in management of acute coronary thrombosis. Frequently an adjunct to heparin, q.v.

The dose is determined by periodically testing the prothrombin time. If heparin is being given, it is important that three to four hours elapse between the last dose of heparin and the time the blood is drawn for the prothrombin test.

CONTRAINDICATIONS: Subacute bacterial endocarditis, recent brain, spinal, or eye surgery, purpura and blood dyscrasias in vitamin K deficiency and in absence of prothrombin determination. The drug is excreted in the mother's milk. Thus infants whose mothers are receiving dicumarol should be carefully observed for bleeding tendency.

In cases of hemorrhage due to this drug, stop the drug immediately and give vitamin K intravenously; whole fresh blood may be needed.

    RS: heparin; vitamin K.

didactylism (dī-dak'tĭ-lizm) [Gr. *dis,* two, + *daktylos,* finger]. The congenital condition of having only two digits on a hand or foot.

didelphic (di-del'fĭk) ["+ *delphys,* uterus]. Having or pertaining to a double uterus.

didymalgia (did-ĭ-mal'jĭ-ă) [Gr. *didymos,* twin, + *algos,* pain]. Pain in a testicle. SYN: *didymodynia.*

didymitis (did-ĭ-mī'tis) ["+ *-itis,* inflammation]. Inflammation of a testicle. SYN: *orchitis.*

didymodynia (did"ĭ-mō-dĭn'ĭ-ă) ["+ *odynē,* pain]. Pain in a testicle. SYN: *didymalgia.*

didymus (dĭd'ĭ-mŭs) [Gr. *didymos,* twin, testis]. 1. A twin. 2. A congenital abnormality involving joined twins. 3. A testicle.

diechoscope (dī-ĕk'ō-skōp) [Gr. *dis,* two, + *ēchō,* echo, + *skopein,* to examine]. A stethoscope for simultaneous auscultation from two different sites.

di"elec'tric [Gr. *dia,* through, + *ēlektron,* amber]. An insulating substance offering great resistance to passage of electricity by conduction through which electric force may act by induction.

dielectrolysis (di"e-lek-trol'ĭsĭs) ["+ "+ *lysis,* loosening]. The forcing of a drug or medicinal compound to a particular part of the body by osmosis brought about or accelerated with an electric current.

diencephalon (di"en-sef'ă-lon) ["+ *enkephalos,* brain]. Second portion of the brain or that lying between the telencephalon and mesencephalon. It includes the epithalamus, thalamus, metathalamus, and hypothalamus. SYN: *thalamencephalon; between brain; 'tween-brain.*

dienestrol (di"ēn-es'trol). A nonsteroid, synthetic estrogen used for estrogen therapy.

Dientamoeba (di"ĕn-tă-mē'bă). A genus of parasitic protozoa characterized by possession of two similar nuclei. They belong to the class Sarcodina.

    D. fragilis. A species of parasitic amebae inhabiting the intestine of man. There is strong evidence that it may sometimes be pathogenic, producing symptoms such as intestinal colic and diarrhea.

dieresis (di-er'ĕ-sis) [Gr. *diairesis*, a division]. 1. Breaking up or dispersion of things normally joined, as by an ulcer. 2. Mechanical separation of parts by surgical means.

dieret'ic. Pert. to dieresis; dissolvable or separable.

diet [Gr. *diaita*, way of living]. 1. Food substances, liquid and solid, regularly consumed in the course of normal living. 2. A prescribed allowance of food adapted for a particular state of health or disease, as a diabetic diet. 3. To cause to eat or drink sparingly in accordance with prescribed rules.

   d., balanced. One adequate in energy-providing substances (carbohydrates and fats); tissue-building compounds (proteins); inorganic chemicals (water and mineral salts); agents which regulate or catalyze metabolic processes (vitamins); substances for certain physiological processes such as bulk for promoting peristaltic movements of the digestive tract.

diet, words pert. to: alkaline-ash d.; bland d.; calcium (high and low) d.; cellulose (high) d.; colostomy d.; elimination d.; fat (low) d.; feeding; fluid d.; ketogenic d.; light d.; liquid (full) d.; residue d. (high and low); roughage d.; salt-free d.; Sippy d.; soft d.; water-balance d.

dietary (di'ĕ-ta″rĭ). A regulated diet.

dietetic (di-ĕ-tet'ik). Pert. to diet.

dietet'ics [Gr. *diaitetikos*]. The science of the use of foods in health and disease. Some fundamental principles and facts of this science will be summarized here.

   CONSERVATION OF ENERGY: In order to obtain metabolic balance, there must be as much caloric value (energy and heat) in the food as will equal the amt. of work done by the subject or patient plus the heat which he constantly loses. The number of calories in his daily food must in the long run equal his basal metabolic rate plus his additional metabolism due to muscular work and added heat losses. Thus a subject whose basal rate is 1700 Calories (kilogram calories) per 24 hours may, during the day, do work and lose heat adding, say, 2000 Calories to his output; he must, therefore, obtain 3700 Calories in his diet.

     1 gm. of fat gives about 9.3 Cal.
     1 gm. of carbohydrate   4.0 Cal.
     1 gm. of protein   4.0 Cal.

   CONSERVATION OF MATTER: Everything that leaves the body, whether exhaled as carbon dioxide and water, or excreted as urea and minerals, must be replaced in the food. Thus if a man excretes 10 gm. of nitrogen daily he must receive 10 gm. of it in his diet, for the element can neither be created nor destroyed. This metabolic balance may be monitored by the use of careful chemical analysis of all that is eaten and excreted.

   DIFFICULTY OF SOME ORGANIC SYNTHESES: The power of the body to build tissue is limited, and for a given purpose only certain raw materials can be used. Thus proteins are "made up" of carbon, hydrogen, oxygen, and nitrogen; but eating charcoal and inhaling the gases would not enable one to make tissue protein. For instance, hemoglobin cannot be synthesized unless the body is supplied with proteins containing one of the essential building blocks, the pyrole ring, for this complex molecule. This group occurs in the amino acids tryptophan, proline, and hydroxyproline; proteins which do not contain these amino acids therefore are insufficient for needs of the body.

   SUMMARY: A diet should contain water; carbohydrates; fats; proteins; minerals; roughage (indigestible residue); vitamins.

diethylstilbestrol   (di-eth″il-stil′bĕs′trol). USP. A synthetic preparation possessing estrogenic properties. It is several times more effective than natural estrogens and may be given orally. It is used therapeutically in the treatment of menopausal disturbances and other disorders due to estrogen deficiencies. SYN: *stilbestrol.*

dietitian (di-ĕ-tish'an) [Gr. *diaita*, way of living]. One scientifically trained in dietetics (which includes nutrition).

Dietl's crisis (dē'tlz). [Joseph Dietl, Pol. physician, 1804-1878] Renal colic due to kinking and partial obstruction of the ureter; accompanied by scanty, bloodstained urine.

Dieulafoy's triad (dyuh-lä-fwahz'). [Georges Dieulafoy, Fr. physician, 1839-1911] Tenderness, muscular contraction, and skin hyperesthesia in acute appendicitis at McBurney's point.

differential (dif″er-en'shal) [L. *differre*, to carry apart]. Marked by differences.

   d. blood count. Determination of the number of each variety of leukocytes in a cubic millimeter of blood. SEE: *blood count.*

   d. diagnosis. Diagnosis based on comparison of symptoms of two or more similar diseases to determine which the patient is suffering from. SEE: *diagnosis.*

differentia'tion. Acquirement of functions different from those of the original type.

diffraction (di-frak'shun) [L. *diffringere*, to break to pieces]. The change which occurs in light when it passes through crystals, prisms, or parallel bars in a grating in which the rays are deflected and thus appear to be turned aside producing dark or colored bands or lines, or other phenomena. Term is also applied to similar phenomena in sound and electricity.

diffusate (dif ū-sāt) [L. *dis*, apart, + *fundere*, to pour]. In the process of dialysis, that portion of a liquid which passes through a membrane and which contains crystalloid matter in solution. SYN: *dialysate.*

diffuse (dĭ-fūs'). Spreading, scattered, spread.
    d. inflammation. One not localized.

diffusible (dĭ-fūz'ĭ-bl). Capable of being diffused.

diffusion (dĭ-fū'zhŭn) [L. *dis*, apart, + *fundere*, to pour]. 1. Absorption of a liquid such as the absorption, by cells, of water from lymph when the percentage of salt is less in lymph than in the cells. When the percentage is greater in the lymph than in the cells, water is withdrawn from the latter. SEE: *osmosis.*

2. A process whereby different gases interpenetrate and become mixed, due to the incessant motion of their molecules. Similarly, if aqueous solutions of different materials stand in contact, mixing occurs on standing, even if the solutions be separated by thin membranes.

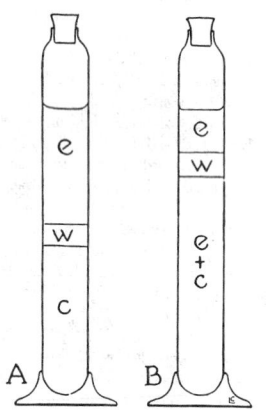

DIFFUSION

A, Beginning of the experiment. A thin layer of water (w) separates a large volume of ether (e) above from an equal volume of the much heavier carbon tetrachloride (c) below. B, Three weeks later the layers are still distinct, but the lowest layer has visibly increased in volume at the expense of the uppermost layer. Ether has passed through the water into the carbon tetrachloride.

3. The tendency of molecules of a substance (gaseous, liquid, or solid) to move from a region of high concentration to one of lower concentration.

digastric (di-gas'trĭk) [Gr. *dis*, twice, + *gastēr*, belly]. Having two bellies; said of certain muscles.

digen'esis ["+ *genesis*, production]. Reproduction in which alternate generations are asexual.

Digenetica (di-jĕ-nĕt'ĭ-kă). An order of parasitic flatworms belonging to the class Trematoda and characterized by having an asexual generation, living usually in molluscs, alternating with a sexual generation living in vertebrates as their final host. It includes all the flukes parasitic in man. These include four groups of flukes. SEE: *fluke.*

digest' [L. *dis*, apart, + *gerere*, to carry]. 1. To undergo digestion. 2. To make a condensation of a subject.

diges'tant. 1. An agent that will digest food or aid in digestion. Ex: pepsin, pancreatin. 2. A preparation made from the digestive glands or lining membrane of the stomach, classified according to the foods it digests, such as carbohydrate or protein.

diges'tible. Pert. to that which may be digested.

diges'tion [L. *digestio*, a taking apart]. The process by which food is broken down, mechanically and chemically, in the gastrointestinal tract and is converted into absorbable forms.

Salt, the simplest sugars (such as glucose), crystalloids in general, and water can be absorbed unchanged; but starches, fats, and proteins for the most part are not absorbable until disintegrated by the digestive fluids, and even the sugar, sucrose (a disacchararose, q.v.), must first undergo inversion.

The chemical actions are chiefly hydrolytic; they are brought about by a variety of enzymes, each of which acts in an acid or alkaline or neutral juice according to its peculiar properties.

The higher carbohydrates are converted into monosaccharoses, q.v.; proteins (through successive stages of peptones and polypeptides) ultimately into amino acids, and fats into fatty acids and glycerine. In the stomach the soluble casein of milk is converted into insoluble paracasein, resulting in its coagulation or clotting. This is brought about by the enzyme, pepsin. The rennin and acid are responsible for the clotting (curdling) of milk, which normally occurs in the stomach. An enzyme, lipase, is able to attack fats in emulsified form. It liberates, for instance, butyric acid from the fats in milk, and thus causes the characteristic odor of vomitus. The chemical actions are facilitated by the churning, wavelike motions of the stomach walls. When the chyme is ready to leave the stomach, the pylorus opens from time to time and the chyme is quickly propelled into the duodenum.

d., artificial. D. outside the living organism by a ferment.

d., duodenal. The acid, chyme, is made alkaline, and the fats it contains are emulsified by the action of bile. A fresh set of enzymes adapted to these new conditions are supplied by the pancreatic juice which enters by two ducts, and by the intestinal juice which comes from small glands in the wall of the intestine itself. The hydrolysis of starches, fats, and proteins is carried to its physi-

ological completion here, and in the remainder of the small intestine.

d., extracellular. That occurring outside the body of the cell.

d., gastric. Portion of the digestive process taking place in the stomach.

d., intestinal. Hydrolytic processes continue here, and absorption of the products is active. From the ileum the food residues pass in a nearly liquid state through a small opening into the ascending colon. A sphincter muscle prevents backflow. True digestive processes in the colon are slight, but there is normally much bacterial action (the products of which are mostly absorbed) and reabsorption of water. The remaining substances, now colored by pigments which entered with bile and changed to a firm consistency by the loss of water, pass on through the transverse colon, the descend-

Action of Digestive Juices
On Proteins, Fats, and Carbohydrates

Digestive Juice	Proteins	Fats	Carbohydrates
Saliva			Changes cooked starch into maltose
Gastric Juice	Curdles milk Changes proteins into peptones		
Pancreatic Juice	Changes peptones to simpler substances	Changes fats to fatty acids and glycerol	Changes sugars into simpler forms
Bile		Emulsifies fats	
Intestinal Juice	Completes the changes of peptones into amino acids		Completes the change of all sugars into the simplest form, glucose

On Foods

Food	Ferment or Enzyme	Digestive Juice	Where Juice Acts
Protein	Pepsin	Gastric juice, acid	Stomach
	Trypsin	Pancreatic juice, alkaline	Small intestine
	Erepsin	Succus Entericus, alkaline	Small intestine
Fats	Lipase	Pancreatic juice	Small intestine
Carbohydrates	Ptyalin	Saliva, alkaline	Mouth and in stomach
	Amylopsin	Pancreatic juice, alkaline	Small intestine
	Invertase	Succus Entericus	Small intestine

ing colon, and the sigmoid flexure into the rectum. They are retained in the rectum by the action of sphincters until defecation occurs. SEE: *absorption.*

d., intracellular. D. within cell body.

d., oral. Portion of the digestive process taking place in the mouth.

d., pancreatic. Portion of digestive process influenced by pancreatic juice.

d., peptic. Gastric d.

d., primary. Portion of digestive process taking place in the gastrointestinal tract.

d., salivary. Digestive action by the saliva. SEE: *salivary digestion.*

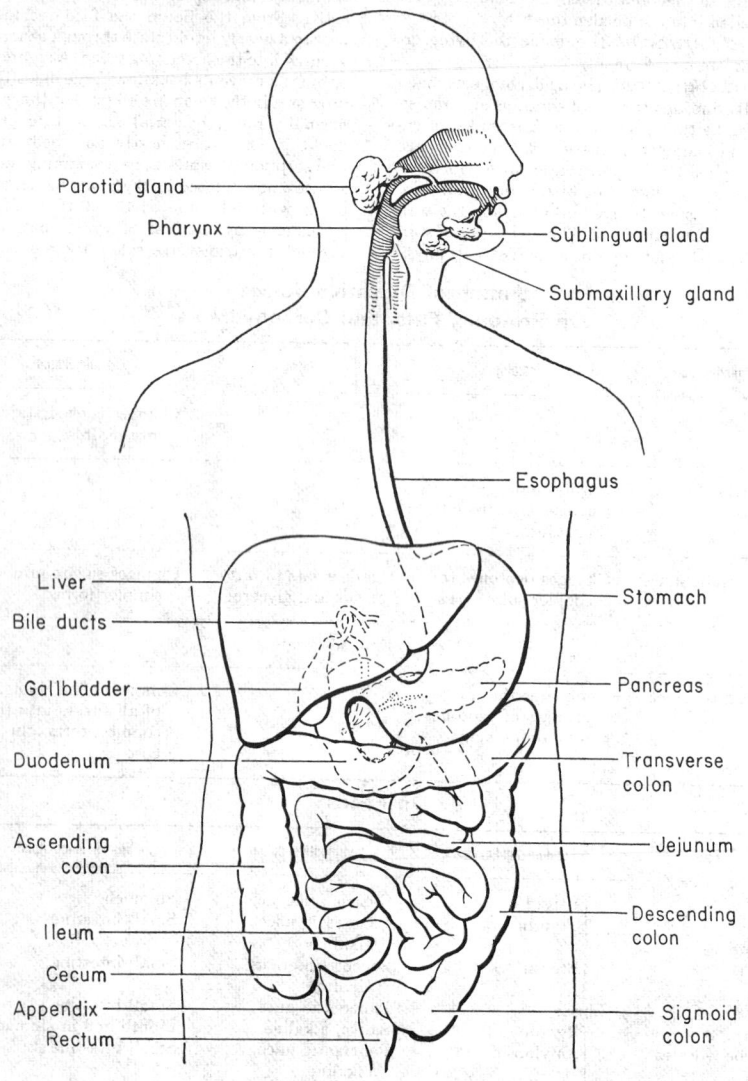

Parotid gland

Pharynx

Sublingual gland

Submaxillary gland

Esophagus

Liver

Bile ducts

Gallbladder

Duodenum

Ascending colon

Ileum

Cecum

Appendix

Rectum

Stomach

Pancreas

Transverse colon

Jejunum

Descending colon

Sigmoid colon

THE DIGESTIVE SYSTEM

d., secondary. Cellular assimilation of nutritive material.

digestive (dĭ-jes'tĭv). Pert. to digestion.

d. juice. One of several secretions which aid in processes of digestion.

d. system. All the organs and glands associated with ingestion and digestion of food; the tract from the mouth to the anus.

digit (dij'it) [L. *digitus*, finger]. (pl. *digits*) A finger or toe.

digital (dij'ĭ-tal). Pert. to or resembling a finger or toe.

d. reflex. Sudden flexion of terminal phalanx of a finger or thumb when nail is suddenly tapped.

digitalis (dij'ĭ-tal'ĭs) [L. *digitus*, finger, because of its finger-shaped corolla]. USP. Foxglove. The dried leaves of Digitalis purpurea used in powdered form as tablets or capsules. Cardiotonic glycosides, esp. digitoxin and digoxin, are obtained from various species of the Digitalis plant.

ACTION AND USES: Increases the force of muscular contraction of the heart. All other beneficial effects which occur in congestive heart failure—increased cardiac output, decreased heart size, diuresis and relief of edema—all are due to the increased contractile force of the heart.

POISONING: A valuable drug, widely used in treatment of cardiac diseases, toxicity may develop acutely or chronically from its cumulative effect.

SYM: Digestive disturbances, as nausea, and vomiting. Frequently distressing headache. Cardiac irregularities are common, esp. slowing of heart with ventricular extrasystoles or partial heart block.

F. A. TREATMENT: Evacuate stomach, administer diffusible stimulants; cathartics and sedatives are desirable. Because these patients are usually chronically ill, special care is necessary in their management.

digitalism (dij'ĭ-tal-izm). The poisonous effects produced by digitalis.

digitalization (dij'ĭ-tal-ĭ-zā'shun). Subjection of an organism to the action of digitalis.

dig'itate [L. *digitus*, finger]. Having fingerlike impressions or processes.

digitation (dij-ĭ-tā'shun). A fingerlike process.

digiti (dij'ĭ-tī). Pl. of digitus; toes or fingers.

digitoxin (dij-ĭ-tok'sĭn). USP. A cardiotoxic glycoside obtained from various species of the Digitalis plant. A heart stimulant, administered orally or by injection. SEE: *digitalis.*

dig'itus [L]. (pl. *digiti*) A finger or toe.

diglossia (dī-glos'ĭ-ă) [Gr. *dis*, double, + *glōssa*, tongue]. Having a double tongue.

digoxin (dī-jok'sĭn). USP. A cardiotonic glycoside obtained from Digitalis lanata. A heart stimulant administered orally or by injection.

dihydrostreptomycin (dī-hī''drō-strĕp-tō-mī'sĭn). Derivative of streptomycin and originally thought to be less toxic. Uses and dosage same as with parent drug.

dihydrotachysterol (dī-hī''drō-tăk-ĭ-ster'-ol). A hydrogenated tachysterol; a steroid, obtained by irradiation of ergosterol. In hypoparathyroidism, aids absorption of calcium from digestive tract.

dihydrotheelin (dī-hī''drō-thē'ĕl-ĭn). Estradiol, q.v.

dihysteria (dī''hĭs-tēr'ĭ-ă) [Gr. *dis*, double, + *hystera*, the uterus]. State of having a double uterus.

diiodohydroxyquin (dī''ī-o''dō-hī-drok'sĭ-qwin). USP. $C_9H_5I_2NO$. An anti-amebic agent, it is used in treatment of amebiasis and Trichomonas hominis infection of intestines. Proprietary name: Diodoquin.

diktyoma (dik-tĭ-o'mä) [Gr. *diktyon*, net, + *ōma*, tumor]. A ciliary epithelium tumor. Dictyoma.

dilaceration (dī''las-er-ā'shun) [L. *dilacerāre*, to tear apart]. A tearing apart, as of a cataract. SEE: *discission.*

Dilantin (dī-lăn'tĭn). Proprietary name for diphenylhydantoin sodium. A derivative of glyceryl urea. An anti-convulsant used esp. in the treatment of epilepsy.

dilatant (dī-lā'tant) [L. *dilātāre*, to enlarge]. Anything that causes dilation.

dilatation (dil-ă-tā'shun). 1. Expansion of an organ or vessel. 2. Expansion of an orifice with a dilator. SYN: *dilation.*

d., digital. D. of an opening or a cavity by use of the fingers.

d., heart. Abnormal increase in the size of the cavities of the heart, a common result of valvular disease or hypertension.

d., stomach. Condition in which the stomach is extremely dilated. Acute d. of the stomach or acute gastromesenteric ileus may occur as a postoperative or postpartum condition and usually results from obstruction of the duodenum.

dila'tion. 1. Expansion of an orifice with a dilator. 2. Expansion of an organ, orifice or vessel. SYN: *dilatation.*

dilator (dī-lā'tor) [L. *dilātāre*, to expand]. Instrument for dilating muscles, stretching cavities or openings.

d., Barnes'. Rubber bag that is filled with fluid for dilatation of the cervix uteri.

d., Bossi's. A multiple pronged instrument that dilates by separation of the prongs. Used for dilation of the cervix uteri.

d., Goodell's. Similar to the Bossi except that it has three prongs.

d., gynecologic. An instrument for dilating the cervix uteri.

d., Hegar's. Graduated metal sounds that are inserted into the cervical canal and cause a graded dilatation.

d.'s, tent. Small cones made of seaweed, sponge, or tree roots which are inserted into the uterine canal dry and, on absorbing moisture, expand to cause a slow dilatation.

d., vaginal. A glass, plastic, or metal device for dilating the vagina.

dildo, dildoe. Object used to simulate a penis. Artificial penis.

dil'uent [L. *diluere*, to wash away]. That which dilutes.

dilution (di-lu'shun). 1. Process of rendering a substance attenuated or diluted. 2. A diluted substance.

dim. Reduced light or action of decreasing light present.

dimenhydrinate (di''men-hi'drin-āt). USP. A drug occurring as an odorless, crystalline, white powder. It is used to prevent or treat motion sickness and to control nausea, vomiting, and dizziness in other conditions. Proprietary name: Dramamine.

dimercaprol (di-mer-kăp'rŏl). USP. $C_3H_8OS_2$ A compound, 2,3-dimercaptopropanol, used as an antidote in poisoning from heavy metals as arsenic, gold, and mercury. It occurs as a colorless liquid with a disagreeable odor. Mixed with benzyl benzoate and oil, it is administered intramuscularly. It is marketed under its proprietary name, BAL (British Anti-Lewisite).

dimetria (di-me'tri-ă) [Gr. *dis*, double, + *mĕtra*, uterus]. A double uterus.

dimorphous (di-mor'fus) [" + *morphē*, form]. Occuring in two different forms.

dimpling. The formation of a dimple or dimples due to retraction of the subcutaneous tissue. Occurs in certain carcinomas. SEE *peau d'orange.*

dineuric (di-nū'rik) [Gr. *dis*, twice, + *neuron*, nerve]. Having two axis-cylinder processes.

dinical (din'i-kal) [Gr. *dinos*, vertigo]. Pert. to giddiness or vertigo or to their relief.

dioctyl sodium sulfosuccinate (di-ok'til so'dĭ-um sul''fo-suk'sin-āt). USP. A wetting agent or an agent which lowers surface tension. Used as a fecal softener in treatment of constipation.

diodrast (di'o-drast). Proprietary name for iodopyracet, a radiopaque medium used in x-ray studies, esp. of the urinary tract.

diodoquin (di''o-dō'kwin). Proprietary name for diiodohydroxyquin, an antiamebic drug.

diop'ter [Gr. *dia*, through, + *optos*, visible]. Refractive power of lens with focal distance of 1 meter, used as unit of measurement in refraction.

dioptometer (di''op-tom'i-ter) [" + "+ *metron*, measure]. Device for measuring ocular refraction.

dioptom'etry. The determination of refraction and accommodation of the eye.

dioptral (di-op'tral). Pert. to a diopter.

dioptre (di-ŏp'ter). Diopter, q.v.

dioptric (di-ŏp'trik). Dioptral; pert. to refraction of light.

diop'trics. The science of refraction of light.

diorthosis (di-or-thō'sis) [Gr. *dia*, through, + *orthos*, straight]. Reduction of a fracture or dislocation. SYN: *diaplasis.*

diosmosis (di-oz-mō'sis) [" + *ōsmos*, a pushing]. Passage of a fluid through a membrane. SEE *dialysis; osmosis.*

dioxide (di-oks'id) [Gr. *dis*, twice, + *oxys*, sharp]. A compound having two oxygen atoms per molecule.

dipeptid(e (di-pep'tid, -tid) [" + *peptein*, to digest]. A derived protein obtained by hydrolysis of proteins or condensation of amino acids.

dipeptidase (di-pĕp'tĭ-dās). An enzyme that hydrolyzes dipeptids to amino acids.

diphallus (di-fāl'ŭs) [Gr. *dis*, twice, + *phallos*, penis]. A condition in which there is either a complete or incomplete doubling of the penis or clitoris.

diphasic (di-fā'zik) [" + *phasis*, a phase]. Having two phases.

diphenhydramine hydrochloride (di''fen-hi'drā-min hi-dro-klo'rid). USP. An antihistaminic agent. It is an odorless, white, crystalline powder.

diphenylhydantoin sodium (di-fen''il-hi-dan'to-in). USP. A white odorless powder, freely soluble in water. An anticonvulsant used esp. in the treatment of epilepsy.

diphonia (di-fō'ni-ă) [Gr. *dis*, twice, + *phōnē*, voice]. Simultaneous production of two different voice tones.

diphtheria (dif-thē'ri-ă) [Gr. *diphthera*, a skin]. An acute infectious disease characterized by the formation of a false membrane on any mucous surface and occasionally on the skin. Usually accompanied by great prostration.

ETIOL: Causative organism Corynebacterium diphtheriae, a gram-positive nonmotile, non-spore-forming, club-shaped bacillus. In stained smears the bacilli are usually arranged at sharp angles with each other. This gives the characteristic Chinese-letter appearance. The disease is rare under one year of age. The vast majority of cases occur before the age of 10, but older children and adults are not exempt. Both sexes equally susceptible. Esp. prevalent in fall and winter months. Transmission through direct contact with a human carrier, or as a result of exposure through contact with articles that have been contaminated by the d. patient. INCUBATION: two to five days, occasionally longer.

SYM: Onset gradual. Usually slight headache and malaise. Temperature 100° F. to 101° F. (37.8 to 38.3° C.), and sore throat with presence of yellowish-white membrane adherent to tonsils and pharyngeal walls. Cervical adenitis may develop early in severe types. In nasal d., fever is a much more evident symptom. Adenitis often severe, serous discharge from nostrils which may be blood tinged; strong fetid odor of breath common.

d. antitoxin. The antibody which counteracts the diphtheria toxin; the blood serum of a horse or some other animal which has been immunized against diphtheria toxin.

d. carrier. A person harboring in his body the causative organism without manifest symptoms, thus acting as a potential distributor of the infection.

The bacillus usually disappears from the throat of carrier within four weeks, even without treatment. However, administration of penicillin or erythromycin is the most effective treatment for acute or chronic carrier.

d., laryngeal. Considered to be a complication of diphtheria. Results from extension of the membrane from the pharynx with gradual occlusion of the airway. Signs are restlessness, use of accessory respiration muscles, and development of cyanosis. If this is not remedied effectively, death results.

d., surgical. Diphtheric membrane formation on wounds. SYN: *wound d.*

d. toxin. An exotoxin produced by the d. bacillus. A thermolabile substance capable of producing in susceptible animals the same symptoms brought about by inoculation with the living organism.

d. toxin-antitoxin. A mixture of diphtheria toxin and antitoxin. Formerly used in the treatment of diphtheria to produce active immunity. It has been relaced by d. toxoid, q.v., or d. antitoxin; the latter is administered to patients exposed to the disease but who have not been immunized previously.

d. toxoid. D. toxin which has been detoxified. Used to produce active immunity against d.

DIFFERENTIAL DIAGNOSIS: Tonsillitis; scarlet fever; acute pharyngitis; streptococcus sore throat; peritonsillar abscess; infectious mononucleosis; Vincent's angina; acute moniliasis; and staphylococcous infections in the respiratory tract following chemotherapy. Examination of a smear from infected area is advisable, but cultures should be obtained in every instance for the purpose of confirming the diagnosis. In the laryngeal type, edema of the glottis, foreign bodies, and retropharyngeal abscess may require consideration.

PROG: Favorable when antitoxin in sufficient amounts is administered within three days from time of onset. If given on 1st day, death should hardly ever occur. In laryngeal diphtheria, intubation or, rarely, tracheotomy, is usually necessary, as well as an adequate dose of diphtheria antitoxin. Age is important factor, with death more frequent in very young or very old patients than in intermediate age group.

When therapy is not given promptly the incidence of nerve damage is quite high.

ACTIVE IMMUNIZATION: Since all individuals are not susceptible to diphtheria, and because this doubtful factor may be determined by means of the Schick test, it is usually advisable to make use of this test in adults before administering either toxin-antitoxin or toxoid. Routine immunization should begin at age three months, d. toxoid being administered in combination with pertussis vaccine and tetanus toxoid; this is then followed by booster doses. D. toxoid, following a subcutaneous test for hypersensitivity, is used for immunization of adults.

GENERAL MEASURE: Strict bed rest during acute and convalescent stages of disease. In cases with myocardial involvement, prolonged rest in bed may be as important as the early administration of diphtheria antitoxin.

TREATMENT: Specific treatment consists of diphtheria antitoxin after determination of sensitivity to horse serum. No interference with diphtheria membrane is advisable. Gargles should not be used, although cleansing mouthwashes are permissible. On the other hand, the use of suction in nasal cases is sometimes of distinct advantage. A liquid diet (consisting of plenty of water, fruit juices, and nourishing broths) or a soft diet is recommended. In the acute stage, stimulants of any description are rarely necessary. In fact, they are more likely to do harm than good.

In laryngeal diphtheria, surgical interference is sometimes a necessity. Intubation is always to be preferred to tracheotomy, provided an experienced operator is available, and furthermore that the patient is safeguarded by hospitalization which will make possible any attention required within a moment's notice.

SEE: *anatoxin; antitoxin; diphtheria carrier; Klebs-Loeffler bacillus; Schick test.*

diphthe′rial. Pert. to diphtheria.

diphtheriaphor   (dif-thē′rǐ-ă-for)   [Gr. *diphthera*, a skin, + *pherein*, to carry]. A diphtheria carrier or vector.

diphtheric (dǐf-thē′rǐk). Pert. to diphtheria. SYN: *diphtheritic.*

diphtherin (dǐf′thě-rǐn). The toxin of diphtheria, from Corynebacterium diphtheriae.

diphtheritic (dǐf-thěr-ǐt′ǐk). Pert. to diphtheria.

diphtheroid (dǐf′thě-royd) [Gr. *diphthera*, membrane, + *eidos*, appearance]. 1. Resembling diphtheria or the bacteria which cause diphtheria. 2. The formation of a false or pseudomembrane not due to the diphtheria bacillus.

diphtherotox′in ["+ *toxikon*, poison]. The specific toxin of the diphtheria bacillus.

diphthongia (dǐf-thŏn′jǐ-ă) [Gr. *dis*, double, + *phthongos*, voice]. The simultaneous utterance of two vocal sounds of different pitch in pathological conditions of the larynx.

Diphyllobothrium (di-fǐl″ō-bǒth′rǐ-um) ["+ *phyllon*, leaf, + *bothrion*, pit]. A genus of tapeworms belonging to the order Pseudophyllidea and characterized by possession of a scolex possessing two slit-like grooves or bothria. Formerly called Dibothriocephalus.

D. cordatum. The heart-shaped tapeworm, a small species infesting carnivores in Greenland, formerly known as D. mansoni. The plerocercoids are occasionally found in man.

D. erinacei. A species infesting dogs, cats, and other carnivores. Larval stages are occasionally found in man.

D. latum. The broad or fish tapeworm. The adult lives in the intestine of fish-eating mammals and man. It is the largest human tapeworm and may reach a length of 50 to 60 feet or 15.2 to 18.3 meters (average 20 feet or 6.1 meters). The eggs develop into ciliated larvae called coracidia which are eaten by certain species of copepods in which each becomes an onchosphere which develops into a procercoid. Further development occurs in a fish where it develops into a worm-like plerocercoid or sparganum larva.

Infection of the final host occurs following eating improperly cooked fish. Pathological effects are abdominal pain; loss of weight; digestive disorders; progressive weakness; and a severe type of anemia which is clinically identical with pernicious anemia.

diphyodont (dǐf′ǐ-ō-dŏnt) [Gr. *dis*, double, + *phyein*, to produce, + *odous*, tooth]. Having two sets of teeth; as man.

diplacusis (dǐp″lă-ku′sis) [Gr. *diplous*, double, + *akousis*, hearing]. Variety of disturbed perception of pitch characterized by hearing two tones for every sound produced.

diplegia (dī-plē′jǐ-ă) [Gr. *dis*, twice, + *plēgē*, a stroke]. Paralysis of similar parts on both sides of the body. SYN: *double hemiplegia.*

d., infantile. Birth palsy.

d., spastic. Congenital spastic stiffness of the limbs.

diplegic (dī-plē′jik). Pert. to diplegia.

diploalbuminuria (dǐp″lō-al-bu″mǐn-u′rǐ-ă) [Gr. *diplous*, double, + L. *albūmen*, white of egg, + Gr. *ouron*, urine]. Coexistence of physiologic and pathologic albuminuria.

diplobacil′lus ["+ L. *bacillus*, a little stick]. A double bacillus, two being linked end to end.

diplobacte′rium ["+ *baktērion*, little rod]. An organism made up of two adherent bacteria.

diploblastic (dǐp-lō-blas′tǐk) ["+ *blastos*, germ]. The ectoderm and endoderm having two germ layers.

diplocar′dia ["+ *kardia*, heart]. Having the two lateral halves of the heart somewhat separated by a groove.

diplocephaly (dǐp″lō-sěf′ă-lǐ) [Gr. *diplores*, double, + *kephalē*, head]. State of having two heads.

diplococcemia (dǐp″lō-kǒk-sē′mǐ-ă) ["+ *kokkos*, berry, + *haima*, blood]. Diplococci in the blood.

Diplococcus (dǐp-lō-kǒk′us) ["+ *kokkus*, berry]. A genus of bacteria belonging to the family Lactobacillaceae. They are gram-positive organisms occuring in pairs.

D. pneumoniae. A species of bacteria, oval or spherical in shape, gram positive, nonmotile. They possess a capsule. The species is made up of a number of distinct strains of which more than 80 serological types have been isolated. It is the causative agent of certain types of pneumonia, esp. lobar pneumonia and is associated with other infectious diseases such as cerebrospinal meningitis, otitis media, amd septicemia. SYN: *D. lanceolatus; Micrococcus lanceolatus; M. pneumoniae; pneumococcus; Streptococcus pneumoniae.*

diplocoria (dĭp″lō-kō′rĭ-ă) [Gr. *diplous*, double, + *korē*, pupil]. Double pupil in the eye.

diploe (dĭp′lō-ē) [Gr. *diploē*, fold]. Cancellated tissue between the tables of the skull.

diploet′ic, diplo′ic. Pert. to the diploe or cancellated tissue between cranial tables.

diplogen′esis [Gr. *diplous*, double, + *genesis*, production]. Having two parts or producing two substances; production of double fetus or the doubling of some fetal parts.

diploid (dĭp′loyd) [″+ *eidos*, form]. Having double the haploid number of chromosomes. Said of somatic cells which contain twice the number of chromosomes present in the egg or sperm.

diplokaryon (dĭp″lō-kar′ĭ-ŏn) [Gr. *diplous*, double, + *karyon*, nucleus]. A nucleus containing twice the diploid number of chromosomes.

diplomellituria (dĭp″lō-mĕl′ĭ-tūr′ĭ-ă) [″+ *meli*, honey, + *ouron*, urine]. Condition in which diabetic and nondiabetic glycosuria occur either simultaneously or alternately in the same individual.

diplomyelia (dĭp″lō-mī-ē′lĭ-ă) [″+ *myelos*, marrow]. Condition in certain types of spina bifida in which the spinal cord is doubled.

diploneu′ral [″+ *neuron*, nerve]. Having two nerves from different origins, as certain muscles.

diplopagus (dĭp-lŏp′ă-gus) [″+ *pagos*, a thing fixed]. Conjoined twins which share some organs.

diplophonia (dĭp-lō-fō′nĭ-ă) [″+ *phōnē*, voice]. Having two different voice tones at the same time. SYN: *diphonia*.

diplopia (dĭp-lō′pĭ-ă) [Gr. *diplous*, double, + *ōpē*, sight]. Double vision; monocular (astigmatism, subluxated lens, incipient cataract); binocular (due to derangement of extraocular muscles).

    d., binocular. Double vision occurs when both eyes are used but not in focus. Seen in disease of the eyeballs, cranial nerve affections, disease of the cerebellum, cerebrum, and meninges.

    d., crossed. Binocular vision in which the images are reversed.

    d., direct. D., homonymous, q.v.

    d., heteronymous. D., crossed, q.v.

    d., homonymous. Double vision in which right-hand image appears on right side and left-hand image on left side. SEE: *d., crossed.*

    d., monocular. Double vision with one eye.

    d., unocular. D., monocular, q.v.

    d., vertical. D. with one of two images higher than the other.

diplopiometer (dĭp-lō″pĭ-om′ĕ-ter) [″+ ″+ *metron*, measure]. Device for estimating double vision.

dip′loscope [″+ *skopein*, to examine]. Device for study of binocular vision.

diplosoma′tia [Gr. *diplous*, double, + *sōma*, body]. Twins joined at one or more points. SYN: *diplosomia*.

diploso′mia. Twins joined together. SYN: *diplosomatia*, q.v.

dip′ping. 1. Palpation of the liver by a quick depression movement of the fingers while the hand is held flat on the abdomen. 2. The act of immersing an object in a solution, esp. applied to the dipping of cattle in a solution for the control of cattle ticks.

diprosopus (dĭp-rō-sōp′ŭs) [Gr. *dis*, twice, + *prosōpon*, face]. A malformed fetus characterized by possession of a double face.

dipsesis (dĭp-sē′sis) [Gr. *dipsēsis*, a thirst]. Extreme thirst or craving for abnormal liquids.

dipsomania (dĭp″sō-mā′nĭ-ă) [Gr. *dipsa*, thirst, + *mania*, madness]. A morbid and uncontrollable craving for alcoholic beverages. SEE: *alcoholism*.

dipsopathy (dĭp-sŏp′ă-thĭ) [″+ *pathos*, disease]. Dipsomania.

dipsophobia (dĭp-so-fō′bĭ-ă) [Gr. *dipsa*, thirst, + *phobos*, fear]. Morbid fear of drinking.

dipsosis (dĭp-sō′sis) [″+ *-ōsis*, condition]. Abnormal thirst.

dipsotherapy (dĭp″so-ther′ă-pĭ) [″+ *therapeia*, treatment]. Limitation of water intake as a means of treatment.

Diptera (dĭp′ter-ă) [Gr. *dipteros*, having two wings]. An order of insects characterized by having sucking or piercing mouth parts, one pair of wings, and complete metamorphosis. It includes the flies, gnats, midges, and mosquitos. It contains many species involved in the transmission of pathogenic organisms.

dipterous (dĭp′ter-ŭs). Having two wings; characteristic of the order Diptera.

dipylidiasis (dĭp′ĭ-lĭ-dī′ă-sis). Infestation with the tapeworm, Dipylidium caninum.

Dipylidium (dĭp′ĭ-lĭd′ĭ-um) [Gr. *dipylos*, having two entrances]. A genus of tapeworms belonging to the family Dipyliidae which infests dogs and cats.

    D. caninum. A species of Dipylidium, a common parasite of dogs and cats. Occasionally human infestation may occur through the accidental ingestion of lice or fleas which serve as the intermediate host.

direct′ [L. *dīregere*, to direct]. Immediate; uninterrupted; straight.

    d. current. An electric current flowing in one direction only.

d. light reflex. One in which response occurs on same side as the stimulus.

d. murmur. That due to stenosis of cardiac orifices.

d. reflex. Prompt contraction of sphincter of iris when light entering through pupil strikes retina of eye.

director (di-rek'tor). Grooved device for guiding a knife in surgery.

dirigomotor (dir''ĭ-go-mo'tor) [L. *dirigere*, to direct, + *motor*, mover]. Controlling or directing muscular activity.

dis-. 1. [L. *dis*, apart] Prefix indicating free of, to undo. 2. [Gr. *dis*, twice] Prefix meaning double or twice.

disaccharide (di-sak'ĭ-rĭd) [Gr. *dis*, twice, + *sakkharon*, sugar]. A member of the disaccharose, q.v., group of carbohydrates. SEE: *carbohydrates*.

disaccharose (di-sak'ă-rōs). A complex sugar that may be split into two molecules of monosaccharides. The two monosaccharoses resulting from the decomposition may be different or identical. Thus the maltose, $C_{12}H_{22}O_{11}$, for each molecule yields two molecules of glucose, $C_6H_{12}O_6$, while the sucrose, $C_{12}H_{22}O_{11}$, yields a molecule each of glucose and fructose.

The d.'s consist of the following: *Levulose:* same as fructose. In the body this is formed in the digestion of sucrose. It is found in fruits, plants, and in honey. *Maltose:* is found in malt and malt products, and in germinating seeds. It is acted upon in the intestines by maltase, resulting in production of two molecules of glucose. It is a reducing sugar. Commercial maltose is a mixture of maltose and dextrins. *Sucrose:* Cane sugar or table sugar. A nonreducing sugar. It comes from sugar cane, sorghum, maple sugar, sugar beets, and honey. An increase in temperature while heating sucrose results in caramel. It is acted upon in the intestines by sucrase, an enzyme converting it into one molecule each of glucose and fructose.

ACTION: Some sugars undergo fermentation by yeasts, or decomposition is brought about by bacteria or molds which oxidize sugars into carbon dioxide and water. Alcohol is produced when dextrose ferments.

Most of the sugar on the market consists of beet and cane sugar. Ripe fruits and vegetables contain sucrose. The starch of green fruits is changed to a mixture of sucrose, glucose, and levulose.

Sucrose gives the sweet flavor to ripe fruits. It has the following chemical characteristics: (1) Extremely soluble. Cold water will hold in solution almost twice its weight of sucrose. Hot water will dissolve even more. (2) It crystallizes very easily. (3) It melts at about 160° C., changes to an amber hue and becomes less sweet; when heated to about 200° C., it becomes a brown, syrupy mass with a distinctive flavor called caramel.

SEE: *carbohydrates; monosaccharide; polysaccharide.*

disarticula'tion [L. *dis*, apart, + *articulus*, joint]. Amputation through a joint.

disassimila'tion ["+ *ad*, to, + *similāre*, to make like]. Changing assimilated material into less complex compounds for the production of energy.

disc [Gr. *diskos*, quoit]. A round, flat, platelike structure. SEE: *disk.*

discharge (dĭs-charj', dĭs'charj) [ME. *dischargen*, to discharge]. 1. The escape (esp. by violence) of pent up or accumulated energy or of explosive material. 2. The flowing away of a secretion or excretion of pus, feces, urine, etc. 3. The material thus ejected.

d., cerebral cortical. The violent action of an injured or malfunctioning portion of the cerebral cortex that gives rise to an epileptic paroxysm.

d., convective. One from a high potential source in the form of electrical energy passing through the air to the patient.

d., disruptive. A passage of current through an insulating medium due to the breakdown of the medium under electrostatic stress.

d., electric. A slow or instantaneous bringing back to a neutral electric condition, by which every highly electrified body loses its surplus electricity, giving it up to surrounding bodies less highly electrified.

d., lochial. Uterine excretion following childbirth. SEE: *lochia.*

discharg'ing. The emission of or the flowing out of material as the discharge of pus from a lesion. Excreting.

d. lesion. A lesion of nerve center in brain suddenly discharging motor impulses.

dischrona'tion [L. *dis*, apart, + Gr. *chronos*, time]. Lack of a sense of relativity in the consciousness of time.

discission (dĭs-sizh'un) ["+ *scindere*, to cut]. Rupture of the capsule of the crystalline lens in operation for cataract.

discitis (dis-ki'tis) [Gr. *diskos*, disk, + *-itis*, inflammation]. Diskitis, q.v.

discoblas'tic ["+ *blastos*, germ]. Pert. to discoid segmentation of yolk in an impregnated ovum.

discoblastula (dĭs''kō-blas'tū-lă). A modified blastula found in highly telolecithal eggs, as in birds in which the blastomeres form a cellular cap (germinal disc or blastoderm) which is separated from the yolk by a space, the blastocoele.

dis'coid. Like a disc.

discoplacen'ta [Gr. *diskos*, quoit, + *plakous*, a flat cake]. A disklike placenta.

discrete (dis-krēt') [L. *discretus*, separated]. Separate; said of certain eruptions on the skin. SEE: *confluent.*

discrimina'tion [L. *discriminãre*, to divide]. The process of distinguishing or differentiating.

   d., one-point. The ability to locate specifically a point of pressure on the surface of the skin.

   d., tonal. The ability to distinguish one tone from another. This is dependent upon the integrity of the transverse fibers of the basilar membrane of the organ of Corti.

   d., two-point. The ability to localize two points of pressure on the surface of the skin and to identify them as discrete sensations. SYN: *tactile.*

dis'cus [Gr. *diskos*, quoit]. (pl. *discuses* or *disci*) [NA] A disk.

   d. articularis. [NA]. An interarticular fibrocartilage; an articular disk.

   d. proligerus. The cumulus oophorus, q.v.

discuss' [L. *discutere*, to dissipate]. To disperse, scatter, or cause to disappear.

discussion (dis-kush'un). Dispersal of a tumor or swelling.

discussive (dis-kus'iv). An agent which causes a disease process to disperse or undergo resolution.

discutient (dis-ku'shent) [L. *discutere*, to dissipate]. Agent which disperses a lesion or tumor.

disdiaclast (dis-di'ä-klast) [Gr. *dis*, twice, + *diaklan*, to break through]. A doubly refracting element in the tissues of striated muscles.

disdiadochokinesia (dis-di''ä-do''ko-kī-ne'zī-ä) [L. *dis*, apart, + Gr. *diadochos*, succeeding, + *kinēsis*, motion]. Inability to make finely coordinated movements of a part in opposite directions. For example, quickly supinating and pronating the hand. SEE: *diadochokinesia.*

disease (dī-zēz') [Fr. *dēs*, from, + *aise*, ease]. Literally the lack of ease; a pathological condition of the body that presents a group of symptoms peculiar to it and which sets the condition apart as an abnormal entity differing from other normal or pathological body states.

   d., acute. D. having a rapid onset and of relatively short duration.

   d., anticipated. A d., which by its known ability to occur in individuals or groups who have certain genetic, biochemical, physical, or geographical characteristics, may be predicted to occur in those persons.

   d., chronic. One having a slow onset and lasting for a long period of time.

   d., communicable. D., the causative organism of which is transmissible from one person to another, either directly, or indirectly through a carrier or vector.

   d., congenital. D. which is present at birth. May be due to hereditary factors, or prenatal infection, injury or the effect of a drug the mother took during pregnancy.

   d., constitutional. 1. D. due to an individual's hereditary make-up. 2. A disease involving the body as a whole in contrast to one involving specific organs. SEE: *diathesis.*

   d., contagious. An infectious d. readily transmitted from one person to another.

   d., deficiency. A d. resulting from inadequate intake or absorption of essential dietary factors such as vitamins or minerals.

   d., degenerative. A d. resulting from degenerative changes that occur in tissues and organs, characteristic of old age.

   d., endemic. A d. which is present more or less continously or recurs in a community.

   d., epidemic. D. which attacks a large number of individuals in a community at the same time.

   d., familial. A d. which occurs in several individuals of the same family.

   d., functional. A d. in which no anatomical changes can be observed to account for the symptoms present.

   d., hereditary. D. due to hereditary factors transmitted from parent to offspring.

   d., hypokinetic. Physical and mental illness produced by lack of or by insufficient exercise.

   d., idiopathic. D. for which no causative factor can be recognized.

   d., infectious. D. resulting from the presence in the body of a pathogenic organism.

   d., malignant. 1. Cancer, q.v. 2. D., including cancer but not limited to that, in which the progress is extremely rapid, generally threatening or resulting in death within a short time.

   d., molecular. A hereditary d. that may be caused by a defective molecule.

   d., occupational. D. resulting from factors associated with the occupation engaged in by the patient.

d., organic. D. resulting from recognizable anatomical changes in an organ, or tissue of the body.

d., pandemic. An epidemic d. which is extremely widespread, involving an entire country, continent, or possibly the entire world.

d., parasitic. D. resulting from the growth and development of parasitic organisms (plants or animals) in or upon the body.

d., psychosomatic. D. in which structural changes in or malfunctioning of organs are due to the mind, esp. the emotions. *NOTE:* It is not possible for a human being to be consciously sick without there being some interplay between the emotions and the bodily functions.

d., sporadic. D. in which only occasional cases occur; not epidemic or endemic.

d., subacute. D. in which symptoms are less pronounced but more prolonged than in an acute disease; intermediate between acute and chronic disease.

d., venereal. Includes syphilis, gonorrhea, lymphogranuloma venerum, and chancroid. D. usually acquired through sexual relations, either heterosexual or homosexual. ABBR: V.D.

disengage'ment [Fr.]. The emergence of the fetal head from within the maternal pelvis.

disequilibrium (dis-ē''kwǐ-lib'rǐ-um) [L. *dis,* apart, + *aequus,* equal, + *libra,* balance]. On unequal and unstable equilibrium.

disinfect (dis-in-fekt') ["+ *inficere,* to corrupt]. To free from infection by physical or chemical means.

disinfec'tant. 1. A chemical which kills bacteria. Common disinfectants are the halogens: chlorine, fluorine, iodine; salts of heavy metals: mercuric chloride (bichloride of mercury), silver nitrate; acids: sulphurous acid; alkalies: chloride of lime; organic compounds: formaldehyde, alcohol 70%, iodoform, organic acids, phenol (carbolic acid), cresols, benzoic and salicylic acids and their sodium salts; miscellaneous substances: thymol, hydrogen peroxide, potassium permanganate, boric acid. SYN: bactericide; germicide.

2. An agent that frees from infection. Term is usually applied to a chemical or physical agent which kills vegetative forms of microorganisms.

disinfecting agents. SEE: *alcohol; borax; boric acid; chlorine preparations; cresol; formaldehyde; hydrogen dioxide; mercuric chloride; nitric acid; phenol; potassium permanganate; sulfur.*

disinfec'tion. The application of disinfectants. It is not possible to insure a 100% d. of a room unless the entire room and its contents are treated with a gaseous agent such as ethylene oxide. Disinfestation, or the killing of vermin by chemicals and their vapors, however, is possible.

d. of blankets and woolens. May be steam-disinfected, or soaked for two hours in 5% carbolic acid solution and then washed and rinsed thoroughly. Cotton goods may also be so treated, or boiled before washing. Materials which might be harmed by conventional methods of d. may be treated in a chamber with ethylene-oxide gas.

d. of excreta. Should be soaked in 5% carbolic acid solution for one hour before disposal. All infected excreta should be burned, but sputum may be treated as excreta if impossible to burn.

d. of field of operation. A safe rule is to make the d., if anything, too extensive. Thus, in operations of any magnitude upon scalp and large wounds of this structure, and in all operations on the skull and its contents the entire scalp must be shaved and disinfected.

In operations upon the breast, the axilla and half of the chest must be prepared, and if glands of neck are involved the entire neck must be included in field of operation.

In amputation of foot and lower third of leg the d. must extend as far as knee, and in all higher amputations it should include the whole limb and corresponding side of pelvis.

In all abdominal operations below the umbilicus the pubic area must be shaved, and the surface d. must include the whole anterior surface and both sides as far as the breasts.

In operations on the stomach, liver, and bile ducts the field extends from the pubic area to the breasts. A general warm bath with liberal use of tincture of green soap should precede d. of the field of operation in all abdominal and pelvic operations, including hernia and varicocele.

In operations upon parts of the body difficult to disinfect, as scalp, palm of hand, and sole of foot, it is advisable to scrub with hot water and tincture of green soap then rinse; then use 70- per-cent solution of alcohol, benzalkonium chloride, hexachlorophene, or other disinfectant. Alcohol is universally useful in hand and surface d.

The mucous membranes are active, absorbing surfaces so that the use of solutions of carbolic acid, mercuric bichloride, and other potent antiseptics is prohibited. The

Methods of Disinfection*

Method	Concentration or Intensity	Use	Limitations
Moist heat			
Autoclaving	250–270° F. (121–132° C.)	Sterilize instruments not harmed by heat and water	Moisture will not permeate some materials Cannot be used for heat-sensitive items
Boiling water	212° F. (100° C.)	Kill nonspore-forming pathogenic organisms	Does not kill spores Probably not effective against hepatitis virus
Radiation			
Ultraviolet light		Air and surface disinfection	Penetrates poorly Harmful to unprotected skin and eyes
Ionizing		Sterilize medicines, some plastics, sutures, and biologicals	Expensive
Filtration			
Membrane		Water purification	Slow and expensive
Fiberglass filters		Air disinfection	Only cleans incoming air; does not prevent recontamination
Physical cleaning			
Ultrasonic		Disinfect instruments	Aids in cleaning but not effective alone
Washing		Disinfect hands and surfaces	Does not remove all organisms
Chemicals			
Alcohols	70–90%	Skin degerming	Sometimes irritating Does not kill spores
Chlorines	100–200 parts per million	Water disinfection Food surface sanitization	Inactivated by inorganic matter Does not kill spores Ineffective at certain pH values
Iodines, tincture	2%	Skin degerming	Not sporocidal Sometimes irritating
Iodines, iodophors	74–450 parts per million	General disinfectant	Not sporocidal
Phenols	1–4%	General disinfectant	Ineffective against some bacteria May be irritating or corrosive
Quarternary ammonia compounds, tincture	0.1%	Skin degerming	Neutralized by soap Not sporocidal

* Adapted from Benarde, M. A. (ed.): Disinfection: A Treatise. Dekker, Marcel Inc., New York, 1970.

Methods of Disinfection* *(Continued)*

Method	Concentration or Intensity	Use	Limitations
Quarternary ammonia compounds, aqueous	Diluted one part to 750 parts	General disinfectant	May be incompatible with some water Ineffective against some bacteria
Mercurials	0.1%	Skin degerming	Slow acting May be irritating
Formaldehyde (formalin)	5%	Drastic disinfection	Irritating, corrosive
Gluteraldehyde	2%	Instrument sterilization	Irritates mucous membranes Unstable
Germicidal soaps (hexachlorophene)	2–3%	Skin degerming	Bacteriostatic rather than bactericidal
Gaseous Ethylene oxide	450 mg./liter	Sterilization of heat-sensitive materials	Temperature, time, humidity critical Treated materials need to air for varying periods of time (depending on composition) following treatment
Formaldehyde gas		Fumigation Sterilization of heat-sensitive materials	Irritating, corrosive

free use of any of these agents in the vagina, uterus, or rectum has frequently resulted in serious poisoning, and in some instances death.

In grave operations, such as excision of superior or inferior maxilla, and amputation of tongue, the employment of a disinfecting solution is preceded by thorough cleansing of the teeth, and the mucous membrane is swabbed with hydrogen peroxide.

In operations upon the rectum the procedure in common use consists of shaving perianal area, and giving enemas.

Vaginal d. is more satisfactory. After a thorough cleansing with warm water and tincture of green soap, a douche of warm water with a suitable disinfectant is recommended. The vaginal d. is preceded by shaving and d. of the external genitals.

Catheterization should always be preced-ed by d. of the meatus with green soap and rinsing thoroughly with sterile water.

The ear should be mechanically cleansed of wax, dirt, blood clot, etc., and then be carefully disinfected by a low-pressure stream of warm hydrogen peroxide, until it is absolutely clean.

disinfestation (dis"in-fes-tā'shun) [L. *dis,* apart, + *infestāre,* to strike at]. The process of killing infesting insects or parasites.

disinsected. Freed of insects.

disintegra'tion [L. *dis,* apart, + *integer,* entire]. The product of catabolism; the falling apart of the constituents of a substance.

disjoint. To disarticulate or to separate bones from their natural positions in a joint.

disk [Gr. *diskos,* a disk]. A round, flat, plate-like structure.

d., anisotropic. A dark, shining, highly refractile d. forming a part of the striation of the myofibril of a striated muscle fiber. Also called A or Q stripe.

d., articular. A d. of dense fibrous tissue or fibrocartilage found in the structure of certain joints, esp. the temporomandibular joint.

d., Bowman's. Segment of a muscle fiber.

d., choked. A swollen optic d. due to inflammation or edema. SYN: *papilledema.*

d., diameter. Optic-disk diameter.

d., embryonic. An oval d. of cells in the blastocyst of a mammal from which the embryo proper develops. Its lower layer, the endoderm, forms the roof of the yolk sac; its upper layer, the ectoderm, forms the floor of the amniotic cavity. The primitive streak develops on the upper surface of the d.

d., epiphyseal. Disklike epiphysis at vertebral centrum's ends.

d., germinal. A d. of cells on the surface of the yolk of the eggs of reptiles and birds from which the embryo develops; the blastoderm.

d., Hensen's. A pale d. occurring in the middle of a muscle fiber.

d., herniated. Rupture or herniation of the intervertebral d., esp. between the 4th and 5th lumbar vertebrae. This usually causes pain in the affected side. SYN: *herniated nucleus pulposus.*

d. holder. Joint for microscope stand to enable mobility in every direction.

d., intercalated. A highly refractive band which extends transversely across the fiber of cardiac muscle. It is bounded on each side by Z lines.

d., intermediate. Myofibrils. Also called Z line or Krause's membrane.

d., interpubic. D. of cartilage between the pubic bones at their symphysis.

d., intervertebral. A fibrocartilage substance between vertebral surfaces.

It may rupture but it does not slip. It serves as a shock absorber. The gelatinous mass in the center is called the nucleus pulposus. When the d. material protrudes into the neural canal, pressure on the adjacent nerve root is manifested by pain. This is called herniation of an intervertebral d. Symptoms will depend upon the location of the herniation. Those in the cervical area produce distinctive signs and symptoms in the upper extremities and cervical area. Those in the lumbar area cause symptoms of lumbar nerve root pressure.

d., isotropic. A d. lying between the A d. of a striated muscle myofibril. Also called I or J d. It extends across the entire muscle fiber.

d., M. A thin line lying in the center of Hensen's d.

d., Merkel's. A disklike expansion found at the end of sensory nerve fibers in the epidermis. It is a touch receptor. SYN: *tactile disk.*

d., optic. Area of the retina where optic nerve enters it.

d., proligerous. D., germinal, q.v.

d., Q. The anistropic or A d. of a striated muscle myofibril.

d., tactile. D., Merkel's, q.v.

d., Z. The intermediate d. of a striated muscle fiber. SEE: *striate muscle.*

diskitis (disk-i'tis). Inflammation of a disk, esp. an interarticular cartilage. SYN: *meniscitis.*

dis"loca'tion [L. *dis,* apart, + *locāre,* to place]. The displacement of any part, esp. the temporary displacement of a bone from its normal position in a joint.

d., closed. D., simple, q.v.

d., complete. One which completely separates the surfaces of a joint.

d., complicated. One which is associated with other important injuries.

d., compound. One in which the joint communicates with the external air.

d., congenital. One which exists from or before birth.

d., consecutive. One in which the luxated bone has changed its position since its first displacement.

d., divergent. One in which the ulna and radius are dislocated separately.

d., habitual. One which often recurs after replacement.

d., incomplete. A subluxation; a slight displacement.

d., intrauterine. One which occurs to the fetus in utero.

d., metacarpophalangeal joint. D. of finger.

This is usually complicated by an interposition of tendons or other structures, and if reduced tends to slip out immediately. In many instances manipulating of this region only tends to make it more difficult for a subsequent reduction; therefore, immobilize the disturbed area with well-placed and padded splints of hand and wrist. Send patient to doctor promptly.

d., Monteggia's. D. of hip joint in which head of femur is near anterosuperior spine of the ilium.

d., Nelaton's. D. of the ankle in which the astragalus is forced up between the end of the tibia and the fibula.

d., old. A d. in which no reduction has been accomplished, even after many days, weeks, or months.

d., partial. Same as incomplete.

d., pathologic. One which results from paralysis or disease of joint or supporting tissues.

d., primitive. One in which the bones remain as originally displaced.

d., recent. One seen shortly after it occurred.

d., simple. One in which the joint is not penetrated by a wound.

d., subastragalar. Separation of the calcaneum and the scaphoid from the astragalus.

d., thyroid. Displacement of the head of the femur into the thyroid foramen.

d., traumatic. One due to injury or violence.

dismemb'er. To remove an extremity or a portion of it.

disomus (dī-sō'mus) [Gr. *dis,* twice, + *sōma,* body]. A malformed fetus with a double trunk.

disorganiza'tion [L. *dis,* apart, + Gr. *organon,* a unified organ]. Alteration in an organic part, causing it to lose most or all of its distinctive characteristics.

disorientation (dis-o''rī-en-tā'shun) [L. *dis,* apart, + *oriens,* arising]. Inability to estimate direction or location, or to be cognizant of time or of persons.

disparate points (dis'par-at, dis-par'at) [L. *disparāre,* to separate]. Points on the two retinas which are not corresponding or identical, causing objects to appear double.

dispen'sary [L. *dispensāre,* to give out]. Place or clinic for dispensation of medicines and treatment.

dispense (dis-pens'). To prepare or deliver medicines.

disperse (dis-pers') [L. *dis,* apart, + *spargere,* to scatter]. 1. To scatter, esp. applied to the scattering of light rays. 2. To dissipate or effect the disappearance of, as of a tumor or the particles of a colloidal system.

dispersion (dis-per'zhun). 1. Act of dispersing. 2. That which is dispersed.

d., coarse. Mechanical suspension.

d., colloidal. Colloid solution.

d., medium. Liquid in which a colloid is dispersed.

d., molecular. A true solution.

d., particles. Colloid particles in a colloid system.

d. system. A colloid solution.

dispersonalization (dis-per''son-al-ī-zā'-shun). Mental state in which the individual

denies the existence of his personality or parts of the body.

dispireme (dī-spī'rēm) [Gr. *dis,* twice, + *speirēma,* coil]. Stage that succeeds the diaster and precedes division of cell body, when threads of daughter cell are convoluted.

displace'ment [Fr. *déplacer,* to lay aside]. 1. Removal from the normal or usual position or place. 2. Adding to a fluid one of greater density causing the first fluid to be dispersed. 3. Transfer of emotion from repressed conflict to some apparently indifferent idea. In psychoanalysis, this would be the transfer of an emotion pert. to one set of ideas to an inappropriate idea; although properly thus associated in the unconscious.

disposi'tion [L. *dispōnere,* to arrange]. A natural tendency or aptitude exhibited by an individual or group of individuals. This may be manifested toward acquiring a certain disease, presumably due to hereditary factors. SEE: *diathesis.*

dissect (dis-sekt') [L. *dissecāre,* to cut up]. To separate tissues and parts of a cadaver for anatomical study.

dissection (dis-sek'shun). The cutting of parts for purpose of separation and studying of the same.

dissem'inated [L. *dis,* apart, + *semināre,* to sow]. Scattered or distributed over a considerable area, esp. applied to disease organisms; scattered throughout an organ or the body.

d. sclerosis. A degenerative disease of the nervous system.

disseminated intravascular coagulation. Clinical condition of altered blood coagulation. It is secondary to a variety of diseases. SYN: *consumption-coagulopathy,* q.v.

dissipation (dis-ī-pā'shun) [L. *dissipāre,* to scatter]. 1. Dispersion of matter. 2. Act of being wasteful and living a dissolute life, esp. drinking alcoholic beverages to excess.

dissociation (dis-so''sī-ā'shun) [L. *dis,* apart, + *sociatiō,* union]. Separation, as the separation by heat of a complex compound into simpler molecules.

d., microbic. Substrains arising from pure strains.

d. of personality. Split in consciousness resulting in two different phases of personality, neither being aware of the words, acts, and feelings of the other. SEE: *dual personality; multiple personality.*

d., psychological. Disunion of mind of which the person is not aware. Dual personalities, fugues, somnambulism, selective amnesia are examples.

d. symptoms. Anesthesia to heat, cold, and pain, without loss of muscular sense or tactile sensibility.

dissolu'tion [L. *dissolvere,* to dissolve]. 1. Death. 2. Pathological resolution or breaking up of the integrity of an anatomical entity.

dissolve (dĭ-zolv') [L. *dissolvere,* to dissolve]. To cause absorption of a solid in and by a liquid.

dissolvent (diz-ol'vent). 1. Having the power to dissolve. 2. That which is capable of being dissolved.

dissol'ving. To cause to enter into a solution.

distad (dis'tad) [L. *distāre,* to be distant]. Away from the center.

distal (dis'tal) [L. *distāre,* to be distant]. Farthest from the center, from a medial line, or from the trunk. SEE: *proximal.*

distend' [L. *distendere,* to stretch out]. 1. To stretch out. 2. To become inflated.

disten'tion. The state of being distended. SEE: *goblet cell.*

distichiasis (dis"tĭ-kĭ'ă-sis) [Gr. *dis,* twice, + *stikhos,* row]. Two rows of eyelashes, one or both of which are directed inward toward the eye.

distill (dis-til') [L. *destillāre,* to drop from]. To vaporize by heat, condensing and collecting the volatilized products.

distillate (dis'til-āt). That which has been derived from the distillation process.

distilla'tion. Condensation of a vapor which has been obtained from a liquid heated to the volatilization point, as the condensation of steam from boiling water.

D. is used for the purification of water and for other purposes. Distilled water should not be exposed as it readily takes up impurities from the atmosphere.

d., destructive. The process of decomposing complex organic compounds by heat in the absence of air, and condensing the vapor of the liquid products.

d., dry. D. of solids without adding liquids.

d., fractional. Separation of liquids based upon the difference in their boiling points.

distinctometer (dis"tink-tom'ĭ-ter) [L. *distinguere,* to mark out, + Gr. *metron,* measure]. Device for palpation of abdomen along its borders.

distobuccal (dis"tō-buk'al) [L. *distāre,* to be distant, + *bucca,* cheek]. Pert. to the distal and buccal walls of bicuspid and molar teeth.

Distoma, Distomum (dis'tō-mă, -mum) [Gr. *dis,* two, + *stoma,* mouth]. Former name of genus of trematode worms. Its members have been placed in many new genera.

dis'tome. A fluke with two suckers, an oral and a ventral sucker or acetabulum.

distomiasis (dīs"tō-mī'ă-sis). Infestation with flukes which may infest the intestine, liver, bile ducts, gallbladder, blood vessels, or lungs.

distor'tion [L. *dis,* apart, + *torsio,* a twisting]. 1. A twisting or bending out of regular shape. 2. A writhing or twisting movement as of the muscles of the face. 3. A deformity in which the part or structure is altered in shape. 4. In ophthalmology, visual perception of an image which does not provide a true picture. This is due to astigmatism or to retinal abnormalities. 5. In psychiatry, adapting an idea to conform with a patient's wishes, esp. in dreams.

distractibil'ity. A condition of mental wandering in which the thoughts are attracted by extraneous conditions or influenced by a dissociation of consciousness.

distraction (dis-trak'shun) [L. *dis,* apart, + *tratiō,* a drawing]. 1. State of mental confusion or derangement. 2. Separation of the surfaces of a joint by extension without injury or dislocation of the parts.

distraught (dis-trawt') [L. *distrahere,* to perplex]. The mental state of being in doubt, deeply troubled, and having conflicting thoughts. Patient may be frantic and have need to be continuously occupied.

distress (dis-tres') [L. *distringere,* to draw apart]. Physical or mental trouble or suffering.

distribution [L. *dis,* apart, + *tribuere,* to allot]. 1. The dividing and spreading of anything, esp. blood vessels and nerves, to tissues. 2. The presence of entities at various sites or in particular patterns throughout the body such as hair, fat, nutrients, etc.

districhiasis (dis-trik-ĭ'ă-sis) [Gr. *dis,* double, + *thrix,* hair]. Two hairs growing from the same hair follicle.

distrix (dis'triks). The splitting of ends of the hairs.

disulfiram (dī-sul'fĭ-ram). A drug administered orally to deter ingestion of alcohol. If alcohol is ingested following taking of drug, there occurs an unpleasant reaction which includes nausea and vomiting. Proprietary name: Antabuse. SYN: *tetraethylthiuram disulfide.*

Dittrich's plugs (dĭt'rĭk). [Franz Dittrich, Ger. pathologist, 1815-1859]. Small particles in fetid sputum composed of pus, detritus, bacteria, and fat globules.

diuresis (dī″u-rē′sis) [Gr. *diourein*, to urinate]. Secretion and passage of abnormally large amounts of urine.

This occurs in diabetes mellitus. It is an early sign of chronic interstitial nephritis. May also be due to: hysteria or as a result of fear and anxiety; ingestion of large quantities of liquids; diabetes insipidus; the action of drugs which have the ability to cause diuresis.

diuretic (dī″u-ret′ik). Increasing or an agent which increases the secretion of urine.

Diuretics act in two ways: (1) by increasing glomerular filtration or (2) by decreasing reabsorption from the tubules. An increase in blood flow in the renal vessels increases urine formation by increasing glomerular filtration-pressure and by increasing the number of glomeruli functioning.

Diuretics act on the kidney cells, increasing permeability, and also on the circulation to the kidneys. Alcohol dilates the blood vessels of the kidneys and thus increases circulation to them.

Cold applications have a diuretic action by contracting superficial vessels and raising blood pressure. SEE: *diuresis.*

diuril (dī′u-rīl). Proprietary name for chlorothiazide, a diuretic agent.

diur′nal [L. *diēs,* day]. 1. Daily. 2. Happening in the daytime or pert. to it. SEE: *nocturnal.*

divagation (dī-vă-gā′shun) [L. *divagāri,* to wander about]. Disconnected and incoherent speech.

divergence (dī-ver′jens) [L. *divergere,* to turn aside]. Separation from a common center, esp. that of the eyes.

diver′gent. Radiating in different directions.

diver′s paralysis. Occupational disease due to returning too suddenly to normal atmosphere after working under high air pressure. SYN: *bends; caisson disease; tunnel disease.*

divertic′ula [L. *dēvertere,* to turn aside]. Pl. of diverticulum, q.v.

diverticulec′tomy [″ + Gr. *ektomē,* excision]. Surgical removal of a diverticulum.

diverticuli′tis [″ + Gr. *-itis,* inflammation]. Inflammation of a diverticulum or of diverticula in the intestinal tract, esp. in the colon, causing stagnation of feces in little distended sacs of the colon (diverticula).

    d., acute. SYM: Similar to appendicitis: inflammation of peritoneum, formation of an abscess, and, finally, gangrene accompanied by perforation may ensue.

    d., chronic. SYM: Constipation growing worse, mucus in stools, griping abdominal pains at intervals. Wall of bowels may thicken, which may produce chronic intestinal

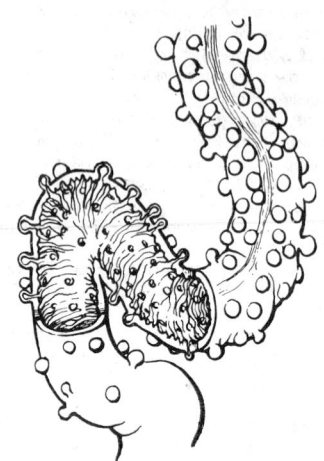

MULTIPLE DIVERTICULA OF THE COLON

obstruction.

diverticulo′sis [″ + Gr. *-ōsis,* condition]. Diverticula in the colon without inflammation or symptoms. Only a small per cent of persons with diverticulosis go on to develop diverticulitis.

diverticulum (dī″ver-tik′u-lum). (pl. *diverticula)* A sac or pouch in the walls of a canal or organ.

    d., false. D. without muscular coats in wall or pouch. This type of d. is acquired.

    d., Meckel′s. Caused by continued existence of the omphalomesenteric duct. Its occurrence is fairly common. Usually located on ileum close to ileocecal valve.

    d. of duodenum. D. commonly located near entrance of common and pancreatic ducts.

    d. of jejunum. D. marked usually by severe pain in upper abdomen, followed occasionally by massive hemorrhage from intestine.

    d. of stomach. D. of wall of stomach.

    d., true. D. involving all the coats of muscle in the pouch wall. Usually congenital.

division (dī-vizh′un) [L. *dividere,* to divide]. 1. A separation into parts. 2. That which separates, as anatomical boundary, partition, or wall.

    d., cell. The formation of two daughter cells from the original cell.

divulsor (dī-vul′sor) [L. *dis,* apart, + *vellere,* to pluck]. Device for dilatation of a part, esp. the urethra.

d., pterygium. Instrument for separating corneal portion of the pterygium.

d., tendon. Device for separating tendon from surrounding tissue.

dizygotic twins (dī″zǐ-got′ǐk) [Gr. *dis*, two, + *zygon*, yoke]. Twins who are the product of two ova. Fraternal twins. SEE: *twin, monozygotic.*

diz′ziness [AS. *dysig*, foolish]. Giddiness, vertigo.

DMF Index. The total number of decayed, missing, and filled teeth.

DNA. Abbr. for *deoxyribonucleic acid*, q.v.

Dobell's solution (dō′bĕl). [Horace B. Dobell, Brit. physician, 1828-1917]. Carbolic acid, borax, sodium bicarbonate, glycerine, and water in solution.

Dobie's globule (dō′bēs). [William M. Dobie, Brit. physician, 1828-1915]. A very tiny spherical body in a striated muscle fiber's light band.

DOCA. Proprietary name for desoxycorticosterone.

dochmiasis, dochmiosis (dok-mī′as-is, -mī-o′sis) [Dochmius, a nematode parasite]. Hookworm disease. SYN: *ankylostomiasis, uncinariasis.*

Dochmius (dok′mī-us). A species of parasite. SYN: *ankylostoma.*

doctor [L. *docēre*, to teach]. 1. The recipient of an advanced degree, i.e., doctor of medicine (M.D.); doctor of philosophy (Ph.D.); doctor of science (D.Sc.); doctor of divinity (D.D.); etc. 2. One who, after being licensed to do so, practices medicine.

The use of the word doctor is sometimes confusing. This may be remedied when writing or speaking of those who possess an M.D. degree by using the word physician.

In some countries persons are, after college, awarded the degree of Doctor of Jurisprudence and are referred to thereafter as doctor.

dog bite. Lacerated wound by a dog.

Preserve the dog alive if possible. Animal should be observed for 10 days to determine the presence of rabies.

TREATMENT: Thorough cleansing of bite wounds with strong soap or detergent solutions (as 1:1000 solution of benzalkonium hydrochloride), followed by infiltration of the wound areas with antirabies serum. SEE: *Rabies.*

dol. Symb. for degree of pain registered on the dolorimeter.

dolichocephalic (dol″ĭ-ko-sĭ-fal′ĭk) [Gr. *dolichos*, long, + *kephalē*, head]. Having a skull with a long anterior-posterior diameter.

dolichocolon (dol″ĭ-ko-ko′lon) [" + *kolon*, colon]. Abnormally long colon.

dolichohieric (dol″ĭ-ko-hī-er′ĭk) [" + *hieron*, sacred]. Having a long, slender sacrum.

dolichopellic, dolichopelvic (dol″ĭ-ko-pel′-ĭk, -pel′vĭk) [Gr. *dolichos*, long, + *pyelos*, an oblong trough]. Having an abnormally long or narrow pelvis.

dolichosigmoid (dol″ĭ-ko-sig′moyd) [" + *sigma*, 18th letter of the Greek alphabet, + *eidos*, form]. Having an abnormally long sigmoid flexure.

dolor (do′lor) [L.]. Pain; one of the principal indications of inflammation. SEE: *calor; rubor; tumor.*

d. cap′itis. Headache.

dolorific (do″lor-if′ik) [L. *dolor*, pain]. Causing pain.

dolorimeter (do″lor-ĭm′ĭ-ter) [" + Gr. *metron*, measure]. SYMB: *dol.* Device for measuring degree of pain.

dolorogen′ic [" + Gr. *gennan*, to produce]. Causing pain.

domatophobia (do-măt-ō-fō′bĭ-ă) [Gr. *dōma*, house, + *phobos*, fear]. A form of claustrophobia; abnormal aversion to being in a house.

domicil′iary (dom″ĭ-sil′ē-ār″ĭ) [L. *domus*, house]. Pert. to or carried on in a house.

dom′inant [L. *dominăns*, ruling]. In genetics a trait or characteristic which will develop in the offspring even though it is present in the genetic material of only one of the parents. SEE: *recessive.*

donee (do-nē′) [L. *donăre*, to give]. One who receives something, such as a blood transfu-

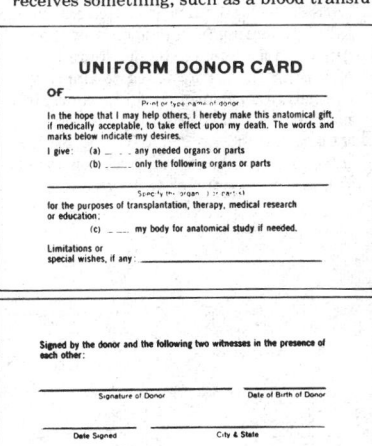

UNIFORM DONOR CARD

OF_____
Print or type name of donor

In the hope that I may help others, I hereby make this anatomical gift, if medically acceptable, to take effect upon my death. The words and marks below indicate my desires.

I give: (a) ___ ... any needed organs or parts

(b) _____ only the following organs or parts

_____
Specify the organ(s) or part(s)

for the purposes of transplantation, therapy, medical research or education:

(c) ___ ... my body for anatomical study if needed.

Limitations or special wishes, if any : _____

Signed by the donor and the following two witnesses in the presence of each other:

_____ _____
Signature of Donor   Date of Birth of Donor

_____ _____
Date Signed   City & State

_____ _____
Witness   Witness

This is a legal document under the Uniform Anatomical Gift Act or similar laws.

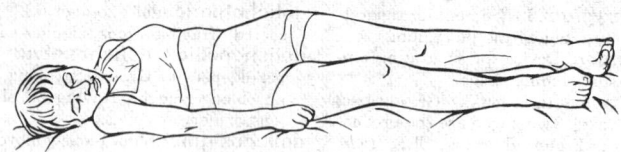

DORSAL INERTIA POSTURE

sion, from a donor.

do'nor. One who furnishes blood, tissue, or an organ to be used in another person.

 d. card. A document used by a person who wishes to make an anatomical gift, at the time of his death, of an organ needed for transplantation. SEE: *transplantation.*

 d., universal. One whose blood is of Group O, and whose blood is therefore usually compatible with most other blood types. In actual practice this compatibility rarely occurs because of the many factors other than the major blood antigens (A, B, AB) which determine blood compatibility.

Don'ovan bodies. [Charles Donovan, Ir. physician in India, 1863 —] Leishmania donovani, a small protozoan parasite occurring as a small oval or round body in bone marrow or in spleen or liver. The causative agent in kala-azar.

dopa. A chemical substance, 3,4-dihydroxyphenylalanine, produced by the oxidation of tyrosine to typosinase.

dopamine (dō'pă-mēn). Compound which increases blood pressure. It is used experimentally in treating hypotension and shock.

doping. In athletic medicine, administration of a drug that is designed to improve the competitor's performance, remaining in the body at the time of competition.

doraphobia (dō"ră-fō'bĭ-ă) [Gr. *dora,* hide, + *phobos,* fear]. Abnormal aversion to touching the hair or fur of animals.

Dorel'lo's canal. A bony canal in tip of temporal bone enclosing abducens nerve.

Dorendorf's sign. [Hans Dorendorf, Ger. physician, 1866 —] A filling up or fullness of the supraclavicular groove in aneurysm of the aortic arch.

dorsa. Pl. of dorsum.

dorsabdom'inal [L. *dorsum,* back, + *abdōmen,* belly]. Pert. to the back and abdomen.

dor'sad ["+ *ad,* toward]. Toward the back.

dor'sal [L. *dorsum,* back]. 1. Pert. to the back. 2. Indicating a position toward a rear part.

 d. elevated postion. Patient is on the back with head and shoulders elevated at an angle of 30° or more. Employed for digital examination of genitalia, and in bimanual examination.

 d. inertia posture. In which patient rests on the back and shows a tendency to turn to either side or to slip down in bed if head of bed is elevated.

 This may be seen in great weakness; in acute infectious diseases such as typhoid; mental apathy; and in muscular weakness.

 d. nerves. Nerves emerging from the dorsal vertebrae, q.v.

 d. recumbent position. Same as dorsal elevated, except extremities are moderately flexed and rotated outward, the soles of the feet resting upon bed or table, or legs may be extended. With legs not flexed, this position is used for examination of chest, ab-

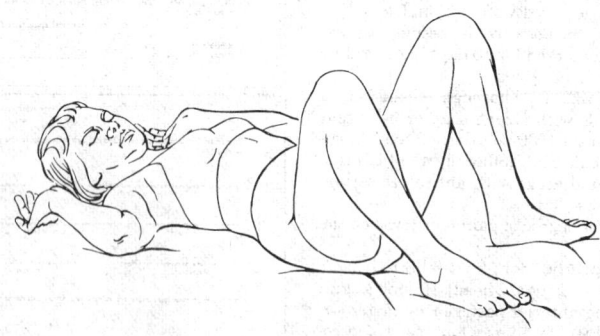

DORSAL RECUMBENT POSITION

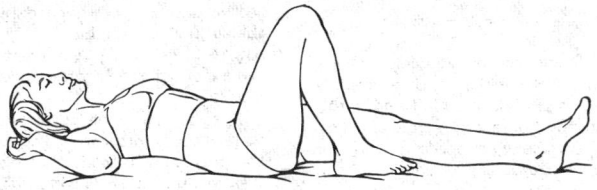

DORSAL RIGID POSTURE
With right leg drawn up

domen, and lower limbs. With legs flexed, it is used in giving douches, for bathing, for catheterizing, and for applying abdominal compresses. The patient may be placed in this position for bimanual palpation, or for vaginal examinations and repair of lesions following parturition.

d. reflex. Irritation of the skin over the erector spinal muscles, causing contraction of muscles of the back.

d. rigid posture. One in which both legs (or the right one only) are drawn up; observed in peritonitis, meningitis, ascites, and tympanites. The right leg is drawn up in appendicitis, pelvic inflammation, renal calculus in right ureter, psoas abscess, or peritonitis on the right side.

d. slit. A surgical method of making the foreskin of the penis easily retractable. The foreskin is cut in the d. midline but not far enough to extend into the mucous membrane next to the glans. D. slit can be used as a simple substitute for circumcision.

d. vertebrae. Twelve bones of the spinal column between the cervical and lumbar vertebrae. SEE: *position; posture.*

dorsalgia (dor-sal'ji-ä) ["+ Gr. *algos,* pain]. Pain in the back. SYN: *notalgia; rachialgia.*

dorsi-, dorso-, dors-. Combining form for L. *dorsum,* back.

dor'siduct [L. *dorsum,* back, + *ducere,* to lead]. To draw toward the back or backward.

dorsiduc'tion. Drawing toward the back.

dorsiflect (dor'si-flekt) [L. *dorsum,* back, + *flectere,* to bend]. To bend backward.

dorsiflex'ion. Movement of a part at a joint so as to bend the part toward the dorsum or posterior aspect of the body. Thus d. of the foot indicates movement of the foot backward at the ankle. D. of the toes indicates moving the toes toward the sole of the foot. When the hand is overextended and bent backward, it is dorsiflexed. Opposed to plantar flexion, q.v.

dorsimesad (dor"si-mes'ad). In the direction of the dorsimeson.

dorsimeson (dor-si-mes'on) [L. *dorsum,* back, + Gr. *meson,* middle]. The median plane of the back.

dorsispinal (dor'si-spi'nal) ["+ *spina,* thorn]. Pert. to the back and spine.

d. veins. Veins around the vertebrae.

dorsocephalad (dor"so-sef'ä-lad) ["+ Gr. *kephalē,* head, + L. *ad,* toward]. Situated toward the back of the head.

dorsodynia (dor"so-din'i-ä) ["+ Gr. *odynē,* pain]. Pain in the muscles of upper part of back.

dorsosa'cral ["+ *sacrum,* sacred, "sacred bone"]. Pert. to lower back.

d. position. Patient lies upon the back, as in the dorsal recumbent position, q.v., except that thighs are flexed upon abdomen and legs upon thighs, which are abducted. Leg holders are used to support legs in position.

Used for gynecological examinations and treatments; in plastic operations in genital tract; in vaginal hysterectomy; and in diagnosis and treatment of diseases of urethra and bladder. SYN: *lithotomy position.* SEE: lithotomy position for illustration.

dor'sum [L.]. (pl. *dorsa*). The back or posterior surface of a part.

dos'age [Gr. *dosis,* a giving]. The amt. of medicine to be administered to a patient at one time.

d., calculation of, for children. There is no absolutely reliable formula for calculating the dose of a medicine an infant or child should receive. Several rules for calculating a child's dose are given here.

Young's rule for children:
  for Children from 1 to 12 Years:
      Formula:

$$\frac{\text{Age in yr.}}{\text{Age} + 12} \times \text{Adult dose} = \text{child's dose.}$$

Ex. The adult dose of a substance is 500 mg. How much should a 4-year-old child receive?

$$\frac{4}{4+12} \times 500 = 125$$

The child should receive 125 mg.

Body surface area: The surface area in square meters is divided by 1.7 and multiplied by the adult dose. Ex: A child of 0.4 sq. meters of surface who needs a drug for which the adult dose is 500 mg.:

$$\frac{0.4}{1.7} \times 500 = 117$$

Thus the dose would be 117 mg. Obviously medicines are not packaged in 117 mg. doses; so either 100 mg. or 125 mg. could be safely given. If the medicine were in liquid form, the dose could be easily determined by using the same formula.

d. meter. An instrument designed to estimate the quantity of radiation, so as to determine the duration of exposure when using roentgen rays. SYN: *dosimeter.*

dose (dōs). Amt. of a medicinal preparation to be taken at one time.

d., divided. Fractional portions administered at short intervals.

d., erythema. Smallest amount of X rays that will produce erythema within two weeks following treatment.

d., lethal. A fatal dose.

d., maximum. Largest dose it is safe to administer.

d., minimum. Smallest dose that will be effective.

dosimeter (dō-sim′ĭ-ter) [Gr. *dosis,* a giving, + *metron,* measure]. Device for measuring x-ray output.

dosimetric (dō″sĭ-met′rik). Pert to dosimetry.

d. system. One of regular dosage.

dosimetry (dō-sim′ĕt-rĭ) [Gr. *dosis,* a giving, + *metron,* measure]. Measurement of doses.

do′tage [ME. *doten,* to be silly]. Senility; feeblemindedness of very old age.

double (dŭb′l) [L. *duplus,* twofold]. Combining two things or qualities.

d. consciousness. Expression of two phases of personality.

d. personality. A split in consciousness, neither personality being aware of acts and words of other. SEE: *dual personality; multiple personality.*

d. touch. Exploration with a finger in one cavity and thumb in another.

d. uterus. State of having a double uterus. SYN: *dihysteria.*

d. vision. Seeing two images of an object at the same time. SYN: *diplopia.*

double blind technique. A method of investigation in which neither the subject nor the investigator working with the subject or data knows what treatment, if any, the subject is receiving.

douche (doosh) [Fr.]. A current of vapor or stream of hot or cold water directed against a part.

D.'s may be made up of plain water or water that is medicated. The d. may be for the purpose of personal hygiene or for the treatment of a local condition. A vaginal douche following sexual intercourse does not provide an effective method of contraception.

d., air. Air current directed on body for therapeutic purposes.

d., alternating. D., Scotch, q.v.

d., astringent. One containing substances for shrinking the mucous membrane, such as alum or zinc sulfate.

d., circular. Needle spray or application of water to body through horizontal jets the size of a needle from a number of small rows of sprays so placed that the water is projected against the skin of bather from four directions simultaneously.

d., cleansing. An external or perineal d. for cleansing genitalia following defecation or following operations such as hemorrhoidectomy; curettement; rectal surgery; circumcision; perineorrhaphy, etc. Mild antiseptic or disinfectant solution, 98° to 104° F., poured or sprayed over the parts, followed by gentle drying and inspection for cleanliness. SYN: *external d.; perineal d.*

d., deodorizing. One to deodorize the vagina and vaginal secretions when they have an offensive odor.

d., high. One where the bag is at least four feet above the hips of the patient.

d., jet. A solid stream from the douche hose.

d., low. One where the bag is 1-1 1/2 feet (31-46 cm.) above the hips of the patient.

d., medicated. One containing a medicinal substance for the treatment of local conditions.

d., neutral. D. given at average surface temperature of body—90-97° F. (32.2-36.1° C.).

d., perineal. One projected upward from a bidet, q.v., placed just above the floor; patient sits on the seat of the bidet and receives d. upon perineum. SYN: *cleansing d.,* q.v.

d., rain. Overhead shower.

d., Scotch. Alternating of hot and cold jets of water against local area of skin.

d., vaginal. D. of vagina ordered for deodorant, antiseptic, stimulating, or hemostatic purposes. Temperature of solutions: antiseptic or deodorant d., 105° to 112° F.

(40.6° to 44.4° C.); stimulating or hemostatic d., 118° to 120° F. (47.8° to 48.9° C.). Solution should flow slowly with little pressure, the douche solution container being elevated up to two feet above patient's pelvis. Quantity generally two to three quarts of solution unless otherwise ordered.

The vagina, like many other areas of the body, has the ability to cleanse itself. Thus there is very little reason for a normal healthy woman to use a vaginal douche. Also there is no evidence that a postcoital vaginal douche is effective as a contraceptive.

Douglas' cul-de-sac. [James Douglas, Scot. anatomist, 1675-1742]. Peritoneal sac which lies behind uterus and in front of rectum. SYN: *D.'s pouch.*

douglasitis (dug-las-i′tis). Inflammation of the cul-de-sac of Douglas.

dow′el [ME. *dowle*, peg]. Metal pin for fastening an artificial crown to a tooth root.

Down's syndrome. [J. Langdon Down, Brit. physician, 1828-1896] Mongolism, a variety of congenital, moderate to severe mental retardation. Marked by sloping forehead; presence of epicanthal folds causing an Oriental appearance of eyes; bridge of nose flat or sometimes absent; low-set ears; and generally dwarfed physique.

Doyère's eminence (dwah-yair). [Louis Doyère, Fr. physiologist, 1811-1863]. Elevation where a nerve filament enters a muscle.

D.P. Abbr. for *Doctor of Pharmacy.*

dr. Abbr. for *dram; drachm.*

DR. Abbr. for *reaction of degeneration.*

drachm (dram) [Gr. *drachmē*, a Greek unit of weight]. A unit of weight in apothecaries' system. SYMB: ℨ. ABBR: *dr.* SEE: *dram.*

dracontiasis (drak″on-ti′ă-sis) [Gr. *drakontion*, little dragon]. Dracunculiasis.

dracunculiasis (dră-kung″ku-li′ă-sis). Infestation with the nematode, Dracunculus medinensis.

dracunculosis (dră-kung″ku-lo′sis). Dracunculiasis.

Dracunculus (dră-kung′ku-lus). A genus of parasitic nematodes.

 D. medinensis. The guinea worm or "fiery serpent." A species of nematode which is a common human parasite, esp. in Africa and India. Adult female parasite burrows under skin of leg of human beings. Larvae are discharged into environment, esp. when legs are in water. Fleas in water swallow larvae and become infective. Man becomes infected after drinking contaminated water.

drain (drān) [AS. *drēahnian*, to draw off]. 1. Exit or tube for discharge of a morbid matter. 2. To draw off a fluid.

 d., capillary. Drawing off by capillary attraction.

 d., cigarette. D. made by covering a small strip of gauze with rubber.

 d., Mikulicz's. Single layer of gauze pushed into the wound cavity, to which is added thick gauze wicks that project from the cavity.

 d., nonabsorbable. One made from horsehair, gauze, rubber, glass, or metal. Types are abdominal, antrum, perineal, suprapubic, etc.

 d., Penrose. A cigarette d. made with a piece of small rubber tubing through which gauze has been pulled.

drainage (drān′ij). The free flow or withdrawal of fluids, as pus from a cavity or wound. SEE: *autodrainage; drain.*

 d., capillary. D. by method of capillary attraction.

 d., funnel. D. with glass funnels.

 d., postural. D. for draining nasal area, bronchi, and the sinuses. The patient lies on his back on a bed with shoulders over the side and head hanging down.

 d., tidal. A method, controlled mechanically, of filling the bladder with solution by gravity, and periodically emptying the vesicle by siphonage. Usually used when the patient lacks control of the bladder, as in injuries or lesions of the spinal cord.

 d. tube. Device for allowing escape of pus, serum, blood, or other fluids from a wound, abscess, etc.

 d. t. carrier. Device for placing drainage tube in position.

 d. t. trocar. Device to introduce drainage tube without making a large incision.

dram [Gr. *drachmē*]. A unit of weight in apothecaries' system. Sixty gr. or 1/8 oz. apothecary weight; 3.888 gm., 27.34 gr. or 1/16 oz., avoirdupois.

 d., fluid. A teaspoonful or 1/8 of a fluid ounce or 57.1 gr. of distilled water, the equivalent of 3.70 cc. or ml. In Great Britain 54.8 gr. of distilled water or 3.5 ml.

dramamine (dram′ă-mēn). Proprietary name for dimenhydrinate, an antihistamine.

dram′atism [Gr. *drama*, acting, + *ismos*, state of]. Dramatic behavior and lofty speech in insanity.

drapetomania (drăp″ĕt-o-mā′ni-ă) [Gr. *drapetēs*, runaway, + *mania*, madness]. Insane impulse to wander from home.

dras′tic [Gr. *drastikos*, effective]. 1. Acting strongly. 2. A very active cathartic, usually producing many explosive bowel movements accompanied by pain and tenesmus. The use of this type of cathartic is not advisable.

draught (draft) [ME. *draught,* a pulling]. 1. A drink. 2. Drawing liquid into the mouth. 3. Breeze produced by wind or fan. 4. A liquid medicinal dose to be taken all at once.

draw sheet. Historically, the term "draw sheet" was given to a long roll or bolt of muslin with the free end placed under the patient's buttocks. When this became soiled, it was drawn from under the patient and rolled up on the opposite side of the cot or bed, allowing the patient to lie on a clean section of the roll of muslin.

The draw sheet is now used to cover a rubber sheet which protects the mattress from soiling and drainage. A crib sheet or one-half a regular sheet is the usual size, but it must be wide enough to extend from the patient's shoulders to below the knees and long enough to tuck under both sides of mattress. SEE: *bed.*

dream [AS. *drēam,* joy]. Occurence of ideas, emotions, and sensations during sleep. Some dreams may be recalled upon awakening, others may not be. SEE: *R.E.M.*

    d., wet. Involuntary discharge of semen during sleep. Usually occurs during an erotic dream.

drepanocyte (drep"ă-no-sīt) [Gr. *drepanē,* sickle, + *kytos,* cell]. Sickle or crescent cell.

drepanocytemia (drep"ă-no-sī-tē'mĭ-ă) ["+ "+ *haima,* blood]. Sickle-cell anemia.

drepanocytic (drep"ă-no-sit'ik). Pert. to or resembling a sickle cell.

dressing [O.Fr. *dresser,* to prepare]. Covering, protective or supportive, for diseased or injured parts.

    NP: These rules should be followed when preparing to dress any type of wound: Assemble all necessary articles, either on a tray or surgical-dressing cart. Scrub hands thoroughly with soap under hot running water. Use sterile rubber gloves for procedure if doctor so advises. Also the nurse, physician, and patient may be required to wear surgical-type masks. Tell the patient what is going to be done; then drape with a sheet or bath blanket, exposing only the area necessary to be dressed. Place sterile towel beside the wound and, using sterile forceps, place upon the towel the sterile instruments, gauze, etc., from their sterile containers.

Using clean forceps, remove soiled d.'s and place in paper bag for burning. Follow doctor's instructions as to use of antiseptics, powders, petroleum, gauze, etc. If drainage is profuse, reinforce the d. with absorbent cellulose pads. Make the patient comforta-

ble; remove all articles from room; take tray or cart to area for cleaning and replenishing supplies.

    RS: bandage; compress.

    d., absorbent. Gauze, sterilized gauze, absorbent cotton.

    d., antiseptic. D. consisting of gauze permeated with an antiseptic solution.

    d., dry. D. consisting of dry gauze, absorbent cotton, or other dry material.

    d., fixed. D. permeated with starch, silicate of soda, or plaster of Paris. When this d. dries it provides fixation of the part so treated.

    d., hot moist. Most common form is hot normal saline solution, hot as can be borne by bare forearm of nurse. Sterile towel unfolded, gauze d.'s dropped into it; towel immersed in solution at middle, wrung out by turning dry ends in opposite directions. D. is then applied, with sterile forceps, directly to the wound and a dry, sterile towel is sometimes used over it, to keep d. in place. Heat is best maintained by infrared lamp. *CAUTION:* Do not burn patient.

    d., non-adherent. One which has little or no tendency to adhere to dried secretions from the wound.

    d., occlusive. D. that seals a wound completely to prevent infection from without and to prevent mositure from escaping from the d.

    d., pressure. One which is used to apply pressure to the wound. May be used following skin grafting.

    d., protective. D. applied for purpose of preventing injury or infection to the part so treated.

    d., water. D. consisting of gauze, cotton, or similar dressing material which is kept wet by the application of sterilized water.

Drinker respirator. [Philip Drinker, Amer. engineer in industrial hygiene, 1894 —]. Apparatus in which alternating positive and negative air pressure upon the patient's thoracic area, by allowing the air in the otherwise immobile lung to be alternately inspired and exhaled, acts to produce artificial respiration. Commonly called the iron lung.

drip [ME. *drippen,* to drip]. 1. To fall in drops. 2. To instill drop by drop.

    d., intravenous. Slow injection of a solution (glucose, saline, etc.), a drop at a time, intravenously.

    d., Murphy. Slow rectal instillation of a fluid drop by drop. SEE: *Murphy's drip.*

    d., nasal. Method of administering fluid slowly to dehydrated babies by means of a catheter with one end placed through the nose into the esophagus.

   d., postnasal. A condition due to chronic sinusitis in which a discharge flows from the postnasal region into the pharynx.

drip sheet. Modified sheet bath.

drive (drīv) [AS. *drifan*]. The force or impulse to act.

dromomania (drŏ″mō-mā′nĭ-ă) [Gr. *dromos*, a running, + *mania*, madness]. Insane impulse to wander.

dromotrop′ic ["+ *tropikos*, a turning]. Pert. to supposed fibers in cardiac nerves which influence conductivity of muscles.

drop [AS. *dropa*]. 1. A minute spherical mass of liquid. 2. Falling of a part from paralysis or injury.

   d., culture. A bacterial culture in a d. of culture media.

   d.'s ear. Medication administered by d.'s placed in the external canal of the ear.

   d. foot. Toes dragging in walking, with falling of foot due to paralysis of dorsal flexor muscles.

   d., hanging. Application of a d. of solution to a small glass cover-slip. This is then inverted over a glass slide with a depression in it. The contents of the suspended solution can then be examined microscopically.

   d.'s, knockout. A drug to cause unconsciousness; usually administered for criminal purposes.

   d. wrist. Paralysis of extensor muscles causing hand to hang down from forearm.

droplet. Very small drop.

   d. infection. That conveyed by means of infective particles, as when carried in a spray from the nose or mouth. Usual mode of infection from common cold.

dropsy (drop′sĭ) [Gr. *hydōr*, water]. A condition rather than a disease. Morbid accumulation of fluid and edema in the tissues and cavities; hydrops.

   ETIOL: Heart disease, kidney disease, cirrhosis of the liver, and other causes such as excess sodium retention. SEE: *nephritis.*

   DIET: Sufficient proteins, carbohydrates, fats, vitamins, and iron; reduction of sodium intake; a salt-free diet with an acid base. Salt substitutes may be used.

   d. of amnion. Abnormal increase in amt. of amniotic fluid. SYN: *polyhydramnios.*

   d. of the belly. Ascites.

   d. of brain. Hydrocephalus.

   d., cardiac. That due to cardiac disease.

   d. of chest. Hydrothorax.

   d. of peritoneum. Hydroperitoneum.

   d., tubal. A collection of fluid in the fallopian tube. SYN: *hydrosalpinx.*

   d., uterine. A collection of fluid in the uterine cavity. SYN: *hydrometra.*

Drosophila (drō-sŏf′ĭ-lă). A genus of flies belonging to the order Diptera. Includes the common fruit flies.

   D. melanogaster. A genus of fruit flies used extensively in the study of genetics. The development of the chromosome theory of heredity was largely the outcome of research on this species.

drowning [ME. *dr(o)unen*, to drown]. A special type of asphyxia resulting from the body being submerged in water. External respiration is blocked by a spasm of the larynx or the filling of the lungs with fluid.

   SYM: Unconsciousness, cessation of respiration, cyanosis, etc., depending upon duration of submersion. Due to action of the epiglottis, there is very little, if any, water in the lung.

   F. A. TREATMENT: Artificial respiration at once. Do not waste time trying to get water out of lungs. Use oxygen or oxygen-carbon dioxide mixtures with resuscitation. May have to be kept up for several hours. Cardiac resuscitation may also be required.

   RS: artificial respiration; asphyxia; shock; syncope; unconsciousness.

drownproofing. A method of staying afloat by using a minimum amount of energy. May be kept up for hours even by nonswimmers, whereas only the most fit and expert of swimmers could stay afloat for more than 30 minutes. Details of the drownproofing technique may be obtained from local chapters of the American Red Cross.

   TECHNIQUE: *Rest:* Take a deep breath and sink vertically beneath the surface, relax your arms and legs, keep chin down and allow fingertips to brush against knees. Keep neck relaxed and back of head above the surface. *Get set:* Gently raise arms to a crossed position with back of wrists touching forehead. At the same time step forward with one leg and backward with the other. *Lift head, exhale:* Without moving your arms and legs from the previous position, raise your head quickly but smoothly to the vertical and exhale through your nose.

   Stroke and kick, inhale: To support your head above the surface while you inhale through your mouth—gently sweep the arms outward and downward and step downward with both feet. *Head down, press:* As you drop beneath the surface put your head down and press downward with your arms and hands to arrest your fall. *Rest:* Important to relax completely as in the first step for six to ten seconds. Always breathe from choice—never from necessity.

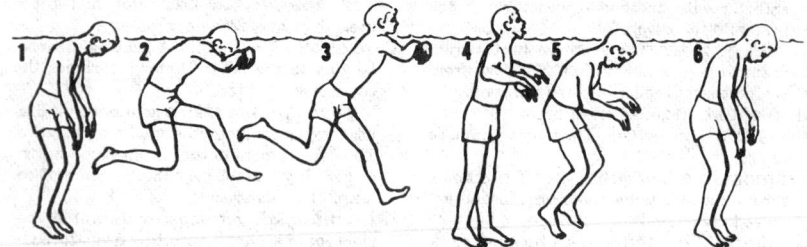

DROWNPROOFING TECHNIQUE
1, Rest. 2, Get set. 3, Lift head, exhale. 4, Stroke and kick, inhale. 5, Head down, press. 6, Rest.

drug [O. Fr. *drogue,* chemical material]. Any substance that when taken into the living organism may modify one or more of its functions.

d. abuse. The use, usually by self administration, of any drug in a manner that deviates from the approved medical or social patterns within a given culture.

d. action. *Local:* When the drug is applied locally or directly to a tissue or organ it may combine to form an albuminate with the cells' albumins. This action may be (1) Astringent when the drug cannot act because the albuminate does not dissolve; (2) Corrosive when the drug is strong enough to destroy cells; (3) Irritating when too much of the drug combines with cells to impair them.

General or Systemic Action: When the drug enters the blood stream by absorption or direct injection affecting tissues and organs not near the site of entry. Systemic action may be (1) Specific when specific in the cure of a certain disease; (2) Substitutive when it supplies substances deficient in the body; (3) Physical when some of the constituents of a cell are dissolved by the action of the drug in the blood stream; (4) Chemical when the drug or some of its principles combine with the constituents of cells or organs to form a new chemical combination; (5) Salt action by osmosis, q.v., caused by dilution of salt (also acids, sugars, and alkalies) in the stomach or intestines by fluid withdrawn from the blood and tissues, or by diffusion, q.v., when water is absorbed by cells from the lymph; (6) Selective, action produced by drugs which only affect certain tissues or organs; (7) Synergistic, the stimulating of the action of one drug by another drug; (8) Antagonistic, counteraction of one drug by another; (9) Physiological, the effect of a drug similar to that which the body normally produces; (10) Therapeutic, the effect upon diseased organs or tissues; (11) Side ac-

tion, creating an effect not desired; (12) Empiric, an effect produced but not proved by laboratory experiment; (13) Toxicological, a toxic or undesired effect generally from result of an overdose.

Cumulative: The effect of drugs that are too slowly excreted or absorbed so that with repeated doses an accumulation of the drug in the body produces a toxic effect. Such drugs should not be administered continuously.

Incompatible: Ill effects produced by two or more drugs antagonistic to each other.

RS: active principles; alkaloids; antidotes; dosage; medical preparations; names of individual drugs; names of poisons; names of preparations; preparations given rectally; prescription writing.

d. addiction. A condition caused by excessive or continued use of habit-forming drugs.

Illicit drugs may or may not contain the kind and amount of drug the user thought was purchased. For this reason a user may have a serious reaction (even death) to the unknown substance present in the material.

SYM: The symptom pattern may be changed according to the drug used. In general there may be a change in personality, loss of appetite, dulled appetite, disturbance in normal sleep-rhythm, generally a weight loss. The addict may be dull, sleepy, and incoordinated in movement, having the appearance of intoxication. The eyes often tearing and bloodshot; a watery fluid at times dripping from the nose. When intramuscular or intravenous injection is used there may be scars, hardening and swelling of the arm tissues. Serum hepatitis may occur when narcotic addicts use dirty needles and syringes for adminstering drugs to themselves or fellow addicts. SEE: *hepatitis, homologous serum.*

d. dependence. A psychic (and sometimes physical) state resulting from interaction of a living organism and a drug. Characterized by behavioral and other responses that include a compulsion to take the drug on a continuous or periodic basis in order to experience its psychic effects or to avoid the discomfort of its absence. Tolerance may or may not be present and a person may be dependent on more than one drug.

d. interaction. Effects of drugs altered by other drugs present in the body. May be due to altered absorption, excretion, or metabolism of the drug.

d. rashes. Rashes produced in some patients by application or ingestion of drugs. In general, drug rashes are not specific for certain drugs. Therefore the following should be used only as a rough guide.

Antipyrin: Papular, erythematous rash, sometimes accompanied by edema and much irritation. *Arsenic:* Papular or erythematous rash, sometimes urticarial. Prolonged use many produce pigmentation of skin. *Belladonna:* Erythematous rash, usually accompanied by intense itching. *Bromides:* Usually like acne vulgaris. Sometimes erythema.

Chloral: Papular erythema. *Iodides:* Usually papular erythema, sometimes with acnelike pustules. *Phenolphthalein:* Macular rash, sometimes purpuric. *Quinine:* Very irritable erythema or urticaria. *Salicylate:* Erythematous rash, possibly morbilliform. *Serum:* Usually urticaria.

d. reaction. Adverse and undesired reaction to a substance taken for its pharmacological effects. An estimated 15% of hospitalized patients will develop toxic or allergic drug reactions.

drug-fast. Resistance, as of bacteria, to action of a drug or drugs.

drugs and their administration. *Acids:* When acids are administered orally they should be given well diluted through a glass tube or by stomach tube because they are corrosive to the enamel and dentine of the teeth. They should be given with much water and the drinking tube should be placed well back in the mouth to prevent the fluid coming in contact with the teeth before passing into the throat. Hydrochloric acid is one preparation that should always be given using this technique.

Barbituric Acid Derivatives: All such preparations should be given from one-half to one hour before sleep is desired. All procedures should be taken care of before the medicament is given in order that nothing shall disturb the patient after the drug is administered.

Habit-Forming Drugs: These should be given as ordered by the physician. *Insulin:* When this is administered, it should be given hypodermically according to the instructions of the attending physician. The type of insulin, dosage, and frequency of dosage vary greatly with each patient. *Laxatives:* These are best given in the evening because it usually takes 6 or 8 hours for them to produce an effect. Saline purgatives are usually given well diluted on an empty stomach in the morning. Other purgatives usually are given as ordered and needed.

Mouthwash: Stock solutions used for mouthwash should be diluted one-half or more before being given to the patient. Only enough for the immediate mouth washing

Comparison of Toxic and Allergic Drug Reactions

Differences may be indistinct. Shock from drug overdose may be no different than allergic shock.

	Toxic	Allergic
Incidence	May occur with any drug	Occurs infrequently
Dosage	Usually high	Therapeutic
Reaction time	May occur with first dose, or may be due to cumulative effect	Usually only upon re-exposure, but some drugs cross-react with chemicals of similar structure
Symptoms	Similar to pharmacological action of drug	Not related to pharmacological action of drug
Associated disorders	None	Asthma, hay fever

should be given to the patient at a particular time.

Horse Serum: When injections containing it are administered, information should be obtained as to whether the patient has ever received horse serum and what his reaction to it was, because a reaction is liable to occur. If the patient is allergic to horse serum, a test for sensitivity should always be done by injecting a few drops of the greatly diluted material containing horse serum hypodermically, and within a short time a reaction will occur. A small spot appears at the site of the injection if the patient has a tendency toward an unfavorable reaction. If the person is allergic to horse serum the physician will provide instructions for desensitizing him.

Oxygen: The most commonly used method for the administration of oxygen consists of inserting a catheter into a nostril, or into each nostril. Oxygen may also be given from a tank by means of a mask over the patient's nose and mouth, or the patient may be placed in an oxygen tent, an oxygen chamber, or room. The last two methods are not only expensive but also extremely dangerous and must be used cautiously as the danger from fire hazard is very great.

Saline Purgatives: Should always be given to the patient when the stomach is empty, preferably in the morning. *Vaccines:* Most of these are administered subcutaneously. Pertussis vaccine (USP) may be given subcutaneously or intramuscularly while adsorbed pertussis vaccine (USP) is given via the intramuscular route.

drugs, handling of. Carefully read the label or other printed instruction issued with medicine. Measure the ordered doses (quantities) accurately and never guess.

A measuring glass or spoon should be used, marked either in drams and ounces only, or with teaspoons and tablespoons also.

One drop equals 1 minim, symbol ♏. One teaspoonful equals 1 dram, symbol Ʒ. Two teaspoonfuls equal 2 drams; four teaspoons equal 1/2 ounce or 1 tablespoonful. Two tablespoons equal 1 ounce, symbol Ʒ.

When giving a dose of medicine be sure to whom it has to be given, what has to be given, when it has to be given, and the amount to be given. The nurse should not leave the bedside until she sees the patient actually swallow oral medicine.

NOTE: The cover must never be left off the container because a necessary property may evaporate, the drug may become dangerously concentrated, or the medicine may absorb moisture from the air and become difficult to handle or dilute. The drug compartment must be kept locked.

drugs, words pert. to: absorbent, action, alkaloids, alterative, ampule, analeptic, analgesic, anesthetic, anodyne, antacid, anthelmintic, antiarthritic, antidiuretic, antiemetic, antipyretic, antiseptic, antisialagogue, antispasmodic, antizymotic, aperient, aromatic, balsam, bitters, cachet, calmant, capsule, carminative, cathartic, caustic, chemical compounds, cholagogue, confection, convulsant, correctant, corrosive, counterirritant, decoction, demulcent, deodorant, depilatory, depressant, detergent, diaphoretic, digestant, disinfectant, diuretic, ecbolic, element, elixir, emetic, emmenagogue, emollient, emulsion, enzyme, escharotic, evacuant, expectorant, extract, febrifuge, ferment, fluidextract, galactagogue, glucoside, hematinic, hemostatic, hormone, hydragogue, hypnotic, idiosyncrasy, infusion, irritation, laxative, liniment, lozenge, mixture, mucilage, mydriatic, myotic, oil, ointment, oleate, oleoresin, oxytocics, paper, pharmacognosy, pharmacology, pill, plaster, powder, prophylactic, purgative, refrigerant, resins, rubefacient, saline purgative, saponins, sedative, sensitization, serum therapy, sialagogue, solution, somnifacient, soporific, specific, spirit, stimulant, stomachic, styptic, sudorific, suppository, synergism, tablet, tincture, tonic, vaccine, vasoconstrictor, vasodilator, vermicide, vermifuge, vesicant, vinegar, water, wine.

drum. The ear drum of tympanic cavity; the tympanum or cavity of the middle ear.

drunkenness [AS. *drincan,* to drink]. Alcoholic intoxication. In legal medicine, intoxication or being "under-the-influence" of alcohol is defined according to the concentration of alcohol in the blood or exhaled air.

drusen (dru′zen) [Ger. *Druse,* weathered ore]. Small, hyaline, globular pathological growths formed on optic papilla or on Descemet's membrane.

dry diet. A high-carbohydrate diet, with measured liquid given between meals only.

dry ice. Proprietary name for solidified carbon dioxide used for commercial refrigeration. Also used in the form of a pencil-shaped block for treating certain skin lesions such as warts. The temperature of solid carbon dioxide is −78.5° C. For this reason it is extremely important to use gloves when handling it. Momentary skin contact with dry ice can cause severe frostbite and blisters. SYN: *carbon dioxide snow.*

dry measure. A measure of volume for dry commodities. SEE: *weights and measures* in *Appendix*.

Drys'dale's corpuscles. [Thomas M. Drysdale, Amer. gynecologist, 1831-1904] Nonnucleated, granular cells present in the fluid of certain ovarian cysts.

dualism (du'ă-lizm) [L. *duo*, two]. 1. The condition of being double or two-fold. 2. The theory that the human individual consists of two entities, mind and matter, which are independent of each other. 3. The theory that blood corpuscles arise from two types of stem cells: myeloblasts giving rise to the myeloid elements, and lymphoblasts giving rise to the lymphoid elements.

dual personality. A form of multiple personality seen in hysteria and schizophrenia which results in the expression of two different phases of personality at various intervals, neither personality, as a rule, being aware of the words, acts, and feelings of the other. When this occurs in schizophrenia the individual psychic function is split off from the personality as a whole and becomes autonomous. This may be unrelated to and contradictory of the main personality. SEE: *dissociation of personality; multiple personality; vigilambulism.*

Dubini's disease (dū-bě'nē). [Angelo Dubini, It. physician, 1813-1902]. Rhythmic, rapid contractions of a group or groups of muscles. SYN: *electric chorea; spasmus Dubini.*

duboisine (du-boy'sēn). Alkaloid derivative of plant Duboisea myoporoides. It is a form of hyoscyamine.

    d., poisoning from. Resembles atropine sulfate poisoning, q.v.

Duchenne's disease (dū-shěn'). [Guillaume B. A. Duchenne, Fr. neurologist, 1806-1875] 1. Bulbar paralysis. 2. Tabes dorsalis.

Ducrey's bacillus (du-krā'). [Augusto Ducrey, It. dermatologist, 1860-1940] Hemophilus ducreyi. The cause of chancroid or soft chancre; small, rod-shaped organism found in pairs.

duct [L. *ducere*, to lead]. 1. A narrow tubular vessel or channel, esp. one serving to convey secretions from a gland. 2. A narrow enclosed channel containing a fluid, as the semicircular d. of the ear.

    d., accessory pancreatic. D. of the pancreas, leading into the pancreatic d. or the duodenum near the mouth of the common bile d. SYN: *ductus pancreaticus accessorius* [NA].

    d., alveolar. A branch of a respiratory bronchiole which leads to the alveolar sacs of the lungs. SYN: *ductulus alveolaris* [NA].

    d., Bartholin's. The major d. of the sublingual gland. SYN: *ductus sublingualis major* [NA].

    d.'s, biliary. The canals which carry bile. The intrahepatic d.'s include the bile canaliculi and interlobular d.'s; the extrahepatic d.'s include the hepatic d., cystic d., and common bile d. SYN: *bile ducts.*

    d., cochlear. Canal of the cochlea. SYN: *ductus cochlearis* [NA].

    d., common bile. D. formed by the confluence of the hepatic and cystic d.'s. Conveys bile to the duodenum opening at the papilla of Vater. SYN: *ductus choledochus* [NA].

    d., cystic. Excretory d. of the gallbladder. SYN: *ductus cysticus* [NA].

    d., efferent. Any d. conveying secretion from a gland.

    d., ejaculatory. Conveys semen into urethra. SYN: *ductus ejaculatorius* [NA].

    d., endolymphatic. In the embryo, a tubular projection of the otocyst ending in a blind extremity, the endolymph sac. In the adult, it connects the endolymphatic sac with the utricle and saccule. SYN: *ductus endolymphaticus* [NA].

    d., excretory. Any d. which conveys a product from an organ, as the excretory d. of a salivary gland.

    d., galactophorous. D. carrying milk in lobes of mammary glands. SYN: *ductus lactiferi* [NA].

    d., Gartner's. A remnant of the wolffian d. extending from the parovarium through the broad ligament into the vagina. SYN: *ductus epoophori longitudinalis* [NA].

    d.'s, hepatic. Right and left d.'s receive bile from right and left lobes of liver and carry bile to common bile d. SYN: *ductus hepaticus dexter* [NA] and *ductus hepaticus sinister* [NA].

    d.'s, interlobular. One of the d.'s carrying bile. SEE: *biliary duct.*

    d., lacrimal. One of two short d.'s, inferior and superior, which conveys tears from the lacrimal lake to the lacrimal sac. Their openings are on the margins of the upper and lower eyelids. SYN: *canaliculus lacrimalis* [NA].

    d.'s, lactiferous. A group of 15 to 20 d.'s which drain the lobes of the mammary gland. Each opens in a slight depression in the tip of the nipple. SYN: *ductus lactiferi* [NA].

    d., Leydig's. Mesonephric duct, q.v.

d., lymphatic. One of two main d.'s conveying lymph to the blood stream: the left lymphatic d. (thoracic d.) and the right lymphatic d.

d., lymphatic, left. Thoracic d.

d., lymphatic, right. A d., smaller than the left lymphatic d., draining the right side of the body above the diaphragm. Discharges into the right innominate vein. SYN: *ductus lymphaticus dexter* [NA].

d., mammary. Lactiferous d.

d., mesonephric. The d. which, in the embryo, connects the mesonephros with the cloaca. In the male it develops into the ductus deferens. SYN: *ductus mesonephricus* [NA]; *wolffian d.*

d., metanephric. Ureter.

d., milk. D., lactiferous, q.v.

d., Muller's; mullerian d. Bilateral d.'s in the embryo that form the uterus, vagina, and fallopian tubes. SYN: *ductus paramesonephricus* [NA].

d., nasolacrimal. The d. which conveys tears from the lacrimal sac to the nasal cavity. It opens beneath the inferior nasal concha. SYN: *ductus nasolacrimalis* [NA].

d., omphalomesenteric. D., vitelline, q.v.

d., pancreatic. Conveys pancreatic juice to the duodenum. SYN: *d. of Wirsung; ductus pancreaticus* [NA].

d.'s, paraurethral. Skene's d.'s.

d., parotid. Duct through which secretions from the parotid gland enter into mouth. SYN: *ductus parotideus* [NA].

d.'s, prostatic. About 20 d.'s which discharge prostatic secretion into the urethra. SYN: *ductus prostatici* [NA].

d.'s of Rivinus. Five to 15 d.'s (the minor sublingual d.'s) which drain the posterior portion of the sublingual gland. SYN: *ductus sublinguales minores* [NA].

d., salivary. Any of the d.'s which drain a salivary gland. SYN: *ductus pancreaticus accessorius* [NA].

d. of Santorini. Accessory pancreatic d. SYN: *ductus pancreaticus accessorius* [NA].

d., secretory. The smaller canals of a gland.

d., segmental. A pair of embryonic tubes located between visceral and parietal layers of mesoblast on each side of the body.

d.'s, semicircular. Three membranous tubes forming a part of the membranous labyrinth of the inner ear. They lie within the semicircular canals and bear corresponding names, anterior, posterior, and lateral. SYN: *ductus semicircularis* [NA].

d., seminal. Any of the d.'s which convey semen, specifically the ductus deferens and the ejaculatory d.

d.'s, Skene's. Paraurethral d.'s. Two slender d.'s of Skene's glands which open on either side of the urethral orifice in the female. SYN: *ductus paraurethrales* [NA].

d., spermatic. Excretory d. of the testicle which later joins the d. of the seminal vesicle to become the ejaculatory d. SYN: *vas deferens; ductus deferens* [NA].

d., Stensen's; Steno's d. Parotid d.

d.'s, sublingual. The excretory d.'s of the sublingual gland. SEE: *Bartholin's d.; d.'s of Rivinus.*

d., submandibular. D. of the submandibular gland. It opens on a papilla at the side of the frenulum linguae. SYN: *submaxillary d.; Wharton's d.; ductus submandibularis* [NA].

d., submaxillary. Submandibular d.

d., sudoriferous. Sweat d.

d., tear. A d. that conveys tears, including excretory d.'s of lacrimal glands, lacrimal and nasolacrimal d.'s.

d., testicular. Spermatic d.

d., thoracic. The left lymphatic d. Drains the left side of the body above the diaphragm and all of the body below the diaphragm. Discharges into the left innominate vein. SYN: *ductus thoracicus* [NA].

d., umbilical. D., vitelline, q.v.

d., utriculosaccular. A narrow tube emanating from the utricle and opening into the endolymphatic d. SYN: *ductus utriculosaccularis* [NA].

d., vitelline. The narrow d. which, in the embryo, connects the yolk sac (umbilical vesicle) with the intestine. SYN: *umbilical d.; yolk stalk.*

d., of Wirsung. Pancreatic d.

duct'less [L. *ducere*, to lead, + AS. *loessa*, less]. Having no duct, secreting only internally.

d. glands. Ductless glands secrete internally one or more hormones which have a specific action upon the body. SEE: *endocrine; exocrine.*

ductule (duk'tūl). A very small duct.

d., aberrant. One of a group of small tubules associated with the epididymis. They are blindly ending, representing the vestigial remains of the caudal group of mesonephric tubules.

ductus (dŭk'tŭs). (pl. *ductus*) [NA] Duct. SEE: *duct.*

d. arteriosus. [NA]. A channel of communication between main pulmonary artery of the fetus and aorta.

d. arteriosus, patent. Persistence after birth of the foramen ovale. A treatable form of congenital heart defect.

d. choledochus. [NA]. The common bile duct, q.v.

d. cochlearis. [NA]. The cochlear duct, q.v. Also called scala media.

d. communis. One about three in. long, formed by union of cystic and hepatic d.; carries the bile to the intestine.

d. deferens. [NA] Excretory duct of the testicle. Conveys sperm from the epididymis to the ejaculatory duct. SYN: *vas deferens.*

d. efferent. One of a group of 12-14 small tubes which constitute the efferent ducts of the testis. They lie within the epididymis and connect the rete testis with the d. epididymis. Their coiled portions constitute the lobulus epididymis.

d. hemithoracicus. [NA]. Ascending branch of thoracic duct, opening either into right lymphatic duct or close to angle of union of right subclavian and right internal jugular veins.

d. hepaticus dexter. [NA]. One issuing from the right lobe of the liver, uniting with the d. hepaticus sinister and forming the hepatic duct.

d. hepaticus sinister. [NA]. One issuing with d. hepaticus dexter to form hepatic duct.

d. prostatici. [NA]. Ducts for secretion of prostate into the urethra.

d. sacculo-utricularis. Small tube connecting saccule of internal ear with utricle.

d. venosus. [NA]. Smaller, shorter, and posterior of two branches into which umbilical vein divides after entering the abdomen; empties into the inferior vena cava.

duipara (dū-ip'ă-ră) [L. *duo*, two, + *parēre*, to bear]. A female pregnant for the second time. SYN: *secundipara.*

dulcite (dul'sit) [L. *dulcis*, sweet]. A sugar, $C_6H_{14}O_6$, found in certain plants. SYN: *dulcin; dulcitol; dulcose.*

dull [ME. *dul*]. 1. Not resonant on percussion. 2. Not mentally alert.

dullness, dulness (dul'nes). 1. Lack of normal resonance on percussion. 2. State of being dull.

dumb [AS.]. Mute. Unable to speak.

d. ague. Latent malaria not expressed by ordinary signs.

dumb'ness. Muteness.

dumping syndrome. A syndrome characterized by sweating and weakness after eating. Occurs in patients who have had gastric resections. Exact cause is unknown but rapid emptying (i.e., dumping of the stomach

contents) into the small intestine is associated with the symptoms.

duodenal (dū-ō-dē'năl) [L. *duodeni*, twelve]. Pert. to the duodenum.

d. bulb. Area of duodenum just beyond the pylorus.

d. delay. Delay in the movement of food through the duodenum due to conditions such as inflammation of lower portion of the intestine which reflexly inhibits duodenal movements.

d. papilla. Raised surface near entrance of ductus choledochus communis into duodenum.

d. papilla major. Slight elevation in descending portion of the duodenum bearing openings of the common bile duct and main pancreatic duct.

d. papilla minor. Slight elevation about 2 cm. above the papilla major bearing opening of the accessory pancreatic duct.

d. ulcer. Broken mucus membrane, usually accompanied by suppuration. Sometimes a sore which bleeds is present. This creates danger of perforation.

A d. ulcer heals slowly due to constant passage of irritating fluids and food over it. DIET: SEE: *peptic ulcer.*

duodenectasis (dū″ō-děn-ěk'tă-sĭs) [L. *duodeni*, twelve, + Gr. *ektasis*, expansion]. Chronic dilatation of the duodenum.

duodenectomy (du″o-den-ek'tō-mĭ) [″+ Gr. *ektomē*, excision]. Excision of part or all of the duodenum.

duodenitis (du″od-ĕ-nī'tĭs) [L. *duodeni*, twelve, + Gr. *-ītis*, inflammation]. Inflammation of the duodenum.

duodenocholecystostomy (du″o-de″no-ko-lĭ-sis-tos'to-mĭ) [″+ Gr. *cholē*, bile, + *kystis*, bladder, + *stōma*, mouth]. Formation by surgical means of a fistula between duodenum and gallbladder.

duodenocholedochotomy (du″o-de″no-ko-led-o-kot'o-mĭ) [″+ Gr. *choledochos*, bile duct, + *tomē*, incision]. Surgical incision of the duodenum to reach the gallbladder.

duodenocystostomy (du″o-de″no-sis-tos'-to-mĭ). Duodenocholecystostomy.

duodenoenterostomy (du″o-de″no-en″ter-os'to-mĭ) [L. *duodeni*, twelve, + Gr. *enteron*, intestine, + *stōma*, opening]. Formation of passage between the duodenum and intestine.

duodenogram (du-od'ĕ-no-gram″) [″+ Gr. *gramma*, a writing]. A roentgenogram of the duodenum.

duodenohepatic (du-od″e-no-he-pat'ik) [″+ Gr. *hēpatos*, liver]. Pert. to duodenum and liver.

duodenojejunostomy (du″o-de″no-jĕ-joo-nos′to-mĭ) ["+ *jejunum,* empty, + Gr. *stoma,* opening]. Making a passage between the duodenum and jejunum.

duodenoscopy (du″od-ĕ-nos′ko-pĭ) [L. *duodeni,* twelve, + Gr. *skopein,* to examine]. Inspection of the duodenum with an endoscope.

duodenostomy (du″od-ĕ-nos′to-mĭ) ["+ Gr. *stoma,* opening]. Operation of making a permanent opening into the duodenum through the wall of the abdomen.

duodenotomy (du″od-ĕ-not′o-mĭ) ["+ Gr. *tomē,* incision]. An incision into the duodenum.

duodenum (dū″ō-dē′nŭm) [L. *duodeni,* twelve]. [NA] The first part of the small intestines connecting with the pylorus of the stomach and extending to the jejunum.

The d. receives hepatic and pancreatic secretions through the same duct. It is 8 to 11 inches (20-28 cm.) long, the average length being 10 inches (25 cm.). Brunner's glands and Lieberkühn's glands are found in the d. Chyle is formed here.

It is a crucial section of the alimentary canal since in it occurs the mixing of acid chyme from the stomach, bile from the liver and gallbladder, pancreatic juice entering by way of two ducts, and intestinal juices secreted by the glands of Brunner and the crypts of Lieberkühn.

The nerve supply comes from the celiac plexus. Pancreaticoduodenal branches of the hepatic and superior mesenteric arteries and the right gastric artery supply blood. SEE: *digestive system* for illustration.

ACTION: The entry of acid chyme into the duodenum brings about discharge of bile from the gallbladder and the secretion of pancreatic juice by the pancreas. These enter through the common bile duct. Bile salts alkalinize the chyme and emulsify the fats. Through the action of pancreatic enzymes, the following changes occur: steapsin (pancreatic lipase) hydrolyzes neutral fats to fatty acids and glycerol; amylopsin (pancreatic amylase) hydrolyzes starch to maltose; maltase hydrolyzes maltose to glucose. Three proteolytic enzymes (trypsin, chymotrypsin, and peptidase) act on proteins hydrolyzing them to proteoses, peptones, and amino acids.

Secretory Phenomena: Two substances are secreted by the duodenum. One of these, secretin, q.v., excites the pancreas to increased production of its juice. The other, cholecystokinin, causes the gallbladder to contract and force its contents through the ductus choledochus into the duodenum. In addition, nervous mechanisms contribute to the coordination which exists here, regulating the rate of discharge of chyme from the stomach, varying both quality and quantity of the various secretions, and determining the rate of passage through the duodenum.

Motor Phenomena: The first part of the d. (pars superior, duodenal cap, d. bulb) is the small portion immediately following the pylorus. It is regularly full of material and consequently visible in roentgenograms as a spade-shaped shadow. The next part (pars descendens) is that into which the common bile duct (ductus choledochus) and pancreatic ducts open. Movement through it and through the pars inferior and the pars ascendens is rapid so that they are normally inconspicuous on x-ray film. Throughout the duodenum the mucosa is thrown into folds (plicae circulares) and shows the active projections called villi. The folds are permanent and inactive. The villi, which stud the surface of the folds as well as the spaces between them, exhibit waving and thrusting movements.

RS: bile; Brunner's glands; choledochoduodenostomy; digestion; duodenal ulcer; enzyme; gallbladder; intestines; juice, gastric; juice, pancreatic; Lieberkühn crypts; liver; pancreas; succus entericus.

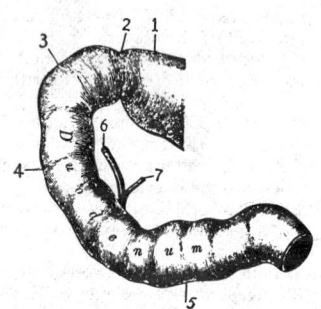

THE DUODENUM
1, Pyloric end of the stomach. 2, Pyloric valvule. 3, Upper transverse part. 4, Descending part. 5, Lower transverse part. 6, Choledochus duct. 7, Pancreatic duct.

duplica′tion, du′plicature [L. *duplicāre,* to double]. A doubling or folding, or state of being folded.

duplicitas (du-plis′ĭ-tas). Fetal abnormality in which the cephalic and/or the pelvic end is doubled.

dupp (dŭp). Part of the word lubb-dupp, denoting 2nd sound at cardiac apex heard in aus-

cultation. It is due to the closing of the pulmonary and aortic semilunar valves.
The 1st sound is longer and pitched lower. SEE: *heart, auscultation of; lubb; lubb-dupp.*

Dupuytren's contracture (dū-pwē-trăn'). [Baron G. Dupuytren, Fr. surgeon, 1777-1835]. Contracture of palmar fascia causing ring and little fingers to bend into palm so that they cannot be extended.

dura (du'rā) [L. *durus*, hard]. Dura mater.

dural (du'ral) [L. *durus*, hard]. Pert. to the dura.

dura mater [L., hard mother]. The outer membrane covering the spinal cord (d. m. spinalis [NA]) and brain (d. m. cerebri [NA] or d. m. encephali [NA]). SEE: *pia mater; tentorium.*

durama'tral. Pert. to the dura. SYN: *dural.*

du'raplasty ["+ Gr. *plassein*, to form]. Plastic repair of the dura mater.

durematoma (dū″rem-ă-tō′mă) ["+ Gr. *haima*, blood, + *-oma*, tumor]. Accumulation of blood between arachnoid and dura.

duritis (du-ri'tis) [L. *durus*, hard, + Gr. *-itis*, inflammation]. Inflammation of the dura. SYN: *pachymeningitis.*

duroarachnitis (dū″ro-ăr″ak-nī′tis) ["+ Gr. *arachnē*, spider, + *-itis*, inflammation]. Inflammation of dura and arachnoid membrane.

Durorziez' murmur (dūrō″zī-ē′). [Paul Louis Duroziez, Fr. physician, 1826-1897] The systolic and diastolic murmur heard over a large artery when pressure is applied to the area just distal to the stethoscope.

dust. Minute, fine particles of earth; any powder.

d., blood. Hemoconia.

d. cells. Reticuloendothelial cells in the walls of the alveoli of the lungs which ingest or destroy dust particles.

d., ear. Fine calcareous bodies found in the gelatinous substance of the otolithic membrane of the ear; otoconia or otoliths.

dust'ing powder. Any fine powder for dusting on skin.

Duverney's gland (dū-ver-nā'). [Joseph G. Duverney, Fr. anatomist, 1648-1730] The vulvovaginal gland.

dwarf [AS. *dweorg*, dwarf]. An abnormally short or undersized person; a pygmy.

d., achondroplastic. One with normal trunk but possessing shortened extremities, with a large head, and protruding buttocks.

d., asexual. One with deficient sexual development.

d., hypophyseal. One due to hypofunction of anterior lobe of the hypophysis.

d., infantile. One showing marked physical, mental and sexual underdevelopment.

d., Levi-Lorain. An hypophyseal or pituitary d.

d., micromelic. One with very small limbs.

d., ovarian. An undersized female due to absence or underdevelopment of the ovaries.

d., phocomelic. One with abnormally short diaphyses of either pair of extremities or of all four.

d., physiologic. A person normally developed except for stature.

d., pituitary. An hypophyseal one.

d., primordial. One in whom there is a selective deficiency of growth hormone but with otherwise normal endocrine function.

d., rachitic. One due to rickets.

d., renal. One due to renal osteodystrophy.

d., thanatophoric. SEE: *thanatophoric dwarfism.*

dwarfism. Condition of being abnormally small. May be hereditary, or a result of endocrine dysfunction; deficiency diseases; renal insufficiency; diseases of the skeleton or other causes.

dy'ad [Gr. *duas*, pair]. 1. A pair. 2. A pair of chromosomes formed by the division of a tetrad in miosis. A dyad represents a single chromosome split precociously for a subsequent division. 3. In chemistry, a bivalent element or radical.

dynamia (dī-nam'ĭ-ă) [Gr. *dynamis*, power]. Vital energy or ability to combat disease.

dynamic (dī-nam'ik). Pert. to vital force or inherent power, opposite of static.

dynam'ics. The science of bodies in motion and their forces.

dynamization (dī″nam-ĭ-zā′shun). The attempt to add to the potency of medicine by agitation or comminution, q.v. SEE: *attenuation.*

dynamogenesis (dī″nă-mo-jen′ē-sis) [Gr. *dynamis*, power, + *genesis*, growth]. The capacity to call forth increased energy.

dynamogen'ic ["+ *gennan*, to produce]. Pert. to, or caused by, an increase of energy.

dynamograph (dī-nam'o-graf) ["+ *graphein*, to write]. Device for recording muscular strength.

dynamometer (dī″nă-mom′ē-ter) ["+ *metron*, measure]. 1. A device for measuring muscular strength. 2. A device for giving the magnifying power of a lens.

dynamoneure (dī-nam'o-nūr) ["+ *neuron*, nerve]. A motor, spinal nerve cell.

dynamoscope (dī-nam′o-skōp) [″+ *skopein*, to examine]. Instrument for auscultation of muscles.

dynamoscopy (di-nam-os′ko-pī). Auscultation of muscles.

dyne (dīn) [Gr. *dynamis*, power]. Force needed for imparting an acceleration of 1 cm./sec./ sec. to a 1-gm. mass.

dys- [Gr.]. Prefix meaning bad, difficult, painful.

dysacousia, dysacousma (dis″ă-koo′zī-ă, -kooz′mă) [Gr. *dys*, bad, + *akousis*, hearing]. 1. Discomfort caused by loud noises. 2. Difficulty in hearing.

dysadrenia (dis″ă-drē′nī-ă) [″+ L. *ad-*, toward, + *ren*, kidney]. Functional disorder of the kidneys.

dysalbumose (dis-al′bū-mōs) [″+ L. *albumen*, white of egg]. A variety of albumose insoluble in water or hydrochloric acid.

dysantigraphia (dis″an-tī-graf′ī-ă) [Gr. *dys*, bad, + *anti*, against, + *graphein*, to write]. Inability to copy writing or printed letters.

dysaphia (dis-af′ī-ă) [″+ *haphē*, touch]. Dullness of the sense of touch.

dysarteriotony (dis″ar-tē″rī-ot′o-nī) [″+ *arteria*, artery, + *tonos*, tension]. Abnormal blood pressure, either too low or too high.

dysarthria (dis-ar′thrī-ă) [″+ *arthroun*, to utter distinctly]. 1. Difficulty in articulation of joints, as in amyostasia. 2. Incorrectly applied to imperfect speech; stammering.

dysarthro′sis [″+ *arthrōsis*, joint]. Joint malformation.

dysautonomia (dis″aw-tō-no′mī-ă) [″+ *autonomia*, freedom to use own laws]. A rare hereditary disease involving the autonomic nervous system with mental retardation, motor incoordination, vomiting, frequent infections, and convulsions.

dysbarism (dis-bar′izm) [Gr. *dys*, bad, + *barys*, heavy, + *ismos*, condition]. Symptom complex following exposure of body to less-than-atmospheric pressure in air flight or altitude chamber. When occurring in severe form, sometimes called decompression sickness or bends.

dysbasia (dis-bā′zī-ă) [″+ *basis*, a step]. Difficulty in walking, esp. when due to disease of the brain or spinal cord.

dysbolism (dis′bo-lizm) [″+ *ballein*, to change]. Disordered metabolism.

dysbulia (dis-bu′lī-ă) [″+ *boulē*, will]. 1. Inability to fix the attention; difficulty experienced in thinking; mind weariness. 2. Weak and uncertain willpower.

dyschezia (dis-kē′zī-ă) [″+ *chezein*, go to defecate]. Painful or difficult bowel movements.

dyschiria (dis-kī′rī-ă) [″+ *cheir*, hand]. Inability to tell which side of the body has been touched.

If referred to the wrong side it is called allochiria, q.v.; to both sides, synchiria, q.v. SYN: *achiria*.

dyscholia (dis-kō′lī-ă) [Gr. *dys*, bad, + *cholē*, bile]. Morbid condition of the bile.

dyschondroplasia (dis″kŏn-drō-plā′zī-ă) [″+ *chondros*, cartilage, + *plassein*, to form]. Disease, usually hereditary, resulting in disordered growth. Characterized by multiple exostoses of growth of the epiphyses, esp. of the long bones, metacarpals, and phalanges. SYN: *dyschondroplasia; Ollier's disease*.

dyschroa, dyschroia (dīs-krō′-ă, dis-kroy′ă) [″+ *chroia*, complexion]. Discolored skin, esp. of the face; poor or bad complexion.

dyschromatopsia (dis″kro-mă-top′sī-ă) [″+ *chrōma*, color, + *opsis*, vision]. Imperfect color vision.

dyschro′mia. Discoloration, as of the skin.

dyschronism (dis-kro′nizm) [Gr. *dys*, bad, + *chronos*, time]. 1. Disturbed time relation, esp. that which occurs when one is transported from one time zone to one that is five to 10 hours ahead of or behind the original. This leads to disturbances of biological rhythms. 2. Separate as to time.

dyscinesia (dis-sĭ-nē′zī-ă). Dyskinesia.

dyscoimesis (dis″koy-me′sis). Dyskoimesis.

dyscoria (dis-ko′rī-ă) [Gr. *dys*, bad, + *korē*, pupil]. Abnormal form of the pupil.

dyscrasia (dis-kra′zī-ă) [Gr. *dyserasia*, bad temperament]. An old term meaning abnormal mixture of the four "humors." The word is now used as a synonym for disease.

d., blood. A general nonspecific term for blood disease.

dyscrasic (dis-krā′sik). Pert. to dyscrasia.

dyscrinism (dis-krī′nizm) [Gr. *dys*, bad, + *krinein*, to secrete, + *ismos*, condition of]. Any disorder of secretions, esp. of an endocrine gland.

dysdiadochokinesia (dis″di-ad″o-ko-kī-ne′sī-ă) [″+ *diadochos*, succeeding, + *kinēsis*, movement]. Inability to quickly substitute antagonistic motor impulses to produce antagonistic muscular movements.

dysdiemorrhysis (dis″di-em-or′ī-sis) [″+ *dia*, through, + *haima*, blood, + *rhysis*, a flowing]. Sluggish circulation of capillary blood.

dyse′mia [″+ *haima*, blood]. Any blood disease.

dysendocriniasis (dis-en″dō-krin-i′ă-sis) [″+ *endon*, within, + *krinein*, to secrete]. Faulty function of the endocrine glands.

dysendocrinism (dis''en-dok'rĭ-nizm). Faulty function of the endocrine glands; dysendocriniasis.

dysendocrisi'asis. Dysendocriniasis.

dysenteric (dis''en-ter'ĭk). Pert. to dysentery.

dysentery (dis'en-ter'ĭ) [Gr. *dys,* bad, + *enteron,* intestine]. A term applied to a number of intestinal disorders, esp. of the colon, characterized by inflammation of the mucous membrane.

ETIOL: Bacterial or viral infection; infestation by protozoa or parasitic worms; chemical irritants.

SYM: Abdominal pain, tenesmus, diarrhea with passage of mucus or blood.

    d., amebic. Due to amebas.

    d., bacillary. An acute infectious disease caused by bacteria of the genus Shigella, esp. Sh. dysenteriae, Sh. boydii, Sh. flexneri, and Sh. sonnei. It may occur sporadically or in epidemics. In addition to intestinal symptoms, a severe toxemia may occur due to exo- and endotoxins produced by the organisms.

    d., balantidial. D. caused by ciliate protozoan, Balantidium coli.

    d., malignant. A form in which symptoms are very pronounced and progress rapid, usually terminating fatally.

    d., viral. D. caused by virus.

dysepulotic (dis''ep-u-lot'ik) ["+ *epoulōtikos,* promoting scarring]. Slow formation of a scar.

dysergasia (dis''er-gā'zĭ-ă) ["+ *ergon,* work]. Inability to function properly. In psychiatry, a behavior disorder characterized by disorientation, hallucinations, dream states, and delirium. May sometimes be due to toxic conditions such as uremia, or alcohol intoxication. SYN: *neurasthenia.*

dysergastic (dis-er-gas'tik). Pert. to dysergasia.

    d. reaction. Hallucinations, fears, disorientation, dream states, and other mental disorders resulting from poor circulation and metabolism of the brain.

dysergia (dis-er'jĭ-ă) [Gr. *dys,* bad, + *ergon,* work]. Lack of coordination in muscular voluntary movements.

dysesthesia (dis''es-thē'zĭ-ă) ["+ *aisthēsis,* sensation]. 1. Sensations, as of the pricks of pins and needles, or of crawling. SYN: *formication.* 2. Failing sensitivity, esp. of touch. 3. Painfulness of any sensation which is not normally painful.

    d., auditory. Abnormal discomfort from loud noises. SYN: *dysacusia.*

    d., pedis. Severe itching and burning of the plantar surface of the feet and toes. May occur as a reaction to heparin therapy.

dysfunction (dis-funk'shun) ["+ L. *functio,* a performance]. Abnormal, inadequate or impaired function of an organ or part.

dysgalac'tia ["+ *gala,* milk]. Defective milk secretion.

dysgammaglobulinemia. Disproportion in the concentration of immunoglobulins in the blood. May be congenital or acquired.

dysgenesia, dysgenesis (dis-jen-ē'sĭ-ă, -jen'ĕ-sis) ["+ *genesis,* procreation]. Impairment or loss of procreative powers.

dysgen'ic ["+ *gennan,* to produce]. 1. Pert. to dysgenesis. 2. Causing racial deterioration.

dysgen'italism ["+ L. *genitalia,* organs of reproduction, + Gr. *ismos,* state of]. Condition caused by abnormal genital development.

dysgerminoma (dis''jer-min-o'mă) ["+ L. *germen,* a sprout, + Gr. *-ōma,* tumor]. A malignant neoplasm of the ovary.

dysgeusia (dis-gu'zĭ-ă) ["+ *geusis,* taste]. Impairment or perversion of the gustatory sense such that normal tastes are interpreted as being unpleasant or completely different from the characteristic taste of a particular food or chemical compound. SEE: *hypogeusia, idiopathic.*

dysglan'dular [Gr. *dys,* bad, + L. *glans,* acorn]. Abnormal functioning of glands, esp. those of internal secretion.

dysglycemia (dis''glī-se'mĭ-ă) ["+ *glykys,* sweet, + *haima,* blood]. Faulty blood sugar metabolism.

dysgnosia (dis-no'sĭ-ă) [Gr. *dysgnōsia,* difficulty of knowing]. Any anomaly of intellect. SYN: *dysthymia.*

dysgonesis (dis''go-nē'sis) [Gr. *dys,* bad, + *gonē,* seed]. 1. Functional disorder of the genital organs. 2. Poor growth of bacterial culture.

dysgon'ic. Bacterial cultures of sparse growth.

dysgraph'ia (dĭs-grăf'ĭ-ă) [Gr. *dys,* bad, + *graphein,* to write]. 1. Inability to write properly. Usually the result of a brain lesion. 2. Writer's cramp.

dyshematopoiesia (dis-hem''ă-to-poy-e'sĭ-ă) ["+ *haima,* blood, + *poiein,* to make]. Imperfect blood formation.

dyshidria (dis-hid'rĭ-ă) ["+ *hidrōs,* sweat]. Dyshidrosis.

dyshidrosis (dis-hĭ-dro'sis). 1. Disorder of the sweating apparatus. 2. A recurrent vesicular eruption on skin of hands and feet marked by intense itching. SYN: *pompholyx.*

dyshor'monal ["+ *hormaein,* to excite]. Caused by endocrine disturbance.

dyshor'monism ["+ "+ -ismos, state of]. Deficiency or excessive production of hormones or any internal secretions.

dysidrosis (dis-ĭ-drō'sĭs) ["+ hidrōs, sweat, + -ōsis, condition]. Dyshidrosis.

dysin'sulinism ["+ L. insula, island, + Gr. -ismos, state of]. Imperfect secretion of insulin.

dyskerato'sis [Gr. dys, bad, + keras, horn, + -ōsis, process]. Epithelial alterations in which a certain number of isolated malpighian cells become differentiated. Any alteration in the keratinization of the epithelial cells of the epidermis. Characteristic of many skin disorders.

dyskine'sia ["+ kinēsis, movement]. Defect in voluntary movement.

    d. al'gera. Condition in which active movement is painful if done quickly, but not so for slow movement. Due to hysteria.

    d. intermit'tens. Limb disability occurring intermittently.

    d., tardive. Slow, rhythmical, automatic stereotyped movements, either generalized or in single muscle groups. These occur as an undesired effect of therapy with certain psychotropic drugs, esp. the phenothiazines.

    d., uterine. Pain in the uterus on movement.

dyskinet'ic. Concerning dyskinesia.

dyskoimesis (dis"koy-mē'sis) [Gr. dys, bad, + koimēsis, sleeping]. Difficulty in going to sleep.

dyslalia (dis-lal'ĭ-ă) ["+ lalein, to talk]. Impairment of speech due to defect of speech organs.

dyslexia (dis-leks'ĭ-ă) ["+ lexis, diction]. An imprecise term used to indicate a variety of reading, writing and learning disorders.

dyslochia (dis-lo'kĭ-ă) ["+ lochia, lochia]. Disordered lochial discharge, or premature cessation.

dyslogia (dis-lo'jĭ-ă) ["+ logos, understanding]. Difficulty in expression of ideas.

dysmasesis (dis"mă-sē'sis) ["+ masēsis, mastication]. Difficulty in masticating. SYN: dysmastesis.

dysmegalop'sia ["+ megas, big, + opsis, vision]. Inability to visualize correctly the size of things, which appear larger than they really are.

dysmelia (dis-mē'lĭ-ă) [Gr. dys, bad, + melos, limb]. Congenital deformity or absence of a portion of one or more limbs.

dysmenorrhea (dis"men-o-rī'ă) ["+ mēn, mouth, + rhein, to flow]. Painful or difficult menstruation, either primary or secondary.

    d., congestive. Condition caused by pelvic congestion.

    d., inflammatory. Condition caused by pelvic inflammation.

    d., membranous. A severe spasmodic d. which is accompanied by the passage of a cast of the uterine cavity. Treated by curettage, and if not relieved, hysterectomy.

    d., neurotic. Form caused by neurosis.

    d., primary. Difficult menstruation starting from the first period and for which there is no obvious pathological cause.

    d., secondary. When periods were, at the outset, normal, but, because of the development of some pathological state in the pelvis, painful menstruation develops. Frequently associated with pelvic inflammatory disease, endometritis, or uterine myomata.

    d., spasmodic. D. caused by uterine contractions of spasmodic form.

dysmetria (dis-mē'trĭ-ă) [Gr. dys, bad, + metron, measure]. An inability to fix the range of a movement. Rapid and brusk movements are made with more force than necessary. Seen in cerebellar affections. RS: adiadochokinesis; asynergia; gait.

dysmetrop'sia ["+ "+ opsis, vision]. Inability to visualize correctly the size and shape of things.

dysmimia (dis-mim'ĭ-ă) ["+ mimia, imitation]. 1. Inability to express oneself by gestures or signs. 2. Inability to imitate.

dysmnesia (dis-nē'zĭ-ă) [Gr. dys, bad, + mnēmē, memory]. Any impairment of memory.

dysmorphophobia (dis"mor-fo-fo'bĭ-ă) [Gr. dysmorphas, deformed, + phobos, fear]. Morbid fear of deformity.

dysmorphosis (dis"mor-fo'sis) ["+ -ōsis, condition]. Not normal in form.

dysmyoto'nia [Gr. dys, bad, + mys, muscle, + tonos, tone]. 1. Muscle atony; abnormal muscle tonicity.

dysneuria (dis-nu'rĭ-ă) ["+ neuron, nerve]. Impairment of nerve function.

dysodontiasis (dis"o-don-tī'ă-sis) ["+ odous, tooth, + -iasis, process]. Painful or difficult dentition.

dysontogenesis (dis"ŏn-to-jĕn'ĭ-sis) ["+ ōn, being, + gennan, to produce]. Defective development of an organism, esp. of an embryo.

dysontogenet'ic. Pert to dysontogenesis.

dysopia, dysopsia (dis-o'pĭ-ă, -op'sĭ-a) ["+ opsis, vision]. Defective or painful vision.

dysorexia (dis"o-rek'sĭ-ă) ["+ orexis, appetite]. Perverted or lessened appetite.

dysosmia (dis-oz'mĭ-ă) ["+ osmē, smell]. Impairment of the sense of smell.

dysostosis (dis"os-tō'sis) ["+ osteon, bone]. Defective bone formation.

d., cleidocranial. A congenital ossification of the skull with partial atrophy of clavicles.

d., mandibulofacial. Hypoplasia of the facial bones; downward sloping of the palbebral tissues; defects of the ear; macrostomia; and a fish-face appearance. It is supposed to be a sex-linked recessive trait. SYN: *Treacher-Collins syndrome.*

dysovarism (dis-o'var-izm) [Gr. *dys*, bad, + L. *ovarium*, ovary, + Gr. *-ismos*, condition]. Defective ovarian internal secretion.

dysox'idizable ["+ L. *oxidum*, oxide]. Not easy to oxidize.

dyspan'creatism ["+ *pankreas*, pancreas, + *-ismos*, condition of]. Impaired pancreatic function.

dyspareunia (dis"pā-ru'nī-ă) [Gr. *dyspareunos*, unhappily mated as bedfellows]. Painful coitus experienced by women.
  ETIOL: May be due to physical or mental causes.

dyspepsia (dis-pep'sĭ-ă) [Gr. *dys*, bad, + *peptein*, to digest]. Imperfect digestion. Not a disease in itself, but symptomatic of other diseases or disorders. Characterized by vague abdominal discomfort; a sense of fullness after eating; eructation; heartburn; nausea and vomiting; and loss of appetite. These symptoms may occur irregularly and in different patterns from time to time. The symptoms are increased in times of stress.

d., acid. Due to excessive acid.

d., alcoholic. Caused by excessive use of alcoholic beverages.

d., biliary, bilious. Form in which there is insufficient quantity or quality of bile secretion.

d., cardiac. Form occurring during heart disease.

d., gastric. D. caused by faulty stomach function.

d., gastrointestinal. D. caused by faulty function of stomach and intestines.

d., hepatic. D. caused by liver disease.

d., hysterical. D. present during hysterical attacks.

dyspeptic (dis-pep'tik). 1. Affected with or pert. to dyspepsia. 2. One afflicted with dyspepsia.

dysperma'sia ["+ *sperma*, seed]. Dysspermia, q.v.

dysper'matism. Dysspermia, q.v.

dysper'mia. Dysspermia, q.v.

dysphagia (dis-fā'jī-ă) [Gr. *dys*, bad, + *phagein*, to eat]. Inability or difficulty in swallowing.

d. constricta. D. due to narrowing of the pharynx or esophagus.

d. lusoria. D. caused by pressure exerted on the esophagus by an anomaly of the right subclavian artery.

d. paralytica. D. due to paralysis of muscles of deglutition.

d. spastica. D. resulting from a spasm of pharyngeal or esophageal muscles.

dysphagy (dis'fā-jī). Dysphagia, q.v.

dysphasia (dis-fā'zī-ă) [Gr. *dys*, bad, + *phasis*, speech]. Impairment of speech resulting from a brain lesion.

dysphemia (dis-fē'mī-ă) ["+ *phēmē*, speech]. Stammering of psychoneurotic origin.

dysphonia (dis-fō'nī-ă) ["+ *phōnē*, voice]. Difficulty in speaking; hoarseness.

d. clerico'rum. Clergyman's sore throat.

d. pu'berum. Change of voice in boys during puberty.

dysphoria (dis-fo'rĭ-ă) [Gr. *dysphoria*, excessive anguish]. Exaggerated feeling of depression and unrest without apparent cause.

dysphrasia (dis-frā'zī-ă) [Gr. *dys*, bad, + *phrasis*, speech]. Impairment of speech due to a brain lesion. SYN: *dysphasia.*

dysphrenia (dis-frē'nī-ă) ["+ *phrēn*, mind]. Functional or constitutional psychosis; the opposite of the organic type.

dysphylaxia (dis-fi-laks'ī-ă) ["+ *phylaxis*, watching]. Waking too early from sleep.

dyspinealism (dis-pin'ī-al-izm) ["+ L. *pinealis*, shaped like a pine cone, + Gr. *-ismos*, condition of]. Functional impairment of pineal gland.

dyspitu'itarism ["+ L. *pituīta*, mucus]. Condition due to disorder of the pituitary body.

dyspla'sia [Gr. *dys*, bad, + *plassein*, to form]. Abnormal development of tissue. SYN: *alloplasia; heteroplasia.*

d., anhidrotic. A congenital condition marked by few, absent or deficient sweat glands; intolerance of heat; and abnormal development of teeth and nails.

d., cervical. Abnormal changes in the tissues covering the cervix uteri.

d., chondroectodermal. Condition marked by defective development of bones, nails, teeth and hair, and by congenital heart disease. SYN: *Ellis-Van Creveld syndrome.*

d., hereditary ectodermal. Hereditary defect marked by few or absence of sweat glands and hair follicles; smooth shiny skin; abnormalities or absence of teeth; nail deformities; cataracts or alterations of cornea; absence of mammary glands; concave face; prominent eyebrows; conjunctivitis; deficient hair growth; and mental retardation. SYN: *congenital ectodermal defect; Siemen syndrome.*

d., monostotic fibrous. Replacement of bone by fibrous tissue. Marked by pain usually in tibia or femur. Cause is unknown.

d., polyostotic fibrous. Replacement of bone by avascular fibrous tissue. Marked by difficulty in walking, and multiple bone deformities and fractures. Usually commences in childhood. Cause is unknown.

dyspnea (disp-nē'ă, disp'nĭ-ă) ["+ *pnoē,* breathing]. Air hunger resulting in labored or difficult breathing, sometimes accompanied by pain. Is normal when due to vigorous work or athletic activity.

ETIOL: Insufficient oxygenation of the blood resulting from disturbances in the lungs, low oxygen pressure of air, circulatory disturbances, hemoglobin deficiency. Other causes may be: acidosis; excessive CO_2 content of blood; lesions of the respiratory center; emotional excitation; hyperexcitability of Hering-Breuer reflex; cardiac asthma; and orthopnea. It may be a subjective feeling.

SYM: Audible, labored breathing; distressed, anxious expression; dilated nostrils; protrusion of abdomen and expanded chest; gasping; marked cyanosis.

d., cardiac. D. due to cardiac insufficiency.

d., expiratory. As in asthma and bronchitis; wheezing and painful expiration. Secretions in respiratory tract cause of sound.

d., inspiratory. D. due to interference in passage of air to the lungs.

dyspneic (disp-nē'ik). Affected with or due to dyspnea.

dyspragia (dis-prā'jĭ-ă). Dyspraxia.

dyspraxia (dis-prax'ĭ-ă) [Gr. *dyspraxia,* ill success]. Difficulty or pain in performing any function. SYN: *dyspragia.*

dysprosium (dis-pro'sĭ-um). SYMB: Dy. At. wt. 162.50; at. no. 66. A metallic element of the yttrium group of rare earths.

dysraphia, dysraphism (dis-rā'fĭ-ă, -izm) [Gr. *dys,* bad, + *rhaphē,* a seam]. In the embryo, failure of raphe-formation, or failure of fusion of parts which normally fuse.

d. spinal. A general term applied to failure of fusion of parts along the dorsal midline. May involve any of the following structures: skin, vertebrae, skull, meninges, brain and spinal cord.

dysspermatism (dis-sper'mă-tizm). Dysspermia.

dysspermia (dis-sper'mĭ-ă) [Gr. *dys,* bad, + *sperma,* seed]. Difficult or painful emission of sperm during coitus.

dyssta'sia ["+ *stasis,* standing]. Difficulty in standing.

dysstat'ic. Exhibiting difficulty in standing.

dyssyner'gia [Gr. *dys,* bad, + *synergia,* cooperation]. Failure of muscular co-ordination. SYN: *ataxia.*

dyssystole (dis-sis'tō-lĭ) ["+ *systolē,* contraction]. Asystole; incomplete cardiac systole.

dystaxia (dis-tax'ĭ-ă) ["+ *taxis,* arrangement]. Partial ataxia.

dystectia (dis-tek'shĭ-ă) ["+ L. *tectum,* roof]. In the embryo, failure of closure of the neural tube. Thus deformities such as spina bifida or meningocele are produced.

dysteleology (dis"tē-lē-ol'o-jĭ) [Gr. *dys,* bad, + *telos,* end, + *logos,* knowledge]. A theory, esp. in biology, that rudimentary organs have no useful purpose to life or organism.

dysthymia (dis-thim'ĭ-ă) ["+ *thymos,* mind]. 1. Mental perversion; melancholia. 2. Condition resulting from malfunctioning of the thymus gland during childhood.

dysthyreosis (dis"thĭ-re-o'sis) ["+ *thyreos,* shield, + *-ōsis,* condition]. Impaired functional activity of thyroid gland. SYN: *dysthyroidism.*

dysthyroidism (dis-thi'roy-dizm) ["+ "+ *eidos,* form, + *ismos,* condition]. Imperfect development and function of the thyroid gland.

dystith'ia ["+ *tithēnē,* a nurse]. Difficulty or inability to nurse at breast.

dystocia (dĭs-tō'sĭ-ă) ["+ *tokos,* birth]. Difficult labor. May be produced by either the passenger (the fetus) or the passage (the pelvis of the mother).

FETAL CAUSES: Usually large babies. Other causes are: malpositions of the fetus (transverse presentation, face, brow, breech, or compound presentations); abnormalities of the fetus (hydrocephalus, tumors of the neck or abdomen, hydrops; multiple pregnancy (interlocked twins).

MATERNAL CAUSES: *Uterus:* Primary and secondary uterine inertia; congenital anomalies of the uterus (bicornuate uterus); tumors of the uterus (fibroids, carcinoma of the cervix); abnormal fixation of the uterus by previous operation.

Bony Pelvis: Contracted pelves, the commoner clinical types of which are flat pelvis, rachitic and nonrachitic; generally contracted pelvis; flat and generally contracted pelvis; funnel pelvis; exostoses of the pelvic bones; tumors of the pelvic bones.

Cervix Uteri: Bandl's contraction ring; rigid cervix that will not dilate; stenosis and stricture preventing dilatation. *Ovary:* Ovarian cysts that block the pelvis. *Vagina and Vulva:* Cysts; tumors; atresias and stenoses.

DIAG: Can generally be made by vaginal examination and external pelvimetry before the patient goes into labor.

TREATMENT: Varies according to the condition present that causes the dystocia. In general it aims toward the correction of the abnormality in order to allow the fetus to pass. If this is not possible, operative delivery is necessary. SEE: *cesarean section.*

dystonia (dĭs-tō'nĭ-ă) [Gr. *dys,* bad, + *tonos,* tone]. Impaired or disordered tonicity, esp. muscle tone.

d. musculum deformans. A symptom characterized by distorted twisting or movement of a part or all of the body. May be caused by toxic or infectious diseases of the nervous system, or its cause may be unknown. It is important that the patient not be treated as if the disease were due to hysteria or mental illness. Treatment usually is successful but remissions do occur. SYN: *torsion dystonia.*

dyston'ic. Pert. to distonia or hyper- or hypotonicity of tissues.

dysto'pia [Gr. *dys,* bad, + *topos,* place]. Malposition; displacement of any organ.

dystopic (dis-top'ĭk). Not in place.

dys'topy [Gr. *dys,* bad, + *topos,* place]. Dystopia, q.v.

dystro'phia ["+ *trephein,* to nourish]. Disorder caused by defective nutrition. SYN: *dystrophy,* q.v.

dystrophic (dis-trof'ĭk). Pert. to dystrophia.

dystrophoneurosis (dis-trof''o-nu-ro'sis) [Gr. *dys,* bad, + *trephein,* to nourish, + *neuron,* nerve, + *-ōsis*]. Defective nutrition accompanied by a nervous disease.

dystrophy (dis'tro-fĭ). Disorder caused by defective nutrition. SYN: *dystrophia.*

d., adiposogenital. A condition characterized by a peculiar type of obesity and hypogenitalism due to a disturbance in the hypothalamus which controls food intake and of the pituitary which controls gonadal development. SYN: *Fröhlich's syndrome; sexual infantilism.*

d., Landouzy-Dejerine. A form of d., in which there is marked atrophy of facial muscles, shoulder girdle and arm. Facial atrophy produces a peculiar expression called myopathic facies.

d., progressive muscular. A familial disease characterized by progressive atrophy and wasting of muscles. Onset is usually at an early age and it occurs more frequently in males than females. Its cause is thought to be a genetic defect in muscle metabolism.

d., pseudohypertrophic muscular. An hereditary disease usually beginning in childhood in which muscular ability is lost. At first there is muscular pseudohypertrophy followed by atrophy.

dystrypsia (dis-trip'sĭ-ă) [Gr. *dys,* bad, + *tripsis,* rubbing]. Impaired secretion of pancreas.

dysuria (dis-u'rĭ-ă) ["+ *ouron,* urine]. Painful or difficult urination, symptomatic of numerous conditions. D. may be indicative of cystitis; urethritis; urethral stricture; hypertrophied, cancerous, or ulcerated prostate in the male; prolapsus of uterus in the female; pelvic peritonitis and abscess; metritis; cancer of the cervix, or dysmenorrhea. Pain and burning may also be caused by concentrated acid urine.

dysu'riac. One affected with dysuria.

dyszooamylia (dĭs-zō''ō-ăm-ĭl'ĭ-ă) [*dys,* bad, + *zōon,* animal, + *amylon,* starch]. Failure to transform dextrose into glycogen.

dyszoospermia (dis'zo-o-sperm'ĭ-ă) ["+ "+ *sperma,* seed]. Imperfect formation of spermatozoa.

E

E. Abbr. for *electromotive force; emmetropia; energy; Escherichia; eye;* chem. symb. for einsteinium.

e. Abbr. for *electric charge; electron;* L. *ex,* from.

ea. Abbr. for *each.*

ead. Abbr. for L. *eadem,* the same.

Eales' disease (ēlz). [Henry Eales, Brit. physician, 1852-1913]. Repeated hemorrhages into the retina and vitreous.

ear [AS. *ēar*]. Organ of hearing. Consisting of external, middle, and internal e.

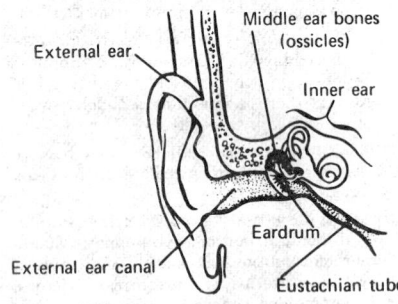

THE EAR

    e., Blainville's. Congenital asymmetry of the two e.'s.

    e. bones. Ossicles of tympanic cavity; malleus, incus, and stapes.

    e., Cagot. An e. without a lower lobe.

    e., cauliflower. A deformity consisting of a thickening of the external e. resulting from trauma which caused a hematoma. Commonly seen in prize fighters.

    e. drum. The tympanum, or cavity in middle e.

    e. dust. Calcareous concretions in membranous labyrinth. SYN: *otoconia; otolith.*

    e., examination of. Watch test for hearing; color, size, and shape; discharge from middle or inner e.; tenderness upon pressure in front or back of e.; inflammation or bulging of drum; perforations, or scars of drum.

    Acute hearing sometimes precedes delirium. Deafness may indicate wax in external e. passage, disorders of 8th (acoustic) nerve, disease of the middle ear or the toxic effect of drugs. Pallor of ears, tongue, and gums indicates shock or anemia. Ringing in ears is noted in cerebral hyperemia and anemia, in disease of e., Ménière's disease, and after use of certain drugs like quinine and salicylic acid.

    e., external. Comprises auricle and external auditory canal; is separated from middle e. by tympanic membrane or eardrum.

    e., foreign bodies in. These are usually insects, pebbles, beans, or peas. Insects in the e. cannot be attracted from the e. by a bright light. They may be stimulated to crawl in deeper by the bright light.

    SYM: Pain, ringing or buzzing in the e. and, if an insect, there is a great noise.

    TREATMENT: Drop in bland oil and so float insect out of e. In case of a solid foreign body, oil or water should not be used, because they either might push the object further in the e. or cause it to swell and become firmly embedded. Such foreign bodies in the e. do not constitute an emergency and should be left untreated until seen by a physician.

    Swimmers sometimes find that water enters the e. and will not flow out spontaneously. This may occasionally be dislodged by a sudden tap on the side of the head above the e., or by introducing a long wisp of cotton which will draw out the water by capillarity. Also a few drops of 70% alcohol instilled in the canal will hasten evaporation of the so-called trapped water. Occasionally this sensation of water in the e. is not due to water but to swelling of the cerumen, q.v., that is usually present. In such instances a physician should be consulted.

    e., internal. Consists of the cochlea containing the sensory receptors for hearing and the vestibule and semicircular canals which contain the receptors for equilibrium and the sense of position. Innervated by the vestibulocochlear nerve.

    e., middle. An irregular cavity in temporal bone. In front it communicates with eustachian tube which forms an open channel between middle e. and cavity of nasopharynx. Behind, middle e. opens into mastoid antrum, and this in turn communicates with the mastoid cells. There are two openings into the inner e., both of which are covered with membrane. Three ossicles (small bones), joined together, extend from the tympanic membrane to the fenestra vestibuli; these are the malleus, incus, and stapes.

    e., nerve supply of. External: branches of facial, vagus, and mandibular nerves and from cervical plexus. Middle: tympanic plexus and branches of mandibular, vagus, and facial nerves. Internal: vestibulocochlear nerve.

e. oximeter. A device which determines the oxygen content of the blood flowing through the e.

e., pierced. E. lobes which have been pierced with a needle so that a permanent channel will remain. Done in order to permit the wearing of earrings.

e. plug. A device for helping to prevent sound from entering the ear by occluding the external auditory canal. Should not be used while swimming because the device may interfere with pressure equalization.

e., swelling in front or behind. ETIOL: Mumps, mastoid disease, scurvy, anthrax, or gangrenous stomatitis.

e. wax. Wax in the ear. SYN: *cerumen.*

ear, words pert. to: acoustic meatus; aditus; angiotitis; annulus; antihelix; antitragus; antrotympanitis; auricle; "auris-" words; binaural; cavum tympani; cerumen; cochlea; concha; crista ampullaris; cupola; deafness; endolymph; epitympanum; eustachian; foreign bodies; helix; hydrotis; incus; labyrinth; labyrinthitis; malleus; ossicle; "ot-" or "oto-" words; pinna; scala tympani; tinnitus aurium; tympanum; "utri-" words; vestibule; vitreous.

earache. Aural pain. SYN: *otalgia.*

earth eating. Eating clay or dirt. Sometimes done by children as a form of pica, q.v.

ear trumpet. A conically shaped device held to the ear to aid the deaf in hearing.

eat [AS. *etan*]. 1. To devour as food. 2. To take solid food. 3. To corrode.

eat, words pert. to: acoria; apastia; appetite; bradyphagia; bulimia; dysphagia; fastidium; fasting; geophagia; hunger; hyperorexia; mastication; parorexia; pica; polyphagia.

Eberthella (e″ber-thel′ä). [K.J. Eberth, Ger. pathologist, 1835-1926]. Formerly a genus of bacteria. Now classified under Salmonella.

E. typhosa. Salmonella typhosa.

Eb′ner′s glands. [A. G. Victor von Ebner, Austrian histologist, 1842-1925]. Serous glands of the tongue usually found in the vicinity of the circumvallate papillae.

ebonation (e″bo-nā′shŭn) [L. *ē*, out, + AS. *ban*, bone]. Removal of bony fragments from a wound.

Ebstein's anomaly of tricuspid valve (eb′stīn). [Wilhelm Ebstein, Ger. physician, 1836-1912]. A congenital condition of the heart, symptoms of which are fatigue, palpitation and dyspnea, resulting from downward displacement of the tricuspid valve from the annulus fibrosus. SYN: *downward displacement of tricuspid valve.*

ebullism (ĕb′u-lĭzm) [L. *ebullire*, to boil over]. Spontaneous boiling of body fluids which occurs when the body is exposed to atmospheric pressure below that of the boiling point of the fluids.

ebullition (ĕb-ŭ-lĭsh′ŭn). 1. Boiling. 2. Effervescence.

eburnation (ĕb″ŭr-nā′shŭn) [L. *eburnus*, made of ivory]. Changes in bone causing them to become dense like ivory and hardened.

eburneous (ē-bŭr′nē-ŭs). Resembling ivory; ivory-colored.

ecaudate (e-kaw′dāt) [L. *e*, without, + *cauda*, tail]. Without a tail.

ecbolic (ĕk-bol′ik) [Gr. *ekbolikos*, throwing out]. 1. Hastening labor by causing contractions of the uterine muscles. 2. Causing abortion. 3. Any agent producing or hastening labor or abortion. SYN: *oxytocic.*

eccentric (ĕk-sĕn′trĭk) [Gr. *ek-*, out, + *kentron*, center]. 1. Peculiar, abnormal in action or ideas. 2. Proceeding away from a center. 3. Peripheral.

e. atrophy. Atrophy with dilatation.

e. convulsion. One caused by peripheral irritation.

e. hypertrophy. Hypertrophy of a hollow organ with dilatation.

e. limitation. Having smaller visual field than normal.

eccentro-osteochondrodysplasia (ĕk-sĕn″trŏ-ŏs″te-o-kŏn″dro-dĭs-plā′zhĭ-ä) [Gr. *ekkentros*, from the center, + *osteon*, bone, + *chondros*, cartilage, + *dys-*, bad, + *plassein*, to form]. A pathological condition of bones due to imperfect bone formation. Ossification occurs in eccentric centers instead of one common center.

eccentropiesis (ĕk-sĕn″tro-pi-e′sis) ["+ *piēsis*, pressure]. Pressure from within exerted outward.

ecchondroma, ecchondrosis (ĕk-on-dro′mä, -dro′sis) [Gr. *ek-*, out, + *chondros*, cartilage, + *-ōma*, tumor]. A chondroma or cartilaginous tumor.

ecchondrotome (ĕk-on′dro-tōm) ["+ "+ *tomē*, incision]. Knife for excision of cartilage.

ecchymoma (ĕk-ĭ-mō′mä) ["+ *chymos*, juice, + *ōma*, tumor]. An extravasated blood tumor. A swelling due to the accumulation of blood in subcutaneous tissues such as occurs following a bruise.

ecchymosis (ĕk-ĭ-mō′sĭs) ["+ "+ *ōsis*, condition]. (pl. *ecchymoses*) A form of macula appearing in large irregularly-formed hemorrhagic areas of the skin. The color is blue-black, changing to greenish brown or yellow.

ETIOL: Extravasation of blood into skin or mucous membrane.

ecchymotic (ĕk-ĭ-mot'ĭk) ["+ *chymos,* juice]. Resembling or rel. to an ecchymosis.

eccrine (ĕk'rin) [Gr. *ekkrinein,* to secrete]. Excretory. SYN: *exocrine.*

    e. sweat. Sweat from the eccrine sweat glands. These glands are important in regulating body temperature. SEE: *apocrine.*

eccrinology (ĕk-rĭn-ŏl'ō-jĭ) ["+ "+ *logos,* study]. The science of excretions and glandular secretions.

eccrisis (ĕk'krĭs-is) [Gr. *ek-,* out, + *krisis,* separation]. The excretion of waste products. SYN: *excretion.*

eccritic (ĕk-krit'ĭk). Promoting or that which promotes excretion.

eccyclomastopathy (ĕk-si''klo-mas-top'ā-thĭ) [Gr. *ek-,* out, + *kyklos,* circle, + *mastos,* breast, + *pathos,* disease]. A mass of lesions of the breast made up of connective tissue and/or epithelial cells. SYN: *cyclomastopathy.*

eccyesis (ek''si-e'sis) ["+ *kyēsis,* pregnancy]. Extrauterine or ectopic pregnancy.

ecdemic (ĕk-dĕm'ĭk) [Gr. *ekdēmos,* foreign]. Neither endemic nor epidemic, as a disease carried to a region from without.

ecdemomania (ĕk''de-mo-mā'nĭ-ā) ["+ *mania,* madness]. Wanderlust; abnormal desire to wander. SYN: *drapetomania; dromomania; vagabondage.*

ecderon (ek'dĕ-ron) [Gr. *ek-,* out, + *deros,* skin]. Epidermis, or outer portion of skin, as distinguished from enderon, q.v., or inner portion.

ecdysis (ĕk'dĭ-sĭs) [Gr. *ek-,* out, + *dyein,* to put on]. (pl. *ecdyses*) 1. The shedding or sloughing off of the epidermis of the skin; desquamation. 2. The shedding of the outer covering of the body as occurs in certain animals such as insects, crustaceans, and snakes; molting.

ECG., ecg. Abbr. for *electrocardiogram.*

echidnase (ĕ-kĭd'nās) [Gr. *echidna,* viper, + *-ase,* suffix denoting enzyme]. An enzyme present in snake venom which produces inflammation.

echidnin(ĕ-kĭd'nĭn). 1. The venom of poisonous snakes. 2. The active principle present in snake venom.

Echidnophaga (ĕ''kĭd-nof'ă-gă). A genus of fleas belonging to the family Pulicidae.

    E. gallinacea. The sticktight flea which is the most important flea pest of poultry. It collects in clusters on the heads of poultry and in the ears of mammals. It may infest humans, esp. children.

echinate (ĕk'ĭ-nāt) [Gr. *echinos,* hedgehog]. 1. Spiny. 2. In agar streak, a growth with pitted or toothed margins along the inoculation line; in stab cultures, coiled growth with pointed outgrowths. SYN: *echinulate.*

echinococcosis (ĕ-kĭ''no-kok-ō'sis, ek''ĭ-no-kok-ō'sis) ["+ *kokkos,* berry, + *-ōsis,* condition]. Infestation with echinococcus.

echinococcotomy (ĕ-kĭ''no-kok-ŏt'ō-mĭ) ["+ "+ *tomē,* incision]. Operation for evacuation of an echinococcus cyst.

Echinococcus (ĕ-kĭ''no-kŏk'us). (pl. *Echinococci*) A genus of tapeworms. They are minute forms consisting of a scolex and three or four proglottids.

    E. granulosus. A species of tapeworms that infests dogs and other carnivores. Its larva, called a hydatid, develops in other mammals including man and causes the formation of hydatid cysts in the liver and/or lungs. SEE: *hydatid.*

    E. hydatidosus. Variety of E. characterized by development of daughter cysts from the mother cyst. SEE: *hydatid.*

echinosis (ĕk'i-nō'sis) [Gr. *echinos,* hedgehog, + *-ōsis,* condition]. Blood corpuscles appearing like a sea urchin, having lost their smooth outlines. Crenation of red blood cells.

Echinostoma (ĕk'ĭ-nos'tō-mä) ["+ *stoma,* mouth]. A genus of flukes characterized by a spiny body and the presence of a collar of spines near the anterior end. They are found in the intestines of many vertebrates, esp. aquatic birds. They occasionally occur as accidental parasites in man.

echinulate (ĕ-kĭn'ū-lāt). A bacterial growth having pointed processes or spines. SYN: *echinate.*

echo (ĕk'ō) [Gr. *ēkhō,* echo]. A reverberating sound.

    e. acou'sia. Subjective echoes of sounds just normally heard.

    e., amphor'ic. Amphoric sound sometimes heard in auscultation of chest. SEE: *chest.*

    e. sign. Repetition of closing word of a sentence, a sign of epilepsy or other brain conditions.

    e. speech. Echolalia.

ECHO virus. One of the viruses belonging to the group known as Enteric Cytopathogenic Human Orphan group. Cause of nonbacterial viral meningitis, enteritis, and various infections with or without fever or rash. At first more than 30 viruses were assigned to this group. Later it was realized that some of these should be reclassified. Thus several types (9, 10, and 28) were removed from the ECHO group.

echography (ĕk-ŏg′ră-fĭ) ["+ *graphein*, to write]. The use of ultrasonic technique to produce a photograph of the echo produced when sound waves are reflected from tissues of different density.

echokinesia (ĕk″ō-kĭn-ē′sĭ-ă) [Gr. *ēkhō*, echo, + *kinēsis*, movement]. Involuntary repetition of another's gestures.

echolalia (ĕk-ō-lā′lĭ-ă) ["+ *lalia*, talk, babble]. An involuntary, parrotlike repetition of words spoken by others, often accompanied by twitching of muscles. Frequently seen in catatonic schizophrenia.

echomatism (ĕ-kō′mă-tĭzm) ["+ *-matos*, willing, striving, + *-ismos*, condition]. Automatic repetition of another's actions.

echomimia (ĕk″ō-mim′ĭ-a) [Gr. *ēkhō*, echo, + *mimēsis*, imitation]. The imitation of the actions of others without meaning as seen in schizophrenia.

echomotism (ĕk″ō-mo′tizm) ["+ L. *motus*, moving]. Imitation of movements. SYN: *echomatism*.

echopathy (ĕ-kop′ă-thĭ) ["+ *pathos*, disease]. Imitation of another's actions and repetitions of his words; a neurosis.

echophotony (ĕk″ō-fot′o-nĭ) [Gr. *ēkhō*, echo, + *phos*, light, + *tonos*, tone]. Mental association of certain sounds with particular colors.

echophrasia (ĕk″ō-fra′sĭ-ă) ["+ *phrasis*, speech]. Echolalia, q.v.

echopraxia (ĕk″ō-prăk′sĭ-ă) ["+ *prassein*, to perform]. Imitation, without meaning, of motions made by others. SYN: *echomimia*.

echoprax′is. Echopraxia, q.v.

eclabium (ĕk-la′bĭ-um) [Gr. *ek-*, out, + L. *labium*, lip]. Eversion of a lip.

eclampsia (ĕ-klamp′sĭ-ă) ["+ *lampein*, to shine]. A major toxemia of pregnancy accompanied by high blood pressure, albuminuria, oliguria, tonic and clonic convulsions, and coma. May occur during pregnancy or shortly after delivery. SEE: *preeclampsia*.

ETIOL: Unknown. Occurs more often in primiparae. Hypertension and glomerulonephritis contribute to cause.

PATH: Seen most frequently in the kidney, liver, brain, and placenta. The kidney shows degenerated tubal nephritis, the tubal epithelium showing cloudy swelling, fatty degeneration, and coagulation necrosis. The liver is enlarged and mottled, there are portal vein thrombosis and degeneration of the periphery of the lobules with subcapsular hemorrhages. The brain shows edema, hyperemia, thrombosis, and hemorrhages. The placenta shows infarcts, thromboses,

and hemorrhages. There is also retinal edema.

SYM: Edema of the legs and feet, puffiness of the face, hyperpiesis, q.v., and albuminuria, q.v. Severe headaches, dizziness, spots before the eyes, epigastric pain and nausea, convulsions (beginning with fixation of the eyeballs, rolling of the eyes, twitchings of the face, arms, and hands; the paroxysms then involve the entire body), and coma. There may be one or many convulsions. The pulse is rapid and bounding, the temperature usually rises to 103° or 104° F. (39.4-40° C.), and the blood pressure may be quite elevated. The patient may continue in coma until death.

TREATMENT: Prophylactic: The most important. Good prenatal care, with careful watching of the patient's blood pressure, urine, and weight; instituting medical management as soon as any abnormal findings are presented, and terminating pregnancy if unsuccessful in reducing the signs of danger.

Convulsions: Prevent the patient from doing herself bodily harm (restrain her in bed, protect the tongue by keeping the teeth separated). Relieve vasoconstriction; promote diuresis. Sedatives only on order by physician. Tracheostomy may be required to maintain an airway.

Delivery: This should not be instituted until the general condition of the patient has improved unless the patient is in active labor, in which case the labor should be conducted by most conservative methods. Cesarean section should not be done unless there is some other obstetrical reason. If medical management effects no improvement, then labor must be instituted by one of the recognized methods, but local rather than general anesthesia is preferred.

NP: During a convulsion the patient must not be left alone. Restrain only enough to keep her in bed. Side boards or some type of restraint must be used after the convulsion to make certain the patient will not fall out of bed during the coma, delirium, and restless stage. Use mouth gag to keep patient from biting her tongue. See that the physician is notified immediately. Have the fetal heart checked frequently, in cases of convulsion before delivery, because the fetal circulation is interfered with and the infant may register signs of distress.

e., infantile. A convulsion occurring in children. It is of reflex origin being associated with teething, acute digestive disorders, worm infestation, or cerebral congestion.

e. nutans. E. characterized by nodding movements. SYN: *nodding spasm, salaam convulsion.*

e., puerperal. A convulsion occurring near the end of pregnancy, during labor, or immediately following labor.

eclampsism (ĕ-klamp'sĭzm) ["+ "+ *ismos,* state of]. Puerperal eclampsia without convulsive seizures.

eclamp'tic. Rel. to, or of the nature of, eclampsia.

eclamptogenic (ĕk-lamp"to-jĕn'ĭk) [Gr. *ek-,* out, + *lampein,* to shine, + *gennan,* to produce]. Causing convulsions.

eclamptogenous. Producing convulsions. SYN: *eclamptogenic.*

eclectic (ĕk-lĕk'tĭk) [Gr. *ek-,* out of, + *legein,* to choose]. Selecting from various sources what seems to be the best.

e. school of medicine. One employing a selected method, as indigenous plants or "specifics" according to patient's symptoms.

eclecticism (ĕk-lĕk'tĭ-sĭzm) ["+ "+ *ismos,* state of]. A system of medicine treating disease through specific remedies for individual pathological conditions, rather than by treating body as a whole. Remedies principally botanical.

eclysis (ĕk-lĭ'sĭs). A mild syncope.

ecmnesia (ĕk-nē'zĭ-ă) [Gr. *ek-,* out, + *mnēsis,* memory]. Inability to remember recent events as seen in senility. The memory of before and after events not affected.

ecocide [Gr. *oikos,* house, + L. *caedere,* to kill]. Willful destruction of some portion of the environment.

ecoid (e'koyd) [Gr. *oikos,* house, + *eidos,* form]. The framework of a red blood corpuscle.

E. Coli. Partial abbr. for *Escherichia coli,* q.v.

ecology (ē-kŏl'ō-jĭ) ["+ *logos,* study of]. Science of the relations and interactions of the totality of organisms to their environment, including the relations and interactions of organisms to each other in that environment. SYN: *bionomics.*

ecomania (e"ko-ma'nĭ-ă) ["+ *mania,* madness]. Obsolete term for extreme humbleness manifested before those in authority but a dominating, irritable attitude towards members of the family.

ecosphere (ĕk'ō-sfīr") ["+ L. *sphēra,* ball]. Portions of the universe habitable by living organisms and plant life.

ecostate (e-kŏs'tāt) [L. *e,* without, + *costa,* rib]. Without ribs.

ecosystem (ĕk'ō-sĭs"tĕm) [*ecology* + *system*]. The smallest ecology unit. The living organisms and plants and their environment in a defined area.

écouvillonage (ā-koo"vĭ-yŏ-nŏhzh') [Fr. *écouvillon,* a stiff brush or swab]. The cleansing and application of remedies to a cavity by means of a brush or swab.

ecphoria (ĕk-fōr'ĭ-ă) [Gr. *ek-,* out of, + *pherein,* to bear]. An engram, or the reestablishment of a memory trace or engram.

ecphyadectomy (ĕk-fĭ-ă-dĕk'tō-mĭ) [Gr. *ekphyas,* appendix, + *ektomē,* excision]. Removal of vermiform appendix. SEE: *appendectomy.*

ecphyaditis (ĕk-fĭ-ă-dī'tĭs) ["+ *-itis,* inflammation]. Inflammation of vermiform appendix. SYN: *appendicitis.*

ecphylactic (ĕk-fĭ-lăk'tĭk) [Gr. *ek-,* out, + *phylaxis,* guarding]. Pert. to ecphylaxis.

ecphylax'is. Impotent antibodies or phylactic agents in the blood.

ecphyma (ĕk-fī'mă) [Gr. *ek-,* out of, + *phyma,* growth]. An outgrowth or excrescence, as a wart.

écrasement (ā-kräz-mon'). Excision by means of an écraseur, q.v.

écraseur (ā-krä-zer') [Fr. *écraser,* to crush]. A wire loop used for excisions.

ecstasy (ĕk'stă-sĭ) [Gr. *ekstasis,* a standing out]. An exhilarated, trancelike condition or state of exalted delight.

ecstrophy (ĕk'stro-fĭ) [Gr. *ekstrophe,* a turning out]. Turning an organ inside out. SYN: *exstrophy.*

ECT. Abbr. for *electroconvulsive therapy.*

ec'tad [Gr. *ektos,* outside, + L. *ad,* toward]. Toward the surface; outward; externally.

ec'tal. External, outer, on the surface.

ectasia, ectasis (ĕk-tā'sĭ-ă, ek'tă-sĭs) [Gr. *ek-,* out, + *teinein,* to stretch]. Dilatation of any tubular vessel.

e., hypostatic. Dilatation of a blood vessel from the pooling of blood in dependent parts, especially the legs.

e. iridis. Smallness of the pupil of the eye caused by displacement of the iris.

e. ventriculi paradoxa. Hourglass stomach.

ectat'ic. Distensible or capable of being stretched.

ecten'tal [Gr. *ektos,* without, + *entos,* within]. Pert. to entoderm and ectoderm.

e. line. Point of entodermal and ectodermal junction in the gastrula.

ectethmoid (ĕk-teth'moyd) ["+ *ēthmos,* sieve, + *eidos,* form]. Lateral mass of the ethmoid bone.

ecthyma (ĕk-thī'mă) [Gr. *ek-,* out, + *thyein,* to rush]. An infection of the skin. Usually a result of neglected treatment of impetigo, q.v. It is marked by shallow lesions with adherent crusts or scabs. May be followed by pigmentation and scarring. Treatment is the same as that for impetigo.

ecthyreosis (ĕk-thī″rē-ō′sĭs) ["+ *thyreos,* shield, + *-ōsis,* condition]. Loss of thyroid gland or its function.

ectiris (ĕk-tī′rĭs) [Gr. *ektos,* outside, + *īris,* iris]. The external portion of the iris.

ecto- [Gr. *ektos,* outside]. Prefix meaning outside.

ectoantigen (ĕk″to-ăn′tĭ-gĕn) [Gr. *ektos,* out, + *anti,* against, + *gennan,* to produce]. 1. Any toxin or stimulator of antibody formation. 2. An antigen assumed to have its origin in ectoplasm of bacterial cells or one loosely attached to the surface of bacteria and capable of being separated from the bacterial cell.

ectoblast (ĕk′to-blăst) ["+ *blastos,* germ]. 1. Wall of a cell. 2. Ectoderm. 3. Any outer membrane.

ectocardia (ĕk-to-kăr′dĭ-ā) ["+ *kardia,* heart]. Having the heart out of normal position.

ectochoroidea (ĕk″to-ko-roy′de-ā) ["+ *khorioeidēs,* choroid]. Outer layer of choroid coat of the eye.

ectocinerea (ĕk″to-sĭn-e′re-ā) [Gr. *ektos,* outside, + L. *cinereus,* ashen]. The outer gray matter of the brain.

ectocolostomy (ĕk″to-kŏ-lŏs′tō-mĭ) ["+ *kolon,* colon, + *stoma,* opening]. Formation through the abdominal wall of an opening into the colon.

ectocondyle (ĕk″to-kŏn′dĭl) ["+ *kondylos,* knuckle]. The outer condyle of the bone.

ectocornea (ĕk-to-kŏr′nē-ā) ["+ L. *corneus,* horny]. External layer of the cornea.

ectocuneiform (ĕk-to-kū′nē-ĭ-fŏrm) [Gr. *ektos,* outside, + L. *cuneus,* wedge, + *forma,* form]. External cuneiform bone.

ectocytic (ĕk″to-si′tĭk) ["+ *kytos,* hollow vessel]. Outside of the cell.

ectodactylism (ĕk-to-dăk′tĭl-ĭzm) ["+ *daktylos,* finger, + *ismos,* state of]. Lack of a digit or digits.

ectoderm (ek′to-derm) ["+ *derma,* skin]. The outer layer of cells in a developing embryo. From it are developed skin structures, the nervous system, organs of special sense, and pineal and part of pituitary and suprarenal glands. SYN: *epiblast.* SEE: *entoderm.*

ectoder′mal. Rel. to the ectoderm.

ectodermatosis (ĕk″to-dĕr″mă-tō′sĭs) [Gr. *ektos,* outside, + *derma,* skin, + *ōsis,* diseased condition]. Illness resulting from congenital maldevelopment of ectodermal structures.

    e. pluriorificialis. A form of erythema multiforme characterized by fever, chills, profuse salivation, small blisters on tongue, lips and cheeks, and erythematous lesions on the hands. The disease is rare, occurring in children and young persons. SYN: *dermatostomatitis.*

ectoder′mic. Pert. to the ectoderm. SYN: *ectodermal.*

ectodermoidal (ĕk″to-dĕr-moyd′ăl) [Gr. *ektos,* outside, + *derma,* skin, + *eidos,* form]. Pert. to or resembling the ectoderm.

ectoentad (ĕk″to-en′tăd) ["+ *entos,* within]. From without inward.

ectoenzyme (ĕk″to-ĕn″zīm) ["+ *en-,* in, + *zymē,* leaven]. An extracellular enzyme, or one that acts outside of the cell that secretes it.

ectogenous (ĕk-tŏj′ĕ-nŭs) ["+ *gennan,* to produce]. Having its origin outside of a body or structure, as infection.

ectoglia (ĕk-tŏg′lĭ-ă) [Gr. *ektos,* outside, + *glia,* glue]. Superficial embryonic layer in beginning of stratification of the medullary tube.

ectoglobular (ĕk″to-glŏb′ū-lăr) ["+ L. *globulus,* globule]. Not within blood cells or globular bodies.

ectogony (ĕk-tog′o-nĭ) ["+ *gonos,* seed]. Influences on the mother's body and metabolism caused by the developing zygote.

ectokelostomy (ĕk″to-ke-lŏs′tō-mĭ) ["+ *kēlē,* hernia, + *stoma,* opening]. Making an external opening into a hernial sac to prepare for a radical operation.

ectolecithal (ĕk″to-les′ĭ-thăl) [Gr. *ektos,* outside, + *lekithos,* yolk]. Pert. to ovum having food yolk placed near the surface.

ectol′ysis ["+ *lysis,* dissolution]. Ectoplasmic lysis.

ectomere (ĕk′tō-mēr) ["+ *meros,* part]. One of the blastomeres forming the ectoderm.

ectomesoblast (ĕk″to-mĕs′ō-blast) [Gr. *ektos,* outside, + *mesos,* middle, + *blastos,* germ]. Cells from which the ectoblast and mesoblast will develop.

ectomorphy (ĕk′to-mor″fĭ) ["+ *morphe,* form]. Body build characterized by predominance of tissues derived from the ectoderm. SEE: *endomorphy; mesomorphy; somatotype.*

ectomy (ĕk′tō-mĭ) [Gr. *ektomē*]. Excision of any organ or gland.

ectonuclear (ĕk-to-nū′klē-ăr) [Gr. *ektos,* outside, + L. *nucleus,* kernel]. Occurring outside a cell nucleus.

ectopagus (ĕk-top′ă-gŭs) ["+ *pagos,* something fixed]. An abnormal fetus consisting of twins fused at the thorax.

ectoparasite (ĕk″tō-păr′ă-sīt″) ["+ *parasite*]. A parasite that lives on the outer surface of the body.

ectoperitonitis (ĕk″to-pĕr′ĭ-to-nī′tĭs) ["+
peritonaion, peritoneum, + *itis,* inflamma-
tion]. Inflammation of the parietal layer of
peritoneum (layer lining the abdominal
wall).

ectopia (ĕk-tō′pĭ-ă) [Gr. *ek-,* out, + *topos,*
place]. Malposition or displacement, especially congenital, of an organ or structure.
   e. cordis. Malposition of the heart in
which heart lies outside the thoracic cavity.
   e. lentis. Displacement of the crystalline lens of the eye.
   e., pupillae. Displacement of the pupil.
SYN: *corectopia.*
   e. renis. Displacement of the kidney.
   e. testis. Displacement of the testis.
   e. vesicae. Displacement of the bladder, esp. exstrophy of the bladder.
   e., visceral. An umbilical hernia.

ectopic (ĕk-tŏp′ĭk). In an abnormal position;
said of a fetus.
   e. beat. Cardiac beat beginning at a
point other than sinoatrial node.
   e. gestation. Implantation of the fertilized ovum outside of the uterine cavity.
There is usually a poorly developed decidual
reaction in the uterus. SYN: *e. pregnancy.*
   LOCATIONS: *Abdominal:* In the free abdominal cavity and attached to one of the
abdominal viscera, usually secondary to tubal. *Interstitial:* In the interstitial portion of
the tube. *Ovarian:* In the ovary. The ovarian
and primary abdominal types are very rare.
Tubal: In the fallopian tube, the most frequently encountered. The pregnancy may be
situated in the interstitial, ampullar, or isthmic portion of the tube, the isthmic type being the most common.
   ETIOL: Most commonly associated with
inflammatory conditions of the tube and
other conditions which mechanically interfere with the downward passage of the
ovum, such as diverticula, polypi in the tubal lumen, peritoneal adhesions, and a large
migrating ovum. Any variety of pregnancy
or any combination of varieties may occur
(uterine plus ectopic, bilateral ectopic, etc.).
   SYM: Missed menstruation; tenderness,
soreness, pain on affected side; pallor, weak
pulse, signs of shock or hemorrhage; pain
may be reflected to shoulder; perhaps bluish
discoloration of umbilicus.
   Unruptured: Amenorrhea may or may
not be present; vague pains in the abdomen
usually on one side; irregular hemorrhage.
The diagnosis at this stage can be made by
the usual biological tests for pregnancy.
   Ruptured: Without a severe hemorrhage:
Severe pain in the lower abdomen with
fainting spells which occur repeatedly. Diag-

nosis made by transvaginal needle puncture
of the peritoneal cavity. This will reveal free
blood. If bleeding is severe and surgical
therapy is not instituted without delay,
death may result.
   DIFFERENTIAL DIAGNOSIS: Ectopic
must be differentiated from uterine pregnancy, acute salpingitis, twisting of the pedicle of an ovarian cyst or pedunculated
fibroid tumor, and hemorrhage from a ruptured graafian follicle or corpus luteum cyst.
   TREATMENT: Once the diagnosis of ectopic pregnancy is made, operative treatment is indicated. In those cases where there
is profound shock from hemorrhage, the patient should be supported by blood transfusion and saline infusions before major
surgery is attempted.
   e. rhythm. Any cardiac rhythm that is
abnormal or irregular.

ec′toplasm [Gr. *ektos,* outer, + *plasma,* a
thing formed]. The outermost layer of cell
protoplasm.

ec″toplas′mic. Pert. to ectoplasm.

ectoplas′tic [Gr. *ektos,* outside, + *plassein,*
to form]. Formed at the periphery; ectoplasmic.

ectopotomy (ĕk-tō-pŏt′ō-mĭ) [Gr. *ek-,* out, +
topos, place, + *tomē,* incision]. Removal of
the fetus in ectopic pregnancy.

ectopterygoid (ĕk″to-tĕr′ĭ-goyd) [Gr. *ektos,*
outside, + *pteryx,* wing, + *eidos,* form]. External or lateral pterygoid muscle. Acts to
bring jaw forward. SYN: *musculus pterygoideus lateralis* [NA].

ectopy (ĕk′tō-pĭ) [Gr. *ek-,* out, + *topos,* place].
Displacement. SYN: *ectopia,* q.v.

ectoretina (ĕk″to-rĕt′ĭ-nă) [Gr. *ektos,* outside, + L. *rete,* net]. Outer layer of retina.

ectoscopy (ĕk-tŏs′ko-pĭ) ["+ *skopein,* to ex-
amine]. Diagnosis by study of thoracic movements when patient speaks, or by abdominal
movements.

ectostosis (ĕk-tŏs-tō′sis) ["+ *osteon,* bone, +
-ōsis, condition]. Formation of bone beneath
the periosteum.

ectotoxemia (ĕk″to-tŏk-sē′mĭ-ă) ["+ *toxikon,* poison, + *haima,* blood]. Toxemia from
introduction of a toxin into the body.

Ectotrichophyton (ĕk-tō-trī-kŏf′ĭ-tŏn) [Gr.
ektos, outside, + *thrix,* hair, + *phyton,*
plant]. Term applied to Trichophyton mega-
losporon ectothrix, a genus of parasitic fungi, causing tinea or ringworm of the hair.

ectozoon (ĕk-to-zō′ŏn) ["+ *zōon,* animal].
Parasitic animal that infests the outer integument of the body.

ectrodactylism (ĕk″trō-dăk′tĭl-izm) [Gr.
ektrōma, abortion, + *daktylos,* finger, + *is-*

mos, state of]. Congenital absence of one or more fingers or toes.

ectromelia (ĕk″tro-me′lĭ-ă) [″+ *melos,* limb]. Congenital absence of one or more limbs.

ectropic (ĕk-trō′pĭk) [Gr. *ek-,* out, + *trepein,* to turn]. Pert. to complete or partial eversion of a part, generally the eyelid.

ectropion (ĕk-trō′pĭ-ŏn). Eversion of an edge or margin, as the edge of an eyelid.

ETIOL: Old age; relaxation of skin; cicatrix following trauma; infection; palsy of facial nerve.

e. of the cervix uteri. In gynecology, a turning out of the edges of the cervix following laceration.

ectro′pionize. To evert, or cause an eversion.

eczema (ek′zĕ-mă) [Gr. *ekzein,* to boil out]. This word has become synonymous with chronic dermatitis caused by a number of external and internal factors acting singly or in combination. It has therefore no specific connotation, particularly with respect to etiology. Acute or chronic cutaneous inflammatory condition with erythema, papules, vesicles, pustules, scales, crusts, or scabs alone or in combination; they may be dry or with watery discharge, with thickening, infiltration, and more or less itching or burning. More a symptom than a disease.

ETIOL: No class, age, or sex is exempt, but those with thin, dry skins are more susceptible. Not infectious. Two classes of causes: (1) External or exciting (irritation, allergic contact, reaction to exposure to certain microorganisms, occupational and nonoccupational, chemicals, etc.). (2) Constitutional or predisposing; this includes eczema due to genetic and psychological factors.

SYM: Primary type characterized by erythematous, papular, vesicular, or pustular lesions. In secondary type, the lesions evolve from primary variety. Invasion by pathogenic organisms may cause suppuration.

e., erythematous. Dry, pinkish, ill-defined patches with itching and burning; slight swelling with tendency to spread and coalesce; branny scaling; roughness and dryness of skin. May become generalized.

e. fissum. Form of e. with painful fissures.

e. herpeticum. Massive crops of vesicles which become pustular, occurring when infection with herpes simplex virus takes place in a person, usually an infant, with pre-existing e.

e. hypertrophicum. E. with a permanent enlargement of papillae of the skin, or with skin growths.

e., lichenoid. E. with a thickened condition of the skin.

e. marginatum. E. caused by ringworm. SYN: *tinea cruris.*

e., nummular. Discoid e. Lesions are coin- or oval-shaped.

e., pustular. Includes many forms: Follicular, impetiginous, or consecutive types including e. rubrum (red, glazed surface with little oozing), e. madidans (raw, red, and covered with moisture), e. crustosum (more or less crusting with exudate), e. fissum (thick, dry, inelastic skin with cracks and fissures), squamous e. (chronic, on soles, legs, scalp; multiple, circumscribed infiltrated patches with thin, dry scales), e. sclerosum (marked thickening, elephantiasis-like papillary hypertrophy resulting in rough, horny, verrucose patches on legs, soles, and palms with fissuring), furrowed e. (slightly erythematous skin, harsh and dry, with innumerable cracks on outer epidermal layer).

PROG: Chronic, amenable to treatment but prone to relapse and recurrence.

TREATMENT: Depends upon the etiology and will therefore be highly individualized according to the causative agent, organism, or condition. SEE: *allergy; dermatitis, contact.*

e., seborrheic. Form marked by excessive secretion from the sebaceous glands. SYN: *seborrhea.*

e. vaccinatum. Generalized vaccinial lesions or local lesions elsewhere than at vaccination site in persons who have eczema and have been vaccinated. Also may occur as result of accidental contact with a recently vaccinated parent or sibling.

eczematous (ĕk-zĕm′ă-tŭs). Marked by or resembling eczema.

ED. Abbr. for *effective dose; erythema dose.*

edema (ĕ-dē′mă) [Gr. *oidēma,* swelling]. (pl. *-mas* or *-mata*) In England, spelled *oedema.* A condition in which the body tissues contain an excessive amount of tissue fluid. It may be local or general. Generalized edema is sometimes called dropsy or anasarca.

ETIOL: May result from increased permeability of the capillary walls; increased capillary pressure due to venous obstruction or heart failure; lymphatic obstruction; disturbances in renal functioning; reduction of plasma proteins; inflammatory conditions; fluid and electrolyte disturbances, particularly those causing sodium retention; malnutrition; starvation; chemical substances such as bacterial toxins, venoms, caustic substances, and histamine.

May occur by diffusion, q.v., osmosis, q.v., or dialysis, q.v.

TREATMENT: Bed rest desirable. Salt intake restricted; may be moderate or severe restriction, depending upon degree of edema. Fluid intake restricted; may be as low as 600 ml. in 24 hours. This proscription may be relaxed when free diuresis has been attained. Diuretics are effective when renal function is good, e. mild, and when underlying abnormality of cardiac function, capillary pressure, or salt retention is being corrected simultaneously. Diuretics contraindicated in the true nephritic e. of acute diffuse glomerulonephritis. They are often useless in cardiac e. associated with advanced renal insufficiency. One of a variety of effective diuretics may be used. The diet in e. should be adequate in protein, high in calories, rich in vitamins, and low in salt. When diuresis appears, the patient may resume a normal diet.

e., acute circumscribed. Form with localized swelling, usually on the face.

e., angioneurotic. Large areas of swelling of subcutaneous tissues, mucous membranes, and occasionally viscera. May be due to allergic sensitivity to drugs, food, or physical agents such as cold or wind, but in many cases the cause is unknown. SYN: *angioedema.*

e., blue. Hysteric paralysis inducing a swollen, bluish condition of a limb.

e. bullosum vesicae. Form affecting the bladder.

e. of glottis. An infiltration of the submucosa of the larynx with cough, loss of voice, and feeling of suffocation.

e., inflammatory. E. of inflamed tissues.

e., malignant. E. characterized by a rapid course and speedy destruction of tissue.

e. neonatorum. E. in newborn, especially premature infants. Condition is usually transitory, involving hands, face, feet, and genitalia, and it rarely becomes generalized.

e., purulent. E. caused by purulent infiltration.

e., salt. Form caused by increase of salt in the diet.

edema, words pert. to: angioedema; cephaledema; chemosis; giant urticaria; hives; lung; nephritis; phlegmasia alba dolens.

edematous (ĕ-dĕm′ăt-ŭs) [Gr. *oidēma*, swelling]. Pert. to, or affected with, edema.

edentia (ē-dĕn′shĭ-ă) [L. *e*, without, + *dens*, tooth]. Absence of teeth.

edentulous (ē-dĕnt′ū-lŭs). Without teeth.

edible (ĕd′ĭ-bl) [L. *edere*, to eat]. Suitable for food; fit to be eaten, i.e, non-poisonous.

e. portion. That fraction of food which is ordinarily considered edible.

edulcorant (e-dul′ko-rant) [L. *e*, out, + *dulcorāre*, to sweeten]. Sweetening.

edulcorate (ē-dŭl′ko-rāt). 1. To sweeten. 2. To wash out salts or acids.

EEE. Abbr. for *Eastern equine encephalitis.*

EEG. Abbr. for *electroencephalogram.*

effect (ĕ-fĕkt′). Result of an action or force.

e., additive. A therapeutic effect of a combination of two or more drugs which is greater than the sum of the individual drug effects.

e., cumulative. E. of a drug which is apparent only after a number of doses have been given. Caused by excretion or metabolic degradation of only a fraction of each dose given. Though this type of effect is usually avoided, sometimes it is therapeutically desirable.

effect′or [L. *effectus*, accomplishing]. One of the nerve endings having the efferent process end in a gland or muscle cell. The terminal arborizations of efferent or motor nerves. Also applied to effector organs (muscles and glands).

e. organ. A structure, specifically muscles and glands, which when stimulated produces an effect.

effemination (ĕ-fĕm-ĭ-nā′shŭn) [L. *effeminare*, to make feminine]. The state or condition of a male having the mental and physical characteristics of a female; the production of such characteristics in a male.

ef′ferent [L. *ex*, away from, + *ferre*, to carry]. Carrying away from a central organ or section, as efferent nerves which conduct impulses from the brain or spinal cord to the periphery, efferent lymph vessels which convey lymph from lymph nodes, and efferent arterioles which carry blood from glomeruli of the kidney.

e. nerves. Motor nerves. They can carry impulses having the following effects: (1) Motor, causing contraction of muscles; (2) secretory, causing glands to secrete, and (3) inhibitory, causing some organs to become quiescent.

effervesce (ĕf′ĕr-vĕs′) [L. *effervescere*, to boil up]. To boil, or form bubbles on the surface of a liquid.

effervescence (ĕf-ĕr-vĕs′ĕns). Formation of bubbles of gas rising to surface of fluid.

efferves′cent. Bubbling. Rising in little bubbles of gas.

effleurage (ef-flūr-ahzh′) [Fr. *effleurer*, to touch lightly]. In massage, deep or gentle stroking.

efflorescence (ĕf-flor-ĕs'ĕns) [L. *efflorescere*, to bloom]. A rash; a redness of the skin. SYN: *exanthem*, q.v.

efflorescent. Becoming powdery or drying from loss of water of crystallization.

effluent (ĕf'lu-ent) [L. *effluere*, to flow out]. 1. A flowing out. 2. Fluid material discharged from a sewage treatment plant or an industrial plant.

effluvium (ĕf-lu'vĭ-um). (pl. *effluvia*) A malodorous exhalation, particularly one that is toxic.

effuse (ĕ-fūs') [L. *ex*, out, + *fundere*, to pour]. Thin; widely spreading. Applied to a bacterial growth which forms a very delicate film over a surface.

effusion (ĕ-fū'zhŭn). Escape of fluid into a part, as the pleural cavity, such as pyothorax (pus), hydrothorax (serum), hemothorax (blood), chylothorax (lymph), pneumothorax (air), hydropneumothorax (serum and air), and pyopneumothorax (pus and air).

    e., pleural. Fluid in the pleural space.

egersis (ē-ger'sĭs) [Gr., a waking]. Extreme or abnormal wakefulness; extremely alert.

egesta (ē-jĕs'tā) [L. *e*, out of, + *gerere*, to bear]. Waste matter eliminated from the body, especially excrement.

egg [AS. *aeg*]. 1. The female sex cell or ovum, applied especially to a fertilized ovum which is passed from the body and develops outside, as in fowls. 2. The mammalian ovum.

    Food value of 100 gm. (two large chicken eggs, raw or hard-boiled): Cal. 163; protein 12.9 gm.; fat 11.5 gm.; carbohydrate 0.9 gm.; calcium 54 mg.; iron 2.3 mg.; vitamin A, 1180 I.U.

    e. albumen. The white of an e. SEE: *sac, yolk; vitellin; vitellus.*

ego (ē'go, ĕg'ō) [L. *ego*, I]. In psychoanalysis, one of the three major divisions in the model of the psychic apparatus. The others are id and superego. The ego possesses consciousness and memory and serves to mediate between the primitive instinctual or animal drives (the id), internal social prohibitions (the superego), and reality. Thus the ego allows one to adapt to what might otherwise be a very unpleasant situation. The psychiatric use of the term should not be confused with its common usage in the sense of "self-love" or "selfishness." SEE: *id; superego.*

    e. ideal. The unconscious perfection of an individual's pattern or standard of character, usually identified with one greatly admired.

    The social standards of the individual in contrast to his instinctive unsocial desires. While undoubtedly there is an inherent difference in the child's capacity to attain an e. ideal as definitely as to attain mature intelligence, much of its formulation depends upon teaching and example in the early years.

    Organic disease modifies its evolution, and even more definitely may effect its involution. The later experiences of life, each in turn, add some little modification. E. ideal constitutes one phase of "conflict." Overdevelopment or compensatory overemphasis may lead to manifestations desirable from neither the social nor personal viewpoints.

    e. instincts. All instincts not of a sexual nature.

    e. libido. Drive concentrated in and upon the e. and not manifested toward external objects. Manifested in narcissistic disorders.

    e. super-. SEE: *superego.*

egobronchophony (ē"gō-brŏn-kŏf'ō-nĭ) [Gr. *aix, aig-*, goat, + *bronkhos*, windpipe, + *phōnē*, voice]. A bleating sound with bronchophony. SEE: *egophony.*

egocentric (ē"gō-sĕn'trĭk) [L. *ego*, I, + *centrum*, center]. Pert. to a withdrawal from the external world with concentration upon inner self.

egomania (ē"gō-mā'nĭ-ă) ["+ Gr. *mania*, madness]. Abnormal self-esteem and self-interest.

egophony (ē-gŏf'o-nĭ) [Gr. *aix, aig-*, goat, + *phōnē*, voice]. A nasal sound somewhat like the bleat of a goat heard in auscultation of the chest when the subject speaks in a normal tone. Heard in pleural effusion.

egotropic (ē"go-trŏp'ĭk) [L. *ego*, I, + Gr. *tropos*, a turning]. Interested chiefly in oneself; self-centered.

Ehrenritter's ganglion (ār'ĕn-rĭt"ĕr). [Johann Ehrenritter, Austrian anatomist, — 1790] The superior ganglion of the glossopharyngeal nerve.

Ehrlich's side-chain theory (ār'lĭk). [Paul Ehrlich, Ger. bacteriologist, 1854-1915] So named because the protoplasmic cell is said to possess certain receptors or "side chains" which are capable of becoming fixed to certain protein groups with which they have a chemical affinity. This "fixation" is of value to the cell in that it enables it to attach the various food substances which it needs for nourishment. The molecules of a toxin, according to this theory, contain two groups for attachment to the cell.

    Haptophore Group: It becomes fixed to a suitable cell receptor. When this happens, the receptor detaches from the cell and floats off in the blood stream. The cell responds to this loss by producing more effectors, which are again liberated into the blood, where they combine with toxins and thereby render them inert, and so form free antitoxin.

Toxophore Group: Toxicity results when this becomes attached to certain receptors of the cell called toxophiles, and this union is prevented by rendering the haptophore group inert. SEE: *immunity.*

Ehrlich's theory of immunity. A theory which attempts to explain the formation of antitoxin in the blood. SYN: *E.'s side-chain theory,* q.v.

eidetic (ī-dĕt'ĭk) [Gr. *eidos,* form]. Relating to or having the ability of total visual recall of anything previously seen.

eidoptometry (ī-dŏp-tom'ē-trĭ) [Gr. *eidos,* form, + *optein,* to see, + *metron,* measure]. Determination of ability to visually perceive form.

eighth cranial nerve. Acoustic nerve, q.v.

eikonometry (ī"ko-nŏm'ē-trĭ) [Gr. *eikōn,* image, + *metron,* measure]. Determination of distance of an object by measuring the image produced by a lens of known focus.

eiloid (ī'loyd) [Gr. *eilein,* to coil, + *eidos,* appearance]. Having a coil-like structure.

Eimeria (ī-mē'rĭ-ă). A genus of sporozoan parasites belonging to the class Telosporidea, subclass Coccidia. They are intracellular parasites living in the epithelial cells of vertebrates and invertebrates. They rarely are parasitic to man.

   E. hominis. A species which has been found in empyema in man.

einsteinium (īn-stīn'ĭ-um). [Albert Einstein, German-born Amer. physicist, 1879-1955]. SYMB: *Es.* At. no. 99. A radioactive element.

eisodic (ī-sŏd'ĭk) [Gr. *eis,* into, + *hodos,* way]. Centripetal or afferent, as nerve fibers of a reflex arc.

ejaculatio (ē-jăk"ū-la'shĭ-o) [L.]. Sudden expelling, as of semen.

   e. precox. Premature ejaculation. Inability to prevent ejaculation of semen at the beginning of copulation, or prior to it.

ejaculation (ē-jăk"ū-lā'shŭn) [L. *ejaculāri,* to throw out]. Ejection of the seminal fluids from the male urethra.

   e., mechanism of. E. consists of two phases: (1) the passage of semen and the secretions of the accessory organs (bulbourethral and prostate glands and seminal vesicles) into the urethra and (2) the expulsion of the seminal fluid from the urethra. The former is brought about by contraction of the smooth muscle of the ductus deferens and the increased secretory activity of the glands; the latter by the rhythmical contractions of the bulbocavernosus and ischiocavernosus muscles and the levator ani.

The prostate discharges its secretions before those of the seminal vesicle. The sensations associated with e. constitute the male orgasm.

E. is a reflex phenomenon. Afferent impulses arising principally from stimulation of the glans penis pass to the spinal cord by way of the internal pudendal nerves. Efferent impulses arising from a reflex center located in the upper lumbar region of the cord pass through sympathetic fibers in the hypogastric nerves and plexus to the ductus deferens and seminal vesicles. Other impulses arising from the 3rd and 4th sacral segments pass through the internal pudendal nerves to the ischiocavernous and bulbocavernous muscles.

Erection of the penis usually precedes e. E. occurs normally during copulation or it may occur as a nocturnal emission. The seminal fluid normally contains 60 to 150 million sperm/ml. The volume of the ejaculation is from two to five ml. SEE: *semen.*

   RS: coitus; excitation; orgasm; semen.

ejac'ulatory. Pert. to ejaculation.

   e. duct. The terminal portion of the seminal duct formed by the union of the ductus deferens and the excretory duct of the seminal vesicle.

ejecta (ē-jĕk'tă) [L. *ejectus,* thrown out, ejected]. Material, esp. waste material, excreted by the body. SYN: *dejecta; egesta.*

EKG. Abbr. for *electrocardiogram.* Also ECG.

ekphorize (ĕk'fō-rīz) [Gr. *ek-,* out, + *phorein,* to bear]. In psychiatry, a bringing back of the effect of a psychic experience in an attempt to experience it again in memory. SEE: *engram.*

elaiopathy (ē"lā-ŏp'ă-thī) [Gr. *elaion,* oil, + *pathos,* disease]. Swelling of joints due to contusion, followed by fatty deposits. SYN: *eleopathy.*

elastic (e-lăs'tĭk) [Gr. *elastikos,* elastic]. Capable of being stretched and returning to its original state; having elasticity.

   e. bandage. Bandage which can be stretched.

   e. cartilage. Yellow cartilage such as is found in the epiglottis, pharynx, external ears, and auditory tube.

   e. lamina. Descemet's membrane.

   e. skin. Rare condition in which there is unusual elastic state of the skin.

   e. stocking. One worn to place pressure on surface of the foot, or portion of the leg.

   e. tissue. Connective tissue supplied with elastic fibers as found in the middle coat of arteries.

elasticity (e-lăs-tĭs'ĭ-tĭ). The quality of returning to original size and shape after compression or stretching.

elastin (e-lăs'tĭn). 1. An albuminoid substance forming the principal constituent of yellow elastic tissue, comprising about 30% of this tissue. 2. A protein which can be prepared from various connective tissues.

elastinase (e-lăs'tĭn-ās) [Gr. *elastikos*, elastic]. An enzyme that dissolves elastin.

elastoid (e-lăs'toyd) ["+ *eidos*, form]. Pert. to a substance formed by hyaline degeneration.

elasto'ma ["+ *-ōma*, tumor]. A chronic disease of the skin; pseudoxanthoma.

elastomer ["+ *meros*, a part]. A polymeric substance which has elastic properties similar to rubber.

elastometer (e"las-tōm'ē-ter) [Gr. *elastikos*, elastic, + *metron*, measure]. Device for measuring elasticity.

elastom'etry. The measurement of elasticity of tissues.

elastose (e-lăs'tōs). A peptone resulting from gastric digestion of elastin.

elation (e-lā'shŭn) [L. *elatus*, borne out of]. Joyful emotion. It is of pathological origin when out of accord with patient's actual circumstances.

elbow (ĕl'bō) [AS. *eln*, forearm, + *boga*, bend]. Joint of arm and forearm.
RS: anconad; anconeus; anconitis; tennis elbow.

e. jerk. Involuntary bending of elbow caused by striking tendon of biceps or triceps muscle.

e. joint. Joint between arm and the forearm. Includes the humeroulnar, humeroradial, and proximal radioulnar articulations.

e. reflex. Sharp extension of forearm resulting from tapping of triceps tendon while arm is held loosely in bent position.

elective surgery, elective therapy. A treatment or surgical procedure not requiring immediate attention and therefore planned for the patient's convenience.

Electra complex. [Gr. *Elektra*, Agamemnon's daughter, who helped assassinate her mother because of love for her father, whom the former had slain.] In psychoanalysis, a group of symptoms due to suppressed sexual love of daughter for father. SEE: *Oedipus complex.*

elec'tric [Gr. *ēlektron*, amber]. Pert. to, caused by, or resembling electricity.

e. baker. Device for placing intense heat on a part, as in arthritis. SEE: *baker.*

e. contacts and injuries. Injuries from electricity vary with type and strength of current, length of contact, location of con-

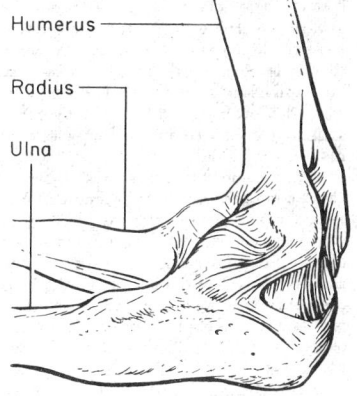

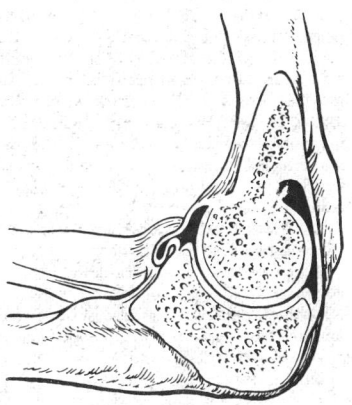

ELBOW JOINT
Above, medial side; Below, cross section through humeroulnar joint.

tact such as legs, arms, etc.; and hence vary from trivial burns to complete charring; or unconsciousness from either paralysis of the respiratory center, fibrillation of the heart, or both.

Direct currents of less than 300 volts are seldom fatal, but alternating currents of 15 to 60 cycles may be fatal, even when below 100 volts. Ordinary household or office currents vary from 30 to 220 volts.

Insulation: Protection against such currents may be made with dry nonconductors such as folded newspapers, magazines, cardboard, wood, rubber, clothing, etc. These may be used to move patient from the contact or to remove wire from patient. It is always preferable to turn off the current if possible. If patient is in water, remember that it is electrically charged and special precautions must be taken. On a humid or rainy day ordinary insulators may contain sufficient moisture to conduct electricity. Make sure insulators are dry.

High tension currents, such as those used about x-ray equipment or in conducting currents for long distances or for special industrial locations cannot be insulated by such means. Such currents may jump through rubber, paper, or strips of wood. A safe procedure is to ascertain the source of current and have it shut off, otherwise multiple tragedies result. TREATMENT: SEE: *electric shock.*

e. shock. SYM: Burns, with loss of consciousness; contact or proximity to source of current are principal symptoms.

F. A. TREATMENT: Carefully free victim from source of current with nonconductors such as dry wood, paper, rubber, etc., or shut off current. Prolonged artificial respiration may be necessary. SEE: *resuscitation; shock.*

electric'ity. A form of energy which exhibits magnetic, chemical, mechanical, and thermal effects. Composed of two parts: positive which is protons and negative which is electrons.

e., frictional. Generation of static e. by rubbing two articles together.

e., galvanic. E. generated by chemical action.

e., induced. E. generated in a body from another body close by, without contact.

e., magnetic. E. induced by means of a magnetic device.

e., negative. Electric charge caused by an excess of electrons negatively charged.

e., positive. Electric charge caused by loss of negative electrons.

e., static. E. generated by friction of certain materials.

e., unit of. SEE: *ampere; coulomb; farad; ohm; volt.*

elec'trify [Gr. *ēlektron,* amber, + L. *facere,* to make]. To charge a body with electricity.

electriza'tion. The act of charging or treating by use of electricity.

electro-, electr- [Gr. *ēlektron,* amber]. Prefix indicating relationship to electricity.

electroanalgesia ["+ *analgesia,* want of feeling]. Producing relief from pain by using low intensity electrical currents applied locally or through implanted electrodes.

electroanesthesia (e-lĕk″trō-ăn″ĕs-thē′zĭ-ă) ["+ *an,* not, + *aisthēsis,* sensation]. 1. Local anesthesia induced by an anesthetiz-

ing substance injected into tissues by electricity. 2. General anesthesia produced by a device which passes electricity of a certain frequency, amplitude, and wave form through the brain. Has been used experimentally in both the U.S.S.R. and U.S.A.

electrobiol'ogy ["+ *bios,* life, + *logos,* study of]. Science of electric phenomena in the living body.

electrobios'copy ["+ "+ *skopein,* to examine]. Electric test to determine if life is present.

electrocardiogram (e-lĕk″trō-kăr′dĭ-o-grăm″) ["+ *kardia,* heart, + *gramma,* writing]. A record of the electrical activity of the heart; shows certain waves called P, Q, R, S, and T waves. Sometimes a U wave is seen. The first or P wave is caused by contraction of the atria. During this time the heart muscle is electrically polarized and then depolarized. The Q, R, S, and T waves are related to contraction of the ventricles. The cause of the U wave is unknown. The electrocardiogram gives important information concerning the spread of excitation to the different chambers of the heart and it is of value in the diagnosis of cases of abnormal cardiac rhythm and myocardial damage. ABBR: ECG; EKG.

electrocardiograph (e-lĕk″trō-kăr′dĭ-o-grăf) ["+ "+ *graphein,* to write]. Device for recording electrical variations in action of heart muscles.

electrocardiog'raphy. The making and study of graphic records (electrocardiograms) produced by electrical currents originating in the heart.

electrocardiophonograph (e-lĕk″trō-kăr″dĭ-o-fō′no-grăf) [Gr. *ēlektron,* amber, + *kardia,* heart, + *phōnē,* sound, + *graphein,* to write]. Device for recording heart sounds.

electrocatalysis (e-lĕk″trō-kă-tăl′ĭ-sĭs) ["+ *kata,* down, + *lysis,* loosening]. Chemical decomposition produced by electricity.

electrocautery (e-lĕk″trō-kaw′tĕr-ĭ) ["+ *kautērion,* branding iron]. Cauterization by means of an apparatus consisting of a holder containing a wire, which may be heated to a red or white heat by a current of electricity, either direct or alternating.

electrochem'istry ["+ *chēmeia,* chemistry]. Science of chemical changes produced by electricity.

electrochem'y. Therapy concerned with physical applications, such as electricity, which produce chemical effects in the tissues.

electrocision (e-lĕk″trō-sĭzh′ŭn) [Gr. *ēlektron,* amber, + L. *caedare,* to cut]. Excision by electric current.

electrocoagulation (e-lĕk″trō-kō-ăg″ū-lā′shŭn) [″ + L. *coagulare*, to thicken]. Coagulation of tissue by means of a high frequency electric current. The heat producing the coagulation is generated within the tissue to be destroyed.

electrocontractility (e-lĕk″tro-kŏn-trăk-tĭl′ĭ-tĭ) [″ + L. *contrahere*, to contract]. Contraction of muscular tissue by electrical stimulation.

electrocryptectomy (e-lĕk″tro-krĭp-tĕk′tō-mĭ) [″ + *kryptos*, concealed, + *ektomē*, excision]. Destruction of tonsillar crypts by diathermy.

electrocu′tion [Gr. *ēlektron*, amber, + *execute*]. The destruction of life by means of electric current.

electrocystoscopy (e-lĕk″tro-sĭs-tŏs′kō-pĭ) [″ + *kystis*, bladder, + *skopein*, to examine]. The use of electric light to see the interior of the bladder.

electrode (e-lĕk′trōd) [″ + *hodos*, way]. A medium intervening between an electric conductor and the object to which the current is to be applied. In electrotherapy an e. is an instrument with a point or a surface from which to discharge current to the body of a patient.

    e., brush. A wire brush used to apply electricity to a part of the body.

    e., depolarizing. E. with greater resistance than the part of the body in the circuit.

    e., disper′sive. When e.'s may be applied in pairs dissimilar in size and shape, then the smaller e. is called the active, and the larger, the dispersive, indifferent, or inactive e.

    e., hydrogen. Form absorbing hydrogen gas.

    e., indifferent. SEE: *e., dispersive.*

    e., multiple point. Several sets of terminals providing for the use of several electrodes. SEE: *multiterminal.*

    e., negative. Cathode.

    e., point. An e. with an insulating handle at one end and a metallic point at the other for use in applying static sparks.

    e., positive. Anode.

    e., spark ball or point. An insulating handle having on one end a metallic ball or point. Used in giving static sparks.

    e., therapeutic. E. for introduction of medicines through the skin by ionization. SEE: *iondophoresis.*

electrodesiccation (e-lĕk″trō-dĕs″ĭ-kā′shŭn) [Gr. *ēlektron*, amber, + L. *desiccāre*, to dry up]. The destructive drying of cells and tissue by means of short high-frequency electric sparks, in contradistinction to fulguration, which is the destruction of

tissue by means of long high-frequency electric sparks.

electrodiagnosis. Use of electric and electronic devices for diagnostic purposes. Their use is helpful in almost all branches of medicine, but particularly in investigating function of nerves and muscles.

electrodialysis(e-lĕk″trō-dī-ăl′ĭ-sĭs)[″ + *dia-*, apart, + *lysis*, dissolving]. (pl. *-ses*) A method of separating electrolytes from colloids by passing a current through a solution containing both.

electrodynamometer (e-lĕk″trō-dī″nă-mŏm′ĕ-tĕr) [″ + *dynamis*, power, + *metron*, measure]. An instrument to measure the strength of an electric current.

electroencephalogram (ē-lĕk″trō-ĕn-sĕf′ă-lō-grăm) [Gr. *ēlektron*, amber, + *enkephalos*, in the head, brain, + *gramma*, a writing]. A tracing on an electroencephalograph. ABBR: EEG.

electroencephalograph (e-lĕk-trō-ĕn-sĕf′ă-lō-grăf) [″ + ″ + *graphein*, to write]. An instrument for recording electrical activity of the brain. SEE: *electroencephalography.*

electroencephalography. Amplification, recording, and analysis of the electrical activity of the brain. The record obtained is called an electroencephalogram (EEG).

    Electrodes are placed on the scalp in various locations. The difference between the electrical potential of two sites is recorded. The potential between a pair at a time or between many pairs can be obtained simultaneously. The most frequently seen pattern in the normal adult under resting conditions is the alpha rhythm of 8 1/2-12/seconds. A characteristic change in the wave occurs during sleep, upon opening the eyes, and during mental attention.

    Some persons who have intracranial disease will have a normal EEG and others with no otherwise demonstrable disease will have an abnormal EEG. Nevertheless the use of this diagnostic technique has proven to be very helpful in studying epilepsy and convulsive disorders and in localizing lesions in the cerebrum. SEE: *rhythm, alpha; rhythm, beta.*

electrohemostasis (e-lĕk″tro-hē-mŏs′tă-sĭs) [″ + *haima*, blood, + *stasis*, standstill]. The arrest of bleeding by means of a high-frequency current.

electrol′ogy [″ + *logos*, science]. The branch of science that deals with the phenomena and properties of electricity.

electrolysis (e′lĕk-trŏl′ĭ-sĭs) [″ + *lysis*, dissolution]. The decomposition of a substance by passage of an electrical current through it.

Hair follicles may be destroyed by use of this method.

electrolyte (e-lĕk'trō-līt) ["+ *lytos*, soluble]. 1. A solution which is a conductor of electricity. 2. A substance which, in solution, conducts an electric current and is decomposed by the passage of an electric current.

Acids, bases, and salts are common electrolytes.

   e., amphoteric. One which produces both hydrogen (H+) and hydroxyl (OH−) ions.

electrolytic (e-lĕk''trō-lĭt'ĭk). Caused by or rel. to electrolysis.

   e. conduction. In metals the electrical charges are carried by the electrons of inappreciable mass.

   In solutions the electrical charges are carried by e. ions, each one of a mass several thousand times as great as the electron. When a direct current passes through an e. solution between metallic electrodes immersed in it, the positive ions move to the cathode, the negative ions to the anode.

electromag'net [Gr. *ēlektron*, amber, + *magnēs*, magnet]. A magnet consisting of a length of insulated wire wound around soft iron core.

electromagnet'ic. Pert. to an electromagnet.

   e. induc'tion. Generation of an electromotive force in an insulated conductor moving in an electromagnetic field, or in a fixed conductor in a moving magnetic field.

electromag'netism. Magnetism produced by an electrical current.

electromassage [Gr. *ēlektron*, amber, + Fr. *masser*, to massage]. Massage combined with electrical treatment.

electrom'eter ["+ *metron*, measure]. An instrument for measuring differences in electric potential.

electromo'tive ["+ L. *motor*, mover]. Pert. to passage of electricity in a current, or motion produced by it.

   e. force. That effect of differences of potential which, on the closing of a circuit, causes a flow of electricity from one place to another, giving rise to an electric current. The strength of an electric current is directly proportional to the impressed electromotive force, and inversely proportional to the resistance in the case of direct current and to the impedance in the case of alternating current. Electromotive force is measured in volts or in some convenient multiple or fraction of a volt. Microvolt, millivolt and kilovolt are, respectively, one-millionth volt, one-thousandth volt and 1000 volts. ABBR: EMF.

electromyogram (e-lĕk''trō-mī'o-grăm) ["+ *mys*, muscle, + *gramma*, writing]. A graphic record of the contraction of a muscle as a result of electrical stimulation.

electromyography (e-lĕk''tro-mī-ŏg'rā-fĭ) ["+ "+ *graphein*, to write]. The preparation, study of, and interpretation of electromyograms.

elec'tron [Gr. *ēlektron*, amber]. An extremely minute corpuscle or charge of negative electricity which revolves about the central core or nucleus of an atom. They are the smallest known particles that exist, their mass being 1/1838 that of a hydrogen atom. When emitted from radioactive substances, they are known as beta particles or rays.

electronarcosis (e-lĕk''trō-năr-kō'sĭs). The induction of narcosis or unconsciousness by the application of electricity to the brain. Used in the treatment of schizophrenia.

electro''neg'ative [Gr. *ēlektron*, amber, + L. *negāre*, to deny]. Condition of being charged with negative electricity which results in the attraction of bodies positively charged and the repulsion of bodies negatively charged.

electron'ic. Pert. to electrons.

electroniza'tion [Gr. *ēlektron*, amber]. The use of radiation to restore electrical equilibrium to diseased cells.

electropathology (e-lĕk''trō-pā-thŏl'ō-gĭ) ["+ *pathos*, suffering, + *logos*, study of]. Determining electrical reaction of muscles and nerves as means of diagnosis.

electrophoresis (e-lĕk''trō-fōr-ē'sĭs) ["+ *phorēsis*, bearing, transmission]. The movement of charged colloidal particles through the medium in which they are dispersed as a result of changes in electrical potential. Electrophoretic methods are useful in the analysis of protein mixtures as protein particles move with different velocities dependent principally on the number of charges carried by the particle. SEE: *phoresis*.

   RS: diathermy; iontophoresis.

electrophorus (ē-lĕk''trŏf'ō-rŭs) ["+ *phorein*, to bear]. An instrument for obtaining static electricity by means of induction. SYN: *electrophore*.

electrophototherapy (e-lĕk''trō-fō''tother'ă-pī) ["+ *phōs*, light, + *therapeia*, treatment]. Treatment by means of electric light.

electrophrenic (e-lĕk''tro-frĕn'ĭk). Pert. to stimulation of the phrenic nerve by electricity.

electrophysiology (e-lĕk''tro-fĭz''ĭ-ŏl'ō-gĭ) ["+ *physis*, nature, + *logos*, study of]. A branch of physiology which deals with the relations of body functions to electrical phenomena such as the effects of electrical stimulation upon the tissues, the production of electrical currents by organs and tissues, and the therapeutic use of electric currents.

electropos'itive [Gr. *ēlektron*, amber, + L. *positivus*, emphatic]. The condition of being subject to repulsion by bodies positively electrified, and to attraction by bodies negatively electrified.

elec'tropuncture ["+ L. *punctura*, a piercing]. Piercing tissues with an electric needle.

electropyrexia (e-lĕk"trō-pī-rĕks'ĭ-ă) ["+ *pyressein*, to be feverish]. Elevation of temperature by electricity.

electroradiometer (e-lĕk"trō-rā-dī-ŏm'ĕ-tĕr) ["+ L. *radius*, ray, + Gr. *metron*, measure]. An electroscope for differentiation of radiant energy.

electroretinogram (e-lĕk"tro-rĕt'ĭ-no-grăm). A record of the action currents of the retina produced by visual or light stimuli.

electroscission (e-lĕk'tro-sĭ'zhun) [Gr. *ēlektron*, amber, + L. *scindere*, to cut]. Division of tissues by electrocautery.

electroscope (e-lĕk'trō-skōp) ["+ *skopein*, to see]. An instrument which detects positive or negative static electricity.

elec'troshock. Shock produced by an electric current.

    e. therapy. The induction of convulsive seizures by the passing of an electric current through the brain. Used in the treatment of certain types of psychoses.

electrosleep. Sleep production as a result of the passage of mild electrical impulses through parts of the brain. Has been used experimentally in treating insomnia and mental illness.

electrostat'ic [Gr. *ēlektron*, amber, + *statikos*, causing to stand]. Pert. to static electricity.

    e. generator. A device that generates static electricity.

    e. unit. Any unit of electrical measurement based on the attraction or repulsion of a static charge, as distinguished from an electromagnetic unit, which is defined in terms of the attraction or repulsion of magnetic poles.

electrosurgery (e-lĕk"tro-sūr'jē-rĭ) ["+ *kheir*, hand, + *ergon*, work]. Surgery accomplished by means of an electrical knife.

electrotaxis (e-lĕk"trō-tăk'sĭs) ["+ *taxis*, arrangement]. The movement of a cell or an organism toward or away from an electrical stimulus.

electrothanasia (e-lĕk"tro-thă-nā'zĭ-ă) ["+ *thanatos*, death]. Death resulting from elec-

electrotherapeutics (e-lĕk"trō-thĕr-ă-pū'tĭks) ["+ *therapeutikē*, treatment]. The use of electricity in the treatment of disease.

electrotherapist (e-lĕk"trō-thĕr'ă-pĭst) [Gr. *ēlektron*, amber, + *therapeia*, treatment]. A physician who has had special training in and has acquired skill in the therapeutic use of electricity. The term is sometimes used incorrectly to designate anyone who administers electrical treatments.

elec"trother'apy. Use of electricity in treating disease. SYN: *electrotherapeutics*.

elec'trotherm [Gr. *ēlektron*, amber, + *thermē*, heat]. An electrical apparatus for the therapeutic application of heat to the surface of the body. Used for relief of pain.

electrothermotherapy (e-lĕk"trō-thĕr"mo-thĕr'a-pĭ) ["+ "+ *therapeia*, treatment]. The production of heat within the living tissues for therapeutic purposes by means of bodily resistance to the passing of an electric current.

electrotome (e-lĕk'trō-tōm) ["+ *tomē*, a cut]. An electrocautery device used for surgical procedures.

electroton'ic ["+ *tonos*, tension]. Of or pert. to electrotonus.

electrotonus (e-lĕk-trŏt'ŏ-nŭs). The change in the irritability of a nerve or muscle during the passage of an electric current.

electrotropism (e-lĕk-trŏt'ro-pĭzm) [Gr. *ēlektron*, amber, + *tropē*, a turning, + *ismos*, condition of]. Reaction of cells to an electrical current.

electuary (e-lĕk'tū-ă-rĭ) [Gr. *ekleikhein*, to lick up]. Medicinal substance mixed with honey or sugar to form a paste suitable for oral consumption.

eleidin (ē-lē'ĭ-din) [Gr. *elaion*, oil]. An acidophil substance present in the stratum lucidum of the epidermis.

el'ement [L. *elementum*, a rudiment]. In modern chemistry, a substance which cannot be separated into substances different from itself by ordinary chemical processes. They exist in a free and in a combined state. More than 100 have been identified. SEE: *Table of Chemical Elements* in *Appendix*.

    Some of the e.'s found in the human body are: oxygen; silicon; aluminum; carbon; cobalt; hydrogen; nitrogen; calcium; phosphorus; potassium; sulfur; sodium; chlorine; magnesium; iron; fluorine; iodine; copper; manganese; and zinc.

    e.'s, trace. Chemical e.'s, extremely small amounts of which are present in the body or in the diet. Some are necessary in metabolism.

Elements Having Medicinal Uses

Element	Compound Form	Some Medicinal Uses
Aluminum (Al)	Alum	Astringent to contract mucous membranes; as a gargle and a douche
	Aluminum acetate	Astringent and antiseptic in surgical dressings
	Aluminum hydroxide	Antacids for gastric hyperchlorhydria
	Aluminum phosphate	
Barium (Ba)	Barium sulfate	Coats the stomach and intestines for taking x-ray pictures
Bismuth (Bi)	Bismuth subnitrate	Insoluble compounds used as dusting powders on the skin
	Bismuth subcarbonate	Astringent, antacid, and coating in diarrhea and gastroenteritis
Calcium (Ca)	Calcium carbonate (chalk)	Antacid
	Calcium chloride Calcium gluconate Calcium phosphate	Electrolyte replacement
	Calcium hydroxide (lime water)	Antacid; calcium replacement; antidote in acid poisonings
Chlorine (Cl)	Sodium chloride	Common salt
	Chlorinated lime	Disinfectant for urinals and excreta; a deodorant
Copper (Cu)	Copper sulfate (blue vitriol)	Removes granulations on the eyelids in trachoma; produces vomiting; used as an astringent
Hydrogen (H)	Hydrogen peroxide	Antiseptic
Iodine (I)	Potassium Iodide	Expectorant
Iron (Fe)	Ferrous salts	Hematinic in treatment of anemia; astringent
Magnesium (Mg)	Magnesium carbonate	Antacid
	Magnesium hydroxide suspension (milk of magnesia)	Antacid and laxative
	Magnesium oxide	Antacid
	Magnesium silicate, hydrous (talc)	Dusting powder
	Magnesium sulfate (Epsom salt)	Cathartic; local anti-inflammatory agent
	Magnesium trisilicate	Antacid
Nitrogen (N)	Nitrous oxide (laughing gas)	General anesthetic
	Ammonia water	Cleanser; reflex stimulant by inhalation

Elements Having Medicinal Uses (*Continued*)

Element	Compound Form	Some Medicinal Uses
Oxygen (O)		Used in resuscitation in anoxemia and in determination of basal metabolic rate
Phosphorus (P)	Sodium phosphate	Saline purgative
Potassium (K)	Potassium acetate	Diuretic
	Potassium bicarbonate	Electrolyte replacement
	Potassium chloride	Electrolyte replacement
	Potassium iodide	Expectorant; also source of iodine
	Potassium permanganate	In solution, as a topical anti-infective agent in various skin affections, or for gastric lavage in certain poisonings
	Potassium sodium tartrate (Rochelle salts)	Mild cathartic
Radium (Ra)	Radium salts	Treatment of neoplasms
Silver (Ag)	Silver nitrate	In dilute form, as prophylactic for ophthalmia neonatorum (gonococcal conjunctivitis of the newborn); to cauterize; for nose an throat inflammations
Sodium (Na)	Sodium bicarbonate (baking soda)	In intravenous fluids for electrolyte replacement
Sulfur (S)		Used in ointments for skin diseases; may be used as a laxative
Zinc (Zn)	Zinc oxide	Astringent and protective for skin conditions
	Zinc peroxide	Anti-infective and deodorant for skin diseases
	Zinc stearate	Dusting powder (irritating if inhaled)
	Zinc sulfate	In dilute solution, as an ophthalmic astringent

element, words pert. to: atom; body; chemical e.; mineral e.; monad; name of each element; oxidation; oxide; radical.

eleoma (el″e-ō′mă) [Gr. *elaion*, oil, + *ōma*, tumor]. A swelling in tissue produced by the injection of oil.

eleometer (el″e-ŏm′ĕ-tĕr) [″ + *metron*, measure]. Instrument for determining quality and specific gravity of oils.

eleomyenchysis (el″e-o-mī-en′kĭs-ĭs) [″ + *mys*, muscle, + *enchysis*, infusion]. 1. The intramuscular injection of oils for chronic local spasms. 2. Prosthesis, q.v., by paraffin injection.

eleopathy (el″e-op′ă-thĭ) [Gr. *elaion*, oil, + *pathos*, disease]. Swelling of joints due to fatty deposits. SYN: *elaiopathy*.

eleoptene (el-e-op′tēn) [″ + *ptēnos*, fleeting]. The fluid part of a volatile oil.

eleosaccharum (el″e-o-sak′ă-rum) [″ + *sakcharon*, sugar]. A mixture of powdered sugar with a volatile oil.

eleotherapy (el″e-o-thĕr′ă-pĭ) [Gr. *elaion*, oil, + *therapeia*, treatment]. The use of oil for therapeutic purposes.

eleotho′rax [″ + *thōrax*, chest]. The injection of oil into the pleural cavity to compress a tuberculous lung.

elephantiasis (ĕl″ĕ-făn-tī′ăsĭs) [Gr. *elephas*, elephant]. A chronic condition characterized by pronounced hypertrophy of the skin and subcutaneous tissues resulting from obstruction of the lymphatic vessels. The lower extremities and the scrotum are parts most frequently involved.

ETIOL: E. may be congenital (Milroy's disease), or the result of metastatic invasion of the lymph nodes by tumor cells; inflammatory e. results from filariasis or local infection of the lymph nodes. E. is most common in tropical countries and is caused by infestation by Wuchereria bancrofti, a filarial worm.

e. arabum. SYN: *elephantiasis.*

e. graecorum. Leprosy.

e. telangiectodes. E. which affects only a limited area of skin.

el'evator [L. *elevāre,* to lift]. 1. Curved retractor for holding lid away from the globe of the eye. 2. One for raising depressed bones by levers or screws.

eleventh cranial nerve. Accessory nerve, q.v.

eliminant (e-lĭm′ĭ-nănt) [L. *e,* out, + *līmen,* threshold]. 1. Effecting evacuation. 2. Agent aiding in elimination.

eliminate (e-lĭm′ĭ-nāte). To expel; to rid the body of waste material.

elimina′tion. Excretion of waste body products by the skin, kidneys, and intestines.

e. diet. Based on patient's history of food sensitiveness and results of skin tests. The "elimination diet" found to relieve the patient's symptoms is increased by gradual addition of foods to which patient has been found to be nonsensitive, until insofar as possible all the essentials of an adequate diet are included.

elimination, words pert. to: constipation; defecation; dejecta; ejecta; evacuate; feces; names of excretions.

elinguation (e′′lin-gwā′shun) [L. *e,* out, + *lingua,* tongue]. The operation of removing the tongue from the oral cavity.

elixir [Arabic *al-iksir,* philosopher's stone]. A sweetened, aromatic, hydro-alcoholic liquid used in the compounding of oral medicines. Elixirs constitute one of the most commonly used types of medicinal preparation taken orally in a liquid form.

El'liott treatment. [Charles R. Elliott, Amer. gynecologist]. Treatment given by means of rubber bag that distends vagina when attached to machine delivering water at temperature of 115° to 128° F. maintained for 45 to 60 minutes; used in pelvic inflammatory disease.

Ellis-Van Creveld syndrome. SEE: *dysplasia.*

elutriation (e-lū-trĭ-ā′shŭn) [L. *elutriāre,* to cleanse]. The separation of insoluble particles from finer ones by decanting the fluid.

elytritis (ĕl′′ĭ-trī′tis) [Gr. *elytron,* sheath (vagina), + *itis,* inflammation]. Inflammation of the vagina. SYN: *colpitis.*

elytrocele (ĕl′ĭ-tro-sēl) ["+ *kēlē,* hernia]. Hernia into the vagina. SYN: *colpocele.*

elytroclasia (ĕl′′ĭ-tro-kla′sĭ-a) ["+ *klasis,* rupture]. Rupture of the vagina.

elytrocleisis (ĕl′′ĭ-tro-kli′sis) [Gr. *elytron,* sheath (vagina), + *kleisis,* closure]. Surgical closure of the vagina. SYN: *colpocleisis.*

elytroplasty (ĕl′ĭ-tro-plas′′tĭ) ["+ *plassein,* to form]. Plastic operation upon the vagina. SYN: *colpoplasty.*

elytroptosis (ĕl′′ĭ-trŏ-tō′sĭs) ["+ *ptōsis,* a dropping]. Prolapse of the vagina. SYN: *colpoptosis.*

elytrorrhaphy (ĕl-ĭ-tror′rä-fĭ) [Gr. *elytron,* sheath (vagina), + *raphē,* suture]. Suture of vaginal wall. SYN: *colporrhaphy.*

elytrostenosis (ĕl′′ĭ-tro-sten-ō′sĭs) ["+ *stenōsis,* narrowing]. Narrowing of the vagina. SYN: *colpostenosis.*

elytrotomy (ĕl-ĭ-trot′ō-mĭ) ["+ *tomē,* incision]. Incision into vaginal wall. SYN: *colpotomy.*

emaciate (e-mā′sĭ-āt) [L. *ēmaciāre,* to grow thin]. To cause to become excessively lean.

ema′ciated. Excessively lean.

emacia′tion. State of being extremely lean.

ETIOL: Malnutrition; diseases of gastrointestinal canal. If rapid: Marasmus, Addison's d., tuberculosis, cancer, diabetes, suppuration, hyperthyroidism, chronic diarrhea, stricture of esophagus, pyloric obstruction; parasites; loss of sleep, exophthalmic goiter, starvation. SEE: *lean; tabes; wasting.*

emaculation (em-ak′′ū-lā′shŭn) [L. *ēmaculāre,* to remove spots]. Removal of spots from the skin.

emailloid (e-ma′loyd) [Fr. *émail,* enamel, + Gr. *eidos,* form]. Tumor having its origin in tooth enamel.

emana′tion [L. *e,* out, + *manāre,* to flow]. 1. Something given off; radiation; emission. 2. A gaseous product of radioactive disintegration.

e., actinium. One given off by actinium. SYN: *actinon.*

e., radium. A radioactive gas given off by radium. SYN: *niton.*

e., thorium. One given off by thorium. SYN: *thoron.*

emansio mensium (em-an′sĭ-o men′sĭ-um) [L. Absence of the menses]. Amenorrhea in which menstruation has never occurred.

emasculation (e-măs-kū-lā'shŭn) [L. *ēmasculāre*, to castrate]. 1. Castration. 2. Excision of the entire male genitalia.

embalming (em-bahm'ing) [L. *im-*, put on, + *balsamum*, balsam]. Preservation of a dead body against putrefaction.

embed'ding [" + AS. *bedd*, to bed]. In histology, the process by which a piece of tissue is placed in a firm medium such as paraffin or celloidin in order to support it and keep it intact during the subsequent cutting into thin sections for microscopic examination.

embolalia (em″bo-la'lĭ-ă) [Gr. *embolos*, thrown in, + *lalia*, babble]. Meaningless language of the insane. SYN: *embolophrasia*.

embole (em'bo-lē) [Gr. a throwing in, insertion]. 1. Reduction of a dislocation. 2. Formation of the gastrula by invagination. SYN: *emboly*.

embol'ic. Pert. to or caused by embolism.

embol'iform [Gr. *embolos*, thrown in, inserted, + L. *forma*, form]. 1. Resembling a nucleus. 2. Wedge-shaped, as the nucleus emboliformis.

embolism (ĕm'bŏ-lĭzm) [Gr. *embolē*, a throwing in, + *ismos*, condition]. Obstruction of a blood vessel by foreign substances or a blood clot.

    RS: embolus, thrombosis, thrombus.

    Diagnosis depends upon the factors predisposing. Arteriosclerosis favors a diagnosis of thrombosis, while atrial fibrillation, bacterial endocarditis, or thrombophlebitis points to embolism. Embolism is usually due to blood clots.

    NP: Postoperative cases must be handled with great care. Sudden sitting up or turning over may displace an embolus into the circulation and cause sudden death. Fat embolism is not uncommon in bone injuries and fractures, and bacterial emboli may be present in so-called blood poisoning.

    e., air. One caused by air bubble. SEE: *air embolism.*

    e., fat. Globules of fat obstructing blood vessels.

    e., pulmonary. Obstruction of the pulmonary artery or one of its branches. Usually caused by an embolus from thrombosis in lower extremities.

    e., pyemic. E. caused by purulent matter.

embolophrasia (ĕm″bol-o-fra'zĭ-ă) [" + *phrasis*, utterance]. Meaningless speech. SYN: *embolalia.*

em'bolus [Gr. *embolos*, plug]. (pl. *emboli*) A mass of undissolved matter present in a blood or lymphatic vessel brought there by the blood or lymph current. Emboli may be solid, liquid, or gaseous. Other emboli may consist of bits of tissue, tumor cells, globules of fat, air bubbles, clumps of bacteria, and foreign bodies such as bullets. Emboli may arise within the body or they may gain entrance from without. Occlusion of vessels from emboli usually results in the development of infarcts, q.v. SEE: *thrombosis; thrombus.*

    e., air. An air bubble in the veins, the right atrium or ventricle, or in the capillaries. SEE: *air embolism.*

    e., coronary. May be complication of arteriosclerosis and cause angina pectoris. SYM: Similar to pulmonary e.

    e., pulmonary. E. in pulmonary artery or one of its branches.

em'boly [Gr. *embolē*, a throwing in]. Formation of the gastrula from invagination. SYN: *embole.*

embrace reflex (ĕm-brās') [L. *em-*, in, + *brachium*, arm]. A variety of defensive reflex. The throwing out of the arms in an attitude of embrace, in fearful response. SYN: *Moro's reflex.*

embrasure (ĕm-brā'zhŭr) [Fr. opening in wall for firing cannon]. An opening widening outwardly or inwardly.

    e., buccal. Opening spreading toward the buccal aspect.

    e., labial. E. opening toward the labial aspect.

    e., lingual. E. spreading to the lingual aspect.

    e., occlusal. Space mesially and distally between marginal ridges of approximating teeth.

embroca'tion [Gr. *embrochē*, moistening with lotion]. 1. Application of a liniment to the skin, esp. one that acts as a counterirritant to the skin. For example, turpentine; methyl salicylate. 2. A drug rubbed into the skin.

embryectomy (ĕm-brī-ĕk'tō-mĭ) [Gr. *embryon*, embryo, + *ektomē*, excision]. Removal of an extrauterine embryo.

embryo (ĕm'brĭ-ō) [Gr. *embryon*, from *en-*, in, + *bryein*, to grow]. 1. The young of any organism in an early stage of development. 2. Stage in prenatal development of a mammal between the ovum and the fetus. In humans, stage of development between the 2nd and 8th weeks, inclusive.

    Stages of Development: Following fertilization, cells multiply (cleavage) resulting in formation of a morula which develops into a blastocyst, consisting of a trophoblast and inner cell mass. Two cavities (amniotic cavity and yolk sac) arise within the inner cell mass. These are separated by the embryonic disk which gives rise to the three germ layers (ectoderm, mesoderm, and endoderm) which develop into the embryo proper; the blastocyst wall of trophoblast gives rise to auxiliary structures.

During the period of the embryo (2nd through 8th weeks) the germ layers of the embryonic disk give rise to the principal organ systems and the body acquires a somewhat human form. After the 2nd month, the developing young is called a fetus.

e., development of. (1) Period of the ovum (1st week): Blastocyst forms. Embryo enters uterus and implantation occurs. (2) Period of the embryo (2nd through 8th weeks): Embryo increases in length from about 1.5 mm. to 23 mm. Organ systems arise and embryo acquires human form. (3) Period of the fetus (3rd to 9th month).

The alimentary canal, liver, pancreas, and lungs develop from endoderm; muscle, all connective tissues, blood, lymphatic tissue and the epithelium of blood vessels, body cavities, kidney, gonads, and suprarenal cortex develop from mesoderm; the epidermis nervous tissue, hypophysis, and the epithelium of the organs, nasal cavity, mouth, salivary glands, bladder, and urethra develop from ectoderm.

embryocardia (ĕm-brĭ-ō-kăr'dĭ-ă) ["+ kardia, heart]. Heart action in which first and second sounds are equal, and resemble the fetal heart sounds. A sign of cardiac distress. SYN: *tic-tac rhythm.*

embryoctony (ĕm'brĭ-ok'tō-nĭ) ["+ kteinein, to kill]. Destroying the fetus in utero, as in cases where delivery is impossible, or for abortion. SEE: *craniotomy.*

embryogenet'ic, embryogen'ic [Gr. embryon, embryo, + gennan, to originate]. Pert. to or giving rise to an embryo.

embryogeny (ĕm-brĭ-ōj'ē-nĭ). The growth and development of an embryo.

embryog'raphy [Gr. embryon, embryo, + graphein, to write]. A treatise on the embryo.

embryol'ogy ["+ logos, study]. The science which deals with the origin and development of an individual organism.

embryoma (ĕm-brĭ-ō'mă) ["+ ōma, tumor]. A tumor consisting of derivatives of the embryonic germ layers but lacking in organization; a dermoid cyst.

em'bryonal. Pert. to or resembling an embryo.

embryonic (ĕm-brĭ-ŏn'ĭk) [Gr. embryon, embryo]. Pert. to or in condition of an embryo.

embryoniza'tion. Reversion of a cell or tissue to an embryonic structure.

embryonoid (em'brĭ-o-noyd) [Gr. embryo, embryo, + eidos, form]. Having the appearance of an embryo.

embryoplas'tic ["+ plassein, to form]. Having a part in the formation of an embryo; said of cells.

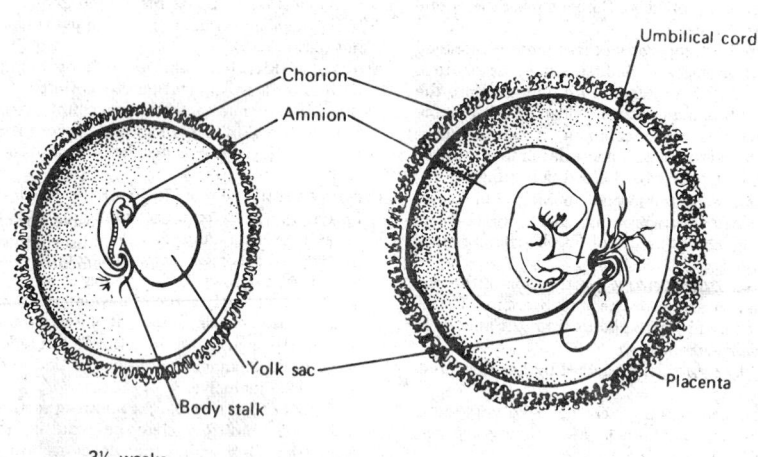

HUMAN EMBRYO
Left, at 3½ weeks; Right, at 5½ weeks.

embryotocia (ĕm″brĭ-ō-to′sĭ-ă) ["+ *tokos,* birth]. An abortion; delivery of an embryo.

embryotome (em′brĭ-o-tōm″) ["+ *tomē,* incision]. Instrument used in dismemberment of fetus in utero.

embryotomy (ĕm″brĭ-ŏt′ō-mĭ). The dissection of a fetus to aid its delivery.

embryotoxon (ĕm″brĭ-ō-tŏk′sŏn) ["+ *toxon,* bow]. Congenital marginal opacity of the cornea. SYN: *arcus juvenilis.*

embryotroph (ĕm′brĭ-ō-trŏf) ["+ *trophē,* nourishment]. A fluid resulting from the enzyme action of the trophoblasts upon the neighboring maternal tissue and which nourishes the embryo from the time of implantation into the uterus.

embryotrophy (ĕm″brĭ-ŏt′ro-fĭ). Nutrition of the fetus.

embryulcia (ĕm″brĭ-ul′sĭ-ă) [Gr. *embryon,* embryo, + *elkein,* to draw]. Forcible removal of the fetus by instruments, as in embryotomy.

embryulcus (ĕm″brĭ-ul′kŭs) [Gr. *embryoulkos*]. Instrument for extracting a dead fetus from the uterus.

emedullate (e-med′ū-lāt) [L. *e,* out, + *medulla,* marrow]. To remove the marrow from a bone.

emer′gency [L. *emergere,* to raise up]. An unexpected serious happening, demanding immediate action.

  e. light reflex. Marked pupillary contraction, frowning, and closure of eyelids, resulting from sudden powerful light stimulus of retina.

  e. theory. Formulated by Cannon: Adrenal secretion is stimulated by sympathetic nervous system activity to meet bodily emergencies, as emotional excitement, pain, etc.

emergency, words pert. to: asphyxia; asphyxiation; bites or stings; choking; convulsion; dislocation; drowning; fainting; fire emergencies; foreign bodies; fumes; gas; gases, war; poisoning; shock; sting; unconsciousness.

emer′gent [L. *emergere,* to raise up]. 1. Growing from a cavity or other part. 2. Sudden, unforeseen.

emesis (ĕm′ĕ-sĭs) [Gr. *emein,* to vomit]. Vomiting.

  May be of gastric, systemic, nervous, or reflex origin, or due to irritation of vomiting center.

  NP: The relation and timing of vomiting to eating is important, and the nurse should determine how it is affected by pain, by soft or solid foods, by liquids, by odors before or after eating or drinking. Note the type, character, and color of vomitus.

If patient is extremely weak, barely conscious, or comatose while vomiting, then great care must be exercised to prevent aspiration of food into the lungs. Elevate foot of bed and have suction apparatus available for removing vomitus from hypopharynx if necessary. Tracheotomy may be required. SEE: *antemetic; emetic; vomit; vomitus.*

  e., gastric. In gastric ulcer, gastric carcinoma, acute gastritis, chronic gastritis, hyperacidity and hypersecretion, Asiatic cholera, pressure upon stomach.

  e. gravidarum. Vomiting of pregnancy.

  e., irritation. Drugs, uremia, nephritis, some brain tumors, chloroform, ether.

  e., nervous. Tumor or abscess of brain, sea sickness, acute myelitis, meningitis, anemia and hyperemia of brain, concussion and contusion of brain, fracture of skull, Meniere's disease, migraine.

  e., reflex. Irritation of fauces and pharynx; coughing, removal of viscous secretion from nasopharynx, unpleasant odors and sights, shock, nervousness, anticipation, anxiety, hysteria, morning sickness, gastric crisis of tabes, hiccough.

  e., systemic. Pulmonary tuberculosis, whooping cough, peritonitis, irritations of bowels, acute obstruction of bowels, renal or biliary colic, Addison's disease.

emetic (e-mĕt′ĭk) [Gr. *emein,* to vomit]. Medicine that produces vomiting. Ex: *apomorphine; a. hydrochloride; ipecac; mustard; sodium chloride.*

  e., direct. Those acting by their presence in the stomach, e.g., mustard.

  e., indirect. Those acting on vomiting center of brain, as apomorphine.

  Procedure to Induce Vomiting: Dilute contents of stomach before giving any e. E.'s may be dangerous because of their own toxic effect, as in severe cardiovascular diseases, tuberculosis, advanced pregnancy, hernia, ulcers of the stomach, or corrosive poisoning. For these reasons the indiscriminate use of chemical e.'s is contraindicated.

  Vomiting may be induced by drinking generous amounts of warm water, preferably warm soapy water and by stimulating the uvula or posterior pharynx. Gastric lavage is preferable to emetics in poisoning. E.'s may induce vomiting by their local effect, as copper sulfate or zinc sulfate, mustard and ipecac, in small doses diluted in water; or by their effect on the central nervous system, such as apomorphine hydrochloride which works by hypodermic injection. Emesis is much more likely to take place when the stomach is distended.

emetine (ĕm'ĕ-tēn) [Gr. *emein*, to vomit]. Powdered, white alkaloid emetic obtained from ipecac, q.v.

e. bismuth iodide. A combination of emetine and bismuth containing about 20% emetine and 20% bismuth. Action and uses same as emetine.

e. hydrochloride. USP. The hydrated hydrochloride of an alkaloid obtained from ipecac. It is used for the treatment of both intestinal and extratestinal amebiasis. It should be used cautiously in old or debilitated patients. Children, pregnant women and patients with serious organic disease should not receive emetine.

em'etism ["+ *ismos*, condition of]. Poisoning from overdose of ipecac.

SYM: Acute inflammation of pylorus, hyperemesis, diarrhea, and perhaps coughing and suffocation.

emetocathar'tic (ĕm''ĕ-to-kă-thăr'tĭk) ["+ *katharsis*, a purging]. Producing both emesis and catharsis.

emetol'ogy ["+ *logos*, study of]. Study of emetics and their action.

E.M.F. Abbr. for *electromotive force; erythrocyte maturation factor.*

emiction (e-mik'shun) [L. *e*, out, + *mingere*, to urinate]. The act of urination.

emigra'tion ["+ *migrāre*, to move]. Passage of white blood corpuscles through the walls of capillaries and veins during inflammation.

em'inence ["+ *minēre*, to hang on]. A prominence or projection, esp. of a bone.

e., arcuate. A rounded e. on upper surface of petrous portion of temporal bone. SYN: *eminentia arcuata* [NA].

e., articular, of the temporal bone A rounded e. forming anterior boundary of the glenoid fossa. SYN: *tuberculum articulare* [NA].

e., auditory. A collection of gray matter on floor of 4th ventricle of brain at its lower part, forming the deep origin of the auditory nerve.

e., bicipital. A tuberosity for insertion of biceps muscle on radius.

e., blastodermic. An elevated mass of cells of a developing ovum forming the blastoderm.

e., canine. A vertical ridge on the external surface of the superior maxilla.

e., collateral. One between middle and posterior horns in lateral ventricle of brain. SYN: *eminentia collateralis* [NA].

e. of Doyère. Slight elevation of muscular fiber corresponding to entrance of a nerve fiber.

e., frontal. A rounded prominence on either side of median line, a little below center of frontal bone. SYN: *tuber frontale* [NA].

e., germinal. Cumulus oophorus, q.v.

e., hypothenar. E. on ulnar side of palm, formed by muscles of little finger.

e., iliopectineal; e., iliopubic. E. on upper aspect of pubic bone above the acetabulum, marking the junction of bone with the ilium. SYN: *eminentia iliopubica* [NA].

e., intercondyloid. A process on the head of the tibia lying between the two condyles. SYN: *eminentia condyloidea; eminentia intercondylaris* [NA]; intercondylar e.

e., mamillary. Projection of inner pillars of fornix. SYN: *corpus mamillare* [NA]; *mammillary body.*

e., median. Anterior bodies of medulla oblongata separated by anterior median fissure. SYN: *eminentia medialis* [NA].

e., nasal. A prominence on vertical portion of frontal bone above the nasal notch and between the two superciliary ridges.

e., occipital. Protuberance on occipital bone.

e., olivary. Oval projection at upper part of medulla oblongata above extremity of lateral column. SYN: *oliva* [NA]; *olivary body.*

e., parietal. The marked convexity on outer surface of parietal bone. SYN: *parietal tuber; tuber parietale* [NA].

e.'s, portal. The small median lobes on lower surface of liver.

e., pyramidal. An elevation on the mastoid wall of the tympanic cavity. It contains a cavity in which lies the stapedius muscle. SYN: *eminentia pyramidalis* [NA]; *pyramid of tympanum.*

e., thenar. E. formed by muscles, below the thumb on the palm of the hand.

eminentia (ĕm''ĭn-ĕn'shĭ-ă) [L.]. (pl. *-entiae*) An eminence, q.v.

emissary (ĕm'ĭ-sā-rī) [L. *e*, out, + *mittere*, to send]. 1. Providing an outlet. 2. An outlet.

e. veins. Small veins piercing the skull, carrying blood from the sinuses within the skull to the veins without.

emissio (e-mis'sĭ-o) [L.]. A discharge; emission, q.v.

e. seminis. Discharge of semen.

emission (e-mĭsh'ŭn) [L. *e*, out, + *mittere*, to send]. An issuance or discharge; the sending forth or discharge, such as of an atomic particle, exhalation, or of a light or heat wave.

e., nocturnal. Involuntary discharge of semen during sleep. SYN: *wet dream.*

emmenagogue (em-ĕn'ă-gŏg) [Gr. *emmēna*, menses, + *agōgos*, leading]. A substance which promotes or assists the menstrual flow. SEE: *ecbolic*.

     e., direct. That which has a direct effect on the reproductive tract, such as a hormone.

     e., indirect. An agent which alters the menstrual function by changing the general state of health.

emmenia (em-me'nĭ-ă) [Gr. *emmēna*]. The menstrual flow.

emmen'ic. Pert. to the menses.

emmeniopathy (em-me''nĭ-ŏp'ă-thĭ) [Gr. *emmēna*, menses, + *pathos*, disease]. Any disorder of menstruation.

emmenology (ĕm''ĕn-ŏl'ō-jĭ) [" + *logos*, science]. Science of menstruation.

emmetrope (em'mĕ-trōp) [Gr. *emmetros*, in due measure, + *opsis*, sight]. One endowed with normal vision.

emmetropia (ĕm-mĕ-trō'pĭ-ă). Normal condition of eye in refraction; with eye at rest parallel rays are focused on retina; ability to focus on the retina a luminous point from 3.9 to 4.7 in. from the eye. SEE: *astigmatism; myopia.*

emmetrop'ic. Normal in vision. SEE: *hypermetropic; myopic.*

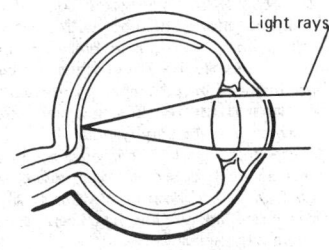

Light rays

EMMETROPIC EYE
Light rays focus on retina.

Em'met's operation. [Thomas A. Emmet, Amer. gynecologist, 1828-1919] 1. Uterine trachelorrhaphy, i.e., suture of torn uterine cervix. 2. Suturing of a lacerated perineum. 3. Converting a sessile submucous tumor of the uterus into a pedunculated one. 4. Operation for prolapse of uterus.

emollient (e-mŏl'yĕnt) [L. *e*, out, + *mollire*, to soften]. An agent that will soften and soothe the part when applied locally. The term is usually confined to agents affecting the surface of the body. Ex: ointment of rose water; olive oil; petrolatum. SEE: *demulcent.*

emotion (e-mō'shŭn) [L. *ēmovēre*, to stir up]. 1. A mental state or strong feeling affect

usually accompanied by physical changes in the body such as alteration in heart rate and respiratory activity, vasomotor reactions, and changes in muscle tone. 2. A mental state or feeling such as fear, hate, love, anger, grief, joy. These constitute the "drive" which brings about the emotional or mental adjustment necessary to satisfy instinctive needs.

Frustration is normally associated with displeasure and the intensifying of need; the process of gratification is accompanied by pleasurable feeling which persists for a variable period in less intense form. Physiologic changes invariably accompany alteration in the emotions but such change may not be apparent to either the person experiencing the emotion or an observer.

Anxiety, or fear, arises when one doubts his ability adequately to meet a situation; neutralization consists of "flight" from the danger, and a struggle (fight) to remove the threat. The physical changes are those favorable to success and during biological evolution may well have antedated the psychic phase of the fear. Civilized man may find an instinctive goal unattainable because his conditioned (moral) reactions regard the goal as socially objectionable (or even deny the goal entirely). Here arise the conflict and the starting point of psychogenic disease.

     e., disorders of. An e. is not felt in the same way by healthy persons as by one suffering from schizophrenia. In the latter, there is a decrease of pleasure, hate, love, and other e.'s. There is loss of ability to feel and express e.'s such as love or hate. The patient is said to be blunted. The e.'s he does show are not in harmony with his ideas; for example, he may smile while describing tortures and terrors.

Unhappiness is marked in manic depressive psychosis. It varies in degree and may lead to suicide. In the excited stage undue happiness is marked. Depressions and elations have no apparent cause.

E.'s are easily aroused in aged persons and in alcoholics.

Depressed patients are so wrapped up in their own misery they take no notice of anything else. Excited patients cannot concentrate their attention. Confused ones may not realize they are not in the proper place for their actions. Hallucinating patients are influenced by imaginary voices, visions, places and persons. Deluded ones have unreasonable fears.

emotion, words pert. to: affective; amor; cathexis; mania; psychiatry; sex.

emo′tional [L. *ēmovēre*, to stir up]. Relat. to any of the emotions.

   e. attitudes. Those which express any of the emotions, such as joy, sorrow. Seen in hysteroepilepsy.

   e. disturbance. Mental illness.

   e. instability. In psychology, given to easy rage, brooding, and vastly fluctuating moods.

emotivity (e-mo-tĭv′ĭ-tĭ). One's capability for emotional response.

em′pasm, empas′ma [Gr. *en-*, in, + *passein*, to sprinkle]. A powder, usually perfumed, for external application to the body.

empath′ic ["+ *pathos*, feeling]. Pert. to, or characterized by, empathy.

empathy (ĕm′pă-thĭ). Objective awareness of and insight into the feelings, emotions, and behavior of another person and their meaning and significance. Not the same as sympathy which is usually nonobjective and noncritical.

emphlysis (em′flĭs-is) [Gr. *en-*, in, + *phlysis*, an eruption]. (pl. *emphlyses*) Any vesicular or exanthematous eruption.

emphractic (ĕm-frăk′tĭk) [Gr. *emphraxis*, an obstruction]. 1. Obstructive, as clogging of pores of skin. 2. Anything that obstructs a function.

emphraxis (ĕm-frăk′sĭs). A stoppage, or obstruction; an infarction.

emphysatherapy (ĕm″fĭz-ă-thĕr′ă-pĭ) [Gr. *emphysan*, to inflate, + *therapeia*, treatment]. Injection of gas into a cavity for therapeutic purposes.

emphysema (ĕm″fĭ-sē′mă) [Gr. *emphysan*, to inflate]. 1. Distention of tissues by gas or air in the interstices. 2. A condition in which the alveoli of the lungs become distended or ruptured. Usually the result of an interference with expiration, or loss of elasticity of the lung. SYN: *pulmonary emphysema.*

   e., atrophic. Senile e.

   e., chronic hypertrophic. E. accompanied with bony changes resulting in the so-called barrel chest.

   e., compensatory. E. which results from overstretching of a functional part of the lung when another portion fails to function. A secondary condition seen in tuberculosis or pneumonia. SYN: *complemental e.*

   e., interstitial. Rupture of pulmonary alveoli with escape of air to interstices of the lung and then to the mediastinum to produce mediastinal emphysema.

   e., obstructive pulmonary. Emphysema which affects predominantly men between the ages of 45 and 65. Associated with a history of chronic bronchitis, cigarette smoking, or exposure to cold, damp weather and a dusty working or city environment. The disease may develop without any of these conditions having been experienced. The most helpful, diagnostic clinical sign is breathlessness. Treatment is directed to the basic cause, such as bronchitis, a dusty environment, or cigarette smoking.

   e., subcutaneous. Presence of air or gas in subcutaneous tissues, with consequent distention. Often caused by infection by gas-producing organisms, esp. Clostridium perfringens.

   e., surgical. Subcutaneous emphysema caused by surgery, esp. after wounds of respiratory tract.

   e., vesicular. Overdistention of alveoli and smaller bronchial tubes with air. SYM: Dyspnea upon exertion; accelerated pulse, cough, and expectoration of whitish mucus. Short inspiration, prolonged expiration.

emphysematous (ĕm″fĭ-sĕm′ă-tus). Affected with or pert. to emphysema.

empiric (ĕm-pĭr′ĭk) [Gr. *empeirikos*, skilled, experienced]. 1. Based on experience. SEE: *empirical*. 2. A practitioner whose skill or art is based upon what has been learned through experience.

empirical (ĕm-pĭr′ĭk-al). Based on experience and usually without respect to scientific principles.

empiricism (ĕm-pĭr′ĭs-ĭzm) [Gr. *empeirikos*, skilled, experienced, + *ismos*, condition of]. 1. Experience, not theory, as basis of medical science. 2. Quackery.

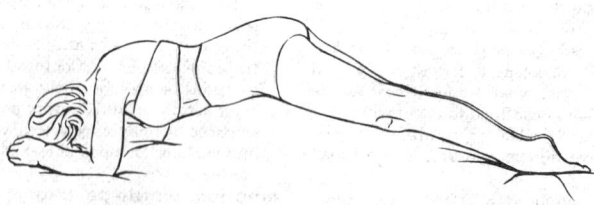

EMPROSTHOTONOS

emplastic (em-plăs′tik) [Gr. *emplastikos*, clogging]. 1. A constipating medicine. 2. Adhesive or able to be used as a plaster.

emplas′trum [L.]. (pl. *emplastra*) A plaster or preparation for external application; adheres to the skin when applied. SEE: *plaster.*

emprosthotonos (ĕm″prŏs-thŏt′ō-nŏs) [Gr. *emprosthen*, forward, + *tonos*, tension]. Lying with body incurved and resting upon forehead and feet with face downward.

Sometimes seen in tetanus and strychnine poisoning. Opposed to opisthotonos. SEE: *posture.*

emptysis (ĕmp′tĭ-sĭs) [Gr., a spitting]. Expectoration of blood or blood-stained mucus; hemoptysis.

empyema (em″pĭ-ē′ma) [Gr. from *en*, within, + *pyon*, pus]. Pus in a body cavity, esp. in the pleural cavity (pyothorax). Usually result of a primary infection in the lungs.

SYM: Chills, fever, and sweating. Skin is gray, malar flush, appetite poor, marked malaise, pain in chest, cough, emaciation. Dyspnea may ensue.

TREATMENT: Antibiotic therapy, aspiration of pleural fluid. Treatment of primary condition. Surgical drainage may be necessary.

NP: Postoperative: Patient should sit up inclined to affected side to facilitate drainage, then to opposite side to aid expansion of lung; high protein, high vitamin diet; breathing exercises. SEE: *resection.*

     e., interlobular. Form with pus between lobes of lung.

     e. necessitatis. Form in which pus can escape spontaneously.

     e., pulsating. Form with cardiac beats causing pulsation of chest wall.

empyesis (em″pĭ-ē′sĭs) [Gr. *empyein*, to suppurate]. A pustular eruption on the skin.

empyocele (ĕm″pĭ-ō-sēl) [″ + *kēlē*, tumor]. A collection of pus in a sacculated cavity, especially in the scrotum; a suppurating hydrocele.

emul′gent [L. *ēmulgere*, to drain out]. Extracting or draining.

     e. vessel. Blood vessel of the kidney.

emulsification (e-mŭl′sĭ-fĭ-kā′shŭn) [L. *emulsio*, emulsion, + *facere*, to make]. 1. Process of making an emulsion. 2. The breaking down of large fat globules in the intestine to smaller, uniformly distributed particles, accomplished largely through the action of bile acids which lower surface tension.

emul′sifier. Anything used to make an emulsion.

emulsify (e-mŭl′sĭ-fī). To form into an emulsion.

emul′sion [L. *emulsio*, from *e*, out of, + *mulgēre*, to milk]. A mixture of two liquids not mutually soluble.

If they are thoroughly shaken, one will divide into globules and is called the discontinuous or dispersed phase; the other is then the continuous phase. Milk is an emulsion in which butter fat is the discontinuous and the liquid portion the continuous phase.

emulsoid (ē-mŭl′soyd) [″ + Gr. *eidos*, form]. A colloid in an aqueous solution in which the colloid has a marked attraction for water to the extent that the dispersoid contains large quantities of water. Also called hydrophilic or lyophilic colloids. Protoplasm, starch, soap, gelatin, and egg white are common examples.

emulsum (e-mul′sum) [L.]. A fluid in which oil or resin is suspended by means of a mucilaginous substance.

emunctory (e-mŭnk′tō-rĭ) [L. *e*, completely, + *mungēre*, to blow the nose]. 1. Pert. to organ or duct having an excretory function. 2. An excretory duct, i.e., pores of skin.

E.N.A. Abbr. for *extractable nuclear antigen,* q.v.

enamel (en-ăm′ĕl) [O. Fr. *esmail*, enamel]. The hard, white, dense substance forming a covering for the crown of the teeth. It is the hardest substance in the body. SYN: *enamelum* [NA]; *substantia adamantina.*

     e., mottled. Condition in which the enamel acquires a mottled appearance as a result of the ingestion of excessive amounts of fluorides in water or foods.

     e. organ. A cup-shaped structure which forms on the dental lamina of an embryo. It produces the enamel and serves as a mold for the remainder of the tooth.

enam′elum. [NA]. Enamel, q.v., of teeth.

enanthem, enanthema (en-an′them, -an-the′ma) [Gr. *en*, in, + *anthēma*, blossoming]. Eruption of mucous membrane. Ex: Koplik's spots. SEE: *exanthem; rash.*

enanthematous (en″an-them′ă-tus). Of the nature of an enanthema.

enanthesis (en″an-the′sis) [Gr. *en-*, in, + *anthein*, to bloom]. A skin eruption due to internal disease.

enanthrope (ĕn′an-thrōp) [″ + *anthrōpos*, man]. Any disease originating within the body.

enantiobiosis (en-an″tĭ-o-bĭ-o′sis) [Gr. *enantios*, opposite, + *bios*, life]. The condition in which associated organisms are antagonistic to each other. SEE: *symbiosis.*

enantiopathy (en-an″tĭ-op′ă-thĭ) [″ + *pathos*, disease]. Treatment of one disease by another disease antagonistic to it, as malaria in general paresis.

enarkyochrome (en-ar'kī-o-krōm) [Gr. *en*, in, + *arkus*, network, + *chrōma*, color]. A nerve cell arranged like a network, taking a stain best in the cell body.

enarthritis (ĕn"ăr-thrī'tĭs) ["+ *arthron*, joint, + *itis*, inflammation]. Inflammation of a ball-and-socket joint.

enarthrosis (en"ar-thro'sis) ["+ *arthrōsis*, joint, + *-ōsis*, condition]. (pl. *enarthroses*) A ball-and-socket joint such as the hip joint; a form of diarthrosis.

RS: amphiarthrosis; condylarthrosis; diarthrosis; synarthrosis; synchondrosis.

encan'this [Gr. *en*, in, + *kanthos*, angle of the eye]. An excrescence or new growth at the inner angle of the eye.

encapsula'tion [L. *en*, in, + *capsula*, a little box]. 1. Enclosure in a sheath not normal to the part. 2. The process of the formation of a capsule or a sheath about a structure.

encatarrhaphy (en"kat-ar'ā-fĭ) [Gr. *enkatarrhaptein*, to sew in]. Insertion of an organ or tissue into a part where it is not normally found.

enceinte (on-sănt') [Fr.]. Pregnant.

encelialgia (en"se-le-al'jĭ-ă) [Gr. *en*, in, + *koilia*, belly, + *algos*, pain]. Abdominal pain.

encephalalgia (ĕn-sĕf-ăl-ăl'jĭ-ă) [Gr. *enkephalos*, brain, + *algos*, pain]. Deep-seated head pain. SYN: *cephalalgia.*

encephalasthenia (ĕn-sĕf'ăl-ăs-the'nĭ-ă) ["+ *asthenia*, weakness]. Deficiency in brain power.

encephalatrophy (ĕn-sĕf-ăl-ăt'rō-fĭ) ["+ *a-*, not, + *trophē*, nourishment]. Cerebral atrophy.

encephalic (ĕn"sĕf-ăl'ĭk) [Gr. *enkephalos*, brain]. Pert. to the brain or its cavity.

encephalitis (ĕn-sĕf'ă-lī'tĭs) ["+ *itis*, inflammation]. Inflammation of the brain.

ETIOL: It may be a specific disease entity due to an arthropod-borne (arbor) virus, or it may occur as a sequela of influenza, measles, German measles, chickenpox, smallpox, vaccinia, or other diseases.

e., cortical. E. of brain cortex only.

e., epidemic. Any form of e. which occurs as an epidemic.

e., equine. Originally isolated as an e. affecting horses, it has been found to be transmitted to man by vectors also.

e., equine, Eastern. Primarily a disease of birds and wild animals, transmitted to horses and man by mosquitoes. More severe than other types of e. Outbreaks have occurred in the Eastern and Gulf Coast states.

e., equine, Western. A mild type of e., having occurred in Western United States and Canada.

e., hemorrhagic. Hemorrhage in brain inflammation.

e. hyperplastica. Acute e. without suppuration.

e., infantile. Brain inflammation in the young which may cause cerebral palsy.

e., Japanese B. Similar to St. Louis e., it is caused by a different strain of virus. Occurs in summer and fall.

e., lead. E. due to lead poisoning.

e. lethargica. Epidemic neurotaxis, epidemic stupor. An infective disease believed to be of viral origin which first appeared pandemically in 1916-1917. It appeared pandemically in various regions of the world up to 1925 usually following epidemics of influenza. Since that time, it has occurred sporadically. Occurs usually in winter months. SYN: *Economo's disease; sleeping sickness.*

e., meningo-. E. combined with meningitis.

e. neonato'rum. A form occurring within the first several weeks of life.

e. periaxialis. Inflammation of the white matter of the cerebrum, occurring mainly in the young.

e., postinfection. E. occurring following a smallpox vaccination or one of the common communicable diseases, as chickenpox.

e., purulent. E. characterized by abscesses in the brain.

e., St. Louis. A virus disease which first occurred epidemically in the summer of 1933 in and around St. Louis. Now endemic in America. Occurs most frequently during summer and early fall.

e., toxic. That resulting from metal poisonings, as lead poisoning.

encephalocele (ĕn-sĕf'ă-lō-sēl) ["+ *kēlē*, hernia]. Protrusion of the brain through a cranial fissure. SYN: *hydrencephalocele.*

encephalocystocele (ĕn-sĕf'ă-lo-sĭs'tō-sēl) ["+ *kystis*, a bladder, + *kēlē*, hernia]. Protrusion of brain distended by hernial sac containing fluid.

encephalodialysis (ĕn-sĕf'ă-lo-dī-ăl'ĭ-sĭs) [Gr. *enkephalos*, brain, + *dialysis*, loosening]. Softening of the brain.

encephalogram (ĕn-sĕf'ă-lō-grăm) ["+ *gramma*, a writing]. X-ray picture of the brain. Usually done with air having been injected in the ventricles in order to provide contrast in the picture.

encephalography (ĕn-sĕf'ă-lŏg'ră-fĭ) ["+ *graphein*, to write]. X-ray examination of head, esp. examination following the introduction of air into the ventricles through a lumbar or cisternal puncture.

encephaloid (ĕn-sĕf'ă-loyd) [" + *eidos*, form]. 1. Resembling the cerebral substance. 2. A malignant neoplasm of brainlike texture.

   e. cancer. Malignant tumor of the brain. SYN: *encephaloma.*

encephalolith (ĕn-sĕf'ă-lo-lĭth) [" + *lithos*, stone]. A calculus of the brain.

encephalology (ĕn"sĕf-ă-lŏl'ŏ-jĭ) [Gr. *enkephalos*, brain, + *logos*, study of]. That division of medical science which deals with the structure, function, and pathology of the brain.

encephaloma (ĕn-sĕf'ă-lō'mă) [" + *ōma*, tumor]. Tumor of the brain.

encephalomalacia (ĕn-sĕf'ă-lō-mă-la'sĭ-ă) [" + *malakia*, softening]. Brain softening.

encephalomeningitis (ĕn-sĕf'ă-lō-mĕn"ĭn-jī'tĭs) [" + *mēninx*, membrane, + *itis*, inflammation]. Inflammation of the brain and its membranes.

encephalomeningocele (ĕn-sĕf'ă-lō-mĕ-nĭng'go-sēl) [" + " + *kēlē*, hernia]. Protrusion through the cranium of membranes and brain substance.

encephalomere (ĕn-sĕf'ă-lo-mēr) [Gr. *enkephalos*, brain, + *meros*, part]. A primitive segment of the embryonic brain; a neuromere.

encephalometer (ĕn-sĕf'ă-lŏm'ĕ-ter) [" + *metron*, measure]. An instrument for measuring the cranium and locating brain regions.

encephalomyelitis (ĕn-sĕf'ă-lō-mī-ĕl-ī'tĭs) [" + *myelos*, marrow, + *itis*, inflammation]. An acute inflammation of the brain and spinal cord.

   e., acute disseminated. Acute disorder of the brain and spinal cord due to causes such as vaccination or acute exanthema. SYN: *postinfectious encephalomyelitis.*

   e., equine. Virus disease of horses that may be communicated to man. Includes Eastern and Western equine encephalitis, q.v.

encephalomyelopathy (ĕn-sĕf'ă-lō-mī"ĕl-ŏp'ă-thĭ) [" + " + *pathos*, disease]. Any disease of brain and spinal cord.

encephalon (ĕn-sĕf'ă-lŏn) [Gr. *enkephalos*, brain]. The brain, including the cerebrum, cerebellum, medulla oblongata, and pons, diencephalon and mid-brain.

encephalopathy (ĕn-sĕf'ă-lŏp'ă-thĭ) [" + *pathos*, disease]. Any dysfunction of the brain.

   e., lead. Neuronal degeneration and cerebral edema, apparently due to presence of lead in the brain.

encephalopuncture (ĕn-sĕf'ă-lō-pŭnk'tūr) [" + L. *punctura*, a piercing]. Puncture into the brain substance.

encephalopyosis (ĕn-sĕf'ă-lo-pi-ō'sĭs) [" + *pyōsis*, suppuration]. Abscess of the brain.

encephalorrhagia (ĕn-sĕf'ă-lō-ra'jĭ-a) [Gr. *enkephalos*, brain, + *rhēgnynai*, to burst forth]. Hemorrhage of the brain.

encephalosclerosis (ĕn-sĕf'ă-lō-sklē-rō'sĭs) [" + *sklērōsis*, hardening]. Brain hardening.

encephalo'sis [" + -*ōsis*, diseased condition]. A degenerative process of the brain.

encephalospi'nal [" + L. *spina*, thorn, spine]. Pert. to brain and spinal cord.

   e. axis. Cerebrospinal axis.

encephalothlipsis (ĕn-sĕf'ă-lō-thlip'sĭs) [" + *thlipsis*, pressure]. Compression of the brain.

encephalotome (ĕn-sĕf'ă-lo-tōm) [Gr. *enkephalos*, brain, + *tomē*, incision]. Instrument for incising brain tissue.

encephalotomy (ĕn-sĕf'ă-lŏt'ō-mĭ). 1. Brain dissection. 2. Surgical destruction of the brain of a fetus to facilitate delivery.

enchondroma (ĕn"kŏn-drō'mă) [Gr. *en*, in, + *chondros*, cartilage, + -*ōma*, tumor]. A benign cartilaginous tumor occurring generally where cartilage is absent or within a bone where it expands the diaphysis. SYN: *true chondroma.*

enchondrosarcoma (ĕn-kŏn"drō-săr-kō'mă) [" + " + *sarx*, flesh, + -*ōma*, tumor]. Sarcoma made up of cartilaginous tissue.

enchondrosis (ĕn-kŏn-drō'sĭs) [" + " + -*ōsis*, diseased condition]. A benign cartilaginous outgrowth from bone or cartilaginous tissue; an enchondroma.

enclave (ĕn'klāv) [Fr. *enclavér*, to enclose]. A mass of tissue which becomes enclosed by a tissue of another kind.

enclavement (ĕn-klāv'ment) [Fr.]. An impaction of the fetus in the pelvic strait.

enclitic (ĕn-klĭt'ĭk) [Gr. *enklinein*, to lean on]. Having the planes of the fetal head inclined to those of the maternal pelvis.

encolpism (ĕn-kŏl'pĭzm) [Gr. *en*, in, + *kolpos*, vagina, + *ismos*, condition]. Medication by vaginal suppositories and injections.

encolpitis (ĕn-kŏl-pī'tĭs) [" + " + *itis*, inflammation]. Inflamed condition of the vaginal mucosa. SYN: *endocolpitis.*

encopresis (ĕn-kŏp-re'sĭs) [Gr. *en*, in, + *kopros*, excrement]. Fecal incontinence not due to illness or organic defect.

encra'nial [" + *kranion*, cranium]. Intracranial or within the cranium.

encyesis (ĕn"sĭ-ē'sĭs) [" + *kyēsis*, pregnancy]. Normal uterine pregnancy.

encysted (ĕn-sĭst′ed) [L. *in-*, put into, + Gr. *kystis*, bladder, pouch]. Surrounded by membrane; encapsulated.

end [AS. *ende*]. A termination; extremity.

e. artery. An artery which does not anastomose directly or indirectly with other arteries, e.g., in kidney and spleen.

e. brain. The telencephalon.

e. bud, bulb, capsule. The terminal of a sensory nerve.

e. bulb of Krause. An encapsulated nerve ending found in the skin and mucous membranes.

e. organ. An encapsulated sensory nerve ending.

e. organ, neuromuscular. Spindle-shaped bundle of specialized muscle fibers in which sensory nerve fibers terminate in muscles; muscle spindle.

e. organ, neurotendinous. Specialized tendon fasciculi in which sensory nerve fibers terminate in tendons; a tendon spindle.

e. product. The final waste or excretory product of digestion that passes from the system.

e. result. The ultimate or final result.

Endamoeba (en″dă-mē′bă). Entamoeba, q.v.

endangeitis, endangiitis (ĕnd″an-jī-ī′tĭs) [Gr. *endon*, within, + *angeion*, vessel, + *itis*, inflammation]. Inflammation of the endangium or inner coat of blood vessels.

endangium (ĕn-dăn′jĭ-ŭm). Innermost coat or intima of blood vessels.

endaortitis (ĕnd″a-or-tĭtĭs) [Gr. *endon*, within, + *aortē*, aorta, + *itis*, inflammation]. Inflammation of inner coat of the aorta.

endarterial (ĕnd″ăr-te′rĭ-al) ["+ *artēria*, artery]. 1. Pert. to the inner portion of an artery. 2. Within an artery.

endarteritis (ĕnd-ăr-ter-ī′tĭs) ["+ "+ *itis*, inflammation]. Inflammation of innermost coat or intima of an artery resulting from syphilis, trauma, pyogenic bacteria, or infective thrombi.

e., acute. Of large arteries. Rare.

e., chronic. Degeneration of arterial coats in the aged. SYN: *atheroma.*

e. deformans. Thickening of intima or replacement with atheromatous or calcareous deposits.

e. obliterans. Chronic progressive thickening of intima leading to stenosis or obstruction of lumen.

e. syphilitic. E. caused by syphilis. SYN: *syphilitic vasculitis.*

endeictic (en-dīk′tĭk) [Gr. *endeixis*, a pointing out]. Symptomatic.

endem′ic [Gr. *en*, in, + *dēmos*, people]. Said of a disease peculiar to and more or less

recurring continuously in a particular locality or population, but only in a small number of cases. Used in contrast to sporadic, q.v., or epidemic, q.v.

e. neuritis. A form of polyneuritis. SYN: *beriberi.*

endemoepidemic (ĕn-dĕm″o-ĕp-ĭ-dĕm′ĭk) ["+ "+ *epi*, on, among, + *dēmos*, people]. Endemic, but becoming epidemic periodically.

endermat′ic, enderm′ic [Gr. *endon*, within, + *derma*, skin]. Administering medicine by absorption through the skin.

endermo′sis ["+ "+ *ōsis*, condition]. 1. Administration of medicines through the skin. 2. Herpetic affection of any mucous membrane.

en′deron ["+ *deros*, skin]. The dermis or corium; the portion of a mucous membrane underlying the epithelial layer.

endive (ĕn′dĭv). Plant cultivated for its crown of leaves, used in salads.

Food value of 100 gm. (raw, curly, including escarol): Cal. 20; protein 1.7 gm.; fat 0.1 gm.; carbohydrate 4.1 gm.; calcium 81 mg.; vitamin A, 3300 I.U.; ascorbic acid 10 mg.

endoaneurysmorrhaphy (en″do-an″ū-rismor′af-ĭ) [Gr. *endon*, within, + *aneurysma*, aneurysm, + *rhaphē*, suture]. Opening an aneurysmal sac and suturing its orifice.

endoangiitis (ĕn″do-ăn-jī-ī′tĭs) ["+ *angeion*, vessel, + *itis*, inflammation]. Inflammation of the coat of blood vessels. SYN: *endangiitis; endoarteritis; endophlebitis.*

endoantitoxin (ĕn″do-ăn-tĭ-tŏk′sĭn) ["+ *anti*, against, + *toxikon*, poison]. An antitoxin within a cell.

endoappendicitis (ĕn″do-ă-pĕn″dĭ-sī′tĭs) [Gr. *endon*, within, + L. *appendere*, to hang, + Gr. *itis*, inflammation]. Inflammation of mucosa of the vermiform appendix.

endoarteritis (ĕn″do-ăr″tĕr-ī′tĭs) [Gr. *endon*, within, + *arteria*, artery, + *itis*, inflammation]. Endarteritis, q.v.

endoauscultation (ĕn″do-aws″kŭl-tā′shŭn) ["+ L. *auscultāre*, to listen to]. Auscultation by esophageal tube passed into the stomach.

endobiotic (ĕn″do-bī-ŏt′ĭk) ["+ *bios*, life]. Pertaining to an organism living parasitically in the host.

endoblast (ĕn′do-blăst) [Gr. *endon*, within, + *blastos*, germ]. 1. The nucleus cell. 2. Inner layer of the blastoderm. SYN: *endoderm; hypoblast.*

endobronchitis ["+ *bronchos*, windpipe, + *itis*, inflammation]. Inflammation of bronchial mucosa.

endocar′diac, endocar′dial ["+ *kardia*, heart]. Within the heart or arising from the endocardium.

endocarditis (ĕn″do-kăr-dĭ′tĭs) ["+ "+ *itis,* inflammation]. Inflammation of the lining membrane of the heart or endocardium.

It is usually confined to the external lining of the valve, sometimes to the lining membrane of its chambers. Generally of bacterial origin.

NP: Practically the same as that for pericarditis and other heart conditions. Rest in bed essential, but during symptoms of dyspnea patient should be propped up in bed and supported by pillows with arms resting on pillows. All bodily activities should be kept at a minimum. Patient should not reach for anything. Pulse should be taken before and after any exertion and if it does not return to original pulse within two minutes after the effort it indicates strain as a result. Maintain proper elimination.

TREATMENT: Antibiotic therapy for at least one month. Procaine penicillin in large doses is usually employed, although other antibiotics may be required.

  e., acute bacterial. E. that progresses rapidly; usually caused by staphylococci or the pneumococcus.

  e., chronic. E., ulcerative, q.v.

  e., malignant. Usually secondary to suppurative inflammation elsewhere. SEE: *e., ulcerative.*

  e., subacute bacterial. A condition caused by lodgment of the Streptococcus viridans group (mainly S. salivarius, S. mitis, S. bovis, S. fecalis, S. sanguis) in an abnormal heart or in valves damaged previously by rheumatic fever.

  e., ulcerative. A rapidly destructive form of acute bacterial e., characterized by necrosis or ulceration of the valves and the deposition of colonies of micrococci. Usually fatal.

  e., vegetative. Fibrinous clots on ulcerated valvular surfaces.

  e., verrucous. Nonbacterial e. occurring frequently in lupus erythematosus. SYN: *Libman-Sacks disease; nonbacterial verrucous e.*

  e. viridans. Subacute bacterial endocarditis.

endocar′dium [Gr. *endon,* within, + *kardia,* heart]. [NA]. Lining (serous) membrane of inner surface and cavities of the heart.

It is continuous with the intima or interior coat of arteries.

endocervical (ĕn″do-sĕr′vĭ-kal) ["+ L. *cervix,* neck]. Pert. to the endocervix.

endocervicitis (ĕn″dō-sĕr′vĭ-sĭ′tĭs) ["+ "+ *itis,* inflammation]. Inflammation of mucous lining of the cervix uteri. Usually chronic and due to infection, and accompanied by cervical erosion.

SYM: White or yellow mucoid discharge.

TREATMENT: Electrocauterization of cervical lesion. An antibiotic for local application may be prescribed.

endocervix (ĕn-do-sĕr′vĭks) [Gr. *endon,* within, + L. *cervix,* neck]. The lining of the canal of the cervix uteri.

endochondral (ĕn″do-kŏn′drăl) ["+ *chondros,* cartilage]. Within a cartilage.

endochorion (en″do-kō′rĭ-ŏn) ["+ *khorion,* afterbirth]. The inner chorion; vascular layer of allantois.

endochrome (ĕn′do-krōm) ["+ *chrōma,* color]. The coloring matter of a cell's endoplasm.

endocolitis [Gr. *endon,* within, + *kōlon,* colon, + *itis,* inflammation]. Inflammation of the mucosa of colon. SEE: *colitis.*

endocolpitis (ĕn″do-kŏl-pī′tĭs) ["+ *kolpos,* vagina, + *itis,* inflammation]. Inflammation of the vaginal mucosa. SYN: *encolpitis.*

endocom′plement ["+ L. *complēre,* to fill]. An intracellular complement or one contained within the erythrocyte.

endocorpuscular (ĕn″do-kŏr-pŭs′kū-lăr) ["+ L. *corpusculum,* small body (corpuscle)]. Within a corpuscle.

endocra′nial [Gr. *endon,* within, + *kranion,* cranium]. 1. Intracranial or within the cranium. 2. Pert. to the endocranium.

endocranitis ["+ "+ *itis,* inflammation]. Inflammation of endocranium. SYN: *external pachymeningitis.*

endocra′nium. The dura mater of the brain which forms the lining membrane of the cranium.

endocrinasthenia (ĕn″do-krĭn″ăs-thē′nĭ-ă) ["+ *krinein,* to secrete, + *astheneia,* weakness]. Neurasthenia due to dysfunction of the endocrine system.

endocrine (ĕn′do-krĭn, -krĭn, -krēn) ["+ krīnein, to separate, secrete]. 1. An internal secretion. 2. Endocrinous. 3. Pert. to a gland that produces an internal secretion.

  e. gland. A ductless gland which produces an internal secretion discharged into the blood or lymph and circulated to all parts of the body. Hormones, the active principles of the glands, produce effects on tissues more or less remote from their place of origin. In addition to their e. function, some glands also produce an external secretion (Ex: pancreas, testes).

The e. glands include: hypophysis (pituitary gland); thyroid gland (the thymus and pineal body have not been shown to produce any hormones); parathyroid glands; adrenal (suprarenal) glands; islands of Langerhans of the pancreas; and the gonads (ovaries and testes). Other structures such as the gastrointestinal mucosa and the placenta have an e. function.

The hormones secreted by the ductless glands may have a specific effect on an organ or tissue, while in some cases the effect is general affecting the entire body, as in the case of the thyroid hormone which affects the rate of metabolism. Among the physiological processes affected by hormones are rate of metabolism and the metabolism of specific substances such as carbohydrates and calcium; growth and developmental processes; the secretory activity of other endocrine glands; the development and functioning of the reproductive organs; sex-

Principal Endocrine Glands

Name	Position	Function	Endocrine Disorders
Thyroid	Two lobes in anterior portion of neck	Influences basal metabolic rate; indirectly influences growth and nutrition	Hypofunction—Cretinism in young; myxedema in adult Goiter in hyperfunction and hypofunction
Parathyroid	Four or more small glands near thyroid	Calcium and phosphorus metabolism; indirectly affect muscular irritability	Hypofunction—Tetany Hyperfunction—Resorption of bone; renal calculi
Adrenal Cortex	One above each kidney	Steroid hormones regulating carbohydrate metabolism and salt and water balance; some effects on sexual characteristics	Hypofunction—Addison's disease Hyperfunction—Adrenogenital syndrome; Cushing's syndrome
Adrenal Medulla	Embedded in adrenal surrounded by cortex	Effects on sympathetic nervous system and carbohydrate metabolism	Hypofunction—Almost unknown Hyperfunction—Pheochromocytoma
Anterior Pituitary	Small gland at base of brain	Influences growth, sexual development, skin pigmentation, thyroid function, adrenalcortical function through effects on other endocrine glands (except for growth factor which acts directly on cells)	Hypofunction—Dwarfism in child; decrease in all other endocrine gland functions except parathyroids Hyperfunction—Acromegaly in adult; diabetes, gigantism in child
Posterior Pituitary	Attached to anterior pituitary	Oxytocic factor influencing some aspects of uterine contraction Antidiuretic factor influencing absorption of water by kidney tubule	Unknown Hypofunction—Diabetes insipidus
Testes and Ovaries	Testes—in the scrotum Ovaries—in the pelvic cavity	Development of secondary sex characteristics; some effect on metabolism	Hypofunction—Lack of sex development or regression in adult Hyperfunction—Abnormal sex development

ual characteristics and libido; the development of personality and higher nervous functions; the ability of the body to meet conditions of stress; resistance to disease.

E. dysfunction may result from hyposecretion in which an inadequate amount of the hormone(s) is secreted; or hypersecretion in which excessive amounts of hormones are produced. Secretion of e. glands may be under nervous control, or it may be controlled by chemical substances in the blood; or in some cases, by other hormones. Many pathological conditions are the result of, or associated with, the malfunctioning of the e. glands.

endocrinic (ĕn″do-krĭn′ĭk). Same as endocrinous, q.v.

endo′crinism [Gr. *endon*, within, + *krīnein*, to separate, secrete, + *ismos*, condition]. Disease due to malfunction of one or more of the endocrine glands. SYN: *endocrinopathy*.

endocrino-. Combining form for endocrine.

endocrinology (ĕn″do-krĭn-ŏl′ŏ-jĭ) [Gr. *endon*, within, + *krīnein*, to separate, secrete, + *logos*, study of]. The science of the endocrines, or ductless glands, and their functions.

endocrinopath (ĕn″do-krĭn′o-path) [″ + ″ + *pathos*, disease]. Person affected by a disorder of one or more glands of internal secretion.

endocrinopath′ic. Of the nature of endocrinopathy.

endocrinop′athy. Any disease due to disorder of an endocrine gland or glands.

endocrinosis (en″do-krĭn-ō′sĭs) [Gr. *endon*, within, + *krīnein*, to separate, secrete, + *-ōsis*, condition]. Condition resulting from dysfunction of an endocrine gland.

endocrinotherapy (ĕn″do-krĭn-o-thĕr′ă-pĭ) [″ + ″ + *therapeia*, treatment]. Treatment with endocrine preparations.

endocrinous (ĕn-dŏk′rĭn-ŭs) [Gr. *endon*, within, + *krīnein*, to separate, secrete]. Pert. to internal secretions or endocrine glands.

endocrit′ic. Pert. to internal secretions.

en′docyst [Gr. *endon*, within, + *kystis*, bladder, pouch]. The innermost layer of any hydatid cyst.

endocystitis (ĕn-do-sĭs-tī′tĭs) [″ + ″ + *itis*, inflammation]. Inflammation of mucous membrane of bladder. SEE: *cystitis*.

endoderm (ĕn′do-dĕrm) [″ + *derma*, skin]. Inner layer of cells of an embryo. SYN: *entoderm*, q.v.; *hypoblast*.

endoderm′al. Pert. to the entoderm. SYN: *entodermal*.

Endodermophyton (ĕn″do-dĕr-mŏf′ĭ-ton) [Gr. *endon*, within, + *derma*, skin, + *phy-*

ton, a growth]. Former name of a genus of parasitic fungi growing in the epidermis of the skin. Now included in the genus Trichophyton, q.v.

endodiascope (ĕn″do-dī′ă-skōp) [″ + *dia*, through, + *skopein*, to examine]. X-ray tube that may be placed within the body for radiological examination and radiation therapy.

endodiascopy (ĕn″do-di-ăs′kō-pĭ). X-ray examination with an endodiascope of a body cavity.

endodontia (ĕn″do-dŏn′shĭ-ă) [Gr. *endon*, within, + *odous*, tooth]. Endodontics.

endodontics (ĕn″do-dŏn′tĭks). A branch of dentistry concerned with diagnosis, treatment, and prevention of diseases of the dental pulp and its surrounding tissues.

endodon′tist. A specialist in the practice of endodontics.

endodontitis (ĕn″do-dŏn-tī′tĭs) [Gr. *endon*, within, + *odous, odont-*, tooth, + *itis*, inflammation]. Inflammation of the dental pulp. SYN: *pulpitis*.

endodon′tium. Obsolete term for pulp of a tooth. SEE: *pulp*.

endodontol′ogist. An endodontist.

endodontol′ogy. Endodontics, q.v.

endoectothrix (ĕn″do-ĕk′to-thrĭks) [Gr. *endon*, within, + *ektos*, outside, + *thrix*, hair]. Any fungus growth on and in the hair.

endoenteritis (ĕn″do-en″tĕr-ĭ′tĭs) [″ + *enteron*, intestine, + *itis*, inflammation]. Inflammation of mucous membrane of intestines.

endoenzyme (ĕn″do-ĕn′zĭm) [″ + *en*, in, + *zymē*, leaven]. An intracellular enzyme.

endogamy (ĕn-dŏg′ă-mĭ) [″ + *gamos*, marriage]. 1. Inbreeding; the custom or tribal requirement of marriage within a tribe or group. 2. In biology, reproduction by joining together gametes descended from the same ancestral cell.

endogastrectomy (en″do-găs-trĕk′tō-mĭ) [″ + *gastēr*, belly, + *ektomē*, excision]. Excision of the gastric mucosa.

endogastric (ĕn″do-găs′trĭk). Pert. to the stomach's interior.

endogastritis (ĕn″do-găs-trī′tĭs) [Gr. *endon*, within, + *gastēr*, belly, + *itis*, inflammation]. Inflammation of the lining membrane of the stomach.

endogenic (ĕn″do-jĕn′ĭk) [″ + *gennan*, to produce]. Having origin within the organism. SYN: *endogenous*, q.v.

endogenous (ĕn-dŏj′ĕ-nŭs). 1. Produced or arising from within a cell or organism. 2. Concerning spore formation within the bacteria cell. SYN: *endogenic*.

endogeny (ĕn-dŏj′ĕ-nĭ). Formation or growth within the cell.

endoglobar (ĕn″do-glōb′är). Endoglobular, q.v.

endoglob′ular [Gr. *endon*, within, + L. *globulus*, a globule]. Within the blood corpuscles, as malarial germs.

endointoxication (ĕn″do-ĭn-tŏk″sĭ-kā′shŭn) [″+ L. *in*, into, + Gr. *toxikon*, poison]. Poisoning due to an endogenous toxin.

endolabyrinthitis (ĕn″do-lăb″ĭ-rĭn-thī′tĭs) [″+ *labyrinthos*, labyrinth, + *itis*, inflammation]. Inflamed condition of the membranous labyrinth.

endolaryngeal [″+ *larynx*, larynx]. Within the larynx.

endolemma (ĕn-dō-lĕm′ă). Neurilemma, q.v. SYN: *sheath of Schwann.*

Endolimax na′na (ĕn″do-lī′maks) [Gr. *endon*, within, + *leimax*, meadow]. A minute species of ameba inhabiting the intestine of man, monkeys, and other mammals. It is nonpathogenic in man and is found in the intestines of healthy persons.

endolum′bar [″+ L. *lumbus*, loin]. In the lumbar portion of the spinal cord.

endolymph (ĕn′do-lĭmf) [″+ L. *lympha*, clear fluid]. Pale, limpid fluid within the labyrinth of the ear. SYN: *endolympha* [NA].

endolymphat′ic. Rel. to the endolymph.

    e. duct. A slender duct extending from posterior surface of the saccule of the inner ear. It ends blindly in the petrous portion of temporal bone as a dilated pouch, the endolymphatic sac.

endolysin (ĕn-dōl′ĭ-sĭn) [Gr. *endon*, within, + *lysis*, a loosening]. Bacterial substance within a leukocyte which destroys bacteria.

endol′ysis. Disintegration of cell cytoplasm.

endomastoiditis (ĕn″do-măs″toy-dī′tĭs) [Gr. *endon*, within, + *mastos*, breast, + *eidos*, form, + *itis*, inflammation]. Inflammation of mucosa lining the mastoid cavity and cells.

endometrectomy (ĕn″dō-mē-trĕk′tō-mĭ) [″+ *metra*, uterus, + *ektome*, excision]. Excision of uterine mucosa. SEE: *curettage.*

endometrial (ĕn″dō-mē′trĭ-al) [″+ *metra*, uterus]. Pert. to the lining mucosa of the uterus.

    e. cyst. An ovarian cyst or tumor that bleeds. Usually seen in ovarian endometriosis. SYN: *chocolate cyst of ovary.*

    e. jet washing. Collection of fluid which has been used to irrigate the uterine cavity. Cells present in the fluid are examined for evidence of malignancy. Method is used as a screening test for endometrial carcinoma.

endometrioma (ĕn″dō-mē″trĭ-ō′mă) [″+ ″+ *oma*, tumor]. A tumor containing shreds of ectopic endometrium; found most frequently in the ovary, cul-de-sac, rectovaginal septum, and the peritoneal surface of the posterior portion of the uterus.

endometriosis (ĕn″do-mē″trĭ-ō′sĭs) [″+ ″+ *osis*, condition]. Ectopic endometrium located in various sites throughout the pelvis or in the abdominal wall.

    e., direct. Invasion, by the mucous membrane lining the uterus, of the myometrium. SYN: *adenomyoma of the wall of the uterus.*

    e., implantation. E., peritoneal, q.v.

    e., internal. E., direct, q.v.

    e., metastatic. Extraperitoneal lesions in circumstances resembling metastatic pelvic carcinoma.

    e., peritoneal. Endometrial tissue found throughout the pelvis.

    e., primary. E., direct, q.v.

    e., transplantation. E. taking place within abdominal incision scar following pelvic surgery.

endometritis (ĕn″dō-me-trī′tĭs) [″+ ″+ *itis*, inflammation]. Inflammation of the endometrium, the inner mucous lining of the uterus.

    ETIOL: Produced by bacterial invasion. May be acute, subacute, or chronic, the acute cases most commonly resulting from infection by staphylococci, colon bacilli, or gonococci; trauma; septic abortion. The subacute type is the result of repeated acute attacks as is the chronic type. Occasionally the chronic type may be a tuberculous infection. There are many other conditions which are labeled as e. but which are of either vascular or endocrine origin. Some of these conditions are senile e.; hyperplastic e.; hypertrophic e.

    SYM: In acute cases the symptoms are usually low back and low abdominal pain; dysmenorrhea; menorrhagia; sterility; constipation. In chronic e., there is scant serosanguineous vaginal discharge. A positive diagnosis cannot be made without a curettage and a histological study of the recovered material. SEE: *cervix uteri; endometrium; uterus.*

    e., cervical. Inflammation of the inner portion of the cervix uteri.

    e., decidual. Inflammation of the mucous membrane of a gravid uterus.

    e. dissecans. E. accompanied by development of ulcers and shedding of the mucous membrane.

    e., puerperal. Acute e. following childbirth.

endometrium (ĕn-dō-mē′trĭ-ŭm) [Gr. *endon*, within, + *metra*, uterus]. [NA] The mucous membrane lining the inner surface of the uterus. Histologically, it consists of a surface epithelium made up of a single layer of columnar cells, a few of which bear cilia. Invaginations of the epithelium form simple, branched tubular glands which extend to the myometrium. The glands are separated by connective tissue resembling mesenchyme which forms the stroma. There is no submucosa, the mucosa lying closely attached to the myometrium.

The e. is supplied by two types of arteries: straight arteries which supply the deeper third or basal layer of the e. and spiral arteries which supply the spongy and compact layers. They penetrate between the glands and form a subepithelial capillary plexus. These arteries show marked changes in response to hormonal stimulation during the menstrual cycle.

Beginning with menarche and ending at menopause, the uterine e. passes through cyclic changes which constitute the menstrual cycle, q.v. These changes are related to the development and maturation of the graafian follicle in the ovary, the discharge of the ovum, and the subsequent development of the corpus luteum in the ovary.

Following fertilization of the ovum, the e. serves as nesting place and implantation occurs. The e. fuses with the developing chorion of the embryo and at birth there is a splitting off and shedding of the uterine lining or decidua. During pregnancy, the decidua basalis, the e. lying between the chorionic vesicle and the myometrium, develops into the maternal portion of the placenta, q.v.

If the ovum is not fertilized, or if the fertilized ovum does not implant, then the endometrial lining is shed. When this is completed, the cycle begins again.

endom'etry ["+ *metron*, measure]. Measurement of the interior of a cavity or organ.

endomorphy (ĕn"do-mŏr'fĭ) ["+ *morphē*, form]. Body build characterized by predominance of tissues derived from the endoderm. SEE: *ectomorphy; mesomorphy; somatotype.*

endomyocarditis (ĕn"do-mĭ-o-kăr-dī'tĭs) ["+ *mys*, muscle, + *kardia*, heart, + *itis*, inflammation]. Inflammation of the endocardium and myocardium.

endomysium (ĕn"do-mĭs'ĭ-ŭm) [Gr. *endon*, within, + *mys*, muscle]. A thin sheath of connective tissue consisting principally of reticular fibers which invests each striated muscle fiber and binds the fibers together within a fasciculus.

endoneuri'tis ["+ *neuron*, nerve, + *itis*, inflammation]. Inflammation of the endoneurium, q.v.

endoneurium (ĕn"do-nū'rĭ-ŭm). Henle's sheath. A delicate connective tissue sheath which surrounds nerve fibers within a fasciculus.

endoparasite (ĕn"dō-păr'ă-sīt) [Gr. *endon*, within, + *parasitos*, parasite]. Any parasite living within its host.

endopathy (ĕn-dŏp'ă-thĭ) [Gr. *endon*, within, + *pathos*, disease]. Any endogenous disease.

endopelvic (ĕn"do-pĕl'vĭk) ["+ L. *pelvis*, basin]. Within the pelvis.

    e. fasciae. The downward continuation of the parietal peritoneum of the abdomen to form the pelvic fasciae which have a very important part in the support of the pelvic viscera.

endopericarditis (ĕn"do-pĕr"ĭ-kăr-dī'tĭs) ["+ *peri*, around, + *kardia*, heart, + *itis*, inflammation]. Endocarditis complicated by pericarditis.

endoperimyocarditis (ĕn"do-pĕr"ĭ-mī'o-kăr-dī'tĭs) ["+ "+ *mys*, muscle, + *kardia*, heart, + *itis*, inflammation]. Inflammation of the pericardium, myocardium, and endocardium.

endoperitonitis (ĕn"do-pĕr"ĭ-to-nī'tĭs) ["+ *peritonaion*, peritoneum, + *itis*, inflammation]. Superficial inflammation of the peritoneum.

endophasia (ĕn"do-fā'zĭ-ă) [Gr. *endon*, within, + *phasis*, utterance]. Formation of words by the lips without producing sound.

endophlebitis (ĕn"do-fle-bī'tĭs) ["+ *phleps*, vein, + *itis*, inflammation]. Inflammation of inner coat of a vein.

    e. obliterans. E. causing obliteration of a vein.

    e. portalis. Inflammation of the portal vein.

en'doplasm ["+ *plasma*, matter formed]. The internal, more fluid protoplasm of a cell which lies within the ectoplasm which forms the peripheral layer.

end organ. The expanded end of a nerve fiber in a peripheral structure.

    e. o., sensory. An encapsulated termination of a nerve fiber which serves as a receptor.

endorhinitis (ĕn"do-ri-nī'tĭs) ["+ *rhis, rhin-*, nose, + *itis*, inflammation]. Inflammation of the mucous membranes of the nose. SYN: *coryza.*

endorrhachis (ĕn"do-rā'kĭs) [Gr. *endon*, within, + *rhachis*, spine]. Membrane lining the spinal cord dura mater.

endosalpingitis (ĕn"do-săl"pĭn-jĭ'tĭs) ["+ *salpinx*, trumpet (tube), + *itis*, inflammation]. Inflammation of lining of fallopian tubes.

endoscope (ĕn'dō-skōp) ["+ *skopein*, to examine]. A device consisting of a tube and optical system for observing the inside of an organ or cavity. This may be done through a natural body opening or through a small incision.

endoscopy (ĕn-dŏs'kō-pĭ). Inspection of body organs or cavities by use of the endoscope.

endosep'sis [Gr. *endon*, within, + *sēpsis*, decay]. Septicemia having its origin within the body.

endoskel'eton ["+ *skeleton*, skeleton]. Internal bony framework of the body. SEE: *exoskeleton*.

endosmometer (ĕn'dŏs-mŏm'ē-ter) ["+ *ōsmos*, a thrusting, + *metron*, measure]. Device for estimating passage by osmosis of a substance through a membrane or tissue.

endosmosis (ĕn'dŏs-mō'sĭs) ["+ "+ *ōsis*, condition]. Osmosis in which flow of water is from the outside liquid to the solution within a membranous cell.

en'dospore [Gr. *endon*, within, + *sporos*, a seed]. In biology, thick walled spore within the bacterium.

endosteitis (ĕn'dŏs-tē-ī'tĭs) ["+ *osteon*, bone, + *itis*, inflammation]. Inflammation of the endosteum or of medullary cavity of a bone.

endosteo'ma ["+ "+ *ōma*, tumor]. A tumor in the medullary cavity of a bone.

endos'teum ["+ *osteon*, bone]. Membrane lining bone in the medullary cavity.

endostitis (ĕn'dŏs-tī'tĭs) ["+ "+ *itis*, inflammation]. Inflammation of the endosteum or the medullary cavity of a bone. Also endosteitis.

endostoma (ĕn-dŏs-tō'mă) [Gr. *endon*, within, + *osteon*, bone, + *ōma*, tumor]. Osseous tumor within a bone.

endostosis (ĕn'dŏs-tō'sĭs) ["+ "+ *ōsis*, condition]. The development of an endostoma.

endothelial (ĕn'dō-thē'lĭ-ăl) [Gr. *endon*, within, + *thēlē*, nipple]. Pert. to or consisting of endothelium.

endotheliocyte (ĕn'dō-thē'lĭ-o-sīt) ["+ "+ *kytos*, cell]. Large, phagocytic, wandering cell found in circulating blood and in tissue.

endotheliocytosis (ĕn'dō-thē'lĭ-o-sī-tō'sĭs) ["+ "+ "+ *ōsis*, condition of increase]. Abnormal increase in endothelial cells.

endothelioinoma (ĕn'dō-thē'lĭ-o-ĭ-nō'mă) ["+ "+ *is*, *inos-*, fiber, + *ōma*, tumor]. Tumorous growth arising from endothelium containing fibrous substance.

endotheliolysin (ĕn'dō-thē-lĭ-ol'ĭ-sin) [Gr. *endon*, within, + *thēlē*, nipple, + *lysis*, dissolution]. An antibody found in snake venom which dissolves endothelial cells.

endotheliolytic (ĕn'dō-thē-lĭ-o-lĭt'ĭk). Capable of destroying endothelial tissue.

endothelioma (ĕn'dō-thē-lĭ-ō'mă) [Gr. *endon*, within, + *thēlē*, nipple, + *ōma*, tumor]. Malignant growth of lining cells of the blood vessels.

endotheliomyoma (ĕn'dō-thē''lĭ-o-mī-ō'mă) ["+ "+ *mys*, muscle, + *ōma*, tumor]. Muscular tumor with elements of endothelium.

endotheliomyxoma (ĕn'dō-thē''lĭ-o-mĭk-sō'mă) ["+ "+ *myxa*, mucus, + *ōma*, tumor]. Myxoma with element from endothelium.

endotheliotoxin (ĕn'dō-thē-lĭ-o-tŏks'ĭn) ["+ "+ *toxikon*, poison]. A specific toxin which acts on endothelial capillary cells, causing hemorrhages.

endothelium (ĕn'dō-thē'lē-ŭm) [Gr. *endon*, within, + *thēlē*, nipple]. [NA] A form of squamous epithelium consisting of flat cells which line the blood and lymphatic vessels, the heart, and various other body cavities. It is derived from mesoderm.

endother'mal [Gr. *endon*, within, + *thermē*, heat]. Endothermic, q.v.

endother'mic. 1. Storing up potential energy or heat. 2. Absorbing heat. 3. Absorption of heat during chemical reactions. SYN: *endothermal.*

en'dotherm knife. A knife devised for using a high frequency current.

endothermy (ĕn'dō-thĕr''mĭ). A term used as a synonym for surgical diathermy, q.v.

en'dothrix [Gr. *endon*, within, + *thrix*, hair]. Any fungus growing inside the hair.

endothyreopexy (ĕn'do-thī'rē-o-pĕks'ĭ) ["+ *thyreos*, shield, + *pēxis*, fixation]. Displacing the thyroid gland and fixing it to the side of the neck.

endothyroidopexy (ĕn'do-thī'royd-o-peks'-ĭ) ["+ "+ *eidos*, form, + *pēxis*, fixation]. Operative displacement of the thyroid gland and fixing it to the side of the neck. SYN: *endothyreopexy.*

endotoscope (ĕn-dō'to-skōp) ["+ *ous, ot-*, ear, + *skopein*, to examine]. An ear speculum. SYN: *otoscope.*

endotoxicosis (ĕn'do-tŏk''sĭ-kō'sĭs) ["+ *toxikon*, poison, + *-ōsis*, condition]. Poisoning due to an endotoxin.

en'dotoxin. Bacterial toxin confined within the body of a bacterium, freed only when the bacterium is broken down.

    SEE: *cytotoxin; erythrotoxin; exotoxin; leukotoxic; neurotoxin.*

endotracheitis (ĕn'do-tra-ke-ī'tĭs) [Gr. *endon*, within, + *tracheia*, trachea, + *-itis*, inflammation]. Inflammation of the tracheal mucosa.

endotrachelitis (ĕn″do-trā-kĕl-ī′tĭs) ["+ *trachēlos*, neck, + *ītis*, inflammation]. Inflammation of the endocervical tissues of the uterine cervix. SYN: *endocervicitis.*

endovasculitis (ĕn″do-văs″kū-lī′tĭs) ["+ L. *vasculum*, vessel, + Gr. *ītis*, inflammation]. Inflammation of the endangium or inner coat of a blood vessel. SYN: *endangeitis.*

endove′nous ["+ L. *vēna*, vein]. Within a vein. SYN: *intravenous.*

endplate. The terminal mass of a nerve fiber ending on a muscle cell.

     e., motor. An ending in a striated muscle fiber; a myoneural junction.

endyma (ĕn′dĭm-ă) [Gr. a garment]. Membranous lining of cerebral ventricles. SYN: *ependyma.*

enema (ĕn′ĕ-mă) [Gr. *en-*, in, + *hienai*, to send, throw]. Injection of water, either plain or containing various drugs, etc., into the rectum and colon to empty the lower intestine or to introduce food or medicine for therapeutic purposes.

     e., antispasmodic. One to counteract spasms.

     e., barium. Administration of barium sulfate in solution as a diagnostic aid in x-ray examination of colon.

     e., carminative. One given to relieve distention caused by flatus and to stimulate peristalsis.

     e., cleansing. One to empty the lower intestine or the colon.

     PROCEDURE: Bring all equipment to bedside. Screen bed and explain to patient what is to be done and why it is being done; take time to gain patient's cooperation. Turn patient on left side, with right leg flexed, in as comfortable a position as possible. Place small rubber sheet covered with large towel under buttocks. Cover patient with bath blanket while fan-folding top covers; drape to expose required area. Hang enema can on stand, having it about two feet above patient (not more), and see that stopcock is working properly. See that solution is the proper temperature. Lubricate rectal or enema tube for about two inches at end. Run a little of the solution through tube into bedpan to warm tube; close stopcock. Insert tube into rectum. If you meet with resistance wait a few seconds, then proceed gently. Open stopcock and let fluid run in. If it seems to be flowing too fast pinch the tube with your finger and thumb. If patient complains of sharp pain, or is unable to retain fluid, stop flow for a minute. When all fluid has been run in slowly remove tube and place bedpan. Detach e. or rectal tube and place it in emesis basin; do not put it into the

can. See that patient is comfortable on pan, covered with the bath blankets and the signal within reach. Remove and care for e. tray. When patient has finished expelling e. remove pan and do perineal toilet as usual. Remove bath blankets and replace upper bedding. If patient has used toilet paper himself provide soap and water for his hands. Chart e. as directed.

     e., double-contrast. An e. of barium or other radiopaque material is injected and evacuated. This is followed by injection of air. X-rays of the lower intestinal tract are then taken.

     e., emollient. One given to soothe and protect the intestinal mucosa by making a coating over membranes, allaying local pain and irritation, and to act as a vehicle for the rectal administration of drugs.

     It should be given at a temperature of about 105° F. (40.6° C.). After giving, the record must show if the patient felt relieved, and to what extent; also if the solution was retained in its entirety.

     e., high. One to reach the colon. Insertion of rubber tube into rectum to carry water as far as possible.

     e., lubricating. Administered after an operation for hemorrhoids, and in order to soften the feces and lubricate the passage or anal canal to the external orifice or anus. When there is an impaction of feces, a lubricating e. may be given, followed in two hours by a cleansing e.

     Olive oil, four to six ounces (180 ml.), warmed, may be given, or cottonseed oil warmed in quantities of from four to six ounces in the evening. The patient should remain in a prone position with hips elevated for half an hour following the e. in order to help retain the oil and thus aiding it in passing higher in the colon.

     e., medicinal. An e. to which some drug or medication has been added on order of attending physician. It is necessary that this e. be retained and absorbed. It may be given to medicate diseased conditions of the rectum, sigmoid, or colon, or for absorption for its general effects. Although substances (other than fluids) are not absorbed in the large intestine as extensively as in the small intestine, the chemical changes that may occur must be very simple if any absorption may be expected. SEE: *preparations often given rectally.*

     e., nutrient or nutritive. One to give sustenance to a patient unable to be fed otherwise.

e., one-two-three. Magnesium sulfate, one ounce (30 ml.); glycerine, two ounces (60 ml.), and hot water, three ounces (90 ml.).

This mixture must be given with a small tube because of the small quantity, and the action desired. The results following the injection are more satisfactory if given very carefully with assistance to help the patient retain it.

e., physiological salt solution. One teaspoonful of salt to a pint of water is a normal salt solution. It may be abbreviated as N. S. Sol. The distention made by this enema excites peristalsis and evacuation. There is no harm in retaining this enema. Often ordered when there is dehydration.

e., quantity of. For retention, 100 to 240 ml. Cleansing: For a child: 240 to 360 ml.; infants: 15 to 60 ml.; adults: 960 to 1930 ml. (approx. one to two liters).

e., retention. May be used to provide nourishment, to medicate a diseased mucous membrane, or for absorption purposes, or for general, local, or systemic action. This e. must be of constituents which will not stimulate the nerve endings and reflexly promote peristalsis. It necessarily must consist of a small amt. of solution. The rectum and lower bowel must first be well cleansed, and all irritation resulting from evacuation must subside before giving, or the purpose will be defeated. The patient should be placed on left side with knees flexed, and the rectal tube inserted high; six inches or more. Before inserting, allow the fluid to flow through the tube to expel air. Pressure on tube should be made with fingers to prevent loss of liquid. Lubricate tube before inserting, and introduce with a twisting motion, slowly pushing it in so as not to bring discomfort to the patient. Unless absolutely necessary, the tube should not be slipped forward or backward to make the solution flow. Pushing may stimulate peristalsis. If the fluid does not readily flow, grasp tube in one hand, squeezing, compressing, and relaxing, so that suction will cause solution to flow. Allow fluid to run very slowly, stopping occasionally to aid retention. If the least desire to expel is manifested fluid should be stopped until the desire to evacuate has passed. Upon withdrawal of tube, which should be done quickly, pressure with a pad of cotton should be made over anus for a minute or two to prevent evacuation. The patient should be informed of the purpose of this enema so that cooperation may be secured.

e., saline. One with solution salt or magnesium sulfate in warm water.

e., soapsuds. The soapsuds are either ready prepared, or may be made by placing soap particles in a shaker and agitating the water until the right consistency is obtained. If liquid soap is used, one ounce to one quart (30 to 1000 ml.) of water is the right proportion. A milky solution is of sufficient strength. Strong soapsuds should not be used, as there is danger of injuring the intestinal mucosa. The mild white soaps, such as castile, are best for suds.

Incompatibilities: magnesium sulfate.

enema, words pert. to: clyster; coloclyster; colonic irrigation; enteroclysis; medication routes, rectal.

enepidermic (ĕn″ep-ĭ-dĕr′mĭk) [Gr. *en*, in, + *epi*, upon, + *derma*, skin]. Applied to or placed upon the surface of the skin. A term used in connection with application of medicinal agents to the skin without friction. SEE: *inunction.*

energometer (ĕn″ĕr-gŏm′ĕ-tĕr) ["+ *ergon*, work, + *metron*, measure]. An instrument for measuring blood pressure. Especially one used in studying pulse pressure.

energy (ĕn′ĕr-jĭ) [Gr. *en-*, at, + *ergon*, work]. The capacity of a system for doing work or its equivalent in the strict physical sense. E. is manifested in various forms: Motion (kinetic e.), position (potential e.), light, heat, sound, and so on. These forms are mutually interchangeable according to certain laws. Thus, the chemical e. residing in one gram of glucose can be liberated in the form of heat, so that if complete oxidation (to carbon dioxide and water) is carried out at 20° C. and atmospheric pressure, one obtains 3.74 Calories (or kilocalories, abbr: *kcal*) of heat. This fact is fundamental in the science of dietetics. SEE: *calorie.*

e. changes. These may be physical or chemical, or both. Movement of a part of the body, as the arm, shortens and thickens the muscles involved and changes the position and size of cells, temporarily, but the intake of oxygen in the blood, combining with sugar and fat, creates a chemical change, producing heat (i.e. energy) and waste products within the cells, which in turn produce fatigue.

e., conservation of. The theory that no e. can be lost, but that it may be transformed into other forms.

e., latent. That which exists but which is not being used.

e., potential. SEE: *e., latent.*

e., radiant. That form of e. which is transmitted through space without the support of a sensible medium. Radio waves, infrared waves, visible rays, ultraviolet waves, x-rays, gamma rays and cosmic rays are e. in this form.

e., static. SEE: *e., latent.*

energy, words pert. to: "chemo-" words; dietetics; kinesis; kinetic; metabolism; radiant; synergic; unit.

enerva'tion [L. *ex-*, removal, + *nervus*, nerve, sinew]. 1. Deficient in nervous strength; weakness. 2. Resection or removal of a nerve.

engagement. In obstetrics, the entrance of the fetal head or the part being presented into the superior pelvic strait.

En'gelmann's disk. [Theodor W. Engelmann, Ger. physiologist, 1843-1909] A narrow zone of transparent material lying on each side of the intermediate disk in the isotropic or I disk of a striated muscle fiber.

englobe [Gr. *en*, in, + L. *globus*, a ball]. To absorb within a spherical body, as the ingestion of bacteria by the phagocytes.

engorged (ĕn-gŏrjd') [O.Fr. *engorgier*, to obstruct, to devour]. Distended, as with blood.

engorge'ment. Vascular congestion; distention.

engram (ĕn'grăm) [Gr. *en*, in, + *gramma*, mark]. 1. In neurology, a pattern of nervous activity established in performing a skilled act. 2. In psychiatry, a loose term referring to the memory or psychical trace produced by an experience.

engraphia (ĕn-grăf'ĭ-ă) ["+ *graphein*, to write]. The process of making engrams, q.v.

enhematospore (ĕn-hem'ă-to-spōr") ["+ *haima*, blood, + *sporos*, spore]. A spore of the malarial parasite.

enhemospore (ĕn-hem'o-spōr). Enhematospore, q.v.

enissophobia (ĕn-is"o-fō'bĭ-ă) [Gr. *enissein*, to reproach, + *phobos*, fear]. Fear of criticism, esp. for having committed a sin.

enkatarrhaphy (ĕn"kăt-ar'af-ĭ) [Gr. *enkatarrhaptein*, to sew in]. Burying of structure by suturing adjacent tissue over it.

enolase (ē'no-lās). An enzyme present in muscle tissue which converts phosphoglyceric acid to phosphopyruvic acid.

enomania (e"no-mā'nĭ-ă) [Gr. *oinos*, wine, + *mania*, madness]. Craving for alcoholic beverages; delirium tremens.

enophthalmus (en"of-thăl'mŭs) [Gr. *en*, in, + *ophthalmos*, eye]. Recession of eyeball into orbit.

enosimania (ĕn"os-ĭ-mā'nĭ-ă) [Gr. *enosis*, a quaking, + *mania*, madness]. A mental state characterized by excessive and irrational terror.

enostosis (en"os-tō'sĭs) [Gr. *en-*, in, + *osteon*, bone, + *ōsis*, condition]. An osseous tumor within the cavity of a bone.

ensiform (ĕn'sĭ-form) [L. *ensis*, sword, + *forma*, form]. Swordlike structure.

e. cartilage. Lower part of sternum, below the gladiolus. SYN: *xiphoid cartilage* or *process.* SEE: *xiphodynia.*

ensisternum (ĕn"sĭ-ster'num) ["+ Gr. *sternon*, sternum]. The tip of the sternum; ensiform or xiphoid appendix. SYN: *metasternum.*

enstrophe (en'stro-fe) [Gr. *en*, in, + *strephein*, to turn]. Inversion; a turning inward, esp. of eyelids.

en'tad ["+ L. *ad*, toward]. Toward the inside; inwardly.

en'tal [Gr. *entos*, within]. Pert. to the interior; inside, central.

entamebiasis (ĕnt"ă-me-bī'ă-sĭs) ["+ *amoibē*, change]. Infestation with Entamoeba.

Entamoeba (ent-ă-me'bă). A genus of ameba several of which live in the intestine of man. Some are parasitic. Characterized by the presence of 4 or 8 nuclei in their cysts.

E. buccalis. E. gingivalis, q.v.

E. coli. Found normally in the upper intestinal tract. Nonpathogenic to man.

E. gingivalis. Nonpathogenic species which inhabits the mouth.

E. histolytica. A pathogenic form of ameba, the cause of amebic dysentery and tropical abscess.

E. kartulisi. Found in the pus of necrotic bone abscesses.

E. tetrage'na. Now considered identical with E. histolytica, q.v.

E. un'dulans. A species found in the intestine.

entasia, entosis (en-ta'sĭ-ă, en'tō-sĭs) [Gr. *entasis*, a straining]. Spasmodic muscular contraction.

entelechy (ĕn-tĕl'ĕ-kĭ) [Gr. *entelekheia*, actuality]. 1. The complete realization or expression of a vital function. 2. In philosophy, a vital force urging someone to complete fulfillment.

enteradenitis (ĕn"tĕr-ad"e-nī'tĭs) [Gr. *enteron*, intestine, + *adēn*, gland, + *-itis*, inflammation]. Inflammation of intestinal glands.

en'teral [Gr. *enteron*, intestine]. Within the intestine as distinguished from *parenteral*, q.v.

enteralgia (ĕn"tĕr-ăl'jĭ-ă) ["+ *algos*, pain]. Neuralgia or pain in the intestines. Intestinal cramps or colic.

enterectasia (ĕn"tĕr-ĕk-tā'sĭ-ă) ["+ *ektasis*, dilatation]. Dilatation of the small intestines.

enterectomy (ĕn"tĕr-ĕk'tō-mĭ) [Gr. *enteron*, intestine, + *ektomē*, excision]. Excision of a portion of the intestines.

enterelcosis (ĕn″tĕr-el-kō'sis) ["+ *elkōsis*, ulceration]. Intestinal ulceration.

enterepiplocele (ĕn″tĕr-ep-ip'lo-sēl) ["+ *epiploon*, omentum, + *kēlē*, hernia]. Hernia involving the bowel and omentum.

enteric (ĕn-tĕr'ĭk) [Gr. *enteron*, intestine]. Pert. to the intestinal tract.

    e. -coated tablets. Tablets which are coated with a substance that does not dissolve until reaching the intestine where the drug is then released.

    e. fever. Typhoid fever.

enter'icoid ["+ *eidos*, resemblance]. Resembling typhoid fever.

enteritis (ĕn-tĕr-ī'tĭs) ["+ *-itis*, inflammation]. Inflammation of the intestines, more particularly of the mucous and submucous tissues usually of the small intestines.

entero-, enter- [Gr. *enteron*, intestine]. Prefix: Noting some relation to the intestines.

enteroanastomosis (ĕn″tĕr-o-ăn-ăs″to-mō'sĭs) ["+ *ana*, up, + *stomōsis*, a mouth]. Intestinal anastomosis.

enteroan'tigen ["+ *anti*, against, + *gennan*, to form]. An antigen derived from the intestines.

enteroapokleisis (ĕn″tĕr-o-ap″o-kli'sis) ["+ *apokleisis*, a shutting out]. Operation for exclusion of a part of the intestine.

enterobacteriotherapy (ĕn″tĕr-o-băk-tē″rĭ-o-thĕr'ă-pī) ["+ *bakterion*, little rod, + *therapeia*, treatment]. Use of vaccines containing intestinal bacteria.

enterobi'asis [Gr. *enteron*, intestine, + *bios*, life]. Infestation with pinworms (Enterobius vermicularis).

enterobil'iary ["+ L. *bilis,* bile]. Pert. to the intestines and the bile passages.

Enterobius (ĕn″tĕr-ō'bĭ-us) ["+ *bios*, life]. A genus of parasitic nematode worms, formerly Oxyuris vermicularis.

    E. vermicularis. A species of nematode worms which inhabits the cecum, appendix, and neighboring regions of the intestine. In females, the genital organs and bladder may become infected. Female worms average 8 to 13 mm. in length, male worms, 2 to 5 mm. Distribution is worldwide. Infestations characterized by irritation of the anal region and allergic reaction of the neighboring skin, accompanied by intense itching which may result in loss of sleep, excessive irritability, and a secondary infection of the area around the anus as a result of the scratching. SYN: *pinworm.*

enterobro'sia [Gr. *enteron*, intestine, + *brōsis*, an eating]. Perforation of the intestine.

enterocęle (ĕn'tĕr-o-sēl) ["+ *kēlē*, hernia]. 1. A hernia of the intestine. 2. Posterior vaginal hernia.

enterocentesis (ĕn″tĕr-o-sen-te'sis) ["+ *kentēsis*, puncture]. Puncture of intestine to withdraw gas or fluids.

enterochirurgia (ĕn″tĕr-o-ki-rur'jĭ-ă) ["+ *cheir*, hand, + *ergon*, work]. Intestinal surgery.

enterocholecystostomy (ĕn″tĕr-o-ko″le-sĭs-tōs'tō-mĭ) [Gr. *enteron*, intestine, + *cholē*, bile, + *kystis*, a bladder, + *stōma*, opening]. Making an opening between the gallbladder and small intestine. SYN: *cholecystenterostomy.*

enterocholecystotomy (ĕn″tĕr-o-ko″le-sĭs-tōt'ō-mĭ) ["+ "+ *tomē*, incision]. Incision of both gallbladder and intestine.

enterocinesia (ĕn″tĕr-o-sĭn-ē'sĭ-ă) ["+ *kinēsis*, movement]. Intestinal movement. SYN: *peristalsis.*

enterocinetic (ĕn″tĕr-o-sĭn-ĕt'ĭk). Pert. to or promoting peristalsis.

enteroclysis (ĕn″tĕr-ok'lĭ-sĭs) [Gr. *enteron*, intestine, + *klysis*, a washing out]. 1. Injection of a nutrient or medicinal liquid into bowel. 2. Irrigation of colon with large amt. of fluid intended to fill the colon completely and flush it. SYN: *enteroclysm.*

en'teroclysm. A high enema. SYN: *enteroclysis.*

enterococcus (ĕn″tĕr-o-kŏk'ŭs). Any species of streptococcus inhabiting the intestine.

enterocoele (ĕn'tĕr-ō-sēl) [Gr. *enteron*, intestine, + *koilia*, hollow]. The abdominal cavity.

enterocolitis (ĕn″tĕr-o-kō-lī'tĭs) ["+ *kōlon*, colon, + *itis*, inflammation]. Inflammation of intestines and colon. This serious condition may be so acute as to require immediate treatment of shock, regulation of electrolyte balance, and antibiotics if ordered by physician.

enterocrinin (ĕn″tĕr-ok'rĭ-nin) ["+ *krinein*, to separate]. Hormone from animal intestines which aids digestion by stimulating the secretion of intestinal juice by the intestinal glands.

enterocyst (ĕn'tĕr-o-sĭst) ["+ *kystis,* bladder]. A cyst of the intestinal wall.

enterocystocele (ĕn″tĕr-o-sĭs'to-sēl) [Gr. *enteron*, intestine, + "+ *kēlē*, hernia]. Hernia of the bladder wall and intestine.

enterocysto'ma ["+ "+ *ōma*, tumor]. Cystic tumor of the intestinal wall. SYN: *enterocyst.*

enterodyn'ia ["+ *odynē*, pain]. Pain in the intestine. SYN: *enteralgia.*

enteroenterostomy (ĕn″tĕr-o-ĕn″tĕr-ŏs'tō-mĭ) [Gr. *enteron*, intestine, + *enteron*, intestine, + *stōma,* opening]. Formation of a communication between two segments (not continuous) of the intestine.

enteroepiplocele (ĕn″tĕr-ō-ē-pĭp′lō-sēl) ["+ *epiplōon,* omentum, + *kēlē,* hernia]. Hernia of small intestine and omentum.

enterogastritis (ĕn″tĕr-o-găs-trī′tĭs) ["+ *gastēr,* belly, + *ītis,* inflammation]. Inflammation of stomach (gastritis) and of the intestines (enteritis).

enterogastrone (ĕn″tĕr-ō-găs′trōn). A hormone secreted by the intestinal mucosa which, by depressing gastric motility and secretion, controls the release of food from the stomach into the duodenum. A meal high in fat content will cause greater secretion of this hormone than will a normal feeding.

enterogenous (ĕn″tĕr-ŏj′ĕ-nŭs) [Gr. *enteron,* intestine, + *gennan,* to produce]. Originating in the intestines.

en′terogram ["+ *gramma,* mark]. Tracing or graph of intestinal movements.

enterog′raphy ["+ *graphein,* to write]. 1. A description of the intestines. 2. Making of an enterogram.

enterohepatic (ĕn″tĕr-o-hĕ-păt′ĭk) ["+ *hēpar, hēpat-,* liver]. Pert. to intestines and the liver.

enterohepatitis (ĕn″tĕr-o-hĕp-ă-tī′tĭs) ["+ "+ *ītis,* inflammation]. Inflamed condition of both intestine and liver.

enterohydrocele (ĕn″tĕr-o-hī′dro-sēl) ["+ *hydōr,* water, + *kēlē,* hernia]. Hydrocele with loop of intestine in the sac.

enteroidea (ĕn″tĕr-oyd′e-ă) [Gr. *enteron,* intestine, + *eidos,* form]. The intestinal fevers; those caused by intestinal bacilli including typhoid fever.

enterokinase (ĕn″tĕr-ō-ki′nās) ["+ *kinēsis,* movement]. A substance or hormone occurring in the mucosa of the duodenum, necessary for the activation of the trypsinogen of the pancreatic juice which is converted into trypsin. One of the enzymes of the succus entericus. It has no fat-splitting properties.
RS: enzyme; trypsin; trypsinogen.

enterolith (ĕn′tĕr-o-līth) ["+ *lithos,* stone]. An intestinal concretion.

enterolithiasis (ĕn″tĕr-o-lĭ-thī′ă-sĭs). The formation or existence of intestinal calculi.

enterol′ogy [Gr. *enteron,* intestine, + *logos,* study]. The study of the intestinal tract.

enteromegalia, enteromegaly (ĕn″tĕr-o-mĕ-ga′lĭ-a, ĕn″tĕr-o-mĕg′ă-lĭ) ["+ *megas,* large]. Abnormal enlargement of the intestines. SYN: *megacolon; megaloenteron.*

Enteromonas hominis (ĕn″tĕr-ŏm′ŏ-nās). A minute flagellated, protozoan parasite

which lives in the intestine of man. It is rare and considered nonpathogenic.

enteromycosis (ĕn″tĕr-o-mī-kō′sĭs) [Gr. *enteron,* intestine, + *mykēs,* fungus, + *-ōsis,* diseased condition]. Disease of intestine due to bacteria or fungi.

enteromyiasis (ĕn″tĕr-ō-mī-ī′ă-sĭs) ["+ *myia,* fly]. Disease due to the presence of maggots (the larvae of flies) in the intestines.

enteron (ĕn′tĕr-ŏn) [Gr.]. The intestine.

enteroneuritis (ĕn″tĕr-o-nū-rī′tĭs) [Gr. *enteron,* intestine, + *neuron,* nerve, + *ītis,* inflammation]. Inflammation of nerves of the intestines.

enteronitis (ĕn″tĕr-on-ī′tĭs) ["+ *ītis,* inflammation]. Inflammation of the small intestine. SYN: *enteritis.*

enteroparesis (ĕn″tĕr-o-par′ē-sis) ["+ *paresis,* relaxation]. Flaccidity of the intestinal walls with diminished peristalsis.

enteropathy (ĕn″tĕr-ŏp′ă-thĭ) ["+ *pathos,* disease]. Any intestinal disease.

enteropexy (ĕn′tĕr-o-pĕks′ĭ) [Gr. *enteron,* intestine, + *pēxis,* fixation]. Fixation of the intestine to the abdominal wall.

enteroplasty (ĕn′tĕr-o-plăs-tĭ) ["+ *plassein,* to form]. Plastic operation on intestines. NP: Watch diet and fluid orders. Care of mouth. SEE: *laparotomy.*

enteroplegia (ĕn″tĕr-o-plē′jĭ-ă) ["+ *plēgē,* stroke]. Paralysis of intestines. SEE: *paralytic ileus.*

enteroplex (ĕn′tĕr-o-plĕks) ["+ *plexis,* a weaving]. Instrument for joining cut edges of intestines.

en′teroplexy. Union of divided parts of the intestine.

enteroproctia (ĕn″tĕr-o-prŏk′shĭ-ă) [Gr. *enteron,* intestine, + *proktos,* anus]. The condition of having an artificial anus.

enteroptosis (ĕn″tĕr-ŏp-tō′sĭs) ["+ *ptōsis,* a dropping]. Prolapse of the intestine or abdominal organs.

enterorrhagia (ĕn″tĕr-o-ra′jĭ-ă) ["+ *rēgnunai,* to burst forth]. Hemorrhage from the intestines.

enterorrhaphy (ĕn″tĕr-or′ă-fĭ) ["+ *raphē,* suture]. The stitching of the lips of an intestinal wound, or of the intestines to some other structure.

enterorrhexis (ĕn″tĕr-o-rĕks′ĭs) [Gr. *enteron,* intestine, + *rhēxis,* rupture]. Rupture of the intestine.

enteroscope (ĕn′tĕr-o-skōp) ["+ *skopein,* to examine]. Device for examination of intestines.

enterosep′sis ["+ *sēpsis,* decay]. Intestinal toxemia; sepsis developed from the intestinal contents.

enterosite (ĕn'tĕr-o-sīt) [Gr. *enteron*, intestine, + *parasite*]. Any parasite which inhabits the intestinal tract.

enterospasm (ĕn'tĕr-o-spăzm) ["+ *spasmos*, spasm]. Intermittent painful contractions of the intestines.

enterosta'sis ["+ *stasis*, a standing]. Intestinal stasis. Cessation of or delay in the passage of food through the intestine.

enterostenosis (ĕn"tĕr-o-ste-nō'sĭs) ["+ *stēnōsis*, a narrowing]. Narrowing or stricture of the intestine.

enterostomy (ĕn"tĕr-ŏs'tō-mĭ) [Gr. *enteron*, intestine, + *stoma*, opening]. Surgical formation of a permanent opening into the intestine through the abdominal wall.

enterotome (ĕn'tĕr-o-tōm) ["+ *tomē*, incision]. Instrument for incision of intestines.

enterotomy (ĕn-tĕr-ŏt'ō-mĭ). Incision or dissection of the intestines.

enterotoxin (ĕn"tĕr-o-tŏk'sĭn) [Gr. *enteron*, intestine, + *toxikon*, poison]. 1. A toxin produced in or originating in the intestinal contents. 2. A toxin specific for the cells of the mucosa. 3. A toxin produced by certain species of bacteria which produces symptoms characteristic of food poisoning.

enterotox'ism. Absorption of toxins from the intestinal contents. SYN: *enterosepsis.*

enterotrop'ic [Gr. *enteron*, intestine, + *tropē*, a turning]. Affecting or attracted by the intestines.

enterovaccine (ĕn"tĕr-o-văk'sēn) ["+ L. *vacca*, a cow]. A vaccine composed of fecal bacteria.

enterovi'rus. A virus which multiplies in the human gastrointestinal tract. Includes Coxsackie viruses, polioviruses, ECHO viruses, rhinoviruses, and others which are unclassified.

enterozo'ic [Gr. *enteron*, intestine, + *zōon*, animal]. Pert. to parasites inhabiting the intestines.

enterozo'on. Any intestinal animal parasite.

entheomania (ĕn"the-o-mā'nĭ-ā) [Gr. *entheos*, inspired, + *mania*, madness]. Religious insanity.

enthesis (en'thē-sis) [Gr. a putting in]. The use of metallic or other inorganic substances to substitute for or replace lost tissue.

enthetic (en-thĕt'ik). 1. Pert. to enthesis, q.v. 2. Introduced from outside. SYN: *exogenous.*

enthlasis (en'thlă-sis) [Gr. a dent]. Depressed fracture of the skull.

entity (ĕn'tĭ-tē") [L. *ens*, being]. 1. A thing existing independently, containing in itself all the conditions necessary to individuality. 2. That which forms a complete whole, denoting a distinct condition or disease.

ento- [Gr. *entos*, within]. Prefix indicating within, inside.

en'toblast ["+ *blastos*, germ]. 1. The entoderm, q.v., or hypoblast. 2. The cell nucleolus.

entocele (ĕn'to-sēl) ["+ *kēlē*, hernia]. 1. Internal hernia. 2. Displacement of a part, inward.

entochondrostosis (ĕn"to-kŏn"dros-tō'sĭs) ["+ *chondros*, cartilage, + *ōsis*, formation of]. The development of bone within cartilage.

entochoroidea (ĕn"to-ko-roy'de-ă) ["+ *chorioeidēs*, choroid]. The inner layer of the choroid; coat of the eye.

entocineria (ĕn"to-sĭn-e'rĭ-ă) [Gr. *entos*, within, + L. *cinereus*, ashen]. The internal gray matter of nerve centers, esp. of the brain.

entocone (ĕn'to-kōn) ["+ *kōnos*, cone]. The inner posterior cusp of an upper molar tooth.

entocor'nea ["+ L. *corneus*, horny]. Posterior or inner lining membrane of cornea. SYN: *Descemet's membrane.*

entocyte (ĕn'to-sīt) ["+ *kytos*, hollow vessel]. Interior part of a cell within the ectoplasm. SYN: *endoplasm.*

entoderm (ĕn'to-dĕrm) ["+ *derma*, skin]. Inner layer of cells in the blastoderm, q.v. Innermost of the three primary germ layers of a developing embryo. It gives rise to the epithelium of the digestive tract and its associated glands, the respiratory organs, bladder, vagina and urethra. SYN: *endoderm; hypoblast.*

entoectad (ĕn"to-ĕk'tăd) [Gr. *entos*, within, + *ektos*, without, + L. *ad*, toward]. From within outward.

entome (ĕn'tōm) [Gr. *en*, in, + *tomē*, a cut]. Knife for division of urethral stricture.

entomion (ĕn-tō'mĭ-on) [Gr. *entomē*, notch]. The tip of mastoid angle of the parietal bone.

entomol'ogy [Gr. *entomon*, insect, + *logos*, science]. The study of insects.

   e., medical. That branch of entomology which deals with insects and their relationship to disease.

entophyte (ĕn'to-fit) [Gr. *entos*, within, + *phyton*, plant]. Any vegetable parasite living within the body.

entopic [Gr. *en*, in, + *topos*, place]. Normally situated; in a normal place.

entoptic (ĕn-tŏp'tĭk) [Gr. *entos*, within, + *optikos*, seeing]. Pert. to the interior of the eye.

   e. phenomena. Visual phenomena arising from within the eye, characterized by seeing floating bodies, circles of light, black spots, and transient flashes of light. May be due to person seeing his own blood cells move through the retinal vessels or floaters which are small specks of tissue floating in the vitreous fluid. SEE: *photopsia.*

entoptoscopy (ĕn″tŏp-tos′ko-pĭ) [" + *ōps,* eye, + *skopein,* to examine]. Visual examination of the interior of the eye. SEE: *ophthalmoscopy.*

entoret′ina [" + L. *rete,* a net]. Internal layer of the retina.

entorrhagia (ĕn-tor-ā′jĭ-ă) [" + *rhēgnynai,* to burst forth]. Enterorrhagia.

entotic (ĕnt-ō′tĭk, ĕnt-ŏt′ĭk) [Gr. *entos,* within, + *ous, ot-,* ear]. Pert. to interior of ear or to perception of sound due to condition of the auditory apparatus.

entozoon (ĕn″to-zō′ŏn) [" + *zōon,* animal]. (pl. *entozo′a)* Any animal parasite living within the body of another animal.

entrophia (ĕn-trō′fĭ-ă) [Gr. *en,* in, + *trophē,* nourishment]. Normal growth and nourishment.

entro′pion [" + *trepein,* to turn]. Inward curling of eyelid, esp. lower lid, with lashes.

e., cicatricial. An e. resulting from scar tissue on the inner surface of the lid.

e., spastic. An e. resulting from a spasm of the orbicularis oculi muscles.

entro′pionize. To invert or correct by turning in.

entro′pium. Entropion, q.v.

entropy (ĕn′trō-pĭ). That portion of energy within a system which cannot be utilized for mechanical work but is available for internal use.

enucleate (ē-nū′klē-āt) [L. *enucleāre,* to remove the kernel of]. 1. To remove a tumor or a structure from the body without rupturing; to remove a part in its entirety. 2. To destroy or take out the nucleus of a cell.

enucleation (ē-nū″klē-ā′shŭn). 1. Removal of a tumor or structure from its capsule. 2. Removal of the eyeball.

enu′cleator. Instrument for separating a tumor mass, as a myoma.

enuresis (ĕn″ū-rē′sĭs) [Gr. *enourein,* to void urine]. Incontinence. Involuntary urination, complete or partial, diurnal or nocturnal, dependent upon pathological or functional causes, although it may be voluntary as representative of a behavior pattern.

A child, for instance, may feel neglected or feel a desire for attention, and attempt to center attention upon himself by deliberately wetting his bed. Urinary control, however, is generally established after the second year, although incontinence may be reestablished as a pathological manifestation.

Condition in adults is called incontinence, q.v.

e., diurnal. Urinary incontinence during the day. Its etiology is of a pathological nature. It may be caused by muscular contractions brought about by laughing, coughing, or crying. Often persists for long periods of time, esp. after protracted illness, but more frequently in the female.

ETIOL: Enuresis may result from urethral irritation, and fecal incontinence is sometimes associated with it. Excessive water drinking may contribute to e. There may be a neurological basis due to injury to the spinal cord, cystitis may be present, and it may be associated with various diseases such as diabetes insipidus and mellitus, epilepsy, or mental deficiency.

Children suffering from enuresis may be shy and sensitive; sometimes gloomy. These nervous manifestations may result from the reaction to the condition, or they may be a part of the behavior pattern of which the enuresis is a symptom.

Devices which awaken the child the moment the bed is wet are available. The value of this type of therapy is unknown.

NP: Examine the urine for evidence of infection. Great concern or censure should be avoided as it adds to apprehensiveness on part of child. If the result of a behavior pattern, the condition should be ignored as much as possible, but the cause of the behavior difficulty needs to be found and corrected.

Fluid should be restricted late in day, and diurnal voidings should be spaced at more than ordinary intervals. The child may be awakened once or twice in the night and when fully awake, robed and walked to the bathroom. As improvement is noticed the number of awakenings may be lessened. The foot of the bed may also be elevated.

e., nocturnal. Urinary incontinence during the night. Wetting is irregular and unaccompanied by urgency or frequency. Incontinence may cease for several weeks only to return. This type is more common in boys than in girls.

envi′ronment [O. Fr. *en-,* in, + *viron,* circle]. The surroundings, conditions, or influences which affect an organism, or the cells within an organism.

e., external. Those influences which are outside the body.

e., internal. Those influences within the body. Specifically, the tissue fluid constitutes the internal environment.

enzygotic (ĕn″zĭ-gŏt′ĭk) [Gr. *en,* in, + *zygon,* yoke]. Developed from the same ovum.

e. twins. Identical twins; those developed from one ovum. SEE: *dizygotic twins.*

enzyme (ĕn′zīm) ["+ *zymē*, leaven]. An organic catalyst produced by living cells but capable of acting independently. They are complex proteins which are capable of inducing chemical changes in other substances without being changed themselves in the process.

E.'s are found particularly in digestive juices acting upon food substances, causing them to break down into simpler compounds. They are capable of accelerating greatly the speed of chemical reactions.

The reactions effected by the digestive e.'s are chiefly decompositions of a hydrolytic nature, but e.'s are equally important in the synthetic reactions of assimilation.

Each hydrolytic e. has been given a name indicating the substance upon which it acts with the addition of the suffix -*ase*. Ex: lipases indicate fat-splitting e.'s; amylases starch-splitting ones; and proteases, protein-splitting e.'s. Some of them take a qualifying adjective, as salivary or pancreatic e.'s. Some of the best-known enzymes such as rennin, pepsin, trypsin, and thrombin do not end in -*ase*.

Summary of the Main Enzymatic Processes in Digestion*

Site	Secretion	Enzyme	Substrate	Degree of Digestion	Products of Digestion
Mouth	Saliva	Ptyalin	Starch	Slight	Dextrins, maltose
		Maltase	Maltose	Very slight	Glucose
Stomach	Gastric juice	Pepsin	Protein	Incomplete	Proteoses, peptones
		Rennin	Casein	Nearly complete	Paracasein
		Lipase	Emulsified fats	Very slight	Fatty acids, glycerol
Intestine	Pancreatic juice	Trypsin Chymo-trypsin Carboxy-peptidase	{ Proteins Proteoses Peptones Peptides }	Nearly complete	Amino acids
		Steapsin	Fats	Nearly complete	Insoluble fatty acids, glycerol
		Amylopsin	Starch	Nearly complete	Dextrins, maltose
Intestine	Intestinal juice and intestinal mucosa	Erepsin	Ordinary peptides	Nearly complete	Amino acids
		Amylase	Starch	Nearly complete	Dextrins, maltose
		Enterokinase	Trypsinogen		Trypsin
		Maltase	Maltose	Complete	Glucose
		Lactase	Lactose	Complete	Glucose, galactose
		Sucrase	Sucrose	Usually complete	Glucose, fructose
		Nucleosidases (in mucosa)	Nucleosides	Usually complete	Purine bases, carbohydrates

*Adapted from Biddle, H. C., and Floutz, V. W.: Chemistry in Health and Disease, ed. 6. F. A. Davis Company, Philadelphia, 1965.

The substance acted upon by an e. is called the substrate. Zymogen is the name given to the precursor of an e. The more common groups of e.'s are: Hydrolytic e.'s; fat-, protein-, starch-, and sugar-splitting e.'s; coagulating e.'s or those which cause clotting, such as rennin or thrombin; oxidases or oxidizing e.'s; deamidizing e.'s, those which are important in removing amines or amino groups during oxidation; reductases or reducing e.'s; splitting enzymes; joining enzymes.

E.'s are specific in their action, i.e., they will act only upon a certain substance or a group of closely-related chemical substances and no other; each e. has an optimum temperature at which it acts with greatest efficiency; each e. is influenced by the reaction of the medium in which it acts, there being an optimum degree of acidity or alkalinity.

E. activity can be retarded or inhibited by low temperatures; high temperatures; presence of salts of heavy metals (copper, mercury); dehydration; ultraviolet radiation.

E.'s sometimes require the presence of additional substances in order to make them active. Nonspecific substances which activate enzymes are called activators (Ex: HCl for pepsin); specific substances which act selectively with certain enzymes only are called coenzymes (Ex: enterokinase for trypsinogen). More than 650 known enzymes.

e., amylolytic. E. changing starch to sugar.

e., autolytic. E. producing autolysis, or cell digestion.

e., bacterial. E. developed by bacteria.

e., coagulating. E. converting soluble proteins into insoluble ones. Ex: rennin. A coagulase.

e., deamidizing. E. dividing amino acids into ammonia compounds.

e., decarboxylating. E. which separates CO_2 from organic acids. (Ex: carboxylase).

e., digestive. E. which is involved in digestive processes in the alimentary canal.

e., extracellular. E. which produces its effects outside the cell that produces it.

e., fermenting. E. produced by bacteria or yeasts which bring about the fermentation of substances, esp. carbohydrates.

e., glycolytic. E. oxidizing sugar.

e., hydrolytic. E. which reacts on a substance to form smaller molecules by the addition of water.

e., inorganic. A metallic colloidal solution, acting somewhat like an e.

e., intracellular. An e. that acts within the cell which produces it.

e., inverting. E. that converts a double sugar (sucrose) into simple sugars.

e., lipolytic. E. that acts on fats hydrolyzing them to glycerol and fatty acids; a lipase.

e., oxidation. E., deamidizing, q.v.

e., oxidizing. E. that catalyzes oxidative reactions; an oxidase or dehydrogenase.

e., polypeptolytic. E. having a hydrolytic action on the polypeptides.

e., proteolytic. E. changing proteins into peptones.

e., reducing. Reductase. E. that removes oxygen.

e., respiratory. E. that acts within tissue cells catalyzing oxidative reactions with the release of energy. Ex: cytochromes; flavoproteins.

e., uricolytic. E. converting uric acid into urea.

e., yellow. A flavoprotein. One of a group of e.'s involved in cellular oxidations.

enzymolysis (ĕn-zĭm-ŏl′ĭ-sĭs) [Gr. *en*, in, + *zymē*, leaven, + *lysis*, dissolution]. Chemical change or disintegration caused by an enzyme.

enzymo′sis ["+ "+ *ōsis*, condition]. Enzymolysis.

enzymuria (ĕn″zĭm-ū′rĭ-ă) ["+ "+ *ouron*, urine]. Enzymes in the urine.

eonism (ē′ō-nĭzm). [Chevalier d'Eon, Fr. political adventurer, 1728–1810]. Desire to dress in the clothing of the opposite sex. SYN: *transvestism*, q.v.

eosin (ē′ō-sĭn) [Gr. *ēōs*, dawn (rose colored)]. 1. A dye derived from action of bromine on fluorescein, $C_{20}H_8Br_4O_5$. An acid dye much used for staining tissues for microscopic examination. SYN: *tetrabromfluorescein*. 2. Any of several similar dyes. 3. Rosy-red; dawn colored.

eosin′oblast ["+ *blastos*, germ]. A bone marrow cell which develops into a myelocyte. SYN: *myeloblast*.

eosinopenia (ē″ō-sĭn-o-pe′nĭ-ă) ["+ *penia*, poverty]. Abnormally small number of eosinophil cells in the peripheral blood.

eosinophil (ē″ō-sĭn′ō-fĭl) ["+ *philein*, to love]. A cell or cellular structure that stains readily with the acid stain, eosin; specifically an eosinophil leukocyte.

e. leukocytes. Spherical cells having a diameter of 9 to 14 microns found in blood and sometimes in connective tissues. The nucleus is polymorphic usually having two lobes connected by a thin strand. The cytoplasm contains numerous coarse, highly refractile granules which stain intensely with eosin or other acid stains. They constitute 1% to 3% of the white cell count.

E. leukocytes originate in the red bone marrow. Their function is not well established. They are ameboid but do not exhibit phagocytic activity. They increase in number in certain diseases such as asthma and in certain infestations with animal parasites. They decrease in number in circulating blood following the administration of ACTH or cortisone.

eosinophile (ē″ō-sīn′ō-fil). 1. Eosinophilic. 2. Eosinophil, q.v.

eosinophilia (ē″ō-sīn-ō-fīl′ī-ă) [Gr. *ēōs*, dawn, + *philein*, to love]. 1. Accumulation of un-unusual number of eosinophils in the blood. 2. Condition of being eosinophilic with respect to staining characteristics.

eosinophilic (ē″ō-sīn-ō-fīl′ĭk). Readily stainable with eosin.

eosinophilous (ē″ō-sīn-ŏf′ĭ-lŭs) [Gr. *ēōs*, dawn, + *philein*, to love]. 1. Easily stainable with eosin. 2. Having eosinophilia.

eosinotactic (ē″ō-sīn-ō-tăk′tĭk) ["+ *taktikos*, arranged]. Attraction or repulsion of eosinophil cells.

epacmastic (ep″ak-mas′tĭk) [Gr. *epi*, upon, + *akmē*, point, summit]. Denoting increase of symptoms.

epactal (ē-păk′tăl) [Gr. *epaktos*, added to]. Supernumerary.

    e. bone. Wormian bone.

eparsalgia (ep″ar-săl′jĭ-ă) [Gr. *epairein*, to lift, + *algos*, pain]. Any disorder due to overstrain of a part.

eparterial (ēp″ăr-tē′rĭ-ăl) [Gr. *epi*, over, upon, + *artēria*, artery]. Located over or above an artery.

epaxial (ēp-ăk′sĭ-al) ["+ L. *axis*, axis]. Situated above or behind any axis.

epencephalon (ēp″en-sēf′ă-lŏn) ["+ *enkephalos*, brain]. The metencephalon; the anterior portion of the embryonic hindbrain (rhombencephalon) from which arise the pons and cerebellum.

ependyma (ēp-en′dĭ-mă) [Gr. *ependyma*, an upper garment, wrap]. [NA]. Membrane lining the cerebral ventricles and central canal of spinal cord.

    e. medullae spinalis. The spinal portion of the e.

    e. ventriculorum cerebri. The ventricular portion of the e.

ependymal (ēp-en′dĭ-măl). Pert. to the ependyma.

    e. cells. Cells of the developing neural tube which give rise to the ependyma. They arise from spongioblasts derived from the neural epithelium.

    e. layer. The innermost of three layers which form the neural tube of an embryo.

ependymitis (ēp″en-dĭ-mī′tĭs) [Gr. *ependyma*, an upper garment, wrap, + *itis*, inflammation]. Inflammation of the ependyma.

ependymoblast (ĕp-en′dĭ-mo-blăst) ["+ *blastos*, germ]. An embryonic ependymal cell or ependymocyte.

ependymocyte (ĕp-en′dĭ-mo-sīt) ["+ *kytos*, hollow vessel (cell)]. A cell of the ependymal region.

ependymo′ma ["+ *ōma*, tumor]. A tumor arising from fetal inclusion of ependymal elements.

ephebiatrics (ĕ-fē-bĭ-ăt′rĭks) [Gr. *epi*, at, + *hēbē*, youth, + *iatrikos*, medical]. A branch of medicine dealing with adolescents.

ephebic (ĕ-fē′bĭk) [Gr. *ephēbikos*, pert. to puberty]. Pert. to adolescence.

ephebology (ĕf-ē-bŏl′ō-jī) [Gr. *epi*, at, + *hēbē*, youth, + *logos*, study of]. The study of puberty and its changes.

ephedrine (ĕ-fēd′rĭn, ĕf′ĕ-drēn). An alkaloid originally obtained from species of Ephedra; first isolated by Nagai in 1887. In ancient Chinese medicine it was used as a diaphoretic and antipyretic. It was not until recent times, however, that its action was studied and its valuable therapeutic properties made known. It is a sympathomimetic drug, and is usually produced synthetically.

Action is similar to that of adrenalin. Its effects, although less powerful, are more prolonged, and it exerts an action when given orally, whereas adrenalin is effective only by injection. Ephedrine orally (or by injection) dilates the bronchial muscles, contracts the nasal mucosa, and raises the blood pressure. Chiefly used for its bronchodilator effect in asthma, and for its constricting effects on the nasal mucosa in hay fever.

INCOMPATIBILITIES: Calcium chloride; iodine; tannic acid.

    e. hydrochloride. A more soluble salt of the alkaloid, having the same action and uses as e.

    e. sulfate. USP. The sulfate of e. It occurs as fine white crystals or as a powder. Its action and uses are the same as those for e.

ephelis (ĕf-ē′lĭs) [Gr. *ephēlis*, freckle]. (pl. *ephelides*). Freckle, lentigo, q.v.

ephemeral (ĕ-fĕm′ĕr-ăl) [Gr. *epi*, on, + *hēmera*, day]. Of brief duration.

ephidrosis (ĕf′ĭ-drō′sĭs) [Gr., a sweating]. Abnormal amt. of sweating.

    e. cruenta. Sweat containing blood.

    e. tincta. Colored sweat. SYN: *chromidrosis.*

epi-, ep- [Gr.]. Prefix meaning upon, over, at, in addition to, after.

epiblast (ĕp′ĭ-blăst) [Gr. *epi*, upon, + *blastos*, germ]. Outer layer of cells of the blastoderm. SYN: *ectoderm*, q.v.

epiblastic (ĕp-ĭ-blas′tik). Pert. to the epiblast.

epibole, epiboly (ĕ-pĭb′ō-lĭ) [Gr. *epibolē*, cover]. Inclusion of the hypoblast within the epiblast, due to swifter growth of the latter. SEE: *emboly*.

epibulbar (ĕp′ĭ-bul′bar). Lying upon the bulb of any structure; more specifically, located upon the eyeball.

epican′thus [Gr. *epi*, upon, + *kanthos*, canthus]. A fold of skin extending from the root of the nose to the median end of the eyebrow, covering the inner canthus and caruncle. It is a characteristic of certain races and may occur as a congenital anomaly in Caucasians.

epicardia (ĕp′ĭ-kărd′ĭ-ă) [″+ *kardia*, heart]. The abdominal portion of the esophagus extending from the diaphragm to the stomach, about two cm. in length.

epicar′dium. [NA]. The inner or visceral layer of the pericardium, q.v., which forms a serous membrane forming the outermost layer of the wall of the heart.

epichordal (ĕp′ĭ-kŏrd′ăl) [Gr. *epi*, upon, + *khordē*, cord]. Located dorsad to the notochord.

epicomus (ĕ-pik′o-mus) [″+ *komē*, hair]. A congenital malformation consisting of a parasitic twin, or head attached to the summit or vertex of the skull.

epicondylalgia (ĕp′ĭ-kŏn-dĭ-lăl′jĭ-ă) [″+ *kondylos*, condyle, + *algos*, pain]. Pain in the elbow joint in the region of the epicondyles.

epicondyle (ĕp-ĭ-kŏn′dil) [″+ *kondylos*, condyle]. The eminence at the articular end of a bone above a condyle.

epicra′nium [Gr. *epi*, upon, + *kranion*, cranium]. Soft parts covering the cranium.

epicranius (ĕp′ĭ-krā′nĭ-us). Occipitofrontal muscle and scalp.

epicrisis (ĕp′ĭ-krī′sĭs) [Gr. *epi*, after, + *krisis*, crisis]. A secondary crisis following the initial critical stage of a disease.

epicritic (ĕp-ĭ-krĭt′ĭk) [Gr. *epikritikos*, judging]. 1. Pertaining to extreme sensibility, such as that of the skin when it discriminates between degrees of sensation caused by touch or temperature. 2. Pertaining to an epicrisis, q.v.

epicysti′tis [Gr. *epi*, upon, + *kystis*, bladder, + *itis*, inflammation]. Inflammation of cellular tissue above the bladder.

epicystotomy (ĕp′ĭ-sĭs-tŏt′ō-mĭ) [″+ ″+ *tomē*, incision]. Opening above the symphysis pubis into the bladder.

epicyte (ĕp′ĭ-sīt) [Gr. *epi*, around, covering, + *kytos*, hollow vessel (cell)]. 1. An epithelial cell. 2. A cell membrane.

epidemic (ĕp′ĭ-dĕm′ĭk) [Gr. *epi*, among, on, + *dēmos*, people]. Appearance of an infectious disease or condition which attacks many people at the same time in the same geographical area.

　e. jaundice. Infectious or spirochetal jaundice; Weil's disease. An infectious disease caused by a spirochete, Leptospira icterohaemorrhagiae. SYM: Onset of sudden fever, in a few days followed by jaundice, hemorrhage into skin, and anemia. SEE: *endemic; pandemic.*

　e. neuromyasthenia. A poorly defined condition including severe muscle and joint pain, transient gastrointestinal symptoms, usually lack of fever, and a prolonged course.
　ETIOL: Unknown. TREATMENT: Symptomatic. PROG: Complete recovery.

epidemiography (ĕp′ĭ-dē″mĭ-ŏg′ră-fĭ) [″+ ″+ *graphein*, to write]. Study of epidemics and epidemic diseases. Originally more or less limited to infectious diseases; the principles employed in studying those diseases can and have been successfully applied to a variety of disorders including cardiovascular diseases, drug toxicity, suicide, mental illness, accidents, and malnutrition.

epidemiologic (ĕp′ĭ-dē-mĭ-o-lŏj′ĭk) [″+ ″+ *logos*, study]. Pert. to the study of epidemics.

epidemiologist (ĕp′ĭ-dē-mĭ-ŏl′o-jĭst). One who applies his knowledge in the field of epidemiology.

epidemiology (ĕp-ĭ-dē-mĭ-ŏl′ō-jĭ). The division of medical science concerned with defining and explaining the interrelationships of the host, agent, and environment in causing disease; medical ecology.

epider′mal, epider′mic [Gr. *epi*, upon, over, + *derma*, skin]. Pert. to the epidermis.

epidermatoplasty (ĕp′ĭ-dĕr-măt′o-plăs-tĭ) [″+ ″+ *plassein*, to mold]. Grafting with pieces of epidermis with the underlying layer of the corium.

epidermic (ĕp-ĭ-dĕr′mĭk) [Gr. *epi*, over, + *derma*, skin]. Pert. to the external layer of the skin or epidermis.

epidermidolysis (ĕp′ĭ-dĕr″mĭ-dŏl′ĭ-sĭs) [″+ ″+ *lysis*, loosening]. Epidermolysis, q.v.

epidermidosis (ĕp′ĭ-dĕrm″mĭ-dō′sĭs) [″+ ″+ *ōsis*, condition]. Epidermosis, q.v.

epidermis (ĕp′ĭ-dĕr′mĭs) [Gr. *epi*, over, + *derma*, skin]. Cuticle, or outer layer of skin;

scarf skin. It is nonvascular and is formed from within outward.

It consists of four layers or strata; (1) stratum germinativum (stratum mucosum; malpighian layer), the innermost layer; (2) stratum granulosum epidermis [NA], located immediately above the stratum germinativum; (3) stratum lucidum [NA], the clear layer; (4) stratum corneum [NA], the outermost layer of the e.

epidermi'tis ["+ "+ *itis*, inflammation]. Inflammation of the superficial layers of the skin.

epidermization (ĕp'ĭ-dĕr''mĭ-zā'shŭn). 1. Skin grafting. 2. Conversion of deeper germinative layer of cells into outer layer of epidermis.

epidermoid (ĕp'ĭ-dĕr'moyd) [Gr. *epi*, over, + *derma*, skin, + *eidos*, form]. 1. Resembling or pert. to the epidermis. 2. A tumor arising from aberrant epidermal cells. SYN: *cholesteatoma*.

epidermolysis (ĕp'ĭ-dĕr-mŏl'ĭ-sĭs) ["+ "+ *lysis*, loosening]. Loosening of the epidermis.

e. bullosa. A form characterized by formation of deep-seated bullae appearing after irritation or rubbing of a part.

epidermo'ma ["+ "+ *ōma*, growth]. An excrescence on the skin.

epidermomycosis (ĕp-ĭ-dĕr''mo-mĭ-kō'sĭs) ["+ "+ *mykēs*, fungus, + *ōsis*, condition]. Skin disease caused by a fungus.

Epidermophyton (ĕp'ĭ-dĕr-mŏf'ĭ-tŏn) [Gr. *epi*, over, + *derma*, skin, + *phyton*, plant]. A genus of fungi, similar to Trichophyton but affecting the skin and nails, instead of the hair.

E. floccosum. The causative agent of certain types of tinea, esp. tinea pedis (athlete's foot), tinea cruris, tinea unguium, and tinea corporis.

epidermophytosis (ĕp'ĭ-dĕr-mo-fĭ-tō'sĭs) ["+ "+ "+ *ōsis*, condition]. Infection by a species of Epidermophyton.

epidermo'sis ["+ "+ *ōsis*, condition]. Any disease affecting the skin, esp. the epidermis.

epidiascope (ĕp'ĭ-dĭ'ă-skōp) [Gr. *epi*, upon, + *dia*, through, + *skopein*, to examine]. Lantern used for projection of images on a screen. SYN: *episcope*.

epididymectomy (ĕp'ĭ-dĭd-ĭ-mĕk'tō-mĭ) [Gr. *epi*, upon, + *didymos*, testis, + *ektomē*, excision]. Removal of the epididymis.

epididymis (ĕp'ĭ-dĭd'ĭ-mĭs) [Gr. *epi*, at, near, + *didymos*, testis]. (pl. *epididymides*). A small, oblong body resting upon and beside the posterior surface of the testes, consisting of a convoluted tube 13 to 20 ft. long, enveloped in the tunica vaginalis, ending in the ductus deferens.

It consists of (1) the head (caput or globus major) which contains 12 to 14 efferent ducts of the testis, (2) the body, and (3) the tail (cauda or globus minor). It constitutes the first part of the excretory duct of each testis. The epididymis is supplied by the internal spermatic, deferential, and external spermatic arteries; it is drained by corresponding veins.

epididymitis (ĕp'ĭ-dĭd''ĭ-mĭ'tĭs) ["+ "+ *itis*, inflammation]. Inflammation of the epididymis.

ETIOL: May be complication of gonorrhea, syphilis, tuberculosis, mumps, prostatitis, urethritis, prostatectomy, or following prolonged use of indwelling catheter.

SYM: Fever and chills, pain in inguinal region, swollen epididymis.

TREATMENT: Bed rest, support of scrotum, and appropriate antibiotic.

epididymodeferentectomy (ĕp'ĭ-dĭd'ĭ-mo-dĕf'er-en-tĕk'tō-mĭ) ["+ "+ L. *deferens*, carrying away, + Gr. *ektomē*, excision]. Excision of epididymis and ductus deferens.

epididymodeferential (ĕp'ĭ-dĭd'ĭ-mo-dĕf''ĕr-ĕn'shăl). Concerning both the epididymis and ductus deferens.

epididymoorchitis (ĕp'ĭ-dĭd''ĭm-o-ŏr-kī'-tĭs) [Gr. *epi*, at, near, + *didymos*, testis, + *orchis*, testis, + *itis*, inflammation]. Epididymitis with orchitis, q.v.

epididymotomy (ĕp'ĭ-dĭd'ĭ-mŏt'ō-mĭ) ["+ "+ *tomē*, incision]. Incision into the epididymis.

epididymovasostomy (ĕp-ĭ-dĭd'ĭ-mo-văs-ŏs'tō-mĭ) ["+ "+ L. *vas*, vessel, + Gr. *stoumoun*, to provide with an opening or mouth]. Making an anastomosis between the epididymis and the vas.

epidu'ral [Gr. *epi*, over, +L. *durus*, hard]. Located over or upon the dura.

e. space. Space outside of dura mater of brain and spinal cord.

epifascial (ĕp'ĭ-fash'ĭ-al). On or upon a fascia.

epifolliculitis (ĕp'ĭ-fŏl-lĭk''ū-lī'tĭs) [Gr. *epi*, upon, + L. *folliculus*, follicle, + Gr. *itis*, inflammation]. Inflammation of hair follicles of the scalp.

epigas'ter ["+ *gastēr*, belly]. Embryonic structure which develops into the large intestine. SYN: *hindgut*.

epigastralgia (ĕp'ĭ-găs-trăl'jĭ-ă) ["+ "+ *algos*, pain]. Pain in the epigastrium.

epigas'tric. Pert. to the epigastrium. SEE: *precordia*.

e. reflex. Contraction of the upper portion of the rectus abdominis muscle when skin of the epigastric region is scratched.

epigastrium (ĕp'ĭ-găs'trĭ-um) [Gr. *epi,* over, upon, + *gastēr,* belly]. Region over the pit of the stomach. SEE: *Auenbrugger's sign.*

epigastrocele (ĕp'ĭ-găs'tro-sēl) ["+ "+ *kēlē,* hernia]. Hernia in the epigastrium.

epigastrorrhaphy (ĕp'ĭ-găs-trŏr'ă-fĭ) ["+ "+ *rhaphē,* suture]. Suture of an abdominal wound in the epigastric area.

epigenesis (ĕp'ĭ-jĕn'ĕ-sĭs) [Gr. *epi,* after, + *genesis,* formation]. In embryology, the theory that parts of an organism arise by a process of progressive development from simple to complex structures through the utilization of cells as building units; in contrast to preformation which holds that parts exist in the ovum preformed.

epiglottidean (ĕp'ĭ-glŏ-tĭd'ē-ăn) [Gr. *epi,* upon, over, + *glōttis,* glottis]. Pert. to the epiglottis.

epiglottidectomy (ĕp'ĭ-glŏt'ĭd-ĕk'tō-mĭ) ["+ "+ *ektomē,* excision]. Excision of the epiglottis.

epiglottiditis (ĕp'ĭ-glŏt''tĭd-ī'tĭs) ["+ "+ *itis,* inflammation]. Inflammation of the epiglottis. SYN: *epiglottitis.*

epiglottis (ĕp'ĭ-glŏt'ĭs) [Gr. *epi,* over, + *glōttis,* glottis]. (pl. *epiglottidēs*) [NA] A thin leaf-shaped structure located immediately posterior to the root of the tongue which covers the entrance of the larynx when swallowing, thus preventing food or liquids from entering the airway. It consists of the epiglottic cartilage, an impaired laryngeal cartilage, and is covered with mucous membrane.

epiglottitis (ĕp'ĭ-glŏt-ī'tĭs) ["+ "+ *-itis,* inflammation]. Inflammation of the epiglottis. If untreated, may be so severe as to cause death. Appears most commonly in young children.

SYM: Sore throat, fever, croupy cough, drooling, cyanosis, and even coma.

TREATMENT: Establishment of airway by tracheostomy if necessary. Administration of appropriate antibiotic.

epihy'al [Gr. *epi,* over, + *hy,* upsilon, the Greek letter *u.*]. Pert. to the arch of the hyoid.

e. bone. Ossified stylohyoid ligament.

epilate (ep'ĭ-lāt) [L. *e,* out, + *pilus,* hair]. To extract the hair by the roots.

ep'ilating. Depilating; extracting a hair.

e. dose. The quantity of roentgen rays or radium necessary to cause temporary loss of hair.

e. forceps. Tweezers for pulling out hairs.

epilation (ep-ĭ-la'shun). Extraction of hair. SYN: *depilation.*

epilatory (e-pĭl'ă-tor-ĭ). Pert. to removal of hairs, or that which removes them. SYN: *depilatory.*

epilemma (ep-ĭ-lem'ă) [Gr. *epi,* upon, + *lemma,* husk]. Neurilemma of small branches of nerve filaments.

epilepsy (ĕp'ĭ-lĕp''sĭ) [Gr. *epilēpsia,* seizure, from *epi,* besides, in addition to, + *lēptos,* seized]. Recurrent transient attacks of disturbed brain function. Characterized by various combinations of the following: motor, sensory, or psychic malfunction; with or without convulsions; altered or complete loss of consciousness. Because convulsions are not a consistent finding in e., it is best to speak of epileptic seizures to describe all types of attacks.

Next to stroke, e. is the most frequent neurological disease.

ETIOL: May be due to one of many causes; electroencephalographic studies reveal a direct relationship between changes in electrical brain potentials and the occurrence of seizures. Heredity plays an important role.

SYM: Often a peculiar sensation or feeling (the aura) precedes loss of consciousness. The patient falls during the attack, often injuring himself. He may bite his tongue, pass urine, and awake to realize something has happened because of muscular soreness. There is a tendency to sleep following the attack; indeed attacks may occur only during sleep.

Grand Mal: Often preceded by a peculiar sensation known as an aura, beginning in finger or toe and rising until head is involved. At this time the patient gives a shrill cry and falls unconscious; tonic spasm followed by clonic movements; face cyanosed; frothing at mouth; coma. Prognosis is unfavorable but not fatal.

Petit Mal: Seizure consists of momentary unconsciousness.

NP: Do not attempt to stop attack. During attack position head so as to facilitate breathing. Prevent tongue from being bitten or from obstructing windpipe. Place pad between teeth during attack. Afterward allow patient to sleep. Dilantin is used as an anticonvulsant without depressive action, but signs of toxicity must be watched for.

TREATMENT: Remove causative or precipitating factors. Regular well-balanced diet; no alcoholic beverages. Avoid constipation. Regular amounts of sleep. Anticonvulsant drugs.

e., cortical. SEE: *e., jacksonian.*

e., focal. E., jacksonian, q.v.

e., hemiplegic. E., jacksonian, q.v.

e., idiopathic. Presence of e. without known cause.

e., jacksonian. E. in which convulsions tend to be restricted to certain groups of muscles, or limited to one side of the body, due to disease involving the cortex. Also called cortical, focal, hemiplegic, partial, or symptomatic e.

e., menstrual. Form in which attacks coincide with menstruation.

e., myoclonic. E. in which clonic contractions of muscles, esp. those of the extremities, occur between seizures.

e., nocturnal. Occurs only during sleep. Symptoms similar to grand mal. PROG: Favorable.

e., partial. E., jacksonian, q.v.

e., reflex. E. in which attacks are induced by sensory stimuli.

e., sleep. Spasmodic uncontrollable desire to sleep. SYN: *narcolepsy.*

e., traumatic. E. caused by trauma to the brain.

e., uncinate. E. due to a lesion of the uncinate gyrus of the temporal lobe. Preceded by aura of smell.

epilepsy, words pert. to: analepsis; aura; fit; ictus; status epilepticus.

epilep'tic [Gr. *epilēptikos,* pert. to a seizure]. 1. Concerning epilepsy. 2. Individual suffering from epileptic attacks.

epilep'tiform [Gr. *epilēpsia,* seizure, + L. *forma,* form]. Having the form of epilepsy.

epileptogenic, epileptogenous (ĕp'ĭ-lĕp-to-jĕn'ik, -tŏj'ĕ-nus) ["+ *gennan,* to produce]. Giving rise to epileptoid convulsions.

e. zone. Certain motor areas in cerebral cortex, irritation of which gives rise to an epileptic seizure.

epilep'toid ["+ *eidos,* resemblance]. Resembling epilepsy. SYN: *epileptiform.*

epileptol'ogy ["+ *logos,* study]. Study of epilepsy.

epileptosis (ĕp'ĭ-lĕp-to'sĭs) ["+ *ōsis,* condition]. Any mental disease due to epilepsy.

epiloia (ĕp'ĭ-loy'ă). A syndrome consisting of progressive mental deficiency, adenoma sebaceum, convulsions, hypertrophic sclerosis of the brain, tumors in the kidneys, and nodules on floor of lateral ventricle. SYN: *tuberous sclerosis.*

epilose (ep'ĭ-lōs) [L. *e,* without, + *pilus,* hair]. Bald; without hair.

epimandibular (ĕp'ĭ-măn-dĭb'ū-lăr) [Gr. *epi,* upon, above, + L. *mandibulum,* jaw]. Above or upon the lower jaw.

epimenorrhagia (ĕp'ĭ-mĕn''ō-rā'jĭ-ă) ["+ *mēn,* month, + *rhēgnynai,* to burst forth]. Too much and too frequent menstruation.

epimenorrhea (ĕp'ĭ-mĕn-ō-rē'ă) ["+ "+ *rhoia,* flow]. Menstruation occurring too frequently.

epimerite (ĕp'ĭ-mer'ĭt) ["+ *meros,* part]. An organ of certain protozoa by which they attach themselves to epithelial cells.

epimorphosis (ĕp'ĭ-mŏr'fō-sĭs) [Gr. *epi,* upon, after, + *morphoun,* to give shape, + *-ōsis,* formation of]. Regeneration of a part of an organism by growth at the cut surface.

epimysium (ĕp'ĭ-mĭz'ĭ-um) ["+ *mys,* muscle]. Outermost sheath of connective tissue which surrounds a skeletal muscle. Consists of irregularly distributed collagenous, reticular, and elastic fibers, connective tissue cells, and fat cells.

ep'inasty ["+ *nastos,* pressed close]. More vigorous growth on the upper than on the under surface, leading to a downward curvature of an organ.

epinephrectomy (ĕp'ĭ-nĕ-frĕk'tō-mĭ) ["+ *nephros,* kidney, + *ektomē,* excision]. Excision of the suprarenal gland. SYN: *adrenalectomy.*

epinephrine (ĕp'ĭ-nĕf'rĭn) [Gr. *epi,* upon, + *nephros,* kidney]. USP. $C_9H_{13}NO_3$. This substance and norepinephrine are the two active hormones produced by the adrenal medulla. Epinephrine, which has been synthesized, is also produced by tissues other than the adrenal. It is employed therapeutically as a vasoconstrictor, cardiac stimulant, and to relax bronchioles. Its effects are similar to those brought about by stimulation of the sympathetic division of the autonomic nervous system. SYN: *adrenaline.*

Used to check local hemorrhage and to relieve asthmatic attacks. Also to prolong action of local anesthetics by constricting blood vessels. This prevents rapid absorption.

INCOMPATIBILITIES: Light; heat; air; iron salts; and alkalies.

e. bitartrate. USP. A white or grayish white crystalline powder ($C_9H_{13}NO_3C_4H_6O_6$). It is a sympathomimetic agent used for topical application to the eye.

epinephrinemia (ĕp'ĭ-nĕf'rĭ-nē'mĭ-ă) ["+ "+ *haima,* blood]. Epinephrine in the blood.

epinephritis (ĕp'ĭ-nĕf-rī'tĭs) [Gr. *epi,* upon, + *nephros,* kidney, + *-itis,* inflammation]. Inflammation of an adrenal gland.

epinephro'ma ["+ "+ *ōma,* tumor]. A lipomatoid tumor of the kidney. SYN: *Grawitz's tumor; hypernephroma.*

epineural (ĕp'ĭ-nū'răl) ["+ *neuron,* nerve]. Located upon a neural arch.

epineurium (ĕp'ĭ-nū'rĭ-ŭm). The general connective tissue sheath of a nerve. SEE: *nerve.*

ep″iot′ic [Gr. *epi,* above, + *ous, ot-,* ear].
Located above the ear.

   e. center. Ossification center of temporal bone forming upper and posterior part of
the auditory capsule.

epipas′tic [″+ *passein,* to sprinkle]. Resembling a dusting powder.

epipharynx (ĕp′ĭ-far′inks) [″+ *pharynx,*
pharynx]. Nasal portion of pharynx. SYN:
rhinopharynx.

epiphenom′enon [″+ *phainomenon,* phe-
nomenon]. An exceptional symptom or occurrence in a disease which is not always
present and may be unrelated to the usual
course of the disease.

epiphora (ĕ-pĭf′o-rā) [Gr. downpour]. Abnormal overflow of tears down the cheek due to
excess secretion of tears or to obstruction of
the lacrimal duct.

epiphylactic (ĕp″ĭ-fĭ-lăk′tĭk) [Gr. *epi,* upon,
+ *phylaxis,* protection]. Pert. to epiphylaxis.

epiphylaxis (ĕp″ĭ-fĭ-lăk′sĭs). Increase of defensive powers of the body.

epiphyseal (ĕp″ĭ-fĭz′e-al) [Gr. *epi,* upon, +
physis, growth]. Pert. to or of the nature of
an epiphysis. Also spelled *epiphysial.*

epiphyseolysis (ĕp″ĭ-fĭz″e-ŏl′ĭ-sĭs) [″+ ″+
lysis, loosening]. Separation of an epiphysis.

epiphyseopathy (ĕp″ĭ-fĭz-e-ŏp′ă-thĭ) [″+ ″+
pathos, disease]. Any disease of an epiphysis
or of the pineal gland.

epiphysial (ĕp″ĭ-fĭz′-ĭ-ăl). Of the nature of or
concerning an epiphysis. Also spelled epiphyseal.

epiphysis (ĕ-pĭf′ĭ-sĭs) [Gr. a growing upon].
(pl. *epiphyses*) [NA] 1. In the developing infant and child, a secondary boneforming (ossification) center separated from a parent
bone in early life by cartilage. As growth
proceeds and at a different time for each
epiphysis, it becomes a part of the larger (or
parent) bone. By use of x-ray studies, it is
possible to judge the age of a child from the
development of these ossification centers. 2.
A center for ossification at each extremity of
long bones. SEE: *diaphysis.*

   e. cerebri. The pineal body.

epiphysitis (ĕ-pĭf″ĭ-sī′tĭs) [″+ *-itis,* inflam-
mation]. Inflammation of an epiphysis, esp.
that at the hip, knee, and shoulder in infants.

epipial (ĕp″ĭ-pī′ăl) [Gr. *epi,* upon, + L. *pia,*
tender]. Situated above or upon the pia mater.

epiplocele (ĕ-pĭp′lo-sēl) [Gr. *epiploon,* omentum, + *kēlē,* hernia]. Hernia containing
omentum.

epiploenterocele (ĕ-pĭp″lo-ĕn′tĕr-o-sēl) [″+
enteron, intestine, + *kēlē,* hernia]. Hernia
consisting of omentum and intestine.

epiploic (ĕp′ĭ-plo′ik) [Gr. *epiploon,* omen-
tum]. Pert. to the omentum.

   e. foramen. The opening between the
greater and lesser peritoneal cavities.

epiploitis (ĕ-pĭp″lo-i′tĭs) [″+ *-itis,* inflamma-
tion]. Inflammation of the omentum.

epiplomerocele (ĕ-pĭp″lo-me′ro-sēl) [″+
mēros, thigh, + *kēlē,* hernia]. Femoral
hernia containing omentum.

epiplomphalocele (ĕ-pĭp″lom-fal′o-sēl) [″+
omphalos, navel, + *kēlē,* hernia]. Umbilical
hernia with omentum protruding.

epiploon (ĕ-pĭp′lŏ-ŏn) [Gr. omentum]. The
omentum, esp. the greater omentum. SEE:
omentum.

epiplopexy (ĕ-pĭp′lo-peks″ĭ) [Gr. *epiploon,*
omentum, + *pēxis,* fixation]. Suturing of
omentum to the anterior abdominal wall.

epiplosarcomphalocele (ĕ-pĭp″lo-sar″-
kom-fal′o-sēl) [″+ *sarx,* flesh, + *omphalos,*
navel, + *kēlē,* hernia]. An umbilical hernia
with protruding omentum. SYN: *epiplomphalocele.*

epiploscheocele (ĕ-pĭp″los-ke′o-sēl) [″+
oscheon, scrotum, + *kēlē,* hernia]. Omental
hernia into the scrotum.

epipygus (ĕp″ĭ-pi′gus) [″+ *pygē,* buttocks]. A
developmental anomaly in which an accessory limb is attached to the buttocks;
pygomelus.

episclera (ĕp″ĭ-skle′rā) [Gr. *epi,* upon, +
sklēros, hard]. Outermost superficial layer
of the sclera of the eye.

episcleral (ĕp″ĭ-skle′ral). 1. Pertaining to the
episclera. 2. Overlying the sclera of the eye.

episcleritis (ĕp″ĭ-skle-ri′tĭs) [Gr. *epi,* upon, +
sklēros, hard, + *-itis,* inflammation]. Inflammation of the subconjunctival layers of
the sclera.

ep′iscope [″+ *skopein,* to examine]. Projection lantern for examination of an object on
a screen. SYN: *epidiascope.*

episioclisia (ĕ-pis″ĭ-o-klis′ĭ-ă) [Gr. *episeion,*
pudenda, + *kleisis,* closure]. Surgical closure of the vulva.

episioelytrorrhaphy (ĕ-pis″ĭ-o-el″ĭ-trŏr′ră-
fĭ) [″+ *elytron,* vagina, + *rhaphē,* suture].
Narrowing of vagina and vulva.

episioperineorrhaphy (ĕ-pis″ĭ-o-per″ĭ-ne-
or′ă-fĭ) [″+ *perinaion,* perineum, + *raphē,*
suture]. Suturing the vulva and perineum
for the support of a prolapse of the uterus.

   NP: Prevent necessity for straining on
defecation by providing stool softeners and a
diet which will help to produce soft bowel
movements; routine perineal care.

episioplasty (ĕ-pis″ĭ-o-plăs′tĭ) [Gr. *episeion,*
pudenda, + *plassein,* to form]. Plastic surgery on the vulva.

episiorrhaphy (e-pis″ĭ-or′a-fĭ) ["+ *rhaphē*, suture]. Sewing of a lacerated perineum.

episiostenosis (ĕ-pis″ĭ-o-stĕ-nō′sis) ["+ *stenōsis*, narrowing]. Narrowing of the vulvar slit.

episiotomy (ĕ-pis″ĭ-ŏt′ŏ-mĭ) [Gr. *episeion*, pudenda, + *tomē*, incision]. Incision of perineum at end of second stage of labor to avoid laceration of perineum and to facilitate delivery.

epispadias (ep″ĭ-spa′dĭ-as) [Gr. *epi*, upon, + *spadōn*, a rent]. Congenital opening of urethra on dorsum of penis; in the female, opening by separation of the labia minora and a fissure of the clitoris.

epispas′tic [Gr. *epi*, after, + *span*, to draw]. 1. An agent that, applied locally, will produce a serous discharge. 2. Causing a blister.

episplenitis (ĕp″ĭ-sple-nī′tis) [Gr. *epi*, upon, + *splēn*, spleen, + *-itis*, inflammation]. Inflammation of the splenic capsule.

epistasis (ĕ-pĭs′tă-sĭs) [Gr. stoppage, from *epi*, upon, + *stanai*, to set, place]. 1. A film which forms on urine which has been allowed to stand. 2. The suppression of any discharge. SEE: *hypostasis*.

epistaxis (ĕp″ĭ-stăk′sĭs) [Gr. dropping, from *epi*, upon, + *stazein*, to drip]. Hemorrhage from nose; nosebleed.

ETIOL: Trauma, picking the nose with finger, direct blow, postoperative, foreign bodies, diseases (local and general), violent exertion, basilar skull fracture, vicarious menstruation, and high altitudes.

TREATMENT: Lie quietly propped up in bed, cold compresses, epinephrine locally, followed by cautery of bleeding vessel, packing.

NP: Simple nosebleed may be stopped ordinarily by elevating head of patient and pinching nostrils. Refrain from breathing through or blowing nose. Pressure across upper lip or cold cloths placed over nose and on back of neck are beneficial.

In severe nose bleeding, if necessary, pack entire nose or upper pharynx (retrograde packing). Occasionally epinephrine, styptics, or astringents may be used. However, for most first-aid purposes, these are unsatisfactory.

episternal (ĕp″ĭ-stĕr′năl) [Gr. *epi*, upon, + *sternon*, chest]. Situated above the sternum.

epister′num. Upper portion of the sternum. SYN: *manubrium*.

epistropheus (ĕp″ĭ-stro′fe-us). (pl. *epistropheī*) Former term for axis.

epitendineum (ĕp″ĭ-ten-din′e-um) [Gr. *epi*, around, covering, + L. *tendere*, to stretch]. The fibrous sheath enveloping a tendon.

epitenon (ep-ĭ-ten′on) ["+ *tenōn*, tendon]. The connective tissue holding a tendon within its sheaths. SYN: *epitendineum*.

epithalamus (ĕp″ĭ-thăl′ă-mus) [Gr. *epi*, on, at, + *thalamos*, chamber]. [NA]. The uppermost portion of the diencephalon. It includes the pineal body, trigonum habenulae, habenula, and the habenular commissure.

epithalaxia (ĕp″ĭ-thă-lăk′sĭ-ă) ["+ *thēlē*, nipple, + *allaxis*, exchange]. Desquamation of epithelial cells, esp. of lining of the intestine.

epithe′lia ["+ *thēlē*, nipple]. (pl. of *epithelium*, q.v.) Epithelial layer of cells.

epithelial (ĕp″ĭ-thē′lĭ-al). Pert. to or composed of epithelium.

   e. cancer. Carcinoma composed of e. cells. SYN: *epithelioma*.

   e. casts. Aggregations of renal epithelium, with cells filled with granules or fat droplets. They often preserve their original form in the e. tubes.

   e. cells. Cells which are irregular in shape, having a single nucleus. Frequently two or three are joined together.

   e. tissue. Those cells which form the outer surface of the body, and line the body cavities and the principal tubes and passageways leading to the exterior. They form the secreting portions of glands and their ducts, and important parts of certain sense organs. The cells of e. tissues lie closely approximated to each other and contain very little intercellular substance. They are arranged in one or a few layers and are devoid of blood vessels. SEE: *tissue.*

epithelioblastoma (ĕp″ĭ-thē″lĭ-o-blăs-tō′mă) [Gr. *epi*, at, + *thēlē*, nipple, + *blastos*, germ, + *-ōma*, tumor]. Epithelial cell tumor.

epitheliogenic, epitheliogenetic (ĕp″ĭ-thē″lĭ-o-jĕn′ik, -jĕ-nĕt′ik) ["+ "+ *gennan*, to produce]. Caused by epithelial proliferation.

epithelioid (ĕp″ĭ-thē′lĭ-oyd) ["+ "+ *eidos*, form]. Resembling epithelium.

epitheliolysin (ĕp″ĭ-thē-lĭ-ŏl′ĭ-sĭn) ["+ "+ *lysis*, dissolution]. A specific lysin formed in blood serum of an animal in which epithelial cells of an animal of a different species were injected. E. destroys the cells of an animal of the same species as that from which the epithelial cells were derived.

epitheliolysis (ĕp″ĭ-thē-lĭ-ŏl′ĭ-sĭs). Death of epithelial tissue. The destruction or dissolving of epithelial cells by an epitheliolysin.

epithelioma (ĕp″ĭ-thē-lĭ-ō′mă) [Gr. *epi*, at, + *thēlē*, nipple, + *-ōma*, tumor]. A malignant tumor consisting principally of epithelial cells; a carcinoma. A tumor originating in the epidermis of the skin or in a mucous membrane.

e. adamantinum. An adamantinoma, q.v.

e. adenoides cysticum. A basal cell carcinoma of low malignancy, occurring on the surface of the body, esp. the face. Characterized by formation of cysts.

e., basal cell. One derived from cells in the basal layer of the epidermis (stratum germinativum). SYN: *e. adenoides cysticum; rodent ulcer.*

e., deep seated. Involving lymphatic glands; irregular rounded ulcers, occurring after several months.

e. molluscum. Molluscum contagiosum, q.v.

epitheliomatous (ĕp″ĭ-thē-lĭ-o′mă-tus). Pert. to epithelioma.

epitheliosis (ĕp″ĭ-thē″lĭ-ō′sĭs) [Gr. *epi,* at, + *thēlē,* nipple, + *-ōsis,* condition]. Trachomatous proliferation of the conjunctival epithelium.

epithelium (ĕp″ĭ-thē′lĭ-ŭm) [″ + *thēlē,* nipple]. (pl. *epithelia*) [NA] The layer of cells forming the epidermis of the skin and the surface layer of mucous and serous membranes. The cells rest on a basement membrane and lie closely approximated to each other with little intercellular material between them. E. may be simple, consisting of a single layer, or stratified, consisting of several layers. Cells comprising e. may be flat (squamous), cube-shaped (cuboidal) or cylindrical (columnar). Modified forms of e. include ciliated, pseudostratified, glandular, and neuroepithelium. E. may include goblet cells, which secrete mucus. Squamous e. is classified as endothelium, which lines the blood vessels and the heart, and mesothelium, which lines the serous cavities. E. serves the general functions of protection, absorption, secretion, and specialized functions such as movement of substances through ducts, production of germ cells, and reception of stimuli. Its ability to regenerate is excellent.

e., ciliated. Epithelial cells with fine hair-like protuberances, called cilia, on their free border. These cells are able to sweep particles in a certain direction.

e., columnar. E. composed of cells shaped like pillars.

e., cuboidal. E. consisting of cube-shaped or prismatic cells with height approximately equal to width.

e., germinal. The e. which covers the surface of the genital ridge of the urogenital folds of an embryo. It gives rise to seminiferous tubules of the testes and the surface layer of the ovary. It is thought to give rise to the germ cells (spermatozoa and ova).

e., glandular. E. consisting of cells which secrete.

e., laminated. Stratified e.

e., maternal. Uterine e. contrasted with that of the embryo.

e., mesenchymal. E. of the squamous type which lines the subarachnoid and subdural cavities, the chambers of the eye, and the perilymphatic spaces of the ear.

e., neuro-. E. terminating the nerves of special sense.

e., pavement. E. of flat, platelike cells.

e., pigmented. E. consisting of cells containing pigment granules.

e., pseudostratified. E. in which the bases of cells rest on the basement membrane but the distal ends of some do not reach the surface. Nuclei of the cells lie at different levels giving the appearance of stratification.

e., squamous. E., pavement, q.v.

e., stratified. E. with the cells in layers.

e., transitional. A form of stratified e. in which the cells have the ability to adjust themselves to mechanical changes such as stretching and contracting. Found only in the urinary system (pelvis and kidney, ureter, bladder, and a part of the urethra).

epitonic (ĕp″ĭ-ton′ĭk) [Gr. *epitonos,* strained]. Increased tonus.

epitox′oid [Gr. *epi,* upon, + *toxikon,* poison, + *eidos,* form]. Any toxoid which has less affinity for an antitoxin than is possessed by the toxin. SYN: *toxon.*

epitrichium (ĕp″ĭ-trĭk′ĭ-um) [″ + *trichion,* hair]. Superficial layers of the epidermis of the fetus.

epitrochlea (ĕp″ĭ-trok′le-ă) [″ + *trochalia,* pulley]. The inner condyle of the humerus.

epitrochlear (ĕp″ĭ-trok′le-ar). Pert. to the inner condyle of the humerus.

epitur′binate [Gr. *epi,* upon, + L. *turbo,* top]. The tissue upon or covering the turbinate bone.

epitympanum (ĕp″ĭ-tĭm′pă-num) [″ + *tympanon,* drum]. The attic of middle ear; area above the drum membrane.

epityphlitis (ĕp″ĭ-tif-lĭ′tis) [″ + *typhlon,* cecum, + *itis,* inflammation]. Appendicitis.

epizoic (ĕp″ĭ-zō′ĭk) [″ + *zōon,* animal]. Living as a parasite on the exterior of an animal.

epizoicide (ĕp″ĭ-zō′ĭ-sĭd) [″ + ″ + L. *caedere,* to kill]. That which destroys epizoa. SEE: *epizoon.*

epizoon (ĕp″ĭ-zō′ŏn) [″ + *zōon,* animal]. (pl. *epizoa*) An animal organism living as a parasite on the exterior of the host animal.

epluchage (ā″plū-shazh′) [Fr., cleaning]. Wound excision for removing damaged and macerated tissue. SEE: *debridement.*

eponychium (ĕp″ō-nĭk′ĭ-um) [Gr. *epi*, upon, + *onyx, onych-*, nail]. 1. The horny embryonic structure from which the nail develops. 2. Perionychium [NA].

eponym (ĕp′ō-nĭm) [Gr. *epōnymos*, named after]. A name for anything (diseases, organs, functions, places) adapted from the name of a particular person.

eponym′ic. Pert. to eponym. SYN: *eponymous*.

epon′ymous. Named after a person.

epoophorectomy (ĕp″ō-ō-fō-rĕk′tō-mī) [Gr. *epi*, upon, + *ōophoron*, ovary, + *ektomē*, excision]. Removal of the parovarium.

epoophoron (ĕp″ō-ōf′o-ron). A rudimentary structure located in the mesosalpinx consisting of a longitudinal duct (duct of Gartner) and ten to fifteen transverse ducts. It is the remains of the upper portion of the mesonephros and is the homologue of the head of the epididymis in the male. SYN: *organ of Rosenmüller; parovarium.*

epsilon-amino-caproic acid. A synthetic substance used to correct an overdose of certain fibinolytic agents. Also useful in treating excessive bleeding due to increased fibrinolytic activity in the blood.

epsom salt (ep′sŭm). Magnesium sulfate, q.v.

EPSP. Abbr. for *excitatory postsynaptic potential.*

epulis (ĕp-u′lis) [Gr. *epoulis*, a gumboil]. (pl. *epulides*) A fibrous, sarcomatous tumor having its origin in the periosteum of the lower jaw.

e., malignant. Jaw sarcoma made up of giant cells.

epuloid (ĕp′u-loyd) [" + *eidos*, form]. 1. Like an epulis. 2. Tumor of the jaw or gum appearing like an epulis.

epulosis (ĕp″u-lō′sis) [" + *-ōsis*, condition]. Cicatrization; a cicatrix.

epulot′ic [Gr. *epoulis*, gumboil]. Promoting cicatrization.

equa′tion [L. *aequāre*, to make equal]. 1. State of being equal. 2. In chemistry, a symbolic representation of a chemical reaction.

e., personal. The potential for error in experimental studies due to the emotional and intellectual differences between observers responsible for supervising the research.

equa′tor. Line encircling a round body and equidistant from both poles.

e. of a cell. The boundary of a plane through which the division of a cell occurs.

e. of crystalline lens. Line which marks the junction of the anterior and posterior surfaces; the equator lentis. To it are attached the fibers of the suspensory ligament.

e. oculi. An imaginary line encircling the bulb of the eye midway between anterior and posterior poles.

equato′rial. Pert. to an equator.

e. plate. Mass of chromosomes at equator of the nuclear spindle during karyokinesis.

equi- [L. *aequus*, equal]. Prefix meaning equal.

equilibrating (ē-kwĭl′ĭ-brāt-ing) [L. *aequilibris*, in perfect balance]. Maintaining equilibrium.

e. operation. Section of the antagonist of a paralyzed ocular muscle. SEE: *tenotomy.*

equilib′rium [L. *aequus*, equal, + *libra*, balance]. State of balance or rest. Condition in which contending forces are equal.

e., nitrogenous. Having amt. of nitrogen in egesta equal to that of ingesta.

e., physiological. Having egesta equal to the ingesta.

e., sense of. The complex and interrelated nervous and muscular control which is responsible for maintaining body posture or position without falling.

equilin (ĕk′wĭl-ĭn) [L. *equus*, horse]. Crystalline estrogenic hormone derived from pregnant mares' urine, which affects growth of female sex organs. SYN: *theelin.*

equinia (ē-kwĭn′ĭ-ä) [L. *equus*, horse]. Infectious disease of horses which can also affect man. SYN: *glanders.*

equinovarus (ē-kwī′nō-vā′rus) [L. *equinus*, equine, + *varus*, bent inward]. A form of clubfoot with a combination pes equinus and pes varus, i.e. walking without touching the heel to the ground and with the sole turned inward.

equivalence (ē-kwĭv′ā-lĕns) [L. *aequus*, equal, + *valere*, to be worth]. 1. Quality of being equivalent. 2. Condition in which two radicals reacting are of the same valence and one displaces the other in a compound.

equivalent (ē-kwĭv′a-lent). 1. Equal in power, force, or value. 2. Amount of weight of any element needed to replace a fixed weight of another body.

e., epilepsy. Any mental or physical disturbance, which may take the place of an epileptic seizure.

Er. Chem. symb. for erbium.

E.R. Abbr. for *external resistance.*

erasion (ē-rā′zhŭn) [L. *e*, out, + *radere*, to scrape]. Laying open a diseased part and scraping away diseased tissue.

Erben's reflex (erb′en). [Siegmund Erben, Austrian physician, 1863- —] Retardation of pulse when head and trunk are forcibly bent forward.

er'bium. SYMB: *Er.* At. wt. 167.26; at. no. 68; sp. gr. 9.051. A rare metallic element.

Erb's paralysis, palsy. [Wilhelm H. Erb, Ger. neurologist, 1840-1921]. Paralysis of group of muscles of shoulder and upper arm involving cervical roots of 5th and 6th spinal nerves.

The arm hangs limp, the hand rotates inward and normal movements are lost. SEE: *palsy, Erb's.*

erectile (e-rĕk'til) [L. *erigere,* to erect]. Able to become erect.

    e. tissue. Vascular tissue which, when filled with blood, becomes erect or rigid, as the clitoris, penis, or nipples.

erec'tion. The state of swelling, hardness, and stiffness observed in the penis and to a lesser extent in the clitoris of the female, generally due to sexual excitement.

    Due to engorgement with blood of the corpora cavernosa and the corpus spongiosum of the penis and the c. cavernosa clitoridis of the female.

    E. is necessary in the male for the intromission of the penis into the vagina of the female and for the emission of semen. After ejaculation the blood withdraws from the penis and the e. is reduced. E. of the penis may occur as the result of sexual excitement, during sleep, or due to physical stimulation of the penis. Abnormal, persistent e. of the penis not due to sexual excitement is called priapism, q.v. SEE: *nocturnal emission.*

    e. center. This is in lumbar and sacral region; responds to organic and psychic stimuli and with the genitalia responding to peripheral irritation of the sensory nerves. This center is not directly under control of the will. The nervi erigentes in the first three sacral nerves under excitation convey their impulse to the corpora cavernosa. Reflex stimuli also affect it.

erec'tor [L. *erigere,* to erect]. A muscle that raises a part.

    e. spinae reflex. Irritation of the skin over the erector spinae muscles causing contraction of muscles of the back. SYN: *dorsal reflex; lumbar reflex.*

erect posi'tion. One having the occiput and heels in line with nose, groin, and great toes in same relative plane.

eremacausis (er''ĕm-ă-kaw'sis) [Gr. *ērema,* slowly, + *kausis,* burning]. Slow oxidation of organic matter exposed to moisture, air, and heat.

eremophobia (er''ĕm-o-fō'bĭ-ă) [Gr. *erēmos,* solitary, + *phobos,* fear]. Dread of being alone.

erepsin (ē-rĕp'sĭn). Term applied to a peptide-splitting enzyme found in the succus entericus (intestinal juice). The peptide-splitting action is due to the action of several peptidases which act on peptides which have escaped pancreatic digestion. This action converts polypeptides to amino acids.

erethism (ĕr'ĕ-thĭzm) [Gr. *erethismos,* irritation]. Abnormal mental excitability or sensitivity to sensory stimulation.

erethis'mic. Pert. to or causing erethism. SYN: *erethitic.*

erethisophrenia (ĕr''ĕ-thĭ-zo-fre'nĭ-ă) [Gr. *erethizein,* to irritate, + *phrēn,* mind]. Unusual mental excitability.

erethistic (ĕr''ĕ-thĭs'tĭk) [Gr. *erethismos,* irritation]. Erethismic, exciting.

erethitic (ĕr''ĕ-thĭt'ĭk). Causing erethism; irritable, excited.

ereuthrophobia (er''u-thro-fō'bĭ-ă) [Gr. *erythros,* red, + *phobos,* fear]. Pathological fear of blushing. SYN: *erythrophobia.*

erg [Gr. *ergon,* work]. In physics, the amount of work done when a force of one dyne acts through a distance of one centimeter.

    One erg is roughly 1/980 gram-centimeter; that is, to raise a load of one gram against gravity the distance of one centimeter requires that a force of 980 dynes operate through a distance of one centimeter and hence that 980 ergs of work be done.

ergasia (er-gā'sĭ-ă) [Gr., work]. Functions of the mind and behavior resulting therefrom in contrast to those depending upon physiological functions.

ergasiomania (er-gā''sĭ-o-mā'nĭ-ă) ["+ *mania,* madness]. An abnormal desire to be busy at work.

ergasiophobia (er-ga''sĭ-o-fō'bĭ-ă) ["+ *phobos,* fear]. Abnormal dislike for work of any kind, or for assuming responsibility.

ergasthenia (er''gas-thē'nĭ-ă) [Gr. *ergon,* work, + *astheneia,* weakness]. A symptom, condition, or weakness due to overwork.

ergas'tic [Gr. *ergon,* work]. Possessing potential energy.

ergograph (ĕr'go-grăf) ["+ *graphein,* to write]. An apparatus for recording the contractions of muscles and measuring the amount of work done.

ergom'eter [Gr. *ergon,* work, + *metron,* measure]. An apparatus for measuring the amount of work done by a human or animal subject.

ergonomics ["+ *nomikos,* law]. The science which is concerned with the problem of how to fit a job to man's anatomical, physiological, and psychological characteristics in such a way as to enhance human efficiency and well-being.

ergopho'bia ["+ *phobos,* fear]. Morbid dread of working.

ergophore (ĕr'go-fōr) [Gr. *ergon,* work, + *pherein,* to bear]. That part of an antigen on which the specific properties of the substance depend. SYN: *toxophore.*

er'gostat ["+ *statos,* standing]. A machine for measuring work done by a contracting muscle.

ergos'terol. A substance derived from yeast, ergot, and other fungi, and resembling cholesterol in composition.

    e., irradiated. E. subjected to ultraviolet radiation, vitamin D₂. May be used in treating rickets. SYN: *viosterol.*

ergot (ĕr'gŏt). A drug obtained from Claviceps purpurea, a fungus which grows parasitically on rye. Several valuable alkaloids, as ergotamine, q.v., are obtained from ergot.

    e. poisoning. May come from eating bread made with diseased grain or by taking overdoses of the drug.

    SYM: Appear several hours after ingestion. Vomiting, burning, and cramping in abdomen; great thirst; profound weakness; diarrhea; slow, weak pulse; anesthesia, tingling, and twitching in extremities; dilated pupils; occasionally convulsions, anuria. If patient survives may develop gangrene of fingers, toes, or limited areas of skin, and cataracts.

    F.A. TREATMENT: Slurry of activated charcoal by mouth, followed by emesis or gastric lavage, and instillation of a saline cathartic, external heat. SEE: *Table of Poisons and Poisoning* in *Appendix.*

ergotamine (ĕr-got'ă-mēn). A crystalline alkaloid (C₃₃H₃₅O₅N₅) derived from ergot.

    e. tartrate. A white crystalline substance which stimulates smooth muscle of blood vessels and the uterus, inducing vasoconstriction and uterine contractions. Used in the treatment of migraine.

ergotherapy (er''go-thĕr'ă-pī) [Gr. *ergon,* work, + *therapeia,* treatment]. Work used as a treatment of disease.

    e., passive. Generalized muscular exercise by faradic current.

ergotism (ĕr'gŏ-tĭzm). Poisoning resulting from excessive use of ergot or from eating food made from rye or wheat infected with the fungus Claviceps purpurea. May be acute or chronic. SEE: *ergot poisoning.*

ergotrate (ĕr'go-trāt). An active principle isolated from ergot. Used to obtain several alkaloids.

ergotrop'ic [Gr. *ergon,* work, + *tropos,* a turning]. Pert. to ergotropy, q.v.

ergotropy (ĕr-gŏt'ro-pī). Injection of nonspecific proteins to increase body resistance.

eriom'eter [Gr. *erion,* wool, + *metron,* measure]. Device for measuring size of minute particles.

Eristalis (ĕr-ĭs'tă-lĭs). A genus of flies belonging to the family Syrphidae. The larva, called rat-tailed maggot (E. tenax), may cause intestinal myiasis in man.

erode (e-rōd) [L. *erodere,* to gnaw away]. 1. To wear away. 2. To eat away by ulceration.

erogenous (e-rŏj'ĕ-nus) [Gr. *erōs,* love, + *gennan,* to produce]. Causing sexual excitement. SYN: *erotogenic,* q.v.

    e. zone. Any part of the body, touching or stroking of which causes sexual excitement.

erosion (e-rō'zhŭn) [L. *erodere,* to gnaw away]. An eating away of tissue. External or internal destruction of a surface layer by physical or inflammatory processes.

    e. of the cervix uteri. The alteration of the epithelium on a portion of the cervix as a result of irritation by infection.

    SYM: In the early stages, the epithelium shows necrosis which nature tries to heal by a downgrowth of epithelium from the endocervical canal. If this is accomplished by a single layer of tissue having a grossly granular appearance, it is called a simple granular e. If the downgrowth is excessive and shows papillary tufts, it is called a papillary e.

    Histologically, the papillary e. shows many glands of the branching racemose type whose epithelium is the mucus-bearing cell with the nucleus at the base. In the healing process, squamous epithelium grows over the eroded area with the following results: the squamous cells take the place of the tissue beneath it completely, giving a complete healing, or the glands fill with squamous plugs and remain in that state, or the mouths of the glands are occluded by the squamous cells and cysts are formed (nabothian cysts). In the congenital type of e. the portio is covered by high columnar epithelium.

    TREATMENT: Prophylaxis, proper care of the cervix following delivery. Cauterization of the early e. with electrocautery is usually curative.

    e., dental. The wearing away of the surface layer (enamel) of a tooth.

erosive (e-rō'sĭv). 1. Able to produce erosion. 2. An agent that erodes anything.

erotic (e-rŏt'ĭk) [Gr. *erōtikos,* pert. to love]. Pert. to sexual passion. SYN: *lustful.*

erot'icism ["+ *ismos,* condition]. Excessive libido; also intense sex desire.

    e., allo-. E. directed to an external object rather than to self. SEE: *erotomania.*

e., anal. Sensations of pleasure experienced by the child through defecation.

e., auto-. 1. Self-gratification of the sexual instinct. 2. Self-admiration combined with sexual emotion, such as that obtained from viewing one's naked body, or one's genitals. SEE: *erotomania.*

e., oral. Sensation of pleasure experienced when nursing at the breast, modified and sublimated but continuing into adult life through normal contacts of the lips, mouth, and throat.

er'otism. In psychology, eroticism.

erotogenic (ĕ-rŏ″to-jĕn′ĭk) [Gr. *erōs*, love, + *gennan*, to produce]. Producing sexual excitement. SEE: *zone, erogenous.*

erotology (ĕr″ŏ-tŏl′ō-jĭ) [″+ *logos*, study]. The study of love and its manifestations.

erotomania (e-rō″tŏ-, e-rŏt″ō-mā′nĭ-ă) [″+ *mania*, madness]. Pathological exaggeration of sexual behavior. SEE: *eroticism.*

erotopathia (e-rō″to-, e-rŏt″o-păth′ĭ-ă) [″+ *pathos*, disease]. Any abnormal or perverted sex impulse.

erotophobia (e-rō″to-, e-rŏt″o-fō′bĭ-ă) [″+ *phobos*, fear]. Aversion to sexual love or its manifestations.

erotopsychic (e-rō″to-, e-rŏt″o-sī′kik) [″+ *psychē*, mind]. Having abnormal sexual desires.

errat'ic [L. *errāre*, to wander]. Wandering, having an unpredictable or fluctuating course or pattern. SYN: *eccentric.*

errhine (ĕr′ĭn) [Gr. *en*, in, + *rhis, rhin-*, nose]. 1. Causing increased nasal discharge. 2. An agent that will increase the secretion of the mucous membrane lining the nose.

erubes'cence [L. *erubēscere*, to grow red]. Reddening of the skin; a blush.

eructa'tion [L. *eructāre*, to belch]. Producing gas or fluid from the stomach, usually with the production of a characteristic sound; belching.

eruption (e-rŭp′shŭn) [L. *eruptio*, a breaking out]. 1. A breaking out and becoming visible, esp. applied to the appearance of a skin lesion or rash accompanying a disease such as measles or scarlet fever. 2. The appearance of a lesion such as redness or spotting on the skin or mucous membrane. 3. The breaking through of a tooth through the gum; the cutting of a tooth.

e., creeping. A skin lesion characterized by a tortuous elevated red line which progresses at one end while fading out at the other. It is caused by the migration of the larvae of certain nematodes, esp. Ancylostoma braziliense and other cat and dog nematodes which occur as accidental invaders of man. SYN: *larva migrans.*

e., drug. Dermatitis medicamentosa; skin reaction resulting from the ingestion of certain drugs, such as iodides.

e., serum. That which occurs following the injection of a serum. May be accompanied by chills and fever.

erup'tive. Breaking out, as with a rash.

erysipelas (ĕr″ĭ-sĭp′ĕ-lăs) [Gr. *erythros*, red, + *pella*, skin]. Acute febrile disease with localized inflammation and swelling of skin and subcutaneous tissue accompanied by systemic disturbance of variable degree.

ETIOL: Streptococcus pyogenes.

SYM: Fever; chills; nausea; vomiting; painful and warm skin; face and head lesions that are hot and red usually seen within 24-48 hours. Bullae may develop.

TREATMENT: Penicillin or erythromycin. Cool magnesium sulfate solution compresses for skin. Aspirin for pain.

PROG: Excellent with treatment. If untreated, nephritis, abscesses and septicemia may develop.

erysipelatous (ĕr″ĭ-sĭ-pĕl′ă-tus). Of the nature of or pert. to erysipelas.

erysipeloid (ĕr-ĭ-sĭp′ĕ-loyd) [Gr. *erythros*, skin, + *pella*, skin, + *eidos*, form]. An infective dermatitis resembling erysipelas usually limited to the hands and characterized by hyperemia, edema, and occasionally systemic complications.

ETIOL: It is caused by Erysipelothrix rhusiopathiae, usually acquired by handling of fish products.

Erysipelothrix (ĕr-ĭ-sī-pel′o-thriks). A genus of bacteria belonging to the family Corynebacteriaceae. They are branching filamentous, rod-shaped, nonmotile organisms.

E. rhusiopathiae. The causative agent of swine erysipelas and erysipeloid in man.

erysipelotoxin (ĕr′ĭ-sĭp″ĕ-lo-tŏk′sĭn). The toxin produced by Streptococcus pyogenes, the causative agent of erysipelas.

erythema (ĕr″ĭ-thē′mă) [Gr. redness]. A form of macula showing diffused redness over the skin.

ETIOL: Caused by capillary congestion, usually due to dilatation of the superficial capillaries as a result of (1) some nervous mechanism within the body, (2) inflammation, (3) as a result of some external influence, such as heat, sunburn, etc.

e. ab igne. Localized e. due to exposure to heat.

e. annulare. E. with rounded, raised marginal lesions.

e. circinatum. In red circles.

e. congestivum. E. with congestive state of skin.

e., diffuse. Widely spread over body.

e. dose. The amount of radiant energy sufficient to evoke perceptible redness of the skin.

e. hyperaemicum. Caused by heat or cold (e. caloricum, chilblain), sun (e. solare), artificial heat as from hot water bottle or electric pad (e. ab igne, q.v.).

e. infectiosum. Contagious form with rose-colored eruption.

e. intertrigo. Chafing of opposing surfaces, with e. and often with maceration and abrasion.

e. multiforme. A macular eruption with dark red papules or tubercles. Usually on extremities appearing in successive eruptions of short duration. No itching, burning or rheumatic pains. May appear in separate rings, concentric rings, disk-shaped patches, distributed elevations, and figured arrangements.

Eruptive, Infective, and Contagious Diseases

Name	Period of Incubation	Time of Eruption	Duration of Eruption	Period of Quarantine or Isolation
Scarlet Fever	1–3 days	12–24 hr. after onset	7–10 days	7 days isolation
Smallpox	8–17 days	3rd or 4th day of fever	14–21 days	21 days or until all scabs disappear
Measles (Rubeola)	8–13 days	4th day of fever	4–6 days	Isolation from diagnosis until 7 days after appearance of rash. Strict isolation from children under 3 years
Rubella	14–21 days	2nd day of fever	1–3 days	None, but avoid contact with nonimmune pregnant women
Mumps	12–26 days			Until all swellings have subsided
Whooping Cough	About a week			Isolation for 3 weeks after onset of spasmodic cough
Chickenpox	14–21 days	2nd day of fever	7–21 days	7 days after onset
Diphtheria	2–5 days			7 days and until 2 successive nose and throat cultures, 24 hr. apart, are negative; to be taken after cessation of antibiotic therapy
Typhus Fever	7–14 days	3rd to 8th day of fever	14 days	None
Typhoid Fever	7–21 days	4th day of fever	3–5 days for each crop of spots	Release after 3 successive negative cultures of urine and feces not less than 24 hr. apart and not earlier than one month after onset

e. nodosum. Red and painful nodules on legs associated with rheumatism. Also caused by certain drugs and food poisoning.

e., punctate. In minute points, as scarlet fever rash.

e. venenatum. Form caused by contact with an irritating substance.

erythemat'ic, erythem'atous [Gr. *erythēma*, redness]. Pert. to or marked by erythema.

erythemogen'ic ["+ *gennan*, to produce]. Pert. to erythema.

erythemomegalalgia (er-ĭ-thē'mo-mĕg-al-ăl'jĭ-ă) ["+ *megas*, great, + *algos*, pain]. Painful redness of skin. SYN: *erythromelalgia.*

erythralgia (ĕr'ĭ-thral'jĭ-ă) [Gr. *erythros*, red, + *algos*, pain]. A condition of painful redness of the skin. SYN: *erythromelalgia.*

erythrasma (ĕr'ĭ-thrăz'mă). Reddish-brown eruption in patches in the axillae and groins formerly thought to be due to a fungus, but now considered to be bacterial in origin.

erythredema (ĕ-rĭth"rĕ-dē'mă) [Gr. *erythros*, red, + *oidēma*, swelling]. An infantile disease characterized by lesions of the skin on the hands and feet, swelling of the extremities, digestive disturbances. It is frequently followed by arthritis involving multiple joints and muscle weakness. Its cause is unknown. SYN: *acrodynia; pink disease.*

erythre'mia ["+ *haima*, blood]. Excessive increase of red blood corpuscles with cyanosis. SYN: *polycythemia rubra.*

erythrism (ĕ-rĭth'rĭzm) ["+ *ismos*, condition of]. Redness of the hair and beard with ruddy complexion.

erythristic (ĕr'ĭ-thrĭs'tik) [Gr. *erythros*, red]. Ruddy complexion. Having reddish hair.

erythro-. Prefix meaning red.

erythroblast (ĕ-rĭth'ro-blăst) [Gr. *erythros*, red, + *blastos*, germ]. Any form of nucleated red corpuscles. The earliest stages in the development are pronormoblast; basophilic normoblast; polychromatic normoblast; and orthochromatic normoblast. Nucleated red cells are not normally seen in the circulating blood. E's possess hemoglobin.

In the embryo they are found in blood islands of the yolk sac, body mesenchyma, liver, spleen, and lymph nodes; after the third month they are restricted to the bone marrow.

erythroblaste'mia ["+ "+ *haima*, blood]. An excessive number of erythroblasts in the blood.

erythroblas'tic. Pert. to erythroblasts.

erythroblasto'ma [Gr. *erythros*, red, + *blastos*, germ, + *-ōma*, tumor]. A tumor (myeloma) with cells resembling megaloblasts.

erythroblasto'sis ["+ "+ *-ōsis*, condition]. A condition marked by many erythroblasts in the blood.

e. fetalis. A hemolytic disease of the newborn characterized by anemia, jaundice, and enlargement of the liver and spleen, generalized edema (hydrops fetalis). ETIOL: It is due to the development in an Rh negative mother of antibodies against an Rh positive fetus. This occurs following a preceding pregnancy in which the fetus was Rh positive or following transfusion of Rh positive blood.

erythrochloropia (ĕ-rĭth"ro-klōr-ō'pĭ-ă) [Gr. *erythros*, red, + *chlōros*, green, + *ōps*, eye]. Partial color blindness with ability to see only red and green.

erythrochromia (ĕ-rĭth"ro-krō'mĭ-ă) ["+ *chroma*, color]. Hemorrhagic red pigmentation of the spinal fluid.

erythroclas'tic ["+ *klasis*, a breaking]. Destructive to red blood cells.

erythrocyano'sis ["+ *kyanos*, blue, + *-ōsis*, condition]. Red or bluish discoloration on the skin with swelling, itching and burning.

erythrocyte (ĕ-rĭth'ro-sit) [Gr. *erythros*, red, + *kytos*, hollow vessel (cell)]. Red blood corpuscle.

Each is a non-nucleated, biconcave disk averaging 7.7 microns in diameter. The body of the cell consists of a spongelike stroma containing a respiratory pigment, hemoglobin, enclosed in a cell membrane of proteins in combination with lipoid substances. Hemoglobin is a conjugated protein consisting of a colored iron-containing portion, hematin, and a simple protein, globin. It combines readily with oxygen to form an unstable compound oxyhemoglobin.

The total surface area of the red cells of an average man is 3820 square meters or about 2000 times greater than his total body surface area.

NUMBER: In a normal person, the number of erythrocytes averages about 5,000,000 per cubic millimeter (5,500,000 for males 4,-500,000 for females). The total number in an average-sized person is about 35 trillion. The number per cubic millimeter varies with age, being higher in infants; time of day, being lower during sleep; activity and environmental temperature, increasing in both conditions; and altitude. Persons living at altitudes of 10,000 ft. (3,048 meters) or more may have a red cell count of 8,000,000 per cubic mm. or more.

If an individual has a normal blood volume of 5 liters, 5,000,000 red blood cells per cubic millimeter of blood, and the erythrocytes have an average life span of 120 days, then the body needs to produce 2,400,-000 red blood cells per second in order to maintain this concentration of blood.

The primary function of the red blood cells is to carry oxygen and carbon dioxide. They also play a role in the regulation of the acid-base balance of the blood and in the formation of bile pigments which are derived from decomposition products of hemoglobin.

Red cell formation (erythropoiesis) in the adult takes place in the red bone marrow, principally in the vertebrae, ribs, sternum, diploe of cranial bones, and proximal ends of the humerus and femur. They arise from large nucleated stem-cells (promegaloblasts) which give rise to pronormoblasts in which hemoglobin appears. These give rise to normoblasts which extrude their nuclei. Red cells at this stage possess a fine reticular network and are known as reticulocytes. This reticular structure is lost before the cells enter circulation as mature e.'s.

The proper formation of e.'s depends upon several factors, among them: healthy condition of the bone marrow; dietary substances such as iron, cobalt, and copper, all essential for the formation of hemoglobin, plus essential amino acids, and certain vitamins, esp. B_{12} and folic acid (pteroylglutamic acid).

Life History and Fate: The average length of life of a red blood cell is estimated to be about 120 days. Cells are continuously dying and disintegrating. The cellular debris is picked up by the cells of the reticuloendothelial system, esp. those of the spleen, liver, and bone marrow. Hemoglobin is broken down, and proteins and iron are stored and utilized in the formation of new e.'s. The iron-containing portion, hematin, gives rise to bilirubin, which is excreted in the bile as one of the bile pigments.

Variations: On microscopic examination e.'s may reveal variations in the following respects: Size (anisocytosis); shape (poikilocytosis); staining reaction (achromia, hypochromia, hyperchromia, polychromatophilia); structure (possession of bodies such as Cabot's rings, Howell-Jolly bodies, Heinz bodies, parasites such as malaria, a reticular network, or nuclei); number (anemia, polycythemia).

e., achromatic. A phantom corpuscle or one from which the hemoglobin has been dissolved; a colorless corpuscle.

e., basophilic. E. in which cytoplasm stains blue indicating the presence of basophilic material. May be diffuse (basophilic material uniformly distributed) or punctate (material appearing as pin point dots).

e., crenated. E. with a serrated or indented edge usually the result of withdrawal of water from the cell as occurs when cells are placed in hypertonic solutions.

e., immature. An erythroblast.

e., orthochromatic. E. that stains with acid stains only, cytoplasm appearing pink.

e., polychromatic. E. that does not stain uniformly.

erythrocythemia (ĕ-rĭth″ro-sĭ-the′mĭ-ă) [Gr. *erythros,* red, + *kytos,* hollow vessel (cell), + *haima,* blood]. Enormous increase in red blood cells. SYN: *erythremia; polycythemia.*

erythrocytolysis (ĕ-rĭth″ro-sĭ-tŏl′ĭ-sis) ["+ "+ *lysis,* dissolution]. Dissolution of red blood corpuscles with the escape of hemoglobin; hemolysis.

erythrocytometer (ĕ-rĭth″ro-sĭ-tŏm′ĕ-tĕr) ["+ "+ *metron,* measure]. Instrument for counting red blood corpuscles.

erythrocytoopsonin (ĕ-rĭth″ro-sī″to-ŏp-sō′-nĭn) ["+ "+ *opsōnein,* to prepare food for]. A substance opsonic for red corpuscles.

erythrocytorrhexis (ĕ-rĭth″ro-sī″to-rĕk′sis) ["+ "+ *rhēxis,* rupture]. The breaking up of red blood cells with particles or fragments of the cell escaping into the plasma; plasmorrhexis.

erythrocytoschisis (ĕ-rĭth″ro-sĭ-tŏs′kĭ-sis) [Gr. *erythros,* red, + *kytos,* hollow vessel (cell), + *schisis,* division]. The breaking up of red blood cells into small disk-like particles resembling blood platelets.

erythrocytosis (ĕ-rĭth″ro-sĭ-tō′sis) ["+ "+ -*ōsis,* increasing condition]. Abnormal increase in the number of red blood cells in circulation; polycythemia; erythemia; erythrocytothemia.

erythroderma (ĕ-rĭth″ro-dĕr′mă) ["+ *derma,* skin]. Erythema, erythrodermia, q.v.

e. desquamativum. A disease, resembling seborrhea, of breast-fed infants characterized by redness of skin and development of scales; Leiner's disease.

e. ichthyosiforme congenitum. A congenital condition characterized by thickening and redness of the skin; may resemble ichthyosis or lichen.

e., maculopapular. A condition of the skin characterized by redness and eruption of macules and papules.

e. squamosum. An eruption of the skin consisting of groups of papules covered by scales; parapsoriasis.

erythrodermia (ĕ-rĭth″ro-dĕr′mĭ-ă). Abnormal redness in the skin. SYN: *erythema.*

erythrodextrin (ĕ-rĭth″ro-dĕx′trĭn) [Gr. *erythros*, red, + L. *dexter*, right]. Form of dextrin from splitting of a polysaccharide molecule. SEE: *achroodextrin.*

erythrogen′esis [″+ *genesis*, development]. The development of red blood corpuscles.

erythroleukemia (ĕ-rĭth″ro-lū-kē′mĭ-ă) [Gr. *erythros*, red, + *leukos*, white, + *haima*, blood]. Malignant growth of both the red- and white-blood-cell-forming tissues. Rapid and progressive disorder accompanied by severe anemia and many abnormal white and red cells in the blood. Changes similar to those of pernicious anemia and myelocytic leukemia.

erythroleukosis (ĕ-rĭth″ro-lū-kō′sĭs) [″+ ″+ *ōsis*, condition of increase]. Abnormal increase of red cells and granulocytes.

erythrolysin (ĕr″ĭ-thrŏl′ĭ-sin) [″+ *lysis*, dissolution]. An agent causing erythrolysis. SYN: *erythrocytolysin; hemolysin.* SEE: *lysin.*

erythrol′ysis. Dissolution of red blood corpuscles. SYN: *erythrocytolysis.*

erythromelalgia (ĕ-rĭth″ro-mel-ăl′jĭ-ă) [Gr. *erythros*, red, + *melos*, limb, + *algos*, pain]. A skin neurosis accompanied by burning and throbbing which come and go, affecting any one of the extremities, esp. the feet.

erythrome′lia [″+ *melos*, limb]. Erythema of extensor surfaces of extremities but without pain.

erythromycin (ĕ-rĭth″ro-mī′sĭn) [″+ *mykēs*, fungus]. An antibiotic from Streptomyces erythreus. It is effective orally against many gram positive and some gram negative organisms.

erythron (ĕr′ĭ-thrŏn) [Gr. *erythros*, red]. The concept of blood as a body system including the circulating red cells and the organ from which they arise, i.e., the bone marrow.

erythroneocytosis (ĕ-rĭth″ro-nē″o-sī-tō′sĭs) [″+ *neos*, new, + *kytos*, cell, + *-ōsis*, forming]. Regenerative forms of red blood cells in the blood.

erythronoclastic (ĕr-ĭ-thrŏn-o-klăs′tĭk) [″+ *klan*, to break]. Destructive to the erythron.

erythropar′asite [Gr. *erythros*, red, + *parasitos*, parasite]. A red blood corpuscle parasite.

erythrop′athy [″+ *pathos*, disease]. Disease of the red blood corpuscles.

erythropenia (ĕ-rĭth″ro-pē′nĭ-ă) [″+ *penia*, poverty]. Deficiency in number of red blood corpuscles.

erythrophage (ĕ-rĭth″ro-fāj) [″+ *phagein*, to eat]. A phagocyte which destroys red corpuscles.

erythropha′gia. Destruction of red blood cells by phagocytes.

erythrophile, erythrophilous (ĕ-rĭth′ro-fĭl, ĕr″ĭ-thrŏf′ĭ-lus) [Gr. *erythros*, red, + *philein*, to love]. Readily staining red.

erythrophobia (ĕ-rĭth″ro-fō′bĭ-ă) [″+ *phobos*, fear]. 1. Abnormal dread of blushing or fear of being diffident or of being embarrassed. 2. A morbid fear of, or aversion to, anything colored red.

erythrophose (ĕ-rĭth′ro-fōz) [″+ *phōs*, light]. Any red subjective perception of a bright spot. SEE: *phose.*

erythrophthisis (ĕ-rĭth″ro-thī′sĭs) [″+ *phthisis*, wasting]. Serious damage to the restorative power of the red corpuscles.

erythrophthoric (ĕ-rĭth″ro-thor′ĭk) [Gr. *erythros*, red, + *phtheirein*, to destroy]. Rapid destruction of erythrocytes by a process other than hemolysis.

erythropia, erythropsia (er″ĭ-thro′pĭ-ă, -throp′sĭ-ă) [″+ *opsis*, vision]. Condition in which objects appear to be red.

erythroplasia (ĕ-rĭth″ro-plā′zĭ-ă) [″+ *plasis*, molding, forming]. A condition considered to be precancerous characterized by the appearance of erythematous lesions involving the junctions of the epithelium of the skin and mucous membranes at the mouth, anus, penis, and vulva.

erythropoiesis (ĕ-rĭth″ro-poy-ē′sĭs) [″+ *poiēsis*, making]. The formation of red blood corpuscles.

erythropoietic (ĕ-rĭth″ro-poy-ĕt′ĭk). Pert. to red blood cells.

erythroprosopalgia (ĕ-rĭth″ro-pro-so-păl′-jĭ-ă) [Gr. *erythros*, red, + *prosōpon*, face, + *algos*, pain]. A neuropathy characterized by redness and pain in the face.

erythropsia (ĕr-ĭ-thrŏp′sĭ-ă) [″+ *opsis*, vision]. Perversion of color vision in which all objects look red.

erythrop′sin [″+ *opsis*, vision]. Pigment in the external portion of the rods of the retina. SYN: *rhodopsin; visual purple.*

erythrorrhexis (ĕ-rĭth″ro-rĕks′ĭs) [Gr. *erythros*, red, + *rhexis*, rupture]. Rupture of a red cell and escape of its plasma. SYN: *erythrocytorrhexis; plasmorrhexis.*

erythrosis (ĕr-ĭ-thrō′sĭs) [″+ *-ōsis*, condition]. A reddish-purple discoloration of the skin and mucous membranes in polycythemia.

erythrotoxin (ĕ-rĭth″ro-tŏk′sĭn) [″+ *toxikon*, poison]. An exotoxin that attacks red blood cells. SEE: *leukotoxic.*

erythruria (ĕr-ĭ-thrū′rĭ-ă) [″+ *ouron*, urine]. Red color of the urine.

escape [O.Fr. *escaper*, to emerge from restraint]. 1. To escape from confinement; leak or seep out. 2. The act of attaining freedom.
 e. mechanism. In psychiatry, the reaction of a person in adjusting temporarily to

difficult, unpleasant, or intolerable situations by unconsciously employing another means of adaption which is less difficult or more pleasant.

e., vagal. Occurrence of a ventricular contraction when the normal rhythmical beat of the heart has been stopped or inhibited by stimulation of the vagus nerve. SYN: *escape from inhibition; escape of the heart; vagus escape.*

e., ventricular. Occurrence of single or repeated ventricular contractions from impulses arising in the atrioventricular node rather than the sino-auricular node. SYN: *nodal extrasystole.*

eschar (ĕs'kär) [Gr. *eschara,* scab]. A slough, esp. one following a cauterization or burn. SEE: *escharotic.*

escharotic (ĕs-kăr-ŏt'ĭk). Agent used to destroy tissue and to cause sloughing which produces what is known as an eschar. The third degree of counterirritation.

The agents are caustics, the mild ones being used in the treatment of skin diseases; the stronger being employed to destroy infected tissue and to counteract the bites of animals and insects, caustic soda and antimonial ointment being applied for this purpose. Escharotics may be acids, alkalies, metallic salts, phenol or carbolic acid, carbon dioxide, or electric cautery.

escharotomy. Removal of the eschar formed on the skin and underlying tissue of severely burned areas. Procedure is particularly helpful in restoring circulation to the extremities of patients in which the eschar forms a tight swollen band around the circumference of the limb.

Escherich's reflex (ĕsh'ĕr-ĭk). [Theodor Escherich, Ger. physician, 1857-1911] Pursing or muscular contraction of lips resulting from irritation of mucosa of lips.

Escherichia (ĕsh-ĕr-ĭk'ĭ-ă). A genus of bacteria belonging to the family Enterobacteriaceae, tribe Eschericheae. They are common inhabitants of the alimentary canal of man and other animals.

E. coli. The colon bacillus; Short, plump, gram-negative, nonspore-forming motile bacillus almost constantly present in the alimentary canal of humans and some animals. They are normally nonpathogenic in the intestinal tract. Outside the body and under certain conditions, particularly in the urinary tract, E. coli is responsible for infections in other systems and for enteritis in infants. The presence of the bacilli in milk or water is an indicator of fecal contamination.

eschrolalia (ĕs-krō-lā'lĭ-ă) [Gr. *aischros,* indecent, + *lalia,* babble]. Meaningless utterance of obscene words. SYN: *coprolalia.*

es'culent [L. *esculentus,* edible]. Suitable to be eaten.

escutcheon (ĕs-kŭch'ŭn) [L. *scutum,* shield]. The coarse pubic hair in the adult.

ESF. Abbr. for *erythropoietic stimulating factor.*

Esmarch's bandage (ĕs'märk). [Johannes F. A. von Esmarch, Ger. surgeon, 1823-1908] A rubber bandage for controlling bleeding. Before operation commences, bandage is applied tightly to limb, commencing at distal end and reaching above site of operation, where a rubber tourniquet is firmly applied. The bandage is then removed. This renders operative area virtually bloodless. Caution: Tourniquet must not be applied so tightly as to cause nerve damage. Also it must be removed in time to prevent injury due to lack of blood flow to the distal tissues. SEE: *bandage.*

esodic (ē-sŏd'ĭk) [Gr. *es,* toward, + *hodos,* way]. Centripetal or afferent; pert. to sensory nerves conducting impulses toward the brain and spinal cord.

esoethmoiditis (ĕs"ō-ĕth"moy-dĭ'tĭs) ["+ *ēthmos,* sieve, + *eidos,* form, + *-itis,* inflammation]. Inflammation of membrane of ethmoid cells.

esogastri'tis ["+ *gastēr,* belly, + *-itis,* inflammation]. Inflammation of the gastric mucus membrane.

esophagalgia (ē-sŏf-ă-găl'jĭ-ă) [Gr. *oisophagos,* esophagus, + *algos,* pain]. Pain in the esophagus.

esophageal (ē-sŏf'ă-jē'al). Pert. to the esophagus.

esophagectasia, esophagectasis (ē-sŏf'ă-jĕk-tā'sĭ-ă, -jĕk'tă-sis) [Gr. *oisophagos,* esophagus, + *ektasis,* distention]. Dilatation of the esophagus.

esophagec'tomy ["+ *ektomē,* excision]. Excision of a part of the esophagus.

esophagismus (ē-sŏf-ă-jĭs'mŭs) ["+ *-ismos,* condition]. Esophageal spasm.

esophagitis (ē-sŏf-ă-jī'tĭs) ["+ *-itis,* inflammation]. Inflammation of the esophagus.

esophagocele (ē-sŏf'ă-gō-sēl) ["+ *kēlē,* hernia]. Hernia of the esophagus.

esophagodynia (ē-sŏf'ă-gōn'ĭ-ă) [Gr. *oisophagos,* esophagus, + *odynē,* pain]. Pain in the esophagus.

esophagoenterostomy (ē-sŏf'ă-gō-ĕn-tĕr-ŏs'tō-mī) ["+ *enteron,* intestine, + *stoma,* mouth]. Formation of communication between the esophagus and intestine following excision of stomach.

esophagogastroscopy (ē-sŏf-ă-gō-gas-trŏs'kō-pī) ["+ *gastēr,* belly, + *skopein,* to examine]. Inspection of esophagus and stomach by using a type of endoscope capable of viewing both the esophagus and stomach.

esophagogastrostomy (ē-sŏf'ă-gō-găs-trŏs'tō-mī) ["+ "+ *stoma*, mouth]. Formation of a communication between the esophagus and stomach.

esophagomalacia (ē-sŏf'ă-gō-mă-lā'sǐ-ă) [Gr. *oisophagos*, esophagus, + *malakia*, softness]. Softening of the esophageal walls.

esophagomycosis (ē-sŏf'ă-gō-mī-kō'sǐs) ["+ *mykēs*, fungus, + *ōsis*, condition]. Bacterial or fungus disease of esophagus.

esophagoplasty (ē-sŏf'ă-gō-plăs"tī) ["+ *plassein*, to form]. Repair of the esophagus by a plastic operation.

esophagoplication (ē-sŏf'ă-gō-plǐ-kā'shŭn) ["+ L. *plicāre*, to fold]. The surgical procedure of reducing dilation of the esophagus by taking tucks in its walls.

esophagoptosia, esophagoptosis (ē-sŏf'ă-gŏp-tō'sǐ-ă, -sǐs) [Gr. *oisophagos*, esophagus, + *ptōsis*, a falling]. Relaxation and prolapse of the esophagus.

esophagoscope (ē-sŏf'ă-gō-skōp) ["+ *sko-pein*, to examine]. A type of endoscope for examination of esophagus.

esoph'agospasm ["+ *spasmos*, spasm]. Spasm of the esophagus.

esophagostenosis (ē-sŏf'ă-gō-stěn-ō'sǐs) ["+ *stenōsis*, contraction]. Stricture or narrowing of the esophagus.

esophagostomy (ē-sŏf-ă-gŏs'tō-mī) [Gr. *oisophagos*, esophagus, + *stoma*, opening]. Surgical formation of an opening into the esophagus.

esophagotome (ē-sŏf'ă-gō-tōm) ["+ *tomē*, incision]. Instrument for forming an esophageal fistula.

esophagotomy (ē-sŏf-ă-gŏt'ō-mī). Surgical incision into esophagus.

esophagus (ē-sŏf'ă-gŭs) [Gr. *oisophagos*]. (pl. *esophagi*) [NA]. A muscular canal extending from the pharynx to the stomach. Length about 23-25 cm. (9-9 3/4 in.). SYN: *gullet*.

    e., foreign bodies in. F. A. TREATMENT: The patient may complain of pain or an uncomfortable feeling deep in the chest. The article often can be dislodged by making the patient vomit by using the finger to stimulate the oral pharynx or back part of the throat.

    A physician should always be called. Foreign bodies in the stomach are ordinarily not dangerous and usually pass through the alimentary tract in a few days without danger. However, it may be dangerous to give cathartics or enemas. These patients should always be under the care of a physician.

esophoria (ĕs-ō-fō'rǐ-ă) [Gr. *esō*, inward, + *phorein*, to bear]. In ophthalmology, tenden-

cy of visual lines to converge. Inward turning or amount of inward turning of the eye. SEE: *esotropia; exophoria; heterotropia*.

esophylac'tic ["+ *phylaxis*, protection]. That which is phylactic or protective.

esophylaxis (ĕs"ō-fī-lăks'ĭs). The protective biological action against disease exercised by the fluids and cells of the body. SEE: *exophylaxis*.

esosphenoiditis (ĕs"ō-sfē-noyd-ī'tĭs) [Gr. *esō*, inward, + *sphēn*, wedge, + *eidos*, form, + *-itis*, inflammation]. Osteomyelitis of the sphenoid bone.

esoteric (ĕs-ō-tĕr'ĭk) [Gr. *esōterikos*, inner]. 1. Secret, hidden, or understood only by a small group. 2. In physiology, arising from within the organism.

esotropia (ĕs-ō-trō'pǐ-ă) [Gr. *esō*, inward, + *tropos*, turning]. Marked turning inward of eye, crossed eyes.

ESP. Abbr. for *extrasensory perception*.

ESR. Abbr. for *electron spin resistance; erythrocyte sedimentation rate*.

-ess [O.Fr. *-esse*]. Suffix noting female sex.

es'sence [L. *essentia*, being or quality]. 1. The spirit or principle of anything. 2. An alcoholic solution of volatile oil.

essen'tial [L. *essentialis*]. 1. Pert. to an essence. 2. Indispensable. 3. Specific; independent of a local morbid condition. SYN: *idiopathic*.

    e. oil. Any volatile oil of vegetable or animal origin.

es'ter [L. *aethēr*, ether]. In organic chemistry, a compound formed by the combination of an organic acid with an alcohol.

    Ex: Ethyl acetate is an ester formed by combining acetic acid with ethyl alcohol. Esters are commonly liquids with characteristic fruity or flowery odors.

esterase (ĕs'tĕr-ās). Generic term for an enzyme that catalyzes the hydrolysis of esters.

    e., acetylcholine. Cholinesterase, an enzyme that quickly hydrolyzes acetylcholine to acetic acid and choline.

es'terize. To convert into an ester.

esthematology (ĕs"thĕm-ă-tŏl'ō-gī) [Gr. *aisthēma*, sensation, + *logos*, science]. Science of the sense organs and their function.

esthesia (ĕs-thē'zǐ-ă) [Gr. *aisthēsis*, sensation]. 1. Perception, feeling, sensation. 2. Any disease that affects sensation or perception.

esthesioblast (ĕs-thē'zǐ-ō-blast) ["+ *blastos*, germ]. An embryonic ganglion cell. SYN: *ganglioblast*.

esthesiol'ogy ["+ *logos*, science]. Science of sensory phenomena. SYN: *esthematology*.

esthesiomania (ĕs-thē″zĭ-ō-mā′nĭ-ă) [Gr. *aisthēsis*, sensation, + *mania*, madness]. Insanity with sensory hallucinations and perverted moral sensibilities.

esthesiometer (ĕs-thē-zĭ-ŏm′ĕ-ter) ["+ *metron*, measure]. Device for measuring tactile sensibility.

esthesioneurosis (ĕs-thē′zĭ-ō-nū-rō′sĭs) ["+ *neuron*, nerve, + *ōsis*, condition]. A loss of feeling without any apparent organic lesion.

esthesiophysiology (ĕs-thē″sĭ-ō-fĭs-ĭ-ōl′ō-jĭ) [Gr. *aisthēsis*, sensation, + *physis*, nature, + *logos*, study]. Physiology of the sense organs.

esthesioscopy (ĕs-thē′zĭ-ŏs′kō-pĭ) ["+ *skopein*, to examine]. Testing tactile and other forms of sensibility.

estheticokinetic (ĕs-thĕt″ĭ-kō-kĭn-ĕt′ĭk) ["+ *kinēsis*, motion]. Being both sensory and motor.

esthiomene (ĕs″thĭ-ŏm′ĕ-nē) [Gr. *esthiomenos*, eating]. A chronic hypertrophic ulcerative vulvovaginitis. A complication of lymphogranuloma venereum. SYN: *esthiomenus*.

estival (ĕs′tĭ-văl) [L. *aestivus*]. Rel. to or occurring in summer.

estivoautumnal ["+ *autumnalis*, pert. to autumn]. 1. Pert. to summer and autumn. 2. A term applied to form of malaria.

estradiol (ĕs-tră-dī′ŏl). $C_{18}H_{24}O_2$, a crystalline steroid produced by the ovary and possessing estrogenic properties. Large quantities are found in the urine of pregnant women and mares and in the urine of stallions, the latter two serving as sources of the commercial product. Estradiol is effective when given subcutaneously or intramuscularly but not when administered by mouth. In the body it is converted to estrone. SEE: *estrogen*.

   e. dipropionate. An ester of estradiol.

estriol (ĕs′trĭ-ōl). Estrogenic hormone considered to be the metabolic product of estrone and estradiol. It is found in the urine of the female.

estrogen (ĕs′trō-jĕn) [Gr. *oistros*, mad desire, + *gennan*, to produce]. Any natural or artificial substance that induces estrogenic activity; more specifically the estrogenic hormones, estradiol and estrone, produced by the ovary; the female sex hormones. Estrogens are responsible for the development of secondary sexual characteristics, cyclic changes in the vaginal epithelium and endothelium of the uterus. They are used in the treatment of menopausal symptoms. Natural estrogens include estrodiol, estrone, and their metabolic product, estriol. When used therapeutically, estrogens are usually given in the form of a conjugate such as ethinyl estradiol, conjugated estrogens (USP), or the synthetic estrogen diethylstilbestrol. These preparations are effective when given by mouth.

estrogenic (ĕs-trō-jĕn′ĭk). Causing estrus; acting to produce the effects of an estrogen, q.v.

es′trone. An estrogenic hormone, $C_{18}H_{22}O_2$, found in the urine of pregnant women and mares. It is also prepared synthetically. Used in the treatment of estrogen deficiencies. It is less active than estradiol but more active than estriol.

es′trual [Gr. *oistros*, mad desire]. Pert. to estrus of animals.

estrua′tion. The sexually fertile period in animals; the so-called period of heat.

es′trus, oestrus [Gr. *oistros*, mad desire]. The recurrent period of sexual activity in mammals other than primates, called heat, characterized by congestion of and secretion by the uterine mucosa, proliferation of vaginal epithelium, swelling of the vulva, ovulation, and acceptance of the male by the female.

   e. cycle. The cycle from the beginning of one e. period to the beginning of the next. Includes proestrus, estrus, and metestrus followed by a short period of quiescence called diestrus.

estua′rium [L.]. Vapor bath.

état mamelonné (ā-tä′mä-mĕl-ŏn-ā′) [Fr., knobby state]. Condition of gastric mucosa in chronic inflammation with nodular projections.

ethanol (ĕth′ă-nŏl). Ethyl alcohol. SEE: *alcohol.*

e′ther [Gr. *aithēr*, air]. 1. Hypothetic substance once regarded as permeating all space and capable of transmitting electromagnetic waves. 2. Any organic compound in which an oxygen atom links together with carbon chains.

   The general formula is R′OR″. The ether used for anesthesia is diethyl ether, $C_4H_{10}O$. As an anesthetic it causes postoperative nausea and profuse salivation.

   CAUTION: Ether is highly flammable and should be handled with great care. Also it should not be stored once the can is opened because toxic products form when ether is exposed to light.

   e. anesthesia. Ethyl oxide, or diethyl ether, $C_4H_{10}O$, the common ether used in anesthesia. It is a thin, colorless, highly volatile, and highly flammable liquid with a sp. gr. of 0.7077 at 25° C. It has a characteristic sweetish pungent odor and produces a burning sensation when tasted. It is widely used for general anesthesia. The action of ether is slower than other general anesthetics and the margin of safety is greater.

For 10-15 minutes after e. anesthesia is discontinued the exhaled air may be flammable.

PHYS. ACTION: In the early stages of anesthesia, ether stimulates the respiratory mucus membranes and the respiratory center in the medulla oblongata. It stimulates and accelerates the action of the heart. It lowers body temperature and raises blood pressure unless given in large doses or continued over a long period, when it lowers blood pressure. Compared to other inhalation anesthetics it produces excellent muscular relaxation.

CONTRA: Its use is contraindicated in diabetes, liver damage, kidney disease, chronic pulmonary conditions (tuberculosis), surgical shock, or following recent severe blood loss.

AFTER EFFECTS: Excitement with desire to talk follows e. anesthesia; the patient perspires freely, exhibits signs of nausea and begins to vomit, all before the return to consciousness which may not be regained for several hours. Upon awakening he feels dizzy, complains of headache and thirst. These effects may last for hours. The flow of saliva and the secretion of mucus may be increased. It is usually excreted from the body within 24 hr. Pneumonia is the most common complication following e. anesthesia. Gas pains and inability to urinate may occur. The latter symptom may be aggravated by the use of morphine or its derivatives for pain.

NP: Warm or cold water; the quantity permitted to relieve thirst depends upon the surgeon. Foot of bed elevated and the head should be turned to one side when vomiting to prevent vomitus from passing into the trachea. Apparatus for aspiration of secretions and vomitus from the pharynx should be available at the bedside or in the recovery room. Cold compresses may be placed to head. A rectal irrigation may be given or a rectal tube may be inserted to relieve gas pressure. SEE: *chloroform anesthesia.*

e. asphyxia. Suffocation during ether anesthetization. SEE: *e. anesthetic; gases; resuscitation.*

e. bed. Bed prepared to receive patient immediately following an operative procedure requiring anesthesia.

ARTICLES NECESSARY: Bedding for making an ordinary closed bed; two small rubber sheets; two draw sheets or special ether sheets; two bath blankets; two pieces of bandage about 3 in. wide; two towels; two emesis basins; pad and pencil; small pieces of gauze or paper wipes; paper bags; safety pins; shock blocks; rubber pillow case; hot water bottles filled and covered (if they are to be used).

PROCEDURE: Make up bottom part of bed as usual. Place one small rubber sheet where region of operation will come; place another across head of mattress where patient's head will lie. Cover each with a draw sheet, tucking it firmly under mattress. Spread the two bath blankets one over the other with tops 6 in. from top of mattress; hot water bottles placed between these; tuck lower blanket in at sides. Place top bedding as usual but do not tuck in; fan-fold top sheet over bed blanket to protect it. Fold all top bedding together, including the top bath blanket, even with mattress edge all around, then fold toward side of bed away from the door, or where the stretcher will be placed, until it lies in a neat fold. Tie one pillow upright on its side against the headboard with a bandage. Put rubber pillow case on other pillow and have it ready to put under patient's knees if needed. Place shock blocks at foot of bed on each side ready for instant pushing into position. Place pad, pencil, emesis basin, wipes, and one towel on bedside table, other towels over headbar of bed. Place chairs and table out of way of the stretcher. Have necessary stands and equipment available for administering intravenous fluids and blood or blood components.

e. drunkenness. Intoxication produced by imbibing e.

ethereal (ē-thē′rĭ-ăl) [Gr. *aithēr,* air]. Pert. to or made with ether.

e. oil. A volatile oil.

etherization (ē″thĕr-ĭ-zā′shŭn). Administering ether to induce anesthesia.

e′therize. To anesthetize by use of ether.

etheromania (e″thĕr-ō-mā′nĭ-ă) [Gr. *aithēr,* air, + *mania,* madness]. Addiction to use of ether.

ethics [Gr. *ēthos,* moral custom]. A system of moral principles or standards governing conduct.

e., medical. A system of principles governing medical conduct. It deals with the relationship of a physician to the patient, the patient's family, his fellow physicians, and society at large.

e., nursing. A system of principles governing conduct of a nurse. It deals with the relationship of a nurse to the patient, the patient's family, her associates and fellow nurses, and society at large.

ethiopification (ē″thǐ-ŏp″ǐ-fǐ-kā′shŭn) [Gr. *Aithiops,* Ethiopian, + L. *facere,* to make]. Pathological blackening of the skin from use of silver or other metals.

eth″mocardi′tis [Gr. *ēthmos,* sieve, + *kardia,* heart, + *-itis,* inflammation]. Chronic inflammation and proliferation of cardiac connective tissue. SYN: *cardiosclerosis.*

ethmoid (ĕth′moyd) [″+ *eidos,* form]. Sievelike; cribriform.

    e. bone. Sievelike spongy bone which forms a roof for the nasal fossae and part of floor of anterior fossa of skull. It contains a number of thin-walled cellular cavities, the ethmoidal cells, which are arranged in three groups. They open into the nasal cavity.

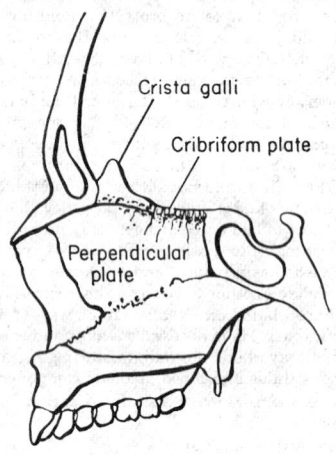

Crista galli

Cribriform plate

Perpendicular plate

ETHMOID BONE

    e. sinus. Air cells or space inside ethmoid bone, opening into nasal cavity.

ethmoi′dal. Pert. to the ethmoid bone or sinuses.

ethmoidectomy (ĕth-moy-dĕk′tō-mǐ) [Gr. *ethmos,* sieve, + *eidos,* form, + *ektomē,* excision]. Excision of ethmoid cells.

    NP: Patient in sitting position, ice packs to nose often ordered.

ethmoidi′tis [″+ ″+ *-itis,* inflammation]. Inflammation of ethmoidal cells. May be acute or chronic. SYM: Headache, acute pain between eyes, nasal discharge.

ethmyphitis (ĕth″mǐf-i′tǐs) [″+ *hyphē,* tissue, + *-itis,* inflammation]. Diffuse inflammation of cellular tissue. SYN: *cellulitis.*

ethnography (ĕth-nŏg′ră-fǐ) [Gr. *ethnos,* race, + *graphein,* to write]. The description of the human race.

ethnology (ĕth-nŏl′ō-jǐ) [″+ *logos,* science]. Study of social and economic systems and the cultural origins of various peoples and races.

ethology (ĕ-, ē-thŏl′ō-jǐ) [Gr. *ēthos,* moral customs, + *logos,* science]. Scientific study of animal customs and behavior.

ethyl (ĕth′il) [Gr. *aithēr,* air, + *hylē,* matter]. In organic chemistry, the radical C_2H_5 which enters into the constitution of many compounds such as ethyl ether, ethyl alcohol, and ethyl acetate.

    e. acetate. $CH_3COOC_2H_5.$ A colorless flammable liquid used as a solvent.

    e. alcohol. $C_2H_5OH.$ Grain alcohol. SEE: *alcohol, e.*

    e. aminobenzoate. Same as benzocaine, a topical anesthetic.

    e. chaulmoograte. The e. esters of the fatty acids of chaulmoogra oil. Used in the treatment of leprosy.

    e. chloride. $CH_3CH_2OH,$ hydrochloric ether. A very volatile liquid with a pleasant odor. When sprayed on the skin, it evaporates so quickly that the tissue is cooled immediately. Because of this property the skin is anesthetized.

    USES: Local anesthetic in minor surgery. It is a topical anesthetic and is used only for very short periods of anesthesia.

ethylamine (ĕth″ǐl-ăm′ǐn). $CH_3CH_2NH_2.$ An amine formed in the decomposition of certain proteins.

ethylene (ĕth′ǐl-ēn). A colorless gas (CH_2CH_2) prepared from alcohol by dehydration and found in illuminating gas to the extent of 4%. It is colorless and has a sweetish taste, but a pungent, foul odor. It is lighter than air and diffusible when liberated. It is flammable and explosive.

    e. anesthesia. Since e. is a rather weak anesthetic, it usually is given in a combination of oxygen 20%, cyclopropane 10%, and ethylene 70%.

    PHYS. EFFECTS: It causes less alteration in the blood gases than does nitrous oxide. E. alone causes very little muscular relaxation; the blood pressure may rise and respiration is not depressed. Analgesia results before loss of hearing or before complete unconsciousness. Nausea and vomiting seldom persist as long as 24 hr., but generally disappear before consciousness has returned.

    ADVANTAGES: Slightly stimulating to cardiac and respiratory systems. It is not irritating to mucus glands and kidneys. It has a short period of induction and makes possible a very rapid recovery. There is an absence of cyanosis and a minimum of emesis.

The difference between e. and any other anesthetic known today is that there is a less marked effect on all the systems of the body. It is the choice anesthetic for elderly patients, for poor surgical risks, when moderate anesthesia is desired, or where complete relaxation is not required.

DISADVANTAGES: Has an objectionable smell. Relaxation is not so complete or as perfect as from the use of ether anesthetics. It is highly flammable and explosive; many lives have been lost because someone was careless and a spark was emitted from some immediate source.

PRECAUTIONS: E. should be stored where there is plenty of air. The administration must be done away from fire, electric appliances, or x-ray apparatus. To prevent sparks, all lights should be turned on before bringing the tanks into the room. Furniture should never be dragged into the room or rolled into the room while the anesthetic is being given. The humidity of the room should be checked during the administration of this anesthetic. Nylon clothing or undergarments should not be worn by anyone in the room; friction from the material may generate static electricity.

E. does not combine as readily with air as do other anesthetics but floats around as clouds. The vapor rises in a cloudlike form and any gust of air may carry it out of the room; a devastating explosion will result if someone on the outside is smoking or if an elevator causes a spark.

E. always is stored in red tanks; oxygen in green tanks; nitrous oxide in blue tanks; carbon dioxide in gray tanks. SEE: *chloroform anesthesia; ether anesthesia.*

e. oxide. A chemical, C_2H_4O, which in its gaseous state is used to sterilize materials that can't withstand heat or steam. Also used as a fumigant.

ethylmorphine hydrochloride. A white bitter powder used in spasmodic respiratory diseases, insomnia, and neuralgia.

etiocholanolone (ē''tǐ-ō-kō-lǎn'ō-lōn). A urinary steroid produced by testosterone catabolism.

etiolate (ē'tǐ-ō-lāt'') [Fr. *étioler*]. Pale or sickly looking from lack of light or from continued illness.

etiologic, etiological (ē''tǐ-ō-lŏj'ǐk, -ǐ-kǎl) [Gr. *aitia,* cause, + *logos,* study]. Pert. to the cause or causes of disease.

etiology (ē''tǐ-ŏl'ō-jǐ). The study of the causes of disease.

etiotropic (ē''tǐ-ō-trŏp'ǐk) [Gr. *aita,* cause, + *tropos,* turning]. Directed against the cause of a disease, said of a drug or treatment that

destroys or inactivates the causal agent of a disease. Opposed to nosotropic, q.v.

etrohysterectomy (ē''trō-hǐs-tēr-ēk'tō-mǐ) [Gr. *ētron,* hypogastrium, + *hystera,* uterus, + *ektomē,* excision]. Excision of the uterus through the abdominal wall in the hypogastric region.

etymology (ĕt''ǐ-mŏl'ō-jǐ) [Gr. *etymologia*]. The science of the origin and development of words.

Most medical words are derived from Latin and Greek, but many of those from the Greek have reached us through the Latin, being modified by that language. Generally when two Greek words are used to form one word, they are connected by the letter "o."

Many medical words have been formed from one or more roots, forms used or adapted from the Latin or Greek, and many of them are modified either by a prefix or a suffix, or both. A knowledge of important Latin or Greek roots and prefixes will reveal the meaning of a great many other words. SEE: *Prefixes and Suffixes* in *Appendix.*

Eu. Chem. symb. for europium.

eu- [Gr. *eus,* good]. Prefix meaning healthy, normal, good, well.

Eubacteriales (ū''bǎk-tē-rǐ-ā'lēz) [Gr. *eus,* good, + *baktērion,* little rod]. An order of bacteria which includes many of the microorganisms pathogenic to man.

eubiotics (ū-bī-ŏt'ǐks) ["+ *bios,* life]. The science of healthy and hygienic living.

eu'bolism. Normal metabolism.

eucalyptol (ū''kǎ-lǐp'tōl) [Gr. *eus,* good, + *kalyptein,* to cover]. A substance obtained from oil of eucalyptus. Has an aromatic odor and has been used in expectorants.

eucalyptus, oil of (ū-kǎ-lǐp'tǔs). Oil distilled from fresh leaves of the plant. Used as an expectorant.

eucapnia (ū-kǎp'nǐ-ǎ) [Gr. *eus,* good, + *kapnos,* smoke]. Presence of normal amounts of carbon dioxide in the blood.

euchlorhydria (ū''klor-hǐ'drǐ-ǎ). Presence of the normal amount of free hydrochloric acid in the gastric juice.

eucholia (ū-kō'lǐ-ǎ) [Gr. *eus,* good, + *cholē,* bile]. Normal condition of bile regarding its constituents and amount secreted.

euchylia (ū-kǐ'lǐ-ǎ) ["+ *chylos,* chyle]. Normal condition of the chyle.

eucrasia (ū-krā'sǐ-ǎ) ["+ *krasis,* mixture]. Condition of normal health; state of the body in which all activities are in normal balance.

eudiaphoresis (ū''dǐ-ǎ-fō-rē'sǐs) [Gr. *eus,* good, + *dia,* through, + *pherein,* to carry]. Normal secretion of perspiration.

eudiemorrhysis (ū″dĭ-ē-mōr′ĭ-sĭs) ["+ "+ *haima*, blood, + *rhysis*, flow]. The normal blood flow through the capillaries.

eudiometer (ū″dĭ-ŏm′ē-tĕr) [Gr. *eudia*, good weather, + *metron*, measure]. An instrument for testing purity of air and analysis of gases.

euesthesia (ū-ĕs-thē′sĭ-ă) [Gr. *eus*, good, + *aisthēsis*, sensation]. Having normal senses.

eugenics (ū-jĕn′ĭks) ["+ *gennan*, to produce]. The science which deals with the physical, moral, and intellectual improvement of the human race by genetic control.

   e., negative. Those measures which seek to restrict the numbers of offspring with genetically undesirable traits.

   e., positive. Those measures which seek to bring about an increase in the numbers of offspring of families with genetically desirable traits.

eugenism (ū′jĕn-ĭzm) ["+ "+ *ismos*, condition]. The circumstances of environment and heredity which tend to bring about happy and healthy existence.

euglobulin (ū-glŏb′ū-lĭn). A true globulin, or one soluble in distilled water and dilute salt solution. SEE: *pseudoglobulin.*

eugonic (ū-gŏn′ĭk) [Gr. *eus*, good, + *gonē*, seed]. Pert. to a luxuriant growth of bacteria.

eukinesia (ū-kĭn-ē′sĭ-ă) ["+ *kinēsis*, motion]. Normal power of movement.

eumenorrhea (ū″mĕn-ō-rē′ă) ["+ *mēn*, menses, + *rhoia*, flow]. Normal menstruation.

Eumycetes (ū″mi-sē′tēz) [Gr. *eus*, good, + *mykes*, fungus]. A class of Thallophyta including all the true fungi.

eunoia (ū-noy′ă) ["+ *nous*, mind]. Soundness of mind.

eunuch (ū′nŭk) [Gr. *eunē*, bed, + *echein*, to guard]. Castrated male; one who has had his testicles removed. Absence of the male hormone produces certain symptoms, such as a female type of voice and loss of hair on the face.

   In some countries eunuchs were employed to guard the women of a harem.

eunuchism (ū′nŭk-ĭzm) ["+ "+ *ismos*, condition]. Condition resulting from complete lack of male hormone. This may be due to atrophy or removal of testicles.

eunuchoid (ū′nŭ-koyd) ["+ "+ *eidos*, form]. Having the characteristics of a eunuch such as retarded development of external and accessory sex organs, absence of beard and bodily hair, high-pitched voice, and striking lack of muscular development.

   e., pituitary. One produced by failure of the anterior lobe of the pituitary to secrete

gonadotrophic hormones; secondary hypogonadism.

eunuchoidism (ū-nŭk′oyd-ĭsm) ["+ "+ "+ *ismos*, condition]. Deficient production of male hormone, androgen, by the testes.

eupancreatism (ū-pān′krē-ă-tĭzm) [Gr. *eus.* good, + *pankreas*, pancreas, + *ismos*, condition]. Normal condition of the pancreas.

eupep′sia ["+ *pepsis*, digestion]. Normal digestion as distinguished from dyspepsia.

eupep′tic. Pert. to good digestion.

euphonia (ū-fōn′ĭ-ă) [Gr. *eus*, good, + *phōnē.* voice]. Having a normal clear voice.

euphoria (ū-for′ĭ-ă) ["+ *phoros*, bearing]. 1. A condition of good health. 2. In psychiatry, an exaggerated feeling of well-being; mild elation.

euplas′tic ["+ *plastikos*, formed]. Healing quickly and well.

eupnea (ūp-nē′ă) [Gr. *eus*, good, + *pnein*, to breathe]. Normal breathing as distinguished from dyspnea and apnea.

eupraxia (ū-prāks′ĭ-ă) ["+ *prassein*, to do]. Normal capacity to execute a motor pattern. SEE: *paralysis.*

eupraxic (ū-prāks′ĭk). Contributing to proper functioning.

europium (ū-rō′pĭ-ŭm). SYMB: *Eu.* At. no. 63; at. wt. 151.96. An element of the lanthanide series.

Eurotium (ū-rō′shĭ-ŭm) [Gr. *eurōs*, mold]. A genus of molds.

   E. malig′num. A species causing inflammation in external auditory meatus.

euryon (ū′rĭ-ŏn) [Gr. *eurys*, broad]. Either end of bilateral diameter of head.

eustachian (ū-stā′kĭ-ăn, -shĕn). [Bartolommeo Eustachio, It. anatomist, 1524-74] Pert. to the auditory tube.

   RS: salpingemphraxis, syringitis, syrinx.

   e. catheter. Instrument for insertion into e. tube.

   e. tube. The auditory tube (from the middle ear to the pharynx 3-4 cm. long and lined with mucus membrane).

   e. valve. Valve at the entrance of the inferior vena cava. SYN: *valvula venae cavae inferioris.*

eustachitis (ū-stā-kĭ′tĭs). Inflammation of the eustachian tube.

eusystole (ū-sĭs′tō-lĭ) [Gr. *eus*, good, + *systellein*, to draw together]. A state of the systole of the heart that is normal in time and force.

eutectic (ū-tĕk′tĭk) [Gr. *eutēktos*]. Easily melted.

   e. mixture. A mixture of two or more substances which has a melting point lower than that of any of its constituents.

euthanasia (ū-thă-nā′zĭ-ă) [Gr. *eus*, good, + *thanatos*, death]. 1. Dying easily, quietly, and painlessly. 2. The proposed practice of ending of life in case of incurable disease.

euthenics (ū-thĕn'ĭks) [Gr. *euthēnia*, well-being]. The science of improvement of the race through modification of the environment; in contrast to eugenics, q.v.

euthyroid (ū-thī'royd). Normal thyroid gland function.

eutocia (ū-tō'sĭ-ă) [Gr. *eus*, good, + *tokos*, birth]. Normal or natural labor and childbirth.

eutrophication (ū-trŏf'ĭ-kā'shŭn) [Gr. *eutrophein*, to thrive]. Alteration of the aquatic environment by increasing the mineral and organic nutrients to the extent that plant growth is favored over animal life.

evacuant (ē-văk'ū-ănt) [L. *evacuans*, making empty]. Drug that stimulates the bowels to move.

evac'uate [L. *evacuatio*, emptying]. 1. To discharge, esp. from the bowels; to empty the uterus. 2. To move patients from place or site of accident to a hospital.

evacuation (ē-văk-ū-ā'shŭn). 1. Emptying, esp. the bowels. 2. The material discharged from the bowels; stool. 3. Removal of air from a closed container; the production of a vacuum.

RS: absorption; feces; stool.

evacuator (ē-văk'ū-ā-tor). Device for emptying, as of the bowels, or for irrigating the bladder and removing calculi.

evaginate (ē-văj'ĭ-nāt) [L. *ēvāgīnāre*, to unsheath]. Pert. to protrusion of some part or organ from its normal place.

evagination (ē-văj-ĭ-nā'-shŭn). 1. Emergence from a sheath. 2. Protrusion of an organ or part. SEE: *invagination*.

evanescent (ĕv''ă-nĕs'ĕnt) [L. *evanescere*, to vanish]. Not permanent; of brief duration; passing gradually.

Evans blue. [Herbert M. Evans, Amer. anatomist, 1882 —] USP. A diazo dye occurring as a bluish-green powder, very soluble in water. It is used intravenously as a diagnostic agent.

evapora'tion [L. *ē*, out, + *vaporāre*, to steam]. 1. Change from liquid form to vapor. 2. Loss in volume due to conversion of a liquid into a vapor.

evectics (ē-věk'tĭks) [L. *evehere*, to lift up]. Acquiring good body vigor and habits.

eventra'tion [L. *ē*, out, + *venter*, belly]. 1. Partial protrusion of the abdominal contents through an opening in the abdominal wall. 2. Removal of contents of the abdominal cavity.

e. of the diaphragm. Elevation of the diaphragmatic dome into the thoracic cavity.

eversion ["+ *vertere*, to turn]. Turning outward. SEE: *chilectropion*.

e. of the cervix. A turning out of the cervical edges subsequent to laceration. SYN: *ectropion of cervix*.

Eve's method. [F. C. Eve, Brit. physician, 1871-1952] Resuscitation in drowning. *NOTE:* This method of artificial respiration is presented mostly for historical reasons. Mouth-to-mouth method of artificial respiration is much more effective.

Place the victim face down on a stretcher with ankles and wrists tied to handles, arms extending away from the body beyond the head. Support stretcher on a trestle about 34 in. (76.4 cm.) high. Rock the patient back and forth about 12 full cycles per minute. The head is lowered to an angle of 45° and the feet to the same extent. SEE: *artificial respiration; resuscitation*.

évidement (ā-vēd-mŏn') [Fr., a scooping out]. Scraping away diseased tissue.

evil [AS. *yfel*]. Disease or illness.

eviration (ē''vĭ-rā'shŭn) [L. *ē*, out, + *vir*, man]. 1. Castration. 2. Loss of masculine characteristics. 3. In psychiatry, delusion in a male who thinks he has become a woman.

evisceration (ē-vĭs''ĕr-ā'shŭn) ["+ *viscera*, viscera]. 1. Removal of the viscera. 2. Removal of the contents of a cavity. 3. Protrusion of the viscera.

e., obstetrical. Removal of the thoracic and abdominal contents of a fetus to facilitate delivery.

evisceroneurotomy (ē-vĭs''ĕr-ō-nū-rŏt'ō-mī) ["+ "+ Gr. *neuron*, nerve, + *tomē*, incision]. Scleral evisceration of the eye with division of optic nerve.

evolu'tion [L. *ē*, out, + *volvere*, to roll]. A process of orderly and gradual change or development. More generally, any orderly and gradual process of modification whereby a system, whether physical, chemical, social, or intellectual, becomes more highly organized.

e., doctrine of. The view that all present-day species of plants and animals, including man, have come into existence by gradual continuous change from earlier preexisting forms. It considers that life first came into existence as a simple primordial mass of protoplasm from which, through a series of progressive changes, the highly complex specialized forms of today arose.

e., spontaneous. Spontaneous birth of a child in transverse presentation.

evul'sion ["+ *vellere*, to pluck]. 1. Tearing away of a part or new growth. 2. Forcible extraction as of teeth.

ex- [Gr. *ex*, out]. Prefix indicating out, away from, completely.

exacerbation (ĕks-ās″ĕr-bā′shŭn) [″+ *acerbus*, harsh]. Aggravation of symptoms or increase in the severity of a disease.

exacrinous (ĕks-ăk′rĭn-ŭs) [″+ *krinein*, to secrete]. Concerning a gland's external secretion.

exaltation [L. *exaltāre*, to lift up]. A mental state characterized by feelings of grandeur, excessive joy, elation, and optimism; an abnormal feeling of personal well-being or self-importance.

examina′tion, phys′ical [L. *examināre*, to examine]. The act or process of examining the body to determine the presence or absence of disease.

Local examination includes specific parts and organs. Four procedures utilized are inspection, palpation, percussion and auscultation. Laboratory examination includes urinalysis, tests, cultures, basal metabolism, etc.

Terms employed indicating type of examination are physical, bimanual, digital, oral, rectal, O.B. (obstetrical), roentgenological, cystoscopic.

exangia (ĕks-ăn′jĭ-ă) [Gr. *ex*, out, + *angeion*, vessel]. Any dilatation of a blood vessel. Ex: aneurysm, varix.

exanthem (ĕks-ăn′thĕm) [Gr. *exanthēma*, eruption]. (pl. exanthems) Any eruption of the skin accompanied by inflammation, e.g. measles, scarlatina, erysipelas, q.v.

e. subitum. An acute disease of infants Probably due to a virus. Marked by high fever for three or four days and sometimes convulsions at the onset. A diffuse maculopapular rash usually appears just at the time the fever suddenly subsides. Treatment is symptomatic. SYN: *roseola infantum*. SEE: *convulsion.*

exanthema (ĕks-ăn-thē′mă) [Gr.]. (pl. *exanthemas*, *-mata*) Exanthem.

exanthematous (ĕks″ăn-thĕm′ă-tŭs). Pert to an eruption or rash.

exanthrope (ĕks′ăn-thrōp) [Gr. *ex*, out, + *anthrōpos*, man]. A cause or source of a disease originating outside the body.

exarteritis (ĕks″ăr-tĕr-ī′tĭs) [″+ *artēria*, artery, + *itis*, inflammation]. Inflammation of the outer coat of an artery.

exarticula′tion [″+ *articulus*, joint]. 1. Amputation of a limb through a joint. 2. Excision of a part of a joint.

excavation [″+ *cavus*, hollow]. 1. A hollow or depression. 2. Formation of a cavity.

e., dental. The preparation of a cavity in a tooth prior to filling.

e. of the optic nerve. A slight depression in the center of the optic papilla or disk from which retinal vessels emerge. Depression is total in glaucoma as a result of high intraocular pressure.

e., rectouterine. The rectouterine pouch or pouch of Douglas.

excentric (ĕk-sĕn′trĭk) [Gr. *ex*, out, + *kentron*, center]. Eccentric.

excerebration (ĕk″sĕr-ĕ-brā′shŭn) [″+ *cerebrum*, brain]. 1. Removal of brain of the dead fetus in order to facilitate delivery. 2. In anatomy, removal of the brain.

excernant (ĕk-sĕr′nănt) [L. *excernere*, to excrete]. Bringing about an evacuation or excretion. SYN: *excretory.*

excipient (ĕk-sĭp′ĭ-ĕnt) [L. *excipiēns*, excepting]. Any substance added to a medicine to permit it to be formed into the proper shape and consistency. The excipient should have no action of its own and should not interfere with the solubility of the medicine.

excise (ĕk-sīz′) [Gr. *ex*, out, + *caedere*, to cut]. To cut out or remove surgically.

excision (ĕk-sĭ′zhŭn) [L. *excisiō*]. An act of cutting away or taking out.

excitabil′ity [L. *excitāre*, to arouse]. Sensitiveness to being stimulated.

e., independent. Power of a muscle to respond to a stimulus without intervention of motor nerves.

e., reflex. Sensitiveness to reflex irritation.

excitant (ĕk-sĭt′ănt). An agent that will excite a special function of the body; subdivided, according to action, as motor, cerebral, etc. Ex: alcohol, cocaine, strychnine.

excitātion [L. *excitatio*]. 1. The act of exciting. 2 Condition of being stimulated or excited.

e., direct. Stimulation of a muscle by placing an electrode in it or physically stimulating it.

e., indirect. Stimulation of a muscle via its nerve.

e. wave. The wave of irritability originating in the atrioventricular node which sweeps over the conductile tissue of the heart and induces contraction of the atria and ventricles.

excit′ing. Causing excitement.

e. cause. Acting immediately as a cause of disease.

excitoglandular (ĕk-sĭt″ō-glăn′dū-lăr) [L. *excitāre*, to arouse, + *glans, gland-*, kernel]. Increasing glandular function.

excitometabolic (ĕk-sĭt″ō-mĕt′ă-bŏl′ĭk) [″+ Gr. *metabolē*, change]. Inducing metabolic changes.

excit″omo'tor ["+ *motor,* moving]. Increasing rapidity of muscular activity.

excit″omus'cular [L. *excitāre,* to arouse, + Gr. *mys,* muscle]. Causing muscular activity.

excitonutrient (ĕk-sĭt″ō-nū'trĭ-ĕnt) ["+ *nutrīre,* to nourish]. Stimulating nutrition.

exci'tor [L. *excitāre,* to arouse]. That which incites to greater activity. SYN: *stimulant.*

excitosecretory (ĕk-sĭt″ō-sē'krĕ-tor-ĭ) ["+ *secretiō,* a hiding]. Tending to bring about secretion.

excitovas'cular ["+ *vasculāris,* pert. to a vessel]. Increasing circulation activity.

exclave (ĕks'klāv) [Gr. *ex,* out, + *clavis,* key]. Detached part of an organ.

excochleation (ĕks-kŏk-lē-ā'shŭn) ["⊥ *cochlea,* spoon]. Scraping out or curetting a cavity.

excoriation (ĕks-kō-rĭ-ā'shŭn) ["+ *corium,* skin]. Abrasion of the epidermis, or of the coating, of any organ of the body by trauma, chemicals, burns, or other causes.

excrement (ĕks'krĕ-mĕnt) [L. *excrementum*]. Waste material passed out of the body, esp. feces. SEE: *excretion.*

excrementitious (ĕks″krĕ-mĕn-tĭsh'ŭs). Of the nature of excrement.

excrescence (ĕks-krĕs'ĕns) [Gr. *ex,* out, + *crescere,* to grow]. 1. Normal outgrowth from the surface of a part such as hair. 2. Diseased or useless growth on the surface of a part as a wart or mole.

excreta (ĕks-krē'tă) [L.]. Waste matter excreted from the body. Includes feces, sweat, and urine.

DISINFECTION OF: When using these disinfecting materials, be certain they do not come in contact with skin or eyes.

Carbolic acid: A 5% solution to be used in quantity at least equal to the amount of the material to be disinfected.

Caustic lime: Prepared by mixing one part of calcium hydroxide (slaked lime) with eight parts of water, to be used in an amount equal to that of the excreta to be disinfected.

Chloride of lime: Dissolve in the proportion of four ounces (120 ml.) to one gallon (3.8 liters) of water. One quart (946 ml.) of this solution for disinfection of each liquid discharge. For solid fecal matter a stronger solution or a larger quantity of above solution will be required.

It will be prudent to use a large quantity of the standard solution recommended for a copious liquid discharge. With a spatula the formed material should be broken up and covered with chlorinated lime. The container should be set aside and the feces or urine, with the coating of lime, covered with a lid

or newspapers. Let the mixture stand for one hour, stirring the lime into the contents from time to time, then it may be emptied into the sewer.

Cupric sulfate: Is used as chloride of lime but in a 4% solution.

Involuntary discharges: These should be cared for by placing cellulose pads under the patient. The pads should be wrapped thoroughly in strong paper after being soiled to prevent scattering of the feces. In handling all infected discharges, the nurse should wear rubber gloves.

excrete (ĕks-krēt') [L. *excrētus,* sifted out]. To expel or eliminate waste material from the body, blood, or organs.

excre'tin. A crystalline substance found in the feces. A fraction of the hormone, secretin, which stimulates pancreatic secretion.

excre'tion [L. *excretiō*]. 1. Waste matter, excreta. 2. The elimination of waste products from the body.

ORGANS OF: *Intestines:* Indigestible residue, water, and bacteria. *Kidneys:* Filter from the blood, water, nitrogenous substances (urea, uric acid, creatine, creatinine) mineral salts. *Respiratory system:* Carbon dioxide, water vapor, and other gases. *Skin:* Small amt., through perspiration, of water, salts, minute quantities of urea. Its excretory function is stimulated by kidney inactivity. Diaphoretics, hot packs, and warm blankets stimulate skin and aid kidneys, thus helping to avoid uremic coma.

excretion, words pert. to: defecation; dejecta; elimination; excrement; excreta; expectoration; feces; hydragogue; incontinence; lung; perspiration; pore; respiration; skin; sputum; sweat; urine; void.

ex'cretory [L. *excrētus,* sifted out]. Pert. to or bringing about excretion.

excur'sion [L. *excursiō*]. 1. Wandering from the usual course. 2. Extent of movement of a part such as the extremities or eyes.

excurva'tion [Gr. *ex,* out, + *curvus,* bend]. A curvature outward.

excystation (ĕk″sĭs-tā'shŭn) ["+ *kystis,* cyst]. Pert. esp. to the escape of certain organisms (parasitic, worms, protozoa) from an enclosing cyst wall or envelope. Process which occurs in the life cycle of an intestinal parasite after encysted form is ingested.

exencephalia (ĕks-ĕn-sĕf-ā'lĭ-ă) [Gr. *ex,* out, + *enkephalos,* brain]. A congenital anomaly in which the brain is located outside the skull. A term for encephalocele, hydrencephalocele, meningocele, and synencephalocele.

exenteration (ĕks-ĕn-tĕr-ā'shŭn) ["+ *enter-on*, intestine]. 1. Evisceration. 2. Removal of viscera of fetus in embryotomy.

exercise [L. *exercitus*, having drilled]. Functional activity of the muscles, voluntary or otherwise.

   e., active. A form of bodily movement which the patient performs with or without the personal supervision of the operator.

   e., assistive. A form of bodily movement which the patient performs assisted by the operator or by some mechanical means such as a pulley or weight.

   e., blowing. E. in which water is blown from one bottle to another, thus increasing intrabronchial pressure which tends to aid in expansion of the lung. It is by this means that obliteration of an empyema cavity is facilitated. SEE: *empyema.*

   e., Buerger's postural. E. used for circulatory disturbances of the extremities.

   e., corrective. Use of specific exercises to correct deficiencies caused by trauma or inactivity.

   e., crawling. E. devised for treatment of scoliosis, q.v., essentially for children.

   e., free. Form of bodily movement which is carried through by patient against least possible resistance.

   e., Master's. E. consisting of ascending and descending two steps a variable number of times. Used as a tolerance test for circulatory efficiency and as an exercise in heart disease. SYN: *Master two-step test.*

   e., Mosher's. E. for dysmenorrhea. Lie on back on floor with knees bent, feet on floor. Raise abdomen, relax it, contract it forcibly and relax. Repeat 10 times. This should be done daily.

   e., muscle-setting. Contracting and relaxing a muscle or group of muscles without moving the part or changing the muscle length. SYN: *isotonic contraction; static exercise.*

   e., passive. Form of bodily movement which is carried through by the operator without the assistance or resistance of the patient. Same as relaxed movement.

   e., resistive. Form of supervised bodily movement, with or without apparatus, which offers resistance to muscle action.

   e., rhythm. E. to song or music. Used in obstetrical paralysis.

   e., sling suspension. Method of supporting arm or leg to be exercised in a sling suspended from overhead, thus eliminating the weight of the extremity as a hindrance during movement.

   e., static. Alternate contraction and relaxation of a muscle or group of muscles

without movement of the joint. SYN: *muscle setting.* SEE: *e., muscle-setting.*

   e., therapeutic. Scientific supervision of bodily movement, with or without apparatus, for purpose of restoring normal function to diseased or injured tissues.

   e., water. Hydrogymnastics.

exercise bone. Bony growth developing in a muscle due to overexercise.

exeresis (ĕks-ĕr'ĕ-sĭs) [Gr. *exairesis*, taking out]. Excision of any part.

exfetation (ĕks-fē-tā'shŭn) [Gr. *ex*, out, + L. *fetus*, fetus]. Ectopic gestation.

exflagellation (ĕks"flăj-ĕ-lā'shŭn) ["+ L. *flagellum*, whip]. The formation of microgametes (flagellated bodies) from the microgametocytes. Occurs in the malarial organism (Plasmodium) in the stomach of a mosquito.

exfolia'tion ["+ L. *folium*, leaf]. The scaling off of dead tissue. RS: apostasis.

exhala'tion ["+ L. *hālāre*, to breathe]. The process of breathing outward; emanation of a gas or vapor. Opposed to inhalation.

exhaus'ter [L. *exhaustus*, drawn out]. A cataract evacuator for removal of loosened or fluid matter by vacuum pressure through a hollow needle.

exhaus'tion. 1. State of being exhausted, extreme fatigue, or weariness; loss of vital powers; inability to respond to stimuli. 2. Process of removing the contents of or using up a supply of anything. 3. To draw or let out.

   e., heat. Heat prostration; a condition resulting from exposure to high temperatures. Characterized by drowsy state of mind, rapid breathing, paleness, cold and sweaty skin, and normal or below normal temperature. May be due to salt deficiency, failure of the sweating mechanism, deficient water intake, or a combination of these factors.

exhibit (ĕgs-hĭb'ĭt) [L. *exhibere*, to display]. 1. To show. 2. To administer a drug. 3. Collection of objects for public inspection.

exhibi'tionism ["+ Gr. *ismos*, condition]. 1. Tendency to attract attention to oneself by any means. 2. An abnormal impulse that causes one to expose the genitals to one of the opposite sex. A psychoneurosis.

exhibitionist. 1. One with an abnormal desire to attract attention. 2. One who yields to an impulse to expose the genitals to the view of one of the opposite sex.

exhilarant (ĕg-zĭl'ăr-ănt) [L. *exhilarāre*, to gladden]. That which is mentally stimulating.

exhuma'tion [Gr. *ex*, out, + *humus*, earth]. Removal of the dead body from the grave after it has been buried.

exitus (ĕk'sĭ-tŭs) [L., going out]. Death.

Exner's nerve (ĕks'nĕr). [Siegmund Exner, Austrian physiologist, 1846-1926] Nerve from the pharyngeal plexus to the cricothyroid membranes.

Exner's plexus. A plexus of nerve fibers forming a layer near the surface of the cerebral cortex.

exo- [Gr. *exō*, outside]. Prefix indicating without; outside of.

exocar'dia [Gr. *exō*, outside, + *kardia*, heart]. Congenitally abnormal position of the heart.

exocar'dial. Occurring outside of the heart.

exocataphoria (ĕks″ō-kăt-ă-for'ĭ-ă) [Gr. *exō*, outside, + *kata*, down, + *phoros*, bearing]. A downward and outward turning of the visual axes.

exocoli'tis ["+ *kōlon*, colon, + *itis*, inflammation]. Inflammation of the peritoneal coat of the colon.

exocrine (ĕks'ō-krĭn) ["+ *krinein*, to separate]. 1. The external secretion of a gland. Opposed to endocrine. 2. Term applied to glands whose secretion reaches an epithelial surface either directly or through a duct.

exodic (ĕks-ŏd'ĭk) [Gr. *exō*, outside, + *hodos*, way]. Efferent, centrifugal. Transmitting nerve impulses out from the central nervous system.

exodontia (ĕks-ō-dŏn'shĭ-ă) ["+ *odous, odont-*, tooth]. 1. Extraction of a tooth. 2. Protrusion of teeth forward.

exodontol'ogy ["+ "+ *logos*, study]. Branch of dentistry concerned with extraction of teeth.

exoenzyme (ĕk-sō-ĕn'zīm) [Gr. *exō*, outside, + *en*, in, + *zymē*, leaven]. Enzyme that does not function within the cells from which it is secreted.

exogamy (ĕks-ŏg'ă-mĭ) ["+ *gamos*, marriage]. 1. Marriage outside of same family; outbreeding. 2. In biology, conjugation between gametes of different ancestry, as in some protozoans. SEE: *heterosexuality.*

exogastri'tis ["+ *gastēr*, belly, + *itis*, inflammation]. Inflammation of the peritoneal coat of stomach.

exogenous (ĕks-ŏj'ĕ-nŭs) [Gr. *exō*, outside, + *gennan*, to produce]. Originating outside an organ or part.

exohysteropexy (ĕks″ō-hĭs″tĕr-ō-pĕks'sĭ) ["+ *hystera*, uterus, + *pēxis*, fixation]. Fixation of the uterus by implanting the fundus into the abdominal wall.

exometritis (ĕks″ō-mē-trī'tĭs) ["+ *mētra*, womb, + *itis*, inflammation]. Inflammation of the peritoneal coat of the uterus.

exomphalos (ĕks-ŏm'fă-lŭs) [Gr. *ex*, out, + *omphalos*, navel]. 1. Umbilical protrusion. 2. Umbilical hernia.

exopath'ic [Gr. *exō*, outside, + *pathos*, disease]. Pert. to a disease originating outside of the body.

exophoria (ĕks″ō-fō'rĭ-ă) ["+ *phoros*, bearing]. In ophthalmology, tendency of visual axes to diverge outward. SEE: *esophoria.*

exophthalmia (ĕks″ŏf-thăl'mĭ-ă) [Gr. *ex*, out, + *ophthalmos*, eye]. Abnormal protrusion of the eyeball. SYN: *exophthalmos.*

> **e. cachectica.** Exophthalmic goiter, q.v.

> **e. fungosa.** Late state of glioma retinae.

exophthalmic (ĕks″ŏf-thăl'mĭk). Pert. to protrusion of the eyeball.

> **e. goiter.** A condition marked by protrusion of the eyeballs, increased heart action, enlargement of the thyroid gland, weight loss, nervousness. SYN: *thyrotoxicosis.* SEE: *hyperthyroidism.*

exophthal'mos, exophthal'mus. Abnormal protrusion of eyeball. May be due to thyrotoxicosis, tumor of the orbit, orbital cellulitis, leukemia, or aneurysm.

> **e., pulsating.** E. accompanied by pulsation and bruit due to an aneurysm behind the eye.

exophylac'tic [Gr. *exō*, out, + *phylaxis*, guarding]. Pert. to exophylaxis.

ex″ophylax'is. Protection from disease originating outside the body. Ex: protection by the skin.

ex'oplasm [Gr. *exō*, outside, + *plasma*, matter]. Outer protoplasm of a cell. SYN: *ectoplasm.*

exorbitism (ĕks-or'bĭ-tĭzm) [Gr. *ex*, out, + L. *orbita*, eye]. Protrusion of eyeball. SYN: *exophthalmos.*

exormia (ĕks-or'mĭ-ă) ["+ *hormē*, rash]. Any papular skin disease.

exosep'sis [Gr. *exō*, outside, + *sēpsis*, decay]. Septic poison of external origin.

exoserosis (ĕks″ō-sēr-ō'sĭs) ["+ *serum*, whey, + Gr. *ōsis*, condition]. An oozing of serum or discharging of an exudate.

exoskel'eton ["+ *skeleton*, skeleton]. 1. The hard outer covering of certain invertebrates such as the molluscs and arthropods. Composed of chitin, calcareous material, or both. 2. In vertebrates, the hard outer covering such as the shell of a turtle, or more specifically, the hard parts of the body surface derived principally from the ectoderm.

These include such structures as hair, hooves, horns, nails, feathers, and scales.

exosmo'sis [Gr. *ex*, out, + *ōsmos*, a thrusting, + *ōsis*, condition]. Diffusion of a fluid from within outward, as from a blood vessel.

exosplenopexy (ĕks-"ō-splēn'ō-pĕks-ĭ) [Gr. *exō*, outside, + *splēn*, spleen, + *pēxis*, fixation]. Suturing the spleen to opening in the abdominal wall.

exostosis (ĕks"ōs-tō'sĭs) [Gr. *ex*, out, + *osteon*, bone]. A bony growth which arises from the surface of a bone, often involving the ossification of muscular attachments.

    e. **bursata.** An e. arising from the epiphysis of a bone and covered with cartilage and a synovial sac.

    e. **cartilaginea.** E. consisting of cartilage underlying the periosteum.

    e., dental. E. on the root of a tooth.

    e., multiple osteocartilaginous. A disorder of growth characterized by the development of multiple exostoses, usually located on the diaphyses of long bones near the epiphyseal lines. Results in irregularities of growth of the epiphyses and often secondary deformities. Etiology unknown; tends to be hereditary. SYN: *dyschondroplasia*, q.v.

exoter'ic [Gr. *exōterikos*, outer]. Pert. to causes developing outside the body. SYN: *exopathic.*

exother'mal, exother'mic [Gr. *exō*, outside, + *thermē*, heat]. Chemical reaction with production of heat.

exothy'mopexy ["+ *thymos*, thymus, + *pēxis*, fixation]. Suturing of an enlarged thymus gland to the sternum.

exothyreopexy (ĕks"ō-thī'rē-ō-pĕks'ĭ) ["+ *thyreos*, shield, + *pēxis*, fixation]. Exothyropexy.

exothy'ropexy. Suture of the thyroid and external fixation to induce atrophy. SYN: *exothyreopexy.*

exotic (ĕg-zŏt'ĭk) [Gr. *exōtikos*]. Originating in another part of the world, i.e., a foreign country.

    e. disease. A disease which normally would not be expected to be seen or to occur in a certain area or locality. Ex: malaria in an area that has no mosquitoes.

exotoxin (ĕks"ō-tŏks'ĭn) [Gr. *exō*, outside, + *toxikon*, poison]. A toxin produced by a microorganism and excreted into its surrounding medium. It can usually be recovered from the liquid medium in which the toxin-producing organisms have developed. Exotoxins usually are unstable, being sensitive to the effects of chemicals, light, and heat. Exotoxins are produced by diphtheria and tetanus organisms.

Exotoxins differ with regard to the particular tissues of the host that may be affected.

    RS: cytotoxin; endotoxin; erythrotoxin; leukocidin; leukotoxic; neurotoxin.

exotro'pia ["+ *tropos*, turning]. Divergent strabismus; abnormal turning of one or both eyes outward.

expansion (ĕks-păn'shŭn) [L. *expandere*, to spread out]. Increase of volume; spreading out.

    e., muscle. Degree a muscle may be stretched by an attached weight.

expansive delusion. Belief in one's power and wealth, accompanied by a feeling of well-being. These beliefs are not consistent with reality. SEE: *megalomania.*

expec'tant [Gr. *ex*, out, + L. *spectāre*, to watch]. Waiting.

    e. treatment. Treatment of symptoms as they arise.

expecta'tion. Hoping, anticipation.

    e. of life. Probable duration of life after a given age.

expec'torant [Gr. *ex*, out, + L. *pectus, pector-*, breast]. An agent that facilitates the removal of the secretions of the bronchopulmonary mucus membrane.

Expectorants are classed as sedative expectorants and stimulating expectorants.

Ex: Ammonium carbonate; ammonium chloride; ipecac.

expectoration. Expulsion of mucus or phlegm from the throat or lungs. It may be mucous, mucopurulent, serous, or frothy.

In pneumonia it is viscid and tenacious, sticks to anything, and is rusty in appearance. In bronchitis it is frothy, often streaked with blood, and greenish-yellow because of pus. In tuberculosis it varies from small amt. of frothy fluid to abundant offensive greenish-yellow sputum often streaked with blood.

SEE: *anacatharsis; sputum; vomica.*

expel (ĕks-pĕl') [L. *expellere*]. To drive out.

experiment [L. *experimentum*, to test]. The scientific procedure used to test the validity of a hypothesis, to gain further evidence or knowledge, or to test the usefulness of a drug or type of therapy which has not been tried previously.

    e., controlled. E. wherein part of a group of similar entities, animals, or human beings is tested or treated; the others do not receive the test or treatment.

expira'tion [Gr. *ex*, out, + L. *spirāre*, to breathe]. The expulsion of air from the lungs in breathing. Its sound is the shortest breath sound heard. In general, if the duration of expiration is longer than inspiration a pathological condition such as emphysema or asthma is present.

Muscles used in expiration are the internal intercostal muscles, m. rectus abdominis, m. transversus abdominis, the triangularis sterni and possibly the iliocostalis, serratus posterior inferior, and quadratus lumborum. SEE: *inspiration; respiration.*

e., active. E. accomplished as a result of muscular activity, as in forced respiration. The muscles used in respiration are the muscles of the abdominal wall (external and internal oblique, rectus, and transversus abdominis); the internal intercostals, serratus posterior inferior, and quadratus lumborum.

e., passive. E. during quiet respiration in which no muscular effort is required. It is brought about by the elasticity of the lung, recoil of the elastic tissues of the chest such as the costal cartilages, and the weight of the thoracic wall.

expiratory (ĕks′pĭ′ră-tor′ĭ). Pert. to expiration.

e. center. The part of the respiratory center in the medulla controlling e. movements.

expire. 1. To breathe out or exhale. 2. To die.

explant [Gr. *ex,* out, + L. *planta,* sprout]. To remove a piece of living tissue from the body and transfer to an artificial culture medium for growth as in tissue culture. Opposed to implantation, q.v.

explora′tion [L. *explorāre,* to search out]. Examination of an organ or part by various means.

explo′ratory. Pert. to an exploration.

explorer. An instrument used in diagnosis.

explo′sive speech. Sudden and explosive utterance. SEE: *speech.*

express′ [L. *expressāre*]. To squeeze out.

expres′sion. 1. Expelling anything by pressure. 2. Facial disclosure of feeling or emotion. SYN: *facies.* SEE: *face.*

expressivity. The extent to which the effect of a gene is manifest in the individual carrying the gene.

expul′sive [L. *expellere,* to drive out]. Having a tendency to expel.

e. pains. Labor pains which are effective, contracting the uterine muscle.

exsanguinate (ĕks-săn′gwĭn-āt) [Gr. *ex,* out, + *sanguis,* blood]. 1. To deprive of blood. 2. Bloodless.

exsanguination (ĕks-săn″gwĭn-ā′shŭn). The process of expressing blood from a part.

exsanguine (ĕks-săn′gwĭn). Anemic; bloodless.

exsec′tion [L. *exsectus,* having cut]. Excision.

exsiccant (ĕk-sĭk′ănt) [L. *exsiccāre,* to dry out]. 1. Absorbing or drying up a discharge. 2. An agent that absorbs moisture. 3. A dusting or drying powder.

exsicca′tion. 1. To make dry. 2. In chemistry, removing the water from compounds or solutions. SYN: *desiccation.*

exsic′cative. Causing to dry up or that which dries. SYN: *desiccative.*

exso′matize [Gr. *ex,* out, + *sōma,* body]. To remove from the body.

exstrophy (ĕks′trō-fĭ) ["+ *strephein,* to turn"]. Eversion; turning inside out of a part.

e. of the bladder. A congenital malformation in which the lower portion of the abdominal wall and anterior wall of the bladder are missing and the bladder is everted through the opening; ectopia vesicae.

exsufflation (ĕk″sū-flā′shŭn) ["+ *sufflatio,* blown up"]. Forceful expulsion of air from the lungs either by natural means or by use of a mechanical exsufflator.

ext. Abbr. of L. *extractum,* extract.

extempora′neous [LL. *extemporaneus*]. Not prepared according to formula but devised for the occasion.

e. mixture. A preparation to be taken at once because of tendency to deteriorate.

extension (ĕks-tĕn′shŭn) [L. *extensio*]. 1. The movement by which both ends of any part are pulled apart. A movement which brings the members of a limb into or toward a straight condition. Opposed to flexion. 2. The application of a pull (traction) to a fractured or dislocated limb.

e., Buck′s. A method of producing traction by applying adhesive tape or moleskin to the skin and keeping it in smooth close contact by means of circular bandaging of the part to which it is applied. The adhesive strips are placed longitudinal to the member, the superior ends being about 1 in. from fracture site. Weights sufficient to produce the required extension are fastened to the inferior end of the adhesive strips, by means of a rope which is run over a pulley to permit free motion.

exten′sor [L.]. A muscle that extends a part.

exte′rior [L.]. Outside of; external.

exte′riorize. 1. To temporarily expose a part in surgery; marsupialization, q.v. 2. In psychiatry, the process of turning one's interests outward.

extern(e (ĕks′turn) [L. *externus,* outside]. A medical student, living outside of a hospital, who assists in the medical and surgical care of patients. SEE: *intern.*

external. Exterior; lateral; opposed to medial or internal.

externalia (ĕks″tĕr-nā′lī-ă) [L. *exter*, outside, + *genitalis*, genital]. External genitalia.

exteroceptive (eks″ter-o-sep′tiv) [L. *exterus*, outside, + *receptus*, having received]. Pert. to end organs receiving impressions from without.

exteroceptor (ĕks″tĕr-ō-sĕp′tor). A sense organ, as the eye, adapted for the reception of stimuli from outside the body.

ex″terofec′tive [L. *exterus*, outside, + *facere*, to make]. Pert. to responses to stimuli mediated by the central nervous system and somatic nerves in contrast to those mediated through the autonomic nervous system.

extima (ĕks′tī-mă) [L., outermost]. The outer layer of a blood vessel; the tunica adventitia.

extinc′tion [L. *exstinctus*, having extinguished]. 1. The process of extinguishing or putting out. 2. The complete inhibition of a conditioned reflex as a result of failure to reinforce it.

    e. of mercury. Causing the disappearance of mercury by rubbing with lard or some other agent.

extirpation (ĕks-tĭr-pā′shŭn) [L. *extirpāre*, to root out]. Excision of a part; taking out by the roots.

extor′sion [Gr. *ex*, out, + L. *torsio*, twisting]. Rotation of an organ or limb outward.

extra- [L. *exter*, outward]. Prefix meaning outside of, in addition to, beyond.

extra-artic′ular [L. *exter*, outward, + *articulus*, joint]. Outside a joint.

ex′tract [L. *extractum*]. 1. To pull out or remove forcibly, as to e. a tooth. 2. A solid or semisolid preparation made by extracting the soluble portion of a compound by using water or alcohol and evaporating the solution. 3. Active principle of a drug obtained by distillation or chemical processes.

    e., alcoholic. E. in which alcohol acts as the solvent.

    e., aqueous. E. in which water is the solvent.

    e., aromatic fluid. E. made from an aromatic powder.

    e., compound. E. prepared from more than one drug or substance.

    e., ethereal. E. using ether as the vehicle.

    e., fluid. E. made into a solution from a vegetable drug which contains medicinal components.

    e., powdered. A crushed, dried e.

    e., soft. E. of the consistency of honey.

    e., solid. E. made by evaporating the fluid part of a solution.

extractable nuclear antigen. An antigen present in the cells of patients with a certain type of rheumatic syndrome. Corticosteroids are very helpful in treating patients with high concentrations of E.N.A. ABBR: E.N.A.

extrac′tion [L. *extractum*, drawing out]. 1. Pulling out, as a tooth. 2. The removing of the active portion of a drug.

extract′or. Instrument for removing foreign bodies. Varieties include esophageal, throat, shot, tympanum, tissue.

    e., tissue. Needles, trocars, or pointed instruments with a form of barb for extracting soft tissue for examination.

    e., tube. Device for removing an intubation tube from trachea.

extrac′tum [L., a drawing out]. (pl. *extrac′ta*) Solid or semi-solid preparations produced by evaporating solutions of vegetable principles.

    The official extracts are either powders or soft solids. The majority can be obtained in powdered form and many physicians prefer them that way. Extracts are usually about five times the strength of the crude drug. ABBR: ext. SEE: *fluidextract.*

extracystic (ĕks″tră-sĭs′tĭk) [L. *exter*, outward, + Gr. *kystis*, bladder]. Outside of or unrelated to a bladder or cystic tumor.

extradu′ral [″+ *durus*, hard]. 1. On outer side of the dura mater. 2. Unconnected with the dura mater.

extragenital (ĕks″tră-jĕn′ĭ-tăl) [″+ *genitalis*, genital]. Outside of or unrelated to the genital organs.

extrahep′atic [L. *exter*, outward, + Gr. *hēpatos*, liver]. Outside of or unrelated to the liver.

ex″traligamen′tous [″+ *ligāre*, to bind]. Outside of or unrelated to a ligament.

extramalleolus (ĕks″tră-măl-lē′ō-lŭs) [″+ *malleōlus*, little hammer]. The external or lateral malleolus.

extramar′ginal [L. *exter*, outward, + *margō*, margin]. Pert. to subliminal consciousness.

extramastoiditis (ĕks″tră-măs″toyd-i′tĭs) [″+ Gr. *mastos*, breast, + *eidos*, form, + *-itis*, inflammation]. Inflammation of outside tissues contiguous to the mastoid process.

extramedullary (ĕks″tră-mĕd′ū-lă-rĭ) [″+ *medulla*, marrow]. Outside or unrelated to any medulla, esp. the medulla oblongata.

extraneous (ĕks-trā′nē-ŭs) [L. *extraneus*, external]. Outside and unrelated to an organism.

extranu′clear [L. *exter*, outward, + *nucleus*, kernel]. Outside of a nucleus.

extrapo'lar ["+ *polus,* pole]. Outside instead of between poles, as the electrodes of a battery.

extrasensory. Pert. to forms of perception not dependent upon the five primary senses; e. g., thought transference.

    e. perception. Perception, esp. of another person's thoughts or actions not received by use of the senses. ABBR: ESP.

extrasys'tole [L. *exter,* outward, + Gr. *systole,* contraction]. Premature contraction of the heart. In humans it is the result of some factor that initiates an impulse in the impulse-conducting system. It may occur in either the presence or absence of organic heart disease. It may be of reflex origin being initiated by stimuli from almost any part of the body or it may be of central origin. It may be induced experimentally by stimulating the heart at any time except during the absolute refractory period.

    e., atrial. Premature contraction of the atrium at some point outside the S-A node.

    e., nodal. E. occurring as a result of the origin of an impulse in the A-V node.

    e., ventricular. E. which occurs after the normal contraction of the ventricle has ceased. Usually followed by a long compensatory pause.

extrau'terine [L. *exter,* outward, + *uterus,* womb]. Outside the uterus.

extravag'inal ["+ *vagina,* vagina]. Outside the vagina.

extravasate (ĕks-trăv'ă-sāt) ["+ *vas,* vessel]. 1. To escape from a vessel into the tissues, said of serum, blood, or lymph. 2. Fluids so escaping.

extravasation (ĕks-trăv"ă-sā'shŭn). The escape of fluids into the surrounding tissue.

extravas'cular [L. *exter,* outward, + *vasculum,* vessel]. Outside a vessel.

extraventric'ular ["+ *ventriculus,* little belly]. Outside of any ventricle, esp. one of the heart.

extremital (ĕks-trĕm'ĭ-tăl) [L. *extrēmus,* outermost]. Pert. to an extremity. SYN: *distal.*

extrem'ity. 1. The terminal part of anything. 2. An arm or leg.

    RS: "acro-" words; dactyl; dactylus.

    e., lower. The lower limb including the hip, thigh, leg, ankle, and foot.

    e., upper. The upper limb including the shoulder, arm, forearm, wrist, and hand.

extrin'sic [LL. *extrinsecus,* outer]. From, or coming from, without.

    e. muscles. Those partly attached to the trunk and partly to a limb.

extrospection (ĕks"trō-spĕk'shŭn) [L. *exter,* outward, + *spectare,* to look]. Continual inspection by the patient of his skin for evidence of dirt. Caused by mysophobia, compulsive fear of dirt.

extroversion (ĕks"trō-vĕr'zhŭn) ["+ *vertere,* to turn]. 1. Eversion; turning inside out. 2. In psychology, the direction of attention and energy outward from the self. SEE: *introversion.*

ex'trovert. A personality-reaction type; one who is interested mainly in external objects and actions.

    The extreme pathological extrovert reaction is seen in manic-depressive insanity. Opposed to introvert, q.v. SYN: *extravert.*

extrude (ĕks-trūd') [L. *extrūdere,* to squeeze out]. To push out of a normal position or situation.

extru'sion. 1. Occupying an abnormal external position. 2. Position of a tooth pushed forward from line of occlusion.

extubation (ĕks"tū-bā'shŭn) [Gr. *ex,* out, + L. *tuba,* tube]. Removal of a tube, as the laryngeal tube.

exudate (ĕks'ū-dāt) [L. *exsūdāre,* to sweat out.]. Accumulation of a fluid in a cavity, or matter that penetrates through vessel walls into adjoining tissue, or the passing out of pus or serum, or the matter so passed.

    In comparison to a transudate, there are more cells, protein, and solid material in an e. Exudates may be classified as catarrhal, fibrinous, hemorrhagic, diphtheritic, purulent, and serous, the fluids being different in various affections. A fibrinous exudate may wall off a cavity, resulting in adhesions following an operation, as in empyema and appendicitis. Inflammatory processes tend to wall off the injured area to localize the inflammation and to prevent its spread. SEE: *empyema; exudation; infection; inflammation; pus; resorption; transudate.*

exudation (ĕks"ū-dā'shŭn). Morbid oozing of fluids, usually the result of inflammatory conditions. SEE: *exudate.*

exudative (ĕks'ū-dā"tĭv). Having the property of exudation.

exude (ĕg-zūd', ĕk-sūd') [L. *exsūdāre,* to sweat out]. To pass off slowly through the tissues; said of a semisolid or fluid.

exumbilication (ĕks"ŭm-bĭl"ĭ-kā'shŭn) [Gr. *ex,* out, + L. *umbilicus,* navel]. Protrusion of navel. SYN: *exomphalos.*

exuviae (ĕg-zū'vĭ-ē) [L., stripped-off clothing]. (sing. *exuvium*) Cast-off parts, as desquamated epidermis; a slough.

eye [AS. *ēage*]. Organ of vision.

    ANAT: Composed of three coats. From inside the e. out they are retina, sensory for light; uvea (choroid, ciliary body, and iris), nutritional; sclera and cornea, serve to protect delicate retina.

These layers enclose two cavities, the more anterior or ocular chamber being the space lying in front of the lens. It is divided by the iris into an anterior chamber and a posterior chamber, both of which are filled with a watery aqueous humor. The cavity behind the lens is much larger and filled with a jelly-like vitreous body. The lens is suspended behind the iris by the ciliary zonule. Anteriorly, the cornea is covered by the conjunctiva which continues and forms the inner layer of the eyelids.

Movements of the eyeball are brought about by six muscles: the superior, inferior, medial and external rectus muscles, and the superior and inferior oblique muscles.

Nerve supply: 2nd or optic nerve; *eye muscles,* 3rd or oculomotor, 4th or trochlear, and 6th or abducens; *lid muscles,* facial to orbicularis oculi and oculomotor to levator palpebrae. Sensory fibers to orbit furnished by ophthalmic and maxillary fibers of the 5th or trigeminal. Sympathetic postganglionic fibers are derived from the carotid plexus, their cell bodies lying in the superior cervical ganglion. They supply the dilator muscle of the iris, lacrimal gland, and smooth muscle fibers in the eyelid; parasympathetic fibers from the ciliary ganglion pass to the ciliary muscle and constrictor muscles of the iris.

FUNCTION: Light entering the eye passes through the cornea, then through the pupil, an opening in the iris, and on through the crystalline lens and the vitreous body to the retina. The aqueous humor, lens, and vitreous body constitute the refracting media of the e. Through changes in the curvature of the lens brought about by its elasticity and contraction of the ciliary muscles, light rays are focused on the retina where they stimulate the rods and cones, the sensory receptors. The cones are concerned with color vision; rods with vision in dim light. Sensory impulses are conveyed over the optic nerve to the brain where, in the visual area of the cerebral cortex located in the occipital lobe, they register as visual sensations. The amount of light entering the eye is regulated by the pupil, its size being controlled by the dilator and constrictor muscles of the iris.

DIAG: The diagnosis of disease which the physician makes from an examination depends largely upon symptoms manifested by the pupils of the eyes.

Contracted Pupils: May denote irritative lesions of the 3rd nerve in early stages of anesthesia from chloroform or during alcoholic excitement, or may result from opium poisoning. Contraction of one pupil indicates irritative lesion of the opposite side of the brain, situated at the 3rd nerve nuclei, or a paralysis of the sympathetic nerve fibers due to a lesion somewhere in their course.

Dilated Pupils: May result from belladonna or atropine, or from irritation of the sympathetic. May occur during attacks of dyspnea in the last stages of anesthesia. Dilation of one pupil indicates a paralysis of the 3rd nerve from some brain lesion, or an irritation of the cervical sympathetic.

Floating Specks: Most individuals see little specks of materials which are small pieces of tissue floating in the vitreous humor. These are called muscae volitantes which is Latin for flying flies. These specks are the remainder of intraocular embryonic tissue which did not completely disappear. This is not an abnormal condition. *Squinting:* This is an unfavorable symptom in the course of a brain disease.

USE OF COMPRESSES: *Cold compresses:* Used to relieve congestion of eyelids; to control intraocular hemorrhage; occasionally

THE EYE

for conjunctivitis and early lid injuries to prevent hemorrhage into tissues.

Use the following procedure: scrub hands, wring out compresses of isotonic saline solution with forceps and place on ice to chill; place compresses over lids and extend over cheek; change every 30 seconds. Each compress may be used over and over if there is no pus. When pus is present, may be used only once.

Hot compresses: Used to increase the blood supply to the eyelids and eyeballs, and to relieve pain.

Scrub hands, apply petroleum jelly with clean swab to area to which compresses are to be applied; wring compresses dry with forceps, test on wrist, and apply as hot as patient can tolerate. To increase blood supply to eyelids, place compresses over lids and extend over cheek; to increase blood supply to eyeballs, place compresses over lids and extend over brow. Use new compresses for each application if pus is present; dry the eyelid when last compress is removed.

e., aphakic. An e. from which the crystalline lens has been removed.

e. bank. Depository for corneas to be used in transplantations.

e., black. Ecchymosis of the tissues surrounding the eye.

e. closure reflex. Contraction of orbicularis palpebrarum with closure of lids resulting from percussion above supraorbital nerve. SYN: *McCarthy's reflex; supraorbital reflex.*

e., cross-. Strabismus, q.v.

e., dark-adapted. An e. which has become adjusted for viewing objects in dim light; one adapted for scotopic or rod vision. Depends upon the regeneration of a light sensitive substance, visual purple.

e., dominant. The e. which a person unconsciously gives preference to as a source of stimuli for visual sensations.

e., exciting. In sympathetic ophthalmia, the damaged eye which is the source of sympathogenic influences.

e., fixing. In strabismus, the eye that is directed toward the object of vision.

e., foreign body in. Manifested by pain, lacrimation, spasm of the eye; later there is redness, swelling, and occasionally headache.

F. A. TREATMENT: Tearing often washes dust from the eye. Bringing the upper lid over the lower, and directing patient to roll eye, often deposits dust on the margin of the lower lid.

Great care is necessary in removing larger particles, which should be done in a quiet,

well lighted place with clean, preferably sterile, materials. Follow by instillation of 1 or 2 drops of a bland oil into the eye. A mild antiseptic, as 5-10% mild silver proteinate, is desirable. If inflamed, use repeated hot compresses.

If for any reason patient cannot be taken care of at once, the eye should be bandaged to keep it closed and thus avoid scratching the lid. There should be no delay in having the speck removed, as serious injury to the eyeball or to the vision may result. The longer the foreign body remains in the eye the deeper it becomes embedded

Infection may be carried into the eye, resulting in an ulcer of the cornea. Metal produces a chemical effect as it disintegrates which affects the eyeball. The X ray is sometimes used to detect any tiny particles of metal, and the electromagnet to remove them. Sympathetic ophthalmia, q.v., the transference of inflammation from an injury to the normal eye, may be produced by wounds which pierce the eyeball. Loss of vision in both eyes may result.

e., hare's. Lagophthalmos; condition in which the eye cannot be completely closed.

e., light-adapted. An e. that has become adjusted to viewing objects in bright light; one adapted for phototic or cone vision; one in which visual purple has been bleached.

e., pink-. Acute epidemic conjunctivitis.

e., refracting media of. Aqueous humor, lens, and vitreous body.

e., refracting surfaces of. Cornea and anterior and posterior surfaces of the lens.

e., squint. Strabismus, q.v.

e., squinting. The e. affected in strabismus.

e., sympathizing. In sympathetic ophthalmia, the uninjured e. which responds to sympathogenic influences.

e., watery. Epiphora; abnormal secretion of tears.

e. worm, African. Loa Loa, a genus of nematode which frequently infests the eye.

eyeball. The body of the eye.

It has three humors: aqueous, lens or crystalline, and vitreous. Tension and position in relationship to orbit should be noted.

PATH: *Exophthalmos:* (protrusion) If bilateral may be due to goiter. E. may appear to protrude in fright, asthma, and spasmodic croup. It is noted in thrombosis of superior longitudinal sinus, cardiac atrophy, laryngeal stenosis, and paralysis of ocular movements. One or both may be affected by hemorrhage in orbit, aneurysm, exostosis, or tumor of orbit, or enlarged lacrimal glands. *Enophthalmos:* Bilateral or unilateral recession of eyeball.

eyebrow. The arch over the eye; also its covering, esp. the hairs.

eyecup. 1. The optic vesicle, evagination of the embryonic brain from which the retina develops. 2. A small cup which fits over the eye, used for bathing the surface of the eye.

eyeglass. A glass lens used to aid the defective eye in seeing.

eyeground. Fundus of eye, seen with ophthalmoscope.

eyelash. Cilium, q.v. A stiff hair on the margin of the eyelid. SEE: *capsulociliary; "cili-" words; trichiasis.*

eyelid. One of two movable protective folds which when closed cover the anterior surface of the eyeball. They are separated by the palpebral fissure. The upper (palpebrae superior) is the larger and more movable. It is raised by contraction of the levator palpebrae superioris muscle. Angles formed by the lids at inner and outer ends are known as the canthi. The cilia, or eyelashes, arise from the edges of the eyelids. The posterior surface is lined by the conjunctiva, a mucus membrane.

   e. dropping. Ptosis.

   e., fused. A congenital anomaly resulting from failure of the fetal eyelids to separate.

eyestrain. Tiredness of the eye due to overuse. SYN: *asthenopia.*

eyetooth. A cuspid or upper canine tooth.

F

F. 1. Abbr. for *Fahrenheit; field of vision; formula; Fusiformis.* 2. Chem. symb. for fluorine.

F₁. In genetics, the first filial generation, the offspring of a cross between two unlike individuals.

F₂. The second filial generation or the offspring of a cross between two individuals of the F₁ generation.

FA., F.A. Abbr. for *fatty acid; filterable agent; first aid; fluorescent antibody.*

fabel'la [L., little bean]. (pl. *fabellae*) Fibrocartilages or bones which sometimes develop in the head of the gastrocnemius muscle.

fabrication (fab″rĭ-ka'shŭn) [L. *fabricatus,* having built]. A deliberately false statement told as if it were true. Present in Korsakoff's syndrome.

F.A.C.D. Abbr. for *Fellow of the American College of Dentists.*

face [L. *facies*]. Anterior part of the head from forehead to chin and extending laterally to but not including the ears; the visage or countenance.

ANAT: Arteries include left common carotid with exterior and interior branches, right common carotid with exterior and interior branches and circle of Willis. The face has 14 bones. The veins include exterior and interior jugular. SEE: *skeleton.*

DIAGNOSIS: The following conditions affect the features: mouth breathing, chronic alcoholism, narcotic drug use, abdominal diseases, facial hemiplegia, cretinism, myxedema, congenital syphillis, exophthalmic goiter, paralysis agitans, encephalitis lethargica, locomotor ataxia, acromegaly, mongolian idiocy, acute diffuse peritonitis, dyspnea, hysteria, late stages of pulmonary tuberculosis, lobar pneumonia, renal diseases, typhoid fever, hippocratic facies.

Brownish-yellow spots: Liver spots. Seen in pregnancy, malignancies of liver or uterus, and in exophthalmic goiter. Cosmetics and facial irritants, sunburn, and exposure to weather also factors. Occur in many diseases including Addison's disease, diabetes, hemochromatosis, pellagra, acanthosis nigricans, and others. Also occurs in arsenic poisoning.

Yellowish discoloration: Jaundice due to presence of excess of bile pigments in the blood. *Cyanosis:* Deficient oxygenation of the blood which may be due to acquired or congenital malformations of the heart, to asthma, whooping cough, pulmonary tuberculosis, croup, obstruction of trachea, aneurysm, tumor, asphyxia, drug poisoning, emphysema, dilation of right side of the

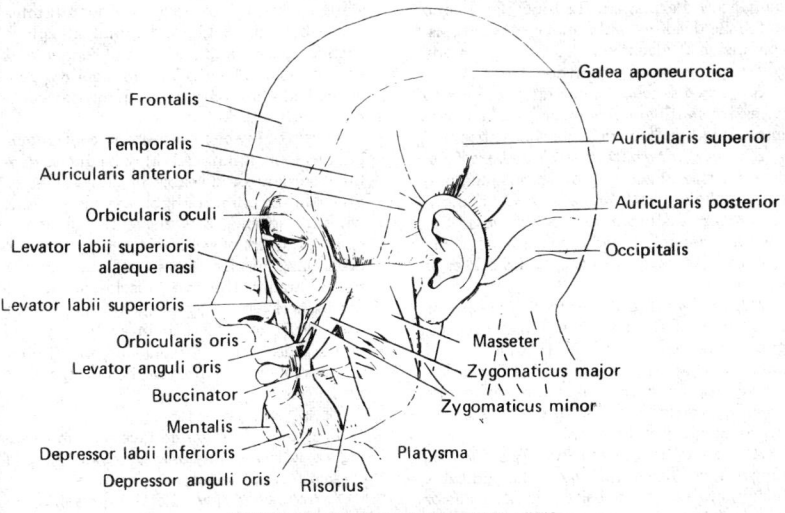

MUSCLES OF THE FACE—SIDE VIEW

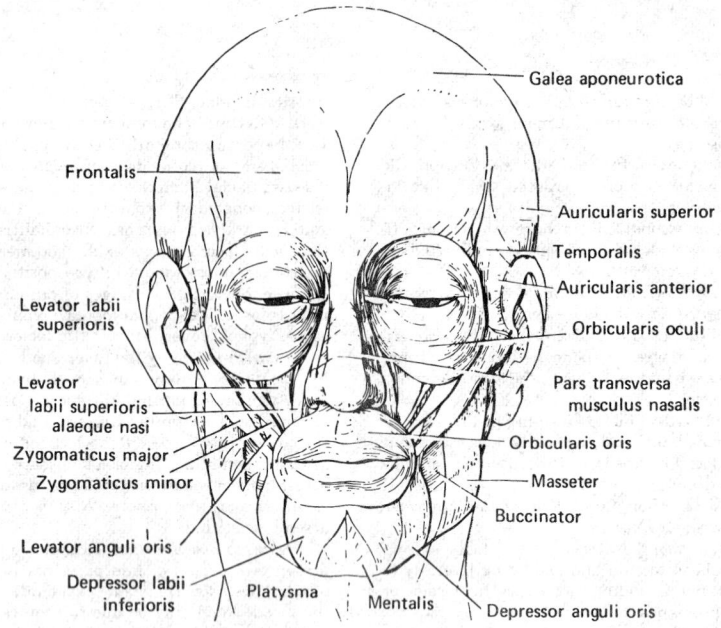

Galea aponeurotica

Frontalis

Auricularis superior

Temporalis

Auricularis anterior

Orbicularis oculi

Levator labii superioris

Levator labii superioris alaeque nasi

Zygomaticus major

Zygomaticus minor

Pars transversa musculus nasalis

Orbicularis oris

Masseter

Buccinator

Levator anguli oris

Depressor labii inferioris

Platysma

Mentalis

Depressor anguli oris

MUSCLES OF THE FACE—ANTERIOR VIEW

heart.

Flushing (hyperemia): May be permanent or evanescent. If due to emotions will be temporary. Permanent flushing may be due to febrile diseases, pulmonary tuberculosis, convulsions, alcoholism, ovarian tumors, goiter, plethora, hypertension.

Pallor: Absence of color. May be due to excessive confinement indoors, malnourishment, anemia, hemorrhage, shock, fright.

Redness, alternating with pallor: Emotion such as anger, cerebrospinal meningitis, typhoid, menopause, and general vasomotor disturbances. *Sallowness:* Cachexia, cancer, lead poisoning, some anemias, Addison's disease, and diseases of the liver.

Edema: Swelling of the face from edema is noted in cardiac, renal, and blood diseases, pneumothorax, mediastinal tumors, and aneurysm. It may be localized and evanescent due to urticaria, angioneurotic edema, or anaphylaxis. Seen in thrombosis of superior longitudinal sinus.

Absence of expression from half the face downward, drawn and distorted: Indicates facial paralysis of opposite side. *Anxious or pinched look:* Anxiety and mental unrest.

Hippocratic facies: A cadaverous appearance seen in cholera and acute general peritonitis. *Risus sardonicus:* A sardonic smile caused by contraction of mouth muscles which indicates abdominal affections such as spasms and peritonitis. *Sudden lack of expression:* Apathy and immobility, generally bad symptoms except in mental weakness and hysteria.

Spasms: May be intermittent, continuous, bilateral, or unilateral. May be due to dental disorders or diseases of skin, nose, or eyes. May be mimic or habit spasms; choreic, winking spasms; convulsive tic; blepharospasm. Closure of eyelids caused by spasm of orbicular muscles due to affection of the nerve supply, the eye muscles, or to eye diseases. Spasm of eyelids, chin, upper lips, or muscles of face seen in early stages of meningitis. Tonic spasms due to tetanus, spasms following paralysis, hysteria, and tic douloureux.

SEE: *cyanosis.*

f., moon. Full round face seen in Cushing's syndrome. May also be a side effect of corticosteroid therapy.

f. presentation. Fetal f. presentation in childbirth.

facet, facette (făs'ĕt) [Fr. *facette*, small face]. A small, smooth area on a bone or other hard surface.

fa'cial [L. *facialis*,]. Pert. to the face.

   f. center. Brain center causing facial movements.

   f. nerve. Seventh cranial nerve, a mixed nerve consisting of efferent fibers supplying the facial muscles, the platysma muscle, the submaxillary and sublingual glands; afferent fibers from taste buds of the anterior two thirds of the tongue and from the muscles. Afferent fibers originate from geniculate ganglion; motor and secretory fibers from nuclei in pons. They are distributed throughout the ear, face, palate, tongue. Branches are tympanic, chorda tympani, posterior auricular, digastric, stylohyoid, temporal, malar, infraorbital, buccal, supramaxillary, inframaxillary. SYN: *nervus facialis* [NA]. SEE: *cranial nerves*.

   f. paralysis. Affecting the muscles of the face. The 7th cranial nerve is involved.

   f. reflex. Contraction of f. muscles following pressure on eyeball.

   f. spasm. Tic. SEE: *cranial nerves; face*.

facies (fā'shĭ-ēz) [L]. (pl. *fa'cies*) [NA] 1. Face. 2. Surface of an organ or tissue.

   f. abdomina'lis. Pinched, anxious, shrunken, and drawn expression seen in abdominal troubles.

   f., adenoid. Dull lethargic appearance with open mouth.

   f. aor'tica. Expression seen in aortic valve insufficiency, bluish sclerae, cheeks sunken, face sallow.

   f. hepat'ica. Seen in liver affections. Skin is sallow, conjunctivae yellow, and eyeballs sunken.

   f. hippocrat'ica. Seen in those dying from long-continued illness or from cholera; cheeks and temples hollow, eyes sunken, complexion leaden, and lips relaxed.

   f. leontina. Lion-like face seen in certain forms of leprosy.

   f., mask-like. Expressionless face with little or no animation seen in parkinsonism.

   f. mitralis. Seen in mitral insufficiency. Capillaries more or less visible, cheeks pink, more or less cyanosis.

   f., myopathic. Due to muscular weakness, esp. that of the face. Lids drop and lips protrude.

   f. ovari'na. Seen in women with ovarian tumor; face drawn and pinched. SYN: *ovarica*.

   f., typhoid. Dusky complexion, injected conjunctivae, and dull expression.

facilitation (fā-sĭl'ĭ-tā'shŭn) [L. *facilis,* easy]. Making an action or process easier, the energy of an impulse being added to that of other impulses activated at the same time.

fa'cing [L. *facies*, face]. An inlay to form the outer surface of a tooth.

faciobrachial (fā''shĭ-ō-brā'kĭ-ăl) ["+ Gr. *brachion*, arm]. Pert. to the face and arm, esp. to juvenile muscular dystrophy.

faciocephalalgia (fā''shĭ-ō-sĕf'ă-lăl'jĭ-ă) ["+ Gr. *kephalē*, head, + *algos*, pain]. Neuralgia of the face and head.

faciocervical (fā''shĭ-ō-sĕr'vĭ-kăl) ["+ *cervix*, neck]. Pert. to the face and neck, esp. to progressive dystrophy of facial muscles.

faciolingual (fā''shĭ-ō-lĭn'gwal) [L. *facies*, face, + *lingua*, tongue]. Pert. to the face and the tongue, esp. a paralysis of them.

facioplasty (fā''shĭ-ō-plăs'tĭ) ["+ Gr. *plassein*, to form]. Plastic surgery of the face.

facioplegia (fā''shĭ-ō-plē'jĭ-ă) ["+ Gr. *plēge*, stroke]. Facial paralysis. SYN: *prosopoplegia*.

facioscapulohumeral (fā''shĭ-ō-skăp''ū-lō-hū'mĕr-ăl) ["+ *scapula*, shoulder blade, + *humerus*, shoulder]. Pert. to the face, the scapula, and the upper arm.

F.A.C.P. Abbr. for *Fellow of the American College of Physicians*.

F.A.C.S. Abbr! for *Fellow of the American College of Surgeons*.

factitious (făk-tĭsh'ŭs) [L. *facticius,* made by art]. Something produced artificially.

   f. fever. Fever produced artificially, usually by the patient in order to feign illness.

   f. illness. Illness which is feigned. SEE: *Munchhausen syndrome*.

factor [L., maker]. A condition, element, influence, or circumstance that contributes to a result.

   f., accessory food. A substance in food which does not serve as a source of energy but is essential for normal growth and development or normal metabolic activities; a vitamin, q.v.

   f., antianemic. A substance stored in the liver, essential for the normal development of red blood cells in the bone marrow. It is formed in the stomach and intestine by the interaction of an extrinsic factor, vitamin B_{12}, and an intrinsic factor present in gastric juice. It is used in the treatment of pernicious anemia.

   f., lethal. A gene which, when homozygous, causes the death of an individual before development is complete.

   f., milk. A substance present in certain strains of mice which is transferred to offspring through milk from the mammary glands. It is capable of inducing the development of mammary cancer in suckling mice exposed to the f.

f., Rh. SEE: *Rh blood factor.*

fac'ulta"tive [L. *facultas,* capability]. 1. Having the capacity to do something, but doing it is not compulsory. 2. In biology and particularly bacteriology, having the ability to live under certain conditions. Thus a microorganism may be f. with respect to oxygen and be able to live with or without oxygen.

fac'ulty. 1. A mental attribute or sense. 2. Ability to function.

f., affective. Capacity for expressing emotions.

f., germinative. Power of a germ to develop.

fagopyrism (făg-ō-pīr'ĭzm, -ŏp'ĭ-rĭzm) [L. *fagopyrum,* buckwheat]. Buckwheat poisoning.

Fahrenheit scale (făr'ĕn-hīt"). [Gabriel D. Fahrenheit, Ger. physicist, 1686-1736]. The temperature scale used in the U.S.A. and England. The freezing point of water is 32° and the boiling point 212°. Indicated by F. SEE: *thermometer.*

Fahrenheit and Centigrade Scales

F.	C.	F.	C.	F.	C.
500°	260°	248°	120°	95°	35°
401	205	239	115	86	30
392	200	230	110	77	25
383	195	212	100	68	20
374	190	203	95	50	10
356	180	194	90	41	5
347	175	176	80	32	0
338	170	167	75	23	− 5
329	165	140	60	14	−10
320	160	122	50	+ 5	−15
311	155	113	45	− 4	−20
302	150	105	40.56	−13	−25
284	140	104	40	−22	−30
275	135	100	37.8	−40	−40
266	130	98.5	36.9	−76	−60

1° F. = .54° C.
1.8° F. = 1° C.
3.6° F. = 2° C.
4.5° F. = 2.5° C.
5.4° F. = 3° C.

failure-to-thrive syndrome. Failure of a child to develop mentally and physically as he should. May be due to a variety of causes but often is associated with a disturbed mother-child relationship.

faint [O.Fr. *faindre,* to feign]. 1. To feel weak as though about to lose consciousness. 2. Weak. 3. Syncope. SEE: *fainting.*

fainting (fănt'ing). Loss of consciousness due to cerebral anemia or insufficient blood to the brain.

SYM: Prior to onset patient may be pale, weak, dizzy, have cold perspiration and uncomfortable abdominal sensation. He may fall on the ground unconscious. Pulse is usually weak, rapid, often irregular.

F.A. TREATMENT: If a patient is sitting, lower head between the knees or preferably have patient lie down with the head lower than the body. Elevate lower extremities. Rub extremities toward the heart. Stimulate by allowing patient to smell aromatic spirits of ammonia at intervals.

When able to swallow, give hot black coffee, strong tea, or other hot drinks. Twenty drops of aromatic spirits of ammonia in hot water may be given by mouth.

RS: apoplexy; asphyxia; coma; shock; swoon; syncope; unconsciousness.

faint'ness. 1. A sensation of impending loss of consciousness. 2. A sensation due to lack of food.

falcate (făl'kāt) [L. *falx,* sickle]. Sickle-shaped.

falcial (făl'shăl). Pert. to the falx.

falciform (făl'sĭ-form) [L. *falx,* sickle, + *forma,* form]. Sickle-shaped.

f. ligament. The triangular ligament attached to sides of the sacrum and coccyx by its base. SYN: *sacrotuberous ligament.*

f. ligament of liver. That portion of the peritoneum reflected around the ligamentum teres, and attaching the upper surfaces of the liver to the diaphragm and abdominal wall. SYN: *ligamentum falciforme hepatis* [NA].

f. process. That portion of the f. ligament along the inner margin of the ramus of the ischium.

fal'cula [L., little sickle]. The falx cerebelli.

fal'cular. 1. Sickle-shaped. 2. Pert. to the falx cerebelli, q.v.

fallec'tomy. Cutting away part of the fallopian tube.

falling drop. 1. A metallic tinkle heard over the normal stomach and bowel when inflated. 2. The same sound heard over large cavities containing fluid and air, as observed in hydropneumothorax.

falling sickness. Epileptic condition.

falling womb. Dropping of the uterus, so that it protrudes into vagina. SYN: *descensus uteri.*

fallopian canal (fă-lō'pī-ăn). [Gabriele Falloppio, It. anatomist, 1523-62] Canal in petrous bone for nervus facialis.

fallopian ligament. Round ligament of the uterus.

fallopian tube. The tube or duct which extends laterally from the lateral angle of the uterus, terminating near the ovary. It serves to convey the ovum from the ovary to the uterus and spermatozoa from the uterus towards the ovary. Medially each tube opens into the uterus; distally each opens into the peritoneal cavity. Each lies in the superior border of the broad ligament.

ANAT: The narrow region near the uterus, the isthmus, continues laterally as a wider ampulla. The latter expands to form the terminal funnel-shaped infundibulum, at the bottom of which lies a small opening, the ostium, through which the ovum enters the oviduct. Surrounding each ostium are a number of fingerlike processes called fimbria, one of which, the fimbria ovarica, is considerably longer than the others, extending towards and may be connected to the ovary. Each tube averages about 4 1/2 in. (11.5 cm.) in length and 1/4 in. (6 mm.) in diameter. Its wall consists of three layers: mucosa, muscular layer, and serosa. The epithelium of the mucosa consists of ciliated and non-ciliated cells. Ciliary action aids in the movement of the ovum towards the uterus. The muscular layer consists of an inner circular and an outer longitudinal layer of smooth muscle. The serosa consists of connective tissue underlying the outermost layer of peritoneum.

The blood supply is derived from branches of the uterine and ovarian arteries. The nerve supply from pelvic, ovarian, and uterine nerve plexuses, sending fibers to the tubes. SYN: *oviduct; tuba uterina* [NA]; *uterine tube.*

fallostomy (făl-ŏs'tō-mī). Surgical opening of the fallopian tube. SYN: *salpingostomy.*

Fallot, tetralogy of (fălō'). [Etienne L. A. Fallot, Fr. physician, 1850-1911] A congenital condition characterized by defect in the interventricular septum, stenosis of the pulmonary artery, dextroposition of the aorta, and hypertrophy of the right ventricle. Modern surgical therapy has made it possible to treat this condition effectively.

fallot'omy. Division of the fallopian tubes. SYN: *salpingotomy,* q.v.

fallout. Settling of radioactive fission products from the atmosphere after explosion of an atomic bomb.

false [L. falsus]. That which is untrue or incorrect.

f. **-negative.** A test or examination which indicates that a condition or disease is not present when it is in fact present. This may produce dire consequences when, for example, a patient is told that a malignancy is not present when it is.

f. **-positive.** A test or examination indicating that a condition or disease is present when in fact it is not. Several diseases including malaria, infectious mononucleosis, leprosy, and spirochetal diseases such as yaws and pinta may cause certain serological tests for syphilis to give a positive reaction when the patient does not have syphilis.

f. **ribs.** The lower five pairs of ribs which do not unite with the sternum. SEE: *ribs; vertebrae.*

falx [L.]. (pl. *fal'ces*) [NA] Any sickle-shaped structure.

f. **cerebelli.** [NA] A fold of the dura mater which forms a vertical partition between the hemispheres of the cerebellum.

f. **cerebri.** [NA] A fold of the dura mater which lies in the longitudinal fissure and separates the two cerebral hemispheres.

f. **inguinalis.** [NA] The conjoined or conjoint tendon which forms the origin of the transversus abdominis and internal oblique muscles.

f. **ligamento'sa.** The broad ligament of the liver. SYN: *falciform ligament of liver.*

famil'ial [L. *familiā,* family]. Pert. to or common to the same family, as f. symptoms.

family. 1. A group consisting of parents and their children. 2. In biological classification, the division between order and genus.

f., degenerate. F. that produces offspring of low or subnormal mentality.

f., Jukes. A family whose history covers five generations of degeneracy.

f., Kallikak. An Amer. family with one branch mentally unfit and another of average intelligence.

f. **planning.** The planning and spacing of conception of children according to the wishes of the couple rather than to chance. This is accomplished by practicing some form of birth control.

F. and R., F & R. Abbr. for *force and rhythm* (of pulse).

fang [AS., to plunder]. 1. A sharp-pointed tooth. 2. The root of a tooth.

f.'s, poison. Two teeth in upper jaw adjacent to their poison glands in poisonous reptiles.

far'ad. [Michael Faraday, Brit. physicist, 1791-1867] A unit of electrical capacity. The capacity of a condenser which, charged with 1 coulomb, gives a difference of potential of 1 volt. This unit is so large that one-millionth part of it has been adopted as a practical unit called a microfarad.

farad'ic. Pert. to induced electricity.

far'adism. The therapeutic use of an interrupted current to stimulate muscles and nerves. Such a current is derived from the secondary or induction coil.

faradization. 1. The treatment of nerves or muscles with the faradic current. 2. The condition of nerves or muscles so treated.

faradother'apy. Treatment of disease by the faradic current.

far'cy [L. *farcire,* to stuff]. A form of glanders.

    f. bud. A glanderous tumor.

    f., button. F. marked by dermal tubercular nodules.

farina (fā-rē'nă) [L.]. Finely ground meal commonly made from wheat or other grain. Used as cereal and flour.

farinaceous (făr''ĭ-nā'shŭs). 1. Starchy. 2. Pert. to flour.

farpoint. The farthest point of vision at which objects can be seen distinctly with eyes in complete relaxation.

Farre's tubercles (făr). [John R. Farre. Brit. physician, 1775-1862] Carcinomatous masses on surface of the liver.

farsight'ed. Pert. to far-sightedness, q.v. SYN: *hypermetropic; hyperopic.*

farsight'edness. An error of refraction in which, with accommodation completely relaxed, parallel rays come to a focus behind the retina. SYN: *hypermetropia; hyperopia.*

fascia (făsh'ĭ-ă) [L., a band]. (pl. *fasciae*) 1. [NA] A fibrous membrane covering, supporting, and separating muscles. It also unites the skin with underlying tissue. Fascia may be superficial, a nearly subcutaneous covering permitting free movement of the skin, or deep, enveloping and binding muscles. 2. A bandage.

    f., Abernethy's. SEE: *Abernethy's fascia.*

    f., anal. F. of connective tissue covering levator ani muscle from the perineal aspect.

    f., Buck's. A fascial covering of the penis, derived from Colles' f.

    f., cerivical, deep. F. of the neck covering the muscles, vessels, and nerves.

    f., cervical, superficial. F. of the neck just inside the skin.

    f., Cloquet's. Femoral f.

    f., Colles'. Inner layer of the perineal f.

    f., cremasteric. F. covering the cremaster muscle of the spermatic cord. SYN: *f. cremasterica* [NA].

    f., cribriform. The f. of the thigh covering the saphenous opening. SYN: *f. cribrosa* [NA].

    f., dentate. Gray matter in the cerebral dentate convolution. SYN: *gyrus dentatus* [NA].

    f., infundibuliform. Funnel-shaped f., derived from interior abdominal wall, encasing the spermatic cord and testis. SYN: *f. spermatica interna* [NA].

    f., intercolumnar. F. derived from external abdominal ring sheathing the spermatic cord and testis.

    f., ischiorectal. F., anal, q.v.

    f. lata. [NA] Wide covering encasing thigh muscles.

    f., lumbodorsal. Deep investing membrane covering deep muscles of the trunk and back.

    f., pectineal. Pubic section of f. lata.

    f., pelvic. Fascial tissues of extreme importance in the maintenance of normal strength in the pelvic floor. SEE: *diaphragm, pelvic.*

    f., thyrolaryngeal. F. covering thyroid gland.

    f. transversalis. F. located between perineum and transversalis muscle; lines the abdominal cavity.

fasciae (făsh'ĭ-ē). Pl. of fascia.

fascial (făsh'ĭ-ăl) [L. *fascia,* band]. Pert. to or of the nature of fascia.

    f. reflex. Muscular contraction resulting from percussing facial fascia.

fasciaplasty (făsh'ĭ-ă-plăs''tĭ) ["+ Gr. *plassein,* to form]. Plastic surgery of fascia.

fascicle (făs'ĭ-kl) [L. *fasciculus,* little bundle]. A fasciculus.

fascicular (fă-sĭk'ū-lăr). 1. Arranged like a bundle of rods. 2. Pert. to a fasciculus.

fasciculus (fă-sĭk'ū-lŭs). (pl. *fascic'uli*) [NA] A bundle of nerve or muscle fibers. More specifically a division of a funiculus of the spinal cord consisting of fibers of one or more tracts. Sometimes the term is used as a synonym for tract. SYN: *fasciola.*

    f. cuneatus. A triangular-shaped bundle of nerve fibers lying in the dorsal funiculus of the spinal cord. Its fibers enter the cord through the dorsal roots of spinal nerves and terminate in the medulla. SYN: *tract of Burdach.*

    f., fundamental. Portion of anterior column of spinal cord continuing into medulla oblongata.

    f. gracilis. A bundle of nerve fibers lying in the dorsal funiculus of the spinal cord medial to the f. cuneatus. Conducts sensory impulses from the periphery to the medulla.

    f., longitudinal, dorsal. A bundle of association fibers connecting the frontal lobe with the occipital and temporal lobes.

f., longitudinal, inferior. A bundle of association fibers connecting the occipital and temporal lobes of the brain.

f., longitudinal, medial. A bundle of fibers running from the spinal cord to the upper portion of the midbrain.

f., longitudinal, posterior. Nerve fiber bundle running between corpora quadrigemina and nuclei of 4th and 6th nerves.

f. teres. Column on both sides of median furrow in floor of 4th ventricle.

f., unciform. Fibers within sylvian fissure connecting frontal and temporosphenoid lobes. SYN: *f. uncinatus* [NA]; *uncinate f.*

fasciectomy (făsh″ĭ-ĕk′tō-mĭ) [L. *fascia*, band, + Gr. *ektomē*, excision]. Excision of strips of fascia.

fasciodesis (făsh′ĭ-ŏd′ē-sĭs) ["+ Gr. *desis*, binding]. Operation of attaching a fascia to a tendon or another fascia.

Fasciola (fă-sī′ō-lă) [L. *fasciola*, a band]. A genus of flukes belonging to the class Trematoda.

F. hepatica. A species of flukes infesting the liver and bile ducts of cattle, sheep, and other herbivores; the common liver fluke. An occasional parasite of man. Intermediate hosts are snails belonging to the genus Limmeus.

fasciola (fă-sī′ō-lă) [L., little band]. (pl. *fasciolae*) A bundle of nerve or muscle fibers. SYN: *fasciculus,* q.v.

f. cine′rea. Upper portion of dentate fascia.

fasciolar (fă-sī′ō-lăr). Pert. to the fasciola cinerea.

fascioliasis (făs″ĭ-ō-lī′ă-sĭs) [L. *fascia*, band, + Gr. *-iasis*, condition]. Infection of the body with a genus of trematode worms. SYN: *distomiasis.*

fascioplasty (făsh′ĭ-ō-plăs″tĭ) ["+ Gr. *plassein*, to form]. Plastic operation on a fascia.

fasciorrhaphy (făsh-ĭ-or′ă-fĭ) ["+ Gr. *rhaphē*, suture]. Suturing a fascia.

fasciotomy (făsh-ĭ-ŏt′ō-mĭ) ["+ Gr. *tomē*, incision]. Surgical incision and division of a fascia.

fascitis (fă-sī′tĭs) ["+ Gr. *itis*, inflammation]. Inflamed condition of a fascia.

fast. 1. [AS. *faest*, fixed] Resistant to the effects or action of a chemical substance. 2. [AS. *faestan*] Fasting.

f., acid. Term applied to bacteria, esp. the tuberculosis group, which after staining are not decolorized when treated with acid.

f., drug. Term applied to bacteria or other organisms which become resistant to drugs such as penicillin.

fastidium (făs-tĭd′ĭ-ŭm) [L., aversion]. Aversion to food or to eating. Sometimes seen in hysteria but not as the result of delusions.

fastigatum (făs″tĭ-gā′tŭm) [L., pointed]. The gray matter on both sides of the inferior vermiform process of the cerebellum. SYN: *nucleus fastigii.*

fastigium (făs-tĭj′ĭ-ŭm) [L., ridge]. 1. The highest point. The full period of development of acute, infectious diseases when the temperature reaches the maximum or stadium and all symptoms have developed. 2. The most posterior portion of the 4th ventricle formed by the junction of the anterior and posterior medullary vela projecting into the medullary substance of the cerebellum.

fast′ing [AS. *faestan*, to hold fast]. Going without food for a stated period.

Energy requirements of body metabolism during fasting are supplied by the oxidization of fats which, if glucose is not supplied, results in the products of incomplete fat combustion such as fatty acids, diacetic acid, and acetone, producing ketosis or a mild acidosis. This condition occurs quickly in children as they have little glycogen reserve.

fast′ness [AS. *faest*, fixed]. Resistance to stains or destructive agents.

fat [AS. *faett*]. 1. Adipose, obese, corpulent. 2. Greasy, oily. 3. In chemistry, triglyceride ester of fatty acids; one of a group of organic compounds closely associated in nature with the phosphatides, cerebrosides, sterols. The term lipid or lipide, q.v., is applied in general to a fat or fatlike substance.

Fats are insoluble in water but soluble in ether, chloroform, benzene, and other fat solvents. Upon hydrolysis, fats break down into fatty acids and glycerol (an alcohol). Fats are hydrolyzed by the action of acids, alkalies, lipases (fat-splitting enzymes) and superheated steam.

CHEM. STRUCTURE: In the fat molecule, one molecule of glycerol is combined with three of fatty acids. Three fatty acids, oleicacid($C_{18}H_{34}O_2$), stearic acid ($C_{18}H_{36}O_2$), and palmitic acid ($C_{18}H_{32}O_2$), comprise the bulk of fatty acids present in neutral fats found in body tissues. According to the fatty acid (oleic) with which the glycerol is combined, corresponding fats are triolein, tristearin, and tripalmitin. These three fats are the principal fats present in foods.

PHYSIOLOGICAL FUNCTIONS: Fats serve as a source of energy. Subcutaneous fats form an insulating layer which prevents loss of heat. Fat acts to support and protect certain organs such as the eye and kidney; provides a concentrated reserve of food; provides essential fatty acids necessary for normal growth and development; and is a vehicle for natural fat-soluble vitamins. In conjunction with carbohydrates, fats serve as protein sparers. They are an important constituent of cell structure, forming an integral part of the cell membrane. When properly distributed, fat gives a pleasing contour to the body.

DIGESTION AND ABSORPTION: In the stomach, emulsified fats such as cream or egg yolk are acted on by gastric lipase; however, most fats undergo digestion in the intestine where they are acted on by a pancreatic lipase, steapsin, which hydrolyzes them to fatty acids and glycerol. Although containing no lipolytic enzymes, bile is essential for the digestion of fats. It aids in the emulsification of fats and has a hydrotropic action, i.e., renders substances such as fatty acids, which are normally insoluble in water, readily soluble in the fluids of the intestine. Bile salts also act as specific activators of the pancreatic lipase. Bile salts react with fatty acids forming water-soluble, diffusible soaps which facilitate the emulsification of fats. Glycerol and fatty acids enter the epithelial cells where they recombine to form neutral fats most of which enter the lacteals. The fats are carried by the lymph through lymph vessels to the thoracic duct from which they enter the blood stream. After a meal rich in fats the mesenteric lymph vessels are filled with a milklike fluid, the chyle containing finely emulsified fat particles called chylomicrons.

METABOLISM: Absorbed fats are utilized in the following ways: oxidized with the release of energy; deposited in adipose tissue as storage fat; incorporated in the cells of tissues as an integral part of the protoplasm; desaturated and stored in the liver; excreted in the secretions of the mammary and sweat glands and in the feces.

Intermediary metabolism: In the oxidation of fat to carbon dioxide and water, several intermediary substances (ketones) are formed. The principal ones are acetoacetic acid, beta-hydroxybutyric acid, and acetone. Excessive production of ketone bodies which occurs when fats are incompletely oxidized is called ketosis. This especially occurs when there is an interference in carbohydrate metabolism, as in diabetes. Ketosis also occurs in certain fevers, toxemias of pregnancy, and hyperthyroidism. Ketosis results in acidosis.

SOURCES: In addition to fat being absorbed from the intestine, body fat may arise from the conversion of carbohydrates (glucose) or proteins into fat. Fatty acids cannot be converted directly to glucose in the body, but a portion of the molecule of fatty acids of certain length can be utilized as carbohydrate.

NUTRITION: Fats have a high caloric value yielding 9 Cal. per gm. as compared with 4.0 Cal. for carbohydrates and proteins. (These values are given in round numbers.) The average diet of 3000 Cal. should contain 30-40% of its caloric value in fats. The average diet contains 50-130 gm. of fat. Quantities in excess of 150 gm. are repulsive and difficult to digest. In addition to their nutritive values, fats improve the taste and odor of foods, provide a feeling of satiety, and because of their high caloric content, are of especial importance in high-caloric diets.

CONTRA: Fat intake should be reduced in certain diseases such as hepatitis and in low-caloric diets.

RS: bile; fatty acid; gallbladder; glycerol; ketones; lipase; liver.

f. depot. Accumulations of fat in certain regions of the body such as the buttocks or abdominal wall.

f., low-, diet. Approx. 40-50 gm. fat daily. SEE: *reduction diet.*

f., neutral. Compounds of the higher fatty acids (palmitic, stearic, and oleic) with glycerol. They are the common fats of animal and plant tissues.

f.-free and protein-free diet. Carbohydrates, high-water-content fruits such as citrus, melons, cucumbers, marmalades and jellies, rhubarb, fresh tomatoes.

f. -pad. The buccal pad of fat seen in cheeks of nursing infants.

f.- soluble. Soluble in fat as in the case of certain vitamins.

fat, words pert. to: absorption; acid; "adip-" words; calorie; chondrolipoma; chromolipoid; digestion; fatty acid; fuel value; hydrogenation; ketogenic diet; "lip-" words; obesity; palmitic acid; palmitin; stearin.

fatal (fāt'l) [L. *fātālis*]. 1. Inevitable. 2. Causing death.

fatigue (fā-tēg') [L. *fatigāre*, to tire]. 1. A feeling of tiredness or weariness resulting from continued activity. 2. The state or condition of an organ or tissue in which its response to stimulation is reduced or lost as a result of overactivity. 3. To bring about a condition of fatigue.

Fatigue may be the result of excessive activity which results in the accumulation of metabolic waste products such as lactic acid; malnutrition (deficiency of carbohydrates, proteins, minerals, or vitamins); circulatory disturbances such as heart disease or anemia which interfere with the supply of oxygen and energy materials to tissues; respiratory disturbances which interfere with the supply of oxygen to tissues; infectious diseases in which toxic products are produced or body metabolism altered; endocrine disturbances such as occur in diabetes, hyperinsulinism, and menopause; psychogenic factors such as emotional conflicts, frustration, anxiety, neurosis, boredom; physical factors such as incorrect posture or flat feet.

f., acute. F. with sudden onset such as occurs following excessive exertion; relieved by rest.

f., chronic. Long-continued f. not relieved by rest. Indicative of disease such as tuberculosis or diabetes or other conditions of altered body metabolism.

f., muscular. The reduced capacity of a muscle to perform work as a result of repeated contractions. F. may be partial or complete.

f. reaction. In tuberculosis, an elevation of temperature following exertion.

f. stance. F. resulting from standing for long periods of time.

f. syndrome. Neurasthenia, q.v.

fatty. Of, or pert. to, fats or fatty substances; adipose. SEE: *fat; heart.*

f. acid. A hydrocarbon in which one of the hydrogen atoms has been replaced by a carboxyl (COOH) group; a monobasic aliphatic acid made up of an alkyl radical attached to a carboxyl group.

Saturated fatty acids are those which have no double bonds (i.e. $C = C$) between carbon atoms. They include acetic, butyric, caproic, caprylic, capric, lauric, formic, myristic, palmitic, and stearic acids, all of which contain an even number of carbon atoms. Saturated fatty acids have the general formula $C_nH_{2n}O_2$. The unsaturated fatty acids include those of the oleic series (oleic, tiglic, hypogeic, palmitoleic, and physetoleic acids) and the linoleic or linolic series (linoleic, linolenic, clupanodonic, arachidonic, hydrocarpic, and chaulmoogric acids). Fatty acids are insoluble in water. This would prevent their being absorbed from the intestines were it not for the action of bile salts on the fatty acids to enable them to be absorbed.

f. acid, essential. The unsaturated fatty acids, linoleic, linolenic, and arachidonic, cannot be synthesized in the body. Therefore they have been considered to be essential to maintain health. This is true for most mammals but has not been proven for adult humans.

Unsaturated fatty acids are important in relation to the metabolism of cholesterol. SEE: *digestion.*

f. casts. Casts seen in the urine sediments. They are usually abnormal and consist of a mass of fat globules.

f. degeneration. A change involving the deposition of fat in the cytoplasm.

fauces (fŏ'sēz) [L.]. [NA] The constricted opening leading from the mouth and the oral pharynx. It is bounded by the soft palate, base of the tongue, and the palatine arches.

The anterior pillars of the fauces are known as the glossopalatine arch, and the posterior pillars, as the pharyngopalatine arch. SEE: *fossa.*

faucial (fŏ'shāl) [L. *fauces,* throat]. Pert. to the fauces.

f. reflex. Gagging or vomiting resulting from irritation of fauces.

faucitis (fŏ-sī'tīs) ["+ Gr. *-itis,* inflammation]. Inflammation of the fauces.

faveolate (fā-vē'ō-lāt) [L. *faveolus,* little honeycomb]. Honeycombed. SYN: *alveolate.*

faveolus (fā-vē'ō-lŭs) [L., little honeycomb]. A depression or small pit, esp. on the skin.

favism (fā'vĭzm) [It. *fava,* bean]. A condition common in Sicily and Sardinia resulting from sensitivity to a species of bean, Vicia faba. It is characterized by fever, acute hemolytic anemia, vomiting, diarrhea, and may lead to prostration and coma. It is caused by ingestion of the beans, or inhalation of the pollen of the plant by persons who have congenital absence of the enzyme glucose-6-phosphate dehydrogenase.

favus (fā'vŭs) [L., honeycomb]. Contagious skin disease characterized by pinhead to pea-sized, saucer-shaped, yellowish crust (scutulum) over hair follicles and accompanied by musty odor and itching. It may spread all over the body. SYN: *crusted ringworm; honeycomb ringworm. SEE: scutulum*

ETIOL: Fungus, Trichophyton schönleinlii

PROG: Good. TREATMENT: Grisofulvin.

F.D. Abbr. for *fatal dose; focal distance.*

Fe. Chem. symb. for L. *ferrum,* iron.

fear [AS. *faer*]. Fright, dread. Primitively, the emotional reaction to an environmental threat; it now also presents itself frequently as an indicator of inner problems.

A partial fear reaction may be considered the expression of somatic disease. Fear is met clinically in anxiety neuroses, anxious psychotic pictures (e.g., depression), and in toxic deliria (e.g., delirium tremens). At the somatic level, hyperthyroidism and hyperadrenalism may strongly simulate the fear state. SEE: *emotion; phobia* for table.

febricide (fĕb'rĭ-sĭd) [L. *febris,* fever, + *cidus,* killing]. Destructive to fever. SYN: *antipyretic.*

febrifacient (fĕb-rĭ-fā'sĭ-ĕnt) [L. *febris,* fever, + *facere,* to make]. Producing fever.

febrific (fĕ-brĭf'ĭk). Producing or conveying fever.

febrifugal (fĕb-rĭf'ū-găl) [L. *febris,* fever, + *fugare,* to put to flight]. Reducing fever.

febrifuge (fĕb'rĭ-fūj). That which lessens fever. SYN: *antipyretic.*

febrile (fĕ'brĭl, fĕ'brĭl, fĕb'rĭl) [L. *febris,* fever]. Feverish; pert. to a fever. SEE: *fever.*

 f. convulsions. A convulsion occurring during fever but not due to an infection in the brain. Occurs almost exclusively between the ages of six months and five years and more commonly in boys. In addition to symtomatic and specific therapy for the cause of the fever, children with high fever should be sedated in order to attempt to prevent convulsions.

 f. state. A term used to describe constitutional symptoms which accompany a rise in temperature. Pulse and respiration usually rise with headache, pains, malaise, loss of appetite, concentrated and diminished urine, constipation, restlessness, not dry skin, insomnia, irritability.

febriphobia (fĕb''rĭ-fō'bĭ-ă) [L. *febris,* fever, + Gr. *phobos,* fear]. Anxiety or fear induced by a rise in body temperature.

febris (fĕ'brĭs) [L.]. Fever.

 f. enterica. Typhoid fever.

 f. flava. Yellow fever.

 f. undulans. Brucellosis.

 f. variolosa. A form of smallpox.

fecal (fē'kăl) [L. *faeces,* refuse]. Pert. to, or of the nature of, feces.

 f. vomit. Feces in vomitus. Occurs in strangulated hernia or intestinal obstruction preventing anal outlet.

fecalith (fē'kă-lĭth) ["+ Gr. *lithos,* stone]. A fecal concretion. SYN: *coprolith.*

fecaloid (fē'kă-loyd) ["+ Gr. *eidos,* form]. Resembling feces.

fecaloma (fē''kăl-ō'mă) [L. *faeces,* refuse, + Gr. *ōma,* tumor]. A large mass of accumulated feces in the rectum resembling a tumor. SYN: *Coproma; scatoma; stercoroma.*

fecaluria (fē''kăl-ū'rĭ-ă) ["+ Gr. *ouron,* urine]. Fecal matter in the urine.

feces (fē'sēz) [L. *faeces*]. Stools; excreta; dejecta; excrement. Body waste such as food residue, bacteria, epithelium, and mucus, discharged from the bowels by way of the anus. SYN: *stool.*

COMPOSITION: The total weight of the stool in a healthy adult male on a normal diet will be 100-200 gm. daily. Of this, 65% will be water and the remainder dry matter. Excreted nitrogen will be less than 1.7 gm. daily.

The stool is composed of residue of food, water, products of secretions, bacterial decomposition, indole, skatole, cholesterol, mucus and epithelial cells, purine bases, pigment, microorganisms, inorganic salts, and sometimes foreign substances.

The normal reaction is neutral or slightly alkaline. An acid reaction usually indicates some fermentation in the gut or an excess of vegetables in the diet. The stools of infants usually are acid.

DIAG: Inspection should include color, formation, odor, and the presence of any observable foreign substances, including calculi.

The color of the feces may be indicative of various disorders. *Black:* May follow intestinal hemorrhage or the use of drugs such as bismuth, iron, tannin, manganese, or charcoal. *Bloody:* May indicate hemorrhoids, cancer of the rectum, ulcers, fissures, abraded rectal membrane from dry feces, eroded rectal polypus, acute proctitis, foreign bodies, colitis, intussusception or strangulated hernia in children, cancer of the colon, rupture of abdominal aneurysm, typhoid fever, phosphorus poisoning. *Clay-colored:* May denote impaired bile formation or obstruction, phosphorus poisoning, or yellow atrophy of the liver. *Green:* In general this indicates in children and infants that the bowel contents have passed quickly through the intestinal tract.

Form and Consistency: Normally soft and formed. Hard, nodular, or scybalous in constipation. Fluid or mushy in diarrhea. Flattened or ribbonlike in rectal obstruction or spastic colitis. Frothy in fermentative conditions. Greasy in jaundice.

Mucus: Amount should be noted. Present in both abnormal as well as normal circumstances. May occur as superficial gelatinous streaks or blobs; mixed with the stool and only apparent on making a thin paste with water; mixed with blood as in dysentery; composing almost the entire stool, sometimes as firm bands or cords.

Odor: This varies much with disease and dietary differences. It is most marked on a meat diet and almost absent on a milk diet. Variations, such as sour, pungent, putrid, etc., occur in different diseases. *Offensive odor:* In jaundice, acute indigestion, enteritis, typhoid fever, and occasionally in constipation. *Putrid odor:* May be the result of syphilitic or carcinomatous ulceration of the rectum or gangrenous dysentery. *Sour odor:* Normal stools of infants.

Parasites: The presence of various intestinal parasites can be determined by examination of the feces. Gross examination may reveal the presence of nematodes (roundworms) or tapeworms; however, microscopic examination is necessary to determine the presence of protozoa, helminth ova, or larvae. In examination of feces, stools are collected in clean, dry, containers. For microscopic examination, representative bits of feces, or mucus are emulsified in saline solution on a clean slide, then spread evenly, and covered with a coverglass. Enterobiasis (pinworms) is best diagnosed by examination of scrapings from the anal and perianal regions.

f., sheep. Small masses broken off from stonelike feces remaining in colon too long.

feces, words pert. to: acoprosis; acoprous; anus; colon; constipation, defecation; dejecta; elimination; excreta; excretion; hypostasis; impaction; intestine; meconium; melanorrhea; melana; rectum; scatology; scybalum; sigmoid; steatorrhea; stool.

Fe(C₃H₅O₃)₂. Ferrous lactate; lactate of iron.

Fechner's law (fĕk'nĕr). [Gustav T. Fechner, Ger. philosopher, 1801-87] A theory stating that the magnitudes of sensation produced by given stimuli form an arithmetical progression, the stimuli forming a geometrical progression. SYN: *psychophysical law.*

FeCl₂. Ferrous chloride.

FeCl₃. Ferric chloride.

FeCO₃. Ferrous carbonate.

fecula (fĕk'ū-lă) [L. *faecula,* dregs]. 1. Sediment. 2. Starch.

feculent (fĕk'ū-lĕnt) [L. *faeculentus*]. Having sediment.

fecundate (fē'kŭn-dāt) [L. *fēcundāre,* to bear fruit]. To fertilize or impregnate or render fertile.

fecundation (fē-kŭn-dā'shŭn). Impregnation; fertilization.

f., artificial. Impregnation by injecting the seminal fluid into the uterus by mechanical means. SYN: *artificial insemination.*

fecundity (fē-kŭn'dĭ-tĭ). Ability to produce offspring; fertility.

feeblemind'edness. Arrested mental development as distinguished from temperamental abnormality. Mental deficiency, q.v.

feedback. In medical electronics or in biology, the return of information to the place of origin of the information by the system that receives the information. To a certain degree, blood pressure and blood sugar are regulated by feedback mechanisms. Feedback may be negative or positive. Thus a positive feedback signal indicates that more blood glucose needs to be made available when blood sugar level falls. Conversely, there will be a negative feedback signal when the blood sugar level rises to normal, indicating that production of blood sugar should be reduced or stopped.

feed'ing [AS. *fēdan,* to give food to]. Taking or giving nourishment, esp. extra-orally. The latter is sometimes necessary because the patient either refuses or is unable to eat.

f., artificial. 1. This is accomplished by providing liquid food preparation through a tube passed into the stomach or the rectum; also through gastrostomy or duodenostomy. 2. Feeding of a baby with food other than mother's milk.

f., breast. Feeding of an infant at the breast.

f., colonic. Less useful with psychotic than with physically sick patients but at times it can be utilized. The limited ability for absorption in the colon limits the usefulness of this method of feeding.

f., esophageal. Used after operations on tongue or jaw, diseases of mouth, in mental cases, for test meals, and forcible feedings.

f., forcible. This is by way of esophagus or rectum.

f., nasal. Largely used for children, and when patient is unable to take nourishment normally such as in delirium, coma, and stupor, diseases of mouth and pharynx. The tube is passed through the nose into the esophagus and stomach. Any strained liquid food that will pass through catheter can be used. Temperature of feeding, 100° F. (37.8° C.). Olive oil and swabs needed for cleaning nostrils.

f., rectal. Commonest form used, although little nourishment can be absorbed through colon. Normal saline often used with glucose, making a 5-10% solution by adding 1/2 to 1 oz. (45 ml.) of glucose to 10 oz. (300 ml.) of normal saline.

f., tube. Done through the mouth or nostril, the latter requiring a much smaller tube and a little more dexterity, but less likely to be successfully resisted. If the patient is delirious or insane the procedure is best done with patient lying, arms bound to body by encircling sheets, the lubricated (glycerine) tube is gently passed into pharynx and, avoiding the larynx, it is passed into the stomach. Entry into the larynx may produce struggling and cyanosis.

CAUTION: Be certain tube is in stomach and not in the bronchus prior to feedings. This can be determined by aspirating the tube and observing for gastric contents, or by listening to the end of the tube. If air comes out of the tube with each expiration, the tube is not in the stomach. Foods or nutritional substances as ordered by the physician are fed slowly.

feel'ing [AS. *fēlan,* to feel]. The conscious phase of nervous activity. The emotions or centrally stimulated f.'s and those sensations peripherally produced by excitation of peripheral nerves, including those of the special senses.

feet [AS. *fēt*]. (sing. *foot*) The pedal extremities of the legs. SEE: *foot.*

Fehl'ings solution (fā'ling). [Hermann von Fehling, Ger. chemist, 1812-85] A solution used for detecting the presence of sugar in urine. It consists of equal parts of Solutions A and B prepared as follows: Solution A (copper solution): dissolve 34.66 gm. of copper sulfate crystals in an amount of water to make 500 ml. Solution B (alkaline tartrate solution): dissolve 173 gm. of crystallized potassium sodium tartrate and 50 gm. of sodium hydroxide in an amount of water to make 500 ml. Mix equal portions of Solutions A and B immediately before using.

fel (fēl) [L.]. Bile

fellatorism (fēl-ă'tor-īzm) [L. *fellātus,* having sucked]. A form of sex perversion in which gratification is accomplished by buccal intromission of the penis; buccal coitus.

fel'on [ME. *feloun,* malignant]. Suppuration of terminal joint of a finger. SYN: *paronychia,* q.v.; *runaround; whitlow.*

felt'work. 1. Fibrous network. 2. A plexus of nerve fibrils.

fe'male [L. *fēmella,* little woman]. 1. A woman or girl-child. 2. Pert. to a woman. SEE: *genitalia, female.*

f. sex hormone. Hormone secreted by the ovaries which cause development of the uterus, vagina, and breasts at puberty, aids in regeneration of mucosa following menstruation, stimulates uterine contraction. SYN: *estrin; estrogen.*

fem'inism [L. *fēmininus*]. 1. The female character. 2. Possession of female characteristics by the male. 3. Social movement for female independence and equality.

feminiza'tion. Acquiring or adoption of female characteristics.

fem'oral [L. *femoralis*]. Pert. to the thigh bone or femur.

f. artery. [NA] Artery beginning at external iliac artery, terminating behind the knee as the popliteal artery, on inner side of femur. SYN: *arteria femoralis.*

f. reflex. Extension of knee and flexion of foot resulting from irritation of skin over upper anterior third of thigh.

f. vein. [NA] Continuation of the popliteal vein upward toward the external iliac vein. SYN: *vena femoralis.*

femorocele (fēm'ō-rō-sēl) [L. *femur,* thigh, + Gr. *kēlē,* hernia]. Femoral hernia.

femorotibial (fēm"ō-rō-tīb'ĭ-ăl) ["+ *tibia,* pipe]. Rel. to the femur and tibia.

femur (fē'mur) [L.]. [NA] The thigh bone. It extends from the hip to the knee and is the longest and strongest bone in the skeleton.

RS: calcar femorale; cavalry bone; cotyloid cavity; femoral; trochanter.

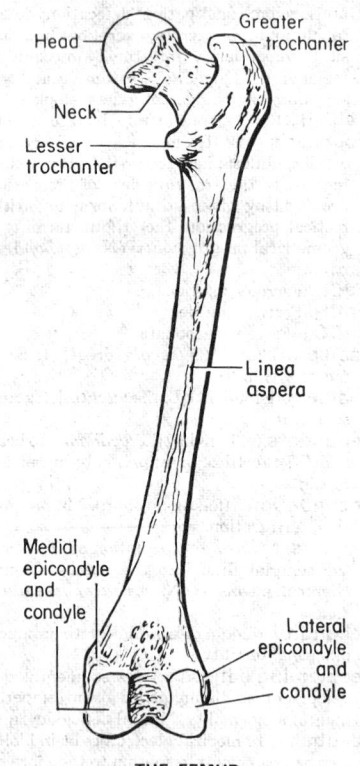

THE FEMUR

fenes'tra [L., window]. (pl. *fenestrae*) 1. An aperture frequently closed by a membrane. 2. An open area, as in the blade of a forceps.

f. cochleae. [NA] Leading into the cochlea. It is closed by a membrane, the secondary tympanic membrane. SYN: *f. rotunda.*

f. vestibuli. [NA] An oval opening on the inner wall of the middle ear or tympanum leading to the vestibule, into which the base of the stapes fits. SYN: *f. ovalis.*

fenestrated (fĕn'ĕs-trāt''ĕd) [L. *fenestra,* window]. Having openings.

f. membrane of Henle. Elastic tissue layer in intima of larger arteries.

fenestra'tion. 1. Condition of having a fenestra. 2. An operation in which an artificial opening is made into the labyrinth of the ear. Performed in cases of otosclerosis.

ferment (fĕr-mĕnt', fĕr'mĕnt) [L. *fermentum*]. 1. To decompose. 2. A substance capable of producing fermentation in other substances. 3. A catalytic agent which is capable of inducing fermentation in substances with which it comes in contact. SYN: *enzyme,* q.v.

RS: enzyme; hydrolyst; pancreatin; papain; steapsin; trypsin; trypsinogen; tyrosinase; yeast.

fermenta'tion. The oxidative decomposition of complex substances through the action of enzymes or ferments, produced by microorganisms. Bacteria, molds, and yeasts are the principal groups of organisms involved in fermentation. Fermentations of economic importance are those involved in the production of alcohol, alcoholic beverages, lactic and butyric acids, and the baking of bread.

f., acetic. The production of acetic acid by the bacterial oxidation of ethyl alcohol under aerobic conditions.

f., alcoholic. The production of ethyl alcohol from carbohydrates, usually through the action of yeasts.

f., amylolyt'ic. The process of hydrolyzation of starch with the formation of sugar.

f., autolyt'ic. Disintegration of tissues after death due to enzymes present in the tissues.

f., butyric. Formation of butyric acid from bacterial action on carbohydrates under anaerobic conditions.

f., citric acid. Formation of citric acid from action of molds on carbohydrates.

f., invertin. F. that converts cane sugar into dextrose and levulose.

f., lactic. F. which sours milk.

f., lactic acid. Formation of lactic acid from carbohydrates by action of lactic acid bacteria. The genera Streptococcus and Lactobacillus are the forms usually involved. Lactic acid is responsible for the souring of milk.

f., oxalic acid. Formation of oxalic acid from carbohydrates from the action of certain molds, esp. Aspergillus.

f., propionic acid. Formation of propionic acid from carbohydrates from action of certain bacteria.

f. test. A confirmation test for sugar in the urine. Gas forms in the f. tube if sugar is present.

f., viscous. Production of gelatinous material by different forms of bacilli.

fermen'toid [L. *fermentum,* decompose, + Gr. *eidos,* form]. A ferment without fermentive power.

fermentum (fĕr-mĕn'tŭm) [L]. Yeast; a ferment.

fermium (fĕr'mĭ-ŭm). [Enrico Fermi, winner of the Nobel Prize in physics in 1938] SYMB: *Fm.* At. no. 100. Radioactive element.

fern [AS. *fearn*]. A flowerless plant belonging to the class Filicinae of the division Tracheophyta. At one time a substance derived from male f. was used in treating certain kinds of intestinal parasites.

fern pattern. The palm leaf pattern which cervical mucus assumes under microscope during certain stages of the menstrual cycle. The pattern, caused by crystallization of the mucus as it dries, is dependent upon the concentration of electrolytes present, esp. sodium chloride.

Usually seen at midcycle in normal menstruating women; therefore it is used as a test in determining ovulation in women who have difficulty becoming pregnant. The mucus has a beaded pattern at other times in the cycle and during pregnancy.

-ferous [L.]. Suffix meaning producing.

ferrated (fĕr-āt'ĕd) [L. *ferrum,* iron]. Combined with iron or containing iron.

ferri-, ferro- [L. *ferrum,* iron]. Prefix used to indicate presence of iron.

fer'ric. 1. Pert. to or containing iron. 2. Denoting a compound containing iron in its trivalent form. SYN: *ferruginous.*

f. ammo'nium cit'rate. Thin, garnet-red crystals, containing about 17% of iron. Used in hypochromic anemia.

f. chlo'ride. (FeCl$_3$) Used principally in form of tincture as an astringent application to throat and as a hematinic.

ferricyanide. A salt of hydroferricyanic acid.

ferrihemoglobin. Methemoglobin, a reduced form of hemoglobin.

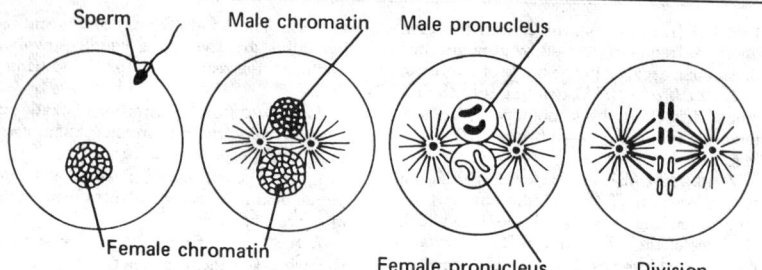

STAGES IN FERTILIZATION PROCESS

fer'rin. An iron-containing compound isolated from liver tissue.

ferritin (fĕr'ĭ-tĭn). An iron-phosphorus-protein complex containing about 23% iron. It is formed in the intestinal mucosa by the union of ferric iron with a protein, apoferritin. Ferritin is the form in which iron is stored in the tissues, principally in the reticuloendothelial cells of the liver, spleen, and bone marrow.

ferrom'eter [L. *ferrum,* iron, + Gr. *metron,* measure]. Device for estimating proportion of iron in the blood.

ferropectic (fĕr"ō-pĕk'tĭk) ["+ Gr. *pĕxis,* fixation]. Pert. to fixing iron.

ferropexia (fĕr-ō-pĕks'ĭ-ă). Iron fixation.

ferroprotein. A protein combined with an iron-containing radical. Ferroproteins are important oxygen-transferring enzymes (e.g., Warburg's enzyme, cytochrome, oxidase).

ferrous (fĕr'ŭs) [L. *ferrum,* iron]. 1. Pert. to iron. 2. Denoting a compound containing iron of a lower valence than three. SYN: *ferruginous.*

    f. fumarate. USP: ($C_4H_2FeO_4$) A form of iron used to treat anemias.

    f. gluconate. USP. Occurs as a yellowish powder or granules. Used as a hematinic.

    f. sulfate. USP. ($FeSO_4$) Iron sulfate. Pale, bluish-green crystals. Used internally, same as other preparations of iron. Incompatible with alkalies, chlorides, tannic acid, and oxidizing agents.

ferruginous (fĕr-ū'jĭ-nŭs) [L. *ferrugo,* iron rust]. 1. Pert. to or containing iron. 2. Of the color of iron rust.

ferrule (fĕr'ŭl) [L. *viriola,* little bracelet]. A band or ring of metal applied to the end of root or crown of a tooth to strengthen it.

fer'rum [L., iron]. SYMB: *Fe.* Iron.

fertile (fĕr'tĭl) [L. *fertilis*]. Capable of reproduction.

fertility (fĕr-tĭl'ĭ-tĭ). Quality of being productive or fertile.

fertiliza'tion [L. *fertilis,* reproductive]. 1. Fecundation; impregnation of an ovum with the spermatozoon of the male, the male sex cell being carried in the seminal discharge. This usually takes place in the fallopian tube. Spermatozoa have been found in the tube alive 48 hours after the last coitus. On meeting the ovum the head of the spermatozoon penetrates it and its tail drops off. Cell division begins and the fertilized ovum enters the uterus.

Development of Fetal Tissue

Ectoderm
Epidermis
Epithelium of:
External and internal ear,
Nasal cavity,
Mouth,
Anus,
Amnion, chorion,
Distal part of male urethra
Nervous tissue

Mesoderm
Connective tissues
Male and female reproductive tracts
Blood vessels, lymphatics
Kidneys, ureters, trigone of bladder
Pleura, peritoneum, pericardium
Muscles

Entoderm
Respiratory tract except nose
Digestive tract except mouth and anus
Bladder except trigone
Male urethra, proximal portion
Female urethra

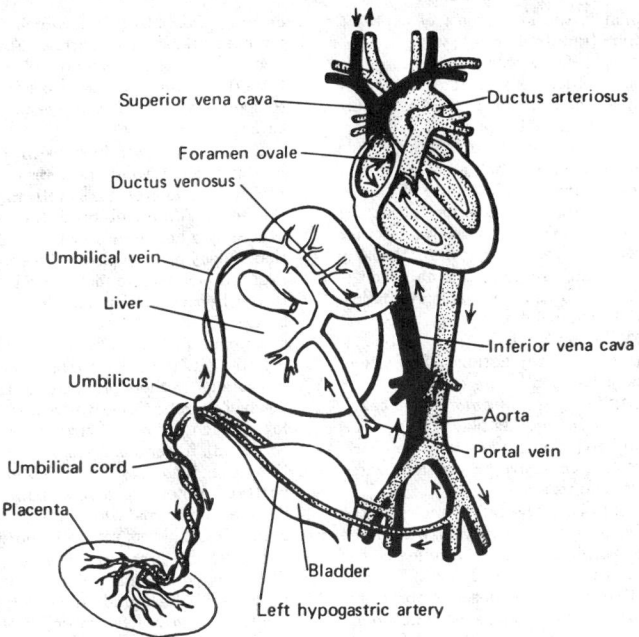

FETAL CIRCULATION
Vessels indicated in black carry venous blood; white, arterial blood; gray, mixture of both.

2. In botany, the union of the male and female gametes. In higher plants, when the pollen tube enters the ovule, two gametes emerge, one uniting with the egg to form the zygote, from which the embryo develops; the other uniting with two endosperm nuclei to form a primary endosperm cell from which the endosperm (reserve food) develops.

RS: coitus; conception; impregnation; ovum; spermatozoa; sterile; sterility.

fertilizin (fĕr″tĭ-lī′zin). A substance, possibly a glycoprotein, extracted from eggs which when added to a suspension of sperms causes agglutination of the sperms. It probably aids in fertilization by fixing sperm to the egg membrane. It is complementary to antifertilizin, a substance extracted from sperm which agglutinates eggs.

fervescence (fĕr-vĕs′ĕns) [L. *fervescere*, to grow hot]. Increase of fever.

fes′ter [L. *fistula*, ulcer]. To become inflamed and suppurate.

festina′tion [L. *festinatio*]. Abnormal and involuntary increase in speed of walking in an attempt to catch up with the displaced center of gravity. Seen in certain neurological diseases.

festoon (fĕs-tūn′) [L. *festus*, festal]. The wreathlike curvature of the gums around the necks of the teeth.

fe′tal [L. *fetus*, fetus]. Pert. to fetus.

f. circulation. The course of the flow of blood in a fetus. Significant differences between f. and postnatal circulation are the presence in the fetus of umbilical arteries and veins which carry blood to and from the placenta; foramen ovale, an opening in the interatrial septum; and ductus arteriosus, a vessel connecting the pulmonary artery with the aorta. The latter two enable the blood to by-pass the lungs which are nonfunctional in the fetus.

fetalism (fe′tal-izm) [" + Gr. *ismos*, condition]. Retention of fetal structures after birth.

feta′tion [L. *fetus*, fetus]. Pregnancy.

feticide (fe′tĭ-sĭd) [" + *cidus*, kill]. Intentional destruction of fetal life. SEE: *infanticide*.

fetid (fĕt′ĭd) [L. *fētidus*, stink]. Rank or foul in odor.

fetish, fetich (fĕ′tĭsh, fĕt′ĭsh) [Portug. *feitico*, charm, sorcery]. 1. An object, such as an idol or charm, which is thought to have mysterious, magical, and supernatural power. 2.

In psychiatry, the love object of a person who suffers from fetishism, q.v.

fe'tishism ["+ Gr. *ismos,* condition]. 1. Belief in some object as possessing power, or being capable of inspiring a stimulus. 2. Substitution for a normal love object (a person) of parts or possessions of such a one. Libido gratification from contact with articles of dress, braid of hair, etc. 3. A form of mental illness which finds a sex stimulus at the sight of a woman's shoe or glove, or other article of apparel, or of some part of the body such as the hair, esp. the pubic hair. To the masochist, q.v., all such symbols are indicative of the woman's domination.

fetometry (fē-tŏm'ĕ-trĭ) [L. *fetus,* fetus, + Gr. *metron,* measure]. Estimation of size of the fetus or its head before delivery.

fe'toplacen'tal ["+ *placenta,* a flat cake]. Pert. to the fetus and its placenta.

fetor (fē'tor) [L.]. Stench; an offensive odor.

   f., ex ore. Offensive breath, halitosis.

   f. oris. Halitosis.

fe'tus [L. *fetus*]. 1. The latter stages of the developing young of an animal within the uterus or within an egg. 2. In humans, the child in utero from the third month to birth. Prior to that time it is called an embryo, q.v.

   f. amorphus. A shapeless fetal anomaly, one scarcely recognizable as a fetus.

   f., calcified. A lithopedion, q.v.

   f. compressus. F. papyraceus, q.v.

   f. in fetu. Condition in which a small imperfect f., called parasite, is contained within the body of another f., the autosite.

   f., mummified. A dead f. that has assumed a mummified form upon failure of resorption to occur.

   f., paper doll. F. papyraceus, q.v.

   f. papyraceus. In twin pregnancy, the dead f. pressed flat by the development of the living twin.

fe'ver [L. *febris*]. 1. Pyrexia, or elevation of temperature above the normal. The normal temperature taken orally is 98.6° F. (37° C.). However, it may be within the range of normal if it is 1° above or 2° below this value. On the other hand, if a person whose normal temperature is 97.8° F. (36.5° C.) has become ill, 98.8° F. (37° C.) could represent fever in that individual. Thus it is not practical to attempt to designate a precise level of normal body temperature. Rectal temperature will be 0.5°-1.0° higher than oral temperature. 2. A disease which is characterized by an elevation of body temperature, such as typhoid fever, yellow fever.

CLASSIFICATION: *Intermittent:* A temperature curve which returns to normal during the day and reaches its peak in the evening. *Remittent:* A f. which fluctuates but does not return to normal. *Sustained:* A temperature which remains elevated with little fluctuation. *Relapsing:* Periods of f. interspersed with periods of normal temperature.

ETIOL: Moderate increase in body temperature in the young may result from minor causes and is of less significance than in the adult. After childhood, fevers may be caused by a hot environment or the generation of body heat by physical means such as exercise; neurogenic factors such as injury to the hypothalamus; dehydration such as occurs after excessive diuresis; chemical substances such as caffeine or cocaine when injected into the blood stream; the injection of proteins or their products, or the breakdown of necrotic tissue (these are the aseptic fevers such as follow surgery or coronary occlusion); infectious diseases or inflammation (fever is the result of the breakdown of bacterial proteins or toxins liberated by the disease organisms which affect the heat-regulating centers); severe hemorrhage.

PERIODS: *Invasion or onset of fever:* While temperature is rising and until maximum is reached, gradual, as in typhoid, or sudden, as in scarlet fever. *Fastigium or stadium:* When the fever is more or less stationary with variations often reaching the maximum observed in that illness. This highest point in the f. is known as the fastigium. *Defervescence:* During which the fever declines until normal. When sudden it is known as crisis, as in lobar pneumonia; when gradual, lysis, as in measles.

SYM: Face flushed; hot, dry skin; anorexia; headache; nausea and sometimes vomiting; constipation and sometimes diarrhea; aching all over; scant, highly-colored urine; tissue waste. Delirium possible if temperature is over 105° F. (40.5° C.) or in some cases with less fever. Convulsions may follow, esp. in children; coma. SEE: *febrile convulsions.*

   f., childbed. Puerperal sepsis. An infection of the genital tract following childbirth. SEE: *puerperal sepsis.*

   f., continuous. As in scarlet fever, typhus, or pneumonia, in which there is a slight diurnal variation.

   f., induced. That artificially produced to favorably modify the course of a disease, as in central nervous system syphilis. Sustained fever of 105° F. (40.5° C.), or even higher, maintained for 6 to 8 or 10 hours may be induced by the use of medical diathermy or injection of malarial parasites.

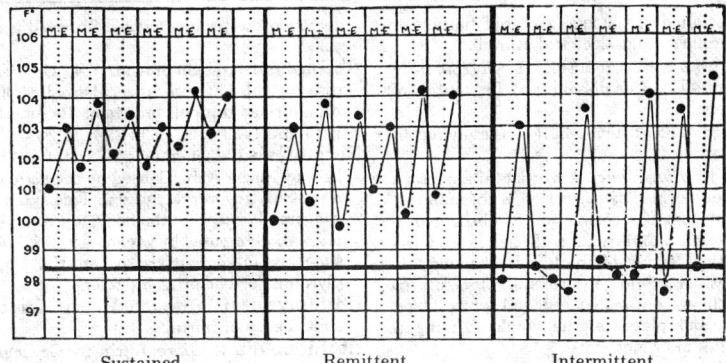

Sustained Remittent Intermittent

FEVER

f., relapsing. Any one of a group of acute infectious diseases caused by a variety of Borrelia. There are alternating periods of fever and normal temperature; the typical temperature curve being a characteristic of the disease. SEE: *relapsing fever.*

f., remittent. As in typhoid fever, septic fever, or remittent fever, with minimum temperature above normal, and with marked diurnal variation.

f., septic. F. due to septic matter in the body.

fever, words pert. to: ague; antifebrile; apyrexia; crisis; dengue; febrifacient; febrifuge; lysis; pulse; "pyr-" words; quartan; quintan; quotidian; respiration; temperature.

fiat (fī′ăt) [L.]. Let there be made, a term used in writing prescriptions.

fi′ber [L. *fibra*]. Threadlike or filmlike element, as a nerve f. A neuron or the axonal portion of a neuron.

RS: chondrofibroma; cilia; cimbia; cingulum; "fibr-" words; filament; filum.

f., accelerator. Fiber causing increased heart rate.

f., afferent. F. carrying incoming impulses to nerve cells.

f., efferent. F. carrying outgoing impulses.

f., inhibitory. F. causing slower heart action.

f., medullated; myelinated. Nerve f. in which axis cylinder is sheathed in myelin.

f., nerve. The part of a nerve cell which carries impulses. SEE: *nerve.*

f., nonmedullated; unmyelinated. Nerve f. in which there is no myelin sheath between axis cylinder and neurilemma.

f.'s, Purkinje. SEE: *Purkinje fibers.*

fiberoptic. A flexible material made of glass or plastic which transmits light along its course by reflecting it from the side or wall of the fiber. Use of this principle permits transmission of light and therefore visual images around corners. Devices utilizing fiberoptic materials are quite useful in endoscopic examinations.

fi′bra [L.]. [NA] (pl. *fibrae*) A fiber.

fibralbumin (fī-brăl-bū′mĭn) ["+ *albumen*, white of egg]. Globulin.

fibremia (fī-brē′mĭ-ă) ["+ Gr. *haima*, blood]. Fibrin formed in the blood, causing embolism or thrombosis. SYN: *inosemia.*

fi′bril [L. *fibrilla*, little fiber]. A small fiber. A very small filamentous structure, oftentimes the component of a cell or a fiber.

f., muscle. A myofibril; an extremely minute fibril found within the cytoplasm of smooth muscle cells and in the sarcoplasm of striated and cardiac muscle fibers.

f., nerve. A neurofibril; delicate fibrils found in the cell body and processes of a neuron.

fibril′la [L.]. (pl. *fibrillae*) A fibril or small fiber.

fibril′lar, fib′rillary. Pert. to, or consisting of, fibrils.

fib′rillated [L. *fibrilla*, little fiber]. Composed of minute fibers. SYN: *fibrillar; fibrous.*

fibrillation (fī″brĭl-ā′shŭn). 1. The formation of fibrils. 2. Quivering or spontaneous contraction of individual muscle fibers.

f., atrial. Extremely rapid, incomplete, contractions of the atria resulting in fine, rapid, irregular, and uncoordinated movements. SYN: *auricular f.*

f., ventricular. A condition similar to atrial f. resulting in rapid, tremulous, and ineffectual contractions of the ventricles. May result from mechanical injury to the heart, occlusion of coronary vessels, effects of certain drugs such as excess of digitalis or chloroform, and electrical stimuli.

fibrillolysis (fĭ″brĭl-ŏl′ĭ-sĭs) [L. *fibrilla*, little fiber, + Gr. *lysis*, dissolution]. Dissolution of fibrils.

fibrillolyt′ic (fĭ″brĭl-o-lĭt′ĭk). Dissolving fibrils.

fibrin [L. *fibra*, fiber]. A whitish, filamentous protein formed by the action of thrombin on fibrinogen. The conversion of fibrinogen, a hydrosol, into fibrin, a hydrogel, is the basis for the clotting of the blood. The fibrin is deposited as fine interlacing filaments in which are entangled red and white blood cells and platelets, the whole forming a coagulum or clot.

RS: blood clot; clotting; fibrinogen; prothrombin; thrombin.

    f. foam. A spongelike substance prepared from human f. When impregnated with thrombin it is used in surgery as a hemostatic agent. It is especially useful in neurosurgery and in injuries to parenchymatous organs. It is slowly absorbed.

fibrination (fĭ″brĭ-nā′shŭn). Abnormal amt. of fibrin in the blood.

fibrinemia (fĭ″brĭ-nē′mĭ-ă) [L. *fibra*, fibrin, + Gr. *haima*, blood]. Presence of fibrin in the blood. SYN: *fibremia.*

fibrinogen (fĭ-brĭn′ō-jĕn) [″+ Gr. *gennan*, to produce]. A protein present in the blood plasma which through the action of thrombin in the presence of calcium ions is converted into fibrin; this is essential for clotting of blood. SEE: *blood, clotting of; coagulation.*

fibrinogen′ic, fibrinog′enus. Producing fibrin.

fibrinogenopenia (fĭ-brĭn″ō-jĕn″ō-pē′nĭ-ă) [L. *fibra*, fibrin, + Gr. *gennan*, to produce, + *penia*, poverty]. Reduction in the amount of fibrinogen in the blood, usually the result of a liver disorder.

fi′brinoid (″+ Gr. *eidos*, form). Resembling fibrin.

    f. change. Alteration in connective tissues in response to immune reactions. The tissue becomes swollen, homogenous, and bandlike in appearance.

    f. material. A fibrinous substance which develops in the placenta, increasing in quantity as the placenta becomes older. Its origin is attributed to the degenerating decidua and trophoblast. It forms an incomplete layer in the chorion and decidua basalis and also occurs in the form of small irregular patches on the surface of the chorionic villi. In late pregnancy, the material may have a striated or canalized appearance

to which the term canalized fibrinoid is applied.

fibrinolysin (fĭ-brĭn-ŏl′ĭ-sĭn) [″+ Gr. *lysis*, dissolution]. The substance, also called plasmin, formed from plasminogen. Its function is to dissolve fibrin. SEE: *fibrinolysis.*

fibrinolysis (fĭ-brĭn-ŏl′ĭ-sĭs). Dissolution of fibrin by fibrinolysin. Caused by the action of a proteolytic enzyme system. This sytem is continually active in the body, but its action is greatly increased by various stress stimuli such as intense exercise, anoxia, hypoglycemia, or bacterial infections.

fibrinolytic (fĭ-brĭn-ō-lĭt′ĭk). Pert. to the splitting up of fibrin.

fibrinope′nia [L. *fibra*, fibrin, + Gr. *penia*, poverty]. Fibrin and fibrinogen deficiency in the blood.

fibrinoplas′tic [″+ Gr. *plassein*, to form]. Of the nature of fibrinoplastin.

fi″brinopu′rulent [″+ *purulentus*, festering]. Consisting of pus and fibrin.

fibrinos′copy [″+ Gr. *skopein*, to examine]. Physical and chemical examination of the fibrin of blood clots and exudates. SYN: *inoscopy.*

fibrino′sis (″+ Gr. *ōsis*, condition). Excess of fibrin in the blood.

fibrinous (fĭ′brĭn-ŭs) [L. *fibra*, fiber]. Pert. to, of the nature of, or containing fibrin.

fibrinuria (fĭ-brĭn-ū′rĭ-ă) [″+ Gr. *ouron*, urine]. Passage of fibrin in the urine.

fibro- [L. *fibra*]. Prefix indicates relationship to fibers or fibrous tissues.

fibroadenia (fĭ″brō-ă-dē′nĭ-ă) [″+ Gr. *adēn*, gland]. Fibrous degeneration of glandular tissue.

fibroadenoma (fĭ-brō-ăd-ĕ-nō′mă) [″+ ″+ *ōma*, tumor]. Adenoma with fibrous tissue forming a dense stroma.

fibroad′ipose [″+ *adeps, adip-*, fat]. Being fibrous and fatty.

fibroangio′ma [L. *fibra*, fiber, + Gr. *angeion*, vessel, + *ōma*, tumor]. A fibrous tissue angioma.

fibroareolar (fĭ″brō-ă-rē′ō-lăr) [″+ *areola*, little space]. With fibrous tissue and areolar arrangement.

fi′broblast [″+ Gr. *blastos*, germ]. Any cell or corpuscle from which connective tissue is developed. SYN: *desmocyte; fibrocyte.*

fibroblastoma (fĭ″brō-blăs-tō′mă) [″+ ″+ *ōma*, tumor]. Tumor of connective tissue or fibroplastic cells.

fibrobronchi′tis [L. *fibra*, fiber, + Gr. *bronchia*, air tubes, + *itis*, inflammation]. Croupous or fibrinous bronchitis.

fibrocarcino′ma [″+ Gr. *karkinos*, cancer, + *ōma*, tumor]. A carcinoma in which the trabeculae are resistant and thickened with granular degeneration of the cells.

f. cysticum. A f. with enclosed cysts.

fibrocar'tilage ["+ *cartilago,* gristle]. A type of cartilage in which the matrix contains thick bundles of white or collagenous fibers. Found in the intervertebral disks.

fibrocell'ular ["+ *cellula,* little cell]. Both fibrous and cellular. SYN: *fibroareolar.*

fibrochondritis (fī″brō-kŏn-drī′tĭs) [L. *fibra,* fiber, + Gr. *chondros,* cartilage, + *-itis,* inflammation]. Inflammation of fibrocartilage.

fibrochondro'ma ["+ "+ *ōma,* tumor]. Tumor of fibrous tissue and cartilage.

fi'brocyst ["+ Gr. *kystis,* cyst]. A fibrous tumor that has undergone cystic degeneration or one which has accumulated fluid in the interspaces.

fibrocystic (fī″brō-sĭs′tĭk). 1. Consisting of fibrocysts. 2. Fibrous with cystic degeneration.

f. disease of pancreas. SEE: *cystic fibrosis.*

fibrocysto'ma [L. *fibra,* fiber, + Gr. *kystis,* cyst, + *ōma,* tumor]. Fibroma combined with cystoma.

fibrocyte (fī′brō-sīt) ["+ *kytos,* cell]. A fibroblast.

fibroelas'tic ["+ Gr. *elastikos,* elastic]. Pert. to connective tissue containing both white, nonelastic, collagenous fibers and yellow elastic fibers.

fibroelastosis. Overgrowth of fibroelastic tissue.

f., endocardial. F. of the endocardium, leading to cardiac failure.

fibroenchondroma (fī″brō-ĕn″kŏn-drō′mă) [L. *fibra,* fiber, "+ Gr. *en,* in, + *chondros,* cartilage, + *ōma,* tumor]. An enchondroma containing fibrous elements.

fibroglioma (fī-brō-glī-ō′mă) ["+ Gr. *glia,* glue, + *ōma,* tumor]. A fibroma partly glioma.

fi'broid ["+ Gr. *eidos,* form]. 1. Containing or resembling fibers. SEE: *degeneration.* 2. A colloquial term for fibroma, esp. fibroma of the uterus. SYN: *fibroma,* q.v.

f., interstitial. Tumor in muscular wall of uterus which may grow inward and form a polypoid f., or outward and become a subperitoneal f.

f., uterine. F. in uterus. SEE: *fibroma, uterine.*

fibroidectomy (fī-broyd-ĕk′tō-mī) ["+ "+ *ektomē,* excision]. Surgical removal of a fibroid tumor.

fibrolipo'ma [L. *fibra,* fiber, + Gr. *lipos,* fat, + *ōma,* tumor]. A lipoma having much fibrous tissue.

fibro'ma ["+ Gr. *ōma,* tumor]. (pl. *fibromata*) A fibrous, encapsulated, connective tissue tumor.

A f. is irregular in shape, slow in growth, with a firm consistency. Painless except by pressure or cystic degeneration. May be found in the periosteum. May affect the jaws, the occiput, pelvis, vertebrae, ribs, long bones, and sternum.

f. of breast. A benign tumor non-ulcerative and painless.

f., intramural. Tumor located in muscle tissue of uterus between peritoneal coat and endometrium.

f. molluscum pedunculum of vulva. A pedunculated fibroid tumor of the vulva.

f., submucous. F. encroaching upon endometrial cavity; sessile or pedunculated.

f., subserous. F. lying beneath peritoneal coat of uterus, often pedunculated.

f., uterine. A fibroid tumor of the uterus. SEE: *fibrosis uteri.*

PATH: A benign tumor varying in size from a few millimeters in diameter to a size large enough to fill the entire abdominal cavity. May be single or multiple. These tumors are completely encapsulated by a fibrous connective tissue capsule in which the blood vessels that supply the tumor are found. They are subjected to numerous benign degenerations such as necrobiotic changes (red and gray degeneration), hyaline changes, telangiectatic and lymphangiectatic changes, calcareous degeneration, fatty degeneration, and infection. Occasionally, a fibroid will show sarcomatous degeneration.

SYM: Fibromata rarely cause symptoms before the age of 30. The occurrence is common after the age of 30, esp. in the Negro race. Although the cardinal symptoms of fibromata are supposed to be dysmenorrhea, menorrhagia, and leukorrhea, these symptoms are found only infrequently and the symptomatology is directly related to the location of the tumors in the uterus. Thus tumors that encroach upon the bladder region cause frequency and dysuria; those pressing on the rectum cause a rectal tenesmus; those that encroach upon the endometrium cause menorrhagia and dysmenorrhea, and very large subserous growths may be absolutely symptomless. SEE: *dysmenorrhea; dysuria; menorrhagia; tenesmus.*

TREATMENT: Fibromata producing no symptoms should be left in place and the patient kept under observation. If unusually rapid growth is evidenced, they should be removed.

Tumors that produce symptoms need intervention. The type of treatment depends upon age of patient, location and size of tumor, and symptoms present. In general, wherever possible, conservation of the menstrual function should be considered. Tumors larger than a fetal head are best treated by surgical removal. Fibromectomy is clearly indicated in patients who hope subsequently to become pregnant.

fibromatosis (fī″brō-mă-tō′sĭs) [L. *fibra*, fiber, + Gr. *ōma*, tumor, + *ōsis*, condition]. The simultaneous development of many fibromas. SYN: *fibrosis*.

fibromatous (fĭ-brō′mă-tŭs). Pert. to, or of the nature of, a fibroma.

fibromectomy (fī″brō-mĕk′tō-mī) [L. *fibra*, fiber, + Gr. *ōma*, tumor, + *ektomē*, excision]. Removal of a fibroid tumor.

fibromem′branous ["+ *membrana*, web]. Having both fibrous and membranous tissue.

fibromus′cular ["+ *musculus*, muscle]. Consisting of muscle and connective tissue.

fibromyitis (fī″brō-mī′ī-tĭs) [L. *fibra*, fiber, + Gr. *mys, my-*, muscle, + *-itis*, inflammation]. Inflammation of the muscular system followed by fibrous degeneration of muscular fibers and atrophy.

fibromyoma (fī″brō-mī-ō′mă) ["+ "+ *ōma*, tumor]. 1. Fibrous tissue myoma. 2. A fibroid tumor of the uterus that contains more fibrous than muscle tissue.

fibromyomectomy (fī″brō-mī″ō-mĕk′tō-mī) ["+ "+ *ektomē*, excision]. Removal of a fibromyoma from the uterus, leaving that organ in place.

fibromyositis (fī″brō-mī″ō-sī′tĭs) [L. *fibra*, fiber, + *mys, my-*, muscle, + *-itis*, inflammation]. Chronic muscular inflammation with hyperplasia of connective tissue. SYN: *inomyositis*.

fibromyotomy (fī″brō-mī-ŏt′ō-mī) ["+ "+ *tomē*, incision]. Opening of a fibroid tumor.

fibromyxoma (fī″brō-mĭks-ō′mă) ["+ Gr. *myxa*, mucus, + *-ōma*, tumor]. A fibroma that has undergone partial myxomatous degeneration.

fibromyxosarco′ma ["+ "+ *sarkos*, flesh, + *ōma*, tumor]. 1. A sarcoma containing fibrous and myxoid tissue. 2. A sarcoma which has undergone mucoid degeneration.

fibroneuroma (fī″brō-nū-rō′mă) [L. *fibra*, fiber, + Gr. *neuron*, nerve, + *ōma*, tumor]. A mixed neuroma and fibroma. SYN: *inoneuroma*.

fibro-osteoma (fī″brō-ŏs-tē-ō′mă) ["+ Gr. *osteon*, bone, + *ōma*, tumor]. Tumor containing bony and fibrous elements.

fibropapilloma (fī″brō-păp-ĭ-lō′mă) ["+ *papilla*, nipple, + Gr. *ōma*, tumor]. A mixed fibroma and papilloma sometimes occurring in the bladder.

fibropericardi′tis ["+ Gr. *peri*, around, + *kardia*, heart, + *-itis*, inflammation]. Fibrinous pericarditis.

fibropla′sia [L. *fibra*, fiber, + Gr. *plasis*, a molding]. The development of fibrous tissue, as in wounds.

   f., retrolental. Fibrous overgrowth of the vascular tissue of the eye. Occurs in some premature infants who have been exposed to excess oxygen concentration while in an incubator.

fibroplas′tic ["+ Gr. *plassein*, to form]. Giving formation to fibrous tissue.

   f. tumor. small spindle-celled sarcoma.

fibroplastin (fĭ-brō-plăs′tĭn). A globulin in blood serum and other body fluids. SYN: *fibrinoplastin; paraglobulin.*

fibropsammoma (fĭ-brō-sŏ-mō′mă) [L. *fibra*, fiber, + Gr. *psammos*, sand, + *ōma*, tumor]. A tumor containing fibromatous and psammomatous tissue.

fibropu′rulent ["+ *purulentus*, festering]. Pus containing flakes of fibrous tissue.

fibrosarco′ma ["+ Gr. *sarkos*, flesh, + *ōma*, tumor]. A spindle-celled sarcoma containing much connective tissue.

fibrosis (fĭ-brō′sĭs) ["+ Gr. *ōsis*, condition]. Abnormal formation of fibrous tissue.

   f., arteriocapillary. Arteriolar and capillary fibroid degeneration.

   f. of lungs. Formation of scar tissue in connective tissue framework of lungs following inflammation or pneumonia and in pulmonary tuberculosis.

   f. uteri. A condition of the uterus manifested by excess of fibrous tissue, predominating symptom being menorrhagia, q.v.

   The uterus may be large or small. The endometrium, q.v. may be normal, atrophic, or in the larger number show hyperplastic and hypertrophic glandular and interstitial endometritis of vascular origin.

   ETIOL: Not definitely known, but it is seen in patients with syphilis, those who have had a number of pregnancies, and in conditions where venous stasis has been present over a long period, such as in chronic retroversion with or without infection and procidentia.

fibrositis (fĭ-brō-sī′tĭs) ["+ Gr. *itis*, inflammation]. Nonsuppurative inflammation of white fibrous connective tissue anywhere in the body. SYN: *muscular rheumatism.*

   f., bursal. F. of a bursa; bursitis.

f., intramuscular. F. of fibrous sheaths of muscles; muscular rheumatism; interstitial myositis.

f., periarticular. F. of the fibrous tissue of the articular capsule.

f., perineural. F. of the fibrous sheath surrounding nerves, esp. the sciatic nerve; sciatica.

f., subcutaneous. F. of the subcutaneous tissue; panniculitis.

fibrot'ic. Marked by or pert. to fibrosis.

fibrous (fī-brŭs) [L. *fibra,* fiber]. Composed of or containing fibers. Opposed to osseous (bony) composition.

fib'ula. [NA] Calf bone, peroneal bone. One of the longest and thinnest bones of the body. The outer and smaller bone of the leg from the ankle to the knee, articulating above with the tibia, and below with the tibia, and talus (astragalus). SEE: *peroneal; peroneus; tibia.*

fib'ular. Rel. to the fibula.

fibulocalcaneal (fīb″ū-lō-kăl-kā′nĭ-ăl) [L. *fibula,* pin, + *calcaneus,* pert. to the heel]. Pert. to the fibula and calcaneus, or os calcis.

field [AS. *feld*]. A specific area in relationship to an object.

f., au'ditory. The space or distance within the limit of hearing.

f. of vision. That portion of space which the fixed eye can see.

fifth cranial nerve. Trigeminal or trifacial n.

fifth ventricle. Space separating layers of septum lucidum.

fig [L. *ficus*]. A sweet, pear-shaped fruit of Ficus carica.

Food value of 100 gm. (raw): Cal. 80; protein 1.2 gm.; trace of fat; carbohydrate 20 gm.; calcium 35 mg.; potassium 194 mg.; vitamin A, 80 I.U.

100 gm. (dried): Cal. 274; protein 4.3 gm.; fat 1.3 gm.; carbohydrate 69 gm.; calcium 126 mg.; potassium 640 mg.; vitamin A, 80 I.U.

fig'ure [L. *figūra*]. A body; form, shape, or outline.

f., achromatic. In mitosis or meiosis, the spindle fibers and the asters.

f., chromatic. The chromosomes or the chromatin material.

fila (fī′lă) [L. *filum,* thread]. Pl. of filum, q.v.

filaceous (fī-lā′shŭs). Composed of filaments. SYN: *filamentous.*

fil'ament [L. *filamentum*]. A fine thread.

f., axial. A fine f. forming the central axis of the tail of a spermatozoon.

filamen'tous. In biology, made up of long, interwoven or irregularly placed filaments.

Filaria (fĭl-ā′rĭ-ă) [L. *filum,* thread]. Term formerly applied to a genus of nematodes belonging to the superfamily Filarioidea.

F. bancrofti. Wuchereria bancrofti, q.v.

F. loa. Loa loa, q.v.

F. medinensis. Dracunculus medinensis, q.v.

F. sanguinis hominis. Wuchereria bancrofti, q.v.

filaria (fĭl-ā′rĭ-ă) [L. *filum,* thread]. A long filiform nematode belonging to the superfamily Filarioidea. The adults live in vertebrates including man. In man they may be found in the lymphatic vessels and lymphatic organs, circulatory system, connective tissues, esp., subcutaneous tissues, and serous cavities. Typically, the female produces larvae called microfilariae which may be sheathed or sheathless. These reach the peripheral blood or lymphatic vessels where they may be ingested by a blood sucking arthropod (mosquitos, gnats, flies). In the intermediate host, they transform into rhabditoid larvae, which metamorphose into infective filariform larvae. These migrate to the proboscis and are deposited in or on the skin of the vertebrate host.

fila'rial. Pert. to or caused by filariae.

filariasis (fĭl-ă-rī′ă-sĭs) [L. *filum,* thread, + Gr. *-iasis,* condition]. A chronic disease due to one of the filariae.

filarici'dal ["+ *caedere,* to kill]. Pert. to that which is destructive to Filaria.

filial generation. In genetics, the first offspring of a specific mating or cross mating. This is abbreviated F$_1$. Descendants resulting from F$_1$ matings are known as the F$_2$ or second filial generation.

fil'iform ["+ *forma,* form]. In biology, pert. to a growth that is uniform along the inoculation line in stab or streak cultures. 2. Hairlike, filamentous.

f. papillae. Smallest tongue papillae.

fil'ipuncture ["+ *punctura,* a piercing]. Insertion of a slender wire or thread in an aneurysm to induce coagulation.

fil'let [Fr. *filet,* a band]. 1. A loop of thread, cord, or tape used for providing traction or suspension of tissue during surgery. 2. Two bundles of sensory fibers in the medulla, pons, and brain. SYN: *lemniscus.*

f. of corpus callosum. Fibers forming white substance of the gyrus fornicatus.

f., olivary. Nerve fasciculus surrounding olivary body.

filling (fĭl′ĭng) [AS. *fyllan,* to fill]. 1. The material for insertion in a tooth cavity; usually gold, amalgam, or cement. 2. The operation of filling tooth cavities.

film. 1. A thin skin, membrane, or covering. 2. A thin sheet of material, usually cellulose, coated with a light-sensitive emulsion used in taking photographs. 3. In microscopy, a thin layer of blood or other material spread on a slide or cover slip.

filopressure (fī'lō-prĕ"shūr) [L. *filum*, thread, + *pressura*, pressure]. Pressure on a blood vessel caused by a ligature.

filovaricosis (fī"lō-văr-ĭ-kō'sĭs) ["+ *varix*, a dilated vein, + Gr. *ōsis*, condition]. Dilatation or thickening of the axis cylinder of a nerve fiber.

filter [L. *filtrare*, to strain through]. 1. To pass a liquid through any porous substance that prevents particles larger than a certain size to pass through. 2. Device for filtering liquids, light rays, or radiations. SEE: *absorption; osmosis*.

f. bed. Large-scale filter to purify the water supply.

f., Berkefeld. F. of diatomaceous earth which will not allow bacteria to pass through.

f., infrared. Cell of water and red glass which confines radiation to spectral region from 600 to 1400 mu, red glass alone from 600 to 4000 mu.

f., Kitasato's. Suction variety of f. using porcelain dilator.

f. paper. Coarse form of paper used in filtering solutions.

f., Pasteur-Chamberland. Filters of unglazed porcelain capable of retaining bacteria and some viruses; either pressure or suction is required to force or draw the liquid through the f.

f., Wood's. A glass ·creen allowing passage of ultraviolet rays and absorbing rays of visual light. Used in diagnosing certain dermatological conditions, esp. tinea capitis.

filterable [L. *filtrare*, to strain through]. Capable of passing through the pores of a porcelain filter, through which bacteria cannot pass.

fil'trate. The fluid which has been passed through a filter. The residue is the precipitate.

f., glomerular. The fluid which passes from the blood through the capillary walls of the glomeruli of the kidney. It is a protein-free plasma from which urine is formed.

filtra'tion. Removal of particles from a solution by allowing the liquid portion to pass through a membrane or other partial barrier. This barrier contains holes or spaces through which the liquid may pass but which are too small to permit the solid particles to pass. SEE: *filter*.

f. of roentgen rays. The absorption of some of the relatively longer wave lengths of roentgen radiation by placing in the path of the rays some absorbing medium, such as aluminum, copper, or zinc.

filtratometer (fĭl"tră-tŏm'ē-ter) [L. *filtrare*, to strain through, + Gr. *metron*, measure]. Device for measuring gastric filtrates.

fil'trum [L.]. A filter.

filum (fī'lŭm) [L.]. (pl. *fī'la*) [NA] A threadlike structure.

f. coronaria. A fibrous band extending from the base of the medial cusp of the tricuspid valve to the aortic annulus.

f. olfactoria. Groups of fibers consisting of the axons of olfactory cells which form the olfactory nerves. These pass from the olfactory epithelium through the cribriform plate and terminate in the olfactory bulb.

f. terminale. A long slender filament forming one end of spinal cord.

fimbria (fĭm'brĭ-ă) [L., fringe]. (pl. *fimbriae*) Any structure resembling fringe.

f. ova'rica. The longest fringelike extremity of the fallopian tubes; extending from the infundibulum close to the ovary.

f. tubae. Fringelike portion at abdominal end of the fallopian tubes.

fimbriate (fĭm'brĭ-āt"). 1. Having fingerlike projections. 2. Fringed.

f. body. Corpus fimbriatum.

fim'briated [L. *fimbria*, fringe]. Fringed.

fimbriocele (fĭm'brĭ-ō-sēl") ["+ Gr. *kēlē*, hernia]. Hernia including the fimbriated portion of the oviduct.

fin'ger [AS]. One of the five digits of the hand.

f., baseball. SEE: *baseball f.*

f., dislocation of the. First, be certain that there is no fracture. Dislocations occur only at a joint. If there has been a crushing injury, assume that a fracture is present until an x-ray picture has been made. Dislocations of a finger usually are easily diagnosed and quite easily reduced. They may be caused by blows, falls, and similar accidents.

If there is no fracture, the dislocation may be treated by asking the patient to steady and support his own wrist (or getting somebody else to do so) for countertraction. Then take hold of the finger beyond the dislocated muscles and tendons, and with the free hand slip the dislocated bone into place.

This is to be followed by an application of a splint from the tip of the finger well into the palm of the hand. This may be made of plastic, tongue depressors, heavy cardboard, etc.

NOTE: Do not under any circumstances attempt to reduce a dislocation of the thumb joint nearest to the palm of the hand until x-ray examination has ruled out the possibility of fracture.

f. stall. A finger cot.

finger, words pert. to: acroataxia; acrodynia; arachnodactyly; camptodactylia; dactyl; dactylus; digit; nail; phalanx.

fingerprint. An imprint made by the cutaneous ridges of the fleshy portion of the distal end of a finger. Fingerprints are used for purposes of identification.

fire [AS. *fyr*]. Flame producing heat.

f. emergencies. If a person's clothing catches fire, he should be rolled in a rug or blanket to smother flames. Running only fans the flames. It may be necessary to trip a burning person in order to prevent his running about. If an individual is outdoors, rolling in the dirt will smother flames.

If patient is trapped in a burning building, this particular room should have doors closed to prevent cross breezes from increasing the fire. The window should be opened if patient is to be rescued by lowering him. Do not open any door more than a few inches to ascertain possibility of escape. A burst of flame or hot air may push door in and asphyxiate anyone in the room. Wet cloths or towels should be held over mouth and nostrils to keep out smoke and gases. SEE: *burn; flames; gases; transportation.*

f., St. Anthony's. Erysipelas. SYN: *St. Francis' fire.*

first aid. The administration of emergency assistance to individuals who have been injured or otherwise disabled, prior to the arrival of a doctor or transportation to a hospital or doctor's office. F.a. should never be the substitution for definitive medical care. SEE: *Medical Emergencies* in *Appendix.*

RS: antidote; apoplexy; artifical respiration; asphyxia; bites; burn; coma; dislocation; drowning; emetic; fainting; flames; food poisoning; foreign bodies; fracture; freezing; frostbite; fumes; gases; insect bites; laceration; poison; shock; snake bite; triage; unconsciousness.

first cranial nerve. Olfactory nerves, q.v.

fish poisoning. A form of food poisoning caused by eating poisonous fish. Some fish are inherently poisonous; others become poisonous through decomposition, infection, by feeding on other poisonous forms, or by poisonous metabolic substances produced during the spawning season.

SYM: When poisoning is due to a toxin, the principal signs are vomiting and muscular paralysis. These occur within thirty minutes to four hours after eating the fish.

Convulsions may occur along with diarrhea, abdominal cramps, and shock.

TREATMENT: Removal of toxic fish from stomach by gastric lavage, emetics, and then cathartics. Treat convulsions with appropriate sedative, and treat shock with fluid replacement, whole blood, and plasma expanders.

fishskin disease. A disease of the skin characterized by increase of the horny layer and deficiency of the skin secretions. SYN: *ichthyosis,* q.v.

fission (fĭsh'ŭn) [L. *fissiō*]. 1. Splitting into two or more parts. 2. A method of asexual reproduction seen in bacteria, protozoa, and other lower forms of life in which the cell or the body divides into two or more parts, each of which develops into a complete individual. 3. Splitting of the nucleus of an atom into smaller nuclei, SYN: *nuclear fission.*

fissip'arous [L. *fissus,* cleft, + *parere,* to bring forth]. Reproducing by fission.

fissura (fĭs-ū'rǎ) [L.]. (pl. *fissurae*) [NA] Fissure. SYN: *cleft; sulcus.*

fis'sural. Pert. to a fissure.

fissure (fĭsh'ur) [L. *fissura*]. 1. A groove or natural division, cleft or slit, deep furrow in the brain, liver, spinal cord, and other organs. 2. Ulcer or cracklike sore. 3. A break in the enamel of a tooth.

f., anal. A linear ulcer on the margin of the anus.

f., auricular. F. of petrous portion of the temporal bone.

f. of Bichat. A f. below the corpus callosum in the cerebellum.

f., Broca's. F. encircling the third left frontal convolution of the brain.

f., Burdach's. F. connecting lateral surface of insula and inner surface of operculum of the brain.

f., calcarine. F. extending from the cerebrum's occipital end to the occipital f.

f., callosomarginal. A conspicuous sulcus in mesial surface of cerebral hemisphere running above and concentric with the curved upper surface of the corpus callosum.

f., central. F., Rolando's, q.v.

f., Clevenger's. Inferior temporal sulcus.

f., collateral. F. on the inferior surface of cerebral hemisphere separating subcalcarine and subcollateral gyri.

f.'s, Henle's. Connective tissue areas between the muscular fibers of heart.

f., hippocampal. F. of brain extending from posterior part of corpus callosum to the tip of temporal lobe.

f., inferior orbital. A f. at the apex of the orbit through which pass the infraorbital blood vessels and maxillary branch of the trigeminal nerve; the sphenomaxillary f.

f., interparietal. Intraparietal sulcus.

f., longitudinal. A f. on the lower surface of the liver.

f., occipitoparietal. The f. between the occipital and parietal lobes of the brain.

f., palpebral. Opening separating the upper and lower eyelids.

f., portal. The opening into the liver on its under surface; continues into the liver as the portal canal.

f., Rolando's. F. separating frontal and parietal lobes.

f., sphenoidal. F. separating the wings and body of the sphenoid.

f. of Sylvius. The lateral cerebral f. A f. separating the frontal and parietal lobes from the temporal lobe of the brain.

f., transverse. 1. The f. between the cerebellum and cerebrum of the brain. 2. A f. on lower surface of the liver which serves as the hilum transmitting vessels and ducts to the liver.

f., umbilical. Anterior portion of liver's longitudinal fissure which contains the round ligament, the obliterated umbilical vein.

f., Wernicke's. F. dividing the temporal and parietal lobes from the occipital lobe.

fistula (fĭs'tū-lă) [L., pipe]. An abnormal tubelike passage from a normal cavity or tube to a free surface or to another cavity. May be congenital due to incomplete closure of parts or may result from abscesses, injuries, or inflammatory processes.

f., anal. F. near the anus.

f., biliary. F. through which bile is discharged after a biliary operation.

f., blind. F. open at only one end.

f., branchial. An open branchial cleft.

f., cervical. 1. An abnormal opening into the cervix uteri. 2. An opening in the neck leading to the pharynx, resulting from incomplete closure of the brachial clefts.

f., complete. F. with both external and internal opening.

f., enterovaginal. F. between the bowel and vagina.

f., fecal. F. in which there is a discharge of feces through the opening.

f., metroperitoneal. F. between uterine and peritoneal cavities.

f., parotid. F. from the parotid gland to the skin surface.

f., perineovaginal. Opening from vagina through the perineum.

f., rectovaginal. Opening between rectum and vagina.

f., ureterovaginal. Opening between ureter and vagina.

f., vesicouterine. Opening between uterus and bladder.

f., vesicovaginal. Opening from bladder into the vagina.

fistulatome (fĭs'tū-lă-tōm) [L. *fistula*, pipe, + Gr. *tomē*, incision]. Instrument for incising a fistula.

fistulectomy (fĭs-tū-lĕk'tō-mĭ) ["+ Gr. *ektomē*, excision]. Excision of a fistula.

fistulization (fĭs"tū-lĭ-zā'shŭn) [L. *fistula*, pipe]. Becoming fistulous.

fistuloenterostomy (fĭs"tū-lō-ĕn-tĕr-ŏs'tō-mĭ) ["+ Gr. *enteron*, intestine, + *stoma*, opening]. Operative closure of a biliary fistula and formation of new passage of bile into the intestine.

fistulous (fĭs'tū-lŭs). Pert. to, or containing, a fistula.

fit (fĭt) [AS. *fitt*]. A sudden attack, convulsion, or paroxysm. SEE: *convulsion.*

F.A. TREATMENT: Do not try to stop attack. Prevent patient from hurting or injuring self. Place a pad between teeth to prevent biting tongue or cheeks. Allow patient to sleep. *CAUTION:* When placing object between teeth do not pry the mouth open in such manner as to break the teeth, and be careful not to have your finger bitten.

fixa'tion [L. *fixatio*]. 1. The act of holding or fastening in a f. position. The condition of being fixed. Immobilizing, making rigid. 2. A phase of psychosexual development in which the libido is arrested at an inferior or presexual level. Ex: father or mother f.

f., complement. The action of a complement, a constituent of fresh blood serum, on an antigen which in turn has been acted on by its antibody. During the uniting of antigen, antibody, and complement, the complement is rendered inactive or destroyed, and this process is known as f. of complement. The basis of the Wassermann and Kolmer tests for syphilis and other tests for infectious diseases.

f. of eyes. The movement of the eyes for the most acute vision in which they are directed toward an object so that the visual axes meet and the image of the object falls on corresponding points of each retina. SYN: *binocular f.*

f., father. Unrestrained attachment to the male parent.

f., field of. The widest limits of vision in all directions within which the eyes can fixate.

f. forceps. Forceps for holding a part.

f., mother. Abnormal attachment to the female parent.

f. point. The fovea or the point on the retina where the visual axes (lines) meet the point of clearest vision.

fix′ative [L. *fixus,* fastened]. 1. A substance that serves to make firm or fixed. 2. A substance used to harden and preserve pathological specimens.

fix′ing. Rapid killing of tissue elements so that their normal living form is preserved.

Fl. 1. Abbr. for *fluid.* 2. Chem. symb. for fluorine.

flabel′lum [L., fan]. White fibers in form of a fan-shaped bundle in corpus striatum.

flaccid (flăk′sĭd) [L. *flaccidus,* flabby]. Relaxed, flabby, having defective or absent muscular tone.

flagella (flă-jĕl′ă) [L.]. Pl. of flagellum, q.v.

flagellant (flăj′ē-lănt) [L. *flagellum,* whip]. 1. Pert. to flagella. 2. Pert. to stroking in massage. 3. One who practices flagellation.

flagellate (flăj′ē-lāt). 1. With one or more flagella. 2. A protozoon with one or more flagella.

    f. cell. Cell with long cilia for propulsion.

flagella′tion. 1. Whipping. 2. Massage by strokes. 3. Applying electricity by tapping the body. 4. A form of sexual aberration in which the libido is stimulated by whipping oneself, being whipped, or whipping someone else.

flagellum (flă-jĕl′ŭm) [L., whip]. (pl. *flagella*) A hairlike, motile process on the extremity of a bacterium or protozoon.

flail joint. A joint with excessive mobility usually due to paralysis of the muscles which control it.

flames, inhalation of. SYM: Intense irritation of nose, throat, pharynx, windpipe and lungs with choking, coughing, interference with respiration; intense swelling of throat; breathing is markedly limited. Shock.

    TREATMENT: Administration of oxygen; occasionally tracheotomy necessary. Pain relieved by spraying nose and throat with a local anesthetic of low toxicity. Follow with oil sprays. Steam inhalations are very soothing and may have to be kept up for long periods of time. SEE: *burn; fire; gases.*

flank [O.Fr. *flanc*]. The part of the body between ribs and upper border of ilium. Also loosely used to refer to the outer side of the thigh, hip, and buttock. SEE: *latus.*

flap [Dutch *flappen,* to strike]. A mass of partly detached tissue attached at the base after resection.

    f., amputation. A f. covering the end of a part left after an amputation.

f., extraction. Removal of cataract so as to make a flap in the cornea.

flare. A flush or spreading area of redness which surrounds a line made by drawing a pointed instrument across the skin. It is the second reaction in the triple response, q.v., and due to dilatation of the arterioles.

flashbacks. The return of imagery and hallucinations after the immediate effects of hallucinogens have worn off. These may occur for an extended period. Usually they are of a frightening or threatening form, but may consist only of perceptual distortion.

flash method. Means of pasteurizing milk by rapidly raising temperature of milk to 178° F. (80.1° C.), maintaining it there for a few minutes, and rapidly chilling it until the temperature is 40° F. (4.4° C.).

flash point. The temperature at which a substance will burst into flame.

flask [LL. *flasco*]. A small bottle with a narrow neck.

flatfoot. Abnormal flatness of sole and arch of foot. This condition may exist without causing symptoms or interfering with normal function of the foot.

    The inner longitudinal and anterior transverse metatarsal arches are those that may be depressed. It may be acute, subacute, or chronic. SYN: *pes planus; splayfoot.*

    f., spasmodic. The foot is held everted by spasmodic contraction of the peroneal muscle.

flat′ness. Resonance heard on percussing over solid organs, or when there is fluid in the thoracic cavity.

flatulence (flăt′ū-lĕns) [NL. *flatulentus*]. Excessive gas in the stomach and intestines.

    NP: *Stomach:* Seat patient upright, administer carbonated beverage. Silicone antifoam compounds may help by decreasing foam in stomach.

    Intestines: Have patient lie down for one-half hour before and after meals. No fluids with meals but hot water may be sipped afterwards. Give carminatives, carminative enema if needed, or institute intestinal suction by applying mild suction to a tube leading into the intestines.

    Rectum: Pass rectal tube.

    SEE: *distention; gastrointestinal decompression; Wangensteen's method.*

flatulent (flăt′ū-lĕnt). Affected with or caused by gas in the alimentary tract.

fla′tus [L., a blowing]. 1. Gas in digestive tract. 2. Expiration of air; eructation. SEE: *borborygmus.*

    f. tube. A rectal tube to procure expulsion of flatus in distention and before a saline enema.

NP: Patient on back or side. Lubricate tube and insert gently. It may be passed 6-8 inches (15.2-20.3 cm.). It may be left in position for 20-30 minutes.

f. vaginalis. Expulsion of air from vagina.

flatworm. A worm belonging to the phylum Platyhelminthes, q.v.

flavedo (flă-vē'dō) [L.]. Yellowness, as of the skin; sallowness; jaundice.

flavescent (flă-věs'ĕnt). Yellowish.

flavin (flā'vĭn). One of a group of natural water-soluble pigments occurring in milk, yeasts, bacteria, and some plants. All contain the flavin or isoalloxazine nucleus and are yellow in color. Present in riboflavin and in Warburg's yellow enzyme.

fla'vism [L. *flāvus*, yellow, + Gr. *ismos*, condition]. Having a yellow tinge to the hair.

flavo- [L. *flāvus*, yellow]. Prefix indicating yellow.

Flavo"bacter'ium. A genus of rod-shaped bacteria belonging to the Achromobacteriaceae. They are found in soil and water and produce an orange-yellow pigment in cultures.

fla"vopro'tein. One of a group of conjugated proteins which constitute the yellow enzymes essential in cellular respiration.

flax'seed. Seed of Linum usitatis simum. SYN: *linseed.*

fl. dr. Abbr. of *fluidram.*

flea (flē) [AS. *flēa*]. Any insect of the order Siphonaptera. Fleas are wingless, suck blood, and have legs adapted for jumping. Usually they are parasitic on warm-blooded animals including man.

Fleas of the genus Xenopsylla transmit the bacillus of plague (Pasteurella pestis) from rats to humans. Fleas may transmit other diseases such as tularemia, endemic typhus, and brucellosis, and they serve as intermediate hosts for the cat and dog tapeworms.

f. bites. Hemorrhagic puncta, q.v., surrounded by erythematous and urticarial patches as the result of the injection of flea saliva.

PREVENTION: Treat the skin with an insect repellent available in form of a powder, spray or oil for topical use.

f., cat. Ctenophalides felis.

f., chigger. Tungra penetrans. SYN: *chigger; jigger; sand flea.*

f., dog. Ctenophalides canis.

f., human. Pulex irritans.

f., rat. Xenopsylla cheopis.

fleam (flēm) [Fr. *flieme*]. Lancet used in venesection.

Flechsig's areas (flěk'zĭg). [Paul E. Flechsig, Leipzig neurologist, 1847-1929] Anterior, lateral, and posterior areas of each lateral half of the medulla.

fleece of Stilling. Meshwork of white fibers that surrounds the dentate nucleus of the cerebellum.

flesh [AS. *flaesc*]. The soft tissues of the animal body, esp. the muscles. SEE: *carnivorous; carnophobia; meat.*

f., examination of animal. Examine for color, consistency, proportion of fat, odor, and taste. In general, it should be neither very pale nor dark purple; marbled; of firm and elastic consistency; hardly moistening the finger; free from odor.

NOTE: *Yellow:* May be produced by food eaten by animal. In disease, due to animals having been jaundiced. *Brown:* Rare except in old meat undergoing decomposition. *Dark Purple:* May indicate animal died a natural death or suffered from acute fever, tuberculosis, or rinderpest. Avoid. *Dark Reddish-Brown:* May indicate animal was hunted or overdriven, poisoned, drowned, or suffocated. Avoid. *Scarlet:* Rare. Indicates arsenic or carbon monoxide poisoning. *Diffused redness:* Indicates that animal may have been poisoned or the meat frozen. *Green or Violet:* Indicates the beginning of putrefaction. Dangerous. *Saffron:* Indicates artificial coloring of smoked pork. *Brilliant Red:* Due to poisonous bacteria. *Gray:* Usually in sausages. Due to bacteria. *Phosphorescent:* Not due to putrefaction. Usually found in fish and shellfish. Increased by heat. Sometimes in meat, esp. veal, caused by bacteria, and generally transmitted from fish kept in the same place with meat. *White:* Rare except in calves. Found in certain diseases. Avoid.

f., goose. Cutis anserina, q.v.

f., proud. 1. Fungus growth. 2. Excessive granular tissue in a wound or ulcer.

fletch'erism. [Horace Fletcher, Amer. dietitian, 1849-1919] Taking small amounts of food at a time without excessive mastication.

flex [L. *flexus*, bent]. To bend upon itself, as a muscle; flexion, bending.

flexibilitas cerea (flěks-ĭ-bĭl'ĭ-tăs sē'rē-ă) [L.]. A cataleptic state in which limbs retain any position in which they are placed. Characteristic of catatonic patients.

flexibil'ity [L. *flexus*, bent]. Quality of being bent without breaking; adaptability. SYN: *pliability.*

flex'ible. Capable of being bent without breaking.

flexile (flěks'ĭl) [L. *flexus*, bent]. Pliant, flexible.

flexion (flĕk'shŭn) [L. *flexio*]. The act of bending, or condition of being bent, in contrast to extending. SEE: *antecurvature; clawfoot; clawhand.*

flexor (flĕks'or) [L]. A muscle that bends a part, in a generally proximal direction. Opposed to extensor.

flexure (flĕk'shĕr) [L. *flexura,* a bending]. A bend. SYN: *flexura* [NA].

   f., duodenojejunal. Curve at meeting point of jejunum and duodenum.

   f., hepatic. The bend on right side forming junction of the ascending with the transverse colon.

   f., sigmoid. The s-like loop (in left iliac fossa) of the descending colon as it meets the rectum. SEE: *colon.*

   f., splenic. Bend at junction of transverse with descending colon.

flick'er. The sensation of alternating intervals of brightness caused by interruptions in light stimuli.

flight of ideas. In psychoanalysis, continuous but fragmentary stream of talk.

   The general train of thought can be followed but direction is frequently changed, often by chance stimuli from the environment. May be seen in acute manic states.

flint disease. Deposit of fine particles in the lungs. SYN: *chalicosis.*

floaters (flō'ters) [AS. *flotian,* float]. Translucent specks of various sizes and shapes that float across the visual field. These are due to small bits of protein or cells floating in the vitreous. SEE: *muscae volitantes.*

floating [AS. *flota,* a raft]. Moving about. Out of normal location.

   f. kidney. Kidney movable from its normal bed of fat.

   f. ribs. The 11th and 12th ribs which do not articulate with the sternum.

floats. Glass capsules containing labels to float in an exposed liquid to designate its nature.

floccillation, floccitation (flŏk-sĭ-lā'shŭn, -tā'shŭn) [L. *floccilatio*]. Semiconscious picking at bedclothes in fevers and stupors. SYN: *carphologia; carphology.*

floccose (flŏk'ōs) [L. *floccōsus,* full of wool tufts]. In biology, pert. to a growth made up of short and densely but irregularly interwoven filaments.

floccular (flŏk'ū-lăr) [L. *flocculus,* little tuft]. Pert. to the flocculus of the cerebellum.

flocculence (flŏk'ū-lĕns") State of being flocculent or resembling shreds or tufts of cotton.

flocculent (flŏk'ū-lĕnt). Resembling the white portion of floating island or a fluid or culture containing whitish shreds of mucus.

flocculoreaction (flŏk"ū-lō-rē-ăk'shŭn) [L. *flocculus,* little tuft, + *rē,* again, + *agere,* to act]. Flocculation of a serum reaction.

flocculus (flŏk'ū-lŭs) [L., little tuft]. (pl. *flocculi*) 1. A small tuft of wool-like fibers. 2. [NA] A lobe below and behind the middle peduncle of the cerebrum on each side of the median fissure.

   f. retinae. Ciliary process of retina.

flooding (flŭd'ĭng) [AS. *flōd*]. Profuse uterine bleeding.

Flood's ligament. [Valentine Flood, Ir. surgeon, 1800-1847] A band of ligaments attached to lower part of lesser tuberosity of the humerus.

floor [AS. *flōr*]. The surface which forms the lower limit of a cavity or space, as the floor of the cranial cavity, fourth ventricle, mouth, nasal fossa, or pelvis.

flora (flor'ă) [L. *flos, flor-,* flower]. 1. Plant life as distinguished from animal life. 2. Plant life occurring or adapted for living in a specific environment. Thus one speaks of the intestinal, vaginal, or skin flora.

florid (flor'ĭd) [L. *floridus,* blossoming]. Having a bright deep-red color. Used to describe skin coloration.

floss, dental. A waxed or unwaxed tape or thread used to clean between the teeth.

flour [L. *flos, flor-,* flower]. Finely ground meal obtained from wheat or other grain; any soft fine powder. SEE: *bread; cereals.*

flow [AS. *flōwan,* to flow]. 1. Action of flowing; said of liquids. 2. The menstrual discharge.

flower [L. *flōs, flor-,* flower]. That part of a plant which comprises the organs of reproduction. Ex: anthemis, arnica, matricaria. A complete flower includes a calyx, corolla, stamens which produce pollen, and a pistil which produces the ovule.

flowmeter. Device for measuring the flow of a gas or liquid. Used esp. in monitoring flow of anesthetic gases.

flucticuli (flŭk-tĭk'ū-lĭ) [L., little waves]. (sing. *flucticulus*) Wavelike markings on lateral wall of 3rd ventricle.

fluctuation [L. *fluctuatio*]. A wavy impulse felt in palpation and produced by vibration of body fluid.

   DIAG: If felt over lower abdomen, ascites usually is present. May be caused by peritoneal hemmorrhage. If confined to limited portion of abdomen, tuberculous peritonitis may be indicated; over central portion, bladder distention. In lower abdomen in women, an ovarian cyst or pregnancy. In right hypochondria, a hydatid cyst; abscess of liver, distended gallbadder; over left hypochondria, cysts or abscess. Above umbilicus, dilated colon or stomach partly filled with fluid and gas.

flu′id [L. *fluidus*]. A nonsolid, liquid, or gaseous substance. SEE: *secretion*.

  f., amniotic. A clear yellowish fluid that fills the fetal membranes in pregnancy. Spec. grav. approx. 1.006. It is composed of albumin, salts (chiefly urea), and water, and suspended in it are lanugo, epidermal cells, vernix caseosa, and meconium. It is derived from the amnion. Its chief function is protection for the fetus. SEE: *amnion; meconium.*

  f. balance. Regulation of amount of water in the body by its controlling mechanism. The balance is upset when fluids are lost by vomiting, diarrhea, bleeding, or when dehydration occurs. Treatment of fluid imbalance depends upon the cause, the kind and quantity of fluids lost, and the state of renal function.

  f., cerebrospinal. F. found in central canal of spinal cord and in the ventricles of the brain, and in the subarachnoid space about the brain and spinal cord. It is formed by the choroid plexuses of the ventricles.

  f. diet. Diet for postoperative cases: carbonated water, ginger ale, tea, albumin, water, beef tea, broth, coffee. Raw fruit juices and milk should not be given unless ordered. SEE: *liquid diet.*

  f., extracellular. Tissue f. or f. occupying spaces between the tissue cells; interstitial f.

  f., extravascular. All the body fluids outside the blood vessels; includes tissue f., fluids within the serous and synovial cavities, the cerebrospinal f., and lymph.

  f., interstitial. Tissue f.

  f., intracellular. The f. contained within cells and comprising about 50% of body weight.

  f., intraocular. The f. within the anterior and posterior chambers of the eye.

  f. repair. Solution in water of electrolytes and usually glucose, given I.V. to correct or repair fluid and electrolyte imbalance.

  f. retention. Failure to eliminate f. from the body due to renal, cardiac, or metabolic disease, or combinations of these disorders.

  Retention of salt is another cause of f. retention. Excess salt in the body requires retention of water to maintain the proper chemical and physical properties of body fluids. A salt-free diet is indicated in f. reten-

tion. The use of diuretics will depend upon the functional state of the kidneys.

  f., serous. A f. in the serous cavities.

  f., synovial. The f. contained within synovial cavities, bursae, and tendon sheaths. SYN: *synovia.*

  f., tissue. The interstitial or extracellular fluid.

fluidextract, fluidextractum [L. *fluidus,* fluid, + *extractum,* extract]. Solution of the soluble constituents of vegetable drugs of such strength that each cc. or ml. represents 1 gm. of the drug.

  Fluidextracts contain alcohol as a solvent and/or preservative, and many of these give precipitates with water.

  f., aromatic cascara. USP. Liquid preparation of cascara sagrada, magnesium oxide, glycyrrhiza extract, saccharin, anise oil, coriander oil, methyl salicylate, alcohol, and water. Used as a cathartic.

  f., glycyrrhiza. USP. A liquid preparation of glycyrrhiza.

  f., ipecac. USP. A fluid preparation of the powdered rhizome and roots of Cephaelis ipecacuana or C. acuminata. It is used as an emetic and expectorant.

fluidounce. Measure of apothecaries fluid volume, equal to eight fluidrams or 29.57 ml. SYMB: f℥.

fluidram. Apothecaries measure of fluid volume, equal to 3.697 ml. SYMB: f℥.

fluke (flūk) [AS. *flōc,* flatfish]. A parasitic worm belonging to the class Trematoda, phylum Platyhelminthes. Those parasitic in man belong to the order Digenea. Most flukes have complex life cycles which include asexual generations that live in a mollusc (snail or bivalve). Stages of a typical fluke include adult, egg, miracidium, sporocyst, redia, cercaria, and metacercaria.

  f., blood. A schistosome. Flukes of the genus Schistosome, S. haematobium, S. mansoni, and S. japonicum. Adults live principally in the mesenteric and pelvic veins. They cause schistosomiasis and schistosome dermatitis (swimmer's itch).

  f., intestinal. Species of intestinal flukes infesting man include Gastrodiscoides hominis, Fasciolopsis buski, Heterophyes heterophyes, Metagonimus yokogawai.

  f., liver. Species living in the liver and bile ducts. Species infesting man include Clonorchis sinensis, Fasciola hepatica, Dicrocoelium dendriticum, and Opisthrochis felineus.

  f., lung. Only one species is common in man, namely Paragonimus westermani.

flumina pilorum (flū″mĭ-nă-pĭ-lō″rŭm) [L., rivers of hair]. [NA] The curved lines along which the hairs of the body are arranged, esp. in the fetus.

fluor albus (flū″or-ăl′bŭs) [L., white flow]. White discharge from the uterus or vagina. SYN: *leukorrhea*.

fluorescein (flū″ō-rĕs′ē-ĭn). A red crystalline powder. Used chiefly in diagnostic purposes, detecting foreign bodies in the eye, or corneal lesions.

fluorescence (flū″ō-rĕs′ĕnts). Property of certain substances to emit light when exposed to certain types of light radiation.

    Usually ultraviolet, first noted in fluorspar; caused by absorption of certain wave lengths and simultaneous emission of a longer wave length which terminates simultaneously with the cessation of the incident exciting radiation.

fluorescent (flū-ō-rĕs′ĕnt). 1. In biology, having one color by transmitted light and another by reflected light. 2. Luminous when exposed to other light rays.

    f. antibody. An antibody which has been stained or marked by a fluorescent material. Use of the FA technique permits rapid diagnosis of various kinds of infections. ABBR: FA.

    f. screen. 1. A sheet of cardboard, paper, or glass coated with a material which fluoresces visibly, such as calcium tungstate, used as the chief part of a fluoroscope when roentgen rays, radium rays, or electrons impinge upon it; a substitute for a fluoroscope in a darkened room. 2. A sheet of cardboard, paper, or glass, coated with anthracene or other fluorescing materials to observe ultraviolet radiations.

    f. treponemal antibody-absorption test. Test for syphilis using fluorescent antibody, q.v., technique.

fluoridation (flū″ōr-ĭ-dā′shŭn). The addition of fluorides to a water supply as a means of reducing dental caries.

fluoride (flū-ō-rĭd). A compound of fluorine with a radicle; a salt of hydrofluoric acid.

fluorine (flū′ō-rēn flūr′ēn). SYMB: F. At. wt. 18.9984; at. no. 9. Gaseous, chemical element.

    F. is found in the soil in combination with calcium. It seems absolutely necessary to plant life and in animal life it helps to form the bones and teeth. Insoluble mineral elements must be absorbed by plant life and taken into the animal body as food before they can be assimilated. It is found in cow's milk, egg yolk, and brain.

fluorometer (flū-or-ŏm′ĕ-ter). 1. Device for determining the amount of radiation produced by X rays. 2. Device for adjusting a fluoroscope in order to better establish the location of the target and to produce an undistorted image or shadow.

fluoroscope (flū′or-ō-skōp). A device consisting of a fluorescent screen suitably mounted, either separately or in conjunction with a roentgen tube, by means of which the shadows of objects interposed between the tube and the screen are made visible.

fluoros′copy. The use of a fluoroscope for medical diagnosis or for testing various materials by roentgen rays.

fluorosis (flū-or-ō′sĭs). Chronic fluorine poisoning, sometimes marked by mottling of tooth enamel. Often results from too much fluoride in drinking water.

flush [ME. *flusshen*, to fly up]. 1. Sudden redness of the skin. 2. Irrigating of a cavity with water.

    f., hec′tic. Redness of the cheeks seen in some chronic affections, such as pulmonary tuberculosis, and due to rise of temperature.

    f., hot. F. accompanied with sensation of heat; common in neuroses, psychoneuroses, and during menopause.

flut′ter [AS. *floterian*, to fly about]. A tremulous movement, esp. of the heart as atrial and ventricular flutter.

    f., atrial. Condition in which contractions of the atrium become extremely rapid (200-400 per min.). In pure flutter, a regular rhythm is maintained; in impure flutter, the rhythm is irregular. SYN: *auricular f.*

flux [L. *fluxus*, a flow]. 1. An excessive flow or discharge from an organ or cavity of the body; diarrhea. 2. Discharge from the bowels.

    f., bloody. Dysentery.

    f., menstrual. Menstrual flow.

fly [AS. *flēoge*]. An insect belonging to the order Diptera, characterized by possessing sucking mouth parts, one pair of wings, and incomplete metamorphosis. Term is sometimes applied to insects belonging to other orders. Ex: May fly, dragon fly. SEE: *Diptera.*

    f., black. Simulium, q.v.

    f., blow. Flies of the family Calliphoridae. They breed in dung or the flesh of dead animals. SYN: *bluebottle flies.* SEE: *Calliphora vomitoria.*

    f., bot. Botfly, q.v.

    f., flesh. The Sarcophagidae, q.v.

    f., house. Musca domestica, q.v.

    f., sand. Phlebotomus, q.v.

    f., screwworm. A fly belonging to the families Calliphoridae and Sarcophagidae, q.v.

    f., Spanish. Cantharides, q.v.

f., tsetse. Glossina palpalis. F. which transmits African sleeping sickness or trypanosomiasis.

f., warble. Dermatobia, q.v.

fm. Abbr. for *fermium.*

f.m. Abbr. for L. *fiat mistura,* make a mixture.

foam (fōm) [AS. *fām*]. A mixture of finely-divided gas bubbles interspersed in a liquid.

fo'cal [L. *focus,* hearth]. Pert. to a focus.

f. infection. Infection occurring near a focus, such as the cavity of a tooth.

f. lesion. A limited central lesion.

foci (fō'sī) [L.]. Pl. of focus, q.v.

fo'cus (L., hearth). (pl. *foci*) The point of convergence of light rays or waves of sound.

f., real. Point at which convergent rays intersect.

f., virtual. The point at which divergent rays would intersect if prolonged backward.

fog'ging. A method of testing vision, used particularly in testing astigmatism and in postcycloplegic examination. SYN: f. system.

fold [AS. *fealdan,* to fold]. A ridge; a doubling back. SYN: *plica.*

f., amniotic. Folded edge of the amniotic membrane where it rises over and finally encloses the embryo of birds, reptiles, and some mammals.

f., genital. F. of skin in the embryo on each side of the genital tubercle which develops into the labia minora in the female.

f., mesouterine. F. of peritoneum supporting the uterus.

folia (fō'lī-ā) [L.]. Pl. of folium, q.v.

foliaceous (fō-lī-ā'shĭ-ŭs) [L. *folia,* leaves]. Resembling or pert. to a leaf.

folic acid (fō'lik). Pteroylglutamic acid. Found in liver, yeast, and green leaves. Used in treating macrocytic anemia due to folic acid deficiency, celiac syndrome, and sprue. Pernicious anemia should not be treated with folic acid, but with vitamin B_{12}.

folie (fō-lē') [Fr.]. Mania; psychosis.

f. à deux. Occurrence of psychosis at the same time in two closely associated persons.

f. du doute. Abnormal doubts about ordinary acts and beliefs; inability to decide upon definite course of action or conduct.

folium (fō'lī-ŭm) [L., leaf]. (pl. *folia*) Thin, broad, leaflike structure.

f. vermis. [NA] A fold on the posterior part of the upper surface of the vermis of the cerebellum. SYN: *f. cacuminis.*

foll'icle [L. *folliculus,* little bag]. A small secretory sac or cavity.

f., aggregated. Peyer's patch, q.v.

f., atretic. An ovarian f. that has undergone degeneration or involution.

f., graafian. The complete development of the primary oocyte in the cortex of the ovary to the stage where the ovum is fully developed. SEE: *ovary.*

f., growing. A developing f. of the ovary.

f., hair. An invagination of the epidermis from which a hair develops.

f., nabothian. Dilated cyst of the glands of the cervix uteri.

f., ovarian. A spherical structure in the cortex of the ovary consisting of an oogonium or an oocyte and its surrounding epithelial (follicular) cells.

Follicles are of three types: primary, consisting of an oogonium and a single layer of follicular cells; growing, in which the f. cells proliferate forming several layers and the first maturation division occurs; vesicular, or graafian f. which possesses a cavity (antrum) containing the follicular fluid (liquor folliculi). The oocyte lies in the cumulus oophorus, a mass of cells on the inner surface. The cells lining the f. constitute the stratum granulosum. The f. is a secretory structure producing estrogens.

f., sebaceous. Oil gland of the skin.

f., solitary. A single lymph nodule of the intestine.

f., thyroid. Spherical or ovoid structure found in the thyroid gland lined with a single layer of cuboidal epithelial cells which secrete the thyroid hormone. The follicles are filled with colloid, a viscid substance rich in iodine.

f., vesicular. F. containing a cavity; a mature ovarian or graafian f.

folliclis (fōl'ĭk-lĭs) [L. *folliculus,* little bag]. Indolent papulonecrotic lesion, esp. on the extremities and possibly the face, due to tuberculosis.

follic'ular. Pert. to a follicle or follicles.

f. tonsillitis. Inflammation of follicles on surface of the tonsil which become filled with pus.

f. tumor. A sebaceous cyst.

folliculitis (fō-lĭk"ū-lī'tĭs) [L. *folliculus,* little bag, + Gr. *-itis,* inflammation]. Inflammation of a follicle or follicles.

f. barbae. Tinea barbae, q.v.

f. decalvans. Purulent follicular inflammation of the scalp resulting in irregular alopecia and scarring.

ETIOL: Essential cause unknown. Believed to be caused by staphylococci. Affects mostly males between 2nd and 4th decades.

SYM: Initial inflammatory papule or pustule at mouth of follicle pierced by a hair is followed by crusting and desiccation, when it drops off along with loosened hair. Bald patches with slight depressed whitish center surrounded by inflamed margin. Extends peripherally.

PATH: Sebaceous gland atrophy and flattened papillae.

PROG: Baldness is permanental though extension may be arrested.

TREATMENT: Externally, topical antibiotics or corticosteroids, frequent shampoos, and daily antiseptic.

folliculoma (fō-līk″ū-lō′mă) [L. *folliculus*, little bag, + Gr. *ōma*, tumor]. A tumor of the ovary originating in a graafian follicle, in which the cells resemble the cells of the stratum granulosum.

folliculose (fō-līk′ū-lōs). Composed of follicles.

folliculo′sis [L. *folliculus*, little bag, + Gr. *-ōsis*, condition]. Presence of an abnormal quantity of lymph follicles.

folliculus (fō-līk′ū-lŭs) [L.]. (pl. *fol′liculi*) [NA] A follicle.

   f. oophorus vesiculosus. A graafian follicle, q.v.

fomentation (fō″mĕn-tā′shŭn) [L. *fomentatio*]. A hot, wet application for the relief of pain or inflammation. SEE: *dressing, hot moist; stupe.*

fomes (fō′mēz) [L., tinder]. (pl. *fomites*) Any substance that absorbs and transmits infectious material.

fomites (fō′mī-tēz). Pl. of fomes, q.v.

Fontana's spaces. [Felice Fontana, It. scientist, 1730-1805] Spaces between the processes of ligamentum pectinatum of the iris. These convey the aqueous humor.

fontanel, fontanelle (fŏn″tă-nĕl′) [Fr. *fontanelle*, little fountain]. An unossified space or soft spot lying between the cranial bones of the skull of a fetus.

   f., anterior. F. at the junction of the coronal, frontal, and sagittal sutures.

   f., posterior. F. at the junction of the sagittal and lambdoid sutures.

fonticulus (fŏn-tīk′ū-lŭs) [L., little fountain]. [NA] Fontanel, q.v.

food [AS. *fōda*]. (pl. *foods*) Nutritive substance which provides heat, energy, minerals, and vitamins for maintenance of well-being of the body. SEE: names of foods.

COURSE: *Alimentary canal:* Foods enter the mouth and in the buccal area are reduced to a pulp or semifluid mass through the processes of mastication and insalivation (the mixing of f. with saliva). Swallowing or deglutition then occurs. In swallowing, the f. mass or bolus passes into the pharynx and then through the esophagus to the stomach, the entrance to which is controlled by the cardiac sphincter.

Stomach: In the stomach the f. is stored and mixed with gastric juice. After it attains a certain fluid consistency, it passes through the pyloric sphincter into the small intestine.

Small intestine: In the first portion or duodenum, the intestinal contents (now called chyme) are mixed with bile secreted by the liver and the pancreatic juice, both of which enter through the opening of the common bile duct. In the next two portions, the jejunum and ileum, the chyme is mixed with the intestinal juice secreted by the intestinal glands or crypts of Lieberkuhn. In the small intestine, digestion is completed and the end products of digestion (simple sugars, amino acids, fatty acids and glycerol) are absorbed into the capillaries and lacteals of the intestinal mucosa.

Large intestine: Undigestible material passes from the small intestine into the large intestine (colon) through the ileocecal valve located at the junction of the ascending colon and the cecum, a blind pouch which terminates in the vermiform appendix. The material continues through the colon (ascending, transverse, descending, and

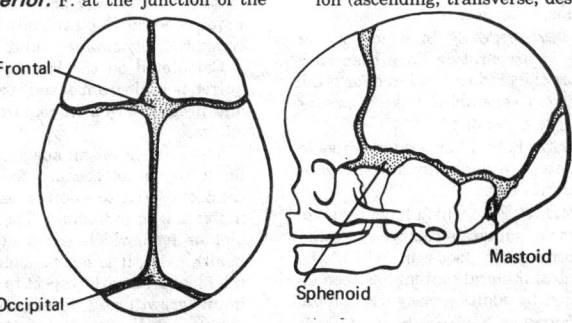

FONTANELS OF INFANT'S SKULL

Frontal

Occipital

Mastoid

Sphenoid

sigmoid) to the rectum from which it is discharged as feces through the anal canal at the anus or anal orifice. In the large intestine, the major portion of the water of the intestinal contents is absorbed. Digestive changes are limited to the action of bacteria which brings about putrefaction and fermentation of incompletely digested foods. No enzymes are secreted by the glands of the large intestine.

f. additives. Substances or a mixture of substances, other than basic foodstuff, which are present in a food as a result of any aspect of production, processing, storage, or packaging. Accidental contaminants are not considered to be food additives.

f. adulterant. A substance which makes f. impure or inferior, i.e. toxic organisms, filth, pesticide residues, radioactive fallout, any poisonous or deleterious substance, or any substance added to increase bulk or weight in a f. product.

f. allergies. Allergic reactions resulting from ingestion of foods to which a person has become sensitized. One may become sensitive to almost any f. However, certain foods such as milk, eggs, wheat, seafood, chocolate, and oranges are frequent offenders.

SYM: Urticaria (hives), certain eczemas, nausea, vomiting, diarrhea, and intestinal cramps. A syndrome (angioneurotic edema) characterized by a transient swelling of various parts of the body and spasm of the intestine may result.

f. ball. Gastric stone made up of fruit and vegetable skins, seeds, and fibers. SYN: *phytobezoar.*

f., contamination of. F. may be the cause of illness due to its acting as the carrier of pathogenic organisms such as those which cause enteritis (Salmonella) or tuberculosis; parasites such as those which cause trichinosis; or certain types of worms (roundworms, tapeworms).

f., convenience. F. in which one or more steps in preparation have been completed before the product is offered for retail sale. Ex: frozen vegetables, bake mixes, or heat-and-serve types of f.

f., dietetic. F. that has been modified in nutrient content in some way in order to be used in special diets.

f., enriched. F. to which have been added vitamins or minerals removed in refining and processing; foods in which the vitamin and/or mineral content has been increased either by addition or by irradiation.

f. exchanges. Commonly used foods grouped according to similarities in composition so that such foods may be used interchangeably in diet planning.

f., nutrient substances of. Substances which in the body serve as a source of energy or provide material for the growth and repair of tissue. Foods are organic substances (proteins, carbohydrates, fats) present in animal and plant tissues. The term "food" is commonly used to refer to any substance taken into the body which serves a nutrient function. Thus any discussion of f. would include vitamins, minerals, water, and trace of elements (zinc, chromium, cobalt, manganese, molybdenum, selenium).

f. poisoning. An imprecise term indicating an illness resulting from the ingestion of foods containing poisonous substances. True f. poisoning includes mushroom poisoning, shellfish poisoning, poisoning resulting from foods contaminated with poisonous insecticides or toxic substances such as lead or mercury, milk sickness (due to milk from cows that have fed on certain poisonous plants). Also occasionally poisoning resulting from eating foods that have undergone putrefaction or decomposition or poisoning from bacteria.

f. requirements. It is assumed that an average healthy man (158 pounds or 72 kilograms), performing light to moderate muscular work, requires 2950 Cal./day. This would be supplied in part by protein, but mostly by fat and carbohydrates. Persons in sedentary occupations require smaller amounts. In general adults require one gram of protein per day for each kilogram of their adult weight.

A diet made up of ordinary foods and supplying the necessary amounts of protein and energy undoubtedly supplies an abundance of mineral matter. The assumption is usually made that, provided a woman is engaged in some moderately active occupation, she requires fewer Cal. each day because of her comparatively smaller build.

Calculated on the basis of f. energy required per kilogram of body weight, children and pregnant women require more f. than adults.

The criteria for an adequate diet are difficult to define because food habits vary from one area to another as well as from individual to individual. There is no single diet or food which is essential for life or health. Also, it is not possible to state that the ideal diet, with respect to assuring maximum growth and development, would be the one which would assure maximum longevity. SEE: *dietetics* in *Appendix.*

Food Requirements
Organic Composition of Proteins

Elements	Symbol	Per Cent	Metabolic End Products
Carbon	C	53 %	Urea, uric acid, H_2SO_4, CO_2, H_2O
Hydrogen	H	7 %	Formation of salts
Oxygen	O	22 %	Proteins are tissue, including muscle and
Nitrogen	N	16 %	nerve builders, and also furnish heat and
Sulfur	S	1½%	energy
Phosphorous	P	½%	
Other Minerals		trace	
		100%	

Classification of Proteins

Albumen	Casein	Gluten	Myosin
Eggs	Milk	Cereals	Fowls
Meat	Cheese	Beans	
		Peas	
		Lentils	
		Nuts	

Composition of Carbohydrates (Cx(H$_2$O)y)

Elements	Symbol	Per Cent	Metabolic End Products
Carbon	C	76%	Formation of salts
Hydrogen	H	12%	CO_2 and H_2O
Oxygen	O	12%	Energy
		100%	

Classification of Carbohydrates

Glucose	Cane Sugar	Cellulose
$C_6H_{12}O_6$	$C_{12}H_{22}O_{11}$	$C_6H_{10}O_5$

Carbohydrates as well as fats are heat and energy producers, but neither can take the place of proteins as they contain no nitrogen. They consist principally of sugars, starch, and cellulose.

Composition of Fats

Elements	Symbol	Per Cent	Metabolic End Products
Carbon	C	45%	CO_2 and H_2O
Hydrogen	H	06%	Fats produce heat and energy but do not
Oxygen	O	49%	build tissues or cells.
		100%	

Food Requirements (*Continued*)
Origin of Fats

Animal	Oils	Nuts	Fruits
Butter, Oleomargarine, Lard, Meat, Dairy Products	Cottonseed, Corn, Sunflower	Peanuts	Palm, Olive

Additional Dietary Requirements

Water, Minerals (Iodine, Iron, Magnesium, Calcium, Copper, Chromium, Cobalt, Zinc, Selenium, Manganese, and Molybdenum), Vitamins

foot [AS. *fōt*]. 1. The terminal portion of the lower extremity. The bones of the foot include the tarsus, metatarsus, and phalanges. ABBR: ft. SEE: *skeleton.* 2. A unit of measurement.

f.-and-mouth disease. A virus disease of cattle and horses which is rarely transmitted to man.

SYM: Fever, headache, malaise with dryness and burning sensation of the mouth. Vesicles develop on the lips, tongue, mouth, palms, and soles. TREATMENT: Symptomatic. Full recovery occurs in 2-3 weeks.

f. arches. Four arches: Internal longitudinal; outer longitudinal, and two transverse ones.

f., athlete's. An imprecise term indicating almost any dermatitis of the feet. SEE: *athlete's foot.*

f. -candle. Amount of light radiated one ft. from a standard candle.

f., cleft. Condition in which a cleft extends between the digits to the metatarsal region, usually due to a missing digit.

f., contracted. Clawfoot, q.v., or pes cavus, q.v.

f., flat. Flatfoot, q.v.; pes planus.

f., immersion. Condition resulting from prolonged immersion of the feet in water.

f., Madura. Bone hypertrophy and degeneration, frequently followed by suppuration or gangrene.

f. plate. Base of the stapes; an ossicle of the tympanum. It fits into, and closes, the fenestra vestibuli (oval window).

f. pound. Amount of energy required to lift one pound a vertical distance of one foot.

f., splay. Flatfoot accompanied by extreme eversion of the f.

f., weak. Condition resulting from weakened muscles, or from faulty walking habits. Results in chronic eversion of the f.

footdrop. Failure to maintain the foot in a normally flexed position, or dragging of the foot. Usually due to trauma or paralysis of the muscles which flex the foot.

foot'ling presentation. Presentation of feet foremost in labor.

footprint. An impression of the foot, esp., an ink impression used for identification of infants.

forage (fō-rŏzh') [Fr., boring]. Creating a channel through an enlarged prostate by diathermy.

foramen (for-ā'mĕn) [L.]. (pl. *foram'ina*) [NA] A passage or opening; an orifice, a communication between two cavities of an organ, or a hole in a bone for passage of vessels or nerves.

f., intervertebral. Opening between every two articulated vertebrae for passage of nerves to and from spinal cord.

f. magnum. Opening of the occipital bone through which passes the spinal cord from the brain.

f. of Monro. Opening between third and lateral ventricles of the brain.

f., obturator. Large oval f. below acetabulum bounded by the pubis and ischium. SEE: *Magendie's f.*

f., olfactory. An opening in the ethmoid bone for passage of the olfactory nerves.

f. ova'le. 1. An opening between the two atria of the heart in the fetus. The opening closes shortly before or after birth in most cases. If it remains open it is possible to surgically repair the defect. 2. Oval opening in posterior margin of great sphenoidal wing, for inferior maxillary nerve and small meningeal artery.

force, unit of. Arbitrary definition of a certain amount of force. Ex: a dyne is the amount of force necessary to move a 1 gm. weight the distance of 1 cm. in 1 second.

forceps (for'sĕps) [L.]. Pincers for holding, seizing, or extracting. There are many distinct types of f., varying according to the

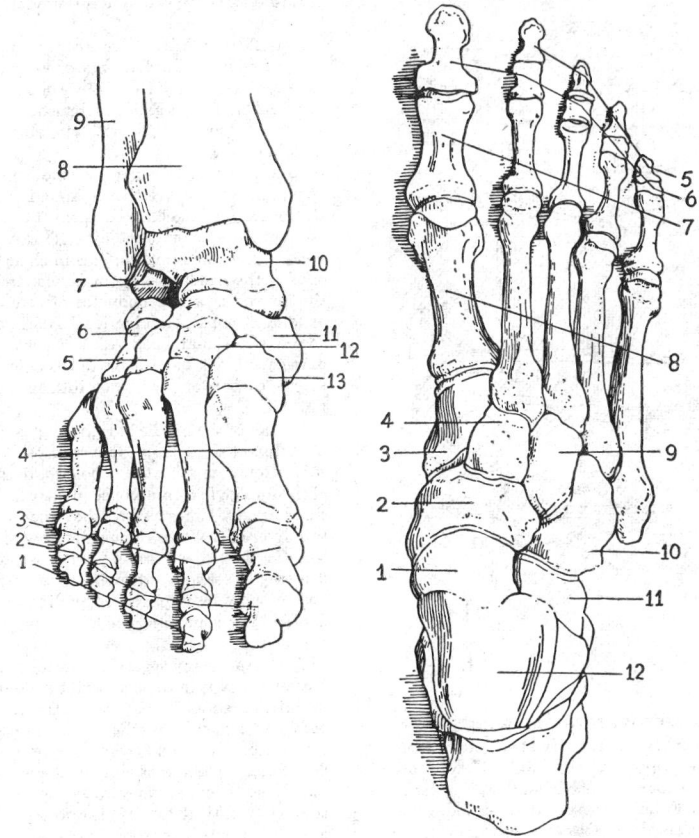

FOOT

TARSAL AND METATARSAL BONES AND PHALANGES

1, 3rd phalanges. 2, 2nd phalanges. 3, 1st phalanges. 4, Metatarsals. 5, External cuneiform. 6, Cuboid. 7, Os calcis. 8, Tibia. 9, Fibula. 10, Astragalus. 11, Scaphoid. 12, Middle cuneiform. 13, Internal cuneiform.

1, Astragalus. 2, Scaphoid. 3, Internal cuneiform. 4, Middle cuneiform. 5, 3rd phalanges. 6, 2nd phalanges. 7, 1st phalanges. 8, Metatarsals. 9, External cuneiform. 10, Cuboid. 11, Os calcis. 12, Astragalus (talus).

operation for which they are intended.

f., artery. F. for holding ends of an artery in order to perform ligation.

f., bone. F. used for cutting bone and removal of bone fragments.

f., dressing. F. for general use in dressing wounds—removing dead tissue, drainage tubes, etc.

f., needle. F. for grasping and holding a needle.

f., rongeur. F. used for cutting bone.

forcipate (for'sĭ-pāt) [L. *forceps*, tongs]. Shaped like forceps.

for'cipressure [" + *pressura*, pressure]. Arresting hemorrhage by pressure on an artery with forceps.

fore- [AS.]. Prefix meaning before or in front of.

forearm (for'arm) [AS. *fore*, in front, + *arm*, arm]. The part of arm between elbow and

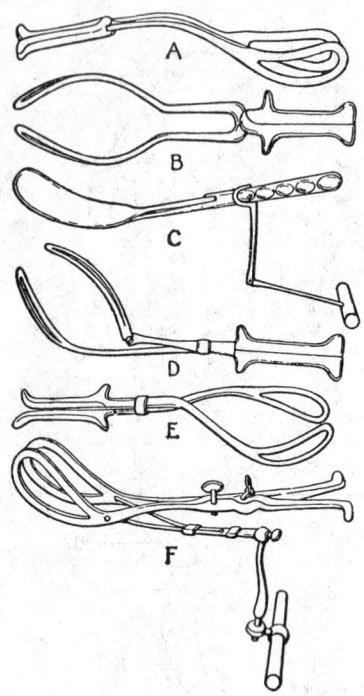

SOME OBSTETRICAL FORCEPS

A, Piper. B, Simpson (DeLee modification).
C, Tucker-McLean with Bill's axis traction
handle. D, Barton. E, Kielland. F, Tarnier axis
traction. From Bryant and Overland: Wood-
ward and Gardner's Obstetric Management and
Nursing, ed. 7. 1964.

wrist.

forebrain (for'brān) ["+ *bregen*, brain]. Anterior portion of the brain of the embryo.
SYN: *prosencephalon.*

fore'finger. The first or index finger.

fore'gut [AS. *fore*, in front, + *gut*, a pouring].
First part of the embryonic digestive tube
whence pharynx, esophagus, stomach, and
duodenum are formed. SYN: *protogaster.*

forehead (for'ĭd, ·for'hĕd) [AS. *forhēafod*].
The anterior part of the head below the hairline and above the eyes. SYN: *frons; meto-
pon.*

foreign bodies. Slivers, cinders, dirt, or
small objects in the skin, ears, eyes, nose, or
internal. They frequently lead to infection,
and if not removed lead to unsightly marks

or tattooing of the skin and inflammation of
the tissue involved.

F.A. TREATMENT: Carefully clean the
areas involved. Foreign material can be
removed carefully piece by piece or by vigorous swabbing with gauze or brush, using a
soapy solution. Follow with an antiseptic
dressing.

In attempting to remove a small foreign
body, first cover area with an antiseptic;
sterilize a clean needle by heating it to a dull
or bright red color in a flame. This can be
done with a single match; inasmuch as both
ends of the needle get hot it is wise to hold
the far end in a nonconductor of heat such
as folds of paper, sticking it in a cork, or in
the edge of a small book. Allow it to cool and
disregard black deposit on the needle; it is
sterile carbon and will not interfere with
procedure.

Introduce the needle at right angles to the
direction of sliver and lift it out. Most persons attempt to stick the needle in direction
of the foreign body and consequently have to
thrust many times before they manage to
lift sliver out. When removed, apply an antiseptic and cover wound with a sterile
dressing. Tetanus antitoxin or a tetanus
booster may be required depending on the
depth of the wound and the history of immunization.

In the ear: If any vegetable matter such as
a bean or pea is in the ear, water should not
be introduced as it may cause the foreign
body to be pushed further into the ear or
cause it to swell and become firmly embedded. Place a globule of glue on the end of a
match stick or an applicator; gently introduce it until it touches the foreign body
and then remove gently.

If an insect is in the ear, the patient may
experience loud buzzing, pain, and dizziness.
Flood ear with warm oil or water, letting
insect float out.

In wounds: F. b. are often present in
wounds and generally should be left undisturbed if a surgeon is available within a
short time. If small, as a sliver, it may be
desirable to remove it. If large, it may be
very dangerous to try any method of removing inasmuch as it might be embedded in
large blood vessels, muscles, etc. Removing
it might result in much loss of blood or might
cause breaking off of splinters, particles of
rust, dirt, etc. Within a few moments, blood
and the natural reaction of swelling would
tend to fill in the wounds and cover this foreign material, making it exceedingly difficult for the doctor to care for the patient.
In such instances, it is much wiser, when

possible, to leave the large foreign body in position and obtain the services of a doctor promptly.

SEE: *ear; esophagus; eye; nose; stomach; throat.*

forensic (for-ĕn'sĭk) [L. *forēnsis,* public]. Pert. to the law; legal.

f. medicine. Legal medicine or medicine in relation to the law.

f. pathology. The use of information obtained from the pathological examination of biological materials in legal proceedings.

fore'pleasure [AS. *fore,* in front, + L. *placere,* to please]. Sexual pleasure preceding orgasm.

fore'skin ["+ O.Norse *skinn,* skin]. Prepuce, q.v., or loose skin at and covering the end of the penis or clitoris.

Excision of the prepuce constitutes circumcision. Smegma praeputii, q.v., is secreted by Tyson's glands and collects under foreskin. SEE: *circumcision.*

NP: In infant cases the nurse must see that the prepuce is not adherent or interfering with urination. Abnormalities must be reported to the doctor.

-form [L. *forma*]. Suffix meaning having the form of.

formaldehyde (for-măl'dĕ-hĭd). USP. CH_2O. A colorless, pungent, irritant gas commonly made by oxidation of methyl alcohol; the simplest member of the group of aldehydes. It is used in medicinal form as f. solution which contains 37% of f. with methanol added.

ACTION AND USES: A disinfectant, preservative, or fumigant. A 10% solution is useful as an astringent.

A 1% or 2% solution used for cleansing dishes, instruments, or fabrics. F. is a powerful disinfectant, esp. in the form of gas, because of its penetrating power, but it is active only in the presence of an abundance of moisture. The solution is germicidal in the strength of 1-2%, but the action may be delayed 20-30 minutes. It hardens tissues and is often used in histology for this purpose. It has a similar hardening effect on the living skin; it is very irritating to mucous membranes and produces reddening, inflammation, and necrosis, if applied repeatedly or continuously. It is sometimes used in soap for disinfection of the hands. A 10% solution is used for sterilizing feces, urine, and sputum; 5-10% for clothing and towels. SEE: *aldehyde; fumigation.*

POISONING SYM: Local irritation of eyes, nose, mouth, throat, respiratory and gastrointestinal tracts, and central nervous system, causing vertigo, stupor, abdominal pain, convulsions, unconsciousness, renal damage.

F.A. TREATMENT: The immediate objective is to delay absorption of ingested f. Give tap water, milk, or activated charcoal by mouth and remove by gastric lavage or emesis. If available, either 1% ammonium carbonate or 2% sodium bicarbonate is preferable to tap water. Treat shock and anuria symptomatically.

for'malin. Aqueous solution of 37% of formaldehyde with methanol added. SEE: *aldehyde.*

formate (for'māt). A salt of formic acid.

formatio (for-mā'shĭ-ō) [L]. (pl. *formationes*) [NA] A structure with definite arrangement and shape.

f. reticula'ris. Dorsal part of the medulla oblongata.

forma'tion. 1. A structure, shape, or figure. 2. The giving of form or shape to, or the development of, a structure.

f. reaction. Development of attributes that hold in check and repress unconscious impulses.

f., reticular. A reticular structure formed of gray matter and interlacing fibers of white matter found in the medulla oblongata (i.e., part of brain stem) between the pyramids and the floor of the 4th ventricle. It is also present in the spinal cord, midbrain, and pons. Fibers from this structure are believed to be able to activate the cortex of the brain independently of specific sensory or other neural systems. Thus reticular f. is part of the reticular activating or alerting system. SEE: *reticular activating system.*

forme fruste (form früst) [Fr., defaced]. (pl. *formes frustes*) An aborted form of disease arrested before running its course. Thus the disease appears in an atypical and indefinite form.

for'mic [L. *formica,* ant]. Pert. to ants, or to f. acid.

f. acid. (H.COOH) A clear, pungent liquid obtained from the oxidation of formaldehyde or wood alcohol. Originally it was obtained from the distillation of the bodies of red ants. Probably it is the cause of the pain and swelling resulting from the bites or stings of certain insects or the irritation from nettles.

f. aldehyde. Formaldehyde.

f. ether. Volatile anesthetic liquid ethyl formate.

formica'tion. A sensation as of ants creeping upon the body; a form of paresthesia.

formiciasis (for"mĭs-ĭ'ă-sĭs) [L. *formica,* ant, + Gr. *iasis,* condition]. Symptoms caused by ant bites.

formilase (for'mĭ-lās). An enzyme which converts acetic acid into formic acid.

for'mula [L., a little form]. (pl. *forulas, -lae*) 1. A rule prescribing ingredients and proportions for the preparation of a compound. 2. In chemistry, an expression by symbols of the constitution of a molecule consisting of letters, each denoting one atom of one elementary substance, with figures, written as subscripts, denoting the number of atoms present. Ex: water consists of two molecules of the element hydrogen and one of oxygen. The formula is H_2O. It may also be written HOH or H—O—H.

Collections of atoms which constitute a group by themselves (radical) are often separated by periods or parentheses, and in this case figures prefixed or appended to the parentheses or placed before an expression contained within periods apply to all the symbols embraced by the parentheses or periods.

In all other cases, a figure prefixed to a symbolical expression for a molecule, like a coefficient in an algebraical f., is understood to be a multiplier of all the symbols following.

f., Arneth's. Method of estimating number of immature leukocytes by means of an elaborate differential blood count, based upon their shape and number of lobes in the nucleus. It is seldom used.

f., dental. F. showing the number and arrangement of the teeth. For the permanent teeth.

$$\left(i\frac{2}{2},\ c\frac{1}{1},\ pm\frac{2}{2},\ m\frac{3}{3}=\frac{8}{8}\right)2 = 32.$$

In this f. the numerators indicate the number in the maxilla and the denominators those in the mandible; *i, c, pm,* and *m* indicate incisor, canine, premolar, and molar respectively. Thus if one upper incisor was missing that portion of the f. would be written i 1/2.

f., empirical. The f. of a compound which shows the atoms and their numbers in a molecule, as H_2O.

f., official. F. in a pharmacopeia.

f., structural. The f. of a compound which shows the relationship of the atoms to each other in a molecule. The atoms are shown joined by valence bonds, for example: H—O—H.

form'ulary [L. *formula,* a little form]. A book of formulas.

f., national. A book issued by the American Pharmaceutical Association.

formyl. The radical of formic acid, HCO.

for'nicate [L. *fornicatus,* arched, brothel]. 1. Arched or vaultlike. 2. To have sexual intercourse with a partner to whom one is not married.

fornica'tion. Sexual intercourse between unmarried partners.

fornices (for'nĭ-sēz) [L]. Pl. of fornix, q.v.

for'nicolumn [L. *fornix,* arch, + *columna,* column]. The anterior pillar of the fornix.

fornicommissure (for-nĭ-kŏm'ĭ-sūr) ["+ *commissura,* a joining together]. The commissure or body of the fornix uteri.

for'nix [L., arch]. (pl. *fornices*) [NA] 1. A fibrous vaulted band connecting the cerebral lobes. 2. Any body with vaultlike or arched shape.

f. conjunctivae. [NA] Loose fold connecting palpebral and bulbar conjunctivae.

f. uteri. Anterior and posterior spaces into which the upper vagina is divided. These recesses are formed by protrusion of the cervix uteri into the vagina.

f. vaginae. The f. uteri, q.v.

fortifica'tion spectrum. Appearance of dark patch with zigzag outline in visual field. SYN: *scintillating scotoma; teichopsia.*

Foshay's serum. [Lee Foshay, 20th century Amer. physician] Serum used in the treatment of tularemia.

fossa (fŏs'ă) [L]. (pl. *fossae*) [NA] A furrow or shallow depression.

f., amygdaloid. Depression containing the tonsil.

f., axillary. The armpit.

f., Claudius'. Triangular area harboring the ovary.

f., iliac. One of the concavities of the iliac bones of pelvis. SYN: *f. iliaca* [NA].

f. lacrimalis. Hollow of frontal bone holding the lacrimal gland.

f. navicularis. F. between the vulva and fourchette. SYN: *f. vestibuli vaginae* [NA].

f. ovalis. Opening in thigh through which the large saphenous vein passes.

f. ovalis cordis. [NA] Remnant of embryonic foramen ovale in right cardiac atrium.

f., Rosenmüller's. Depression in pharynx posterior to opening of eustachian tube.

f. supratonsillaris. [NA] Space between anterior and posterior pillars of the fauces above the tonsil.

fossae (fŏs'ē) [L]. Pl. of fossa, q.v.

fossette (fŏ-sĕt') [Fr]. 1. A small depression or fossa. 2. A small, but deep, corneal ulcer.

foulage (fū-lŏzh') [Fr]. Kneading with pressure of the muscles.

fourchet, fourchette (fūr-shĕt') [Fr. *fourchette*, a fork]. A tense band or transverse fold of mucous membrane at the posterior commissure of the vagina, connecting the posterior ends of the labia minora.

The fossa navicularis, a more or less deep cul-de-sac anterior to the fourchette, separates it from the hymen. It disappears after defloration or parturition, leaving a more open vulva below and behind. SYN: *frenulum labiorum pudendi.*

fourth cranial nerve. Trochlear nerve, q.v.

fovea (fō'vē-ă) [L]. (pl. *foveae*) [NA] A pit or cuplike depression. SEE: *fossa.*

f. centralis retinea. [NA] Pit in the middle of macula lutea.

foveate (fō'vē-āt) [L. *foveatus*]. Pitted; having depressions.

foveation (fō''vē-ā'shŭn). Pitting, as in smallpox.

foveola (fō-vē'ō-lă) [L., little pit]. (pl. *foveolae*) A minute pit or depression.

Fow'ler's position. [George R. Fowler, Amer. surgeon, 1848-1906] A semi-sitting position.

The head of bed may be raised on blocks, pins, or other support, or the back rest may be elevated, or patient may rest upon four or five pillows. It is more easily maintained if the patient sits in a swing or hammock, made by folding a bedsheet lengthwise, placing center of sheet tightly across the buttocks, with one end on each side. The ends are fastened securely at head of the bed, or as high as ends will reach.

This position may be ordered if patient is suffering from dyspnea, q.v., or after a thyroid or an abdominal operation and where drainage is expected. Some pneumonia patients are placed in this position.

Fowler's solution. [Thomas Fowler, Brit. physician, 1736-1801] An arsenical solution containing 0.95-1.5 gm. of arsenic trioxide for each 100 ml. of solution. SYN: *potassium arsenite solution.*

Fr. Chem. symb. for francium.

fraction [L. *fractiō*, act of breaking]. In biological chemistry the separable part of a substance such as blood or plasma.

fractional. Pert. to a fraction or a portion of a whole.

f. test meal. F. examination of stomach contents. The method for collection and examination of stomach contents follows: First the residual contents are removed and then the test meal given; after the meal, samples are removed every 15 min. for two hours, examined, and submitted to chemical tests.

Free hydrochloric acid, bile, blood, starch, mucus, and the total of acids are looked for. Free hydrochloric and total acids are normally small in amount.

In peptic ulcers there is a high acid curve; there is a low one in carcinoma; and an absence of acid in pernicious anemia.

fracture (frăk'chĕr) [L. *fractūra*, break]. 1. A sudden breaking of a bone. 2. A broken bone.

CAUSE: In certain diseases and conditions bones break spontaneously without trauma. Ex: osteomalacia, syphilis, osteomyelitis.

Direct violence: The bone is broken directly at the spot where the force was applied, as in fracture of the tibia by being run over. *Indirect violence:* The bone is fractured by a force applied at a distance from the site of fracture and transmitted to the fractured bone, as in a clavicle fractured by falling on the outstretched hand. *Muscular contraction:* The bone is broken by a sudden violent contraction of the muscles.

VARIETIES: *Simple:* The bone is broken, but there is no external wound. *Compound:* The bone is broken, and there is an external wound leading down to the site of fracture, or fragments of bone protrude through the skin. *Complicated:* The bone is broken, and has injured some internal organ, e.g., a broken rib piercing a lung. *Comminuted:* The bone is broken or splintered into pieces.

Impacted: The bone is broken, and one end is wedged into the interior of the other.

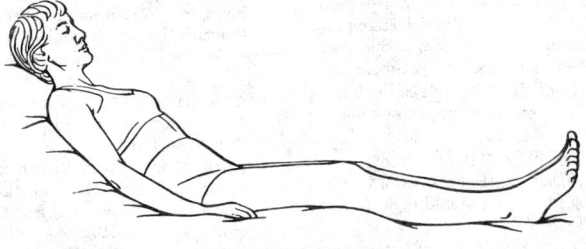

FOWLER'S POSITION

Incomplete: The line of fracture does not include the whole bone. *Green Stick:* The bone is partially bent and partially broken, as when a green stick breaks. It occurs in children, esp. in those with rickets. *Depressed:* When a piece of the skull is broken and driven inwards. *Separation of an epiphysis:* Takes place between the shaft of a bone and its growing end, and occurs only in young patients.

SIGNS: Loss of power of movement; pain with acute tenderness over the site of fracture; swelling and bruising; deformity and possible shortening; unnatural mobility; crepitus or grating which is heard when the ends of the bone rub together. The nurse should never try to obtain these last two signs. To find out the kind of fracture and its exact position, x-ray picture are used.

F.A. TREATMENT: In simple fractures the limb or part must be kept immovable by means of splints. If proper wooden, plastic, or metal splints are unavailable they may be improvised by using magazines or folded newspapers. The clothing should not be removed unless there is dangerous hemorrhage. If it is necessary to remove clothing, do so by cutting the cloth away so as to cause a minimum of motion of the affected part.

If it is an upper extremity it should be supported in a sling, and the patient may then walk. If a lower limb is injured the patient should remain lying, and make no attempt to walk.

TREATMENT: Reduce the fracture, i.e., place the fragments in proper position. Keep the bone in position by means of splints until union has taken place. Restore the limb to complete function by physical therapy and exercise.

In compound fractures, any bleeding must be arrested before treating the fracture. The wound is then washed and cleaned with sterile saline. If the area is grossly contaminated, mild soap solution may be used provided it is thoroughly washed away by using generous amounts of sterile saline. When quite clean, a sterilized dressing is put on and secured by a bandage. Splints are then applied as in simple fractures.

RS: buttonhole f.; cerclage; extension; green stick f.; malunion; name of bone fractured; splint.

fragilitas (frä-jĭl′ĭ-tăs) [L.]. Fragility.

   f. crin′ium. Brittleness, as of the hair, showing splitting and breaking of the shaft. Cause unknown.

   f. oss′ium. Brittleness of bones.

   f. sanguinis. Red blood cell fragility.

   f. unguium. Abnormal brittleness of nails.

fragil′ity. State of brittleness.

   f. of the blood. Tendency of red blood cells to rupture. This is determined by subjecting the cells in laboratory tests to different concentrations of saline.

   f., capillary. Breaking down of capillaries with hemorrhage into almost any site but most noticeably in the skin.

   f. test. If red blood cells are placed in distilled water, they swell rapidly and burst because they normally are suspended in a solution of much greater osmotic pressure. This phenomenon is called hemolysis. If they are suspended in a solution of normal saline, the cells retain their normal shape and do not burst. If they are placed in successively weaker solutions of saline, a point is reached at which some of the cells burst and liberate their hemoglobin within a given length of time, while others do not (partial hemolysis). Finally, at a given dilution, all of the cells have burst within the allotted time, which is usually two hours. The cells of normal blood begin to hemolyze in about 0.44%, and complete hemolysis occurs in about 0.35% saline. If the cells are abnormally fragile, hemolysis occurs in stronger solutions of saline.

fragmenta′tion [L. *fragmentum,* detached part]. Breaking up into fragments.

frambesia (frăm-bē′zĭ-ă) [Fr. *framboise,* raspberry]. Infectious tropical disease. SYN: *yaws,* q.v. SEE: *frambesioma.*

frambesioma (frăm-bē-zĭ-ō′mă) ["+ Gr. *ōma,* swelling]. Primary lesion of yaws in the form of a protruding nodule. This mother yaw appears at the site of inoculation of the causative agent, Treponema pertenue.

francium (frăn′sĭ-ūm). [Named for France, the country in which it was discovered] SYMB: *Fr.* At. no. 87. The at. wt. of the most stable isotope is 233. A metallic element occurring as a natural isotope.

Frankenhäuser's ganglion (frang′kĕn-hoy″zer). [Ferdinand Frankenhäuser, 19th Century Ger. gynecologist] A nerve ganglion sometimes found in lateral walls of the cervix uteri.

Frank′lin glasses. [Benjamin Franklin, Amer. statesman and inventor, 1706-90] Bifocal spectacles.

Fraunhofer's lines (frown′hŏf-er). [Joseph von Fraunhofer, Ger. optician, 1787-1826] Absorption bands or lines seen in a spectrum, caused by the absorption of groups of light rays in their passage through solids, liquids, or gases.

freckle (frĕk'l) [O.Norse *freknur*]. Small local brownish or yellowish pigmentation of the skin. SYN: *ephalis; lentigines; lentigo.*

ETIOL: Exposure to sun in majority. Universal types are probably symptomatic (anemia, abdominal disorders, etc.).

SYM: Minute circumscribed brownish pigmentary macules appearing chiefly on face and dorsal surfaces of hands, more marked in spring and summer. In lentigo senilis the forearms are affected in individuals showing other senile skin changes.

TREATMENT: Protection from the sun.

free associa'tion. 1. Uncontrolled ideas when not under mental restraint or direction. 2. The procedure in psychoanalysis which requires the patient to speak aloud his thought flow, word for word, without censorship.

free medical clinics. Clinics which are established by the community rather than a hospital and provide low cost, if not free, medical care. They are unusual in that their purpose is to deal with illnesses and conditions that are both medical and social. Ex: drug use, run-away young people, political action, birth control, and illegitimate pregnancy. The clinics are supported by individuals, foundations, volunteers, and professionals who may work for nothing or for very low pay.

free standing clinic. Medical outpatient clinic which is community based and not a part of a hospital.

freez'ing [AS. *frēosan*]. Frigidity of a limb due to cold.

Most common in the debilitated, the exhausted, and those alcoholics who fall asleep in a location exposed to extreme cold.

SYM: Paleness, cyanosis, coldness. Unconsciousness usually develops.

F. A. TREATMENT: Protect part with a cradle and apply dry heat at room temperature. Sudden applications of heat undesirable. SEE: *frostbite; wind chill factor.*

    f. microtome. One for cutting frozen objects.

    f. mixtures. For ice bags, 5 oz. (150 ml.) each of ammonium chloride and potassium nitrate, and one part water.

    f. point. Temperature at which liquids freeze.

Frei's disease (frī). [William S. Frei, Ger. dermatologist, 1885-1943] Venereal disease chiefly affecting the inguinal area with formation of buboes. SYN: *lymphogranuloma inguinale; lymphogranuloma venerea; Nicolas-Favre disease.*

Frei's test. Test given to confirm diagnosis of lymphogranuloma inguinale.

Consists of injecting an extract from the lymph nodes of a lymphogranulomatous patient into the skin. Positive reaction is evidenced by marked reddening and thickening of the skin about the site of the injection.

fremitus (frĕm'ĭ-tŭs) [L]. Vibratory tremors, esp. those felt by palpation through the chest wall.

Varieties are vocal or tactile, friction, hydatid, rhonchal or bronchial, cavernous or succussion, pleural, pericardial, tussive, thrills. SEE: *palpation.*

    f., vocal. Vibrations of the voice transmitted to the ear on auscultation of the chest of a person speaking. In determining the vocal f. observe following precautions: Palpate symmetrical parts of chest; make firm pressure; when comparing use the same pressure on both sides; apply hands as nearly parallel to ribs as possible; remember the fremitus normally increases over the right apex. Is decreased in pleural effusions (air, pus, blood, serum, or lymph); emphysema; pulmonary collapse from an obstructed bronchus; pulmonary edema; morbid growths of the lung.

fre'nal [L. *fraenum*, bridle]. Pert. to the frenum.

French scale. A system used to indicate the diameter of catheters and sounds. Each unit on the scale is approx. equivalent to 1/3 mm.; thus a 21 French sound is 7 mm. in diameter.

frenosecretory (frē-nō-sē'krĕ-tor-ī) ["+ *secernere,* to secrete]. Exercising an inhibitory power over secretions.

frenotomy (frē-nŏt'ō-mī) ["+ Gr. *tomē,* incision]. Division of any frenum, esp. for tongue-tie.

frenulum (frĕn'ū-lŭm) [L., a little bridle]. (pl. *frenula*) 1. [NA] A small frenum. SYN: *vinculum.* 2. A small fold of white matter on the upper surface of the anterior medullary velum extending to the corpora quadrigemina.

    f. clitoridis. [NA] The union of inner parts of the labia minora on undersurface of the clitoris, q.v.

    f. labiorum pudendi. [NA] Fold of membrane connecting posterior ends of labia minora.

    f. linguae. [NA] A fold of mucus membrane which extends from the floor of the mouth to the inferior surface of the tongue along its midline.

    f. prepu'tii. [NA] One that unites the foreskin (prepuce) to the glans penis.

    f. of tongue. F. attaching lower side of tongue to the gum.

frenum (frē'nŭm) [L. *fraenum*, bridle]. (pl. *fre'na*) A fold of mucus membrane which connects two parts, one more or less movable, and serves to check the movement of this part. SEE: *frenulum*.

frenzy [ME. *frenesie*]. A state of violent mental agitation; maniacal excitement.

fre'quency [L. *frequēns*, often]. 1. The number of repetitions of a phenomenon in a certain period of time as the f. of heart beat, f. of sound vibrations. 2. In biometry, the ratio of the number of individuals falling into a single group (having a certain characteristic, disease, or condition) to the total number of individuals in the population being studied. This is usually expressed for a definite period of time. SEE: *incidence*.

  3. The rate of oscillation or alternation in an alternating current circuit, in contradistinction to periodicity in the interruptions or regular variations of current in a direct current circuit. F. is computed on the basis of a complete cycle, a complete cycle being one in which the current rises from zero to a maximum, returns to zero, and rises to an opposite maximum and returns to zero.

Freud, Sigmund (froyd). A famous Austrian neurologist and psychoanalyst (1856-1939) whose teachings stress the theory:

  (1) Of the existence of a subconscious mind.

  (2) That emotional processes have the attributes of quantity and can be displaced from one idea to another.

  (3) That the child experiences a rich sexual life and from this is derived the later stages of narcissism or self-love, homosexuality or attraction to the same sex, or heterosexuality which is the normal attraction to the opposite sex.

  (4) That dreams are fulfillments of wishes which find no realization in waking hours; theories are also formulated with regard to the importance of sex in dreams.

  (5) That forgetting, misplacing articles, and slips of the tongue or pen are the outward manifestation of repression.

  RS: abreaction; complex; consciousness; heterosexuality; homosexuality; narcissism; Oedipus complex; psychoanalysis; subconsciousness.

freudian (froy'dĭ-ăn). Pert. to Sigmund Freud or his theories of unconscious or repressed libido or past sex experiences or desires as the cause of various neuroses, the cure for which is the restoration of such conditions to consciousness through psychoanalysis. SEE: *Freud, Sigmund.*

fri'able [L. *friabilis*]. Easily broken or pulverized.

fric'tion [L. *frictio*]. In massage, strong circular manipulations always followed by centripetal stroking.

  In hydrotherapy, friction is used in drying patients after tonic baths, shampoos, salt glows, wet mitten friction, and drip sheet rubs.

  f., dry. F. using no liquid.

  f., moist. F. using a liquid or oil.

  f. murmur. A frictional sound heard in pleurisy. SYN: *f. sound.*

fric'tional electric'ity. Electricity produced by friction. SEE: *electricity, static.*

Friedländer's bacillus (frēd'lĕn-dĕr). [Karl Friedländer, Ger. physician, 1847-87] Klebsiella pneumoniae, q.v.

Fried'man's test. [Maurice H. Friedman, Amer. physiologist, 1903—]. Pregnancy test. The injection of the urine of a woman suspected of pregnancy into an unmated female rabbit will cause the formation of corpora lutea and corpora hemorrhagica in the rabbit at the end of two days if the woman is pregnant.

Friedreich's ataxia (frēd'rĭks). [Nikolaus Friedreich, Ger. neurologist, 1825-82]. Rare disease, resembling locomotor ataxia, occurring in children, esp. girls of the same family. SYN: *hereditary ataxia.*

Friedreich's disease. Friedreich's ataxia, q.v.

Friedreich's sign. 1. Sudden collapse of the cervical veins previously distended, at each diastole, caused by an adherent pericardium. 2. Lowering of the pitch of the percussion note during inspiration which occurs over an area of cavitation.

fright [AS. *fryhto*]. Extreme sudden fear.

  f. neuroses. Traumatic hysteria.

  f., precordial. Nausea and fear felt before the onset of manic-depressive illness.

frigid (frĭj'ĭd) [L. *frigidus*]. 1. Cold. 2. Irresponsive to emotion, applied esp. to the inability on the part of a woman to feel sexual desire.

frigidity (frĭ-jĭd'ĭ-tĭ). In the female, absence of sexual desire. Inability to have an orgasm.

frigolabile (frĭg''ō-lā'bĭl) [L. *frigor*, cold, + *labilis*, unstable]. Capable of being destroyed by low temperature.

frigorific (frĭg''ō-rĭf'ĭk) [L. *frigorificus*,]. Generating cold.

frig'orism [L. *frigor*, cold, + Gr. *ismos*, condition]. A condition due to long exposure to cold.

frigostabile (frĭg''ō-stā'bl) [" + *stabilis*, firm]. Incapable of being destroyed by low temperature.

frigotherapy (frĭg''ō-thĕr'ă-pĭ) [" + Gr. *therapeia*, treatment]. The use of cold in treatment of disease.

frit [It. *fritta,* fry]. 1. The material from which glass or the glazed portion of pottery is made. 2. A similar material for making the glaze of artificial teeth.

frog belly. Flaccid abdomen in children afflicted by rickets, and atony of abdominal cells resulting from dyspepsia, accompanied by flatulence.

frog face. Flatness of face resulting from intranasal disease.

Fröhlich's syndrome (frā'lĭk). [Alfred Fröhlich, Austrian neurologist, 1871-1953]. A condition characterized by adiposity of the female type, atrophy or hypoplasia of the gonads, and altered secondary sex characteristics. Due to disturbance of the hypothalamus and hypophysis. SYN: *adiposogenital dystrophy; sexual infantilism.*

Froin's syndrome (frō-an'). [Georges Froin, Fr. physician, 1874—]. Yellow cerebrospinal fluid which rapidly coagulates. It contains an excess of lymphocytes, and protein, particularly globulin.

frolement (frōl-mŏn') [Fr.]. 1. Very light friction with the hand in massage. SEE: *massage.* 2 A sound resembling rustling heard in auscultation.

Frommann's lines (frŏm'än). [Carl Frommann, Ger. anatomist, 1831-92]. Transverse lines in the axis cylinder of medullated nerve fibers. Demonstrated by staining with silver nitrate.

frons (frŏnz) [L.]. [NA] The forehead.

fron'tad [L. *frons, front-,* brow, + *ad,* toward]. Toward the frontal aspect.

fron'tal [L. *frontalis*]. 1. Anterior. 2. Pert. to the forehead bone.

     f. bone. Forehead bone.

     f. lobe. Four main convolutions in front of the central sulcus of the cerebrum.

     f. plane. A plane parallel with the long axis of the body and at right angles to the median sagittal plane.

     f. sinuses. A pair of hollow spaces in the frontal bone lying above the orbits. They are lined with mucus membrane, contain air, and communicate with the middle nasal meatus by means of the nasofrontal duct.

fronto- [L. *frons,* brow]. Prefix indicating anterior position or relationship with the forehead.

frontomalar (frŏn"tō-mā'lär) ["+ *mala,* cheek]. Rel. to the frontal and malar bones.

frontomaxillary (frŏn"to-măks'ĭ-lär"ĭ) ["+ *maxilla,* jaw]. Rel. to the frontal bone and maxillary bones.

frontoparietal (frŏn"tō-pă-rī'ĕ-tăl) ["+ *parietalis,* pert. to a wall]. Pert. to the frontal and parietal bones.

frontotem'poral ["+ *tempora,* the temples]. Pert. to frontal and temporal bones.

front-tap reflex. Contraction of gastrocnemius muscles resulting from percussing stretched muscles of extended leg.

frost [AS.]. Frozen vapor deposit.

     f., urea. Deposit of urea crystals on the skin in a patient whose kidneys are severely impaired, such as in uremia.

frostbite. Freezing or effect of freezing of a part of the body. The nose, fingers, and toes are usually the parts affected.

     SYM: Tingling, redness, followed by paleness and numbness of affected area. It is of three degrees: Transitory hyperemia following numbness; formation of vesicles; and gangrene.

     F.A. TREATMENT: Do not rub part with snow. Slow rewarming or rapid rewarming in water at 103°-105° F. (39.4-40.6° C.), rapid rewarming to be used if it is certain that the vascular tissues are not injured. Stimulate with tea, coffee, beef tea. Patient should not be allowed to smoke. Artificial respiration if unconscious. Patients have been known to recover when parts were black and the necessity of amputation seemed clear.

frost-itch. Itching skin disease in cold climates. SYN: *pruritus hiemalis.*

frottage (frō-tŏzh') [Fr., rubbing]. 1. A condition of hyperesthesia sexualis often associated with lowered virility inducing an irresistible impulse of pressing up behind women in crowds, thus producing an orgasm. 2. Massage technique using rubbing.

frotteur (frō-ter') [Fr. *frottage,* rubbing]. One who practices frottage, q.v.

fruc'tose [L. *frūctus,* fruit]. Levulose; fruit sugar.

     A monosaccharose and a hexose, having the same empirical formula as glucose, $C_6H_{12}O_6$, and found in corn syrup, honey, fruit juices, and in the syrup resulting from the inversion of sucrose; an invert sugar. It produces glycogen and maintains normal content of glucose in the blood. In the liver, it may be converted into glycogen, which in turn may be converted into glucose. SEE: *disaccharose.*

fructosuria (frŭk"tō-sū'rĭ-ă) ["+ Gr. *ouron,* urine]. Fructose in the urine.

fruit [L. *fructus,* fruit]. A ripened ovary of seed-bearing plants and the surrounding tissue. Ex: pod of a bean, nut, grain, pome, or berry. The edible product of a plant consisting of ripened seeds and the enveloping tissue.

     Fruits in general tend to add bulk to the diet. This quality, as well as in some cases their containing specific laxative substances, makes fruits quite helpful in treating constipation.

COMP: Carbohydrates in the form of f. sugar form the chief nutritive value of fruits. Seventy-five per cent of it is a mixture of dextrose and levulose. Proteins and energy factors are variable. Good source of vitamins and mineral elements. Iodine content, 6-120 parts/billion.

Pectose bodies: The principle in fruits that causes them to jell. Pectose is found in unripe f.; pectin is found in ripe f. Pectosic acid, from pectose, is found in cooked fruit; pectic acid, from pectin, is found in fruit cooked a long time.

Principal acids: Acetic in wine and vinegar. Citric in lemons, oranges, limes, and citron. Malic in apples, pears, apricots, peaches, currants, gooseberries. Tannic in gallnuts. Oxalic in rhubarb, sorrel, cranberries. Tartaric in grapes, pineapples, and tamarinds. Salicylic in currants, cranberries, cherries, plums, grapes, crabapples, and berries.

Combined acids: Citric and malic in raspberries, strawberries, gooseberries, cherries. Citric, malic, and oxalic in cranberries. They contain iron and other mineral substances.

f. sugar. Fructose, levulose, q.v.

frumentaceous (frū-mĕn-tā'shŭs) [L. *frumentum,* grain]. Resembling or belonging to grain.

frumenti, spiritus [L., essence of grain]. Whiskey.

frumentum (frū-mĕn'tŭm) [L.]. Wheat or other grain.

frustration [L. *frūstrātus,* disappointed]. 1. The failure of libido to find adequate outlet. 2. The condition which results from the thwarting or prevention of acts which if performed would bring satisfaction or gratification of physical or personality needs.

FSH. Abbr. for *follicle-stimulating hormone,* secreted by the anterior lobe of the hypophysis.

ft. Abbr. for L. *fiat* or *fiant,* let there be made; *florentium,* former name for promethium; *foot.*

FTA-ABS. Abbr. for *fluorescent treponemal antibody-absorption test for syphilis.*

fuel value. Energy to be produced by oxidation of edible foods after eating. SEE: *calorie; energy; food requirements.*

-fuge [L. *fugāre,* to put to flight]. Suffix meaning to expel or drive away.

fugitive (fū'jĭ-tĭv) [L. *fugitivus*]. 1. Temporary, transient. 2. Wandering; pert. to inconstant symptoms.

fugue (fyūg) [L. *fuga,* flight]. Serious personality dissociation. Leaving home or surroundings on impulse. Upon recovering from the fugue state there usually is loss of memory for actions occurring while in the state.

fulgurant (fŭl'gū-rănt) [L. *fulgurans*]. Severe and sudden coming and going like a flash of light, as a f. pain.

ful'gurating [L. *fulgurāre,* to lighten]. Pert. to fulguration. SYN: *fulgurant.*

fulguration (fŭl-gū-rā'shŭn). Destruction of tissue by means of long high frequency electric sparks. SEE: *electrodesiccation.*

fuliginous (fū-lĭj'ĭ-nŭs) [L. *fuligō,* soot]. Resembling soot, esp. in color.

full'ing [O. Fr. *fauler,* to fill]. A movement in massage; kneading with the limb held between the hands, rolling it backward and forward.

full term. Normal end of pregnancy, when the fetus is 20-21 in. (51-53 cm.) long, has well-developed finger- and toenails, and if a boy, with both testicles descended. The fetus should weigh 2500 gm. or more.

fulminant (fŭl'-, fŭl'mĭ-nănt) [L. *fulmināns*]. Fulgurant. Coming in lightninglike flashes of pain, as in tabes dorsalis.

ful'minating. Fulgurant; occurring with very great rapidity, said of certain pains.

fumes [L. *fūmus,* smoke]. Vapors, esp. those having irritating qualities.

f., nitric acid. Used in various chemical processes.

SYM: Choking, gasping, swelling of mucus membranes, tightness in chest, pulmonary edema, cough, and shock. Symptoms may last for one week or more.

TREATMENT: Should be directed at maintaining good ventilation of lungs. Therapy for shock. Administration of oxygen under pressure by using a mask may be required along with analgesics for anxiety. Cortisone may be helpful in diminishing inflammatory response in lungs.

fu'migant [L. *fūmigāre,* to make smoke]. An agent used in disinfecting a room. The substance used produces fumes which are lethal to insects and rodents.

fumiga'tion. 1. The use of poisonous fumes or gases to destroy living organisms, esp., rats, mice, insects, and other vermin. Fumigants are relatively ineffective against bacteria and viruses, consequently the practice of terminal disinfection of the sick room, formerly a common practice, has been discontinued. 2. The disinfecting of rooms by gases.

fu'ming [L. *fūmus,* smoke]. Having a visible vapor.

function (fŭng'shŭn) [L. *functiō,* performance]. 1. The action performed by any structure. In a living organism this may pertain to a cell or a part of a cell, tissue, organ, or system of organs. 2. The act of carrying on, or performing, a special activity. Normal f. is the normal action of an organ. Abnormal functioning or the failure of an organ to perform its f. are the bases of disease or disease processes. Structural changes in an organ constitute pathological changes and are common causes of malfunctioning, although an organ may f. abnormally in the absence of observable structural changes.

function, words pert. to: absorption; anabolism; analogue; assimilation; catabolism; digestion; excretion; metabolism; secretion.

func'tional. 1. Pert. to function. 2. A word applied to disturbances of function in a variety of ways.

The disturbance of function of one organ by structural change in another is at times termed f., but incorrectly, as it represents organic change. Disturbances of function resulting from unfortunate conditioning of the organism to an external situation may more suitably be called f., although this conditioning may be purely structural.

f. disease. Inorganic disease, or one in which changes of an organ are not in evidence; a disturbance of any organ's functions.

f. overlay. The emotional response to physical illness. This may take the form of a conversion or hysterical response, affective overreaction, prolonged symptoms of physical illness after signs of the illness have subsided, or combinations of these reactions.

F. overlay may appear to be the primary disease and require skillful diagnosis to determine the actual cause of illness.

f. psychosis. One exhibited in psychosis, in which no pathology of the central nervous system is apparent.

functioning tumor. A tumor which is capable of synthesizing the same product as the normal tissues from which they arise, esp. endocrine or nonendocrine tumors which produce hormones.

funda (fūn'dă) [L., sling]. A four-tailed bandage.

fundal (fŭn'dăl) [L. *fundus*, base]. Pert. to a fundus.

fundament (fŭn'dă-měnt) [L. *fundamentum*]. 1. A foundation. 2. The anus.

fundic (fŭn'dĭk). Pert. to a fundus.

fun'diform [L. *fundus*, sling, + *forma*, shape]. Sling-shaped or looped.

fun'dus [L., base]. (pl. *fundi*) [NA] 1. The larger part, base, or body of a hollow organ. 2. The portion of an organ most remote from its opening.

f. glands. Minute tubelike glands of the gastric mucosa in the cardiac section.

f. oculi. Posterior inner part of eye as seen with ophthalmoscope.

f. uteri. The body of the uterus from the internal os of the cervix upward above the fallopian tubes.

fundusectomy (fŭn"dŭs-ěk'tō-mĭ) [L. *fundus*, base, + Gr. *ektomē*, excision]. Excision of the fundus of the stomach. SYN: *cardiectomy*.

fungal septicemia. Presence of pathogenic fungi in the blood. May be seen as a complication of parenteral hyperalimentation SYN: *fungemia*.

fun'gate [L. *fungus*, mushroom]. To grow like a fungus.

fungating (fŭn'gāt-ing). Growing rapidly like a fungus, applied to certain tumors.

fungemia (fŭn-jē'mĭ-ă) [L. *fungus*, mushroom, + Gr. *haima*, blood]. Presence of fungi in the blood.

Fungi (fŭn'jī) [L. *fungus*, mushroom]. A division of plants which includes slime molds, sac fungi, club fungi, and imperfect fungi. They were formerly considered as a subdivision of the Thallophytes. Fungi are simple dependent plants lacking chlorophyll. Their bodies show little differentiation and they have relatively simple life cycles. They include the molds, rusts, mushrooms, toadstools, lichens, and yeasts. Many forms are pathogenic to plants and animals.

fungi. Pl. of fungus, q.v.

f. fission. The bacteria or Schizomycetes.

f. imperfect. The Fungi Imperfecti, or Deuteromycetes, a class of fungi so-called because their life cycles are only partly known, the sexual stage being absent. Many species are parasitic, causing disease.

f. slime. The slime molds, Myxomycetes.

f. true. F. with a plant body composed of hyphae. Include the algal fungi (Phycomycetes), sac fungi (Ascomycetes), club fungi (Basidiomycetes), and imperfect fungi (Fungi Imperfecti).

fungicide (fŭn'jĭ-sīd) [L. *fungi*, mushroom, + *cidus*, killing]. Bactericide; that which destroys bacteria or fungi.

fungiform (fŭn'jĭ-form) [" + *forma*, shape]. Fungus-shaped.

f. papillae. Small, rounded eminences on middle and anterior parts of dorsum and esp. along sides of tongue.

fungistasis (fŭn-jĭ-stā'sĭs) [" + Gr. *stasis*, a halting]. A condition in which the growth of fungi is inhibited. SEE: *fungicide*.

fungistat (fŭn'jĭ-stăt) ["+ Gr. *statikos,* standing]. That which inhibits the growth of fungi.

fungistatic. Inhibiting the growth of fungi.

fungoid (fŭn'goyd) [L. *fungus,* mushroom, + Gr. *eidos,* form]. Having the appearance of a fungus.

   f., chignon. Bacterial growth of the hair.

fungosity (fŭn-gŏs'ĭ-tĭ). A soft, spongy funguslike growth.

fungous (fŭn'gŭs). Fungus, q.v.

fungus (fŭn'gŭs) [L., *mushroom*]. (pl. *fungi)* 1. A vegetable cellular organism that subsists on organic matter. 2. A plant belonging to the division Fungi. 3. A sponge-like morbid growth on the body resembling fungus. SEE: *actinomycosis.*

fu'nic (fū'nĭk) [L. *funis,* cord]. Pert. to the umbilical cord.

   f. souffle. The purring sound heard over the pregnant uterus, and having the same rate as the fetal heart beat.

funicle (fū'nĭ-kl) [L. *funiculus,* little cord]. A small, threadlike structure. SYN: *funiculus.*

funicular (fū-nĭk'ū-lăr). Pert. to the spermatic or umbilical cord.

   f. process. That part of the tunica vaginalis that covers the spermatic cord.

funiculitis (fū-nĭk"ū-lī'tĭs) [L. *funiculus,* little cord, + Gr. *-itis,* inflammation]. Inflammation of the spermatic cord.

funiculopexy (fū-nĭk'ū-lō-pĕks-ĭ) ["+ Gr. *pēxis,* fixation]. Suturing the spermatic cord to the tissues in cases of undescended testicle.

funiculus (fū-nĭk'ū-lŭs) [L., little cord]. (pl. *funic'uli)* 1. [NA] Any small structure resembling a cord. 2. A division of the white matter of the spinal cord consisting of fasculi or fiber tracts lying peripherally to the gray matter. Differentiated into dorsal, lateral, and ventral funiculi.

fu'niform [L. *funis,* cord, + *forma,* shape]. Cordlike.

funis (fū'nĭs) [L., cord]. 1. A cordlike structure. 2. The umbilical cord.

fun'nel [L. *fundere,* to pour]. Conical, wideopen-mouthed device for pouring through its open tube at end into another vessel.

   f. breast. Sternal depression of chest walls resembling a f.

   f. drainage. Drainage by funnels.

funny bone. The internal condyle of the humerus.

F.U.O. Abbr. for *fever of unknown origin.*

furacin. Trade name for nitrofurazone, q.v.

fur'cal [L. *furca,* fork]. Forked.

furcula (fŭr'kū-lă) [L., little fork]. The hypobranchial eminence, an elevation in the floor of the embryonic pharynx at the level of the 3rd and 4th branchial arches. It gives rise to the epiglottis and the aryepiglottic folds.

furfur (fŭr'fŭr) [L., bran]. (pl. *fur'fures)* Scurf, dandruff.

furfuraceous (fŭr-fū-rā'shŭs). Scaly or resembling scales.

furibund (fū'rĭ-bŭnd) [L. *furibundus*]. Maniacal; raging, as in certain types of insanity.

fu'ror [L., rage]. Extremely violent outbursts or anger, often without provocation.

   f. amatorius. Insatiable sexual desire.

   f. epilepticus. Epileptic insanity or sudden anger as expressed by epileptics.

   f. feminius. Nymphomania, q.v.

   f. genitalis. Erotomania, q.v.

furred (ferd) [O.F. *forre,* lining]. Said of the tongue on which a dustlike deposit has formed.

furrow [AS. *furh*]. A groove.

furuncle (fū'rŭng-kl) [L. *furunculus*]. A boil. SYN: *furunculus.*

furuncular (fū-rŭng'kū-lăr). Pert. to a boil.

furunculoid (fū-rŭng'kū-loyd) [L. *furunculus,* boil, + Gr. *eidos,* form]. Resembling a furuncle or boil. SYN: *furunculous.*

furunculosis (fū-rŭng"kū-lō'sĭs) ["+ Gr. *ōsis,* condition]. A condition resulting from boils.

furunc'ulous. Pert. to or of the nature of a boil or boils.

furunculus (fū-rŭng'kū-lŭs) [L., a boil]. (pl. *furun'culi)* Boil, furuncle. Acute, deep-seated phlegmonous inflammation formed in the skin usually ending in suppuration and necrosis.

   ETIOL: Staphylococcal infection of follicular or sebaceous glands.

   SYM: Neck, axillae, face, buttocks and breasts are common sites of predilection, beginning in hair follicle or sudoriparous gland as subcutaneous swelling or acuminate pustule around hair shaft, skin smooth and shining, with pain and tenderness. Lesion may come to head, or become boggy and fluctuant, or regression may take place before suppuration, resulting in disappearance by absorption (blind boil). Lesion ruptures spontaneously or following incision, discharging core, necrotic tissue, and pus; healing follows.

   TREATMENT: Moist heat, incision or pointing of lesion, systemic antibiotic.

Fusarium (fū-zā'rĭ-ŭm) [L. *fusus,* spindle]. A genus of fungi.

fuscin (fŭs'ĭn) [L. *fuscus,* brown]. A brown pigment, a melanin, present in the outermost layer (pigmented epithelium) of the retina.

fuse (fūz) [L. *fūsus*, poured]. A safety device comprising a strip of wire of easily fusible metal, the conductance of which is predetermined. The metal fuses and breaks circuit when excess of current passes through. Convenient forms mounted in plugs, between hard metal ends under screwheads.

fu'sible. Capable of being melted.

fu'siform [L. *fūsus*, spindle, + *forma*, shape]. Tapering at both ends; spindle-shaped.

fusion (fū'shŭn) [L. *fūsiō*]. Meeting and joining together through liquefaction by heat. The process of fusing or uniting.

    f. faculty. Blending of the images of binocular vision into a single perception having the quality of depth.

    f., spinal. Surgical fusion of two or more vertebrae. SYN: *spondylosyndesis.*

Fus"obacter'ium. A genus of nonspore-forming, nonencapsulated, nonmotile, gram-negative bacteria usually found in necrotic lesions of the mouth and bowel.

    F. fusiforme. The causative òrganism of Vincent's infection. It is also found in the normal mouth. SYN: *fusiform bacillus.*

    F. plauti-vincenti. F. fusiforme.

fusocel'lular [L. *fūsus*, spindle, + *cellulus*, little cell]. Spindle celled.

fusospirillosis (fū"sō-spĭr-ĭl-ō'sĭs) ["+ *spirillum*, coil, + Gr. *-ōsis*, condition]. Vincent's angina.

fusospirochetal (fū"sō-spī-rō-kē'tăl) ["+ Gr. *speira*, coil, + *chaitē*, hair]. Pert. to fusiform bacilli and spirochetes such as found in Vincent's angina.

fusospirocheto'sis ["+ "+ "+ *-osis*, condition]. Infection with fusiform bacilli and spirochetes.

fusostreptococcosis (fū"sō-strĕp"tō-kŏk-kō'sĭs) [L. *fūsus*, spindle, + Gr. *streptos*, twisted, + *kokkos*, berry, + *-ōsis*, condition]. Infection with fusiform bacteria and streptococcus.

fustiga'tion [L. *fustigatio*]. In massage, beating with light rods.

fututrix (fū-tū'trĭks). A girl or woman who practices tribadism, q.v.

G

G. 1. The force of gravity. It causes bodies falling free to be accelerated at the rate of 32.17 feet/sec./sec. (980.62 cm./sec./sec.). 2. In aviation physiology, G. is a unit of force resulting from acceleration or centrifugal motion. 3. Abbr. for *gingival; gram(s)*.

G-6-PD. Glucose-6-phosphate dehydrogenase. An enzyme of the red blood cells. A deficiency of the enzyme may cause the red cells to hemolyze more rapidly than normal following administration of certain drugs to or ingestion of fava beans by patients; there are several variants of this disease.

Ga. Chem. symb. for gallium.

GABA. Abbr. for *gamma-aminobutyric acid.*

gad′fly. An insect which lays eggs under the skin of its victim, causing swellings simulating a boil. Multiple furuncles appear with hatching of larva. A fly belonging to the family Tabanidae, q.v. Includes horseflies, deerflies, and other bloodsucking flies. SEE: *botfly.*

gadolinium (găd″ō-lĭn′ĭ-ŭm). SYMB: *Gd.* At. wt. 157.25; at. no. 64. A very rare element.

Gaffkya (găf′kĭ-ă). [Georg T. A. Gaffky, Ger. bacteriologist, 1850-1918] A genus of bacteria of the family Micrococcaceae.

G. tetrag′ena. A species which occasionally causes arthritis, meningitis, pneumonia, soft-tissue abscesses, or endocarditis. SYN: *Micrococcus tetragenus.*

gag. 1. Device for keeping the jaws open or forcibly opening the mouth. 2. To retch or cause to retch.

g. reflex. Gagging and vomiting resulting from irritation of fauces.

Gaisböck′s disease (gīs′beks). [Felix Gaisböck, Ger. physician] Abnormal number of red corpuscles in blood with cardiac hypertrophy and elevated blood pressure, without splenic enlargement. SYN: *polycythemia hypertonica.*

gait (gāt) [ME. *gait,* passage]. Manner of walking.

Characteristic of certain anomalies: Body leans backward and feet are widely separated in pregnancy, obesity, ascites, and large abdominal tumors. Limping or hobbling g. is seen in rheumatism, sciatica, hip- or knee-joint disease or injury, metatarsal neuralgia, and affections of lower extremities such as poliomyelitis. When standing with feet close together in locomotor ataxia, aural vertigo, and disease of middle cerebellar lobe, patient sways and may fall. G. is slovenly in the weak, anemic, or apathetic and in patients with chronic mental or physical defects. SEE: *adiadochokinesis; asynergia; dysmetria; walking.*

g., ataxic. Raising foot high, striking ground suddenly with entire sole.

g., brachybasic. Shuffling g. of partial paraplegia.

g., cerebellar. A staggering movement.

g., cow. Swaying due to knock-knees.

g., equine. Raising foot by flexing thigh on abdomen. Characteristic of peroneal paralysis. Slow, awkward.

g., festinating. Body bent forward and rigid. Patient walks on toes as though pushed. Starts slowly, increases and may continue until he forces himself to stop by grasping some object for support.

g., flat-footed. Toes everted, legs often bowed.

g., frog. That of infantile paralysis: hopping.

g., hemiplegic. Patient abducts paralyzed limb, swings it around and brings it forward so foot comes to ground in front of him.

g., Huntington′s chorea. A few normal paces, a long slow one, and then one or two hops.

g., multiple neuritis. That of a high-stepping horse. Steppage g., q.v.

g., paralysis agitans. Tendency to begin slowly, then rapidly, falling forward. SYN: *festinating g.*

g., paralytic. Feet dragged with slow movements. Stumbles easily. Seen in chronic myelitis.

g., scissor. One in which legs cross in walking.

g., spastic. A stiff movement, toes seeming to catch and drag, legs held together, hips and knee joints slightly flexed. Seen in spastic paraplegia, sclerosis of lateral pyramidal columns of cord, tumor of spinal cord, and arachnoiditis.

g., steppage. Foot and toes lifted high, heel brought down first. Seen in peripheral neuritis, late stages of diabetes, alcoholism, chronic arsenical poisoning.

g., waddling. Feet wide apart and walk resembling that of a duck. Seen in coxa vara and double congenital displacement of hip when lordosis is present.

galact-, galacto- [Gr. *gala,* milk]. Combining forms, pert. to milk.

galactacrasia (gă-lăk″tă-krā′zĭ-ă) [Gr. *gala*, milk, + *akrasia*, bad mixture]. An abnormal composition of milk from the breast.

galactagogue (gă-lak′tă-gog) [″+ *agō-gos*, leading]. Agent that promotes the flow of milk.

galactan (gă-lak′tan). A complex carbohydrate forming galactose upon hydrolysis.

galac′tase. An enzyme or proteolytic ferment of milk.

galactemia (gă-lak-tē′mĭ-ă) [Gr. *gala*, milk, + *haima*, blood]. Milky condition of the blood.

galactic (gă-lak′tik). Pert. to flow of milk.

galactidrosis (gă-lăk″tĭ-drō′sĭs) [Gr. *gala*, milk, + *hidrōs*, sweat]. A milklike sweat.

galactin (gă-lak′tin). 1. A basic amorphous substance in milk. 2. Old term for prolactin, q.v.

galactischia (gal″ak-tisk′ĭ-ă) [Gr. *gala*, milk, + *ischein*, to suppress]. Suppression of the secretion and flow of milk. SYN: *galactoschesia.*

galactoblast (gă-lak′tō-blast) [″+ *blastos*, germ]. Body found in mammary acini; contains fat globules.

galactocele (gă-lak′tō-sēl) [″+ *kēlē*, hernia]. 1. A tumor caused by occlusion of a milk duct. 2. Hydrocele containing a milklike liquid.

galac′toid. Resembling milk.

galactolip′in [Gr. *gala*, milk, + *lipos*, fat]. A phosphorus-free lipid combined with galactose; a cerebroside.

galactoma (gal-ak-to′ma) [″+ *ōma*, tumor]. Cystic tumor of female breast. SYN: *galactocele*, def. 1.

galactom′eter [″+ *metron*, measure]. Device for measuring the specific gravity of milk. SYN: *lactometer.*

galactop′athy [″+ *pathos*, disease]. 1. Treatment of nursing infants by drugs administered to the mother. 2. Therapeutic use of milk. SYN: *galactotherapy.*

galactopex′ic [Gr. *gala*, milk, + *pēxis*, fixation]. Holding galactose. SEE: *galactopexy.*

galac′topexy. The fixation of galactose by the liver.

galactophagous (găl″ăk-tŏf′ă-gŭs) [″+ *phagein*, to eat]. Feeding upon milk.

galactophlysis (găl″ăk-tŏf′lĭ-sĭs) [Gr. *gala*, milk, + *phlysis*, eruption]. Eruption of vesicles containing milklike contents.

galac′tophore [″+ *pherein*, to bear]. A milk duct.

galactophoritis (găl-ăk″tō-fō-rī′tĭs) [″+ ″+ *-itis*, inflammation]. Inflammation of a milk duct.

galactophorous (gal″ak-tŏf′or-us). Giving milk.

g. ducts. Excretory ducts of the mammae.

galactophthisis (gal″ak-tof′thĭ-sis) [Gr. *gala*, milk, + *phthisis*, a wasting]. Debility and emaciation as result of excessive or prolonged milk secretion.

galactophygous (găl-ăk-tŏf′ĭ-gŭs) [″+ *phygē*, flight]. Arresting flow of milk.

galactoplania (gă-lăk″tō-plā′nĭ-ă) [″+ *planē*, wandering]. Secretion of milk in some part of the body other than the mammary gland.

galactopoietic (gă-lăk″tō-poy-ĕt′ĭk) [″+ *poiein*, to make]. 1. Having to do with the production of milk. 2. A substance which promotes the secretion of milk.

galactopyra (gă-lak″tō-pi′ră) [″+ *pyr*, fire]. Milk fever.

galactorrhea (gă-lak″tō-rī′ă) [″+ *rhoia*, flow]. 1. Continuation of lactation, or flow of milk at intervals after cessation of nursing. 2. Excessive flow of milk.

galactoschesia, galactoschesis (gal″ak-tō-skē′zĭ-ă, -tos′kĭ-sis) [″+ *schesis*, suppression]. A stopping of the milk secretion.

galactose (gă-lak′tōs). $C_6H_{12}O_6$ a monosaccharide or simple hexose sugar.

Galactose is an isomer of glucose and is formed, along with glucose, in the hydrolysis of lactose. It is dextrorotatory and reduces alkaline copper solutions such as Fehling's solution. It is a component of cerebrosides. In the digestive tract, galactose is readily absorbed; in the liver it is converted into glycogen.

galactosemia (gă-lăk″tō-sē′mĭ-ă) [galactose, + Gr. *haima*, blood]. An inborn error of metabolism characterized by decreased ability to convert galactose to glucose. It is due to congenital absence of the enzyme which is required for conversion of galactose to glucose and its derivatives. This enzyme is galactose 1-phosphate uridyl transferase.

In the past, galactose tolerance test was used to diagnose this disorder, but tests for galactose in the urine have made the test obsolete.

galactosis (gal-ak-tō′sis). The secretion of milk.

galactostasis (gal″ak-tos′tă-sis) [Gr. *gala*, milk, + *stasis*, a stopping]. Cessation or checking of milk secretion. SYN: *galactoschesia.*

galactosu′ria [″+ *ouron*, urine]. Galactose in the urine.

galactotherapy (gă-lak″tō-ther′ă-pĭ) [″+ *therapeia*, treatment]. 1. Treatment of a nursing infant by drugs administered to the mother. 2. Therapeutic use of milk, as a milk diet.

galactotoxin (gă-lak″tō-toks′in) ["+ *toxikon*, poison]. A toxic substance in milk. It is produced by bacteria.

galactotox′ism. Poisoning due to drinking milk which contains toxic substances.

galactotrophy (gal″ak-tot′ro-fĭ) [Gr. *gala*, milk, + *trophē*, nourishment]. Feeding with nothing but milk.

galactoxism (gal-ak-toks″izm) ["+ *toxikon*, poison, + *-ismos*, state of]. Poisoning by milk containing toxic substances. SYN: *galactotoxism.*

galactozymase (gă-lak″tō-zī′mās) ["+ *zymē*, leaven]. A starch-hydrolyzing enzyme in milk.

galactu′ria ["+ *ouron*, urine]. The passing of milky urine. SYN: *chyluria*, q.v.

galea (gā′lĭ-ă) [L. *galea*, helmet]. 1. The epicranial aponeurosis which connects the bellies of the occipitofrontal muscle. 2. A type of head bandage.

galeanthropy (gā″lē-an′thro-pĭ) [Gr. *galē*, cat, + *anthrōpos*, man]. A delusion that one has become transformed into a cat.

Ga′len, Claudius. A noted Greek physician and medical writer, 130?-200? A.D., born in Pergamum and later residing in Rome. Recognized as the authority on medicine through the Middle Ages. Called the father of experimental physiology.

   G.'s veins. The veins running through the tela chorioidea formed by the joining of the terminal and choroid veins, and forming the vena cerebri magna which empties into the straight sinus.

galena (gă-lē′nă). Lead sulfide ore.

galen′ic. Pert. to Galen or his teachings.

galenicals, galenics (gă-lĕn′ĭ-kăls, -ĭks). 1. Herb and vegetable medicines. 2. Crude drugs and medicinals as distinguished from pure active principles contained in them. 3. A medicine prepared according to an official formula.

galeophilia (gal″e-o-fil′ĭ-ă) [Gr. *galē*, cat, + *philein*, to love]. Fondness for cats.

galeophobia (gal″e-o-fo′bĭ-ă) ["+ *phobos*, fear]. Abnormal aversion to cats.

galeropia, galeropsia (gal-er-o′pĭ-ă, -op′-sĭ-ă) [Gr. *galeros*, cheerful, + *opsis*, vision]. Unusual clearness of vision.

gall [AS. *gealla*, sore place]. 1. An excoriation. 2. The bitter secretion of the liver stored in the gallbladder; bile. It has no ferments and it assists in the emulsifying of fats. It also stimulates intestinal action and multiplies the action of the pancreatic juice three-fold. It is discharged through the cystic duct into the duodenum.

   RS: bile ducts; calculus; "chol-" words; colic, biliary; cystic duct.

gallate (gal′lāt). A salt of gallic acid.

gall′bladder [AS. *gealla*, sore place + *blǣedre*, bladder]. Pear-shaped sac on undersurface of right lobe of liver holding bile from the liver until discharged through cystic duct; 3-4 in. (7.6 to 10.2 cm.) long, 1 in. (2.54 cm.) greatest diameter; capacity 50-75 ml. concentrated bile equivalent to 1 1/2 pt. (710 ml.) liver bile.

gall duct ["+ L. *ductus*, a passage]. Tube carrying bile from the liver and gallbladder.

gallium (gal′ĭ-um). SYMB: *Ga*. At. wt. 69.72; at. no. 31. A rare metal, small amounts of which are found in bauxite and zinc blende.

gal′lon [Med. L. *galleta*, jug]. Four liquid measure quarts; 231 cubic inches or 3.79 liters. In England the Imperial liquid gallon is 277.4 cubic inches or 4.55 liters.

gall′stone [AS. *gealla*, sore place + *stān*, stone]. Concretion formed in the gallbladder or bile ducts.

   Traditionally g.'s have been classified according to their composition. This information was then used to demonstrate the cause of the stone formation. This is no longer considered valid. Generally the core of all g.'s contains a mixture of cholesterol, bilirubin and protein.

   SYM: Stone may remain dormant and give little distress unless inflammation and distention of the gallbladder take place or unless it enters and is unable to pass through the biliary ducts, when colic ensues. The pain may radiate to the back and right shoulder, usually several hours after eating and when the stomach is empty; flatulence, jaundice usually absent.

   TREATMENT: Morphine under physician's directions. If attacks of biliary colic or cholecystitis persist, surgical treatment is indicated.

   NP: Postoperative position, propped up in bed to prevent pneumonia, to permit free drainage, and to relieve pressure on diaphragm. Lavage if vomiting is persistent. Only liquids in small amt. given. Note character of drainage and stools for color and nature of contents, and for proper discharge of bile. Protect drainage from all areas. Use cradle if no dressing is permitted, and absorbent pad at side for discharge.

   RS: bilifuscin; calculus; cholelithiasis.

Gal′ton's whistle. [Sir Francis Galton, Brit. scientist, 1822-1911] A whistle with which a note may be changed, used to test the hearing.

galvan′ic. [Luigi Galvani, It. physiologist, 1737-1798] Pert. to galvanism.

g. battery. A series of cells, giving a combined effect of all the units, and generating electricity by chemical reaction.

g. cell. One of a series of cells generating electricity through chemical reaction.

gal'vanism. Therapeutic use of direct current of electricity.

galvanization (gal-van-ĭ-za'shun). Employment of a galvanic current as a therapeutic measure.

galvanocau'tery [galvanism + Gr. *kautērion*, cautery]. Cauterization of tissue by means of an electric current. SEE: *electrocautery*.

galvanocontractil'ity ["+ L. *contractus*, drawn together]. Capability of a muscle of contracting under a galvanic stimulation.

galvanofaradiza'tion. Combined use of continuous and interrupted electrical current in treating a nerve or a muscle.

galvanom'eter [galvanism + Gr. *metron*, measure]. An instrument that measures current by electromagnetic action.

galvanopalpa'tion ["+ L. *palpāre*, to touch]. A method of measuring tactile sensibility of the nerves of the skin by use of electric current.

galvanopunc'ture ["+ L. *punctura*, puncture]. Introduction of needles to complete a galvanic current.

galvanoscope (găl-văn'ō-skōp) [galvanism + Gr. *skopein*, to examine]. Instrument which shows the presence and direction of a galvanic current.

galvanosur'gery ["+ Gr. *cheir*, hand, + *ergon*, work]. Use of galvanism in surgery.

galvanotax'is ["+ Gr. *taxis*, a drawing up in rank and file]. The tendency of a living organism to arrange itself in a medium so that its axis bears a certain relation to the direction of the electric current in the medium.

galvanotherapeu'tics, galvanother'apy ["+ Gr. *therapeia*, treatment]. Treatment by means of electricity. SYN: *electrotherapy*.

gal"vanotherm'y ["+ Gr. *thermē*, heat]. Treatment by the heat from a galvanic battery.

galvanot'onus ["+ Gr. *tonos*, tension]. Tonic contractions caused by a galvanic current.

galvanot'ropism ["+ Gr. *tropos*, a turn]. The tendency of an organism to grow, turn, or move into a certain relation with an electric current.

gamete (găm'ēt) [Gr. *gamein*, to marry]. A mature male or female reproductive cell; the spermatozoon or ovum. SEE: *chromosome*.
RS: conception; embryo; fertilization; gene; maturation; ovum; spermatozoon.

gamet'ic. Pert. to gametes.

gametocide (gam'ē-tō-sīd) ["+ L. *caedere*, to kill]. An agent destructive to gametocytes, particularly those of malaria.

gametocyte (gă-me'to-sīt) ["+ *kytos*, cell]. The sexual cell forming the gamete. An oocyte or spermatocyte.

gametogen'esis [Gr. *gamein*, to marry, + *genesis*, production]. Development of gametes: oogenesis or spermatogenesis. SEE: *maturation*.

gametog'ony. The phase in the life cycle of the malarial parasite (Plasmodium) in which male and female gametocytes, which infect the mosquito, are formed.

gamet'ophyte [Gr. *gamein*, to marry + *phyton*, plant]. In plants, the sexual or gamete-producing generation which alternates with the asexual or spore-producing generation.

Gam'gee tissue. [Sampson Gamgee, Brit. surgeon, 1826-1886] A dressing made of a thick layer of absorbent cotton between two layers of absorbent gauze; used for surgical dressing.

gam'ic [Gr. *gamein*, to marry]. Sexual, esp. as applied to eggs which develop only after fertilization in contrast to those which develop parthenogenetically.

gam'ma [Gr. letter g.]. 1. Third letter of the Gr. alphabet, γ. 2. In chemistry it is used to designate the third of a series, as the third carbon atom in an aliphatic chain. 3. One microgram; or one thousandth of a milligram (0.001 mg.); or one millionth of a gram.

g. globulin. A protein formed in the blood. Ability to resist infection is related to concentration of such proteins.

g. rays. Electromagnetic waves of extremely short wave length emitted by radioactive substances. They are thought to be of the same nature as x-rays. They have greater penetrating power than alpha or beta rays. SEE: *ray*.

gam'macism. Inability to pronounce correctly g and k sounds.

Gamna's disease. [Carlos Gamna, It. physician, 1896 —] Splenomegaly with slow, progressive enlargement of the spleen.

Gamna's nodules. Nodules stained yellow or brown in certain varieties of splenic enlargement. SEE: *G.'s disease*.

gamo- [Gr. *gamos*, marriage]. Combining form indicating relationship to marriage or sexual union.

gam'ont ["+ *ōn*, being]. A sexual form of certain protozoons.

gamophobia (gam"o-fo'bĭ-ă) ["+ *phobos*, fear]. Neurotic fear of marriage.

gampsodactylia (gamp"so-dak-til'ĭ-ă) [Gr. *gampsos*, curved, + *daktylos*, digit]. Deformity of the toes causing them to resemble claws. SYN: *clawfoot.*

ganglial (gang'lĭ-ăl) [Gr. *ganglion,* knot]. Pert. to a ganglion. SYN: *ganglionic.*

gangliated (gang'lĭ-at-ed). 1. Having ganglia. 2. Intermixed.

     g. cord. Main trunk of sympathetic nervous system.

gangliec'tomy [Gr. *ganglion,* knot, + *etomē,* excision]. Excision of a ganglion.

gangliform (gang'lĭ-form) ["+ L. *forma,* shape]. Formed like a ganglion.

ganglioform (gang'lĭ-o-form). Gangliform.

ganglioglio'ma (Gr. *ganglion,* knot, + *glia,* glue, + *ōma,* tumor). A ganglion-cell glioma.

ganglioglioneuroma (gang"glĭ-o-glī"o-nu-ro'ma) ["+ "+ *neuron,* nerve, + *ōma,* tumor]. Ganglion cells, glia cells, and nerve fibers in a nerve tumor.

ganglioma (gang-lĭ-o'mă) ["+ *ōma,* tumor]. 1. Tumor of a lymphatic gland. 2. A swelling of lymphoid tissue.

ganglion (gang'lĭ-ŏn) [Gr.]. (pl. *ganglia* or *ganglions*) 1. A mass of nervous tissue composed principally of nerve-cell bodies and lying outside the brain or spinal cord: e.g. the chain of ganglia which form the main sympathetic trunks; the dorsal root g. of a spinal nerve. 2. Cystic tumors developing on a tendon or aponeurosis; sometimes occur on the back of the wrist.

     g., abdominal. Any one of the abdominal ganglia.

     g., anterior cerebral. Corpus striatum. Corpus striatum and corpus lenticulare considered together.

     g., aorticore'nal. A g. lying near to the lower border of the celiac g. It is located near the origin of the renal artery.

     g., Arnold's auricular. Tiny g. located beneath foramen ovale. SYN: *otic g.; otoganglion.*

     g., auricular. G., Arnold's auricular, q.v.

     g., autonomic. A g. of the autonomic division of the nervous system.

     g., basal. Mass of gray matter beneath 3rd ventricle. Consisting of the caudate, lentiform, and amygdaloid nuclei and the claustrum.

     g., basal optic. Mass of gray matter beneath 3rd ventricle.

     g., cardiac. Tiny g. toward which converge the fibers of superficial cardiac plexus. It lies on the right side of the ligamentum arteriosus. SYN: *ganglion of Wrisberg.*

     g., carotid. G. formed by filamentous threads from the carotid plexus beneath the carotid artery.

     g., celiac. One of a pair of prevertebral or collateral ganglia located near the origin of the celiac artery. They form a part of the celiac plexus. SYN: *semilunar g.*

     g., cerebral. Main cerebral nerve centers.

     g., cervical. Three pairs of ganglia (superior, middle, inferior) located in the neck region. They are the ganglia of the cervical portion of the sympathetic trunk.

     g., cervicouterine. G. near the uterine cervix. SYN: *Frankenhauser's ganglion.*

     g., ciliary. Tiny g. located in the rear portion of the orbit.

     g., coccygeal. A g. located in the coccygeal plexus and forming the lower termination of the two sympathetic trunks; sometimes absent.

     g., collateral. A prevertebral g.

     g., dorsal root. A g. located on the dorsal root of a spinal nerve. Contains the cell bodies of sensory neurons. SYN: *posterior root g.; spinal g.*

     g., gasserian. It lies on the sensory root of the trigeminal nerve and from it arise the three branches (ophthalmic, maxillary, mandibular). SYN: *semilunar g.*

     g., geniculate. A g. on the pars intermedia, the sensory root of the facial nerve. It lies in the anterior border of the anterior geniculum of the facial nerve.

     g., inferior mesentric. A prevertebral sympathetic g. located in the inferior mesenteric plexus near the origin of the inferior mesenteric artery.

     g., interpeduncular. SEE: *nucleus, interpeduncular.*

     g., intervertebral. A spinal g., q.v.

     g., jugular. A g. located on the root of the vagus nerve and lying in upper portion of jugular foramen.

     g., lateral. One of a chain of ganglia forming the main sympathetic trunk. SYN: *vertebral g.*

     g., lenticular. G., ciliary, q.v.

     g., lumbar. G. usually four in number in the lumbar portion of the sympathetic trunk.

     g., nodose. G. of the trunk of the vagus nerve. Located immediately below jugular g. It makes connections with the spinal accessory nerve, hypoglossal nerve, and the superior cervical g. of the sympathetic trunk.

     g., ophthalmic, g., optic. G., ciliary, q.v.

     g., otic. A small g. located deep in the zygomatic fossa immediately below the foramen ovale. It lies medial to the mandibular nerve. It supplies postganglionic parasympathetic fibers to the parotid gland. SYN: *Arnold's auricular g.*

g., petrous. G. located on lower margin of temporal bone's petrous portion.

g., pharyngeal. G. in contact with the glossopharyngeal nerve.

g., phrenic. One of a group of ganglia joining the phrenic plexus.

g., renal. One of a group of ganglia joining the renal plexus.

g., sacral. Four small ganglia located in the sacral portion of the sympathetic trunk. They lie on the anterior surface of the sacrum and are connected to the spinal nerves by gray rami.

g., semilunar. 1. G., gasserian, q.v. 2. G., ciliac, q.v.

g., sphenopalatine. A g. associated with the great superficial petrosal nerve (branch of facial) and the maxillary nerve. It transmits both sympathetic and parasympathetic fibers to the nasal mucosa, palate, pharynx and orbit.

g., spinal. Ganglionic enlargement of spinal nerves' dorsal roots. SYN: *dorsal root g.; posterior root g.*

g., spiral. A long coiled g. in the cochlea of the ear. It contains bipolar cells, the peripheral processes of which terminate in the organ of Corti. The central processes form the cochlear portion of the acoustic nerve and terminate in the cochlear nuclei of the medulla.

g., submaxillary. A g. lying between the mylohyoideus and hyoglossus muscles and suspended from the lingual nerve by two small branches. Peripheral fibers pass to the submandibular, sublingual, lingual, and adjacent salivary glands. SYN: *submandibular g.*

g., superior mesenteric. A prevertebral g. of the sympathetic nervous system which lies close to the celiac g. and with it forms a part of the celiac plexus. It lies close to the base of the superior mesenteric artery.

g., suprarenal. G. situated in the suprarenal plexus.

g., sympathetic. Those of the thoracolumbar (sympathetic) division of the autonomic nervous system. Include vertebral or lateral ganglia (those forming the sympathetic trunk) and prevertebral or collateral ganglia, more peripherally located.

g., temporal. Tiny g. joining the anterior branches of superior cervical g.

g., terminal. A g. of the autonomic division of the nervous system which lies close to or within the organ innervated.

g., thoracic. One of 11 or 12 ganglia of the thoracic area of sympathetic trunk.

g., tympanic. On tympanic portion of the glossopharyngeal nerve.

g., vestibular. A bilobed g. located on the vestibular branch of the acoustic nerve at the bottom of the internal acoustic meatus. Its peripheral fibers arise in the maculae of the sacculus and utriculus and the cristae of the ampullae of the semicircular ducts. SYN: *g. of Scarpa.*

gang'lionated. Having or consisting of ganglia.

ganglionectomy (gang'lĭ-ō-nĕk'tō-mĭ) [Gr. *ganglion,* knot, + *ektomē,* excision]. Excision of a ganglion.

ganglioneuroma (gang'lĭ-o-nū-ro'mă) [" + *neuron,* nerve, + *ōma,* tumor]. A neuroma containing ganglion cells.

ganglionic (gang-lĭ-on'ik). Pert. to or of the nature of a ganglion.

ganglionitis (gang'lĭ-on-ī'tis) [Gr. *ganglion,* knot, + *-itis,* inflammation]. Inflamed condition of a ganglion.

gang'lioside. A cerebroside present in the brain and containing neuraminic acid, a particular type of fatty acid.

gangosa (gang-go'să) [Sp. *gangosa,* muffled voice]. A lesion of the nose and hard palate, regarded as a late stage of yaws. SYN: *rhinopharyngitis mutilans.*

gangrene (gang'grēn) [Gr. *gangraina,* an eating sore]. A necrosis, or death, of tissue, usually due to deficient or absent blood supply.

ETIOL: Usually results from cutting off of blood supply to an organ or tissue, which may have resulted from inflammatory processes, injury, or degenerative changes such as arteriosclerosis. It is commonly a sequela of boils, frostbite, crushing injuries, or diseases such as diabetes, and Raynaud's disease. Emboli in large arteries in almost any part of the body will, due to cutting off of the blood supply, cause gangrene of the area distal to that point. The part that dies is known as a slough if the soft tissues are involved, or a sequestrum if it is a bone that dies. The dead matter must be removed before healing can take place.

g., anemic. G. resulting from an obstructed circulation in the part.

g., angioneurotic. State resulting from thrombotic arteries and veins.

g., diabetic. Moist gangrenous condition arising in some diabetics.

g., dry. This results when the part that dies has little blood and when it remains aseptic. The arteries but not the veins are obstructed. The tissues dry and drop off, the process continuing for weeks or months.

SYM: Pain in early stages. The part is cold and black and begins to wither. The toes are generally first affected, the necrosis then spreading upward. Usually seen in advanced diabetes and arteriosclerosis.

g., embolic. Gangrenous condition arising subsequent to an embolic obstruction.

g., gas. This is g. in a wound infected by a gas bacillus, the most common etiologic agent being clostridium perfringens. TREATMENT: Antibiotics, clostridial antitoxin. In some cases surgical intervention may be necessary.

g., hospital. Moist g. due to wound contamination by putrefactive bacteria. It was common in hospitals in the days when overcrowding and lack of cleanliness were the rule.

g., humid. G., moist, q.v.

g., idiopathic. When the cause is unknown.

g., inflammatory. That associated with acute infections and inflammation.

g., moist. This occurs after a crushing injury, usually at distal part of an extremity, or when dry gangrene is infected with putrefactive bacteria, and when the part is full of blood. SYM: The part is hot, red; later cold and bluish, commencing to slough. It spreads rapidly and there is an offensive odor. The process is known to the layman as mortification. Death may result in a few days.

g., primary. G. developing in a part without previous inflammation.

g., secondary. G. developing subsequent to local inflammation.

g., symmetric. G. on opposite sides of the body in corresponding parts. Usually the result of vasomotor disturbances. Characteristic of Raynaud's and Buerger's disease.

g., traumatic. Result of extensive injuries.

gangrenosis (gang″grĕn-ō'sĭs) [" + -ōsis, condition]. Condition of mortification or gangrene.

gang'renous. Of the nature of gangrene.

gan'oblast [Gr. ganos,·brightness, + blastos, cell]. The cell which forms enamel of a tooth. SYN: ameloblast.

Ganser's syndrome (găn'zĕr). [Sigbert J. M. Ganser, Ger. phychiatrist, 1853-1931] Nonsense syndrome. Absurd acts and speech seen in prison psychosis, hysteria, and other states. In many cases it appears that the patient is attempting to act out what he imagines psychotic behavior to be like.

gap [Old Norse, gap, chasm]. An opening or a break; an interruption in continuity.

g., auscultatory. A period of silence which occurs in the determination of blood pressure by the auscultatory method. Exact cause unknown. May cause a false reading of the blood pressure. SEE: blood pressure.

g., cranial. A congenital fissure in the skull.

gargarism (gar'gar-izm) [Gr. gargarisma, a gargle]. A gargle or throat wash.

gargle (gar'gl) [L. gurgulio, windpipe]. 1. A wash for the throat. 2. To wash out the mouth and throat by tipping the head back so that the fluid runs to the tonsils and is there agitated by expired air that is forced out of the lungs.

gargoylism. A condition, usually congenital, characterized by dwarfism, kyphosis, and other skeletal abnormalities, disturbances in lipoid metabolism, and usually mental deficiency. SYN: Hurler's disease; lipochondrodystrophy.

garlic [AS. gār, spear, + lēac, the leek]. An edible, strongly flavored bulb of Allium sativum used mainly for seasoning. COMP: The active principle of garlic is allyl sulfide.

gar'rot [Fr. garroter, to tie fast]. A form of tourniquet.

Gart'ner's duct. [Hermann T. Gartner, Danish surgeon and anatomist, 1785-1827] A small duct, the mesosalpinx lying parallel to the uterine tube. It is a vestigial structure representing the persistent mesonephric duct. SYN: duct of the epoophoron; ductus epoophori longitudinalis.

G.A.S. Abbr. for general adaptation syndrome.

gas. 1. One of the basic forms of matter. The molecules are free and move swiftly in all directions. Thus a g. not only takes the shape of the containing vessel but expands and fills the vessel no matter what its volume.

Among the common important g.'s are oxygen; nitrogen; hydrogen; helium; sewer g., which contains carbon monoxide (q.v.), carbon dioxide (q.v.); the anesthetic g.'s; ammonia (q.v.); the poison war g.'s etc. Liquids and solids when heated often give off fumes which may be poisonous; among the more common are the mineral acids; ammonia water; mercury and its compounds; cyanides; zinc-containing metals, etc. SEE: anesthesia; gases.

g. bacillus. SEE: gangrene.

g., digestive tract. Among the g.'s in the digestive tract are: oxygen; nitrogen; hydrogen; carbon dioxide; methane; and in decomposition of proteins, hydrogen sulfide, indole, skatole.

g., distention. Abdominal distention is result of abnormal gaseous, fluid, or solid accumulation in abdominal cavity. It may be: acute; chronic; local, or general. The abdominal wall, the cavity, or the intra-abdominal viscera may be involved. *Postoperative:* Result of complication following an operation. Limited to lower part of small, and all of large intestines. Careless administration of anesthesia may be a cause, as is degree of peritonitis. *Preoperative:* Enema may prevent.

TREATMENT: No cold fluids, change of posture, insertion of rectal tube; enemata only as advised by surgeon.

g. excretions. Metabolic processes produce carbon dioxide which is excreted through the lungs. The amount produced increases as physical activity increases.

g., gangrene. That caused by the g. bacillus. SEE: *gangrene.*

g., illuminating. This is a mixture of various combustible gases including hydrogen and carbon monoxide. Its poisonous effects are largely due to carbon monoxide, q.v. TREATMENT: Resuscitation, q.v.

g., inert. G. such as helium, argon, neon or krypton, which react little if at all with other substances.

g. in the blood. The principal g.'s found in the blood are oxygen, nitrogen, and carbon dioxide. They may be dissolved in the plasma or they may exist in loose chemical combination with other compounds, as oxygen combined with hemoglobin.

g., laughing. Nitrous oxide.

g., marsh. Methane.

g., mustard. Poisonous gas used in warfare (dichlorethyl sulfide).

g., noble. SEE: *inert gas.*

g., refrigerant. A number of these gases are used in ordinary household mechanical refrigerators. Poisoning may be caused by leaks, faulty connections or breakage, with gas dissipated into the atmosphere. Among these gases are methyl chloride, ammonia, sulfur dioxide and more than 20 other gases. Most of these are toxic. Careful researches are now being carried on to develop nontoxic gases. Warning agents mixed with these gases are not a guarantee of protection to infants, children, hospital patients, firemen and refrigerator workers; therefore, instead of merely adding a protective agent, it would be wiser to have a nontoxic refrigerant. Methyl chloride is the most common cause of poisoning due to refrigerant g.'s. Sulfur dioxide, because it is an irritant to the respiratory tract, is easily detected.

g., tear. A g. that irritates the conjunctiva, producing a flow of tears.

gaseous (gas'ĭ-us). Of the nature or form of gas.

gases, war. Any chemical substances, whether solid, liquid, or vapor, used to produce poisonous g.'s with irritant effects. They can be classified as lacrimators, sternutators, (i.e., sneeze-causing), lung irritants, vesicants, and those that act as a systemic poison, such as nerve g.'s. Some g.'s have multiple effects.

They are known as persistent or nonpersistent, i.e., those which diffuse and are dispersed fairly rapidly, and those which linger and evaporate slowly.

It is of the greatest importance that persons rendering first aid should avoid becoming casualties; precautions must be taken, masks worn, as well as being fitted to the patients. Strict discipline must be maintained during g. raids in order to avoid panic. If g. training has been thorough and if organization is good, much may be done to lessen the effect, and maintain a good morale.

Decontamination centers are essential and nurses must understand that thorough decontamination of clothing, boots, ambulances, etc., is vitally necessary, and they should make themselves familiar with the necessary procedures.

It is also important to remove all clothing which is contaminated with the g. prior to bringing the patient into the hospital emergency room. If this precaution is not taken the unaffected persons in the area may become casualties.

g., lewisite. Contains arsenic and smells of geraniums.

SYM: Similar to those of vesicant gas, q.v., but come on at once and as a rule are not so severe. Arsenic can be recovered from the serum of the blisters and symptoms of arsenic poisoning may occur.

TREATMENT: Similar to that for vesicant gas, q.v.

g., lung irritant. Ex: Chlorine and phosgene.

SYM: Burning sensation of the eyes, nose, and throat, bronchitis and pneumonia, sometimes followed by edema of the lungs and probably death.

TREATMENT: Remove patient from exposure, apply respirator; if there has been exposure to phosgene (smells like musty hay), the symptoms may be delayed and the patient may collapse later. It is important, therefore, to provide complete rest, remove patient on a stretcher, and provide warmth; oxygen may be required in large quantities over a fairly long period.

g., mustard. Dichlorethyl sulfide. SEE: *g., vesicant.*

g., nerve. One which acts by interfering with or preventing transmission of nerve impulses.

g., nose irritant. Diphenylchloroarsine. An irritant smoke.

SYM: Intense pain in the nose, throat, and air passages; sneezing followed by headache and aching in teeth and jaws; acute mental depression, and sometimes vomiting.

TREATMENT: Casualties must be reassured that no permanent harm is done and should be warned against removing respirator in spite of the fact that the symptoms may get worse after donning it. This is a g. likely to lead to panic. Nasal douching with warm sodium bicarbonate is helpful.

g., suffocating. Made from chlorine compounds.

g., tear. Substance which, when dispersed into the air, interferes with seeing due to sudden and excessive production of tears. Ex: bromoacetone.

TREATMENT: As a rule, none is necessary, for upon removal from the contaminated area, the symptoms tend gradually to subside. Irrigating the eyes with large amounts of clear water or physiological saline will hasten recovery.

g., toxic. Hydrocyanic acid type.

g., vesicant. Also known as blister gas because of its effect on the skin. Attacks every part of body; clothing and boots are infected and a source of danger. Ex: mustard g., lewisite.

SYM: Do not appear at once; may be six hours or longer before the patient is aware of anything wrong. Pain in the eyes, lacrimation, and discharge may be the first evidence, the eyelids swelling and the patient being unable to see; there is a diffuse redness of the skin, followed by blistering and ulceration.

PROG: Healing is very slow, but generally follows if treatment is prompt and efficient.

TREATMENT: Decontamination is essential and must be thorough. Bathe eyes freely with normal saline or plain water; a drop or two of castor oil will prevent lids sticking; no bandage should be worn. The patient should be scrubbed, if possible, under a hot or warm shower for 10 minutes. Bleach cream or powder, if ordered, should be applied first, and left in contact with the skin for five minutes. If, in spite of these precautionary measures, blisters arise, they may be successfully treated with tannic acid.

g., vomiting. G. which induces emesis, specifically chloropicrin.

gas'oline. A product of the destructive distillation of petroleum.

Commercial gasolines may contain additives such as tetraethyl lead or tricresyl phosphate which are toxic.

POISONING SYM: Giddiness; headache; intoxication; nervous disturbance; muscular tremors; difficulty in respiration; paralyses; convulsions; cyanosis; unconsciousness; pulmonary hemorrhage. Usually no local disturbance of stomach unless the gasoline has been swallowed.

F.A. TREATMENT: Fresh air, inhalation of oxygen and carbon dioxide; artificial respiration when necessary. Otherwise treat symptoms. If clothing and skin have been grossly contaminated all precautions to prevent sparks and open flames must be taken. Gasoline is highly inflammable and when mixed with air is also explosive.

gasomet'ric. Pert. to measurement of gases.

gasometry (gas-om'ĕ-trĭ) [Gr. *metron*, measure]. Estimation of amount of gas present in a mixture.

gasp [Old Norse *geispa,* gasp]. To catch the breath; to inhale and exhale with quick, difficult breaths; the act of gasping.

gasserectomy (gas''er-ek'tō-mĭ). Excision of the gasserian ganglion.

gas'sing. The use of war gases, q.v.

gaster-, gastero-, gastro-. Combining forms meaning "pertaining to the stomach or the region of the stomach."

gasteral'gia [Gr. *gastēr,* belly, + *algos,* pain]. Gastralgia, q.v.

gasterangiemphraxis (gas''ter-an''jĭ-em-fraks'is) ["+ *angeion,* vessel, + *emphraxis,* obstruction]. 1. Congestion of blood vessels of stomach. 2. Pyloric obstruction.

gasterasthenia (gas''ter-as-thē'nĭ-ă) ["+ *asthenēs,* weak]. Gastrasthenia, q.v.

gasterhysterotomy (gas''ter-his''ter-ot'o-mĭ) ["+ *hystera,* uterus, + *tomē,* incision]. Incision of uterus through abdomen. SEE: *cesarean section.*

Gasterophilus (gas''ter-of'ĭ-lus). A genus of botflies belonging to the family Oestridae, order of Diptera. The larvae infest horses.

G. hemorrhoidalis. A species which infests horses.

G. intestinalis. Infest stomach of horses.

G. nasalis. The chin fly. Eggs are laid on shafts of hairs on lower lip and jaw of horses.

gastorrhagia (găs-tōr-ā'jĭ-ă) [Gr. *gastēr,* belly, + *rhēgnynai,* to burst forth]. Gastrorrhagia, q.v.

gastradenitis (gas″trad-en-i′tis) ["+ *adēn*, gland, + *-itis*, inflammation]. Inflammation of the stomach glands.

gastralgia (gas-tral′ji-ă) ["+ *algos*, pain]. Pain in the stomach from any cause.

gastralgocenosis (găs-trăl″gō-sĕn-ō′sĭs). Gastralgokenosis, q.v.

gastralgokenosis (gas-tral″go-ken-o′sis) [Gr. *gastēr*, stomach, + *algos*, pain, + *kenō-sis*, emptiness]. Gastric pain due to emptiness of stomach; hunger pangs due to hunger contractions, powerful peristalic contractions which sweep over the stomach.

gastraneuria (gas″tra-nu′rĭ-ă) ["+ *neuron*, nerve]. Defective action of nerves of the stomach.

gastrasthe′nia ["+ *asthenēs*, weak]. Debility of the stomach. SYN: *gasterasthenia.*

gastratrophia (gas″tră-tro′fĭ-ă) ["+ *atrophia*, atrophy]. Atrophy of the stomach.

gastrecta′sia, gastrec′tasis ["+ *ektasis*, dilatation]. Dilatation of the stomach. May be acute or chronic.

ETIOL: Obstruction of pylorus; atony, overeating, congenital weakness, imperfect peristalsis, omental hernia, periduodenal adhesions, gastroptosis.

SYM: *Chronic:* Vomiting of food taken several days before, vomitus sour, contains fatty acids, mucus, bacteria. *Acute:* Severe, sudden pain accompanied by collapse. Small, rapid pulse, temperature subnormal, upper abdominal pain resembling angina pectoris. Distended and tympanic abdomen. Vomiting of fluids and eructation of gas.

gastrectomy (gas-trek′tōmĭ) [Gr. *gastēr*, belly, + *ektomē*, excision]. Surgical removal of a part or the whole of the stomach.

gas′tric [Gr. *gastēr*, stomach]. Pert. to the stomach. SEE: *digestion; stomach.*

g. analysis. Determines quality of secretion, amount of free and combined hydrochloric acid, absence or presence of blood, bile, bacteria, fatty acids. The test is particularly helpful in suspected cases of gastric bleeding, gastric carcinoma or pernicious anemia.

g. digestion. The stomach serves as a temporary storage and mixing place for food. While there the semisolid mass of food known as chyme is mixed with the salivary juices, and certain other substances are added from the stomach, including hydrochloric acid, mucus, pepsin and some lipase. Infants also secrete remin which digests milk proteins.

CHEMICAL ASPECTS: During the meal, nervous impulses from the brain are carried to the stomach by way of the vagi; they result from the sensations of sight, smell, and taste. In addition, the stretching of the stomach wall excites the g. glands by local nervous mechanisms. This causes the hormone gastrin to be discharged from the pyloric region into the blood. The circulating gastrin reaches the g. glands and causes them to secrete.

The following changes occur in the food while in the stomach. Pepsin acts on proteins of high molecular weight hydrolyzing them to proteoses and peptones. Pepsin also coagulates milk. Hydrochloric acid is essential for the activity of pepsin. It also dissolves collagen, disintegrates nucleoproteins, hydrolyzes double sugars, and is responsible for the antiseptic action of the g. juice. G. lipase acts on emulsified fats, reducing them to fatty acids and glycerol but its action is limited.

MOTOR ASPECTS: After the initial relaxation, the stomach increases its pressure upon its contents. The cardiac sphincter closes firmly to prevent regurgitation into the esophagus. The pyloric part of the stomach begins to exhibit wavelets of contraction which run toward the pylorus. They become deeper, and their focus of origin shifts in the direction of the cardia.

At first the pylorus, like the cardia, remains firmly closed, and the wavelets result only in mixing and in facilitating the chemical comminution and solution. Now the pylorus begins to open occasionally, allowing the acid chyme to spurt at intervals into the duodenum. The further course of the chyme is described under duodenal digestion. How quickly the chyme leaves the stomach is influenced by the amount of the feeding, its osmotic character and the amt. of fat present. In general a high-fat-content meal will leave the stomach at a slower rate than a low-fat one.

g. fever. Fever accompanied by gastric disturbances.

g. glands. Cardiac, fundic or oxyntic, and pyloric glands of the stomach.

These are tubular glands lying in the mucosa of the wall; the g. juice exudes from them just as sweat drips from one's forehead. the general result of g. digestion is the reduction of the ingested mass to a mushy, gray mixture called acid chyme. G. glands contain Zymogenic, or peptic cells, which secrete pepsinogen, the inactive form of pepsin; parietal border, or oxyntic cells, which secrete hydrochloric acid, and mucous cells found in the neck of the gland, which secrete mucin.

g. juice. The digestive juice of the g. glands of the stomach. It is a thin colorless fluid containing pepsin, hydrochloric acid, mucin, small quantities of inorganic salts, and the "intrinsic factor" of the antianemic principle. It is strongly acid, having a pH of 0.9 to 1.5, its total acidity being equivalent to 10 to 50 ml. of tenth-normal (10%) hydrochloric acid; free HCl is from 0 to 30 ml. of tenth-normal HCl. The amount secreted in 24 hours varies greatly.

The mixture of acid and pepsin has effects which neither substance has alone, and dissolves some proteins with remarkable speed. Rennin, present in the g. juice of infants, is the cause of the normal clotting or curdling of milk in the stomach. There is also a lipase which can release butyric fat from butter fat and this gives the characteristic odor to vomitus.

DIAG: *Achlorhydria:* Pernicious anemia is the most common cause of this finding in persons who do not have gastric cancer. *Carcinoma:* Boas-Oppler bacilli, sarcinae, blood, and sometimes tumor cells are present; frequently no hydrochloric acid is found. *Hyperacidity:* May indicate gastric ulcer. *Lactic Acid:* Present in carcinoma. *Pus Cells:* Indicate severe inflammation of the stomach. *Red Cells:* Same significance as pus cells.

RS: digestion; gastric analysis; hydrochloric acid; hyper-and hypochlorhydria; stomach.

g. lavage. Washing out of the stomach. USES: To empty stomach when contents are irritating, as in prolonged postanesthetic vomiting, and in some cases of regurgitant vomiting in acute intestinal obstruction; to clean cavity before an operation is preformed upon it; to remove poison in cases in which this method of treatment is indicated; for removal of a test meal.

METHOD: If possible patient is propped up in bed; a rubber sheet and towel are placed around neck and arranged to protect clothing in front. The apparatus required is an esophageal tube with plastic or glass connection; a length of rubber tubing and a funnel; several pints of solution and a solution thermometer; glycerine to lubricate tube; a towel and receiver for vomitus (patient may hold this); a container for measuring amount of returned fluid; a receiver for stomach contents; and sodium bicarbonate solution, four grams to a pint (473 ml.) of water should be prepared at a temperature of 100° F. (37.8° C.).

The procedure is explained to the patient if he is capable of understanding. His mouth is cleaned and he is asked to swallow the lubricated tube which is placed in his mouth. He is encouraged to control the desire to retch. As the tube is swallowed the nurse will gently help to pass it along. When a special mark on the tube is on a level with the patient's lips the tube may be expected to be in the stomach, and the funnel is attached to glass connection by short length of rubber tubing and is then inverted to empty the stomach of its contents; if nothing is seen, the tube should be passed farther in until it is found to be in the stomach.

CAUTION: Prior to attempting to pour liquids into the stomach via the tube, be certain that end of tube is in stomach and not in bronchus.

If possible collect stomach contents in receiver provided. Then pinch the tube below funnel and fill the funnel with solution, expel air from the tube by pinching and rubbing it upward toward the funnel. Let fluid run in very slowly, using from 1/2 to 1 pint (237 to 473 ml.) at a time; invert funnel and let this run out; repeat until all fluid has been used or until it returns clear. When the treatment is finished, pinch tube and withdraw it quickly, giving patient a mouthwash immediately, and then place soiled tube in a basin of tepid water.

The siphoned gastric contents should be examined, and the amount of returned solution measured and inspected for blood, bile, and mucus. If necessary, it should be saved for the doctor's inspection or labeled and specimen sent to laboratory if so ordered.

g. motor meals. These meals are used to test the motor activity of the stomach and intestines.

g. mucin. A fine, straw-colored powder, prepared from hog stomach. Used as a protective in peptic ulcer.

g. ulcer. An ulcer of the stomach. SYN: *peptic ulcer,* q.v.

gastricism (gas'trĭ-sizm) [Gr. *gastēr,* belly, + *ismos,* state]. Any gastric disorder.

gas'trin. A hormone that stimulates secretion of the glands in the main body of the stomach. It is formed at the pyloric end of the stomach in response to the stimulus produced by the presence of food in the stomach.

gastritis (găs-trī'tĭs) [Gr. *gastēr,* belly, + *-itis,* inflammation]. Inflammation of the stomach.

Characterized by epigastric pain or tenderness, nausea, vomiting, and systemic electrolyte changes if vomiting persists. The mucosa may be atrophic or hypertrophic.

ETIOL: Generally unknown. May result from infection, excessive indulgence in alcoholic beverages, dietary indiscretions. Pain in the region of the stomach may be due to causes other than gastritis, such as cancer. G. may be due to an excess or a deficiency of hydrochloric acid, and a remedy suitable for one would not be proper for the other condition. The type must first be determined before medication.

g., acute. SYM: Moderate fever; anorexia, coated tongue; intense pain in epigastrium; persistent vomiting; thirst; prostration. PROG: Good. TREATMENT: Symptomatic, because the process heals spontaneously. If massive bleeding persists, surgery may be required.

g., atrophic. Chronic g. with atrophied mucosa and glands.

g., chronic. SYM: Usually asymptomatic but one or more of the following may be present: mild nausea and anorexia; sense of distention or fullness after eating a small meal; bad taste in mouth; pain over epigastrium may be mild or acute. PROG: Good. TREATMENT: Antispasmodics, antacids, reassurance and sedatives.

g., hypertrophic. G. combined with glandular hypertrophy and infiltration.

gastro- [Gr. *gastēr,* stomach]. Used as a combining form to denote the stomach.

gastroanastomosis (gas″tro-an-as″to-mo′sis) [″+ *anastomōsis,* outlet]. Formation of passage between two pouches of stomach for relief of hour-glass contraction.

gastroblennorrhea (gas″tro-blen″o-rī′ā) [″+ *blennos,* mucus, + *rhoia,* flow]. Excessive secretion of gastric mucus.

gastrobrosis (gas″tro-bro′sis) [Gr. *gastēr,* stomach + *brōsis,* eating]. Perforating ulcer of the stomach.

gastrocamera (gas″tro-kam′ē-rā). A camera small enough to be swallowed. Used to photograph inside of stomach.

gastrocele (gas′tro-sēl) [Gr. *gastēr,* stomach, + *kēlē,* hernia]. Hernia of the stomach.

gastrochronorrhea (gas″tro-kron″o-rē′ā) [″+ *chronos,* time, + *rhoia,* flow]. Chronic gastric disease marked by permanent hypersecretion with dilatation and thickening of stomach walls and hypertrophy of glands.

gastrocnemius (gas″trok-nē′mĭ-us) [″+ *knēmē,* leg]. The large muscle of the posterior portion of the lower leg. It is the most superficial of the calf muscles. Extends foot and helps to flex knee upon thigh.

gastrocol′ic [″+ *kōlon,* colon]. Pert. to stomach and colon.

g. omentum. The great omentum. SYN: *epiploon.*

g. reflex. Peristaltic wave in colon induced by entrance of food into fasting stomach.

gastrocoli′tis [″+ ″+ *-itis,* inflammation]. Inflammation of stomach and colon.

gastrocoloptosis (gas″tro-kol″op-tō′sis) [″+ ″+ *ptōsis,* dropping]. Downward prolapse of stomach and colon.

gastrocolostomy (gas″tro-kol-os′tō-mĭ) [″+ ″+ *stoma,* opening]. Establishment of permanent passage between stomach and colon.

gastrocolotomy (gas″tro-ko-lot′o-mĭ) [″+ ″+ *tomē,* incision]. Incision into stomach and colon.

gastrocolpotomy (gas″tro-kol-pot′o-mĭ) [Gr. *gastēr,* belly, + *kolpos,* vagina, + *tomē,* incision]. An incision through the abdominal wall into upper part of vagina.

gastrodiaphane (gas″tro-dī′ă-fān) [″+ *dia,* through, + *phainein,* to show]. Device for electrically illuminating stomach interior, making visible its outlines through the abdomen.

gastrodiaphanos′copy, gastrodiaph′any [″+ ″+ *skopein,* to examine]. Examination of interior of the stomach by rendering its walls translucent by an electric light introduced through the esophagus into the stomach.

gastrodisciasis (gas″tro-dis-kī′ă-sis). Infestation by a fluke, Gastrodiscoides hominis.

Gastrodiscoides (gas″tro-dis-koy′dēz). A genus of flukes belonging to family Gastrodiscidae, suborder Amphistomata.

G. hominis. A species of flukes commonly infesting hogs but occasionally found in man.

gastroduodenal (gas″tro-du″o-dēn′al) [Gr. *gastēr,* stomach, + L. *duodeni,* twelve]. Rel. to the stomach and duodenum.

gastroduodenitis (gas″tro-dū-od″en-ī′tis) [″+ ″+ Gr. *-itis,* inflammation]. Inflammation of stomach and duodenum.

gastroduodenostomy (gas″tro-du″o-den-os′to-mĭ) [″+ ″+ Gr. *stoma,* mouth]. Formation of an artificial opening between the stomach and duodenum.

gastrodynia (gas″tro-din′ĭ-ă) [″+ *odynē,* pain]. Pain in the stomach, SYN: *gastralgia,* q.v.

gastroelytrotomy (gas-tro-el-ĭ-trot′o-mĭ) [Gr. *gastēr,* stomach + *elytron,* vagina, + *tomē,* incision]. Cesarean section through linea alba into upper portion of vagina. SYN: *gastrocolpotomy.*

gastroenteralgia (gas″tro-en″ter-al′jĭ-ă) [″+ *enteron,* intestine, + *algos,* pain]. Pain in stomach and intestines.

gastroenter′ic [″+ *enteron,* intestine]. Pert. to stomach and intestines or to a condition involving them both.

gastroenteritis (gas"tro-en-ter-i'tis) ["+ "+ -*itis*, inflammation]. Inflammation of the stomach and intestinal tract.

gastroenterocolitis (gas"tro-en"ter-o-kol-i'tis) ["+ "+ *kōlon*, colon, + -*itis*, inflammation]. Inflammation of stomach, small intestine, and colon.

gastroenterocolostomy (gas"tro-en"ter-o-ko-los'to-mi) ["+ "+ "+ *stoma*, opening]. Creation of a passage between the stomach, small intestine, and colon.

gastroenterol'ogy ["+ "+ *logos*, study]. The branch of medical science concerned with study of the physiology and pathology of the stomach, intestines, and related structures such as the esophagus, liver, gallbladder, and pancreas.

gastroenteroptosis (gas"tro-en"ter-op-to'-sis) ["+ "+ *ptōsis*, a dropping]. Prolapse of stomach and intestines.

gastroenterostomy (gas"tro-en-ter-os'to-mi) [Gr. *gastēr*, stomach, + *enteron*, intestine, + *stoma*, opening]. Surgical anastomosis between the stomach and small bowel.

This operation is required for patients who are suffering from carcinoma or cicatricial stricture of pyloric orifice of the stomach.

gas"troenterot'omy ["+ "+ *tomē*, incision]. Incision of stomach and intestine through abdominal wall.

gas"troepiplo'ic [Gr. *gastēr*, belly, + *epiploon*, omentum]. Pert. to stomach and great omentum.

gastroesophagitis (gas"tro-e-sof"ā-ji'tis) ["+ *oisophagos*, gullet, + -*itis*, inflammation]. Inflammation of stomach and esophagus.

gastroesophagostomy (gas"tro-e-sof"ā-gos'to-mi) ["+ "+ *tomē*, incision]. Formation of passage from the esophagus into the stomach.

gastrogastrostomy (gas"tro-gas-tros'to-mi) ["+ *gastēr*, belly, + *stoma*, opening]. Formation of passage in hourglass contraction between the two gastric pouches. SYN: *gastroanastomosis*.

gastrogavage (gas"tro-gă-vazh') ["+ Fr. *gavage*, cramming]. Artificial feeding through an opening into the stomach.

gastrogen'ic [Gr. *gastēr*, belly, + *gennan*, to produce]. Having its origin in the stomach.

gastrohelcosis (gas"tro-hel-ko'sis) ["+ *helkos*, ulcer]. Ulcer of the stomach.

gas"trohepat'ic ["+ *hēpar*, liver]. Pert. to stomach and liver.

gastrohepatitis (gas"tro-hep-ā-ti'tis) ["+ "+ -*itis*, inflammation]. Combination of gastritis and hepatitis at same time.

gastrohydrorrhea (gas"tro-hi"dro-rē'ā) [Gr. *gastēr*, belly, + *hydōr*, water, + *rhoia*, flow]. Excretion of much watery fluid, other than gastric juice, into the stomach.

gastrohysterectomy (gas"tro-his"ter-ek'to-mi) ["+ *hystera*, uterus, + *ektomē*, excision]. Removal of the uterus through an abdominal incision.

gastrohysteropexy (gas"tro-his'ter-o-peks'i) ["+ "+ *pēxis*, fixation]. Ventrofixation of the uterus.

gastrohysterorrhaphy (gas"tro-his"ter-or'-ă-fi) ["+ "+ *rhaphē*, suture]. Fixation of uterus to the abdominal wall. SYN: *gastrohysteropexy*.

gastrohysterotomy (gas"tro-his"ter-ot'o-mi) ["+ "+ *tomē*, incision]. Incision of uterus through abdomen; cesarean section. SYN: *gasterhysterotomy*.

gastroiliac (gas-trō-īl'ī-ak) ["+ L. *ilium* groin]. Pert. to stomach and ileum.

   g. reflex. Physiologic relaxation of ileocecal valve resulting from food in stomach.

gastrointes'tinal [Gr. *gastēr*, stomach, + L. *intestinalis*, intestine]. Pert. to stomach and intestine.

   g. decompression. Drainage of gases from the intestinal tract by use of suction through a tube inserted through the nostrils and into the digestive tract. SEE: *Wangensteen's apparatus.*

gastrojejunostomy (gas-tro-je-ju-nos'to-mi) ["+ L. *jejunum*, empty, + Gr. *stoma*, opening]. Surgical anastomosis between the stomach and jejunum.

gastrolith (gas'tro-lith) [Gr. *gastēr*, belly, + *lithos*, stone]. A concretion in the stomach.

gastrolithiasis (gas"tro-lith-i'ā-sis) ["+ *lithos*, stone]. Formation of calculi in the stomach.

gastrology (gas-trol'o-ji) ["+ *logos*, study]. Study of function and diseases of the stomach.

gastrol'ysis ["+ *lysis*, loosening]. Breaking adhesions between stomach and adjoining structures.

gastromalacia (gas-tro-ma-lā'shī-ā) ["+ *malakia*, softening]. Softening of the stomach walls.

gastromegaly (gas"tro-meg'ā-lī) [Gr. *gastēr*, belly, + *megas*, large]. Enlargement of the stomach.

gastromenia (gas"tro-mē'nī-ā) ["+ *mēniaia*, menses]. A form of vicarious menstruation through the stomach.

gastromycosis (gas"tro-mi-ko'sis) ["+ *mykēs*, fungus, + *ōsis*, condition]. Disease of the stomach due to fungi.

gastromyotomy (gas"tro-mī-ot'o-mī) ["+ *mys*, muscle, + *tomē*, incision]. Incision of circular muscle fibers of stomach.

gastromyxorrhea (gas"tro-miks"o-rē'ä) [Gr. *gastēr*, belly, + *myxa*, mucus, + *rhoia*, flow]. Excessive secretion of gastric mucus.

gastronephritis (gas"tro-nĕ-frī'tis) ["+ *nephros*, kidney, + *-itis*, inflammation]. Inflammation of the stomach and kidney at same time.

gastronesteostomy (gas"tro-nes"tē-os'tō-mī) ["+ *nēstis*, fasting, + *stoma*, opening]. Formation of communication between jejunum and stomach. SYN: *gastrojejunostomy.*

gastropancreatitis (gas"tro-pan"krē-ă-tī'-tis) ["+ *pan*, all, + *kreas*, flesh, + *-itis*, inflammation]. Inflammation of the stomach and pancreas at same time.

gastroparalysis (gas"tro-par-al'ī-sis) ["+ *para*, beyond, + *lyein*, to loosen]. Paralysis of the stomach.

gastroparesis (gas"tro-par'ēsis) ["+ *paresis*, paralysis]. Mild form of gastroparalysis.

gastropathy (gas-trop'ă-thī) [Gr. *gastēr*, belly, + *pathos*, disease]. Any disorder of the stomach.

gastroperiodynia (gas"tro-per"ī-o-din'ī-ä) ["+ *periodos*, period, + *odynē*, pain]. Periodic pain in the stomach SYN: *gastralgia.*

gastropexy, gastropexis (găs"trō-pĕk"sī, -sis) ["+ *pēxis*, fixation]. Suture of the stomach to the abdominal walls for correction of displacement.

gastrophrenic (gas"tro-fren'īk) ["+ *phrēn*, diaphragm]. Rel. to the stomach and diaphragm.

gastroplasty (gas'tro-plas"tī) [Gr. *gastēr*, belly, + *plassein*, to form]. Plastic operation on the stomach.

gastroplegia (gas"tro-plē'jī-ä) ["+ *plēgē*, stroke]. Paralysis of the stomach.

gastroplication (gas"tro-plī-ka'shun) ["+ L. *plicāre*, to fold]. Stitching the walls of the stomach to reduce dilatation.

gastroptosia, gastroptosis (găs"trŏp-tō'sī-ä, -sīs; găs"trŏ-tō'sī-ä, -sīs) ["+ *ptōsis*, a dropping]. Abnormal falling of the stomach, Glénard's disease.

Usually accompanied by the displacement of other organs, the abdomen being pendulous.

gastroptyxis, gastroptyxy (găs"trŏp-tīks'īs, -ī; găs"trŏ-tīk'sīs, -ī) ["+ *ptyxis*, a folding]. Reduction of a dilated stomach by surgery. SYN: *gastroplication.*

gastropylorectomy (gas"tro-pi"lor-ek'tō-mī) ["+ *pylōros*, pylorus, + *ektomē*, excision]. Excision of stomach at pyloric end.

gastropylor'ic. Rel. to stomach and pylorus.

gastroradiculitis (gas"tro-ră-dik"u-li'tis) [Gr. *gastēr*, belly, + L. *radix*, root, + Gr. *-itis*, inflammation]. Inflammation of the posterior spinal nerve roots, the sensory fibers of which supply the stomach.

gastrorrhagia (gas"tro-rā'jī-ä) ["+ *rhēgnynai*, to burst forth]. Hemorrhage from stomach.

gastrorrhaphy (gas-tror'ă-fī) [Gr. *gastēr*, belly, + *raphē*, suture]. 1. Suture of an injured stomach wall. 2. Gastroplication.

gastrorrhea (gas-tro-rē'ä) ["+ *rhoia*, flow]. An excessive secretion of gastric juice.

gastrosalpingotomy (gas"tro-sal"pin-got'o-mī) ["+ *salpinx*, tube, + *tomē*, incision]. Incision of the oviduct by abdominal section.

gastroschisis (gas-tros'kī-sis) ["+ *schisis*, cleft]. A congenital fissure in wall of abdomen which remains open.

gastroscope (gas'tro-skōp) ["+ *skopein*, to examine]. An endoscope for inspecting stomach's interior.

gastros'copy. Examination of the stomach and abdominal cavity.

gastro'sis [Gr. *gastēr*, belly, + *ōsis*, condition]. Any disease of the stomach.

gas'trospasm ["+ *spasmos*, spasm]. A spasm of the stomach.

gastrosplen'ic ["+ *splēn*, spleen]. Of or pert. to stomach and spleen.

gastrostaxis (gas"tro-stak'sis) ["+ *staxis*, trickling]. Oozing of blood from membrane of the stomach.

gastrostenosis (gas"tro-sten-o'sis) ["+ *stēnōsis*, narrowing]. Contracted state of the stomach.

   g. cardiaca. Stenosis of cardiac orifice.

   g. pylorica. Stenosis of pylorus.

gastrostogavage (gas-tros"to-gă-vazh') ["+ *stoma*, opening, + Fr. *gaver*, to stuff]. Feeding by means of a tube leading from outside the body into the stomach through a gastric fistula. SEE: *gavage.*

gastros'toma [Gr. *gastēr*, belly, + *stoma*, opening]. A fistula of the stomach.

gastros'tomize. To perform a gastrostomy.

gastrostomy (gas-tros'to-mī). Surgical creation of a gastric fistula through the abdominal wall.

It is necessary in carcinoma, and in some cases of cicatricial stricture of the esophagus; made for purpose of introducing food into stomach.

NP: Teach patient to care for self after hospitalization. Help patient to make mental adjustment. Mouth should receive special care because it is not being used for the normal purpose of chewing.

gastrosuccorrhea (gas"tro-suk"or-ē'ă) [Gr. *gastēr*, belly, + L. *succus*, juice, + Gr. *rhoia*, flow]. An excessive secretion of gastric juice with increased acidity; hypersecretion.

gastrother'apy ["+ *therapeia*, treatment]. 1. Treatment of gastric diseases. 2. Treatment with extract of gastric mucosa of hogs; used esp. in pernicious anemia.

gastrotome (gas'tro-tōm) ["+ *tomē*, incision]. Instrument for incising stomach or abdomen.

gastrotomy (gas-trot'o-mī) ["+ *temnein*, to cut]. Gastric or abdominal incision.

gastrotonometer (gas"tro-to-nom'ī-ter) ["+ *tonos*, tension, + *metron*, measure]. Instrument for measuring intragastric pressure by insufflation of air or carbonic acid gas.

gastrotrachelotomy (găs"trō-trā"kĕl-ŏt'ō-mī) ["+ *trachēlos*, neck, + *tomē*, incision]. Cesarean section in which the uterus is opened by a transverse incision across the cervix.

gastrotrop'ic [Gr. *gastēr*, belly, + *tropos*, turning]. Attracted to or affecting the stomach.

gastrotubotomy (găs"trō-tŭb-ō-mī) ["+ L. *tubus*, tube, + Gr. *tomē*, incision]. Incision into fallopian tube through abdomen. SYN: *gastrosalpingotomy.*

gastrotympanites (găs"trō-tĭm"păn-ī'tēz) ["+ *tympanon*, drum]. Distention of the stomach caused by gas.

gastroxynsis (găs"trŏks-ĭn'sĭs) ["+ *oxynein*, to sharpen]. Excessive hydrochloric-acid secretion by stomach. SYN: *hyperchlorhydria.*

gastrula (gas'tru-lă) [L. dim. of Gr. *gastēr*, belly]. Stage in embryonic development following the blastula in which the embryo assumes a two-layered condition. The outer layer is the ectoderm or epiblast; the inner layer, the endoderm or hypoblast. The latter lines a cavity, the gastrocoele or archenteron, which opens to the outside through an opening, the blastopore.

gastrula'tion. The development of the gastrula.

Gatch bed. [Willis D. Gatch, Amer. surgeon, 1878 —] A bed in which the patient can be raised and held in a half-sitting position.

gath'ering [AS. *gaderian*, to collect]. Colloquial term for abscess or swelling.

ga'tism [Fr. *gâter*, to spoil]. Vesical or rectal incontinence.

gatophilia (gat"o-fil'ī-ă) [Gr. *gatos*, cat, + *philein*, to love]. Abnormal love for cats. SYN: *ailurophilia.*

gatophobia (gat"o-fo'bĭ-ă) ["+ *phobos*, fear]. Aversion to cats. SYN: *ailurophobia; galeophobia.*

Gaucher's disease (gō-shā'). [Philippe C. E. Gaucher, Fr. physician, 1854-1918] A rare chronic congenital disorder of lipid metabolism. Fatty substances called cerebrosides accumulate in the reticuloendothelial cells. Associated with enlarged spleen, increased skin pigmentation, and bone lesions.

gauge (gāj). Device for measuring size, capacity, amount or power of an object or substance; a standard of measurement.

Gault's reflex (galt). Contraction of orbicularis palpebrarum muscle to produce a blinking of the eye following a loud noise close to the ear. The reflex is tested in cases of suspected malingering to feign deafness. SEE: *malingerer.*

gauntlet (gawnt'let) [Fr. *gant*, glove]. A glovelike bandage which fits the hand and fingers.

gauss (gows). [Johann Karl F. Gauss, German physicist, 1777-1855] The unit of intensity of a magnetic flux.

Gauss' sign (gows). [Carl J. Gauss, Ger. gynecologist, 1875-1957] Unusual mobility of the uterus in the early weeks of pregnancy.

gauze (gawz) [O. Fr. *gaze*, gauze]. Thin, transparent fabric used in surgery.

　g., antiseptic. G. containing antiseptic substance.

　g., aseptic. 1. A gauze sterilized and packaged in an aseptic container and ready for surgical use. 2. A gauze rendered free of microorganisms.

gavage (gă-vazh') [Fr. *gaver*, to stuff]. Feeding with a stomach tube, or with a tube passed through the nares, pharynx, and esophagus into the stomach; the food is in liquid or semiliquid form at a temperature of about 100° F. (37.8° C.). SEE: *gastrostogavage.*

Gavard's muscle (gă-vār'). [Hyacinthe Gavard, Fr. anatomist, 1753-1802] The oblique muscular fibers of the stomach's coat.

Gay-Lussac's law (gā"lū-săk'). [Joseph L. Gay-Lussac, Fr. naturalist, 1778-1850] If pressure remains constant the volume of a gas will vary directly with change in the absolute temperature. SEE: *Charles' law.*

Geigel's reflex (gī'gĕl). [Richard Geigel, Ger. physician, 1859-1930] Reflex in females resembling cremasteric reflex, q.v., in males.

Geiger counter (gī'ger). [Hans Geiger, Ger. physicist in England, 1882-1945] An instrument for detecting ionizing radiation.

gel (jel) [L. *gelāre*, to congeal]. 1. A semisolid condition of a precipitated or coagulated colloid. Jelly. A jellylike colloid. 2. Coagulum of a sol.

g., aluminum hydroxide. A white, viscous suspension; antacid.

gelatin (jel′ă-tin) [L. *gelatina*, gelatin]. A derived protein obtained by the hydrolysis of collagen present in the connective tissues of the skin, bones, and joints of animals.

USES: As a food, in preparation of pharmaceuticals, as a medium for culture of bacteria.

g. culture. Gelatinous base for bacterial growth.

g., nutrient. SEE: *g. culture.*

g. peptone. Digestive product of g.

g. sponge. A spongy sheet of g. prepared for use as a hemostatic.

gelat′inase. An enzyme that liquefies gelatin.

gelatiniferous (jel″at-in-if′er-us) [L. *gelatina*, gelatin, + *ferre*, to bear]. Producing gelatin.

gelatinize (jel-at′in-īz) [L. *gelatina*, gelatin]. To convert into gelatin.

gelatinoid (jel-at′in-oyd) [″+ Gr. *eidos*, form]. Resembling gelatin.

gelatinolytic (jel-at″in-o-lit′ĭk) [″+ Gr. *lysis*, dissolution]. Dissolution or splitting up of gelatin.

gelat″inotho′rax [″+ Gr. *thōrax*, chest]. Injection of gelatin solution intrapleurally.

gelatinous (jĕl-ăt′ĭn-ŭs). Containing or of the consistency of gelatin.

gelation (jel-ā′shun). The transformation of a colloid from a sol into a gel.

gelfoam. Proprietary name for absorbable gelatin sponge. It is used as a surgical sponge in operative wounds.

Gellé's test (zhĕl-ā′). [Marie Ernst Gellé, Fr. physician, 1834-1923] A tuning fork is connected with a rubber tube inserted in the ear. Pressure or suction in the tube is produced by an attached bulb and, if ear is normal, vibrations are felt.

gelodiagno′sis [L. *gelāre*, to congeal, + Gr. *dia*, through, + *gnōsis*, knowledge]. Identification of bacteria by means of a culture medium which turns red when coliform bacteria ferment the lactose present, thus producing acid. Other enteric bacteria grow but do not alter the color of the medium.

gelose (jĕ′lōs) [L. *gelāre*, to congeal]. 1. Gelatinous element of agar ($C_6H_{10}O_5$)n. 2. Bacterial-culture medium.

gelosis (jel-o′sis). A hard lump which is so firm as to appear frozen. Occurs esp. in muscle tissue.

gelotherapy (jel″o-ther′ă-pī) [Gr. *gelōs*, laughter, + *therapeia*, treatment]. Inducing

hilarity in treatment of certain forms of mental illness.

gelotripsy (jel′o-trip″sī) [L. *gelāre*, to congeal, + Gr. *tripsis*, a rubbing]. The massaging away of indurated swellings.

-gels. A termination to indicate colloids in a solid state.

gemellus (jem-el′us) [L. *gemellus*, twin]. Either of two muscles inserted in the obturator internus tendon.

geminate (jem′ĭ-nāt) [L. *geminātus*, paired]. In pairs.

gemination. 1. Development of two teeth within a single alveolus. 2. Production of twins.

gem′ma [L. *gemma*, bud]. 1. A small budlike, reproductive structure, produced by lower forms of life. 2. Any small budlike structure such as a taste bud or end bulb.

gemmation (jem-mā′shun) [L. *gemmāre*, to bud]. Fission by budding.

Budlike processes or daughter cells, each containing chromatin, separate from the mother cell from which the bud is projected.

gemmule (jem′ŭl) [L. *gemmula*, little bud]. 1. A gemma, q.v. 2. One of numerous minute processes present on the dendrites of a neuron.

gena (je′nă) [L. *gena*, cheek]. The side of the face or cheek.

genal (je′nal) [L. *gena*, cheek]. Pert. to the cheek. SYN: *buccal.*

gender [L. *genus*, kind]. The sex of an individual, i.e., male or female.

g. identity. The sex classification of an individual.

g. identity, mistaken. Assignment of incorrect sex to a newborn. This may lead to the individual's having a g. role opposite of the chromosomal sex.

g. role. The behavior and appearance of an individual with respect to the cultural classifications male and female. G. role may, due to congenital or developmental abnormalities, be in contrast to the chromosomal sex.

gene (jēn) [Gr. *gennan*, to produce]. (pl. *genes*) The basic unit of heredity. Each g. occupies a certain place on a chromosome. They are self-producing, ultramicroscopic particles capable under certain circumstances of giving rise to a new character, such a change being called a mutation.

Heredity traits are controlled by pairs of genes in the same position on a pair of chromosomes. These g. pairs, or alleles, may both be dominant or both be recessive. In either of those cases the individual is said to be pure or homozygous for the trait controlled by that g. pair. If the g. pair (alleles) consist of one dominant and one recessive g. the individual is heterozygous for the trait controlled by that g. pair.

g., holandric. A g. located in the non-homologous portion of the Y-chromosome.

g., inhibiting. A g. which prevents the expression of another gene.

g., lethal. A g. which when in a homozygous condition brings about an effect which results in the death of an individual.

g., modifying. A g. which influences or alters the effect of another gene.

g., sex-linked. A g. contained within the X or sex chromosome.

gen'era. Pl. of genus.

gen'eralize [L. *generālis*, relating to all]. 1. To become or render general. 2. To become systemic, as a local disease.

generation (jen"er-a'shun) [L. *generāre*, to beget]. 1. An act of forming a new organism. 2. A group of animals or plants the same distance removed from an ancestor, as the first filial (F₁) generation. SEE: *filial generation.* 3. The average period of time between the birth of parents and the birth of their children. This could be 16 to 20 years in some cultures and 20 to 25 years in others. Also the time would be different if only female parents were considered in computing this average unless all marriages occurred between persons of the same age. 4. The production of an electric current.

g's., alternation of. A mode of reproduction in which a sexual g. alternates with an asexual g., characteristic of all plants above the Thallophytes. It also occurs in some of the lower animals.

g., asexual. Reproduction which occurs without the union of sexual elements or gametes, such as reproduction by fission, or spore production.

g., F₁. The first filial g.; the offspring of a given mating or cross.

g., sexual. Reproduction by the union of male and female cells.

g., spontaneous. The theory that living things can originate from nonliving matter. SYN: *abiogenesis.*

g., viviparous. Normal method of g. among higher animals.

generative (jen'er-a-tiv). Concerned in reproduction of or affecting the species.

generic (jen-er'ik) [L. *genus*, kind]. 1. General. 2. Pert. to a genus. 3. Distinctive.

g. name. The nonproprietary name of a drug or pharmaceutical preparation.

genesiology (jen-e-zī-ol'o-jī) [Gr. *genesis*, generation, + *logos*, science]. The science of reproduction.

genesis (jen'ĕ-sis). 1. Act of reproducing; generation. 2. The origin of anything.

genetic (jen-et'ik). Pert. to generation.

g. counseling. The application of what is known about human genetics in providing advice to those who are concerned about the possibility of their offspring being free of hereditary abnormality.

geneticist (jen-et'ī-sist) [Gr. *gennan*, to produce]. One who specializes in genetics.

genet'ics. The science that accounts for natural differences and resemblances among organisms related by descent. 2. The study of heredity and its variation.

genetopathy (jĕn-ĕ-tŏp'ă-thī) [Gr. *genesis*, generation, + *pathos*, disease]. Disease affecting reproductive function.

genetous (jĕn'ĕ-tŭs). From birth. SYN: *congenital*, q.v.

genial (je'nĭ-al) [Gr. *geneion*, chin]. Rel. to the chin.

genic [Gr. *gennan*, to produce]. Rel. to or caused by genes.

-genic. Suffix indicating generation or production.

geniculate (jen-ik'u-lāt) [L. *geniculāre*, to bend the knee]. 1. Kneed. 2. Bent as a knee. 3. Pert. to the ganglion or geniculum of the facial nerve.

g. otalgia. Pain transmitted from the facial nerve to the ear.

geniculum (jĕn-ĭk'ū-lŭm) [L. *geniculum*, little knee]. A structure resembling a knot, or a knee. Indicates an abrupt bend or angle in a small structure.

genion (je'nĭ-ŏn) [Gr. *geneion*, chin]. Apex of the spina mentalis.

genioplasty (je'nĭ-ō-plăs"tī) [" + *plassein*, to form]. Plastic surgery of the chin or cheek.

genital (jĕn'ĭ-tăl) [L. *genitalis*, belonging to birth]. Pert. to the genitals.

genitalia, gen'itals (jen-ĭ-tal'ĭ-ă). Organs of generation; reproductive organs.

g., female. Those concerned with reproduction.

The external genitalia collectively are termed the vulva or pudendum and include the mons veneris; labia majora; labia minora; clitoris; fourchet; fossa navicularis; vestibule; vestibular bulb; Skene's glands; glands of Bartholin; hymen and vaginal introitus; and perineum.

The internal genitalia are the two ovaries; fallopian tubes; uterus; and vagina.

g., male. Two bulbourethral (Cowper's) glands; two ejaculatory ducts; two glandular organs producing spermatozoa (the testes or gonads): penis with urethra: two seminal ducts (vasa deferentes or ductus deferentes);

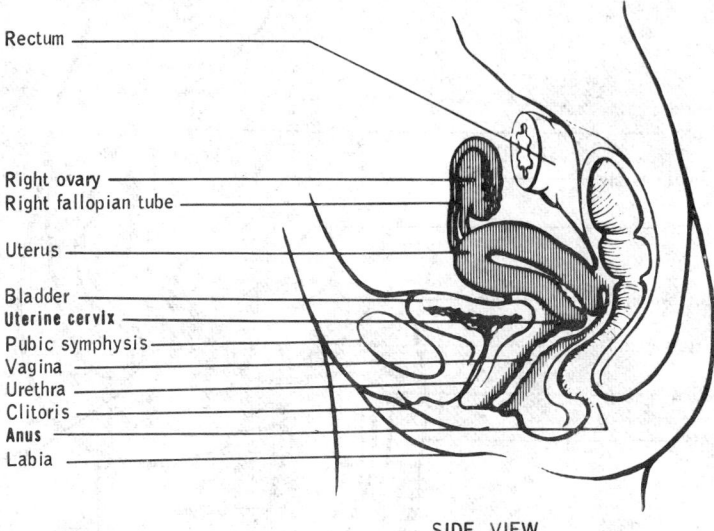

Rectum

Right ovary
Right fallopian tube

Uterus

Bladder
Uterine cervix
Pubic symphysis
Vagina
Urethra
Clitoris
Anus
Labia

SIDE VIEW

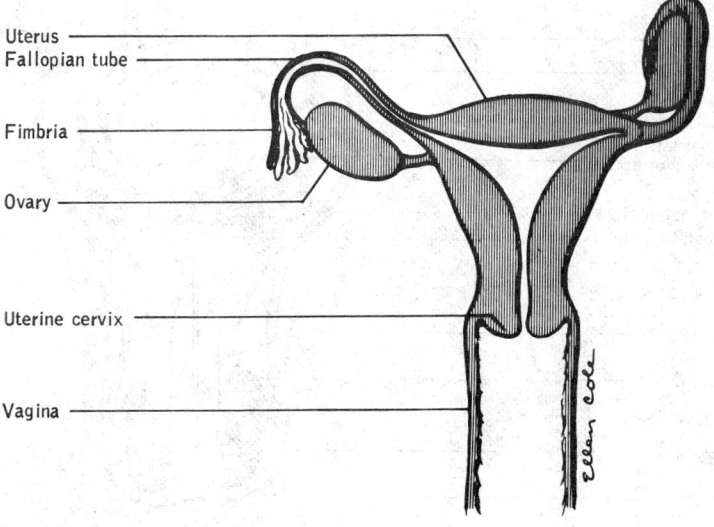

Uterus
Fallopian tube

Fimbria

Ovary

Uterine cervix

Vagina

FRONT VIEW

FEMALE GENITOURINARY SYSTEM

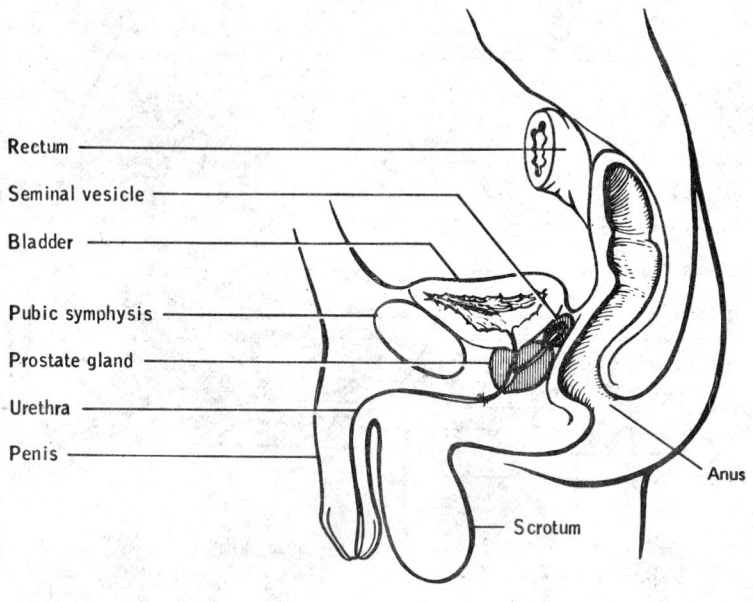

Rectum
Seminal vesicle
Bladder
Pubic symphysis
Prostate gland
Urethra
Penis
Anus
Scrotum

SIDE VIEW

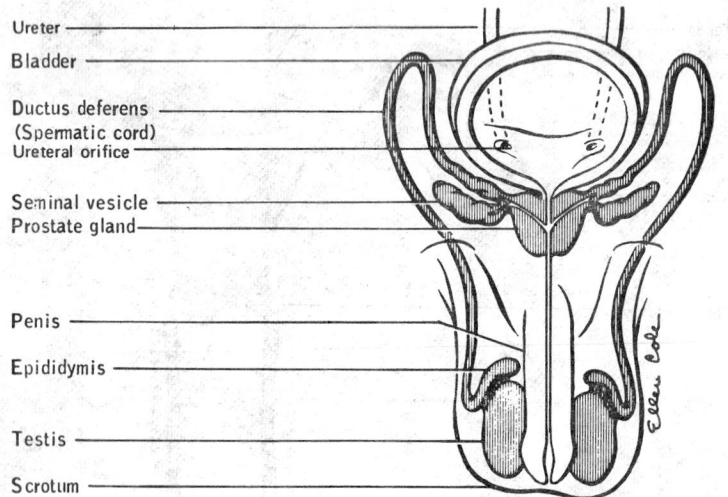

Ureter
Bladder
Ductus deferens
(Spermatic cord)
Ureteral orifice
Seminal vesicle
Prostate gland
Penis
Epididymis
Testis
Scrotum

FRONT VIEW

MALE GENITOURINARY SYSTEM

two seminal vesicles; two spermatic cords; scrotum; and prostate gland. SEE: *prostate.*

gen″itoplas″ty [L. *genitalis,* genital, + Gr. *plassein,* to form]. Reparative surgery on the genital organs.

gen″itou′rinary ["+ Gr. *ouron,* urine]. Pert. to the genitals and the urinary organs.

     g. system. Organs and parts concerned with the kidneys, urinary bladder, and organs of generation and their accessories.

genocide (jĕn″ō-sīd′) [Gr. *genos,* race, + L. *caedere,* to kill]. Willful and planned murder of a group, esp. pert. to human beings.

genodermatosis (jĕn″o-der-mă-to′sis) [Gr. *gennan,* to produce, + *derma,* skin, + *-ōsis,* morbid process]. Any congenital disease of the skin.

genotype (jĕn′o-tīp) [Gr. *gennan,* to produce, + *typos,* type]. 1. Basic hereditary combination of genes of an organism. 2. A type species. 3. Group marked by same hereditary characteristics. SEE: *phenotype.*

gentian (jĕn′shun). Dried rhizome roots of the plant Gentiana lutea.

     g. violet. USP. A dye derived from coal tar. Widely used as a stain in histology, cytology, and bacteriology. Used therapeutically as a topical anti-infective. Its chemical name is hexamethylpararosaniline chloride ($C_{25}H_{30}ClN_3$).

gentianophil(e, gentianophilous (jĕn′-shăn-ō-fīl; jĕn″shăn-ŏf′ī-lŭs). Easily and readily staining with gentian violet.

genu (jē′nu) [L.]. [NA] 1. The knee. 2. Any structure of angular form resembling a bent knee.

     g. extrorsum. g. varum, q.v.

     g. introrsum. g. valgum, q.v.

     g. recurvatum. Hyperextension at the knee joint.

     g. val′gum. Knock-knee.

     g. va′rum. Bowleg.

genuclast (jĕn′u-klăst) [L. *genu,* knee + Gr. *klan,* to break]. Instrument for breaking knee-joint adhesions.

genucu′bital ["+ *cubitus,* elbow]. Pert. to the elbows and knees.

     g. position. Knee-elbow position. One with the patient on the knees, thighs upright, body resting on elbows, head down on hands; employed when not possible to use the knee-chest position.

genupectoral (jĕn″u-pek′tor-al) ["+ *pectus,* breast]. Pert. to the chest and knees.

     g. position. Knee-chest position.

A position assumed by the female patient in which the patient is supported upon her knees and chest. This position is used for purposes of examination and treatment.

genus (jē′nus) [L. *genus,* kind]. In biology, the division between the species and the family.

genyantralgia (jen″ī-an-tral′jī-ă) [Gr. *genys,* jaw, + *antron,* cave, + *algos,* pain]. Pain in the antrum of Highmore or frontal nasal sinuses.

genyantritis (jen″ī-an-trī′tis) ["+ "+ *-itis,* inflammation]. Inflammation of the antrum of Highmore or frontal nasal sinuses.

genyplasty (jen′ī-plas″tī) ["+ *plassein,* to form]. Any plastic operation on the jaw.

geode (jē′ōd) [Gr. *geōdēs,* earthlike]. A dilated lymph space connected with the lymphatic system.

geograph′ic tongue. Numerous denuded patches on dorsal surface of tongue coalescing into freeform, shapes similar to geographic presentations or maps.

geophagia, geophagism, geophagy (je-o-fa′jī-ă, -of′ă-jĭzm, -of′ă-jī) [Gr. *gē,* earth, + *phagein,* to eat]. A condition in which the patient eats inedible substances, as chalk or earth. SYN: *chthonophagia.* SEE: *pica.*

geotragia (jē″o-trā′jī-ă) ["+ *trōgein,* to chew]. Earth eating. SYN: *chthonophagia; geophagism.*

geo″tricho′sis. Infection by a fungus, Geotrichum, which usually attacks the lungs. Symptoms resemble those of chronic bronchitis or tuberculosis. May also infect the mouth or intestine.

Geot′richum. A genus of fungi belonging to the family Eremascaceae; the causative agent of geotrichosis, q.v.

gephyrophobia (jē″fī″rō-fō′bī-ă) [Gr. *gephyra,* bridge, + *phobos,* fear]. Aversion to bodies of water, or to crossing on bridges over water, or to traveling on boats.

geratic (je-rat′ik) [Gr. *gēras,* old age]. Rel. to old age.

geratology (jer″ă-tol′o-jī) ["+ *logos,* study]. The study of old age. SYN: *gerontology.*

Gerdy's fibers (zher′dēz). [Pierre N. Gerdy, Fr. physician, 1797-1856] The superficial transverse ligament of the palm.

gereology (jer″e-ol′o-jī) [Gr. *gēras,* old age, + *logos,* study]. The science of old age and aging.

geriatrics (jer″ī-at′riks) ["+ *iatrikē,* medical treatment]. Study and treatment of the diseases of old age.

Gerlach's valve (gĕr′läk). [Joseph von Gerlach, Ger. anatomist, 1820-1896] An inconstant valve present at the opening of the vermiform process (appendix) into the cecum.

Gerlier's disease (zhĕr-lē-ā′). [Felix Gerlier, Swiss physician, 1840-1914] Paralyzing vertigo.

SYM: Pains in head and neck, disturbance of vision, vertigo, ptosis, weakness of muscles of the neck and of extremities.

germ [L. *germen*, sprout, fetus]. 1. A microorganism, esp. one that causes disease. 2. The first rudiment of an organism. 3. An ovum.

g. cell. An ovum or spermatozoon.

g., dental. The rudimentary structure from which a tooth develops; includes the dental papilla and the enamel organ. SYN: *tooth germ.*

g. disease. A disease which is caused by a microorganism.

g. epithelium, g. ridge. Ridge of epithelium in the embryo from which develops the sexual portions of the body.

g., hair. The rudimentary structure from which a hair develops. Consists of an ingrowth of epidermal cells called hair peg which pushes into the corium.

g. layers. Three primary layers of cells in an embryo from which the organs and tissues develop. They are the ectoderm, mesoderm, and entoderm, q.v.

g. plasm. The reproductive tissues, in contrast to the non-reproductive tissues which constitute the remainder of the body, the soma.

g. theory. The hypothesis that disease is the result of the presence of microorganisms or their products in the body.

germanium (jer-ma'nĭ-um). SYMB: *Ge.* At. wt. 72.59; at. no. 32; sp. gr. 5.323 (25° C). A grayish white metallic element of the silicon group.

German measles. Acute contagious disease with rash of short duration, resembling measles and scarlet fever. The disease is important because of the effect it may have on the fetus if it occurs in the first trimester of pregnancy. The risk of the fetus so exposed being born with a severe congenital defect is quite high. Women who are pregnant and have not had a proven case of rubella should be protected from this disease. At one time immune serum globulin was thought to provide sufficient protection to warrant its use. The antibody titer against rubella virus present in the original immune globulin was much lower than that in those currently available. Thus an immune serum globulin with a known high titer of antibody against rubella virus should be given to women who are pregnant and are known not to have had rubella. *Note:* Pregnant women should not be given rubella virus vaccine. SYN: *rötheln; rubella.*

germicidal (jerm"ĭ-sī'dal) [L. *germen*, sprout, + *caedere*, to kill]. 1. Destructive to germs. 2. Pert. to an agent destructive to germs.

germicide (jer'mĭs-id). A substance that destroys germs. SEE: *bactericide; disinfectant.*

Bacteria and spores may be killed by boiling for 30 minutes; by dry heat at 160° to 170° C. for an hour; by steam at 121° C. for 20 minutes.

germ'inal [L. *germen*, sprout]. Pertaining to a germ or reproductive cells. (egg or sperm), or to germination.

g. center. A light area of lymphocytopoietic cells which occupies the center of lymphatic nodules of the spleen, tonsils, and lymph nodes.

g. disk. A disk of cells on the surface of the yolk of a teloblastic egg from which the embryo develops; the blastoderm.

g. epithelium. 1. The epithelium which covers the surface of the genital ridge of an embryo. 2. The epithelium which covers the surface of a mature mammalian ovary.

g. vesicle. Nucleus of oocyte, q.v.

germina'tion [L. *germināre*, to sprout]. 1. Development of an impregnated ovum into an embryo. 2. The sprouting of the spore or seed of a plant.

gerocomia (jer"o-ko'mĭ-ă) [Gr. *gerōn*, old man, + *komein*, to care for]. The hygiene of old age, or care of old men.

geroder'ma, gerodermia (jer-o-der'mĭ-ă) ["+ *derma*, skin]. An appearance of senility brought about by premature loss of hair, wrinkling of the skin, and general atrophy.

geromaras'mus [Gr. *gerōn*, old man, + *marasmos*, a wasting]. Emaciation which accompanies extreme old age.

geromorphism (jer"o-mor'fizm) ["+ *morphē*, form, + *ismos*, state of]. Appearance of age in youth.

gerontal (jĕ-ron'tal) [Gr. *gerōn*, old man]. Pert. to an old man or to the aged. SYN: *senile.*

gerontology (je-ron-tol'o-jĭ) ["+ *logos*, study of]. The study of the phenomena of old age. SYN: *geriatrics.*

gerontophil'ia ["+ *philein*, to love]. Fondness or love for old people.

gerontopia (jer"on-to'pĭ-ă) ["+ *opsis*, vision]. Change in vision of elderly persons, by which they go back to the sight of their youth. SYN: *senopia.*

gerontoxon (jĕ-ron-toks'on) ["+ *toxon*, bow]. Degenerative circle about corneal exterior surface seen in the aged. SYN: *arcus senilis.*

Gerota's capsule (gā-rō'tahz). [Dumitru Gerota, Rumanian anatomist, 1867-1939] The perirenal fascia.

gestaltism (ges-talt'izm) [Ger. *Gestalt*, form]. The theory that the objects of mind come as wholes which cannot be split up into parts and which are, therefore, unanalyzable.

gestation (jes-tā'shun) [L. *gestāre,* to bear]. Period of intrauterine fetal development from conception to birth.

    g., abdominal. Ectopic g. in which the product of conception develops in the peritoneal cavity.

    g., cornual. G. in an ill-developed cornu of a bicornuate uterus.

    g., ectopic. Fetus develops outside the uterus.

    g., interstitial. Tubal g. in which the ovum is developed in portion of oviduct that traverses wall of uterus.

    g., ovarian. A form of ectopic g. in the ovary.

    g., plural. G. with more than one embryo.

    g., prolonged, g., protracted. G. prolonged beyond the usual period.

    g. sac. The amnion and its contents.

    g., secondary. The ovum becomes dislodged from original seat of implantation, and continues to develop in a new situation.

    g., secondary abdominal. Extrauterine g. in which the fetus, originally situated in oviduct or elsewhere, has developed in abdominal cavity because of the rupture of the fetal sac.

    g. time. The duration of normal pregnancy for a species.

    g., tubal, g., tubarian. Ectopic g. in which the product of conception grows in the oviduct.

    g., tuboabdominal. Extrauterine g. in which fetal sac is formed partly of the abdominal extremity of the oviduct and partly of plastic exudation in the area.

    g., tubo-ovarian. Extrauterine g. in which the fetal sac is made up of the ovary and the abdominal end of the oviduct.

    g., uterotubal. G. in which the ovum is developed partly in uterine portion of oviduct and partly within cavity of uterus.

gestosis (jes-tō'sis) [L. *gestāre,* to bear, + Gr. *ōsis,* condition]. Any disorder of pregnancy.

geumaphobia (gū″mă-fo'bĭ-ă) [Gr. *geuma,* taste, + *phobos,* fear]. Abnormal dislike or fear of tastes.

GH. Growth hormone.

gher'kin. A form of small cucumber used for pickling. It is more of a condiment than a vegetable or a food.

Ghon's primary lesion, tubercle. [Anton Ghon, Czechoslovakian pathologist, 1866-1936] A bean-shaped shadow in the x-ray film of the lung seen in certain cases of pulmonary tuberculosis in children. It is usually the primary lesion of tuberculosis in children.

ghost corpuscle. Depigmented red blood corpuscle. SYN: *phantom corpuscle.*

giant (ji'ant) [Gr. *gigas,* giant]. An individual or structure much larger than normal.

    g. cell. One of large size with several nuclei, appearing to be made up of many cells, but not clearly outlined; found in both kinds of marrow, esp. in red marrow and spleen; a megakaryocyte. Also found in tissues which are healing; around foreign bodies; and in the inflammatory reaction to tuberculosis.

    g. c. tumor. Rare, benign, encapsulated tumor in lower jaw or on alveolar process of upper jaw in the young.

giantism (ji'an-tizm). Abnormal development of the body or its parts. SYN: *gigantism.*

Gianuzzi's cells or **crescents** (jän-ūt'sē). Crescent-shaped groups of serous cells found in the mixed salivary glands. They appear as darkly staining cells forming a caplike structure on the alveoli. SYN: *demilunes of Heidenhain.*

Giardia (jē-är'dĭ-ă). [Alfred Giard, Fr. biologist, 1846-1908] A genus of protozoa possessing flagella. They inhabit the small intestine of man and other animals; are pear-shaped; and have two nuclei and four pairs of flagella. They attach themselves to the cells of the intestinal mucosa, from which they absorb their nourishment.

    G. lamblia. Species of G. found in man. They were formerly considered nonpathogenic but evidence indicates that they interfere with the absorption of fats, their presence having been connected with recurring attacks of diarrhea and the passage of stools containing large amounts of unabsorbed fats and quantities of yellow mucus. They form cysts intermittently.

giardiasis (jĭ″är-dĭ'ă-sĭs). Infection with Giardia lamblia. SYN: *lambliasis.*

Gibbon's hydrocele (gĭb'ŏn). [Q. V. Gibbon, Amer. surgeon, 1813-1894] A hydrocele and large hernia combined.

gibbos'ity [LL. *gebbōsus,* humped]. 1. Condition of having a humpback. 2. A hump or gibbus, as the deformity of Pott's disease.

gibbous (gĭb'bus). Humped; protuberant or humpbacked.

gid'diness [AS. *gydig,* insane]. State of dizziness. SYN: *vertigo.*

Giemsa's stain (gēm'zŏ). [Gustav Giemsa, Ger. chemist, 1867-1948] A stain for staining blood smears. Used for differential leukocyte counts and for the detection of parasitic microorganisms.

Gifford's reflex (gĭf'ford). [Harold Gifford, Amer. oculist, 1858-1929] Pupillary contraction resulting from endeavoring forcibly to close eyelids which are held apart.

gigantism (jī'gan-tizm) [Gr. *gigas*, giant, + *ismos*, state of]. Abnormal development of the body or of a part. SYN: *giantism*.

   g., acromegalic. G. in which acromegalic features (overgrowth of the bones of the hands, feet, and face) are present. Due to excessive production of the growth hormone after full skeletal growth has been attained.

   g., eunuchoid. G. accompanied by eunuchoid features and sexual insufficiency.

   g., normal. G. of the body in which the bodily proportions and functional activities are normal. Usually the result of hypersecretion of the growth hormone.

gigan'toblast ["+ *blastos*, germ]. A very large nucleated red corpuscle.

gigantocyte (ji-gan'to-sīt) ["+ *kytos*, cell]. 1. A giant cell. 2. A very large erythrocyte.

gigantosoma (ji-gan''to-so'mä) ["+ *sōma*, body]. Abnormal size of the body. SYN: *giantism; gigantism.*

Gigli's saw (gēl'yē). [Leonardo Gigli, It. gynecologist, 1863-1908] A wire saw originally used to cut the pubis. Now used in removing the scalp in craniotomy.

Gilles de la Tourette's syndrome. [Georges Gilles de la Tourette, Fr. neurologist, 1857-1904] Convulsive tic with echolalia, coprolalia and motor incoordination. The movements cease during sleep. Etiology unknown.

Gimbernat's ligament (hĭm-bĕr-nät'). [Antonio de Gimbernat, Sp. surgeon, 1734-1790] Pectineal portion of the inguinal ligament. Its lateral free edge forms the medial portion of the femoral ring. SYN: *ligamentum lacunare* [NA].

gin'ger [L. *zinziberi*, ginger]. Dried rhizome of the plant Zingiber officinale found in many tropical countries.

   ACTION AND USES: Used chiefly as a flavoring agent.

gingiva (jin-jī'vă, jin'jī-vă) [L.]. The gum; the tissue which surrounds the necks of the teeth and covers the alveolar processes of the maxilla and mandible.

   g., labial. G. covering labial surfaces of the teeth.

   g., lingual. G. covering lingual surface of the teeth.

gingival (jin'jiv-al) [L. *gingiva*, gum]. Rel. to the gums.

gingival'gia ["+ Gr. *algos*, pain]. Pain in the gums.

gingivally (jin'jī-văl''lī). Toward the gums.

gingivectomy (jin''jī-vek'to-mī) [L. *gingiva*, gum, + Gr. *ektomē*, excision]. Excision of gum tissue in pyorrhea. SYN: *ulectomy.*

gingivitis (jin-jī-vī'tis) [L. *gingiva*, gum, + Gr. *-itis*, inflammation]. Inflammation of the gums, characterized by redness, swelling, and tendency to bleed. SYN: *ulitis.*

   ETIOL: May be local, due to improper dental hygiene; poorly fitting dentures or appliances; poor occlusion; or it may accompany generalized stomatitis associated with mouth and upper respiratory infections. May also occur in deficiency diseases such as scurvy, blood dyscrasias, or metallic poisoning.

   g., acute ulcerative. SEE: *Vincent's g.*

   g., expulsive. Osteoperiostitis of a tooth in which the tooth is expelled from its socket.

   g. gravidum. G. of pregnancy. Characterized by generalized hypertrophy of the gums which may progress to the state of tumor formation.

   g., interstitial. Inflammation of the gums and alveolar processes which precede pyorrhea.

   g., phagedenic. A rapidly spreading ulceration of the gums accompanied by extensive ulceration and sloughing of tissue.

   g., Vincent's. An ulcerative necrotizing inflammation. Both fusobacteria and spirochetes are found in the lesions. TREATMENT: Hydrogen peroxide mouthwash twice daily, penicillin or tetracycline or metronidazole. SYN: *trench mouth; Vincent's stomatitis.*

gingivoglossitis (jĭn''jī-vō-glŏs-sī'tĭs) [L. *gingiva*, gum, + Gr. *glōssa*, tongue, + *-itis*, inflammation]. Inflammation of the gums and tongue. SYN: *stomatitis.*

ginglyform (jing'lī-form) [Gr. *ginglymos*, hinge, + L. *forma*, shape]. In the form of a hinged joint. SYN: *ginglymoid.*

ginglymoarthrodial (jing'lī-mo-ar-thrō'dī-al) ["+ *arthrōdia*, gliding joint]. Pert. to a joint that is both hinged and arthrodial. SEE: *arthrodia.*

ginglymoid (jing'lī-moyd) ["+ *eidos*, form]. Pert. to or shaped like a hinged joint.

ginglymus (jing'lī-mus) [Gr. *ginglymos*, hinge]. A hinge joint; diarthrosis, q.v. SEE: *joint.*

Giraldés' organ (hir-al-däs'). [Jachim A. C. C. Giraldés, Portuguese surgeon in Paris, 1808-1875] A vestige of the wolffian body at posterior side of the testicle. SYN: *paradidymis.*

girdle (gŭr'dl) [AS. *gyrdel,* girdle]. 1. A zone or belt; cingulum, the waist. 2. A structure which resembles a circular belt or band.

　　g. **anesthesia.** A portion around the body, without sensation.

　　g., **Neptune.** Stimulating or heating compress of linen covered by flannel encircling trunk from lower end of sternum to pubes.

　　g. **pain.** Painful sensation around the body.

　　g., **pelvic.** The portion of the lower extremities to which the lower limbs are attached. Composed of the two innominate or hip bones.

　　g. **sensation.** G. pain, q.v.

　　g., **shoulder.** The portion of the upper extremities to which the upper limbs are attached. Composed of the two clavicles and two scapulae.

　　g. **symptom.** A symptom in tabes as of a tight girdle, such as a feeling of constriction about the chest; also found in compression of the cord due to collapse of the vertebrae as in Pott's disease. SYN: *Hitzig's g.*

gitalin (jĭt'ă-lĭn). A cardiac glycoside from digitalis.

gitter cell. A honeycombed cell packed with a number of lipoid granules.

glabel'la [L. *glaber,* smooth]. The smooth surface of the frontal bone lying between the superciliary arches; the portion directly above the root of the nose.

gla'brate [L. *glaber,* smooth]. 1. Bald. 2. Smooth.

glabrificin (glăb-rĭf'ĭ-sĭn) ["+ *facere,* to make]. A variety of antibody which exposes a capsulated bacterium to the action of lysin.

gla'brous [L. *glaber,* smooth]. 1. Bald. 2. Smooth. SYN: *glabrate.*

glacial (glā'shal) [L. *glacialis,* icy]. Glassy; resembling ice.

gladiate (glā'dĭ-āt) [L. *gladius,* sword]. Swordshaped. SYN: *ensiform; xiphoid.*

gladi'oline. An alkaloid from tissue of the brain.

gladiolus (glă-dĭ'o-lus) [L. *gladiolus,* little sword]. The intermediate and principal segment of the sternum, q.v.

glairin (glār'in) [L. *clārus,* clear]. Gelatinous substance in water of some sulfur springs.

glair'y. Viscous; albuminous; mucoid.

gland [L. *glans,* acorn]. 1. A secretory organ or structure. 2. A cell or a group of cells which has the ability to manufacture a secretion which is discharged and used in some other part of the body.

　　On the basis of complexity of structure, g.'s may be simple (consisting of one or a few

secreting units) or compound (consisting of many secreting units whose secretions leave the g. by a common duct). Simple tubular g.'s may be straight, coiled or branched.

　　G.'s consisting of one cell are called unicellular; those of more than one cell, multicellular.

　　On the basis of their secretion, g.'s are mucous (those producing a viscous, slimy secretion); serous (those producing a clear watery secretion); or mixed (those producing both).

　　On the basis of the presence or absence of ducts, g.'s are exocrine (those which possess ducts which carry the secretions to an epithelial surface) and endocrine (those without ducts and whose secretions enter the blood or lymph). The latter are gonads or sex g.'s; pineal, pituitary, thyroid, parathyroid, thymus, and adrenal g.'s.

　　On the basis of the shape of the secreting units, g.'s are tubular (secreting portion elongated with a narrow lumen) or saccular (secreting portion in the form of a sac or flask). If the lumen of the secreting portion is wide, it is termed an alveolus; if narrow, an acinus. G.'s composed of these types of units are termed alveolar and acinar respectively.

　　On the basis of the manner by which secretion is accomplished, g.'s are merocrine (secretion forms within cells and is passed through cell membranes into excretory ducts); apocrine (secretion forms in apical ends of cells which break off and form a part of the secretion), e.g., mammary g.; and holocrine (entire cell with its contents is extruded as the secretion), e.g., sebaceous g.'s.

　　g., **absorbent.** Any one of the lymphatic g.'s.

　　g., **accessory.** G. functioning as an accessory to another g. of similar structure some distance removed.

　　g., **acinotubular.** A g. structurally midway between an acinous and a tubular g.

　　g., **acinous.** A g. whose secreting units are composed of saclike structures each possessing a narrow lumen.

　　g., **adrenal.** An endocrine g. lying above each kidney. SEE: *adrenal g.*

　　g.'s, **aggregate.** Lymphatic g.'s in patch formation found mainly in ileum. SYN: *Peyer's patches.*

　　g.'s, **agminated.** G., aggregate, q.v.

　　g.'s, **albuminous.** Digestive tract g.'s secreting a fluid containing albumin.

　　g., **anal.** G.'s in the region of the anus.

　　g., **aprocrine.** A g. whose cells lose some of their cytoplasmic contents in the formation of the secretion. Ex: mammary g., some sweat g.'s.

g.'s, areolar. Large sebaceous and rudimentary milk g.'s present in the areola surrounding the nipple of the female breast. SYN: *Montgomery's g.'s.*

g.'s, auricular. External otic lymph nodes.

g.'s, axillary. Axillary lymph nodes.

g.'s, Bartholin's. Numerous g.'s which open into the vestibule of the female. Homologous to bulbourethral g.'s of the male. SYN: *major vestibular g.'s.*

g.'s, Blandin's; g.'s, Blandin-Nuhn's. Tiny racemose g.'s secreting mucus and saliva, near the tip of the tongue on the undersurface.

g.'s, Bowman's. Simple, branched, tubular g.'s present in the olfactory mucosa of the nasal cavity.

g.'s, brachial. Lymph g.'s in the arm and forearm.

g.'s, bronchial. Mixed g.'s lying in the submucosa of the bronchi and bronchial tubes.

g.'s, Bruch's. Conjunctival lymph nodes in lower lids.

g.'s, Brunner's. G.'s in the duodenal submucosa secreting intestinal juice.

g.'s, buccal. Acinous g.'s in the cheek tissue.

g., bulbourethral. Cowper's g. Two small g.'s above the bulb of corpus spongiosum, whose secretion forms part of seminal fluid.

g.'s, cardiac. G.'s of the stomach near the cardiac orifice of the esophagus.

g., carotid. Tiny g. at bifurcation of the common carotid artery. SYN: *carotid body.*

g.'s, cecal. Cecal lymph nodes.

g.'s, ceruminous. G.'s in auditory canal excreting cerumen.

g.'s, cervical. Lymph g.'s situated in the neck.

g.'s, ciliary. G.'s, Moll's, q.v.

g.'s, circumanal. The anal g.'s, q.v.

g.'s, Cobelli's. G.'s in the esophageal mucosa.

g.'s, coccygeal. G., Luschka, q.v.

g., compound. A g. consisting of a number of branching duct systems which open into the main excretory duct.

g., compound tubular. G. composed of numerous minute tubules leading to a lone duct.

g., conglobate. Lymphatic g.

g., conglomerate. G., acinous, q.v.

g., Cowper's. G., bulbourethral, q.v.

g.'s, cutaneous. G.'s of the skin, esp. the sebaceous and sudoriferous g.'s. Also includes modified forms such as the ciliary, ceruminous, anal, preputial, areolar, meibomian g.'s.

g., cytogenic. A g. whose product is living cells, such as the testis or ovary.

g.'s, decidual. G.'s possessing no secretory duct.

g., ductless. A g. which lacks an excretory duct; an endocrine g., q.v.

g.'s, duodenal. G.'s, Brunner's g.'s, q.v.

g., Ebner's. Serous g.'s of the tongue located in the region of the vallate papillae, their ducts opening into the furrows surrounding the papillae. SYN: *g. of von Ebner.*

g., endocrine. An organ or structure which secretes a hormone that is absorbed into the blood or lymph; a ductless g. The principal endocrine g.'s are the hypophysis, thyroid, and testes, q.v. SEE: *endocrine g.'s.*

g.'s, female. Bartholin's, nabothian, ovaries, Skene's, uterine, glans clitoridis, mammary.

g.'s, Frankel's. Tiny g.'s located below the margin of the vocal cords.

g., fundic. G.'s of the body and fundus of the stomach; gastric g.'s which secrete gastric juice.

g.'s, Gay's. Multiple sweat g.'s developed to a great extent in the perianal area.

g., genal. G. in buccal submucosa.

g.'s, genital. Ovaries (in female) and testes (in male).

g.'s, gingival. G.'s at gum margins.

g.'s, hair. Sebaceous g.'s opening into each hair follicle.

g.'s, haversian. G.'s secreting synovial fluid.

g.'s, hematopoietic. G.'s participating in blood production.

g.'s, hemolymph. Modified g.'s containing blood and lymph sinuses, which probably participate in the formation of the leukocytes and the destruction of red blood corpuscles.

g.'s, hepatic. Lymph nodes located in front of the portal vein.

g.'s, inguinal. Lymph nodes in the inguinal region.

g., interscapular. Embryonic lymphatic tissue.

g., interstitial. G. in connective tissue of seminiferous tubules of testes and which produce internal secretions. SYN: *interstitial* or *Leydig's cells.*

g.'s, intestinal. Simple or branched tubular g.'s of the intestine which secrete the succus entericus. Include Brunner's g.'s, and crypts of Lieberkühn.

g.'s, jugular. G.'s, cervical, q.v.

g.'s, Krause's. Small g.'s in the conjunctiva of the eyelids, also called accessory lacrimal glands.

g.'s, labial. Multiple acinous g.'s between the mucosa of the lips and the opening on the inner lip.

g., lacrimal. A compound tubuloalveolar g. located in the roof of the orbit which secretes tears.

g.'s, lactiferous. G., mammary, q.v.

g.'s, Lieberkühn's. Tiny tubular g.'s on the intestinal mucosa. SYN: *intestinal g.'s.*

g., lingual. G.'s of the tongue, includes the anterior lingual g.'s (g.'s of Nuhn), posterior lingual g.'s (g.'s of von Ebner) and mucous g.'s at the root of the tongue.

g.'s, Littré's. Tiny mucous g.'s in the urethral mucosa in the cavernous portion.

g.'s, lumbar. Lymphatics located behind the peritoneal region and the lower section of the diaphragmatic posterior part.

g., Luschka's. G. located near the coccygeal tip.

g., lymph; g., lymphatic. Nodule of lymphatic tissue, found along the path of a lymphatic vessel.

g.'s, male. Cowper's, seminal, prostate, Tyson's.

g., mammary. A compound alveolar g. which secretes milk. SEE: *mammary g.'s.*

g., mandibular. The submaxillary g., q.v.

g.'s, meibomian. G.'s, tarsal, q.v.

g., merocrine. A g. in which the cells remain intact in the process of the elaboration and discharge of their secretion.

g.'s, Mery's. G., bulbourethral, q.v.

g.'s, Moll's. Modified sweat g.'s in the eyelid.

g.'s, Montgomery's. G.'s, areolar, q.v.

g.'s, Morgagni's. G.'s, Littré's, q.v.

g.'s, muciparous; g.'s, mucous. G.'s secreting mucus.

g.'s, nabothian. Dilated mucous g.'s in the uterine cervix.

g.'s, odoriferous. G.'s exuding odoriferous materials, as those around the prepuce or anus.

g.'s, oxyntic. Gastric g.'s usually found in the abdominal cardiac region.

g.'s, pacchionian. Small masses along the surface of the dura mater in the cranium.

g.'s, palatine. Mucous g.'s in the tissue of the palate.

g., palpebral. Tarsal g.'s, q.v.

g., parathyroid. SEE: *parathyroid*

g.'s, paraurethral. Small rudimentary g.'s which open on either side of the posteri-

or portion of the urethral orifice in the female; Skene's g.'s.

g., parotid. Largest salivary g., located in front of the ear. It is a compound tubuloacinous, serous g.

g.'s, Peyer's. G.'s, aggregate, q.v.

g., pineal. Tiny glandular body of conical shape located between two superior quadrigeminal bodies, connected with the thalamus, but not a part of the brain.

g., pituitary. The hypophysis cerebri, q.v. SEE: *pituitary.*

g.'s, preputial. G.'s, Tyson's, q.v.

g., prostate. G. surrounding male bladder neck and urethra. SEE: *prostate.*

g.'s, pulmonary. G.'s in lung tissue.

g.'s, pyloric. Gastric g.'s near the pylorus secrete gastric juice.

g., racemose. G., acinous, q.v.

g.'s, Rivini's. G.'s, sublingual, q.v.

g., saccular. An alveolar g.

g., salivary. Any g. secreting saliva, as parotid, sublingual and submaxillary. SEE: *salivary.*

g., sebaceous. A simple or branched alveolar g. which secretes sebum. They are found in the skin. Their ducts usually open into hair follicles.

g.'s, serous. G.'s, albuminous, q.v.

g., sex. Old term for the ovary or testis.

g.'s, Skene's. The paraurethral g.'s, q.v.

g.'s, solitary. G.'s, intestinal, q.v.

g.'s, sublingual. Tiny salivary g.'s situated on either side of the tongue.

g.'s, submaxillary. Tiny salivary g.'s on either side of the tongue in the submaxillary triangles.

g.'s, sudoriferous. G.'s secreting perspiration; situated in the skin. SYN: *sudoriparous g.'s; sweat g.'s.* SEE: *sweat.*

g., suprarenal. The adrenal g., q.v.

g.'s, sweat. G.'s, sudoriferous, q.v.

g.'s, synovial. G.'s secreting synovial fluid. SYN: *haversian g.'s.*

g.'s, tarsal. G.'s situated in the eyelid secreting sebaceous substance which keeps the lids from adhering to each other. SYN: *meibomian g.'s.*

g., thymus. The thymus body or thymus, q.v.

g., thyroid. Ductless g. situated in the neck in front of the trachea. SEE: *thyroid.*

g.'s, tracheal. Acinous g.'s of the tracheal mucosa.

g., tubular. A g. whose terminal secreting portions are narrow tubes.

g.'s, Tyson's. Tiny sebaceous g.'s found on the inner surface of the prepuce and on the glans of the penis.

g.'s, urethral. G.'s, Littré's, q.v.

g.'s, vaginal. Acinous g.'s in the vaginal mucosa. These are found only in uppermost portion near the cervix. The major portion of the vaginal mucosa is devoid of g.'s.

g.'s, vestibular. G.'s of the vaginal vestibule. They include the minor vestibular g.'s and the major vestibular g.'s (g.'s of Bartholin).

g.'s, vulvovaginal. G.'s, Bartholin's, q.v.

g.'s, Waldeyer's. G.'s in the eyelid.

g.'s, Weber's. G.'s in the tongue mucosa.

g.'s of Zeis. Large sebaceous g.'s found in the eyelids. They are associated with the follicles of the eyelashes.

g., Zuckerkandl's. Tiny yellowish lobe occasionally seen between geniohyoid muscles. An accessory thyroid g.

gland, words pert. to: "aden-" words, "adreno-" words, bulbourethral, endocrine, gastric, holocrine, name of each gland, seborrhea, "sial-" words.

glanders (glan'derz). Contagious infection by Malleomyces mallei in horses, donkeys and mules, communicable to man.

SYM: Fever, inflammation of the skin and mucous membranes, esp. those of the nasal cavity, with formation of ulcers and abscesses. Small subcutaneous nodules (farcy buds) develop which break down, giving rise to ulcers. Beginning as small areas, these tend to spread and coalesce and finally involve large areas which exude a viscid, mucopurulent discharge with a foul odor. May occur in acute or chronic form. In the acute septicemic form, prognosis is grave. It is almost invariably fatal.

TREATMENT: Experience with the disease is limited, but sulfonamides with streptomycin are the recommended therapy.

glandula (glan'du-lă). (pl. *glandulae*) A small gland. SYN: *glandule.*

glan'dular [L. *glandula,* little acorn]. Pert. to or of nature of a gland.

g. therapy. Treatment of disease with endocrine glands or their extracts. SYN: *organotherapy.*

glandule (glan'dūl). A small gland. SYN: *glandula.*

glans [L. *glans,* acorn]. (pl. *glandes*) 1. A gland. 2. Goiter.

g. clitoridis. [NA] The head of the clitoris. SEE: *clitoris.*

g. penis. [NA] Bulbous end of the penis. SYN: *g. phalli.* SEE: *penis.*

glare [ME. *glaren,* to gleam]. Temporary blurring of vision, with possible permanent injury to retina from intense light (visible radiation) emanating from highly reflecting objects, such as sunlight reflected from water or snow, or projected by automobile headlight, or by a therapeutic lamp.

glase'rian artery. [Johann Heinrich Glaser, Swiss anatomist, 1629-1675] A branch of internal maxillary artery; goes to tympanum. SYN: *tympanic artery.*

glaserian fissure. A fissure in the temporal bone. SYN: *petrotympanic fissure.*

glass [AS. *glaes*]. A hard, brittle, transparent material composed of silica and various bases.

g. polarized. A medium that permits the exiting light waves to vibrate in only one direction.

g., safety. A type of laminated g. which meets specific requirements concerning the force necessary to break it, and is so designed that it breaks without shattering. Its use in automobiles reduces the risk of injury in accidents which result in broken glass.

g., tempered. G. which has been treated with heat so that the force required to break it is increased in comparison to ordinary g.

g., ultraviolet transmitting. G. designed to admit ultraviolet radiation through it. The best transmits 50-60% of the solar radiation, between 290 and 320 millimicrons. With age the transparency to these rays drops off 50%.

glass'es [AS. *glaes,* glass]. 1. Transparent refractive device worn to correct eye defects. 2. Device worn to protect eyes from glare or particles in the air.

g., bifocal. Those in which the refracting power of the lower portion differs from that in the upper portion, the lower portion being used for viewing near objects or reading, the upper portion for distant objects. SYN: *Franklin g.*

g., safety. Those using heat-treated glass or impact-resistant plastic lenses. Their use serves to protect the eyes from dangerous slivers of glass which are produced when ordinary lenses are broken in an accident. Use of g. of this kind is mandatory in some states and in the U.S. Armed Forces.

g., sun. G. with tinted lenses for decreasing the intensity of light seen through them.

g., trifocal. G. with three different corrections in each lens: one each for near, intermediate and far vision.

glas'sy. Hyaline; vitreous; like glass, smooth and shiny.

Glau'ber's salt (glō'bĕr). [Johann Rudolf Glauber, Ger. physician, 1604-1668] Sodium sulfate.

glaucoma (glaw-kō'mä) [Gr. *glaukos*, gray, + *ōma*, swelling]. Disease of eye characterized by increase in intraocular pressure which results in atrophy of optic nerve and blindness. There are two types: primary, which occurs without known cause, and secondary in which there is an increase in intraocular pressure due to other eye disease. The acute type often attended by acute pain. The chronic type has an insidious onset. Normal tonometer reading is 13 to 22.

An early sign of glaucoma is subjective complaint that lights appear to have halos around them.

ETIOL: Closing of the canal of Schlemm due to a variety of conditions.

TREATMENT: *Nonoperative:* Miotics (eserine, pilocarpine); phospholine iodide. Control of associated disorders, as diabetes.

Operative: Paracentesis of cornea; iridectomy (broad peripheral); cyclodialysis; anterior sclerotomy; sclerotomy with inclusion of iris as iridotasis or iridocleisis; sclerectomy. SEE: *ciliarotomy.*

    g. absolutum. Eye completely blind; cornea insensitive; anterior chamber shallow; excavated optic disk; eye as hard as stone; extremely painful.

    g., chronic. Tonometer indicates intraocular pressure reading of up to 45-50; enlargement of anterior ciliary veins; cornea clear; dilated pupil; pain; poor vision during attacks; visual field may be normal; cupping of the optic disc is not present in the early stages.

    g., infantile. Increased intraocular tension occurring in infancy and producing uniform enlargement of eye.

    g. simplex. Pressure not high; contracted visual field; glaucomatous cupping; blindness; no acute attacks. TREATMENT: Neostigmine.

glaucomatous (glaw-ko'mä-tus). Pert. to glaucoma.

gleet [L. *glithus*, sticky]. A mucous discharge from the urethra in chronic gonorrhea.

Glénard's disease (glā-narz'). [Frantz Glénard, Fr. physician, 1848-1920] Prolapse of one or more of the internal organs. SYN: *enteroptosis; splanchnoptosis.*

glenohumeral (gle''no-hu'mer-al) [Gr. *glēnē*, socket, + L. *humerus,* humerus]. Pert. to the humerus and the glenoid cavity.

    g. ligaments. Three ligaments in shoulder.

gle'noid ["+ *eidos,* form]. Having the appearance of a socket.

    g. cavity. The socket which receives the head of the humerus, below the acromium at the junction of the superior and axillary borders.

    g. fossa. The mandibular fossa, which receives the capitulum of the mandible.

gli'a [Gr. *glia*, glue]. The neuroglia, q.v.; the non-nervous or supporting tissue of the brain and spinal cord.

    g. cells. Neuroglia cells, includes astrocytes, oligodendroglia (oligoglia), and microglia. SEE: *cell; neuroglia.*

gliacyte (gli'ă-sīt) ["+ *kytos,* cell]. A neuroglia cell.

gli'adin. A protein separable from the gluten of wheat.

It is deficient in the essential amino acid lysine. The sticky mass which results when wheat flour and water are mixed is due to g.

glial (gli'al). Concerning glia or neuroglia.

gliarase (gli'ă-rās) [Gr. *glia*, glue]. Astrocytic mass with incomplete fission of cytoplasm.

gliobacte'ria ["+ *baktērion*, little rod]. A zoogleal mass (bacteria imbedded in a gelatinous mass) containing bacilli.

glioblasto'ma ["+ *blastos*, germ, + *-ōma,* tumor]. A neuroglia cell tumor. SYN: *glioma.*

    g. multiforme. A neoplasm of the central nervous system, esp. the cerebrum, consisting of a variety of cellular types.

gliococ'cus [Gr. *glia,* glue, + *kokkos,* berry]. A micrococcus in a mass of zooglea.

gliocyte (gli'ō-sit) ["+ *kytos,* cell]. A neuroglia cell. SYN: *gliacyte.*

gliocyto'ma ["+ "+ *-ōma,* tumor]. A neuroglia cell tumor.

gliogenous (gli-ōj'ĕ-nŭs) [Gr. *glia*, glue, + *gennan,* to produce]. Of the nature of neuroglia.

glio'ma ["+ *-ōma,* tumor]. (pl. *glio'mata*) 1. A sarcoma of neuroglial origin. 2. Neoplasm or a tumor composed of neuroglia cells.

    g. retinae. Malignant tumor of retina; occurs in children; metastasizes late. SEE: *pseudoglioma.*

gliomatosis (gli''o-mă-tō'sis) ["+ "+ *-ōsis,* increase]. Formation of a glioma, esp. a large one.

gliomatous (gli'o-mă-tus). Affected with or of the nature of a glioma.

gliomyoma (gli''o-mi-o'mä) [Gr. *glia,* glue, + *mys,* muscle, + *-ōma,* tumor]. A mixed glioma and myoma.

glioneuroma (gli''o-nū-ro'mä) ["+ *neuron,* nerve, + *-ōma,* tumor]. A tumor having the characteristics of glioma and neuroma.

gliosarco'ma ["+ *sarx*, flesh, + *-ōma,* tumor]. Glioma combined with fusiform cells of sarcoma.

gliosis [Gr. *glia*, glue, + *-ōsis*, condition]. Proliferation of neuroglial tissue in the central nervous system.

gliosome (gli'o-sōm) ["+ *sōma*, body]. One of the rounded bodies seen in neuroglia cells.

gliotoxin (gli"o-tok'sin). An antibiotic obtained from several different fungi, esp. Trichoderma.

glischrin (glis'krin) [Gr. *glischros*, gluey]. Mucinous substance produced in urine by bacterial activity.

glischruria (glis-krū'rĭ-ă) ["+ *ouron*, urine]. Glischrin in the urine.

glisso'nian cirrhosis. Inflammation of peritoneal coat of the liver. SYN: *perihepatitis*.

glissoni'tis. Inflammation of Glisson's capsule.

Glisson's capsule (glis'ŭn). [Francis Glisson, Brit. physician, 1597-1677] The outer capsule of fibrous tissue investing the liver. SYN: *capsula fibrosa hepatis.*

glo'bin [L. *globus*, globe]. 1. A protein constituent of hemoglobin. 2. One of a particular group of proteins.

g. insulin. SEE: *insulin, globin.*

globinom'eter ["+ Gr. *metron*, measure]. Device for determining the amount of oxyhemoglobin in the blood.

glo'boid ["+ Gr. *eidos*, form]. Spheroid; resembling a globe.

globular (glob'u-lar) [L. *globus*, a globe]. Resembling a globe or globule; spherical.

globule (glob'ūl) [L. *globulus*, globule]. Any small rounded body.

globulim'eter ["+ Gr. *metron*, measure]. Device for determining the number of red cells in a measured volume of blood. SYN: *cytometer.*

globulin (glob'u-lin) [L. *globulus*, globule]. One of a group of simple proteins insoluble in pure water but soluble in neutral solutions of salts of strong acids with strong bases.

Ex: serum globulin; fibrinogen; myosinogen; lactoglobulin.

g., Ac. Accelerator g.; a g. present in blood serum which speeds up the conversion of prothrombin to thrombin in the presence of thromboplastin and calcium ions.

g., antihemophiliac. A clotting component present in the plasma which is essential for the normal agglutination and disintegration of blood platelets. It is deficient in the blood of hemophiliacs.

g., gamma. That fraction of serum g. with which most of the immune antibodies are associated. Most of the antibodies to viruses, bacterial agglutinogens, exotoxins, and injected foreign proteins are contained

in the g. g. fraction. It is thought to arise from plasma cells.

g., placental. A preparation of g.'s, antibodies obtained from the human placenta. It contains the antibodies or immune factors against measles and is used in the prevention, modification, and treatment of measles.

g., serum. G.'s present in blood plasma or serum; the fraction of the blood serum with which antibodies are associated. By electrophoresis, they can be separated into alpha, beta, and gamma globulins, which differ in their isoelectric points.

glob'ulism [L. *globulus*, globule, + Gr. *-ismos*, state]. Abnormal amt. of red corpuscles in the blood.

globulolysis (glŏb"ū-lŏl'ĭ-sĭs) ["+ Gr. *lysis*, dissolution]. Red blood corpuscle destruction. SYN: *hemolysis.*

globulolytic (glŏb"ū-lō-lĭt'ĭk). Capable of destroying red blood corpuscles.

globulose (glob'u-lōs) [L. *globulus*, globule]. Albumose or protein produced by the digestion of globulins.

globu'lysis [L. *globulus*, globule, + Gr. *lysis*, dissolution]. Destruction of red blood corpuscles. SYN: *globulolysis; hemolysis.*

globus [L.]. A globe or sphere.

g. hystericus. A lump in the throat in hysteria and other neuroses.

g. major. Head of epididymis.

g. minor. Lower end of epididymis.

g. pallidus. [NA] Pale section within the lenticular nucleus of the brain. SEE: *paleostriatum.*

glomangioma (glo-man" jĭ-o'mă) [L. *glomus*, a ball, + Gr. *angeion*, vessel, + -ōma, tumor]. A benign tumor which develops from an arteriovenous glomus (cluster of blood cells) of the skin.

glom'erate [L. *glomerāre*, to wind into a ball]. Conglomerate, clustered, grouped.

glomer'ular [L. *glomerulus*, little ball]. Clustered. Pert. to a glomerulus.

glomerule (glom'er-ūl) [L. *glomerulus*, little ball]. A glomerulus.

glomer'uli [L. *glomerulus*, little ball]. (sing. *glomerulus*) 1. Small structures in the malpighian body of the kidney made up of capillary blood vessels in a cluster and enveloped in a thin wall, giving off uriniferous tubules. 2. Plexuses of capillaries. Twisted secretory parts of sweat glands.

glomerulitis (glo-mer"u-li'tis) ["+ Gr. *-itis*, inflammation]. Inflammation of glomeruli, esp. of the renal glomeruli. SYN: *glomerulonephritis.*

glomerulonephritis (glo-mer"u-lo-nĭ-fri'tis) [L. *glomerulus*, little ball, + Gr. *nephros*, kidney, + -*itis*, inflammation]. A form of nephritis in which the lesions involve primarily the glomeruli. May be acute, subacute, or chronic. Etiology is unknown but it frequently follows other infections, esp. those of the upper respiratory tract. Characterized by hematuria, edema, hypertension, and, in severe cases, dyspnea, delirium, convulsions, and coma. SYM: *glomerulitis.*

glomerulus (glō-mĕr'ū-lŭs). (pl. *glomeruli*) 1. A small rounded mass or spherical structure. 2. One of the small structures in the malpighian body of the kidney made up of capillary blood vessels in a cluster and enveloped in a thin wall, giving off uriniferous tubules.

　　g., olfactory. A rounded body found in the olfactory bulb, formed by the numerous terminal branches of the dendrites of a mitral cell intertwining with the terminal fibers of several olfactory receptor cells.

glomus (glo'mus) [L. *glomus*, a ball]. A small, round swelling made up of tiny blood vessels and found in a stroma containing many nerve fibers.

　　g. caroticum. [NA] The carotid body, q.v.

　　g. choroideum. [NA] An enlargement of the choroid plexus at its entrance into the inferior corum of the lateral ventricle.

　　g. coccygeum. [NA] The coccygeal body.

glos'sa [Gr. glōssa, tongue]. The tongue.

glos'sal. Rel. to the tongue.

glossalgia (glos-sal'jĭ-ă) [Gr. *glōssa*, tongue, + *algos*, pain]. Pain in the tongue. SYM: *glossodynia.*

glossectomy (glos-ek'to-mĭ) ["+ *ektomē*, excision]. Partial or complete excision of tongue. SYM: *elinguation.*

Glossina (glos-sī'nă). A genus of flies called tsetse flies. Includes about 20 species of bloodsucking flies which are confined principally to central and southern Africa. They transmit the trypanosomes (Trypanosoma gambiense, T. rhodesiense), the causative agents of sleeping sickness in man, and other trypanosomes which infect wild and domestic animals. Important species are Glossina palpalis, G. morsitans, G. tachinoides, and G. swynnertoni. SEE: *Trypanosoma; sleeping sickness.*

glossi'tis [Gr. *glōssa*, tongue, + -*itis*, inflammation]. Inflammation of the tongue.

　　g., acute. Associated with stomatitis, q.v. The tongue is covered with ulcers and is tender and painful. Another form affects the parenchyma of tongue and is characterized by edema, which may spread to surrounding

structures, producing asphyxia and necessitating tracheotomy operation.

SYM: Tongue is painful; saliva thick and viscid, rendering swallowing difficult. Marked malaise, and often a rise in temperature.

TREATMENT: Oral cleanliness by frequent use of antiseptic mouthwashes. Anesthetic solution as oral rinse for pain. Bland or liquid diet.

　　g. areata exfoliativa. Geographic tongue, q.v.

　　g., chronic. Sometimes while suffering from chronic ill health, chronic dyspepsia, and septic teeth, this condition arises.

SYM: Tongue is large, pale, and flabby, and shows indentation marks from teeth pressure. Mouth is uncomfortable and there may be an unpleasant taste or foul odor.

TREATMENT: Improvement of the general health, relief of constipation, careful attention to oral hygiene.

　　g. desic'cans. A painful, raw, and fissured tongue.

　　g., median rhomboidal. An inflammatory area, somewhat diamond shaped, found on the dorsum of the tongue anterior to the vallate papillae.

　　g., Moeller's. Glossodynia exfoliativa, q.v.

　　g. parasit'ica. Black tongue. SYM: *glossophytia.*

glosso- [Gr. *glōssa*, tongue]. Prefix pert. to the tongue.

glossocele (glos'so-sēl) [Gr. *glōssa*, tongue, + *kēlē*, swelling]. Swelling and protrusion of the tongue due to disease or malformation.

glossodynamometer (glos''so-dī''nă-mom'ĕ-ter) ["+ *dynamis*, power, + *metron*, measure]. Device for measuring contractile power of the tongue muscles.

glossodynia (glos''o-din'ĭ-ă) ["+ *odynē*, pain]. Pain in the tongue. SYM: *glossalgia.*

　　g. exfoliativa. Moeller's glossitis. A chronic superficial inflammation of the tongue characterized by burning or pain and increased sensitivity to hot and spicy foods.

glossoepiglottic (glos''o-ĕp-ĭ-glŏt'ĭk) [Gr. *glōssa*, tongue, + *epi*, upon, + *glōttis*, back of tongue]. Pert. to the ligament between base of tongue and epiglottis.

glossoepiglottidean (glos''o-ĕp-ĭ-glŏ-tĭd'ē-ăn). Rel. to the tongue and epiglottis.

　　g. folds. Three mucous membrane folds from base of tongue to the epiglottis. SYM: *plicae epiglotticae.*

　　g. ligament. Elastic band from base of tongue to the epiglottis in middle g. fold.

glossograph (glŏs'o-grăf) [Gr. *glōssa*, tongue, + *graphein*, to write]. An instrument for recording the tongue's movements in speaking.

glossohyal (glŏs''o-hī'ăl) ["+ *yoeidēs*, U-shaped]. Rel. to tongue and hyoid bone. SYN: *hyoglossal.*

glossokinesthetic (glŏs''o-kĭn''ĕs-thĕt'ĭk) ["+ *kinēsis*, movement, + *aisthētikos*, perceptive]. Pert. to movements of the tongue, esp. those in speech.

glossolabial (glŏs''ō-lā'bĭ-ăl) [Gr. *glōssa*, tongue, + L. *labium*, lip]. Pert. to the tongue and lips.

glossolalia (glŏs''ō-lā'lĭ-ă) ["+ *lalia*, babble]. Repetition of senseless remarks not related to the subject or situation involved.

glossology (glŏ-sŏl'ō-jĭ) ["+ *logos*, study]. Study of the tongue and its diseases. SYN: *glottology.*

glossolysis (glŏ-sŏl'ĭ-sĭs) [Gr. *glōssa*, tongue, + *lysis*, loosening]. Paralysis of tongue. SYN: *glossoplegia.*

glossopalatine (glŏs''ō-păl'a-tīne). Pert. to the tongue and the palate.

glossopathy (glŏ-sŏp'ă-thĭ) [Gr. *glōssa*, tongue, + *pathos*, disease]. Disease of the tongue.

glossopharyngeal (glŏs''o-fă-rĭn'jĭ-ăl) ["+ *pharynx*, pharynx]. Rel. to tongue and pharynx.

g. nerve. Ninth cranial n. Function: Special sensory (taste), visceral sensory, motor. Origin: By several roots from the medulla oblongata. Distribution: Pharynx, ear, meninges, posterior third of tongue, parotid gland. Branches: Carotid, tympanic, pharyngeal, lingual, tonsillar, and sinus nerve of Hering.

glossophytia (glŏs''o-fĭ'tĭ-ă) ["+ *phyton*, plant]. Black or hairy tongue, characterized by the appearance on the dorsum of the tongue of a dark furlike patch consisting of hypertrophied filiform papillae, pigment, and shed epithelial cells. SYN: *hyperkeratosis linguae.*

glossoplasty (glŏs'o-plăs''tĭ) ["+ *plassein*, to form]. Reparative surgery of the tongue.

glossoplegia (glŏs''ō-plē'jĭ-ă) [Gr. *glōssa*, tongue, + *plēgē*, stroke]. Paralysis of tongue, usually unilateral. ETIOL: Cerebral hemorrhage, disease, or injury which involves the hypoglossal nerve. SYN: *glossolysis.*

glossoptosis (glŏs''ŏp-tō'sĭs) ["+ *ptōsis*, a dropping]. A dropping of the tongue downward out of normal position.

glossopyrosis (glŏs''o-pī-rō'sĭs) ["+ *pyrōsis*, a burning]. A burning sensation of the tongue.

glossorrhaphy (glŏ-sŏr'ă-fĭ) [Gr. *glōssa*, tongue, + *raphē*, suture]. Suture of wound of the tongue.

glossoscopy (glŏ-sŏs'kŏ-pĭ) ["+ *skopein*, to examine]. Inspection of the tongue.

glossospasm (glŏs'o-spăzm) ["+ *spasmos*, spasm]. Spasmodic contraction of muscles of the tongue.

glossotomy (glŏ-sŏt'ō-mĭ) [Gr. *glōssa*, tongue, + *tomē*, incision]. Incision of tongue.

glossotrichia (glŏs''o-trĭk'ĭ-ă) ["+ *thrix*, hair]. Hairy tongue, due to greatly elongated filiform papillae which give the tongue a hairy appearance.

gloss'y. Smooth and shining.

g. skin. Shiny appearance of the skin due to atrophy or injury to nerves.

glot'tic [Gr. *glōttis*, back of tongue]. Of or pert. to the tongue, or the glottis.

glottis (glŏt'ĭs) [Gr., back of tongue]. (pl. *glottises* or *glottides*) [NA] The sound-producing apparatus of the larynx consisting of the two vocal folds and the intervening space, the rima glottidis. A leaf-shaped lid of fibrocartilage (the epiglottis) protects this opening.

g., edema of. The accumulation of fluid in the tissues lining the larynx. It may result from irritation of the larynx from improper use of the voice, excessive use of tobacco or alcohol, chemical fumes, acute infections, or more serious conditions such as tuberculous or syphilitic laryngitis.

SYM: Hoarseness, and later complete aphonia, extreme dyspnea at first on inspiration, but later on expiration also. Stridulous respiration, barking cough when epiglottis is involved.

glotti'tis [Gr. *glōttis*, back of tongue, + *-itis*, inflammation]. Inflammation of the tongue. SYN: *glossitis.*

glottol'ogy ["+ *logos*, study]. The study of the tongue and its diseases. SYN: *glossology.*

glucagon (glū'kă-gŏn). USP. A substance secreted by the alpha cells of the pancreas. It stimulates the breakdown of glycogen and the release of glucose by the liver, thereby causing an increase in blood sugar.

glucatonia (glū-kă-tō'nĭ-ă) [Gr. *gleukos*, sweet (new wine), + *a*, not, + *tonos*, tone, tension]. Reduction of blood sugar by administering insulin to the extent that symptoms result. Insulin shock.

gluciphore (glū'sĭ-fŏr). Glucophore, q.v.

glucocorticoid (glū''ko-kŏrt'ĭ-koyd) [Gr. *gleukos*, sweet, + L. *cortex*, cortex, + Gr. *eidos*, form]. A general classification of adrenal cortical hormones which are primarily active in protecting against stress and in affecting protein and carbohydrate metabolism. SEE: *mineralocorticoid.*

glucohemia (glū″ko-hē′mĭ-ă) [″+ *haima,* blood]. Sugar in the blood. SYN: *glycosemia.*

gluconeogenesis (glū″ko-nē″o-jĕn′ĕ-sĭs) [Gr. *gleukos,* sweet (new wine), + *neos,* new, + *genesis,* origin]. The formation of glucose from noncarbohydrate sources such as proteins, and possibly fats. It occurs in the liver under such conditions as low carbohydrate intake or starvation. SYN: *glyconeogenesis.*

glucophore (glū′ko-fōr) [″+ *phorein,* to carry]. An atomic group which, when combined with other tasteless atoms called auxoglucs, forms sweet compounds. SEE: *auxogluc.*

glucose (glū′kōs) [L. *glucosum* from Gr. *gleukos,* sweet (new wine)]. 1. A sugar. In medicine, the word is used to indicate the sugar dextrose. This is also called d-glucose. 2. An intermediate in metabolism of carbohydrates in the body. Formed during digestion.

G. is the most important carbohydrate in body metabolism. It is formed during digestion from the hydrolysis of di- and polysaccharides, esp. starch, and absorbed from the intestines into the blood of the portal vein. In its passage through the liver excess g. is converted into glycogen (glycogensis). The concentration of sugar in the blood is approximately 0.1% (100 mg.), the amount being maintained at a fairly constant level (80-120 mg.) through the action of insulin produced by the islets of Langerhans of the pancreas. Failure of the pancreas to produce adequate insulin results in hyperglycemia in which the blood sugar (glucose) level may rise to 200 mg. or higher. When above the renal threshold (about 160-180 mg./100 ml.), g. appears in the urine (glycosuria), a symptom of diabetes. Overproduction of insulin or injection of insulin as in insulin shock treatment reduces the blood sugar below normal, a condition known as hypoglycemia, q.v.

In the tissue, g. may be converted into glycogen, converted into fat, or oxidized to carbon dioxide and water. Free g. is not used in the tissues until phosphorylated by ATP (adenosinetriphosphate). This occurs through the action of an enzyme, hexokinase, with the resultant production of glucose-6-phosphate. Through a complex series of reactions involving several enzymes, the action of certain hormones, and the formation of several intermediate products including lactic and pyruvic acids, oxidation to carbon and water is brought about. Hormones of the anterior lobe of the hypophysis, the adrenal gland (cortex and medulla), thyroid and the gonads play a role in carbohydrate metabolism.

When the blood sugar is below normal, fats are consumed. Incomplete combustion leads to the formation of ketone bodies, also a symptom of diabetes. Blood sugar acts as a protein sparer, q.v. Nervous tissue is especially dependent upon g. as its source of energy, the brain being able to oxidize it directly.

g. conditions which change blood
The g. found in the blood stream has a dual origin. First, g. is present normally in both the whole blood and plasma; secondly, the greater percentage of the normal g. concentration has an exogenous origin—that is, from the food intake. The normal g. concentration in the blood is 80-120 mg./100 cc. Increased concentration is associated with the following conditions: acromegaly; adrenal tumors; increased intercranial pressure; diabetes mellitus; hemochromatosis; hyperthyroidism; hyperpituitarism; hyperadrenalism. Decreased concentration is associated with Addison's disease; adenoma or carcinoma of islets of Langerhans; cretinism; hyperinsulinism; hypopituitarism; hypothyroidism; insulin shock; muscular dystrophy; myxedema.

g., liquid. USP. A liquid obtained from the incomplete hydrolysis of starch. It is a thick syrupy liquid, sweet in taste, containing d-glucose (dextrose), dextrins, and other carbohydrates. It is used for nutritive purposes and in various pharmaceutical and food preparations.

g. 6-phosphate dehydrogenase.
An enzyme present in the liver and kidney which is important in converting glycerol to glucose.

g. 6-phosphate dehydrogenase deficiency anemia. Hemolytic anemia which is produced when persons who have a deficiency of glucose 6-phosphate are given certain drugs. SYN: *G6PD anemia.*

g. tolerance test. A test done by giving a certain amount of g. to the patient orally or intravenously. Blood samples are drawn at specified intervals and the blood g. determined in each sample. By this means, the ability of the patient to metabolize g. can be determined. In suspected cases of hyperinsulinism, the test is prolonged to six hours with samples of blood being drawn hourly and analyzed for sugar content. If the blood-sugar level continues to drop after three hours, falling below 80 mg./100 cc., hyperinsulinism is indicated although other conditions may produce a deficiency in blood sugar (hypoglycemia).

g. tolerance test, cortisone oral. A test which involves administering a dose of cortisone 8 1/2 hours and 2 1/2 hours prior to giving the glucose. The cortisone increases the demand for insulin and thus reveals deficiency in insulin response.

glucosidase (glŭ'kō-sī-dās). An enzyme which catalyzes the hydrolysis of a glucoside.

glucoside (glū'kō-sīd) [Gr. *gleukos,* sweet (new wine)]. A glycoside which upon hydrolysis yields a sugar, glucose, and one or two additional products. G.'s are numerous and widely distributed in plants. Many g.'s have medicinal properties, for example digitalin and strophanthin, present in digitalis and strophanthus respectively, which have a specific effect upon the heart. SEE: *glycoside.*

glucosin (glū'kō-sĭn). Any one of a series of bases derived by action of ammonia on glucose.

glucosuria (glū″kō-su'rĭ-ā) [Gr. *gleukos,* sweet (new wine), + *ouron,* urine]. Abnormal amt. of sugar in the urine. SYN: *glycosuria.*

glue ear. A descriptive term for chronic accumulation of a high viscosity fluid in the middle ear. Occurs principally in children 5-8 years old. It causes deafness which can be treated by removal of the exudate.

Gluge's corpuscles (glü'gĭ). [Gottlieb Gluge, Ger. pathologist, 1812-1898] Granular cells containing fat droplets, usually found in degenerating nervous tissue.

glutamic acid (glū-tăm'ĭk) [L. *glūten,* glue, + *am*monium]. An amino acid

$$COOH(CH_2)_2CH(NH_2)COOH$$

formed in the hydrolysis of proteins. It is the only amino acid metabolized by the brain.

glutaminase (glū-tam'ĭ-nās). An enzyme which catalyzes the breakdown of glutamine into glutamic acid and ammonia.

glutamine (glū'tă-mĭn, -mēn″). The monoamide of amino-glutaric acid. It is present in the juices of many plants and is essential in the hydrolysis of proteins.

glutathione (glū-tă-thi'ōn) [L. *gluten,* glue, + Gr. *theion,* sulfur]. A tripeptide of glutamic acid, cysteine, and glycine.

Found in small quantities in active animal tissues; takes up and gives off hydrogen; fundamentally important in cellular respiration.

gluteal (glū'tē-ăl) [Gr. *gloutos,* buttock]. Pertaining to the buttocks.

 g. fold. Crease between the thigh and the buttocks. SEE: *rump.*

 g. reflex. Contraction of g. muscles from stimulation of their skin.

glutelin (glū'tē-lin) [L. *gluten,* glue]. A simple protein found in grain seeds, soluble in al-

kalies and dilute acids, but not in neutral solutions. SEE: *protein.*

glu'ten [L., glue]. Vegetable albumin, a protein which can be prepared from wheat and other grain.

 g. enteropathy. Adult celiac disease. A condition associated with malabsorption of food from the intestinal tract. The symptoms of diarrhea and malnutrition are usually controlled by eliminating gluten from the diet. SEE: *gluten-free diet.*

 g. -free diet. Elimination of g. from the diet by avoiding all products containing wheat, rye, oats, or barley and vegetables such as beans, cabbage, turnips, dried peas, and cucumbers. Rice, potatoes, corn, and cornmeal are allowed.

glu'tin. The viscid portion of wheat gluten. SYN: *gliadin.*

glutinous (glū'tĭn-ŭs) [L. *glutinosus,* glue]. Adhesive; sticky.

gluti'tis [Gr. *gloutos,* buttock, + *-itis,* inflammation]. Inflammation of muscles of buttocks.

glycase (glī'kās) [Gr. *glykys,* sweet]. The enzyme that converts maltose into dextrose. SEE: *enzyme.*

glycemia (glī-sē'mĭ-ā) ["+ *haima,* blood]. Sugar or glucose in the blood. SYN: *glycosemia, q.v.*

glyceride (glĭs'ĕr-ĭd) [Gr. *glykys,* sweet]. An ester of glycerin compounded with an acid.

glycerin (glĭs'ĕr-ĭn). USP. $C_3H_8O_3$. A trihydric alcohol, trihydroxy-propane present in chemical combination in all fats. It is a syrupy, colorless liquid, soluble in all proportions in water and alcohol. It is made commercially by the hydrolysis of fats, esp. during the manufacture of soap. SYN: *glycerol.*

 Used extensively as a solvent, as a preservative, as an emollient in various skin diseases.

glycerol (glĭs'ĕr-ōl) [Gr. *glykys,* sweet]. A synonym for glycerine, q.v.

glyceryl (glĭs'ĕr-ĭl). The trivalent radical C_3H_5 of glycerol.

 g. trinitrate. Nitroglycerin (USP). Made by action of nitric acid on glycerin in presence of sulfuric acid.

 Used to dilate blood vessels in some cases of angina pectoris. Commonly in tablet form for sublingual use. *NOTE:* Tablets should be stored in tight containers to prevent loss of potency.

glycine (glī'sēn, sĭn) [Gr. *glykys,* sweet]. The simplest of amino acids, alpha aminoacetic acid.

glyco-, glyc- (gli-ko) [Gr. *glykys,* sweet]. Prefix used in chemical compounds to indicate

(1) relationship to sugar or (2) presence of glycerol or similar substance.

gly'cocin. Glycine, q.v.

glycoclastic (glī″ko-klăs'tĭk) [Gr. *glykys*, sweet, + *klan*, to break]. Pert. to the hydrolysis and digestion of sugars.

glycogen (glī'kŏ-jĕn) ["+ *gennan*, to produce]. A polysaccharide ($C_6H_{10}O_{5x}$) commonly called animal starch, a whitish powder which can be prepared from mammalian liver and muscle and other animal tissues.

Formation of g. from carbohydrate sources is called glycogenesis; from noncarbohydrate sources, glyconeogenesis. The conversion of g. to glucose is called glycogenolysis.

G. is the form in which carbohydrate is stored in the animal body for future conversion into sugar, and for subsequent use in performing muscular work or for liberating heat.

It is formed from sugar and a part of the fat and protein in the blood. It is converted when needed by the tissues into glucose. It is a muscle food, and with the contraction of the muscles it breaks down into lactic acid, causing fatigue. Oxygen is then needed to convert lactic acid back into g., at which time some of the lactic acid is burned, producing carbonic acid and heat. Sugar from the blood takes the place of the lactic acid consumed.

Oxygen and sugar are necessary to prevent fatigue from muscular exertion long continued.

glycogenase (glī-kŏ'jĕn-ās). An enzyme in the liver which hydrolyzes glycogen. Its end product is dextrose.

glycogenesis (glī″kŏ-jĕn'ĕ-sĭs) [Gr. *glykys*, sweet, + *genesis*, formation]. The formation of glycogen, as occurs in man after the eating of a carbohydrate meal.

glycogenet'ic. Pert. to the formation of glycogen.

glycogen'ic. Rel. to glycogen.

glycogenolysis (glī″ko-jĕn-ŏl'ĭ-sĭs) [Gr. *glykys*, sweet, + *gennan*, to produce, + *lysis*, dissolution]. Conversion of glycogen into glucose in body tissues.

glycogenolytic (glī″ko-jĕn″ŏ-lĭt'ĭk) ["+ "+ *lysis*, dissolution]. Pert. to the hydrolysis of glycogen.

glycogenosis (glī″kŏ-jĕn-ō'sĭs) ["+ "+ -*ōsis*, diseased condition]. Glycogen retention or storage disease. Due to the inability of the liver to convert glycogen to dextrose, glycogen is retained in the liver. SYN: *von Gierke's disease.*

glycogeusia (glī″ko-ju'sĭ-ă) ["+ *geusis*, taste]. A sweet taste.

glycohemia (glī″ko-hē'mĭ-ă) [Gr. *glykys*, sweet, + *haima*, blood]. Abnormal amt. of sugar in the blood. SYN: *glycosemia.*

glycol (glī'kŏl, -kōl) [Gr. *glykys*, sweet, + alco*hol*]. Any one of the dihydric alcohols related to ethylene glycol, $C_2H_4(OH)_2$.

glycolipid(e (glī″ko-lĭp'id) ["+ *lipos*, fat]. Compound of fatty acids with a carbohydrate, containing nitrogen, but no phosphoric acid. Found in myelin sheath of nerves.

glycolysis (glī-kŏl'ĭ-sĭs) ["+ *lysis*, dissolution]. Hydrolysis of sugar by an enzyme in the body.

glycolyt'ic. Pert. to hydrolyzing sugar.

    g. enzyme. An enzyme which catalyzes the hydrolysis of sugars.

glycometabolic (glī″ko-mĕt-ă-bŏl'ĭk) [Gr. *glykys*, sweet, + *metabolē*, change]. Rel. to metabolism of sugar.

glycometabolism (glī″ko-mĕ-tăb'ŏ-lĭzm). Utilization of sugar, q.v., by the body. SYN: *saccharometabolism.* SEE: *metabolism.*

glyconeogenesis (glī″ko-nē-ō-jĕn'ĕ-sĭs) [Gr. *glykys*, sweet, + *neos*, new, + *genesis*, formation]. The formation of carbohydrates from noncarbohydrates, such as fat or protein. SYN: *gluconeogenesis.*

glyconucleoprotein (glī″ko-nū″klē-ō-prō'tē-ĭn) ["+ L. *nucleus*, kernel, + Gr. *prōtos*, first]. A nucleoprotein so named to emphasize the presence of sugar units in the substance.

glycopenia (glī-ko-pē'nĭ-ă) ["+ *penia*, poverty]. Having a tendency to hypoglycemia.

glycopex'ic [Gr. *glykys*, sweet, + *pēxis*, fixation]. Pert. to the fixing or storing of sugar.

glycopex'is. The storing of glycogen in the liver.

glycophilia (glī″ko-fĭl'ĭ-ă) [Gr. *glykys*, sweet, + *philein*, to love]. A condition in which there is a marked tendency to hyperglycemia.

glycopolyuria (glī″ko-pŏl'ĭ-ū'rĭ-ă) ["+ *polys*, much, + *ouron*, urine]. Diabetes mellitus with moderately increased sugar in the urine but greatly increased uric acid.

glycopri'val, glycopri'vous ["+ L. *privus*, deprived of]. Lacking in or without carbohydrates.

glycoprotein (glī″kŏ-prō'tē-ĭn) [Gr. *glykys*, sweet, + *prōtos*, first]. A compound consisting of a carbohydrate and protein. The carbohydrate is hexosamine, an amino sugar.

glycoptyalism (glī″ko-tī'ăl-ĭzm) ["+ *ptyalon*, saliva, + *ismos*, state of]. Excretion of glucose in the saliva.

glycoregulation (glī″ko-rĕg″ū-lā'shŭn) ["+ L. *regula*, rule]. The regulation of sugar metabolism.

glycoreg'ulatory. Rel. to glycoregulation.

glycorrhachia (glī-ko-rak'ĭ-ă) [Gr. *glykys*, sweet, + *rhachis*, spine]. Sugar in the cerebrospinal fluid.

glycorrhea (glī''ko-rē'ă) ["+ *rhoia*, flow]. Discharge of sugar from the body as in urine.

glycosecretory (glī''ko-sē-krē'tō-rī) ["+ L. *secretus*, from *secernere*, to separate]. Pert. to or determining the formation of glycogen.

glycosemia (glī-ko-sē'mĭ-a) ["+ *haima*, blood]. Abnormal amount of sugar in the blood.

glycosialia (glī''ko-sī-āl'ĭ-ă) [Gr. *glykys*, sweet, + *sialon*, saliva]. Sugar in the saliva.

glycosialorrhea (glī''ko-si''āl-o-rē'ă) ["+ "+ *rhoia*, flow]. Excessive secretion of saliva containing sugar.

gly'coside. A substance derived from plants which upon hydrolysis yields a sugar and one or more additional products. Depending on the sugar formed, glycosides are designated glucosides, galactosides, etc. SEE: *glucoside.*

glycosom'eter [Gr. *glykys*, sweet, + *metron*, measure]. Device for determining proportion of sugar in urine in glycosuria.

glycosuria (glī''kō-sū'rĭ-ă) ["+ *ouron*, urine]. The presence of sugar (glucose) in the urine.

Traces of sugar, particularly glucose, may occur in normal urine, but are not detected by ordinary qualitative methods. In routine urinalyses the presence of a reducing substance is suspicious of diabetes mellitus. It is found when the blood sugar level exceeds the renal threshold (about 170 mg./100 ml. of blood). Fasting level of blood glucose is usually between 80 and 120 mg./100 ml. of blood.

Glycosuria may result from pancreatic (insulin) insufficiency; disorders of the endocrine glands, esp. hypophysis, adrenals, thyroid, or ovaries; excessive carbohydrate intake; excessive glycogenolysis; reduction of renal threshold.

    g., alimentary. G. following ingestion of large amounts of starches or sugars.

    g., diabetic. G. resulting from hyposecretion of insulin.

    g., emotional. G. resulting from emotional states such as worry or anxiety.

    g., phloridzin. G. resulting from the injection of phloridzin which reduces the renal threshold for glucose.

    g., pituitary. G. resulting from dysfunction of the anterior pituitary.

    g., renal. Condition occurring when glucose is persistent and not accompanied by hyperglycemia. It occurs when the renal threshold for glucose is decreased.

glycuresis (glī''kū-rē'sĭs) [Gr. *glykys*, sweet, + *ourēsis*, urination]. Presence of sugar (glucose) in the urine. SYN: *glycosuria*, q.v.

glycuronuria (glī-kū''rō-nū'rĭ-ă). Glycuronic acid in the urine.

glycylglycine (glīs''īl-glīs'ĭn). The simplest form of a polypeptide.

glycyltryptophan (glīs''īl-trĭp'tō-fān). A dipeptide of glycine and tryptophan.

glycyrrhiza (glīs-ĭ-rī'ză) [Gr. *glykys*, sweet, + *rhiza*, root]. USP. The dried root of Glycyrrhiza glabra known commercially as Spanish licorice. Used as an ingredient of glycyrrhiza fluidextract (USP) and glycyrrhiza syrup (USP), both of which are used as flavoring agents in compounding medicine. SEE: *licorice.*

glyoxalase (glī-ŏk'să-lās). An enzyme which catalyzes the conversion of methylglyoxal to lactic acid by the addition of water.

gm., Gm. Abbr. for *gram*.

gnat (năt). Any of a number of small insects belonging to the order Diptera, suborder Orthorrhapha. Term applied generally to insects smaller than mosquitoes. Includes black flies, midges, and sand flies.

    g., buffalo. A small dipterous insect belonging to the family Simuliidae. SEE: *Simulium.*

gnathalgia (năth-ăl'jĭ-ă) [Gr. *gnathos*, jaw, + *algos*, pain]. Pain in the jaw. SYN: *gnathodynia.*

gnathic (năth'ĭk) [Gr. *gnathos*, jaw]. Pert. to an alveolar process or to the jaw.

gnathion (năth'ĭ-ŏn). Lowest point of middle line of lower jaw; a craniometric point.

gnathitis (năth-ī'tĭs) [Gr. *gnathos*, jaw, + *-itis*, inflammation]. Inflammation of the jaw or adjacent soft parts.

gnatho- (nă-th'o) [Gr. *gnathos*, jaw]. Prefix pert. to jaw or cheek.

gnathocephalus (năth-o-sēf'ă-lus) [Gr. *gnathos*, jaw, + *kephalē*, head]. A malformed fetus in which the head consists principally of the jaws.

gnathodynamometer (năth''ō-dī'nă-mŏm'ĕ-tĕr) [Gr. *gnathos*, jaw, + *dynamis*, power, + *metron*, measure]. Device for measuring biting force.

gnathodynia (năth-ō-dīn'ĭ-ă) ["+ *odynē*, pain]. Pain in the jaw. SYN: *gnathalgia.*

gnathoplasty (năth'ō-plăs''tĭ) ["+ *plassein*, to form]. Reparative surgery of jaws or cheek.

gnathoschisis (năth-ŏs'kĭ-sĭs) [Gr. *gnathos*, jaw, + *schizein*, to split]. Congenital jaw cleft.

Gnathostoma (năth-ŏs'tō-mă) ["+ *stoma*, mouth]. A genus of nematode worms which infest the stomach walls of domestic and wild animals. They occasionally accidentally infest man.

gnathostomiasis (năth″o-sto-mǐ′ă-sǐs). Infestation with Gnathostoma, q.v.

gnosia (no′sǐ-ă) [Gr. *gnōsis*, knowledge]. The perceptive faculty of recognizing persons, things, and forms.

gnotobiotics (nō″to-bǐ-ŏt′ǐks) [Gr. *gnotos*, known, + *bios*, life]. Study of animals that have been raised in germ-controlled or germ-free surroundings.

goat-leap pulse. An irregular and bounding pulse. SEE: *pulse*.

goat milk. Food value of 100 gm. (fluid; whole): Cal. 67; protein 3.2 gm.; fat 4.0 gm.; carbohydrate 4.6 gm.; calcium 129 mg.; vitamin A, 160 I.U.

goblet cell. A type of secretory cell found in the epithelium of the intestinal and respiratory tracts; a unicellular gland which secretes mucus. Mucin droplets accumulate in the distal end of the cell, forming a large ovoid mass which causes the cell to become swollen and distorted in shape. The free surface of the cell finally ruptures liberating the mucus. SYN: *mucous cell.* SEE: *cell; gland; mucus; secretion.*

gog′gle-eyed. Having an abnormally protruding eye. SYN: *exophthalmic.*

goiter (goy′tĕr) [L. *guttur*, throat]. An enlargement of the thyroid gland.

ETIOL: May be due to lack of iodine in diet; thyroiditis; inflammation from infection; tumors; or hyper- or hypofunction of the thyroid gland. SYN: *struma.*

   g., aberrant. Supernumerary thyroid enlargement.

   g., acute. G. growing rapidly.

   g., adenomatous. Thyroid enlargement due to growth of encapsulated adenomata. Nodular g.

   g., colloid. One in which there is a great increase of follicular contents.

   g., congenital. One present at birth.

   g., cystic. A g. in which a cyst or a number of cysts are formed. May result from the degeneration of tissue or liquification within an adenoma.

   g., diffuse. G. in which the thyroid tissue is diffuse in contrast to its nodular form as in adenomatous g.

   g., diver; g., diving. G. which is movable, located sometimes below and at other times above the sternal notch.

   g., endemic. G. development in certain geographic localities, especially those in which iodine is deficient in food and water.

   g., exophthalmic. G. with exophthalmos. SYN: *Graves' disease; hyperthyroidism; thyrotoxicosis.*

ETIOL: Unknown. Occurs in constitutionally predisposed individuals. Incidence higher in females.

SYM: Bulging eyeballs generally present, enlarged thyroid, tremor of fingers and muscles of hands, tachycardia, increased metabolism, vomiting and diarrhea, profuse perspiration, nervous irritability, skin eruptions, emaciation, anemia, hyperglycemia. G.'s are more prevalent in fresh water and lake countries, and less so on the sea coast, due to the lack of iodine in fresh water. Iodine and iodized salt are used as remedies and preventives.

   g., fibrous. G. with hyperplastic capsule and stroma of the thyroid gland.

   g., follicular. G., parenchymatous, q.v.

   g., hyperplastic. G., parenchymatous, q.v.

   g., intrathoracic. G. in which a portion of the thyroid tissue lies within the thoracic cavity.

   g., lingual. Hypertrophied mass forming a tumor at posterior portion of dorsum of tongue.

   g., parenchymatous. G. characterized by multiplication of cells lining the follicles or alveoli. There is usually a reduction in colloid and the follicular cavities assume various sizes and are often obliterated by infoldings of their walls. Fibrous tissue may increase markedly. Iodine content of gland is low. G. usually of a diffuse nature.

   g., perivascular. G. surrounding a large blood vessel.

   g., retrovascular. G. development behind a large blood vessel.

   g., simple. Thyroid gland hyperplasia unaccompanied by constitutional symptoms.

   g., substernal. Enlargement of lower part of thyroid isthmus.

   g., suffocative. G. causing shortness of breath due to pressure.

   g., toxic. Exophthalmic g. or g. in which there is an excessive production of the thyroid hormone.

   g., vascular. G. due to distention of blood vessels of thyroid gland.

goitrogens [L. *guttur*, throat, + *gennan*, to produce]. Any substance which causes goiter. These occur in nature in certain foods including turnips, rutabaga, and cabbage.

gold. SYMB: *Au* (from L. *aurum*, shining down). At. wt. 196.967; at. no. 79; sp. gr. 19.32. A metallic element, yellow in color. Its salts are used in early rheumatoid arthritis and in nondisseminated lupus erythematosus. Radioactive gold, gold Au 198 injection (USP), is used in treatment of certain types of cancer and as an aid in outlining certain organs, as in liver scanning. SEE: *scanning.*

goldbeater's skin. A membrane from the cecum of the ox for surgical use.

Gold'flam's disease. [Samuel V. Goldflam, Polish physician, 1852-1932] Excessive tiring of voluntary muscles and rapid decrease of contractility. SYN: *myasthenia gravis pseudoparalytica.*

Golgi apparatus (gol'jī). [Camillo Golgi, It. histologist, 1844-1926] A lamellar membranous structure near the nucleus of almost all cells. It contains curved parallel series of flattened saccules which are often expanded at their ends. The structure is best seen by electron microscopy. In secretory cells the apparatus functions to concentrate and package the secretory product. Its function in other cells, though apparently important, is poorly understood.

Golgi's cells. Multipolar nerve cells in the cerebral cortex and posterior horns of spinal cord. There are two types: Type I, those that possess long axons and Type II, those that possess short axons.

Golgi's corpuscle. A sensory nerve ending or receptor found in tendons, or aponeuroses; an end organ of muscle sense. Also called organ of Golgi.

Goll's tract. [Friedrich Goll, Swiss anatomist, 1829-1904] One in posterior white column of spinal cord. SYN: *faciculus gracilis* [NA].

gomphiasis (gŏm-fī'ă-sĭs) [Gr.]. An abnormal condition in which the teeth become loose.

gomphosis (gŏm-fō'sĭs) [Gr. *gomphos*, bolt, tooth, + *-ōsis*, condition]. A conical process fitting into a socket in immovable joint. A tooth in its bony socket is an example of this type joint.

gonad (gō'năd, gŏn'ăd) [Gr. *gonos*, procreation, genitals]. A generic term referring to both the female sex glands, or ovaries, and the male sex glands, or testes. The embryonic sex gland before differentiation into definitive testis or ovary.

Each forms the cells necessary for human reproduction, spermatozoa from the testes, ova from the ovaries.

INTERNAL SECRETIONS: *Female:* The vesicular follicles of the ovaries secrete estrogen, which is important in regulating and controlling female reproductive function including the development of secondary sex characteristics; also the corpus luteum, producing the luteal secretion (progesterone) which helps to prepare the lining of the uterus (endometrium) to receive and assist

in the implantation of the fertilized ovum. *Male:* The interstitial cells of the testes secrete the androgen, testosterone, which stimulates metabolism, increases muscular strength, and influences the development of secondary sex characteristics.

Hormones from both sexes have been isolated and standardized, and are used in the treatment of conditions arising from an insufficiency of these hormones. SEE: *estrogen; ovary; testicle; testosterone.*

gonadal (gon'ă-dal). Pert. to a gonad. SYN: *gonadial.*

  g. dysgenesis. Congenital endocrine disorder caused by failure of the ovaries to respond to pituitary hormone (gonadotropin) stimulation. Clinically there is amenorrhea, failure of sexual maturation, and usually short stature. About a third of these patients have webbing of the neck and many have marked cubitus valgus, q.v. Intelligence may be impaired. SYN: *Turner syndrome.*

gonadectomy (gŏn-ă-dĕk'tō-mī) [Gr. *gonos,* genitals, + *ektomē,* excision]. Excision of a testis or ovary.

gonad'ial [Gr. *gonos,* genitals, procreation]. Pert. to a reproductive gland. SYN: *gonadal.*

gonadop'athy [" + *pathos,* disease]. Any disease of the sexual glands.

gonadother'apy [" + *therapeia,* treatment]. Treatment by injection of extracts containing testicular or ovarian hormones.

gonadotrope (gŏn-ăd'o-trōp) [Gr. *gonos,* genitals, + *trope,* turning]. 1. A person whose body constitution is dominated by gonadal hormones. 2. A gonadotrophic hormone.

gonadotrophic (gŏn''ă-dō-trŏf'ĭk) [" + *trophē,* nourishment]. Rel. to stimulation of the gonads.

  g. hormones. Gonadotrophins, q.v. or gonad-stimulating hormones.

gonadotrophin (gŏn''ă-dō-trō'fĭn). A gonad-stimulating hormone.

  g.'s anterior pituitary. Those produced by the anterior lobe of the hypophysis. Include follicle-stimulating hormone (FSH); leuteinizing hormone (LH): In the male this is called the interstitial cell stimulating hormone (ICSH); luteotrophic hormone (LTH).

  g., chorionic. G.'s produced by the chorionic villi of the placenta. They are present in the blood and urine of pregnant women and in the blood of pregnant mares. Their presence in urine is the basis of the Ascheim-Zondeck, Friedman, and other pregnancy tests. SYN: *anterior pituitary-like hormone; pregnancy hormone.*

gonadotropism (gŏn″ăd-ŏt′ro-pizm) [Gr. *gonos*, genitals, + *tropē*, turning, + *ismos*, state of]. Body constitution in which the gonads exert a dominant influence.

gon'aduct ["+ L. *ductus*, canal]. The seminal duct or the oviduct.

gonagra (gŏn-ag′ră) [Gr. *gony*, knee, + *agra*, seizure]. Gout in the knee.

gonal'gia ["+ *algos*, pain]. Pain in the knee.

gonangiectomy (gŏn″ăn-jĭ-ĕk′tō-mĭ) [Gr. *gonos*, genitals, + *angeion*, vessel, + *ektomē*, excision]. Excision of the vas deferens or a part of it. SYN: *vasectomy*.

gonarthritis (gon″ăr-thrī′tĭs) [Gr. *gony*, knee, + *arthron*, joint, + *-itis*, inflammation]. Inflammation of knee joint.

gonarthrocace (gon″ar-thrŏk′ă-se) ["+ "+ *kakos*, bad]. Swelling of knee joint due to tuberculosis. The skin over the inflamed joint is white.

gonarthromeningitis (gŏn-ăr″thro-mĕn-ĭn-jĭ′tĭs) ["+ "+ *mēninx*, membrane, + *-itis*, inflammation]. Snyovitis of the knee joint.

gonarthrotomy (gŏn″ăr-thrŏt-o-mĭ) ["+ "+ *tomē*, incision]. Incision of knee joint.

gonatag'ra [Gr. *gony*, knee, + *agra*, seizure]. Gout in the knee.

gonatocele (gon-at′o-sēl) ["+ *kēlē*, tumor, swelling]. White swelling; tumor of the knee.

gonecyst, gonecystis (gŏn′ĕ-sĭst, gŏn-ĕ-sĭs′tĭs) [Gr. *gonos*, genitals, + *kystis*, a bladder]. A seminal vesicle.

gonecystitis (gŏn″e-sĭs-tī′tĭs) ["+ "+ *-itis*, inflammation]. Inflammation of seminal vesicles.

gonecystolith (gŏn″ĕ-sĭs′to-lĭth) ["+ "+ *lithos*, stone]. A concretion or calculus in a seminal vesicle.

gonecystopyosis (gŏn″e-sĭst″o-pī-ō′sĭs) ["+ "+ *pyōsis*, suppuration]. Suppuration in a seminal vesicle or gonecyst.

goneitis (go-ne-ī′tis) [Gr. *gony*, knee, + *-itis*, inflammation]. Inflammation of the knee.

gonepoiesis (gŏn″e-poy-ē′sis) [Gr. *gonos*, offspring, genitals, + *poiein*, to make]. The secretion of the semen.

Gongylonema (gŏn″jĭ-lo-nē′mă) [Gr. *gongylos*, round, + *nēma*, thread]. A genus of nematode worms belonging to the suborder Spirurata. They are parasitic in wall of the esophagus and stomach of domestic animals. Occasionally, they are accidental parasites in man. G. pulchrum is the species most frequently involved.

goniometer (gō″nĭ-ŏm′ĕ-ter) [Gr. *gōnia*, angle, + *metron*, measure]. Apparatus to measure joint movements and angles.

gonion (gō′nĭ-ŏn) [Gr. *gōnia*, angle]. Point of angle of the mandible or lower jaw.

gonioscope (gō′nĭ-o-skōp) ["+ *skopein*, to examine]. An instrument for inspecting angle of anterior chamber of eye and for determining ocular motility and rotation.

gono-, gon- (gŏn′ō) [Gr. *gonos*]. Prefix meaning generation, genitals, offspring, semen.

gonoblast (gŏn′ō-blăst). SEE: *ganoblast*.

gonocide (gŏn′ō-sĭd) [Gr. *gonos*, genitals, + L. *caedere*, to kill]. Destructive to the gonococcus.

gonococ'cal ["+ *kokkos*, berry]. Rel. to or caused by gonococci.

gonococcemia (gŏn″o-kŏk-sē′mĭ-ă) ["+ "+ *haima*, blood]. Gonococci in the blood.

gonococ'ci (gŏn″o-kŏk′sī). Pl. of *gonococcus*.

gonococcic (gŏn″o-kŏk′sĭk) [Gr. *gonos*, genitals, + *kokkos*, berry]. Pert. to the gonococcus.

g. smears. Gonococci are in pairs and tetrads, never in chains. They are biscuit-shaped with concave adjacent surfaces, gram-negative and intracellular. Stains: Gram's method, methylene blue.

gonococcide (gŏn″o-kŏk′sĭd) ["+ "+ L. *caedere*, to kill]. An agent which kills gonococci.

gonococcocide (gŏn″o-kŏk′o-sĭd). Gonococcide.

gonococcus (gon″o-kŏk′ŭs) [Gr. *gonos*, genitals, + *kokkos*, berry]. (pl. *gonococci*) The organism causing gonorrhea. Neisseria gonorrhoeae.

It is an intracellular biscuit-shaped diplococcus and tends to occur in pairs. It is classified as a gram-negative bacterium and may be found in or on the genitals, in the blood, the eye, urine, feces, and in boils.

gonocyte (gŏn′o-sit) ["+ *kytos*, cell]. The primitive reproductive cell.

gonohemia (gŏn″o-hē′mĭ-ă) [Gr. *gonos*, genitals, + *haima*, blood]. Gonococcal septicemia. SYN: *gonococcemia*.

gonophage (gŏn′o-fāj) ["+ *phagein*, to eat]. The bacteriophage produced by the gonococcus.

gon'ophore ["+ *phorein*, to carry]. Any body that stores up, transports, or activates sex cells, as the spermatic duct, seminal vesicle, oviduct, or uterus.

gonorrhea (gŏn″ō-rē′ă) [Gr. *gonos*, genitals, + *rhoia*, flow]. A specific, contagious, catarrhal inflammation of the genital mucus membrane of either sex.

ETIOL: Infection by the gonococcus, Neisseria gonorrhoeae.

The disease also may affect other structures of the body, such as the conjunctiva, the oral mucosa, the rectum, or the joints. In the female the parts involved may be the urethra, vulva, vulvovaginal glands, vagina, endocervix, Skene's glands, Bartholin's glands, or fallopian tubes.

SYM: *Male:* Yellow mucopurulent discharge from the penis due to inflammation of the urethra. May become deep-seated and affect the prostate. Slow, difficult and painful urination, and sometimes painful induration of the penis.

Female: G. in the female may be asymptomatic, and even when symptoms are present they may not be uncomfortable enough to cause the patient to seek medical care. Symptoms include one or more of the following: urethral or vaginal discharge; painful or frequent urination; lower abdominal pain; tenderness in the area of Bartholin's and Skene's glands; acute pelvic inflammatory disease.

DIAG: Gram's stain of the urethral discharge is almost 100% accurate in diagnosing gonorrhea in the male. This not true for the female. The material for diagnosis in the female should be obtained from multiple sites including the cervix, vaginal vault, urethra, and by milking of Bartholin's and Skene's glands. The material should be inoculated without delay on Thayer-Martin medium.

NOTE: It is important to obtain a serological test for syphilis prior to starting antibiotic therapy. Penicillin therapy may mask a case of syphilis. Also it is important to test all sexual contacts of the patient for presence of either g. or syphilis.

PROG: It may clear up without serious results, or become chronic (involving deeper tissues and producing urethral stricture), or produce complications (prostatitis, epididymitis, orchitis, cystitis, arthritis and endocarditis). No case of acute g. in the female should be considered as cured until three successive negative smears from the cervix, Bartholin's and Skene's glands are obtained, at least two of which should be examined immediately after a menstrual period. Even then the patient must be regarded with suspicion.

NP: Every precaution for self-protection. Rubber gloves and a gown should be worn. The latter should not be worn in caring for another patient, and gloves should be sterilized after treatment. All linens and equipment should be sterilized after using and dressings immediately disposed of. Always wash hands after caring for patient. The danger of the nurse developing an eye infection is considerable.

PROPHYLAXIS: Avoidance of contact with infected persons; immediate penicillin as a preventive following contact. In new-born, instillation of silver nitrate or penicillin solution in both eyes. SEE: *opthalmia neonatorum.*

TREATMENT: Local measures, including urethral instillations, having largely given way to penicillin therapy. Penicillin is specific, and is regarded as the drug of choice. Strains of gonococcus resistant to some forms of penicillin have developed. These may be treated with ampicillin, tetracyclines or erythromycin. Local therapy may be required for eradication of foci of infection in the female, involving such structures as Skene's duct, Bartholin's glands, and the cervix.

gonorrhe'al. Of the nature of or pert. to gonorrhea.

   g. arthritis, g. rheumatism. Arthritis or rheumatism resulting from gonorrheal infection.

gonycamp'sis [Gr. *gony,* knee, + *kampsis,* bending]. Abnormal curvature of the knee or ankylosis.

gonycrotesis (gŏn″ĭ-kro-te′sĭs) ["+ *krotēsis,* knocking]. Knock-knee, genu valgum.

gonyectyposis (gŏn″ĭ-ĕk-tĭ-pō′sĭs) ["+ *ektypōsis,* modelling in relief]. Bowlegs. SYN: *genu varum.*

gonyocele (gŏn′ĭ-ō-sēl) ["+ *kēlē,* swelling]. Tuberculous synovitis of the knee. SYN: *white swelling.*

gonyoncus (gŏn″ĭ-ŏn′kŭs) ["+ *onkos,* tumor]. Tumor of the knee.

goose flesh. A skin reaction caused by erection of skin papillae from cold or shock due to contraction of the arrector pili muscles. This causes transient roughness of the skin. SYN: *cutis anserina.*

Gordon's reflex (gord′on). [Alfred Gordon, Amer. neurologist, 1874-1953] Extension of great toe when sudden pressure is made on deep flexor muscles of calf of leg. It is present in pyramidal tract disease. SEE: *Babinski's reflex.*

gorget (gŏr′jĕt) [Fr. *gorge,* throat, because of shape of instrument]. A grooved instrument to protect soft tissues from injury from point of knife.

Gossypium (gŏ-sĭp′ĭ-um) [L.]. A genus of perennial shrub of the Malvaceae family. Widely grown because of cotton fiber derived from the covering of seeds. Bark of some species is diuretic, emmenagogic, and oxytocic. SEE: *cotton.*

gouge (gowj). Instrument for cutting away hard tissue of bone.

gout (gowt) [L. *gutta,* drop]. Paroxysmal metabolic disease marked by acute arthritis and inflammation of the joints. Joints affected may be at any location but gout usually begins in the knee or foot.

ETIOL: Excessive uric acid in blood and deposits of urates of sodium in and around joints. Several different metabolic abnormalities may cause hyperuricemia.

SYM: Most persons with hyperuricemia are asymptomatic. When an attack of acute gouty arthritis does develop, it usually begins at night with moderate pain which increases in intensity to the point where no body position provides relief.

NP: The painful joints may be wrapped in cotton. They should be elevated and supported on a pillow. The weight of the bedclothes should be carried on a cradle. Hot formentations may afford some relief. Massage and radiant energy may be employed. Watch for vomiting and purgation resulting from the use of colchicine. Force fluids to prevent urine from becoming concentrated. Colchicine will cause fewer side effects if given intravenously.

DIET: Should be well-balanced and devoid of purine-rich foods.

TREATMENT: Acute g. responds to colchicine. Long-term therapy is directed to preventing hyperuricemia. This can be accomplished by giving probenecid, or allopurinol.

g., abarticular. G. which involves structures other than the joints.

g., chronic. Persistent form of g.

g., tophaceous. G. marked by the development of tophi (deposits of sodium urate) in the joints, the external ear, and about the fingernails.

gout'y. Of the nature of, or rel. to gout.

g. diathesis. Predisposition to gout.

Gowers' tract (gow'erz). [Sir William R. Gowers, Brit. neurologist, 1845-1915] One formed of fibers from posterior roots of lateral tract of the spinal cord reaching the cerebellum by way of the superior peduncle. SYN: *anterior spinocerebellar tract.*

gr. Abbr. for *grain.*

graaf'ian fol'licle. [Regnier de Graff, Dutch physician and anatomist, 1641-1673] A mature, vesicular follicle of the ovary.

Beginning with puberty and continuing until the menopause, except during pregnancy, a graafian follicle develops at approximately monthly invervals. Each follicle contains a nearly mature ovum (an oocyte) which, upon rupture of the follicle, is discharged from the ovary, a process called ovulation. Ovulation occurs usually about the 13th day of the menstrual cycle, dated from the first day of the next menstrual period. Within the ruptured graafian follicle, the corpus luteum develops. Both the follicle and the corpus luteum are glands of internal secretion, the former secreting estrogens, the latter, estrogen and progesterone.

gracile (grăs'ĭl) [L. *gracilis,* delicate]. Slender; slight.

g. nucleus. Mass of medullary gray matter terminating the funiculus gracilis.

gracilus (grăs'ĭ-lŭs). A long slender muscle on the medial aspect of the thigh.

grada'tim [L.]. Gradually or by degrees.

Gradenigo's syndrome (grä-dĕn-e'gō). [Giuseppe Gradenigo, It. physician, 1859-1926] Suppurative otitis media with abducens paralysis and pain in temporal region.

gradient (grā'dĭ-ent). A slope or grade; an increase or decrease of varying degrees; or the curve which represents such.

g., axial. A g. of physiological or metabolic activity exhibited by embryos and many adult animals, the principal one of which follows the main axis of the body, being highest at the anterior end and lowest at the posterior end.

graduate (grăd'ū-āt) [L. *gradus,* a step]. 1. A vessel marked by lines for measuring liquids. 2. One who has been awarded an academic or professional degree from a college or university.

grad'uated. Marked by a series of lines indicating degrees of measurement, weight, or volume.

g. tenotomy. Partial surgical division of tendon of an eye muscle.

Graefe's, von, sign. [Albrecht von Graefe, Ger. ophthalmologist, 1828-1870] Failure of the upper lid to follow a downward movement of the eyeball when the patient changes his vision from upward, downward. Seen in Graves' disease (hyperthyroidism) with exophthalmos.

graft [L. *graphium,* grafting knife]. Skin or other living substance inserted into a similar substance to supply an absence or defect by attachment and growth into an integral part of the original substances.

Homograft involves grafting material from another individual of the same species. Heterograft indicates the grafted tissue or organ was obtained from a species different from the recipient.

RS: autograft; transplantation; zoografting.

g., autogenous. One taken from another part of the patient.

g., bone. A piece of bone generally taken from the tibia and inserted elsewhere in the body to replace another osseous structure. Banks for storage of bone have been established.

g., cadaver. Grafting tissue, including skin, cornea, or bone, obtained from a body immediately after death.

g., heteroplas'tic. One taken from another person.

g., nerve. Healthy nerve, usually from an animal, implanted to join a degenerated nerve in a human being.

g., ovarian. Implantation of a section of an ovary into the muscles of the abdominal wall.

g., pinch. A g. consisting of small bits of skin.

g., postmortem. Tissue taken from body after death and stored under proper conditions to be used later on a patient requiring a g. of such tissue.

g., skin. Removal of small sections of skin to a raw, clean surface such as a large superficial burn.

g., sponge. Small piece of sponge placed over an ulcerating part to stimulate epidermal growth.

g., Thiersch's. One in which only epidermis and small amt. of dermis are used.

g., Wolfe's. One in which the whole thickness of the skin is used.

g., zooplas'tic. One taken from an animal.

grafting. Implantation of skin or tissue from a healthy site to an injured site.

graft-versus-host reaction. The pathological reaction between the host and tissue grafted. Occurs when the host's immune response is deficient because of faulty immunosuppressive therapy.

grain [L. *granum*]. 1. The seed or seedlike fruit of many members of the grass family, esp. corn, wheat, oats, and other cereals. 2. A weight; 0.065 of a gram. 3. Direction of fibers or layers.

gram. A unit of weight (mass) of the metric system. It equals approximately the weight of a cubic centimeter or one milliliter of water. It is equal to 15.432 grains. ABBR: gm., Gm., g.

grammeter. A unit of work energy equivalent to that expended in raising a weight of

Gram Conversion into Ounces (Avoirdupois)*

Gm.	Oz.	Gm.	Oz.	Gm.	Oz.	Gm.	Oz.
1	0.03	30	1.06	59	2.08	88	3.10
2	0.07	31	1.09	60	2.12	89	3.14
3	0.11	32	1.13	61	2.15	90	3.17
4	0.14	33	1.16	62	2.18	91	3.21
5	0.18	34	1.20	63	2.22	92	3.24
6	0.21	35	1.23	64	2.26	93	3.28
7	0.25	36	1.27	65	2.29	94	3.31
8	0.28	37	1.30	66	2.33	95	3.35
9	0.32	38	1.34	67	2.36	96	3.38
10	0.35	39	1.37	68	2.40	97	3.42
11	0.39	40	1.41	69	2.43	98	3.46
12	0.42	41	1.44	70	2.47	99	3.49
13	0.45	42	1.48	71	2.50	100	3.53
14	0.49	43	1.51	72	2.54	125	4.41
15	0.53	44	1.55	73	2.57	150	5.30
16	0.56	45	1.59	74	2.61	175	6.18
17	0.60	46	1.62	75	2.64	200	7.05
18	0.63	47	1.65	76	2.68	250	8.82
19	0.67	48	1.69	77	2.71	300	10.58
20	0.70	49	1.73	78	2.75	350	12.34
21	0.74	50	1.76	79	2.79	400	14.11
22	0.77	51	1.80	80	2.82	450	15.87
23	0.81	52	1.83	81	2.85	453.6	16.00
24	0.84	53	1.87	82	2.89	500	17.64
25	0.88	54	1.90	83	2.93	600	21.16
26	0.91	55	1.94	84	2.96	700	24.69
27	0.95	56	1.97	85	3.00	800	28.22
28	0.99	57	2.01	86	3.03	900	30.75
29	1.02	58	2.04	87	3.07	1000	35.27

* One gram is equal to 0.03527 ounce (Avoirdupois)

The Chief Gram-negative Bacteria

Genus	Species	Colloquial or Old Names	Disease Caused in Man
Actinobacillus	P. mallei	Bacillus mallei or the glanders bacillus	Glanders
Pseudomonas	P. aeruginosa	Bacillus pyocyaneus	Suppuration ("blue pus")
Vibrio	N. meningitidis	Comma bacillus	Cholera
Neisseria	V. comma	Meningococcus	Cerebrospinal meningitis
	N. gonorrhoeae N. catarrhalis	Gonococcus Micrococcus catarrhalis	Gonorrhea Nasopharyngeal catarrh
Proteus	P. vulgaris	Bacillus proteus	Suppuration
Escherichia	E. coli	Bacillus coli	Occasionally suppuration, cystitis, and pyelitis
Klebsiella	K. pneumoniae	Pneumobacillus or Bacillus mucosus capsulatus	Occasionally pneumonia
Salmonella	S. typhosa S. paratyphi (A&B) S. enteritidis S. typhimurium	Typhoid bacillus Bacillus paratyphosus, etc. (Salmonella group)	Typhoid fever Paratyphoid fever, gastro-enteritis (food poisoning)
Shigella	S. dysenteriae	The dysentery bacilli	Bacillary dysentery
Pasteurella	Past. pestis	Bacillus pestis; plague bacillus	Plague
Hemophilus	H. influenzae	Pfeiffer's bacillus	Meningitis conjunctivitis, and influenza
Bordetella	B. pertussis	Bordet-Gengou bacillus	Whooping cough
Brucella	Br. melitensis Br. abortus Br. suis	Micrococcus melitensis Bang's bacillus	Undulant fever
Borrelia	13 species B. vincentii	Vincent's bacillus	Relapsing fever Vincent's angina (trench mouth)
Leptospira	L. icterohaemor-rhagiae		Weil's disease (infectious jaundice)
Treponema	T. pallidum T. pertenue		Syphilis Yaws

one gram vertically a height of one meter.

gram mol'ecule. The weight in grams of a substance equal to its molecular weight.

gram-negative. Losing the stain and taking the color of the counterstain in Gram's method of staining. A primary characteristic of certain microorganisms. SEE: *Gram's method.*

gram-positive. Retaining the color of the gentian violet stain in Gram's method of staining. SEE: *Gram's method.*

Gram's method. [Hans C. J. Gram, Danish physician, 1853-1938] A method for staining bacteria. It is of importance in the identification of bacteria.

PROCEDURE: Prepare a film on a slide, dry and fix with heat. Stain with aniline gentian violet or ammonium oxalate crystal violet one minute. Rinse in water, then immerse in Gram's iodine solution for one minute. Rinse off iodine solution then decolorize in 95% ethyl alcohol or acetone. Counterstain with dilute carbolfuchsin or safranine, 30 seconds. Rinse with water, blot dry, and examine.

NOTE: In order to provide a simple means of checking on the accuracy of the staining materials, a small amount of material from between one's teeth can be placed on the slide at the opposite end from that of the specimen being examined. Gram-negative and gram-positive organisms are always present in the mouth. Thus that end of the slide is examined first. If both types of organisms are seen, proceed to examine the specimen.

Gran'cher's disease. [Jacques J. Grancher, Fr. physician, 1843-1907] Massive pneumonia. SYN: *splenopneumonia.*

Gran'cher's sign. Raised pitch of expiratory murmur in pulmonary consolidation.

The Chief Gram-positive Bacteria

Genus	Species	Colloquial or Old Names	Disease Caused in Man
Actinomyces	*A. bovis* *A. israelii*	Nocardia actinomyces; ray fungus	Actinomycosis
Mycobacterium	*M. tuberculosis* *M. leprae*	Tubercle bacillus Leprosy bacillus	Tuberculosis Leprosy (Hansen's disease)
Corynebacterium	*C. diphtheriae*	Diphtheria bacillus Klebs-Löeffler bacillus	Diphtheria
Streptococcus	*Str. pyogenes*		Suppuration, scarlet fever, septicemia
	Str. viridans	*Str. mitis*	Subacute bacterial endocarditis
Staphylococcus	*Staph. aureus, albus, etc.*		Suppuration, pyemia, osteomyelitis
Sarcina	*Sarcina lutea*		Rarely suppuration
Bacillus	*B. anthracis* *B. subtilis*	Anthrax bacillus Hay bacillus	Anthrax Eye infections (rarely)
Clostridium	*Cl. tetani* *Cl. botulinum* *Cl. perfringens*	Tetanus bacillus Bacillus botulinus Cl. welchii	Tetanus Botulism Gas gangrene
Diplococcus	*D. pneumoniae*	Streptococcus pneumoniae	Lobar and bronchopneumonia; other infections

grand mal (grahn mal) [Fr., great evil]. The typical epileptic attack with or without coma. SEE: *epilepsy.*

gran'ular [L. *granulum*, little grain]. Of the nature of granules. Roughened by prominences like those of seeds.

  g. cast. Coarse or fine granule, short and plump, sometimes yellowish, similar to hyaline cast.

  Soluble in acetic acid. Seen in inflammatory and degenerative nephropathies. SEE: *cast.*

granula'tion. 1. Formation of granules, or state or condition of being granular. 2. Fleshy projections formed on the surface of a gaping wound that is not healing by first intention, q.v., or indirect union.

  Each g. represents the outgrowth of new capillaries by budding from the existing capillaries and then joining up into capillary loops supported by cells which will later become fibrous scar tissue. G.'s bring a rich blood supply to the healing surface.

  g., arachnoidal. Villus-like projections of the subarachnoid layer of the meninges which project into the superior sagittal sinus and other venous sinuses of the brain. Through them cerebrospinal fluid reenters the blood stream. SYN: *arachnoid villi; pacchionian bodies.*

  g., exuberant. An excessive mass of g. tissue formed in the healing of a wound or ulcer; proud flesh.

gran'ule [L. *granulum*, little grain]. 1. A small, grainlike body. 2. In histology, a minute mass in a cell which has an outline but no apparent structure; any minute mass; or the crossing points of an intracellular reticulum end-wise.

  g., acidophil. Alpha g., q.v.

  g., agminated. Small round or angular particle of disintegrated red blood corpuscle in the blood.

  g., albuminous. Cytoplasmic g. in many normal cells, not affected by ether or chloroform, but disappears from view when acetic acid is added.

  g., aleuronoid. Pigment cell g.; colorless, myeloid, and colloidal.

  g., alpha. Albuminous g. in leukocytes. Coarse, eosinophil, and highly refractive. SYN: *acidophil g.; eosinophil g.; oxyphil g.*

  g., Altmann's. Mitochondria, q.v.

  g., amphophil. One which stains with both acid and basic dyes; beta g., q.v.

  g., azurophil. One which takes a stain with azure dyes easily. Found in lymphocytes and monocytes; small and red or reddish-purple in color; they are inconstant in number being present in about 30% of the cells.

  g., basal. A small deeply staining g. found in certain protozoa from which the flagellum arises. SYN: *blepharoplast,* q.v.

  g., beta. An azurophil g. found in beta cells of the hypophysis or islets of Langerhans of the pancreas. SYN: *amphophil g.*

  g., chromatin. Small masses of deeply staining substance suspended within the meshes of the linin network of the nucleus of a cell.

  g., chromophil. A g. of chromophil substance present in the cytoplasm of neurons; Nissl g.'s.

  g.'s, cone. The nuclei of the cones, sensory cells of the retina. They form the outer zone of the outer nuclear layer of the retina.

  g.'s, delta. Small g.'s in the delta cells of the pancreas.

  g., eosinophil. Alpha g., q.v.

  g., Fauvel's. Peribronchitic abscess.

  g., glycogen. Minute particles of glycogen seen in liver cells following fixation.

  g., Grawitz's. Found in lead poisoning basophilia, in the red blood corpuscles.

  g., iodophil. Found in polymorphonuclear leukocytes and staining easily with iodine. Seen in various acute infectious diseases.

  g., metachromatic. Found in protoplasm of numerous bacteria. Stains deeply; irregular in size.

  g., neutrophil. G.'s such as those found in neutrophil leukocytes which stain with both basic and acid dyes, assuming a neutral tint.

  g., Nissl. Chromophil g.'s found in the cell bodies of neurons; Nissl's bodies. q.v.

  g., oxyphil. G., alpha, q.v.

  g., pigment. Particle of coloring matter seen esp. in pigment cells.

  g., Plehn's. Basophilic and seen in conjugating form of Plasmodium vivax.

  g., protein. Protein particles of minute size in cells.

  g., rod. Nucleus of the rod visual cell found in the external nuclear layer of the retina; connected with the rods.

  g., Schüffner's. Polychrome methylene blue-staining g. found in parasitized erythrocytes of tertian malaria; coarse and red.

  g., secretory. G., zymogen, q.v.

  g., seminal. Minute particles in semen, supposed to derive from disintegrated nuclei in nutritive cells from seminiferous tubules.

  g., vitelline. G., yolk, q.v.

g., yolk. Minute particles of fatty and albuminous nutritive substances present in the yolk (deutoplasm) of ova.

g., zymogen. G.'s present in gland cells esp. secretory cells of pancreas, chief cells of the gastric glands, and serous cells of the salivary glands. They are the precursors of the enzymes secreted.

granulitis (grăn-ū-lǐ'tĭs) [L. *granulum,* little grain, + Gr. *-itis,* inflammation]. Acute miliary tuberculosis.

gran'uloblast ["+ Gr. *blastos,* germ]. Mother cell of a granulocyte. A myeloblast, found in bone marrow.

granulocyte (grăn'ū-lo-sīt) [L. *granulum,* little grain, + Gr. *kytos,* hollow vessel (cell)]. A granular leukocyte. A polymorphonuclear leukocyte (neutrophil, eosinophil, or basophil).

granulocytopenia (grăn"ū-lo-sī"to-pē'nĭ-ă) ["+ "+ *penia,* poverty]. Abnormal reduction of granulocytes in the blood. SYN: *granulopenia.*

granulocytopoiesis (grăn"ū-lo-sī"to-poy-ē'-sĭs) ["+ "+ *poiein,* to form]. The formation of granulocytes.

granulo'ma [L. *granulum,* + Gr. *-ōma,* tumor]. A granular tumor or growth, usually of lymphoid and epithelioid cells. They occur in various diseases such as leprosy, cutaneous leishmaniasis, yaws, and syphilis.

    g., annulare. A condition of the skin characterized by development of reddish nodules arranged in the form of a circle.

    g., apical. G., dental, q.v.

    g., coccidioidal. A chronic, generalized granulomatous disease caused by Coccidioides immitis. SEE: *coccidioido-mycosis.*

    g., dental. G. developing at the root of a tooth. May contain epithelial rests or colonies of bacteria.

    g., eosinophilic. G. containing eosinophils and usually accompanied by eosinophilia.

    g., fungoides. Mycosis fungoides, q.v.

    g., infectious. Any infectious disease in which g.'s are formed, such as tuberculosis or syphilis. G.'s are also formed in mycoses, protozoan infections, and in certain metazoal diseases.

    g. inguinale. A granulomatous disease common in the tropics caused by Donovan bodies (Leishmania donovani). Characterized by purulent lesions of the skin in region of the groin and often involving external genitalia.

    g. iridis. G. which develops on the iris.

    g., malignant. Lymphogranulomatosis; Hodgkin's disease.

    g. pyogenicum. G. containing pyogenic organisms, which develop at the site of a wound. They may also occur at the tip of the fingers along the sides of the nails or beneath the free edge of the nail. They bleed easily and are usually painful to touch. Also called septic granuloma.

    g., venereal. Lymphogranuloma venereum, q.v.

granulomatosis (grăn"ū-lō"mă-tō'sĭs) [L. *granulum,* little grain, + Gr. *-ōma,* tumor, + *-ōsis,* diseased condition]. The development of multiple granulomas.

    g., lipoid. Xanthomatosis, q.v.

granulopenia (grăn"ū-lo-pē'nĭ-ă) ["+ Gr. *penia,* poverty]. Abnormal decrease of granulocytes in the blood. SYN: *granulocytopenia.*

granuloplastic (grăn"ū-lo-plăs'tĭk) ["+ Gr. *plassein,* to form]. Developing granules.

granulopoiesis (grăn"ū-lo-poy-ē'sĭs) ["+ Gr. *poiein,* to make]. The formation of granulocytes.

granulopo'tent [L. *granulum,* little grain, + *potentia,* power]. Potentially capable of forming granules.

granulosa (grăn"ū-lō'să). The membrana granulosa.

gran'ulose. The soluble portion of starch. It is converted into sugar by hydrolysis.

granulo'sis [L. *granulum,* little grain, + Gr. *-ōsis,* condition]. A mass of minute granules.

    g. ru'bia na'si. Disease of the skin of the nose.

    ETIOL: Inflammatory infiltration about nose with slightly elevated papules, and dilated sweat glands.

    SYM: Moist erythematous patch on numerous macules.

grapefruit. A citrus fruit. Food value of 100 gm. of pulp (fresh): Cal. 41; protein 0.5 gm.; fat 0.1 gm.; carbohydrate 10.6 gm.; calcium 16 mg.; vitamin A, 440 I.U. (pink and red varieties only); ascorbic acid 38 mg.

    Food value of 100 gm. of juice (canned, sweetened): Cal. 39; fat 0.1 gm.; carbohydrate 9.2 gm.; calcium 9 mg.; vitamin A, 80 I.U.; ascorbic acid 38 mg.

grapes. 1. The fruit of the genus Vitis. Contains acid potassium tartrate. Acidity decreases with the age of the grape and sugar increases. The sugar is nearly all glucose and is more abundant than in any other fruit. Mannite, dulcite, and saccharose also represented. Rasins (sweet dried g.'s) contain more sugar and less water. 2. Structure or growth resembling a g. or bunch of g.'s.

    Food value 100 gm. (American type, raw): Cal. 69; protein 1.3 gm.; carbohydrate 15.7 gm.; calcium 16 mg.; vitamin A, 100 I.U.

grape sugar. Dextrose, q.v.

graph (grăf). A presentation of statistical, clinical, or experimental data by dots and lines.

-graph [Gr. -graphos, written, from graphein, to write]. Suffix indicating a writing or treatise.

graphesthesia (grăf'ĕs-thē'zĭ-ă) ["+ aisthēsis, perception]. The sense by which outlines, numbers, words, or symbols traced or written upon the skin are recognized.

graphite (grăf'ĭt) [Gr. graphein, to write]. A soft form of carbon. SYN: plumbago.

grapho- [Gr. graphein, to write]. Prefix meaning to write.

graphology (grăf-ŏl'ō-jĭ) ["+ logos, study]. Examination of handwriting in diseases of the nerves as a means of diagnosis.

graphomotor (grăf'o-mō'tŏr) ["+ L. motor, mover]. Pert. to movements involved in writing.

graphophobia (grăf'o-fō'bĭ-ă) ["+ phobos, fear]. Abnormal fear of writing.

graphorrhea (grăf'o-rē'ă) [Gr. graphein, to write, + rhoia, flow]. Writing of many meaningless words and phrases.

graphospasm (grăf'o-spăzm) ["+ spasmos, spasm]. Writer's cramp.

GRAS List. Indicates food additives generally recognized as safe by the U.S. Food and Drug Administration. SEE: food additives.

grattage (gra-tăhzh') [Fr., a scraping]. Removal of morbid growths by rubbing with a brush or harsh sponge.

grave [L. gravis, heavy]. Serious; dangerous; severe.

   g. wax. Waxlike matter on flesh caused by exposure to moisture with exclusion of air, as a body in the water or underground. SYN: adipocere.

grav'el [Fr. gravelle, coarse sand]. Crystalline dust, or concretions of crystals from the kidneys.

   Generally made up of phosphates, calcium, oxalate, and uric acid.

Graves' disease. [Robert J. Graves, Irish physician, 1797-1853] Exopthalmic goiter.

gravid (grăv'ĭd) [L. gravida, pregnant, from gravis, heavy]. Pregnant; heavy with child.

gravida (grăv'ĭd-ă) [L.]. A pregnant woman.

grav'idism [L. gravida, pregnant woman, + Gr. ismos, state of]. State of being pregnant.

gravidity (gră-vĭd'ĭ-tĭ) [L. gravida, pregnant]. Pregnancy.

gravidocardiac (grăv'ĭd-o-kăr'dĭ-ăk) ["+ Gr. kardia, heart]. Pert. to cardiac disorders resulting from pregnancy.

gravimet'ric [L. gravis, heavy, + Gr. metron, measure]. Determined by weight.

   g. method. Examination of blood by weighing.

gravistatic (grăv-ĭ-stăt'ĭk) ["+ Gr. statikos, causing to stand, skilled in weighing]. Resulting from gravitation, as in a form of congestion.

gravita'tion [L. gravitas, weight]. Force and movement tending to draw every particle of matter together, esp. the attraction of the earth for bodies at a distance from its center.

grav'ity. Property of possessing weight. The force of the earth's gravitational attraction.

   g., specific. Weight of a substance compared with a known standard such as that of water, air, or hydrogen. ABBR: sp. gr.

gray. Color without hue between extremes of black and white.

   g. matter. Nervous tissues of a grayish color, in which myelinated nerve fibers do not predominate. It contains large numbers of cell-bodies of neurons.

   The term is generally applied to gray portions of the central nervous system, which include the cerebral cortex, basal ganglia, and nuclei of the brain and the gray columns of the spinal cord which form an H-shaped region surrounded by white matter. Sympathetic ganglia and nerves may also be gray. SYN: substantia grisea [NA[.

green. A color intermediate between blue and yellow, afforded by rays of wave length between 4920 and 5750 angstrom units. SEE: words beginning with chloro.

   g. blindness. Aglaucopsia; a type of color-blindness in which g. colors cannot be distinguished.

   g., malachite. A dye used as a stain and antiseptic.

   g. sickness. A form of anemia in adolescent girls, perhaps due to faulty diet during puberty. SYN: chlorosis.

   g. soap. A solution of soft soap in alcohol, molded and dried.

   g. soft'ening. Cranial abscess with pus of a greenish hue.

   g. vit'riol. Ferrous sulfate. SYN: copperas.

greenstick fracture. Fracture involving only part of the thickness of a bone. SEE: fracture.

greffotome (grĕf'o-tōm) [Fr. greffe, graft, + Gr. tomē, incision]. Instrument for making tissue grafts.

grenz rays [Ger. Grenze, boundary]. Roentgen rays with an average wave length of two angstroms. SEE: ray.

griffe des orteils (grĕf dăz ŏr-ta') [Fr.]. Muscular atrophy of foot with contraction. SYN: clawfoot.

grinder (grin'der) [AS. *grindan,* to gnash]. A molar tooth. SYN: *dens molaris* [NA].

grind'ers' disease. Chronic lung disease due to dust inhalation. SYN: *pneumoconiosis; siderosis.*

grip, grippe (grĭp) [Fr. *gripper,* to seize]. Acute, infectious disease marked by fever, prostration, pains in head and back, and upper respiratory tract symptoms such as cough and nasal congestion. SYN: *influenza,* q.v.

gripes (grĭps) [AS. *grīpan,* to grasp]. Intermittent severe pains in bowels. SYN: *colic.*

griseofulvin. An antifungal antibiotic for oral administration. Especially effective in ringworm.

gristle (grĭs'ĕl) [AS.]. Cartilage.

grits. Coarsely ground corn.

Food value of 100 gm. (degermed, enriched, cooked): Cal. 51; protein 1.2 gm.; carbohydrate 11 gm.

grocers' itch. Eczema or psoriasis of the hands due to irritation from handling flour, sugar, etc.

Groff electrosurgical knife. Device for use of cutting current. Utilizes a high frequency current which seals vessels as it divides them.

groin [AS. *grynde,* abyss]. The depression between the thigh and trunk. The inguinal region. SEE: *venereal bubo.*

groove [Middle Dutch, *groeve,* ditch]. Long narrow channel, depression, or furrow. SYN: *sulcus.*

g., biciptal. Depression for long tendon of the triceps located on anterior surface of humerus. SYN: *intertubercular g.*

g., branchial. In the embryo, a g. lined with ectoderm which lies between two branchial arches. SEE: *branchial arches; branchial g.'s.*

g., carotid. A broad g. on the inner surface of the sphenoid bone lateral to the body. It lodges the carotid artery and the cavernous sinus. SYN: *cavernous g.*

g., costal. A g. on the lower internal border of a rib. It lodges the intercostal vessels and nerve. SYN: *subcostal g.*

g., costovertebral. A broad g. extending along each side of the vertebrae. It lodges the sacrospinalis muscle and its subdivisions. SYN: *vertebral g.*

g., infraorbital. A g. on the orbital surface of the maxilla which transmits the infraorbital vessels and nerve.

g., intertubercular. G., bicipital, q.v.

g., labial. A g. which develops in each of the primitive jaws. It gives rise to the vestibule separating the lips from the gums.

g., lacrimal. 1. A g. on posterior surface of frontal process of the maxilla. 2. A g. on anterior surface of the posterior lacrimal crest of the lacrimal bone. The two g.'s serve to lodge the lacrimal sac.

g., laryngotracheal. A g. along the ventral surface of the anterior portion of the embryonic gut which gives rise to the respiratory organs.

g., malleolar. G. on anterior surface of distal end of tibia which lodges tendons of the tibialis posterior and flexor digitorum longus musculi.

g., medullary. G., neural, q.v.

g., musculospiral. G., radial, q.v.

g., mylohyoid. G. on inner surface of the mandible which runs obliquely forward and downward lodging the mylohyoid nerve and artery. In the embryo it lodges Meckel's cartilage.

g., nasolacrimal. In the embryo, a g. extending from inner angle of the eye to the primitive olfactory sac. It separates the maxillary and lateral nasal processes and its epithelial lining gives rise to the nasolacrimal duct.

g., nasopalatine. G. on vomer lodging nasopalatine nerve and vessels.

g., neural. A longitudinal g. on dorsal surface of the embryo lying between the neural folds. Upon closure of the folds to form the neural tube, the g. becomes the cavity of the neural tube, eventually giving rise to the ventricles of the brain and the central canal of the spinal cord.

g., obturator. A g. at the superior and posterior angle of the obturator foramen through which pass the obturator vessels and nerve.

g., olfactory. A shallow g. on superior surface of cribriform plate of the ethmoid on each side of the crista galli. It lodges the olfactory bulb.

g., palatine. One of a number of g.'s on the inferior surface of the palatine process of the maxilla. They lodge the palatine vessels and nerves.

g., peroneal. 1. A shallow g. on lateral aspect of the calcaneus. 2. A deep g. on inferior surface of the cuboid bone. Each transmits the tendon of the peroneus longus muscle.

g., pharyngeal. G., branchial, q.v.

g., primitive. In the embryo, a shallow g. in the primitive streak of the blastoderm and bordered by the primitive folds.

g., pterygopalatine. The pterygopalatine sulcus. A g. on the maxillary surface of the perpendicular portion of the palatine bone which, with corresponding g.'s on the maxilla and pterygoid process of the sphenoid, transmits the palatine nerve and descending palatine artery.

g., radial. The musculospiral g.; a broad shallow g. running in a spiral direction on posterior surface of the humerus. It transmits radial nerve and the profunda branchi artery.

g., rhombic. One of seven transverse g.'s in the floor of the developing rhombencephalon. They separate the neuromeres.

g., sagittal. The sagittal sulcus; a shallow g. on inner surface of the parietal bones which lodges the superior sagittal sinus.

g., sigmoid. G. on inner surface of the mastoid portion of temporal bone. It transmits the transverse sinus.

g., subcostal. G., costal, q.v.

g., tympanic. A g. at the bottom of the exterior auditory meatus which receives the inferior portion of the tympanic membrane.

g., urethral. A g. on caudal surface of the genital tubercle or phallus bordered by the urethral folds. The latter close, transforming the g. into the cavernous urethra.

g., vertebral. G., costovertebral, q.v.

g., visceral. G., branchial, q.v.

gross (grōs) [L. *grossus,* thick]. 1. Consisting of large particles or components; coarse or large. 2. Being quite large or obese. 3. Having an insensitiveness or lack of refinement.

g. anatomy. Study of organs and parts seen without the aid of a microscope.

g. lesion. Lesion visible to the eye without the aid of a microscope.

Grotthuss, law of. Only those light rays which are absorbed are biologically active.

ground. Basic substance or foundation; reduced to a powder; pulverized.

g. bundle. Fasciculus proprius, a bundle of nerve fibers which immediately surrounds the gray matter of the spinal cord. It is divided into three regions, the anterior, lateral, and posterior bundles which lie in the corresponding funiculi. These consist principally of short descending fibers.

g., itch. Ancylostomiasis cutis. Inflammation of the skin resulting from the invasion of the larvae of hookworms (Ancylostoma or Necator).

g. substance. The fluid, semifluid, or solid material which occupies the intercellular spaces in fibrous connective tissue, cartilage, or bone. SYN: *interstitial substance; matrix.*

group [It. *gruppo,* knot]. A number of similar objects or structures taken or considered together; thus bacteria with similar metabolic characteristics are considered together as a g. Atomic molecules and compounds with similar structures or properties are classified within certain groups.

g. therapy. A form of simultaneous psychotherapy involving two or more patients and one or more psychotherapists.

group'ing. Classification.

g., blood. Classifying blood of different individuals according to agglutinating and hemolyzing qualities before making a blood transfusion. SEE: *blood groups; blood transfusion.*

g. serum. A serum used for determining the blood group to which unknown cells belong. The g. serums commonly used are human serums secured from donors and rabbit antiserums prepared commercially.

grow'ing pains. An imprecise term indicating ill-defined pain in the musculo-skeletal system of young persons. There is no evidence that the pain is related to rapid growth.

growth [AS. *grōwan,* to grow]. The progressive development or increase in size of a living thing. This may be normal as in growth of an embryo or child, or pathological as in a cyst or benign or malignant tumor.

METHODS: (1) By the synthesis of new protoplasm and multiplication of cells. (2) By the manufacture and deposition of nonliving substances either within or outside of cells.

TYPES: (1) Organs of the lymphoid type, such as the thymus and the lymph nodes, grow fastest early in life, reach their peak of development at the age of about 12, and then regress.

(2) The neural type of organ, such as the brain, cord, eye, and meninges, grows in childhood, but is close to its adult size by the age of 8 years. This size is maintained without regression.

(3) The general type of growth is seen in the weight of the body, the height of the body, and lengths of various bones, the total weight of the muscles and various internal organs. It is a slower and steadier growth than the first two, but has a marked acceleration just after birth and at the time of puberty.

(4) The genital type of growth is seen in the testes, ovaries, and other genitourinary structures. Their growth is the slowest of these four types in infancy, but at puberty they grow faster than the others and cause the striking changes in appearance noted in the secondary sex characteristics and the reproductive organs.

Not all of the organs of the body are included in the above four types. Some structures, such as the mammary glands, have several cycles of growth and regression in a lifetime, and many other pecularities of particular organs might be mentioned.

g. hormone. Hormone liberated by the anterior pituitary which is important in regulating g.

g., new. A neoplasm or tumor.

g., postnatal. G. subsequent to birth.

g. prenatal. G. occurring before birth.

gru'el [L. *grutum*, meal]. Any cereal boiled in water.

gru'mose, gru'mous [L. *grumus*, heap]. 1. Made up of coarse granular bodies in the center. 2. Lumpy, clotted.

Grünfelder's reflex (grün'fēld-ēr). Fanlike spreading of toes with upward flexion of great toe resulting from pressure over posterior fontanel.

grutum (grü'tüm) [L. meal]. 1. Small pink and white patches most frequently on skin of face and scrotum caused by inspissated sebum beneath the horny epidermis. SYN: *milium.* 2. Oaten grits.

GSR. Abbr. for *galvanic skin response.*

G-suit. A coverall-type garment designed for use by aviators. The suit contains compartments which inflate and bring pressure on the legs and abdomen so as to prevent blood from pooling there. In aviators this helps to prevent unconsciousness due to positive acceleration.

The suit has been used in medicine to treat postural hypotension.

gt. Abbr. of L. *gutta*, a drop. SEE: *gtt.*

gtt. Abbr. of L. *guttae*, drops.

guaiacol (gwī'ȧ-kōl). A substance similar to phenol obtained by fractional distillation of creosote or by synthetic means.

Used as antiseptic and germicide, intestinal antiseptic and expectorant.

guanase (gwan'ās) [Sp. *guano*, from Quechua *huanu*, dung]. An enzyme in a number of glands; it converts guanine into xanthine.

guanethidine (gwăn-ĕth'ĭ-dēn). A drug which depresses the function of postganglionic adrenergic nerves. Thus sympathetic nerve activity is inhibited. G. is used in treating hypertension.

guanidine (gwăn'ĭ-dēn). A crystalline organic compound, $NH: C(NH_2)_2$, found among the decomposition products of proteins.

guanidinemia (gwăn''ĭd-ēn-ē'mĭ-ȧ) [*guanidine*, + Gr. *haima*, blood]. Guanidine in the blood.

guanine (gwā'nēn). An organic compound, $C_5H_5N_5O$, which occurs as a natural constituent of animal and vegetable nucleic acids. It is abundant in liver, muscle, glandular tissue such as pancreas, and seeds. Uric acid is its metabolic end point.

gubernaculum (gu''ber-nak'u-lum) [L. helm]. A structure which guides; a cordlike structure uniting two structures.

g. dentis. A connective tissue band which connects the tooth sac of an unerupted tooth with the overlying gum.

g. testis. [NA] A fibrous cord in the fetus which extends from the caudal end of the testis through the inguinal canal to the scrotal swelling. It plays a role in the descent of the testis into the scrotum.

Gubler's line (gūb'ler). [Adolphe Gubler, Fr. physician, 1821-1879] The level of superficial origin of the trigeminus or 5th nerve.

Gubler's paralysis. Hemiplegia affecting parts on opposite sides of the body. SYN: *alternate hemiplegia; crossed hemiplegia.*

Gubler's tumor. A fusiform swelling on wrist in lead palsy.

Gudden's inferior commissure (gūd'en). [Bernard A. von Gudden, Ger. neurologist, 1824-1886] Fibers of optic tract. SYN: *arcuate c.*

Gudden's law. When a nerve is divided, degeneration in the proximal portion is toward the nerve cell.

guillotine (gĭl'ō-tēn) [Fr., instrument for beheading]. Instrument for excising tonsils and laryngeal growths.

Guinea worm. Dracunculus medinensis, q.v.

gul'let [L. *gula*, throat]. The esophagus, q.v.

Gull's disease. [Sir William W. Gull, Brit. physician, 1816-1890] Atrophy of the thyroid gland and resulting myxedema.

gum. 1. A substance which is given out or extracted from certain plants. It is sticky when moist but hardens upon drying. Roughly, any resinlike substance given out by plants. 2. The fleshy substance or tissue covering the alveolar processes of the jaws. SYN: *gingiva.*

DIAG: *Bleeding easily:* Indicates scurvy or inflammation as in trench mouth or pyorrhea. *Bluish red:* Indicates mercurial stomatitis or lead poisoning, if bluish line is at edge of teeth. *Greenish line:* At edge of teeth may indicate copper poisoning. *Purplish line or color:* Scurvy. *Red line:* In youth, indicates gingivitis, pyorrhea, scurvy. *Spongy g. and ulceration:* Gingivitis; scurvy; stomatitis; leukemia; tuberculosis; diabetes; and digestive disturbances.

RS: diagnosis; gingiva; ulatropia; ulemorrhagia; uletic; ulitis; uloglossitis; uloncus; ulorrhea.

gumboil (gum'boyl). Gum abscess. SYN: *parulis.*

ETIOL: Subperiosteal infection associated with a carious tooth, irritation or injury by a denture.

SYM: Gum is red, swollen, tender, and very painful. A fluctuating swelling may appear containing pus. It may point and break or require incision.

TREATMENT: Hot mouthwashes and applications over gum or externally. Warn patient not to swallow pus. Frequent mouthwashes after being evacuated. SEE: *gum.*

gumma (gum'mă) [L. *gummi,* gum]. A soft tumor of the tissues characteristic of the tertiary stage of syphilis. It is a granuloma varying in size from a millimeter to a centimeter or more in diameter. May be single or multiple, and tend to be encapsulated. Each consists of a central necrotic mass surrounded by an inflammatory zone and fibrosis. The necrotic portion may be firm or elastic, gelatinous or hyalinized. Infectious organisms may be present. They occur most frequently in the liver but may occur in other organs such as the brain, testis, heart, bone, and skin.

SYM: Depend upon location. Bursting of a g. leads to a gummatous ulcer, painless, but slow to heal. The base is formed by a "washleather" slough but surrounding tissues are healthy. SEE: *syphilis.*

gummose (gŭm'ōs). A sugar from animal gum. $C_6H_{12}O_6$.

gum'my [L. *gummi,* gum]. Sticky, swollen, puffy.

gun'shot wound. Penetrating or perforating wound which may contain a foreign body, as a bullet. SEE: *wound.*

gun'stock deform'ity. Deformity in which the long axis of the extended forearm turns outwardly from the arm, caused by fracture at the elbow.

gustation (gŭs-tā'shun) [L. *gustāre,* to taste]. Sense of taste.

gustatory (gŭs'tă-tō-rĭ). Pert. to sense of taste.

g. sweating. Sweating and flushing over the distribution of the auriculotemporal nerve in response to chewing. SYN: *auriculotemporal syndrome.*

gustom'etry (L. *gustāre,* to taste, + Gr. *metron,* measure). Measurement of acuteness of the sense of taste.

gut [AS.]. 1. The bowel or intestine. 2. The primitive gut or embryonic digestive tube which includes the foregut, midgut, and hindgut. 3. Short term for catgut.

g., blind. Cecum.

gut'ta [L. a drop]. (pl. *guttae*) 1. A drop. The amount in a drop varies with the nature of

the liquid and its temperature. It is therefore not advisable to use the number of drops per minim of a solution as anything more than a general guide to the amount of material being administered intravenously. ABBR: gt. (pl. gtt.). 2. A lesion in the form of a drop.

g. rosacea. Acne rosacea. SEE: *rosacea.*

g. serena. Blindness. SEE: *amaurosis.*

gutt'ate [L. *gutta,* drop]. Resembling a drop, said of certain cutaneous lesions.

gutta'tim [L.]. Drop by drop.

gut'tur [L.]. The throat.

guttural (gŭt'ŭ-răl). Pert. to the throat.

gutturotetany (gŭt"ŭr-o-tĕt'ă-nĭ) [L. *guttur,* throat, + Gr. *tetanos,* tension]. Laryngeal spasm of throat with temporary stutter.

Guyon's sign (gū-on'). [Felix J. C. Guyon, Fr. surgeon, 1831-1920] Ballottement of kidney.

Gwath'mey's method or technique. [James T. Gwathmey, Amer. surgeon, 1863-1944] Use of anesthetic consisting of ether and olive oil solution. This is placed in the rectum and colon where it is absorbed. SEE: *anesthesia.*

gymnas'tics [Gr. *gymnastikos,* pert. to nakedness]. Systematic body exercise, with or without special apparatus.

g., ocular. Systematic exercise of the eye muscles to improve muscular coordination and efficiency.

g., Swedish. A system of movements made by a patient against a resistance provided by the attendant.

gymnophobia (jĭm-no-fō'bĭ-ă) [Gr. *gymnos,* naked, + *phobos,* fear]. Abnormal aversion to viewing a naked body.

gynander (jĭ-năn'dĕr, ji-, gī) [Gr. *gynē,* woman, + *anēr, andr-,* man]. A gynandromorph, q.v. A pseudohermaphrodite; an individual possessing both male and female characteristics.

gynandroid (jĭ-nan'droyd, jĭ-, gī-) ["+ "+ *eidos,* form]. An individual having sufficient hermaphroditic sexual characteristics to be mistaken for a person of the opposite sex.

gynandromorph (jĭ-nan'dro-morf, jĭ-, gī-) ["+ "+ *morphē,* form]. An individual in which certain parts of the organism are male and certain parts female. SYN: *gynander.*

gynandromor'phous. Having the characteristics of both the male and female.

gynandry (jĭ-nan'dri, jĭ-, gī-) [Gr. *gynē,* woman, + *anēr, andr-,* man]. Condition of pseudohermaphroditism.

gynatresia (jĭ-nă-tre'zĭ-ă, jĭ-, gī-) ["+ *a-,* not, + *trēsis,* perforation]. Atresia, q.v., of the vagina.

gynecic (jĭ-nē'sĭk, jĭ-, gī-) [Gr. *gyne,* woman]. Pert. to women.

gyneco-, gyno- [Gr.]. Prefix meaning woman, female.

gynecologic, gynecological (gī''nĕ-kŏ-lŏj'ĭk, jī'',- jĭn''ē-; -ĭ-kăl) [Gr. *gynē,* woman, + *logos,* study]. Pert. to gynecology, or study of diseases peculiar to women.

   g. operative procedures. NP: Preoperative: SEE: *preoperative preparation.*

   Postoperative: Count and chart pulse every 15 minutes for first few hours. Report immediately any change in rate or volume. Watch for shock or internal hemorrhage. Keep warm and quiet; no visitors. Fluids when tolerated, tap water being best. Hypodermoclysis or infusions in excessive vomiting instead of fluids by mouth.

   Care must be taken to prevent retention of urine. Sterile, closed, continuous drainage of the bladder may be preferable to repeated catheterization.

   Patient catheterized every 12 hours after operation, then every 8 hours until able to void. Catheterization after voiding to prevent retention, until less than one-half ounce urine is thus obtained after two successive voidings. Thrombophlebitis with embolism is a dreaded complication which is to be avoided. This is best done by having the patient exercise her legs quite frequently. Also elastic stocking up to the knee, not circular elastic bandages, should be worn continuously while a bed patient.

gynecologist (gī''nĕ-kol'o-jĭst, jī'',- jĭn''ē-). Physician who specializes in diseases peculiar to women.

gynecology (gī''nĕ-kŏl'ō-jĭ, jī'',- jĭn''ē-) [Gr. *gynē,* woman, + *logos,* study]. The study of the diseases of the female, particularly of the genital, urinary or rectal organs.

gynecomania (jĭ''-nĕ-ko-mā'nĭ-ă, gī'',- jĭn''ē-) [''+ *mania,* madness]. Abnormal sex desire in the male. SYN: *satyriasis,* q.v.

gynecomastia, gynecomasty, gynecomazia (jĭ''nĕ-ko-mas'tĭ-ă, gī'',- jĭn''ē-; tĭ, -ma'zĭ-ă) [''+ *mastos,mazos,* breast]. Abnormally large mammary glands in the male; sometimes may secrete milk.

gynecopathy (jĭ-nĕ-kop'ă-thĭ, gī'',- jĭn''ē) [Gr. *gyne,* woman, + *pathos,* disease]. Diseases peculiar to women.

gynecophonus (jĭ''nĕ-kof'on-us, gī'',- jĭn''ē-) [''+ *phōnē,* voice]. Having an effeminate voice.

gynephobia (jĭ''nĕ-fo'bĭ-ă, gī'',- jĭn''ē-) [''+ *phobos,* fear]. Abnormal aversion to the company of women, or fear of them.

gynesic (gĭ-nē'sik, jĭ-, jĭn-ē') [Gr. *gynē,* women]. Pert. to the diseases of women.

gyniatrics (jī''nĭ-at'riks, gī''-, jĭn''ī-) [''+ *iatrikos,* medical treatment]. Treatment of diseases of women.

gynopath'ic [''+ *pathos,* disease]. Pert. to disease of women.

gynoplastic [Gr. *gyne,* woman, + *plassein,* to form]. Pertaining to gynoplasty.

gynoplastics (jī''no-plas'tiks, gī''-). Reparative surgery of female genitalia.

gynoplasty. Gynoplastics, q.v.

gyrate (jī'rāt) [Gr. *gyros,* circle]. 1. Ring-shaped, convoluted. 2. To revolve.

gyration (jī-rā'shŭn). A rotary movement.

gyre (jir) [Gr. *gyros,* circle]. Convolution. SYN: *gyrus.*

gyrencephalic (jī-rĕn-sĕ-făl'ĭk) [''+ *enkephalē,* head]. Having a brain marked by numerous convolutions.

gyri (jī'rī). Pl. of gyrus, q.v.

gyri breves insulae. [NA] Preinsular g.

gyro- [Gr.]. Combining form meaning a circle, spiral, ring.

gyrochrome (jī'rō-krōm) [Gr. *gyros,* circle, + *chrōma,* color]. A nerve cell in which the stainable substance occurs in rings.

gyroma (jī-rō'mă) [Gr. *gyros,* circle, + *-ōma,* tumor]. Ovarian tumor consisting of a convoluted mass.

gyromele (jī'rō-mĕl) [''+ *mēlē,* a probe]. Revolving stomach tube for massage and cleansing of stomach, determining its location, size and condition.

gyrometer (jī-rŏm'ĕ-ter) [''+ *metron,* measure]. A device for measuring the cerebral gyri.

gyrosa (jī-rō'să) [Gr. *gyros,* circle, + *-ōsis,* diseased condition]. Gastric vertigo causing one to close one's eyes to prevent falling, as everything turns round when standing.

gyrose (jī'rōs). In bacteriology, marked by wavy lines or circles. Applied to bacterial colonies.

gyrospasm (jī'rō-spăzm) [Gr. *gyros,* circle, + *spasmos,* spasm]. Spasmodic rotary head movement.

gyrotrope (jī'rō-trōp) [''+ *tropē,* a turning]. Cord connecting an electrode with source of an electric current. SYN: *rheotrope.*

gyrous (jī'rŭs) [Gr. *gyros,* circle]. Marked by circular lines. SYN: *gyrose.*

gyrus (jī'rŭs). (pl. *gyri)* [NA] One of the convolutions of the cerebral hemispheres of the brain. They are separated by shallow grooves (sulci) or deeper grooves (fissures).

   g., angular. G. of the parietal lobe embracing posterior end of the superior temporal sulcus.

   g., annectent. Any of many short folds of gray matter which are formed as a result of short branches or twigs of sulci extending into adjacent gyri. They are not always present.

g., anterior central. G. of the frontal lobe extending vertically between precentral and central sulci.

g., Broca's. G., frontal, inferior, q.v.

g., callosal. A large g. on medial surface of cerebral hemisphere which lies directly above the corpus callosum, and arches over its anterior end.

g., cerebelli. Layer of the cerebellum.

g., dentate. A g. marked by indentations which lie on the upper surface of the hippocampal g.

g., fornicatus. G. on medial surface of cerebrum which includes the g. cinguli, the isthmus, the hippocampus, hippocampal g. and uncus.

g., frontal, inferior. Convolution on external surface of frontal lobe of cerebrum located between the sylvian fissure and the inferior frontal sulcus.

g., frontal, middle. G. between the superior and inferior frontal sulci.

g., frontal, superior. Convolution of cerebral frontal lobe situated above the superfrontal fissure.

g., fusiform. G. beneath the collateral fissure joining the occipital and temporal lobes.

g., Heschl's. Transverse temporal g.

g., hippocampal. G. situated between the hippocampal and collateral fissures.

g., lingual. G. between the calcarine and collateral fissures.

g., longus insulae. [NA] Lengthy g. composing the postinsula.

g., marginal. G., frontal, superior, q.v.

g., middle temporal. G. located between middle temporal sulcus and superior temporal sulcus.

g., occipital. Any of the gyri on the lateral surface of the occipital lobe. They are

not always present. Classified roughly in two groups, the inferior or lateral occipital gyri and the superior occipital gyri.

g., occipitotemporal. G., fusiform, q.v.

g., orbital. One of four g. (anterior, posterior, lateral and medial) forming inferior surface of the frontal lobe.

g., paracentral. Area on mesial aspect of the cerebrum; the paracentral lobule. Lies above cingulate sulcus.

g., parietal. G. on lateral aspect of parietal lobe. Include posterior central gyrus, superior and inferior parietal gyri.

g., postcentral. G. situated between the central and postcentral fissures.

g., primary. Fetal cerebral regions marked by the primary fissures.

g., profundi cerebri. Very deep gyri of the cerebrum.

g., rectus. [NA] G. on the orbital aspect of the frontal lobe, located between the mesial margin and the olfactory sulcus.

g., Retzii, g., sagittal. The supra- and subcallosal gyri.

g., subcallosal. A narrow band of gray matter on medial surface of hemisphere below the rostrum of the corpus callosum.

g., subcollateral. G., fusiform, q.v.

g., supracallosal. A rudimentary g. on the upper surface of the corpus callosum.

g., supracallosus. Gray matter layer covering the corpus callosum.

g., supramarginal. G. in the inferior parietal lobule twisting about the upper terminus of the sylvian fissure.

g., temporal. Three gyri (superior, middle, inferior) on lateral surface of temporal lobe.

g., transitivus. G., annectent, q.v.

g., uncinate. Anterior hooked portion of the hippocampal g.

H

H. Chem. symb. for hydrogen.

H., h. Abbr. for *haustus*, a draft of medicine; *height; henry; hora* or *hour; horizontal; hypermetropia.*

H+. Chem. symb. for hydrogen ion.

H^1. Chem. symb. for protium.

H^2. Chem. symb. for deuterium, an isotope of hydrogen.

Haab's reflex. [Otto Haab, Swiss ophthalmologist, 1850-1931] Contraction of pupils without alteration of accommodation or convergence when gazing at a bright object. A sign of a cortical lesion.

habena (hă-bē'nă) [L., rein]. (pl. *habenae*) 1. A frenum. 2. Bandage for a wound. 3. Pineal gland peduncle. SYN: *habenula* [NA].

habe'nal, habe'nar [L. *habena*, rein]. Pert. to the habena or habenula.

habenula (hă-ben'u-lă) [L. little rein, strap]. 1. A frenum, or any rein- or whiplike structure. 2. [NA] A peduncle or stalk attached to the pineal body of the brain. Fibers which travel posteriorly along the dorsomedial border of the thalamus to the habenular ganglia (epithalamus) resemble reins. 3. A narrow bandlike stricture.

h. urethra'lis. One of two whitish bands between the clitoris and meatus urethra in young females.

habenul'ar. Pert. to the habenula, esp. the stalk of the pineal body.

h. commissure. A band of transverse fibers connecting the two habenular areas.

h. trigone. A depressed triangular area located on the lateral aspect of the posterior portion of the third ventricle. Each contains a medial and lateral habernacular nucleus.

habit [L. *habēre, habitus*, to have, hold]. 1. A motor pattern executed with facility following constant or frequent repetition; an act at first performed in a typical voluntary manner but which after sufficient repetition is performed as a reflex action. H.'s result from the passing of impulses through a particular set of neurons and synapses many times. 2. A particular type of dress or garb. 3. Mental or moral constitution or disposition. 4. Bodily appearance or constitution, esp. as related to a disease or predisposition to a disease, as the apoplectic h. 5. Addiction to the use of drug or beverage as the drug h., alcoholic h. SYN: *habitus*, q.v.

h., chorea. H., spasm, q.v.

h., full. Habitus apoplecticus, q.v.

h., spasm. A spasmodic voluntary movement that has become involuntary.

Often due to something irritating; sometimes from mimicry. SYN: *tic*, q.v.

h. training. Development by young children of specific behavior patterns concerning basic activities such as eating, dressing, using the toilet, and sleeping.

habitua'tion. Act of becoming accustomed to anything from frequent use. In drug addiction, the mental equivalent of physical tolerance and dependence on drugs.

hab'itus [L. habit]. (pl. *habitus*) Indications in appearance of tendency to disease or abnormal conditions.

h. apoplecticus. The supposed body build and appearance of one predisposed to develop apoplexy: short, thicknecked with flushed face and prominent temporal arteries.

h. enteroptoticus. Physical state marking enteroptosis. The abdomen is long and narrow and the angle between the ribs and the long axis of the body is less than 90°.

habromania (hab''ro-mā'nĭ-ă) [Gr. *habros*, cheerful, + *mania*, madness]. Obsolete term for a psychosis accompanied by pleasant delusions.

hachement (hăsh-mŏn') [Fr., chopping]. Strokes with edge of hand in massage. SYN: *hacking*.

hack'ing [AS. *haccian*, to chop]. Strokes with edge of hand in massage. SYN: *hachement*.

h. cough. A frequent, short cough.

haem. Heme, q.v.

haem-. SEE: words beginning with *hem-*.

Haemadipsa (hē''mă-dĭp'să). A genus of terrestrial leeches found in Asia which attack man and animals.

H. ceylonica; H. japonica. Species found in Ceylon and Japan, respectively.

Haemagogus (he''mă-gog'us). A genus of mosquitoes. Includes the species H. capricorni which serves as a vector of yellow fever.

Haemophilus (hē-mof'ĭl-ŭs) [Gr. *haima*, blood, + *philein*, to love]. Chiefly Brit. spelling for a genus of Bacteriaceae. SEE: *Hemophilus.*

Haemosporidia (hē''mō-spō-rĭd'ĭ-ă). An order of sporozoa which live in the blood cells of vertebrates and reproduce sexually in invertebrates; includes the genus Plasmodium, four species of which cause malaria in man.

haf'nium. SYMB: *Hf.* At wt. 178.49; at no. 72; sp. gr. 13.29. A rare chemical element.

Hagedorn needle (hä′gĕ-dorn). [Werner Hagedorn, Ger. surgeon, 1831-1894] A curved surgical needle with flattened sides.

hahnium (hŏ′nĭ-ŭm). [Otto Hahn, Ger. physicist, 1879-1968] An element, No. 105, first synthesized in 1970 at the University of California, Berkeley.

hair [AS. *haer*]. 1. A keratinized, threadlike outgrowth from the skin of mammals. 2. Collectively, the threadlike outgrowths which form the fur of animals, or which grow on the human body.

A h. is a thin flexible shaft of cornified cells which develops from a cylindrical invagination of the epidermis, the h. follicle. Each consists of a free portion or shaft (scapus pili) and a root (radix pili) embedded within the follicle. The shaft consists of three layers of cells: the cuticle or outermost layer; the cortex, forming the main horny portion of the h.; and the medulla, the central axis. H. color is due to pigment in the cortex.

H. in each part of the body have a definite period of growth after which they are shed. In man there is a constant gradual loss and replacement of h. H. of the eyebrows last only three to five months; that of the scalp two to five years. Baldness or alopecia re-

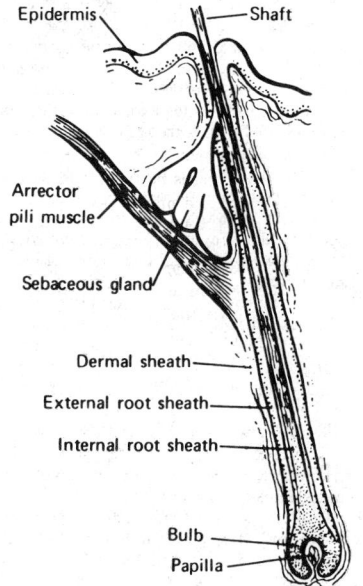

Epidermis — Shaft
Arrector pili muscle
Sebaceous gland
Dermal sheath
External root sheath
Internal root sheath
Bulb
Papilla

**HAIR FOLLICLE AND
RELATED STRUCTURES**

sults when replacement fails to keep up with h. loss. It may be due to hereditary factors or pathological conditions such as infections or injury from irradiation.

h., beaded. Swellings and constrictions in the h. shaft due to a developmental defect known as monilethrix.

h., bulb. Lower expanded portion of a h. root. Growth of a h. results from the proliferation of cells of the h. bulb. SYN: *bulbus pili* [NA].

h. cell. An epithelial cell possessing fine nonmotile cilia found in the maculae and the organ of Corti of the membranous labyrinth of the inner ear. They are receptors for the senses of position and hearing.

h. dye. May contain silver nitrate or aniline dyes which are often irritating to the skin or eyes, causing severe dermatitis or conjunctivitis. Occasionally results in blindness.

F.A. TREATMENT: Wash with sterile salt solution, followed by soap and water, and sponge with alcohol; cover with bland ointment, as cold cream or lanolin. The eye should be washed with normal saline and then instill paraffin oil, olive oil, or other bland oil.

h. follicle. An invagination of the epidermis which forms a cylindrical depression, penetrating the corium into the connective tissue which holds the h. root.

Sebaceous glands which secrete an oily fluid, and tiny muscles which cause the h. to stand (arrectores pili), are attached to these follicles.

h., gustatory. A taste h. One of several fine hairlike processes extending from the ends of gustatory cells in a taste bud. They project through the inner pore of a taste bud.

h. kinky. Short, sparse, kinky hair which may be poorly pigmented. Associated with kinky hair disease, q.v.

h. papilla. A projection of the corium which extends into the h. bulb at the bottom of a h. follicle. It contains capillaries through which a h. receives nourishment.

h., pubic. That over the pubes. SYN: *escutcheon.* SEE: *pubic.*

h. transplantation. Surgical procedure for transplanting h. follicles from one body site to another. This technique, which is very time consuming, has been used to treat alopecia of the scalp.

h., woolly. The distinctive hair type of the Negroid race. May be present as the only Negroid feature in persons of mixed Caucasian and Negroid race. The hair type is not linked to hair color.

hairball. A mass in the stomach consisting of hair. SYN: *trichobezoar.*

hairy tongue. One covered with hairlike papillae entangled with threads produced by the fungus Aspergillus niger or Candida albicans. Usually seen as the result of antibiotic therapy which inhibits growth of bacteria normally present in the mouth. This permits overgrowth of fungi. SYN: *black tongue; furry tongue.*

hala'tion [Gr. *alōs*, a halo]. Blurring of vision due to light from a wrong direction.

half-life. 1. Time required for half the nuclei of a radioactive substance to lose its activity by undergoing radioactive decay. 2. In biology and pharmacology, the time required by the body, tissue, or organ to metabolize or inactivate half the amount of a substance taken in. This is an important consideration in determining the proper amount and frequency of dose of drug to be administered. SYN: *biological half-life.* 3. Time required for radioactivity of material taken in by a living organism to be reduced to half its initial value by a combination of radioactive decay and biological elimination. SYN: *effective half-life.*

half-value layer. SEE: *half-value thickness.*

half-value thickness. The thickness of a substance which, when placed in the path of a given beam of rays, will lower its intensity to one half of the initial value.

halisteresis (hă-lĭs″tĕr-ē′sĭs) [Gr. *hals,* salt, + *sterēsis,* deprivation]. Lack of calcium (lime salt) in bone. SYN: *osteomalacia.*

halistere'tic. Rel. to or affected with halisteresis, q.v.

halitosis (hăl-ĭ-tō′sĭs) [L. *halitus,* breath, + Gr. *-ōsis,* condition]. Offensive breath.

halituous (hăl-ĭt′ū-ŭs) [L. *halitus,* exhalation]. Covered with moisture. SYN: *vaporous.*

hal'itus. 1. The breath. 2. Warm vapor.

Hal'ler's anastomatic circle. [Albrecht von Haller, Swiss physiologist, 1708-1777] Circle of arteries around the intraocular portion of the optic nerve. Made up of branches of the posterior ciliary arteries. SYN: *Haller-Zinn circle.*

hal'lex [L.]. (pl. *hal'lices*) The great toe. SYN: *hallus; hallux.*

hallucination (hă-lū-sĭ-nā′shŭn) [L. *hallūcināri,* to wander in mind]. In psychology, false perception having no relation to reality and not accounted for by any exterior stimuli. May be visual, auditory, olfactory, etc.

Commonly, the patient is unable to consider it as not constituting reality, but judgment may at times recognize discrepancies, and even at times deny the hallucination entirely. Usually, then, the patient reacts emotionally and behaves as one would to a real situation. An indifferent attitude strongly suggests deterioration. Any sense may be involved, or elaborate combinations may occur. As in dreams, here the patient might be terrified at seeing an approaching assaulter, hear his threats, and feel his blows, and struggle in desperate defense. Emotional tone, delusions, and hallucinations tend to harmonize and this may be ascribed to the last, reflecting rather than determining the others.

Structural disease of the sensory organ and conducting mechanism may favor the formation of hallucinations, e.g., the deafness of an old otitis media often is associated with tinnitus, and at times the paresthesia is associated with phonemes. An irritative lesion of the visual cortex may produce more directly the hallucination, but even here an intact mind probably quickly would recognize the perception as unreal.

RS: acousma; delusion; hallucinosis; hypnagogic; illusion.

h., extracampine. H. which arises from outside the normal sensory field or range, as someone having the sensation of seeing something which is behind him.

h., haptic. One pert. to touching the skin, or to sensations of temperature or pain.

h., hypnagogic. Pre-sleep phenomena having the same practical significance as a dream but experienced while consciousness persists. Includes sense of falling, sinking, or of the ceiling moving.

h., kinetic. Sensation of flying or moving the body or a part of it.

h., microptic. One in which things seem reduced in size. SYN: *lilliputian h.*

h., motor. Imaginary perceptions of movement.

h., olfactory. One involving smell.

h., somatic. Sensation of pain attributed to visceral injury.

h., teleologic. One which advises or guides the subject, such as those of Jeanne d'Arc.

hallucinogen (hă-lu′sĭ-nō-jĕn) [″+ Gr. *-genēs,* born]. Drug which produces hallucinations. Ex: LSD, marihuana, peyote, and sometimes ethyl alcohol.

hallucinosis (hă-lū″sĭn-ō′sĭs) [″+ Gr. *-ōsis,* condition]. The state of having hallucinations more or less persistently. SEE: *hallucination.*

h., acute. In psychiatry, alcoholic psychosis. SYM: Fear or anxiety and auditory hallucinations.

hallus. Hallux, q.v.

hallux (hăl'ŭks) [L.]. (pl. *hal'luces*) [NA] The great toe.

h. doloro'sus. Pain in the metatarso-phalangeal joint of the great toe due to flatfoot.

h. flexus. Hammertoe.

h. valgus. Displacement of great toe toward other toes.

h. varus. Displacement of great toe away from other toes.

halmatogenesis (hal"ma-to-jen'ĕ-sis) [Gr. *halma,* jump, + *genesis,* development]. A sudden deviation of type from one generation to the other one. SYN: *saltatory variation.*

ha'lo [Gr. *halōs,* a halo]. 1. The areola, esp. of the nipple. 2. A ring surrounding the macula lutea in ophthalmoscopic images. 3. A circle of light surrounding a shining body.

h., glaucomatous. A whitish ring surrounding the optic disk; seen in glaucoma.

h. symptom. Colored circle or circles around lights. These are seen by patients with glaucoma and also by those with punctate lens opacities.

halogen (hăl'ō-jĕn) [Gr. *hals,* salt, + *gennan,* to form]. A salt former; one of a group of elements (chlorine, Cl; bromine, Br; iodine, I; and fluorine, F) having very similar chemical properties.

They combine with hydrogen to form acids and with metal to form salts.

haloid (hăl'oyd) ["+ *eidos,* form]. Resembling salt.

h. salt. A salt made up of a base and a halogen, resembling common salt.

halometer (hă-lŏm'ĕ-tĕr) [Gr. *halōs,* a halo, + *metron,* measure]. 1. Device for measuring diffraction halo of a red blood cell. 2. Device for measuring the halo around optic disk.

halosteresis (hă-lŏs"tĕr-ē'sĭs) [Gr. *hals,* salt, + *sterēsis,* privation]. Deficiency of lime salts in the bones. SYN: *halisteresis.*

halothane (hal'o-thān). A fluorinated hydrocarbon used as a general anesthetic.

Hal'sted's operation. [William Stewart Halsted, Amer. surgeon, 1852-1922] Operation for inguinal hernia and for amputation of breast with carcinoma.

Halsted's suture. An interrupted one for intestinal wounds.

ham [AS. *haum,* haunch]. 1. The popliteal space or region behind the knee. 2. Common name for the thigh, hip, and buttock. 3. The thigh of an animal, esp. the hog, prepared for food.

hamartia (hăm-ăr'shĭ-ă) [Gr. defect]. Error in development due to imperfect tissue combination.

hamartoma (ham-ar-tō'mă) [Gr. *hamartia,* defect, + *-ōma,* tumor]. 1. A tumor due to new growth of blood vessels, as opposed to dilatation of pre-existing vessels. 2. A tumor due to failure of development.

hamartomatosis (ham"ar-to-mă-tō'sis) ["+ "+ *-ōsis,* condition]. Existence of multiple hamartomas.

hamatum (hă-mā'tŭm) [L. *hamatus,* hooked]. The unciform bone, os hamatum.

hammer. 1. An instrument with a head attached crosswise to the handle for striking blows. 2. Common name for the malleus, the middle ear bone.

h., percussion. A h. with a rubber head used for tapping surfaces of the body in order to produce sounds for diagnostic purposes. SEE: *plexor.*

h., reflex. A h. used for tapping parts of the body such as a muscle, tendon, or nerve in order to initiate certain reflex responses.

ham'mertoe. A toe with dorsal flexion of 1st phalanx and plantar flexion of 2nd and 3rd phalanges.

hamster. A rodent Cricetus cricetus belonging to the family Cricetidae, common in Europe and W. Asia. It is extensively used as a laboratory animal.

ham'string [AS. *haum,* haunch]. One of the tendons which form the medial and lateral boundaries of the popliteal space.

h.'s, inner. Tendons of the semimembranosus, semitendinosus, and gracilis muscles.

h.'s, outer. The tendon of the biceps femoris.

hamstrings. Three muscles on the posterior aspect of the thigh, the semitendinosus, semimembranosus, and biceps femoris. They flex the leg and adduct and extend the thigh.

ham'ular [L. *hamulus,* a small hook]. Unciform; hook-shaped.

hamulus [L., a small hook]. 1. Any hook-shaped structure. 2. Hooklike process on the hamate bone.

h. cochleae. A hooklike process at the tip of the osseous spiral lamina of the cochlea.

h. lacrimalis. [NA] Hooklike process on the lacrimal bone.

h. pterygoideus. [NA] Hooklike process at tip of medial pterygoid process of the sphenoid bone.

hand [AS. *hand*]. That part of the body attached to the forearm at the wrist.

It includes the wrist (carpus) with its 8 bones, the metacarpus, or body of the h. (ossa metacarpalia) having five bones, and the phalanges (fingers) with their 14 bones.

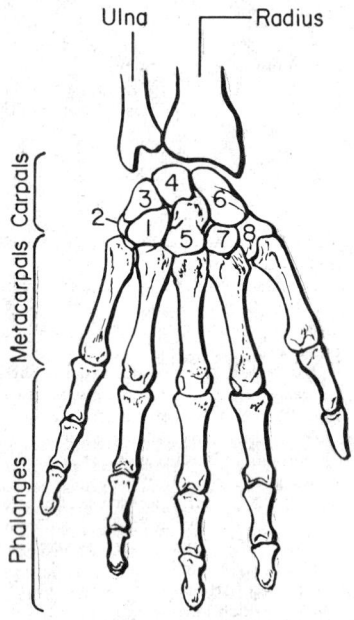

Ulna　　　Radius

Carpals

Metacarpals

Phalanges

BONES OF THE HAND AND WRIST

h., ape. Deformity of h. in which thumb is permanently extended.

h., claw. SEE: *clawhand.*

h., cleft. Deformity of h. in which the division between the fingers, particularly between the third and fourth, extends into the carpus.

h., opera-glass. Deformity of h. due to chronic absorptive arthritis. The phalanges appear to be telescoped into one another like an opera glass.

H. and E. Abbr. for *hematoxylin* and *eosin,* a staining method much used in histology.

hand'edness. The tendency to use one hand in preference to the other.

h., left-. Sinistrality; preferential use of the left hand.

h., right-. Dextrality; preferential use of the right hand.

Hand-Schüller-Christian syndrome or disease. [Alfred Hand, Jr., Amer. pediatrician, 1868-1949; Artur Schüller, Austrian neurologist, 1874 —; Henry A. Christian, Amer. pathologist, 1876-1951] A condition of unknown cause. Pathological lesion is that of a histiocytic granuloma. These lesions are found in bone (particularly the skull), the skin, and viscera. The disease is seen in children and young adults. Adrenal cortical hormones have been of some help in treating the illness. SYN: *histiocytosis X; Schüller-Christian disease; xanthoma disseminatum.*

hang'ing drop culture. A method of culturing microorganisms by placing a drop of the culture medium containing organisms on a coverslip, then inverting the coverslip over a concavity of a hanging drop slide.

hang'nail [AS. *hangian,* to hang, + *naegel,* nail]. Partly detached piece of skin at root of fingernail. SYN: *agnail.*

Hanot's disease (ă-nō'). [Victor C. Hanot, Fr. physician, 1844-1896] Hypertrophic cirrhosis of liver with jaundice.

Hansen's bacillus. [Gerhard H. A. Hansen, Norwegian physician, 1841-1912] Mycobacterium leprae, the cause of leprosy, which Hansen discovered in 1871.

Hansen's disease. Leprosy.

hapalonychia (hăp″ăl-ō-nĭk′ĭ-ă) [Gr. *hapalos,* soft, + *onyx, onych-,* nail]. Lack of rigidity of the nails. SYN: *onychomalacia.*

haphalgesia (haf″al-ge′zĭ-ă) [Gr. *haphē,* touch, + *algēsis,* pain]. A sensation of pain upon touching the skin lightly or with an object which is not an irritant.

haphephobia (haf″e-fō′bĭ-ă) ["+ *phobos,* fear]. Aversion to being touched by another person.

haplodermatitis (hap″lo-der″mă-tī′tis) [Gr. *haplous,* simple, + *derma,* skin, + *-itis,* inflammation]. Simple inflammation of the skin. SYN: *haplodermitis.*

haplodermitis (hap″lo-der-mī′tis). Uncomplicated inflammation of the skin.

hap'loid [Gr. *haplous,* single, simple, + *eidos,* form]. Possessing half the diploid or normal number of chromosomes found in somatic or body cells. Such is the case of the germ cells, ova or sperm, following the reduction divisions in gametogenesis, the haploid number being 23 in man.

haplop'ia ["+ *ōps,* vision]. Single vision; condition in which an object viewed by two eyes appears as a single object in contrast to diplopia, in which it appears as two objects.

hap'ten(e [Gr. *haptein,* to seize]. The portion of an antigen containing the grouping on which the specificity depends.

haptic (hăp′tik) [Gr. *haptein,* to touch]. Pert. to touch. SYN: *tactile.*

hap'tics [Gr. *haptein,* to touch]. The science of the touch sense.

haptin (hăp′tin). Haptene, q.v.

haptoglobin. A mucoprotein to which hemoglobin released into plasma is bound. It is increased in certain inflammatory conditions and decreased in hemolytic disorders.

haptophil(e (hăp'tō-fĭl, -fīl) [Gr. *haptein,* to touch, + *philein,* to love]. That portion of a receptor that unites with the haptophore group of a toxin.

haptophore (hăp'to-fōr) ["+ *pherein,* to bring]. The atom group of an antigen causing a combination with its corresponding antibody. SEE: *Ehrlich's sidechain theory.*

haptophor'ic, haptoph'orous. Pert. to the action of a haptophore.

har'dening [AS. *heardian,* to harden]. 1. Rendering a pathological or histological specimen firm or compact for making thin sections for microscopic study. 2. The development of increased resistance to extremes of environmental temperature. SEE: *acclimation.*

hard'ness. 1. Quality of water containing certain substances, esp. soluble salts of calcium and magnesium. These react with soaps forming insoluble compounds which are precipitated out of solution, thus interfering with their cleansing action. 2. That quality of X rays determining their penetrating power. Hardness lessens as wave lengths become longer.

h. of a gas tube. A term used to qualify the condition of a tube according to the degree of rarefaction of the residual gas.

The higher the vacuum, the harder the tube and the rays emitted, the higher the voltage required to cause a discharge with a cold cathode, and hence the shorter the wave length of the resulting roentgen rays.

harelip [AS. *hara,* hare, + *lippa,* lip]. A vertical cleft or clefts in the upper lip. It is congenital resulting from the faulty fusion of the median nasal process and the lateral maxillary processes. It is usually unilateral and on the left side although it may be bilateral. It may involve the lip or the upper jaw alone or both together, and often occurs with cleft palate. SYN: *cheiloschisis.*

h. suture. A twisted figure-of-eight suture.

harlequin fetus (hăr'lĕ-kwĭn). A newly-born infant with abnormal skin which resembles a thick horny armor. The skin is divided into areas by deep red fissures. These infants die within a few days. This condition has been known by many names including ichthyosis foetalis and ichthyosiform erythroderma. These were at one time regarded as separate diseases but are now known to represent different degrees of severity of the same entity.

Har'rison's groove. [Edwin Harrison, Brit. physician, 1779-1847] Depression on lower edge of the thorax caused by tug of the diaphragm; seen in rickets and any disease of infants which tends to obstruct inspiration. The chest is pressed in by the labored inspiration at its weakest point.

Hashimoto's struma. [Hakura Hashimoto, Jap. surgeon, 1881-1934] A chronic form of thyroiditis.

hashish (hăsh'ĭsh) [Arabic, hemp, dried grass]. A more or less purified extract prepared from the flowers, stalks, and leaves of the marihuana plant Cannabis sativa. The gummy substance is smoked or chewed for its hallucinogenic effects. Its use and sale in most countries including the U.S.A. are illegal.

Has'ner's valve or fold. [Joseph R. Hasner, Prague ophthalmologist, 1819-1892] A fold of the mucous membrane at the opening of the nasolacrimal duct in the inferior meatus of the nasal cavity. SYN: *plica lacrimalis.*

Has'sall's corpuscles or bodies. [Arthur H. Hassall, Brit. chemist and physician, 1817-1894] Spherical or oval bodies present in the medulla of the thymus. Each consists of central area of degenerated cells surrounded by concentrically arranged flattened or polygonal cells. They are characteristic of the thymus. SYN: *thymic corpuscle.*

Hatchcock's sign. Tenderness just beyond the angle of the jaws when the finger follows on the under surface of the mandible towards the angle. Found in mumps before any swelling can be detected.

haunch (hawnsh) [Fr. *hanche*]. The hips and buttocks.

h. bone. The ilium. SYN: *os coxae* [NA].

haustra (haws'tra) [L. *haurire,* to draw, drink]. (sing. *haustrum*) The sacculated pouches of the colon.

h. coli. Sacculations of the colon resembling tucks caused by the fact that the gut is longer than the longitudinal bands or taeniae.

haustral (haw'stral). Pert. to the colonic haustra.

h. churning. Agitation of the intestinal contents.

haustrum (haw'strum) [L. *haurire,* to draw, drink]. (pl. *haus'tra*) One of the sacculations of the colon caused by longitudinal bands shorter than the gut which causes formation of pouches in the colon. SYN: *haustra coli.*

haus'tus [L., a drink]. A swallow, or draft, of medicine.

haut-mal (ō-măl) [Fr., high evil]. Grand mal when at its height.

haver'sian canal. [Clopton Havers, Brit. physician and anatomist, 1650-1702] Minute vascular canals found in osseous tissue.

haversian canaliculi. Delicate canals extending from the lacunae into the matrix of bone. They anastomose with canaliculi of adjacent lacunae forming a network of fine channels which communicate with haversian and Volkmann's canals. They transmit nutrient materials.

haversian gland. A mass of fatty tissue lodged in the acetabular fossa of the innominate bone. Also called synovial gland.

haversian system. Architectural unit of bone consisting of a central tube (h. canal) with alternate layers of intercellular material (matrix) surrounding it in concentric cylinders. Alternating layers of matrix and cells are called h. lamellae. SEE: *bone.*

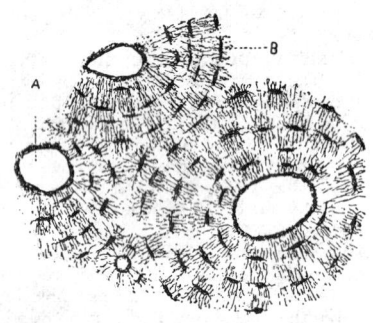

HAVERSIAN SYSTEM OF BONE
Magnified cross section of a dog's femur. A, Haversian canal. B, Lacunae and canaliculi.

hay fever. An allergic disease of mucous passages of nose and upper air passages induced by external irritation. SYN: *allergic coryza; pollinosis; vasomotor rhinitis.*

SYM: Inflammation, catarrh, watery discharges from the eyes, cold in the head, coryza, headache, asthmatic symptoms.

ETIOL: Air-borne pollens. Spring type due to pollens of trees such as oak, elm, hickory, ash; Summer type due to pollens of plants such as grasses, plantain, and sorrel; Fall type due principally to the pollen of ragweeds. Non-seasonal hay fever may result from inhalation of irritating substances such as the danders of animals, or dust such as hay, straw, or house dust; or from ingestion of substances such as drugs or foods to which the subject is allergic.

TREATMENT: Change of climate, sea voyage. Filtration of air by air conditioning, masks, and nasal filters. Drug therapy in which epinephrine, antihistamines, or other drugs are given orally or used as nose drops, or nasal sprays. Prophylactic treatment consisting of desensitization by injection of pollen extracts made from pollen to which the subject is sensitive.

Hay'garth's deformities. [John Haygarth, Brit. physician, 1740-1827] Exostoses or bony tumors on joints in rheumatoid arthritis. SYN: *Haygarth's nodes; Haygarth's nodosities.*

Hb. Abbr. for *hemoglobin.*

HCG. Abbr. for *human chorionic gonadotrophin.*

H.D. Abbr. for *hearing distance.*

h.d. Abbr. for L. *hora decubitus,* the hour of going to bed.

He. Chem. symb. for helium.

head [AS. *heafod*]. 1. Caput. That part of the animal body containing the brain and organs of sight, hearing, smell, and taste. It includes the facial bones. 2. The proximal end of a bone. 3. The larger extremity of any structure or body.

h., abnormal fixity of. May be caused by postpharyngeal abscess, occipitocervical myelalgia, arthritis deformans, swollen cervical glands, rheumatism, traumatism of neck, sprains of cervical muscles, congenital spasmodic torticollis, caries of a molar tooth, burn scars, eye muscle imbalance (hyperphoria).

h., abnormal movement of. Habit spasms, such as nodding.

h., aftercoming. The head of a fetus in a breech presentation.

h. fold. A fold of the blastoderm of a chick which grows caudad under the anterior portion of the neural plate. It brings about the establishment of the h. and the foregut.

h. gut. Part of embryo which develops into stomach, duodenum, and esophagus.

h., inability to move the. May be due to caries of cervical vertebrae and diseases of articulation between occiput and atlas or paralysis of neck muscles.

h. kidney. Embryonic kidney.

h. lock. Interlocking of chins in twin birth.

h., nerve. The optic disk.

h. process. A strand of cells in the embryo extending forward from the primitive knot. Also called notochordal plate.

h., retracted. Seen in acute meningitis, cerebral abscess, tumor, thrombosis of superior longitudinal sinus, acute encephalitis, laryngeal obstruction, tetanus, hydrophobia, epilepsy, spasmodic torticollis, strychnine poisoning, hysteria, and rachitic conditions. Also in painful neck lesions at the back.

h., rhythmical nodding of. Seen in aortic regurgitation, chorea, torticollis, q.v.

h. scald. Affection of scalp accompanied by crusts or scales.

head, words pert. to: acromegaly; caput; "ceph-" words; coryza; face; gyrospasm; macrocephalous; nutation; occipital; sinciput; skeleton; temple; vertex.

head'ache [AS. *hēafod*, head, + *acan*, to ache]. A diffuse pain in different portions of the head and not confined to any nerve distribution area. May be acute or chronic.

It may be frontal, temporal, or occipital; confined to one side of head or to region immediately over one eye. The character of pain may vary; may be dull ache; acute, almost unbearable pain; intermittent, intense pain; throbbing pain; pressure pain when head feels as if it will burst, or penetrating pain driving through head. SYN: *cephalgia.*

ETIOL: Transient acute headaches may be due to a variety of causes including diseases of the eye, ear, nose, or throat; acute infections; or trauma to the head.

Chronic headaches may be caused by a variety of conditions including physical, emotional, psychosomatic, or psychogenic factors; fevers; metabolic conditions; endocrine imbalance; or exposure to toxic chemicals.

The exact cause can be determined by thorough analysis of the data obtained from history, physical examination, tests, and laboratory studies which may include x-ray pictures of skull, electroencephalography, and metabolic studies.

Toxic Factors: (1) Exogenous origin: Foul air from poor ventilation, etc.; poisonous gases, including fumes from furnaces or gas fires; drugs (quinine, morphine, atropine, histamine); alcohol; tobacco; wines with high histamine content. (2) Endogenous origin: Any absorption of the toxins of bacterial infection will cause headache. Includes, chronic infections (nose and sinuses, teeth, middle ear, pharynx, tonsils, appendix, gallbladder, pelvic viscera); fever; bacteremias (typhoid fever, malaria, smallpox, tuberculosis, grippe and influenza, puerperal fever).

Systemic diseases: Nephritis with uremia, biliary tract disease including acute yellow atrophy of the liver, rheumatism, diabetes, anemia, polycythemia, eclampsia, central nervous system syphilis.

Gastrointestinal Disturbances: Dyspepsia, gastric hyper- and hypoacidity, intestinal stasis, and constipation. *Physicochemical Disturbances:* Acidosis, alkalosis. *Cardiovascular Disturbances:* High blood pressure; low blood pressure; myocardial and valvular insufficiency causing congestive heart failure; constriction, dilatation, or edema of intracranial blood vessels.

Endocrine Disorders: Pituitary, thyroid, adrenal, and ovarian tumors; carcinoid tumors. *Gynecological Factors:* due to functional disturbances of one or more of the endocrine glands; puberty, dysmenorrhea, premenstrual tension, pregnancy, menopause. *Neurological Factors:* Nervous shock; nervous exhaustion; worry, excitement, anger, or nervous tension; migraine; hysteria; epilepsy; psychoneuroses.

Diseases of Special Sense Organs: Iritis, glaucoma, conjunctivitis; adenoids, deviated septum; middle ear affections. *Organic Disease of Brain:* Causing pressure such as tumor, abscess, gumma, cyst, hydrocephaly, intracranial hemorrhage; intracranial vascular disease; arteriosclerosis; embolism, thrombosis, or aneurysm; encephalitis. *Various Forms of Meningitis:* Including meningismus.

Miscellaneous Causes: Almost any disturbance of body function may cause headache. Other causes are external pressure and constriction of head; trauma to head; sunstroke; any form of motion sickness; irritation of mucous membrane of nose and sinuses by dust, pollen; fatigue (physical or mental); insomnia; eyestrain (uncorrected defects, overwork). Spinal puncture or diagnostic examination involving injecting dyes or radioactive substances into cranial arteries or air into the ventricles of the brain may be followed by headache.

TREATMENT: Depends entirely upon cause. *IMPORTANT:* A h. which may be the symptom of a serious disease should not be treated symptomatically without attempting to find its cause.

h., cluster. A headache similar to migraine, recurring as often as two or three times a day over a period of weeks. After this cluster of headaches, the patient may be free of symptoms for weeks or months. The headaches come on abruptly and are characterized by intense throbbing pain behind the nostril and one eye. The eye and nose water, the skin over the throbbing area becomes red, and the pupil of the eye may become constricted. An attack rarely lasts longer than two hours. Ergotamine tartrate is useful for both treatment and prophylaxis.

h., histamine. H. resulting from injection of histamine or excessive histamine in circulating blood. Due to dilatation of branches of the carotid artery.

h., sick. A nervous headache occurring periodically, usually on one side of the head, accompanied by nausea and vomiting. SEE: *migraine.*

heal (hēl) [AS. *hael,* whole]. To cure; to make whole or healthy.

heal'ing. The restoration to a normal condition, esp. of an inflammation or a wound.

H. by first intention: This process closes the edge of a wound with little or no inflammatory reaction, and in such a manner that little or no scar is left to reveal the site of the injury. New cells are formed to take the place of dead ones, and the capillary walls stretch across the wound to join themselves to each other in a smooth surface. New connective tissue may form an almost imperceptible scar which proves temporary.

H. by second intention: This is h. by granulation or indirect union. Granulation tissue is formed to fill the gap between the edges of the wound with a thin layer of fibrinous exudate. It bars out bacteria and aids in checking bleeding by the coagulation of the new blood. Connective tissue cells support the new capillaries. This form of h. is slower than that by first intention and its grayish-red surface may become pale and flabby if the h. is too long delayed. If the granulations show above the surface they may have to be removed with caustics. If the granulations first form at the top instead of the bottom of the wound, it may have to be kept open by drainage.

H. by third intention: Of an ulcer, wound, or cavity by filling with granulations. It generally results in the formation of a scar.

COMPLICATIONS: These may result from the formation of a scar interfering with functioning of the part, and possible deformity; the formation of a keloid, q.v., the result of overgrowth of connective tissue forming a tumor in the surface of a scar; necrosis of the skin and mucus membrane producing a raw surface that results in an ulcer; a sinus or fistula which may be due to bacteria or some foreign substance remaining in the wound; proud flesh. This represents excessive growth of granulation tissue.

health (hĕlth) [AS. *hǣlth,* wholeness]. A condition in which all functions of body and mind are normally active. The World Health Organization defines health as a state of complete physical, mental, or social well-

being and not merely the absence of disease or infirmity.

h., bill of. Public h. certificate certifying that passengers on a public conveyance or ship are free of infectious disease.

h., board of. A public body in charge of the h. of a community.

h. certificate. An official statement signed by a physician attesting to the state of h. of a particular individual.

h., department of. Branch of a government (city, county, or nation) for regulation and protection of the people's h.

h., industrial. The h. of employees of industrial firms.

h. nurse, public. Nurse employed by a board or dept. of h. to serve the public.

h., public. The state of health of the population of a particular community, as opposed to individual or personal health. SYN: *community health.*

healthful. Conducive to good health.

health'y. Being in a state of health or enjoying it.

hear'ing [AS. *hiēran*]. The act or power of perceiving sound.

h., after. Perception of sound after the stimulus producing it has ceased to act.

h. aid. An apparatus used by those with impaired hearing for amplifying sound.

h. distance. Distance at which a given sound can be heard. On the prairies a voice may be heard for two miles or more.

h., functional tests for. Hearing acuity can be determined by: (1) The distance at which a person can hear a certain sound, such as a watch tick. (2) The use of audiometers, in which electrically produced sounds are conveyed by wires to a receiver applied to the subject's ear. Intensity and pitch of sound can be altered and is indicated on dials. Results are plotted on a graph known as an audiogram. (3) Bone conduction tests in which a device such as tuning fork or an apparatus which converts an electrical current into mechanical vibrations is applied to the skull. This is of value in distinguishing between perceptive and transmission deafness.

h. hallucinations. Subjective sensations of sound such as hearing voices when none actually exists.

heart (hărt) [AS. *heorte*]. A hollow, muscular, contractile organ, the center of the circulatory system. Its wall possesses three layers: the outer epicardium, a serous layer; the middle myocardium, composed of cardiac muscle; and the inner endocardium, a layer which lines the four chambers of the heart and covers the valves. The heart is enclosed in a fibroserous sac, the pericardium, the space between the pericardium and the epicardium forming the pericardial cavity.

CHAMBERS: Each lower cavity is the ventriculum or ventricle; each upper one the atrium, or auricle. The right auricle is called the atrium dexter, and the left one the atrium sinistrum, the two ventricles being known as ventriculus dexter (right) and v. sinister (left) respectively.

Contraction of the heart chambers is called systole; relaxation with accompanying dilation, diastole. The complete series of events which occurs in a single heart beat is known as the cardiac cycle. In a heart beating at the rate of 72 per minute, each cycle lasts about 0.85 sec. The heart is divided perpendicularly from base to apex by the interatrial and interventricular septa, the right side having no communication with the left. The right side receives deoxygenated blood from the tissues and pumps it to the lungs; the left side receives oxygenated blood from the lungs and pumps it to the tissues.

The atria, serving as receiving chambers, are thin walled; the ventricles, serving as pumping chambers, are thick walled.

Accelerator impulses are conveyed over nerves and ganglia of the sympathetic division. Preganglionic neurons which lie in the thoracic portion of the spinal cord synapse with postganglionic neurons located in the cervical ganglia of sympathetic trunk whose axons pass to the heart. Impulses from these nerves increase rate and force of heart beat. Impulses regulating the heart arise in the cardiac center in the medulla oblongata.

Afferent fibers pass through the vagus trunks to the medulla. Some are depressor fibers originating in receptors in the base of the aorta. Impulses over these fibers reflexly slow the heart rate. Others are pressor fibers originating in receptors in the vena cavae and right atrium. These reflexly increase heart beat. Fibers conveying pain impulses are also present.

VALVES: The atrioventricular orifice between each atrium and ventricle. Valvula tricuspidalis (tricuspid) guards the opening between the atrium dexter and the ventriculus dexter. Valvula bicuspidalis (bicuspid or mitral valve), between the atrium sinistrum (left atrium) and the ventriculus sinister (left ventricle). Valvulae semilunares (semilunar valves) guard the orifice

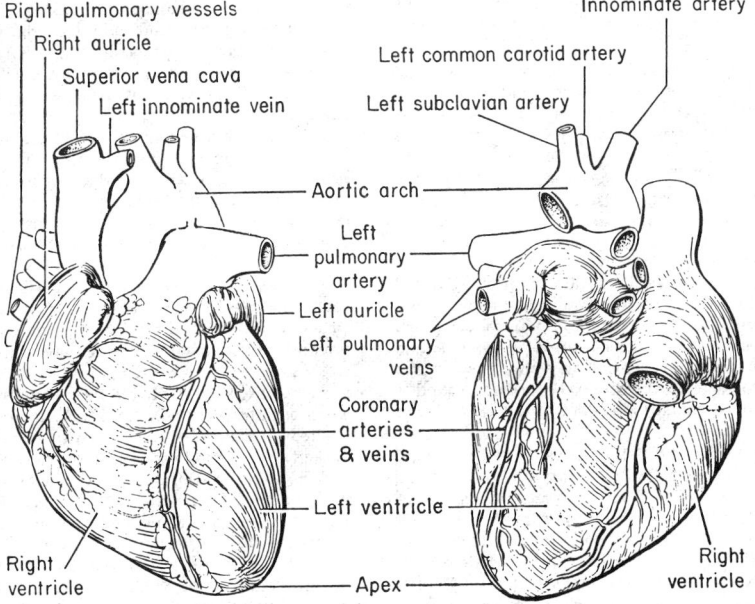

Right pulmonary vessels

Right auricle

Superior vena cava

Left innominate vein

Innominate artery

Left common carotid artery

Left subclavian artery

Aortic arch

Left pulmonary artery

Left auricle

Left pulmonary veins

Coronary arteries & veins

Left ventricle

Right ventricle

Apex

Right ventricle

HEART
Left, anterior view; Right, posterior view.

between the ventriculus dexter and the pulmonary artery. Valvulae semilunares aortae (aortic valves) guard the orifice between the ventriculus sinister and the aorta.

NERVE SUPPLY: *Inhibitory:* (Vagus or pneumogastric, acceleratory): by way of the sympathetic ganglia of the autonomic system and phrenic nerve. *Afferent:* A depressor nerve running from the heart to a cardioinhibitory center in the medulla, through the sheath of the vagi nerves, causing reflex inhibition of the heart. *Efferent fibers:* Inhibitory impulses are conveyed by preganglionic fibers of the vagus nerve, which synapse with postganglionic neurons located in terminal ganglia in the wall of the heart. They are distributed to the S-A node and other conductile tissue of the heart.

FUNCTION: Two to three ounces (60-90 ml.) of blood are driven into the arteries by each heartbeat. The power exerted by the heart is said to equal that necessary to lift 80 lb. (36.4 kg.) one foot (.31 meters) each minute. At the rate of 72 times each minute, the human heart beats 104,000 times a day, 38,000,000 times during a year. At every stroke 5 cu. in. (82 ml.) of blood are forced out into the body, or 500,000 cu. in. (8,193 liters) a day. In terms of work this is the equivalent of raising one ton (907 kg.) to a height of 41 ft. (12.5 meters) every 24 hr.

AUSCULTATION: Shows intensity, quality, and rhythm of heart sounds and detects the presence of any adventitious sounds, as murmurs. Both sounds over the heart have been represented by the syllables "lubb," "dupp." The first sound (systolic) results from the contraction of the ventricle, tension of the atrioventricular valves, and the impact of the heart against the chest wall, and is synchronous with the apex beat and carotid pulse. This sound is prolonged and dull; after the first sound is a short pause, then the second sound (diastolic), which results from the closure of the aortic and pulmonary valves. This sound is short and high pitched. After the second sound a longer pause follows before the first is heard again.

Intensity: Both sounds are either heard better or actually accentuated in increased heart action from any cause; anemia; cardiac hypertrophy; subjects with thin chest walls; consolidation of the lung, as in pneumonia. Accentuation of the aortic second sound results from hypertrophy of the left ventricle; increased arterial resistance, as in arteriosclerosis with hypertension; aortic aneurysm. Accentuation of the pulmonary

second sound results from pulmonary obstruction, as in emphysema, pneumonia; hypertrophy of the right ventricle. Both heart sounds are poorly heard or actually decreased in intensity in general obesity; general debility; degeneration or dilatation of the heart; pericardial or pleural effusion; emphysema.

Reduplication of Heart Sounds: Probably due to a lack of synchronous action in the valves of both sides of the heart, and results from many conditions, but notably from increased resistance in the systemic or the pulmonary circulation, as in arteriosclerosis and emphysema. Frequently noted in mitral stenosis and pericarditis.

Murmurs: A murmur is an abnormal sound heard over the heart or blood vessels and may result from obstruction or regurgitation at the valves following endocarditis; dilatation of the ventricle or relaxation of its walls rendering the valves relatively insufficient; aneurysm; a change in the blood constituents, as in anemia; roughening of the pericardial surfaces, as in pericarditis; irregular action of the heart. Murmurs produced within the heart are termed endocardial, those outside exocardial; those produced in aneurysms, bruits; those produced by anemia, hemic murmurs.

Hemic murmurs: Soft and blowing in character, usually systolic in time, heard best over pulmonary valves. Associated with symptoms of anemia, and disappear with the latter.

Aneurysmal murmur or bruit: Usually loud, booming in character, systolic in time, heard best over the aorta or base of heart, often associated with an abnormal area of dullness and pulsation, and with symptoms resulting from pressure on neighboring structures.

Pericardial friction sounds: Superficial, rough, and creaking in quality, to and fro in time, not transmitted beyond the precordium and may be modified by pressure of the stethoscope.

Procedure: Patient should be recumbent when beginning examination; then, having elicited all the signs possible, repeat with patient sitting, standing, or leaning forward, and note any variations from change of position. First listen while patient is breathing naturally, then while holding breath in both deep inspiration and expiration, and finally have patient take three or four forced inspirations. Explore whole thoracic cavity and endeavor to localize the points at which heart sounds, both normal and abnormal, are heard with the greatest intensity. Proceed from below upward, from left to right.

Normal Location of Valves for Auscultation: Aortic, 3rd intercostal space, close to left side of sternum; pulmonary, in front of aorta, behind junction of 3rd costal cartilage with sternum, left side; tricuspid, behind middle of sternum about level of 4th of costal cartilage; mitral, behind 3rd intercostal space about one in. to the left of sternum.

PALPATION: Not only determines position, force, extent, and rhythm of apex beat, but also detects existence of any fremitus or thrill. A thrill is a vibratory sensation likened to that received when the hand is placed on the back of a purring cat. Thrills at base of heart may result from valvular lesions, atheroma of aorta, aneurysm, and from roughened pericardial surfaces as in pericarditis. A presystolic thrill at apex is almost pathognomonic of mitral stenosis.

PERCUSSION: Determines shape and extent of cardiac dullness. The normal area of superficial or absolute percussion-dullness (part uncovered by lung) is detected by light percussion and extends from the 4th left costo-sternal junction to the apex beat; from the apex beat to the juncture of the xiphoid cartilage, with the sternum, and thence up left border of the sternum. The normal area of deep percussion dullness (the heart projected on the chest wall) is detected by firm percussion and extends from 3rd left costo-sternal articulation to the apex beat; from

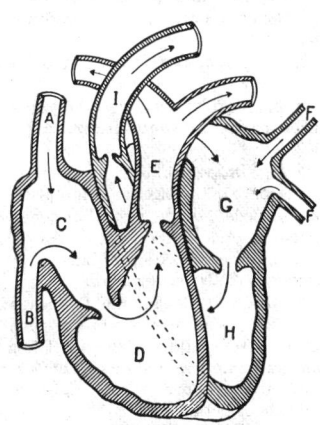

**CIRCULATION OF BLOOD
THROUGH THE HEART**

A, Superior vena cava. B, Inferior vena cava. C, Right atrium. D, Right ventricle. E, Pulmonary artery. F, Pulmonary veins. G, Left atrium. H, Left ventricle. I, Aorta.

apex beat to junction of the xiphoid cartilage with the sternum; and hence up right border of sternum to the 3rd rib. The lower level of the cardiac dullness fuses with the liver dullness and can rarely be determined. The area of cardiac dullness is increased in hypertrophy and dilation of the heart; pericardial effusion. The area of detectable cardiac dullness is diminished in emphysema; pneumothorax; pneumocardium.

h., abdominal. A h. that is displaced into the abdominal cavity.

h., armoured. Condition characterized by deposit of calcareous matter in the pericardium.

h., athletic. Supposed hypertrophy of the heart as a result of strenuous physical activity. There is no evidence that this condition exists.

h. attack. A seizure of abnormal heart functioning, as a coronary thrombosis, q.v.

h., beriberi. H. failure due to vitamin deficiency.

h., boatshaped. H. in which one ventricle is dilated and hypertrophied as a result of aortic regurgitation.

h., bony. A h. having calcareous patches in its walls and pericardium.

h., cervical. A h. that is located in the neck.

h., dilatation of. Enlargement of h. due to stretching of its walls. Varieties are dilatation with thickening of walls; dilatation with thinning walls.

SYM: So long as the associated hypertrophy keeps pace with the dilatation no symptoms result, but otherwise dyspnea, edema, cough.

h. disease. Any pathological disorder of the h.

h., fatty degeneration of. Myocardium has undergone fatty degeneration.

SYM: All signs of heart failure, i.e., dyspnea; asthma; cough; weak, irregular pulse; dyspepsia; attacks of syncope. PROG: Unfavorable. Death may occur on slight exertion.

h., fatty infiltration of. Abnormal amount of fat deposited in and upon heart.

SYM: Shortness of breath increased by exertion; weak but regular pulse; precordial distress; tendency to pulmonary congestion with resulting bronchitis. PROG: Depends upon cause. If due to a correctable condition, it is favorable.

h., fibroid. Chronic myocarditis in which fibrous tissue develops within the muscular tissue of the h.

SYM: Same as fatty degeneration, condition dependent upon atheroma or sclerosis of coronary arteries.

h., frosted. A h. covered with a thick, white coating that resembles frosting on a cake. Appearance due to thickening of the pericardium.

h., hairy. H. in which pericardium possesses a hairy appearance resulting from deposit of an exudate or shreds of fibrin. Occurs in pericarditis. SYN: *cor villosum; shaggy heart.*

h., hypertrophy of. Enlargement due to increased size of myocardium. Varieties are simple, thickened muscle and cavities normal size; eccentric, thickened muscle and cavities dilated; concentric, thickened muscle and cavities diminished in size, always congenital.

SYM: Unless advanced, no symptoms. Extreme hypertrophy, precordial distress, palpitation, strong pulse. Sometimes flushed face, ringing in ears, flashes of light, headache, and disturbed sleep.

TREATMENT: Graduated exercise, light diet, sedatives.

h., icing. H., frosted, q.v.

h., irritable. Neurocirculatory asthenia, or effort syndrome. Syndrome characterized by breathlessness, palpitation, weakness, and exhaustion. SYN: *soldier's heart.*

h., left. The left atrium and ventricle. This is the portion of the heart that receives the aerated blood from the lungs and propels it into the systemic circulation.

h., palpitation of. May result from dyspepsia; mental or physical excitement; organic heart disease; hyperthyroidism; anemia; hysteria; an independent neurosis; or endocarditis, myocarditis and pericarditis due to infection and trauma, circulatory disturbances, disorders of metabolism, nutrition, and growth.

h., pulmonary. H., right, q.v.

h. reflex. A cardiac reflex; any reflex in which the stimulation of a sensory nerve brings about an increase or decrease in heart rate. Ex: Bainbridge's reflex in which stimulation of sensory receptors in right atrium by increased venous return results in increase of heart rate.

h., right. The right atrium and ventricle. This portion of the heart receives the venous blood and propels it to the lungs.

h. sounds. SEE: auscultation under *heart.*

h. test. Various methods of clinical testing of the heart have been devised. These are usually based upon the ability of the healthy h. to return to a normal rate within a specified time following exertion. The amount of exercise is usually measured precisely.

heart block. Condition in which the conductile tissue of the heart (S-A node, A-V node, bundle of His, Purkinje fibers) fails to conduct impulses normally from the atrium to the ventricles. This causes altered rhythm of the heart beat. Known as arrhythmia, the condition may be present in several forms.

ETIOL: Structural changes as from tumor or damage of the myocardium due to coronary artery occlusion. Toxic effects of drugs or the toxins of infections. Nutritional or endocrine factors.

h. b., atrioventricular. A form in which impulses are impeded at the A-V node.

h. b., bundle branch. Condition in which impulses are blocked in one of the branches of the bundle of His, resulting in ventricles beating out of rhythm with each other so that one ventricle is stimulated to beat slightly before the other.

h. b., complete. Condition in which there is a complete dissociation between atrial and ventricular systoles. Ventricles may beat at a rate of 30-40/min. while atria are beating the normal 70 beats/min.

h. b., congenital. H. b. present at birth due to improper development of the impulse-conducting system.

h. b., incomplete. H. b. in which conduction time of impulses is prolonged; usually recognized only by electrocardiograph; partial h.b.

h. b., interventricular. H. b., bundle branch, q.v.

h. b., partial. One of two or three impulses passes to ventricle; pulse is thus 40-50.

h. b., sinoatrial. H. b. in which there is interference in the passage of impulses from the S-A node. May be partial or complete.

heartburn. Acid liquid raised from the stomach, causing sensation of burning in the esophagus. SYN: *water brash.*

heart failure. 1. Cessation of the beat of the heart. 2. A syndrome or clinical condition resulting from failure of the heart to maintain adequate circulation of blood. May result from failure of the right or left ventricle or both.

ETIOL: Hypertension, infections, valvular insufficiency, coronary disease, congenital malformations, arteriosclerosis, atherosclerosis.

SYM: Dyspnea, cardiac asthma, stasis in systemic or portal circulation, edema, cyanosis, hypertrophy of heart. Symptoms vary depending on which side of the heart is affected.

h. f., backward. H. f. in which venous return to the heart is reduced with resulting venous stasis and congestion. Due principally to failure of the right ventricle.

h. f., congestive. Condition characterized by weakness, breathlessness, abdominal discomfort, edema in lower portions of body resulting from venous stasis and reduced outflow of blood. SYN: *cardiac decompensation; myocardial insufficiency.*

h. f., forward. H. f. in which forward flow of blood to the tissues is inadequate due either to inability of left ventricle to pump sufficient blood or to insufficient blood arriving at the ventricle.

heart pump, nuclear powered. An artificial heart pumped by nuclear energy. It has been used experimentally in cows and may eventually be developed sufficiently to use in humans.

heat [AS. *haētu*]. 1. Condition of being hot; warmth. 2. High temperature. 3. A form of energy manifested to the senses, as in the effects of fire, sun's rays, etc. 4. Sexual excitement in lower mammals; period of such excitement. SYN: *estrus.* 5. To make hot. 6. To become warm.

H. is constantly being produced within the body as a result of exothermic chemical processes occurring in metabolic activities. Ultimately all h. produced in the body results from oxidative processes. Body temperature (normally 98.6° F. or 37° C.) is the result of a balance between h. produced (thermogenesis) and h. loss (thermolysis).

The temperature of the body is not uniform. Oral temperatures range from 96.6° F. to 100° F. (37°-37.8° C.). Axillary temperature is somewhat lower and rectal temperature is somewhat higher.

Reducing the temperature of the skin reflexly brings about a constriction of the blood vessels, thus reducing h. loss and conserving h. within the body. The application of h. reflexly induces the dilation of blood vessels, thus increasing blood flow to the skin with consequent increase in h. loss.

The application of h. to the skin reflexly produces effects in the deeper portions of the body. It induces muscle relaxation, increases blood supply, and stimulates metabolic activity. Physiological effects resulting are hyperemia and sedation of sensory or motor activity. Application of moderate cold tends to produce the opposite effects.

Relaxation of muscular tissue results in relief of pain, which may be due to rigidity and spasm in tissues. Local hot applications may have some reflex effect on deep organs. This is the basis of treating certain conditions by means of counterirritation such as that produced by liniments or mustard plaster. SEE: *fever.*

h., acclimatization to. Adjustment of an organism to h. Exposure to high environmental temperature requires a period of adjustment in order for the body to function efficiently. The amount of time required will depend upon the temperature, humidity, and duration of exposure each day. Significant physiological adjustments will occur in five days and will be completed within two weeks to a month.

h., application of. *General:* May be dry or moist. The effect is first to produce a slight contraction of vessels in skin, thus increasing blood pressure; this makes patient feel that his head is full and bursting. However, this effect is only of very short duration, and discomfort can be avoided by application of cold compress or ice bag to head.

The true effect follows immediately when blood vessels in skin are dilated due to relaxation of involuntary muscle contained in their walls. The skin is reddened, increased blood supply to the sweat glands causes them to act freely, and h. loss is accelerated.

During a general application of h. it is necessary to watch the patient carefully, noting any apparent discomfort, state of pulse and respiration, and color; and to be certain patient does not become dehydrated or suffer h. exhaustion, q.v.

Local: May be dry or moist. Dry applications include rubber hot-water bottles; bags of hot salt previously heated in an oven; radiant heat; electric pads; and diathermy.

Moist: Considered more penetrating than dry heat but this is due more to the fact that water-soaked materials loose h. slower than dry ones. The application should be approx. 120° F. (48.9° C.). Compresses may be kept warm by keeping hot water bottles at proper temperature next to them. Do not use electric heating devices next to moist dressings.

Devices which force hot water at a selected temperature through soft flexible tubing are available. These may be used to h. wet or dry compresses.

h., conductive. A term applied to h. transferred by conduction from a h. source to an object which is cold. The two materials are in contact with each other.

h., convective. Flow of h. to an object or part of the body by passage of heated particles, gas, or liquid from the h. source to the colder body.

h., conversive. H. generated in the tissues by a current of electricity or by some form of radiant energy.

h. cramps. Acute painful spasms of voluntary muscles following hard work in hot environment without adequate fluid and salt intake. SYN: *fireman's or miner's cramps.*

F.A. TREATMENT: Remove to cool place and give salt solution (one-quarter teaspoon of table salt in a glass of water) by mouth. Repeat at 5- to 30-minute intervals until cramping ceases. May be prevented by adding salt to drinking water on hot days.

PREVENTIVE: One to two gr. of salt taken three or four times a day with at least two glasses (16 ounces or 1/2 liter) of water with each dose. SEE: *cramps; salt.*

h., diathermy. Electrical energy is converted into h. by the use of diathermy and short wave.

h., dry. May be administered in form of hot, dry pack; hot water bottle; electric light bath; heliotherapy; hot bricks; resistance coil; electric pad or blanket; hot air bath; or therapeutic lamp.

h. exhaustion. Must not be mistaken for h. hyperpyrexia, q.v. Acute reaction to h exposure. SYN: *h. collapse; h. prostration*

SYM: Weakness, dizziness, nausea, headache, and finally collapse. Skin is cold and clammy, pupils dilated. Body temperature usually is normal; blood pressure may be decreased.

PROG: Favorable under proper treatment.

F. A. TREATMENT: Remove to cool place, loosen clothes, place in a head-low position, give intravenous isotonic saline solution slowly to avoid overloading the circulatory system.

h. hyperpyrexia. An acute and dangerous reaction to h. exposure. Characterized by high body temperature, usually

higher than 105° F. (40.6° C.); cessation of sweating; headache, numbness, tingling, and confusion prior to sudden delirium or coma; fast pulse; rapid respiratory rate; usually elevated blood pressure. The basic defect is failure of the h. regulating mechanisms of the body. SYN: *h. stroke; h. pyrexia; sunstroke.*

TREATMENT: Effective therapy may save the patient's life. Thus there should be absolutely no delay in placing the nude patient in an ice water filled bathtub. This will not cause pain, shock, or cutaneous vasoconstriction. The patient's temperature will need to be monitored carefully. Remove from bath when temperature falls to 103° F. (39.4° C.). If ice water and a bathtub are not available, place wet sheets on nude body, fan vigorously, and massage the skin. The use of sedatives may be required to control convulsions. Careful observation of patient for signs of fluid imbalance and renal failure will be required for several days.

h., initial. Muscular h. produced during contraction when tension is increasing, during maintenance of tension, and during relaxation when tension is diminishing.

h., latent. H. which is required to convert a solid into a liquid or a liquid into a gas at the same temperature.

h., latent, of fusion. H. which is required to convert 1 gm. of a solid into liquid at the same temperature, e.g., when 1 gm. of ice at 0° C. is converted into water at 0° C.; this process requires 80 cal., and until it is completed there will be no rise of temperature.

h., latent, of vaporation. H. required to change 1 gm. of a liquid at its boiling point to vapor at the same temperature. The latent h. of steam is 540 cal.; therefore, when steam cools to liquid, each gm. gives out 540 cal. This explains why it is that a scald from steam is much more severe than one caused by boiling water.

h., luminous. H. derived from light. This form may be tolerated better than

The mode of elimination of body heat and the per cent of heat lost through each of the following is:

Radiation	55%	
Convection and Conduction	15%	94%
Evaporation through skin and lungs	24%	
Warming inspired air	2%	
Elimination of CO_2 from lungs	3%	6%
Warming ingested food and water and loss through feces and urine	1%	

Figures are approximate and vary with physiological activity of the body, type of clothing worn, relative humidity, and degree of acclimatization to a particular environment.

Comparison of Heatstroke and Heat Exhaustion

Heat or Sunstroke. *Definition:* A condition or derangement of the heat-control centers due to exposure to the rays of the sun or very high temperatures

History: Exposure to sun's rays or extreme heat

Differential Symptoms:
Face: Red, dry, and hot
Skin: Hot, dry, and no diaphoresis

Temperature: High, 106° to 110° F. (41.1° to 43.3° C.)
Pulse: Full, strong, bounding
Respirations: Dyspneic and sonorous
Muscles: Tense and possible convulsions
Eyes: Pupils are dilated but equal

Treatment: Absolute rest with head elevated; cold packs to promote heat loss

Drugs: Allow no stimulants; give infusions of normal saline (to force fluids)

Heat Exhaustion. *Definition:* A state of very definite weakness produced by the loss of normal fluids and sodium chloride of the body

History: Exposure to heat, usually indoors

Differential Symptoms:
Face: Pale, cool, and moist
Skin: Cool, clammy, with profuse diaphoresis
Temperature: Slight elevation to subnormal
Pulse: Weak, thready, and rapid
Respirations: Shallow and quiet
Muscles: Tense and contracted
Eyes: Pupils are normal, eyeballs may be soft

Treatment: Keep patient quiet; head should be lowered; keep body warm to prevent shock symptoms
Drugs: Aromatic spirits of ammonia; Salt tablets and fruit juices in abundant amounts. Intravenous isotonic saline will be required if patient is unconscious.

---

other forms of radiation. Light may be converted into h. Short infrared rays penetrate subcutaneous tissues to a greater extent than long, invisible rays.

h., mechanical equivalent of. The value of h. units in terms of work units. H. used or produced at the rate of one Cal. (kcal.) per minute is equal to 3088 footpounds of work per minute or one kilogrammeter per minute.

h., moist. May be applied as hot bath pack, hot wet pack, hot foot bath, fomentations, poultices or vapor bath. Watch for chill, fainting, dizziness, headache, collapse, faintness, increased pulse, weakness. Cold applications to head should be used during and after treatment. Opinion regarding therapeutic use of h. or cold differs.

h., molecular. Result of multiplying a substance's molecular weight by its specific h.

h., prickly. Vesicles due to obstruction or acute inflammation of sweat glands. SYN: *miliaria.*

h., radiant. H. given off from a heated body; it passes through the air in form of waves.

h. rays. Visible rays, 4000-7000 A. U.; and infrared rays, 6000-14,000 A. U.

h. recovery. Muscular h. produced after relaxation is complete.

h., sensible. H. producing a temperature rise when absorbed by a body.

h., specific. The h. or number of cal. needed to raise the temperature of 1 gr. of a substance 1° C.

h. therapy. Use of h. in treatment of the body.

h. therapy, wet. Application of h. by hot water, steam, and mud baths, and hot pack.

h. unit. A calorie, q.v.

heatstroke. SEE: *heat hyperpyrexia.*

heaves (hēvs). Vomiting.

h., dry. Attempting to vomit without producing vomitus.

hebeosteotomy (hē″bē-os″tē-ŏt′ō-mī) [Gr. *hēbē,* youth, + *osteon,* bone, + *tomē,* incision]. Section of the pubic bone in order to enlarge the pelvic opening for facilitation of delivery. SYN: *pubiotomy.*

hebephrenia (hē″bĕ-frē′nĭ-ă) ["+ *phrēn,* mind]. A chronic form of schizophrenia characterized by bizarre, illogical and senseless thought processes and actions, delusions, and hallucinations. Wild excitement at one moment may be replaced by depression and crying. Patient may laugh often without cause and talk incoherently and excessively. Onset usually before age 20. Prognosis poor.

hebephrenic (hē″bĕ-frĕn′ĭk). Pert. to hebephrenia.

Heberden's disease (he′ber-dĕn). [William Heberden, Brit. physician, 1710-1801] Arthritis deformans.

Heberden's nodes. Hard nodules or enlargements of tubercles of last phalanges of fingers; seen in osteoarthritis.

hebetic (hē-bĕt′ĭk) [Gr. *hēbē*, youth]. Pert. to or occurring at the time of puberty.

hebet′omy ["+ *tomē*, incision]. Surgical division of the pubis. Usually done, lateral to the midline, to facilitate delivery. SYN: *pubiotomy*.

hebetude (heb′ē-tūd) [LL. *hebetūdo*, dullness of mind]. Emotional dullness and disinterest. Patient is withdrawn and has no interest in his surroundings. In late stages indifference to personal comfort is marked. Seen in schizophrenia.

hebosteotomy (hē-bŏs″tē-ŏt′ō-mĭ) [Gr. *hēbē*, youth, + *osteon*, bone, + *tomē*, incision]. Enlargement of pelvic diameter by section of the pelvis to aid delivery. SYN: *hebotomy;*

pubiotomy.

hebot′omy. Section through the pubis to facilitate labor. SYN: *hebosteotomy; pubiotomy.*

hecateromeric, hecatomeric (hĕk″ă-tĕr″ō-mĕr′ĭk, hĕk″ă-tō-mĕr′ĭk) [Gr. *hekateros*, each of two, + *meros*, part]. Having two processes on a spinal neuron, one supplying each side of the spinal cord.

hectic (hĕk′tĭk) [Gr. *hektikos*, habitual]. 1. Habitual. 2. An afternoon rise of fever. Seen in active tuberculosis.

hec′togram [Gr. *hekaton*, hundred, + *gramma*, weight]. One hundred grams, or 3.527 avoirdupois ounces.

hectoliter (hĕk′tō-lē″ter) ["+ *litra*, a pound]. One hundred liters.

hec′tometer ["+ *metron*, measure]. One hundred meters.

hedonia (hē-dō′nĭ-ā) [Gr. *hēdonē*, pleasure]. Excessive cheerfulness.

hedonism (hēd′n-izm) ["+ *ismos*, condition]. A theory or standard of conduct in which the

Height and Weight Table*

Person	Age From	Age To	Height Without Shoes Inches	Height Without Shoes Centimeters	Weight Pounds	Weight Kilograms
Infants	Months 0	2	22	55	9	4
	2	6	25	63	15	7
	6	12	28	72	20	9
Children	Years 1	2	32	81	26	12
	2	3	36	91	31	14
	3	4	39	100	35	16
	4	6	43	110	42	19
	6	8	48	121	51	23
	8	10	52	131	62	28
Men	10	12	55	140	77	35
	12	14	59	151	95	43
	14	18	67	170	130	59
	18	22	69	175	147	67
	22	35	69	175	154	70
	35	55	68	173	154	70
	55	75+	67	171	154	70
Women	10	12	56	142	77	35
	12	14	61	154	97	44
	14	16	62	157	114	52
	16	18	63	160	119	54
	18	22	64	163	128	58
	22	35	64	163	128	58
	35	55	63	160	128	58
	55	75+	62	157	128	58

* National Research Council: Recommended Dietary Allowances, ed. 7. Publication 1694, National Academy of Sciences, Washington, D.C., 1968.

principal object of life is pleasure.

hedrocele (hĕd′rō-sēl) [Gr. *hedra*, anus, + *kēlē*, hernia]. Hernia; prolapse through the anus. SYN: *proctocele*.

heel [AS. *huela*, heel]. Rounded posterior portion of the foot under and behind the ankle. SYN: *calx*.

 h. bone. Bone at back of tarsus. SYN: *calcaneum; calcaneus; os calcis.*

Hegar's sign (hā′gar). [Alfred Hegar, Freiburg gynecologist, 1830-1914] Sign which may be present during 2nd and 3rd month of pregnancy. On bimanual examination, the lower part of the uterus is easily compressed between fingers placed in the vagina and those of the other hand over the pelvic area. This is due to the softening of lower segments of the uterus and to the fact that the ovum does not fill the uterine cavity at this stage, leaving an empty space in the lower part.

 The sign is not a positive one for pregnancy.

Heidenhain's demilunes (hī′dĕn-hīnz). [Rudolph P. Heidenhain, Ger. physiologist, 1834-97] Crescent-shaped groups of serous cells at the base of, or along the sides of, the mucous alveoli of the salivary glands, esp. sublingual and submaxillary. SYN: *crescents of Gianuzzi*.

height (hīt) [AS. *hiehthu*]. Vertical distance from the bottom to the top of an organ or structure.

Heine-Medin disease (hī′nĕ-mā′dĭn). [Jacob Heine, Ger. physician, 1800-79; Karl O. Medin, Swedish physician, 1847-1928] Acute anterior poliomyelitis. SEE: *poliomyelitis.*

Heinz bodies. [Robert Heinz, Ger. pathologist, 1865-1924] Granules in red blood cells due to damage of the hemoglobin molecules. Seen in premature infants, in certain forms of drug sensitivity, and in a certain type of hereditary hemolytic anemia. The bodies are best seen when the blood is stained with a special stain. SEE: *Heinz body anemia.*

Heinz body anemia. Hemolytic anemia of infancy associated with the finding of Heinz bodies in the red cells.

Heister, spiral valve of (hī′ster). [Lorenz Heister, Ger. anatomist, 1683-1758] A spiral fold of the mucous membrane lining the cystic duct. It serves to keep the lumen open.

helcoid (hĕl′koyd) [Gr. *helkos*, ulcer, + *eidos*, form]. Resembling an ulcer.

helcology (hĕl-kŏl′ō-jĭ) [″+ *logos*, study]. The study of ulcers.

helcoplasty (hĕl′kō-plăs-tĭ) [″+ *plassein*, to form]. Grafting healthy skin on ulcers. SEE: *dermatoplasty.*

helco′sis [″+ *ōsis*, condition]. The development of an ulcer. SYN: *ulceration.*

helicine (hĕl′ĭ-sīn) [Gr. *helix*, coil]. 1. Spiral. 2. Pert. to a helix or coil.

 h. arteries. Tortuous arteries in cavernous tissue of the penis and clitoris, and in the uterus.

helicoid (hĕl′ĭ-koyd) [″+ *eidos*, resemblance]. Resembling a helix or spiral.

helicopodia (hĕl′ĭ-kō-pō′dĭ-ă) [″+ *pous, pod-*, foot]. A peculiar movement in which the foot, when brought forward, drags and describes a partial arc. Results in a gait such as seen in spastic hemiplegia.

helicotrema (hĕl-ĭ-kō-trē′mă) [″+ *trema*, a hole]. The opening at the tip of the cochlear canal where the scala tympani and scala vestibuli unite.

heliophobia (hē″lĭ-ō-fō′bĭ-ă) [Gr. *hēlios*, sun, + *phobos*, fear]. Abnormal fear of the sun's rays esp. by one who has suffered a sunstroke.

helio′sis [″+ *-ōsis*, condition]. Sunstroke.

heliotherapy (hē″lĭ-ō-thĕr′ă-pĭ) [″+ *therapeia*, treatment]. Exposure to sunlight for therapeutic purposes.

heliotropism (hē″lĭ-ŏt′rō-pĭzm) [″+ *trepein*, to turn, + *ismos*, condition]. Tendency of living organisms to turn or grow towards the sun.

helium (hē′lĭ-ŭm) [Gr. *hēlios*, sun]. SYMB: *He.* At. wt. 4.0026; at. no. 2. A gaseous element. It is given off by radium and other radioactive elements as charged h. ions known as alpha rays.

 Because of its low density, it being next to the lightest element known, it is mixed with air or oxygen and used in the treatment of various respiratory disorders. Because of its low solubility, it is mixed with air supplied to workers laboring under high atmospheric pressure, as in caissons. When so used, it reduces time required in adjusting to increasing or decreasing air pressure and reduces the danger of bends.

helix (hē′lĭks) [Gr., coil]. 1. A coil or spiral. 2. [NA] Margin of the external ear.

 h., Watson-Crick. A double h. named after the two scientists who established its existence. Each half of the h. contains chemical compounds arranged in a specific sequence. Variation in the sequence of these compounds enables genetic information to be transmitted. The double h. is DNA or deoxyribonucleic acid.

Hel′ler's test. [Johann F. Heller, Austrian pathologist, 1813-1871] A test for the presence of albumin in urine.

 Pour pure nitric acid into a clean test tube to a depth of one-half inch (13 mm.) and carefully overlay it with an equal quantity of urine. The presence of albumin is indicated by the appearance of an opaque white ring at the junction of the fluids. Certain drugs in the urine, and urates in highly-concentrated specimens, may give false-positive tests.

RS: albumin; urine.

Hel'lin's law. [Dyonizy Hellin, Polish pathologist, 1867-1935] Occurrence of twins once in 80 pregnancies, triplets once in 6400, (i.e. 80^2) pregnancies, quadruplets once in 512,000 (i.e., 80^3) pregnancies.

hel'minth [Gr. *helmins*, worm]. 1. A worm-like animal. 2. More specifically any animal, either free-living, or parasitic, belonging to the phyla Platyhelminthes (flatworms), Acanthocephala (spiney-headed worms), nemathelminthes (threadworms or roundworms) or Annelida (segmented worms).

helminthagogue (hĕl-mĭnth'ă-gŏg) ["+ *agōgos*, leading]. A medicine or treatment which causes parasitic worms to be expelled from the intestinal tract. SYN: *vermifuge.*

helminthemesis (hĕl-mĭn-thĕm'ĕ-sĭs) ["+ *emesis*, vomiting]. The vomiting of intestinal worms.

helminthiasis (hĕl-mĭn-thī'ă-sĭs) [Gr. *helmins*, worm, + *iasis*, condition]. Having intestinal parasites or worms.

helmin'thic. 1. Pert. to worms. 2. Pert. to that which expels worms. SYN: *anthelmintic; vermifugal.*

helminthicide (hĕl-mĭn'thĭ-sīd) [Gr. *helmins*, worm, + L. *cidus*, kill]. A medicine which kills worms. SYN: *vermicide.*

helminthoid (hĕl-mĭn'thoyd) ["+ *eidos*, form]. Wormlike or resembling a worm.

helminthol'ogy ["+ *logos*, study]. The study of parasitic intestinal worms.

helmintho'ma [Gr. *helmins*, worm, + *ōma*, tumor]. A tumor caused by parasitic worms.

helminthophobia (hĕl-mĭn"thō-fō'bĭ-ă) ["+ *phobos*, fear]. Morbid dread of worms or delusion of being infested by them.

heloma (hē-lō'mă) [Gr. *hēlos*, nail, + *ōma*, tumor]. A callosity or corn. SYN: *clavus.*

helosis (hē-lō'sĭs) ["+ *-ōsis*, condition]. The state of having corns.

helotomeia (hē"lō-tō-mī'ă) ["+ *tomē*, incision]. Helotomy.

helotomon (hē-lŏt'ō-mŏn). Surgical knife for cutting corns.

helotomy (hē-lŏt'ō-mĭ). Surgical treatment of corns.

Helweg's bundle (hĕl'vĕg). [Hans K. S. Helweg, Danish physician, 1847-1901] A small tract passing from the olive body to the anterior horn cells in the cervical region.

Part of the extrapyramidal motor system. SYN: *olivospinal tract.*

hema- (hē'mă, hĕm'ă) [Gr. *haima*, blood]. Combining form indicating blood.

hemabarometer (hē"mă-, hĕm"ă-bă-rŏm'ĕ-tĕr) [Gr. *haima*, blood, + *baros*, weight, + *metron*, measure]. Device for determining specific gravity of blood.

hemachro'sis ["+ *chrōsis*, coloring]. Abnormal redness of blood.

hemacytom'eter (hē"mă-, hĕm"ă-sī-tŏm'ī-tĕr) ["+ *kytos*, cell, + *metron*, measure]. Apparatus used in counting blood cells.

hemacytozoon (hē"mă-, hĕm"ă-sī-tō-zō'ŏn) ["+ "+ *zōon*, animal]. A protozoan parasite infesting red blood corpuscles.

hemad (hē'măd) [Gr. *haima*, blood, + L. *ad*, toward]. 1. Pert. to blood or blood vessels. 2. Toward the ventral or hemal aspect of the body. Opposed to neural or dorsal. SYN: *hemal.*

hemadostenosis (hē"mă-, hĕm"ă-dō-stĕn-ō'sĭs) ["+ *stenōsis*, narrowing]. Contraction of blood vessels.

hemadromometer (hē"mă-, hĕm"ă-drō-mŏm'ī-tĕr) ["+ *dromos*, course, + *metron*, measure]. Device for recording rapidity of flow of blood. SYN: *hemodromometer.*

hemadynamometer (hē"mă-, hĕm"ă-dī"nă-mŏm'ī-tĕr) ["+ *dynamis*, power, + *metron*, measure]. Device for determining blood pressure.

hemadynamometry (hē"mă-, hĕm"ă-dī-nă-mŏm'ĭtrĭ). Measurement of blood pressure.

hemafa'cient [Gr. *haima*, blood, + L. *facere*, to make]. A substance which increases the quality and quantity of blood. SYN: *hematopoietic.*

hemafecia (hē"mă-, hĕm-ăfē'sĭ-ă) ["+ L. *faex, faec-*, dregs]. Feces containing blood.

hemagglutination (hĕm"ă-glū-tĭn-ā'shŭn) ["+ L. *agglutināre*, to paste to]. The clumping of red blood corpuscles.

hem"agglu'tinin. An antibody that induces clumping of red blood corpuscles.

 h., cold. Agglutination of erythrocytes (usually of sheep) at low temperatures by the serum of patients with certain diseases.

hemagogue (hē"mă-, hĕm'ă-gŏg) [Gr. *haima*, blood, + *agōgos*, leading]. An agent that promotes the flow of blood, esp. menstrual flow. SYN: *emmenagogue.*

he'mal. 1. Pert. to the blood or blood vessels. 2. Pert. to side of the body in which the heart is located.

 h. arch. The ribs, breastbone, and that part of the vertebrae which, together, enclose the heart and viscera.

 h. gland. A h. or hemolymph node.

h. node. A body resembling a lymph node in structure but associated with blood vessels instead of lymph vessels. Present in certain ungulates. SYN: *hemal gland; hemolymph gland or node.*

hemanal'ysis [Gr. *haima,* blood, + *analysis,* a dissolving]. A blood analysis. SEE: *blood.*

hemangiectasis (hē''măn-, hĕm''ăn-jĭ-ĕk'tā-sĭs) ["+ *angeion,* vessel, + *ektasis,* dilatation]. Dilatation of blood vessels.

hemangioblastoma (hē-măn''jĭ-ō-blăs-tō'mă) ["+ "+ *blastos,* germ, + *ōma,* tumor]. Hemangioma of the brain of a capillary nature.

hemangioendothelioma (hē''măn-jĭ-ō-ĕn''dō-thē-lĭ-ō'mă) ["+ "+ *endon,* within, + *thēlē,* nipple, + *ōma,* tumor]. An overgrowth of the endothelium of the minute capillary vessels. They are variable in size and are commonly seen in the capillary net of the cerebral meninges.

hemangioma (hē-măn''jĭ-o'mă) [Gr. *haima,* blood, + *angeion,* vessel, + *ōma,* tumor]. (pl. *hemangiomata*) A benign tumor of dilated blood vessels.

hemangiomatosis (hē-măn''jĭ-ō-mă-tō'sĭs) ["+ "+ "+ *-ōsis,* condition]. Multiple angiomata of blood vessels.

hemangiosarcoma (hē-man''jĭ-ō-sar-kō'mă) ["+ "+ *sarkos,* flesh, + *ōma,* tumor]. A mixed sarcoma and hemangioma. SYN: *angiosarcoma.*

hemaphein (hĕm-ă-fē'ĭn) [Gr. *haima,* blood, + *phaios,* tawny]. Brown coloring matter in the blood; a decomposition product of hematin.

hemapoiesis (hĕm''ă-poy-ē'sĭs) ["+ *poiēsis,* formation]. Blood formation. SYN: *hematopoiesis.*

hemapoietic (hĕm-ă-poy-ĕt'ĭk) ["+ *poiein,* to form]. Pert. to hemapoiesis. SYN: *hematopoietic.*

hemapophysis (hĕm-ă-pŏf'ĭ-sĭs) ["+ *apo,* from, + *physis,* growth]. Portion of a developing vertebra which forms a rib and costal cartilage.

hemarthros (hĕm-ăr'thrōs) [Gr. *haima,* blood, + *arthron,* joint]. Bloody effusion into cavity of a joint. SYN: *hemarthrosis.*

hemarthrosis (hĕm-ăr-thrō'sĭs) ["+ "+ *-ōsis,* condition]. Effusion of blood in a joint cavity.

hematachometer (hĕm-ă-tă-kŏm'ĕ-ter) ["+ *tachus,* swift, + *metron,* measure]. Device for determining speed of blood flow.

hematapostema (hĕm''ă-tă-pŏs-tē'mă) ["+ *apostēma,* abscess]. (pl. *hematapostemata*) Abscess containing extravasated blood.

hematemesis (hĕm-ăt-ĕm'ē-sĭs) [Gr. *haima,* blood, + *emesis,* vomiting]. Vomiting of blood.

SYM: Blood often clotted and mixed with food; acid in reaction. Subsequent stools may be tarry. If of gastric origin, the blood is generally dark and acid. If of pharyngeal origin, it is bright red and alkaline in reaction. If loss of blood is severe enough, shock and collapse may occur.

TREATMENT: Absolute rest, nothing by mouth. Feed intravenously if necessary. No stimulants. Have patient lie down; cold applications-ice bag to abdominal region. Keep patient quiet. Surgery may be necessary. SEE: *hemoptysis; hemorrhage.*

hematencephalon (hĕm''ăt-ĕn-sĕf'ă-lŏn) ["+ *enkephalos,* brain]. Cerebral hemorrhage.

hematherapy (hĕm''ă-thĕr'ă-pī) ["+ *therapeia,* treatment]. Administration of fresh blood in treatment of disease.

hemathermal (hĕm''a-, hē''mă-thĕr'măl) ["+ *thermē,* heat]. Warm blooded, applied to animals whose blood remains at a fairly constant temperature. SYN: *hematothermal.*

hemather'mous. Warm blooded. SYN: *hemathermal; hematothermal.*

hemathidrosis, hematidrosis (hē-măt''hĭ-drō'sĭs) [Gr. *haima,* blood, + *hidros,* sweat, + *-ōsis,* condition]. Condition in which sweat contains blood.

hematic (hē-măt'ĭk). 1. Rel. to the blood. 2. A drug used in treating anemia. SYN: *hematinic.*

hematimeter (hĕm-ă-tĭm'ē-ter) [Gr. *haima,* blood, + *metron,* measure]. Apparatus used in counting blood corpuscles in a cu.mm. of blood. SYN: *hematometer; hemocytometer.*

hem'atin. The old term for heme. It is the iron-containing nonprotein portion of the hemoglobin molecule.

hematinemia (hē-mă-, hĕm-ă-tĭn-ē'mĭ-ă). Heme in the circulating blood.

hematinic (hē-mă-, hĕm-ă-tĭn'ĭk) [Gr. *haima,* blood]. 1. Pert. to blood. 2. An agent which increases the amount of hemoglobin in the blood.

hematinuria (hē''mă-tĭn-ū'rĭ-ă) ["+ *ouron,* urine]. Heme in the urine. SYN: *hemoglobinuria.*

hematischesis (hĕm-ă-tĭs'kĭ-sĭs) ["+ *schesis,* checking]. Arrest of bleeding or hemorrhage.

hemato- (hē''mă-tō, hĕm''ă-tō) [Gr. *haimatos,* blood]. Prefix indicating blood.

hemato'bium (hē''mă-, hĕm''ă-tō'bĭ-ŭm) ["+ *bios,* life]. A parasite that lives in the blood. SYN: *hematozoon.*

hematoblast (hē″mă-, hĕm′ă-tō-blast) [Gr. *haimatos*, blood, + *blastos*, germ]. 1. A hemocytoblast, q.v. 2. Old term for blood platelet.

hematocele (hē″mă-, hĕm′ă-tō-sēl) ["+ *kēlē*, hernia]. 1. A blood cyst. 2. Effusion of blood into a cavity. 3. Swelling due to effusion of blood into the tunica vaginalis testis.

h., parametric. Tumor formed by blood effusion in the cul-de-sac of Douglas walled off by adhesions. SYN: *pelvic h., retrouterine h.*

h., pudendal. A blood-filled swollen area of the labium.

hematocelia (hĕm″ă-tō-sē′lĭ-ă) ["+ *koilia*, cavity]. Hemorrhage into the peritoneal cavity.

hematocephalus (hē″mă-, hĕm″ă-tō-sĕf′ă-lŭs) ["+ *kephale*, head]. Fetus born with infusion of blood in the head.

hematochezia (hĕm″ă-tō-kē′zĭ-ă) [Gr. *haimatos*, blood, + *chezein*, to go to stool]. Passage of stools containing blood.

hematochromato′sis ["+ *chrōma*, color, + *-ōsis*, condition]. A condition showing staining of tissues with blood pigment due to abnormal and excessive deposition of iron from hemoglobin or excessive ingestion of iron. SYN: *hemochromatosis.*

hematochyluria (hē″mă-, hĕm″ă-tō-kī-lū′rĭ-ă) ["+ *chylos*, juice, + *ouron*, urine]. Blood and chyle in the urine.

hematocolpometra (hē″mă-, hĕm″ă-tō-kol″pō-me′tră) ["+ *kolpos*, vagina, + *mētra*, uterus]. Retention of menstrual blood in the vagina and uterus.

hematocolpos (hē″mă-, hĕm″ă-tō-kol′pŏs). Retained menstrual blood in the vagina from an imperforate hymen.

hematocrit (hē-măt′ō-krĭt) [Gr. *haimatos*, blood, + *krinein*, to separate]. 1. Centrifuge for separating solids from plasma in the blood. 2. The volume of erythrocytes packed by centrifugation in a given volume of blood. The h. is expressed as the percentage of total blood volume which consists of erythrocytes or as the volume in cubic centimeters of erythrocytes packed by centrifugation of blood. Normal values at sea level: men, average 47%, range 40-54%; women, average 42%, range 37-47%; children, varies with age from 35-49%; newborn, 49-54%.

hematocryal (hē″mă-tŏk′rĭ-ăl, hĕm-ăt″ō-krī′ăl) ["+ *kryos*, cold]. Possessing cold blood.

hematocyst (hē″mă-, hĕm′ă-tō-sĭst) ["+ *kystis*, a bladder]. 1. Hemmorhage into a cyst or the urinary bladder. 2. A blood-filled cyst.

hematocyte (hē′mă-, hĕm′ă-tō-sīt) [Gr. *haimatos*, blood, + *kytos*, cell]. 1. A red blood cell. 2. Any blood cell.

hematocytolysis (hē″mă-, hĕm″ă-tō-sī-tŏl′ĭ-sĭs) ["+ "+ *lysis*, dissolution]. Dissolution of blood corpuscles freeing hemoglobin. SYN: *hemolysis.*

hematocytometer (hē″ma-, hĕm″ă-tō-sī-tŏm′ĕ-ter) ["+ "+ *metron*, measure]. Device for counting number of blood cells in given quantity of blood.

hematocytozoon (hē″mă-, hĕm″ă-tō-sī-tō-zō′ŏn) ["+ "+ *zōon*, animal]. A parasite which lives in red blood cells.

hematocyturia (hē″mă-, hĕm″ă-tō-sī-tū′rĭ-ă) ["+ "+ *ouron*, urine]. Red blood cells in urine; hematuria, q.v., as differentiated from hemoglobinuria, q.v.

hematogenesis (hē″mă-, hĕm″ă-tō-jĕn′ĕ-sĭs) [Gr. *haimatos*, blood, + *genesis*, formation]. The development of blood cells. SYN: *hematopoiesis.*

hematogenic, hematogenous (hē″mă-, hĕm″ă-to-jĕn′ĭk, -tŏj′ĕ-nŭs) ["+ *gennan*, to produce]. 1. Pert. to formation of blood. SYN: *hematopoietic.* 2. Pert. to or originating in the blood.

hematohidrosis (hē″mă-, hĕm″ă-tō-hī-drō′sĭs) ["+ *hidrōs*, sweat, + *-ōsis*, condition]. Secretion of sweat containing blood. SYN: *hemathidrosis.*

hematoid (hē′mă-, hĕm′ă-toyd) ["+ *eidos*, resemblance]. Resembling blood.

hematoidin (hē″mă-, hĕm-ă-toy′dĭn). The yellow crystalline substance, biliverdin, which remains when red blood cells are destroyed in bruised tissue.

hematokolpos. Hematocolpos, q.v.

hem′atolith [Gr. *haimatos*, blood, + *lithos*, stone]. Concretion in a blood vessel wall. SYN: *hemolith.*

hematologist (hē″mă-, hĕm″ă-tŏl′ō-jĭst) ["+ *logos*, study]. One who specializes in the study of the blood.

hematology (hē″mă-, hĕm″ă-tŏl′ō-jĭ). The science concerned with blood and the blood-forming tissues.

hematolymphangioma (hē″mă-, hĕm″ă-tō-lĭmf-ăn″jĭ-ō′mă) [Gr. *haimatos*, blood, + L. *lympha*, lymph, + Gr. *angeion*, vessel, + *ōma*, tumor]. A tumor consisting of dilated blood vessels and lymphatics.

hematolysis (hē″mă-, hĕm-ă-tŏl′ĭ-sĭs) ["+ *lysis*, dissolution]. Hemolysis, q.v.

hematolytic (hĕm-ă-tō-lĭt′ĭk). Pert. to hemolysis, q.v.

hematoma (hē″mă-, hĕm-ă-tō′mă) [Gr. *haimatos*, blood, + *ōma*, tumor]. A tumor or swelling which contains blood.

h. auris. H. beneath perichondrium of ear cartilage.

h., pelvic. H. present in cellular tissue of pelvis.

h., subdural. H. located beneath the dura, usually the result of head injuries.

h., vulvar. H. occurring on the vulva.

hematomediastinum (hē″mă-, hĕm″ă-tō-mē″dĭ-ă-stī′nŭm) ["+ L. *mediastinus*, in the middle]. Blood effusion into the mediastinum.

hematometer (hē-mă-tŏm′ĕ-ter) ["+ *metron*, measure]. Hemoglobinometer, q.v.

hematometra (hē″mă-, hĕm″ă-tō-mē′tră) [Gr. *haimatos*, blood, + *mētra*, uterus]. 1. Hemorrhage in the uterus. 2. Accumulation of menstrual blood in the womb. SEE: *hematocolpos; hydrometra; pyometra.*

hematom′etry ["+ *metron*, measure]. Determination of varieties and number of blood cells and amount of hemoglobin in the blood.

hematomphalocele (hē″mă-, hĕm″ăt-ŏm-făl′ō-sēl) ["+ *omphalos*, navel, + *kēlē*, hernia]. Effusion of blood into an umbilical hernia.

hematomyelia (hē″mă-, hĕm″ă-tō-mĭ-ē′lĭ-ă) [Gr. *haimatos*, blood, + *myelos*, marrow]. Hemorrhage of blood into the spinal cord.

hematomyelitis (hē″mă-, hĕm″ă-tō-mī″ĕl-ī′tĭs) ["+ "+ *itis*, inflammation]. Inflammation of spinal cord with bloody effusion.

hematomyelopore (hē″măt-, hĕm″ăt-ō-mī′ĕl-ō-pōr) ["+ "+ *poros*, opening]. Formation of cavities and channels in the spinal cord as a result of hemorrhage.

hematonephrosis (hē″mă-, hĕm″ă-tō-nĕ-frō′sĭs) ["+ *nephros*, kidney, + *ōsis*, condition]. Accumulation of blood in the pelvis of the kidney.

hematopathol′ogy [Gr. *haimatos*, blood, + *pathos*, disease, + *logos*, study]. The study of pathological conditions of the blood.

hematopericar′dium ["+ *peri*, around, + *kardia*, heart]. Bloody effusion into the pericardial sac.

hematoperitone′um ["+ *peritonaion*, peritoneum]. Bloody effusion into the peritoneal cavity. SYN: *hemoperitoneum.*

hematopex′in ["+ *pēxis*, fixation]. Any substance that causes blood to coagulate. SYN: *hemopexin.*

hematopex′is. Coagulation of the blood. SYN: *hemopexia.*

hem′atophage [Gr. *haimatos*, blood, + *phagein*, to eat]. A phagocytic cell which destroys red blood cells.

hematopha′gia. 1. Subsistence on blood. 2. Administration of blood as a treatment. 3. Destruction of blood cells by phagocytes.

hematophagous (hĕm-ă-tŏf′ă-gŭs). Living on blood. SYN: *hematophagia.*

hematophilia (hĕm″ă-tō-fĭl′ĭ-ă) [Gr. *haimatos*, blood, + *philein*, to love]. Hemophilia, q.v.

hematophobia (hē″mă-, hĕm″ă-tōfō′bĭ-ă) ["+ *phobos*, fear]. Hemophobia, q.v.

hematophyte (hē″mă-, hĕm″ă-tō-fīt) [Gr. *haimatos*, blood, + *phyton*, plant]. Plant organism or bacteria in the blood.

hematopla′nia ["+ *planē*, wandering]. Condition of vicarious menstruation.

hematoplas′tic ["+ *plassein*, to form]. Pert. to formation of blood. SYN: *hematopoietic.*

hematopneic (hē″mă-, hĕm-ă-tō-nē′ĭk) ["+ *pnein*, to breathe]. Rel. to oxygenation of the blood.

hematopoiesis (hē″mă-, hĕm″ă-tō-poy-ē′sĭs) [Gr. *haimatos*, blood, + *poiein*, to form]. The production and development of blood cells, normally in the bone marrow. Tissues which produce blood cells are said to be hematopoietic.

h., extramedullary. Production of blood cells in tissues other than bone marrow. This occurs in severe anemia and other diseases affecting the blood.

hematopoietic (hē″mă-, hĕm″ă-tō-poy-ĕt′ĭk). 1. Pert. to the production and development of blood cells. 2. A substance that assists in or stimulates the production of blood cells. SYN: *hematogenic; hematoplastic.*

h. system. The blood-making organs, esp. bone marrow and lymph nodes.

hematoporphyrin (hē″mă-, hĕm″ă-tō-por′fĭ-rĭn) [Gr. *haimatos*, blood, + *porphyra*, purple]. Iron-free heme, a decomposition product of hemoglobin in the urine in certain conditions.

hematoporphyrinuria (hē″mă-, hĕm″ă-tō-por″fĭ-rĭn-ū′rĭ-ă) ["+ "+ *ouron*, urine]. Hematoporphyrin in urine.

hematorrhachis (hĕm-ă-tor′ă-kĭs) ["+ *rhachis*, spine]. Hemorrhage into the spinal cord.

hematorrhea (hĕm″ă-tō-rē′ă) ["+ *rhoia*, flow]. Profuse hemorrhage.

hematosalpinx (hē″mă-, hĕm″ă-tō-sal′pĭnks) [Gr. *haimatos*, blood, + *salpinx*, tube]. Retained menstrual fluid in the fallopian tube.

hematoscheocele (hĕm-ă-tŏs′kē-ō-sēl) ["+ *oscheon*, scrotum, + *kēlē*, hernia]. Blood accumulated in the scrotum.

hematoscope (hē′mă-, hĕm″ă-tō-skōp) ["+ *skopein*, to examine]. Device for optical or spectroscopic examination of blood.

hematoscopy (hē″mă-, hĕm-ă-tŏs′kō-pī). Examination of the blood.

hematose (hē′mă-, hĕm′ă-tōs) [Gr. *haimatos,* blood, + *-ōsis,* condition]. Full of blood.

hematosep′sis [″+ *sēpsis,* putrefaction]. Septicemia, q.v.

hematospec′troscope [″+ L. *spectrum,* image, + Gr. *skopein,* to examine]. Spectroscope for inspecting blood.

hematospectros′copy. Examination of blood with the hematospectroscope.

hematospermatocele (hĕm″ă-tō-sper-măt′ō-sēl) [Gr. *haima,* blood, + *sperma,* seed, + *kēlē,* tumor]. A blood filled spermatocele.

hematospermia (hĕm″ă-tō-sper′mĭ-ă). Semen which contains blood. SYN: *hemospermia.*

h. spuria. H. coming from the prostatic urethra.

h. vera. H. coming from the seminal vessels.

hematostatic (hĕm″ă-tō-stăt′ĭk) [Gr. *haimatos,* blood, + *stasis,* standing]. 1. Retaining blood in a part. 2. Pert. to the arrest of blood flow in a hemorrhage. SYN: *hemostatic.*

hematosteon (hĕm-ă-tŏs′tē-ŏn) [″+ *osteon,* bone]. Bleeding into the medullary cavity of a bone.

hematother′mal [″+ *thermē,* heat]. Warmblooded. SYN: *hemathermal; hemathermous.*

hematothorax (hĕm″ă-tō-thō′răks) [″+ *thōrax,* chest]. Blood in the chest. SYN: *hemothorax.*

hematotox′ic [Gr. *haimatos,* blood, + *toxikon,* poison]. 1. Pert. to septicemia. 2. Something which is toxic to blood cells.

hematotrachelos (hĕm″ă-tō-tră-kē′lŏs) [″+ *trachēlos,* neck]. Retained menstrual blood in cervix uteri, causing distention.

hematotympanum (hĕm″ă-tō-tĭm′păn-ŭm) [″+ *tympanon,* drum]. Blood in the middle ear.

hematoxylin. A colorless crystalline compound, $C_{16}H_{14}O_6$, obtained by extraction with ether from logwood. Upon oxidation it is converted into hematein, an oxidation product of hematoxylin, which stains certain structures a deep blue color. It is an excellent nuclear stain, and widely used in histological work.

hematozoon (hē″mă-, hĕm″ă-tō-zō′ŏn) [Gr. *haimatos,* blood, + *zōon,* animal]. Any living organism in the blood.

hematozymosis (hē″mă-, hĕm″ă-tō-zī-mō′sĭs) [″+ *zymōsis,* fermentation]. Blood fermentation.

hematuria (hē″mă-, hĕm″ă-tū′rĭ-ă) [Gr. *haima,* blood, + *ouron,* urine]. Blood in the urine.

NOTE: The occurrence of bright red blood in the urine and its appearance in the toilet bowl is quite frightening to the patient. Both the patient and the nurse should realize that a very small amount of blood may cause the entire toilet bowl contents to appear to be full of pure blood.

SYM: Urine may be slightly smoky, reddish, or very red.

ETIOL: Lesion of urinary tract; blood dyscrasia; contamination during menstruation or puerperium; prostatic disease; tumors; poisoning, esp. carbolic acid and cantharides; malaria; toxemias; and calculus.

DIAG: If blood is well mixed with urine, probably from kidneys. If clotted in tubular casts of ureters, from kidneys or ureters. If passed at beginning of urination, from the urethra; if at the end, from bladder.

h., renal. Urine smoky, sometimes bright red.

h., urethral. Always bright red. Precedes urination.

h., vesical. Urine bright red, not uniform.

hemaurochrome (hē″mă-, hĕm″ă-ū′rō-krōm) [″+ *ouron,* urine, + *chrōma,* color]. A heme derivative found in the urine in sarcoma and carcinoma, malaria, anemias, and other disorders. Supposed to result from dissolution of red blood corpuscles.

heme (hēm). An iron-containing nonprotein portion of the hemogloblin molecule. Formerly called hematin.

hemeralopia (hĕm″ĕr-ăl-ō′pĭ-ă) [Gr. *hēmera,* day, + *alaos,* blind, + *ōps,* eye]. Diminished vision in bright light.

Term formerly erroneously applied to night blindness or nyctalopia. Nyctalopia indicates inability to see in dim light, though otherwise vision is normal.

In day blindness, the sight is poor in sunlight and in good illumination; it is good at dusk, at twilight, and in poor illumination. This is noted in albinism, retinitis with central scotoma, toxic amblyopia, coloboma of the iris and choroid, opacity of the crystalline lens or cornea, and in conjunctivitis with photophobia.

hemi- [Gr.]. Prefix meaning half.

hemiacephalus (hĕm″ĭ-ă-sĕf′ă-lŭs) [″+ *a-,* not, + *kephalē,* head]. A malformed fetus with a markedly defective head. SEE: *anencephalus.*

hemiachromatopsia (hĕm″ĭ-ă-krō-mă-tŏp′-sĭ-ă) [″+ ″+ *chrōma,* color, + *opsis,* vision]. Color blindness in one half, or in corresponding halves, of the visual field.

hemialbumin (hĕm''ĭ-ăl-bū'mĭn) [" + L. *albumen*, white of egg]. A product resulting from the digestion of albumin. SYN: *antialbumin*.

hemialbumose (hĕm''ĭ-ăl'bū-mōs). An albumoid product from the digestion of certain proteins. It occurs in bone marrow.

hemialbumosuria (hĕm''ĭ-ăl-bū''mō-sū'rĭ-ă) [Gr. *hemi-*, half, + L. *albumen*, white of egg, + Gr. *ouron*, urine]. Hemialbumose in the urine.

hemialgia (hĕm-ĭ-ăl'jĭ-ă) [" + *algos*, pain]. Pain in one half of the body.

hemiamaurosis (hĕm''ĭ-ăm''ō-rō'sĭs) [" + *amaurosis*, darkness]. Blindness in half the visual field. SYN: *hemianopsia*.

hemiamblyopia (hĕm''ĭ-ăm''blĭ-ō'pĭ-ă) [" + *amblys*, dim, + *ōps*, sight]. Blindness in half the visual field. SYN: *hemianopsia*.

hemiamyosthenia (hĕm''ĭ-ă''mĭ-ŏs-thē'nĭ-ă) [Gr. *hemi-*, half, + *a-*, not, + *mys, myo-*, muscle, + *sthenos*, strength]. Absence of normal muscular power on one side of the body. SYN: *hemiparesis*.

hemianacusia (hĕm''ĭ-ăn''ă-kū'zĭ-ă) [" + *an-*, not, + *akousis*, hearing]. Deafness in one ear.

hemianalgesia (hĕm''ĭ-ăn-ăl-jē'zĭ-ă) [" + " + *algos*, pain]. Lack of sensibility to pain (analgesia) on one side of the body.

hemianesthesia (hĕm''ĭ-ăn-ĕs-thē'zĭ-ă) [" + " + *aisthēsis*, sensation]. Anesthesia of half of the body.

hemianopia, hemianopsia (hĕm''ĭ-ă-nō'pĭ-ă, -nŏp'sĭ-ă) [Gr. *hemi-*, half, + *an-*, not, + *ōps*, eye]. Blindness for one-half field of vision in one or both eyes.

  h., altitudinal. Blindness in upper or lower half in each eye.

  h., binasal. Affection of nasal half of visual field in each eye.

  h., bitemporal. Affection of temporal half of visual field in each eye.

  h., complete. Blindness in half the visual field.

  h., crossed. Bitemporal or binasal h.

  h., heteronymous. H., crossed, q.v.

  h., homonymous. Blindness of nasal half of one eye and temporal half of the other or right-sided or left-sided h. of corresponding sides in both eyes.

  h., incomplete. Blindness in less than half of the visual field of each eye.

  h., quadrant. Blindness of symmetrical quadrant of the field in each eye.

  h., unilateral. Heminaopsia affecting only one eye. SYN: *uniocular h.*

hemianosmia (hĕm''ĭ-ăn-ŏs'mĭ-ă) [Gr. *hemi-*, half, + *an-*, not, + *osmē*, smell]. Loss of smell in one nostril.

hemiapraxia (hĕm''ĭ-ă-prăks'ĭ-ă) [" + *a-*, not, + *prassein*, to do]. Incapacity to exercise purposeful movements on one side of the body.

hemiarthroplasty of the hip. Replacement of the femoral head with a metal ball held in place by a stem extending into the shaft of the femur. The acetabulum is not altered. Particularly useful in patients with necrosis of the femoral head.

hemiarthrosis (hĕm''ĭ-ăr-thrō'sĭs) [" + *arthron*, joint, + *ōsis*, condition]. A false articulation between two bones. SYN: *synchondrosis*.

hemiasynergia (hĕm''ĭ-ă''sĭn-er'jĭ-ă) [" + *a-*, not, + *syn*, with, + *ergon*, work]. Lack of coordination of parts affecting one side of the body.

hemiataxia (hĕm''ĭ-ă-tăks'ĭ-ă) [Gr. *hemi-*, half, + *ataxia*, lack of order]. Impaired muscular coordination causing awkward movements of the affected side of the body.

hemiathetosis (hĕm''ĭ-ăth''ĕ-tō'sĭs) [" + *athetos*, without fixed position, + *-ōsis*, condition]. Slow change of position; athetosis of one side of the body.

hemiatrophy (hĕm-ĭ-ăt'rō-fĭ) [" + *atrophia*, atrophy]. Impaired nutrition resulting in atrophy of one side of the face or other part; marked by white or yellow macules on affected side.

hemiballism (hĕm-ĭ-băl'ĭzm) [" + *balismos*, jumping]. Jerking and twitching movements of one side of the body. SYN: *hemichorea*.

hemic (hē'mĭk, hĕm'ĭk) [Gr. *haima*, blood]. Pert. to blood. SYN: *hemal*.

hemicanities (hĕm''ĭ-kăn-ĭsh'ĭ-ēz) [Gr. *hemi-*, half, + L. *canitiēs*, gray hair]. Grayness of hair on one side only.

hemicardia (hĕm-ĭ-kar'dĭ-ă) [" + *kardia*, heart]. Half of a four-chambered heart.

hemicellulose (hĕm-ĭ-sĕl'ū-lōs) [Gr. *haima*, blood, + L. *cellula*, little cell]. One of a group of polysaccharides which differ from cellulose in that they may be hydrolyzed by dilute mineral acids and from other polysaccharides in that they are not readily digested by amylases. Includes pentosans, galactosans (agar agar), and pectins.

hemicentrum (hĕm-ĭ-sĕn'trŭm) [Gr. *hemi-*, half, + *kentron*, center]. Either lateral half of the centrum of a vertebra.

hemichorea (hĕm-ĭ-kō-rē'ă) [" + *choreia*, a dancing]. Convulsive movements of one side of the body.

hemichromatopsia (hĕm''ĭ-krō-mă-tŏp'sĭ-ă) [" + *chrōma*, color, + *opsis*, vision]. Blindness to color in one half of the visual field. SYN: *hemiachromatopsia*.

hemicrania (hĕm-ĭ-krā′nĭ-ă) [Gr. *hemi-*, half, + *kranion*, skull]. 1. Unilateral head pain, usually migraine. 2. Malformed fetus having only one half of the skull developed.

hemicraniectomy (hĕm′′ĭ-krā-nĭ-ĕk′tō-mĭ) [″ + ″ + *ektomē*, excision]. Surgical division of cranial vault from front backward, exposing half of the brain.

hemicraniosis (hĕm′′ĭ-krā-nĭ-ō′sĭs) [″ + ″ + *ōsis*, condition]. Enlargement of half of cranium or face.

hemidiaphoresis (hĕm′′ĭ-dī′′ă-fŏr-ē′sĭs) [″ + *dia*, through, + *pherein*, to carry]. Sweating on one side of the body. SYN: *hemidrosis; hemihidrosis.*

hemidiaphragm (hĕm′′ĭ-dī′ă-frăm) [Gr. *hemi-*, half, + *dia*, through, + *phragma*, wall]. Paralysis affecting only half of the diaphragm.

hemidro′sis 1. [Gr. *hemi-*, half, + *hidrosis*, sweating] Sweating on one side of the body. SYN: *hemidiaphoresis; hemihidrosis.* 2. [Gr. *haima*, blood, + *hidrosis*, sweating] Secretion of sweat containing blood. SYN: *hemathidrosis.*

hemidysergia (hĕm′′ĭ-dĭs-ĕr′jĭ-ă) [″ + *dys*, bad, + *ergon*, work]. Lack of coordination of muscles on one side of the body.

hemidysesthesia (hĕm′′ĭ-dĭs-ĕs-thē′zĭ-ă) [″ + ″ + *aisthēsis*, sensation]. Impaired sensation of one half of the body.

hemidystrophy (hĕm′′ĭ-dĭs′trō-fĭ) [″ + ″ + *trophē*, nourishment]. Inequality in development of the two sides of the body.

hemiep′ilepsy [″ + *epilēpsia*, seizure]. Epilepsy with convulsions confined to lateral half of the body.

hemifa′cial [Gr. *hemi-*, half, + L. *faciēs*, face]. Pert. to one side of the face.

hemigastrectomy (hĕm′′ĭ-găs-trĕk′tō-mĭ) [″ + *gastēr*, belly, + *ektomē*, excision]. Excision of one half of the stomach.

hemiglossi′tis [″ + *glōssa*, tongue, + *-itis*, inflammation]. Vesicular eruption on one half of the tongue and inner surface of cheek. Herpetic in character.

hemiguesia (hĕm-ĭ-gū′sĭ-ă) [″ + *geusis*, taste]. Loss of sense of taste on one side of the tongue.

hemihidro′sis [Gr. *hemi-*, half, + *hidrōsis*, perspiration]. Sweating on only one side of the body. SYN: *hemidiaphoresis; hemidrosis.*

hemihyperesthesia (hĕm′′ĭ-hī-per-ĕs-thē′-zĭ-ă) [″ + *hyper*, over, + *aisthēsis*, sensation]. Abnormal tactile and painful sensitiveness of one side of the body.

hemihyperidrosis (hĕm′′ĭ-hī-per-ĭ-drō′sĭs) [″ + ″ + *hidrosis*, sweating]. Excessive perspiration confined to one side of the body.

hemihyperto′nia [Gr. *hemi-*, half, + *hyper*, over, + *tonos*, tone]. Exaggerated tonicity of muscles on lateral half of the body.

hemihyper′trophy [″ + ″ + *trophē*, nourishment]. Hypertrophy of muscles of half of the body or face.

hemihypesthesia (hĕm′′ĭ-hī′′pĕs-thē′zĭ-ă) [″ + *hypo*, under, + *aisthēsis*, sensation]. Diminished sensibility on one side of the body.

hemihypotonia (hĕm′′ĭ-hī-pō-tō′nĭ-ă) [″ + ″ + *tonos*, tone]. Partial loss of tonicity of muscles on one side of the body.

hemilat′eral [Gr. *hemi-*, half, + L. *latus*, side]. Rel. to one side only.

hemimelia (hĕm′′ĭ-mē′lĭ-ă) [″ + *melos*, limb]. A malformed fetus with defective development of the extremities, esp. the distal portion.

hemin (hē′mĭn) [Gr. *haima*, blood]. A brownish-red crystalline salt of heme formed when hemoglobin is heated with glacial acetic acid and sodium chloride. Used in testing for presence of blood. SYN: *heme hydrochloride.*

h. crystals. Teichmann's crystals, formed when the above test is made.

heminephrectomy (hĕm′′ĭn-ē-frĕk′tō-mĭ) [Gr. *hemi-*, half, + *nephros*, kidney, + *ektomē*, excision]. Excision or removal of a portion of a kidney.

hemineurasthenia (hĕm′′ĭ-nū-răs-thē′nĭ-ă) [″ + *neuron*, nerve, + *astheneia*, weakness]. Neurasthenia affecting one side of the body only.

hemiopia (hĕm-ĭ-ō′pĭ-ă) [″ + *ōps*, eye]. Blindness in half of the visual field. SYN: *hemianopia,* q.v.

hemiopic (hĕm-ĭ-ōp′ĭk) [″ + *ōps*, eye]. Pert. to hemiopia.

hemiparal′ysis [Gr. *hemi-*, half, + *paralyein*, to loosen from the sides]. Paralysis of one side of the body only.

hemiparanesthesia (hĕm′′ĭ-păr-ăn-ĕs-thē′-zĭ-ă) [″ + *para*, beyond, + *an-*, not, + *aisthēsis*, sensation]. Anesthesia of one lower extremity or lower half of one side.

hemiparaplegia (hĕm′′ĭ-păr-ă-plē′jĭ-ă) [″ + ″ + *plēgē*, stroke]. Paralysis of the lower half of one side or of one leg.

hemiparesis (hĕm′′ĭ-păr′ē-sĭs, hĕm-ĭ-păr-ē′sĭs) [″ + *paresis*, paralysis]. Paralysis affecting only one side of the body.

hem′′iparesthe′sia [″ + *para*, beyond, + *aisthēsis*, sensation]. Numbness of one side of the body.

hemiplegia (hĕm-ĭ-plē′jĭ-ă) [Gr. *hemi-*, half, + *plēgē*, a stroke]. Paralysis of only one half of the body.

ETIOL: A brain lesion involving upper motor neurons and resulting in paralysis of the opposite side of the body. May result from disturbed blood flow to a portion of the brain. This may be due to hemorrhage, cerebral thrombosis, or embolism, or to a tumor of the cerebrum.

NP: Elevate head and shoulders. See that tongue does not obstruct breathing. Avoid stimulants. Do not move patient until arrival of doctor.

Chart nursing care and observations every four hours for the first two days. Turn patient frequently to avoid hypostatic pneumonia. Watch for bedsores and retention of urine. Urine should be measured and tested for albumin and sugar. Avoid burning patient with hot water bottles. Do not discuss patient's condition in his presence, even if he appears to be unconscious.

SEE: *Benedikt's syndrome; paralysis; thalamic syndrome.*

h., alternate. H. affecting one side of face and trunk, and of extremities of opposite side.

h., capsular. H. resulting from a lesion of the internal capsule of the brain.

h., cerebral. Due to brain lesion.

h., crossed. Alternate h.

h., facial. Paralysis of muscles of one side of face.

h., spastic. H. accompanied by spasms, usually occurring in infants.

h., spinal. H. resulting from a lesion of the spinal cord. SEE: *Brown-Sequard's paralysis.*

hemiplegic (hĕm-ĭ-plē′jĭk). Pert. to hemiplegia.

Hemiptera (hĕm-ĭp′tĕr-ă). The true bugs; an order of insects characterized by piercing and sucking mouth parts; 1st pair of wings leathery at base and membranous at tip, 2nd pair of wings membranous; incomplete metamorphosis. Includes bedbugs, kissing bugs, and several other species which are pests or transmitters of pathogenic organisms.

hemirachischisis (hĕm′′ĭ-ră-kĭs′kĭ-sĭs) [Gr. *hemi-*, half, + *rhachis*, spine, + *schisis*, cleft]. Rachischisis in which protrusion of the spinal meninges does not occur. SYN: *spina bifida occulta*, q.v.

hemisec′tion ["+ L. *sectio*, a cutting]. In surgery or anatomy, cutting an organ or tissue in half. SYN: *bisection.*

hemisomus (hĕm′′ĭ-sō′mŭs) ["+ *soma*, body]. Fetus with lateral half of body missing or malformed.

hemispasm (hĕm′′ĭ-spăzm) ["+ *spasmos*, spasm]. Spasm of only one side of the body or face.

hemisphere (hĕm′ĭ-sfĕr) ["+ *sphaira*, sphere]. Either half of the cerebrum or cerebellum.

h., dominant. The cerebral h. in which the higher cortical functions, esp. those rel. to speech and certain motor activities, are associated; the left one in right-handed individuals. Results in phenomenon known as cerebral dominance.

Hemis′pora stella′ta. A variety of fungus causing mycosis.

hemispore (hĕm′ĭ-spōr) [Gr. *hemi-*, half, + *sporos*, seed]. A spore which reproduces by division of terminal part of a hyphus.

hemisporosis (hĕm-ĭ-spō-rō′sĭs) ["+ "+ *ōsis*, condition]. Infection with a fungus, Hemispora stellata, resulting in swellings of bone and other tissue of a gummatous nature. May later ulcerate.

hemistrumectomy (hĕm′′ĭ-strŭ-mĕk′tō-mĭ) ["+ L. *struma*, goiter, + Gr. *ektomē*, excision]. Excision of about one half of a goiter.

hemisyndrome (hĕm′′ĭ-sĭn′drōm) ["+ *syndromē*, a running with]. One indicating a unilateral lesion of the spinal cord.

hemisystole (hĕm-ĭ-sĭs′tō-lē) [Gr. *hemi-*, half, + *systole*, a contracting]. One pulse beat to every two heart beats. Results from failure of the ventricle to contract every other time.

hemiterata (hĕm-ĭ-tĕr′ă-tă) ["+ *teras*, monster]. Individuals possessing congenital malformations but not to such a degree as to cause severe disability or disfigurement.

hemiteric, hemiteratic (hĕm-ĭ-tĕr′ĭk, -tĕr-ăt′ĭk). Congenitally deformed, but not severely so.

hemivertebra (hĕm′′ĭ-ver′tĕ-bră). Congenital absence of one half of a vertebra.

hem′lock [AS. *hemléac*]. 1. A species of evergreen plant. 2. Volatile oil extracted from dried, unripe fruit of Conium maculatum, poison hemlock.

POISONING SYM: Weakness, drowsiness, nausea, vomiting, difficult breathing, paralysis, and death.

TREATMENT: Empty stomach by means of a stomach pump or an emetic. Give cathartic. Treat respiratory failure with artificial respiration and oxygen.

hemo-. Prefix meaning blood. SEE: Words beginning with *haemo-, haem-, hem-, hema-,* and *hemato-.*

he′′moagglutina′tion [Gr. *haima*, blood, + L. *agglutinans*, gluing]. The clumping of red blood corpuscles.

he″moagglu′tinin. An agglutinin which clumps the red blood corpuscles.

he″moalkalim′eter (Gr. *haima*, blood, + Arab. *alkali*, the kali plant, + Gr. *metron*, measure). A device for estimating degree of alkalinity of blood.

hemobilinuria (hē″mō-bĭl-ĭn-ū′rĭ-ă) ["+ L. *bilis*, bile, + Gr. *ouron*, urine]. Urobilin in the blood and urine.

hemocatharsis ["+ *katharsis*, cleansing]. Process of cleansing the blood of impurities.

hemocatheresis (hē″mō-kăth-ĕr-ē′sĭs) ["+ *kathairesis*, destruction]. Destruction of blood cells.

hemocatheretic (hē″mō-kăth-ĕr-ē′tĭk) [Gr. *haima*, blood, + *kathairetikos*, destructive]. Destructive to blood cells.

hemochorial (hē″mō-kor′ĭ-al) ["+ *chorion*, envelope]. Pert. to the relationship between blood of the mother and the chorionic ectoderm. SEE: *placenta.*

hemochromatosis (hē′mō-krō″mă-tō′sĭs) ["+ *chrōma*, color, + *-ōsis*, condition]. A disease characterized pathologically by excess deposits of iron throughout the body. The liver becomes enlarged; the skin is pigmented so that it has a bronze hue; and there is diabetes and frequently cardiac failure. It is a rare disease seen ten times as frequently in males as females. The majority of cases develop after the 4th decade. SYN: *bronzed diabetes.*

he′mochrome. Hemoglobin, q.v.

he″mochro′mogen [Gr. *haima*, blood, + *chrōma*, color, + *gennan*, to produce]. General term applied to compounds of heme with nitrogen-containing substances such as a protein.

hemochromometer (hē″mō-krō-mŏm′ĕ-tĕr) ["+ "+ *metron*, measure]. A colorimeter used for estimating the amount of hemoglobin in the blood.

hemoclasia (hē″mō-klā′sĭ-ă) ["+ *klasis*, a breaking]. Hemolytic crisis.

hemoc′lasis. Disintegration of red blood cells. SYN: *hemolysis.*

hemoclas′tic. Destructive of erythrocytes. SYN: *hemolytic.*

he″moconcentra′tion. An increase in the number of red blood cells resulting from a decrease in the volume of plasma. SYN: *anhydremia.*

hemoconia (hē″mō-kō′nĭ-ă) [Gr. *haima*, blood, + *konis*, dust]. Minute colorless bodies in blood thought to be the products of disintegration of red blood cells. SYN: *blood dust; hemokonia.*

hemoconio′sis ["+ "+ *-ōsis*, condition]. Having an abnormal amt. of hemoconia in the blood. SYN: *hemokoniosis.*

he′moculture ["+ L. *cultura*, development]. A bacteriological blood culture.

hemocyte (hē′mō-sīt) [Gr. *haima*, blood, + *kytos*, cell]. 1. Any blood cell. 2. Red blood cell.

he″mocy′toblast ["+ "+ *blastos*, germ]. The primitive reticuloendothelial stem cell found in bone marrow from which all blood cells are thought to arise.

hemocytoblasto′ma ["+ "+ "+ *ōma*, tumor]. A tumor containing embryonic blood cells.

hemocytocatheresis (hē″mō-sī″tō-kă-thĕr′ē-sĭs) ["+ "+ *kathairesis*, destruction]. Hemolysis, q.v.

hemocytogenesis (hē″mō-sī″tō-jĕn′ē-sĭs) [Gr. *haima*, blood + *kytos*, cell, + *genesis*, development]. The formation of blood cells. SYN: *hematopoiesis.*

hemocytology (hē″mō-sī-tŏl′ō-jĭ) ["+ "+ *logos*, study]. Study of structure and function of blood cells.

hemocytolysis (hē″mō-sī-tŏl′ĭ-sĭs) ["+ "+ *lysis*, dissolution]. Dissolution of the blood corpuscles. SYN: *hematocytolysis; hemolysis*, q.v.

hemocytometer (hē″mō-sī-tŏm′ĕ-ter) ["+ "+ *metron*, measure]. Device for determining relative number of cells in the blood.

hemocytopoiesis (hē″mō-sī″tō-poy-ē′sĭs) [Gr. *haima*, blood, + *kytos*, cell, + *poiein*, to form]. The development of blood cells.

hemocytotripsis (hē″mō-sī″tō-trī′sĭs) ["+ "+ *tripsis*, a crushing]. Fragmentation of the red blood cells.

hemocytozoon (hē″mō-sī″tō-zō′ŏn) ["+ "+ *zōon*, animal]. An animal microparasite of the blood cells. SYN: *hematobium.*

hemodia (hē-mō′dĭ-ă) [Gr. *haimōdia*]. Extreme sensitivity of the teeth.

hemodiagno′sis [Gr. *haima*, blood, + *dia*, through, + *gnōsis*, knowledge]. Examination of the blood for diagnostic purpose.

hemodialysis (hē″mō-, hĕm″ō-dĭ-al′ĭ-ĭs) ["+ "+ *lysis*, dissolve]. Removal of chemical substances from the blood by passing it through tubes made of semipermeable membranes. The tubes are continually bathed by solutions which selectively remove unwanted material.

    Used to cleanse the blood of patients in whom one or both kidneys are defective or absent and to remove excess accumulation of drugs or toxic chemicals in the blood.

hemodi′astase ["+ *diastasis*, separation]. An amylolytic ferment in the blood.

he″modilu′tion. An increase in the volume of blood plasma resulting in reduced concentration of red blood cells.

hemodromometer (hē″mō-drō-mŏm′ĕ-ter) [Gr. *haima*, blood, + *dromos*, course, + *metron*, measure]. Device for determining the blood's velocity.

hemodynam′ics ["+ *dynamis*, power]. A study of the forces involved in circulating blood through the body.

hemodynamometer (hē″mō-dī′nă-mŏm′ĕ-ter) ["+ "+ *metron*, measure]. Device for measuring blood pressure.

hemodystrophy (hē″mō-dĭs′trō-fĭ) ["+ *dys*, bad, + *trophē*, nutrition]. Blood disease due to malnutrition. SYN: *hematodystrophy.*

he″moendothe′lial. Pert. to the relationship between blood of the mother and the endothelium of chorionic vessels. SEE: *placenta.*

hemoflagellate (hē″mō-flăj′ĕ-lāt″) [Gr. *haima*, blood, + L. *flagellum*, whip]. Any flagellate protozoan of the blood. The most important genera are Trypanosoma and Leishmania.

hemofuscin (hē″mō-fū′sĭn) ["+ L. *fuscus*, brown]. Brown pigment derived from hemoglobin. In urine it produces a reddish color.

hemogenesis (hē″mō-jĕn′ĕ-sĭs) ["+ *genesis*, formation]. Blood formation. SYN: *hemopoiesis.*

hemogen′ic ["+ *gennan*, to produce]. Rel. to the production of blood.

hemoglobin (hē″mō-, hĕm″ō-glō′bĭn) [Gr. *haima*, blood, + L. *globus*, globe]. The iron-containing pigment of the red blood cells. Its function is to carry oxygen from the lungs to the tissues.

The amount of h. in the blood averages 12-16 gm./100 ml. of blood in adult females; 14-18 in males; and somewhat less in children. One gm. of h. can combine with 1.36 cc. of oxygen, the resulting compound being oxyhemoglobin.

H. is a crystallizable, conjugated protein consisting of an iron-containing pigment called heme or hematin, and a simple protein, globin. In the lungs it combines readily with oxygen to form a loose, unstable compound called oxyhemoglobin, a process called oxygenation. In the tissues where oxygen tension is low and carbon dioxide tension is high, oxyhemoglobin liberates its oxygen in exchange for carbon dioxide.

H. liberated from disintegrating red blood cells is removed from circulation by the cells of the reticuloendothelial system, esp. those of the liver and spleen. The globin is converted to amino acids and reutilized. Iron from the iron-containing portion is stored in the liver and spleen and reutilized; the noniron-containing pigment is converted to bilirubin which is excreted as one of the bile pigments.

H. combines with carbon monoxide to form the stable compound carboxyhemoglobin. Oxidation of the ferrous iron of h. to the ferric state produces methemoglobin.

A large number of different types of h. have been discovered. Study of these has facilitated investigating human genetics. H. is named according to the way the amino acid components of the globin move when studied by electrophoresis. There are more than a hundred different types of abnormal h. H. S is the abnormal form of h. found in persons with sickle-cell disease.

h., fetal. H. found in the erythrocytes of the fetus. It is capable of taking up and giving off oxygen at lower oxygen tensions than that in the erythrocytes of the adult.

hemoglobinemia (hē″mō-glō-bĭn-ē′mĭ-ă) [Gr. *haima*, blood, + L. *globus*, globe, + Gr. *haima*, blood]. Presence of hemoglobin in the blood plasma.

hemoglobinocholia (hē″mō-glō″bĭn-ō-kō′lĭ-ă) ["+ "+ Gr. *cholē*, bile]. Hemoglobin in the bile.

hemoglobinolysis (hē″mō-glō-bĭn-ŏl′ĭ-sĭs) ["+ "+ Gr. *lysis*, dissolution]. Dissolution of hemoglobin.

hemoglobinometer (hē″mō-glō-bĭn-ŏm′ĕ-ter) ["+ "+ Gr. *metron*, measure]. Device for determining the amount of hemoglobin in the blood.

hemoglobinopepsia (hē″mō-glō″bĭn-ō-pĕp′-sĭ-ă) [Gr. *haima*, blood, + L. *globus*, globe, + Gr. *pepsis*, digestion]. Destruction of hemoglobin. SYN: *hemoglobinolysis.*

hemoglobinophilic (hē″mō-glō-bĭn-ō-fīl′ĭk) ["+ "+ Gr. *philein*, to love]. Pert. to organisms which grow better in presence of hemoglobin.

hemoglo′binous. Pert. to or containing hemoglobin.

hemoglobinuria (hē″mō-glō-bĭn-ū′rĭ-ă) [Gr. *haima*, blood, + L. *globus*, globe, + Gr. *ouron*, urine]. The presence of hemoglobin in the urine, but free from red blood cells. Occurs when hemoglobin from disintegrating red blood cells or from rapid hemolysis of red cells exceeds the ability of the blood proteins to combine with the hemoglobin.

ETIOL: Hemolytic anemia; scurvy; purpura; certain drugs such as arsenic, phosphorus; typhus fever; or septicemia.

h., cold. H. following local or general exposure to cold. SYN: *paroxysmal cold h.*

h., epidemic. H. of the newborn characterized by jaundice, cyanosis, and fatty degeneration of heart and liver. SYN: *Winckel's disease.*

h., malarial. Blackwater fever.

h., march. H. occurring following strenuous exercise.

h., paroxysmal. Intermittent, recurring attacks of h. following exposure to cold (cold h.) or strenuous exercise (march h.). Results from increased fragility of red blood cells, or presence of a thermolabile autohemolysin.

h., toxic. H. resulting from toxic substances such as muscarine or snake venom; toxic products of infectious diseases such as yellow fever, typhoid fever, syphilis, and certain forms of hemolytic jaundice; organisms such as Plasmodium which destroy red blood cells; foreign proteins in blood as may follow blood transfusion or serum therapy.

he″moglo″binu′ric. Rel. to or marked by hemoglobinuria.

he′mogram [Gr. *haima,* blood, + *gramma,* a writing]. A graph of the differential blood count. SEE: *Schilling's classification.*

he′moid [″+ *eidos,* resemblance]. Having the appearance of blood. SYN: *hematoid.*

hemoko′nia [″+ *konis,* dust]. (pl. *hemokoniae*) Minute, highly refractive body in the blood, said to be disintegrated particle of blood cell. SYN: *blood dust; hemoconia.*

hemokoniosis (hē″mō-kō-nĭ-ō′sĭs) [″+ ″+ -*ōsis,* condition]. Abnormal amount of hemokoniae in the blood. SYN: *hemoconiosis.*

he′molith [Gr. *haima,* blood, + *lithos,* stone]. A calculus in the wall of a blood vessel.

he′molymph (hē′mō-lĭmf′) [″+ L. *lympha,* lymph]. Blood and lymph.

hemolysin (hē-mŏl′ĭ-sĭn) [″+ *lysis,* dissolution]. An agent in a serum destructive of erythrocytes, q.v.

hemolysis (hē-mŏl′ĭ-sĭs) [Gr. *haima,* blood, + *lysis,* dissolution]. The destruction of red blood cells with the liberation of hemoglobin which diffuses into the fluid surrounding them. May occur as a result of the effects of bacterial toxins, snake venoms, immune bodies (hemolysins), and hypotonic saline solutions.

    Their stroma is ruptured or dissolved and the hemoglobin is liberated into the plasma. As a result, the blood, examined grossly, appears to be more transparent and to have a richer, red color; under the microscope the dissolution of the red corpuscles can be observed.

    When h. occurs within the blood vessels, the body is unable to retain the hemoglobin, which is lost through the kidneys and imparts a red color to the urine, a condition called hemoglobinuria, q.v.

    Injection of a hypotonic saline solution or distilled water into the blood stream induces

h. and may result in death. The red blood cells swell and become globular; their membranes rupture and hemoglobin is liberated. All solutions injected intravenously must be isotonic to the blood. H. may result from infection by certain disease organisms, e.g. certain streptococci, staphylococci and the tetanus bacillus. H. also occurs in smallpox, diphtheria, and following severe burns. SEE: *fragility test.*

hemolytic (hē″mō-lĭt′ĭk). Pert. to the breaking down of red blood cells.

hemolytopoietic (hē-mŏl″ĭ-tō-poy-ĕt′ĭk) [Gr. *haima,* blood, + *lysis,* dissolution. + *poiein,* to form]. Rel. to processes of production and destruction of blood cells.

he′molyze. To produce hemolysis.

hemomediastinum (hē″mō-mē″dĭ-ă-stī′nŭm) [Gr. *haima,* blood, + L. *mediastinus,* in the middle]. Effusion of blood into mediastinal spaces. SYN: *hematomediastinum.*

hemometra (hē″mō-mē′trä) [″+ *mētra,* uterus]. Retention of blood within the uterus. SYN: *hematometra.*

hemonephro′sis [″+ *nephros,* kidney, + *ōsis,* condition]. Blood in pelvis of the kidney. SYN: *hematonephrosis.*

hemopath′ic [Gr. *haima,* blood, + *pathos,* disease]. Rel. or due to disease of the blood.

hemopathol′ogy [″+ ″+ *logos,* study]. The science of blood disorders.

hemop′athy. A disease of the blood.

hemoperitone′um [Gr. *haima,* blood, + *peritonaion,* peritoneum]. Effusion of blood into the peritoneal cavity.

hemopexin (hē″mō-pĕks′ĭn) [″+ *pēxis,* fixation]. A globulin of high carbohydrate content which is capable of combining with heme.

hemopex′is (hē″mo-pĕks′ĭs). Blood coagulation.

hemophage (hē′mō-fāj) [Gr. *haima,* blood, + *phagein,* to eat]. A cell destroying red blood cells by phagocytosis.

hemophagocyte (hē″mō-fag′ō-sĭt) [″+ ″+ *kytos,* cell]. A phagocyte that ingests red blood cells.

hemophilia (hē″mō-, hĕm″ō-fĭl′ĭ-ä) [Gr. *haima,* blood, + *philein,* to love]. An hereditary blood disease characterized by greatly prolonged coagulation time. The blood fails to clot and abnormal bleeding occurs. It is a sex-linked hereditary trait, being transmitted by normal heterozygous females who carry the recessive gene. It occurs almost exclusively in males.

    The term h. has been used to designate a variety of coagulation disorders of blood. This has led to confusion which can be prevented by using the word h. to mean what it originally meant and to designate conditions resembling it by the name of the specific coagulation factor which is lacking.

ETIOL: The cause of true h. is deficiency of a factor in plasma necessary for coagulation of blood. This factor is called by several names including factor VIII, antihemophilic globulin, and antihemophilic factor.

SYM: Abnormal tendency to bleed. May cause swelling of the joints.

PROG: Unfavorable; depends upon severity of the disease.

TREATMENT: There is no cure for h. In an emergency, transfusion of fresh whole blood or plasma is required. This provides factor VIII. Hemophiliacs should avoid trauma. Excellent pamphlets concerning home care of the hemophiliac child are available from the National Hemophilia Foundation, 25 West 39th Street, New York, N. Y. 10018.

Subject should carry notice on person that he or she is a hemophiliac so that in case of accident requiring an operation the surgeon may be forewarned and take necessary precautions. SEE: *blood.*

h. B. This term refers to Christmas disease which is a hemophilia-like disease, caused by a lack of factor IX which is the plasma thromboplastin component. Named for the surname of one of the first families in which the disease was recognized.

hemophiliac (hē″mō-fĭl′ĭ-ăk). One afflicted with hemophilia.

he″mophil′ic. 1. Fond of blood, said of bacteria which grow well in culture media containing hemoglobin. 2. Pert. to hemophilia or hemophilics.

Hemophilus (hē-mŏf′ĭl-ŭs) [Gr. *haima,* blood, + *philein,* to love]. A genus of bacteria which require either the growth factor X or V, or both, provided by blood. The small, nonmotile, gram-negative bacilli are aerobic and do not form spores.

The V factor is destroyed by enzymes present in unheated red blood cells. Thus chocolate agar is the preferred culture medium.

H. aegyptius. Koch-Weeks bacillus; the cause of one form of conjunctivitis.

H. ducreyi. The causative organism of chancroid or soft chancre.

H. influenzae. An organism found in respiratory infections and formerly thought to be the cause of influenza, but now considered to be a primary and a secondary invader. It is the causative organism of influenzal meningitis, conjunctivitis, septicemia, and respiratory infections.

H. pertussis. Former name for Bordetella pertussis, the causative organism of whooping cough.

hemophobia (hē″mō-fō′bĭ-ă) [Gr. *haima,* blood, + *phobos,* fear]. Aversion to seeing blood or to bleeding.

hemophor′ic [″+ *phoros,* bearing]. Conveying blood.

hemophthalmia,   **hemophthalmus** (hē″mŏf-thăl′mĭ-ă,   hē″mŏf-thăl′mus) [″+ *ophthalmos,* eye]. Effusion of blood into the eye.

he″moplas′tic [″+ *plassein,* to form]. Blood-forming. SYN: *hemopoietic.*

hemopneumothorax   (hē″mō-nū-mō-thō′răks) [Gr. *haima,* blood, + *pneuma,* air, + *thōrax,* chest]. Blood and air in the pleural cavity.

hemopoiesis (hē″mō-poy-ē′sĭs) [″+ *poiein,* to make]. Formation of blood cells. SYN: *hematopoiesis.*

hemoptysis (hē-mŏp′tĭ-sĭs) [″+ *ptyein,* to spit]. Expectoration of blood arising from hemorrhage of the larynx, trachea, bronchi, or lungs.

Comparison of Hemoptysis and Hematemesis

Hemoptysis	**Hematemesis**
Probable previous history of tuberculosis.	Probable previous history of gastric or duodenal trouble.
Blood is coughed up.	Blood is vomited.
Blood is frothy, bright red, and alkaline in reaction.	Blood is usually (not always) dark, usually not frothy, and acid in reaction. Often clotted.
Blood may be mixed with sputum.	Blood may be mixed with food.
There is some dyspnea, pain, and a tickling sensation in the chest.	There is often nausea and pain referred to stomach.

SYM: Attack sudden. Salty taste. Blood frothy, bright red.

TREATMENT: Cold applications over chest.

NP: Patient must be kept perfectly quiet in bed in a semirecumbent position with head of bed slightly elevated. No movement or excitement permitted and no visitors. Patient should be reassured and kept as quiet as possible. No hot drinks. Light diet.

In tuberculosis, in absence of doctor in case of hemorrhage, follow these rules: Support the patient's head and shoulders with pillows; patient in a semirecumbent position. If the bleeding side is known, incline him towards that side, and, if any feeling of suffocation, loosen clothing about throat and chest. If there be thirst, give chipped ice in small amounts.

Keep patient warm but not hot. Keep patient calm and comforted. Do not adm. any drugs until doctor comes, and on no account give stimulants. An injection of morphine may be prescribed. Should patient faint, hemorrhage may cease. This is often nature's means of cure.

SEE: *bleeding; hematemesis; hemorrhage.*

h., endemic. Paragonimiasis. SEE: *h., parasitic.*

h., parasitic. Spitting of blood resulting from infection of the lungs by Paragonimus westermani, q.v., a parasitic fluke.

hemorrhage (hĕm′ĕ-rĭj) [Gr. *haima*, blood, + *rhĕgnynai*, to burst forth]. Abnormal internal or external discharge of blood. May be venous, arterial, or capillary from blood vessels into tissues, into or from the body.

Venous blood is dark red; flow is continuous. Arterial blood is bright red; flows in jets. Capillary blood is of a reddish color; exudes from tissue.

SYM: Diagnosis is obvious when h. is visible. When internal, diagnosis may be made from the general condition. Patient is in shock; pulse weak, rapid and irregular; face pale; skin cold and moist.

NP: Depends upon location. Remove all dirt with absorbent cotton, using moisture of the blood, not water; apply sterilized qauze sponge; bandage firmly; elevate limb. Patient should recline. Very cold water contracts vessels; warm water increases bleeding. Do not use alum, iron solutions, or other caustics or astringents. If an open wound, apply sterile dressing and a firm bandage. In an emergency, when bleeding is from a small vessel, firm pressure over the actual site of bleeding may be sufficient to stop the bleeding. Continue to apply pressure until definitive treatment can be provided. In the case of a ruptured varicose vein, pressure may be best applied with a flat firm object such as a coin of suitable size.

h., accidental. In obstetrics and gynecology, a h. caused by premature rupture of the placenta. SEE: *ablatio placentae.*

h., antepartum. H. appearing before the onset of labor.

h., armpit. Place sterile gauze sponge into wound; apply pressure over pad. Bandage over shoulder and under armpit of both arms.

h., armpit and elbow, between. Insert sterile gauze sponge into wound; apply pressure over pad, or use tourniquet.

h., arterial. In arterial bleeding (red) the blood ordinarily comes through in waves or spurts. The flow may be steady if the torn artery is deep or buried.

F. A. TREATMENT: It is usually necessary to make pressure along the course of artery somewhere between heart and bleeding point by means of fingers (digitals pressure) on the pressure points and then pressure by a tourniquet above the point of injury. Tourniquet should be used only if absolutely required after other means failed to stop the bleeding. When used, apply only the pressure required to stop the bleeding. Improperly applied, a tourniquet may cause permanent damage to nerves. Elevate the part. Apply a sterile dressing and a firm bandage. Gradually release tourniquet after 12 to 15 minutes; if bleeding begins again, retighten. Do not give stimulants until bleeding is controlled. SEE: *tourniquet.*

h., capillary. Bleeding from minute blood vessels, present in all bleeding. When large vessels are not injured they may be controlled by simple elevation and pressure with a sterile dry compress.

h., carotid artery. Usually accompanied by bleeding from the jugular veins. May be fatal in a short time.

F. A. TREATMENT: Compression with the thumbs transversely across the neck, both above and below the wound, the fingers directed around the back of the neck to aid in compression. It may be more desirable to pack the wound with sterile gauze and compress it with the closed fist. Wounds of the jugular vein are sometimes the cause of air embolism.

h., cerebral. Escape of blood into tissues of brain.

ETIOL: hypertension, arteriosclerosis or atherosclerosis, infections.

SYM: Unconsciousness, slow pulse, stertorous breathing; hemiplegia, death. May be

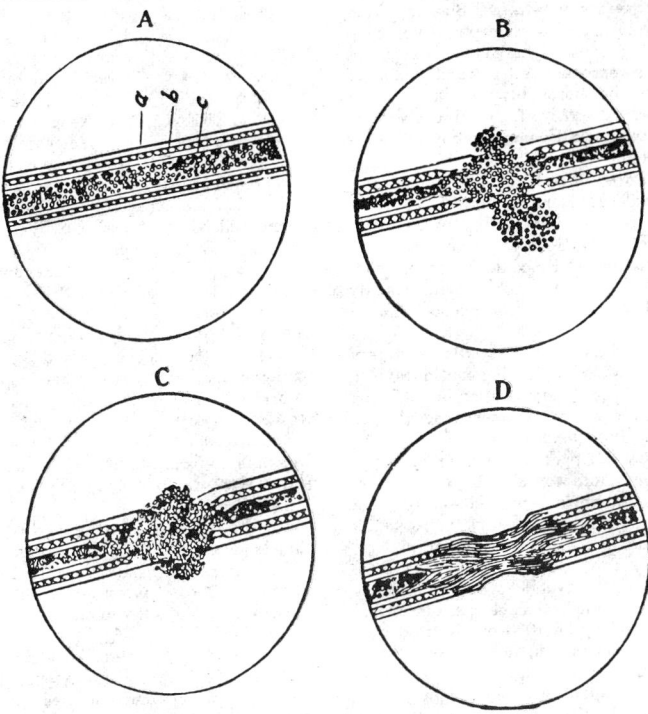

ARREST OF HEMORRHAGE

Temporary and permanent, diagrammatic. A, Normal small artery: a, outer coat, adventitia; b, middle coat, muscular; c, inner coat, intima. B, Artery torn across with retraction of middle and inner coats; contraction of muscular coat. C, Clotting of blood outside and inside the vessel; temporary arrest. D, Obliteration of the lumen of the vessel with fibrous tissue; permanent arrest.

speech disturbance, incontinence of bladder and rectum, or constipation according to location of damaged brain tissue.

TREATMENT: Supportive therapy to maintain airway and oxygenation. Be certain patient is positioned properly to prevent nerve compression of arms. Maintain hydration and fluid and electrolyte balance.

h., consecutive. H. some time after an injury, 20-24 hours after an operation.

TREATMENT: Compress applied to main artery and wound. Elevate parts. Reopen and tie bleeding vessels.

h., contact. H. from the cervix uteri coming on as a result of exertion, contact during coitus, douching, or instrumentation.

h., elbow and hand, between. Apply pad and pressure; bandage over it as a tourniquet.

h. of foot. Apply pad, pressure, and bandage.

h. of hand. If from palmar area, fill hand with large firm pad of sterile gauze and have patient make firm fist around it. Then bandage firmly.

h. of knee. At the knee or below, apply pad with pressure. If behind knee, apply pad at site and bandage leg firmly. Follow same precautions as with tourniquet with respect to loosening at 12-15 minute intervals.

h., lung. Blood bright red and frothy, frequently coughed up.

TREATMENT: Rest in cool bed, shoulders and head raised. Small pieces of ice to swallow. SEE: *hemoptysis.*

h., pancreas. H. of dark blood in vomitus with slimy mucus, coming from pancreas, usually occurring in inflammation of pancreas. SEE: *pancreatitis, hemorrhagic.*

h., petechial. H. in form of small rounded spots or petechiae occurring in the skin or mucous membranes.

h., postmenopausal. Bleeding from the vagina after the menopause has been established. This may be a sign of malignancy of the reproductive tract and should be carefully and thoroughly investigated.

h., postpartum. H., uterine, q.v.

h., primary. H. immediately following any trauma.

h., secondary. H. occurring some time after primary h. It may occur after 24 hrs. or at time of separation of ligature, usually between 7th and 10th day. Due to sepsis.

h., stomach. Blood dark, perhaps clotted or mixed with stomach contents, usually vomited. May be from rupture of esophageal varices.

TREATMENT: Ice to swallow. Surgery may be required if bleeding continues. If h. from esophagus, compression of bleeding site with a special intraesophageal tube balloon may be helpful.

h., thigh. Upper part near groin. Insert pad of gauze into wound and apply pressure or press thumb in center of fold of groin against bone until bleeding stops below groin. Pad, or tourniquet with pad under.

h., typhoid. Gross h. occurs in approx. 10% of cases of typhoid which progress to the stage of ulceration of gastrointestinal tract. Loss may be 1000 ml. It may occur singly or in succession, the latter being more serious than large hemorrhages. H.'s take place at the end of the 2nd week and during the 3rd week of the disease.

h., unavoidable. Ceaseless, painless bleeding from placenta previa, q.v.

h., uterine. H. into cavity of uterus. There are three types of uterine h. *Essential uterine h.:* Occurs in connection with pelvic, uterine, or cervical diseases. SYN: *metropathia haemorrhagica. Intrapartum h.:* during labor. *Postpartum h.:* Occurs after 3rd stage of labor. Due to inversion, rupture, lacerations, relaxation of the uterus, or hematoma.

SEE: *fibrosis uteri.*

ETIOL: Common causes are trauma; congenital abnormalities; pathological processes such as tumors; infections, esp. of alimentary, respiratory, and genitourinary tracts; generalized vascular disorders such as various purpuras; coagulation defects; retained products of conception following criminal or therapeutic abortion.

TREATMENT: Application of umbrella pack, q.v., will apply pressure to uterine arterial supply. A retained placenta, when present and causing hemorrhage, should be removed with uterine forceps. A relaxed uterus may need a hypodermic injection of posterior pituitary extract. The patient may need transfusion and, in some cases, surgery will be required to prevent fatal h.

h., venous. Characterized by steady, profuse bleeding of rather dark blood.

F. A. TREATMENT: Keep patient quiet and try to relieve anxiety; elevate the bleeding part if possible. Apply a sterile dressing and make pressure directly over the wound. Elevation and pressure will control most venous bleeding. Observe closely for signs of shock. SEE: *tourniquet.*

h., vicarious. H. from a part due to suppression in another part. SEE: *vicarious menstruation.*

hemorrhage, words pert. to: anthemorrhagic; autotransfusion; bleeding; clotting; coagulation; hematorrhea; hemophilia; rhinorrhagia; Werlhoff's disease; wound.

hemorrhagenic   (hĕm″o-rä-jĕn′ĭk)   [Gr. *haima,* blood, + *rhēgnynai,* to burst forth, + *gennan,* to form]. Producing hemorrhage.

hemorrhagic (hĕm-ō-răj′ĭk). Pert. to or marked by hemorrhage.

h. disease of the newborn. Due to inadequate supply of prothrombin received from mother or delay in establishment of bacterial flora of intestine which produces vitamin K. Adm. of vitamin K. corrects the condition.

h. fever, epidemic. An acute h. illness characterized by thrombocytopenia, acute vascular injury, and impaired renal function. There is nausea, vomiting, headache, high fever, and chills. The disease is thought to be caused by a virus. It occurs in Europe and Asia. There is no specific treatment.

h. fevers. A group of diseases due to arthropod-borne viruses. This includes yellow fever, Omsk h. fever, Crimean h. fever, North and South Vietnam h. fever, Argentinian h. fever, Bolivian h. fever, and Kyasanur Forest disease (India).

hemorrhagiparous   (hĕm″ō-răj-ĭp′ă-rŭs)   [Gr. *haima,* blood, + *rhēgnynai,* to burst forth, + L. *parēre,* to produce]. Producing hemorrhage. SYN: *hemorrhagenic.*

hemorrhea (hĕm″ō-rē′ă) [″+ *rhioa,* flow]. Hemorrhage, q.v.

hemorrhoid (hĕm′ō-royd) [Gr. *haimorrhois*]. A mass of dilated, tortuous veins in the anorectum involving the venous plexuses of that area. There are two kinds: external, those involving veins distal to the anorectal line; internal, those involving veins proximal to the anorectal line.

TREATMENT: Depends upon the severity of the symptoms, not the extent of the hemorrhoids. In many instances, the only therapy required is improvement in anal hygiene and administration of stool softeners to prevent straining to have a bowel movement. The decision concerning the necessity of surgery should not be made until acute symptoms and inflammation have subsided. This allows tissues to regain their usual shape. SEE: *hemorrhoidectomy; piles.*

hemorrhoidal (hĕm-ō-roy'dăl). Rel. to hemorrhoids. 2. Pert. to certain anal arteries; arteria hemorrhoidalis.

hemorrhoidectomy (hĕm''ō-royd-ĕk'tō-ī) [Gr. *haimorrhois,* vein liable to bleed, + *ektomē,* excision]. Surgical excision of hemorrhoids.

NP: In order to prevent difficult bowel movements postoperatively, give cleansing enema preoperatively and start stool softeners three days prior to surgery and keep them up for at least one week postoperatively.

Preoperative: Patient in lithotomy position. A towel, wet with antiseptic solution, is placed over external genitalia. The operating field is thoroughly scrubbed with soap and water and flushed with a topical antiseptic. The patient is draped with leggings; lithotomy sheet.

Postoperative: Knees tied together until anesthetic has worn off. Head and shoulders elevated on pillows. After each bowel movement cleanse anus gently, but thoroughly, with physiological saline solution and renew dressing. Repack as necessary. Redress 2nd day with petrolatum gauze or dry dressing. Watch for retention of urine and possibility of hemorrhage.

DRESSING: Petrolatum, gauze, sponges, gauze strips 3 and 8 in. (7.62 cm. and 20.32 cm.) wide, cotton and T bandages, leg holders, solution for irrigation.

hemosal'pinx [Gr. *haima,* blood, + *salpinx,* tube]. Blood accumulated in an oviduct. SYN: *hematosalpinx.*

hemosiderin (hē''mō-sĭd'ĕr-ĭn) [''+ *sidēros,* iron]. An iron-containing pigment derived from hemoglobin from disintegration of red blood cells. It is one method whereby iron is stored until it is needed for making hemoglobin.

he''mosidero'sis [''+ ''+ *ōsis,* condition]. Condition characterized by the deposition, esp. in liver and spleen, of hemosiderin. Occurs in diseases in which there is marked red cell destruction, such as hemolytic anemias, pernicious anemia, and chronic infection.

hemosozic (hē''mō-, hĕm''ō-sō'zĭk) [''+ *sozein,* to save]. That which protects red blood cells from hemolysis.

hemospasia (hē''mō-spā'zĭ-ă) [Gr. *haima,* blood, + *spaein,* to draw]. Withdrawal of blood by cupping or leeching.

hemosper'mia [''+ *sperma,* seed]. Bloody semen. SYN: *hematospermia.*

Hemosporidia (hē-mō-spōr-ĭ'dĭ-ă) [''+ *sporos,* seed]. An order of parasites found in the blood of various animals, including man.

hemostasis (hē-mŏs'tă-sĭs) [''+ *stasis,* stopping]. 1. Arrest of bleeding or of circulation. SYN: *hemostasia.* 2. Stagnation of blood.

he'mostat [''+ *statikos,* standing]. 1. Device or medicine which arrests the flow of blood. 2. Compressor for controlling hemorrhage of the tonsils.

he''mostat'ic. 1. Checking hemorrhage. 2. Any drug, medicine, or blood component that serves to stop bleeding. Ex: vitamin K, whole blood, or epinephrine applied locally.

hemostyp'tic [Gr. *haima,* blood, + *styptikos,* astringent]. An astringent that stops bleeding; chemically hemostatic.

hemotachometer (hē''mō-tă-kŏm'ē-ter) [''+ *tachos,* swiftness, + *metron,* measure]. Device for measuring velocity of the blood.

hemotherapeu'tics [''+ *therapeutikē,* medical practice]. The use of blood, by transfusion or otherwise, in treatment of disease.

hemother'apy [''+ *therapeia,* treatment]. Blood transfusion as a therapeutic measure. SYN: *hematotherapeutics.*

hemothorax (hē''mō-thō'răks) [Gr. *haima,* blood, + *thōrax,* chest]. Bloody fluid in the pleural cavity caused by rupture of small blood vessels, due to inflammation of the lungs in pneumonia, pulmonary tuberculosis, or a malignant growth.

hemothymia (hē''mō-thī'mĭ-ă) [''+ *thymos,* anger]. An irrestible impulse to murder.

hemotoxin (hē''mō-tŏks'ĭn) [''+ *toxikon,* poison]. A toxin destructive of red blood cells. SYN: *hemolysin.*

hemotrip'sia [''+ *tripsis,* a rubbing]. Hemorrhage in one part that induces hemorrhage in another part.

hemotrophic (hē-mō-trŏf'ĭk) [Gr. *haima,* blood, + *trophē,* nourishment]. Pert. to nutrient substances carried in the blood.

h. nutrition. Nutrition of the fetus by substances in the maternal blood which pass to the blood of the fetus through vessels within the villi.

hemotropic (hē-mō-trŏp'ĭk) [''+ *tropos,* turning]. Attracted to or having an affinity for blood or blood cells.

hemotympanum (hē''mō-tĭm'pă-nŭm) [''+ *tympanon,* drum]. Blood in the middle ear.

hemozoin (hē''mō-zō'ĭn). A dark pigment found within malarial organisms (plasmodia). It is derived from the disintegration of hemoglobin.

he'mozoon. A hematozoon, q.v.

henbane. Hyoscyamus, q.v.

Henle's ampul'la. [Freidrich G. J. Henle, Ger. anatomist, 1809-85] A ductus deferens dilatation just above the ejaculatory duct.

Henle's layer. Outer layer of cells of inner root sheath of hair follicle.

Henle's loop. A U-shaped portion of a renal tubule lying between the proximal and distal convoluted portions. Consists of a thin descending limb and a thicker ascending limb.

Henle's membrane. Bruch's layer forming inner boundary of the choroid of the eye.

Henle's sheath. Connective tissue support of individual nerve fibers in a funiculus. SYN: *endoneurium.*

Henoch-Schönlein purpura (hĕn'ŏk-shän'lĭn). [Edouard H. Henoch, Ger. pediatrician, 1820-1910; Johann L. Schönlein, Ger. physician, 1793-1864] A form of allergic purpura with erythema, urticaria, effusions of serum into subcutaneous or submucous tissue or viscera, accompanied by gastrointestinal and joint symptoms. Syndrome seen mostly in children.

henry (hĕn'rĭ). [Joseph Henry, Amer. physicist, 1797-1878] Unit designating electrical inductance.

Hensen's cells. [Victor Hensen, Ger. anatomist and physiologist, 1835-1924] Tall columnar cells which form the outer border cells of the organ of Corti of the cochlea.

Hensen's disk. Band in center of the A disk of a sarcomere of striated muscle. During contraction it appears lighter than the remaining portion and in its center, a dark stripe, the M stripe, is seen.

Hensen's stripe. A dark band on the under surface of the tectorial membrane of the inner ear.

he'par [Gr. *hēpar,* liver]. The liver, q.v.

heparin (hĕp'ă-rĭn). A mucoitin polysulfuric acid which has been isolated from the liver, lung, and other tissues. It is produced by the mast cells of the liver and by basophil leukocytes. It inhibits coagulation by preventing conversion of prothrombin to thrombin by forming an antithrombin, and by preventing liberation of thromboplastin from blood platelets. The action of heparin requires the presence of a co-factor found in serum albumin of the plasma. Available as sodium heparin (USP).

USES: An anticoagulant in prevention and treatment of thrombosis and embolism and in treating frostbite. Sometimes employed concurrently with dicumarol, q.v.

The antagonist for an overdose is protamine sulfate.

hep'arinize. To inhibit coagulation of blood with heparin.

hepatalgia (hĕp″ă-tal′jĭ-ă) [Gr. *hēpar, hēpat-,* liver, + *algos,* pain]. Pain in the liver. SYN: *hepatodynia.*

hepatal′gic. Pert. to hepatalgia.

hepatatrophia (hĕp″at-ă-tro′fĭ-ă) [Gr. *hepat-,* liver, + *atrophia,* atrophy]. Atrophied condition of the liver.

hepatauxe (hĕp″at-awk′se) ["+ *auxē,* increase]. Enlargement or hypertrophy of the liver.

hepatectomy (hĕp″ă-tĕk′tō-mĭ) ["+ *ektomē,* excision]. Excision of part or all of liver.

hepat′ic [Gr. *hēpar, hēpat-,* liver]. Pert. to the liver.

  h. amebiasis. Infection of the liver by Entamoeba histolytica resulting in hepatitis and abscess formation. Usually a sequel to amebic dysentery. SEE: *amebiasis.*

  h. duct. The canal that receives bile from the liver. It unites with cystic duct to form the common bile duct.

  h. flexure. The right bend of colon under the liver. The junction of the ascending and transverse colon.

  h. lobes. Divisions of the liver.

  h. veins. The three vessels returning blood from the liver and discharging into the inferior vena cava.

  h. zones. Venous, arterial, and portal regions.

hepaticoduodenostomy (hĕ-păt″ĭ-ko-du″o-dĕ-nos′to-mĭ) ["+ L. *duodenum,* duodenum, + Gr. *stoma,* opening]. Making an artificial opening between hepatic duct and duodenum.

hepaticoenterostomy (hĕ-păt″ĭ-ko-en-ter-os′to-mĭ) ["+ *enteron,* intestine, + *stoma,* opening]. Operation for artificial opening between hepatic duct and intestine.

hepaticogastrostomy (hĕ-păt″ĭ-ko-gas-tros′to-mĭ) ["+ *gastēr,* stomach, + *stoma,* opening]. The operation for a passage between the hepatic duct and the stomach.

hepaticolithotripsy (hĕ-păt″ĭ-ko-lĭth′o-trip-sĭ) [Gr. *hēpar, hēpat-,* liver, + *lithos,* stone, + *tripsis,* a crushing]. The crushing of a biliary calculus in the hepatic duct.

hepaticostomy (hĕ-păt″ĭ-kŏs′tō-mĭ) ["+ *stoma,* opening]. Establishment of permanent fistula into hepatic duct.

hepaticot′omy ["+ *tomē,* incision]. Incision into the hepatic duct.

hepatitis (hĕp″ă-tī′tĭs) [Gr. *hēpar, hēpat-,* liver, + *-itis,* inflammation]. Inflammation of the liver of virus or toxic origin. It is usually manifest by jaundice and, in some instances, liver enlargement. Fever and other systemic disorders are usually present.

h., acute anicteric. H. marked by slight fever, gastrointestinal upset and anorexia, but no jaundice.

h., cholangiolitic. H. characterized by jaundice, tiredness, pruritus, vomiting of bile, and hepatomegaly. SYN: *cholestatic h.*

h., fulminant. H. marked by sudden onset of nausea and vomiting, chills, high fever, severe and early jaundice, convulsions, shock, deep coma, and death usually within 10 days. SYN: *massive necrosis of liver.*

h., homologous serum. H. in which the virus is transmitted parenterally by blood transfusion, plasma, needles or other parenteral instruments. Incubation period varies from six weeks to six months. Marked by sudden onset of headache, fever, chills, general weakness, nausea, vomiting, abdominal pain, prostration, jaundice, pruritus, enlarged and tender liver. SYN: *homologous serum jaundice; inoculation h.; serum h.; transfusion jaundice.*

h., infectious. H. occurring sporadically and in epidemics. Transmitted by oral or parenteral route. Incubation period is two to six weeks. Gastrointestinal and respiratory disturbances followed by sudden onset of jaundice, enlarged and tender liver, pruritus, muscle pain, splenomegaly, loss of weight. SYN: *epidemic h.; epidemic jaundice.*

h., toxic. H. caused by exposure to certain poisons (as carbon tetrachloride) or drugs (as sulfonamides), the latter causing hypersensitivity in some patients.

hepatitis-associated antigen. An antigen found in the serum of some of the persons who have had either serum or infectious hepatitis. At one time called the Australian antigen (AU antigen). ABBR: HAA.

hepatization (hep″ă-tĭ-zā'shŭn) [Gr. *hēpar, hēpat-,* liver]. The second and third stages in consolidation in lobar pneumonia. The surface of the lung has the appearance of liver tissue.

hepato- [Gr.]. Prefix indicating the liver.

hepatocele (hep′ă-to-sēl) [Gr. *hēpar, hēpat-,* liver, + *kēlē,* hernia]. Hernia of the liver.

hepatocholangiocystoduodenostomy (hĕp″ă-to-ko-lan″jĭ-o-sis″to-du″o-dē-nos′to-mĭ) [″+ *cholē,* bile, + *angeion,* vessel, + *kystis,* bladder, + L. *duodenum,* + Gr. *stoma,* opening]. Establishment of drainage of bile ducts into the duodenum through the gallbladder.

hepatocholangioduodenostomy (hĕp″-ă-to-ko-lan″jĭ-o-du-o-dē-nos′to-mĭ) [″+ ″+ ″+ L. *duodenum,* + Gr. *stoma,* opening]. Establishment of drainage of bile ducts into the duodenum.

hepatocholangioenterostomy (hĕp″ă-to-ko-lăn″jĭ-o-en″ter-ŏs′tō-mĭ) [″+ ″+ ″+ *enteron,* intestine, + *stoma,* opening]. Establishment of a passage between the liver and intestine.

hepatocholangiogastrostomy (hĕp″ă-to-ko-lan″jĭ-o-gas-tros′to-mĭ) [″+ ″+ ″+ *gastēr,* belly, + *stoma,* opening]. Establishment of drainage of bile ducts into the stomach.

hepatocholangiostomy (hĕp″ă-to-ko-lan-jĭ-os′to-mĭ) [″+ ″+ ″+ *stoma,* opening]. Establishment of free drainage by opening into the gall duct.

hepatocirrhosis (hĕp″ă-to-sĭ-ro′sis) [Gr. *hepat-,* liver, + *kirrhos,* tawny, + *-ōsis,* condition]. Cirrhosis of liver.

hepatocol'ic [″+ *kōlon,* colon]. Rel. to both liver and colon.

hepatocys'tic [″+ *kystis,* bladder]. Rel. to the liver and gallbladder, or the gallbladder.

hepatoduodenostomy (hĕp″ă-to-du″o-dē-nŏs′tō-mĭ) [″+ L. *duodenum,* + Gr. *stoma,* opening]. Establishment of an opening from the liver into the duodenum. SYN: *hepaticoduodenostomy.*

hepatodynia (hĕp″ă-tō-dīn′ĭ-ă) [Gr. *hepat-,* liver, + *odynē,* pain]. Pain in the liver.

hepatodysentery (hĕp″ă-to-dĭs′ĕn-tĕr-ĭ) [″+ *dys,* bad, + *enteron,* intestine]. Inflammation of the liver causing dysentery.

hepatoenteric (hĕp″ă-to-en-tĕr′ĭk) [″+ *enteron,* intestine]. Rel. to the liver and intestines.

hepatogas'tric [″+ *gastēr,* belly]. Rel. to the liver and stomach.

hepatogenic (hĕp-ă-to-jĕn′ik) [″+ *gennan,* to produce]. Having its origin in the liver.

hepatogenous (hĕp-ă-tŏj′ĕ-nus). Originating in the liver.

hepatog'raphy [Gr. *hēpar, hēpat-,* liver, + *graphein,* to write.]. 1. Treatise on human liver. 2. Roentgenography of the liver.

hepatohemia (hĕp″ă-to-hē′mĭ-ă) [″+ *haima,* blood]. Liver congestion.

hep'atoid [″+ *eidos,* form]. Having the structural form of the liver.

hepatolenticular (hĕp″ă-to-len-tik′u-lăr) [Gr. *hepat-,* liver, + L. *lenticula,* lentil, lens]. Rel. to lenticular nucleus and the liver.

h. degeneration. Progressive lenticular degeneration in cirrhosis of the liver. SEE: *Wilson's disease.*

h. disease. Wilson's disease, q.v.

hepatolith (hĕp′ă-to-lĭth) ["+ *lithos*, stone]. A biliary concretion in the liver.

hepatolithiasis (hĕp″ă-to-lĭ-thī′ă-sis) ["+ *lithos*, stone, + *-iasis*, diseased condition]. Calculi or concretions in the liver.

hepatol′ogist ["+ *logos*, study]. A specialist in diseases of the liver.

hepatolysin (hĕp″ă-tol′ĭ-sin) [Gr. *hepat-*, liver, + *lysis*, dissolution]. A cytolysin destructive to hepatic cells.

hepatol′ysis. Liver cell destruction.

hepatolyt′ic. Destructive to tissues of the liver.

hepatoma (hĕp-ă-tō′mă) [Gr. *hepat-*, liver, + *-ōma*, tumor]. A tumor of the liver.

hepatomalacia (hĕp″ă-to-mă-la′sĭ-ă) ["+ *malakia*, softening]. Softening of the liver.

hepatomegaly (hĕp″ă-to-mĕg′ă-lĭ) ["+ *megas*, large]. Enlargement of the liver.

hepatomelanosis (hĕp″ă-to-mel″ă-nō′sis) ["+ *melas*, black, + *ōsis*, condition]. Pigmented deposits or melanosis in the liver.

hepatonephri′tis [Gr. *hepat-*, liver, + *nephros*, kidney, + *-itis*, inflammation]. Inflammation of both liver and kidneys.

hepatonephromegaly (hĕp″ă-tō-nĕf′rō-mĕg′ă-lĭ) ["+ " + *megas*, large]. Hypertrophy of both liver and kidney or kidneys.

    h. glycogenica. Von Gierke's disease, characterized by hypertrophy of liver and excess accumulation of glycogen resulting from failure of glycogenolysis to occur.

hepatopathy (hĕp-ă-tŏp′ă-thĭ) ["+ *pathos*, disease]. Disease of the liver.

hepatoperitonitis (hĕp″ă-to-per″ĭ-to-nī′tis) ["+ *peritonaion*, peritoneum, + *-itis*, inflammation]. Inflammation of the peritoneal covering of the liver. SYN: *perihepatitis.*

hep′atopexy [Gr. *hēpat*, liver, + *pēxis*, fixation]. Fixation of a movable liver to abdominal wall.

hepatophage (hep′ă-to-fāj) ["+ *phagein*, to eat]. A phagocyte that attacks liver cells.

hepatoportogram. X-ray examination of the portal vein and its branches in the liver.

hepatoptosia, hepatoptosis (hĕp″ă-tŏp-tō′sĭ-ă, -tō′sĭs) ["+ *ptōsis*, a dropping]. Downward displacement of the liver.

hepatopulmonary (hĕp″ă-to-pŭl′mo-năr″ĭ) ["+ L. *pulmō*, lung]. Rel. to both liver and lungs.

hepatorenal (hĕp″ă-to-rē′năl) ["+ L. *renalis*, kidney]. Pert. to both liver and kidneys.

hepatorrhaphy (hĕp″ă-tŏr′ă-fĭ) [Gr. *hēpat-*, liver, + *raphē*, suture]. The suturing of a wound of the liver.

hepatorrhea (hĕp″ă-to-rē′ă) ["+ *rhoia*, flow]. 1. Bilious diarrhea. 2. Morbid flow from the liver.

hepatorrhexis (hĕp″ă-to-rĕks′is) ["+ *rhēxis*, rupture]. Rupture of the liver.

hepatos′copy ["+ *skopein*, to examine]. Inspection of the liver.

hepatosplenitis (hĕp″ă-to-splĕ-nī′tĭs) [Gr. *hēpat-*, liver, + *splēn*, spleen, + *-itis*, inflammation]. Inflamed condition of both liver and spleen.

hepatosplenomegaly (hĕp″ă-to-splĕ″no-mĕg′ă-lĭ) ["+ " + *megas*, large]. Enlargement of both liver and spleen.

hepatostomy (hĕp″ă-tŏs′tō-mĭ) ["+ *stoma*, opening]. The making of an artificial fissure into the liver.

hepatotherapy (hĕp″ă-to-thĕr′ă-pĭ) ["+ *therapeia*, treatment]. 1. Treatment of liver disease. 2. The use of liver or liver extract.

hepatotomy (hĕp″ă-tŏt′ō-mĭ) [Gr. *hēpat-*, liver, + *tomē*, incision]. Incision into the liver.

hepatotoxemia (hĕp″ă-to-tŏks-ē′mĭ-ă) ["+ *toxikon*, poison, + *haima*, blood]. Autointoxication due to malfunctioning of the liver.

hepatotoxin (hĕp″ă-to-tŏk′sĭn). A cytotoxin specific for liver cells.

heptachromic (hĕp″tă-krō′mĭk) [Gr. *hepta*, seven, + *chrōma*, color]. Possessing normal color vision.

hep′tad ["+ L. *ad*, to]. Any element with a valence of seven.

heptose (hĕp′tōs). Any sugar containing seven carbon atoms in its molecule.

heptosuria (hĕp″to-sū′rĭ-ă) [Gr. *hepta*, seven, + *ouron*, urine]. Heptose in the urine.

herb (erb) [L. *herba*, grass]. A plant with a soft stem containing little wood, esp. one of the aromatic plants used in medicine or as seasoning.

herbivorous (hĕr-bĭv′o-rus) ["+ *vorāre*, to eat]. Vegetarian; feeding on grasses and herbs.

herd [AS. *heord*]. Any large aggregation of people or animals.

    h. instinct. The urge to remain one of the social group and to conform to social patterns and general opinions. An aversion to excessive individualism.

hered′itary [L. *hereditarius*, an heir]. Transmitted or inherited from one's ancestors.

    h. ataxia. H. spinal ataxia. SYN: *Friedreich's ataxia.* SEE: *ataxia, h.*

heredity (hĕ-rĕd′ĭ-tĭ) [L. *hereditas*, heir]. Innate capacity of an individual to develop traits and characteristics (body size and form, skin and hair color, intellectual capacity, tendency to certain diseases) possessed by its ancestors. Such is dependent upon the presence of genes (hereditary factors or determiners) in the chromosomes of the fertilized ovum from which the individual develops.

RS: chromosome; gene; genetics; linkage; sex.

heredo- [L. *hered-*, heir]. Prefix meaning heredity.

heredoataxia (hĕr″ē-do-ă-tăks′ĭ-ă) [L. *heres, hered-*, heir, + Gr. *ataxia*, lack of order]. Hereditary spinal ataxia. SYN: *Friedreich's ataxia.* SEE: *ataxia, hereditary.*

Hering-Breuer reflex (hĕr′ĭng-broy′ĕr). [Carl Ewald K. Hering, Ger. physiologist, 1834-1918, and Josef Breuer, Ger. physician, 1842-1925] Reflex inhibition of inspiration resulting from stimulation of pressoreceptors by inflation of the lungs.

Hering's nerves. [Heinrich Ewald Hering, Austrian physician, 1866 —] Afferent nerve fibers leading from carotid sinus via glossopharyngeal nerve to the brain. They are pressoreceptor nerves responding to changes in blood pressure which reflexly control heart rate. An increase in pressure diminishes heart rate.

Her'ing's theory. [Carl Ewald K. Hering, Ger. physiologist, 1834-1918] A theory of color vision in which it is assumed that the retina possesses three photochemical substances which, depending on their decomposition or resynthesis, produce different color sensations by their stimulation of different nerve endings.

heritage (hĕr′ĭ-tĭj) [L. *heres*, heir]. All the characteristics transmitted by parents to their children.

hermaphrodism (hĕr-măf′ro-dizm). Hermaphroditism, q.v.

hermaphrodite (hĕr-măf′rō-dīt) [Gr. *Hermaphroditos*, son of Hermes and Aphrodite, who was man and woman combined]. One possessing genital and sexual characteristics of both sexes. The clitoris is usually enlarged, resembling the penis of the male. SYN: *androgyne.*

RS: gynandry.

hermaphroditism (hĕr-măf′ro-dīt-izm). Condition in which both ovarian and testicular tissue exist in the same individual. Occurs rarely in humans. SYN: *hermaphrodism.*

    h., **complex.** Having internal and external organs of both sexes.

    h., **dimidiate.** Lateral h., q.v.

    h., **false.** Pseudohermaphroditism; possession of the sex glands of one sex (ovary or testis) but accompanied by secondary sexual characteristics and external genitalia of the opposite sex.

    h., **lateral.** Possession of a testis on one side and an ovary on the other.

    h., **spurious.** False h.

    h., **transverse.** Having the outward organs indicating one sex, and the internal ones the other.

    h., **true.** H. in which the individual possesses both ovarian and testicular gonads.

    h., **unilateral.** H. in which an ovary and a testis or an ovotestis are present on one side and either an ovary or testis present on the other side.

hermet'ic. Airtight.

hermetical (hĕr-mĕt′ĭk-ăl). Airtight.

hernia (hĕr′nĭ-ă) [L.]. The protrusion or projection of an organ or a part of an organ through the wall of the cavity which normally contains it. SYN: *rupture.*

    ETIOL: Failure of certain normal openings to close during development; weakness resulting from debilitating illness, old age, or injury; prolonged distention as from tumors, pregnancy, or corpulence; increased intraabdominal pressure resulting from lifting heavy loads, or coughing.

    TREATMENT: 1. Surgery. 2. Mechanical reduction. 3. In very large hernias, mechanical devices or trusses may be used.

    RS: herniotomy; rupture.

    h., **abdominal.** H. through the abdominal wall.

    h., **acquired.** H. which develops any time after birth in contrast to one present at birth (congenital h.). Usually the result of excessive strain on the muscular wall. Frequently occurs following injuries or operations.

    h., **bladder.** Protrusion of the bladder or a part of bladder through normal or abnormal orifice.

    h., **cerebral.** H. of the brain through the cranial wall.

    h., **Cloquet's.** A type of femoral h.

    h., **complete.** H. in which sac and its contents have passed through the aperture.

    h., **concealed.** H. that is imperceptible when palpated.

    h., **congenital.** H. existing from birth.

    h., **crural.** SEE: *h., femoral.*

    h., **cystic.** Bladder h. SYN: *cystocele.*

    h. **of diaphragm.** There are three groups: congenital, acquired or traumatic, and esophageal. In the latter, a portion of the diaphragm is pushed through the esophageal hiatus into the stomach; or h. protruding through the diaphragm.

    h., **direct.** SEE: *h., inguinal.*

    h., **diverticular.** Protrusion of intestinal congenital diverticulum.

    h., **encysted.** Scrotal protrusion which, enveloped in its own sac, passes into the tunica vaginalis.

h., epigastric. H. of the intestine through an opening in the midline above the umbilicus.

h., fascial. Protrusion of muscular tissue through its fascial covering.

h., femoral. Descending of intestines through femoral ring.

h., funicular. H. into the umbilical or spermatic cord.

h., hiatus. Protrusion of the stomach upward into the mediastinal cavity through the esophageal hiatus of the diaphragm.

h., Holthouse's. SEE: *h., inguinocrural.*

h., incarcerated. H. completely obstructing the bowels.

h., incomplete. H. which has not gone completely through the aperture.

h., indirect. SEE: *h., inguinal.*

h., inguinal. Protrusion of the hernial sac containing the intestine at the inguinal opening. In indirect lateral or oblique inguinal h., the sac protrudes through the internal inguinal ring into the inguinal canal often descending into the scrotum; in direct medial inguinal h., the hernial sac protrudes through the abdominal wall in the region of Hesselbach's triangle, a region bounded by the rectus abdominus muscle, inguinal ligament, and inferior epigastric vessels. Inguinal h. accounts for about 80% of all h.'s.

h., inguinocrural. H. which is femoral and inguinal.

h., internal. H. which occurs within the abdominal cavity. May be intraperitoneal or retroperitoneal.

h., interstitial. Form of inguinal h. in which the hernial sac lies between layers of the abdominal muscles. SYN: *intermuscular hernia.*

h., irreducible. H. which cannot be returned to its orignal position out of its sac by manual methods.

h., labial. Protrusion of a loop of bowel into the labium majus.

h., lateral. SEE: *h., inguinal.*

h., lumbar. In lumbar regions or loins.

h., medial. SEE: *h., inguinal.*

h., mesocolic. H. between the layers of the mesocolon.

h., nuckian. H. into canal of Nuck.

h., oblique. SEE: *h., inguinal.*

h., obturator. H. through the obturator foramen.

h., omental. H. containing a portion of the omentum.

h., ovarian. Presence of an ovary in a hernial sac.

h., phrenic. Projecting through the diaphragm into one of the pleural cavities.

h., posterior vaginal. H. of Douglas' sac downward between rectum and posterior vaginal wall. SYN: *enterocele,* q.v.

h., properitoneal. Protrusion through the peritoneum and into the abdominal wall.

h., reducible. H. which can be replaced by manipulation.

h., retroperitoneal. H. into peritoneal sac extending behind the peritoneum into the iliac fossa.

h., Richter's. H. in which only a portion of wall of intestine protrudes, the main portion of the intestine being excluded from the hernial sac and the lumen remaining open.

h., scrotal. One that descends into the scrotum.

h., strangulated. One so tightly constricted that gangrene results if operation does not relieve. Not reducible by ordinary means.

h., umbilical. Occurring at the navel. More frequent in women than men. Treated by surgery.

h., uterine. Presence of the uterus in the hernial sac.

h., vaginal. Hernial protrusion of the vagina.

h., vaginolabial. H. of a viscus into the posterior end of the labium majus.

h., ventral. H. through the abdominal wall. If stretching and thinning of an abdominal scar occur, pressure from the abdomen may cause protrusion of part of the gut. It is then protected only by a layer of thin scar tissue.

her′nial [L. *hernia,* rupture]. Pert. to a hernia.

h. sac. The pouch of peritoneum pushed before a hernia and into which it descends.

her′niated. Having a hernia.

h. disk. Rupture or herniation of the intervertebral disk, esp. between lumbar vertebrae. This usually causes pain in the affected side. SYN: *herniated nucleus pulposus.*

herniation (hĕr-nĭ-ā′shŭn). Development of a hernia.

hernioenterotomy (hĕr″nĭ-o-ĕn″tĕr-ŏt′ō-mĭ) [L. *hernia,* rupture, + Gr. *enteron,* intestine, + *tomē,* incision]. Herniotomy at same time as enterotomy.

her′nioid ["+ Gr. *eidos,* resemblance]. Resembling a hernia.

herniolaparotomy (hĕr″nĭ-o-lăp″ă-rŏt′ō-mĭ) ["+ Gr. *lapara,* loin, + *tomē,* incision]. Abdominal surgery for the cure of hernia.

herniol′ogy ["+ Gr. *logos,* study]. The science of hernia.

her′nioplasty [″+ Gr. *plassein*, to form]. Surgical operation for hernia.

herniopuncture (hĕr′nĭ-o-pŭnk′chur) [″+ *punctura*, puncture]. Puncture of a hernia with hollow needle for withdrawal of fluid or gas.

herniorrhaphy (hĕr-nĭ-or′ă-fĭ) [L. *hernia*, rupture, + Gr. *rhaphē*, a suture]. Surgical operation for hernia.

herniotomy (hĕr-nĭ-ŏt′ō-mĭ) [″+ Gr. *tomē*, incision]. Surgery for the relief of hernia; an operation for the correction of irreducible hernia, esp. strangulated hernia.

NP: Paint area with topical antiseptic as ordered. Place sterile towel over chest and abdomen, place lap ring (small sheet about a yard square, with opening in center) over area of incision. Place an open regular lap sheet on abdomen. Place four towels around area of incision, two lengthwise and two crosswise.

When the operator is finished with an instrument, discard it and remove from sterile field. While the skin is being sutured prepare final dressing. The operating nurse washes off her gloves thoroughly before removing them. She then assists in replacing the dressing. In bilateral hernias, each side should be draped and treated as a separate operation.

Towels, gauze sponges, gauze compresses, safety pins, bandages, and cotton are used for dressing. One pillow under head until otherwise ordered, elevate legs to prevent strain on abdominal muscles—assist in turning, etc.

heroin (hĕr′ō-ĭn). A narcotic derived from morphine. Importation of this drug is illegal in the United States. SYN: *diacetylmorphine.* SEE: *drug addiction.*

   h. toxicity. Poisoning by heroin.

TREATMENT: Acute. Establish and maintain an airway. Remove false teeth, and clean mouth and pharynx of mucus, blood, etc. Give mouth-to-mouth or mouth-to-nose artificial respiration if necessary.

Assess and treat any abnormality of cardiac function. Use cardiac massage, defibrillator, or cardiac pacer as needed. Treat pulmonary edema with continuous positive pressure respiration.

Administer I.V. (may have to use femoral or jugular vein) opiate antagonist such as levallorphan tartrate or nalorphine hydrochloride according to directions in package. Also administer a respiratory stimulant such as 3-5 ml. of doxapram hydrochloride I.V.

Stay with patient until he is fully responsive. A long-acting narcotic may continue to act after short-acting antagonist has worn off. If patient fails to respond look for another cause for the coma.

heroinism (hĕr′ō-ĭn-ĭzm) [heroin + Gr. *ismos*, condition]. Addiction to use of heroin. SEE: *drug addiction.*

herpangina (hĕrp-ăn-jī′nă, hĕrp-ăn′jĭ-nă) [Gr. *herpēs*, shingles, a creeping, + L. *angina*, a choking]. A benign, infectious disease of children and, less commonly, of young adults. Occurs in epidemic form throughout the world, most often in summer and early fall.

ETIOL: One of several strains of Coxsackie virus.

SYM: Sudden onset of fever, severe sore throat, nausea, vomiting, excess salivation, and malaise. The throat and posterior area of the mouth are covered with vesicles 1 to 2 mm. in diameter which rupture and form ulcers.

TREATMENT: Symptomatic and supportive. There is no specific therapy.

herpes (hĕr′pēz) [Gr. *herpēs*, shingles, a creeping, from *herpein*, to creep]. A word which at one time was used to indicate a vesicular eruption due to a virus, esp. herpes simplex or herpes zoster. Also it indicated what lay people call a "cold sore" or "fever blister." Its use as a single word is imprecise. SEE: subentries below, esp. *h. simiae; h. simplex; h. zoster.*

   h. facialis. A form of h. simplex, q.v., which occurs on the face.

   h. genitalis. Herpetic lesions on the male or female genitalia.

   h. labialis. H. simplex, q.v., occurring on the lips. SYN: *cold sore; fever blister.*

   h. menstrualis. Herpetic lesions appearing at the time of the menstrual period.

   h., mouth. H. marked by appearance of multiple whitish areas on soft palate and mucosa of mouth. SYN: *gingivostomatitis.*

   h. praeputialis. H. of the male genitals.

   h. progenitalis. H. simplex of vulva.

   h. simiae. Spread from monkeys to man. Almost always fatal. SYN: *B virus.*

   h. simplex. An infectious disease caused by the virus of that name. Characterized by thin-walled vesicles which tend to recur in the same area of the skin, usually at a site where the mucous membrane joins the skin; but may be limited to the gingiva, oropharynx, or conjunctiva. In newborn infants meningoencephalitis or a panvisceral infection may occur. In adults 5 to 7% of cases of aseptic meningitis are due to h. simplex virus.

TREATMENT: Idoxuridine is particularly beneficial in early infections of the eye. Interferon topically has been useful. Antibiotics may be helpful in treating secondary infection. Eye lesions should be treated by an ophthalmologist.

h. zoster. An acute infectious disease due to the varicella-zoster virus. It is limited to man and is characterized by inflammation of the posterior root ganglia of only a few segments of the spinal or cranial nerves. A painful vesicular eruption occurs along the course of the nerve and is almost always unilateral. The incubation period is from 7 to 21 days. The total duration of the disease from onset to complete recovery varies from 10 days to 5 weeks. In general, the disease lasts longer in adults than in children. Also, if all of the vesicles appear within 24 hours the total duration is usually short.

The virus which causes reactivation of h. zoster is the same as that which causes chicken pox, i.e. varicella. Treatment is directed towards making the patient comfortable. If the eye is affected, idoxuridine should be used and the treatment supervised by an ophthalmologist. SYN: *shingles.*

h. zoster ophthalmicus. H. zoster affecting the 1st division of the 5th cranial nerve. The area of the face, eye, and nose supplied by this nerve is affected. The ocular complications can be quite serious. It is important that the eye be treated early with idoxuridine and that therapy be supervised by an ophthalmologist.

herpesvirus [Gr. *herpein,* to creep]. A family of viruses including that which causes herpes simplex, herpes zoster, and varicella (chicken pox). The latter two diseases are caused by the same virus, which is called the varicella-zoster virus. Another form, herpes simiae or B virus, is spread from monkeys to man and is almost always fatal.

h. hominus. Carcinoma of the cervix is thought to be associated with HVH, type 2. ABBR: HVH.

h. simiae encephalomyelitis. A severe, almost always fatal, encephalomyelitis due to the H. simiae (also called B virus). It is seen in veterinarians, laboratory workers, and others who have come in contact with infected monkeys.

herpet'ic [Gr. *herpēs,* herpes, a creeping]. Pert. to herpes.

h. neuralgia. Neural pain with herpes zoster.

h. sore throat. H. tonsillitis.

herpet'iform ["+ L. *forma,* form]. Resembling herpes.

her'petism ["+ *ismos,* state of]. Predisposition to herpetic eruption.

hersage (ār-sazh') [Fr., a harrowing]. Splitting of a nerve trunk into separate fibers.

Herter's infantilism. [Christian A. Herter, Amer. physician, 1865-1910] Celiac disease; a form of infantilism resulting from defective fat and calcium absorption. Resembles sprue in adults.

Hertig-Rock embryos. [Arthur T. Hertig, Amer. pathologist, 1904 —; John Rock, Amer. gynecologist, 1890 —] Very beautifully preserved and dated embryos obtained experimentally in 1952.

Hertig-Rock ovum. Fertilized human ovum 7 to 7 1/2 days old, described in 1945.

Hesselbach's hernia (hĕs'ĕl-bŏk). [Franz K. Hesselbach, Ger. surgeon, 1759-1816] A lobated hernia which passes through the cribriform fascia.

Hesselbach's triangle. The triangular space bounded by Poupart's ligament below, exterior border of rectus muscle internally, and epigastric artery exteriorly.

heteradenia (het-er-ă-de'nĭ-ă) [Gr. *heteros,* other, + *adēn,* gland]. 1. Glandular substance in a part which does not normally contain glands. 2. Abnormal glandular tissue.

heteradenic (hĕt-ĕr-ă-dĕn'ik). Pert. to Heteradenia.

heteradenoma (hĕt''ĕr-ad-ĕ-nō'mă) [Gr. *heteros,* other, + *adēn,* gland, + *-ōma,* tumor]. (pl. *heteradenomata*) A glandular tumor arising from an area which does not usually contain glands.

heterecious (hĕt''ĕr-ē'shŭs) ["+ *oikos,* house]. Living upon different hosts at different stages of development.

heterecism (hĕt''ĕr-ē'sīzm). Development of different cycles of existence on different hosts, said of certain parasites.

heteresthesia (hĕt''ĕr-ĕs-thē'zĭ-ă) [Gr. *heteros,* other, + *aisthēsis,* sensation]. Variation in degree (plus or minus) of sensory response to cutaneous stimuli.

hetero-, heter- [Gr. *heteros,* other]. Prefix indicating different, or relationship to another.

heteroagglutinin (hĕt''ĕr-o-ă-glū'tĭ-nĭn). An agglutinin formed as result of injection of an antigen from an animal of a different species; an agglutinin capable of agglutinating blood cells of other species of animals.

heteroalbumose (hĕt''ĕr-o-al'bu-mōs) [Gr. *heteros,* other, + L. *albumen,* white of egg]. Albumose insoluble in water but soluble in saline solutions, in acid or alkaline solutions. SYN: *hemialbumose.*

heteroautoplasty (hĕt″ĕr-o-aw′to-plas-tĭ) ["+ *autos*, self, + *plassein*, to form]. Grafting skin from one person to another.

heteroblas′tic ("+ *blastos*, germ). Having origin in tissue of another kind. Opposed to homoblastic.

heterocel′lular. Composed of different kinds of cells.

heterochiral (hĕt″ĕr-ō-kī′ral) [Gr. *heteros*, other, + *cheir*, hand]. Reversed as to right and left, but otherwise of the same form and size; said of images in a plane mirror.

heterochromatin (hĕt″ĕr-o-krō′mä-tĭn) ["+ *chrōma*, color]. A type of chromatin that stains less distinctly than the euchromatin, forming clear disks interposed between dark bands on chromosomes. In interphasic nuclei it constitutes the chromocenters. It is thought that it controls certain metabolic activites of cells. It is genetically inert. SEE: *euchromatin.*

heterochromatosis (hĕt″ĕr-ō-krō-mä-tō′sĭs) ["+ "+ *-ōsis*, condition]. 1. Pigmentation of skin from foreign substances. 2. Difference in color. SYN: *heterochromia.*

heterochromia (hĕt″ĕr-ō-krō′mĭ-ä). A difference in color.

    h. iridis. Different color of iris or sector of iris in the two eyes. This may occur naturally or be due to previous disease in the lighter-colored eye.

heterochromosome (hĕt″ĕr-ō-krō′mo-sōm). 1. The X and Y or sex chromosomes. 2. A chromosome which contains material, heterochromatin, which stains differently from the remainder of the chromatin material.

heterochromous (hĕt″ĕr-o-krō′mŭs) [Gr. *heteros*, other, + *chrōma*, color]. With abnormal difference in coloration.

heterochro′nia ["+ *chronos*, time]. Denoting an abnormal time for the occurrence of a phenomenon or production of a structure.

heterochron′ic. Occurring at different or at abnormal times.

heterochylia (hĕt″ĕr-o-kī′lĭ-ä) [Gr. *heteros*, other, + *chylos*, juice]. A change in character of the gastric juice without apparent cause.

heterocinesia (hĕt″ĕr-o-sĭ-nē′zĭ-ä) ["+ *kinēsis*, movement]. Movements different from those the patient is instructed to make.

heterocladic (hĕt″ĕr-o-klăd′ik) ["+ *klados*, branch]. Pert. to an anastomosis between branches of two different arteries, in contrast to homocladic.

heterocri′sis ["+ *krisis*, division]. Irregular crisis with abnormal symptoms.

heterocyclic (hĕt″ĕr-o-sī′klĭk) ["+ *kyklos*, circle]. In chemistry, pert. to ring compounds which contain one or more elements other than carbon in the ring.

heteroder′mic ["+ *derma*, skin]. Pert. to a method of skin grafting when grafts are taken from another person. SEE: *dermatoheteroplasty.*

het′erodont ["+ *odous, odont-*, tooth]. Having teeth of various shapes.

heteroecious. Heterecious, q.v.

heteroecism. Heterecism, q.v.

heteroerotism (hĕt″ĕr-ō-ĕr′ō-tĭzm) [Gr. *heteros*, different, + *erōs*, love, + *ismos*, state of]. Sexual desire for another person.

heterogametic (hĕt″ĕr-ō-gă-mĕt′ĭk) [Gr. *heteros*, different, + *gamōs*, marriage]. Pertaining to the production of unlike gametes, applied esp. to a male which produces two types of sperm, one containing the X chromosome, the other the Y chromosome.

heterogamy (hĕt″ĕr-ōg′ă-mĭ). The union of gametes which are dissimilar in size and structure. Occurs in higher plants and animals. SEE: *isogamy.*

heterogeneous (hĕt″ĕr-o-jē′nē-us) [Gr. *heteros*, other, + *genos*, type]. Of unlike natures; composed of unlike substances. In contrast to homogeneous, q.v.

    h. vaccine. That made from some source other than patient's own organism. Opposite of autogenous vaccine.

heterogenesis (hĕt″ĕ-rō-jĕn′ĕ-sĭs) ["+ *genesis*, production]. Production of offspring which have different characteristics in alternate generations. An example would be alternation of an asexual generation with a sexual one. SYN: *metagenesis.*

heterogenet′ic. Rel. to heterogenesis.

heterogeusia. Perception of an inappropriate quality of taste when food is present in the mouth or chewed. The taste sensation is unexpected and unusual but not necessarily unpleasant.

het′erograft [Gr. *heteros*, other, + L. *graphium*, grafting knife]. A graft taken from another individual or an animal of a different species from the one for whom it is intended. SEE: *autograft; graft; isograft.*

heterog′raphy ["+ *graphein*, to write]. Writing different words from those the writer intended.

heteroinfec′tion ["+ L. *in*, in, + *facere*, to make]. Infection by a microorganism from outside the body. SYN: *exogenous infection.*

heteroinoculation (hĕt″ĕr-ō-ĭn-ŏk″ū-lā′shŭn) ["+ "+ *oculus*, bud]. Inoculation with a microorganism from a source outside the body.

heterolalia (hĕt″ĕr-o-lā′lĭ-ä) ["+ *lalia*, babbling]. The use of meaningless words instead of those intended.

heterologous (hĕt″ĕr-ŏl′o-gŭs) [Gr. *heteros*, other, + *logos*, relation]. 1. Made up of cell tissue not normal to the part. 2. A tissue, cells, or blood obtained from a different individual or species.

heterol′ogy. Different from the normal in structure or method of growth.

heterolysin (hĕt-ĕr-ŏl′ĭ-sĭn) [Gr. *heteros*, other, + *lysis*, solution]. Lysins formed from an antigen from an animal of a different species. SEE: *autolysin; hemolysin.*

heterolysis (hĕt″ĕr-ŏl′ĭ-sĭs). Hemolytic action of blood serum of an animal upon corpuscles of another species. SEE: *isolysis.*

heteromeric (hĕt″ĕr-o-mĕr′ik) [Gr. *heteros*, other, + *meros*, a part]. 1. Pert. to spinal neurons with processes to opposite side of cord. 2. Possessing a different chemical composition.

heterometaplasia (hĕt″ĕr-o-mĕt″ă-plā′zĭ-ă) [″+ *meta*, beyond, + *plassein*, to form]. Transformation of tissue to a tissue foreign to the part where produced.

heteromorphous (hĕt″ĕr-ō-mŏr′fŭs) [″+ *morphē*, form]. Deviating from the normal type.

heteronomous (hĕt″ĕr-ŏn′o-mus) [″+ *nomos*, law]. Abnormal; differing from type.

heteronymous (hĕt″ĕr-ŏn′ĭ-mŭs) [Gr. *heteros*, other, + *onyma*, name]. 1. Having different names but correlated. Ex.: parent and child. 2. In opposite relation.

   h. diplopia. Having a false image on same side as the sound eye.

hetero-osteoplasty (hĕt″ĕr-o-ŏs′tē-o-plăs″tĭ) [″+ *osteon*, bone, + *plassein*, to form]. Grafting of bone, esp. with a graft from an animal.

heteropathy (hĕt″ĕr-ŏp′ă-thĭ) [″+ *pathos*, disease]. 1. Abnormal reaction to irritation or to stimuli. 2. Creation of a pathological condition to neutralize another disorder. SEE: *allopathy.*

heterophany (hĕt″ĕr-ŏf′ă-nĭ) [″+ *phainein*, to appear]. Having different expressions of the same disorder.

heterophasia (hĕt″ĕr-o-fā′zĭ-ă) [″+ *phasis*, speech]. Expression of meaningless words instead of those intended. SYN: *heterolalia.*

heterophe′mia, heteroph′emy [″+ *phēmē*, speech]. Expressing one thing when another is intended. SYN: *heterolalia; heterophasia.*

heterophil(e (hĕt′ĕr-o-fĭl; fĭl) [Gr. *heteros*, other, + *philein*, to love]. 1. Pert. to an antibody reacting with other than the specific antigen. 2. Pert. to a tissue or microorganism that takes a stain other than the ordinary one.

heterophonia (hĕt″ĕr-o-fō′nĭ-ă) [″+ *phōnē*, voice]. Change of voice, esp. that which occurs at puberty.

heterophoralgia (hĕt″ĕr-o-for-ăl′jĭ-ă) [″+ *phoros*, bearing, + *algos*, pain]. Deviation of one eye accompained by pain.

heteropho′ria [Gr. *heteros*, other, + *phoros*, bearing]. The tendency of the eyes to deviate from their normal position for visual alignment, esp. when one eye is covered; latent deviation or squint.

   ETIOL: Imbalance or insufficiency of ocular muscles.

heterophthalmos (hĕt″ĕr-ŏf-thăl′mŏs) [″+ *ophthalmos*, eye]. Difference in appearance of the eyes due to the irides differing in color. SEE: *heterochromia.*

Heterophyes (hĕt″ĕr-ŏf′ĭ-ēz) [″+ *phyē*, stature]. A genus of flukes belonging to the family Heterophyidae, q.v.

   H. heterophyes. A species of intestinal fluke commonly infesting man. In heavy infestations may cause diarrhea, nausea, and abdominal discomfort.

heterophyiasis (hĕt″ĕr-o-fī-ī′ă-sis). Infestation by any fluke belonging to the family Heterophyidae, q.v.

Heterophyidae. A family of Trematoda (flukes) which infests the intestines of dogs, cats and other mammals including humans. Infestations are common in Egypt and in the Far East. Includes the genera Heterophyes, Haplorchis, Diorchitrema and Metagonimus. Intermediate hosts are snails, the cercaria encysting in fishes, esp. mullets, or frogs.

heteroplasia (hĕt″ĕr-o-plā′zĭ-ă) [Gr. *heteros*, other, + *plassein*, to mold]. The development of normal tissue in a place where that tissue would not normally be found.

heteroplastic (hĕt″ĕr-o-plăs′tĭk). Rel. to heteroplasia.

het′eroplasty. Grafting with tissue from another person or an animal.

heteroploid (hĕt′ĕr-o-ployd) [Gr. *heteros*, other, + *-ploos*, -fold]. Possessing a chromosome number that is not a multiple of the haploid number common for the species.

heteroprosopus (het″ĕr-o-prō′sō-pŭs) [″+ *prosōpon*, face]. A congenitally deformed fetus having one head and two faces.

heteropsia (hĕt″ĕr-ŏp′sĭ-ă) [″+ *opsis*, vision]. Inequality of vision in the two eyes.

heteroptics (hĕt″ĕr-ŏp′tĭks). Perversion of vision such as seeing objects that do not exist or misinterpreting what is seen.

heteropyknosis (hĕt″ĕr-o-pĭk-nō′sis) [Gr. *heteros*, other, + *pyknos*, dense, + *-ōsis*, condition]. The property whereby various parts of a chromosome stain with varying degrees of intensity; thought to be due to variations in concentration of nucleic acid.

heteros'copy ["+ *skopein*, to examine]. 1. Finding range of vision in strabismus. 2. Unequal vision in the eyes.

heteroserotherapy (hĕt″ĕr-o-sē″rō-thĕr′-ă-pĭ) ["+ L. *serum*, whey, + Gr. *therapeia*, treatment]. Treatment by serum from another person.

heterosexual (hĕt″ĕr-ō-sĕk′shŭ-ăl) ["+ L. *sexus*, sex]. 1. Having normal attraction for the opposite sex. 2. Belonging to the opposite sex.

het″erosexual′ity. The normal state of love for one of the opposite sex.

heterosis (hĕt-ĕr-ō′sĭs) [Gr. *heteros*, other, + *-ōsis*, condition]. Greater strength, size, vigor and growth rate as a result of crossbreeding of genetically different members of the same species. Referred to as hybrid vigor.

heterosmia ["+ *osme*, smell]. Consistent perception of an inappropriate smell when an odorant is inhaled. The smell perceived is unusual and unexpected but not unpleasant.

heterotax'ia [Gr. *heteros*, other, + *taxis*, arrangement]. Abnormal position of organs or parts. SEE: *dextrocardia; situs inversus viscerum.*

heteroto'pia ["+ *topos*, place]. 1. Development of a normal tissue in an abnormal location. 2. Displacement of an organ or part from its normal location.

heterotop'ic. Misplaced; pert. to heterotopia.

 h. grafts. Grafts placed in unnatural position. Ex: use of a piece of small bowel to repair a ureter.

heterotopy (hĕt″ĕr-ŏt′ō-pĭ) [Gr. *heteros*, other, + *topos*, place]. Displacement of an organ or a portion of the body.

heterotox'in ["+ *toxikon*, poison]. A toxin introduced from without the patient's body.

heterotrans'plant [Gr. *heteros*, other, + L. *trans*, across, + *plantare*, to plant]. An organ, tissue, or structure taken from an animal and grafted into, or on, another animal of a different species. Such transplants usually atrophy.

heterotrichosis (hĕt″ĕr-o-trĭ-kō′sĭs) ["+ *trichōsis*, growth of hair]. Growth of different kinds or color of hairs on the scalp or body.

heterotroph (hĕt′ĕr-ō-trŏf) ["+ *trophē*, food]. An organism such as man which requires complex organic food in order to grow and develop. In contrast to plants which can synthesize food from inorganic materials.

heterotro'pia ["+ *tropos*, a turning]. Manifest deviation of the eyes due to absence of binocular equilibrium. SEE: *strabismus.*

heterovaccine (hĕt″ĕr-o-văk′sēn) [Gr. *heteros*, other, + L. *vaccinus*, pert. to a cow]. A vaccine from a source other than that of the disease for which it is intended.

heteroxanthine (hĕt″ĕr-o-zăn′thin) ["+ *xanthos*, yellow]. Methyl xanthine found in the urine.

heterozygosis (hĕt″ĕr-ō-zī-gō′sĭs) ["+ *zygon*, yoke, pair, + *-ōsis*, condition]. Condition in which the two members of a pair of genes in the zygote differ from each other; the result of crossbreeding. SEE: *homozygosis.*

heterozygote (hĕt″ĕr-ō-zī′gōt). An individual in which the members of one or more pairs of genes are unlike.

heterozygous (hĕt″ĕr-ō-zī′gŭs). Genetically impure, not breeding true. Having one or many pairs of genes in the phase of heterozygosis resulting from crossbreeding. Having unlike genes. SEE: *homozygous.*

hettocyrtosis (hĕt″o-sĭr-tō′sis) [Gr. *hēttōn*, less, + *kyrtōsis*, curvature]. A slight curvature.

Heubner's disease (hoyb′ner). [Johann Otto L. Heubner, Ger. pediatrician, 1843-1926] Syphilitic endarteritis of the brain.

heurteloup (hert-loo′). [Charles Louis Stanislaus Baron Heurteloup, Fr. surgeon, 1793-1864] An artificial leech; a cupping apparatus.

hex-, hexa- [Gr. *hex*, six]. Prefix indicating six.

hexaba'sic [Gr. *hex*, six, + *basis*, base]. Having six replaceable hydrogen atoms.

hexachlorophene (hĕks″ā-klō′rō-fēn). USP. A bactericidal and bacteriostatic compound, used in emulsions and soaps for preoperative cleansing of skin and for scrubbing the nurse's and surgeon's hands prior to surgery.

hexachro'mic [Gr. *hex*, six, + *chrōma*, color]. Not being able to distinguish more than six of the seven colors of the spectrum or to distinguish violet from indigo.

hexad (hĕks′ăd) [Gr. *hex*, six]. The atom of an element having a valence of six.

hexadactylism (hĕks″ā-dăk′tĭl-ĭzm). Possession of six fingers or six toes.

hexamethonium (hĕks″ā-mē-thō′nĭ-um). A compound which acts as a ganglionic blocking agent. Used in the treatment of hypertension.

Hexapoda (hĕks-ăp′o-dă) [Gr. *hex*, six, + *pod-*, foot]. The insects or six-legged arthropods.

hexatomic (hĕks″ā-tŏm′ĭk) [Gr. *hex*, six, + *atomos*, indivisible]. Pert. to a compound consisting of six atoms, or a compound having six replaceable hydrogen or univalent atoms.

hexavaccine (hĕks″a-vak′sēn) ["+ L. *vaccinus*, pert. to a cow]. A vaccine made from six different microorganisms.

hexavalent (hĕks″ă-vā′lĕnt) ["+ L. *valere*, to have power]. Having a valence of six. SYN: *sexivalent.*

hexokinase (hĕks″o-kī′nās) ["+ *kinein*, to move, + diast*ase*, denoting an enzyme]. An enzyme present in muscle tissue which catalyzes the phosphorylation of glucose. It has also been isolated from yeast.

hex′one [Gr. *hex*, six]. One of the amino acids, as histidine, arginine and lysine, so called because they contain chains of six carbon atoms. SYN: *hexone base.*

hexon′ic. Rel. to hexone bases.

hex′ose. Any monosaccharide of the general formula $C_6H_{12}O_6$; the group includes particularly dextrose and levulose, q.v.

hexosephosphate (hĕks″ōs-fōs′fāt) [Gr. *hex*, six, + *phosphoros*, phosphorus]. A phosphoric acid ester of glucose. One of several esters (Cori, Robison, et al.) formed in the muscles and other tissues in the metabolism of carbohydrates.

hexylresorcinol (hĕks″ĭl-rĕ-sŏr′sĭ-nōl). USP. $C_{12}H_{18}O_2$. White needle-shaped crystals. Used as an anthelmintic.

Hey′s lig′ament. [William Hey, Brit. surgeon, 1736-1819] The semilunar lateral margin (falciform margin) of the fossa ovalis which lies between iliac and pubic portions of the fascia lata.

Hg. Chem. symb. for mercury.

HgCl₂. Chem. symb. for mercuric chloride; corrosive sublimate.

Hg₂Cl₂. Chem. symb. for mercurous chloride; calomel.

HgI₂. Chem. symb. for mercuric iodide.

HgO. Chem. symb. for mercuric oxide.

HgS. Chem. symb. for mercuric sulfide.

HgSO₄. Chem. symb. for mercuric sulfate.

hiatus (hī-ā′tŭs) [L., an opening]. 1. An opening, a foramen. 2. The vulva. 3. An aperture.

　　h. aorticus. [NA] Opening in diaphragm through which pass the aorta and the thoracic duct.

　　h. canalis facialis. H. canalis nervi petrosi majoris, q.v.

　　h. esophageus. [NA] Opening in diaphragm through which the esophagus passes.

　　h. fallopii. H. canalis facialis, q.v.

　　h. maxillaris. [NA] Opening of maxillary sinus into the nasal cavity, located on nasal surface of maxillary bone.

　　h. semilunaris. [NA] The groove in the external wall of middle meatus of nasal fossa into which the frontal sinus, maxillary sinus, and anterior ethmoid cells drain.

hiccough, hiccup (hĭk′ŭp) [Probably of imitative origin]. Spasmodic periodic closure of the glottis following spasmodic lowering of the diaphragm, causing a short, sharp, inspiratory cough. SYN: *singultus.*

　　ETIOL: It may be caused by indigestion, irritation of diaphragm, alcoholism, new growths of the pleura, certain cerebral lesions, or hysteria. May be due to a disturbance of the phrenic nerve. If prolonged it has serious significance.

　　TREATMENT: Antiemetic drugs, rebreathing in a paper bag, carbon dioxide breathing, gastric suction. Stimulation of the nasopharynx with a soft rubber tube should also be tried. If these are not effective, anesthetization of the phrenic nerve may be helpful.

Hicks′ sign. [John Braxton Hicks, Brit. gynecologist, 1825-1897] Uterine intermittent contractions at end of 3rd month of pregnancy.

hide′bound disease′ [AS. *hyd*, a skin, + *bindan*, to tie up]. Hardening and thickening of the skin with loss of elasticity. SYN: *scleroderma.*

hidradenitis (hī-drăd-ĕ-nī′tĭs) [Gr. *hidrōs*, sweat, + *adēn*, gland, + *-itis*, inflammation]. Inflammation of sweat glands.

hidradenoma (hī-drăd-ĕ-nō′mă) ["+ "+ *-ōma*, tumor]. Adenoma of the sweat glands.

hidroa (hī-drō′ă) [Gr. *hidrōs*, sweat]. Vesicles due to retention of sweat. Not to be confused with hydroa, q.v. SYN: *sudamina.*

hidrocystoma (hī-drō-sĭs-tō′mă) ["+ *kystis*, cyst, + *-ōma*, tumor]. A cystic tumor of a sweat gland.

hidropoiesis (hī-drō-poy-ē′sĭs) ["+ *poiēsis*, formation]. The formation of sweat.

hidropoiet′ic. Pert. to hidropoiesis. SYN: *sudorific.*

hidrorrhea (hī-drō-rē′ă) [Gr. *hidrōs*, sweat, + *rhoia*, flow]. Abnormal sweating.

hidrosadenitis (hī-drōs-ăd-ĕ-nī′tĭs) ["+ *adēn*, gland, + *-itis*, inflammation]. Inflammation of sweat glands. SYN: *hidradenitis.*

hidroschesis (hī-drōs′kĕ-sĭs) ["+ *schesis*, a holding]. 1. Retention of perspiration. 2. Suppression of perspiration.

hidrosis (hī-drō′sĭs) [Gr. *hidrōs*, sweat, + *-ōsis*, condition]. 1. Formation and excretion of sweat. 2. Excessive sweating.

hidrot′ic. 1. Causing the secretion and excretion of sweat. SYN: *diaphoretic; sudorific.* 2. Any drug or medicine that induces sweating.

hieralgia (hī-ĕr-ăl′jĭ-ă) [Gr. *hieron*, sacred, sacrum, + *algos*, pain]. Pain in the region of the sacrum.

hierarchic principle. An organism's striving to achieve, restore, or maintain a state of equilibrium with the least possible effort.

hierophobia (hī''ēr-ō-fō'bī-ā) [Gr. *hieron*, sacred, + *phobos*, fear]. Abnormal fear of sacred things, or persons connected with religion.

high. An imprecise colloquial term for the hallucinogenic experience or intoxication-like phenomenon produced by use of certain drugs, esp. drugs of abuse such as LSD. SYN: *stoned.*

high blood pressure. Increased blood pressure. A diagnostic judgment or opinion which must be considered with respect to the person's age, body build, previous blood pressure, and state of mental and physical health at the time the blood pressure is obtained. In general it is not advisable to declare that a person has elevated blood pressure if the opinion is based on one determination of the blood pressure.

RS: blood; blood pressure; hypertension; hypotension; pulse pressure.

high calorie diet. One that includes more calories than would be normally required for that person's metabolic and energy needs. *Indicated:* To prevent loss of weight; in wasting diseases; in high basal metabolism; after long illness; in deficiency caused by anorexia, poverty, poor dietary habits; during lactation when 1000 to 1200 extra Calories are indicated.

Three meals plus between-meal feedings. Fermentable and bulky foods to be avoided.

high cellulose diet. The general diet plus the following: *Breakfast:* Bran muffin or a tablespoon of bran added to a cereal, and extra large serving of fruit. *10 A.M.:* Fruit juice. *Dinner:* Salad, extra serving of vegetables, fruit. *Supper:* Salad, extra serving of vegetables and fruits.

high frequency treatment. High frequency current passed through the body to produce heat in the tissues. RS: circuit; current; diathermy.

High'more, antrum of. [Nathaniel Highmore, Brit. surgeon, 1613-1685] The maxillary sinus. SEE: *antracele; antrum.*

Highmore's body. Fibrous tissue mass, a prolongation of albuginea testis, projecting forward along posterior border of testis. SYN: *mediastinum testis* [NA].

highmori'tis. Inflammation of the maxillary sinus or antrum of Highmore. SYN: *antritis; sinusitis maxillaris.*

hill'ock. A small eminence or projection.

   h., anal. One of two small eminences which lie lateral and posterior to the cloacal membrane, and later, the anal fissure in the embryo.

   h., axon. A small conical elevation on the cell body of a neuron from which the axon arises.

   h., seminal. The colliculus seminalis [NA], q.v.

Hil'ton's law. [John Hilton, Brit. surgeon, 1804-1878] The trunk of a nerve, which sends branches to a particular muscle, also sends branches to the joint moved by that muscle and to the skin overlying the insertion of the muscle.

Hilton's line. A white one at junction of skin of perineum and anal mucosa.

Hilton's muscle. The aryepiglottic muscle.

Hilton's sac. Pit along external portion of false vocal cords. SYN: *sacculus laryngis.*

hi'lum. (pl. hila) Hilus, q.v.

hi'lus [L. a trifle]. (pl. *hili*) [NA] 1. Depression or recess at exit or entrance of duct into a gland, or of nerves and vessels into an organ. 2. The root of the lungs at level of 4th and 5th dorsal vertebrae.

himantosis (hi-man-to'sis) [Gr. *himantōsis*, a long strap]. Abnormal lengthening of the uvula.

hind'brain [AS. *hindan*, behind, + *bragen*, brain]. The most caudal of the three divisions of the embryonic brain; the rhombencephalon. It differentiates into the metencephalon which gives rise to the cerebellum and pons, and the myelencephalon which gives rise to the medulla oblongata.

hindgut. The caudal portion of the entodermal tube which develops into the alimentary canal. It gives rise to the ileum, colon, and rectum.

hind kidney. The metanephros, the most caudal of three embryonic kidneys. It persists and develops into the permanent kidney. SEE: *metanephros.*

hinge joint. An articulation which permits flexion and extension about a single axis; ginglymus.

Hin'ton's test. [William A. Hinton, Amer. bacteriologist, 1883-1959] A serological test for syphilis.

hip [AS. *hype*]. 1. Upper part of thigh, formed by the femur and innominate bones. 2. The region on each side of the pelvis. SEE: *hip joint.*

   h. bone. Os coxae. Its three portions are the ilium (pl. ilia), ischium (pl. ischia), and pubis (pl. pubes).

   h., dislocation of. Dislocations of the hip are very often accompanied by a fracture and it is extremely difficult even for a well-trained surgeon to distinguish a pure dislocation from a fracture dislocation without an x-ray.

DIAG: Person has great difficulty in straightening the hip following an accident. It is always accompanied by pain. The knee on the injured side resistantly points inwardly toward the other knee and it is difficult to straighten the leg.

SYM: Pain, rigidity, loss of function, and the dislocation may be obvious by the abnormal position in which the leg is held, or by seeing or feeling the head of the femur in an abnormal position.

F.A. TREATMENT: Place the patient on a large splint as in a fractured back. In addition, place a large pad, such as a pillow, under the knee of the affected side. Treat for shock if required.

h., dislocation of, backward. Onto the dorsum ilii or sciatic notch. SYM: Inward rotation of thigh, with flexion, inversion, adduction, shortening; pain, tenderness; loss of function and immobility.

TREATMENT: Patient anesthetized. Dorsal position, leg flexed on thigh, latter upon abdomen. Adduct thigh, rotate outward; circumduction outwardly across abdomen, back to straight position. Traction may be required.

h., dislocation of, downward. Rare. TREATMENT: Traction in flexed position. Outward rotation and extension.

h., dislocation of, forward. Through obturator foramen, on pubis, in perineum, or through fractured acetabulum. SYM: Pain, tenderness, and immobility. Shortening in pubic and suprapubic forms; lengthening in obturator and perineal forms. TREATMENT: Hyperextension and direct traction. Flexion, abduction with inward rotations, adduction.

h. replacement, total. SEE: *total hip replacement.*

hip joint. Articulation between femur and innominate bone. A ball and socket (enarthrosis) formed by the head of the femur fitting into a concavity, the acetabulum. SYM: *articulatio coxae* [NA].

h.j., arthritis of. Usually occurring before age of 14 years. Varieties: Arthritic, acetabulum, femoral. SYM: wasting, spasm, lameness, pain, swelling, deformity. PROG: Influenced by circumstances. Tendency toward recovery. TREATMENT: Determined by cause and extent of disease at the time it is diagnosed.

h.j. disease. May be tubercular; fracture; congenital deformities; dislocation of; Perthe's disease, q.v. SYM: Early—pain, limp, muscle spasm. Later—muscle wasting,

swelling, deformity. TREATMENT: Build up patient's general health by proper diet and exercise as permitted. Specific drug or surgical therapy will depend upon the cause of the disease.

h.j., snapping. A slipping around of the hip joint, sometimes producing an audible snapping sound.

hippocam'pal [Gr. *hippokampos,* seahorse]. Pert. to the hippocampus.

h. commissure. A thin sheet of fibers passing transversely under posterior portion of the corpus callosum. They connect the medial margins of the crura of the fornix. SYN: *commissura fornicis* [NA]; *commissure of the fornix.*

h. fissure. Fissure above the temporal lobe on mesial surface of cerebrum. SYN: *sulcus hippocampi* [NA].

h. formation. Olfactory structures lying along the medial margin of the pallium. It includes the hippocampus, dentate gyrus, supracallosal gyrus, longitudinal striae, subcallosal gyrus, diagonal band of Broca, and h. commissure. SYN; *formatio hippocampalis.*

hippocam'pus ma'jor. Elevation of floor of inferior horn of lateral ventricle of the brain, occupying nearly all of it.

h., digitations of. Three or four shallow grooves on anterior portion of hippocampus.

hippocampus minor. A small elevation on medial wall of lateral ventricle formed by end of the calcarine fissure. SYN: *calcar avis* [NA].

Hippocrates (hǐ-pŏk'rǎ-tēz). [5th and 4th centuries B.C.] Greek physician who is referred to as the Father of Medicine. SEE: *Hippocratic oath.*

hippocrat'ic fa'cies. The appearance of the face at the time of impending death.

SYM: Dark brown, livid, or lead colored skin; hollow appearance of eyes, collapse of temples, sharpness of nose, lobes of ears contracting and turning outward. SEE: *facial.*

Hippocratic oath. Oath exacted of his students by Hippocrates: "I swear by Apollo the physician, and Aesculapius, and Hygeia, and Panacea, and all the gods and goddesses, that according to my ability and judgment, I will keep this oath and its stipulation—to reckon him who taught me this art equally dear to me as my parents, to share my substance with him, and to relieve his necessities if required; to look upon his offspring in the same footing as my own brothers, and to teach them this art if they shall wish to learn it, without fee or stipulation, and that by precept, lecture, and every other mode of instruction, I will impart a knowledge of the art to my own sons, and those of my teachers, and to disciples bound by a stipulation and oath according to the law of medicine, but to none other.

"I will follow that system of regimen which, according to my ability and judgment, I consider for the benefit of my patients, and abstain from whatever is deleterious and mischievous. I will give no deadly medicine to anyone if asked, nor suggest any such counsel; and in like manner I will not give to a woman a pessary to produce abortion. With purity and with holiness I will pass my life and practice my art. I will not cut persons laboring under the stone, but will leave this to be done by men who are practitioners of this work. Into whatever houses I enter, I will go into them for the benefit of the sick, and I will abstain from every voluntary act of mischief and corruption; and, further, from the seduction of females or males, of freemen and slaves. Whatever, in connection with my professional practice, or not in connection with it, I see or hear, in the life of men, which ought not to be spoken of abroad, I will not divulge, as reckoning that all such should be kept secret.

"While I continue to keep this Oath unviolated, may it be granted to me to enjoy life and the practice of this art, respected by all men, in all times. But should I trespass and violate this Oath, may the reverse be my lot."

In part, some of these points are still the accepted standard for the ethical physician today. RS: Declaration of Geneva; Prayer of Maimonides.

hippu'ria [Gr. *hippos,* horse, + *ouron,* urine]. Large quantities of hippuric acid in the urine.

hippu'ric acid. An acid formed and excreted by the kidneys. It is formed in the human body from the combination of benzoic acid and glycine, the synthesis taking place in the liver and to a limited extent by the kidney.

The ability of the kidneys to excrete hippuric acid can be tested by administering six grams of sodium benzoate orally and then determining amt. of hippuric acid in the urine four hours later. The normal value is three to 3.5 grams. If the test is done intravenously, 1.77 grams are given and 0.7 gram of hippuric acid would normally be present in the urine one hour after the intravenous dose.

hippur'icase. An enzyme found in the liver, kidney, and other tissues which catalyzes the synthesis of hippuric acid from benzoic acid and glycine. SYN: *hippurase; histozyme.*

hippus (hĭp'ŭs) [Gr. *hippos,* horse]. Rhythmical and rapid dilatation and contraction of the pupils. Tremor of iris, spasmodic in character.

   h., respiratory. Dilatation during inspiration, and contraction of pupil during expiration.

hirci (hĭr'sī) [L. pl. goat]. (sing. *hircus)* Axillary hairs.

hircismus. A malodorous condition of the axillae. The odor resembles that present on the male goat.

Hirschberg's reflex (hirsh'berg). [Leonard Keene Hirschberg, Amer. physician, 1877—] Adduction of foot when sole at base of great toe is irritated.

Hirschsprung's disease (hirsh'sprung). [Harold Hirschsprung, Dan. physician, 1830-1916] Megacolon due to failure of development of the myenteric plexus of the recto-sigmoid area of the large intestine. The colon above the inactive area of the sigmoid dilates and there is chronic constipation, abdominal distention and fecal impaction.

   TREATMENT: Surgical excision of affected bowel is the treatment of choice. The remaining normal colon is anastomosed to the anus. SYN: *megacolon.*

hirsute (hur'sūt) [L. *hirsutus,* shaggy]. Hairy.

hirsuties (hur-sū'shĭ-ēz). Hirsutism.

hirsutism (hur'sūt-izm). Condition characterized by the excessive growth of hair or the presence of hair in unusual places.

hirudicide (hĭ-rū'dĭ-sĭd) [L. *hirūdo,* a leech, + *caedere,* to kill]. Any substance that destroys leeches.

hir'udin. A substance present in the secretion of the buccal glands of the leech which prevents coagulation of the blood. It inactivates thrombin.

Hir"udin'ea. A class of annelida. They are hermaphroditic, lack setae or appendages, and usually possess two suckers. Includes the blood-sucking leeches. A number of species, including H. medicinalis, were formerly used extensively for blood-letting.

hir"udini'asis. Infestation by leeches. In external h., leeches attach themselves to the skin and suck blood. After the leeches drop off, bleeding may continue as a result of the action of hirudin. Bites may become infected or ulcerate.

   h., internal. Results from accidental ingestion of leeches in drinking water, which may attach to wall of pharynx, nasal cavity, or larynx.

Hiru'do. A genus of leeches belonging to the family Gnathobdellidae.

His, bundle of. [Wilhelm His, Jr., Ger. physician, 1863-1934] The atrioventricular bundle, A-V bundle, a group of modified muscle fibers, Purkinje fibers forming a part of the impulse conducting system of the heart. It arises in the atrioventricular node and continues in the interventricular septum as a single bundle, the crus commune which divides into two trunks which pass respectively to the right and left ventricles, fine branches passing to all parts of the ventricles. It conducts impulses from the atria to the ventricles which initiate ventricular contraction.

histaffine (hĭs'tă-fēn) [Gr. *histos,* tissue, + L. *affīnis,* having affinity for]. Having affinity for tissues.

histaminase (hĭs-tăm'ĭ-nās). An enzyme widely distributed in the body which inactivates histamine.

histamine (hĭs'tă-mĭn, -mēn). A substance normally present in the body. It exerts its pharmacological action when tissues are injured. Red flush of a burn is due to the local production of histamine. It is produced from the amino acid histidine.

Injected under the skin, if the circulation is normal, it produces a small red spot which appears within a few seconds, reaches a maximum in about a minute and then becomes bluish. This is followed by a wheal surrounded by a flare, suggesting a mosquito bite. Given intravenously, causes gastric secretion, flushing of skin, lowered blood pressure, and headache.

   h. headache. When histamine is given by injection an intense headache may appear. The precise relationship of this to histaminic cephalalgia is not clear. Some persons will experience headache after drinking certain wines. This appears to be related to the histamine content of those wines.

   h. phosphate. USP. Water soluble colorless crystals. Sometimes called histamine acid phosphate or histamine diphosphate.

   Used most frequently as a diagnostic agent in determining the acid-secreting power of the stomach.

histamine'mia [*histamine* + Gr. *haima,* blood]. Histamine in the blood.

histamin'ia. Shock induced by histamine in the body.

his'tase [Gr. *histos,* tissue, + diast*ase,* suffix denoting an enzyme]. An enzyme which digests tissue.

histen'zyme ["+ *en,* in, + *zymē,* leaven]. An enzyme in renal tissues which splits up hippuric acid into benzoic acid and glycocol. SYN: *histozyme.*

his'tidase. An enzyme present in the liver which acts on 1-histidine. It splits the imidazole ring with the resultant formation of glutamic and formic acids and ammonia.

histidine (hĭs'tĭ-dĭn, -dēn). An amino acid, $C_6H_9N_3O_2$, obtained by hydrolysis from tissue proteins and necessary for tissue repair and growth.

histiocyte (hĭs'tĭ-o-sīt) [Gr. *histos,* web, tissue, + *kytos,* cell]. A cell present in all loose connective tissues. It may exhibit active ameboid movement and show marked phagocytic activity. These cells easily ingest trypan blue, colloidal carbon, and other foreign substances of a particulate nature. Histiocytes belong to the reticuloendothelial system. SYN: *adventitial cells; clasmatocyte; macrophage; resting wandering cells.*

histiocytoma (hĭs''tĭ-o-sī-tō'mă) ["+ "+ *-ōma,* tumor]. A tumor containing histiocytes.

histiocytosis (hĭs''tĭ-o-sī-tō'sis) [Gr. *histion* dim. of *histos,* web, + *kytos,* cell, + *-ōsis,* condition]. Histocytes in the blood in unusual numbers.

   h., lipoid. Niemann-Pick disease, q.v.

histiogenic (hĭs-tĭ-o-jēn'ĭk) ["+ *gennan,* to form]. Formed by the tissues. SYN: *histogenous.*

his'tioid ["+ *eidos,* form]. Resembling or composed of one of the body tissues. SYN: *histoid.*

his''tioir'ritative ["+ L. *irritāre,* to excite]. Irritative to connective tissue.

histio'ma ["+ *-ōma,* tumor]. A tissue tumor.

histo- [Gr. *histos,* web]. Prefix indicating rel. to tissue.

his'toblast [Gr. *histos,* tissue, + *blastos,* germ]. A tissue cell.

histochemistry (hĭs''tō-kĕm'ĭs-trī). Study of chemistry of cells and tissues. This is done by using both light and electron microscopy and by use of special chemical tests and stains.

histochromatosis (hĭs''tō-krō''mă-tō'sis) [Gr. *histos,* web, tissue, + *chrōma,* color, + *-osis,* diseased condition]. Name of disorders of reticuloendothelial system.

histoclas'tic ["+ *klastos,* breaking]. Decomposing tissue.

histocompatibility. The ability of cells to survive without immunological interference. Esp. important in blood transfusion and transplantation.

histocyte (hĭs'tō-sīt) [Gr. *histos*, tissue, + *kytos*, cell]. A tissue cell. SYN: *histiocyte.*

his"todiagno'sis ["+ *dia*, through, + *gnōsis*, knowledge]. Diagnosis made from examination of the tissues, esp. by use of microscopy.

histodial'ysis ["+ *dialysis*, a loosening]. Disintegration of tissue. SYN: *histolysis.*

histogenesis (hĭs-tō-jĕn'ĕ-sĭs) [Gr. *histos*, tissue, + *genesis*, formation]. Development into differentiated tissues of the germ layer; origin and development of tissue.

histogenetic (hĭs"tō-jĕ-nĕt'ĭk). Pert. to histogensis.

histogenous (hĭs-tŏj'ĕ-nus). Made by the tissues.

histogram (hĭs'tō-gram) [L. *historia*, observation, from Gr. *histōr*, learned man, + Gr. + *gramma*, a writing]. A graph showing frequency distributions.

histog'raphy [Gr. *histos*, tissue, + *graphein*, to write]. A written description of the tissues.

histohem'atin ["+ *haima*, blood]. A hemoglobin pigment in various tissues.

histohematogenous (hĭs"tō-hem"ă-tōj'ĕ-nus) ["+ "+ *gennan*, to form]. Arising from both the tissues and the blood.

histoid (hĭs'toyd) ["+ *eidos*, form]. 1. Resembling one of the tissues. 2. Developed from a single tissue, as fibroma.

histokinesis (hĭs-to-kĭ-nē'sĭs) [Gr. *histos*, tissue, + *kinēsis*, movement]. Movement in the tissues of the body.

histolog'ical ["+ *logos*, knowledge]. Pert. to histology, q.v.

histol'ogy. Study of the microscopic structure of tissue.

   h., normal. Study of healthy tissue.

   h., pathologic. Study of diseased tissue.

histolysis (hĭs-tŏl'ĭ-sĭs) [Gr. *histos*, tissue, + *lysis*, dissolution]. Disintegration of tissues.

histolyt'ic. Pert. to histolysis.

histo'ma [Gr. *histos*, tissue, + *-ōma*, tumor]. A tumor composed of tissue. SYN: *histioma.*

his'ton(e [Gr. *histos*, web, tissue]. A class of simple proteins derived from cell nuclei which interferes with coagulation, yielding certain amino acids (the histone or hexone bases) as a result of hydrolysis.

   Histones are found in the thymus, sperm, and blood cells.

histonec'tomy ["+ *ektomē*, excision]. Periarterial excision of parts of the sympathetic nerve.

histon'omy ["+ *nomos*, law]. The law governing development and structure of tissues.

histonu'ria ["+ *ouros*, urine]. Excretion of histones in the urine.

histopathol'ogy [Gr. *histos*, tissue, + *pathos*, disease, + *logos*, study]. Histology of diseased tissues.

histophysiol'ogy ["+ *physis*, nature, + "]. Study of functions of cells and tissues.

Histoplas'ma ["+ *plasma*, thing formed]. A genus of parasitic fungi.

   H. capsulatum. The causative agent of histoplasmosis, q.v.

histoplas'min. An antigen prepared from cultures of *Histoplasma capsulatum* and used as a skin test for the diagnosis of histoplasmosis.

histoplasmo'sis [Gr. *histos*, tissue, + *plasma*, plasma, + *-ōsis*, diseased condition]. A systemic, fungal, respiratory disease due to Histoplasma capsulatum.

   SYM: The signs and symptoms vary from those of a mild self-limited infection to a severe fatal disease. In the severe form there is fever, anemia, enlargement of spleen and liver, leukopenia, pulmonary involvement, adrenal necrosis, and ulcers of the gastrointestinal tract.

   TREATMENT: amphotericin B intravenously.

historeten'tion [Gr. *histos*, tissue, + L. *rē*, back, + *tenēre*, to hold]. Retention of substances in the tissues.

historrhexis (hĭs-tō-rek'sĭs) ["+ *rhēxis*, rupture]. Disintegration of tissue by a noninfectious agent.

histother'apy ["+ *therapeia*, treatment]. Administration of animal tissues. SYN: *cytotherapy; organotherapy.*

histothrom'bin ["+ *thrombos*, a clot]. A thrombin derived from connective tissue.

histotome (hĭs'to-tōm) [Gr. *histos*, tissue, + *tomē*, incision]. Instrument for cutting tissue into very thin slices for microscopic study of its minute structure. SYN: *microtome.*

histotomy (hĭs-tŏt'ō-mĭ) ["+ *tomē*, incision]. 1. Dissection of tissue. 2. The cutting of thin sections of tissue for microscopic study. SYN: *microtomy.*

histotox'ic ["+ *toxikon*, poison]. Pertaining to a poisonous condition within the cells.

   h. anoxia. Anoxia in which oxidative processes of tissues are depressed or abolished, as in cyanide poisoning.

his'totribe ["+ *tribein*, to crush]. Instrument for crushing the tissues to stop bleeding.

his'totroph [Gr. *histos*, tissue, + *trophē*, nourishment]. Nutritive substances other than the mother's blood which the embryo utilizes in early development. These include endometrial tissues which have been destroyed during implantation, extravasated blood, and glandular secretions. SYN: *embryotroph.*

histotrophic (hǐs-tō-trof'ik). 1. Pert. to or favoring the formation of tissue. 2. Pert. to histotroph, q.v.

h. nutrition. Nutrition of the embryo in which histotroph serves as a source of nourishment. SEE: *hemotrophic nutrition.*

histotrop'ic [Gr. *histos,* tissue, + *tropē,* a turning]. Having attraction for tissue cells, as certain parasites, stains, or chemicals.

histozo'ic ["+ *zōē,* life]. Living within or on tissues, said of certain protozoan parasites.

histozyme (hǐs'to-zīm) ["+ *zymē,* leaven]. A renal enzyme which converts hippuric acid into benzoic acid and glycocoll, causing fermentation.

histrion'ic [L. *histriō,* an actor]. Theatrical, dramatic.

h. mania. Dramatic gestures, expressions and speech in certain psychiatric states.

h. spasm. Facial spasm, tics.

hives [of uncertain origin]. Eruption of very itchy wheals, caused by an allergic substance or food. Sudden sharp changes in climate may produce hives in some persons who are allergic to heat or cold. SYN: *nettle rash; urticaria,* q.v.

Hl. Abbr. for *latent hyperopia; hectoliter.*

Hm. Abbr. for *manifest hyperopia.*

HMD. Abbr. for *hyaline membrane disease,* q.v.

HMG. Abbr. for *human menopausal gonadotrophin.*

HNO₂. Chem. symb. for nitrous acid.

HNO₃. Chem. symb. for nitric acid.

Ho. Chem. symb. for holmium.

H₂O. Chem. symb. for water.

H₂O₂. Chem. symb. for hydrogen peroxide.

hoarse'ness [AS. *hās,* harsh]. A rough quality of the voice.

ETIOL: Simple chronic inflammations secondary to chronic nasopharyngitis (infected teeth, chemical irritants, tobacco, alcohol, etc.). Specific chronic laryngitis, syphilis, tuberculosis, leprosy. Neoplasms, papilloma, angioma, fibroma, singer's nodes, carcinoma. Paralyses. Prolapse of ventricle of larynx.

hob'nail liv'er. One with irregular surface. ETIOL: Cirrhosis from one of a variety of causes.

Hochsinger's sign (hōk'zing-er). [Karl Hochsinger, Austrian pediatrician, born 1860] Closure of fist in tetany when the inner side of biceps muscle is pressed.

Hodara's disease. [Menahem Hodara, Turkish physician, — 1926] Trichorrhexis nodosa, q.v.

hodegetics (hod''e-jĕt'iks) [Gr. *hodēgētikos,* suitable for guiding]. Medical ethics and etiquette.

Hodgkin's disease (hoj'kin). [Thomas Hodgkin, Brit. physician, 1798-1866] A disease of unknown etiology producing enlargement of lymphoid tissue, spleen and liver, with invasion of other tissues.

SYM: Enlargement of lymph nodes beginning in the cervical region, then the axillary, inguinal, mediastinal and mesenteric. There are signs due to pressure caused by lymphoid infiltration of blood vessels, bone marrow (with consequent anemia), and organs such as the liver and spleen. It may appear in several forms: acute, localized, latent with relapsing pyrexia, splenomegalic form, and lymphogranulomatosis.

hodoneuromere (hod-o-nū'ro-mēr) [Gr. *hodos,* path, + *neuron,* nerve, + *meros,* part]. Portion of the primitive trunk including neurons and processes.

hof [Ger., court]. The hollow area of the cell cytoplasm in which the nucleus is imbedded.

Hofbauer cell. [J. Isfred Isidore Hofbauer, Amer. gynecologist, 1878 —] A histiocyte found in the connective tissue of chorionic villi. It is thought to be phagocytic.

Hoffmann's atrophy. [Johann Hoffmann, Ger. neurologist, 1857-1919] A form of progressive muscular atrophy with characteristic changes in the forearm, hands, and lower legs. A familial condition which occurs in children.

holarthritis (hol-ar-thri'tis) [Gr. *holos,* entire, + *arthron,* joint, + *-itis,* inflammation]. Inflammation of all or many joints.

Hol'den's line. [Luther Holden, Brit. anatomist, 1815-1905] A wrinkle or indistinct furrow in the groin at the junction of the thigh and the abdomen.

holergasia (hol''er-ga'zī-ă) [Gr. *holos,* entire, + *ergon,* work]. A psychiatric disease of such degree as to affect the whole person.

holergastic (hol'er-gas'tik) [Gr. *holos,* entire, + *ergon,* work]. Pert. to holergasia.

hol'ism. The philosophy that, in nature, entities such as individuals and other complete organisms function as complete units which cannot be reduced to the sum of their parts. Originally discussed by Jan C. Smuts.

holis'tic. Pert. to holism.

hol'low-back. Anterior posterior spinal curvature. SYN: *lordosis.*

Holm'gren's test. [Alarik F. Holmgren, Swedish physiologist, 1831-1897] Matching colored skeins of yarn for testing color blindness.

holmium (holm´ĭ-um). SYMB: *Ho*. At. wt. 164.930; at. no. 67. An element, a rare earth metal.

holoblas´tic ova [Gr. *holos*, whole, + *blastos*, germ]. Cleavage with segmentation of the entire yolk. Complete division of the egg as opposed to partial or meroblastic cleavage.

holocrine (hol´o-krin) ["+ *krinein*, to secrete]. Pert. to a secretory gland or its secretions consisting of altered cells of the same gland. Opposite of merocrine, q.v.

holodiastol´ic ["+ *diastellein*, to expand]. Rel. to the entire diastole, esp. a murmur which occurs during all of diastole.

holography (hō-lŏg´rā-fĭ) [Gr. *holos*, whole, + *graphein*, to write]. A method of producing pictures in which the image appears as a three-dimensional representation of the original object. The picture obtained is called a hologram, i.e., "whole message."

holomastigote (hol´´o-măs´tĭ-gōt) ["+ *mastix, mastig-*, lash]. Having flagella all over the surface.

holorrachischisis (hol´´o-rā-kīs´kĭ-sis) ["+ *rachis*, spine, + *schisis*, fissure]. Complete spina bifida.

holosystol´ic [Gr. *holos*, entire, + *systellein*, to draw together]. Rel. to the entire systole.

holotetanus (hol-o-tĕt´ă-nus) ["+ *tetanos*, tetanus]. General tetanus. SYN: *holotonia, q.v.*

holoto´nia ["+ *tonos*, tension]. Muscular spasm of the entire body. SYN: *holotetanus.*

holoton´ic. Pert. to or affected by holotonia.

holotrichous (hōl-ŏt´rĭ-kus) [Gr. *holos*, entire, + *thrix*, hair]. Covered entirely with cilia, said of certain protozoa and bacteria.

holozo´ic ["+ *zōion*, animal]. Resembling an animal as to its method of nutrition in which organic materials serve as a source of energy.

Holt´house's hernia. [Carsten Holthouse, Brit. surgeon, 1810-1901] Inguinal hernia protruding along folds of the groin.

Holtz static machine. Machine for producing static electricity by induction.

Homan's sign. [John Homan, Amer. surgeon, 1877-1954] Pain in the calf when the toe is passively dorsiflexed. An early sign in venous thrombosis of the deep veins of the calf.

homax´ial [Gr. *homos*, the same, + L. *axis*, axis]. Having all axes alike, as a sphere.

homeo- [Gr. *homoios*, like, similar]. Prefix indicating likeness or resemblance.

homeomorphous (hō-mē-ō-mor´fŭs) ["+ *morphē*, form]. Of like shape but not of same composition.

hom´´eo-os´teoplasty ["+ *osteon*, bone, + *plassein*, to form]. Grafting of a piece of bone like the one upon which it is grafted.

homeopathic (hō-mē-ō-păth´ĭk) ["+ *pathos*, disease]. Pert. to homeopathy.

homeopathist (hō-mē-ŏp´ă-thĭst). One who practices homeopathy.

homeopathy (hō-mē-ŏp´ă-thĭ) [Gr. *homoios*, like, + *pathos*, disease]. School of medicine founded by Dr. S.C.F. Hahnemann (1755-1843) in 1796 in Philadelphia, which assumes that medicines which cure disease produce similar symptoms in the healthy. The drugs used are given in extremely small doses.

homeoplasia (hō-mē-ō-plā´zĭ-ă) ["+ *plassein*, to form]. Formation of new tissue similar to that already existing in a part.

homeoplas´tic. Rel. to or resembling the structure of adjacent parts.

homeostasis (hō´´mē-ō-stā´sis) [Gr. *homoios*, like, + *stasis*, a standing]. 1. State of equilibrium of the internal environment. 2. The state of relative constancy of the body fluids (blood, lymph, tissue fluid) as to their chemical and physical properties.

homeostat´ic. Pert. to homeostasis.

homeotherapy (hō´´mē-ō-thĕr´ă-pĭ) [Gr. *homoios*, like, + *therapeia*, treatment]. Treatment or prevention of disease with a substance similar to but not identical with the active causative agent. Ex: *jennerian vaccination.*

homeotransplant (hō´´mē-ō-trăns´plănt) ["+ L. *trans*, across, + *plantāre*, to plant]. Tissue from one individual transplanted into another of the same species.

homeotransplantation (hō´´mē-ō-trăns-plăn-tā´shŭn). Tissue transplantation from one to another of the same species.

homergy (hōm´ĕr-jĭ) [Gr. *homos*, same, + *ergon*, work]. Normal metabolism and its results.

homesickness [AS. *hām*, home, + *seōc*, ill]. Abnormal desire to return home. SYN: *nostalgia.*

homicide (hom´ĭ-sīd) [L. *homō*, man, + *caedere*, to cut]. 1. Murder. 2. A murderer.

homiculture (hom´ĭ-kult-chur) ["+ *cultura*, cultivation]. Application of the laws of breeding to the human species. SYN: *eugenics.*

hominid (hŏm´ĭ-nĭd) ["+ *eidos*, form]. A primate of the Hominidae family. Man is the only surviving species.

homo- [Gr. *homos*, same]. Prefix: Likeness.

homocen´tric [Gr. *homos*, same, + *kentron*, center]. Having the same center.

    h. rays. Light rays from the same center.

homochronous (hō-mō-krŏn′ŭs) ["+ *chronos*, time]. Occurring at the same time, or at the same age in each generation.

homogamet′ic ["+ *gamos*, marriage]. Producing one kind of gamete as regards the sex chromosome. In humans, the XX female is the homogametic sex as all ova produced contain the X chromosome. SEE: *heterogametic*.

homogenate (hō-mŏj′ĕ-nāt). The material obtained when something is homogenized.

homogeneous (hō-mō-jē′nē-ŭs) ["+ -*genēs*, born]. Uniform in structure, composition or nature.

homogenesis (hō-mō-jĕn′ē-sis) [Gr. *homos*, same, + *genesis*, development]. Reproduction of offspring similar to the parents. Opposite of heterogenesis.

homogenize (ho-mŏj′ĕ-nīz). To make homogeneous; to produce a uniform emulsion or suspension of two substances normally immiscible.

homogentis′ic acid. Alkaptone; an acid in the urine due to incomplete oxidation of tyrosine.

homogeny (hō-mŏj′ĕ-nī) [Gr. *homos*, same, + -*genēs*, born]. Reproduction of offspring similar to parents.

homoglandular (ho″mō-glăn′dū-lăr) ["+ L. *glandula*, a little acorn]. Rel. to the same gland.

homoiopodal (hō″moy-ŏp′o-dal) [Gr. *homoios*, like, + *pous, pod-*, foot]. With only one kind of process, as nerve cells.

homoiotherm (hō-moy′ō-thŭrm) ["+ *thermē*, heat]. A warm-blooded organism.

homolat′eral [Gr. *homos*, same, + L. *latus*, side]. Pert. to or on the same side. SYN: *ipsilateral*. SEE: *contralateral*.

homologous (hō-mŏl′o-gŭs) ["+ *logos*, proportion]. Similar in fundamental structure and in origin but not necessarily in function: e.g., the arm of man, forelimb of a dog, and the wing of a bird are homologous structures.

   h. **organs.** Structures which are morphological equivalents as the arm of man and forelimb of quadrupeds; penis of male and clitoris of female.

   h. **series.** Compounds with a similar chemical structure and properties, arranged in order of their molecular complexity, such as methane and ethane.

   h. **tissues.** Those identical in structure.

   h. **vaccine.** One from the microorganism infecting the patient. SYN: *autogenous vaccine.*

homologue (hŏm′ō-lŏg). 1. An organ or part common to a number of species. 2. One that

corresponds to a part or organ in another structure.

homology (hō-mŏl′o-jī) [Gr. *homos*, same, + *logos*, proportion]. Similarity in structure and in origin.

   h., **serial.** Anterior-posterior correspondence of parts of an organism which occur in a serial fashion, as the appendage of a crayfish, or the fore- and hind limbs of quadrupeds.

homolysin (ho-mŏl′ĭ-sin) ["+ *lysis*, dissolution]. An agent in a serum destructive of erythrocytes. SYN: *isolysin*.

homonomous (hō-mŏn′o-mus) ["+ *nomos*, law]. Pert. to parts arranged in a series which are similar in form and structure as metameres of a segmented animal or the fingers and toes.

homonymous (hō-mŏn′ĭ-mus) ["+ *onyma*, name]. Having the same name.

   h. **diplopia.** D. in which the image seen by the right eye is on the right side and vice versa.

homophil (hō′mō-fīl) ["+ *philein*, to love]. Pert. to an antibody reacting only with a specific antigen.

homophile (hō-mō-fīl′). Homosexual, q.v.

homoplas′tic [Gr. *homos*, same, + *plassein*, to form]. Having similar form and structure.

ho′moplasty. Repair by tissue similar to the one replaced.

Homo sapiens (hō′mō sā′pē-ĕnz) [L. *homo*, man, + *sapiens*, wise, sapient]. The species to which all races of modern man belong.

homosex′ual [Gr. *homos*, same, + L. *sexus*, sex]. 1. One sexually attracted to another of the same sex. 2. Pert. to attraction to another of same sex. SEE: *asexual; heterosexual.*

ho″mosexual′ity. A condition in which the libido is directed toward one of the same sex.

homostim′ulant [Gr. *homos*, same, + L. *stimulāre*, to arouse]. Stimulating the organ from which an extract is derived.

homotherm′al ["+ *thermē*, heat]. Condition in which the body temperature is maintained at a fairly constant level regardless of the temperature of the environment. SYN: *warm-blooded.*

homotonic (hō″-mō-tŏn′ik) ["+ *tonos*, tension]. Of uniform tension.

homotype (hō′mō-tīp) ["+ *typos*, type]. One organ or part similar in form and function to another, as one of two paired parts or organs.

homotypic (hō-mō-tīp′ik). Of the same form and type.

homozygosis (hō″mō-zī-gō′sis) [Gr. *homos*, same, + *zygon*, yoke, pair, + -*ōsis*, condition]. Formation of a zygote by the union of

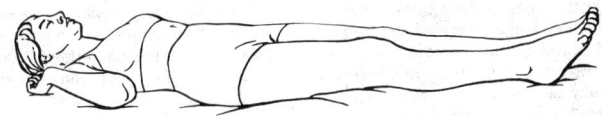

HORIZONTAL POSITION

genetically identical gametes. SEE: *heterozygosis.*

homozygote (hŏ″mō-zī′gōt). A homozygous individual; an individual developing from like gametes and thus possessing like pairs of genes for any hereditary characteristic.

homozygous (hŏ″mō-zī′gŭs). 1. Produced by similar gametes. 2. Pure bred. 3. Said of an organism when all germ cells transmit identical genes resulting from inbreeding.

homunculus (hō-mŭn′kū-lŭs) [L. diminutive of *homo,* man]. A dwarf in which the parts of the body develop in their normal proportions.

honey. A sweet thick liquid substance produced by bees from the nectar gathered from flowers and stored by them for food. The color and flavor is determined by the flowers used. H. has been used by man as a food since ancient times when it was early man's principal source of sugar. About 80% of h. is levulose and dextrose, the remainder mostly water.

Food value of 100 gm. (strained): Cal. 304; protein 0.3 gm.; carbohydrate 82.3 gm.; calcium 5 mg.; phosphorus 6 mg.; sodium 5 mg.; potassium 51 mg.; riboflavin .04 mg.; niacin 0.3 mg.; vitamin C content, minimal and decreases with age of the h.

hook [AS. *hōk,* an angle]. A curved instrument.

   h., blunt. One used in extraction of fetus or in embryotomy.

hook-up. Term used in speaking of the method of arranging circuits, appliances and electrodes in the giving of any particular treatment.

hook′worm. A parasitic nematode belonging to the superfamily Strongyloidea, esp. Ancylostoma duodenale and Necator americanus, q.v.

hook′worm disease. A condition brought about by the presence of the hookworm in the intestinal tract. SYN: *ancylostomiasis; uncinariasis.*

hordeolum (hor-de′o-lum) [L. barleycorn]. Inflammation of a sebaceous gland of the eyelid. SYN: *sty,* q.v.

   h. internum. Suppuration of Zeiss or meibomian glands.

horismascope (hor-is′mă-skōp) [Gr. *orizma,*

a boundary, + *skopein,* to examine]. A U-shaped tube for an acid test for albumin in the urine.

horizocardia (hŏ-rǐ″zo-kăr′dǐ-ă) [Gr. *horizōn,* horizon, + *kardia,* heart]. Horizontal position of the heart.

horizon′tal posi′tion [Gr. *horizōn,* horizon]. Lying supine and parallel to the floor. Employed in palpitation and auscultation of fetal heart beat and in operative procedures.

   h. p., abdominal. The patient lies flat on the abdomen. Employed in the examination of back and spinal column.

hormion (hor′mĭ-on) [Gr. *hormion,* a little chain]. Junction of posterior border of the vomer with the sphenoid bone.

hormone (hŏr′mōn) [Gr. *horman,* to urge on]. 1. A substance originating in an organ, gland, or part, which is conveyed through the blood to another part of the body, stimulating it by chemical action to increased functional activity and increased secretion. Contains amino acids which may be the precursors of h.'s. 2. The secretion of the ductless glands, such as insulin, by the pancreas.

   H.'s are active in minute quantities and do not supply energy. A h. that induces an excitatory effect is called an autacoid.

   h., adrenocortical. H. secreted by the cortex of the adrenal gland. SEE: *adrenal gland.*

   h., adrenocorticotropic. A h. secreted by the anterior lobe of the hypophysis (pituitary gland) which stimulates the adrenal cortex. SYN: *ACTH: corticotropin.*

   h., androgenic. Includes testosterone, androsterone, and dehydroandrosterone. H. which regulates the development and maintenance of the male secondary sexual characteristics; an androgen, q.v. Androgens are secreted by the interstitial tissue of the testis and by the adrenal cortex of both sexes. SYN: *male sex hormones.*

   h., anterior pituitary. H. secreted by anterior lobe of the hypophysis. Includes the somatotropic (SH) (also called human growth hormone (HGH)); thyrotropic (TH); gonadotropic; follicle-stimulating (FSH); interstitial-cell stimulating (ICSH); luteotropic (LH); prolactin; melanocyte stimulating; and adrenocorticotropic (ACTH) h.'s.

h., A.P.L. Anterior pituitary-like h. A chorionic gonadotropin secreted by the placenta and found in the urine of pregnant women and serum of pregnant mares. Used in pregnancy tests.

h., calcitonin. H. which in man is produced in the thyroid gland. Important in regulating calcium and bone metabolism.

h., corpus luteum. Progesterone, q.v.

h., corticoadrenal. Adrenocortical h., q.v.

h., estrogenic. A h., as estrogen, which stimulates the development and maintenance of female sexual characteristics. Estrogens are secreted by the ovary, the placenta, and the adrenal cortex in both sexes. Female h.'s. Include estradiol, estrone, estriol.

h., follicle, h., follicular. H. secreted by the ovarian follicles; an estrogen.

h., follicle-stimulating. (FSH). H. secreted by the anterior lobe of hypophysis which stimulates development of the ovarian follicles.

h., gastric. Gastrin, q.v.

h., gonadotropic. Anterior pituitary h. affecting the gonads. SEE: *follicle-stimulating h.; luteinizing h.; luteotropic h.*

h., human growth. Anterior pituitary h. promoting normal growth. ABBR: HGH. SYN: *somatotropin.*

h., interstitial cell-stimulating. (ICSH). SEE: *luteinizing h.*

h., intestinal. A h. produced by the mucosa of the intestine. SEE: *cholecystokinin; secretin.*

h., lactogenic. Former name for prolactin, q.v.

h., luteal. H. produced by the corpus luteum. SYN: *progesterone,* q.v.

h., luteinizing. H. produced by the anterior lobe of hyphophysis which induces ovulation and the formation of the corpus luteum. Also stimulates development of interstitial cells of the testes. SYN: *interstitial cell-stimulating hormone (ICSH).*

h., luteotropic. H. produced by anterior lobe of hypophysis which stimulates the secretion of progesterone by the corpus luteum and secretion of milk by the mammary gland. ABBR: LH. SYN: *lactogenic h.; prolactin.*

h., melanocyte stimulating. One that darkens the skin in man.

h., ovarian. A h. produced by the ovary. SEE: *estradiol; estriol; estrone; progesterone.*

h., pancreatic. H. produced by the islets of Langerhans of the pancreas. SEE: *insulin.*

h., parathyroid. H. secreted by the parathyroid glands which regulates calcium and phosphorus metabolism. Deficiency results in tetany. SEE: *parathormone.*

h., placental. H. secreted by the placenta. Includes estrogens and chorionic gonadotropin.

h., posterior pituitary. H. secreted by posterior lobe of hypophysis. Includes pitressin, which produces vasopressor and antidiuretic effects and oxytocin, which causes contraction of smooth muscles of the uterus.

h., prolactin. H. of the anterior pituitary which is important in lactation.

h.'s, sex, female. Estrogenic h.'s, q.v.

h.'s, sex, male. Androgenic h.'s, q.v.

h., testicular. H. produced by the interstitial tissue of the testis, e.g. testosterone, androsterone, and dehydroandrosterone, q.v.

h., thyroid. Thyroxine, the h. secreted by follicles of the thyroid gland.

h., thyrotropic. H. produced by anterior lobe of hypophysis which regulates development and functioning of the thyroid gland.

hormon'ic [Gr. *horman*, to urge on]. Rel. to or acting as a hormone. SYN: *hormonal.*

hormonogenesis (hŏr''mō-nō-jĕn'ĕ-sĭs) ["+ *genesis*, production]. Production of an internal secretion. SYN: *hormonopoiesis.*

hormonogenic (hŏr''mō-nō-jĕn'ik) ["+ *gennan*, to produce]. Producing hormones. SYN: *hormonopoietic.*

hormonol'ogy ["+ *logos*, study]. The study of hormones. SYN: *clinical endocrinology.*

hormonotropic. Stimulation of production of a hormone.

hormopoiesis (hŏr''mō-poy-ē'sĭs) [Gr. *horman*, to urge on, + *poiēsis*, formation]. The production of hormones. SYN: *hormonopoiesis.*

hormopoietic (hŏr-mō-poy-ĕt'ĭk). Rel. to hormones and their formation. SYN: *hormonopoietic.*

horn. A cutaneous outgrowth composed chiefly of keratin. A horn-like projection. SYN: *cornu,* q.v.

h. of Ammon. Hippocampus, q.v.

h., dorsal. Posterior projection of gray matter of the spinal cord. SYN: *posterior column.*

h., ventral. Anterior projection of gray matter of the spinal cord. SYN: *anterior column.*

Hor'ner's syndrome. [Johann F. Horner, Swiss ophthalmologist, 1831-1886] Contraction of the pupil, partial ptosis of the eyelid, enophthalmos, and sometimes loss of sweating over the affected side of the face. Due to paralysis of the cervical sympathetic nerve trunk.

hor′net sting. Sting by a hornet.

A general urticaria may result from the sting of this insect.

TREATMENT: Remove the stinger; apply cold compresses. Household ammonia in 10% solution applied to the area is beneficial and subsequent soothing lotions such as calamine lotion may be used. If pain is intense a local anesthetic may be injected.

If the systemic reaction is intense, 1 ml. of epinephrine of 1:1000 concentration may be given subcutaneously to adults. An injectable antihistamine may be administered subcutaneously or intravenously if given quite slowly.

hor′ny [AS. horn]. Resembling or consisting of horn.

   h. epithelium. The horny granulations in trachoma of the skin.

   h. layer. Horny layer of the skin. SYN: *stratum corneum* [NA].

horopter (hor-op′ter) [Gr. *horos*, limit, + *optēr*, observer]. Sum of all points in the binocular vision.

horripilation (hor′ĭ-pĭ-lā′shun) [L. *horrere*, to bristle, + *pilus*, hair]. Goose flesh. SYN: *cutis anserina.*

horse′shoe fis′tula. A fistulous tract in a semicircle in front of or behind the anus.

   h. kidney. A congenital abnormality. Both kidneys are united at their lower poles forming a horseshoe mass generally at a lower level than normal.

hos′pital [L. *hospitālis*, pert. to a guest]. Institution for medical and surgical treatment of the sick and injured.

   h., base. A h. unit within the lines of an army for reception from the front of wounded and sick patients as well as for those within the line.

   h., camp. An immobile military unit for care of sick and wounded in camp.

   h., cottage. A collection of detached cottages for care of the sick.

   h., evacuation. A mobile advance h. unit to take the place of field h.'s, and to supplement base h.'s.

   h., field. A portable military h. behind the zone of conflict and beyond the dressing stations. SYN: *mobile h.*

hos′pitalism [L. *hospitalis*, pert. to a guest, + Gr. *ismos*, state]. 1. The air of depression and apathy which often surrounds a group of seriously ill patients, esp. if they are in the same ward and overcrowded. 2. A neurotic tendency to seek hospitalization and, once hospitalized, to resist being discharged.

hospitalization. Removal of a patient to and confinement in a hospital.

host [L. *hospes*, a stranger]. 1. The organism from which a parasite obtains its nourishment. 2. In embryology, the larger and relatively normal of conjoined twins. 3. In transplantation of tissue, the individual who receives the graft.

   h., accidental. A h. other than the usual or normal host.

   h., alternate. H., intermediate, q.v.

   h., definitive. 1. The final h. or h. in which the parasite reaches sexual maturity. 2. The vertebrate, when the intermediate h. is an invertebrate.

   h., final. H., definitive, q.v.

   h., intermediate. 1. H. in which a parasite passes through its larval or asexual stages of development. 2. The invertebrate host, when final host is a vertebrate.

   h., primary. H., final, q.v.

   h., reservoir. A h. other than the usual or normal one, in which a parasite is capable of living and serving as a source of infestation.

   h., secondary. H., intermediate, q.v.

hot [AS. *hāt*, hot]. 1. Possessing a high temperature. 2. Actively conducting an electrical current. 3. Contaminated with dangerous radioactive material.

   h. flashes. Crises of vasodilation in skin of head, neck, and chest, accompanied by sensation of suffocation and sweating. Occurs commonly during menopause.

Hot′tentot ap′ron. Excessive elongation of the labia minora seen in Hottentot women. SYN: *velamen vulvae.*

Hottentot deformity. Abnormal fatness of the buttocks. SYN: *steatopygia.*

hot′tentotism. Abnormal form of stuttering.

hot water bag. Rubber or plastic bag of various shapes and sizes for applying dry heat to circumscribed areas and for keeping moist applications warm.

hourglass contrac′tion. Excessive, irregular contraction of an organ at its center, as the pregnant uterus during 3rd stage of labor.

The placenta is held in upper part of uterus by a tightly constricting band between lower and upper uterine segments. SYN: *ectasia.*

hourglass stomach. Division of stomach (in form of an hourglass) by a muscular constriction; often associated with gastric ulcer.

house fly. Musca domestica, a fly belonging to the order Diptera. Serves as a transmitter of organisms of many infectious diseases.

house'maid's knee. A traumatism resulting from kneeling, which produces a swelling of the bursa anterior to the patella.

house physician. A physician, esp. an intern or resident, who is responsible for caring for patients under the direction of the medical and surgical staff.

house staff. The interns and externs of a hospital acting under direction of the general staff.

house surgeon. The senior surgical member of the hospital staff who acts for the attending surgeon in his absence.

Houston's muscle (hūs'tonz). [John Houston, Irish surgeon, 1802-1845] The anterior part of the musculus bulbocavernosus.

Houston's valves. The folds of mucous membrane or valves formed by them in rectum. They are cresent-shaped. SYN: *plica transversalis recti.*

Howell-Jolly bodies. [William H. Howell, American physiologist, 1860-1945; Justin Jolly, French histologist, 1870-1953] Spherical granules seen in erythrocytes in slides of stained blood. They are thought to be nuclear particles. The bodies are seen in cases of congenital absence of the spleen; following splenectomy; in hemolytic anemia; in pernicious anemia; in thalassemia, and leukemia.

Howship's lacunae. [John Howship, English surgeon, 1781-1841] Small pits, grooves or depressions found where resorption of bone is occurring. They are usually occupied by osteoclasts. SEE: *osteoclast.*

Howship's symptom. Paresthesia, or pain in obturator hernia, on inner side of thigh.

HPO₃. Metaphosphoric acid.

H₃PO₂. Hypophosphorous acid.

H₃PO₃. Phosphorous acid.

H₃PO₄. Orthophosphoric acid.

H₄P₂O₆. Hypophosphoric acid.

Hr factors. Structures including Hr agglutinogens and Hr antigens, on surface of the red blood cells responsible for reactions with Hr antiserums. A number of related factors of human blood, so named because of their reciprocal relationship to the Rh factors. The factors, Hr', Hr'', and Hr₀ have been identified. These blood factors are important because sensitization may give rise to dangerous blood transfusion reactions. The baby of a sensitized Hr-negative pregnant woman may develop the blood disease, erythroblastosis fetalis, just as with sensitized Rh-negative mothers.

H.S. Abbr. for *house surgeon.*

h.s. Abbr. for *hora somni*, at bedtime.

H₂S. Hydrogen sulfide.

H₂SO₃. Sulfurous acid.

H₂SO₄. Sulfuric acid.

H-substance. A substance similar to or identical with histamine, q.v.

Ht. Abbr. for *total hypermetropia.*

Hub'bard tank. One used for underwater exercises.

Huguier's canal (ē-gǐ-äz). [Pierre C. Huguier, French surgeon, 1804-1873] A canal through which the chorda tympani nerve exits from the cranium.

Huguier's diseases. Lupus of vulva, and uterine fibroma.

Huguier's glands. Two tiny vaginal glands.

Huhner test. [Max Huhner, American urologist, 1873-1947] One for sterility in the male. SEE: *test.*

hum. A soft continuous sound.

    h., venous. Sound from large veins in certain anemias. SYN: *bruit de diable.*

hu'man [L. *hūmānus*, human]. Pert. to or characterizing man or mankind.

    h. bite. Wound caused by human teeth. SYM: Intense swelling, edema, and foul discharge may develop. The organisms which may be found in wounds from such bites are staphgloccus; steptococcus; anaerobic streptococcus; Vincent's bacillus; spirochete; fusiform bacillus; and gas-gangrene bacillus. The fusiform bacillus and the spirochete are believed to cause the gangrenous nature of the wounds.

    TREATMENT: If lymphangitis, moderate fever, and leukocytosis occur, a wide incision may be necessary with debridement and irrigation. Bacterial examination of pustular material taken from the wound will permit appropriate antibiotic therapy. Victims of a h. b. need the immediate attention of a physician.

    h. placental lactogen. A hormonal substance produced by the placenta. Its actions include stimulating the metabolism of glucose and converting it to fat. ABBR: HPL.

humectant (hu-mek'tant) [L. *humectus*, moist]. A moistening agent.

humeral (hū'mer-al) [L. *humerus*, upper arm]. Pert. to the humerus.

humeroradial (hū"mer-o-rā'dī-ăl) ["+ *radius*, wheel spoke, ray]. Pert. to humerus and radius, esp. in comparison of their length.

humeroulnar (hū"mer-o-ul'nar) ["+ *ulna*, elbow]. Pert. to the humerus and ulna, esp. in comparison to their length.

hu'merus [L., upper arm]. Upper bone of arm from the elbow (articulating with the ulna and radius) to the shoulder joint, where it articulates with the scapula.

    h., fracture of. 1. If the fracture is of the upper end the arm is abducted on a wire

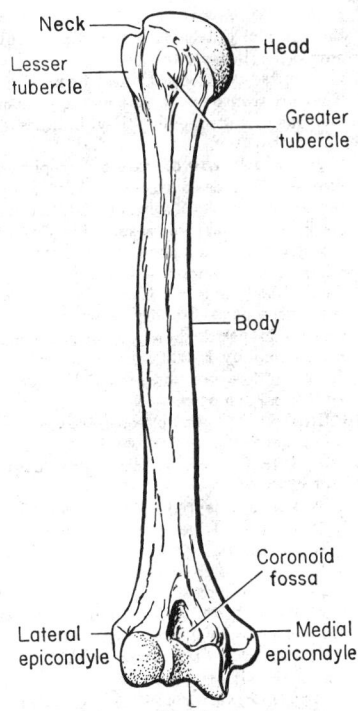

RIGHT HUMERUS, ANTERIOR VIEW

Neck — Head
Lesser tubercle
Greater tubercle
Body
Coronoid fossa
Lateral epicondyle — Medial epicondyle
Trochlea

Air Is Completely Saturated With Water Vapor

At		If it Contains
F.	C.	grams
50°	10°	9.6 water/cubic meter
60°	15.5°	13.3 water/cubic meter
70°	21°	18.1 water/cubic meter
90°	32°	32.7 water/cubic meter

ic pressure. Air which is fully saturated with moisture has 100% relative h. When air which is fully saturated is cooled, the excess moisture condenses as in the case of dew or moisture on a cold glass in the summer.

If air was saturated at a temperature of 70° F. (21.1° C.), water would condense on all objects if the temperature fell to 68° F. (20° C.). Air can contain at 90° F. (32.2° C.) almost twice as much water as at 70° F. (21.1° C.).

humor [L. *humor,* fluid]. 1. Any fluid or semifluid substance in the body. 2. In ancient medicine, the four 'juices' or fluids (blood, phlegm, black bile, yellow bile) of which the body was thought to be composed.

  h., aqueous. The clear watery fluid in the anterior and posterior chambers of the eye.

  h., crystalline. The fluidlike substance of the crystalline lens of the eye.

  h., vitreous. The vitreous body, q.v. A semifluid, transparent substance occupying the space between the lens and retina of the eye.

hu'moral [L. *humor,* fluid]. Pertaining to body fluids or substances contained in them.

  h. control or correlation. The control of various bodily activites by chemical substances, esp. hormones transported by the blood or lymph. In contrast to nervous control brought about through nerve impulses.

humpback. 1. Curvature of the spine to such an extent that the back appears to have a lump or protuberance on it. 2. An individual with a humpback. SYN: *kyphosis.*

hung'er [AS. *hungur,* hunger]. 1. A sensation resulting from lack of food, characterized by dull or acute pain referred to the epigastrium or lower part of chest. Usually accompanied by weakness and an overwhelming desire to eat. H. pains coincide with powerful contractions of the stomach. H. is distinguished from appetite in that the latter is a pleasant sensation based on previous experience which causes one to seek food for the

splint for about four weeks. Movements of the elbow and wrist are started early and movements (active) of shoulder in about three weeks.

2. Fracture of shaft and lower end: The limb is put in plaster in a position midway between pronation and supination with the h. at right angles to the forearm. Movement of the shoulder, wrist, and finger is allowed at once.

  RS: acromiohumeral; capitellum; cubitus; glenoid cavity.

hu'mid [L. *humidus,* moist]. Moist, damp, esp. when pert. to air.

  h. gangrene. G. with serous exudation and rapid decomposition. SEE: *gangrene.*

humidifier (hū-mid'ĭ-fī"er). Apparatus to increase moisture content of the air in a room.

humid'ity [L. *humiditās*]. Moisture in the atmosphere.

  The moisture content of air usually is expressed as relative h. This indicates the amount of water vapor in the air compared to the total amount of moisture the air could contain at that temperature and atmospher-

purpose of tasting and enjoying. 2. To have a strong desire.

h., air. Dyspnea, breathlessness.

h. contractions. Those occurring in the normal empty stomach. They may be painful. A series of such contractions is followed by a period of rest, after which they may return with great intensity unless food is taken. Digestion may be activated under such conditions.

h. cure. Restricted diet or fasting for cure of disease. SYN: *nestitherapy.*

hungry. Craving food.

hunte'rian chancre. Indurated, syphilitic chancre. SEE: *chancre.*

Hun'ter's canal. [John Hunter, English anatomist and surgeon, 1728-1793] Canalis adductorius.

Hurler's syndrome. [Gertrud Hurler, Austrian pediatrician] Lipochondrodystrophy, q.v.

Huschke's auditory teeth (hoosh'kĕz). [Emil Huschke, Ger. anatomist, 1797-1858] Tiny, toothlike protuberances at edge of cochlear labium vestibulare.

Huschke's canal. Canal formed by juncture of the annulus tympanicus tubercules. Usually present only during early childhood.

Huschke's foramen. Perforation found in arrested development near inner extremity of tympanic plate.

Huschke's valve. Plica lacrimalis, q.v.

Hutchinson's patch (hŭtsh'ĭn-sŏn). [Sir Jonathan Hutchinson, English surgeon, 1828-1913] Salmon-colored area in the cornea seen in syphilitic keratitis. SYN: *salmon patch.*

Hutchinson's teeth. A congenital condition; pegged, lateral incisors and notched central incisors along the cutting edge.
  A sign of congenital syphilis.

Hux'ley's layer. [Thomas H. Huxley, English physiologist and naturalist, 1825-1895] Inner layer of nucleated cells forming the inner root sheath of a hair follicle.

HVH. Abbr. for *herpesvirus hominus.*

hyalin (hī'ă-lin) [Gr. *hyalos,* glass]. 1. A substance obtainable from the products of amyloid, colloid, or hyaloid degeneration. 2. Basement substance of hyaline cartilage.

hyaline (hī'ă-lin) [Gr. *hyalos,* glass]. Crystalline, glassy, translucent. SEE: *casts; degeneration.*

h. alcoholic. Acidophilic staining material in the liver cells in certain forms of cirrhosis.

h. bodies. Homogeneous substance; the result of colloid degeneration and found in degenerated cells.

h. cartilage. The true cartilage. Smooth and pearly. It covers the articular surfaces of bones.

h. casts. The commonest form of cast. They are transparent, pale, and have homogeneous rounded ends; they indicate nephropathy.

h. membrane disease. A respiratory disease of the newborn infant. It is characterized by dyspnea, expiratory grunt, cyanosis, limpness and rapid respiration. Severity varies greatly. In some cases it is mild; in others the symptoms subside within four days. If death occurs it is usually within the first three days. Etiology is unknown and there is no specific therapy, only supportive. Approximately 25,000 infants in the U. S. die of this disease each year. SYN: *respiratory distress syndrome.*

hyalino'sis ["+ *ōsis,* increase]. Waxy or hyaline degeneration.

hyalinu'ria ["+ *ouron,* urine]. Hyalin present in the urine.

hyalitis (hi-ă-li'tis) ["+ *-itis,* inflammation]. Inflammation of the vitreous humor.

h., asteroid. Spherical or star-shaped bodies in the vitreous of the eye. Due to inflammation.

h. puncta'ta. A form marked by minute opacities in the vitreous humor.

h. suppurati'va. A purulent inflammation of the vitreous humor.

hyalo- [Gr. *hyalos,* glass]. Prefix indicating resemblance to glass.

hyaloenchondroma (hi''ă-lo-en''kon-dro'mă) ["+ *en,* in, + *chondros,* cartilage, + *ōma,* tumor]. A chondroma composed of hyaline cartilage.

hyalogen (hi-al'o-jen) ["+ *gennan,* to produce]. A protein substance in cartilage and the vitreous humor.

hyaloid (hī'ă-loyd) ["+ *eidos,* form]. Hyaline, glassy.

h. artery. Present in the fetus. Supplies nutrition to lens. Disappears in later months of gestation.

h. canal. Lymph channel in vitreous extending from optic disk to posterior capsule of lens; contains hyaloid artery in fetus.

h. membrane. That which envelops the vitreous humor.

hyaloiditis (hi''ă-loyd-i'tis) ["+ "+ *-itis,* inflammation]. Inflammation of the hyaloid membrane of the vitreous humor. SYN: *hyalitis.*

hyaloma (hi-ă-lōmă) [Gr. *hyalos,* glass, + *ōma,* tumor]. A small yellow papule which develops in the corium of the skin as a result of colloid degeneration. SYN: *colloid milium.*

hyalomere (hī'ă-lo-mīr) ["+ *meros*, part]. Homogeneous part of a blood platelet, pale in color, as contrasted with the chromomere.

hyalomu'coid ["+ L. *mucus*, mucus, + Gr. *eidos*, form]. Mucoid in vitreous body.

hyalonyxis (hī"ă-lo-nik'sis) ["+ *nyxis*, puncture]. The surgical procedure of puncturing the vitreous body.

hyalophagia (hī"ă-lo-fa'jī-ă) ["+ *phagein*, to eat]. The eating of glass by the demented.

hyalophagy (hī"ă-lof'ă-jī). Eating of glass by the demented. SYN: *hyalophagia.*

hyalopho'bia [Gr. *hyalos*, glass, + *phobos*, fear]. Fear of touching glass.

hyaloplasm (hī'ă-lo-plazm) ["+ *plasma*, a thing formed]. The fluid portion of protoplasm. The basic ground substance; also called basic or fundamental protoplasm. SYN: *hyalomitome.*

h., nuclear. Clear substance filling the meshes of the nuclear reticulum. SYN: *karyolymph; nuclear sap.*

hyaloserositis (hī"ă-lo-se"ro-si'tis) ["+ L. *serum*, whey, + Gr. *-itis*, inflammation]. Inflammation of a serous membrane with fibrinous exudate undergoing hyaline transformation.

h., progressive multiple. Phthisis of serous membranes.

hyalotome (hi-al'o-tōm) [Gr. *hyalos*, glass]. Fluid portion of protoplasm. SYN: *hyaloplasm.*

hyaluron'ic acid. An acid mucopolysaccharide found in the ground substance of connective tissue which acts as a binding and protective agent. Also found in the synovial fluid, vitreous and aqueous humors.

hyaluronidase (hī"ă-lur-on'ĭ-dās). An enzyme found in the testes and other tissues and present in semen. It depolymerizes hyaluronic acid thereby increasing the permeability of connective tissues by dissolving the substances that hold body cells together. It acts to disperse the cells of the corona radiata about the newly ovulated ovum. SYN: *Duran-Reynals spreading factor.*

hybrid [L. *hybrida*, mongrel]. The offspring of parents from unlike races, cultures, species, etc.

hybridization (hī'brid-i-zā'shun). The production of hybrids by cross breeding.

hydantoin (hi-dan'to-in). A colorless base, glycolyl urea, $C_3H_4N_2O_2$, from urea or allantoin.

hydatid (hi'dă-tid) [Gr. *hydatis*, watery vesicle]. 1. A cyst formed in the tissues, esp. liver, resulting from the development of the larval stage of the dog tapeworm, Echinococcus granulosus. The cysts develop slowly forming a hollow bladder from the inner surface of which hollow brood capsules are formed. These are attached to the mother cyst by slender stalks or they may fall free into the fluid-filled cavity of the mother cyst. Scolices form on the inner surface of the older brood capsules. In older cysts there is a granular deposit of brood capsules and scolices called hydatid sand. Hydatids may grow for years, sometimes attaining an enormous size. 2. A small cystic remnant of an embryonic structure.

TREATMENT: Surgical.

h. fremi'tus. A tremulous sensation felt on palpating a hydatid tumor.

h. mole. Degenerative process in chorionic villi, which gives rise to multiple cysts and rapid growth of uterus with hemorrhage. DIAG: Indicated by the hemorrhaging and expulsion of some of the cysts.

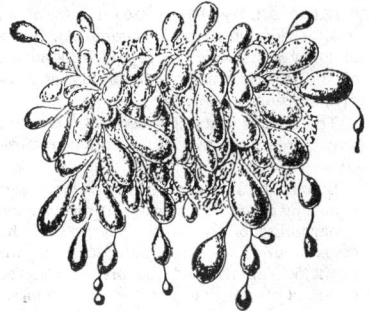

HYDATID MOLE
The entire placenta is transformed into a large number of edematous vesicles which resemble a bunch of grapes. Only a small part of the placenta is represented in this picture.

h. of Morgagni. Cystlike remnant of the mullerian duct which is attached to the fallopian tube.

h., sessile. Morgagnian h. connected with a testicle.

h., stalked. Morgagnian h. connected with a fallopian tube.

hydatidiform (hi"dă-tid'ĭ-form) ["+ L. *forma*, shape]. Having the form of a hydatid.

hydatidocele (hi"dă-tid'o-sēl) ["+ *kēlē*, tumor]. Hydatid cyst of scrotum or testicle.

hydatido'ma ["+ *ōma*, tumor]. A tumor consisting of hydatids.

hydatidosis (hī"dă-tĭd-ō'sĭs) [Gr. *hydatis*, watery vesicle, + *-ōsis*, increase]. Condition caused by infestation with hydatids.

hydatidostomy (hi″dă-tid-os′to-mĭ) ["+ *stoma*, opening]. Evacuation of a hydatid cyst by means of surgery.

hydat′iform ["+ L. *forma*, form]. Hydatidiform, q.v.

hy′datism ["+ *ismos*, state of]. The sound produced by fluid in a cavity.

hydradenitis (hi″drad-ĭ-ni′tis) [Gr. *hydrōs*, sweat, + *adēn*, gland, + *-itis*, inflammation]. Inflammation of a sweat gland.

hydradeno′ma ["+ "+ *ōma*, tumor]. Tumor of a sweat gland.

hydraeroperitoneum (hi-dra″er-o-per′ĭ-to-ne′um) [Gr. *hydōr*, water, + *aēr*, air, + *peritonaion*, peritoneum]. Collection of fluid and gas in the peritoneal cavity.

hydragogue (hi′dră-gog) ["+ *agōgos*, leading]. Drug promoting watery evacuation of the bowels.

Ex: Magnesium sulfate, sodium phosphate.

hydramnion, hydramnios (hi-dram′nĭ-on, -os) ["+ *amnion*, a caul on a lamb]. An excess of liquor amnii which leads to overdistention of the uterus and the possibility of malpresentation.

The normal amount is 500 to 1,000 ml. It may increase to 2,500 ml. and not be regarded as abnormal.

Liquor amnii is secreted by the fetus, and abnormal amounts are probably due to some abnormality of the fetus. Nearly half the cases occur in twin pregnancies. H. begins about 5th month and the pressure of the enlarged uterus gives rise to breathlessness, edema, cyanosis, and varicose veins in the mother. The uterus is large for the length of pregnancy and the fetus may be felt bobbing about in the liquor and the fetal heart is not easily heard.

hydrargyrum (hi-drar′jir-um) ["+ *argyros*, silver]. Mercury or quicksilver. SEE: *mercury*.

hydrarthrosis (hi″drar-thrō′sis) ["+ *arthron*, joint, + *-ōsis*]. Serous effusion in a joint cavity; white swelling.

hydrase. An enzyme which catalyzes the addition or withdrawal of water from a compound without hydrolysis occurring.

hydrate (hi′drāt) [Gr. *hydōr*, water]. A crystalline substance formed by water combining with various compounds.

hydrated (hi′dră-ted). Combined chemically with water.

hydra′tion. The chemical combination of a substance with water.

hydrazine (hi′dră-zin). 1. A colorless gas, H₄-N₂, with peculiar odor; soluble in water. 2. One of a class derived from hydrazine.

hydre′mia [Gr. *hydōr*, water, + *haima*, blood]. Excess of watery fluid in the blood.

hydrencephalocele (hi″dren-sef′ă-lo-sēl) ["+ *enkephatos*, brain, + *kēlē*, tumor]. A hernia through a cranial defect of brain substance and meninges, in which fluid occupies the space between the two.

hydrencephalus (hi″dren-sef′ă-lus). Accumulation of fluid in the cerebral ventricles or outside of the brain. SYN: *hydrocephalus*.

hydrepigastrium (hi″drep-ĭ-gas′trī-um) ["+ *epi*, upon, + *gastēr*, belly]. Accumulation of fluid between the peritoneum and the abdominal muscles.

hydriatric (hi-drī-at′rik) ["+ *iatrikos*, healing]. Pert. to treatment of disease with water, as hydriatic procedures or hydriatric institutions.

hydriatrics (hi-drī-at′riks). Application of water in treatment of disease. SYN: *hydrotherapeutics*.

hydriat′rist. One who practices hydrotherapy.

hy′dride. Chemical compound containing hydrogen and an element or radical.

hy′drion. The hydrogen ion (H⁺).

hydro- [Gr. *hydōr*, water]. Prefix pert. to water or to hydrogen.

hydro′a. Chronic inflammatory skin disease. Not to be confused with hidroa, q.v.

SYM: Bullae, erythema, itching, papules, pustules, and vesicles.

hydroappen′dix [Gr. *hydōr*, water, + L. *appendere*, to hang upon]. Watery fluid distending the vermiform appendix.

hydrobilirubin (hi″dro-bil″ĭ-ru′bin) ["+ L. *bilis*, bile, + *ruber*, red]. A brownish-red bile pigment perhaps identical with stercobilin and urobilin.

hydrobromate (hi″dro-bro′māt) ["+ *brōmos*, stench]. A salt of hydrobromic acid.

hydrocarbon [Gr. *hydōr*, water, + L. *carbo*, coal]. A compound made up only of hydrogen and carbon.

Hydrocarbons may exist as aliphatic chain compounds in which the carbon atoms are arranged in the form of a chain, or as aromatic or cyclic compounds in which the carbon atoms form one or more rings.

h., saturated. H. in which the carbon atoms are linked by a single electron pair and in which all valences are satisfied.

h., unsaturated. H. in which carbon atoms share two or three pairs of electrons.

hydrocele (hi′dro-sēl) ["+ *kēlē*, tumor]. The accumulation of serous fluid in a saclike cavity, esp. in the tunica vaginalis testis; serous tumors of the testes or associated parts.

h., acute. Most common, majority of cases present between 2nd and 5th years, h. occurring suddenly, usually the result of inflammation of the epididymis or testis.

h., cervical. H. in the neck resulting from accumulation of serous fluid in persistent cervical duct or cleft.

h., chronic. H. usually seen in men of middle age. May result from filariasis.

h., congenital. That present at birth, resulting from failure of closure of the vaginal process.

h., encysted. H. in the vaginal process in which openings to the scrotal and peritoneal cavities are closed.

h. feminae. H. in labium majus or canal of Nuck.

h. hernialis. When hernia accompanies infantile or congenital h. and there is an accumulation of peritoneal fluid in a hernia sac.

h., infantile. Peritoneal fluid in the tunica vaginalis and vaginal process with the latter closed at the abdominal ring.

h. muliebris. H. feminae, q.v.

h., spermatic. Spermatic fluid in the tunica vaginalis of the testes.

h. spinalis. Spina bifida.

hydrocenosis (hi″dro-sen-o′sis) ["+ *kenōsis,* an emptying]. Evacuation of accumulation of peritoneal fluid by tapping or by a hydragogue. SYN: *paracentesis.*

hydrocephal′ic [Gr. *hydōr,* water, + *kephalē,* head]. Pert. to hydrocephalus.

hydrocephalocele (hi″dro-sef′ă-lo-sēl) ["+ "+ *kēlē,* tumor]. Watery hernia of the brain. SYN: *hydrencephalocele.*

hydroceph′aloid ["+ "+ *eidos,* resemblance]. Resembling or pert. to hydrocephalus.

hydrocephalus (hi-dro-sef′ă-lus) [Gr. *hydōr,* water, + kephalē, head]. The increased accumulation of cerebrospinal fluid within the ventricles of the brain. Results from interference with normal circulation and with absorption of the fluid and, esp., from destruction of the foramina of Magendie and Lushka. This may result from developmental anomalies, infection, injury, or brain tumors.

In severe cases in children, the head is usually globular or pyramidal in shape. Face disproportionately small. Eyes hidden in sockets and turned upward. Sutures separated, with bulging fontanels and thin cranial bones.

In older individuals, after skull has formed, there are headache, vomiting, choked disks, atrophy of optic nerve, mental disturbances.

h., communicating. H. in which normal communication between 4th ventricle and subarachnoid space is maintained.

h., congenital. Chronic type occurring in infancy. SYN: *infantile h.*

h., external. Accumulation of fluid in subdural spaces.

h., internal. Accumulation of fluid within ventricles of the brain.

h., normal pressure. Type of h. with enlarged ventricles of the brain with no increase in the spinal fluid pressure or no demonstrable block to the outflow of spinal fluid.

h., secondary. H. following injury or infections such as meningitis or syphilis.

hydrochlorate (hi″dro-klo′rāt) ["+ *chlōros,* green]. Any salt of hydrochloric acid.

hy′drochlo′ric acid. An aqueous solution of hydrogen chloride (HCl), containing 35 to 38% HCl. Crude commercial hydrochloric acid is known as muriatic acid.

It is a normal constituent of gastric juice, amounting to 0.4 to 0.5% and is produced by the parietal cells of gastric glands. It serves the following functions: Converts pepsinogen into pepsin and produces an acid medium favorable for the activity of pepsin; dissolves and disintegrates nucleoproteins and collagen; hydrolyzes sucrose; precipitates caseinogen; inhibits multiplication of bacteria, esp. putrefactive organisms which ferment lactic acid and certain pathogenic forms; stimulates secretion by the duodenum. It inhibits the action of ptyalin and thus stops salivary digestion in the stomach.

Average amount found in the food content of stomach is only about 0.2%, due to dilution and neutralization by alkaline contents. In pernicious anemia there is an absence of this acid (achlorhydria).

h. a., dilute. Aqueous solution of 10% HCl.

hydrocholecystis (hi″dro-ko″lī-sis′tis) [Gr. *hydōr,* water, + *cholē,* bile, + *kystis,* bladder]. Dropsy of gallbladder.

hydrocholeresis (hi″dro-ko″ler-ē′sis) ["+ "+ *hairesis,* a taking]. Choleresis in which water content of the bile is increased resulting, in production of bile with reduced specific gravity, viscosity, and total solid content.

hydrocirsocele (hi″dro-sir′so-sēl) ["+ *kirsos,* varix, + *kēlē,* tumor]. Hydrocele combined with varicose veins of spermatic cord.

hydrocollidine (hi″dro-kol′ĭ-din) ["+ *kolla,* glue]. A toxic substance from putrefying fish or animal flesh.

hydrocolpos (hi-dro-kol′pos) [Gr. *hydōr,* water, + *kolpos,* vagina]. Retention cyst of the vagina containing watery, nonsanguineous fluid, or mucus.

hydroconion (hi″dro-ko′nĭ-on) ["+ *konis,* dust]. An atomizer which emits a fine spray.

hy′drocyst ["+ *kystis,* a bladder]. A cyst containing watery fluid.

hydrocysto′ma ["+ "+ *ōma,* tumor]. Disease marked by small cysts which originate in the sweat gland. Sudamina on the face, esp. in women after middle age. SYN: *hidrocystoma.*

hydrodiascope (hi″dro-di′ă-skōp) ["+ *dia,* through, + *skopein,* to examine]. Device to treat astigmatism.

hydrodictiotomy (hi″dro-dik″tĭ-ot′o-mĭ) ["+ *diktyon,* retina, + *tomē,* incision]. A surgical procedure to correct displacement of the retina.

hydroencephalocele (hi″dro-en-sef′ă-lo-sēl) [Gr. *hydōr,* water, + *enkephalos,* brain, + *kēlē,* tumor]. Brain substance expanded into a watery sac protruding through a cleft in the cranium. SYN: *hydrencephalocele.*

hydrogel (hi′dro-jel) ["+ L. *gelāre,* to congeal]. A colloid containing water that solidifies in gelatinous form.

hy′drogen [Gr. *hydōr,* water, + *gennan,* to produce]. SYMB: *H.* At. wt. 1.0080; at no. 1; sp. gr. 0.069. An element existing as a colorless, odorless, tasteless gas. It possesses one valence electron. Three isotopes of hydrogen (protium, deuterium, and tritium) exist having atomic weight of 1, 2, and 3, respectively.

OCCURRENCE: H. occurs in its free state (in natural gases and volcanic eruptions) only in minute quantities. It is present in the sun and stars; on the earth it comprises about 1% of all known terrestrial matter. It occurs principally as hydrogen oxide (water, H_2O) and is a constituent of all hydrocarbons. It is present in all acids and in ionic form is responsible for the properties characteristic of acids. It is present in nearly all organic compounds and is a component of all carbohydrates, proteins, and fats.

USES: It is highly inflammable and used in the oxyhydrogen flame in welding, in hydrogenation of oils for solidifying purposes, as a reducing agent, and in many syntheses.

    h. acceptor. In oxidation reduction reactions a substance which receives hydrogen atoms from another substance. SEE: *coenzyme.*

    h. donator. In oxidation-reduction reactions a substance which gives up hydrogen atoms to another substance, the acceptor.

hy′drogenate. To bring about a combination with hydrogen.

hydrogenation (hi″dro-jen-a′shun). A process of changing an unsaturated fat to a solid saturated fat by the addition of hydrogen in the presence of a catalyst, as olein and stearin.

hydrogen dioxide (di-oks′ĭd) [Gr. *hydōr,* water, + *gemman,* to produce, + *dis,* twice, + *oxys,* sharp]. Hydrogen peroxide (H_2O_2), q.v.

hydrogen ion. The positively charged nucleus of a hydrogen atom.

    h. ion concentration. The relative proportion of hydrogen ions in a solution, the factor responsible for the acidic properties of a solution.

    h. ion (pH) scale. A scale used to express the degree of acidity or alkalinity of a solution. It extends from 0.00 (total acidity) to 14 (total alkalinity), the numbers running in reverse order of H-ion concentration. The pH value is the negative logarithm of the H-ion concentration of a solution, expressed in gram ions (moles) per liter.

As the hydrogen ion concentration decreases, a change of 1 pH unit means a ten-fold increase in hydrogen-ion concentration or true acidity. Thus a solution with a pH of 1.0 is ten times more acid than one with a pH of 2.0 and 100 times more acid than one with a pH of 3.0. A pH of 7.0 indicates neutrality.

As the hydrogen-ion concentration varies in a definite reciprocal manner with the hydroxyl-ion (OH–) concentration, a pH reading above 7.0 indicates alkalinity. The blood and body fluids are slightly alkaline, having a pH of 7.35 to 7.45.

hydrogen peroxide [Gr. *hydōr,* water, + *gennan,* to form, + L. *per,* through, + Gr. *oxys,* sharp]. H_2O_2, a colorless, syrupy, liquid with an irritating odor and acrid taste. It decomposes readily, liberating oxygen. Light is particularly effective in activating H_2O_2; therefore it should be stored in tightly sealed glass jars in a dark place.

USES: As a commercial bleaching agent, as an oxidizing and reducing agent. In a 3% solution, as a mild antiseptic, germicide, and cleansing agent.

    h. p., solution of. In a 3% aqueous solution h. p. has the ability to kill bacteria, and this is the most important use of s. of h. p. However, its germicidal activity has been greatly overrated. Organic matter has a tendency to decompose it and as long as there is effervescence when the solution is applied to a wound, there is no great destruction of bacteria.

S. of h. p. has value as a cleansing agent for suppurating wounds and inflamed mucous membranes. It is esp. useful for this purpose because of its development of gas which tends to loosen adherent deposits and organic detritus, q.v., which might form a breeding place for microrganisms.

S. of h. p. is sometimes injected into deep cavities to determine the presence of pus, which will be indicated by effervescence. Because of its lack of toxicity it is a favored disinfectant for application to various mucous membranes, esp. those of the nose and throat. Diluted with equal parts of water it is used as a gargle in pharyngitis, or mouthwash in stomatitis.

hydroglossa (hi″dro-glos′ă) [″+ *glōssa,* tongue]. Cystic tumor beneath the tongue. SYN: *ranula.*

hydrogymna′sium [Gr. *hydōr,* water, + *gymnazein,* to train naked]. Pool for underwater excercises.

hydrogymnas′tics. Underwater exercises.

hydrohematonephrosis (hi″dro-hem″ă-to-nef-ro′sis) [Gr. *hydōr,* water, + *haima,* blood, + *nephros,* kidney, + *-ōsis,* increase]. Blood and urine distending pelvis of the kidney.

hydrohymenitis (hi″dro-hi″men-i′tis) [″+ *hymēn,* membrane, + *-itis,* inflammation]. Any inflammation of a serous membrane.

hydrokinet′ics [Gr. *hydōr,* water, + *kinēsis,* motion]. Science of fluids in motion.

hydrolase (hi′dro-lās). An enzyme that causes hydrolysis.

hydrology (hi-drol′o-jī) [Gr. *hydōr,* water, + *logos,* science]. The science of water in all its aspects.

hydrolysis (hi-drol′ĭ-sis) [Gr. *hydōr,* water, + *lysis,* dissolution]. Any reaction in which water is one of the reactants, more specifically the combination of water with a salt to produce an acid and a base, one of which is more dissociated than the other. The reverse of neutralization. A chemical decomposition in which a substance is split into simpler compounds by the addition of and the taking up of the elements of water.

Reactions of this kind are extremely frequent in life processes. The conversion of starch to maltose, of fat to glycerol and fatty acid, and of protein to amino acids, are examples of hydrolysis, as are other reactions involved in digestion. A simple example is the reaction in which the hydrolysis of ethyl acetate yields acetic acid and ethyl alcohol: $C_2H_5C_2H_3O_2 + H_2O = HC_2H_3O_2 + C_2H_5OH$. Such reactions can be reversed, usually; the reversed reaction is called neutralization, esterification, or condensation. SEE: *assimilation; enzyme.*

hydrolyst (hi′dro-līst). Any substance which catalyzes hydrolysis.

hydrolyt′ic. Rel. to hydrolysis.

hydrolyze. To cause to undergo hydrolysis.

hydroma (hi-dro′mă) [Gr. *hydōr,* water, + *ōma,* tumor]. 1. Hygroma, q.v. 2. Any cyst containing a watery substance.

hydromeningitis (hi″dro-men″in-ji′tis) [″+ *mēninx,* membrane, + *-itis,* inflammation]. 1. Inflammation of membranes of brain with serous effusion. 2. Inflammation of Descemet's membrane.

hydromeningocele (hi″dro-men-in′go-sēl) [″+ ″+ *kēlē,* hernia]. Protrusion of meninges or spinal cord in a sac of fluid.

hydrom′eter [″+ *metron,* measure]. An instrument which measures the density of a liquid by the depth to which a graduated scale sinks into the liquid.

hydrometra (hi″dro-mē′tră) [″+ *mētra,* uterus]. Collection of watery fluid or mucus in the uterus.

hydromphalus (hi-drom′fă-lus) [″+ *omphalos,* navel]. Watery tumor at the umbilicus.

hydromyelia (hi″dro-mi-e′lĭ-ă) [Gr. *hydōr,* water, + *myelos,* marrow]. Increased fluid in central canal of spinal cord. SYN: *hydrorrhachis.*

hydromyelocele (hi″dro-mi-el′o-sēl) [″+ ″+ *kēlē,* hernia]. Protrusion of sac with cerebrospinal fluid through a spina bifida.

hydromyoma (hi″dro-mi-o′mă) [″+ *mys,* muscle, + *ōma,* tumor]. Cystic fibroid, usually uterine, filled with fluid.

hydronephrosis (hi″dro-nef-ro′sis) [″+ *nephros,* kidney, + *ōsis,* increase]. Collection of urine in the kidney pelvis due to obstructed outflow, forming a cyst by production of distention and atrophy of organ.

DIAG: Large, fluctuating, soft mass in region of kidney, appearing and disappearing as retained urine passes into the ureters and bladder.

TREATMENT: Aspiration, nephrectomy, or nephrotomy depending on the severity of the disease. Medical or surgical removal of the cause of the retention is indicated.

hydroparasalpinx (hi″dro-par″ă-sal′pinks) [Gr. *hydōr,* water, + *para,* beside, + *salpinx,* tube]. Accumulation of serous fluid in the accessory tubes of the fallopian tube.

hydroparoti′tis [″+ ″+ *ous,* ear, + *-itis,* inflammation]. Accumulation of fluid in the parotid gland.

hydropath′ic [″+ *pathos,* disease]. Rel. to hydropathy.

hydropathy (hi-drop′ă-thī). A treatment regimen involving the use of large amounts of water internally and externally. It is falsely claimed that such treatment will cure a great variety of diseases. SEE: *hydrotherapy.*

hydropenia (hi″dro-pē′nĭ-ă) ["+ *penia,* poverty]. Deficiency in body water.

hydropericardi′tis ["+ *peri,* around, + *kardia,* heart, + *-itis,* inflammation]. Serous effusion accompanying pericarditis.

hydropericardium (hi″dro-per′ĭ-kar′dĭum). Pericardial dropsy. Accumulation of water in pericardial sac without inflammation.

SYM: Distress in region of heart; diminished cardiac function with signs of heart failure; dysphagia, and dyspnea.

TREATMENT: Paracentesis. Definitive therapy depends upon cause of disease.

hydroperinephrosis (hi″dro-per′ĭ-nĭ-fro′sis) [Gr. *hydōr,* water, + *peri,* around, + *nephros,* kidney, + *-ōsis,* increase]. Accumulation of serum of connective tissue surrounding the kidney.

hydroperion (hi″dro-per′ĭ-on) ["+ "+ *ōon,* egg]. Fluid present between decidua capsularis and decidua parietalis; occurs early in pregnancy.

hydroperitone′um ["+ *peritonaion,* peritoneum]. Accumulation of fluid in peritoneal cavity. SYN: *ascites.*

hydropexis (hi″dro-pek′is) ["+ *pēxis,* fixation]. The retaining or fixing of water.

hydroph′ilism [Gr. *hydōr,* water, + *philein,* to love]. Tendency of tissues to attract and hold water.

hydrophilous (hi-drof′ĭ-lus). Taking up moisture. SYN: *bibulous.*

hydrophobia (hi-dro-fo′bĭ-ă) [Gr. *hydōr,* water, + *phobos,* fear, + *ia,* condition]. 1. Morbid fear of water. 2. Common name for rabies, q.v. resulting from bite of a rabid animal. SYN: *lyssa.*

hydrophobophobia (hi″dro-fo″bo-fo′bĭ-ă) ["+ "+ *phobos,* fear, + *ia,* condition]. Morbid fear of contracting hydrophobia (rabies), sometimes resulting in a hysterical condition resembling hydrophobia.

hydrophthalmos (hi″drof-thal′mos) ["+ *ophthalmos,* eye]. Distention of the eyeball due to accumulation of fluid within it. SYN: *infantile glaucoma.*

hydrophysometra (hi″dro-fĭ″so-me′tră) ["+ *physa,* air, + *metra,* uterus]. Presence of water and gas in the uterus.

hydrop′ic [Gr. *hydrōpikos,* pert. to dropsy]. Dropsical or pert. to dropsy.

hydropigenous (hi″dro-pij′ĕ-nus) [L. *hydrops,* dropsy, + *gennan,* to produce]. Producing dropsy, e.g., cardiac or renal disease.

hydropneumatosis (hi″dro-nu″mă-to′sis) [Gr. *hydōr,* water, + *pneumatōsis,* infla-

tion]. Liquid and gas in the tissues producing combined edema and emphysema.

hydropneumogony (hi″dro-nu-mō′go-nĭ) [Gr. *hydōr,* water, + *pneuma,* air, + *gony,* knee]. Diagnosis of joint effusion by injecting air in joint.

hydropneumopericardium (hi″dro-nu″mo-per-ĭ-kar′di-um) ["+ "+ *peri,* around, + *kardia,* heart]. Serous effusion with gas in the pericardium.

hydropneumoperitoneum (hi″dro-nu″mo-per″ĭ-to-ne′um) ["+ "+ *peritonaion,* peritoneum]. Gas and serous fluid in the peritoneal cavity.

hydropneumothorax (hi″dro-nu″mo-tho′raks) ["+ "+ *thōrax,* chest]. Gas and serous effusion in pleural cavity. SYN: *pneumohydrothorax.*

hy′drops, hydrop′sy [Gr.]. Dropsy or edema.

   h. abdominis. Dropsy of the abdominal cavity; ascites.

   h., endolymphatic. H., labyrinthine, q.v.

   h. fetalis. Erythroblastosis fetalis, q.v.

   h. folliculi. Accumulation of fluid in graafian follicle of ovary.

   h. gravidarum. Edema accompanying pregnancy.

   h., labyrinthine. Dilatation due to an accumulation of fluid in the endolymphatic space of the ear. A characteristic of Meniere's disease, q.v.

   h. tubae. Collection of fluid in an oviduct. Hydrosalpinx.

   h. tubae profluens. A h. of the tube in which the distention becomes so great that the tube is forced to empty itself by the pressure, the emptying taking place via the uterine cavity. SYN: *intermittent hydrosalpinx.*

   h. vesi′cae fel′leae. Fluid in the gallbladder causing distention.

hydropyonephrosis (hi″dro-pī″o-nef-ro′sis) [Gr. *hydōr,* water, + *pyon,* pus, + *nephros,* kidney, + *ōsis,* increase]. Dilatation of kidney pelvis with pus and urine.

hydrorheostat (hi″dro-rē′o-stat) ["+ *rheos,* current, + *histanai,* to place]. A device used to control the flow of electrical current by changes in water resistance.

hydrorrhachis (hi-dror′ă-kis) ["+ *rhachis,* spine]. Condition of increased cerebrospinal fluid between membranes and spinal cord or its central canal or cavities.

hydrorrhachitis (hi-dror-ă-ki′tis) ["+ "+ *-itis,* inflammation]. Serous effusion from the spinal cord or its membranes with inflammation of the cord.

hydrorrhea (hi"dro-rē'ă) ["+ *rhoia,* flow]. Copious watery discharge from any part, as from the nose.

   h. gravidarum. Discharge of a watery fluid from the vagina during pregnancy, sometimes mistaken for amniotic fluid.

hydrosalpinx (hi"dro-sal'pinks) ["+ *salpinx,* tube]. Distention of fallopian tube by clear fluid.

   h., intermittent. A discharge of watery fluid from the oviduct. SYN: *hydrops tubae profluens.*

hydrosarcocele (hi"dro-sar'ko-sēl) ["+ *sarx,* flesh, + *kēlē,* tumor]. Hydrocele with chronic swelling of testis.

hydro'sis. Hidrosis.

hydrosol. The fluid state of a colloidal solution; a sol. State of a colloidal solution in which, the colloid particles, separated by water in a continuous phase, are free to move about. SEE: *hydrogel.*

hydrosphygmograph (hi-dro-sfig'mo-graf) [Gr. *hydōr,* water, + *sphygmos,* pulse, + *graphein,* to write]. A sphygmograph with indicator consisting of a column of water.

hydrostat'ic ("+ *statikos,* standing). Pert. to the pressure of liquids in equilibrium and that exerted on liquids.

   h. test. Putting lungs of a dead infant in water. If they float, the infant has breathed prior to death.

hydrostat'ics. Science of properties of fluids in equilibrium.

hydrosudotherapy (hi"dro-su"do-ther'ă-pī) [Gr. *hydōr,* water, + L. *sudor,* sweat, + Gr. *therapeia,* treatment]. Treatment of disease by sweating and hydrotherapy.

hydrosyringomyelia (hi"dro-sir-ing"o-mi-e'lī-ă) ["+ *syrinx,* tube, + *myelos,* marrow]. Distention of central canal of spinal cord with effusion of fluid and formation of cavities.

hydrotaxis (hi"dro-tak'sis) ["+ *taxis,* arrangement]. The response of an organism or cell toward or away from moisture. SEE: *hydrotropism.*

hydrotherapeu'tics ("+ *therapeia,* treatment). Treatment of disease with water. SYN: *hydrotherapy.*

hydrotherapist (hi"dro-ther'ă-pist). One who practices hydrotherapy.

hydrotherapy (hi-dro-ther'ă-pī) [Gr. *hydōr,* water, + *therapeia,* treatment]. Scientific application of water in treatment of disease.

   The therapeutic effects of hydrotherapy are as follows:

   Brief Hot Tub and Shower Baths: Relieve fatigue, produce general relaxation.

   Cold Baths and Applications: Cool the body or part and stimulate, esp. if followed by friction and percussion. They contract the small blood vessels when applied locally.

   Cold and Hot Applications: One followed by the other stimulate the cardiovascular system both generally and locally.

   Gradually Elevated Temperature of Hot Tub and Vapor Baths: Relax all muscles of the body.

   Hot Baths: Relax tissues, including capillaries of skin, drawing blood from deeper tissues; also relieve pain.

   Warm and Hot Baths and Applications: They soothe cutaneous nerves, and nerves of internal organs in reflex relation with skin areas to which heat is applied. SEE: *Kneipp cure.*

hydrothionammonemia (hi"dro-thi"o-nam-o-ne'mī-ă) ["+ *theion,* sulfur, + *ammōniakos,* of Amen, from near whose temple it came, + *haima,* blood]. Ammonium sulfide in the blood.

hydrothionemia (hi"dro-thi"o-ne'mī-ă) ["+ "+ *haima,* blood]. Condition caused by hydrogen sulfide in the blood.

hydrothionuria (hi"dro-thi"o-nu'rī-ă) ["+ "+ *ouron,* urine]. Condition caused by hydrogen sulfide in the urine.

hydrothorax (hi"dro-tho'raks) [Gr. *hydōr,* water, + *thōrax,* chest]. A non-inflammatory collection of fluid in the pleural cavity.

   SYM: Dyspnea; absence of vesicular breath sounds; murmur; flatness over location of fluid.

   TREATMENT: According to cause. Aspiration of fluid.

hydro'tis (Gr. *hydōr,* water, + *ous,* ear). Serous effusion in the internal ear or tympanum.

hydrotomy (hi-drot'o-mī) ["+ *tomē,* a cutting]. Dissection of tissue by forcible injection of water into the vessels.

hydrotropism (hi"dro-tro'pizm) ["+ *tropē,* a turning]. Response of plants toward (positive h.) or away (negative h.) from moisture.

hydrotym'panum ("+ *tympanon,* drum). Edema fluid in the middle ear.

hydroure'ter ("+ *ourētēr,* ureter). Distention of ureter with fluid due to obstruction.

hydrovarium (hi"dro-va'rī-um) ["+ L. *ovarium,* ovary]. Edema or cyst of the ovary.

hydroxide (hi-droks'id) [Gr. *hydōr,* water, + *oxys,* sour]. A compound which contains the hydroxyl (OH) group. Ex.: NaOH (sodium hydroxide, or caustic soda).

hydroxy acids (hi-droks'ī). Acids containing one or more hydroxyl groups in addition to the carboxyl group. Ex: lactic acid.

hydroxybutyric dehydrogenase. A serum enzyme which is increased in myocardial infarction.

hydrox'yl. The univalent radical OH, which, when combined with a metallic ion or a radical which acts as a metal (e.g., NH₄), forms a hydroxide. Commonly called a base or alkali.

hydruria (hi-dru'rĭ-ă) [Gr. *hydōr*, water, + *ouron*, urine]. Excessive secretion and discharge of urine. As a rule the urine does not contain abnormal constituents.

hygeiolatry (hi″jĭ-ol″ă-trĭ) [Gr. *Hygieia*, goddess of health, + *latreia*, servitude]. Excessive concern with one's own health.

hygiene (hi'jēn) [Gr. *hygieinos*, healthful]. The study of health and observance of health rules. Study of the methods and means of preserving health.

     h., community. That branch of h. which deals with the health of a large group of individuals such as city, state, or nation, and esp. with the control of communicable diseases.

     h., industrial. That branch of h. which deals primarily with health of industrial workers, esp. study, treatment and prevention of occupational diseases.

     h., mental. Science of developing and maintaining mental health and preventing mental illness.

     h., military. That branch of h. which deals with the health of men in military service.

     h., oral. Scientific care of teeth and mouth.

hygienic (hi″jiĭ-en'ik). 1. Pert. to health or its preservation. 2. In a healthy condition.

hygien'ics. A system for promoting health.

hygienist (hi'jĭ-en-ist). A specialist in hygiene.

     h., dental. One trained in dental prophylaxis.

hygienization (hi″jĭ-en-ĭ-za'shun). The establishment of sanitary conditions and rules of hygiene.

hy'gric [Gr. *hygros*, moisture]. Pert. to moisture.

hy'gro-. Prefix indicating relationship to moisture.

hygroma (hi-gro'mă) [Gr. *hygros*, moisture, + *ōma*, tumor]. (pl. *hygromas* or *hygromata*) A sac or bursa containing fluid.

     h., cystic. A rapidly growing hygroma of lymphatic origin. Usually located in the neck but may be in the thorax.

hygrometer (hi-grom'ĕ-ter) [″+ *metron*, measure]. An instrument for measuring the amount of moisture in the air.

hygroscopic (hi-gro-skop'ik) [″+ *skopein*, to examine]. 1. Pert. to hygroscopy. 2. Absorbing moisture readily. SYN: *bibulous; hydrophilous.*

hygros'copy. Estimation of the quantity of moisture in the atmosphere.

hygrostomia (hi-gro-stō'mĭ-ă) [Gr. *hygros*, moist, + *stoma*, mouth]. Excess flow of saliva. SYN: *ptyalism; salivation.*

hyla (hi'lă). A lateral extension of the aquaeductus cerebri. SYN: *paraqueduct.*

hylo'ma (Gr. *hylē*, matter, + + *ōma*, tumor). A tumor composed of or in the hylic tissues, such as hypohyloma, and mesohyloma.

hymen (hi'měn) [Gr. *hymēn*, membrane]. A fold of mucous membrane which normally partially covers the entrance to the vagina. Contrary to folklore, presence or absence of the hymen cannot be used to prove or disprove virginity or history of sexual intercourse.

     Its rupture or absence is not evidence of loss of virginity. Conversely, pregnancy has occurred even though the hymen has not been entered.

     RS: defloration; hymenorrhaphy; hymenotomy.

     h. annularis. H. with a ringshaped opening in the center.

     h. biforis. One with two parallel openings with a thick septum between.

     h. cribriformis. One with many small perforations.

     h. denticulatis. One with an opening with serrated edges.

     h., fenestrated. Same as cribriform.

     h. imperforatus. A h. with no opening in it.

     h., lunar. H. shaped like the moon.

     h., ruptured. H. that has been torn by coitus, injury or operation.

     h. septus or h., septate. H. in which the opening is separated by a thin septum.

     h., unruptured. Imperforate h.

hymenal (hi'men-al). Pert. to the hymen.

hymenectomy (hi″men-ek'tō-mĭ) [Gr. *hymēn*, membrane, + *ektomē*, excision]. 1. In surgery and gynecology, incision or removal of the hymen. 2. Excision of a membrane.

hymenitis (hi-men-i'tis) [″+ *-itis*, inflammation]. Inflammation of the hymen or a membrane.

Hymenolepis (hi″men-ol'ĕ-pis) [″+ *lepis*, rind]. A genus of tapeworm. Parasitic in birds and mammals.

     H. nana. The dwarf tapeworm, a parasite in the intestine of rats and mice; also commonly found in man. It averages about 1 in. (2.5 cm.) in length and differs from other tapeworms in that it is capable of completing its life cycle within a single host. It causes severe toxic symptoms, esp. in children.

hymenology (hi″men-ol′o-jĭ) [Gr. *hymēn,* membrane, + *logos,* science]. Science of the membranes and their diseases.

hymenorrhaphy (hi″men-or′ă-fĭ) [″+ *raphē,* suture]. Plastic operation on the hymen to produce partial or complete closure of the vagina.

hymenotome (hi-men′o-tōm) [″+ *tomē,* incision]. Knife used to divide membranes.

hymenotomy (hi″men-ot′o-mi). 1. Incision of the hymen. 2. Dissection of a membrane.

hyo- [Gr. *hyoeides,* U-shaped]. Prefix indicating connection with hyoid bone.

hyobasioglossus (hi″o-ba″sĭ-o-glos′us) [″+ *basis,* base, + *glōssa,* tongue]. The part of hyoglossal muscle attached to the hyoid bone. SYN: *basioglossus.*

hyoepiglottic (hi″o-ep′ĭ-glot′ik) [″+ *epiglōttis,* epiglottis]. Rel. to hyoid bone and epiglottis.

hyoepiglottidean (hi″o-ep′ĭ-glot-id′ĭ-an). Rel. to hyoid bone and epiglottis. SYN: *hyoepiglottic.*

hyoglos′sal (Gr. *hyoeides,* U-shaped, + *glōssa,* tongue). 1. Pert. to the hyoglossus. 2. Extending to the tongue from the hyoid bone.

hyoglossus. A muscle arising from body and greater cornu of hyoid bone and inserted into dorsum of tongue.

ACTION: Draws down sides and retracts tongue.

hy′oid (Gr. *hyoeides,* U-shaped). 1. Shaped like the Gr. letter U. 2. Pert. to the h. bone, q.v.

   h. **arch.** Second branchial arch.

   h. **bone.** Horseshoe-shaped bone lying at base of tongue.

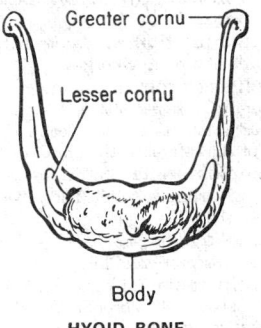

Greater cornu

Lesser cornu

Body

HYOID BONE

hyopharyngeus (hi″o-far-in′jĭ-us) [″+ *pharynx,* gullet]. Middle pharyngeal constrictor.

hyoscine (hi′o-sin). Scopolamine.

   h. **hydrobromide.** Scopolamine hydrobromide.

Hyoscyamus (hi″o-sī′ă-mus) [Gr. *hys,* a pig, + *kyamos,* bean]. Dried leaves of the plant Hyoscyamus niger. A narcotic.

POISONING: Related to atropine, q.v.

hypacousia, hypacusia, hypacusis (hi″pă-koo′sĭ-ă, -ku′sĭ-ă, -sis) [Gr. *hypo,* under, + *akousis,* hearing]. Impaired hearing.

hypalbuminosis (hi″pal-bu-min-o′sis) [″+ L. *albumen,* white of egg, + Gr. *-ōsis,* increase]. Deficiency in proportion of albumin in blood.

hypalgesia (hi-pal-jē′zĭ-ă) [Gr. *hypo,* under, + *algēsis,* pain]. Lessened sensitivity to pain. SEE: *hyperalgesia.*

hypalgia (hi-pal′jĭ-ă) [″+ *algos,* pain]. Lessened sensitivity to pain. SYN: *hypalgesia.*

hypamnios (hi-pam′nĭ-os) [″+ *amnion,* caul of a lamb]. Deficiency in amt. of amniotic fluid.

hypanakinesis (hi-pan″ă-kin-e′sis) [″+ *anakinēsis,* exercise]. Lowered rate of movement.

hypaphrodisia (hi-paf″ro-diz′ĭ-ă) [Gr. *hypo,* under, + *aphrodisia,* sexual pleasure]. Decreased or deficient sexual desire.

hypaxial (hi-paks′ĭ-al) [″+ *axōn,* axle]. Situated beneath the body axis.

hyper- [Gr. *hyper,* above]. Prefix meaning above, excessive, or beyond.

hyperacidaminuria (hi″per-as″id-am-in-u′rĭ-ă) [Gr. *hyper,* above, + L. *acidus,* sour, + *amine,* + Gr. *ouron,* urine]. Presence of an excess of amino acids in the urine. SYN: *acidaminuria.*

hyperacid′ity [″+ L. *acidus,* sour]. 1. An excess of acid. 2. An excess of acid in the stomach. SEE: *hyperchlorhydria.*

hyperacuity (hi″per-a-ku′ĭ-tĭ) [″+ L. *acuitas,* sharpness]. Abnormal acuteness of one of the special senses such as hearing or sight.

hyperacusis (hi″per-ă-ku′sis) [″+ *akousis,* hearing]. Abnormal sensitivity to sound. Sometimes found in hysteria.

hyperadenosis (hi″per-ad″ĭ-no′sis) [″+ *adēn,* gland, + *-ōsis,* increase]. Lymph gland enlargement. SEE: *Hodgkin's disease.*

hyperadiposis, hyperadiposity (hi″per-ad″ĭ-po′sis, -pos′ĭ-tĭ) [″+ L. *adeps,* fat, + Gr. *-ōsis,* increase]. Excessive fatness.

hyperadrenalemia (hi″per-ad-rē″nal-e′-mĭ-ă) [″+ L. *ad,* toward, + *ren,* kidney, + Gr. *haima,* blood]. Excess of adrenal secretion in the blood.

hyperadre′nalism. Excess of adrenal secretion.

hyperadre′nia. Condition caused by abnormal activity of adrenal glands.

hyperalbuminosis (hi″per-al-bu″min-o′sis) [Gr. *hyper*, above, + L. *albumen*, white of egg, + Gr. *ōsis*, increase]. Increased albumin in the blood.

hyperalgesia (hi″per-al-jē′zĭ-ă) [Gr. *hyper*, above, + *algēsis*, pain]. Excessive sensibility to pain; opposite of hypalgesia.

hyperalgia (hi-per-al′jĭ-ă) ["+ *algos*, pain]. Excessive sensitivity to pain.

hyperaminoacidemia (hi″per-am″ĭ-no-as′ĭ-dē′mĭ-ă). An abnormal amount of amino acids in the blood.

hyperanacinesia, hyperanacinesis (hi″per-an″ă-sin-e′zĭ-ă, -sis) [Gr. *hyper*, above, + *anakinēsis*, exercise]. Hyperanakinesis, q.v.

hyperanakine′sis. Excessive function or movement activity of an organ or part such as of the stomach or intestines.

hyperaphia (hi″per-ā′fĭ-ă) [Gr. *hyper*, above, + *haphē*, touch]. Excessive sensitiveness to touch.

hyperaphic (hi-per-af′ĭk). Marked by extreme sensitiveness to touch.

hyperazoturia (hi″per-az″o-tū′rĭ-ă) [Gr. *hyper*, above, + Fr. *azote*, nitrogen, + Gr. *ouron*, urine]. Excessive amt. of nitrogenous matter in the urine.

hyperbaric oxygen. Oxygen under greater pressure than at normal atmospheric pressure. Pressure chambers in which the oxygen is hyperbaric have been used in treating gas gangrene and carbon monoxide poisoning, and experimentally in surgery of congenital cyanotic heart disease. It is usually used at 1 1/2 to 3 times absolute atmospheric pressure.

hyperbilirubinemia (hi″per-bil″ĭ-ru-bin-e′mĭ-ă) [Gr. *hyper*, above, + L. *bilis*, bile, + *ruber*, red, + Gr. *haima*, blood]. Excessive amt. of bilirubin in the blood.

hyperbrachycephaly (hi″per-brak″ĭ-sef′ă-lĭ) ["+ *brachys*, short, + *kephalē*, head]. Excessive degree of brachycephaly; having a cephalic index over 85.

hyperbu′lia [Gr. *hyper*, above, + *boulē*, will]. Abnormal degree of will power.

hypercalcemia (hi″per-kal-sē′mĭ-ă) ["+ L. *calx*, lime, + Gr. *haima*, blood]. An excessive amt. of calcium in the blood.

hypercalciuria (hi″per-kal″sĭ-u′rĭ-ă) ["+ "+ Gr. *ouron*, urine]. An excessive quantity of calcium in the urine.

hypercap′nia ["+ *kapnos*, smoke]. Increased amt. of carbon dioxide in the blood.

hypercatharsis (hi″per-kă-thar′sis) [Gr. *hyper*, above, + *katharsis*, purge]. Excessive bowel movement in response to administration of cathartics.

hypercementosis (hi″per-sē″men-tō′sis) ["+ L. *cementum*, cement, + Gr. *-ōsis*, increase]. Overgrowth of tooth cement (cementum).

hypercenesthesia (hi″per-sē″nes-thē′zĭ-ă) ["+ *koinos*, common, + *aisthēsis*, sensation]. Exaggerated feeling of well-being. SYN: *euphoria*.

hyperchloremia (hi″per-klo-rē′mĭ-ă) [Gr. *hyper*, above, + *chlōros*, green, + *haima*, blood]. Increase in chloride content of the blood.

hyperchlorhydria (hi″per-klor-hi′drĭ-ă) ["+ "+ *hydor*, water]. An excess of hydrochloric acid in the gastric secretion. It causes a burning sensation in the stomach in the absence of ingested foods.

The amount secreted above what is needed to combine with albumoid and basic substances is known as free HCl.

The ability of the stomach to produce hydrochloric acid can be evaluated clinically. A tube is carefully placed in the stomach and the contents aspirated prior to, and at 15 minute intervals for an hour after, stimulation of the parietal cells of the stomach. This is accomplished by giving the histamine analogue, betazole, 2.0 mg./kg. body weight subcutaneously. If the pH of the aspirate obtained 30 minutes later is six or above, the patient has achlorhydria. The production of more than 24 millequivalents of hydrochloric acid in the four specimens obtained following the injection of betazole is considered abnormal and consistent with the presence of hyperchlorhydria.

SYN: *gastrosuccorrhea*. SEE: *achlorhydria; gastritis; hydrochloric acid; hypochlorhydria*.

hyperchlorida′tion. A dosing with large amounts of sodium chloride.

hypercholesterolemia (hi″per-ko-les″ter-ol-e′mĭ-ă) [Gr. *hyper*, above, + *cholē*, bile, + *stereos*, solid, + *haima*, blood]. Excessive amt. of cholesterol in the blood.

hypercholesterolia (hi″per-ko-les″ter-o′lĭ-ă) ["+ "+ *stereos*, solid]. Excessive cholesterol in the bile.

hypercholia (hi″per-ko′lĭ-ă) ["+ *cholē*, bile]. Abnormal secretion of bile.

hyperchromasia (hi″per-kro-mā′zĭ-ă) [Gr. *hyper*, above, + *chrōma*, color]. Hyperchromatism, q.v.

hyperchromatic (hi″per-kro-mat′ĭk) ["+ *chrōma*, color]. Overpigmented.

   h. cell. A cell or a part of a cell which contains more than the normal number of chromosomes and hence stains more densely.

hyperchro'matism ["+ "+ -*ismos*, state of]. 1. Excessive pigmentation. 2. Increased staining capacity of any structure. SYN: *hyperchromatosis.*

hyperchromatopsia (hi″per-kro″ma-top′sĭ-ă) ["+ "+ *opsis*, vision]. Defect of vision in which all objects appear colored.

hyperchromatosis [Gr. *hyper*, above, + *chrōma*, color, + -*ōsis*, increase,]. 1. Excessive pigmentation, esp. of the skin. 2. Increased staining capacity.

hyperchromemia (hi″per-kro-me′mĭ-ă) ["+ "+ *haima*, blood]. Condition of a high color index of the blood due to increased amount of hemoglobin in red cells.

hyperchromia (hi″per-kro′mĭ-ă) ["+ *chrōma*, color]. Excessive pigmentation. SYN: *hyperchromatism.*

hyperchromic (hi-per-krŏ′mic) ["+ *chrōma*, color]. 1. Pert. to excessive pigmentation. 2. Intensely colored.

hyperchylia (hi″per-kī′lĭ-ă) [Gr. *hyper*, above, + L. *chylus*, juice]. Abnormal secretion of gastric juice.

hypercinesia (hi″per-sin-e′zĭ-ă) ["+ *kinēsis*, motion]. Increased function or motion.

hypercri'nism ["+ *krinein*, to separate, + -*ismos*, state of]. Condition due to excessive activity of any endocrine gland.

hypercryalgesia (hi″per-kri″al-jē′zĭ-ă) [Gr. *hyper*, above, + *kryos*, cold, + *algēsis*, pain]. Excessive sensitivity to cold. SYN: *hypercryesthesia.*

hypercryesthe'sia ["+ "+ *aisthēsis*, sensation]. Excessive sensitivity to cold. SYN: *hypercryalgesia.*

hypercyanosis (hi″per-sī″ă-no′sis) [Gr. *hyper*, above, + *kyanos*, dark blue, + -*ōsis*, increase]. Extreme cyanosis.

hypercyanotic (hi″per-sī″ă-not′ik). Denoting extreme cyanosis.

hypercyesis (hi″per-sī-e′sis) [Gr. *hyper*, above, *kyēsis*, gestation]. Presence of more than one fetus in a uterus because of fertilization of a second ovum within a short time. SYN: *superfetation.*

hypercythemia (hi″per-sī-thē′mĭ-ă) ["+ *kytos*, cell, + *haima*, blood]. Condition of having an excessive number of red blood corpuscles.

hypercytosis (hi″per-sī-tō′sis) ["+ "+ -*ōsis*, increase]. Abnormal increase in leukocytes in the blood. SYN: *leukocytosis.*

hyperdactyl'ia [Gr. *hyper*, above, + *daktylos*, finger]. State of having supernumerary fingers or toes.

hyperdiastole (hi′per-di-as′tō-lĭ) ["+ *diastellein*, to draw apart]. Extreme cardiac diastole.

hyperdicrot'ic ["+ *dikrotos*, beating double]. Abnormally dicrotic. SEE: *dicrotic.*

hyperdistention (hi″per-dis-ten′shun) ["+ L. *distendere*, to stretch out]. Excessive inflation or distention.

hyperdiure'sis ["+ *dia*, through, + *ourein*, to urinate]. Excessive formation of urine. SYN: *polyuria.*

hyperdyna'mia [Gr. *hyper*, above, + *dynamis*, force]. Muscular restlessness or extreme violence.

   h. uteri. Abnormal uterine contractions in labor.

hypereccrisia, hypereccrisis (hi″per-ek-kris′ĭ-ă, -ek′kris-is) ["+ *ekkrisis*, excretion]. Abnormal amt. of excretion.

hypereccritic (hi-per-ek-krit′ik). Pert. to hypereccrisis.

hyperemesis (hi″per-em′ĭ-sis) [Gr. *hyper*, above, + *emesis*, vomiting]. Excessive vomiting.

   h. gravidarum. Nausea and vomiting during pregnancy of such severity and duration that systemic effects such as acidosis and weight loss occur.

   ETIOL: Occurs most frequently in highly sensitive, neurotic individuals, but although it may begin on a neurotic basis the constant vomiting brings on pathological changes.

   SYM: The condition may start as a simple vomiting of early pregnancy, but with combined vomiting first of gastric contents, and later of bile, there is developed a chloride depletion, an acidosis, and, finally, with severe and continued vomiting, pathological changes in the liver take place.

   TREATMENT: In early cases, rest in bed; small amounts of carbohydrates taken frequently; moderate restriction of fluids; mild sedation and antiemetic drugs are usually effective. In the average case where nervous irritability is a factor the patient should be kept in a darkened, quiet room free from all visitors.

   With careful management of this type, and no relief from symptoms, and if the pulse and temperature rise and there is definite evidence of liver damage (jaundice), therapeutic abortion should be resorted to.

   The necessity for emptying the uterus should occur only rarely if the patient is seen early, and the proper treatment instituted at once. When the patient improves, food taken by mouth should consist of a light solid diet given in frequent small feedings, with fruit juice, milk, etc. between feedings.

   h. lactentium. Vomiting in nursing infants.

hyperemia (hi″per-e′mĭ-ă) [Gr. *hyper*, above, + *haima*, blood]. 1. Congestion. An unusual amount of blood in a part. 2. A form of macula; red areas on skin which disappear on pressure. 3. In physical therapy, increase in the quantity of blood flowing through any part of the body, shown by redness of the skin caused by the application of heat.

h., active, h., arterial. H. caused by increased blood inflow.

h., Bier's, h., constriction. Passive h., q.v., produced by application of an elastic bandage and by suction.

h., leptomeningeal. Pia-arachnoid congestion.

h., passive, h., venous. H. caused by decreased blood outflow.

hyperemization (hi″per-e″mi-za′shun). Hyperemia produced artificially for therapeutic purposes.

hyperemotiv′ity [Gr. *hyper*, above, + L. *emovere*, to disturb]. Excessive emotivity or response to stimuli.

hyperendocrin′ia [Gr. *hyper*, above, + *endon*, within, + *krinein*, to separate]. Hyperendocrinism.

hyperendocrinism (hi″per-en-dok′rĭ-nizm). Abnormal increase of endocrine gland secretion.

hyperendocrisia (hi″pĕr-ĕn″dō-krĭs′ĭ-ă). Excessive increase of internal secretions. SYN: *hyperendocrinism*.

hypereosinophilia (hi″pĕr-ē″ō-sĭn-ō-fĭl′ĭ-ă) [Gr. *hyper*, above, + *ēōs*, dawn, + *philein*, to love]. Marked increase in number of eosinophils in the blood.

hyperephidrosis (hi″pĕr-ĕf′ĭ-drō′sĭs) [″+ *epi*, upon, + *hidrōs*, sweating]. Abnormal sweating.

hyperepinephria (hi″pĕr-ĕp′ĭ-nĕf′rĭ-ă) [″+ ″+ *nephros*, kidney]. Excessive production of epinephrine with arterial tension.

hyperepinephrine′mia [″+ ″+ *nephros*, kidney, + *haima*, blood]. Abnormally large amt. of adrenalin in the blood. SYN: *hyperadrenalemia*.

hy″perequilib′rium [″+ L. *aequus*, equal, + *libra*, balance]. A tendency to vertigo when making even slight turning movements.

hypererethism (hi″pĕr-ĕr′ĭ-thĭzm) [″+ *erethisma*, stimulation]. Excessive irritability.

hyperergasia (hi″pĕr-ĕr-gă′sĭ-ă) [″+ *ergasia*, work]. Unusual functional activity.

hyperergia (hi″pĕr-ĕr′jĭ-ă). 1. Excessive or increased functional activity. SYN: *hyperergasia*. 2. Abnormal sensitivity to allergens.

hyperergy (hi′pĕr-ĕr″jĭ) [Gr. *hyper*, above, + *ergon*, energy]. Hypersensitivity or condition in which there is an exaggerated response.

hypererythrocythemia (hi″pĕr-e-rĭth″rō-sĭ-thē′mĭ-ă) [Gr. *hyper*, above, + *erythros*, red, + *kytos*, cell, + *haima*, blood]. Excess of red blood cells in the blood.

hyperesophoria (hi″pĕr-ĕs″ō-fō′rĭ-ă) [″+ *esō*, inward, + *phorein*, to bear]. Tendency of the visual axis to deviate upward and inward due to muscular imbalance. A form of heterophoria, q.v.

hyperesthesia (hi″pĕr-ĕs-thē′zĭ-ă) [″+ *aisthēsis*, sensation]. Unusual sensibility to sensory stimuli, such as pain or touch. SYN: *algesia*.

h., acoustic, h., auditory. Abnormal sensitivity to sound.

h., cerebral. H. caused by a cerebral lesion.

h., gustatory. Oversensitivity of taste.

h., muscular. Muscular sensitivity to pain and tiredness.

h., optic. Abnormal sensitivity to light.

h. sexualis. Abnormal increase in libido.

h., tactile. Abnormal sensitivity of touch.

hyperesthet′ic. Pert. to hyperesthesia.

hyperexophoria (hi″pĕr-ĕks″ō-fō′rĭ-ă) [″+ *exō*, outward, + *phorein*, to bear]. Tendency of visual axis to deviate upward and outward due to muscular imbalance. A form of heterophoria, q.v.

hyperextension (hi″pĕr-ĕks-tĕn′shŭn) [″+ L. *extendere*, to stretch out]. Extreme or abnormal extension.

hyperfunction [Gr. *hyper*, above, + L. *functio*, performance]. Excessive activity.

hypergalactia (hi-pĕr-găl-ăk′shĭ-ă) [″+ *gala*, milk]. Excessive milk secretion.

hypergenesis (hi″pĕr-jĕn′ĭ-sĭs) [″+ *genesis*, development]. Redundancy of organs or parts; overproduction. SYN: *hyperplasia*.

hypergenitalism (hi″pĕr-jĕn′ĭt-ăl-ĭzm) [Gr. *hyper*, above, + L. *genitalis*, genital]. Excessive development of the genital organs. SYN: *precocious puberty*.

ETIOL: Disturbances in endocrine secretions of the adrenal gland or gonads, or hypothalamic disorders.

hypergeusesthesia,   hypergeusia (hi″pĕr-gŭ-sĕs-the′sĭ-ă, -gū′sĭ-ă) [″+ *geusis*, taste, + *aisthēsis*, perception]. Excessive acuteness of sense of taste.

hyperglan′dular [″+ L. *glandula*, a little acorn]. Having excessive glandular secretions.

hyperglobulinemia (hi″pĕr-glŏb″ū-lĭn-ē′mĭ-ă) [″+ L. *globulus*, a globule, + Gr. *haima*, blood]. Excessive globulin in the blood.

hyperglycemia (hī"pĕr-gli-sē'mĭ-ă) ["+ *glykys*, sweet, + *haima*, blood]. Increase of blood sugar as in diabetes.

This condition increases susceptibility to infection and it often precedes diabetic coma. SEE: *hypoglycemia.*

hyperglycistia (hī"pĕr-gli-sĭs'tĭ-ă) [Gr. *hyper*, above, + *glykys*, sweet, + *istos*, tissue]. Excess of glucose in the tissues.

hyperglycogenolysis (hī"pĕr-gli"kō-jĕn-ŏl'ĭ-sĭs) ["+ "+ *gennan*, to form, + *lysis*, dissolution]. Excessive conversion of glycogen into glucose by hydrolysis.

hyperglycoplasmia (hī"pĕr-gli"kō-plăz'mĭ-ă) ["+ "+ *plasma*, matter formed]. Excessive sugar in the plasma of the blood.

hyperglycorrhachia (hī"pĕr-gli"kō-rā'kĭ-ă) [Gr. *hyper*, above, + *glykys*, sweet, + *rhachis*, spine]. Excess of sugar in the cerebrospinal fluid.

hyperglycosemia (hī"pĕr-gli-kō-sē'mĭ-ă) ["+ "+ *haima*, blood]. Excessive sugar in the blood. SYN: *hyperglycemia.*

hyperglycosuria (hī"pĕr-gli"kō-sū'rĭ-ă) ["+ "+ *ouron*, urine]. Excessive sugar in the urine. SEE: *glycosuria.*

hypergonadism (hī"pĕr-gō'năd-ĭzm) ["+ *gonē*, seed, + *ismos*, state of]. Excessive internal secretion of the sexual glands.

hyperguanidinemia (hī"pĕr-gwan"ĭ-dĭn-ē'mĭ-ă) ["+ Sp. *guano*, dung, + *haima*, blood]. Abnormal amt. of guanidine in blood.

hyperhedonia, hyperhedonism (hī"pĕr-hē-dō'nĭ-ă, -hē'dŏn-ĭzm) [Gr. *hyper*, above, + *hēdonē*, pleasure, + *-ismos*, state of]. 1. Abnormal pleasure in anything. 2. Abnormal sexual excitement.

hyperhidrosis (hī"pĕr-hi-drō'sĭs) ["+ *hidrōs*, sweat, + *-ōsis*, condition]. Excessive sweating.

ETIOL: Functional overactivity of sweat glands caused by debilitating disease or stimulants. Increased in rheumatic, malarial, relapsing and septic fever. Occurs in neuralgia, migraine and follows certain drugs and hot drinks. Locally (hands and feet), in hysteria, fright, nervous irritability, and hyperthyroidism. SEE: *sweat.*

   h. oleosa. Increased and altered sebaceous secretion. SYN: *seborrhea.*

hyperhor'monism ["+ *hormaein*, to arouse, + *-ismos*, state of]. Excessive activity of the endocrine glands.

hyperinose'mia ["+ *inos*, fiber, + *haima*, blood]. Abnormal coagulability of the blood; excess of fibrinogen in the blood.

hyperino'sis [Gr. *hyper*, above, + *inos*, fiber, + *-ōsis*, condition]. Excessive fibrinogen in the blood. SYN: *hyperinosemia.*

hyperinsulinism (hī"pĕr-ĭn'sū-lĭn-ĭzm) ["+ L. *insula*, island, + Gr. *-ismos*, state of]. An excessive amount of insulin in the blood.

ETIOL: Tumor on islets of Langerhans, or excessive sensitivity of the islet tissue to an increase in blood-sugar level. May also occur following injection of excessive dosage of insulin.

SYM: The hypoglycemic picture: hunger; weakness; sweating; staggering; diplopia; rarely convulsions; coma; and death. Occasionally spontaneous in which case symptoms are similar to but more chronic than in insulin shock. SEE: *insulin; insulin shock; shock.*

hyperinvolution (hī"pĕr-ĭn"vō-lū'shŭn) [Gr. *hyper*, above, + L. *involvere*, to enwrap]. 1. Reduction in size of uterus below normal after childbirth. 2. Reduction in size below normal of any organ following hypertrophy. SYN: *superinvolution.*

   h. uteri. Extreme atrophy of the uterus seen following prolonged lactation or severe puerperal sepsis.

hyperisoton'ic ["+ *isos*, equal, + *tonos*, tension]. Said of one of two solutions which has the greater osmotic pressure. SYN: *hypertonic.*

hyperkalemia (hī"per-kă-lē'mĭ-ă) [Gr. *hyper*, above, + L. *kalium*, potassium, + Gr. *haima*, blood]. Excessive amount of potassium in blood.

hyperkeratomycosis (hī"pĕr-kĕr"ă-tō-mĭ-kō'sis) ["+ *keras*, horn, + *mykēs*, fungus, + *-ōsis*, condition]. Hypertrophy of horny layer of the epidermis due to a parasitic fungus.

hyperkerato'sis ["+ "+ *-ōsis*, condition]. 1. Overgrowth of the cornea. 2. Overgrowth of the horny layer of the epidermis. SYN: *keratodermia; keratosis.*

   h. congenitalis. Hyperkeratosis in the harlequin fetus.

hy"perketonur'ia. Excessive quantity of ketones in urine.

hyperkine'sia, hyperkine'sis [Gr. *hyper*, above, + *kinesis*, motion]. Excessive amt. of mobility. SYN: *hypercinesia.*

hyperlacta'tion ["+ L. *lactare*, to suckle]. Excessive milk secretion. SYN: *superlactation.*

hyperleukocyto'sis ["+ *leukos*, white, + *kytos*, cell, + *-ōsis*, increase]. Excessive quantity of leukocytes. SYN: *leukocytosis.*

hyperlipemia (hī"pĕr-lĭp-ē'mĭ-ă) [Gr. *hyper*, above, + *lipos*, fat, + *haima*, blood]. Excessive quantity of fat in the blood.

hyperlipoproteinemia (hī"pĕr-lĭp"ō-prō"tē-ĭn-ē'mĭ-ă). An increase in the concentration of the three fatty substances of the blood —cholesterol, phospholipid, and triglyceride. These substances do not circulate freely in the blood but are combined with the plasma proteins; they are called lipoproteins.

By using paper electrophoresis the various forms of h. have been classified into five major types.

hyperlipo'sis [Gr. *hyper*, above, + *lipos*, fat, + *-osis*, condition]. 1. Abnormal amt. of fat; adiposity. 2. Excessive fatty degeneration.

hyperlithuria (hī″pĕr-līth-ū′rī-ă) ["+ *lithos*, stone, + *ouron*, urine]. Excessive excretion of lithic (uric) acid in the urine.

hypermas'tia ["+ *mastos*, breast]. 1. Excessively large mammary gland. SYN: *gynecomastia*. 2. Presence of abnormal number of mammary glands. SYN: *polymastia; polymazia*.

hypermature (hī″pĕr-mă-tūr′) [Gr. *hyper*, above, + L. *maturus*, ripe]. 1. Pert. to anything which has passed the stage of maturity. 2. Overripe, as a cataract; or abscess which has gone past the optimum time for incision.

hypermegasoma (hī′pĕr-mĕg″ă-sō′mă) ["+ *megas*, large, + *sōma*, body]. Excessive bodily development. SYN: *giantism*.

hypermenorrhea (hī″pĕr-mĕn″ō-rē′ă) ["+ *mēn*, month, + *rhoia*, flow]. 1. Too frequent menstrual periods. 2. Abnormal increase in the duration and/or amount of menstrual flow.

hypermetaplasia (hī″pĕr-mĕt″ă-plā′sī-ă) ["+ *meta-*, after, + *plassein*, to form]. Overactivity in tissue replacement or transformation from one type of tissue to another, as cartilage to bone.

hyperme'tria [Gr. *hyper*, above, + *metron*, measure]. Unusual range of movement; state in which muscular movement overreaches the objective.

hypermetrope (hī″pĕr-mĕt′rōp) ["+ " + *ōps*, eye]. One who is farsighted. SYN: *hyperope*.

hypermetro'pia. Farsightedness. Opposed to myopia. SYN: *hyperopia*.

hy″permetrop'ic. Pert. to farsightedness.

hypermimia (hī″pĕr-mīm′ī-ă) [Gr. *hyper*, above, + *mimēsis*, imitation]. Use of a great number of gestures while speaking.

hypermnesia (hī″pĕrm-nē′zī-ă) ["+ *mnēmē*, memory]. 1. Great ability to remember names, dates, and details. 2. An exaggeration of memory involving minute details of a past experience. It occurs in manic phase of manic-depressive psychosis; in delirium, hypnoses; at the moment of shock and fright in life-threatening situations; with fever; during neurosurgical procedures where the temporal lobe is stimulated, and following some brain injuries.

hypermorph (hī′pĕr-morf) ["+ *morphē*, form]. One whose length of limb and consequent standing height is high in proportion to the sitting height. SEE: *hypomorph; mesomorph; somatotype*.

hypermotil'ity ["+ L. *motiō*, motion]. Unusual motility. SYN: *hyperkinesia*.

hypermyatrophy (hī″per-mi-at′ro-fī) [Gr. *hyper*, above, + *mys*, muscle, + *atrophia*, atrophy]. Unusual wasting of muscle.

hypermyesthesia (hī″pĕr-mī″ĕs-thē′sī-ă) ["+ " + *aisthēsis*, sensation]. Muscular hyperesthesia.

hypermyotonia (hī″pĕr-mī″ō-tō′nī-ă) ["+ " + *tonos*, tone]. Excessive muscular tonus.

hypermyotrophy (hī″pĕr-mī-ŏt′rō-fī) ["+ " + *trophē*, nourishment]. Abnormal muscular development.

hyperneocytosis (hī″pĕr-nē″ō-sī-tō′sĭs) [Gr. *hyper*, above, + *neos*, new, + *kytos*, cell, + *-ōsis*, condition]. Abnormal increase of leukocytes in the blood (leukocytosis) including an abnormal amt. of immature forms. SYN: *hyperleukocytosis*.

hy″pernephro'ma ["+ *nephros*, kidney, + *ōma*, tumor]. A tumor of the kidney which to the naked eye resembles adrenal tissue.

hyperneurotization (hī″pĕr-nū-rŏt′ī-zā′-shun) ["+ *neuron*, nerve]. Grafting of a motor nerve into a muscle to increase its energy.

hypernitremia (hī″pĕr-nī-trē′mī-ă) ["+ *nitron*, niter, + *haima*, blood]. Excess of nitrogen in the blood.

hypernoia (hī-pĕr-noy′ă) ["+ *nous*, mind]. Excessive mental activity or imagination. SYN: *hyperpsychosis*.

hypernor'mal [Gr. *hyper*, above, + L. *norma*, rule]. Abnormal.

hypernormocytosis (hī″pĕr-nor″mō-sī-tō′-sĭs) ["+ " + Gr. *kytos*, cell, + *-ōsis*, condition]. An increased proportion of neutrophils in the blood.

hypernutri'tion ["+ L. *nutrīre*, to nourish]. Supernutrition; overfeeding.

hyperonychia (hī″pĕr-ō-nĭk′ī-ă) ["+ *onyx*, nail]. Overgrowth (hypertrophy) of the nails.

hyperope (hī′pĕr-ōp) ["+ *ōps*, eye]. One who is farsighted. SYN: *hypermetrope*.

hypero'pia [Gr. *hyper*, above, + *ōps*, eye]. Farsightedness.

Parallel rays come to a focus behind the retina due to flattening of the globe of the eye, or to error in refraction. SYM: Ocular fatigue and poor vision. SYN: *hypermetropia*.

> ***h., absolute.*** H. in which the eye cannot accommodate.

> ***h., axial.*** H. caused by shortness of the eye's anteroposterior axis.

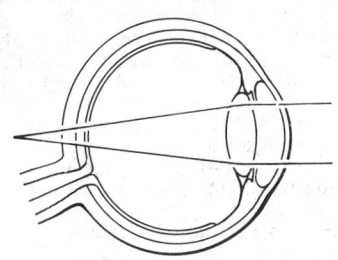

HYPEROPIA

h., facultative. H. which can be corrected by accommodation.

h., latent. H. in which the error of refraction is overcome and disguised by ciliary muscle action.

h., manifest. Total amount of h. which can be neutralized by a convex lens without interfering with clarity of vision.

h., relative. H. in which vision is clear only when excessive convergence is made.

h., total. Complete h. combining both latent and manifest types; the amt. of hyperopia present when accommodation is completely suspended by paralyzing the ciliary muscle. This is done by use of a cycloplegic drug.

hyperorchidism (hī″pĕr-or′kĭd-ĭzm) [Gr. *hyper,* above, + *orchis,* testicle, + *-ismos,* state of]. Abnormal activity of testicular secretion.

hyperorexia (hī″pĕr-ō-rĕks′ĭ-ă) [″+ *orexis,* appetite]. Abnormal hunger.
Usually satisfied by frequent small meals, as in gastric diseases, diabetes, hysteria, psychosis, hyperthyroidism and brain tumors.
It is found in heminthiasis, diabetes, hysteria, convalescence from acute diseases, psychosis, hyperthyroidism, brain tumors, diseases of the stomach in which hypermotility and hypersecretion are present. SYN: *bulimia.*

hyperorthocytosis (hī″pĕr-or″thō-sī-tō′sīs) [″+ *orthos,* straight, + *kytos,* cell, + *-osis,* increase]. Increased white blood cells with normal proportion of various forms and without immature forms.

hyperos′mia [Gr. *hyper,* above, + *osmē,* smell]. Abnormal sensitiveness to odors.

hyperosto′sis [″+ *osteon,* bone, + *-osis,* condition]. Abnormal growth of osseous tissue. SYN: *exostosis.*

h., infantile cortical. Increased growth of subperiosteal bone occurring most frequently in the mandible and clavicles,

with fever and other systemic manifestations.

hyperova′ria [″+ L. *ovarium,* ovary]. Precocity of sexual development in young girls due to excessive ovarian secretion as the result of unusual and premature development of the ovaries.

hyperpancreatism (hī″pĕr-păn′krē-ă-tĭzm) [″+ *pankreas,* pancreas, + *-ismos,* state of]. Abnormal amount of secretion from the pancreas.

hy″perpar′asitism. Condition in which a parasite lives in or upon another parasite.

hyperparathyroidism (hī″pĕr-păr″ă-thī′-roy-dizm) [Gr. *hyper,* above, + *para,* beyond, + *thyreos,* shield, + *eidos,* form, + *-ismos,* state of]. Condition due to increased activity of the parathyroid glands.

hyperpep′sia [″+ *pepsis,* digestion]. Indigestion due to hyperchlorhydria.

hyperpepsinia (hī″pĕr-pĕp-sīn′ī-ă) [″+ *pepsis,* digestion]. Excess of pepsin in the gastric secretion.

hyperperistalsis (hī″pĕr-pĕr′ī-stăl′sĭs) [″+ *peri,* around, + *stalsis,* contraction]. Overactive peristalsis.

hyperphalangism (hī″pĕr-făl-ăn′jĭzm) [″+ *phalanx,* a line, + *-ismos,* state of]. Having an extra phalanx on a finger or toe. SYN: *polyphalangism.*

hyperphasia (hī″pĕr-fā′zĭ-ă) [Gr. *hyper,* above, + *phasis,* speech]. Abnormal desire to talk.

hyperphonesis (hī″pĕr-fō-nē′sĭs) [″+ *phōnēsis,* sounding]. Increase in voice or percussion sound in auscultation.

hyperphonia (hī″pĕr-fō′nĭ-ă) [″+ *phōnē,* voice]. 1. Stuttering or stammering due to irritability of the vocal cords. 2. Explosive speech exhibited by those who stammer.

hyperphoria (hī″pĕr-fō′rĭ-ă) [″+ *phorein,* to bear]. Tendency of one eye to turn upward.

hyperphosphatemia (hī″pĕr-fŏs″fā-tē′mĭ-ă) [″+ L. *phosphās,* phosphate, + Gr. *haima,* blood]. Abnormal amt. of phosphorus in the blood.

hyperphosphaturia (hī″pĕr-fŏs-fā-tū′rĭ-ă) [Gr. *hyper,* above, + L. *phosphās,* phosphate, + Gr. *ouron,* urine]. Increased amt. of phosphates in the urine.

hyperphospheremia (hī″pĕr-fŏs-fĕr-ē′mĭ-ă) [″+ ″+ Gr. *haima,* blood]. Abnormal amt. of phosphorous compounds in the blood. SYN: *hyperphosphatemia.*

hyperphrenia (hī″pĕr-frē′nĭ-ă) [″+ *phrēn,* mind]. 1. Excessive mental activity. Seen in the manic phase of manic-depressive psychosis. 2. Mental ability and capacity much greater than normal.

hyperpiesia, hyperpiesis (hī″pĕr-pī-ē′zĭ-ă, -pī′ĭ-sĭs) ["+ *piesis*, pressure]. Abnormally high blood pressure.

hyperpietic (hī″pĕr-pī-ĕt′ĭk). Rel. to extremely high blood pressure.

hyperpituitarism (hī″pĕr-pĭ-tū′ĭ-tar-ĭsm) [Gr. *hyper*, above, + L. *pituita*, mucus, + Gr. *-ismos*, state of]. Condition resulting from overactivity of the anterior lobe of the pituitary. SEE: *acromegaly; gigantism.*

hyperplasia (hī″pĕr-plā′zĭ-ă) ["+ *plassein*, to form]. Excessive proliferation of normal cells in the normal tissue arrangement of an organ.

    h., fibrous. Connective-tissue cell increase following any inflammation or in chronic visceral fibrosis.

    h., lipoid. Increase in cells containing lipoid.

hyperplastic (hī″pĕr-plăs′tĭk) ["+ *plassein*, to form]. Rel. to hyperplasia.

hyperpnea (hī″pĕrp-nē′a) [Gr. *hyper*, above, + *pnoia*, breath]. An increased respiratory rate or breathing which is deeper than that usually experienced during normal activity. A certain degree of hyperpnea is normal after exercise.

    ETIOL: Pain, respiratory disease, febrile or cardiac disease, or due to certain drugs, hysteria, or atmospheric conditions experienced at high altitude.

hyperporo'sis ["+ *pōrōsis*, callosity]. Excessive callous formation after a bone fracture.

hyperpragic (hī″pĕr-prā′jĭk) ["+ *praxis*, action]. Denoting excessive activity.

hyperprax'ia. Excessive activity and restlessness seen in some mental disorders.

hyperprochoresis (hī″pĕr-prō″kŏ-rē′sĭs) [Gr. *hyper*, above, + *prochōrēsis*, a going forth]. Unusually rapid passage of food through the alimentary tract due to increased peristalsis. SYN: *hyperperistalsis.*

hyperprosexia (hī″pĕr-prō-sĕks′ĭ-ă) ["+ *prosechein*, to heed]. In psychoanalysis, fixation of an idea to the exclusion of other ideas, as in compulsion states.

hyperproteinemia (hī″pĕr-prō″tĭ-ĭn-ē′mĭ-ă) ["+ *prōtos*, first, + *haima*, blood]. Excess of protein in the blood plasma.

hy″perpro″teinu'ria ["+ "+ *ouron*, urine]. Excess of protein in the urine.

hyperproteosis (hī″pĕr-prō″tē-ō′sĭs) ["+ "+ *-ōsis*, increase]. A condition resulting from an excess of protein in the diet.

hyperpselaphesia (hī″pĕrp-sĕl″ă-fē′zĭ-ă) ["+ *psēlaphēsis*, touch]. Abnormal sensitivity to touch. SYN: *hyperaphia.*

hyperpsycho'sis [Gr. *hyper*, above, + *psychē*, mind, + *-ōsis*, condition]. Overfunctioning of the mind.

hyperpyretic (hī″pĕr-pī-rĕt′ĭk). Pert. to high body temperature (hyperpyrexia).

hyperpyrexia (hī″pĕr-pī-rĕks′ĭ-ă) [Gr. *hyper*, above, + *pyressein*, to be feverish]. Elevation of body temperature above 106° F. (41.1° C.).

    Produced by physical agents such as hot baths, diathermy, hot air; or by reaction to infection caused by microorganisms.

hyperpyrex'ial. Denoting high body temperature.

hyperreflex'ia [Gr. *hyper*, above, + L. *reflexus*, bent back]. Increased action of the reflexes.

hyperres'onance ["+ L. *resonāre*, to resound]. Increased resonance produced when the area is percussed.

hy″persaliva'tion [Gr. *hyper*, above, + L. *salivatio*, salivation]. Excessive secretion of saliva.

hypersecretion (hī″pĕr-sē-krē′shŭn) ["+ L. *secernere*, to secrete]. Abnormal amt. of secretion.

hy″persensibil'ity ["+ L. *sensibilitas*, sensibility]. Hypersensitivity of the body to a foreign protein or drug. SYN: *anaphylaxis, q.v.*

hypersensitiveness (hī″pĕr-sĕn′sĭ-tĭv-nĕs) ["+ L. *sensitivus*, sensitive]. Excessive and abnormal susceptibility to the action of a given agent, as pollen or foreign protein. SEE: *allergy; anaphylaxis; hay fever.*

hy″persensitiv'ity. Abnormal sensitivity to a stimulus of any kind.

hypersensitiza'tion. 1. Producing or inducing increased sensitivity to an organism or drug. 2. The condition of being sensitive to an abnormal degree to something.

hyperskeocytosis (hī″pĕr-skē″ō-sĭ-tō′sĭs) [Gr. *hyper*, above, + *skaios*, left, + *kytos*, cell, + *-ōsis*, condition]. Leukocytosis with many immature forms of leukocytes. SYN: *hyperneocytosis.*

hypersom'nia ["+ L. *somnus*, sleep]. Sleeping for pathological lengths of time. Occurs in certain types of encephalitis.

hypersthenia (hī″pĕr-sthē-nĭ-ă) ["+ *sthenos*, strength]. Abnormal strength or excessive tension of the entire body or of part of it.

hypersthen'ic. Denoting excessive strength, or tension.

hypersthenuria (hī″pĕr-sthĕn-ū′rĭ-ă) [Gr. *hyper*, above, + *sthenos*, strength, + *ouron*, urine]. Passage of abnormally concentrated urine. Usually due to dehydration or excess loss of fluids in sweat.

hy″persuscep″tibil'ity ["+ L. *suscipere*, to take up, + *-bilis*, able]. Unusual susceptibility to a disease or to pathological conditions. SEE: *allergy; anaphylaxis; anatoxic.*

hypersystole (hī″pĕr-sĭs′tō-lĭ) ["+ *systolē,* contraction]. Unusual force or duration of the systole, q.v.

hypersystol′ic. Pert. to hypersystole.

hypertarachia (hī″pĕr-tă-rāk′ĭ-ă) [Gr. *hyper,* above, + *tarachē,* disorder]. Excessive irritability of the nervous system.

hypertelorism (hī-pĕr-tĕl′or-ĭzm) ["+ *tēlouros,* distant]. Abnormal width between two paired organs.

   h., ocular. Abnormal width between the eyes.

hy″pertensin′ogen. A globulin present in blood plasma which when acted upon by the enzyme renin forms angiotensin, q.v.

hyperten′sion [Gr. *hyper,* above, + L. *tensiō,* tension]. 1. Tension or tonus above normal. 2. A condition in which patient has a higher blood pressure than that judged to be normal.

   ETIOL: The primary factor in hypertension is an increase in peripheral resistance resulting from vasoconstriction or narrowing of peripheral blood vessels. The specific etiology for this condition can be determined in not more than 10% of patients with h. However, it is important to attempt to define the exact etiology because, if the disease is due to certain pathological states, definitive and curative therapy can be obtained. Causes in this category include coarctation of the aorta; hyperthyroidism with thyrotoxicosis; patent ductus arteriosis; pheochromocytoma; psychogenic causes; certain forms of renal disease, particularly when limited to one kidney; adrenal tumors; primary aldosteronism; and polycythemia.

   There are no precise rules concerning what blood pressure reading is considered to represent h. In general, if the systolic pressure is above 140 mm. of mercury or the diastolic above 90 mm., the person is considered to have elevated blood pressure. It is not a fact that normal systolic blood pressure is 100 plus the individual's age. Coronary artery disease and cerebral vascular disease, the great causes of death and disability, are much more frequent in those who have elevated blood pressure than those who are normotensive. On the other hand, a patient's blood pressure may register high merely because he is excited over having his pressure taken. For this reason it is advisable to take the pressure on separate occasions to be certain that the true blood pressure is being obtained.

   h., benign. H. that progresses slowly. The basic disease process may progress to

the same endpoint as in malignant h. but at a slower rate.

   h., essential. H. that develops without apparent cause. SYN: *primary h.*

   h., Goldblatt. H. that resembles renal h. produced in experimental animals by decreasing the blood flow to the kidney.

   h., malignant. A form of h. that progresses rapidly, accompanied by severe vascular damage. It may progress to the point of death.

   h., renal. H. resulting from kidney disease. H. produced experimentally by constriction of renal arteries. It is due to a humoral substance, renin, produced in an ischemic kidney.

   RS: blood pressure; diastolic p.; hypotension; pulse; pulse pressure; systolic p.

hyperten′sive. Marked by a rise in blood pressure.

hyperthe′lia [Gr. *hyper,* above, + *thēlē,* nipple]. The presence of more than two nipples.

hyperthermalgesia (hī″pĕr-thĕrm″ăl-jē′zĭ-ă) ["+ *thermē,* heat, + *algēsis,* pain]. Unusual sensitiveness to heat.

hyperther′mia ["+ *thermē,* heat]. 1. Unusually high fever. SYN: *hyperpyrexia.* 2. Treatment of disease by raising bodily temperature, accomplished by introduction of the malaria organism, injection of foreign proteins, or by physical means.

hyperthermoesthesia (hī″pĕr-thĕrm″ō-ĕs-thē′zĭ-ă) ["+ "+ *aisthēsis,* sensation]. Unusual sensitiveness to heat. SYN: *hyperthermalgesia.*

hyperthrombinemia (hī″pĕr-thrŏm″bĭn-ē′mĭ-ă) [Gr. *hyper,* above, + *thrombos,* clot, + *haima,* blood]. Excess of thrombin in the blood. This tends to promote intravascular clotting.

hyperthymia (hī″pĕr-thī′mĭ-ă) ["+ *thymos,* mind]. 1. Pathological sensitiveness or excitability. 2. Sudden cruelty or foolhardiness.

hyperthyreosis (hī″pĕr-thī″rē-ō′sĭs). Overactivity of the thyroid. SYN: *hyperthyroidism.*

hyperthyroidism (hī″pĕr-thī′royd-ĭzm) [Gr. *hyper,* above, + *thyreos,* shield, + *eidos,* form, + *-ismos,* state of]. A condition caused by excessive secretion of the thyroid glands which increases the basal-metabolic rate, causing an increased demand for food to support this metabolic activity.

   SYM AND SIGNS: Exophthalmos goiter, fine tremor of the extended fingers and tongue, increased nervousness, weight loss, increased bowel activity, heat intolerance, excessive sweating, increased heart rate.

   TREATMENT: Surgical, by removal of the thyroid gland following proper medical preparation. Medical, by use of antithyroid drugs (as propylthiouracil, methimazole, or carbimazole), iodide or radioactive iodine (I^{131}).

NP: Mental and physical rest with freedom from worry and excitement imperative. Exercise during hot weather aggravates symptoms. Winter months often bring improvement.

Visitors should not be permitted prior to operation or in severe cases, and the nurse should attempt to allay all nervousness on part of patient. Simple diversions help to allay restlessness. Bedclothes during hot weather reduced to a minimum. Encourage patient to drink plenty of water.

RS: cretinism; goiter; myxedema; thyroid.

hyperthyro'sis. Hyperthyroidism.

hyperto'nia [Gr. *hyper*, above, + *tonos*, tension]. Abnormal tension of arteries or muscles.

hyperton'ic. 1. Having a higher osmotic pressure than a compared solution. Pert. to a solution of higher osmotic pressure than another. 2. Being in a state of greater than normal tension or of incomplete relaxation. Said of muscles. Opposed to hypotonic, q.v.

hypertonicity (hi″pĕr-tŏn-ĭ′sĭ-tĭ). Excess muscular tonus or intraocular pressure. SYN: *hypertonia.*

hypertonus (hĭ′pĕr-tō′nŭs). Increased tension, as muscular tension in spasm.

hypertoxic'ity [Gr. *hyper*, above, + *toxikon*, poison]. The state of being excessively poisonous.

hypertrichiasis (hĭ″pĕr-trĭk-ĭ′ă-sĭs) [Gr. *hyper*, above, + *thrix, trich-*, hair, + *-iosis*, diseased condition]. Hypertrichosis, q.v.

hypertrichophobia (hĭ″pĕr-trĭk″o-fō′bĭ-ă) ["+ "+ *phobos*, fear]. Fear of hair on the body.

hypertrichophrydia (hĭ″pĕr-trĭk″ō-frĭd′ĭ-ă) ["+ "+ *ophrys*, eyebrow]. Undue length of the eyebrows.

hypertrichosis (hĭ″pĕr-trĭ-kō′sĭs) ["+ "+ *-ōsis*, condition]. Growth of hair in excess of normal.

ETIOL: Congential or obscure causes. May be due to adrenal or gonad disturbances.

hypertrophia (hĭ″pĕr-trō′fĭ-ă) [Gr. *hyper*, above, + *trophē*, nourishment]. Increased size of an organ, or of the body, due to growth. SYN: *hypertrophy.*

hypertrophic (hĭ″pĕr-trōf′ik) ["+ *trophē*, nourishment]. Pert. to hypertrophy.

hypertrophy (hĭ″pĕr′trō-fĭ) [Gr. *hyper*, above, + *trophē*, nourishment]. Increase in size of an organ or structure which does not involve tumor formation. Term is generally restricted to an increase in size or bulk not resulting from an increase in number of cells or tissue elements, as in the hypertrophy of a muscle. Term sometimes used to apply to any increase in size as a result of functional activity. SYN: *hypertrophia.* SEE: *hyperplasia.*

h., adaptive. H. in which an organ increases in size to meet increased functional demands, as h. of the heart which accompanies valvular disorders.

h., cardiac. H. of the heart; increase in size of the heart resulting from h. of muscle tissue but without increase in size of cavities.

h., compensatory. H. resulting from increased function of an organ due to a defect, or due to impaired function of the opposite of a paired organ.

h., concentric. H. in which the walls of an organ become thickened, with no enlargement, but with diminished capacity.

h., eccentric. H. of an organ with dilatation.

h., false. H. with degeneration of one constitutent of an organ and its replacement by another.

h., Marie's. Chronic arthral enlargement subsequent to chronic periostitis.

h., numerical. H. caused by increase in structural elements.

h., physiological. That due to natural rather than pathological factors.

h., pseudomuscular. A disease usually of childhood, characterized by paralysis, depending upon degeneration of the muscles which, however, become enlarged from a deposition of fat and connective tissue. SYN: *pseudohypertrophic muscular dystrophy.*

SYM: Weakness of muscles, child is awkward, stumbles and seeks support in walking. As paralysis increases, the muscles, particularly those of the calf, thigh, buttocks and back, enlarge. Upper extremities less frequently affected. In erect posture feet are wide apart, abdomen protrudes and spinal column shows a marked curvature with convexity forward. Patient rises from recumbent position by grasping the knees or by resting the hands on the floor in front of him, extending the legs and pushing the body backwards. Gait is waddling. In course of few years paralysis becomes so marked patient is unable to leave his bed; atrophy of muscles follows.

PROG: Unfavorable.

TREATMENT: Physical therapy helps to prevent contractures, but there is no effective therapy.

h., simple. H. due to increase in size of structural parts.

h., true. H. caused by increase in size in all the different tissues composing a part.

h., vicarious. H. of an organ when another organ of allied function is disabled or destroyed.

hypertro'pia [Gr. *hyper*, above, + *trope*, a turning]. Vertical strabismus upward.

hyperuresis (hī″pĕr-ū-rē′sĭs) ["+ *ouresis*, urination]. 1. Excess of urinary secretion. SYN: *polyuria*. 2. Enuresis.

hyperuricemia (hī″pĕr-ū″rĭs-ē′mĭ-ă) ["+ ouron, urine, + *haima*, blood]. Abnormal amt. of uric acid in the blood.

hyperuricuria (hī″pĕr-ū″rĭk-ū′rĭ-ă) ["+ "+ *ouron*, urine]. Abnormal amt. of uric acid in the urine.

hypervas′cular ["+ L. *vasculus*, vessel]. Excessively vascular.

hypervenosity (hī″pĕr-vĕ-nŏs′ī-tĭ) ["+ L. *venosus*, pert. to a vein]. Excessive development of the venous system.

hy″perventila′tion [Gr. *hyper*, above, + L. *ventilatio*, ventilation]. Hyperpnea as occurs in forced respiration; increased inspiration and expiration of air as a result of increase in rate or depth of respiration, or both. Results esp. in carbon dioxide depletion (acapnia) with accompanying symptoms (fall in blood pressure, vasoconstriction, and sometimes syncope). This is usually accompanied by marked anxiety. The immediate treatment involves having the patient breathe into a paper bag until the CO_2 content of the blood has an opportunity to return to normal. Just as effective is to close one nostril and be certain the patient breathes with mouth closed. In both cases the patient needs to be reassured and calmed.

hyperviscos′ity ["+ L. *viscosus*, gummy]. Excessive viscosity or exaggeration of adhesive properties. Seen in anemias and inflammatory diseases.

hypervitaminosis (hī″pĕr-vī″tă-mĭn-ō′sĭs) ["+ L. *vita*, life, + amine + *-osis*, condition]. A condition caused by an excessive amount of vitamin. Occurs in cases of administration of massive doses of vitamins A or D.

hypervolemia (hī″pĕr-vŏl-ē′mĭ-ă) ["+ L. *volumen*, volume, + Gr. *haima*, blood]. Plethora of blood; abnormal increase in the volume of circulating blood.

hypesthesia (hĭ-pĕs-thē′zĭ-ă) [Gr. *hypo*, under, + *aisthesis*, sensation]. Lessened sensibility to touch. (Variant of hypoesthesia.)

hypha (hī′fă) [Gr. *hyphe*, web]. (pl. *hyphae*) A filament of mold, or part of a mold mycelium.

hyphedonia (hĭp″hĕ-dō′nĭ-ă) [Gr. *hypo*, under, + *hedone*, pleasure]. Abnormal diminution in gratification of desires.

hyphemia (hĭ-fē′mĭ-ă) ["+ *haima*, blood]. 1. Blood in the anterior chamber of the eye in front of iris. 2. Oligemia, a deficiency of blood.

hyphidrosis (hĭp-hĭd-rō′sĭs) ["+ *hidros*, sweat]. Diminished secretion of sweat.

Hyphomycetes (hī″fō-mĭ-sē′tēz) [Gr. *hyphe*, web, + *mykes*, fungus]. The Fungi Imperfecti. Filamentous fungi with branched or unbranched threads. Do not have sexual spores.

hypinosis (hĭp″ĭn-ō′sĭs) [Gr. *hypo*, under, + *is*, *in-*, fiber, + *-osis*, condition]. Deficiency of fibrin in the blood; hypoinosemia.

hypnagogic (hĭp-nă-gŏj′ĭk) [Gr. *hypnos*, sleep, + *agogos*, leading]. 1. Inducing sleep or induced by sleep. SYN: *hypnotic*. 2. In psychology, pert. to hallucinations or dreams just before loss of consciousness. SEE: *hypnogenic zones*.

h. state. A transitional state between sleeping and awaking and delusions which may result therefrom.

hypnalgia (hĭp-năl′jĭ-ă) ["+ *algos*, pain]. False sense of pain experienced in a dream.

hypnic (hĭp′nĭk) [Gr. *hypnos*, sleep]. Causing sleep. SYN: *somnifacient; somniferous*.

hyp′nocyst ["+ *kystis*, a cyst]. A quiescent cyst or one in which the activity is in abeyance.

hypnogenetic (hĭp″nŏ-jĕ-nĕt′ĭk) ["+ *gennan*, to produce]. Producing sleep.

h. spots. Areas which, on being stimulated, produce sleep. SYN: *hypogenic zones*, q.v.

hypnogenic zones (hĭp″nŏ-jĕn′ĭk) ["+ *gennan*, to produce]. Areas on the body which, when stimulated, produce sleep, esp. a sleep resembling somnambulism.

The area may be the elbow or the popliteal spaces. SEE: *hypnagogic*.

hypnoidal (hĭp-noy′dăl) [Gr. *hypnos*, sleep, + *eidos*, resemblance]. Pert. to a condition between sleep and waking, resembling sleep.

hypnoidiza′tion ["+ *eidos*, form]. Induction of hypnosis.

hypnolepsy (hĭp′nŏ-lĕp-sĭ) ["+ *lepsis*, seizure]. Irresistible sleepiness. SYN: *narcolepsy*.

hypnology (hĭp-nŏl′o-jĭ) ["+ *logos*, study]. Scientific study of sleep.

hyp″nophob′ia ["+ *phobos*, fear]. Morbid fear of falling asleep.

hypnopompic (hĭp″nŏ-pŏm′pĭk) [Gr. *hypnos*, sleep, + *pompe*, procession]. Pert. to dreams or visual images persisting after sleep prior to complete awakening.

hypnosis (hĭp-nō'sĭs) ["+ -ōsis, condition]. A subconscious condition in which the objective manifestations of mind are more or less inactive, accompanied by abnormal sensibility to suggestions made by the hypnotist. SEE: *autohypnosis; hypnotism; sleepwalking.*

hypnosophy (hĭp-nŏs'o-fĭ) ["+ sophia, wisdom]. The study of sleep.

hypnother'apy ["+ therapeia, treatment]. Treatment by hypnotism, or by inducing prolonged sleep.

hypnot'ic [Gr. hypnos, sleep]. 1. Pert. to sleep or hypnosis. 2. An agent that induces sleep or which dulls the senses. Ex: chloral hydrate.

hypnot'ics [Gr. hypnos, sleep]. Drugs which cause insensibility to pain by inhibiting afferent impulses, or the cortical centers of the brain receiving sensory impressions, and thus causing partial or complete unconsciousness.

They include sedatives, analgesics, anesthetics, and intoxicants. They should yield not unpleasant aftereffects and result in natural sleep.

They are sometimes called somnifacients and soporifics when used to induce sleep.

NP: They should not be administered without a physician's order.

RS: analgesic; anesthetic; intoxicant; sedative; somnifacient; soporific.

hypnotism (hĭp'nō-tĭzm) ["+ ismos, state of]. An induced sleeplike state during which patient is peculiarly susceptible to the suggestions of the hypnotist.

hyp'notist [Gr. hypnos, sleep]. One who practices hypnotism.

hypnotize (hĭp'nō-tiz). To put under hypnotism.

hypo (hī'pō) [Gr. hypo, under]. Popular name for hypodermic syringe or injection.

hypo-, hyp- [Gr. hypo, under]. Prefix: Less than, below, under.

hypoacidity (hī''pō-ă-sĭd'ĭ-tĭ) [Gr. hypo, under, + L. acidus, sour]. A condition caused by lowered hydrochloric secretion. Secondary to other disorders, such as pernicious anemia.

TREATMENT: Dilute HCl by mouth.

hypoade'nia (hī''pō-ă-dē'nĭ-ă) ["+ adēn, gland]. Defective activity of the glands.

hypoadrenalism (hī''pō-ăd-rē'năl-izm, -nĭ-ă) ["+ L. ad, to, + rēnalis, pert. to kidney, + Gr. ismos, state of]. Adrenal insufficiency.

hypoalimenta'tion ["+ L. alimentum, nourishment]. Insufficient nourishment.

hypoalonemia (hī''pō-ăl-ō-nē'mĭ-ă) [Gr. hypo, under, + hals, salt, + haima, blood]. Lack of salts in the blood.

hypoazoturia (hī''pō-ăz-ō-tū'rĭ-ă) ["+ azotum, nitrogen, + ouron, urine]. Diminished urea in the urine.

hypobaropathy (hī''pō-băr-ŏp'ă-thĭ) ["+ baros, pressure, + pathos, disease]. Symptoms produced by diminished air pressure, anoxia, mountain sickness, aviator's sickness.

hypoblast (hī'pō-blăst) [Gr. hypo, under, + blastos, germ]. The inner cell layer or entoderm which develops during gastrulation. The external layer is called epiblast.

hypoblastic (hī-pō-blăs'tĭk). Pert. to the inner layer of the blastoderm.

hypobulia (hī''po-bū'lĭ-ă) ["+ boulē, will]. Lack of will power.

hypocalcemia (hī''pō-kăl-sē'mĭ-ă) ["+ L. calx, lime, + Gr. haima, blood]. Abnormally low blood calcium.

hypocalcia (hī''po-kăl'sĭ-ă) [Gr. hypo, under, + L. calx, lime]. Lack of calcium in the system.

hypocap'nia ["+ kapnos, smoke]. Lack of carbon dioxide in the blood.

hypochloremia (hī''pō-klō-rē'mĭ-ă) ["+ chlōros, green, + haima, blood]. Having deficiency of the chloride content of the blood.

hypochlorhydria (hī''pō-klŏr-hī'drĭ-ă) ["+ " hydōr, water]. Diminished secretion of hydrochloric acid.

Small amount and low acid may be indicative of carcinoma or anemia. May be found in subacute and chronic gastritis, early carcinoma. SEE: *achlorhydria; hyperchlorhydria.*

hy''pochloriza'tion ["+ chlōros, green]. Reduction of sodium chloride in the diet in nephritis.

hypochloruria (hī''pō-klŏr-ū'rĭ-ă) [Gr. hypo, under, + chlōros, green, + ouron, urine]. Diminution of chlorides in the urine.

hypocholesteremia (hī''pō-lĕs-tĕr-ē'mĭ-ă) ["+ cholē, bile, + stereos, solid, + haima, blood]. Decreased blood cholesterol.

hypochon'dria ["+ chondros, cartilage]. Abnormal concern about health with false belief of suffering from some disease. SYN: *hypochondriasis.*

hypochon'driac. 1. Pert. to the region of the hypochondrium, q.v., or upper lateral region on each side of the body and below the thorax; beneath the ribs. 2. One having interest in and fear of disease.

h. region. Part of abdomen beneath lower ribs on both sides of epigastrium. SYN: *hypochondrium.*

hypochondriacal (hī''pō-kŏn-drĭ'ă-kăl) [Gr. hypo, under, + chondros, cartilage]. Affected with a pathological interest in health and disease.

hypochondrial reflex (hī″pō-kŏn′drĭ-ăl). A sudden inspiratory act resulting from sudden pressure below costal border.

hypochondriasis (hī″pŏ-kŏn-drī′ă-sĭs) [Gr. *hypo*, under, + *chondros*, cartilage, + *iosis*, diseased condition]. Abnormal anxiety about one's health; a frequent symptom of depressed states. SYN: *hypochondria*.

hypochon′drium. That part of the abdomen beneath the lower ribs on each side of the epigastrium.

hypochromasia (hī″po-krō-mā′sĭ-ă) [Gr. *hypo*, under, + *chrōma*, color]. Lack of hemoglobin in the red blood cells.

hypochromatosis (hī″pō-krō-mă-tō′sĭs) ["+ "+ *-ōsis*, condition]. Disappearance of the chromatin or nucleus in a cell. SYN: *chromatolysis*.

hy″pochrom′ia. Condition of the blood in which the red blood cells have a reduced hemoglobin content.

hypochromic (hī″pō-krōm′ĭk). Pert. to hypochromia.

hypochylia (hī″po-kī′lĭ-ă) [Gr. *hypo*, under, + *chylos*, juice]. Lack of normal secretion of gastric juice.

hypocinesia (hī″pō-sĭn-ē′zĭ-ă) ["+ *kinēsis*, motion]. Diminished power of movement. SYN: *hypokinesia*.

hypocolasia (hī″pō-kō-lā′zĭ-ă) ["+ *kolasis*, hindering]. Functional weakness of the inhibiting mechanism.

hypocondylar (hī″pō-kŏn′dĭ-lar) ["+ *kondylos*, condyle]. Below a condyle.

hy″pocone ["+ *kōnos*, cone]. The distolingual cusp of an upper molar tooth.

hy″pocon′id. The distobuccal cusp of a lower molar tooth.

hypocrinism (hī″pō-krī′nĭzm) ["+ *krinein*, to separate, + *ismos*, state of]. Deficient secretion of any gland, esp. an endocrine.

hypocyclosis (hī″pō-sī-klō′sĭs) [Gr. *hypo*, under, + *kyklos*, circle]. Deficient accommodation.

 h., ciliary. Weakness of ciliary muscle.

 h., lenticular. Lack of elasticity in crystalline lens.

 Both forms interfere with accommodation.

hypocystotomy (hī″po-sĭs-tŏt′ō-mĭ) ["+ *kystis*, a bladder, + *tome*, incision]. Perineal opening of the bladder.

hypocytosis (hī-po-sī-tō′sĭs) ["+ *kytos*, cell, + *-ōsis*, condition]. Lack of normal number of blood corpuscles.

hypodactylia (hī″pō-dăk-tĭl′ĭ-ă) ["+ *daktylos*, finger]. Having a decreased number of fingers or toes.

hypodermatomy (hī″po-dĕr-măt′ō-mĭ) ["+ *derma*, skin, + *tome*, incision]. Subcutaneous incision or section, as of a muscle or tendon.

hypoder′mic [Gr. *hypo*, under, + *derma*, skin]. Under, or inserted under the skin, as a hypodermic injection.

 It may be given subcutaneously (under the skin), intracutaneously (into the skin), intramuscularly (into a muscle), intraspinally (into the spinal canal), or intravenously (into a vein).

 It is given to secure prompt action of a drug when the drug cannot be taken by mouth, when it may not be readily absorbed in the stomach or intestines, when it might be changed by action of the gastric secretions, or to act as an anesthetic about the site of injection.

 CAUTION: Pull back on the syringe plunger after the needle is inserted to determine if the needle is in a vein or artery. Because medicines produce serious undesired effects when given intravascularly, do not inject the medicine if the needle is in a vessel.

 h., antitoxin, serum, and vaccine. Usually given subcutaneously in area over the deltoid muscle of the arm. May also be administered intramuscularly.

 h., intracutaneous. Into the skin.

 h., intramuscular. Given in gluteal or in lumbar region. Used when a drug is not easily absorbed or when it is irritating and when large quantity of liquid is to be used.

 h., intravenous. Into a vein, the usual site being median basilic, or median cephalic vein of the arm.

 h., subcutaneous. Given just under the skin, usually in outer surface of arms and forearm.

hypodermoclysis, hypodermatoclysis (hī″po-dĕr-mŏk′lĭ-sĭs, -mă-tŏk′lĭ-sĭs) ["+ "+ *klysis*, a washing out]. The injection of fluids into the subcutaneous tissues to supply the body with liquids quickly, as after shock, hemorrhage, or diarrhea; it may be given in any condition in which it is impossible to give sufficient water by mouth or by rectum.

 When it is necessary to maintain a larger amount of water in the tissues in order to keep up proper metabolism, hypodermoclysis may be ordered. The purpose is about the same as that of intravenous infusions.

 Physiological salt solution (normal salt solution) is generally used because it is one of the principal constituents of the blood.

 There are other solutions given by this method as preferred by the attending physician. If the solution is not of the correct osmolarity, hemolysis, q.v., may occur.

It is essential that solution be of the proper temperature, which should be from 108°-115° F. (42.2°-46.1° C.) in the flask, as it cools rapidly while passing through the tubing.

Site of injection may be: In the loose tissues at the base of the breasts; in the thighs or buttocks (care being taken to avoid the large blood vessels); in the axillary line (esp. for men); beneath the skin of the abdomen (half way between the navel and the anterior superior spine); and intraperitoneally in children. The thighs should be used as site of injection only with great caution because of the closeness of the femoral vein.

hypodynamia (hī″pō-dĭ-nā′mĭ-ă) [Gr. *hypo,* under, + *dynamis,* power]. Diminished muscular power or energy. SYN: *adynamia.*

hypoeccrisia (hī″po-ĕk-krĭs′ĭ-ă) [″+ *ek,* out, + *krisis,* separation]. Diminished excretion of waste material.

hypoeccritic (hī″pō-ĕk-krĭt′ĭk). 1. Retarding normal excretion. 2. Pert. to insufficient or defective excretion.

hypoendocrinism (hī″pō-ĕn-dōk′rĭ-nĭzm) [Gr. *hypo,* under, + *endon,* within, + *krinein,* to separate, + *ismos,* state of]. Insufficiency of internal secretion in one or more glands.

hypoendocrisia (hī″pō-ĕn″dō-krĭz′ĭ-ă). Insufficiency of endocrine secretion. SYN: *hypoendocrinism.*

hypoeosinophilia (hī″po-ē″ō-sīn″o-fĭl′ĭ-ă) [Gr. *hypo,* under, + *eōs,* dawn, + *philein,* to love]. Diminished quantity of eosinophil leukocytes of the blood.

hypoepinephria (hī″po-ĕp′ĭ-nĕf′rĭ-ă) [″+ *epi,* upon, + *nephros,* kidney]. Diminished secretion of epinephrine.

hypoergy (hī″po-ĕr′jĭ) [″+ *ergon,* work]. Hyposensitiveness to allergens.

hypoesophoria (hī″po-ĕs″o-fō′rĭ-ă) [″+ *esō,* inward, + *phorein,* to bear]. Downward and inward deviation of the eye.

hypoesthe′sia [Gr. *hypo,* under, + *aisthēsis,* sensation]. Dulled sensitivity to touch.

hypoexophoria (hī″po-ĕks-o-fō′rĭ-ă) [″+ *exō,* outward, + *phorein,* to bear]. Downward and outward deviation of the eye.

hypogas′tric [″+ *gastēr,* belly]. Pert. to lower middle of the abdomen or hypogastrium.

   h. artery. Arteria iliaca interna.

   h. plexus. Sympathetic nerve plexus in the pelvis.

   h. region. The hypogastrium. SEE: *abdominal regions.*

hypogas′trium. Region below the umbilicus, or navel, between the right and left inguinal regions.

hypogen′esis [Gr. *hypo,* under, + *genesis,* development]. Cessation of growth or development at an early stage, causing defective structure. SYN: *ateliosis.*

hypogenitalism (hī″po-jĕn′ĭ-tăl-izm) [″+ L. *genitalis,* a genital, + Gr. *ismos,* state of]. Condition in which the genital organs are underdeveloped. Characterized by reduced size of genital organs, failure of testes to descend in some cases, and incomplete development of secondary sex characters. SEE: *hypogonadism.*

hypogeusia (hī″po-gū′sĭ-ă) [″+ *geusis,* taste]. Blunting of sense of taste.

   h., idiopathic. A syndrome consisting of decreased taste and olfactory acuity, and with or without perverted taste (dysgeusia, q.v.) and smell. Cause of the syndrome is unknown. In experimental studies certain trace elements added to the diet appear to correct some of the symptoms.

hypoglos′sal [″+ *glōssa,* tongue]. Situated under the tongue.

   h. alternating hemiplegia. Medulla lesion paralyzing the tongue by involving the 12th nerve fibers as they course through the uncrossed pyramid. The pathology may extend across the midline or dorsally, involving the medial fillet, causing contralateral anesthesia.

   h. nerve. A mixed nerve, the 12th cranial. It carries afferent proprioceptive impulses as well as efferent motor impulses. Originates in the medulla oblongata. Distribution: Extrinsic and intrinsic muscles of tongue.

hypoglot′tis [″+ *glōssa,* tongue]. Undersurface of tongue.

hypoglyce′mia [Gr. *hypo,* under, + *glykos,* sweet, + *haima,* blood]. Deficiency of sugar in the blood. A condition in which the glucose in the blood is abnormally low.

   ETIOL: Hyperfunction of the islets of Langerhans may cause it or injection of excessive quantity of insulin. SEE: *coma; hyperglycemia; hyperinsulinism.*

   SYM: Acute fatigue, restlessness, malaise, marked irritability and weakness. In severe cases, mental disturbances, delirium, coma, and possibly death.

hypoglycemic (hī″po-glī-sē′mĭk). Pert. to or causing hypoglycemia.

   h. shock. Production of shock by artificial production of hypoglycemia by intramuscular administration of insulin in the treatment of schizophrenia. RS: insulin; schizophrenia; shock.

hypoglycogenolysis (hī″po-glī-ko-jĕn-ŏl′ī-sis) [Gr. *hypo*, under, + *glykos*, sweet, + *gennan*, to produce, + *lysis*, loosening]. Defective hydrolysis of glycogen (glycogenolysis).

hypognathous (hī-pŏg′nă-thus) [″+ *gnathos*, jaw]. Having a lower jaw longer than the upper one.

hypogonadism (hī″po-gō′năd-izm) [″+ *gonē*, semen, + *ismos*, state of]. Defective internal secretion of the gonads.

hypohepatia (hī″po-hě-pā′tī-ă) [″+ *ēpar*, *ēpat-*, liver]. Deficient liver function.

hypohidrosis (hī-po-hī-drō′sis) [″+ *hidrōs*, sweat, + *-ōsis*, condition]. Diminished perspiration. SYN: *hyphidrosis.*

hypohyloma (hī″po-hī-lō′mă) [Gr. *hypo*, under, + *hylē*, matter, + *-ōma*, tumor]. A tumor formed by embryonic tissue. Derived from hypoblast tissue.

hypoinosemia (hī″po-īn″o-sē′mī-ă) [″+ *is*, *in-*, fiber, + *haima*, blood]. Decreased amount of fibrin in the blood.

hypoin′sulinism [″+ L. *insula*, island, + Gr. *ismos*, state of]. Insufficient secretion of insulin. SYN: *diabetes mellitus.*

hypoisotonic (hī″po-ī″so-tŏn′ĭk) [″+ *isos*, equal, + *tonos*, tension]. Hypotonic, q.v.

hypokalemia (hī″po-kă-lē′mī-ă) [″+ Mod. L. *kalium*, potash, + Gr. *haima*, blood]. Extreme potassium depletion in the circulating blood, commonly manifested by episodes of muscular weakness or paralysis, tetany, and postural hypotension. SYN: *hypopotassemia.*

hypokinesia (hī″po-kīn-ē′zī-ă) [″+ *kinēsis*, motion]. Decreased motor reaction to stimulus.

hypokinet′ic. Pert. to hypokinesia.

hypokolasia (hī″po-kŏl-ā′zī-ă) [Gr. *hypo*, under, + *kolasis*, hindrance]. Imperfect inhibitory power.

hypolem′mal [″+ *lemma*, sheath]. Situated below a sheath or membrane.

hypolepidoma (hī″po-lĕp′ĭ-dō′mă) [″+ *lepis*, *lepid-*, flake, + *-ōma*, tumor]. A hypoblastic tissue tumor.

hypoleukocytosis (hī″po-lū″ko-sī-tō′sis) [Gr. *hypo*, under, + *leukos*, white, + *kytos*, cell, + *-ōsis*, condition]. Diminished number of leukocytes in blood. SYN: *leukopenia.*

hypoliposis (hī″po-lī-pō′sis) [″+ *lipos*, fat, + *-ōsis*, condition]. Deficiency of fat in the tissues.

hypologia (hī-po-lō′jī-ă) [Gr. *hypo*, under, + *logos*, word]. A cerebral symptom marked by inadequate speech.

hypolymphemia (hī-po-līm-fē′mī-ă) [″+ L. *lympha*, lymph, + Gr. *haima*, blood]. De-creased lymphocytes in the blood with normal number of leukocytes.

hypomania (hī″po-mā′nī-ă) [″+ *mania*, madness]. Mild mania and excitement with moderate change in behavior.

hypomastia, hypomazia (hī-po-măs′tī-ă, -mā′zī-ă) [″+ *mastos*, *mazos*, breast]. Condition of having abnormally small breasts.

hy″pomelanchol′ia [Gr. *hypo*, under, + *melas*, black, + *cholē*, bile]. Melancholia without delusions.

hypomenorrhea (hī″po-mĕn-or-rē′ă) [″+ *mēn*, month, + *rhoia*, flow]. Deficient menstrual flow.

hypomere (hī′po-mēr) [″+ *meros*, part]. That portion of the mesoderm that later forms the pleuroperitoneal walls.

hypometabolism (hī″po-mĕ-tăb′o-lizm) [″+ *metabolē*, change, + *ismos*, state of]. Lowered metabolism.

hypometria (hī″po-me′trī-ă) [Gr. *hypo*, under, + *metron*, measure]. Shortened range of movement.

hypometropia (hī″pō-mĕ-trōp′ī-ă) [″+ ″+ *ōps*, eye]. Myopia or shortsightedness.

hypomnesia, hypomnesis (hī″pŏm-nē′zī-ă, -nē′sĭs) [″+ *mnēsis*, memory]. Impaired memory.

hypomorph (hī′po-mŏrf) [″+ *morphē*, form]. One with short limbs who is short when standing in proportion to when sitting. The opposite of hypermorph, q.v. SEE: *mesomorph.*

hypomotility (hī″po-mō-tĭl′ĭ-tī) [″+ L. *mōtus*, moved]. Hypokinesia, q.v.

hypomyotonia (hī″po-mī″o-tō′nī-ă) [Gr. *hypo*, under, + *mys*, *myo-*, muscle, + *tonos*, tension]. Lacking in muscular tonus.

hypomyxia (hī″po-mīks′ī-ă) [″+ *myxa*, mucus]. Diminished secretion of mucus.

hyponanosoma (hī″pō-năn-ō-sō′mă) [″+ *nanos*, dwarf, + *sōma*, body]. Extreme dwarfism.

hyponatremia (hī″po-nă-trē′mī-ă) [″+ Arabic *natrūn*, carbonate of soda, + Gr. *haima*, blood]. Decreased concentration of sodium in the blood.

hyponeocytosis (hī″pō-nē″ō-sī-tō′sīs) [″+ *neos*, new, + *kytos*, cell, + *-ōsis*, condition]. Decreased number of leukocytes (leukopenia) with immature cells in the blood.

hyponoia (hī″po-noy′ă) [″+ *nous*, mind]. Sluggish mental activity or imagination. SYN: *hypopsychosis.*

hyponychium (hī-po-nīk′ī-um) [Gr. *hypo*, under, + *onyx*, *onych-*, nail]. [NA] The nail bed. SYN: *matrix unguis.*

hypopallesthesia (hī″po-păl″ĕs-thē′zī-ă) [″+ *pallein*, to shake, + *aisthēsis*, perception]. Decreased ability to perceive vibratory sense.

hypopancreatism (hī″po-păn′krē-ă-tizm) ["+ *pankreas*, pancreas, + *ismos*, state of]. Diminished activity of the pancreas.

hypoparathyreosis (hī″po-păr-ă-thī-rē-ō′-sis) ["+ *para*, beside, + *thyreos*, shield, + *-ōsis*, condition]. A condition due to lessened or absent secretion of the parathyroids. SYN: *hypoparathyroidism.*

hypoparathyroidism (hī″po-păr-ă-thī′-royd-izm) ["+ "+ "+ *eidos*, form, + *ismos*, state of]. Insufficient secretion of the parathyroid glands.

hypopep′sia ["+ *pepsis*, digestion]. Impaired digestion due to lack of pepsin.

hypopepsinia (hī″po-pĕp-sĭn′ĭ-ă). Deficient pepsin in the gastric juice.

hypophar′ynx [Gr. *hypo*, under, + *pharynx*, pharynx]. The laryngopharynx; the lowermost portion of the pharynx which leads to the larynx and esophagus.

hypophonesis (hī″po-fō-nē′sis) ["+ *phōnē*, voice]. A diminished sound in auscultation or in percussion fainter than usual.

hypophonia (hī″po-fō′nĭ-ă). Abnormally weak voice due to incoordination of speech muscles.

hypophoria (hī″po-fō′rĭ-ă) [Gr. *hypo*, under, + *phorein*, to bear]. Tendency of one visual axis to fall below the other one.

hypophosphatemia (hī″po-fŏs″fă-tē′mĭ-ă) ["+ L. *phosphas*, phosphate, + Gr. *haima*, blood]. Phosphates below normal in the blood.

hypophrenia (hī″po-fre′nĭ-ă) [Gr. *hypo*, under, + *phrēn*, mind]. Mental deficiency.

hypophyseal (hī″po-fīz′ē-al) ["+ *physis*, growth]. Pert. to the hypophysis or pituitary.

hypophysectomy (hī″po-fĭ-sĕk′tō-mī) ["+ "+ *ektomē*, excision]. Excision of the hypophysis cerebri.

hypophysis (hī-pŏf′ĭ-sis) [Gr. an undergrowth]. (pl. *hypophyses*) 1. Any undergrowth. 2. [NA] The pituitary body.

h. cerebri. A gland of internal secretion lying in the sella turcica of the sphenoid bone. It consists of two portions, the adenohypophysis and the neurohypophysis. These are differentiated into the anterior and posterior lobes which are attached to the hypothalamus of the brain by the hypophyseal stalk. SYN: *pituitary gland*, q.v.

hypophysitis (hī-pŏf′ī-sī′tis) [Gr. *hypo*, under, + *physis*, growth, + *-itis*, inflammation]. Inflammation of the pituitary body.

hypopiesis (hī″po-pī-ē′sis) ["+ *piesis*, pressure]. Lower than normal blood pressure.

hypopinealism (hī″po-pĭn′ē-al-izm) ["+ L. *pineus*, pert. to pine cone, + Gr. *ismos*, state of]. Diminished secretion of the pineal gland.

hypopituitarism (hī″po-pĭ-tū′ĭ-tă-rizm) [Gr. *hypo*, under, + L. *pituita*, mucus, + Gr. *ismos*, state of]. A condition resulting from diminished secretion of pituitary hormones, esp. those of the anterior lobe.

hypoplasia (hī″po-plā′zĭ-ă) ["+ *plasis*, formation]. Defective development of tissue. RS: tissue.

hypoporosis (hī″po-pō-rō′sis) ["+ *pōros*, callus, + *-ōsis*, condition]. Deficient development of a callus at site of a bone fracture.

hypopotassemia (hī″po-pō″tăs-sē′mĭ-ă) ["+ New Latin *potassium*, + Gr. *haima*, blood]. Hypokalemia, q.v.

hypopraxia (hī″po-prăk′sĭ-ă) [Gr. *hypo*, under, + *praxis*, action]. Decreased and inefficient activity.

hypoproteinemia (hī″po-prō″tē-īn-ē′mĭ-ă) ["+ *prōtos*, first, + *haima*, blood]. Decrease in the amount of protein in the blood.

hypoproteino′sis. Condition of deficient proteins in the body or diet.

hypoprothrombinemia (hī″po-prō-thrŏm″bĭn-ē′mĭ-ă) [Gr. *hypo*, under, + L. *pro*, for, + Gr. *thrombos*, clot, + *haima*, blood]. Deficiency of blood clotting factor II (prothrombin) in the blood.

hypopselaphesia (hī″pŏp-sĕl-ă-fē′zĭ-ă) ["+ *psēlaphēsis*, touch]. Blunted tactile sense.

hypopsychosis (hī″po-sī-kō′sis) [Gr. *hypo*, under, + *psychē*, mind, + *-ōsis*, condition]. Weakness of the function of thought. SYN: *hyponoia.*

hypoptyalism (hī″po-tī′ăl-izm) ["+ *ptyalon*, saliva, + *ismos*, state of]. Decreased salivary secretion.

hypopyon (hī-po′pī-on) ["+ *pyon*, pus]. Pus in anterior chamber of the eye in front of iris but behind cornea, seen in corneal ulcer.

hyporeflex′ia ["+ L. *reflexus*, bent back]. Diminished function of the reflexes.

hyposalemia (hī″po-săl-ē′mĭ-ă) ["+ L. *sal*, salt, + Gr. *haima*, blood]. Decreased amt. of salts in the blood. SYN: *hypochloremia.*

hypo″saliva′tion. Abnormal decrease in flow of saliva.

hyposar′ca [Gr. *hypo*, under, + *sarx*, flesh]. Extreme dropsy (anasarca) of subcutaneous connective tissue.

hyposecre′tion ["+ L. *secrētus*, from *secernere*, to separate]. Lowered amt. of secretion.

hy′posen′sitive [Gr. *hypo*, under, + L. *sentīre*, to feel]. Having reduced ability to respond to stimuli.

hy″posensitiza′tion. Production of hyposensitiveness.

hyposialadenitis (hī″po-sī″ăl-ăd-ĕ-nī′tis) [Gr. *hypo*, under, + *sialon*, saliva, + *adēn*, gland, + *-itis*, inflammation]. Submaxillary salivary gland inflammation.

hyposmia (hī-pŏz′mĭ-ă) ["+ *osmē*, smell]. Defect in sense of smell.

hypospadia, hypospadias (hī″po-spā′dĭ-ă, -ăs) ["+ *span*, to draw]. Congenital opening of the male urethra upon the undersurface of the penis; also an urethral opening into vagina.

hyposphresia (hī″pŏs-frē′sĭ-ă) ["+ *osphrēsis*, smell]. Hyposmia, q.v.

hyposphyxia (hī″pŏs-fĭk′sĭ-ă) ["+ *sphyxis*, pulse]. Sluggish circulation due to abnormally low blood pressure.

hypostasis (hī″pŏs′tă-sis) ["+ *stasis*, a standing]. 1. Diminished blood flow or circulation. 2. Deposit of sediment due to decreased flow of a body fluid such as blood or urine.

hypostatic (hī″po-stăt′ik) [Gr. *hypo*, under, + *statikos*, standing]. 1. Of or pertaining to hypostasis. 2. In genetics, hidden or suppressed, said of a gene whose effect is suppressed by the presence of another gene.

hyposteatolysis (hī″po-stē-ă-tŏl′ĭ-sis) ["+ *stear*, fat, + *lysis*, loosening]. Diminished emulsification of fats during digestion.

hyposthenia (hī″pŏs-thē′nĭ-ă) ["+ *sthenos*, strength]. Subnormal strength; an enfeebled state; weakness.

hypostheniant (hī″pŏs-thē′nĭ-ant). Reducing vital forces; debilitant.

hyposthenic (hī-pŏs-thĕn′ĭk). Debilitant.

hyposthenuria (hī″pŏs-thĕn-ū′rĭ-ă) [Gr. *hypo*, under, + *sthenos*, strength, + *ouron*, urine]. The secretion of urine of low specific gravity, chiefly in chronic nephritis.

   h., tubular. H. resulting from disease of renal tubule epithelial cells.

hypostypsis (hī″po-stĭp′sis) ["+ *stypsis*, a contracting]. State of being slightly astringent.

hypostyptic (hī″po-stĭp′tĭk). Slightly astringent.

hyposynergia (hī″po-sĭn-ĕr′jĭ-ă) [Gr. *hypo*, under, + *syn*, together, + *ergon*, work]. Poor coordination.

hyposystole (hī″po-sĭs′to-lĭ) ["+ *systolē*, contraction]. A weak or lowered systolic contraction.

hypotaxia (hī″po-tăks′ĭ-ă) ["+ *taxis*, arrangement]. State of reduced control over voluntary actions such as occurs in early stages of hypnotism.

hypoten′sion [Gr. *hypo*, under, + L. *tensiō*, tension]. 1. Decrease of systolic and diastolic blood pressure below normal. 2. Deficiency in tonus or tension.

   It occurs in shock and collapse; in hemorrhages, infections, fevers, cancer, anemia, neurasthenia, Addison's disease; in other debilitating or wasting diseases; and approaching death.

   h., orthostatic. H. occurring when a person assumes an erect position.

   h., postural. H. occurring upon suddenly arising from a recumbent position or from standing still.

hypoten′sive. Denoting low blood pressure.

hypotensor (hī″po-tĕn′sor). Agent that lowers blood pressure.

hypothalamus (hī″pō-thăl′ă-mus) [Gr. *hypo*, under, + *thalamos*, chamber]. [NA] The portion of the diencephalon comprising the ventral wall of the third ventricle below the hypothalamic sulcus and including structures forming ventricular floor, including the optic chiasma, tuber cinereum, infundibulum, and mammillary bodies. It lies beneath the thalamus and laterally is continuous with the subthalamic regions. It contains neurosecretions which are of importance in the control of certain metabolic activities, such as maintenance of water balance, sugar and fat metabolism, regulation of body temperature and secretion of endocrine glands. It is the chief subcortical region for the integration of sympathetic and parasympathetic activities.

   The hypothalamus is the source of the hormones vasopressin and oxytocin stored and released by the neural lobe of the hypophysis.

hypothenar (hī-pŏth′ĕ-nar) ["+ *thenar*, palm]. The fleshy prominence on inner side of the palm next to the little finger.

   h. eminence. Prominence on palm below little finger.

hypother′mal ["+ *thermē*, heat]. 1. Tepid. 2. Subnormal temperature.

hypother′mia. 1. Having a body temperature below normal. 2. A technique of lowered body temperature, usually between 78° and 90° F. (26° and 32.5° C.), to reduce oxygen need during surgery (esp. cardiovascular and neurological procedures) and in hypoxia, to reduce blood pressure, and to remedy hyperpyrexia.

hypothesis (hī-pŏth′ĕ-sis) [Gr. *hypo*, under, + *thesis*, a placing]. (pl. *hypotheses*) 1. An assumption not proved by experiment or observation. It is assumed for the sake of testing its soundness or to facilitate investigation of a class of phenomena. 2. A conclusion drawn before all the facts are established and tentatively accepted as a basis for further investigation.

hypothrombinemia (hī″po-throm-bĭn-ē′mĭ-ă) ["+ *thrombos*, clot, + *haima*, blood]. Deficiency of thrombin in the blood.

hypothymergasia (hī″po-thī″mĕr-gā′sĭ-ă) ["+ *thymos*, mind, + *ergasia*, energy]. A condition of physical and mental depression.

hypothymia (hī″po-thī′mĭ-ă) ["+ *thymos*, mind]. Decreased emotional response to stimuli.

hypothymism (hī″po-thī′mizm) ["+ "+ *ismos*, state of]. Decreased activity of the thymus.

hypothyroid (hī″pō-thī′royd) [Gr. *hypo*, under, + *thyroidēs*, shield-shaped, + *eidos*, form]. Marked by insufficiency of thyroid secretion.

hypothyroida′tion. Condition causing insufficient thyroid secretion.

hypothyroidism (hī″po-thī′royd-izm). A condition due to deficiency of the thyroid secretion, resulting in a lowered basal metabolism. A lesser degree of cretinism.

SYM: May be obesity; dry skin and hair, both of which become lusterless. Low blood pressure, slow pulse, sluggishness of all functions, depressed muscular activity, goiter.

TREATMENT: Replacement therapy with thyroid hormone preparations either natural or synthetic. Increase iodine in diet if iodine is deficient.

NP: Constipation is a marked feature of this disease, as is decreased metabolic rate, with a subnormal temperature. Guard against chilling, as the patient is abnormally sensitive to cold. If thyroid extract is ordered, watch for signs of hyperthyroidism. Observe the patient carefully and watch for overexertion during treatment with thyroid extract.

hypotonia (hī″po-tō′nĭ-ă) [Gr. *hypo*, under, + *tonos*, tone]. 1. Reduced tension; relaxation of arteries. 2. Loss of tonicity of the muscles or intraocular pressure.

hypotonic (hī-po-tŏn′ik). 1. Pert. to defective muscular tone or tension. 2. A solution of lower osmotic pressure than another.

hypotoxicity (hī″po-tŏks-ĭs′ĭ-tĭ) [Gr. *hypo*, under, + *toxikon*, poison]. A reduced toxic quality; only slightly poisonous.

hypotrichosis (hī″po-trĭ-kō′sis) ["+ *thrix*, *trich-*, hair, + *-osis*, condition]. Abnormal deficiency of hair.

hypotrophy (hī-pŏt′rŏ-fĭ) ["+ *trophē*, nourishment]. Progressive degeneration and functional loss of cells and tissues. SYN: *abiotrophy*; *atrophy*.

hypotropia (hī″po-trō′pĭ-ă) ["+ *tropē*, a turning]. Vertical strabismus downward.

hypouresis (hī″po-ū-rē′sis) [Gr. *hypo*, under, + *ourēsis*, urination]. Diminished output of urine.

hypouricuria (hī″po-ū-rĭ-kū′rĭ-ă) ["+ *ouron*, urine, + *ouron*, urine]. Deficient uric acid in the urine.

hypourocrin′ia ["+ "+ *krinein*, to separate]. Deficient urinary secretion.

hypovaria (hī″po-va′rĭ-ă) ["+ L. *ovarium*, ovary]. Deficient internal secretion of the ovary and consequent retardation of growth and development in girls.

hypovenosity (hī″po-vĕn-ŏs′ĭ-tĭ) [Gr. *hypo*, under, + L. *venōsus*, pert. to a vein]. Incomplete development of the venous system in an area, resulting in atrophy or degeneration.

hy″poventila′tion ["+ L. *ventilātiō*, ventilation]. Reduced rate and depth of breathing.

hypovitaminosis (hī″po-vī″tă-mĭn-ō′sis) ["+ L. *vita*, life, + *amine*, + Gr. *-ōsis*, condition]. A condition due to a lack of vitamins in the diet.

hypovolemia (hī″po-vō-lē′mĭ-ă) ["+ L. *volumen*, volume]. Diminished blood supply. SYN: *oligemia*; *oligohemia*.

hypoxanthine (hī″pō-zăn′thĭn, -thēn) ["+ *xanthos*, yellow]. A purine derivative, C_5H_4-N_4O, in muscles and tissues in a stage of urea and uric acid formation. It is formed during protein decomposition. In small amts. it is normal in urine.

hypoxemia (hī-pŏks-ē′mĭ-ă) ["+ *oxys*, acid, + *haima*, blood]. Insufficient oxygenation of the blood. SYN: *hypoxia*.

hypoxia (hī″pŏks′ĭ-ă). Anoxia; lack of an adequate amount of oxygen in inspired air such as occurs at high altitudes; reduced oxygen content or tension.

hypsarrhythmia (hĭp″săr-ĭth′mĭ-ă) [Gr. *hypsi*, high, + *a-*, not, + *rhythmos*, rhythmn]. An abnormal electroencephalographic pattern of persistent generalized slow waves and very high voltage. Clinically it is often associated with infantile spasm and progressive mental deterioration. Etiol. is unknown.

hypsibrachycephalic (hĭp″sĭ-brăk-ĭ-sĕ-fāl′ik) [Gr. *hypsi*, high, + *branchys*, broad, + *kephalē*, head]. Having a broad and high skull.

hypsicephalic (hĭp″sĭ-sĕ-fāl′ĭk) ["+ *kephalē*, head]. Having a skull with a cranial index above 75.1°.

hypsicephaly (hĭp-sĭ-sĕf′ă-lĭ). The condition of having a skull with a cranial index over 75.1°.

hypsiconchous (hĭp-sĭ-kŏng′kus) [Gr. *hypsi,* high, + *konchē,* shell]. Having an orbital index about 85°.

hypsiloid (hĭp′sĭ-loyd) [Gr. *ypsilon,* U or Y, + *eidos,* form]. U- or Y-shaped. SYN: *hyoid.*

h. ligament. Ligamentum iliofemorale.

hypsistaphylia (hĭp-sĭ-stăf-ĭl′ĭ-ā) [Gr. *hypsi,* high, + *staphylē,* uvula]. Having a narrow, high palatal arch.

hypsistenocephalic   (hĭp″sĭ-stĕn″o-sĕ-fāl′ĭk) ["+ *stenos,* narrow, + *kephalē,* head]. Having a cranial index over 75.1°. SYN: *hypsicephalic.*

hypsoceph′alous ["+ *kephalē,* head]. Having a cranial index over 75.1°. SYN: *hypsicephalic.*

hypsokine′sis [Gr. *hypsos,* height, + *kinēsis,* motion]. Tendency to fall backward when standing; seen in paralysis agitans.

hypsonosus (hĭp-sŏn′o-sus) ["+ *nosos,* disease]. Mountain sickness; balloon sickness. SYM: Epistaxis, headache, nausea.

hypsophobia (hĭp″so-fō′bĭ-ă) ["+ *phobos,* fear]. Fear of being at great heights. SYN: *aerophobia.*

hypurgia (hī-pŭr′jĭ-ă) [Gr. *hypourgia,* help]. Any minor factors which change the course of a disease, esp. for the better.

hysteral′gia [Gr. *hystera,* uterus, + *algos,* pain]. Uterine pain.

hysterectomy (hĭs-tĕr-ĕk′tō-mĭ) ["+ *ektomē,* excision]. Removal of the uterus. The presence of tumors, both benign and malignant, is a common cause. The uterus may be removed through the abdominal wall or through the vagina.

  NP: The patient is placed in dorsal position. The table is ready to be tipped into the Trendelenburg position. As soon as incision is made through the peritoneum, table should be put into Trendelenburg position. This procedure is the same for all abdominopelvic surgery.

  This position allows the intestines and abdominal organs to fall backwards from pelvis, so that they may be easily packed off with large pads or with a large roll of packing. Postoperatively, watch intake and output of patient closely, prevent bladder distention, turn frequently. SEE: *laparotomy.*

    h., abdominal. Removal of the uterus through an abdominal incision.

    h., Porro. Subtotal hysterectomy following cesarean section.

    h., subtotal. Removal of the uterus, leaving the cervix uteri in place.

    h., supracervical. Same as subtotal.

    h., supravaginal. Same as subtotal.

    h., total. Removal of body and cervix.

    h., vaginal. Removal of the uterus through the vagina.

hystere′sis [Gr. *hysterēsis,* a coming too late]. 1. Failure of related phenomena to keep pace with each other. 2. Failure of the manifestation of an effect to keep up with its cause.

hystereurynter (hĭs″tĕr-ū-rĭn′tĕr) [Gr. *hystera,* uterus, + *eurynein,* to stretch]. An instrument for dilating the os uteri.

hysteria (hĭs-tĕ′rĭ-ă) [Gr. *hystera,* uterus]. A condition presenting somatic symptoms, simulating almost every type of physical disease, and a series of mental manifestations. The condition occurs in the absence of organic disease to account for the symptoms.

  The mental attitude is calm; there is a not unfriendly aloofness, but psychotic indifference is quite another matter, and not seen in h. There may be easy laughing and crying-episodes of emotionalism possibly without any apparent explanation, and even occurring in sleep. Episodic states known as fugues (sleepwalking is similar, occurring in sleep). In these, certain dissociated (repressed) ideas, emotions and goals develop a reality sufficient to constitute a secondary personality which now functions apart from the primary personality.

  When the primary consciousness reasserts itself, there is a forgetting (amnesia) of the secondary state. The multiplication or alternation of personalities is quite distinct from schizophrenic splitting in which incongruities and confusion result from the coexistence of each phase of the personality more or less continuously.

  An accurate definition is difficult because of extreme diversity of symptoms; a psychoneurosis found in a patient of low vitality, characterized by psychic weakness and undue susceptibility to autosuggestion.

  ETIOL: Variable, as in most psychic disturbances. It occurs in both sexes before and after adolescence and at periods of emotional and physical stress, as alternating crying and laughing.

  SYM: Emotional instability, various sensory disturbances and a marked craving for sympathy which sometimes leads to fraud.

  TREATMENT: Place patient in a quiet place devoid of spectators. Cold applications to head, face, and neck are helpful. Quiet, firm suggestions are important. Sedatives are to be used under the direction of a physician.

    h., anxiety. H. combined with an anxiety neurosis.

    h., major. Very severe h. accompanied by epileptiform convulsions.

h., minor. Mild form of h. without loss of consciousness.

hyste'riac [Gr. *hystera,* uterus]. A hysterical person.

hyster'ic, hyster'ical. Pert. to hysteria.

   h. ataxia. Loss of sensation in leg muscles and skin in h.

   h. chorea. A form of h. with choreiform movements.

hystericoneuralgic (hĭs-tĕr″ik-o-nū-răl′jik) [Gr. *hystera,* womb, + *neuron,* nerve, + *algos,* pain]. Pert. to pain of hysterical origin, but resembling neuralgia.

hysteritis (hĭs-tĕr-ī′tĭs) ["+ *-itis,* inflammation]. Inflammation of the uterus.

hystero-, hyster- [Gr. *hystera,* womb]. Prefix: womb; hysteria.

hysterobubonocele (hĭs″tĕr-o-bū-bŏn′o-sēl) [Gr. *hystera,* womb, + *boubōn,* groin, + *kēlē,* hernia]. Inguinal hernia surrounding the uterus.

hysterocat'alepsy ["+ *kata,* down, + *lēpsis,* seizure]. Major hysteria with cataleptic symptoms.

hysterocele (hĭs′tĕr-o-sēl) ["+ *kēlē,* hernia]. Hernia of the uterus, esp. when gravid.

hysterocervicotomy (hĭs″tĕr-o-sĕr-vĭ-kŏt′o-mĭ) ["+ L. *cervix,* neck, + Gr. *tomē,* incision]. Cesarean section through the vagina. SYN: *hysterotrachelotomy.*

hysterocleisis (hĭs″tĕr-o-klī′sĭs) ["+ *kleisis,* closure]. Surgical closure of the os uteri.

hysterocystocleisis (hĭs″tĕr-o-sĭs″to-klī′-sĭs) ["+ *kystis,* a bladder, + *kleisis,* a closure]. Operation fastening the cervix uteri in the wall of the bladder.

hysterodynia (hĭs′tĕr-o-dĭn′ĭ-ă) [Gr. *hystera,* uterus, + *odynē,* pain]. Uterine pain. SYN: *hysteralgia.*

hysteroepilepsy (hĭs″tĕr-o-ĕp′ĭ-lĕp″sĭ) ["+ *epilēpsia,* seizure]. Major hysteria with violent epileptiform convulsions.

   In addition to usual symptoms of epilepsy, anger, disgust, joy, surprise and other emotions are dramatically expressed when final stage (delirium) is reached.

hysterofrenic (hĭs″tĕr-o-frĕn′ik) ["+ L. *frenāre,* to restrain]. 1. Arresting an attack of hysteria. 2. Application of pressure to certain areas of the body to produce hysteria.

hysterogastrorrhaphy (hĭs″tĕr-o-găs-trŏr′ă-fĭ) ["+ *gastēr,* belly, + *rhaphē,* suture]. Fixation of uterus to gastric wall. SYN: *hysteropexy.*

hysterogen'ic [Gr. *hystera,* womb, + *gennan,* to produce]. Causing a hysterical attack.

hysteroid (hĭs′tĕr-oyd) ["+ *eidos,* resemblance]. 1. Resembling hysteria. 2. Pert. to hysteria.

hysterolaparotomy (hĭs″tĕr-o-lăp″ă-rŏt′ŏ-mĭ) ["+ *lapara,* flank, + *tomē,* incision]. Uterine incision through abdominal wall; abdominal hysterectomy.

hysterolith (hĭs′tĕr-o-lĭth) ["+ *lithos,* stone]. A calculus in the uterus.

hysterology (hĭs-tĕr-ŏl′ŏ-jĭ) [Gr. *hystera,* womb, + *logos,* knowledge]. Sum of what is known about the uterus.

hysterolysis (hĭs″tĕr-ŏl′ĭ-sĭs) ["+ *lysis,* loosening]. Operation of lossening the uterus from its adhesions.

hysteroma'nia ["+ *mania,* madness]. 1. Hysterical mania. 2. Nymphomania, q.v.

hysterometer (hĭs″tĕr-ŏm′ē-ter) ["+ *metron,* measure]. Device for measuring the uterus.

hysterom'etry. Measurement of the size of the uterus.

hysteromyoma (hĭs″tĕr-o-mī-ō′mă) [Gr. *hystera,* womb, + *mys, myo-,* muscle, + *-ōma,* tumor]. Myoma or fibromyoma of the uterus.

hysteromyomectomy (hĭs″tĕr-o-mī″o-mĕk′tō-mĭ) ["+ "+ *ektomē,* excision]. Excision of a uterine fibroid.

hysteromyotomy (hĭs″tĕr-o-mī-ŏt′ō-mĭ) ["+ "+ *tomē,* incision]. Uterine incision for removal of a solid tumor.

hysteroneurosis (hĭs″tĕr-o-nū-rō′sĭs) ["+ *neuron,* nerve, + *-ōsis,* condition]. A neurosis related to disease of the uterus.

hystero-oophorectomy (hĭs″tĕr-ō-ō″ō-fōrĕk′tō-mĭ) ["+ *ōion,* egg, + *phoros,* bearing, + *ektomē,* excision]. Removal of the uterus and one or both ovaries.

hysteropathy (hĭs″tĕr-ŏp′ă-thĭ) [Gr. *hystera,* womb, + *pathos,* disease]. Any uterine disorder.

hysteropexy (hĭs′tĕr-o-pĕks′ĭ) ["+ *pēxis,* fixation]. Surgical fixation of uterus.

hystero'pia ["+ *ōps,* eye]. A hysterical visual defect.

hysteropsychosis (hĭs″tĕr-o-sī-kō′sĭs) ["+ *phychē,* mind, + *-ōsis,* condition]. Mental disorder due to uterine disease.

hysteroptosia, hysteroptosis (hĭs″tĕr-ŏp-tō′sĭ-a, -sĭs) ["+ *ptōsis,* a dropping]. Prolapse of the uterus. SYN: *procidentia.*

hysterorrhaphy (hĭs-tĕr-ŏr′ă-fĭ) [Gr. *hystera,* womb, + *rhaphē,* sewing]. Suture of womb.

hysterorrhexis (hĭs″tĕr-o-rĕks′ĭs) ["+ *rhēxis,* rupture]. Rupture of the uterus, esp. when pregnant.

hysterosalpingography (hĭs″tĕr-o-săl″pĭn-gŏg′ră-fĭ) ["+ *salpinx,* tube, + *graphein,* to write]. X-ray study of the uterus and oviducts after injecting radiopaque material into those organs.

hysterosalpingo-oophorectomy (hĭs"-těr-o-săl-pĭng"gō-ō"ō-fŏr-ĕk'tō-mĭ) ["+ "+ ōion, egg, + phoros, bearing, + ektomē, excision]. Surgical removal of uterus, oviducts and ovaries.

hysterosalpingostomy (hĭs"těr-o-săl"-pĭng-ŏs'tō-mĭ) ["+ "+ stoma, opening]. Anastomosis of the uterus with the distal end of the fallopian tube after excision of a strictured portion of the tube.

hysteroscope (hĭs'těr-o-skōp) [Gr. hystera, womb, + skopein, to examine]. Instrument for examining the uterine cavity.

hysteroscopy (hĭs-těr-ŏs'kō-pĭ). Inspection of the uterus by use of a special endoscope. SEE: hysteroscope.

hys'terospasm [Gr. hystera, uterus, + spasmos, a spasm]. Uterine spasm.

hysterostomatocleisis (hĭs"těr-o-stō"mă-tō-klĭ'sĭs) ["+ stoma, opening, + kleisis, closure]. Operation for vesicovaginal fistula. Closure of the cervix uteri, making the vesical and uterine cavities into a common cavity by means of the opening between them.

hysterostomatomy (hĭs"těr-o-stō-măt'ō-mĭ) ["+ "+ tomē, incision]. Surgical enlargement of the os uteri; incision of the os or cervix uteri.

hysterosyph'ilis. A hysterical manifestation due to syphilis.

hysterosystole (hĭs"těr-o-sĭs'tō-lĭ) [Gr. hystera, womb, + systolē, contraction]. A delayed contraction of the heart after its normal time, as opposed to extrasystole.

hysterotabetism (hĭs"těr-o-tā'bĕt-ĭzm) ["+ L. tabes, a wasting away, + Gr. -ismos, state of]. Condition of hysteria and tabes combined.

hysterotokotomy (hĭs"těr-o-tō-kŏt'ō-mĭ)

["+ tokos, birth, + tomē, incision]. Cesarean operation.

hys'terotome ["+ tomē, incision]. Instrument for incision of the uterus.

hysterotomotokia (hĭs"těr-o-tōm"o-tō'kĭ-ă) ["+ "+ tokos, birth]. Cesarean section.

hysterotomy (hĭs-těr-ŏt'ō-mĭ) [Gr. hystera, womb, + tomē, incision]. 1. Incision of the uterus. 2. Cesarean section, q.v.

hysterotrachelorrhaphy (hĭs"těr-o-trā"kĕl-or'ă-fĭ) ["+ trachēlos, neck, + rhaphē, sewing]. A plastic operation for a lacerated cervix by paring the edges and suturing them together.

hysterotrachelotomy (hĭs"těr-o-trā"kĕl-ŏt'ō-mĭ) ["+ "+ tomē, incision]. Surgical incision of neck of uterus.

hysterotraumatic (hĭs"těr-o-träw-măt'ĭk) ["+ trauma, wound]. Pert. to traumatic hysteria.

hysterotraumatism (hĭs"těr-o-träw'mă-tĭzm) ["+ "+ ismos, state of]. Hysteric symptoms due to or following traumatism.

hysterotris'mus [Gr. hystera, womb, + trismos, a spasm]. Uterine spasm.

hysterovagino-enterocele (hĭs"těr-ō-văj"ĭn-o-ĕn'těr-o-sēl) ["+ L. vagina, sheath, + Gr. enteron, intestine, + kēlē, hernia]. Hernia surrounding uterus, vagina, and intestines.

hystriciasis, hystricism (hĭs-trĭ-sī'ă-sĭs, his'trĭ-sizm) [Gr. hystrix, hedgehog]. 1. Erection of hairs like the spines of a hedgehog. 2. A skin disease.

SYM: Thickened epidermis, warty growths, elongated and hypertrophied papillae. SYN: ichthyosis hystrix.

hyther (hī'thĕr) [Gr. hydōr, water, + thermē, heat]. The combined effect of humidity and temperature of atmosphere upon the body.

I

I. Chem. symb. for iodine.

I[131]. Radioactive iodine. At. wt. 131.

I[132]. Radioactive iodine. At. wt. 132.

i. Abbr. for *optically inactive.*

iamatology (ī″ăm-ă-tŏl′ō-jĭ) [Gr. *iama*, remedy, + *logos*, science]. Study of therapeutics and remedies.

ianthinopsia (ĭ-ăn-thĭ-nŏp′sĭ-ă) [Gr. *ianthinos*, violet colored, + *opsis*, vision]. Abnormality of vision in which all objects appear to be violet.

-iasis [Gr.]. Suffix, same as *-ōsis*, meaning the state or condition of, particularly a pathological condition.

iatraliptics (ĭ-ă-tră-lĭp′tĭks) [Gr. *iatreia*, cure, + *aleiphein*, to anoint]. Treatment by inunction or friction.

iatric (ĭ-ăt′rĭk) [Gr. *iatros*, physician]. Medical. Referring to the medical profession or physicians.

iatrochem′istry ["+ *chēmeia*, chemistry]. Seventeenth century opinion that chemistry is the basis of all physiological phenomena.

iatrogenic disorder (ĭ″ăt-rō-jĕn′ĭk) ["+ *gennan*, to produce]. An abnormal mental or physical condition induced in a patient by effects of treatment by a physician or surgeon. Term implies that such effects could have been avoided by proper and judicious care on the part of the physician. Ex: drug habituation; anxiety neuroses.

iatrogeny (ĭ″ă-trŏj′ĕ-nĭ). Abnormal state or condition induced by a physician. SEE: *iatrogenic disorder.*

iatrology (ĭ-ă-trŏl′ō-jĭ) [Gr. *iatros*, physician, + *logos*, science]. Medical science.

iatropic stimulus (ĭ″ă-trŏp′ĭk) ["+ *tropē*, turning]. The stimulus or event which makes a person seek medical attention. If the person is sick, it is called the chief complaint.

However, there are many reasons for apparently healthy people to seek medical care voluntarily, i.e., an armed forces draft examination, health screening survey, or pre-employment or premarital examination. Thus it is possible for disease to be discovered prior to the time when it would make itself known to the individual. When evidence of disease is discovered in a patient who did not know he had the disease, it is said to be a lanthanic disease.

iatrotechniques (ĭ-ăt-rō-tĕk-nēks′) ["+ *technē*, art]. The art and technique of medicine and surgery.

ice (ĭs) [AS. *ĭs*]. Water frozen solid. Water becomes i. at a temperature of 32° F. (0° C.). I. may be chilled to any degree lower than the freezing point.

   i. bag, i. cap, i. collar. Devices for holding i. to be applied to a patient to obtain the effect of continuous cold in a circumscribed area.

The affected part should always be covered with several thicknesses of cloth to prevent freezing.

   i. cravat. I. pack applied around the neck.

   i., dry. Carbon dioxide cooled to the point where it is a solid. This occurs at –110° F. (–78.9° C.). Used as a commercial refrigerant; also for therapeutic refrigeration in the treatment of warts. SEE: *carbon dioxide.*

   i. treatment. Use of i. applied either directly or in a suitable container to cool an injured area. It is believed that i. therapy, at least in the first 24-48 hours following injury, is much more beneficial than heat in treating superficial bruises, contusions, and sprains. The use of i. water in immediate treatment of a burn helps to reduce the extent of inflammation and pain.

Iceland moss. An edible lichen containing a form of starch; a slightly tonic demulcent. SYN: *Cetraria.*

ichnogram (ĭk′no-grăm) [Gr. *ichnos*, footstep, + *gramma*, mark]. A footprint taken while standing.

ichor (ī′kŏr) [Gr. *ichōr*, serum]. Thin, fetid discharge from an ulcer or from a wound.

ichoremia (ĭ-kŏr-ē′mĭ-ă) ["+ *haima*, blood]. Septicemia or blood poisoning.

ichorous (ī′kŏr-ŭs) [Gr. *ichōr*, serum]. Resembling ichor or watery pus.

ichthammol (ĭk′thă-mŏl). A reddish brown, viscous fluid obtained by the destructive distillation of certain bituminous shale.

Used as a mild antiseptic and local stimulant in certain skin diseases.

ichthyism, ichthyismus (ĭk′thĭ-izm, ĭk″-thĭ-iz′mus) [Gr. *ichthys*, fish, + *-ismos*, state of]. Poisoning from eating decomposed or toxic fish.

ichthyo- [Gr. *ichthys*, fish]. Combining form meaning fish.

ichthyoid (ĭk′thĭ-oyd) [Gr. *ichthys*, fish, + *eidos*, form]. Fishlike.

ichthyophobia (ĭk-thĭ-o-fō′bĭ-ă) ["+ *phobos*, fear]. Aversion to fish.

ichthyosis (ĭk″thĭ-ō′sis) ["+ *-ōsis*, condition]. Condition in which the skin is dry and scaly, resembling fish skin. Because i. is so easily recognized, a variety of diseases have been called by this name.

i. hystrix. An hereditary form which is extremely rare. Characterized by gross keratosis with quill-like projections involving the entire body except the face, genitalia, palms, and soles.

i. vulgaris. Diagnosis includes two genetically distinct types of i.: Dominant ichthyosis vulgaris, which is also called xeroderma and ichthyosis simplex, which is produced by an autosomal dominant gene. It is not present at birth and is usually noticed between the ages of one and four. Characterized by dry, rough, scaly skin. Many cases improve in later life. Sex-linked i. vulgaris is present only in males and is transmitted by the female as a recessive gene. Onset of scattered large brown scales is in early infancy. The scalp may be involved but the face is spared except for the sides and in front of the ear. There is little tendency to improve with age.

There is no satisfactory therapy for either form of i. vulgaris.

ichthyotic (ik-thī-ot'ik) [Gr. *ichthys,* fish]. Rel. to ichthyosis.

ICN. Abbr. for *International Council of Nurses.*

iconolagny (ĭ-kŏn″ō-lag'nī) [Gr. *eikōn,* image, + *lagneia,* lewdness]. Sexual stimulation produced by suggestive pictures, statues, or objects.

ICSH. Abbr. for *interstitial cell stimulating hormone.* In male, this hormone stimulates the production of testosterone from the interstitial cells of the testes. Same as LH (luteinizing hormone).

ictal (ĭk'tăl) [L. *ictus,* a blow or stroke]. Pert. to or caused by a sudden attack or stroke such as acute epilepsy.

icterepatitis (ĭk-tĕr-ĕ-pă-tī'tis) [Gr. *ikteros,* jaundice, + *hēpar,* liver, + *-itis,* inflammation]. Hepatitis associated with jaundice.

icteric (ĭk-tĕr'ĭk) [Gr. *ikteros,* jaundice]. Pert. to jaundice.

i. index. A number obtained by matching blood serum in a colorimeter against a standard solution of potassium dichromate (1:10,000), which gives a color approximately same as bilirubin.

A test for determining the intensity of the yellow color of blood serum. Since serum color depends upon bile pigment, the index is an indication of the concentration of this pigment in the blood. Valuable in study of jaundice.

The serum is diluted to known strength and then compared; the reading of the standard, divided by the reading of the serum and multiplied by the dilution gives the icteric index. Normal serum gives a value of between four and seven. In patients with visible jaundice values above 15 are obtained.

icteritious (ĭk-tĕr-ĭsh'us). Yellowish; resembling jaundice. SYN: *icteroid.*

icteroane'mia [Gr. *ikteros,* jaundice, + *an-,* not, + *haima,* blood]. Icterus associated with anemia, hemolysis and splenic enlargement.

icterogenic, icterogenous (ĭk″tĕr-o-jĕn'ĭk, -ŏj'en-us) ["+ *gennan,* to produce]. Causing jaundice.

icterohepatitis (ĭk″tĕr-o-hĕp-ă-tī'tis) ["+ *hēpar,* liver, + *-itis,* inflammation]. Liver inflammation with jaundice.

icteroid (ĭk'tĕr-oyd) ["+ *eidos,* form]. Resembling jaundice; yellow-hued.

icterus (ĭk'tĕr-us) [Gr. *ikteros,* jaundice]. Jaundice, q.v. Pigmentation of the tissues, membranes and secretions with bile pigments.

i. gravis. Acute yellow atrophy of liver with cerebral disorders.

i., hemolytic; nonobstructive. Rare chronic form, frequently congenital, with periodic attacks of intense hemolysis.

SYM: Much the same as in obstructive icterus, q.v., but staining not so intense. Sometimes found in acute yellow atrophy, the anemias and infectious fevers. Enlarged spleen.

i. neonatorum. Hemolytic jaundice of the newborn.

i., obstructive. Jaundice caused by obstruction to the flow of bile in the common or hepatic duct.

ETIOL: Cholangitis, carcinoma, gallstones, cirrhosis of liver, cysts, parasites in ducts, pressure by tumors, hepatic abscess.

SYM: Skin, mucous membrane and secretions stained yellow; first noticed in the conjunctivae. Stool light or clay-colored, urine dark, pulse low, temperature slightly subnormal. In extreme cases, delirium, convulsions, coma.

ic'tus [L., stroke]. 1. A beat or stroke. 2. An attack.

i. cordis. A term applied to heartbeat.

i. epilepticus. Epileptic convulsion.

i. sanguinis. Apoplexy.

i. solis. Sunstroke.

I.C.U. Abbr. for *intensive care unit.*

ID. Abbr. for *identification; inside diameter; intradermal.*

id. 1. [Gr. *idios,* own] In biology, a hypothetical structure carrying the heredity qualities; "an ancestral germ plasm." 2. [L. *id,* it] In psychiatry, one of the three divisions of the psyche, the others being the ego, q.v., and superego, q.v. The i. is the obscure, inaccessible part of our personality which serves as the repository of instinctual drives which are continually striving for expression. Expression is manifest as an impulsion to obtain satisfaction for the instinctive needs in accordance with the pleasure-pain principle.

-id [Gr. *eidos*, form, shape]. Suffix indicating certain secondary skin eruptions which appear some distance from site of primary infection. If etiologic agent of primary infection is known, the secondary lesion is designated by adding "-id", as tuberculid, tricophytid.

-ide [Fr. ac*ide*, acid]. In chemistry, an ending indicating a binary compound, as *sodium chloride*.

ide'a [Gr. form, from *idein*, to see]. A mental image; a concept.

> *i., autochthonous.* An unaccountable i.

> *i., compulsive.* A persistent, obsessional impulse or thought.

> *i., dom'inant.* I. controlling all one's actions and thoughts.

> *i., fixed.* I. that completely dominates the mind, as a delusion.

> *i., flight of.* Rapid speech, often disconnected and incoherent, in certain mental diseases.

> *i. of reference.* An impression that the conversation or actions of others have reference to oneself.

ideation (ī-dē-ā'shŭn). The process of thinking; formation of ideas. It is slow in dementias, depressions, and other organic brain diseases, and in narcotic intoxications, but quickened in early stage of intoxications. It is unduly active in manic-depressive insanity.

idée fixe (ē-dā-fēks') [Fr.]. An obsession; a fixed idea. SEE: *idea.*

iden'tical [L. *identicus*, the same]. Exactly alike.

> *i. twins.* Twins developed from one fertilized cell. SEE: *Hellin's law; twin.*

identifica'tion ["+ *facere*, to make]. 1. A kind of daydream, as when one indentifies himself with the hero of a book or play. 2. The process of determining the sameness of a thing or person with that described or known to exist.

> *i., anthropometric.* The Bertillon system of i., q.v.

> *i., Bertillon system of.* A system based on physical characteristics.

> *i., Galton system of.* A system based on fingerprints.

> *i., palm and sole system of.* A system based on prints of the palmar surface of hand and the plantar surface of the foot.

ideo- [Gr. *idea*, form]. Prefix pert. to mental images.

ideogenous (ī-dē-ŏj'ĕn-us) [Gr. *idea*, form, + *gennan*, to produce]. Stimulated by an idea.

ideometabolism (ī''dē-o-mĕ-tăb'o-lizm). Metabolic changes induced by mental or emotional factors.

ideomo'tion [Gr. *idea*, form, notion, + L. *motus*, moving]. Muscular automatic movement activated by a dominant idea.

ideomo'tor. Pert. to ideomotion.

ideophrenic (ĭd''ē-ō-frĕn'ĭk) [Gr. *idea*, form, notion, + *phrenitikos*, insane]. Marked by abnormal ideas of a perverted nature.

ideoplastia (ĭd-ē-o-plăs'tĭ-ä) ["+ *plassein*, to form]. Condition of the mind of a hypnotized person in which he is capable of receiving and responding to suggestions of the hypnotist.

ideovascular (ĭd''ē-o-văs'kū-lar). Pert. to vascular changes induced by ideas, memories, or emotions.

idio- [Gr. *idios*, own, personal, distinct]. Prefix indicating individual, distinct.

idiocrasy (ĭd''ī-ŏk'ră-sĭ) [Gr. *idios*, own, + *krasis*, temperament]. Peculiarity which renders one susceptible to certain habits or drugs. SEE: *idiosyncrasy.*

idiocratic (ĭd''ī-o-krăt'ĭk). Pert. to idiocrasy.

id'iocy [Gr. *idiōtēs*, ignorant person]. Mental deficiency usually congenital. SEE: *mental deficiency.*

> *i., amaurotic familial.* Term for a group of related familial diseases marked by dementia and impaired vision. SEE: *amaurotic familial idiocy.*

> *i., complete or profound.* I. in which primitive instincts are lacking, even that of self-preservation.

> *i., cretinoid.* Endemic i. accompanied by goiter.

> *i., diplegic.* I. marked by paralysis of all extremities in infants.

> *i., epileptic.* I. accompanied by epilepsy.

> *i., genetous.* I. of congenital origin.

> *i., hemiplegic.* Hemiplegic manifestations in infants.

> *i., hydrocephalic.* I. accompanied by chronic hydrocephalus.

> *i., intrasocial.* I. in which mentality permits some occupation.

> *i., microcephalic.* I. accompanied by microcephalia.

> *i., mongolian.* Congenital form of i. in which person has mongolian features, the nose being broad, the eyes slanting and the skull flat. SYN: *Down's syndrome*, q.v.

i., paralytic. I. combined with paralysis.

i., paraplegic. I. combined with paraplegia.

i., sensorial. Mental deficiency caused by loss of one of the special senses.

i., traumatic. I. caused by an injury received in infancy or in early childhood.

idiogenesis (ĭd-ĭ-o-jĕn'ĕ-sis) [Gr. *idios*, own, + *gennan*, to produce]. Of self-origin or origin without known cause, esp. with reference to idiopathic disease.

idioglos'sia ["+ *glōssa*, tongue]. Inability to articulate properly so that the sounds emitted are like those of an unknown language.

idioisolysin (ĭd"ĭ-o-ĭ-sŏl'ĭ-sin) ["+ *isos*, equal, + *lysis*, solution]. A hemolysin active against the cells of an individual of the same species.

idiolysin (ĭd"ĭ-ŏl'ĭ-sin) [Gr. *idios*, own, separate, + *lysis*, solution]. A lysin in the blood not formed in response to injection of an antigen.

idiometritis (ĭd"ĭ-o-mē-trī'tis) ["+ *mētra*, uterus, + *-itis*, inflammation]. Inflammation of the uterine parenchyma.

idiomus'cular ["+ L. *musculus*, a muscle]. Pert. to the muscles independent of nerve control.

i. contraction. Motion produced by degenerated muscles without nerve stimulus.

idioneurosis (ĭd"ĭ-ō-nū-rō'sĭs) ["+ *neuron*, nerve, + *-ōsis*, condition]. Any functional neurosis arising without stimuli.

idiopathic (ĭd"ĭ-ō-păth'ĭk) [Gr. *idios*, own, personal, + *pathos*, disease]. Pert. to conditions without clear pathogenesis, or disease without recognizable cause, as of spontaneous origin.

idiopathy (ĭd-ĭ-ŏp'ă-thĭ). A primary disease without apparent external cause.

idiophrenic (ĭd"ĭ-o-frĕn'ĭk) [Gr. *idios*, own, personal, + *phrēn*, mind]. Pert. to or originating in the mind alone.

idioreflex (ĭd"ĭ-o-rē'flĕks) ["+ L. *reflexus*, reflected]. A reflex resulting from a stimulus which arises within the organ in which the reflex takes place.

idiosyncrasy (ĭd"ĭ-o-sĭn'kră-sĭ) ["+ *syn-*, together, + *krasis*, mixture]. 1. Special characteristics by which persons differ from each other. 2. That which makes one react differently from others. A peculiar or individual reaction to an idea, an action, a drug, a food, or some other substance through unusual susceptibility.

i. to drug. When no effects are produced from large doses of a drug, or unusual effects from small doses or from certain drugs.

i. of effect. When doses of a drug which would have a known and predictable effect cause a toxic or opposite effect, or an unusual or no effect.

idiosyncratic (ĭd"ĭ-ō-sĭn-krăt'ĭk). Pert. to an idiosyncrasy.

id'iot [Gr. *idiōtēs*, an ignorant person]. Former term for severe mental deficiency. SEE: *idiocy; mental deficiency.*

idiot'ic. Like an idiot; said of an idea or action.

idiotrophic (ĭd"ĭ-o-trŏf'ĭk) [Gr. *idios*, own, + *trophē*, nourishment]. Capable of securing its own nourishment.

idiotrop'ic ["+ *tropē*, a turning]. Turning inward mentally. Individual.

i. type. An introvert type satisfied by his own emotions, and by inner contemplation and pursuits, who is content to live apart from social contacts.

idiotypic (ĭd"ĭ-o-tĭp'ĭk) ["+ *typos*, type]. Rel. to heredity.

idioventricular (ĭd"ĭ-o-vĕn-trĭk'ū-lar) ["+ L. *ventriculus*, little belly]. Pert. to the cardiac ventricle alone when dissociated from the atrium.

idrosis (ĭ-drō'sis) [Gr. *hidrōs*, sweat, + *-ōsis*, condition]. Excessive sweating. SYN: *hidrosis.*

IDU. Abbr. for *5-iodo-2'deoxyuridine.* Used to treat herpes virus infections of the eye. SEE: *mace.*

IgE. Abbr. for *immunoglobulin gamma E.* The exact role of this protein in immunological mechanisms has not been defined.

igniextirpation (ĭg"nĭ-ĕks"tĭr-pā'shŭn) [L. *ignis*, fire, + *exstirpāre*, to root out]. Cautery excision.

ignioperation (ĭg"nĭ-ŏp"ĕr-ā'shŭn) ["+ *operarī*, to operate]. An operation by cautery.

ignipuncture (ĭg"nĭ-pŭnk'chūr) ["+ *punctura*, a piercing]. The use of heated needles in cauterization by puncture.

ignis (ĭg'nĭs) [L., fire]. Fire; cautery. SYN: *moxa.*

i. infernalis. Ergotism.

i. sa'cer. An inflammatory skin disease. SYN: *herpes zoster.*

i. Sanc'ti Anto'nii. Acute febrile disease with localized inflammation. SYN: *erysipelas; St. Anthony's fire.*

I.H. Abbr. for *infectious hepatitis.*

ileac (ĭl'ē-ăk). 1. Pert. to the ileum. 2. Pert. to ileus.

ileal (ĭl'ē-ăl). Pert. to the ileum.

i. bypass. Surgical procedure for decreasing absorption of nutrients from the small intestine by anastomosing one portion of the upper portion of the small intestine to another portion some distance farther along the intestine. Method has been used experimentally in treating obesity.

i. conduit. Method of diverting the urinary flow by transplanting the ureter into a prepared and isolated segment of the ileum which is sutured closed on one end. The other end is connected to an opening in the abdominal wall. The urine is collected there in a special receptacle. SYN: *cutaneous ureteroileostomy.*

ileectomy (ĭl″ē-ĕk′tō-mĭ) [L. *ileum,* groin, flank, + Gr. *ektomē,* excision]. Excision of the ileum.

ileitis (ĭl″ē-ī′tis) [L. *ileum,* flank, + Gr. *-itis,* inflammation]. Inflammation of the ileum. The membrane becomes inflamed and ulcerates, the affected portion becoming thick, rigid, and edematous and the lumen progressively narrowed. The lymph glands enlarge and the adjacent mesentery becomes thickened. Most often found in the terminal ileum, but it may spread to other parts of the bowel and to the cecum. Adhesions may be formed. Pain is centered around the umbilicus and right lower quadrant with general distention. Diarrhea alternates with constipation. Vomiting may occur. The stools show occult blood, and mucous shreds if bowels are loose.

i., regional. A nonspecific inflammatory, granulomatous lesion involving the terminal ileum. It is nontuberculous. May be acute or chronic. The acute form simulates appendicitis. The chronic form may extend over many years, with diarrhea, abdominal pain, anemia, loss of weight, fistula formation, and eventually obstructive intestinal symptoms. Stools are soft and grayish or brown in color with abundant fecal particles.

ileocecal (ĭl″ē-o-sē′kăl) [″+ *caecus,* blind]. Rel. to the ileum and cecum.

i. valve. Sphincter muscles which serve to close the ileum at the point where the small intestines open into the ascending colon. It prevents food material from reentering the small intestines.

ileocecum (ĭl″ē-o-sē′kŭm). The ileum and cecum combined.

ileocol′ic [L. *ileum,* groin, flank, + Gr. *kōlon,* colon]. Pert. to the ileum and colon. SEE: *ileocecal.*

ileocolitis (ĭl″ē-o-kō-lī′tis) [″+ ″+ *-itis,* inflammation]. Inflammation of mucous membrane of the ileum and colon.

ileocolostomy (ĭl″ē-o-kō-lŏs′tō-mĭ) [″+ ″+ *stoma,* opening]. Anastomosis between ileum and colon.

ileocolotomy (ĭl″ē-o-kō-lŏt′ō-mĭ) [″+ ″+ *tomē,* incision]. Incision of ileum and colon.

ileoproctostomy (ĭl″ē-o-prŏk-tŏs′tō-mĭ) [L. *ileum,* groin, flank, + Gr. *prŏktos,* rectum, + *stoma,* opening]. Establishment of opening between ileum and rectum.

ileorectostomy (ĭl″ē-o-rĕk-tŏs′tō-mĭ) [″+ *rectum,* rectum, + Gr. *stoma,* opening]. Formation of passage between ileum and rectum. SYN: *ileoproctostomy.*

ileosigmoidostomy (ĭl″ē-o-sĭg″moyd-ŏs′tō-mĭ) [″+ Gr. *sigma,* letter S, + *eidos,* form, + *stoma,* opening]. Surgical opening between the ileum and sigmoid flexure.

ileostomy (ĭl″ē-ŏs′tō-mĭ) [L. *ileum,* groin, flank, + Gr. *stoma,* opening]. Creation of a surgical passage through abdominal wall into ileum.

ileotomy (ĭl″ē-ŏt′ō-mĭ) [″+ Gr. *tomē,* incision]. Incision into the ileum. SYN: *ileostomy.*

ileotransversostomy (ĭl″ē-o-trăns″vĕr-sŏs′tō-mĭ) [″+ *transversus,* crosswise, + Gr. *stoma,* opening]. Connection of the ileum with the transverse colon.

ileum (ĭl′ē-ŭm) [L., groin, flank]. (pl. *ilea*) [NA] Lower three-fifths of the small intestines, from the jejunum to the ileocecal valve. It varies in the adult male from 31 feet six inches (9.6 meters) to 15 feet six inches (4.72 meters). SEE: *digestive system* for illustration.

ileus (ĭl′ē-ŭs) [Gr. *eileos,* a twisting]. Intestinal obstruction.

Originally meant colic due to intestinal obstruction.

SYM: Acute obstruction; sudden pain, paroxysmal, then continuous; constipation; persistent fecal vomiting; abdominal distention; collapse.

RS: intussusception; occlusion; strangulation; torsion; volvulus.

i., adynamic. That caused by intestinal muscle paralysis.

i., dynamic. That caused by intestinal muscle contraction. SYN: *hyperdynamic i.*

i., mechanical. That produced by an obstruction.

i. paralyticus. I., adynamic, q.v.

il′iac [L. *iliacus,* pert. to ilium]. Rel. to the ilium.

i. crest. The hip. Upper free margin of the ilium. SYN: *crista iliaca* [NA].

i. fascia. Transversalis fascia over anterior surface of the iliopsoas muscle.

i. fossa. Fossa iliaca, q.v.

i. region. Inguinal region on either side of hypogastrium.

i. roll. Sausage-shaped mass in left i. fossa. Caused by induration of sigmoidal walls.

i. spine. Spina iliaca.

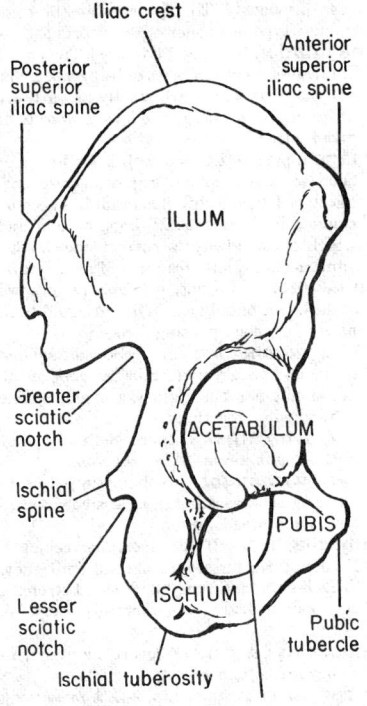

Iliac crest

Anterior superior iliac spine

Posterior superior iliac spine

ILIUM

Greater sciatic notch

ACETABULUM

Ischial spine

PUBIS

Lesser sciatic notch

ISCHIUM

Pubic tubercle

Ischial tuberosity

Obturator foramen

THE ILIUM—LATERAL VIEW

iliocolotomy (ĭl″ĭ-o-kō-lŏt′ō-mĭ) [L. ilium + Gr. *kōlon*, colon, + *tomē*, incision]. Opening into the colon in the iliac or inguinal region.

iliofemoral (ĭl″ĭ-o-fĕm′ōr-al) ["+ *femoralis*, pert. to femur]. Pert. to the ilium and femur.

ilioinguinal (ĭl″ĭ-o-ĭn′gwĭ-năl) ["+ *inguinalis*, pert. to groin]. Pert. to the groin and iliac regions.

iliolumbar (ĭl″ĭ-o-lŭm′băr) ["+ *lumbus*, loin]. Rel. to the iliac and lumbar regions.

iliometer (ĭl″ĭ-ŏm′ĕ-ter) [L. ilium + Gr. *metron*, measure]. Device for measuring the iliac spines.

iliopectineal (ĭl″ĭ-o-pĕk-tĭn′ē-al) ["+ *pecten*, a comb]. Rel. to the ilium and the pubes.

iliopsoas (ĭl″ĭ-o-sō′ăs) ["+ Gr. *psoa*, loin]. The compound iliacus and psoas magnus muscles.

   i. abscess. An abscess in the psoas and iliacus muscles.

iliosacral (ĭl″ĭ-o-sā′krăl) ["+ *sacralis*, pert. to sacrum]. Pert. to the sacrum and ilium.

iliotib′ial ["+ *tibialis*, pert. to tibia]. Pert. to the ilium and tibia.

   i. band. A thick, wide fascial layer from the iliac crest to the knee joint.

ilium (ĭl′ĭ-ŭm) [L., groin, flank]. (pl. *ilia*) 1. One of the bones of each half of the pelvis. It is the superior and widest part. Serves to support the flank. In the child it is a separate bone. SYN: *os ilium* [NA]. 2. The flank. SEE: *hip bone; sacroiliac.*

ill (ĭl) [Old Norse *illr*, bad]. Sick; not healthy; diseased.

illaqueation (ĭl″ăk-wē-ā′shun) [L. *illaqueāre*, to ensnare]. Turning an inverted eyelash by drawing a loop of thread behind it.

illegal (ĭl-lē′găl) [L. *in-*, not, + *lēgalis*, pert. to law]. Contrary to authorized law.

illegitimate (ĭl″lē-jĭt′ĭ-mĭt) ["+ *legitimus*, according to law]. 1. Not according to law; not authorized. 2. Born out of wedlock.

illness (ĭl′nĭs) [Old Norse *illr*, bad, + AS. -*ness*, state of]. 1. State of being sick. 2. Ailment.

illu′minating gas. A mixture of various combustible gases, including hydrogen and carbon monoxide. Its poisonous effects are largely due to carbon monoxide, q.v.

   TREATMENT: Resuscitation, q.v.

illumination (ĭl-lū-mĭn-ā′shun) [L. *illumināre*, to light up]. 1. The lighting up of a part for examination or of an object under a microscope. 2. Amt. of light thrown upon anything.

   i., axial. Light transmitted along the axis of a microscope.

   i., central. Axial i., q.v.

   i., darkfield. I. of an object under a microscope in which the central or axial light rays are stopped and the object illuminated by light rays coming from the sides, the object then appearing light against a dark background. Used to observe extremely small objects such as spirochetes, colloid particles, etc.

   i., direct. I. of an object under a microscope by directing light rays upon its upper surface.

   i., focal. The concentration of light upon an object by means of a mirror or a system of lenses.

   i., oblique. I. of an object from one side.

   i. (by) transmitted light. I. in which the light is directed through the object. Light may come directly from a light source or be reflected by a mirror.

illum′inism. Condition in certain psychotic states in which the patient has delusions of talking or communing with supernatural or exalted beings.

illu'sion [L. *illusiō,* from *illudere,* to mock]. In psychology, inaccurate perception; misinterpretation of sensory impressions, whereas a hallucination has no source in fact.

Vague stimuli favor i.'s, but essentially it is a disorder of ideation, as in toxic and exhaustive deliria. If an i. becomes fixed it is said to be a delusion.

i., optical. A visual impression which is inaccurate with respect to what was available to be seen.

illu'sional. Pert. to, or of the nature of, an illusion.

I.M. Abbr. for *intramuscular(ly).*

image (ĭm'ĭj) [L. *imagō,* likeness]. 1. A mental picture representing a real object. 2. A more or less accurate likeness of a thing or person. 3. The picture of an object such as that produced by a lens or mirror.

i., after-. SEE: *afterimage.*

i., direct; i., erect. Picture from rays not yet focused.

i., double. Condition occurring in strabismus when the visual axes of the eyes are not directed toward the same object. The false i. is formed in the eye that deviates; the true i. in the other eye. SEE: *diplopia.*

i., false. I., double, q.v.

i. intensifier. Device used in radiology to increase the intensity of brightness of an image produced in x-ray and x-ray fluoroscopy studies. This technique permits discrimination of much smaller objects in the image and greatly decreases the exposure of the patient and the examiner to radiation.

i., inverted. I. that is turned upside down.

i., real. I. formed by convergence of rays of light from an object.

i., true. I., double, q.v.

i., virtual. I., direct, q.v.

imagery (ĭm'ĭj-rĭ) [L. *imagō,* likeness]. Imagination; the calling up of events or mental pictures.

Mental imagery may be of various types.

i., auditory. When sounds can be recalled to mind, as thunder, wind, etc.

i., motor. When movement only is recalled, as the passing of a train. Motormindedness is recognized in the mastery of spelling. The constant repetition of movements in writing make for automatic habit formation and fixation of the visual word-image.

i., tactile. When the feel of an object can be readily recalled.

i., taste; i., smell. Mental conception of taste or odor sensations previously experienced. Often very weak.

i., visual. Mental conception of an object seen previously. This is probably the commonest type of imagery. RS: afterimage.

imagination [L. *imagō,* likeness]. The power of forming mental images of things, persons, or situations which are wholly or partially different from those previously known or experienced.

imago (ĭ-mā'gō) [L., likeness]. 1. An image or shadow. 2. A memory, esp. of a loved one, developed during childhood that has become clouded by idealism and imagination, and which is not always a correct one. 3. The adult, sexually mature form of an insect.

imbal'ance [L. *in-,* not, + *bilanx, bilanc-,* two scales]. Out of balance. Without equality in power between opposing forces.

i., autonomic. An i. between sympathetic and parasympathetic divisions of the autonomic nervous system, esp. as pertains to vasomotor reactions.

i., sympathet'ic. Increased excitability of the vagus nerve. SYN: *vagotonia.*

i., vasomotor. Involving impulses to blood vessels resulting in excessive vasoconstriction or vasodilation.

imbecile (ĭm'bĕ-sĭl) [L. *imbecillus,* feeble]. 1. Former term for severe mental deficiency. SEE: *mental deficiency.* 2. Without strength of mind or body; esp. mentally weak. 3. Stupid.

imbecil'ity. A state of severe mental deficiency. SEE: *imbecile.*

imbed' [L. *in,* in, (put) into, + AS. *bedd,* bed]. In histology, to surround with a firm substance, such as paraffin or collodium, preparatory to cutting sections. SEE: *embedding.*

imbibition (ĭm″bĭ-bĭsh'un) [L. *in,* in, + *bibere,* to drink]. The absorption of fluid by a solid body or gel.

imbricate, imbricated (ĭm'brĭ-kāt, -ĕd) [L. *imbricāre,* to tile]. Overlapping, as tiles or fish scales; overlapping aponeurotic layers.

imbrication (ĭm″brĭ-kā'shun) [L. *imbricāre,* to tile]. 1. Overlapping, as tiles. 2. The overlapping of aponeurotic layers in abdominal surgery.

imidazole; iminazole (ĭm″ĭd-āz'ōl″, -ă-zōl′; ĭm″ĭn-). An organic compound characterized structurally by the presence of the heterocyclic ring which occurs in histidine and histamine.

imide (ĭm'ĭd). A compound with the bivalent atom group (NH).

immature (ĭm''mă-tūr') [L. *in-*, not, + *maturus*, ripe]. Not fully developed or ripened.

imme'diate ["+ *mediāre*, to be in middle]. Direct; without intervening steps.

   i. agglutination. Healing by first intention.

   i. auscultation. A. by ear applied to the body. SEE: *auscultation.*

   i. cause. A cause directly originating a disease.

   i. contagion. Contagion by direct contact.

   i. union. Healing by first intention.

immedicable (ĭ-mĕd'ĭ-kă-bl) ["+ *medicabilis,* curable]. Incurable.

immersion (ĭm-ĕr'shun) ["+ *mergere,* to dip]. Placing a body under water, or another fluid.

In microscopy, the act of immersing the objective (then called an i. lens) in water, oil, etc., preventing total reflection of rays falling obliquely upon peripheral portions of the objective.

   i., homogeneous. I. in which the stratum of air between objective and cover glass is replaced by a medium which deflects as little as possible the rays of light passing through the cover glass.

   i. lens, oil. A special lens used with oil and producing a high magnification; useful in studying bacteria.

immiscible (ĭ-mĭs'ĭ-bl) [L. *in-*, not, + *miscere,* to mix]. Pert. to that which cannot be mixed, as oil and water.

immobiliza'tion ["+ *mobilis,* movable]. The making of a part or limb immovable.

NP: Watch for loosening of splints and prevent pressure sores.

immune (ĭm-ūn') [L. *immunis,* safe]. 1. Protected or exempt from a disease. 2. Exempt from a certain disease by vaccination or inoculation.

   i. bodies. Substances in those afflicted with an infectious disease formed by the tissues and possessing power to destroy or injure the disease-producing agent, or to neutralize its toxins.

They are found in the serum of coagulated blood, in blood plasma, and in lymph; they are also called antibodies.

Each is the result of a specific antigen or disease-producing factor which acts only upon the same antigen. They are determined by the effect they cause. If the antigen is poisonous it is called a toxin, and its antibody is called an antitoxin.

RS: anaphylaxis; antibody; ceptor; immunity; immunology; opsonin; precipitin; proteolysis; toxin.

immunifacient (ĭ-mū''nĭ-fa'shent) ["+ *facere,* to make]. Making immune.

immun'ity [L. *immunitas*]. The state of being resistant to noxious agents or organisms due to previous exposure to the same agent or organism.

Such resistance may be due in specific instances to the presence in the blood of antibodies such as antitoxins which counteract bacterial toxins; precipitins which render a foreign protein insoluble; opsonins which increase the ability of leukocytes to ingest bacteria; agglutinins which cause clumping of foreign cells; lysins which dissolve such cells.

   i., acquired. I. resulting from the development of active or passive i.; opposite of natural or innate i.

   i., active. I. resulting from the development within the body of substances which render a person immune. This may result from having the disease or by the injection of the infectious organism, usually attenuated, or products produced by the organism. SEE: *vaccination.*

   i., congenital. I. present at birth. It may be natural or acquired, the latter being dependent upon antibodies received from the blood of the mother.

   i., local. I. which is limited to a given area or tissue of the body.

   i., natural. A more or less permanent i. to disease with which an individual is born, the result of natural inherent factors. It may be the heritage of an individual, a race, or a species. It may be due to the natural presence of immune bodies, but other factors such as diet, differences in metabolism or temperature or adaptive features of infective organisms may be involved.

   i., passive. Produced by actual injection of sera containing the antibodies into the subject to be protected.

immunity, words pert. to: antianaphylaxis; aphylactic; immunoglobulins.

immuniza'tion [L. *immunitas,* immunity]. Becoming immune or the process of rendering a patient immune. SEE: *autoimmunization; immunity.*

immunizing unit. A unit which expresses an antitoxin's strength. It varies with different antitoxins.

immunochemistry (ĭm''mū-nō-kĕm'ĭs-trĭ) [L. *immunis,* safe, + Gr. *chēmeia,* chemistry]. The chemistry of immunization. The chemistry of antigens, antibodies, and their relation to each other.

immunoelectrophoresis. A method of investigating the amount and character of proteins and antibodies in body fluids by using electrophoresis.

immunofluorescence. Method of detecting antibodies and bacteria in infected materials by introducing fluorescent materials into proteins.

immunofluorescent method. Detection of antibodies by using special proteins labeled with fluorescein. If the specific organism or antibody which is being searched for is present it is observed as a fluorescent material when examined microscopically while illuminated with a fluorescent light source.

immunogen (ĭ-mū'nō-jĕn) [L. *immunis*, safe, + Gr. *gennan*, to produce]. A substance which stimulates the formation of an antibody.

immunogenic (ĭm″ū-nō-jĕn′ĭk). Inducing immunity.

immunogenicity (ĭm″mū-nō-jĕ-nĭs′ĭ-tĭ). The capacity to stimulate the formation of antibodies. Not an inherent property of the substance but a condition which exists in a particular biological system. Thus a substance may act to produce antibodies in some individuals and not others.

immunoglobulins (ĭm″mū-nō-glŏb′ū-lĭnz). The system of closely related though not identical proteins which are capable of acting as antibodies. Five different i.'s are normally present in the human adult: IgG (γG), with a molecular weight of 145,000; IgA (γA), with a molecular weight of approximately 160,000; IgM (γM), with a molecular weight of 900,000; IgD (γD), with molecular weight of approximately 160,000; and IgE (γE), with a molecular weight of 200,000. Use of either system of naming the immunoglobulins is acceptable.

immunologic (ĭm″mū-no-lŏj′ĭk) [L. *immunis*, safe, + Gr. *logos*, science]. Pert. to immunology.

i. diseases. Those due to the action of antibodies, as in allergic hypersensitiveness to antigens, or to specific reactivity of the tissues. SEE: *anaphylaxis; serum sickness.*

immunol'ogy ["+ Gr. *logos*, study]. The study of immunity to diseases. SEE: *serology; serum; toxin; vaccination.*

immunopathology. Study of tissue alterations that result from immune or allergic reactions.

immunopro'tein [L. *immunis*, safe, + Gr. *prōtos*, first]. Any protein immune body or substance that confers immunity.

immunosuppression. Prevention of formation of immune response.

immunosuppressive. Acting to suppress the body's natural immune response to an antigen.

i. agent. A substance that suppresses or interferes with normal immune response. Such are used in controlling autoimmune diseases and in enhancing the chances for survival of foreign tissue grafts and transplants. A wide variety of drugs and X rays are used as i. agents.

immunotherapy (ĭm″mū-no-thĕr′ă-pĭ) [L. *immunis*, safe, + Gr. *therapeia*, treatment]. The production of immunity.

immunotox'in ["+ Gr. *toxikon*, poison]. An antitoxin.

immunotransfusion (ĭ-mū″no-trăns-fū′-zhun) ["+ *trans*, across, + *fusus*, poured]. Transfusion of blood from one who has been immunized by an autogenous vaccine.

immunprotein (ĭ-mūn-prō′tē-ĭn) ["+ Gr. *prōtos*, first]. A bacteriolytic substance formed by the injection of attenuated bacterial cultures.

impac'ted [L. *impactus*, pressed on]. Pressed firmly together so as to be immovable. Term may be applied to a fracture in which ends of bones are wedged together; a tooth so placed in jaw bone that eruption is impossible; a fetus wedged in birth canal; cerumen; calculi, or accumulation of feces in the rectum.

impaction (ĭm-păk′shun) [L. *impactiō*, a pressing together]. 1. Condition of being tightly wedged into a part; overloading of an organ, as the feces in the bowels.

impal'pable [L. *in-*, not, + *palpāre*, to touch]. Felt with difficulty; hardly perceptible to the touch.

impal'udism [L. *in*, into, + *palus*, marsh, + Gr. *-ismos*, state of]. Malaria. SYN: *paludism.*

im'par [L., unequal]. Unpaired. SYN: *azygous.*

imparidigitate (ĭm-păr″ĭ-dĭj′ĭ-tāt) ["+ *digitus*, finger]. Having uneven number of fingers or toes.

impatent (ĭm-pā′tĕnt) [L. *in-*, not, + *patere*, to be open]. Closed, not patent.

impedance (ĭm-pē′dăns) [L. *impedīre*, to hinder]. Resistance met by alternating currents in passing through a conductor; consists of resistance, reactance, inductance, or capacitance.

The resistance due to the inductive and condenser characteristics of a circuit is called reactance.

imper'ative [L. *imperatīvus*, commanding]. Obligatory; not controlled by the will; involuntary.

i. concept. An idea which dominates one, as a fear or doubt.

impercep'tion [L. *in-*, not, + *percipere*, to perceive]. Inability to form a mental picture; lack of perception.

imper'forate ["+ *per*, through, + *forare*, to bore]. Without an opening.

i. hymen. A hymen without an opening. Menstruation occurs but the blood cannot escape from the vagina because of the obstruction of the hymen. The treatment is surgical incision of the hymen. SEE: *hymen.*

imperfora'tion [L. *imperforātus*, not open]. State of being closed or occluded. SYN: *atresia.*

imperious acts. Tics and motions not under control of the will. Urges of compulsion states. SEE: *impulsion.*

imper'meable [L. *in-*, not, + *permeāre*, to pass through]. Not allowing passage, as of fluids; impenetrable.

imper'vious ["+ *per*, through, + *via*, way]. Unable to be penetrated.

impetiginous (ĭm″pĕ-tĭj′ĭn-ŭs) [L. from *impetere*, to attack]. Rel. to impetigo.

impetigo (ĭm-pĕ-tī′gō, -tē′gō) [L. from *impetere*, to attack]. Inflammatory skin disease marked by isolated pustules which become crusted and rupture. Occurs principally around mouth and nostrils. Usually caused by either staphylococcal or streptococcal or a combined infection.

i. contagiosa. A contagious form. Children esp. afflicted.

SYM: Discrete, thin-walled vesicles and bullae which become pustular and thin-crusted, appearing in crops. They may be flat and umbilicated with no tendency to rupture, and they are filled with a straw-colored fluid. They dry up as thin yellow crusts.

ETIOL: Streptococcic or staphylococcic.

TREATMENT: Soaking off crusts with soapy water; warm compresses of potassium permanganate solution; topical antibiotics as neomycin sulfate.

i. herpetiformis. Rare form occurring usually in puerperal women and accompanied by serious systemic disturbance.

i. syphilit'ica. A pustular syphilide.

implant [L. *in-*, into, + *plantare*, to plant]. 1. (ĭm-plănt′) To transfer a part, to graft, to insert. 2. (ĭm′plănt) That which is implanted, such as a piece of tissue, a pellet of medicine, or a tube or needle of radioactive substance.

implantation (ĭm″plăn-tā′shun) [L. *in-*, into, + *plantāre*, to plant]. 1. Grafting. 2. Artificial placing of a substance under the skin into the blood, into the uterine canal, etc. 3.

Embedding of the developing blastocyst in the uterine mucosa.

i., hypodermic. Introduction of an implant under the skin. Usually a solid substance placed by use of the hypodermic needle.

i., parenchymatous. Introduction of medicinal substance into a neoplasm.

i., teratic. Union of an abnormal fetus with a nearly normal fetus.

implosion. A violent collapse inward.

i. flooding. A method of treating fear due to a phobia by exposing the person to the worst possible phobic situation. The fear is experienced at maximum intensity for up to an hour until the patient is no longer capable of experiencing further fear. The phobic situation is imagined in the first sessions and later produced in reality. SEE: *phobic desensitization.*

impon'derable [L. *in-*, not, + *pondus*, weight]. Having no appreciable weight; incapable of being weighed.

im'potence, im'potency ["+ *potentiā*, power]. Weakness, esp. inability of the male to copulate.

i., anatomic; i., organic. I. caused by a defect in the genitalia.

i., atonic. I. resulting from paralysis of nervi erigentes which convey impulses bringing about erection.

i., functional. I. not due to an organic or anatomical defect; usually of psychogenic origin.

i., psychic. Due to mental disturbance.

i., symptomatic. Due to poor health, drugs, presence of disease, etc.

impotent (ĭm′pō-tĕnt). 1. Unable to copulate. 2. Sterile; barren.

impotentia (ĭm″pō-tĕn′shĭ-ă). Impotence.

i. coeun'di. Inability on part of the male to perform the sexual act.

i. erigen'di. I. due to inability to produce an erection.

impregnate (ĭm-prĕg′nāt) [L. *impregnāre*, to make pregnant]. 1. To render pregnant. To fertilize an ovum. 2. To saturate.

impreg'nated. 1. Rendered pregnant. 2. Saturated.

i. carbon. Electrode having a carbon shell with core of various metals or salts of metals for use in a carbon arc lamp.

impregnation (ĭm″prĕg-nā′shun) [L. *impregnāre*, to make pregnant]. Fertilization of an ovum; fecundation.

i., artificial. Artificial implantation of semen in the female reproductive tract.

impres'sio [L., impression]. [NA] A mark, as of one part upon another.

i. cardi'aca. [NA] Depression on surface of liver corresponding to position of the heart.

i. col'ica. [NA] Depression on under surface of right lobe of liver.

i. digitatae. [NA] A depression on the inner cranial surface.

i. duodena'lis. [NA] Depression on under surface of liver beside the gallbladder indicating position of duodenum.

i. gas'trica. [NA] Hollow under left lobe of liver indicating position of stomach.

i. rena'lis. [NA] Hollow on under surface of right lobe of liver adjacent to the right kidney.

impres'sion [L. *impressiō*]. 1. A hollow or depression in a surface. 2. Effect produced upon the mind by external stimuli. 3. Plastic imprint of the jaw and teeth for making a denture.

i., digitate. I. on inner surface of frontal bone for convolutions of the cerebrum.

impulse (ĭm'pŭls) [L. *impulsus,* from *impellere,* to drive out]. 1. Act of driving onward with sudden force. 2. An incitement of the mind, prompting an unpremeditated act. 3. In physiology, a change transmitted through certain tissues, esp. nerve fibers and muscles, resulting in physiological activity or inhibition.

i., cardiac. 1. The heart beat felt at the left side of the chest over the apex of the heart. This is a physical i. 2. I. transmitted over conducting pathway of the heart and responsible for the contraction of the muscular tissue of the heart. This is an electrical i. SEE: *heart.*

i., ectopic. A cardiac i. arising in some part of the heart other than the sinoatrial node.

i., enteroceptive. Afferent nerve i.'s arising from stimuli originating in receptors located in internal organs.

i., excitatory. One which stimulates activity.

i., exteroceptive. Afferent nerve i.'s arising from stimuli originating in sense organs located on the body surface.

i., inhibitory. One which lessens activity.

i., morbid. An uncontrollable desire to perform an abnormal act.

i., nervous. A self-propagated excitatory state transmitted along a nerve fiber. It is the result of physicochemical changes occurring in the membrane of the nerve fiber. The impulse on reaching the termination of the fiber may: Induce an impulse in another nerve cell; induce activity in a tissue such as in muscles (contraction) or in glands (secre-

tion); or give rise to a sensation in the higher nervous centers.

i., proprioceptive. Afferent nerve i.'s arising from stimuli originating in joints, muscles, or tendons, or other sensory endings which respond to pressure or stretch.

impul'sion. Idea to do something or commit some act or crime suddenly imposed upon the subject which tortures him until the act is accomplished.

Clear consciousness of the proposed act followed by an agonizing struggle, defeat, and sense of relief following the act are characteristics of impulsions, obsessions, and of inhibitions. Impulsions may include Folie du doute or doubting mania (Ex: repeatedly checking to determine whether something has been done); obsessive fears of contact or delirium of touch; agoraphobia; dipsomania; pyromania; kleptomania; homicidal or suicidal impulsion; onomatomania; arithmomania; exhibitionism. SEE: *cerebrifugal; cerebripetal; imperious acts.*

In. Chem. symb. for indium.

in- [L.]. Prefix indicating not; in, inside, within; also intensive action.

inac'tivate [L. *in-,* not, + *activus,* acting]. To make inactive.

inactiva'tion. Rendering anything inert by using heat or other means.

i. of complement. Loss of activity caused by heating serum to about 55° C. (131° F.) for half an hour.

inadequacy (ĭn-ăd'ĕ-kwă-sĭ) [L. *in-,* not, + *adaequare,* to be equal]. Insufficiency; incompetence.

i., renal. Inability of kidney to perform its physiological functions.

inan'imate ["+ *animatus,* alive]. 1. Not alive; not animate. 2. Dull, lifeless.

inani'tion [L. *inanis,* empty]. A condition due to lack of sufficient food material essential to the body, such as general underfeeding, undernutrition, or caloric insufficiency.

ETIOL: It may be due to causes other than the food supply, such as malabsorption, or other disease of the gastrointestinal system which prevents absorption of food.

inappetence (ĭn-ap'ĕ-tens) [L. *in-,* not, + *appetere,* to long for]. Lack of craving or desire, esp. for food.

inartic'ulate ["+ *articulus,* joined]. 1. Not jointed; without joints. 2. Unable to pronounce distinct syllables or express oneself intelligibly. 3. Not given to expressing oneself verbally.

in artic'ulo mor'tis [L.]. At the very moment of death.

inassim'ilable [L. *in-*, not, + *assimilis*, to make similar]. Not capable of being utilized by the body for nutrition.

inborn. 1. Innate or inherent, said of characteristics both structural and functional which are inherited or developed during intrauterine development. 2. Inherited, as in inborn error of metabolism.

in'breeding [L. *in*, into, + AS. *brēdan*, to cherish]. Producing offspring from those closely related.

incandes'cent [L. *incandescere*, to glow]. Glowing with light; white hot.

Incaparina. A mixture of cereal grains and oilseed meals of a given range of protein and quality, fortified with vitamins and minerals. Developed at INCAP (Institute of Nutrition of Central America and Panama). Distributed in Latin-American countries for feeding young children.

incar'cerated [L. *in*, into, + *carcer*, prison]. Imprisoned, confined, constricted, as an irreducible hernia.

incarcera'tion. Legal confinement. 2. Imprisonment of a part; constriction.

incarial bone (ĭn-kā'rĭ-ăl). Os incae; interparietal bone.

incep'tion [L. *inceptiō*, taking in, beginning]. 1. The beginning of anything. 2. Ingestion. 3. Intussusception.

incest (ĭn'sĕst) [L. *incestus*, unchaste, incest]. Coitus between those of near relationship. The persons are usually so closely related that a legal marriage would not be possible.

in'cidence [L. *in*, on, + *cadere*, to fall]. 1. The frequency of occurrence of any event or condition over a period of time and in relation to the population in which it occurs, as i. of a disease. SEE: *prevalence*. 2. The falling or impinging upon, touching, or affecting in some way.

in'cident [L. *incidere*, to happen to]. 1. A happening, event, or occurrence. 2. Apt to happen, esp. in connection with some other event. 3. Falling or striking, as a ray of light.

incineration (ĭn-sĭn''ĕr-ā'shun) [L. *in*, into + *cinis, ciner-*, ash]. Destruction by fire. SYN: *cremation.*

incipient (ĭn-sĭp'ĭ-ent) [L. *incipere*, to begin]. Beginning.

incise' [L. *incisus*, from *in*, into, + *caedere*, to cut]. To cut, as with a sharp instrument.

incised (ĭn-sīzd'). Cut with a knife.

   i. wound. One clearly cut.

incision (ĭn-sĭzh'un) [L. *incisiō*, from *in*, into, + *caedere*, to cut]. A cut made with a knife, esp. for surgical purposes.

incisive (ĭn-sī'sĭv). 1. Cutting; having the power of cutting. 2. Rel. to the incisor teeth.

   i. bone. Anterior or medial part of the superior maxilla.

incisor (ĭn-sī'zŏr) [L. *incisor*, a cutter]. 1. That which cuts. 2. That which applies to the incisor teeth. 3. One of the cutting teeth. The four front teeth in each jaw of the adult. SEE: *dentition.*

   i., prostatic. Surgical knife for incision of an enlarged prostate.

incisu'ra [L. a cutting into]. (pl. *incisurae*) 1. An incision. 2. [NA] Incisure; notch; emargination; indentation at the edge of any structure.

incisure (ĭn-sī'ūr) [L. *incisura*, a cutting into]. A notch or slit.

   i.'s of Schmidt and Lantermann. Oblique lines on medullated nerve fiber sheaths.

inclina'tion [L. *inclinere*, to slope]. Leaning from the normal, or from the vertical, as a tooth.

inclinometer (ĭn''klĭ-nŏm'et-er) ["+ Gr. *metron*, measure]. Device for measuring ocular diameter from vertical and horizontal lines.

inclu'sion [L. *inclusus*, enclosed]. Being enclosed or included.

   i. blennorrhea. An inflammatory disease of the conjunctiva of newborn infants. SYN: *opthalmia neonatorum.*

   i. bodies. Bodies present in the nucleus of cytoplasm of certain cells in cases of infection by filtrable viruses. SEE: *Negri bodies.*

   i., cell. Lifeless, temporary, constituent of the protoplasm of a cell. SEE: *cell.*

   i., fetal. Malformed twins in which one, the parasite, is completely enclosed within its host, the autosite.

incoercible (ĭn''kō-ĕr'sĭb-l) [L. *in-*, not, + *coercere*, to restrain]. Uncontrollable; not able to be held in check.

   i. vomiting. Uncontrollable vomiting.

incoherence (ĭn''kō-hēr'ĕns) ["+ *cohairens*, adhering]. Inability to express oneself coherently, or to present ideas in a related order.

incoherent (ĭn''kō-hē'rĕnt). Not coherent or understandable.

incombus'tible [L. *in-*, not, + *combustus*, burned]. Incapable of being burnt.

incompatibil'ity ["+ *compatī*, to sympathize with]. State which renders admixture of remedies unsuitable through chemical action or interaction, insolubility, formation of poisonous or explosive compounds; difference in solubility, or opposite action.

   The quality of not being mixed without chemical changes, or without antagonizing the action of ingredients in a compound.

   i., physiological. A condition in which one or more substances in a mixture have a physiological action antagonistic to that of one of the other compounds.

incompat'ible. 1. Not capable of uniting in solution. 2. Antagonistic in action, said of some drugs.

   i. transfusion. A transfusion in which the isoagglutinins of the recipient react with the red blood cells of the donor resulting in intravascular agglutination and hemolysis.

incom'petence, incom'petency [L. *in-*, not, + *competere*, to be suitable]. Inadequate ability to perform the function or action normal to an organ or part.

   i., aortic. Regurgitation of blood through the aortic valves.

   i., ileocecal. Inability of ileocecal valve to stop the return of the material from the colon to the ileum.

   i., mental. Mental inability to retain charge of one's self or possessions.

   i., muscular. Imperfect closure of the cardiac valve due to weak action of papillary muscles.

   i., pyloric. Weakness of pylorus which permits undigested food to leave the stomach and enter the duodenum.

   i., relative. Excessive dilatation of a cardiac cavity which makes perfect closure of opposite cardiac valve impossible.

   i., valvular. Leaky condition of one or more cardiac valves permitting the return of blood at the time the valves should be completely closed.

incom'petent. 1. One legally unable to execute a contract, such as a feebleminded or insane person. 2. Incapable.

   i. palatal syndrome. Incomplete or ineffective separation by the soft palate of the nasopharynx from the oropharynx characterized by hypernasality and distortion of speech called whinollalia.

   ETIOL: May be due to congenital or acquired defects of the palate, or to psychiatric disorders.

incompres'sible [L. *in-*, not, + *compressus*, pressed together]. Compact; not compressible.

incon'tinence ["+ *continere*, to stop]. 1. Inability to retain urine, semen, or feces, through loss of sphincter control, cerebral or spinal lesions. 2. Absence of restraint with respect to sexual activity. SEE: *continence.*

   i., active. Discharge of feces and urine in the normal way at regulated intervals but involuntarily.

   i., intermittent. Loss of control of bladder on sudden pressure or movement, because of interruption of voluntary path above the lumbar center.

   i. of milk. Excessive milk flow. SYN: *galactorrhea.*

   i., overflow. I. caused by pressure of urine retained in the bladder.

   i., paralytic. Constant voiding of small amt. of urine and feces due to defective nervous control of sphincters.

   i., passive. Urinary i. of a form in which there is a full bladder that doesn't empty normally, but urine drips away upon pressure.

   i., urinary stress. Inability to prevent escape of urine during stress such as laughing, coughing, sneezing, lifting, or sudden movement. Occurs frequently enough in young women to be classed as normal. Nevertheless it should be investigated to be certain it is not caused by a structural abnormality.

   i. of urine. Inability to control urination. Sphincter muscle always relaxed. SEE: *enuresis.*

incontinen'tia. Incontinence.

   i. alvi. Fecal incontinence.

   i. urinae. Involuntary continual dripping of urine.

incoor'dinate ["+ *coordinare*, to arrange]. 1. Not able to make coordinate muscular movements. 2. Unable to adjust one's work harmoniously with others.

incoordination (ĭn"kō-ŏr"dĭ-nā'shun). Inability to produce harmonious, rhythmic, muscular action, but not due to weakness.

   ETIOL: The condition may be sensory, due to failure of afferent impulses to be transmitted from muscles, bones, and joints to coordination centers, or motor, due to disturbance in tone or harmony between simultaneously acting muscle groups. SYN: *asynergy.* SEE: *disdiadokokinesia.*

incorporation (ĭn-kŏr"pŏ-rā'shun) [L. *in-*, (intensive), + *corporare*, to form into a body]. Combining two ingredients to form a homogenous mass.

increment (ĭn'krē-mĕnt) [L. *incrementum*]. 1. Increase or addition. 2. To increase or add to.

incre'tion [L. *incrētus*, sifted in]. Internal secretion. 2. Functional activity of an endocrine gland.

incretogenous (ĭn"kre-tŏj'ĕn-us) [L. *in*, in, + Gr. *gennan*, to produce]. Pert. to the internal secretions.

incrusta'tion [L. *in*, on, + *crusta*, crust]. Formation of crusts or scabs.

incubation (ĭn"kū-bā'shŭn) [L. *incubare*, to lie on]. 1. The interval between exposure to infection and the appearance of the first symptom. 2. In bacteriology, the period of culture development. 3. The care of a prema-

Incubation and Isolation Periods in Common Infections

	Incubation Period	Isolation of Patient
Brucellosis (undulant fever)	Usually 5 to 21 days	None
Chickenpox	2 to 3 weeks	1 week after onset
Common cold	12 hours to 3 days	None
Diphtheria	Usually 2 to 5 days	Until 2 cultures taken at least 24 hrs. apart from nose and throat are negative. Cultures to be taken after cessation of antibiotic therapy
Dysentery, amebic	5 days to 4 weeks	None
Dysentery, bacillary (shigellosis)	1 to 7 days	As long as stools remain positive
Encephalitis, mosquito-borne	7 to 14 days	None
Gonorrhea	3 to 9 days	No sexual contact until cured
Influenza	1 to 3 days	As practical
Malaria	Usually 2 weeks	Protected from mosquitoes
Measles (rubeola)	8 to 13 days	From diagnosis to 7 days after appearance of rash. Strict isolation from children under 3 years
Meningitis, meningococcal	2 to 10 days	Until 24 hours after start of chemotherapy
Mumps	12 to 26 days	Until the glands recede
Paratyphoid fevers	1 to 10 days	Until 3 stools are negative
Pneumonia, pneumococcal	Believed to be 1 to 3 days	Until 24 hrs. after administration of antibiotics
Poliomyelitis	3 to 21 days	1 week from onset
Puerperal fever, streptococcal	1 to 3 days	Transfer from maternity ward
Rabies	Usually 2 to 6 weeks	Strict for duration of illness; danger to attendants
Rubella (German measles)	14–21 days	None, but avoid contact with non-immune pregnant women

Incubation and Isolation Periods in Common Infections (*Continued*)

	Incubation Period	Isolation of Patient
Scarlet fever	1 to 3 days	7 days; may be terminated in 24 hrs.
Smallpox	8 to 17 days	Strict; in screened hospital wards until all scabs have disappeared
Syphilis	2 days to 10 weeks, usually 3 weeks	Should be enforced until surface lesions are healed in noncooperative patients
Tetanus	4 days to 3 weeks	None
Trachoma	5 to 12 days	Until lesions disappear, but usually not practical
Tuberculosis	4 to 6 weeks to primary lesion	In "open" cases until properly educated
Tularemia	1 to 10 days	None
Typhoid fever	Usually 1 to 3 weeks	Until 3 cultures of feces and urine are negative, to be taken not earlier than 1 month after onset
Typhus fever	7 to 14 days	None
Whooping cough	Usually a week	For 3 weeks after onset of spasmodic cough
Vincent's angina	2 to 5 days	Preferably during the acute stage

ture infant in an incubator. 4. The development of an impregnated ovum. SYN: *latent period.*

in′cubator [L. *incus.*]. 1. Apparatus for rearing premature babies in which the temperature may be regulated. 2. Apparatus for providing suitable atmospheric conditions for culturing bacteria or for maintaining eggs until they hatch.

incubus (ĭn′kū-bŭs) [L. *incubāre,* to lie upon]. 1. A burden. 2. A nightmare.

in′cudal [L. *incus,* anvil]. Rel. to the incus.

incudectomy (ĭng″kū-dĕk′tō-mĭ) ["+ Gr. *ektomē,* excision]. Surgical removal of the incus.

incudiform (ĭn-kū′dĭ-form) ["+ *forma,* shape]. Like an anvil in shape.

in″cudomal′leal ["+ *malleus,* a hammer]. In the middle ear relating to the incus and malleus and articulation of the anvil and hammer in the tympanum.

incudostapedial (ĭn″kū-do-stă-pē′dĭ-ăl) ["+ *stapes,* a stirrup]. In the middle ear pertaining to the incus and stapes and articulation between anvil and stirrup in the tympanum.

incu′rable [L. *in,* not, + *curāre,* to care for]. 1. Not capable of being cured. 2. A person with an incurable disease. SYN: *immedicable.*

in′cus [L., anvil]. (pl. *incudes*) [NA] In the middle ear, the middle of the three ossicles in the tympanum; the anvil.

incyclophoria (ĭn-sī″klō-fō-rī′a) [L. *in,* not, + Gr. *kyklos,* circle, + *phoros,* bearing]. Median or negative cyclophoria; the affected eye, when covered, turns inward about its anteroposterior axis.

incyclotropia (ĭn-sī″klō-trō′fĭ-ă) [L. *in,* within, + "+ *tropos,* turning]. Cyclotropia in which the eye turns inward toward the nose even when both eyes are open.

in d. Abbr. for L. *in dies,* daily.

indagation (ĭn″dă-gā′shun) [L. *indagāre*, to search]. A careful, searching investigation, esp. examination of the genitalia at termination of puerperium.

indenization (ĭn-dĕn″ĭ-zā′shun) [L. *in*, into, + O. Fr. *deinzein*, from L. *de intus*, from within]. Arrest and development of cells in a part to which they have been carried by metastasis. SYN: *innidiation*.

indenta′tion ["+ *dens, dent-*, tooth]. A depression or hollow.

index (ĭn′dĕks) [L., an indicator]. (pl. *indexes* or *indices*) 1. The forefinger. 2. The ratio between the measurement of a given substance compared with that of a fixed standard.

  i., alveolar. Degree of jaw prominence.

  i., cephalic. Skull breadth multiplied by 100 and divided by its length.

  i., cerebral. Ratio of greatest transverse to the greatest anteroposterior diameter of the cranium.

  i., color. The ratio of hemoglobin present in red blood cells compared to the normal of 100.

  i., gnathic. Degree of jaw prominence expressed by a number.

  i., gonoopsonic. Opsonic i. in gonococcal infection.

  i., hemorenal. Ratio of blood's electrical resistance to urine's.

  i., icteric. The ratio of bilirubin in the blood to a standard.

  i., opsonic. The ratio of number of bacteria which are ingested by leukocytes contained in normal serum, compared with the number ingested by leukocytes in the patient's own blood serum.

  i., pelvic. Ratio of pelvic conjugate and transverse diameters.

  i., phagocytic. Average of bacteria ingested per leukocyte of blood.

  i., refractive. Refraction coefficient.

  i., thoracic. Ratio of thoracic anteroposterior diameter to transverse diameter.

indican (ĭn′dĭ-kăn). Potassium salt of indoxylsulfate, found in sweat and urine, and formed when intestinal bacteria convert tryptophan to indole.

indicanemia (ĭn″dĭ-kăn-ē′mĭ-ă) [indican + Gr. *haima*, blood]. Indican in the blood.

indicanu′ria ["+ Gr. *ouron*, urine]. Excess of indoxyl-sulfate of potassium, a derivative of indol, in urine.

  In normal urine it is found in small quantities.

indica′tion [L. *indicāre*, to point out]. That which indicates the proper treatment.

  i., causal. That shown by a knowledge of the cause of a disease.

  i., symptomatic. That shown by symptoms.

in′dicator [L. *indicāre*, to show]. A substance which can be used to distinguish acid from alkali. (In a more general sense, any substance which can be used to determine the completeness of a chemical reaction, as in volumetric analysis.)

  USES: 1. In titration of ammonia and other weak bases. 2. Topfer's reagent, for determining free acid in gastric juice. 3. In titrating weak acids and for determining combined acid in gastric juice.

Colors of Indicators

	Color		
	Toward Acid	Toward Alkali	Range of pH
Methyl yellow	red	yellow	2.9–4.0
Congo red	blue	red	3.0–5.2
Methyl orange	red	yellow	3.1–4.4
Methyl red	red	yellow	4.2–6.2
Litmus	red	blue	4.5–8.3
Bromcresol purple	yellow	purple	5.2–6.8
Bromothymol blue	yellow	blue	6.0–7.6
Phenol red	yellow	red	6.8–8.4
Phenolphthalein	colorless	pink	8.2–10.0

indif′ferent [L. *in-*, not, + *differre*, to differ]. 1. Neutral; tending in no specific direction. 2. Not responsive to normal stimuli; apathetic. 3. Pert. to cells which have not differentiated.

indigenous (ĭn-dĭj′ĕn-ŭs) [L. *indigenus*, born in]. Native to a country or region.

indigestible (ĭn″di-jĕs′tĭ-bl) [L. *in-*, not, + *digerere*, to separate]. Not digestible.

indiges′tion [L. *in-*, not, + *digerere*, to separate]. Incomplete or imperfect digestion, usually accompanied by one or more of the following symptoms: pain, nausea, and vomiting, heartburn and acid regurgitation, accumulation of gas and belching. SYN: *dyspepsia.*

indigitation (ĭn-dĭj″ĭ-tā′shun) [L. *in*, in, + *digitus*, finger]. Displacement of intestines by intussusception, q.v. SYN: *invagination.*

indigouria (ĭn″dĭ-gō-ū′rĭ-ă) [Gr. *indikon*, Indian dye, + *ouron*, urine]. Indigo in the urine.

indirect′ [L. *indirectus*, not kept straight]. Not direct.

  i. cell division. Amitosis. Single cell division in which a mitotic figure is not formed.

i. reflexes. 1. Passive flexion of one part following flexion of another. 2. Passive flexion of one leg causing similar movement of opposite leg.

indisposi'tion [L. *in-*, not, + *dispositus*, arranged]. Disorder; any slight or temporary illness.

indium (ĭn'dĭ-um) [from *indigo*]. SYMB: *In.* At. wt. 114.82; at. no. 49; sp. gr. 7.31. A rare metallic element.

indolaceturia (in''do-las''ē-tū'rĭ-ă) [indol + L. *acetum*, vinegar, + Gr. *ouron*, urine]. Excretion of a considerable amount of indolacetic acid in the urine.

in'dole. A solid, crystalline substance, C_8H_7N, found in feces. It is the product of bacterial decomposition of tryptophan and is largely responsible for the odor of feces. In intestinal obstruction it is absorbed and eliminated in the urine in the form of indican, q.v. SYN: *ketol.*

in'dolent [L. *in-*, not, + *dolere*, to feel pain]. 1. Indisposed to action. 2. Inactive; not developing; sluggish.

i. ulcer. One that is slow to heal but not painful.

indologenous (ĭn''do-lŏj'ĕn-us) [indol + *gennan*, to produce]. Causing the production of indole.

indolu'ria. The presence of indol in urine.

indoxyl (ĭn-dŏk'sĭl) [Gr. *indikon*, indigo, + *oxys*, sharp]. An oily substance, C_8H_7NO, sometimes found in urine of the apparently healthy, formed from the decomposition of tryptophan by intestinal bacteria.

indoxylemia (ĭn-dŏk''sĭl-ē'mĭ-ă) ["+ "+ *haima*, blood]. Indoxyl in the blood.

indoxyluria (ĭn''dŏk-sĭl-ū'rĭ-ă) ["+ "+ *ouron*, urine]. Excretion of indoxyl in urine.

induced (ĭn-dūsd') [L. *inducere*, to lead in]. Produced; caused.

i. abortion. One brought about intentionally.

induc'tance. That property of an electric circuit by virtue of which a varying current induces an electromotive force in that circuit or a neighboring circuit.

It is susceptible of measurement. The unit of inductance, or "self-induction" is the henry.

induction (ĭn-dŭk'shun). 1. The process of causing or producing, as labor. 2. The generation of electric current in a body by electricity in another body near it. 3. In embryology the production of a specific morphogenic effect by a chemical substance from one part of the embryo to another. Also called evocation.

inductor'ium. An induction coil.

inductotherm (ĭn-dŭk'to-therm) [L. *inducere*, to lead, + Gr. *thermē*, heat]. Device for producing pyrexia by electricity.

inductothermy. Treatment of disease by artificial production of fever by electromagnetic induction.

in'durate [L. *in*, in, + *durus*, hard]. 1. To harden. 2. Hardened.

in'durated. Hardened.

indura'tion. 1. The act of hardening. 2. An area of hardened tissue. SEE: *sclerosis; skin.*

i., cyanotic. An i. from long continued venous hyperemia, pressure on vessels causing transudation of blood and serum and formation of a dark, hard mass.

In the liver, spleen, etc., it leads to absorption of more or less of the parenchyma and to formation of new connective tissue.

i., fibrous, of the lung. A form of interstitial pneumonia. Hardened pigment forms red points on the lung.

in'durative. Pert. to induration.

indu'sium (L., tunic]. 1. A membranous covering. 2. The amnion.

i. griseum. The supracallosal gyrus, a rudimentary gyrus located on the upper surface of the corpus callosum.

inebriant (ĭn-ē'brĭ-ănt) [L. *inebrius*, drunken]. 1. Any intoxicant. 2. Making drunk.

ine'briate. To make drunk or to become intoxicated.

inebriation (ĭn-ē'brĭ-ā'shun). State of intoxication, q.v. SYN: *drunkenness; intoxication.*

inelas'tic [L. *in-*, not, + Gr. *elastikos*, elastic]. Not elastic.

inemia (ĭn-ē'mĭ-ă) [Gr. *is*, fiber, + *haima*, blood]. Fibrin in the blood. SYN: *inosemia.*

inert' [L. *iners, inert-*, unskilled, idle]. 1. Not active; sluggish. 2. In chemistry, having little or no tendency or ability to react with other chemicals.

inertia (ĭn-ĕr'shĭ-ă) [L., inactivity]. 1. Tendency of a body to remain in repose. 2. Sluggishness; lack of activity.

i., uterine. Absence or weakness of uterine contractions in labor.

in extremis (ĭn ĕks-trē'mĭs) [L.]. At the point of death.

in'fant [L. *infans*]. 1. A babe. 2. A child not over two years of age. 3. In law, a minor, or one under legal age.

i., artificial feeding of. An exact time schedule is not considered necessary. Temperature of feeding should be 100° F. (37.8° C.). Test heat by shaking some on the back of the hand. See that bottle is not overheated and that it does not burn i. through contact.

Nipples should be kept clean and not fitted to bottle until ready to use. They should not be handled more than necessary, and before touching them one should be assured that the hands are clean. See that the hole in nipple permits a free, but not too rapid, flow of milk. The hole may be enlarged with a heated needle. Change i. before feeding.

In administering feeding, i.'s head and shoulders should be raised higher than his abdomen, but it is better to hold i. while giving the feeding. See that the child is properly protected from drafts or cold. If being fed when in a reclining position, the formation of gas may result in belching of the feeding. Change position of bottle as level of the fluid changes. See that nothing disturbs the child while being fed and that the feeding is not interrupted. Close observation is essential because the baby must receive all the feeding, which will not be the case if it is regurgitated or lost from belching. Interruptions may cause air-swallowing, which results in gas distention and a feeling of fullness that may cause a rejection of necessary nourishment.

If an accumulation of gas interferes with the feeding, the usual methods of expelling the gas should be employed, such as holding the child over the shoulder and patting it on the back. This should also be done after each feeding in order to expel any air. Do not rock a baby after it has been fed. Water should be given between feedings to maintain required fluid intake.

Care of nipples and bottles: Bottles and nipples should be soaked in cold water. Wash bottles with hot water and mild soap, using a brush for the purpose. Sterilize them by boiling in hot water. The nipples after being boiled may be kept in a covered sterile container.

i. development. For three days after birth a baby loses weight; in the next four days, however, it should regain its loss and weigh as much as it weighed at birth.

Average weekly weight gain in the first three months is 210 gm. for boys and 195 for girls; from three to six months it is 150 gm. for both girls and boys; from six to nine months, 90 gm. for boys and 105 for girls; from 9 to 18 months 60 gm. for both sexes; and from 18 to 24 months 45 gm.

By the 4th week lifts head momentarily; by 16th week holds head erect, coos, or laughs; walks with hands held by 52nd week; by 15th month toddles alone and may have a vocabulary of a few words.

i. feeding. The infant should have nothing by mouth for the first 12 to 24 hours. Then if the mother's condition permits he should be placed at the breast. The regular nursing schedule is not necessary until the milk comes in. Water should be offered every four hours. The three- or four-hour nursing interval depends upon the physician, hospital, and the condition of the mother and the baby. The three-hour interval is advocated by some physicians during the first two or three weeks. This keeps the breasts emptied, thereby relieving congestion, and increases the amount of the baby's fluid intake in 24 hours. Others prefer the four-hour interval, esp. if the infant is large. Breast-fed infants need vitamins C and D added to their food intake. This can be accomplished by feeding liquid vitamin preparations to the infant daily by use of a medicine dropper.

The early cessation of night feedings is an advantage of the three-hour schedule rarely attained in the four-hour régime. The individual breast is stimulated by the 15-minute nursing period. Followed by the six-hour rest period, this combination provides for maximum functioning.

Complementary feeding: An artificial feeding used to round out a breast feeding that is inadequate. It is better given immediately after the breast feeding rather than before it. It abets the utilization of breast milk without interfering with it, while providing for breast milk deficiency that may exist.

Supplemental feeding: An artificial feeding replacing breast feeding, one or several times daily. It is not as generally used as the complementary, since it operates against the stimulation of breast milk production, and so tends to reduce it further.

Composition of artificial food: The basis of artificial infant feedings is cow's milk, which is modified by the addition of water and a carbohydrate. Estimation of the composition of the formula should be based upon the physiological requirements of the infant. No less than 1 1/2 oz. (45 ml.) of milk per lb. (450 gm.) of body weight are sufficient for this purpose, and may be increased to 2 oz. (60 ml.) per lb. of body weight within a week or 10 days. Calculation is based upon a 4% fat milk and allows for introducing a weak but sustaining food.

Daily caloric requirements for infants less than one year of age are 90 to 130 Cal./kilogram of body weight (41-59 Cal./pound). Premature and undernourished children will require somewhat more food.

Fluid requirements up to two years of age are 150 ml./kg. of body weight (68 ml./pound) daily.

Food components: The infant's diet would normally contain 10-15% protein, 65-85% carbohydrate, and 10-20% fat. The requirements are met when two thirds of the Cal. are derived from milk and one third from added carbohydrate.

Mineral requirements: The diet adequate in fluids, Cal., and various food components will provide sufficient minerals except iron and in some cases iodine. Five mg. of iron daily is required to supplement the diet. If iodine is required, iodized salt may be used. Iron may be obtained by including it with a vitamin supplement.

Vitamins: All infants under two years of age whether breast fed or artificially fed should be given daily sufficient aqueous vitamin preparations by mouth to prevent scurvy, rickets, and tetany.

i., post term. One born after beginning of the 43rd week of gestation (longer than 295 days).

i., preterm. One born from beginning of 20th week through 38 weeks of gestation (134-266 days).

i. respiration. At birth, 30-80 per min.; 1st year, 20-40; 5th year, 20-25; 15th year, 15-20. SEE: *pulse; respiration; temperature.*

i. temperature. Normal (rectal) temperature may have a daily variation of one to 1.5° C. (1.8 to 2.7 ° F.). It is usually highest between five and eight p.m. and lowest between 3 and 6 a.m. There is therefore no specific normal temperature, but the values given should be regarded as ranging around the value of 37.6° C. (99.6° F.) when the temperature is taken rectally.

i., term. One born between the beginning of the 39th week through the 42nd week of gestation (267-294 days).

infanticide (ĭn-făn'tĭs-īd) [L. *infans,* infant, + *caedere,* to kill]. 1. The killing of an infant. 2. One who takes the life of an infant.

infantile (ĭn'făn-tĭl). Pert. to infancy or infant.

infantilism (ĭn-făn'tĭl-ĭzm) [L. *infans,* infant, + Gr. *-ismos,* condition]. A condition in which the mind and body make slow development. Failure to attain adult characteristics, physical or psychic.

i., angioplastic. I. due to defective development of vascular system.

i., Brissaud's. Infantile myxedema.

i., cachectic. I. caused by chronic infection or poisoning.

i., celiac. I. caused by celiac disease.

i., dysthyroidal. I. caused by defective thyroid.

i., hepatic. I. combined with cirrhosis of liver.

i., Herter's. I. of the intestines.

i., hypophyseal. Dwarfism resulting from hyposecretion of growth promoting and gonadotrophic hormones of anterior lobe of the hypophysis. SYN: *pituitary i.*

i., idiopathic. Variety of arrested physical development, of unknown cause.

i., intestinal. I. associated with chronic intestinal disorder, causing the child to gain no weight nor to grow.

i., lymphatic. A form of i. associated with lymphatism.

i., myxedematous. SYN: *cretinism.* SEE: *Brissaud's i.*

i., partial. Arrest in development of a lone tissue or part.

i., pituitary. Hypophyseal i., q.v.

i., renal. I. caused by defect in renal function.

i., sex. Continuation of childish traits, esp. sex characteristics, beyond the age of puberty.

i., symptomatic. I. caused by poor tissue development.

i., toxemic. I., toxemic, q.v.

i., universal. Drawfed stature, otherwise fairly normal development, except for absence of secondary sexual characteristics.

in'farct [L. *infacire,* to stuff into]. An area of tissue in an organ or part which undergoes necrosis following cessation of blood supply. May result from occlusion or stenosis of supplying artery or more rarely occlusion of vein draining tissue.

i., anemic. I. in which blood pigment is lacking or decoloration had occurred. Also called white or pale infarct.

i., bland. I. in which infection is absent.

i., calcareous. I. in connective tissue in which calcareous salts have been deposited.

i., cicatrized. I. which has been replaced or encapsulated by fibrous tissue.

i., pale. An anemic infarct, q.v.

i., red. An i. which is swollen and red as a result of hemorrhage. Also called hemorrhagic infarct.

i., uric acid. I. in kidney of a newborn infant due to obstruction of renal tubules by uric acid crystals.

i., white. I., anemic, q.v.

infarc'tion [L. *infarcire,* to stuff into]. 1. Formation of an infarct. 2. An infarct.

i., cardiac. Myocardial infarction, q.v.

i., myocardial. I. in cardiac muscle, usually resulting from formation of a thrombus in the coronary arterial system.

i., pulmonary. I. in lung usually resulting from pulmonary embolism.

infect. To cause pathogenic organisms to be present in or upon, as to infect a wound.

infection (ĭn-fĕk'shŭn) [L. *inficere,* to taint].
The state or condition in which the body or
a part of it is invaded by a pathogenic agent
(microorganism or virus) which, under favorable conditions, multiplies and produces
effects which are injurious.

Localized i. is usually accompanied by
inflammation, but inflammation may occur
without i.

ETIOL: The principal causes of i.'s are
agents belonging to the following groups of
microorganisms: viruses, bacteria, Rickettsias, fungi, and animal parasites.

SYM: The symptoms of i. are those of
inflammation. The five classical symptoms
listed by early medical writers are: *Dolor,*
pain; *calor,* heat; *rubor,* redness; *tumor,*
swelling; and *functio laesa,* disordered function.

Pain: This is esp. prominent when the i. is
confined within closed cavities. The pain is
in proportion to the virulence and extent of
the infection. *Redness and Swelling:* Not evident when infection is within some rigid
tissue or deep within some cavity; more
apparent when superficial structures are
involved. Discoloration would be a better
term than "redness," as the color is more
bluish or purple in advanced infections,
while tuberculosis infections have long been
called "white swellings."

Heat: Heat may not be evident on the
surface, but there may be considerable elevation of body temperature even with small
infections. *Disordered Function:* This depends upon the part affected as well as upon
the virulence. With almost all acute infections there is an increase of polymorphonuclear leukocytes either absolute or relative.

The degree of prostration is out of proportion to the extent of the injury. There have
been many deaths from infection following
pricks of needles, small splinters of bone, a
trifling cut, or an infection from the bristle
of a brush, in which streptococcus was the
inciting cause. In this type of infection, a red
streak may be seen running up the extremity from the site of injury, and following the
superficial lymphatics. This red line is absent in staphylococcus infections of the lymphatic vessels.

Infection may be local or general. Local
infections may be at the portal of entry, or
remote if transferred by the blood or lymph.

SITE OF: Microorganisms may gain entry
to the tissues through the gastrointestinal
tract, as in typhoid fever, or through the
respiratory tract, as in tuberculosis and
common colds, or through wounds, as in
rabies, or from contaminated objects, as in
tetanus, or from bites of insects, as in
malaria and yellow fever.

Some medicines, but especially adrenal
cortical hormones and certain antibiotics,
upset either the immume mechanism or the
bacterial interrelations so that the growth of

The Commoner Protozoal Infections of Man

Disease	Primary Site of Infection	Parasite	Mode of Transmission
Malaria: Benign tertian Benign quartan Malignant tertian	Erythrocytes	*Plasmodium vivax* *Plasmodium malariae* *Plasmodium falciparum*	Mosquito (*Anopheles*)
Sleeping sickness	Blood plasma	*Trypsanosoma gambiense*	Tsetse fly (*Glossina palpalis*)
Rhodesian sleeping sickness	Blood plasma	*T. rhodesiense*	Tsetse fly (*Glossina morsitans*)
Leishmaniasis, vis- ceral (Kala-azar)	Reticulo- endothelial cells and plasma	*Leishmania donovani*	The sand fly (*Phlebotomus argentipes*)
Amebic dysentery	Wall of large in- testine	*Entamoeba histolytica*	Fecal (cyst) contami- nation of food and water

Fungus Infections

Disease	Causative Organisms	Structures Infected	Microscopic Appearances
Ringworm (tinea, otomycosis)	*Microsporum (audouini, etc.)*	Horny layer of epidermis and hairs, chiefly of scalp	Fine septate mycelium inside hairs and scales; spores in rows and mosaic plaques on hair surface
	Trichophyton (tonsurans, etc.)	Hairs of scalp, beard, and other parts; nails	Mycelium of chained cubical elements and threads in and on hairs; often pigmented
Favus (tinea favosa)	*Trichophyton schönleini*	Yellow disks in epidermis around a hair; all parts of body; nails	Vertical hyphae and spores in epidermis; sinuous branching mycelium and chains in hairs
Epidermophytosis (Dhobie itch, etc.)	*Epidermophyton (inguinale, etc.)*	Inflamed patches in inguinal, axillary, and interdigital folds; hairs not affected	Long, wavy, branched and segmented hyphae and spindle-shaped cells in stratum corneum

Some Systemic Infections

Disease	Causative Organisms	Structures Infected	Microscopic Appearances
Thrush and other forms of moniliasis	*Candida albicans*	White patches on tongue, mouth, throat; also may cause lesions of vagina and skin	Yeastlike budding cells and oval thick-walled bodies in lesion
Actinomycosis	*Actinomyces bovis, A. israelii*	Chronic, usually in neck	Branched filaments on radiating rods, forming colonies
Nocardiosis	*Nocardia asteroides*	Lower extremities or lung	Closely resemble bacteria; found in pus
Blastomycosis	*Blastomyces brasiliensis, B. dermatitidis*	Skin and/or lungs	Yeastlike cells demonstrated in lesion
Coccidioidomycosis	*Coccidioides immitis*	Respiratory tract	Nonbudding spheres containing many endospores, in sputum
Cryptococcosis	*Cryptococcus neoformans*	Meninges; sometimes lungs	Yeastlike fungus having gelatinous capsule; demonstrated in spinal fluid

certain microorganisms is encouraged. The resulting superinfection may be quite difficult to control and may be so severe as to cause death. Cortisone therapy encourages the recurrence or resurgence of tuberculosis.

METHODS OF: *Air-borne Infection:* Pathogenic organisms in the respiratory tract, discharged from the mouth or nose, may be borne on the air and settle on food, clothing, walls and floors, and if they are of the type which resists drying for a long period they may remain virulent until transmitted to another person. Coughing, sneezing, and expectorating may be responsible for "droplet infection," as bacteria are expelled into the air.

Animal Carriers: Some microorganisms may be carried from an animal to man by direct contact, indirect transfer, or by intermediary hosts. *Contact Infection:* This is the result of transmission from person to person, as in kissing, coming in contact with those afflicted with communicable diseases, or with utensils handled by one with an infection. *Food-borne Infection:* Bacteria may be communicated through food. Root and salad vegetables may carry bacteria from the soil or from manure used as fertilizer. Cooking safeguards by destroying microorganisms on food.

Human Carriers: Some parasites may live in or upon the bodies of those who themselves do not suffer from them, but may be carried by them to others. Carriers may be: Contact carriers, or those who never show symptoms; incubationary carriers, or those in whom the infection is starting but has not completed the incubation period; and convalescent carriers, or those who have recovered but who still harbor the organism causing their disease. *Insect Vectors:* An insect may act as a physical carrier, as the housefly, which may transmit the typhoid bacillus from one point to another, or one that acts as an active intermediate host, such as the Anopheles mosquito, which transmits malaria by injecting the causative agent into the host while biting that person or animal. *Prenatal Infection:* This is the result of the fetus being infected from the mother's blood stream, or from contiguity with the maternal membranes.

Soil-borne Infections: Soil-borne, spore-forming organisms commonly enter the body through wounds, as in tetanus and gas gangrene. *Water-borne Infection:* Organisms producing typhoid, dysentery, cholera, and amebic infections may be carried through a water supply, or water in public pools used for bathing. These organisms may pass into the water from the feces of an infected person and be communicated to others.

i., acute. Appears suddenly and may be of brief or prolonged duration.

i., acute exacerbation. Recurrence after a period of quiescence.

i., apical. I. located at the tip of root of a tooth.

i., chronic. One having a protracted course.

i., concurrent. Existence of two or more i.'s at the same time. SEE: *superinfection.*

i., droplet. Acquired by inhalation of a microorganism in the air. Esp. one added to the air by someone's breath or cough.

i., endogenous. I. caused by bacteria, normally nonpathogenic inhabiting the digestive tract.

i., food. SEE: *food, contamination of.*

i., local. I. caused by germs lodging and multiplying at one point in a tissue and remaining there, as a boil.

i., low grade. Loosely used term for a subacute or chronic infection with only mild inflammation and without pus formation.

i., metastatic. Local i. caused by microorganisms circulated from a focus of infection.

i., mixed. Caused by two or more organisms.

i., pyogenic. I. resulting from pus-forming organisms.

i., secondary. I. by a different organism added to the one already present.

i., simple. Due to a single species of organism.

i., subacute. Intermediate between acute and chronic.

i., terminal. One occurring in the late stage of a disease. Generally acute and septic, usually causing death.

infectious (in-fek'shus) [L. *inficere,* to make into, dye, taint]. 1. Capable of being transmitted with or without contact. 2. Pert. to a disease due to a microorganism. 3. Producing infection. SEE: *eruptive.*

i. disease. Any disease caused by growth of pathogenic microorganisms in the body. May or may not be contagious.

NOTE: Period of quarantine varies in different states. SEE: *quarantine;* names of infectious diseases.

infecundity (īn-fē-kŭn'dĭ-tĭ) [L. *infecunditās,* sterility]. Barrenness; sterility in women.

inferior (ĭn-fē'rĭ-or) [L. *inferus,* below]. Beneath; lower.

inferiority complex. In psychology, a repressed state of mind in which one feels himself inferior to others. Such a group of ideas may be manifested by the assumption of superiority, often resulting in over-compensation. Opposed to superiority complex. RS: complex.

infertility. Inability or diminished ability to produce offspring; unproductivity. Condition may be present in either or both sexual partners and is not necessarily irreversible.

Diagnosis includes many tests and thorough investigation. Some factors responsible for i. are immature or abnormal reproductive systems; anomalies of other organs in that vicinity; endocrine dysfunction; immunological antagonisms; general nutrition; and emotional problems.

i., abortion. Condition in which pregnancy is initiated but terminated in spontaneous abortion before 24th week of gestation.

i., primary. I. in which pregnancy has never occurred.

i., secondary. I. in which there have been one or more pregnancies prior to the present condition of i.

infest' [L. *infestāre,* to attack]. To overrun to a harmful extent. Said esp. of parasites.

infesta'tion. The harboring of animal parasites, esp. macroscopic forms such as ectoparasites and arthropod endoparasites.

infibulation (ĭn-fĭb-ū-lā'shun) [L. *in,* in, + *fibula,* clasp]. 1. Fastening the labia of the vagina together, or the prepuce over the glans penis to prevent sexual intercourse. 2. Joining the lips of wounds by clasps.

infiltrate (ĭn-fĭl'trāt, ĭn'fĭl-trāt) [" + *filtrare,* to strain through]. 1. To pass into or through a substance or a space. 2. The material that has infiltrated.

infiltration (ĭn''fĭl-trā'shun) [L. *in,* into, + *filtrare,* to strain through]. The process of a substance passing into and being deposited within the substance of a cell, tissue, or organ. Ex: i. of a tissue or organ with blood corpuscles, or of a cell by fatty particles.

It must not be confused with degeneration, as in the latter condition the foreign substances are from changes within the cell.

i., amyloid. I. of tissue or viscera with a glycoprotein.

i., anesthesia. Injection of an anesthetic solution directly into the tissue. SEE: *anesthesia.*

i., calcareous. Deposits of calcium or magnesium salts within a tissue.

i., cellular. I. of cells, esp. blood cells, into tissues; invasion by cells of malignant tumors into adjacent tissue.

i., fatty. Deposit of fat in the tissues, or oil or fat globules in the cells.

i., glycogenic. Glycogen deposit in cells.

i., pigmentary. Of pigments.

i., purulent. Pus cells in a tissue.

i., serous. With diluted lymph.

i., urinous. With urine.

i., waxy. Amyloid degeneration.

in'finite distance. 1. A distance without limits. 2. In vision, light rays coming from a point of any distance beyond 20 feet (6.1 meters) are practically parallel and accommodation is unnecessary.

infirm. Weak or feeble, esp. from old age or disease.

infir'mary [L. *infirmarium*]. A hospital; a place for the care of sick or infirm persons.

infirmity. 1. Weakness. 2. A sickness or illness.

inflamma'tion [L. *inflammāre,* to flame within]. Tissue reaction to injury. The succession of changes which occur in living tissue when it is injured.

The inflamed area undergoes continuous change as the body repair processes start to heal and replace injured tissue.

Inflammation is a conservative process modified by whatever produces the reaction, but it should not be confused with infection; the two are relatively different conditions, although one may arise from the other.

ETIOL: The reaction of tissue to injury of any kind may be the result of: Blows and foreign bodies; chemicals; electricity; heat and cold (thermic causes); microorganisms; surgical operations (traumatic causes); or ionizing radiation.

SYM: *Dolor,* pain; *calor,* heat; *rubor,* redness; *tumor,* swelling, and *functio laesa,* disordered function. In addition to the symptoms mentioned, the absorption of some of the constituents of inflammatory lymph may cause a slight rise of temperature (99° to 101° F. or 37° to 38° C.), headache, loss of appetite, and a general feeling of discomfort.

Pathological Changes: Vascular dilatation within 30 minutes of the injury and greatly increased blood flow. This may last for hours; exudation of fluid from blood vessels into tissues with comcomitant swelling; migration of leukocytes into the tissues; gelation of fibrinogen in intercellular spaces. Depending upon the severity of the injury, some red blood cells will escape into the tissue. If the injury is not too severe, these processes reach their maximum in six to eight hours, after which reparative processes take place. Blood vessels return to normal size, normal blood flow is reestablished. Leukocytes degenerate or reenter circulation, cellular disintegration or proliferation occurs in which injured cells are replaced; swelling disappears with resorption of tissue fluid and digestion of fibrin.

The lymphatic system plays an active and important part in the healing of inflamed tissues.

Each type of cell has a particular role to play in the inflammatory process. The monocytes, q.v., and macrophages, q.v., are great scavengers for all kinds of dead tissue. The neutrophils or polymorphonuclear leukocytes are active in autolysis, q.v., and the destruction of bacteria. These cells appear in inflammatory conditions at stated intervals, and in a definite order or succession; the macrophage, for instance, antedating the polymorph by a week.

Lymphocytes both large and small are ever present in inflamed and healing tissues but the precise role they play is not clear. Small lymphocytes, particularly, are important in systemic immune reactions.

NOMENCLATURE: Most words denoting inflammation end with the suffix *-itis,* which in itself pertains to inflammatory conditions. The principal inflammations of the various systems are: *Ear:* Otitis externa, interna and media; mastoiditis. *Eye:* Conjunctivitis; dacryocystitis; iritis; keratitis; optic neuritis; panophthalmitis; uveitis. *Gastrointestinal Tract:* Appendicitis; colitis; cholangitis; cholecystitis; duodenitis; enteritis; gastritis; hepatitis; pancreatitis; peritonitis; periproctitis; peridontitis; parotitis; proctitis. *Miscellaneous Organs:* Arthritis; carbuncle; dermatitis; furuncle; myositis; osteitis; osteomyelitis; periostitis; cellulitis; tendovaginitis.

Nervous System: Encephalitis; leptomeningitis; myelitis; neuritis; pachymeningitis; polyneuritis. *Respiratory System:* Bronchitis; empyema; laryngitis; pharyngitis; pleurisy; pleuritis; pneumonia; rhinitis. *Urinary System:* Balanitis; cystitis; cervicitis; epididymitis; endometritis; myometritis; nephritis; oophoritis; pyelitis; prostatitis; perimetritis; parametritis; pyometra; pyosalpinx; orchitis; seminal vesiculitis; salpingitis; salpingo-oophoritis; urethritis. *Vascular System:* Aortitis; endarteritis; endocarditis; epicarditis; lymphangitis; lymphadenitis; myocarditis; pericarditis.

i., acute. I. in which the onset is rapid and the course relatively short.

i., adhesive. One characterized by opposing tissues or sides of a cavity adhering to each other.

i., bacterial. I. induced by the growth of bacteria.

i., catarrhal. I. of a mucous membrane characterized by the excessive secretion of mucus.

i., chronic. I. which progresses slowly, is of long duration, and usually results in the formation of scar tissue.

i., exudative. One in which there is a large accumulation of blood cells and serum.

i., fibrinous. I. in which the exudate is rich in fibrin.

i., hemorrhagic. I. in which red blood cells are conspicuous in the exudate.

i., interstitial. I. involving principally the noncellular or supporting elements of an organ.

i., purulent. I. in which pus is formed.

i., reactive. One about a foreign body or dead tissue.

i., serous. I. in which the exudate is composed principally of serum.

i., suppurative. Purulent i., q.v.

i., toxic. This is one due to toxin or poison.

inflam'matory [L. *inflammāre,* to flame within]. Rel. to or marked by inflammation.

inflation (ĭn-flā'shŭn) [L. *in,* into, + *flāre,* to blow]. Distention of a part by air, gas, or liquid.

inflection (ĭn-flĕk'shun) ["+ *flectere,* to bend]. 1. An inward bending. 2. Change of tone or pitch of the voice; nuance.

influenza (ĭn"flū-ĕn'za) [It., influence]. Grippe, an acute, contagious respiratory infection characterized by sudden onset, fever, chills, headache, myalgia, and sometimes prostration. Coryza, cough and sore throat are common. It is usually a self-limited disease which lasts from two to 7 days. SYN: *la grippe.*

ETIOL: The causative agent is a virus, of which several types and subtypes, AO, A1, A2, B and C, have been identified.

EPIDEMIOLOGY: Usually more prevalent in winter and spring. Young adults, in robust health, appear to be particularly susceptible. The disease is contagious and is spread by discharges from the mouth and nose of infected persons. It may occur sporadically, epidemically, or pandemically.

INCUBATION: One to three days.

SYM: Begins abruptly with lassitude, malaise, chilliness, severe pain in head and back, fever from 101°-103° F. (38.3°-39.4° C.). Prostration out of proportion to the fever. Eyes injected, sneezing, hoarseness, and hard paroxysmal cough. Coryza is moderate to severe. Less frequently, gastrointestinal symptoms including anorexia, nausea, and vomiting, but not diarrhea, are present.

COURSE: Ordinarily runs from four to five days, and may terminate by crisis or speedy lysis. Pulse rate is usually not increased in proportion to fever; may be 90 to 100. Blood pressure low; nosebleed not uncommon. Examination of blood demonstrates a leukopenia. Urinalysis generally demonstrates presence of albumen and casts.

The principal complications are secondary bacterial infections of the nasal sinuses, middle ear and lungs.

Even though fairly rapid recovery is the rule some patients will experience lassitude for weeks or even months after the acute phase has disappeared.

Death may occur but mostly in infants under one year and in those over 60 or in persons who have a chronic disease.

DIFFERENTIAL DIAGNOSIS: Typhoid fever, smallpox in the prodromal stage, cerebrospinal meningitis, and, rarely, pulmonary tuberculosis.

PROG: As a rule, outcome is favorable in absence of pulmonary complications. In patients with cyanosis, severe nerve disturbances, or bloody expectoration, prognosis must be extremely guarded.

NP: *Prophylactic:* Isolation of patients, disinfection of sputum, and application of aseptic methods in handling sufferers by attendants is of utmost importance; also, sometimes, the wearing of suitable masks. The avoidance of public gatherings and general application of hygienic methods deserve consideration. A vaccine containing influenza viruses types A, B, and the Asian variant strain is available for prophylaxis. In recent years, however, epidemics have been due to serologically new subtypes. This requires a new vaccine which may take so long to prepare that it becomes available only after the epidemic has ended.

Active: Isolation, absolute rest, good ventilation, and a selected diet. No specific treatment; care largely symptomatic.

i., Asian. Influenza caused by a variant strain of influenza virus type A. SEE: *influenza.*

influenzal (ĭn″flū-ĕn′zăl) [It. *influenza,* influence]. Relating to influenza.

infolding. Process of enclosing within a fold; an operation employed in the treatment of stomach ulcer in which the walls on either side of the lesion are sutured together.

infra- [L.]. Prefix meaning below; under; beneath; inferior to; after.

infraaxillary (ĭn″fră-ăks′ĭl-ă-rĭ) [L. *infrā,* beneath, + *axilla,* little axis]. Below the axilla.

in″fraclavic′ular ["+ *clavicula,* little key]. Below the clavicle.

infracostal (ĭn″fră-kŏs′tal) ["+ *costa,* rib]. Below a rib.

infraction (ĭn-frăk′shŭn) [L. *infractus,* to destroy]. An incomplete fracture of a bone in which parts do not become displaced.

infraglenoid (ĭn″fră-glē′noyd) [L. *infrā,* beneath, + Gr. *glēnē,* cavity, + *eidos,* form]. Beneath the glenoid fossa. SYN: *subglenoid.*

infrahyoid (ĭn″fră-hī′oyd) ["+ Gr. *hyoeides,* U-shaped]. Below the hyoid bone.

inframam′mary ["+ *mamma,* breast]. Below the mammary gland.

inframar′ginal ["+ *margō,* a margin]. Below any edge or margin.

i. convolution. The superior temporal one of the brain.

inframax′illary ["+ *maxilla,* little jaw]. Below the jaw; submaxillary.

infraocclu′sion ["+ *occlusiō,* a shutting up]. Location of a tooth below the line of occlusion.

infraorbital (in-fră-or′bĭ-tal) [L. *infrā,* beneath, + *orbita,* track]. Beneath the orbit.

infrapatellar (ĭn″fră-pă-tel′ăr) ["+ *patella,* a small plate]. Below the patella.

infrapu′bic ["+ *pubēs,* hair on genitals]. Below the pubis.

in′frared rays. Invisible heat rays beyond red end of spectrum.

Their wave length ranges from 7,700 Angstrom units to 1 mm. Long-wave infrared rays (15,000-150,000 A.U.) are emitted by all heated bodies and exclusively by bodies of low temperature such as hot-water bottles and electrical heating pads; shortwave infrared rays (7,200-15,000 A.U.) are those emitted by all incandescent bodies.

SOURCES: The sun, electric arc, incandescent globe, and so-called infrared burners.

USES: Their energy is transformed into heat in a superficial layer of the tissues. They are used therapeutically to stimulate local and general circulation and for relief of pain.

The use of a device, infrared thermograph, for detecting and photographing infrared rays has been useful in studying the heat of tissues. This device has many applications such as in investigation of the rate of blood flow through a part. SEE: *radiation; ray.*

infrascap′ular [L. *infrā,* below, + *scapula,* shoulder blade]. Beneath the shoulder blade.

infraspi'nous ["+ *spīna*, a thorn]. Beneath the scapular spine.

infraster'nal ["+ Gr. *sternon*, chest]. Beneath the sternum.

infratrochlear (ĭn″frā-trŏk'lĭ-ăr) ["+ *trochlea*, pulley]. Beneath the trochlea.

infric'tion [L. *in*, on, + *frictio*, rubbing]. Rubbing of ointments into the skin. SYN: *inunction*.

infundibuliform (ĭn″fŭn-dĭb'ū-lĭ-form) [L. *infundibulum*, funnel, + *forma*, form]. Funnel-shaped.

   i. fascia, i. process. The membranous layer investing the spermatic cord.

infundibulum (ĭn″fŭn-dĭb'ū-lŭm) [L.]. 1. Funnel-shaped passage or structure. 2. Tube connecting the frontal sinus with the middle nasal meatus. 3. Stalk of the pituitary gland. 4. Any renal pelvis division. 5. Cavity formed by fallopian fimbriae. 6. Terminus of a bronchiole. 7. Terminus at upper end of cochlear canal. 8. Conelike upper anterior angle at right cardiac ventricle, from which the pulmonary artery arises. SYN: *conus arteriosus.*

infu'sible [L. *in*, into, + *fundere*, to pour]. 1. Not capable of being fused or melted. 2. Capable of being made into an infusion.

infusion (ĭn-fū'zhŭn). 1. A liquid substance introduced into the body via a vein for therapeutic purposes. 2. Steeping a substance in hot or cold water in order to obtain its active principle. 3. Product obtained from process of def. 2.

   RS: infiltration; intravenous.

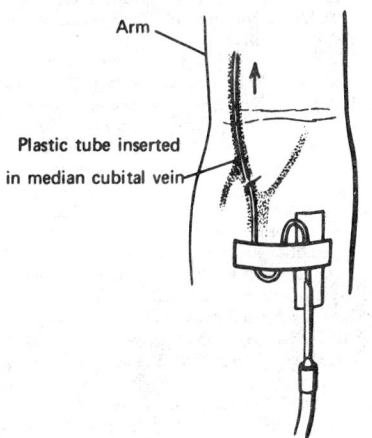

Arm

Plastic tube inserted in median cubital vein

INTRAVENOUS (I.V.) INFUSION

i., intravenous. Injection of a solution directly into a vein, usually the cephalic or median basilic vein of the arm.

infusodecoction (ĭn-fū″sō-dē-kŏk'shŭn) [L. *infusio*, infusion, + *dē*, down, + *coquere*, to boil]. 1. Infusion followed by decoction. 2. A medicine made from a crude drug steeped in cold water and then in boiling water.

infusoria (ĭn-fū-sō'rĭ-ă). Name formerly applied to a class of Protozoa, now called Ciliata.

infu'sum [L., infusion]. Product obtained from steeping a substance in hot or cold water. SYN: *infusion.*

ingesta (ĭn-jĕs'tă) [L. *in*, into, + *gerere*, to carry]. Food and drink received into the body through the mouth.

inges'tion. The process of taking material (particularly food) into the gastrointestinal tract, or by which a cell takes in foreign particles.

ingrassia's apoph'yses. [Giovanni Filippo Ingrassia, It. anatomist, 1510-1580] The lesser wings of the sphenoid.

ingravescent (ĭn″grăv-ĕs'ĕnt) [L. *in*, upon, + *gravesci*, to grow heavy]. Becoming more severe.

ingredient (ĭn-grē'dĭ-ent) [L. *ingredi*, to enter]. Any part of a compound or a mixture; a unit of a more complex substance.

in'growing [L. *in*, into, + AS. *grōwan*, to grow]. Growing inward.

   i. nail. One growing into the flesh. SYN: *onyxia.*

inguen (ĭn'gwĕn) [L.]. The groin.

inguinal (ĭng'gwĭ-nal) [L. *inguinalis*, pert. to the groin]. Pert. to the region of the groin.

   RS: bubo; bubononcus; groin; hernia.

   i. canal. The one carrying the spermatic cord in the male, and the round ligament in the female. It is 1 1/2 in. (3.8 cm.) long; a potential source of weakness; may be the site of a hernia.

   i. glands. Those of the groin.

   i. hernia. Hernia in i. region.

   i. ligament. A fibrous band extending from anterior, superior, iliac spine to the pubic tubercle. SYN: *Pouport's ligament.*

   i. reflex. One in females resembling cremasteric, q.v., reflex in males.

   i. region. The groin. The iliac region on either side of the pubes.

   i. ring. Interior opening of the i. canal (abdominal i. ring), and the end of the i. canal (subcutaneous i. ring).

inguinodynia (ĭn″gwĭ-nō-dĭn'ĭ-ă) [L. *inguen*, groin, + Gr. *odynē*, pain]. Pain in the groin or inguinal region.

inhal'ant [L. *inhalare*, to inhale]. A medication or compound suitable for inhaling.

inhalation (ĭn″hă-lā′shŭn). 1. Act of drawing in of breath, vapor, or gas into the lungs; inspiration. 2. Introduction of dry or moist air or vapor into the lungs for therapeutic purposes, such as aromatic spirits of ammonia used to overcome fainting.

SUBSTANCES INHALED: Mixture of oxygen and carbon dioxide to relieve depressed breathing.

Steam inhalations are given to reduce dryness of mucous membranes and to provide heat and moisture to the membranes of the lungs.

i. therapy. Administration of medicines, water vapors, gases (such as oxygen, carbon dioxide, or helium), or anesthetics by inhalation. The medicines usually are nebulized by using an aerosol or spray apparatus. SEE: *intermittent positive pressure breathing.*

inhale′. To draw in the breath; to inspire.

inhaler. 1. Device for administering medicines by inhalation. 2. One who inhales.

inhe′rent [L. *inhaerēre,* to inhere]. Intrinsic; belonging to anything naturally, not as a result of circumstances.

i. cauterization. Deep cauterization.

inheritance (ĭn-hĕr′ĭ-tăns) [L. *heres,* heir]. The sum total of all that is inherited; that which is the result of hereditary factors within the egg and sperm.

i., blending. Type of i. in which characteristics of male and female parents appear to be blended in offspring. May result from lack of dominance or equal contributions of several pairs of multiple factors.

inherited. Received from one's ancestors; not acquired.

inhibition (ĭn″hĭ-bĭsh′ŭn) [L. *inhibere,* to restrain]. 1. Repression or restraint of a function. 2. In physiology, a stopping of an action or function of an organ. An example of this is the slowing or stopping of the heart produced by electrical stimulation of the vagus. 3. In psychiatry, restraint of one mental process almost simultaneously by another opposed mental process; an inner impediment to free activity.

i., psychic. Arrest of an impulse, thought, action, or speech. The term is commonly applied to the denial of the sex instinct. SYN: *suppression.*

inhib′itor. That which inhibits. For example: A chemical substance which stops enzyme activity or a nerve which suppresses activity of an organ innervated by it.

inhibitory (ĭn-hĭb′ĭ-to-rĭ). Restraining, preventing.

i. nerve. A nerve which carries impulses which act to slow down or inhibit action in the organ or tissue supplied by its fibers.

inhibitrope (ĭn-hĭb′ĭ-trōp) [L. *inhibere,* to restrain, + Gr. *tropos,* a turning]. One in whom certain stimuli cause partial arrest of function.

iniac, inial (ĭn′ĭ-ak, -ăl) [Gr. *inion,* back of the head]. Pert. to the inion.

inion (ĭn′ĭ-ŏn). External occipital protuberance.

initial (ĭn-ĭsh′ăl) [L. *initium,* beginning]. Incipient; rel. to the beginning, or commencing.

initis (ĭn-ī′tĭs) [Gr. *is,* fiber, + *-itis,* inflammation]. 1. Inflammation of fibrous tissue. SYN: *fibrositis.* 2. Inflammation of a tendon. SYN: *tendinitis.* 3. Inflamed condition of a muscle. SYN: *myositis.*

inject′ [L. *injicere,* to throw in]. To introduce fluid into the body or its parts artificially.

injec′ted [L. *injectus,* thrown in]. Filled by injection of fluid; congested.

injection (ĭn-jĕk′shŭn). 1. Forcing of a fluid into a vessel or cavity or under the skin. 2. Substance introduced in this manner. 3. State of being injected; congestion.

NP: All equipment to be used must be sterilized and preferably autoclaved if heat sterilization is used. Boiling alone does not destroy the virus of serum hepatitis. The nurse must wash her hands before assembling the syringe and securing the needle. Expel air and measure dosage accurately. Cleanse site of injection with alcohol and sterile cotton before injection and after withdrawal of needle. Rinse syringe and needle, sterilize.

Caution: Neither the needle nor the syringe should be reused until each of them has been thoroughly cleaned and resterilized. Failure to observe this rule permits transmission by inoculation of the virus of serum hepatitis from person to person.

RS: douche; enema.

i., epidural. Injection of anesthetic solution or other medicine into the epidural space of the spinal cord.

i., hypodermic. Originally indicated injection of a substance beneath the skin. Now used to indicate a medicine by injection with a hypodermic syringe or needle without respect to whether it is beneath the skin or intramuscular.

i., intracardial. Into the heart.

i., intracutaneous. I. into the skin, a method employed in giving of serums and vaccines when a local reaction is desired.

i., intralingual. I. of medicines into the tongue. Usually done as an emergency measure when a vein suitable for use is not available because of circulatory collapse.

i., intramuscular. Into intramuscular tissue usually in front of thigh or in one of the buttocks.

i., intraperitoneal. I. into the peritoneal cavity.

i., intravenous. Into a vein.

i., jet. Technique of injecting medicines and vaccines through the skin without puncturing it. This is done by the use of a nozzle which ejects a fine spray of liquid at such speed as to penetrate the skin. The skin is not harmed and the procedure is harmless. Esp. useful in immunizing a great number of persons quickly and economically.

i., rectal. Into the rectum; an enema.

i., sclerosing. I. into a vessel or into a tissue of a substance which will bring about obliteration of the vessel or hardening of the tissues.

i., spinal. I. into the spinal canal.

i., subcutaneous. I. beneath the skin. SYN: *hypodermic i.*

i., vaginal. A douche.

inject′ors. Various instruments for injecting medicinal fluids, making hypodermic injections and for transfusion of blood and intravenous injection.

in′jury [L. *in*, not, + *jus*, right]. Damage to some part of the body.

SYM: These will depend on the nature, extent and severity of the damage. If severe there may be signs of shock with progressive fall in blood pressure; subnormal temperature; shallow, rapid breathing; cold, clammy, pale skin.

NP: Avoid rough handling, the loss of fluids and body heat, and exposure of tissue in burns. Cover all wounded surfaces, keep warm but do not apply heat to the injured area. Treatment of shock will be determined by the fluid and blood needs. This will be quite different for the person who is severely burned as compared to the one whose i. was received in an automobile accident. One to two pints of hot coffee or tea if patient is conscious and there are no abdominal injuries. In case of broken bones and laceration, stop hemorrhage, make comfortable, but do not move patient until physician arrives.

SEE: *transportation of the injured.*

i., egg-white. I. resulting from biotin deficiency. It is produced in experimental animals by feeding raw egg white or its antibiotin component, avidin.

i., steering wheel. I. following automobile accidents in which driver is thrown forward against steering wheel resulting in contusion of heart.

ink poisoning. Many of the poisonings ascribed to ink are forms of dermatitis. Several types of materials may be responsible. Ordinary ink may cause irritation, either because of irritating nature, or because of susceptibility of particular skins. Sometimes cleaning materials used in removing ink stains have been found to be causative agents.

SYM: Redness, occasionally small pustules and cracking.

F. A. TREATMENT: Wash with alcohol, soap and water. Rinse carefully, apply a bland dressing, as cold cream, etc.

in′lay [L. *in*, in, + AS. *lecgan*, to lay]. A solid filling made to the shape of a cavity of a tooth and cemented into it.

in′let. Passage leading to a cavity.

i. of the pel′vis. The upper opening into the pelvic cavity.

innate′ [L. *in*, in, + *natus*, born]. Inborn; inherent.

innervate (ĭn-nŭr′vāt, in′ur-) ["+ *nervus*, nerve]. To stimulate a part as the nerve supply of an organ.

innervation (ĭn″ĕr-vā′shŭn). 1. Stimulation of a part through the action of nerves. 2. The distribution and function of the nervous system. 3. The nerve supply of a part.

i., collateral. Development of nerve supply in a nerve tract adjacent to original nerve supply which has been injured or destroyed.

i., double. I. of an organ with both sympathetic and parasympathetic fibers.

i., reciprocal. I. of antagonistic muscles of a limb by which impulses of central origin which induce an action such as flexion bring about inhibition of the opposing extensors.

innidiation (ĭ-nĭd-ĭ-ā′shŭn) [L. *in*, in, + *nidus*, nest]. Multiplication of cells in a part to which they have been carried by metastasis.

innocent (ĭn′ō-sĕnt) [L. *in*, not, + *nocere*, to injure]. Benign; not malignant. SYN: *innocuous.*

innoc′uous [L. *in*, not, + *nocuus*, harmful]. Harmless or benign.

innominate (ĭ-nŏm′ĭ-nāt) [L. *innominatus*, unnamed]. Nameless.

i. artery. Right artery arising from the arch of the aorta, dividing into the right subclavian and right common carotid arteries.

i. bone. Os innominatum. The hip bone, composed of the ilium, ischium, and pubis; united to form the pelvis by the sacrum and coccyx.

i. veins. Right and left vein, each formed by union of internal jugular with subclavian veins.

innoxious (ĭ-nŏk′shŭs) [L. *in*, not, + *noxius*, harmful]. Not harmful. SYN: *innocuous.*

inochondritis (ĭn″ō-kŏn-drī′tĭs) [Gr. *inos*, fiber, + *chondros*, cartilage, + *-itis*, inflammation]. Inflammation of a fibrocartilage.

inochondroma (ĭn″ō-kŏn-drō′mă) [″+ ″+ *ōma*, tumor]. A chondroma or tumor with much fibrous tissue; fibrochondroma.

inoculability (ĭn-ŏk″ū-lă-bĭl′ĭ-tĭ) [L. *in*, into, + *oculus*, bud]. State of being inoculable.

inoc′ulable. 1. Transmissible by inoculation. 2. Susceptible to a transmissible disease. 3. Capable of being inoculated.

inoc′ulate. To inject a microorganism, serums, or toxic materials into the body. This can be accomplished by using a needle and syringe, by scarification of the skin, or by some special technique such as a very high-speed jet of air capable of a force sufficient to carry a liquid solution into the skin.

inoculation (ĭn-ŏk″ū-lā′shŭn). The process of being inoculated. SEE: *inoculate.*

i., animal. The injection of serums, microorganisms, or viral organisms into laboratory animals for the purpose of immunizing them or for the purpose of investigating the effects of the inoculated material upon the animals.

inoc′ulum. The substance introduced by inoculation.

inocyst (ĭn′ō-sĭst) [Gr. *inos*, fiber, + *kystis*, a bladder]. A fibrous capsule.

inocystoma (ĭn″ō-sĭs-tō′mă) [″+ ″+ *ōma*, tumor]. Fibrous tumor undergoing cystic degeneration.

inoepithelioma (ĭn″ō-ĕp′ĭ-thē″lĭ-ō′mă) [″+ *epi*, upon, + *thēlē*, nipple, + *ōma*, tumor]. Epithelioma containing fibrous tissue.

inogenous (ĭn-ŏj′ĭ-nŭs) [Gr. *inos*, fiber, + *gennan*, to produce]. Forming tissue or produced from it.

inohymenitis (ĭn″ō-hī″mĕn-ī′tĭs) [″+ *hymen*, membrane, + *itis*, inflammation]. Inflammation of any fibrous membrane or of an aponeurosis.

inoleiomyoma (ĭn″ō-lī″ō-mī-ō′mă) [″+ *leios*, smooth, + *mys*, muscle, + *ōma*, tumor]. A smooth muscle tissue tumor.

in′olith [″+ *lithos*, stone]. A concretion formed from fibrous tissue.

inoma (ĭn-ō′mă) [Gr. *inos*, fiber, + *ōma*, tumor]. A fibrous tumor. SYN: *fibroma.*

inomyoma (ĭn″ō-mī-ō′mă) [″+ *mys*, muscle, + *ōma*, tumor]. A fibrous tissue myoma. SYN: *fibromyoma.*

inomyositis (ĭn″ō-mī″ō-sī′tĭs) [″+ ″+ *-itis*, inflammation]. Chronic muscular inflammation with connective tissue hyperplasia. SYN: *fibromyositis.*

inomyxo′ma [″+ *myxa*, mucus, + *ōma*, tumor]. A mixed myxoma and fibroma. SYN: *fibromyxoma.*

inoneuroma (ĭn″ō-nū-rō′mă) [″+ *neuron*, nerve, + *ōma*, tumor]. A mixed neuroma and inoma. SYN: *fibroneuroma.*

inop′erable [L. *in*, not, + *operāri*, to work]. Unsuitable for being operated upon because of one or more reasons. In the case of a tumor, the disease may have spread so extensively as to make surgery useless; or the patient's general condition may be so poor that surgery could cause death.

inopex′ia [Gr. *inos* fiber, + *pēxis*, fixation]. Tendency of blood to coagulate spontaneously in the vessels.

inorgan′ic [L. *in*, not, + Gr. *organon*, an organ]. 1. In chemistry, occurring in nature independently of living things. Sometimes considered to indicate chemical compounds which do not contain carbon. 2. Not pert. to living organisms.

i. acid. An acid composed of inorganic constituents. SYN: *acid, mineral.*

i. chemistry. C. dealing only with inorganic compounds.

i. compound. One without carbon.

inosclerosis (ĭn″ō-sklĭ-rō′sĭs) [Gr. *inos*, fiber, + *sklēros*, hard]. Increased fibrous-tissue density.

inos′copy [″+ *skopein*, to examine]. Diagnosis by examining fibrinous deposits in body fluids.

inos′culating [L. *in*, in, + *osculum*, little mouth]. Directly communicating; anastomosing.

inosculation (ĭn-ŏs″kū-lā′shŭn). Union of two vessels; anastomosis, q.v.

inosemia (ĭn-ō-sē′mĭ-ă) [Gr. *inos*, fiber, + *haima*, blood]. 1. An excessive amount of fibrin in the blood. 2. The presence of inositol in the blood.

inosin′ic acid [″+ L. *acidus*, sour]. A mononucleotide (present in muscular tissue and also a product of nucleic acid) which, upon hydrolysis, yields hypoxanthine and d-ribose-5-phosphoric acid.

inosite (ĭn′ō-sīt). Inositol, q.v.

inositis (ĭn″ō-sī′tĭs) [Gr. *inos*, fiber, + *-itis*, inflammation]. Inflammation of fibrous tissue.

inositol (ĭn-ŏs′ĭ-tōl). Hexahydroxycyclohexane, a sugar-like crystalline substance, $C_6H_6(OH)_6$, found in the liver, kidney, skeletal and heart muscle; and also present in the leaves and seeds of most plants. It is part of the vitamin B complex, deficiency of which in experimental animals results in loss of hair, eye defects, and retardation of growth. Its significance in human nutrition has not been established.

inosituria (ĭn″ō-sĭ-tū′rĭ-ă) [Gr. *inos,* fiber, + *ouron,* urine]. Inositol in the urine.

inosteotoma (ĭn″ō-stē″ă-tō′mă) ["+ *stear,* fat, + *ōma,* tumor]. Fatty tumor with fibroma.

inosuria (ĭn-ō-sū′rĭ-ă) [Gr. *inos,* fiber, + *ouron,* urine]. 1. Fibrinous excess in urine. 2. Inositol in the urine. SYN: *inosituria.*

inotropic (ĭn″ō-trŏp′ĭk) [Gr. *inos,* fiber, + *trepein,* to influence]. Influencing the force of muscular work.

in′quest [L. *in,* into, + *quaerere,* to seek]. 1. In legal medicine, official examination and investigation into the cause, circumstance and manner of sudden, unexpected, violent, or unexplained death. 2. The act of inquiring.

insaliva′tion ["+ *saliva,* spittle]. The process of mixing saliva with food, as in chewing.

insalu′brious [L. *in,* not, + *salus,* health]. Not healthy; not contributing to health.

insane (ĭn-sān′) ["+ *sanus,* sound]. Mentally deranged; pert. to insanity.

insan′itary. Not conductive to health; unhealthful, esp. pert. to filth.

insan′ity [L. *insanitās,* insanity]. A severe mental disorder such as a psychosis as distinguished from a neurosis. A general term for unsoundness of mind or any mental disorder. In legal medicine, the state or mental condition characterized by inability to distinguish between right and wrong; possession of delusions or hallucinations which prevent an individual from looking after his own affairs with ordinary prudence or which render him a menace to others; and actions resulting from impulses of such intensity that they cannot be resisted.

LUCID INTERVALS: During lucid intervals an insane person may enter into a legal contract, marriage, business, or buying and selling providing at the time he or she is capable of entering into such matters with an understanding of all that is implied. The mental capacity at the time determines the validity of such acts and not the condition before or after.

RS: neurosis; phobia; psychosis; restraint.

i., alternating. Manic-depressive psychosis, q.v.

i., climacteric. Mental illness occurring during or near the time of the menopause.

i., communicated. Folie a deux in which delusions of one person are transmitted to and accepted by a second person.

i., compulsive. I. in which the actions of a person are the result of obsessions or impulses over which he has no control.

i., delusional. I. in which delusions or hallucinations are characteristic.

i., impulsive. I. characterized by the commission of acts, usually of a violent nature, as a result of sudden uncontrollable impulses.

i., manic-depressive. Manic-depressive psychosis, q.v.

i., moral. I. characterized by the commission of immoral acts although reasoning and intellectual processes are normal.

i., toxic. I. resulting from the effects of a poisonous or toxic substance such as alcohol, opium, or other drugs.

insatiable (ĭn-sā′shĭ-ă-bl) [L. *insatiabilis*]. Incapable of being satisfied or appeased.

inscriptio (ĭn-skrĭp′shĭ-o) [L.]. Inscription.

i. tendin′ea. Tendinous band traversing a muscle.

inscription (ĭn-skrĭp′shŭn) [L. *in,* upon, + *scribere,* to write]. Body of a prescription which gives the names of the drugs prescribed and dosage.

in′sect [L. *insectum*]. Common name for any of the class Insecta of the phylum Arthropoda. Insects of medical importance are flies, mosquitoes, lice, fleas, ticks, spiders, scorpions, bees, hornets, wasps, and the true bugs.

i. bites and stings. In some cases the venom of a stinging insect may be more toxic than that of a poisonous snake. Fortunately the insect injects a very small amount of venom into the body.

FA: Remove the stinger if it is present, and cool the area as quickly and efficiently as possible to prevent the venom from gaining access to the general circulation. To prevent injecting further venom, gently tease the stinger out by grasping the stinger with fingernails or forceps. If a specific therapy or antiserum is available it should be administered.

An antivenin for black widow spiders (Latrodectus mactans) of North America is available from Merck Sharp and Dohme, West Point, Pa. 19486.

There is no antiserum for the bite of the brown recluse spider (Loxosceles reclusus), but hydrocortisone in a dose of 1-3 mg./kg. of body weight every six hours for 4-8 doses is beneficial.

For bees, wasps, and hornets 0.2-0.5 ml. of epinephrine subcutaneously and an antihistamine suitable for intravenous injection should be given slowly. If shock and collapse appear to be imminent, hydrocortisone should be given. Apply ice pack to sting. If muscle spasms are present, intravenous infusion of calcium lactate or calcium gluconate should be given. In some cases curare (dimethyl tubocurarine chloride) will be required to relieve muscle spasms.

Insecta. A class of the phylum Arthropoda characterized by three distinct body divisions (head, thorax, abdomen), three pairs of jointed legs, trachea, and usually two pairs of wings. Insects are of medical significance in that some are parasitic, some serve as carriers or vectors of pathogenic organisms, and some are annoying pests causing injury by their bites or their stings. SYN: *Hexapoda.*

insecticide (ĭn-sĕk'tĭ-sīd) [L. *insectum,* insect, + *caedere,* to kill]. 1. An agent used to exterminate insects. 2. Destructive to insects.

insemination (ĭn-sĕm''ĭn-ā'shŭn) [L. *in,* into, + *semen,* seed]. 1. Discharge of semen from the penis into the vagina during coitus. 2. Fertilization of an ovum.

i., artificial. Introduction by artificial means of viable sperm into the vagina, cervical canal or uterus. SEE: *impregnation.*

i., heterologous artificial. Artificial i. in which the semen is obtained from a donor other than the husband.

i., homologous artificial. Artificial i. in which the semen is obtained from the husband.

insen'sible [L. *in,* not, + *sensibilis,* appreciable]. 1. Unconscious; without feeling or consciousness. 2. Not preceptible.

inser'tion [L. *in,* into, + *serere,* to join]. 1. The manner or place of attachment of a muscle to the bone that it moves. 2. A putting into.

i., velamentous. Attachment of the umbilical cord to the edge of the placenta.

insheathed (ĭn-shēthd') [L. *in,* into, + AS. *scēath,* sheath]. Enclosed, as by a sheath or capsule; encysted.

insidious (ĭn-sĭd'ĭ-ŭs) [L. *insidiōsus,* cunning]. Used to indicate a disease which comes on in such a manner (lacking symptoms) as to make the patient unaware of the onset of the disease.

in'sight. A patient being aware that the symptoms of his illness indicate an abnormal condition.

insipid (ĭn-sĭp'ĭd) [L. *in,* not, + *sapidus,* tasty]. Without taste; lacking in spirit or animation.

in si'tu [L.]. In position.

insolation (ĭn''sō-lā'shŭn) [L. *insolāre,* to expose to the sun]. 1. Any exposure to the rays of the sun. 2. Heat- or sunstroke.

In the past it was felt that exposure to the sunlight was a powerful therapeutic measure. It is now known that persons who expose themselves to excess sunlight on either an acute or a chronic basis may be unwise. Acute overexposure leads to severe sunburn of the skin. Caucasians who experience chronic exposure to the sun have an increased chance of developing malignant neoplasms of the skin. SEE: *heat; heat exhaustion; heatstroke; heat therapy.*

insoluble (ĭn-sŏl'ū-bl) [L. *in,* not, + *solvere,* to dissolve]. Incapable of solution or of being dissolved.

insomnia (ĭn-sŏm'nĭ-ă) ["+ *somnus,* sleep]. Inability to sleep, or sleep prematurely ended or interrupted by periods of wakefulness. Insomnia is not a disease but may be the symptom of many diseases. It may be associated with a trivial or serious illness; the persistence and severity of the insomnia is of little help in diagnosing the condition which causes it. The most frequent causes of insomnia are anxiety and pain.

NP & TREATMENT: Do not try to sleep if too wakeful. Sit up and read until tired. Hot foot bath, drink of warm milk or a mild sweet wine before retiring may be of help.

Change of occupation if necessary and possible. Physical exercise during day, and a walk in fresh air at night after dinner. The several hours prior to bedtime should be as anxiety-free as possible. Peace of mind is essential to falling asleep. Those complaining about insomnia generally secure more sleep than they realize. Some require much less sleep than others. Inability to sleep continuously through the night is not a pathological condition. If the insomnia is due to pain it is important to relieve that symptom and to attempt to cure the cause of the pain. SEE: *narcolepsy; somnambulism; vigil.*

inspect' [L. *inspicere,* to examine]. To examine visually.

inspec'tion. Visual examination of the external surface of the body as well as of its movements and posture. SEE: *abdomen; chest; circulatory system.*

inspersion (ĭn-spĕr'zhŭn) [L. *in,* upon, + *spargere,* to sprinkle]. Sprinkling with powder or a fluid.

inspiration (ĭn''spĭr-ā'shŭn) [L. *in,* in, + *spirāre,* to breathe]. Inhalation; drawing air into the lungs. Opposed to expiration, q.v.

Inspiration may be costal or abdominal, the latter being deeper. The breaking point for breath holding is quite variable. Some professional divers are able to prolong this for more than two minutes.

Rate: 16-18 respirations per minute in a normal adult at rest. SEE: *respiration.*

MUSCLES OF: External intercostals; diaphragm; levatores costarum; pectoralis minor; scaleni; serratus posterior; and superior sternocleidomastoid.

RS: air; apnea; asphyxia; breathing; Cheyne-Stokes respiration; dyspnea; hyperpnea; lungs; respiration; ventilation.

i., crowing. Peculiar noise in laryngismus stridulus, q.v., or spasmatic croup, q.v.

i., external. Interchange of gases in the lungs.

i., forcible, difficult, labored. I. in which the muscles of i. are assisted by inspiratory auxiliaries (i.e., muscles attached to chest which by contraction increase the volume of the thoracic cavity directly or indirectly by furnishing fixed support whereby other muscles may act more advantageously). If movements become excessively labored, there is brought into coordinate action every muscle in the body which can either directly or indirectly increase the capacity of the thorax.

i., full. I. in which lungs are filled as completely as possible (voluntarily, as in determining the amount of complemental air or involuntarily, as in cardiac dyspnea).

i., internal. Interchange of gases in the tissues. SEE: *respiration, cell.*

inspirator (ĭn′spĭ-rā″tor). A type of respirator or inhaler.

inspiratory (ĭn-spī′rä-tor-ĭ). Pert. to inspiration.

inspissate (ĭn-spĭs′āt) [L. *in,* within, + *spissare,* to thicken]. To thicken by evaporation or absorption of fluid.

inspissated (ĭn-spĭs′ă-ted). Thickened by absorption, evaporation or dehydration.

inspissation (ĭn-spĭ-sā′shŭn). 1. Thickening by evaporation or absorption of fluid. 2. Diminished fluidity or increased thickness.

in′step. Arch on upper surface of foot in the middle, in front of ankle.

instillation (ĭn″stĭl-ā′shŭn) [L. *in,* into, + *stillāre,* to drop]. Slowly pouring or dropping a liquid into a cavity or onto a surface.

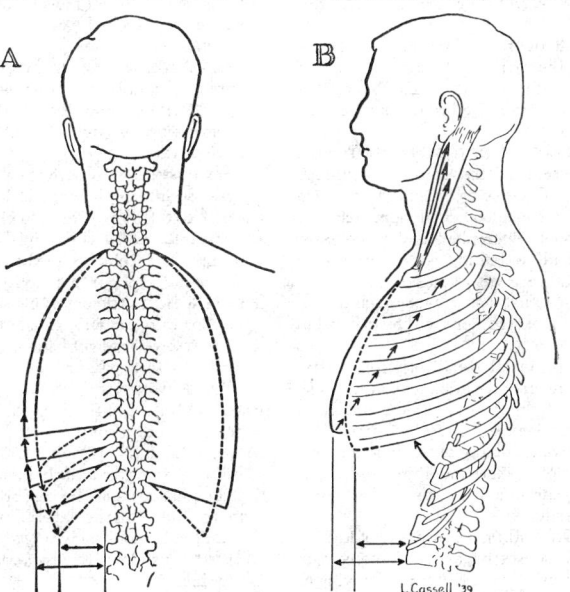

A   B

L.Cassell '39

CHANGES IN SIZE OF THORAX DURING INSPIRATION

A, Back view. The contraction of the external intercostal muscles raises the ribs, makes them flare laterally, and so increases the transverse diameter of the thorax.

B, Side view. The contraction of the sternocleidomastoid muscle aids the external intercostals in raising the ribs, and so increases the anteroposterior diameter of the thorax. (Highly schematic.)

in'stillator. An apparatus for introducing, drop by drop, liquids into a cavity.

instinct (ĭn'stĭngkt) [L. *instinctus*, instigation]. The inherited tendency for the members of specific species, including man, to react to certain environmental conditions and stimuli in a particular way. The nature of the reaction is that which has through many generations enabled the individuals and species involved to adapt and survive. Instincts are best understood when considered against the evolutionary background of the individuals and species being observed.

Freud spoke of instinct, but present-day psychoanalytical terminology would refer to the forces Freud described as being drive instead of instinct.

instinct'ive [L.]. Determined by instinct.

instrument (ĭn'strŭmĕnt) [L. *instrumentum*, tool]. 1. A mechanical device. 2. A special tool for accomplishing specific tasks. Thus a reflex hammer, a microscope, stethoscope, cystoscope, and the surgeon's scalpel are all examples of instruments.

instrumen'tal. 1. Pert. to instruments. 2. Being the cause of anything.

i. delivery. Delivery of a child with forceps.

instrumenta'tion. 1. The use of instruments, and their care. 2. Accomplishment of a task by use of instruments. Ex: Removal of a foreign body from the bronchus by means of a bronchoscope.

instruments, care and sharpening of. After operation collect, count and unlock instruments. Cleanse by rinsing with warm water to remove blood, and next, use hot water and soap. Then place under hot-water faucet and allow boiling water to run on them, dry at once with gauze.

To remove rust use cleanser sparingly, else surface of instrument will be injured in course of time.

Reliable bacterial sterilization of instruments before an operation can always be assured by boiling in a 1% solution of sodium bicarbonate for 15 minutes. This helps to prevent rusting of the instruments. The dipping of an instrument into alcohol or even pure carbolic acid cannot be relied upon to sterilize it.

CAUTION: Boiling water does not kill the virus which causes hepatitis. To be certain this virus is destroyed, either autoclaving or the use of some chemical method of sterilization such as ethylene oxide gas is required.

Washita stone is best for sharpening dull instruments as it cuts away the metal faster. Arkansas stone is better for finishing. Glycerin is best lubricant. Entire edge of knife should be covered in one sweep. Hold knife at angle of 30°. All knives should be honed before being used. Blunt instruments should be kept highly polished. Rub with fine emery paper and polish with rouge and chamois skin or gauze. Do not use emery paper on saws. Sharpen with three-cornered files. Silver instruments should not come in contact with rubber, or be exposed to atmosphere. Wrap in dry gauze.

insufficiency (ĭn"sŭ-fĭsh'ĕn-sĭ) [L. *in*, not, + *sufficiens*, sufficient]. The condition of being inadequate for its purpose.

i., aortic. An imperfect closure of the aortic valve.

i., cardiac. Inability of heart to function normally.

i., gastric. Inability of the stomach to empty itself.

i., hepatic. Inability of the liver to function properly.

i., mitral. Condition in which the mitral valve closes inefficiently with rhythmic action of the heart.

i., muscular. Condition in which a muscle is unable to exert its normal force and bring about normal movement of the part to which it is attached. Term applied esp. to eye muscles.

i. of the ocular muscles. Absence of dynamic equilibrium of ocular muscles.

i., renal. Inability of the kidney to remove waste products from the blood at the normal rate.

i., valvular. Imperfect cardiac valve closure, permitting leakage of blood.

insuf'flate [L. *insufflāre*, to blow into]. 1. To blow into, as in the lungs of a newborn infant. 2. To blow a medicated powder or medicinal vapor into a cavity.

insuffla'tion. The act of blowing a vapor or powder into a cavity, as the lungs.

i., tubal. Transuterine i. with carbon dioxide to test patency of fallopian tubes. SYN: *Rubin's test.*

insufflator (ĭn'sŭ-flā-tor). Device for blowing powders into a cavity.

in'sula [L.]. 1. [NA] The central lobe (island of Reil) of the cerebral hemisphere. It is a triangular area of the cerebral cortex lying in the floor of the lateral fissure. 2. Any round cutaneous body or patch.

insular (ĭn'sŭ-lăr) [L. *insula*, island]. Rel. to any insula.

insula'tion [L. *insulāre*, to make into an island]. 1. The protection of a body or substance with a nonconducting medium to prevent the transfer of electricity, heat, or sound. 2. The material or substance which insulates.

The electrical resistance of an insulator is expressed in megohms, a unit representing a million ohms.

in'sulator. That which insulates; specifically, a substance or body that interrupts the transmission of electricity to surrounding objects by conduction; anything that exerts great resistance to the passage of an electric current by conduction. SEE: *nonconductor.*

in'sulin [L. *insula,* island]. 1. A hormone secreted by the beta cells of the islets of Langerhans of the pancreas. It can be readily crystallized as a zinc salt although nickel, calcium, and cobalt also are effective. It is a protein with a molecular weight of approx. 35,000. I. is essential for the proper metabolism of blood sugar (glucose) and for maintenance of the proper blood sugar level. Inadequate secretion of i. results in improper metabolism of carbohydrates and fats and brings on diabetes characterized by hyperglycemia and glycosuria. The secretion of i. is primarily dependent upon the concentration of blood glucose, an increase of blood sugar bringing about an increase in the secretion of i. SYN: *antidiabetic hormone.*

2. A preparation used in medical treatment of diabetes. Prepared from animal pancreas, usually pork or beef. First discovered and used successfully in diabetes by Sir F. G. Banting. Not a cure, and not necessary in every case. I. when injected (it is not active orally) into a diabetic produces the following effects: normal storage of glycogen in the liver and muscle tissue; reduction in blood sugar level; disappearance of ketosis and hyperlipemia; prevention of excessive breakdown of protein; and increase in respiratory quotient.

DOSAGE: Should always be expressed in units rather than in milliliters or minims. There is no average dose of i. for diabetics; each case must be studied individually. In general, it is advisable to keep the volume per injection at from one-half to three-quarter ml., choosing the strength which will give the required number of units in this volume or less.

ADM: I. preparations are divided into three categories according to how quickly they act and their potency and duration following subcutaneous administration. The three types are fast-, intermediate-, and long-acting. Examples of these are listed below. SEE: *i. injection* (fast-acting); *i. suspension, isophane* (intermediate-acting); *i. suspension, protamine zinc* and *i. zinc suspension, extended* (long-acting).

Duration of Effect of Various Insulins When Given by Subcutaneous Injection

Type of Insulin	Synonym or Trade Name	Onset	Maximum	Duration
			(Given in Hours)	
Insulin Injection (USP)	Insulin, Insulin Hydrochloride, Regular Insulin, Unmodified Insulin	0.5–1.0	3	6–8
Prompt Insulin Zinc Suspension (USP)	Semilente Insulin	0.5–0.75	5–7	12–18
Globin Zinc Insulin Injection (NF)	Globin Insulin	1–2	8–10	24
Isophane Insulin Suspension (USP)	Isophane Insulin, NPH Insulin	0.5–1	7–11	24–28
Insulin Zinc Suspension (USP)	Lente Insulin	1–1.5	14–18	28–32
Protamine Zinc Insulin Suspension (USP)	Protamine Zinc Insulin	6–8	10–18	20–36
Extended Insulin Zinc Suspension	Ultralente	5–8	22–26	34–36

i. injection. USP. A fast-acting i., acting within one hour of injection and lasting approx. six hours. SYN: *regular insulin.*

i. NPH. Abbr. for neutral-protamine-Hagedorn. SEE: *i. suspension, isophane.*

i. shock. Condition resulting from an overdose of i. resulting in reduction of blood sugar level below normal (hypoglycemia).

SYM: Excessive hunger, thirst, and nervousness, fear, and excitability. Rapid pulse, flushing, pallor and sweating, fainting, convulsions, coma.

TREATMENT: Eating sugar or candy, orange juice, glucose, other carbohydrates and injections of strong glucose solution intravenously. Adrenalin is of great though transient value.

i. shock therapy. The treatment of schizophrenia and other mental disorders by the injection of i. Sufficient i. is injected to produce unconsciousness, the dosage being carefully regulated during course of treatment. When a deep coma is reached, the patient is brought out of the comatose condition by the administration of glucose followed by a meal rich in carbohydrates.

Because it is a potentially dangerous procedure it should be employed only by those who are fully equipped, fully qualified, and thoroughly familiar with all aspects of this method. It is essential to have available at all times suitable solutions of dextrose for intravenous use for interrupting the hypoglycemic state which is artificially created.

i. suspension, isophane. USP. Intermediate-acting i. with onset in two hours and duration of 24 hours. SYN: *NPH i.*

i. suspension, protamine zinc. USP. Long-acting i. with onset in seven hours and duration of 36 hours.

i. tolerance. The degree to which the body responds to the injection of i.

i. zinc suspension, extended. USP. Long-acting i. with onset in seven hours and duration of 36 hours.

i. zinc suspension, prompt. USP. Fast-acting i. with onset in one hour and duration of 14 hours.

insulinemia (ĭn-sū-lĭn-ē'mĭ-ă) [L. *insula*, island, + Gr. *haima*, blood]. An undue amt. of insulin in the blood.

insulinogenic (ĭn″sū-lĭn″ō-jĕn′ĭk) ["+ Gr. *gennan*, to produce]. 1. Caused by insulin whether administered or produced by the pancreas. 2. Pert. to production of insulin.

insulinoid (ĭn′sū-lĭn-oyd) ["+ Gr. *eidos*, resemblance]. Resembling or having the properties of insulin.

insulo'ma [L. *insula*, island, + Gr. *ōma*, tumor]. A tumor of the islands of Langerhans.

insulopath'ic ["+ Gr. *pathos,* disease]. Rel. to or caused by abnormal insulin secretion.

insusceptibility (ĭn″sŭ-sĕp″tĭ-bĭl′ĭ-tĭ) [L. *in*, not, + *suscipere*, to take up]. Immunity or lack of susceptibility to infection or disease.

integration (ĭn″tĭ-grā′shŭn) [L. *integrāre*, to make whole]. The bringing together of various parts or functions so that they function as a harmonious whole.

i., primary. Early recognition of the body and its psyche as apart from one's environment.

i., secondary. The process involved in developing the adult personality so that the individual coordinates components into unified and socialized action.

integrator (ĭn′tĕ-grā″tor). Device for measuring body surfaces.

integument (ĭn-tĕg′ū-mĕnt) [L. *integumentum*, a covering]. 1. A covering. 2. The skin, consisting of the corium or dermis, and epidermis.

integumentary (ĭn-tĕg-ū-mĕn′tă-rĭ). Rel. to the integument. SYN: *cutaneous; dermal.*

i. system. The skin and its appendages, including the hair and nails.

in'tellect [L. *intelligere,* to understand]. The mind, or understanding; conscious brain function.

intellec'tual. 1. Pert. to the mind. 2. Possessing intellect.

intel'ligence [L. *intelligere,* to understand]. The capacity to comprehend relationships. The ability to think; the ability to solve problems and to adjust to new situations.

It is doubtful that using a single test to estimate the intelligence of persons from different social, racial, cultural, or economic backgrounds is reliable.

i. quotient. An index of intelligence determined through the subject's answers to arbitrarily chosen questions. IQ is merely a standard score which places an individual in

Classification of IQ's

IQ	Classification
Above 140	"Near" genius or genius
120–140	Very superior intelligence
110–120	Superior intelligence
90–110	Normal or average intelligence
80–90	Dull normal
70–80	Borderline deficiency
50–70	Educable mentally retarded
30–50	Trainable
20–30	Severe mentally retarded
Below 20	Profoundly mentally retarded

reference to the scores of others within his age group. ABBR: IQ.

i. test. A test designed to determine the intelligence of an individual. A number of tests have been devised including the Binet t., Babcock-Levy t., Stanford-Binet t., and others. Tests are used as a basis for determining intelligence quotient (IQ), q.v.

intem'perance [L. *in*, not, + *temperare*, to moderate]. Excess in the use of anything; lack of moderation.

inten'sifying [L. *intensus*, intense, + *facere*, to make]. Making intense.

i. screen. A thin sheet of celluloid or other substance coated with a finely divided substance which fluoresces under the influence of roentgen rays and is intended to be used in close contact with the emulsion of a photographic plate or film for the purpose of reinforcing the image. A fluorescent screen.

intensimeter (in″ten-sim′ĭ-ter) [″+ Gr. *metron*, measure]. An instrument, often a selenium cell or ionization chamber, designed to measure the intensity of x-rays.

intensity (in-těn′sĭ-tĭ). 1. The degree or extent of activity, strength, force, electric current, etc. 2. The state or quality of being intense.

i. of roentgen rays. The attribute of a beam of roentgen rays which determines the rate of ionization of air at a given point, under the conditions stipulated in the definition of roentgen. It is expressed in roentgens per unit of time. SEE: *ray.*

intensive (in-těn′sĭv). Rel. to or marked by intensity.

intention (in-těn′shŭn) [L. *in*, upon, + *tendere*, to stretch]. 1. A natural process of healing. 2. Goal or purpose.

i., first. Healing without granulation or suppuration.

i., second. Healing by adhesion of two granulated surfaces with suppuration.

i., third. Healing of an ulcer, wound, or cavity by filling by granulation and followed by cicatrization. SEE: *first i.; granulation; resolution; second i.*

i. tremor. One exhibited or intensified when attempting coordinated movements.

inter- [L.]. Prefix meaning in the midst, between.

interartic'ular [L. *inter*, between, + *articulus*, joint]. 1. Between two joints. 2. Situated between two articulating surfaces.

interatrial (in″ter-ā′trĭ-ăl) [″+ *atrium*, hall]. Located between the atria of the heart. SYN: *interauricular.*

interauricular (in″tĕr-ŏ-rĭk′ū-lăr) [″+ *auricula*, little ear]. 1. Situated between the auricles or pinnae. 2. Interatrial.

in'terbrain [″+ AS. *braegen*, brain]. The hinder original part of the forebrain including the thalamus, pineal body (epithalamus) and geniculate bodies (metathalamus). SYN: *diencephalon; thalamencephalon.*

intercadence (in″tĕr-kā′dĕns) [L. *inter*, between, + *cadere*, to fall]. A supernumerary pulse wave between two regular beats.

intercalary (in-tĕr′kă-ler″ĭ) [″+ *calare*, to call]. 1. Inserted between as something in addition; extraneous. 2. Pert. to an upstroke on a pulse tracing which comes between two pulse beats, intercalated.

intercalated (in-tĕr′kăl-āt-ĕd). 1. Inserted between as something in addition; extraneous. 2. Pert. to an upstroke on a pulse tracing which comes between two pulse beats, intercalary.

i. disks. SEE: *disk, intercalated.*

i. ducts. Short, narrow ducts which lie between secretory ducts and the terminal alveoli in the parotid and submaxillary glands and in the pancreas.

intercarot'ic [L. *inter*, between, + Gr. *karōs*, deep sleep]. Between the external and internal carotid arteries.

in″tercartilag'inous [L. *inter*, between, + *cartilago*, cartilage]. Connecting or between cartilages.

intercellular (in″tĕr-sĕl′ū-lăr) [″+ *cella*, compartment]. Between the cells of a structure.

interchondral (in″tĕr-kŏn′drăl) [″+ Gr. *chondros*, cartilage]. Between cartilages. SYN: *intercartilaginous.*

intercilium (in″tĕr-sĭl′ĭ-ŭm) [″+ *cilium*, eyelash]. The space between the eyebrows. SYN: *glabella.*

interclavic'ular [L. *inter*, between, + *clavicula*, clavicle]. Between the calvicles.

intercolumnar (in″tĕr-kō-lŭm′năr) [″+ *columna*, column]. Between columns.

i. fascia. A membrane between pillars of the abdominal ring, enclosing the spermatic cord.

i. fibers. Intercrural fibers.

intercon'dylar, intercon'dyloid, intercon'dylous [″+ Gr. *kondylos*, knuckle]. Between two condyles (the rounded eminence at the articular end of a bone).

intercos'tal [″+ *costa*, rib]. Between the ribs.

i. muscles, external. Outer layer of muscles between the ribs, originating on the lower margin of each rib, being inserted on the upper margin of the next rib. They elevate the ribs, enlarging the thorax and thus functioning in inspiration.

i. muscles, internal. Those between the ribs lying beneath the external intercostals; function uncertain.

intercostobrachial (ĭn″tĕr-kŏs″tō-brā′kĭ-al) ["+ "+ *brachium,* arm]. Pert. to the intercostal space and the arm, as the posterior lateral branch of the second intercostal nerve supplying the skin of the arm, or a similar branch of the third intercostal nerve. Formerly called intercostohumeralis.

intercos″tohumera′lis. Term formerly used for intercostobrachial, q.v.

in′tercourse [L. *intercursus,* running between]. Social interaction between individuals or groups. Communication.

i., sexual. The sexual act. SYN: *coitus.*

intercris′tal ["+ *crista,* crest]. Between two crests of a bone, organ, or process.

intercrural (ĭn″tĕr-krū′rãl) [L. *inter,* between, + *crus,* limb]. Between two crura.

intercur′rent ["+ *currere,* to run]. 1. Intervening. 2. Pert. to a disease attacking a patient with another malady.

intercusp′ing ["+ *cuspis,* point]. The fitting together of the surfaces of opposing teeth.

interden′tal ["+ *dens,* tooth]. Between the teeth.

interdentium (ĭn″tĕr-dĕn′shĭ-ŭm). The space between any two contiguous teeth.

interdigita′tion [L. *inter,* between, + *digitus,* digit]. 1. Interlocking of toothed or fingerlike processes. 2. Processes so interlocked.

interfascicular (ĭn″tĕr-făs-ĭk′ū-lãr) ["+ *fasciculus,* bundle]. Between fasciculi.

interfem′oral ["+ *femoralis,* pert. to the thigh]. Between the thighs.

interfer′ence [L. *inter,* between, + *ferire,* to strike]. Clashing or colliding.

i. of impulses. Condition in which two excitation waves, upon approaching each other and meeting in any part of the heart, are mutually extinguished.

interferon (ĭn-tĕr-fēr′ŏn). A protein or proteins formed when cells are exposed to viruses. Noninfected cells exposed to interferon are protected against viral infection.

interfib′rillar, interfib′rillary [L. *inter,* between, + *fibrilla,* a small fiber]. Between fibrils.

interfi′lar ["+ *filum,* thread]. Between the fibrils of a recticulum.

i. mass. The fluid portion of the protoplasm.

interganglion′ic [L. *inter,* between, + *ganglion,* a swelling]. Between ganglions.

interglob′ular ["+ *globulus,* globule]. Between globules.

i. spaces. Gaps in dentin due to failure of calcification. SYN: *Czermak's spaces.*

interlo′bar ["+ *lobus,* lobe]. Between lobes.

interlobi′tis ["+ "+ Gr. *itis,* inflammation]. Inflammation of the pleura separating the pulmonary lobes.

interlob′ular [L. *inter,* between, + *lobulus,* lobule]. Between lobules of an organ.

i. emphysema. Air between the lobes of the lung.

intermar′riage ["+ *maritare,* to marry]. 1. Marriage between persons of two different races or tribes. SYN: *miscegenation.* 2. Marriage between blood relations.

intermax′illary [L. *inter,* between, + *maxilla,* jawbone]. Between two maxillae.

intermediary (ĭn″tĕr-mē′dĭ-ar-ĭ) ["+ *medius,* middle]. 1. Situated between two bodies. 2. Occurring between two periods of time.

i. metabolism. The series of intermediate compounds formed during digestion before the final excretion or oxidation products are formed or eliminated from the body.

intermediolat′eral ["+ "+ *latus,* side]. Intermediate but not central.

i. tract of spinal cord. A lateral tract between the dorsal and ventral horns.

intermeningeal (ĭn″tĕr-mĕn-ĭn′jē-ăl) ["+ *mēninx,* membrane]. Between the meninges.

intermenstrual (ĭn″tĕr-mĕn′strū-al) [L. *inter,* between, + Gr. *mēn,* month]. Between the menses, or menstrual periods.

intermis′sion ["+ *mittere,* to send]. 1. Interval between two paroxysms of a disease. 2. Temporary cessation of symptoms.

intermit′tence. 1. Condition marked by intermissions in the course of a disease or of a process. 2. A loss of one or more pulse beats.

intermittent (ĭn″tĕr-mĭt′ĕnt). Suspending activity at intervals. Coming and going.

i. fever. One in which there is complete absence of symptoms between paroxysms of the fever. SEE: *malaria; undulant fever.*

i. pulse. One in which a beat is dropped at intervals.

i. temperature. One that reaches the normal line at intervals during the course of a fever.

intermittent positive pressure breathing. Method used to assist breathing. The patient breathes through a mask connected to a device which produces intermittent positive air pressure. When the pressure is increased the lungs are inflated, and then the pressure is released and the patient exhales. ABBR: IPPB.

intermus′cular [L. *inter,* between, + *musculus,* muscle]. Between muscles.

intern (ĭn′tern) [L. *internus,* within]. Physician or surgeon on a hospital staff, usually a recent graduate receiving a year of postgraduate training prior to being eligible to be licensed to practice medicine. SEE: *externe.*

inter'nal [L. *internus,* within]. Within the body. Within or on the inside; enclosed, inward. Opposed to external.

i. bleeding. Internal hemorrhage.

i. ear. The vestibule, semicircular canals, and cochlea.

i. injury. Any injury not visible from the outside, as injury to the organs occupying the thoracic, abdominal, or cranial cavities.

SYM: Vary with structures involved. Ordinarily, profound shock. Patient is pale, cold, perspiring freely, has an anxious expression, may be semicomatose. Pain usually intense at first, and may continue or gradually diminish as patient grows worse.

In severe injuries, pain may not be manifested. The pulse is very feeble, fast, often irregular. Patient may be very restless, breathless, and usually has shallow respiration.

F.A. TREATMENT: Above all, patient should be kept very quiet and comfortably warm but not hot. Do not give anything by mouth, and do not give stimulants, as they may exaggerate bleeding. Transportation must be done very cautiously. If patient is in shock shoulders should be lowered and extremities elevated at least 45°. This may be done by placing patient on a chair, box, or a folded coat.

i. medicine. That branch of medicine that deals with diseases not usually treated surgically.

i. secretion. That of the ductless glands which, entering the blood stream, activates other glands and organs. SYN: *hormones,* q.v.

SEE: *ductless glands; endocrine; secretion.*

International unit. One defined and adopted by the International Conference for Unification of Formulae.

in'terne [L. *internus,* within]. Intern, q.v.

intern'ist. One who specializes in internal medicine.

in'ternode [L. *inter,* between, + *nodus,* knot]. Space between adjacent nodes.

internun'cial ["+ *nuncius,* messenger]. Acting as a connecting medium.

i. neuron. One between two other neurons in a neural pathway.

interocep'tive [L. *inter,* within, + *capere,* to take]. In nerve physiology, concerned with sensations arising within the body itself, as distinguished from those (e.g., sight) arising outside the body.

interoceptor (ĭn''tĕr-ō-sĕp'tor). A receptor activated by stimuli within the body.

i., general. An end organ carrying sensations of hunger, thirst, visceral pain, nausea, sexual and circulatory sensations.

i., special. One for smell and taste.

interofec'tive [L. *inter,* within, + *afficere,* to influence]. 1. Pert. to that which concerns the interior of an organism. 2. Cannon's term concerning the autonomic nervous system.

in''teroinfe'rior. Pert. to an inward and downward position.

interol'ivary [L. *inter,* between, + *oliva,* olive]. Between the olivary bodies.

interor'bital ["+ *orbita,* orbit]. Between the orbits.

inteross'eous ["+ *os,* bone]. Situated or occurring between bones, as some muscles and ligaments.

interosseus (ĭn''tĕr-ŏs'ĭ-ŭs). (pl. *interossei*) A muscle lying between bones.

interpalpebral (ĭn''tĕr-păl'pĭ-brăl) [L. *inter,* between, + *palpebra,* eyelid]. Between the eyelids.

interpari'etal ["+ *paries,* wall]. 1. Between walls. 2. Between the parietal bones. 3. Between the parietal lobes of the cerebrum.

i. bone. SEE: *incarial bone.*

i. suture. Sagittal suture.

interparoxys'mal [L. *inter,* between, + Gr. *paroxysmos,* spasm]. Between paroxysms.

interpeduncular (ĭn''tĕr-pĭ-dŭnk'ū-lăr) ["+ *pedunculus,* peduncle]. Between peduncles.

interphalangeal (ĭn''tĕr-fă-lăn'jē-ăl) ["+ Gr. *phalanx,* phalanx]. In a joint between two phalanges.

interpolar (ĭn''tĕr-pō'lăr) ["+ *polus,* pole]. Between two poles.

i. path. Path of galvanic current through tissues between poles.

interprox'imal ["+ *proximus,* next]. Between two adjoining surfaces.

i. space. Triangular space between two adjacent teeth.

interpu'bic ["+ *pubes,* pubes]. Between the pubic bones.

interpu'pillary [L. *inter,* between, + *pupilla,* pupil]. Between the pupils.

i. distance. Distance between centers of the pupils of the eyes.

interre'nal ["+ *rēn,* kidney]. Between the kidneys.

interrupt'er ["+ *ruptus,* broken]. A device, usually automatic, for making and breaking (closing and opening alternately) an electric circuit. Such a device is ordinarily employed in low-voltage, direct-current circuits.

interscapil′ium ["+ *scapula,* shoulder blade]. Area between the shoulders or scapulae. SYN: *interscapulum.*

interscap′ular. Between the scapulae.

   i. reflex. Scapular muscular contraction following percussion or stimulus between the scapulae.

interscap′ulum. Section of back between shoulder blades. SYN: *interscapilium.*

intersex (in′ter-seks). An individual having both male and female characteristics. The term has some descriptive but little or no diagnostic value. Determination of sex in individuals who appear to have both male and female characteristics is a complex task. The diagnosis should be made after careful study of the chromosomes and of the gross and microscopic anatomical findings. SEE: *hermaphroditism.*

in′terspace. The space between two similar parts, as between two ribs.

inter′stice [L. *intersistere,* to stand in the middle of]. A space or gap in a tissue or structure of an organ.

interstitial (īn″tĕr-stĭsh′ăl). 1. Placed or lying between. 2. Pert. to interstices or spaces within an organ or tissue.

   i. cells of testes. Cells of Leydig, located in groups between the seminiferous tubules. They produce the internal secretion (testosterone) of the testes.

intersystole (īn″tĕr-sĭs′tō-lĭ) [L. *inter,* between, + Gr. *systolē,* contraction]. The period between the end of the atrial systole and the commencement of the ventricular systole.

intertrigo (īn″tĕr-trī′gō) ["+ *terere,* to rub]. A superficial dermatitis in the folds of the skin. SEE: *erythema intertrigo.*

intertrochanteric (īn″tĕr-trō″kăn-tĕr′ĭk) ["+ Gr. *trochantēr,* trochanter]. Between the femur's two trochanters.

   i. line. The ridge between the greater and lesser trochanters of femur on posterior aspect of the bone.

intertubular (īn″tĕr-tū′bū-lăr) ["+ *tubulus,* tubule]. Between or among tubules.

interureteral (īn″tĕr-ū-rē′tĕr-ăl) ["+ Gr. *ourētēr,* ureter]. Between the two ureters. SYN: *interureteric.*

interureteric (īn″tĕr-ū-rī-tĕr′ĭk). Between the ureters. SYN: *interureteral.*

intervaginal (īn″tĕr-văj′ĭ-năl) [L. *inter,* between, + *vagina,* sheath]. Between sheaths.

in′terval ["+ *vallum,* a breastwork]. 1. The space or time between two objects or periods. 2. Break in the course of a disease or between paroxysms.

   i., a-c., atriocarotid i., auriculocarotid i. In a venous pulse-tracing, the i. between onset of the presystolic wave (a) and the systolic (c) wave. It indicates the time required for impulses to travel from S-A node to ventricle, normally about 0.2 sec.

   i., A-V. That between beginning of atrial systole and ventricular systole, measured in man from an electrocardiogram.

   i., c-a., cardio-arterial i. The time between apex beat and radial pulsation.

   i., focal. Distance between anterior and posterior focal point of the eyes.

   i., isometric. Between onset of ventricular systole and opening of the semilunar valves. SYN: *presphygmic,* q.v.

   i., lucid. Brief remission of symptoms in a psychosis.

   i., passive. The rest period of the heart.

   i., postsphygmic. I. between closure of the semilunar valves and opening of semilunar valves and opening of atrioventricular valves.

   i., presphygmic. Brief period between the ventricular systole and opening of the semilunar valves.

   i., QRST. The ventricular complex of the electrocardiogram.

intervas′cular [L. *inter,* between, + *vasculum,* a vessel]. Situated between blood vessels.

interventric′ular ["+ *ventriculum,* a small cavity]. Between the ventricles.

interver′tebral ["+ *vertebra,* joint]. Situated between two adjacent vertebrae.

   i. disk. Broad and flattened disk of fibrocartilage between the bodies of vertebrae.

intes′tinal [L. *intestinum,* intestine]. Pert. to the intestines. SEE: *digestion; intestine.*

   i. flora. The bacteria present in the intestines. The chemical nature of the contents of the intestines varies considerably with respect to the portion of the tract being considered.

   At birth no bacteria are present in the intestines but are found there very shortly therafter. Favorable bacteria may protect the body from invasion by unfavorable ones, which cannot thrive in an acid condition. Also, certain medicines, particularly antibiotics, may cause drastic alterations in the number and kinds of bacteria present.

   i. gases. Carbon dioxide; hydrogen; methane; methylmercaptan; and sulfurated hydrogen.

   i. juice. An imprecise term used to denote the liquid substances secreted into the intestine, esp. the small intestine. It contains a number of enzymes, peptidases, lipase, maltase, and sucrase. Each is important in digesting food.

i. obstruction. *Acute:* Small intestine usually involved. Due to intussusception, strangulation, volvulus (twists), foreign bodies, knots, adhesions, tumors, stricture, and gallstones in intestines. Auscultation of the abdomen may reveal a high-pitched tinkle or no sound at all. SYM: Pain localized and intense. Temperature subnormal or normal; vomiting, constipation and distention of abdomen.

Chronic: Involves large intestine. Due to stricture, inflammation, abscesses, tumors, fecal matter or chronic peritonitis; gallstones may obstruct feces. Gradual constipation, pain becoming more severe in few days followed by acute symptoms.

i. perforation, test for. Administration of 50-60 ml. of diatrizoate by mouth. If there is an i. perforation the substance will enter the peritoneal cavity, be absorbed and excreted in the urine. If the gastrointestinal tract is intact diatrizoate will not be absorbed. The test is negative if the i. perforation sealed off prior to administration of the dye.

Diatrizoate is detected in the urine by adding concentrated hydrochloric acid one drop at a time. Some antibiotics, particularly penicillin, will also cause a precipitation in the urine when hydrochloric acid is added. However diatrizoate in the urine causes a greater increase in specific gravity than penicillin.

i. putrefaction. The chemical changes by bacteria in the intestine, forming the following: indole; skatole; paracresol; phenol; phenylpropionic acid; phenylacetic acid; paraoxyphenylacetic acid; hydroparacumaric acid; fatty acids; carbon dioxide; hydrogen; methane; methylmercaptan; and sulfurated hydrogen.

i. reflex. I. contraction and relaxation above a portion of bowel which is stimulated.

intestine (ĭn-tĕs′tĭn) [L. *intestinum*]. The alimentary canal extending from the pylorus to the anus.

It is approx. 7.3 meters (24 feet) long, and is divided into the small i. and large i. or colon. The length of the i. given is based on measurements made at autopsy. During life the small i. is approx. three meters (9 feet, 10 inches) long.

The total surface of the inside of the small i. is estimated to be 800 square meters (8,611 square feet or 956.8 square yards).

PALPATION: Fecal accumulations feel like tumor but hard and resistant; but if one finger be pressed steadily upon them for one

or two minutes will indent; most frequently collect in descending colon.

PERCUSSION: In normal condition large i. furnishes a more amphoric percussion sound than the stomach. When filled with liquid or solid accumulations, the situation of these accumulations can be marked out on the surface by dullness on percussion. Because these accumulations most frequently occur in the descending colon, the percussion sound over this portion is usually less resonant than over the ascending or transverse colon.

i., large. The large i. extends from the ileum to the anus, and consists of cecum with vermiform appendix, colon, and rectum.

Mucous coat resembles that of small i., q.v., although glands are smaller.

The beginning of the large i. is the cecum, a pouch situated on right side, adjoining the ascending colon.

Attached to the cecum is the vermiform appendix about 7.5 to 10.4 cm. (3 to 4 inches) long.

The colon is approx. 1.5 meters (5 feet) in length. The first portion of ascending colon extends from the cecum to the under surface of the liver where it turns to the left as the transverse colon. Its bend is the right colic or hepatic flexure. The transverse colon passes horizontally to the left to the region of the spleen where it turns downward as the descending colon. This turn is the splenic flexure. The descending colon continues downward on the left side of the abdomen until it reaches the pelvic brim and curves like the letter S and is placed in front of the sacrum to become the rectum. This S-shaped section is known as the "sigmoid colon." The rectum, about 10.2 to 12.7 cm. (4 to 5 inches) long, passes downward to terminate in the lower opening of the tract, the anus or anal opening.

i., small. This begins with the duodenum, approx. 20.3 cm. to 25.4 cm. (8 to 10 inches) long, which receives the food mass from the stomach through the pylorus, the bile from the liver and gallbladder, and the pancreatic juice from the pancreas. It connects with the jejunum, about 2.5 meters (8 feet) long. The jejunum, in turn, joins the ileum or twisted intestine, about 3.7 meters (12 feet) long, which is attached to the large intestine by the ileocecal or colic valve that controls passage of food into large i.

In the wall of the small i. are found Brunner's glands, intestinal glands (crypts of Lieberkühn), blood and lymph vessels (lacteals), and lymphatic tissue in the form of solitary nodules or aggregated nodules (Peyer's patches).

Inner surface is thrown into folds (circular folds), and lining the entire surface are minute fingerlike villi through which the products of digestion (simple sugars, amino acids, and fatty acids and glycerol) are absorbed. The villi are from 0.5 to 1.5 mm. long and there are from 10 to 40 per sq. mm. of intestinal mucosa. SEE: *digestive system* for illustration.

intestinum (ĭn″tĕs-tĭ′nŭm) [L.]. Intestine.
> *i. crassum.* [NA] The large intestine.
> *i. rectum.* The rectum.
> *i. tenue.* [NA] The small intestine.

in′tima [L.]. Innermost coat of a structure, as a blood vessel. SYN: *tunica intima.*

intimal (ĭn′tĭm-ăl). Pert. to the inner coat of a blood vessel, the intima.

intimi′tis [L. *intima,* innermost, + Gr. *-itis,* inflammation]. Inflammation of an intima.

intol′erance [L. *in,* not, + *tolerare,* to bear]. Inability to endure or incapacity for bearing, as pain, or the effects of a drug or other substance.

intoxicant (in-toks′ĭ-cant). An agent which produces intoxication.

intoxica′tion [L. *in,* in, + Gr. *toxikon,* poison]. 1. State of being intoxicated, esp. of being poisoned by a drug or toxic substance. 2. Intoxicated from overindulgence in alcoholic beverages. 3. Drunk.

The determination of alcohol content of the blood (i.e., ethyl alcohol, the alcohol present in commercial beverages such as beer, wine, and whiskey) is frequently of value in the diagnosis of i. from alcohol, esp. in differentiating other disorders. Normally the alcohol content of body tissues and fluids is negligible. Upon ingestion, alcoholic fluids are absorbed slowly or quickly depending upon the amount swallowed, presence of food in the stomach, and rate of gastric emptying. The amount of alcohol found in each ml. of blood will also depend upon body size. Thus if 70 kg. (154 pound) and 90 kg. (198 pound) individuals drink the same amount of alcohol in the same time and under similar conditions, the concentration of alcohol in each ml. of blood will be least in the person who weighs the most. Results of blood alcohol determinations are expressed in mg. of alcohol present per ml. of blood.

The amount of alcohol present in expired air will also provide an estimate of the alcohol content of the blood. The amount of alcohol present in the blood does not provide completely valid information about the degree of i. because of the ability of the central nervous system to adapt to alcohol. SEE: *alcoholism; breatholyzer.*

> *i., water.* I. resulting from excessive intake or undue retention of water.

intra- [L.]. Prefix meaning within.

in″tra-abdom′inal [L. *intra,* within, + *abdomen,* belly]. Within the abdomen.
> *i. pressure.* Pressure within the abdomen.

intra-arte′rial ["+ Gr. *artēria,* artery]. Within the artery(ies).

intra-articular (ĭn″tră-ăr-tĭk′ū-lăr) ["+ *articulus,* little joint]. Within a joint.

intra-atrial (ĭn″tră-ā′trĭ-al) [L. *intra,* within, + Gr. *atrion,* hall]. Within the atrium or atria of the heart.

intracap′sular ["+ *capsula,* little box]. Within a capsule.
> *i. fracture.* One occurring within the capsule of a joint.

intracartilaginous (ĭn″tră-kăr″tĭ-lăj′ĭn-ŭs) ["+ *cartilago,* gristle]. Within a cartilage or cartilaginous tissue.

intracellular (ĭn″tră-sĕl′ū-lăr) ["+ *cellula,* cell]. Within cells.

intracra′nial ["+ Gr. *kranion,* skull]. Within the cranium or skull.

intracuta′neous [L. *intra,* within, + *cutis,* skin]. Within the substance of the skin. SEE: *intradermal.*
> *i. reaction.* One following injection of tuberculin into the skin.

intracys′tic ["+ Gr. *kystis,* bladder]. Inside a bladder or cyst.

intrad (ĭn′trăd). Inwardly; toward the inner part.

intrader′mal [L. *intra,* within, + Gr. *derma,* skin]. Within the substance of the skin. SYN: *intracutaneous.*

intradermoreaction (ĭn″tră-derm″ō-rē-ăk′shŭn) ["+ "+ L. *re,* back, + *agere,* to do]. Reaction resulting from the injection of a reagent into substance of the skin. SYN: *intracutaneous reaction.*

intraduct (ĭn′tră-dŭkt) ["+ *ductus,* a canal]. Inside a duct.

in″traduode′nal ["+ *duodeni,* twelve]. Within the duodenum.

intradu′ral ["+ *durus,* hard]. Within or enclosed by the dura mater.

intrafeb′rile ["+ *febris,* fever]. During the febrile stage.

intrafi′lar [L. *intra,* within, + *filum,* thread]. Within a network. or reticulum.

intragas′tric ["+ Gr. *gastēr,* belly]. Within the stomach.

intragem′mal ["+ *gemma,* bud]. Within a bud or the expanded ending of a nerve, as a taste bud.

intraglan'dular ["+ *glans*, acorn]. Within a gland.

intraintes'tinal [L. *intra*, within, + *intestinus*, internal]. Within the intestine.

intraligamen'tary ["+ *ligamentum*, a binding]. Within the leaves of a ligament.

Usually used in referring to fibroid tumors or cysts of the ovary that have grown within the broad ligament.

intraligamen'tous. Within a ligament.

intralo'bar [L. *intra*, within, + *lobus*, a lobe]. Within a lobe.

intralob'ular ["+ *lobulus*, a lobule]. Within a lobule.

intraloc'ular ["+ *loculus*, a cavity]. Within the cavity of any structure.

intralum'bar ["+ *lumbus*, loin]. Within the lumbar region or portion of the spinal cord.

intraluminal (ĭn″trä-lŭ'mĭ-năl) ["+ *lumen*, light]. Within any tubular structure. SYN: *intratubal.*

intramastoiditis (ĭn″trä-măs″toyd-ī'tĭs) ["+ Gr. *mastos*, breast, + *eidos*, form, + *-itis*, inflammation]. Inflammation of the antrum and mastoid process. SYN: *endomastoiditis.*

intramu'ral [L. *intra*, within, + *murus*, a wall]. Within the walls of a hollow organ or cavity.

intramus'cular ["+ *musculus*, a muscle]. Within a muscle.

    i. injection. Hypodermic injection of drugs into a muscle.

intranas'al ["+ *nasus*, nose]. Within the nasal cavity.

intraoc'ular ["+ *oculus*, eye]. Within the eyeball.

intraor'al ["+ *oralis*, pert. to the mouth]. Within the mouth.

intraor'bital ["+ *orbita*, mark of a wheel]. Within the orbit.

intraosseous (ĭn″trä-ŏs'ĭ-ŭs) [L. *intra*, within, + *os*, bone]. Within the bone substance.

intraparietal (ĭn″trä-pä-rī'ĕ-tăl) ["+ *pariēs*, wall]. 1. Within the parietal lobe of the cerebrum. 2. Intramural.

intraperitone'al ["+ Gr. *peritonaion*, peritoneum]. Within the peritoneal cavity.

intrapleu'ral ["+ Gr. *pleura*, rib]. Within the pleural cavity.

intrapon'tine ["+ *pons*, bridge]. Within the pons Varolii.

intrapsychic, intrapsychical (ĭn″trä-sī'kĭk, kī-kăl) [L. *intra*, within, + Gr. *psychē*, mind]. Having a mental origin or basis, such as conflicts and complexes.

intrapul'monary ["+ *pulmō*, lung]. Within the lung substance.

intrapyretic (ĭn″trä-pī-rĕt'ĭk) ["+ Gr. *pyretos*, fever]. During the period of fever. SYN: *intrafebrile.*

intraspi'nal [L. *intra*, within, + *spina*, spine]. 1. Ensheathed, within a sheath. 2. Within the spinal canal. SYN: *intrathecal.*

intrathecal (ĭn″trä-thē'kal) ["+ Gr. *thēkē*, sheath]. 1. Within spinal canal. 2. Within a sheath. SYN: *intraspinal.*

intrathoracic (ĭn″trä-thō-răs'ĭk) ["+ Gr. *thōrax*, chest]. Within the thorax.

intratracheal (ĭn″trä-trāk'ī-ăl) ["+ Gr. *tracheia*, trachea]. Introduced into, or inside, the trachea.

    i. anesthesia. A. administered through a catheter passed down the trachea.

in″tratu'bal [L. *intra*, within, + *tubus*, hollow tube]. Within a tube, esp. the fallopian tube.

in″tratympan'ic ["+ Gr. *tympanon*, drum]. Within the tympanic cavity.

intrauterine (ĭn″trä-ū'tĕr-ĭn) ["+ *uterus*, womb]. Within the uterus.

intravasation (ĭn-trăv″ä-zā'shŭn) ["+ *vas*, vessel]. Passage into the blood vessels of matter formed outside of them through traumatic or pathological lesions.

intravas'cular. Within blood vessels.

intravenous (ĭn-trä-vē'nŭs) [L. *intra*, within, + *vena*, vein]. Within or into a vein. ABBR: IV.

    i. department. A hospital department responsible for initiating intravenous therapy after it has been ordered by a physician. Services provided include administration of parenteral fluids, drugs in solution, blood or its components; hypodermoclysis collection of venous blood samples for laboratory studies, bacteriology, or blood bank.

    i. feeding. Providing total nutritional requirements intravenously; essential in treating some diseases. This is accomplished by carefully controlling the composition of fluid given with respect to total calories derived from protein hydrolysate and dextrose, and the electrolytes, minerals, and vitamins. Patients have been maintained for months on nothing but the nutrients and fluids given intravenously. SEE: *parenteral hyperalimentation.*

    i. infusion. Injection into a vein of a solution to secure an immediate result as in hemorrhage, shock, or collapse.

    SOLUTIONS: Many liquid preparations are given by i. infusion. Those commonly used include isotonic saline, Ringer's solution, 1/6 molar sodium lactate, dextrose 5% in water, potassium chloride 0.2% in 5% dextrose.

    QUANTITY: Depends on needs of patient. May be given 100 ml. or be given continuously at the rate of from 1 to 2 or more liters per day.

SITE: Median basilic or median cephalic vein.

Preparation same as for i. injection but a needle or cannula is used. The vein must be exposed if cannula is used. Introduction of solution should be very slow, usually from 60 drops/minute (using a 19-gauge needle) to 120 drops/minute (using a 26-gauge needle).

i. infusion pump. A special pump designed to provide constant but adjustable rate of flow of solutions given intravenously. The pump may work by applying intermittent pressure on the tubing carrying the solution so that the fluid is not actually in contact with the pump itself.

i. injection. Surface over skin is sterilized, tourniquet or bandage applied to middle of arm, the median cephalic or median basilic vein at front of elbow being used. Hypodermic needle is inserted in the vein, pointing upward. Pressure should be released before injection, which should be given very slowly.

i. medication. The injection of a sterile solution of a drug or an infusion into a vein.

i. treatment. This may consist of intravenous injection or intravenous infusion. The *injection* is usually known as the introduction of a small amount of solution into a vein with a hypodermic syringe. An *infusion* is usually known as the introduction of a solution in a larger quantity—250-500 ml. by means of a bottle connected to the needle by a plastic or rubber tubing. The rate of infusion may be regulated by adjusting the number of drops per minute. Flow is usually by gravity but can be given under pressure.

CAUTION: I.V. infusions should be discontinued or infusion fluid replenished when the bottle being administered is depleted. If this is not done it is possible for air to be introduced into the blood stream.

in″traventric′ular [L. *intra,* within, + *ventriculus,* ventricle]. Within a ventricle.

intravi′tal [″+ *vita,* life]. During period of living.

i. stain. One which when introduced into a living organism is taken up by living cells.

in′tra vi′tam [L.]. During life.

intravitelline (ĭn″tră-vĭ-tĕl′ĭn) [L. *intra,* within, + *vitellus,* yoke]. Within the vitelline or yolk.

intrin′sic [L. *intrinsicus,* on the inside]. Located entirely within or pertaining exclusively to a part.

i. factor. A substance prepared from animal intestines which, in humans, increases absorption of vitamin B complex.

i. muscles. Those which have their origin and insertion entirely within a struc-

ture, as the intrinsic muscles of the tongue, larynx, or eye.

intro- [L.]. Prefix meaning in or into.

introdu′cer [L. *intro,* into, + *ducere,* to lead]. Device for controlling, directing and placing an intubation tube within the trachea. SYN: *intubator.*

introflexion (ĭn″trŏ-flĕks′shŭn) [L. *intro,* into, + *flexus,* bent]. A bending inward.

introitus (ĭn-trŏ′ĭ-tŭs) [″+ *ire,* to go]. The opening or entrance into a canal or cavity, as the vagina.

i. canalis sacralis. Terminal opening of spinal canal at end of sacrum.

i. laryngis. Upper opening of larynx.

i. vaginae. Exterior orifice of vagina.

introjec′tion [″+ *jacere,* to throw]. In psychoanalysis, identification of the self with another, or with some object, the victim assuming the supposed feelings of the other personality.

intromission (ĭn″trŏ-mĭsh′ŭn) [″+ *mittere,* to send]. An insertion or placing of one part into another.

intromittent (ĭn-trŏ-mĭt′ĕnt). Conveying or injecting into a cavity or body.

introspec′tion [L. *intro,* within, + *spicere,* to look]. Looking within, esp. examination of one's own mind.

introsusception (ĭn″trŏ-sŭ-sĕp′shŭn) [″+ *suscipere,* to receive]. Intussusception, q.v.

introversion (ĭn″trŏ-vĕr′shŭn) [″+ *versio,* a turning]. 1. Turning inside out of a part or organ. 2. Condition of an introvert, q.v. Preoccupation with one's self.

in′trovert. A personality-reaction type characterized by withdrawal from reality; fantasy formation, and stress on the subjective side of life adjustments, seen pathologically in extreme form in schizophrenia. Opposed to extrovert, q.v.

intubate (ĭn′tū-bāt) [L. *in,* into, + *tuba,* a tube]. To insert a tube in a part, esp. the larynx. SEE: *catheterization.*

intubation (ĭn-tū-bā′shŭn). Insertion of a tube into any hollow organ, as into the larynx through the glottis for entrance of air, or to dilate a stricture.

POSITION: Patient held upright in lap of assistant, head upon assistant's left shoulder, arms secured by wrapping sheet about patient's body or being grasped by elbows. Another assistant stands behind patient with hands firmly grasping the head and holding gag in place. Patient so held that body, neck, and head are kept naturally in a straight line.

NP: Never leave patient alone, do not feed for two or three hours after intubation; nursing infants may go to breast, soft diet to others; keep on back with head and shoulders elevated to position of greatest comfort in breathing.

in'tubator. Device used in inserting a tube into the larynx. SYN: *introducer.*

intumesce (ĭn-tū-mĕs') [L. *intumescere*, to swell up]. To enlarge or swell.

intumes'cence. A swelling or the process of enlarging. SYN: *tumefaction.*

intumescent (ĭn-tū-mĕs'ĕnt). Swelling or becoming enlarged.

intussusception (ĭn"tŭ-sŭ-sĕp'shŭn) [L. *intus*, within, + *suscipere*, to receive]. Invagination. The slipping of one part of an intestine into another part just below it. Noted chiefly in children—usually in the ileocecal region.

PROG: Good, if surgery is performed immediately. High mortality rate if untreated within 24 hours. SEE: *ileus.*

intussuscep'tum. The inner segment of intestine which has been pushed into another segment.

intussuscipiens (ĭn"tŭ-sŭ-sĭp'ĭ-ĕns). That portion of intestine which receives the intussusceptum.

inulase (ĭn'ū-lās). An enzyme that converts inulin into levulose.

in'ulin. A polysaccharide found in plants. Yields levulose when hydrolyzed. It is used to study renal function.

inunction (ĭn-ŭngk'shŭn) [L. *in*, into, + *unguere*, to anoint]. Ointment or medicated substance rubbed into the skin, to secure a local or a more general systemic effect.

inustion (ĭn-ŭs'chŭn) ["+ *urere*, to burn]. 1. To apply cautery. 2. Deep cauterization.

in u'tero [L.]. Within the uterus.

in vac'uo. Within a cavity or a space from which air has been exhausted.

invaginate (ĭn-văj'ĭn-āt) [L. *in*, into, + *vagina*, sheath]. 1. To ensheath. 2. To insert one part of a structure within a part of the same structure; intussusception. 3. In embryology, to grow in or from an ingrowth or inpocketing, esp. the ingrowth of the wall of the blastula which results in the formation of the gastrula.

invag'inated. Enclosed in a sheath; ensheathed.

invagina'tion. The process of becoming ensheathed. SYN: *intussusception.* SEE: *evagination.*

in'valid [L. *in*, not, + *validus*, strong]. 1. Not well; weak. 2. A sickly person, particularly one who is confined to a bed or wheelchair.

inva'sion [L. *in*, in, + *vadere*, to go]. 1. That period of a disease following entrance of infective organisms and preceding the appearance of symptoms. 2. The entrance of

bacteria or other infectious organisms into the body and their distribution to the tissues.

invermina'tion ["+ *vermis*, worm]. Infestation by intestinal worms.

inverse-square law. The intensity of radiation at any distance is inversely proportional to the square of the distance between the irradiated surface and a point source. Thus a light with a certain intensity at four feet distance will have only one fourth that intensity at 8 feet and would be four times as intense at two feet distance.

inversion (ĭn-vĕr'zhŭn) [L. *in*, into, + *vertere*, to turn]. 1. Reversal of normal relationship. 2. Turning inside out of an organ, e.g., the uterus. 3. In chemistry, the process of converting sucrose (which rotates the plane of polarized light to the right) into a mixture of dextrose and levulose, which mixture rotates the plane to the left. The resulting mixture is called invert sugar, and the enzyme which catalyzes this conversion is called invertase. SEE: *enzyme.*

i., sexual. Deviation from normal sex relationship, diametrically opposite, i.e., sexual interest in one of the same sex. SYN: *homosexuality.*

i., uterine. A condition in which the fundus of the uterus protrudes through the cervix, and in some cases through the vaginal introitus. May be acute or chronic, the acute type usually occurring immediately postpartum as a result of too vigorous placental expression or pulling on the placental cord when the placenta is fixed in the uterus. The chronic type is usually due to tumors of the fundus uteri that pull themselves and the uterus through the cervix.

invert. 1. (ĭn'vert) One who, or that which, is opposite the normal. SEE: *homosexual.* 2. (ĭn-vert') To turn inside out or upside down.

i. sugar. A term usually applied to a mixture of levulose and dextrose, formed by inversion of sucrose by enzyme, invertase. SEE: *carbohydrates; inversion; sugar.*

invertase (ĭn-vĕr'tās). A sugar-splitting ferment or enzyme found in the intestinal juice. It causes the inversion of sugar. SYN: *invertin.*

inver'tebrate [L. *in*, not, + *vertebratus*, vertebrate]. Without a backbone; species of animals which do not have a backbone.

invertin (ĭn-vĕr'tĭn). An intestinal ferment which converts cane sugar into invert sugar. SYN: *invertase.*

invest'ing [L. *in*, in, + *vestire*, to clothe]. Ensheathing, encircling with a sheath or coating, as tissue; surrounding.

invest'ment. A covering or sheath.

invet'erate [L. *in*, into, + *vetus*, old]. Chronic; firmly seated, as a disease or a habit.

in vitro (in vī'trō) [L., in glass]. In glass, as in a test tube. Thus an in vitro test is one done in the laboratory rather than in a living organism as is the case with an in-vivo test or procedure.

in vivo (in vī'vō) [L., in the living body]. In the living body or organism. SEE: *in vitro.*

involucre, involucrum (in'vo-lu"ker, in"-vo-lu'krum) [L. *in*, in, + *volvere,* to wrap]. 1. A sheath or covering. 2. The covering of newly formed bone enveloping sequestrum in infection of bone.

invol'untary [L. *in*, not, + *voluntas*, will]. Independent of or even contrary to volition.

involution (ĭn"vō-lŭ'shŭn) [L. *in*, into, + *volvere*, to roll]. 1. A turning or rolling inward. 2. The reduction in size of the uterus following delivery. 3. The retrogressive change in vital processes after their functions have been fulfilled, such as the change which follows the menopause. 4. A backward change. 5. Diminishing of an organ in vital power or in size. 6. In bacteriology, digression from the usual morphological type such as occurs in certain bacteria, esp. when grown under unfavorable conditions; degeneration.

   i. forms. Bacteria possessing abnormal and unusual forms.

   i. of uterus. Return of uterus by absorption to normal size after childbirth.

   i., senile. Atrophy of an organ or part from old age.

   i., sexual. Cessation of menstrual function. SYN: *climacteric; menopause,* q.v.

involutional (ĭn-vō-lŭ'shŭn-ăl). Concerning involution or a turning inward.

   i. melancholia. Depressive psychosis which occurs during the involutional period (40 to 55 years of age in women; 50 to 65 in men). There is usually no previous history of mental illness. Characteristic symptoms include depression; delusions of sin, guilt or poverty; an obsession with death; imagined gastrointestinal-tract disease; and sometimes delusions of being persecuted. The patient manifests agitation and dejection.

   The condition may be successfully treated with antidepressant drugs or electroconvulsive therapy.

I. & O. Abbr. for *intake and output.*

Iodamoeba (ī"ō-dă-mē'bă). A genus of amebas found in the intestinal tract. Their cysts are peculiar in that they are irregular in shape, nucleus usually single, and they possess a vacuole filled with glycogen which stains brown in iodine.

   I. bütschlii. A small, sluggish ameba found in the large intestine of man. Also found in monkeys and pigs. It is usually nonpathogenic. SYN: *Endolimax williamsi.*

iodide (ī'ō-dīd). A compound of iodine containing another radical or element, as potassium iodide.

iodine (ī'ō-dīn, ī'o-dēn) [Gr. *ioeides,* violet colored]. SYMB: *I.* At. wt. 126.904; at. no. 53.; sp. gr. (solid, 20° C.) 4.93. A nonmetallic element belonging to the halogen group. It is a black, crystalline substance having a melting point of 113.5° C.; it boils at 184.4° C., giving off a characteristic violet vapor.

   FUNCTIONS: I. aids in development and functioning of the thyroid gland, formation of thyroxine and prevention of goiter; regulation of basal metabolic rate. The amount of iodine in the entire body averages 50 mg., of which one-third to one-fifth (10-15 mg.) is found in the thyroid. Butanol-extractable-iodine content of the serum varies from 3.5 to 6.5 micrograms per 100 ml. Protein-bound-serum iodine varies from 3.5 to 8.0 micrograms per 100 ml. Daily requirement for iodine is 50 to 75 micrograms. A growing child or a pregnant woman needs more than this amount. Those under emotional strain and adolescents likewise need more iodine.

   SYM. OF DEFICIENCY: I. deficiency in diet may lead to simple goiter characterized by thyroid enlargement and hypothyroidism. This may result in retardation of physical, sexual, and mental development in the young, a condition called cretinism.

   SOURCES: In vegetables, esp. those growing near the seacoast, and in seafoods, esp. in liver of halibut and cod or the fish-liver oils.

   POISONING SYM: Brown stains on lips and mouth; burning pain in mouth, throat and stomach; vomiting (blue vomitus if stomach contained starches, otherwise yellow vomitus); bloody diarrhea.

   F.A. TREATMENT: Give immediately by mouth a cornstarch or flour solution, 15 gm. in 500 ml. (2 cups) of water. Lavage with starch solution or 2% sodium-thiosulfate solution. Morphine for pain and mild stimulants as indicated. Following this therapy promote catharsis with 30 gm. of sodium sulfate and 15 gm. of starch in 250 ml. (one cup) of water. INCOMPATIBILITIES: Alkaloids.

   USES: Tincture of iodine (a 2 or 3% solution in alcohol) is used as a disinfectant and germicide. It is used as a preventative of simple goiter and, in the form of Lugol's solution, is invaluable in the treatment of exophthalmic goiter.

i., radioactive. I[131] an isotope of I with an at. wt. of 131. Used in diagnosis of thyroid disorders and in the treatment of toxic goiter and thyroid carcinoma.

i., tincture of. A 2% solution of iodine and sodium iodide in dilute alcohol.

iodism (ī′ō-dĭzm). Condition induced by prolonged and excessive use of iodine or its compounds. SEE: *iodine poisoning.*

i′odize. To administer or impregnate with iodine.

i′odized. Impregnated with iodine.

i. salt. Salt containing 0.5 to one part sodium or potassium iodide to 10,000 parts of sodium chloride. SEE: *salt.*

io′doform [Gr. *ioeides,* violet colored, + L. *forma,* form]. CHI₃. Yellow crystals having a disagreeable odor. Produced by the action of iodine on acetone in the presence of an alkali. Has mild antibacterial action. Is seldom used because its effectiveness has not been demonstrated.

io′doformism ["+ "+ Gr. *ismos,* state of]. Poisoning caused by iodoform.

iodophilia (ī′′ō-dō-fĭl′ĭ-ă) ["+ *philein,* to love]. Condition in which certain cells, when stained, esp. polymorphonuclear leukocytes, show a pronounced affinity for iodine, the cells acquiring a brownish-red color. Seen in pathologic conditions such as acute infections and anemia.

i., intracellular. I. in which color changes occur within the cells.

i., extracellular. I. in which substances in the plasma outside the cells are colored.

iodophor (ī′′ō-dō-for′). A combination of iodine and a solubizing agent or carrier which liberates free iodine in solution. Some forms are used as general antiseptics; they are less irritating than tincture of iodine. SYN: *tamed iodine.*

iodopyracet (ī′′ō-dō-pī′ră-sĕt). A radiopaque medium used in intravenous pyelography and urography. Proprietary name is Diodrast.

iodother′apy [Gr. *ioeides,* violet colored, + *therapeia,* treatment]. Use of iodine medication.

i′on [Gr. *iōn,* going]. Molecular constituent, i.e., one or more atoms, carrying an electric charge.

A particle carrying an electric charge, consisting of an atom or group of atoms into which the molecules of an electrolyte are divided; or one of the electrified particles into which the molecules of a gas are divided by ultraviolet rays, gamma rays, or X rays, or by other ionizing agents.

Ions occur in gases, esp. at low pressures, under the influence of strong electrical discharges, X rays, and radium; in solutions of acids, bases, and salts. Such moving particles render the gas or solution capable of conducting the electric current, and on reaching the electrodes they are discharged.

Ions which carry *positive* charges and which consequently discharge at the negative electrode (cathode) are called cations; examples are the hydrogen in aqueous solutions of acids and the sodium in aqueous solutions of sodium chloride.

Ions which carry *negative* charges will appear at the positive electrode (anode) and are, therefore, called anions; an example is the chlorine in aqueous solutions of hydrochloric acid or of sodium chloride. Thus the reaction in ionization of hydrogen chloride (hydrochloric acid) when dissolved in water is represented as

$$HCl \longrightarrow H^+ + Cl^-$$

It means that when the electric current is passed through the solution hydrogen gas will appear as bubbles at the cathode, while chlorine will appear at the anode.

ion-exchange resins. Synthetic organic substances of high molecular weight. They replace certain negative or positive ions which they encounter in solutions. Have been used to replace sodium ions in cases of edema, or to reduce the acidity of gastric juice.

ion′ic [Gr. *iōn,* going]. Pert. to ions.

i. medication. The introduction of chemical ions into the superficial tissues for medicinal purposes by means of a direct current.

The basic rules are: Substances of like electric charge repel each other; unlike forms attract each other. Bases, metallic radicals, and alkaloids are electropositive and should be placed at the positive pole. Acids and acid radicals are electronegative and should be placed at the negative pole. Ex: Potassium iodide for the introduction of free iodine should be placed at the negative pole, cocaine hydrochloride for local anesthesia at the positive pole. SYN: *iontophoresis 2,* q.v.

ioniza′tion. The dissociation of compounds (acids, bases, salts) into their constituent ions.

i′onize. To separate into ions; ionization, q.v.

i″onom′eter [Gr. *iōn,* going, + *metron,* measure]. An instrument consisting of an ionization chamber, an electroscope and an electric charging current designed to measure the amount of radiation used by roentgen rays or radium and to measure the intensity of the rays themselves.

ionotherapy (ī″ŏn-ō-thĕr′ă-pī) ["+ *therapeia*, treatment]. Introduction of ions into the body. SYN: *iontophoresis*.

iontophoresis (ī-ŏn″tō-fō-rē′sĭs) ["+ *phorein*, to carry]. 1. Process of electrical current traveling through salt solution causing migration of metal (positive) ion to negative pole and radical (negative) ion to positive pole. 2. Introduction of various ions into tissues through the skin by means of electricity. SYN: *ionic medication*.

iontoquantimeter (ī-ŏn″tō-kwŏn-tĭm′ĕtĕr) ["+ L. *quantus*, how much, + Gr. *metron*, measure]. Instrument used to measure the amount of radiation used by, and the intensity of, roentgen rays. SYN: *ionometer; iontoradiometer*.

iontoradiometer (ī-ŏn″tō-rā″dī-ŏm′ī-tĕr) ["+ L. *radius*, ray, + Gr. *metron*, measure]. Instrument for measuring the amount and intensity of roentgen rays. SYN: *ionometer*.

iontotherapy (ī-ŏn″tō-thĕr′ă-pī) ["+ *therapeia*, treatment]. Treatment by introducing ions into the body electrically.

IOP. Abbr. for *intraocular pressure*.

iophobia (ī″ō-fō′bĭ-ă) [Gr. *ios*, poison, + *phobos*, fear]. 1. Fear of being poisoned. SYN: *toxicophobia*. 2. Fear of touching any rusty object.

iotacism (ī-ō′tă-sĭzm) [Gr. *iōta*, letter i]. Defective utterance marked by constant substitution of an ē sound (Greek iota) for other vowels.

ipecac (ĭp′ē-kăk). USP. A dried root of the plant ipecacuanha grown in Brazil. It is the source of emetine.
   ACTION AND USES: Emetic.

IPPB. Abbr. for *intermittent positive pressure breathing, q.v.*

IPPV. Abbr. for *intermittent positive pressure ventilation*.

ipsilateral, ipselateral (ĭp″sĭ-lăt′ĕr-ăl) [L. *ipse*, same, + *latus*, side]. On the same side. Affecting the same side of the body.
   Thus, when the right patellar tendon is tapped, a knee-jerk is observed on the same side. Said of findings (paralysis) appearing on same side of body as brain or spinal cord lesion producing them. Opposed to crossed, contralateral. SYN: *homolateral*.

IPSP. Abbr. for *inhibition*.

IQ. Abbr. for *intelligence quotient*, q.v.

IR. Abbr. for *infrared*.

I.R. Abbr. for *internal resistance*.

Ir. Chem. symb. for iridium.

iral′gia [Gr. *iris*, rainbow, + *algos*, pain]. Pain felt in the iris. SYN: *iridalgia*.

irascible (ĭ-răs′ĭ-bl) [L. *irasci*, to be wrathful]. Marked by hot temper or ease of becoming angered.

iridadenosis (ĭr′ĭ-dăd-ĭ-nō′sĭs) [L. *iris*, iris, + Gr. *adēn*, gland, + *-ōsis*, increase]. A glandular affection of the iris.

iridal (ī′rĭd-ăl). Rel. to the iris.

iridalgia (ī″rĭd-al′jī-ă) [Gr. *iris*, iris, + *algos*, pain]. Pain felt in the iris. SYN: *iralgia*.

iridauxesis (ĭr′ī-dŏk-sē′sĭs) ["+ *auxēsis*, increase]. Increase in thickness of the iris.

iridectome (ĭr′ĭd-ĕk′tōm) ["+ *tomē*, a cutting]. Instrument for cutting the iris in iridectomy.

iridectomesodialysis (ĭr′ī-dĕk″tō-mēs″ō-dī-al′ī-sĭs) ["+ *ektomē*, excision, + *mesos*, middle, + *dialysis*, loosening]. Formation of an artificial pupil, by separating adhesions on inner margin of iris.

iridectomize (ĭr′ĭd-ĕk′tō-mīz) ["+ *ektomē*, excision]. To excise a portion of the iris.

iridec′tomy. Surgical removal of a portion of iris.
   i., optical. I. done for purpose of making an artificial pupil.

iridectropium (ĭr-ĭ-dĕk-trō′pĭ-ŭm) [Gr. *iris*, iris, + *ektropē*, a turning aside]. Partial eversion of the iris.

iride′mia ["+ *haima*, blood]. Bleeding from the iris.

iridencleisis (ĭr′ĭd-ĕn-klī′sĭs) ["+ *enklein*, to lock in]. Iris-inclusion operation; the iris being incarcerated in the wound, thereby forming a fistula lined with iris tissue. Performed in glaucoma.

iridentropium (ĭr′ĭ-dĕn-trō′pĭ-ŭm) ["+ *en*, in, + *tropein*, to turn]. Partial inversion of the iris.

irideremia (ĭr′ĭd-ĕr-ē′mĭ-ă) ["+ *erēmia*, lack]. Partial or total congenital absence of the iris. SYN: *aniridia*.

iridesis (ĭ-rĭd′ĕ-sĭs) ["+ *desis*, a binding]. Formation of an iris artificially, by ligation. SYN: *iridodesis*.

iridic (ĭ-rĭd′ĭk) [Gr. *iris*, iris]. Rel. to the iris. SYN: *iridal*.

iridis, rubeosis. A condition in which new blood vessels form on the anterior surface of the iris, associated with vascular disease which affects the retinal vein of the eye. Seen most frequently in diabetics although it is not limited to these patients. Leads to painful, hemorrhagic glaucoma.

iridium (ĭ-rĭd′ĭ-ŭm) [Gr. *iris*, rainbow]. SYMB: *Ir*. At. wt. 192.2; at. no. 77. A white, hard metallic element.

ir′ido- [Gr. *iris*, iris]. Combining form pert. to the iris.

iridoavulsion (ĭr′ĭ-dō-ăv-ŭl′shŭn) [Gr. *iris*, iris, + L. *avulsiō*, a pulling away from]. Tearing away (avulsion) of the iris.

iridocapsulitis (ĭr′ĭd-ō-kăp-sū-lī′tĭs) ["+ L. *capsula*, little box, + Gr. *-itis*, inflammation]. Iritis with inflammation of the capsule of the lens.

iridocele (ĭ-rĭd'ō-sēl) ["+ *kēlē*, hernia]. Protrusion of a portion of the iris through a defect in the cornea.

iridochorioiditis, iridochoroiditis (ĭr''ĭ-dō-kō''rĭ-oy-dĭ'tĭs, ĭr''ĭ-dō-kō-roy-dĭ'tĭs) ["+ *chorioeidēs*, skinlike]. Inflamed condition of both iris and choroid.

ir''idocolobo'ma ["+ *kolobōma*, mutilation]. Congenital defect or fissure of the iris.

iridocyclectomy (ĭr''ĭ-dō-sī-klĕk'tō-mĭ) [Gr. *iris*, iris, + *kyklos*, circle, + *ektomē*, excision]. Surgical removal of iris and ciliary body.

iridocyclitis (ĭr''ĭd-ō-sī-klī'tĭs) ["+ "+ *-itis*, inflammation]. Inflammation of iris and ciliary body.

iridocystectomy (ĭr''ĭ-dō-sĭs-tĕk'tō-mĭ) ["+ *kystis*, bladder, + *ektomē*, excision]. An operation for removal of a cyst from the iris.

iridodesis (ĭr-ĭ-dŏd'ĭ-sĭs) [Gr. *iris*, iris, + *desis*, a binding]. Ligature of part of iris to form an artificial one. SYN: *iridesis*.

ir''idodiagno'sis ["+ *dia*, through, + *gnōsis*, knowledge]. Diagnosis of disease by examination of the iris.

iridodialysis (ĭr''ĭd-ō-dī-ăl'ĭ-sĭs) ["+ *dialysis*, loosening]. The separation of the outer margin of the iris from its ciliary attachment.

iridodila'tor ["+ L. *dilatāre*, to dilate]. Substance causing dilatation of the pupil.

iridodonesis (ĭr''ĭd-ō-dō-nē'sĭs) ["+ *donēsis*, tremor]. Tremulousness of iris, seen in an aphakic eye or one with subluxated lens. SYN: *hippus*.

iridokeratitis (ĭr''ĭ-dō-kĕr''ă-tī'tĭs) [Gr. *iris*, iris, + *keras*, horn, + *-itis*, inflammation]. Inflammation of the iris and the cornea.

iridokinesis (ĭr''ĭd-ō-kĭn-ē'sĭs) ["+ *kinēsis*, motion]. The contracting and expanding movements of the iris.

iridoleptynsis (ĭr-ĭ-dō-lĕp-tĭn'sĭs) ["+ *leptynsis*, attenuation]. Thinning or atrophy of the iris.

iridology (ĭr-ĭ-dŏl'ō-jĭ) ["+ *logos*, study]. The study of changes in the iris during course of a disease.

iridomalacia (ĭr''ĭd-ō-mă-lā'shĭ-ă) ["+ *malakia*, softness]. Softening of the iris.

iridomedialysis (ĭr''ĭd-ō-mēd-ĭ-al'ĭ-sĭs) [Gr. *iris*, iris, + L. *medius*, in middle, + Gr. *dialysis*, loosening]. Separation of inner marginal adhesions of iris. SYN: *iridomesodialysis*.

iridomesodialysis (ĭr''ĭd-ō-mĕs''ō-dĭ-ăl'ĭ-sĭs) ["+ *mesos*, middle, + *dialysis*, loosening]. Separation of adhesions around the inner border of iris. SYN: *iridomedialysis*.

iridomo'tor ["+ L. *motor*, that which moves]. Rel. to movements of the iris.

iridon'cus [Gr. *iris*, iris, + *onkos*, bulk]. Tumefaction of the iris or development of a tumor.

ir''idoparal'ysis ["+ *paralysis*, a loosening]. Paralysis of the iris. SYN: *iridoplegia*.

iridoparelkysis (ĭr''ĭ-dō-păr-ĕl'kĭ-sĭs) ["+ *parelkysis*, protraction]. Dislocation of pupil due to prolapse of the iris. This is done surgically in order to displace the pupil.

iridoperiphacitis, iridoperiphakitis (ĭr''-ĭ-dō-pĕr''ĭ-fă-sī'tĭs, -pĕr''ĭ-fă-kī'tĭs) ["+ *peri*, around, + *phakos*, lens, + *-itis*, inflammation]. Inflammation of the iris and anterior portion of capsule of the lens.

iridoplegia (ĭr''ĭd-ō-plē'jĭ-ă) [Gr. *iris*, iris, + *plēgē*, stroke]. Paralysis of sphincter of iris.

i., accommodative. Inability of iris to contract when stimulated by accommodation.

i., complete. I. in which the iris fails to respond to any stimulation.

i., reflex. Absence of light reflex with retention of accommodation reflex (Argyll Robertson pupil, q.v.).

iridoptosis (ĭr''ĭ-dŏp-tō'sĭs) ["+ *ptōsis*, a falling]. Prolapse of the iris.

iridorrhexis (ĭr''ĭd-ō-rĕks'ĭs) ["+ *rhēxis*, rupture]. Rupture of or a tearing of the iris away from its attachment.

iridosclerotomy (ĭr''ĭd-ō-sklē-rŏt'ō-mĭ) ["+ *sklēros*, hard, + *tomē*, incision]. Piercing of the sclera and of the border of the iris.

iridosteresis (ĭr''ĭ-dō-stē-rē'sĭs) ["+ *sterēsis*, loss]. Removal of the iris or a portion of it.

iridot'asis ["+ *tasis*, a stretching]. Stretching the iris in treatment of glaucoma.

iridotomy (ir-ĭ-dot'ō-mĭ) ["+ *tomē*, incision]. Incision of iris without excising a portion, done for the purpose of making a new aperture in the iris when the pupil is closed. Indicated in eyes that had been operated on for cataract but which have lost their sight through subsequent iridocyclitis. Also done in seclusio pupillae. SYN: *iritomy; irotomy.*

i'ris [Gr.]. (pl. *irides*) The colored contractile membrane suspended between the lens and the cornea in the aqueous humor of the eye, separating the anterior and posterior chambers of the eyeball and perforated in the center by the pupil. It regulates by contraction and dilatation the entrance of light.

ANAT: The free inner edge rests on the lens when the pupil is contracted or partially dilated. The i. contains two muscles, the sphincter pupillae (circular fibers) about one millimeter wide, and the dilator pupillae (meridionally arranged fibers) extending from sphincter pupillae to root of i. The former is supplied through the oculomotor nerve with parasympathetic fibers derived from the ciliary ganglion; the latter by sympathetic fibers from the superior cervical ganglion.

The color of the iris depends on the pigment in the stroma cells and in the cells of the retinal layers.

SEE: *aniridia; choroidoiritis; heterochromia iridis; "irid-" words.*

i. bombé. Seen in annular posterior synechia (seclusio pupillae). The i. is bulged forward by the pressure of the aqueous humor which cannot reach the anterior chamber.

i., chromatic asymmetry of. Difference in color of the two irides (heterochromia). One may be blue or gray and the other brown. May occur in early iritis or cyclitis.

i. contraction reflex. Normal contraction on exposure to light.

i., piebald. Dark discoloration in irregularly shaped area. May be in one or both eyes.

I'rish moss. A genus of seaweeds: Chondrus crispus; a demulcent used in pharmacologic preparations. SYN: *carrageen.*

iritic (ī-rĭt'ĭk) [Gr. *iris,* iris]. Rel. to the iris.

iri'tis ["+ *-itis,* inflammation]. Inflammation of the iris.

SYM: Pain, photophobia, lacrimation, diminution of vision; the iris appears swollen, dull, and muddy; the pupil is contracted, irregular and sluggish in reaction.

TREATMENT: One per cent atropine is used, as an ointment or in drop form, frequently enough to keep the pupil dilated. Cortisone or hydrocortisone is used systemically as well as topically. If the primary disease causing the i. is known it should be treated. However, the etiology of i. is usually not known.

i., plastic. I. in which the fibrinous exudate forms new tissue.

i., primary. When the process develops in the iris itself. Seen in general diseases as syphilis, tuberculosis; metastatic in infectious diseases, gonorrhea and focal infections; also occurs in trauma and sympathetic ophthalmia.

i., purulent. One with a purulent exudate.

i., secondary. When the inflammation spreads from neighboring parts as diseases of cornea and sclera.

i., serous. Serum forming the exudate.

iritomy (ī-rĭt'ō-mī) ["+ *tomē,* incision]. Formation of an artificial pupil. SYN: *iridotomy; irotomy.*

iron (ī'ern) [AS. *iren;* L. *ferrum*]. SYMB: *Fe.* At. wt. 55.847; at. no. 26. A metallic element widely distributed in nature. Compounds (oxides, hydroxides, salts) exist in two forms: ferrous, in which i. has a valence of two, and ferric, in which it has a valence of three. It is widely used in the treatment of certain forms of anemia.

I. is essential for the formation of chlorophyll in plants, although it is not a constituent of chlorophyll. It is part of the hemoglobin molecule.

FUNCTIONS: Because it is essential to hemoglobin formation it is essential to life. I. is also present in enzymes which permit cellular respiration to occur. It plays a role in the nutrition of epithelial tissues. There are approximately four to five gm. of iron in the adult body, distributed as follows: 60-70% in hemoglobin, 15% in the iron-protein compound ferritin. The remainder is present in enzymes and myoglobin. I. is stored in the tissues principally as ferritin. I. is absorbed from the food in the small intestine; it passes, in the blood, to the bone marrow; here it is used in making hemoglobin which is incorporated in the red corpuscles. A corpuscle, after circulating in the blood for approximately 120 days, is destroyed, and its i. is used over again. The adult male requires from 0.5 to 1.0 mg. of i. a day. A female of menstrual age will require about double this amount. During pregnancy and lactation from two to four mg. of i. per day will be required. Prior to puberty and after menopause the female requires no more i. than the male.

Copper in the food is necessary for the utilization of i. It is stored in the body and is reused repeatedly. The infant's food is poor in i. so it draws upon its store to such an extent that the reserve supply may be exhausted before the child is six months old.

Because only a fraction of the i. present in food is absorbed, it is necessary to provide from 15 to 30 mg. of iron in the diet to be certain that 1.0 to 4.0 mg. will be absorbed.

Manganese and cobalt, in addition to copper, are necessary for proper utilization of iron.

Iron, as a component of hemoglobin, is essential in the transportation of oxygen. It is needed for tissue respiration and the development of blood cells.

DEFICIENCY SYM: Anemia, lowered vitality, pale complexion, retarded development, decreased amt. of hemoglobin in each red cell.

NOTE: Sometimes a disturbance in iron metabolism occurs in which an iron-containing pigment, hemosiderin, and hemofuscin are deposited in the tissues. This gives rise to hemochromatosis. Excessive deposition of hemosiderin in the tissues, such as may occur as a result of excessive breakdown of red cells, is called hemosiderosis.

SOURCES: Almonds; asparagus; bran; beans; cauliflower; celery; chard; dandelions; Boston brown bread; graham bread; egg yolk; kidney; lettuce; liver; oatmeal; oysters; soy beans; whole wheat. Other good sources are apricots; greens; beets; beef; cabbage; cucumbers; currants; dates; duck; goose; lamb; molasses; oranges; parsnips; peppers; peas; potatoes; prunes; radishes; raisins; rhubarb; pineapple; tomatoes; peanuts; turnips; cornmeal; mushrooms. There is less i. in carrots and milk than in other foods. Only 50% of the i. in spinach and similar vegetables is assimilable by the body.

irot'omy [Gr. *iris,* iris, + *tomē,* incision]. Formation of an artificial pupil. SYN: *iridotomy; iritomy.*

irra'diate [L. *in,* into, + *radiare,* to emit rays]. To administer X rays or other forms of radiation.

irra'diating. Diverging or spreading out from a common center.

irradia'tion. 1. Therapeutic application of roentgen rays, radium rays, ultraviolet rays or other radiation to a patient. 2. Application of form of radiation to an object or substance to give it therapeutic value, or increase that which it already has. 3. Phenomenon in which a bright object on a dark background appears larger than a dark object of the same size on a bright background. 4. The spreading in all directions from a common center, as nerve impulses, the sensation of pain.

RS: heliotherapy; radium; ray; roentgen; roentgen; ultraviolet.

i., interstitial. Therapeutic i. by the insertion into the tissues of capillary tubes containing radon.

i. of reflexes. The spread of a reflex to an increasing number of motor units upon increasing the strength of the stimulus.

irreducible (ĭr″rē-dū′sĭ-bl) [L. *in,* not, + *rē,* back, + *ducere,* to lead]. Not capable of being reduced or made smaller.

irrel'evance ["+ *relevans,* raising]. Inappropriate to or unrelated to that which was asked or being discussed.

irrespirable (ĭr″rē-spī′rā-bl) ["+ *respirare,* to breathe again]. Unfit for breathing, as a gas, or incapable of being breathed.

ir'rigate [L. *in,* into, + *rigare,* to carry water]. To wash out with a fluid.

ir″riga'tion. The cleansing of a canal (as the throat, ear, or colon) by flushing with water or other fluids; the washing of a wound.

Solutions should be sterile and have an approx. temperature slightly warmer than body temperature (100° to 115° F. or 37.8° to 46.1° C.).

i., bladder. Washing out of bladder for treatment of inflammation.

NP: *Articles Needed:* The same as for a catheterization plus: Sterile funnel about three in. diameter; solution ordered, in sterile pitcher, covered and warmed to 105° F. (40.6° C.); bedpan.

If medication is ordered for instillation following i. have it ready in medicine glass covered with fold of sterile gauze.

Procedure: The patient may be placed on the bedpan and catheterized or she may be catheterized first and the pan put in place after that. Catheterize but do not remove catheter. Attach funnel to free end of catheter; do not put your fingers inside funnel. Hold funnel up and pour full of solution, allowing almost all of it to run in; then refill. Do this three times and the 4th time fill funnel and turn it down quickly toward bedpan. This will siphon off contents of bladder. Repeat until amount of solution ordered has been used or until solution returns clear. If irrigating can is used, attach small end of connector to catheter and let four oz. of solution flow in gently. Detach catheter and allow fluid to run out into bedpan. Repeat. If return-flow catheter is used just keep solution running gently, as it will return by other side of catheter. Run medication ordered through catheter as soon as i. is finished. Remove catheter so that medicine does not drain out of the bladder. Care for patient and equipment.

Record treatment including the following information: *Bladder Irrigation:* Time. By whom done. Solution used: kind; amount; temperature. Appearance of return flow: bloody; mucus shreds; etc. Medication instilled. Reaction of patient.

i., colonic. The flushing of the colon with water. SEE: *colonic i.*

ir″riga'tor. Device with hose attachment used for purpose of flushing or washing a part or cavity with fluids.

ir″ritabil'ity [L. *irritare,* to tease]. 1. Excitability. 2. The ability to respond in a specific way to a change in environment, a property of all living tissue. 3. Condition in which a person, organ, or a part responds excessively to a stimulus. 4. Quick response to annoyance; impatience.

i., muscular. Normal response of muscle to a stimulus.

i., nervous. Response of a nerve to stimulus.

ir'ritable. 1. Capable of reacting to a stimulus. 2. Sensitive to stimuli.

i. colon syndrome. SEE: *colon syndrome, i.*

i. heart. A syndrome characterized by forceful uncomfortable heart beats; tachycardia; atrial flutter and fibrillation; faintness; fatigue and other symptoms. SYN: *anxiety neurosis; effort syndrome; neurocirculatory asthenia.*

ir'ritant. An agent which, when used locally, produces more or less local inflammatory reaction. Anything which induces or gives rise to irritation. Ex: iodine.

i. poisons. These include a large number of poisons of great variety, not including the corrosive acids or alkalies. They cause pain in the mouth, esophagus, and stomach; nausea; vomiting; great thirst; abdominal cramping; bloody diarrhea; diminished urine.

TREATMENT: Varies. SEE: *Table of Poisons and Poisoning* in *Appendix.*

irrita'tion. 1. Reaction to that which is irritating. 2. Extreme reaction to pain or pathological conditions. 3. Normal response to stimulus of a nerve or muscle.

i., spinal. A neurasthenic condition characterized by tenderness along the spinal column, numbness and tingling in the limbs, and susceptibility to fatigue.

i., sympathetic. The response of an organ to i. in another organ.

ir'ritative. Pert. to that which causes irritation.

I.S. Abbr. for *intercostal space.*

ischemia (ĭs-kē'mĭ-ă) [Gr. *ischein,* to hold back, + *haima,* blood]. Local and temporary anemia due to obstruction of the circulation to a part.

ischesis (ĭs-kē'sĭs). Suppression of a discharge, esp. a normal one.

ischiac, ischiadic (ĭs'kĭ-ăk, ĭs-kĭ-ăd'ĭk). Ischiatic.

ischial (ĭs'kĭ-al) [Gr. *ischion,* hip]. Pert. to the ischium.

ischialgia (ĭs''kĭ-al'jĭ-ă) [" + *algos,* pain]. Neuralgic pain in the hip. SYN: *sciatica.*

ischiatic (ĭs-kĭ-at'ĭk) [Gr. *ischion,* hip]. Pert. to ischium or hip bone. SYN: *sciatic.*

ischiatitis (ĭs''kĭ-ă-tī'tĭs) [" + *itis,* inflammation]. Sciatic nerve inflammation.

ischidrosis (ĭs-kĭ-drō'sĭs) [Gr. *ischein,* to hold back, + *hidrōsis,* sweat]. Suppression of perspiration.

ischio- [Gr. *ischion,* hip]. Prefix pert. to the ischium.

ischiobulbar (ĭs''kĭ-ō-bŭl'băr) [" + L. *bulbus,* bulb]. Rel. to the ischium and urethral bulb.

ischiocavernosus (ĭs''kĭ-ō-kăv-ĕr-nō'sŭs) [" + L. *cavernosus,* cavernous]. A muscle extending from the ischium to the penis or clitoris. It assists in the erection of these structures.

ischiocele (ĭs'kĭ-ō-sēl) [" + *kēlē,* hernia]. Hernia through the sciatic notch.

ischiococcygeus (ĭs''kĭ-ō-kŏk-sĭj'ĭ-us) [" + *kokkyx,* coccyx]. 1. Coccygeus muscle. 2. Posterior portion of the levator ani.

ischiofemoral (ĭs''kĭ-ō-fĕm'or-ăl) [Gr. *ischion,* hip, + L. *femur,* thigh]. Rel. to the ischium and femur.

ischiofib'ular [" + L. *fibula,* buckle]. Rel. to the ischium and fibula.

ischiohebotomy (ĭs''kĭ-ō-hē-bŏt'ō-mī) [" + *hēbē,* pubes, + *tomē,* incision]. Surgical division of the ascending ramus of the pubes and the ischiopubic ramus. SYN: *ischiopubiotomy.*

ischiomenia (ĭs''kĭ-ō-mē'nĭ-ă) [Gr. *ischein,* to suppress, + *mēniaia,* menses]. Ischomenia, q.v.

ischioneuralgia (ĭs''kĭ-ō-nū-răl'jĭ-ă) [Gr. *ischion,* hip, + *neuron,* nerve, + *algos,* pain]. Neuralgic pain in the hip. SYN: *sciatica.*

ischiopubic (ĭs''kĭ-ō-pū'bĭk) [" + L. *pubes,* the pubes]. Rel. to the ischium and pubes.

ischiopubiotomy (ĭs''kĭ-ō-pū''bĭ-ŏt'ō-mī). Ischiohebotomy, q.v.

is''chiorec'tal [Gr. *ischion,* hip, + L. *rectus,* straight]. Pert. to the ischium and rectum.

i. abscess. Collection of pus in fatty tissue on either side of rectum.

ischium (ĭs'kĭ-ŭm) [Gr. *ischion,* hip]. (pl. *is'chia*) Lower portion of the innominate or hip bone.

ischo- (ĭs'kō) [Gr. *ischein,* to hold back]. Prefix meaning to suppress or restrain.

ischogalactic (ĭs''kō-gă-lăk'tĭk) [" + *gala,* milk]. 1. Causing suppression of breast milk. 2. Agent which checks milk secretion. SYN: *antigalactic.*

ischomenia (ĭs''kō-mē'nĭ-ă) [" + *mēniaia,* menses]. Menstrual suppression or retention.

ischuretic (ĭs''kū-rĕt'ĭk) [" + *ouron,* urine]. 1. Relieving or pert. to ischuria. 2. That which relieves urinary retention or suppression.

ischuria (ĭs-kū'rĭ-ă) [" + *ouron,* urine]. Suppression or retention of the urine.

island (ī'land) [AS. *igland,* island]. A structure detached from surrounding tissues, or characterized by difference in structure; an islet.

i.'s of Calleja. Groups of densely packed, small cells in the cortex of the gyrus hippocampi.

i.'s of Langerhans. Clusters of cells in the pancreas. The cells are of three types: alpha, beta, and delta cells. The beta cells are found in greatest abundance and produce insulin. Destruction or impairment of function of the i's may result in diabetes or hypoglycemia.

   i., pancreatic. I.'s of Langerhans, q.v.

   i. of Reil. The insula, a lobe of the cerebral cortex comprising a triangular area lying in the floor of the lateral or sylvian fissure. It is overlapped and hidden by the gyri of the fissure which constitute the operculum of the insula.

islet (ī'lĕt). A tiny isolated mass of one kind of tissue within another type.

   i.'s of Calleja. SEE: *islands of Calleja.*

   i.'s of Langerhans. SEE: *islands of Langerhans.*

-ism [Gr. *ismos*]. Suffix meaning condition or theory of; principle or method.

iso- [Gr. *isos*, equal]. Combining form meaning equal.

isoagglutinin (ī″sō-ă-glū'tĭn-ĭn) [Gr. *isos*, equal, + L. *agglutinare*, to glue to]. Antibody in a serum which agglutinates the blood cells of those of the same species from which it is derived.

   RS: agglutinin; blood grouping; isohemagglutinin.

isoagglutinogen (ī″sō-ă-glū-tĭn'ō-jěn). One of two substances designated A and B which may be present in red blood cells. Cells containing these substances become agglutinated when mixed with serum containing corresponding isoagglutinins (*a* or *b*).

isobar (ī'sō-băr) [Gr. *isos*, equal, + *baros*, weight]. In chemistry, one of two or more chemical bodies having same atomic weight, but with different atomic numbers.

isobaric (ī″sō-băr'ĭk). Specific gravity equal to that with which it is being compared. Thus an anesthetic solution used in spinal anesthesia if isobaric would be of the same specific gravity as the spinal fluid.

isocel'lular [Gr. *isos*, equal, + L. *cellula*, cell]. Composed of equal and similar cells.

isochromatic (ī″sō-krō-măt'ĭk) [″+ *chrōma*, color]. 1. Having the same color. 2. Of uniform color.

isochromatophil(e (ī″sō-krō-măt'ō-fĭl, -fīl) [″+ ″+ *philein*, to love]. Having the same affinity for a dye.

isochronal (ī-sŏk'rō-năl) [″+ *chronos*, time]. Acting in uniform time, or taking place at regular intervals. SYN: *isochronic; isochronous.*

isochroous (ī-sŏk'rō-ūs) [″+ *chroa*, color]. Of uniform color. SYN: *isochromatic.*

isocitric dehydrogenase. An enzyme present in serum. Its serum level is increased in diseases which cause liver cell necrosis. The level in cerebrospinal fluid is increased in meningitis and in patients with cerebral tumors.

isocolloid (ī-sō-kŏl'oyd) [Gr. *isos*, equal, + *kollōdēs*, glutinous]. A colloid having the same composition in various transformation.

isocom'plement [″+ L. *complere*, to complete]. One from the same individual or species which provides the amboceptor.

isocoria (ī″sō-kō'rī-ă) [″+ *korē*, pupil]. Equality of size of both pupils. SEE: *anisocoria.*

i″so-cort'ex [″+ L. *cortex*, bark]. The neopallium or non-olfactory portion of the cerebral cortex. It is composed of six layers of fibrous and cellular tissue having a similar distribution pattern. SYN: *neopallium.*

isocytotoxin (ī″sō-sī″tō-tŏk'sĭn) [″+ *kytos*, cell, + *toxikon*, poison]. A cytotoxin destructive to homologous cells of the same species.

isodactylism (ī-sō-dăk'tĭl-ĭzm) [Gr. *isos*, equal, + *daktylos*, finger]. Condition of having fingers or toes of equal length.

isodiametric (ī″sō-dī-ă-mět'rĭk) [″+ *dia*, across, + *metron*, measure]. Having equal diameters.

isoelectric (ī″sō-ĭ-lĕk'trĭk) [″+ *ēlektron*, amber]. Having equal electric potentials.

i″soenerget'ic [″+ *energeia*, energy]. Showing equal force or activity.

isoenzyme (ī″sō-ĕn'zīm) [Gr. *isos*, equal, + *en*, in, + *zymē*, leaven]. One of several forms in which an enzyme may exist in various tissues. Although the i.'s are similar in catalytic qualities, they may be separated from each other by special chemical tests. SYN: *isozyme.* SEE: *lactic dehydrogenase.*

isogam'ete [″+ *gametē*, wife, *gametēs*, husband]. 1. A cell which, through conjugation or fusion with a similar cell, reproduces. 2. A gamete of the same size as the one with which it fuses or unites.

isogenesis (ī″sō-jěn'ĭ-sĭs) [″+ *genesis*, production]. Similarity in morphological development.

i'sograft [Gr. *isos*, equal, + L. *graphium*, grafting shoot]. A graft taken from another individual or animal of the same genotype as the recipient. SEE: *autograft.*

isohemagglutinin (ī″sō-hěm″ă-glū'tĭn-ĭn) [″+ *haima*, blood, + L. *agglutinare*, to glue to]. Substance normally present in most human blood serum; responsible for the clumping of corpuscles observed when incompatible bloods are mixed.

The clumping is ascribed to the interaction of an agglutinogen in the corpuscles with a specific agglutinin in the foreign serum. In transfusions, the corpuscles of the donor are exposed to an overwhelming quantity of the recipient's plasma; therefore the agglutinogen content of the donor's corpuscles and the agglutinin content of the recipient's serum are the factors which determine compatibility.

Assuming that there are but two possible agglutinogens, red corpuscles from a given donor may contain both, either, or neither. If the agglutinin, alpha, can react only with agglutinogen A, one can construct a table from which compatibilities can be deduced (Jansky system). SEE: *agglutinin; blood groups* for table.

i"**sohemol′ysin** ["+ "+ *lysis,* dissolution]. Substance destroying red blood corpuscles of animals of same species from which it is obtained. SYN: *isolysin.* SEE: *hemolysin.*

i"**sohemol′ysis.** Action of an isohemolysin. SYN: *isolysis.*

isohypercytosis (ī″sō-hī′pĕr-sī-tō′sĭs) [Gr. *isos,* equal, + *hyper,* over, + *kytos,* cell, + *-ōsis,* increase]. Increase of leukocytes, the proportion of varieties being unchanged.

isohypocytosis (ī″sō-hī′pō-sī-tō′sĭs) ["+ *hypo,* under, + *kytos,* cell, + *-ōsis,* increase]. Decrease in number of leukocytes with proportion of varieties unchanged.

isoiconia (ī″sō-ī-kō′nĭ-ă) [Gr. *isos,* equal, + *eikōn,* image]. Equality of both retinal images.

isoiconic (ī″sō-ī-kŏn′ĭk). Having equal retinal images.

i"**soimmuniza′tion** [Gr. *isos,* equal, + L. *immunis,* safe]. Immunization of an individual against the blood of an individual of the same species, esp. the development of Rh-agglutinins in an Rh-mother in response to agglutinogens present in transfused Rh + blood or developed in an Rh + fetus.

i′**solate** [It. *isolato,* isolated]. 1. To separate or detach from other persons, as during an infectious disease. 2. In chemistry, to obtain a substance in pure form from the mixture or solution which contains it.

isola′tion. Limitation of movement and social contacts of patient suffering from, or a known carrier of, communicable disease, in contradistinction to quarantine, which limits the movements of exposed or contact persons. SYN: *sequestration.* SEE: *quarantine.*

NP: A patient is placed in i. to prevent the spread of the disease-causing agents. These general rules should be followed in order to confine the organisms to the isolated area

and to protect those caring for the isolated patient: Consider as contaminated everything in the room or area with which the patient is in direct or indirect contact. The hands of the nurse or attendant are the commonest means of carrying the infection. Therefore, thorough scrubbing, rinsing, and keeping them away from the face are the most important means of control.

Burn, boil, or disinfect all contaminated material such as dishes, uneaten food, linens, all body discharges, and utensils. Upon leaving the patient, gowns, masks, and caps used in the sickroom should be removed and left at the entrance to the area. Contact the local health authorities, and the doctor or hospital in charge of the case for specific imformation about procedure to be followed in individual cases.

i. ward. Hospital ward where patients suffering from communicable diseases may be kept apart from the rest of the patients.

isoleucine (ī″sō-lū′sēn). An amino acid formed during hydrolysis of fibrin and other proteins. It is essential in the diet.

isolophobia (ī″sō-lō-fō′bĭ-ă) [It. *isolato,* isolated, + Gr. *phobos,* fear]. Fear of being alone.

isolysin (i-sŏl′ĭ-sĭn) [Gr. *isos,* equal, + *lysis,* dissolution]. Substance which dissolves red corpuscles of animals of the same species from which it is obtained. SYN: *isohemolysin.*

isol′ysis. Destruction of red blood corpuscles produced by an isolysin. SYN: *isohemolysis.* SEE: *hemolysis.*

isolyt′ic. Rel. to isolysis.

isomer (ī′sō-mĕr) [Gr. *isos,* same, + *meros,* part]. One of two or more chemical substances which have the same molecular formula but different chemical and physical properties due to different arrangement of the atoms in the molecule. Dextrose is an isomer of levulose. SEE: *metamere; polymer.*

isomeric (ī″sō-mĕr′ĭk). Pertaining to isomerism, q.v.

isomerism (i-sŏm′ĕr-ĭzm). State of being composed of compounds of the same number of atoms, but having different atomic arrangement in the molecule. SEE: *metamerism, polymerism.*

isomet′ric [Gr. *isos,* equal, + *metron,* measure]. Having equal dimensions. SEE: *isotonic.*

i. contraction. C. of a muscle in which shortening or lengthening is prevented. Tension is developed but no mechanical work performed, all energy being liberated as heat.

i. contraction phase. The first phase in contraction of the ventricle in which ventricular pressure increases but there is no decrease in volume of contents because semilunar valves are closed.

i. muscle. Contraction in which a muscle increases its tension without shortening.

isometro'pia ["+ "+ ōps, eye]. Same refraction of the two eyes.

isomor'phism ["+ morphē, form, + ismos, state of]. Condition marked by possession of the same form.

isomorphous (ī"sō-mor'fūs). Possessing the same shape.

isoniazid (ī"sō-ni'ă-zĭd). USP. C₆H₇N₃O. An odorless compound occurring as colorless or white crystals or as a white crystalline powder. An antibacterial, used principally in treating tuberculosis. SYN: *isonicotinic acid hydrazide.*

isonormocytosis (ī"sō-nor"mō-sī-tō'sīs) [Gr. *isos,* equal, + L. *norma,* rule, + Gr. *kytos,* cell, + *-ōsis,* condition]. State of having leukocytes of the blood normal in number and proportion of varieties.

isop'athy ["+ pathos, disease]. Therapeutic administration of the causative agent of the disease or its products. SYN: *isotherapy.*

isophoria (ī"sō-fō'rĭ-ă) ["+ phorein, to carry]. Equal tension of vertical muscles of the eyes with visual lines in same horizontal plane both hyperphoria, q.v., and hypophoria, q.v., being absent.

isoplastic (ī"sō-plăs'tĭk) [Gr. *isos,* equal, + *plastos,* formed]. Term applied to a graft taken from one individual and transplanted to another of the same species. SEE: *isograft.*

isoserother'apy (ī"sō-sē"rō-thĕr'ă-pĭ) ["+ L. *serum,* whey, + Gr. *therapeia,* therapy]. Treatment with serum from one having had the same disease as the patient.

isose'rum. A serum from one having had the disease for which a patient is to receive treatment.

isosmotic (ī"sŏs-mŏt'ĭk) [Gr. *isos,* equal, + *ōsmos,* impulsion]. Having the same total concentration of osmotically active molecules or ions in solution as the solution or body fluid to which it is being compared. SEE: *isotonic.*

Isospora. A genus of Sporozoa belonging to the order Coccidia.

I. hominis. A parasitic protozoon inhabiting the small intestine of man. It is nonpathogenic.

isosthenuria (ī"sōs-thĕn-ū'rĭ-ă) [Gr. *isos,* equal, + *sthenos,* strength, + *ouron,* urine]. Condition of the urine being of a uniform specific gravity and osmolarity despite

variations in fluid intake. A sign of marked impairment of renal function.

isostimula'tion ["+ L. *stimulare,* to goad]. Stimulation of an animal by the use of antigenic material derived from another animal of the same species.

isother'apy ["+ therapeia, treatment]. Treatment of disease by active causative agent of the same disease. SYN: *isopathy.*

isother'mal ["+ thermē, heat]. Being at or having equal temperature.

isothermognosis (ī"sō-thĕrm"ŏg-nō'sīs) ["+ "+ gnōsis, knowledge]. Abnormal perception in which stimulation by pain, heat, and cold are all felt as heat.

isoto'nia ["+ tonos, tone]. The state of equal osmotic pressure of two or more solutions or substances.

isotonic (ī"sō-tŏn'ĭk). 1. Having the same tension or tone. Said of muscles in physiology. An isotonic muscle contraction occurs when equal tension on the muscle is maintained while the length of the muscle is decreased during the performance of work or exercise. SEE: *isometric.* 2. Having the same osmotic pressure.

i. solution. A solution which has a concentration of electrolytes, nonelectrolytes, or a combination of the two which will exert equivalent osmotic pressure as that solution with which it is being compared. Ex: Either 0.16 molar sodium chloride solution (approx. 0.95% salt in water) or 0.3 molar nonelectrolyte solution is approx. isotonic with human red blood cells.

isotonicity (ī"sō-tō-nĭs'ĭ-tĭ). The state or condition of being isotonic.

isotope (ī'sō-tōp) [Gr. *isos,* equal, + *topos,* place]. One of a series of chemical elements which have nearly identical chemical properties but which differ in their atomic weights and electric charge. Many isotopes are radioactive.

i. cisternography. Use of a radioactive tracer to investigate the circulation of cerebrospinal fluid. A tracer such as I¹³¹ serum albumin is injected in the lumbar subarachnoid space. Flow of the tracer toward the head and into areas of the brain can be recorded by means of serial scintillation scanning. This technique is useful in studying hydrocephalus.

isotropic (ī"sō-trŏp'ĭk) ["+ tropos, a turning]. 1. Possessing similar qualities in every direction. 2. Having equal refraction.

isotyp'ical ["+ typos, mark]. Belonging to the same variety or classification.

issue (ĭsh'ū) [L. *exīre,* to go out]. 1. Offspring. 2. A suppurating sore maintained by a

Rocky Mountain spotted fever, relapsing fever, and tularemia.

ixomyelitis (īks″ō-mī-ĕ-lī′tĭs) [Gr. *ixōdes*, like birdlime, + *myelos,* marrow, + *-itis,* inflammation]. Inflammation of the spinal cord in the lumbar region.

J

J. Symb. for *joule.*

Jaboulay's button (zŏ″bū-lă′). [Mathieu Jaboulay, Fr. suregon, 1860-1913] Two cylinders which may be screwed together for lateral intestinal anastomosis.

jack′et [O.Fr. *jacquet,* jacket]. A plaster-of-Paris or leather bandage applied to the trunk to immobilize spine or correct deformities.

    j., Sayre′s. Plaster-of-Paris jacket used as a support for deformity of the spinal column.

    j., strait. Device for restraining a patient or criminal who is violent. It has sleeves which extend beyond the hands. The ends of these may be secured, thereby preventing movement of the arms and trunk. SYN: *camisole.*

jack-knife position. Position in which the patient lies on the back with shoulders elevated, thighs flexed on abdomen, legs on thighs, the thighs being at right angles to the abdomen. Employed when passing a urethral sound. SYN: *reclining position.*

jackscrew. A threaded screw used for expanding the dental arch.

jackson′ian ep′ilepsy. [John Hughlings Jackson, Brit. neurologist, 1835-1911] A localized form of epilepsy with spasms confined to one part or one group of muscles. SEE: *epilepsy.*

Jacob's mem′brane. [Arthur Jacob, Irish opthalmologist, 1790-1874] Retinal layer of rods and cones.

Jacob's ulcer. Epithelioma, usually of the face, which slowly destroys soft tissue and bones. SYN: *rodent ulcer,* q.v.

Ja′cobson's car′tilage. [Ludwig Jacobson, Dan. anatomist, 1783-1843] One of two narrow longitudinal cartilages lying along anterior portion of inferior border of nasal septum. They are rudimentary in man.

Jacobson's nerve. Nervus tympanicus.

Jacobson's organ. Rudimentary sac in nasal septum. SYN: *vomeronasal organ.*

Jacobson's sulcus. Portion of middle ear containing branches of tympanic plexus.

Jacquemier's sign (zhŏk-mē-ā′). [Jean Jacquemier, Fr. obstetrician, 1806-79] Blue or purplish color of the vaginal mucosa. A presumptive sign of pregnancy.

jactitation (jăk″tĭ-tā′shŭn) [L. *jactitāre,* to toss]. Convulsive movements; restless tossing. Changing from one posture to another, usually characteristic of severe mental and febrile affections.

    j., periodic. Chorea.

Jadelot's lines (zhŏd-lŏ′). [Francois N. Jadelot, Fr. physician, 1791-1830] Lines on the face, said to indicate disease in children. SYN: *Jadelot's furrows; Jadelot's traits.*

    Ocular line: Down from corner of mouth; seen in respiratory diseases.

    Nasal line: From lower border of ala nasi about outer side of orbicularis oris muscle; seen in abdominal disorders.

    Labial line: From inner canthus toward glenoid fossa; observed in cerebral disease.

Jaeger's test types (yā′gĕr). [Edward Jaeger von Jastthal, Viennese ophthalmologist, 1818-84] Lines of type of various sizes, printed on a card for testing near vision. The smallest type read at the closest distance is recorded.

jalap (jăl′ăp) [Jalapa, a city in Mexico]. The dried tuberous root of Exogonium purga. Formerly used as a cathartic. Now considered to be unapproved for this use.

jargon (jar′gŭn) [O.Fr. a chattering]. Unintelligible speech. SYN: *paraphasia.*

jar″gonapha′sia ["+ Gr. *a-,* not, + *phasis,* speech]. A form of aphasia, q.v., in which words are jumbled so that speech is unintelligible. SYN: *paraphasia.*

Jar′vis′ snare. [William C. Jarvis, Amer. laryngologist, 1855-95] A snare for removing growths.

jaundice (jŏn′dĭs) [L. *galbinus,* greenish yellow]. A condition characterized by yellowness of skin; whiteness of eyes, mucous membranes, and body fluids, due to deposition of bile pigment resulting from excess bilirubin (hyperbilirubinemia) in the blood. It may be caused by obstruction of bile passageways, excess destruction of red blood cells (hemolysis), or disturbances in functioning of liver cells.

    J. is a symptom which may be the indicator of a benign and curable disease, such as a gallstone blocking the common duct. It may be due to carcinoma of the head of the pancreas involving the opening of the bile duct into the duodenum. It is therefore important to attempt to make a diagnosis by employing certain tests. Sometimes diagnosis can be made only after exploratory surgical procedures. SYN: *icterus,* q.v.

    j., acholuric. J. without bile pigment in the urine.

    j., catarrhal. J. resulting from inflammation of the liver. Now considered identical with infectious hepatitis. SEE: *hepatitis, infectious.*

j., cholestatic. J. due to failure of bile to reach the duodenum, whether due to blockage of the flow of bile or to liver cell changes.

j., congenital. J. occurring at or shortly after birth due to maldevelopment of biliary apparatus.

j., hematogenous. J., hemolytic, q.v.

j., hemolytic. Any one of several disease states which cause j. due to increased destruction of red blood cells. The serum bilirubin may be only slightly elevated even though bile pigment production may be increased as much as six times normal. The bilirubin which is mostly unconjugated and therefore insoluble in water does not appear in the urine. The spleen usually is enlarged.

j., hepatocanalicular. J. resulting from changes in the bile canaliculi, the liver cells remaining relatively normal.

j., hepatocellular. J. resulting from changes in liver cells.

j., hepatogenous. J. due to disease of the liver.

j., homologous serum. A form resembling infectious hepatitis. Follows injection of homologous serum containing the virus which causes serum hepatitis.

j., infectious. Infectious hepatitis. SEE: *hepatitis, infectious.*

j., malignant. Acute yellow atrophy of the liver.

j. of newborn. J. affecting newborn infants. SYN: *icterus neonatorum.*

j., obstructive. J. due to a mechanical impediment in the flow of bile from the liver to the duodenum.

j., parenchymatous. J., hepatocellular, q.v.

j., posthepatic. J. resulting from obstruction of flow of bile ducts. May be incomplete or complete.

j., regurgitation. J. due to bile entering lymph channels of the liver and thence being conveyed to the blood. May result from biliary obstruction or lesions involving bile capillaries.

j., retention. J. resulting from inability of liver cells to remove bile pigment from circulation.

j., spirochetal. An acute infectious disease due to a spirochete, Leptospira icterohaemorrhagiae. SYN: *Weil's disease.*

j., surgical. J. due to a cause which requires surgical therapy. Ex: blockage of bile duct by a gallstone.

j., toxic. J. resulting from bacterial toxins or poisons such as phosphorus, arsphenamine, carbon tetrachloride, etc.

j., xanthochromic. J. without bile pigment in the urine, but with yellowish discoloration of soles and palms.

Javelle water (zhŭ-vĕl′) [Javel, a city now part of Paris]. An aqueous solution of potassium or sodium hypochlorite used as a bleach and a disinfectant. SYN: *javel water.*

jaw [ME. *iawe*]. Either or both the maxillary and mandibular bones, bearing the teeth and forming mouth framework. SEE: *lockjaw.*

j., dislocation of the. Such dislocations are uncomfortable and extremely embarrassing to the patient. They may occur on either side, in which instance the tip of the jaw is pointed away from the dislocation.

On the normal side, just in front of the ear, may be felt a little hollow or depression which is often tender. If both sides of the jaw are dislocated, the jaw is pushed downward and forward. In either event, there is pain and difficulty in speech and the condition is often accompanied by shock. Backward dislocation of the jaw is rare.

CAUSES: Dislocations of the jaw are most often caused by a blow to the face or a fall on the chin, but occasionally they are caused by chewing large chunks of food, by yawning, or by hearty laughing.

REDUCTION OF: These dislocations are reduced by placing well padded thumbs inside of the mouth on the lower molar (back) teeth with the fingers running along the jawbone as a lever. The thumbs should be pressed downward toward the patient's lips and the fingers upward toward the patient's nose. Give a twisting motion to the jaw and at the same time with the wrist and elbows press backward toward the neck. The jaw gliding over the ridge of bone may be felt and just as this occurs the jaw usually snaps into place. When this motion is noted, move the thumbs laterally toward the cheeks to avoid the thumbs being crushed between the molars.

This snapping into place is due to an involuntary spasm of the muscles pulling the jaw as though an overstretched rubber band were attached to it. Following the reduction, an immobilizing bandage or double cravat should be applied.

j. jerk reflex. Clonic movement resulting from percussing or stroking lower jaw.

j., lumpy. Fungus disease affecting the jaw, brain, lungs, and gastrointestinal tract. Common in cattle and sometimes affecting humans. SYN: *actinomycosis,* q.v.

j., swelling of. Lower: May be due to alveolar abscess, a cyst, gumma, sarcoma, or actinomycosis. *Upper:* Occurs in alveolar abscess, parotid tumor, parotitis, carcinoma, sarcoma, necrosis of bone, or disease of antrum.

j. winking. Elevation of the upper eyelid when there is depression of the lower jaw.

jaw, words pert. to: alveolar; alveolate; alveolus; anisognathous; epulis; gnathic; hypognathous; mandible; maxilla; ramus; submaxillary; tetanus; trismus.

jecur (jē'kŭr) [L.]. The liver.

jejunal (jē-jū'năl) [L. *jejunum,* empty]. Rel. to the jejunum.

jejunectomy (jē"jū-něk'tō-mĭ) ["+ Gr. *ek-tomē,* excision]. Excision of part or all of the jejunum.

jejunitis (jē"jū-nī'tĭs) ["+ Gr. *-itis,* inflammation]. Inflammation of the jejunum.

jejuno- [L.]. Combining form referring to the jejunum.

jejunocolostomy (jē-jū"nō-kōl-ŏs'tō-mĭ) [L. *jejunum,* empty, + Gr. *kōlon,* colon, + stoma, mouth]. Formation of artificial passage between jejunum and colon.

jejunoileitis (jē-jū"nō-īl"-ē-ī'tĭs) ["+ *ileum,* small intestine, + Gr. *-itis,* inflammation]. Inflamed condition of the jejunum and ileum.

jejunoileostomy (jē-jū"nō-īl"ē-ŏs'tō-mĭ) ["+ "+ Gr. stoma, mouth]. Formation of a passage between jejunum and ileum.

jejunojejunostomy (jē-jū"nō-jē"jū-nŏs'tō-mĭ) [L. *jejunum,* empty, + *jejunum,* empty, + Gr. stoma, mouth]. Formation of a passage between two parts of the jejunum.

jejunostomy (jē"jū-nŏs'tō-mĭ) ["+ Gr. stoma, mouth]. Surgical creation of a permanent opening into the jejunum.

jejunotomy (jē"jū-nŏt'ō-mĭ) ["+ Gr. tomē, incision]. Surgical incision into the jejunum.

jejunum (jē-jū'nŭm) [L., empty]. The second portion of the small intestine extending from the duodenum to the ileum. It is about 8 feet (2.4 meters) in length, comprising about two fifths of the small intestine.

j., inflammation of. SYM: Absence of diarrhea; colic, distention of abdomen, borborygmus; flocculent or semisolid stools containing undigested food, unchanged bile, and some mucus.

jel'ly [L. *gelāre,* to freeze]. A thick semisolid, gelatinous mass.

j., contraceptive. A j. introduced into the vagina for the prevention of conception. It may act as an occlusive agent or it may serve as a vehicle for spermicidal substances.

j., mineral. Petrolatum, petroleum j.

j., petroleum. Petrolatum.

j., vaginal. A j. introduced into the vagina for therapeutic or contraceptive purposes.

j., Wharton's. Soft gelatinous connective tissue that constitutes the matrix of the umbilical cord.

Jen'ner's stain. [Louis Jenner, Brit. physician, 1866-1904] Eosin methylene blue stain.

jerk (jŭrk). 1. A sudden muscular movement. 2. Certain reflex actions resulting from striking or tapping a muscle or tendon. SEE: *reflex.*

j., elbow. Involuntary extension of forearm produced by external stimulation of stretched triceps.

j., jaw. Result of tapping the mandible when the jaw is half open. It may be increased when there are bilateral supranuclear cerebral lesions.

j., knee. Forward j. of lower leg upon striking patellar tendon when knee is flexed at right angles. Absent in locomotor ataxia, infantile paralysis, meningitis, diabetes, destructive lesions of lower part of cord, and certain forms of paralysis. Increased in affections of pyramidal areas, brain tumors, spinal irritability, and lateral or cerebrospinal sclerosis. SYN: *patellar-tendon reflex.*

jig'ger. Common name for parasitic fleas belonging to the species Tunga penetrans, q.v. SYN: *chigger; chigoe.* SEE: *chiggers.*

jim'son weed. Stramonium, q.v.

Jocasta complex (jō-kăs'tă) [Jocasta, mother in the Oedipus complex, who was the wife and mother of Oedipus]. A term implying a mother-son complex.

Joffroy's reflex (zhŏf-rwä'). [Alexis Joffroy, Fr. physician, 1844-1908] Twitching of gluteal muscles when pressure is made against buttocks.

Joffroy's sign. 1. Absence of facial muscle contraction when eyes turn upward in exophthalmic goiter. 2. Inability to do simple sums in arithmetic. An early sign of general paralysis.

jogger's heel. Irritation of the fibrous and fatty tissue covering the heel. Due to the type of running characteristic of jogging wherein the heel strikes the surface first, rather than the toes as in sprinting. Persons prone to develop this may diminish the risk by wearing pads on their heels and by running on surfaces softer than wood, concrete, or asphalt.

joint [L. *junctio,* a joining]. An articulation. The point of juncture between two bones.

A j. is usually formed of fibrous connective tissue and cartilage. It is classified as being immovable (synarthrosis), slightly movable (amphiarthrosis), and freely movable (diarthrosis).

Synarthrosis: J. in which the two bones are separated only by an intervening membrane, as the cranial sutures. *Amphiarthrosis:* (1) J. having a fibrocartilaginous disk between the bony surfaces (symphysis), as the symphysis pubis, or a j. with a ligament uniting the two bones (syndesmosis), as the tibiofibular articulation. *Diarthrosis:* J. in which the adjoining bone ends are covered with a thin cartilaginous sheet and joined by ligament lined by a synovial membrane, which secretes a lubricant.

Grouping is according to motion: ball and socket (enarthrosis); hinge (ginglymus); condyloid, pivot (trochoid); gliding (arthrodia); and saddle joint.

MOVEMENT: Movements of joints are of four kinds: *gliding* in which one bony surface glides on another without angular or rotatory movement; *angular* occurring only between long bones, increasing or decreasing the angle between the bones; *circumduction* occurring in joints composed of the head of a bone and an articular cavity, the long bone describing a series of circles, the whole forming a cone; and *rotation* in which a bone moves about a central axis without moving from this axis. In angular movement, if it occurs forward and backward, it is called flexion and extension; away from the body, abduction; and toward the median plane of the body, adduction.

INJURIES: Contusions, sprains, dislocations, and penetrating wounds.

j., amphidiarthrodial. J. both ginglymoid and arthrodial.

j., arthrodial. Diarthrosis permitting a gliding motion. SYN: *gliding j.*

j., ball and socket. J. in which round end of one bone fits into cavity of another bone. SYN: *enarthrosis; multiaxial joint.*

j., biaxial. J. possessing two chief movement axes at right angles to each other.

j., bilocular. J. separated into two sections by interarticular cartilage.

j., bleeders'. J. hemorrhage in hemophiliacs.

j., Brodie's. Arthrodial neuralgia due to hysteria.

j., Budin's. Congenital cartilaginous band between squamous and condylar parts of the occipital bone.

j. capsule. The saclike structure that encloses the ends of bones in a diarthrodial joint. Consists of an outer fibrous layer and an inner synovial layer and contains synovial fluid.

j. cavity. The articular cavity or space enclosed by the synovial membrane and articular cartilages. It contains synovial fluid.

j., Charcot's. A disease in tabes dorsalis or syringomyelia. Joint enlargement owing to wasting away of muscles below the joint.

j., Chopart's. Union of remainder of tarsal bones with os calcis and astragalus.

j., cochlear. Hinge j. permitting lateral motion.

j., compound. J. made up of several bones.

j., condyloid. J. permitting all forms of angular movements except axial rotation.

j., Cruveilhier's. Atlanto-odontoid j.

j., diarthrodial. A j. characterized by the presence of a cavity within the capsule separating the bony elements, thus permitting considerable freedom of movement.

j., dry. Arthritis of chronic villous type.

j., ellipsoid. J. having two axes of motion through the same bone.

j., enarthrodial. J., ball and socket, q.v. SYN: *multiaxial j.*

j., false. False j. formation subsequent to a fracture.

j., flail. J. which is extremely relaxed, the distal portion of limb being almost beyond the control of the will.

j., ginglymoid. J. having only forward and backward motion as a hinge. SYN: *hinge j.*

j., gliding. Diarthrosis permitting a gliding motion.

j., hemophiliac. J., bleeders', q.v.

j., hinge. J. having only a forward and backward motion, as a hinge. SYN: *ginglymoid j.*

j., immovable. J. in which a cavity is lacking between the bones. SYN: *synarthrosis.*

j.'s, intercarpal. Articulations which the carpal bones form in relation to one another.

j., irritable. Inflamed spasmodic condition of j. of unknown cause.

j., midcarpal. J. separating the navicular, lunate, and triangular bones from the distal row of carpal bones.

j., mixed. J. with surfaces joined by fibrocartilaginous disks.

j. mouse. Loose cartilage or other body in a j.

Comparison of Joint Diseases[*]

	Rheumatic Fever	Rheumatoid Arthritis	Osteoarthritis	Gout
Age	Children and young adults	25 and over	Middle and old age	Middle and old age
Sex	Either	Chiefly women	Either	Chiefly men
Cause	Unknown. Autoimmune reaction to streptococci	Unknown. Autoimmune (Collagen) disease	Trauma, old age, degenerative changes	Uric acid in blood due to disordered purine metabolism
Joints	Usually large joints, subsiding in one and commencing in another	Multiple, including small joints of hands and feet	Usually one large joint, e.g. hip, knee, shoulder	Several, e.g. great toe, knee, elbow, hands
Pyrexia	At onset	In acute stages	None	During acute attack
Permanent Deformity	None	Spindle-shaped joints; often gross deformity	Often slight	Deformity mainly from "chalky" deposits
Heart	Often affected	Infrequently affected	Not affected	Often arteriosclerosis
Treatment	Salicylates; steroids; rest in bed	Local heat, etc. Physiotherapy. Gold. Steroids. Phenylbutazone. Indomethacin. Antimalarials. Analgesics.	Analgesics, physiotherapy + Orthopedic measures	Colchicine. Probenacid. Phenylbutazone. Steroids. Local applications. Diet

[*] Sears, W. G., Winwood, R. S.: Medicine for Nurses, ed. 11. Edward Arnold Publishers Ltd., London, 1970.

j., movable. Slightly movable or freely movable joint. SYN: *amphiarthrosis* and *diarthrosis*, respectively.

j., multiaxial. J., ball and socket, q.v. SYN: *enarthrodial j.; polyaxial j.*

j., pivot. A j. which permits rotation of a bone, the j. being formed by a pivot-like process which turns within a ring, or by a ringlike structure which turns on a pivot. SYN: *rotary j.; trochoid j.*

j., polyaxial. J., ball and socket, q.v. SYN: *enarthrodial j.; multiaxial j.*

j., receptive. J., saddle, q.v. SYN: *reciprocal j.*

j., rotary. J., pivot, q.v.

j., saddle. A j. in which the opposing surfaces are reciprocally concavoconvex.

j., simple. J. composed of two bones.

j., spheroid. Multiaxial j. with spheroid surfaces.

j., spiral. J., cochlear, q.v.

j., synarthrodial. J., immovable, q.v.

j.'s, tarsometatarsal. Made up of three arthrodial joints, the bones of which articulate with the bases of the metatarsal bones.

j., trochoid. J., pivot, q.v.

j., uniaxial. J. moving on a single axis.

j., unilocular. J. with a single cavity.

joule (jūl). [James P. Joule, Brit. physicist, 1818-99] Work done in one second by current of one ampere against a resistance of one ohm. One kilogram calorie (kcal. or Calorie) is equal to 4185.5 joules. One calorie (small calorie) is equal to 4.1855 joules.

Joule's law. Law that states that at a constant temperature the internal energy of a gas does not vary with its volume.

jugal [L. *jugalis*]. 1. Connected or united as by a yoke. 2. Pert. to the malar or zygomatic bone.

j. bone. Malar or zygomatic bone.

j. process. Temporal bone process forming zygomatic arch. SYN: *zygomatic process.*

jugale (jū-gā'lē) [L. *jugum*, yoke]. The point at the margin of zygomatic process.

jugate (jū'gāt) [L. *jugatus*, joined]. 1. Coupled, yoked. 2. Having ridges.

jugular (jŭg'ū-ler) [L. *jugularis*]. Pert. to the throat.

j. foramen. Opening formed by j. notches of the occipital and temporal bones.

j. fossa. Depression in the petrosal portion of the temporal bone for the j. vein.

j. ganglion. Nodes of vagus root and glossopharngeal nerve in j. foramen.

j. process. Projection from occipital bone toward the temporal bone.

j. veins. External, receives the blood from the exterior of the cranium and the deep parts of the face. It lies superficial to the sternocleidomastoid muscle as it passes down the neck to join the subclavian vein. *Internal,* receives blood from the brain and superficial parts of the face and neck. It is directly continuous with the transverse sinus, accompanying the internal carotid as it passes down the neck, and joins with the subclavian vein to form the innominate vein.

They are more prominent during expiration than during inspiration. Also during cardiac decompensation.

jugulate (jŭg'ū-lāt) [L. *jugulāre*, to cut the throat]. To arrest quickly a process or disease by therapeutic measures.

jugula'tion. Sudden arrest of a disease by therapeutic means.

jug'ulum [L.]. Neck or throat.

ju'gum [L., a yoke]. (pl. *ju'ga*) 1. Ridge or furrow connecting two points. 2. A type of forceps.

j. penis. Forceps for temporarily compressing the penis.

j. petrosum. Eminence on petrous section of temporal bone showing the position of superior semicircular canal. SYN: *arcuate eminence.*

juice [L. *jus*, broth]. Liquid that exudes or is expressed from any part of an organism.

j., alimentary. The digestive juices.

j., gastric. Secretions of the stomach, consisting of water, salts, pepsin, and free hydrochloric acid. SEE: *gastric j.*

j., intestinal. A clear, yellowish, viscid fluid; alkaline in reaction, secreted by Lieberkühn's crypts. SYN: *succus entericus.* SEE: *intestinal j.*

j., pancreatic. A clear, viscid, alkaline digestive juice of the pancreas poured into the duodenum. It contains the enzymes trypsin, amylase, and lipase or steapsin.

jujitsu, jiujitsu (jū-jĭt'sū) [Jap.]. A system of physical training for developing the art of self-defense without weapons in which the opponent's weight and strength are used to his disadvantage. Esp. developed in Japan.

jumentous (jū-měn'tŭs) [L. *jumentum*, beast of burden]. Like that of a horse, said of odor of urine in certain diseased conditions.

jum'per. One with nervous disorder who is startled easily or who jumps at sound of a loud noise. SEE: *palmus.*

junction (jŭnk'shŭn) [L. *junctĭō*, a joining]. The place of union or coming together of two parts.

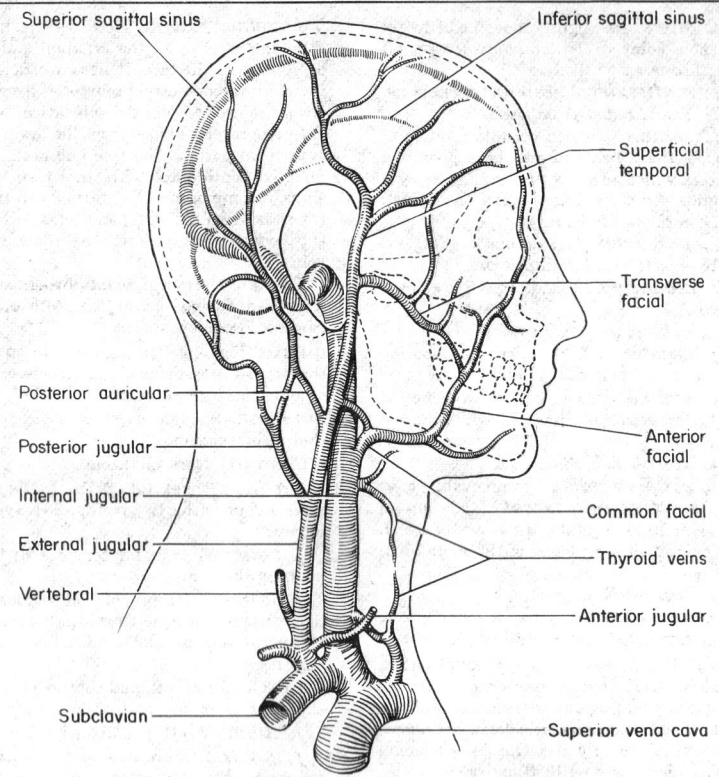

VEINS OF RIGHT SIDE OF HEAD AND NECK

j., mucocutaneous. A j. between the skin and a mucous membrane.

j., myoneural. Meeting point of a nerve with the muscle to which it is distributed. SYN: *motor end-plate.*

j., sclerocorneal. Meeting point between the sclera and the cornea marked on the external surface of the eyeball by the outer scleral sulcus.

junctura (jŭnk-tū′rǎ) [L., a joining]. (pl. *juncturae*) Suture of bones. Articulation.

junk′et [L. *juncus*]. 1. Curds and whey; a type of cream cheese. 2. Commonly, a flavored and sweetened custard set by rennet.

jurymast (jūr′ī-mast) [L. *jurāre*, to be right, + AS. *masc,* a stick]. Apparatus for support of head in disease of the spine.

jusculum (jŭs′kū-lŭm) [L.]. Broth or soup.

Juster's reflex. Finger extension instead of flexion when palm of hand is irritated.

jus′to ma′jor [L., larger than normal]. Bigger than normal, as a pelvis.

jus′to mi′nor [L., smaller than normal]. Smaller than normal, as a pelvis.

jute (jūt) [Sanskrit *jūta*, matted hair]. Fiber used in dressings.

juvantia (jū-văn′shǐ-ā) [L.]. Adjuvant medicines which intensify action of other drugs or assist them.

juvenile (jū′vĕ-nĭl″) [L. *juvenis*, young]. 1. Pert. to youth or childhood. 2. Young; immature.

j. cell. The early developmental form of white blood cells.

juxta- [L., near]. Prefix indicating close proximity.

juxta-articular (jŭks″tă-ăr-tĭk′ū-lăr) [″+ *articulus,* joint]. Situated close to a joint.

juxtaglomerular (jŭks″tă-glō-mĕr′ū-lăr) [″+ *glomus,* ball]. Near or adjacent to a glomerulus.

j. apparatus. A structure consisting of myoepithelioid cells forming a cuff surrounding the arteriole leading to a glomerulus of the kidney.

j. cells. Myoepithelioid cells resembling those of the carotid body present in the juxtaglomerular apparatus. Their function is unknown.

juxtangi'na [L. *juxta*, near, + *angina*, a choking]. Inflamed condition of pharyngeal muscles.

juxtaposition (jŭks"tă-pō-zĭ'shŭn) ["+ *positiō*, place]. Position that is adjacent or side by side. SYN: *apposition; contiguity.*

juxtapyloric (jŭks"tă-pi-lor'ĭk) ["+ Gr. *pylōros*, pylorus]. Near the pylorus or pyloric orifice.

juxtaspinal (jŭks"tă-spī'năl) ["+ *spina*, thorn]. Near the spinal column.

K

K. 1. Chem. symb. for potassium. 2. Symb. for Gr. letter *kappa.* 3. Used in some formulae in chemistry and physics to indicate a constant or value which does not change.

Ka. Abbr. for *cathode;* also Ca.

Kader's operation (kŏ'der). [Bronislaw Kader, Polish surgeon, 1863-1937] Surgical formation of a gastric fistula with feeding tube inserted through valvelike flap.

Kaes' feltwork (kīz). [Theodor Kaes, Ger. neurologist, 1852-1913] Nerve fiber network in cerebral cortex.

Kahn test (kŏn). [Reuben L. Kahn, Amer. bacteriologist, 1887 —] A flocculation test for the diagnosis of syphillis.

Positive reaction based upon appearance of a white precipitate when an alcoholic extract of normal heart muscle is added to the blood serum of one afflicted with syphilis.

kaif (kīf) [Arabic, quiescence]. A dreamy, tranquil state induced by drugs.

kainophobia (kī-nō-fō'bĭ-ă) [Gr. *kainos,* new, + *phobos,* fear]. Abnormal aversion to new situations and things. SYN: *neophobia.*

kais'erling, Kais'erling's solution. [Karl Kaiserling, Ger. pathologist, 1869-1942] Liquid used in preserving pathological specimens.

kakidrosis (kăk-ĭ-drō'sĭs) [Gr. *kakos,* bad, + *hidrōsis,* sweat]. Unpleasant odor of the sweat. SYN: *bromidrosis.*

kakke (kŏk'kā) [Jap.]. Endemic form of polyneuritis. SYN: *beriberi.*

kakosmia (kăk-ŏz'mĭ-ă) [Gr. *kakos,* bad, + *osmē,* smell]. Perception of bad odors which do not exist. SYN: *cacosmia; parosmia.*

kakotrophy (kăk-ŏt'rō-fĭ) ["+ *trophē,* nourishment]. Malnutrition. SYN: *cacotrophy.*

kala-azar (kă'lă ă'-zăr) [Hindi, black fever]. An infectious disease, common in the rural parts of tropical and subtropical areas of the world. There are several types which differ as to preference for children or adults, incidence in domestic animals, and transmitting agent. The disease is characterized by lesions of the reticuloendothelial system, esp. the liver and spleen. It is often fatal. SYN: *visceral leishmaniasis.*

ETIOL: Leishmania donovani, a flagellated protozoon. The organism is transmitted by the bite of infected sandflies of the genus Phlebotomus. TREATMENT: Pentavalent compounds of antimony.

kaliemia (kă-lĭ-ē'mĭ-ă) [L. *kali,* potash, + Gr. *haima,* blood]. Potassium in the blood.

kaligenous (kă-lĭj'ĕ-nŭs) ["+ Gr. *gennan,* to produce]. Forming potash.

kalimeter (kă-lĭm'ĕ-ter) ["+ Gr. *metron,* measure]. Device for determining degree of alkalinity of a substance. SYN: *alkalimeter.*

ka'lium [L.]. Potassium; a mineral element necessary to the growth of cells, esp. those of the muscles and blood. SYMB: K. SEE: *potassium.*

kallidin (kăl'ĭ-dĭn). A plasma kinin. SEE: *kinin.*

kallikrein (kăl-ĭ-krē'ĭn) [Gr. *kallikreas,* pancreas]. An enzyme normally present in blood plasma, urine, and body tissue in an inactive state. When activated, kallikrein is one of the most potent vasodilators. It forms kinin, q.v.

kallikreinogen ["+ *gennan,* to produce]. The precursor in blood plasma of kallikrein, q.v.

kaolin (kā'ō-lĭn) [Fr. from Mandarin Chinese *kao,* high, + *ling,* mountain]. A yellowish-white or gray clay powder, occurring in a natural state as a form of hydrated aluminum silcate. Used internally as an absorbent; externally, as a protective by absorbing moisture. SYN: *China clay.*

kaolinosis (kā"ō-lĭn-ō'sĭs). Pneumokoniosis caused by inhaling kaolin particles.

Kaposi's varicelliform eruption (kăp'ō-sē"). [Moritz K. Kaposi, Austrian dermatologist, 1837-1902] Skin disease which results from infection with virus of either herpes simplex or vaccinia in the presence of another skin disease such as eczema. SYN: *eczema herpeticum; eczema vaccinatum.*

karyo- [Gr. *karyon,* nucleus]. Prefix referring to a cell's nucleus.

kar"yochromat'ophil ["+ *chrōma,* color, + *philein,* to love]. Having a nucleus which stains.

karyochrome (kăr'ĭ-ō-krōm). The cell of a nerve with an easily staining nucleus.

karyoclasis (kăr-ĭ-ŏk'lă-sĭs) [Gr. *karyon,* nucleus, + *klasis,* a breaking]. The fragmentation of a cell nucleus. SYN: *karyorrhexis.*

karyogamy (kăr-ĭ-ŏg'ă-mĭ) ["+ *gamos,* marriage]. Union of nuclei in cell conjugation.

karyogen (kăr'ĭ-ō-jĕn") ["+ *gennan,* to produce]. A compound of iron in certain cell nuclei.

karyogenesis (kăr'ĭ-ō-jĕn'ĕ-sĭs) [Gr. *karyon,* nucleus, + *genesis,* production]. Formation and development of a cell nucleus.

karyogram (kăr'ĭ-ō-grăm) ["+ *gramma*, mark]. A picture of the interphase of mitosis in somatic chromosomes.

karyokinesis (kăr'ĭ-ō-kĭn-ē'sĭs) ["+ *kinēsis*, movement]. The equal division of nuclear material which occurs in cell division. SEE: *cytokinesis; mitosis.*

karyokinetic (kăr'ĭ-ō-kĭ-nĕt'ĭk). 1. Pert. to karyokinesis. 2. Ameboid.

karyolobism (kăr'ĭ-ō-lō'bĭzm) [Gr. *karyon*, nucleus, + L. *lobus*, lobe, + Gr. *ismos*, state of]. Condition in which the nucleus of a cell is lobed as in polymorphonuclear leukocytes.

kar'yolymph ["+ L. *lympha*, lymph]. Fluid in meshes of the nucleus.

This fluid is now known to contain active submicroscopic granular components of the nucleoplasm. Thus the terms karyolymph and nuclear sap do not describe clearly definable entities and should not be used. SEE: *cell; organelle.*   (

karyolysis (kăr-ĭ-ōl'ĭ-sĭs) ["+ *lysis*, dissolution]. The destruction of a nucleus or loss of affinity for basic dyes. SYN: *chromatolysis.*

karyolyt'ic. Producing or rel. to karyolysis.

karyomitosis (kăr'ĭ-ō-mĭ-tō'sĭs) [Gr. *karyon*, nucleus, + *mitos*, thread, + -*ōsis*, condition]. Nuclear changes in cell division. SYN: *karyokinesis.*

karyomorphism (kăr-ĭ-ō-mor'fĭzm) ["+ *morphē*, form, + *ismos*, state of]. The form of a cell nucleus.

karyon (kăr'ĭ-ŏn) [Gr.]. Obsolete term for cell nucleus.

karyophage (kăr'ĭ-ō-fāj) ["+ *phagein*, to eat]. An intracellular protozoan parasite which destroys the nucleus of a cell.

karyorrhexis (kăr'ĭ-ō-rĕk'sĭs) ["+ *rhēxis*, rupture]. Fragmentation of the chromatin in nuclear disintegration.

karyosome (kăr'ĭ-ō-sōm) [Gr. *karyon*, nucleus, + *soma*, body]. Irregular clumps of chromatin material seen in the nuclei of cells which are not dividing. SYN: *chromatin particles.*

karyotheca (kăr'ĭ-ō-thē'kă) ["+ *thēkē*, sheath]. The enveloping membrane of a cell nucleus.

karyotype (kăr'ĭ-ō-tĭp) ["+ *typos*, mark]. A systematic array of the chromosomes of a single cell in the matephase stage. The human male k. consists of 22 pairs of chromosomes plus the XY pair. The female also has 22 pairs but has the XX pair in place of XY. SEE: *chromosome* for illustration.

kata- [Gr.]. Prefix meaning down, reversing process, according to, entirely, wrongly, back, against. SEE: words beginning with *cata-*.

katab'olism ["+ *ballein*, to throw, + *ismos*, state of]. Catabolism, q.v.

kataphraxis (kăt"ă-frăks'ĭs) ["+ *phraxis*, a blocking]. Surgical formation of metallic supports for an organ.

kataplasia (kăt-ă-plā'sĭ-ă). Cataplasia, q.v.

katathermometer (kăt"ă-thĕr-mŏm'ē-ter) [Gr. *kata*, down, + *thermē*, heat, + *metron*, measure]. A thermometer for measuring the efficiency of ventilation and cooling and drying processes, i.e., the measurement of the cooling power (or, in a very warm atmosphere, of the warming power) of the atmosphere exerted on surface of two thermometers, one a dry bulb and the other wet bulb. Both are heated to 110° F. (43.3° C.) and the time required for each thermometer to fall from 100° to 90° F. (37.8° to 32.2° C.) is noted.

The dry kata gives the cooling power by radiation and convection. The wet kata gives the cooling power by radiation, convection, and evaporation.

katatonia (kăt-ă-tō'nĭ-ă) ["+ *tonos*, tension]. Catatonia, q.v.

kathisophobia (kăth"ĭ-sō-fō'bĭ-ă) [Gr. *kathizein*, to sit down, + *phobos*, fear]. Fear of sitting down, and subsequent inability to sit still.

kation (kăt'ĭ-ŏn) [Gr., descending]. Cation, q.v.

katotro'pia [Gr. *katō*, below, + *tropos*, a turning]. Tendency of the eyeball to drop too far downward. SYN: *katophoria.*

KBr. Potassium bromide.

KC₂H₃O₂. Potassium acetate.

KCl. Potassium chloride.

KClO. Potassium hypochlorite.

KClO₃. Potassium chlorate.

K₂CO₃. Potassium carbonate.

kefir, kefyr (kĕf'ẽr) [Caucasus region of Russia]. A preparation of curdled milk made originally in the Caucasus by adding kefir grains to milk.

kelectome (kē'lĕk-tōm) [Gr. *kēlē*, tumor, + *tomē*, incision]. Instrument for removing specimen of tumor tissue.

kelis (kē'lĭs) [Gr., blemish]. Keloid, q.v.

Kelly's pad. [Howard A. Kelly, Amer. surgeon, 1858-1943] A drainage pad for the operating table or bed made by wrapping one end of a rubber sheet over a rolled small blanket, forming a bolster; the bolster is twisted round like a horseshoe to form the pad, the free part of the sheet forming the apron. Also commercial inflatable rubber pad of horseshoe shape used in same way.

keloid (kē'loyd) [Gr. *kēlē*, tumor, + *eidos*, form]. Scar formation in the skin following trauma or surgical incision. The tissue response is out of proportion to the amount of scar tissue required for normal repair and healing. The result is a raised, firm, thickened red scar which may grow for a prolonged period of time. Negroes are esp. prone to developing k.'s.

k., acne. K. which develops at site of acne pustule.

keloidosis (kē″loy-dō′sĭs) ["+ "+ -ōsis, condition]. The formation of keloids.

kelotomy (kē-lŏt′ō-mĭ) [Gr. kēlē, hernia, + tomē, incision]. Operation for strangulated hernia through tissues of the constricting neck.

Kenny treatment. [Sister Elizabeth Kenny, Australian nurse, 1886-1952] Treatment for poliomyelitis. Consists of application of hot, moist packs to affected muscles and early re-education of muscles, first through passive exercise and then by active movements as soon as possible. Rigid fixation of paralyzed limbs is disparaged.

kenophobia (kĕn″ō-fō′bĭ-ā) [Gr. kenos, empty, + phobos, fear]. Fear of empty spaces.

kephalin (kĕf′ă-lĭn) [Gr. kephalē, head]. Cephalin, q.v.

kerasin (kĕr′ă-sĭn). A cerebroside isolated from brain tissue.

keratalgia (kĕr″ă-tăl′jĭ-ā) [Gr. keras, horn, + algos, pain]. Neuralgia of the cornea.

keratectasia (kĕr″ă-tĕk-tā′sĭ-ā) ["+ ektasis, extension]. Conical protrusion of the cornea.

keratectomy (kĕr-ă-tĕk′tō-mĭ) ["+ ektomē, excision]. Excision of portion of cornea.

keratiasis (kĕr-ă-tī′ă-sĭs) [Gr. keras, horn, + -iasis, condition]. Horny wart formations on the skin.

kerat′ic. Rel. to horn. SYN: horny.

ker′atin. An extremely tough protein substance in hair, nails, and horny tissue, insoluble in water, weak acids, or alkalis, and unaffected by most proteolytic enzymes.

keratinize (kĕr′ă-tĭn-īz) [Gr. keras, horn]. To become hard or horny. Usually said of tissue.

keratinous (kĕr-ăt′ĭ-nŭs). Pert. to or composed of keratin.

keratitic precipitates. Inflammatory cells of the anterior chamber of the eye which adhere to the endothelial surface of the corner. These may be large, heavy, fat precipitates, or small and punctate.

keratitis (kĕr-ă-tī′tĭs) [Gr. keras, horn, + -itis, inflammation]. Inflammation of cornea.

k., band-shaped. Whitish or grayish band extending across the cornea.

k. bullosa. The formation of large, quite resistant blebs in the cornea of blind trachomatous eyes with increased tension.

k., deep. K., interstitial, q.v.

k., dendritic. Superficial branching corneal ulcers.

k., disciformis. Gray disk-shaped opacity in middle of cornea.

k., fascicular. Corneal ulcer resulting from phlyctenules which spread from limbus to center of cornea accompanied by fascicle of blood vessels.

k., herpetic. Vesicular k. in herpes zoster.

k., hypopyon. Serpiginous ulcer with pus in anterior chamber.

k., interstitial. Deep form of nonsuppurative k. with vascularization, occurring usually in syphilis and rarely in tuberculosis. Commonly found between 5th and 15th years.

SYM: Pain, photophobia, lacrimation, and loss in vision.

k., lagophthalmic. Desiccation of cornea due to defective closure of lids.

k., mycotic. Produced by mold fungi.

k., neuroparalytic. Dull and slightly cloudy insensitive cornea seen in lesions of fifth nerve.

k., parenchymatous. K., interstitial, q.v.

k., phlyctenular. Circumscribed inflammation of conjunctiva and cornea accompanied by formation of small projections called phlyctenules which consist of accumulations of lymphoid cells. The phlyctenules soften at the apices, forming ulcers.

k., punctate. Cellular deposits on posterior surface of cornea seen in diseases of uveal tract.

k., purulent. K. with formation of pus.

k., sclerosing. Triangular opacity in deeper layers of cornea, associated with scleritis.

k., superficial punctate. Small gray spots in superficial layers of cornea, beneath Bowman's membrane, occurring in young persons.

k., trachomatous. K. with abnormal membrane on cornea. SYN: pannus.

k., traumatic. K. caused by wound of the cornea.

k., xerotic. Softening, desiccation, and ulceration of cornea due to dryness of the conjunctiva.

kerato-, kerat- [Gr. keras, horn]. Combining form indicating rel. to horny substances or to the cornea.

keratoacanthoma (kĕr″ă-tō-ăk″ăn-thō′mă) ["+ akantha, thorn, + ōma, tumor]. A papular lesion filled with a keratin plug. It is benign and usually subsides spontaneously. SYN: molluscum sebaceum.

keratocele (kĕr-ăt'ō-sēl) ["+ *kēlē*, hernia]. Protrusion or herniation of Descemet's membrane through the floor of corneal ulcer.

keratoconjunctivitis (kĕr"ă-tō-kŏn-jŭnk"tĭ-vĭ'tĭs). Inflammation of the cornea and the conjunctiva.

   k., epidemic. An acute, self-limited k. due to a virus.

   k., flash. K. resulting from exposure of the eyes to intense ultraviolet irradiation.

   k., virus. K., epidemic, q.v.

keratoconus (kĕr-ă-tō-kō'nŭs) [Gr. *keras*, horn, + *kōnos*, cone]. Conical protrusion of center of cornea without inflammation.

keratoderma (kĕr"ă-tō-dĕr'mă) ["+ *derma*, skin]. A localized or disseminated disease of the horny layer of the skin.

   k. blennorrhagica. Prominent cone-shaped hyperkeratosis. As new lesions develop they tend to merge and produce a relief map appearance.

   ETIOL: Not clear; probably due to a virus. May be associated with non-specific urethritis or gonorrhea, but is not considered to be caused by bacteria. SEE: *Reiter's syndrome.*

keratodermatitis (kĕr"ă-tō-dĕr"mă-tī'tĭs) ["+ "+ *-itis*, inflammation]. Inflammation of the horny layer of the skin with proliferation.

ker"atoder'mia. Hypertrophy of the stratum corneum or horny layer of the epidermis, esp. on the palms of hands and soles of feet producing a horny condition of the skin.

keratogenous (kĕr-ă-tŏj'ĕ-nŭs) [Gr. *keras*, horn, + *gennan*, to produce]. Causing horny tissue development.

ker"atoglo'bus ["+ L. *globus*, circle]. Globular protrusion and enlargement of cornea seen in congenital glaucoma.

keratohelcosis (kĕr"ă-tō-hĕl-kō'sĭs) ["+ *helkōsis*, ulceration]. Corneal ulceration.

keratohyalin. A substance present in the form of granules in the cytoplasm of cells in the stratum granulosum of the skin.

ker'atoid [Gr. *keras*, horn, + *eidos*, form]. Horny or resembling horn or corneal tissue.

keratoiditis (kĕr"ă-toyd-ī'tĭs) ["+ "+ *-itis*, inflammation]. Inflammation of the cornea.

keratoiritis (kĕr"ă-tō-ī-rī'tĭs) ["+ *iris*, iris, + *-itis*, inflammation]. Inflammation of the cornea and iris.

keratoleptynsis (kĕr"ă-tō-lĕp-tĭn'sĭs) [Gr. *keras*, horn, + *leptynein*, to make thin]. Removal of the corneal surface, then covering the area with bulbar conjunctiva. A cosmetic operation performed on a sightless eye.

keratoleukoma (kĕr"ă-tō-lū-kō'mă) ["+ *leukos*, white, + *ōma*, tumor]. White corneal opacity.

keratolysis (kĕr-ă-tōl'ĭ-sĭs) ["+ *lysis*, loosening]. 1. Loosening of horny layer of the skin. 2. Shedding of the skin at regular intervals.

keratolyt'ic. Rel. to or causing keratolysis. SYN: *desquamative.*

kerato'ma [Gr. *keras*, horn, + *ōma*, tumor]. 1. A callosity. 2. A horny growth. SYN: *keratosis.*

keratomalacia (kĕr"ă-tō-mă-lā'sĭ-ă) ["+ *malakia*, softness]. Softening of the cornea seen in early childhood due to deficiencies of vitamin A. SYN: *xerotic keratitis.*

keratome (kĕr'ă-tōm) ["+ *tomē*, incision]. Knife for incising the cornea.

keratometer (kĕr-ă-tŏm'ĕ-ter) [Gr. *keras*, horn, + *metron*, a measure]. An instrument for measuring the curves of the cornea.

keratomycosis (kĕr"ă-tō-mĭ-kō'sĭs) ["+ *mykes*, fungus, + *ōsis*, condition]. Fungus growth on the cornea.

ker"atono'sis ["+ *nosos*, disease]. Any noninflammatory disease or deformity of the horny layer of the skin.

keratonyxis (kĕr"ă-tō-nĭks'ĭs) [Gr. *keras*, horn, + *nyssein*, to puncture]. Corneal puncture, esp. surgical puncture.

keratoplasty (kĕr'ă-tō-plăs"tĭ) ["+ *plassein*, to form]. Plastic operation on the cornea.

ker"atopro'tein ["+ *prōtos*, first]. The protein of the hair, nails, epidermis, etc.

keratorrhexis (kĕr"ă-tō-rĕks'ĭs) [Gr. *keras*, horn, + *rhēxis*, rupture]. Corneal rupture.

keratoscleritis (kĕr"ă-tō-sklĕr-ī'tĭs) ["+ *sklēros*, hard, + *-itis*, inflammation]. Inflammation of both cornea and sclera.

keratoscope (kĕr'ăt-ō-skōp) ["+ *skopein*, to examine]. An instrument for examination of the cornea.

keratos'copy. Examination of the cornea and its reflection of light.

keratose (kĕr'ă-tōs) [Gr. *keras*, horn]. Horny.

keratosis (kĕr-ă-tō'sĭs) [Gr. *keras*, horn, + *ōsis*, condition]. (pl. *keratoses*) 1. Horny growth. 2. Any condition of the skin characterized by the formation of horny growths or excessive development of the horny growth.

   k. climatericum. A skin disease occurring in women during the menopause, characterized by a circumscribed hyperkeratosis of the palms and soles.

   k. follicularis. Darier's disease.

   k. nigricans. Acanthosis nigricans, q.v.

   k. pilaris. Chronic inflammatory disorder of area surrounding the hair follicles.

   SYM: Accumulation of horny material at follicular orifices, giving to affected surfaces a nutmeg-graterlike appearance, commonly in those with rough, dry skin. Most pronounced in winter, on lateral aspects of thighs and upper arms, with possible extension to legs, forearms and scalp.

TREATMENT: There is no specific therapy. Keratolytic lotions may be of some value.

k., seborrheic. A benign skin tumor which may be pigmented. Quite common in the elderly. It is composed of immature epithelial cells. SYN: *acanthotic nevus; seborrheic wart; senile wart.*

ETIOL: Unknown.

SYM: Keratoid, nevoid, acanthoid, or verrucose types occurring in elderly and in those with long-standing dry seborrhea, on face, scalp, interscapular or sternal regions, and backs of hands. Yellowish, grayish, brownish sharply circumscribed lesions covered with a firmly adherent scale, greasy or velvety on trunk or scalp, but harsh, rough, and dry on face or hands. The tendency as time passes is for the lesions to increase in number. It is doubtful that they ever become malignant.

TREATMENT: Thorough curretage is quite effective. This leaves a flat surface which becomes covered with normal skin within a week. Pedunculated lesions can be removed surgically. Cautery may produce scarring, thus it should not be used.

k. seni'lis. Dry, harsh skin of the aged.

keratotome (kĕr-ăt'ō-tōm) [Gr. *keras*, horn, + *tomē*, incision]. A knife for incising the cornea. SYN: *keratome.*

keratotomy (kĕr-ă-tŏt'ō-mĭ). Incision of cornea.

keraunoneurosis (kē-rŏ"nō-nū-rō'sĭs) [Gr. *keraunos*, lightning, + *neuron*, nerve, + *ōsis*, condition]. A neurosis caused by fear of a thunderstorm or stroke of lightning.

keraunophobia (kē-rŏ"nō-fō'bĭ-ă) ["+ *phobos*, fear]. Dread of thunder and lightning.

Kerck'ring's folds. [Theodorus Kerckring, Dutch anatomist, 1640-93] Transverse folds of mucous membrane of small intestine. SYN: *Kerckring's valves; plicae circulares; valvulae conniventes.*

kerectomy (kē-rĕk'tō-mĭ) [Gr. *keras*, horn, + *ektomē*, excision]. Excision of a portion of the cornea.

kerion (kē'rĭ-ŏn) [Gr., honeycomb]. A form of tinea capitis due to Trichophyton tonsurans. SEE: *tinea capitis.*

kerither'apy [Gr. *keros*, wax, + *therapeia*, treatment]. Treatment of burns and denuded surfaces with liquid paraffin.

kernicterus (kĕrn-ĭk'tĕr-ŭs) [Ger.]. A form of icterus neonatorum occurring in infants. The basal ganglia and other areas of the brain and spinal cord are infiltrated with a yellow pigment. Develops during the 2nd to 8th day of life. Prognosis is quite poor.

Ker'nig's sign. [Vladimir Kernig, Russ. physician, 1840-1917] A symptom of meningitis evidenced by reflex contraction and pain in the hamstring muscles when attempting to extend the leg after flexing the thigh upon the body.

ketamine hydrochloride. A nonbarbiturate general anesthetic agent which is administered parenterally. Used experimentally.

ketogenesis (kē-tō-jĕn'ē-sĭs) [ketone + Gr. *genesis*, production]. Production of ketones or acetone substances.

ketogenic diet (kē-tō-jĕn'ĭk) ["+ Gr. *gennan*, to produce]. One that produces acetone or ketone bodies, or mild acidosis. Has been used in treatment of epilepsy.

This is accomplished by providing a diet wherein the ratio of fatty acid to available carbohydrate is from 3 to 1 to 4 to 1.

ketohex'ose. A nonsaccharide consisting of a six-carbon chain and containing a ketone group, in addition to alcohol groups. Fructose is an example.

ketolysis (kē-tŏl'ĭ-sĭs) [ketone + Gr. *lysis*, dissolution]. The dissolution of acetone or ketone bodies.

ketolyt'ic. Pert. to ketolysis.

ketone (kē'tōn). A substance containing the carbonyl group ($=$CO). Oxidation product of a secondary alcohol. Organic chemical substance of the general formula

$$\begin{matrix} R \\ R \end{matrix} \!\! >\!\! CO.$$

Acetone is an example of a simple k. The k. acids in the body are the end products of fat metabolism.

k. bodies. A group of compounds produced during the oxidation of fatty acids, including acetoacetic acid, β-hydroxybutyric acid, and acetone. SEE: *ketosis.*

k. threshold. Level of k. in the blood above which k. bodies appear in the urine.

ketonemia (kē"tō-nē'mĭ-ă) [ketone + Gr. *haima*, blood]. Acetone bodies in the blood. SYN: *acidosis.*

ketonuria (kē-tō-nū'rĭ-ă) ["+ Gr. *ouron*, urine]. Acetone bodies in the urine.

ketopla'sia ["+ Gr. *plassein*, to form]. The formation or excretion of ketones.

ketoplas'tic ["+ Gr. *plastikos*, formed]. Pert. to ketoplasia or formation of ketones.

ke'tose. A carbohydrate containing the ketones.

ketosis (kē-tō'sĭs) [ketone + Gr. -ōsis, condition]. The accumulation in the body of the ketone bodies: acetone, betahydroxybutyric acid, and acetoacetic acid.

It is frequently associated with acidosis and is often miscalled acidosis. Ketosis results from the incomplete metabolism of fatty acids, generally from carbohydrate deficiency or inadequate utilization, and is commonly observed in starvation, high fat diet, pregnancy, following ether anesthesia, and most significantly in diabetes mellitus. Large quantities of these ketone bodies may be eliminated in the urine (ketonuria). The presence of ketosis is easily determined by testing for the presence of acetone or diacetic acid in the urine. Ketonuria is an early sign of acidosis in patients with diabetes mellitus.

17-ke'tosteroid. One of a group of neutral steroids having a ketone group in position 17. They are produced by the adrenal cortex and gonads and appear normally in the urine. Among them are androsterone, dehydroisoandrosterone, corticosterone, compound E, and 11-hydroxyisoandrosterone. A greater than normal or less than normal excretion in the urine is indicative of certain endocrine disorders. SEE: *perhydrocyclopentanophenanthrene.*

Key-Retzius foramina (kē'rĕt'zĭ-ŭs). [Ernst A. H. Key, Swedish physician, 1832-1901; Magnus G. Retzius, Swedish histologist, 1842-1919] Passages in the pia mater carrying the choroid plexus to the fourth ventricle. SYN: *Luschka's foramen.*

kg. Abbr. for *kilogram.*

KHCO₃. Potassium bicarbonate.

KHSO₄. Potassium bisulfate.

KI. Potassium iodide.

kibe (kīb) [Welsh *cibi,* chilblain]. Inflamed patch on hands or feet caused by exposure to cold. SYN: *chilblain,* q.v.

kid'ney [ME. *kidenei*]. One of two organs, purplish-brown in color, situated at the back (retroperitoneal area) of the abdominal cavity, one on each side of the spinal column. Their function is to excrete urine which contains the end products of metabolism and to help regulate the water, electrolyte, and acid base content of the blood.

The upper level is opposite the 12th thoracic (dorsal) vertebra, the lower level opposite the 3rd lumbar vertebra. The right kidney is slightly lower than the left one.

Weight: 113-170 gm. (4-6 oz.). Size: about 11.4 cm. (4 1/2 in.) long, 5-7.5 cm. (2-3 in.) broad, and 2.5 cm. (1 in.) thick. The kidneys in the newborn are about three times as large in proportion to body weight as in the adult.

ANAT: Each kidney is embedded in fatty tissue known as an adipose capsule, and surrounded by the renal fascia, a sheath of fibrous tissue, which helps to hold the kidney in place. The concave border of the kidney faces the median line, the center of the concave border opening into a fissure called the hilum, q.v.

The ureter enters the kidney through the hilum into the pelvis of the kidney. The outer portion of the kidney is the cortex, a mass of cortical substance; the inner portion (medullary substance) is the medulla.

Within the cortical substance are found the arteries, veins, convoluted tubules, and glomerular capsules, while the medulla contains the renal pyramids, conical masses with papillae projecting into the cuplike cavities (calyces) of the pelvis.

Each kidney contains 8-18 pyramids made up of collecting tubules, lymphatics, and blood vessels, the pyramids being penetrated by the cortical substance and supporting them; these extensions are known as the renal columns, or columns of Bertini.

The cortical and medullary substance is composed of renal tubules, connective tissue, blood vessels, nerves, and lymphatics. The renal tubule or nephron constitutes the structural and functional unit of the kidney. Each consists of a capsule, proximal convoluted portion, loop of Henle and distal convoluted portion, which leads to a collecting duct. The capsule, called the glomerular or Bowman's capsule, encloses a globular mass of capillaries, the glomerulus. The capsule and the enclosed glomerulus comprise the malpighian or renal corpuscle. The renal corpuscles are located principally in the cortex.

URINE FORMATION: Urine consists of water (95%) and solids (5%), the latter being in solution. The solids include organic constituents (urea, hippuric acid, uric acid, creatinine) and inorganic constituents, principally salts of sodium and potassium. The kidneys remove these substances from the blood thus acting to maintain homeostasis of the blood and body fluids. Urine is formed by the processes of filtration and reabsorption. As blood passes through the glomerulus, water and dissolved substances are filtered through the capillary walls and the inner or visceral layer of Bowman's capsule, resulting in formation of the glomerular filtrate. Blood cells and colloidal substances such as proteins are retained within the capillaries. The glomerular filtrate passes through the renal tubules to the collecting ducts, during the course of which all of the sugar and some of the salts and other substances are selectively reabsorbed into the capillaries surrounding the tubule. Substances such as uric acid and hydrogen ions may be added to the urine by the cells of the tubules through the process of secretion. The final product now known as urine passes through straight collecting ducts into larger collecting ducts (papillary ducts) which open on the tips of the renal papillae. There urine is discharged into the minor calyces of the renal pelvis, and then is conveyed by the ureters to the bladder. Periodically the bladder is voluntarily emptied and discharges its contents to the outside through the urethra (micturition).

Substances which are entirely or almost entirely reabsorbed during passage through the tubule are known as high threshold substances. These include glucose and chlorides of sodium, potassium, calcium, and magnesium. These are important blood constituents and excreted only when their concentrations in the blood are above normal. Low or nonthreshold substances are those which are reabsorbed only in limited quantities or not at all. These are usually end products of metabolism such as urea, uric acid, and creatine which appear in considerable quantities in the urine.

The formation of urine is a continuous process, the rate of filtration being dependent primarily upon the blood pressure within the glomeruli and the daily fluid intake. Osmotic pressure exerted by proteins within the blood plasma tends to hold water and dissolved substances within the blood vessels so that the effective filtration pressure (25 mm. Hg) is the difference between capillary blood pressure (70 mm. Hg) and the osmotic pressure of the plasma (25 mm. Hg) and the pressure inside the capsular space (15 mm. Hg). General blood pressure and the velocity of blood flow are primary factors in the rate of urine formation.

The volume of urine excreted daily varies from 1000 to 2000 ml. (av. 1500 ml.). The amount varies with water intake, nature of diet, degree of body activity, environmental and body temperature, age, blood pressure, and many other factors. Pathological conditions may affect the volume and nature of the urine excreted.

NERVE SUPPLY: From renal plexuses forming rich networks about renal vessels. Include both sympathetic and parasympathetic (vagal) fibers.

SYMPTOMS OF KIDNEY DISORDER: Lumbar pain, renal colic, fever, disturbances in micturition (anuria, oliguria, or pain on micturition), presence of blood or pus in the urine, tenderness or swelling in costovertebral region, enlargement or diminution in size of kidney, edema.

KIDNEY EXAMINATION: By palpation, intravenous pyelography, cystoscopy, retrograde cystoscopy, panendoscopy.

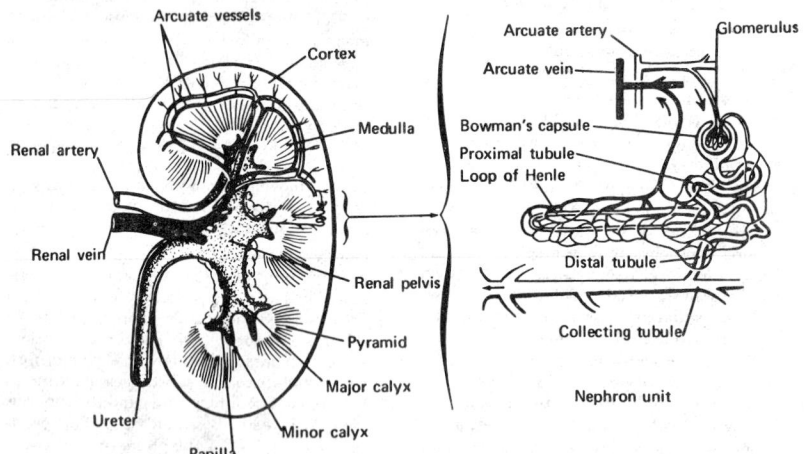

KIDNEY
Left, cross section of kidney; right, enlarged view of nephron unit.

k. amyloid. K. infiltrated with amyloid.

k., contracted. The small k. of chronic interstitial or diffuse nephritis.

k., cystic. K. that has undergone cystic degeneration.

k., embolic contracted. A contracted k. in which embolic infarction of the renal arterioles produces degeneration of renal tissue, and hyperplasia of fibrous tissues produces irregular contraction.

k., fatty. K. with fatty infiltration or degeneration of tubular, glomerular, or capsular epithelium, or of vascular connective tissue.

k., floating. K. which is displaced and movable.

k., granular. A slow form of chronic nephritis, in which the size is diminished, and color is red with hard, fibrous, and granular texture.

k., horseshoe. Congenital malformation with superior or inferior extremities united by an isthmus of renal or fibrous tissue, in the form of a horseshoe.

k., lardaceous. K. infiltrated with amyloid.

k., movable. A k. which is not firmly attached due to lack of support of fatty tissue and perinephric fascia. SYN: *nephroptosis.*

k., polycystic. K. bearing many cysts.

k., red contracted. K., granular, q.v.

k., sacculated. A condition in which the organ has been absorbed and only the distended capsule remains.

k., small red granular. K., granular, q.v.

k. stones. Concretions present in the pelvis of the k. They are composed principally of oxalates, phosphates, and carbonates and vary in size from small granular masses to an inch (2.5 cm.) in diameter. SYN: *renal calculus; renal lithiasis.* SEE: *colloid.*

k., syphilitic. K. with fibrous bands running across it, also caseating gummata, due to syphilis.

k., waxy. K. infiltrated with amyloid.

Kiernan's spaces (kēr'năn). [Francis Kiernan, Brit. physician, 1800-74] The spaces between the lobes of the liver.

Kiesselbach's area (kē'sĕl-bŏk). [Wilhelm Kiesselbach, Ger. laryngologist, 1839-1902] An area on the anterior inferior portion of the nasal septum, the commonest site of nosebleed origin.

Kilian's pelvis (kĭl'ĭ-ăn). [Hermann F. Kilian, Ger. gynecologist, 1800-63] Pelvis affected with osteomalacia. SYN: *pelvis spinosa.*

kilo- [Fr.]. Combining form indicating 1,000.

kil'ogram [Fr. *kilo,* a thousand, + *gramme,* a weight]. One thousand gm. or 2.2 lbs. avoirdupois. ABBR: kg.

kiloliter (kĭl'ō-lē''ter) [Fr. *kilolitre*]. One thousand liters. ABBR: kl.

kil'ometer [Fr. *kilomètre*]. One thousand meters, or 3281 feet (roughly 0.6 of a mile). ABBR: km.

kil'ovolt [Fr. *kilo,* a thousand, + volt]. One thousand volt unit. ABBR: kv.

kil'owatt. A unit of electrical energy equal to one thousand watts. ABBR: kw.

kinanesthesia (kĭn-ăn-ĕs-thē'zĭ-ă) [Gr. *kinēsis,* movement, + *an-,* not, + *aisthēsis,* sensation]. Inability to perceive extent of movement or direction, resulting in ataxia.

kinase (kĭn'ās). An organic substance which activates an enzyme.

kinekard [Gr. *kinesis,* motion, + *kardia,* heart]. A polypeptide substance found in plasma. Acts to stimulate cardiac and vascular muscle; inhibits smooth muscle of the alimentary canal.

kinemat'ics [Gr. *kinēmatos,* movement]. Science of motion.

kineplastic (kĭn''ĭ-plăs'tĭk) [Gr. *kinein,* to move, + *plastikos,* formed]. Pert. to kineplasty.

kin'eplasty. A form of amputation so that motion is imparted to an artificial limb.

kinergety (kĭn'ĕr-jĕt-ĭ) [Gr. *kinein,* to move, + *ergon,* energy]. The potential capacity for kinetic energy.

kinesalgia (kĭn''ē-sal'jĭ-ă) [Gr. *kinēsis,* movement, + *algos,* pain]. Pain attending muscular movement.

kinesia (kĭ-nē'sĭ-ă). Sickness caused by motion, as seasickness, car sickness. SYN: *kinectosis.*

kinesialgia (kĭn-ē-sĭ-ăl'jĭ-ă) [Gr. *kinēsis,* movement, + *algos,* pain]. Pain caused by muscular movements. SYN: *kinesalgia.*

kinesiatrics (kĭ-nē''sĭ-ăt'rĭks) ["+ *iatrikos,* curative]. Treatment involving active and passive movements. SYN: *kinesitherapy.*

kinesics. Systematic study of the body and the use of its static and dynamic position as a means of communication.

kinesim'eter [Gr. *kinēsis,* movement, + *metron,* measure]. An apparatus for determining the extent of movement of a part.

kinesiodic (kĭ-nē''sĭ-ŏd'ĭk) ["+ *hodos,* path]. Pert. to paths through which motor impulses pass.

kinesiology (kĭ-nē''sĭ-ŏl'ō-jĭ) [Gr. *kinēsis,* motion, + *logos,* study]. The study of muscles and muscular movement.

kinesioneurosis (kĭ-nē''sĭ-ō-nū-rō'sĭs) ["+ *neuron,* nerve, + *-ōsis,* condition]. Functional disorder marked by tics and spasms.

k., external. K. affecting external muscles.

k., vascular. K. of the vasomotor system.

k., visceral. K. affecting muscles of internal organs.

kinesiotherapy (kĭ-ne″sĭ-ō-thĕr′ă-pĭ) ["+ _therapeia,_ therapy]. Therapeutic exercises. SYN: _kinesitherapy._

kinesis (kĭn-ē′sĭs) [Gr.]. Motion.

kinesither'apy ["+ _therapeia,_ therapy]. Treatment by movements. SYN: _kinetotherapy._

kinesodic (kĭn″ē-sŏd′ĭk) ["+ _hodos,_ path]. Rel. to the conveyance of motor impulses.

kinesthesia (kĭn″ēs-the′zĭ-ă) [Gr. _kinēsis,_ movement, + _aisthēsis,_ sensation]. Ability to perceive extent, direction, or weight of movement.

kinesthesiometer (kĭn″ēs-thē-zĭ-ŏm′ĕ-ter) ["+ "+ _metron,_ measure]. Instrument for testing ability to determine the position of the muscles.

kinesthet'ic. Rel. to kinesthesia.

kinetic (kĭ-nĕt′ĭk) [Gr. _kinēsis,_ motion]. Pert. to or consisting of motion.

kinetosis (kĭn″ē-tō′sĭs) ["+ _-ōsis,_ condition]. Any disorder caused by motion, such as seasickness, car sickness. SYN: _kinesia._

kinetotherapy (kĭ-nĕt″ō-thĕr′ă-pĭ) ["+ _therapeia,_ treatment]. Treatment that employs active and passive movements. SYN: _kinesitherapy._

king's evil. Constitutional condition characterized by glandular swellings in neck and inflammation of joints and mucosa. So called, because it was thought curable by touch of a king. SYN: _scrofula,_ q.v.

kinin [Gr. _kinēsis,_ movement]. A general term for a group of polypeptides which have considerable biological activity. They are capable of influencing smooth muscle contraction; inducing hypotension; increasing blood flow in, and permeability of, small blood capillaries; and inciting pain. Their clinical usefulness has not been demonstrated.

kininases, plasma. Plasma carboxypeptidases which inactivate plasma kinins.

kink [Low Ger. _kinke,_ a twist in rope]. Unnatural angle or bend in a duct or tube such as the intestine or ureter.

kinky hair disease. Congenital syndrome due to an autosomal recessive gene, consisting of short, sparse, kinky hair which is frequently poorly pigmented. Both physical and mental development are retarded. The disease is due to a metabolic defect which causes an abnormality in the fatty acid composition of the grey matter of the brain.

Death follows progressive severe degenerative changes in the central nervous system.

kinomom'eter. Device which measures degree of motion in a joint.

kiotome (kĭ′ō-tōm) [Gr. _kiōn,_ column, + _tomē,_ incision]. Instrument for amputating the uvula.

kiotomy (kĭ-ŏt′ō-mĭ). Use of the kiotome in amputating the uvula.

Kisch's reflex (kĭsh). [Bruno Kisch, Ger. physiologist, 1890 —] Closure of an eye resulting from stimulation of heat or some tactile irritant on the auditory meatus. SYN: _auriculopalpebral reflex._

Kite apparatus. [Joseph H. Kite, Amer. orthopedic surgeon, 1891 —] Apparatus for reeducation of weak muscles and for assistance in overcoming contractures of forearm, wrist, and fingers.

KJ. Abbr. for _knee jerk._

KK. Abbr. for _knee kick_ (knee jerk).

kl. Abbr. for _kiloliter._

Klebsiella (klĕb-sĭ-ĕl′ă). [Edwin Klebs, Ger. bacteriologist, 1834-1913] A genus of bacteria of the family Enterobacteriaceae. They are short, plump, gram-negative bacilli which form capsules, but not spores. Frequently associated with respiratory infections and may cause urinary tract infections.

    K. ozenae. Species found in ozena, q.v.

    K. pneumoniae. A cause of pneumonia. Also found as a secondary invader in other respiratory infections such as bronchitis or sinusitis. SYN: _Friedländer's bacillus; pneumobacillus._

    K. rhinoscleromatis. The cause of rhinoscleroma, a destructive granuloma of the nose and pharynx.

Klebs-Loeffler bacil'lus (klĕbs-lĕf′lĕr). [Edwin Klebs; Friedrich Loeffler, Ger. bacteriologist, 1852-1915] The bacillus of diphtheria. SYN: _Corynebacterium diphtheriae._ SEE: _diphtheria._

klepto- (klĕp′tō) [Gr. _kleptein,_ to steal]. Combining form meaning to steal.

kleptolagnia (klĕp″tō-lăg′nĭ-ă) ["+ _lagneia,_ lust]. Sexual gratification derived from stealing.

kleptomania (klĕp-tō-mā′nĭ-ă) ["+ _mania,_ madness]. Impulsive stealing, the motive not being in the intrinsic value of the article to the patient. There is often deep regret following the act.

kleptoma'niac. 1. Pert. to kleptomania. 2. A psychopathic personality suffering from impulsive stealing.

kleptophobia (klĕp-tō-fō′bĭ-ă) [Gr. _kleptein,_ to steal, + _phobos,_ fear]. Morbid fear of stealing.

Klieg eye (klēg). Conjunctivitis, lacrimation, and photophobia from exposure to the intense lights used in making motion pictures or television films.

Klinefelter's syndrome (klin'fĕl-tĕr). [Harry F. Klinefelter, Jr., Amer. physician, 1912 —] Congenital endocrine condition of primary testicular failure which usually is not evident prior to puberty. In the classical form the testes are small and firm. Gynecomastia, abnormally long legs, and subnormal intelligence usually are present. In variant forms, the severity and number of abnormal findings are diversified. The syndrome is estimated to occur once in each 500 births.

Diagnosis may be confirmed by chromosomal analysis of tissue culture.

Kline test. [Benjamin Kline, Amer. pathologist, 1886 —] A microscope slide precipitation test for presence of syphilis. SYN: *Kline-Young test.*

Klon'dike bed. Outdoor sleeping bed that protects patient from drafts.

Klumpke's paralysis (klŭmp'kĕ). [Madame A. Dejerine Klumpke, Fr. neurologist, 1859-1927] Atrophic paralysis of forearm.

km. Abbr. for *kilometer.*

KMnO₄. Potassium permanganate.

Knapp's forceps (năp). [Herman J. Knapp, Amer. opthalmologist, 1832-1911] A forceps with blades like rollers for expressing trachomatous granulations on the palpebral conjunctiva.

kneading (nēd'ing) [AS. *cnedan*]. A form of massage consisting of grasping, wringing, lifting, rolling, or pressing part of a muscle or group of muscles. SYN: *pétrissage.*

knee [AS. *cnēo*]. The anterior aspect of the leg at the articulation of the femur and tibia and the articulation itself, covered anteriorly with the patella or kneecap. Formed by the femur, tibia, and patella.

RS: geniculate; geniculum; "genu-" words; "gon-" words; housemaid's k.; patella; popliteal.

k., Brodie's. A chronic, fungoid synovitis of the knee joint in which the affected parts become soft and pulpy.

k. -chest position. Resting upon the knees and chest with forearms supporting the head. SEE: *position.*

k., dislocation of the. Displacement of the knee.

Dislocations of the knee in themselves are unusual. The so-called dislocation of the knee is usually due to various injuries of the joint and of the complicating structures of the knee, such as the tearing of the crushed tendons or ligaments, or slipping of the cartilages. They should be treated either by a straight splint, as in a fracture of the kneecap; or two splints, one on either side of the knee, as in a fracture; and the patient should be transported to a hospital as quickly as possible.

k., game. A lay term for internal derangement of knee joint.

PATH: Usually a torn internal cartilage, a fracture of the tibial spine, or an injury to the collateral or cruciate ligaments.

SYM: Pain or instability, locking, and weakness. F.A. TREATMENT: Immobilize with a posterior splint. Surgical exploratory arthrotomy may be necessary.

k., housemaid's. Inflamed condition of the bursa in front of the patella with accumulation of fluid therein. May be seen in those who have to kneel frequently or continually while working.

k., in-. The condition in which the knees come together while the ankles are far apart, caused by an outward distortion of the leg throwing knee inside the normal line. SYN: *genu valgum; knock-k.*

k. -jerk reflex. The reflex contraction or clonic spasm of the quadriceps muscle, produced by sharply striking the ligamentum patellae when the leg hangs loosely flexed at right angles. It is seen normally in health, but is usually absent in locomotor ataxia, multiple neuritis, lesions of the lower portion of the spinal cord, lesions of the

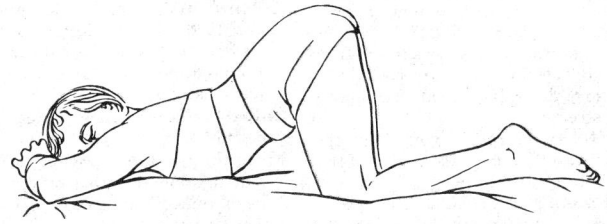

KNEE-CHEST OR GENUPECTORAL POSITION

anterior gray horns of the cord, meningitis, infantile paralysis, pseudohypertrophic paralysis, atrophic paralysis, etc., and increased in spinal irritability, lesions of the pyramidal tract, cerebral tumors, sclerosis of the brain and cord, etc. SYN: *patellar reflex.* SEE: *jerk.*

k. joint. The articulation of the femur and tibia.

k., knock-. In-knee, q.v.

k., locked. Condition in which the leg cannot be extended. Usually due to displacement of semilunar cartilage.

k. of the internal capsule. The curve at the meeting place of the anterior and posterior limbs of the internal capsule of the brain.

k., out-. Bowleg. SYN: *genu varum.*

knee'cap. The patella, q.v.

Kneipp cure (nĭp). [Rev. Father Sebastian Kneipp, Ger. priest, 1821-97] Application of water in various forms and degrees of temperature in the cure of disease, esp. wading in cold, dewy grass. SYN: *hydrotherapy.*

kneippism (nĭp'ĭzm). Walking barefoot in dewy grass, bathing in cold water, etc., as a cure of disease.

knife (nīf) [AS. *cnīf*]. A cutting instrument.

k., electric. A knife carrying a high frequency cutting current.

knismogenic (nĭs''mō-jĕn'ĭk) [Gr. *knismos,* tickling, + *gennan,* to produce]. Producing a tickling sensation.

knit'ting [AS. *cnyttan,* to make knots]. The process of healing by union of pieces of a fractured bone.

KNO₃. Potassium nitrate, niter, saltpeter.

knob (nŏb) [ME. *knobbe*]. A protuberance on a surface or extremity; a mass, q.v., or nodule, q.v.

knock-knee. Condition of having the knees turned inward. SYN: *genu valgum; in-knee,* q.v.

knockout drops. Slang term for chloral hydrate given in alcoholic beverages to produce rapid coma. Does not cause immediate loss of consciousness.

knot [AS. *cnotta*]. 1. An intertwining of a cord or cordlike structure to form a lump or knob. 2. In surgery, the intertwining of the ends of a suture, ligature, bandage, or sling so that the ends will not slip or become separated. 3. In anatomy, an enlargement forming a knoblike structure.

k., false. An external bulging of the umbilical cord resulting from the coiling of the umbilical blood vessels.

k., Hensen's. A knoblike structure at the anterior end of the primitive streak. SYN: *Hensen's node.*

k., primitive. K., Hensen's, q.v.

k., syncytial. A protuberance formed by many nuclei of the syntrophoblast and found on surface of a chorionic villus.

k., true. A knot formed by the fetus slipping through a loop of the umbilical cord.

knuckle (nŭk'el) [Middle Low Ger. *knökel*]. Prominence of the dorsal aspect of any of the phalangeal joints, esp. of the distal heads of the metacarpals when the fist is clenched.

k. pads. Discrete fibromatous pads overlaying the finger joints. Usually appear between ages of 15 and 30. Etiol. is unknown but trauma is not a significant factor.

K.O.C. Abbr. of *cathodal opening contraction.* SYN: *COC.*

Kocher's reflex (kō'kĕr). [Theodor Kocher, Swiss surgeon, 1841-1917] Contraction of abdominal muscles following moderate compression of testicle.

Koch's bacil'lus (kōk). [Robert Koch, Ger. bacteriologist, 1843-1910] The bacillus of tuberculosis. SYN: *Mycobacterium tuberculosis.*

Koch's law or postulates. Criterion used in proving an organism is the cause of a disease or lesion: (1) microorganism in question is regularly found in the lesions of the disease; (2) pure cultures can be obtained from it; (3) pure cultures when inoculated into susceptible animals can reproduce the disease or pathological condition; and (4) the organism can be obtained again in pure culture from the inoculated animal.

Koch's phenomenon. Local inflammatory reaction resulting from injection of tuberculin into the skin of a person who has been previously exposed to the tubercle bacillus.

KOH. Potassium hydroxide.

Kohlrausch's fold (kōl'rowsh). [Otto L. B. Kohlrausch, Ger. physician, 1811-54] Horizontal folds of the mucosa of the rectum; rectal valve. SYN: *Houston's valves; Kohlrausch's valve; plica transversales recti.*

koilonychia (koy-lō-nĭk'ĭ-ă) [Gr. *koilos,* hollow, + *onyx, onych-,* nail]. Malformation of the fingernails; outer surface is concave.

Kol'mer test. [John Kolmer, Amer. pathologist, 1886 —] 1. A modification of the Wassermann test, a serological test for syphilis. 2. Complement fixation test for some infectious diseases.

kolp-. Prefix indicating vagina. SEE: words beginning with *colp-.*

kolpi'tis [Gr. *kolpos,* vagina, + *-itis,* inflammation]. Inflammation of vaginal mucous membrane. SYN: *colpitis.*

kolpot'omy ["+ *tomē,* incision]. A vaginal operation. SYN: *colpotomy; elytrotomy.*

kolyone (kŏ'lĭ-ōn) [Gr. *kōlyein*, to hinder]. An organic secretion carried in the blood to other organs. It functions to inhibit growth and function. SYN: *chalone; colyone.*

kolypeptic (kŏ"lĭ-pĕp'tĭk) ["+ *pepsis*, digestion]. Retarding digestion.

kolyphrenia (kŏ"lĭ-frē'nĭ-ă) ["+ *phrēn*, mind]. Exaggerated mental inhibition.

kolyseptic (kŏ"lĭ-sĕp'tĭk) ["+ *sēpsis*, putrefaction]. Antiseptic.

kolytic (kō-lĭt'ĭk) [Gr. *kōlyein*, to hinder]. Temperament control by inhibiting, hindering, or checking a reaction to a stimulus.

Kondoleon's operation (kŏn-dō'lē-ōn). [Emmanuel Kondoleon, Gr. surgeon, 1879-1939] Surgical removal of layers of subcutaneous tissue to relieve elephantiasis.

koniocortex (kō"nĭ-ō-kor'tĕks) [Gr. *konis*, dust, + *metron*, measure]. The cortex of the sensory areas, so named because of its granular appearance.

koniol'ogy ["+ *logos*, study]. Science of dust and its effects. SYN: *coniology.*

koniometer (kō-nĭ-ŏm'ĕ-ter) ["+ *metron*, measure]. Device for estimating amt. of dust in the air.

koniosis (kō-nĭ-ō'sĭs) ["+ *-ōsis*, condition]. Any morbid condition caused by dust. SYN: *coniosis.*

kopf-tet'anus. Tetanus developing subsequent to head wounds.

kopiopia (kŏ"pĭ-ō'pĭ-ă) [Gr. *kopos*, fatigue, + *opsis*, sight]. Eyestrain. SYN: *copiopia.*

Kop'lik's spots. [Henry Koplik, Amer. pediatrician, 1858-1927] Small red spots with bluish-white centers on the oral mucosa, particularly in the region opposite the molars.

A diagnostic sign in measles before the rash appears. Not infrequently, the spots disappear as the eruption develops.

kopophobia (kŏp"ō-fō'bĭ-ă) [Gr. *kopos*, fatigue, + *phobos*, fear]. Abnormal fear of fatigue or exhaustion.

Kopp's asthma. [Johann Heinrich Kopp, Ger. physician, 1777-1858] Spasm of the glottis in infants not over two years of age. Thought to be due to an enlarged thymus. SYN: *laryngismus stridulus.*

koronion (kō-rō'nĭ-ōn) [Gr. *korōnē*, crest]. Apex of coronoid process of the mandible.

koroscopy (kor-ŏs'kō-pĭ) [Gr. *korē*, pupil, + *skopein*, to examine]. Shadow test for refraction of the eye.

Korsakoff's syndrome (kor'să-kŏf). [Sergei S. Korsakoff, Russ. neurologist, 1854-1900] Personality characterized by a psychosis with polyneuritis, disorientation, muttering delirium, insomnia, illusions and hallucinations. Painful extremities, rarely a bilateral wrist drop, more frequently bilateral foot drop with pain or pressure over the long nerves. Occurs as a sequel to chronic alcoholism but may be due to other intracranial pathology. SYN: *K.'s psychosis, polyneuritic psychosis.*

kosher (kō'shĕr) [Hebrew *kāshēr*, proper]. Food prepared and served according to Jewish dietary laws.

koumiss (kū'mĭs) [Tartar *kumyz*]. Fermented milk beverage. Also spelled kumiss, kumyss.

Kr. Chem. symb. for krypton.

Kraepelin's classification (krā'pā-lĭn). [Emil Kraepelin, Ger. psychiatrist, 1856-1926] A classification of mental disease into two groups: the manic-depressive and the schizophrenic.

kraurosis (krŏ-rō'sĭs) [Gr. *krauros*, dry]. Atrophy and dryness of skin and any mucous membrane, esp. of the vulva.

The subcutaneous fat of the mons pubis and labia disappears, clitoris and prepuce atrophy, and stenosis of the vaginal orifice is common. Fissures may develop. Epithelioma is prone to occur most frequently in postmenopausal women or those who have had ovaries removed.

ETIOL: Probably hypoestrinism.

k. penis. Condition in which the glans penis atrophies and becomes shriveled.

k. vul'vae. An atrophy of the skin and mucosa which pathologically consists of a marked atrophy of the vulvar skin, and which is characterized clinically by severe itching. Seen in elderly women.

The skin has a white marblelike appearance, and frequently shows excoriations as a result of the scratching. In a large percentage of these patients, the skin, if allowed to go on without operative interference, may undergo malignant degeneration. SYN: *leukoplakic vulvitis.*

Krause's end bulb. [Wilhelm Krause, Ger. anatomist, 1833-1910] An encapsulated sensory receptor found widely distributed in connective tissue underlying the skin and mucous membranes. It is the end organ for cold sensations.

Krause's glands. [Karl Krause, Ger. anatomist, 1797-1868] Small mucous acinous glands located beneath the fornix conjunctiva. They are accessory lacrimal glands and open into the fornix.

Krause's membrane. [Wilhelm Krause] Thin, dark disk transversely crossing through and bisecting clear zone of a striated muscle and bisecting the clear zone (isotropic disk) of a striated muscle fiber.

The portion between two disks constitutes a sarcomere. SYN: *Z disk.*

Krause's valve. [Karl Krause] Mucous membrane fold at juncture where lacrimal sac narrows into nasal duct.

Krompecher's tumor (krŏm'pĕk-er). [Edmund Krompecher, Hung. pathologist, 1870-1926] Rodent ulcer.

Krönig's area (krā'nĭg). [Georg Krönig, Ger. physician, 1856-1911] Resonant region in the thorax over the apices of the lungs. SYN: *K.'s field.*

Krukenberg's tumor (krü'kĕn-berg). [Frederick Krukenberg, Ger. pathologist, 1871-1946] A malignant tumor of the ovary, usually bilateral, and frequently secondary to malignancy of the gastrointestinal tract.

Histologically these tumors consist of myxomatous connective tissue and cells having a signet ring arrangement of their nuclei. The epithelial tissue resembles malignancy of the original site.

krypton (krĭp'tŏn) [Gr. *kryptos,* hidden]. SYMB: *Kr.* At. wt. 83.80; at. no. 36. A gaseous element found in small amts. in the atmosphere.

K₂SO₄. Potassium sulfate.

Kufs' disease. A rare form of amaurotic idiocy with onset of symptoms between 21 and 26 years of age. Diagnosed by the development of dementia, myoclonic jerks in a young adult, and associated with blindness and retinitis pigmentosa.

kumiss, kumyss (kū'mis) [Tartar *kumyz*]. 1. Cow's milk with sugar and yeast after fermentation. 2. Fermented mare's milk. Also spelled koumiss.

Kund'rat's lymphosarco'ma. [Hans Kundrat, Ger. pathologist, 1845-93] Lymphosarcoma which affects adjacent glands, but rarely invades neighboring organs.

Kupffer's cells (kŭp'fer). [Karl N. Kupffer, Ger. anatomist, 1829-1902] SEE: *cell, Kupffer.*

kuru (kū'rū). A rapidly progressive neurological disease which is invariably fatal. The disease affects mostly adult women and children of both sexes of members of the Fore tribe of New Guinea.

Probably due to a slow-acting virus. It is believed that the disease may be transmitted by cannibalism.

kwashiorkor (kwăsh-ĭ-or'kor) [African, golden boy]. A disease resulting from a deficiency of protein in infancy or early childhood.

kyestein, kyesthein (kĭ-ĕs'tē-ĭn) [Gr. *kyēsis,* conception]. A scum or film on stale urine; formerly throught to be a sign of pregnancy. SYN: *cyesthein.*

kyllosis (kĭl-lō'sĭs) [Gr., crippling]. Clubfoot.

ky'matism [Gr. *kyma,* wave, + *ismos,* state of]. Twitching of isolated segments of muscle. SYN: *myokymia.*

ky'mogram. A tracing or recording made by a kymograph.

ky'mograph [Gr. *kyma,* wave, + *graphein,* to write]. An apparatus for recording movements of a writing pen. The apparatus is designed so that the pen moves in response to force applied to it. Widely used in physiology to record activities such as blood pressure changes, muscle contractions, respiratory movements, etc. Consists of a drum rotated by a spring or electric motor. Drum is covered by a paper upon which the record is made.

ky'moscope ["+ *skopein,* to examine]. Device for measuring variations in blood flow and pressure.

kyogenic (kī''ō-jĕn'ĭk) [Gr. *kyēsis,* pregnancy, + *gennan,* to produce]. Inducing pregnancy.

kypho- [Gr. *kyphos,* a hump]. Prefix indicating humped.

kyphorachitis (kī''fō-răk-ī'tĭs) ["+ *rhachis,* spine, + *-itis,* inflammation]. Rachitic deformity involving thorax and spinal column. Results in development of anteroposterior hump.

kyphoscoliosis (kī''fō-skō''lĭ-ō'sĭs) ["+ *skoliōsis,* curvation]. Lateral curvature of the spine accompanying anteroposterior hump.

kyphosis (kĭ-fō'sĭs) [Gr., humpback]. Exaggeration or angulation of normal posterior curve of spine. Gives rise to condition commonly known as humpback, hunchback, or Pott's curvature. Also refers to excessive curvature of the spine with convexity backward. The former may be due to congenital anomaly, disease (tuberculosis, syphilis), malignancy, or compression fracture. The latter may result from faulty posture, osteo- or rheumatoid arthritis, rickets, or other conditions. SYN: *humpback; spinal curvature.*

kyphotic (kĭ-fŏt'ĭk). Affected by or pert. to kyphosis.

kyrtorrhachic (kĭr''tō-răk'ĭk) [Gr. *kyrtos,* curved, + *rhachis,* spine]. Spinal curvature with concavity backward.

kysthitis (kĭs-thī'tĭs) [Gr. *kysthos,* vagina, + *-itis,* inflammation]. Inflammation of the vagina. SYN: *colpitis; vaginitis.*

kysthoptosis (kĭs-thŏp-tō'sĭs) ["+ *ptōsis,* a falling]. Prolapse of the vagina.

kyto- [Gr. *kytos,* hollow vessel]. Prefix denoting a cell. SEE: words beginning with *cyto-.*

L

L. Abbr. for *Latin; Lactobacillus; left; length; light sense; liter.*

l. Abbr. for *left; left eye; lethal; liter.*

L₊ Symb. for limes death, q.v.

L₀. Symb. for limes zero, q.v.

L-. Chem. prefix using a small capital to indicate a compound structurally related to L-glyceraldehyde. Opposed to D-.

l-. Chemical abbr. for *levo,* left or counterclockwise.

La. Chem. symb. for lanthanum.

Labbe's vein (lăb-ā'). [Leon Labbe, Fr. surgeon, 1832-1916] Vein connecting lateral to superior longitudinal sinus. SYN: *superior anastamotic vein.*

la belle indifference [Fr., beautiful indifference]. An unrealistic degree of indifference to, or complacency about, startling and gross symptoms of hysterical anesthesia or paralysis. Seen in conversion reaction.

labia (lā'bĭ-ă) [L.]. (sing. *labium*) 1. Lips. 2. The lips of the vulva.

l. oris. [NA] The skin and muscular tissue surrounding the mouth; lips of the mouth.

l. majora. The two folds of cellular adipose tissue lying on either side of the vaginal opening and forming the lateral borders of the vulva.

Their medial surfaces unite anteriorly above the clitoris to form the anterior commissure; posteriorly they are connected by a poorly defined posterior commissure. They are separated by a cleft, the rima pudendi, into which the urethra and vagina open. In young girls, their medial surfaces are in contact with each other, concealing the labia minora and vestibule. In older women, the labia minora may protrude between them.

l. minora. Two thin folds of integument which lie within the labia majora and enclose the vestibule. Anteriorly each divides into two smaller folds which unite with similar folds from the other side and enclose the clitoris, the more anterior one forming the prepuce (preputium clitoridis) of the clitoris, the posterior one forming the frenulum clitoridis. In young children they are entirely hidden by the labia majora.

RS: clitoris; Hottentot's apron; mons veneris; nympha; nymphoncus; smegma; vagina.

labial (lā'bĭ-al) [L. *labialis*]. Pert. to the lips.

l. glands. Many racemose glands between labial mucosa and orbicularis muscle opening on lip's inner surface.

labialism (lā'bĭ-al-ĭzm) ["+ Gr. *ismos,* state of]. Defective speech in which labial sounds are stressed.

labile (lā'bĭl) [L. *labi,* to glide]. Not fixed; unsteady; easily disarranged.

l., heat. Easily altered or decomposed by heat. SYN: *thermolabile.*

lability (lă-bĭl'ĭ-tĭ). State of being unstable or changeable.

labioalveolar (lā'bĭ-ō-ăl-vē'ō-lar) [L. *labium,* lip, + *alveolus,* little hollow]. Pert. to lips and tooth sockets.

labiocervical (lā'bĭ-ō-sĕr'vĭ-kl) ["+ *cervix, cervic-,* neck]. Pert. to the buccal surface of the lips and the neck of a tooth.

labioglossolaryngeal (lā'bĭ-ō-glŏs''ō-lăr-ĭn'jĭ-ăl) ["+ Gr. *glōssa,* tongue, + *larynx,* larynx]. Pert. to lips, tongue, and larynx.

labioglossopharyngeal (lā'bĭ-ō-glŏs''ō-făr-ĭn'jĭ-ăl) ["+ "+ *pharynx,* throat]. Pert. to the lips, tongue, and pharynx.

labiograph (lā'bĭ-ō-grăf) [L. *labium,* lip, + Gr. *graphein,* to write]. Device for registering lip movements in speaking.

labiology (lā-bĭ-ŏl'ō-jĭ) ["+ Gr. *logos,* study]. Study of lip movements in speaking or singing.

labiomancy (lā'bĭ-ō-măn''sĭ) ["+ Gr. *manteia,* foretelling]. Interpreting speech by reading lip movements.

labiomental (lā-bĭ-ō-měn'tăl) ["+ *mentum,* chin]. Pert. to the lower lip and chin.

labiomycosis (lā'bĭ-ō-mī-kō'sĭs) [L. *labium,* lip, + Gr. *mykes,* fungus, + *-ōsis,* condition]. Any disease of the lips due to presence of a fungus.

labiopalatine (lā'bĭ-ō-păl'ă-tĭn) ["+ *palatum,* palate]. Rel. to the lips and palate.

labioplasty (lā'bĭ-ō-plăs''tĭ) ["+ Gr. *plassein,* to form]. Plastic surgery of the lips. SYN: *cheiloplasty.*

labiotenaculum (lā''bĭ-ō-těn-ăk'ū-lŭm) ["+ *tenaculum,* a hook]. Instrument for holding lips during an operation.

labium (lā'bĭ-ŭm) [L.]. (pl. *labia*) [NA] A lip or a structure like one. SEE: *labia.*

l. cerebri. Margin of the cerebral hemispheres overlapping the corpus callosum.

l. inferius oris. [NA] Lower lip.

l. majus. Labia majora, q.v.

l. minus. Labia minora, q.v.

l. superius oris. [NA] The upper lip.

l. tympanicum. Outer edge of organ of Corti.

l. urethrae. Lateral margin of meatus urinarius externus.

l. uteri. Thickened margin of the cervix uteri.

l. vestibulare. Vestibular or inner edge of organ of Corti.

la'bor [L., work]. The physiological process by which the fetus is expelled from the uterus. SYN: *childbirth; delivery; parturition.*

Approx. 95% of normal full-term babies are born 265-300 days from the first day of the last menstrual period. Average duration of normal pregnancy is 282 days.

Traditionally labor is divided into three stages, but *lightening* is noticed prior to that. Lightening occurs several weeks before the onset of labor. The shape of the abdomen changes with the lower portion becoming more pendulous and the costal area looking flatter. This change is due to the fetal head's having descended into the pelvis. Lightening is most noticeable in primigravidas and may not occur in multiparas until the onset of labor.

FIRST STAGE: Period from the onset of regular contractions of the uterus until the cervix is fully dilated. Averages 12 hours in primigravidas and eight in multiparas.

Identification of this stage is particularly important to the woman who is having her first baby. Diagnosis is complicated by the fact that many persons experience *false labor pains.* These may begin as early as three to four weeks before onset of true labor. False labor pains are quite irregular, usually confined to the lower part of the abdomen and groin, and do not extend from the back around the abdomen as in true labor. False labor pains do not increase with time and are not made more intense by walking. The conclusive distinction is made by determining the effect of the pains on the cervix. False labor pains do not cause effacement and dilatation of the cervix as do true labor pains.

A reliable sign of impending labor is *show.* The appearance of a slight amount of vaginal blood-tinged mucus is a good indication that labor will begin within the next 24 hours. Loss of more than a few milliliters of blood at this time must be regarded as being due to a pathological process.

SECOND STAGE: Period from complete dilatation of the cervix through the birth of the fetus. Averages 50 minutes duration in primigravidas and 20 minutes in multigravidas. Labor pains are severe, occur at two or three minute intervals, and last from a little less than one minute to a little more than a minute and a half.

Rupture of the membranes (bag of waters) usually occurs during the early part of this stage, accompanied by a gush of amniotic fluid from the vagina. The muscles of the abdomen contract involuntarily during this portion of labor. The patient directs all her strength to *bearing down* during the pains. She may be quite flushed during the pains and perspire. As labor continues the perineum bulges and, in a head presentation, the scalp of the fetus appears through the vulvar opening. With cessation of each pain the fetus recedes from its position and then advances a little more when the pains return. This continues until more of the head is visible and the vulvar ring encircles the head. This is called *crowning.*

At this time the decision is made concerning an incision in the perineum to facilitate delivery. If done it is most commonly a midline posterior episiotomy. When the head is completely removed from the vagina it falls posteriorly; later the head rotates as the shoulders turn to come through the pelvis. There is a gush of amniotic fluid as the shoulders are delivered.

THIRD STAGE: Period from birth of the fetus through explusion of the placenta and membranes.

As soon as the fetus is delivered the remainder of the amniotic fluid escapes. This will contain a small amount of blood. Uterine contractions and pains begin, and usually within eight to ten minutes the placenta and membranes are delivered. Following this there is a certain amount of bleeding from the uterus. The amount may vary from 100 to 500 ml. or more, but the average is 200 ml.

Amount of blood loss will vary directly with the size of the fetus. The probability that blood loss will exceed 500 ml. is less than 5% if the fetus weighs five pounds (2268 gm.) or less. The chances that blood loss will exceed 500 ml. is 25% if the fetus weighs more than nine pounds (4082 gm.). Other factors such as episiotomy or perineal laceration will also affect the amount of blood loss.

NP: In preparing for labor at home or in the hospital it is essential to reassure the patient, provide a calm environment, and dispel any anxiety. The more tense and fearful the patient, the more prolonged and difficult will be the labor. This is esp. true of the primipara who may have more misinformation than facts.

Upon admission to the hospital, or at home, the usual data will be obtained and the patient prepared for examination. Blood pressure, pulse, weight and height, and initial laboratory studies will be done. If labor is in progress, maintain an accurate record of frequency and duration of contractions as well as examinations and medications.

The Rh status of the mother will probably be known. If it is not, the following has to be done. If the mother is Rh negative and the Rh status of the conceptus is unknown or found to be Rh positive, the mother will be given Rh immune globulin. This should be done within 72 hours after delivery.

First stage: In the past it has been customary to shave the perineum, upper and inner aspects of the thighs, and lower abdominal area in preparation for labor. This is still done for convenience of the nursing and medical staff, but it is not mandatory. It has also been customary to give an enema and catheterize a patient in order to prepare for labor. Rather, the patient should be asked to urinate and have a bowel movement voluntarily. Catheterization is indicated if she is unable to urinate.

As soon as labor begins the perineal area is thoroughly prepared, using swabs and sponges. While the area is exposed to soap and water the introitus is protected by a sponge. This prevents water from running into the vagina. After the vulva has been cleansed the labia are separated and the introitus flushed out with a suitable antiseptic solution.

Second stage: The patient is in lithotomy position, covered with sterile drapes. During this stage it is common for small bits of feces to be expelled from the anus. These are removed, soiling the area as little as possible, and the area sponged or swabbed with an antiseptic solution, always moving down and away from the vagina.

Just after delivery the cord is clamped in two places, cut between the clamps, and the side nearest the infant tied. The actual tie is made about 2 cm. from the umbilicus. Alternatively a plastic cord clamp may be used. It is applied the same distance from the umbilicus. The clamp may be removed on the 2nd or 3rd day by cutting through one end, or it may be left in place to drop off with the cord.

The infant's nose and pharynx are aspirated, and prophylaxis for gonococcal infection of the eye is given. Physical condition of the infant is judged by use of the Apgar score, q.v.

Third stage: An injection to cause contraction of the uterus may be used during this stage although this is not mandatory. The placenta and membranes are carefully examined to determine if any portion has

remained in the uterus. The hour immediately following the end of the third stage is extremely important because it is in this time that postpartum hemorrhage is most likely to occur. The uterus must be carefully watched during this period. This is done by the nurse's maintaining her hand on the fundus and massaging it as often as necessary to maintain contractions. If the uterus becomes soft and fails to contract, the physician or nurse in charge should be notified promptly.

l. **active.** Regular uterine contractions with increasing dilatation of the cervix and descent of the presenting part.

l. **arrested.** Failure of labor to proceed through the normal stages. May be due to uterine inertia, obstruction of the pelvis, or systemic disease.

l., **artificial.** Induction of labor, q.v.

l., **complicated.** Labor occurring with an accompanying abnormal condition, i.e., hemorrhage or inertia.

l., **dry.** Labor after most of the amniotic fluid has been drained away. Usually associated with premature rupture of the membranes.

l., **false.** Uterine contractions coming on before the onset of actual labor.

l., **induction of.** Use of oxytocics or other methods to stimulate uterine contractions prior to the time they normally would occur.

l., **instrumental.** Labor completed by mechanical means, such as the use of forceps.

l., **missed.** Labor which begins normally, but contractions stop.

l., **normal.** Progressive dilatation and effacement of the cervix with descent of the presenting part.

l., **precipitate.** Labor which lasts less than 2-3 hours from onset to delivery.

l., **premature.** Labor which begins before the normal time. Usually between the 28th and 38th week of gestation.

l., **spontaneous.** Labor that is completed without mechanical or operative interference.

l., **trial of.** Permitting labor to continue long enough to determine if normal birth appears to be possible.

labor, words pert. to: abortion; "amni-" words; ante partum; bag, hydrostatic; bag of waters; ballotement; bipara; biparous; bradytocia; breech presentation; brow presentation; bruit, placental; caput succedaneum; caul; cephalhematoma; cephalic version; cephalotomy; cesarean section; cesarotomy; cleidotomy; conception; conjugate; Crede's method; cross birth; delivery; disengagement; dystocia; ecbolic; eclampsia; embryectomy; embryo; embryoctony; embryotocia; eutocia; fetus; gestation; Hegar's sign; hourglass contraction; impetigo herpetiformis; maneuver; obstetrician; obstetrics; placenta; puerpera; puerperal; puerperium; quintuplet; restitution; show.

laboratory (lăb′rā-tor″ĭ) [L. *laboratorium*]. A room or building equipped for scientific experimentation, research, testing, or clinical studies of materials, fluids, or tissues obtained from patients.

Laborde's method (lŏ-bordz′). [Jean B. V. Laborde, Fr. physician, 1830-1903] Stimulation of the respiratory center in asphyxiation by a series of rhythmical traction movements upon the tongue.

labrum (lā′brŭm) [L., lip]. (pl. *labra*) Lip, or liplike structure; the upper lip of an insect.

labyrinth (lăb′ĕ-rĭnth) [Gr. *labyrinthos*]. 1. Intricate communicating passages. 2. The internal ear consisting of osseous and membranous labyrinths.

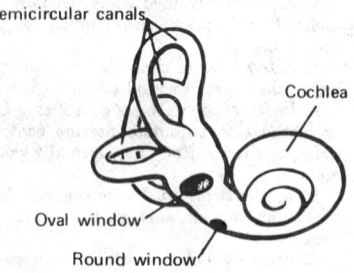

Semicircular canals
Cochlea
Oval window
Round window

BONY LABYRINTH (PERILYMPH)

l., bony. L., osseous, q.v.

l., ethmoidal. The lateral mass of the ethmoid bone. Includes the superior and middle conchae and encloses the ethmoidal air cells.

l., membranous. Structure in osseous l. consisting of utricle and saccule of vestibule, three semicircular ducts, and the cochlear duct. All are filled with endolymph.

l., olfactory. L., ethmoidal, q.v.

l., osseous. Consists of vestibule, three semicircular canals, and cochlea. Channeled out of petrous portion of temporal bone.

labyrinthectomy (lăb-ĭ-rĭn-thĕk′tō-mĭ) [″ + *ektomē*, excision]. Excision of the labyrinth.

labyrinthine (lăb-ĭ-rĭn′thĭn). 1. Pert. to a labyrinth. 2. Intricate or involved, as a labyrinth.

labyrinthitis (lăb″ĭ-rĭn-thī′tĭs) [Gr. *labyrinthos*, maze, + *-itis*, inflammation]. Inflammation (acute or chronic) of labyrinth.

ETIOL: Primary infection, complication of influenza, otitis media, or of meningitis.

SYM: Vertigo, vomiting, nystagmus.

RS: Meniere's disease.

labyrinthotomy (lăb″ĭ-rĭn-thŏt′ō-mĭ) [″ + *tomē*, incision]. Incision of the labyrinth.

lac (lăk) [L.]. 1. Milk. 2. Milky medicinal substance.

lacerate (lăs′ĕr-āt) [L. *lacerare*, to tear]. To tear, as into irregular segments.

lac′erat″ed. Torn; broken.

lacera′tion. A wound or irregular tear of the flesh.

l. of cervix. Bilateral, stellate, or unilateral tear of the cervix uteri caused by childbirth.

l. of perineum. Injury to perineum caused by childbirth. If extending through sphincter ani muscle it is complete.

lacertus (lă-sĕr′tŭs) [L., lizard]. 1. Muscular part of the arm. 2. A muscular or fibrous band.

l. cordis. Muscular tissue bands on inner cardiac surface. SYN: *trabecula carneae.*

l. fibro′sus. Aponeurotic band from the biceps tendon to the bicipital or semilunar fascia of forearm.

lacrimal (lăk′rĭm-ăl) [L. *lacrima*, tear]. Pert. to the tears.

l. apparatus. Structures concerned with secretion and conduction of tears. Includes l. gland and its excretory ducts, l. canaliculi, l. sac, and nasolacrimal duct which empties into nasal cavity.

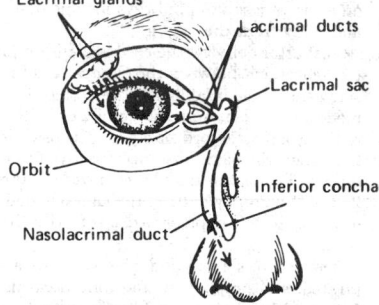

Lacrimal glands
Lacrimal ducts
Lacrimal sac
Orbit
Inferior concha
Nasolacrimal duct

LACRIMAL APPARATUS

l. bone. Bone at inner side of the orbital cavity.

l. duct. One of two ducts, superior and inferior, which convey tears from lacrimal lake to the lacrimal sac. SYN: *canaliculus.*

l. gland. Gland which secretes tears. A tubuloalveolar gland located in orbit, superior and lateral to the eyeball. Consists of a large superior portion (pars orbitalis) and a smaller inferior portion (pars palpebralis).

l. reflex. Secretion of fluid resulting from irritation of corneal conjunctiva.

l. sac. Upper dilated portion of nasolacrimal duct situated in groove of l. bone. Upper part is behind internal tarsal ligament. Measures 12-15 mm. in length.

lacrima'tion [L. *lacrima,* tear]. Secretion and discharge of tears.

lacrimator. A substance which induces the secretion of tears.

lacrimotomy (lăk″rĭm-ŏt′ō-mĭ) [L. *lacrima,* tear, + Gr. *tomē,* incision]. Incision of lacrimal duct.

lactacidase (lăk-tăs′ĭ-dās) [L. *lac,* milk, + *acidus,* sour, + *ase,* enzyme]. Enzyme in lactic acid bacteria which causes fermentation of lactic acid.

lactacidemia (lăkt-ăs-ĭ-dē′mĭ-ă) ["+ "+ Gr. *haima,* blood]. Lactic acid in the blood. SYN: *lacticemia.*

lactaciduria (lăkt-ă-sĭd-ū′rĭ-ă) ["+ "+ Gr. *ouron,* urine]. Lactic acid excreted in the urine.

lactagogue (lăk′tă-gŏg) [L. *lac,* milk, + Gr. *agōgos,* leading]. Agent which induces secretion of milk. SYN: *galactagogue.*

lactalase (lăk′tă-lās) ["+ *ase,* enzyme]. Ferment converting dextrose into lactic acid.

lactalbu'min ["+ *albumen,* coagulated white of egg]. The albumin of milk and cheese; a soluble simple protein. L. is present in higher concentration in human milk than in cow's milk.

When milk is heated, the l. coagulates and appears as a film over the top of the milk.

lac'tase [L. *lac,* milk, + *ase,* enzyme]. An intestinal sugar-splitting enzyme converting lactose into dextrose and galactose; found in intestinal juice.

SEE: *enzyme; maltase; sucrase; sugar.*

lactate (lăk′tāt). A salt derived from lactic acid.

lactation (lăk-tā′shŭn) [L. *lactatiō,* a sucking]. 1. The period of suckling in mammals. 2. The function of secreting milk.

DIET: During this period the mother needs additional calcium to offset its loss of milk. One qt. of milk, an egg, and meat are needed once a day. Fruits, vegetables, and whole grain cereal should also be included.

lacteal (lăk′tē-ăl) [L. *lacteus,* of milk]. 1. Pert. to milk. 2. An intestinal lymphatic that takes up chyle and passes it to the lymph circulation, and by way of the thoracic duct to the blood vascular system.

SEE: *absorption; lymphatic.*

lactescence (lăk-tĕs′ĕns) [L. *lactescere,* to become milky]. Condition of becoming, or resembling milk.

lac'tic [L. *lac,* milk]. Pert. to milk.

l. acid. A colorless syrupy liquid ($C_3H_6O_3$) formed in milk, sauerkraut, and in certain types of pickles by the fermentation of the sugars by microorganisms. It is also formed in muscles during activity by the breakdown of glycogen (glycolysis). Medicinally, lactic acid is used as a spermicidal agent and as a dietary constituent. SYN: *hydroxypropionic acid.*

l. acid fermentation. The production of lactic acid from carbohydrates by the action of various bacteria. Occurs commonly in milk and milk products.

l. dehydrogenase. An enzyme present in various tissues and serum which is important in catalyzing the oxidation of lactate.

In man LDH is present in several molecular forms called isoenzymes. Some LDH isoenzymes are present in certain tissues to a greater extent than in others. When one of these particular tissues is damaged, an isoenzyme of LDH is released into the blood. In that case determination of the pattern of LDH isoenzymes in serum may help to identify which tissue has been damaged. ABBR: LDH.

lacticemia (lăkt-ĭ-sē′mĭ-ă) [L. *lac,* milk, + Gr. *haima,* blood]. Lactic acid in the blood. SYN: *lactacidemia.*

lactiferous (lăkt-ĭf′ĕr-ŭs) ["+ *ferre,* to bear]. Secreting and conveying milk.

l. ducts. Ducts of the mammary gland.

l. glands. 1. The mammary glands. 2. Montgomery's glands consisting of 20-24 glands in the areola of the nipples.

lactification (lăk″tĭ-fĭ-kă′shŭn) ["+ *facere,* to make]. Lactic acid production.

lactifuge (lăk′tĭ-fūj) [L. *lac,* milk, + *fugāre,* to expel]. 1. Stopping milk secretion. 2. Agent stopping milk secretion.

lactigenous (lăk-tĭj′ĕn-ŭs) ["+ Gr. *gennan,* to produce]. Producing milk.

lactigerous (lăk-tĭj′ĕr-ŭs) ["+ *gerere,* to carry]. Secreting or conveying milk.

lac'tin [L. *lac,* milk]. Lactose, sugar of milk.

lactinated (lăkt′ĭn-āt-ĕd). Containing or prepared with milk sugar.

lactivorous (lăk-tĭv′or-ŭs) [L. *lac,* milk, + *vorāre,* to devour]. Living upon milk.

lactobacillin(e (lăkt-ō-băs′ĭl-ĭn) ["+ *bacillus,* little rod]. A preparation of lactic acid bacilli used to counteract intestinal putrefaction and to cause lactic acid fermentation.

Lactobacillus (lăkt-ō-bă-sĭl′ŭs) [L. *lac*, milk, + *bacillus*, little rod]. A genus of bacteria belonging to the family Lactobacillaceae. They are gram-positive, nonmotile, rod-shaped organisms which do not produce spores and are acid resistant. They produce lactic acid from carbohydrates. They are responsible for the souring of milk.

L. acidophilus. An organism which produces lactic acid by fermenting the sugars in milk. Found in milk, feces of infants fed by bottle, and adults. Also present in carious teeth and the saliva.

L. bulgaricus. The bacillus found in fermented milk. Milk fermented with this organism is known as Bulgarian milk.

L. casei. A type found in milk and cheese.

L. helveticus. Type found in Swiss cheese.

L. panis. Type occurring in sour dough.

lactobutyrometer (lăkt″ō-bū-tĭ-rŏm′ē-tĕr) [L. *lac*, milk, + Gr. *boutyron*, butter, + *metron*, measure]. Instrument for estimating the cream content of milk.

lactocele (lăkt′ō-sēl) ["+ Gr. *kēlē*, hernia]. Cystic tumor of breast due to occlusion of a milk duct. SYN: *galactocele.*

lactocrit (lăkt′ō-krĭt) ["+ *kritēs*, judge]. Instrument for determining the fat content of milk.

lactodensimeter (lăkt-ō-dĕn-sĭm′ē-ter) [L. *lac*, milk, + *densus*, thick, + Gr. *metron*, measure]. Instrument for determining specific gravity of milk.

lac′tofla″vin ["+ *flavus*, yellow]. Riboflavin, q.v.

lac″togen′ic ["+ Gr. *gennan*, to produce]. Inducing the secretion of milk.

l. hormone. Prolactin, q.v.

lactoglobulin (lăk″tō-glŏb′ū-lĭn) [L. *lac*, milk, + *globulus*, globule]. A protein found in milk.

lactolase (lăk′tō-lās) ["+ *ase*, enzyme]. An enzyme forming lactic acid. SYN: *lactacidase.*

lactometer (lăk-tŏm′ē-ter) ["+ Gr. *metron*, measure]. Device for determining the specific gravity of milk.

lactophosphate (lăkt″ō-fŏs′făt) [L. *lac*, milk, + *phosphās*, phosphate]. A salt derived jointly from lactic and phosphoric acid.

lactorrhea (lăkt-ō-rē′ă) ["+ Gr. *rhoia*, flow]. Discharge of milk between nursings and after weaning of offspring. SYN: *galactorrhea.*

lactoscope (lăk′tō-skōp) ["+ Gr. *skopein*, to examine]. Device for determining quality of milk.

lac′tose. $C_{12}H_{22}O_{11}$ + H_2O. 1. A disaccharide which on hydrolysis yields glucose and galactose.

Bacteria can convert it into lactic and butyric acids, as in the souring of milk. The milk of mammals contains 4-7% lactose. Its presence in the urine may be indicative of obstruction to flow of milk after cessation of nursing. Commercially, a fine powdered, white substance that will not dissolve in cold water.

2. USP. Crystalline sugar obtained from evaporation of cow's milk. Used in manufacturing tablets.

l. intolerance. Intolerance to milk characterized by gastrointestinal symptoms.

ETIOL: Deficiency of the enzyme lactase which is essential to the absorption of lactose from the intestinal tract. The deficiency may be present in the newborn, or it may be acquired as an adult.

lactoserum (lăkt-ō-sēr′ŭm) [L. *lac*, milk, + *serum*, whey]. Blood serum of an animal inoculated with milk; used to precipitate specific caseins from milk.

lactosuria (lăk-tō-sū′rĭ-ă) ["+ Gr. *ouron*, urine]. Occurrence of milk sugar (lactose) in the urine.

Frequent during pregnancy and lactation. Identified by osazone crystals.

lactotherapy (lăkt-ō-thĕr′ă-pĭ) ["+ Gr. *therapeia*, therapy]. 1. Treatment with milk diet. 2. Medicinal treatment of nursing infant with drugs given to mother to be excreted in milk. SYN: *galactotherapy.*

lac″totox′in ["+ Gr. *toxikon*, poison]. Any toxic substance occurring in milk that has decomposed.

lactovegetarian. 1. Pert. to milk and vegetables. 2. One who lives on a diet of milk and vegetables.

lactulose. A synthetic disaccharide, β-1, 4-galactosido-fructose, which is not hydrolyzed or absorbed in man. It is metabolized by bacteria in the colon with the production of acid and diarrhea.

Used in treating the encephalopathy which develops in patients with advanced cirrhosis of the liver. It probably acts by preventing the absorption of ammonia from the colon.

lacuna (lă-kū′nă) [L., a pit]. (pl. *lacunae*) [NA] 1. A small hollow space, such as that found in bones, in which lie the osteoblasts. 2. A gap or hiatus found in cartilage or bone in which lie cartilage or bone cells.

l., absorption. L., Howship's, q.v.

l., blood. L., trophoblastic, q.v.

l., bone. One of the isolated ovoid spaces between osseous lamellae, connected by canaliculi, containing a protoplasmic body or bone cell.

l., Howship's. A pit or groove in bone where resorption or dissolution of bone is occurring. Usually containing osteoclasts.

l., intervil'lous. A space in the placenta occupied by maternal blood and into which fetal placenta villi project. SYN: *intervillous space.*

l. laterales. Irregular diverticula on either side of the superior sagittal sinus of the brain into which the arachnoidal granulations project.

l. magna. The largest pitlike recess in the fossa navicularis of the distal end of the male urethra.

l. pharyngis. Pit at pharyngeal end of eustachian tube.

l., trophoblastic. Irregular cavities in the syntrophoblast which develop into intervillous spaces or lacunae, q.v.

l. of the urethra. One of those in mucous membrane of the urethra, esp. along the floor and in the bulb. They compose the openings of the urethral glands.

l. vasorum. Internal aperture of femoral canal.

l., venous. Endothelial lined spaces in the dura mater which communicate with the meningeal veins and blood sinuses, esp. the superior sagittal sinus.

lacunae (lă-kū'nē) [L.]. Pl. of lacuna.

lacunar (lă-kū'năr) [L. *lacuna*, pit]. Pert. to lacunae.

lacunes. Small irregularly-jagged cavities in the brain ranging in size from 0.5 to 15 mm. in diameter. They are believed to be small, deep, cerebral infarcts. Principal locations are the lenticular nucleus, pons, thalamus, caudate nucleus, internal capsule, and corona radiata. They are absent from the cerebral and cerebellar cortex. Even though they are undoubtedly important in explaining cerebral pathology, they are incompletely understood.

lacunula (lă-kū'nū-lă) [L., little pit]. Small or minute lacuna.

lacus (lā'kŭs) [L., lake]. Collection of fluid in small hollow or cavity.

l. lacrimalis. [NA] Space at inner canthus of eye where tears collect.

Laënnec's cirrhosis (lā''ĕ-nek'). [René T. H. Laënnec, Fr. physician, and the inventor of the stethoscope, 1781-1826] Atrophic cirrhosis of liver. SYN: *hobnail liver.*

Laënnec's pearls. Round gelatinous masses in asthmatic sputum.

Laënnec's rale. Modified subcrepitant rale due to mucus in bronchioles.

Laënnec's thrombus. Globular thrombus in heart.

lag. 1. Period of time between application of stimulus and resulting reaction. 2. Early period following bacterial inoculation into culture medium. Growth is slow during this time. SYN: *lag phase.*

lageniform (lă-jĕn'ĭ-form) [L. *lagena*, flask, + *forma*, shape]. Flask-shaped.

lagophthalmos, lagophthalmus (lăg''ŏf-thăl'mŏs, -mŭs) [Gr. *lagōs*, hare, + *opthalmos*, eye]. Incomplete closure of palpebral fissure when an attempt is made to shut the eyelids. This results in exposure and injury to bulbar conjunctiva and cornea.

ETIOL: Contraction of a scar of eyelid, facial nerve injury, atony of orbicularis palpebrarum, exophthalmos. Incomplete closure of the lids during sleep is seen in hysteria, in exhausted adults, and often in healthy children. SYN: *hare's eye.*

la grippe (lă grĭp') [Fr., the grip]. Influenza, q.v.

laity (lā'ĭ-tĭ) [Gr. *laos*, the people]. The great portion of people as distinguished from those who are members of a particular profession such as law, medicine, or the ministry.

lake [L. *lacus*]. A small cavity of fluid. SEE: *lacus.*

laked. Said of the blood in hemolysis, q.v., or disintegration of the red blood corpuscles, freeing the hemoglobin into the blood plasma.

lak'ing. Freeing of hemoglobin from red blood corpuscles.

laliatry (lăl-ī'ă-trĭ) [Gr. *lalia*, talk, + *iatria*, therapy]. Study and treatment of speech disorders and defects.

lalla'tion, lal'ling [L. *lallatio*]. A babbling form of stammering. Infantile form of speech. The constant use of "l" instead of "r."

lalognosis (lăl-ŏg-nō'sĭs) [Gr. *lalia*, talk, + *gnōsis*, understanding]. Science of understanding speech, particularly lallation.

laloneurosis (lăl''ō-nū-rō'sĭs) ["+ *neuron*, nerve, + *-ōsis*, condition]. Speech impairment of neurotic origin.

lalop'athy ["+ *pathos*, disease]. Any disorder affecting the speech.

lalophobia (lăl''ō-fō'bĭ-ă) [Gr. *lalia*, talk, + *phobos*, fear]. Morbid reluctance to speak due to fear of stammering or committing errors.

laloplegia (lăl-ō-plē'jĭ-ă) ["+ *plēgē*, a stroke]. A paralysis of speech muscles without affecting action of tongue.

lalorrhea (lăl''ō-rē'ă) ["+ *rhoia*, flow]. Abnormal flow of speech.

Lamarck's theory (lă-mark'). [Jean Baptiste P. A. Lamarck, Fr. naturalist, 1744-1829] Theory that evolutionary changes are the result of environmental changes; that basic inherent needs or changes necessitated by environmental modifications bring about the development of an organ; that use accentuates the development of a structure, disuse brings about its loss or atrophy; that acquired characters are inherited and passed on to descendents. Theory lacks experimental proof and is not generally accepted by Western scientists. SYN: *lamarckism*.

lamb (lăm) [AS.]. A young sheep.

Food value of 100 gm. (Leg of lamb, prime grade, cooked, roasted): Cal. 319; protein 24 gm.; fat 24 gm.; calcium 10 mg.; iron 1.6 mg.; niacin 5.2 mg.

lambda (lăm'dă) [Gr.]. 1. Letter in Gr. alphabet (Λ, λ). Also signified by letter L or l. 2. Point or angle of junction of lambdoid and sagittal sutures.

lambdacism (lăm'dă-sĭzm) [Gr. *lambdakismos*]. 1. Stammering of "l" sound. 2. Inability to pronounce "l" sound properly.

lambdoid, lambdoidal (lăm'doyd, lămdoyd'ăl) [Gr. *lambda*, L, + *eidos*, form]. Shaped like Gr. letter Λ.

l. suture. Suture between the occipital and two parietal bones.

lambert. [Johann H. Lambert, Ger. physicist, 1728-77] A unit of brightness equal to that seen when a perfectly diffusing surface radiates or reflects one lumen of light per square centimeter.

Lamblia intestinalis (lăm'blĭ-ă). [Wilhelm D. Lambl, Bohemian physician, 1824-95] Flagellate protozoan parasite found in intestine. Giardia lamblia, q.v.

lambliasis (lăm-blĭ'ă-sĭs) Giardiasis, q.v.

lame [AS. *lama*]. Disabled in limb, esp. in leg or foot; also applied to weak or painful condition as a lame back.

lamella (lă-mĕl'ă) [L. a little plate]. (pl. *lamellae*) 1. A thin plate or scale. 2. A medicated disk of gelatin inserted under lower eyelid and against the eyeball; used as a local application to eye.

l., bone. Thin layer of ground substance of osseous tissue.

l., circumferential. L. found on the external surface or lining the marrow cavity of a bone. SYN: *basic lamella; general lamella*.

l., concentric. Plate of bone surrounding a haversian canal.

l., intermediate. Bone l. filling irregular spaces between concentric lamellae.

l., interstitial. Bone lamella filling irregular spaces between concentric lamellae. SYN: *ground lamella*.

l., medullary. The osseous lamella surrounding and forming wall of medullary cavity of tubular bones.

l., periosteal. Bone lamella next to and parallel with the periosteum, forming external portion of bone.

l., triangular. Small fibrous lamina between choroid plexuses of 3rd ventricle of the brain.

l., vitreous. Innermost layer of the choroid next to the retina. SYN: *Bruck's membrane; lamina basalis*.

lamellar (lă-mĕl'ăr). Arranged in thin plates or scales.

lameness. Limping, abnormal gait, or hobbling resulting from partial loss of function in a leg. May be due to maldevelopment, injury, or disease.

lamina (lăm'ĭ-nă) [L.]. (pl. *laminae*) [NA] 1. A thin, flat layer or membrane. 2. The flattened part of either side of the arch of a vertebra.

l., alar. Alar plate of spinal cord in human embryo; later becomes sensory portion.

l., anterior elastic. Thin, tough membrane just below the corneal epithelium. SYN: *Bowman's membrane*.

l., basal. Basal plate of spinal cord in human embryo; later becomes motor portion.

l. basalis of the choroid. The membrane covering the inner surface of the choroid.

l., Bowman's. Basement membrane beneath epithelium of cornea.

l. cartilaginis cricoideae. [NA] The posterior portion of the cricoid cartilage.

l. choriocapillaris. [NA] Choroid's middle layer containing close mesh of capillaries.

l. cribrosa. [NA] Cribriform plate of the ethmoid bone.

l. cribrosa sclerae. Portion of sclera forming a sievelike plate through which pass fibers of the optic nerve to the retina.

l., dental. An epithelial plate which grows gumward from the labial lamina. From it arise the enamel organs of the future teeth.

l. ganglionaris. Ganglionic layer of the isocortex which is the non-olfactory cerebral cortex.

l. granularis externa. External granular layer of the isocortex.

l. granularis interna. The internal granular layer of the isocortex.

l., interpubic fibrocartilaginous. Part of the articulation of the pubic bones; it connects the opposing surfaces of these bones.

l., labial. A thickened band of epithelium which grows from the ectodermal covering of the primitive jaw. It splits into two sheets by development of the labial groove, thus giving rise to the vestibule of the mouth. From it arises the dental lamina, q.v.

l., medullary, internal. A layer of white substance which divides the gray substance of the thalamus into three parts—anterior, medial, and lateral.

l. multiformis. Polymorphic layer of the isocortex of the cerebral cortex.

l. papyra'cea. A thin, smooth plate of bone on lateral surface of lateral mass of ethmoid bone; forms orbital plate.

l., perpendicular. Thin sheet of bone forming perpendicular plate of the ethmoid bone. Supports upper portion of nasal septum.

l. propria. A thin layer of fibrous connective tissue which lies immediately beneath the surface epithelium of mucous membranes. SYN: *tunica propria.*

l. pyramidalis. The pyramidal cell layer of the isocortex of the cerebral cortex.

l., rostral. Continuation of the rostrum of the corpus callosum and the lamina terminalis of the third ventricle.

l. spiralis. One which divides the interior of spiral canal of cochlea into two scalae and divides into lamina spiralis ossea and lamina spiralis membrana.

l. suprachoroidea. [NA] Outermost layer of the choroid.

l., terminal. Thin sheet of tissue forming the anterior border of the third ventricle.

l. vitrea. Lamina basalis of the choroid, q.v.

l. zonalis. The outer or plexiform layer of the isocortex. SYN: *plexiform layer.*

laminae (lăm'ĭ-nē). Pl. of lamina, q.v.

laminar air flow. Filtered air moving along parallel flow lines to surgical theaters, nurseries, bacteriology work areas, or food preparation areas. This method of air flow helps to prevent bacterial contamination and collection of hazardous chemical fumes in areas where they would pollute the work environment.

laminaria digitata (lăm-ĭ-nār'ĭ-ă dĭj-ĭ-tā'tă). Genus of kelp or seaweed which when dried has the ability to absorb water and expand with considerable force. Has been used to dilate the uterine cervical canal; when so used it is left in the cervical canal for 24 hours.

laminated (lăm'ĭn-āt''ĕd) [L. *lamina*, thin plate]. Arranged in layers or laminae.

lamination (lăm''ĭn-ā'shŭn). 1. Layerlike arrangement. 2. In embryotomy, the slicing of the skull.

laminec'tomy [L. *lamina*, thin plate, + Gr. *ektomē*, excision]. The excision of a vertebral posterior arch.

laminitis (lăm-ĭn-i'tĭs) ["+ Gr. *-itis*, inflammation]. Inflammation of a lamina.

lamp [Gr. *lampein*, to shine]. Device for producing and applying light, heat, radiation, and various forms of radiant energy for the treatment of disease.

l., Gullstrand's. L. constructed so that an intense light is emitted through a slit; used for examination of the eye. SYN: *slit lamp.*

l., infrared. Heat lamp; a lamp which develops a high temperature, emitting infrared rays. Rays penetrate only a short distance (5 to 10 mm.) into the skin. Principal effect is to cause heating of the skin.

lamprophonia (lăm''prō-fō'nĭ-ă) [Gr. *lampros*, clear, + *phōnē*, voice]. Marked distinctness or clearness of voice.

lamprophonic (lăm''prō-fŏn'ĭk). Possessing a clear voice.

lanatoside (lăn-ăt'ō-sīd). Glycoside of Digitalis lanata; an agent used for digitalization.

lance (lăns) [L. *lancea*]. 1. Two-edged surgical knife. 2. To incise with a lancet.

Lancefield classification (lăns'fēld). [Rebecca Lancefield, Amer. bacteriologist, 1895 —] A classification of hemolytic streptococci into various groups by antigenic structure.

lancet (lăn'sĕt) [L. *lancea*, lance]. Pointed surgical knife with two edges.

lancinating (lăn'sĭ-nāt''ing) [L. *lancināre*, to tear]. Sharp or cutting, as pain.

Landouzy-Dejerine atrophy (lăn-dū-zē'dĕ''zhĕ-rēn'). [Louis T. J. Landouzy, Fr. physician, 1845-1917; Joseph Jules Dejerine, Fr. neurologist, 1849-1917] Atrophy of muscles of face and scapulohumeral group.

Landry's paralysis (lăn-drē'). [Jean Baptiste O. Landry, Fr. physician, 1826-65] A form of paralysis in which loss of motor power in lower extremities gradually extends to upper extremities and to circulatory and respiratory centers without sensory manifestations, trophic changes, etc. SYN: *acute ascending paralysis.*

Landsteiner's classification (land'stī-nĕr). [Karl Landsteiner, Austrian biologist in U.S., 1868-1943; Nobel prize winner in medicine in 1930] A classification of blood types designating O, A, B, and AB based on the presence of agglutinogens in the erythrocytes.

Lane's kinks. [Sir W. Arbuthnot Lane, Brit. surgeon, 1856-1943] Bending or twisting of intestine at various points as result of upright position of body.

Langerhans' islands (lŏng'er-hänz). [Paul Langerhans, Ger. pathologist, 1847-88] SEE: *islets of Langerhans*.

Langer's lines. [Carl Ritter von Langer, Austrian anatomist, 1819-1887] The structural orientation of the fibrous tissue of the skin. They form the natural cleavage lines which, though present in all body areas, are visible only in certain sites such as the creases of the palm. These lines are of particular importance in surgery. Incisions made parallel to them make a much smaller scar upon healing than will be the case if the incision has been made at right angles to the lines.

Lange's test (läng'ē). [Carl Lange, Ger. physician, 1883 —] Diagnosis of cerebrospinal syphilis by degree of gold precipitation in varying concentrations of colloidal gold solution and spinal fluid.

Lang'hans' layer. [Theodor Langhans, Ger. pathologist, 1839-1915] The cytotrophoblast, a cellular layer present in chorionic villi of the placenta.

languor (lăng'gĕr) [L. *languēre*, to languish]. Feeling of weariness or exhaustion as from illness; lack of vigor or animation; lassitude.

lanolin (lăn'ō-lĭn) [L. *lana*, wool]. USP. The purified, fatlike substance obtained from the wool of sheep.

Used as an ointment base.

l., anhydrous. USP. Wool fat containing not more than 0.25% water. Used as an ointment base which has the ability to absorb water.

lanthanic disease (lăn-thăn'ĭk) [Gr. *lanthanein*, to hide]. A disease which was discovered in a person or patient who had no knowledge that the disorder existed. SEE: *iatropic stimulus*.

lanthanic patient. A patient whose disease is discovered more or less accidentally in that he did not complain of symptoms referable to the disease. Ex: the discovery of high blood pressure or diabetes during a physical examination for employment.

lanthanum (lăn'thă-nŭm). SYMB: *La.* At. wt. 138.906; at. no. 57. A metallic element. One of a group of elements called lanthanides.

lanuginous (lăn-ū'jĭn-ŭs). Covered with lanugo, q.v.

lanugo (lă-nū'gō) [L. *lana*, wool]. 1. Downy hair covering the body. 2. Fine downy hairs

that cover the body of the fetus, esp. when premature.

laparectomy (lăp''ă-rĕk'tō-mĭ) [Gr. *lapara*, loin, + *ektomē*, excision]. Excision of strips or gores in abdominal wall.

laparo- [Gr. *lapara*, flank, loin, from *laparos*, soft]. Combining form pert. to the flank and to operations through the abdominal wall.

laparocholecystotomy (lăp''ăr-ō-kōl''e-sĭs-tot'o-mĭ) ["+ *cholē*, bile, + *kystis*, bladder, + *tomē*, incision]. Incision into gallbladder through abdominal wall.

laparocolostomy (lăp''ăr-ō-kō-lŏs'tō-mĭ) ["+ *kōlon*, colon, + *stoma*, opening]. Formation of permanent opening into colon through abdominal wall.

laparocolotomy (lăp''ăr-ō-kō-lŏt'ō-mĭ) ["+ "+ *tomē*, incision]. Incision of colon through abdominal wall, forming an artificial opening. SYN: *laparocolostomy*.

laparocolpotomy (lăp''ăr-ō-kŏl-pŏt'ō-mĭ) ["+ *kolpos*, vagina, + *tomē*, incision]. Incision over Poupart's ligament dissecting peritoneum to vagina which is incised transversely, enabling dilation of cervix and extraction of child through os uteri.

laparocystectomy (lă''pă-rō-sĭs-tĕk'tō-mĭ) [Gr. *lapara*, flank, + *kystis*, bladder, + *ektomē*, excision]. Removal of extrauterine fetus or of contents of a cyst through an abdominal incision.

laparocystidotomy (lăp''ăr-ō-sĭst-ĭ-dŏt'ō-mĭ) ["+ "+ *tomē*, incision]. Bladder incision through the abdominal wall.

laparocystotomy (lăp''ăr-ō-sĭs-tŏt'ō-mĭ). Incision of abdomen to remove contents of a cyst or an extrauterine fetus.

laparoelytrotomy (lăp''ăr-ō-ĕl-ĭ-trŏt'o-mĭ) [Gr. *lapara*, flank, loin, + *elytron*, sheath (vagina), + *tomē*, incision]. Abdominal incision to aid in removal of fetus. SEE: *cesarean section*.

laparoenterostomy (lăp''ă-rō-ĕn''tĕr-ōs'tō-mĭ) ["+ *enteron*, intestine, + *stoma*, opening]. Formation of aperture into intestine through abdominal wall.

laparoenterotomy (lăp''ăr-ō-ĕn-tĕr-ōt'ō-mĭ) ["+ "+ *tomē*, incision]. Opening into intestinal cavity by incision through the loins.

laparogastrostomy (lăp''ăr-ō-găs-trŏs'tō-mĭ) [Gr. *lapara*, loin, + *gastēr*, belly, + *stoma*, opening]. Formation of permanent gastric fistula through abdominal wall. SYN: *celiogastrostomy*.

laparogastrotomy (lăp''ă-rō-găs-trŏt'ō-mĭ) ["+ "+ *tomē*, incision]. Abdominal incision into stomach.

laparohepatotomy (lăp''ăr-ō-hĕp-ă-tŏt'ō-mĭ) ["+ *hēpar, hēpat-*, liver, + *tomē*, incision]. Incision of the liver through abdominal wall.

laparohysterectomy (lăp″ăr-ō-hĭs-tĕr-ĕk′tō-mĭ) ["+ *hystera*, uterus, + *ektomē*, excision]. Removal of uterus through an incision in the abdominal wall.

laparohystero-oophorectomy (lăp″ăr-ō-hĭs″tĕr-o-ō″ō-fōr-ĕk′tō-mĭ) ["+ "+ *ōion*, ovum, + *phoros*, bearer, + *ektomē*, excision]. Removal of uterus and ovaries through an abdominal incision.

laparohysteropexy (lăp″ăr-ō-hĭs′tĕr-o-pĕks-ĭ) ["+ "+ *pēxis*, fixation]. Abdominal fixation of the uterus.

laparohysterosalpingo-oophorectomy (lăp″ăr-ō-hĭs″tĕr-ō-săl-pĭn″gō-ō″ō-fō-rek′tō-mĭ) [Gr. *lapara*, loin, + *hystera*, uterus, + *salpinx*, tube, + *ōion*, ovum, + *phoros*, bearer, + *ektomē*, excision]. Removal of uterus, fallopian tubes, and ovaries through abdominal incision. SYN: *celiohysterosalpingo-oothecectomy*.

laparohysterotomy (lăp″ăr-ō-hĭs-tĕr-ŏt′ō-mĭ) ["+ "+ *tomē*, incision]. Incision of uterus through abdominal incision. SEE: *cesarean section*.

laparoileotomy (lăp″ăr-ō-ĭl-ē-ŏt′ō-mĭ) ["+ L. *ileum*, ileum, + Gr. *tomē*, incision]. Abdominal incision into ileum.

laparokelyphotomy (lăp″ăr-ō-kĕl-ĭ-fŏt′ō-mĭ) ["+ *kelyphos*, eggshell, + *tomē*, incision]. 1. Removal of an extrauterine fetus by laparotomy. 2. Suprapubic cystotomy. SYN: *laparocystotomy*.

laparomyitis (lăp″ăr-ō-mĭ-ī′tĭs) [Gr. *lapara*, loin, + *mys*, muscle, + *itis*, inflammation]. Inflammation of muscular portion of abdominal wall.

laparomyomectomy (lăp″ăr-ō-mĭ-o-mĕk′tō-mĭ) ["+ "+ *ōma*, tumor, + *ektomē*, excision]. Abdominal excision of a muscular tumor.

laparonephrectomy (lăp″ăr-ō-nĕ-frĕk′tō-mĭ) ["+ *nephros*, kidney, + *ektomē*, excision]. Renal excision abdominally.

laparorrhaphy (lăp-ăr-or′ră-fĭ) ["+ *raphē*, suture]. Suture of wound in the abdominal wall. SYN: *celiorrhaphy*.

laparosalpingectomy (lăp″ăr-ō-săl-pĭn-jĕk′tō-mĭ) ["+ *salpinx*, tube, + *ektomē*, excision]. Abdominal excision of a fallopian tube.

laparosalpingo-oophorectomy (lăp″ăr-ō-săl-pĭn″gō-ō″ōf-ō-rĕk′tō-mĭ) ["+ "+ *ōion*, ovum, + *phoros*, bearer, + *ektomē*, excision]. Removal of fallopian tubes and ovaries through abdominal incision. SYN: *celiosalpingo-oothecectomy*.

laparosalpingotomy (lăp″ăr-ō-săl-pĭn-gŏt′ō-mĭ) ["+ "+ *tomē*, incision]. Incision of oviduct through abdominal wall. SYN: *celiosalpingotomy*.

laparoscopy (lăp-ăr-os′kō-pĭ) [Gr. *lapara*, loin, + *skopein*, to examine]. Abdominal exploration employing a type of endoscope called a laparascope.

laparosplenectomy (lăp″ăr-o-splēn-ĕk′tō-mĭ) ["+ *splēn*, spleen, + *ektomē*, excision]. Abdominal excision of the spleen.

laparosplenotomy (lăp″ăr-ō-splēn-ŏt′ō-mĭ) ["+ "+ *tomē*, incision]. Incision of the spleen through abdominal wall.

laparotomy (lăp-ăr-ŏt′ō-mĭ) [Gr. *lapara*, loin, + *tomē*, incision]. The surgical opening of the abdomen; an abdominal operation.

PREOPERATIVE PREPARATION: Follow the physician's orders regarding diet, shaving of abdomen and pubic area, enemas, douches and collecting of urine specimens.

POSTOPERATIVE NP: Most patients remain in the hospital's recovery room until they are fully conscious. However, when a patient returns to the room, the nurse shall record her observations regarding the patient's general condition, the pulse and respirations, and blood pressure. The attending physician must be notified at once of any unusual symptoms such as shock or bleeding.

Follow the physician's orders as to the patient's position, fluid intake, diet and medications. If catheterization is necessary, use sterile technique.

laparotrachelotomy (lăp″ăr-ō-trā-kĕl-ŏt′ō-mĭ) [Gr. *lapara*, loin, + *trachēlos*, neck, + *tomē*, incision]. Cesarean section with the incision through the lower segment of the uterus.

laparotyphlotomy (lăp″ăr-ō-tĭ-flŏt′ō-mĭ) ["+ *typhlon*, cecum, + *tomē*, incision]. Incision of cecum through lateral abdominal incision.

laparouterotomy (lăp″ăr-ō-ū-tĕr-ŏt′ō-mĭ) ["+ L. *uterus*, womb, + Gr. *tomē*, incision]. Incision of uterus through abdominal wall. SYN: *laparohysterotomy*.

lapis (lă′pĭs) [L.]. Stone.

laqueus (lăk′wē-ŭs) [L., noose]. A noose-shaped band, fillet, or cord.

lard [L. *lārdum*, fat]. Purified fat from the hog. The sole nutrient is fat. 100 gm. portion contains 902 Cal.

lardaceous (lăr-dā′shŭs) [L. *lardum*, fat]. Resembling lard; waxy, fatty.

larva (lăr′va) [L., ghost, mask]. 1. General term applied to a young animal which differs in form from the parent. 2. An immature stage in insect life after it has emerged from the egg and before it transforms into a pupa from which it emerges as an adult.

l. migrans. Caused by larvae of dog-and-cat hookworm, Ancylostoma braziliense, but may be caused by the larvae of other nematodes or the larvae of flies. SYN: *creeping eruption; sandworm disease.*

l. migrans, visceral. Infestation of viscera by larvae of animal nematodes such as Toxocara canis. These migrate and cause eosinophilia, hepatomegaly, fever and hyperglobulinemia. Occurs mostly in children who play in soil or sand contaminated with dog and cat feces. The ocular symptoms may lead to the clinical diagnosis of retinoblastoma being made erroneously. There is no specific therapy but cortisone may be useful in controlling hypersensitivity reaction.

lar'vate [L. *larva*, mask]. Hidden, concealed.

lar'vicide [" + *caedere*, to kill]. An agent which destroys insect larvae.

laryngalgia (lăr-ĭn-găl'jĭ-ă) [Gr. *larynx*, larynx, + *algos*, pain]. Neuralgia of the larynx.

laryngeal (lăr-ĭn'jĭ-ăl) [Gr. *larynx*, larynx]. Pert. to the larynx.

l. reflex. Cough as result of irritation of larynx or fauces.

laryngectomy (lăr"ĭn-jĕk'tō-mĭ) [" + *ektomē*, excision]. Excision of larynx.

PREPARATION: Similar to tracheotomy, plus additional ligatures, sponge or tampon cannula. Best done in two operations—performing tracheotomy week or two before the main operation.

laryngismal (lăr"ĭn-jĭs'măl) [Gr. *larynx*, larynx, + *-ismos*, condition of]. Concerning or resembling affection with laryngeal spasm.

laryngismus (lăr"ĭn-jĭs'mŭs) [" + *-ismos*, condition of]. Spasm of the larynx.

SYM: Face pale—later cyanosed; eyes rolled up, body arched; thumbs turned into palm, legs extended, soles turned inward. In a few seconds the spasm relaxes.

PROG: Favorable. In very young, death may result from suffocation.

l., infantile. One occurring in children less than one year old, who are poorly nourished.

l. stridulus. A condition characterized by laryngeal stridor of sudden onset, inspiratory dyspnea, temporary apnea, increasing cyanosis, and, in severe cases, unconsciousness, convulsions and possibly death.

ETIOL: Early life (within first two years), male sex, and the rachitic diathesis are predisposing causes; often accompanies tetany. The discharge of motor force apparently

rises in the medulla and may be excited by reflex irritation as in teething and gastrointestinal troubles.

SYM: Attacks often and sudden; may occur on awakening from sleep—are characterized by a sudden arrest in breathing and tonic muscular swelling; can be detected by finger on throat. Spasm relapses, and air is drawn in through glottis with shrill crowing sound—may occur several times a day or weeks apart.

PROG: Extremely grave.

TREATMENT: Correct diet, cod-liver oil, and calcium lactate to prevent attacks. During attacks, cold cloths over thyroid or hot cloths to nape of neck. When dyspnea persists, tracheotomy may be indicated.

laryngitic (lăr-ĭn-jĭt'ĭk) [Gr. *larynx*, larynx]. 1. Resulting from laryngitis. 2. Rel. to laryngitis.

laryngitis (lăr-ĭn-ji'tĭs) [" + *itis*, inflammation]. Inflammation of larynx.

l., acute catarrhal. Acute congestive laryngitis; catarrhal inflammation of laryngeal mucosa and the vocal cords.

SYM: Hoarseness and aphonia and occasionally pain on phonation and deglutition.

ETIOL: Improper use or over-use of voice, exposure to cold and wet, extension from infections in nose and throat, inhalation of irritating vapors and dust, associated with systemic diseases as whooping cough, measles, etc.

TREATMENT: Complete rest of voice, promotion of diaphoresis, liquid or soft diet, medicated steam inhalations such as compound tincture of benzoin, codeine for cough and pain. SEE: *croup.*

l., atrophic. L. leading to diminished secretion and atrophy of the mucous membrane.

SYM: Tickling sensation in throat, hoarseness, cough, dyspnea when crusts are thick and accumulate on vocal cords so as to narrow the breathing aperture.

TREATMENT: Iodides internally, inhalants and medicated sprays to loosen the crusts; strict attention to associated nose and throat pathology.

l., chronic. A type due to a recurrent irritation, or following the acute form. Often secondary to sinus or nasal pathology, improper use of voice, excessive smoking or drinking.

SYM: Tickling in throat, huskiness of voice, dysphonia.

TREATMENT: Correction of preexisting nose and throat pathology, discontinuance of alcohol and tobacco, avoidance of excessive use of voice and proper vocal placement.

l., croupous. Diphtheritic l., q.v.

l., croupous hypertrophic. Hypertrophy of tissues accompanying chronic l.

l., diphtheritic. Invasion of larynx by diphtheria bacilli, usually with formation of membrane.

l., membranous. Characterized by inflammation of larynx with the formation of a false membrane of nondiphtheritic origin.

l., phlegmonous. Inflammed larynx with purulent infiltration or abscesses.

l., syphilitic. ETIOL: Due to syphilis.

SYM: Hoarseness, cough, simple catarrh, formation of broad condylomata, follicular hyperplasia, syphiloma, syphilitic perichondritis.

Secondary stage in form of mucous patches or tertiary in form of gumma. Secondary syphilis is a diffuse infection and one sees luetic patches spread over large areas of larynx.

In tertiary syphilis the gummatous lesion can occur in any part of larynx. There is marked redness over the infiltrated area as well as in the surrounding mucous membrane. When there is breaking down, the resultant ulceration is deep with sharp edges. Pain is usually absent and fixation of the cord is late. Cicatrization and deformity follow healing of gumma.

TREATMENT: Appropriate antibiotic therapy for syphilis.

l., tuberculous. Secondary to pulmonary tuberculosis.

SYM: Hoarseness, aphonia, pain in swallowing, cough. Lesion located in: Interarytenoid area; vocal cords; epiglottis; false cords. Lesions are relatively pale; ulceration occurs early.

laryngo- [Gr. *larynx,* larynx]. Prefix: Pert. to the larynx.

laryngocele (lăr-ĭn'go-sēl) [Gr. *larynx, laryng-,* larynx, + *kēlē,* hernia]. An air sac connected to the larynx. Is normal in some animals but abnormal in man.

laryngocentesis (lăr-ĭn''gō-sĕn-tē'sĭs) ["+ *kentēsis,* puncture]. Incision or puncture of the larynx.

laryngofissure (lăr-ĭng'gō-fĭsh'ūr) ["+ L. *fissura,* a cleft]. The operation of opening the larynx by a median line incision through the thyroid cartilage.

laryngograph (lăr-ĭng'ō-grăf) ["+ *graphein,* to write]. Device for making a record of laryngeal movements.

laryngography (lăr''ĭn-gŏg'ră-fĭ). 1. Description of larynx. 2. X ray of the larynx. Usually done after application of a radio-opaque dye to the larynx.

laryngologist (lăr''ĭn-gŏl'ō-jĭst) ["+ *logos,* study]. Specialist in laryngology.

laryngol'ogy. The practice of medicine dealing with the treatment of diseases of the larynx.

laryngometry (lăr''ĭn-gŏm'-ĕtrĭ) [Gr. *larynx, laryng-,* larynx, + *metron,* measure]. Systematic measurement of larynx.

laryngoparalysis (lăr-ĭn''gō-par-ăl'ĭ-sĭs) ["+ *para,* beside, unfavorably, + *lyein,* to loosen]. Paralysis of muscles of larynx.

laryngopathy (lăr''ĭn-gŏp'ă-thĭ) ["+ *pathos,* disease]. Any disease of the larynx.

laryngophantom (lăr''ĭn-gō-făn'tŏm) ["+ *phantasma,* image]. Plastic model of the larynx.

laryngopharyngeal (lăr-ĭn''gō-far-ĭn'jē-ăl) [Gr. *larynx,* larynx, + *pharynx,* pharynx]. Rel. jointly to larynx and pharynx.

laryngopharyngectomy (lăr-ĭn''gō-făr-ĭn-jek'tō-mĭ) ["+ "+ *ektomē,* excision]. Removal of the larynx and pharynx.

laryngopharyngitis (lăr-ĭn''gō-făr-ĭn-jī'tĭs) ["+ "+ *itis,* inflammation]. Inflammation of the larynx and pharynx.

laryngopharynx (lăr-ĭn''gō-făr'ĭnks). Lower portion of the pharynx that extends from the cornua of the hyoid bone or vestibule of the larynx to the lower border of the cricoid cartilage.

laryngophony (lăr''ĭn-gŏf'ō-nĭ) [Gr. *larynx, laryng-,* larynx, + *phōnē,* voice]. Voice sounds heard in auscultating the pharynx.

laryngoplasty (lăr-ĭn'gō-plăs''tĭ) ["+ *plassein,* to form]. Plastic reparative surgery of larynx.

laryngoplegia (lă-rĭng''gō-plē'jĭ-ă) ["+ *plēgē,* stroke]. Paralysis of laryngeal muscles.

laryngorhinology (lăr-ĭn''gō-rīn-ŏl'ō-jĭ) ["+ *rhis,* nose, + *logos,* study]. The branch of medical science concerned with diseases of the larynx and nose.

laryngorrhagia (lăr''ĭn-gor-rā'jĭ-ă) ["+ *rhēgnynai,* to flow forth]. Laryngeal hemorrhage.

laryngorrhea (lăr''ĭn-gor-rē'ă) [Gr. *larynx,* larynx, + *rhoia,* flow]. Excessive discharge of laryngeal mucus.

laryngoscleroma (lăr-ĭn''gō-sklĕ-rō'mă) ["+ *sklēros,* hard, + *ōma,* tumor]. Scleroma affecting the larynx.

laryngoscope (lăr-ĭn'go-skōp) ["+ *skopein,* to examine]. Instrument for examining the larynx.

laryngoscopic (lăr''ĭn-gō-skŏp'ĭk) [Gr. *larynx, laryng-,* larynx, + *skopein,* to examine]. Pert. to observation with aid of small long-handled mirror for reflecting interior of larynx.

laryngoscopy (lăr″ĭn-gŏs′kō-pī) ["+ *skopein,* to examine]. Examination of interior of larynx.

NP: Instrument should be warmed to help prevent mirror from becoming fogged.

l., direct. That done with laryngeal speculum or laryngoscope.

NP: Tongue, which is covered with a gauze, is protruded and held in that position by the patient or nurse.

l., indirect. That done with a mirror.

NP: Nurse should stand behind the patient with left hand on head, gently holding patient's tongue with right hand to steady it. The tongue is covered with a gauze to prevent its slipping from the fingers.

laryngospasm (lăr-ĭn′gō-spazm) ["+ *spasmos,* spasm]. Spasm of laryngeal muscles.

laryngostenosis (lăr-ĭng″gō-stĕ-nō′sis) ["+ *stenōsis,* a narrowing]. Stricture of larynx.

l., compression. From causes outside the larynx as result of abscesses, tumors, goiter, etc.

l., occlusion. ETIOL: May be due to congenital bands or membranes, foreign bodies, tumors, cicatricial contraction following ulceration as in diphtheria and tertiary syphilis, penetrating wounds or corrosive fluid.

SYM: Dyspnea, esp. on inspiration and exertion. Loud breathing which becomes a stridulous choking respiration; pulse small and frequent; face anxious and cyanotic.

PROG: Grave.

TREATMENT: Depends on cause. Tracheotomy is often necessary.

laryngostomy (lăr-ĭn-gos′tō-mĭ) [Gr. *larynx,* larynx, + *stoma,* opening]. Establishing permanent opening through neck into larynx.

laryngostroboscope (lăr″ĭn-gō-strō′bo-skōp) ["+ *strobos,* whirl, + *skopein,* to view]. Instrument for inspection of vibration of vocal cords.

laryngotomy (lăr-ĭn-gŏt′ō-mĭ) ["+ *tomē,* incision]. Incision of larynx.

laryngotracheitis (lăr-ĭn″gō-trā-kē-ī′tĭs). Inflamed conditon of the larynx and trachea.

laryngotracheotomy (lăr-ĭn″gō-trā-kē-ŏt′ō-mĭ) [Gr. *larynx,* larynx, + *tracheia,* windpipe, + *tomē,* incision]. Incision of larynx, with section of upper tracheal rings.

laryngoxerosis (lăr-ĭn″gō-zĕr-ō′sĭs) ["+ *xeros,* dry, + *-ōsis,* diseased condition]. Abnormal dryness of the larynx.

larynx (lăr′ĭnks) [Gr.]. (pl. *larynges*) The organ of voice, the enlarged upper end of trachea; musculocartilaginous structure lined with mucous membrane.

BLOOD SUPPLY: Inferior thyroid, branch of thyroid axis and superior thyroid, branch of external carotid.

STRUCTURE: Consists of nine cartilages bound together by an elastic membrane and moved by muscles. Cartilages include three single (cricoid, thyroid, and epiglottic) and three paired (arytenoid, corniculate, and cuneiform). The extrinsic muscles include the omohyoid, sternohyoid, sternothyroid, and several others; intrinsic muscles include the cricothyroid, external and internal thyroarytenoid, transverse and oblique arytenoid, and external and internal thyroarytenoid. The cavity of the larynx contains two pairs of folds, the ventricular folds (false vocal cords) and vocal folds (true vocal cords), and is divided into three regions (vestibule, ventricle, and inferior entrance to the glottis). Opening between true vocal folds forms a narrow slit, the rima glottidis or glottis.

NERVES: From interior and external branches of superior laryngeal.

NP IN DISEASES: Patient should stay in bed and avoid changes of atmosphere which may cause an attack of coughing. Room temperature should be maintained at the proper level; drafts avoided. Movements may set up coughing, so patient should rest quietly. The voice is generally affected in abnormal conditions of the larynx, so voice also should be rested. To keep silence, however, may cause patient to become de-

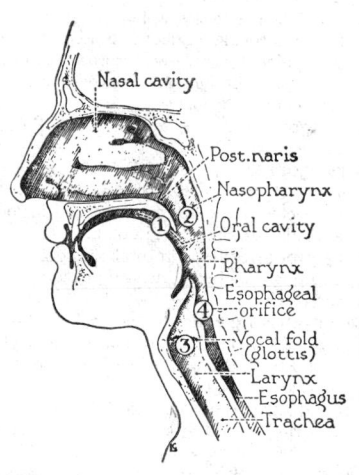

THE LARYNX

Seen in its relationship to: 1, The mouth cavity. 2, Nasopharynx. 3, Glottis. 4, Esophagus.

pressed. The nurse needs to help occupy the patient's time, but she should not ask the patient questions unless they may be answered by a nod of the head. The patient will need encouragement in continuing therapeutic inhalations ordered.

When possible for the patient to use the voice, instructions should be given to use the diaphragm and abdominal muscles rather than the muscles of the throat. In chronic laryngitis cold packs may be applied to the neck continuously.

In edema of the larynx, sucking ice or application of ice to the neck may be helpful. Astringent sprays may be ordered by the doctor.

RS: cricoarytenoid; epiglottis; glottis; "laryng-" words; prominentia laryngea; vestibule; vocal cord.

l., foreign bodies in. Violent spasmodic cough and dyspnea; fixed pain at particular spot; loss of voice.

TREATMENT: Immediately raise patient by the heels and slap him on the back. Search pharynx with finger and extract object. The foreign body will require bronchoscopy for removal if these emergency measures are ineffective. If necessary to maintain an airway, tracheotomy should be done.

lasciv'ia [L. *lascivīre*, to be wanton]. Abnormal sexual desire. SEE: *nymphomania*.

laser (lā'zẽr). Acronym for *l*ight *a*mplification by *s*timulated *e*mission of *r*adiation.

l. cane. An experimental cane which helps a blind person detect objects ahead of, above, and below his path.

Lassa fever. A disease, caused by the Lassa virus, first reported in Africa in 1970 with a mortality of over 50%.

SYM AND SIGNS: High fever, headache, vomiting, diarrhea, cough, epigastric pain and tenderness, severe pharyngitis, dysphagia, and renal and cardiac failure. The liver may be affected sufficiently to cause confusion with yellow fever.

TREATMENT: Specific therapy is not available, but plasma from patients who have recovered should be given.

lassitude (lăs'ĭ-tūd) [L. *lassitūdō*, weariness]. Weariness; exhaustion.

latency (lā'těn-sĭ) [L. *latēre*, to be hidden]. State of being concealed, hidden, inactive, or inapparent.

la'tent [L. *latēre*, to be concealed]. 1. Lying hidden. 2. Quiet; not active.

l. content. In psychology, that part of a dream or unconscious mental content that cannot be brought into the objective con-

sciousness through any effort of will to remember.

l. heat. Caloric or heat energy absorbed by matter changing from solid to liquid or liquid to vapor without a change in temperature.

l. period. 1. Time between a stimulus and its response. SYN: *lag phase*. 2. Time during which a disease is supposed to be existent without manifesting itself; period of incubation.

laterad (lăt'ẽr-ăd) [L. *latus, later-*, side, + *ad*, toward]. Toward a side or lateral aspect.

lateral (lăt'er-al). Pert. to the side.

l. sinus. Transverse and sigmoid portion of two cranial venous sinuses. Extends from occipital protuberance to jugular bulb.

latericeous, lateritious (lăt"ẽr-ĭ'shŭs) [L. *later*, a brick]. Resembling brick dust.

lateroflexion (lăt"ẽr-ō-flĕk'shun) [L. *latus, later-*, side, + *flexus*, from *flectere*, to bend]. Bending or curvature toward a side.

lateroprone, laterosemiprone position (lăt"ẽr-ō-prōn', -sĕm'ĭ-prōn). Patient on left side leaning on chest, right knee and thigh drawn up, left arm back of patient. SYN: *Sims' position*, q.v.

lateropulsion (lăt"ẽr-ō-pŭl'shun) ["+ *pulsus*, driving]. Involuntary tendency in cerebellar and labyrinthine disease to fall to one side.

lateroversion (lăt-ẽr-ō-vẽr'shun) [L. *latus, later-*, side, + *versiō*, a turning]. Tendency or a turning toward one side.

lathyrism (lăth'ĭr-ĭzm) [Gr. *lathyros*, vetch]. Disease presumably caused by eating certain plants of the genus Lathyrus. Characterized by muscular weakness and paraplegia which are irreversible.

latrine (lă-trēn') [L. *latrina*]. A toilet, particularly one in a military camp.

Latrodectus (lăt"rō-dĕkt'ŭs). A genus of small black spiders belonging to the family Theriidae.

L. mactans. The black widow or hourglass spider, a species widely distributed in the United States. The bite of the female produces serious symptoms and may result in death. SEE: *spider, black widow*.

latus (lā'tŭs) [L., broad]. (pl. *latera*) [NA] The side; the flank.

la'tus, la'ta, lat'um [L., broad]. Broad, as the uterine broad ligament.

laud'able [L. *laudabilis*, praiseworthy]. Commendable; healthy; normal; formerly said erroneously of pus.

laudanum (lăw'dăn-ŭm). Tincture of opium. SEE: *morphine*.

laugh (lăf) [ME. *laughen*, to laugh]. 1. Sound produced by laughing. SYN: *risus*. 2. To express emotion, usually happiness or mirth, by a series of inarticulate sounds. Typically the mouth is open and a wide smile is present.

l., sardonic. Spasm of facial muscles producing a grinning effect. SYN: *risus sardonicus.*

laughing gas (laf'ing). Nitrous oxide gas.

laughter, compulsive. L. without cause, occurring in certain psychoses, esp. schizophrenia. SYN: *obsessive laughter.*

laughter reflex (lăf'tĕr). Uncontrollable laughter resulting from tickling or pretense of tickling.

lavage (lă-văzh') [Fr. from L. *lavāre,* to wash]. Washing out of a cavity.

l., gastric. Washing out of the stomach. A stomach tube or catheter is used with a solution of sterile water, or normal saline, or 1-5% sodium bicarbonate.

Quantity of Solution: Not more than 10 oz. at a time repeated until fluid runs clear.

Temperature and time: 105° F. (40.6° C.). Preferably before breakfast.

Position: Semirecumbent or low enough to prevent inhalation of returning fluid. In poisoning, save siphoned fluid for examination. If patient is unconscious use a mouth gag.

Purpose: To remove irritants or poisons, to cleanse the stomach preoperatively or postoperatively. SEE: *colonic irrigation; irrigation, bladder.*

law [AS. *laga,* law]. In the scientific sense, a statement which is found to hold true uniformly for a whole class of natural occurrences.

l., all-or-none. The weakest stimulus capable of producing a response produces the maximum response contraction in cardiac and skeletal muscles and nerves.

l., Avoga'dro's. If temperature and external pressure are the same, all gases contain same number of molecules in equal volumes.

l., Bell's. Anterior spinal nerve roots are motor, and posterior roots are sensory.

l., biogenetic. Ontogeny recapitulates phylogency, i.e., an individual in its development recapitulates stages in its racial development. SYN: *recapitulation theory.*

l., Boyle's. The volume occupied by a fixed quantity of every gas is inversely proportional, and density directly proportional, to pressure applied to the gas.

l., Charles'. When pressure is constant, volume of a gas varies as the absolute temperature.

l., Courvoisier's. When the common bile duct is obstructed by a calculus, dilata-

tion of gallbladder is rare; when otherwise obstructed, dilatation is common.

l. of definite proportions. Two or more elements when united to form a new substance do so in a constant and fixed proportion by weight.

l., Fechner's. The intensity of sensation is proportional to the logarithm of the strength of the stimulus.

l., Graham's. The rate at which a gas diffuses through a porous membrane is inversely proportional to the square root of the density of the gas.

l., Haeckel's. SEE: *l., biogenetic.*

l. of the heart (Starling's). Other things being equal, the stroke volume of the heart varies as the extent of diastolic filling; or, the energy of contraction is a function of the initial length of the muscle fibers.

l., Hilton's. A nerve trunk supplying any joint supplies the muscles which move the joint and skin over insertion of such muscles.

l. of the intestine. Moderate distention of the intestine at a point causes relaxation below (aborally to the point) and contraction above.

l., Koch's, Koch's postulate. To prove an organism to be the cause of a given disease or lesion: The microorganism in question is regularly found in the lesions of the disease; pure cultures can be obtained from it; pure cultures when introduced into susceptible animals reproduce the disease or pathological condition; the organism can be obtained again in pure culture from the inoculated animal.

l. of Magendie. L., Bell's.

l., Marey's. Heart rate varies inversely to arterial blood pressure; that is, a rise or fall in arterial blood pressure brings about, respectively, a slowing or speeding up of heart rate.

l., Mariotte's. Boyle's l., q.v.

l. of mass action. In chemical reactions the amount of change taking place is proportional to action mass of the reacting substance.

l., Mendel's. A number of principles of heredity established by Mendel (1822-1884) which laid the foundation for the modern science of genetics. Includes the principles of unit characters, dominance, segregation, and independent assortment.

l. of multiple proportions. When two substances unite to form a series of chemical compounds the proportions in which they unite are simple multiples of one another or of one common proportion.

l., Murphy's. If something can go wrong, it will. This l. is of the utmost importance in designing and manufacturing apparatus or devices which are so critical that if they fail they will endanger the patient's safety or life. In other words medical devices and apparatus should be so constructed as to make failure, misapplication, or malfunction virtually impossible.

l., Nysten's. Rigor mortis travels progressively from muscles of mastication, through the face, neck, trunk and arms, reaching the legs and feet last.

l., periodic. The physical and chemical properties of chemical elements are periodic functions of their at. wt.

Natural classification of elements according to their at. wt.; when arranged in order of their at. wt. or at. no., elements show regular variations in most of their physical and chemical properties.

l. of reciprocal proportions. In chemistry, the l. that the proportions in which two elementary bodies unite with a third one are simple multiples or simple fractions of the proportions in which these two bodies unite with each other.

l.'s, Rubner's. 1. L. of constant energy consumption: Rapidity of growth is proportional to intensity of the metabolic process. 2. L. of constant growth quotient: The same proportional part, or growth quotient, of total energy is utilized for growth.

l. of specificity of nervous energy. Excitation of a receptor always gives rise to the same sensation regardless of the nature of the stimulus.

l., Waller's, of degeneration. If a spinal nerve is completely divided, the distal portion undergoes fatty degeneration.

l., Weber's. The increase in stimulus necessary to produce the smallest perceptible increase in sensation bears a constant ratio to the strength of the stimulus already acting.

l., Wolff's. Changes in form and function of bones result in definite changes in their internal structure.

lawrencium (lă-rĕn'si-um). [Ernest O. Lawrence, Amer. physicist, 1901-1958] SYMB: *Lw.* At. wt. 257; at. no. 103. A synthetic transuranic chemical element.

lax (lăks) [L. *laxus,* slack]. 1. Without tension. 2. Loose and not easily controlled. Said of bowel movements.

laxative (lăk'să-tĭv) [L. *laxāre,* to loosen]. A mildly purgative medicine; an aperient or mild cathartic.

l. diet. One promoting free intestinal elimination; fresh fruits; lemonade; stewed raisins; prunes; asparagus; cauliflower; spinach; tomatoes; figs; buttermilk; sweet potatoes; sweet corn; pea and bean puree; carrots; greens; nuts; whole grains; yeasts.

layer (lā'ĕr) [ME. *leyer*]. A stratum; a thin sheetlike structure of more or less uniform thickness.

l., bacillary. Rod and cone l. of retina of the eye.

l., basal. The basalis, outermost l. of uterine endometrium lying next to the myometrium.

l., choriocapillary. SEE: *lamina choriocapillaris.*

l., claustral. L. of gray matter between external capsule and insula.

l., compact. The compact surface l. of the uterine endometrium.

l., cuticular, of epithelium. A striated l. secreted by and covering free surface of an epithelial sheet, esp. that on surface of columnar epithelium of the intestine.

l., ependymal. Inner l. of cells of embryonic neural tube.

l., ganglionic. 1. Fifth l. of cerebral cortex. 2. An inner l. of ganglion cells in the retina whose axons form the fibers of the optic nerve.

l., germ. One of the three primary l.'s of the developing embryo from which the various organ systems develop. SEE: *ectoderm; entoderm; mesoderm.*

l., germinative. Stratum germinativum, the innermost l. of the epidermis, consisting of basal l. of cells and a l. of prickle cells (stratum spinosum). SYN: *malpighian l.*

l., granular exterior. Second l. of cerebellar cortex, lying within molecular l. and separated from it by a single row of Purkinje cells. Consists principally of granule cells.

l., granular interior. The fourth l. of the cerebral cortex, consisting principally of closely packed stellate cells.

l., Henle's. A l. of clear cells forming outermost l. of the inner epithelial root sheath of a hair.

l., horny. The stratum corneum, outermost l. of the skin, consisting of clear, dead, scalelike cells, those of the surface l. being constantly desquamated.

l., Huxley's. The middle l. of inner epithelial root sheath of a hair.

l., Langhans' . Cytotrophoblast of a chorionic villus of the placenta.

l., malpighian. SEE: *l., germinative.*

l., molecular. 1. Outermost l. of cerebral or cerebellar cortex. 2. Inner or outer plexiform l. of the retina.

l., osteogenic. Innermost or bone-forming layer of the periosteum.

l., outer-nuclear. A layer of the retina containing the nuclei of the visual cells (rods and cones).

l., papillary. Superficial layer of the corium lying immediately under the epidermis into which it extends, forming dermal papillae.

l., pigment. Outermost l. of the retina. Cells contain a pigment called fuscin.

l., Purkinje. A single row of large flask-shaped cells (Purkinje cells) lying between molecular and granular layers of the cerebellar cortex.

l. of pyramidal cells. The exterior pyramidal l.; third l. of cerebral cortex.

l., reticular. The inner l. of the corium lying beneath the papillary l.

l., somatic. In the embryo, a l. of extra-embryonic mesoderm which forms a part of the somatopleure, the outer wall of the coelom.

l., splanchnic. A l. of extra-embryonic mesoderm, which with the endoderm forms the splanchnopleure.

l., spongy. The stratum spongiosum, the middle l. of the uterine endometrium. Contains dilated portions of uterine glands.

l., subendocardial. L. of loose connective tissue immediately under the endocardium which binds it to the myocardium. Contains fibers of the conducting system of the heart.

l., subendothelial. L. of fine fibers and fibroblasts lying immediately under the endothelium of the tunica intima of larger arteries and veins.

lazaret'to [It. *lazzaro*, a leper]. 1. A quarantine station. 2. Hospital for treatment of contagious diseases. SYN: *pesthouse.*

lb. Abbr. for *pound.*

LD. Abbr. for *lethal dose.*

LD₅₀. Abbr. for the median *lethal dose* of a substance, which will kill 50% of the animals which receive that dose. Dose is usually calculated on amount of material given per gram or kilogram; or on the basis of amount per unit of body surface area.

LDH. Abbr. for *lactic dehydrogenase.*

L-Dopa. L-3,4-dihydroxyphenylalanine. A drug used in the treatment of Parkinson's disease. SYN: *levodopa.*

leaching (lēch'ing) [AS. *leccan*, to wet]. Extraction of a substance from a mixture by washing the mixture with a solvent in which only the desired substance is soluble. SYN: *lixiviation.*

lead (lĕd). SYMB: *Pb.* [L. *plumbum*] At. wt. 207.2; at. no. 82; sp. gr. 11.35. A metallic element. Its compounds are poisonous. Accumulation and toxicity occur if more than 0.5 mg. per day is absorbed. Most cases of lead poisoning occur in children who live in homes where lead was used in the paint. Children eat the paint and thus develop signs of lead toxicity. SEE: *pica.*

l. colic. That due to l. poisoning.

l. encephalopathy. Disease of brain caused by l. poisoning.

l. line. Bluish line on gums in l. poisoning.

l. pipe contraction. Cataleptic condition during which limbs remain in any position in which placed.

l. poisoning, acute. ETIOL: From large overdosage.

SYM: Metallic taste in mouth, burns in throat and gullet. Later abdominal cramps and prostration.

F.A. TREATMENT: Wash out stomach. Administration of magnesium sulfate (epsom salts) or sodium sulfate which precipitates the lead and helps remove the lead by purging. Give 10% dextrose in water intravenously to initiate urine flow. If this isn't successful, give mannitol, 20% solution, at the rate of one ml. per minute for a total dose of one to two grams/kg. of body weight.

If children have signs of lead encephalopathy give dimercaprol 4 mg./kg. intramuscularly every four hours for 30 doses. Four hours after the last of that series of doses give calcium disodium edetate, 12.5 mg./kg. intramuscularly every four hours in a 20% solution with 0.5% procaine added for a total of 30 doses. Adults with signs of acute encephalopathy should be given the same therapy. In either adults or children, if convulsions occur treat with appropriate anticonvulsant. Complete recovery may take as long as a year.

l. poisoning, chronic. ETIOL: Exceedingly common. Exposure in the industries; from food when lead vessels are used in its preparation; from cosmetics; or in children from nipple shields, chewing lead toys or objects covered with lead paints, such as walls or window sills.

SYM: Anorexia, nausea, vomiting, salivation, anemia, the lead line on the gums, abdominal pains, muscle cramps and pains in the joints. One of the most typical findings is the abdominal pain known as lead colic. There may be impairment of any part of the nervous system, often leading to muscle atrophy and the characteristic foot or wrist drop. Various blood changes may be found, especially the "stippling" of the red cells.

TREATMENT: Depends on severity of symptoms. If severe, treatment outlined above will be required.

lead (lēd) [AS. *lǣdan,* to guide]. An electrocardiograph record.

The three common l.'s are: lead I, right arm to left arm; lead II, right arm to left leg; lead III, left arm to left leg. These are known as standard l.'s, bipolar limb l.'s or indirect l.'s.

l., precordial. Record taken when one electrode is placed over the precordium, the other over an indifferent region.

l., unipolar. Record made when one electrode is placed on chest wall overlying the heart, where potential changes are of considerable magnitude and the other (distant or indifferent electrode) placed where potential changes are of small magnitude.

leaf (lēf) [AS.]. A plant organ usually shooting out from the side of a stem or branch; somewhat flattened and oval in shape, and green in color. SEE: *belladonna; digitalis; hyoscyamus.*

lean (lēn) [AS. *hlaene,* without flesh]. Without flesh, emaciated.

l. body mass. The weight of the body devoid of fat. Because some lipid substances are essential to body function the term is better replaced by the concept of fat-free body.

Leber's disease (lā'bĕr). [Theodor Leber, Ger. ophthalmologist, 1840-1917] Hereditary form of atrophy of the optic nerve which usually affects young males.

Leber's plexus. Plexus of venules in eye between Schlemm's canal and Fontana's spaces.

Lecat's gulf (lā-kăts'). [Claude N. Lecat, Fr. surgeon, 1700-1768] Bulbous portion of the urethra.

lechery (lĕtch'ĕr-ĭ) [Fr. *lecher,* to lick]. Lewdness; sensualism.

lecithin (lĕs'ĭth-ĭn) [Gr. *lekithos,* egg yolk]. A fatty substance, of the group called phospholipins, found in blood, bile, brain, egg yolk, nerves, and other animal tissues, and yielding stearic acid, glycerol, phosphoric acid, and choline on hydrolysis.

lec"ithin'ase. An enzyme that catalyzes the decomposition of lecithin.

l., cobra. An enzyme present in certain snake venoms.

lectual (lekt'ū-ăl) [L. *lectus,* bed]. Pert. to a bed or couch.

leech (lētch) [AS. *laece*]. A bloodsucking water worm, belonging to the phylum Annelida, class Hirudinea. It is parasitic on

man and other animals, producing a condition known as hirudiniasis, q.v. Leeches were at one time used as a means of bloodletting, a practice common up to the middle of the 19th century, but which now has been almost completely abandoned. They are a source of hirudin, an anticoagulating principle secreted by their buccal glands. SEE: *Hirudo.*

l., artificial. Cup and suction pump or syringe for drawing blood.

lees. The sediment obtained by allowing a solution to settle. Esp. the dregs at the bottom of a wine bottle.

Lee's ganglion (lē). Cervical uterine ganglion formed from 3rd and 4th sacral nerves and hypogastric and ovarian plexuses.

left. The opposite of right. SYN: *sinistral.*

left-handedness. Condition of being more adept in use of left hand. SYN: *sinistrality.*

left lateral recumbent position. Patient on left side, right knee and thigh drawn up. Used in rectal operations and sometimes in obstetrics.

leg (lĕg) [ME.]. One of the two lower extremities, including the femur, tibia, fibula, and patella; specifically the part between the knee and ankle.

RS: bayonetleg; bowleg; Buerger's disease; calf; crural; crus; saphena; sura; systremma; tibia.

l., Anglesey. A form of jointed artificial l.

l. badger. Inequality in the length of the l.'s.

l., baker. Genu valgum, or knocknee.

l., bandy. Same as bowleg.

l., Barbadoes. Elephantiasis of the l.'s

l., bayonet. Uncorrected backward displacement of the knee bones, followed by ankylosis at the joint.

l., bird. Reduction in size of the l. from atrophy of the muscles.

l., boomerang. A disease of the l. bones occurring among Australian natives, causing a curvature of the l. resembling a boomerang.

l., bow-. Genu varum; an outward curving of the l.'s at the knees.

l., milk. Phlebitis of the femoral vein occassionally following parturition and typhoid fever. It is characterized by swelling of the l., usually without redness. SYN: *phlegmasia alba dolens; white l.*

l., scissor. Cross l. deformity; a result of double hip disease, in which the patient walks with the l.'s crossed.

l., white. SEE: *l., milk.*

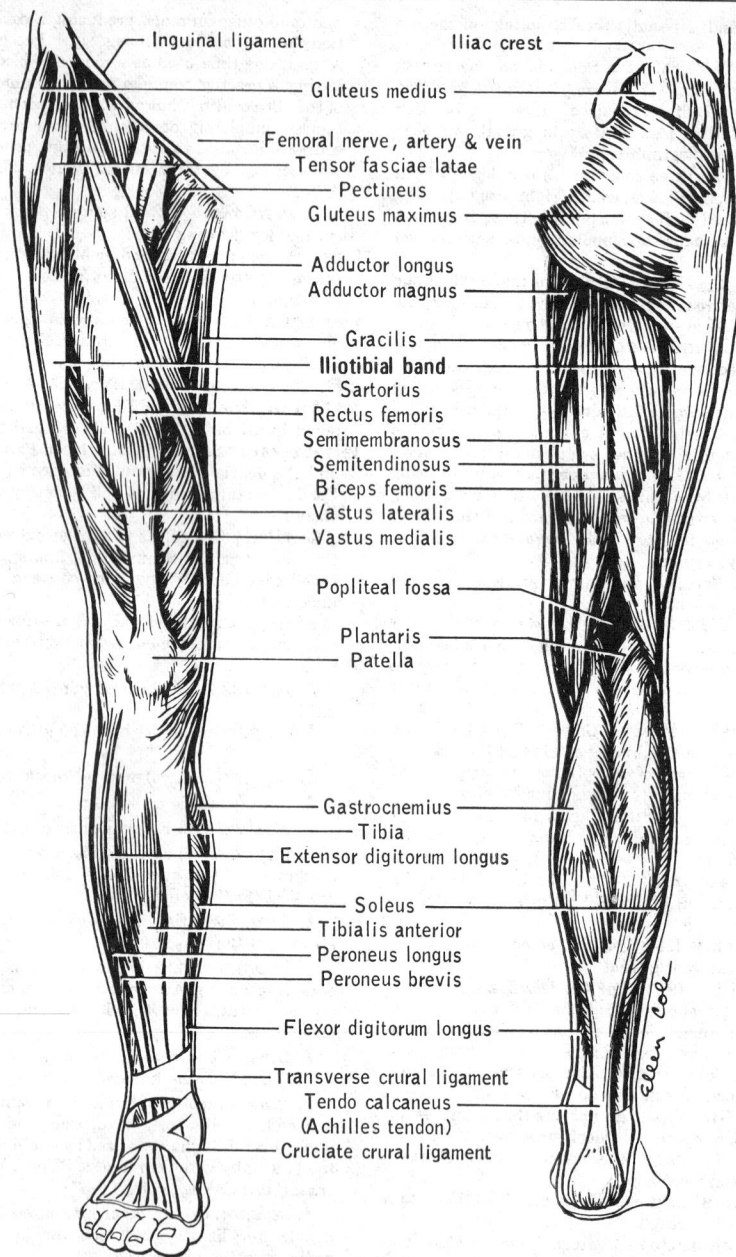

Inguinal ligament

Iliac crest

Gluteus medius

Femoral nerve, artery & vein
Tensor fasciae latae
Pectineus
Gluteus maximus

Adductor longus
Adductor magnus

Gracilis
Iliotibial band
Sartorius
Rectus femoris
Semimembranosus
Semitendinosus
Biceps femoris
Vastus lateralis
Vastus medialis

Popliteal fossa

Plantaris
Patella

Gastrocnemius
Tibia
Extensor digitorum longus

Soleus
Tibialis anterior
Peroneus longus
Peroneus brevis

Flexor digitorum longus

Transverse crural ligament
Tendo calcaneus
(Achilles tendon)
Cruciate crural ligament

ANTERIOR MUSCLES OF LEG

POSTERIOR MUSCLES OF LEG

leggings (lĕg'gĭngs) [ME. *leg,* leg]. Sterile leg coverings used on patient while in operating room.

legitimacy (lĕ-jĭt'ĭm-ă-sĭ) [L. *legitimus,* lawful]. 1. Condition of being legal. 2. Condition of being born in wedlock.

legume (lĕ'gūm) [L. *legumen,* pulse, bean]. Fruit or pod of beans, peas, lentils, etc.

COMP: Nitrogen: Almost equal to that in meat. It is called legumin, q.v., forming with water a paste resembling gluten, but easier to digest.

VITAMINS: (Sprouted beans): A good source of vitamin B complex. Vitamin A and ascorbic acid are present in small amounts.

CARBOHYDRATES: Generally in the form of starch in about the same proportion as the cereals, but with more cellulose.

legumelin (lĕg-ū'mĕl-in) [L. *legumen,* pulse, bean]. An albumin present in many leguminous seeds, as in peas. SEE: *legume, legumin.*

legu'min. A protein globulin contained in legumes; vegetable casein.

leiodermia (lī-ō-dĕr'mĭ-ă) [Gr. *leios,* smooth, + *derma,* skin]. Dermatitis characterized by abnormal glossiness and atrophy of the skin.

leiomyofibroma (lī"ō-mī"ō-fĭ-brō'mă) ["+ *mys,* muscle, + L. *fibra,* fiber, + Gr. *-ōma,* tumor]. A benign tumor composed principally of smooth muscle and fibrous connective tissue.

leiomyoma (lī"ō-mī-ō'mă) ["+ "+ *-ōma,* tumor]. Myoma consisting principally of smooth muscle tissue.

leiomyosarcoma (lī"ō-mī"ō-săr-kō'mă) ["+ "+ *sarx,* flesh, + *-ōma,* tumor]. Combined leiomyoma and sarcoma.

leiotrichous (lī"ōt'rĭ-kŭs) ["+ *thrix,* hair]. Possessing smooth or straight hair.

Leishmania (lēsh-mān'-ĭ-ă). [Sir William B. Leishman, Brit. medical officer, 1865-1926] A genus of parasitic flagellate protozoans which occur as typical leishmanian forms in vertebrate hosts but as leptomonad forms in invertebrate hosts or in cultures. They are transmitted by the sandfly, Phlebotomas.

L. braziliensis. Causative agent of American leishmaniasis.

L. donovani. Causative agent of kala azar (visceral leishmaniasis).

L. tropica. Causative agent of oriental sore (cutaneous leishmaniasis).

leishmaniasis (lēsh"mă-nī'ă-sĭs). Infection with a species of Leishmania, affecting the skin, nasal cavities and pharynx, one form causing oriental boil, another kala azar.

l., American. L. caused by L. braziliensis, involving principally nasopharyngeal

and mucocutaneous membranes. Common in Central and South America.

l., cutaneous. L. due to infection with Leishmania tropica. SYN: *aleppo boil; Delhi ulcer; oriental sore.*

l., visceral. L. caused by L. donovani. SYN: *dumdum fever; kala azar.*

le'ma. The dried secretion of the tarsal glands which collects in the inner canthus of the eye. SYN: *sebum palpebrale.*

lemmocyte (lĕm'mō-sīt) [Gr. *lemma,* husk, + *kytos,* cell]. A cell which becomes a neurilemma cell.

lemniscus (lĕm-nĭs'kŭs) [Gr. *lēmniskos,* a ribbon]. A bundle of sensory fibers (lateral or exterior and median or interior) in the medulla, and pons.

lem'on [Persian *limūn,* lemon]. Fruit of the tree Citrus limonia, containing citrus acid. L.'s contain enough ascorbic acid to prevent or treat scurvy.

Food value of 100 gm. (raw peeled): Cal. 27; protein 1.1 gm.; trace of fat; carbohydrates 8.2 gm.; calcium 26. mg.; ascorbic acid 53 mg. (Ascorbic acid content somewhat less for lemons marketed in winter).

Food value of 100 gm. of lemon juice (fresh): Cal. 25; protein 0.5 gm., carbohydrates 8 gm.; calcium 7 mg.; ascorbic acid 46 mg.

May be used in place of vinegar, spices, and aromatic substances by those who cannot use the latter. Diabetics may use.

CAUTION: Food faddists who drink large quantities of lemon juice by sucking directly from the raw fruit may develop erosion of the enamel of their teeth.

lemoparalysis (le"mo-pă-răl'ĭs-ĭs) [Gr. *laimos,* gullet, + *para,* beside, + *lyein,* to loosen]. Paralysis of esophagus.

lemosteno'sis ["+ *stenōsis,* a narrowing]. Stricture of esophagus.

lenitive (lĕn'ĭ-tĭv) [L. *lenīre,* to soothe]. 1. Demulcent, soothing, slightly laxative. 2. A palliative.

lens (lĕnz) [L. *lens,* lentil, lens (from resemblance of an optical lens to a lentil seed)]. 1. A transparent refracting medium; usually made of glass. 2. [NA] The crystalline lens of the eye.

RS: capsitis; capsulociliary; circle of diffusion; vitreous chamber.

l., achromatic. One for correction of chromatic aberration.

l., bifocal. L. containing in either its upper or lower segment a l. of different power. The main l. is for distant vision; the secondary l. is for near vision.

l., concave spherical. Formed of prisms with their apices together, therefore, thin at the center and thick at the edge. Used in myopia.

l., convex spherical. Formed of prisms with their bases together, therefore, thick at the center and thin at the edge. Used in hyperopia.

l., corneal contact. A type of contact l. which adheres to and covers only the cornea.

l., crystalline. Transparent, colorless structure in eye; biconvex in shape, enclosed in a capsule and held in place just behind the pupil by the suspensory ligament. Consists principally of l. fibers which at the periphery are soft, forming the cortex lentis, and in the center of harder consistency, forming the nucleus lentis. Beneath the capsule on anterior surface is a thin layer of cells, the l. epithelium. Function is to focus rays so they form a perfect image on the retina.

l., cylindrical. Segment of a cylinder parallel to its axis, used in correcting astigmatism.

lenticonus (lĕn″ti-kō′nus) ["+ *conus*, cone]. Conical protrusion of anterior or posterior surface of lens.

lentic′ular [L. *lenticuláris*, pert. to a lens]. 1. Lens shaped. SYN: *lentiform*. 2. Pert. to a lens.

l. fossa. Depression in anterior surface of vitreous for reception of the crystalline lens.

l. glands. Small masses of lymphatic tissue in lamina propria of pyloric region of the stomach.

l. nucleus. Mass of gray matter forming part of the corpus striatum. Consists of the putamen and globus pallidus.

lenticulostriate (lĕn-tĭk″ū-lō-strī′āt) ["+ *striatus*, streaked]. Rel. to the lenticular nucleus and corpus striatum.

lenticulothalmic. Pert. to lenticular nucleus and the thalamus.

lentiform (lĕnt′ĭ-form) [L. *lens, lent-*, lentil, lens, + *forma*, shape]. Lentil or lens shaped. SYN: *lenticular.*

lentiginous (lĕn-tĭj′ĭn-ŭs) [L. *lentigō*, freckle]. 1. Affected by lentigo. 2. Covered with very small dots.

len′tigo [L., freckle]. (pl. *lentigines*) Small brown macules or yellow-brown pigmented areas on skin sometimes caused by exposure to sun and weather. SYN: *ephelis; freckle.*

lentitis (lĕn-tī′tĭs) [L. *lens, lent-*, lentil, lens, + Gr. *itis*, inflammation]. Inflammation of the crystalline lens. SYN: *phakitis.*

leontiasis (lē″ŏn-tī′ä-sĭs) [Gr. *leōn, leont-*, lion]. Lionlike expression about face, accom-

panying certain diseases. May be seen in leprosy.

l. ossea. Enlargement and distortion of facial bones, giving one the appearance of a lion. The condition is rare and not fatal. SYN: *leontiasis.*

leotropic (lē-ō-trop′ĭk) [Gr. *laios*, left, + *tropos*, a turning]. Running from right to left in a spiral form.

leper (lĕp′ĕr) [Gr. *lepros*, scaly]. Person afflicted with leprosy.

lepido- [Gr. *lepis*, scale]. Combining form: Referring to flakes or scales.

Lepidoptera (lĕp′ĭ-dŏp′tĕr-ä) [Gr. *lepsis, lepid-*, scale, + *ptēron*, feather, wing]. An order of the class Insecta which includes the butterflies, moths and skippers. Characterized by scaly wings, sucking mouth parts, and complete metamorphosis.

lepidosis (lĕp′ĭd-ō′sĭs) ["+ *-ōsis*, intensive]. Any scaly or desquamating eruption. An example is pityriasis.

lepothrix (lĕp′o-thriks) [Gr. *lepos*, scale, + *thrix*, hair]. Condition in which shaft of the hair is encased in hardened, scaly, sebaceous matter.

lepra (lĕp′rä) [Gr. *lepra*, leprosy]. A term formerly used for leprosy. Now used to indicate a reaction which occurs in leprosy patients. This can occur in any form of leprosy, may be prolonged, and consists of aggravation of lesions accompanied by fever and malaise.

l. alba. Skin is anesthetic and white, and different forms of paralysis follow.

l. anesthetica. Leprosy with anesthetic areas on body.

l. Arabum. True or nodular leprosy.

l. maculosa. Form with pigmented cutaneous areas.

l. mutilans. Final stage of true leprosy, or mutilation stage.

l. nervorum. Maculo-anesthetic leprosy.

leprid(e (lĕp′rēd) [Gr. *lepra*, leprosy]. Leprous cutaneous lesion.

leprology (lĕp-rol′ō-jī) ["+ *logos*, study]. The study of leprosy and methods of treating it.

leproma (lĕp-rō′mä) ["+ *-ōma*, tumor]. A cutaneous nodule or tubercle characteristic of leprosy.

lep′romin. A substance prepared from lepromatous nodules of leprosy.

l. skin test. One in which l. was introduced intradermally to attempt to diagnose leprosy. The test is of no value.

leprosarium. An institution for the care of lepers.

leprosy (lep′ro-sĭ) [Gr. *lepra*, leprosy]. A chronically communicable disease caused by the acid-fast Mycobacterium leprae. It may occur in various clinical forms. The two principal forms are: (1) Lepromatous, characterized by skin lesions and symmetrical involvement of peripheral nerves with anesthesia, muscle weakness and paralysis. In this form, the lesions are limited to the cooler portions of the body such as skin, upper respiratory tract, and testes. (2) Tuberculoid, which is usually benign. The nerve lesions are asymmetrical and skin anesthesia is an early occurrence. Visceral involvement is not seen.

Lepromatous leprosy is much more contagious than the tuberculoid form. In the latter, Mycobacterium leprae are found only rarely except during reactions.

Between the two major forms are borderline and indeterminate leprosy. In the borderline group, the clinical and bacteriological features represent a combination of the two principal types. In the indeterminate group, there are fewer skin lesions and bacteria are much less abundant in the lesions.

In many respects, this infection resembles tuberculosis and for many years was regarded as incurable, a conclusion no longer considered true. SEE: *Hansen's disease.*

ETIOL: Caused by Mycobacterium leprae. May occur at practically any age.

INCUBATION: From one to 30 years.

SYM: Onset very gradual. The first signs of infection are usually skin changes, but they may be so nonspecific and so slow to progress as to go unrecognized for years.

COMPLICATIONS: Bacterial infections of skin, ulcers, traumatic amputation of fingers due to anesthesia, also fingers may be eaten by rodents while the patient is asleep, tuberculosis is a much more common complication in untreated cases of lepromatous leprosy than in the tuberculoid form. Amyloidosis may be the cause of death in advanced cases.

PROGNOSIS: With proper therapy the outlook for recovery is good.

TREATMENT: Dapsone (4,4'-diamino-diphenyl sulfone, DDS) is the form of sulfone most commonly used.

Segregation of patients in colonies or hospitals until bacterial tests have been negative for six months is not the preferred or effective method of isolating patients. Ambulatory treatment of patients at general clinics has been found to be much more effective. Because they are more susceptible to this disease than adults, children should be removed from contact with leprosy patients.

leprotic (lĕp-rot'ĭk) [Gr. *lepra*, leprosy]. 1. Rel. to leprosy. 2. Affected with leprosy. SYN: *leprous.*

leprous (lĕp'rŭs) [Gr. *lepra*, leper]. 1. Pert. to leprosy. 2. Affected by leprosy. SYN: *leprotic.*

leptocephalia (lĕp″to-sĕ-fa'lĭ-ă) [Gr. *leptos,* fine, small, + *kephalē,* head]. Having an abnormally small head.

leptocephalus. An individual possessing an abnormally small head.

leptodermic (lĕp″to-dĕr'mĭk) [Gr. *leptos,* slender, + *derma,* skin]. Possessing a thin skin.

leptomeninges (lĕp″to-men-ĭn'jēs) ["+ *mēnigx,* membrane]. Pia mater and arachnoid as distinct from dura mater, because of their thinner and more delicate structure.

leptomeningitis (lĕp″to-mĕn-ĭn-ji'tis) ["+ "+ *itis,* inflammation]. Inflammation of the pia and arachnoid memembranes. SEE: *meningitis.*

ETIOL: Tubercle bacillus, spirochete of syphilis, and other organisms.

SYM: Acute headache, pain in back, rigidity of spine, irritability, drowsiness ending in coma.

Clinically, it cannot be distinguished from pachymeningitis, q.v.

leptomeninx. Sing. of leptomeninges. The pia and arachnoid mater of the brain.

leptopellic (lĕp″to-pĕl'ĭk) ["+ *pellis,* a bowl (pelvis)]. Having an abnormally narrow pelvis.

leptophonia (lĕp″to-fo'nĭ-ă) ["+ *phōnē,* voice]. Weakness or feebleness of voice.

leptoprosopia (lĕp″to-prō-sō'pĭ-ă) [Gr. *leptos,* slender, + *prosōpon,* face]. Narrowness of the face.

leptorhine, leptorrhine (lĕp'tor-rīn) ["+ *ris, rin-,* nose]. Having a very thin or slender nose.

leptosome (lĕp'tō-sōm) ["+ *soma,* body]. Person of thin, slight stature.

Leptospira (lĕp-tō-spi'rä) [Gr. *leptòs,* thin, + *spaira,* coil]. Genus of spirochetes; thin, spiral, and hook-ended.

   L. autumnalis. Species first isolated in Japan. Causes a nonicteric infection in man called pretibial or Fort Bragg fever.

   L. hebdomadis. Species causing seven-day fever of Japan.

   L. icterohaemorrha'giae. Species causing infectious, hemorrhagic, spirochetal jaundice (Weil's disease).

leptospirosis (lĕp'tō-spī-rō'sĭs) ["+ "+ -*ōsis,* intensive]. Condition resulting from Leptospira infection.

leptothricosis (lĕp″tō-thri-kō'sĭs) ["+ *thrix,* hair]. Disease from Leptothrix infection.

Leptus autumnalis (lĕp'tūs) [Gr. *leptos,* slender]. Parasitic mite larvae causing itch and sometimes wheals. SEE: *chiggers*.

lere'sis [Gr.]. Loquacity in old age; garrulousness.

les'bian [Gr. *lesbios,* pert. to island of Lesbos]. 1. Pert. to lesbianism, or sexual desire in women for those of their own sex. 2. One who practices lesbianism.

les'bianism. Sexual desire of women for one of their own sex.

Named from the Island of Lesbos wherein the practice of sapphism was reputed to have been general in ancient days. It may be expressed physically or psychically.

lesion (lē'zhŭn) [L. *laesio,* a wound]. 1. A circumscribed area of pathologically altered tissue. 2. An injury or wound. 3. Single infected patch in a skin disease.

Primary or initial lesions include macules; vesicles; blebs, or bullae; chancres; pustules; papules; tubercles; wheals; and tumors, q.v. Secondary lesions are the result of primary lesions. They may be crusts; excoriations; fissures; pigmentations; scales; scars; and ulcers, q.v.

RS: abscess; boil; carbuncle; Cazenave's lupus; cerebropsychosis; chancre; chancroids; felon; gumma; moles; pimples; rash; sebaceous cysts; tumefactions; verruca; wound.

l., degenerative. L. caused by or showing degeneration.

l., diffuse. L. spreading over a large area.

l., discharging. 1. Brain l. discharging nervous impulses. 2. L. discharging an exudate.

l., focal. L. of small definite area.

l., indiscriminate. L. affecting separate systems of the body.

l., initial, of syphilis. Hard chancre.

l., irritative. L. stimulating or exciting activity in part of body where it is situated.

l., local. L. of nervous origin giving rise to local symptoms.

l., peripheral. One of nerve endings.

l., primary. First l. of a disease, esp. used in referring to chancre of syphilis.

l., structural. One causing change in tissue.

l., systemic. L. confined to organs of common function.

l., toxic. One resulting from poisons or toxins from microorganisms.

l., vascular. One of a blood vessel.

le'thal [Gr. *lēthē,* oblivion]. Pert. to or that which causes death.

lethargic (lĕth-ar'jĭk) [Gr. *lēthargos,* drowsiness]. 1. Affected with lethargy. 2. Rel. to lethary. 3. Sluggish.

lethargy (lĕth'ar-jĭ) [Gr. *lēthargos,* drowsiness]. A condition of functional torpor or sluggishness; stupor

RS: noctambulism, personality somnambulism; vigilambulism.

l., African. Sleeping sickness.

l., hysteric. The sleep of hypnotic lethargy, the state in which many cases of apparent death and resurrection are found.

l. induced. Hypnotic trance.

l., lucid. Retention of intellect but loss of will power with a consequent total lack of muscular response. The subject knows what is going on, resents it, perhaps, but is unable to exercise sufficient will to bring about muscular defense.

lethologica (lĕth-ō-loj'ĭk-ă) [Gr. *lēthē,* forgetfullness, + *logos,* word]. Temporary inability to remember a word or name, or an intended action.

Letterer-Siwe's disease. A usually fatal disease of infancy and childhood of unknown cause, with hyperplasia of the reticuloendothelial system. Therapy is limited to supportive measures because of lack of a specific effective agent.

let'tuce. The edible leaves of a plant of the genus Lactuca, esp. L. sativa.

Food value of 100 gm. (crisphead varieties, raw): Cal. 13; protein 0.9 gm.; trace of fat; carbohydrate 22 gm.; calcium 2.9 mg.; vitamin A, 330 I.U.; ascorbic acid 6 mg.

leuc-. For words beginning thus, see 'leuk-' words.

leucine (lū'sēn) [Gr. *leukos,* white]. Alphaamino-isobutyl acetic acid, $C_6H_{13}NO_2$, an amino acid found among the products of digestion of proteins. It is present in body tissues and is essential for normal growth and metabolism.

leucine aminopeptidase. A proteolytic enzyme present in the pancreas, liver, and small intestine. Its serum level is elevated in disease of the pancreas, esp. acute pancreatitis, and in obstruction of the common bile duct. ABBR: LAP.

leucinosis (lū-sĭn-ō'sĭs) ["+ *-ōsis,* intensive]. Excess of leucine in the body producing leucine in the urine.

leucinuria (lū-sin-ū'rĭ-ă) ["+ *ouron,* urine]. Presence of leucine in urine.

leucitis (lū-sī'tĭs) ["+ *itis,* inflammation]. Inflammation of the sclera. SYN: *scleritis.*

leukanemia (lū-kă-nē'mĭ-ă) ["+ *a-,* not, + *haima,* blood]. Rapid and progressive disease with blood changes similar to those of pernicious anemia and myelocytic leukemia. Now called erythroleukemia.

leukasmus (lū-kas′mŭs) [Gr. *leukasmos,* growing white]. Congenital absence of pigment in bands or patches of the skin. SYN: *leukoderma.*

leukemia (lū-kē′mĭ-ă) [Gr. *leukos,* white, growing white, + *haima,* blood]. A disease of unknown cause characterized by rapid and abnormal proliferation of leukocytes in the blood-forming organs (bone marrow, spleen, lymph nodes) and the presence of immature leukocytes in peripheral circulation. May be acute or chronic but inevitably fatal.

NP: Watch for local mouth infections, terminal septicemia, and bronchopneumonia as complications. Good nursing care is very important in all forms of this disease. Hemorrhages from nose and mouth often require packing and hemostatics.

l., acute. L. in which onset is sudden and progress rapid. Usually fatal within a period of two or three months.

l., aleukemic. L. in which the total leukocyte count is normal or below normal and in which immature cells are absent.

l., leukemic. L. in which total leukocyte count in peripheral blood is elevated and immature cells of the series involved are present.

l., lymphatic. That in which there is marked increase in the size of the spleen and lymph glands with a great increase in lymphocytes in blood; acute form occurs in children and young adults.

l., monocytic. A rare form of l. in which monocytes are the predominant cells involved. Involves the reticuloendothelial tissues of bloodforming organs.

l., myelogenous. L. involving the hematopoietic bone marrow, esp. that of the ribs, sternum, and vertebrae. Bone marrow which is normally red in color, becomes gray and assumes a gelatinous consistency. Myeloid elements increase in blood.

SYM: General manifestations of anemia —enlargment of spleen, liver or lymphatic glands. Febrile periods, hemorrhage from mucous membranes, digestive disturbances, dimness of vision. There is marked increase in the leukocytes; proportion to red corpuscles may be 1-50 or even 1-10. This leukocytosis results from an increase in all forms of leukocytes, with a concomitant decrease in red blood cells.

PROG: Death usually results in three to four years.

l., plasma cell. L. in which plasma cells are the predominant cells in the blood.

leukemic (lū-kēm′ĭk) [Gr. *leukos,* white, + *haima,* blood]. 1. Rel. to leukemia. 2. Affected with leukemia.

leukemoid (lū-kē′moyd) ["+ "+ *eidos,* form]. Having symptoms of leukemia, but due to other conditions.

leu′ko-, leuk- [Gr. *leukos,* white, clear]. Combining forms signifying white; colorless; rel. to leukocyte.

leu′koblast [Gr. *leukos,* white, + *blastos,* germ]. General term applied to a cell that gives rise to a leukocyte.

leukoblastosis (lū″kŏ-blăs-tō′sĭs) ["+ "+ *-ōsis,* intensive]. Proliferation of excessive numbers of immature leukocytes.

leukocidin (lū-kō-sid′in) ["+ L. *cidus,* from *caedere,* to kill]. A bacterial toxin which destroys leukocytes.

leukocytal (lū″kŏ-sī′tăl) ["+ *kytos,* cell]. Rel. to leukocytes.

leukocyte (lū′kō-sīt) [Gr. *leukos,* white, + *kytos,* cell]. White blood corpuscle. There are two types; granulocytes (those possessing granules in their cytoplasm) and agranulocytes (those lacking granules). Granulocytes include juvenile neutrophils (3-5%), segmented neutrophils (54-62%), basophils (0-0.75%), and eosinophils (1-3%). Agranulocytes include lymphocytes, large and small (25-33%) and monocytes (3-7%).

The leukocytes act as scavengers and by so doing help to combat infection. They move by ameboid movement and are able to penetrate tissue and then return to the blood stream. The direction of movement is probably due to the stimuli from injured cells. This is called chemotaxis. When invading bacteria destroy them, the dead white blood corpuscles collect in the form of pus, causing an abscess if a ready outlet is not found. Different types combat various kinds of infection.

One cu. mm. of blood contains 5000-10,000 leukocytes normally.

FUNCTIONS: Leukocytes, esp. the granular forms, are markedly phagocytic, i.e., have the power to ingest particulate substances. Neutrophils ingest bacteria and small particles; other cells such as the monocytes and histiocytes in the tissues ingest larger particles. They are important in both defensive and reparative functions of the body. Basophils most probably function by delivering anticoagulants to facilitate blood clot absorption or to prevent blood coagulation. Eosinophils increase in number in certain conditions such as asthma and infestations of animal parasites. Lymphocytes are not phagocytic. They are thought to be a source of serum globulin and possibly certain immune bodies. Their exact role in immunologic reaction is being extensively studied.

A greatly diminished number of erythrocytes is found in the anemias, and a greatly increased number of leukocytes (leukocytosis) is indicative of the presence of inflammatory products. A leukocyte count is usually a preoperative routine if infection is suspected, such as in appendicitis. A count may also be taken following an operation to be sure that no infection from a wound has developed.

How to Recognize: White blood cells are round, edges occasionally broken, nucleated, granular, having a grayish color, sometimes clumped, and can be stained as polynuclears.

Microscopic Examination: They are usually in pieces of mucus and can be stained by ordinary blood stains.

Decrease below normal (5000) is called leukopenia; increase above normal (10,000) is called leukocytosis.

Two determinations are usually made regarding the leukocytes: their total number (total count), and the percentage of each type (differential count). Decrease below the normal is called leukopenia. Relative increase or decrease of any particular type is denoted by adding the suffix "philia" (denoting increase) or "penia" (denoting decrease), as: neutrophilia, granulocytopenia, neutropenia, eosinophilia, etc.

Sometimes immature white cells are discharged into the blood stream and may be observed in blood smears; myelocytes, myeloblasts, or lymphoblasts.

In a smear of blood, the white cells vary in size, shape, appearance, and the color they assume when stained. Some of the cells contain minute granules, and these cells are called granulocytes, the cytoplasm of others is granular. It is seen that the granules in some cells stain bright red, and the cells are called eosinophils; in others, deep blue, and these are called basophils. In most of the cells, however, the granules take a neutral purplish color, and these are called neutrophils. There are two types of nongranular cells, the lymphocytes and the monocytes.

Not all leukocytes are formed in the same place, nor in the same manner. Granulocytes are formed in the bone marrow, arising from large cells called megakaryocytes. Lymphocytes are formed in the lymph nodes; monocytes from the cells lining the capillaries in various organs, perhaps principally in the spleen and bone marrow.

l., acidophil. An eosinophil l., q.v.

l., basophil. L. with cytoplasmic granules which stain with basic dyes. Stain a deep purple with Wright's stain. Comprise 0-0.75% of white cell count.

l., eosinophil. L. with cytoplasmic granules which stain with acid dyes. Appear reddish when stained with Wright's stain. Comprise 1-3% of white cell count.

l., granular. L. containing granules in cytoplasm. SYN: *granulocyte.*

l., heterophilic. Neutrophil l. of certain animals whose granules stain with an acid stain.

l., neutrophil. L. with fine cytoplasmic granules which do not stain with acid or basic stains but have an affinity for neutral stains.

l., nongranular. An agranulocyte; a lymphocyte or monocyte.

Summary of Leukocytes

Cells	Nucleus	Cytoplasmic Granules	Range (in %)
Granulocytes (Polymorphonuclear)			
Juvenile Neutrophils	Unsegmented	Fine; pale stain	3-5
Segmented Neutrophils	Polymorphic	Fine; neutral stain	54-62
Eosinophils	Polymorphic	Coarse; stain with acid dye	1-3
Basophils	Polymorphic	Coarse; stain with basic dye	0-0.75
Agranulocytes			
Lymphocytes, small and large	Spherical (slightly indented)	None	25-33
Monocytes	Kidney-shaped	None	3-7

l., polymorphonuclear. L. with a nucleus consisting of several lobes. One of the granulocytes (neutrophil, eosinophil, basophil).

leukocythemia (lū″kō-sī-thē′mĭ-ă) [Gr. *leukos*, white, + *kytos*, cell, + *haima*, blood]. Blood disease characterized by excess of white blood corpuscles and enlargment of spleen, lymphatic glands and bone marrow. SYN: *leukemia, q.v.*

leukocytic (lū″kō-sĭt′ĭk) ["+ *kytos*, cell]. Pert. to leukocytes.

leukocytoblast (lū″kō-sīt′ō-blast) ["+ "+ *blastos*, germ]. Cell from which leukocytes arise.

leukocytogenesis (lū″kō-sīt″ō-jĕn′ĕ-sĭs) [Gr. *leukos*, white, + *kytos*, cell, + *genesis*, formation]. Leukocyte formation. SYN: *leukopoiesis.*

leukocytoid (lū′kō-sī″toyd) ["+ "+ *eidos*, form]. Resembling a leukocyte.

leu′kocytol′ysin. A lysin which destroys leukocytes. SEE: *leukocidin.*

leukocytolysis (lū-kō-sī-tŏl′ĭ-sĭs) [Gr. *leukos*, white, + *kytos*, cell, + *lysis*, dissolution]. Destruction of leukocytes.

leukocytoma (lū″kō-sī-tō′mă) ["+ "+ *-ōma*, tumor]. 1. Tumor composed of cells resembling leukocytes. 2. Tumorlike mass of leukocytes.

leukocytometer (lū″kō-sī-tŏm′ĕt-ēr) ["+ "+ *metron*, measure]. Device for counting white blood corpuscles.

leukocytopenia (lū″kō-sīt″ō-pē′nĭ-ă) ["+ "+ *penia*, want]. Subnormal number of leukocytes in blood. SYN: *leukopenia.*

leukocytoplania (lū″kō-sīt″ō-plā′nĭ-ă) ["+ "+ *planē*, wandering]. Wandering of leukocytes through blood vessel walls. SYN: *leukopedesis.*

leukocytopoiesis (lū″kō-sī″to-poy′ē′sĭs). Formation of white blood cells.

leukocytosis (lū″ko-sī-to′sis) [Gr. *leukos*, white, + *kytos*, cell, + *-ōsis*, condition of increase]. Increase in number of leukocytes (above 10,000 per cu. mm.) in the blood, generally caused by presence of infection. It may also accompany or occur after the following conditions: hemorrhage; extensive operations; coronary occlusion; malignant growth; pregnancy; certain intoxications; and toxemias. Eosinophilic leukocytosis occurs in certain allergies, infestation with animal parasites, and Hodgkin's disease.

Leukemias, however, release immature leukocytes due to abnormal condition of blood-forming organs. Leukocytosis is present in most infections but not usually in those due to a virus.

In leukocytosis the numbers of white cells may vary from a 50% increase to many times more than normal. In leukemia these may be as many as one million white cells per cu. mm. Leukocytosis is early and marked in severe infections when the patient's resistance is good; if infection and resistance are less marked it appears later to a lesser degree and disappears more quickly. Leukocytosis may occur in unusually virulent infection, such as diphtheria, pneumonia, sepsis, etc.

leukocyturia (lū″ko-sī-tu′rĭ-ă) ["+ "+ *ouron*, urine]. Leukocytes in the urine.

leukoderma (lū-kō-dĕr′mă) ["+ *derma*, skin]. Deficiency of pigmentation of the skin, esp. in patches.

leukodiagnosis (lū″kō-dī″ăg-nō′sĭs) ["+ *dia*, through, + *gnōsis*, knowledge]. Diagnosis by observance of number, variety, or reaction of leukocytes.

leukoencephalitis (lū″kō-ĕn-sĕf-ă-lī′tĭs). Inflammation of the white matter of the brain.

leukokeratosis (lū″kō-kĕr-ă-tō′sĭs) [Gr. *leukos*, white, + *keras*, horn, + *-ōsis*, condition]. White patch formation on the surface of mucosa of tongue, cheek and gums. SYN: *leukoplakia.*

leukolysin (lū-kŏl′ĭ-sĭn) ["+ *lysis*, dissolution]. Serum constituent destructive to leukocytes.

leukolysis (lū-kol′ĭ-sis). Destruction of leukocytes. SYN: *leukocytolysis.*

leuko′ma [Gr. *leukos*, white, + *-ōma*, tumor]. A white, opaque corneal opacity.

l., adherens. Corneal scar with incarcerated iris tissue.

leukomaine (lū-kō′ma-ēn, -ma-ĭn) [Gr. *leukōma*, whiteness]. Toxic nitrogenous alkaloid developed in living tissue as distinguished from one in dead tissue, or one of vegetable origin.

leukomainemia (lū″kō-mā-ĭn-ē′mĭ-ă) ["+ *haima*, blood]. Excess of leukomaines in blood.

leukomatous (lū-kōm′ă-tŭs) ["+ *-ōma*, tumor]. 1. Pert. to leukoma. 2. Suffering from leukoma.

leukomyelitis (lū″ko-mī-ĕ-lī′tis) [Gr. *leukos*, white, + *myelos*, marrow, + *itis*, inflammation]. Inflammation of the white matter of the spinal cord.

leukomyelopathy (lū″kō-mī-ĕl-ŏp′ăth-ĭ) ["+ "+ *pathos*, disease]. Disease involving white matter of spinal cord or myelon.

leukonecrosis (lū″ko-nĕ-krō′sĭs) ["+ *nekrōsis*, deadness]. Dry, light colored or white gangrene, q.v.

leukonychia (lū″kō-nĭk′ĭ-ă) ["+ *onyx, onych-,* nail]. "Gift spots," white spots or streaks on the nails.

leukopathia (lū″kō-păth′ĭ-ă) ["+ *pathos,* disease]. 1. Absence of pigment in skin. 2. Disease involving leukocytes.

leukopedesis (lū″kō-pē-dē′sĭs) ["+ *pēdan,* to leap]. Passage of leukocytes through walls of blood vessels.

leukopenia (lū″kō-pē′nĭ-ă) ["+ *penia,* lack]. Abnormal decrease of white blood corpuscles usually below 5000 per cu. mm.

    l., malignant. An acute infection with extreme leukopenia. SYN: *agranulocytosis.*

leukoplakia (lū″kō-plā′kĭ-ă) [Gr. *leukos,* white, + *plax,* plate]. Formation of white spots or patches on the mucous membrane of the tongue or cheek.

    They are smooth, irregular in size and shape, and hard and occasionally fissured. May become malignant.

    l. buccalis. L. of the mucosa of the cheek.

    l. lingualis. L. of the tongue.

    l. vulvae. L. of the vulva. SEE: *kraurosis vulvae.*

leukoplasia (lū-kō-plā′zĭ-ă) ["+ *plax,* plate]. White patch formation on buccal mucosa. SYN: *leukoplakia,* q.v.

leukopoiesis (lū″kō-poy-ē′sĭs) [Gr. *leukos,* white, + *poiēsis,* formation]. Leukocyte production. SYN: *leukocytogenesis.*

leukopoietic (lū″kō-poy-ĕt′ĭk) ["+ *poiein,* to make]. Forming leukocytes.

leukoprotease (lū-ko-pro′te-ās) ["+ *prōtos,* first, + *-ase,* enzyme]. An enzyme in polynuclear leukocytes that splits protein.

leukopsin. A substance formed in the rods of the retina from rhodopsin under the influence of light.

leukorrhagia (lū″ko-ra′jĭ-ă) ["+ *rhēgnynai,* to flow forth]. Profuse white vaginal discharge. SYN: *leukorrhea,* q.v.

leukorrhea (lū-kŏr-e′ă) ["+ *rhoia,* flow]. White or yellowish mucous discharge from the cervical canal or the vagina.

    There is frequently a normal physiological leukorrhea which may be constantly present but somewhat increased preceding and following menstruation. It may be of considerable concern to the young girl at the time of menarche because she has not been told this white fluid would tend to collect on the vulvae. Leukorrhea may be abnormal because of increase in amount, changes in color, variations in consistency, odors, types of bacterial content, and the appearance of blood.

ETIOL: Pathological states of the endocervix and vagina. Infection by Trichomonas vaginalis.

SYM: Usually indications of acute inflammation, pain, heat, redness of parts involved, which may subside as discharge increases. Pain in groins, hypogastrium, sacral regions and small of back. Urethra often implicated, causing painful micturition. Symptoms which may occur in connection with chronic leukorrhea are innumerable. Reaction of discharge is acid, may be any consistency: thin and watery or viscid and tenacious.

TREATMENT: If due to a specific microorganism, treat with appropriate antibiotic. In general douches are ineffective in curing the cause of this symptom. If due to senile changes in the vagina, estrogen-containing cream or ointment applied locally is quite effective.

leukosarcoma (lū″kō-săr-kō′mă) [Gr. *leukos,* white, + *sarx,* flesh, + *-ōma,* tumor]. An unpigmented sarcoma.

leukosis (lū-kō′sĭs) ["+ *-ōsis,* intensive]. 1. Unnatural pallor. 2. Excessive proliferation of leukocyte-producing tissue. On the basis of type of cell involved, leukosis may be lymphoid, myeloblastic, or myelocytic. SEE: *leukemia.* 3. Increase in leukocyte-forming tissue.

leu″kotac′tic [Gr. *leukos,* white, + *taxis,* arrangement]. Possessing the power of attracting leukocytes.

leu″kotax′is. Possessing the power of attracting (positive l.) or repelling (negative l.) leukocytes.

leukotoxic (lū″kō-toks′ĭk) [Gr. *leukos,* white, + *toxikon,* poison]. Destroying leukocytes.

leukotrichia (lū-kō-trĭk′ĭ-ă) ["+ *thrix, trich-,* hair]. Whiteness of the hair. SYN: *canities.*

leukous (lū′kŭs) [Gr. *leukos,* white]. White, esp. rel. to the skin.

levarterenol bitartrate. A sympathomimetic. SYN: *noradrenalin; norepinephrine.*

levator (lē-vā′tor) [L., lifter]. 1. A muscle that raises a part; opposed to depressor. 2. An instrument which lifts depressed portions.

    l. ani. A broad muscle helping to form the floor of the pelvis.

    l. palpebrae superioris. A muscle which elevates the upper eyelid.

level of activities. Connector neurons are grouped into levels corresponding to different stages of development: spinal cord level; medullary level; midbrain level; basal ganglial level; cortical level. Each level is responsible for certain activities but yet controlled by the one above it.

lever (lĕv'ẽr, lē'vẽr) [L. *levare*, to raise]. Rigid bar used to modify direction, force and motion. A type of simple machine which provides the user with a mechanical advantage. Levers are used to facilitate in moving and lifting of objects too heavy or awkward to move unassisted. There are three classes of levers, only two of which are present in the human musculoskeletal system.

lev"ita'tion. The subjective sensation of rising in the air or moving through the air unsupported. Occurs in dreams and certain mental disorders.

levodopa. L-3,4-dihydroxyphenylalanine. Drug used in the treatment of Parkinson's disease. SYN: *L-Dopa.*

levoduction (lĕv"ō-dŭk'shŭn) [L. *laevus*, left, + *ducere*, to lead]. Movement or drawing toward the left, esp. of an eye.

levogyrous (lĕv"ō-jī'rŭs) ["+ *gyrāre*, to turn]. Causing to turn toward the left, applied esp. to substances that turn polarized light rays to the left. SYN: *levorotatory.*

levophobia (lĕv"ō-fō'bĭ-ă) ["+ Gr. *phobos*, fear]. Morbid dread of objects on the left side of the body.

levorotation (lĕv"ō-rō-tā'shŭn) ["+ *rotāre*, to turn]. Twisting or turning to the left.

levorotatory (lĕv"ō-rō'tă-tō-rī). Causing to turn toward the left, applies esp. to substances that turn polarized light rays to the left.

levotorsion (lĕv"ō-tor'shŭn) [L. *laevus*, left, + *torsiō*, a twisting]. A twisting to the left. SYN: *levorotation.*

levoversion (lĕv"ō-vẽr'shun) ["+ *versiō*, a turning]. A turning to the left. SYN: *levotorsion, levorotation.*

lev'ulose [L. *laevus*, left]. Fructose, or fruit sugar, a monosaccharide and a hexose, having the same empirical formula as dextrose, $C_6H_{12}O_6$.

It is an example of the carbohydrates, q.v. One of the three simple sugars. It is formed in the body by the digestion of sucrose. It is found in plants and fruits, in honey, corn syrup and syrup resulting from the inversion of sucrose.

levulosemia (lĕv"ū-lō-sē'mĭ-ă) ["+ Gr. *haima*, blood]. Presence of levulose in the blood.

levulosuria (lĕv"ū-lō-sū'rĭ-ă) ["+ Gr. *ouron*, urine]. Presence of levulose in the urine.

Leyden jar (lī'dĕn). [Ernst V. von Leyden, Ger. physician, 1832-1910] A glass jar coated partially, inside and out, with metal; it is used as a capacitor or collector of electricity.

Leydig's cells (lī'dĭg). [Franz von Leydig, Ger. anatomist, 1821-1908] Interstitial tissue cells in the testicles, believed to be responsible for internal secretion of the testicles, testosterone.

LH. Abbr. for *luteinizing hormone.*

Lhermitte's sign (lār'mĭt). [Jacques Jean Lhermitte, Fr. neurologist, 1877-1959] The symptom (rather than a sign) of a pain resembling a sudden electric shock throughout the body when the neck is flexed.

    ETIOL: Trauma to the cervical portion of the spinal cord, multiple sclerosis, cervical cord tumor, or cervical spondylosis.

LH-RH/FSH-RH. Abbr. for *luteinizing hormone—releasing hormone/follicle-stimulating hormone—releasing hormone,* q.v.

Li. Chem. symb. for lithium.

liberomotor (lĭb"ẽr-ō-mō'tor) [L. *liber*, free, + *motor*, mover]. 1. Pert. to voluntary movement. 2. Free from motor energy.

libidinous (lĭ-bĭd'ĭ-nŭs) [L. *libidinōsus*, pert. to desire]. 1. Characterized by erotic desires. SYN: *lascivious; salacious.* 2. Rel. to psychic energy.

libido (lĭ-bĭ'dō, -bē-dō) [L., desire]. 1. The sexual drive, conscious or unconscious. 2. In psychoanalysis, the energy or force or affect which is the driving force of human behavior. Variously identified as the sex urge, desire to live, desire for pleasure or satisfaction.

lice. Pl. of louse, q.v.

lichen (lī'kĕn) [Gr. *leichen*, lichen]. 1. Any form of papular skin disease; usually noting l. planus. 2. In botany, any one of numerous plants consisting of a fungus growing symbiotically with certain algae. They form characteristic scaly or branching growths on rocks or barks of trees.

    l. planus. Inflammatory skin disease of many varieties. SYN: *lichen ruber planus.*

    SYM: Begins with pinhead size papules, reddish or violaceous, glistening, then coalescing, forming rough, scaly patches; acute, subacute, or chronic itching situated on extremities. According to type of lesion the disease may be Lichen planus atrophicus, erythematosus, hypertrophicus, linearis, ruber moniliformis, etc.

    ETIOL: Unknown.

    PROG: Prolonged but favorable.

    TREATMENT: Locally, soothing antipruritic ointment. There is no specific therapy. The disease is self-limiting.

    l. spinulosus. Form with spine developing in each follicle. SYN: *keratosis pilaris,* q.v.

    l. tropicus. Form with redness and inflammatory reaction of the skin. SYN: *miliaria rubra, prickly heat.*

lichenification (lĭ-ken'ĭ-fĭ-kā'shun) [Gr. *leichēn*, lichen]. 1. Cutaneous thickening and hardening from continued irritation. 2. Changing of an eruption into resemblance to lichen.

lichenoid (lī'kĕn-oyd) ["+ *eidos*, form]. Resembling lichen.

licorice (lĭk'ŏ-rĭs). A dried root of Glycyrrhiza glabra used as a flavoring agent, demulcent, and mild expectorant. Glycyrrhiza (USP) is prepared from licorice. Ingestion of large amounts of licorice can cause salt retention, excess potassium loss in the urine, and elevated blood pressure. SYN: *glycyrrhiza.*

lid. An eyelid.

l. reflex. Closure of eyelids resulting from direct corneal stimulation. SYN: *corneal reflex.*

Lieben's test (lē'bĕn). [Adolf Lieben, Austrian chemist, 1836-1914] A test for acetone in the urine by caustic and iodine.

Yellow iodoform precipitate indicates presence of acetone.

Lieberkühn crypts (lē'bĕr-kün). [Johann N. Lieberkühn, Ger. anatomist, 1711-1756] Simple tubular glands present in the intestinal mucosa. In their epithelium are found goblet cells, cells of Paneth and argentaffine cells. The glands form minute invaginations opening between the bases of the villi. They lie in the lamina propria, their blind ends extending to the muscularis mucosa. In the large intestine they are longer, contain few if any Paneth cells and more goblet cells. They are arranged vertically with much regularity. SYN: *glands of Lieberkuhn; intestinal glands; Liberkühn's follicles.*

lie detector. A polygraph, an instrument for determining such minor definite physical changes assumed to occur under the stress of lying (or any other emotion) as variations in respiratory rhythm, pulse rate, blood pressure and sweating of the hands. Increased perspiration lessens resistance to passage of electrical current.

The test has popular appeal among law-enforcement departments but results obtained are presumptive and not absolute.

lien (lī'ĕn) [L., spleen]. [NA] The spleen, q.v.

l. accessorius. [NA] Accessory spleen.

lienal (lī-ē'năl) [L. *lien*, spleen]. Rel. to the spleen. SYN: *splenic.*

lienitis (lī''e-nī'tĭs) [L. *lien*, spleen, + Gr. *itis*, inflammation]. Inflammation of the spleen. SYN: *splenitis.*

lienocele (lī-ē'nō-sēl) ["+ Gr. *kēlē*, hernia]. Splenic hernia. SYN: *splenocele.*

lienomalacia (lī-ē''nō-mă-lā'shĭ-ă) ["+ Gr. *malakia*, softening]. Softening of the spleen. SYN: *splenomalacia.*

lienomedullary (lī-ē''nō-mĕd'ū-la-rĭ) ["+ *medulla*, marrow]. Rel. to both spleen and bone marrow.

lienomyelogenous (lī-ē''nō-mī-ĕl-ŏj'ē-nŭs) ["+ Gr. *myelos*, marrow, + *gennan*, to produce]. Derived from both the spleen and bone marrow.

lienomyelomalacia (lī-ē''nō-mī''el-o-mă-lā'-shĭ-ă) ["+ "+ *malakia*, softening]. Softening of the spleen and bone marrow.

lienopancreatic (lī-ē''nō-păn''krē-ăt'ĭk) [L. *lien*, spleen, + Gr. *pankreas*, pancreas]. Rel. to the spleen and pancreas.

lienopathy (lī''ē-nŏp'ă-thĭ) ["+ Gr. *pathos*, a disease]. Any disorder of the spleen. SYN: *splenopathy.*

lienorenal (lī-ē''nō-rē'nal) ["+ *rēnalis*, pert. to kidney]. Rel. to the spleen and kidney.

lienotoxin (lī-ē''nō-tŏks'ĭn) [L. *lien*, spleen, + Gr. *toxikon*, poison]. Cytotoxin having specific action on splenic cells. SYN: *splenotoxin.*

lienteric (lī-ĕn-tĕr'ĭk) [Gr. *leienteria*, smooth intestine]. 1. Pert. to diarrhea with stools containing undigested food. 2. Affected with lientery.

lientery (lī'ĕn-tĕr-ĭ). Diarrhea with undigested foods in the stools.

life (līf) [AS.]. 1. State of being alive; quality manifested by metabolism, growth, reproduction, and adaptation to environment; state in which the organs of an animal or plant are capable of performing all or any of their functions. 2. Time between birth or inception and death of an organism. Biologically, unitary life begins at the moment of conception and ends at death. However, for legal and other reasons the definition of when life begins has been subject to a variety of interpretations. Nevertheless, it is undeniable that life is a continuum which can be arbitrarily but not logically indicated as having begun at some point in time or development past the moment of conception. 3. The sum total of those properties which distinguish living things (animals or plants) from nonliving inorganic chemical matter or dead organic matter.

RS: anima; antibiosis; antibiotic; "bio-" words; vital; vitality.

l., change of. SEE: *menopause.*

l. expectancy. Expectation of life; the number of years that an average person of a given age may be expected to live as determined by mortality tables.

ligament (lĭg'ă-mĕnt) [L. *ligamentum*, a band]. 1. A band or sheet of strong, fibrous connective tissue connecting the articular ends of bones serving to bind them together and to facilitate or limit motion. 2. A thickened portion or fold of peritoneum or mesentery which supports a visceral organ or connects it to another viscus. 3. A band of fibrous connective tissue connecting bones, cartilages, and other structures and serving for support or for attachment of fascia or muscles. 4. A cordlike structure representing the vestigal remains of a fetal blood vessel.

l., accessory. A l. which supplements another one, esp. one on lateral surface of a joint. One outside of and independent of the capsule of a joint.

l., acromioclavicular. One extending from clavicle to the acromial process of the scapula.

l., alar. L. connecting odontoid process of atlas to occipital bone. SYN: *check l.; odontoid l.*

l., annular. A circular l., esp. (1) 1. enclosing head or radius, and (2) l. holding footplate of stapes in fenestra vestibuli.

l., apical. A single median l. extending from odontoid process to occipital bone. SYN: *odontoid l., suspensory l.*

l., arcuate, lateral and medial. L.'s from 12th rib to transverse process of 1st lumbar vertebra to which diaphragm is attached. SYN: *exterior arcuate l.*

l., arcuate popliteal. L. on posterolateral side of knee, extending from head of fibula to joint capsule.

l.'s auricular. The anterior, posterior, and superior auricular l.'s uniting external ear to the temporal bone.

l., broad, of the liver. A wide, sickle-shaped fold of peritoneum, attached to lower surface of diaphragm and internal surface of right rectus abdominis muscle, and to the convex surface of liver.

l., broad, of uterus. Folds of peritoneum attached to lateral borders of uterus from insertion of fallopian tube above to the pelvic wall. It consists of two leaves between which are found the remnants of the wolffian ducts, cellular tissues, and the major blood vessels of the pelvis.

l.'s capsular. Heavy fibrous structures, lined with synovial membrane, surrounding articulations.

l.'s, carpal. Those uniting carpal bones.

l., caudal. Bundles of fibrous tissue uniting dorsal surfaces of the two lower coccygeal vertebrae and superjacent skin.

l., check. One that restrains motion of a joint, esp. the lateral odontoid l.'s.

l., conoid. Posterior portion of coracoclavicular l.

l., coracoacromial. Broad triangular one attached to the outer edge of coracoid

process of the scapula, and to tip of acromion.

l., coracoclavicular. One uniting clavicle and the coracoid process of the scapula.

l., coracohumeral. Broad l. connecting coracoid process of scapula to greater tubercle of the humerus.

l., cornicupharyngeal. L. extending from corniculate cartilage of larynx caudally and attaching to mucosa of the pharynx.

l., coronary, of liver. A fold of peritoneum extending from posterior edge of liver to diaphragm.

l., costocolic. One attaching splenic flexure of colon to diaphragm.

l., costocoracoid. One joining first rib and coracoid process of the scapula.

l's., costotransverse. One uniting ribs with transverse processes of vertebrae.

l., costotransverse, middle. One consisting of parallel fibers extending between a vertebra and its adjacent rib.

l's., costovertebral. Those uniting the ribs and vertebrae.

l., cricopharyngeal. A ligamentous bundle between upper and posterior border of cricoid cartilage and anterior wall of pharynx.

l's., cricothyroid. Ones uniting cricoid and thyroid cartilages.

l., cricotracheal. The ligamentous structure uniting upper ring of trachea and the cricoid cartilage.

l., cruciate. 1. L. of the ankle passing transversely across dorsum of foot which holds tendons of the anterior muscle group in place. 2. A cross-shaped ligament of the atlas consisting of the transverse ligament and superior and inferior bands, the former passing upwards and attaching to margin of foramen magnum, the latter passing downwards and attaching to the body of the atlas. 3. Two l's. of the knee (anterior and posterior), the former passing from tibia to medial aspect of lateral condyle of femur, the latter from tibia to lateral aspect of medial condyle.

l., cruciform. A structure consisting of one l. crossing another.

l., crural. Poupart's l.

l., deltoid. Interior lateral l. of ankle.

l., dentate. Processes of pia mater extending across the subdural space on either side of spinal cord.

l., falciform, of the liver. A wide, sickle-shaped fold of peritoneum, attached to lower surface of diaphragm and internal surface of right rectus abdominis muscle, and to the convex surface of liver.

l., fundiform, of the penis. L. extending from lower portion of the linea alba and Scarpa's fascia to dorsum of penis. SYN: *superficial suspensory l.*

l., gastrophrenic. A fold of peritoneum between esophageal end of stomach and the diaphragm.

l., Gimbernat's. Triangular flat expansion of aponeurosis of abdominal ext. oblique muscle. Forming medial boundary of femoral ring. SYN: *lacunar l.*

l., glenohumeral. Fibers of the coracohumeral l. passing into the joint, and inserted into inner and upper part of bicipital groove.

l., glenoid. One which extends between palmar surfaces of phalanges and corresponding metacarpal bone.

l., hepaticoduodenal. A fold of peritoneum from transverse fissure of liver to vicinity of the duodenum and right flexure of colon, forming anterior boundary of foramen of Winslow.

l., ileopectineal. A portion of the pelvic fascia attached to the ileopectineal line and to capsular l. of hip joint.

l., iliofemoral. Bundle of fibers forming the upper and anterior portion of the capsular l. of the hip joint. L. that extends from ilium to intertrochanteric line.

l., iliolumbar. L. extending from 4th and 5th lumbar vertebrae to iliac crest.

l., infundibulopelvic. The upper free edge of the broad l. in which the ovarian artery is found.

l., inguinal. L. extending from anterior superior iliac spine to pubic tubercle. Forms lower margin of aponeurosis of exterior oblique muscle. SYN: *Poupart's l.*

l., interclavicular. Bundle of fibers between sternal ends of the clavicles, attached to interclavicular notch of sternum.

l.'s, interspinal, interspinous. Those extending from superior margin of a spinous process of one vertebra to lower margin of one above.

l., ischiocapsular. L. extending from ischium to ischial border of acetabulum.

l., lacunar. Gimbernat's l., q.v.

l.'s, lateral, of the liver. Folds of peritoneum extending from lower surface of diaphragm to adjacent borders of right and left lobes of the liver. Also called right and left triangular l's.

l., lateral occipitoatlantal. A ligament on each side between transverse processes of atlas and jugular process of the occipital bone.

l.'s lateral odontoid. Strong l.'s extending between sides of odontoid process of

the axis and inner sides of condyles of the occipital bone.

l., palpebral. Two ligaments medial and lateral, extending from tarsal plates of the eyelids to the frontal process of maxilla and the zygomatic bone respectively.

l., Poupart's. Inguinal l., q.v.

l., pterygomaxillary. Band of fiber extending from apex of internal pterygoid plate of sphenoid bone and the posterior extremity of internal oblique line of inferior maxilla.

l., pubic. Those connecting the pubic bones at the symphysis pubis. Include anterior and superior pubic l's. and the arcuate (inferior) ligament.

l., rhomboid. A strong structure extending from tuberosity of clavicle to outer surface of the cartilage of the first rib. SYN: *costoclavicular l.*

l., round, of the liver. Fibrous cord extending upward from the umbilicus and enclosed in lower margin of the falciform ligament. Represents obliterated left umbilical vein of the fetus. SYN: *ligamentum teres hepatis* [NA] .

l., round, of uterus. L. attached to uterus immediately below and in front of the entrance of the fallopian tube. Each extends laterally in the broad ligament to the pelvic wall where it passes through inguinal ring, terminating in the labium majus. SYN: *ligamentum teres uteri* [NA].

l., sacroiliac. Two ligaments, the anterior and posterior, which connect sacrum and ilium.

l., sacrospinous. L. extending from spine of ischium to sacrum and coccyx in front of the sacrotuberous ligament.

l., sacrotuberous. L. extending from tuberosity of the ischium to posterior superior and inferior iliac spines and to lower part of sacrum and coccyx. SYN: *greater sciatic l.; ligamentum sacrotuberale* [NA].

l., sphenomandibular. L. attached superiorly to spine of sphenoid and inferiorly to lingula of mandible.

l., spiral. The thickened periosteum of the peripheral wall of the osseous cochlear canal. The basilar membrane is attached to its inner surface.

l., stylohyoid. A thin fibroelastic cord between lesser cornu of hyoid bone and apex of styloid process of the temporal bone.

l., stylomandibular. A thin fibrous band of tissue extending between styloid process of temporal bone and lower part of posterior border of ramus of the mandible.

l., stylomaxillary, stylomyloid. A broad fibrous band of tissue extending between styloid process of temporal bone and lower part of posterior border of ramus of the inferior maxilla.

l., suprascapular. A thin fibrous band of tissue extending from base of coracoid process of scapula to inner margin of suprascapular notch.

l., supraspinal, supraspinous. One uniting apices of spinous processes of vertebrae.

l., suspensory. One suspending an organ.

l., suspensory, of lens. The zonula ciliaris (ciliary zonule); the fibers holding the crystalline lens in position.

l., suspensory, of ovary. L. extending from tubal end of ovary laterally to pelvic wall. It lies in layers of the broad ligament. SYN: *infundibulopelvic l.*

l., suspensory, of the penis. A triangular bundle of fibrous tissue extending from anterior surface of the symphysis pubis and adjacent structures to the dorsum of the root of the penis.

l.'s, suspensory, of the uterus. The broad l.'s, the round ones, and the rectouterine folds of the uterus.

l.'s sutural. Thin, fibrous layers interposed between articulating surfaces of bones united by suture.

l., transverse, of atlas. A strong l. passing over odontoid process of the axis.

l., transverse crural. L. lying on anterior surface of leg just above the ankle.

l., transverse, of hip joint. A ligamentous band extending across cotyloid notch of the acetabulum.

l., transverse, of knee joint. A fibrous band extending from anterior margin of external semilunar fibrocartilage of knee to extremity of the internal semilunar fibrocartilage.

l., trapezoid. Anterior exterior portion of the coracoclavicular l.

l., triangular, of liver. Two ligaments, right and left, which connect posterior aspects of right and left lobes with corresponding portions of the diaphragm.

l., umbilical, lateral. Fibrous cord extending from bladder to umbilicus. Represents obliterated interior iliac artery of fetus.

l., umbilical, median. Fibrous cord extending from apex of bladder to umbilicus. Represents the remains of the urachus of fetus.

l., uterorectosacral. Arises from the sides of the cervix and passes upwards and backwards, passing around the rectum, to the second sacral vertebra. They are en-

closed within the recto-uterine folds which demarcate borders of the rectouterine pouch.

l., ventricular, of larynx. The lateral free margin of the quadrangular membrane. It is enclosed within and supports the ventricular fold. SYN: *vestibular ligament.*

l., vocal, of larynx. The thickened free edges of the elastic cone extending from thyroid angle to vocal processes of arytenoid cartilages. They support the vocal fold, q.v.

l., yellow. One of a series of ligaments connecting lamina of adjacent vertebrae. SYN: *ligamentum flavum.*

ligamenta. Pl. of ligamentum, q.v.

ligamentopexis (lĭg-ă-mĕn′tō-peks′ĭs) [L. *ligamentum*, band, + Gr. *pēxis*, fixation]. Suspension of uterus on the round ligament.

ligamentous (lĭg″ă-mĕn′tŭs) [L. *ligamentum*, band]. 1. Rel. to a ligament. 2. Like a ligament.

ligamentum (lĭg″ă-mĕn′tŭm) [L., a band]. (pl. *ligamenta*) [NA] Ligament.

l. arteriosum. [NA] A fibrous cord, from pulmonary artery to arch of aorta, the remains of the ductus arteriosus of the fetus.

l. denticulatum. [NA] A fibrous band of pia mater extending the length of the spinal cord on each side between the spinal nerves. It has a scalloped appearance as it pierces the arachnoid to attach to the dura mater at regular intervals.

l. flavum. [NA] SEE: *ligament, yellow.*

l. nuchae. [NA] The upward continuation of the supraspinous ligament, extending from seventh cervical vertebra to occipital bone.

l. palpebrale. Ligamentous band, external and internal, between outer margin of the orbit and tissues of eyelids.

l. patellae. [NA] A strong, flat band securing the patella to the tibia. It is a continuation of the tendon of the quadriceps femoris muscle.

l. teres femoris. A flat band extending from acetabular fossa to head of femur. SYN: *ligamentum capitis femoris* [NA].

l. teres hepatis. [NA] SEE: *ligament, round, of liver.*

l. teres uteri. [NA] SEE: *ligament, round, of uterus.*

l. venosum. [NA] A solid fibrous cord representing obliterated ductus venosus of the fetus. It lies between the caudate and left lobes of the liver and connects the left branch of the portal vein to the interior vena cava.

ligand. A term employed to indicate a substrate or co-enzyme when discussing enzymes; and to indicate antigens and haptens when discussing antibodies.

ligate (lī′gāt) [L. *ligāre*, to bind]. To apply a ligature.

ligation (li-gā′shun). The application of a ligature.

ligature (līg′a-tūr) [L. *ligatūra*, a binding]. 1. Process of binding or tying. 2. A band or bandage. 3. A thread or wire for tying a blood vessel or other structure in order to constrict it. Cord or material used may be: catgut; synthetic materials such as nylon or dacron; kangaroo gut; silk; or cotton. Sometimes strips of fascia obtained from the patient are used as a ligature. SEE: *catgut*.

light (līt) [AS. *lihtan*, to shine]. The sensation produced by electromagnetic radiation which falls on the retina.

The radiation itself is also called l. over the range of wavelengths which produces sensation, and regarding this range it is also called infrared and ultraviolet l. Radiant energy producing a sensation of luminosity on the retina is limited to a wavelength of from about 3900 to 7700 angstroms. SEE: *ray*.

l. adaptation. Changes which occur in a dark-adapted eye in order for vision to occur in moderate or bright l. Principle changes are contraction of pupil and bleaching of visual purple in the rods.

l., axial. L. with rays parallel to each other and to optic axis.

l. difference. Abbr. L.D. The difference with respect to sensitiveness to intensity of l. between the two eyes.

l., diffused. Rays broken by refraction.

l., polarized. L. in which waves vibrate in one direction only.

l., reflected. L. rays which are thrown back by an illuminated object such as a mirror.

l., reflex. Constriction of the pupil when l. is flashed into the eye.

l., refracted. Rays bent from original course.

l. therapy. Phototherapy; the use of l. rays in the treatment of disease. Includes use of ultraviolet and infrared radiations. SEE: *heliotherapy; lamp.*

l., transmitted. That which passes through an object.

l. unit. A foot candle. This is the amt. of light measured one foot from a standard candle. The ideal amount of light required for work varies with the specific type of work being done. Thus surgery requires a greater intensity of light than would occupations entailing less detailed work. At noon, on a clear day, the sun gives 10,000 candle ft.

of light; under a tree we get 1000; on a porch, 500; on a fairly cloudy day, 200. The term foot candle took the place of candle power, but light intensity is best described by the word lumen, q.v.

light, words pert. to: aclastic; "actin" words; Fraunhofer's lines; heliotherapy; lambert; lumen; lux; "phot-" words; "radi-" words; ray; reflection; reflector; refraction; spectrum.

light (līt) [AS. *lēohte*, not heavy]. 1. Not heavy. 2. Pale.

l. diet. All foods allowed in soft diet, q.v., plus whole grained cereals, easily digested raw fruits and vegetables. Foods not pureed or ground.

lightening [AS. *lēohte*, not heavy]. Uterine descent into pelvis. This usually occurs two to three weeks prior to the beginning of the first stage of labor. It may not occur in multiparas until active labor begins.

ligula (līg′ū-lă) [L., a strap]. Strip of white substance on the margin of the fourth ventricle.

limb (līm) [AS. *lim*]. 1. An arm or leg. 2. An extremity. 3. A limblike extension of a structure.

RS: anisomelia; appendicular; extremity; member.

l., anterior, of internal capsule. The lenticulocaudate portion which lies between lenticular and caudate nuclei.

l., ascending, of renal tubule. Portion between the bend in Henle's loop and the distal convoluted portion.

l., descending, of renal tubule. Portion between proximal convoluted portion and the bend in Henle's loop.

l., pelvic. The lower extremity.

l., thoracic. The upper extremity.

limbic (līm′bĭk) [L. *limbus*, a border]. Pert. to a limbus or border. SYN: *marginal.*

limbus (līm′bŭs) [L., border]. [NA] The edge or border of a part.

l. alveolaris. 1. The upper free edge of the alveolar process of the mandible. 2. The lower free edge of the alveolar process of the maxilla. SYN: *arcus alveolaris.*

l. conjunctivae. The edge of conjunctiva overlapping the cornea.

l. corneae. [NA] The edge of the cornea where it unites with the sclera.

l., corneoscleral. In the eye, a transitional dome 1 to 2 mm. wide where the cornea joins the sclera and conjunctiva.

l. fossa ovalis. [NA] The thickened margin of the fossa ovalis, esp. the rim of the septum secundum bounding the fossa.

l. lamina spiralis. Thickening of the periosteum of the osseous spiral lamina of cochlea to which the tectorial membrane is attached.

l. palpebralis, anterior. The anterior margin of the free edge of the eyelid from which the cilia or eyelashes grow.

l. palpebralis, posterior. The posterior margin of the free edge of the eyelid; the region of transition of skin to conjunctival mucous membrane.

l. sphenoidalis. Ridge on anterior portion of upper surface of sphenoid bone.

lime (līm) [AS. *lim*, glue]. CaO (calcium oxide). A substance obtained from limestone. SEE: *calcium.*

l., chlorinated. Substance resulting from chlorinization of slaked lime, consisting chiefly of calcium chloride and calcium hypochlorite. Used principally as a disinfectant and in aqueous solution as a bleaching agent.

l. liniment. Carron oil.

l., slaked. Calcium hydroxide.

l. water. Solution of calcium hydroxide, Ca(OH)$_2$, in water; a weak base and used as an antacid.

lime [Fr.]. Fruit of Citrus aurantifolia. Its juice is antiscorbutic.

Food value of 100 gm. of l. juice (fresh): Cal. 26; protein 0.3 gm.; carbohydrates 9 gm.; calcium 9 mg.; ascorbic acid 32 mg.

limen (lī'mĕn) [L., threshold]. Edge, threshold.

limes death. The least amount of toxin which when mixed with one unit of antitoxin and injected into a guinea pig weighing 250 gm. will kill it within 96 hours. SYMB: L$_+$.

limes zero. The greatest amount of toxin which when mixed with one unit of antitoxin and injected into a guinea pig weighing 250 gm. will cause no local reaction. SYMB: L$_0$.

liminal (līm'ī-năl) [L. *līmen, limin-*, threshold]. Hardly perceptible; rel. to a threshold as of consciousness.

limitans (līm'ī-tăns) [L. *limitāre*, to limit]. 1. Used in conjunction with other words to denote limiting. 2. Used synonymously to indicate membrane limitans.

limitation (līm'ī-tā'shŭn). Condition of being limited.

l. of motion. The restriction of movement or range of motion of a part or joint. Esp. that imposed by disease or trauma to joints and soft tissues.

limo'sis [Gr. *limos*, hunger]. Abnormal hunger; perverted appetite.

limotherapy (līm-ō-thĕr'ă-pī) ["+ *therapeia*, treatment]. Treatment by restriction of diet or by fasting.

lincture, linctus (līnk'tūr, -tŭs) [L. *linctus*, a licking]. A thick, sweet, syrupy medicinal preparation given for its effect on the throat. Usually taken in sips or may be licked or sucked as with a throat lozenge.

line (līn) [L. *linea*]. 1 Any long, relatively narrow mark. 2. A boundary or an outline. 3. A wrinkle.

l., abdominal. L. indicating abdominal muscle boundaries.

l., alveobasilar. One from nasion to alveolar point.

l., alveolonasal. From alveolar point to nasion.

l., auriculobregmatic. From auricular point to bregma.

l.,axillary.(anterior, posterior and mid-) Downward from axilla.

l., base. From infraorbital ridge through middle of external auditory meatus to midline of occiput.

l., basiobregmatic. From basion to bregma.

l., Baudelocque's. Exterior conjugate diameter of pelvis.

l.'s, Beau's. Transverse lines on the fingernails.

l., biauricular. From one auditory meatus over vertex to other.

l., blue. One on gums in chronic lead poisoning.

l., costoarticular. From sternoclavicular joint to point on 11th rib.

l., costoclavicular. L. midway between nipple and sternum border.

l. of demarcation. Division between healthy and diseased tissue.

l. of femur, internal supracondylar. Inner of two ridges into which linea aspera of femur divides.

l. of fibula, oblique. Prominent ridge on interior surface of shaft of fibula.

l. of fixation. Imaginary l. drawn from subject viewed to the fovea centralis.

l., gingival. 1. Line of junction of cementum and enamel of a tooth. 2. One on neck of tooth where gum is attached.

l.'s, gluteal. Three lines, anterior, posterior, and inferior, on exterior surface of ilium.

l., iliopectineal. Bony ridge marking brim of pelvis.

l. of ilium, intermediate. Ridge upon crest of ilium between inner and outer lip.

l. of inferior maxilla, internal oblique. Ridge on interior surface of lower jaw.

l., interauricular. One joining the two auricular points.

l., intercondylar, intercondylean. Transverse ridge joining condyles of femur above the intercondyloid fossa.

l., intertrochanteric. Ridge upon posterior surface of femur exterior between greater and lesser trochanters.

l., intertuberal. One joining inner borders of ischial tuberosities below small sciatic notch.

l., mammary. Horizontal from one nipple to other.

l., mammillary. Vertical line through center of nipple.

l., median. One joining any two points in the periphery of the median plane of the body, or one of its parts.

l., milk. The mammary ridge, an ectodermal thickening in embryo exterior between bases of limb buds.

l., nasobasilar. Through basion and nasion.

l., nuchal, superior and inferior. Two curved ridges on occipital bone extending laterally from exterior occipital crest.

l., oblique, of fibula. The medial crest of posteromedial border; a l. extending from medial side of head and terminating distally at interosseous crest.

l., oblique, of radius. Faint ridge on anterior surface passing downward and laterally from radial tuberosity.

l., parasternal. L. midway between nipple and border of sternum.

l., pectineal. L. on posterior surface of femur extending downward from lesser trochanter. That portion of iliopectineal l. formed by the os pubis.

l., popliteal. L. of posterior surface of tibia, extending obliquely downward from fibular facet on lateral condyle to medial border about middle of bone.

l., scapular. Downward from lower angle of scapula.

l., semilunar. Curved tendinous condensation of aponeurosis of obliquus abdominis externus.

l., sight. From center of pupil to viewed object, imaginary.

l., sternal. Median line of sternum.

l., sternomastoid. From between heads of sternomastoid muscle to mastoid process.

l., supracondylar, medial and lateral. Two ridges on posterior surface of distal end of femur, formed by diverging lips of the linea aspera.

l., supraorbital. Across forehead above root of exterior angular process of frontal bone.

l., temporal, superior and inferior. Two curved l.'s on lateral surface of skull passing upwards and backwards from zygomatic process of frontal bone and terminating posteriorly at supramastoid crest.

l.'s, test. Those for detecting fracture of shortening of neck of femur.

l., umbilicopubic. That portion of median l. extending from umbilicus to symphysis pubis.

l., visual. One that extends from object to macula lutea passing through the nodal point. SYN: *visual axis.*

linea (lĭn'e-ä) [L., line). (pl. *lineae*) [NA] A anatomical line.

l. alba. [NA] The white line of connective tissue in middle of abdomen from sternum to pubis.

l. aspera. [NA] A longitudinal ridge on posterior surface of middle third of the femur.

l. costoarticularis. A line between the sternoclavicular articulation and point of the 11th rib.

l. ni'gra. Black line or discoloration of the abdomen seen in pregnant women during latter part of term. It runs from above the umbilicus to the pubes.

l. splendens. A thickening of the pia mater extending along anterior median surface of the spinal cord. It ensheaths the anterior spinal artery.

l. sternalis. Median line of the sternum

l. terminalis. [NA] Bony ridge on inner surface of ilium continued on to pubis which divides true and false pelvis.

lineae albicantes. Lines seen on the abdomen. Frequently due to pregnancy but may occur as the result of abdominal distention due to any cause. SEE: *stria.*

lineae transversae ossis sacralis. Ridges formed by lines of union of the 5th sacral vertebrae.

linear (lĭn'e-ar) [L. *linea,* line]. Pert. to or resembling a line.

l. measure. Measure of length.

lingism (lĭng'ĭzm). Treatment or cure of a condition by use of exercise, esp. exercise not involving use of apparatus. SYN: *kinesitherapy.*

Ling's cure (lĭng). [Peter H. Ling, Swed. poet and gymnast, 1776-1839] Treatment by movements. SYN: *Ling's system.*

lingua (lĭng'gwä) [L., tongue). [NA] Tongue or tonguelike structure.

l. fraenata. A tongue with a very short frenum, resulting in tonguetie.

l. nigra. Black tongue, q.v.

l. plicata. A fissured tongue.

lingual (lĭn'gwal) [L. *lingua*, tongue]. 1. Pert. to the tongue. 2. Tongue-shaped.

lingula (lĭn'gū-lă) [L., little tongue]. Tongue-shaped process, esp. lingula cerebelli.

    l. cerebelli. [NA] Tongue of cerebellum prolonged forward on upper surface of superior medullary velum.

    l. of lung. Projection of lung which separates cardiac notch from inferior margin of left lung.

    l. of mandible. Projection of bone forming medial boundary of mandibular foramen.

    l. of sphenoid. Ridge between the body and ala magna of the sphenoid.

    l., Wrisbergi. Connecting fibers of motor and sensory roots of the trifacial nerve.

lin'iment [L. *linimentum*, smearing substance]. A liquid containing a medicament and oil, alcohol or water for use externally, applied by friction method or on a bandage.

linimentum (lĭn-ĭm-en'tum) [L.]. Liquid preparation for external use and usually applied by rubbing. SEE: *liniment.*

linitis (lĭn-i'tĭs) [Gr. *linon*, web, + -*itis*, inflammation]. Inflamed condition of gastric cellular tissue.

    l. plastica. L. with thickening of the wall of the stomach usually due to neoplasmic tissue. Also called leather-bottle stomach.

linkage. In genetics, condition in which two or more genes present in the same chromosome tend to remain together and not assort independently in the formation of gametes.

    l., sex. Condition in which a character is due to a factor located on the X-chromosomes.

lin'seed [AS. *linsāēd*]. Seeds of the common flax, Linum usitatissimum. It is the source of linseed oil. Linseed is used as a demulcent and emollient, and sometimes as a laxative. SYN: *flaxseed.*

    l. poultice. One made from crushed linseed which is heated. Test for heat with hand before applying.

lint (lĭnt) [L. *linteum*, made of linen]. 1. Linen scraped until soft and woolly for dressing wounds. 2. Cotton fiber.

lintin (lin'tĭn). Prepared absorbent cotton; fabric used in dressings.

lip [AS. *lippa*]. 1. Soft external structure around the oral cavity. 2. One of the lips of the pudendum (labium majus or minus). 3. A liplike structure forming border of an opening or groove.

    CONDITIONS: *Chancre:* It is not unusual to have the initial lesion of syphilis appear upon the lip of the mouth as an indurated base, with a thin secretion, accompanied by enlargement of the submaxillary glands. *Condyloma latum:* This appears as a mucous patch, flattened, coated with gray exudate, with strictly delimited area, usually at the angle of the mouth. *Eczema:* Dry fissures, often covered with a crust, bleeding easily, and occurring on both lips. *Epithelioma:* May be confused with chancre. Seldom appears before the age of 40, but there are exceptions. It may appear as a common cold sore, a painless fissure, or other break of the lower lip. Less than 5% occur on upper lip. A crust or scab covers the lesion, leaving a raw surface if removed. Pain does not appear until well advanced. *Herpes:* Appears on the lips in pneumonia, typhoid, common cold, other febrile diseases, and idiopathically. *Tuberculous ulcer:* At inner portion of lip close to angle of mouth. Pathological examination necessary for verification.

    DIAGNOSIS: Examination incomplete unless lips are everted to expose buccal surfaces. *Bluish or purplish:* May appear in the aged, in those exposed to great cold, and in carbon monoxide poisoning. *Dry:* May be seen in fevers or be caused by drugs such as atropine, by thirst, or exhaustion. *Fissured:* May occur after exposure to cold, in avitaminosis, and in children in congenital syphilis. The dribbling of saliva and a toothless condition may cause fissures in the corners of the mouth. *Pale:* May be seen in anemia and wasting diseases, in prolonged fever, and after a hemorrhage. *Rashes:* May be manifestations of typhoid fever, meningitis, or pneumonia. In secondary syphilis, chancre, cancer, and epithelioma, mucous patches may appear.

    RS: buccal; cheilitis; "chil-" words; labia; labium; labrum.

    l., cleft. Harelip, q.v.

    l., glenoid. Thickened fibrocartilaginous structure surmounting margin of acetabulum.

    l.'s, oral. Upper and lower lips which surround mouth opening, and form anterior wall of buccal cavity.

    l. reading. Interpreting what is being said by watching the speaker's lip movements. Used very effectively by deaf persons.

    l. reflex. Reflex movement of lips when angle of mouth is suddenly and lightly tapped during sleep.

    l., tympanic. Lower border of the sulcus spiralis internus of the cochlea.

    l., vestibule. Upper border of the sulcus spiralis internus of the cochlea.

lipacidemia (lĭp″ă-sĭ-dē′mĭ-ă) [Gr. *lipos*, fat, + L. *acidus*, acid, + Gr. *haima*, blood]. Fatty acid in the blood.

lipaciduria (lĭp″ă-sĭ-dū′rĭ-ă) [″ + ″ + Gr. *ouron*, urine]. Fatty acids in the urine.

liparocele (lip′ă-ro-sēl) [″ + *kēlē*, hernia]. 1. Scrotal hernia containing fat. 2. A fatty tumor.

liparomphalus (lĭp″ă-rom′fă-lŭs) [″ + *omphalos*, navel]. Fatty tumor located at, or involving, the umbilical cord.

liparous (lĭp′ăr-ŭs) [Gr. *lipos*, fat]. Obese; fat.

lipase (lĭ′pās, lĭ′pās) [Gr. *lipos*, fat, + *-ase*, enzyme]. A lipolytic or fat splitting enzyme found in the blood, pancreatic secretion and tissues. SEE: *digestive; enzyme.*

Emulsified fats of cream and egg yolk are changed in the stomach to fatty acids and glycerol by gastric lipase.

l., pancreatic. Steapsin, q.v.

lipasuria (lĭp″ās-ū′rĭ-ă) [″ + ″ + Gr. *ouron*, urine]. Lipase in the urine.

lipectomy (lĭ-pĕk′to-mĭ) [″ + *ektomē*, excision]. Excision of fatty tissues.

lipemia (lĭ-pē′mĭ-ă) [″ + *haima*, blood]. Abnormal amt. of fat in the blood.

l. retinalis. Condition in which retinal vessels appear reddish white, or white; found in cases of lipemia.

lipid(e (lĭp′ĭd, -īd) [Gr. *lipos*, fat]. Any one of a group of fats or fatlike substances, characterized by their insolubility in water. Includes true fats (esters of fatty acids and glycerol); lipoids (phospholipids, cerebrosides, waxes); sterols (cholesterol, ergosterol); and hydrocarbons (squalene, carotene). SYN: *lipin; lipoid.* SEE: *fat.*

lipid histiocytosis. Niemann-Pick disease, q.v.

lipido′sis. Any disorder of fat metabolism. SYN: *lipoidosis.*

lipin (lĭp′ĭn) [Gr. *lipos*, fat]. SEE: *lipid.*

lipiodol (lĭp-ĭ′ō-dŏl) [″ + L. *oleum*, oil]. Proprietary name for an iodized oil obtained by fixation of iodine in poppyseed oil.

It contains 40% of pure iodine by weight. It is opaque to X rays and used for radiological diagnosis. It is introduced into cavities by a catheter, into the trachea for outlining the bronchial tree by X ray, and into the spinal canal to locate tumors. It is eliminated completely and does not cause iodism.

l. injection. May be cisternal, lumbar, or both, depending upon whether the suspected block is near the cisterna magna or below it. Two cubic centimeters are injected into spinal canal. There are two forms of lipiodol: ascending and descending. If tumor is near the cisterna, descending lipiodol is given intraspinously; if position is uncertain or halfway between cisterna and lumbar region, both forms are given. If there is a block in the canal, the picture shows a dark mass through which the lipiodol has not passed, and a light streak where the lipiodol is present.

lipo-, lip- [Gr. *lipos*, fat]. Combining forms pert. to fat.

lipoarthritis (lip″ō-arth-rī′tĭs) [Gr. *lipos*, fat, + *arthron*, joint, + *itis*, inflammation]. Inflammation of fatty tissues of joints.

lipoblast (lĭp′ō-blast) [″ + *blastos*, germ]. Immature fat cell.

lipoblastoma (lĭp″ō-blast-ō′mă) [″ + ″ + *-ōma*, tumor]. Tumor of fatty tissue. SYN: *adipoma; lipoma.*

lipocardiac (lĭp″ō-kar′dĭ-ăk) [″ + *kardia*, heart]. 1. Pert. to fatty heart degeneration. 2. Sufferer from fatty degeneration of heart.

lipocele (lĭp′ō-sēl) [″ + *kēlē*, hernia]. Presence of fatty tissue in a hernial sac. SYN: *adipocele; liparocele.*

lipocere (lip′ō-sēr) [″ + L. *cera*, wax]. Waxy substance resulting from exposure of fleshy tissue to moisture with the exclusion of air. SYN: *adipocere.*

lipochondrodystrophy (lĭp″ō-kŏn″drō-dĭs′-trō-fĭ) [Gr. *lipos*, fat, + *chondros*, cartilage, + *dys*, bad, + *trephein*, to nourish]. Congenital abnormality in the skeletal bones and cartilage, with deranged mucopolysaccharide metabolism; kyphosis and other deformity; possible mental deficiency and cloudy corneae. SYN: *Hurler's syndrome.*

lipochondroma (lĭp″ō-kŏn-drō′mă) [″ + ″ + *-ōma*, tumor]. Tumor both fatty and cartilaginous.

lipochrome (lĭp′ō-krōm) [″ + *chrōma*, color]. Colored substance of fatty nature.

Ex: carotene, the fat-soluble yellow pigment found in carrots, sweet potatoes, egg yolk, butter, body fat and corpus luteum. SEE: *carotene.*

lipoclasis (lĭp-ok′lă-sĭs) [″ + *klasis*, breaking]. Splitting up of fat. SYN: *lipolysis.*

lipoclastic (lĭp-ō-klas′tĭk). Rel. to or causing lipoclasis. SYN: *lipolytic.*

lipocyte (lĭp′ō-sīt) [Gr. *lipos*, fat, + *kytos*, cell]. Fat cell.

lipodieresis (lĭp″ō-dī-er′ĭ-sĭs) [″ + *diairesis*, a taking]. Splitting or destruction of fat.

lipodystrophy (lĭp″ō-dĭs′trō-fĭ) [″ + *dys*, bad, + *trophē*, nourishment]. Disturbance or defectiveness of fat metabolism.

l., insulin. Atrophy of subcutaneous fat at site of injection of insulin.

l., intestinal. Disease characterized principally by fat deposits in intestinal and mesenteric lymphatic tissue and by fatty diarrhea, loss of weight and strength, and arthritis.

lipoferous (lĭp-ŏf′ĕr-ŭs) ["+ L. *ferre*, to carry]. Causing or carrying fat.

lipofibroma (lip″ō-fī-brō′mă) [Gr. *lipos*, fat, + L. *fibra*, fiber, + Gr. *-ōma*, tumor]. Tumor indicating lipoma and fibroma. A fibrolipoma, q.v.

lipogenesis (lip″ō-jĕn′ĭ-sĭs) ["+ *genesis*, formation]. Fat formation.

lipogenetic (lip″ō-jĕn-ĕt′ĭk). Fat producing. SYN: *lipogenic; lipogenous.*

lipogenic (lĭp″ō-jĕn′ĭk). Fat producing. SYN: *lipogenetic; lipogenous.*

lipogenous (lip-ŏj′ĕn-ŭs). Producing fat. SYN: *lipogenetic; lipogenic.*

lipogranuloma (lip″ō-gran-ū-lo′mă) [Gr. *lipos*, fat, + L. *granulum*, granule, + Gr. *-ōma*, tumor]. Inflammation of fatty tissue with granulation and development of oily cysts.

lipoid (lĭp′oyd) ["+ *eidos*, form]. 1. Substance resembling fats in appearance and solubility, but containing other groups than the glycerol and fatty acids which make up the true fats. Ex: cholesterol; kephalin; lecithin, q.v. SYN: *lipid.* 2. Similar to fat.

lipoidemia (lĭp″oy-dē′mĭ-ă) ["+ "+ *haima*, blood]. Excess of lipoids in the blood.

lipoidosis (lĭp-oy-dō′sĭs) ["+ "+ *-ōsis*, increase]. Condition in which lipids accumulate in excessive quantities in body tissue. SEE: *Xanthomatosis.*

  l., arterial. Arteriosclerosis, q.v.

  l., cerebral infantile. SEE: *amaurotic familial idiocy, infantile.*

  l., cerebroside. A familial disease characterized by deposition of kerasin, a cerebroside, in cells of the reticuloendothelial system. SYN: *Gaucher's disease.*

  l., primary. L. of unknown etiology in which serum lipids are abnormal in quantity or in quality, or else serum lipids are normal but lipids accumulate intracellularly.

lipoiduria (lĭp″oy-dū′rĭ-ă) ["+ "+ *ouron*, urine]. Lipoids in the urine.

lipolipoidosis (lĭp″ō-lĭp″oy-dō′sĭs) ["+ *lipos*, fat, + *eidos*, form, + *-ōsis*, increase]. Infiltration of fats and lipoids into a tissue.

lipolysis (lĭp-ŏl′ĭ-sĭs) [Gr. *lipos*, fat, + *lysis*, dissolution]. The decomposition of fat.

lipolytic (lĭp-ō-lĭ′-tĭk) ["+ *lysis*, dissolution]. Rel. to lipolysis.

  l. digestion. The conversion of neutral fats by hydrolysis into fatty acids and glycerol; fat splitting.

  l. enzyme. Fat-splitting ferment. SYN: *lipase.* SEE: *enzyme.*

lipoma (lĭ-pō′mă) ["+ *-ōma*, tumor]. A fatty tumor. SEE: *chondrolipoma.*
They are frequently multiple, but not metastatic.

  l. arborescens. An abnormal treelike accumulation of fatty tissue in a joint.

  l., cystic. One containing cysts.

  l., diffuse. One not definitely circumscribed.

  l. diffusum renis. Condition in which fat displaces parenchyma of the kidney.

  l. durum. One in which there is marked hypertrophy of the fibrous stroma and capsule.

  l., hernial. A lipocele.

  l., nasal. A fibrous growth of the subcutaneous tissue of the nostrils.

  l., osseous. One in which the connective tissue has undergone calcareous degeneration.

  l. telangiectodes. A rare form containing a large number of blood vessels.

lipomatosis (lĭp″ō-mă-to′sĭs) [Gr. *lipos*, fat, + *-ōma*, tumor, + *-ōsis*, intensive]. Excessive deposit of fat in the tissues. SYN: *liposis, obesity.*

  l. renis. Fatty infiltration of renal parenchyma. SYN: *lipoma diffusum renis.*

lipomatous (lĭp-ō′mă-tŭs). 1. Of the nature of lipoma. 2. Affected with lipoma.

lipometabolic (lĭp″ō-met″ă-bol′ĭk) [Gr. *lipos*, fat, + *metabolē*, change]. Rel. to metabolism of fat.

lipometabolism (lĭp-ō-mĕ-tab′ol-ĭzm) ["+ "+ *-ismos*, state of]. Fat metabolism.

lipomyoma (lip″o-mī-o′mă) ["+ *mys*, muscle, + *-ōma*, tumor]. A myoma containing fatty tissue.

lipomyxoma (lĭp″ō-miks-ō′mă) ["+ *myxa*, mucus, + *-ōma*, tumor]. A mixed lipoma and myxoma.

lipopectic (lĭp-ō-pek′tĭk) ["+ *pēxis*, fixation]. Characterized by lipopexia.

lipopexia (lĭp″ō-pek′sĭ-ă). Accumulation of fat in the body. SYN: *adipopexia.*

lipophage (lĭp′o-fāj) [Gr. *lipos*, fat, + *phagein*, to eat]. Fat-absorbing cell.

lipophagic (lĭp-ō-fā′jĭk). Consuming, destroying, or absorbing fat.

lipophil (lĭp′o-fĭl) [Gr. *lipos*, fat, + *philein*, to love]. 1. Having an affinity for fat. 2. Absorbing fat.

lipophrenia (lĭp″ō-frē′nĭ-ă) [Gr. *leipein*, to fail, + *phrēn*, mind]. Mental failure or collapse.

lipoproteins. Conjugated proteins consisting of simple proteins combined with lipid components—cholesterol, phospholipid, and triglyceride.

liposarcoma (lĭp-ō-sar-kō′mä) [Gr. *lipos*, fat, + *sarx*, flesh, + -*ōma*, tumor]. Sarcoma with fatty elements.

lipo'sis ["+ -*ōsis*, intensive]. Accumulation of fat in a part.

liposome (lĭp′ō-sōm) [Gr. *lipos*, fat, + *sōma*, body]. A particle of lipoidal substance held in suspension in tissues.

lipostomy (lĭ-pos′tō-mĭ) [Gr. *leipein*, to fail, + *stoma*, mouth]. Congenital absence or extreme smallness of the mouth.

lipothymia (lĭ″po-thī′mĭ-ä) ["+ *thymos*, mind]. Faintness; syncope, q.v.

lipotropic (lĭp-ō-trōp′ĭk) [Gr. *lipos*, fat, + *tropē*, a turning]. Having an affinity for lipids. Ex: certain dyes such as Sudan III which stains fat readily.

l. factors. Compounds which promote the transportation and utilization of fats and help to prevent accumulation of fat in the liver.

lipoxeny (lĭp-oks′ĭ-nĭ) [Gr. *leipein*, to leave, + *xenos*, host]. Desertion of host by parasitic organism after completion of its development.

lipsis (lĭp′sĭs) [Gr. *leiprein*, to fail]. Ending or cessation.

l. animi. Fainting.

lipuria (lĭ-pu′rĭ-ä) [Gr. *lipos*, fat, + *ouron*, urine]. Fat in the urine.

liquefacient (lĭk″wĕ-fā′shent) [L. *liquere*, to flow, + *facere*, to make]. 1. Agent which converts a solid substance into liquid. 2. Converting into liquid.

liquefaction (lĭk″wĕ-fak′shun). 1. The conversion of a solid into a liquid. 2. Conversion of solid tissues to a fluid or semifluid state.

liquescent (lik-wes′sent) [L. *liquescere*, to become liquid]. Becoming liquid. SYN: *deliquescent.*

liqueur (lĭ-ker′) [Fr.]. Alcoholic beverage. Aromatically flavored, often colored, and sweetened. A cordial.

liquid (lĭk′wĭd) [L. *liquere*, to flow]. 1. Flowing easily. 2. Substance which flows without being melted. SEE: *emulsion, liquefacient; liquefaction.*

l. air therapy. Therapeutic application of air which is so cold as to be liquefied. SEE: *refrigeration.*

l. crystals. Substances which alter their color or change from opaque to transparent when subjected to changes in temperature, electric current, pressure, electromagnetic waves, or when impurities are present. They have been used to detect temperature fluctuation in infants.

Liquid crystals are of two general classes: cholestric, which change color, and nematic, which change back and forth from transparent to opaque.

l. di'et. Coffee with hot milk; tea; water; milk in all forms; milk and cream mixtures; cocoa; cream soups strained; fruit juices; meat juices; beef tea; clear broths; gruels; meat soups strained; eggnogs. SEE: *fluid diet.*

l. measure. Measure of liquid capacity.

liquor (lĭk′er) [L.]. 1. Any liquid or fluid. 2. An alcoholic beverage. 3. Solution of medicinal substance in water.

l. amnii. The amniotic fluid, a clear, watery fluid which surrounds the fetus in the amniotic sac.

l. folliculi. The fluid contained in the graafian follicle.

l. puris. Liquid portion of pus.

l. sanguinis. Blood serum or plasma.

l. solutions. Aqueous solutions of nonvolatile substances presenting the greatest variety in strength, character, and method of preparation. They are usually very active medicinal preparations.

lisping (lĭsp′ing) [AS. *wlisp*, lisping]. Substitution of sounds due to defect in speech, as of th sound for s and z.

lissencephalous (lis″sen-sef′ä-lus) [Gr. *lissos*, smooth, + *enkephalos*, brain]. Condition in which the brain is smooth owing to failure of development of cerebral gyri.

lissotrichy (lĭs-sot′rĭ-kĭ) ["+ *thrix*, hair]. Condition of having straight hair.

listeriosis, listerosis (lĭs-tĕr″ĭ-ō′sĭs, lĭs″ter-ō′sĭs). A disease affecting many domestic animals, wild animals, and man. Caused by Listeria monocytogenes, a soil saprophyte which becomes pathogenic for animals or man under favorable circumstances. The most common manifestation in the adult is meningitis. It may be transmitted transplacentally to the fetus in which case it may cause abortion. In newborns the disease, known as granulomatosis infantiseptica, is much more serious than in the adult. Although man has a high degree of resistance to the bacteria, hygienic precautions should be taken when handling infected animals.

liter (lē′tĕr) [Fr. *litre*, liter]. Metric fluid measure; 1000 milliliters (ml.), 270 fl. drams, 61 cu. in., 33.8 fl. oz., 1.0567 qt. The volume occupied by one kilogram of water at 4° C. and 760 mm. pressure. SEE: *metric system.*

NOTE: It is common to define a liter as 1000 cubic centimeters (cc). This is almost but not quite correct because 1 ml. is equal to 1.000028 cubic centimeters.

lithagogue (lĭth′ä-gŏg) [Gr. *lithos*, stone, + *agōgos*, leading]. 1. Agent which expels calculi. 2. Expelling calculi.

lithectasy (lĭth-ĕk'tă-sĭ) ["+ *ektasis*, dilatation]. Removal of a stone from bladder through the dilated urethra.

lithemia (lĭth-ē'mĭ-ă) ["+ *haima*, blood]. Excess of lithic or uric acid in the blood due to imperfect metabolism of the nitrogenous substances.

lithiasis (lĭth-ī'ă-sĭs) ["+ -*iasis*, process]. 1. Formation of calculi and concretions. 2. Uric acid diathesis.

   l. biliaris. Gallstones.

   l. nephritica. Stone formation in the kidneys. SYN: *nephrolithiasis.*

   l. renalis. Kidney stones.

lithicosis (lĭth'ĭ-kō'sĭs) [Gr. *lithikos*, made of stone]. Stone cutters' silicosis; pneumoconiosis.

lithium (lĭth'ĭ-ŭm) [Gr. *lithos*, stone]. SYMB: *Li.* At. wt. 6.941: at. no. 3. A metallic element.

litho-, lith- [Gr.]. Prefixes pert. to stone or calculus.

lithocenosis (lĭth"ō-sēn-ō'sĭs) [Gr. *lithos*, stone, + *kenōsis*, evacuation]. Removal of crushed fragments of calculi.

lithoclast (lĭth'ō-klăst) ["+ *klastos*, broken]. Forceps for breaking up large calculi.

lithoclasty (lĭth'ō-klăs"tĭ). The crushing of a stone into fragments that may pass through natural channels.

lithoclysma (lĭth-ō-klīz'mă) [Gr. *lithos*, stone, + *klysma*, a clyster]. Injection into urinary bladder of substances which have the ability to dissolve calculi. There are no such substances which are both effective and safe to use.

lithocystotomy (lĭth"ō-sĭs-tot'ō-mĭ) ["+ *kystis*, bladder, + *tomē*, incision]. Incision of bladder to remove calculus.

lithodialysis (lĭth"ō-dī-al'ĭ-sĭs) ["+ *dialyein*, to dissolve]. Fragmentation or solution of calculi. SYN: *litholysis.*

lithogenesis (lĭth"ō-jen'ĭ-sĭs) ["+ *gennan*, to produce]. Formation of concretions.

lithokonion (lĭth"ō-kō'nĭ-on) ["+ *konios*, dusty]. Instrument for pulverizing vesical calculi.

litholapaxy (lĭth-ol'a-păks'ĭ) [Gr. *lithos*, stone, + *lapaxis*, evacuation]. The operation of crushing a stone in the bladder followed by immediate washing out of the crushed fragments through a catheter.

lithology (lĭth-ol'ō-jĭ) ["+ *logos*, science]. The science dealing with calculi.

litholysis (lĭth-ol'ĭ-sĭs) ["+ *lysis*, dissolution]. Dissolving of calculi. SYN: *lithodialysis.*

lithometer (lĭth-om'ĭ-tĕr) ["+ *metron*, measure]. Instrument for estimating size of calculi.

lithometra (lĭth-ō-mē'tră) ["+ *mētra*, uterus]. Uterine tissue ossification.

lithomyl (lĭth'ō-mĭl) [Gr. *lithos*, stone, + *mylē*, mill]. Instrument for crushing a vesical stone. SYN: *lithokonion.*

lithonephrotomy (lĭth"ō-nē-frot'ō-mĭ) ["+ *nephros*, kidney, + *tomē*, a cutting]. Incision of kidney for removal of renal calculus.

lithontriptic (lĭth-ŏn-trip'tĭk) ["+ *tribein*, to rub]. An agent that tends to dissolve calculi. There are no drugs, medicines or chemicals which will do this without harming the patient.

lithopedion (lĭth"ō-pe'dĭ-ŏn) ["+ *paidion*, child]. A fetus which has died, remained in uterus, and become calcified.

lithophone (lĭth'ō-fōn) [Gr. *lithos*, stone, + *phōnē*, sound]. Instrument for determining by sound the presence of calculi in the bladder.

lithoscope (lĭth'ō-skōp) ["+ *skopein*, to examine]. Instrument for examining stone in bladder.

lithotome (lĭth'ō-tōm) ["+ *tomē*, incision]. Instrument for performing lithotomy.

lithotomy (lĭth-ŏt'ō-mĭ) ["+ *tomē*, incision]. Incision into bladder for removing a stone.
   NP: See that retention catheter is kept

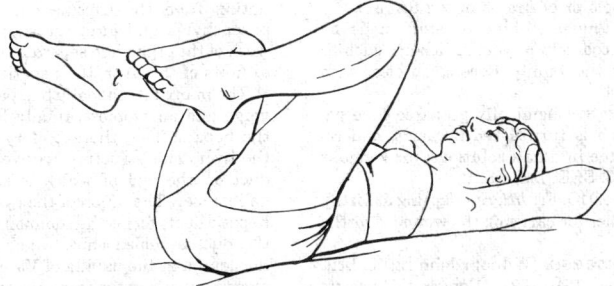

LITHOTOMY OR DORSOSACRAL POSITION

draining at all times. Record intake and output of urine. Keep dressings clean and dry.

l., bilateral. Incision across perineum.

l., high. Suprapubic incision.

l., lateral. Front of rectum to one side of raphe.

l., median. In median line in front of anus.

l. position. Upon the back with thighs flexed upon abdomen and legs upon thighs, which are abducted. SYN: *dorsosacral.*

l., rectal. Through the rectum.

l., vaginal. Through the vaginal wall.

lithotony (lĭth-ot'ō-nĭ) ["+ *teinein,* to stretch]. Removal of a calculus through small incision instrumentally dilated.

lithotresis (lĭth"ō-trē'sĭs) [Gr. *lithos,* stone, + *trēsis,* boring]. Drilling or boring of holes in a calculus to facilitate crushing.

lithotripsy (lĭth'ō-trĭp"sĭ) ["+ *tribein,* to rub]. Crushing of a calculus in bladder or urethra.

lithotriptic (lĭth-o-trĭp'tĭk). 1. An agent that dissolves calculi. There are no substances which have this capability and are harmless to the patient. 2. Pert. to lithotripsy. SYN: *lithontriptic.*

lithotrite (lĭth'o-trĭt) [Gr. *lithos,* stone, + *tribein,* to rub]. Instrument for crushing stone in the bladder. SEE: *lithotrity.*

lithotrity (lith-ot'rĭ-tĭ). Crushing of a stone to small fragments in the bladder.

lithous (lith'us) [Gr. *lithos,* stone]. Rel. to a calculus or stone. SYN: *calculous.*

lithoxiduria (lith"oks-ĭ-dū'rĭ-ă) ["+ L. *oxidum,* oxide, + Gr. *ouron,* urine]. Presence of xanthic oxide in the urine.

lithuresis (lith"u-rē'sis) ["+ *ourēsis,* urination]. Passage of calculus through the urethra during urination.

lithureteria (lĭth"ū-re-tē'rĭ-ă) ["+ *ourētēr,* ureter]. Disease of the ureter due to presence of calculi.

lithuria (lĭth-u'rĭ-ă) ["+ *ouron,* urine]. Excess of uric acid or of urates in the urine.

litmus (lĭt'mus). A blue dyestuff made by treating coarsely powdered lichens, such as those of the family Rocella species, with ammonia.

l. paper. Chemically prepared blue paper which is turned red by acids, and remains blue in alkali solutions; pH range is 4.5 to 8.5. SEE: *indicator.*

litter (lĭt'ter) [O. Fr. *litiere,* offspring at birth]. A stretcher for carrying the wounded or the sick.

Little's disease. [William John Little, Brit. physician, 1810-1894] Congenital spastic paralysis on both sides (diplegia), although it may be paraplegic or hemiplegic in form. Cerebral spastic paralysis.

ETIOL: Possible birth injury.

SYM: Child has urinary incontinence and is mentally deficient. Stiff, awkward movements, legs crossed and pressed together, arm adducted, forearm flexed, hand pronated, scissors gait.

live birth. A term used for statistical purposes indicating an infant born with signs of life such as heartbeat, respiration, or movement of voluntary muscle.

In some countries a live birth is considered not to have occurred if the infant dies in the 24 hours following delivery. Obviously, which of these two definitions is used has considerable effect on various vital statistics concerned with the viability of the fetus at time of delivery.

livedo (lĭv-ē'dō) [L. *livedo,* lividness]. Patchy or general bluish discoloration of the skin. SYN: *lividity.*

l. reticularis. Semipermanent bluish mottling of the skin of the legs and hands. Worse on exposure to cold.

liver (lĭv'ĕr) [AS. *lifer*]. Largest organ in the body, approx. 21-22.5 cm. in its greatest transverse diameter, 15-17.5 cm. in its greatest vertical height, and 10-12.5 cm. in its anterioposterior depth, weighing 1200-1600 gm., situated on right side beneath the diaphragm; occupies the right hypochondrium, epigastrium, and part of left hypochrondrium; level with bottom of sternum; undersurface, concave; covers stomach, duodenum, hepatic flexure of colon, right kidney and suprarenal capsule; secretes bile and is the site of a great many metabolic functions.

ANAT: Completely covered by a tough fibrous sheath, Glisson's capsule, which is thickest at the transverse fissure. At this point the capsule carries the blood vessels and hepatic duct which enter the organ at the hilus. Strands of connective tissue originating from the capsule enter the liver parenchyma and form the supporting network of the organ and separate the functional units of the liver, the hepatic lobules.

The many intrahepatic bile passages converge and anastomose, finally leading into the hepatic duct, the excretory channel of the liver. This structure receives the cystic duct on the end of which is situated the gallbladder. The union of the cystic and the hepatic ducts forms the common bile duct or the ductus choledochus, which enters the duodenum at the papilla of Vater. A ring of smooth muscle at the terminal portion of the choledochus, the sphincter of Oddi, permits the passage of bile into the duodenum by relaxing. Briefly stated, the bile leaving the liver enters the gallbladder where it undergoes concentration principally through loss of fluids by absorption by the gallbladder mucosa. When bile is needed in the small intestine for digestive purposes, the gallbladder contracts and the sphincter relaxes, thus permitting escape of the viscid gallbladder bile. Ordinarily, the sphincter of Oddi is contracted, shutting off the duodenal entrance and forcing the bile to enter the gallbladder after leaving the liver.

Within the sinusoids of the liver and attached to their walls are found the cells of Kupffer, which are highly phagocytic. They remove cellular detritus, bacteria, and other foreign particulate substances from the blood stream.

Has four lobes, five ligaments, five fissures, five sets of vessels, and in the fasting state secretes 500-700 ml. of bile in 24 hours. The amount of bile secreted is greatly increased during digestion.

BLOOD SUPPLY: From the hepatic artery, a branch of the celiac artery and the hepatic portal vein, which drains the intestine.

FUNCTIONS: The liver receives blood from the portal vein and thus is the first organ to receive blood from the intestines where the blood has absorbed the final products of digestion and decomposition products. From this blood the liver removes glucose from which it synthesizes glycogen which it stores. Glucose not stored as glycogen or used to form amino acids is converted to fatty acids, carbon dioxide, and water. It deaminizes amino acids with the resultant formation of ammonia which is converted into urea. Hippuric acid and uric acid are synthesized in the liver. The liver incorporates amino acids into proteins. The liver probably makes such proteins as albumin, prothrombin component, fibrinogen, transferrin, and glycoprotein. The liver is important in the biotransformation (i.e., so-called detoxification) of such substances as indole and skatole which may be absorbed into the blood from the intestine.

The liver excretes bile pigments, bilirubin and biliverdin, formed in the cells of the reticuloendothelial system in various parts of the body from hemoglobin derived from effete (exhausted and no longer functioning) red corpuscles. The liver synthesizes fibrinogen and prothrombin, blood constituents essential for clotting. It is the source of heparin, an anticoagulant. It is the source of red blood cells in the fetus and is the main

site for the production of plasma proteins. Reticuloendothelial cells (Kupffer cells), present in the linings of the sinusoids, act to filter out and destroy bacteria present in the blood stream.

The liver also performs these additional functions: It is a storage place for vitamin B_{12}, the antipernicious anemia factor, and the fat-soluble vitamins A, D, E, and K; it plays a role in the regulation of blood volume and is one of the main sources of body heat; it is important in lipid metabolism. Cholesterol, which is found in most body cells and is a major constituent of bile, is manufactured mainly in the liver.

NERVE SUPPLY: Parasympathetic fibers from the vagi and sympathetic fibers from celiac plexus via hepatic artery.

l., abscess of. ETIOL: Pathogenic bacteria, esp. pyogenic organisms such as Streptococcus, Staphylococcus, and Pneumococcus; traumatism; infection by Entamoeba histolytica.

SYM: Temperature up in evening, low in morning; sweats and chills; liver enlarged, painful, tender, may be bulging and fluctuation. Pus may be detected by aspirating needle.

PROG: Embolic (multiple) abscesses generally fatal. Traumatic abscesses, or those due to an amebic dysentery may terminate favorably after spontaneous or induced evacuation.

l., acute yellow atrophy of. A rare and grave disease, characterized anatomically by a rapid destruction of the liver tissues, and manifested by jaundice and hemorrhages, a reduction in size of liver and marked cerebral phenomena.

SYM: Malaise, slight fever, coated tongue, nausea, vomiting and jaundice. Nervous symptoms follow, as severe headache, tremor, delirium, convulsions and coma; these sometimes precede the jaundice. Urine is scanty, contains albumin, blood, and casts. Hemorrhages are common, the skin may be covered with ecchymoses, and bleeding from the mucous membranes may occur. Hepatic dullness diminished; splenic, increased. PROG: Generally fatal. TREATMENT: Constitutional and palliative.

l., amyloid. An enlargement of liver due to the deposition of an albuminoid substance.

SYM: Failure of general health with anemia. Liver is enlarged, smooth, firm, and painless. Spleen and kidneys share in the degeneration, so the spleen enlarged and urine albuminous. PROG: Unfavorable. TREATMENT: Therapy must be directed to the causal disease, usually prolonged suppuration, syphilis, tuberculosis, or chronic malaria.

l., cancer of. Male sex and heredity are predisposing factors. Malignancy in the liver as a result of spread from a primary source is many times more frequent than primary tumor of the liver. The liver is the most usual site of metastatic spread of tumors which disseminate through the blood stream.

SYM: Severe pain and tenderness; cachexia, i.e., loss of flesh and strength; pressure symptoms; jaundice common; liver enlarged, surface is nodular and the central depression or umbilications can often be detected; symptoms of the primary growth. Fever generally absent, but secondary perihepatitis or suppuration of cancerous nodules may produce it. PROG: Fatal; duration from few months to year. TREATMENT: Palliative, constitutional in first stage.

l., cirrhosis of, atrophic. A chronic disease characterized anatomically by a hyperplasia of the connective tissue and destruction of the secreting cells shown chiefly by symptoms of portal obstruction. In advanced stage, liver small, firm, gray color, and covered with numerous nodular granulations (hobnails).

SYM: Abdominal swelling due to ascites, jaundice, weakness, weight loss, anorexia, nausea, fetor hepaticus, and mild continuous fever. As obstruction becomes greater, portal blood finds new channels, and the superficial abdominal veins enlarge, notably about the umbilicus, forming the so-called caput medusae; hemorrhoids and esophageal varices result from the same cause. In the final stages hepatic encephalopathy develops. This is due in part to substances absorbed from the intestines which have not been metabolized by the liver reaching the brain and producing cerebral intoxication. Clinically the patient is mentally dulled, may have hallucinations and a peculiar type of flapping tremor. PROG: Unfavorable except in first stages.

l., cirrhosis of, hypertrophic. Cirrhosis in which the connective tissue hyperplasia starts from the periphery of the capillary bile ducts instead of from ramifications of portal vein as in atrophic form.

SYM: Marked jaundice; large, yellow liver with surface smooth or finely granular; swollen spleen. Disease may last one or two years, but abrupt termination may occur at any time in convulsions and coma. TREATMENT: Constitutional.

l., cysts of. May be simple cysts, usually small and single; hydatid cysts; or cysts associated with cystic disease of the liver, a rare condition usually associated with congenital cystic kidneys. SEE: *Echinococcus granulosus; hydatid.*

l. extract. A dry, brown powder obtained from mammalian livers which contains the hematinic factor (antianemic factor) which stimulates erythropoiesis. Was important in treatment of pernicious anemia until vitamin B_{12} was discovered. SYN: *extractum hepatis.*

l. flap. A characteristic flapping type of tremor seen in patients with severe impairment of liver function. SYN: *asterixis.*

l. fluke, human. Clonorchis sinensis common in Far East. Adults infest biliary and pancreatic ducts. Eggs pass out with feces and continue development in snails of the subfamily Buliminae (Family Hydrobiidae). Cercaria emerge and infest numerous species of freshwater fishes in which they encyst. Infestation results from eating raw fish containing encysted metacercaria.

l., hobnail. SEE: *l., cirrhosis of, atrophic.*

l., inflammation of. The usual cause of inflammation is the same as that caused by infectious hepatitis (IH) or serum hepatitis (SH) viruses. The clinical picture may be so mild as to be almost unnoticed or may be so severe that the jaundice is followed rapidly by hepatic encephalopathy and death. SYN: *hepatitis.*

TREATMENT: Treated as if the condition were going to progress to the severe form; bed rest; diet as requested by patient but should be high caloric; cortisone should not be given routinely. There is no specific treatment and in general the disease is self-limiting.

l. spots. Yellowish-brown spots on skin. SYN: *Chloasma hepaticum.*

liver, words pert. to: anhepatia; anhepatic; anticholagogue; bile; -acids; -calculi; -colic; -pigments; "bili-" words; capsule, Glisson's; cardiohepatic; choleresis; cirrhosis; facies hepatica; flexure; "glyco-" words; "hepa-" words; jaundice; perihepatitis.

liver. Used as food.

Food value of 100 gm. (beef, fried): Cal. 229; protein 26 gm.; fat 10.6 gm.; carbohydrate 5.3 gm.; calcium 11 mg.; iron 8.8 mg.; vitamin A, approx. 50,000 I.U. but may vary from 100 to 100,000; ascorbic acid 27 mg. The liver stores more vitamin A and D than other parts of the animal.

livid (lĭv'ĭd) [L. *lividus,* lead-colored]. 1. Ashen, cyanotic. 2. Discolored.

lividity (lĭv-ĭd'ĭ-tĭ). 1. Skin discoloration, as from a bruise or venous congestion. 2. State of being livid.

livor (li'vor) [L., a black-and-blue spot]. Lividity, q.v.

   l. mortis. Cutaneous dark spot on dependent portion of a cadaver.

lixiviation (lĭks'ĭv-ĭ-ā'shŭn) [L. *lixivia*, lye]. Separation of soluble from insoluble substances by washing and filtration.

LLQ. Abbr. for *left lower quadrant* (of abdomen).

L.O.A. Abbr. for *left occipitoanterior,* position of fetus.

Loa loa (lō'ä). The African eyeworm, a species of filarial worm which infests the subcutaneous tissues and conjunctiva of man. Its migration causes itching and a creeping sensation. Sometimes causes itchy edematous swellings known as "Calabar swellings." It is transmitted by flies of the genus Chrysops.

lobar (lō'bar) [Gr. *lobos*, lobe]. Pert. to a lobe.

   l. pneumonia. Inflammation of one or more lobes of the lungs. SEE: *pneumonia, acute lobar.*

lobate (lō'bāt) [L. *lobatus*, lobed]. 1. Pert. to a lobe. 2. Having a deeply undulated border. 3. Producing lobes.

lobe (lōb) [Gr. *lobos,* lobe]. A fairly well-defined part of an organ separated by boundaries.

   l., anterior, of hypophysis. Anterior portion of the hypophysis or pituitary gland, consisting of the pars distalis, and pars tuberalis.

   l., caudate. A l. on posterior surface of liver.

   l., central. Island of Reil, which forms floor of lateral cerebral fossa.

   l.'s of the cerebrum. Frontal, parietal, occipital, and temporal l.'s and the insula or island of Reil (central lobe).

   l. of the ear. Lower portion of auricle having no cartilage.

   l., flocculonodular. A l. of the cerebellum consisting of the flocculi, nodulus, and their connecting peduncles.

   l., frontal. That part of a cerebral hemisphere in front of central and sylvian fissures.

   l., insular. SEE: *central l.*

   l.'s, lateral, of the prostate. The portions on each side of the urethra.

   l.'s, lateral, of thyroid gland. The two main portions, one on each side of trachea, united below by thyroid isthmus.

   l., limbic. Marginal section of cerebral hemisphere on medial aspect. SYN: *gyrus fornicatus.*

   l. of the lungs. Large divisions of the lungs: superior and inferior l.'s of the left lung; superior, middle, and inferior l.'s of the right lung.

   l. of the mamma. The 15-20 divisions of the glandular tissue of the breast separated by connective tissue and each possessing a duct (lobar duct) opening on the nipple.

   l., occipital. Caudal region of either hemicerebrum.

   l., olfactory. A series of convolutions below horizontal portion of the intraparietal fissure of cerebrum, containing olfactory bulb. The rhinencephalon, q.v.

   l.'s, orbital. The convolutions above the orbit.

   l.'s of the pancreas. Roundish aggregations of glandular tissue separated by connective tissue.

   l., parietal. Upper and lateral portion of hemisphere of cerebrum.

   l. of the parotid, accessory. A small l., variable in size, on anterior surface of parotid gland superior to exit of parotid duct.

   l., posterior, of hypophysis. The posterior portion of the pituitary gland, consisting of the pars intermedia and the processus infundibuli (pars nervosa).

   l.'s of the prostate. The lateral l.'s and the middle l. of the gland.

   l., pyramidal, of thyroid. A portion of the thyroid gland extending upward from the isthmus. It is extremely variable in size.

   l., quadrate, of liver. An oblong elevation on lower surface of liver.

   l., spigelian. Irregular quadrangular portion of liver behind fissure for portal vein and between fissures for vena cava and ductus venosus. SYN: *caudate lobe.*

   l., temporal. The portion of cerebral hemisphere lying below lateral fissure of Sylvius. It is continuous posteriorly with the occipital lobe.

lobectomy (lō-bĕk'tō-mĭ) [Gr. *lobos,* lobe, + *ektomē,* excision]. Surgical removal of a lobe of any organ or gland.

lobotomy (lō-bot'o-mĭ). A bilateral small trephination in the plane of the coronal suture through which the white matter of the brain is sectioned, disconnecting the diencephalon, esp. the hypothalamic area, from the prefrontal cortex by section of the white fiber connecting pathways subcortically in a plane that passes adjacent to anterior tip of lateral ventricle and posterior margin of sphenoid wing. This operation is performed for relief of mental disturbances.

lob'ular [L. *lobulus,* small lobe]. Composed of small lobes; pert. to a lobule.

lobulate, lobulated (lŏb'ū-lāt, -lāt-ed). 1. Consisting of lobes or lobules. 2. Pert. to lobes or lobules. 3. Resembling lobes. SYN: *lobular.*

lobule (lŏb'ūl) [L. *lobulus,* small lobe]. A small lobe.

   l., central, of the cerebellum. A small lobe at anterior part of the superior vermiform process.

   l. of the epididymis. Conelike divisions of the head of the epididymis formed by the much coiled distal ends of the efferent ducts of the testis.

   l. of the kidney. Subdivision of a renal cortex consisting of a medullary ray and surrounding glandular tissue.

   l. of the liver. Structural unit consisting of hepatic cells arranged in irregular, branching and interconnected groups and anastomosing blood channels (sinusoids) surrounding a central vein. Polyhedral in shape with branches of portal vein, hepatic artery, and interlobular bile ducts at its periphery.

   l. of the lung. Physiological unit of the lung consisting of a respiratory bronchiole and its branches (alveolar ducts, alveolar sacs, and alveoli).

   l., paracentral. Superior convolution of ascending frontal and parietal convolutions, forming a union of both.

   l., parietal. One of two subdivisions of the parietal lobe. The superior parietal l. comprises posterior part of the upper portion; the inferior parietal l. comprises a lateral area continuous with temporal and occipital lobes.

   l. of the testis. One of the pyramidal divisions separated from each other by incomplete partitions called septulae. Each consists of one to three much coiled seminiferous tubules.

   l. of the thymus. Subdivisions of a lobe, each consisting of a cortex and medulla.

lobuli. Plural of lobulus.

lobulus (lŏb'ū-lŭs) [L.]. (pl. *lobuli*) A lobule.

   l. centralis vermis superior. A small lobe at anterior part of superior vermiform process.

   l. epididymidis. Segments into which the epididymis is divided by transverse septa from its tunica albuginea.

   l. parietalis. One of two portions of the parietal lobe.

   l. testiculi. Approx. 250 pyramidal compartments which make up glandular structure of the testicle.

lobus (lŏb'ŭs) [L.]. [NA] Lobe.

   l. cerebelli anteriores. The lobes forming anterior and superior portion of hemisphere of the cerebellum.

   l. pulmonales. Lobes of the lung.

   l. reniculi. Lobes in fetal kidney, later forming malpighian pyramids.

local (lō'kăl) [L. *locus,* place]. Limited to one place or part.

localization (lō-kăl-ĭ-zā'shun). 1. Limitation to a definite area. 2. Determination of the seat of an infection. 3. Relation of a sensation to its point of origin.

   l., cerebral. Determination of centers of various faculties and functions in particular parts of the brain.

localized (lō'kăl-īzd). Restricted to a limited region.

localizer. Apparatus used for locating solid opaque bodies in the eye by roentgenographic examination.

lochia (lō'kǐ-ā) [Gr. *lochia,* pert. to childbirth]. The discharge from the uterus of blood, mucus, and tissue during the puerperal period.

   The first six days it is distinctly blood-tinged and is known as lochia rubra or cruenta; the following three or four days the discharge becomes brownish and is known as lochia serosa; after this it becomes yellowish, turning to white and is known as lochia alba.

   It is diminished or suppressed in high fever. If offensive it is result of contamination with saprophytic organisms. Position should favor drainage.

lochial (lo'kǐ-al). Pert. to the lochia.

lochiocolpos (lō"kǐ-ō-kŏl'pŏs) [Gr. *lochia,* pert. to childbirth, + *kolpos,* vagina]. Retention of lochia in the vagina.

lochiometra (lō"kǐ-ō-mē'trā) ["+ *metra,* uterus]. Retention of lochia in the uterus.

lochiometritis (lō"kǐ-ō-mē-trī'tis) ["+ "+ *itis,* inflammation]. Puerperal inflammation of the uterus.

lochiopyra (lō"kǐ-op'ǐr-ā) ["+ *pyr,* fever]. Puerperal fever.

lochiorrhagia (lo"kǐ-or-rā'jǐ-ā) ["+ *rhēgnynai,* to break forth]. Excessive flow of lochia.

lochiorrhea (lō"kǐ-or-rē'ā) [Gr. *lochia,* pert. to childbirth, + *rhoia,* flow]. Abnormal flow of lochia.

lochioschesis (lō"kǐ-os'kǐ-sǐs) ["+ *schesis,* retention]. Retention or suppression of the lochia.

lochometritis (lō"kō-mǐ-trī'tǐs) [Gr. *lochos,* childbirth, + *metra,* uterus, + *itis,* inflammation]. Puerperal inflammation of uterus.

lock'jaw. Tonic spasm of muscles of jaw. SEE: *tetanus.*

locomotion (lō″kō-mō′shun) [L. *locus*, place, + *movere*, to move]. Movement or power of movement from one place to another

locomotor (lō″kō-mō′tor). Pert. to locomotion.

   l. ataxia. A sclerosis affecting the posterior columns of the spinal cord. SYN: *tabes dorsalis.* SEE: *ataxia; Charcot's arthropathy.*

locular (lŏk′ū-lăr) [L. *loculus*, a small space]. Divided into small cavities.

loculated (lŏk′ū-lāt-ĕd). Containing or divided into loculi. SYN: *locular.*

loculi (lŏk′ū-lī). Pl. of loculus, q.v.

loc′ulus [L.]. (pl. *loculi*) A small space or cavity.

lo′cum ten′ens [L. *locus*, place, + *tenere*, to hold]. A substitute. Physician who substitutes for another temporarily.

lo′cus [L. *locus*, a place]. 1. A spot or place. 2. In genetics the position of a gene on a chromosome.

   l. ceruleus. [NA] A dark-colored depression in floor of 4th ventricle at its upper part. SYN: *l. cinereus; l. ferrugineus.*

   l. niger. Gray matter separating the crusta and tegmentum of the crura cerebri. SYN: *substantia nigra.*

Loeffler's bacillus (lĕf′lĕr). [Friedrich A. J. Loeffler, Ger. bacteriologist, 1852-1915] The bacillus of diphtheria, Corynebacterium diphtheriae. SYN: *Klebs-Loeffler bacillus.*

logadectomy (lŏg″ă-dĕk′tō-mĭ) [Gr. *logades*, the whites of the eyes.]. Excision of a portion of the conjunctiva.

logaditis (lŏg″ă-dī′tĭs) [″+ *-itis*, inflammation]. Inflammation of the sclerotic coat of the eye. SYN: *scleritis.*

logagnosia (lŏg″ăg-nō′sĭ-ă) [Gr. *logos*, word, + *a-*, not, + *gnosis*, knowledge]. Word blindness. SEE: *aphasia.*

logagraphia (lŏg-ă-grăf′ĭ-ă) [″+ ″+ *graphein*, to write]. Loss of ability to express ideas in writing. SYN: *agraphia.*

logamnesia (lŏg-ăm-nē′zĭ-ă) [″+ *amnesia*, forgetfulness]. Aphasia of a sensory character. Inability to recognize spoken or written words.

logaphasia. SEE: *aphasia, motor.*

logoklony (lŏg′ō-klŏn-ĭ) [Gr. *logos*, word, + *klonein*, to agitate]. Intermittent repetition of the last syllable of a word.

logokophosis (lŏg″ō-kō-fō′sĭs) [″+ *kophosis*, deafness]. Inability to understand spoken language; word deafness.

logomania (lŏg-ō-mā′nĭ-ă) [″+ *mania*, madness]. Repetitious, continuous, and excessive flow of speech seen in monomania.

logoneurosis (lŏg″ō-nū-rō′sĭs) [Gr, *logos*, word, + *neuron*, nerve, + *-osis*, condition]. Any neurosis marked by speech disorders.

logopathia (lŏg-ō-păth′ĭ-ă) [″+ *pathos*, disorder]. Any disorder of speech.

logopedia (lŏg″ō-pē′dĭ-ă) [″+ *pais, paid-*, child]. Science dealing with speech defects and their correction. SYN: *logopedics.*

logoplegia (lŏg-ō-plē′jĭ-ă) [Gr. *logos*, word, + *plēgē*, stroke]. Paralysis of the speech organs.

logorrhea (lŏg′o-rē′ă) [″+ *rhoia*, flow]. Unusual loquacity seen in insanity. SYN: *garrulousness; logomania.*

logospasm (lŏg′ō-spăzm) [″+ *spasmos*, spasm]. Spasmodic word enunciation.

-logy [Gr. *logos*, word]. Suffix meaning discourse, science or study of.

loiasis (lō-ī′ă-sĭs). Infestation with Loa loa, q.v.

loimic (loy′mĭk) [Gr. *loimos*, plague]. Pert. to pestilence or plague.

loin (loyn) [O.Fr. *loigne*, long part]. Lower part of back and sides between the ribs and pelvis. SYN: *lumbus* [NA] .

lo′lism. Poisoning by the seeds of Lolium temulentum, darnel ryegrass.

long- [L. *longus*]. Prefix meaning long.

long-acting thyroid stimulator. A serum globulin which causes hyperfunction of the thyroid. Probably there are other similar substances involved in affecting the thyroid gland in thyrotoxicosis.

longevity (lŏn-jĕv′ĭ-tĭ) [L. *longaevus*, aged]. Long duration of life. Age was reckoned by the Romans in six stages: *pueritia*, childhood, to 5 years; *adolescentia*, youth, to 18 years; *juventus*, young man, to 25 years; *majores*, man, to 50 years; *senectus*, old man, to 60 years; *crepita aetas*, decrepit, 60 years to death.

longing. A persistent desire or craving for something, usually that which is remote or unattainable.

longitudinal (lŏn″jĭ-tū′dĭ-năl) [L. *longitudo*, length]. Parallel to the long axis of the body or part.

longsight′edness. Farsightedness. SYN: *hyperopia,* q.v.

loop [ME. *loupe*]. A curve or bend in a cord or cordlike structure, forming roughly an oval.

L.O.P. Abbr. for *left occipitoposterior*, position of fetus.

lophotrichea (lŏf-ō-trĭk′ĭ-ă) [Gr. *lophos*, tuft, + *thrix, trich-*, hair]. Microorganisms possessing flagella in tufts.

lophotrichous (lŏf-ŏt′rĭk-ŭs). Having bunches of flagella at one end.

lordoma (lōr-dō′mă) [Gr.]. Lordosis.

lordoscoliosis (lōr"dō-skō"lĭ-ō'sĭs) [Gr. *lordosis*, bending, + *skoliōsis*, curvation]. Forward curvation of the spine complicated by lateral curvature.

lordosis (lor-dō'sĭs) [Gr.]. Abnormal anterior convexity of the spine.

lotion (lō'shŭn) [L. *lotio*]. Liquid medicinal preparation for local application to, or bathing of, a part.

loupe (lūp) [Fr.]. A convex magnifying lens.

louse [AS. *lūs*]. A small wingless insect which lives as an ectoparasite on birds and mammals. Sucking lice belong to the order Anoplura; biting or chewing lice belong to the order Mallophaga.

Human lice are the primary transmitters of epidemic typhus, trench fever, and relapsing fever. They may also be the mechanical transmitters of other diseases such as plague. SYN: *pediculus*.

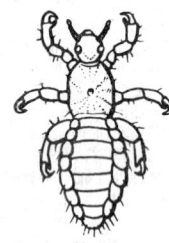

SUCKING BODY LOUSE
Enlarged view of louse .423 cm. in length.

l., body. Pediculus humanus corporis. Lives principally in or on clothing.

l., crab. Phthirus pubis. Lives principally in hair in pubic region, but also found in beard, eyebrows, and eyelashes.

l., head. Pediculus humanus capitus. Lives in hair of the head.

lous'iness. State of being infested with lice. SYN: *pediculosis*, q.v.

love [ME.]. 1. Concern and affection for another person. This may be to such a degree as to cause one individual to risk losing his life in his concern for the safety, care, and well-being of another. 2. In psychiatry, love is equated to pleasure, particularly as it applies to the gratifying experiences between persons of the opposite sex.

Loven's reflex (lō-vān'). [Otto K. Loven, Swed. physician, 1835-1904] Vasodilation with corresponding increase in size of organ resulting from stimulation of afferent nerve of organ.

Low'man bal'ance board. [Charles LeRoy Lowman, Amer. orthopedist, 1879 —] Tilted board for walking with feet inverted to restore proper muscle balance and to correct static faults.

low protein diet. Diet which contains limited amount of protein. The principal sources of food energy are fats and carbohydrates.

low salt diet. Diet in which no salt is allowed on patient's tray and no salty foods are served.

lox. Abbr. for *liquid oxygen.*

loxarthron (lŏks-ăr'thrŏn) [Gr. *loxos*, slanting, + *arthron*, joint]. Oblique deformity of a joint without dislocation.

loxia (lŏks'ĭ-ă) [Gr., slanting]. Wryneck. SYN: *torticollis*.

loxotic (lŏks-ŏt'ĭk) [Gr. *loxos*, slanting]. Distorted in an awry manner.

loxotomy (lŏks-ŏt'ō-mĭ) ["+ *tomē*, a cutting]. Amputation by oblique section.

lozenge (lŏz'ĕnj) [Fr.]. Small, dry, medicinal solid to be held in mouth until it dissolves. SYN: *troche*.

LSD. Abbr. for *lysergic acid diethylamide*, a derivative of an alkaloid in ergot. It is made from a fungus growing on wet grass and grain. LSD is used legally only for experimental purposes. Its illegal use has increased to where it is now a social and legal problem. SYN: *acid*.

LTH. Abbr. for *luteotropic hormone.*

lubb (lub). Word denoting 1st cardiac sound in auscultation. Caused by closure of the atrioventricular valves, the impact of blood rushing into the aorta and pulmonary artery and the contraction of the ventricular muscle. It is pitched low and slightly longer than the 2nd sound. SEE: *dupp; heart, auscultation of.*

lubb-dupp (lŭb-dŭp'). The two sounds heard in auscultation marking a complete cycle of the heart. Pause following the cycle is slightly longer than that between the two sounds.

lubricant (lū'brĭ-kănt) [L. *lūbricāns*]. Agent, usually a liquid oil, which reduces friction between parts which brush against each other as they move. Joints are lubricated by synovial fluid.

lub'ricating en'ema. Enema given to soften feces and lubricate anal canal after hemorrhoidectomy, or to soften fecal impaction. SEE: *enema.*

Lucas-Championnière's disease (lē-kä'-shaw"pē-ŏn-ē-air'). [J. M. M. Lucas-Championnière, Fr. surgeon, 1843-1913] Pseudomembranous bronchitis.

lucid (lū'sĭd) [L. *lucidus*, clear]. Clear, esp. applied to clarity of the mind.

l. interval. Period of normal mental functioning between attacks of mental illness.

lucidity (lū-sĭd'ĭ-tĭ). Quality of clearness or brightness, esp. with regard to mental conditions.

lucotherapy (lū''kō-thĕr'ă-pĭ) [L. *lux*, light, + Gr. *therapeia*, treatment]. Therapeutic use of light rays. SYN: *phototherapy*.

Ludwig's angi'na (lūd'vĭg). [Wilhelm F. von Ludwig, Ger. surgeon, 1790-1865] A suppurative inflammation of subcutaneous connective tissue adjacent to a submaxillary gland. SEE: *angina*.

Luer-Lok syringe (lū'ĕr-lŏk'). A glass syringe made to permit rapid and firm attachment of the needle.

lues (lū'ēz) [L., pestilence]. Any pestilential disease; the plague, esp. syphilis.

   l. venerea. Syphilis.

luetic (lū-ĕt'ĭk). 1. Pert. to syphilis. 2. Affected with syphilis. SYN: *syphilitic.*

Lugol's caustic (lū'gŏl). [Jean G. A. Lugol, Fr. physician, 1786-1851] Aqueous solution of 25% each of iodine and potassium iodide.

Lugol's solution. Iodine, 5 gm.; potassium iodide, 10 gm., and water to make 100 ml. Strong iodine solution used in iodine therapy.

   INCOMPATIBILITIES: Codeine.

lumbago (lŭm-bā'gō) [L. *lumbus*, loin]. A general nonspecific term for dull, aching pain across the loins.

lumbar (lŭm'băr) [L. *lumbus*, loin]. Pert. to the loins. SEE: *lumbago.*

   l. nerves. Five pairs, corresponding with the lumbar vertebrae.

   l. puncture. Puncture made by placing an aspiration needle into the subarachnoid space of the spinal cord. Usually done in the lumbar area at the level of the 4th intervertebral space. SYN: *spinal puncture; subarachnoid puncture.*

   PURPOSE: For the removal of spinal fluid for diagnostic or other purposes, and for the injection of an anesthetic solution. *NOTE:* May be dangerous if done in the presence of increased intracranial pressure. The brain stem may, upon decrease of pressure in the spinal canal, herniate into the foramen magnum of the base of the skull.

   Medication, dissolved in fluid previously removed, or anesthetics for cord blocking, etc., may be cautiously introduced. The part is cleansed and painted with iodine. A sterile puncture needle is then readily passed directly in the midline, to and through the dura. On removing the stylet, spinal fluid will escape and can be collected in two or three tubes for examination. Explain the procedure and reassure patient.

   NP: Patient should be turned on side near edge of bed with back to operator. Thighs flexed on trunk and head lowered to chest, back bowed as far as possible. Nurse holds patient in this position. Alternatively the patient may be in a sitting position with head, neck, and thoracic spine flexed. The legs are allowed to dangle over the side of the bed or table. The nurse stands in front of the patient to support him.

   Articles needed: Sterilized lumbar puncture needles, gloves for physician, alcohol, sterilized gauze and sponge, sterile towel, procaine hydrochloride 0.5% solution, 5 ml., two sterile test tubes. After procedure is completed, patient should remain completely flat, either prone or supine, for 24 hours.

   The use of a small-gauge needle will lessen the chance that spinal fluid will continue to seep from the spinal canal after the needle is removed, and thus the possibility of development of postspinal tap headache will be diminished. SEE: *cerebrospinal fluid; cisternal puncture; spinal puncture; Queckenstedt test.*

   l. reflex. Irritation of the skin over the erector spinal muscles causing contraction of muscles of the back.

   l. region. Each side of umbilical region above the iliac, below the hypochondriac.

   l. vertebrae. Five bones of spinal column between sacrum and thoracic vertebrae.

lumbarization (lŭm''bŭr-ĭ-zā'shŭn) [L. *lumbus*, loin]. Coalescence of the 1st sacral vertebra with the last lumbar vertebra.

lumbo- [L.]. Combining form pert. to the loins.

lumbocolostomy (lŭm''bō-kō-lŏs'tō-mĭ) [" + Gr. *kōlon*, colon, + *stoma*, opening]. Colostomy by lumbar incision.

lumbocolotomy (lŭm''bō-kō-lŏt'ō-mĭ) [" + "+ *tomē*, incision]. Incision into the colon through lumbar region.

lumbocostal (lŭm''bō-kŏs'tăl) [L. *lumbus*, loin, + *costa*, rib]. Rel. to the loins and ribs.

lumbodynia (lŭm''bō-dĭn'ĭ-ă) [" + Gr. *odynē*, pain]. Pain and rigidity in the loins. SYN: *lumbago.*

lumbosa'cral. Pert. to the lumbar vertebrae and the sacrum.

   l. plexus. Nerve plexus formed by union of lumbar, sacral, and coccygeal nerves.

lumbrical (lŭm'brĭ-kăl) [L. *lumbricus*, earthworm]. Like a worm. SYN: *vermiform.*

lumbrica'lis. One of the muscles of the hand or foot which are wormlike in shape.

lum'bus [L.]. [NA] The loin.

lumen (lū'mĕn) [L., light]. (pl. *lu'mina*) 1. The space within an artery, vein, intestine, or tube. 2. Unit of light, the amt. of light emitted in a unit solid angle by a uniform point source of one international candle.

luminal (lū'mĭ-năl). Rel. to lumen of tubular structure, such as a blood vessel.

lunacy (lū'nă-sĭ.) [L. *luna,* moon]. Obsolete term for insanity. Insanity was formerly thought to be affected by the moon.

lu'nar. Pert. to the moon, a month, or silver.
   l. caustic. Silver nitrate.

lu'nate. A bone in the proximal row of the carpus. SYN: *semilunar bone.*

lunatic (lū'nă-tĭk) [L. *luna,* moon]. Obsolete term for an insane person. SEE: *lunacy.*

lunet, lunette (lū-nĕt') [Fr. *lunette,* crescent]. A concavo-convex lens for spectacles.

lung (lŭng) [AS. *lungen*]. One of two cone-shaped, spongy organs of respiration contained within the pleural cavity of the thorax.

ANAT: Connected with the pharynx through the trachea and larynx. The base rests on diaphragm and apex rises from 2.5 to 5 cm. above the sternal end of the first rib, the collarbone, supported by its attachment to the hilum or root structures.

Right lung has three lobes, left one has two. Approx. weight in the adult male: right lung 625 gm., left 570 gm. The lungs contain 300,000,000 alveoli and the respiratory surface is between 70 and 80 square meters. Averages 18 respirations per minute in adult. The total capacity of the lung varies from 3.6 to 9.4 liters in the male and 2.5 to 6.9 in normal females.

The left lung has an indentation for the normal place of the heart, which is called the cardiac depression. Behind this is the hilum through which the blood vessels lymphatics, and bronchi enter and leave the lung.

Air travels from the mouth and nasa passage to the pharynx and the trachea. Two main bronchi, one on each side, extend from the trachea. The main bronchi divide into smaller bronchi, one for each of five lobes These further divide into a great number of smaller bronchioles. The pattern distribution of these into the segments of each lobe is important in lung surgery. There are 10 bronchopulmonary segments in the right lung and eight in the left, but the number is variable. There are 50-80 terminal bronchioles in each lobe. Each of these divide into two respiratory bronchioles which in turn divide to form 2-11 alveolar ducts. The alveolar sacs and alveoli arise from these ducts. The spaces between the alveolar sacs and alveoli are called atria.

The alveolus is the point at which the blood and inspired air are separated only by a very thin wall or membrane which allows O_2 and nitrogen to diffuse into the blood and CO_2 and other gases to pass from the blood into the alveoli. This wall is so thin (0.07 to 2.0 microns) that it is best seen by using an electron microscope. The alveoli contain small pores, 7-10 microns in diameter, which serve to connect adjacent alveoli to each other. Their exact function is unknown.

NERVE SUPPLY: Parasympathetic fibers via vagus nerve and sympathetic fibers from anterior and posterior pulmonary plexuses.

BLOOD VESSELS: Bronchial, pulmonary arteries, and pulmonary veins. Blood passing through lungs gives off carbon dioxide and receives oxygen. The lungs include the lobes, lobules, bronchi, bronchioles, infundibula, and alveoli or air cells.

FUNCTION: The primary purpose of the lung is to bring air and blood into intimate contact so that oxygen can be added to the blood and carbon dioxide can be removed. This is achieved by two pumping systems, one moving a gas and the other a liquid. The blood and air are brought together so closely that only 1.5 micron of tissue separate them. The volume of the pulmonary capillary circulation is 150 ml. but this is spread out over a surface area of approx. 750 sq. feet (69.68 sq. meters). This capillary surface area surrounds 300 million air sacs called alveoli. The blood which is poor in oxygen but high in CO_2 is in contact with the air which is high in oxygen and low in CO_2 for less than one second.

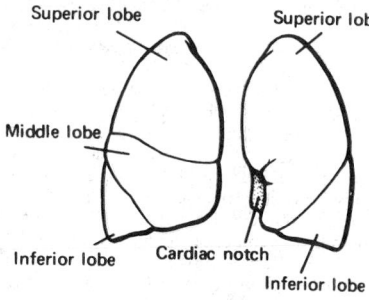

Superior lobe   Superior lobe

Middle lobe

Inferior lobe   Cardiac notch

Inferior lobe

LUNGS—ANTERIOR VIEW

l. abscess. Circumscribed suppuration of lung. SYM: High and irregular fever, rigors, sweats, and pallor. Dyspnea, cough, and purulent expectoration. May be bubbling rales and later cavernous breathing and pectoriloquy.

PROG: Fair, except in embolic abscesses. TREATMENT: Nutritious food. Remedies called for by general condition. Abscess should be opened and drained.

l. cancer. That which may appear in trachea, air sacs, and other lung tubes. It may appear as an ulcer in the windpipe, as a nodule or small flattened lump, or on the surface blocking air tubes. It may invade surface of tubes extending to lymphatics into blood vessels.

l., collapse of. Condition resulting from a lowering of intrapulmonic pressure or an increase in intrathoracic pressure. It may be focal, involving only a few lobules, or massive, in which an entire lobe or the complete lung is involved. It may result from obstruction of the bronchial tubes (obstructive atelectasis) or pressure upon the lung by air or fluid in the pleural cavity, an intrathoracic tumor, or a greatly enlarged heart (compressive atelectasis). Air may be introduced artificially into the pleural cavity (artificial pneumothorax) or it may be derived from emphysematous lesions. Collapse may occur in the newborn as a result of blockage of bronchioles by mucus or from failure of the lung to distend because of weak inspiratory movements. SYN: *atelectasis.*

SYM: In a sudden collapse, there are pronounced dyspnea and circulatory collapse. When collapse occurs gradually, symptoms are less pronounced or may not occur at all. PROG: Depends upon extent of collapse and gravity of preexisting disease. TREATMENT: In the newborn, aspirate the excess mucus from the bronchus and gently inflate lung with a catheter. In acquired varieties, direct remedies to the original disease. SEE: *auscultation; chest; emphysema; tuberculosis.*

l. collapse, hypostatic. Congestion of dependent portions of the lungs occurring in asthenic diseases which necessitate a protracted recumbent position.

SYM: Dyspnea, cough, scanty expectoration. Slight dullness, subcrepitant rales, and feeble bronchial breathing. TREATMENT: Development of congestion should be prevented by frequent change in position and timely use of cardiac stimulants.

l. collapse, passive. Results from obstruction to the flow of blood from the lungs to the heart. SYM: Dyspnea, hard cough, mucous expectoration containing pigmented cells and rales. Slight dullness, feeble breathing.

l.'s, compliance of. A measure of the distensibility of the lungs. It is expressed as the change in volume of the lungs in liters when the transpulmonary pressure is changed by 1 cm. of water pressure. Normally it is between 0.08 and 0.33 liters/cm. H_2O. It is reduced by anything which obstructs the normal flow of air in and out of the lung, whether due to changes in the airway or the mechanical forces which move the ribs and diaphragm.

l., edema of. Effusion of serous fluid into air vesicles and into interstitial tissue of lungs. SYN: *pulmonary edema.*

SYM: Extreme dyspnea; rapid, labored breathing; cough with frothy bloodstained expectoration; cyanosis; cold extremities. PROG: Grave. Often a final symptom of some pulmonary disease.

TREATMENT: Directed toward altering the condition which caused the difficulty. Usually this includes vigorous treatment of the heart condition, oxygen, and morphine; in extreme cases phlebotomy may be required. But prior to this, tourniquets are applied to the limbs in an attempt to have the excess tissue fluid collect in the extremities rather than the lungs. *NOTE:* Tourniquets should be applied to only one limb at a time for 15 minutes and with pressure sufficient to block venous return but not enough to interfere with arterial blood flow to the limb.

l. fluke. Paragonimus westermani, q.v.

l., hemorrhage from. Hemoptysis, q.v.

l. inflammation. Pneumonia, q.v.

l., iron. Device for inducing respiration artificially.

Patient is placed in airtight compartment except for his head and neck, and then atmospheric pressure inside is raised and lowered by a pulmotor. SEE: *Drinker respirator.*

l. motor. An apparatus designed for forcing air or a mixture of air and oxygen into the lungs.

l. surfactant. A substance in the lung which acts to regulate the amount of surface tension of the fluid lining the alveoli.

lung, words pert. to: air; air vesicle; alveobronchitis; alveolar; alveolus; alveolus pulmoneus; anthracosis; anthrax; artificial pneumothorax; asbestosis; atelectasis; atrium of lungs; auscultation; "bronch-" words; byssinosis; cardiopulmonary; chest; emphysema; hilum; pectoriloquy; "pleur-" words; "pneum-" words; pulmonary; rales; siderosis; silicosis; tuberculosis; vesicular resonance.

lunula (lū'nū-lă) [L., little moon]. (pl. *lunulae*) [NA] The semilunar white arch or area near the root of the nail.

lunula of valves of heart. One of two narrow portions on the free edges of the semilunar valves on each side of the nodulus. SYN: *l. valvulae semilunaris.*

lupiform (lū′pĭ-form) [L. *lupus,* wolf, + *forma,* shape]. Resembling lupus.

lupous (lū′pŭs) [L. *lupus,* wolf]. 1. Pert. to lupus. 2. Affected with lupus.

lupus (lū′pŭs) [L., wolf]. Originally any chronic, progressive, usually ulcerating, skin disease. In current usage when the word is used alone, it has no precise meaning. SEE: *l. vulgaris.*

  l., disseminated follicular. L. of face with small and large papules.

  l. erythematosis, discoid. A benign dermatitis characterized by reddish, well-defined, scaly patches which heal and leave atrophic scars. Sensitivity to sunlight is usually present. TREATMENT: Antimalarials such as chloraquine are quite effective.

  l. erythematosus. A chronic and usually fatal systemic disease characterized by pathological changes in the vascular system, esp. the collagen which serves as a binding substance for capillaries and small blood vessels. A skin rash is usually present, the erythema spreading across bridge of nose and face in a butterfly pattern. Marked constitutional symptoms including fever, arthritis, and signs of renal and lung and heart involvement are usually present to varying degree. Etiology is unknown. Incidence highest in females between puperty and menopause. Corticosteroid therapy often helpful.

  l. pernio. Sarcoidosis; Boeck's sarcoid.

  l. vorax. A form of l. vulgaris in which the mucous membranes are invaded and cartilage is destroyed.

  l. vulgaris. Tuberculosis of the skin. Characterized by patches which break down and ulcerate, leaving scars on healing.

LUQ. Abbr. for *left upper quadrant* of abdomen.

Lust's reflex (lŭst). Dorsal flexion and abduction of foot resulting from percussion of external branch of sciatic nerve.

lu′teal [L. *luteus,* yellow]. Pert. to the corpus luteum, its cells, or its hormone.

  l. hormone. Progesterone, q.v. Secreted by the corpus luteum. SEE: *endocrine; hormone; ovary; corpus luteum; estrogen.*

lutein (lū′tē-ĭn). Yellow pigment derived from corpus luteum, egg yolk, and fat cells or lipochromes.

  l. cells. Ovarian cells which contain a yellow pigment and are involved in the formation of the corpus luteum. They are of two types: granulosa lutein cells of follicular origin and theca lutein cells from the theca interna.

luteinization (lū″tē-ĭn-ĭ-zā′shŭn). Process of development of the corpus within a ruptured graafian follicle.

luteinizing hormone. Hormone secreted by anterior lobe of the hypophysis which stimulates development of the corpus luteum. ABBR: LH. SYN: *interstitial-cell stimulating hormone (ICSH).*

luteinizing hormone—releasing hormone/follicle-stimulating hormone—releasing hormone. A hormone which is produced in the hypothalamus and controls the release and synthesis of the two pituitary hormones, the luteinizing and follicle-stimulating hormones.

luteoma (lū-tē-ō′mă) [L. *luteus,* yellow, + Gr. *-ōma,* tumor]. An ovarian tumor containing lutein cells.

luteotropin hormone. Prolactin, q.v.

lutetium (lū-tē′shĭ-ŭm). SYMB: *Lu.* At. wt. 174.97; at. no. 71. A rare element.

luteum (lū′tē-ŭm) [L.]. Yellow.

  l., corpus. Yellow cellular mass which forms after the graafian follicle has erupted. It persists and enlarges if pregnancy occurs.

lutin (lū′tĭn). Hormone of corpus luteum which aids in preparation of endometrium for fertilized ovum. SYN: *progesterone.*

lux (lŭks) [L. light]. A unit of light intensity equivalent to one lumen per square meter.

luxation (lŭks-ā′shŭn) [L. *luxatio,* dislocation]. Displacement of organs or articular surfaces; dislocation of a joint.

luxus (lŭks′ŭs) [L.]. Excess of anything.

Luys′ body (lū-ē′). [Jules B. Luys, Fr. physician, 1828-98] Small mass of gray matter lying on dorsal surface of peduncle dorsolateral to substantia nigra. Luys' nucleus located in the posterior portion of the thalamus. SYN: *centromedian nucleus.*

lycanthropy (lī-kăn′thrō-pī) [Gr. *lykos,* wolf, + *anthrōpos,* man]. Mania in which patient believes himself a wild beast, esp. a wolf. SYN: *lycomania.*

lycomania (lī″kō-mā′nĭ-ă) [″+ *mania,* madness]. Delusion of being a wild animal, esp. a wolf. SYN: *lycanthropy.*

lycoperdonosis (lī″kō-pĕr″dŏn-ō′sĭs) [″+ *perdesthai,* to break wind, + *-ōsis,* condition]. Respiratory disease caused by inhaling large quantities of spores from the mature mushroom commonly called puffball. Lycoperdon is the genus of fungi to which most puffballs belong.

lycopodium (lī-kō-pō′dĭ-ŭm). A yellow powder formed from spores of Lycopodium clavatum, a club moss. Used as a dusting powder, and as a dessicant and absorbent.

lye (lī) [AS. *lēag*]. 1. Liquid from leaching of wood ashes. 2. Any strong alkaline solution, esp. sodium or potassium hydroxide. SEE: *alkalies; NaOH.*

ly'ing-in. 1. The puerperal state. 2. Being in confinement.

lymph (līmf) [L. *lympha*]. The lymph is a body alkaline fluid found in the lymphatic vessels and the cisterna chyli.

Lymph is usually a clear, transparent, colorless fluid; however, in vessels draining the intestines it may appear milky owing to presence of absorbed fats. It differs from blood in that red blood corpuscles are absent and its protein content is lower. Osmotic pressure and alkaline reserve are slightly higher than in blood plasma; viscosity, slightly less. Sp. gr. 1.016-1.023.

Lymph may vary considerably in composition in different parts of the body. In peripheral vessels it is similar to blood plasma except that the protein content is usually much lower. Lymph contains proteins (serum albumin, serum globulin, serum fibrinogen), salts, organic substances (urea, creatinine, neutral fats, glucose), and water. Cells present are principally lymphocytes, formed in lymph nodes and other lymphatic organs. Lymph from the intestine (called chyle) contains fats and other substances absorbed from the intestine.

The lymph is formed in tissue spaces all over the body and is gathered into small vessels which carry it centrally. All lymph eventually enters into either the thoracic duct or right lymph duct, each terminating at the junction of the internal jugular and subclavian veins where the lymph reenters the blood stream. The thoracic duct commences in the abdomen as a dilated sac, the cisterna (receptaculum) chyli, which receives lymph vessels from the lower limbs and pelvis and from the intestines and digestive organs. It continues upward through the thorax receiving intercostal vessels and near its termination it receives the left subclavian trunk, draining left upper extremity, and the left jugular trunk, draining left side of head and neck. The right lymph duct drains the right sides of the thorax, head, and neck.

Lymph, in passing from any region of the body to the main lymph ducts, must pass through lymph vessels which pass through regional lymph nodes. These filter the lymph, freeing it of foreign particulate matter, esp. bacteria.

The absorption of fatty matter chiefly takes place through the epithelial cells of the intestines, and those of the villi. These cells carry it to the lacteals when the particles break up into fat and protein matter.

Absorption is most active in the alimentary canal, the digested material passing into the blood stream through the vessels of the portal circulation and into the lacteals.

l., animal. Lymph from an animal.

l. cell or corpuscle. A lymphocyte.

l. channel. Lymph sinus, q.v.

l. follicle. Old term for lymph node, q.v.

l., inflammatory. Exudate due to inflammation.

l., intercellular. Tissue fluid.

l. node. A lymph node is a rounded body consisting of accumulations of lymphatic tissue found at intervals in the course of lymphatic vessels. Lymph nodes vary in size from a pinhead to an olive; may occur singly or in groups. One side bears an indentation, the hilum, from which blood vessels enter and leave and efferent vessels leave. Afferent vessels enter on side opposite from hilum.

The node is enclosed in a capsule, from which trabeculae project inwardly, dividing node into compartments called ampullae or alveoli. Outer compact region comprises the cortex; the inner diffuse portion, the medulla. The cortex is tightly packed with lymph nodules, which are separated from capsule by the cortical sinus. The lymphatic tissue of the medulla is arranged in the form of medullary cords. Irregular tortuous spaces, called lymph sinuses, are present throughout the node. The nodes are aggregated in regions, the principal ones of which are in the neck (cervical), in the armpit (axillary), in the groin (inguinal). Lymph nodes as well as vessels are divided into superficial and deep groups. Among the deep groups are those draining lymph from the visceral organs of the thorax and abdomen.

FUNCTIONS: Lymph nodes produce lymphocytes and monocytes. They act as filters keeping particulate matter, esp. bacteria, from gaining entrance to the blood stream. They may stop cancer cells, but in turn may be the seat of cancer.

l. nodule. A small, compact, densely staining mass of cells each containing a lighter staining central area in which lymphocytes are formed. They comprise the structural unit of lymphatic tissue. May occur singly, in groups as in Peyer's patches, or in encapsulated organs as lymph nodes.

l. scrotum. Scrotal lymphatic dilatation occurring esp. in elephantiasis.

l. sinus. One of several irregular tortuous vessels found in lymphatic organs. Lined with cells belonging to the reticuloendothelial system.

l. spaces. Those esp. in connective tissue filled with lymph.

lymphadenectasis (lĭm-făd″ē-nĕk′tă-sĭs) [L. *lympha*, lymph, + Gr. *adēn*, gland, + *ektasis*, dilatation]. Dilatation or distention of a lymph node.

lymphade′nia. Hyperplasia affecting lymphatic tissue.

l. ossea. Bone marrow hyperplasia accompanied by Bence-Jones protein in urine.

SYM: Neuralgic pains followed by painful swellings on ribs and skull and possible occurrence of spontaneous fractures. SYN: *multiple myeloma.*

lymphadenitis (lĭm-făd″ĕn-i′tĭs) [L. *lympha*, lymph, + Gr. *adēn*, gland, + *-itis*, inflammation]. Inflammation of a lymphatic gland.

ETIOL: Drainage of bacteria or toxic substances into lymph nodes. May be specific, as by the organisms of typhoid, syphilis, or tuberculosis, or nonspecific, in which causative organism is not identified.

SYM: Marked increase of tissue; possible suppuration. Swelling, pain, tenderness. Usually accompanies lymphangitis.

TREATMENT: Hot, moist dressings; incision and drainage if abscesses occur. Antibiotics as indicated.

l., tuberculous. ETIOL: Myobacterium tuberculosis.

SYM: Possible loss of weight and strength; gradual onset and enlargement of lymph nodes; may become adherent, necrotic, and discharge pus through skin. TREATMENT: Antituberculosis drugs.

lymphadenoma (lĭm-făd″e-nō′mă) [″ + ″ + *-ōma*, tumor]. Hyperplasia of the lymph nodes. SYN: *lymphoma.*

lymphadenopathy (lĭm-făd″e-nŏp′ă-thĭ) [″ + ″ + *pathos*, disease]. Disease of the lymph nodes.

lymphagogue (lĭmf′ă-gŏg) [L. *lympha*, lymph, + Gr. *agōgos*, leading]. An agent that stimulates the production or flow of lymph.

lymphangiectasis (lĭm-făn″jĭ-ĕk′tă-sĭs) [″ + Gr. *angeion*, vessel, + *ektasis*, dilatation]. Dilatation of lymphatic vessels. SYN: *lymphectasia.*

lymphangioendothelioma (lĭm-făn″jĭ-ō-en″dō-thē-lĭ-ō′mă) [″ + ″ + *endon*, within, + *thēlē*, nipple, + *-ōma*, tumor]. Endothelioma originating from lymph vessels. SYN: *lymphendothelioma.*

lymphangiofibroma (lĭm-făn″jĭ-ō-fĭ-brō′-mă) [L. *lympha*, lymph, + Gr. *angeion*, vessel, + L. *fiber*, fiber, + Gr. *-ōma*, tumor]. Fibroma and lymphangioma combined.

lymphangioma (lĭm-făn″jĭ-ō′mă) [″ + ″ + *-ōma*, tumor]. Tumor composed of lymphatic vessels.

lymphangiophlebitis (lĭm-făn″jĭ-ō-flē-bī′-tĭs) [″ + ″ + *phleps*, vein, + *-itis*, inflammation]. Inflammation of lymphatic vessels and veins.

lymphangioplasty (lĭm-făn′jĭ-ō-plăs″tĭ) [L. *lympha*, lymph, + Gr. *angeion*, vessel, + *plassein*, to form]. Formation of artificial lymphatics.

lymphangiosarcoma (lĭm-făn″jĭ-ō-săr-kō′mă) [″ + ″ + *sarx*, flesh, + *-ōma*, tumor]. Lymphangioma and sarcoma combined.

lymphangiotomy (lĭm-făn″jĭ-ŏt′ō-mĭ) [″ + ″ + *tomē*, a cutting]. 1. Dissection of the lymphatics. 2. Anatomy of the lymphatics. SYN: *lymphotomy.*

lymphangitis (lĭm″fan-jĭ′tĭs) [L. *lympha*, lymph, + Gr. *angeion*, vessel, + *-itis*, inflammation]. Inflammation of lymphatic channels or vessels.

ETIOL: May be due to a variety of organisms but is frequently due to streptococci.

SYM: Onset chill and high fever, moderate swelling and pain. Deep general flush with raised border on affected area if infection is in deep layers of skin. The red inflamed area is commonly called blood poisoning by lay persons.

NP: Applications of either moist or dry heat may be ordered. Force fluids. Elevate part. Administration of appropriate antibiotics may be required.

lymphatic (lĭm-făt′ĭk) [L. *lymphaticus*]. 1. Of or pert. to lymph. 2. A lymph vessel.

ANAT: A lymph vessel conveys toward the heart; contains valves like the veins. The intestinal parts of the lymphatics which take up some of the products of digestion are called lacteals.

After the chyle enters the lacteals it is known as lymph. The lymphatics, or lacteals, carry the food material in the form of lymph, which has not hitherto been taken directly into the blood vessels of the alimentary canal, into the blood stream.

Fluids exuded from the blood vessels into the tissues are gathered up and carried back again to the blood by the lymphatics, so that they serve two purposes. They appear like small veins with thin walls, and they are provided with valves. They commence as lymph capillaries, microscopic in size, and empty into two trunks which open into the large veins near the heart.

Unlike the blood, the fluid contained in the lymphatics flows only in one direction from the small capillaries to the main trunk (the thoracic duct and a smaller duct on the right side) and then to the large veins. When the lymph enters the blood it becomes part of its constituents.

PRINCIPAL GROUPS: Right internal jugular vein; right subclavian vein; lymphatics of upper extremities; receptaculum chyli; lymphatics of lower extremities; thoracic duct; right subclavian vein; lacteals; lymphatics of lower extremities.

RS: angiolymphitis; angiolymphoma; bubo; chylangioma; leukosis; varix; "vas-" words.

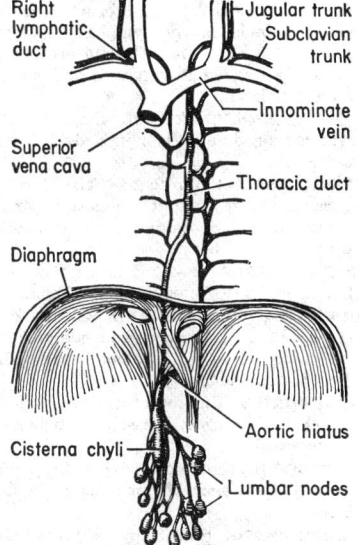

LYMPHATIC DRAINAGE

Labels: Right lymphatic duct; Jugular trunk; Subclavian trunk; Innominate vein; Superior vena cava; Thoracic duct; Diaphragm; Cisterna chyli; Aortic hiatus; Lumbar nodes

l., afferent. Any of the small vessels carrying lymph to a lymph node.

l. blockade. Local defense mechanism in which minute bits of material, such as fibrinous exudate from injured tissue, enter local lymphatic vessels, tending to obstruct them and thus prevent foreign substances, esp. bacteria, from passing to other parts of the body.

l. capillary. The smallest lymph vessels. Minute tubes consisting of a single layer of endothelium ending blindly in swollen or rounded ends. Tissue fluid enters the lymphatic system through the lymph capillaries. In intestinal villi they are called lacteals.

l., efferent. Any of the small vessels carrying lymph from a lymph node.

l. organ. A structure composed principally of lymphatic tissue. Includes lymph nodes, spleen, tonsil, thymus.

l. system. That system including all structures involved in the conveyance of lymph from the tissues to the blood stream. It includes the lymph capillaries, lacteals, lymph nodes, lymph vessels, main lymph ducts (thoracic and right lymphatic duct). SEE: *lymph.*

l. vessels. Thin-walled vessels conveying lymph from the tissues. They resemble veins in structure, possessing three layers: the intima, media, and adventitia. They possess paired valves.

lymphaticostomy (lĭm-făt″ĭ-kŏs′tō-mĭ) [L. *lympha,* lymph, + Gr. *stoma,* opening]. Making of a permanent aperture into a lymphatic duct.

lymphatitis (lĭm″fă-tī′tĭs) ["+ Gr. *-itis,* inflammation]. Inflammation of lymphatic vessel or tissue. SYN: *lymphangitis.*

lymphatolysis (lĭm″fă-tŏl′ĭ-sĭs) ["+ Gr. *lysis,* dissolution]. Destruction of lymphatic vessels or tissue.

lymphatolytic (lĭm″făt-ō-lĭt′ĭk). Destructive to lymphatics.

lymphectasia (lĭmf-ĕk-tā′zĭ-ă) [L. *lympha,* lymph, + Gr. *ektasis,* dilatation]. Dilatation of the lymphatics. SYN: *lymphangiectasis.*

lymphedema (lĭmf-ĕ-dē′mă) ["+ Gr. *oidēma,* swelling]. Edema due to obstruction of lymphatics. SEE: *phlegmasia alba dolens.*

lymphemia (lĭmf-ē′mĭ-ă) ["+ Gr. *haima,* blood]. Presence of an abnormal number of lymphocytes in the blood.

lymphendothelioma (lĭmf-ĕn″dō-thē-lĭ-ō′mă) ["+ Gr. *endon,* within, + *thēlē,* nipple, + *ōma,* tumor]. Tumor from proliferation and dilatation of lymphatics with overgrowth of myxomatous tissue.

lymphenteritis (lĭmf′ĕn-tĕr-ī′tĭs) [L. *lympha,* lymph, + Gr. *enteron,* intestine, + *-itis,* inflammation]. Serous infiltration accompanying inflammation of bowels.

lymphnoditis (lĭmf′nōd-ī′tĭs) ["+ *nodus,* knot, + Gr. *-itis,* inflammation]. Inflamed condition of a lymph node.

lymphoadenoma (lĭm″fō-ăd″ē-nō′mă) ["+ Gr. *adēn,* gland, + *-ōma,* tumor]. 1. A tumor of lymphoid tissue. 2. Hypertrophied condition of the lymphatics. SYN: *lymphadenoma.*

lymphoblast (lĭm′fō-blăst) [L. *lympha,* lymph, + Gr. *blastos,* germ]. A cell which gives rise to a lymphocyte.

lymphoblastoma (lĭm″fō-blăst-ō′mă) ["+ "+ *-ōma,* tumor]. Tumor composed of lymphocytes. SYN: *lymphosarcoma.*

lymphoblasto′sis ["+ "+ -ōsis, condition]. Excessive number of lymphoblasts in the blood.

lymphocele (lĭm′fō-sēl) [L. lympha, lymph, + Gr. kēlē, hernia]. Tumor containing lymph. SYN: lymphocyst.

lymphocyst (lĭm′fō-sist) ["+ Gr. kystis, cyst]. Tumor containing lymph. SYN: lymphocele.

lymphocyte (lĭm′fō-sīt) ["+ Gr. kytos, cell]. Lymph cell or white blood corpuscle without cytoplasmic granules. They normally number from 20 to 50% of total white cells. May increase to 90% in lymphatic leukemia.

Lymphocytes average 10-12 microns in diameter but may be as large as 20 microns. Characterized by deeply staining, compact nucleus taking a dark blue. The nucleus occupies all or most of the cell, either in center or at one side. The cytoplasm is usually clear but in some cells bright reddish-violet granules are seen.

lymphocythemia (lĭm″fō-sī-thē′mĭ-ă) ["+ "+ haima, blood]. Excess of lymph cells in the blood.

lymphocytopenia (lĭm″fō-sīt″ō-pē′nĭ-ă) [L. lympha, lymph, + Gr. kytos, cell, + penia, lack]. Less than normal number of lymphocytes in the blood.

lymphocytopoiesis (lĭm″fō-sīt″ō-poy-ē′sĭs) ["+ "+ poiesis, production]. Lymphocyte production.

lymphocyto′sis ["+ "+ -ōsis, condition]. Excess of lymph cells. SYN: lymphocythemia.

lymphocytotoxin (lĭm″fō-sīt″ō-tŏks′ĭn) ["+ "+ toxikon, poison]. A toxin destructive to lymphocytes.

lymphodermia (lĭm″fō-dĕr′mĭ-ă) [L. lympha, lymph, + Gr. derma, skin]. Disease of cutaneous lymphatics.

lympho″epithelio′ma. A tumor composed of epithelium and lymphatic tissue which develops usually in the nasal cavity or pharynx.

lymphogenous (lĭm-fŏj′ĕn-ŭs) [L. lympha, lymph, + Gr. gennan, to produce]. 1. Forming lymph. 2. Derived from lymph.

lymphogonia (lĭm″fō-gō′nĭ-ă) ["+ Gr. gonos, offspring]. Large lymphocytes with large nuclei appearing in lymphatic leukemia.

lymphogranulomatosis (lĭm″fō-grăn-ū-lō″mă-tō′sĭs) [L. lympha, lymph, + granulum, granule, + Gr. -ōma, tumor, + -ōsis, condition]. 1. Infectious granuloma of the lymphatics. 2. Hodgkin's disease.

lymphogranuloma venereum. A venereal disease characterized by a small primary lesion, usually on genitalia, inflammation of regional lymph nodes, and constitutional symptoms. It is caused by a virus and readily transmitted by sexual contact. SYN: climatic bubo; fourth venereal disease; lymphogranuloma inguinale; lymphopathia venereum.

lymphoidectomy (lĭm″foyd-ĕk′tō-mī) ["+ Gr. eidos, form, + ektomē, excision]. Surgical removal of lymphoid tissue.

lymphoidocyte (lĭm-foyd′ō-sīt) ["+ "+ kytos, cell]. A hemocytoblast, q.v.

lymphology (lĭm-fŏl′ō-jī) ["+ Gr. logos, study]. Science of the lymphatics.

lymphoma (lĭm-fō′mă) [L. lympha, lymph, + Gr. -ōma, tumor]. A general term for growth of new tissue in the lymphatic system. Included in this general group are Hodgkin's disease, lymphosarcoma, and malignant lymphoma.

l. granulomatosum. Small, white lymphatic nodule in liver in Hodgkin's disease.

lymphomatosis (lĭm″fō-mă-tō′sĭs) ["+ "+ -ōsis, condition]. General lymphatic engorgement; general deposition of lymphomata throughout the body.

lymphomatous (lĭm-fō′mă-tŭs). 1. Pert. to a lymphoma. 2. Affected with lymphoma.

lymphopath′ia vene′reum. Venereal disease marked by ulceration and enlargement of lymph nodes in inguinal area. SYN: lymphogranuloma inguinale, q.v.

lymphopathy (lĭm-fŏp′ă-thī) [L. lympha, lymph, + Gr. pathos, disease]. Any lymphatic disease.

lymphopenia (lĭm-fō-pē′nĭ-ă) ["+ Gr. penia, a lack]. Deficiency of lymphocytes in the blood.

lymphopoiesis (lĭm″fō-poy-ē′sĭs) ["+ Gr. poiēsis, production]. Formation of lymphocytes.

lymphopoietic (lĭm-fō-poy-ĕt′ĭk) ["+ Gr. poiein, to produce]. Forming lymphocytes.

lymphoprotease. Protein-splitting enzyme secured from a suspension of lymphatic tissue.

lymphorrhagia (lĭm″fō-rā′jĭ-ă) [L. lympha, lymph, + Gr. rhegnynai, to burst forth]. Flow of lymph from ruptured lymph vessels. SYN: lymphorrhea.

lymphorrhea (lĭm″fō-rē′ă) ["+ Gr. rhoia, flow]. Internal or external discharge of lymph through a wound. SYN: lymphorrhagia.

lymphosarcoma (lĭm″fō-săr-kō′mă) ["+ Gr. sarx, flesh, + -ōma, tumor]. A malignant disease of lymphatic tissue. Clinically may be quite similar to Hodgkin's disease. Diagnosis is made by biopsy rather than by clinical examination.

lym"phosar"comato'sis ["+ "+ "+ -*ōsis,* condition]. Condition characterized by the development of lymphosarcoma.

lymphostasis (lĭm-fŏs'tă-sĭs) [L. *lympha,* lymph, + Gr. *stasis,* a stoppage]. Stoppage of flow of lymph.

lymphotome (lĭm'fō-tōm) ["+ Gr. *tomē,* incision]. Instrument for removing glandular growths from tonsils and adenoids.

lymphotrophy (lĭm-fŏt'rō-fĭ) ["+ Gr. *trophē,* nourishment]. Lymph nourishment of cells in regions devoid of blood vessels.

lymphuria (lĭm-fū'rĭ-ă) [L. *lympha,* lymph, + Gr. *ouron,* urine]. Lymph in the urine.

lymphvascular (lĭmf-văs'kū-lăr) ["+ *vasculus,* a little vessel]. Rel. to the lymphatic vessels.

lyo- [Gr. *lyein,* to dissolve]. Combining form meaning dissolved or loose.

lyochrome (lĭ'ō-krōm) ["+ *chrōma,* color]. Flavin, q.v.

lyogel. A gel containing much water.

lyophilization (lĭ-ŏf'ĭ-lĭ-za'shun). Process of rapidly freezing a substance at an extremely low temperature and then dehydrating in a high vacuum.

ly'ophobe, ly"opho'bic [Gr. *lyein,* to dissolve, + *phobos,* fear]. Tending not to go into solution; applied to colloidal systems in which there is a strong affinity between dispersed phase and dispersion medium.

ly'otrope ["+ *tropos,* a turning]. A substance which goes into solution readily.

lyra (lĭ'ră) [L., Gr., *lyre*]. One of several anatomical structures so called because of their resemblance to the shape of a lyre.

lysimeter (lĭ-sĭm'ē-ter) [Gr. *lysis,* dissolution, + *metron,* measure]. Apparatus for determining solubilities.

lysin (lĭ'sĭn). A specific antibody acting destructively upon cells and tissues. SEE: *immune body.*

lysine (lĭ'sēn). An amino acid which is a hydrolytic cleavage product of protein through digestion. It is essential for growth and repair.

lysis (lĭ'sĭs) [Gr., dissolution]. 1. The gradual decline of a fever or disease. Opposed to crisis, q.v. 2. Destruction of blood cells, etc., by a lysin, as when rabbit's red corpuscles are dissolved by dog's serum.

-lysis. Combining form meaning dissolution or decompositon of. In medicine, reduction or relief of.

lysogenesis (lĭ"sō-jĕn'ē-sĭs) [Gr. *lysis,* dissolution, + *genesis,* production]. The production of cell-dissolving substances known as lysin.

lysogenic (lĭ-sō-jĕn'ĭk) ["+ Gr. *gennan,* to produce.]. Producing lysins.

lysogeny (lĭ-sŏj'ē-nĭ). A special type of virus-bacterial cell interaction maintained by a complex cellular regulatory mechanism. Bacterial strains freshly isolated from their natural environment may contain a low concentration of bacteriophage. This phage will lyse other related bacteria. Cultures which contain these substances are said to be lysogenic.

lysol (lĭ'sŏl). A proprietary preparation of a mixture of cresols. Because of its potential for causing toxicity, its use should be confined to disinfecting inanimate objects, feces, and urine.

POISONING: When swallowed it causes corrosion, edema of the lungs, immobility of pupils, and collapse. Vomiting may occur, death sometimes after symptoms have abated.

TREATMENT: Prompt emptying of the stomach by aspiration through a stomach tube.

lysolec'ithin. A substance obtained from lecithin through the action of an enzyme present in cobra venom. Exerts a powerful hemolytic action.

lysosomes. Parts of an intracellular digestive system which exist as separate particles in the cell. Inside their limiting membrane they contain a number of hydrolytic enzymes capable of breaking down proteins and certain carbohydrates. Even though their importance in health and disease is certain, all of the precise ways lysosomes effect changes are not understood.

lysozyme (lĭ'sō-zĭm) [Gr. *lysis,* dissolution, + *zymē,* leaven]. An enzyme which is now called muramidase, q.v.

lyssa (lĭs'să) [Gr., frenzy]. An acute infectious disease, transferable by inoculation, attacking the nervous system in particular. SYN: *hydrophobia; rabies.*

lyssin (lĭs'sĭn). Virus of lyssa. SYN: *hydrophobin.*

lyssodexis (lĭs-ō-dĕks'ĭs) [Gr. *lyssa,* frenzy, + *dēxis,* a bite]. The bite of an animal infected with rabies virus.

lyssoid (lĭs'oyd) ["+ *eidos,* resemblance]. Resembling lyssa or rabies.

lyssophobia (lĭs-ō-fō'bĭ-ă) ["+ *phobos,* fear]. 1. Hysteria resembling rabies. 2. Fear of rabies.

lyterian (lĭ-tēr'ĭ-ăn) [Gr. *lyein,* to dissolve]. Indicative of the lessening of a disease process.

lytic (lĭt'ĭk). Rel. to lysis or a lysin.

lyze (līz) [Gr. *lysis,* dissolution]. To bring about lysis.

M

M. Abbr. for *master* or *medicine* in professional titles; *mille*, a thousand; *misce*, mix; *molar*.

m. Abbr. for *meter* and *minim;* in chemistry, for *meta-*, and for *mol* or *mole*, q.v.

MA. Abbr. for mental age.

M.A. Abbr. for *Master of Arts*.

Ma. Chem. symbol for masurium.

ma. Abbr. for milliampère.

M.A.C. Abbr. for *maximum allowable concentration*.

macaro'ni [It.]. Food value of 100 gm. (cooked, firm): Cal. 148; protein 5.0 gm.; carbohydrate 30.1 gm.; phosphorous 65 mg.; potassium 79 mg.

mace (mās) [L. *macis*]. A spice from the outer covering of the nutmeg; employed as a condiment.

mace. Acronym for *m* ethylchloroform chloro-*ace* tophenone, a chemical compound used at one time in riot control because of its ability to irritate the eyes. Now it is considered to be too toxic for that purpose.

TREATMENT: Instillation of 0.1% aqueous solution of idoxuridine (IDU) into the eye. SEE: *IDU*.

maceration (măs-ĕr-a'shŭn) [L. *macerāre*, to make soft]. Process of softening a solid by steeping in a fluid.

Mache unit (mä'kĕ). [Heinrich Mache, Austrian physicist, 1876 —] The unit of measurement of concentration of radium emanation. ABBR: *M.u.,* or German, *M.E.* SEE: *unit*.

machonnement (mä-shŏn-mah') [Fr.]. Movement of jaws resembling chewing.

macies (mā'shĭ-ēz) [L. wasting]. Atrophy, wasting, emaciation.

macracusia (măk"-rä-kū'zĭ-ä) [Gr. *makros*, large + *akousis*, hearing]. An auditory illusion in which sounds seem to be louder than they are. May occur at the onset of an epileptic seizure. SEE: *micracusia*.

macrencephalia, macrencephaly (makren"sĕ-fa'lĭ-ä, -sef'a-lĭ) ["+ *enkephalos*, brain]. Abnormal size of the brain.

macro-, macr- [Gr. *makros*, large]. Combining forms meaning large, long.

macrobiosis (mak"rō-bī-ō'sĭs) [Gr. *makros*, large, + *biōsis*, life]. State of surpassing normal span; longevity.

macrobiota (mak"rō-bī-ō'tä). The large living organisms, flora and fauna, of an area. Opposed to microbiota.

macrobleph"ar'ia ["+ *blepharon*, eyelid]. Abnormal largeness of eyelid.

macrobrachia (mak"rō-brā'kĭ-ä) ["+ *brachiōn*, arm]. Abnormal size or length of the arm.

macrocephalia (mak-rō-sĕ-fa'lĭ-ä) [Gr. *makros*, large, + *kephalē*, head]. Abnormal largeness of head.

ETIOL: Found in acromegaly, hydrocephalus, rickets, osteitis deformans, leontiasis ossea, myxedema, sporadic cretinism, idiocy, leprosy, hemiatrophy, and pituitary disturbances.

macrocephalous (mak-ro-sĕf'ä-lŭs). Pert. to or having an excessively large head.

macrocephaly (mak-rō-sĕf'al-ĭ). Abnormal size of head. SYN: *macrocephalia*.

macrocheilia (mak-rō-kī'lĭ-ä) [Gr. *makros*, large, + *cheilos*, lip]. Abnormal size of lip characterized by swelling of glands of lip. It is a congenital condition. SYN: *hypertrophy of lip*.

macrocheiria (mak-rō-kī'rĭ-ä) ["+ *cheir*, hand]. Excessive size of the hands. SYN: *macrochiria*.

macrocornea (mak-rō-kor'nē-ä) [Gr. *makros*, large, + L. *cornu*, horn]. Abnormal size or projection of the cornea. SYN: *keratoglobus, megalocornea*.

mac'rocyte ["+ *kytos*, cell]. Erythrocyte larger than normal, exceeding 10 microns in diameter.

macrocythemia (mak-rō-sī-thē'mĭ-ä) ["+ "+ *haima*, blood]. Abnormal number of macrocytes in the blood.

macrocytosis (mak"rō-sī-tō'sĭs) ["+ "+ -*ōsis*, intensive]. Development of macrocytes, esp. in greater numbers than normal.

macrodactylia (mak"rō-dak-til'ĭ-ä) ["+ *daktylos*, finger]. Excessive size of one or more of the digits.

macrodont (mak'rō-dont) ["+ *odous, odont-*, tooth]. Having abnormally large teeth. SYN: *megadont*.

macroesthesia (mak"rō-ĕs-thē'zĭ-ä) [Gr. *makros*, large, + *aisthēsis*, sensation]. A state in which objects seen or felt appear to be greatly magnified.

macrogam'ete ["+ *gametē*, wife]. A large, immobile reproductive cell formed in certain protozoa and simple plants. Corresponds to the ovum in higher forms. SEE: *anisogamy*.

macrogametocyte. A large nonmotile reproductive cell developing from the merozoite of certain protozoans; the female gametocyte. SEE: *Plasmodium*.

macrogenitosomia praecox (măk-rō-jĕn″ĭ-tō-sō′mĭ-ă prē′kŏks) ["+ L. *genitalis*, genital + Gr. *soma*, body + L. *praecox*, early]. Abnormal size of genitalia due to excess androgens (male hormones) from the fetal adrenal. In the female this causes pseudohermaphroditism and in the male enlarged external genitalia.

macroglia (mak-rog′lĭ-ă) [Gr. *makros*, large, + *glia*, glue]. A type of neuroglia in which cells are called astrocytes, q.v. SEE: *glia cells; neuroglia; spider cells.*

macroglobulinemia (măk-rō-glŏb″ū-lin-ē′-mĭ-ă). Presence of globulins of high molecular weight in serum. SYN: *Waldenstrom's macroglobulinemia.*

macroglobulins (mak″rō-glob′ū-lĭnz). A group of proteins of high molecular weight, about 1,000,000, normally present in the blood but increased in disease states such as multiple myeloma, collagen disorders, cirrhosis of the liver, and amyloidosis.

macroglos′sia [Gr. *makros*, large, + *glōssa*, tongue]. Hypertrophied condition of the tongue; a congenital disorder.

macrognathia (mak-rō-nā′thĭ-ă) ["+ *gnathos*, jaw]. Abnormal size of jaw.

macrogy′ria ["+ *gyros*, circle]. Excessively large size of convolutions (gyri) of cerebral hemispheres.

macrolabia (mak-rō-lā′bĭ-ă) ["+ L. *labium*, lip]. Abnormal size of lip. SYN: *macrocheilia*, q.v.

macrolymphocyte (mak″rō-limf′ō-sīt) ["+ L. *lympha*, lymph, + Gr. *kytos*, cell]. A large lymphocyte.

macromastia (mak-rō-mas′tĭ-ă) ["+ *mastos*, breast]. Abnormal size of the breasts.

macrome′lia [Gr. *makros*, large, + *melas*, limb]. Excessive size of an organ or a part, esp. an extremity.

macrome′lus. An individual possessing limbs of excessive size.

macromere (mak′rō-mēr) [Gr. *makros*, large, + *meros*, a part]. Blastomere of large size.

macronormoblast (mak″rō-nor′mō-blast) ["+ L. *norma*, rule, + Gr. *blastos*, germ]. Large, nucleated red blood corpuscle.

macrophage, macrophagus (mak′rō-fāj, -rof′ă-gus) ["+ *phagein*, to eat]. Cells of the reticuloendothelial system having the ability to phagocytose particulate substances and to store vital dyes and other colloidal substances. They are found in loose connective tissues and various organs of the body. They include Kupffer cells of the liver, splenocytes of the spleen, dust cells of the lung, microglia of spinal cord and brain, and histiocytes of loose connective tissue. SYN: *clasmatocyte; resting wandering cell; adventitial cell.*

    m., fixed. A nonmotile macrophage. SYN: *histiocyte.*

    m., free. A wandering or ameboid macrophage. Found esp. in areas where inflammatory processes are in progress. SYN: *wandering m.*

macrophallus (mak″rō-făl′ūs) ["+ *phallos*, penis]. Abnormally large penis.

macrophthalmia (mak″rof-thal′mĭ-ă) ["+ *ophthalmos*, eye]. Abnormally large eyeballs.

macroplasia (mak″rō-plā′zĭ-ă). Abnormally large size of a part or specific tissue.

macropodia (mak-rō-pō′dĭ-ă). Abnormally large feet.

macroprosopia (mak″rō-prō-sō′pĭ-ă) [Gr. *makros*, large, + *prosōpon*, face]. Large facial features.

macropsia (mak-rop′sĭ-ă) ["+ *opsis*, vision]. Condition in which objects look larger than they really are.

macrorhinia (mak-rō-rīn′ĭ-ă) ["+ *ris, rin-*, nose]. Excessive size of the nose, either congenital or pathological.

macroscelia (mak-rō-sēl′ĭ-ă) ["+ *skelos*, leg]. Abnormal size of the legs.

macroscopic (mak-rō-skop′ĭk) ["+ *skopein*, to examine]. Large enough to be seen by the naked eye. Opposed to microscopic. SYN: *megascopic.*

macroscopy (mak-ros′ko-pĭ). Examination of an object with the naked eye.

macrosomatia (mak″rō-sō-mā′shĭ-ă) [Gr. *makros*, large, + *sōma*, body]. Abnormally large body. SYN: *macrosomia.*

macrosomia (măk-rō-sō′mĭ-ă). Abnormally large body.

macrostomia (mak-rō-stō′mĭ-ă) [Gr. *makros*, large, + *stoma*, mouth]. Excessively wide mouth.

macrotia (mak-ro′shĭ-ă) ["+ *ous, ot-*, ear]. Abnormally large ears.

macrotooth. Abnormally enlarged tooth.

macula (mak′u-lă) [L. spot]. (pl. *maculae*) [NA] A small spot or colored area. SEE: *roseola.* SYN: *macule.*

    m. acusticae. Oval, thickened areas in saccule and utricle in which fibers of vestibular branch of acoustic nerve terminate. They are sensory receptors containing hair cells which respond to movement of the endolymph. They include m. sacculi and m. utriculi.

    m. albida. White mark found on liver in some contagious diseases. SYN: *tache blanche.*

    m. atrophica. Glistening white spot on skin following a circumscribed hemorrhage.

m. caerulea. Steel-gray or blue stain of epidermis, without elevation. It does not disappear on pressure and occurs esp. with pediculosis pubis or bites from fleas.

m., cerebral. Reddened line that becomes deeper and persists for some time when the fingernail is drawn across the skin, esp. in tuberculous meningitis; tache cérébrale, q.v.

m. cornea. Opaque spot in cornea.

m. cribrosa. [NA] One of the tiny foramina in wall of vestibule of bony labyrinth of the ear through which pass filaments of the acoustic nerve.

m. flava. A small yellow spot at ventral end of each vocal cord formed by a small mass of elastic tissue or, sometimes, cartilage.

m. gonorrhoeica. Red spot at orifice of Bartholin's gland. Seen in gonorrheal vulvitis.

m. lutea. A yellow spot in the center of the retina approximately 2 mm. lateral to the optic nerve's exit. Contains a pit, fovea centralis, where the retina is reduced to a layer of closely packed cones, which functions as the area of most acute vision (central vision).

m. sacculi. [NA] SEE: *m. acusticae.*

m. solaris. A freckle.

m. utriculi. [NA] SEE: *m. acusticae.*

macular (mak'ū-lar) [L. *macula,* spot]. 1. Rel. to macules. 2. Having macules.

maculate(d (mak'ū-lāt, -lāt-ĕd). Spotted, as with macules.

maculation (mak-ū-lā'shun) [L. *macula,* spot]. Process of becoming maculate. Development of macules.

macule (mak'ūl). Discolored spot or patch on the skin, neither elevated nor depressed, of various colors, sizes, and shapes.

Macules include hyperemia, roseola, erythema, telangiectasis, nevi vasculosi, areola, achromia, chloasma, purpura, petechiae, ecchymosis, vibices, albinism, vitiligo, lentigines, nevi pigmentosi, nevi spili, discolorations, q.v.

Macules occur in pellagra, pityriasis rosea, pediculosis corporis, rubella, scurvy, serum sickness, peliosis, anemia, leukemia, cancer, Bright's disease, infectious diseases, poisoning, erysipelas, acne rosacea, nevus pigmentosus, vitiligo, leprosy, morphea, facial hemiatrophy, etc. SYN: *macula,* q.v.

maculopap'ular. Consisting of or pertaining to macules and papules.

mad. 1. Not rational. SYN: *insane.* 2. Angry. 3. Rash, foolish, frantic. 4. Suffering from infection with rabies. SYN: *rabid.*

madarosis (mad-ă-ro'sis) [Gr. *madaros,* bald]. Loss of eyelashes or eyebrows.

madescent (mad-es'ent) [L. *madescere,* to become moist]. Slightly moist or becoming so.

madidans (mad'ĭ-dans) [L. *madidus,* wet]. Exuding, moist as in some skin lesions.

Madu'ra foot. Fungus disease of the foot. SYN: *maduromycosis;* q.v.; *mycetoma.*

maduromycosis (măd-ū"rō-mĭ-kō'sĭs) Chronic infection of the foot or hand characterized by marked swelling and development of nodules, vesicles, abscesses, and sinuses.

ETIOL: Various fungi and aerobic actinomycetes.

Magendie's foramen (mă-zhan-de'). [Francois Magendie, French physiologist, 1783-1855] The median of three openings in the roof of the 4th ventricle which is in front of the cerebellum and behind the pons varolii, connecting the ventricle with the subarachnoid space.

magenstrasse (mag"en-stras'ĕ) [Ger. *magen,* stomach, + *strasse,* street]. A groove along lesser curvature of stomach from cardia to pylorus.

mag'got. (origin uncertain). Larva of an insect, esp. the soft-bodied, footless larva of flies (order Diptera). Many are parasitic giving rise to myiasis, q.v.

m. treatment. An obsolete method of treating septic wounds. Meat maggots, introduced into a sloughing septic wound, ingested the necrotic material, leaving the wound with a clean granulating surface. The maggots were then removed and destroyed. SEE: *osteomyelitis.*

magistery (maj'ĭs-tĕr-ĭ) [L. *magister,* master]. 1. Specially compounded remedy. 2. A precipitate.

magistral (măj'ĭs-trăl). Concerning medicines prescribed by a physician for a particular case. SEE: *officinal.*

magma (mag'mă) [Gr. *magma,* from *massein,* to knead]. 1. Mass left after extraction of principal. 2. Salve. 3. A pulpy mass or paste.

magnesia (măg-nē'zĭ-ă). [Magnetic stone found in Magnesia, region of ancient Thessaly] Magnesium oxide. (USP). MgO.

m., milk of. USP. Aperient composed of magnesium hydroxide and water.

magnesium [L.]. SYMB: *Mg.* At. wt. 24.312; at. no. 12; sp. gr. 1.738. A white mineral element found in soft tissue, muscles, bones, and to some extent in the body fluids. It is a naturally occurring element on earth, being extracted from wells and sea water.

The human body contains approximately 25 gm. of magnesium, most of which is in the bones. Muscles contain less of it than they do of calcium. Concentration of Mg in the blood serum is between 1.5 and 2.5 mEq./liter.

Magnesium is widely distributed in foods; therefore deficiency rarely occurs. It is obtained in such sufficient quantities in whole grains, fruits, and vegetables that it is unnecessary to make special dietary planning to include it. A typical diet contains 200-400 mg. but very little of this is absorbed. Deficiency may be present in patients with chronic diarrhea or diseases that interfere with absorption.

FUNCTIONS: Magnesium activates enzymes that catalyze reactions between phosphate ions and adenosine triphosphate (ATP). It is also associated with regulation of body temperature, neuromuscular contraction, and synthesis of protein.

DEFICIENCY SYM: Tetany quite similar to that produced by hypocalcemia, weakness, and mental depression.

    m. *car'bonate.* ($MgCO_3.3H_2O$). A bulky, white, odorless powder.

ACTION AND USES: Taken by mouth to neutralize acid in stomach.

    m. *citrate solution.* A solution containing an amount of magnesium citrate corresponding to approximately 1.6% magnesium oxide.

ACTION AND USES: Purgative.

    m. *hydroxide.* ($Mg[OH]_2$) A bulky white powder which, in aqueous suspension, is milk of magnesia. ACTION AND USES: Laxative and antacid.

    m. *oxide.* USP. (MgO) Calcined magnesia. Light magnesia. A white, very bulky, powder. In Great Britain called light magnesium oxide.

ACTION AND USES: Antacid, laxative.

    m. *phosphate tribasic.* A white, odorless powder.

USES: As an antacid and laxative.

    m. *stearate.* USP. Compound of magnesium and palmitic and stearic acid. Used in manufacture of pharmaceutical tablets.

    m. *sul'fate.* USP. ($MgSO_4.7H_2O$) Small, colorless crystals. Saline bitter taste. SYN: *Epsom salt.*

ACTION AND USES: Cathartic and anticonvulsant.

INCOMPATIBILITIES: Ammonium chloride, soapsuds enema, quinine, ferric chloride, sulfanilamide.

    m. *trisilicate.* USP. Magnesium oxide, silicon dioxide and water. Used as an antacid.

mag'net [Gr. *magnes,* magnet]. Any body which has the property of attracting iron, specifically a mass of iron or steel which has this property given to it artificially. A piece of iron may be magnetized by passage of an electric current through an insulated wire wound around it.

    m. *horseshoe.* M. in shape of a horseshoe.

    m. *operation.* Removal of metal particles with a magnet.

magnet'ic. Pert. to a magnet or having magnetism.

    m. *field.* The space permeated by the magnetic lines of force surrounding a permanent magnet or coil of wire carrying electric current.

    m. *induction.* The production of magnetic properties in magnetic metals, such as iron, by the influence of a magnet or a magnetic field.

    m. *lines of force.* The lines indicating the direction of the magnetic force in the space surrounding a magnet or constituting a magnetic field.

magnetism (măg″ně-tĭzm) ["+ *ismos,* condition]. The property of repulsion and attraction of certain substances.

magnetotherapy (mag″nět-ō-ther′ă-pĭ) ["+ *therapeia,* treatment]. Application of magnets or magnetism in treating diseases.

magnification (mag-nĭ-fĭ-kā′shŭn) [L. *magnus,* great, + *facere,* to make]. Process of increasing apparent size of an object, esp. under microscope.

mag'num [L.]. 1. Large. Ex: foramen magnum. 2. Old term for capitate bone (os magnum), the largest of the carpals.

maidenhead (mād′ĕn-hĕd). Thin, crescentic fold surrounding vaginal opening. At one time considered to be a sign of virginity. However, it may be present in those who have had sexual intercourse and may be absent in those who have never experienced sexual intercourse. SYN: *hymen,* q.v.

maieusiomania (mī-ū-sī-ō-mā′nĭ-ă) [Gr. *maieusis,* childbirth, + *mania,* madness]. Insanity following childbirth.

maieusiophobia (mī-ū-sī-ō-fō′bĭ-ă) ["+ *phobos,* fear]. Extreme fear of childbirth.

maieutics (mī-ū′tĭks) [Gr. *maieusis,* childbirth]. Obstetrics.

maim (mām) [ME. *maymen,* to cripple]. 1. To injure seriously; to disable. 2. To deprive of the use of a part, such as an arm or leg.

main (mān) [Fr.]. Hand.

    m. *en griffe.* Flexion and atrophy of the hand in a claw shape.

    m. *succulente.* Edema of a hand.

Majocchi's disease (mah-yŏk′ē). [Domenico Majocchi, It. physician, 1849-1929] Ring-shaped, purplish eruption of lower limbs; purpura annularis telangiectodes, q.v.

make. In electricity, to complete an electric circuit. Opposed to break.

m. twitch. In physiology, the contraction of a muscle that occurs upon closure of the primary electric circuit.

makro- [Gr.]. SEE: words beginning with *macro-*.

mal-. Combining form meaning ill, bad, poor.

mal (mahl) [Fr. from L. *malum*, an evil]. An evil, a sickness, or a disorder.

m. de Cayenne. Elephantiasis.

m. de la rosa. Pellagra.

m. de mer. Seasickness.

m., grand. A major epileptic attack with convulsions.

m. perforant. A perforating ulcer of the foot.

m. perforant palatin. A perforating ulcer of the palate.

m., petit. A minor attack of epilepsy without convulsions.

mala (ma'lä) [L.]. [NA]. 1. The cheek. 2. The cheekbone.

malabsorption syndrome. Disordered or inadequate absorption of nutrients from the intestinal tract. May be due to a disease which affects the intestinal mucosa, as infections, tropical sprue, gluten enteropathy, pancreatic insufficiency, or due to antibiotic therapy (neomycin).

malachite green (mal'ä-kīt) [Gr. *malakhē*, a mallow]. Dye sometimes used in treating trypanosomiasis, as an indicator, or as a bacteriological stain.

malacia (mä-lā'she-ä) [Gr. *malakia*, softening]. 1. Abnormal softening of tissues of an organ or of tissues themselves. 2. A morbid appetite for some specific food, esp. condiments.

m. cordis. Softening following infarction of the myocardium.

malacoma (mäl-ä-kō'mä). Softening of an organ or part of the body. SYN: *malacia; malacosis.*

malacoplakia (mal-ä-kō-plā'kĭ-ä) [Gr. *malakos*, softening, + *plax, plak-*, plaque]. Existence of soft patches in mucous membrane of a hollow organ.

m. vesical. Soft, fungus-like patches on mucosa of the bladder.

malacosarcosis (mäl-ä-kō-sar-kō'sĭs) [Gr. *malakos*, softening, + *sarx*, flesh, + *-ōsis*, condition]. Softness of tissue, especially muscular.

malacosis (mäl-ä-kō'sĭs) ["+ *-ōsis*, intensive]. Abnormal softening of an organ or tissue. SYN: *malacia.*

malacosteon (mal-ä-kos'tē-ŏn) ["+ *osteon*, bone]. Softening of the bones. SYN: *osteomalacia.*

malacotic (mal-ä-kot'ik). 1. Soft. 2. Affected with malacia. 3. Rel. to malacia.

m. teeth. Those of soft texture easily affected by caries.

malacotomy (mäl-ä-kot'ō-mĭ) [Gr. *malakos*, soft, + *tomē*, incision]. Incision of soft areas of the body, esp. of the abdominal wall.

mal"adjust'ed. Poorly adjusted; unhappy or unsuccessful because of inability or failure to adjust one's desires or needs to one's environment or station in life.

malady (mäl'ä-dĭ) [Fr. *maladie*, illness, from L. *malum*, an evil]. A disease or disorder. SYN: *disease.*

malaise (mä-lāz') [Fr.]. Discomfort, uneasiness, indisposition, often indicative of infection.

malar (mā'lar) [L. *mala*, cheek]. Pert. to the cheek or cheekbones.

m. bone. A 4-pointed bone on each side of the face, uniting the frontal and sup. maxillary bones with the zygomatic process of the maxilla. The zygomatic or cheekbone. SEE: *zygoma.*

malaria (mä-lā'rĭ-ä) [It. *malaria*, bad air]. An acute and sometimes chronic infectious disease due to the presence of protozoan parasites within red blood cells. The parasites undergo an asexual cycle in man and a sexual cycle in the mosquito. Sporozoites injected by the bite of a mosquito go through an exoerythrocytic cycle in tissue cells, such as liver cells where they undergo schizogony. After an interval of 7-10 days, they invade erythrocytes in which they undergo several divisions (schizogony), forming many merozoites. These break free and invade other corpuscles. The destruction of corpuscles with liberation of pigment and waste products brings on the characteristic paroxysms of chills and fever. This occurs at 48-hr. intervals in tertian and 72-hr. intervals in quartan malaria. After several generations of schizonts, some merozoites develop into micro- and macrogametocytes which when sucked up by a mosquito undergo further development. The microgametocytes produce several flagellated bodies which unite with a macrogamete to form a zygote. This elongates forming a vermicule or ookinete which penetrates the stomach wall of the mosquito forming an oocyst in which sporozoites develop. The oocyst bursts when mature, liberating sporozoites into the body cavity through which the sporozoites then make their way to salivary glands. They are discharged through salivary ducts when the mosquito bites a person.

ETIOL: Four species of a sporozoan, Plasmodium (P. vivax, P. falciparum, P. malariae, P. ovale). The causative organism is transmitted through bites of infected mosquitoes of the genus Anopheles; may be transmitted by blood transfusion.

INCUBATION PERIOD: P. falciparum, 12 d.; P. vivax and P. ovale, 14 d.; P. malariae, 30 d. For some strains of P. vivax, may be 8-10 months.

SYM: Various derangements of the digestive and nervous systems. Characterized by periodicity, chills, fever, and sweats in the order mentioned, having pathological manifestations of progressive anemia, splenic enlargement, and deposition in various organs of a melanin, resulting from biological activity of the plasmodia.

TREATMENT: Chloroquine phosphate, primaquine phosphate, and pyrimethamine. In some cases the parasites do not respond to treatment, acting as if they were drug resistant. In this instance treatment with combinations of quinine, pyrimethamine, dapsone, chloroquine, and primaquine may be required. Persons with glucosa-6-phosphate-dehydrogenase deficiency respond poorly to treatment.

m., algid. Cold malaria characterized by coldness of skin. SEE: *m., estivoautumnal.*

m., cephalgic. Unusually severe headache, nausea, vomiting, etc. DIFFERENTIAL DIAG: Meningitis and intracranial lesions.

m., cerebral. Falciparum malaria in which brain is affected due to tendency of corpuscles to agglutinate, resulting in clogging of capillaries which in the brain leads to coma or sometimes sudden death.

m., estivoautumnal. Indistinct chill, usually only a chilly sensation. Intense headache, profound weakness, marked muscular aching. Marked mental depression. Coated tongue, feeble and accelerated pulse, rapid respiration. Febrile stages may be 36 hours long. SEE: *m., falciparum.*

m., falciparum. M. caused by Plasmodium falciparum. More prevalent in tropics; also called malignant tertian, subtertian, estivoautumnal malaria. Symptoms more severe than in other types but runs a shorter course without relapses.

m., latent. Parasites exist within blood stream but give rise to no recognizable symptoms. An individual having this form is a reservoir for the disease.

m., pernicious. Onset may be sudden, resembling apoplexy; however, coma usually comes after obvious, severe, and intense symptoms. Hot skin; petechiae; contracted pupils; Cheyne-Stokes respiration; coated tongue; loss of sphincter control; rapid, irregular, weak pulse; elevated temperature. A remission may occur with profuse perspiration, but other paroxysms follow if treatment is inadequate.

ETIOL: Plasmodium vivax. PROG: In spite of heroic adminstrations, death sometimes occurs. Often general collapse, with death in cases where no treatment is instituted.

m. quartan. Short and less severe paroxysms. Sporulation occurs each 72 hours causing seizures with that interval. Caused by Plasmodium malariae.

m., quotidian estivoautumnal.

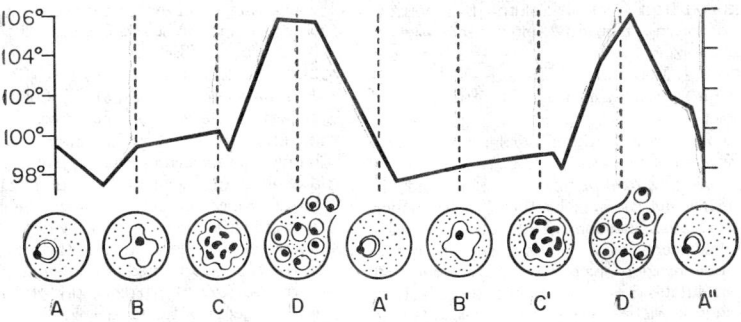

HUMAN CYCLE OF TERTIAN MALARIA

In the circle A, B, C, D, and A′, B′, C′, D′, which represent red blood corpuscles, malarial parasites are shown growing from the little spore in A and A′ to the adult in C and C′ and sporulating in D and D′. Above is a temperature curve, the figures on the left indicating the temperature of the patient (given in the centigrade scale), the vertical lines indicating days. The temperature is highest, i.e. there is a paroxysm, each time the parasite reaches the stage of sporulation, D and D′.

Paroxysms occur with daily periodicity due to 24-hour sporulation. Abrupt rise and fall of temperature. Due to multiple infections with the same organism.

m., tertian. Sporulation each 48 hours. Symptoms more common during the day. Paroxysms divided into chill, fever, and sweating stages. Cold stage usually is 10-15 minutes but may last an hour or more. Febrile stage varies from 4-6 hours.

m., tertian, benign. Caused by Plasmodium vivax; malignant tertian by Plasmodium falciparum.

m., vivax. Malaria caused by Plasmodium vivax. SYN: *benign tertian.*

malarial (mă-lar'ĭ-ăl) [It. *malaria*, bad air]. 1. Affected with malaria. 2. Causing malaria. 3. Resembling malaria. 4. Pert. to malaria. SYN: *malarious.*

malariology (mă-lar-ĭ-ol'ō-jĭ). The scientific study of malaria.

malariotherapy (mă-lar-ĭ-ō-ther'ă-pĭ). A now obsolete method of treating syphilis of the central nervous system by injecting malarial organisms into the body. The organisms produce hyperthermia which is then terminated by administering an antimalarial.

malarious (ma-lar'ĭ-ŭs). Of the nature of, or afflicted with malaria. SYN: *malarial.*

Malasse'zia (mal"ah-se'zi-ah). [Louis C. Malassez, Fr. physiologist, 1842-1910] A genus of fungi.

malassimilation (mal"ă-sim-ĭ-la'shŭn) [L. *malus*, ill, + *assimilāre*, to make like]. Defective, incomplete, or faulty assimilation, esp. of nutritive material. SEE: *malabsorption syndrome.*

malaxation (mal-aks-a'shun) [L. *malaxāre*, to soften]. Kneading movement used in massage.

male. 1. Masculine. 2. The sex which has organs for producing sperm for fertilization of ova.

RS: female; organ; virile; virilescence; virilism.

m. sex hormone. 1. Hormone, found in urine and secreted by the testicles, which regulates development at puberty of male characteristics. SYN: *androsterone,* q.v. 2. An androgen. One of a group of steroids that stimulates the development of secondary sex characteristics and accessory sex organs in the male. It is produced principally by the interstitial cells of the testes, although the adrenal cortex and the ovaries also produce androgenic compounds. It is also found in urine. Principal androgenic hormone is testosterone ($C_{19}H_{30}O_2$). Other androgenic sub-

stances include adrenosterone, androsterone, and isoandrosterone.

malemission (măl"ē-mĭsh'ŭn) [L. *malus,* weak, + *ē,* out, + *mittere,* to send]. Failure of semen to be ejaculated from the urinary meatus during coitus.

maleruption (mal-e-rup'shun). Incorrect eruption of teeth.

malformation (măl-for-mā'shŭn) [L. *malus,* bad, + *formatiō,* a shaping]. Deformity; abnormal shape or structure, esp. congenital.

malic (mā'lĭk, măl'ĭk) [L. *malum,* apple]. Pert. to apples.

m. acid. An acid found in some fruits, such as apples. SEE: *acid.*

malign (mă-lin') [L. *malignus,* of bad kind]. Malignant. Tending to injure or harm.

malignancy (mă-lĭg'năn-sĭ) [L. *malignus,* of bad kind]. 1. State of being malignant. 2. A neoplasm or tumor that is cancerous as opposed to benign. SYN: *virulence.*

malignant (mă-lig'nănt). Virulent. Growing worse; resisting treatment, said of cancerous growths. Tending or threatening to produce death; harmful.

malinger (mă-ling'er) [Fr. *malingre,* weak, sickly]. To feign illness, usually to arouse sympathy, to escape work, or to continue to receive compensation.

malingerer (mă-ling'ger-er). 1. One who pretends to be ill or to be suffering from a non-existent disorder to arouse sympathy. 2. One who pretends slow recuperation from a disease once suffered in order to continue to receive benefits of sick insurance.

malleation (măl-lē-ā'shŭn) [L. *mallere,* to hammer]. Spasmodic action of the hands in which they seem drawn to strike any near object, as spasmodic rapping against thighs, furniture, etc. SEE: *tic.*

malleoincudal (măl"ē-ō-ĭn'kŭ-dăl) [L. *malleus,* hammer, + *incus,* anvil]. Concerning or pert. to the malleus and incus.

malleolar (măl-ē'ō-lar) [L. *malleolus,* little hammer]. Concerning the malleolus.

malleolus (mă-le'o-lus). (pl. *malleolī*) The protuberance on both sides of the ankle joint, the lower extremity of the fibula being known as the lateral m., and the lower end of the tibia as the medial malleolus.

m., external, lateral, outer. Process on outer edge of fibula at lower end.

m., internal, inner, medial. Round process on inner edge of tibia at lower end.

mallet finger (mal'let) [L. *malleus,* hammer]. Loss of power of extension in a finger, causing permanent flexion. SYN: *dropfinger.*

mallet toe (mal'let). Abnormal flexion or loss of power of extension of a toe. SYN: *hammer toe.*

malleus (mal'ē-ŭs). (pl. *mallei*) 1. [NA] The largest of the three auditory ossicles in the middle ear, attached to the eardrum, and articulating with the incus. 2. Glanders, an acute febrile disease with suppuration and necrosis of cartilage and bone.

Mallophaga (măl-ŏf'ă-gă) [Gr. *mallos,* wool, + *phagein,* to eat]. An order of insects that includes biting lice.

malnutrition (măl"nū-trĭ'shŭn). Lack of necessary or proper food substances in the body or improper absorption and distribution of them.

Malnutrition Physical Signs of Deficiency State*

Infants and Children

Lack of subcutaneous fat

Wrinkling of skin on light stroking

Poor muscle tone

Pallor

Rough skin (toad skin)

Hemorrhage of newborn, vitamin K deficiency

Bad posture

Nasal blackheads and whiteheads

Sores—at angles of mouth, cheilosis

Rapid heart

Red tongue

Square head, wrists enlarged, rib beading

Vincent's angina, thrush

Serious dental abnormalities

Corneal and conjunctival changes

Adolescents and Adults

Nasolabial sebaceous plugs

Sores at corners of mouth, cheilosis

Vincent's angina

Minimal changes in tongue color or texture

Red swollen lingual papillae

*Committee on Medical Nutrition, National Research Council.

Glossitis

Papillary atrophy of tongue

Stomatitis

Spongy, bleeding gums

Muscle tenderness, extremities

Poor muscle tone

Loss of vibratory sensation

Increase or decrease of tendon reflexes

Hyperesthesia of skin

Bilateral symmetrical dermatitis

Purpura

Dermatitis; facial butterfly, perineal, scrotal, vulval

Thickening and pigmentation of skin over bony prominences

Nonspecific vaginitis

Follicular hyperkeratosis of extensor surfaces of extremities

Rachitic chest deformity

Anemia not responding to iron

Fatigue of visual accommodation

Vascularization of cornea

Conjunctival changes

mal"occlu'sion. Imperfect occlusion of the teeth. May be due to imperfect development, loss of teeth, abnormal growth of jaws.

malonylurea (mal-ō-nil-ū're-ă). Barbituric acid. SEE: *barbituric.*

malpighian (măl-pĭg'ĭ-ăn). [Marcello Malpighi, It. anatomist, founder of histology, 1628-1694]. Of, related to, or discovered by Malpighi.

    m. body. 1. A malpighian corpuscle, q.v. 2. A splenic nodule, a spherical, ovoid body found in the white pulp of the spleen. Similar in structure to a lymphatic nodule.

    m. corpuscle. A spherical body found in cortex of kidney consisting of a glomerulus and Bowman's capsule. SYN: *renal corpuscle.*

    m. layer. The innermost layer of the epidermis. SYN: *stratum germinativum; stratum mucosum; stratum Malpighii.*

    m. pyramid. A renal pyramid.

malposition (măl-pō-zĭ'shŭn) [L. *malus,* bad, + *positus,* from *ponere,* to place]. Faulty or abnormal position or placement, esp. of the body or one of its parts.

malpractice ["+ Gr. *praxis*, an action]. Incorrect or negligent treatment of a patient by persons responsible for medical care, such as physicians and nurses.

malpresentation ["+ *praesentatiō*, a presenting]. Abnormal position of fetus rendering natural delivery difficult or impossible.

malt [AS. *mealt*]. Germinated grain, usually barley, used in manufacture of ale and beer. Contains carbohydrates (dextrin, maltose), a diastase, and proteins and is used as a food, esp. in wasting diseases.

    m. extract. A viscous, light brown fluid obtained from malt steeped in water.

    m. sugar. Maltose, q.v.

Malta fever. An infectious disease caused by one of three species of Brucella (Br. melitensis from goats, Br. suis from swine, and Br. abortus from cattle). Transmitted principally from animals to man. May occur in acute or chronic form. SYN: *Mediterranean fever; Neapolitan fever; Gibraltar fever; undulant fever.*

    SYM: Swelling of the joints and spleen, excessive perspiration, weakness and anemia, and recurrent febrile attacks. Organisms tend to localize in tissues of the reticuloendothelial system, esp. spleen, liver, bone marrow, and lymph nodes.

maltase (mawl'tās) [AS. *mealt*, grain]. A salivary and pancreatic enzyme which acts on maltose converting it by hydrolysis to glucose. SEE: *digestion; enzyme.*

maltose (mawl'tōs). Malt sugar ($C_{12}H_{22}O_{11}$). A disaccharide present in malt, malt products, and sprouting seeds. It is formed by the hydrolysis of starch and is converted into gluscose by the enzyme maltase, q.v. SEE: *carbohydrates; disaccharose.*

maltosur'ia. Presence of maltose in urine.

malturned. Abnormally turned, said of a tooth turned on its long axis.

malum (mālŭm) [L. an evil]. A disease.

    m. coxae senilis. Hip disease in the aged, esp. osteoarthritis.

    m. perforans pedis. Perforating ulcer of the foot. It begins with thickening of the epidermis.

    m. vene'reum. Syphilis.

malunion [L. *malus*, bad, + *uniō*, oneness]. Growth of the fragments of a fractured bone in a faulty position, forming an imperfect union.

mamelonation (mam-ĕl-ō-nā'shun) [Fr. *mamelle*, from L. *mamma*, breast]. Nipplelike prominences on a part or organ.

mamma (măm'ă) [L. breast]. (pl. *mammae*) [NA]. One of two cutaneous glandular structures which secrete milk in the female; over the anterolateral area between the 3rd and 6th ribs when not pendulous. SYN: *breast; mammary gland.*

mammal (mam'al). An animal of the class Mammalia. Characterized by having breasts from which milk is available for the nourishment of the newborn.

mammalgia (mam-al'jĭ-ă) ["+ Gr. *algos*, pain.]. Pain in the breast. SYN: *mastalgia.*

mammary (mam'ă-rĭ) [L. *mamma*, breast]. Pert. to the breast.

    m. glands. Two compound glands of the female breast that secrete milk. They are made up of lobes and lobules bound together by areolar tissue.

    The main ducts are 15 to 20 in number and are known as lactiferous ducts, each one discharging through a separate orifice upon the surface of the nipple. The dilatations of the ducts form reservoirs for the milk during lactation, q.v. The pink, or dark-colored, skin around the nipple is called the areola, q.v. SYN: *mammae.*

    RS: breast; caked b.; galactagogue; gynecomastia; mammectomy; mastectomy; mastopathy; nipple.

mammectomy (măm-mek'to-mĭ) ["+ Gr. *ektomē*, excision]. Removal of the breast. SYN: *mastectomy.*

mammilla (măm-ĭl'lă) [L. nipple]. 1. Nipple. 2. Any structure resembling a nipple.

mammillary (mam'ĭl-lar-ĭ) [L. *mammilla*, nipple]. Shaped like or concerning a nipple.

mammillated (mam'mĭl-lă-tĕd). Having protuberances like a nipple.

mammillation (măm-ĭl-lā'shŭn). 1. Condition of having a granulated appearance or nipplelike projections. 2. A nipplelike protuberance.

mammilliform (mam-mĭl'ĭ-form) [L. *mammilla*, nipple, + *forma*, shape]. Shaped like a nipple.

mammilliplasty (măm-mĭl'ĭ-plăs-tĭ) ["+ Gr. *plassein*, to form]. Plastic operation on a nipple. SYN: *theleplasty.*

mammillitis (măm''mĭl-ĭ'tĭs) [L. *mamma*, breast, + Gr. *-itis*, inflammation]. Inflammation of a nipple. SYN: *thelitis.*

mammitis (măm-ĭ'tĭs) ["+ Gr. *-itis*, inflammation]. Inflamed condition of the breast. SYN: *mastitis.*

mammography (mam-og'ră-fĭ). Study of the breast by use of X ray.

mammoplasty (mam'o-plas"tĭ). Surgical reconstruction of the breasts; sometimes augmented by substances such as fat tissue or silicone to alter the size and shape.

mammose (mam'ōs) [L. *mamma*, breast]. 1. Having unusually large breasts. 2. Shaped like a breast.

mammotomy (măm-ot'ō-mĭ) ["+ Gr. *tome*, incision]. Surgery of a breast. SYN: *mastotomy*.

man [AS. *mann*]. 1. Member of the human race; a human being. 2. Male member of the species as distinguished from female. 3. The human race, collectively; mankind. SEE: words beginning with *anthrop.*

manchineel (măn″kĭ-nēl′) [Sp. *manzanilla*, small apple]. A tropical tree native to America, Hippomane mancinella, which contains a milky, poisonous sap. Contact with the sap causes blistering of the skin. The fruit is poisonous also.

mancinism (man′sĭn-ĭzm) [L. *mancus*, crippled]. State of being left-handed.

mandelic acid (man-dĕl′ik). A crystalline compound derived from benzaldehyde.

USES: In the treatment of urinary infections, esp. pyelitis and cystitis.

It is necessary that the acidity of the urine be controlled; thus an acidifying agent, as ammonium chloride, usually is required to maintain urine pH of 5.5.

Because of renal irritation it is advised that the drug be used not longer than 12-14 days.

Restriction of fluid intake is essential to keep urine volume below 1500 ml. per day in order that an effective concentration of mandelic acid is obtained.

mandible (man′dĭ-bl) [L. a jaw, from *mando*, to chew]. The horseshoe-shaped bone forming the lower jaw; the inferior maxilla. SYN: *mandibula.*

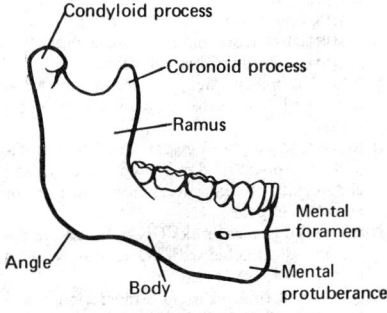

Condyloid process
Coronoid process
Ramus
Mental foramen
Angle
Body
Mental protuberance

MANDIBLE—LATERAL VIEW

mandibula (man-dib′u-la) [L.]. (pl. *mandibulae*) [NA]. The bone of the lower jaw having a horseshoe shape.

mandibular (măn-dib′ū-lar). Rel. to the lower jaw.

   m. reflex. Clonic movement resulting from percussing or stroking lower jaw.

m. and m. enema. One given because its ingredients form gases and distend the bowel, thus causing frequent and copious bowel movements. A mixture of milk and molasses, hence its name. SEE: *enema, m. and m.*

mandrin (man′drĭn) [Fr.]. A guide or stilet for a flexible catheter.

manducation (măn-dū-ka′shŭn) [L. *manducare*, to chew]. The chewing of food. SYN: *mastication.*

maneuver [Fr. *manoeuvre*, from L. *manu operari*, to work by hand]. 1. Any dextrous or skillful procedure. 2. In obstetrics, manipulation of the fetus and placenta to aid in delivery. SEE: *labor.*

   m., Crede's. Method of expressing the placenta in which the hand is placed on the fundus of the uterus with the thumb on the ant. wall and the fingers on the post. wall, the placenta being pushed out by pressure in the direction of the birth canal.

   m., Leopold's. Method of abdominal palpation for the diagnosis of presentation and position of the fetus in utero.

   m., Mauriceau-Smellie-Veit. Method employed to deliver the aftercoming head in breech presentation. Straddling the baby over the right arm, the index finger of that hand is introduced into the mouth of the child and applied over the maxilla; two fingers of the other hand are then hooked over the neck, grasping the shoulders. Downward traction is made until the occiput appears under the symphysis pubis. The body of the child is now raised up toward the mother's abdomen and the mouth, nose, brow, and occiput are successively brought over the perineum.

   m., Muller's. Inspiratory effort with a closed glottis at the end of expiration. This produces negative intrathoracic pressure.

   m., Munro Kerr. A method for determining the presence of disproportion bet. the fetal head and the maternal pelvis. The fetal head is pushed into the pelvis with the right hand on the abdomen, while with two fingers of the left hand in the vagina the possibilities of engagement of the head are noted. At the same time the thumb of the left hand feels over the brim of the pelvis to determine the degrees of overlapping.

   m., Pinard's. Fingers are placed behind the fetal knee, pushing it toward and past the fetal body, causing flexion of knee. Foot is then grasped and brought down in breech presentation.

   m., Prague. A method for the delivery of the aftercoming head in a breech delivery when the occiput is post.

m., Scanzoni. Double application of forceps in post. position of the occiput.

m., Valsalva's. Forcible expiration against the closed glottis. This produces increased intrathoracic pressure.

manganese (man'gă-nēz) [L. *manganesium*]. SYMB: *Mn.* At. wt. 54.938; at. no. 25; sp. gr. 7.21. A metal element found in many foods, in some plants, and in the tissues of the higher animals. An essential element needed for normal bone metabolism and many enzyme reactions. Deficiency in humans has not been demonstrated.

SOURCES: Bananas, bran, beans, beets, blueberries, chard, chocolate, peas, leafy vegetables, and whole grains.

POISONING: A rather uncommon industrial poison found usually after prolonged exposure.

SYM: Muscular weakness, peculiar gait, tremors, central nervous system disturbances, salivation.

F.A. TREATMENT: Removal from source of exposure.

mania (mā'nĭ-ă) [Gr. madness]. 1. Madness, characterized by excessive excitement. 2. A form of psychosis characterized by exalted feelings, delusions of grandeur, elevation of mood, psychomotor overactivity, and overproduction of ideas. SEE: *psychosis, manic-depressive.* 3. Used as combining form to signify obsessive preoccupation.

m. à potu. An obsolete term for several alcoholic psychoses. Used to indicate delirium tremens or alcoholic mania. SEE: *pathological reaction to alcohol.*

m., puerperal. A form of mental derangement that occurs occasionally following childbirth.

m., religious. Mania resulting from excessive religious fervor.

m., transitory. Attacks of severe frenzy, of short duration.

m., unproductive. Behavior characteristic of mania with lack of spontaneity in speech, or muteness sometimes seen in manic-depressive psychosis. SEE: *alcoholism.*

maniac (mā'nĭ-ăk). A person with mental disease, usually one violently disturbed or excited.

maniacal (mă-nī'ăk-l). 1. Related to or characterized by mania. 2. Afflicted with mania.

man'ic-depres'sive psychosis. Cyclic or circular affective psychosis in which there are alternating moods of depression and mania. SEE: *psychosis, manic-depressive.*

man'ikin [D. *manneken,* little man]. 1. A model of the human body or its parts, used esp. in teaching anatomy and nursing procedures.

manipulation [L. *manipulāre,* to handle]. Skillful or dextrous treatment or procedure involving use of the hands.

RS: massage; osteopathy; spondylotherapy; Swedish gymnastics, movements.

manipula'tive surgery. Use of manipulation in surgery, bonesetting, etc.

man'nerism. A peculiar modification or exaggeration of style or habit of dress, speech, or action.

Mann'kopf's sign. [Emil W. Mannkopf, Ger. physician, 1836-1918] Pulse acceleration exhibited on pressing a painful point. Not present in feigned pain.

manometer (măn-om'et-er) [Gr. *manos,* thin, + *metron,* measure]. Device for determining liquid or gaseous pressure.

Mansonia. A genus of mosquito in tropical countries; transmits microfilaria to man.

mantle (man'tl) [AS. *mentel,* a garment]. A covering structure or layer. SYN: *pallium.*

Mantoux's reaction, test (man-tū'). [Charles, Fr. physician, 1877-1947]. Intracutaneous injection of old tuberculin. Within 24-72 hours the area becomes hard (indurated) and red if either an active or inactive tuberculous infection is present.

manual (man'ū-al) [L. *manus,* hand]. 1. Pert. to the hands. 2. Performed by or with the hands.

manubrium (man-u'brĭ-um) [L. handle]. 1. The upper bone of the sternum articulating with the clavicle and first pair of costal cartilages. 2. That portion of the malleus, q.v., resembling a handle. SEE: *umbo.*

m. sterni. [NA]. The upper segment of the sternum.

manus (ma'nus) [L.]. (pl. *manus*) The hand.

manustupration (man"u-stū-prā'shun) ["+ *stupro,* to defile]. Masturbation.

marantic (mă-răn'tĭk) [Gr. *marantikos,* wasting away]. 1. Pert. to marasmus. 2. Wasting away.

marantology ["+ *logos,* study]. Study, care, and treatment of debilitated, elderly, and chronically ill patients whose outlook for recovery is poor.

marasmic (mă-raz'mĭk) [Gr. *marasmos,* a dying away]. Affected with marasmus; wasting away. SYN: *marantic.*

marasmus (măr-ăz'mŭs). Emaciation, wasting. Infantile atrophy which occurs almost wholly as a sequel to acute diseases, esp. diarrheic diseases of infancy.

Most common from 6-18 months of age. Extreme wasting, child becoming a mere living skeleton.

SYM: May be vomiting and diarrhea, restless sleep, general malaise, nervousness, abdominal pain, and headache. Feet edematous, urine scanty, anus and nates chafed and sore from urinal acidity and alkalinity or acidity of evacuations. Prostration becomes extreme, heart weak, abdomen distended, and mesenteric glands enlarged.

PROG: Fair, but recovery is slow.

TREATMENT: Often change of climate or simply from city to country is of great benefit. Keep in fresh air as much as possible. Oil baths.

DIET: Blandest kind of nourishment, as free from starch as possible. Different foods must be tried till one is found to suit the case. Constitutional treatment.

marble bones. Abnormally calcified bones with spotted appearance in a roentgenogram. SYN: *Albers-Schönberg disease, osteopetrosis.*

mareo (măr-ā'ō) [Sp. dizziness]. Seasickness.

   m. de la Cordillera. Mountain sickness.

Marfan's syndrome. [Bernard-Jean Antonin Marfan, Fr. physician, 1858-1942] A hereditary condition of connective tissue, bones, muscles, ligaments, and skeletal structures.

   SYM: Irregular and unsteady gait, lean and tall with stooping shoulders. Lincoln is said by some to have been thus afflicted. SYN: *arachnodactyly; dolichostenomelia.*

margarine. Artificial butter made from refined vegetable oils or a combination of vegetable oils and animal fats. Coloring material and vitamin A are added. Contains about 35 Calories per teaspoonful. SYN: *oleomargarine.*

margin (măr'jĭn) [L. *margo, marginalis*, border, edge.]. A boundary, such as the edge of a structure of the anatomy. SYN: *margo.*

marginal (mar'jĭn-ăl). Concerning a margin or border.

margination (mar-jĭ-nā'shŭn). Adhesion of leukocytes to walls of blood vessel in first stages of inflammation.

margin'oplasty [L. *marginalis*, border, + Gr. *plassein*, to mold]. Plastic surgery of a border, as of an eyelid.

margo (mar'go) [L.]. (pl. *margines*) [NA]. A border or edge.

   m. acutus. A sharp margin of the heart extending from apex to the right.

   m. obtusus. Portion of a line extending from apex to root of pulmonary artery which lies along rounded left side of left ventricle.

Marie's disease (mă-rē'). [Pierre Marie, Fr. physician, 1853-1940]. Chronic condition of enlargement of bones and soft tissues of hands, feet, and face. SYN: *acromegaly, hypertrophic pulmonary osteoarthropathy.*

Marie's sign. Hand tremor seen in exophthalmic goiter.

marijuana (măr'ĭ-wä'nä). Also spelled marihuana. An intoxicating, excitant drug, usually in cigarette form and used illegally in the U.S. and elsewhere. Obtained from leaves and flowers of the Indian hemp plant (Cannabis sativa). Psychologically habituating but not habit-forming. Withdrawal of marijuana causes no such physical symptoms as opiate withdrawal does. Drug is considered to have no medical value.

Mariotte's law (măr''ē-ōt'). [Edme Mariotte, Fr. physicist, 1620-1684]. Boyle's law, q.v.

Mariotte's spot. The blind spot of the eye. SYN: *optic papilla.*

mark [AS. *mearc*]. Any nevus, bruise, cut, or spot on the surface of a body.

   m., birth-. Blemish on the skin at birth. A nevus.

   m., port-wine. A congenital hemangioma or nevus vascularis, q.v.

   m., strawberry. Same as nevus vascularis, q.v.

marker. A device or substance used to indicate or mark something.

   m., fecal. A substance, such as carmine, ingested to mark the beginning and end of fecal collection periods.

Marmo's method (mar'mō). [Serafino Marmo, contemporary It. obstetrician]. A manner of performing artificial respiration in asphyxiated infants. The physician places his hands in the infant's axillae and thereby raises the subject up in the air and suddenly releases the child. A sudden drop of a foot or two will cause inspiration to occur; expiration is effected by pressure of the physician's hands against the chest wall.

mar'row [AS. *mearh*]. The soft tissue occupying the medullary cavities of long bones, some haversian canals, and spaces between trabeculae of cancellous or spongy bone. Of two types, red and yellow, q.v.

   In adult bone there are red and fat (yellow) m. The yellow m. is found esp. in medullary cavity of long bones, and the red in spongy bones.

   It consists of both fat and red marrow; from 20-80% fat marrow, to 100% red marrow. The marrow may be as high as 5% of body weight in an adult.

   RS: giant cell; leukomyelitis.

   m., gelatinous. Yellow marrow of old or emaciated persons, almost devoid of fat and having a gelatinous consistency.

   m., red. Found in cancellous tissue of bone. Concerned with the production of blood cells and hemoglobin.

   m., spinal. Spinal cord.

m., yellow. Found in the medullary canal of long bones. Consists principally of fat cells and thought to have little to do with blood formation.

marsh fever. Malarial fever.

marsh gas. Methane, q.v.

Marsh's test. [James Marsh, Eng. chemist, 1789-1846] A test to detect the presence of arsenic.

marsupialization (mar-sū″pī-al-ĭ-za′shun) [L. *marsupium,* pouch]. Process of raising the borders of an evacuated tumor sac to the edges of the abdominal wound, and stitching them there to form a pouch. The interior of the sac suppurates and gradually closes by granulation.

maschaladenitis (mǎs″kal-ad″ē-ni′tis) [Gr. *maschalē,* armpit, + *adēn,* gland, + *-itis,* inflammation]. Inflammation of axillary glands.

maschaliatry (mas-kal-ĭ-at′rĭ) ["+ *iatreia,* healing]. Medication by axillary inunctions.

masculation (mǎs-kū-lā′shŭn) [L. *masculus,* a male]. Development of male sex characteristics.

masculine (mǎs′kū-lĭn). 1. Pert. to the male sex. 2. Having male characteristics.

masculinovoblastoma (mas″kū-lĭn-o″vō-blas-to′ma). A benign ovarian tumor which resembles, microscopically, adrenal cortical tissue. Usually results in masculinization.

maser. Acronym for *m*icrowave *a*mplification by *s*timulation *e*mission of *r*adiation. A device which produces a small, non-diverging radiation beam.

mask [Fr. *masque*]. 1. A covering for the face, as the gauze mask of a surgeon or nurse. 2. The countenance or appearance of the face such as appears in certain pathologic conditions.

    m., BLB. A mask for administering oxygen to aviators or to patients during anesthesia. Invented by Boothby, Lovelace, and Bulbulian.

    m., death. A plaster cast of the face molded soon after death.

    m., ecchymotic. Cyanotic facies accompanying traumatic asphyxia.

    m., Hutchinson's. A feeling of compression over face as though one is wearing a mask. A symptom of tabes dorsalis.

    m., luetic. Blotchy brown pigmentation of cheeks, forehead, and temples, seen in tertiary syphilis.

    m., Parkinson's. Immobile facial appearance as a result of paralysis agitans (Parkinson's disease). The face is devoid of expression.

    m. of pregnancy. Pigmented areas seen on the face of some pregnant women. SYN: *chloasma gravidarum.*

masked (mǎskd). Concealed, esp. as in masked infection. Ex: Women exposed to rubella during the first trimester of pregnancy may be given immune globulin. This may prevent clinical symptoms of rubella in the mother, yet the fetus may be adversely affected and may be born with congenital defects.

masochism (mas′ō-kizm). [Leopold von Sacher-Masoch, Aust. novelist, 1835-1895] Abnormal sexual passion in which one gains pleasure from the abuse or cruelty of his or her associate; hence any pleasure obtained from being abused or dominated. Opposed to sadism. SEE: *algolagnia; flagellation.*

masochist (mas′ō-kĭst). A person addicted to masochism.

mass [L. *massa*]. 1. A quantity of material, such as cells which unite or adhere to each other. 2. Soft, solid preparation for internal use, and of such consistency that it may be molded into pills. It is frequently prescribed alone or with other agents and may be given in pill form or put into capsules.

    m., cell. An aggregation of cells which serves as the primordium (anlage) of a future organ or part.

    m., epithelial. Inner portion of a developing gonad enclosed within the germinal epithelium.

    m., inner cell. Mass of cells within the blastocyst, q.v., from which the embryo, yolk sac, and amnion develop.

    m., intermediate cell. A plate of nonsegmented mesoderm lying lateral to the segments (somites) and connecting them to the nonsegmented lateral mesoderm. SYN: *nephrotome,* q.v.

mas'sa [L.]. [NA]. Mass.

    m. intermedia. The middle commissure, an inconstant mass of gray matter extending across third ventricle and connecting adjacent surfaces of the thalami.

massage [Gr. *massein,*to knead]. Manipulation; methodical pressure, friction, and kneading of the body. Must always be applied upon the bare skin.

    RS: anatripsis; effleurage; flagellation; friction; frolement; fustigation; kneading; malaxation; masseur; petrissage; Swedish gymnastics, movements; tapotement; vibration.

    m., auditory. Massage of the eardrum membrane.

    m., cardiac. Manual manipulation of the heart to restore heart beat after heart has stopped. Accomplished through an incision in the chest wall.

   m., douche. Massage combined with the application of a douche.

   m., electrovibratory. Massage by means of an electric vibrator.

   m., external cardiac. Accomplished by manual, rhythmic compression of chest wall and infraxiphoid area. This forces blood out of the heart and, when pressure is removed, allows the heart to fill as if the heart were beating. SYN: *external cardiac compression.*

   m., general. Consists of centripetal stroking in connection with some muscular kneading from the toes upward. Principally used for nervousness, being an important part of the well known rest cure. Useful in connection with certain baths, duration 30-40 minutes. As soon as a part is massaged, it should be given a few passive rotary movements and afterwards covered up.

   m., hydropneumatic. Massage by means of air forced through a tube at the end of which is a chamber containing water, the water chamber being applied to the part massaged.

   m., introductory. Consists of centripetal strokings around the affected part; as in an affection of the knee joint, where introductory massage should be used on lower part of thigh and somewhat below the knee. Very useful in cases where it is impossible for operator to apply treatment directly to diseased parts.

   m., local. Treatment confined to particular parts.

   m., tremolo. A type of mechanical massage.

   m., vapor. Treatment of a cavity by a medicated and nebulized vapor under interrupted pressure.

   m., vibratory. Massage by rapidly repeated tapping of the affected surface by means of a vibrating hammer or sound.

masseter (mas-sē'tĕr) [Gr. *masētēr*, chewer]. The muscle which closes the mouth and is the principal muscle in mastication.

masseur (mă-sur') [Fr.]. 1. A man who gives massages. 2. An instrument for massaging.

masseuse (mă-sūz') [Fr.]. A woman who gives massages.

massive (măs'sĭv) [Fr. *massif*]. Bulky; consisting of a large mass; huge.

   m. collapse of the lung. Dyspnea, cyanosis, shock, and pain in chest, esp. in patients who have suffered severe shock and collapse after abdominal operation or thyroidectomy.

Collapse is due to obstruction of a main bronchus by a mucous plug or foreign body.

   TREATMENT: If caused by mucus, CO_2 inhalation and breathing exercises, antibiotics, and oxygen. If due to foreign body, remove it. SEE: *lung.*

massotherapy (măs-ō-ther'ă-pĭ) [Gr. *massein*, to knead, + *therapeia*, treatment]. Use of massage in treatment of disease.

mastadenitis (măst-ad-ĕ-ni'tis) [Gr. *mastos*, breast, + *adēn*, gland, + *-itis*, inflammation]. A mammary gland inflammation.

mastadenoma. A tumor of the breast.

mastalgia (mast-al'jĭ-ă) ["+ *algos*, pain]. Pain in the breast. SYN: *mastodynia.*

mastatrophia (mast-ă-trō'fĭ-ă). Atrophy of breasts. SYN: *mastatrophy.*

mastatrophy (mast-at'rō-fĭ). Atrophy of breasts. SYN: *mastatrophia.*

mastauxe (mas-tawk'se) ["+ *auxē*, increase]. Enlargement of the breast.

mast cells [Gr. *masten*, to feed]. Connective tissue cells that contain heparin and histamine in their granules. Important in cellular defense mechanisms including blood coagulation needed during injury or infection.

mastecchymosis (măs-tĕk'ĭ'mō-sĭs). Ecchymosis of the breast.

mastectomy (mas-tek'to-mĭ) [Gr. *mastos*, breast, + *ektomē*, excision]. Excision of the breast.

   POSTOPERATIVE NP: The doctor will tell the nurse how much information is to be given the patient and her family concerning the physical findings and laboratory reports. One of the nurse's responsibilities will be to recognize the patient's emotional reactions and to reassure her. Fear and anxiety are frequently present after this type of operation. The degree of mobility of the arm and shoulder will be determined by the surgeon and instructions for exercise must be carefully followed. Here again, the nurse is essential to the patient's physical and mental recovery.

Master two-step test. [A. M. Master, contemporary New York physician] A standardized exercise test used to elicit electrocardiographic changes of coronary artery insufficiency.

masthelcosis (măs-thĕl-kō'sĭs) ["+ *elkōsis*, ulceration]. Ulcerated condition of breast.

mastication (măs-tĭ-kā'shŭn) [L. *masticāre*, to chew]. Chewing. The comminution and insalivation of the food in the mouth is the first stage of digestion.

   Certain muscles close the mouth, raise and lower the mandible, tense the cheeks, and accomplish the highly coordinated movements of the tongue.

The smell and taste of food stimulate sensory nerves, which reflexly elicit both motor and secretory activity in various digestive organs. Thus the salivary glands begin to secrete at once, and both the glands and the musculature of the stomach gradually become active. The saliva dissolves some substances, dilutes materials too concentrated for the stomach, hydrolyzes (due to the salivary enzyme, ptyalin) some of the starch to maltose, and lubricates material to be swallowed.

RS: absorption; amasesis; enzyme; gastric and salivary digestion.

masticatory (măs′tĭk-ă-tō″rĭ) [L. *masticāre*, to chew]. 1. Pert. to mastication. 2. Any substance chewed to stimulate secretion of saliva.

Mastigophora (măs-tĭ-gŏf′ō-ră). A class of protozoa characterized by the possession of one or more flagella. Includes both free-living and parasitic forms.

mastitis (măs-tī′tĭs) [Gr. *mastos*, breast, + *-itis*, inflammation]. Inflammation of the breast. Most common in women during lactation, but it may occur at any age.

ETIOL: May be due to entry of disease-producing germs through the nipple. In most cases there is a crack or abrasion of the nipple. Infection begins in one lobule but may extend to other areas.

SYM: The earliest sign is a triangular flush generally underneath the breast. There may be a high temperature and pulse rate.

m., cystic. M. resulting in formation of cysts which give the breast a nodular feeling upon palpation.

m., interstitial. Inflammation of connective tissue of the breast.

m., parenchymatous. Inflammation of the secreting tissue of the breast.

m., puerperal. M. in later portion of puerperium and often accompanied by suppuration. Breast may become indurated owing to retention of milk.

m., stagnation. Caked breast; painful distention occurring during early lactation.

mastocarcinoma (măst″ō-kăr-sĭn-ō′mă) [″+ *karkinos*, crab, cancer, + *-ōma*, tumor]. Carcinoma of the breast.

mastochondroma (mast″ō-kon-drō′mă) [″+ *chondros*, cartilage, + *-ōma*, tumor]. Cartilaginous breast tumor.

mastodynia (măst-ō-dĭn′ĭ-ă) [″+ *odynē*, pain]. Pain in the breast.

mastography [″+ *graphein*, to write]. X-ray study of the breasts.

mastoid (mas′toyd) [″+ *eidos*, form]. 1. Formed like a nipple. 2. Pert. to mastoid process of the temporal bone. 3. The mastoid process of temporal bone.

m. antrum. Small chamber by which the mastoid cells communicate with the tympanic cavity.

m. bone. Mastoid process of temporal bone.

m. cells. Air spaces in the mastoid process of the temporal bone.

m. disease. Inflammation of mastoid.

m. operation. Surgical drainage of mastoid cells.

m. portion of temporal bone. Portion of temporal bone lying behind ext. opening of ear and below temporal line. Contains mastoid cells and antrum and its inner surface bears a deep curved sigmoid groove which transmits a part of the transverse sinus.

m. process. Nipple-shaped process of mastoid portion of temporal bone extending downward and forward behind ext. auditory meatus. Serves for attachment of sternocleidomastoid, splenius capitis, and longissimus capitis muscles.

mastoidal (măs-toy′dăl). Rel. to mastoid process.

mastoida′le. The mastoid process' lowest point.

mastoidalgia (mas-toyd-al′jĭ-ă) [Gr. *mastos*, breast, + *eidos*, form, + *algos*, pain]. Pain in the mastoid.

mastoidec′tomy [″+ ″+ *ektomē*, excision]. Excision of mastoid cells. Rarely indicated since advent of antibiotics. May be simple, involving exenteration of the air cells of the mastoid process alone, or radical, involving the middle ear.

NP: Patient in dorsal position with small sand bag under shoulders. The area of operation is shaved, washed thoroughly, and painted with skin antiseptics. Two sterile towels placed lengthwise under head and shoulders. One is brought up around head and is kept in place with towel clips. The other covers end of table. A laparotomy sheet is placed over patient, with opening over area of operation.

mastoideocentesis (măs-toyd″ē-ō-sen-tē′sĭs) [Gr. *mastos*, breast, + *eidos*, form, + *kentēsis*, puncture]. Surgical puncture of the mastoid process.

mastoiditis (măs-toyd-ī′tis) [″+ ″+ *-itis*, inflammation]. Inflammation of the air cells of the mastoid process.

COMPLICATIONS: Perisinus abscess, periphlebitis, lateral sinus thrombosis. Involvement is metastatic through blood vessels without erosion of sinus plate or extension of suppuration directly through sinus plate into the sinus.

SYM: Fever, chills, tenderness over emissary vein, leukocytosis, sepsis.

TREATMENT: Surgical.

m., Bezold's. Abscess underneath insertion of sternocleidomastoid muscle due to pus breaking through the tip cell.

m., externa. Inflammation of the periosteum of the mastoid process.

m., sclerosing. M. in which there is thickening and hardening of trabeculae between mastoid cells.

mastoidotomy (mas-toyd-ŏt'ō-mĭ) ["+ "+ *tomē*, incision]. Incision into mastoid process.

mastology (mast-ŏl'ō-jĭ) ["+ *logos*, study]. Science or study of the breasts.

mastomenia (mas-tō-mē'nĭ-ă) ["+ *mēnēs*, menses]. Vicarious menstruation from the breast.

mastoncus (mas-tong'kŭs) ["+ *onkos*, bulk]. Any tumor of the breast.

mastooccipital (mas"tō-ŏk-sĭp'ĭ-tăl). Rel. to mastoid process and occipital bone.

mastopathy (măs-tŏp'ă-thĭ). Any disease of the mammary glands.

mastopexy (mas'tō-pĕks-ĭ) [Gr. *mastos*, breast + *pēxis*, fixation]. Surgical correction of a pendulous breast. SYN: *mazopexy*.

mastoplasia (măst-ō-plā'zĭ-ă) ["+ *plassein*, to form]. Hyperplasia of mammary gland tissue. SYN: *mazoplasia*

mastoptosis (mas"tō-tō'sis) ["+ *ptōsis*, fall]. Pendulous breasts.

mastorrhagia (măs-tōr-ā'jĭ-ă) ["+ *rhegnynai*, to burst forth]. Hemorrhage from the breast.

mastoscirrhus (măs-tō-skĭr'ŭs) ["+ *skirros*, hardness]. A hard cancer of breast.

mastos'tomy. Incision into the breast.

mastotomy (mas-tŏt'ō-mĭ). Surgical incision of a breast.

masturbate (mas'ter-bāt) [L. *masturbārī*, to pollute one's self.]. 1. To induce self-excitement through manipulation of the genital organs. 2. To perform masturbation on another.

masturbation (măs"ter-bā'shŭn) [L. *masturbārī*, to pollute one's self]. Stimulation of genitals, usually to orgasm, by some means other than sexual intercourse.

RS: manustupration; onanism.

match'es. Lucifer matches usually are made of phosphorus, q.v., and potassium chlorate and may be lit by friction.

"Safety" matches contain antimony, sulfide, and potassium chlorate and must be lit

by striking on the box which is covered with red phosphorus.

POISONING SYM: Gastrointestinal irritation with blood changes.

F. A. TREATMENT: Wash out stomach with water or very dilute potassium permanganate. Repeated catharsis.

matching. 1. To compare in order to select similar objects. 2. To be identical, equal, or exactly alike.

m. of blood. Technique and procedure for determining the immunologic and genetic characteristics of the patient's blood so that appropriate blood may be used for transfusion. SEE: *blood groups.*

m., cross. Technique of determining the compatibility of the patient's blood with that of blood being considered for use in transfusion. SEE: *blood groups.*

maté (mah-tā') [Sp. *mate*, vessel for preparing leaves]. Paraguay tea made from the leaves of Ilex paraguayensis. Said to contain caffeine and tannin.

USES: Diaphoretic and diuretic.

materia alba (mă-tē'rĭ-ă ăl'bă) [L. white matter]. White cheeselike deposit along gum line about the necks of teeth, consisting of mucus, epithelial cells, food particles, leukocytes, and microorganisms.

materia medica (mă-tē'rĭ-ă mĕd'ĭ-kă) [L., medical matter]. 1. That branch of science dealing with all drugs used in treatment of diseases, their source, preparation, dosage, and use. 2. A substance used to prepare a medicine.

RS: active principle; drug action; drugs and their administration; medical preparations; pharmacognosy; pharmacology.

mater'nal [L. *maternus*, from *mater*, mother]. 1. Rel. to the mother. 2. From a mother.

m. deprivation syndrome. Emotional, physical, and nutritional neglect of an infant or young child. Children suffering from this are emotionally disturbed, withdrawn, apathetic, and retarded in growth and development. The lack of expected growth and development is thought to be due mostly to nutritional neglect rather than emotional neglect.

maternity (mă-ter'nĭ-tĭ). 1. The condition of motherhood. 2. Lying-in hospital or the obstetrical department of a hospital.

matrix (mā'trĭks) [L.]. (pl. *mat'rices*) 1. The womb. 2. The basic substance from which a thing is made; i. e.; tooth or nail. 3. The intercellular material of a tissue. 4. Mold for casting.

m. unguis. [NA]. Nail bed.

matrixitis (mā-trĭks-ī'tĭs). Inflammation of the nail bed. SYN: *onychia.*

matter. 1. Anything that occupies space. May be gaseous, liquid, or solid. 2. Pus.

m., gray. The gray substance of the spinal cord and brain, consisting principally of nerve-cell bodies, dendrites, and portions of axons. Also found in peripheral ganglia and retina of eye. SYN: *substantia grisea.*

m., white. The white substance of spinal cord and brain, consisting principally of nerve fibers (myelinated and unmyelinated). SYN: *substantia alba.*

maturate (măt'ū-rāt) [L. *maturus,* ripe]. 1. To ripen; to mature. 2. To suppurate.

maturation (măt-ū-rā'shŭn). 1. Maturing; ripening, as a graafian follicle. 2. Suppuration. 3. The process in the development of germ cells (spermatozoa and ova) occurring in spermatogenesis or oogenesis in which the number of chromosomes is reduced from the diploid number to the haploid number (one half of diploid). Includes two cell divisions, the first qualitative (meiosis), the second quantitative. SEE: *oogenesis, spermatogenesis.*

mature (ma-tūr'). 1. Fully developed or ripened. 2. To become fully developed.

matu'rity. State of completed growth; fully developed; time when a person becomes capable of reproducing.

matutinal (ma-tū'tĭ-năl) [L. *matutinalis,* morning]. Occurring early in the day, as morning sickness; in the morning.

matzoon (mat-zūn') [Armenian]. Milk with a ferment containing lactic acid, bacilli, and other organisms. SYN: *madzoon.*

maxill'a [L. jawbone]. (pl. *maxillae*) [NA]. A jawbone, esp. the upper one; the superior maxilla. SEE: *skeleton.*

m., inferior. The lower jawbone or mandible.

m., superior. Upper jawbone.

maxillary (măk'sĭ-lĕr"ē). Pert. to the jaw, esp. the upper.

m. bones. Sup. and inf. maxillae; upper and lower jawbones.

m. sinus. The antrum of Highmore, air cavity in sup. maxilla opening into middle meatus of nose.

maxillitis (măks'ĭl-ī'tĭs) [L. *maxilla,* jawbone, +Gr.-*itis,* inflammation]. Inflammation of maxilla.

maxillofacial. Pert. to the maxilla and face.

maximal (maks'ĭ-mal) [L. *maximus,* greatest]. Greatest possible; highest. SEE: *minimal.*

maximum (măks'ĭ-mŭm). 1. The greatest quantity or effect. 2. Height of a disease.

Mayo-Robson's point. [Arthur Mayo-Robson, Eng. surgeon, 1853-1933]. A point just above and to right of the umbilicus, where pressure causes tenderness in pancreatic disease.

mazopexy (mă'zō-pĕk"sĭ) [Gr. *mazos,* breast, + *pēxis,* fixation]. Correction of a pendulous breast by surgical fixation. SYN: *mastopexy.*

mazoplasia (mā-zō-plā'zĭ-ă) ["+ *plassein,* to form]. Degenerative hyperplasia of mammary gland tissue. SYN: *mastoplasia.*

m.b. Abbr. in prescription writing for L. *mis'ce be'ne,* mix well.

Mc. Abbr. for *megacurie.*

mc. Abbr. for *millicurie.*

McBurney's incision. [Charles McBurney, Am. surgeon, 1845-1914] Abdominal incision employed in appendectomy.

An incision is made parallel to path of external oblique muscle, 1-2 inches away from ant. sup. spine of right ilium, cutting through the external oblique to the internal oblique and transversalis, separating their fibers.

McBurney's point. Point of tenderness in acute appendicitis, situated on a line bet. the umbilicus and the right ant. sup. iliac spine, about 1 or 2 inches above the latter.

McCarthy's reflex. [Daniel J. McCarthy, Am. neurologist, 1874—] Contraction of orbicularis palpebrarum with closure of lids resulting from percussion above supraorbital nerve.

McCormac's reflex. Adduction of one leg resulting from percussion of patella tendon of opposite leg.

mcg. Abbr. for *microgram.*

MCH. Abbr. for *mean corpuscular hemoglobin.* The amount of hemoglobin in each red blood cell.

mc.h. Abbr. for *millicurie hour.*

MCHC. Abbr. for *mean corpuscular hemoglobin concentration.* Average hemoglobin concentration in each red blood cell, expressed as a percentage value.

MCV. 1. Abbr. for *mean corpuscular volume-.* Expressed as the average volume of individual cells in cubic microns. 2. Abbr. for *mean clinical value,* obtained by allotting a numerical value to response of patients receiving specific treatment, adding these numbers, and dividing by number of treated patients.

M.D. [L. *Medicinae,* doctor]. Abbr. for *Doctor of Medicine.* Often shortened to Doctor.

This usage leads to confusion. Doctor may mean dentist, veterinarian, or other persons possessing a doctoral degree (e.g., Ph.D., Doctor of Philosophy). Thus, the word physician is preferred over doctor when doctor of medicine is intended.

meal (mēl) [AS. *māēl,* measure, meal]. 1. Portion of food eaten at a particular time to satisfy the appetite. 2. The edible portion of any cereal grain which has been coarsely ground, esp. corn meal. SEE: *test meal.*

mean [L. *medius,* in middle]. In statistics, a number derived from a series of other numbers by a prescribed method of computation. SEE: *median.*

Thus the arithmetic mean (commonly called the average) of a series of n numbers is obtained by adding all the numbers and dividing the sum by n.

   m. corpuscular hemoglobin. A measure of hemoglobin content of red corpuscles. The formula for determining this is

$$\frac{\text{volume of packed red cells, ml. per 1000 ml.}}{\text{red cell count, millions per cmm.}}$$

Ex: if the hemoglobin is 12 gm. and the red cell count is 4,000,000

$$\text{M.C.V.} = \frac{38 \times 10}{4} = 95.$$

This is the weight of hemoglobin in each red cell. ABBR: M.C.H.

   m. corpuscular hemoglobin concentration. ABBR: M.C.H.C. A measure of concentration of hemoglobin in the average red cell. The formula used is

$$\frac{\text{grams of hemoglobin per 100 ml.} \times 10}{\text{red cell count, millions per cmm.}}$$

Ex: if the hematocrit is 38 and the hemoglobin is 12, then

$$\text{M.C.H.} = \frac{120}{4.0} = 44.$$

   m. corpuscular volume. ABBR: M.C.V. A measure of the volume of red corpuscles. The formula for determining this is

$$\frac{\text{grams of hemoglobin per 100 ml.} \times 100}{\text{volume of packed red cells, ml. per 100 ml.}}$$

Ex: if the hematocrit is 38 and the red cell count is 4,000,000, then

$$\text{M.C.H.C.} = \frac{12}{38} \times 100 = 33.7\%.$$

measles (mē′zls) [Dutch *maselen*]. Rubeola. A highly communicable virus disease characterized by catarrhal symptoms and by a typical eruption on the skin and mucous membranes of the mouth (Koplik's spots). It usually occurs before adolescence. The occurrence of measles before the age of six months is relatively uncommon.

An attack of measles almost invariably confers permanent immunity. Active immunization can be produced by administration of measles vaccine, preferably that containing the live attenuated virus, although measles vaccine containing the inactivated virus is available for individuals in whom the live attenuated type is contraindicated. Passive immunization is afforded by administration of gamma globulin.

INCUBATION: About 10 days, varying from 8 to 13.

SYM: Onset gradual; coryza, rhinitis, drowsiness, loss of appetitie, gradual elevation of temperature for first 2 days, when fever may rise to 101-103° F. (38.3°-39.4° C.). Photophobia and cough soon develop, although some recession in the temperature may occur.

About 4th day, fever usually reaches a higher elevation than previously, at times as high as 104-106° F. (40°-41.1° C.). With this recurrence the rash appears.

Eruption first appears on face, being seen early as small maculopapular lesions that increase rapidly in size and coalesce in places, often causing a swollen, mottled appearance. The rash extends to the body and extremities and in some areas may assume a deviousness suggestive of scarlet fever.

A cough, present at this time, is due to bronchitis produced by the inflammatory condition of the mucous membranes which undoubtedly corresponds to the rash seen on the skin. Ordinarily, the rash lasts from 4-5 days and as it subsides the temperature declines. Consequently, by the end of 5 days from appearance of rash, temperature should be normal, or approximately normal in uncomplicated cases. Early in the disease leukopenia, esp. of polymorphonuclear cells, may be present.

COMPLICATIONS: Encephalitis is the most dreaded complication. Of those who develop encephalitis about one in eight will die; approximately half will have permanent central nervous system injury; and the remainder will recover completely. Bronchopneumonia is a serious complication of measles. Otitis media, followed by mastoiditis, brain abscess, or even meningitis, is not rare. Cervical adenitis with marked cellulitis sometimes leads to fatal consequences. Tracheitis and laryngeal stenosis, due to edema of glottis, are sometimes seen in the course of measles. Eye complications are not common in measles, although a marked conjunctivitis usually occurs.

DIFFERENTIAL DIAG: Scarlet fever, German measles, the prodromal rash of smallpox, or even cases of confluent smallpox may have to be considered. If the measles patient is observed prior to appearance of rash, or sometimes even after rash has developed, a definite decision may be based on the presence of Koplik's spots, q.v.

Hemorrhagic spots are also seen on the hard palate and mucous membranes many times before rash is evident on the skin. These spots probably correspond to the typical maculopapular eruption of the disease.

PROG: While usually favorable in the well-nourished child, the seriousness of the possible complications of measles should not be minimized.

TREATMENT AND NP: Patient isolated in a well-ventilated room because ventilation is of utmost importance when a respiratory infection is being dealt with. Although the room frequently is darkened, this is necessary only if the patient appears to have, or complains of, photophobia. Reading need not be prohibited unless photophobia is present.

The average measles patient does not care to eat during first few days of illness. Aside from providing plenty of fluids, no unusual effort should be made to force food upon him. Plenty of water, fruit juices, and milk are desirable. With fading of rash and reduction of temperature, patient soon will regain his appetite.

The eyes should receive careful attention, being cleansed with normal saline solution.

The cough and laryngitis may be controlled to some extent by steam inhalations and cough syrup of physician's choice. Fever controlled by aspirin or cool sponges.

QUARANTINE: It is customary in many states to quarantine until rash has disappeared and temperature has been normal for from 24-48 hours. In the uncomplicated cases, this usually means that the duration of the quarantine will be approximately 10 days from the date of onset. Measles is much more contagious before eruption than it is after eruption has appeared. Consequently, it is not at all likely that the quarantine of measles patients exerts any influence on the control of a measles epidemic. On the other hand, quarantine of susceptible contacts is plainly beneficial in limiting exposures and preventing the spread of infection.

PREVENTION: All children who have not had measles or who have not been vaccinated previously should be immunized with live attenuated measles vaccine at 12 months of age.

Inactivated vaccine is not recommended because of the short-lived protection it produces.

Live attenuated vaccine is contraindicated in pregnancy, leukemia, lymphomas, and other generalized neoplasms; when agents which depress resistance such as steroids and antimetabolites are being given; during severe illness; in active tuberculosis which is not being treated; in individuals with neomycin, duck, or egg sensitivity; and after blood transfusion or injection of immune serum globulin. In these latter two cases wait 12 weeks before administering vaccine.

Measles immune serum globulin is effective in preventing measles if it is given not later than 5 days after exposure.

SEE: *Koplik's spots; rubella; rubeola.*

m., black. A serious form of measles characterized by hemorrhagic areas in the skin and marked constitutional symptoms.

m., German. Rubella, q.v.

m., hemorrhagic. Black measles, q.v.

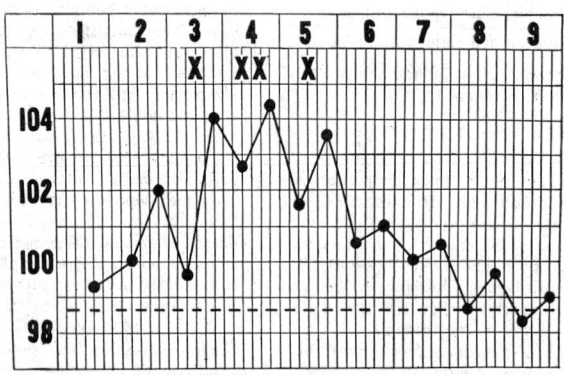

USUAL COURSE OF FEVER IN MEASLES
(Landon, J. F., Sider, H. T.: Communicable Diseases, ed. 8.)

measure (mĕ'zhŭr) [Fr. *mesure*, from L. *mensura*, a measuring]. 1. The dimensions, capacity, or quantity of anything which can be so evaluated. *Length, area, volume,* and *mass* are basic properties of matter and materials which can be measured. 2. To determine the extent of length, area, mass, or volume of a substance or object. 3. A device used in measuring, for ex., a marked tape or a graduated beaker. SEE: In Appendix, *metric system; weights and measures;* and *household measures and weights.*

meat. 1. The edible portion of anything. 2. The flesh of animals, including poultry, which is used for food.

Meat from animals is an important source of vitamins, esp. those of the B complex (thiamine, riboflavin, niacin). Pork is especially rich in thiamine. Liver has an unusually high vitamin content, esp. of vitamin A. The glandular organs such as liver and kidney contain a considerably higher percentage of certain mineral elements and vitamins than are found in other forms of meat.

Most meats have the same nutritive value but differ greatly in flavor and tenderness. Muscle contains about 20% protein, 20% fat, and 60% water. Lean meat is rich in phosphorus, potassium, and iron; it has a good percentage of other minerals but is deficient in calcium. In all meats the acid-forming elements are decidedly in excess of the base-forming.

Many myths about meat have been repudiated. For instance, one kind of meat is as easily digested as another. Also tough meat is just as nutritious as tender meat, but fibrous tissue is less easily digested.

meatal (mē-ā'tăl) [L. *meatus,* passage]. Pert. to a meatus or passage.

meatometer (mē-ă-tŏm'ĕt-ĕr) ["+ Gr. *metron,* measure]. Device for measuring the size of a passage or opening.

meatorrhaphy (mē"at-or'ăf-ĭ) ["+ Gr. *raphē,* a sewing]. Suture of the severed end of the urethra to the glans penis following surgical procedure to enlarge the meatus.

meatoscopy (mē-ă-tŏs'kō-pĭ) ["+ Gr. *skopein,* to examine]. Instrumental examination of a meatus, esp. the meatus of the urethra.

meatotome (mē-ăt'ō-tōm) ["+ Gr. *tomē,* incision]. Knife with probe or guarded point for enlarging meatus by direct incision.

meatotomy (mē-ă-tŏt'ō-mĭ) ["+ Gr. *tomē,* incision]. Incision of urinary meatus to enlarge the opening.

meatus (mē-ā'tŭs) [L.]. (pl. *meatūs*) [NA]. A passage or opening.

m. acusticus externus. [NA]. External auditory canal from the eardrum to the external ear.

m. acusticus internus. [NA]. Canal in the petrous portion of temporal bone, containing facial and auditory nerves and vessels.

m. auditorius. SEE: *m. acusticus, ext.* and *int.*

m. nasi communis. Common nasal cavity on either side of septum, into which three meatus open.

m. nasi inferior. [NA]. Space beneath inf. turbinate.

m. nasi medius. [NA]. Space beneath middle turbinate or concha.

m. nasi superior. [NA]. Space beneath sup. turbinate or concha.

m. nasopharyngeus. [NA]. Posterior portion of nasal cavity which communicates with the nasopharynx.

m. urinarius. External opening of the urethra; usually said of the male.

mechanical rectifier. A device which, by changing contacts at the proper moment in a cycle, changes alternating current into pulsating direct current.

mechanicoreceptor, mechanoreceptor (mē-kan''ĭ-cō-rē-sĕp'tor, mek''ă-nō-rē-sĕp'-tor). A receptor which receives mechanical stimuli such as pressure from sound or touch.

mechanics [Gr. *mēchanē,* machine]. Science of force and matter.

mech'anism. 1. Involuntary and consistent response to a stimulus. 2. A habit or response pattern to achieve a result.

mechanoreceptor, mechanicoreceptor. SEE: *mechanicoreceptor.*

mechanotherapy (mĕk''an-ō-thĕr'ă-pĭ) [Gr. *mēchanē,* machine, + *therapeia,* treatment]. Use of various types of mechanical apparatus to perform passive movements and to exercise various parts of the body.

meckelectomy (mek-el-ek'tō-mĭ) [Gr. *ektomē,* excision]. Excision of Meckel's ganglion.

Meckel's cartilage (Mĕk'ĕl). [Johann Friedrich Meckel (the younger), Ger. anatomist, 1781-1833]. A cartilaginous bar about which the mandible develops.

Meckel's divertic'ulum. [the younger]. A congenital sac or blind pouch sometimes found in lower portion of the ileum. Representing the persistent proximal end of the yolk stalk. Sometimes is continued to the umbilicus as a cord, or as a tube forming a fistulous opening at the umbilicus. Strangulation may cause intestinal obstruction. SEE: *diverticulum, diverticulitis.*

Meckel's ganglion. [Johann F. Meckel (the elder), Ger. anatomist, 1724-1774] Located in the sphenomaxillary fossa giving off nerves to eyes, nose, and palate. SYN: *sphenopalatine g.*

Meckel's space. [the elder]. Area in dura holding the gasserian ganglion.

meclizine hydrochloride (měk'lǐ-zēn). USP. Antiemetic esp. effective for control of nausea and vomiting of motion sickness.

meconium (mǐ-kō'nǐ-ŭm) [Gr. *mēkōnion,* poppy juice]. 1. Opium; poppy juice. 2. First feces of a newborn infant, made up of salts, liquor amnii, mucus, bile and epithelial cells; greenish black to light brown, almost odorless and of a tarry consistency. Present 3 or 4 days after birth.

mecystasis (mē-sis'tǎ-sǐs). Process in which a muscle maintains its original degree of tension although its length is increased.

M.E.D. Abbr. for *minimal effective dose.*

medi- [L.]. Prefix indicating middle.

media (mē'dǐ-ā) [L.]. 1. Plural of medium. 2. Middle or muscular coat of an artery. SYN: *tunica media.*

mediad (mē'dǐ-ăd) [L. *medium,* middle + *ad,* toward]. Toward the median line or plane of the body.

me'dial [L. *medialis*]. 1. Pert. to middle. 2. Nearer the medial plane.

median. 1. Middle; central. 2. In statistics, a number obtained by arranging the given series in order of size and taking the middle number; one then has as many greater as there are less. Thus, in the series 5, 7, 8, 9, 10, the median is 8. SEE: *mean.*

   m. artery. A branch of the volar interosseous artery.

   m. line. An imaginary line extending longitudinally on the ant. or post. surface of the body marking the edges of the median plane, q.v.

   m. nerve. A combined motor and sensory nerve having its origin in the brachial plexus.

   m. plane. The midsagittal plane; a vertical plane through the trunk and head dividing the body into right and left halves. SEE: *plane* for illustration.

mediastinal (mē'dǐ-ăs-tī'năl) [L. *mediastinalis*]. Rel. to the mediastinum.

mediastinitis (mē'dǐ-as''tī-nī'tis). Inflammation of tissue of the mediastinum.

mediastinopericarditis (mē-dǐ-ăs''tǐ-nō-pěr''ǐ-kăr-dī'tǐs) ["+ Gr. *peri,* around, + *kardia,* heart, + *-itis,* inflammation]. Inflammatory condition of mediastinum and pericardium.

mediastinum (mē'dǐ-ăs-tī'nŭm) [L., in the middle]. (pl. *mediastina*) 1. A septum or cavity between two principal portions of an organ. 2. [NA] The folds of the pleura and intervening space between right and left lung. The interpleural space; it contains the thoracic viscera.

   m. testis. [NA] The thickened portion of the tunica albuginea on post. surface of testis. SYN: *corpus Highmori,* or *body of Highmore.*

   m., thoracic. The space between the pleural cavities which encloses the heart and pericardium; large vessels entering and leaving heart, thoracic duct, vagus and phrenic nerves, trachea, esophagus, and thymus. Extends from sternum to vertebral column. Divided into superior, middle, inferior, anterior, and posterior portions.

mediate (mē'dǐ-āt). 1. Accomplished by indirect means. 2. Between two parts or sides.

medic. A member of the medical team in the U.S. Armed Forces. SYN: *medical corpsman.*

medicable (měd'ǐ-kă-bl) [L. *medicāri,* to heal]. Possibly responsive to therapy. Curable.

medical (měd'ǐ-kal). 1. Pert. to medicine or the study of the art and science of caring for those who are ill. 2. Requiring therapy with medicines as distinct from surgical treatment.

   m. assistants. Persons who have had training in some aspect of medical care, i.e., a nurse or corpsman in the armed services. After further training they are capable of assisting a physician in carrying out some of the less difficult medical tasks. SYN: *physician assistants.*

   m. corpsman. An enlisted man in the U.S. Armed Forces who works as a member of the medical team. SYN: *corpsman; medic.*

   m. jurisprudence. Principles of medicine in their application to questions of law.

   m. preparations. SOLID SUBSTANCES: Capsule or capsula; cachet, confection or confectio; cerate or ceratum; extract or extractum; lozenge or trochiscus; lamella, q.v.; ointment or unguentum; plaster or emplastrum; powder or pulvis; pill or pilula; paper or charta; sterule or sterula; suppository or suppositorium; tablet or tabella; vescette.

   FLUIDS: Fluidextract or fluidextractum; tincture or tinctura; infusion or infusum; decoction or decoctum; wine or vinum; oleoresin or oleoresina.

   SUSPENSIONS: Mixture or mixtura; emulsion or emulsum.

   SOLUTIONS: Water or aqua; mucilage or mucilago; solution or liquor; elixir; syrup or syrupus; spirit or spiritus; gylcerite or glyceritum; vinegar or acetum.

MISC. Liniment or linimentum; oleate or oleatum.

RS: alkaloid, active principle, antidote; dosage; drug action; drugs and their administration; names of individual drugs in alphabetical order; names of poisons; *poison; poisoning;* preparations usually given by rectum; *prescription writing.*

m. record. Transcript of information obtained from a patient, guardian, or professionals and presented in tabular, outline, or written form. It may contain history, diagnoses, treatment, prognosis, etc. Utilized by the school, place of employment, personal physician, hospital, etc.

m. record, problem oriented. A technique of clinical record keeping described by Lawrence Weed, a contemporary Amer. physician. The patient's record is organized in a logical and efficient manner including a list of problems and flow charts determining diagnostic and therapeutic plans and indicating what has been done.

Medic Alert. A nonprofit organization which provides a bracelet with an emblem on which is contained information and a warning in case of emergency. The purpose is the prevention of a serious or fatal mistake in rendering aid or medical care to an injured or unconscious person who may have an additional condition or allergy, i.e. diabetes, penicillin allergy.

Applications may be obtained from Medic Alert, Turlock, Calif. Persons wishing to donate organs may also acquire an emblem stating the fact.

med'icament [L. *medicamentum*]. A medicine or remedy.

RS: epispastic, errhine, escharotic, evacuant, medical preparations, rubefacient, saponin, sedative, vesicant, vesicatory.

medicate (měd'ĭ-kāt) [L. *medicatus*]. 1. To treat a disease with drugs. 2. To permeate with medicinal substances.

medication (měd-ĭ-kā'shŭn). 1. Treatment with remedies. 2. Impregnation with medicine.

m., hypodermic. Treatment by injection of medicine into the body through the skin, using a syringe and needle.

m., ionic. Introduction of ions of drugs into the body by cataphoresis, q.v.

m., sublingual. Treatment with an agent, usually in tablet form, placed under the tongue.

m., substitutive. Medical therapy to cause a nonspecific inflammation to counteract a specific one.

medication routes. Various routes by which medicine can be introduced into the body.

m. r., inhalation. By use of masks, atomizers, or vaporizers.

m. r., intra-arterial. Introduction of medicaments or blood into an artery.

m. r., intracardiac. Introduction of a drug into heart muscle or one of the heart chambers.

m. r., intracutaneous. Injection of drug between layers of skin. SYN: *endermic m.r.; intradermal m.r.*

m. r., intramedullary. Introduction of fluids into bone marrow, esp. that of sternum.

m. r., intramuscular. Introduction of drug into muscles. Usual sites are deltoid or triceps muscles, or gluteus maximus. ABBR: I.M.

m. r., intranasal. Introduction of nosedrops or jellies for antiseptic, antihistaminic, or vasoconstrictive effects.

m. r., intrathecal. Introduction into subdural space of spinal cord. Spinal fluid is withdrawn equal to that introduced.

m. r., intravenous. Injection of fluids into a vein, usually the basilic or median cubital vein. ABBR: I.V.

m. r., iontophoresis. Ion transfer. Introduction of drugs into deeper layers of the skin by a galvanic electric current.

m. r., oral. Introduction by mouth. Not available for drugs destroyed by digestion, those incapable of absorption, or drugs that are irritating to mucous membranes.

m. r., rectal. Drugs may be given in form of liquids or suppositories. In diseases of the rectum and adjacent parts, medication is often applied by way of the anus, esp. if medication cannot be adm. by mouth, as in persistent nausea or emesis, during unconsciousness or delirium, or because of the bad taste of the medication. Almost any drug other than those of a corrosive nature may be adm. through the rectum.

Three points must be kept in mind: (1) The rectum must be free of fecal material. A purgative enema should be given an hour before the rectal medicine in order that peristalsis will subside and there will be no fecal contents to absorb the medicated solution.

(2) The medicinal substance must be readily soluble. The solution must have the consistency of thin starch or melt when exposed to body temperature. Medicinal solutions should be warmed to body temperature prior to installation. A normal salt

solution with 5% glucose is a common medicated enema.

(3) The solution is given slowly through a small catheter attached to a funnel. The patient, who remains on his left side for 10 minutes, is assisted in retaining the fluid by pressure on the anus with cotton or tissues.
SEE: *preparations usually given rectally.*

m. r., subcutaneous. Injection of drugs or implantation of pellets under the skin.

m. r., sublingual. Absorption of drugs by the sublingual mucosa.

m. r., vaginal. Drugs may be given in liquid form by douche or in the form of suppository, powder, or paint.

medicinal (mē-dǐ'sǐn-ăl) [L. *medicina,* medicine]. Pert. to medicine.

m. enema. One to which some drug or medication has been added, for retention or absorption, particularly in cases where medication cannot be adm. by mouth. SEE: *enema.*

medicine. 1. A drug or remedy. 2. The art of preventing, caring for, and assisting in the cure of disease, and care of the injured. 3. Treatment of disease medically as distinguished from surgical treatment.

m., aerospace. Branch of medicine concerned with the selection of men for duty as pilots or crew members for flight and space missions and the pathology and physiology of men and animals who travel in airplanes and space craft in the Earth's atmosphere and in outer space.

m., clinical. Observation and treatment at the bedside; the practice of medicine as distinguished from laboratory science.

m., disaster. Large scale application of emergency medical services in a community following a natural or man-made catastrophe. The aim is to save lives and restore every survivor to maximum health as promptly as possible. Its success depends upon prompt sorting of patients according to their immediate needs and prognosis.

m., emergency. That branch of medicine concerned with an individual's resuscitation, transportation, and care from the point of injury or beginning of illness through the hospital or other emergency treatment facility.

m., environmental. Concerned with diseases and conditions peculiar to working conditions. SYN: *occupational medicine, industrial medicine.*

m., experimental. The scientific study of disease or pathologic conditions through experimentation upon laboratory animals or through clinical research.

m., forensic. Application of medical knowledge to legal affairs.

m., group. 1. The practice of medicine by a group of physicians, usually consisting of specialists in various fields who pool their services and share jointly laboratory and x-ray facilities. Such a group is commonly called a clinic. 2. The securing of medical services by a group of individuals who, upon paying definite sums of money, are entitled to certain medical services or hospitalization in accordance to prearranged rules and regulations.

m., internal. 1. That branch of medicine which treats diseases of the internal organs by other than surgical means. 2. Treatment of diseases nonsurgical in nature.

m., legal. Forensic medicine, q.v.

m., man. Person from a primitive culture whose alleged healing powers are derived from mystical and magical sources. SYN: *shaman.*

m., patent. A medicine for which a patent has been granted. May be purchased without a doctor's prescription. SEE: *patent medicine.*

m., physical. Treatment of disease by physical agents such as heat, cold, light, electricity, manipulation, or the use of mechanical devices. SYN: *physiotherapy, physical therapy.*

m., preventive. The study and practice of preventing disease.

m., proprietary. Medicine in which exclusive interests have been secured by patent, copyright of labels, or secrecy of composition. SEE: *proprietary medicine.*

m., psychosomatic. A branch of medicine which recognizes the importance of mind-body interrelationship in all illnesses and in which therapy and management are based on this fact.

m., socialized. Practice of medicine under control and direction of an agency of the government. The cost of medical care under this plan usually is financed by levying taxes or through a national medical insurance program.

m., third party. Medical care plan wherein the costs, particularly those of the physician, are paid by some means other than directly from the patient, i.e., a third party. This third party may be a government agency, an insurer, or an industrial organization. Most plans for socialized medicine also involve this principle of payment through a third party.

m., tropical. Branch of medical science which deals principally with diseases common in tropical or subtropical regions, esp. of parasitic origin.

m., veterinary. That which deals with diagnosis and treatment of diseases of animals.

medicinerea (mĕd″ĭ-sĭn-ē'rē-a) [L. *medius*, middle, + *cinerea*, ashen]. Internal gray matter of the claustrum and lenticula of the brain.

medicochirurgical (mĕd″ĭ-kō-kī-rur'jĭ-kăl). Concerning both medicine and surgery.

medicolegal (mĕd″ĭ-kō-lē'găl) ["+ *legalis*, legal]. Rel. to medical jurisprudence or forensic medicine.

medicopter. Helicopter equipped for emergency care of sick or injured while they are being evacuated to a hospital.

medicornu (med″ĭ-kor'nu). The inferior horn of the lateral ventricle of the brain.

Medina worm. Dracunculus medinensis, q.v.

medio- [L.]. Prefix meaning middle.

mediopontine (mē″dĭ-ō-pon'tĭn) ["+ *pons, pont-*, bridge]. Rel. to center of the pons Varolii.

mediotarsal (mē″dĭ-ō-tăr'săl). Rel. to the middle of the tarsus.

Mediterranean anemia. Thalassemia, q.v. (Cooley's anemia). Also called M. disease.

medium (mĕd'ĭ-ŭm). (pl. *media*) 1. An agent through which an effect is obtained. 2. Substance used for the cultivation of microorganisms or cellular tissue. SYN: *culture medium.* 3. Substance through which impulses are transmitted.

medium-chain triglycerides. Triglycerides with 8 to 10 carbon atoms. They are digested and absorbed differently than the usual dietary fats, and for that reason have been useful in treating malabsorption.

medulla (mĕ-dŭl'lă). [NA]. (pl. *medullae*) 1. The marrow. 2. Inner or central portion of an organ, in contrast to the outer portion or cortex. 3. M. oblonga'ta.

m., adrenal. Inner portion of the adrenal gland composed of chromaffin tissue. Secretes epinephrine. SEE: *adrenal.*

m. of hair. Central axis of a hair.

m. of kidneys. Renal pyramids.

m. nephrica. Pyramids of kidneys.

m. oblongata. [NA]. Enlarged portion of spinal cord in cranium after it enters the foramen magnum at the occipital bone; the lower portion of the brain stem.

m. ossium. [NA]. Marrow in bone.

m. of ovary. Central portion of the ovary composed of loose connective tissue, blood vessels, lymphatics, and nerves.

m. spinalis. [NA]. Spinal cord.

medullary (mĕd'ū-lăr-ĭ) [L. *medularis*]. Concerning marrow or medulla.

medullated (mĕd'ū-lāt-ĕd). Covered by or containing marrow or medulla.

m. nerve fiber. A nerve fiber possessing a myelin or medullary sheath; a myelinated nerve fiber.

medullation. Acquiring a myelin sheath.

medullitis (mĕd-ū-lī'tĭs) [L. *medularis*, marrow, + Gr. *-itis*, inflammation]. Inflammation of marrow. SYN: *myelitis.*

medullization (mĕd-ū-lĭ-zā'shŭn). Conversion to marrow abnormally.

medulloarthritis (mĕ-dūl″ō-ar-thrī'tĭs) [L. *medulla*, marrow, + Gr. *arthron*, joint, + *-itis*, inflammation]. Inflammation of marrow elements of bone ends.

medulloblastoma (mĕ-dūl'ō-blās-tō'mă) [L. *medulla*, marrow, + Gr. *blastos*, germ, + *-ōma*, tumor]. A malignant, soft, infiltrating tumor of the roof of the 4th ventricle and cerebellum. Often invades the meninges.

medullocell (mĕ-dūl'ō-sĕl). Marrow cell. SYN: *myelocyte.*

medulloepithelioma (mĕ-dul'o-ep″ĭ-thĕl-ĭ-ō'mă) [L. *medulla*, marrow, + Gr. *epi*, upon, + *thēlē*, nipple, + *-ōma*, tumor]. Tumor composed of retina epithelium and of neuroepithelium. SYN: *neuroepithelioma, glioma.*

mega- [Gr.]. 1. Combining forms mean great or large. 2. Indicates one million (10^6) when used in combination with terms indicating units of measure; thus megaton is one million tons. SEE: words beginning with *megalo.*

megabladder (mĕg'ă-blăd-ĕr) ["+ AS. *blaedre*]. Permanent abnormal distention of the urinary bladder. SYN: *megalocystis.*

megacardia. Enlargement of the heart. SYN: *cardiomegaly.*

megacephalic (mĕg-ă-sĕf-ăl'ĭk). Having an abnormally large head. SYN: *macrocephalous.*

megacolon (mĕg-ă-ko'lon) [Gr. *mega*, large, + *kōlon*, colon]. Extremely dilated colon. Usually congenital, and occurs also in infancy or childhood. SEE: *Hirschsprung's disease.*

megadont (mĕg'ă-dŏnt) ["+ *odous, odont-*, tooth]. Possessing very large teeth. SYN: *macrodont.*

megadyne (mĕg'ă-dĭn). A unit equal to one million dynes. SEE: *dyne.*

megakaryoblast (mĕg″ă-kăr'ĭ-ō-blăst). An immature megakaryocyte.

megakaryocyte (mĕg″ă-kar'ĭ-ō-sīt) [Gr. *mega*, large, + *karyon*, nucleus, + *cyte*, cell]. Large bone marrow cell with large or multiple nuclei. SYN: *megaloblast, myeloplax.*

megalencephaly (mĕg-ăl-ĕn-sĕf′ă-lĭ). Abnormally large size of the brain, usually accompanied by mental deficiency.

megalgia (mĕg-ăl′jĭ-ă) [Gr. *mega*, large, + *algos*, pain]. Very severe pain.

megalo- [Gr.]. Combining form meaning great size.

megaloblast (mĕg′ă-lō-blăst) ["+ *blastos*, germ]. A large size nucleated red blood corpuscle, from 11-20 microns in diameter, oval and slightly irregular. Found in the blood in cases of pernicious anemia. SYN: *macroblast.*

megalocardia (mĕg″ă-lō-kăr′dĭ-ă) ["+ *kardia*, heart]. Cardiac hypertrophy. SYN: *cardiomegaly.*

megalocephalic (mĕg-ă-lō-sĕf-ăl′ĭk) ["+ *kephalē*, head]. Having an abnormally large skull. SYN: *megacephalic, macrocephalic.*

megalocephaly (mĕg″ă-lō-sĕf′ă-lĭ) [Gr. *megalo*, large, + *kephalē*, head]. 1. Abnormal size of the head. SYN: *macrocephaly.* 2. Leontiasis ossea, a rare disease characterized by hyperostosis of bones of the skull.

megalocornea (mĕg″ă-lō-kor′nē-ă) ["+ L. *cornū*, horn]. An enlarged cornea.

megalocystis (mĕg″ă-lō-sĭs′tĭs) ["+ *kystis*, bladder]. Abnormal, permanent enlargement of the bladder. SYN: *megabladder.*

megalocyte (mĕg′ă-lō-sīt) ["+ *cyte*, cell]. Red blood corpuscle larger than average.

megalodactylous (mĕg″ă-lō-dăk′tĭl-ŭs) ["+ *daktylos*, finger]. Having very large digits.

megalodontia (mĕg″ă-lō-dŏn′shĭ-ă) ["+ *odous, odont-*, tooth]. Abnormally large teeth.

megalogastria (mĕg″ă-lō-gas′trĭ-ă) ["+ *gastēr*, belly]. Excessive size of stomach. SYN: *gastromegaly.*

megaloglossia (mĕg″ă-lō-glŏs′sĭ-ă) ["+ *glōssa*, tongue]. Enlargement of the tongue. SYN: *macroglossia.*

megalohepatia (mĕg″ă-lō-hĕ-păt′ĭ-ă) [Gr. *megalo*, large + *hēpar*, liver]. Abnormal enlargement of the liver. SYN: *hepatomegaly.*

megalokaryocyte (meg-ă-lō-kăr′ĭ-ō-sīt) ["+ *karyon*, nucleus, + *cyte*, cell]. A large bone marrow cell with multiple nuclei. SYN: *megakaryocyte.*

megalomania (mĕg″ă-lō-mā′nĭ-ă) ["+ *mania*, madness]. A psychosis characterized by ideas of personal exaltation and delusions of grandeur.

megalomelia (mĕg″ă-lō-mēl′ĭ-ă) ["+ *melos*, limb]. Abnormally large size of the limbs. SYN: *macromelia.*

megalonychosis (mĕg″ă-lō″nĭ-kō′sĭs) ["+ *onyx, onych-*, nail]. Hypertrophy of the nails.

megalopenis (mĕg″ă-lō-pē′nĭs) ["+ L. *penis*, penis]. Abnormally large penis. SYN: *macrophallus.*

megalophthalmus (mĕg-ă-lŏf-thăl′mŭs) ["+ *ophthalmos*, eye]. Abnormally large eyes.

megalopsia (mĕg-ă-lŏp′sĭ-ă) [Gr. *megalo*, large + *opsis*, vision]. An affection of the eyes in which objects appear enlarged. SYN: *macropsia.*

megaloscope (meg′ă-lō-skōp″) ["+ *skopein*, to examine]. A large magnifying lense. A speculum fitted with a magnifying lense.

megalosplenia (mĕg″ă-lō-splēn′ĭ-ă) ["+ *splēn*, spleen]. Hypertrophy of the spleen. SYN: *splenomegaly.*

megalosyndactyly (mĕg″ă-lō-sĭn-dăk′tĭl-ē) ["+ *syn*, with, + *daktylos*, finger]. A condition of large and webbed digits.

megaloureter (mĕg-ă-lō-ū-rē′tĕr, mĕg-ă-lō-ūr′ĕ-tĕr) ["+ *ourētēr*, ureter]. Increase in diameter of the ureter.

megaprosopous (mĕg″ă-prŏs′ō-pŭs) ["+ *prosōpon*, face]. Possessing a large face.

megarectum (mĕg-ă-rĕk′tŭm) ["+ L. *rectum*, straight]. Excessive dilatation of the rectum.

megaseme (mĕg′ă-sēm) ["+ *sēma*, sign]. 1. Having an orbital aperture with an index exceeding 89, said of a skull. 2. A megaseme skull.

megophthalmos (mĕg-of-thal′mos) ["+ *ophthalmos*, eye]. Abnormally large eyes. SYN: *buphthalmus, megalophthalmus.*

megrim (mē′grĭm) [O. Fr. migraine]. Sick headache. SYN: *migraine*, q.v.

meibomian cyst (mī-bō′mĭ-ăn). [Heinrich Meibom, Ger. anatomist, 1638-1700]. Small tumor on eyelid, the result of inflammation of a meibomian gland. SYN: *chalazion.*

meibomian gland. One of the sebaceous glands between the tarsi and conjunctiva of eyelids. SYN: *tarsal gland.*

meio- [Gr. *meioun*, diminution]. Combining form indicating decrease in size or number. SEE: words beginning with *mio.*

Meissner's corpuscles (mīs′nĕr). [Georg Meissner, Ger. histologist, 1829-1905]. An encapsulated end organ of touch found in dermal papillae close to epidermis. Each is an ovoid body containing endings of myelinated and unmyelinated nerve fibers. Most numerous in hairless portion of skin, esp. volar surface of hands, fingers, feet, and toes; also present in lips, eyelids, tip of tongue, and nipple.

Meissner's plexus. Small aggregations of ganglion cells located in submucosa of intestine.

mel [L.]. Honey, q.v.

melagra (měl-ā'grä) [Gr. *melos,* limb, + *agra,* seizure]. Muscular pain in the limbs. SYN: *melalgia.*

melalgia (měl-ăl'jĭ-ä) ["+ *algos,* pain]. Pain of neural origin in the limbs.

melancholia (měl-an-ko'lĭ-ä) [Gr. *melano-,* black, + *cholē,* bile]. A mental disorder characterized by marked depression, physical and mental apathy, brooding, mournful and doleful notions, and inhibition of activity. Observed in depressed phase of manic-depressive psychoses.

   m., affective. Involving or due to emotions.

   m. agita'ta. M. with much motor excitement.

   m., climacteric. Occurring at the time of menopause.

   m., involutional. Despondency, suicidal tendencies, feelings of unworthiness and mental agitation occurring in the aged.

   m., panphobic. Characterized by dread of everything.

   m., sexual. M. associated with fear of impotence, venereal disease, unsatisfied sexual desires.

   m. simplex. A mild form without delusions or great excitement.

   m. stuporo'sa. M. in which patient lies silent and motionless, indifferent to surroundings.

   m., suicidal. Impulse to commit suicide combined with melancholia.

melanedema (měl-ăn-ě-dě'mä) [Gr. *melano,* black, + *oidēma,* swelling]. Black deposit in the lungs; melanosis of the lungs. SYN: *anthracosis.*

melanemia (měl-ăn-ē'mĭ-ä) ["+ *haima,* blood]. Unnaturally dark color of blood, due to presence of free, dark pigment. Seen mainly in pernicious anemia.

melanephidrosis (měl″ăn-ěf'ĭ-drō'sĭs) ["+ *ephidrosis,* sweating]. A form of chromhidrosis in which the sweat is black. SYN: *melanidrosis.*

melanidrosis (měl″an-ĭd-rō'sĭs) [+ *idrōsis,* sweat]. Discharge of black sweat. SYN: *melanephidrosis.*

melaniferous (měl″ăn-ĭf'ěr-ŭs) ["+ L. *ferre,* to carry]. Containing melanin or some other black pigment.

mel'anin [Gr.]. The pigment which gives color to hair, skin, the substantia nigra of the brain, and the choroid of the eye. It is present in some cancers such as melanoma. Melanin can be prepared chemically.

melanism (měl'ăn-ĭzm) ["+ *ismos,* state of]. Abnormal black pigmentation of the organs and tissues; melanosis.

melano- [Gr.]. Prefix meaning black or darkness.

melanoblast (měl″ăn'ō-blăst) ["+ *blastos,* germ, sprout]. A cell found in basal layers of epidermis and capable of forming melanin.

melanoblastoma (měl″ă-nō-blăs-tō'mä) ["+ "+ *-ōma,* tumor]. A tumor containing melanin.

melanocarcinoma (měl″ă-nō-kar-sĭn-ō'mä). A cancer that has dark pigmentation.

melanocyte (měl″ăn'ō-sīt). A phagocyte that has ingested melanin; responsible for synthesis of melanin. SYN: *chromatophore.*

melanocyte-stimulating hormone. Hormone, located in the posterior pituitary, which influences melanin formation. ABBR: MSH.

mel'anoderm [Gr. *melano,* black, + *derma,* skin]. A person belonging to one of the black races.

melanoderma (měl″ăn-ō-děr'mä) [Gr.]. A patchy or generalized skin discoloration caused by either an increase in the production of melanin by the normal number of melanocytes or an increase in the number of melanocytes.

melanoepithelioma (měl″ăn-ō-ěp″ĭ-thē-lĭ-ō'mä). A malignant epithelioma containing melanin.

melanogenesis (měl″ăn-ō-jěn'ě-sĭs) [Gr. *melano,* black, + *genesis,* production]. Formation of melanin.

melanoglossia (měl″ăn-ō-glōs'sĭ-ä) ["+ *glōssa,* tongue]. Black tongue. SYN: *glossophytia.*

melanoid (měl'ă-noid) ["+ *eidos,* form]. 1. Concerning or resembling melanin. 2. Melanin which is chemically prepared.

melanoleukoderma (měl″ăn-ō-lū″kŏ-der'-mä) ["+ *leukos,* white, + *derma,* skin]. Mottled skin.

   m. col'li. Mottled skin of neck sometimes seen in syphilis. SYN: *collar of Venus; venereal collar.*

melano'ma ["+ *-ōma,* tumor]. A malignant, pigmented mole or tumor. SYN: *nevus pigmentosus.*

melanomatosis (měl″ă-nō″mă-tō'sĭs) ["+ "+ *-ōsis,* intensive]. Formation of numerous melanomas on or beneath the skin.

melanonychia (měl″ă-nō-nĭk'ĭ-ä) [Gr. *melano,* black, + *onyx, onych-,* nail]. Black pigmentation of the nails.

melanopathy (měl″ă-nŏp'ă-thĭ) ["+ *pathos,* disease]. 1. Dark pigmentation of skin. 2. Any disease with dark pigmentation of the skin. SYN: *melanoderma, melasma.*

melanophore (měl'ăn-ō-fōr) ["+ *phoros,* bearing]. Cell carrying dark pigment.

melanoplakia (mĕl″ăn-ō-plā′kĭ-ă) ["+ *plax*, a flat plain]. Condition marked by pigmented patches on the tongue and buccal mucosa.

mel″anorrhag′ia ["+ *rhēgnymi*, to burst forth]. Black feces. SYN: *melanorrhea.*

melanorrhea (mĕl″ăn-ō-rē′ă) ["+ *rhoia*, flow]. Black stools. SYN: *melena.*

melanosarcoma (mĕl″ă-nō-sar-kō′mă). Sarcoma containing melanin. SYN: *malignant melanoma.*

melanoscirrhus (mĕl″ă-nō-skir′ŭs) [Gr. *melano*, black, + *skirros*, hardness]. Black-pigmented cancer; an unusual form of melanoma. SYN: *melanocarcinoma.*

melanosis (mĕl-ăn-ō′sĭs) ["+ *-ōsis*, intensive]. 1. Unusual deposit of black pigments in different parts of body. 2. Disorder of pigment metabolism.

    m. lenticularis. Rare skin disease, beginning in early youth, characterized by scattered pigment discolorations, ulcers, atrophy, etc. SYN: *xeroderma pigmentosum.*

melanot′ic [Gr.]. 1. Black in color. 2. Pert. to melanosis.

melanotrichia linguae (mĕl″ăn-ō-trĭk′ĭ-ă lĭng′gwe) ["+ *thrix, trich,* hair + L. *linguae*, tongue]. Black, hairy tongue. SEE: *tongue.*

melanuria (mĕl-ăn-ū′rĭ-ă) ["+ *ouron*, urine]. Dark pigments in urine.

melasma (mĕl-ăz′mă) [Gr. a black spot]. Any discoloration of the skin. SYN: *nigredo cutis.*

    m. gravidarum. Discoloration of the skin during pregnancy.

    m. suprarenale. Hypofunction of the suprarenals with cutaneous pigmentation and severe anemia. SYN: *Addison's disease,* q.v.

melena (mĕl′ĕ-nă, mĕl-ē′nă) [Gr. *melaina*, black, black bile]. 1. Evacuations resembling tar, due to action of intestinal juices on free blood. Common in the newborn. 2. Black vomitus.

    m. neonatorum. M. in the newborn.

melenemesis (mĕl-ĕ-nĕm′ĕ-sĭs) ["+ *emesis*, vomit]. Black vomitus caused by blood that has been acted upon by the gastric juice. SYN: *melena.*

melicera, meliceris (mĕl-ĭ-sēr′ă, -ĭs) [Gr. *meli*, honey, + *kēros*, wax]. Cyst containing matter of honeylike consistency.

melioidosis (mē″lĭ-oy-dō′sĭs) [Gr.*melis*, a distemper of asses, + *eidos*, resemblance, + *osis*, condition]. An acute or chronic disease due to Pseudomonas pseudomallei (formerly called Malleomyces pseudomallei). Acute form causes pneumonia, multiple abscesses, septicemia and possibly death.

melissopho′bia [Gr. *melissa*, bee, + *phobia*, fear]. Abnormal fear of bee or wasp stings.

melitemia (mel-ĭ-te′mĭ-ă) [Gr. *meli*, honey, + *haima*, blood]. Abnormal amount of sugar in the blood.

melitensis (mĕl-ĭ-tĕn′sĭs). Undulant fever; brucellosis, q.v.

melitis (mĕl-ĭ′tĭs) [Gr. *mēlon*, cheek, + *-itis*, inflammation]. Inflammation of the cheek.

melitoptyalism (mĕl″ĭt-ō-tī′al-ĭzm) [Gr. *meli*, honey, + *ptyalon*, saliva]. Saliva containing glucose. SYN: *glycoptyalism.*

melituria (mĕl-ĭ-tū′rĭ-ă) ["+ *ouron*, urine]. Presence of sugar in the urine.

melodiotherapy (mĕl-ō″dĭ-ō-thĕr′ă-pĭ) [Gr. *melōdia*, music, + *therapeia*, treatment]. Treatment by music. SYN: *musicotherapy.*

melomania (mĕl-ō-mā′nĭ-ă) [Gr. *melos*, song, + *mania*, madness]. Obsessive attachment to music.

melomelus (mē-lŏm′ĕl-ŭs) [Gr. *melos*, limb, + *melos*, limb]. A malformed fetus with rudimentary limb attached to normal limb.

mel′on [Gr. *mēlon*, apple]. COMP: Principally water and carbohydrates, the latter nearly all in the form of sugar. SEE: watermelon.

meloncus (mĕl-on′kŭs) [Gr. *mēlon*, cheek, + *onkus*, bulk]. Tumor of the cheek.

meloplasty (mel′ō-plas-tĭ) [Gr. *melos*, limb, + *plassein*, to form]. Reparative surgery of the extremities.

melting point. Temperature at which conversion of a solid to a liquid begins.

member [L. *membrum*]. An organ or part of the body, esp. a limb.

membrane (mĕm′brăn) [L. *membrana*]. A thin, soft, pliable layer of tissue which lines a tube or cavity, covers an organ or structure, or separates one part from another.

    m., arachnoid. Middle layer of membranes covering brain and spinal cord.

    m., atlantooccipital. A single midline ligamentous structure that extends from the arch of the atlas to borders of the foramen magnum. SYN: *membrana atlantooccipitalis* [NA].

    m., basement. A delicate, noncellular membrane underlying a layer of epithelial cells and serving for their support and attachment.

    m., basilar. M. extending from tympanic lip of osseous spiral lamina to crest of spiral ligament in cochlea of ear. It separates scala tympani from cochlear duct and forms supporting structure for the organ of Corti.

    m., Bowman's. Thin homogeneous m. separating corneal epithelium from proper substance of the cornea.

    m.'s brain and spinal cord. The meninges, pia mater, inner m.; dura mater, outer m.; and arachnoid, middle m.

m., cell. Surface layer of the cytoplasm of a cell.

m., chorioid. The chorioid, the portion of the vascular tunic or uvea of the eye that extends posteriorly from the ora serrata.

m., costocoracoid. Dense fascia bet. the pectoralis minor and subclavius muscles.

m., cricothyroid. M. connecting thyroid and cricoid cartilages of the larynx.

m., croupous. False yellowish-white m. in the larynx during croup.

m., decidual. One of the membranes formed in the endometrium of a pregnant uterus. Includes the decidua basalis, decidua capsularis, and decidua parietalis, q.v.

m., Descemet's. Elastic m. forming lining surface of the cornea.

m., diphtheritic. Fibrinous false m. on mucous surfaces in diphtheria.

m., drum. The tympanic membrane.

m., egg. One of the protective membranes or envelopes enclosing an ovum. May be primary (formed by egg itself, e.g., vitelline membrane); secondary (formed by follicle cells, e.g., zona pellucida); or tertiary (formed by oviduct or uterus, e.g., albumen and shell of hen's egg).

m., elastic. One formed of elastic connective tissue fibers.

m., elastic, of the larynx. Consists of upper quadrangular membrane and lower elastic cone.

m., enamel. 1. Cuticula dentis. 2. Thin calcified internal layer of cells of the enamel organ.

m., false. Fibrinous exudate on a mucous surface of a membrane, as in diphtheria.

m., fenestrated. A layer of elastic connective tissue possessing minute round or oval openings. Found in tunica intima and tunica media of medium-sized and large arteries.

m., fetal. One of the membranous structures that serve to protect and support the embryo. The structures are yolk sac, allantois, amnion, chorion, decidua, and placenta.

m., fibrous. M. composed entirely of connective tissue. Examples are fasciae, aponeuroses, perichondrium, periosteum, dura mater, and capsules of some organs.

m., glassy, of graafian follicle. Transparent capsule which separates membrana granulosa from the theca.

m., glassy, of hair. Internal layer of a hair follicle separating the epithelial and connective tissues.

m., glial. Extremely delicate membrane, formed of foot plates of astrocytes, which surrounds all blood vessels in the brain, spinal cord, and in lining of pia mater separating these vessels from nervous tissue proper. Thought to be one of the components of the blood-brain barrier.

m., Henle's elastic. SEE: *m., fenestrated.*

m., homogeneous. A fine m. covering villi of the placenta.

m., Huxley's. SEE: *layer, Huxley's.*

m., hyaline. 1. Basement m. 2. M. bet. outer root sheath of a hair follicle and inner fibrous layer.

m., hyaloid. One investing the vitreous humor of the eye, seen on longitudinal section. SYN: *membrana vitrea* [NA].

m., hyoglossal. A transverse fibrous lamella uniting tongue to hyoid bone.

m., interosseous. 1. A fibrous m. in the arm connecting ulna to radius. 2. A fibrous m. in the leg connecting tibia to fibula.

m., Krause's. Dark membranous band limiting the sarcomere in striated muscle. Also called Z or intermediate disk.

m., limiting, external. 1. Outer layer of cells of the embryonic neural tube. 2. M. in retina of eye separating rods and cones from their cell bodies.

m., limiting, internal. 1. Inner layer of ependymal cells lining embryonic neural tube. 2. Glial membrane forming innermost layer of the retina and of the iris.

m., meconic. A m. forming a layer in rectum of the fetus.

m., medullary. Endosteum, q.v.

m., mucous. M. lining cavities and canals communicating with the air and kept moist by secretion of mucus.

m., Nasmyth's. A skinlike m. which may cover the teeth after they have erupted. The m. is easily removed by a dentist. SYN: *cuticula dentis.*

m., nictitating. A third eyelid present in lower vertebrates and represented in man by a fold of the conjunctiva, the plica semilunaris.

m., nuclear. A two-layered m. surrounding the nucleus, q.v. Prior to electron microscopy the nucleus was thought to be surrounded by a single thin membrane.

m., obturator. Fibrous m. closing the obturator foramen.

m., oral. Pharyngeal m., q.v.

m., oronasal. A double epithelial layer separating the nasal pits from the embryonic oral cavity. Same as bucconasal membrane.

m., otolithic. A layer of gelatinous substance containing otoconia or otoliths, found on the surface of maculae in inner ear.

m., peridental. Connective tissue between the root of a tooth and the alveolar bone. SYN: *periodontal m.*

m., permeable. A m. which permits the passage of water and certain substances in solution.

m., pharyngeal. M. closing embryonic gut at oral end.

m., plasma. A cell membrane, q.v.

m., pseudoserous. M. resembling a serous m. but differing in structure. Ex: endothelium.

m., pupillary. Transparent m. closing the fetal pupil. If it persists after birth it is known as persistent p. m.

m., pyogenic. Granular lining of an abscess or fistula.

m., pyophylactic. Protective lining of an abscess that prevents reabsorption of injurious matter.

m., quadrangular. Upper portion of the elastic membrane of the larynx, q.v.

m., Reissner's. Delicate membrane separating cochlear canal from scala vestibuli. SYN: *membrana vestibularis.*

m., Ruysch's. Choroid's middle layer composed of a close capillary network. SYN: *lamina choriocapillaris* [NA].

m., schneiderian. Mucosa of the nasal fossae. SYN: *membrana pituitosa.*

m., selectively permeable. A m. that allows a substance such as water to pass through more readily than another, such as salt or sugar.

m., semipermeable. M. allowing passage of water but not substances in solution.

m., serous. M. consisting of mesothelium lying on thin layer of connective tissue which lines the closed cavities (peritoneal, pleural, and pericardial) of the body. Surface is moistened by a thin fluid similar to lymph.

m., Shrapnell's. That portion of the tympanic m. filling the notch of Rivinus.

m., synovial. M. lining a joint and secreting synovia.

m., tectorial. Thin, jellylike membrane projecting from vestibular lip of osseous spiral lamina and overlying the spiral organ of Corti.

m. theory of nerve conduction. Theory that the nerve cell membrane and that of its axon is the seat of the electromotive force establishing the resting potential of a cell; that the breakdown of the membrane such as caused by a threshold stimulus abolishes the membrane potential and

initiates a wave of depolarization which passes along the nerve fiber and is the nerve impulse.

m., thyrohyoid. M. joining the hyoid bone and the thyroid cartilage.

m., tympanic. The drum membrane; membrane separating tympanic cavity from the external auditory canal.

m., virginal. The hymen, q.v.

m., vitelline. Membrane that forms surface layer of an ovum.

m., vitreous. Descemet's membrane, q.v.

m., yolk. A membrane surrounding the ovum; vitelline membrane or zona pellucida, q.v.

membraniform (mĕm-brā′nĭ-form). Resembling or of the nature of a membrane. SYN: *membranoid; membranous.*

membranocartilaginous (mĕm″brăn-ō-kăr-tĭl-aj′ĭ-nŭs). 1. Pert. to both membrane and cartilage. 2. Derived from both membrane and cartilage.

membranoid (mĕm′brā-noid) [L. *membrana*, membrane + Gr. *eidos*, form]. Resembling a membrane. SYN: *membraniform, membranous.*

membranous. Rel. to or resembling a membrane. SYN: *membraniform, membranoid.*

membrum muliebre (mĕm′brum mū-lĭ-ē′-bre) [L. female member]. The clitoris.

membrum virile (mĕm′brŭm vĭr-il′e) [L. male member]. The penis.

memory [L. *memoria*]. The mental registration, retention, and recall of past experience, knowledge, ideas, sensations, and thoughts.

Registration of experience is favored by clear comprehension during intense consciousness. Retention of memory differs greatly with individuals. Memory recall, esp. its intentional recall, means the reproduction of a memory in consciousness. Clear comprehension greatly favors retention. Recall may fail because the memory has been obliterated or because the stream of ideas is that which one does not wish to remember. Various memory defects occur in many diseases.

Memory is confused or obliterated in maniacal states, lively in paranoia, abolished in senile psychosis and organic brain disease, but undisturbed in depressions. In dementia from senile causes there is accurate memory for remote events but none for recent occurrences.

RS: anamnestic; association center; mnemic; mnemonics; retention; retention defect.

m., anterograde. Ability to remember events occurring in the remote past but lacking ability to remember recent events, senile m. SYN: *antegrade amnesia.*

  m., retrograde. Ability to recall events of recent occurrence but lacking ability to recall knowledge with which patient had previously been familiar. SYN: *retrograde amnesia.*

menacme (měn-ăk'mē) [Gr. *mēn,* month, + *akmē,* top]. The pinnacle (acme) of the menstrual life of a woman.

menadiol sodium diphosphate. USP. A synthetic water-soluble vitamin, having same activity as natural vitamin K. Used as an antihemorrhagic agent in hypoprothrombinemia or hemorrhagic disorders due to hypoprothrombinemia.

menarche (měn-ar'kē) [Gr. *mēn,* month, + *archē,* beginning]. Onset of menses. Occurs normally between the 10th and 17th year.

mendelevium (men-dě-lē'vē-um). A transuranium element. SYMB: *Md.* At. wt. 256; at. no. 101.

Mendel's laws. [Gregor Mendel, Austrian monk, 1822-84] Certain principles of heredity established by Mendel. The laws are: *Law of Segregation:* Certain characteristics present in each parent do not combine with or alter each other in the offspring. This accounts for contrasting traits in successive generations. *Law of Independent Combination:* Genes determining pairs of traits combine in the offspring according to chance. *Law of Dominance:* In a pair of genes, one dominant and the other recessive, the recessive trait may appear in an offspring only if both pair of genes are recessive.

  Although Mendel's principles were subsequently shown not to apply universally, his work laid the foundation for the development of modern genetics and the present chromosome theory of heredity (theory of the gene).

Mendel's reflex. [Kurt Mendel, Ger. neurologist, 1874-1946]. Dorsal flexion of 2nd to 5th toes upon percussion of the dorsum of the foot.

menhidrosis (měn-hǐ-drō'sǐs) [Gr. *mēn,* month, + *hidrōs,* sweat]. Vicarious menstruation through the sweat glands. SYN: *menidrosis.*

menidrosis (měn-ǐ-dro'sǐs). Vicarious menstruation through sweat glands. SYN: *menhidrosis.*

Ménière's disease (mān-yair'). [Prosper Meniere, Fr. physician, 1799-1862]. A recurrent and usually progressive group of symptoms including progressive deafness, ringing in the ears, dizziness and a sensation of fullness or pressure in the ears. SYN: *Ménière's syndrome.*

ETIOL: Unknown, but edema of the membranous labyrinth has been found in autopsy studies.

  TREATMENT: In acute attacks bed rest is the most effective treatment. Also antihistamines, discontinuation of smoking, rarely surgical treatment.

meningeal (měn-ĭn'jē-ăl). Rel. to the meninges.

meningeorrhaphy (mě-nĭn-jē-or'ră-fǐ) [Gr. *mēninx,* membrane + *rhaphē,* suture]. Suture of membranes, esp. those of brain and spinal cord.

meninges (měn-ĭn'jēz) [Gr.]. (sing. *meninx)* [NA]. 1. Membranes. 2. The three membranes investing the spinal cord and brain: the dura mater, external; the arachnoid, middle, and pia mater, internal.

meningina (měn-ĭn-jī'nǎ) [Gr. *mēninx,* membrane]. The pia mater and adjacent layer of the arachnoid combined. SYN: *pia-arachnoid.*

meninginitis (měn-ĭn-jǐ-nī'tis) ["+ *-ĭtis,* inflammation]. Inflammation of the pia-arachnoid membrane. SYN: *leptomeningitis; piarachnitis.*

meningioma (měn-ĭn-jǐ-ō'mǎ) ["+ *-ōma,* tumor]. A slow-growing tumor that originates in the arachnoidal tissue.

meningism (měn-ĭn'jĭzm) ["+ *ismos,* state of]. Irritation of the brain and spinal cord with symptoms simulating meningitis, but without actual inflammation.

meningismus. Meningism.

meningitic (měn-ĭn-jĭt'ĭk) [Gr. *mēninx,* membrane]. Pert. to meningitis.

meningitis (měn-ĭn-jī'tis) ["+ *-ĭtis,* inflammation]. Inflammation of the membranes of spinal cord or brain.

  SEE: *chorIomeningitis, Kernig's sign, leptomeningitis, pachymeningitis.*

  m., acute. SYM: Moderate, irregular fever; loss of appetite; constipation; intense headache; intolerance to light and sound; contracted pupils; delirium; retraction of head; convulsions; and coma.

  ETIOL: Caused by bacteria, viruses, or other organisms that reach the meninges from other foci in the body via blood or lymph, through trauma, or from adjacent bony structures (sinuses, mastoid cells).

  PROG: Favorable with prompt diagnosis and appropriate therapy.

  NP AND TREATMENT: The room should be dark and quiet. Retention of urine must be guarded against, as distention is apt to occur. The eyes and mouth must be kept cleansed, and pressure points upon the back should be guarded against. Headache may be relieved by an icebag or cold compresses.

Special nursing technique as may be necessary. Isolation and asepsis are indicated. All discharges should be burned. The eyes should be protected from the light, and all noise and everything that might disturb the patient should be avoided.

A bed cradle may be necessary to relieve pressure and friction. Sudden excitement may cause a convulsion; therefore, quiet is absolutely necessary. Change the patient's position frequently but avoid jarring the bed. Hypostatic pneumonia must be guarded against. A cleansing bath with an alcohol rub should be a daily procedure. All body prominences need special attention to prevent pressure sores. Mouth hygiene is also called for morning and night.

The intake and output of fluids must be recorded. During the acute stage restraints may be necessary.

Sulfonamides are indicated if the organism is sensitive to those drugs. Otherwise intravenous ampicillin is the usual therapy.

DIET: A fluid diet is necessary during the acute stage, but later as much nourishment should be given as possible, as the disease is an exhaustive one. Milk, eggs, beef tea, water, fruit juices, and sugar may be given freely. A more solid diet may be given during convalescence. With stuporous patients, tube feeding is necessary. Children and some adults may have to be fed with a spoon or a medicine dropper.

m., acute aseptic. Lymphocytic choriomeningitis, a nonpurulent form usually running a short, benign course with recovery.

m., basilar. Inflammation at base of brain of the meninges, usually due to tuberculosis.

m., cerebral. Acute or chronic m. of the brain.

m., cerebrospinal. M. of brain and spinal cord.

m., listeria. Listeriosis, q.v.

m., pneumococcal. M. caused by the pneumococcus. Common in young children.

m., serosa circumscripta. M. accompanied by the formation of cystic accumulations of fluid that simulate tumors.

m., serous. Serous exudation in m. into cerebral ventricles.

m., spinal. M. of spinal cord membranes.

m., sterile. M. in which infectious organisms are absent.

m., traumatic. M. resulting from traumatism or injury.

m., tuberculous. An acute inflammation of the cerebral meninges excited by the tubercle bacillus, occurs in children.

SYM: Loss of flesh, gradual wasting of strength, evening rise of temperature, restlessness, irritability, and sleeplessness may exist for some time before acute symptoms come on. These are severe headache, occasional convulsions, delirium, vomiting, fever, optic neuritis.

meningitophobia (měn″ĭn-jĭt″ō-fō′bĭ-ă) [Gr. *mēninx*, membrane, + *phobos*, phobia]. A condition that simulates meningitis and is caused by fear of meningitis.

meningo (měn-ĭn′gō). A combining form that denotes relationship to the membranes covering the spinal cord or brain.

meningoarteritis (men-ĭn″gō-ăr″tĕr-ĭt′ĭs). Inflammatory condition of the meningeal arteries.

meningocele (měn-ĭn′gō-sēl) [Gr. *mēninx*, membrane, + *kēlē*, hernia]. Congenital hernia, the meninges protruding through an opening of the skull or spinal column.

meningococcemia (měn-ĭn″gō-kŏk-sē′mĭ-ă). Meningococci in the circulating blood.

meningococcus (měn-ĭn″-gō-kŏk′ŭs). (pl. *meningococci*). A microorganism of Neisseria meningitidis, the causative agent of epidemic cerebral meningitis (cerebrospinal fever, spotted fever).

meningocortical (měn-ĭn″gō-kor′tĭ-kal). Pert. to the meninges and the cortex of the brain.

meningoencephalitis (měn-ĭn″gō-ěn-sěf′ăl-i′tĭs) [Gr. *mēninx*, membrane, + *enkephalos*, brain, + *-itis*, inflammation]. Inflammation of the brain and its meninges.

meningoencephalocele (měn-ĭn″gō-en-sěf′-ăl-ō-sēl) [″+ ″+ *kēlē*, hernia]. Hernial protrusion of brain and meninges.

meningoencephalomyelitis (měn-ĭn″gō-ĕn-sěf′ăl-ō-mĭ-ěl-ĭ′tĭs) [″+ ″+ *myelos*, marrow, + *-itis*, inflammation]. Inflammation of the brain, spinal cord, and their meninges.

meningomalacia (měn-ĭn″gō-mă-lā′shĭ-ă) [″+ *malakia*, softening]. Softening of any membrane.

meningomyelitis (měn-ĭn″gō-mī″ěl-ĭ′tĭs) [″+ *myelos*, marrow, + *-itis*, inflammation]. Inflammation of spinal cord and its enveloping arachnoid and pia mater; and less commonly of the dura mater.

meningomyelocele (měn-ĭn″gō-mī-ěl′ō-sēl) [″+ ″+ *kēlē*, hernia]. Hernia of spinal cord and membranes through a defect in the vertebral column.

meningopathy (měn-ĭn-gŏp′ă-thī) [″+ *pathos*, disease]. Any pathological condition of the meninges.

meningorrhachidian (měn-ĭn″go-ră-kĭd′-ĭ-an) ["+ *rhachis,* spine]. Concerning the spinal cord and meninges.

meningorrhagia (měn-ĭn″gō-rā′jĭ-ă) ["+ *rhēgnynai,* to burst forth]. Meningeal hemorrhage. SYN: *meningorrhea.*

meningorrhea (men-ĭn″gō-rē′ă) ["+ *rhoia,* flow]. Meningeal hemorrhage. SYN: *meningorrhagia.*

meningotyphoid (men-ĭn″gō-tī′foid). Typhoid fever with symptoms of meningitis.

meningovascular (měn-ĭn″gō-văs′kū-lăr). Pert. to blood vessels of the meninges.

meninguria (měn″ĭn-gū′rĭ-ă) [Gr. *mēninx,* membrane, + *ouron,* urine]. Presence of membraniform shreds in urine.

meninx (mē′ninks) [Gr. membrane]. (pl. *meninges*) [NA] Any membrane, but esp. one of the coverings of the brain or spinal cord.

meniscectomy (měn″ĭ-sĕk′tō-mĭ). Removal of meniscus cartilage of the knee.

menisci (měn-ĭs′ī). Plural of meniscus.

meniscitis (měn-ĭ-sī′tĭs) [Gr. *mēniskos,* crescent, + *-itis,* inflammation]. Inflamed condition of an interarticular cartilage, esp. the semilunar cartilages of the knee joint.

meniscocyte (měn-ĭs′kō-sīt) ["+ *cyte,* cell]. A crescent-shaped red blood cell; sickle cell.

meniscocytosis (měn-ĭs″kō-sī-tō′sĭs) ["+ "+ *-ōsis,* intensive]. Crescent cells in the blood; sickle cell anemia, q.v.

meniscus (měn-ĭs′kŭs) [Gr. *mēniskos,* crescent]. (pl. *menis′ci*) 1. Concavoconvex lens. 2. Interarticular fibrocartilage of crescent shape, found in certain joints, esp. the lateral and medial menisci (semilunar cartilages) of the knee joint. 3. The curved upper surface of a liquid in a container. The surface is convex if the liquid does not wet the container and concave if it does.

    m. articularis. [NA]. Crescent-shaped interarticular fibrocartilage found in certain joints.

menometrorrhagia (měn″ō-mět-rō-rā′jĭ-ă) [Gr. *mēn,* month, + *mētra,* womb, + *rhēgnyna,* to burst forth]. Irregular and excessive menstrual bleeding. RS: menorrhagia, metrorrhagia.

menopause (měn′ō-pawz) ["+ *pausis,* cessation]. That period which marks the permanent cessation of menstrual activity.

    Occurs bet. 35 and 58 years of life. The menses may stop suddenly; there may be a decreased flow each month until there is a final cessation; or the interval bet. periods may be lengthened until complete cessation is accomplished.

    Natural menopause will occur in 25% of women by age 47, in 50% by age 50, 75% by age 52, and in 95% by age 55. Surgical menopause occurs in almost 30% of U.S. women aged 50 to 64.

    SYM: Menopause may be accompanied by hot and cold flashes, feeling of weakness, and in some cases mental depression.

    TREATMENT: Hormone replacement as required. Yearly pelvic examination to include Papanicolaou test for cancer of the cervix. SYN: *change of life; climacteric.*

    RS: involution, menses, menstruation, sexual involution.

    m., artificial. M. occurring subsequent to surgical castration, x-ray irradiation, or radium implantation into the uterus.

    m., premature. M. either natural or artificial occuring before age 35.

menophania (měn-ō-fā′nĭ-ă) ["+ *phainesthai,* to appear]. First appearance of the menses at puberty.

menoplania (měn-ō-plā′nĭ-ă) ["+ *plane,* deviation]. Vicarious menstruation; menstruation through other than the normal outlet, as through the nose.

menorrhagia (měn-ō-rā′jĭ-ă) ["+ *rhēgnynai,* to burst forth]. Excessive bleeding at the time of a menstrual period, either in number of days or amount of blood or both.

    ETIOL: *Endocrine Disturbances:* Pituitary gland, thyroid, and ovary. *General Systemic Diseases:* Hypertension, diabetes mellitus, blood dyscrasias, chronic nephritis. *Malpositions of the Uterus:* Retroversion and retroflexion. *New Growths of the Uterus:* Particularly fibroids of the intramural and submucous types, adenomyosis of the uterus, fibrosis of the uterus with hyperplastic changes of the endometrium. *Conditions of the Cervix Uteri:* Erosions or polypi. *Inflammations in the Pelvis:* Acute salpingitis, acute metritis, acute endometritis, chronic metritis, and endometritis.

    SEE: *hemorrhage, uterine.*

menorrhalgia (men-o-ral′jĭ-ă) ["+ "+ *algia,* pain]. Painful menstruation or pelvic pain accompanying menstruation, sometimes a symptom of endometriosis. SYN: *dysmenorrhea.*

menorrhea (měn-ō-rē′ă). 1. Normal menstruation. 2. Free or profuse menstruation. SYN: *menorrhagia.*

menostaxis (měn″ō-stak′sĭs) [Gr. *mēn,* month, + *staxis,* dripping]. Prolonged menstruation.

menotoxin. A substance present in the menstrual flow. Toxic to certain plants but nontoxic to the menstruant or her associates.

menotropins. Combination of follicle-stimulating and luteinizing hormones (FSH and LH) used to promote growth and maturation of the follicle of the ovary. Menotropins is obtained from the urine of postmenopausal women and is used with human chorionic gondadotropin (HCG) to induce ovulation.

menoxenia (měn-ŏk-sē'nĭ-ă) [Gr. *měn*, month, + *xenos*, strange]. Abnormal menstruation.

menses (men'sēz) [L.]. (pl. of *mensis*, month) Monthly flow of bloody fluid from the uterine mucous membrane; catamenial flow.

menstrual (měn'strŭ-ăl) [L. *menstrualis*]. Pert. to menstruation. SYN: *catamenial*.

m. cycle. The periodically recurrent series of changes occurring in the uterus and associated sex organs (ovaries, vagina) associated with menstruation and the intermenstrual period. The human cycle averages 28 days in length, measured from the beginning of menstruation. The menstrual cycle is, however, quite variable in length even in the same person from month to month.

The menstrual cycle is divided into four phases characterized by histological changes which take place in the uterine endometrium. They are:

Menstruation: Period of uterine bleeding accompanied by shedding of the endometrium. Averages 4 to 5 days in length.

Proliferative Phase: Uterine epithelium is restored to normal; endometrium becomes thicker and more vascular; glands elongate. During this period the ovarian follicle is maturing and secreting estrogens. Period is terminated by rupture of follicle and liberation of ovum at about 14 days before next menstrual period begins. Length of postmenstrual period, 10-13 days.

Luteal or Secretory Phase: Endometrium increases in thickness; glands become more tortuous and produce an abundant secretion containing glycogen. Coiled arteries make their appearance; endometrium becomes edematous; stroma becomes compact. During this period the corpus luteum in ovary is developing and secreting progesterone. Lasts 10 to 14 days.

Premenstrual or Ischemic Phase: A day or two before menstruation, coiled arteries constrict and endometrium becomes anemic and shrinks. Corpus luteum of ovary begins involution. Period lasts about two days and is terminated by opening up of constricted arteries, the breaking off of small patches of necrotic endometrium, and the beginning of menstruation with the flow of menstrual fluid.

Variations in the length of the cycle are due principally to variation in the length of the proliferative phase.

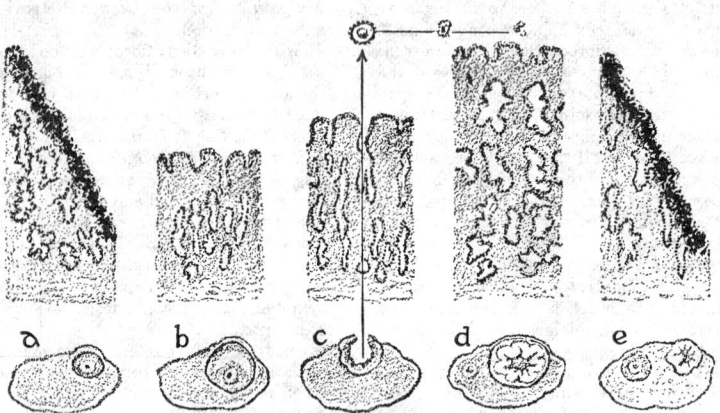

MENSTRUAL CYCLE CHANGES IN THE LINING OF THE UTERUS (ENDOMETRIUM) AND THE OVARY

Above, Endometrium; Below, Graafian follicle. A, Menstrual phase. Lining is shed; graafian follicle begins to develop in ovary. B, Follicular phase. As endometrium is repaired and thickens, the follicle continues to grow. C, Ovulation. Lining of the uterus continues to grow; the graafian follicle ruptures to free the ovum. D, Luteal phase. Endometrium continues to develop in order to provide a suitable place for implantation of the egg if it is fertilized. Corpus luteum begins to develop in ruptured follicle. E, If the ovum is not fertilized the lining is shed and the cycle begins again. The corpus luteum atrophies and a new graafian follicle begins to develop.

m. hygiene. The m. cycle should be thoroughly explained to young girls well before menarche. If this is done, they will not be frightened or alarmed when they first menstruate. The availability of, and directions for using, perineal pads and tampons should also be explained. The m. cycle is a normal physiological event and should be so presented to adolescent girls. There is no medical reason why the m. period should be regarded as being a time of sickness, nor should there be necessity for curtailing the individual's normal activity at work or play.

menstruant (mĕn'strŭ-ănt) [L. *menstruāre*, to discharge the menses]. 1. In the condition of menstruating. 2. One who menstruates.

menstruate (mĕn'strŭ-āt) [L. *menstruāre*]. To discharge menses.

menstruation (mĕn-strŭ-ā'shŭn). The periodic discharge of a bloody fluid from the uterus occurring at more or less regular intervals during the life of a woman from age of puberty to menopause. The discharge contains altered blood with normal, hemolyzed, and sometimes agglutinated, red blood cells; disintegrated endometrial and stroma cells; and secretions of glands. In general, menstrual blood does not coagulate, but the passage of occasional clots is not unusual.

Menstruation is brought on by the reduction in production of ovarian hormones, esp. progesterone, which results from involution of the corpus luteum following failure of the ovum to become fertilized.

Menstruation has its onset at puberty (10-16 years of age). Length of flow varies from 3 to 7 days (av. 4 to 5 days). It occurs on an average every 27 to 28 days, although time may vary from 18 to 40 days. Menstruation ceases temporarily during pregnancy; may or may not cease during lactation; and ceases permanently with onset of menopause. Its failure to occur may result from congenital abnormalities, physical disorders (disease, obesity, malnutrition), emotional or hormonal disturbances, esp. diseases involving the ovaries, hypophysis, thyroid, or adrenal glands.

Menstrual Irregularities: Absence of flow when normally expected is called *amenorrhea;* scanty flow is known as *oligomenorrhea;* painful menstruation is *dysmenorrhea.* Excessive loss of blood is termed *menorrhagia;* loss of blood during intermenstrual periods is known as spotting or *metrorrhagia.*

m., anovulatory. Menstruation occurring without discharge of ovum from ovary.

m., retrograde. Backflow of menstrual fluid through fallopian tubes into peritoneal cavity.

m., suppressed. Failure of menstruation to occur when normally expected.

m., vicarious. Menstruation from site other than the uterus.

menstruous (men'strŭ-ŭs) [L. *menstruāre*, to discharge the menses]. Rel. to menstruation.

menstruum (men'strŭ-ŭm) [L. *menstruus,* menstrual fluid; once it was believed that this fluid had solvent qualities]. A solvent; a medium. SEE: *vehicle.*

mensuration (men-sŭ-rā'shŭn) [L. *mensuro,* to measure]. The process of measuring.

mentagrophyton (men''tă-grŏf'i-ton). The fungus that causes infection in the hair of the scalp and beard, as well as the skin and nails.

mental. 1. [L. *mens, ment-,* mind]. Rel. to the mind. 2. [L. *mentum,* chin]. Rel. to the chin.

m. age. Age of a person with respect to the intellectual development as contrasted with the chronological age. ABBR: MA.

m. deficiency. Deficient intellectual development. The Committee on Nomenclature of the American Psychiatric Association has classified mental deficiency according to intellectual capacity:

Mild: IQ 70-85; functional (vocational) impairment; individual formerly classified as borderline and having lower level of dull normal intelligence; can do laboring jobs.

Moderate: IQ 50-70; intellectual capacity that of 7- to 12-year old; limited social adjustment; special training and guidance required.

Severe: IQ 0-50; intellectual capacity does not exceed that of 7-year old; custodial or complete protective care required.

m. disease. A disorder of the mind or intellect. Mild forms are known as psychoneuroses, q.v.; more severe forms, psychoses, q.v.

m. fog. Clouding of consciousness, usually with some loss of memory.

m. hygiene. Science of maintaining healthy mental and emotional responses and preventing development of psychoses.

m. illness. Any disorder which affects the mind or behavior.

m. retardation. Mental deficiency, q.v.

mentality. Mental power or activity; keenness of breadth of mind.

Men'tha [L.]. Mint; a genus of labiate plants.

M. piperita. Peppermint.

M. pulegium. Pennyroyal.

M. viridis. Spearmint.

menthol. USP. An alcohol ($C_{10}H_{20}O$) obtained from oil of peppermint or other mint oils. May be prepared synthetically. Occurs in crystalline form.

ACTION AND USES: As a counterirritant, antiseptic, and anodyne.

mentulagra (mĕn"tū-lăg'rä) [L. *mentula*, penis, + Gr. *agra*, seizure]. Painful involuntary erection of the penis, sometimes curved. SYN: *chordee; priapism.*

mentulate (mĕn'tū-lāt) [L. *mentula*, penis]. Possessing a large penis.

mentulomania (mĕn"tū-lō-mā'nĭ-ä) ["+ Gr. *mania*, madness]. Mental state characterized by addiction to masturbation.

men'tum [L.]. [NA] The chin. SYN: *genion.*

mephenesin (mĕ-fĕn'ĕ-sin). A skeletal muscle relaxant.

mephit'ic [L. *mephiticus,* mephitis, foul exhalation]. Noxious, foul, as a poisonous odor.

meprobamate (mĕ-prō'bă-māt). A tranquilizing agent, used for relief of anxiety and mental tension.

mEq. Abbr. for *milliequivalent.*

meralgia (mĕr-al'jĭ-ä) [Gr. *meros,* thigh, + *algos,* pain]. Pain in the thigh.

   m. paresthetica. Paresthesia and disturbed sensation of the lateral area of the thigh; due to injury to the external cutaneous femoral nerve.

Mercier's bar (mer-se-ā'). [Louis A. Mercier, Fr. urologist, 1811-1882] A curved fold at neck of bladder forming posterior margin of trigonum vesicae. SYN: *Mercier's barrier.*

mercupurin (mĕr-kū'pū-rĭn). A proprietary diuretic.

mercurial (mĕr-kū'rĭ-al) [L. *mercurialis*]. 1. Pert. to mercury. 2. A substance containing mercury.

   m. diuretics. Organic mercurial compounds that produce diuresis.

   m. palsy. Paralysis induced by mercurial poisoning.

   m. rash. Rash caused by local application of mercurial preparations.

mercurialism (mer-kū'rĭ-al-ĭzm) [L. *mercurius,* mercury, + Gr. *ismos,* state of]. Chronic poisoning by mercury seen as a result of continuous administration of mercury.

Also occurs in workmen who work with the metal or inhale its vapors.

SYM: Soreness of gums and loosening of teeth; increased salivation; fetor of breath; griping, and diarrhea.

mercurialization (mer-kū"rĭ-al-ĭ-zā'shŭn). Condition of influencing with mercury.

mercurialized (mĕr-kū'rĭ-al-ĭzd). 1. Impregnated with mercury. 2. Influenced by or treated with mercury.

mercuric (mer-kū'rĭk). Rel. to bivalent mercury.

   m. chloride. ($HgCl_2$). A common compound of mercury.

This solution used in strength of 1:1000 of water frees the hands or skin from bacteria; in strength of 1:2000 or 1:4000 it may be used for wound irrigation. It should be remembered that this disinfectant coagulates albumen, corrodes metal instruments, and causes local dermatitis. No metallic instrument should ever be placed in contact with mercuric chloride. Since it has been put up in blue coffin-shaped tablets in a notched bottle, poisoning has been less common.

POISONING SYM: *Acute:* Those of any severe gastrointestinal irritation with pain, cramping, constriction of the throat, vomiting, and a metallic taste in the mouth. Stronger solution causes a white coating due to coagulation. Abdominal pain may be so severe as to cause fainting, bloody diarrhea, bloody vomitus, scanty urine, prostration, convulsions, and unconsciousness. Death is the usual outcome unless treatment is begun immediately. *Chronic:* Bad breath, loosening of teeth, fever, urinary difficulties, nausea, diarrhea, sore tongue, paralysis, weakness, and death.

F. A. TREATMENT: Evacuate stomach, wash out with milk or with a baking soda solution made by dissolving a teaspoonful of sodium bicarbonate in 6 oz. (177 ml.) of water. Treatment with BAL (British antilewisite) should begin as soon as possible after poisoning has occurred. Maintain fluid and electrolyte balance.

   m. oxide. (HgO). A powder, usually yellow in color. Used in ointments as an antibacterial agent.

mercurochrome (mer-kū'rō-krōm). A compound containing about 23% mercury, used as an antiseptic in solution.

mercurous (mer-kū'rus, mer'kū-rus). Rel. to monovalent mercury.

   m. chloride. (HgCl) This is a heavy white powder used in small doses in medicine as a laxative; calomel.

It is used in powder form as an application in ulcers and skin rashes.

POISONING: SYM: Salivation, abdominal discomfort, and diarrhea.

F. A. TREATMENT: SEE: *mercuric chloride.*

mercury (mer'kū-rĭ) [L. *mercurius*]. A metallic element. SYMB: *Hg.* At. wt. 200.59; at. no. 80. Insoluble in ordinary solvents but soluble in hydrochloric acid upon boiling. It is a silvery liquid at ordinary temperatures. Forms two series of salts: mercurous in which it has a valence of one (univalent), and mercuric in which it has a valence of two (bivalent). SYN: *quicksilver*.

NOTE: Metallic mercury swallowed in small quantities, as from a broken thermometer, is not harmful.

POISONING SYM: In large doses, increased salivation, abdominal cramps, interference with kidney function, etc. SEE: *Table of Poisons and Poisoning* in *Appendix*.

m., ammoniated. Mercuric chloride ($HgNH_2Cl$); used in anti-infective ointment. SEE: *white precipitate*.

m. bichloride. Corrosive sublimate ($HgCl_2$).

USES: Germicide.

SEE: *mercuric chloride, nephrosis*.

mercuzan'thine. A proprietary name for a preparation of mercurophylline sodium, a diuretic.

meridian. An imaginary line encircling a globular body at right angles to its equator and passing through the poles, or a half of such a line.

m. of eye. A circle passing through ant. and post. poles of the eyeball.

meridrosis (mer-id-rō'sĭs) [Gr. *meros,* part, + *idrōsis,* perspiration]. Local perspiration.

merinthophobia (mĕr-ĭn-thō-fō'bĭ-ă) [Gr. *mērinthos,* a cord, + *phobia,* fear]. Morbid fear of being tied.

merispore (mer'ĭ-spōr) [Gr. *meros,* a part, + *sporos,* seed]. A secondary spore resulting from the division of another spore.

mero- [Gr. *meros*]. Combining form meaning a part.

meroblastic (mer-ō-blăst'ĭk) ["+ *blastos,* germ]. Pert. to a type of ovum containing considerable yolk or a type of cleavage in which cleavage divisions are restricted to the protoplasmic region of the animal pole. Opposed to holoblastic.

merocele (mer'ō-sēl) ["+ *kēlē,* hernia]. Femoral hernia.

merocoxalgia (mer''ō-koks-al'jĭ-ă) ["+ L. *coxa,* hip, + *algia,* pain]. Painful condition of the thigh and hip.

merocrine (mer'o-krĭn) ["+ *krinein,* to separate]. Pert. to a type of secretion in which the glandular cell remains intact during the process of elaborating and discharging its product. SEE: *apocrine, holocrine*.

meroergasia (mĕr''ō-ĕr-gă'zĭ-ă) [Gr. *meros,* a part + *ergasia,* work]. Partial mental disorder with symptoms of emotional instability. SEE: *holergastic*.

merogenesis (mĕr''ō-jĕn'ĕ-sĭs) ["+ *genesis,* production]. Multiplication or reproduction by segmentation.

merology (mer-ŏl'ō-jĭ) ["+ *logos,* study of]. Anatomy of the elementary tissues.

meromicrosomia (mĕr''ō-mī''krō-sō'mĭ-ă) ["+ *micros,* small, + *sōma,* body]. Abnormal smallness of some part or structure of the body.

meronecrosis (mer''ō-nĕk-rō'sĭs) ["+ *nekros,* dead]. Death of cells.

meropia (mer-ō'pĭ-ă) [Gr. *meros,* part, + *ōps,* vision]. Partial blindness.

merorrhachischisis (mē''rō-ră-kis'kĭ-sis) ["+ *rhachis,* spine, + *schisis,* fissure]. Fissure of a portion of the spinal cord.

merosmia (mĕr-ŏs'mĭ-ă) ["+ *osmē,* odor]. Inability to detect certain odors.

merosystolic (mĕr-ō-sĭs-tŏl'ĭk) ["+ *systolē,* a contraction]. Rel. to a portion of the systole.

merotomy (mer-ot'o-mē) ["+ *tomē,* incision]. Division into sections or segments.

merozoite (mer-ō-zō'ĭt) [Gr. *meros,* part, + *zoon,* animal]. A body formed by segmentation or breaking up of schizont in asexual reproduction of certain sporozoans such as Plasmodium. Merozoites when formed are liberated and invade other corpuscles where they repeat the process of schizogony, or develop into gametocytes.

merthiolate (mer-thi'ō-lāt). Proprietary name for thimerosal. An organic combination containing about 50% mercury and less toxic than bichloride, used as a disinfectant in solutions of 1:5000 to 1:1000 aqueous, or in the form of a tincture 1:2000. For ophthalmic use, 1:5000 ointment, or 1:10,000 aqueous.

mesad (mēs'ăd) [Gr. *mesos,* middle, + L. *ad,* toward]. Toward a median point, line, or plane.

mesal (mēs'ăl). In a middle line or plane.

mesaortitis (mēs-ă-or-tī'tĭs). Inflammation of the middle aortic coat.

mesaraic, mesareic (mēs-ar-ā'ĭk, -e'ĭk) [Gr. *mesaraion,* the mesentery]. Rel. to the mesentery. SYN: *mesenteric*.

mesarteritis (mēs-ar-tĕr-ī'tĭs). Inflammation of the tunica media or middle coat of an artery.

mesaticephalic (mēs-ăt'ĭ-sef-al'ĭk) [Gr. *mesatos,* medium, + *kephalē,* brain]. Having a skull with a cephalic index of 75 to 79.9 degrees.

mesatipellic, mesatipelvic (mēs-ăt'ĭ-pĕl'lĭk, -pel'vĭk) ["+ *pella,* bowl]. Having a pelvis with an index bet. 90 and 95 degrees.

mescaline (mēs'kă-lēn). A poisonous alkaloid, the active ingredient of the mescal cactus that causes hallucinations, esp. those involving color and music. SYN: *peyote*.

mesectic (mĕs-ek'tĭk) [Gr. *mesos*, middle, + *echein*, to hold]. Using an average amount of oxygen. SEE: *mionectic, pleonectic.*

mesectoderm (mĕs-ĕk'tō-derm). Migratory cells derived from ectoderm, esp. from the neural crest of the cephalic area in young embryos; become pigment cells.

mesencephalon (mĕs-ĕn-sĕf'ă-lŏn) [Gr. *mesos*, middle, + *enkephalos*, brain]. [NA] The midbrain, one of three primitive cerebral vesicles from which develop the corpora quadrigemina, the crura cerebri, and the aqueduct of Sylvius.

mesenchyme (mĕs'ĕn-kīm) ["+ *enchyma*, infusion]. A diffuse network of cells forming the embryonic mesoderm and giving rise to connective tissues, blood and blood vessels, the lymphatic system, and cells of the reticuloendothelial system.

mesenter'ic. Pert. to the mesentery.

mesenteriolum (mĕs-ĕn-ter-ĭ-ō'lŭm) [L.]. A small mesentery, as that of a diverticulum of the intestine.

mesenteriopexy (mĕs''ĕn-ter'ĭ-ō-pek'sĭ) [Gr. *mesos*, middle, + *enteron*, intestine, + *pēxis*, fixation]. Operation for attaching a torn mesentery.

mesenteriorrhaphy (mĕs''ĕn-ter-ĭ-or'ă- fĭ) ["+ "+ *rhaphē*, suture]. Suturing of the mesentery.

mesenteriplication (mĕs''ĕn-tĕr-ĭ-plĭ-kā'- shun) ["+ "+ L. *plicāre*, to fold]. Shortening the mesentery by taking tucks in it surgically.

mesenteritis (mes''ĕn-tĕr-ī'tĭs). Inflamed condition of the mesentery.

mesenteron (mĕs-ĕn'ter-ŏn). Middle portion of the embryonic digestive tract.

mesentery (mĕs'ĕn-ter'ĭ). A peritoneal fold, encircling the greater part of the small intestines and connecting the intestine to the post. abdominal wall.

mesiad (mē'zē-ăd) [Gr. *mesos*, middle + L. *ad*, toward]. Toward the median plane of a body or part. SYN: *mesad.*

mesial (mē'sī-ăl). Located near the median plane of the body. SYN: *median.*

mesio-. In dentistry, combing form meaning pertaining to or facing the median plane of the mouth.

mesion (mē'sē-ŏn) [Gr. *mesos*, middle]. The imaginary plane dividing the body into right and left symmetric halves. SYN: *meson.*

mesiris (mes-ĭ'ris). Middle portion of the iris.

mesmeric (mes-mer'ĭk). [Franz Anton Mesmer, Austrian physician, 1734-1815] Rel. to or induced by hypnotism; fascinating.

mesmerism (mes'mer-izm). Originally Mesmer's theory of animal magnetism, it now means therapeutics employing hypnotism or hypnotic suggestion.

meso-. Combining form meaning (1) middle; (2) in anatomy, pert. to a mesentery; (3) in medicine, secondary or partial.

mesoaortitis (mes''ō-ā-or-tī'tis). Inflamed condition of aortic middle coat. SYN: *mesaortitis.*

mesoappendicitis. Inflamed condition of the mesoappendix.

mesoappendix (mes''ō-ap-pen'dĭks) [Gr. *mesos*, middle + L. *appendix*, an appendage]. [NA]. Mesentery of the vermiform appendix.

mesobronchitis (mes''ō-bron-kī'tĭs). Inflammation of the middle layer of the bronchi.

mesocardia (mes-ō-kar'dĭ-ă) [Gr. *mesos*, middle, + *kardia*, heart]. Location of the heart in the middle line of the thorax, being a normal position in fetal stage but a malposition in life.

mesocardium (mes-ō-kar'dĭ-ŭm). An embryonic mesentery supporting the heart. The dorsal m. connects heart to the foregut; the ventral m. connects heart to central body wall.

mesocecum (mes-ō-sē'kŭm). Mesentery attaching the cecum.

mesocele (mes'ō-sēl) [Gr. *mesos*, middle, + *koilia*, hollow]. Sylvian aqueduct in the brain.

mesocephalic (mes-ō-sef-al'ik) ["+ *kephalē*, head]. 1. Pert. to the midbrain. 2. Having a medium-sized head. 3. Having a cranial index of 76.0 to 80.9.

mesocolic (mes-ō-kol'ik). Concerning the mesocolon.

mesocolon (mes-ō-kō'lon). [NA]. Mesentery connecting colon with post. abdominal wall.

mesocolopexy (mĕs''ō-kō'lō-pek-sĭ) [Gr. *mesos*, middle, + *kōlon*, colon, + *pēxis*, fixation]. The taking of tucks in the mesocolon and then suturing it to make it shorter in order to correct unneeded mobility and ptosis. SYN: *mesocoloplication.*

mes'ocord. A portion of umbilical cord attached to placenta by means of an amniotic fold.

mesoderm (mĕs'ō-derm) [Gr. *mesos*, middle, + *derma*, skin]. A primary germ layer of the embryo lying between ectoderm and entoderm. From it arise all connective tissues; muscular, skeletal, circulatory, lymphatic, and urogenital systems; and the linings of the body cavities. SEE: *ectoderm; entoderm.*

   m., axial. That giving rise to notochord and prechordal plate.

   m., extraembryonic. That lying outside the embryo proper. It is involved in formation of amnion, chorion, yolk sac, and body stalk.

m., intermediate. M. lying between somite and lateral mesoderm. Gives rise to embryonic and definitive kidneys and their ducts. Also called nephrotome. SYN: *mesomere.*

m., lateral. Unsegmented m. lying lateral to the intermediate mesoderm. In it develops a cavity, the coelom, separating it into layers, the somatic and splanchnic mesoderm. SYN: *hypomere.*

m., paraxial. M. lying immediately lateral to neural tube and notochord. SYN: *epimere.*

m., somatic. Outer layer of lateral mesoderm. Becomes intimately associated with ectoderm, forming somatopleure from which ventral and lateral walls of embryo develop.

m., splanchnic. Inner layer of lateral mesoderm. Becomes intimately associated with entoderm forming splanchnopleure from which the gut and lungs and their coverings arise.

mesoduodenum(mĕs″ō-dū-ō-dē′nŭm). Mesentery connecting duodenum to abdominal wall.

mesogastric (mĕs-ō-gas′trĭk). 1. Pert. to umbilical region. 2. Pert. to the mesogastrium.

mesogastrium (mĕs″ō-gas′trĭ-ŭm) [Gr. *mesos,* middle, + *gastēr,* belly]. 1. [NA] The umbilical region. 2. The part of the mesentery of the embryo attached to the primitive stomach.

mesognathic (mĕs″ŏg-nāth′ĭk) ["+ *gnathos,* jaw]. Having a gnathic index bet. 98 and 103.

mesognathion (mĕs-og-nath′ĭ-on). The intermaxillary or premaxillary bone.

mesohyloma (mes-ō-hī-lō′mă) ["+ *hylē,* matter, + *-ōma,* tumor]. Tumor derived from the mesothelium.

meso-ileum (mes-ō-il′ē-ŭm). Mesentery of the ileum.

mesojejunum (mes-ō-jē-jū′nŭm). Mesentery of the jejunum.

mesomere (mes′ō-mēr) [Gr. *mesos,* middle, + Gr. *meros,* part]. Portion of mesoderm between epimere and hypomere. SYN: *nephrotome; intermediate mesoderm.*

mesometritis (mes-ō-mē-trī′tis) ["+ *mētra,* uterus, + *-itis,* inflammation]. Inflammation of the uterine musculature. SYN: *myometritis.*

mesometrium (mes-o-mē′trī-um). 1. The uterine musculature. 2. [NA]. The broad ligament below the mesovarium.

mesomorph (mes′ō-morf) ["+ *morphē,* form]. A well-proportioned person of medium height. SEE: *somatotype.*

mesomorphy. Body build characterized by predominance of tissues derived from the mesoderm. SEE: *ectomorphy; endomorphy; somatotype.*

meson (mes′ŏn) [Gr. *mesos,* middle]. 1. Particle of mass intermediate between that of the electron and proton. Mesons of more than one variety and of both positive and negative charge occur. SYN: *mesotron.* 2. Mesion, q.v.

mesona′sal. In the middle of the nose.

mesonephric (mĕs-ō-nĕf′rĭk) ["+ *nephros,* kidney]. Pert. to the mesonephros.

m. duct. Embryonic duct which gives rise in the male to reproductive ducts (ductus epididymidis, ductus deferens, seminal vesicle, and ejaculatory duct). In the female, it gives rise to Gartner's duct of the epoophoron, a rudimentary structure. SYN: *wolffian duct.*

m. tubules. Embryonic tubules consisting of two groups, cranial and caudal. The cranial group gives rise in the male to efferent ductules of testes and appendix epididymis; in the female to the epoophoron and vesicular appendices. The caudal group gives rise in the male to the paradidymis and aberrant ductules; in the female to the paroophoron. All structures except the efferent ductules of the testes are vestigial.

mesonephroma (mes″ō-nē-frō′mă). A relatively rare tumor derived from mesonephric cells developing in reproductive organs, esp. ovary or genital tract.

mesonephros (mĕs″ō-nĕf′ros). (pl. *mesonephroi*) [NA]. A type of kidney which develops in all vertebrate embryos of classes above the Cyclostomes. It is the permanent kidney of fishes and amphibians but is replaced by the metanephros in reptiles and mammals. SYN: *wolffian body; middle kidney.*

mesoneuritis (me-sō-nū-ri′tis) [Gr. *mesos,* middle, + *neuron,* nerve, + *-itis,* inflammation]. Inflammation of the substance of a nerve or of its lymphatics.

mesopexy (mes′ō-pĕks-ĭ) ["+ *pēxis,* fixation]. Surgery to attach a torn mesentery.

mesophilic (mes-ō-fil′ĭk) ["+ *philein,* to love]. Preferring moderate temperature, as some bacteria which develop best at temperatures between 15° and 43° C.

mesophryon (mes-ŏf′rī-on) ["+ *ophrys,* eyebrow]. Midpoint in smooth space bet. the eyebrows. SEE: *glabella.*

mesopneumon (mes-ō-nū′mŏn) ["+ *pneumōn,* lung]. Meeting point of two pleural layers at hilus of the lung.

mesopor'phyrin. $C_{34}H_{38}O_4N_4$. An iron-free derivative of hemin.

mesorchium (mes-or'kĭ-um) ["+ *orchis*, testicle]. [NA]. Peritoneal fold which holds fetal testes in place.

mesorectum (mĕs-ō-rĕk'tŭm). Mesentery of the rectum.

mesoropter (mes-ō-rŏp'ter) [Gr. *mesos*, middle, + *horos*, boundary, + *optēr*, observer]. Normal eye position with muscles at rest.

mesorrhachischisis (mĕs''ō-ră-kĭs'kĭ-sĭs) ["+ *rhachis*, spine, + *schisis*, cleft]. Fissure of a portion of the spinal cord. SYN: *merorrhachischisis.*

mesorrhaphy (mes-or'ră-fĭ) ["+ *rhaphē*, suture]. Suture of the mesentery. SYN: *mesenteriorrhaphy.*

mesorrhine (mes'ō-rīn) ["+ *rhis*, nose]. With a nasal index variously quoted to range anywhere bet. 48 and 53.

mesosalpinx (mĕs''ō-sal'pĭnks) [Gr. *mesos*, middle, + *salpinx*, tube]. [NA] The free margin of the upper division of the broad ligament, within which lies the oviduct.

mesoseme (mes'ō-sēm) ["+ *sēma*, sign]. Possessing an orbital index bet. 83 and 89.

mesosigmoid (mĕs-ō-sĭg'moid). Mesentery of the sigmoid flexure.

mesoskelic (mes-ō-skĕl'ĭk) ["+ *skelos*, leg]. Legs of normal length.

mesosternum (mes''ō-ster'nŭm) ["+ *sternon*, chest]. The middle or second section of the sternum. SYN: *gladiolus.*

mesotendon. Tissue lining a fibrous sheath attaching the sheath to the tendon. SYN: *mesotendineum.*

mesothelium (mĕs-ō-thē'lĭ-ŭm). [NA]. The layer of cells, derived from the mesoderm lining the primitive body cavity; in the adult it becomes the epithelium covering the serous membranes.

mesothenar (mes-ō-thē'nar) [Gr. *mesos*, middle, + *thenar*, palm]. The adductor pollicis muscle.

mes'otron. A subatomic particle of weight intermediate between light particles (electrons) and heavy particles (protons). SYN: *meson.*

mesovarium (mĕs-ō-vā'rĭ-ŭm). [NA]. The portion of the peritoneal fold that connects the ant. border of the ovary to the post. layer of the broad ligament.

meta- (mĕt'ă) [Gr. *meta*, after, beyond, over].
1. Prefix denoting change, transformation, or following something in a series. 2. In chemistry, prefix indicating the 1-3 position of benzene derivatives.

metabiosis (mĕt-ă-bĭ-ō'sĭs) ["+ *biōsis*, way of life]. Dependence of an organism for its existence upon another and giving no recompense.

metabolic (mĕt-a-bŏl'ĭk) [Gr. *metaballein*, to turn about, alter]. Pertaining to metabolism.

   m. balance. Comparison of the intake and excretion of a specific nutrient. The balance may be negative when an excess of the nutrient is excreted or positive when more is taken in than excreted.

   m. body size. Body weight in kilograms to the three-fourths power (kg.$^{0.75}$), representative of the active tissue mass or m. mass of an individual. SYN: *physiological size.*

   m. failure. Rapid failure of physical and mental functions ending in death.

   m. gradient. A gradient in metabolic activity that exists in certain structures such as the small intestine from duodenum to ileum or in embryos from animal to vegetal poles in which metabolic activity is highest in one region and becomes progressively lower away from this region.

   m. rate. SEE: *basal metabolism; metabolism, basal.*

metab'olism [Gr. *meta*, change, + *ismos*, state of]. The sum of all physical and chemical changes that take place within an organism; all energy and material transformations that occur within living cells. It includes material changes, i.e., changes undergone by substances furing all periods of life (growth, maturity, senescence) and energy changes, i.e., all transformations of chemical energy of foodstuffs to mechanical energy or heat.

   It involves two fundamental processes: anabolism (assimilation or building-up processes) and catabolism (disintegration or tearing-down processes). Anabolism is the conversion of ingested substances into the constituents of protoplasm; catabolism is the breakdown of substances into simpler substances, the end-products usually being excreted.

   m., basal. Lowest level of energy expenditure. This is determined when the body is at complete rest. For an average person, this is, in terms of Cal., 1500-1800 per day; in terms of body weight, 1 Cal. per kilogram per hour; in terms of body surface, 40 Cal. per sq. meter per hour.

   m., carbohydrate. All carbohydrates are digested to monosaccharides and absorbed as such principally in the form of hexoses, of which glucose is the principal one. In the liver and muscles, glucose is converted to glycogen or it may be oxidized to carbon dioxide and water, the ultimate

Diagram of Normal Metabolic Food Changes

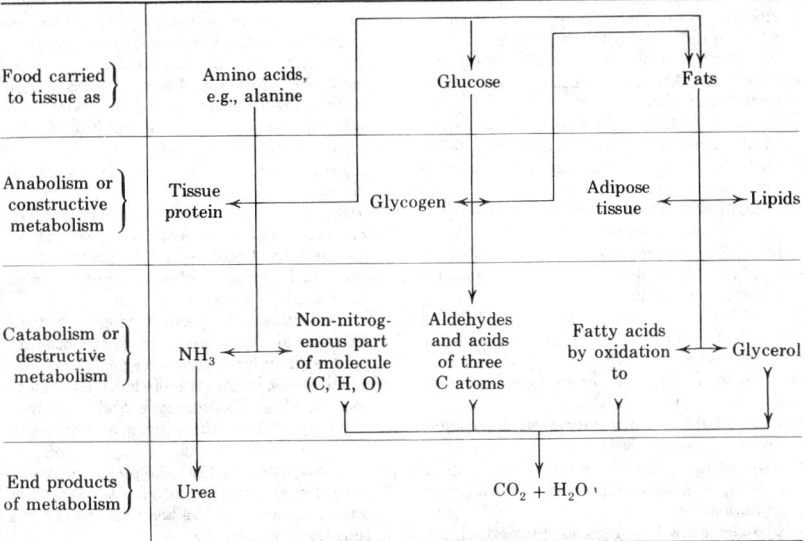

Food carried to tissue as	Amino acids, e.g., alanine		Glucose		Fats	
Anabolism or constructive metabolism	Tissue protein	←	Glycogen ←→		Adipose tissue ←	→Lipids
Catabolism or destructive metabolism	NH_3 ←	→ Non-nitrogenous part of molecule (C, H, O)	Aldehydes and acids of three C atoms	Fatty acids by oxidation to ←→	Glycerol	
End products of metabolism	Urea			$CO_2 + H_2O$		

fate of all carbohydrates. These reactions require the presence of insulin and other hormones. In the process, many intermediate compounds are formed, among them lactic acid.

The basic reaction is $C_6H_{12}O_6 + 6O_2 \rightarrow 6CO_2 + 6H_2O$ which is the basis for the determination of the respiratory quotient (R.Q.). SEE: *quotient, respiratory.*

m., constructive. Anabolism or assimilation. The building-up processes by which complex substances are synthesized.

m., destructive. Catabolism; the breakdown or decomposition of substances into their simple constituents.

m., fat. Fats are digested to fatty acids and glycerol. Following absorption they may be reconverted to neutral fats and stored as adipose tissue or oxidized to CO_2 and H_2O. Fats may be formed from carbohydrates or proteins. In the utilization of fats, the liver plays an important role in the desaturation of fatty acids. Fat metabolism also involves the formation and utilization of substances related to fats, such as sterols and phospholipids.

m., general. Includes all processes involved in utilization of substances entering the body.

m., protein. Proteins are digested to amino acids and absorbed as such. In the

body these are synthesized into body proteins which form an integral part of protoplasm; hence they are essential for normal growth and the repair of tissues. Those not utilized thus are deaminized, i.e., the amino group is removed. This results in the production of urea which is excreted; the remainder, a fatty acid residue (COOH), may be oxidized or converted to glucose, which may be stored as glycogen or converted to fat.

m., purine. M. involving nucleic acids, present in nuclei of cells in which they are combined with proteins to form nucleoproteins. In the breakdown of nucleic acid, uric acid, one of the end products, is formed.

m., special. Applies to all changes involved in utilization of particular substances, such as carbohydrates, proteins, fats, minerals, or water. Referred to as carbohydrate m., protein m., etc.

metabolite (mĕ-tab'ō-līt). Any product of metabolism.

metacar'pal [Gr. *meta,* beyond, + *karpos,* wrist]. Pert. to the bones of the metacarpus, or bones of the hand. SEE: *skeleton.*

metacarpectomy (met"ă-kar-pek'to-mī). Surgical excision or resection of one or more wrist bones.

metacarpus (met-ă-kar'pus). [NA]. The five metacarpal bones of the palm of the hand. SEE: *carpometacarpal.*

metachromasia,   metachromatism (mĕt-ă-krō-mă′zĭ-ă, -krōm′ă-tĭzm) [Gr. *meta,* change, + *chrōma,* color]. Condition in which different substances assume diverse colors or hues when stained by the same dye.

metachromatic (met″ă-krō-mat′ĭk). Pert. to metachromatism.

m. bodies or granules. Granules in protoplasm which stain deeply and differently from the surrounding ones; seen in various bacteria.

metachromophil (met-a-krōm′ō-fĭl) [Gr. *meta,* change, + *chroma,* color, + *philein,* to love]. Not reacting normally to staining.

metachrosis (met-ă-krō′sĭs). Change of color in animal life, e.g., chameleon.

metacone [Gr. *meta,* beyond, + *kōnos,* cone]. The distobuccal cusp of an upper molar tooth.

metaconid. The mesiolingual cusp of a lower molar tooth.

metaconule. The distal intermediate cusp of an upper molar tooth.

metacyesis (met-ă-si-ē′sĭs) [Gr. *meta,* beyond, + *kyēsis,* pregnancy]. Extrauterine gestation.

metagen′esis [″+ *genesis,* formation]. Alternation of generations, esp. involving regular alternation of sexual with asexual reproduction.

metagglutinin (met-ag-glū′tĭn-ĭn) [″+ L. *agglutināre,* to glue]. A partial agglutinin; an agglutinin present in immune serum which acts on organisms closely related to the one acting as the specific antigen.

Metagonimus (mĕt″ă-gŏn′ĭ-mŭs). A genus of flukes belonging to the family Heterophyidae.

M. yokogawai. A species of intestinal flukes common in the Middle and Far East. Normally infests the intestines of dogs, cats, and other animals, but commonly found in man also. Intermediate hosts: snails and fish, esp. a species of trout, Plecoglossus altivelis.

metaicteric (mĕt″ă-ĭk-ter′ĭk) [Gr. *meta,* after, beyond, + *ikteros,* jaundice]. Occurring as a subsequence of jaundice.

metainfective (mĕt-ă-ĭn-fek′tĭv). Occurring subsequent to an infection.

metakaryocyte (met″ă-kar′ĭ-ō-sĭt). A normoblast, q.v.

metakinesis (mĕt″ă-kĭn-e′sĭs) [Gr. *meta,* beyond + *-kinēsis,* motion]. Transition stage in mitosis between prophase and metaphase in which chromosomes move to the equatorial plane. SYM: *metaphase.*

metal fume fever. A syndrome resembling influenza produced by inhalation of excessive concentrations of metallic oxide fumes, such as zinc oxide, or antimony, arsenic, cadmium, cobalt, copper, iron, lead, magnesium, manganese, mercury, nickel, or tin. Occurs in occupations using these metals.

SYM: Come on late. Chills, weakness, lassitude, profound thirst, followed after some hours by sweating and anorexia; occasionally there is mild inflammation of the eyes and respiratory tract.

F.A. TREATMENT: Fresh air and symptomatic treatment.

metallesthesia (mĕt″al-ĕs-thē′sĭ-ă) [Gr. *metallon,* metal, + *aisthēsis,* perception]. Recognition of metals by touching them.

metallic. 1. Pert. to metal. 2. Composed of or resembling a metal.

m. tinkling. A peculiar ringing or bell-like auscultatory sound in pneumothorax over large pulmonary cavities.

metallophobia (mĕ″tal-ō-fō′bĭ-ă) [Gr. *metallon,* metal, + *phobos,* fear]. Abnormal fear of metals and metallic objects and of touching them.

metalloscopy (mĕ-tăl-ŏs′kŏ-pĭ) [″+ *skopein,* to examine]. Determination of the effects of applying metals to the body and the body's sensitivity to them.

metallotherapy (mĕ-tal-ō-ther′ă-pĭ) [″+ *therapeuein,* to heal]. Treatment of disease by applying metals to the affected part.

metallur′gy [″+ *ergon,* work]. Science of obtaining metals from their ores, purifying them, and making them into various shapes and forms.

metamere (met′ă-mēr) [Gr. *meta,* one after the other + *meros,* part]. One of a series of similar segments arranged in a linear series and making up the body of an animal such as an earthworm.

metameric (met-ă-mēr′ĭk). Rel. to metamerism. SYN: *isomeric.*

metamerism (mĕ-tăm′er-izm). 1. Isomerism, q.v. 2. Isomerism consisting of segments or metameres.

metamorphopsia (mĕt″ă-mor-fŏp′sĭ-ă) [Gr. *meta,* beyond, + *morphē,* form, + *opsis,* vision]. In ophthalmology, visual distortion of objects; found in refractive errors, esp. astigmatism, retinal disease, choroiditis, detachment of retina, and tumors of retina and choroid.

metamorphosis (met-ă-mor′fō-sĭs) [″+ *morphōsis,* bringing into shape]. 1. A change in form or structure, esp. the transition from one form to another as in complete metamorphosis of an insect (egg, larva, pupa, adult). 2. In pathology, a degenerative change.

m., fatty. Transformation of fat by infiltration or degeneration.

metamyelocyte (mĕt″ă-mī-ĕl′ō-sīt). A transitional cell intermediate in development between a myelocyte and a mature granular leukocyte. SYN: *juvenile cell.*

metanephros (mĕt-ă-nĕf′ros) [Gr. *meta,* across, + *nephros,* kidney]. (pl. *metanephroi)* The permanent kidney of amniotes (reptiles, birds, and mammals). A portion of it develops from caudal portion of intermediate cell mass or nephrotome; the remaining portion is derived from a bud of the mesonephric duct.

metaneutrophil (met-ă-nū′trō-fil) ["+ L. *neuter,* neither, + Gr. *philein,* to love]. Not reacting normally with neutral dyes.

metaphase (mĕt′ă-fāz) ["+ *phasis,* to appear]. Stage in mitosis in which the chromosomes are arranged in an equatorial plate. Follows the prophase and precedes the anaphase in which longitudinal halves of chromosomes diverge. SYN: *metakinesis.*

metaphen (mĕt′ă-fĕn). A proprietary name of a preparation of nitromersol.

USES: In solution, the agent is used as a disinfectant and antiseptic. It is used especially in preoperative preparation of the skin.

metaphysis (mĕ-tăf′ĭ-sĭs) ["+ *phyein,* to grow]. (pl. *metaphyses)* Portion of a developing long bone between diaphysis or shaft and epiphysis; the growing portion of a bone.

metaplasia (met-ă-plā′zĭ-ă) ["+ *plassein,* to form]. Conversion of one kind of tissue into a form which is not normal for that tissue.

metaplasm (mĕt′ă-plăzm). Reserve material present in protoplasm of a cell, esp. stored nutritive substance. SYN: *cell inclusions; paraplasm.*

metaplastic (met-ă-plas′tik) ["+ *plastikos,* formed]. Pert. to or formed by metaplasia.

metapneumonic (met-ă-nū-mon′ĭk). Succeeding or as a consequence of pneumonia.

metapophysis (met-ă-pŏf′ĭ-sis) [Gr. *meta,* after, + *apophysis,* a process]. Mammillary process on the superior articular processes of a vertebra.

metaprotein. Derived protein resulting from the action of acids or alkalies, in which the molecule is changed to form protein insoluble in neutral solvents but soluble in alkalies and weak acids. SEE: *protein.*

metapyretic (mĕt″ă-pī-rĕt′ĭk) [Gr. *meta,* beyond, + *pyretos,* fever]. Performed or occurring after fever; postpyretic.

metarteriole (mĕt″ar-tē′rī-ōl). A small vessel connecting an arteriole to a venule from which true capillaries are given off. SYN: *precapillary.*

metastable [Gr. *meta,* change, + L. *stabilis,* stable]. Marked by a slight margin of stability. Will change into another phase when conditions change. Term used in chemistry and physics.

metastasis (mĕ-tăs′tă-sis) ["+ *stasis,* stand]. (pl. *metastoses)* 1. Movement of bacteria or body cells (esp. cancer cells) from one part of the body to another. 2. Change in location of a disease or of its manifestations or transfer from one organ or part to another not directly connected.

The usual application is to the manifestation of a malignancy in a secondary growth arising from the primary growth in a new location. Spread is by the lymphatics or blood stream.

metastasize (me-tas′tă-sīz). To invade by metastasis.

metastatic (met-ă-stat′ik). Pert. to metastasis.

metatarsalgia (met-ă-tar-săl′jī-ă). Severe pain or cramp in ant. portion of metatarsus. SYN: Morton's foot; M's neuralgia.

metatarsectomy (met″ă-tar-sĕk′tō-mĭ). Removal of the metatarsus or a metatarsal bone.

metatarsophalangeal (met″ă-tar″sō-fā-lan′jē-ăl). Concerning the metatarsus and phalanges of the toes.

metatarsus (mĕt-ă-tar′sŭs) [Gr. *meta,* beyond, + *tarsos,* tarsus]. [NA]. The region of foot between tarsus and phalanges. Includes the five metatarsal bones.

metathalamus (met-ă-thal′ă-mus) ["+ *thalamos,* a chamber]. [NA]. The post. part of the thalamus including the two geniculate bodies.

metathesis (mĕ-tăth′ĕ-sis) ["+ *thesis,* placement]. 1. A changing of places. 2. Forcible transference of a disease process from one part to another where it will be more accessible for treatment or where it causes less inconvenience. 3. Double decomposition chemically.

metatro′phic ["+ *trophē,* nourishment]. 1. Pert. to metatrophia. 2. Requiring lifeless organic matter for food. SYN: *saprophytic.*

metatuberculosis (mĕt″ă-tū-ber-kū-lō′sīs) ["+ L. *tuberculum,* a small nodule]. A condition of tuberculous reactions with nontuberculous lesions.

Metazoa ["+ *zōon,* animal]. Division of the animal kingdom which includes all multicellular forms, in contrast to unicellular forms or Protozoa.

Metchnikoff's theory. [Elie Metchnikoff, Rus. zoologist in France, 1845-1916]. Microorganisms are ingested by living cells, as by leukocytes and other phagocytes. SEE: *phagocytosis.*

metencephalon (met″ĕn-sĕf′ă-lon) [Gr. *meta*, after, + *enkephalos*, brain]. [NA] The anterior portion of the embryonic rhombencephalon from which the cerebellum and pons arise. SYN: *afterbrain; hindbrain.*

meteorism (mē′tē-or-izm) [Gr. *meteōrizein*, to raise up]. Distention by gas in the abdomen or intestines. SYN: *tympanites.*

meter [Gr. *metron*, measure]. A linear standard of measurement, 39.37 inches.

metergasis (mĕt″er-gā′sis) [″ + *ergon*, work]. Change or alteration in function.

metes′trus. Period following estrus and preceding diestrus.

methadone hydrochloride. USP. A synthetic analgesic drug with potency equal to that of morphine, but the narcotic action is weaker than that of morphine. Methadone is a habit-forming agent and its use should be carefully supervised. Used experimentally in treatment of drug dependence due to use of opium derivatives.

methane. CH_4, marsh gas. A colorless, odorless, inflammable gas. It is produced as a result of putrefaction and fermentation of organic matter.

methanol. A poisonous volatile, inflammable alcohol, CH_3OH, which may be mistaken for ethyl alcohol. If ingested, can cause blindness and death. SYN: *wood alcohol; methyl alcohol.*

methemoglobin (met″hē-mō-glō′bĭn) [Gr. *meta*, across, + *haima*, blood, + L. *globus*, globe.]. A compound closely related to oxyhemoglobin found in the blood following poisoning by certain substances. It gives blood a chocolate-brown color and is useless as a carrier of oxygen.

methemoglobinemia (met‴hē-mō-glōb″ĭ-nē′mĭ-ă). Presence of methemoglobin in the blood.

methemoglobinuria (met‴he-mo-glōb″ĭ-nū′-rĭ-ă). Presence of methemoglobin in the urine.

methenamine (mĕth″ĕn′ă-mēn). $C_6H_{12}N_4$. Colorless crystals with sweetish taste.

    USE: Urinary antiseptic.

    INCOMPATIBILITIES: Ammonium salts, alkalies, ferric salts.

methionine (meth-ĭ′ō-nĭn). A sulfur-bearing compound; an essential amino acid.

method [Gr. *methodos* fr. *meta*, after, + *hodos*, way]. The manner in which a test is made, an operation performed, etc.

methomania [Gr. *methē*, drunkenness, + *mania*, madness]. Pathological craving for intoxicating drinks or other intoxicants.

methyl (meth′ĭl) [Gr. *methy*, wine, + *hylē*, wood]. In organic chemistry, the radical CH_3,

seen, for instance, in the formula for methyl alcohol, CH_3OH.

    m. alcohol. A colorless liquid with an alcoholic odor largely used as a solvent for paints, varnishes, etc.

    POISONING SYM: Different from those of ordinary alcoholism. Depression, weakness, nausea, headache, abdominal cramping, difficult breathing, cold sweats, coma, and convulsions. May be confused with cerebrovascular accident. Blindness which often follows may appear in several hours or not for several days; it may be permanent.

    TREATMENT: Gastric lavage, q.v., or induced vomiting. Intravenous alkali solution (5% sodium bicarbonate) in large amounts, supportive therapy. To prevent formation of formic acid, 10 ml. of ethyl alcohol per hour will prevent metabolism of methyl alcohol.

    m. ether. An anesthetic gas without color.

    m. salicylate. USP. Oil of wintergreen, oil of gaultheria. Produced from distillation of leaves of sweet birch; it has a characteristic odor.

    ACTION AND USES: Commonly used in preparations in the form of liniment or ointment for topical use as an analgesic balm and counterirritant.

    m. violet. Stain employed in histology and bacteriology.

methylcellulose. USP. A tasteless powder which becomes swollen and gummy when wet. Used as a bulk substance in foods and laxatives, also as an adhesive or emulsifier.

methylene blue (meth′ĭ-lēn). USP. Methylthionine chloride. A dark green crystalline powder, producing a distinct blue stain.

    USES: As a urinary antiseptic, as a test for kidney function, and as an antidote for carbon monoxide and cyanide poisoning. It is valuable, also, in the treatment of drug-induced methemoglobinemia (1 mg. of dye per kilogram of body weight).

metopantralgia (met″ō-pan-tral′jĭ-ă) [Gr. *metōpon*, forehead, + *antron*, cavity, + *algia*, pain]. Pain in frontal sinuses.

metopantritis (met-ō-pan-trī′tis). Inflamed condition of frontal sinuses.

metopic (mē-tŏp′ĭk). Rel. to the forehead.

metopion (mē-tō′pĭ-on). Craniometric point in forehead midway bet. frontal eminences.

metopism (mĕt′ō-pĭzm). Persistence of the metopic suture in an adult.

metopodynia (mĕt-ō-pō-dĭn′ĭ-ă) [Gr. *metōpon*, forehead, + *odynē*, pain]. Headache in frontal area of head.

metoxenous (mĕt″ŏk-sē′nŭs) [Gr. *meta*, across, + *xenos*, host]. Denoting a parasite spending each of its two cycles on a different host. SYN: *heterecious*.

metoxeny (mĕt-ŏk'sĕ-nĭ). Condition of being metoxenous, q.v.

metra (mē'tra) [Gr. *mētra*]. Combining form meaning the uterus. SEE: *metro-*.

metralgia (mē-trăl'jĭ-ă) [Gr. *mētra*, uterus, + *algia*, pain]. Pain in the uterus.

metrapectic (met-ră-pek'tĭk) [Gr. *mētēr*, mother, + *apechō*, to avoid]. Denoting a disease that is transmitted by the mother, who herself is unaffected by it, for ex., hemophilia.

metratome (mē'tră-tōm) [Gr. *metra*, uterus, + *tomē*, incision]. Instrument for incising the uterus.

metratomy (mē-trăt'ō-mĭ). Surgical incision of the uterus. SYN: *metrotomy*.

metratonia (mē-tră-tō'nĭ-ă). Uterine atony occurring after childbirth.

metratrophia (mē"tră-trō'fĭ-ă). Atrophy of the uterus.

metrazol (met'ră-zŏl). A proprietary name for a preparation of pentamethylenetetrazole. A white powder, chemically neutral substance.

USES: As a circulatory and respiratory stimulant. Valuable in treating respiratory and circulatory depression due to overdose of barbiturates.

metre (mē'ter) [Gr. *metron*, measure]. Meter, q.v.

metrechoscopy (mĕt"rē-kŏs'kō-pĭ) ["+ *ēchō*, sound, + *skopein*, to examine]. Mensuration and auscultation combined with inspection.

metrectasia (mē"trĕk-tā'zĭ-ă) [Gr. *mētra*, uterus, + *ektasis*, extension]. Uterine dilatation.

metrectomy (mē-trek'to-mĭ) ["+ *ektomē*, excision]. Surgical removal of the uterus. SYN: *hysterectomy*.

metrectopia (mē-trek-tō'pĭ-ă) ["+ *ektopas*, displaced]. Displacement of the uterus.

metrelcosis (mē-trel-kō'sĭs) ["+ *eklōsis*, ulceration]. Uterine ulceration.

metre'mia. Congestion of the uterus.

metreurynter (mē-trŭ-rin'ter) ["+ *eurynein*, to stretch]. An inflatable bag which is inserted in the os uteri and distended to dilate the cervix.

metreurysis (mē-trŭ'rĭ-sĭs). Dilatation of cervix uteri with the metreurynter.

metric system. One based upon the meter (39.37 inches) as the unit of measurement; the gram (15.432 gr.) the unit of weight; the liter (1.057 qt. liquid, or 0.908 qt. dry measure) as the unit of volume.

CONVERSION RULES: (Approximate) To change gm. to gr. multiply by 15 or divide

by 0.064. To change gr. to gm. divide by 15 or multiply by 0.064. To change gm. to avoirdupois oz. divide by 28.3. To change fluid oz. to ml. multiply by 28.3. SEE: *avoirdupois; household measures;* Table in *Appendix; Troy weight.*

metri'tis [Gr. *mētra*, uterus, + *-itis*, inflammation]. Inflammation of the uterus. Designated endometritis if the endometrium is involved and myometritis if the musculature (myometrium) is involved.

     m., chronic. Condition in which there is an increase in fibrous tissue and infiltration of lymphocytes.

metro- [Gr.]. 1. Combining form (*metron*) meaning rel. to measure or measurements. 2. From *metra*, the *uterus*, meaning rel. to the uterus.

metrocarcinoma (mē"trō-kăr-sĭ-nō'mă) [Gr. *mētra*, uterus, + *karkinos*, crab cancer, + *-ōma*, tumor]. Uterine carcinoma.

metrocele (mē'trō-sēl) ["+ *kēlē*, hernia]. Uterine hernia.

metrocolpocele (mē"trō-kol'pō-sēl) ["+ *kolpos*, vagina, + *kēlē*, hernia]. Protrusion of uterus into the vagina which pushes the vaginal wall downward.

metrocystosis (mē"trō-sĭs-tō'sĭs) ["+ *kystis*, cyst, + *-ōsis*, intensive]. Formation of uterine cysts.

metrodynia (mē-trō-dĭn'ĭ-ă) ["+ *odynē*, pain]. Uterine pain.

metrofibroma (mĕt-rō-fĭ-brō'mă) ["+ L. *fibra*, fiber, + *-ōma*, tumor]. Uterine fibroma.

metromalacia (mē"trō-mal-ă-zī-ă) ["+ *malakia*, softness]. Softening of the uterus.

metromalacosis (me"trō-mal-ă-kō'sĭs) ["+ "+ *-ōsis*, intensive]. Malacia or softening of uterine tissues.

metronome (mĕt'rō-nōm) [Gr. *metron*, measure, + *nomos*, law]. Apparatus for recording intervals or periods of time.

metroparalysis (mē"trō-pă-ral'ĭ-sĭs) [Gr. *mētra*, uterus, + *paralysis*, a loosening from the side]. Uterine paralysis during or immediately following childbirth.

metropath'ia haemorrhag'ica ("+ *pathos*, disease, + *haima*, blood, + *rhēgnymi*, to burst forth). Condition of the uterus characterized by hemorrhage, usually accompanied by hypertrophy of the uterine mucous membranes and ovarian cystic disease. SEE: *fibrosis uteri.*

metropathic (mē-trō-path'ĭk). Pert. to or caused by uterine disease.

metropathy (mē-trŏp'ă-thĭ). Any uterine disease.

metroperitonitis (mē"trō-per"ĭ-tō-nĭ'tĭs) ["+ *peritonaion*, peritoneum, + *-ītis*, inflammation]. Inflamed condition of uterus and peritoneum.

metrophlebitis (mē″trō-flē-bī′tĭs) ["+ *phleps, phleb-*, vein, + *-itis*, inflammation]. Inflamed condition of uterine veins.

metroptosis (mē-trō-tō′sĭs) ["+ *ptōsis*, falling]. Dropping of the uterus.

metrorrhagia (mĕt-rō-ra′jĭ-ă) [Gr. *metro*, uterus, + *rhēgnynai*, to burst forth]. Bleeding from the uterus, esp. at any time other than during the menstrual period. May be caused by lesions of the cervix uteri. Its occurrence should lead one to suspect and search for a malignancy in the genital tract, specifically cancer of the cervix. SEE: *menorrhagia.*

metrorrhexis (mē″trō-rĕk′sĭs) ["+ *rhēxis*, rupture]. Rupture of the uterus.

metrorthosis (mē-tror-thō′sĭs) ["+ *orthōsis*, a straightening]. Correction of uterine displacement.

metrosalpingitis (me-trō-săl″pĭn-jī′tĭs) ["+ *salpinx*, tube, + *-itis*, inflammation]. Inflamed condition of uterus and oviducts.

metroscope (me′tro-skōp) ["+ *skopein*, to examine]. Instrument for examining the uterus. SYN: *hysteroscope.*

metrostaxis (mē-tro-stak′sĭs) ["+ *staxis*, a dripping]. Persistent but slight hemorrhage from the uterus.

metrostenosis (mē-trō-stĕn-ō′sĭs) ["+ *stēnōsis*, contraction]. Contraction or narrowing of the uterine cavity.

metrother′apy [Gr. *metron*, measure, + *therapeia*, treatment]. Treatment of a condition by measurement, e.g., in restoration of joint function following injury, measuring the angle of joint motion and recording the progress has a psychologic effect on patient.

metrotome (mē′trō-tōm) [Gr. *mētra*, uterus, + *tomē*, a cutting]. Instrument used in incising the uterus.

metrotomy (mē-trŏt′ō-mĭ). Incision of the uterus. SYN: *hysterotomy.*

metrourethrotome (mĕt-rō-ū-rē′thrō-tōm) [Gr. *metron*, measure, + *ourēthra*, urethra, + *tomē*, incision]. Device for incising the urethra and measuring depth to be incised.

-metry [Gr. *metrein*, to measure]. Suffix meaning to measure.

metycaine (met′ĭ-kān). A white crystalline substance formerly known as neothesin. Proprietary name.

    USES: As a local anesthetic, prompt in action as topical application or subcutaneous injection.

Mev. Abbr. for *million electron volts.*

Meyer's theory. [Adolf Meyer, Amer. psychiatrist, 1866-1950]. That physiologic and psychologic data are considered to be one entity in psychiatry.

Meynert's commis′sure (mī′nert). [Theodor H. Meynert, Aust. neurologist, 1833-1892]. Fibrous tract extending from subthalamic body to base of 3rd ventricle.

M. F. D. Abbr. for *minimum fatal dose.*

Mg. Symb. for *magnesium.*

mg. Abbr. for *milligram.*

mgh. Milligram hour. Dosage obtained by application of 1.0 mg. radium for 1 hr.

miasm, miasma (mī′azm, mī-az′mă) [Gr. *miasma*, stain]. A foul emanation or odor from the earth. Formerly thought to cause disease endemic to certain regions, esp. fevers such as malaria.

miasmatic (mī-az-mat′ĭk). Pert. to miasm.

micella, micelle (mī-sĕl′ă, mī-sĕl′). One of the ultramiscroscopic units of protoplasm.

micracusia (mī″crā-kū′zē-ă) [Gr. *micro*, small, + *akousis*, hearing]. An auditory illusion in which sounds appear to be remote. May occur at the onset of an epileptic seizure.

micrencephalon (mī″krĕn-sĕf′ă-lon) [Gr. *micro*, small, + *enkephalos*, brain]. 1. Cerebellum. 2. Smallness of brain; cretinism, q.v.

micrencephalous (mī″kren-sef′al-ŭs). Possessing a small brain.

micro-, micr- [Gr.]. Combining forms denoting small size or extent. Indicates one millionth of a unit; thus microgram is one millionth of a gram. SYMB: μ.

microaerophilic (mī″krō-ā-er-ō-fĭl′ĭk) ["+ *aēr*, air, + *philein*, to love]. Growing at low oxygen tension.

microanalysis. Analytical examination of tiny granules.

microanatomy. Microscopic anatomy; histology.

microangiitis. Inflammation of very small blood vessels.

Micro″bacter′ium. (pl. *Microbacteria*). A microorganism.

microbe (mī′krōb) [Gr. *micro*, small, + *bios*, life]. 1. A minute one-celled form of life not distinguishable as to its vegetable or animal nature. 2. Bacteria, germs producing fermentation, putrefaction and disease; microorganism.

microbian (mī-krō′bĭ-an). Rel. to a microbe. SYN: *microbic.*

microbic (mī-krōb′ĭk). Concerning microbes. SYN: *microbian.*

microbicidal (mī-krō″bĭ-sī′dal) ["+ "+ L. *cidus*, from *caedere*, to kill]. Lethal to microbes.

microbicide (mī-krō′bis-īd) ["+ "+ L. *cidus*, from *caedere*, to kill]. An agent that kills microbes.

microbiology (mī″krō-bī-ol′ō-jī) ["+ "+ *logos,* study]. Scientific study of microorganisms.

microbiophobia (mī″krō-bī-ō-fō′bī-ă) [Gr. *micro,* small, + *bios,* life, + *phobia,* fear]. An abnormal fear of germs. SYN: *microphobia.*

microbiota (mī″krō-bī-ō′tă). Microscopic organisms of an area. SEE: *macrobiota.*

microbiotic (mī″krō-bī-ot′ik). Of microbic life or origin.

microbism (mī′krōb-īzm) [Gr. *micro,* small, + *bios,* life, + *ismos,* state of]. Infection with microbes.

microblast (mī′krō-blăst) [Gr. *micro,* small, + *blastos,* germ]. Minute red blood corpuscle.

microblepharism, microblephary (mī-krō-blĕf′ar-izm, -ar-ī) ["+ *blepharon,* eyelid]. Condition of having abnormally small eyelids.

microbodies. Small, spherical, cytoplasmic bodies approx. 0.5 μ in diameter. So far they have been found only in the cells of the liver and kidney tubule.

microcalorie (mī″krō-kal′ō-rī) [Gr. *micro,* small, + L. *calor,* heat]. A unit of heat, the amount required to raise the temperature of 1 cc. of distilled water from 0° to 1° C. One thousand microcalories equal one Calorie.

NOTE: A microcalorie is also called calorie (spelled with a small "c"). A thousand calories is equal to one kilocalorie, (kcal.). This is also called a Calorie (spelled with a capital "C").

The energy value of food is expressed in Calories, i.e. kilocalories.

microcardia (mī″krō-kar′dī-ă) ["+ *kardia,* heart]. Unusually small heart.

microcaulia (mī″krō-kaw′lī-ă) ["+ *kaulos,* penis]. Unusually small size of penis.

microcentrum (mī-krō-sĕn′trum) ["+ *kentron,* center]. 1. Centrosome, q.v. 2. Motor or dynamic center of a cell.

microcepha′lia [Gr. *micro,* small, + *kephalē,* head]. Abnormal smallness of the head.

microcephalic (mī-krō-sef-al′ĭk). Having or pert. to a small head; one below 1350 cc. capacity.

microcephalous (mī-kro-sef′al-us). Having an abnormally small head.

microcephalus (mī-krō-sef′a-lŭs). 1. Person with an exceptionally small head; mentally retarded. 2. Fetus with a very small head.

microcephaly, microcephalism (mī-krō-sef′ă-lī, -līzm). Abnormal smallness of head often seen in idiocy; it is congenital.

microcheilia (mī″krō-kī′lī-ă) [Gr. *micro,* small, + *cheilos,* lip]. Abnormal smallness of lips.

microchemistry (mī-krō-kĕm′ĭs-trī) ["+ *chēmeia,* chemistry]. Chemical work in which minute quantities and small instruments are utilized.

microchiria (mī-krō-kī′rī-ă) ["+ *cheir,* hand]. Abnormal smallness of the hand.

Micrococcaceae (mī″krō-kŏk-ā′sē-ē). A family of bacteria belonging to the order Eubacteriales. Contains the genera Micrococcus, Sarcina, and Staphylococcus.

Micrococcus (mī″krō-kŏk′ūs) ["+ *kokkos,* berry]. A genus of spherical, gram-positive bacteria belonging to the family Micrococcaceae. Cells occur singly or in irregular groups.

M. albus. Staphylococcus albus, q.v.

M. melitensis. Cause of undulant fever. SYN: *Brucella melitensis.*

microcolon. Abnormally small colon.

microcor′nea. Abnormally small cornea.

microcoulomb (mī-krō-kū′lom). A microunit of quantity of current electricity; one-millionth part (10^{-6}) of a coulomb, q.v.

microcrystalline (mī-krō-kris′tal-īn, -ēn). Composed of microscopic crystals.

microcurie. Measure of radiation. One-millionth of a curie.

microcyst (mī′krō-sīst). A very small cyst.

microcytase (mī-krō-sī′tās) [Gr. *micro,* small, + *cyte,* cell, + *ase,* enzyme]. Cytase acting on bacteria and formed by leukocytes.

microcyte. 1. A small erythrocyte or red blood corpuscle; one less than 5 microns in diameter. 2. Small, non-nucleated, red blood corpuscle.

microcytosis. Condition characterized by presence of abnormal numbers of microcytes in the blood.

microdactylia (mī″krō-dak-til′ī-ă) [Gr. *micro,* small, + *daktylos,* digit]. Abnormal smallness of the digits.

microdetermination. The chemical examination of extremely minute quantities of a substance.

microdissection (mī″krō-dī-sĕk′shŭn) [Gr. *micro,* small, + L. *dissectio,* a cutting apart]. Dissection with aid of the microscope, esp. by utilization of a micromanipulator.

microdont (mī′krō-dont) ["+ *odous, odont-,* tooth]. Possessing very small teeth.

microdontism (mī-krō-don′tĭzm) ["+ "+ *ismos,* state of]. Unusual smallness of the teeth.

microdose. Minute dose.

microelectrophoresis. Electrophoresis of minute quantities of a solution.

microenvironment. That portion of the environment immediately surrounding an individual.

microfarad (mī-krō-far'ăd). A microunit of electrical capacity; one-millionth of a farad, q.v.

microfiche (mī'krō-fēsh") [Gr. *micro,* small, + Fr. *fiche,* index card]. A sheet of microfilm that enables a large number of library data and medical records to be stored in a small space.

microfilaria (mī"krō-fī-lā'rī-ă). The embryos of filarial worms. They are present in the blood and tissues and are of importance in the diagnosis of filarial infections.

microfilm. A film containing the photograph of something greatly reduced in size.

microgamete (mī-krō-gam'ēt) [Gr. *micro,* small, + *gametēs,* spouse]. Male element in conjugation of protozoa.

microgametocyte (mī-krō-gam-ē'tō-sīt) ["+ "+ *cyte,* cell]. Mother cell of the microgamete.

microgamy (mī-krŏg'ă-mī). Union of male and female cells in certain lower forms.

microgastria (mī-krō-gas'trī-ă) [Gr. *micro,* small, + *gastēr,* stomach]. Unusual smallness of the stomach.

microgenitalism (mī"krō-jĕn'ĭt-ăl-īzm) ["+ L. *genitalia,* genitals, + Gr. *ismos,* state of]. Abnormal smallness of the external genitals.

microglia (mī-krog'lī-ă) ["+ *glia,* glue]. Neuroglia tissue probably derived from the mesoderm, forming a portion of the adventitial structure of the central nervous system.

microglossia (mī-krō-glos'ī-ă) ["+ *glōssa,* tongue]. Abnormally small tongue.

micrognathia (mī-krō-nā'thī-ă) ["+ *gnathos,* jaw]. Abnormal smallness of jaws, esp. lower jaw.

microgram. SYMB: $\mu g.$ or *mcg.* One-millionth part of a gram. One-thousandth of a milligram.

micrograph (mī'krō-graf) [Gr. *micro,* small, + *graphein,* to write]. 1. Apparatus for magnifying and recording minute movements. 2. Photograph of an object through a microscope. SYN: *photomicrograph.*

micrography (mī-krog'ră-fī). 1. Study of physical appearance and characteristics of microscopic objects. 2. Very minute writing, engraving, etc. 3. Study of an object by use of a microscope.

microgyria (mī-krō-jir'ī-ă) [Gr. *micro,* small + *gyros,* circle]. Smallness of cerebral convolutions; polymicrogyria.

microhematocrit. Packed red cell volume of blood determined by using very small

amount of blood collected in a capillary tube and placed in high speed centrifuge.

microhepatia (mī-krō-hĕ-pat'ī-ă) ["+ *hēpar, ēpat-,* liver]. Abnormally small size of the liver.

microhm (mī'krōm). A microunit of electrical resistance; one-millionth of an ohm.

microincineration. Determination of presence and distribution of inorganic matter in tissues by subjecting a microscopic section of tissue to a high temperature which destroys organic matter, leaving mineral matter as ash.

microinjection. Injection of substances into cells or minute vessels by means of a micropipette.

micro"len'tia. Possessing a very small crystalline lens.

microleukoblast [Gr. *micro,* small, + *leukos,* white, + *blastos,* germ]. A small leukoblast. SYN: *myeloblast.*

microliter (mī'krō-lē"ter). One-millionth part of a liter.

microlith (mī'krō-lith) [Gr. *micro,* small, + *lithos,* stone]. A very tiny calculus.

microlithiasis (mī"krō-lī-thī'ă-sīs). The development of very minute calculi.

micrology (mī-krol'o-jī) [Gr. *micro,* small, + *logos,* study]. Science of microscopic investigations.

micromania (mī-krō-mā'nī-ă) ["+ *mania,* madness]. A delusion that one has become small or infantile or insignificant.

micromanipulator. Apparatus by which extremely minute pipettes or needles can be manipulated under a microscope for microinjection or microsurgery.

micromastia (mīk-rō-măs'tī-ă). Micromazia, q.v.

micromazia (mī-krō-mā'zī-ă) [Gr. *micro,* small, + *mazos,* breast]. Abnormally small size of the breasts.

micrometer (mī'krō-mē-ter). A millionth part of a meter (10^{-6}); one-thousandth part of a centimeter (10^{-3}). ABBR: μm. SEE: *micron.*

micrometer (mī-krŏm'ē-tĕr). Device for measuring small distances.

micromillimeter (mī-krō-mīl'ī-mē-ter). One-millionth part of a millimeter. ABBR: μmm. SYN: *millimicron.*

Micromonospora. A genus of fungi belonging to the family Streptomycetaceae.

micromyces (mī-krŏm'ī-sēs) ["+ *mykēs,* fungus]. (pl. *micromycetes*) Minute fungus.

micromyelia (mī-krō-mī-ē'lī-ă) ["+ *myelos,* marrow]. Abnormally small size of spinal cord.

micromyeloblast (mī-krō-mī'ĕl-ō-blăst) [Gr. *micro,* small, + *myelos,* marrow, + *blastos,* germ]. A small, immature myelocyte; often predominating cell in myeloblastic leukemia.

micron. Unit of linear measure; equal to .001 cm. (10⁻³ cm.). In the International System (SI) of units, micron has been designated micrometer. The abbr. for micrometer is μm.

microne (mī′krōn). A colloid particle that is distinguishable with the microscope.

microneedles. Extremely minute needles used in a micromanipulator for microdissection.

micronize. To pulverize a substance into particles only a few micra in size.

micronucleus (mī-krō-nū′klē-us) [Gr. *micro*, small, + L. *nucleus*, kernel]. (pl. *micronuclei*) 1. A small nucleus. 2. The smaller of the two nuclei of infusoria considered as containing the inheritable germ substance.

micronychia (mī-krō″nĭk′ĭ-ă) [″+ *onyx*, nail]. Possessing abnormally small nails.

microorganism (mī-krō-or′găn-ĭzm). Minute living body not perceptible to the naked eye, esp. a bacterium or protozoon.

Microorganisms may be carried from one host to another as follows:

Animal sources: Some organisms are pathogenic for animals as well as man, and may be communicated to man through direct, indirect, or intermediary hosts.

By air: Pathogenic microorganisms in the respiratory tract may be discharged from the mouth or nose and settle on food, dishes, clothing, etc. They may carry infection if they resist drying.

Contact infections: These are the result of direct transmission of bacteria from one to another, as in venereal diseases.

Food-borne: Food and water may contain pathogenic organisms acquired from infected persons handling the food or through fecal or insect contamination.

Human carriers: Persons who have recovered from an infectious disease remain carriers of the organism causing the infection and may transfer the organism to another host.

Insects: They may be the physical carrier, as the housefly or as vectors Anopheles mosquito.

Soil-borne: Spore-forming organisms in the soil may enter the body through a cut or wound. Vegetables and fruits, esp. roots, need thorough cleansing before being eaten raw.

m., pathologic. A disease-causing organism. Includes rickettsias, bacteria, spirochetes, yeasts, molds, protozoons, and some helminths.

micropathology (mī″krō-path-ol′ō-jĭ) [Gr. *micro*, small, + *pathos*, disease, + *logos*, study]. Study of microorganismal disases and their cell and tissue changes.

microphage, microphagus (mī′kro-fāj, -krof′ag-us) [″+ *phagein*, to eat]. A small phagocyte. RS: *bacteria, bacteriolysin, leukocyte, opsonin, phagocyte.*

microphakia (mī″krō-fā′kĭ-ă) [″+ *phakos*, lens]. Abnormally small lens.

microphallus (mī-krō-fal′us) [″+ *phallos*, penis]. Abnormally small size of penis. SYN: *microcaulia.*

microphobia (mī-krō-fō′bĭ-ă) [″+ *phobos*, fear]. 1. Psychopathic fear of microbes. 2. Morbid dread of small objects. SYN: *microbiophobia.*

microphone (mī′kro-fōn) [″+ *phōnē*, voice]. Device for detecting and transmitting sound.

microphonia (mī-krō-fō′nĭ-ă). Weakness of voice.

microphonoscope (mī-krō-fō′nō-skōp) [Gr. *micro*, small, + *phōnē*, voice, + *skopein*, to examine]. Form of binaural stethoscope for magnifying sound.

microphotograph (mī″krō-fō′tō-graf) [Gr. *micro*, small, + *phos, phot-*, light, + *graphein*, to write]. 1. A photograph of extremely small size. 2. A photograph on microfilm. 3. A photomicrograph.

microphthalmia (mī-krŏf-thăl′mĭ-ă) [″+ *ophthalmos*, eye]. Abnormally small size of eyes.

microphthalmus (mī-krŏf-thal′mus). 1. Person with unusually small eyes. 2. Condition characterized by abnormally small eyes.

microphysics (mī-krō-fĭz′ĭks). The branch of science dealing with the forces controlling ultimate structure of matter.

microphyte (mī′krō-fĭt) [Gr. *micro*, small, + *phyton*, plant]. Any microscopic plant, esp. if parasitic.

micropia (mī-krō′pĭ-ă) [″+ *opsis*, vision]. A condition in which objects seem diminished in size. SYN: *micropsia.*

micropipette. An extremely small pipette used for microinjection.

micropodia (mī-krō-pō′dĭ-ă) [″+ *pous, pod-*, feet]. Unusually small size of the feet.

micropolariscope. A microscope with a polarizer.

microprojection. Projection of images of microscopic objects upon a screen.

microprosopia (mī-krō″prō-sō′pĭ-ă). Abnormal smallness of the face.

micropsia (mi-krop′sĭ-ă) [Gr. *micro*, small, + *opsis*, vision]. Condition in which objects seem smaller than they usually are. Seen in paralysis of accommodation, retinitis, and choroiditis. SYN: *micropia.*

micropus (mī-krō'pus) ["+ *pous,* feet]. One with unusually small feet.

micropyle (mī'krō-pīl) ["+ *pylē,* gate]. The opening in the ovum for entrance of the spermatozoon. Seen in ovum of some animals.

microrhinia (mī″krō-rīn'ī-ă) ["+ *rhis,* nose]. Abnormal smallness of the nose.

microscelous (mī-krŏs'kĕ-lŭs) ["+ *skelos,* leg]. Possessing short legs.

microscope (mī'krō-skōp) ["+ *skopein,* to examine]. Optical instrument which greatly magnifies very minute objects.

   m., binocular. M. possessing two eyepieces or oculars.

   m., compound. One with two or more lenses or lens systems for use in observing the minutest bodies.

   m., darkfield. M. using darkfield illumination, q.v. An ultramicroscope.

   m., electron. A m. which utlizes streams of electrons deflected from their course by an electrostatic or electromagnetic field for the magnification of objects. The final image is viewed on a fluorescent screen or recorded on a photographic plate. Because of greater resolving power, images may be magnified up to 400,000 diameters.

   m., fluorescent. SEE: *m., ultraviolet.*

   m., phase, phase-contrast. A compound microscope to which two elements have been added, namely, a diffraction or phase plate and a specialized condenser diaphragm. Such makes visible details of objects characterized by differences in refractive index and thus delineates a change of phase such as brightness or color.

   m., polarization. M. for examining specimens which polarize light or have double refraction.

   m., simple. One with a simple or single lens; magnifying glass.

   m., ultraviolet. M. utilizing ultraviolet radiations as a light source and having an optical system for transmitting them. Used in observing a specimen which fluoresces, such as tissues stained with a fluorescent dye.

   m., x-ray. M. for utilizing x-rays to reveal structure of objects through which light cannot pass.

microscopic, microscopical (mī-krō-skōp'-ik, -ĭ-kal). 1. Pert. to the microscope. 2. Visible only by using the microscope.

microscopy (mī-krŏs'kōp-ī). Inspection with the microscope.

   m., darkfield. M. in which specimens against a dark background are illuminated

by light rays striking from the side. By this means, objects too small to be seen by direct illumination become visible.

microseme (mī'krō-sēm) [Gr. *micro,* small, + *sēma,* sign]. Possessing an orbital index less than 83.

microsoma (mī-krō-sō'mă) ["+ *sōma,* body]. Unusually small stature.

microsome (mī'krō-sōm). Particle derived from the endoplasmic reticulum when cells are broken up by centrifuging with a force 100,000 times that of gravity. It can be seen only by use of electron microscopy.

microsomia (mī-krō-sō'mī-ă). Abnormally small size of body.

microspec″trophotom′etry. Method for the histochemical study of substances present in cells, such as nucleic acid based on absorption in the ultraviolet spectrum. Permits quantitative and qualitative studies of certain cellular components with a high degree of sensitivity.

microspectroscope ["+ L. *spectrum,* image, + Gr. *skopein,* to examine]. A combined spectroscope and microscope.

microspherocyte (mī″krō-sfē′rō-sīt). Red blood cells, small and shaped like spheres. Seen in certain kinds of anemia.

microsphygmia, microsphyxia (mi-krosfĭg′mī-ă, -sfiks′ī-ă) [Gr. *micro,* small, + *sphygmos, sphyxis,* pulse]. Smallness of the pulse.

microsplenia (mī-krō-splē′nī-ă) ["+ *splēn,* spleen]. Abnormal smallness of the spleen.

Microsporon (mī″krō-spō′rŏn) ["+ *sporos,* seed]. Former name of Microsporum, q.v.

Microsporum. A genus of ringworm fungi which causes disease of the skin, hair, and nails.

   M. audouini. Causative agent of tinea capitis (ringworm of scalp).

   M. canis. Cause of ringworm of cats and dogs. May be transmitted to children.

microstomia (mī-krō-stō′mī-ă) [Gr. *micro,* small, + *stoma,* mouth]. Unusual smallness of the mouth.

microstrabismus [Gr. *micro,* small, + *strabismos,* a squinting]. Movement of the eyes in divergent directions or at different speeds. These movements are too small and too quick to be seen, but they have been detected by analyzing high-speed motion pictures of psychiatric patients.

microsurgery. Dissection of tissues under the microscope, usually involving the use of a micromanipulator.

microsyringe. A special syringe for injecting very small quantities of solutions.

microtia (mī-krō'shĭ-ă) [Gr. *micro*, small, + *ous, ot-*, ear]. Unusually small size of the auricle or external ear.

microtome (mī'krō-tōm) [Gr. *micro*, small, + *tomē*, incision]. Instrument for preparing thin sections of tissue for microscopic study.

microtomy (mī-krŏt'ō-mĭ). The process of cutting thin sections of tissues.

microvolt. One-millionth part of a volt.

micturate (mĭk'tū-rāt) [L. *micturire*]. To pass the urine. SYN: *urinate*.

micturition (mĭk-tū-rĭ'shŭn). The voiding of urine. SYN: *urination*.

mid'brain [AS. *mid*, middle, + *braegen*, brain]. The corpora quadrigemina, the crura cerebri, and aqueduct of Sylvius which connect the pons and cerebellum with the hemispheres of the cerebrum. SYN: *mesencephalon*, q.v.

midget. A very small person; an adult who is perfectly formed but has not attained full growth.

midgut (mid'gut) [AS. *mid*, middle, + *gut*, intestine]. The midportion of the embryonic gut which opens ventrally into the yolk stalk.

midriff (mĭd'rĭf) [AS. *mid*, middle, + *hrif*, belly]. The diaphragm.

midwife ["+ *wīf*, wife]. A female who practices the art of aiding in the delivery of children.

midwifery (mid-wĭf'er-ĭ). The art of assisting at childbirth. SYN: *obstetrics*.

migraine (mī'grān) [Fr. from Ger. *hēmikrania*, half skull]. Paroxysmal attacks of headache, frequently unilateral, usually accompanied by disordered vision and gastrointestinal disturbances. Thought to be the result of vasodilation of extracerebral cranial arteries.

ETIOL: Unknown. Frequently hereditary. It may be precipitated by allergic hypersensitivity or emotional disturbances.

SYM: As stated. It is also associated with zigzags of light and vomiting, and at times with diplopia, unilateral sweating, and focal symptoms. Sharp, stabbing pains frequently in temperofrontal region. Susceptible to light and sound.

PROG: It must be distinguished from other types of headache, but the history, the course of the disorder, and the peculiar combination of symptoms rarely permit much uncertainty.

TREATMENT: Rest in quiet, darkened room during attack. Ergotamine tartrate proves efficacious in most cases.

migration (mī-grā'shun) [L. *migrāre*, to move from place to place]. Passage of cells, etc., from one position to another, as the migra-tion of an ovum from the ovary into the fallopian tube or movement of leukocytes through the wall of a blood vessel into surrounding tissues.

   m., internal, of the ovum. Passage of the ovum through the uterine (fallopian) tube to the uterus.

   m. of leukocytes. Passage of white blood corpuscles through walls of capillaries. SYN: *diapedesis*.

   m. of the testicle. Descent of testicle into the scrotum. SYN: *descensus testis*.

migratory. 1. Pert. to migrate. 2. Changing or capable of changing positions.

mikro-. For words beginning thus, see *micro-*.

Mikulicz's drain (mĭk'ū-lĭch). [Johann von M.-Radecki, Polish surgeon, 1850-1905]. A method for draining the abdominal cavity after operating.

Mikulicz's mask. Gauze-covered frame worn over nose and mouth during performance of operation.

Mikulicz's pad. Folded gauze pad for packing off the viscera in abdominal operations and used as a sponge in general.

Mikulicz's syndrome. Chronic infiltration with lymphocytes and painless enlargement of lacrimal and salivary glands.

mil'dew [AS. *mildeāw*]. A discoloration or superficial coating on various materials caused by the growth of fungi. Occurs in damp conditions.

miliaria (mĭl-ĭ-a'rĭ-ă) [L. *milium*, millet]. Vesicles caused by obstruction of ducts of sweat glands. Acute inflammation of the sweat glands will result if the obstruction persists. The three forms of miliaria (sudamina, rubra, and profunda) represent different levels of obstruction of the sweat ducts. Occurs most commonly in infants, the obese, and in those exposed to excessive heat for prolonged periods. Excessive clothing and hyperhidrosis are contributing factors. SYN: *heat rash; prickly heat*.

ETIOL: Exposure to excessive heat, skin irritants, and tendency to hyperhidrosis, q.v.

SYM: Sudden appearance of red patches of small papules. Vesicles are discrete and accompanied by red areolae. They usually appear on the trunk and are accompanied by itching, burning, and fever of short duration. They occur in hot weather, in tropical countries, and in individuals sweating profusely. Papules may become eczematous if irritated.

TREATMENT: The only effective treatment and prevention is avoidance of further sweating. Calamine lotion helps to relieve symptoms.

m. crystallina. Form with clear, thin-walled vesicles 1-2 mm. in diameter. SYN: *sudamina.*

m. profunda. Nearly always follows attacks of m. rubra. Seen almost exclusively in the tropics. Area is covered with pale, firm papules 1-3 mm. across. These are painless and do not cause itching.

m. rubra. Prickly heat; heat rash. An eruption of papulovesicles at the mouth of sweat follicles and accompanied by inflammation, resulting from obstruction to the ducts of the sweat glands. Symptoms oscillate with the heat load of the individual.

miliary (mĭl'ĭ-ă-rĭ) [L. *miliaris,* like a millet seed]. Characterized by presence of small nodules or lesions resembling millet seed.

m. fever. Sudden onset of fever with drenching sweats, followed by miliary vesicles and erythema. May be related to influenza.

m. tubercles. Small gray nodules in first stage of tuberculosis.

m. tuberculosis. Acute, generalized tuberculosis with minute tubercles in the affected part or organ.

milieu (mēl-yew') [Fr.]. Environment.

m. interieur. Internal environment of extracellular fluids of the body.

millium (mĭl'ĭ-ŭm) [L. *milium,* millet seed]. (pl. *milia*) Small pink and white nodule below the epidermis, caused by retention of secretion of sebaceous glands.

TREATMENT: Mechanical keratolytics (pumice stone, soap), salicylic acid and sulfur ointment, or incision and expression of contents.

m., colloid. Tiny papule formed beneath the epidermis due to colloid degeneration.

milk [AS. *meolc*]. A secretion of the mammary glands, sp. gr. about 1.032, for feeding the young.

COMP: Milk consists of water, organic substances, and mineral salts. *Organic substances:* Proteins: The principal proteins are caseinogen, lactoalbumin, and lactoglobu-

lin; in the presence of calcium ions, soluble caseinogen is converted into insoluble casein by the action of acids, rennet, or pepsin. This brings about the curdling of milk. Lactoglobulin is identical with serum globulin of blood and hence contains maternal antibodies. Carbohydrates: Lactose or milk sugar is the principal sugar, although small quantities of other sugars are present. Fats: The principal fats are glycerides of oleic, palmitic, and myristic acid. Smaller quantities of stearic acid and short-chain fatty acids with carbon chains of C_4 to C_{24} are present. Sterols and phosphatides (lecithin and cephalin) are also present. Churning causes the fat globules to unite into a solid mass forming butter. *Mineral salts:* The principal cations are calcium, potassium, and sodium; the principal anions, phosphate, and chloride. Citrates and lactates are present in small quantities. Milk is low in iron and magnesium.

Vitamins: Vitamins A and those of the B complex (thiamine, riboflavin, and pantothenic acid) are present in adequate quantities to meet the needs of a growing child. Milk is low in vitamins C and D.

COW'S, FLUID, WHOLE: 1 cup (244 gm.). Calories: 165. Other main values: 9 gm. protein; 10 gm. fat; 12 gm. carbohydrate; 285 mg. calcium; 390 I.U. vitamin A. Minimum standards for fat content varies from state to state. National average is 3.7% fat.

ACTION: Milk is digested relatively easily.

Milk on standing at room temperature sours as a result of the action of lactic acid bacilli on lactose converting it into lactic acid. When the pH reaches 5.34, coagulation occurs resulting in production of a curd. The remaining watery portion is called whey.

Milk contains antibodies which are present in the mother's blood. Milk also contains a number of enzymes (catalase, oxidase, reductase, phosphatase).

Composition of Milk

	Mother's Milk (%)	Cow's Milk (%)
Water	87–88	85–88
Minerals	0.2	0.7
Protein	1.0–1.5	3.5–4.0
Fat	3.5–4.0	3.5–4.0
Sugar (lactose, carbohydrate)	6.5–7.0	4.5
Reaction	Alkaline	Acid

m., acidophilus. Milk inoculated with Lactobacillus acidophilus, a bacterium which grows best in an acid medium.

m. agent. A carcinogenic substance present in the milk of certain strains of mice capable of inducing the development of cancer in offspring.

m., butter-. That left after removal of butter following churning.

m., casein. M. prepared with a large quantity of casein and fat, but little sugar and salts.

m., certified. That certified by a milk commission as pure.

m., condensed. Partly evaporated and sweetened milk.

m., evaporated. Cows' milk which has been concentrated by evaporating some of the water. It can be canned after pasteurization, q.v., and stored for long periods of time. SEE: *lactic acid evaporated milk.*

m., filled. A product made by combining fats or oils other than milk fat with milk solids. The product resembles milk.

m., fortified. M. enriched by the addition of cream, albumin, or vitamins.

m., homogenized. M. with fats combined with the body of the milk; thus the cream does not separate.

m., instant dry non-fat. Dried skim milk. It may be stored at room temperature until needed. Reconstituted by adding water to the granules.

m., lactic acid evaporated. Evaporated milk to which sugar and lactic acid have been added. It is especially desirable for use in feeding infants because of its availability, cheapness, safety, and digestibility. To prepare this milk add 17 oz. (503 ml.) of water to 13 oz. (384 ml.) of evaporated milk, 2 level tablespoons (1 oz. or 28 gm.) of granulated sugar and 3 tablespoons (45 ml.) of vinegar. This mixture contains 77 Cal. per 100 ml.

May be used for normal infants from birth to 8 months. For older children omit the sugar. This reduces the Cal. to about 67 per 100 ml. (20 per oz.).

m. leg. Thrombosis of the iliac or femoral vein followed by swelling of the leg. So called because it often is a complication of puerperium. SYN: *phlegmasia alba dolens,* q.v.

m. of magnesia. USP. Magnesium hydroxide in permanent suspension.

m., modified. M. altered so that its composition more closely approximates that of human milk.

m., mother's. That from the mammary glands of a woman.

m., non-fat. Same as skimmed milk, q.v.

m., pasteurized. M. heated for 30 minutes at 62° C. to kill the living pathogenic bacteria. SEE: *pasteurization.*

m., protein. M. with high protein, and low carbohydrate and fat content.

m., red. M. contaminated by blood, chromogenic bacteria, or plant pigments.

m., ropy. That which has become viscid due to formation of vegetable gums from carbohydrates or mucinlike substances from proteins as a result of bacterial action.

m., skimmed. M. after removal of cream.

m., sour. M. with lactic acid caused by lactic acid bacteria.

m., sterilized. M. boiled to kill bacteria.

m., sugar of. Lactose.

m. teeth. First or deciduous teeth.

m. tumor. Retention of milk in mammary gland.

m., uterine. Whitish fluid found between villi in placenta of pregnant uterus.

m., uviol. M. sterilized by ultraviolet rays.

m., vegetable. 1. The latex of plants. 2. A synthetic milk prepared from juices expressed from various plants, such as soybean.

m., vitamin D. M. in which vitamin D content had been increased by addition of concentrates, ultraviolet irradiation, or by feeding irradiated yeast to milk-producing animals.

m., witch's. M. secreted in the breasts of the newborn.

Miller-Abbott tube. [T. Grier Miller, Amer. physician, 1886- ; W. Asler Abbott, Amer. physician, 1902-1943] A flexible double lumen tube used for diagnosing and treating intestinal disease. Substances may be placed in the intestinal tract by using one lumen; the other lumen may be used for suction.

milli- [L.]. Prefix used in metric system to denote one-thousandth.

milliam'meter. Ammeter registering in milliamperes. SEE: *ammeter.*

milliampere (mĭl″ē-ăm′pēr). One-thousandth of an ampere. ABBR: ma.

m. minute. An electrical unit of quantity, equivalent to that delivered by 1 milliampere in 1 minute.

millicurie (mĭl″ĭ-kū′rē). One-thousandth of a curie. ABBR: mc.

m. hour. A practical unit of dosage for radon. One millicurie of radon applied for 1 hour. The biologic effect depends on time, filtration, and distance.

milliequiv′alent. Weight of a substance contained in 1 milliliter of a normal solution. ABBR: mEq.

milligram (mil′ĭ-gram). One-thousandth of a gram. ABBR: mg.

milliliter. One-thousandth of a liter. For practical purposes it is equivalent to 1 cc. ABBR: ml.

millimeter. One-thousandth of a meter.

millimicron (mil-i-mi′kron). One-thousandth of a micron; one-millionth of a millimeter. ABBR: mμ or mmm.

millimol (mil′ĭ-mōl). One-thousandth of a mol. ABBR: mM.

milphosis (mĭl-fō′sĭs). Loss of eyebrows or eyelashes.

mime′sis [Gr. *mimēsis,* imitation]. Imitation, mimicry; term applied to a disease which exhibits symptoms of another disease or to conditions in hysteria which simulate organic disease.

mimetic, mimic (mī-mĕt′ĭk, mĭm′ĭk) [Gr. *mimētikos*]. Imitative.

    m. convulsion. Facial convulsion.

    m. labor. False labor.

    m. spasm. Spasm of facial muscles.

min. Abbr. for *minim: minute.*

mind [AS. *gemynd*]. Integration of functions of the brain resulting in the ability to perceive surroundings, to have emotions, imagination, memory, and will, and to process information in an intelligent manner.

mineral [L. *minerale*]. 1. An inorganic element or compound occurring in nature, esp. one that is solid. 2. Inorganic; not of animal or plant origin. 3. Impregnated with minerals, as mineral water. 4. Pertaining to minerals.

    m. compounds. Compounds of mineral elements, excepting carbon, constitute the mineral constituents of the body.

    Minerals serve the following functions: They are essential constituents of all cells; they form the greater portion of the hard parts of the body (bone, teeth, nails); they are essential components of respiratory pigments, enzymes, and enzyme systems; they regulate the permeability of cell membranes and capillaries; they regulate the excitability of muscular and nervous tissue; they are essential for regulation of osmotic pressure equilibria; they are necessary for maintenance of proper acid-base balance; they are essential constituents of secretions of glands; they play an important role in water metabolism and regulation of blood volume.

    Mineral salts and water are excreted daily from the body. These must be replaced through food intake. Daily requirements for principal minerals for a normal adult are as follows: calcium and phosphorous, 0.8-1.4 gm.; sodium, 10-18 mg.; copper, 1-2 mg.; iodine, 50-75 μg (micrograms); magnesium, 20-25 gm.; sodium, about 1 gm. of sodium chloride per kg. of water intake. Requirements are greater for growing children and pregnant women and in certain pathologic conditions.

    SEE: *acid-base balance; body; names of elements; buffer.*

    m. oil. USP. Liquid petrolatum.

    m. spring. A spring in which water contains mineral salts thought to have a therapeutic value in certain diseases, but usually the principal action is as a cathartic. SEE: *spa.*

    m. water. W. charged with inorganic salts.

mineralocorticoid (min″er-al-ō-kor′tĭ-koyd). A biologically active principle of the adrenal cortex effecting the retention or excretion of sodium or potassium. SEE: *glucocorticoid.*

minim (min′im) [L. *minimum,* least]. One-sixtieth part of a fluidram or 0.06 milliliter. ABBR: m., min. SYN: *drop.*

minimal (min′ĭ-mal). Least; the smallest possible.

    m. dose. Smallest dose producing an effect.

minimum (mĭn′ĭ-mŭm). (pl. *min′ima*) Least quantity or lowest limit. SEE: *threshold.*

    m. daily requirements. The daily requirements of vitamins and minerals needed to prevent symptoms of deficiency. ABBR: MDR.

    m. lethal dose. Smallest quantity of a substance producing death.

Minin light (min′in). [A. V. Minin, Russ. surgeon]. A lamp for the administration of violet and ultraviolet light.

minor. Person not of legal age and thus requiring consent for medical, surgical, or dental care. Legal age is not the same in all states.

    m., emancipated. A person not of legal age who is either in the armed services, married, or has left home and is self-sufficient. Some state legislatures do not require such an individual to have parental consent in order to receive medical or surgical care.

Minot-Murphy diet (mī′nŏt). [George R. Minot, Am. physician, 1885-1950; William P. Murphy, Am. physician, 1892 —]. Diet for pernicious anemia containing large quantities of liver.

mio- (mī′ō) [Gr. *meiōn,* less]. Combining form meaning less, smaller.

miocardia (mī-ō-kar'dī-ă) ["+ *kardia*, heart].
Systolic lessening of heart's volume. SYN:
systole.

mionectic (mī-ō-nek'tik) [Gr. *meionektikos*,
disposed to taking too little]. Pert. to or
having or using a subnormal amount of
oxygen, esp. blood. SEE: *mesectic, pleonectic.*

mioplas'mia. Abnormal lessening of the
amount of blood plasma.

miopragia (mī-ō-prā'jī-ă) [Gr. *meĭon*, less, +
prassein, to perform]. Decrease of functional
activity.

miosis, meiosis (mī-ō'sĭs) [Gr. *meiōsis*, a
lessening]. 1. Abnormal contraction of
pupils. 2. Period of diminishing symptoms in
a disease. 3. Method of cell division which
allows each daughter nucleus to receive half
the number of chromosomes present in the
somatic cells.

miot'ic. 1. An agent that causes the pupil to
contract, such as eserine and pilocarpine. 2.
Pert. to or causing contraction of the pupil.
3. Diminishing.

miracidium (mī"ră-sĭd'-ĭ-ŭm). (pl. *miracidia*)
A ciliated free-swimming larva of a digenet-
ic fluke. On emerging from an ovum, it
penetrates a snail of a particular species and
metamorphoses into a sporocyst. SEE: *fluke.*

mire (mēr) [L. *mirari*, to look at]. A test object
on the ophthalmometer, the images of which
denote the amount of astigmatism.

mirror [Fr. *miroir*]. A polished surface that
reflects rays of light and creates visible
images of objects in front of it.

   m. drill. Exercise before a mirror, practicing control of convulsive tics.

   Patient sitting in front of mirror tries to
control movements. When he accomplishes
this, the physician begins to distract the
patient's attention from his reflection by
having him do calisthenics.

   m. speech. That which reverses the order of words in a sentence or pronounces
words backward. SEE: *lalopathy.*

   m. writing. Writing in which the words
are reversed, as seen in a mirror. SEE:
dyslexia.

mis- [AS. *mis*, wrong]. Prefix implying bad,
wrong, improper, negative, etc.

misanthropia (mĭs"an-thrō'pī-ă) ["+ Gr.
anthrōpos, man]. Hatred of mankind.

miscar'riage ["+ L. *carrus*, cart]. Interruption of pregnancy prior to the 7th month.
Usually refers specifically to expulsion of
fetus in period bet. 4th month and viability.
SYN: *abortion.*

misce (mĭs'ē) [L.]. A direction given on prescriptions, instructing the pharmacist to
mix the ingredients. ABBR: M.

miscegenation (mis"ē-jē-nā'shun) [L. *miscere*, to mix, + *genus*, race]. Sex relations or
marriage bet. those of different races.

miscible (mĭs'ī-bl). Capable of being mixed.

misocainia (mĭs-ō-kī'nī-ă) [Gr. *misein*, to
hate, + *kainos*, new]. An aversion to new
ideas. SYN: *misoneism.*

misog'amy ["+ *gamos*, marriage]. Aversion
to marriage.

misogynist (mĭs-oj'ī-nĭst) ["+ *gyne*, woman].
One who hates women.

misogyny (mĭs-oj'īn-ī). Abnormal hatred of
women.

misologia (mĭs-ō-lō'jī-ă) [Gr. *misein*, to hate,
+ *logos*, word]. Aversion to mental work.

misoneism (mī-sō-nē'izm) ["+ *neos*, new].
Aversion to new things or new ideas; con-
servatism.

misopedia (mī-sō-pē'dī-ă) ["+ Gr. *pais, paid-*,
child]. Abnormal dislike for children or the
young.

Mist., mist. Abbr. for *mistura*, q.v.

mistura [L.]. Mixture. Preparation intended
for internal use and containing suspended
insoluble substances which do not unite
chemically. Should always be shaken before
using.

mite (mīt) [AS.]. A minute arachnid, a member of the order Acarina. Some are parasitic
and are the cause of conditions such as
mange and scabies. Some serve as vectors of
disease organisms and as intermediate hosts
for certain Cestodes.

   m., follicle. Demodex folliculorum. M.
which lives in hair follicles and sebaceous
glands.

   m., itch. Sarcoptes scabei.

   m., mange. Mites belonging to the families Sarcoptidae and Psoroptidae. The cause
of mange and scabies in many species of
animals.

   m., red. Redbugs or chiggers, members
of the family Thrombiculidae. SEE: *chiggers.*

mithridatism (mĭth'rĭ-dāt"ĭzm). [Mithri-
dates, king of Pontus, 163-132 B. C., supposed to have acquired immunity in this
fashion]. Immunity to a poison acquired by
taking it in doses of gradually increasing
size.

miticide (mī'tĭ-sīd). A substance that kills
mites.

mitigated (mĭt'ĭ-gāt-ed) [L. *mitigāre*, to soft-
en]. Diminished in severity. SYN: *allayed,
moderated.*

mitochondria (mĭt"ō-kon'drĭ-ă) [Gr. *mitos*,
thread, + *chondros*, cartilage]. (sing. *mitochondrion*) Slender microscopic filaments or
rods 0.5 micron in diameter which can be
seen in cells by using phase-contrast micros-

copy. They are the source of energy in the cell. They are also involved in protein synthesis and lipid metabolism.

mito'ma, mi'tome [Gr. *mitos*, thread]. A fine network support or framework of protoplasm in a cell.

mito'sis. (pl. *mitosēs*) Indirect cell division involving indirect nuclear division (karyokinesis) and division of the cell body (cytokinesis), the process by which all somatic cells of multicellular organisms multiply.

Mitosis is a continuous process divided into four phases: *Prophase:* the chromatin granules of the nucleus stain more densely and become organized into chromosomes which first appear as long, delicate, spiral structures each consisting of two spiral filaments called chromatids. Each chromosome possesses a clear region (centromere) usually in the mid-region. As the prophase progresses, the chromosomes become shorter and more compact and stain densely; the nuclear membrane and the nucleoli disappear. At the same time, the centriole divides and the two daughter centrioles, each surrounded by a centrosphere, move to opposite poles of the cell. They are connected by fine protoplasmic fibrils which form the achromatic spindle. *Metaphase:* the chromosomes (paired chromatids) arrange themselves in an equatorial plane midway between the two centrioles forming the equatorial plate. *Anaphase:* the chromatids (now called daughter chromosomes) diverge and move toward their respective centrosomes. The end of their migration marks the beginning of the next phase. *Telophase:* the chromosomes at each pole of the spindle undergo changes the reverse of those in the prophase, each becoming a long, looselyspiraled thread. The nuclear membrane reforms and nucleoli reappear. Outlines of chromosomes disappear and chromatin appears as granules scattered throughout nucleus and connected by a lightly staining linin net. The cytoplasm becomes separated into two parts, resulting in two complete cells. This is accomplished in animal cells by constriction in the equatorial region; in plant cells a cell plate which gives rise to the cell membrane forms in a similar position. The period between two successive divisions is called interphase.

Mitosis is of particular significance in that the hereditary determiners (genes) are distributed equally to each daughter cell and a constancy in number of chromosomes is maintained in all cells of an organism.

m., heterotypic. The first or reduction

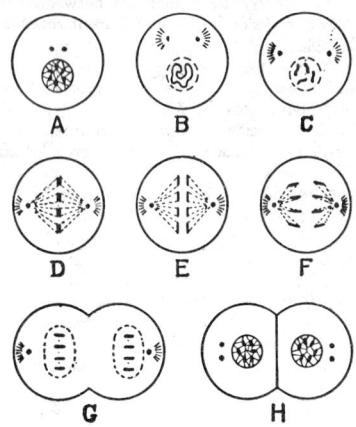

MITOSIS
Four phases of mitotic division in a cell having four chromosomes. A, B, C, Changes in the centrosome and nucleus during prophase. D, Metaphase. E, F, Anaphase. G, H, Telophase.

division in the maturation of germ cells.

m., homeotypic. The second or equational division in the maturation of germ cells.

mitosome (mī'tō-sōm) ["+ *sōma*, body]. 1. A body giving rise to the middle piece of the spermatozoon. 2. Chromatin mass in a cellular nucleus.

mitotic (mī-tŏt'ĭk). Pert. to mitosis.

mitral (mī'tral). Pert. to the bicuspid or mitral valve. SEE: *facies mitralis.*

m. disease. That of the mitral valve. SEE: *heart.*

m. murmur. One produced at the mitral valve.

m. orifice. Left atrioventricular aperture.

m, regurgitation. Due to failure of valve to close completely, blood is allowed to flow back into the auricle.

m. stenosis. Narrowing orifice of the valve obstructing free flow from auricle to ventricle.

m. valve. SYN: *bicuspid valve; valvula bicuspidalis.*

mittelschmerz (mit'el-shmarts) [Ger.]. Pain bet. menstrual periods, occurring at time of ovulation.

mit'tor [L. *mittere,* to send]. A neuron terminal which transmits impulses to ceptors of the adjoining neuron.

mixed [L. *mixtus,* from *miscere,* to mingle]. Consisting of two or more intermingling substances.

m. marriage. Marriage between persons of different races or different religious beliefs.

m. nerves. The spinal nerves containing sensory, or afferent, and motor, or efferent, fibers.

mix″osco′pia [Gr. *mixis,* intercourse, + *skopein,* to examine]. Sexual perversion in which sexual gratification is obtained through observation of others in coition.

mixture (mĭks′tūr) [L. *mistura*]. A combination of two or more substances without chemical union. SEE: *mistura.*

MKS, mks. Abbr. for *meter-kilogram-second.* Indicates measurements used with meter for length, kilogram for weight, and second for time.

M.L.D., m.l.d. Abbr. for *minimum lethal dose.*

mM. Abbr. for *millimole.*

mm. Abbr. for *millimeter.*

mmm. Abbr. for *millimicron.*

Mn. Symb. for *manganese.*

mne″masthe′nia [Gr. *mnēmē,* memory, + *sthenos,* strength]. Poor memory not resulting from organic disease.

mnemic (nē′mĭk). Relating to memory.

mnemonics (nē-mŏn′ĭks). The art of improving or assisting memory. A device to help recall a series of related data, names, or anatomical terms.

Mo. Chemical symbol for *molybdenum.*

mo. Abbr. for *month.*

mo′bile [L. *mobilis*]. Movable.

m. spasm. Tonic spasm with irregular, slow movements of limbs following hemiplegia. Athetosis.

mobility [L. *mobilitas*]. State or quality of being mobile; facility of movement.

mobilization (mo″bĭl-ĭ-zā′shŭn). 1. The making of a fixed or ankylosed part movable. 2. Restoration of motion to a joint. 3. Freeing an organ or making it movable. 4. The freeing, or making available, substances held in reserve as glycogen or fat.

m., stapes. Surgical treatment to restore mobility to the stapes. Used in treatment of deafness.

mobilize (mō′bĭl-īz). 1. To incite to physiological action. 2. To render movable; to put in movement.

Möbius′ sign (me′bĭ-ŭs). [Paul J. Möbius, Ger. neurologist, 1853-1907]. A symptom in Graves′ disease in which one eye converges and the other diverges when looking at the tip of one′s nose.

modal (mōd′l) [L. *modus,* mode]. Pert. to, or characteristic of, a mode. Thus pert. to the most frequent or common or typical. SEE: *mode.*

modal′ity. 1. Quality of being modal. 2. A method of application or the employment of any therapeutic agent; limited usually to physical agents.

mode (mōd). In statistics, the value or item of the class occurring most frequently in a series of variables.

modiolus(mō-dī′ō-lŭs) [L., a small measure]. [NA] Central pillar or axial part of cochlea extending from the base to the apex.

modulus (mōj′ū-lŭs) [L. a small measure]. In physics, a constant or coefficient that indicates to what extent a substance possesses some property.

mo′dus [L.]. A method or a mode.

m. operandi. Method of performing an act.

mogilalia (mōj-ĭ-lā′lĭ-ă) [Gr. *mogis,* with difficulty, + *lalia,* chatter]. Any speech defect, as stuttering.

mogiphonia (mō-jĭ-fō′nĭ-ă) ["+ *phōnē,* voice]. Difficulty in emitting vocal sounds.

Mohrenheim′s space (mor′en-hīm). [Baron J. J. Freiherr von Mohrenheim, Aust. surgeon, —1799]. Space bet. pectoralis major and deltoid just beneath the clavicle.

moist (moyst). Damp, wet.

m. chamber. A vessel for keeping microscopic objects moist.

mo′lar. 1. [L. *molaris,* grinding] A grinding or back tooth, one of three on each side of the jaws. The first permanent molar erupts at the 6th year; the second one about the 12th year. The third molars (wisdom teeth) are extremely variable, usually erupting between 17th and 25th years. However, they may erupt later or not at all. SEE: *dentition, teeth.* 2. [L. *moles,* a mass] Pert. to a mass; not molecular. 3. Pert. to a mole (2). 4. Gram-molecule. SYN: *mole,* q.v.

m. solution. One in which there is one mole of the solute dissolved in each liter of the solution.

molarity. The number of gram molecular weights (moles) of a substance per liter of solution. Thus 1/M (also expressed as 1 M means one mole of a substance per liter, 0.1/M indicates 0.1 mole per liter.

molasses [L. *mellaceus,* honeylike]. Food value of 100 gm. (cane, blackstrap): Cal. 213; carbohydrate 55 gm.; calcium 684 mg.; potassium 2927 mg.

mold. 1. A fuzzy coating of a fungus nature on the surface of decaying vegetable matter. 2. Any one of a group of parasitic or saprophytic fungi which causes mold. Examples are black molds (Mucorales) and blue and green molds (Aspergillales). The latter include Penicillium, the source of the antibiotic, penicillin. 3. To shape a mass, as a pill. 4. To shape the fetal head, adapting it to the pelvic inlet.

mold'ing. 1. Shaping of the fetal head, adapting itself to pelvic inlet. 2. Manual shaping of infant's features following delivery. 3. A protective border, used in plastic surgery. 4. Casting of a reproduction.

mole (mōl) [AS. *māēl*]. 1. A congenital discolored spot elevated above the surface of the skin. ETIOL: Not clear. May arise from local or static condition of circulation in a small area. Harmless unless irritated. TREATMENT: Protect against irritation. Do not tie a thread about a mole. SYN: *nevus.* SEE: *racemose; melanoma.*

2. [Ger. *Mol,* abbr. for *Molekulargewicht,* molecular weight] A quantity of a chemical compound whose weight in grams equals its molecular weight. Thus 18.016 gm. of water would be one mole.

3. [L. *moles,* a shapeless mass] A uterine mass arising from a poorly developed or degenerating ovum.

m., blood. A mass made up of blood clots, membranes, and placenta, retained following abortion.

m., Breus'. Malformation of the ovum, a decidual tuberous subchorional hematoma.

m., carneous. Blood mole which has assumed a fleshlike appearance, when retained in uterus for some time.

m., false. One formed from a uterine tumor or polypus.

m., fleshy. M., carneous, q.v.

m., hydatid, hydatidiform. A polycystic mass in which the chorionic villi have undergone cystic degeneration.

m., pigmented. Nevus pigmentosus, q.v.

m., stone. A fleshy mole which has undergone calcareous degeneration in the uterus.

m., true. Mole representing the degenerated embryo or fetus.

m., vascular. A hemangioma, q.v.

m., vesicular. SEE: *hydatidiform mole.*

molecular (mō-lĕk'ū-lar) [L. *molecula,* little mass]. Pert. to a molecule.

m. disease. Disease due to a defect in a single molecule. The abnormal hemoglobin molecule found in persons with sickle cell anemia causes the abnormally shaped red cells characteristic of this disease.

m. biology. Branch of biology dealing with analysis of the structure and development of biological systems with respect to the chemistry and physics of their molecular constituents.

m. layer. 1. Cortical layer of cerebellar or cerebral substance. 2. (Inner). Inner retinal plexiform layer. 3. (outer). Outer retinal plexiform layer.

m. lesion. One not even visible through a microscope.

m. weight. Weight of a molecule attained by totalling the weight of its constituent atoms. SEE: *atomic weight.*

molecule (mŏl'ĕ-kūl). 1. The smallest quantity into which a substance may be divided without loss of its characteristics. 2. Any small portions of a substance. 3. A chemical combination of two or more atoms which form a specific chemical compound; the chemical elements are formed by the combination of atoms.

Combinations of dissimilar atoms form chemical compounds. In normal molecules the positive and negative electric charges exactly balance. Excess or deficiency of either positive or negative charge by the loss or acquisition of electrons results in the formation of an ion.

The molecule is designated by the number of atoms it contains, as: monatomic (one atom); diatomic (two); triatomic (three); tetratomic (four); pentatomic (five); hexatomic (six), etc. SEE: *cleavage.*

moli'men [L. effort). (pl. *molimina*) Effort to establish any normal function, esp. the monthly effort to establish the menstrual flow.

mollities (mōl-ĭsh'ĭ-ēz) [L.]. Abnormal softening of a part.

m. ossium. Softening of the bones. SYN: *osteomalacia.*

Moll's glands. [Jacob A. Moll, Dutch oculist, 1832-1914]. Modified sweat glands at border of eyelids. SYN: *ciliary glands.*

mol'lusc, mol'lusk. Any member of the phylum Mollusca.

Mollusca. A phylum of animals which includes the bivalves (mussels, oysters, clams), slugs, and snails. Snails serve as intermediate hosts of many parasitic flukes. Oysters and clams may transmit the virus of infectious hepatitis, esp. if improperly cooked.

Molluscous (Mōl-lŭs'kŭs). Concerning molluscum.

molluscum (mŏl-ŭs'kŭm). A mildly infective skin disease characterized by tumor formations on the skin.

m. contagiosum. The usual mildly contagious form of molluscum.

SYM: Characterized by small waxy globular epithelial tumors containing semifluid caseous matter or solid masses, healing without scarring though they may suppurate and break down, commonly on face, eyelids, breasts, genitalia, and inner surface of thigh. On pressure a substance resembling sebum is expressed.

ETIOL: A large virus of the pox group.

TREATMENT: Incision, expression of contents, followed by iodine.

m. fibrosum. A form showing masses of fibrocellular tissue.

m. simplex. SEE: *m. fibrosum.*

mol. wt. Abbr. for *molecular weight.*

molybdenum (mŏ-lĭb'dĕ-nŭm). SYMB: *Mo.* At. wt. 95.94; at. no. 42. A hard, heavy, metallic element.

molysmophobia (mō-lĭz"mō-fō'bĭ-ă) [Gr. *molysma,* stain, + *phobia,* fear]. Morbid fear of contamination or infection. SYN: *mysophobia.*

momentum (mō-mĕn'tŭm) [L.]. 1. Quantity of motion indicated by multiplying the weight of the object in motion by its space. 2. Force of motion acquired by a moving object as a result of continuance of its motion; impetus.

mon'ad [Gr. *monas,* a unit]. 1. A univalent element. 2. A unicellular organism. 3. One of the four components of a tetrad.

monarthritis (mŏn-ar-thrī'tĭs) [Gr. *mono,* single, + *arthron,* joint, + *-itis,* inflammation]. Arthritis affecting a single joint.

monarticular (mŏn-ar-tĭk'ū-lăr). Concerning or affecting one joint.

monaster (mŏn-as'ter) ["+ *astēr,* star]. Single starlike figure formed in mitosis.

monathetosis (mŏn"ăth-ē-tō'sĭs). Athetosis affecting a single part of the body.

Mondonesi's reflex (mŏn-dō-nā'zĭ). [Filippo Mondonesi, It. physician]. In coma, contraction of facial muscles following pressure on eyeball. SYN: *bulbomimic reflex; facial reflex.*

Mondor's disease. [Henri Mondor, Fr. physician, 1885-1962] Thrombosis and sclerosis of a subcutaneous vein or veins in the breast area of either sex. May occur after trauma or appear without apparent cause. The long firm tender cord or stringlike structure extends from the breast up into the axilla or down toward the epigastrium. It is a benign self-limiting disease which is important because its appearance may be confused with cancer of the breast. SYN: *string phlebitis.*

monesthetic (mŏn"ĕs-thet'ĭk) [Gr. *mono,* single, + *aisthēsis,* sensation]. Affecting only one of the senses.

mongolism. Now called Down's syndrome or disease. A severe form of congenital mental deficiency. Children have a characteristic appearance: small head, slanting eyes with inner epicanthal fold (thus the name mon-

gol), and a fissured tongue that usually is large and protruding. About one in eight of all mentally defective infants are afflicted with this syndrome.

About 70% of children with this syndrome are born to women over 30. The risk of a mother who has had one Down's syndrome child having another one is increased four times.

monilethrix (mŏn-ĭl'ĕ-thrĭks) [L. *monile,* necklace, + Gr. *thrix,* hair]. A developmental defect of the hair shaft in which the hair becomes beaded and brittle. The defect usually appears by the second month of life. Etiological factors unknown. No effective treatment.

Monil'ia [L. *monile,* necklace]. Former name for the genus of fungi now called Candida, q.v.

moniliasis (mō"nĭ-lī'ă-sĭs). Infection of the skin or mucous membranes by yeastlike fungi. Usually localized in skin, nails, mouth, vagina, bronchi, or lungs, but may invade blood stream.

ETIOL: Various species of Candida but chiefly C. albicans.

moniliform (mō-nĭl'ĭ-form) [L. *monile,* necklace, + *forma,* shape]. Resembling a necklace or string of beads.

moniliosis (mŏn-ĭl-ĭ-ō'sĭs). Moniliasis, q. v.

monitor (mŏn'ĭ-tur) [L., one who warns]. 1. One who observes an operation, procedure, or apparatus, esp. one who is responsible for detecting and preventing malfunction. 2. A device which provides a warning if that which is being observed fails or malfunctions. 3. To check by using an electronic device.

m., blood pressure. M. providing a record of systolic and diastolic blood pressure.

m., cardiac. M. of heart function, providing visual and audible record of heartbeat.

m., fetal. 1. M. which detects and displays fetal heart beat. 2. Assessment of fetus in utero with respect to its heart rate by use of electrocardiogram, or to chemical analysis of the amniotic fluid or fetal blood.

m., personal radiation. Small device carried by an individual to measure the accumulated radiation dosage over a period of time.

m., temperature. M. for measuring and recording temperature of the body or some particular portion of the body.

mono, mon- [Gr.]. Prefix designating one, single.

mon"oacid'ic. Having one replaceable hydroxyl (OH) group.

monoamine oxidase inhibitors. A group of drugs which are effective in treating depression. Their mode of action in addition to inhibiting monoamine oxidase is not clearly understood.

Because of their toxic potential they should be used with caution. Hypertensive crises have been observed in persons who eat certain kinds of cheese while taking MAO inhibitors. SEE: *tyramine.*

monoanesthesia (mŏn-ō-ăn-ĕs-thē'sĭ-ă). Anesthesia of a single member or organ.

monobasic (mŏn-ō-bā'sĭk) [Gr. *mono,* one + *basis,* a base]. Having one hydrogen atom replaceable by a metal or positive radical.

mon'oblast ["+ *blastos,* germ]. A cell which gives rise to a monocyte.

monoblepsia (mŏn-ō-blĕp'sĭ-ă) [Gr. *mono,* single, + *blepsis,* sight]. 1. Condition in which vision is more distinct when only one eye is used, hence tendency to close one eye to see clearly. 2. A type of color blindness in which only one color can be seen.

monobrachius (mŏn″ō-brā'kĭ-us) ["+ *brachiōn,* arm]. State of having only one arm. 2. Fetus with only one arm.

monobromated (mŏn″ō-brō'māt-ĕd). Pert. to chemical compound with only one atom of bromine in each molecule.

monocalcic (mŏn-ō-kal'sĭk). Pert. to a chemical compound containing only one atom of calcium in the molecule.

monocardian (mŏn-ō-kar'dĭ-ăn) [Gr. *mono,* single, + *kardia,* heart]. Individual possessing a heart with only one atrium and one ventricle.

monocelled (mŏn'ō-sĕld). Composed of a single cell.

monochord (mŏn'ō-kord) [Gr. *mono,* one, + *chordē,* cord]. An instrument for testing upper tone audition by means of friction.

monochorea (mon″ō-kō-rē'ă) ["+ *choreia,* a choral dance]. Chorea which affects but a single part or extremity.

monochorionic (mŏn-ō-kor-ē″ŏn'ĭk). Possessing a single chorion, as in the case of identical twins.

monochromasy (mŏn″ō-krō-mā'sĭ) [Gr. *mono,* single, + *chrōma,* color]. Color blindness in which only one color can be perceived.

monochromatic (mŏn″ō-krō-măt'ĭk). 1. Having but one color. 2. A color-blind person to whom all colors appear to be of one hue.

monochromator (mŏn-ō-krō'mā-tor). Instrument for selective transmission of homogeneous radiant energy.

monococcus (mŏn-ō-kŏk'ŭs) [Gr. *mono,* single, + *kokkos,* berry]. A form of coccus existing singly instead of as part of the usual group or chain.

monocular (mŏn-ŏk'ū-lar) ["+ L. *oculus,* eye]. 1. Concerning or affecting but one eye. 2. Possessing a single ocular or eyepiece.

monoculus (mŏn-ok'ū-lŭs). 1. A bandage for shielding one eye. 2. A fetus with only one eye; cyclops.

monocyesis (mŏn″ō-sī-ē'sĭs) ["+ *kyēsis,* pregnancy]. Pregnancy with a single fetus.

monocyte (mŏn'ō-sīt) ["+ *kytos,* cell]. A large mononuclear leukocyte having more protoplasm than a lymphocyte.

monocytic (mŏn-ō-sĭ'tĭk). Concerning or resembling monocytes.

monocytopenia (mŏn″ō-sī″tō-pe'nĭ-ă) [Gr. *mono,* single, + *kytos,* cell, + *penia,* lack]. Diminished number of monocytes in the blood.

monocytosis (mŏn″ō-sī-tō'sĭs). Excessive number of monocytes in the blood.

monodactylism (mŏn-ō-dak'tĭl-ĭzm) [Gr. *mono,* single, + *daktylos,* digit]. Condition, usually congenital, of having only one digit on a hand or foot.

monodal (mŏn-ōd'ăl) ["+ *hodos,* road]. Connected with one terminal of a resonator so that the patient acts as a capacitor for entrance and exit of high frequency currents.

monodiplopia (mŏn″ō-dī-plō'pĭ-ă) ["+ *diploos,* double, + *ōps,* eye]. Double vision in one eye only.

monodromia. Condition of muscles or nerves in which conduction occurs in one direction only.

monogamy (mo-nog'ă-mĭ) [Gr. *mono,* single, + *gamos,* marriage]. The practice of being married to only one person at a time.

monogony (mō-nŏg'ō-nĭ) ["+ *gonē,* seed]. Asexual reproduction.

monograph (mŏn'ō-grăf) ["+ *graphein,* to write]. A treatise dealing with a single subject.

monohy'brid. Offspring of a cross between parents differing in a single character.

monohydrated (mŏn-ō-hī'drāt-ed) [Gr. *mono,* single, + *hydor,* water]. United with only one molecule of water.

monoideaism, monoideism (mŏn-ō-ī-dē'ă-ĭzm, -dē'ĭzm) ["+ *idea,* idea]. Preoccupation with only one idea; a slight degree of monomania.

monolocular (mŏn″ō-lok'ū-lar) ["+ L. *loculus,* a small chamber]. Having only one cell or cavity. SYN: *unilocular.*

monomania (mŏn-ō-mā'nĭ-ă) ["+ *mania,* madness]. Mental illness characterized by distortion of thought processes concerning a single subject or idea.

monoma'niac. One afflicted with monomania.

monomastigote (mŏn-ō-măs'tĭ-gŏt) [Gr. *mono*, single, + *mastix*, *mastig-*, whip]. Possessing only one flagellum.

monomelic (mŏn-ō-mĕl'ĭk) [Gr. *mono*, single, + *melos*, limb]. Affecting a single limb.

monomer (mŏn'ō-mer). Any molecule that can be bound to similar molecules to form a polymer.

monomeric (mŏn-ō-mĕr'ĭk) [Gr. *mono*, single, + *meros*, part]. Consisting of, or affecting, a single piece or segment of a body.

monomorphic (mŏn-ō-mor'fĭk) ["+ *morphē*, form]. Unchangeable in form; keeping the same form throughout every stage of development.

monomyople'gia [Gr. *mono*, single, + *mys*, *myo-*, muscle, + *plēgē*, stroke]. Paralysis of only one muscle.

monomyositis (mŏn"ō-mi-ō-sī'tĭs) ["+ "+ *-itis*, inflammation]. Inflamed condition of only one muscle.

mononeural (mŏn-ō-nū'răl) ["+ *neuron*, nerve]. Supplied by or concerning a single nerve.

mononeuritis (mŏn"ō-nū-rī'tĭs) ["+ "+ *-itis*, inflammation]. Inflamed condition of a single nerve.

mononuclear (mŏn-ō-nū'klē-ăr) ["+ L. *nucleus*, kernel]. Having one nucleus, particularly a blood cell such as a monocyte or lymphocyte. SYN: *uninuclear*.

mononucleosis (mŏn-ō-nū-klē-ō'sĭs) [Gr. *mono*, single, + *nucleus*, kernel]. Presence of more than normal number of mononuclear leukocytes in the blood.

    m., infectious. An acute infectious disease that affects lymphoid tissue primarily. Characterized by enlarged, often tender, lymph nodes and enlarged spleen with great increase of atypical or abnormal mononuclear leukocytes in the blood. Abnormal liver function test will be found in about 90% of cases. The disease is due to a virus. Incubation period may be as long as 4 to 7 weeks.

    SYM: Constitutional symptoms, fever, sore throat, and generalized lymphadenopathy; hyperplasia of lymphatic tissue. Blood contains heterophile antibodies.

    TREATMENT: There is no specific therapy, but for serious complications (ex: hemolytic anemia, pharyngeal swelling interfering with swallowing) cortisone is indicated.

mononucleotide. A product resulting from hydrolysis of nucleic acid. Contains phosphoric acid combined with a glucoside or pentoside.

monoparesis (mŏn-ō-par'ĕs-ĭs) [Gr. *mono*, single, + *paresis*, weakness]. Paralysis of a single part of body.

monoparesthesia (mŏn"ō-păr-ĕs-thē'sĭ-ă) ["+ *para*, beside, + *aisthēsis*, sensation]. Paresthesia of only one region or limb.

monopathy (mō-nŏp'ăth-ĭ) ["+ *pathos*, disease]. A disease attacking only one part of the body.

monophagia (mŏn-ō-fā'jĭ-ă) ["+ *phagein*, to eat]. 1. Appetite for only one kind of food. 2. The habit of eating of just one meal a day.

monophasia (mŏn-ō-fā'zĭ-ă) ["+ *phasis*, speech]. Inability to utter anything but one word or phrase repeatedly.

monophobia (mŏn-ō-fō'bĭ-ă) ["+ *phobos*, fear]. Abnormal fear of being alone.

monophyletic (mŏn"ō-fĭl-ĕt'ĭk) ["+ *phylē*, tribe]. Originating from a single source.

monoplegia (mŏn-ō-plē'jĭ-ă) [Gr. *mono*, single, + *plēgē*, stroke]. Paralysis of a single limb or a single group of muscles.

monopolar (mŏn-ō-pōl'ăr) ["+ L. *polus*, pole]. Using one terminal only, the ground acting as the 2nd terminal. SEE: *monoterminal*.

monorchid (mŏn-or'kĭd) ["+ *orchis*, testicle]. Person having only one testicle.

monorchidism, monorchism (mŏn-ōr'-kĭd-ĭzm, mŏn'or-kĭzm) ["+ *orchis*, testicle]. Condition in which there is only one descended testicle.

monosaccharide (mŏn-ō-săk'ă-rĭd) [Gr. *mono*, single, + *sakcharis*, sugar]. A simple sugar which cannot be decomposed by hydrolysis. Ex: fructose, galactose, glucose, q.v. These sugars are absorbed directly. They maintain the glucose content of the blood and provide for the production of glycogen. SYN: *monosaccharose*.

monosaccharoses (mŏn-ō-sak'ă-rōs-ĕs). A group name for monosaccharides. SEE: *disaccharose; polysaccharose*.

monosodium glutamate. Sodium salt of glutamic acid, $C_5H_8O_4NaN$. A white crystalline substance that has meatlike taste. Used to flavor foods, esp. in the Orient.

    When ingested in large amounts causes chest pain, facial pressure, headaches, burning sensation, and excessive sweating. This has been termed the Chinese Restaurant syndrome. Suitability of its general use as a food additive is being investigated. Manufactured under various names as Ajinomoto, Accent, Vetsin. ABBR: MSG.

monosome (mŏn'ō-sōm) [Gr. *mono*, single, + *sōma*, body]. An accessory chromosome which, without dividing, goes into only one of the daughter cells. The unpaired sex chromosome.

monospasm (mŏn'ō-spazm). Spasm of a single limb or part.

monosymptomatic (mŏn"ō-sĭmp-tō-mat'-ĭk). Having only one dominant symptom.

monosyphilide (mŏn-ō-sĭf'il-ĭd) [Gr. *mono,* single, + Fr. *syphilide*]. Characterized by only a single syphilitic lesion.

monoter'minal ["+ *terma,* a limit]. Using one terminal only in the giving of treatments, the ground acting as the second terminal for the completion of the electrical circuit.

monothermia (mŏn-ō-therm'ĭ-ă) ["+ *thermē,* heat]. Condition in which body temperature is stable; absence of rise in evening temperature.

Monotricha (mō-nŏt'rĭ-ka) ["+ *thrix, trich-,* hair]. Bacteria having a single flagellum at one pole.

monotrichous (mŏn-ŏt'rĭ-kus). Pert. to or having a single flagellum.

monovalent (mŏn-ō-vā'lent) ["+ L. *valēre,* to have power]. Having the combining power of a single hydrogen atom. SYN: *univalent.*

monox'enous. Said of a parasite that requires only one species as a host.

monoxide (mŏn-ŏk'sĭd). An oxide having only one atom of oxygen.

monozygotic (mŏn"ō-zī-gŏt'ĭk) [Gr. *mono,* single, + *zygōtos,* yoked]. Originating from a single fertilized ovum, said of identical twins.

Monro's foramen (mŏn-rō'). [Alexander Monro, Scot. anatomist, 1737-1817]. Point of communication bet. 3rd and lateral ventricles of the brain.

Monro's sulcus. Sulcus on 3rd ventricle's lateral wall from the foramen interventriculare to the aditus ad aquaeductum cerebri. SYN: *aulix.*

mons (mōns) [L. mountain]. (pl. *mon'tēs*) An anatomical eminence above the surface of the body.

    m. pubis. [NA]. Pubic eminence. SYN: *m. veneris.*

    m. veneris. [L. mount of Venus]. A pad of fatty tissue and coarse skin overlying the symphysis pubis in the woman. After puberty covered with short, curly hair and called pubic escutcheon. Typically triangular in shape. SEE: *pubes.*

mon'ster [L. *monstrum*]. A grossly deformed individual, usually due to faulty development. The term should never be used when discussing such a patient with those who are emotionally attached to him. Terms such as handicapped, congenitally deformed, or abnormal would be more appropriate.

monstripar'ity ["+ *parēre,* to give birth to]. To give birth to a monster.

monstros'ity [L. *monstrositas*]. 1. Monster. 2. Congenital malformation.

Montgomery's glands. [William F. Montgomery, Ir. obstetrician, 1797-1859]. Small prominences around the nipple of the breast which enlarge during pregnancy and lactation. See: *areola; mamma.*

monthlies (mŭnth'lēs). Slang for the menses.

monticulus (mŏn-tĭk'ū-lus) [L. little mountain]. (pl. *monticuli*) A protuberance.

    m. cerebelli. Protuberance of the superior vermis whose ant. portion is called the culmen, the post. portion the declive.

mood [AS. *mōd,* mind, feeling]. Temporary state of mind or feeling manifested by one's thoughts and actions.

morament (mŏr-am'ent) [Gr. *mōros,* stupid, + *amentia,* madness]. A moron of low grade. A person who is mentally defective and without moral sense.

moramentia (mŏr-ă-mĕn'shĭ-ă). State of being without moral sense.

Moraxella (mŏr-ăx-ĕl'ă). Genus of bacteria sometimes confused with Neisseria. Morax-axenfeld species is associated with conjunctivitis.

morbid (mor'bĭd) [L. *morbidus,* sick]. 1. Diseased. 2. Pert. to disease. 3. Preoccupied with unwholesome ideas and circumstances.

morbid'ity [L. *morbidus,* sick]. 1. State of being diseased. 2. The number of sick persons or cases of disease in relationship to a specific population SEE: *incidence.*

    m. rate. Number of cases of a specific disease in a specified period of time, usually a year, per unit of population, usually 1,000 or 10,000, or 100,000 alive.

morbific (mor-bĭf'ĭk) ["+ *facere,* to make]. Causing or producing disease.

morbilli (mor-bil'ī) [L. *morbillus,* little disease]. Measles.

morbil'liform [L. *morbilli,* measles, + *forma,* shape]. Like measles or its rash.

mor'bus [L.]. Disease.

    m. caeruleus. Cyanosis which is congenital.

    m. miseriae. Any condition due to neglect and want.

morcellation, morcellement (mor-sel-ā'-shŭn, -mon') [Fr. *morceller,* to subdivide]. Method of removing a fetus, tumor, or organ by pieces.

mordant (mor'dănt) [L. *mordere,* to bite]. A substance which fixes a stain or dye, as alum and phenol.

mores (mō'rāz) [L. plural of *mos,* custom]. Habits and customs of society. Usually those which come to be regarded as being essential to the survival and wellbeing of the society.

Morgagni (mor-gan'yē). [Giovanni B. Morgagni, It. pathological anatomist, 1682-1771].

    M.'s caruncle. The middle prostatic lobe.

    M.'s cataract. One that is hypermature with a softened cortex and a hard nucleus. SEE: *cataract.*

    M.'s hy'datid. Cystlike remains of müllerian duct attached to testicle or oviduct.

    M.'s ventricle. Ventriculus laryngis. SEE: *ventricle.*

morgagnian (mor-gan'yē-ān). Pert. to or described by Morgagni, q.v.

morgue (morg) [Fr.]. A public mortuary; a place for holding dead bodies for identification and burial. SYN: *mortuary.*

mo'ria [Gr. *mōria,* folly]. 1. Simple dementia. 2. Foolishness.

moribund (mor'ĭ-bŭnd) [L. *moribundus*]. In a dying condition; dying.

morioplasty (mo'rĭ-ō-plas-tĭ) [Gr. *morion,* piece, + *plassein,* to form]. Plastic surgery to restore portions of the body which have been lost through accident or disease:

morning or "A.M." care. AIM: Comfort and cleanliness.

    ARTICLES NECESSARY: Basin with warm water. Washcloth and face towel. Toothbrush, mouthwash, and water for mouth hygiene. Emesis basin. Comb and brush. Fresh linen as needed. Bath blanket. Rubbing alcohol or suitable back-rubbing lotion and talcum powder.

    PROCEDURE: If in ward, screen bed or draw curtains. Offer bedpan before beginning procedure, and supply fresh tampon or perineal pad if necessary. Cover patient with bath blanket and fold top bedding to foot of bed. If very disordered, remove to chair. Remove all but one pillow. Assist patient with care of mouth, or care for it if patient is not able to. Wash face and hands. Turn patient on side and rub back with back-rubbing lotion and powder. Patients whose skin is tender should have back washed before the rubbing. If patient is to have bath later, the linen need not be changed until that is given. Loosen bottom sheet and draw sheet and pull them tight again, brushing out any crumbs that may be on them. Smooth patient's hair. Fluff and rearrange pillows. Rearrange upper bedding neatly. If patient has a hot water bottle or an ice cap refill it. Leave fresh water within patient's reach. Leave fresh washcloth and towel. Before leaving room, adjust bed position, lighting, and ventilation as indicated.

morning sickness. The nausea and vomiting that affect some women during first few months of pregnancy, particularly in the morning. SYN: *hyperemesis gravidarum.*

    Headache, dizziness, and exhaustion also may be experienced. It may clear up after the 3rd month.

    Occurs usually about the 5th or 6th week and symptoms vary from simple morning sickness to pernicious vomiting of pregnancy. Usually clears up without treatment in 1-3 weeks. Occurs in about 50% of pregnancies.

    NP & TREATMENT: Anti-nausea drugs and large doses of B complex vitamins usually are the only treatment necessary; however, the following may be helpful where the drugs are not available: Crackers or vanilla wafers on arising. Three to five small meals per day. Tea helps, some outdoor activities. Psychic causes aggravate condition, so mental hygiene is desirable. Good ventilation during sleep; effervescent drinks.

moron [Gr. *mōros,* stupid]. A feebleminded person, not beyond the Binet age of 12, having the mentality ordinarily attained between 7 and 12. Of greater intelligence than an imbecile. The term implies no moral defect. Possessing an I.Q. of 50 to 70. SEE: *mental deficiency.*

Moro's reflex. [Ernst Moro, Ger. pediatrist, 1874-1951] A defensive reflex, a response consisting of the drawing of the infant's arms across its chest in an embracing manner, in response to stimuli produced by striking the surface on which the infant rests.

morosis (mo-rō'sĭs) [Gr. *mōros,* stupid]. The mental state of a moron; feeblemindedness. SYN: *moronity.*

morphea, generalized (mor-fe'ă) [Gr. *morphē,* form]. A rare skin disease of unknown etiology, characterized by widespread sclerosis of the skin. There is no specific treatment but physiotherapy may help to prevent contractures.

morphea, localized. Localized sclerosis of the skin; cause is unknown. There is no specific therapy. Contractures may be helped by infiltration with cortisone solution.

mor'phia. Morphine.

morphine (mor'fēn) [L. *morphina,* from *Morpheus,* god of sleep]. Main alkaloid found in opium, occurring in bitter, colorless crystals. Widely used as analgesic and sedative.

    POISONING: Brief mental exhilaration; languor; followed by weariness, sleepiness, pinpoint pupils; rapid, forcible pulse that becomes slow and feeble. Respiration slow and shallow. Unconsciousness from which patient may be aroused with difficulty. Muscles become relaxed; reflexes diminished; temperature low; skin pale, cold, and moist; pupils dilated. Coma and death follow.

F. A. AND EMERGENCY TREATMENT: Gastric lavage with 1:10,000 potassium permanganate solution, high enemas, maintenance of airway. Nalorphine hydrochloride, a specific morphine and opiate antagonist, should be administered subcutaneously or intravenously if respiration is depressed. Artificial respiration and inhalation of oxygen may be necessary. SEE: *Table of Poisons and Poisoning* in *Appendix*.

m. sul'fate. USP. $(C_{17}H_{19}NO_3)_2.H_2SO_4$ $+5H_2O$. The sulphate of an alkaloid obtained from opium and occurring as white, feathery crystals, incompatible with alkalies, tannic acid, and iodides. Loses water of crystallization when exposed to air.

ACTION AND USES: Hypnotic and analgesic.

morphinism (mor'fin-izm) [L. *morphina*]. Morbid condition due to habitual or excessive use of morphine. Morphine habit.

morphinomania, morphiomania (mor''-fin-ō-mā'nĭ-ă, fe-ō-mā'nĭ-ă) ["+ *mania*, madness]. 1. Morbid craving for morphine. 2. Insanity resulting from use of morphine.

morphogenesis (mor''fō-jĕn'ĕ-sĭs) [Gr. *morphē*, form, + *genesis*, production]. The various processes occurring during development by which the form of the body and its organs is established.

morphogenetic (mor''fō-jĕn-et'ĭk). Stimulating growth and development of form.

m. processes. Those by which morphogenesis is accomplished. Include cell migration; cell aggregation; localized growth; splitting, including delamination and cavitation; folding, including invagination and evagination.

m. substance. Chemical substances present in eggs or early embryos which induce morphologic differentiation. SEE: *induction*.

morphology (mor-fol'ō-jĭ) [Gr. *morphē*, form, + *logos*, study]. Science of structure and form without regard to function.

morphometry (mōr-fŏm'ĕ-trĭ) ["+ *metron*, measure]. The measurement of forms of organisms.

morpio, morpion (mor'pĭ-ō, -pĭ-ŏn) [L.]. (pl. *morpio'nes*) The crab louse, phthirus pubis, that infests the pubic area.

mors [L.]. Death.

m. putativa. Apparent death.

m. subita. Sudden death.

mor'tal [L. *mors, mort-*, death]. 1. Causing death. 2. Subject to death. 3. Human.

mortality (mor-tal'ĭ-tĭ). 1. State of being mortal. 2. The death rate; ratio of number of deaths to a given population.

mortar (mor'tar) [L. *mortarium*]. Vessel with a smooth interior in which crude drugs are crushed or ground with a pestle.

morti'cian [L. *mors, mort-*, death]. Undertaker; person trained to attend to the dead.

mortification (mor''tĭ-fĭ-kā'shŭn) ["+ *facere*, to make]. Death or failure of a tissue, organ, or part. SYN: *gangrene; necrosis*.

mortinatality (mor''tĭ-nă-tal'ĭ-tĭ) ["+ *natus*, birth]. Ratio of stillbirths to general birth rate. SYN: *natimortality*.

mort'ise joint. Ankle joint.

Mor'ton's disease. [Thomas G. Morton, Amer. surgeon, 1835-1903]. Neuralgia of the metatarsus.

mortuary (mor'tu-a-rĭ) [L. *mortuarium*, a tomb]. 1. Temporary place for keeping dead bodies before burial. SYN: *morgue*. 2. Rel. to the dead or to death.

morula (mor'ū-lă) [L. *morus*, mulberry]. Solid mass of cells, resembling a mulberry, resulting from segmentation of an ovum.

moruloid (mōr'ū-loid) ["+ Gr. *eidos*, form]. 1. A bacterial colony made up of a mass resembling a mulberry. 2. Resembling a mulberry

mosa'ic. 1. A picture or design made of many small colored pieces interspersed in some other material. 2. An individual whose tissues are of different genetic kinds. 3. Spotted condition in plants as in tobacco mosaic, a disease caused by a virus.

m. bone. Bone appearing as small pieces fitted together, characteristic of Paget's disease.

m. development. Type of development exhibited by ova which undergo determinate cleavage in which each blastomere has a characteristic position and unalterable fate.

m., sex. An individual with two or more cell populations derived from the same fertilized ovum or zygote. Each cell population has a different chromosome complement.

mosquito [Sp. little fly]. (pl. *mosquitoes*) 1. A blood-sucking insect belonging to the order Diptera, family Culicidae, q.v. Important species are Anopheles, Culex, Aëes, Haemagogus, Mansonia, and Psorophora. They serve as transmitting agents of many diseases, including malaria, filariasis, yellow fever, dengue, viral encephalitis, and dermatobiasis. 2. Apparatus for drawing blood from a vessel under sterile conditions.

mosquitocide ["+ L. *caedere*, to kill]. An agent that is lethal to mosquitoes or their larvae.

mossy cell. A protoplasmic astrocyte, a neuroglia cell with many branching processes. SEE: *neuroglia.*

mossy fibers. Afferent fibers to the cerebellar cortex. They give off many collaterals each ending in a glomerulus.

moth'er [AS. *mōdor*]. 1. Female parent. 2. A structure which gives rise to others.

　　m. cell. A cell which, by fission or budding, gives rise to similar cells.

　　m. cyst. An echinococcus cyst enveloping smaller ones.

　　m., expectant. One who is pregnant.

　　m. liquor. That left after removal of crystals from a solution.

　　m.'s mark. A birthmark. SEE: *mark.*

motile (mō'tīl) [L. *motilis,* moving]. Able to move spontaneously.

motility (mō-tīl'ĭt-ĭ). Power to move spontaneously.

motion (mō'shun) [L. *motio,* movement]. 1. A change of place or position; movement. 2. Evacuation of bowels. 3. Matter evacuated from bowels. SEE: *movements, circus;* words beginning with *cine; kine.*

　　m., active. Movements caused by the patient's own intention.

　　m., passive. Movements due to an attendant causing the part to be moved.

　　m. sickness. Nausea, vomiting, and vertigo induced by irregular or rhythmic movements. Ex: seasickness, airsickness, car sickness, swing sickness.

motor (mō'tor) [L. *motus,* moving]. 1. Causing motion. 2. A part or center which induces movements, as nerves or muscles.

　　m. aphasia. A condition in which the patient understands but cannot express himself in words or read aloud.

　　m. area. Posterior part of frontal lobe anterior to the central sulcus from which impulses for volitional movement arise.

　　m. end plate. Flat expansion ending a motor nerve fiber where it connects with a muscle fiber.

　　m. fibers. Axons of motor neurons which innervate skeletal muscles.

　　m. nerve. A nerve composed entirely of motor fibers.

　　m. neuron. 1. A neuron which innervates muscle tissue. 2. A neuron which carries impulses initiating muscle contraction.

　　m. points. Points where the motor nerve enters the muscle and where visible contraction can be elicited with a minimal amount of stimulation.

　　m. sense. The kinesthetic sense.

　　m. unit. A single motor neuron and the muscle fibers its branches innervate.

motorial (mō-tor'ĭ-ăl) [L. *motus,* moving]. Concerning motion or a motor center.

motoricity (mō-tor-ĭs'ĭt-ĭ). Capability of movement.

motorium (mō-tōr'ĭ-ŭm) [L. power of motion]. Motor center of a body or organism.

motorius (mō-tōr'ĭ-ŭs). Any motor nerve.

motorpathy (mō-tōr'păth-ĭ) [L. *motus,* moving, + Gr. *pathos,* disease]. Treatment of a condition by prescribed movements. SYN: *kinesitherapy; kinetotherapy.*

mottled enamel. Condition in which the enamel of the teeth becomes discolored. Often associated with excessive fluorine in drinking water. SEE: *fluorosis.*

mottling (mŏt'lĭng) [E. *motley,* many colored]. A condition that is marked by discolored areas.

moulage (moo-lahzh') [Fr.]. 1. A wax model or reproduction of a skin condition. 2. Molding of a wax model.

mould (mōld). SEE: *mold.*

moulding (mōld'ing). SEE: *molding.*

mounding [origin uncertain]. The rising of a lump, as the mounding of a wasting muscle when struck a quick, firm blow.

mountain fever or **m. sickness.** Condition occurring in individuals ascending to high altitudes (over 10,000 ft. or 3,048 meters) or to those subjected to rarefied atmospheres. Due to anoxia resulting from reduced oxygen tension. SYN: *hypobaropathy; mareo de la Cordillera; soreche; puna.*

　　SYM: euphoria, tachycardia, headache, nausea, increased respiratory rate, fatigue, and cerebral disorders (loss of memory, errors of judgment).

mounting (mownt'ing) [L. *mons, mont-,* mountain]. 1. The arrangement of specimens on slides, frames, chart boards, display boards, or any background for study. 2. Sexual activity of lower mammals. Usually indicates male activity but some females, i.e., cows, will attempt to mount males or other females.

mourning. Normal grief usually produced by the death of a loved one. Not synonymous with depression or melancholia.

mouse unit (mows). Least amount of estrus-producing hormone which induces a characteristic desquamation of the vaginal epithelium in a spayed mouse.

mouth (mowth) [AS. *mūth*]. 1. The opening of any cavity. SYN: *buccal cavity; oral cavity.* 2. The cavity within the cheeks, containing the tongue and teeth, and communicating with the pharynx.

　　Some conditions involving the mouth cavity are: *abnormalities of tongue:* dry, coated, smooth, strawberry, large, pigmented, geographic, deviated, tremulous, sore; *conditions involving gums and teeth:* gingivitis, sordes, lead line, pyorrhea, atrophy, hypertrophy, dental caries, alveolar abscesses; *conditions involving mucous membrane or other parts of mouth:* eruptions accompanying exanthematous diseases, stomatitis, canker sores, thrush, trench mouth, cysts, tumors, carcinoma, lesions of syphilis such as chancre, mucous patches, gumma, lesions of tuberculosis, abscesses.

Disorders of the mouth cavity may be indications of purely local disease or they may be symptoms of systemic disturbances such as dehydration, pernicious anemia, nutritional deficiencies, esp. avitaminoses.

RS: agranulocytosis, Ludwig's; antitrismus; astomatous; bucca; buccal; b. glands; cancrum oris; chalinoplasty; chin jerk; fauces; ora; palate; oral; orifice; os; stoma; stomatitis; tongue; xerostomia.

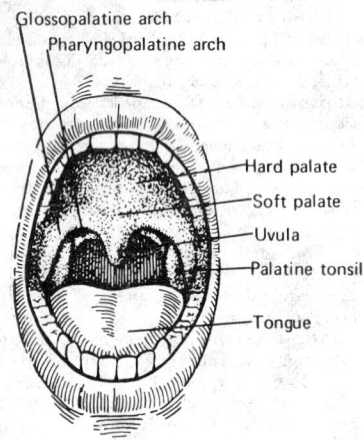

Glossopalatine arch
Pharyngopalatine arch
Hard palate
Soft palate
Uvula
Palatine tonsil
Tongue

MOUTH AND PHARYNX

    m. examination. In addition to visual examination, careful digital examination should be made, as such reveals areas of tenderness and alterations of texture characteristic of leukoplakia, cancer, cystic swellings, and lymphadenopathy.

Excessive moisture of the mouth is seen in stomatitis, irritation of pneumogastric nerve, ingestion of irritating drugs or foods, nervous disorders, teething, seeing appetizing foods, smelling pleasant odors.

    m., rashes in. Stomatitis, measles, scarlet fever. Rashes on lips may indicate typhoid fever, meningitis, pneumonia. In secondary syphilis, chancre, cancer, and

epithelioma mucous patches appear. RS: *canker; catarrh.*

    m., trench. Painful pseudomembranous ulceration of the mucus membranes of the mouth and pharynx.

NP: Keep mouth clean and in good condition. *Articles Necessary:* Small tray with glass of fresh water, glass or cup of mouthwash, applicators, tongue depressors, gauze bandage about 2 in. wide, emesis basin, towel, paper bag, liquid albolene or special ointment, and disposable drinking tube.

Procedure: Have all equipment ready on bedside table. Place towel under patient's chin, across chest. Turn patient's head to side and arrange emesis basin close to corner of mouth. Dip applicators in mouthwash and clean teeth, tongue, gums, and roof of mouth. Discard used applicators into paper bag. Do not dip into mouthwash after using. If teeth are difficult to clean make a larger swab by winding several turns of bandage around tongue depressor. Allow patient to rinse mouth with mouthwash using drinking tube, followed by fresh water. Caution him not to expectorate the fluids forcibly, but to let them run gently out at the corner of his mouth. Keep corner wiped clean. If lips are dry or cracked apply liquid albolene or special ointment. If the patient has a high temperature clean the mouth before each feeding. If he is unconscious hold the mouth open with a tongue depressor padded with gauze. Be gentle and thorough.

SYN: *Vincent's angina,* q.v.

movement (moov′měnt) [L. *movēre,* to move]. 1. Act of passing from place to place or changing position of body or its parts. 2. Evacuation of feces.

    m., active. Accomplished without external assistance.

    m., ameboid. Movement resembling that of an ameba in which the protoplasm of a cell flows into a projection of the cell membrane forming a pseudopodium. Characteristic of leukocytes and certain protozoa.

    m., associated. Involuntary movement of a part occurring coincident with and subsequent to the movement of another part, e.g. the eyes.

    m., autonomic. A spontaneous, involuntary m., independent of ext. stimulation.

    m., brownian. The peculiar jiggling or dancing movement of minute particles suspended in liquids or gases when observed under the microscope, due to bombardment of the particles by molecules of their surrounding medium.

m., ciliary. Rhythmic m. of the cilia of a ciliated cell or epithelium.

m., circus. A phenomenon after injury to a corpus striatum, optic thalamus, or crus cerebri, causing an odd circular gait.

m., disorders of. May be due to injury or disease of muscle, nerve ending, motor nerve, spinal cord, or the brain.

Types are hemiplegia, ataxia, monoplegia, tremors, rigors, choreic, athetosis, convulsions, spasm (clonic or tonic), reflex (hysterical, habit spasm, tics), and spastic paralysis.

m.'s, fetal. Muscular m.'s performed by the fetus in utero.

m., molecular. The movement of molecules of a substance, the basis of the kinetic theory of matter. SEE: *m., brownian.*

m., pendular. Swaying movements of the intestines caused by rhythmic contractions of the longitudinal muscles of the walls of the intestines.

m., peristalic. Peristalsis, q.v.

m., respiratory. Any m. resulting from the contraction of respiratory muscles or occurring passively as a result of elasticity of the thoracic wall or lungs. SEE: *inspiration; expiration; respiration.*

m. of restitution. A partial rotation of the fetal head in cases of head presentation.

m., saccadic. Jerky movements of the eyes as in reading.

m., segmenting. Movement of the intestine in which annular constrictions occur dividing intestine into ovoid segments.

m., vibratile. Ciliary movement, q.v.

moxa (mŏk′sa) [Jap.]. Inflammable substance used as a cautery for the skin or as a counterirritant.

moxibustion (mŏk-sĭ-bŭst′shŭn) ["+ L. *combustus,* burned]. Cauterization by means of a cylinder or cone of cotton wool, called a moxa, placed on the skin and fired at the top. Used to produce counterirritation.

M.P.H. Abbr. for *Master of Public Health.*

M.P.N. Abbr. for *most probable number* (of bacteria present in a quantity of solution, esp. water).

MSH. Abbr. for *melanocyte-stimulating hormone.*

M.T. Abbr. for *medical technologist.*

M. u. Abbr. for *Maché unit.*

m.u. Abbr. for *mouse unit.*

mu (mū) [Greek letter m]. Symb. used for the prefix *micro-* which stands for multiplication by 10^6. Thus μm. would stand for 10^{-6} meter. SYMB: μ; u.

mucedin (mū′sĕ-dĭn) [L. *mucedō,* mucus]. A substance obtained from gluten.

muciferous (mū-sĭf′ĕr-ŭs) ["+ *ferre,* to carry]. Secreting or producing mucus.

muciform (mū′sĭ-form) ["+ *forma,* shape]. Appearing similar to mucus.

mucigen (mū′sĭ-jĕn) ["+ Gr. *gennan,* to produce]. A substance present in mucous cells which upon being extruded from the cell is converted into mucin.

mucigenous (mū-sĭj′ĕn-ŭs). Producing mucus. SYN: *muciferous.*

mucilage (mū′sĭ-lĭj) [L. *mucilago,* moldy juice]. Vegetable preparation used in pharmaceuticals. SEE: *mucilago.*

mucilaginous (mū-sĭl-ăj′ĭn-ŭs). Resembling mucilage; slimy; sticky.

mucila′go. Thick, viscid, adhesive liquid, containing gum or mucilaginous principles dissolved in water, usually employed to hold insoluble substances in suspension in aqueous liquids or as a demulcent.

mucin (mū′sĭn) [L. *mucus,* mucus]. A glycoprotein found in mucus. It is present in saliva and bile and in salivary glands, in the skin, connective tissues, tendon, and cartilage. It is formed from mucigen and in water forms a slimy solution. On decomposition the mucins give dextrose, sulfur, and nitrogen among other products.

m., gastric. A commercial preparation, made from the gastric mucosa of the hog and used in the treatment of ulcers of the digestive tract. It forms a protective coating over the ulcer or erosion, which prevents irritation from the passing of bile and acid secretions in the duodenum and from acid conditions irritating peptic ulcer of the stomach.

mucinemia (mū-sĭn-ē′mĭ-ă) ["+ Gr. *haima,* blood]. Mucin in the blood.

mucinogen (mū-sĭn′ō-jĕn) ["+ Gr. *gennan,* to produce]. A glycoprotein that forms mucin.

mucinoid (mū′sĭn-oid) ["+ Gr. *eidos,* resemblance]. Appearing similar to mucin.

mucinuria (mū-sĭn-ū′rĭ-ă) ["+ Gr. *ouron,* urine]. Presence of mucin in the urine.

muciparous (mū-sĭp′ăr-ŭs) ["+ *parēre,* to bring forth]. Producing or secreting mucus. SYN: *muciferous, mucigenous.*

muco- [L. *mucus,* mucus]. Combining form, indicating relationship to mucus.

mucocele (mū′kō-sēl) ["+ Gr. *kēlē,* tumor]. 1. Enlargement of the lacrimal sac. 2. A mucous cyst. 3. A mucous polypus. 4. Cystic disease of the air cavities of the cranial bones causing erosion of the bone.

mucocolpos (mū″kō-kŏl-pŏs) ["+ Gr. *kolpos,* vagina]. Accumulation of mucus in the vagina.

mucocutaneous (mū″kō-kū-tā′nē-ŭs) ["+ *cutis,* skin]. Concerning a mucous membrane and the skin.

mucodermal (mū-kō-dĕr′măl) ["+ Gr. *derma,* skin]. Pert. to a mucous membrane and the skin. SYN: *mucocutaneous.*

mucoenteritis (mū″kō-ĕn-tĕr-i′tĭs) ["+ Gr. *enteron,* intestine, + -*ītis,* inflammation]. Inflammation of intestinal mucosa.

mucoglobulin (mū″kō-glŏb′ū-lĭn). Any protein group to which plastin belongs.

mucoid (mū′koyd) [L. *mucus,* mucus, + Gr. *eidos,* resemblance]. 1. Glycoprotein similar to mucin. 2. Muciform similar to mucus.

mucopolysaccharide. Polysaccharides which form chemical bonds with water. They contain hexosamine and sometimes proteins. Thick gelatinous material that is found many places in the body, it glues cells together, lubricates joints, and is found in blood group substances.

mucopurulent (mū-kō-pūr′ū-lĕnt) [L. *mucus* + *purulentus,* made up of pus]. Consisting of mucus and pus.

mucopus (mū′kō-pŭs). Mucus combined with or resembling pus.

Mucor (mū′kor) [L.]. A genus of mold fungi seen on dead and decaying matter. Sometimes responsible for infections of external ear, skin, and respiratory passageways.

mucoriferous (mū-kor-ĭf′ĕr-ŭs) [L. *mucor,* mold, "+ *ferre,* to carry]. Covered with mold or a moldlike substance.

mucorin (mū′kor-ĭn). An albuminoid substance derived from molds.

mucormycosis (mū-kor-mĭ-kō′sĭs) [L. *mucus,* mucus, + Gr. *mykēs,* fungus, + -*ōsis,* condition]. A disease due to a fungus of the genus Mucor.

mucorrhea. Increased cervical discharge at ovulation. Usually covers a 3- to 4-day span and has character and appearance of raw egg white. SEE: *spinnbarkheit.*

mucosa (mū-kō′să) [L. mucous]. (pl. *mucosae*) Mucous membrane.

mucosal (mū-kō′săl). Concerning any mucous membrane.

mucosanguineous (mū″kō-san-gwĭn′ē-ŭs) [L. *mucus,* mucus, + *sanguineus,* bloody]. Containing mucus and blood.

mucosedative (mū″kō-sĕd′ă-tĭv) ["+ *sedatīvus,* allaying]. Soothing to mucosae of the body. SYN: *demulcent.*

mucoserous (mū″kō-sēr′ŭs). Composed of mucus and serum.

mucosin (mū′kō-sĭn). Mucin found in thick, sticky mucus.

mucous (mū′kŭs). 1. Having the nature of or resembling mucus. 2. Secreting mucus. 3. Depending on presence of mucus.

RS: mucocele; mucopurulent; mucosa; mucus; words beginning with "myx-."

m. colitis. Inflammation of the mucosa of the colon. SEE: *colitis.*

m. membrane. Membrane lining passages and cavities communicating with the air. Consists of a surface layer of epithelium, a basement membrane, and an underlying layer of connective tissue, the lamina propria. Mucus-secreting cells or glands usually are present in the epithelium but may be absent.

Examination should reveal degree of moisture, cyanosis, pallor, hyperemia, pigmentation, lesions or their absence, and hemorrhage.

Pallor is seen in all anemias. If temporary, may indicate shock, vasomotor spasm, or may occur in severe hemorrhages. Blanching and flushing alternately accompanies aortic regurgitation.

Hyperemia or excessive redness: *Buccal mucous membrane:* Due to decayed teeth, traumatism, stomatitis. SEE: *mouth.*

Nasal mucosa: Ulceration of nose, rhinitis, inflammation. SEE: *nose.*

Eyes (local irritation): Foreign body, ulcer, inflammation. SEE: *jaundice.*

Dryness is seen in fevers, chronic gastritis, some liver disturbances, excitement, shock, prostration, fatigue, thirst, and certain drugs.

m. polypus. Small growth from mucous lining of the cervix or uterus.

mucoviscidosis. SEE: *cystic fibrosis.*

mucus (mū′kŭs) [L.]. A viscid fluid secreted by mucous membranes and glands, consisting of mucin, leukocytes, inorganic salts, water, and epithelial cells. A good example is the almost ropy secretion from the sublingual and submaxillary glands.

RS: amyxorrhea, expectorant, expectoration, glairy, goblet cell, words beginning with "blenn-" and "muc-."

mulatto (mū-lăt′tō) [Sp. *mulato,* of mixed breed, from L. *mulus,* mule]. First generation born of pure negro and white parentage; popularly anyone of mixed white and negro blood.

mulieb′ria [L.]. The female genitalia.

muliebrity (mū-lĭ-ĕb′rĭ-tĭ). Femininity; womanliness. The assumption of womanly qualities at puberty. The assumption of female characteristics by a male.

Müller. [Heinrich Müller, Ger. anatomist, 1820-1864].

M.'s fibers. Fine fibers of neuroglia cells which form supporting elements of the retina. SYN: *radial fibers of M.*

M.'s muscle. 1. Circular fibers of ciliary muscle. 2. The sup. tarsal muscle of the eyelid. 3. Smooth muscle covering over sphenomaxillary fissure.

M.'s trigone. Portion of tuber cinereum folding over the optic chiasm.

Müller. [Johannes B. Müller, Ger. physician, 1801-1858].

M.'s ducts. Embryonic tubes from which the oviducts, uterus, and vagina develop in the female; in the male they become atrophied.

M.'s ring. Muscular ring at junction of cervical canal and the gravid uterus.

M.'s tubercle. Projection on dorsal wall of cloaca at which Müller's ducts terminate.

mult-, multi- [L. *multus*]. Prefixes indicating many or much.

multang'ular. Having many angles.

m. bone, greater. The first or outermost of the distal row of carpal bones. SYN: *trapezium.*

m. bone, lesser. The second in distal row of carpal bones. SYN: *trapezoid.*

multiarticular (mŭl''tĭ-ar-tĭk'ū-lar) [L. *multus,* many, + *articulus,* joint]. Concerning, having, or affecting many joints.

multicapsular (mŭl''tĭ-kap'sū-lar) ["+ *capsula,* a little box]. Composed of many capsules.

multicellular (mŭl''tĭ-sĕl'ū-lar) ["+ *cellula,* small chamber]. Consisting of many cells.

Mul'ticeps. A genus of tapeworms.

multicuspid, multicuspidate (mul''tĭ-kus'-pĭd, -pī-dāt) [L. *multus,* many, + *cuspis,* point]. Having several cusps.

multifactorial. The result of many factors, as in a disease resulting from the combined action of several factors.

multifid (mŭl'tĭf-ĭd) ["+ *fidus,* from *findere,* to split]. Divided into many sections.

multiform (mŭl'tĭ-form) ["+ *forma,* shape]. Having many forms or shapes. SYN: *polymorphous.*

multiglandular (mŭl''tĭ-glănd'ū-lar) [L. *multus,* many, + *glandula,* a little acorn]. Concerning several glands.

multigrav'ida ["+ *gravida,* pregnant]. A woman who has been pregnant two or more times. May be written as Gravida II, III, etc. SEE: *multipara.*

multi-infection (mŭl''tĭ-ĭn-fek'shŭn) ["+ *infectiō,* an infection]. A mixed infection with several organisms developing at the same time.

multilobular (mŭl''tĭ-lŏb'ū-lar) ["+ *lobulus,* a small lobe]. Formed of or possessing many lobules.

multilocular (mŭl''tĭ-lok'ū-lar) ["+ *loculus,* a cell]. Having many cells or compartments. SYN: *multicellular.*

multimammae (mul''tĭ-mam'mē) ["+ *mamma,* breast]. Condition of possessing more than the normal number of breasts. SYN: *polymastia.*

multinodal (mul-tĭ-nō'dāl). Having many nodes or knots.

multinodular (mŭl-tĭ-nŏd'ū-lar) [L. *multus,* many, + *nodulus,* little knot]. Possessing many nodules or small knots.

multinuclear, multinucleate (mul-tĭ-nū'klē-ar, -āt). Possessing several nuclei.

multipara (mul-tĭp'ă-ră) [L. *multus,* many, + *parēre,* to bear]. A woman who has borne more than one offspring, whether or not the offspring were alive at birth. May be written Para II, III, etc. SEE: *multigravida.*

m., grand. A woman who has given birth seven or more times.

multiparity (mul-tĭ-par'ĭ-tĭ). 1. Condition of having borne more than one child. 2. Production of more than one child at birth.

multiparous (mŭl-tĭp'ăr-ūs). 1. Having borne more than one child. 2. Producing more than one child at birth.

multiphasic screening. Determining an individual's health through a variety of methods and techniques. Usually consists of one or more of the following: self-completed medical history, variety of laboratory examinations of urine and blood, chest x-ray pictures, serological test for syphilis, Papanicolaou smear, tonometry, pulmonary vital capacity, electrocardiogram, breast examination, height, weight, vision test, blood pressure.

m.s., automated. Screening tests done with the aid of automated electronic and computer equipment.

multiple (mul'tĭ-pl) [L. *multiplex,* many folded]. 1. Consisting of, or containing more than one; manifold. 2. Occurring simultaneously in various parts of the body.

m. personality. Condition in which the subject may develop two or more personalities. SEE: *dual personality.*

multipolar (mŭl-tĭ-pōl'ar) [L. *multus,* many, + *polus,* a pole]. 1. Possessing more than two poles. 2. Possessing more than two processes, said of neurons.

multiter'minal ["+ Gr. *terma,* a limit]. Providing several sets of terminals, making possible the use of several electrodes.

multivalent (mul-tĭ-vā'lent) ["+ *valēre,* to have power]. Having ability to combine with more than two atoms of a univalent element or radical.

mummification (mum″mĭ-fĭ-kā′shun) [Arabian *mūmiyaa*, mummy, + L. *facere*, to make]. 1. Mortification producing a hard, dry mass. SYN: *dry gangrene*. 2. Drying and shriveling of a body, as a dead fetus.

mumps (mŭmps). An acute, contagious, febrile disease characterized by inflammation of the parotid glands and other salivary glands.

ETIOL: Mumps virus.

SYM: Onset gradual. There may be chilliness, malaise, headache, pain below ears, moderate fever of 101-102° F. (38.3°-38.9° C.) or higher followed by swelling of one or both parotid glands. Usually swelling in one gland is subsiding as other swells. Swelling is below and in front of the ear.

The lobe of the ear is sometimes pushed forward, surrounding tissues are edematous, the features may be greatly distorted. Movements of the jaw are painful and restricted. Saliva may be increased or diminished. In a third of cases only one parotid is involved. Occasionally, the parotid glands seem to escape, and swelling is confined to the submaxillary gland. Swelling usually lasts from 5 to 7 days.

COMPLICATIONS: Complications usually develop about the time the swelling in the parotids subsides. The most common complication in the adult male is orchitis which occurs in about 20 to 30% of cases; in the female oöphoritis and mastitis. Rarely permanent impairment of hearing follows an attack of mumps. Meningoencephalitis has been estimated to occur in 10% of patients.

DIFFERENTIAL DIAGNOSIS: Cases of symptomatic parotitis must be excluded. Instances of trauma, infections about teeth and mouth, or a blocking of Stensen's duct may be suggestive of mumps.

PROG: Favorable, although the possibility of sterility may have to be considered in extremely rare instances of bilateral orchitis.

TREATMENT: Rest in bed, liquid diet; promote elimination; cold, local applications may control swelling of testicles. SYN: *infectious parotitis*.

mump′simus. Blind and irrational adherence to a custom or practice even though to do so has been proven to be inadvisable or even dangerous to the patient.

mumps virus vaccine, live attenuated A vaccine made from the Jeryl Lynn strain of mumps virus for immunization against mumps. Should not be given to pregnant women or to those who are sensitive to eggs, chicken, chicken feathers, or neomycin. Also should not be administered with other vac-

cines, and one month should elapse between its use and the use of other immunizations.

Münchhausen syndrome. A type of malingering in which the patient may practice self-multilation and deception in order to feign illness. When detected he leaves one hospital and appears in the emergency room of another. Patients of this type are seldom recognized in time to receive psychiatric diagnoses and therapy which they need.

mural (mū′ral) [L. *murus*, a wall]. Pert. to a wall of an organ or part.

muramidase. An enzyme found in blood cells of the granulocytic and monocytic series. Its serum and urine level is increased in patients with acute or chronic leukemia. It is also normally present in saliva, sweat, and tears. Formerly called lysozyme.

muriate (mūr′ĭ-āt) [L. *muria*, brine]. An old synonym for chloride.

muriat′ic acid. Commercial hydrochloric acid, q.v.

mur′mur [L. *murmur*]. A soft blowing or rasping sound heard on auscultation. An adventitious sound heard on auscultation of the heart. It results from vibrations produced by movement of the blood within the heart and adjacent large blood vessels. May be heard during systole, diastole, or both.

Two of the valves give forth a "lubb" sound and the other two a "dupp" sound, known as the first and second heart sounds. A blowing sound is heard if the valve does not close tightly, indicating an incompetent valve. A great vessel irregularity, such as an aortic aneurysm, or the flow of blood through a narrowed orifice, as in aortic or mitral stenosis, may produce a murmur.

A murmur does not necessarily indicate organic pathology, and heart disease may not result in any murmur; this may also be true in angina pectoris and coronary disorders. Air in the lungs may simulate sounds similar to heart murmurs.

RS: auscultation, circulation of blood, heart, hum, venous.

m., aneurysmal. Whizzing systolic sound heard over an aneurysm.

m., aortic obstructive. Harsh systolic m. heard with and after the 1st heart sound. Loudest at the base.

m., aortic regurgitant. Blowing and hissing following 2nd heart sound.

m., apex. Inorganic m. over apex of heart.

m., arterial. Soft flowing m., synchronous with pulse.

m., bronchial. M. heard over large bronchi, resembling respiratory laryngeal m.

m., cardiopulmonary. M. caused by movement of heart against lungs.

m., diastolic. M. during dilation of heart.

m., direct. M. caused by obstruction of blood in normal course.

m., endocardial. Abnormal sound produced by any cause and arising within the heart.

m., exocardial. A cardiac m. produced outside the cavities of the heart.

m., friction. M. caused by rubbing of two inflamed mucous surfaces.

m., functional. M. occurring in the absence of any pathological change in structure of heart valves or orifices. It does not indicate organic disease of the heart. It may disappear upon a return to health. It must not be mistaken for true pathological murmurs.

m., hemic. Sound heard on auscultation of anemic persons without a valvular lesion. ETIOL: Abnormal, usually anemic, blood condition.

m., indirect. M. heard when blood flows in abnormal directions.

m., inorganic. M. not due to structural changes.

m., machinery. A continuous rough murmur heard in cases of a patent ductus arteriosus.

m., mitral. M. produced at orifice of mitral or bicuspid valve.

m., organic. M. due to structural changes.

m., pericardial. A friction sound produced within the pericardium.

m., physiologic. A functional murmur, q.v.

m., presystolic. M. occurring just before systole, due to mitral or tricuspid obstruction.

m., pulmonary. M. produced at the orifice of the pulmonary artery.

m., regurgitant. M. due to leakage or backward flow of blood current through a dilated valvular orifice.

m., systolic. M. heard during contraction of heart due to obstruction of flow of blood at one or several of the heart valves or in the aorta.

m., to-and-fro. Pericardial m. heard during both systole and diastole.

m., tricuspid. M. produced at orifice of tricuspid valve, caused by disease.

m., vascular. M. occurring within a blood vessel.

m., vesicular. Normal breathing.

Murphy's button. [John B. Murphy, Amer. surgeon, 1857-1916] Mechanical device used for intestinal anastomosis. Consists of two button-like hollow cylinders, each one sutured to an open end of the intestine and fitted together. After firm union of intestines, cylinders are passed in stools.

Mus [L. mouse]. A genus of rodents including mice and rats.

M. musculus. The common house mouse.

Musca [L. fly]. A genus of flies belonging to the order Diptera, family Muscidae.

M. domestica. The common house fly, the transmitting agent for causative organisms of typhoid fever, bacillary and amebic dysentery, cholera, trachoma, and many other diseases.

muscae volitantes (mŭs'sē vŏl-ĭ-tan'tēz) [L. flitting flies]. Black specks seen floating in the vitreous humor of the eye and visible to the patient; often seen in myopia.

muscle (mŭs'el) [L. *musculus*]. A type of tissue composed of contractile cells or fibers which effects movement of an organ or part of the body. SYN: *musculus.*

The outstanding characteristic of muscular tissue is its ability to shorten or contract. It also possesses the properties of irritability, conductivity, and elasticity. Muscle tissue possesses little intercellular material, hence its cells or fibers lie close together. Three types of muscle differentiated on basis of histologic structure occur in the body, namely, smooth, striated, and cardiac.

Smooth, Nonstriated, Plain: Cells are fusiform or spindle-shaped, each containing a central nucleus. Cells usually arranged in sheets or layers but may occur as isolated units in connective tissue. Called involuntary because they are not under conscious control. Found principally in the internal organs, esp. digestive tract, respiratory passages, urinary and genital ducts, urinary bladder and gallbladder, and walls of blood vessels. Smooth muscle lacks the cross striations characteristic of other types of muscle.

Striated, Striped, Skeletal: The cytoplasm (sarcoplasm) contains numerous myofibrillae. The cytoplasmic cell membrane is called the sarcolemma. Muscle fibers are grouped into bundles called fasciculi, each of which is surrounded by a sheath of connective tissue called perimysium. The fibers within a fasciculus are surrounded by and held together by delicate reticular fibrils forming the endomysium. Striated muscle is found in all skeletal muscles. It also occurs in the tongue, pharynx, and upper portion of esophagus.

Cardiac: Fibers branch and anastomose, forming a continuous network or syncytium.

At intervals, prominent bands or intercalated disks cross the fibers. Certain fibers, called Purkinje fibers, form the impulse-conducting system of the heart.

SHAPE: A contractile organ consisting of muscle tissue which effects movements of parts of the body, esp. a structure composed of striated muscle and attached to a part of the skeleton. A typical muscle consists of a central fleshy portion or belly and its attachments. One end called the head is attached to a fixed structure termed the origin; the other end is attached to a movable part called the insertion. Some muscles are spindle-shaped, others form flat sheets or bands.

Muscles may be attached directly to the periosteum of bones or they may be attached by means of tough cords of connective tissue (tendons) or broad flat sheets (aponeuroses). The connective tissue enclosing a muscle is called epimysium; it is continuous with the deep fascia.

BLOOD SUPPLY: Obtained from small blood vessels which enter the muscular tissue and subdivide into capillaries that permeate throughout.

NERVE SUPPLY: *Voluntary:* From branches of the peripheral cerebrospinal nervous system. It is because of this that the skeletal muscles are under conscious control. *Involuntary:* Smooth and cardiac receive their nerve supply from autonomic nervous system and function involuntarily without conscious control.

FUNCTION: To bring about changes in position.

m., abductor. M. which draws away from the midline.

m., adductor. M. which draws toward the midline.

m., antagonistic. M. which counteracts the action of another muscle. SYN: *agonistic m.*

m.'s, antigravity. M.'s which pull against the force of gravity to maintain posture.

m., appendicular. One of the skeletal muscles of the limbs.

m., articular. M. attached to capsule of a joint.

m., axial. A skeletal m. of the head or trunk.

m., bipennate. M. in which the fibers converge toward a central tendon on both sides.

m., constrictor, of pharynx. A m. which constricts the pharynx.

m., digastric. M. which lowers the jaw.

m., extensor. M. which extends a part.

m., extrinsic. M. whose origin lies outside the part moved.

m. fatigue. The reduced capacity of a muscle to perform work. SEE: *fatigue.*

m., fixation. A m. which acts to steady a part in order that more precise movements in a related structure may be accomplished.

m., flexor. M. which bends a part.

m., fusiform. A m. resembling a spindle.

m., intrinsic. A m. which has both its origin and insertion within a structure, as

Comparison of Properties of Three Types of Muscle

	Smooth	Cardiac	Striped
Synonyms	Involuntary Visceral Plain	Myocardium	Voluntary Skeletal Striated

Fibers:
  Length (in micrometers) . . . .
  Thickness (in micrometers) . . . .
  Shape . . . .
  Marking . . . .
	
	50–200
	4–8
	Spindles
	No striation
		
		Striation
			
			25,000
			75
			Cylinders
			Marked striation

Nuclei	Single	Single	Multiple
Speed of contraction	Very slow	Moderate	Very quick
Effects of cutting related nerve	Slight	Slight	Complete paralysis

intrinsic muscles of the tongue, eye, or limb.

m., involuntary. M. not controlled by the will; mainly smooth.

m., multipennate. M. with several tendons of origin and several tendons of insertion in which fibers pass obliquely from a tendon of origin to a tendon of insertion on each side.

m., nonstriated. Smooth muscle, q.v.

m., papillary. M. on inner surface of ventricle of heart to which chordae tendineae are attached.

m., pectinate. M. on inner surface of rt. atrium giving it a ridged appearance.

m., postaxial. M. on the post. or dorsal aspect of a limb.

m., preaxial. M. on the ant. or ventral aspect of a limb.

m. relaxant. A drug used to provide muscular relaxation necessary for various

medical and surgical procedures and for relief of muscle pain.

m. sense. The proprioceptive or kinesthetic sense.

m., skeletal. M. which is connected with a bone; mainly striated.

m., smooth. Nonstriated muscle; muscle tissue which lacks cross striations on its fibers; involuntary in action and found principally in visceral organs.

m., somatic. M. derived from mesodermal somites. Includes most of skeletal m.

m., sphincter. M. controlling an opening.

m., striated. Muscle fibers which possess alternate light and dark bands or striations; mainly voluntary and comprise skeletal muscles. SYN: *striped m.*

m.'s, synergistic. M.'s aiding one another in function.

m., unipennate. M. whose fibers con-

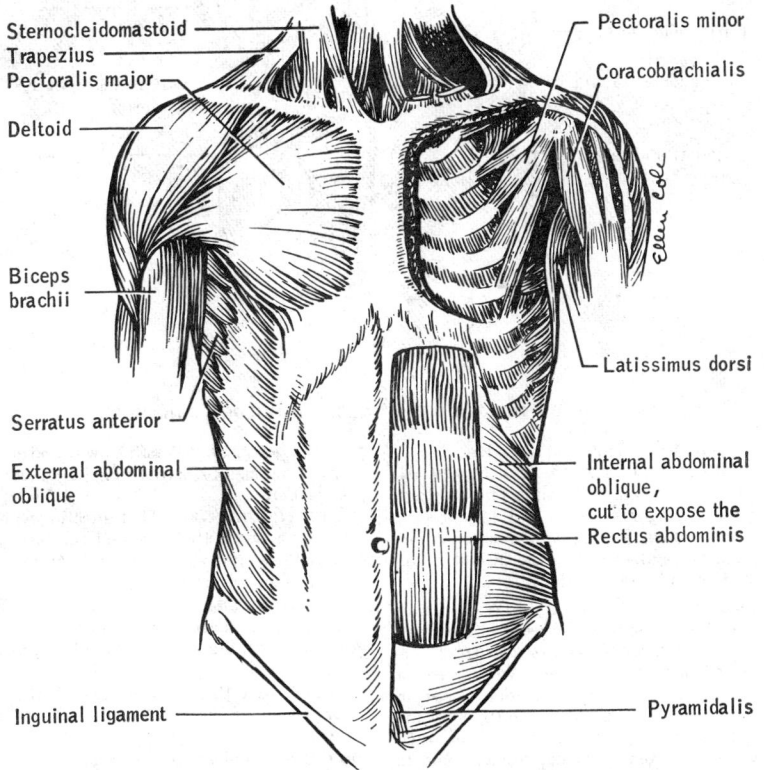

Sternocleidomastoid
Trapezius
Pectoralis major
Deltoid
Biceps brachii
Serratus anterior
External abdominal oblique
Inguinal ligament

Pectoralis minor
Coracobrachialis
Latissimus dorsi
Internal abdominal oblique, cut to expose the Rectus abdominis
Pyramidalis

MUSCLES OF THE ANTERIOR CHEST AND ABDOMINAL WALL

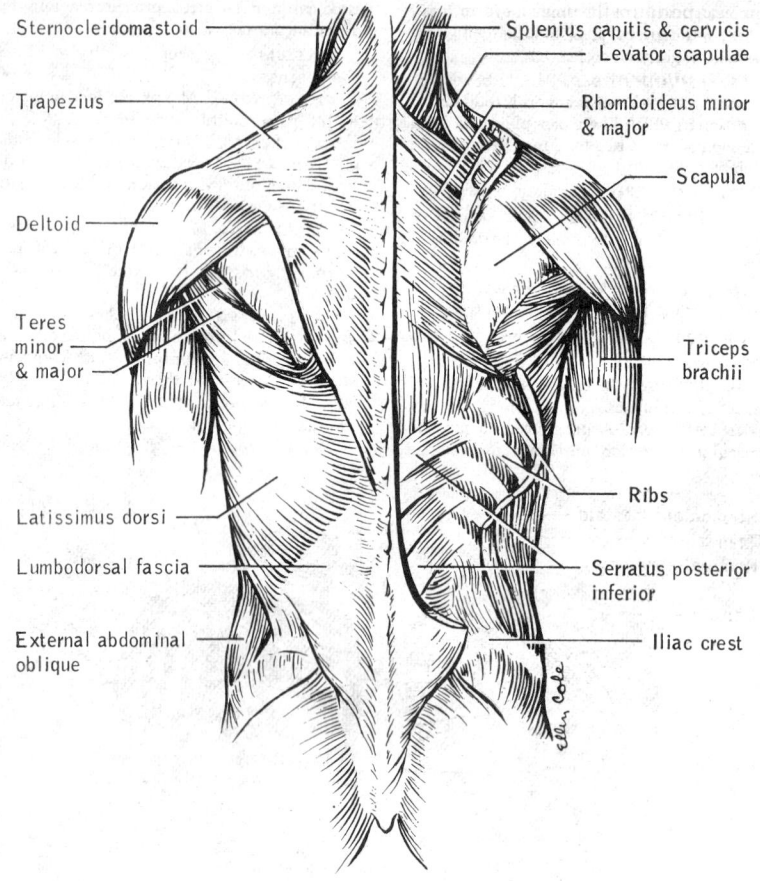

Sternocleidomastoid

Trapezius

Deltoid

Teres minor & major

Latissimus dorsi

Lumbodorsal fascia

External abdominal oblique

Splenius capitis & cervicis

Levator scapulae

Rhomboideus minor & major

Scapula

Triceps brachii

Ribs

Serratus posterior inferior

Iliac crest

MUSCLES OF THE POSTERIOR NECK, SHOULDER, AND BACK

verge on only one side of a tendon.

m., unstriated, m., unstriped. M. without markings; mainly involuntary. SYN: *smooth muscle.*

m., voluntary. M. whose action is controlled by will; excepting the cardiac m., all striated m.'s are voluntary.

mus'cular [L. *muscularis*]. 1. Pert. to muscles. 2. Possessing well-developed muscles.

m. contractions, graduated. Accomplished by use of electrical current of varying strength and duration. Used in muscles with an intact nerve supply when muscles are atonic, wasted away, or when voluntary exercise is not feasible; and in denervated muscles as in cases following nerve injury or poliomyelitis.

m. dystrophy. Wasting away and atrophy of muscles. SEE: *dystrophy, progressive muscular.*

m. rheumatism. That affecting white fibrous tissue of the body. SYN: *fibrositis.*

muscularis (mŭs-kū-la'rĭs) [L.]. Muscular layer of an organ or tubule.

m. mucosae. Unstriated muscular tissue layer of mucous membrane.

muscularity. State or quality of being muscular.

mus'culature [L. *musculus,* muscle]. The arrangement of muscles in the body or its parts.

mus'culin. A globulin in muscle.

musculo- [L.]. Combining form pert. to a muscle.

musculoaponeurotic (mŭs-kŭ-lō-ăp″ō-nū-rŏt′ĭk). Composed of muscle and an aponeurosis of fibrous connective tissue.

musculocutaneous (mŭs″kū-lō-kū-tān′ē-ŭs) [L. *musculus,* muscle, + *cutis,* skin]. 1. Pert. to the muscles and skin. 2. Supplying or affecting the muscles and skin.

musculofascial (mŭs″kū-lō-fash′ē-ăl). Composed of muscle and fascia.

musculomembranous (mŭs″kū-lō-mĕm′-brăn-ŭs). Pert. to or consisting of muscle and membrane.

musculophrenic (mŭs″kū-lō-frĕn′ĭk). Pertaining to muscles of the diaphragm.

mus″culoten′dinous. Composed of both muscle and tendon.

mus′culus [L.]. (pl. *musculi*) [NA]. Muscle, q.v.

mushroom [Fr. *moucheron,* from L. *muscus,* moss]. Umbrella-shaped fungus, belonging to the Basidiomycetes which grows on decaying vegetable matter; common in woods and damp places. Some of the poisonous varieties are commonly called toadstools. SEE: *toadstool.*

COMP: Low in carbohydrates and fats; high in protein but of little alimentary value. Their relationship and similarity to poisonous fungi are so close that only those who are thoroughly capable of distinguishing the poisonous varieties from the edible ones should attempt to gather them. Food value of 100 gm. (canned, solids and liquids): Cal. 17; protein 1.9 gm.; fat 0.1 gm.; carbohydrate 2.4 gm.; calcium 6 mg.; sodium 400 mg.

m. and toadstool poisoning. Poisoning resulting from ingestion of mushrooms, such as Amanita muscaria which contains muscarine or other species which contain phalloidine, a component of the amanita toxin.

Note: Call nearest Poison Control Center for availability and advisability of using thioctic acid in emergency treatment. List appears in Appendix.

SEE: *Muscaria mushrooms* in *Table of Poisons and Poisoning* in *Appendix.*

musicogenic (mū″zĭ-kō-jĕn′ĭk). Caused by music, esp. epileptic convulsions.

musicomania [Gr. *mousikē,* music, + *mania,* madness]. Insane love of music.

musicotherapy [″+ *therapeia,* treatment]. Treatment of mental diseases with music.

musk (mŭsk) [Gr. *moskos,* from Sanskrit *muska,* testicle]. An oily secretion obtained from the musk bag, a gland beneath the abdominal skin of the male musk deer. Has a very strong odor. Used in manufacturing perfume.

musk′melon [″+ Gr. *mēlon,* apple]. One of several varieties of the melon, Cumis melo. Food value of 100 gm.: Cal. 30; protein 0.7 gm.; fat 0.1 gm.; carbohydrate 7.5 gm.; vitamin A content will vary from 280-3400 I.U. being much higher in melons with orange-colored flesh; ascorbic acid 33 mg.

mus′sel. A fresh-water bivalve mollusc belonging to the class Pelecypoda.

m. poisoning. Poisoning common on the Pacific coast resulting from eating mussels or clams which have ingested a poisonous dinoflagellate. Occurs from June to October. The poison is not destroyed by cooking.

mussitation (mŭs-sĭ-tā′shŭn) [L. *mussitāre,* to mutter]. The muttering of delirium or the moving of the lips without sound.

mus′tard [Fr. *moustarde*]. Yellow powder of mustard seed used as a counterirritant, rubefacient, emetic, stimulant, and condiment. SEE: *plaster.*

m. gas. Dichlorodiethyl sulfide, a war gas that causes burns and destruction of tissue internally and externally.

m. greens. Food value of 100 gm.: Cal. 31; protein 3.0 gm.; fat 0.5 gm.; carbohydrate 5.6 gm.; calcium 183 mg.; vitamin A, 7000 I.U.; ascorbic acid 97 mg.

mutagens [L. *mutare,* to change, + Gr. *gennan,* to produce]. Any agent that causes genetic mutations. Many medicines, chemicals, and physical agents such as ionizing radiations and ultraviolet light have this ability.

m., chemical. Chemicals that cause genetic mutations.

mutant (mū′tănt) [L. *mutare,* to change]. A sport or variation that breeds true.

mutase (mū′tās) [″+ *ase,* enzyme]. 1. Enzyme that accelerates oxidation-reduction reactions through activation of oxygen and hydrogen. 2. A food preparation made from leguminous plants high in protein content.

mutation (mū-tā′shŭn). 1. Change; transformation; instance of such change. 2. Sudden, permanent variation with offspring differing from parents in a marked characteristic as differentiated from gradual variation through many generations. Also person showing such change. 3. A change in a gene potentially capable of being transmitted to offspring.

m., induced. M. resulting from experiment or accident with X rays, radioactive substances, etc.

m., natural. M. occurring in nature and without artificial external intervention; thought to be a primary factor in evolutionary change.

m., somatic. M. occurring in somatic cells.

mute (mūt) [L. *mutus,* dumb]. 1. One who is unable to speak. 2. Dumb, without ability to speak.

m., deaf. Individual who is unable to hear or to speak.

mu'tilate [L. *mutilatus,* to maim]. To deprive of a limb or a part; to maim or disfigure.

mutilation (mū″tī-lā′shŭn). Maiming; the act of removing or destroying a conspicuous or essential part or organ.

mutism (mū′tĭzm) [L. *mutus,* dumb]. 1. Condition of being unable to speak. 2. Persistent inhibition to speech; seen in some severe forms of mental disorder.

mutualism (mū′tū-ăl-ĭzm) [L. *mutuus,* exchanged]. A form of symbiosis in which organisms of two different species live in close association to the mutual benefit of each.

my-, myo- [Gr. *mys,* muscle]. Prefix denoting relationship to muscle.

myalgia (mī-ăl′jī-ă) [″+ *algos,* pain]. Tenderness or pain in the muscles; muscular rheumatism.

myasis (mī-ā′sĭs) [Gr. *myia,* a fly]. Condition which arises from larvae of flies or maggots in the body or upon mucous membranes. SYN: *myiasis.*

myasthenia (mī-ăs-thē′nī-ă) [Gr. *mys, my-,* muscle, + *astheneia,* weakness]. Muscular weakness.

m., angiosclerotic. Vascular changes producing excessive muscular fatigue.

m. gastrica. Loss of muscular tone in coats of the stomach.

m. gravis. A disease characterized by great muscular weakness (without atrophy) and progressive fatigability. It is due to a functional abnormality, lack of acetylcholine, or excess of cholinesterase at the myoneural junction in which nerve impulses fail to induce normal muscle contractions.

ETIOL: Unknown. More common in females. Occurs most frequently between ages of 20 and 50.

SYM: Abnormal fatigability and weakness of muscles. Muscles of the face and neck primarily involved, those of the trunk and extremities secondarily. Onset gradual; symptoms worse in the evening. Patient complains of difficulty in chewing, swallowing, and talking. Expressionless facies and ptosis usually present.

PROG: Some cases mild; others rapidly fatal, death resulting from respiratory failure. Course is variable. Prolonged remissions may occur.

TREATMENT: Restricted activity; complete rest in severe cases. Soft or liquid diet; tube feedings sometimes essential. Physostigmine and neostigmine given I.M. or orally are effective. Potassium chloride, ephedrine, and guanidine are also used as adjuvants of neostigmine, the drug of choice.

myasthe'nic. Marked by muscular weakness.

myatonia (mī-ă-tō′nī-ă). Deficiency or loss of muscular tone.

m. congenita. M. of early childhood; it is not hereditary. SYN: *amyotonia congenita.*

myatrophy (mī-at′rō-fī). Muscular wasting away.

myc-, myco- [Gr. *mykēs,* fungus]. Combining form meaning fungus.

mycelioid (mī-sē′lĭ-oid) [″+ *atrophia,* atrophy, + *eidos,* form]. Moldlike; resembling mold colonies in which filaments radiate from a center, said of bacterial colonies.

mycelium (mī-sē′lĭ-ŭm) [Gr. *mykēs,* fungus, + *hēlos,* nail]. The mass of filaments (hyphae) that constitutes the vegetative body of fungi such as molds.

mycetes (mī-sē′tēz). The fungi.

mycethemia (mī-sĕ-thē′mī-ă) [Gr. *mykēs,* fungus, + *haima,* blood]. Fungi in the blood. SYN: *mycohemia.*

mycetism, mycetismus (mī′sĕ-tĭzm, -tĭz′-mŭs) [″+ *ismos,* condition]. Poisoning from eating fungi, esp. poisonous mushrooms.

mycetogenetic, mycetogenic, mycetogenous (mī-sē″tō-jĕn-ĕt′ĭk, -jĕn′ĭk, -toj′-ĕn-ŭs) [Gr. *mykēs,* fungus, + *gennan,* to produce]. Induced by fungi.

mycetoma (mī-sĕ-tō′mă) [″+ *ōma,* tumor]. A disease, induced by fungi, that attacks the foot. SYN: *Madura foot.*

Mycobacte'rium [Gr. *mykēs,* fungus, + *baktērion,* little rod]. A genus of acid-fast organisms belonging to the Mycobacteriaceae which includes the causative organisms of tuberculosis and leprosy. They are slender, nonmotile, gram-positive rods and do not produce spores or capsules.

M. leprae. Believed to be the causative agent of leprosy.

M. marinum. An atypical mycobacterium which produces skin infection resembling sporotrichosis. The organism has been cultured from tropical fish aquariums.

M. tuberculosis. Causative agent of tuberculosis in mammals.

my″cocid'in (mī″kŏ-sī′dĭn). An antibiotic derived from molds of the family Aspergillaceae.

mycoder'ma [Gr. *mykos,* mucus, + *derma,* skin]. Mucous membrane.

mycoid (mī'koyd) [Gr. *mykēs*, fungus, + *eidos*, form]. Funguslike.

mycology (mī-kŏl'ō-jĭ) ["+ *logos*, study]. Science of fungi.

mycomyringitis (mī"kō-mĭr-in-jī'tĭs) ["+ L. *myringa*, drum membrane, + -*itis*, inflammation]. Fungus inflammation of membrana tympani.

mycophthalmia (mī-kŏf-thăl'mĭ-ă). Ophthalmia resulting from fungus infection.

mycoplasmas. Several bacteria of the Mycoplasma genus which are found in the human. Includes M. hominis types 1 and 2, M. salivarium, M. orale, M. fermentans, and M. pneumoniae. Most forms have no cell wall. Mycoplasma which were called pleuropneumonia-like organisms (PPLO) have been proven to be the cause of primary atypical pneumonia (called viral pneumonia at one time). Their relationship to other diseases such as Reiter's syndrome, q.v., has not been proven. T strains, so called because they produce small colonies on agar, inhabit the urogenital tract.

mycosis (mī-kō'sĭs) [Gr. *mykēs*, fungus, + -*ōsis*, intensive]. Any disease induced by a fungus.

   m. fungoides. A rare, poorly understood, malignant disease that originates in the reticuloendothelial cells of the skin. The lymph nodes and internal organs become involved.

   SYM: Urticarial, erythematous, or eczematous patches of irregular shape and size, with well-defined margins usually upon scalp and skin of trunk. Itching intense; frequently the patches become hypertrophic and firm. Hard nodules varying from size of pea to apple, either sessile or pedunculated, develop on them. These eventually break down and form ulcers that contain sensitive, fungating granulation tissue, and discharge thin pus and serum. Death results from progressive cachexia.

   TREATMENT: General supportive measures. Electron beam radiation and cytotoxic agents have been used.

   m., superficial. A dermatomycosis; a fungus infection of the skin or its appendages. Includes erythrasma; tinea barbae, t. capitis, t. corporis, t. cruris, t. favosa, t. pedis, t. unguium; trichomycosis axillaris.

   m., systemic. A deep mycosis; a fungus infection involving various bodily systems or regions. Includes aspergillosis, blastomycosis, chromoblastomycosis, coccidioidomycosis, conidiosporosis, cryptococcosis, geotrichosis, histoplasmosis, maduromycosis, moniliasis, mucormycosis, nocard-

iosis, para-actinomycosis, penicilliosis, rhinosporidiosis, sporotrichosis.

mycotic (mī-kŏt'ĭk). Caused by or affected with microorganisms; concerning mycosis.

mycotoxins. Substances, produced by mold growing in food or animal feed, which cause illness or death when ingested by man or animals.

mycterophonia (mĭk"ter-ō-fō'nĭ-ă) [Gr. *myktēr*, nostril, + *phōnē*, voice]. Phonation in which the voice possesses a nasal quality.

mydaleine (mĭd-ā'le-ēn) [Gr. *mydaleos*, moldy]. A poisonous ptomaine from putrefied visceral organs, acting mainly on the heart.

mydriasis (mĭd-rī'ă-sĭs) [Gr.]. Pronounced or abnormal dilation of the pupil.

   ETIOL: Fright, sudden emotion, 1st and 3rd stages of anesthesia, drugs, coma, hysteria, botulism, or irritation of cervical sympathetic nerve.

   m., alternating. M. which affects one eye, then the other. Also called leaping, springing, or bounding m.

   m., paralytic. M. resulting from paralysis of oculomotor nerve.

   m., spastic. M. resulting from overactivity of dilator muscle of iris or of sympathetic nerves supplying that muscle. Also called spasmodic m.

   m., spinal. M. resulting from a lesion of, or irritation of, ciliospinal center of spinal cord.

mydriatic (mĭd-rī-ăt'ĭk). 1. Causing pupillary dilatation. 2. Any drug that dilates the pupil.

   Ex: atropine, cocaine, ephedrine, euphthalmine, homatropine.

myectomy (mī-ĕk'tō-mĭ) [Gr. *mys*, muscle, + *ektomē*, excision]. Excision of a portion of a muscle.

myectopia (mī-ĕk-tō'pĭ-ă) ["+ *ek*, out, + *topos*, place]. Muscle dislocation.

myelalgia (mī-ĕl-ăl'jĭ-ă) [Gr. *myelos*, marrow, + *algos*, pain]. Pain of the spinal cord or its membranes.

myelanalosis (mī"ĕl-ă-năl-ō'sĭs) ["+ *analōsis*, wasting]. Gradual wasting of spinal cord. SYM: *tabes dorsalis.*

myelapoplexy (mī-ĕl-ăp'ō-plĕks-ĭ) ["+ *apoplēxia*, stroke]. Hemorrhagic effusion into the spinal cord.

myelasthenia (mī-ĕl-ăs-thē'nĭ-ă) [Gr. *myelos*, marrow, + *astheneia*, weakness]. Spinal exhaustion; neurasthenia arising from spinal causes.

myelatelia (mī-ĕl-ă-tē'lĭ-ă) ["+ *ateleia*, imperfection]. Defective development of spinal cord.

myelatrophy (mī-el-at'rōf-ĭ) ["+ *atrophia*, atrophy]. Wasting of the spinal cord.

myelauxe (mī-ĕl-awks'ē) ["+ *auxē*, increase]. Abnormal enlargement of spinal cord.

myelemia (mī-ĕl-ē'mĭ-ă) ["+ *haima*, blood]. Abnormal number of marrow cells in the blood. SYN: *myelocytosis*.

myelencephalon (mī''ĕl-ĕn-sĕf'ă-lŏn) [Gr. *myelos*, marrow, + *enkephalos*, brain]. [NA]. The most post. portion of the embryonic hindbrain (rhombencephalon) which gives rise to the medulla oblongata.

myel'ic. Pert. to the spinal cord.

my'elin. 1. A fatlike substance forming the principal component of the myelin sheath of nerve fibers. Composed of cholesterol, certain cerebrosides, phospholipins, and fatty acids. 2. A complex lipoid substance present in the brain in small quantities.

myelination (mī-ĕl-ĭn-ā'shŭn) [Gr. *myelos*, marrow]. Process of acquiring a myelin sheath. SYN: *myelinization*.

myelinic (mī-ĕl-ĭn'ĭk). Concerning or composed of myelin.

myelinization (mī''ĕl-ĭn-ĭ-zā'shŭn). Acquirement of myelin sheath for nerve fibers. SYN: *myelination*.

myelinogenetic (mī''ĕl-ĭn-ō-jĕn-et'ĭk) [Gr. *myelos*, marrow, + *gennan*, to produce]. Producing myelin or a myelin sheath.

myelinosis (mī''ĕl-ĭn-ō'sĭs) ["+ *-ōsis*, intensive]. Fatty degeneration during which myelin is produced.

myelitic (mī-ĕl-ĭt'ĭk). Concerning myelitis.

myelitis (mī-ĕ-lī'tĭs) [Gr. *myelos*, marrow, + *-itis*, inflammation]. Inflammation of the spinal cord or of bone marrow.

SYM: Moderate fever (101°-103° F. or 38.3°-39.4° C.), loss of appetite, coated tongue and constipation, followed by pain in back radiating into the limbs. Various forms of paresthesia, as numbness, tingling, burning, etc. Frequently a sense of painful constriction, girdle pain at level of the disease. Paralysis soon develops and may become more or less complete. At first may be retention, later frequently incontinence, of feces. Bedsores soon develop. Death may result in few days from extension upward, and involvement of respiratory muscles. In rare cases a spontaneous arrest of inflammation and slow recovery follows, attended with partial paralysis.

SEE: *axophage; osteomyelitis; poliomyelitis.*

m., acute. Simple acute form which develops following injury.

m., acute ascending. M. which moves progressively upward in the spinal cord.

m., bulbar. M. involving the medulla oblongata.

m., central. M. in which the gray matter esp. is involved.

m., central, acute. Resembles acute transverse m., but the trophic disturbances are more marked and duration shorter. Usually fatal in 1 to 2 weeks.

PROG: Always extremely grave.

TREATMENT: If possible place patient on water bed. Continuous closed drainage of bladder is preferable to intermittent catheterization. In incontinence of urine and feces the discharges should be received on cotton or wool, which should be frequently renewed and parts thoroughly cleansed. In the beginning ice bags or wet cups may be applied to the spine. Frequent baths should be given. Milk, eggs, rice, toast, farina, fruit and blanc mange may be given in early stages of disease. Later, more nutritious diet.

m., chronic. Form progressing slowly but steadily.

SYM: Begin with numbness, tingling or burning in lower extremities, followed by loss of power and sensation. Reflexes generally exaggerated. Sphincters soon become involved. Girdle pain at level of disease. Progress slow, 6 months to 10 years.

TREATMENT: Patient should be put at rest. Frequent tepid baths; plenty of sleep; good, nourishing food; moderate exercise that stops short of fatigue. Freedom from mental worry. Constitutional treatment, antisyphilitics where indicated.

m., compression. M. caused by pressure on the cord, as by a hemorrhage or tumor.

m., cornual. M. affecting the spinal cord's horns of gray matter.

m., descending. M. affecting successively lower areas of the spinal cord.

m., diffuse. M. involving large and various sections of the cord.

m., disseminated. M. with several separated foci on the cord.

m., hemorrhagic. M. with hemorrhage.

m., interstitial. Sclerosing m.

m., parenchymatous. M. of nerve substance, differentiated from interstitial m.

m., sclerosing. M. with hardening of cord, and abnormal interstitial tissue growth.

m., systemic. M. affecting only certain tracts of the cord.

m., transverse. M. involving the whole thickness of the cord, but limited longitudinally.

m., transverse, acute. Acute form of m. involving entire thickness of cord, developing subsequent injury to spinal cord.

m., traumatic. M. due to cord injury.

myelo- [Gr.]. Prefix denoting the spinal cord or bone marrow.

myeloblast (mī'el-ō-blăst) ["+ *blastos,* germ]. Bone marrow cell which develops into a myelocyte.

myeloblastemia (mī''ēl-ō-blăst-ē'mī-ă) ["+ "+ *haima,* blood]. Occurrence of myeloblasts in the blood.

myeloblastoma (mī''ēl-ō-blăst-ō'mă) ["+ "+ *-oma,* tumor]. 1. Tumor containing myeloblasts. 2. Myelogenic form of leukemia.

myeloblastosis (mī'ē-lō-blăs-tō'sĭs). Excess production of myeloblasts and their presence in circulating blood; myeloblastic leukemia.

myelocele (mī'ē-lō-sēl). 1. [Gr. *myelo,* spinal cord, + *kēlē,* hernia]. A form of spina bifida with spinal cord protrusion. 2. ["+ *koilia,* hollow]. Central canal of spinal cord.

myelocyst (mī'ēl-ō-sĭst) ["+ *kystis,* bladder]. Cyst arising from the rudimentary medullary canal of the spinal cord.

myelocystocele (mī''ēl-ō-sĭst'ō-sēl) ["+ "+ *kēlē,* hernia]. Cystic tumor of spinal cord substance through a defect in the canal.

myelocystomeningocele (mī''ēl-ō-sĭst''ō-men-ĭn'gō-sēl) [Gr. *myelos,* marrow, + *kystis,* bladder, + *mēning,* membrane, + *kēlē,* hernia]. Combined myelocystocele and meningocele.

myelocyte (mī'el-ō-sīt) ["+ *kytos,* cell]. A large cell in red bone marrow from which leukocytes are derived.

myelocythemia (mī''ēl-ō-sī-thē'mī-ă) ["+ "+ *haima,* blood]. Presence of an excess number of myelocytes in the blood. SYN: *myelocytosis.*

myelocytic (mī''ēl-ō-sit'ĭk). Characterized by prescence of, or pert. to, myelocytes.

myelocytoma (mī''ēl-ō-sī-tō'mă). Leukemia with leukocytes arising from both myeloid and lymphoid substance. SYN: *chronic myelogenous leukemia.*

myelocytosis (mī''ēl-ō-sī-tō'sĭs). Myelocytes in large quantities in the blood. SYN: *myelocythemia.*

myelodiastasis (mī''ēl-ō-dī-as'tă-sĭs) [Gr. *myelos,* marrow, + *diastasis,* separation]. Destruction and disintegration of spinal cord.

myelodysplasia (mī''ēl-ō-dĭs-plā'zī-ă) ["+ *dys,* bad, + *plassein,* to form]. Defective formation of the spinal cord.

myeloencephalic (mī''ēl-ō-ĕn-sĕf-al'ĭk) ["+ *enkephalos,* brain]. Concerning the spinal cord and brain.

myeloencephalitis (mī''ēl-ō-ĕn-sĕf-ă-lī'tĭs) ["+ "+ *-itis,* inflammation]. Inflamed condition of spinal cord and brain.

myelofibrosis (mī''ē-lō-fī-brō'sĭs). Replacement of bone marrow by fibrous tissue.

myelogenesis (mī''ēl-ō-jĕn'ē-sĭs) [Gr. *myelos,* spinal cord, + *genesis,* development]. 1. The development of brain and spinal cord. 2. Development of myelin sheath of nerve fiber.

myelogenic, myelogenous (mī-ē-lō-jen'-ĭk, -loj'ĕn-ŭs) ["+ *gennan,* to produce]. Producing or originating in marrow.

myelography (mī-ē-lŏg'ră-fī) ["+ *graphein,* to write]. Roentgenographic inspection of the spinal cord by use of a radiopaque medium injected into the intrathecal space.

m., air. M. in which oxygen or air is used instead of radiopaque dye.

myeloid (mī'ē-loid) ["+ *eidos,* form]. 1. Medullary; like marrow. 2. Resembling a myelocyte, but not necessarily originating from bone marrow.

myeloidosis (mī''ē-loid-ō'sĭs) ["+ "+ *-ōsis,* intensive]. Formation of myeloid tissue, esp. abnormal tissue formation.

myelolymphangioma (mī''ē-lō-lĭm-făn''jī-ō'mă). Elephantiasis, q.v.

myelolymphocyte (mī''ē-lō-lĭmf'ō-sīt) ["+ L. *lympha,* lymph, + Gr. *kytos,* cell]. Tiny lymphocyte formed abnormally in bone marrow.

myeloma (mī-ē-lō'mă) [Gr. *myelos,* marrow, + *-ōma,* tumor]. A tumor originating in cells of the hematopoietic portion of bone marrow.

m., multiple. A neoplastic disease characterized by the infiltration of bone and bone marrow by myeloma cells forming multiple tumor masses. Usually progressive and generally fatal. Accompanied by anemia, renal lesions, and high globulin levels in blood. Common in 6th decade of life. More frequent in males by ratio of 3:1. SYN: *m. multiplex; Kahler's disease; plasmocytic sarcoma; myeloid m.; lymphadenia ossium; and myelomatosis.*

myelomalacia (mī''ē-lō-mă-lā'sī-ă) ["+ *malakia,* softening]. Abnormal softening of spinal cord.

myelomatosis (mī''ēl-ō-mă-tō'sĭs) [Gr. *myelos,* marrow, + *-ōma,* tumor, + *-ōsis,* intensive]. Disease marked by multiple tumors of the bone marrow, pernicious anemia, and albumosuria. SYN: *multiple myeloma.*

myelomenia (mī-ĕ-lō-mē'nĭ-ă) ["+ *mēn,* month]. Vicarious menstrual discharge in the spinal cord.

myelomeningitis (mī''ĕ-lō-mĕn-ĭn-jī'tĭs) [Gr. *myelos,* marrow, + *mening,* membrane, + *-itis,* inflammation]. Inflamed spinal cord and membranes; spinal meningitis.

myelomeningocele (mī''ĕ-lō-mĕn-ĭn'gō-sēl) ["+ "+ *kēlē,* hernia]. Spina bifida with portion of cord and membranes protruding.

myelomyces (mī-ĕ-lō-mī'sēs) ["+ *mykēs,* fungus]. Malignant growth resembling brain substance. SYN: *encephaloma.*

myelon (mī'ĕ-lŏn) [Gr. *myelos,* marrow]. The spinal cord.

myeloneuritis (mī''ĕ-lō-nū-rī'tĭs) ["+ *neuron,* nerve, + *-itis,* inflammation]. Multiple neuritis and myelitis combined.

myelonic (mī-ĕ-lŏn'ĭk) [Gr. *myelos,* marrow]. Pert. to the spinal cord.

myeloparalysis (mī''ĕ-lō-pă-ral'ĭ-sĭs) ["+ *para,* beside, + *lyein,* to loosen]. Paralysis of the spine.

myelopathy (mī-ĕ-lŏp'ă-thĭ) ["+ *pathos,* disease]. Any pathological condition of the spinal cord.

myelopetal (mī-ĕ-lŏp'ĕt-ăl) ["+ L. *petere,* to seek for]. Proceeding toward the spinal cord, said of certain nerve impulses.

myelophage (mī'ĕ-lō-fāj) ["+ *phagein,* to eat]. A myelin-ingesting macrophage.

myelophthisis (mī-ĕ-lŏf'thĭ-sĭs) [Gr. *myelos,* marrow, + *phthisis,* a wasting]. 1. Atrophy of the spinal cord. SYN: *myelanalosis.* 2. Replacement of the bone marrow by a disease process such as a neoplasm.

myeloplast (mī'ĕ-lō-plast) [Gr. *myelos,* marrow, + *plastos,* formed]. A leukocyte cell of the bone marrow.

my'eloplax ["+ *plax,* plate]. Large, multinuclear, bone marrow cell.

myeloplaxoma (mī''ĕ-lō-plăk-sō'mă) ["+ "+ *-ōma,* tumor]. Tumor composed of myeloplaxes.

myeloplegia (mī''ĕl-ō-plē'jĭ-ă) ["+ *plēgē,* stroke]. Paralysis of spinal origin.

myelopoiesis (mī''ĕl-ō-poy-ē'sĭs) ["+ *poiein,* to form]. The development of bone marrow or formation of cells derived from bone marrow.

> *m., ectopic.* Extramedullary m., q.v.

> *m., extramedullary.* Development of myeloid elements (erythrocytes and granular leukocytes) in regions other than bone marrow.

my'elopore. An opening in the spinal cord.

myeloradiculitis (mī''ĕ-lō-ră-dĭk''ū-lī'tĭs) [Gr. *myelos,* spinal cord, + L. *radiculus,* rootlet, + Gr. *-itis,* inflammation]. Inflam-

mation of spinal cord and dorsal roots of spinal nerves.

myeloradiculodysplasia (mī''ĕ-lō-rā-dĭk''-ū-lō'dĭs-plā'sĭ-ă) ["+ "+ Gr. *dys,* bad, + *plassein,* to form]. Congenital abnormality of spinal cord and spinal nerve roots.

myelorrhagia (mī-ĕ-lō-rā'jĭ-ă) ["+ *rhēgnynai,* to burst forth]. Hemorrhage into myelon.

myelorrhaphy (mī-ĕ-lōr'ă-fī) ["+ *rhaphē,* suture]. Suture of a cut or wound of the spinal cord.

myelosarcoma (mī''ĕl-ō-săr-kō'mă) ["+ *sarx,* flesh, + *-ōma,* tumor]. Sarcoma of bone marrow cells and tissue. SYN: *osteosarcoma.*

myeloschisis (mī''ĕ-lŏs'kĭ-sĭs) ["+ *schisis,* cleft]. Cleft spinal cord resulting from failure of neural tube to close. SEE: *spina bifida; rachischisis.*

myelosclerosis (mī''ĕ-lō-sklĕr-ō'sĭs) [Gr. *myelos,* marrow, + *sklērōsis,* hardening]. Sclerosis of the spinal cord.

myelosis (mī-ĕ-lō'sĭs) ["+ *-ōsis,* intensive]. Formation of a myeloma or medullary tumor.

myelospongium (mī''ĕ-lō-spŏn'jĭ-ŭm) ["+ *spongos,* sponge]. Embryonic network from which the neuroglia arises.

myelotome (mī-ĕl'ō-tōm) ["+ *tomē,* incision]. Instrument used to dissect the spinal cord.

myelotomy (mī-ĕl-ŏt'ō-mī). Surgical severance of nerve fibers of spinal cord.

myelotoxic (mī-ĕl-ō-tŏk'sĭk) ["+ *toxikon,* poison]. 1. Destroying bone marrow. 2. Pert. to or arising from diseased bone marrow.

myelotoxin (mī''ĕl-ō-tok'sĭn) ["+ *toxikon,* poison]. Toxin which destroys marrow cells.

myenteric (mī-ĕn-ter'ĭk) [Gr. *mys,* muscle, + *enteron,* intestine]. Concerning the myenteron, q.v.

> *m. reflex.* Intestinal contraction above and relaxation below the point of stimulation.

myenteron (mī-en'tĕr-ŏn). Muscular coat of the intestine.

myesthesia (mī-ĕs-thē'-zĭ-ă) [Gr. *mys, my-,* muscle, + *aisthēsis,* sensation]. Muscle sense; consciousness of muscle contraction.

myiasis (mī-ī'ă-sĭs) [Gr. *myia,* fly]. Condition resulting from infestation by the larvae (maggots) of flies. Infestation may be cutaneous, intestinal, atrial (within a cavity such as mouth, nose, eye, sinus, vagina, urethra), wound, or external.

myiodesopsia (mī''ī-ō-dĕs -ŏp'sĭ-ă) [Gr. *myiōdēs,* flylike, + *opsis,* vision]. Condition in which spots are seen before the eyes. SEE: *muscae volitantes.*

myitis (mī-ī'tĭs) [Gr. *mys, my-*, muscle, + *-itis*, inflammation]. Inflamed condition of a muscle. SYN: *myositis*.

mylodus. A molar tooth.

mylohyoid (mī''lō-hī'oid) [Gr. *mylē*, mill, + *hyoid* U-shaped]. Pert. to the hyoid bone and the molar teeth.

myo- [Gr. *mys*, muscle]. Combining form pert. to muscle.

myoalbumin (mī''ō-ăl-bū'mĭn) ["+ L. *albus*, white]. Albumin found in muscular tissue.

myoalbumose (mī-ō-al'bū-mōs). A protein derived from muscle.

myoarchitectonic (mī''ō-ar''kĭ-těk-tŏn'ĭk) ["+ *architektōn*, master workman]. Pert. to or resembling structural arrangement of muscle or of fibers.

myoatrophy (mī-ō-ăt'rō-fĭ). Musclar wasting.

myoblast (mī'ō-blast) [Gr. *mys, myo-*, muscle, + *blastos*, germ]. An embryonic cell which develops into muscle fiber cell.

myoblasto'ma. A tumor consisting of cells resembling myoblasts.

myobra'dia ["+ *bradys*, slow]. Slow muscular reaction to stimulation.

myocardiac, myocardial (mī-ō-kar'dĭ-ăk, -ăl) ["+ *kardia*, heart]. Concerning the myocardium.

   m. infarction. Development of an infarct in the myocardium, usually the result of myocardial ischemia following occlusion of a coronary artery.

   SYM: Pain similar to that of angina pectoris, shock, cardiac failure with arrhythmia, and frequently sudden death.

   m. insufficiency. Inability of the heart to perform its usual function. Eventually this results in cardiac failure.

myocardiograph (mī''ō-kar'dĭ-ō-grăf) ["+ "+ *graphein*, to write]. Instrument for recording heart movements.

myocardiosis (mī-ō-kär-dĭ-ō'sĭs) ["+ "+ *-osis*, intensive]. Noninflammatory cardiac disorder. SYN: *myocardia.*

myocarditis (mī-ō-kar-dī'tĭs) [Gr. *mys*, muscle, + *kardia*, heart, + *-itis*, inflammation]. Inflammation of the cardiac muscular tissue.

   ETIOL: Associated with a number of conditions including many types of infections, nephritis, carbon monoxide poisoning, heat stroke, and burns. Occurs commonly after rheumatic fever and diphtheria or may be idiopathic.

   PHYSICAL SIGNS: Apex beat extremely weak and rapid; pulse irregular and weak; tenderness over precordium, percussion negative, auscultation reveals 1st sound of heart resembling 2nd heart sound, high pitched and wanting in muscular quality.

   NP: In acute myocarditis absolute rest is essential. Years may be added to the life of the patient with chronic myocarditis if moderation in all things is observed. Plenty of rest and sleep, light diet, and avoidance of all worry, hurry, and physical strains are very important. High altitudes must be avoided and climbing stairs should be reduced to a minimum, and haste avoided. Proper elimination should be maintained. In some instances graduated exercises may be ordered.

   m., acute, primary. Acute interstitial inflammation of the myocardium.

   m., acute, secondary. Acute inflammation of the heart muscle.

   ETIOL: Secondary to acute inflammation of pericardium or endocardium, or may occur during some infectious disease.

   SYM: Marked by primary disease; great weakness; cardiac palpitation with irregularity; small, feeble pulse, and dyspnea; precordial pain and distress.

   m., acute, septic. Localized, suppurative inflammation of the heart muscle.

   ETIOL: Distant infection, suppurating pericardium or endocardium.

   m., chronic. Characterized by round cell infiltration of interstitial tissue, followed by parenchymatous changes of muscle fibers.

   ETIOL: Nephritis, syphilis, grave anemias, diabetes, rheumatic fever, malaria, toxic substance, or excessive use of alcohol and tobacco. Certain wasting diseases, disease of coronary arteries, joint affections, or extension from endocardium and pericardium.

   SYM: Cardiac insufficiency. Rapid heart which does not immediately recover from exercise. On first exertion the heart and blood pressure rise quickly but become slower with prolonged exertion.

   PHYSICAL SIGNS: Face appears cyanosed, esp. about the lips and ears; also about the fingertips. Apex beat of heart not displaced unless the heart was previously hypertrophied, in which case apex beat will be displaced downward and to the left, or downward if dilatation exists. Pulse weak, blood pressure either low or high. Auscultation reveals a short, feeble 1st sound, lacking in muscular quality with reduplication of that sound. Second sound, esp. the aortic, is accentuated. Systolic murmur at apex over a small area if dilatation exists.

   m., fragmentation. Fragmentation of the myocardium.

m., indurative. Chronic m. causing hardening of muscular walls of the heart.

myocardosis (mī″ō-kär-dō′sĭs) [Gr. mys, myo-, muscle, + kardia, heart, + -osis, intensive]. 1. A noninflammatory disorder of the myocardium. 2. Any degenerative condition (except myofibrosis) of the heart muscle.

myocele (mī′ō-sēl) ["+ kēlē, hernia]. 1. Muscular protrusion through a muscle sheath. 2. Cavity within a somite of an embryo.

myocelialgia (mī″ō-sē-lī-al′jī-ä) ["+ koilia, belly, + algos, pain]. Abdominal muscle pain.

myocelitis (mī-ō-sē-lī′tĭs) ["+ "+ -itis, inflammation]. Inflamed condition of abdominal muscles.

myocellulitis (mī″ō-sēl-ū-lī′tĭs) [Gr. mys, myo-, muscle, + L. cellula, little chamber, + Gr. -itis, inflammation]. Myositis combined with cellulitis.

myocerosis (mī″ō-sē-rō′sĭs) ["+ kēros, wax]. Waxy degeneration of a muscle.

myochorditis (mī″ō-kor-dī′tĭs) ["+ chordē, cord, + -itis, inflammation]. Inflammation of the muscles of the larynx.

myochrome (mī′ō-krōm) ["+ chrōma, color]. Reddish pigment derived from hemoglobin and found in muscle. SYN: myohematin.

myochronoscope (mī″ō-krō′nō-skōp) ["+ chronos, time, + skopein, to examine]. Device for determining time for producing a muscular contraction.

myoclonia (mī-ō-klō′nī-ä) ["+ klonos, tumult]. Condition of intermittent, clonic spasm or twitching of a muscle or muscles.

myoclonus (mī-ŏk′lō-nŭs). Twitching or clonic spasm of a muscle or group of muscles. SYN: paramyoclonus.

m. multiplex. Condition marked by persistent and continuous muscular spasms in unrelated muscles.

myocoele (mi′o-sēl) [Gr. mys, muscle, + koilia, hollow]. SEE: myocele.

myocolpitis (mī″ō-kŏl-pī′tĭs) ["+ kolpos, vagina, + -itis, inflammation]. Inflammation of vaginal muscular tissue.

myocomma (mī-ō-kŏm′mä) ["+ komma, cut]. (pl. myocommata) Septum dividing the myotomes. SYN: myotome.

myocrismus (mī-ō-krĭs′mŭs) ["+ krizein, to creak]. A peculiar crackling sound sometimes heard in auscultation resulting from contraction of a muscle.

myocyte (mī′ō-sīt) ["+ kytos, cell]. A muscular tissue cell.

myocytoma (mī″ō-sī-tō′mä) ["+ "+ -ōma, tumor]. Tumor containing muscle cells.

myodemia (mī-ō-dē′mĭ-ä) ["+ dēmos, fat]. Fatty degeneration of muscular tissue. Mus-

cular fiber cells become filled with fat granules and are ultimately destroyed.

myodesopsia (mī″ō-dēs -ŏp′sĭ-ä) [Gr. myiōdēs, flylike, + opsis, vision]. Myiodesopsia, q.v.

myodiastasis (mī″ō-dī-ăs′tă-sĭs) [Gr. mys, myo-, muscle, + diastasis, separation]. Division or rupture of a muscle.

myodynamia (mī″ō-dī-năm′ĭ-ä) ["+ dynamis, force]. Muscular force or strength.

myodynamometer (mī″ō-dī″nä-mŏm′ĕt-ĕr) ["+ "+ metron, measure]. Device for measurement of muscular strength.

myodynia (mī-ō-dīn′ĭ-ä) ["+ odynē, pain]. Muscle pain. SYN: myalgia.

myoedema (mī″ō-ĕ-dē′mä) [Gr. mys, myo-, muscle, + oidēma, swelling]. 1. Lumping in a wasting muscle when struck. SYN: mounding. 2. Muscular edema.

my″oelast′ic. Pert. to muscle and elastic tissue.

my″oelec′tric. Pert. to electrical properties of muscles.

myoendocarditis (mī″ō-ĕn″dō-kar-dī′tĭs) [Gr. mys, muscle, + endon, within, + kardia, heart, + -itis, inflammation]. Inflammation of the cardiac muscular wall and membranous lining.

myoepithelial (mī″ō-ĕp′ī-thē′lī-ăl). Pert. to contractile epithelial cells.

m. cells. Spindle-shaped or branched contractile epithelial cells found between glandular cells and basement membrane of sweat, mammary, and salivary glands.

myofascitis (mī″ō-făs-ī′tĭs) [Gr. mys, muscle, + L. fascia, band, + Gr. -itis, inflammation]. Inflamed condition of a muscle and its fascia.

myofibril, myofibrilla (mī-ō-fī′brĭl, -fĭ-brĭl′lä) ["+ L. fibrilla, a small fiber]. (pl. myofibrillae) A tiny fibril found in muscular tissue, running parallel to the cellular long axis, from one cell to another. May be the contractile element.

myofibroma (mī″ō-fĭ-brō′mä) ["+ L. fibra, fiber, + Gr. -ōma, tumor]. Tumor containing muscular and fibrous tissue.

myofibrosis (mī″ō-fĭ-brō′sĭs) ["+ "+ Gr. -ōsis, intensive]. Increase of connective or fibrous tissue with degeneration of muscular tissue.

myogelosis (mī-ō-jē-lō′sĭs) ["+ L. gelāre, to congeal]. Hardening of a portion of muscle.

myogen (mī′ō-jĕn) ["+ gennan, to produce]. A protein found in muscle plasma; it is spontaneously coagulable.

myogenesis (mī-ō-jĕn′ē-sĭs) ["+ genesis, development]. Formation of muscular tissue, esp. in embryos.

myogenetic (mī″ō-jĕn-ĕt′ĭk) [Gr. *mys, myo-,* muscle, + *gennan,* to produce]. Having origin in muscle. SYN: *myogenic.*

myogen′ic, myog′enous. Arising from muscle.

myoglia (mī-ŏg′lĭ-ă) [″+ *glia,* glue]. A fibrous network in muscular tissue resembling neuroglia in appearance.

myoglobin. Myohemoglobin, q.v.

myoglobulin (mī″ō-glŏb′ū-lĭn) [Gr. *mys, myo-,* muscle, + L. *globulus,* globule]. A coagulable globulin seen in muscular tissue.

my′ogram [″+ *gramma,* a marking]. A tracing made by the myograph of muscular contractions.

myograph (mī′ō-grăf) [Gr. *mys, myo-,* muscle, + *graphein,* to write]. Instrument for tracing movements caused by muscular contractions.

myographic (mī-ō-grăf′ĭk). Pert. to a myograph, or the tracings made by it.

   m. tracing. A myrogram or muscular tracing.

myography (mī-ŏg′ră-fī). 1. Recording of muscular contractions by a myograph. 2. Description of the muscles and their action.

myohematin (mī″ō-hĕm′-ă-tĭn) [Gr. *mys, myo-,* muscle, + *haima,* blood]. Cytochrome, q.v.

myo″hemoglob′in. A respiratory pigment in muscle tissue which serves as an oxygen carrier. ABBR: MHb. SYN: *myoglobin; myoglobulin.*

myohysterectomy (mī″ō-hĭs-tĕr-ĕk′tō-mī) [Gr. *mys, myo-,* muscle, + *hystera,* uterus, + *ektomē,* excision]. Excision of the body of the uterus, leaving the cervix in place. SYN: *subtotal hysterectomy.*

my′oid [″+ *eidos,* resemblance]. Resembling muscle.

myoidema (mī-oi-dē′mă) [″+ *oidēma,* swelling]. Myoedema, q.v.

myoischemia (mī″ō-ĭs-kē′mĭ-ă) [″+ *ischein,* to hold back, + *haima,* blood]. Localized deficiency of blood supply in muscle tissue.

myokerosis (mī″ō-kē-rō′sĭs) [Gr. *mys, myo-,* muscle, + *kēros,* wax, + *-ōsis,* intensive]. Waxy degeneration of muscle or muscular tissue.

my″okin′ase. An enzyme present in muscle which catalyzes the synthesis of adenosine triphosphate.

myokinesis (mī″ō-kĭn-ē′sĭs) [″+ *kinēsis,* motion]. 1. Muscular activity, 2. Surgical displacement of muscular fibers.

myokymia (mī-ō-kĭm′ī-ă) [″+ *kyma,* wave]. Twitching of fibers of a muscle. It may be functional and is also seen in organic affections and general paresis.

myolipoma (mī″ō-lĭ-pō′mă) [″+ *lipos,* fat, + *-ōma,* tumor]. Muscle tissue tumor containing fatty elements.

myology (mī-ŏl′ō-jī) [″+ *logos,* study]. The science or study of the muscles and their parts.

myolysis (mī-ŏl′ī-sĭs) [Gr. *mys, myo-,* muscle, + *lysis,* destruction]. Fatty degeneration and infiltration with destruction of muscular tissue accompanied by separation and disappearance of muscle cells.

myoma (mī-ō′mă) [″+ *-ōma,* tumor]. (pl. *myomas* or *myomata*) A tumor containing muscle tissue. SEE: *chondromyoma.*

   m., nonstriated. A tumor of unmarked muscle tissue. SYN: *leiomyoma.*

   m. striocellulare. Fibroma with striated muscular fibers. SYN: *rhabdomyoma.*

   m. telangiectodes. Coiled blood vessel tumor in muscular fibers; angiomyoma.

myomalacia (mī″ō-mă-lă′sī-ă) [″+ *malakia,* softening]. Softening of muscular tissue.

   m. cordis. Softening of the heart muscle.

myomatosis (mī-ō-mă-tō′sĭs) [″+ *-ōma,* tumor, + *-ōsis,* intensive]. The development of multiple myomas.

myomatous (mī-ō′mă-tŭs) [″+ *-ōma,* tumor]. Pert. to or resembling a myoma.

myomectomy (mī″ō-mĕk′tō-mī) [″+ ″+ *ektomē,* excision]. 1. Removal of a portion of muscle or muscular tissue. 2. Removal of a myomatous tumor, generally uterine, usually by abdominal section, leaving the uterus in place.

   NP: Same as for cesarean section. Position dorsal, possibly followed by Trendelenburg's.

myomelanosis (mī″ō-mĕl-ă-nō′sĭs) [Gr. *mys, myo-,* muscle, + *melanōsis,* blackening]. Abnormal darkening of muscle tissue.

myomere (mī′ō-mēr) [″+ *meros,* part]. Myotome, q.v.

myometer (mī-ŏm′ĕt-ĕr) [″+ *metron,* measure]. Device for measurement of muscular contractions.

myometritis (mī″ō-mē-trī′tĭs) [″+ *mētra,* uterus, + *-ītis,* inflammation]. Inflamed condition of the muscular wall of the uterus.

myometrium (mī″ō-mē′trī-ŭm). [NA] Muscular wall of the uterus forming the main mass of the uterus.

myomohysterectomy (mī-ō″mō-hĭs-tĕr-ĕk′-tō-mī) [Gr. *mys, myo-,* muscle, + *-ōma,* tumor, + *hystera,* uterus, + *ektomē,* excision]. Hysterectomy performed to remove a myomatous uterus.

myomotomy (mī″ō-mŏt′ō-mī) [″+ ″+ *tomē,* excision]. Excision of a myoma, usually uterine. SYN: *myomectomy.*

my'on [Gr. *mys, myo-*, muscle]. A single muscle.

myonarcosis (mī″ō-năr-kō'sĭs) [″+ *narkosis*, a numbing]. Muscular numbness.

myonephropexy (mī″ō-nef'rō-pĕk″sĭ) [″+ *nephros*, kidney, + *pēxis*, fixation]. Fixation of a movable kidney by attaching it to a portion of muscular tissue with sutures.

my″oneur'al. Pert. to muscle and nerve, esp. nerve terminations in muscles.

    m. junction. Ending of a nerve in a muscle. SEE: *motor end plate.*

myoneurasthenia (mī″ō-nūr-ās-thē'nĭ-ă) [Gr. *mys, myo-*, muscle, + *neuron*, nerve, + *astheneia*, weakness]. Relaxed condition of muscular system associated with neurasthenia.

myoneuroma (mī″ō-nū-rō'mă) [″+ ″+ *ōma*, tumor]. A neuroma partially composed of muscular elements.

myonosus (mī-on'ō-sŭs) [Gr. *mys, myo-*, muscle, + *nosos*, disease]. A disease of muscular tissue. SYN: *myopathy.*

myopachynsis (mī″ō-păk-ĭn″sĭs) [″+ *pachynsis*, thickening]. Abnormal thickening of muscle tissue.

myopalmus (mī-ō-păl'mŭs) [″+ *palmos*, a twitching.]. Twitching of muscles.

myoparalysis (mī″ō-pă-ral'ĭ-sĭs). Paralysis in a muscle; myoparesis.

my″opar'esis. Paralysis of a muscle.

myopathic (mī-ō-păth'ĭk) [Gr. *mys, myo-*, muscle, + *pathos*, disease]. 1. Pert. to muscular disease. 2. One suffering from a muscular disease.

    m. facies. Facial expression caused by relaxation of facial muscles.

myopathy (mī-ŏp'ă-thĭ). Any disease or abnormal condition of striated muscle.

    m., cortisone. Myopathy, especially of the limbs, following high dosage of corticosteroid preparations for an extensive period of time. Recovery takes place upon lowering the dose or discontinuing administration of the drug.

    m., facial. Atrophy of facial muscles. SYM: Lips pouted, smile twisted. Sometimes ptosis of upper eyelids; inability to whistle or to blow out the cheeks, depending upon the muscles affected.

    m., metabolic. Myopathy resulting from enzymatic defects in the muscle walls.

    m., thyrotoxic. A chronic disease characterized by progressive muscular weakness and atrophy and hyperthyroidism.

myope (mī'ōp) [Gr. *myein*, to shut, + *ōps*, eye]. One afflicted with myopia or nearsightedness.

myopericarditis (mī″ō-per-ĭ-kar-dī'tis) [Gr. *mys, myo-*, muscle, + *peri*, around, + *kardia*, heart, + *-itis*, inflammation]. Inflammation of the pericardium and cardiac muscular wall.

myophone (mī'ō-fōn) [″+ *phōnē*, voice]. Device for conveying sound of muscular contractions.

myo'pia [Gr. *myein*, to shut, + *ōps*, eye]. Defect in vision so that objects can only be seen distinctly when very close to the eyes; nearsightedness. Light rays come to a focus in front of the retina.

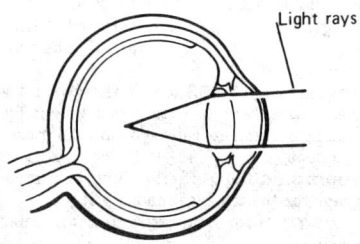

MYOPIA
Light rays do not focus on the retina.

    m., axial. M. due to elongation of the axis of the eye.

    m., chromic. Color blindness only when viewing distant objects.

    m. of curvature. M. due to curvature of the eye's refracting surfaces.

    m., index. M. resulting from abnormal refractivity of the media.

    m., malignant. Disease leading to retinal detachment and blindness. SYN: *pernicious m.; progressive m.*

    m., pernicious. M. with progressive disease of the choroid, terminating in blindness; malignant m.

    m., prodromal. M. in which reading without glasses becomes possible; seen in incipient cataract.

    m., progressive. M. that increases steadily during adult life.

    m., stationary. Myopia that comes to a stop after adult growth is attained.

    m., transient. M. seen in spasm of accommodation, as in acute iritis or iridocyclitis.

myopic (mī-ŏp'ĭk). Pert. to or affected with myopia.

    m. crescent. Posterior crescentic protrusion seen in myopia.

myoplasm (mī'ō-plăzm) [Gr. *mys, myo-*, muscle, + *plasma*, a thing formed]. The contractile part of the muscle cell, as differentiated from the sarcoplasm.

myoplastic (mī-ō-plăst'ĭk) ["+ *plassein*, to form]. Pert. to plastic use of muscle tissue or plastic surgery on muscles.

myoplasty (mĭ'ō-plăs-tĭ). Plastic surgery of muscle tissue.

myoplegia (mī"ō-plē'jĭ-ă) ["+ *plēgē*, stroke]. Muscular paralysis.

my"oportho'sis. Correction of myopia or nearsightedness.

myoprotein (mī"ō-prō'tēn). A protein found in muscle tissue.

myoproteose (mī"ō-prō'tē-ōs). A protein found in muscle plasma. SYN: *myoalbumose.*

myorrhaphy (mī-or'ă-fĭ) [Gr. *mys, myo-*, muscle, + *raphē*, a sewing]. Suture of a muscle wound.

myorrhexis (mī-or-ĕk'sĭs) ["+ *rhēxis*, a rupture]. Rupture of a muscle.

myosalgia (mī-ō-săl'jĭ-ă) ["+ *algos*, pain]. Pain in a muscle. SYN: *myalgia.*

myosalpingitis (mī"ō-săl-pĭn-jī'tĭs) ["+ *salpinx*, tube, + *-itis*, inflammation]. Inflamed condition of muscular tissue of a fallopian tube.

myosarcoma (mī"ō-sar-kō'mă) ["+ *sarx, sark-*, flesh, + *-ōma*, tumor]. Tumor derived from muscular tissue.

myosclerosis (mī"ō-sklĕr-ō'sĭs) ["+ *sklērōs*, hardening]. Hardening of muscle.

my'osin [Gr. *mys, myo-*, muscle]. A protein present in muscle fibrils and comprising about 65% of total muscle protein. It consists of long chains of polypeptides joined to each other by side chains. The molecular structure of myosin is thought to be responsible for the properties of muscle tissue, namely, birefringence, double refraction, contractility, and elasticity. Myosin combines with another muscle protein, actin, to form actomyosin.

m. ferment. A coagulating enzyme in muscle plasma. It converts myosinogen into myosin.

my"osinase'. An enzyme that catalyzes the conversion of myosinogen to myosin.

myosinogen (mī"ō-sĭn'ō-jĕn) [Gr. *mys, myo-*, muscle, + *gennan*, to produce]. A protein present in muscle tissue, the precursor of myosin. SYN: *myogen.*

myosinose (mī-ōs 'ĭn-ōs). A proteose resulting from the hydrolysis of myosin.

myosinuria (mī"ō-sĭn-ū'rĭ-ă). The occurrence of myosin in the urine.

myo'sis [Gr. *myein*, to close]. Contraction of the pupil. SEE: *miosis.*

ETIOL: Irritation of oculomotor system, paralysis of dilators. Occurs in certain fevers, congestion of iris, in typhus, in early stages of meningitis, and from drug poisoning. Seen in brain lesions, sunstroke, and pulmonary congestion.

myositis (mī-ō-sī'tĭs) [Gr. *mys, myo-*, muscle, + *-itis*, inflammation]. Inflammation of muscle tissue, esp. voluntary muscles. SEE: *fibrositis.*

ETIOL: Infection, trauma, diathetic states, or infestation by parasites.

m., interstitial. M. with hyperplasia of connective tissue.

m. ossificans. M. marked by ossification of muscles.

m., parenchymatous. M. of substance of a muscle.

m. purulenta. Suppurative m. with abscesses; caused by bacterial infection.

m., traumatic. May be simple with pain and swelling, or suppurative.

m. trichinosa; m., trichinous. M. due to infestation with trichinae.

myospasm (mī'ō-spăzm) ["+ *spasmos*, spasm]. Spasmodic contraction of a muscle.

myosteo'ma (mī-ŏs"tē-ō'mă) ["+ *osteon*, bone, + *-ōma*, tumor]. A bony growth found in muscle tissue.

myosuria (mī-ō-sū'rĭ-ă) ["+ *ouron*, urine]. Presence of myosin in the urine. SYN: *myosinuria.*

myosuture (mī"ō-sū'chūr) ["+ L. *sutura*, sewing]. Stitching of a muscle.

myosynizesis (mī-ō-sĭn-ĭ-zē'sĭs). [Gr. *mys, myo-*, muscle, + *synizēsis*, sitting together]. Adhesion of muscular layers of tissue.

myotactic (mī"ō-tăk'tĭk) ["+ L. *tactus*, touch]. Pert. to muscle or kinesthetic sense.

m. reflex. The stretch reflex, q.v.

myotasis (mī-ŏt'ă-sĭs) ["+ *tasis*, stretching]. Stretching of a muscle.

myotat'ic. Pert. to the stretching of muscles.

myotenontoplasty (mī"ō-tĕn-ŏn'tō-plăst-ĭ) [Gr. *mys, myo-*, muscle, + *tenōn, tenot-*, tendon, + *plassein*, to form]. Plastic operation involving muscles and tendons. SYN: *tenontomyoplasty.*

myotenositis (mī"ō-tĕn-ō-sī'tĭs) ["+ "+ *-itis*, inflammation]. Inflamed condition of a muscle and its tendon.

myotenotomy (mī"ō-tĕn-ŏt'ōmĭ) ["+ "+ *tomē, incision*]. Division of the tendon of a muscle.

myothermic (mī"ō-thĕrm'ĭk) ["+ *thermē*, heat]. Pert. to rise in muscle temperature due to its activity.

myot'ic [Gr. *myō*, to close the eyes]. 1. An agent that will contract the pupil of the eye. Ex: physostigmine, pilocarpine. 2. Producing contraction of a pupil.

myotility (mī-ō-tĭl'ĭ-tĭ) [Gr. *mys, myo-*, muscle]. Contractility of a muscle.

myotome (mī'ō-tōm) ["+ *tomē*, incision]. 1. Knife for cutting muscles. 2. That portion of an embryonic somite which gives rise to somatic (striated) muscles. SYN: *muscle plate*.

myotomy (mī-ŏt'ō-mĭ). Division or anatomical dissection of muscles.

myotonia (mī-ō-tō'nĭ-ă) ["+ *tonos*, tension]. Tonic spasm of a muscle, or temporary rigidity after muscular contraction.

   m. atrophica. M. dystrophica, q.v.

   m. congenita. A disease characterized by tonic spasms of the muscles induced by voluntary movements; usually congenital and transmitted from one generation to another.

   SYM: Disease appears in early childhood, is manifested by a tonic spasm of the muscles every time they are put in use. In a few minutes, rigidity wears away and the movements become free from repeated contractions, the muscles becoming firm and extremely well developed; under electrical treatment the muscles contract and relax slowly. SYN: *Thomsen's disease*.

   PROG: Incurable.

   TREATMENT: Quinine or procaineamide for relief of myotonia. Avoid obesity, prolonged bed rest, and inactivity. Neostigmine is contraindicated.

   m. dystrophica. An hereditary disease, it is characterized by muscular wasting, myotonia, and cataract. SYN: *m. atrophica; Steinert's disease*.

myoton'ic. Pert. to tonic muscular spasm, as differentiated from myokinetic spasm.

myotonometer (mī''ō-tō-nŏm'ĕt-ĕr) ["+ "+ *metron*, measure]. Instrument used to measure muscular tonus.

myot'onus ["+ *tonos*, tension]. A tonic muscle spasm with temporary rigidity.

myot'rophy ["+ *trophē*, nourishment]. Nutrition of the tissues of muscle.

Myriapoda (mĭr-ĭ-ăp'ō-dă) [Gr. *myrios*, numberless, + *pous, pod-*, foot]. Group of arthropods including millepedes and centipedes.

myriapodiasis (mĭr''ĭ-ăp-ō-dī'ă-sĭs). Infestation with one of the Myriapoda.

myringa (mĭr-ĭn'gă) [L.]. The tympanic membrane.

myringectomy (mĭr-ĭn-jĕk'tō-mĭ) ["+ Gr. *ektomē*, excision]. Myringodectomy, q.v.

myringitis (mĭr-ĭn-jī'tĭs) [L. *myringa*, drum membrane, + Gr. *-ītis*, inflammation]. Inflammation of the tympanum or eardrum.

   m. bullosa. M. with serous or hemorrhagic blebs or vesicular inflammation of the eardrum and adjacent wall.

myringodectomy (mĭr-ĭn-gōdĕk'tō-mĭ) [L. *myringa*, drum membrane + Gr. *ektomē*,

excision]. Excision of a part or the entire tympanic membrane. SYN: *myringectomy*.

myringomycosis (mĭr-ĭn''gō-mĭ-kō'sĭs) ["+ Gr. *mykes*, fungus, + *ōsis*, intensive]. Inflammation of the tympanic membrane resulting from infection by parasitic fungi. SYN: *mycomyringitis; otomycosis; mycotic otitis externa*.

myringoplasty (mĭr-ĭn'gō-plăst-ĭ) ["+ Gr. *plassein*, to form]. Plastic operation on membrana tympani.

myringoscope (mĭr-ĭn'gō-skōp) ["+ Gr. *skopein*, to examine]. Instrument used for examination of the eardrum.

myringotome (mĭ-rĭn'gō-tōm) ["+ Gr. *tomē*, incision]. Knife for incising the tympanic membrane.

myringotomy (mĭr-ĭn-gŏt'ō-mĭ). Incision of tympanic membrane.

myrrh (mur) [Gr. *myrra*]. A gum resinous substance used by man for many centuries. In antiquity, cherished as a constituent of incense and perfume; most important use today is as an aromatic, astringent mouthwash. Tincture of m. provides symptomatic relief when applied to canker sores.

mysophobia (mī-sō-fō'bĭ-ă) [Gr. *mysos*, filth, + *phobos*, fear]. Abnormal aversion to dirt or contamination.

mytacism (mī'tă-sĭzm) [Gr. *mytakismos* from Gr. letter μ]. Excessive or incorrect use of the letter *m* or the *m* sound, in writing or speaking.

mythomania (mĭth''ō-mā'nĭ-ă) [Gr. *mythos*, myth, + *mania*, madness]. Abnormal tendency to lie and exaggerate.

mythophobia (mĭth''ō-fō'bĭ-ă) ["+ *phobos*, fear]. Abnormal dread of making a false or incorrect statement.

myxadenitis (mĭks-ad-en-ī'tĭs) [Gr. *myxa*, mucus, + *adēn*, gland, + *-ītis*, inflammation]. Inflammation of mucous gland or glands.

   m. labialis. Painless m. of the lips. SYN: *Baelz's disease; cheilitis glandularis*.

myxadenoma (mĭks''ăd-ē-nō'mă) ["+ "+ *-ōma*, tumor]. 1. A tumor with the structure of a mucous gland. SYN: *myxoadenoma*. 2. A tumor of glandular structure containing mucous elements.

myxangitis (mĭks-ăn-jī'tis) ["+ *angeion*, vessel, + *-ītis*, inflammation]. Inflammation of mucous gland ducts.

myxasthenia (mĭks-ăs-thē'nĭ-ă) ["+ *asthēneia*, weakness]. Imperfect or insufficient secretion of mucus.

myxedema (mĭks-ĕ-dē'mă) [Gr. *myxa*, mucus, + *oidēma*, swelling]. Condition resulting from hypofunction of the thyroid gland. Occurs in older children and adults. SYN: *Gull's disease.*

ETIOL: Iodine deficiency in diet, surgical excision or atrophy of thyroid gland, excessive use of antithyroid drugs. May occur secondary to hypofunction of anterior pituitary and is complicated by adrenal and gonadal deficiencies.

SYM: Low B.M.R. (–35 to –40), low radioactive iodine uptake by thyroid, decreased protein-bound iodine, anemia, myxedematous facies, large tongue, slow speech, puffiness of hands and face, coarse and thickened edematous skin, loss and dryness of hair, mental apathy, drowsiness, and sensitivity to cold.

TREATMENT: Desiccated thyroid.

m., childhood. M. occurring before puberty.

m., operative. M. following removal of thyroid gland. SYN: *cachexia strumipriva.*

m., pituitary. M. occurring secondary to anterior pituitary hypofunction.

myxedematoid (mĭks-ĕ-dēm'ă-toid) ["+ "+ *eidos,* resemblance]. Resembling myxedema.

myxedematous (mĭks-ĕ-dēm'ă-tŭs) ["+ *oidēma,* swelling]. Marked by or concerning myxedema.

myxemia (mĭk-sē'mĭ-ă) [Gr. *myxa,* mucus, + *haima,* blood]. Accumulation of mucin in the blood. SYN: *mucinemia.*

myxidiotie (mĭks-ĭd-ĭ-ot'ĭk) ["+ *idiōtēs,* private]. Myxedema with marked mental defects.

myxiosis (mĭks-ĭ-ō'sĭs) [Gr. *myxa,* mucus]. A mucous discharge or secretion.

myxo-, myx- [Gr. *myxa*]. Combining form designating relationship to mucus.

myxoadenoma (mĭks"ō-ăd-ē-nō'mă) ["+ *adēn,* gland, + *-ōma,* tumor]. Myxadenoma.

Myxobacterales (mix"ō-băk-tĕ-rā'lēz). An order of bacteria found in soil and dung. Characterized by a slimy spreading colony.

myx"ochon"drofibrosar"co'ma. A malignant tumor composed of myxomatous, chondromatous, fibrous, and sarcomatous elements.

my"xochondro'ma. A benign tumor composed of myxomatous and chondromatous elements.

myxocystoma (mĭk"sō-sĭs-tō'mă) ["+ *kystis,* cyst, + *-ōma,* tumor]. A benign cystic tumor containing mucus.

myxoedema (mĭks-ĕ-dē'mă) [Gr. *myxa,* mucus, + *oidema,* swelling]. Myxedema, q.v.

myxoenchondroma (mĭks"ō-ĕn-kŏn-drō'mă) ["+ *en,* in, + *chondros,* cartilage, + *-ōma,* tumor]. A cartilaginous tissue tumor which has undergone partial mucous degeneration.

myxofibroma (mĭks"ō-fĭ-brō'mă) ["+ L. *fibra,* fiber, + Gr. *-ōma,* tumor]. Tumor composed of mucous and fibrous elements.

myxoglioma (mĭk"sō-glĭ-ō'mă) [Gr. *myxa,* mucus, + *glia,* glue, + *-ōma,* tumor]. Tumor composed of myxomatous and gliomatous elements.

myxoid (mĭk'soid) ["+ *eidos,* resemblance]. Similar to or resembling mucus.

myxoinoma (mĭk"sō-ĭn-ō'mă). A myxofibroma, q.v.

myxolipoma (mĭk"sō-lĭ-pō'mă) ["+ *lipos,* fat, + *-ōma,* tumor]. Mucous tumor with fatty tissue elements in it. SYN: *lipomyxoma.*

myxoma (mĭk-sō'mă) [Gr. *myxa,* mucus, + *-ōma,* tumor]. (pl. *myxomas* or *myxomata*) A tumor composed of mucous connective tissue similar to that present in the embryo or umbilical cord. Cells are stellate or spindle-shaped and separated by mucoid. The tumors are usually soft, gray, lobulated, and translucent and are not completely encapsulated. May be pure or of mixed types involving other types of tissue.

m., cartilaginous. Chondromyxoma, q.v.

m., cystic, cystoid. One with parts fluid enough to resemble cysts.

m., enchondromatous. One with nodules of hyaline cartilage.

m., erectile. M. containing an excess of vessels, resembling an angioma.

m., fibrous. Fibromyxoma, q.v.

m., intracanalicular, of the mamma. One developing in the interstitial connective tissue of the mamma.

m., telangiectatic, vascular. One of highly vascular structure.

myxomatosis (mĭk"sō-mă-tō'sĭs). 1. Formation of multiple myxomas. 2. Degeneration of myxomatous type.

myxomycetes (mĭk"sō-mī-sē'tēz) [Gr. *myxa,* mucus, + *mykēs,* fungus]. A group of organisms of uncertain classification, but thought to be fungus-like. Includes slime molds. SEE: *Myxobacterales*

myxomyoma (mĭk-sō-mī-ō'mă) ["+ *mys, myo-,* muscie, + *-ōma,* tumor]. Muscle tissue tumor that has undergone mucous degeneration.

myxoneuroma (mĭks"ō-nū-rō'mă) ["+ *neuron,* nerve, + *-ōma,* tumor]. Tumor composed of mucous and nerve tissue elements.

myxopapilloma (mĭk"sō-păp'ĭl-ō'mă) ["+ L. *papilla,* nipple, + Gr. *-ōma,* tumor]. Combination myxomatous and papillomatous tumor or tumors.

myxorrhea (mĭk-sō-rē'ă) ["+ *rhoia,* flow]. Free discharge from mucous surfaces. SYN: *blennorrhea.*

*m. **gastrica.*** Excessive mucous secretion in the stomach.

*m. **intestinalis.*** Secretion of mucus from the bowel in neurotic persons in times of mental stress.

myxosarcoma (mĭk″sō-săr-kō′mă) [Gr. *myxa*, mucus, *sarx, sark-*, flesh, + *-ōma*, tumor]. Mixed tumor, partly myxomatous and partly sarcomatous, having undergone partial degeneration.

myxosarcomatous (mĭk″sō-săr-kō′măt-ŭs) ["+ "+ *-ōma*, tumor]. Pert. to or of the nature of myxosarcoma.

myxospore (mĭk′sō-spor) [Gr. *myxa*, mucus, + *sporos*, seed]. Spore embedded in a gelatinous mass, seen in some fungi and protozoa.

Myxosporidia (mĭk-sō-spor-ĭd′ĭ-ă). Parasitic sporozoans, most commonly found in epithelial cells of lower vertebrates.

myxoviruses. Family of viruses including those which cause influenza. SEE: *paramyxoviruses.*

myzesis (mĭ-zē′sĭs) [Gr. *myzain*, to suck]. Sucking.

N

N. 1. Chem. symb. for *nitrogen.* 2. Abbr. for *normal,* esp. with reference to solutions.

n. 1. Symbol for *index of refraction.* 2. Abbr. for *nasal; number.*

N¹⁵. Symb. for radioactive isotope of *nitrogen.*

NA. Abbr. for *nicotinic acid; Nomina Anatomica; numerical aperture; Nurse's Aid.*

Na. Sodium.

nabothian cysts (na-bō'thǐ-ăn). Retention cysts formed by the n. follicles at neck of uterus. SYN: *n. follicles; n. glands.* SEE: *cyst.*

ETIOL: Due to closing of mouths of glands by new epithelium of a healed erosion. They always denote an erosion has been present.

NaBr. Sodium bromide

NaCl. Sodium chloride.

NaClO. Sodium hypochlorite.

Na₂CO₃. Sodium carbonate.

nacreous (nā'krē-ŭs) [L. *nacer,* pearl shell]. Having an iridescent pearl-like luster, as bacterial colonies.

NAD. Abbr. for *nicotinamide àdenine dinucleotide.*

N.A.D. Abbr. for *no appreciable disease.*

Naegele's obliquity. [Franz Carl Naegele, Ger. obstetrician, 1777-1851] Inclination of fetal head, laterally in a flat pelvis.

Naegele's pelvis. An obliquely contracted pelvis, caused by disease in infancy.

Naegele's rule. To estimate the day labor will begin, count back 3 months from the day the last menstrual period began and add 7 days.

NaF. Sodium fluoride.

NaHCO₃. Sodium bicarbonate.

NaHSO₃. Sodium bisulfite.

nail [AS. *naegel*]. 1. A rod made of metal, bone, or solid material used to attach the ends or pieces of broken bones. 2. A horny cell structure of the epidermis forming flat plates upon the dorsal surface of the terminal phalanges. SYN: *unguis* (L.); *onyx* (Gr.).

A nail consists of a body, the exposed portion, and a root, the proximal portion hidden by the nail fold, both of which rest on the nail bed or matrix. The latter consists of epithelium and corium continuous with the epidermis and dermis of the skin of the nail fold. The crecent-shaped white area near the root is the lunula. The epidermis extending from the margin of the nail fold over the root is called eponychium; that underlying the free border of the distal portion is called hyponychium.

A nail grows in length and thickness through activity of cells in the stratum germinativum in region of the root. Average rate of growth in fingernails is about 1 mm. per week. It is slower in toenails and slower in summer than in winter. It varies with age and is affected by disease and certain hormone deficiencies.

Changes in the nails, such as ridges, may occur in defective nutrition or after a serious illness. In achlorhydria and hypochromic anemia, excessive spoon-shaped nails with center depression may occur. In chronic pulmonary conditions and congenital heart disease excessive curving of the nails may be associated with clubbed fingers.

ATROPHY: May occur as a result of hereditary or congenital tendencies. Permanent atrophy may follow injuries, scars from disease, frostbite, nerve injuries and hyperthyroidism. Nail shedding is due to the same causes.

Nails that are fragile or split often may be congenital or due to prolonged contact with chemicals or to too frequent manicuring.

DISCOLORATIONS: *Black:* In diabetes and other forms of gangrene. *Blueblack:* Common condition, usually due to hemorrhage, bleeding diseases such as hemophilia, and trauma. May be painful and can be relieved by drilling a small hole in the nail at the site of hemorrhage. This may be done by using a dental drill or the heated tip of a paper clip or similar rigid wire. *Brown:* May be due to arsenical poisoning. *Brownish-black:* This discoloration often indicates chronic mercurial poisoning due to formation of sulfide of mercury in the tissues. *Cyanosis:* Usually indicates anemeia, poor circulation, or venous stasis. *Slate:* This is an early manifestation of argyria and administration of silver should be stopped at once. *White spots:* Striate lesions may be due to trauma and are more frequent in women. Transverse white bands in all nails may be a sign of acute or chronic arsenical poisoning, or rarely of thallium acetate poisoning. SYN: *leukonychia.*

DRY, MALFORMED: May result from trophic changes resulting from injury to nerve or finger, neuritis, Raynaud's disease, pulmonary osteoarthropathy, syphilis, onychia, scleroderma, acrodermatitis and granuloma fungoides of the fingers.

STRIATIONS, LONGITUDINAL: Often found in those past middle life; frequently associated with onychorrhexis, splitting at the free margins. Note in association with a focus of infection in the bowel or at root of a tooth. Vitamin deficiency may be a cause. Microscopic examination of nail clippings should be made for ringworm. When hard and brittle, gouty conditions are indicated.

Transverse lines (Beau's lines) may result from previous interference of nail matrix growth. May be caused by local or systemic conditions. Approximate date of lesion may be determined, as it takes 4-6 months for the nail to grow.

ULCERS AND ECCHYMOSIS: Chancre may be suspected if a small, indolent ulcer appears near the nail, esp. if indurated and associated with enlarged lymph glands above the inner condyle.

QUINCKE'S CAPILLARY PULSATION: Rhythmic flushing and blanching most frequent in aortic regurgitation and often in anemia.

n. bed. The end of a finger or toe covered by the nail. SYN: *nail matrix.*

n. biting. A nervous affliction or neurosis in which the free edges of the nails are bitten down to the quick. SYN: *onychophagia.*

n., eggshell. Nail plate is soft, semitransparent, bends easily, and splits at end. Associated with arthritis, peripheral neuritis, leprosy, and hemiplegia. May be the only visible sign of late syphilis.

n. fold. Groove in the cutaneous tissue surrounding the margins and proximal edges of the nail.

n. groove. The space between nail wall and the nail bed.

n., hang. Broken epidermis at edge of the nail. SYN: *agnail.*

n., ingrowing. Nail with tissue overgrowing its edges causing a pyogenic neoplasm.

n. matrix. The nail bed, q.v.

n., reedy. One marked by longitudinal fissures.

n. root. Proximal portion of nail covered by nail fold.

n., spoon. A nail with central portion depressed and lateral edges elevated.

n. wall. Epidermis covering edges of the nail. SYN: *vallum unguis.*

naked (nā'kĕd) [AS. *naced,* nude]. Uncovered, exposed to view, nude, bare.

nalorphine (nal-or'fēn). Generic name for N-allylnormorphine. Used in treatment of certain kinds of narcotic overdose especially morphine.

nanism (na'nizm) [L. *nanus,* dwarf]. Condition of being dwarflike in build.

n., symptomatic. N. with deficient dentition, sexual development, and ossification.

nano- (nā'nō) [L. *nanus,* dwarf]. Prefix indicating 1 billionth of the unit following. Thus a nanogram is 1 billionth of a gram.

nanocephalism (nan-ō-sef'ăl-ĭzm) ["+ *kephalē,* head]. Condition of having an abnormally small head.

nanocephalous (nan-ō-sĕf'ă-lŭs). Having an abnormally small head.

nanocormia (nā"nō-kor'mĭ-ā) ["+ *kormos,* trunk]. Abnormally dwarfed thorax or body.

nanoid (nā'noid) ["+ *eidos,* like]. Dwarflike.

nanomelus (nā-nŏm'ē-lus). Fetus with congenital deformity characterized by undersized extremities.

nanosoma. Nanosomia, q.v.

nanosomia (nā-nō-sō'mĭ-ā) [L. *nanus,* dwarf, + *sōma,* body]. State of being a dwarf. SEE: *nanism.*

nanosomus (nā-nō-sō'mŭs). A person of stunted size; a dwarf.

nanous (nan'ŭs) [L. *nanus,* dwarf]. Dwarfed or stunted.

na'nus. 1. A dwarf. 2. Stunted; dwarflike.

NaOH. Sodium hydroxide.

nap (năp) [AS. *hnappian,* nap]. 1. To slumber. 2. A short sleep; a doze.

napalm (na'palm) [from *na*phthene + *palm*itate]. Gasoline made thick or jelly-like for use in incendiary bombs and flame throwers.

n. burn. Burn due to use of napalm, usually during war.

nape (nāp; năp) [origin uncertain]. Back of neck.

napex (na'peks) [origin uncertain]. Scalp beneath the occipital protuberance.

naphtha (naf'thă). 1. A volatile inflammable liquid distilled from carbonaceous substances. 2. Petroleum, esp. more volatile varieties.

naphthalene (naf'thă-lēn). $C_{10}H_8$. A hydrocarbon, one of principal constituents of coal tar.

USES: As a disinfectant, in moth balls, and in manufacture of dyes and explosives.

naphthol (năf'thōl). $C_{10}H_7OH$. Coal tar substance used as an antiseptic and in certain dyes. Also prepared from naphthalene.

napiform (na'pĭ-form) [L. *napus,* turnip, + *forma,* shape.]. In bacteriology, formed like a turnip, as gelatin liquefaction in a culture.

naprapathy (nă-prăp'ăth-ĭ) [Bohemian *napravit,* correction, + Gr. *pathos,* disease]. Method of therapeutic manipulation based upon the assumption that all disease is caused by faulty functioning of ligaments.

narcism, narcissism (nar'sĭzm, nar-sĭs'-izm). [Narcissus, a Gr. mythical character who fell in love with his own image]. 1. Self-love or self-admiration. 2. Sexual pleasure derived from observing one's own naked body.

narcissistic (nar-sĭs-sĭst'ĭk). Pert. to narcissism.

    n. object choice. Selection of another like one's own self as the object of love, friendship, or liking.

narco- [Gr. *narkē*, numbness]. Combining form meaning numbness, stupor.

narcoanesthesia (nar″kō-ăn-ĕs-thē'zĭ-ă). Anesthesia produced by a narcotic, as scopolamine and morphine.

narcohypnia (nar″kō-hĭp'nĭ-ă) [Gr. *narkē*, numbness, + *hypnos*, sleep]. Numbness following sleep.

narcohypnosis (när-cō″hĭp-nō'sĭs). Stupor or deep sleep produced by hypnosis. SYN: *hypnonarcosis.*

narcolepsy (nar'ko-lĕp-sĭ) [″+ *lēpsis*, seizure]. A chronic ailment consisting of recurrent attacks of drowsiness and sleep. The patient is unable to control these spells of sleep but he is easily awakened. About three quarters of persons with narcolepsy also experience cataplexy, q.v. Except for frequent sleep patterns, the electroencephalogram is normal. SYN: *sleep epilepsy; paroxysmal sleep.*

    TREATMENT: Symptomatic with stimulants.

    ETIOL: Unknown.

narcoleptic (nar-ko-lĕp'tĭk) [″+ *lēpsis*, seizure]. Pert. to or marked by an overwhelming desire to sleep.

narcoma (nar-kō'mă) [″+ *kōma*, coma]. Coma or stupor from use of a narcotic.

narcomania (nar-kō-mā'nĭ-ă) [Gr. *narkē*, numbness, + *mania*, madness]. 1. Abnormal craving for alcohol or narcotics. 2. Insanity due to use of alcohol or narcotics.

narcomaniac (nar-kō-mā'nĭ-ăk). 1. Pert. to narcomania. 2. One affected by narcomania.

narcomatous (nar-kō-mā'tus) [″+ *kōma*, coma]. Pert. to a state of stupor from use of narcotics.

nar'cose [Gr. *narkē*, stupor]. In a stuporous state.

narco'sis [Gr. *narkōsis*, a benumbing]. Unconscious state due to narcotics.

    n., basal. Initial n. produced by sedatives used prior to administration of a general anesthetic.

    n., medullary. General anesthesia induced by a local anesthetic injected in the sheath of the spinal cord in lumbar region. SYN: *spinal anesthesia.*

narcosomania (nar-kō″sō-mā'nĭ-ă) [″+ *mania*, madness]. Morbid craving for narcotics or insanity produced by narcotics. SYN: *narcomania.*

narcot'ic [Gr. *narkōtikos*, benumbing]. 1. Producing stupor or sleep. 2. A drug which in moderate doses depresses the central nervous system thus relieving pain and producing sleep but which in excessive doses produces unconsciousness, stupor, coma, and possibly death. Examples are opium, morphine, codeine, papaverine, heroin, and many synthetics. Most are habit forming. 3. Anything that soothes, relieves or lulls. 4. One addicted to the use of narcotics.

    Narcotics are more powerful than hypnotics. Ex: chloral hydrate, sulfonal, trional, veronal.

    RS: drug addiction.

    n. addict. One who has become physiologically or psychologically dependent upon narcotics.

narcotism (nar'kō-tizm) [Gr. *narkē*, stupor, + *ismos*, condition]. 1. State of stupor induced by a narcotic. SYN: *narcosis.* 2. An addiction to the use of narcotics.

    Addiction may be said to exist when discontinuance causes abstinence symptoms relieved speedily by a dose of the drug. It is this addition to the original purpose in taking the drug that so readily aggravates the need.

    TREATMENT: Ordinarily successful only during hospitalization. Experimental use of drugs, even though they are narcotics, has fewer undesired effects and has resulted in some success. Relapses are frequent and the building up of a new philosophy of life is of prime importance.

    POISONING: Narcotic or sleep producing poisons as opium and its derivatives, chloral combinations, barbital and its myriad subvarieties, etc.

    SYM. AND SIGNS: Depression, slowing of heart and respiration, sleep, followed by coma.

    F. A. TREATMENT: Remove poison by vomiting, purging, diuretics, intravenous hypertonic glucose. Administer stimulants by appropriate routes.

nar'cotize (Gr. *narkōtikos*, benumbing). To place under the influence of a narcotic.

naris (nā'ris) [L.]. (pl. *nares*) [NA]. The nostril.

    n., anterior. External nostril.

    n., posterior. The opening between the nasal cavity and the nasopharynx.

    RS: anosmia; epistaxis; hyperosmia; nose; parosmia; septum; smell.

nasal (nā'zl) [L. *nasus*, nose]. 1. Pert. to the nose. 2. Uttered through the nose. 3. A nasal bone.

n. bones. The two small bones forming the arch of the nose.

n. cartilages. C. forming principal portion of framework of external nose.

n. cavity. C. between floor of cranium and roof of mouth.

n. conchae. SEE: *concha, nasal.*

n. douche. Injection of fluid into nostril, with fluid escaping by way of the nasopharynx out of the mouth.

Patient should keep mouth open to prevent fluid from entering the throat. Force must not be great. Atomized spray is safer. Container should not be suspended over 6 inches (9.2 cm.) above patient, who should not blow the nose during treatment.

n. feeding. N. gavage, q.v.

n. fossa. One of the two halves of the nasal cavity.

n. gavage. Feeding through a tube in the nasal passage. This is resorted to when it is the only route available to the stomach or when the patient refuses to eat. Quite often in the latter case, nasal feeding is necessary to make him realize that it is much easier to eat.

NP: Throughout a course of tube feedings in mental cases, the nurse should frequently experiment to see if the patient will eat. Try him with a fully prepared tray. Also offer the tube feeding in a glass that he may drink it. Again, it should be remembered that suggestion is a very powerful factor in the care of the mental patient, so the nurse may see the reflection of her own attitude in the patient's behavior.

ARTICLES NECESSARY: Tray with feeding (consisting usually of milk, eggs, sugar and malted milk, concentrated broths, purées with milk, cream, and orange juice) at room temperature. Pitcher of water (about 100 ml.). Basin with ice and nasal tube and funnel. Medicine glass with glycerine. Gowns for doctor and nurse. Rubber draw sheet to protect patient. Face towel. Bowl of water to invert funnel in. Any medication ordered.

PROCEDURE: Have patient in bed or in chair according to the doctor's wishes, usually in a chair however. Restrain if a mental patient with a blanket sheet or restraining jacket. Protect patient with rubber draw sheet. Attach nasal tube to funnel, pour water into it, and clamp tube so no air will enter. Dip end of nasal tube in glycerine. After tube is inserted, note color of face, invert funnel in water and if air bubbles appear, tube is in the trachea and should be removed immediately. If certain tube is in stomach, fill funnel with feeding and hold slightly above patient's head to allow flow by gravity. Give any medication, also water. Hold towel over patient's mouth and keep head raised slightly as patient is more apt to retain the feeding. Remove tube quickly and keep patient quiet for a few minutes, until desire for regurgitation has passed. Entire amount of fluid given at one feeding should not exceed 500 ml. Three or four feedings of this size are preferable to one large feeding.

n. height. Distance bet. lower border of nasal aperture and the nasion.

n. index. The greatest width of the nasal aperture in relation to a line from the lower edge of the n. aperture to the nasion.

n. line. L. from lower edge of the ala nasi curving to outer side of the orbicularis oris muscle. SYN: *Jadelot's furrow* or *line.*

n. meatus. SEE: *meatus.*

n. obstruction. Commonest causes: Irregular septum; enlarged turbinates; nasal polypi; in children foreign bodies such as food, buttons, or pins. Many complications result.

TREATMENT: Nasal douches, inhalations and operative care: resection of septum; turbinectomy; removal of polypi; opening and draining sinuses; removal of foreign body.

n. reflex. Sneezing resulting from irritation of nasal mucosa.

n. sinuses, accessory. The paranasal sinuses, q.v. SEE: *sinuses, accessory nasal.*

n. width. Maximum width of nasal aperture.

nascent (năs'ĕnt; nā'sĕnt) [L. *nascens*, born]. 1. Just born; incipient or beginning. 2. Pert. to a substance being set free from a compound.

nasion (nā'zĭ-ŏn) [L. *nasus*, nose]. The point where the nasofrontal suture is cut across by the median anteroposterior plane.

nasitis (nā-zī'tĭs) ["+ Gr. -*itis*, inflammation]. Inflammation of the nose. SEE: *rhinitis.*

Nasmyth's membrane (năz'mĭth). [Alexander Nasmyth, Scotch dental surgeon, —1847]. Epithelial m. enveloping enamel of a tooth for short period after birth.

naso- [L. *nasus,* nose]. Combining form indicating relationship to the nose.

nasoantritis (nā"zō-ăn-trī'tĭs) [L. *nasus,* nose, + Gr. *antron,* cavity, + -*itis,* inflammation]. Inflammation of nose and antrum of Highmore.

nasociliary (nā"zō-sĭl'ĭ-ār-ĭ). Pert. to nose, eyebrow, and eyes. Applied esp. to nerve supplying these structures.

nasofron'tal [L. *nasus,* nose, + *frons, front-,* forehead]. Pert. to nasal and frontal bones.

nasola'bial ["+ *labium,* lip]. Connected with or rel. to the nose and lip.

nasolacrimal (nā″zō-lăk ′rĭm -ăl) ["+ *lacrima,* tear]. Pert. to nose and lacrimal apparatus.

nasology (nā-zōl′ō-jĭ) ["+ Gr. *logos,* study]. Study of the nose and its diseases.

nasomental (nā″zō-mĕn ′tăl) ["+ *mentum,* chin]. Pert. to the nose and chin.

n. reflex. Contraction of mentalis muscle with elevation of lower lip and wrinkling of skin of chin. Elicited by percussion of side of nose.

nasopalatine (nā″zō-păl′ă-tīn) [L. *nasus,* + *palatum,* palate]. Pert. to both nose and palate.

nasopharyngeal (nā″zō-făr-ĭn′jē-ăl) ["+ Gr. *pharynx,* pharynx]. Pert. to the pharynx and nose.

nasopharyngitis (nā″zō-făr-ĭn-jī′tĭs) ["+ "+ *-itis,* inflammation]. Inflamed condition of the nasopharynx.

nasopharynx (nā″zō-far′ĭnks) ["+ Gr. *pharynx,* pharynx]. Part of pharynx situated above the soft palate (postnasal space).

nasoscope (nā′zō-skōp) ["+ Gr. *skopein,* to examine]. Electrical device for examination of the nasal cavity.

nasoseptitis (nā″zō-sĕp-tī′tĭs) ["+ *saeptum,* partition]. Inflamed condition of the nasal septum.

nasosinuitis, nasosinusitis (nā″zō-sĭn-ū-ī′-tĭs, -sī-nū-sī′tĭs) ["+ *sinus,* cavity]. Inflammation of the nasal accessory sinuses and cavities.

nasospinale (nā″zō-spīn′-ăl-ē). Point at which med. sagittal plane intersects line joining lowest points on nasal margins.

nasus (nā′sŭs) [L.]. [NA]. The nose, organ for respiration and sense of smell. SEE: *nose.*

natal (nā′tăl). 1. [L. *natus,* birth]. Pert. to birth or the day of birth. 2. [L. *nates,* buttocks]. Pert. to the buttocks.

natal'ity [L. *natus, natalis,* birth]. The birth rate, ratio of births to population of a given community.

natant (nā′tănt) [L. *natāre,* to swim]. Floating; swimming.

nates (nā′tēz) [L.]. (pl. of *natis*) 1. [NA]. region; fleshy prominences on the lower back formed by the gluteal muscles with a covering of fat and skin. SYN: *buttocks.* 2. The ant., sup. or upper two corpora quadrigemina.

natimortality (nā″tĭ-mor-tăl′ĭ-tĭ) [L. *natus,* one born, + *mortalitās,* death.]. Rate of stillbirths in proportion to birth rate.

National Formulary. Formulary issued by the Amer. Pharmaceutical Assn. ABBR: N.F.

native (nā′tĭv) [L. *nativus*]. 1. Born with; inherent. 2. Natural, normal. SYN: *indigenous.* 3. Belonging to, as place of one's birth.

n. albumin. Albumin normally found in the body. SEE: *albumin.*

natremia (nă-trē′mĭ-ă) [L. *natrium,* sodium, + Gr. *haima,* blood]. Sodium in the blood.

natrium (nā′trĭ-um) [L.]. SYMB: Na. Sodium. This is found abundantly in plants, animal fluids, and minerals, as common salt.

natriuresis (nā″trē-ū-rē′sĭs) ["+ Gr. *ouresis,* make water]. Sodium normally excreted in the urine.

natriuretic. A drug which causes loss of sodium in the urine. SEE: *diuretic.*

na'tron. Sodium carbonate

na'trum. Homeopathic name for soda or sodium.

natural [L. *natura,* nature]. Not abnormal or artificial.

n. selection. A theory of evolution proposed by Chas. Darwin to account for the origin of species. Essential points are that all species tend to overproduce. As food supply is limited, there is a struggle for existence. Variations occur, hence individuals possessing favorable variations would tend to survive; those with unfavorable ones would die out. Through heredity, such variations would be transmitted to successive generations and, in time, new types or species differing from their ancestors would come into existence.

na'turopath ["+ Gr. *pathos,* suffering]. One who practices naturopathy.

naturopathy (nā″tŭr-op′ă-thĭ). A therapeutic system which does not use drugs or therapy, but employs natural forces such as light, heat, air, water and massage.

nausea (naw′sē-ă) [Gr. *nausia,* seasickness]. Inclination to vomit; usually preceding emesis.

It is present in seasickness, early pregnancy, diseases of the central nervous system, neurasthenia, hysteria. It may be due to the sight or odor of obnoxious matter or conditions or to mental images of same. It may be present, without vomiting, in certain gallbladder disturbances and in carsickness.

NP: Report the nature of vomitus, if it occurs, frequency and time, effect of food and sleep, bilious, fecal, profuse, purulent, watery, mucous, and hematemesis. Be prepared to maintain airway if patient is stuporous. SEE: *vomitus.*

n. gravidarum. Morning sickness of pregnancy.

n. navalis. Seasickness. SYN: *mal de mer.*

nauseant (naw'shē-ănt; naw'sē-ănt). 1. Provoking nausea. 2. That which causes nausea.

nauseate (naw'shē̯-āt; naw'sē-āt). To cause nausea.

nauseous (naw'shus; naw'shē-ŭs). Producing nausea, disgust, or loathing. Also to be nauseated.

navel (nā'vĕl) [AS. *nafela*]. The depression or scar in center of abdomen, where the umbilical cord was attached to fetus. SYN: *umbilicus,* q.v.

RS: umbilical cord; umbilicate.

    n. string. Umbilical cord.

navicula (nă-vīk'ū-lă) [L. *navicula,* boat]. Fossa navicularis, q.v.

navicular (nă-vīk'ū-lar). 1. Shaped like a boat. 2. Scaphoid bones in the carpus and in the tarsus. SEE: *skeleton.*

    n. fossa. SEE: *fossa navicularis.*

Nb. Chem. symb. for the element *niobium* (columbium).

N.C.A. Neurocirculatory asthenia.

Nd. Chem. symb. for neodymium.

Ne. Chem. symb. for neon.

near point. Closest point of distinct vision with maximum accommodation. It recedes with age, varying from 3 in. (7.62 cm.) at 2 yr. to 40 in. (101.60 cm.) at 60 yr. ABBR: n.p. SYN: *punctum proximum.*

    n. p., absolute. For either eye.

    n. p., relative. For both eyes taken together.

nearsight. Ability to see clearly only those objects held close to the eye. SYN: *myopia.* SEE: *nearsighted.*

nearsighted. Ability to see clearly only those objects held close to the eye.

This is caused by inability of the image to be focused on the back of the eye. A negative (concave) lense will correct myopia. SYN: *myopic.* RS: hypermetropia; farsighted; presbyopia; eye.

nearsightedness. Ability to see distinctly only a short distance. SYN: *myopia.*

nearthrosis (nē''ar-thrō'sĭs) [Gr. *neos,* new, + *arthron,* joint]. A false joint or abnormal articulation.

nebula (nĕb'ū-lă) [L. mist, cloud). (pl. *nebulae*) 1. Slight haziness on the cornea. 2. Cloudiness in urine. 3. Aqueous or oil substance for use in an atomizer.

    n. corneae. Grayish opacity of the cornea.

nebulization. 1. Treatment with spray method. 2. Conversion into a vapor. SYN: *vaporization.*

nebulizer (nĕb 'ū-lĭ-zĕr) [L. *nebula,* mist]. An atomizer or sprayer.

Ne"ca'tor [L. *murderer*]. A genus of nematode hookworms belonging to the family Ancylostomidae.

    N. americanus. A species of hookworm widely distributed in tropical regions, and common in the southern United States. Called the American hookworm. Adults live in small intestine attached to mucosa by their buccal capsules. Adults lay eggs which pass out with feces and under proper conditions of warmth and moisture hatch within 24 hrs. into rhabditiform larvae. After two molts, the larvae become strongyliform. After two more molts occurring within five days, they become infective larvae. They enter the body through the skin, pass into the lymph or blood stream and are carried to the lungs. Here they burrow into air spaces from which they pass via bronchial tubes and trachea to the pharynx from which they are expectorated or swallowed. If swallowed, they reach the intestine, bury themselves among the villi, molt again, acquire a mouth capsule and attach themselves to the mucosa. Worms may live 5 years.

Disease is contracted by walking barefoot or otherwise exposing the skin to soil which has been contaminated by feces of persons who are infected with the worm. SYM: Anemia, weakness, failure to grow. DIAG: Microscopic examination of preparation of feces reveals eggs of the worm. RS: hookworm; ancylostoma.

necatoriasis (nē-kā''tō-rī'ă-sĭs). Infestation by Necator americanus, q.v.

neck [AS. *hnecca,* nape]. 1. Part of body bet. head and shoulders. 2. The constricted portion of an organ, or that resembling a neck. 3. Region between crown and root of a tooth.

    n., anatomical. Constriction just below the head of the humerus.

    n., back of. Nape. SYN: *nucha, scruff.*

    n., Madelung's. Diffuse lipoma of the neck.

    n., surgical. Narrow part of humerus below the tuberosity. Fracture here is common.

    n. of womb. The cervix uteri.

    n., wry. Torsion of the neck caused by contracted muscles. SYN: *torticollis.*

necrectomy (nĕ-krĕk'to-mĭ) [Gr. *nekros,* dead, + *ektomē,* excision]. Surgical removal of necrosed tissue.

necro- [Gr. *nekros,* dead]. Combining form meaning pertaining to death.

necrobiosis (nĕk-rō-bī-ō'sĭs) ["+ *biosis,* life]. Gradual degeneration and death of tissue. SEE: *necrosis.*

    n. lipoidica diabeticorum. A skin disease common in diabetics characterized by necrosis of connective tissue and discoloration of skin. SYN: *Oppenheim-Urbach disease.*

necrobiotic (nĕ″krō-bī-ŏt′ĭk). Pert. to or affected by necrosis. SYN: *necrotic.*

necrocytosis (nĕ″krō-sī-tō′sĭs) [Gr. *nekros,* death, + *kytos,* cell, + *-ōsis,* condition]. Cellular death or decomposition.

necrocytotoxin (nĕk″rō-sī″tō-tŏks′ĭn). A toxin which causes death of cells.

necrogenic, necrogenous (nĕ-krō-jĕn′ĭk, -krŏj′ĕn-ŭs) [″+ *gennan,* to produce]. Caused by, pert. to, or originating in dead matter.

necrologist (nĕk-rŏl′ō-jĭst) [″+ *logos,* study]. A student of mortality statistics.

necrology (nĕk-rŏl′ō-jĭ) [″+ *logos,* study]. The study of mortality statistics.

necromania (nĕk-rō-mā′nĭ-ă) [Gr. *nekros,* dead, + *mania,* madness]. 1. Abnormal interest in dead bodies or in death. 2. Mania with desire for death.

necrometer (nĕk-rom′ĕt-ĕr) [″+ *metron,* measure]. Device for measurement of dead organs.

necromimesis (nĕk″rō-mī-mē′sĭs) [″+ *mimēsis,* imitation]. A delusion in which a person believes himself to be dead or acts as though he were dead.

necronectomy (nĕk-rō-nĕk′tō-mĭ) [″+ *ektomē,* excision]. Excision of a necrotic part, esp. of necrotic ossicles.

necrophagous (nĕ-krŏf′ă-gŭs) [″+ *phagein,* to eat]. Feeding or existing on dead bodies or matter.

necrophile (nĕk′rō-fīl) [″+ *philein,* to love]. One who has a morbid interest in or violates dead bodies.

necrophilism (nĕk-rŏf′ĭl-ĭzm). 1. Sexual perversion in which there is insane love for, or violation of, the dead. 2. Strong desire for death.

necrophilous (nĕk-rŏf′ĭl-ŭs). 1. Having a morbid fondness for, or feeding on, dead tissue. 2. Pert. to or affected with necrophilism.

necrophobia (nĕk-rō-fō′bĭ-ă) [Gr. *nekros,* dead, + *phobos,* fear]. 1. Abnormal aversion to dead bodies. 2. Insane dread of death. SYN: *thanatophobia.*

necropneumonia (nĕk″rō-nū-mō′nĭ-ă) [″+ *pneumōn,* lung]. Pulmonary gangrene.

necropsy (nĕk′rŏp-sĭ) [″+ *opsis,* view]. The scientific examination of a dead body to determine cause of death or pathological conditions. SYN: *autopsy; necroscopy; postmortem.*

necrosadism (nĕk″rō-sā′dĭzm) [″+ *sadism*]. Sexual gratification derived from the mutilation of dead bodies.

necroscopy (nĕ-krŏs′kō-pĭ) [Gr. *nekros,* death, + *skopein,* to examine]. Scientific inspection of a dead body to find cause of death or pathological condition. SYN: *autopsy; necropsy.*

necrose (nĕk-rōs′) [Gr. *nekros,* dead]. To cause or to undergo necrosis.

nec′rosin. A substance obtained from inflamed tissues which induces inflammatory changes in normal tissue.

necrosis (nē-krō′sĭs) [Gr. *nekrōsis,* a killing]. (pl. *necroses*) Death of areas of tissue or bone surrounded by healthy parts; death in mass as distinguished from necrobiosis, a gradual degeneration.

The dead part in bone is called sequestrum; in soft tissue, a slough or sphacelus. Term is usually applied to bone destruction or small areas of tissue, while gangrene is generally applied to destruction of specific parts or larger areas. SYN: *gangrene; mortification.*

ETIOL: Cessation of blood supply; physical agents such as trauma, radiant energy (electricity, infrared, ultraviolet, roentgen and radium rays); chemical agents (exogenous substances acting locally or acting internally following absorption and endogenous substances), or products (toxins) of bacteria.

n., anemic. N. caused by disturbed circulation in a part.

n., Balser's fatty. Pancreatitis with gangrenous areas in the fatty tissues.

n., caseous. N., cheesy, q.v.

n., central. N. which affects only the center of a part.

n., cheesy. N. with soft, dry, cheeselike formation. Usually seen in tuberculosis or syphilis.

n., coagulative. N. occurring esp. in infarcts in which coagulation occurs in necrotic area converting it into a homogenous mass depriving the organ or tissue of blood.

n., colliquative. N. caused by liquefaction of tissue due to autolysis or bacterial putrefaction.

n., dry. N. with dryness of the sequestrum.

n., embolic. N. resulting from an embolus which causes anemic n.

n., fat. N. in small scattered areas in the fatty tissue.

n., fibrinous. N., coagulative, q.v.

n., focal. Coagulative n. in small scattered areas.

n., gummatous. N. resulting from syphilis forming a dry rubbery mass.

n., ischemic. N. resulting from interference in blood supply to a part. Results in development of an infarct, decubitus, or gangrene.

n., liquefactive. N., colliquative, q.v.

n., medial. N. of cells in tunica media of arteries.

n., moist. N. with softening and moist condition of the dead tissue.

n., putrefactive. N. caused by bacterial decomposition.

n., superficial. N. affecting only the outer layers of bone or any tissue.

n., thrombotic. N. due to thrombus formation.

n., total. N. affecting an entire organ or part.

n. ustilaginea. Dry n. due to ergot poisoning.

necrospermia [Gr. *nekros*, death, + *sperma*, seed]. Condition in which spermatozoa in the ejaculate are immobile or lifeless.

necrot'ic [Gr. *nekrōsis*, a killing]. Rel. to death of a portion of tissue.

necrotomy (nĕ-krŏt'ō-mĭ) [Gr. *nekros*, dead, + *tomē*, a cutting]. 1. Dissection of a cadaver. 2. Excision of a sequestrum or other necrotic tissue.

nectarine (nek"ter-ēn'). A variety of peach.
Food value of 100 gm. (raw): Cal. 64; protein 0.6 gm.; carbohydrate 17.1 gm.; 1,650 I. U. vitamin A.

needle [AS. *naedl*]. A pointed instrument for stitching, ligaturing, or puncturing.

It may be straight, half curved, full curved, semicircular, double curved, (sometimes called "S" or sigmoid-shaped), or double ended. There are two classifications: cutting edge and round point. Cutting edge type is used in skin and dense tissue work, while round point needles are used for more delicate operations. All curved needles are used with a holder, straight usually without a holder.

CARE OF: Wash off; scrub with mild cleanser, benzene, and ether; sharpen; and sterilize.

n., hypodermic. A hollow needle for hypodermic injections.

needling. Treatment by puncturing with a needle. SYN: *discission.*

n. of aneurysm. Insertion of needles into an aneurysm in an effort to thicken and strengthen walls of the sac. Several fine needles are introduced into sac and left to be played upon by the blood stream, so that the farther wall becomes scratched and irritated, thus setting up an inflammatory thickening.

n., cataract. Puncturing of capsule of lens to allow entrance of aqueous fluid in order to bring about absorption of lens substance. SYN: *discission.*

n. of heart. Cardiocentesis, q.v.

n. of kidney. Insertion of a needle into the kidney.

NEFA. Abbr. for *nonesterified fatty acids.*

negative (neg'ă-tiv) [L. *negāre*, to deny]. 1. Without positive statement. 2. Lacking results. 3. Marked by resistance or retreat, as to a suggestion. 4. Directed away from a source of stimulation. 5. Not affirming presence of an organism, as a negative diagnosis.

n. culture. One not revealing the suspected organism.

n. electricity. Static e. in which elementary unit is the electron, and which is produced by friction.

n. electrode. The pole by which currents leave. SYN: *negative pole.*

n. glow. The luminous glow that is adjacent to the cathode in a vacuum tube through which an electrical discharge is passing.

n. reaction. Absence of a positive indication of disease, as a negative serologic test for syphilis.

n. sensation. One caused by stimulus not perceived in consciousness.

n. sign. Minus sign (–) used in subtraction and to indicate a lack.

negativism. Behavior peculiarity marked by not performing suggested actions (passive negativism) or in doing the opposite (active negativism), as seen in dementia praecox.

A patient may refuse to respond to suggestions because of sluggish mental reflexes or from fear. Retardation may be slow, or sudden and intense, as in manic depressive insanity. Opposition from fear must be considered apart from dementia praecox, in which the patient performs acts directly contrary to those suggested.

Negri bodies (na'gre). [Adelchi Negri, It. physician, 1876-1912]. Very minute bodies formed in nerve cells of the brain of one affected by rabies.

Neisseria (nī-sē'rī-ă). A genus of bacteria belonging to the family Neisseriaceae. They are gram-negative and usually occur in pairs with flattened sides but may occur singly or in irregular groups. The two species most often associated with disease in man are N. meningitis and N. gonorrhoeae which cause meningitis and gonorrhea respectively.

N. catarrhalis. Species of N. found in catarrhal inflammations of the upper respiratory tract. They may be confused with meningococci.

N. gonorrhoeae. Species causing gonorrhea. SYN: *gonococcus.*

N. meningitidis. Species causing epidemic cerebrospinal meningitis, usually called meningococcal meningitis. SYN: *N. intracellularis; Micrococcus meningitidis; M. intracellularis meningitidis.*

N. sicca. Species found in mucous membrane of respiratory tract. Occasionally may cause bacterial endocarditis.

Nelaton's line (na-lä-ton'). [Auguste Nelaton, Fr. surgeon, 1807-1873]. Line from anterior superior spine of the ileum to tuberosity of the ischium.

nemathelminth (něm-ă-thěl'mǐnth) [Gr. *nēma,* thread, + *helmins,* worm]. A roundworm belonging to the phylum Nemathelminthes.

Nemathelminthes (něm-ă-thěl-mǐn'thēz). The phylum of the roundworm.

nematocide (nem'ă-tō-sīd) ["+ L. *caedere,* to kill]. An agent that kills nematode worms.

Nematoda (něm"ă-tō'dǎ) ["+ *eidos,* form]. A class of the phylum Nemathelminthes which includes the true roundworms or threadworms, many species of which are parasitic. They are cylindrical or spindle-shaped worms possessing a resistant cuticle, have a complete alimentary canal, lack a true coelom, sexes usually separate, development usually direct and simple.

nematode (něm'ă-tōd) [Gr. *nema,* thread, + *eidos,* like]. A member of the class Nematoda, q.v.

nematodiasis (něm"ă-tō-dī'ă-sis) ["+ "+ *iasis,* infection]. Infestation by a parasite belonging to the class Nematoda.

nematoid (něm'ă-toid). Threadlike, like a nematode.

nematology (něm"ă-tōl'ō-jǐ). The division of parasitology which deals with worms belonging to the class Nematoda.

nembutal (něm'bū-tal). Proprietary name for pentobarbital sodium. Used as a preanesthetic, sedative, and hypnotic.

neo- [Gr. *neos*]. Combining form meaning new or recent.

neoarthrosis (nē"ō-ar-thrō'sīs) ["+ *arthron,* joint, + *-ōsis,* intensive]. A false joint. SYN: *nearthrosis.*

neoblas'tic ("+ *blastos,* germ). Pert. to, or constituting, a new growth of tissue.

neocerebellum (nē"ō-sěr-ě-běl'ŭm) [Gr. *neos,* new, + L. *cerebellum,* little brain]. The portion of the corpus cerebelli of the cerebellum which lies between the primary and prepyramidal fissures. Consists principally of the ansiform lobules. Phylogenetically it develops last in conjunction with cerebral cortex and is concerned with the integration of voluntary movements. The posterior lobe of the cerebellum.

neocortex (nē"ō-kor'těks). The neopallium, q.v.

neodymium (ne"o-dim'e-um). SYMB: *Nd.* At. wt. 144.24; at. no. 60. A shiny, silvery, rare-earth chemical element.

neofetus (nē-ō-fē'tŭs) ["+ L. *foetus,* offspring]. Embryo during 8th or 9th week of intrauterine existence.

neoformation (nē"ō-for-mā'shŭn) ["+ L. *formātiō,* a shaping]. 1. Regeneration. 2. A neoplasm or new growth.

neogala (nē-ōg'ă-lă) [Gr. *neos,* new + *gala,* milk]. The first milk following childbirth. SEE: *colostrum.*

neogenesis (nē-ō-jěn'ě-sǐs) ["+ *genesis,* formation]. Regeneration or re-formation, as of tissue.

neogenetic (nē"ō-jěn-ět'ǐk). Newly formed; relating to new formations.

neohydrin (nē-ō-hī'drǐn). Proprietary name for chlormerodrin, a diuretic.

neohymen (nē-ō-hī'měn) [Gr. *neos,* new, + *hymēn,* membrane]. A false or new membrane. SYN: *pseudomembrane.*

neologism (nē-ōl'ō-jǐzm) ["+ *logos,* study, + *ismos,* state]. 1. A new work or phrase, or a new meaning attached to an old word or phrase. 2. A mental condition in which the patient coins new words which are meaningless, or words to which he gives special significance without being aware of their normal significance. SEE: *lalopathy.*

neomembrane (nē-ō-měm'brān) ["+ L. *membrana,* membrane]. A false or a new membrane. SYN: *neohymen.*

neomorph (nē'ō-mōrf) ["+ *morphē,* form]. A new formation or development which is not inherited from a similar structure in an ancestor.

neomycin (nē"ō-mī'sǐn) [Gr. *neos,* new, + *mykes,* fungus]. An antibiotic from a species of Streptomyces, isolated from soil. Active against gram-positive and gram-negative bacteria, as well as streptomycin-resistant strains of Mycobacterium tuberculosis. Toxic to kidneys and eighth nerve, and may affect hearing.

neon (nē'ŏn) [Gr. *neos,* new]. SYMB: Ne. At. wt. 20.183; at. no. 10. A rare, inert, gaseous element in the air. Only 18 parts per million parts of air are neon.

n. gas. Colorless gas but it makes a reddish-orange glow when an electric charge strikes it.

neonatal (nē"ō-nā'tǎl) ["+ L. *natus,* born]. Concerning the first four weeks after birth.

neonate (nē'ō-nāt). A newborn infant.

neopallium (nē″ō-păl′ĭ-ŭm) [Gr. *neos*, new, + L. *pallium*, cloak]. That portion of cerebral hemisphere not belonging to the rhinencephalon or corpus striatum, comprising most of the convoluted cortex and its associated white fibers.
Phylogenetically, it is the new part of the pallium. SYN: *neocortex; isocortex.*

neopathy (nē-ŏp′ă-thĭ) ["+ *pathos*, disease]. 1. A newly found disease. 2. A new complication or new condition of a disease.

neophilism (nē-ŏf′ĭl-ĭzm) ["+ *philein*, to love, + *ismos*, state]. Morbid love of novelty and new persons and scenes.

neophobia (nē″ō-fō′bĭ-ă) [Gr. *neos*, new, + *phobos*, fear]. Fear of new scenes or novelties; aversion to all that is unknown or not understood. SYN: *cainotophobia.*

neophrenia (nē″ō-frē′nĭ-ă) ["+ *phrēn*, mind]. Mental deterioration in early youth.

neoplasia (nē″ō-plā′zĭ-ă) ["+ *plassein*, to form]. The development of new tissues or neoplasms.

neoplasm (nē′ō-plăzm) ["+ *plasma*, a thing formed]. A new and abnormal formation of tissue, as a tumor or growth. It serves no useful function, but grows at the expense of the healthy organism.

    n., benign. A growth not spreading by metastases or infiltration of tissue.

    n., histoid. A n. in which structure resembles the tissues and elements which surround it.

    n., malignant. A growth that infiltrates tissue, metastasizes, and often recurs after attempts at surgical removal. SYN: *cancer.*

    n., mixed. A n. composed of tissues from two of the germinal layers.

    n., multicentric. A growth arising from a number of distinct groups of cells.

    n., organoid. A n. in which the structure is similar to some organ of the body.

    n., unicentric. A growth having origin in one group of cells.

neoplastic (nē″ō-plas′tĭk) [Gr. *neos*, new, + *plastikos*, formed]. Pert. to, or of the nature of, new, abnormal tissue formation.

neoplasty (nē′ō-plăs-tĭ) ["+ *plassein*, to form]. Surgical formation or restoration of parts.

neosalvarsan (nē″ō-săl′var-săn). A proprietary name for neoarsphenamine.

neostigmine (ne-o-stig′min). A cholinergic drug used clinically in the form of a bromide or methylsulfate.

    n. bromide. USP. A preparation of neostigmine used for oral administration in the treatment of myasthenia gravis. Ophthalmic solution used for glaucoma.

    n. methylsulfate. USP. A preparation of neostigmine used for parenteral administration in treatment of myasthenia gravis.

neostomy (nē-ŏs′tō-mĭ) [Gr. *neos*, new, + *stoma*, opening]. Surgical formation of artificial opening into an organ or bet. two organs.

neostriatum (nē″ō-strĭ-ā′tŭm) ["+ L. *striatum*, grooved]. The caudate nucleus and the putamen considered together.

neo-synephrine hydrochloride (nē″ō-sĭn-ef′rĭn). Proprietary name for phenylephrine hydrochloride (USP).

nephelometer (nĕf-ĕl-ŏm′ĕ-ter) [Gr. *nephelē*, mist, + *metron*, measure]. Apparatus for measuring the turbidity of a fluid. This apparatus also may be used in estimating the degree of contamination of air by particulate matter.

nephelometry (nĕf-ĕl-ŏm′ĕ-trĭ). The employment of the nephelometer.

nephelopia (nĕf-ĕ-lō′pĭ-ă) [Gr. *nephelē*, mist, + *ōps*, eye]. Dim or cloudy vision from lessened transparency of the ocular media.

nephradenoma (nĕf′răd-ĕ-nō′mă) [Gr. *nephros*, kidney, + *adēn*, gland, + *-ōma*, tumor]. Renal adenoma.

nephralgia (nē-fral′jĭ-ă) ["+ *algos*, pain]. Renal pain. In absence of other symptoms, may alone be symptomatic of an obstructive renal process, but commonly presents a problem in differential diagnosis.

nephralgic (nē-frăl′jĭk). Pert. to renal pain.

nephrapostasis (nĕf′ră-pŏs′tă-sĭs) ["+ *apostasis*, suppuration]. Renal abscess or purulent inflammation of the kidney.

nephratony (nē-frăt′ō-nĭ). Lack of normal renal tone. SYN: *nephrotonia.*

nephrauxe (nĕf-rawks′ē) [Gr. *nephros*, kidney, + *auxē*, increase]. Renal enlargement.

nephrectasia, nephrectasis, nephrectasy (nĕf-rĕk-tā′zĭ-ă, -rĕk′tă-sĭs, -tă-sĭ) [Gr. *nephros*, kidney, + *ektasis*, distention]. Distention of the kidney.

nephrectomy (nē-frek′tō-mĭ) ["+ *ektomē*, excision]. Removal of a kidney.

    NP: *Operative:* Patient is placed on nonoperative side. Lower thigh is flexed to a right angle at hip and heel is drawn up to buttocks. Other leg is in straight relaxed position on table. Arms are in relaxed position in front of patient. A kidney bridge or sandbag is placed under the loin. The procedure is routine.

    The wound should be redraped after kidney is removed and instruments used in its removal discarded. Plenty of heavy drainage tubing, both of plain and cigarette types, should be ready.

Postoperative: Patient should be kept on back without a pillow. Urine is measured each day. Bland diet throughout illness. Dressing watched for signs of bleeding and changed often. Drainage tube left in for a few days, removed, and dressings changed. Stitches removed in 10-12 days.

COMPLICATIONS: Suppression of urine and secondary hemorrhage.

nephrelcosis (něf-rěl-kō'sĭs) ["+ *elkōsis,* ulceration]. Ulceration of the mucosa of the kidney.

nephrelcus (něf-rěl'kŭs). Renal ulcer.

nephremia (něf-rē'mǐ-ă) ["+ *haima,* blood]. Congested state of kidney. SYN: *nephrohemia.*

nephremphraxis (něf'rěm-frăks'ĭs) [Gr. *nephros,* kidney, + *emphraxis,* obstruction]. Obstruction in the renal vessels.

nephric (něf'rĭk) [Gr. *nephros,* kidney]. Pert. to the kidney or kidneys. SYN: *renal.*

nephritic (ne-frĭt'ĭk). 1. Rel. to the kidney. 2. Pert. to nephritis. 3. An agent used in nephritis.

nephritis (ne-frī'tĭs or něf-rī'tĭs) [Gr. *nephros,* kidney, + *-itis,* inflammation]. (pl. *nephritides*) Inflammation of the kidney.

ETIOL: Bacteria or their toxins; scarlet fever; diphtheria; septicemia; or toxic drugs, such as mercury, arsenic, alcohol. The glomeruli, tubules, and interstitial tissue may be affected. It may be either acute or chronic.

RS: arteriosclerosis, glomerulonephritis, kidney, nephrosis, nephrotic syndrome, pyelonephritis, nephrosclerosis.

n., acute. An inflammatory form involving the glomeruli, the tubules, or the entire kidney. It is of various types, depending on the portion of the kidney involved, degenerative, diffuse, suppurative, hemorrhagic, interstitial, and parenchymatous.

n., chronic. Progressive form in which entire structure of kidney may be affected, or affection may be confined to the glomerular or tubular processes. One variety of nephritis may merge with another, causing a diffuse nephritis. Symptoms depend upon the tissues involved.

n., diffuse, acute. An inflammatory process involving the entire kidney structure.

SYM: Acute onset; moderate fever; dull lumbar pain; marked edema and anasarca; hypertension; rapid pulse; vomiting; delirium; scanty, highly colored urine, containing large quantities of albumin and blood; bloody, hyaline and granular casts; uremic symptoms may develop.

PROG: Poor. May become chronic or death through exhaustive uremia or dropsy.

TREATMENT: Absolute rest in bed until albumin has disappeared from urine. Severe cases in pregnancy may require therapeutic abortion or induction of premature labor.

DIET: Milk, buttermilk, citrus fruit juices; later add cereals, fruits, vegetables. Cream and sugar allowed. Limit proteins, salt, and fluids.

n., diffuse, chronic. SEE: *interstitial n.; chronic n.*

n., focal. N. with foci of inflammation distributed throughout the kidney.

n., glomerular. A form involving the renal glomeruli. It may be acute or chronic. SEE: *glomerulonephritis.*

n., glomerular, acute. Acute form in which the pulse is rapid; and hypertension, edema, and urine containing albumin, blood, and casts are present. There is retention of urea and salt.

n., glomerular, chronic. Form almost always following acute glomerular n. It is marked by hyalinization of the glomeruli, arteriosclerosis, hypertension, albuminuria, edema, and later uremic symptoms. Usually fatal. SEE: *glomerulonephritis.*

n., glomerular, focal, embolic. N. in which emboli lodge in the capillary loops of the glomeruli, occluding them.

ETIOL: Subacute bacterial endocarditis due to Streptococcus viridans.

Glomerulus becomes hyalinized and there is blood in the lumen of tubules. Marked by blood, albumen, and hyaline and granular casts in urine. There is no edema or hypertension.

TREATMENT: That of endocarditis.

n., hemorrhagic. Acute n. with tubular hemorrhage and subsequent hematuria.

n., idiopathic. N. of unknown etiology.

n., interstitial, chronic. Glomeruli and interstitial tissue involved.

ETIOL: May follow parenchymatous n., alcoholism, lead poisoning, irritating toxins, bacterial infection, syphilis.

SYM: Headache, weakness, digestive disturbances, retinal hemorrhages and eye disturbances, dry skin. Vasomotor disturbances, such as tingling in fingers, with blanching. Hypertension marked. Low sp.gr. of urine, the quantity of which is considerable; as much by night as by day. Trace of albumin, few narrow hyaline casts, and sometimes granular casts. Retention of urea, uric acid, creatinine and protein waste products in blood.

NP: Rest and general hygienic care. Observe diet strictly; care for skin. Treat symptoms as they arise.

n., lipomatous. Fatty infiltration of the renal parenchyma. SYN: *lipomatosis renis.*

n., parenchymatous, acute. Acute glomerular nephritis with associated changes in tubules.

n., parenchymatous, chronic. Chronic glomerular nephritis, q.v., with associated changes in renal tubules.

n., saturnine. N. from lead poisoning.

n., saturnine, acute. Purulent form with abscess formation. Usually a result of genito-urinary surgery.

n., saturnine, chronic. Cheesy and tubercular form of n.

n., suppurative. Purulent form of n.

n., transfusion. Renal damage following blood transfusion of incompatible blood.

n., tubal, n., tubular. N. affecting the renal tubules with little change in glomerular structure.

n., tuberculous. Chronic n. due to presence of tubercle bacilli.

nephro-, nephr- [Gr. *nephros*, kidney]. Prefix pert. to the kidney.

nephroabdominal (něf'rō-ăb-dom'ĭ-năl) ["+ L. *abdominalis*, abdomen]. Concerning the kidney and abdomen.

nephrocalcinosis (něf-rō''kăl'sĭn-ō'sĭs). Calcinosis of the kidney characterized by deposits of calcium phosphate in renal tubules.

nephrocapsectomy (něf'rō-kăp-sěk'tō-mǐ) [Gr. *nephros*, kidney, + L. *capsula*, capsule, + Gr. *ektomē*, excision]. Renal decapsulation.

nephrocardiac (něf'rō-kar'dǐ-ăk) ["+ *kardia*, heart]. Concerning the heart and kidney.

nephrocele (něf'rō-sēl) ["+ *kēlē*, hernia]. 1. Renal hernia. 2. Embryonic cavity of a nephrotome.

nephrocolic (něf'rō-kŏl'ĭk) ["+ *kōlikon*, colon]. 1. Severe colicky pain in ureter due to passage of stone. 2. Concerning the colon and kidney.

nephrocolopexy (něf'rō-kŏl'ō-pĕks'ĭ) ["+ "+ *pēxis*, fixation]. Surgical suspension of kidney and colon using the nephrocolic ligament.

nephrocoloptosis (něf'rō-kō-lŏp-tō'sĭs) ["+ "+ *ptōsis*, a dropping]. Condition in which the kidney and colon are displaced downward.

nephrocystanastomosis (něf'rō-sĭst-ă-năs''-to-mō'sĭs) ["+ *kystis*, bladder, + *anastomōsis*, outlet]. Surgical formation of an artificial connection bet. kidney and the bladder, in permanent ureteral obstruction.

nephrocystitis (něf'rō-sĭs-ti'tĭs) [Gr. *nephros*, kidney, + *kystis*, a bladder, + *-itis*, inflammation]. Inflamed condition of kidneys and bladder.

nephrogenetic, nephrogenic, nephrogenous (něf'rō-jěn-ět'ĭk, -jěn'ĭk, -rō'jěn-ŭs) ["+ *gennan*,to produce]. Arising in or from the renal organs; capable of giving rise to kidney tissue.

n. cord. The intermediate mesoderm, q.v.

nephrogram. X-ray picture of the kidney.

nephrohydrosis (něf'rō-hi-drō'sĭs) [Gr. *nephros*, kidney, + *hydōr*, water, + *-ōsis*, intensive]. Accumulation of urine in renal pelvis and calyces due to obstruction. SYN: *hydronephrosis.*

nephrohypertrophy (něf'rō-hi-pěr'trō-fǐ) ["+ *hyper*, over, + *trophē*, nourishment]. Increased size of kidneys.

nephroid (něf'roid) ["+ *eidos*, form]. Resembling a kidney; kidney-shaped. SYN: *reniform.*

nephrolith (něf'rō-lǐth) ["+ *lithos*, stone]. Stone in the kidney.

nephrolithiasis (něf'rō-lǐth-i'ă-sĭs). The formation of renal stones. SYN: *lithiasis nephritica, lithiasis renalis.* SEE: *calculus, renal.*

nephrolithotomy (něf'rō-lǐth-ŏt'ō-mǐ) [Gr. *nephros*, kidney, + *lithos*, stone, + *tomē*, incision]. Renal incision for removal of calculus.

nephrology (nē-frŏl'ō-jǐ) [Gr. *nephros*, kidney, + *logos*, study]. Science of the structure and function of the kidney.

nephrolysis (nē-frŏl'ĭs-ĭs) ["+ *lysis*, loosening]. 1. Surgical detachment of an inflamed kidney from paranephric adhesions. 2. Destruction of kidney tissue by action of a nephrotoxin.

nephroma (nē-frō'mă) ["+ *-ōma*, tumor]. Renal tumor or one of renal tissue.

nephromalacia (něf'rō-mă-lā'sǐ-ă) ["+ *malakia*, softening]. Abnormal renal softness or softening.

nephromegaly (něf'rō-měg'ă-lǐ) ["+ *megas*, great]. Extreme enlargement of one or both kidneys.

nephromere (něf'rō-mēr) [Gr. *nephros*, kidney, + *meros*, part]. Segment in embryo from which kidney develops. The intermediate mesoderm in an embryo from which the kidney develops. SYN: *nephrotome.*

nephron (něf'ron) [Gr. *nephros*, kidney]. The structural and functional unit of the kidney consisting of a renal (malpighian) corpuscle (a glomerulus enclosed within Bowman's capsule) and its attached tubule consisting of the proximal convoluted portion, loop of Henle, and distal convoluted portion. These connect by arched collecting tubules with straight collecting tubules. Urine is formed by filtration in renal corpuscle and selective reabsorption and secretion by cells of the renal tubule. There are approximately one million nephrons in each kidney. SYN: *renal tubule; uriniferous tubule.* SEE: *kidney; malpighian corpuscle; urine.*

nephroncus (nĕf-rŏn'kŭs) ["+ *onkos,* tumor]. A renal tumor.

nephroparalysis (nĕf'rō-păr-ăl'ĭ-sis) ["+ *paralysis,* a loosening]. Paralyzed renal function.

nephropathy (nē-frŏp'ă-thĭ) ["+ *pathos,* disease]. Disease of the kidney. This term includes inflammatory (nephritis), degenerative (nephrosis), and sclerotic (arteriosclerotic) lesions of the kidney.

nephropexy (nĕf'rō-pĕks-ĭ) ["+ *pēxis,* fixation]. Surgical attachment of a floating kidney.

nephrophthisis (nē-frŏ'thĭ-sĭs) ["+ *phthisis,* a wasting]. 1. Tuberculosis of the kidney with caseous degeneration. 2. Suppurative nephritis with wasting of the kidney substance.

nephroptosis (nĕf-rŏp-tō'sĭs) ["+ *ptōsis,* a dropping]. Prolapse or downward kidney displacement.

ETIOL: Shape of lumbar recess, pregnancy, emaciation, and enteroptosis are predisposing factors.

SYM: None. If any, not referable to kidney (nervous and digestive disorders or pain). Painful paroxysms simulating renal colic; albuminuria; painful, scanty, and frequent micturition.

TREATMENT: May require surgery or no therapy, depending upon symptoms and functional capacity of the kidney. SEE: *nephrectomy; nephropexy.*

nephropyelitis (nĕf'rō-pī-ĕl-ī'tĭs) [Gr. *nephros,* kidney, + *pyelos,* pelvis, + *-itis,* inflammation]. Inflammation of the renal pelvis and parenchyma of kidney. SYN: *pyelonephritis.*

nephropyosis (nĕf'rō-pī-o'sĭs) ["+ *pyōsis,* suppuration]. Purulence of a kidney.

nephrorrhagia (nĕf-ror-ā'jĭ-ă) ["+ *rhēgnynai,* to burst forth]. Renal hemorrhage into pelvis and tubules.

nephrorrhaphy (nĕf-ror'ă-fĭ) ["+ *rhaphē,* suture]. Surgical procedure of suturing the kidney.

nephros (nĕf'rŏs) [Gr.]. The kidney.

nephrosclerosis (nĕf'rō-sklĕ-rō'sĭs) ["+ *sklērōsis,* a hardening]. Renal sclerosis or

hardening. SEE: *nephritis, chronic interstitial.*

n., arterial. Arteriosclerosis of kidney arteries. Results in ischemia, atrophy of parenchyma, and fibrosis of kidney.

n., arteriolar. Sclerosis of the smaller renal arterioles, esp. the afferent glomerular arterioles with resulting fibrosis, ischemic necrosis, and glomerular degeneration and failure. Occurs in most cases of essential hypertension.

n., malignant. N. which develops rapidly in patients with severe hypertension. SEE: *hypertension, malignant.*

nephrosis (nĕf-rō'sĭs) [Gr. *nephros,* kidney]. (pl. *nephroses*) Condition in which there are degenerative changes in the kidneys without the occurrence of inflammation.

n., acute. N. accompanying acute infectious disease or resulting from poisoning or metabolic disturbances such as toxemias of pregnancy or obstructive jaundice. Marked by scanty urine.

n., amyloid. N. due to deposition of amyloid within the walls of the renal blood vessels and at the base of the cells of the tubules. Marked degeneration of kidney tissue results.

n., lipoid. A chronic disease of unknown etiology in which large amounts of albumin are lost in urine, resulting in depletion of the plasma protein and development of nephrotic edema. It probably is due to disordered metabolism. Occurs mainly in children and young adults.

SYM: Gradual development of edema, which reaches a high degree. Oliguria, albumin, casts of hyaline and granular type and lipids in urine. Blood serum proteins markedly reduced, but nitrogenous constituents remain normal. Blood cholesterol and globulin elevated. Hypertension absent. Anemia occurs.

PROG: Guarded.

TREATMENT: Prolonged bed rest is not required. High-protein and low-sodium diet, cortisone may help.

nephrostoma, nephrostome (nē-frŏs'tō-mă, nĕf'ros-tōm) [Gr. *nephros,* kidney, + *stoma,* mouth]. The internal orifice of a wolffian tubule, connected with the celom in the human embryo.

nephrostomy (nē-frŏs'to-mĭ). Formation of an artificial fistula into the renal pelvis.

nephrotic (nē-frŏt'ĭk) [Gr. *nephros,* kidney]. Rel. to, or caused by, nephrosis.

n. syndrome. Term applied to renal disease of whatever cause, characterized by massive edema, proteinuria, and usually elevation of serum cholesterol and lipids.

nephrotome (nĕf'rō-tōm) ["+ *tome*, a section]. Embryonic bridge of cells, connecting primitive segments along neural tube to the somatic and splanchnic mesoderm from which arises the urogenital system. SYN: *intermediate cell mass; mesomere; nephromere.*

nephrotoxin (nĕf'rō-tŏks'ĭn) ["+ *toxikon*, poison]. A specific toxin which destroys renal cells.

nephrotresis (nĕf-rōtrē'sĭs) ["+ *trēsis*, piercing]. Formation of a permanent excretory opening in the kidney through the loin.

nephroureterectomy (nef'rō-ū-rē"tĕr-ĕk'-tō-mĭ) ["+ *ourētēr*, ureter, + *ektomē*, excision]. Surgical excision of kidney with the ureter or part of it.

nephrydrosis (nĕf-rĭ-drō'sĭs) ["+ *hydōr*, water, + *-ōsis*, intensive]. Distention and dilation of renal pelvis resulting from obstruction. SYN: *hydronephrosis; nephrohydrosis.*

Nep'tune gir'dle. Compress of linen covered by flannel which encircles the trunk from lower end of sternum to the pubes. Used in applying wet packs, esp. cold.

NP: First, patient should be given a foot bath of 104°-110° F. (40°-43.3° C.) for five minutes with cold compress over forehead. Forehead compress should be continued throughout treatment. Then linen is soaked in water of 42°-50° F. (5.6°-10° C.), wrung out, and placed on patient. Girdle remains 1-6 hours; however, linen should be changed when necessary to maintain 42°-50° F. (5.6°-10° C.) temperature. Cover with blanket.

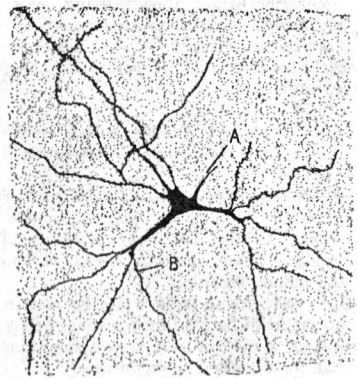

NERVE CELL FROM CEREBRAL CORTEX
A, Axis cylinder, directed towards periphery.
B, Dendrites.

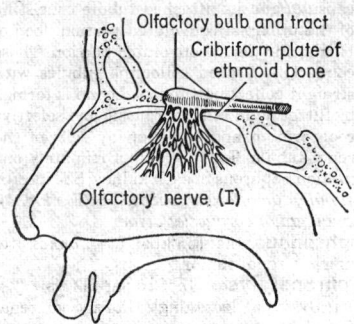

Olfactory bulb and tract
Cribriform plate of ethmoid bone
Olfactory nerve (I)

OLFACTORY NERVE (1st Cranial)

neptun'ium. SYMB: *Np.* At. wt. 237; at. no. 93. An element obtained by bombarding uranium with neutrons.

nerve [L. *nervus*, sinew; probably from Gr. *neuron*, sinew]. A bundle or a group of bundles of nerve fibers outside the central nervous system which connects the brain and spinal cord with various parts of the body. Nerves conduct afferent impulses centrally from receptor organs and efferent impulses peripherally to effector organs. The fibers of peripheral nerves are the processes of neurons whose cell bodies are located within the brain, spinal cord, or in ganglia.

A bundle of nerve fibers is called a fasciculus. The fibers within a fasciculus are surrounded and held together by delicate connective tissue fibers forming the endoneurium. Each fasciculus is surrounded by a sheath of connective tissue, the perineurium. The entire nerve is enclosed in a thick sheath of connective tissue, the epineurium which may contain numerous fat cells. Small nerves may lack an epineurium.

n., accelerator. N. to the heart carrying sympathetic fibers conveying impulses which, when stimulated, accelerate the heart beat.

n., afferent. One which transmits impulses from the periphery to a nerve center.

n., autonomic. A n. of the autonomic nervous system.

n. block. The induction of regional anesthesia by preventing sensory nerve impulses from reaching centers of consciousness. Accomplished by injecting an anesthetic solution, such as procaine, about the nerve some distance from the region or by anesthetizing nerve endings in the region itself (infiltration).

n. cell. A neuron, q.v; consists of a cell body and its processes, an axon and one or more dendrites.

n., cerebrospinal. A n. originating from the brain or spinal cord.

n., cranial. One of the 12 parts of nerves arising from the brain. Makes its exit through a foramen of the cranium. SEE: *Table* in *Appendix.*

n., depressor. Any afferent n. which when stimulated depresses the activity of an organ or nerve center.

n., efferent. One transmitting impulses from a nerve center to the periphery.

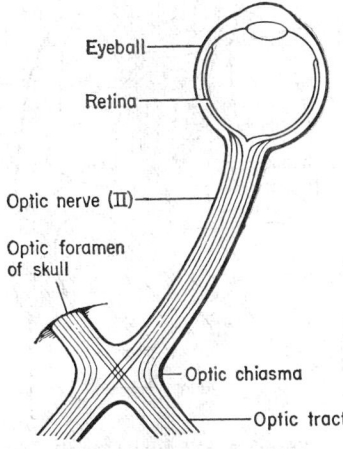

OPTIC NERVE (2nd Cranial)

n. ending. The termination of a nerve fiber (axon or dendrite) in a peripheral structure. May be sensory (receptor) or motor (effector). Sensory endings are nonencapsulated (Ex: free nerve endings, peritrichal endings, tactile corpuscles of Merkel) or encapsulated (Ex: end-bulbs of Krause, Meissner's corpuscles, Vater-Pacini corpuscles, Golgi-Mazzoni corpuscles, neuromuscular and neurotendinous spindles).

n., excitatory. N. transmitting impulses which stimulate function.

n. fiber. SEE: *nerve fiber(s).*

n. fibril. A fine fiber in the cytoplasm and cell processes of a neuron. SYN: *neurofibrilla.*

n., frigorific. A sympathetic n. causing a lowering in temperature on stimulation.

n. impulse. Name for the excitatory process which travels along a nerve fiber

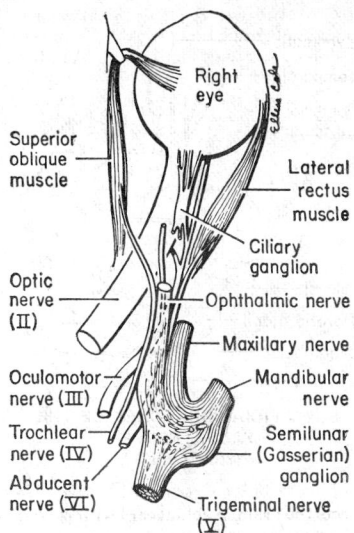

OCULOMOTOR, TROCHLEAR, AND ABDUCENT NERVES
(3rd, 4th, and 6th Cranial)

when stimulated.

n., inhibitory. One which, upon stimulation, lessens activity in a part.

n., mixed. One containing both afferent (sensory) and efferent (motor) fibers.

n., motor. One containing motor fibers and conveying motor impulses. SYN: *efferent n.*

n., parasympathetic. A n. of the parasympathetic division of the autonomic nervous system.

n., peripheral. Any nerve which con-

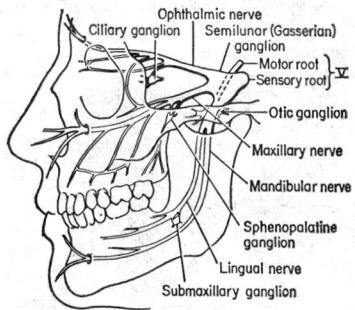

LEFT TRIGEMINAL NERVE
(5th Cranial)

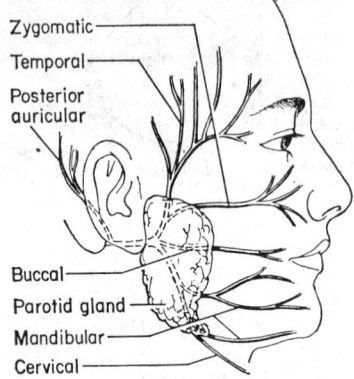

**SUPERFICIAL BRANCHES OF THE
FACIAL NERVE**
(7th Cranial)

nects the brain or spinal cord with peripheral receptors or effectors.

n., pilomotor. A nerve which innervates the arrectores pilorum muscles of hair follicles.

n. plexus. A group of nerves intertwined.

n., pressor. An afferent n. which when stimulated excites the vasoconstrictor center thus increasing blood pressure.

n., secretory. N. whose stimulation excites secretion in a part.

n., sensory. A nerve that conducts afferent impulses from sensory receptors to the brain or spinal cord.

n., somatic. A n. which innervates somatic structures, i.e., those comprising the body wall and extremities.

n., spinal. One of 31 pairs of nerves

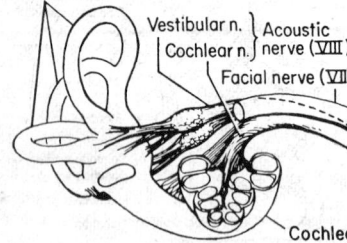

RIGHT ACOUSTIC NERVE
(8th Cranial)—**FRONT VIEW**

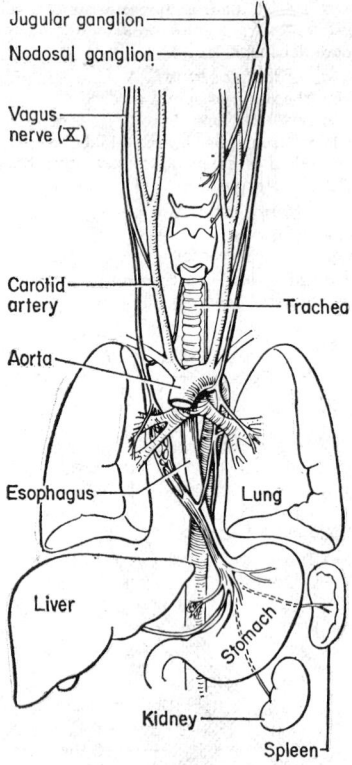

VAGUS NERVE (10th Cranial)

which connect with the spinal cord. Includes 8 cervical, 12 thoracic, 5 lumbar, 5 sacral, 1 coccygeal.

n., sympathetic. N. of the sympathetic division of the autonomic nervous system. SEE: *autonomic nervous system.*

n. trunk. The main stem of a peripheral nerve.

n., vasoconstrictor. A n. which conducts impulses that bring about constriction of a blood vessel.

n., vasodilator. A n. which conducts impulses that bring about dilation of a blood vessel.

n., vasomotor. N. which controls the caliber of a blood vessel. A vasoconstrictor or vasodilator nerve, q.v.

nerve fiber(s). An elongated process of a nerve cell or neuron, usually the axon, concerned primarily with the conduction of impulses. Nerve fibers form the major portion of the white matter of the brain and

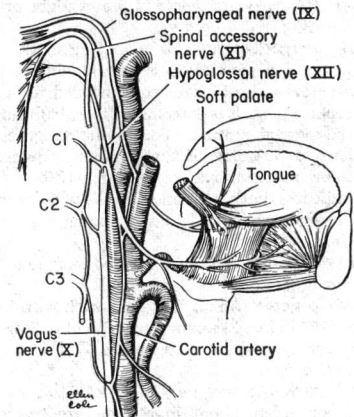

Glossopharyngeal nerve (IX)
Spinal accessory
nerve (XI)
Hypoglossal nerve (XII)
Soft palate
C1
Tongue
C2
C3
Vagus
nerve (X)
Carotid artery

ellen
cole

**RIGHT GLOSSOPHARYNGEAL,
SPINAL ACCESSORY, AND
HYPOGLOSSAL NERVES**
(9th, 11th, and 12th Cranial)

spinal cord and all nerves. Most fibers in peripheral nerves are myelinated (medullated, i. e., they are covered by a noncellular sheath of myelin, a fatty substance). The myelin sheath is interrupted at intervals by the nodes of Ranvier. Outside the myelin sheath and closely investing it is another sheath, the neurilemma or sheath of Schwann. Between the two sheaths are Schwann cells, thin cells having flat, oval-shaped nuclei. One Schwann cell occurs at each internode length. Fibers lacking a myelin sheath are called nonmedullated (unmyelinated). The neurilemma is lacking in all fibers of the central nervous system.

   n. f., adrenergic. Nerve fiber that liberates an adrenaline-like substance (sympathin) at its ending. Include most postganglionic fibers of the sympathetic division.

   n. f., arcuate. Arch-shaped n. f. in the medulla. Comprise three groups, the ext. dorsal, ext. ventral, and internal.

   n. f., association. N. f. which connects one region of the cerebral cortex with another region in the same hemisphere.

   n. f., cholinergic. N. f. which liberates acetylcholine at its ending. Includes preganglionic fibers ending in sympathetic ganglia, postganglionic parasympathetic fibers, and efferent somatic fibers ending in skeletal muscle.

   n. f.'s, climbing, of cerebellum. 1. Afferent n. f.'s entering cortex and synapsing with dendrites of Purkinje cells. SYN: *mossy fibers.* 2. Collateral branches of Purkinje cell axons which return to molecular layer terminating about Purkinje or basket-cell dendrites.

   n. f., collateral. A small branch extending at a right angle from an axon.

   n.f., commissural. N. f. which passes from one cerebral hemisphere to the other.

   n. f., mossy. SEE: *n. f.'s, climbing, of cerebellum.*

   n. f., myelinated. One possessing a myelin sheath.

   n. f., nonmedullated. N. f. containing only an axis cylinder and a neurilemma.

   n. f., postganglionic. N. f. of the autonomic nervous system which terminates in smooth or cardiac muscle or a gland. Its cell body lies in an autonomic ganglion.

   n. f., preganglionic. N. f. of the autonomic nervous system which terminates and synapses in one of the autonomic ganglia. Its cell body lies in the brain or spinal cord.

   n. f., projection. N. f. arising in the diencephalon and passing to the cerebral cortex or a fiber arising in cerebral cortex and terminating in lower portions of the brain or in the spinal cord.

nervi. Plural of *nervus.*

   n. terminales. [NA]. Terminal nerves, accompanying the olfactory nerve to the brain. Consists principally of sensory fibers from mucosa of nasal septum.

nervo- [L.]. Combining form pertaining to a nerve.

nervomuscular ["+ *musculus,* a muscle]. Rel. to nerve supply of muscles.

nerv'one. A cerebroside present in brain tissue; contains nervonic acid.

nervosism (ner'vō-sĭzm) ["+ Gr. *ismos,* state of]. 1. Neurasthenia or nervousness. 2. The idea that morbid conditions depend upon alterations of nerve force.

nervosity. Nervosism, q.v.

nervous (ner'vus) [L. *nervosus*]. (pl. *nervi*) 1. Characterized by instability of nerve action: excitability. 2. Pert. to the nerves.

   n. debility. Nervous fatigue with resultant physical exhaustion. SYN: *neurasthenia.*

   n. exhaustion. SEE: *nervous debility.*

   n. impulse. The excitatory process set up in nerve fibers by stimuli. It is probably in the nature of a wave of electrochemical disturbance traveling at the comparatively slow rate (even in fastest conducting mammalian nerves) of 50-80 meters per second. The velocity varies in different fibers according to the diameter.

   n. prostration. SEE: *nervous debility.*

n. system. A system of extremely delicate nerve cells, elaborately interlaced with each other. Made up collectively of the brain, cranial nerves, spinal cord, spinal nerves, autonomic ganglia, ganglionated trunks and nerves, maintaining the vital function of reception and response to stimuli.

The nervous system regulates and coordinates body activities and brings about responses by which the body adjusts to changes of environment, either external or internal. These changes constitute stimuli which initiate impulses in receptors or sense organs. The principal organs of this group are the eye, ear, the organs of taste and smell, and sensory receptors located in the skin, joints, muscles, and various parts of the body.

The nervous system is divided into two divisions: the central nervous system, which includes the brain and spinal cord, and (2) the peripheral nervous system, which includes the craniosacral nerves, the organs of special sense, and the sympathetic nervous system. SEE: *autonomic n.s.; central n.s.; parasympathetic n.s.; sympathetic n.s.*

n. tissue. The tissue which comprises the nervous system. Includes the nervous elements proper (neurons) and the interstitial tissue (neuroglia, neurilemma cells, and satellite cells).

nervousness (nĕr'vŭs-nĕs) [L. *nervus,* sinew]. Excitability of the nervous system associated with unrest.

nervus (ner'vus). (pl. *nervi*) [NA]. Nerve, q.v.

n. erigens. [NA]. The pelvic nerve. A scattered bundle of craniosacral autonomic fibers originating from the 2nd to 4th sacral nerves and passing to terminal ganglia from which postganglionic fibers pass to the pelvic organs (bladder, colon, rectum, prostate gland, seminal vesicles, ext. genitalia).

n. intermedius. [NA]. The pars intermedia (intermediate nerve of Wrisberg), a branch of the facial nerve consisting principally of sensory fibers.

n. nervorum. Nerve fibers which innervate sheaths of nerves.

n. vasorum. Nerve fibers which innervate the walls of blood vessels.

nest. A small mass of cells, resembling a bird nest, alien to its surroundings.

n., cancer. A mass of cells extending from a common center; seen in cancerous growths.

n., cell. A small mass of epithelial cells set apart from surrounding cells by connective tissue.

n. et m. Abbr. for *nocte et mane,* night and morning.

net reproductive rate. A measure of whether a population is reproducing at a greater or lesser rate than needed for its replacement. It is determined by calculating the average number of surviving daughters born to the women in that population during their reproductive years. An NRR of 1 indicates that each woman in the population has one surviving daughter during her lifetime. ABBR: NRR.

ne tr. s. num. Abbr. for *ne tradas sine nummo,* do not deliver unless paid.

net'tle rash [AS. *netel*]. Skin rash with intense itching, resembling condition produced by stinging with nettles. SYN: *hives; urticaria.*

net'work [AS. *net,* net, + *wyrcan,* to work]. Fiber arrangement in a structure resembling a net. SYN: *rete; reticulum.*

Neumann's disease (noi'măn). [Isidor Neumann, Austrian dermatologist, 1832-1906]. Pemphigus vegetans, q.v.

neuragmia (nū-răg'mĭ-ă) [Gr. *neuron,* sinew, + *agmos,* break]. The tearing or rupturing of a nerve trunk.

neural (nū'răl). Pert. to nerves or connected with the nervous system.

n. crest. A band of cells extending longitudinally along the neural tube of an embryo from which cells forming cranial, spinal, and autonomic ganglia arise.

n. fold. One of two longitudinal elevations of the neural plate of an embryo which unite to form the neural tube.

n. plate. A thickened band of ectoderm along the dorsal surface of an embryo, from which the nervous system develops.

n. spine. Spinous vertebral process.

n. tube. Tube formed from fusion of the neural folds from which the brain and spinal cord arise.

neuralgia (nū-ral'jĭ-ă) [Gr. *neuron,* sinew, + *algos,* pain]. Severe, sharp pain along the course of a nerve.

ETIOL: Pressure on nerve trunks, faulty nerve nutrition, toxins, neuritis. Usually no morphologic changes can be detected.

SYM: According to the part affected. SEE: *geniculate; sciatica.*

n., cardiac. Angina pectoris.

n., degenerative. N. caused by degenerative changes in the nerves or nerve cells; occurs in the elderly.

n., epileptiform. Spasmodic facial n. SYN: *tic douloureux.*

n., facial. SEE: *n., trigeminal.*

n., facialis vera. Geniculate n.

n., Fothergill's. Trigeminal n., q.v.

n., geniculate. N. characterized by pain over all or any part supplied by sensory fibers of facial nerve. Pain may be deep in facial muscles, within the ear, or in pharynx. SYN: *herpes zoster auricularis; herpes zoster oticus; Hunt neuralgia or syndrome; Ramsay-Hunt syndrome.*

n., glossopharyngeal. N. along the course of the glossopharyngeal nerve characterized by severe pain in back of throat, tonsils, and middle ear.

n., hallucinatory. Impression of local pain without actual peripheral pain.

n., Hunt's. Geniculate n.

n., idiopathic. N. without structural lesion or pressure from a lesion.

n., intercostal. Pain follows course of intercostal nerves, frequently associated with eruption of herpes zoster. Spots of tenderness near vertebral column, in middle of nerve, and near sternum. May be dependent upon spinal caries or thoracic aneurysm.

n., mammary. N. of the breast. SYN: *mastodynia.*

n., Morton's. N. of joint of 3rd and 4th toes. SYN: *metatarsalgia.*

n., nasociliary. N. of eyes, brows, and root of nose.

n., occipital. Involves upper cervical nerves. A spot of tenderness found bet. mastoid process and upper cervical vertebrae. May be due to spinal caries.

n., otic. Geniculate n.

n., reminiscent. Continued mental impression of pain after n. has ceased.

n. of sphenopalatine ganglion. Neuralgia of the sphenopalatine ganglion. SYN: *Sluder's n.*

SYM: Pain on one side of face radiating to eyeballs, ear, occipital and mastoid areas of skull; sometimes to nose, upper teeth, and shoulder of same side.

PROG: good.

n., stump. Pressure on nerves at site of amputation, causing pain.

n., symptomatic. N. not primarily involving the nerve structure, but occurring as a symptom of local or systemic disease.

n., trifacial. Old term for trigeminal neuralgia, q.v.

n., trigeminal. N. involving the gasserian ganglion or one or more branches of the trigeminal nerve.

ETIOL: Unknown. Attacks often precipitated by initiation of pain by obvious stimuli on certain hypersensitive areas, called trigger zones of face, lips, or tongue.

SYM: Tender points correspond to supraorbital, infraorbital, and mental foramina. Often violent spasm of muscles. In long standing cases hair on affected side sometimes becomes coarse and bleached.

PROG: Good.

TREATMENT: Alcohol injection or cutting of the nerve. Symptomatic treatment may permit spontaneous remission to occur.

SYN: *tic douloureux; Fothergill disease.*

neuralgic (nū-ral′jĭk) [Gr. *neuron,* sinew, + *algos,* pain]. Of, or concerning, neuralgia.

neuramebimeter (nū″răm-ē-bĭm′ĕt-ẽr) [″ + *amoibē,* response, + *metron,* a measure]. Device for determining rate of response of a nerve to a stimulus.

neurapophysis (nū-rȧ-pŏf′ĭ-sĭs) [″ + *apo,* from, + *physis,* growth]. Either of the two sides of a vertebra which unite to form the neural arch.

neurapraxia (nū-rȧ-prăks′ĭ-ȧ) [″ + *apraxia,* nonactive]. Cessation in function of a peripheral nerve without degenerative changes occurring. Recovery is the usual outcome.

neurasthenia (nū-răs-thē′nĭ-ȧ) [Gr. *neuron,* sinew, + *astheneia,* weakness]. An ill-defined disease commonly following depressed states characterized by a sense of weakness or exhaustion, or by the symptoms of various types of organic disease without the existence of organic disease in a degree sufficient to justify the subjective complaints of the patient.

SYM: Fatigue; weakness; headache; sweating; polyuria; tinnitus and vertigo; photophobia; fear; easy exhaustion on the slightest effort; inability to concentrate; irritability and complaint of poor memory; poor sleep; numerous, constantly varying aches and pains; vasomotor disturbances.

The neurasthenic is often physically asthenic with a long, narrow thorax, small muscles, and undernourished. The face is thin, alert, and often suggests chronic suffering. Much of this is the result of the neurasthenia, but it suggests also a physical type, inherently predisposed to develop the disease.

Freud believes the disease is probably a frustration (esp. sexual) which possibly complicates the symptoms by an element of renunciation as well.

PROG: Favorable if cause can be removed.

TREATMENT: Attempt to determine cause. If no specific illness, such as anemia or chronic infection can be discovered, intensive psychotherapy is indicated.

neurastheniac, neurasthenic (nū-răs-thē′-nĭ-ăk, -nĭk). 1. Individual suffering from neurasthenia. 2. Suffering from or concerning neurasthenia.

neuratrophia, neuratrophy (nū-rǎ-trō'fǐ-ǎ, -rǎt'rō-fǐ) ["+ *atrophia*, a wasting]. Atrophy of the nervous tissue or deficient nutrition of the nervous system.

neuraxitis (nū-rǎks-i'tǐs) ["+ *axon*, axis, + *-itis*, inflammation]. Encephalitis.

  n., epidemic. Epidemic encephalitis.

neuraxon(e (nū-rǎks'ōn). The axis cylinder process of a nerve cell. SYN: *axon.* SEE: *nerve fiber.*

neurectasia, neurectasis, neurectasy (nū''rěk-tā'sǐ-ǎ, -rěk'tǎ-sǐs, -rěk'tǎ-sǐ) ["+ *ektasis*, a stretching]. Surgical nerve stretching.

neurectomy (nū-rěk'tō-mǐ) ["+ *ektomē*, excision]. Partial or total excision or resection of a nerve.

neurectopia, neurectopy (nū-rěk-tō'pǐ-ǎ, nūr-ek'tō-pǐ) ["+ *ek*, out, + *topos*, place]. Displacement or abnormal position of a nerve.

neurenteric (nū-rěn-těr'ǐk) [Gr. *neuron*, sinew, + *enteron*, intestine]. Rel. to the neural canal and intestinal tube of the embryo.

  n. canal. Temporary canal of the embryo, between the neural and intestinal tubes. In human development, the temporary communication between cavities of the yolk sac and the amnion.

neurepithelium (nūr''ěp-ǐ-thē'lǐ-ŭm) ["+ *epi*, upon, + *thēlē*, nipple]. 1. Epithelial structures forming the terminations of nerves of special sense. 2. Embryonic layer from which arises the cerebrospinal axis. SYN: *neuroepithelium.*

neurergic (nū-rer'jǐk) ["+ *ergon*, work]. Concerning the activity of a nerve.

neurexeresis (nū''rěks-ē-rē'sǐs) ["+ *exairein*, to draw out]. Ripping or tearing out of a nerve to relieve neuralgia.

neuriatry (nū-rī'a-trǐ) ["+ *iatreia*, treatment]. Study and treatment of diseases of nervous system. SYN: *neurology.*

neurilemma, neurolemma [Gr. *neuron*, sinew, + *lemma*, husk]. A thin membranous sheath enveloping a nerve fiber. SYN: *sheath of Schwann.* SEE: *nerve fiber.*

neurilemmitis (nu''rǐ-lěm-mǐ'tǐs) ["+ "+ *-itis*, inflammation]. Inflamed condition of a neurilemma.

neurilemmoma (nū''rǐ-lě-mō'mǎ) ["+ *eilēma*, tight sheath, *-ōma*, tumor]. A firm, encapsulated fibrillar tumor of peripheral nerves. SYN: *neurinoma; schwannoma; peripheral glioma.*

neurilemosarcoma (nū''rǐ-lěm-ǎ-sar-kō'mǎ). A malignant neurilemmoma.

neurimo'tor [Gr. *neuron*, nerve + L. *motor*, a mover]. Concerning a motor nerve.

neurinoma (nū-rǐ-nō'mǎ) ["+ *-oma*, swelling]. A tumor of a peripheral nerve arising from endoneurium or sheath of Schwann. SYN: *neurilemmoma; neurofibroma; schwannoma.*

neurinomatosis (nū''rǐ-nō-mǎ-tō'sǐs). Condition of having multiple neurinomas on nerve fibers. SYN: *neurofibromatosis.*

neurite (nu'rǐt) [Gr. *neuron*, sinew]. The axis cylinder process of a neuron. Both axites and dendrites are neurites. SYN: *neuraxon.*

neuritis (nū-rī'tǐs) [Gr. *neuron*, sinew or nerve, + *-itis*, inflammation]. Inflammation of a nerve or nerves, usually associated with a degenerative process.

ETIOL: Mechanical factors: compression, contusion, trauma. Infections: localized involving direct infection of nerves or may accompany diseases such as leprosy, tetanus, tuberculosis, malaria, measles, etc. Toxins: esp. poisoning by heavy metals (arsenic, lead, mercury), alcohol, carbon tetrachloride, etc. Metabolic factors: as in thiamine deficiency, gastrointestinal dysfunction, diabetes, toxemias of pregnancy, etc. Vascular: as in n. accompanying peripheral vascular disease.

SYM: Neuralgia in part affected; hyperesthesia, paresthesia, dysesthesia, hypesthesia, or anesthesia; muscular atrophy of part supplied by affected nerve; paralysis; lack of reflexes.

NP: Rest in bed (water or air bed). Uniformity of pressure on body. Temperature of water in water bath must be maintained by frequent replacement of cooling water with warm water. Hot water bags or electric heating pads under covers but not next to skin, as lack of sensibility to heat on part of patient may lead to burns. Cradles may be necessary. Padded splints with little bandage compression to affected parts. No sudden change of position. Place limb in suspended towel to move it. No rubbing. Later diathermy under direction of physician, also massage using mildest of manipulations. Avoid all strain on patient. SEE: *polyneuritis.*

  n., adventitial. Inflammation of nerve sheath.

  n., ascending. N. moving upward along a nerve trunk away from periphery.

  n., axial. Inflammation of inner portion of a nerve.

  n., degenerative. N. with rapid degeneration of nerve.

  n., descending. N. that leads away from the central nervous system.

  n., dietetic. Same as beriberi, q.v.

n., diphtheritic. N. following diphtheria.

n., disseminated. N. involving a large group of nerves.

n., endemic. Same as beriberi.

n., interstitial. N. involving connective tissue of a nerve.

n., intraocular. N. of retinal fibers of optic nerve.

SYM: Disturbed vision, contracted field, enlarged blind spot, fundus findings such as exudates, hemorrhages, and abnormal condition of blood vessels.

TREATMENT: Depends on etiology such as brain tumors, meningitis, syphilis, nephritis, diabetes, etc.

n. migrans. N. which passes along a nerve trunk, affecting one area and then another. May be ascending or descending, q.v.

n., multiple. Simultaneous impairment of a number of peripheral nerves. SYN: *polyneuritis*

SYM: Related to suddenness of onset and severity, usually lower limbs are affected first with weakness which may progress until the entire body is affected. Muscle strength, deep tendon reflexes, sensory nerves, and autonomic nerves become involved.

ETIOL.: Infectious diseases such as diphtheria; metabolic disorders including alcoholism, diabetes, pellagra, beriberi, and sprue; various poisons. In some instances the disease arises without apparent cause.

TREATMENT: Remove causative factors if possible. Skilled nursing with particular care taken to prevent bed sores. Dietary therapy depending upon the etiology.

n. nodosa. N. with formation of nodes on nerves.

n., optic. N. of optic nerve.

n., parenchymatous. N. of nerve fiber substance.

n., peripheral. N. of terminal nerves or of end organs.

n., retrobulbar. N. of optic nerve behind eyeball.

SYM: Acute loss of vision in one or both eyes. Pain may be absent or unbearable and may last for days or only a brief period.

ETIOL: May be caused by a variety of illnesses but is most frequently caused by multiple sclerosis, pernicious anemia, diabetes, alcohol ingestion, or excessive use of tobacco.

n., rheumatic. N. with symptoms of rheumatism.

n., sciatic. Inflammation of the sciatic nerve. SEE: *sciatica.*

n., segmental. N. affecting segments of a nerve interspersed with healthy segments.

n., senile. N. in the elderly, usually affecting the extremities.

n., sympathetic. N. of opposite nerve without attacking nerve center.

n., tabetic. N. in locomotor ataxia. Caused by syphilis.

n., toxic. N. resulting from poisons-metallic poisons (such as arsenic, mercury, thallium) or nonmetallic poisons (various hydrocarbons and organic solvents).

n., traumatic. N. following an injury.

neuro- [Gr. *neuron,* sinew, nerve]. Combining form indicating relationship to a nerve, nervous tissue, or nervous system.

neuroanastomosis (nū″rō-ă-năs″tō-mō′sĭs). Surgical attachment of one end of a severed nerve to the other end.

neu″roanat′omy. Study of anatomy of the nervous system.

neuroarthritism (nū″rō-ăr′thrĭ-tĭzm) [Gr. *neuro,* nerve, + *arthron,* joint, + *ismos,* condition]. Tendency toward contraction of nervous and gouty disorders.

neuroarthropathy (nū″rō-ar-thrŏp′ăth-ĭ) ["+ "+ *pathos,* disease]. Disease of a joint combined with disease of the central nervous system.

neurobion (nū-rō-bī′ŏn) ["+ *bios,* life]. A hypothetical particle connected with renewal of nerve tissue.

neurobiotaxis (nū-rō-bī-ō-tăk′sĭs) [Gr. *neuron,* sinew, + *bios,* life, + *taxis,* order]. The phenomenon involving growth of dendrites and migration of nerve-cell bodies during development toward the region from which their dominant impulses are initiated.

neuroblast (nū′rō-blăst) ["+ *blastos,* germ]. An embryonic cell derived from neural tube or neural crest, giving rise to a neuron.

neuroblastoma (nū-rō-blăst-tō′mă) ["+ "+ *ōma,* tumor]. A malignant hemorrhagic tumor composed principally of cells resembling neuroblasts which give rise to cells of the sympathetic system, esp. adrenal medulla. Occurs chiefly in infants and children. Primary sites are in the mediastinal and retroperitoneal regions. SYN: *neuroblastoma sympatheticum.*

neurocanal (nū″rō-kă-năl′) [Gr. *neuron,* nerve + L. *canalis,* passage]. The central canal of the spinal cord.

neurocardiac (nū″rō-kar′dĭ-ăk) ["+ *kardia,* heart]. 1. Pert. to the nerves supplying the heart or nervous system and the heart. 2. Concerning a cardiac neurosis.

neurocele (nū′rō-sēl) ["+ *koilia,* cavity]. Ventricles and cavities in the cerebrospinal axis.

neurocentral (nū″rō-sĕn′trăl) ["+ *kentron,* center]. Pert. to the centrum of a vertebra and the neural arch.

neurochemistry (nū″rō-kĕm′ĭs-trĭ). Physiological chemistry dealing with nervous tissue.

neurochorioretinitis (nū″rō-kō″rĭ-ō-rĕ-tĭn-ī′tĭs) ["+ *chorion,* skin, + L. *rētē,* a net, + Gr. *-itis,* inflammation]. Inflammation of choroid and retina combined with optic neuritis.

neurochoroiditis (nū″rō-kō-roi-dī′tĭs) ["+ "+ *eidos,* like, + *-itis,* inflammation]. Inflamed condition of the choroid coat and optic nerve.

neurocirculatory (nū″rō-sŭr′kŭ-lă-tō″rĭ) ["+ L. *circulatiō,* circulation]. Pert. to circulation and the nervous system.

    n. asthenia. A combination of nervous and circulatory disturbances with fatigue and precordial pain, usually seen in soldiers. SYN: *irritable heart; soldier's heart.* SEE: *asthenia.*

neuroclonic (nū″rō-klŏn′ĭk) [Gr. *neuron,* nerve, + *klonos,* spasm]. Marked by spasms of nervous origin.

neurocoele (nū′rō-sēl) ["+ *koilia,* cavity]. System of cavities in cerebrospinal axis. SYN: *neurocele.*

neurocranium (nū″rō-krā′nĭ-ŭm) ["+ *kranion,* skull]. The part of the skull enclosing the brain.

neurocutaneous (nū″rō-kū-tā′nē-ŭs) ["+ L. *cutis,* skin]. Pert. to the nervous system and skin.

neurocyte (nū′rō-sīt) [Gr. *neuron,* sinew, + *kytos,* cell]. A nerve cell. SYN: *neuron.*

neurocytoma (nū″rō-sī-tō′mă) ["+ "+ *-ōma,* tumor]. A tumor formed of cells, usually ganglionic, of nervous origin. SYN: *neuroma.*

neurodealgia (nū-rō″dē-ăl′jĭ-ă) [Gr. *neurōdēs,* retina, + *algos,* pain]. Pain in the retina.

neurodendrite, neurodendron (nū″rō-dĕn′drīt, -dron) [Gr. *neuron,* sinew, + *dendron,* tree]. Protoplasmic branched process of a nerve cell. SYN: *dendrite; dendron.*

neurodermatitis (nū″rō-dĕr-mă-tī′tĭs) [Gr. *neuron,* nerve, + *derma,* skin, + *-itis,* inflammation]. Cutaneous inflammation with itching that is associated with, but not entirely due to, emotional disturbance. Circumscribed neurodermatitis is used as a synonym for lichen simplex.

    n., disseminated. Chronic superficial inflammation of skin characterized by thickening, excoriation, and lichenification, beginning usually in infancy. Common in families with high familial incidence of allergic diseases. SYN: *atopic dermatitis; atopic eczema; Brocq disease.*

neurodermatosis (nū″rō-dĕr-mă-tō′sĭs) ["+ "+ *-ōsis,* condition]. Any skin disease of neural origin. Includes neurofibromatosis (von Recklinghausen's disease), von Hippel-Lindau disease, Sturge-Weber syndrome, and tuberous sclerosis.

neurodermatrophia (nū-rō-derm-ă-trŏf′-ĭ-ă). Atrophy of the skin from nervous disease.

neurodiagnosis (nū″rō-dĭ-ăg-nō′sĭs). Diagnosis of nervous disorders.

neurodocitis (nū″rō-dō-sī′tĭs) ["+ *-itis,* inflammation]. Lesion of nerve roots due to pressure.

neurodynamia (nū″rō-dĭ-năm′ĭ-ă) ["+ *dynamis,* power]. Nervous energy or force.

neurodynamic (nū″rō-dĭ-năm′ĭk). Concerning nervous force or energy.

neurodynia (nū″rō-dĭn′ĭ-ă) [Gr. *neuron,* sinew or nerve, + *odynē,* pain]. Pain in a nerve or nerves. SYN: *neuralgia.*

neuroendocrine (nū′rō-ĕn′dō-krĭn). Pertaining to the nervous and endocrine system as an integrated functioning mechanism.

neuroepidermal (nū″rō-ĕp-ĭ-dŭr′măl) ["+ *epi,* upon, + *derma,* skin]. Pert. to or giving rise to nervous system and epidermis.

neuroepithelioma (nū″rō-ĕp″ĭ-thē-lĭ-ō′mă) ["+ "+ *thēlē,* nipple, + *-ōma,* tumor]. A relatively rare tumor of neuroepithelium in a nerve of special sense.

neuroepithelium (nū″rō-ĕp″ĭ-thē′lĭ-ŭm). 1. A specialized epithelial structure forming the termination of a nerve of special sense. Includes gustatory cells, olfactory cells, haircells of inner ear, and rods and cones of retina. 2. Embryonic layer of the epiblast from which the cerebrospinal axis is developed.

neurofibril, neurofibrilla (nū-rō-fī′brĭl, -fī-brĭl′ă) [Gr. *neuron,* sinew, + L. *fibrilla,* a small fiber]. (pl. *neurofibrils, neurofibrillae*) Many tiny fibrils that extend in every direction in the cytoplasm of the nerve cell body. They extend into the axon and dendrites of the cell. SEE: *neuron.*

neurofibroma (nū″rō-fī-brō′mă) ["+ L. *fibra,* fiber, + Gr. *-ōma,* tumor]. (pl. *neurofibromata* or *-mas*) A tumor of connective tissue of a nerve including medullated layer of a nerve fiber. May occur in mouth, pleura, or stomach.

    SYN: *neuroma, false; pseudoneuroma.*

neurofibromatosis (nū″rō-fī-brō″mă-tō′sĭs) ["+ "+ "+ *-ōsis,* increase]. Condition in which there are tumors of various sizes on peripheral nerves. They may be neuromas or fibromas.

n., multiple. SYN: *von Recklinghausen's disease,* q.v., *multiple neurofibroma.*

neurofibrosarcoma (nū-rō-fĭ-brō-săr-kō'mă). A malignant neurofibroma. SYN: *neurogenic sarcoma.*

neurofibrositis (nū″rō-fĭ″brō-sī'tĭs) ["+ "+ Gr. *-itis,* inflammation]. Inflammation of nerve fibers and sensory nerve fibers in muscular tissue.

neurogangliitis (nū″rō-gan-glĭ-ī'tis) [Gr. *neuron,* sinew, + *ganglion,* knot, + *-itis,* inflammation]. Inflamed condition of a neuroganglion.

neuroganglion (nū″rō-găn'glē-ŏn). A knotted mass of nervous matter.

neurogenesis (nū″rō-jĕn′ē-sĭs) ["+ *genesis,* production]. 1. Growth or development of nerves. 2. Development from nervous tissue.

neurogenetic (nūr″ō-jĕn-et'ĭk). 1. Pert. to nerve formation. 2. Pert. to origin in nerves.

neurogenic, neurogenous (nū-rō-jĕn'ĭk, -rōj'ĕn-ŭs). 1. Originating from nervous tissue. 2. Due to or resulting from nervous impulses.

neurogeny (nū-rŏj'ĕn-ĭ). SEE: *Neurogenesis.*

neuroglia (nū-rŏg'lĭ-ă) [Gr. *neuron,* sinew, + *glia,* glue]. The tissue which forms the interstitial or supporting elements—cells and fibers—of the nervous system. Neuroglia, also called glia includes: astrocytes, oligodendroglias, microglia (mesoglia), ependyma, neurilemma sheath cells or nerve fibers (cells of Schwann), and satellite (capsule) cells surrounding cranial and spinal ganglia. All except the microglia are of ectodermal origin. Neuroglia acts as connective or supporting tissue and also plays an important role in the reaction of the nervous system to injury or infection.

n. cell. Any of the cells of neuroglia; a neurogliacyte. SYN: *Glial cell.*

n. proper. Astroglia (astrocytes) and oligodendroglia (oligodendrocytes) of the central nervous system.

neurogliacyte (nū-rŏg'lĭ-ă-sīt) ["+ "+ *kytos,* cell]. Any one of the cells found in neuroglial tissue.

neuroglial (nū-rŏg'lē-ăl). Pertaining to the neuroglia.

neuroglioma (nū″rō-glĭ-ō'mă) [Gr. *neuron,* nerve, + *glia,* glue, + *-ōma,* tumor]. Tumor of neuroglial tissue. SYN: *glioma.*

n., ganglionar, n., gangliona're. Glioma with ganglion cells.

neurogliosis (nū-rŏg″lē-ō'sis) ["+ "+ *-ōsis,* condition]. Development of numerous neurogliomas.

neurogram (nū″rō-grăm) ["+ *gramma,* a mark]. The impression made upon the physi-

cal brain following any mental experience, thus retained as unconscious memory. SEE: *engram.*

neurography (nū-rog'ră-fĭ) [Gr. *neuron,* sinew, + *graphein,* to write]. 1. A study or description of the nervous system. 2. Formation of neurograms in the brain.

neurohematology (nū″rō-hem″at-ol'ō-jĭ) ["+ *haima,* blood, + *logos,* study]. The study of hemic changes in neural diseases.

neurohistology (nū″rō-hĭs-tŏl'ō-jĭ) ["+ *istos,* tissue, + *logos,* study]. Study of the microscopic anatomy of nervous tissue.

neurohumor (nū-rō-hū'mŏr). A chemical substance liberated at a nerve-ending that excites or activates an adjacent structure (neuron or muscle fiber). Ex: acetylcholine and sympathin (epinephrine). These substances are essential for transmission of impulses across synapses or myoneural junctions.

neurohypophysis (nū″rō-hĭ-pŏf'ĭs-ĭs) ["+ *hypo,* under, + *physis,* growth]. Posterior portion or pars nervosa of the pituitary gland.

neuroinduction (nū″rō-ĭn-dŭk'shŭn) ["+ L. *inductus,* leading]. Mental suggestion.

neurokeratin (nū″rō-kĕr'ă-tĭn) [Gr. *neuron,* sinew or nerve, + *keras, kerat-,* horn]. The variety of keratin found in myelinated nerve fibers.

neuroleptic drugs. Medicines which produce symptoms resembling those of diseases of the nervous system.

neurologic, neurological (nū-rō-lŏj'ĭk, -ĭ-kal) ["+ *logos,* study]. Pert. to the study of nervous diseases.

neurologist (nū-rŏl'ō-jĭst). A specialist in diseases of the nervous system.

neurology (nū-rŏl'ō-jĭ) [Gr. *neuron,* sinew, + *logos,* study]. The branch of medicine that deals with the nervous system and its diseases.

neurolymph (nū′rō-lĭmf) ["+ L. *lympha,* fluid]. The cerebrospinal fluid.

neurolysin (nū-rol′ĭs-ĭn) ["+ *lysis,* destruction]. A substance which destroys nerve cells.

neurolysis (nū-rol'ĭs-ĭs). 1. Stretching of a nerve to relieve tension. 2. Loosening of adhesions surrounding a nerve. 3. Disintegration of nerve tissue.

neurolytic (nū-rō-lĭt'ĭk). Concerning neurolysis.

neuroma (nū″rō-mă) [Gr. *neuron,* sinew, + *-ōma,* tumor]. A tumor along the course of a nerve or at the end of a divided nerve, consisting of coiled masses of axis cylinders, Schwann cells, and fibrous tissue.

n., amputation. N. occurring on a stump after amputation.

n., amyelinic. N. composed principally of unmyelinated nerve fibers.

n., appendiceal. N. found in mucosa and submucosa of the appendix.

n. cutis. N. in the skin.

n., cystic. N. with cystic formations.

n., false. Tumor arising from connective tissue of nerves, including the myelin sheath. SYN: *neurofibroma; pseudoneuroma.*

n., ganglionated. N. composed of true nerve cells.

n., myelinic. N. composed of medulated nerve fibers.

n., plexiform. N. of nerve trunks that appear to be twisted.

n. telangiectodes. N. with an abundance of blood vessels contained within it.

n., traumatic. Unorganized mass of nerve fibers occurring in wounds or on an amputation stump; result of accidental or intentional cutting of the nerve.

neuromalacia (nū″rō-măl-ā'sĭ-ă) [Gr. *neuron*, sinew, + *malakia*, softening]. Pathological softening of neural tissue.

neuromatosis (nū-rō″mă-tō'sĭs) ["+ -*ōma*, tumor, + *ōsis*, increase]. Multiple neuromas occurring in the body.

neuromatous (nū-rō'mă-tŭs). Rel. to a neuroma.

neuromechanism (nū″rō-měk′ăn-ĭzm). The neural structure controlling organic and systemic function.

neuromere (nū′rō-mēr) [Gr. *neuron*, sinew, + *meros*, part]. One of a series of segmental elevations on the ventrolateral surface of the rhombencephalon. SYN: *rhombomere.*

neuromimesis (nū-rō-mī-mē'sĭs) ["+ *mimēsis*, imitation]. Hysterical or neurotic activation of organic disease.

neuromuscular (nū″rō-mus′kū-lăr) ["+ L. *musculus*, a muscle]. Concerning both nerves and muscles.

neuromyelitis (nū-rō-mī-ĕl-ī'tĭs) [Gr. *neuron*, sinew, + *myelos*, marrow, + -*itis*, inflammation]. Inflammation of nerves and the spinal cord.

n. optica. A syndrome resulting from demyelinization occurring in the spinal cord, optic nerves, and chiasma. Etiology is unknown. May be a variant form of multiple sclerosis. SYN: *neuropticomyelitis; Devic's disease.*

neuromyopathic. Pert. to pathologic conditions involving both muscles and nerves.

neuromyositis (nū″rō-mī″ō-sī'tĭs) [Gr. *neuron*, nerve, + *mys*, muscle, + -*itis*, inflammation]. Neuritis complicated by inflammation of muscles which come in contact with affected nerves.

neuron (nū′rŏn) [Gr. *neuron*, nerve, sinew]. A nerve cell, the structural and functional unit of the nervous system. A n. consists of a cell body or perikaryon and its processes, an axon, and one or more dendrites. Neurons function in initiation and conduction of impulses. SEE: *nerve; nerve impulse; nervous system; nervous tissue.*

n., afferent. N. conducting impulses toward brain or spinal cord; a sensory neuron.

n., associative (association). N. which mediates impulses between a sensory and a motor neuron; a central neuron.

n., bipolar. N. bearing two processes, an axon and a dendrite.

n., central. N. confined entirely to central nervous system; an association n.

n., commissural. N. whose axon crosses to opposite side of brain or spinal cord.

n., efferent. N. which conducts impulses away from the brain or spinal cord.

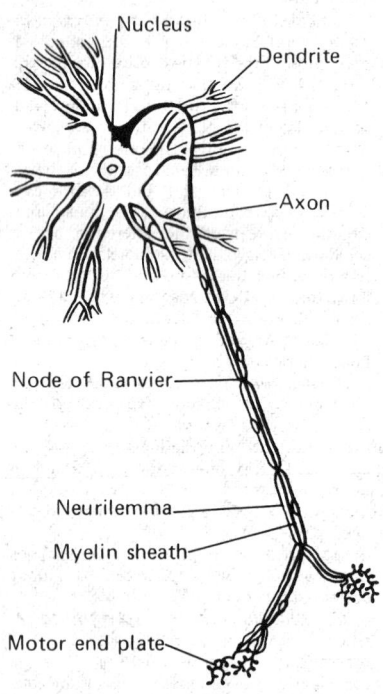

MOTOR NEURON

n., motor. N. that conveys impulses initiating muscle contraction.

n., motor, lower. N. whose cell body lies in anterior gray column of spinal cord. Its axon innervates striated muscle fibers. SYN: *ventral horn cells.*

n., motor, upper. N. whose cell body lies in motor area of cerebral cortex. Its axon passes down spinal cord and synapses with lower motor neurons.

n., multipolar. N. with one axon and many dendrites.

n., peripheral. N. whose process constitutes a part of the peripheral nervous system (cranial, spinal, or sympathetic nerves).

n., postganglionic. N. whose body lies in an autonomic ganglion and its axon terminates in an effector organ (smooth or cardiac muscle or glands).

n., preganglionic. N. of autonomic nervous system whose cell body lies in central nervous system and axon terminates in peripheral ganglia.

n., sensory. An afferent n. which conveys impulses that give rise to sensations.

n., unipolar. N. whose cell body bears one process.

neuronal (nū'rō-năl). Pertaining to one or more neurons.

neurone (nū'rōn). Neuron, q.v.

neuronevus (nū"rō-nē'vŭs). Intradermal nevus.

neuronitis (nū-rōn-ī'tĭs) [Gr. *neuron*, nerve, + *-itis*, inflammation]. Inflammation or degenerative inflammation of nerve cells.

neuronophage (nū-rŏn'ō-fāj) ["+ *phagein*, to eat]. A phagocyte that destroys tissue in the nervous system.

neuronophagia, neuronophagy (nū-rŏn-ō-fā'jĭ-ă, -ŏf'ă-jĭ). Destruction of nerve cells by phagocytes.

neuronyxis (nū-rō-nĭk'sĭs) ["+ *nyxis*, a piercing]. Therapeutic or diagnostic neural puncture.

neuropathic (nū-rō-păth'ĭk) [Gr. *neuron*, nerve, + *pathos*, disease]. Rel. to neuropathy.

neuropathogenesis (nū"rō-păth"ō-jĕn'ē-sĭs) ["+ "+ *genesis*, production]. The origin and development of a neural disease.

neuropathology (nū"rō-pă-thŏl'ō-jĭ) ["+ "+ *logos*, study]. The study of diseases of the nervous system and structural and functional changes occurring in them. The diseases are divided into (1) congenital defects in development, those in which an inherent tendency to degeneracy reveals itself only after a period of time, and (2) those in which destructive influences act upon a brain which was normal initially. The last-named

are mainly inflammatory, toxic, traumatic, mechanical, or neoplastic in type. Circulatory impairment, disuse, and overactivity also contribute to the development of nervous diseases.

neuropathy (nū-rŏp'ă-thĭ). Any disease of the nerves.

neurophonia (nū"rō-fō'nĭ-ă) [Gr. *neuron*, nerve, + *phōnē*, voice]. A tic or spasm of muscles of speech resulting in an involuntary cry or sound.

neurophysiology (nū"rō-fĭz-ĭ-ol'ō-jĭ) ["+ *physis*, growth, + *logos*, study]. Physiology of the nervous structure of the body.

neuropil (nū'rō-pĭl) [Gr. *neuron*, sinew, + *pilos*, felt]. Network of unmyelinated fibrils into which nerve processes of central nervous system divide.

neuroplasm (nū'rō-plăzm) ["+ *plasmos*, a thing formed]. The undifferentiated cytoplasmic substance of a neuron which surrounds and separates the neurofibrils. SYN: *interfibrillar* or *perifibrillar substance.*

neuroplasmic (nū"rō-plaz'mĭk). Concerning the protoplasm of a neuron.

neuroplasty (nū'rō-plăs'tĭ) ["+ *plassein*, to form]. Reparative surgery of the nerves.

neu"ropo'dia [Gr. *neuron*, nerve, + *podion*, little feet]. (pl. of *neuropodium*). Small bulblike expansions of axon terminals at a synaptic junction. SYN: *end feet; terminal buttons.*

neuropore (nū'rō-pōr) ["+ *poros*, an opening]. Embryonic opening from neural canal to exterior.

neuropsychiatry (nū"rō-sī-kī'ă-trĭ) ["+ *psychē*, mind, + *iatreia*, healing]. The branch of medicine pertaining to study and treatment of nervous and mental diseases.

neuropsychopathy (nū"rō-sī-kop'ăth-ĭ) ["+ "+ *pathos*, disease]. Psychiatric disease combined with mental disorder.

neurorelapse (nū"rō-rē-lăps") [Gr. *neuron*, sinew, + L. *relapsus*, fallen back]. Nervous symptoms in syphilis subsequent to an injection of salvarsan.

neuroretinitis (nū"rō-rĕt"ĭn-ī'tĭs) ["+ L. *rētē*, net, + Gr. *-itis*, inflammation]. Inflamed condition of optic nerve and retina.

neurorrhaphy (nū-rŏr'ă-fĭ) ["+ *raphē*, a sewing]. Suturing of ends of a severed nerve.

neurosarcokleisis (nū"rō-săr"kō-klī'sĭs) [Gr. *neuron*, nerve, + *sarx, sark-*, flesh, + *kleisis*, closure]. Operation for relief of neuralgia by resection of a wall of the osseous canal carrying a nerve and transplanting the nerve to soft tissues.

neurosarcoma (nū"rō-săr-kō'mă) ["+ "+ *-ōma*, tumor]. A sarcoma containing neuromatous components.

neurosclerosis (nū″rō-sklē-rō′sĭs) ["+ *sklērōsis*, a hardening]. Hardening of nervous tissue.

neurosecretion (nū″rō-sē-krē′shŭn). The elaboration and discharge of a chemical substance by a neuron. Ex: secretion of hormones by cells of the hypothalamus.

neurosensory (nū″rō-sĕn′sō-rĭ) ["+ L. *sēnsōrius*, pert. to a sensation]. Concerning a sensory nerve.

neurosis (nū-rō′sĭs) [Gr. *neuron*, sinew, + *-ōsis*, disease]. (pl. *neuroses*) A disorder of the thought processes not due to demonstrable disease of the structure of the central nervous system. Probably due to unresolved internal conflicts which make for an uneasy adjustment to life. Contact with reality is maintained which is not the case in psychosis, q.v. The neuroses are usually classified as fatigue (or neurasthenia); simple nervousness (or anxiety); phobic; obsessive compulsive (or psychasthenia); hysteria; hypochondriasis; reactive depression. The disease rarely occurs in one of these pure forms. Thus most neurotic persons would be classed as having mixed psychoneuroses. SYN: *psychoneurosis*.

TREATMENT: Psychotherapy, tranquilizers, and sedatives. It must be remembered that in general a symptom due to a neurotic reaction to a situation is just as real to the patient as if it were due to organic disease. Usually such a symptom is much more difficult to treat than it would be if due to organic disease.

n., accident. A nervous disorder caused by injury or an accident.

n., anxiety. N. in which fear or apprehension is the essential symptom. SEE: *anxiety n.*

n., association. N. in which association of ideas causes mental repetition of an experience.

n., cardiac. SEE: *asthenia, neurocirculatory.*

n., compensation. N. developing after an accident in people who think they can obtain compensation by being ill.

n., compulsion. N. marked by overpowering impulse to perform acts against the will.

n., craft. N., occupational, q.v.

n., expectation. Condition in which anticipation of an occurrence produces nervous symptoms.

n., fatigue. Neurasthenia, q.v.

n., obsessional. Uncontrollable obsessions dominating the victim's behavior.

n., occupational, n., professional. N. due to the occupation or profession of a patient.

n., pension. Compensation n., q.v.

n., sexual. N. involving sexual function.

n., traumatic. N., accident, q.v.

n., war. N. brought on by conditions of war, seen in soldiers. SYN: *shell shock.*

neurospasm (nū′rō-spăzm) [Gr. *neuron*, nerve, + *spasmos*, spasm]. Spasmodic muscular twitching due to a nervous disorder.

Neuros'pora. Pink bread-mold, a fungus belonging to the Ascomycetes. Used for research in studies of genetics and in bio-assays.

neurosurgery (nū″rō-sur′jĕ-rĭ) [Gr. *neuron*, sinew, + L. *chirurgia*, hand, + *ergon*, work]. Surgery of the nervous system.

neurosuture (nū″rō-sū′chŭr) ["+ L. *sutura*, a stitch]. Stitching of ends of a cut nerve. SYN: *neurorrhaphy.*

neurosyphilis (nū″rō-sĭf′ĭ-lĭs). Syphilis affecting the nervous structures. SEE: *dementia paralytica.*

n., asymptomatic. N. preceding symptomatic neurosyphilis but showing no symptoms. Diagnosed by changes in spinal fluid.

n., meningovascular. A form of n. involving the meninges and vascular structures in the brain or spinal cord or both.

neurotension (nū″rō-tĕn′shŭn) [Gr. *neuron*, nerve, + L. *tensiō*, a stretching]. Operative stretching of a nerve. SYN: *neurectasis.*

neurothecitis (nū″rō-thē-sī′tĭs) ["+ *thēkē*, sheath, + *-itis*, inflammation]. Inflamed condition of a nerve sheath.

neurotherapeutics (nū″rō-thĕr-ă-pū′tĭks) ["+ *therapeutikē*, treatment]. Treatment of disorders of the nervous system. SYN: *neurotherapy.*

neurotherapy (nū-rō-ther′ă-pĭ) [Gr. *neuron*, nerve, + *therapeia*, treatment]. Treatment of nervous disorders.

neurothlipsis (nū″rō-thlĭp′sĭs) ["+ *thlipsis*, pressure]. Irritation or pressure on a nerve.

neurotic (nū-rŏt′ĭk) [Gr. *neuron*, sinew, nerve]. 1. One suffering from a neurosis. 2. Pert. to neurosis. 3. Nervous.

neuroticism (nū-rŏt′ĭ-sĭzm) ["+ *ismos*, state of]. A condition or trait of neurosis.

neurotization (nū″rŏt-ĭ-zā′shŭn) [Gr. *neuron*, sinew]. 1. Acquisition of nervous substance. 2. Regeneration of a nerve after division. 3. Surgical introduction of a nerve into a paralyzed muscle.

neurotmesis (nū″rŏt-mē′sĭs). Nerve injury with complete loss of function of the nerve even though there is little apparent damage anatomically.

neurotology (nū″rō-tŏl′ō-jĭ) ["+ *ous, ot-*, ear, + *logos*, study]. The division of otology which deals with the inner ear, esp. its nerve supply, nerve connections with the brain, and auditory and labyrinthine pathways and centers within the brain.

neurotome (nū′rō-tōm) ["+ *tome*, a cut]. Fine knife used in the division of a nerve.

neurotomy (nū-rŏt′ō-mĭ) ["+ *tome*, an incision]. Division or dissection of a nerve.

neurotonic (nū″rō-tŏn′ĭk) ["+ *tonos*, tension]. 1. Concerning neural stretching. 2. Having a stimulating effect upon nerves or the nervous system.

neurotony (nū-rŏt′ō-nĭ). Nerve stretching, usually to ease pain.

neurotoxic (nū″rō-tŏks′ĭk) [Gr. *neuron*, nerve, + *toxikon*, poison]. Poisonous to the nerve cells.

neurotoxin (nū″rō-tŏks′ĭn). A toxin that attacks nerve cells. SYN: *neurolysin*.

neurotrauma (nū-rō-traw′mă) ["+ *trauma*, wound]. Injury of a nerve.

neurotripsy (nū′rō-trĭp′sĭ) ["+ *tripsis*, a rubbing]. Surgical crushing of a nerve.

neurotrophasthenia (nū″rō-trŏf-ăs-thē′nĭ-ă) ["+ *trophe*, nourishment, + *astheneia*, weakness]. Malnutrition of the nervous system.

neurotroph′ic. Pert. to the influence of nervous impulses upon the well-being of an organ or structure.

neurotrophy (nū-rŏt′rō-fĭ). Nutrition and maintenance of nervous tissue.

neurotropism (nū-rŏt′rō-pĭzm) [Gr. *neuron*, nerve, + *trope*, a turning, + *ismos*, condition]. Attraction which nutritive elements, basic dyes, and microorganisms have for nervous tissue.

neurotropy (nū-rŏt′rō-pĭ). Neurotropism, q.v.

neurotrosis (nū″rō-trō′sĭs) [Gr. *neuron*, nerve, + *trōsis*, a wound]. Injury of a nerve. SYN: *neurotrauma*.

neurovaccine (nū″rō-văk′sĭn). A standardized vaccine virus of specific strength. Usually secured by cultivation in a rabbit's brain.

neurovaricosis (nū″rō-văr″ĭ-kō′sĭs) ["+ L. *varicōsus*, pert. to a swollen vein]. Multiple swellings along the pathway of a nerve.

neurovascular (nū″rō-văs′kū-lăr) ["+ L. *vasculus*, a small vessel]. Concerning both the nervous and vascular systems.

neurovirus (nū″rō-vī′rŭs). Virus which has been modified by its growing in nervous tissue. Used in preparing a vaccine.

neurula (nū′rū-lă). Stage in development of an embryo, esp. amphibian embryos, during which the neural plate develops and axial embryonic nervous structures are elaborated.

neutral (nū′trăl) [L. *neutralis, neuter*, neither]. 1. Neither alkaline nor acid. 2. Indifferent; having no positive qualities.

   n. fat. One of the fats commonly found in the tissues; an ester of fatty acids with glycerol. Ex: tristearin; triolein; tripalmitin.

   n. point. pH7, a point on the pH scale which represents neutrality, i.e., the solution is neither acid or alkaline in reaction.

   n. red. A dye used as an indicator and as a vital stain.

neutralization (nū-trăl-ĭ-zā′shŭn). 1. The opposing of one force or condition with an opposite force or condition to such degree as to cause counteraction that permits neither to dominate. 2. In chemistry, the process of destroying the peculiar properties or effect of a substance, i.e., the neutralization of an acid with a base or vice versa. 3. In medicine, the process of checking or counteracting the effects of any agent which produces a morbid effect.

neutralize (nū′trăl-īz). 1. To counteract and make ineffective. 2. In chem. to destroy peculiar properties or effect; to make inert.

neutroclusion (nū″trō-klū′zhŭn) [L. *neuter*, neither, + *occludo*, to close]. State in which the anteroposterior occlusal positions of the teeth or the mesiodistal positions are normal, but malocclusion of the other positions exists.

neutron (nū′trŏn) [L. *neuter*, neither]. Subatomic particle equal in mass to a proton but without an electric charge. A constituent of the atomic nucleus, it has a mass 1,839 times that of an electron. As a free particle it has an average life of little less than 17 minutes.

neutropenia (nū-trō-pē′nĭ-ă) ["+ Gr. *penia*, lack]. Abnormally small number of neutrophil cells in the blood.

neutrophil(e (nū′trō-fĭl, -fīl) ["+ Gr. *philein*, to love]. 1. Staining easily with neutral dyes. 2. A leukocyte that stains easily with neutral dyes. SEE: *polymorphonuclear leukocyte*.

neutrophilia (nū″trō-fĭl′ĭ-ă). Increase in the number of neutrophil leukocytes in the blood.

neutrophilic, neutrophilous (nū-trō-fĭl′-ĭk, -trŏf′ĭ-lŭs) [L. *neuter*, neither + Gr. *philein*, to love]. Staining readily with neutral dyes.

nevoid (nē′voyd) [L. *naevus*, birthmark, + Gr. *eidos*, form]. Resembling a nevus.

nevolipoma (nē-vō-lĭ-pō′mă) ["+ Gr. *lipos*, fat, + *-ōma*, tumor]. Rare lipoma containing numerous blood vessels, probably a degenerated nevus.

nevose (nē'vōs) [L. *naevus*, birthmark]. Spotted or marked with nevi. SEE: *nevus*.

nevus (nē'vŭs) [L. *naevus*, birthmark]. (pl. *nevi*). A congenital discoloration of a circumscribed area of the skin due to pigmentation. SYN: *birthmark; mole*. 2. Circumscribed vascular tumor of the skin, usually congenital, due to hyperplasia of the blood vessels. SEE: *angioma*.

    n. angiectodes. N. vascularis, q.v.

    n. angiomatodes. Extensive diffuse angiomatous condition of the subcutaneous tissues.

    n. araneus. Acquired or congenital dilatation of the capillaries, marked by red lines radiating from a central red dot. SYN: *spider n.*

    n., capillary. N. of dilated capillary vessels, elevated above the skin.

    TREATMENT: Ligature, excision.

    n., cutaneous. N. formation on the skin.

    n. flammeus. Reddish discoloration of the face or neck, usually not elevated above the skin. A serious deformity due to large size and color.

    n. lipomatodes. Fatty connective tissue tumor, probably a degenerated nevus containing numerous blood vessels. SYN: *nevolipoma.*

    n. maternus. A birthmark; congenital angioma.

    n. pigmentosus; pigmented n. Congenital pigment spot varying in color from light yellow to black. Intradermal, or common moles, are benign. Other types are or may become malignant.

    TREATMENT: Malignant or suspicious lesions should be treated by wide surgical excision. Benign lesions do not require treatment except when located at sites of friction causing bleeding, ulceration, etc. Some are removed for cosmetic reasons.

    n. pilosus. A n. covered with hair.

    n., spider. N. araneus, q.v.

    n. spilus. Pigmented n. with smooth surface.

    n., strawberry. N. vascularis, q.v.; strawberry mark.

    n., telangiectatic. N. containing dilated capillaries.

    n. vascularis, n. vasculosus. N. in which superficial blood vessels are enlarged. Nevi are usually congenital and of variable size and shape; slightly elevated; reddish or purplish; on face, head, neck, and arms though no region is exempt. Usually disappear spontaneously but wrinkling, pigmentation, and scarring are sometimes seen.

    SYN: *strawberry n.; strawberry mark.*

    n., venosus, n. venous. N. formed of dilated venules.

    n. verrucosus. N. with a raised wartlike surface.

new growth. Any new growth of tissue. Usually considered to be abnormal but not always so; the normal fetus is in fact a new growth. SYN: *neoplasm.*

nexus (nĕk'sŭs) [L. bond]. (pl. *nexus*) A connection or link; a binding together. Used to designate a bond between components of a group.

N. F. Abbr. for *National Formulary,* q.v.

NH₃. Ammonia.

NH₄Br. Ammonium bromide.

NH₄Cl. Ammonium chloride (USP).

NH₄NO₃. Ammonium nitrate.

NH₄OH. Ammonium hydroxide. SYN: *aqua ammonia* or *ammonia water.*

Ni. Symb. for *nickel.*

niacin (nī'ă-sĭn). Nicotinic acid.

niacinamide (nī''a-sĭn-ăm'ĭd). Nicotinamide.

niche (nĭch) [Fr.]. A depression or recess on a smooth surface. Esp. an erosion in the wall of a hollow organ, detected by roentgenogram.

    n., enamel. One of two depressions which develop between the dental lamina and the enamel organ. SYN: *enamel crypt.*

nickel (nĭk'el) [L. *niccolum*]. SYMB: *Ni.* At. wt. 58.71, at. no. 28. Metallic element.

    n. arc. One that emits strongly at 230 and esp. at 350 millimicrons.

Nicolas-Favre disease (nē''kō-lă făv'r) Venereal disease marked by involvement of inguinal lymph glands with an exuding lesion. SYN: *Frei's disease; lymphogranuloma venerea.*

nicotinamide (nĭk''ō-tĭn'ă-mĭd). Member of vitamin B complex, used in management or prevention of pellagra. The peripheral flush that often accompanies therapy with nicotinic acid, q.v., is avoided with nicotinamide. SYN: *niacinamide.*

nicotine (nĭk'ō-tēn, -tĭn) [L. *nicotiana,* tobacco]. A poisonous alkaloid found in all parts of the tobacco plant, but esp. in the leaves. When pure, it is a colorless oily fluid with little odor, but a sharp, burning taste. On exposure to air or in crude materials, it becomes deep brown with the characteristic tobacco-like smell.

    N. is one of the most toxic of all poisons. Cigarette tobacco contains from 15 to 30 mgm. of n. per cigarette, but since smoke contains less than 10 mgm. of this amount only a few milligrams are absorbed. SEE: *n. poisoning, acute.*

    n. poisoning, acute. SYM: Excitement, restlessness, clonic convulsions, confusion, weakness, increased salivation, nausea and vomiting, abdominal cramps and diarrhea, rapid and irregular pulse, rapid and labored respiration.

TREATMENT: If patient is conscious, oral administration of universal antidote, q.v., tannic acid, activated charcoal, or strong tea, followed by gastric lavage or an emetic. In unconsciousness use gastric lavage. Keep patient warm with external heat and maintain the airway. Artificial or mechanical respiration and oxygen therapy if necessary. If convulsions are severe or persist, intravenous barbiturates in small doses are indicated.

nicotinic acid (nĭk″ō-tĭn′ĭk). The antipellagra principle of vitamin B complex. Occurs as a white crystal or powder. Used orally or parenterally as a preventive, and specifically as therapy in pellagra. SYN: *niacin.*

nicotinism (nĭk′ō-tĭn-ĭzm). Poisoning from excessive use of tobacco or nicotine.

nictation, nictitation [L. *nictitare,* to wink]. Involuntary winking.

nictitate (nĭk′tĭ-tāt). To wink.

nictitating (nĭk′tĭ-tāt-ĭng). Winking or blinking.

    n. spasm. Clonic spasm of eyelid with continuous winking.

nidal (nī′dal) [L. *nidus,* nest]. Pert. to a nidus.

nidation (nī-da′shun). Implantation of the fertilized ovum in the lining of the uterus (endometrium).

nidus (nī′dŭs) [L. nest]. (pl. *ni′di*) 1. A cluster; nestlike structure. 2. Focus of infection. 3. A nucleus or origin of a nerve.

    n. avis cerebelli. A deep sulcus on each side of the inferior vermis separating it from adjacent lobes of hemispheres.

Niemann-Pick disease (nē′man-pĭk). [Albert Niemann, Ger. pediatrician, 1880-1921; Ludwig Pick, Ger. physician, 1868-]. A disturbance of lipoid metabolism characterized by enlargement of liver and spleen (hepatosplenomegaly), anemia, lymphadenopathy, and progressive mental and physical deterioration. A hereditary disease, its onset is in early infancy with death usually before the third year. Typical cell, having a foamy appearance and filled with a lipoid believed to be sphingomyelin, can be found in bone marrow, spleen, or lymph nodes and aids in establishing the diagnosis. SYN: *lipid histiocytosis.*

night blindness [AS. *nyht,* night]. Absence of, or defective, vision in the dark. SYN: *nyctalopia; nyctotyphlosis.*

    ETIOL: Due to lack of visual purple in the rods or to its slowness in regenerating after

exposure to light. May result from vitamin A deficiency or hereditary factors.

Nightingale, Florence (nit′ĭn-gāl). [Eng. philanthropist, 1820-1910]. Founder of modern nursing and reformer of hospital conditions. Served as a nurse in Crimean War. Founded a training school for nurses.

    N. oath or pledge. "I solemnly pledge myself before God and in the presence of this assembly to pass my life in purity and to practice my profession faithfully. I will abstain from whatever is deleterious and mischievous, and will not take or knowingly administer any harmful drug. I will do all in my power to elevate the standard of my profession, and I will hold in confidence all personal matters committed to my keeping, and all family affairs coming to my knowledge in the practice of my calling. With loyalty will I endeavor to aid the physician in his work and devote myself to the welfare of those committed to my care."

nightmare (nīt′mār) [AS. *nyht,* night, + *mara,* a demon]. A bad dream accompanied by great fear and a feeling of suffocation. Once believed to be caused by a female monster or spirit that sat upon the dreamer. SYN: *oneirodynia.* SEE: *antephialtic.*

nightshade (nīt′shād) [AS. *nihtscada*]. Any of several of the plants of the genus Solanum.

    n., deadly. Belladonna, q.v.

night sweat [AS. *nyht,* night, + *swat,* sweat]. Profuse sweating during sleep at night. Often it is an early sign of disease, esp. with intermittent temperature. In children it occurs in rickets in debilitated states. Patient should be rubbed down, sponged, and changed into dry clothing.

night terrors ["+ L. *terror,* state of fear]. Form of nightmare in children causing them to awaken in terror, screaming. Fear continues for a period after the return to consciousness. SYN: *pavor nocturnus.*

night vision. The ability to see at night or in light of low intensity. Results from dark adaptation in which pupil dilates, visual purple increases, and intensity threshold of the retina is lowered. Any decrease in oxygen content of the blood is accompanied by some loss of night vision. Thus smoking cigarettes or being in an atmosphere with decreased oxygen pressure decreases night vision. SYN: *scotopic vision.*

nightwalking ["+ *wealcan,* to revolve]. State in which individual habitually walks about while sleeping. SYN: *somnambulism.*

nigra (nī′gră) [L. black]. Mass of gray matter bet. the dorsal and pedal parts of the crus cerebri. SYN: *substantia nigra.*

nigri-, nigro- [L.]. Combining forms pert. to blackness.

nigricans (nī'grĭ-kăns) [L.]. Blackened.

nigrities (nĭ-grĭsh'ĭ-ēz) [L. blackness]. Blackness; black pigmentation.

n. linguae. A black pigmentation of the tongue. SYN: *glossophytia.*

NIH. Abbr. for *National Institutes of Health.*

nihilism (nī'ĭ-lĭzm) [L. *nihil,* nothing, + Gr. *ismos,* state of]. 1. Disbelief in power of medicine in modifying disease. 2. A delusion in which everything is unreal.

Nikolsky's sign (nĭ-kŏl'skĭ). [Pyotr Nikolsky, Rus. dermatologist, 1855-]. Condition of the external layer of the skin in which it can be rubbed off by slight friction or injury. Seen in pemphigus.

ninth cranial nerve. Glossopharyngeal nerve. SEE: *Table of Cranial Nerves* in *Appendix.*

niobium (nī-ō'bē-ŭm). [Legendary Gr. woman, Niobe, who was turned into stone]. SYMB: Nb. At. wt. 92.906; at. no. 41. A chemical element formerly called columbium.

niphablepsia (nĭf'ă-blĕp'sĭ-ă) [Gr. *nipha,* snow, + *ablepsia,* blindness]. Blindness caused by light glare on snow.

niphotyphlosis (nĭf'ō-tĭf-lō'sĭs) ["+ *typhlōsis,* blindness]. Snow blindness. SYN: *niphablepsia.*

nipple (nĭp'l) [AS. *neb.,* a little protuberance]. 1. The conical protuberance in each breast of the female from which the lactiferous ducts discharge. SYN: *mammilla; papilla mammae* [NA]; *teat.* 2. Artificial substitute for female n. to be used on a nursing bottle.

The nipple contains erectile tissue and is surrounded by a pigmented area called the areola. The areola is pink in those who have never borne children and darker in those who have. It is supplied with a row of small sebaceous glands around its base called areolar glands which secrete an oily substance to keep it supple. SEE: *breast* for illustration.

NP: During postpartum nipples should be washed well with soap and water and dried with a rough towel. Excessively dry nipples may be massaged with cold cream or lanolin. Cracked and sore nipples result from misuse of the nipple due to the baby's chewing.

RS: acromastitis, halo, mammary, mammillation, Paget's disease of n., thelalgia, thelitis.

n., crater. N., retracted, q.v.

n. line. A vertical line passing through the nipple. SYN: *mammillary line.*

n., retracted. N. whose tip lies below level of mammary gland. Caused by deficiency of muscle tissue or flattening of erectile tissue.

n. shield. Mechanical device to protect the nipple during lactation period.

Nissl's bodies or granules (nĭs'l). [Franz Nissl, Ger. neurologist, 1860-1919]. Chromophil substance in the form of granules found in the cell bodies and dendrites of neurons but lacking in the most peripheral region of the nerve cell cytoplasm and the area where the axis cylinder (axon hillock) originates and from the axon cylinder. They are stained selectively by toluidin and other basic aniline dyes. They consist principally of the ribose type of nucleic acid and nucleoprotein.

They are concerned with protein synthesis and metabolism; their condition varies with physiologic and pathologic conditions. In fatigue and certain pathologic states they may dissolve and disappear, a phenomenon called chromatolysis. SYN: *tigroid bodies.*

nisus (nī'sŭs) [L. effort]. Effort, exertion, or a strong force.

nit (nĭt) [AS. *hnitu*]. The egg of a louse or any other parasitic insect. SEE: *pediculosis.*

niter (nī'ter) [Gr. *nitron,* soda]. Sodium nitrate or potassium nitrate (saltpeter). SEE: *nitre.*

niton (nī'tŏn). Radon, q.v.

nitrate (nī'trāt) [L. *nitratum*]. A salt of nitric acid.

ni'trated. Combined with nitric acid or a nitrate.

nitra'tion. Combination with nitric acid or a nitrate.

nitre (nī'tĕr) [Gr. *nitron,* soda]. Br. spelling of niter, q.v.

ni'tric acid. HNO_3. A colorless, corrosive, poisonous liquid in concentrated form, employed as a caustic. It is widely used in industry and in chemical laboratories.

POISONING SYM: Essentially same as those produced by sulfuric acid. Pain, burning, vomiting, thirst, and shock.

TREATMENT: Dilute with large volumes of water. Neutralize with weak alkalies; give magnesium oxide, milk of magnesia, milk or egg white in large amounts. Avoid emetics and stomach tubes because either may cause rupture of the stomach.

n. a., fuming. Nitric acid which emits fumes of a choking nature. SEE: *fumes.*

nitride (nī'trĭd). A binary compound formed by direct combination of nitrogen with another element, as lithium nitride Li_3N.

nitrification (nī"trĭ-fĭ-kā'shŭn). The process by which the nitrogen of ammonia or other compounds is oxidized to nitric or nitrous acid or their salts (nitrates, nitrites). Takes place continually in the soil through the action of nitrifying bacteria.

nitrifying (nī′trĭ-fī″ĭng). The process of nitrification, q.v.

   n. bacteria. Bacteria which induce nitrification. Include the nitrite bacteria Nitrosomas which convert ammonia to nitrites and nitrate bacteria Nitrobacter which convert nitrites to nitrates.

nitrile (nī′trĭl). An organic compound in which the nitrogen of ammonia exists with all three of the displaced hydrogen atoms.

nitrite (nī′trīte) [Gr. *nitron,* salt]. A salt of nitrous acid. Nitrites dilate blood vessels, reduce blood pressure, depress motor centers of the spinal cord, and act as antispasmodics. Principal nitrites used in medicine are amyl, ethyl, potassium, and sodium nitrite, q.v.

nitritoid (nī′trĭ-toyd) ["+ *eidos,* resemblance]. Resembling a nitrite.

   n. crisis. A syndrome resembling symptoms produced by the use of a nitrite, usually occurring after arsphenamine injection.

nitrituria (nī-trĭ-tū′rĭ-ă) ["+ *ouron,* urine]. Nitrites present in the urine.

nitro-, nitr- [Gr.]. Combining form denoting combination with nitrogen or presence of the group NO_2.

nitrofurazone (nī-trō-fu′ră-zōn). A synthetic antibiotic for topical application in some skin diseases.

nitrogen (nī′trō-jĕn) [Gr. *nitron,* niter, + *gennan,* to produce]. SYMB: *N.* At. wt. 14.0067; at. no. 7. A colorless, odorless, tasteless gaseous element occurring free in the atmosphere, forming 4/5 of its volume.

One of the important elements in all proteins, n. is essential to plant and animal life for tissue building. Generally it is found in organic nature only in the form of compounds, as ammonia, nitrites, and nitrates. These are transformed by plants into proteins, and, being consumed by animals, are converted into animal proteins of the blood and tissues.

RS: azotation; azote; azotification; azotized.

   n. balance. The difference between the amount of nitrogen ingested and that excreted each day. If intake is greater, a positive balance exists; if less, there is a negative balance. SEE: *n. equilibrium.*

   n. cycle. N. discharged from animal life into the soil; n. is then taken up from soil into plants for their nourishment; and in turn n. returns to animal life through plants eaten.

   n. equilibrium. Condition during which nitrogen excreted in the urine, feces, and sweat equals amount taken in by the body in food.

   n. fixation. Conversion of atmospheric n. into nitrates through the action of bacteria in the soil.

   n. lag. Extent of time required after a given protein is ingested before an amount of n. equal to that in protein has been excreted.

   n. monoxide. N_2O. Nitrous oxide. Also referred to as laughing gas.

   n. mustards. 1. A term embracing certain therapeutic mustard compounds. Used because they destroy lymphoid tissue in Hodgkin's disease, lymphosarcoma, giant follicular lymphoblastoma, chronic lymphoid, myeloid leukemia, rheumatoid arthritis, and nephritis. 2. Used in chemical warfare.

   n. narcosis. Condition of euphoria, impaired judgement, decreased coordination, and motor ability seen in persons exposed to high air pressure such as divers and submariners. The effects are similar to those produced by alcoholic intoxication, caused by the increased concentration of n. gas in body tissues, including the brain. Once the condition passes, it is harmless.

   n., nonprotein. That n. which appears in food, blood, or other substance but is not present as a protein.

nitrogenous (nī-trŏj′ĕn-ŭs) [Gr. *nitron,* soda, + *gennan,* to produce]. Pert. to or containing nitrogen. Foods which contain nitrogen are the proteins; those which do not contain nitrogen are the fats and carbohydrates. The retention of nitrogenous products in the blood is marked in kidney diseases.

nitroglycerin (nī″trō-glĭs′ĕr-ĭn) ["+ *glycerin*]. Any nitrate of glycerol. Specifically the trinitrate—a heavy, oily, explosive, colorless liquid obtained by treating glycerol with nitric and sulfuric acids. It is the explosive constituent of dynamite. In medicine it has the action of nitrites and is a vasodilator. Used esp. in angina pectoris. SYN: *glyceryl trinitrate.*

nitromuriatic acid (nī″trō-mū-rī-ăt′ĭk) ["+ L. *muriaticus,* briny]. A mixture of 1 part nitric acid and 3 parts hydrochloric acid used in commercial industries because it dissolves all the metals including platinum and gold. SYN: *aqua regia*

   POISONING SYM: Same as those of nitric acid poisoning.

   TREATMENT: Same.

nitrous (nī′trŭs) [Gr. *nitron,* soda]. Containing nitrogen in its lowest valency.

n. oxide. N_2O. Colorless sweet-tasting gas with pleasing smell causing temporary general anesthesia when inhaled. Noninflammable, it is given in various amounts with oxygen or other anesthetic agents. Its action as an anesthetic can be potentiated by other classes of drugs—barbiturates, narcotics, tranquilizers, and inhalation agents. SYN: *laughing gas.*

N.o. has little or no effect on body temperature, blood pressure, volume or composition of blood, metabolism, or the genitourinary system. Diaphoresis, increased muscle tone, or both may occur with induction of anesthesia with n.o.

Asphyxiation may occur if n.o. is not administered properly. Prolonged administration of n.o. will cause depression of bone marrow.

CONTRAINDICATIONS: Not to be given in advanced conditions of anemia, in patients with hypertension or hypotension, decompensated heart lesions, diabetes, dyspnea, alcoholism, or in advanced pulmonary tuberculosis.

SYM: Signs of deep n.o. anesthesia are a slight increase in respirations, some dyspnea. Cyanosis becomes deeper; eyeballs are fixed either upward or downward. There is muscular rigidity; cyanosis increases to a grayish pallor; pupils become fixed in a dilated form; and respirations become paralyzed.

TREATMENT: The patient who suffers from an overdosage should be given oxygen under pressure. A respiratory stimulant should be administered. Carbon dioxide may also be given.

N.L.N. Abbr. for *National League of Nursing.*

N.L.N.E. Abbr. for *National League of Nursing Education.*

NMRI. Abbr. for *Naval Medical Research Institute* (U.S. Navy).

N. N. D. Abbr. for *New and Nonofficial Drugs,* a publication previously issued annually by the Council on Drugs of the American Medical Association, listing and describing the articles that are proposed for use. Since 1965 has been called *New Drugs.*

No. Abbr. for L. *numero,* to the number of.

N₂O. Nitrous oxide.

N₂O₃. Nitrogen trioxide.

N₂O₅. Nitrogen pentoxide.

nobelium (nō-bēʹlĭ-ŭm). [Named for Nobel Institute where it was first prepared] SYMB: *No.* At. wt. of the most stable isotope in 254 (other isotopes vary in weight from 252 through 256); at. no. 102. Element obtained from bombardment of curium.

Nocardia. [Edmund I. E. Nocard, Fr. veterinary pathologist, 1850-1903] Gram-positive, aerobic bacteria. Some species are acid-fast and thus may when stained be confused with the causative organism for tuberculosis. Species pathogenic for man cause the disease Nocardiosis which is sometimes called actinomycosis.

N. asteroides. Species of Nocardia pathogenic for man. The invasion site may be the lungs or skin. Abscesses called mycetomas arise in the skin.

N. brasiliensis. Species of Nocardia pathogenic for man. Chronic subcutaneous abscesses are formed.

nocardioʹsis. Pathologic condition resulting from infection by any species of Nocardia. May occur as a pulmonary infection which may spread, resulting in abscesses in the skin, brain, or other areas. May also give rise to fungus tumors (mycetomas) which occur most frequently in lower extremities, esp. the foot, in which case it is called maduromycosis or Madura foot. Nocardiosis is distinguishable from actinomycosis by identification of organism.

TREATMENT: Sulfadiazine daily. This may be supplemented by an antibiotic after laboratory determination of the antibiotic agents to which the strain of the causative organism is sensitive.

nociceptive (nō″sĭ-sĕpʹtĭv) [L. *nocere,* to hurt, + *ceptus,* receiving]. Pert. to stimuli to the brain.

n. impulses. Impulses giving rise to sensations of pain.

n. reflex. A reflex initiated by painful stimuli.

nociperception (nō″sĭ-pĕr-sĕpʹshŭn) ["+ *perceptiō,* apprehension]. The perception by the nerve centers of injurious influences or painful stimuli.

Noct. Abbr. for L. *nocte,* night.

noctalbuminuria (nŏk″tăl-bū-mĭn-ūʹrĭ-ă) [L. *nox, noct-,* night, + *albumen,* white of egg, + Gr. *ouron,* urine]. Excess of albumin voided in urine at night. SYN: *nyctalbuminuria.*

noctambulism (nŏk-tămʹbū-lĭzm) ["+ *ambulāre,* to walk, + Gr. *ismos,* state of]. Sleep walking. SYN: *somnambulism.*

noctiphobia (nŏk″tĭ-fōʹbĭ-ă) ["+ Gr. *phobos,* fear]. Fear of the night and darkness. SYN: *nyctophobia.*

nocturia (nŏk-tūʹrĭ-ă) ["+ Gr. *ouron,* urine]. Urination, esp. excessive, during the night. SYN: *nycturia.* SEE: *enuresis.*

noctur'nal [L. *nocturnus,* at night]. Pert. to or occurring in the night. Opposed to diurnal. SEE: words beginning with *nyct.*

n. emission. Involuntary discharge of semen during sleep. Usually occurs in conjunction with an erotic dream. SYN: *wet dream.*

n. enuresis. Urinary incontinence during sleep at night. SYN: *bedwetting.* SEE: *enuresis.*

no'cuous. Noxious, injurious, harmful.

nodal (nō'dăl) [L. *nodus,* knot]. Pert. to a protuberance.

n. points. One of two points situated on axis of a lens so that any incident ray sent through one will produce a parallel emergent ray sent through the other.

n. rhythm. Cardiac rhythm with origin at auriculoventricular node.

nodding (nŏd'ing). Involuntary allowing of head to fall downward as when momentarily dozing. SYN: *nutation.*

n. spasm. Nodding of the head due to spasm of the sternomastoid muscles. SYN: *salaam convulsion.*

node (nōd) [L. *nodus,* knot]. 1. A knot, knob, protuberance, or swelling. 2. A constricted region. 3. A small rounded organ or structure.

n., atrioventricular. A tangled mass of Purkinje fibers located in lower part of interatrial septum from which the atrioventricular bundle (b. of His) arises. SYN: *A-V node.*

n., A-V. Abbr. for *atrioventricular node;* q.v.

n.'s, Haygarth's. Swelling of joints in arthritis deformans.

n.'s, Heberden's. N. on fingers seen in osteoarthritis.

n., Hensen's. A mass of rapidly proliferating cells at anterior end of primitive streak of embryo. SYN: *Hensen's knot; primitive knot.*

n., lymph. Mass of lymphoid tissue along the course of lymphatic vessels.

n.'s, Meynet's. Those in capsules of joints and in tendons in rheumatism, esp. in children.

n.'s, Parrot's. Osteophytes around anterior fontanel seen in hereditary syphilis.

n., piedric. Node on the hair shaft seen in piedra, q.v.

n.'s of Ranvier. Constrictions of the myelin sheath of a myelinated nerve fiber.

n., sentinal. A signal node, q.v.

n., signal. Enlargement of one of the supraclavicular lymph nodes. Usually indicative of primary carcinoma of thoracic or abdominal organs. SYN: *Virchow's node; Virchow's signal node.*

n., singer's. Small white node which develops on vocal cords caused by over-use or improper use. SEE: *chorditis nodosa.*

n., sinoatrial. N. in wall of rt. atrium near entrance of superior vena cava, consisting of dense network of Purkinje fibers. Source of impulses initiating heart beat. Also called pacemaker of the heart. SYN: *S-A node.*

n., sinoauricular. Sinoatrial node, q.v.

n., sinus. Sinoatrial node, q.v.

n., syphilitic. Circumscribed swelling at end of long bones due to congenital syphilis. Sensitive and painful during inflammation, esp. at night. SEE: *Parrot's n.*

nodose (nō'dōs) [L. *nodosus,* knotted]. Swollen or knotlike at intervals; marked by nodes or projections.

nodosity (nō-dōs'ĭ-tĭ) [L. *nodositas,* a knot]. 1. A protuberance or knot. 2. Condition of having nodes.

nodular (nŏd'ū-lăr). Containing or resembling nodules.

nodule (nŏd'ūl) [L. *nodulus,* little knot]. 1. A small node. 2. A small aggregation of cells. SEE: *chalarosis; cladosporiosis.*

n.'s, aggregate. A group of solitary lymph nodules. Ex: Peyer's patches of small intestine.

n., Albini's. N.'s sometimes seen on free edges of auriculoventricular valves in infants.

n.'s, Arantius'. Central fibrous tubercles in segments of semilunar valves. SYN: *corpora Arantii.*

n., Aschoff's. N. found in myocardium, a characteristic lesion of rheumatic carditis.

n. of cerebellum. SEE: *nodulus.*

n.'s, cortical. Lymph nodules located in cortex of a lymph node.

n.'s, Gamna. Yellowish-brown n.'s. in the spleen in certain enlargements. SYN: *tabac n.'s.*

n., lymph. A mass of densely packed lymphocytes forming the structural unit of lymphatic tissue. Each contains a germinal center where new lymphocytes are formed.

n., lymphatic, lymphoid. A lymph nodule, q.v.

n.'s, Morgagni. N.'s, Arantius, q.v.

n., Schmorl's. N. formed by herniation of nucleus pulposus of intervertebral disc.

n. of semilunar valve. N.'s, Arantius, q.v.

n.'s, siderotic. Small brown n.'s, seen in spleen and other organs, consisting of necrotic tissue encrusted by iron salts.

n., solitary. An isolated nodule of lymphatic tissue such as occurs in mucous membranes.

n.'s, typhoid. N.'s characteristic of typhoid fever found in the liver.

nodulus (nŏd'ū-lŭs) [L.]. (pl. *noduli*) 1. Nodule. 2. [NA]. Anterior portion of vermis of the cerebellum.

nodus (nō'dŭs) [L.]. (pl. *nodi*) [NA]. Node; anatomically a small circumscribed mass of undifferentiated tissue.

noematachograph (nō-ē"mă-tăk'ō-grăf) [Gr. *noēma*, thought, + *tachys*, swift, + *graphein*, to write]. Device for recording time taken in mental activity.

noematachometer (nō-ē"mă-tăk-ŏm'ē-tĕr) *[*" + "+ *metron*, measure]. Device for measurement of the time taken in a simple perception. SYN: *noematachograph.*

noise [O.Fr. *noise*, strife, brawl]. Sound of any sort. Loud, harsh, confused, or senseless.

noli-me-tangere (nō"lī-mē-tăn'jĕ-rē) [L. touch me not]. Cancerous ulcer, generally of the face, which eats away bone and soft tissue; rodent ulcer.

noma (nō'mă) [Gr. *nomē*, a spreading.]. A gangrenous progressive condition, generally found in undernourished children, spreading rapidly from the mucous membrane of the cheek or gum to the cutaneous surface. SYN: *cancrum oris; gangrenous stomatitis.*

n. pudendi, n. vulvae. A similar ulcerative condition affecting the labia majora, esp. in young children.

no'madism [Gr. *nomas*, roaming about]. Impulse to wander about aimlessly; restlessness.

nomenclature (nō'mĕn-klā"chur) [L. *nomen*, name, + *calare*, to call]. Classified system of technical or scientific names. SYN: *terminology.*

nomogram (nŏm'ō-gram) [Gr. *nomos*, law, + *gramma*, mark]. Representation by graphs, diagrams, or charts of the relationship bet. numerical variables.

nomography (nō-mŏg'ră-fī) ["+ *graphein*, to write]. A graphic representation of the relation bet. numerical variables.

nomotopic (nō-mō-tŏp'ĭk) ["+ *topos*, place]. Occurring at the normal site.

non- [L.]. Prefix denoting negation.

nona-, non- [L.]. Prefix meaning ninth.

nona (nō'nă) [L. *nonus*, ninth]. Old term for acute or chronic infectious disease of central nervous system. SYN: *encephalitis lethargica; sleeping sickness.*

nonan (nō'năn). Having increased symptoms or reappearing every 9th day, as the paroxysms of malaria.

non compos mentis (nŏn kŏm'pŏs mĕn'tĭs) [L.]. Not of sound mind, mentally incompetent to handle one's affairs.

nonconductor (nŏn"kŏn-dŭk'tŏr) [L. *non*, not, + *con*, with, + *ductor*, a leader]. Any substance that does not transmit heat, sound, or electricity; or conducts it with difficulty. Strictly speaking, there is no perfect nonconductor. On the application of a sufficiently high voltage, current may be caused to flow through materials usually spoken of as nonconductors. SYN: *insulator.*

non"disjunc'tion. 1. The condition in which one or more pair of homologous chromosomes fail to separate following synapsis. 2. Term also applied to failure of daughter chromosomes to separate during mitosis.

nonelectrolyte [L. *non*, not, + *ēlectron*, amber, + *lytos*, dissolved]. A solution which will not conduct electricity because its chemical constituents are not sufficiently dissociated into ions.

nonigravida (nŏ"nē-gră'vī- dă) [L. *nonus*, ninth, + *gravida*, pregnant]. A woman pregnant for the ninth time. Written Gravida IX. SEE: *nonipara*, q.v.

nonipara (nō-nĭp'ăr-ă) ["+ *parēre*, to bring forth]. A woman who has given birth 9 times. Written Para IX.

nonlaxative diet. Low residue diet, q.v., with boiled milk and toasted crackers. No strained oatmeal, vegetable juice, or fruit juice given. Fats and concentrated sweets are restricted.

nonopaque (nŏn"ō-pāk'). Not opaque, esp. to X rays.

nonpolar (nŏn-pō'lĕr) [L. *non*, not + *pōlus*, a pole]. Not having separate poles; sharing electrons.

n. compound. One formed by the sharing of electrons.

nonprotein ["+ Gr. *prōtos*, first]. Any substance not a protein.

n. nitrogen. 1. A nitrogenous constituent of blood that is not a protein. 2. Sum of all nonprotein nitrogen in the blood. SEE: *nitrogen.*

non repetat [L.]. Do not repeat.

nonrestraint (nŏn"rē-strănt') [L. *non*, not, + *rē*, back, + *stringere*, to bind back]. Treatment of the insane without using mechanical repression.

nonseptate (nŏn-sĕp'tāt) ["+ *septum*, a partition]. Having no dividing walls.

nonsexual (nŏn-sĕk'shū-ăl). Without sex. SYN: *asexual.*

nontoxic (nŏn-tŏk'sĭk) [Gr. *non*, not, + Gr. *toxikon*, poison]. Not poisonous or productive of poison.

nonunion (nŏn-ūn'yŭn) ["+ *uniō*, oneness]. Failure of fragments of a fractured bone to knit together.

no'nus [L.]. 1. Ninth. 2. Hypoglossal nerve, formerly regarded as ninth cranial nerve.

nonviable (nŏn-vī'ā-bl) ["+ *via*, life]. Incapable of life or of living; frequently used to indicate a dead fetus, born prior to 20th week of gestation.

nookleptia (nō-ō-klep'tī-ă) [Gr. *nous*, mind, + *kleptein*, to steal]. An obsession that one's thoughts are being stolen by others.

norepinephrine (nor-ĕp''ĭ-nĕf'rĭn). A hormone produced by the adrenal medulla, similar in chemical and pharmacologic properties to epinephrine, but it is chiefly a vasoconstrictor and has little effect on cardiac output. SYN: *noradrenalin; levarterenol bitartrate.*

norethindrone. A steroid hormone similar in action to progesterone. Used in progestation agents for birth control.

norm [L. *norma*, rule]. 1. A standard or ideal for a specific group. 2. Normal.

nor'ma [L. rule]. A view or aspect, esp. with reference to the skull.

n., anterior. N. facialis or n. frontalis.

n. basilaris. N. inferior or ventralis. View of underneath surface of skull.

n. facialis. View directed towards the face.

n. frontalis. Outline of the skull viewed from the front; n. facialis.

n., inferior. View of underneath surface of the skull.

n. lateralis. View as seen from the side; a profile view.

n. occipitalis. View of the skull as seen from behind.

n. sagittalis. View as seen in sagittal section.

n., superior. N. verticalis, q.v.

n. ventralis. View of inferior surface of skull.

n. verticalis. View of skull as seen from above.

normal (nor'măl) [L. *normalis*, according to pattern]. 1. Standard; performing proper functions; natural; regular. 2. In biology, not affected by experimental treatment; occurring naturally and not because of disease or experimentation. 3. In psychology, free from mental disorder; or of average development or intelligence. 4. In chemistry, a term used to describe a solution so made that 1 liter contains 1 gram equivalent to the solute. In the case of acids and bases formed by univalent radicals, a normal solution is the same as molar, as in the case of HCl. In the case of H_2SO_4, however, the normal solution would be half as strong as the molar, and in the case of H_3PO_4 it would be one third.

n. body temperature. 98.6° F. (37.0° C.).

n. pulse. For adults at rest 60-80 beats per minute, but may be greater than this in children.

n. respiration. In adults at rest 18-24 per minute.

n. salt. An ionic compound containing no replaceable hydrogen or hydroxyl ions. SYN: *neutral salt.*

n. solution. 1. Solution containing 1 gm. molecular weight of dissolved substance divided by the hydrogen equivalent of the substance per liter of solution. 2. A solution which neutralizes an equal volume of a normal solution of any base or acid.

normalization (nŏr-māl-ĭ-zā'shŭn) [L. *normalis*, according to pattern]. Modification or reduction to the normal standard.

normergic (nor-mĕr'jĭk). Reacting, or pertaining to that which reacts, in a normal manner.

normoblast (nor'mō-blăst) [L. *norma*, rule, + Gr. *blastos*, germ]. A nucleated red blood corpuscle similar in size to an ordinary erythrocyte.

normochromasia (nŏr''mō-krō-mā'zĭ-ă) ["+ Gr. *chrōma*, color]. Average staining capacity in a cell or tissue.

normochromia (nor''mō-krō'mĭ-a). Blood possessing normal color and hemoglobin content.

normocyte (nor'mō-sīt) [L. *norma*, rule, + Gr. *kytos*, cell]. An average-sized red blood corpuscle. SYN: *erythrocyte.*

normocytosis (nor''mō-sī-tō'sĭs) ["+ "+ *-ōsis*, condition]. A normal state of the corpuscular elements of the blood.

normoglycemia (nor''mō-glĭ-sē'mĭ-ă) ["+ Gr. *glykus*, sweet, + *haima*, blood]. Normal state of sugar content of the blood.

normoglycemic (nor''mō-glĭ-sē'mĭk). Having a normal amount of sugar in the blood.

normoorthocytosis (nor''mō-or''thō-sī-tō'-sĭs) [L. *norma*, rule, + Gr. *orthos*, correct, + *kytos*, cell, + *-ōsis*, increase]. Increase in the blood of the number of leukocytes, but with normal proportion of the different varieties.

normoskeocytosis (nor''mō-skē''ō-sī-tō'sĭs) ["+ *skaios*, left, + *kytos*, cell, + *-ōsis*, condition]. Normal number of the leukocytes of the blood with deviation to the left, i.e., with immature forms present.

normosthenuria (nor''mō-sthĕn-ū'rĭ-ă) [L. *norma*, rule, + Gr. *sthenos*, strength, + *ouron*, urine]. Urination of normal amount and specific gravity.

normotensive (nor''mō-tĕn'sĭv). Normal blood pressure; a person with normal blood pressure.

normotonic (nor″mō-tŏn′ĭk) ["+ Gr. *tonos*, tension]. 1. Having normal muscular tonus. 2. One who has normal muscle tonus.

normotopia (nor″mō-tō′pĭ-ă) ["+ Gr. *topos*, place]. Situation in the regular place.

normotopic (nor″mō-tŏp′ĭk). In the right location; pert. to the normal situation.

normovolemia (nor″mō-vō-lē′mĭ-ă) ["+ *volūmen*, volume, + Gr. *haima*, blood]. Normal state of blood volume.

Norwegian itch. Severe form of scabies marked by pustules and crusts.

nose [AS. *nosw*]. Projection in center of face; the organ of olfaction and the entrance which warms, moistens, and filters the air for the respiratory tract.

The external portion of the nose is a triangle of cartilage and bone covered with skin and lined with mucous membrane. Internally, a septum divides nose into two chambers. Each chamber contains three meatuses which are found underneath the corresponding turbinates. Orifices of frontal, anterior, ethmoid and maxillary sinuses are in middle meatus. Orifices of posterior ethmoids and sphenoids are in superior meatus. SYN: *nasus* [NA]; *organon olfactus*.

Sinuses, Communicating: Ethmoidal, frontal, maxillary, and sphenoidal. *Nerves:* Facial, olfactory, ophthalmic, and maxillary. *Blood Supply:* External and internal maxillary arteries from the external carotid and ethmoidal artery from the internal carotid.

EXAM: Note shape, size, color, state of the alae nasi, discharge, interference with respiration, evidences of injury, deflected or perforated septum, enlarged turbinates, and tenderness over frontal and maxillary sinuses.

DIAG: *Chronic red n.:* Dilated capillaries as a result of alcoholism, lupus erythematosus, acne rosacea, pustules, boils, and digestive disorders. *Superficial ulceration:* Tuberculous ulcer, epithelioma, syphilis. *Broad and coarse:* Cretinism, myxedema, acromegaly. *Sunken:* Syphilis or injury. *Pinched with Small Nares:* Hypertrophied adenoid tissue or chronic obstructions; also tumors. *Inoffensive watery discharge:* Present in nasal catarrh, early stages of measles, hay fever, acute irritation of lining membranes. *Offensive discharge:* Nasopharyngeal diphtheria, lupus, local infection, impacted foreign bodies, caries, rhinitis, glanders, syphilitic infection.

FOREIGN BODY IN THE NOSE: Irritation of nose resulting in coughing or watery or purulent discharge. Occasionally pain and obstruction of nose. If not recognized immediately it often causes a foul discharge on the affected side of the nose. There may be obstruction to breathing in one nostril. If the foreign body is very small, symptoms may be absent.

TREATMENT: Take the patient to a physician. Vigorous blowing of the nose is dangerous because it may spread infection to the various cavities and sinuses about the nose or to the ear. Do not attempt to fish the body out; attempts to dislodge it may cause it to slip further into the nose, or down the throat and into the windpipe.

n., bridge of. Superior portion of external nose formed by union of the two nasal bones.

n., hammer. Rhinophyma, q.v.

n., saddle. Nose with depressed bridge seen in tertiary syphilis due to gummatous destruction of septal supporting structure, and following operations which are com-

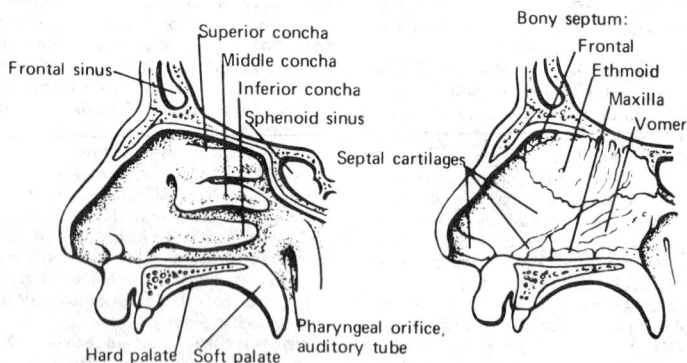

Superior concha
Middle concha
Inferior concha
Sphenoid sinus
Frontal sinus
Septal cartilages
Pharyngeal orifice, auditory tube
Hard palate   Soft palate

LATERAL WALL OF RIGHT NASAL CAVITY

Bony septum:
Frontal
Ethmoid
Maxilla
Vomer

SEPTUM OF LEFT NASAL CAVITY

plicated by suppuration and destruction of supporting framework.

nose, words pert. to: agger nasi; ala nasi; alinasal; anosmia; bulb, olfactory; bulla ethmoidalis; choana; columella nasi; epistaxis; hyperosmia; naris; nostril; parosmia; rhinalgia; rhinitis; septum; sinus, accessory nasal; sinusitis; smell; vestibule of nose; vibrissae; vomer; xeromycteria; and words beginning with "nas," "rhino."

nosebleed. Hemorrhage from nose. SYN: *epistaxis.*

Nosema (nō-sē'mă). A genus of Microsporidia.

nosema (nō-sē'mă) [Gr. *nosēma,* disease]. (pl. *nose'mas* or *nosem'ata*) Any ailment or disease.

noso- [Gr. *nosos,* disease]. Combining form pert. to disease.

nosochthonography (nŏs"ŏk-thō-nŏg'ră-fĭ) ["+ *chthōn,* earth, + *graphein,* to write]. Study of geographical distribution of diseases; medical geography. SYN: *nosogeography.*

nosocomial (nŏs"ō-kō'mĭ-al) ["+ *komeion,* to care for]. Pert. to a hospital or infirmary.

   n. infection. Infection acquired in a hospital.

nosogenesis, nosogeny (nŏs"ō-jĕn'ĕ-sĭs, nō-sŏj'ĕn-ĭ) [Gr. *nosos,* disease, + *gennan,* to produce]. The development and progress of a disease.

nosogeography (nŏs"ō-jē-ŏg'ră-fĭ) ["+ *gē,* earth, + *graphein,* to write]. Study of medical geography. SYN: *nosochthonography.*

nosography (nō-sŏg'ră-fĭ) ["+ *graphein,* to write]. The description of a disease.

nosohemia (nŏs-ō-hē'mĭ-ă) [Gr. *nosos,* disease, + *haima,* blood]. Disease of the blood.

nosology (nō-sŏl'ō-jĭ) ["+ *logos,* study]. The science of description or classification of diseases.

nosomania (nŏs"ō-mā'nĭ-ă) ["+ *mania,* madness]. The delusion that one is diseased.

nosomycosis (nŏs"ō-mī-kō'sĭs) ["+ *mykēs,* fungus, + *-ōsis,* condition]. Any disease caused by a parasitic fungus or Schizomycete.

nosonomy (nŏs-on'ō-mĭ) [Gr. *nosos,* disease, + *nomos,* law]. The science of disease classification.

nosophobia (nō"sō-fō'bĭ-ă) ["+ *phobos,* fear]. Abnormal aversion to illness or to a particular affection.

nosophyte (nŏs'ō-fīt) ["+ *phyton,* plant]. A disease-causing plant microorganism.

nosopoietic (nŏs"ō-poy-ĕt'ĭk) ["+ *poiein,* to form]. Producing or causing disease.

Nosopsyllus (nŏs"ŏp-sĭl'us) ["+ *psylla,* flea]. A genus of fleas belonging to the order Siphonaptera.

   N. fascia'tus. A species of rat fleas responsible for transmission of murine typhus and perhaps of plague.

nosotherapy (nŏs"ō-thĕr'ă-pĭ) ["+ *therapeia,* treatment]. Treatment of one disease by voluntarily introducing another microorganism into the body.

nosotrophy (nō-sŏt'rō-fĭ) [Gr. *nosos,* disease, + *trophē,* nourishment]. Nursing care and feeding of the sick.

nosotropic (nō"sō-trŏp'ĭk) ["+ *tropos,* turning]. Directed against the symptoms or effects of a disease. SEE: *etiotropic.*

nostalgia (nŏs-tăl'jĭ-ă) [Gr. *nostos,* a return home, + *algos,* pain]. Homesickness; longing to return to one's native land. SEE: *cainotophobia.*

nostomania (nŏs"tō-mā'nĭ-ă) ["+ *mania,* madness]. Nostalgia verging on insanity.

nos'tril [AS. *nosu,* nose, + *thyrel,* a hole]. One of the external apertures of the nose. SYN: *naris.* SEE: *nose.*

   n. reflex. Reduction of opening of naris on affected side in lung disease in proportion to lessened alveolar air capacity on affected side.

nostrum (nŏs'trŭm) [L., our]. A patent or quack remedy.

notal (nō'tăl) [Gr. *nōton,* back]. Concerning the back. SYN: *dorsal.*

notalgia (nō-tal'jĭ-ă) ["+ *algos,* pain]. Painful condition of the back. SYN: *dorsalgia.*

notch (nŏch). A rather deep indentation or narrow gap in the edge of a structure. SYN: *incisura.*

   n., acetabular. Notch in inferior border of acetabulum.

   n., aortic. N. in sphygmogram from rebound at aortic valve closure.

   n., cardiac. Concavity on anterior border of left lung into which the heart projects.

   n., cerebellar, anterior, and posterior. A deep notch separating the hemispheres of the cerebellum.

   n., clavicular. One at the upper angle of the sternum with which the clavicle articulates.

   n., costal. One of seven pairs of indentations on lateral surfaces of the sternum, for articulation with costal cartilages.

   n., cotyloid. N., acetabular, q.v.

   n., ethmoidal. N. separating the two orbital portions of frontal bone.

   n., frontal. N. on supraorbital arch which transmits frontal artery and nerve.

n., greater sciatic. Large n. on posterior border of hip bone between posterior inferior iliac spine and spine of ischium.

n., interclavicular. A rounded one at top of manubrium of sternum, between surfaces articulating with the clavicles.

n., jugular (of occipital bone). One which forms the posterior and middle portions of jugular foramen.

n., jugular (of sternum). N. on upper surface of manubrium between the two clavicular notches.

n., lesser sciatic. N. immediately below spine of ischium on posterior border of hip bone. Converted into a foramen by the sacrotuberous ligament.

n., mandibular. N. on superior border of ramus of mandible separating coronoid and condyloid processes.

n., nasal. 1. Deep notch on anterior surface of maxilla and forming lateral border of piriform aperture. 2. N. between internal angular processes of frontal bone.

n., pancreatic. N. on lateral surface of head of pancreas for superior mesenteric artery and vein. It separates uncinate process of head from remaining portion.

n., radial. N. on lateral surface of coronoid process of ulna for receiving circumference of head of radius.

n. of Rivinus. Tympanic notch, q.v.

n., scapular. A deep n. on superior border of scapula. Transmits suprascapular nerve.

n., sciatic. SEE: *sciatic n.*

n., semilunar. N. on anterior aspect of proximal end of ulna for articulation with trochlea of humerus.

n., sphenopalatine. N. between orbital and sphenoidal processes of palatine bone.

n., suprasternal. Jugular n. of the sternum, q.v.

n., tentorial. N. in free border of tentorium cerebelli through which brain stem passes.

n., thyroid. Deep n. on superior border of thyroid cartilage of larynx separating the two laminae.

n., tympanic. N. in superior portion of the tympanic ring. SYN: *n. of Rivinus.*

n., ulnar. N. on distal end of radius for receiving head of ulna.

n., umbilical. N. on anterior border of liver where it is crossed by falciform ligament.

n., vertebral. Concavity on inferior surface of root of vertebral arch. When two vertebrae are in position, the notches form the intervertebral foramina.

note [L. *nota,* a mark]. 1. A sound of definite pitch. 2. A brief comment or condensed report.

     n. blindness. Inability to recognize musical notes; due to a central lesion.

notencephalocele (no″tĕn-sef′al-ō-sēl) [Gr. *nōton,* back, + *enkephalos,* brain, + *kēlē,* hernia]. Protrusion of brain substance at the back of the head.

notifi'able diseases. The laws of the various states require that certain diseases when existing shall be reported to the local health authorities, such as a Board of Health. A fine may be levied for not doing so. Among the diseases generally required to be reported are all communicable or contagious diseases, such as smallpox; scarlet fever; relapsing fever; diphtheria; enteric fevers, such as typhoid fever; puerperal fever; cholera; typhus; meningococcal meningites; acute anterior poliomyelitis; polioencephalitis; encephalitis lethargica; tuberculosis; epidemic of acute diarrheal disease; chickenpox; gonorrhea; syphilis. SEE: *quarantine; reportable diseases.*

notochord (nō′tō-kord) [Gr. *nōton,* back, + *chordē,* cord]. A rod of cells lying dorsal to intestine and extending from anterior to posterior end which forms axial skeleton in embryos of all chordates. In vertebrates it is replaced partially or completely by centra of vertebrae. A remnant persists in man as a portion of nucleus pulposus of intervertebral disk.

no″togen'esis [″+ *genesis,* production]. Development of the notochord.

noumenal (nū′mē-n* * *l) [Gr. *nooumenon,* a thing perceived]. Pert. to noumenon, q.v. Pert. to that which arises because of intellectual intuition rather than sensory perception.

noumenon (nū′mē-nŏn). That which one knows or perceives by intellectual intuition alone, as distinguished from something perceived through sensory perception.

nourishment (nur′ĭsh-mĕnt) [L. *nutrire,* to nurse]. 1. Act of nourishing or of being nourished. 2. Sustenance; nutriment. SEE: *center, trophic; trophic.*

Novocain (nō′vō-kān). A proprietary name for procaine hydrochloride, q.v.

noxa (nok′sä) [L. injury]. (pl. *nox′ae*) Anything harmful to health.

noxious (nok′shus) [L. *noxius,* injurious]. Harmful; not wholesome.

NP. Abbreviation for *nucleoprotein; nursing procedure; neuropsychiatrist; neuropsychiatry.*

Np. Chemical symbol for *neptunium.*

NPH insulin. Abbr. for *neutral protamine Hagedorn insulin.* SEE: *insulin, NPH.*

NPN. Abbr. for *nonprotein nitrogen.*

n.p.t. Abbr. for *normal pressure and temperature.*

NSD. Abbr. for *nominal standard dose* in ret. Ret indicates *r*adiation *e*quivalent *t*herapy which is analogous to the rem *r*oentgen *e*quivalent *m*an) used in radiation protection.

Nt. Symbol for *niton.*

nth (enth). Used in medical statistics to indicate the continuation of data or subjects to large numbers in that progression or series. Thus, one would indicate patients numbered beginning P1, P2, P3, and so forth through P nth. P nth would be the last patient indicated.

nubecula (nū-bĕk'ū-la) [L., little cloud]. Cloudiness of the cornea or the urine.

nubile (nū'bĭl) [L. *nubere,* to marry]. Pert. to a girl who has attained puberty and who is thus able to marry,

nubility (nū-bĭl'ĭ-tĭ). Marriageableness, said of female at puberty, the final state of sex development.

nucha (nū'kă) [L.]. [NA]. Nape of neck.

nuchal (nū'kal) [L. *nucha,* back of neck]. Pert. to the neck or nucha.

Nuck's canal or diverticulum (nook). [Anton Nuck, Dutch anatomist, 1650-1692] An anomalous peritoneal pouch extending for a variable distance into the labium. Homologous to processus vaginalis of the male.

nuclear (nū'klē-ăr) [L. *nucleus,* a kernel]. Resembling or concerning a nucleus.

   n. arc. Region of equator of crystalline lens where cells undergo transition into lens fibers. SYN: *nuclear zone; lens vortex.*

   n. envelope. Consists of two parallel membranes enclosing a narrow perinuclear space, enveloping the nucleus. Prior to electron microscopy the nucleus of a cell was thought to be surrounded by a single, thin membrane.

   n. family. The parents or parent and child or children considered as a unit.

   n. medicine. That branch of medicine concerned with the diagnostic, therapeutic, and investigative use of radionuclides, q.v.

   n. powered heart pump. An artificial heart pump powered by nuclear energy. It has been used experimentally in cows and may eventually be developed sufficiently to use in humans.

nuclease (nū'klē-ās) [L. *nucleus,* kernel, + *ase,* enzyme]. Any enzyme in animals and plants that facilitates hydrolysis of nuclein and nucleic acids.

nucleate (nū'klē-āt) [L. *nucleatus,* having a kernel]. 1. Having a nucleus. 2. To form a nucleus. 3. A salt or ester of nucleic acid.

nucleic acid. An important group of substances of large molecular weight, found in cells, esp. the nuclei. They have a complex chemical structure being formed of sugars (pentoses), phosphoric acid, and nitrogen bases (purines and pyrimidines). Most important are deoxyribonucleic acid and ribonucleic acid, q.v. SYN: *nucleinic acid.*

nuclein (nū'klē-ĭn) [L. *nucleus,* a kernel]. A normal chemical constituent of a cell nucleus; a colorless, shapeless substance obtained by hydrolysis of nucleoproteins or cells containing nucleic acid and proteins rich in phosphorus.

   n. bases. Bases formed from decomposition of nuclein. Ex: adenine, guanine, xanthine, hypoxanthine.

nucleinase. Nuclease, q.v.

nucleo- [L.]. Pert. to a nucleus.

nucleoalbumin (nū''klē-ō-ăl-bū'mĭn) [L. *nucleus,* kernel, + *albus,* white]. A complex of nucleic acid and albumin. SYN: *paranuclein; pseudonuclein.*

nucleoalbuminuria (nū''klē-ō-al-bū''mĭ-nū'rĭ-ă) ["+ "+ Gr. *ouron,* urine]. The presence of nucleoalbumin in urine.

nucleoalbumose (nū''klē-ō-ăl'bū-mōs) ["+ "]. Partly hydrated nucleoalbumin found in the urine of patients with osteomalacia.

nucleofugal (nū-klē-ŏf'ū-găl) [L. *nucleus,* kernel, + *fugere,* to flee]. Directed or moving away from a nucleus in the cell.

nucleohiston (e) (nū''klē-ō-hĭs'ton, -tōn) ["+ *istos,* tissue]. A substance composed of nuclein and histone, found in sperm of various animals.

nucleoid (nū'klē-oyd) ["+ Gr. *eidos,* resemblance]. Resembling a nucleus.

nucleolar (nū-klē'ō-lăr) [L. *nucleolus,* a little kernel]. Pert. to a nucleolus.

nucleoliform (nū-klē-ō'lĭ-form) ["+ *forma,* shape]. Like a nucleolus.

nucleolin (nū-klē'ō-lĭn). The substance composing the nucleolus.

nucleolonucleus (nū''klē-ōl-ō-nū'klē-ūs). Nucleololus; a minute point within the nucleolus.

nucleolus (nū-klē'ō-lūs) [L. little kernel]. (pl. *nucle'oli*) A spherical body within the cell nucleus.

   n., chromatin. A false nucleolus, q.v.

   n., false. Dense bodies of chromatin found on chromonemata. SYN: *karyosome,* q.v.

nucleomicrosome (nū''klē-ō-mĭ'krō-sōm) [L. *nucleus,* kernel, + Gr. *mikros,* tiny, +

sōma, body]. Any one of the minute granules making a nucleoplasmic fiber.

nucleons (nū′klē-ŏnz). Collective name of the particles that make up the nucleus of an atom.

nucleopetal (nū-klē-ŏp′ē-tăl) ["+ *petere*, to seek]. Seeking or moving toward the nucleus.

nu″cleoplas′mic. Pert. to nucleoplasm.

    n. index. The ratio of nuclear volume to cytoplasmic volume, expressed thus:

$$NP = \frac{\text{vol. of nucleus}}{\text{vol. of cell} - \text{vol. of nucleus}}$$

nucleoprotein (nū″klē-ō-prō′tē-ĭn) [L. *nucleus*, kernel, + Gr. *prōtos*, first]. The combination of one of the proteins with nucleic acid to form a conjugated protein found in cell nuclei.

nucleoreticulum (nū″klē-ō-rē-tĭk′ū-lŭm) ["+ *reticulum*, network]. Any mesh framework in a nucleus.

nucleosidase (nū″klē-ō′sī-dās). An enzyme that catalyzes the hydrolysis of nucleosides.

nu′cleoside. A glycoside formed by the union of a purine or pyrimidine base with a sugar (pentose).

nucleospindle (nū″klē-ō-spĭn′dl). Spindle-shaped body occurring in karyokinesis, q.v.

nucleotidase (nū″klē-ōt′ĭ-dās). An enzyme (nucleophosphatase) that splits phosphoric acid from nucleotides leaving a nucleoside.

5-nucleotidase. An enzyme present in serum. Its serum level is increased in carcinoma of the pancreas when there is common bile duct obstruction or metastasis to the liver.

nucleotide (nū′klē-ō-tīd) [L. *nucleus*, kernel]. A compound formed of phosphoric acid, a sugar, and a base (purine or pyrimidine), all of which constitute the structural unit of nucleic acid. SYN: *mononucleotide*.

nu″cleotox′in ["+ Gr. *toxikon*, poison.]. A toxin acting upon or produced by cell nuclei.

nucleus (nū′klē-ŭs) [L. little kernel]. (pl. *nuclei*) 1. A central point about which matter is gathered, as in a calculus. 2. The vital body in the protoplasm of a cell; the essential agent in growth, metabolism, reproduction, and transmission of characteristics of a cell. SEE: *cell structure.* 3. [NA] group of nerve cells or mass of gray matter in the central nervous system, esp. the brain. 4. In chemistry, a heavy central atomic particle in which most of the mass and total positive electric charge are concentrated.

    n., abducent. A gray n., the origin of abducens nerve, on floor of 4th ventricle, behind trigeminal n. SYN: *abducens nucleus; nucleus of abducens nerve.*

    n. ambiguus. [NA]. N. of the glossopharyngeal and vagus nerves in medulla oblongata. Lies in lateral half of reticular formation. SYN: *ambiguous nucleus.*

    n., amygdaloid. N. projecting into inferior cornua of lateral ventricle. Constitutes part of basal ganglia.

    n., angular. The superior vestibular nucleus. SYN: *Bechterew's n.*

    n., anterior, of thalamus. N. located in rostral part of thalamus. Receives fibers of mammillothalamic tract.

    n., arcuate. 1. N. located on basal aspect of pyramid of medulla. 2. The posteromedial ventral n. of the thalamus. SYN: *semilunar n.*

    n., auditory. Nest of nerve cells where auditory nerves arise.

    n. of von Bechterew. The superior vestibular nucleus, q.v.

    n. of Burdach. N., cuneate, q.v.

    n., caudate. A comma-shaped mass of gray matter forming part of the corpus striatum. Constitutes part of the basal ganglia.

    n., central, of thalamus. A group of nuclei in middle part of thalamus. SYN: *centromedian n.*

    n., centromedian. The central nucleus of the thalamus, q.v. SYN: *n. of Luys.*

    n., cerebellar. One of the nuclei of the cerebellum: *n. fastigii, n. emboliformis, n. globosus,* and *n. dentatus.*

    n., cochlear, dorsal. N. in medulla oblongata lying dorsal to restiform body. Receives fibers of cochlear nerve. SEE: *nucleus, cochlear, ventral.*

    n., cochlear, ventral. N. in medulla oblongata lying anterior and lateral to restiform body. Receives fibers from cochlear nerve. SEE: *nucleus, cochlear, dorsal.*

    n., cornucommissural, posterior. A column of cells extending entire length of spinal cord lying along medial border of posterior column near posterior gray commissure.

    n., cuneate. N. in inferior portion of medulla oblongata in which fibers of the fasciculus cuneatus terminate. SYN: *nucleus cuneatus* [NA]; *nucleus of Burdach.*

    n., Deiter's. Lateral vestibular nucleus, q.v.

    n., dentate. Large convoluted mass of gray matter in lateral portion of cerebellum. It is folded so as to enclose some of the central white matter. Gives rise to fibers of the superior cerebellar peduncle. SYN: *n. dentatus cerebelli* [NA].

    n., dorsal, of spinal cord. A column of gray matter lying at base of dorsal horn of gray matter and extending from 7th cervical to 3rd lumbar segments. Cells give rise to fibers of the dorsal spinocerebellar tract. SYN: *Clarke's column.*

n., dorsal motor, of vagus. A column of cells in medulla oblongata lying lateral to hypoglossal nucleus. Its cells give rise to most of efferent fibers of vagus nerve.

n., dorsal sensory, of vagus. N. lying lateral to dorsal motor nucleus of vagus. Receives fibers of solitary tract.

n., ectoblastic. One in cells of the epiblast.

n., Edinger-Westphal. N. of midbrain located dorsomedially to oculomotor nucleus. Gives rise to visceral efferent fibers terminating in ciliary ganglion, axons from which innervate ciliary muscle and sphincter iridis.

n., emboliform. N. of cerebellum lying between dentate and globose nuclei. Receives axons of Purkinje cells and sends efferent fibers into brachium conjunctivum.

n., facial motor. N. in medulla oblongata in floor of 4th ventricle giving rise to efferent fibers of facial nerve. SYN: *nucleus nervi facialis* [NA]; *nucleus of facial nerve.*

n., fastigial. N. in medullary portion of cerebellum. Receives afferent fibers from vestibular nerve and superior vestibular nucleus. Afferent fibers form fasciculus uncinatus and fastigiobulbar tract.

n. funiculi gracilis. Elongated mass of gray matter in dorsal pyramid of medulla oblongata.

n., germinal. N. resulting from union of male and female pronuclei.

n., globose. N. of the cerebellum located medial to the emboliform nucleus.

n. gracilis. [NA]. N. in medulla oblongata in which fibers of the fasciculus gracilis terminate.

n. habenular. N. of the diencephalon located in the havenular trigone. Functions as an olfactory correlation center. SYN: *nucleus of the habenula; nucleus habenulae* [NA].

n., hypoglossal. An elongated mass of gray matter in the medulla oblongata in floor of 4th ventricle. Gives rise to motor fibers of hypoglossal nerve. SYN: *nucleus of hypoglossal nerve; nucleus nervi hypoglossi* [NA].

n., hypothalamic. One of the nuclei occurring in four groups found in hypothalamus. Includes the following nuclei: dorsomedial, intercalatus, lateral, mamillary (lateral and medial), paraventricular, posterior, supraoptic, tuberal, ventromedial. Cells of these nuclei, esp. the supraoptic and paraventricular, in addition to serving a neural function, are secretory and produce the vasopressor, oxytocic, and antidiuretic principles of the hypophysis. These hormones pass through efferent fibers of the infundibular stalk to the pars nervosa (posterior lobe) of the hypophysis where they are stored and liberated. SYN: *nucleus hypothalamicus; nucleus subthalamicus* [NA].

n., interpeduncular. N. of the midbrain near superior border of pons. Receives fibers of the habenulopeduncular tract.

n., interstitial, of Cajal. N. in superior portion of midbrain. Receives fibers from vestibular nuclei, basal ganglia, and occipital regions of cerebral cortex. Efferent fibers pass to ipsi- and contralateral fasciculi and interstitiospinal tracts.

n., intraventricular. N., caudate, q.v.

n., lenticular. One of the n. forming part of the basal ganglia of the cerebrum. Consists of globus pallidus and putamen. With the caudate nucleus, it forms the corpus striatum.

n. lentis. [NA]. The core or inner dense section of the crystalline lens.

n., mother. One that divides into two or more parts called daughter nuclei.

n., motor. N. giving rise to motor fibers of a nerve.

n., motor, of trigeminal nerve. N. in medulla oblongata near 1st margin of superior part of 4th ventricle. Gives rise to motor fibers of trigeminal nerve. SYN: *nucleus motorius nervi trigemini* [NA].

n., oculomotor. N. in central gray matter of midbrain lying below rostral end of cerebral aqueduct.

n., olivary, inferior. A large convoluted mass of cells lying in ventral part of medulla oblongata and forming part of the reticular system. Gives rise to fibers of the olivocerebellar tract. SYN: *olivary nucleus; nucleus olivaris inferior; nucleus olivaris* [NA].

n., olivary, superior. A small n. located in mid-lateral tegmental region of pons. Receives fibers from ventral cochlear nucleus. SYN: *nucleus dorsalis corporis trapezoidei* [NA].

n. of origin. Any collection of nerve cells giving rise to fibers of a nerve or nerve tract.

n., paraventricular. N. of hypothalamus lying in supraoptic portion. Its axons with those of supraoptic n. form supraopticohypophyseal tract. SEE: *n. hypothalamic.*

n., pontine. One of several groups of nerve cells located in the pons. Receives

n., vesicular. N. having deeply stainin membrane and pale center.

n., vestibular. One of four nuclei medulla oblongata in which fibers of ve tibular nerve terminate. Include medi (Schwalbe's), superior (Bechterew's), later (Deiter's), and inferior. SYN: *nuclei ve tibulares* [NA]; *nuclei nervi vestibularis.*

n., vitelline. One formed by union male and female pronuclei within the vite lus. SYN: *yolk n.*

n., white. Central white substance corpus dentatum of olive.

n., yolk. A part of the cytoplasm of a ovum in which the initial process of accum lation of food supplies probably is located

nuclide (nū'klīd). Any atomic nucleus ident fied by its atomic number, mass, and energ state.

nude [L. *nudus,* naked]. 1. Bare; naked; u. clothed. 2. An unclothed body.

nud'ism. 1. In psychiatry, morbid desire remove clothing. 2. The cult or practice living in a nude condition.

nudo [L. *nudus*]. Combining form denotin uncovered, naked.

nudomania (nū"dō-ma'nī-ă) [L. *nudu* naked, + Gr. *mania,* madness]. Abnorma desire to be nude.

nudophobia (nū"dō-fō'bĭ-ă) ["+ Gr. *phobc* fear]. Abnormal fear of being unclothe SEE: *gymnophobia.*

Nuel's space (nū'ĕl). [Jean P. Nuel, Be oculist, 1847-1920]. S. in organ of Cor between outer pillar and outer phalange cells (Deiter's cells).

Nuhn's gland (noon). [Anton Nuhn, Ge anatomist, 1814-1889]. Mucous gland c each side of frenum of the tongue. SY Blandin's gland.

null hypothesis. The assumption hypothesis that the observed difference b tween two groups of patients studied accidental or due to chance, and is not d to one of the groups having received specific treatment.

nullipara (nŭl-ĭp'ă-ră) [L. *nullus,* none, *parēre,* to bear]. A woman who has borne n children.

nulliparity (nŭl'ī-par'ī-tĭ). Condition of ne having given birth to a child.

nulliparous (nŭl-lĭp'ăr-ŭs). Never havin borne a child.

numb (nŭm). 1. Insensible; lacking in feelin as from cold. 2. Deadened or lacking power to move as *numb* with cold.

number (nŭm'bĕr) [L. *numerus,* number]. A total of units. 2. A symbol graphical representing an arithmetical sum.

---

afferent fibers from cerebral cortex; efferent fibers pass through brachium pontis to cerebellum.

n. pulposus. [NA]. The center cushioning of gelatinous mass lying within an intervertebral disk; remains of the notochord.

n., pyramidal. Band of gray matter near olivary n. in the medulla.

n., red. Large oval pigmented mass in upper portion of midbrain and extending upward into subthalamus. Receives fibers from cerebral cortex and cerebellum; efferent fibers give rise to rubrospinal tracts.

n., reticular. A column of neurons in spinal cord, brain stem, and thalamus affecting local reflex activity, muscle tone, and wakefulness.

n. ruber. [NA] Mass of red-colored gray matter in crus cerebri located in the anterior portion of the tegmentum and extending into the posterior portion of the subthalamic region.

n., salivatory, inferior. N. located in pons near level of dorsal motor nucleus of the vagus. Gives rise to preganglionic parasympathetic fibers which pass to otic ganglion via hypoglossal nerve. Impulses regulate secretion of parotid gland.

n., salivatory, superior. An ill-defined n. in pons lying dorsomedial to facial nucleus. Gives rise to preganglionic parasympathetic fibers passing through chorda tympani and lingual nerve to submaxillary ganglion. Impulses regulate secretion of submaxillary and sublingual glands.

n., segmentation. N. of zygote formed by fusion of male and female pronuclei.

n., sensory. A n. of termination, q.v., of afferent fibers of a peripheral nerve.

n., sensory, of trigeminal nerve. A group of nuclei in pons and medulla oblongata consisting of spinal nucleus that extends inferiorly into spinal cord, the main nucleus lying dorsal and lateral to motor nucleus, and the mesencephalic nucleus lying in lateral wall of 4th ventricle.

n., subthalamic. N., hypothalamic, q.v.

n., supraoptic. N. of the hypothalamus lying above rostral ends of optic tracts and lateral to optic chiasma. SEE: *n., hypothalamic.*

n. of termination. Clusters of cells in the brain and medulla in which fibers of a nerve or nerve tract terminate.

n., thalamic. Any of the nuclei of the thalamus. Include a large number belonging to the following groups: anterior, intralaminar, lateral, and medial thalamic nuclei.

RS: mean; median; modality; mode; numeral.

numbness (nŭm'nĕs). Lack of sensation in a part, esp. from cold. SEE: *narcohypnia; obdormition.*

numeral (nū'mĕr-ăl) [L. *numerus*, number]. 1. Denoting or pert. to a number. 2. A conventional symbol expressing a number.

num'miform, num'mular [L. *nummus*, a coin, + *forma*, shape]. 1. Coin-shaped, said of some mucous sputum. 2. Arranged like a stack of coins.

nummulation (nŭm-ū-lā'shŭn). The formation of a coinshaped mass.

nunnation (nŭn-ā'shŭn) [Heb. *nun*, letter N]. Frequent and abnormal use of the n sound.

Nupercaine (nū'pĕr-kān). Proprietary name for dibucaine, a white powder or crystals manufactured from cinchoninic acid. Used as a local anesthetic of prolonged action.

nurse [L. *nutrix*, nurse]. 1. One who cares for the sick, wounded, or feeble, esp. one who makes a profession of it after successfully completing a prescribed course in a school of nursing. 2. To feed an infant at the breast. 3. To perform the duties of caring for an invalid. 4. To care for a young child.

    n., charge. One in charge of a hospital ward.

    n. clinician. A registered nurse with general knowledge of nursing theory and practice, esp. skilled in the clinical specialty in which he or she works. This nurse is capable of working independently in solving patient-care problems and is able to teach and work successfully with others on the medical-care team. Term first used by Frances Reiter, R.N., M.A., Dean, Graduate School of Nursing, New York Medical College.

    n., community, n., district. A visiting nurse whose duties are limited to a certain community or district.

    n., dry. An infant's nurse who does not suckle the child.

    n., flight. N. who cares for patients being transported in airplanes.

    n., general duty. One not specializing in a particular field of nursing, but available for any duty.

    n., graduate. One who is a graduate of an accredited school of nursing.

    n., head. A supervisor at the head of a hospital nursing staff.

    n., health. A community or visiting nurse whose duty is to give information on hygiene and prevention of disease. SEE: *n., public health.*

    n., practical. One who is licensed to administer care, usually working under direction of a licensed physician or a registered nurse. May be a graduate of an accredited school for practical nursing or one who has practical experience only.

    n., private. A nurse who cares for a single patient.

    n., private duty. One who is not a member of the hospital staff but is called upon to care for an individual patient in the hospital.

    n., probationer. A student nurse who during the first part of training is under observation.

    n., public health. A graduate nurse who has had additional training in the methods of promoting health and preventing disease. SEE: *n., health.*

    n., registered. A graduate nurse who has been registered and legally licensed to practice by state authority. ABBR: R.N.

    n., school. A registered nurse whose duties are to supplement the work of the physician in providing for the medical needs of students while they are in school.

    n., scrub. N. who is a member of the surgical team in an operating room. She has prepared for the procedure by scrubbing just as the physicians have. She is gowned and wears sterile gloves. Her duty is to hand instruments to the surgeon and assist in any other way necessary.

    n., special. A private nurse taking special care of one patient or one who specializes in the care of certain types of diseases.

    n., student. An individual who is enrolled in a school of nursing.

    n., trained. A registered nurse.

    n., visiting. A registered nurse, employed by an association to care for the sick poor in their homes.

    n., wet. A woman who breast feeds the infants of others.

nursery. Department of a hospital where the newborn are cared for.

    n., day. A nursery in which children, usually of preschool age, are cared for during the day.

nur'sing [L. *nutrix*, nurse]. 1. Scientific care of the sick by a graduate, registered nurse. 2. Loosely applied to any care of the sick. 3. Breast feeding. 4. Lactation.

nursing histories. Used by nurses to improve nursing care and patient communication. Valuable information can be obtained from this history, and reactions to previous hospitalization can be recorded and utilized in managing the patient's care during the current stay. SEE: *Nursing History Form.*

nutation (nū-tā'shŭn) [L. *nutatio*]. Nodding, as of the head.

Nursing History Form

Admission date _____ History taken by _____ Date _____

Diagnosis _____ Date of injury/illness _____

Special circumstances of present illness _____

Previous hospitalization _____

List nursing activities or omissions which were helpful or deleterious to the patient during previous

hospitalization _____

Expected result from present hospitalization _____

Is patient transient? _____

Family background

married ____ single ____ widowed ____ divorced ____ estranged ____ common law ____

Religion _____

Does patient wish visitors excluded? _____ If so, give reason _____

Daily living habits:

Food and fluid likes and dislikes _____

Sleeping habits: preferred time of retiring and arising _____

dreams _____ nightmares _____ insomnia _____

Television, radio, and phone preference _____

Bowel and urinary habits _____

Medicines taken regularly _____ Known allergies _____

Female patients: Is a personal supply of pads or tampons available? _____

Interests, hobbies, pastimes _____

List wounds or special medical care _____

Cultural factors, vocabulary, education _____

Questions patient asked _____

Additional observations _____

*Adapted from Shaw, J. S., McLaughlin, M.: Nursing Histories in a Naval Hospital, U.S. Navy Medical News Letter. 54:43–46, 1969.

nutrient (nū'trĭ-ĕnt) [L. *nutriens*]. 1. Food that supplies the body with its necessary elements. 2. Nourishing.

Certain nutrients (carbohydrates, fats, proteins, and alcohol) provide energy; other nutrients (water, electrolytes, minerals, and vitamins) are essential to the metabolic process. Those containing carbon are organic food nutrients. Organic food nutrients may or may not contain nitrogen.

RS: calorie; carbohydrate; fat; food; mineral; nitrogen; protein; vitamin.

nutriment (nū'trĭ-mĕnt) [L. *nutrimentum*, nourishment]. That which nourishes; nutritious substance.

nutrition (nū-trĭsh'ŭn) [L. *nutritio*, nourish]. The sum total of the processes involved in the taking in and utilization of food substances by which growth, repair, and maintenance of activities in the body as a whole in any of its parts are accomplished. Includes ingestion, digestion, absorption, and metabolism (assimilation). Nutrients are stored by the body in various forms and drawn upon when the food intake is not sufficient.

nutritional (nū-trĭsh'ŭn-ăl). Rel. to nutrition.

nutritious (nū-trĭsh'ŭs) [L. *nutritius*]. Affording nutriment. SYN: *nutritive*.

nutritive (nū'trĭ-tĭv). Pert. to the process of assimilating food; having the property of nourishing.

　　n. enema. One of predigested foods to give sustenance to a patient unable to take nourishment in the usual way. SEE: *enema*.

nutriture (nū'trĭ-tūr). The state of body nutrition.

nux vomica (nŭks vŏm'ĭ-kă). A poisonous seed from an East Indian tree, containing several alkaloids, the principal ones being brucine and strychnine, q.v.

nyctalbuminuria (nĭk''tăl-bū''mĭn-ū'rĭ-ă) [Gr. *nyx, nykt-*, night, + L. *albus*, white, + Gr. *ouron*, urine]. A cyclic albuminuria occurring at night. SYN: *noctalbuminuria*.

nyctalgia (nĭk-tal'jĭ-ă) ["+ *algos*, pain]. Pain during the night.

nyctalopia (nĭk-tă-lō'pĭ-ă) ["+ *alaos*, blind, + *ōps*, eye]. 1. A condition in which person cannot see well in a faint light or at night. Occurs in retinitis pigmentosa and choroidoretinitis. Also may be due to vitamin A deficiency. Smoking tobacco impairs ability to see at night. SYN: *night blindness*. 2. Used incorrectly as having better sight at night or in semidarkness than by day; night vision. SEE: *hemeralopia*.

nyctamblyopia (nĭk''tăm-blĭ-ō'pĭ-ă) [Gr. *nyx, nykt-*, night + *amblyōpia*, poor sight].

Poor vision at night without visible eye changes.

nyctaphonia (nĭk-tă-fō'nĭ-ă). Hysterical loss of voice during the night.

nycterine (nĭk'tĕr-ĭn) [Gr. *nykterinos*, by night]. 1. Taking place at night. 2. Obscure.

nycthemerus (nĭk-them'ĕ-rŭs) [Gr. *nychthemeros*]. 1. Space of a day and a night. 2. Pert. to a night and day.

nyctohemeral (nĭk''tō-hĕm'er-al) ["+ *hēmera*, day]. Rel. to both day and night.

nyctophilia (nĭk''to-fil'ĭ-ă) [Gr. *nyx, nykt-*, night, + *philein*, to love]. Abnormal predilection for darkness or night. SYN: *scotophilia*.

nyctophobia (nĭk''tō-fō'bĭ-ă) ["+ *phobos*, fear]. Abnormal dread of the night or of darkness. SYN: *scotophobia*.

nyctophonia (nĭk''tō-fō'nĭ-ă) ["+ *phōnē*, voice]. Hysterical loss of voice only during the day.

nyctotyphlosis (nĭk''tō-tĭf-lō'sĭs) ["+ *typhlōsis*, blindness]. Poor vision at night. SYN; *night blindness; nyctalopia*.

nycturia (nĭk-tū'rĭ-ă) ["+ *ouron*, urine]. Urination, esp. excessive, during the night. SYN: *nocturia*. SEE: *enuresis*.

nygma (nĭg'mă) [Gr. *nygma*, a puncture]. A puncture wound.

nym'pha [Gr. *nymphē*, a maiden]. (pl. *nymphae*) One of the labia minora, q.v., the small folds of mucous membrane forming the inner lips of the vulva. So called from the nymphs or goddesses of the fountain. SYN: *labium minus pudendi*.

　　n. pendulae. Stretched pendulous nymphae.

nymphectomy (nĭm-fĕk'tō-mĭ) ["+ *ektomē*, excision]. Excision of hypertrophied nymphae.

nymphitis (nĭm-fī'tĭs) [Gr. *nymphē*, a maiden, + *-itis*, inflammation]. Inflamed condition of the nymphae.

nymphocaruncular sulcus (nĭm''fō-kăr-ŭn'-kū-lăr sŭl'kŭs) ["+ L. *caruncula*, little mass of flesh, + *sulcus*, a groove]. The depression bet. the caruncula of the hymen and the labium minus.

nymphohymenal sul'cus (nĭm''fō-hī'mĕn-ăl) ["+ *hymēn*, membrane, + *sulcus*, a groove]. Trench bet. labium minus and the hymen on either side.

nympholepsy (nĭm'fō-lĕp''sĭ) [Gr. *nymphē*, a maiden, + *lēpsis*, a seizure]. 1. Frenzied ecstasy usually erotic in nature. 2. Obsession for something which is unattainable.

nymphomania (nĭm''fō-mā'nĭ-ă) ["+ *mania*, madness]. Abnormally excessive sexual desire in the female. SYN: *furor femininus; furor uterinus*. SEE: *satyriasis*.

nymphomaniac (nĭm''fō-ma'nĭ-ăk) [Gr. *nymphē*, maiden, + *mania*, madness]. 1. Woman who is afflicted with excessive sexual desire. 2. Affected by excessive sexual desire.

nymphoncus (nĭm-fon'kŭs) ["+ *onkos*, a swelling]. Swelling or tumor of the nymphae.

nymphotomy (nĭm-fot'ō-mĭ) ["+ *tomē*, incision]. 1. Removal of the nymphae. SYN: *nymphectomy*. 2. Incision into a nympha or clitoris.

nystagmic (nĭs-tăg'mĭk) [Gr. *nystagmos*, to nod]. Rel. to or suffering from condition of involuntary eyeball movements.

nystagmiform (nĭs-tăg'mĭ-form) ["+ L. *forma*, shape]. Like or resembling nystagmus. SYN: *nystagmoid*.

nystagmograph (nĭs-tăg'mō-grăf) ["+ *graphein*, to write]. Apparatus for recording the oscillations of the eyeball in nystagmus.

nystagmoid (nĭs-tag'moyd) ["+ *eidos*, resemblance]. Similar to or resembling nystagmus.

nystagmus (nĭs-tag'mŭs) [Gr. *nystagmos*, to nod]. Constant, involuntary, cyclical movement of the eyeball. Movement may be in any direction.

ETIOL: *Congenital*, seen in bilateral amblyopia; *occupational*, as in miners and train dispatchers; *labyrinthine irritability;* neurologic diseases.

n., aural. N. due to disorder in the labyrinth of the ear. Eye movement is spasmodic.

n., convergence. Slow abduction of eyes followed by rapid adduction. Usually accompanies other types of nystagmus.

n., end-position. Occurs when eyes are turned to extreme positions. May occur normally in debilitation or fatigue. May be due to pathology of the subcortical centers for conjugate gaze.

n., jerk. N., rhythmic, q.v.

n., labyrinthine. N. due to disease of the labyrinthine vestibular apparatus.

n., lateral. Horizontal movement of eyes from side to side.

n., miner's. N. occuring in those who work in comparative darkness for long periods.

n., opticokinetic. A rhythmic jerk nystagmus occurring while looking at constantly moving objects, such as telephone poles, from a moving car or train.

n., pendular. Characterized by movement which is approximately equal in both directions. Usually seen in those who have congenital absence of central vision or who lost it prior to the age of two.

n. rhythmic. N. in which the eyes move slowly in one direction and then are jerked back rapidly. SYN: *jerk nystagmus*.

n., rotatory. Rotation of the eyes about the visual axis.

n., vertical. Up and down ocular movements.

n., vestibular. That due to ear disturbances.

n. voluntary. A rare type of pendular n. in persons who have learned to oscillate their eyes rapidly, usually by extreme convergence. It is an acquired art which has no clinical significance.

Nysten's law (nē-stă'). [Pierre - Hubert Nysten, Fr. pediatrician, 1774-1817]. Rigor mortis begins with muscles of mastication and progresses from the head down the body, affecting legs and feet last. SEE: *rigor mortis.*

nyxis (nĭk'sĭs) [Gr.]. Puncture or piercing. SYN: *paracentesis.*

O

O. 1. Chem. symb. for oxygen. 2. Abbr. for *oculus*, eye; *octarius*, pint. 3. Symb. for a particular blood type.

o-. Abbr. for the prefix *ortho-*, most commonly used in chemical terminology.

O₂. Symb. for the molecular formula of oxygen.

O₃. Chem. symb. for ozone.

oakum (ō'kŭm) [AS. *ācumba*, tow]. Loose fiber obtained from old hemp ropes, formerly used as a surgical dressing.

oarialgia (ō"ār-ĭ-ăl'jĭ-ă) [Gr. *ōarion*, little egg, + *algos*, pain]. Ovarian pain. SYN: *oothecalgia; ovarialgia.*

oario-, oari- [Gr.]. Prefix pert. to the ovary. SEE: words beginning with *ovario-* or *oophor-.*

oasis (ō-ā'sĭs) [Gr. a fertile area in an arid region]. (pl. *oa'ses*) Area of healthy tissue surrounded by a diseased portion.

oat [AS. *āte*, oat]. Grain or seed of a cereal grass used as an article of diet.

oath [AS. ooth]. A solemn attestation or affirmation. SEE: *Hippocratic oath.*

RS: Declaration of Geneva; Prayer of Maimonides.

oatmeal ["+ *mele*, meal]. Rich in fats and lecithins. Food value of 100 gm. (cooked): Cal. 55; protein 2 gm.; fat 1 gm.; carbohydrate 9.7 gm.; calcium 9 mg.

ACTION: Stimulating, laxative, fattening, and nutritive.

O.B., OB. Abbr. for *obstetrics.*

ob- [L.]. Combining form meaning towards, against, in the way of.

obcecation (ŏb"sē-kā'shŭn). Partial blindness.

obdormition (ŏb-dor-mĭsh'ŭn) [L. *ob*, towards, + *dormīre*, to sleep]. Numbness followed by tingling in an extremity produced by pressure of the nerve trunk supplying it. Limb is commonly referred to as being asleep.

obduction (ŏb-dŭk'shŭn) ["+ *ducere*, to lead]. Scientific inspection of a dead body to learn pathological conditions and cause of death. SYN: *autopsy; necropsy.*

obelion (ō-bē'lĭ-ŏn) [Gr. *obelos*, a spit]. A craniometric point on the sagittal suture between the two parietal foramina.

obese (ō-bēs') [L. *obesus*]. Extremely fat. SYN: *corpulent.*

obesity (ō-bē'sĭ-tĭ) [L. *obesitas*, corpulence]. Abnormal amount of fat on the body. Term usually not employed unless individual is from 20-30% over average weight for his age, sex, and height. Obesity is the result of an imbalance between food eaten and energy expended, but the underlying cause usually is quite complex and difficult to treat. SYN: *adiposity; corpulence.*

There are two general classifications: exogenous, that caused by excessive food intake, and endogenous, that caused by some abnormality within the body (endocrine or faulty metabolism).

ENDOCRINE CAUSES: *Hypothyroidism*, producing a decreased metabolic rate and insufficient energy output to balance the caloric intake; not a very frequent cause; *adrenal hyperfunction, testicular and ovarian hypofunction*, the most important of the endocrine factors causing obesity.

ETIOL: Sex, obesity being more frequent in the female; race; heredity, and occupation. Common past middle age.

TREATMENT: Prophylaxis in children of families with a tendency to obesity, in the form of moderate eating and exercise; dieting; dextroamphetamine in combination with a relatively low calorie diet. Dextroamphetamine stimulates nervous energy, produces a sense of well being, and reduces the desire for food.

Diet should be below maintenance requirements so far as energy units are concerned and must be provided with all other essential nutrients. Maintenance requirements are based on what the average weight should be. 1200-1600 Cal. per day is a slow reduction regimen; 1000-1200 Cal. is more rapid.

DIET: The average basic reducing diet is about 9 Cal. per pound of ideal body weight per day. Thus a 160 pound person whose ideal wt. is 135 should eat a diet of about 1000 Cal. a day. These calories should be obtained from foods which would provide adequate protein, carbohydrates, fats, minerals, and vitamins and not from a fad diet. Adherence to this diet should cause the person to lose the excess weight. After that the diet is adjusted in that caloric intake is just equal to total energy output. Obviously this is different for each individual.

Losing weight by fasting is effective but is not recommended unless done under strict medical and nursing supervision.

RS: carbohydrate, emaciation, fat, height, protein, starch, sugar, vitamin, weight.

*o., **endogenous.*** O. caused by some abnormality within the body, endocrine or metabolic.

*o., **exogenous.*** O. due to excessive intake of food.

*o., **hypothalamic.*** O. resulting from dysfunction of hypothalamus, esp. the appetite-regulating center.

obex (ō'běks) [L. a band]. [NA]. A thin, crescent-shaped band of tissue covering the calamus scriptorius at the point of convergence of nervous tissue at the caudal end of 4th ventricle.

obfuscation (ŏb-fŭs-kā'shŭn) [L. *obfuscāre,* to darken]. 1. The act of making obscure or confusing. 2. Mental confusion.

ob'ject [L. *objectus*]. That which is visible or tangible to the senses.

*o. **blindness.*** Affection in which brain fails to recognize things seen correctly by eyes. SEE: *apraxia.*

*o. **choice.*** Selection of love object decided by a fixation developed in pregenital stage.

*o. **libido.*** Love or interest expressed external to oneself upon persons, objects, causes. SEE: *anaclitic choice.*

objective (ŏb-jĕk'tĭv). 1. Perceptible to other persons, said of symptoms. SEE: *subjective.* 2. Directed toward external things. 3. The lens of a microscope which is closest to the object.

*o. **symptoms.*** Those apparent to physical means of diagnosis.

obligate (ŏb'lĭ-gāt) [L. *obligatus*]. 1. To make necessary or to require. 2. Compulsory, bound.

*o. **aerobe.*** A microbe that must have oxygen in order to live.

*o. **anaerobe.*** A microorganism that lives only without oxygen.

*o. **parasite.*** One that can exist only at the expense of another plant or organism.

oblique (o-blēk', o-blīk') [L. *obliquus*]. Slanting, diagonal.

*o. **muscles.*** Two muscles of the eye, two of the abdomen, two of the head, and two of the ears.

obliquimeter (ŏb'lĭ-kwĭm'ĕt-ĕr) ["+ Gr. *metron,* measure]. Apparatus for indicating the angle of the pelvic brim with the upright body.

obliquity (ŏb-lĭk'wĭ-tĭ) [L. *obliquus,* slanting]. The state of being oblique.

*o., **Litzmann's.*** Inclining of the fetal head until the posterior parietal bone presents to the uterine canal.

*o., **Nägele's.*** Presentation of the fetal head with anterior parietal bone toward the uterine canal with oblique biparietal diameter in relation to the pelvic brim.

*o. **of pelvis.*** Inclination of pelvis.

*o., **Roederer's.*** Presentation of fetal head with occiput at pelvic brim.

obliquus (ŏb-lĭk'wŭs). A name applied to several muscles. SEE: *Table of Muscles* in *Appendix.*

*o. **reflex.*** Contraction of ext. obliquus muscle in toto on application of stimulus to skin of thigh below Poupart's ligament.

obliteration (ŏb-lĭt"ĕr-ā'shŭn) [L. *obliterāre,* to remove]. Extinction or complete occlusion of a part by degeneration, disease, or surgery.

oblongata (ŏb"lon-gā'tä) [L. *oblongus,* long]. The medulla oblongata; the cylindrical extension of the spinal cord as it enters the brain, about an inch long, reaching to the pons, and forming part of base of 4th ventricle.

obmutescence (ŏb-mū-těs'ěns) [L. *obmutescere,* to become dumb]. Loss of vocal power. SYN: *aphonia.*

obnubilation (ŏb-nū-bĭl-ā'shŭn) [L. *obnubilatus,* to befog or darken]. An impaired or confused state of mind.

obscure (ŏb-skūr') [L. *obscurus,* hide]. 1. Hidden, indistinct, as the cause of a condition. 2. To make less distinct or to hide.

observerscope (ob-zer'ver-skōp). Type of endoscope having two branches so that two persons can inspect the same place simultaneously.

obses'sion [L. *obsessus,* besiege]. An uncontrollable desire to dwell on an idea or an emotion, or to perform a specific act. It is not uncommon among normal persons, but if not banished may become all compelling, developing into a compulsion neurosis. A dominating condition in certain psychoses.

*o.'s, **impulsive.*** Those accompanied by action. They sometimes become manias, q.v.

*o.'s, **inhibitory.*** O.'s accompanied by impediments to action. They represent the phobias, q.v.

obses'sional neuro'sis. A psychoneurosis marked by obsessions controlling the behavior of the individual. SYN: *compulsion neurosis.*

obsessive-compulsive. Marked by an inclination to perform certain rituals repetitiously in order to relieve anxiety.

obstetric, obstetrical (ŏb-stĕt'rĭk, -rĭ-kăl) [L. *obstetrix,* midwife]. Pert. to obstetrics or midwifery.

*o. **forceps.*** Instrument used to facilitate delivery of the fetus.

obstetrician (ŏb-stĕt-rĭsh'ăn). A physician who treats women during pregnancy and parturition. SYN: *accoucheur.*

obstetrics (ŏb-stĕt'rĭks) [L. *obstetrix,* midwife]. Branch of medicine that concerns management of women during pregnancy, childbirth, and the puerperium. SYN: *maieutics.*

RS: childbirth; delivery; labor; maneuver; midwife; parturition; pregnancy.

obstipation (ŏb"stĭ-pā'shŭn) [L. *obstipatio*]. 1. The act or condition of obstructing. 2. Obstinate or extreme constipation due to an obstruction.

obstruction (ŏb-strŭk'shŭn). 1. Blocking of a structure that prevents it from functioning normally. 2. A thing that impedes; an obstacle.

o., aortic. Blocking of the aorta, thereby preventing flow of blood.

o., intestinal. Blockage of the lumen of the intestine. SEE: *intestinal o.*

obstructive lung disease, chronic. Increased resistance to the passage of air in and out of the lung due to narrowing of the bronchial tree. It is diagnosed by determining that the amount of air forcibly expired from the lung in one second is less than normal. The disease process may be caused by a number of irritants or diseases which damage the bronchial tree, including pulmonary tuberculosis, cigarette smoking, and silicosis.

obstruent (ŏb'strū-ĕnt) [L. *obstruens*]. 1. Blocking up. 2. That which closes a normal passage in the body.

obtund (ŏb-tŭnd') [L. *obtundere,* to beat against]. To dull or blunt, as sensitivity or pain.

obtundent (ŏb-tŭn'dĕnt) [L. *obtundens*]. 1. Having the capacity to deaden sensibility of a part or reduce irritability. 2. A soothing remedy.

obturation (ŏb-tūr-ā'shun) [L. *obturāre,* to stop up]. Closure of a passage or opening, as in intestinal obstruction.

obturator (ob'tū-rā"tor). 1. Anything that obstructs or closes a cavity or opening. 2. Rel. to the o. membrane. 3. Bridge for spanning the gap in the cleft palate.

o. foramen. O. in the anterior part of the os innominatum between pubis and ischium.

o. membrane. Strong o. occluding the o. foramen.

o. muscles. Two muscles on each side in the pelvic region which rotate the thighs outward. SEE: *Table of Muscles* in *Appendix; psoas* for illustration.

obtuse (ŏb-tūs') [L. *obtusus*]. 1. Not pointed or acute; dull or blunt. 2. Stupid; dull mentally.

obtusion (ŏb-tū'zhŭn). Blunting or weakening of normal sensation, as in certain diseases.

Occam's razor (ŏck-hăm). [Sir William of Occam, or Okham, Eng. philosopher, 1300-1349] The concept that entities do not have to be proven beyond the point of proof.

occipital (ŏk-sĭp'ĭ-tăl) [L. *occipitalis*]. Concerning the back part of the head.

o. bone. Bone in lower back part of skull between the parietal and temporal bones.

o. lobe. Posterior lobe of the cerebral hemisphere which is shaped like a three-sided pyramid.

occipitalis (ŏk-sĭp"ĭ-tā'lĭs) [L.]. The posterior portion of the occipitofrontalis muscle at back of the head.

occipito- [L.]. Combining form showing relationship between the occiput and another part.

occiput (ŏk'sĭ-pŭt) [L.]. [NA]. The back part of the skull.

occlude (ŏ-klūd') [L. *occludere,* to shut up]. To close up, obstruct, or join together, as bringing the biting surfaces of opposing teeth together.

occlus'al (ŏ-klū'zal). Pert. to the closure of an opening.

o. surface. The masticating surface of a tooth.

occlusion (ŏ-klū'zhŭn) [L. *occlusio*]. 1. The closure, or state of being closed, of a passage. May be acquired or congenital. SYN: *imperforation.* 2. Adsorption of gas by a substance which does not thereby lose its characteristic property. 3. Relation of the teeth when the jaws are closed.

o., coronary. Coronary thrombosis; obstruction of a coronary vessel by thrombosis or as a result of spasm.

oc'cult (ŭ-kŭlt') [L. *occultus*]. Obscure; concealed, as a hemorrhage.

o. blood. Blood in such minute quantity that it can only be recognized by microscopic or chemical means.

occupation neurosis. A functional disorder of a part caused by certain occupations, as writer's cramp.

occupational therapy. Treatment based on utilization of activities calculated to encourage the physically or mentally disabled patient to contribute to his own recovery. On the request of the patient's physician a registered occupational therapist selects and directs the patient's activities.

ochlesis (ŏk-lē'sĭs) [Gr. *ochlēsis,* crowding]. Any disease caused by conditions of overcrowding.

ochlophobia (ŏk"lō-fō'bĭ-ă) [Gr. *ochlos*, crowd, + *phobos*, fear]. Abnormal dread of crowds or populated places.

ochrodermia (ō"krō-der'mĭ-ă) [Gr. *ōchros*, pale yellow, + *derma*, skin]. A yellow state of the skin.

ochrometer (ō-krŏm'ĕt-ĕr) ["+ *metron*, measure]. Device for estimating the capillary blood pressure by compression of a finger until its skin becomes blanched.

ochronosis, ochronosus (ō-krō-nō'sĭs, -sŭs) ["+ *nosos*, disease]. A rare condition marked by dark pigmentation of the ligaments, cartilage, fibrous tissues, skin, and urine. May be caused by an inborn error of metabolism, alkaptonuria. This allows formation of homogentisic acid, part of which is excreted in the urine and part of which is stored in the tissues. The condition also may be caused by chronic phenol poisoning.

octa-, octo- [Gr. *oktō*, L. *octo*]. Combining forms meaning eight.

octahedron (ŏk-tă-hē'drŏn). An eight-sided solid figure.

octan (ŏk'tăn) [L. *octo*, eight]. Reappearing on every 8th day, as a fever.

octane (ŏk'tăn). C_8H_{18}. A hydrocarbon of the paraffin series.

octarius (ŏk-tā'rĭ-ŭs) [L.]. Pint. ABBR: O.

octavalent (ŏk"tăv-ā'lĕnt) [L. *octo*, eight, + *valeo*, to have power]. Having a valency of 8.

octipara (ŏk-tĭp'ă-ră) ["+ L. *parere*, to bear]. A woman who has given birth to eight children.

octogenarian (ŏk-tō-jĕn-ĕr'ĭ-ĕn) [L. *octogenarius*, containing eighty]. A person who is in his eighties.

octoroon (ŏk-tō-roon'). One who has one-eighth negro blood and seven-eighths white blood; progeny of a white person and a quadroon.

ocular (ŏk'ū-lăr) [L. *oculus*, eye]. 1. Concerning the eye or vision. 2. Eyepiece of a microscope.

oculist (ŏk'ū-lĭst). Old term for ophthalmologist, a physician who is a specialist in diseases of the eye.

oculocephalogyric reflex (ŏk"ū-lō-sĕf'ă-lō-jī'rĭk). Associated movements of eye, head, and body in focalizing vision upon an object.

oculogyration (ŏk"ū-lō-jĭ-rā'shŭn) [L. *oculus*, eye, + Gr. *gyros*, circle]. Motions of the eyeball.

oculogyric (ŏk"ū-lō-jī'rĭk). Producing or concerning movements of the eye. SYN: *ophthalmogyric.*

    o. crisis. Attack of involuntary deviation and fixation of the eyeballs, usually upwards. The crisis may last for several minutes or hours. May be seen with postencephalitic parkinsonism or encephalitis lethargica.

oculomotor (ŏk"ū-lō-mō'tor) [L. *oculus*, eye, + *motor*, mover]. Rel. to eye movements. SYN: *oculogyric.*

    o. nerve. The 3rd cranial nerve. Originates in the medial surface of the cerebral peduncle of the midbrain and consists of general somatic efferent, general visceral efferent, and general somatic afferent fibers. It is distributed through all extrinsic muscles of the eye except exterior rectus and superior oblique; through levator palpebrae superioris of eyelid; through the ciliary muscle; and through the sphincter muscle of iris. It has primarily a motor function, but it also contains proprioceptive fibers. SYN: *nervus oculomotorius* [NA].

    SEE: *Table of Cranial Nerves* in *Appendix.*

oculomycosis (ŏk"ū-lō-mī-kō'sĭs) ["+ Gr. *mykēs*, fungus, + *-ōsis*, condition]. Any disease of the eye or its parts caused by a fungus.

oculonasal (ŏk"ū-lō-nā'sal) ["+ *nasus*, nose]. Concerning both eye and nose.

oculoreaction (ŏk"ū-lō-rē-ăk'shŭn) [L. *oculus*, eye, + *rē*, back, + *actus*, acting]. A reaction in the eye when toxins of tuberculosis and typhoid are instilled into the eye. More severe in persons suffering from the disease. SYN: *ophthalmic reaction; Calmette's reaction.*

oculozygomatic (ŏk"ū-lō-zī-gō-măt'ĭk) ["+ Gr. *zygon*, yoke]. Pert. to the eye and zygoma.

    o. line. Line between inner canthus of eye and cheek supposedly indicating neural disorders.

oculus (ŏk'ū-lŭs) [L.]. (pl. *oc'uli*) [NA]. Eye; the organ of vision made up of the eyeball and optic nerve.

    o. dexter. The right eye. ABBR. O.D.

    o. sinister. The left eye. ABBR. O.S.

    o. uterque. Each eye. ABBR. O.U.

O.D. Abbr. for *oculus dexter*, right eye; *Doctor of Optometry.*

odaxesmus (ō"dăk-sez'mŭs) [Gr. *odaxēsmos*, an irritation]. The biting of the tongue, lip, or cheek during an epileptic attack.

odaxetic (ō-dăk-sĕt'ĭk). Producing a stinging or itching sensation.

Oddi's sphincter (ŏd'ĭ). [Ruggero Oddi, It. physician]. A sphincter at the opening of the common bile duct into the duodenum at the papilla of Vater.

odogenesis (ō"dō-jĕn'ĕ-sĭs) [Gr. *hodos*, pathway, + *genesis*, formation]. The reestablishment of connections between the divided ends of a nerve by nerve process attraction. SYN: *neurocladism*.

dontagra (ō-dŏn-tă'grä) [Gr. *odous, odont-*, tooth, + *agra*, seizure]. Toothache, esp. when originating from gout.

dontalgia (ō-dŏn-tăl'jĭ-ă) ["+ *algos*, pain]. Toothache. SYN: *odontia; odontodynia*.

    o., phantom. Pain felt in the area from which a tooth has been pulled.

dontatrophy (ō"dŏn-tăt'rō-fĭ) [Gr. *odous, odont-*, tooth, + *atrophia*, atrophy]. Imperfect development of the teeth.

dontectomy (ō-dŏn-tek'tō-mĭ) ["+ *ektomē*, excision]. Surgical removal of a tooth.

donterism (ō-dŏn'tĕr-ĭzm) ["+ *erismos*, quarrel]. Chattering of the teeth.

dontia (ō-dŏn'shĭ-ă) [Gr. *odous, odont-*, tooth]. 1. Pain in a tooth. SYN: *odontalgia*. 2. Condition or abnormality of the teeth.

dontiasis (ō"dŏn-tī'ă-sĭs) ["+ *iasis*, disease]. 1. Cutting of the teeth. SYN: *dentition; teething*. 2. Disease caused by teething.

dontitis (ō-dŏn-tī'tĭs) ["+ *-itis*, inflammation]. Inflammation of a tooth.

donto-, odont- [Gr. *odous*, tooth]. Combining form relating to the tooth or teeth.

dontoblast (ō-dŏn'tō-blăst) [Gr. *odous, odont-*, tooth, + *blastos*, germ]. One of the cells forming the surface layer of the dental papilla which is responsible for the formation of the dentine of a tooth. After a tooth is formed the odontoblasts line the pulp cavity and continue to produce dentine for years after the tooth has erupted. From their distal ends Tomes' fibers extend to the periphery of the dentine.

dontoblasto'ma. A tumor composed principally of odontoblasts.

dontobothrion (ō-dŏn"tō-bŏth'rĭ-ŏn) ["+ *bothrion*, pit]. Socket of a tooth.

don"tobothri'tis. Inflammation of the socket of a tooth.

dontocele (ō-dŏn'tō-sēl) [Gr. *odous, odont-*, tooth, + *kēlē*, hernia]. An alveolodental cyst.

dontochirurgical (ō-dŏn-tō-kĭ-rŭr'jĭ-kăl) ["+ *cheirourgia*, surgery]. Pert. to dental surgery.

dontoclasis (ō-dŏn-tōk'lă-sĭs) ["+ *klasis*, fracture]. The breaking or fracture of a tooth.

don'toclast. A cell which brings about the absorption of the roots of deciduous teeth.

dontodynia (ō-dŏn"tō-dĭn'ĭ-ă) ["+ *odynē*, pain]. Toothache. SYN: *odontalgia; odontia*.

dontogenesis, odontogeny (ō-dŏn"tō-jĕn'ĕ-sĭs, -tŏj'ĕn-ĭ) ["+ *genesis*, production]. The origin and formation of the teeth.

dontoid (ō-dŏn'toyd) [Gr. *odous, odont-*, tooth + *eidos*, resemblance]. Toothlike.

    o. process. The toothlike projection from upper surface of the body of the 2nd cervical vertebrae.

odon'tolith. The accretion of a calcareous substance on the teeth; tartar.

odontol'ogist. A dentist or dental surgeon.

odontology (ō"dŏn-tol'ō-jĭ) [Gr. *odous, odont-*, tooth + *logos*, study]. The science of dealing with the teeth and their care. SYN: *dentistry*.

odontoma (ō-dŏn-tō'mă) ["+ *-oma*, tumor]. Tumor of a tooth or of the dental tissue.

    o., coronary. Bony tumor at crown of a tooth.

    o., follicular. Bony shell in gums below tooth margin, usually after 2nd dentition.

    ETIOL: Excessive number of dental follicles.

    SYM: Crepitating to pressure. Tumor often contains one or more teeth. SYN: *dentigerous cyst*.

    o., radicular. Bony tumor at root of a tooth.

odontonecrosis (ō-dŏn"tō-nē-krō'sĭs) ["+ *nekros*, dead, + *-ōsis*, intensive]. Extensive decay of a tooth.

odontopathy (ō-dŏn-top'ăth-ĭ) [Gr. *odous, odont-*, tooth, + *pathos*, disease]. Any disease of the teeth.

odontophobia (ō-dŏn"tō-fō'bĭ-ă) ["+ *phobos*, fear]. 1. Abnormal aversion to the sight of teeth. 2. Abnormal fear of dental surgery.

odontoplerosis (ō-dŏn"tō-plē-rō'sĭs) [Gr. *odous, odont-*, tooth, + *plērōsis*, filling]. The filling of a dental cavity.

odontoprisis (ō-dŏn"tō-prī'sĭs) ["+ *prisis*, sawing]. Grinding of the teeth. SYN: *bruxism*.

odontorrhagia (ō-dŏn"tō-rā'jĭ-ă) ["+ *rhēgnynai*, to burst forth]. Hemorrhage from a tooth socket following extraction.

odontorthosis (ō-dŏn"tō-tŏr-thō'sĭs) ["+ *orthos*, straight]. Operation of straightening irregular teeth.

odontosis (ō-dŏn-tō'sĭs) [Gr. *odous, odont-*, tooth, + *-ōsis*, intensive]. 1. Development of teeth. 2. Eruption of teeth.

odontotherapy (ō-dŏn"tō-ther'ă-pĭ) ["+ *therapeia*, treatment]. Care of diseased teeth.

odontotripsis (ō-dŏn"tō-trĭp'sĭs) ["+ *tripsis*, a rubbing]. Natural abrasion of the teeth.

odontotrypy (ō-dŏn-tŏt'rĭ-pĭ) ["+ *trypan*, to bore]. Drilling of a tooth.

odor (ō'der) [L.]. 1. That quality of a substance which renders it perceptible to sense of smell. 2. Any smell, esp. a sweet scent. 3. Any sensation of sense of smell.

    Each odoriferous substance causes its own sensation. Odors have been classed as (1) pure odors, (2) those mixed with sensations from the mucous membrane, and (3) those mixed with the sensation of taste.

Pure odors are aromatic, burning, fragrant, fetid, nauseating, or repulsive.

Another classification is spicy, flowery, fruity, resinous, foul, scorched.

RS: antibromic; "brom-" words; deodorant; effluvium; olfactory; osmolagnia; osphresiolagnia; pungent; smell.

odoriferous (ō″dor-ĭf′ē-rŭs) [L. *odor*, smell, + *ferre*, to bear]. Bearing scent, having an odor; fragrant; perfumed.

odorim′etry. The measurement of the ability of a substance to induce olfactory sensations.

o′dorous [L. *odor*, smell]. Having an odor, scent, or fragrance.

odynacusis (ō-dĭn-ă-kū′sĭs) [Gr. *odynē*, pain, + *akousis*, hearing]. A condition in which noises cause pain in the ear.

odynometer (ō-dĭn-om′ĕt-ĕr) ["+ *metron*, measure]. Device for measuring pain.

odynophagia (ŏd′ĭn-ō-fā′jĭ-ă) ["+ *phagein*, to eat]. Pain upon swallowing.

odynophobia (ŏd′ĭn-ō-fō′bĭ-ă) ["+ *phobos*, fear]. Abnormal dread of pain.

Oedipus com′plex (ēd′ĭ-pŭs). [Oedipus, a character in Gr. tragedy who fell in love with his mother, killed his father in jealousy, and married his mother]. Abnormally intense love of the child for parent of the opposite sex retained in adulthood. Usually involves jealous dislike of the other parent. Most commonly love of a son for his mother. SEE *Electra complex*.

Oertel's terrain cure (er′tel). [Max J. Oertel, Ger. physician, 1835-1897]. Graduated exercise, mountain climbing, diet, and reduction of fluids for patients with some types of heart disease, obesity, circulatory diseases, etc. SYN: *Oertel's treatment*.

Oesophagos′tomum (ē-sof″ă-gŏs′tō-mŭm). A genus of nematodes belonging to the suborder Strongylata; parasitic in the intestinal walls of animals and men.

O. apiostomum. The nodular worm of monkeys. Occasionally infests man.

offi′cial. Said of medicines authorized as standard in the U.S. Pharmacopeia and in the National Formulary.

officinal (ŏf-ĭs′ĭn-al) [L. *officina*, shop]. Regularly kept in a druggist's stock. See *magistral.*

Oguchi's disease (o-goot′chē). [Chuta Oguchi, Jap. ophthalmologist, 1875—]. Recessive hereditary night blindness. Onset is in infancy. Commonly found in Japan; rare in United States.

-OH. Chemical formula for the hydroxyl ion.

ohm (ōm). Unit of electrical resistance equ. to that of a conductor in which a current one ampere is produced by a potential of or volt across the terminals.

-oid [Gr. *eidos*, form]. Suffix indicating resen blance to the item designated in the fir part of the word.

oikofugic (oy″kō-fū′jĭk) [Gr. *oikos*, house, L. *fugere*, to flee]. Having a compulsion t leave home.

oikomania (oy-kō-mā′nĭ-ă) ["+ *mania*, ma. ness]. Nervous disorder induced by unhapp home surroundings. SEE *ecomania.*

oikophobia (oy″kō-fō′bĭ-ă). Morbid dislike o the home.

oil (oyl) [L. *oleum*]. A greasy liquid not misc ble with water, usually obtained from, an classified as mineral, vegetable, or anima According to character, oils are subdivide principally as fixed or fatty and volatile o essential.

Ex: Fixed: Castor oil, olive oil, cod liver oi Volatile: Oils of mustard, peppermint, rose

RS: oleaginous; oleate; oleic; olein; oleum unctuous.

ointment (oynt′mĕnt) [Fr. *oignement*]. A medicated, fatty, soft substance having an tiseptic, cosmetic, or healing properties Usually its base is petroleum jelly, lard, o lanolin to which the medicament is added These forms are not water soluble. Howeve some ointments are composed of ingredient which are water soluble. SYN: *salve; un guent.*

okra (ō′kra). A tropical and semitropical plant and its edible sticky green pods.

Food value of 100 gm. (cooked): Cal. 29 protein 2 gm.; trace of fat; carbohydrate 6 gm.; calcium 92 mg.; vitamin A, 490 I.U.

ol. Abbr. for L. *oleum*, oil.

O.L.A. Abbr. for L. *occipito laevo anterior* fetal presentation with the occiput toward the maternal left acetabulum. SYN: *L.O.A* SEE: *position.*

olea (ō′lē-ă) [L.]. 1. Olive. 2. Pl. of oleum.

oleaginous (ō-lē-ăj′ĭ-nŭs) [L. *oleaginus*]. Greasy; oily; unctuous.

oleate (ō′lē-āt) [L. *oleatum*]. 1. Any salt of oleic acid. 2. Salt of oleic acid dissolved in an excess of the acid. Used as an ointment.

oleatum (ō-lē-ā′tŭm) [L.]. Preparation made by dissolving metallic salts or alkaloids in oleic acid, SYN: *oleate.*

olecranal (ō-lĕk′răn-ăl) [Gr. *ōlekranon*, elbow]. Concerning the elbow.

olecranarthritis (ō-lĕk″răn-ar-thrī′tĭs) ["+ *arthron*, joint, + *-itis*, inflammation]. Inflamed condition of the elbow joint.

olecranarthrocace (ō-lĕk″răn-ar-thrŏk′ă-sĭ) ["+ "+ *kakē*, badness]. Tuberculous ulceration of the elbow joint.

olecranarthropathy (ō-lĕk″răn-ar-thrŏp′-ă-thĭ) ["+ "+ *pathos*, disease]. Any disease of the elbow joint.

olecranoid (ō-lĕk′ră-noyd) ["+ *eidos*, resemblance]. Similar to the olecranon.

olecranon (ō-lĕk′răn-ŏn) [Gr., elbow]. [NA]. A large process of the ulna projecting behind the elbow joint and forming the bony prominence of the elbow.

FRACTURE: Prevent spasm of triceps muscle to avoid separation of fragments. Latter may have to be wired.

TREATMENT: Similar to that for fracture of patella, q.v. SEE: *elbow* for illustration; *skeleton.*

oleic (ō-lē′ĭk) [L. *oleum*, oil]. Derived from or pert. to oil.

   o. acid. USP. A colorless, oily liquid prepared from tallow and other fats, the salts of which are oleates. Formula $C_8H_{34}O_2$.

olein (ō′lē-ĭn) [L. *oleum*, oil]. An oleate of glyceryl found in nearly all fixed oils and fats; an important part of oils. SYN: *triolein.*

oleo- [L. *oleum*, oil]. Combining form meaning oil.

oleoarthrosis (ō″lē-ō-ar-thrō′sĭs) [L. *oleum*, oil, + Gr. *arthron*, joint, + *-ōsis*, condition]. Therapeutic introduction of oil into a joint.

oleoinfusion (ō″lē-ō-ĭn-fū′zhŭn) ["+ *in*, into, + *fusus*, poured]. Combination of a drug and oil.

oleomargarine (ō″lē-ō-mar′jă-rĭn) ["+ *margarine*]. Artificial butter made from refined vegetable and animal fats. Vitamins, preservatives, and coloring agents usually are included. SYN: *margarine.*

oleoresin (ō″lē-ō-rĕz′ĭn) ["+ *resina*, resin]. Extract of plant containing resinous substance and oil, prepared by dissolving the crude drug in ether, acetone, or alcohol.

oleosaccharum (ō-lē-ō-săk′ă-rŭm) [L. *oleum*, oil, + *saccharum*, sugar]. A substance compounded of sugar and volatile oil.

oleotherapy (ō″lē-ō-ther′ă-pĭ) ["+ Gr. *therapeia*, treatment]. Therapeutic injection of oil. SYN: *eleotherapy.*

oleothorax (ō-lē-ō-thō′răks) ["+ Gr. *thōrax*, chest]. Therapeutic injection of oil into the pleural cavity, as in pulmonary tuberculosis.

oleum (ō′lē-ŭm) [L.]. (pl. *o′lea*) Oil.

   o. morrhuae. Cod liver oil.

   o. olivea. Olive oil. ABBR: ol. oliv.

   o. percomorphum. Mixture of oils from livers of various members of order Percomorphi. More potent than cod liver oil in vitamins A and D.

   o. ricini. Castor oil.

olfactie (ŏl-făk′tĭ) [L. *olfacere*, to smell]. Unit of smell; the threshold of olfactory stimulation.

olfaction (ŏl-făk′shŭn) [L. *olfacere*, to smell]. The sense of smell. Smelling.

olfactive (ŏl-făk′tĭv) [L. *olfacere*, to smell]. Pert. to the sense of smell. SYN: *olfactory.*

olfactology (ŏl-făk-tŏl′ō-jĭ) ["+ Gr. *logos*, study]. Scientific investigation of sense of smell.

olfactometer (ŏl″fak-tom′et-ĕr) [L. *olfactus*, smell, + Gr. *metron*, measure]. Apparatus for testing the power of the sense of smell.

olfactory (ŏl-făk′tō-rĭ). Pert. to smell.

   o. area. Area in the hippocampal convolution. Anterior portion of the callosal gyrus and the uncus. SYN: *anterior perforated substance.*

   o. bulb. Enlarged anterior extremity of the o. tract.

   o. cortex. Portion of the cerebral cortex concerned with the olfactory sense. Includes the pyriform lobe and the hippocampal formation. SYN: *archicortex; allocortex.*

   o. esthesioneuroma. Slowly-growing malignant tumor of the nasal fossa, developing from epithelial and neural tissues of the olfactory mucosa.

   o. lobe. A cranial lobe projecting from anterior lower part of each cerebral hemisphere.

   o. membrane. M. in upper part of nasal cavity which contains olfactory receptors.

   o. nerves. The first pair of cranial nerves supplying the nasal olfactory mucosa. Consists of delicate bundles of unmyelinated fibers, the fila olfactoria, which pass through cribriform plate and terminate in olfactory glomeruli of olfactory bulb. The fila are central processes of bipolar receptor neurons of olfactory mucous membrane.

   o. organ. The nose.

   o. striae. Three bands of fibers, lateral, intermediate, and medial, which form the roots of the olfactory tract.

   o. tract. Band of fibers extending posteriorly from o. bulb to anterior perforated substance. Here it enlarges and divides into the olfactory striae.

   o. trigone. Small triangular area between lateral and medial olfactory striae.

   o. tubercle. An elevation at rostral end of anterior perforated substance. Well developed in lower mammals, rudimentary in man.

oligemia (ŏl-ĭg-ē″mĭ-ă) [Gr. *oligos*, little, + *haima*, blood]. Deficient volume of blood in the body. SYN: *oligohemia.*

oligergasia (ŏl-ĭ-gĕr-gā'sĭ-ă). Psychic disorder from brain deficiency caused by imperfect development.

olighidria (ŏl-ĭ-gĭd'rĭ-ă) [Gr. *oligos*, little, + *hidrōs*, sweat]. Deficient perspiration. Also spelled oligidria.

olighydria (ŏl-ĭ-gĭd'rĭ-ă). Deficiency of body fluids.

oligo-, olig- [Gr. *oligos*, little]. Combining form meaning small or few.

oligocholia (ŏ-lĭ-gō-kō'lĭ-ă) [Gr. *oligos*, little, + *cholē*, bile]. Lack or deficiency of bile.

oligochromemia (ol'ĭg-ō-krō-mē'mĭ-ă) ["+ *chrōma*, color, + *haima*, blood]. Reduction of total amount of hemoglobin in the blood.

oligochylia (ŏl-ĭ-gō-kī'lĭ-ă) ["+ *chylos*, juice]. Deficiency of gastric juice.

oligochymia (ŏl-ĭg-ō-kī'mĭ-ă) ["+ *chymos*, juice]. Deficiency of chyme.

oligocystic (ŏl-ĭ-gō-sĭs'tĭk) [Gr. *oligos*, little, + *kystis*, a bladder]. Having just a few cysts, as a tumor.

oligocythemia (ŏl'ĭ-gō-sī-thē'mĭ-ă) ["+ *kytos*, cell, + *haima*, blood]. Deficiency in number of red blood corpuscles.

oligocytosis (ol'ĭ-gō-sī-tō'sĭs) ["+ "+ *-osis*, intensive]. Deficiency of red blood corpuscles. SYN: *oligocythemia*.

oligodactylia (ol-ĭ-gō-dăk-tĭl'ĭ-ă) ["+ *daktylos*, digit]. Subnormal number of fingers or toes.

oligodendrocyte [Gr. *oligos*, little, + *dendron*, tree, + *cyte*, cell]. Neuroglial cells having few and delicate processes.

oligodendroglia (ŏl'ĭ-gō-dĕn-drŏg'lĭ-ă) ["+ "+ *glia*, glue]. Adventitial cells found in central nervous system with characteristic vinelike processes. SYN: *mesoglia*.

oligodendroglioma (ol'ĭ-gō-dĕn"drō-glĭ-ō'mă). A malignant tumor occurring principally in the cerebrum, consisting mostly of oligodendrocytes. Frequently calcification occurs. Etiology is unknown.

oligodipsia (ŏl-ĭ-gō-dĭp'sĭ-ă) [Gr. *oligos*, little, + *dipsa*, thirst]. Abnormal absence of desire for fluids.

oligodon'tia ["+ *odont*, tooth]. A hereditary developmental anomaly characterized by fewer teeth than normal.

oligodynamic (ŏl'ĭ-gō-dī-năm'ĭk) [Gr. *oligos*, little, + *dynamis*, power]. Effective in a small quantity.

oligoerythrocythemia (ŏl'ĭ-gō-ĕ-rith"rō-sī-thĕm'ĭ-ă) ["+ *erythros*, red, + *kytos*, cell, + *haima*, blood]. Deficiency of hemoglobin or red blood corpuscles.

oligogalactia (ŏl'ĭ-gō-găl-ăk'tĭ-ă) ["+ *gala*, *galakt-*, milk]. Deficient milk secretion.

oligogenics (ŏl-ĭ-gō-jĕn'ĭks) [Gr. *oligos*, little, + *gennan*, to produce]. Limitation of the number of offspring by utilizing some form of birth control. SYN: *birth control*.

oligohemia (ŏl'ĭ-gō-hē'mĭ-ă) ["+ *haima*, blood]. Insufficiency in the amount of blood in the body. SYN: *oligemia*.

oligohydramnios (ŏl'ĭg-ō-hī-dram'nĭ-ŏs) [Gr. *oligos*, little, + *hydor*, water, + *amnion*, amnion]. Abnormally small amount of amniotic fluid.

oligohydruria (ŏl'ĭ-gō-hī-drū'rĭ-ă) ["+ "+ *ouron*, urine]. Highly concentrated urine.

oligoleukocythemia (ŏl'ĭ-gō-lū"kō-sī-thē'mĭ-ă) [Gr. *oligos*, little, + *leukos*, white, + *kytos*, cell, + *haima*, blood]. Reduction in leukocytic content of blood. SYN: *leukopenia*.

oligomania (ŏl-ĭ-gō-mā'nĭ-ă) ["+ *mania*, madness]. Insanity involving only a few mental faculties.

oligomastigate (ŏl-ĭ-gō-măs'tĭ-gāt) ["+ *mastix*, *mastig-*, whip]. Characterized by two flagella.

oligomenorrhea (ŏl'ĭ-gō-mĕn-ō-rē'ă) [Gr. *oligos*, little, + *mēn*, month, + *rhoia*, flow]. Scanty or infrequent menstrual flow.

oligopepsia (ŏl-ĭ-gō-pĕp'sĭ-ă) ["+ *pepsis*, digestion]. Insufficient digestive tone.

oligophosphaturia (ŏl'ĭ-gō-fŏs-fā-tū'rĭ-ă) ["+ *phosphas*, phosphate, + *ouron*, urine]. Scanty amount of phosphates in the urine.

oligophrenia (ŏl'ĭg-ō-frē'nĭ-ă) [Gr. *oligos*, few, + *phrēn*, mind]. Mental deficiency due to faulty development. SYN: *mental deficiency*.

oligoplasmia (ŏl'ĭg-ō-plăz'mĭ-ă) ["+ *plasmos*, a thing formed]. Insufficient amount of blood plasma.

oligopnea (ŏl-ĭ-gŏp'nĭ-ă) ["+ *pnoia*, breath]. Infrequent respiration. Respiration shallow or abnormally deep; rate as slow as 6-10 per minute. Usually accompanied by slow pulse, although high in some conditions. SYN: *hypopnea*.

   ETIOL: Cerebral compression, meningeal or pontine hemorrhage, cerebral or cerebellar tumors, abscess, gumma of meninges, osteoma of cranium, some forms of meningitis, trauma of brain, drug poisoning, shock, constitutional diseases, etc.

oligoposy (ŏl-ĭ-gŏp'ō-sĭ) ["+ *posis*, drink]. Insufficient intake of liquids.

oligoptyalism (ŏl-ĭ-gō-tī'ă-lĭzm) ["+ *ptyalon*, saliva]. Insufficient secretion of saliva. SYN: *oligosialia*.

oligoria (ŏl-ĭ-gōr'ĭ-ă) [Gr. negligence]. A form of melancholia in which there is apathy toward things and people.

oligosialia (ŏl'ĭ-gō-sī-ă'lĭ-ă) [Gr. *oligos*, few, + *sialon*, saliva]. Scanty salivary secretion. SYN: *oligoptyalism*.

oligospermia (ŏl″ĭ-gō-spĕr′mĭ-ă) ["+ *sperma*, seed]. Deficient amount of spermatozoa in seminal fluid. It may be temporary or permanent. SYN: *hypospermatogenesis.*

oligotrichia (ŏl-ĭ-gō-trĭk′ĭ-ă) ["+ *thrix*, hair]. Congenital scantiness of hair.

oligotrophy (ŏl-ĭ-gŏt′rō-fĭ) ["+ *trophē*, nourishment]. Inadequate nutrition.

oliguresis (ŏl-ĭg-ū-rē′sĭs) ["+ *ourēsis*, urination]. Scantiness of urine; infrequent urination.

oliguria (ŏl-ĭg-ū′rĭ-ă) ["+ *ouron*, urine]. Diminished amount of urine formation.

ETIOL: Seen after profuse perspiration, bleeding, and diarrhea. Also in retention of urine due to brain disease, drug poisoning, and deep coma.

oliva (ō-lī′vă) [L. olive]. (pl. *oli′vae*) [NA] An oliveshaped gray body behind the anterior pyramid of the medulla oblongata. SEE: *olivary body.*

ol′ivary [L. *oliva*, olive]. Shaped like an olive; oval.

    o. body. A rounded mass located in anterolateral portion of the medulla oblongata. Consists of a convoluted sheet of gray matter enclosing white matter. SYN: *oliva; inferior olivary nucleus; inferior olive.*

olive. Olive tree or its fruit.

Food value of 100 gm. (pickled, green): Cal. 116; protein 1.4 gm.; fat 12.7 gm.; carbohydrate 1.3 gm.; calcium 61 mg.

100 gm. (ripe): Cal. 129; protein 1.1 gm.; fat 13.8 gm.; carbohydrate 2.6 gm.

olive (ŏl′ĭv) [L. *oliva*, olive]. Oliva, q.v.

    o., accessory. Two masses of gray matter lying adjacent to the inferior olive. SYN: *accessory olivary nuclei, dorsal* and *medial.*

    o., inferior. Olivary body, q.v., inferior olivary nucleus.

    o., superior. The superior olivary nucleus, q.v.

olive oil. USP. Oil obtained by pressing the ripe fruit of olives (olea europaea). Used as an emollient in treating skin diseases.

-ology [Gr. *logos*, study]. Suffix pert. to study of, knowledge, or science of.

olophonia (ŏl-ō-fōn′ĭ-ă) [Gr. *oloos*, destroyed, + *phōnē*, voice]. Malformation of vocal organs with resultant unnatural speech.

O. L. P. Abbr. for L. *occipito laeva posterior*, fetal presentation with its occiput toward the left posterior quadrant of the pelvis. SYN: *L.O.P.* SEE: *position.*

o.m. Abbr. for L. *omni mane*, every morning.

-oma [Gr.]. Suffix denoting a tumor.

omagra (ō-mă′grä) [Gr. *ōmos*, shoulder, + *agra*, seizure]. Attack of gout in the shoulder.

omalgia (ō-mal′jĭ-ă) ["+ *algos*, pain]. Neuralgia of shoulder.

omarthritis (ō″mar-thrī′tĭs) ["+ *arthron*, joint, + *-ītis*, inflammation]. Inflamed condition of the shoulder joint.

ombrophobia (ŏm-brō-fō′bĭ-ă) [Gr. *ombros*, rain, + *phobos*, fear]. Fear and anxiety induced by storms, threatening clouds, or rain.

omenta (ō-mĕn′tä) [L.]. Plural of omentum.

omental (ō-mĕn′tăl) [L. *omentum*, covering]. Pert. to the omentum, the peritoneal fold supporting the viscera.

    o. bursa. A cavity within the layers of peritoneum forming the great omentum. Its opening into the main peritoneal cavity is the epiploic foramen (foramen of Winslow). SYN: *lesser peritoneal sac.*

omentectomy (ō-mĕn-tĕk′tō-mĭ) ["+ Gr. *ektomē*, excision]. Surgical removal of a portion of the omentum.

omentitis (ō-mĕn-tī′tĭs) ["+ Gr. *-ītis*, inflammation]. Inflamed condition of omentum.

omentopexy (ō-mĕn′tō-pĕks″ĭ) [L. *omentum*, covering + Gr. *pēxis*, fixation]. Fixation of the omentum to the abdominal wall or adjacent organ.

omentorrhaphy (ō-mĕn-tor′ră-fĭ) ["+ Gr. *rhaphē*, suture]. Suturing of the omentum.

omentosplenopexy (ō-mĕn″tō-splē′nō-pĕks-ĭ) ["+ Gr. *splēn*, spleen, + *pēxis*, fixation]. Fixation of the spleen and omentum. Combined omentopexy and splenopexy.

omentotomy (ō-mĕn-tot′ō-mĭ) ["+ Gr. *tomē*, incision]. Incision of the omentum.

omentum (ō-mĕn′tŭm) [L. a covering]. (pl. *omenta*) A double fold of peritoneum attached to the stomach and connecting it with certain of the abdominal viscera. It contains a cavity, the omental bursa (lesser peritoneal cavity).

The omenta are the great o., or gastrocolic; and the lesser, or gastrohepatic o.

PALPATION OF: Cancerous and tubercular enlargements are distinguished by the fact that they extend across the abdomen; cannot be traced backward; do not ascend behind the ribs; are rough, hard, and uneven.

RS: abdomen, caul, epiploon, kidney, ovary, spleen.

    o., great. Portion of the o. suspended from greater curvature of the stomach and covering the intestines like an apron. It dips in among the folds of the intestines and is attached to the transverse colon and mesocolon. It contains fat; aids in keeping the intestines warm, prevents friction, and aids in localizing infections. SYN: *o. majus* [NA].

    o., lesser. It passes from the lesser cur-

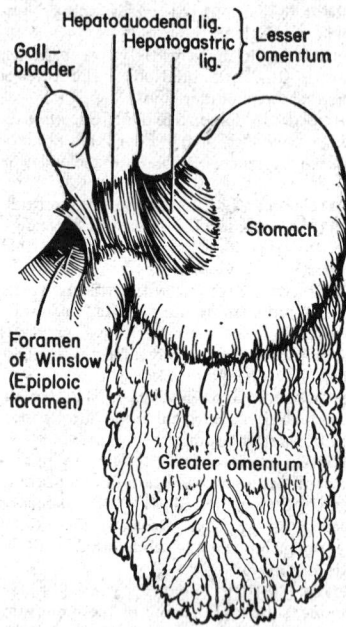

ANATOMIC RELATIONSHIPS OF THE GREATER AND LESSER OMENTUM

vature of stomach to transverse fissure of the liver. SYN: *o. minus* [NA].

omitis (ō-mī'tĭs) [Gr. *ōmos*, shoulder, + *-itis*, inflammation]. Inflamed condition of the shoulder.

omn. bih. Abbr. for L. *omni bihora*, every two hours.

omn. hor. Abbr. for L. *omni hora*, every hour.

omni- (ŏm'nī) [L. *omnis*]. Prefix designating all.

omnipotence of thought. Infantile concept of reality whereby one expects all his wishes to be instantly accomplished.

    Ex: A child who gains his objectives through crying comes to believe in his own omnipotence because of a parent's surrender to his demands.

omnivorous (ŏm-nĭv'ō-rŭs) [L. *omnis*, all, + *vorāre*, to eat]. Living on all kinds of food.

omn. noct. Abbr. for L. *omni nocte*, every night.

omn. quad. hor. Abbr. for L. *omni quadrante hora*, every quarter of an hour.

omo- [Gr. *ōmos*, shoulder]. Combining form pert. to the shoulder.

omodynia (ō-mō-dĭn'ĭ-ă) [Gr. *ōmos*, shoulder, + *odynē*, pain]. Pain of the shoulder.

omohyoid (ō-mō-hī'oyd). 1. Concerning the scapula and the hyoid bone. 2. Muscle attached to the hyoid bone and the scapula. SEE: *Table of Muscles* in *Appendix.*

omophagia (ō-mō-fā'jĭ-ă) [Gr. *ōmos*, raw, + *phagein*, to eat]. The custom of eating raw foods, esp. flesh.

OMPA. Abbr. for *octamethyl pyrophosphoramide;* used as cholinesterase inhibitor.

omphal-, omphalo [Gr. *omphalos*, the naval]. Combining form designating relationship to the navel.

omphalectomy (ŏm-făl-ĕk'tō-mĭ) [Gr. *omphalos*, naval, + *ektomē*, excision]. Surgical removal of the umbilicus.

omphalic (ŏm-făl'ĭk) [Gr. *omphalikos*]. Concerning the umbilicus.

omphalitis (ŏm-făl-ī'tĭs) [Gr. *omphalos*, navel, + *-itis*, inflammation]. Inflamed condition of the navel.

omphalocele (ŏm-făl'ō-sēl) [Gr. *omphalos*, navel, + *kēlē*, hernia]. Congenital hernia of the navel. SEE: *hernia.*

omphalomesenteric (ŏm''făl-ō-mĕs-ĕn-ter'ĭk) ["+ *mesenterion*, mesentery]. Concerning the umbilicus and mesentery.

omphaloncus (ŏm-făl-ŏn'kŭs) ["+ *onkos*, tumor]. Umbilical tumor or swelling.

omphalophlebitis (ŏm''făl-ō-flē-bī'tĭs) ["+ *phleps*, vein, + *-itis*, inflammation]. Inflamed condition of umbilical veins.

omphalorrhagia (ŏm''făl-ō-rā'jĭ-ă) [Gr. *omphalos*, navel, + *rhēgnynai*, to burst forth]. Umbilical hemorrhage.

omphalorrhea (ŏm-făl-ō-rē'ă) ["+ *rhoia*, flow]. Discharge of lymph at the navel.

omphalorrhexis (ŏm-făl-ō-rĕk'sĭs) ["+ *rhēxis*, rupture]. Rupture of the navel.

omphalos (ŏm'făl-ŏs) [Gr.]. Umbilicus. SYN: *navel.*

omphalosotor (om-fal-ō-sō'tor) [Gr. *omphalos*, navel, + *sōtēr*, preserver]. Device used in replacing the prolapsed umbilical cord at childbirth.

omphalospinous (ŏm-făl-ō-spī'nŭs) ["+ L. *spina*, thorn]. Concerning the navel and the anterior superior spine of the ilium.

omphalotomy (ŏm-făl-ŏt'ō-mĭ) ["+ *tomē*, incision]. Division of umbilical cord at birth. The navel should be dressed with sterile cotton that should be changed on second day of life.

omphalotripsy (ŏm'făl-ō-trĭp'sĭ) ["+ *tripsis*, a rubbing]. Severing of the umbilical cord by a crushing method.

ON. Abbr. for *orthopedic nurse.*

o.n. Abbr. for L. *omni nocte*, every night.

onanism (ō'năn-ĭzm). [So named because it was practiced by the Biblical character Onan, son of Judah]. Coitus interruptus; withdrawal before completion of sexual act. Erroneously used to designate masturbation, q.v.

onanist (ō'nă-nĭst). One who practices coitus interruptus. Erroneously used to indicate one who masturbates.

Onanoff's reflex (ŏn-ăh-nŏf'). [Jacques Onanoff, Fr. physician, 1859 -]. Contraction of bulbocavernous muscle resulting from compression of glans penis.

Onchocerca (ŏng-kō-ser'kă) [Gr. *onkos,* hook, + *kerkos,* tail]. A genus of filarial worms. They live in subcutaneous and connective tissues and usually are enclosed in fibrous cysts or nodules.

O. caecutiens. A species of O. that causes cutaneous filariasis in man.

O. volvulus. A species of O. that infests man, frequently invading the tissues of the eye. Transmitted by species of the blackfly; Simulium and Eusimulium.

onchocerciasis (ŏng-kō-ser-kī'ă-sĭs) [" + "+ *iasis,* infestation]. Condition produced by infestation with one of the worms of Onchocerca. It is characterized by a nodular swelling over the coiled parasite. SYN: *onchocercosis.*

onco- [Gr. *onkos,* mass, bulk]. Combining form indicating relationship to a tumor, swelling, or mass.

Oncocerca. Onchocerca, q.v.

oncocercosis. Onchocerciasis, q.v.

oncogenesis (ong''kō-jĕn'ĕ-sĭs) [Gr. *onkos,* mass, + *genesis,* production]. Tumor formation and development.

oncogenous (ŏng-kŏj'ĕ-nŭs). Forming or producing tumors.

oncograph (ŏng'kō-grăf) [Gr. *onkos,* mass, + *graphein,* to write]. Device attached to oncometer for making record of the internal organs' size.

oncology (ŏng-kŏl'ō-jĭ) [" + *logos,* study]. The branch of medicine dealing with tumors.

oncolysis (ŏng-kŏl'ĭ-sĭs) [" + *lysis,* dissolution]. The absorption or dissolution of tumor cells.

oncolytic (ong-kō-lĭt'ĭk). Destructive to tumor cells.

oncometer (ŏng-kŏm'ĕt-ĕr) [Gr. *onkos,* mass, + *metron,* measure]. Apparatus for measurement of variations in size of internal organs. SEE: *plethysmograph.*

oncometric (ong-kō-mĕt'rĭk). Pertaining to oncometry.

oncom'etry. The measurement of variations in size of internal organs.

oncosis (ŏng-kō'sĭs) [Gr. *onkos,* mass, + *-ōsis,* intensive]. 1. A condition characterized by the development of tumors. 2. A swelling or tumor.

oncosphere (ŏng'kō-sfēr) [Gr. *onkos,* hook, + *sphaira,* sphere]. Embryonic stage of a tapeworm in which it has hooks.

oncothlipsis (ŏng-kō-thlĭp'sĭs) [Gr. *onkos,* tumor, + *thlipsis,* pressure]. Pressure caused by presence of a tumor.

oncotic (ŏng-kŏt-ĭk) [Gr. *onkos,* tumor]. Concerning, caused, or marked by swelling.

oncotomy (ŏng-kŏt'ō-mĭ) [" + *tomē,* incision]. The incision of a tumor, abscess, or boil.

oncotropic (ŏng-kō-trŏp'ĭk) [" + *tropos,* a turning]. Possessing special attraction for tumor cells. SYN: *tumoraffin.*

Ondine's curse. Condition in which the respiratory center in the brain is unable to stimulate breathing in response to the increased amount of carbon dioxide in the blood. SYN: *hypothalamic alveolar hypoventilation syndrome.*

oneiric (ō-nī'rĭk) [Gr. *oneiros,* dream]. Resembling, rel. to, or accompanied by dreams.

oneirism (ō-nī'rĭzm) [" + *ismos,* state of]. Dreamlike hallucination in a waking state.

oneirodynia (ō-nī-rō-dīn'ĭ-ă) [Gr. *oneiros,* dream, + *odynē,* pain]. Painful dreaming; nightmare, q.v.

oneirology (ō''nī-rol'ō-jĭ) [" + *logos,* study of]. The scientific study of dreams.

oneiroscopy (ō''nī-rŏs'kō-pĭ) [" + *skopein,* to examine]. Analysis of dreams in order to diagnose the individual's emotional state.

oniomania (ō-nī-ō-mă'nī-ă) [Gr. *ōnios,* for sale, + *mania,* madness]. A psychoneurotic urge to spend money.

onion (ŭn'yŭn) [AS. *oignon*]. L. name for the common onion is alium cepa. May be important in increasing the fibrinolytic activity of blood.

The characteristic odor of onions is due to several volatile chemicals, some of which contain sulfur. The ability of onions to cause persons who peel them to shed tears probably is caused by a derivative of cysteine containing sulfur and oxygen.

Food value of 100 gm. (raw mature): Cal. 38; protein 1.5 gm.; trace of fat; carbohydrate 8.7 gm.; calcium 27 mg.

onkinocele (ŏng-kĭn'ō-sēl) [Gr. *onkos,* mass, + *in-,* fiber, + *kēlē,* swelling]. Inflammation with swelling of a tendon sheath.

onomatology (ŏn-ō-mă-tŏl'ō-jĭ) [Gr. *onoma,* name, + *logos,* study]. Science of names. SYN: *nomenclature; terminology.*

onomatomania (ŏn''ō-mă''tō-mā'nī-ă) [" + *mania,* madness]. A mental derangement characterized by an abnormal impulse to dwell upon or repeat certain words, by attaching significance to their imagined hidden meanings, or by trying frantically to recall a particular word.

onomatophobia (ŏn″ō-mă″tō-fō′bĭ-ă) ["+ *phobos*, fear]. Abnormal fear of hearing a certain name or word because of an imaginary dreadful meaning attached to it.

onomatopoiesis (ŏn″ō-mă″tō-poy-ē′sĭs) [Gr. *onoma*, name, + *poiein*, to make]. Created, usually meaningless, imitative words and sounds formed by the insane.

ONP. Abbr. for *operating nursing procedure*.

ontogenesis (ŏn″tō-jĕn′ĕ-sĭs). Ontogeny, q.v.

ontogeny (ŏn-tŏj′ĕn-ĭ) [Gr. *ōn*, being, + *gennan*, to produce]. The history of the development of an individual. SYN: *ontogenesis*.

onychalgia (ŏn″ĭ-kal′jĭ-ă) [Gr. *onyx*, *onych-*, nail, + *algos*, pain]. Pain in the nails.

　o. nervosa. Extreme sensitivity of nails. SYN: *hyperesthesia unguium*.

onychatrophia (ŏn″ĭ-kăt′rō-fĭ-ă) [Gr. *onyx*, *onych-*, nail, + *trophē*, nourishment]. Atrophy of the nails.

onychauxis (ŏn″ĭ-kawk′sĭs) ["+ *auxein*, to increase]. Overgrowth of the nails.

onychectomy (ŏn″ĭ-kĕk′tō-mĭ) ["+ *ektome*, to cut]. Surgical removal of the nail of a finger or toe.

onychia (ō-nĭk′ĭ-ă) [Gr. *onyx*, *onych-*, nail]. Inflammation of the nail bed with suppuration and frequently loss of the nail. SYN: *matrixitis; onychitis; onyxitis*. SEE: *paronychia*.

　o. craquele. Fragility of nails.

　o. lateralis. Suppuration of tissues in the area lateral to fingernail. SYN: *paronychia*.

　o. maligna. Type of o. in debilitated persons in which there is fetid ulceration and loss of the nail.

　o. parasitica. Any parasitic disease of the nails. SYN: *onychomycosis*.

　o., piannic. Hyperkeratotic plaques which occur in the periungual region and cause deformities of the nail fold.
　ETIOL: yaws.

　o. punctata. Condition in which a nail possesses small punctiform depressions.

onychitis (ŏn-ĭ-ki′tĭs) ["+ *-itis*, inflammation]. Inflammation of the nail bed. SYN: *onychia*.

onychocryptosis (ŏn″ĭ-kō-krĭp-tō′sĭs) ["+ *kryptein*, to conceal"]. Ingrowing of the toenail.

onychograph (ŏn-ĭk′ō-grăf) ["+ *graphien*, to write]. Device for making record of capillary blood pressure under the fingernails.

onychogryposis (on″ĭ-kō-grĭ-fō′sĭs) [Gr. *onyx*, *onych-*, nail, + *grypōsis*, a curving].

Abnormal overgrowth of the nails with inward curvature.

onychoid (ŏn′ĭ-koyd) ["+ *eidos*, resemblance]. Similar to a nail, esp. a fingernail.

onycholysis (ŏn-ĭ-kŏl′ĭ-sĭs) ["+ *lysis*, destruction]. Loosening or detachment of the nail from the nail bed.

onychoma (ŏn-ĭ-kō′mă) [Gr. *onyx*, *onych-*, nail, + *-ōma*, tumor]. Tumor of the nail or nail bed.

onychomalacia (ŏn″ĭ-kō-mă-lā′sĭ-ă) ["+ *malakia*, softening]. Unnatural softening of the nails. SEE: *hapalonychia*.

onychomycosis (ŏn″ĭ-kō-mĭ-kō′sĭs) ["+ *mykēs*, fungus, + *-ōsis*, condition]. Disease of the nails due to a parasitic fungus.

onychonosus (ŏn-ĭ-kŏn′ō-sŭs) ["+ *nosos*, disease]. Any disease of the nails.

onychopathy (ŏn-ĭ-kŏp′ăth-ĭ) [Gr. *onyx*, *onych-*, nail + *pathos*, disease]. Any disease of the nails. SYN: *onychonosus*.

onychophagy (ŏn-ĭ-kŏf′ă-jĭ) ["+ *phagein*, to eat]. The practice of nail biting.

onychophosis (ŏn-ĭk-ō-fō′sĭs). Accumulation of horny layers of epidermis under the toenail.

onychophyma (ŏn″ĭ-kō-fī′mă) [Gr. *onyx*, *onycho*, nail, + *phyma*, a growth]. Painful degeneration of the nails with hypertrophy.

onychoptosis (ŏn″ĭk-ŏp-tō′sĭs) [Gr. *onyx*, *onych-*, nail, + *ptōsis*, a falling]. Dropping off of the nails.

onychorrhexis (ŏn″ĭ-kō-rĕk′sĭs) ["+ *rēxis*, a rupture]. Abnormal brittleness and nail splitting. SYN: *brittle nails; fragilitas unguium*.

onychosis (ŏn-ĭ-kō′sĭs) ["+ *-ōsis*, disease]. Any diseased condition of the nails. SYN: *onychopathy*.

onychotomy (ŏn″ĭ-kŏt′ō-mĭ) [Gr. *onyx*, *onych-*, nail, + *tomē*, incision]. Surgical incision of a fingernail or toenail.

onychotrophy (ŏn-ĭ-kŏt′rō-fĭ) ["+ *trophē*, nourishment]. Nourishment of the nails.

onyx (ŏn′ĭks) [Gr., nail]. 1. A fingernail or toenail. 2. Pus collection between the corneal layers of the eye. SYN: *hypopyon*.

onyxis (ō-nĭk′sĭs). Ingrowing of the nails.

onyxitis (ŏn-ĭk-sī′tĭs) ["+ *-itis*, inflammation]. Onychia, q.v.

oo- (ō-ō) [Gr. *ōon*, egg]. Combining form denoting an egg or the primordial cell that develops into an ovule. SEE: words beginning with *ovo-*.

oocyesis (ō″ō-sĭ-ē′sĭs) ["+ *kyēsis*, pregnancy]. Ectopic pregnancy in the ovary.

oocyst (ō′ō-sĭst) [Gr. *ōon*, egg, + *kystis*, bladder]. The encysted form of a fertilized gamete (zygote) occurring in certain Sporozoa. SEE: *ookinete*.

oocyte (ō'ō-sīt) ["+ *kytos*, cell]. The early or primitive ovum before it has developed completely.

    o., primary. Cell at end of growth period of oogonium and before 1st maturation division has occurred.

    o., secondary. The larger of two cells resulting from first maturation division. SEE: *body, polar.*

oogenesis (ō''ō-jĕn'ĕ-sĭs) [Gr. *ōon*, egg, + *genesis*, formation]. Formation and development of the ovum. SYN: *ovigenesis.*

oogonium (ō''ō-gō'nĭ-ŭm) ["+ *gone*, generation]. (pl. *oogonia*) 1. The primordial cell from which an oocyte originates. 2. Descendant of primordial cell from which the oocyte arises.

ookinesis (ō'ō-kĭn-ē'sĭs) [Gr. *ōon*, egg, + *kinēsis*, movement]. Mitotic phenomena taking place within an ovum during maturation and fertilization.

ookinete (ō''ō-kĭ-nēt') ["+ *kinētos*, motile]. An elongated motile zygote occurring in the life cycle of certain sporozoan parasites, esp. Plasmodium. It penetrates stomach wall of a mosquito and gives rise to an oocyst.

oophor- [Gr. *ōophoros*, bearing eggs]. Combining form indicating relationship to the ovary.

oophoralgia (ō''ŏf-ō-ral'jĭ-ă) [Gr. *ōon*, egg, + *phoros*, bearing, + *algos*, pain]. Pain in an ovary.

oophorauxe (ō''ŏf-ō-rawks'ē) ["+ "+ *auxein*, to increase]. Ovarian enlargement.

oophorectomy (ō''ŏf-ō-rĕk'tō-mĭ) ["+ "+ *ektomē*, excision]. Excision of an ovary. SYN: *ovariectomy.*

oophoritis (ō''ŏf-ō-rī'tis) ["+ "+ *-itis*, inflammation]. Inflamed condition of the ovary. SYN: *ovaritis*, q.v.

    o., follicular. Inflammation of the graafian follicles.

oophorocystosis (ō-ŏf''ō-rō-sĭs-tō'sĭs) [Gr. *ōon*, egg, + *phoros*, bearing, + *kystis*, cyst, + *-ōsis*, condition]. Development of an ovarian cyst.

oophorohysterectomy (ō-ŏf''ō-rō-hĭs-tĕr-ĕk'tō-mĭ) ["+ "+ *hystera*, uterus, + *ektomē*, excision]. Surgical removal of the uterus and ovaries. SYN: *oothecohysterectomy; ovariohysterectomy.*

oophoroma (ō-ŏf''ō-rō'mă) ["+ "+ *-ōma*, tumor]. Malignant ovarian tumor.

oophoron (ō-ŏf'ō-rŏn) [Gr. *ōon*, egg, + *phoros*, bearing]. An ovary. SYN: *ootheca.*

oophoropathy (ō-ŏf''ō-rŏp'ă-thĭ) ["+ "+ *pathos*, disease]. Any pathologic condition of the ovary.

oophoropeliopexy (ō-ŏf''ō-rō-pē'lĭ-ō-pĕk''sĭ) [Gr. *ōon*, egg, + *phoros*, bearing, + *pellis*,

pelvis, + *pēxis*, fixation]. Suture of a displaced ovary to the pelvic wall.

oophoropexy (ō-ŏf''ō-rō-pĕk'sĭ) ["+ " *pēxis*, fixation]. Fixation of a displaced ovary. SYN: *oophoropeliopexy.*

oophorosalpingectomy (ō-ŏf''ō-rō-săl-pĭn-jĕk'tō-mĭ) ["+ "+ *salpinx*, tube, + *ektomē*, excision]. Excision of an oviduct and ovary. POSITION: Dorsal. SYN: *ovariosalpingectomy.*

oophorosalpingitis (ō-ŏf''or-ō-săl''pĭn-jī'tĭs). Inflammation of the ovary and oviduct.

oophorostomy (ō-ŏf-ō-rŏs'tō-mĭ) [Gr. *ōon*, egg, + *phoros*, bearing, + *stoma*, opening]. Creation of artificial opening into ovarian cyst for drainage.

oophorrhagia (ō''ŏf-ō-rā'jĭ-ă) ["+ "+ *rhegnynai*, to burst forth]. Hemorrhage from an ovulatory site severe enough to cause clinical symptoms or signs.

oophorrhaphy (ō-ŏf-or'ă-fĭ) ["+ "+ *raphē*, suture]. Suture of a displaced ovary to the pelvic wall.

ooplasm (ō'ō-plăsm). The cytoplasm of an ovum.

oosperm (ō'ō-spĕrm) [Gr. *ōon*, egg, + *sperma*, seed]. The cell formed by union of the spermatozoon with the ovum; the fertilized ovum.

ootheca (ō-ō-thē'kă) [Gr. *ōothēkē*, ovary]. An ovary. SYN: *oophoron.*

oothecohysterectomy (ō-ō-thē''kō-hĭs-tĕr-ĕk'tō-mĭ) [Gr. *ōothēkē*, ovary, + *hystera*, uterus, + *ektomē*, excision]. Excision of the uterus and ovaries. SYN: *oophorohysterectomy.*

ootherapy (ō''ō-ther'ă-pĭ) [Gr. *ōon*, egg, + *therapeia*, treatment]. Treatment with ovarian substance.

OP. Abbr. for *operative procedure; outpatient.*

opacity (ō-păs'ĭ-tĭ) [L. *opacitas*, shadiness]. 1. State of being opaque. 2. An opaque area or spot.

opaque (ō-pāk') [L. *opacus*, dark]. 1. Impenetrable by visible light rays or by other forms of radiant energy such as X rays. 2. Not transparent. 3. Dense or slow to learn.

OPC. Abbr. for *outpatient clinic.*

OPD. Abbr. for *outpatient department.*

open (ō'pĕn) [AS.]. 1. Not shut. 2. Uncovered, exposed, as a wound to air. 3. To puncture, as to open a boil. 4. Interrupted, said of an electric circuit, when current cannot pass.

operable (ŏp'ĕr-ă-bl) [L. *operor*, to work]. 1. Practicable. 2. Admitting of treatment by operation with reasonable expectation of cure.

operant conditioning. Conditioning or influencing behavior by rewarding an individual for certain forms of behavior. This reward, also called reinforcement, induces the person to act in such a way as to receive the award.

operate (ŏp'ĕr-āt) [L. *operatus*, worked]. 1. To perform an excision or incision or to make a suture on the body or any of its organs or parts to restore health. 2. To produce an effect, as a drug.

operation (ŏp-ĕr-ā'shŭn) [L. *operatio*, a working]. 1. The act of operating. 2. A surgical procedure to restore health. 3. Action of a drug.

PREPARATION FOR:

Abdominal: Shave entire abdomen and pubic hair. Cleanse umbilicus.

Anal and perineal: Shave genital area.

Arm: Shave axilla and area from shoulder to below elbow.

Breast: Shave axilla and well around the breast. If radical operation, also chest from sternum to spine and area from costal margin to clavicle.

Cerebellar: In males and children, shave the whole head and back of neck to scapulae; in females, back of head from above ears down to scapulae.

Cerebral: Shave entire head unless otherwise ordered.

Chest: Shave from median line to median line, including back.

Elbow: Shave from middle of upper arm to fingers; also axilla.

Forearm: Shave from hand to shoulder.

Hernia: Shave genital area and lower abdomen to umbilicus; also down front of thighs to middle of thighs.

Kidney: Shave from scapula to sacrum, and spine to anterior median line.

Knee: Shave from thigh to foot.

Leg: Shave from thigh to ankle.

Neck lateral: Shave two inches behind ear on side indicated; cheek in males.

Rectal: Shave genital area.

Spine: Shave entire back if necessary.

Thigh: Shave from groin to foot, also genital area.

Thyroid: Shave lower neck in front if necessary.

SEE: Name of individual operation.

PREPARATION FOR, IN HOME: If it is impossible for an operation to be performed in a hospital, it may be necessary to set up a room in a home as an operating room. The area should be near a water supply and have facilities for boiling surgical instruments, water, and other necessary articles such as pans and basins.

On the day before the operation, remove curtains, rugs, and all unnecessary furniture. Wash the windows, walls, woodwork, tables, and floor by scrubbing with plenty of hot water and soap. Supplies of sterile sheets, towels, handbrushes, masks, caps, and gauze sponges must be prepared in the following manner: Make separate packets of each type of supply and label in pencil on the outside cover. The sheets, towels, gowns, etc., should be washed and ironed, folded compactly, wrapped in squares of sterile muslin, pinned with straight pins, and labeled in pencil. Bake these packets in a moderate oven (350° F. or 176.70° C.) for 30 minutes or until the outside wrapping shows a light tinge of scorching.

For an operating table, select a kitchen table of the proper height for the surgeon to work comfortably. Cover top with a clean blanket for padding; cover the padding with a sterile sheet. The surgeon will indicate the instruments, which are to be boiled for 10 minutes in a pan with a tight lid.

Everyone in the operating room must wear a sterile gown (nightshirts may be used), a cap to cover the head and hair, and a gauze mask.

Proper ventilation in the room is necessary but there must be no drafts. Keep the temperature of the room at 72°-75° F. (22.3°-23.9° C.).

   o., ablative. O. in which a part is removed.

   o., exploratory. O. performed for diagnostic purposes.

   o., major. One involving danger to life.

   o., minor. O. not serious or risking life.

   o., plastic. O. for reconstruction and repair of surface structures.

   o., radical. O. performed to effect complete cure.

   o., reconstructive. O. to repair a loss or defect.

   o., subtotal. One in which only a portion of the organ is removed, as subtotal removal of thyroid gland.

operative (op'ĕr-ā-tĭv) [L. *operativus*, working]. 1. Effective, active. 2. Pert. to or brought about by an operation. 3. A drug that is acting.

   o. procedure. A surgical operation.

opercular (ō-pur'kū-lăr) [L. *operculum*, a cover]. Concerning a covering structure.

operculum (ō-pur'kū-lŭm) [L., a covering]. (pl. *oper'cula*) 1. Any covering. 2. Plug of mucus which fills up the opening of the cervix upon impregnation. 3. [NA]. Convolutions of the cerebrum, the margins of which are separated by the lateral cerebral (Sylvian) fissure. The opercula cover the insula.

ophiasis (ō-fī'ă-sĭs) [Gr. *ophis*, snake]. Baldness occuring in winding streaks across the head.

ophidiophobia (ō-fĭd''ĭ-ō-fō'bĭ-ă) [Gr. *ophidion*, snake, + *phobos*, fear]. Abnormal fear of snakes.

ophidism (ō'fĭd-ĭzm) ["+ *ismos*, condition]. Poisoning from snake bite.

ophiotoxemia (ō''fĭ-ō-tŏk-sē'mĭ-ă) ["+ *toxikon*, poison, + *haima*, blood]. Poisoning due to venom injected by a snake.

ophritis, ophryitis (ŏf-rī'tĭs, -rē-ī'tĭs) [Gr. *ophrys*, eyebrow, + *-itis*, inflammation]. Inflammation of the eyebrow.

ophryon (ŏf're-on). Meeting point of the facial median line with a transverse line across the forehead's narrowest portion.

ophthalmagra (ŏf'thăl-măg'ră) [Gr. *ophthalmos*, eye, + *agra*, seizure]. Gouty or rheumatic inflammation of the eye, with pain.

ophthalmalgia (ŏf'thăl-măl'jĭ-ă) ["+ *algos*, pain]. Pain in the eye. SYN: *ophthalmodynia.*

ophthalmatrophy (ŏf-thăl-măt'rō-fĭ) ["+ *atrophia*, a wasting]. Atrophy of eyeball.

ophthalmectomy (ŏf-thăl-mĕk'tō-mĭ) [Gr. *ophthalmos*, eye, + *ektomē*, excision]. Surgical excision of an eye.

ophthalmia (ŏf-thăl'mĭ-ă) [Gr. *ophthalmos*, eye]. Severe inflammation of the eye, usually including the conjunctiva.

  o., catarrhal. Conjunctivitis of a severe, frequently purulent, form.

  o., Egyptian. Granular conjunctivitis. SYN: *trachoma.*

  o., electric. Ophthalmia marked by pain in the eye, intolerance to light, and tearing (lacrimation). Occurs following exposure, usually prolonged, to intense light as that in arc welding.

  o., gonorrheal. Severe, purulent form due to infection with gonococcus.

  o., granular. Severe purulent conjunctivitis with formation of granules on the eyelids. SYN: *trachoma.*

  o., metastatic. Sympathetic inflammation of the choroid due to pyemia or metastasis.

  o. neonatorum. Severe purulent conjunctivitis in the newborn.

  ETIOL: Infection of the birth canal at the time of delivery. Gonococcus is responsible for great majority of cases. Symptoms present 12-48 hrs. after birth when due to gonorrhea.

  PROPHYLAXIS: Introduction of a few drops of a silver nitrate solution or penicillin ophthalmic ointment into each eye of newborn at birth.

  o., neuroparalytic. One resulting from injury or disease involving semilunar ganglion or branches of trigeminal nerve supplying eyeball.

  o., phlyctenular. Vesicular formations on epithelium of conjunctiva or cornea.

  o., purulent. Purulent inflammation of eye, usually due to gonococcus.

  o., scrofulous. Phlyctenular o., q.v.

  o., spring. Conjunctivitis in the spring of the year, usually an allergic reaction to tree pollen. SYN: *vernal conjunctivitis.*

  o., sympathetic. Rare bilateral granulomatous inflammation of the entire uveal tract of both eyes. Occurs in the untraumatized eye following perforation of the globe of the other eye.

  SYM: Photophobia, lacrimation, pain, blurring of vision, eyeball tenderness, deposits on posterior surface of cornea. Exudate appears in pupillary area with posterior synechia, seclusio pupillae, secondary atrophy with blindness.

  TREATMENT: Mydriatics, analgesics, steroid or other anti-inflammatory therapy. Sympathetic ophthalmia does not occur immediately following injury; thus it is not necessary to remove the injured eye as an emergency procedure.

  o., varicose. O. seen in varicose veins of the conjunctiva.

ophthalmiatrics (ŏf-thăl-mĭ-at'rĭks) [Gr. *ophthalmos*, eye, + *iatreia*, treatment]. The treatment of eye diseases.

ophthalmic (ŏf-thăl'mĭk). Pert. to the eye.

  o. nerve. A branch of the trigeminal or trifacial nerve (5th cranial n.). It is sensory and its branches are the lacrimal, frontal, and nasociliary.

  o. reaction. Reaction of the eye following instillation into the eye of toxins of typhoid or tuberculosis. SYN: *Calmette's reaction; oculoreaction; ophthalmoreaction.*

ophthalmitis (ŏf-thăl-mī'tĭs) ["+ *-itis*, inflammation]. Inflamed condition of the eye.

ophthalmo- [Gr. *ophthalmos*, eye]. Combining form pert. to the eye.

ophthalmoblennorrhea (ŏf-thăl''mō-blĕn''ō-rē'ă) [Gr. *ophthalmos*, eye, + *blenna*, mucus, + *rhoia*, flow]. Purulent inflammation of the eye or conjunctiva, usually due to the gonococcus.

ophthalmocele (ŏf-thăl'mō-sēl) ["+ *kēlē*, swelling]. Abnormal protrusion of the eyeballs. SYN: *exophthalmos.*

ophthalmocopia (ŏf-thăl-mō-kō'pĭ-ă) ["+ *kopos*, fatigue]. Ocular fatigue; eyestrain. SYN: *asthenopia.*

ophthalmodesmitis (ŏf-thăl''mō-dĕs-mī'tĭs) [Gr. *ophthalmos*, eye, + *desmos*, ligament,

+ *-itis,* inflammation]. Inflammation of tendons of the eye.

ophthalmodiagnosis (ŏf-thăl″mō-dī″ăg-nō′sĭs) ["+ *dia,* through, + *gnōsis,* knowledge]. Diagnosis of eye conditions by means of the ophthalmoreaction, q.v.

ophthalmodynamometer ["+ *dynamis,* power, + *metron,* measure]. Instrument for determining pressure in ophthalmic arteries. Device is placed against conjunctiva of eye. If pressure is higher on one side than the other appropriate studies to attempt to define the cause are indicated.

ophthalmodynamometry. Determination of pressure in the ophthalmic artery by use of an instrument which produces pressure on the eyeball until pulsations in the ophthalmic artery are seen through the ophthalmoscope. That pressure is diastolic. As the pressure is increased the vessel collapses; this is systolic pressure.

ophthalmodynia (ŏf-thăl-mō-dĭn′ĭ-ă) ["+ *odynē,* pain]. Pain in the eye. SYN: *ophthalmalgia.*

ophthalmofundoscope (ŏf-thăl″mō-fŭn′dō-skōp) [Gr. *ophthalmos,* eye, + L. *fundus,* base, + Gr. *skopein,* to examine]. Apparatus used in examining the fundus of the eye.

ophthalmography (ŏf′thăl-mŏg′răf-ĭ) ["+ *graphein,* to write]. Description of the eye.

ophthalmogyric (ŏf-thăl″mō-jī′rĭk) ["+ *gyros,* circle]. Causing or concerning concentric ocular movements. SYN: *oculogyric.*

ophthalmolith (ŏf-thăl′mō-lĭth) ["+ *lithos,* stone]. A calculus of the lacrimal duct.

ophthalmologist (ŏf-thăl-mŏl′ō-jĭst) [Gr. *ophthalmos,* eye, + *logos,* study]. A physician who specializes in the treatment of disorders of the eye; an oculist.

NOTE: The preferred term for a physician who treats and studies diseases of the eye is ophthalmologist. An optometrist is not a physician, but one who is skilled in testing visual acuity and prescribing corrective lenses. An optician sells or makes optical materials.

ophthalmology (ŏf-thăl-mŏl′ō-jĭ) [Gr. *ophthalmos,* eye, + *logos,* study]. The science dealing with the eye and its diseases.

ophthalmomalacia (ŏf-thăl″mō-măl-ā′sĭ-ă) ["+ *malakia,* softening]. Abnormal shrinkage or softening of the eye.

ophthalmometer (ŏf-thăl-mŏm′ĕt-ĕr) [Gr. *ophthalmos,* eye, + *metron,* measure]. Instrument for making measurements of corneal astigmatism.

ophthalmometry (ŏf-thăl-mŏm′ĕt-rĭ). Measurement of the ocular defects and refractive powers.

ophthalmomycosis (ŏf-thăl″mō-mī-kō′sĭs) [Gr. *ophthalmos,* eye, + *mykēs,* fungus, + *-ōsis,* condition]. Any fungus disease of the eye.

ophthalmomyitis (ŏf-thăl″mō-mī-ī′tĭs) ["+ *mys, my-,* muscle, + *-itis,* inflammation]. Inflammation of the ocular muscles.

ophthalmomyositis (ŏf-thăl″mō-mī-ō-sī′-tĭs). Ophthalmomyitis, q.v.

ophthalmomyotomy (ŏf-thăl″mō-mī-ŏt′ō-mĭ) [Gr. *ophthalmos,* eye, + *mys, my-,* muscle, + *tomē,* incision]. Surgical section of the muscles of the eyes.

ophthalmoneuritis (ŏf-thăl″mō-nū-rī′tĭs) ["+ *neuron,* sinew, + *-itis,* inflammation]. Inflamed condition of the optic nerve.

ophthalmopathy (ŏf′thăl-mŏp′ă-thĭ) ["+ *pathos,* disease]. Any eye disease.

ophthalmophlebotomy (ŏf-thăl″mō-flē-bŏt′ō-mĭ) ["+ *phleps, phleb-,* vein, + *tomē,* incision]. Incision of the eye to overcome congestion of conjunctival veins.

ophthalmophthisis (ŏf′thăl-mŏf′thĭ-sĭs) [Gr. *ophthalmos,* eye, + *phthisis,* wasting]. Ophthalmomalacia, q.v.

ophthalmoplasty (ŏf-thăl′mō-plăs″tĭ) ["+ *plassein,* to form]. Ocular plastic surgery.

ophthalmoplegia (ŏf-thăl″mō-plē′jĭ-ă) ["+ *plēgē,* stroke]. Paralysis of ocular muscles.

　　o. externa. Paralysis of extraocular muscles.

　　o. interna. Paralysis of iris and ciliary muscle.

　　o., nuclear. O. due to lesion of nuclei of origin of the ocular motor nerves.

　　o. partialis. Incomplete paralysis, involving only one or two of the ocular muscles.

　　o. progressiva. Form in which all muscles become involved slowly, caused by deterioration of the motor nerve nuclei.

　　o. totalis. Paralysis that affects both internal and external ocular muscles.

ophthalmoptosis (ŏf-thăl″mŏp-tō′sĭs) [Gr. *ophthalmos,* eye, + *ptōsis,* fall]. Protrusion of the eyeball. SYN: *exophthalmos.*

ophthalmoreaction (ŏf-thăl″mō-rē-ăk′shŭn) ["+ L. *rē,* back, + *actus,* acted]. Reaction of the conjunctiva following instillation of a drop of tuberculin or typhoid fever toxin into the eye of persons suffering from tuberculosis or typhoid diseases. Of diagnostic value. SYN: *Calmette's reaction; oculoreaction; ophthalmic reaction.*

ophthalmorrhagia (ŏf-thăl-mō-rā′jĭ-ă) [Gr. *opthalmos,* eye, + *rhegnynai,* to burst forth]. Ocular hemorrhage.

ophthalmorrhea (ŏf-thăl-mō-rē′ă) [Gr. *ophthalmos,* eye, + *rhoia,* flow]. Discharge from the eye.

ophthalmorrhexis (ŏf-thăl-mō-rĕk'sĭs) ["+ *rhēxis*, rupture]. Rupture of an eyeball.

ophthalmoscope (ŏf-thăl'mō-skōp) ["+ *skopein*, to examine]. Instrument for examining interior of the eye.

ophthalmoscopy (ŏf-thăl-mŏs'kō-pĭ). The examination of the interior of the eye.

   o., direct. Examination in which image in interior of eye is upright.

   o., indirect. Examination in which image in interior of eye is inverted.

ophthalmospasm (ŏf-thăl'mō-spăsm). Spasm of ocular muscles.

ophthalmostat (ŏf-thăl'mō-stăt) [Gr. *ophthalmos*, eye, + *statos*, made to stand]. Instrument used to hold the eye still during an operation.

ophthalmostatometer (ŏf-thăl''mō-stăt-om'ĕt-ĕr) ["+ "+ *metron*, measure]. Instrument for ascertaining position of eyes.

ophthalmosynchysis (ŏf-thăl''mō-sĭn'kĭ-sĭs) ["+ *synchisis*, a mixing]. Effusion into one of the cavities of the eye.

ophthalmothermometer (ŏf-thăl''mō-thĕr-mom'ĕt-ĕr). Instrument for determining local temperature in eye diseases.

ophthalmotonometer (ŏf-thăl''mō-tō-nŏm'ĕt-ĕr) ["+ *tonos*, tension, + *metron*, measure]. Instrument for determining tension within globe of eye.

ophthalmotoxin (ŏf-thăl''mō-tok'sĭn) [Gr. *ophthalmos*, eye, + *toxikon*, poison]. Cytotoxin derived on injection of emulsions of the ciliary body.

ophthalmotrope (ŏf-thăl'mō-trōp) ["+ *tropē*, a turning]. Instrument or model of the eye used to demonstrate the movements of the extraocular muscles.

ophthalmotropometer (ŏf-thăl''mō-trō-pŏm'ĕt-ĕr) ["+ "+ *metron*, measure]. Instrument for measuring the eye movements.

ophthalmovascular (ŏf-thăl''mō-văs'kū-lar). Pert. to blood vessels of eye.

ophthalmoxyster (of-thal''mŏks-is'ter) ["+ *xystēr*, scraper]. Instrument used to scrape the conjunctiva.

opiate (ō'pĭ-āt). 1. A drug derived from opium. 2. A drug that induces sleep. 3. To deaden, to put to sleep.

The principal opiates are opium and its derivatives, such as morphine. They are all habit-forming.

   o. abstinence syndrome. Symptoms induced by withdrawal of opiate from an addict. In a mild addict, they are restlessness, depression, and mild disturbances in functioning of autonomic nervous system. In a strong addict, an acute illness develops, lasting several days. Emotional reactions may be pronounced.

opiomania (ō''pĭ-ō-mā'nĭ-ă). Insane craving for opium or its derivatives.

opiophagism (ō-pĭ-ŏf'ă-jizm). Addiction to the use of opium, esp. the eating of it.

opisthenar (ō-pĭs'the-när) [Gr. *opisthen*, behind, + *thenar*, palm]. Back of the hand.

opisthion (ō-pĭs'thĭ-ŏn) [Gr., rear]. Craniometric point at middle of lower border of foramen magnum.

opistho-, opisth- [Gr. *opisthen*]. Combining form meaning backward or indicating relationship to the back.

opisthognathism (ō''pĭs-thō'nă-thizm) ["+ *gnathos*, jaw, + *ismos*, state of]. Skull abnormality marked by a receding lower jaw.

opisthoporeia (ō-pĭs''thō-pō-rē'ä) ["+ *poreia*, walk]. Involuntary walking backward due to loss of motor control.

opisthorchiasis (ō''pĭs-thor-kī'ă-sĭs). Infestation of the liver by flukes of the genus Opisthorchis.

Opisthorchis (ō''pĭs-thor'kĭs) [Gr. *opisthen*, behind, + *orchis*, testicle]. A genus of parasitic flukes characterized by having testicles near the posterior end of the tapered body.

   O. felineus. A species of liver flukes in dogs, cats, foxes. Occasionally infest man through raw or partially cooked fish.

   O. sinensis. A common liver fluke in man, esp. in the Far East, through eating inadequately cooked fish. SYN: *Clonorchis sinensis.*

opisthotic (ō''pĭs-thŏt'ĭk) [Gr. *opisthen*, behind, + *ous, ot-*, ear]. Located behind the ear or in the interior ear.

opisthotonos (ō''pĭs-thŏt'ō-nŏs) ["+ *tonos*, tension]. An arched position of the body with feet and head on the floor caused by a tetanic spasm. Seen in severe cases of

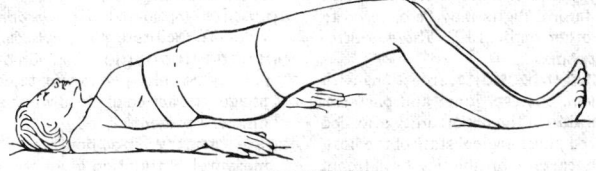

OPISTHOTONOS

meningitis and tetanus. SEE: *empros-thotonos; pleurothotonos; posture.*

opium (ō′pĭ-ŭm). USP. The substance obtained by air drying the juice from the unripe capsule of the poppy, Papaver somniferum. It has a number of important alkaloids such as morphine, codeine, heroin, and papaverine.

ACTION: Opium is a narcotic, soporific, and astringent. In therapeutic doses, it relieves pain and discomfort and induces a deep sleep.

USES: (1) As a sedative. (2) Given to suppress ineffective coughing, it diminishes secretions of the bronchial tubes and relieves spasm. Caution indicated because it is a respiratory depressant. (3) A heart depressant, but it is administered in some heart cases to produce sleep and so improve condition of heart by relieving anxiety and permitting sleep. It slows the pulse. (4) Sedative to the nervous system; promotes rest and sleep by relieving excitability and fear. It relieves pain. (5) Inhibits all secretions of the body except perspiration which it increases. It also contracts the pupils, even in small doses.

POISONING: SEE: *morphine* in *Table of Poisons and Poisoning* in *Appendix.*

opiumism (ō′pĭ-ŭm-ĭzm). 1. Opium habit; addiction to use of opium. 2. Physical condition resulting from overuse of opium.

opo- [Gr. *opos,* juice]. Prefix meaning derived from juice; used in trade names of some organic extracts.

Oppenheim's disease (ŏp′ĕn-hīm). [Hermann Oppenheim, Ger. neurologist, 1858-1919]. A noninherited but sometimes familial disease, characterized by absence of muscular development with the lower extremities being the first involved. It is first seen at, or shortly after, birth. SYN: *amyotonia congenita.*

oppilation (ŏp′ĭ-lā′shŭn) [L. *oppilatio*]. 1. An obstruction. 2. Act or state of being obstructed. 3. Constipation.

oppilative (ŏp′ĭ-lā′tĭv) [L. *oppilare,* to stop up]. 1. Closing the pores. 2. Constipating. 3. Obstructive. 4. A constipating agent.

opponens (ō′pō′nĕns) [L.]. Opposing, a term applied to muscles of hand or foot by which one of the lateral digits may be opposed to one of the other digits. SEE: *Table of Muscles* in *Appendix.*

opportunistic infections. Infections with any organism, but esp. fungi and bacteria, which occur due to the opportunity afforded by the altered physiological state of the host. Thus when certain antibiotics or adrenal cortical steroids are given for long periods,

certain microorganisms which would otherwise be nonpathogenic become pathogenic.

opsialgia (ŏp″sē-al′jĭ-ā) [Gr. *ōps,* face, + *algos,* pain]. Neuralgic pain of the face.

opsinogenous (ŏp″sĭn-ŏj′ĕn-ŭs) [″+ *gennan,* to produce]. Capable of forming opsonins.

opsiometer (ŏp-sĭ-ŏm′ĕt-ĕr) [Gr. *opsis,* vision, + *metron,* measure]. Apparatus for measuring refractive power of the eye. SYN: *optometer.*

opsionosis (ŏp″sĭ-ō-nō′sĭs). A disease or disorder of the eye or vision.

opsiuria (ŏp-sĭ-ū′rĭ-ā) [Gr. *opse,* late, + *ouron,* urine]. Condition in which excretion of urine is more rapid during fasting than after a meal.

opsoclonus. Irregular and nonrhythmical jerking movements of the eyes. Seen in comatose patients with lesions of the brain stem. SYN: *opsoclonia.*

opsomania (ŏp″sō-mā′nĭ-ā) [Gr. *opson,* food, + *mania,* madness]. Craving for some special article of food.

opsonic (ŏp-sŏn′ĭk) [Gr. *opsōnein,* to prepare food for]. Pert. to opsonins or their use in therapy.

    o. index. A measure of the resistance of a patient to bacterial invasion. Determined by the ratio between the number of bacteria destroyed and ingested by the leukocytes in normal blood serum, as compared with the number ingested by leukocytes under the influence of the patient's own serum.

    A special technique is followed. The white corpuscles are fixed, stained, and examined under the microscope. The number of bacteria in 100 leukocytes are counted. The total is then divided by 100, showing the patient's phagocytic index. This is divided by average from normal blood serum and result is the opsonic index.

opsonification (ŏp-sŏn″ĭ-fĭ-kā′shŭn). Effect of opsonins in rendering cells or bacteria phagocytized more readily.

opsonin (ŏp-sō′nĭn) [Gr. *opsōnein,* to provide]. Substance in blood serum which acts upon microorganisms and other cells, facilitating phagocytosis.

opsonization (ŏp″sō-nī-zā′shun). Action of opsonins to facilitate phagocytosis. SYN: *opsonification.*

opsonize (ŏp′sō-nīz) [Gr. *opsōnein,* to provide]. To facilitate phagocytosis.

opsonocytophagic (op″sŏn-ō-sī″tō-fā′jĭk) [″+ *kytos,* cell, + *phagein,* to eat]. Pert. to phagocytic action of blood when serum opsonins are present.

opsonometry (ŏp-sō-nŏm′ĕt-rĭ) [″+ *metron,* measure]. Estimation of amt. of opsonins in the blood serum. SEE: *opsonic index.*

opsonophilia (ŏp″sō-nō-fĭl′ĭ-ă) ["+ *philein*, to love]. Attraction for opsonins.

opsonophil′ic. Attractive to opsonins.

opsonotherapy (ŏp″sō-nō-thĕr′ă-pĭ). Treatment by stimulation of a specific opsonin with bacterial vaccines. SYN: *vaccine therapy.*

Optacon. Proprietary name of a portable electronic reading assistance device for use by the blind. It translates printed material to patterns of raised pins under the user's finger.

optesthesia (ŏp″tĕs-thē′zĭ-ă) [Gr. *optikos*, optical, + *aisthēsis*, sensation]. Visual sensibility; perception of visual stimuli.

optic (ŏp′tik) [Gr. *optikos*]. Pert. to the eye or the sight.

    o. chiasm, o. commissure. An x-shaped crossing of the optic nerve fibers in the brain. Past this point the fibers travel in optic tracts. Fibers which originated in the outer half of the retina end up on the same side of the brain, those from the inner half cross over.

    o. disk. Area in retina for entrance of optic nerve; the blind spot.

    o. foramen. Groove for optic nerve and ophthalmic artery at the orbit's apex.

    o. nerve. Second cranial n. FUNCT: Special sense of sight. ORIG: Lateral geniculate body of thalamus via optic tract and optic chiasma. DIST: Retina. SEE: *Table of Cranial Nerves* in *Appendix.*

    o. papilla. SEE: *optic disk.*

    o. tract. Fibers of optic nerve which continue beyond optic chiasma, most of which terminate in lateral geniculate body of thalamus. Some continue to superior colliculus of midbrain, others enter hypothalamus and terminate in supraoptic and medial nuclei.

optical (ŏp′tĭ-kăl) [L. *opticus;* Gr. *optikos*]. Pert. to vision, the eye, or optics.

    o. activity. In chemistry, the property of rotating the plane of polarized light. Measurement of this property is called polarimetry, and is useful in the determination of optically active substances like dextrose. Particularly the sugars are classified according to this criterion. Optical activity in a substance can be detected by placing it between polarizing and analyzing prisms.

optician (ŏp-tĭsh′ăn). 1. One who makes optical apparatus. 2. One skilled in the grinding of lenses and fitting glasses.

    o., dispensing. One who deals in ophthalmic lenses.

optico- [Gr. *optikos*]. Combining form indicating relationship to the eye or vision.

opticociliary (ŏp″tĭ-kō-sĭl′ĭ-ăr-ĭ) ["+ L. *ciliaris*, pert. to eyelash]. Concerning the optic and ciliary nerves.

opticonasion (op″tĭ-ko-na′sĭ-on). Length of an imaginary line drawn from the posterior edge of the optic foramen to the nasion.

opticopupillary (ŏp″tĭ-kō-pū′pĭl-ĕr-ĭ) ["+ L. *pupilla*, pupil]. Concerning optic nerve and the pupil.

optics (ŏp′tĭks) [Gr. *optikos*, pert. to vision]. The science dealing with light and its relationship to vision.

optimum (ŏp′tĭm-ŭm) [L. *optimus*, best]. (pl. *optima*) (adj. *optimal*) The condition which is most conducive to a function or functions such as growth and development.

    o. temperature. That temperature which is most suitable for an operation, esp. the development of bacterial cultures.

opto- [Gr. *optos*, seen]. Combining form meaning vision or eye.

optogram (ŏp′tō-grăm) [Gr. *optos*, seen, + *gramma*, mark]. Image of ext. object fixed on the retina by photochemical bleaching action of light on the visual purple.

optometer (ŏp-tŏm′ĕt-ĕr) ["+ *metron*, measure]. Instrument for measurement of the eye's refractive power. SYN: *opsiometer.*

optometrist (ŏp-tŏm′ĕ-trĭst). A person specifically trained and licensed to examine the eyes in order to determine the presence of vision problems and to prescribe and adapt lenses to preserve or restore maximum efficiency of vision. The optometrist's professional degree is Doctor of Optometry (O.D.).

optometry (ŏp-tom′ĕt-rĭ). Measurement of the visual refractive power; correction of visual defects with eyeglasses.

optomyometer (ŏp″tō-mī-ŏm′ĕt-ĕr) [Gr. *optos*, seen, + *mys, my-*, muscle, + *metron*, a measure]. Instrument for determining strength of the muscles of the eye.

optophone (ŏp′tō-fōn) ["+ *phōnē*, voice]. Instrument converting light energy into sound waves. Used by the blind.

optostriate (ŏp-tō-strī′āt) ["+ L. *striatus*, grooved]. Concerning the optic thalamus and the corpus striatum.

OR. Abbr. for *operating room.*

ora (ō′ra) [L.]. 1. Pl. of **os**, mouth, opening. 2. (pl. *orae*). A border or margin.

    o. serrata retinae. [NA] Notched anterior edge of sensory portion of retina.

orad (ō′răd) [L. *os, oris*, mouth, + *ad*, toward]. Toward the mouth or oral region.

oral (or′ăl) [L. *oralis*]. Concerning the mouth.

orale (ō-rā′lĕ). Point on hard palate in midsagittal plane where lines drawn tangent to

lingual margins of alveoli of medial incisor teeth intersect.

oralogy (ō-răl'ō-jĭ) [L. *oralis*, mouth, + Gr. *logos*, study of]. 1. The science of dental and medical hygiene. 2. Study of diseases of the mouth.

orange (ŏr'ĕnj) [Persian *nārang*, orange]. Fruit of a tropical tree. Contains citric acid, sugar, and considerable cellulose.

Food value of 100 gm. (raw): Cal. 49; protein 1.0 gm.; fat 0.2 gm.; carbohydrate 12.2 gm.; calcium 41 mg.; vitamin A, 200 I.U.; ascorbic acid 115 mg.

100 gm. (fresh juice): Cal. 45; protein 0.7 gm.; carbohydrate 10.4 gm.; calcium 11 mg.; vitamin A, 200 I.U.; ascorbic acid 50 mg.

orb [L. *orbis*, circle, disk]. A spherical body, esp. the eyeball.

orbicular (ŏr-bĭk'ū-lăr) [L. *orbiculus*, a small circle]. Circular.

    o. bone. Ossicle frequently becoming attached to the incus. SYN: *orbiculare*. SEE: *o. process*, *orbiculare*.

    o. muscle. Muscle encircling an opening.

    o. process. End of long process of the incus. SYN: *lenticular process.*

orbiculare (or-bĭk"ū-lā'rē). Orbicular bone; ear ossicle that frequently becomes attached to the incus at the end of its long process.

orbicularis (ŏr"bĭk-ū-la'rĭs) [L. *orbiculus*, little circle]. Muscle surrounding an orifice; a sphincter muscle.

    o. ciliaris. The ciliary muscles of the eye. SYN: *ciliary ring.*

    o. oculi. Muscle encircling the opening of orbit of the eye.

    o. oris. Circular muscle surrounding the mouth.

    o. palpebrarum. SEE: *o. oculi.*

orbit (or'bĭt) [L. *orbita*, track]. The bony pyramid-shaped cavity of the skull which holds the eyeball. It is pierced posteriorly by the optic foramen, which transmits the optic nerve and ophthalmic artery, the superior and inferior orbital fissures, and several foramina.

It is formed by the frontal, malar, ethmoid, maxillary, lacrimal, sphenoid, and palatine bones.

orbita (or'bĭ-tă) [L.]. (pl. *orbitae*) [NA]. Latin term for orbit.

orbital (or'bĭ-tăl) [L. *orbitalis*]. Concerning the orbit.

orbitotomy (or-bĭ-tŏt'ō-mĭ) ["+ Gr. *tome*, incision]. Surgical incision into the orbit.

orchectomy (ŏr-kĕk'tō-mĭ) [Gr. *orchis*, testicle, + *ektome*, excision]. Surgical removal of a testicle. DRESSINGS: Small drainage tube

and sterile gauze. SYN: *orchidectomy*; *orchiectomy.*

orcheoplasty (or'kē-ō-plăs"tĭ) ["+ *plassein*, to form]. Plastic repair work of the testicle.

orchialgia (or-kĭ-ăl'jĭ-ă) ["+ *algos*, pain]. Pain in the testes. SYN: *orchiodynia*, *orchioneuralgia.*

orchichorea (or"kĭ-kō-rē'ă) ["+ *choreia*, a dance]. Involuntary jerking movements of the testicles.

orchidalgia (or-kĭ-dal'jĭ-ă) [Gr. *orchis*, *orchid-*, testicle, + *algos*, pain]. Neuralgia in the testicles. SYN: *orchialgia.*

orchidectomy (or"kĭ-dek'tō-mĭ) ["+ *ektome*, excision]. Removal of a testicle surgically. SYN: *orchectomy*; *orchiectomy.*

orchidic (or-kĭd'ĭk). Concerning or rel. to the testes.

orchido- [Gr. *orchidion*]. Combining form indicating relationship to the testicle SEE: words beginning with *orchio-*.

orchidoncus (or-kĭ-dong'kŭs) [Gr. *orchis*, testicle, + *onkos*, mass]. A neoplasm of the testicle. SYN: *orchioncus.*

orchidopexy (or'kĭd-ō-pĕk"sĭ) ["+ *pexis*, fixation]. Surgical transfer of an imperfectly descended testicle into the scrotum and suturing it there. SYN: *orchiopexy.*

orchidoplasty (or'kĭd-ō-plăs"tĭ) ["+ *plassein*, to form]. Operative transfer of an undescended testicle to the scrotum.

orchidoptosis (or"kĭd-ŏp-tō'sĭs) ["+ *ptosis*, a falling]. Dropping of the testicle.

orchidotomy (or-kĭd-ŏt'ō-mĭ) [Gr. *orchis*, *orchid-*, testicle, + *tome*, incision]. Incision into the testes.

orchiectomy (or"kĭ-ĕk'tō-mĭ) ["+ *ektome*, excision]. Surgical excision of a testicle. SYN: *orchectomy*; *orchidectomy*. SEE: *castration.*

orchiencephaloma (or"kĭ-ĕn-sĕf-ă-lō'mă) ["+ *enkephalos*, brain, + *-oma*, tumor]. Tumor of brainlike substance in the testicle. SEE: *orchiomyeloma.*

orchiepididymitis (or"kĭ-ep"ĭ-dĭd'ĭ-mi'tĭs) ["+ *epi*, upon, + *didymos*, testis, + *-itis*, inflammation]. Inflamed condition of a testicle and epididymis.

orchiocele (or'kĭ-ō-sēl) ["+ *kele*, hernia]. 1. Scrotal hernia. SYN: *orchidocele*. 2. A tumor of the testicle.

orchiodynia (ŏr"kĭ-ō-din'ĭ-ă) ["+ *odyne*, pain]. Testicular pain. SYN: *orchialgia*; *orchidalgia.*

orchiomyeloma (or"kĭ-ō-mĭ"ē-lō'mă) [Gr. *orchis*, testicle, + *myelos*, marrow, + *-oma*, tumor]. Tumor of the testicle composed of marrowlike cells.

orchioncus (ŏr″kĭ-ong′kŭs) ["+ *onkos*, tumor]. Neoplasm of the testicle. SYN: *orchidoncus.*

orchioneuralgia (or″kĭ-ō-nū-răl′jĭ-ă) ["+ *neuron*, sinew, + *algos*, pain]. Neuralgia of the testicles. SYN: *orchialgia.*

orchiopathy (ŏr″kĭ-op′ăth-ī) ["+ *pathos*, disease]. Any diseased condition of the testes.

orchiopexy (or″kĭ-ō-pek′sĭ) [Gr. *orchis*, testicle, + *pēxis*, fixation]. The suturing of an undescended testicle in the scrotum. SYN: *orchidopexy; orchiorrhaphy.*

orchioplasty (or′kĭ-ō-plas″tĭ) ["+ *plassein*, to form]. Plastic repair of the testicle.

orchiorrhaphy (ŏr″kĭ-or′ră-fĭ) ["+ *rhaphē*, suture]. The suturing of an undescended testicle to surrounding tissue in the scrotum. SYN: *orchidopexy; orchiopexy.*

orchioscheocele (or″kĭ-ō-ske′ō-sēl) ["+ *oscheon*, scrotum, + *kēlē*, hernia]. Scrotal hernia with enlargement or tumor of testicle.

orchioscirrhus (or″kĭ-ō-skĭr′rŭs) [Gr. *orchis*, testicle, + *skirros*, hard]. Testicular hardening due to tumor formation.

orchis (ōr′kĭs) [Gr.]. A testicle.

orchitic (or-kĭt′ĭk) [Gr. *orchis*, testicle, + *-itis*, inflammation]. Concerning or caused by orchitis.

orchitis (ŏr-kī′tĭs) [Gr. *orchis*, testicle, + *-itis*, inflammation]. Inflammation of a testis due to trauma, metastasis, mumps, or infection elsewhere in the body.

   SYM: Swelling, severe pain, possibly gangrene, chills, fever, vomiting, hiccough, delirium. May end in atrophy of organ.

   TREATMENT: In mumps, confine patient to bed first 8 days, immobilize organ, and use ice bag.

   o., gonorrheal. O. due to gonococcus.

   o., metastatic. O. due to infection from organisms in blood stream.

   o., syphilitic. SYM: Usually begins painlessly in body of gland but apt to be bilateral; causes dense, irregular, knotty induration but not much increase in size.

   o., tuberculous. Form generally arising in the epididymis. It may be accompanied by formation of chronic sinuses, and destruction of tissues.

   SYM: Little or no pain. Begins as hard, irregular enlargement at lower and posterior aspect of gland, gradually increases, and sometimes extends along vas deferens. Later whole gland undergoes caseous degeneration.

orchitolytic (or″kĭt-ō-lĭt′ĭk) ["+ *lysis*, destruction]. Destructive to testicular tissue.

orchotomy (ŏr-kŏt′ō-mĭ) ["+ *tomē*, incision]. Incision, but not excision, of a testicle.

orcin, orcinol (or′sĭn, -ol). A white, crystalline substance derived from lichens and used as an external treatment of skin disorders.

order [L. *ordo*, a row, series]. In biological classification, the main division under class and superior to family.

orderly (or′dĕr-lĭ). Male attendant in a hospital who does general work to assist nurses. Responsible for lifting patients, transporting patients, and preparing male patients for surgery (shaving, catheterizing, etc.).

ordure (or′dūr). Feces or other excrement.

orexigenic (ō-rĕk-sī-jĕn′ĭk) [Gr. *orexis*, appetite, + *gennan*, to produce]. Stimulating the appetite.

oreximania (ō-rĕk-sī-mā′nĭ-ă) ["+ *mania*, madness]. Abnormal desire for food because of fear of becoming thin.

orf. A contagious pustular dermatitis mainly affecting lambs and occurring in the spring. The disease rarely occurs in humans. When it does it usually is confined to a single pustular lesion on a finger, which encrusts and finally heals.

   ETIOL: Orf virus which is related to the vaccinia-variola subgroup of pox viruses.

   SYN: *contagious pustular dermatitis; ecthyma contagiosum.*

organ (or′găn) [Gr. *organon;* L. *organum*]. A part of the body having a special function. Most organs are in pairs. Any one organ may be extirpated and the remaining one will perform all necessary functions peculiar to it. Even half of the brain may be removed without being fatal. From one-third to two-fifths of some organs may be removed without interference with their functions.

   o., accessory. One having a subordinate function.

   o., acoustic. O. of Corti, q.v.

   o. of Corti. Terminal acoustic apparatus in the cochlea. SEE: *Claudius' cells; ear.*

   o., enamel. A knoblike thickening which develops on dental lamina, giving rise to a double-walled, cup-shaped organ that encloses the dental papilla. It functions in the shaping of the tooth and the formation of enamel.

   o., end. The specialized termination of a sensory nerve fiber which serves as a receptor. May be nonencapsulated or encapsulated.

   o., endocrine. An organ yielding internal secretions. SEE: *endocrine.*

   o., excretory. An organ which is concerned with the excretion of waste products from the body.

   o.'s of generation. The reproductive

Size, Weight, and Capacity of Various Organs
and Parts of the Body ♂ male ♀ female*

Description	Size	Weight	Capacity
Adrenal gland	3 to 5 cm. long, 4 to 6 cm. thick	3.5 to 5.0 gm.	
Bladder	12 cm. in diameter		500 ml. (when moderately full)
Blood volume			♂ 4200 ml. ♀ 5000 ml.
Brain		♂ 1430 gm. ♀ 1294 gm.	
Esophagus	23 to 25 cm.		
Fallopian tube	10 cm.		
Gallbladder	7 to 10 cm. long 2.5 cm. wide		30 to 35 ml.
Heart	12 x 8 to 9 x 6.0 cm.	♂ 280 to 340 gm. ♀ 230 to 280 gm.	
Intestines—small	Quite variable 472 to 970 cm. long		
Intestines—large	150 cm. long		
Intestines—vermiform appendix	2 to 20 cm. long Average 8.3 cm.		
Intestines—rectum	12 cm. long		
Kidney	11.25 cm. long, 5 to 7.5 cm. broad, 2.5 cm. thick	♂ 125 to 170 gm. ♀ 115 to 155 gm.	
Liver		♂ 1400 to 1600 gm. ♀ 1200 to 1400 gm.	
Lung		Rt. 625 gm. Lt. 567 gm.	6500 ml.
Ovaries	4 x 2 x 0.8 cm.	2 to 3.5 gm.	
Pancreas	12.5 to 15 cm. long	♂ 74 to 106 gm. ♀ 70 to 100 gm.	
Pharynx	12.5 cm. long		
Prostate	2 x 4 x 3 cm.	20 gm.	
Skeleton		Average adult male, 4957 gm.	
Skull		Average (without teeth), 642 gm.	
Spinal cord	42 to 45 cm. long	30 gm.	
Spleen	12 x 7 x 3 to 4 cm.	100 to 250 gm. Decreases with age	
Stomach	Quite variable 25 cm. long, 10 cm. wide		Quite variable 1000 ml.

* Gray's Anatomy, ed. 27. Lea & Febiger, Philadelphia, 1959; Growth Federation of American Societies for Experimental Biology, Washington, D.C., 1962.

Size, Weight, and Capacity of Various Organs and Parts of the Body ♂ male ♀ female* (Continued)

Description	Size	Weight	Capacity
Testes	4 to 5 x 2.5 x 3.0 cm.	10.5 to 14 gm.	
Thoracic duct	38 to 45 cm. long		
Thymus		Newborn, 10.9 gm. 10–15 yrs., 29.5 gm. 20–25 yrs.. 18.6 gm.	
Thyroid	Each lobe 5 x 3 x 2 cm.	30 gm. total	
Trachea	11 cm. long, 2 to 2.5 cm. in diameter		
Ureter	28 to 34 cm. long		
Urethra	♂ 17.5 to 20 cm. long ♀ 4 cm. long		
Uterus	7.5 x 5.0 x 2.5 cm.	30 to 40 gm. (nonpregnant)	

organs, external and internal. SEE: *genitalia, male and female.*

o. of Giraldès. A small body on the spermatic cord, above the epididymis. SYN: *paradidymis.*

o., Golgi's. A spindle shaped structure at junction of a muscle and tendon. Functions as a receptor for proprioceptive sense. SYN: *neurotendinous spindle; Golgi's corpuscle.*

o., gustatory. The organ controlling the sense of taste; a taste bud. SYN: *organum gustus* [NA].

o. of Jacobson. A blind tubular sac which develops in medial wall of nasal cavity; becomes a functional olfactory organ in lower animals but degenerates or remains rudimentary in man. SYN: *vomeronasal o.*

o., reproductive. Any organ concerned with the production of offspring. Includes the primary organs (testes and ovaries) and accessory structures (penis and spermatic cord in the male and fallopian tubes, uterus, and vagina in the female).

o. of Ruffini. Sensory receptor of warmth located principally at tips of fingers. SYN: *corpuscle of Ruffini.*

o., sense. A sensory receptor. A structure consisting of specialized sensory nerve endings which are capable of reacting to a stimulus (an environmental change) by giving rise to nerve impulses which pass through afferent nerves to the central nervous system. These impulses may give rise to sensations or reflexly bring about responses in the body. SYN: *organa sensuum* [NA].

o., sex. A reproductive organ, q.v.

o., special sense. The organs of smell, taste, sight, and hearing.

o., vomeronasal. O. of Jacobson, q.v.

o., Weber's. Residual prostatic pouch in the male, the remains of the müllerian ducts.

o.'s of Zuckerkandl. A pair of o's, appearing in the embryo and persisting until shortly after birth. Located under anterior surface of abdominal aorta.

organelle (or″găn-ĕl′). A specialized part of a cell which performs a definite function. Ex: mitochondria, Golgi apparatus, endoplasmic reticulum, lysosomes, and cell centriole.

organic (or-găn′ĭk) [Gr. *organikos*]. 1. Pert. to an organ or organs. 2. Structural. 3. Pert. to or derived from animal or vegetable forms of life.

o. acid. Any acid containing one or more -COOH or carboxyl groups. Ex: acetic, formic, lactic, and all fatty acids.

o. chemistry. Branch of c. dealing with substances containing carbon compounds.

o. disease. A disease associated with observable or detectable changes in the organs or tissues of the body.

o. psychoses. A general term applied to those psychoses induced by structural brain changes. In general, a character change is manifested in behavior and disposition. The patient is less stable than before; emotional instability, irritability and anger outbursts being frequent. His attention fluctuates widely; gradually he deteriorates; early or later, memory, comprehension, ideation, and orientation become defective.

ETIOL: Alcohol, narcotics, trauma, syphilis, drugs, poisons, chronic infections, encephalitis, and brain tumors among many others.

organism (or'găn-ĭzm) [Gr. *organon,* organ, + *ismos,* condition]. Any living thing, plant, or animal. May be unicellular (bacteria, yeasts, protozoa) or multicellular (all complex organisms including man).

organization (or''găn-ĭ-zā'shŭn). 1. Process of becoming organized. 2. Systematic arrangement. 3. That which is organized; an organism.

o. center. 1. A group of cells in an embryo which induces the development of another structure. 2. A region in an ovum which is responsible for the mode of development of the fertilized ovum.

organize (or'găn-īz). To develop from an amorphous state to that having structure and form.

organogenesis, organogeny (or-găn-ō-jen'-ĕ-sĭs, -oj'ĕn-ĭ) [Gr. *organon,* organ, + *genesis,* production]. The formation and development of body organs from embryonic tissues.

organography (or-găn-ŏg'ră-fĭ) [" + *graphein,* to write]. The description of the body organs.

organoid [" + *eidos,* form]. 1. Resembling an organ. 2. An organelle, q.v.

organoleptic (or-găn-ō-lep'tĭk) [Gr. *organon,* organ, + *lepsis,* a seizure]. 1. Affecting an organ, esp. the organs of special sense. 2. Susceptible to sensory impressions.

o. test. Subjective test (taste, odor, consistency) of drugs, foods, and beverages.

organology (or-gă-nŏl'ō-jĭ) [" + *logos,* study]. The science dealing with the body organs.

organon (or'gă-nŏn) [Gr.]. (pl. *or'gana*) Organum, q.v.

organopexy (or'găn-ō-pĕk''sĭ) [Gr. *organon,* organ, + *pēxis,* fixation]. Surgical fixation of an organ that is detached from its proper position.

organoscopy (or-gă-nos'kō-pĭ) [" + *skopein,* to examine]. Examination of abdominal organs of the body by means of an endoscope.

organotherapy (or''găn-ō-thĕr'ă-pĭ) [Gr. *organo,* organ, + *therapeia,* treatment]. The treatment of disease by preparations of the endocrine glands of animals or by extracts made from the same.

organotrope, organotropic (or-găn'ō-trōp, -trŏp'ĭk) [" + *tropos,* turning]. Having affinity for tissues or certain organs.

organ perfusion system. A mechanical device equipped to supply metabolic, oxygen, and electrolyte needs in order to keep viable for transplantation an organ obtained from a cadaver or donor.

The organ and the perfusion solution pumped through it can be kept at the ideal temperature for organ survival. Together they can be transported by any means required to deliver the organ to the patient.

or'ganum [L.]. (pl. *organa*) [NA]. An organ.

o. auditus. O. vestibulocochleare, q.v.

o. gustus. [NA]. Organ of taste.

o. olfactus. [NA]. Organ of smell; olfactory region in the nasal cavity.

o. spirale. [NA]. Spiral organ in the cochlea. SYN: *o. of Corti.*

o. vestibulocochleare. [NA] Organ of hearing. SEE: *ear.*

o. visus. [NA]. The organ of sight; the eye and its adnexa.

o. vomeronasale. [NA] Canal opening into nasal septum. SYN: *organ of Jacobson,* q.v.

orgasm (or'găzm) [Gr. *orgasmos,* swelling, lustful]. A state of paroxysmal emotional excitement, esp. that which occurs at the climax of sexual intercourse. In the male it is accompanied by the ejaculation of semen.

orgastic. Concerning or related to sexual orgasm. SYN: *orgasmic.*

orien'tal sore. An ulcerating, chronic, nodular skin lesion prevalent in the Orient and tropics, due to infection with Leishmania tropica. SYN: *cutaneous leishmaniasis; Aleppo boil; Delhi boil.*

orientation (or''ĭ-ĕn-tā'shŭn) [L. *oriens,* to arise]. Ability to comprehend and to adjust one's self in an environment with regard to time, location, and identity of persons. Partially or completely absent in some psychoses.

orifice (or'ĭ-fĭs) [L. *orificium*]. Mouth, entrance, or outlet to any aperture.

o., anal. The anus.

o., atrioventricular. The opening between the atrium and the ventricle on each side of the heart.

o., auriculoventricular. The atrioventricular orifice, q.v.

o., cardiac. Opening of esophagus into stomach.

o., mitral. Opening between atrium and ventricle.

o., pyloric. Opening from stomach into the duodenum. SEE: *pylorus.*

o., ureteric. Opening of ureter into bladder.

o., urethral, external. Exterior opening of the urethra. In male, located at tip of glans penis; in female, located anterior and cephalad to vaginal opening.

o., urethral, internal. Opening from which urethra makes its exit from bladder.

orificial (or-ĭ-fĭ'shăl) [L. *orificium,* outlet]. Pert. to or forming an orifice.

origin (or'ĭ-jĭn) [L. *origo,* beginning]. 1. The source of anything; a starting point. 2. The beginning of a nerve. 3. The more fixed attachment of a muscle.

o., deep, ental. The region within the brain where the fibers comprising a cranial nerve terminate.

o., superficial, ectal. Point where a cranial nerve makes its exit from the brain.

orinase (or'ĭ-nās). Proprietary brand of tolbutamide (1-butyl-3-[p-tolysulfonyl]urea). An antidiabetes agent used in treatment of diabetes mellitus. Administered orally.

Ornithodoros (or''nĭ-thŏd'ō-rŏs). A genus of ticks belonging to the family Argasidae, which infest mammals including man. Several species serve as transmitters of the causative agents of disease including spotted fever, tick fever, Q fever, tularemia, Russian encephalitis, and relapsing fever.

ornithosis (or''nĭ-thō'sĭs) [Gr. *ornithos,* bird, + *ōsis,* condition]. A virus disease of birds and domesticated fowls, communicated to man.

SYN: *psittacosis,* q.v.; *parrot fever.*

SYM: Headache, chills and fever, anorexia, sore throat, nausea, and vomiting.

orodiagnosis (or''ō-dī-ăg-nō'sĭs) [Gr. *oros,* serum, + *dia,* through, + *gnōsis,* knowledge]. Diagnosis by using serums or serum reactions.

orolingual (ōr''ō-ling'gwăl) [L. *os, or-,* mouth, + *lingua,* tongue]. Concerning the mouth and tongue.

oronasal (ōr''ō-nā'zăl) ["+ *nasus,* nose]. Concerning the mouth and nose.

oropharynx (ōr''ō-far'ĭnks) ["+ Gr. *pharynx,* pharynx]. Central portion of pharynx lying between the soft palate and upper portion of epiglottis.

orotherapy (ōr''ō-thĕr-ă-pĭ) [Gr. *oros,* serum, + *therapeia,* treatment]. 1. Treatment of

disease with injection of blood serum from immune persons or animals. SYN: *serotherapy.* 2. Use of whey in treatment.

oro'ya fever [Oroya, a region of Peru]. An acute infectious disease endemic in Peru and other S.A. countries. The first clinical stage of bartonellosis, q.v. SYN: *verruca peruviana; bartonellosis; Carrion's disease.*

SYM: Intermittent fever; lymphadenopathy; severe anemia; and pains in joints and long bones.

orrhology (or-ŏl'ō-jĭ) [Gr. *orrhos,* blood serum, + *logos,* study]. The study of serums and their reactions. SYN: *serology.*

orrhomeningitis (or''ō-men''ĭn-jĭ'tĭs) ["+ *mēninx,* membrane, + *-itis,* inflammation]. Inflammation of a serous membrane.

orrhoreaction (or''ō-rē-ăk'shŭn) ["+ L. *rē,* back, + *actus,* acted]. A reaction from injection of serum. SYN: *seroreaction.*

orrhorrhea (or''ō-rē'ă) [Gr. *orrhos,* blood serum, + *rhoia,* flow]. Any watery, thin, colorless discharge from a body structure. Usually it is the result of inflammation.

orrhotherapy (or''rō-thĕr'ă-pĭ) ["+ *therapeia,* treatment]. Serotherapy; therapeutic use of serums.

O.R.T. Abbr. for *operating room technician.*

ortho- [Gr. *orthos,* straight]. Combining form meaning straight, correct, normal, in proper order.

orthobiosis ["+ *bios,* life]. Right living. A term used by Metchnikoff to encompass all the factors that may affect longevity and well-being.

orthocephalic (or''thō-sē-făl'ĭk) [Gr. *orthos,* correct, + *kephalē,* head]. Having a well-proportioned head; a head with a height-length index between 70 and 75.

orthochorea (or''thō-kō-rē'ă) [Gr. *orthos,* straight, + *choreia,* dance]. A type of chorea in which attacks appear mainly when the person is in an erect position.

orthochromatic (or''thō-krō-măt'ĭk) [Gr. *orthos,* normal, + *chrōma,* color]. Having normal color or staining normally.

orthochromophil (or''thō-krō'mō-fĭl) ["+ "+ *philein,* to love]. Staining normally with neutral dyes.

orthocrasia (or''thō-krā'sĭ-ă) ["+ *krasis,* temperament]. Condition in which the body reacts normally to drugs, proteins, and treatment in general.

orthodiagraph (or''thō-dĭ'ă-grăf) ["+ *dia,* through, + *graphein,* to write]. An instrument for accurate recording of the outlines and positions of organs or foreign bodies as seen by radiographic apparatus.

or''thodig'ita ["+ L. *digitus,* finger or toe]. The division of podiatry which deals with the correction of deviated toes; the prevention and correction of deformities of the fingers or toes.

orthodontia (or″thō-dŏn′shĭ-ă) ["+ *odous, odont*-, tooth]. Division of dentistry dealing with prevention and correction of abnormally positioned or aligned teeth. Ex: malocclusion. SYN: *orthodontics.*

orthodontist. A dentist who is an expert in orthodontia, q.v.

orthogenesis (or″thō-jĕn′ĕ-sĭs) [Gr. *orthos*, straight, + *genesis*, development]. A biological principle that evolution of an animal species is in a given direction, governed by intrinsic factors and independent of external factors.

orthogenic. Pert. to, or related to, the correction, treatment, or rehabilitation of children with mental or emotional difficulties.

orthognathous (or-thŏg′nă-thŭs) ["+ *gnathos*, jaw]. Having straight jaws with a gnathic index of 97.9 or less.

orthograde (or′thō-grād) ["+ L. *gradi*, to walk]. Walking with the body vertical or upright; pert. to bipeds, esp. man. Opposed to pronograde.

orthometer (or-thŏm′ĕ-tĕr) ["+ *metron*, measure]. Device for determining the degree of protrusion or retraction of the eyeballs.

orthopedia (orthopaedia) (or″thō-pē′dĭ-ă) [Gr. *orthos*, straight, + *pais, paid*-, child]. Orthopedics, q.v.

orthopedic (orthopaedic) (or″thō-pē′dĭk). Concerning orthopedics; prevention or correction of deformities.

o. surgery. Surgical prevention and correction of deformities.

orthopedics (orthopaedics) (or″thō-pē′-dĭks) [Gr. *orthos*, straight, + *pais, paid*-, child]. Branch of medical science that deals with prevention or correction of disorders involving locomotor structures of the body, esp. the skeleton, joints, muscles, and fascia.

orthopedist (or″thō-pē′dĭst). A specialist in orthopedics.

orthopercussion (or″thō-pĕr-kŭsh′ŭn) ["+ L. *percussiō*, a striking through]. Percussion with the distal phalanx of the percussing finger held perpendicularly to the surface percussed.

orthophoria (or″thō-fō′rĭ-ă) [Gr. *orthos*, normal, + *pherein*, to bear]. Parallelism of visual axes, the normal muscle balance.

orthophrenia (or″thō-frē′nĭ-ă) ["+ *phrēn*, mind]. The normal mental state in social relations.

orthopnea (or-thŏp-nē′ă) [Gr. *orthos*, straight, + *pnoia*, breath]. Respiratory condition in which there is discomfort in breathing in any but erect sitting or standing position.

ETIOL: Seen in grave cardiac diseases, bronchial and cardiac asthma, pulmonary edema, severe emphysema, pneumonia, angina pectoris, spasmodic croup.

SYM: Respiratory rate, slow or rapid; sitting or standing posture necessary; muscles of respiration forcibly used; patient feels necessity of bracing himself in order to breathe. Anxious expression, face cyanosed. Struggle to inhale and exhale.

RS: dyspnea; hyperpnea; oligopnea; posture; respiration.

orthopraxy (or′thō-prăk-sĭ) ["+ *prassein*, to make]. Correction and prevention of deformities by mechanical means. SYN: *orthopedics.*

orthopsychiatry (or″thō-sī-kī′ă-trĭ) ["+ *psychē*, soul, + *iatreia*, treatment]. The study and treatment of borderline emotional and behavioral disorders, esp. in the young.

orthoptic (or-thŏp′tĭk) [Gr. *orthos*, straight, + *optikos*, pert. to vision]. Pert. to or producing normal binocular vision.

o. training. Eye muscle exercises for the purpose of correcting squint; orthoptics.

orthop′tics. 1. The science of correcting defects in binocular vision resulting from defects in optic musculature. 2. The technique of eye exercises for correcting faulty eye coordination affecting binocular vision.

orthoroentgenography (or″thō-rĕnt-gĕn-og′ră-fĭ). Measurement of size and position of internal organs accurately, using radiographic apparatus. SEE: *orthodiagraph.*

orthoscope (or′thō-skōp) [Gr. *orthos*, straight, + *skopein*, to examine]. Instrument for examining the eyes through a layer of water.

orthoscopic (or″thō-skōp′ĭk). 1. Having correct and undistorted vision. 2. Made to correct optical distortion.

orthoscopy (or-thŏs′kō-pĭ). Ocular examination with an orthoscope.

ortho′sis [Gr., making straight]. The straightening or correction of a deformity or disability.

orthostatic (or″thō-stăt′ĭk) [Gr. *orthos*, straight, + *statikos*, causing to stand]. Concerning an erect position.

orthostatism (or′thō-stăt″ĭzm) ["+ "+ *ismos*, condition]. An upright standing position of the body.

orthotast (or′thō-tăst) ["+ *tassein*, to arrange]. Instrument for straightening bone curvatures.

orthotic [Gr. *orthosis*, making straight]. 1. Rel. to orthosis, q.v. 2. Orthostatic, q.v.

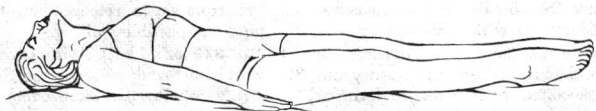

ORTHOTONOS

orthotics (or-thŏt′ĭks). 1. The science pert. to mechanical appliances for orthopedic use. SYN: *orthopedics.* 2. The use of orthopedic appliances.

orthotist (or′thō-tist) [Gr. *orthosis,* making straight]. One skilled in orthosis, q.v.

orthotonos, orthotonus (or-thŏt′ō-nŏs, -nŭs) [Gr. *orthos,* straight, + *tonos,* tension]. Tetanic spasm marked by rigidity of the body in a straight line.

orthropsia (or-thrŏp′sĭ-ă) [Gr. *órthros,* time near dawn, + *opsis,* sight]. Characteristic of human vision by which sight is better at dawn or dusk than in bright sunlight.

orthuria (orth-ū′rĭ-ă) [Gr. *orthos,* normal, + *ouron,* urine]. Average frequency of urination.

O. S., o. s. Abbr. for L. *oculus sinister,* left eye.

Os. Symb. for osmium.

os (ŏs) [L]. (pl. *ō′ra*) [NA]. Mouth, opening.
   o. uteri. Mouth of the uterus.
   o. uteri externum. The opening of cervical canal of uterus into the vagina.
   o. uteri internum. The internal opening of the cervical canal into the uterus.
   o. ventriculi. The cardia of the stomach.

os (ŏs) [L]. (pl. *os′sa*) [NA]. Bone.
   o. calcis. [NA]. Heel bone. SYN: *calcaneus.*
   o. coxae. [NA]. Hip bone.
   o. hamatum. [NA]. Hooked bone in second row of carpus. SYN: *unciform bone.*
   o. hyoideum. [NA]. U-shaped bone at the base of the tongue; hyoid bone.
   o. ilium. [NA]. The ilium.
   o. innominatum. Hip bone.
   o. magnum. A carpal bone, the third in the second distal row. SYN: *capitate.*
   o. orbiculare. Tiny bone in the ear which becomes attached to the incus, forming the lenticular process.
   o. peroneum. Bone occasionally found in tendon of peroneus longus muscle.
   o. planum. [NA]. 1. Flat bone. 2. Orbita plate of ethmoid bone.
   o. pubis. [NA]. The pubic bone; anterior inferior part of the hip bone.
   o. scaphoideum. [NA] SEE: *scaphoid.*
   o. trigonum. [NA] Triangular bone;

bone which develops from an extra center of ossification along posterior surface of talus.
   o. unguis. Lacrimal bone.
   o. vesalianum. Bone which develops from ossification of the posterior tubercle of the fifth metatarsal.

osazone (ō′să-zōn). Any of a series of compounds resulting from heating sugars with acetic acid and phenylhydrazine.

oscedo (ŏs-sē′dō) [L]. 1. Yawning. 2. White spots on the mucosa of the mouth. SYN: *aphthae.*

oscheal (ŏs′kē-ăl) [Gr. *oscheon,* scrotum]. Concerning the scrotum.

oscheitis (ŏs-kē-i′tĭs) ["+ *-itis,* inflammation]. Inflamed condition of the scrotum. SYN: *oschitis.*

oscheo- [Gr.]. Combining form meaning the scrotum.

oscheocele (ŏs′kē-ō-sēl) ["+ *kēlē,* swelling]. 1. A scrotal swelling or tumor. SYN: *oscheoma.* 2. Scrotal hernia.

oscheohydrocele (ŏs″kē-ō-hī′drō-sēl) ["+ *hydōr,* water, + *kēlē,* hernia]. Scrotal hydrocele; collection of fluid in the sac of a scrotal hernia.

oscheolith (ŏs′kē-ō-lĭth) [Gr. *oscheon,* scrotum, + *lithos,* stone]. A concretion in the scrotal sebaceous glands.

oscheoma (ŏs-kē-ō′mă) ["+ *-ōma,* tumor]. Scrotal tumor. SYN: *oscheoncus.*

oscheoncus (ŏs″kē-ŏn′kŭs) ["+ *onkos,* tumor]. A tumor of the scrotum.

oscheoplasty (os′kē-ō-plăs″tĭ) ["+ *plassein,* to form]. Plastic surgical repair of the scrotum.

oschitis (ŏs-kī′tĭs). Oscheitis, q.v.

oscillation (ŏs″sĭl-ā′shŭn) [L. *oscillare,* to swing]. A swinging, pendulum-like movement; a vibration; fluctuation.

oscillogram (ŏs′il-ō-grăm) ["+ Gr. *gramma,* a mark]. Graphic record made by the oscillograph.

oscillograph (ŏs′il-ō-grăf) ["+ Gr. *graphein,* to write]. An instrument (either electronic, mechanical, or combined) for recording electric vibrations, as of the heart or blood pressure.

oscillometer (ŏs-ĭl-om′ĕt-ĕr) ["+ Gr. *metron,* measure]. Machine to measure oscillations, esp. those of the blood stream.

oscillometry (ŏs-ĭl-ŏm'ĕ-trĭ). The measurement of oscillations with a machine.

oscillopsia. Sensation of oscillation or swinging of the visual field. It is illusory and may be associated with a severe form of labyrinthine nystamus.

oscilloscope (ŏ-sĭl'ō-skōp) [L. *oscillare*, to swing, + Gr. *skopein*, to examine]. An instrument for making visible the presence, nature, and form of oscillations or irregularities of an electric current.

Oscinidae. The eye flies. A family of small hairless flies that includes the genera Hippelates, Siphunculina, and Oscinis. They are serious pests and transmit a number of infectious diseases. SYN: *Chloropidae.*

oscitation (ŏs-ĭ-ta'shŭn) [L. *oscitatio*]. Yawning, gaping.

oscula'tion [L. *osculum*, little mouth, kiss]. 1. The union of two vessels or structures by their mouths. 2. Kissing.

osculum (ŏs'kū-lŭm) [L.]. (pl. *os'cula*) Any tiny aperture or pore.

-ose. 1. Chemical suffix indicating that the substance is a carbohydrate, as glucose. 2. Suffix indicating a primary alteration product of a protein, as proteose.

-osis [Gr.]. Suffix indicating a process, increase, or invasion by parasites.

Osler's disease (ŏs'lĕr). [Sir William Osler, Canadian-born physician, 1849-1919]. Disease of the blood in which the red cells are increased in number, the spleen becomes enlarged and the face is a deep red rather than truly cyanotic. SYN: *erythremia; polycythemia vera; Vaquez's disease.*

Osler-Weber-Rendu disease. [W.O.; Henri J.L.M. Rendu, Fr. physician, 1844-1902; Frederick P. Weber, Eng. physician, 1863-1962] An hereditary disease of capillaries. SEE: *telangiectasia, hereditary hemorrhagic.*

os'mate. A salt of osmic acid.

osmatic (ŏz-măt'ĭk) [Gr. *osmasthai*, to smell]. Pert. to, or having, a keen sense of smell.

osmesis (ŏz-mē'sĭs) [Gr. *osmēsis*, smelling]. The sense of smell; act of smelling.

osmesthesia (ŏz"mĕs-thē'zĭ-ă) [Gr. *osmē*, odor, + *aisthēsis*, sensation]. Olfactory sensibility; power of perceiving and distinguishing odors.

osmic acid (ŏz'mĭk). OsO4. Volatile, colorless compound formed by heating osmium in air; used as a caustic, stain for fats, tissue fixative for electron microscopy. SYN: *osmium tetroxide.*

CAUTION: Vapors are extremely toxic to eyes, skin, and respiratory tract. Container must not be opened without safeguarding eyes from vapors released both from uncapping and possible spilling.

osmicate (ŏz'mĭ-kāt). To impregnate or stain with osmic acid.

osmics (ŏz'mĭks) [Gr. *osmē*, odor]. The science of odors.

osmidrosis (ŏz-mĭ-drō'sĭs) ["+ *hidrōs*, perspiration]. Condition in which perspiration has a very strong odor. SYN: *bromidrosis.*

osmium (ŏz'mĭ-ŭm) [Gr. *osmē*, smell]. SYMB. *Os.* At. wt. 190.2; at. no. 76. A metallic element.

    o. tetroxide. OsO4. SEE: *osmic acid.*

osmo- [Gr. *osmē*, odor]. 1. Combining form indicating relationship to odor or smell. 2. [Gr. *ōsmos*, impulse]. Combining form indicating a thrusting forth. 3. [Gr. *ōsmos*, impulse]. Pert. to osmosis.

osmodysphoria (ŏz-mō-dĭs-fō'rĭ-ă) [Gr. *osmē*, odor, + *dys*, bad, + *pherein*, to bear]. Deep-seated and abnormal dislike of certain odors.

osmolagnia (ŏz"mō-lăg'nĭ-ă) ["+ *lagneia*, lust]. Erotic satisfaction derived from odors, usually of the body.

osmolality (ŏs"mō-lal'ĭ-tĭ). Osmotic concentration, the characteristic of a solution determined by the ionic concentration of the dissolved substance per unit of solvent.

osmologically clean. Control of obnoxious odors.

osmology (ŏz-mŏl'ō-jĭ). 1. ["+ *logos*, study]. The study of odors. SYN: *osphresiology.* 2. [Gr. *ōsmos*, impulse, + *logos*, study]. Study of osmosis.

osmometer (ŏz-mŏm'ĕt-ĕr). 1. [Gr. *osmē*, smell, + *metron*, measure]. Device for measuring acuity of sense of smell. 2. [Gr. *ōsmos*, impulse, + *metron*, measure]. A device for measuring osmotic pressure.

osmonosology (ŏz"mō-nō-sŏl'ō-jĭ) [Gr. *osmē*, smell, + *nosos*, disease, + *logos*, study]. Branch of medicine dealing with diseases and disorders of the organs of smell.

osmopho'bia ["+ *phobia*, fear]. Morbid fear of odors.

osmose (ŏz'mōs) [Gr. *ōsmos*, thrusting]. 1. To subject to osmosis. 2. To undergo osmosis.

osmosis (ŏz-mō'sĭs) [Gr. *ōsmos*, impulse, + *-ōsis*, intensive]. The passage of solvent through a semipermeable membrane separating solutions of different concentrations. The solvent, usually water, passes through the membrane from the region of lower concentration of solute to that of a higher concentration of solute, thus tending to equalize the concentrations of the two solutions.

    The rate of osmosis is dependent primarily upon the difference in osmotic pressures of the solutions on the two sides of a membrane, the permeability of the membrane, and the electric potential across the membrane and charge upon walls of the pores in it.

RS: absorption; dialysis; diffusion; diosmosis; hypotonic; isotonic.

osmotic (ŏz-mŏt'ĭk) [Gr. *ōsmos*, thrusting]. Pert. to osmosis.

   o. pressure. 1. The pressure which develops when two solutions of different concentrations are separated by a semipermeable membrane. 2. The pressure which would develop if a solution were enclosed in a membrane impermeable to all solutes present and surrounded by pure solvent.

   Osmotic pressure varies with concentration of the solution and with temperature increase. Animal cells have an osmotic pressure approximately equal to that of the circulating fluid, the blood. Solutions exerting this osmotic pressure are said to be isotonic or isosmotic; stronger solutions which cause cells to shrink are hypertonic; weaker solutions which cause cells to swell are hypotonic.

osphresiolagnia (ŏs-frē''zĭ-ō-lag'nĭ-ă) [Gr. *osphrēsis*, smell, + *lagneia*, lust]. Excitement of an erotic nature produced by odors. SYN: *osmolagnia.*

osphresiology (ŏs-frē-zĭ-ŏl'ō-jĭ) ["+ *logos*, study]. Science of odors and the sense of smell. SYN: *osmology.*

osphresiometer (ŏs-frē-zĭ-ŏm'ĕt-ĕr) ["+ *metron*, measure]. Apparatus for measuring the acuteness of the sense of smell. SYN: *osmometer.*

osphresis (ŏs-frē'sĭs) [Gr.]. The sense of smell. SYN: *olfaction.*

osphretic (ŏs-frĕt'ĭk). Concerning the sense of smell. SYN: *olfactory.*

osphus (os'fŭs) [Gr. *osphys*]. Loin.

osphyalgia (ŏs-fĭ-al'jĭ-ă) ["+ *algos*, pain]. Pain in the loins or hips. SEE: *lumbago; sciatica.*

osphyitis (ŏs-fĭ-ĭ'tĭs) ["+ *-itis*, inflammation]. Inflammation of the lumbar region.

osphyomyelitis (ŏs''fĭ-ō-mĭ''ĕl-ĭ'tĭs) ["+ *myelos*, marrow, + *-itis*, inflammation]. Inflamed condition of the lumbar region of the spinal cord.

os pubis (ŏs pū'bĭs) [L. *os*, bone, + *pubis*, pubes]. A bone that in adult life unites the innominate or hip bone with the ilium and ischium to form the pelvis. Irregular shape, divided into a horizontal, ascending, and descending ramus. The outer extremity constitutes approximately one fifth of the acetabulum. The inner unites in middle line with corresponding part of the bone of opp. side, forming the symphysis pubis.

ossa (ŏs'ă) [L.]. (sing. *os*) Bones.

ossein (ŏs'ē-ĭn) [L. *ossa*, bones]. The organic substance of bones. SYN: *ostein.*

osseofibrous (ŏs''ē-ō-fī'brŭs) ["+ *fibra*, fiber]. Composed of bone and fibrous tissue.

osseous (ŏs'ē-ŭs) [L. *osseus*, bony]. Bonelike; concerning bones. SYN: *bony.*

ossicle (ŏs'ĭ-kl) [L. *ossiculum*, little bone]. Any small bone, esp. one of the three bones of the ear, the malleus, incus, or stapes.

ossicula (ŏ-sĭk'ū-lă) [L.]. (sing. *ossiculum*) Little bones.

ossiculectomy (ŏs''ĭk-ū-lĕk'tō-mĭ) [L. *ossiculum*, little bone, + Gr. *ektomē*, excision]. Excision of an ossicle, esp. one of the ear.

ossiculotomy (ŏ''sĭk-ū-lŏt'ō-mĭ) ["+ Gr. *tomē*, incision]. Surgical incision of one or more of the ossicles of the ear.

ossiculum (ŏ-sĭk'ū-lŭm) [L.]. (pl. *ossic'ula*) Tiny bone, esp. one of the three in the middle ear.

ossiferous (ŏs-ĭf'ĕr-ŭs) [L. *os*, bone, + *ferre*, to bear]. Composed of, or forming, bone or bony tissue.

ossific (ŏs-ĭf'ĭk) ["+ *facere*, to make]. Producing or becoming bone.

ossification (ŏs''ĭ-fĭ-kā'shŭn) ["+ *facere*, to make]. 1. Formation of bone substance. 2. Conversion of other tissue into bone. SEE: *center, epiotic.*

   o., endochondral. The formation of bone in cartilage, as in formation of long bones. It involves the destruction and removal of cartilage and the formation of osseous tissue in space occupied by the cartilage. SYN: *intracartilaginous o.*

   o., intramembranous. The formation of bone in or underneath a fibrous membrane, such as occurs in formation of the cranial bones.

   o., pathologic. Formation of bone in abnormal sites or abnormal development of bone.

ossifluence (ŏ-sĭf'lu-ens). Osteolysis or softening of bone.

ossiform (ŏs'ĭ-form). Resembling bone. SYN: *osteoid.*

ossify (ŏs'ĭ-fī) [L. *os*, bone, + *facere*, to make]. To turn into bone.

ostalgia (ŏs-tăl'jĭ-ă) [Gr. *osteon*, bone, + *algos*, pain]. Pain in a bone. SYN: *osteodynia.*

osteal (ŏs'tĭ-ăl). Pert. to bone.

ostealleosis (ŏs''tē-ăl''lē-ō'sĭs). A change in the substance of bone.

osteanabrosis (ŏs''tē-ăn-ă-brō'sĭs) [Gr. *osteon*, bone, + *anabrōsis*, eating up]. Wasting away of bone.

osteanagenesis (ŏs″tē-ăn-ă-jĕn′ē-sĭs) ["+ *anagenesis*, reproduction]. Regeneration or re-formation of bone.

ostearthrotomy (ŏs″tē-ăr-thrŏt′ō-mĭ) ["+ *arthron*, joint, + *tomē*, incision]. Surgical excision of the articular end of a bone. SYN: *osteoarthrotomy.*

ostectomy, osteectomy (ŏs-tek′tō-mĭ, -tē-ĕk′tō-mĭ) [Gr. *osteon*, bone, + *ektomē*, excision]. Surgical excision of a bone or a portion of one.

osteectopia (ŏs″tē-ĕk-tō′pĭ-ă) ["+ *ektopos*, out of place]. Displacement of a bone.

osteitis (ŏs-tē-ī′tĭs) ["+ *-itis*, inflammation]. Inflammation of a bone.

   o., **condensing.** O. in which the marrow cavity becomes filled with osseous tissue. Bone becomes denser and heavier.

   o. **deformans.** Skeletal disease of older people. Chronic form of o. with thickening and hypertrophy of the long bones and deformity of the flat bones. SYN: *Paget's disease of bone.*

   ETIOL: Unknown.

   SYM: Slow and insidious in onset. Pain in lower limbs, esp. the tibia. Frequent fractures. Waddling gait. Skull becomes enlarged, so that the face appears small and triangular in shape with the head pushed forward. Stature shortens.

   TREATMENT: Constitutional and palliative. There is no known specific therapy.

   o. **fibrosa cystica generalisata.** A condition resulting from over-activity of the parathyroid glands with resulting disturbances in calcium and phosphorus metabolism. Characterized by decalcification and softening of bone, nephrolithiasis, and elevation of blood calcium and lowering of blood phosphorus. Cysts form and tumors may develop. SYN: *hyperparathyroidism.*

   o., **gummatous.** Chronic o. associated with syphilis and characterized by the formation of gummas.

   o., **rarefying.** Form in which inorganic matter is lessened and bone tissue becomes lattice-like in structure. SYN: *osteoporosis.*

   o., **sclerosing.** O., condensing, q.v.

ostembryon (ŏs-tĕm′brĭ-ŏn) [Gr. *osteon*, bone, + *embryon*, fetus]. A fetus which has become ossified.

ostemia (ŏs-tē′mĭ-ă) [Gr. *osteon*, bone, + *haima*, blood]. Congestion of blood in a bone.

ostempyesis (ŏs″tĕm-pī-ē′sĭs) ["+ *empyēsis*, suppuration]. Purulent inflammation within a bone.

osteo- [Gr. *osteon*, bone]. Combining form indicating relationship to a bone.

osteoaneurysm (ŏs″tē-ō-an′ū-rĭzm) [Gr. *osteon*, bone, + *aneurysma*, a widening]. Aneurysm, or dilatation of a blood vessel filled with clotted blood, occurring within a bone.

osteoarthritis (ŏs″tē-ō-ăr-thrī′tĭs) ["+ *arthron*, joint, + *-itis*, inflammation]. A chronic disease involving the joints, esp. those bearing weight. Characterized by destruction of articular cartilage, overgrowth of bone with lipping and spur formation, and impaired function. SYN: *degenerative joint disease; hypertrophic arthritis.*

osteoarthropathy (ŏs″tē-ō-ar-thrŏp′ă-thĭ) ["+ "+ *pathos*, disease]. Any disease involving the joints and bones, accompanied by severe pain.

   o., **hypertrophic pulmonary.** An affection characterized by enlargement of distal phalanges of fingers and toes and a thickening of their distal ends, accompanied by a peculiar longitudinal curving of nails. Wrist and interphalangeal joints may become enlarged as well as distal ends of tibia and fibula and the jaw.

   ETIOL: Found in pulmonary tuberculosis, chronic bronchitis, bronchiectasis, congenital heart disease, and chronic cardiac affections.

osteoarthrotomy (ŏs″tē-ō-ar-thrŏt′ō-mĭ) ["+ "+ *tomē*, incision]. Excision of joint end of a bone. SYN: *ostearthrotomy.*

osteoblast (ŏs′tē-ō-blăst) [Gr. *osteon*, bone, + *blastos*, germ]. A cell of mesodermal origin which is concerned with the formation of bone.

osteocampsia (ŏs″tē-ō-kămp′sĭ-ă) ["+ *kamptein*, to bend]. Curvature of a bone, as in osteomalacia.

osteocarcinoma (ŏs″tē-ō-kăr-sĭn-ō′mă) ["+ *karkinos*, crab, cancer, + *-ōma*, tumor]. 1. Osteoma and carcinoma combined. 2. Carcinoma of a bone.

osteocephaloma (ŏs″tē-ō-sĕf-ă-lō′mă) ["+ *enkephalē*, head, + *-ōma*, tumor]. Encephaloma, a malignant neoplasm of brainlike texture in a bone.

osteochondritis (ŏs″tē-ō-kŏn-drī′tĭs) [Gr. *osteon*, bone, + *chondros*, cartilage, + *-ītis,* inflammation]. Inflammation of bone and cartilage.

   o. **deformans juvenile.** Chronic inflammation of head of femur in childhood resulting in atrophy and shortening of neck of femur and wide, flat head.

   o. **dissecans.** Condition affecting a joint in which a fragment of cartilage and its underlying bone become detached from articular surface. Occurs commonly in the knee joint.

osteochondrodystrophy (ŏs″tē-ō-kŏn″drō-dĭs′trō-fĭ) ["+ "+ *dys*, bad, + *trephein,* to nourish]. A disorder of skeletal growth resulting from bone and cartilage malformation. Produces a form of dwarfism. SYN: *Morquio's disease.*

osteochondroma (ŏs"tē-ō-kŏn-drō'mă) ["+ "+ -ōma, tumor]. Tumor composed of both cartilaginous and bony substance.

osteoclasia, osteoclasis (ŏs"tē-ō-klā'zĭ-ă, -ōk'lă-sĭs) [Gr. *osteon*, bone, + *klasis*, a breaking]. 1. Surgical fracture of a bone in order to remedy a deformity. 2. Bony tissue absorption and destruction.

osteoclast (ŏs'tē-ō-klăst) ["+ *klan*, to break]. 1. Device for fracturing bones for therapeutic purposes. 2. Giant multinuclear cell formed in bone marrow of growing bones. Found in depressions (called Howship's lacunae) on the surface of the bone. Concerned with absorption and removal of unwanted tissue.

osteocope (ŏs'tē-ō-kōp) [Gr. *osteon*, bone, + *kopos*, pain]. Extreme pain in the bones, esp. in syphilitic bone disease.

osteocopic (ŏs"tē-ō-kŏp'ĭk). Concerning severe pain in the bone.

osteocranium (ŏs"tē-ō-krā'nĭ-ŭm) [Gr. *osteon*, bone, + *kranion*, skull]. The portion of the cranium formed of membrane bones in contrast to that formed of cartilage (chondrocranium).

osteocystoma (ŏs"tē-ō-sĭs-tō'mă) ["+ *kystic*, sac, bladder, + *-ōma*, tumor]. Cystic tumor of a bone.

osteodensitometer. Device for determining the density of bones. Usually x-ray technique is used.

osteodermia (ŏs"tē-ō-der'mĭ-ă) ["+ *derma*, skin]. The formation of bony deposits in the skin.

osteodynia (ŏs"tē-ō-dĭn'ĭ-ă) [Gr. *osteon*, bone, + *odynē*, pain]. Persistent pain in a bone. SYN: *ostealgia.*

osteodystrophia (ŏs"tē-ō-dĭs-trō'fĭ-ă) ["+ *dys*, ill, + *trophē*, nourishment]. Defective bone development. SYN: *asteodystrophy.*

osteodystrophy (ŏs"tē-ō-dĭs'trō-fĭ). Defective bone development.

osteoepiphysis (ŏs"tē-ō-ē-pĭf'ĭs-ĭs) [Gr. *osteon*, bone, + *epi*, upon, + *physis*, growth]. A small piece of bone which is separated in childhood from the larger bone by cartilage; during later growth the two bones join.

osteofibroma (ŏs"tē-ō-fī-brō'mă) ["+ L. *fibra*, fiber, + Gr. *-ōma*, tumor]. Tumor of bony and fibrous tissues. SYN: *fibroosteoma.*

osteogen (ŏs'tē-ō-jĕn) ["+ *gennan*, to produce]. Substance of the inner periosteal layer from which bone is formed.

osteogenesis, osteogeny (ŏs"tē-ō-jĕn'ē-sĭs, -ōj'ē-nĭ). Formation and development of

bone taking place in connective tissue or in cartilage. Ossification.

   o. imperfecta. A congenital bone disease causing the bones to fracture easily.

osteogen'ic. Pertaining to osteogenesis.

osteography (ŏs"tē-og'raf-ĭ) [Gr. *osteon*, bone, + *graphein*, to write]. Descriptive treatise on the bones.

osteohalisteresis (ŏs"tē-ō-hăl-ĭs-tĕr-ē'sĭs) ["+ *hals*, salt, + *sterein*, to deprive]. Softening of the bones, caused by deficiency of mineral constituents of the bone.

osteoid (ŏs'tē-oyd) ["+ *eidos*, resemblance]. Resembling bone; ossiform.

osteology (ŏs-tē-ŏl'ō-jĭ) ["+ *logos*, study]. The science of structure and function of bones.

osteolysis (ŏs"tē-ol'ĭ-sĭs) ["+ *lysis*, dissolution]. Softening and destruction of bone, as in caries.

osteoma (ŏs-tē-ō'mă) [Gr. *osteon*, bone + *-ōma*, tumor]. (pl. *osteomata, osteomas*) A benign bony tumor; a bonelike structure that develops on a bone or, occasionally, at other sites.

   o., cancellous. One that is soft and spongy. Its thin and delicate trabeculae enclose large medullary spaces similar to cancellous bone.

   o., cavalryman's. Bony outgrowth of femur at the insertion of the adductor femoris longus.

   o. dentale. A bony outgrowth from the jawbone.

   o. medullare. An osteoma containing medullary spaces.

   o., osteoid. A benign tumor of bone composed of sheets of osteoid tissue partially calcified and ossified. Occurs esp. in extremities of young; rare.

   o. spongiosum. Spongy tumor in the bone.

osteomalacia (ŏs"tē-ō-măl-ā'sĭ-ă) ["+ *malakia*, softening]. Softening of the bones. A disease marked by increasing softness of the bones, so that they become flexible and brittle, thus causing deformities. Occurs in adults and chiefly in women. SYN: *malacosteon; mollities ossium.*

   SYM: Rheumatic pains in the limbs, spine, thorax, and esp. the pelvis; anemia and signs of deficiency disease; progressive weakness. Finally death occurs from exhaustion.

   ETIOL: Deficiency or loss of calcium salts; vitamin D deficiency.

osteomalacic (ŏs"tē-ō-măl-ā'sĭk) [Gr. *osteon*, bone, + *malakia*, softening]. Concerning or characterized by softening of the bone.

osteomatoid (ŏs-tē-ō′mă-toyd) [Gr. *osteon*, bone, + *-ōma*, tumor, + *eidos*, resemblance]. Resembling a bonelike tumor.

osteomatosis (ŏs″tē-ō-mă-tō′sĭs) [″ + ″ + *-osis*, condition]. Formation of multiple osteomas.

osteomere (ŏs′tē-ō-mēr) [″ + *meros*, part]. One in a series of similar bony segments, as the vertebrae.

osteometry (ŏs-tē-ŏm′ĕt-rĭ) [″ + *metron*, measure]. The study of the measurement of parts of the skeletal system.

osteomyelitis (ŏs″tē-ō-mī-ĕl-ī′tĭs) [Gr. *osteon*, bone, + *myelos*, marrow, + *-itis*, inflammation]. Inflammation of bone, esp. the marrow, caused by a pathogenic organism.

SYM: Pain in the affected part, fever, sweats, leukocytosis, overlying muscles usually rigid, skin inflamed, pain on pressure over affected part. Suppuration may occur.

TREATMENT: Prompt and adequate doses of antibiotics; sedation for pain and anxiety; aspiration of abscess; immobilization of affected extremity; surgery if abscess persists.

osteoncus (ŏs-tē-ŏn′kŭs) [″ + *onkos*, tumor]. A bone tumor. SYN: *exostosis; osteoma*.

osteonecrosis (ŏs″tē-ō-nĕ-krō′sĭs) [Gr. *osteon*, bone, + *nekrōsis*, death]. Death of bone tissue in mass.

osteoneuralgia (ŏs″tē-ō-nū-ral′jĭ-ă) [″ + *neuron*, nerve, + *algos*, pain]. Pain of a bone.

osteopath (ŏs′tē-ō-păth) [″ + *pathos*, disease]. A practitioner of osteopathy, q.v.

osteopathic (ŏs″tē-ō-păth′ĭk). Concerning therapeutic bone manipulation.

osteopathology (ŏs-tē-ō-path-ol′ō-jĭ) [Gr. *osteon*, bone, + *pathos*, disease, + *logos*, study]. 1. Any bone disease. SYN: *osteopathy*. 2. Study of bone diseases. SYN: *osteopathy*.

osteopathy (ŏs-tē-op′ă-thĭ) [Gr. *osteon*, bone, + *pathos*, disease]. 1. Any bone disease. 2. A school of medicine based upon the theory that the normal body is a vital mechanical organism whose structural and functional states are of equal importance and that the body is able to rectify itself against toxic conditions when it has favorable environmental circumstances and satisfactory nourishment. Therefore it is the osteopathic physician's responsibility to establish and remove any internal or external peculiarities to the system. Although using manipulation for the most part to restore structural and functional balance, he also relies upon physical, medicinal, and surgical methods.

osteopecilla (ŏs″tē-ō-pĕ-sĭl′ĭ-ă) [″ + *poikilia*, spottedness]. Osteosclerosis fragilis generalisata, q.v.

osteopedion (ŏs″tē-ō-pĕ′dĭ-ŏn) [″ + *paidion*, child]. A calcified or hardened fetus. SYN: *lithopedion; ostembryon*.

osteoperiosteal (ŏs″tē-ō-per′ĭ-os′tē-ăl) [Gr. *osteon*, bone, + *peri*, around, + *osteon*, bone]. Concerning bone and its periosteum, the protective connective tissue covering bone.

osteoperiostitis (ŏs″tē-ō-per-ĭ-ōs-tī′tĭs) [″ + ″ + ″ + *-itis*, inflammation]. Inflammation of a bone and its protective membrane, the periosteum.

osteopetrosis (ŏs″tē-ō-pĕ-trō′sĭs) [Gr. *osteon*, bone, + *petra*, stone, + *-osis*, disease]. Excessive calcification of bones causing spontaneous fractures and marblelike appearance. SYN: *marble bones*.

osteophage (ŏs′tē-ō-fāj) [″ + *phagein*, to eat]. Large multinuclear cell which causes absorption of bone. SEE: *osteoclast*.

osteophagia (ŏs″tē-ō-fā′jĭ-ă). Craving for bones caused by a mineral deficiency.

osteophlebitis (ŏs″tē-ō-flē-bī′tĭs) [Gr. *osteon*, bone, + *phleps, phleb-*, vein, + *-itis*, inflammation]. Inflammation of veins of a bone.

osteophone (ŏs′tē-ō-fōn″) [″ + *phōnē*, voice]. Device used by the deaf for conducting sound through facial bones.

osteophyma (ŏs″tē-ō-fī′mă) [″ + *phyma*, growth]. A swelling or growth of bone.

osteophyte (ŏs′tē-ō-fit) [Gr. *osteon*, bone, + *phyton*, plant]. A bony excrescence or outgrowth, usually branched in shape.

osteoplastic (ŏs″tē-ō-plăs′tĭk) [″ + *plastikos*, formed]. 1. Pert. to bone repair by plastic surgery or grafting. 2. Concerning bone formation.

osteoplasty (ŏs′tē-ō-plăs′tĭ) [Gr. *osteon*, bone, + *plassein*, to form]. Plastic repair of the bones.

osteopoikilosis (ŏs″tē-ō-poy-kĭ-lō′sĭs) [″ + *poikilos*, spotted]. Disease of bones marked by excessive calcification in spots less than one cm. in diameter. It is a benign disease not associated with symptoms.

osteoporosis (ŏs″tē-ō-por-ō′sĭs) [″ + *poros*, passage + *-osis*, condition]. Increased porosity of bone.

SYM: Softening of bone, widening of haversian canals, absorption of calcareous matter. SEE: *osteomalacia*.

o., parachitic. O. with tendency to develop into rickets. Congenital.

osteoporotic (ŏs″tē-ō-pōr-ot′ĭk). Concerning a porous condition of the bones.

osteopsathyrosis (ŏs″tē-ōp-săth′ĭ-rō′sĭs) [Gr. *osteon*, bone, + *psathyros*, fragile].

Osteogenesis imperfecta, q.v.; fragility or brittleness of bones. Hereditary condition of unknown etiology in which the long bones seem normal in appearance and chemical composition, but are extremely brittle.

SYM: Breaks may occur upon bathing infant or turning him over, following minor injuries, chewing, bending the knee, etc. Breaks almost painless with slight swelling and only evidence is unwillingness of the child to use his injured limb.

PROG: Condition tends to improve after puberty but may return in later life.

TREATMENT: Good hygiene, nourishing diet, supports to prevent breaks. Bones knit quickly with normal amount of callus. SYN: *fragilitas ossium; osteogenesis imperfecta.*

osteoradionecrosis (ŏs″tē-ō-rā-dĭ-ō-nĕ-krō′sĭs). Death of bone following irradiation.

osteorrhagia (ŏs″tē-ō-rā′jĭ-ă) [Gr. *osteon,* bone, + *rhēgnynai,* to burst forth]. Hemorrhagic flow of blood from a bone.

osteorrhaphy (ŏs-tē-or′ă-fĭ) [″+ *rhaphē,* a sewing]. Suture of bone or the wiring of bone fragments.

osteosarcoma (ŏs″tē-ō-sar-kō′mă) [Gr. *osteon,* bone, + *sarx, sark-,* flesh, + *-ōma,* tumor]. A malignant sarcoma of the bone.

osteosarcomatous (ŏs″tē-ō-sar-kō′măt-ŭs). Concerning or like an osteosarcoma.

osteosclerosis (ŏs″tē-ō-sklē-rō′sĭs) [″+ *sklēros,* hard, + *-ōsis,* intensive]. Hardening of bone with increased heaviness.

o. fragilis generalisata. Abnormal calcification of the bones causing spontaneous fractures and spotted marble-like appearance in the roentgenogram.

osteoscope (ŏs′tē-ō-skōp) [Gr. *osteon,* bone, + *skopein,* to examine]. Appliance used to test x-ray machines by observing certain bones of the forearm which are considered as a standard.

osteoseptum (ŏs″tē-ō-sĕp′tŭm) [″+ L. *septum,* a partition]. The bony area of the nasal septum.

osteosis (ŏs″tē-ō′sĭs) [Gr. *osteon,* bone, + *-ōsis,* condition]. Presence of bone-containing nodules in the skin.

o. cutis. Diffuse thickening of skin and subcutaneous tissue. Rare.

osteospongioma (ŏs″tē-ō-spon″jĭ-ō′mă) [″+ *spongos,* sponge, + *-ōma,* tumor]. A spongy neoplasm of bone. SYN: *osteoma spongiosum.*

osteosteatoma (ŏs″tē-ō-stē″ă-tō′mă) [″+ *stear, steat-,* fat, + *-ōma,* tumor]. A benign fatty tumor with bony elements.

osteostixis (ŏs″tē-ō-stik′sĭs) [Gr. *osteon,* bone, + *stixis,* a puncture]. Therapeutic puncture of a bone.

osteosuture (ŏs″tē-ō-sū′chŭr) [″+ L. *sutura,* a stitch]. Suture or wiring of bone fragments. SYN: *osteorrhaphy.*

osteosynovitis (ŏs″tē-ō-sin″ō-vī′tĭs) [″+ *syn,* with, + *ōon,* egg, + *-itis,* inflammation]. Inflammation of a synovial membrane and the surrounding bones.

osteosynthesis (ŏs″tē-ō-sĭn′thē-sĭs) [″+ *synthēsis,* a joining]. Surgical fastening of the ends of a fractured bone by mechanical means.

osteotabes (ŏs″tē-ō-tā′bēz) [Gr. *osteon,* bone, + L. *tabes,* wasting]. Atrophy of the bone in infants, beginning with wasting of the marrow and gradually including the rest of the bone.

osteotelangiectasia (ŏs″tē-ō-tĕl-ăn″jĭ-ĕk-tā′zĭ-ă) [″+ *telos,* end, + *angeion,* vessel, + *ektasis,* a stretching]. Sarcomatous tumor of the bone containing dilated blood vessels.

osteothrombosis (ŏs″tē-ō-thrŏm-bō′sĭs) [″+ *thrombōsis,* a clotting]. Clot formation in the veins of a bone.

osteotome (ŏs′tē-ō-tōm) [″+ *tomē,* a cutting]. A chisel bevelled on both sides for cutting through bones.

osteotomy (ŏs-tē-ot′ō-mĭ) [Gr. *osteon,* bone, + *tomē,* incision]. The operation for cutting through a bone.

o., cuneiform. The excision of a wedge of bone.

o., linear. Lengthwise division of a bone.

o., Macewen's. Supracondylar section of the femur for correction of knock-knee.

o., subtrochanteric. Gant's operation, division of shaft of femur below lesser trochanter to correct ankylosis of hip joint.

o., transtrochanteric. Section of the femur through the lesser trochanter for deformity about the hip joint.

osteotrite (ŏs′tē-ō-trīt) [″+ *tribein,* to grind or rub]. Instrument used to scrape away diseased bone.

osteotrophy (ŏs-tē-ot′ro-fĭ) [″+ *trophē,* nutrition]. Bone nutrition.

osthexia (ŏs-thĕk′sĭ-ă) [Gr. *osteon,* bone, + *hexis,* condition]. Excessive ossification, esp. in abnormal places.

ostial (os′tĭ-ăl) [L. *ostium,* a little opening]. Concerning an orifice.

ostitis (ŏs-tī′tĭs) [Gr. *osteon,* bone, + *-itis,* inflammation]. Inflammation of a bone. SYN: *osteitis,* q.v.

ostium (os′tĭ-ŭm) [L. a small opening]. (pl. *ostia*) [NA] Small opening, esp. one into a tubular organ.

o. abdominale tubae uterinae. [NA]. Fimbriated end of fallopian tube. SYN: *o. abdominale.*

o. arteriosum. [NA]. Arterial orifice of ventricle of the heart into the aorta or pulmonary artery.

o. internum. Uterine end of a fallopian tube. SYN: *o. uterinum tubae internum.*

o. pharyngeum. Pharyngeal opening of the auditory (eustachian) tube.

o. tympanicum. Tympanic opening of the auditory (eustachian) tube.

o. urethrae externum. [NA]. Ext. opening of the urethra.

o. vaginae. [NA]. Ext. opening of the vagina.

ostraco, ostrac- [Gr.]. Combining form meaning hard shell.

ostreotoxismus (ŏs″trē-ō-tŏks-ĭz′mŭs) [Gr. *ostreon*, oyster, + *toxikon*, poison]. Poisoning from eating contaminated oysters.

O.T. Abbr. for *old term*, in contrast to BNA or NA term; *old tuberculin; occupational therapy.*

otacoustic (ō″tă-koo′stĭk) [Gr. *ōtakousteō*, to listen]. 1. Aiding or concerning the hearing. 2. Device to aid hearing; an ear trumpet.

otalgia (ō-tăl′jĭ-ă) [Gr.]. Pain in the ear. SYN: *earache; otodynia; otoneuralgia.*

TREATMENT: *Local:* Heat in the form of compresses, hot water bottle, or warm glycerin dropped in ear. Incision of drum if bulging is present. *General:* Nasal astringents to help maintain patency of the eustachian tube; relieve pain.

otantritis (ō″tăn-trī′tĭs) [Gr. *ous, ot-*, ear, + L. *antrum*, sinus, + Gr. *-itis*, inflammation]. Inflammation of the mastoid antrum.

OTD. Abbr. for *organ tolerance dose*, limitation of radiation tolerated by particular tissues.

otectomy (ō-tĕk′tō-mī) [Gr. *ous, ot-*, ear, + *ektomē*, excision]. Surgical excision of the contents of the middle ear.

othelcosis (ō-thĕl-kō′sĭs) ["+ *helkōsis*, ulceration]. Ulceration or suppuration of the ear.

othematoma (ō″thē-mă-tō′mă) ["+ *haima*, blood, + *-ōma*, tumor]. Effusion of blood, causing a hard swelling between perichondrium and cartilage of pinna. Common in fighters or wrestlers. SYN: *hematoma auris.* SEE: *cauliflower ear.*

othemorrhea (o-thĕm″ō-rē′ă) ["+ "+ *rhoia*, flow]. Excessive bleeding from the ear.

othygroma (ō-thī-grō′mă) [Gr. *ous, ōt-*, ear, + *hygros*, moist, + *-ōma*, tumor]. Edema of ear lobe.

otic (ō′tĭk) [Gr. *ōtikos*]. Concerning the ear.

oticodinia (ō″tĭ-kō-dĭn′ĭ-ă) [Gr. *ōtikos*, aural, + *dinē*, whirl]. Vertigo due to ear disease. RS: *Meniere's disease; vertigo.*

otitic (ō-tĭt′ĭk) [Gr. *ous, ot-*, ear + *-itis*, inflammation]. Concerning inflammation of the ear.

otitis (ō-tī′tĭs) [Gr. *ous, ot-*, ear, + *-itis*, inflammation]. Inflamed condition of the ear. It is differentiated as *externa, media,* and *interna,* depending upon the portion of the ear which is inflamed.

o., aero-. O. resulting from pressure changes when auditory tubes are obstructed. Occurs commonly in aviators or divers.

o., furuncular. Furuncle formation in ext. meatus.

o. labyrinthica. Inflammation of the labyrinth.

o. mastoidea. Inflamed condition of the middle ear which involves the mastoid spaces.

o. mycotica. Fungus inflammation.

o. parasitica. Inflammation caused by a parasite.

o. sclerotica. Inflammation of inner ear accompanied by hardening of the aural structures.

oto-, ot- (Gr. *ous, ōtos,* ear). Combining form relating to the ear.

otoantritis (ō″tō-ăn-trī′tĭs) ["+ *antron,* cavity, + *-itis,* inflammation]. Inflamed condition of mastoid antrum and the tympanic attic.

otoblennorrhea (ō″tō-blĕn″o-rē′ă) ["+ *blenna,* mucus, + *rhoia,* flow]. Mucous discharge from the ear.

otocatarrh (ō″tō-kă-tar′) ["+ *katarrhein,* to flow down]. Catarrhal discharge of the ear.

otocleisis (ō-tō-klī′sĭs) [Gr. *ous, ōtos,* ear, + *kleisis,* closure]. Occlusion of any auditory passages.

otoconium (ō″tō-kō′nĭ-ŭm) ["+ *konis,* dust]. (pl. *otoconia*) Minute particles, composed chiefly of calcium carbonate, found in otolithic membrane on surface of maculae of inner ear. SYN: *otolith; ear dust.*

otocyst (ō′tō-sĭst) ["+ *kystis,* sac, bladder]. Primordial chamber from which arises the membranous labyrinth. SYN: *auditory vesicle.*

otodynia (ō″tō-dĭn′ĭ-ă) ["+ *odynē,* pain]. Pain in the ear; earache. SYN: *otalgia; otoneuralgia.*

otogenic, otogenous (ō″tō-jĕn′ĭk, ō-tŏj′ĕn-ŭs) [Gr. *ous, ōtos,* ear, + *gennan,* to produce]. Having its origin in the ear.

otolaryngologist (ō″tō-lar″ĭn-gŏl′ō-jist) ["+ *larynx,* larynx, + *logos,* study]. A specialist in otolaryngology.

otolaryngology (ō″tō-lar″ĭn-gŏl′ō-jī). The division of medical science which includes otology, rhinology, and laryngology.

otolith (ō'tō-lĭth) [Gr. *ous, otos,* ear, + *lithos,* stone]. Otoconium, q.v.

otological (ō''tō-lŏj'ĭ-kl) ["+ *logos,* study]. Rel. to study of diseases of the ear.

otologist (ō-tŏl'ō-jĭst). One versed in the anatomy, physiology, and pathology of the ear. SYN: *aurist.*

otology (ō-tŏl'ō-jĭ) [Gr. *ous, otos,* ear, + *logos,* study]. The science dealing with the ear, its function, and its diseases.

otomyasthenia (ō''tō-mī''ăs-thē'nĭ-ă) ["+ *mys, my-,* muscle, + *astheneia,* weakness]. 1. Weakened condition of the ear muscles. 2. Defective hearing caused by paresis of the tensor tympani and stapedius muscles.

otomyces (ō''tō-mī'sēz) ["+ *mykēs,* fungus]. Any fungus infesting the ear.

otomycosis (ō''tō-mī-kō'sĭs) ["+ "+ *-ōsis,* condition]. An infection of ext. auditory meatus of the ear caused by a fungus infestation. SYN: *otitis mycotica; mycomyringitis; myringomycosis.*

otoncus (ō-tŏng'kŭs) [Gr. *ous, otos,* ear, + *onkos,* tumor]. An aural tumor.

otonecrectomy,   otonecronectomy (ō''tō-nē-krĕk'tō-mĭ, -nĕk'to-mĭ) ["+ *nekros,* dead, + *ektomē,* excision]. Excision of necrosed areas from the ear.

otoneuralgia (ō''tō-nū-răl'jĭ-ă) ["+ *neuron,* sinew, + *algos,* pain]. Pain in the ear. SYN: *otalgia; otodynia.*

otoneurasthenia (ō''tō-nū''răs-thē'nĭ-ă) ["+ "+ *astheneia,* weakness]. Neurasthenia caused by ear disease.

otoneurology (ō''tō-nū-rŏl'ō-jĭ) ["+ "+ *logos,* study]. Study of ear conditions in conjunction with neural complications. SYN: *neurotology.*

otopathy (ō-tŏp'ă-thĭ) [Gr. *ous, otos,* ear + *pathos,* disease]. Any diseased condition of the ear.

otopharyngeal (ō''tō-far-ĭn'jē-ăl) ["+ *pharynx,* pharynx]. Concerning the ear and pharynx.

o. tube. Passage between tympanic cavity and the pharynx. SYN: *eustachian tube.*

otophone (ō'tō-fōn) [Gr. *ous, otos-,* ear, + *phōnē,* voice]. Device for assisting deaf to hear.

otopiesis (ō''tō-pī'ē-sĭs) ["+ *piesis,* a pressing]. Abnormal pressure in the ear which produces depression or bulging of the tympani membrane and causes defective hearing.

otoplasty (ō'tō-plăs''tĭ) ["+ *plassein,* to form]. Plastic surgery of the ear to correct defects and deformities.

otopolypus (ō''tō-pŏl'ĭ-pŭs) ["+ *polypous,* a morbid excrescence]. Smooth growth occurring in the ear.

otopyorrhea (ō''tō-pī''ō-re'ă) [Gr. *ous, otos,* ear, + *pyon,* pus, + *rhein,* to flow]. Purulent discharge from the ear.

otopyosis (ō''tō-pī-ō'sĭs) ["+ "+ *-ōsis,* infection]. Ear disease marked by discharge of pus.

otorhinolaryngology (ō''tō-rī''nō-lăr''ĭn-gŏl'ō-jĭ) ["+ *rhis, rhin-,* nose, + *larynx,* larynx, + *logos,* study]. The science of ear, nose, and larynx and their functions and diseases.

otorhinology (ō''tō-rī-nŏl'ō-jĭ) ["+ "+ *logos,* study]. Branch of medicine dealing with the ear and nose and their diseases.

otorrhagia (ō-tō-rā'jĭ-ă) [Gr. *ous, otos-,* ear + *rhēgnynai,* to burst forth]. Discharge of blood from the ear.

otorrhea (ō''tō-rē'ă) ["+ *rhoia,* flow]. Inflammation of ear with purulent discharge. SEE: *otitis.*

otosalpinx (ō''tō-săl'pĭnks) ["+ *salpinx,* trumpet]. Passage connecting pharynx and tympanic cavity. SYN: *eustachian tube; otopharyngeal tube; tuba auditive* [NA].

otoscleronectomy (ō''tō-sklē''rō-nĕk'tō-mĭ) ["+ *sklēros,* hard, + *ektomē,* excision]. Surgical excision of sclerosed and ankylosed ear ossicles.

otosclerosis (ō''tō-sklē-rō'sĭs) [Gr. *ous, ōtos,* ear, + *sklerosis,* hardening]. Condition characterized by chronic progressive deafness esp. for low tones. Caused by formation of spongy bone, esp. around the oval window with resulting ankylosis of stapes. In late stages atrophy of the organ of Corti may occur. More common in females. May be made worse by pregnancy.

ETIOL: Unknown. In some cases, condition is familial.

otoscope (ō'tō-skōp) ["+ *skopein,* to examine]. Device for examination of the ear.

otosis (ō-tō'sĭs) ["+ *-ōsis,* intensive]. Mishearing or misunderstanding of spoken sounds.

otosteal (ō-tŏs'tē-ăl) [Gr. *ous, otos,* ear, + *osteon,* bone]. Concerning the bones or ossicles of the ear.

ototomy (ō-tŏt'ō-mĭ) ["+ *tomē,* incision]. Incision into or dissection of the ear.

O. U., o.u. Abbr. for L. *oculus uterque,* for each eye.

ouabain (wăh-băh'ĭn). USP. A glycoside prepared from Strophanthus gratus. USES: Cardiotonic.

oulitis (oo-lī'tĭs) [Gr. *oulon,* gum, + *ītis,* inflammation]. Ulitis, q.v.

oulorrhagia (oo-lō-rā'jĭ-ă) ["+ *rhēgnynai,* to burst forth]. Hemorrhage from the gums. SYN: *ulorrhagia.*

ounce (ouns) [L. *uncia*, a twelfth]. A measure of weight used in both the avoirdupois and apothecaries' system. ABBR: oz.

Apothecary or *troy* weight: SYMB: ℥. Equivalent to 1/12 lb., 480 gr., 31.103 gm. When used in USP, 1 oz. contains 8 drams.

Avoirdupois measure: Equivalent to 1/16 lb., 437.5 gr., 28.349 gm.

    o., fluid. Apothecaries' measure for liquid medicines, 8 fluid drams (1/16 pint, 29.6 ml.).

outflow. In neurology, the passage of impulses outwardly from the central nervous system.

    o., craniosacral. Impulses passing through parasympathetic nerves.

    o., thoracolumbar. Impulses passing through sympathetic nerves.

outlet. A vent or opening for something to escape.

    o., pelvic. The inferior aperture of the true pelvis.

out'patient. One who receives treatment at a hospital, clinic, or dispensary but is not hospitalized.

ova (ō'vă) [L. *ovum*, egg]. (pl. of *ovum*, q.v.) RS: ovary.

oval (ō'văl) [L. *ovalis*, egg shaped]. 1. Concerning an ovum, the reproductive cell of the female. 2. Having an elliptical shape like an egg.

    o. window. Oval-shaped aperture in the middle ear into which fits the base of the stapes.

ovalbumin (ō″văl-bū′mĭn) ["+ *albumen*, albumin]. Albumin occurring in egg white.

ovalocyte (o'văl-ō-sīt) ["+ Gr. *kytos*, cell]. Elliptical red blood corpuscle.

ovalocytosis (ō-văl″ō-sī-tō′sĭs) ["+ " + *-ōsis*, intensive]. Abnormally large amount of elliptical red blood corpuscles in the blood.

ovaralgia, ovarialgia (o″var-ăl′jĭ-ă, -ĭ-ăl′jĭ-ă) [L. *ovarium*, ovary, + Gr. *algos*, pain]. Ovarian pain. SYN: *oothecalgia; oophoralgia.*

ovarian (ō-vā′rĭ-ăn) [L. *ovarium*, ovary]. Concerning or resembling the ovary.

    o. cyst. A sac that develops in the ovary proper. It consists of one or more chambers containing fluid. These loculi, or chambers, may contain an enormous amt. of fluid. Although nonmalignant, the cyst may prove fatal if not removed because of twisting of the pedicle, which causes gangrene, or because of pressure.

    o. follicle. SEE: *follicle, o.*

ovariectomy (ō-vā-rĭ-ĕk′tō-mĭ) ["+ Gr. *ektomē*, excision]. Excision of an ovary or a portion of it. SYN: *oophorectomy.*

ovario- [Gr. *ovarium*, ovary]. Combining form indicating relationship to the ovary.

ovariocele (ō-vā′rĭ-ō-sēl) [L. *ovarium*, ovary, + Gr. *kēlē*, mass]. Ovarian tumor or hernia.

ovariocentesis (ō-vā-rĭ-ō-sĕn-tē′sĭs) ["+ Gr. *kentēsis*, puncture]. Surgical puncture and drainage of an ovarian cyst.

ovariocyesis (ō-vā″rĭ-ō-sī-ē′sĭs) ["+ Gr. *kyēsis*, pregnancy]. Pregnancy in the ovary.

ovariodysneuria (ō-vā″rĭ-ō-dĭs-nū′rĭ-ă) ["+ Gr. *dys*, ill, + *neuron*, sinew]. Neuralgia in an ovary.

ovariohysterectomy (ō-vā″rĭ-ō-hĭs″tĕr-ĕk′tō-mĭ) ["+ Gr. *hystera*, uterus, + *ektomē*, excision]. Excision of the ovaries and uterus. SYN: *oophorohysterectomy; oothecohysterectomy.*

ovariorrhexis (ō-vā″rĭ-ō-rĕk′sĭs) [L. *ovarium*, ovary, + Gr. *rhēxis*, a rupture]. Rupture of an ovary.

ovariosalpingectomy (ō-vā″rĭ-ō-săl″pĭn-jĕk′tō-mĭ) ["+ Gr. *salpinx*, tube, + *ektomē*, excision]. Removal of an ovary and oviduct. SYN: *oophorosalpingectomy.*

ovariosteresis (ō-vā″rĭ-ō-ster-ē′sĭs) [L. *ovarium*, ovary, + Gr. *sterēsis*, loss]. Removal of an ovary.

ovariostomy (ō-vā-rĭ-ŏs′tō-mĭ) ["+ Gr. *stoma*, opening]. Creation of an opening in an ovarian cyst for drainage purpose.

ovariotexy. Surgical procedure for encompassing the ovaries in a Silastic bag in order to prevent contact of the ovum with sperm.

ovariotomy (ō-vā″rĭ-ŏt′ō-mĭ) ["+ Gr. *tomē*, incision]. 1. Incision into, or removal of, an ovary. 2. Removal of a tumor of the ovary.

ovariotubal (ō-vā″rĭ-ō-tū′băl) ["+ *tuba*, a narrow duct.]. Concerning the ovary and the oviducts.

ovariprival (ō-vā″rĭ-prī′văl) ["+ *privāre*, to remove]. Resulting from loss of the ovaries.

ovaritis (ō-vă-rī′tĭs) [L. *ovarium*, ovary, + Gr. *-itis*, inflammation]. Inflamed condition of an ovary. Usually involved secondarily in inflammation of the oviducts or pelvic peritoneum. May involve the substance of the organ (oophoritis) or its surface (perioophoritis), and may be acute or chronic.

    o., acute. Acute, severe inflammation of the ovary.

    o., chronic. Inflammation of ovary over a long period of time.

ovarium (ō-vā′rĭ-ŭm) [L.]. (pl. *ova′ria*) [NA]. Ovary, q.v.; sexual gland in the female.

ovary (ō′vă-rĭ) [L. *ovarium*, ovary, egg holder]. One of two glands in the female; produces the reproductive cell, the ovum, and two known hormones. The ovaries are almond-shaped bodies lying in the fossa ovarica on either side of the pelvic cavity, attached to the uterus by the utero-ovarian ligament and lying close to the fimbria ovarica of the fallopian tube. About 4 cm. long, 2 cm. wide, and 1.5 cm. thick. Each ovary is attached to the broad ligament by the mesovarium. It is also attached to the side of the uterus by the ovarian ligament and to the side of the pelvis by the suspensory ligament. The surface of the ovary in early life is smooth and in later life is markedly pitted as an end result of the atrophy of corpora lutea.

STRUCTURE: Each ovary consists of two parts, an outer portion or cortex which encloses a central medulla. The medulla consists of a stroma of connective tissue containing nerves, blood, and lymphatic vessels, and some smooth muscle tissue at region of hilus. The cortex consists principally of follicles in various stages of development (primary, growing, and mature or graafian). Its surface is covered by a single layer of cells, the germinal epithelium beneath which is a layer of dense connective tissue, the tunica albuginea. Other structures (corpus luteum, corpus albicans, q.v.) may be present.

BLOOD SUPPLY: Mainly derived from the ovarian artery which reaches the ovary through the infundibulopelvic ligament.

FUNCTION: 1. The production of ova. 2. The production of hormones among which are estrogen, female sex hormones secreted by the follicles, and progesterone, secreted by the corpus luteum. These hormones are responsible for development and maintenance of secondary sexual characteristics, preparation of uterus for pregnancy, and development of the mammary gland.

Functional activity of the ovary is controlled primarily by gonadotrophins of the hypophysis, esp. the follicle stimulating hormone (FSH) and luteinizing hormone (LH) or interstitial cell hormone (ICH).

ovary, words pert. to: adnexitis; albuginea; castrate; cell, interstitial; conception; corpus albicans; dysovarism; facies ovarica; fimbria ovarica; folliculoma; graafian follicle; hyperovaria; Krukenberg's tumor; menstruation; mesosalpinx; mesovarium; oarialgia; pyoovarium; spay; spermatozoon; stroma; teratoma; tunica albuginea; and words beginning with "oophor-" and "ov-".

overbite. The vertical extension of the upper teeth over the lower anterior teeth when the jaws are in centric occlusion.

overcompensation. The process by which a person substitutes an opposite trait or in which he exerts effort in excess of that needed to compensate for, or conceal, a psychological feeling of guilt, inadequacy, or inferiority. May lead to maladjustment.

overcorrection. The use of too powerful a lens to correct the defect in refractive power of the eye.

overdetermination. The idea in psychoanalysis that every symptom and dream may have several meanings, being determined by more than a single association.

overexertion. Physical exertion to a state of exhaustion.

overextension. Hyperextension; extension beyond that which usually occurs.

overflow. The continuous escape of fluid from a vessel or viscus, as of urine or tears.

overgrowth. Excessive growth; hypertrophy or hyperplasia. In bacteriology, the growth of one type of microorganism on a culture plate so that it covers and obscures the growth of other types.

overlay. An addition superimposed upon an already existing state.

    o., psychiatric. Mental symptoms added to those initially present because of the basic disease or defect.

overproduction. Excessive output of an organic element during the reparative process, as excessive callous development after a bone fracture.

overriding. The slipping of one end of a fractured bone past the other part.

overtone. In music and acoustics, a harmonic.

    o., psychic. An awareness of additional impressions associated with any stimulus.

overweight. Weighing more than is generally accepted to be normal. SYN: *obesity.*

overwork. Excessive work causing exhaustion. SEE: *ergasthenia.*

ovi- [L. *ovum*]. Combining form meaning egg.

ovi albumen (ō″vĭ ăl-bū′mĭn) [L.]. White of egg. SYN: *ovalbumin.*

oviduct (ō′vĭ-dŭkt) [L. *ovum*, egg, + *ductus*, a path]. One of two tubes extending laterally from superior angles of the uterus; serves to convey the ovum from the ovary to the uterus. Each o. consists of the infundibulum, expanded portion surrounding the ostium or opening through which the ovum enters, bearing many fingerlike processes called fimbria; the ampulla, the tube itself; and the isthmus, a straight narrow portion that connects with the uterus.

Each oviduct is a muscular tube consisting of three layers-mucosa, muscular layer, and serosa. The mucosa consists of columnar epithelial cells, some ciliated, others glandular. In addition to conveying the ovum, the oviduct provides a passageway through which sperm travel from the uterus toward the ovary. It is the usual site of fertilization of the ovum. SYN: *uterine tube; fallopian tube.*

oviferous (ō-vĭf'ĕr-ŭs) ["+ *ferre*, to bear]. Containing or producing ova. SYN: *ovigerous.*

ovification (ō-vĭ-fĭ-kā'shŭn) ["+ *facere*, to make]. The production of ova. SYN: *ovulation.*

oviform (ō'vĭ-form) [L. *ovum*, egg, + *forma*, shape]. 1. Having the shape of an egg. SYN: *ovoid.* 2. Resembling an ovum.

ovigenesis ["+ Gr. *gennan*, to produce]. Oogenesis, q.v.

ovigenous (ō-vij'ĕn-us). Giving rise to ova.

ovigerm (ō'vĭ-jĕrm) [L. *ovum*, egg, + *germen*, a bud]. The cell which produces or develops into an ovum.

ovigerous (ō-vĭj'ĕr-ŭs) ["+ *gerere*, to bear]. Producing or carrying ova. SYN: *oviferous.*

oviparous (ō-vĭp'ăr-ŭs) ["+ *parere*, to produce]. Producing eggs which are hatched outside the body; egg laying. Opposed to ovoviviparous.

oviposition ["+ *ponere*, to place]. The laying of eggs as in oviparous reproduction.

ovipositor (o''vĭ-pŏs'ĭ-tor). A specialized tubular structure found in many female insects, through which they lay their eggs in plants or soil.

ovo- [L. *ovum*, egg]. Combining form indicating relationship to an egg.

ovocenter. The centrosome of a fertilized ovum.

ovoflavin (ō''vō-flā'vin) [L. *ovum*, egg, + *flavus*, yellow]. A flavin derived from eggs; identical to riboflavin.

ovogenesis (ō''vō-jĕn'ĕ-sĭs) ["+ Gr. *genesis*, production]. Production of ova. SYN: *oogenesis.*

ovoglobulin (ō''vō-glŏb'ū-lĭn) ["+ *globulus*, globule]. The globulin found in egg white. SEE: *albumin; protein, simple.*

ovoid (ō'voyd) [L. *ovum*, egg, + Gr. *eidos*, form]. Egg shaped. SYN: *oviform.*

ovomucoid (ō''vō-mū'koyd) ["+ *mucus*, mucus, + Gr. *eidos*, form]. A glycoprotein principle derived from egg white.

ovoplasm (ō'vō-plazm) ["+ Gr. *plasma*, anything formed]. Protoplasm of an unfertilized egg. SEE: *ooplasm.*

ovovitellin (ō''vō-vī-tĕl'ĭn) ["+ *vitellus*, yolk]. Protein found in an egg yolk.

ovoviviparous (ō''vō-vī-vip'ă-rŭs) [L. *ovum*, egg, + *vivus*, a live, + *parere*, to bear]. Reproducing by eggs which have a well-developed shell and which hatch inside the maternal organism. Opposed to oviparous.

ovula (ŏv'ū-lă) [L.]. (sing. *ovulum*) Little eggs.

o. nabothi. Distended mucous glands in tissues of the cervix uteri.

ovular (ō'vū-lăr) [L. *ovulum*, little egg]. Concerning an ovule or ovum.

ovulation (ōv''ū-lā'shŭn) [L. *ovulum*, little egg]. The periodic ripening and rupture of the mature graafian follicle and the discharge of the ovum from the cortex of the ovary. Ovulation occurs approximately 14 days before the next menstrual period. It is virtually impossible to determine when ovulation will occur by counting from the first day of the preceding menstrual period. Following ovulation, a corpus luteum develops within the collapsed follicle. SEE: *corpus luteum.*

The ovum, being liberated from the follicle, enters the fallopian tube and is transported slowly toward the uterus. If sperm are present, it may become fertilized; if not, the ovum degenerates within the oviduct and is passed out of the body with the menstrual flow.

RS: anovular; conception; menstruation; ovary; ovum; spermatozoon; fertilization; follicle; corpus luteum.

ovulatory (ōv'ū-lă-tō''rĭ). Concerning ovulation.

ovulogenous (ō-vū-lŏj'ĕn-ŭs). 1. Giving rise to ovules or ova. 2. Originating from an ovule or ovum.

ovum (ō'vum) [L., egg]. (pl. *ova*) [NA] The female reproductive or germ cell; a cell which is capable of developing into a new organism of the same species. Usually fertilization by a spermatozoon is necessary, although in some lower animals ova develop without fertilization (parthenogenesis).

The various parts of the ovum have been named as follows: The protoplasm is known as the *vitellus* or *yolk;* the outer layer is referred to as the *ectoplasm, zona pellucida,* or *zona radiata;* the inner layer, the cell membrane, is the *vitelline membrane;* the nucleus is called the *germinal vesicle;* and the nucleolus is the *germinal spot.*

The cellular layers proliferate, becoming cuboid in shape, and in the center a clear albuminous fluid, the liquor folliculi, forms. The follicular cells surrounding the fluid-filled cavity are known as the membrana granulosa. The layer surrounding the egg cell, or oocyte, is known as the discus proligerus or cumulus oophorus.

As the follicular layer enlarges to form the *graafian follicle,* the term for the developed ovum before it leaves the ovary, there is a slight protrusion of the ovarian surface. Rupture through the ovarian surface frees the ovum, which then proceeds through the fallopian tube and into the uterus. This process is known as ovulation, q.v. It usually takes the ovum from 5 to 7 days to go from the ovary to the uterus. SEE: *menstruation.*

Normally, only one graafian follicle matures each month, not necessarily in alternate ovaries.

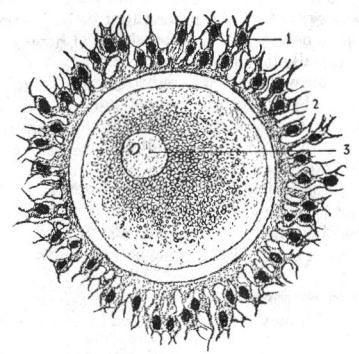

**MATURE HUMAN OVUM AFTER
DISCHARGE FROM FOLLICLE**

1, Cells of corona radiata. 2, Zone pellucida. 3, Nucleus or germinal vesicle.

o., alecithal. One in which there is little or no food yolk.

o., centrolecithal. One having a large central food yolk, as in a bird's egg.

o., holoblastic. O. that undergoes complete cleavage.

o., human. The female reproductive cell which develops within the graafian follicle of the ovary. It develops from an oogonium that undergoes a process of maturation (oogenesis) during which primary and secondary oocytes are produced, finally giving rise to the mature ovum. During this process the number of chromosomes is reduced from 46 to 23 and the egg is prepared for fertilization.

A mature ovum is approximately 0.130 mm. to 0.140 mm. in diameter .0051 to .0055 inch. Each contains a spherical nucleus, bounded by a nuclear membrane, enclosing chromatin material and one or more nucleoli. The cytoplasm is granular and contains yolk granules or deutoplasm and other characteristic organoids of cells. Its surface layer is the vitelline membrane. When liberated from the ovary as a primary oocyte it is surrounded by a clear layer, zona pellucida, and several layers of adhering follicular cells, the latter constituting the corona radiata.

The length of time a human ovum retains its ability to be fertilized and develop is not known precisely but it is probably at least 48 hours. If fertilized, it undergoes development. If not fertilized, it degenerates. SEE: *embryo, development of; cleavage; follicle; conception; fertilization; menstruation; ovulation; spermatozoa.*

o., isolecithal. O. in which the yolk is uniformly distributed.

o., meroblastic. O. in which only the protoplasmic region undergoes cleavage; characteristic in ova containing a large amount of yolk.

o., permanent. O. ready for fertilization.

o., primordial. Germ cells that arise very early in development of embryo, usually in yolk sac endoderm, and migrate into urogenital ridge and possibly serve as progenitors of functional sex cells.

o., telolecithal. O. in which yolk is fairly abundant and tends to concentrate in one hemisphere.

ox. Abbr. for *oxymel.*

ox-. Combining form indicating presence of oxygen.

oxa-. Combining form indicating presence of oxygen in place of carbon.

oxacid (ŏks'ă-sĭd) [Gr. *oxys,* sour, + L. *acidum,* acid]. An acid of which oxygen is a constituent.

oxacillin (oks"ă-sil'in). A semisynthetic penicillin.

oxal-, oxalo-. Combining forms indicating derivation from oxalic acid.

oxalacetic acid (ŏks"ăl-ă-sē'tĭk). A product of carbohydrate metabolism resulting from oxidation of malic acid. May be derived from other sources. SYN: *oxyaloacetic acid.*

oxalate (ŏk'să-lāt) [Gr. *oxalis,* sorrel]. A salt of oxalic acid.

oxalic acid (ŏks -ăl'ĭk). A white crystalline powder often used about the home as a stain remover or bleach, resembling Epsom salts in appearance. O. a. rapidly reduces blood coagulation time, thus its value in treating hemorrhage, jaundice, etc. SYN: *ethanedioic acid.*

SOURCES: Cranberries, chard, rhubarb, gooseberries, spinach, beet leaves. When these are eaten they should be accompanied by liberal portions of calcium foods, such as eggs, beans, and milk.

POISONING SYM: Erosive action on swallowing; sour taste; burning in mouth, throat, and stomach; great thirst; bloody vomitus; collapse; sometimes convulsions and coma.

TREATMENT: Prompt treatment with any soluble calcium salt such as powdered chalk in water or milk, lime water, or calcium lactate. This procedure inactivates the acid by precipitating it as an insoluble calcium salt. Careful gastric lavage with dilute lime water. Do not induce vomiting. Intravenous calcium gluconate or calcium chloride to treat tetany. Morphine may be required for pain. SEE: *Table of Poisons* in *Appendix.*

    o. a. diathesis. Chronic state of oxalemia.

oxalism (ok'săl-izm) [Gr. *oxalis*, sorrel, + *ismos*, state of]. Poisoning from oxalic acid or an oxalate.

oxaluria (ok-sa-lū'rĭ-ă) ["+ *ouron*, urine]. Excess excretion of oxalates in the urine, esp. calcium oxalate.

oxalylurea (ŏk″să-lĭl-ū-rē'ă). An oxidation product of uric acid.

oxidase (ŏk'sĭ-dās) [Gr. *oxys*, sour]. An enzyme present in animal and vegetable life which catalyzes an oxidation reaction; a respiratory enzyme.

    o., cytochrome. Enzyme present in most cells which oxidizes reduced cytochrome back to cytochrome.

oxidation (ok'sĭ-dā'shŭn) [Gr. *oxys*, sour]. 1. The process of a substance combining with oxygen. 2. The loss of electrons in an atom with an accompanying increase in positive valence.

oxide (ŏk'sīd). Any chemical compound in which oxygen is the negative radical.

oxidize (ŏk'sĭ-dīz). 1. To combine with oxygen. 2. To increase the positive valence, or to decrease the negative valence, by bringing about a loss of electrons.

oximeter (ŏk-sĭm'ĕ-ter) [Gr. *oxys*, sour, + *metron*, measure]. Photoelectric apparatus for determining the amount of oxygen in the blood. Usually done by measuring the amount of light transmitted through a translucent part of the skin.

    o., ear. O. attached to pinna of the ear to determine blood flow.

oxonemia (ŏk″sō-nē'mĭ-ă) [L. *oxone*, acetone, + Gr. *haima*, blood]. Excess of acetone bodies found in the blood. SYN: *acetonemia.*

oxophenarsine hydrochloride. USP. An antitrypanosomal compound containing 30% arsenic.

oxy- [Gr. *oxys*]. Combining form indicating (1) sharp, keen, acute, acid, pungent; (2) presence of oxygen in a compound; (3) presence of a hydroxyl group.

oxyacusis (ŏk″sĭ-ă-kū'sĭs) [Gr. *oxys*, acute, + *akousis*, hearing]. Abnormally acute hearing. SYN: *hyperacusis.*

oxybenzene (ŏk″sĭ-bĕn'zēn). Phenol, q.v.

oxyblepsia (ŏk″sĭ-blĕp'sĭ-ă) [Gr. *oxys*, acute + *blepsis*, vision]. Extraordinary acuteness of vision.

oxybutyria (ŏk″sĭ-bū-tĭr'ĭ-ă). Oxybutyric acid in the blood or in the urine.

oxycalcium (ok″sĭ-kal'sĭ-ŭm). Of or pertaining to oxygen and calcium.

oxycephalia (ŏk″sĭ-sĕf-ă'lĭ-ă) [Gr. *oxys*, sharp, + *kephalē*, head]. State of having a high and pointed skull.

oxycephalous (ŏk-sĭ-sef'ă-lŭs). Denoting a head that is pointed and conelike.

oxychloride (ŏk″sĭ-klō'rĭd) [Gr. *oxys*, sharp, + *chlōros*, green]. A compound consisting of an element or radical combined with oxygen and chlorine or the hydroxyl radical (OH) and chlorine.

oxychromatic (ŏk″sĭ-krō-măt'ĭk) ["+ *chrōma*, color]. Staining readily with acid dyes.

oxychromatin (ŏk″sĭ-krō'mă-tĭn). That part of chromatin that stains readily with acid dyes.

oxycinesia (ŏk″sĭ-sĭ-nē'zĭ-ă) [Gr. *oxys*, keen, + *kinēsis*, movement]. Pain experienced on moving.

oxydase (ŏk'sĭ-dās) ["+ *ase*, enzyme]. Old spelling of oxidase, q.v.

oxyecoia (ok″sĭ-ē-koy'ă) ["+ *akoē*, hearing]. Abnormal sensitivity to noises.

oxyesthesia (ŏk″sĭ-ĕs-thē'zĭ-ă) ["+ *aisthēsis*, sensation]. Abnormal acuteness of sensation. SYN: *algesia; hyperesthesia.*

oxygen (ŏk'sĭ-jĕn) [Gr. *oxys*, sour, + *gennan*, to produce]. USP. SYMB: *O*. At. wt. 15.9994; at. no. 8. A nonmetallic element occurring free in the atmosphere as a colorless, odorless, tasteless gas. It is a constituent of animal, vegetable, and mineral substances, comprising by weight 3/4 of the animal, 4/5 of the vegetable, and 1/2 of the mineral world; and by volume 1/5 of the atmosphere; and by weight 8/9 of water.

O. is essential to respiration of most forms of animal and plant life, and is the most important and abundant element. It represents 65% of the elements in the body: 10-16% in venous and 17-21% in arterial blood at sea level.

It is the only element that enters the animal organism in a free state. It is absorbed by plants in the form of water and carbon dioxide, converted by them into organic substances which are used as food by man, and returned to the atmosphere by man in form of waste products of water and carbon dioxide. Thus the balance of oxygen and carbon dioxide in the atmosphere is maintained.

When O. combines with another substance, the process is called oxidation. When combination takes place rapidly enough to produce light and heat, the process is called burning or *combustion.* O. combines readily with other elements to form oxides.

USES: In conditions in which there is insufficient oxygen carried by the blood to the tissues. Therefore O. is used in cases of severe anemia, shock or circulatory collapse, pulmonary edema, pneumonia; or by mountain climbers, astronauts, or aviators when at heights where the amount of oxygen present in the atmosphere is insufficient to support life.

Oxygen is administered by mask, nasal tube, tent, or by placing the patient in an airtight chamber in which pressure may be increased. No matter how much O. is given it is important to have it adequately humidified. It is desirable to administer O. at whatever rate is necessary to increase the O. content of inspired air to 50%.

Frequently O. is employed with ether or other agents used for the induction of general anesthesia. Following extensive surgery it reduces reactions to anesthetic. Also employed in septicemia, gas gangrene, peritonitis, and intestinal obstruction.

Oxygen is used under pressure in chambers for cardiac surgery; in treating aerobic infections such as gas gangrene, vascular disorders, carbon monoxide poisoning; and in connection with radiation therapy of tumors. When oxygen is used in this manner it is called hyperbaric oxygenation.

CAUTION: Inhalation of high concentrations of oxygen, esp. at pressures of more than one atmosphere, may produce deleterious effects such as irritation of respiratory tract, reduced vital capacity, and sometimes neurological symptoms. Serious eye defects may result in premature infants. SEE: *retrolental fibroplasia.*

O will explode. Prohibit smoking, open flames, or static electricity in the vicinity of O apparatus.

o. capacity. The maximum amount of oxygen expressed in volume per cent (cc. per 100 cc.) which a given amount of blood will absorb. For normal blood it is about 20 cc.

o. content. The amount of oxygen in volume per cent which is present in the blood at any one moment.

o. debt. The amount of oxygen required after muscular activity for the removal of lactic acid and other metabolic products which accumulate when the supply of oxygen is below the needs of the organism.

o. dissociation curve. A curve which shows relationship between partial pressure of oxygen and the percentage saturation of hemoglobin with oxygen, i.e., the proportion of oxyhemoglobin to reduced hemoglobin. Factors which favor shift of curve to the right, accelerating the decomposition of hemoglobin, are a rise in temperature and an increase of H ions that results from liberation of CO_2 and formation of lactic acid.

o. saturation. Oxygen content of blood divided by oxygen capacity and expressed in volume per cent.

o. tent. An airtight enclosure for a patient's head and shoulders in which the oxygen content of the air can be raised above normal.

o. therapy. The administration of oxygen for the treatment of conditions resulting from oxygen deficiency. It is used to combat acute arterial anoxia that may result from pneumonia, pulmonary edema, or obstruction to breathing. It is also employed in congestive heart failure, coronary thrombosis, and following surgery. It may be administered by nasal catheter, mask (nasal or oronasal), funnel or cone, oxygen tent, or special oxygen chamber, and usually in a concentration of 70-100%.

o. toxicity. Progressive failure of ventilation of the lungs which develops when pure oxygen is breathed for a prolonged period. Failure of ventilation leads to decreased oxygen tension in the blood.

o. want. Anoxia, oxygen lack.

oxygenase (ŏk'sĭ-jĕn-ās) [Gr. *oxys,* sharp, + *gennan,* to produce, + *ase,* enzyme]. An enzyme which enables an organism to use atmospheric oxygen in respiration.

oxygenate (ŏk'sĭ-jĕn-āt). To combine or supply with oxygen.

oxygenation (ŏk"sĭ-jĕn-a'shŭn). Saturation or combination with oxygen, as the aeration of the blood in the lungs.

o., hyperbaric. Administration of oxygen under increased pressure while patient is in an airtight chamber. Used for certain surgical procedures, treatment of aerobic infections such as gas gangrene, and in conjunction with radiation therapy of tumors.

oxygenic (ŏk"sĭ-jĕn'ĭk) [Gr. *oxys,* oxygen, + *gennan,* to produce]. Concerning, resembling, containing, or consisting of oxygen.

oxygenize. To oxidize, q.v.

oxygeusia (ŏk"sĭ-gū'sĭ-ă) [Gr. *oxys,* keen, + *geusis,* taste]. Abnormally keen sense of taste.

oxyhematin. An iron compound which constitutes the coloring matter in oxyhemoglobin. When oxidized it yields hematinic acid; when reduced, hematoporphyrin.

oxyhemoglobin (ŏk″sĭ-hē″mō-glō′bĭn) ["+ *haima,* blood, + L. *globus,* a sphere]. The combined form of hemoglobin and oxygen. Hemoglobin with oxygen is found in arterial blood and is the oxygen carrier to the body tissues.

oxyhemoglobinometer (ŏk″sĭ-hē″mō-glō″-bĭn-ŏm′ĕt-ĕr) ["+ "+ "+ Gr. *metron,* a measure]. Apparatus for measurement of amount of oxygen in the blood.

oxyhydrocephalus (ŏk″sĭ-hī-drō-sĕf′ăl-ŭs) [Gr. *oxys,* sharp, + *hydōr,* water, + *kephalē,* brain]. Type of hydrocephalus in which the head has a pointed shape.

oxyiodide (ŏk″sĭ-ĭ′ō-did) [Gr. *oxys,* oxygen, + *ioeides,* violet colored]. Compound of iodine and oxygen with an element or radical.

oxylalia (ok″sĭ-lā′lĭ-ă) [Gr. *oxys,* swift, + *lalein,* to speak]. Abnormal rapidity of speech.

oxyntic (ŏk-sĭn′tĭk) [Gr. *oxynein,* to make acid]. Producing or secreting acid. SEE: *cell.*

oxyopia (ŏk″sĭ-ō′pĭ-ă) [Gr. *oxys,* sharp, + *ōps,* sight]. Unusual acuteness of vision.

oxyopter (ŏk″sĭ-ŏp′tĕr). A unit of measuring visual acuity; the reciprocal of the visual angle expressed in degrees.

oxyosmia (ŏk″sĭ-ŏz′mĭ-ă) ["+ *osmē,* odor]. Unusual acuity of sense of smell.

oxyosphresia (ok″sĭ-ŏs-frē′zĭ-ă) ["+ *osphrēsis,* smell]. Abnormal acuity of the sense of smell.

oxypathia, oxypathy (ok″sĭ-păth′ĭ-ă, -sĭp′ăth-ĭ) [Gr. *oxys,* sharp, + *pathos,* feeling]. 1. Unusual acuity of sensation. 2. An acute condition. 3. Condition in which the body is unable to eliminate unoxidizable acids which combine with fixed alkalies of the tissues and harm the organism.

oxyperitoneum (ŏk″sĭ-pĕr-ĭ-tō-nē′ŭm) [Gr. *oxys,* oxygen + *peritonaion,* peritoneum]. Introduction of oxygen into the peritoneal cavity.

oxyphil(e (ok′sĭ-fĭl, -fĭl) ["+ *philein,* to love]. 1. Staining readily with acid dyes. 2. A cell which stains readily with acid dyes.

oxyphilous (ŏk-sĭf′ĭl-ŭs). Having an affinity for acid dyes. SYN: *oxyphil.*

oxyphonia (ok″sĭ-fō′nĭ-ă) [Gr. *oxyphōnia*]. An abnormally sharp or shrill pitch to the voice.

oxypurine (ŏk″sĭ-pū′rĕn) [Gr. *oxys,* sharp, + L. *purus,* pure, + *urina,* urine]. An oxidation product of purine. Includes hypoxanthine, xanthine, and uric acid.

oxyrhine (ŏk′sĭ-rĭn) ["+ *rhis,* nose]. 1. Having a sharp-pointed nose. 2. Possessing an acute sense of smell.

oxytetracycline (ŏks″ĭ-tĕt″ră-sī′klēn). One of a group of broad-spectrum antibiotic substances called tetracyclines. Originally obtained from a strain of Streptomyces, it is now prepared synthetically.

oxytocia (ŏk″sĭ-tō′sĭ-ă) [Gr. *oxys,* swift, + *tokos,* childbirth]. Unusual rapidity of childbirth.

oxytocic (ŏk″sĭ-tō′sĭk). 1. Agent which stimulates uterine contractions. 2. Accelerating childbirth.

     o. principle. A hormone stored in the posterior lobe of hypophysis which acts specifically on smooth musculature of the uterus increasing tone of, and inducing, uterine contractions. SYN: *oxytocin,* q.v.

oxytocin (ŏk″sĭ-tō′sĭn). A pituitary hormone that stimulates the uterus to contract, thus inducing parturition. It also acts on the mammary gland to stimulate the release of milk.

     o. injection. USP. An aqueous solution containing the oxytocic principle of the posterior pituitary gland.

oxyuriasis (ŏk″sĭ-ū-rī′ăs-ĭs) [Gr. *oxys,* sharp, + *oura,* tall, + *iasis,* infection]. Infestation with Enterobius vermicularis (pinworm), q.v.

oxyuricide (ŏk″sĭ-ū′rĭ-sĭd) ["+ "+ L. *caedere,* to kill]. Destructive to pinworms, such as an agent that destroys them.

oxyurid. Pinworm or seatworm. SEE: *Enterobius vermicularis.*

Oxyuris [Gr. *oxys,* sharp, + *oura,* tail]. Old name for genus of nematode intestinal worms which includes the pinworms or seatworms. SEE: *Enterobius.*

     o. vermicularis. Enterobius vermicularis, q.v.

oyster (oi′ster) [AS. *oistre*]. Shellfish eaten raw or cooked. When eaten raw or partially cooked may be source of infectious hepatitis virus.

     Food value of 100 gm. (raw, meat only, Eastern): Cal. 66; protein 8.4 gm.; fat 1.8 gm.; carbohydrate 3.4 gm.; sodium 73 mg.; calcium 94 mg.; vitamin A, 310 I.U.

oz. Abbr. for *ounce.*

oz. ap. Abbr. for the pharmaceutical term *ounce apothecary's.*

oz. av. Abbr. for the term *ounce avoirdupois.*

ozena (ō-zē′nă) [Gr. *ozē,* stench]. Disease of the nose characterized by atrophy of the turbinates and mucous membrane accompanied by considerable crusting, discharge, and a very offensive odor. It is present in various forms of rhinitis.

ozochrotia (ō″zō-krō′shĭ-ă) ["+ *chrōs*, skin]. Strong odor given off by the skin. SYN: *bromidrosis*.

ozonator (ō′zō-nā″tor). Device for generating ozone.

ozone (ō′zōn) [G. *ozein*, to smell]. A form of oxygen in which three atoms of the element combine to form the molecule O_3.

ozonization (ō″zō-nĭ-zā′shŭn). The act of converting to, or impregnating with, ozone.

ozonize (ō′zō-nīz) [Gr. *ozein*, to smell]. 1. To convert oxygen to ozone, q.v. 2. To impregnate the air of a substance with ozone.

ozonometer (ō″zō-nom′ĕt-ĕr) [Gr. *ozē*, stench, + *metron*, a measure]. An apparatus for estimating the quantity of ozone in the atmosphere.

ozonoscope (ō-zō′nō-skōp) ["+ *skopein*, to examine]. A device for showing the presence or amount of ozone.

ozostomia (ō″zō-stō′mĭ-ă) [Gr. *ozē*, stench, + *stoma*, mouth]. Fetid breath, halitosis.

P

P. Symb. for *phosphorus.* Abbr. for *position, posterior, postpartum, pressure, pulse, pupil, probability* (in statistics).

P₁. Symb. for *first parental generation* (in genetics). Abbr. for *first pulmonic heart sound.*

P₂. Abbr. for *pulmonic second sound.*

P³²; ³²P. Symb. for *radioactive isotope of phosphorus.*

p. Abbr. for *page, pupil.*

p-. Abbr. for *para-* in chemical formulas.

P & A. Abbr. for *percussion and auscultation.*

Pa. Chemical symb. for *protactinium.*

P-A, p-a. Abbr. for *posteroanterior.*

PABA. Abbr. for *para-aminobenzoic acid,* q.v.

pablum (păb'lŭm). Proprietary or trade name for a cereal food for infants.

pabular (păb'ū-lar) [L. *pabulum,* food]. Pert. to nourishment.

pabulum (păb'ū-lŭm) [L.]. Food; nourishment.

PAC. Abbr. for *phenacetin, aspirin,* and *caffeine.*

pacchionian (păk″ē-ō'nĭ-ăn). [Antonio Pacchioni, It. anatomist, 1665-1726]. Used as an adjective.

   p. bodies. Enlarged villi, small pedunculated or rounded growths of fibrous tissue along longitudinal fissure of the cerebrum growing on arachnoid membrane.

   p. depressions. Small pits produced on inner surface of skull by protuberance of p. bodies.

   p. glands. SEE: *p. bodies.*

pacemaker (pās'māk-ĕr) [L. *passus,* a step, + AS. *macian,* to make]. 1. The sinoatrial node, so named because cardiac rhythm commences here, taking place near the spot where the large veins empty into the atrium. 2. An object that influences the rate of occurrence of an event.

   cardiac p., artificial or electric. An electrical device which can substitute for a defective natural pacemaker and control the beating of the heart by a series of rhythmic electrical discharges. If the electrodes which deliver the discharges to the heart are placed on the outside of the chest, the device is called an *external pacemaker.* If the electrodes are placed within the chest wall, it is called an *internal pacemaker.*

pacer. Pacemaker.

pachismus (păk-ĭz'mŭs) [Gr. *pachys,* thick, + *ismos,* condition]. Condensation or thickening of an organ or part.

pachy-, pach- [Gr. *pachys,* thick, clotted]. Combining form meaning thick, large, heavy, massive.

pachyacria, pachyakria (păk″ĭ-ā'krĭ-ā) [Gr. *pachys,* thick, + *akron,* end]. Hypertrophy of soft portions of the extremities.

pachyblepharon (păk″ĭ-blĕf'ă-rŏn) [″+ *blepharon,* eyelid]. A thickening of the border of the eyelid.

pachyblepharosis (păk″ĭ-blĕf'ă-rō'sĭs). Chronic thickening of the eyelid.

pachycephalic (păk″ĭ-sĕ-fal'ĭk) [Gr. *pachys,* thick, + *kephalē,* brain]. Possessing an abnormally thick skull. SYN: *pachycephalous.*

pachycephalous (păk″ĭ-sĕf'a-lŭs). Thick skulled. SYN: *pachycephalic.*

pachycephaly (păk″ĭ-sĕf'ă-lĭ). Unusual thickness of the walls of the skull.

pachychilia (păk″ĭ-kī'lĭ-ā) [Gr. *pachys,* thick, + *cheilos,* lip]. Unusual thickness of the lips.

pachycholia (păk″ĭ-kō'lĭ-ā) [″+ *cholē,* bile]. Thickening or inspissation of the bile.

pachychromatic (păk″ĭ-krō-măt'ĭk) [″+ *chrōma,* color]. Possessing a coarse chromatin network.

pachycolpismus (păk″ĭ-kŏl-pĭz'mŭs) [Gr. *pachys,* thick, + *kolpos,* vagina, + *ismos,* condition]. Chronic inflammation of vagina with thickened vaginal walls. SYN: *pachyvaginitis.*

pachydactylia, pachydactyly (păk″ĭ-dăk-til'ĭä, -dak″tī-lĭ) [″+ *daktylos,* digit]. Condition marked by unusually large fingers and toes.

pachyderma (păk-ĭ-der'mä) [″+ *derma,* skin]. Unusual thickness of the skin. SYN: *pachydermia.*

pachydermatocele (păk″ĭ-dĕr-măt'ō-sēl) [″+ ″+ *kēlē,* swelling]. 1. A pendulous state of the skin with thickening. SYN: *dermatolysis; cutis laxa.* 2. Huge neurofibroma. SYN: *elephantiasis neuromatosa.*

pachydermatosis (păk″ĭ-dĕr″mă-tō'sĭs) [″+ ″+ *-ōsis,* condition]. Chronic hypertrophy of the skin. SYN: *pachydermia.*

pachydermatous (păk-ĭ-der'mă-tŭs) [Gr. *pachys,* thick, + *derma,* skin]. Possessing a thick skin.

pachydermia (păk-ĭ-der'mĭ-ä). 1. Excessive thickening of the skin. 2. Elephantiasis, q.v.

   p. laryngis. Irregular thickening and hypertrophy of mucous membrane in the larynx seen in chronic laryngitis.

p. lymphangiectatica. A diffuse form of skin thickening due to blocked or defective lymph drainage.

p., occipital. A disease in which the skin of the scalp, esp. in occipital region, falls into thickened folds.

p. vesica. Condition in which there is a thickened mucous membrane in the urinary bladder.

pachydermoperiostosis. Hereditary form of osteoarthropathy with marked thickening of the skin over the face and extremities. It is self-limiting with an active progressive phase during adolescence.

pachyemia (păk-ĭ-ē'mĭ-ă) [Gr. *pachys*, thick, + *haima*, blood]. Thickness of the blood.

pachyglossia (păk''ĭ-glŏs'sĭ-ă) ["+ *glossa*, tongue]. Unusual thickness of the tongue.

pachygnathous (pă-kĭg'năth-ŭs) ["+ *gnathos*, jaw]. Having a thick or large jaw.

pachygyria (păk-ĭ-jĭ'rĭ-ă) ["+ *gyros*, a circle]. Flat, broad formation of the cerebral convolutions.

pachyhematous (păk-ĭ-hĕm'ă-tŭs) [Gr. *pachys*, thick, + *haima*, blood]. Having, or pert. to, thickened blood.

pachyhemia (păk-ĭ-hē'mĭ-ă). A thickened state of the blood.

pachyleptomeningitis (păk-ĭ-lĕp''tō-mĕn''ĭn-jī'tĭs) [Gr. *pachys*, thick, + *leptos*, thin, + *mēninx*, membrane, + *-itis*, inflammation]. Inflammation of pia and dura of the brain and spinal cord.

pachylosis (păk-ĭ-lō'sĭs) [Gr. *pachylos*, thick, + *-osis*, condition]. A chronic condition of rough, dry, thickened skin. SYN: *xerosis.*

pachymenia (păk-ĭ-mē'nĭ-ă) [Gr. *pachys*, thick, + *hymen*, membrane]. Thickening of the skin or membranes.

pachymeningitis (păk-ĭ-mĕn''ĭn-jī'tĭs) ["+ *mēninx*, membrane, + *itis*, inflammation]. Inflamed condition of the dura mater. Inflammation of the pia, dura, or arachnoid membranes is sure to extend to one or both of the others, and the consequence in any form is suppuration, abscess, effusion into the ventricles, and softening of cerebral tissue if brain is involved.

p. externa. Inflammation of outer layer of dura mater.

p., hemorrhagic. Circumscribed effusion of blood on inner surface of dura with inflammation. SYN: *chronic subdural hematoma.*

SYM: Intermittent headache, choked disks, hemiparesis, dilated pupil, unconsciousness in varying degrees.

ETIOL: Usually the result of trauma, such as a blow, resulting in a venous tear. Blood oozes into subdural space; a blood clot

is formed which becomes encysted, giving rise to a hematoma.

p. interna. Inflammation of inner layer of dura mater.

p., spinal. Inflammation of the dura of the spinal cord.

pachymeningopathy (păk''ĭ-mĕn''ĭn-gŏp'ă-thĭ) ["+ "+ *pathos*, disease]. Any disease of the dura mater.

pachymeninx (păk-ĭ-mē'nĭnks) [Gr. *pachys*, thick, + *mēninx*, membrane]. Membrane known as the dura mater.

pachymeter (păk-ĭm'ē-tĕr) ["+ *metron*, measure]. Instrument for measuring thickness of objects, esp. thin objects.

pachynsis (pă-kĭn'sĭs) [Gr.]. Thickening of a substance or part, usually abnormal.

pachyntic (pă-kĭn'tĭk) [Gr. *pachynsis*, a thickening]. Pert. to abnormal thickening.

pachyonychia (păk''ĭ-ō-nĭk'ĭ-ă) [Gr. *pachys*, thick, + *onyx, onych-*, nail]. Abnormal thickening of finger or toe nails.

p. congenita. A congenital condition characterized by thickening of the nails, thickening of the skin on palms of hands and soles of feet, follicular keratosis at knees and elbows, and corneal dyskeratosis.

pachyostosis (păk''ĭ-ŏs-tō'sĭs) ["+ *osteon*, bone, + *-ōsis*, disease]. A benign condition of thickening of the bones.

pachyotia (păk-ĭ-ō'shĭ-ă) ["+ *ous, ōt-*, ear]. Abnormal thickness of the ears.

pachypelviperitonitis (păk''ĭ-pĕl''vĭ-pĕr''ĭ-tō-nī'tĭs) ["+ L. *pelvis*, basin, + Gr. *peritonaion*, peritoneum, + *-itis*, inflammation]. Inflammation of the pelvic and peritoneal membranes with hypertrophy and thickening of their surfaces.

pachyperitonitis (păk''ĭ-pĕr''ĭ-tō-nī'tĭs) ["+ *peritonaion*, peritoneum, + *-itis*, inflammation]. Inflammation of the peritoneum with thickening of the membrane.

pachypleuritis (păk-ĭ-plū-rī'tĭs) [Gr. *pachys*, thick, + *pleura*, side, + *-itis*, inflammation]. Inflamed condition of the pleura with thickening.

pachypodous (pă-kĭp'ō-dŭs) ["+ *pous*, pod-, foot]. Having abnormally thick feet.

pachyrhinic (păk''ĭ-rī'nĭk). Having a thick, flat nose.

pachysalpingitis (păk''ĭ-săl''pĭn-jī'tĭs) [Gr. *pachys*, thick, + *salpinx*, tube, + *-itis*, inflammation]. Chronic inflammation of an oviduct with thickening of the walls.

pachysalpingoovaritis (păk''ĭ-săl-pĭn''gō-ō''văr-ĭ'tĭs) ["+ "+ L. *ovarium*, ovary, + Gr. *-itis*, inflammation]. Chronic inflamed condition of an ovary and oviduct with thickening of the membranes.

pachysomia (păk-ĭ-sō'mĭ-ă) [Gr. *pachys*, thick, + *sōma*, body]. Pathological thickening of the soft parts of the body.

pachyvaginalitis (păk''ĭ-văj'ĭn-ă-lī'tĭs) [" + L. *vagina*, sheath, + Gr. *-itis*, inflammation]. Inflamed condition of the tunica vaginalis of the testes.

pachyvaginitis (păk''ĭ-văj'ĭn-ī'tĭs). Chronic inflammation of the vagina with thickening of the membranes. SYN: *pachycolpismus.*

pacing (pās'ing) [L. *passus*, a step]. Setting the rate or pace of an event, esp. the heartbeat.

pacinian corpuscles (pă-sĭn'ĭ-ăn). [Filippo Pacini, It. anatomist, 1812-1883]. Encapsulated sensory nerve endings found in subcutaneous tissue and many other parts of the body (pancreas, penis, clitoris, nipple). These corpuscles are sensitive to deep or heavy pressure. SYN: *Vater-Pacini corpuscles.*

pack (păk) [AS. *pak*]. 1. A dry or moist, hot or cold, blanket or sheet wrapped around a patient. Used for treatment. 2. The procedure in which one enwraps a person. 3. To fill up a cavity with cotton, gauze, or a similar substance.

p., cold wet sheet. This pack is a physiological sedative and hypnotic employed for relief of restlessness and insomnia; used extensively in psychiatric conditions. Patient is wrapped in two or more sheets that have been placed in cold water and wrung out before application. The patient's body is then wrapped in heavy blankets to prevent loss of cooling and evaporation of moisture.

p., dry. Procedure used in combination with hot bath to induce perspiration. When patient leaves hot bath he is placed in a dry, warm sheet and wrapped in several warm blankets.

p., full. SEE: *pack, wet sheet.*

p., half. Wet sheet pack extending from the axillae to below the knees.

p., hot bath. SEE: *pack, dry.*

p., hot blanket. The envelopment of a patient in moist blanket wrung from very hot water (150° to 160° F. or 65.6°-71.1° C.). Given to relax contracted muscles, relieve convulsions, or induce profuse perspiration.

p., ice. A substitute for an ice bag; a local cold application made by folding a soft towel so it will fit the area and filling it with crushed ice.

p., neutral wet sheet. SEE: *pack, wet sheet.*

p., one sheet. A wet sheet pack in which only one large sheet, 84 × 96 in. (213.36 × 243.84 cm.), is used.

p., partial. SEE: *p., half; p., three-quarter.*

p., three-quarter. Pack using same temperatures as wet sheet pack, but the body is enveloped upward as far as the armpits.

p., umbrella. A p. inserted through the abdominal incision following hysterectomy. The p. itself consists of a piece of cotton or nylon cloth about 24 inches (61 cm.) square into the middle of which is placed about 60 feet (18.28 meters) of 2 inch (5 cm.) gauze. The tails of the p. are pulled through the vagina from below. The corners of the cloth are then brought together to form the tail of the p. After placement the tail is pulled firmly, and the bolus of gauze in the cloth exerts enough pressure against the blood vessels to stop arterial bleeding.

In Greece this is known as the Logothetopulos tampon, named after the physician who developed it in 1926.

p., wet sheet. The envelopment of patient in one, two, or three linen or soft cotton sheets that have been wrung out of water. These are held against the body by large woolen blankets. Temperature of the water used for the sheets varies, depending upon the purpose.

packer (păk'ĕr). Device for packing a cavity or a wound.

packing (păk'ĭing). 1. The process of filling a cavity or wound with gauze, sponges, etc. 2. Material used to fill a cavity or wound.

pad (păd). Cushion of soft material used to apply pressure, relieve pressure, support an organ or part, etc. Usually cotton, oakum, jute, or wood wool. Surgical cotton is not suitable for open wounds or broken surfaces. Oakum or marine lint is too irritating to place in direct contact with skin.

p., abdominal. Dressing for absorbing discharges from surgical wounds, etc., of abdomen.

p., dinner. Pad placed on stomach prior to application of a plaster cast. Pad is then removed, leaving space for abdominal distention after meals.

p., kidney. Air or water pad fixed on abdominal belt for compression over a movable kidney.

p.'s, knuckle. Congenital condition in which small nodules appear on dorsal side of fingers.

p., Malgaigne's. Mass of fat in knee joint on either side of the patella's upper end.

p., Mikulicz's. P. of folded gauze used in surgery.

p., perineal. Pad covering the perineum. Used to cover a wound or to absorb the menstrual flow.

p., sucking. A pad of fat seen inside the cheeks of infants.

p., surgical. Soft rubber pad with apron and inflatable rim for drainage of escaping fluids, used in operations and obstetrics.

P.ae. Abbr. in prescription writing for L. *partes aequales,* in equal parts.

paed-, paedo-. For words beginning with this spelling, refer to ped-, pedia-, pedo-.

Paget's disease (păj'ět). [Sir James Paget, Eng. surgeon, 1814-1899]. Skeletal disease of elderly with chronic inflammation of bones, resulting in thickening and softening of bones, and bowing of long bones. SYN: *osteitis deformans.*

P.d. of nipple. Carcinoma of the mammary ducts.

pagophagia [Gr. *pagos,* frost, + *phagein,* to eat]. A form of pica, q.v., characterized by the deliberate eating of large quantities of ice.

pain (pān) [L. *poena,* a fine, a penalty]. 1. A sensation in which a person experiences discomfort, distress, or suffering, due to provocation of sensory nerves. 2. In the plural, refers to contractions of the uterus in childbirth, or labor pains.

Pain is one of the cardinal symptoms of inflammation. Pain may vary in intensity from that which produces mild discomfort to that of intolerable agony. In most cases, pain stimuli are harmful to the body and tend to bring about reactions by which the body protects itself. Adaptation to pain stimuli does not readily occur.

Later in life, if one had always been well, definite pain may be a danger signal. In a chronic complainer, a new pain may not mean much.

p., abdominal. Increased with respiration; experienced in appendicitis, broken ribs, intercostal neuralgia, wounds, herpes zoster, pleurisy, pleurodynia, myalgia, periostitis, acute peritonitis, colic; hepatic, gastric, or renal ulcer; gallbladder disorders; carcinoma in late stages; and gummata of this region.

p., aching. Generalized aching may be ushered in with infectious disease such as influenza, smallpox, or rheumatic fever. It is also found in myalgia and various headaches.

p., acute. Same as lancinating pain. Usually associated with acute inflammation or inflammation of serous membranes as in pleurisy and pericarditis; also posterior spinal-root pains.

p., after-. That following labor, caused by contraction of uterine muscles during involution.

p., agonizing. May be due to coronary thrombosis, angina pectoris, aortic aneurysm, mediastinitis. May occur in milder form in asthma, tracheobronchitis, or it may be due to referred pain from gallbladder, intestinal obstruction, diaphragmatic hernia, pancreatitis, or a perforated ulcer.

p., angina pectoris. Paroxysmal, severe pain due to decreased blood supply to the myocardium, radiating through the shoulder down arm, or rarely from the heart to the abdomen, ear, or back. At the same time the patient may experience a feeling that the chest is being crushed or compressed. Lasts from a few seconds to several minutes. SEE: *angina pectoris.*

p., appendicitis. If acute, abdominal pain, usually severe, generally throughout the abdomen, followed by localization of pain in lower right quadrant of abdomen with tenderness over right rectus muscle with rigidity.

p., bearing-down. Straining with uterine contractions. Usually occurs in second stage of labor.

p., Brodie's. P. caused near a joint affected with neuralgia when the skin is folded near it.

p., burning. Experienced in heat burns, superficial skin lesions, herpes zoster, and in circumscribed neuralgias. SYN: *causalgia.*

p., cardiac. Angina pectoris, q.v.

p., causalgic. A spontaneous pain, esp. burning in character, when associated with anesthesia or hyperesthesia in a given nerve. SEE: *causalgia.*

p., central. P. due to a lesion in the brain or spinal cord.

p., cephalgic. Head p., q.v.

p., chest. Severe pain in chest from exercise may be due to heart disease. If due to pleurisy it comes with a deep breath. If pain accompanies stiff shoulder or neck, it may be due to arthritis or fibrositis. If it comes when bending over after a meal, it may be due to diaphragmatic or hiatus hernia.

p., continuous. May indicate persistent obstruction; also a tendency to suppuration.

p., cramplike. Muscular spasm such as epigastric pain. Significance depends upon location of pain.

p., degree of. SEE: *dol; dolorimeter.*

p., dilating. P. occuring during the first stage of labor accompanying dilatation of the cervix.

p., dull. Continuous mild throbbing.

p., ear. May indicate inflammation of the ext. auditory canal, except in young children. Also may indicate a furuncle in the meatus; or middle ear disease. SYN: *otodynia.*

p., eccentric. P. occurring in peripheral structures due to a lesion involving posterior roots of spinal nerves.

p., ecstatic. Unreasonable desire for excitement, pleasurable or painful. A martyrlike situation, or a feeling of being unfairly treated, may be experienced with satisfaction.

p., epigastric. Severe pain occurring in paroxysms in gastric disorders. In general, may accompany any gastric or intestinal disorder, as well as pleural and some cardiac affections. SEE: *cardialgia.*

p., expulsive. That of the second and third stages of labor.

p., false. One mistaken for a true labor pain; an ineffective pain of labor.

p., fixed. Indicates derangement at some special point.

p., fulgurant. Sudden, brief, intense p., esp. experienced in tabes dorsalis due to syphilis. SYN: *shooting p.*

p., gallbladder. In upper right abdominal quadrant, dull pain just below the last rib in infection, or sharp pain in same area radiating to the back and up under right shoulder, esp. if calculi are present.

p., gastralgic. Severe pain occurring in paroxysms in gastric disorders. SYN: *epigastric p.*

p., girdle. One resembling sensation of a constricting cord around the waist, occurring in spinal cord disease.

p., growing. That felt in the joints or limbs of growing children; may be rheumatic. An imprecise term indicating ill-defined pain in the musculo-system of young persons. There is no evidence that the pain is related to rapid growth.

p., head. An ache or pain located in the head, esp. one experienced in region of cranial vault. Headache may be a symptom of acute systemic infections; intracranial tumors, infections, or vascular lesions; hypertension; acute and chronic infections of the nose, sinuses, pharynx, eye, and ear; and toxic states such as alcoholism, uremia, etc. Headache may occur after the injection of histamine, following a lumbar puncture, in infections of the meninges, and in subarachnoid hemorrhages. Headache occurs in many febrile diseases, in anemia and oxygen want, and following head injuries (post-traumatic). Migraine, q.v., is a common type, of unknown etiology. Many headaches are psychogenic such as those occurring in conversion hysteria, anxiety states, etc. SYN: *headache; cephalalgia.*

p., heterotopic. Referred pain, q.v.

p., homotopic. P. felt at the point of injury.

p., hunger. Pain due to need for food; coincide with powerful contractions of the stomach. May be an evidence of gastric disorder. SEE: *hunger.*

p., hypogastric. Pain in the hypogastrium.

p., ideogenous. Pain of mental origin.

p., imperative. A persistent sensation of pain occurring in psychasthenia.

p., inflammatory. Pain in presence of inflammation which is increased by pressure.

p., intermenstrual. Pelvic p. arising during the cycle between the menses; accompanies eruption of ovum from ovary. SYN: *mittelschmerz.*

p., intractable. Pain that cannot be easily relieved, as that occurring from certain neoplastic invasions.

p., joy. Apparent enjoyment of pain during hysterical conditions.

p.'s, labor. Rhythmical uterine contractions at childbirth; increasing in frequency and severity, climaxing in vaginal delivery.

p., lancinating. A short, sharp, cutting pain.

p., lightning. The cutting, darting p. associated with tabes dorsalis.

p., lingual. Pain in tongue which may be due to local lesions, glossitis, fissures, or pernicious anemia.

p., lung. SEE: *pain, pulmonary.*

p., menstrual. Pain, usually cramping, occurring just prior to onset and/or during the menstrual period. SYN: *dysmenorrhea.*

p., mental. One of psychic origin such as mental distress or grief. If persistent may cause true physical pain (psychosomatic pain).

p., middle. Pain between menstrual periods. SYN: *mittelschmerz.*

p., migraine. Headache accompanied by nausea and vomiting. It may arise from a number of causes, esp. those of neurological origin.

p., mind. P. of mental origin or p. occurring subsequent to mental effort, noted esp. in melancholia.

p., mobile. P. that moves from one area to another.

p., movement. Kinesalgia, q.v.

p., neuralgic. Pain, frequently paroxysmal, occurring along the branches of a nerve. Temporarily relieved by heat or pressure. May be rheumatic in origin, a tic, inflammation of nerves, or nerve trauma.

p., niggling. The early p.'s of puerperal labor; persistently nagging, petty.

p., night. Pain in hip or knee during muscular relaxation in sleep.

p., noise. Pain of ear caused by a noise. SEE: *odynacusis.*

p., objective. P. induced by some external or internal irritant, by inflammation, or by injury to nerves, organs, or other tissues which interfere with the function, nutrition, or circulation of the affected part. Usually traceable to a definite pathological process.

p., organic. Somatalgia, q.v.

p., osteocopic. Pain in bones. SEE: *osteocope.*

p., parenchymatous. P. felt at the peripheral end of a nerve.

p., paresthesic. Stinging or tingling sensation manifested in central and peripheral nerve lesions. SEE: *paresthesia.*

p., phantom. Pain which seems to be in a certain limb following amputation of that limb. SEE: *phantom limb.*

p., postprandial. Abdominal pain after eating.

p., premonitory. Ineffective contractions of the uterus prior to the beginning of true labor.

p., pseudomyelic. False sensation of movement in a paralyzed limb or of no movement in a moving limb. Not a true pain.

p., psychic. Mental suffering such as that resulting from a sense of unworthiness or from feelings of guilt.

p., psychogenic. P. having mental origin as opposed to organic origin.

p., psychosomatic. P. due to mental or emotional disorders.

p., pulmonary. Sharp pain in the region of the lungs.

p., rectal, constant. Usually aggravated by defecation. May be due to ischiorectal abscess, anal abscess, inflamed or strangulated hemorrhoids, carcinoma, periproctitis, prostatic abscess, seminal vesiculitis, fecal impaction, acute salpingitis, tabes dorsalis, irritation from diarrhea, foreign bodies, fissures, rectal polyps, or adenoma. P. during defecation may result from fissure in ano, ulcer, hemorrhoids, anal abscess, stenosis, stricture, dysentery, impaction, foreign body, or any inflammation.

p., referred. P. seeming to arise in an area other than its origin, as pain from appendicitis which often seems to occur in areas other than that of the appendix. SYN: *synalgia.*

p., reflex. A reflex action resulting from a painful stimulus. Pain reflexes are protective and tend to take precedence over less urgent reflexes.

p., regional. Pain in a specific area and its significance.

p., remittent. P. with temporary abatements in severity. Characteristic of neuralgia and colic.

p., root. Cutaneous pain caused by disease of sensory nerve roots.

p., shifting. P. which seems to arise from different sites from time to time. Present in rheumatism, hysteria, and locomotor ataxia.

p., shooting. SEE: *p., fulgurant.*

p., sick headache. Migraine, q.v.

p.'s, spot. Pains which seem to be located in patches of the skin.

p.'s, starting. P.'s accompanied by muscular spasm during early stages of sleep.

p., subdiaphragmatic (pleurisy). A sharp, stitchlike pain occurring during breathing. When the breath is held, the pain ceases. Pressure against the lower costals eases the pain.

p., subjective. One that has no apparent physical basis for its existence. It may be found among the highly imaginative neurotics in whom mild sensations are translated into pain sense.

p., sympathetic. See: *p., referred.*

p., tenesmic. P. accompanying urination or defecation. SEE: *tenesmus.*

p., terebrant, p., terebrating. A boring or piercing type of pain.

p., thermalgesic. Pain caused by heat.

p., thoracic. A sharp pain over the sternum, often running down the arm to the elbow. May be indicative of angina pectoris, although it must not be confused with pain from gastric pressure in the region of the heart, caused by an accumulation of gas. It is increased with respiration. It is experienced in broken ribs; intercostal neuralgia; wounds; herpes zoster; pleurisy; pleurodynia; myalgia; periostitis; acute peritonitis; colic; hepatic, gastric, or renal ulcer; gallbladder disorders; carcinoma in late stages; and gumma of this region.

p., threshold of. Ascertained by a low amount of controlled heat to a square centimeter of skin surface for three seconds. The pain threshold is reached when sensation starts to be painful, or when 220 millicalories or heat units are reached.

p., throbbing. Found in dental caries, headache, and associated with phlegmonous inflammation and suppuration.

p., tongue. SEE: *p., lingual.*

p., tracheal. Trachealgia.

p., wandering. P. which changes its location repeatedly.

p., worry and anxiety. Worry and anxiety cause muscular tension resulting in pain which if long continued may interfere with nerve and blood circulation.

paint (pānt). 1. A solution of medication for application to skin. 2. To apply a medicated liquid to the skin.

p., Castellani's. A germicide consisting of phenol, resorcinol, boric acid, acetone, and basic fuchsin.

painters' colic. Colic accompanying lead poisoning. SEE: *Lead* in *Table of Poisons* in *Appendix.*

PAL. Abbr. for *posterior axillary line; pathology laboratory* (test).

palatable (păl″ăt-ă-bl) [L. *palatum,* palate]. Pleasing to the palate or taste, as food.

palatal (păl′ă-tăl). Pert. to the roof of the mouth, the palate.

p. reflex. Swallowing induced by stimulation of soft palate.

palate (păl′ăt) [L. *palatum,* palate]. The horizontal structure separating the mouth and the nasal cavity; the roof of the mouth. SEE: *mouth* for illustration.

DISORDERS: *Koplik's Spots:* A rash frequently seen upon the palate in measles. *Secondary Syphilis:* Indicated by mucous patches on the palate. *Herpes of the Throat:* Shown by vesicles in circles upon the pharyngeal walls and soft palate. *Swelling of Uvula:* Noted in inflammations of pharynx and tonsil, in nephritis, severe anemia, angioneurotic edema, and general debility. In diphtheria and Vincent's angina, a membranous exudate appears. In purpura hemorrhagica and some hemorrhagic diatheses, bloody extravasation appears. *Paralysis:* May result from diphtheria, bulbar paralysis, neuritis, basal meningitis, tumor at base of brain. *Anesthesia:* Seen in involvement of 2nd division of the 5th nerve.

RS: Avellis' paralysis syndrome; Bednar's aphthae; cheilognathopalatoschisis; cleft; words beginning with "palat-," "staphyl-," "uran-," "uvul-."

p., artificial. Hard substance molded to fill a cleft in the palate.

p. bones. Bones forming posterior part of hard palate and lateral nasal wall between the interior pterygoid plate of sphenoid bone and superior maxilla.

p., cleft. One with congenital opening between two parts of palate.

p., falling. Abnormally long uvula.

p., gothic. An excessively high palate arch.

p., hard. Anterior part supported by the maxillary and palatine bones.

p., soft. Posterior muscular, membranous fold partly separating the mouth and pharynx. SYN: *velum.*

palatine (păl′ă-tīn) [L. *palatinus*]. 1. Concerning the palate. 2. The palate bones, q.v.

p. arches. Two archlike folds of mucous membrane (*glossopalatine* and *pharyngopalatine arches*) which form the lateral margins of faucial and pharyngeal isthmuses. They are continuous above with the soft palate. SYN: *pillars.*

p. artery, greater. A branch of the maxillary artery which supplies the palate, upper pharynx, and pharyngotympanic tube.

p. bone. Palate bones, q.v.

palatitis (păl-ăt-i′tĭs) [L. *palatum,* palate, + Gr. *-itis,* inflammation]. Inflamed condition of the palate.

palatoglossus (păl″ă-tō-glŏs′ŭs) ["+ Gr. *glōssa,* tongue]. Muscle arising from sides and under surface of tongue. Fibers pass upward through glossopalatine arch and are inserted in palatine aponeurosis. It constricts faucial isthmus by raising root of tongue and drawing sides of soft palate downward. SYN: *glossopalatinus.*

palatognathous (păl″ă-tog′nă-thŭs) ["+ Gr. *gnathos,* jaw]. Having a congenital cleft in the palate.

palatography (păl″ă-tog′ră-fe) ["+ Gr. *graphein,* to write]. The recording of the movements of the palate in speech.

palatopharyngeus (păl″ăt-ō-far′ĭn-jē′ŭs) [L. *palatum,* palate, + Gr. *pharynx, pharyng-,* pharynx]. Muscle arising from thyroid cartilage and pharyngeal wall, extending upward in posterior pillar, and inserting into aponeurosis of soft palate. Constricts pharyngeal isthmus, raises larynx, and depresses soft palate.

palatoplasty (păl′ăt-ō-plăs″tĭ) [L. *palatum,* palate, + Gr. *plassein,* to form]. Plastic surgery of the palate, usually to correct a cleft. SYN: *staphylorrhaphy; uranoplasty.*

palatoplegia (păl″ă-tō-plē′jĭ-ă) ["+ Gr. *plēgē,* stroke]. Paralysis of muscles of the soft palate. SEE: *palate.*

palatorrhaphy (păl-ă-tor′ă-fĭ) ["+ Gr. *rhaphē,* a sewing]. Operation for uniting of a cleft palate. SYN: *staphylorrhaphy.*

palatoschisis (păl-ă-tŏs′kĭ-sĭs) ["+ *schisis,* fissure]. Palate with cleft in it.

palatum (păl-ă′tŭm) [L.]. (pl. *pala′ta*) [NA] The palate.

paleencephalon, paleoencephalon (pā″-lē-ĕn-sĕf′ă-lŏn, -ō-ĕn-sef′ă-lŏn) [Gr. *palaios,* old, + *enkephalos,* brain]. Phylogenetically older portion of the brain; includes all of it except the cerebral cortex and its allied structures.

paleo- [Gr. *palaios,* old, ancient]. Combining form meaning old or ancient.

paleocerebellum (păl″e-ō-sĕr″e-bĕl′ŭm) [Gr. *palaios,* old, + L. *cerebellum,* little brain]. Phylogenetically, the older portion of the cerebellum including the flocculi, certain parts of the vermis (lingula, nodulus, uvula), and the lobulus centralis (culmen, pyramis, uvula, and simple lobule). These parts are concerned primarily with equilibrium and movements of locomotion.

paleogenesis (pā″lē-ō-jĕn′e-sĭs) [″+ *genesis,* production]. Reproduction of ancestral characteristics without change in a later generation, esp. abnormalities.

paleogenetic (pā″lē-ō-jĕn-ĕt′ĭk) [″+ *gennan,* to produce]. Having origin in a previous generation.

paleokinetic (pā″lē-ō-kĭ-nĕt′ĭk) [″+ Gr. *kinētikos,* concerning movement]. Noting a peripheral motor nervous system controlling automatic associated movements. It is older phylogenetically than system controlling voluntary movement.

paleontology (pā″lē-ŏn-tŏl′ō-jĭ) [Gr. *palaios,* old, + *onta,* existing things, + *logos,* study]. Branch of biology dealing with ancient plant and animal life of the earth. SEE: *phylogeny.*

paleopathology (pā″lē-ō-pă-thŏl′ō-jĭ) [″+ *pathos,* disease, + *logos,* study]. The study of diseases in remains of bodies and fossils of ancient times.

paleostriatal (pā″lē-ō-strī-ā′tăl) [″+ L. *striatus,* ridged]. Concerning the primitive portion of the corpus striatum.

paleostriatum (pā″lē-ō-strī-ā′tŭm). Primitive portion of corpus striatum, the globus pallidus. SEE: *neostriatum.*

paleothalamus (pā″lē-ō-thăl′ă-mŭs) [″+ *thalamos,* chamber]. Medial portion of thalamus—the medullary or noncortical part—which is older phylogenetically. SEE: *thalamus.*

palikinesia (păl″ĭ-kĭn-ē′zĭ-ă) [Gr. *palin,* again, + *kinēsis,* motion]. Continued, involuntary, repetitious movements.

palilalia (păl-ĭ-lā′lĭ-ă) [″+ *lalein,* to speak]. Pathological repetitious use of words and phrases.

palinal (păl′ĭn-ăl) [Gr. *palin,* backward]. Moved or moving backward.

palindromia (păl-ĭn-drō′mĭ-ă) [″+ *dromos,* a running]. The recurrence of a disease or a relapse.

palindromic (păl-ĭn-drŏm′ĭk). Recurring, as the symptoms of a disease. SYN: *relapsing.*

palinesthesia (păl″ĭn-ĕs-thē′zĭ-ă) [Gr. *palin,* again, + *aisthēsis,* sensation]. Return of power of sensation, as after recovery from anesthesia or coma.

palingenesis (păl″ĭn-jĕn′e-sĭs) [″+ *genesis,* formation]. 1. Regeneration or restoration of an organism or part of one. 2. Reappearance of ancestral characteristics, esp. abnormal ones. SYN: *atavism; paleogenesis.*

palingraphia (păl″ĭn-grăf′ĭ-ă) [″+ *graphein,* to write]. Pathological repetition of words or phrases in writing.

palinopsia [Gr. *palin,* again, + *opsis,* vision]. Persistence or recurrence of visual images after the stimulus of the image has been removed. Occurs in visual field defects, in acute mental and visual defects, and in association with auditory or somatic hallucinations.

palinphrasia, paliphrasia (păl-ĭn-frā′zĭ-ă, -ĭ-frā′zĭ-ă) [″+ *phrasis,* speech]. Pathological condition in which there is coherent speech but certain words or phrases frequently are repeated. SYN: *palilalia.*

palladium (pă-lā′dē-ŭm) [L.]. SYMB: *Pd.* At. wt. 106.4; at. no. 46. Metallic element. Used in dentistry and surgical instruments.

pallanesthesia (păl″ăn-ĕs-thē′zĭ-ă) [Gr. *pallein,* to shake, + *anaisthēsia,* anesthesia]. Loss of vibration sensation of skin and bones. SYN: *apallesthesia.* SEE: *pallesthesia.*

pallescence (păl-lĕs′ĕns) [L. *pallescere,* to grow pale]. Diminution of body color; a pale appearance. SYN: *pallor.*

pallesthesia (păl-ĕs-thē′zĭ-ă) [Gr. *pallein,* to shake, + *aisthēsis,* sensation]. The sensation of vibration felt in skin or bones, as that produced by a tuning fork when held against the body.

palliate (păl′ĭ-āt) [L. *palliatus,* cloaked]. To ease or reduce in violence; to allay temporarily, as pain, without curing.

palliative (păl′ĭ-a″tĭv). 1. Serving to relieve or alleviate, without curing. 2. An agent which alleviates or eases.

pallid (păl′ĭd) [L. *pallidus,* pale]. Lacking color; pale, wan.

pallidal (păl′ĭ-dăl). Concerning the pallidum of the brain.

pallidum (păl′ĭ-dŭm) [L.]. The globus pallidus of the lenticular nucleus in the corpus striatum.

pallium (păl′ĭ-ŭm) [L., cloak]. [NA]. The cerebral cortex with its adjacent white substance, considered as a cover for rest of the brain. SYN: *brain mantle.*

pallor (păl′or) [L.]. Lack of color; paleness. SEE: *skin.*

palm [L. *palma*, hand]. Anterior or flexor surface of the hand from wrist to fingers. SYN: *vola manus*. SEE: *antithenar; thenar*.

palmar (păl'mar). Concerning the palm of the hand.

p. or darwinian reflex. A grasping reflex in infants, more highly developed in some than in others. It gradually disappears and is absent after 4 or 5 months.

palmaris (păl-mā'rĭs). [NA]. One of two muscles, p. brevis and p. longus. SEE: *Table of Muscles* in *Appendix*.

palm-chin reflex. Scratching the thenar eminence of the hand with a sharp object causes contraction of the chin muscles on the same side.

palmic (pal'mĭk) [Gr. *palmikos*]. 1. Concerning palpitation or pulse. 2. Concerning palmus, q.v.

palmitic acid (pal-mĭt'ĭk). $CH_3(CH_2)_{14}$ COOH. A fatty acid found in palm oil, solid fats, some waxes, and many fatty oils.

palmitin (pal'mĭ-tĭn). An ester of glycerol and palmitic acid, derived from fat of both animal and vegetable origin.

palmomen'tal reflex. SEE: *palm-chin reflex.*

palmoplantar (păl"mō-plăn'tar). Pert. to the palms of the hands and soles of the feet. SYN: *volar.*

palmoscopy (pal-mŏs'kō-pĭ) [Gr. *palmos*, vibration, + *skopein*, to examine]. Observation and study of pulsation of heart.

palmus (păl'mŭs) [Gr. *palmos*, pulsation, quivering]. 1. Palpitation; a throb. 2. Jerking; a disease with convulsive nervous twitching of the leg muscles, similar to jumping. 3. Heart beat.

palpable (păl'pă-bl) [L. *palpabilis*, stroke, touch]. Perceptible, esp. by touch.

palpate (păl'pāt) [L. *palpare*, to touch]. To examine by touch; to feel.

palpation (păl-pā'shŭn) [L. *palpatio*]. Process of examining by application of the hands or fingers to the external surface of the body to detect evidence of disease in the various organs.

palpebra (păl'pē-bră) [L. *palpebra*, eyelid]. (pl. *pal'pebrae*) An eyelid.

p. inferior. [NA] The lower eyelid.

p. superior. [NA] The upper eyelid.

palpebral (păl'pē-brăl). Concerning an eyelid.

p. cartilages. Thin plates of condensed tissue forming the framework of the eyelid. SYN: *tarsal cartilages.*

p. commissure. The union of the eyelids at each end of palpebral fissure.

p. fissure. The opening between the eyelids.

p. ligament. One of two ligamentous structures (medial and lateral) which fix the two ends of the tarsi to the orbital wall.

p. muscles. 1. Palpebral portion of m. orbicularis oculi. 2. Levator palpebra muscle.

palpebrate (păl'pē-brāt). 1. [L. *palpebrare*]. To wink. 2. [L. *palpebra*, eyelid]. Possessing eyelids.

palpitant (păl'pĭ-tănt) [L. *palpitāre*, to quiver]. Throbbing; trembling.

palpitate (păl'pĭ-tāt) [L. *palpitatus*, throbbing]. 1. To cause to throb. 2. To throb or beat intensely or rapidly, usually said of the heart.

palpitation (păl-pĭ-tā'shŭn). Rapid, violent, or throbbing pulsation, as an abnormally rapid throbbing or fluttering of the heart. SEE: *heart.*

p., arterial. That felt in course of an artery.

palsy (pawl'zĭ) [ME. *palesie*, from L. *paralysis*]. Temporary or permanent loss of sensation or loss of ability to move or to control movement. SYN: *paralysis.*

p., Bell's. Paralysis of the facial nerve in its peripheral distribution. Muscles of unaffected side of face pull the face into a distorted position.

p., birth. P. arising from an injury received at birth.

p., cerebral. Bilateral, symmetrical, nonprogressive paralysis resulting from developmental defects in brain or trauma at birth. SYN: *cerebral spastic infantile paralysis; Little's disease.*

p., crutch. P. resulting from pressure on nerves in the axilla from use of a crutch.

p., Erb's. A paralysis of the deltoid, biceps, long supinator, and brachialis anticus muscles due to a lesion of the brachial plexus or of the 5th and 6th cervical nerves.

p., lead. Paralysis of extremities in lead poisoning.

p., night. Form of paresthesia in which numbness is a symptom, esp. at night.

p., scrivener's. Writer's cramp.

p., shaking. Progressive muscular weakness and tremor with impaired voluntary motion. SYN: *paralysis agitans; Parkinson's disease.*

p., wasting. Chronic condition in which there is atrophy and paralysis of muscles; grows progressively worse. SYN: *progressive muscular atrophy.*

paludal (păl'ū-dăl) [L. *palus*, a marsh]. Concerning, or originating in, marshes. SYN: *malarial.*

paludism (păl'ū-dĭzm) ["+ Gr. *ismos*, condition]. Swamp fever. SYN: *malaria*, q.v.

pampiniform (păm-pĭn′ĭ-form) [L. *pampinus*, tendril, + *forma*, shape]. Convoluted like a tendril.
   p. plexus. 1. A mesh of spermatic or ovarian veins. 2. Network of nerves supplying the testicles.

pampinocele (păm-pĭn′ō-sēl) ["+ Gr. *kēlē*, swelling]. A swollen, painful condition of the veins of the spermatic cord. SYN: *varicocele*, q.v.

pan- [Gr.]. Combining form indicating all.

panacea (păn-ă-sē′ă) [Gr. *panakeia*, universal remedy]. A remedy for all ills; cure-all. Obviously no such treatment exists.

panagglutinin (păn″ă-glū′tĭn-ĭn) [Gr. *pan*, all, + L. *agglutināre*, to glue to]. Substance capable of agglutinizing corpuscles of every blood group.

panaris (pan′ă-rĭs) [L. *panaricium*, disease of the fingernail]. Inflammation of the skinfold surrounding the nail. SYN: *paronychia*.

panarthritis (păn-ar-thrī′tĭs) [Gr. *pan-*, all, + *arthron*, joint, + *-itis*, inflammation]. 1. Inflammation of all parts of a joint. 2. Inflamed condition of all the joints of the body.

panasthenia (păn″ăs-thē′nĭ-ă) ["+ *astheneia*, weakness]. Generalized weakness or exhaustion without evidence of organic disease. SYN: *neurasthenia*, q.v.

panatrophy (păn-ăt′rō-fĭ) ["+ *atrophy*, wasting away]. Wasting away of an entire structure; generalized wasting away of the body.

pancarditis (păn-kăr-dī′tĭs) ["+ *kardia*, heart, + *-itis*, inflammation]. Inflamed condition involving all the structures of the heart.

panchreston (păn-krē′stŏn) ["+ *chrēstos*, useful]. A remedy for every disease. SYN: *panacea.*

panchromia (păn-krō′mĭ-ă) ["+ *chrōma*, color]. Power of staining with numerous dyes.

pancreas (păn′krē-ăs) [Gr. *pan-*, all, + *kreas*, flesh]. (pl. *pan′creata*) [NA]. A compound tubuloacinar or racemose gland situated behind the stomach in front of the 1st and 2nd lumbar vertebrae in a horizontal position, its head attached to the duodenum and its tail reaching to the spleen. The portion between the head and the tail constitutes the body.
   The gland is composed of lobules that form lobes connected by strands of tissue with ducts which lead from the lobules into a main one, the *pancreatic duct* or *duct of Wirsung.* This duct is connected with the duodenum. Scattered throughout the substance are differentiated masses of cells which are the *islets of Langerhans.* An *accessory pancreatic duct* or *duct of Santorini* frequently is present. It is smaller than the main duct and opens into the duodenum cephalad to the main duct with which it communicates.
   FUNCTIONS: The pancreas produces both an external and an internal secretion. The external secretion, called *pancreatic juice*, q.v., is produced by the cells of the acini. It passes through the pancreatic ducts into the duodenum where it plays an important role in the digestion of all classes of foods. The internal secretion, which is elabo-

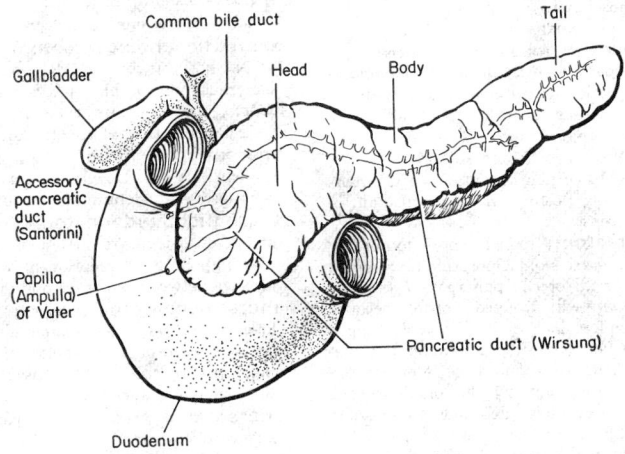

Common bile duct   Tail

Gallbladder   Head   Body

Accessory pancreatic duct (Santorini)

Papilla (Ampulla) of Vater

Pancreatic duct (Wirsung)

Duodenum

THE PANCREAS, DUCTS, AND DUODENUM

rated by the islets of Langerhans, includes the hormones *insulin* and *glucagon* (hyperglycemic-glycogenolytic factor). These hormones in conjunction with hormones from other endocrine glands (adrenal cortex, medulla, anterior hypophysis), play a primary role in the regulation of carbohydrate metabolism.

Diminished secretion of insulin by the islets of Langerhans results in a clinical entity called *diabetes mellitus,* q.v. In this disease there are disturbances in the metabolism of carbohydrates and fats resulting in the elevation of blood glucose, cholesterol, and ketone bodies. Urinary output is greatly increased and the urine usually contains glucose and ketone bodies.

Excessive secretion of insulin (*hyperinsulinism*) may sometimes occur. This results in the lowering of blood sugar (*hypoglycemia*).

RS: diabetes mellitis; secretin; pancreatic juice; insulin.

p., accessory. Small mass of pancreatic tissue close to the pancreas but detached from it.

p., annular. An anomalous condition in which a portion of the pancreas encircles the duodenum.

p., dorsal. A dorsal outpocketing of the embryonic gut which gives rise to the body and tail of the adult pancreas.

p., fibrocystic disease of. SEE: *cystic fibrosis.*

p., little or lesser. Semidetached lobular part of posterior surface of head of the p., sometimes having a separate duct opening into the principal one. SYN: Willis' p.

p., ventral. An outgrowth at the angle of the hepatic diverticulum and the embryonic gut which migrates and fuses with the dorsal pancreas. It forms the head of the definitive organ.

p., Willis'. SEE: *pancreas, little.*

pancreatalgia (păn″krē-ă-tăl′jĭ-ă) [Gr. *pan-,* all, + *kreas,* flesh, + *algos,* pain]. Pain in the pancreas.

pancreatectomy (păn″krē-ăt-ĕk′tŏ-mĭ) ["+ "+ *ektomē,* excision]. Operation for removal of part or all of the pancreas. *Total pancreatectomy* will produce diabetes because of a complete lack of insulin. Following a *subtotal* (or partial) *pancreatectomy,* diabetes will develop some time later because the remaining islets will be unable to take care of the excessive demands placed upon them. SEE: *diabetes.*

pancreatemphraxis (păn″krē-ăt-ĕm-frăk′sĭs) ["+ "+ *emphraxis,* stoppage]. Con-

gestion of pancreas due to obstruction of pancreatic duct causing .swelling of the gland.

pancreathelcosis (păn″krē-ăth″ĕl-kō′sĭs) ["+ "+ *helkōsis,* ulceration]. Ulcerated condition of the pancreas or its suppurative inflammation.

pancreatic (păn″krē-ăt′ĭk) [Gr. *pancreaticus*]. Concerning the pancreas.

p. cystic fibrosis. SEE: *cystic fibrosis.*

p. juice. Its secretion is brought about by two hormones, *secretin* and *pancreozymin,* which are secreted by the duodenal mucosa. P.j. is discharged into the duodenum through the duct of Wirsung. The pancreas secretes 500-800 cc. every 24 hr. P.j. begins to flow when the acid contents of the stomach pass through the pylorus. It is a clear, viscid, alkaline fluid (pH 8.4-8.9) resembling saliva in consistency. It contains water, protein, inorganic salts, and enzymes. Among the enzymes are *trypsinogen* which by the action of intestinal enterokinase is converted into trypsin, a proteolytic enzyme; *chymotrypsinogen* which is converted by trypsin into chymotrypsin, a milkcurdling enzyme; *amylopsin,* a maltase which acts on carbohydrates; and *steapsin,* a lipase which acts on fats.

Amylopsin hydrolyzes starch to maltose; steapsin hydrolyzes fats to fatty acids and glycerol; trypsinogen, by the action of enterokinase in the duodenum, is converted into the active form trypsin which hydrolyzes proteins to amino acids. The alkali neutralizes the acidity of the chyme entering the duodenum from the stomach.

RS: enzyme; pancreas; secretion.

pancreaticocholecystostomy (păn″krē-ăt″ĭ-kō-kō″le-sĭs-tŏs′tō-mĭ) [Gr. *pancreaticus,* pancreas, + *cholē,* bile, + *kystis,* bladder, + *stoma,* opening]. Surgical creation of passage between the gallbladder and pancreas.

pancreaticoduodenal (păn″krē-ăt′ĭ-kō-dū-ō-dē′năl) ["+ L. *duodeni,* twelve]. Concerning the duodenum and pancreas.

pancreaticoduodenostomy (păn″krē-ăt′ĭ-kō-dū″ŏ-dē-nŏs′tō-mĭ) ["+ "+ Gr. *stoma,* opening]. Surgical creation of an artificial passage between pancreas and duodenum.

pancreaticoenterostomy (păn″krē-ăt′ĭ-kō-en″ter-ŏs′to-mĭ) [Gr. *pancreaticus,* pancreas, + *enteron,* intestine, + *stoma,* opening]. Surgical creation of a passage between the pancreatic duct and the intestine.

pancreaticogastrostomy (păn″krē-ăt′ĭ-kō-găs-trŏs′to-mĭ) ["+ *gastēr,* belly, + *stoma,* opening]. Surgical creation of a passage between pancreas and the stomach.

pancreaticojejunostomy (păn″krē-ăt′ĭ-kō-jē″jū-nos′tō-mĭ) ["+ L. *jejunum*, empty, + Gr. *stoma*, opening]. Surgical creation of a passage between the pancreatic duct and the jejunum.

pancreatin (păn′krē-ă-tĭn) [Gr. *pan-*, all, + *kreas*, flesh]. 1. One of the active ferments of the pancreas. 2. A mixture of enzymes obtained from pancreas of ox or hog.

ACTION AND USES: Chiefly as a digestant. Inactive in presence of acid, should be administered in combination with an alkali such as sodium bicarbonate.

pancreatitis (păn″krē-ă-tī′tĭs) [Gr. *pan-*, all, + *kreas*, flesh, + *-itis*, inflammation]. Inflamed condition of the pancreas.

p., acute. Form characterized by necrosis, suppuration, gangrene, and hemorrhage.

SYM: Sudden and intense pain in epigastric region, vomiting, belching of gas, sometimes hiccough, collapse. Rigidity and tenderness over umbilicus. Constipation, slow pulse, possible jaundice.

p., calcareous. P. occurring with calculi formation.

p., centrilobar. P. located around divisions of the pancreatic duct.

p., chronic. Form marked by formation of scar tissue in pancreas associated with malfunction. SEE: *pancreas.*

SYM: Pain, mild or severe. Pain has tendency to radiate to the back. Jaundice, weakness, emaciation, diarrhea.

p., hemorrhagic. Form with hemorrhage into pancreatic tissue.

SYM: Paroxysms of deep-seated pain in epigastrium, nausea, retching, constipation. Slight rise in temperature, blood and mucus in vomitus, delirium, tympanites jaundice, hiccough, cyanosis, collapse.

p., interstitial. P. with overgrowth of inter- and intra-acinar connective tissue.

p., perilobar. Fibrosis of the pancreas between acinous groups.

p., purulent. P. with suppuration.

p., suppurative. Form marked by development of many small abscesses. Sym. may be those of acute or chronic form.

pancreatoduodenectomy (păn″krē-ă-tō-dū″ō-dē-nĕk′tō-mĭ) [Gr. *pan-*, all, + *kreas*, flesh, + L. *duodeni*, twelve, + Gr. *ektomē*, excision]. Excision of the head of the pancreas and the adjacent portion of the duodenum.

pancreatogenic, pancreatogenous (păn″krē-ă-tō-jĕn′ĭk, -tŏj′ĕ-nŭs) ["+ "+ *gennan*, to produce]. Produced in or by the pancreas; having origin in the pancreas.

pancreatolith (păn″krē-ăt′ō-lĭth) [Gr. *pan-*, all, + *kreas*, flesh, + *lithos*, stone]. A calculus of the pancreas.

pancreatolithectomy (păn″krē-ăt-ō-lĭth-ĕk′tō-mĭ) ["+ "+ "+ *ektomē*, excision]. Removal of a concretion from the pancreas. SYN: *pancreatolithotomy.*

pancreatolithotomy (păn″krē-ăt-ō-lĭth-ŏt′-ō-mĭ) ["+ "+ "+ *tome*, an incision]. Removal of a concretion from the pancreas. SYN: *pancreatolithectomy.*

pancreatolysis (păn″krē-ă-tŏl′ĭ-sĭs) [Gr. *pan-*, all, + *kreas*, flesh, + *lysis*, dissolution]. Destruction of the pancreatic substance.

pancreatolytic (păn″krē-ăt-ō-lĭt′ĭk). Destructive to the pancreatic tissues. SYN: *pancreolytic.*

pancreatomy (păn-krē-ăt′ō-mĭ) [Gr. *pan-*, all, + *kreas*, flesh, + *tome*, incision]. Operation into the pancreas. SYN: *pancreatotomy.*

pancreatoncus (păn-krē-ăt-ong′kŭs) ["+ "+ *onkos*, tumor]. A pancreatic tumor.

pancreatopathy (păn″krē-ă-top′ă-thĭ) ["+ "+ *pathos*, disease]. Any pancreatic disease.

pancreatotomy (păn″krē-ă-tŏt′ō-mĭ) ["+ "+ *tome*, incision]. Surgical incision into the pancreas. SYN: *pancreatomy.*

pancreectomy (păn″krē-ĕk′tō-mĭ) ["+ "+ *ektomē*, excision]. Partial or total excision of the pancreas.

pancreolithotomy (păn″krē-ō-lĭth-ŏt′ō-mĭ) [Gr. *pan-*, all, + *kreas*, flesh, + *lithos*, stone, + *tome*, incision]. Surgical removal of a pancreatic concretion.

pancreolytic (păn″krē-ō-lĭt′ĭk) ["+ "+ *lysis*, dissolution]. Destructive to the pancreas.

pancreopathy (păn″krē-ŏp′ă-thĭ) ["+ "+ *pathos*, disease]. Any diseased condition of the pancreas. SYN: *pancreatopathy.*

pancreozymin (păn′krē-ō-zī′mĭn). A hormone, extracted from the duodenal mucosa, that stimulates the secretion of pancreatic juice, esp. increasing its enzymatic concentration. Opposed to secretin, which stimulates secretion of water and salts.

pancytopenia (păn″sī-tō-pē′nĭ-ă) [Gr. *pan-*, all, + *-cyte*, cell, + *penia*, poverty]. A reduction in all cellular elements of the blood. SEE: *anemia, aplastic.*

pandemia (păn-dē′mĭ-ă) [Gr. *pan-*, all, + *dēmos*, the people]. Epidemic affecting the major portion of the population of a district.

pandemic (păn-dĕm′ĭk). A disease affecting the majority of the population of a large region, or which is epidemic at the same time in many different parts of the world.

pandiculation (păn″dĭk-ū-lā′shŭn) [L. *pandiculāri*, to stretch one's self]. Stretching of the limbs and yawning, as on awakening from normal sleep.

Paneth, cells of (pă'năt). [Josef Paneth, Ger. physician, 1857-1890]. Large secretory cells, containing coarse granules, found at the blind end of the crypts of Lieberkuhn (the intestinal glands).

pang. 1. A paroxysm of extreme agony. 2. A sudden attack of any emotion.

pangenesis (păn-jĕn'ĕ-sĭs) [Gr. *pan-*, all, + *genesis*, production.]. The discredited hypothesis that each cell of the parent is represented by a particle in the reproductive cell, and thus each part of the organism reproduces itself in the progeny.

panglossia (păn-glŏs'sĭ-ă) [Gr.]. Excessive talkativeness, esp. in psychotic persons.

panhidrosis (păn''hĭd-rō'sĭs) [Gr. *pan-*, all, + *hidrōs*, perspiration]. Perspiration over the entire surface of the body. SYN: *panidrosis*.

panhydrometer (păn''hī-drŏm'ĕt-ĕr) ["+ *hydor*, water, + *metron*, measure]. Apparatus for obtaining specific gravity of any fluid.

panhysterectomy (păn''hĭs-tĕr-ĕk'tō-mĭ) [Gr. *pan-*, all, + *hystera*, uterus, + *ektomē*, excision]. Excision of entire uterus including the cervix uteri.

NP: Preparation same as for ovariohysterectomy. SEE: *hysterectomy*.

panhysterocolpectomy (păn-hĭs''tĕr-ō-kŏl-pĕk'tō-mĭ) ["+ "+ *kolpos*, vagina, + *ektomē*, excision]. Total excision of the uterus and vagina.

panhystero-oophorectomy (păn-hĭs''ter-ō-o-of'-ō-rĕk'tō-mĭ) ["+ "+ *ōophoros*, bearing eggs, + *ektomē*, excision]. Excision of uterus, cervix uteri, and one or both ovaries.

panhysterosalpingo - oophorectomy (pan-his''ter-o-sal''ping-go-ō''ōf-ō-rĕk'tō-mĭ) ["+ "+ *salpinx*, tube, + *ōophoros*, bearing eggs,+ *ektomē*, excision]. Excision of entire uterus, ovaries, and uterine tubes.

panic (pan'ĭc). A sudden overwhelming fright, esp. one without a reasonable cause.

panidrosis (păn''ĭd-rō'sĭs) [Gr. *pan-*, all, + *hidrōs*, perspiration]. Panhidrosis, q.v.

panis (păn'ĭs) [L.]. Bread.

    p., mica. Breadcrumb.

panmyelophthisis (păn''mī-ĕl-of'thĭ-sĭs) [Gr. *pan-*, all, + *myelos*, marrow, + *phthisis*, a wasting]. General wasting away of the bone marrow.

panmyelosis (păn''mī-ĕl-ō'sĭs) ["+ "+ *-ōsis*, intensive]. Increase in all the elements of the bone marrow.

panneuritis (păn''ū-rī'tĭs) ["+ *neuron*, sinew, + *-itis*, inflammation]. Generalized neuritis.

    p. endemica, p. epidemica. Deficiency disease in which there is lack of vitamin B_1. SYN: *beriberi*.

panniculitis (pan-īk''ū-lī'tĭs) [L. *panniculus*, a small piece of cloth, + *-itis*, inflammation]. Inflamed condition of a layer of fatty connective tissue in the anterior wall of the abdomen.

SYM: Pain and tenderness and hypertrophy of tissue in parts where fat is the thickest.

panniculus (păn-ik'ū-lŭs) [L., a small piece of cloth]. Any clothlike sheet or layer of tissue.

    p. adiposus. [NA]. The subcutaneous layer of fat, esp. where fat is abundant; the superficial fascia which is heavily laden with fat cells.

    p. carnosus. Thin layer of muscular tissue in superficial fascia. SEE: *platysma myoides*.

pannus (păn'nŭs) [L., cloth]. Newly formed vascular tissue involving the upper half of the front of the cornea. The area is cloudy, and its surface is uneven as it is covered with a film of new capillary blood vessels. May cover entire cornea. Seen in trachoma, acne rosacea, eczema, and as a result of irritation in granular conjunctivitis.

    p. carateus. Pinta, q.v.

    p. carnosus. P. crassus, q.v.

    p. crassus. P. which is highly vascularized, thick, and opaque.

    p. degenerativus. P. siccus, q.v.

    p. siccus. P. accompanying xerophthalmia; composed principally of connective tissue; poorly vascularized and dry.

    p. tenuis. P. which is thin, poorly vascularized, and with slight opacity.

panophobia (păn-ō-fō'bĭ-ă) [Gr. *pan-*, all, + *phobos*, fear]. Morbid fear of some unknown evil or of everything in general; general apprehension. SYN: *pantophobia*.

panophthalmia, panophthalmitis (păn-ŏf-thăl'mĭ-ă, -mī'tĭs) ["+ *ophthalmos*, eye, + *-itis*, inflammation]. Inflammation of entire eye.

panoptic (păn-ŏp'tĭk) ["+ *optikos*, vision]. Making every part visible.

    p. stain. Stain which causes every part of the tissue to be differentiated.

panoptosis (păn-ŏp-tō'sĭs) ["+ *ptōsis*, falling]. General prolapse of the abdominal organs.

panosteitis (păn''ŏs-tē-ī'tĭs) [Gr. *pan-*, all, + *osteon*, bone, + *-itis*, inflammation]. Inflammation of every structure of a bone.

panotitis (păn-ō-ti'tĭs) ["+ *ōt-*, ear, + *-itis*, inflammation]. Inflammation involving all the parts of the ear.

panphobia (păn-fō'bĭ-ă) ["+ *phobos,* fear]. Groundless fear of everything. SYN: *pantophobia.*

pansinusitis (pan"si-nus-i'tis) [Gr. *pan-,* all + *sinus,* cavity, + *-itis,* inflammation]. Inflammation of all of the paranasal sinuses.

pansphygmograph (păn-sfĭg'mō-grăf) ["+ *sphygmos,* pulse, + *graphein,* to write]. Apparatus for registering cardiac movements, the pulse wave, and chest movements at the same time.

Panstrongylus (păn-strŏn'jĭ-lŭs). A genus of insects belonging to the order Hemiptera, family Reduviidae.

 P. megistus. Species which serves as vector for Trypanosoma cruzi, the causative agent of Chagas' disease.

pant [ME. *panten*]. 1. To breathe hard; to gasp for breath. 2. A short or labored breath.

 ETIOL: Produced by physical overexertion, as in running, or from fear.

pant-, panto- [Gr. *pantos,* all]. Combining form indicating all or the whole of something.

pantachromatic (păn"tă-krō-măt'ĭk) [Gr. *pant-,* all, + *achromatic,* colorless]. Entirely colorless.

pantalgia (păn-tăl'jĭ-ă) ["+ *algos,* pain]. Pain felt over the entire body.

pantatrophia, pantatrophy (păn-tă-trō'-fĭ-ă, -tat'rō-fĭ) ["+ *atrophia,* atrophy]. General wasting and atrophy.

panthodic (păn-thŏd'ĭk) ["+ *hodos,* way]. Radiating to all parts of the body, esp. applied to nervous impulses.

panting (pănt'ĭng) [ME. *panten*]. 1. Breathing hard; gasping for breath. 2. Labored breathing.

pantophobia (păn-tō-fō'bĭ-ă) [Gr. *pant-,* all, + *phobos,* fear]. Morbid, groundless fear of everything in general. SYN: *panophobia.*

pantoscopic (păn"tō-skŏp'ĭk) ["+ *skopein,* to examine]. Adjusted to view everything, both close and distant objects.

 p. glasses. Glasses with two segments of different focal lengths for near and far objects. SYN: *bifocal lenses.*

pantothenic acid (păn-tō-thĕn'ĭk). A vitamin of the B-complex group widely distributed in nature, occurring naturally in yeast, liver, heart, salmon, eggs, and various grains. It was synthesized in 1940.

pantothermia (păn"tō-thĕr'mĭ-ă) [Gr. *panto-,* all, + *thermē,* heat]. Condition in which there is a variation in bodily temperature without any apparent reason.

pantropic (pan-tro'pik, -trop'ik) [Gr. *pan-,* all, + *tropos,* turning]. Showing affinity to many organs, as pantropic viruses. SYN: *polycytotropic.*

panturbinate (păn-tur'bĭ-nāt) ["+ L. *turbinatus,* shaped like a top]. All of the turbinate structure of the nose; the nasal concha.

pap (păp) [L. *pappa,* infant's sound for food]. Any soft, semiliquid food.

papain (pă-pā'ĭn). Proteolytic enzyme obtained from the fruit of the papaya, Carica papaya. Used to tenderize meat.

Papanicolaou test. [George Papanicolaou, Amer. scientist, 1883-1962]. A study for early detection of cancer cells. It involves collecting material from areas of the body which shed cells or in which shed cells collect, esp. the cervix and vagina. This material is then prepared for microscopic study by special staining test. Analysis of the cells is extremely helpful in diagnosing cancer. ABBR: Pap smear; Pap test.

papaverine hydrochloride (pă-păv'ĕr-ēn) [L., poppy]. The salt of an alkaloid obtained from opium. Used as an antispasmodic, esp. in gastric and intestinal distress, and recommended in bronchial spasm.

papaya (pă-pā'yă) [Sp. AmerInd.]. 1. A tropical tree, Carica papaya. 2. Large, oblong, edible fruit from that tree. Source of papain, q.v.

paper (pā'per) [L. *papyrus,* paper]. 1. Cellulose pulp prepared in thin sheets from fibers of wood, rags, and other substances. 2. A piece of paper prepared with a medicinal solution. SYN: *charta.*

 p., bibulous. P. which absorbs water readily.

 p., blistering. A paper saturated with a substance, such as cantharides, that causes vesiculation.

 p., chromatography. Analysis of biological fluids by use of special papers that permit selectively the fluid constituents to migrate up the paper.

 p., filter. A porous, unglazed paper used for filtration.

 p., indicator. P. saturated with an indicator solution of known strength and then dried. Used for testing the pH (acidity or alkalinity) of a solution.

 p., litmus. An indicator paper impregnated with litmus, which in alkalies turns blue, in acids red.

 p., test. An indicator paper, q.v.

papilla (pă-pĭl'ă) [L.]. (pl. *papil'lae*) [NA]. A small, nipplelike protuberance or elevation.

 p., circumvallate. One of the large papillae near the base on the dorsal aspect of the tongue, arranged in a V-shape. The taste buds are located in the epithelium of the trench surrounding the papilla.

 p., dental. A mass of connective tissue that becomes enclosed by the developing enamel organ. It gives rise to dentine and dental pulp.

p., dermal. Small elevations of the corium that indent the inner surface of the epidermis.

p., duodenal. SEE: *p. of Vater.*

p., filiform. One of the very slender papillae at tip of the tongue.

p., fungiform. One of the broad, flat papillae resembling a fungus, chiefly found on dorsal central area of tongue.

p., gustatory. Taste papilla of tongue; one of those possessing a taste bud.

p. of hair. A conical process of the corium which projects into undersurface of a hair bulb. It contains capillaries through which a hair receives its nourishment.

p., lacrimal. An elevation in medial edge of each eyelid, in the center of which is the opening of the lacrimal duct.

p., lenticular. A small rounded elevation underlying lymphatic nodules in mucosa of root of tongue. SYN: *papillae lenticularis.*

p., lingual. Any one of the tiny eminences covering anterior two-thirds of tongue, including circumvallate, filiform, fungiform, and conical papillae.

p. mammae. [NA]. The nipple of the mammary gland. SYN: *mammary p.*

p., optic. Point at which optic nerve fibers leave the eyeball. SYN: *blind spot; optic disk; papilla nervi optici.*

p., renal. Apex of a malpighian pyramid in the kidney.

p., tactile. A dermal papilla that contains a sensory end-organ for touch.

p., taste. SEE: *gustatory p.*

p. of Vater. The duodenal end of the drainage systems of the pancreatic and common bile ducts. Commonly, but inaccurately, called ampulla of Vater. SYN: *duodenal papilla.*

papillary (păp′ĭ-lar-ĭ) [L. *papilla*, nipple]. 1. Concerning a nipple or papilla. 2. Resembling or composed of papillae.

p. ducts of Bellini. Short ducts which open on tip of renal papilla. They are formed by union of the straight collecting tubules.

p. layer. The layer of the corium that adjoins the epidermis. SYN: *stratum papillare.*

p. muscles. Muscular eminences in ventricles of the heart.

p. tumor. Neoplasm composed of or resembling enlarged papillae. SEE: *papilloma.*

papillate (păp′ĭ-lāt) [L. *papilla*, nipple]. Having nipplelike growths on the surface, as a culture in bacteriology.

papillectomy (păp′ĭ-lĕk′tō-mĭ) [″ + Gr. *ektomē*, excision]. Excision of any papilla or papillae.

papilledema (păp′ĭl-ĕ-dē′mă) [″ + Gr. *oidēma*, swelling]. Edema and inflammation of the optic nerve at its point of entrance into the eyeball. SYN: *choked disk.*

ETIOL: Intracranial pressure, often caused by tumor of the brain pressing on optic nerve.

PROG: Blindness may result very rapidly unless relieved.

papilliferous (păp′ĭ-lĭf′ĕr-ŭs) [″ + *ferre*, to carry]. Having or containing papillae.

papilliform (pă-pĭl′ĭ-form) [L. *papilla*, nipple, + *forma*, shape]. Having the characteristics or appearance of papillae.

papillitis (păp-ĭ-lī′tĭs) [″ + Gr. *-itis*, inflammation]. Inflammation of optic disk with edema. SYN: *choked disk.*

papilloadenocystoma (păp′ĭl-ō-ăd′ē-nōsĭs-tō′mă) [″ + Gr. *adēn*, gland, + *kystis*, a cyst, + *-ōma*, tumor]. A tumor composed of elements of papilloma, adenoma, and cystoma.

papillocarcinoma (păp′ĭl-ō-kăr-sĭ-nō′mă) [″ + Gr. *karkinos*, crab cancer, ″ + *-ōma*, tumor]. 1. A malignant tumor of hypertrophied papillae. 2. Carcinoma with papillary growths.

papilloma (păp-ĭ-lō′mă) [L. *papilla*, nipple, + Gr. *-ōma*, tumor]. 1. Any benign epithelian tumor. 2. Epithelial tumor of skin or mucous membrane consisting of hypertrophied papillae covered by a layer of epithelium. Included in this group are *warts, condylomas,* and *polyps.* SEE: *acanthoma.*

p. durum. A hardened p., as a wart or corn.

p., hard. P. which develops from squamous epithelium. SYN: *p. durum.*

p. molle. A p. with only a thin, horny layer covering it; condyloma.

p., soft. P. formed from columnar epithelium; applies to any small, soft growth.

papillomatosis (păp′ĭ-lō-mă-tō′sĭs) [L. *papilla*, nipple, + Gr. *-ōma*, tumor, + *-ōsis*, disease]. 1. Widespread formation of papillomas. 2. Condition of being afflicted with many papillomas.

papilloretinitis (păp′ĭ-lō-rĕt-ĭn-ī′tĭs) [″ + *rētē*, net, + Gr. *-itis*, inflammation]. Inflamed condition of the papilla and retina extending to the optic disk.

pappataci fever. SEE: *sandfly fever.*

pap′pose [L. *pappus*, down]. Covered with fine, downy hair.

pap′pus [L.]. The first growth of beard hair appearing on the cheeks and chin as a fine, downy hair.

paprika (păp'rĭ-ka, păp-rē'kă) [Gr. *peperi,* pepper]. A mild, powdered seasoning made from sweet red peppers. Also used to color food.

Pap smear; Pap test. Abbr. for Papanicolaou test, q.v.

papula (păp'ū-lă) [L.]. A small, inflammatory, congested spot on the skin; a pimple. SYN: *papule.*

papular (păp'ū-ler). Concerning an eruption of the nature of papules.

　　p. fever. Mild fever with maculopapular eruptions and rheumatoid pains.

papulation (păp-ū-lā'shŭn). 1. The development of papules. 2. The stage of pimple formation in a disease.

papule (păp'ūl) [L. *papula,* pimple]. Red elevated area on the skin, solid and circumscribed.

　　P.'s often precede vesicular or pustular formation and may appear in erythema multiforme, eczema papulosum, prurigo, syphilis, measles, smallpox, and they may develop after use of bromides, iodides, coal tar preparations, etc.

　　In *measles* they are small and run together. In *smallpox* they are hard and feel like shot, terminating in umbilicated vesicles that itch. In *prurigo* they are small, pale, deep seated, and accompanied by intense itching. In *syphilis* they are dark colored and widely distributed, esp. on the trunk and surfaces of the extremities; they do not cause itching. In *eczema* they are small, often associated with pustules and vesicles, and are closely aggregated; there is intense itching and the skin is thickened. In *erythema multiforme* they are found with macules and tubercles and are bright red or purple and flat, appearing esp. on the extremities; they do not suppurate or cause itching.

　　p., dry. Chancre; hard p. which is primary lesion of syphilis, occurring at site of infection.

　　p., moist; p., mucous. A syphilitic eruption of papules with flat tops. SYN: *condyloma latum.*

papuliferous (păp'ū-lĭf'ĕr-ŭs) [L. *papula,* pimple, + *ferre,* to bear]. Having papules or pimples.

papulo- [L. *papula,* pimple]. Combining form indicating a pimple or a papule.

papyraceous (păp-ĭ-rā'shŭs) [L.]. Parchmentlike. In obstetrics it denotes a fetus retained in the uterus beyond natural term, thus assuming a mummified appearance.

par [L., equal]. A pair, esp. a pair of cranial nerves.

p. vagum. The vagus or 10th pair of cranial nerves.

para [L. *parere,* to bring forth, to bear]. Used as a combining form to indicate a woman who has produced viable offspring. Ex: A woman who has been delivered of two or more living children is a multipara; one who has not delivered a living child is a nullipara. 2. Used as a prefix (Para-O or Para-1) to indicate the number of living children a woman has delivered.

para-, par- [Gr. *para,* beyond; L. *par,* equal, pair]. Combining forms meaning near, beside, past, beyond, the opposite, abnormal, irregular, or two like parts. ABBR: p- when used in chemistry to indicate *para-.*

para-aminobenzoic acid (păr''ă-ăm-ĭ-nō-bĕn-zō'ĭk). Inhibits bacteriostatic action of sulfonamides; hence contraindicated during sulfonamide therapy. ABBR: PABA.

para-aminosalicylic acid (păr''ă-ăm-ĭ-nō-săl-ĭ-sĭl'ĭk). An adjuvant to streptomycin or dihydrostreptomycin in treatment of tuberculosis. Valuable both for inhibitory effect on tubercle bacillus and for ability to delay development of streptomycin-resistant organisms. ABBR: PAS.

para-anesthesia (păr''ă-ăn-ĕs-thē'zĭ-a) [Gr. *para,* two like parts, + *an-,* negative, + *aisthēsis,* sensation]. Anesthesia of two corresponding sides, esp. of lower half of body.

para-appendicitis (păr''ă-ă-pĕn''-dĭ-sī'tĭs) [Gr. *para,* beside, + L. *appendix,* + Gr. *-itis,* inflammation]. Inflammation involving the connective tissue adjacent to the appendix. SYN: *perityphlitis.*

parabionts ["+ *bioun,* to live]. Two individuals living in the condition of parabiosis, q.v.

parabiosis (păr''ă-bĭ-ō'sĭs) [Gr. *para,* two like parts, + *biōsis,* living]. 1. Joining together of two individuals. This may occur congenitally as with Siamese twins or by surgical means. 2. Temporary suppression of excitability of a nerve.

parabiotic (păr''ă-bĭ-ŏt'ĭk). Concerning parabiosis.

parablepsia, parablepsis (păr''ă-blĕp'sĭ-ă, -sĭs) [Gr. *para,* irregular, + *blepsis,* vision]. Abnormality of the visual sensations.

parabulia (păr''ă-bū'lĭ-ă) ["+ *boulē,* will]. Perversion or abnormality of will power.

paracanthoma (păr''ă-kăn-thō'mă) [Gr. *para,* beside, + *akantha,* thorn, + *-ōma,* tumor]. A tumor involving the prickle-cell layer of the epidermis.

paracasein (păr-ă-kā'sē-ĭn). A substance formed when rennin or pepsin acts on the casein of milk. In the presence of calcium ions, an insoluble protein is formed resulting in the curdling of milk.

Paracelsus (păr-ă-sĕl'sŭs). [Philippus Aureolus Theophrastus Bombastus von Hohenheim, 1493-1541] Swiss alchemist and physician who introduced several chemicals (lead, sulfur, iron, and arsenic) into pharmaceutical chemistry. Remembered because of his independent spirit, observant mind, and his fearlessness in breaking with traditional practice.

paracentesis (păr''ă-sĕn-tē'sĭs) [Gr. *para*, beside, + *kentēsis*, a puncture]. Puncture of a cavity with removal of fluid, as in pleural effusion or ascites.

NP: Watch pulse and respirations for signs of collapse during and following procedure.

    p., abdominal. Tapping of the abdomen.

    p. capitis. P. of the cranium.

    p. cordis. Surgical puncture of the heart.

    p. pericardii. Puncture of the pericardial sac.

    p. pulmonis. Removal of fluid from a lung.

    p. thoracis. Drainage of fluid from the cavity of the chest. SEE: *aspiration.*

    p. tunicae vaginalis. Puncture of the tunica vaginalis.

    p. tympani. Drainage or irrigation through incision of the tympanic membrane.

    p. vesicae. Puncture of the wall of the urinary bladder.

paracentetic (păr''ă-sĕn-tĕt'ĭk). Concerning paracentesis.

paracentral (păr''ă-sĕn'trăl) [Gr. *para*, near, + L. *centralis*, center]. Located near the center.

    p. lobule. Cerebral convolution on mesial surface joining the upper terminations of the ascending parietal and frontal convolutions.

paracholia (păr''ă-kō'lĭ-ă) [Gr. *para*, abnormal, + *cholē*, bile]. Condition of disturbed bile secretion.

parachordal (păr-ă-kor'dăl) [Gr. *para*, beside, + *chordē*, cord]. Lying alongside the anterior portion of the notochord in the embryo.

    p. cartilage. One of a pair of cartilages in head of embryo which in man unite to form a single basal plate which is the forerunner of the occipital bone.

parachroma (păr''ă-krō'mă) [Gr. *para*, abnormal, + *chrōma*, color]. Unusual coloration of the skin.

parachromatopsia (păr''ă-krō-mă-tŏp'sĭ-ă) ["+ "+ *opsis*, vision]. Color blindness.

parachromatosis (păr''ă-krō-mă-tō'sĭs) ["+ "+ *-ōsis*, disease]. Any one of the diseases in which the skin is pigmented.

parachromophoric (păr''ă-krō''mō-for'ĭk) ["+ "+ *phoros*, bearing]. Excreting pigment, but retaining it within the organism.

paracinesia, paracinesis (păr''ă-sĭ-nē'zĭ-ă, -sĭs) [Gr. *para*, abnormal, + *kinēsis*, motion]. Condition in which there is perversion of motor powers; motor abnormality. SYN: *parakinesia.*

paracme (par-ăk'mĭ) [Gr. *par-*, beyond, + *akmē*, point]. Denoting the stage at which symptoms or a fever begin to decline.

Paracoccidioides (par''ă-kŏk-sĭd''ē-oy'dēz). A genus of yeastlike fungi.

    P. brasiliensis. The causative agent of paracoccidioidomycosis.

paracoccidioidomycosis (par''ă-kŏk-sĭd''ē-oy''dō-mĭ-kō'sĭs). A chronic granulomatous disease of the skin caused by Paracoccidioides brasiliensis. SYN: *South American blastomycosis.*

paracolitis (par''ă-kō-lī'tĭs). Inflammation of the tissue surrounding the colon.

paracolon bacilli. Colonlike bacilli which ferment lactose. They can cause urinary tract infections, and occasionally gastroenteritis.

paracolpitis (păr''ă-kŏl-pī'tĭs) [Gr. *para*, beside, + *kolpos*, vagina, + *-itis*, inflammation]. Inflammation of tissues surrounding the vagina.

paracolpium (păr''ă-kŏl'pī-ŭm). The connective tissue adjacent to the vagina.

paracrisis (păr-ak'rĭ-sĭs, păr''ă-krī'sĭs) [Gr. *para*, abnormal, + *krinein*, to secrete]. Any abnormality of body secretions.

paracusia (par''ă-kū'sĭa) ["+ *akousis*, a hearing]. Any abnormality or disorder of the sense of hearing.

    p. acris. Excessively acute hearing.

    p. duplicata. The hearing of one sound as two. SYN: *diplacusis.*

    p. loci. Difficulty in locating the direction of sound.

    p. willisiana. An apparent ability to hear better in a noisy place, found in deafness due to stapes fixation and adhesive processes. SYN: *paracusis of Willis.*

paracusis (par''ă-kū'sĭs). Impaired hearing.

    p. of Willis. SEE: *paracusia willisiana.*

paracyesis (păr-ă-sī-ē'sĭs) [Gr. *para*, abnormal, + *kyēsis*, pregnancy]. Extrauterine pregnancy.

paracystitis (păr''ă-sĭs-tī'tĭs) [Gr. *para*, beside, + *kystis*, bladder, + *-itis*, inflammation]. Inflamed condition of connective tissues and other structures around the urinary bladder.

paracystium (păr-ă-sĭs'tĭ-ŭm). The connective tissue surrounding the urinary bladder.

paradenitis (păr''ăd-ĕn-i'tĭs) [Gr. *para*, beside, + *adēn*, gland, + *-itis*, inflammation]. Inflammation of tissues around a gland.

paradidymis (păr-ă-dĭd'ĭ-mĭs) ["+ *didymos*, testicle]. [NA]. The atrophic remnants of the tubules of the wolffian body, situated on the spermatic cord above the epididymis.

paradione (par-ă-di'ŏn). Proprietary name for a preparation of paramethadione, an anticonvulsant drug.

paradoxic, paradoxical (păr''ă-dŏk'sĭk, -sĭ-kal) [Gr. *paradoxos*, conflicting with expectation]. Seemingly contradictory, but demonstrably true.

paraffin (păr'ă-fĭn) [L. *parum*, little, + *affinis*, neighboring]. 1. A waxy, white, tasteless, odorless mixture of solid hydrocarbons obtained from petroleum. Used as ointment base or wound dressing. 2. One of a series of saturated aliphatic hydrocarbons having the formula C_nH_{2n+2}. Paraffins constitute the methane or paraffin series.

p., hard. Solid p. with a melting point between 45° C. and 60° C.

p., liquid. Liquid hydrocarbon. SYN: *liquid petrolatum*.

p., soft. A semisolid p. SEE: *petrolatum*.

paraffinoma (păr''ă-fĭn-ō'mă) ["+ "+ Gr. *-ōma*, tumor]. A tumor which arises at site of injection of paraffin.

paraffinum (păr-ă-fē'nŭm) [L.]. Paraffin, q.v.

paraformaldehyde (par''ă-fŏr-măl'dě-hĭd). A white, powdered antiseptic and disinfectant, a polymer of formaldehyde.

paragammacism (păr''ă-găm'mă-sĭzm) [Gr. *para*, irregular, + *gamma*, Gr. letter G, + *ismos*, condition]. Inability to pronounce "g," "k," and "ch" sounds, with substitution of other consonants such as "d" or "t."

paraganglia (păr''ă-găng'lĭ-ă) [Gr. *para*, beside, + *ganglion*, knot]. (sing. *paraganglion*). [NA]. Groups of chromaffin cells, similar in staining reaction to cells of the adrenal medulla, associated anatomically and embryologically with the sympathetic system. They are located in various organs and parts of the body.

paraganglioma (păr''ă-găng-lĭ-ō'mă) ["+ "+ *-ōma*, tumor]. A tumor derived from chromaffin cells. Includes tumors of the adrenal medulla and the paraganglia. SYN: *pheochromocytoma*.

paraganglion (păr''ă-găng'lĭ-ŏn) [Gr. *para*, beside, + *ganglion*, knot]. (pl. *paraganglia*). SEE: *paraganglia*.

parageusia, parageusis (păr-ă-gū'sĭ-ă, -sĭs) [Gr. *para*, abnormal, + *geusis*, taste].

Disorder or abnormality of the sense of taste.

paraglobulin (păr''ă-glŏb'ū-lĭn) [Gr. *para*, near, + L. *globulus*, a small sphere]. A globulin found in blood plasma, lymph, and other body fluids; associated with coagulation.

paraglobulinuria (păr''ă-glŏb''ū-lĭn-ū'rĭ-ă) ["+ "+ Gr. *ouron*, urine]. Excessive excretion of paraglobulin in the urine.

paraglossa (păr-ă-glŏs'să) [Gr. *para*, abnormal, + *glōssa*, tongue]. 1. Enlargement of the tongue. 2. Congenital hypertrophy of the tongue.

paraglossia (par''ă-glŏs'sĭ-ă). Inflammation of the tissues underlying the tongue.

paragomphosis (par''ă-gŏm-fō'sĭs) [Gr. *para*, abnormal, + *gomphoun*, to fasten, + *-osis*, condition]. Impaction of the fetal head in the pelvic canal.

Paragonimus (păr''ă-gŏn'ĭ-mŭs). Genus of trematode worms.

P. westermani. The lung fluke, a common parasite of certain mammals including man, dog, cat, pig, and mink. Human infestation occurs through eating raw crabs or crayfish, the second intermediate host. Infestation endemic in certain parts of Orient.

par'agram'matism. A speech defect characterized by improper use of words and inability to arrange them grammatically.

paragraphia (păr-ă-grăf'ĭ-ă) [Gr. *para*, opposite, + *graphein*, to write]. The writing of letters or words other than those intended.

parahemophilia (par''ă-hē''mō-fĭl'ĭ-ă) [Gr. *para*, irregular, + *haima*, blood, + *philein*, to love]. A rare, congenital, idiopathic disorder due to deficiency of factor V characterized by prolonged prothrombin and coagulation times.

parahepatitis (păr''ă-hĕp''ă-ti'tĭs) [Gr. *para*, beside, + *hēpar, hēpat-*, liver, + *-itis*, inflammation]. Inflamed condition of parts immediately adjacent to the liver.

par'ahor'mone [Gr. *para*, beyond, + *hormaein*, to set in motion]. A substance which is conveyed through the circulatory system and exerts a stimulating effect like hormones, yet not originating in endocrine tissue. Ex: carbon dioxide.

par'ahypno'sis [Gr. *para*, abnormal, + *hypnos*, sleep]. Abnormal or disordered sleep.

par'ainfec'tion [Gr. *para*, beside, + L. *in*, into, + *facere*, to make]. The symptomatology of an infectious disease without evidence of the presence of the microorganisms causing the disease.

parakeratosis (păr''ă-kĕr''ă-tō'sĭs) ["+ *keras, kerat-*, horn, + *-osis*, infection]. Any disorder affecting the horny layer of the epidermis.

p. psoriasiformis. Scab formation resembling that of psoriasis.

p. scutularis. Scalp disease with hairs encircled by epidermic crust formation.

parakinesia. SEE: *paracinesia.*

paralalia (păr″ă-lā′lī-ă) [Gr. *para,* abnormal, + *lalein,* to babble]. Any speech defect characterized by sound distortion.

p., literalis. Stammering, q.v.

paralambdacism (păr″ă-lăm′dă-sĭzm) [Gr. *para,* irregular, + *lambda,* Gr. letter L, + *ismos,* condition]. Inability to sound the letter "l" correctly, substituting some other letter for it.

paralbumin (păr″ăl-bū′mĭn) [Gr. *para,* beside, + L. *albumen,* white of egg]. An albumin found in fluid content in ovarian cysts and in ascites.

paraldehyde (păr-ăl′dĕ-hīd). USP. $C_6H_{12}O_3$. A liquid polymer of acetaldehyde that is colorless with unpleasant taste and characteristic, but not unpleasant odor. Made by action of hydrochloric acid on acetic aldehyde.

ACTION AND USES: Hypnotic, having low toxicity and prompt action as a sedative. Sometimes used as an analgesic in obstetrics, esp. in combination with rectal ether.

POISONING SYM: Resemble those of chloral hydrate—cardiac and respiratory depression, dizziness, collapse with partial or complete anesthesia. Odor on the breath is a constant distinct sign.

F. A. TREATMENT: Same as for chloral hydrate, q.v.

CAUTION: Do not dispense paraldehyde from a bottle that has been open longer than 24 hours. Oxidation occurs in partially-filled containers to form acetic acid.

paraldehydism (păr-ăl′dĕ-hīd″ĭzm). Poisoning from an overdose of paraldehyde, q.v.

paralepsy (păr′ă-lĕp″sĭ) [Gr. *para,* abnormal, + *lēpsis,* seizure]. Temporary attack of mental inertia and hopelessness, or sudden alteration in mood or mental tension. SYN: *psycholepsy.*

paralexia (păr″ă-lĕk′sĭ-ă) ["+ *lexis,* speech]. Inability to comprehend printed words or sentences with substitution of meaningless combinations of words.

paralgesia (păr″ăl-jē′zĭ-ă) ["+ *algēsis,* sense of pain]. Any unusual sensation that is painful.

paralgia (păr-al′jĭ-ă) ["+ *algos,* pain]. Sensation both abnormal and painful.

parallagma (păr″ăl-ăg′mă) [Gr. *parallagma,* alternation]. Overlapping or displacement of the fragments of a fractured bone.

parallax (păr′ă-lăks) [Gr. *parallaxis,* change of position]. The apparent movement or displacement of objects caused by change in observational position or by movement of the head or eyes.

paralogia (păr″ă-lō′jĭ-ă) [Gr. *para,* abnormal, + *logos,* understanding]. A disorder of the reasoning.

p., benign. Disordered thinking and communication of thought. Delusions, bizarre thoughts, hallucinations, and regressive behavior are absent. The patient is not severely incapacitated and should not be considered to have schizophrenia.

paralutein cells. Theca lutein cells. SEE: *lutein cells.*

paralysis (pă-răl′ĭ-sĭs) [Gr. *paralyein,* to disable at one side]. (pl. *paralyses*) Temporary suspension or permanent loss of function, esp. loss of sensation or voluntary motion.

Any voluntary movement depends on the integrity of two motor neurons—one arising in the motor cortex, coursing across the brain stem and ending in the anterior gray horn of the spinal cord; and the lower neurons arising in the anterior horn cell and passing to the muscle. If the latter are destroyed, the muscle loses tone, atrophies (withers away), and shows reaction of degeneration (R. D.).

The flaccidity and absent muscular reflexes reveal the loss of tonus. If the upper neuron is paralyzed, the patient is equally unable to move the affected part, but the intact lower neuron may permit other motor centers to act on the muscle. In addition, tone is increased, there is no R.D., and no atrophy except that of disuse. So-called pathological reflexes may appear in addition to the increase of normal deep reflexes.

Paralyses are divided into two groups—*spastic* when due to lesion of upper motor neuron, and *flaccid* when due to lesion of lower motor neuron.

Psychic inhibition of motor function occurs most characteristically in hysteria, but the evidence of organic disease is always lacking in these hysterical paralyses.

p. of accommodation. Inability of the eye to adjust itself to various distances due to paralysis of ciliary muscles.

p., acoustic. Deafness, q.v.

p., acute ascending. Rapidly progressing form of paralysis which begins in the feet and slowly ascends. Fatal within one to three weeks. SYN: *Landry's p.*

p., acute atrophic. SEE: *p., infantile.*

p., acute infectious. SEE: *p., infantile.*

p. agitans. A disease of middle and late life producing a picture of rigid tremulousness progressive in its course, and marked by weakness, delay of voluntary motion, a peculiar festinating gait, and muscular contraction, causing peculiar and characteristic positions of the limbs and head. While movement is slow, there is no true paralysis. The face appears expressionless, there is general flexion attitude, the balance tends to be lost (in a forward direction). Sometimes occurs following encephalitis lethargica; others are due to an unknown cause. SYN: *Parkinson's disease, q.v.*

p., alcoholic. P. due to habitual drunkenness.

p., anesthesia. P. which develops following administration of anesthesia.

p., anterior spinal. SEE: *p., infantile.*

p., arsenical. P. following poisoning from arsenic.

p., ascending. P. beginning with the lower limbs and progressing upward.

p., association. SEE: *p., bulbar.*

p., Bell's. Facial paralysis.
ETIOL: Lesion of the facial nerve or of its nucleus; a neuritis of this nerve. Pressure on nerve as it reaches the face through its bony canal near the ear.
SYM: One side of entire face may be affected, corner of mouth may drop, or eyelid may droop or be unable to close, patient may be unable to close lips or to speak, or lose control of eye.

p., Bernhardt's. Pain and hyperesthesia on the outer femoral surface from lesion or disease of the external cutaneous nerve of the thigh.

p., birth. P. caused by injury received at birth.

p., brachial. P. of one or both arms.

p., brachiofacial. P. of the face and an arm.

p., Brown-Sequard's. P. due to a cutting through of the spinal cord. On the side of the lesion there is paralysis with loss of position and vibration sense. On the opposite side there is loss of sensation of pain and temperature.

p., bulbar. P. caused by changes in the motor centers of the brain stem.

p., central. Any p. from a lesion of the brain or spinal cord.

p., cerebral spastic infantile. Nonprogressive p. resulting from developmental defects in brain or from trauma at birth. SYN: *cerebral palsy; Little's disease.*

p., complete. P. in which there is total loss of function and sensation.

p., compression. P. due to prolonged pressure on a nerve, as by a crutch or during sleep.

p., crossed. P. affecting one side of the face and limbs of the opp. side of the body.

p., crutch. P. due to pressure in the armpit.

p., decubitus. P. due to pressure on a nerve from lying in one position for a long time, as in sleep.

p., diver's. P. due to decrease in pressure after a deep-sea diver has been exposed to pressure greater than atmospheric pressure. SYN: *caisson disease; bends.*

p., Erb's. 1. SEE: *p., birth.* 2. Partial p. of the brachial plexus.

p., exhaustion. P. due to prolonged voluntary movements involving exhaustion of the nerve centers.

p., facial. SEE: *p., Bell's.*

p., flaccid. P. in which there is loss of muscle tone, loss of or reduction of tendon reflexes, atrophy and degeneration of muscles, and reaction of degeneration. Due to lesions of lower motor neurons of spinal cord.

p., general. Progressive loss of power and mental faculties resulting eventually in dementia and death. SYN: *paresis.*

p., ginger. P. of the limbs after drinking Jamaica ginger. SYN: *Jamaica ginger polyneuritis,* q.v.

p., glossolabial. P. of the tongue and lips. Occurs in bulbar paralysis, q.v.

p., histrionic. P. of certain facial muscles, producing a fixed facial expression of a certain emotion.

p., hysteric. One that may simulate any form of p.; it appears to have no adequate causative lesion.

p., incomplete. Partial p. of the body or a part.

p., infantile. Motor p. in children with atrophy of a group of muscles, following an acute infectious disease which is transmitted by a filtrable virus. SYN: *acute anterior poliomyelitis.*

p., ischemic. P. resulting from impaired blood supply.

p., jake. SEE: *p., ginger.*

p., Klumpke's. Wasting p. of the arms and hands; often resulting from birth injury.

p., Kussmaul's; p., Landry's. SEE: *p., acute ascending.*

p., lead. P. following poisoning by lead.

p., local. P. of a single muscle or one group of muscles.

p., muscular. Loss of the capacity of muscles to contract. May be due to a structural or functional disorder in the muscle, at the myoneural junction, in efferent nerve fibers, in cell bodies of nuclei of origin of brain or gray matter of spinal cord, in conducting pathways of brain or spinal cord, or in motor centers of the brain.

p., nuclear. P. caused by lesion of a nerve nucleus in the central nervous system.

p., obstetrical. SEE: *p., birth.*

p., periodic. P. which recurs and abates temporarily.

p., phonetic. P. of the vocal cords.

p., progressive bulbar. SEE: *p., bulbar.*

p., pseudobulbar. P. caused by cerebral center lesions, simulating the bulbar types of paralysis.

p., sensory. Loss of sensation. May be due to a structural or functional disorder of the sensory end-organs, sensory nerves, conducting pathways of spinal cord or brain, or sensory centers in the brain.

p., sleep. Condition of being unable to speak or move even though fully aware of external events. Most commonly occurs upon awakening but may appear just prior to falling asleep. The attack usually is of short duration but to the patient the elapsed time may seem like hours. The exact cause or explanation of this condition is unknown.

p., spastic. P. usually involving groups of muscles. Characterized by excessive tone and spasticity of muscles, exaggeration of tendon reflexes but loss of superficial reflexes, positive Babinski response, no atrophy or wasting except from prolonged disuse, and absence of reaction of degeneration. Due to lesions of upper motor neurons or cerebrum.

p., spinal. P. due to injury or disease of the spinal cord.

p., supranuclear. P. resulting from disorders in pathways or centers above nuclei of origin.

p., tick-bite. P. resulting from bites of certain species of ticks, esp. of the genera Ixodes and Dermacentor, presumably due to a toxin present in saliva of tick. Affects domestic animals and humans, esp. children. Causes a progressive ascending, flaccid, motor paralysis. Recovery usually occurs after removal of ticks.

p., Todd's. A transitory paralysis following an epileptic seizure.

p., tourniquet. P., esp. of the arm, resulting from a tourniquet being applied for too long a time.

p., vasomotor. P. of vasomotor centers resulting in lack of tone and dilation of blood vessels.

p., Volkmann's. SEE: *p., ischemic.*

p., wasting. Progressive wasting away of the muscles. SEE: *progressive muscular atrophy.*

paralytic (păr″ă-lĭt′ĭk) [Gr. *paralyein*, to disable at one side]. 1. Concerning paralysis. 2. One afflicted with paralysis.

p. dementia. Progressive paralysis with mental deterioration. SYN: *paresis.*

p. ileus. P. of intestinal wall with distention and symptoms of acute obstruction and prostration.

ETIOL: It may occur after any abdominal operation.

paralyzant (păr″ă-lĭz″ănt) [Fr. *paralyser*, paralyze]. 1. Causing paralysis. 2. A drug or other agent that induces paralysis.

paralyze (păr″ă-līz) [Fr. *paralyse*]. 1. To cause temporary or permanent loss of muscular power or sensation. 2. To render ineffective.

paramastitis (păr″ă-măs-tī′tĭs) [Gr. *para*, beside, + *mastos*, breast, + *-itis*, inflammation]. Inflammation around the breast.

paramedic (par″ă-mĕd′ĭk) [Gr. *para*, beyond, + L. *medicus*, doctor]. A military physician or trained medical assistant who parachutes to areas where medical services are needed, or participates in rescue operations.

paramedical. Supplementing the work of medical personnel in related fields: social work; physical, occupational, and speech therapy.

paramenia (păr″ă-mē′nĭ-ă) [Gr. *para*, abnormal, + *mēniaia*, menses]. Irregular, abnormal, or difficult menstruation.

parameter (păr-ăm′ĕ-ter) [Gr. *para*, near, + *metron*, measure]. In mathematics, an arbitrary constant, each value of which determines the specific form of the equation in which it appears. Often misused by biologists to indicate a variable.

paramethadione (par″ă-mĕth″ă-dī′ōn) USP. An anticonvulsant agent used to control petit mal seizures in epilepsy.

parametric (păr″ă-mĕt′rĭk) [Gr. *para*, near + *mētra*, uterus]. 1. Concerning the area near the uterus. 2. Rel. to the parametrium, the tissue surrounding the uterus. 3. Adjective form of parameter.

parametritis (păr″ă-mē-trī′tĭs) ["+ "+ *-itis*, inflammation]. Inflamed condition of parametrium, the cellular tissue adjacent to uterus. SYN: *pelvic cellulitis.*

parametrium (păr-ă-mē′trī-ŭm) ["+ *mētra*, uterus]. [NA]. Fat and loose connective tissue, and smooth muscle, around the uterus.

paramimia (păr″ă-mĭm′ĭ-ă) [Gr. *para*, abnormal, + *mimeisthai*, to imitate]. Use of gestures which are inappropriate to the spoken words which they accompany.

paramnesia (păr″ăm-nē′zĭ-ă) [Gr. *para*, the opposite, + *amnēsia*, loss of memory]. 1. The use of words without meaning. 2. The distortion of memory in which there is inability to distinguish imaginary or suggested experiences from those which have actually occurred. 3. Seeming recall of events which never have occurred.

paramorphia (păr″ă-mor′fĭ-ă) [Gr. *para*, abnormal, + *morphē*, form]. Abnormality of shape or structure.

paramusia (păr″ă-mū′zĭ-ă) ["+ *mousa*, music]. A form of aphasia in which the ability to render music correctly is lost.

paramyoclonus multiplex [Gr. *para*, beside, + *mys*, *my-*, muscle, + *klonos*, tumult]. Sudden and frequent shocklike contractions usually affecting muscles of both legs, and trunk muscles particularly. The contractions which disappear during sleep and motion, may occur 10 to 50 times each minute. Usually the condition develops spontaneously but has been known to follow fright, trauma, infectious diseases, and poliomyelitis.

paramyosinogen (păr″ă-mĭ″ŏ-sĭn′ō-jĕn) [Gr. *para*, beside, + *myosin*, protein globin of muscle, + *gennan*, to produce]. Protein derived from muscle plasm.

paramyotonia (păr″ă-mĭ″ŏ-tō′nĭ-ă) [Gr. *para*, irregular, + *mys*, muscle, + *tonos*, tone]. A disorder marked by muscular spasms and abnormal muscular tonicity.

   p. ataxia. Tonic muscular spasm with slight ataxia or paresis when making any attempt at movement.

   p. congenita. Congenital condition of tonic muscular spasms when body is exposed to cold. SYN: *Eulenburg's disease.*

   p., symptomatic. Temporary muscular rigidity when first trying to walk, as in paralysis agitans.

paramyxoviruses. A group of viruses similar in physical, chemical, and biological characteristics. However, they are quite different pathogenetically. Includes parainfluenza, measles, mumps, German measles, Newcastle disease, and respiratory syncytial viruses. SEE: *myxoviruses.*

paranasal (par″ă-nā′săl) [Gr. *para*, near, + L. *nasalis*, pert. to nose]. Situated near or alongside the nasal cavities.

   p. sinuses. Accessory nasal sinuses which open into the nasal cavities. They are the frontal (antrum of Highmore), ethmoidal, sphenoidal, and maxillary. All are lined with a ciliated mucous membrane continuous with that of the nasal cavities. Their significance and function have been the subject of speculation but theories have not been proven.

paraneoplastic syndromes. Indirect effects of neoplasms which may be so severe as to be the actual cause of death rather than the tumor itself. These include endocrine effects of neoplasms of the lungs, kidneys, and various endocrine glands.

paranephritis (păr″ă-ne-fri′tĭs) ["+ *nephros*, kidney, + *-itis*, inflammation]. 1. Inflamed condition of the suprarenal capsules. 2. Inflammation of connective tissue about kidney. SYN: *perinephritis.*

paranephros (păr-ă-nĕf′rŏs). A suprarenal or adrenal capsule.

paranoia (păr″ă-noy′ă) [Gr. *para*, abnormal, + *nous*, mind]. A chronic, psychotic entity characterized by fixed but ever-expanding systematized delusions of persecution. General characteristics are sensitiveness, suspiciousness, jealousy, brooding nature, excessive self-consciousness, fixed ideas developed into well-systematized logical delusions, megalomania, rare hallucinations, and inability to make concessions.

paranoiac (păr-ă-noy′ăk). 1. Concerning or afflicted with paranoia. 2. One suffering from paranoia.

paranoid (păr′ă-noyd) [Gr. *para*, abnormal, + *nous*, mind, + *eidos*, resemblance]. 1. Resembling paranoia. 2. A person afflicted with paranoia.

   p. reaction type. Individual who has fixed systematized delusions, is suspicious, has a persecution complex, is resentful and bitter, and is a megalomaniac. Many states approach true paranoia and resemble it, but lack one or more of its distinguishing features. Some of these are transitory p. states due to toxic conditions; p. type of schizophrenia; and p. states due to alcoholism.

   NP: In dealing with all types of paranoid patients, do not handle without an assistant.

paranomia (păr″ă-nō′mĭ-ă) ["+ *onoma*, name]. Form of aphasia in which there is inability to remember correct name of objects shortly after seeing or using them.

paranorm′al. 1. Pert. to experiences that are not within the range of normal experiences or are not scientifically explainable. 2. Moderately abnormal.

paranuclein (păr″ă-nū′klē-ĭn). A protein which does not yield nitrogenous bases when decomposed. SYN: *nucleoalbumin.*

paranucleus (păr″ă-nū′klē-ŭs) [Gr. *para*, near, + L. *nucleus*, a kernel]. A small body lying close to a cell nucleus.

paraomphalic (păr″ă-ŏm-făl′ĭk) ["+ *omphalos*, navel]. Adjacent to the navel. SYN: *paraumbilical.*

paraoperative (păr″ă-ŏp′ĕr-ă-tĭv) [Gr. *para*, beyond, + L. *operārī*, to work]. Concerning all the details and accessories of operation and preparation of the patient.

paraosteoarthropathy (păr″ă-ŏs″tē-ō-ăr-thrŏp′ăth-ĭ) [Gr. *para*, two like parts, + *osteon*, bone, + *arthron*, joint, + *pathos*, disease]. Paralysis of lower portion of the body in addition to bone and joint disease.

paraparesis (păr″ă-păr-ē′sĭs, -par′ē-sĭs) ["+ *paresis*, paralysis]. Partial paralysis affecting the lower limbs.

parapathia (păr-ă-păth′ĭ-ă) [Gr. *para*, beyond, + *pathos*, disease]. Emotional aspects of a disorder.

parapedesis (păr″ă-pĕd-ē′sĭs) [Gr. *para*, abnormal, + *pēdēsis*, leaping]. Secretion or excretion through other than normal channels.

parapeptone (păr″ă-pĕp′tōn) [Gr. *para*, beside, + *peptein*, to digest]. Intermediate digestion product of albumin. SEE: *peptone*.

paraphasia (păr-ă-fā′zĭ-ă) [Gr. *par*, irregular, + *aphasis*, speech loss]. The misuse of spoken words or word combinations; a form of aphasia.

paraphemia (păr″ă-fē′mĭ-ă) [Gr. *para*, opposite, + *phēmē*, speech]. A disorder marked by consistent use of the wrong words, or mispronunciation of words.

paraphia (păr-ā′fĭ-ă) [Gr. *para*, abnormal, + *haphē*, touch]. Abnormality of the sense of touch.

paraphimosis (păr″ă-fĭ-mō′sĭs) [Gr. *para*, beside, + *phimoun*, to muzzle, + *-osis*, condition]. Strangulation of glans penis due to retraction of narrowed or inflamed foreskin.

   p. oculi. Retraction of eyelid behind the eyeball.

paraphobia (păr″ă-fō′bĭ-ă) [Gr. *para*, irregular, + *phobos*, fear]. A mild form of phobia.

paraphonia (păr″ă-fō′nĭ-ă) [Gr. *para*, abnormal, + *phōnē*, voice]. Partial loss, weakness, or abnormal change of the voice.

   p. puberum. A harsh, deep voice that develops in boys at puberty.

paraphora (păr-ăf′ō-ră) [Gr., a wandering]. A mental disorder of minor degree.

paraphrasia (păr-ă-frā′zĭ-ă) [Gr. *para*, abnormal, + *phrasis*, speech]. Disorder characterized by incoherent speech. SYN: *paraphasia*.

paraphrenia (păr-ă-frē′nĭ-ă) ["+ *phrēn*, mind]. A group of psychoses now called "paranoid conditions."

   p. confabulans. P. marked by memory distortions.

   p. expansiva. P. with delusions of grandeur, exaltation, and moderate excitement.

   p. systematica. P. with progressive delusions of persecution, followed by delu-

sions of grandeur, but intellect shows no deterioration.

paraphrenitis (păr″ă-frē-nī′tĭs) [Gr. *para*, beside, + *phrēn*, diaphragm, + *-itis*, inflammation]. Inflammation of the tissues around the diaphragm.

paraplasm (păr′ă-plăzm) [Gr. *para*, abnormal, + *plasma*, a thing formed]. 1. Any abnormal new formation or malformation. 2. The fluid portion of protoplasm. SYN: *hyaloplasm*.

paraplastic (păr″ă-plăs′tĭk) ["+ *plastikos*, formed]. 1. Misshapen; deformed. 2. Pert. to fluid portion of protoplasm.

paraplectic (păr″ă-plĕk′tĭk) [Gr. *paraplēktikos*, striking at the side]. Afflicted with paralysis of lower extremities. SYN: *paraplegic*.

paraplegia (păr-ă-plē′jĭ-ă) [Gr. *paraplēgia*, stroke on one side]. Paralysis of lower portion of the body and of both legs.

   ETIOL: A lesion involving the spinal cord which may be due to the following: maldevelopment, epidural abscess, hematomyelia, acute transverse myelitis, spinal neoplasms, multiple sclerosis, syringomyelia or trauma.

   p., alcoholic. P. of spinal origin due to excessive use of alcohol.

   p., ataxic. Lateral and posterior sclerosis of spinal cord characterized by slowly progressing ataxia and paresis.

   p., cerebral. P. from bilateral cerebral lesion.

   p. dolorosa. P. due to pressure of a neoplasm on posterior spinal cord and nerve roots. Extremely painful despite paralysis.

   p., peripheral. P. due to pressure on, injury to, or disease of peripheral nerves.

   p., senile. P. resulting from sclerosis of arteries supplying spinal cord.

   p., spastic. P. characterized by increased muscular tone and accentuated tendon reflexes. Seen in multiple sclerosis and other conditions involving the pyramidal tracts.

   p., spastic, primary. P. from degeneration in pyramidal tracts.

   p., tetanoid. SEE: *p., spastic*.

paraplegic (păr-ă-plē′jĭk) [Gr. *paraplēgia*, stroke on one side]. Pert. to, or affected with, paraplegia. SYN: *paraplectic*.

parapleuritis (păr″ă-plū-rī′tĭs) [Gr. *para*, beside, + *pleura*, a side, + *-itis*, inflammation]. 1. Inflammation in the thoracic wall. 2. Mild inflammation of the pleura. 3. Pain in the pleura. SYN: *pleurodynia*.

parapoplexy (păr-ăp′ō-plĕk″sĭ) [Gr. *par*, irregular, + *apoplēxia*, apoplexy]. A mild or slight apoplexy with partial stupor; a stupor resembling apoplexy. SYN: *pseudoapoplexy.*

parapraxia, parapraxis (păr-ă-prăk'sĭ-ă, -sĭs) [Gr. *para,* opposite, + *praxis,* doing]. Disturbed mental processes producing inaccuracy, forgetfulness, and tendency to misplace things and make slips of speech or pen.

paraproctitis (păr''ă-prŏk-tī'tĭs) [Gr. *para,* near, + *prōktos,* anus, + *-itis,* inflammation]. Inflamed condition of tissues near the rectum.

paraproteinemia. A general term for abnormalities of the immunoglobulins, associated with one of several disease states.

parapsia, parapsis (păr-ăp'sĭ-ă, -sĭs) [Gr. *para,* abnormal, + *hapsis,* touch]. Any disorder of touch. SYN: *paraphia.*

parapsoriasis (păr''ă-sō-rī'ă-sĭs) [Gr. *para,* irregular, + *psōriasis,* itching]. A chronic disorder of the skin marked by scaly red lesions.

parapsychology (par''ă-sī-kŏl'ō-jī). The division of psychology which deals with extrasensory perception, telepathy, psychokinesis, clairvoyance, and associated phenomena.

pararenal (păr''ă-rē'năl) [Gr. *para,* near, + L. *rēn,* kidney]. Near the kidneys.

pararhotacism (păr''ă-rō'tă-sĭzm) [Gr. *para,* abnormal, + *rho,* Gr. letter R, + *ismos,* condition]. Constant erroneous use of letter "r" or the placing of undue emphasis on letter "r."

parasalpingitis (păr''ă-săl-pĭn-jī'tĭs) [Gr. *para,* beside, + *salpinx, salping-,* tube, + *-itis,* inflammation]. Inflamed condition of tissues around an oviduct or a eustachian tube.

parasecretion (par''ă-sē-krē'shŭn) [Gr. *para,* abnormal, + L. *secretio,* secretion]. 1. An abnormality in secretion. 2. A substance abnormally secreted.

parasigmatism (păr''ă-sĭg'mă-tĭzm) ["+ *sigma,* Gr. letter S, + *ismos,* condition]. Imperfect pronunciation of the letter "s." SYN: *lisping.*

parasite (păr'ă-sīt) [Gr. *parasitos,* fellow guest]. 1. An organism that lives within, upon, or at expense of another organism, known as the host, without contributing to survival of the host. 2. The smaller or incomplete element of conjoined twins which is attached to and dependent upon the more nearly normal twin, called the autosite.

   p., accidental. One infesting a host that is not its normal host.

   p., external. One which lives on the outer surface of its hosts. EX: fleas, lice, mites, ticks. SYN: *ectoparasite.*

   p., facultative. P. capable of living independently of its host at times. Opposed to obligate p.

   p., incidental. P., accidental, q.v.

   p., intermittent. P. which visits its host at intervals.

   p., internal. P. which lives within the body of the host, occupying the digestive tract or body cavities, or living within body organs, blood, tissues, or even cells. EX: protozoa, worms.

   p., obligate. P. completely dependent on its host. SEE: *p., facultative.*

   p., occasional. P. which seeks its host at intervals to obtain nourishment. SYN: *periodic p.*

   p., periodic. P., occasional, q.v.

   p., permanent. P. which lives upon its host until maturity or spends its entire life upon its host. EX: flukes, itch mites.

   p., specific. P. which requires a specific host in order to complete its life cycle.

   p., temporary. P. which is free-living during a part of its life cycle.

parasitic (păr''ă-sĭt'ĭk) [Gr. *parasitikos*]. Like, caused by, or concerning, a parasite.

parasitic disease drug service. The Center for Disease Control (CDC), Public Health Service, U.S. Department of Health, Education, and Welfare, maintains a supply of antiparasitic agents which otherwise are difficult to obtain. These drugs are available to licensed physicians on an investigational basis by writing the Center for Disease Control, Atlanta, Ga., 30333, U.S.A.

parasiticide (păr''ă-sĭt'ĭ-sīd) [Gr. *parasitos,* fellow guest, + L. *caedere,* to kill]. 1. Destructive to parasites. 2. An agent that will kill parasites.

parasitism (păr'ă-sĭt'ĭzm) ["+ *ismos,* condition]. The state or condition of being infected or infested with parasites.

parasitize (păr''ă-sĭtĭz'). To infest or infect with a parasite.

parasitogenic (păr''ă-sī''tō-jĕn'ĭk) [Gr. *parasitos,* fellow guest, + *gennan,* to produce]. 1. Caused by parasites. 2. Favoring parasite development.

parasitology (păr''ă-sī-tŏl'ō-jī) ["+ *logos,* study]. The study of parasites and parasitism.

parasitophobia (păr''ă-sī''tō-fō'bĭ-ă) ["+ "+ *phobos,* fear]. Unusual fear of parasites.

parasitosis (păr''ă-sī-tō'sĭs) [Gr. *parasitos,* fellow guest, + *-ōsĭs,* condition]. A disease or condition resulting from parasitism.

parasitotropic (păr''ă-sī''tō-trŏp'ĭk) ["+ *tropos,* turning]. Having attraction for parasites, esp. certain drugs that act chiefly upon

Antiparasitic Drugs Available from CDC

Drug	Disease
Pentamide isethionate	Pneumocystis pneumonia, Gambian sleeping sickness
Niclosamide (Yomesan)	Tapeworm infections
Bithionol	Paragonimiasis
Bayer 2502	Chaga's disease
Sodium antimony dimercaptosuccinate (Astiban)	Schistosomiasis
Dehydroemetine	Amebiasis
Suramin	Rhodesian sleeping sickness, onchocerciasis
Sodium antimony gluconate (Pentostan)	Leishmaniasis
Mel B	Sleeping sickness

parasites in the body.

paraspadia (păr-ă-spā'dĭ-ă) [Gr. *paraspadein,* to draw aside]. Condition in which the urethra has an opening through one side of the penis.

paraspasm (păr'ă-spazm) [L. *paraspasmus*]. 1. Muscular spasm of the lower extremities. 2. Spastic paralysis of the lower extremities.

parasteatosis (păr"ă-stē"ă-tō'sĭs) [Gr. *para,* abnormal, + *steatos,* fat, + *-ōsis,* disease]. Any disordered condition of the sebaceous secretions.

parasternal (păr-ă-stern'ăl) [Gr. *para,* beside, + *sternon,* chest]. Beside the sternum.

p. line. Imaginary vertical line running midway between sternal margin and line passing through the nipple.

p. region. Area between sternal margin and parasternal line.

parasthenia (păr"ăs-thē'nĭ-ă) [Gr. *para,* abnormal, + *sthenos,* strength]. Condition characterized by abnormal functioning of organic tissue at odd intervals.

parastruma (păr-ă-strū'mă) ["+ L. *struma,* goiter]. Goiterlike tumor due to hypertrophy of a parathyroid gland.

parasympathetic (păr"ă-sĭm"pă-thĕt'ĭk) [Gr. *para,* beside, + *sympathētikos,* sympathetic nerve]. Of or pertaining to the craniosacral division of the autonomic nervous system.

p. nervous system. The craniosacral division of the autonomic nervous system. Preganglionic fibers originate from nuclei in the midbrain, medulla, and sacral portion of the spinal cord. They pass through cranial nerves III, VII, IX, and X and the second, third, and fourth sacral nerves, and synapse with postganglionic neurons located in auto-

nomic (terminal) ganglia which lie in the walls of or near the organ innervated.

Some effects of parasympathetic stimulation are constriction of pupil, contraction of smooth muscle of alimentary canal, constriction of bronchioles, slowing of heart rate, and increased secretion by glands, except sweat glands. Parasympathetic effects are specific rather than general. SEE: *autonomic nervous system; sympathetic nervous system.*

parasympathicotonia (păr-ă-sĭm-păth-ĭk-ō-tŏn'ĭ-ă) [Gr. *para,* irregular, + *sympathetikos,* sympathetic nerve, + *tonos,* tension]. Condition in which there is an imbalance in functioning of the autonomic nervous system, the parasympathetic division dominating over the sympathetic. SYN: *vagotonia.*

parasympatholytic (păr"ă- sĭm-pă-thō-lĭ-t'ĭk) ["+ "+ *lytikos,* dissolving]. Having a destructive effect on or blocking parasympathetic nerve fibers.

parasympathomimetic (păr"ă-sĭm-pă-thō-mĭm-ĕt'ĭk) ["+ "+ *mimētikos,* imitative]. Producing effects similar to those resulting from stimulation of parasympathetic nervous system.

parasynovitis (păr-ă-sĭn-ō-vī'tis) [Gr. *para,* beside, + *syn,* with, + *ōon,* egg, + *-itis,* inflammation]. Inflamed condition of tissues around a synovial sac.

parasyphilis (par"ă-sĭf'ĭ-lĭs) [Gr. *para,* beyond, + *syn,* with, + *philos,* love]. Any disease condition that is indirectly due to syphilis.

parasyphilitic (păr"ă-sĭf-ĭ-lit'ĭk). Being nonsyphilitic but due to syphilis.

parasystole (păr-ă-sĭs'tō-lē) [Gr. *para*, abnormal, + *systolē*, contraction]. Abnormally prolonged interval of rest between the systole and diastole.

paratarsium (păr-ă-tar'sĭ-ŭm) [Gr. *para*, beside, + *tarsos*, tarsus]. The covering and connective tissues of the tarsus of the feet.

paratenon (păr″ă-tĕn'ŏn) ["+ *tenōn*, tendon]. Fatty and areolar tissue that surrounds the tendon and fills the spaces around the tendon.

paratereseomania (păr″ă-tĕr-ē″sē-ō-mā'nĭ-ă) [Gr. *paratērēsis*, observation, + *mania*, madness]. Insane desire to investigate new scenes and subjects.

paratherapeutic (păr″ă-thĕr′ă-pū'tĭk) [Gr. *para*, beyond, + *therapeutikē*, treatment]. Caused by the treatment used for another disease.

parathormone (păr″ă-thor'mōn) [Gr. *para*, beside, + *thyroid*, + *hormaein*, to excite]. An extract from fresh or frozen parathyroid glands of domestic animals which contains the active principle or principles of these glands.

parathymia (păr″ă-thi'mĭ-ă) [Gr. *para*, abnormal, + *thymos*, mind, spirit]. Disordered state of the emotions.

parathyroid (păr-ă-thi'royd) [Gr. *para*, beside, + *thyreos*, shield, + *eidos*, form]. 1. Located close to the thyroid gland. 2. One of several small endocrine glands about 6 mm. long by 3 to 4 mm. broad on the back of, and at lower edge of, the thyroid gland, or embedded within its substance. These glands secrete a hormone, parathormone, which regulates calcium-phosphorus metabolism.

Hyposecretion, or *hypoparathyroidism*, results in neuromuscular hyperexcitability as manifested in tetany. Blood calcium falls and blood phosphorus rises. Other symptoms include cataract, teeth defects, bone lesions, maldevelopment of hair and nails, and skin disturbances. *Hypersecretion*, or *hyperparathyroidism*, results in a rise in blood calcium and fall in phosphorus. Calcium is removed from bones, resulting in increased fragility. Muscular weakness, reduced muscular tone, and general neuromuscular hypoexcitability occur. Generalized osteitis fibrosa or osteitis fibrosa cystica (von Recklinghausen's disease) is a clinical entity associated with hyperplasia and resulting hypersecretion of the parathyroids. Parathormone, q.v., secreted by these glands contains the active principle or principles. SEE: *thyroid* for illustration.

parathyroidectomy (păr-ă-thi-royd-ĕk'tō-mĭ) ["+ "+ "+ *ektomē*, excision]. Excision of one or more of the parathyroid glands.

parathyroprivia (păr″ă-thi″rō-prĭ'vĭ-ă) ["+ "+ L. *privus*, deprived of]. Condition that results when the parathyroids are removed or cease functioning.

parathyroprivic, parathyroprivous (păr-ă-thi-rō-prĭv'ĭk, -ŭs). Resulting from loss of, function of, or removal of, parathyroid glands.

paratonsilar (păr″ă-tŏn'sĭl-ăr) [Gr. *para*, near, + L. *tonsillaris*, pert. to tonsil]. Near or about the tonsil.

paratrichosis (păr″ă-trĭ-kō'sĭs) [Gr. *para*, abnormal, + *trichōsis*, being hairy]. Abnormality of hair or its location.

paratrimma (păr-ă-trĭm'mă) ["+ *tribein*, to rub]. Chafing; irritation of the skin. SYN: *intertrigo.*

paratripsis (păr″ă-trĭp'sĭs). 1. Rubbing, chafing. 2. A slowing of catabolism.

paratrophic (păr″ă-trō'fĭk) [Gr. *para*, abnormal, + *trophē*, nourishment]. 1. Requiring living substances for food; parasitic. 2. Pert. to abnormal nutrition.

paratrophy (păr-at'rō-fĭ). 1. Localized fatty swellings and nerve lesions in various regions of the body. SYN: *Dercum's disease, adiposis dolorosa.* 2. Defective nutrition. SYN: *dystrophy.*

paratuberculosis (păr″ă-tū-bĕr′kū-lō'sĭs) [Gr. *para*, irregular, L. *tuberculus*, a tubercle, + Gr. *-ōsis*, disease]. A nontuberculous disease thriving in a tuberculous environment.

paratyphlitis (păr″ă-tĭf-lī'tĭs) [Gr. *para*, near, + *typhlos*, blind, + *-ītis*, inflammation]. Inflammation of the connective tissue close to the cecum.

paratyphoid (păr-ă-ti'foyd) ["+ *typhos*, fever, + *eidos*, like]. Similar to typhoid.

p. fever. An infectious fever resembling typhoid.

ETIOL: Bacteria of the genus Salmonella, esp. the species S. paratyphi (A & B strains) and S. schottmulleri. However, any Salmonella pathogenic to man may cause a similar disease.

SYM: Fever with gastroenteritis. Incubation period may be less than in typhoid. Usually patient's condition is less severe than that found in typhoid fever, but symptoms vary from a mild transient diarrhea to those quite similar to typhoid fever, q.v.

paratypic (păr″ă-tĭp'ĭk) [Gr. *para*, irregular, + *typos*, type]. Diverging from a type.

paraumbilical (păr″ă-ŭm-bĭl'ĭk-ăl) [Gr. *para*, near, + L. *umbilicus*, navel]. Close to the navel.

paraurethral (păr″ă-ū-rē′thrăl) ["+ *ourē-thra,* urethra]. Located close to the urethra.

parauterine (păr″ă-ū′těr-īn) ["+ L. *uterus,* womb]. Around the uterus.

paravaginal (păr″ă-văj′ĭn-ăl) [Gr. *para,* beside, *vagina,* sheath]. Around the vagina.

paravaginitis (păr″ă-văj-ĭn-ī′tĭs) ["+ "+ Gr. *-itis,* inflammation]. Inflammation of the tissue surrounding the vagina.

paravertebral (păr″ă-ver′tĕ-brăl) [Gr. *para,* near, + L. *vertebralis,* pert. to vertebrae]. Alongside or near the vertebral column.

p. anesthesia. Injection of a local anesthetic at roots of spinal nerves.

paravesical (păr″ă-věs-ĭk′ăl) ["+ L. *vesica,* bladder]. Near the urinary bladder.

paraxial (păr-ăk′sĭ-ăl) ["+ L. *axis,* axis]. On either side of the axis of the body, or one of its parts.

parazoon (păr″ă-zō′ŏn) ["+ Gr. *zŏon,* animal]. An animal which lives as a parasite upon another animal.

parched (parchd) [ME. *parchen*]. Extremely dry.

parectasia, parectasis (păr″ěk-tā′sĭ-ă, -sĭs) [Gr. *para,* beyond, + *ektasis,* stretching]. Excessive dilatation or stretching of a structure.

paregoric (păr-ĕ-gor′ĭk) [L. *parēgoricus,* soothing]. 1. USP. Camphorated tincture of opium, a narcotic-containing drug which in large doses is poisonous. Used extensively in the symptomatic treatment of diarrhea. 2. Soothing.

TREATMENT FOR POISONING: Same as for morphine, q.v.

parenchyma (păr-ĕn′kĭ-mă) [Gr. *parenkheim,* to pour in beside). [NA]. The essential parts of an organ which are concerned with its function in contradistinction to its framework.

p. disease. Disease affecting the principal tissue of an organ.

p. testis. [NA]. The functional portion of the testis, including the seminiferous tubules within the lobules.

parenchymatitis (păr″ĕn-kĭm″ă-tĭ′tĭs) ["+ *-itis,* inflammation]. Inflamed condition of parenchyma or substance of a gland.

parenchymatous (păr″ĕn-kĭm′ă-tŭs). Concerning the essential substances of an organ.

parent (păr′ĕnt) [L. *parēns*]. A father or a mother; one who begets offspring.

p. fixation. Continuation of the child-parent affiliation into the adult state, so that the person has an abnormal attachment to a parent.

parenteral (păr-ĕn′tĕr-ăl) [Gr. *para,* opposite, + *enteron,* intestine]. Situated or occurring outside of the intestines.

p. digestion. Digestion of foreign substances by body cells as opposed to enteral digestion, which occurs in the alimentary canal.

p. hyperalimentation. Providing the total caloric needs by intravenous route for a patient who is unable to take food orally. Although this is extremely difficult, patients have been maintained in a healthy state for prolonged periods by placing a catheter through the subclavian vein in the superior vena cava.

The daily feeding of 2500-3000 K.Cal. for an adult includes 2500-3000 ml. of water; 100-130 gm. protein hydrolysate (amino acids); 12-18 gm. nitrogen; 525-625 gm. dextrose; 125-150 mEq sodium; 75-120 mEq potassium; 4-8 mEq magnesium; vitamins A, D, E, C, thiamine, riboflavine, niacin, and panthothenic acid. Calcium, phosphorus, and iron given as required; vitamin B_{12}, folic acid, and vitamin K given intramuscularly as needed. Trace elements required after one month of continuous feeding.

p. injection. Injection of substances into the body through any route other than via alimentary canal. Ex: subcutaneous, intravenous, intramuscular, or intrathecal injection.

p. therapy. Introduction of a substance, esp. nutritive material, into the body by means other than the intestinal tract.

parepithymia (păr″ĕp-ĭ-thī′mĭ-ă) [Gr. *para,* abnormal, + *epithymia,* desire]. Abnormal desire or craving.

paresis (păr′ē-sĭs, pă-rē′sĭs) [Gr. *parienai,* to let fall]. 1. Partial or incomplete paralysis. 2. An organic mental disease with somatic, irritative, and paralytic focal symptoms and signs running a slow, chronic, progressive course and tending to a fatal termination. SYN: *general paresis of the insane; dementia paralytica.*

ETIOL: Diffuse and focal involvement of brain and spinal cord due to syphilis, usually occurring 5-15 years after primary infection.

PATH: A diffuse meningoencephalitis with degenerative changes dependent upon vascular and toxic factors.

SYM: May simulate any psychoneuroses or psychoses. Pupillary changes, facial tremors, tremors of the lips and tongue, speech disturbances. Usually Argyll-Robertson pupil, impaired vision, headache, speech slurred with letters and syllables often omitted. Epileptic convulsions. Unequal exaggeration of the reflexes. Always a positive serologic test for syphilis in the spinal fluid with increase of protein and lymphocytes. Colloidal gold curve is abnormal in more than half the cases. Memory defective, expansive delusions, depression, dementia. TREATMENT: Penicillin.

p., juvenile. General p. due to congenital syphilis; seen in children.

paresthesia (păr″ĕs-thē′zĭ-ă) [Gr. *para*, abnormal, + *aisthēsis*, sensation]. Abnormal sensation without objective cause, such as numbness, prickling, and tingling; heightened sensitivity. Experienced in central and peripheral nerve lesions and in locomotor ataxia.

paretic (pă-rĕt′ĭk, pă-rē′tĭk) [Gr. *parienai*, to let fall]. Affected with or concerning paresis.

pareunia (păr-ū′nĭ-ă) [Gr. *pareunos*, lying beside]. Sexual intercourse. SYN: *coition; coitus; copulation.*

paridrosis (păr″ĭ-drō′sĭs) [Gr. *para*, abnormal, + *hidrōsis*, perspiration]. Any disordered secretion of perspiration.

paries (pā′rĭ-ēs) [L., a wall]. (pl. *pari'etes*) [NA]. The enveloping wall of any structure; applied esp. to hollow organs.

parietal (pă-rī′ĕ-tăl) [L. *parietalis*]. Pert. to, or forming, the wall of a cavity. SEE: *suture, sagittal.*

p. bone. One of two bones which together form the roof and sides of the skull.

p. cells. Large cells on margin of the peptic glands of stomach.

p. lobe. The division of each side of the brain lying beneath each p. bone, q.v.

parietes (pă-rī′ĕ-tēs) [L.]. Pl. of paries; walls of an organ or hollow part.

pari passu (par′ē păs′ū) [L., with equal speed]. Occurring at the same time or at the same rate; side by side.

Paris green (păr′ĭs grēn). A compound of copper and arsenic, q.v.; copper acetoarsenite. Poisonous; used as a pigment and insecticide.

parity (păr′ĭ-tĭ). 1. [L. *par*, equal]. Equality, similarity. 2. [L. *parere*, to bear]. The condition of a woman with respect to the number of children she has borne. SEE: *multiparity; nulliparity; primiparity; secundiparity.*

Parkinson's disease (par′kĭn-sŭn). [James Parkinson, Eng. physician, 1755-1824]. A chronic nervous disease characterized by a fine, slowly spreading tremor; muscular weakness and rigidity; and a peculiar gait.

SYM: Onset may be abrupt; generally insidious. First symptom is a fine tremor beginning in hand or foot which may spread till it involves all the members. At first paroxysmal but becomes almost continuous. Face becomes expressionless. Speech slow and measured, later muscular rigidity. Head bowed, body bent forward, arms flexed, thumbs turned into palms, knees slightly bent. Gait characteristic by this time; steps grow faster and faster, body inclines more and more forward until patient falls, seeks some support; this is termed festination. Occasionally a tendency to fall backwards; retropulsion replaces festination. Numbness, tingling, sensation of heat.

PROG: Recovery rarely if ever occurs. Duration indefinite.

TREATMENT: General supportive measures plus medicines to combat muscle rigidity and lethargy. Destruction of a part of the thalamus on one side by producing extreme cold in a very small area. It is not a cure but alleviates tremors. A drug, L-dopa, has produced considerable improvement in some cases. SYN: *palsy, shaking; paralysis agitans.*

Parkinson's mask. Expressionless appearance of the face. Eyebrows are raised, wrinkles are smoothed out, and there is immobility of the facial muscles.

A typical symptom seen in P.'s disease and in postencephalitic states.

Parkinson's syndrome. Symptoms of P.'s disease, q.v. SYN: *parkinsonism.*

paroccipital (păr-ŏk-sĭp′ĭt-ăl) [Gr. *para*, near, + L. *occiput*, occiput]. 1. Close to the occipital bone. 2. The paramastoid process.

parodontitis (păr″ō-dŏn-ti′tĭs) ["+ *odous, odont-*, tooth, + *-itis*, inflammation]. Inflamed condition of tissues around a tooth.

parodynia (păr-ō-dĭn′ĭ-ă) [L. *parere*, to bear, + Gr. *odynē*, pain]. 1. Labor pains. 2. Difficult or abnormal labor or birth. SYN: *dystocia.*

p. perversa. Presentation with fetus lying transversely across the uterus. SYN: *cross birth.*

parolivary (păr-ŏl′ĭ-vă″rĭ) [Gr. *para*, near, + L. *oliva*, olive]. Situated close to the olivary body.

p. bodies. Nuclei in medulla oblongata, lying close to the olivary bodies.

paromphalocele (păr″ŏm-făl′ō-sēl″) ["+ *omphalos*, navel, + *kēlē*, hernia]. Hernia or tumor close to the umbilicus.

paroniria (păr-ō-nĭ′rĭ-ă) [Gr. *para*, abnormal, + *oneiros*, dream]. Abnormal dreaming of a terrifying nature.

p. ambulans. Sleepwalking.

p. salax. Restlessness in sleep with lascivious dreams and nocturnal emissions.

paronychia (păr-ō-nĭk′ĭ-ă) [Gr. *para*, near, + *onyx, onych-*, nail]. Acute or chronic infection of marginal structures about the nail. SYN: *runaround; whitlow.*

ETIOL: Trauma, infection.

SYM: Redness, swelling, and suppuration around nail edge.

TREATMENT: Heat to area unless there is inadequate blood supply; surgery in severe cases.

p. tendinosa. Inflammation of sheath of a digital tendon. ETIOL: Sepsis.

paronychomycosis (păr″ō-nĭ-kō-mī-kō′sĭs). Fungus infection about the nails.

paronychosis (păr-ō-nĭ-kō′sĭs). Growth of a nail in an abnormal position.

paroophoron (păr-ō-ŏf′ō-rŏn) [Gr. *para*, near, + *ōon*, egg, + *phoros*, bearing]. A group of minute tubules located in mesosalpinx between uterus and ovary. It is a vestigial structure consisting of the remains of the caudal group of mesonephric tubules and is a homolog of the paradidymis in the male.

parophthalmia (păr-ŏf-thăl′mĭ-ă) [″+ *ophthalmos*, eye]. Inflamed condition of tissue around the eye.

parophthalmoncus (păr″ŏf-thăl-mŏn′kŭs) [″+ ″+ *onkos*, mass]. A tumor located near the eye.

paropsis (păr-ŏp′sĭs) [Gr. *para*, abnormal, + *opsis*, vision]. Any disorder of sense of sight.

parorchidium (păr-ōr-kĭd′ĭ-ŭm) [″+ *orchis*, *orchid*-, testicle]. Abnormal position, or nondescent, of a testicle. SYN: *ectopia testis.*

parorexia (păr-ō-rĕk′sĭ-ă) [Gr. *para*, abnormal, + *orexis*, appetite]. An abnormal or perverted craving for special or strange foods. SEE: *appetite; taste.*

parosmia (păr-ŏz′mĭ-ă) [″+ *osmē*, odor]. Any disorder or perversion of the sense of smell; a false sense of odors or perception of those which do not exist. Agreeable ones are considered offensive, and disagreeable odors are accepted as pleasant. SYN: *parosphresia.* SEE: *kakosmia.*

parosphresia, parosphresis (păr″ŏs-frē′-zĭ-ă, -sĭs) [″+ *osphrēsis*, smell]. Disordered sense of smell. SYN: *parosmia*, q.v.

parosteitis, parostitis (păr-ŏs-tē-ī′tĭs, -tī′tĭs) [Gr. *para*, beside, + *osteon*, bone, + *-itis*, inflammation]. Inflammation of tissues next to the bone.

parosteosis, parostosis (păr″ŏs-tē-ō′sĭs, -tō′sĭs) [Gr. *para*, abnormal, + ″+ *-ōsis*, disease]. 1. Bone formation outside of the periosteum. 2. Bone development in an unusual location.

parotic (pă-rŏt′ĭk) [Gr. *para*, near, + *ous*, *ōt*-, ear]. Near the ear.

parotid (pă-rŏt′ĭd). Located near the ear; esp. the p. gland, q.v.

p. duct. Approx. 2 in. (5.08 cm.) long. Extends from anterior border of the parotid gland crossing the masseter and piercing the buccinator, and then runs between the buccinator and the mucous membrane. It opens

in the mouth opposite 2nd upper molar. The transverse facial artery is above the duct and buccal branch of 7th nerve below. SYN: *Stensen's duct.* SEE: *saliva.*

p. gland. A nearly pure serous gland, its secreting tubules and acini being long and branched. It is enclosed in a sheath, the parotid fascia. The p. gland is one of the salivary glands of the mouth. Its secretion helps to lubricate food and make it easier to chew and swallow.

parotidectomy (pă-rŏt-ĭ-dĕk′tō-mĭ) [Gr. *para*, near, + *ous*, *ot*-, ear, + *ektomē*, excision]. Excision of parotid gland.

parotiditis (pă-rŏt″ĭ-dī′tĭs) [″+ ″+ *-itis*, inflammation]. Parotitis, q.v.

parotidoscirrhus (pă-rŏt″ĭd-ō-skĭr′ŭs) [″+ ″+ *skirrhos*, hardness]. 1. Hardening of the parotid gland. 2. A scirrhous cancer of the parotid area.

parotitis (pă″rō-tī′tĭs) [Gr. *para*, near, + *ous*, *ot*-, ear, + *-itis*, inflammation]. Inflammation of the parotid gland, either simple or epidemic. SYN: *mumps.*

parous (pā′rŭs) [L. *pario*, to bear]. Parturient; fruitful; having borne at least one child.

parovarian (par-ō-vā′rĭ-ăn) [Gr. *para*, near, + L. *ovarium*, ovary]. 1. Situated near or beside the ovary. 2. Pert. to the parovarium, a residual structure in the broad ligament.

parovariotomy (păr″ō-vā″rĭ-ŏt′ō-mĭ) [″+ ″+ Gr. *tomē*, a cutting]. Removal of a parovarian cyst.

parovarium (păr″ō-vā′rĭ-ŭm). The epoophoron, q.v. SYN: *body of Rosenmuller.*

paroxysm (păr′ŏk-sĭzm) [Gr. *paroxysmos*, irritation]. 1. A sudden, periodic attack or recurrence of symptoms of a disease; an exacerbation of the symptoms of a disease. 2. A sudden spasm or convulsion of any kind. 3. Sudden emotional state, as of fear, grief, or joy.

paroxysmal (păr-ŏk-sĭz′măl). 1. Occurring in or concerning paroxysms. 2. Of the nature of a paroxysm.

parricide (par′ĭ-sīd) [L. *parricida*]. The murdering of one's own parent or a close relative. SYN: *patricide.*

Parrot (păr-ŏ′). [Jules Marie Parrot, Fr. physician, 1839-1883].

P.'s disease. The pseudoparalysis of the extremities in infants; caused by syphilis.

P.'s nodes. Bony nodules on skull of infants with syphilis.

P.'s sign. In meningitis, pupils dilate upon pinching the skin of neck.

P.'s ulcer. Lesions of thrush or stomatitis.

par'rot fever. SYN: *psittacosis*, q.v.

pars (parz) [L.]. (pl. *partes*) [NA] A part; portion of a larger structure.

p. anterior hypophyseos. The anterior lobe of the hypophysis.

p. basilaris ossis occipitalis. [NA] Basilar process of the occipital bone.

p. buccalis hypophyseos. Developmental protrusion in primitive buccal cavity of anterior lobe of hypophysis.

p. caeca oculi. The optic disk.

p. caeca retinae. The parts of the retina not sensitive to light (pars ciliaris retinae and pars iridica retinae, q.v.).

p. cavernosa urethra. Cavernous portion of urethra of male.

p. cephalica nervi sympathici. Plexus, ganglia, and nerves derived from sympathetic nerve.

p. ciliaris retinae. [NA] Portion of retina situated in front of ora serrata and covering the ciliary body.

p. distalis. That part of the hypophysis forming the major portion of the anterior lobe.

p. flaccida. A portion of membrane of the eardrum which fills the notch of Rivinus. SYN: *Shrapnell's membrane.*

p. intermedia. The intermediate lobe of the hypophysis cerebri.

p. iridica retinae. [NA] Portion of retina on posterior surface of iris.

p. membranacea urethrae. The membranous portion of the urethra.

p. nervosa hypophyseos. Posterior lobe of the pituitary gland.

p. optica hypothalami. The optic chiasma.

p. optica retinae. [NA] The sensory portion of the retina extending from optic disc to ora serrata.

p. tensa. The larger portion of the tympanic membrane, a tightly stretched membrane lying inferior to the maleolar folds.

p. tuberalis. The portion of the anterior lobe of the hypophysis cerebri which invests the infundibular stalk.

par'sley [ME. *persely*]. A plant, Petroselinum crispum, belonging to the carrot family. It is used principally in its fresh form as a garnish for foods. It is the source of a volatile oil called apiol.

Food value of 100 gm. (raw): Cal. 44; protein 3.6 gm.; carbohydrate 8.5 gm.; calcium 203 mg.; phosphorus 63 mg.; sodium 45 mg.; potassium 727 mg.; vitamin A, 8500 I.U.

par'snip [ME. *pasnepe*]. A strongly scented herb of the carrot family, cultivated for its white edible root.

Food value of 100 gm. (cooked): Cal. 66; protein 1.5 gm.; fat 0.5 gm.; carbohydrate 15 gm.; calcium 45 mg.

part. aeq. Abbr. for *partes aequales*, equal parts.

partes (pär'tēs). Pl. of pars, q.v.

parthenogenesis (par''thĕn-ō-jĕn'ē-sĭs) [Gr. *parthenos*, virgin, + *genesis*, origin]. Reproduction arising from a female egg which has not been fertilized by the male; unisexual reproduction.

particulate (par-tĭk'ū-lāt) [L. *particula*, small parts]. Made up of particles.

parturient (pär-tū'rĭ-ĕnt) [L. *parturiēns*, in labor]. 1. Concerning childbirth or parturition. 2. Bringing forth; giving birth.

p. canal. Path from uterine cavity to vulva.

parturifacient (pär-tū-rĭ-fā'shĕnt) [" + *facere*, to make]. 1. Inducing or accelerating labor. 2. Drug used to cause or hasten delivery of the fetus.

parturition (pär-tū-rĭsh'ŭn) [L. *parturitio*]. Act of giving birth to young. SYN: *childbirth; delivery.*

parturition, words pert. to: accouchement; accoucheur; accoucheuse; afterbirth; afterpains; axis traction; bradytocia; childbirth; dystocia; labor; multipara; nullipara; obstetrics; oxytocia; parturient; parturifacient; postpartum.

partus (pär'tŭs) [L.]. Labor; parturition.

p. agrippinus. Breech presentation in delivery.

p. caesareus. Delivery by cesarean section.

p. difficilis. Difficult labor. SYN: *dystocia.*

p. immaturus. Premature labor.

p. maturus. Labor at term.

p. precipitat'us. Labor occurring with undue rapidity.

p. serotinus. Prolonged or delayed labor.

p. siccus. Dry labor with little amniotic fluid.

part. vic. Abbr. for *partibus vicibus*, in divided doses.

parulis (pär-ū'lĭs) [Gr. *para*, near, + *oulon*, gum]. Abscess of a gum. SYN: *gumboil.*

parumbilical (pär''ŭm-bĭl'ĭ-kăl) [" + L. *umbilicus*, navel]. Close to the navel.

paruria (pär-ū'rĭ-ă) [Gr. *para*, abnormal, + *ouron*, urine]. Any abnormality in discharge of urine.

parvicellular (pär-vĭ-sĕl'ū-lăr) [L. *parvus*, small, + *cellula*, little box]. Concerning, or composed of, tiny cells.

parvule (pär'vūl) [L. *parvulus*, very small]. A small pill, pellet, or granule.

PAS, PASA. Abbr. for *para-aminosalicylic acid,* q.v.

Paschen bodies (pä′shĕn). [Enrique Paschen, Ger. pathologist, 1860-1936] Particles thought to be the pathogenic virus of vaccinia and variola found in great numbers in skin exanthemas.

passage (păs′aj) [ME., to pass]. 1. A channel between cavities and body structures or with the ext. surface of an organ. 2. Act of passing. 3. An evacuation of the bowels. 4. Introduction of a probe, catheter, etc. 5. Incubation of a pathogenic organism, esp. a virus in one or a series of tissue cultures or living organisms.

passion (păsh′ŭn) [L. *passiō,* suffering]. 1. Suffering. 2. Great emotion, esp. sexual excitement.

passional (păsh′ŭn-ăl). Concerning any passion. SEE: *emotional.*

passive (păs′ĭv) [L. *passivus,* capable of suffering]. 1. Submissive. 2. Acted upon. 3. Not active.

   p. congestion. Congestion due to obstruction in venous return or, if general, due to myocardial insufficiency.

   p. exercise. Muscular exercise without any effort on part of patient; accomplished by use of a machine or an assistant.

   p. hyperemia. Increased blood in an area or part due to decreased outflow.

   p. motion. P. exercise, q.v.

   p. movement. P. exercise, q.v.

passivism (păs′ĭ-vizm) [" + Gr. *ismos,* condition]. 1. Passive behavior or character. 2. Sexual perversion with subjugation of the will to another; usually a male being passive to another male.

paste (pāst) [L. *pasta,* paste]. 1. A moist, doughy, plastic substance. 2. A mixture of flour and water, used as an adhesive. 3. Any ointment whose base is a nonfatty material. 4. To cause to adhere.

Pasteur (pă-stĕr′). [Louis Pasteur, Fr. chemist and bacteriologist, 1822-1895]. Founded the science of microbiology. His greatest accomplishments were in the field of bacteriology and immunology. He developed the technique of immunization and produced vaccines.

   P. treatment. Used for the prevention of rabies. Daily injection of increasingly virulent suspensions prepared from the brain or spinal cord of rabbits which have died of rabies. Suspension is treated so as to kill or inactivate the virus.

   CAUTION: In some cases neurological complications may occur ranging from simple neuritis to serious encephalomyelitis and paralysis which may be fatal. Treat-

ment should be employed only when absolutely necessary. SEE: *rabies.*

Pasteurella (păs-tĕr-ĕl′ă). [Pasteur]. A genus of bacteria belonging to the family Brucellaceae. The organisms are small, nonspore-forming, gram-negative bacilli which are very dangerous to handle in the laboratory. The two most important species to man are P. pestis and P. tularensis, causing human plague and tularemia respectively. P. multocida and P. pseudotuberculosis rarely cause illness in man.

   P. multocida. Organism commonly found in the upper respiratory tract of birds and mammals including man. However, infections in man are rare. P. multocida, unlike P. pestis, is quite sensitive to penicillin.

   P. pestis. Cause of plague, q.v. SYN: *plague bacillus.*

   P. tularensis. Organism causing tularemia, q.v.

pasteurellosis (păs-ter-ĕl-ō′sĭs). Disease caused by infection with bacteria of the *Pasteurella* species.

pasteurization (păs-tūr-ĭ-zā′shŭn). [Louis Pasteur]. The process of heating a fluid at a moderate temperature for a definite period of time in order to destroy undesirable bacteria without changing to any extent its chemical composition.

   In p. of milk, pathogenic bacteria are destroyed by heating at 62°C for 30 minutes, or by "flash" heating to higher temperatures for less than a minute. The p. process, reducing total bacterial count of the milk by 97-99%, is effective because the common milk-borne pathogens (tubercle bacillus, Salmonella, Streptococcus, and Brucella) do not form spores and are quite sensitive to heat.

   Pasteurization should not be considered as a substitute for cleanliness in milk production. SEE: *milk.*

pastille (păs-tēl′, păs-tĭl′) [L. *pastillus,* a little roll]. 1. A medicated disk used for local action on the mucosa of the throat and mouth. 2. A small cone used to fumigate or scent the air of a room. SYN: *lozenge; troche.*

past-pointing. Inability to accurately place finger or some other part of the body on a selected point. Seen in certain neurologic disorders.

patagium (pă-tā′jĭ-ŭm) [L.]. (pl. pata′gia) A weblike membrane extending from one body part to another.

patch (păch) [ME. *pacche*]. A blotch distinct from surrounding surface in character and appearance.

p., herald. Solitary oval p. of efflorescence showing before the general eruption of pityriasis rosea; often several days before.

p., Hutchinson's. Salmon-yellow area seen on cornea in syphilitic keratitis.

p., mucous. A syphilitic eruption having an eroded, moist surface; generally on mucous membrane of mouth or external genitals, or on surface subject to moisture and heat. SYN: *condyloma latum.*

p., opaline. Whitish patch in mouth sometimes observed in syphilis.

p.'s, Peyer's. Masses of lymphoid follicles found on mucous membrane of small intestine. SYN: *noduli lymphatici aggregati.*

p., salmon. Salmon-colored area of cornea seen in interstitial keratitis due to syphilis.

p., smokers'. Leukoplakia, q.v.

p. test. One to detect hypersensitiveness to food, pollen, or other substances by applying suspected substance to an area on the skin. A small square of clean linen cloth should be covered with substance suspected. Cloth is laid on skin of chest or upper arm and another piece of cloth laid over it and fastened with adhesive. Another piece of the cloth containing none of the suspected substance is also applied to the skin. Both pieces are removed at the end of 24 hours. If irritation is present only where the suspected substance was tested, the individual probably is sensitive to it. Substances with which the patient comes in contact may be used for the test. SEE: *allergy; eczema.*

patella (pă-tĕl′ă) [L., a small pan]. (pl. *patellae*) [NA]. A lens-shaped sesamoid bone situated in front of the knee, in the tendon of the quadriceps femoris muscle. SYN: *kneecap; kneepan.*

RS: housemaid's knee; knee.

p., floating. A p. which rides up from the condyles due to a large effusion in the knee.

p., fracture of. TREATMENT: Suture of bone fragments. A plaster cast is applied from the toes to the groin, remaining on 6-8 weeks. Following removal of cast, gradual exercise and weight upon the leg for a few weeks, after which patient may walk.

p., rider's painful. Tenderness and pain in p. from horseback riding.

patellapexy (pă-tĕl′ă-pĕk″sĭ) [L. *patella,* small pan, kneecap, + Gr. *pēxis,* fixation]. Fixation of the patella to the lower end of the femur to stabilize the joint.

patellar (pă-tĕl′ăr). Concerning the patella.

p. reflex. Involuntary jerk of leg due to sudden spasm of quadriceps following percussion of patellar ligament. SYN: *knee-jerk reflex.*

patelliform (pă-tĕl′ĭ-form) ["+ *forma,* shape]. Shaped like the patella.

patellofemoral (pă-tĕl″ō-fĕm′ō-răl). Concerning the patella and the femur.

patency (pā′tĕn-sē) [L. *patens,* open]. The state of being freely open.

patent (păt′ĕnt, pā′tĕnt). Wide open; evident; accessible.

pat′ent med′icine. A drug or medical preparation for public use which is protected by letters patent and sold without a physician's prescription. The law requires that it be labeled with names of active ingredients, the quantity or proportion of the contents, directions for its use, and that it may not have misleading statements as to curative effects on the label. SEE: *prescription.*

paternal (pă-ter′nal) [L. *paternis,* fatherly]. Of, pertaining to, or inherited from the father.

paternity test. Test to determine whether it would be possible for an individual to have fathered a specific child. The results can be used only to exclude the possibility of paternity; they cannot be used to prove paternity. Test results are analyzed with respect to the blood type of the child and that of the suspected father. Thus paternity may be excluded if the child had a blood type it could not have inherited from the mother and the alleged father.

path. SEE: *pathway.*

path-, patho-. Prefix indicating disease.

pathema (pă-thē′mă) [Gr. *pathēma*]. (pl. *pathemas* or *pathemata*) Disease.

pathergasia (păth″ĕr-gā′zĭ-ă) [Gr. *pathos,* disease, + *ergasia,* work]. Adolf Myer's term for personality maladjustment associated with organic, functional, or structural changes.

pathergia (pa-ther′jĭ-ă). Pathergy, q.v.

pathergy (path′er-jĭ). Condition in which the response to a stimulus is either exaggerated or subnormal. SEE: *hyperergy; hypoergy.*

pathetic (pă-thĕt′ĭk) [L. *pathēticus*]. Pert. to, or arousing, the emotions of pity, sympathy, or tenderness.

pathetism (path′ē-tĭzm) [Gr. *pathein,* to suffer, + *ismos,* condition]. State of overcoming another's will by suggestion. SYN: *hypnotism; mesmerism.*

pathfinder (păth′fĭnd-ĕr) [AS. *paeth,* road, + *findan,* to locate]. Instrument for locating stricture of the urethra.

-pathic (pă-thĭk) [Gr. *pathos,* disease]. Suffix indicating a feeling that is affected in a specific way, as in telepathic; a diseased condition, as in cardiopathic; a form of therapy or system of medicine, as allopathic, homeopathic, or osteopathic.

patho- (păth'ō). Combining form indicating disease or suffering.

pathocrine (păth'ō-krĭn, -krēn, -krĭn) [Gr. *pathos*, suffering, + *krinein*, to secrete]. Concerning an endocrine disorder.

pathodixia (păth''ō-dĭk'sĭ-ă) [" + *deixis*, exhibition]. Abnormal exhibitionism in reference to an injury or to disease.

pathodontia (păth''ō-dŏn'shĭ-ă) [" + *odous*, *odont-*, tooth]. Branch of dentistry dealing with diseases of the teeth.

pathogen (păth'ō-jĕn) [Gr. *pathos*, suffering, + *gennan*, to produce]. A microorganism or substance capable of producing a disease.

pathogenesis (păth''ō-jĕn'ĕ-sĭs). Origination and development of a disease.

p. drug. 1. Morbid symptoms of disease produced by a drug. 2. Observation of all symptoms which may be produced by a drug.

pathogenetic, pathogenic (păth''ō-jĕn-ĕt'ĭk, -jĕn'ĭk). Productive of disease. SYN: *morbific*.

p. organism. One that produces disease.

pathogeny (păth-ŏj'ĕn-ĭ). The origin or growth of a disease. SYN: *pathogenesis.*

pathognomonic (păth''ŏg-nō-mŏn'ĭk) [Gr. *pathognōmonikos*, skilled in diagnosing]. Indicative of a disease, esp. its characteristic symptoms.

pathologic, pathological (păth-ō-lŏj'ĭk, -ĭ-kăl) [Gr. *pathos*, disease, + *logos*, study]. 1. Concerning pathology. 2. Diseased; due to a disease. SYN: *morbid.*

p. histology. Histology of diseased tissues.

p. reaction to alcohol. An exceedingly severe reaction to ingestion of alcohol, esp. to small amounts. Manifested by irrational violent behavior followed by exhaustion, sleep, and loss of recall of the event. Patient may not be intoxicated. SYN: *pathological intoxication.*

ETIOL: Unknown, but is associated with hypoglycemia, exhaustion, and stress.

p. reflex. An abnormal reflex indicating an abnormal or diseased state.

pathologist (pă-thŏl'ō-jĭst) [Gr. *pathos*, disease, + *logos*, study]. A specialist in diagnosing the morbid changes in tissues removed at operations and postmortem examinations.

pathology (pă-thŏl'ō-jĭ). 1. Study of the nature and cause of disease which involves changes in structure and function. 2. Condition produced by disease.

p., anatomic. Field of p. that deals with structural changes. SYN: *pathologic anatomy.*

p., cellular. P. which is based upon microscopic changes in body cells during disease.

p., chemical. The study of chemical changes that occur in disease.

p., comparative. The observation of pathological condition, spontaneous or artificial, in the lower animals or in vegetable organisms as compared to those of the human body.

p., experimental. Study of diseases induced artificially and intentionally, esp. in animals.

p., functional. The study of alterations of functions that occur in disease processes without associated structural changes. SYN: *physiologic pathology.*

p., geographical. P. in its relations to climate and geography.

p., medical. The p. of disorders which are not accessible for surgical procedures.

p., special. The p. of particular diseases or organs.

p., surgical. The p. of diseases accessible to surgery.

pathomania (păth-ō-mā'nĭ-ă) [Gr. *pathos*, suffering + *mania*, madness]. Moral insanity; irresistible tendency toward forbidden conduct with retention of reasoning power.

pathometry (pă-thŏm'ĕ-trĭ) [" + *metron*, measure]. The estimate of the incidence of a disease.

pathomimesis (păth''ō-mĭm-ē'sĭs) [" + *mimēsis*, imitation]. Intentional or unconscious as well as conscious imitation of a disease.

pathomimicry (path''ō-mĭm'ĭ-krĭ). Pathomimesis, q.v.

pathomorphism (păth''ō-mor'fĭzm) [" + *morphē*, form, + *ismos*, condition]. Study of abnormal form and structure of organisms.

pathonomy (păth-ŏn'ō-mĭ) [Gr. *pathos*, disease, + *nomos*, law]. Science of the laws of diseased conditions.

pathophilia (păth''ō-fĭl'ĭ-ă) [" + *philein*, to love]. Adjustment of habits to conditions made mandatory by some chronic disease.

pathophobia (păth-ō-fō'bĭ-ă) [" + *phobos*, fear]. Morbid fear of disease.

pathophoresis (păth''ō-for-ē'sĭs) [Gr. *pathos*, disease, + *phoros*, carrying]. The transmission of disease.

pathophoric (păth''ō-for'ĭk). Carrying or transmitting disease, as certain insects.

pathopoiesis (păth''ō-poy-ē'sĭs) [Gr. *pathos*, disease, + *poiēsis*, production]. l. The generation of disease. 2. Tendency to become diseased.

pathopsychology (păth″ō-sĭ-kŏl′ō-jĭ) ["+ *psychē,* soul, + *logos,* study]. The branch of psychology dealing with mental processes during disease.

patho′sis. A diseased state or condition.

pathway. 1. A path or a course; more specifically a p. formed by neurons (cell bodies and their processes) over which impulses pass from their point of origin to their destination. 2. A chemical or metabolic p.; the various chemical reactions that occur in metabolism as specific substances are absorbed, metabolized, and altered as they are utilized in the body.

p., afferent. One leading from a receptor to the spinal cord and/or brain.

p., central. P. within the brain or spinal cord.

p., conduction. A group of fibers in a nerve, spinal cord, or brain over which impulses are conducted.

p., efferent. P. from the central nervous system to an effector.

p., metabolic. The sequence of chemical reactions which occur as a substance is metabolized.

p., motor. P. over which motor impulses are conveyed from a motor center to muscles.

p., sensory. P. over which sensory impulses are conveyed from sense organs or receptors to sensory or reflex centers of the spinal cord or brain.

patient (pā′shĕnt) [L. *patiens*]. 1. Enduring pain or injury. 2. A person who is receiving treatment for disease.

patricide (pat′rĭ-sīd). Parricide, q.v.

patrilineal [L. *pater,* father, + *linea,* line]. Tracing descent through the father.

pattern. 1. A design, figure, model, or example. 2. In psychology, a set or arrangement of ideas or behavior reactions.

patulous (păt′ū-lŭs) [L. *patulus*]. Open, distended, spread apart. SYN: *patent.*

paulocardia (pawl″ō-kar′dĭ-ă) [Gr. *paula,* pause, + *kardia,* heart]. 1. Sensation of momentary stoppage of heartbeat. 2. Undue prolongation of the rest period in the cardiac cycle.

pause (pŏz) [ME.]. An interruption; a temporary cessation of activity.

p., compensatory. The long interval following an extrasystole, so-called because its duration is such that the next beat occurs at the exact time of the succeeding normal beat.

pavement′ing. Condition occurring during inflammation in which leukocytes adhere to the lining of capillaries.

Pavlov (păv′lŏv). [Ivan Petrovich Pavlov, Russian physiologist, 1849-1936]. Winner of Nobel prize in medicine in 1904. He is remembered particularly for his work on conditioned response. SEE: *reflex, conditioned.*

pavor (pā′vor) [L.]. Anxiety, dread.

p. nocturnus. Night terror during sleep in children and the aged.

Pb. Chem. symb. for *plumbum,* lead.

P.B. Abbr. for *Pharmacopoeia Britannica,* British pharmacopeia.

PBI. Abbr. for *protein-bound iodine.*

P.B.W. Abbr. for *posterior bite wing* in dentistry.

PBZ. Abbr. for *pyribenzamine.*

p.c. Abbr. for *post cibos,* after meals.

pCO₂. Symb. for *carbon dioxide pressure* or *tension.*

PCV. Abbr. for *packed cell volume.*

Pd. Chem. symb. for palladium.

P.D. Abbr. for *Doctor of Pharmacy.*

pea (pē) [ME. *pease*]. A climbing annual vine grown in temperate zones and having edible seeds in a green, elongated pod. Richer in proteins than other vegetables except lentils, but poorer in carbohydrates.

Food value of 100 gm. (canned, solids and liquid): Cal. 66; protein 3.5 gm.; fat 0.3 gm.; carbohydrate 12.5 gm.; calcium 20 mg.; vitamin A, 450 I.U.

peach (pēch) [ME. *peche*].

Food value of 100 gm. (raw): Cal. 38; protein 0.6 gm.; trace of fat; carbohydrate 10 gm.; calcium 9 mg.; vitamin A, 1330 I.U. (based on yellow-fleshed varieties; in white-fleshed varieties, value is approx. 50 I.U.).

peanut (pē′nŭt). A vine, Arachis hypogaea, with edible, nutlike, oily seeds used for food and as a source of oil.

Food value of 100 gm. (roasted and shelled): Cal. 582; protein 26 gm.; fat 49 gm.; carbohydrate 26 gm.; calcium 74 mg.

p. butter. Small amount of fat and salt added. Food value of 100 gm.; Cal. 581; protein 28 gm.; fat 49 gm.; carbohydrate 19 gm.; calcium 63 gm.

p. oil. USP. A refined oil obtained from the seed kernels of one or more of the cultivated varieties of Arachis hypogaea. Used as a solvent for intramuscular injections.

pear (pār) [ME. *pere*]. Edible fruit of the widely-cultivated tree, Pyrus communis.

Food value of 100 gm. (raw): Cal. 61; protein 0.7 gm.; fat 0.4 gm.; carbohydrate 15 gm.; calcium 15 mg.

pearl (pĕrl) [ME. *perle*]. 1. Small, tough mass in sputum in asthma. 2. Small, hollow glass capsule containing a medicinal fluid for inhalation. Capsule is crushed in handkerchief and inhaled. 3. Small mass of cells.

p., epithelial. Concentric squamous epithelial cells in carcinoma.

p., gouty. Sodium urate concretion on cartilage of the ear seen in people with gout.

peau d'orange (pō″dō-ränj′) [Fr., orange skin]. Dimpled skin condition which resembles an orange. Seen in lymphatic edema, and may be present over the area of carcinoma of the breast.

pecan (pē-kăn′) [AmerInd. *paccan*]. A tree, *Carya illinoensis*, of the United States with thin-shelled, edible nuts.

Food value of 100 gm. (halves): Cal. 687; protein 9.2 gm.; fat 71 gm.; carbohydrate 15 gm.; calcium 73 mg.; vitamin A, 130 I.U.; ascorbic acid 2 mg.

peccant (pĕk′ănt) [L. *peccāns*, sinning]. Corrupt; producing disease. SYN: *pathogenic; unhealthy; morbid.*

peccatiphobia (pĕk″ăt-ĭ-fō′bĭ-ă) [L. *peccata*, sins, + Gr. *phobos*, fear]. Abnormal dread of sinning.

pecilo-. For words beginning with pecilo-, see words beginning with *poikilo-*.

pectase (pĕk′tās) [Gr. *pēktos*, congealed, + *ase*, enzyme.]. Enzyme facilitating the conversion of pectin to pectic acid and methanol.

pecten (pĕk′tĕn) [L., comb]. (pl. *pec′tines*) 1. A comblike organ. 2. The pubic bone. 3. Middle portion of anal canal.

p. ossis pubis. [NA]. A sharp ridge on superior ramus of pubis which forms pubic portion of the terminal (iliopectineal) line.

pectic acid (pĕk′tĭk) [Gr. *pēktos*, congealed]. An acid, derived from pectin by hydrolyzing the methyl ester group, which is found in many fruits.

pectin (pĕk′tĭn) [Gr. *pēktos*, congealed]. A white, amorphous, plant carbohydrate that forms a gelatinous mass in the cooking of fruits and vegetables, causing them to jell. SEE: *pectose.*

pectinate (pĕk′tĭ-nāt) [L. *pecten*, comb]. Having teeth like a comb.

pectineal (pĕk′tĭn′ē-ăl). Rel. to the os pubis or the pectineus muscle.

p. line. The line or ridge on the os pubis separating the true from the false pelvis. SYN: *iliopectineal line; linea terminalis.*

pectineus (pĕk-tĭn-ē′-ŭs) [L. *pecten*, comb]. A flat, quadrangular muscle at upper and inner part of thigh, arising from superior ramus of pubis and inserted between lesser trochanter and linea aspera of the femur,

which flexes and adducts the thigh. SEE: *Table of Muscles* in *Appendix.*

pectiniform (pĕk-tĭn′ĭ-form) ["+ *forma*, shape]. Toothed like a comb. SYN: *pectinate.*

pectization (pĕk-tĭ-zā′shŭn) [Gr. *pēktos*, congealed]. In colloidal chemistry, the conversion of a substance from sol to gel state.

pectoral (pĕk′tō-răl) [L. *pectoralis*]. 1. Concerning the chest. 2. Efficacious in relieving chest conditions, as a cough.

pectoralgia (pĕk″tō-ral′jĭ-ă) ["+ Gr. *algos*, pain]. Neuralgic pain in the chest.

pectoralis (pĕk″tō-rā′lĭs) [L.]. 1. Pert. to the breast or chest. 2. One of four muscles of the anterior upper portion of the chest.

p. major. A large triangular muscle that extends to the humerus, drawing the arm forward and downward and aiding in chest expansion.

p. minor. Muscle beneath p. major, extending to scapula, which lowers the scapula and depresses the shoulder point.

pectoriloquy (pĕk″tō-rĭl′ō-kwĭ) [L. *pectus, pector-*, chest, + *loqui*, to speak]. The distinct transmission of vocal sounds to the ear through the chest wall in auscultation, q.v. The words seem to emanate from the spot which is ausculted. Heard over cavities which communicate with a bronchus and areas of consolidation near a large bronchus, over pneumothorax when the opening in the lung is patulous, and over some pleural effusions. SEE: *chest.*

p., aphonic. In auscultation, whispered sound heard over a lung with a cavity or pleural effusion.

p., whispering. Sound over a lung with a cavity of limited extent when patient whispers, in auscultation of the chest.

pectorophony (pĕk″tō-rof′ō-nĭ) ["+ Gr. *phōnē*, voice]. Exaggeration of vocal sounds heard on auscultation of the chest. SYN: *pectoriloquy.*

pectose (pĕk′tōs) [Gr. *pēktos*, congealed]. A substance found in some fruits and vegetables, yielding pectin when it is boiled.

pectunculus (pĕk-tŭn′kū-lŭs) [L., little comb]. One of the tiny longitudinal ridges on the sylvian aqueduct of the brain.

pectus (pĕk′tŭs) [L.]. (pl. *pec′tora*) [NA]. The chest, breast, or thorax.

p. carinatum. Abnormal prominence of the sternum. SYN: *chicken* or *pigeon breast.*

p. excavatum. Congenital condition in which sternum is abnormally depressed. SYN: *funnel breast.*

ped- [L.]. Combining form denoting foot.

pedal (pĕd′l) [L. *pedalis*]. Concerning the foot.

pedarthrocace (pē″dăr-thrŏk′ă-sē) [Gr. *pais, paid-,* child, + *arthron,* joint, + *kakos,* bad]. Carious condition of joints of children.

pedatro′phia. SEE: *pedatrophy.*

pedatrophy (pē-dăt′rō-fĭ) [Gr. *pais, paid-,* child, + *atrophia,* want of nourishment]. 1. Marasmus. 2. Any wasting disease in children. 3. Tabes mesenterica.

pederast (pē′dĕr-ăst) [Gr. *paiderastēs,* a lover of boys]. A male who indulges in sexual intercourse with young boys.

pederasty (pē′dĕr-ăs″tĭ). Sexual intercourse between a man and a young boy.

pedes (pē′dēz). Pl. of pes, q.v.

pedesis (pē-dē′sĭs) [Gr., leaping]. The incessant dancing or to-and-fro movements of particles in a colloidal system or minute particles of any substance in a liquid or gaseous medium. SYN: *brownian movement.*

pedi- (ped′ĭ) [L. *pedalis*]. Combining form denoting foot.

pedia- [Gr. *pais, paid-,* child]. Combining form denoting relationship to a child.

pedialgia (pēd-ĭ-ăl′jĭ-ă, pē-dĭ-) [Gr. *pedion,* foot, + *algos,* pain]. Pain of the foot.

pediatric (pē-dĭ-ăt′rĭk) [Gr. *pais, paid-,* child, + *iatreia,* treatment]. Concerning the treatment of children.

pediatrician (pē-dĭ-ă-trĭsh′ăn) [″+ *iatrikos,* healing]. A specialist in treatment of children's diseases. SYN: *pediatrist.*

pediatrics (pē-dĭ-ăt′rĭks) [″+ *iatreia,* treatment]. Medical science relating to hygienic care of children and treatment of diseases peculiar to them. SYN: *pediatry.*

pediatrist (pē″dĭ-ăt′rĭst) [Gr. *pais, paid-,* child, + *iatrikos,* healing]. Physician who specializes in treatment of children's diseases.

pediatry (pĕd′ĭ-ăt′rĭ, pē-dĭ′ăt-rĭ). The treatment of children's diseases. SYN: *pediatrics.*

pedicellation (pĕd″ĭ-sĕl-ā′shŭn) [L. *pediculus,* a little foot; stalk]. Formation and development of a pedicle.

pedicle (pĕd′ĭ-kl). 1. The stem which attaches a new growth. 2. The bony process which projects backward from the body of a vertebra connecting with the lamina on each side. Forms the root of the vertebral arch.

pedicterus (pē-dĭk′tĕr-ŭs) [″+ *ikteros,* jaundice]. Icterus neonatorum or jaundice of the newborn.

pedicular (pē-dĭk′ū-lar). 1. [L. *pediculus,* a louse]. Infested with or concerning lice. 2. [L. *pediculus,* a little foot]. Concerning a stalk or stem.

pediculate (pē-dĭk′ū-lāt) [L. *pediculus,* a little foot]. Having a pedicle or stem. SYN: *pedunculate.*

pediculation (pē-dĭk-ū-lā′shŭn) [L. *pediculatio*]. 1. Infestation with lice. 2. Development of a pedicle.

pediculicide (pē-dĭk′ū-lĭ-sĭd) [L. *pediculus,* a louse, + *caedere,* to kill]. Destroying or that which destroys lice.

Pedicul′idae. A family of lice belonging to the order Anoplura. Includes the species parasitic on primates including man. SEE: *Pediculus.*

pediculophobia (pē-dĭk″ū-lō-fō′bĭ-ă) [L. *pediculus,* a louse, + Gr. *phobein,* to fear]. Abnormal dread of lice. SYN: *phthiriophobia.*

pediculosis (pē-dĭk″ū-lō′sĭs) [″+ Gr. *-ōsis,* infestation]. Lousiness; infestation with lice. SEE: *Pediculus.*

    p. **capitis.** P. due to infestation with the head louse, Pediculus humanus capitis. Transmission is by personal contact or common use of brushes, combs, or headgear.

    SYM: Itching and eczematous dermatitis. In long-standing, neglected cases, scratching may result in marked inflammation and secondary infection by bacteria may occur with formation of pustules, crusts, and suppuration. Hair may become matted and give rise to an unpleasant odor.

    TREATMENT: Rub benzyl benzoate emulsion into scalp at night. A day after treatment hair should be shampooed and then combed with a fine-tooth comb to remove nits. In severe infestations or if hair is matted, hair should be cut short. Treatment should be repeated in ten days to kill newly hatched lice. All possible sources of infection should be examined and treated if necessary. Headgear, combs, brushes should be disinfected by heat or use of disinfection solutions.

    p. **corporis (p. vestimenti).** P. due to infestation with the body louse, Pediculus humanus corporis, q.v. Transmitted by direct contact or use of infested wearing apparel. Occurs as a result of crowding and unhygienic conditions.

    SYM: Intense itching. In heavy infestations there is generalized red skin eruption, mild fever, tiredness, irritability, and in severe cases, weakness and debility.

    TREATMENT: Clothing and bedding should be sterilized by dry heat (140° F. or 60° C. for 5 min.), hot water (150° F. or 65.6° C. for 5 min.), or by dry cleaning. Thorough cleansing of the body and scrubbing with soap followed by a pediculicidal lotion applied to hairy parts of the body.

    p. **pubis.** P. due to infestation with the crab louse, Phthirus pubis, q.v. Generally confined to hairs of genital region but hair of the axilla, eyebrows, eyelashes, beard, and in hairy individuals body surface may be involved. Lice may be acquired through sexual relations, by wearing contaminated clothing, from toilet seats, or from bed clothes.

SYM: Itching, esp. in genital or crural regions. Small pale-blue spots resulting from the action of salivary secretion on hemoglobin are characteristic.

TREATMENT: Cleanse thoroughly with soap and water and treat with a suitable pediculicide. All sources of infestation should be checked and lice eliminated.

Pediculus (pē-dĭk'ū-lŭs). A genus of parasitic insects commonly called lice that infests humans and other primates. Lice are sucking insects belonging to the family Pediculidae, order Anoplura. They are of medical importance in that they are the transmitters of the causative organisms of epidemic typhus, trench fever, and relapsing fever. They may serve as mechanical transmitters of bubonic plague and possibly other diseases. SEE: *louse* for illustration.

    P. humanus capitis. The head louse which lives in fine hair of the head, although beard and eyebrows may be infested. Its eggs, commonly called nits, are glued to hairs and frequently form nests in the vicinity of the ears. Cause of pediculosis capitis, q.v.

    P. humanus corporis. The body louse which inhabits the seams of clothing worn next to the body and feeds on regions of the body covered by that clothing. Eggs are attached to fibers of the clothing. The cause of pediculosis corporis, q.v.

pediculus (pē-dĭk'ū-lŭs) [L.]. (pl. *pedic'uli*) 1. A footlike part. SYN: *pedicle.* 2. Louse. SEE: *Pediculus.*

pedicure (pĕd-ĭ-kūr) [L. *pes, ped-*, foot, + *cura*, care]. 1. Care of the feet. 2. Cosmetic care of the feet and toenails. 3. A podiatrist.

pediform (pĕd'ĭ-form) ["+ *forma*, shape]. Having the shape of a foot.

pediluvium (pĕd-ĭ-lū'vĭ-ŭm) ["+ *luere*, to wash]. A foot bath.

pedionalgia (pē-dĭ-ō'nal'jĭ-ă) [Gr. *pedion*, metatarsus, + *algos*, pain]. Neuralgic pain in the sole of the foot. SYN: *metatarsalgia.*

pediophobia (pē-dĭ-ō-fō'bĭ-ă) [Gr. *pais, paid-*, child, + *phobos*, fear]. Unnatural dread of young children or of dolls.

pedobaromacrometer (pē''dō-băr''ō-mă-krŏm'ĕt-ĕr) ["+ *baros*, weight, + *makros*, long, + *metron*, measure]. Apparatus for determining measurement and weight of infants.

pedobarometer (pē''dō-băr-ŏm'ĕt-ĕr) ["+ "+ *metron*, measure]. Apparatus for weighing infants.

pedodontia, pedodontics (pē''dō-dŏn'shĭ-ă, -tĭks) [Gr. *pais, paid-*, child, + *odous, odnot-*, tooth]. Phase of dentistry dealing with care of children's teeth.

pedodontist (pē''dō-dŏn'tĭst). Dentist who specializes in care of children's teeth.

pedograph (pĕd'ō-grăf) [L. *pēs, ped-*, foot, + Gr. *graphein*, to write]. Imprint of the foot on paper.

pedologist (pē-dŏl'ō-jĭst) [Gr. *pais, paid-*, child, + *logos*, study]. One who has made a study of children and their development.

pedology (pē-dŏl'ō-jĭ). The study of children and their development.

pedometer 1. (pē-dŏm'ĕt-ĕr) [Gr. *pais, paid-*, child, + *metron*, measure] Device for measurement of infants. 2. (pĕd-ŏm'ĕt-ĕr) [L. *pēs, ped-*, foot, + Gr. *metron*, measurement] An instrument that indicates number of steps taken while walking.

pedomorphism (pē''dō-mor'fizm) [Gr. *pais, paid-*, child, + *morhpē*, form, + *ismos*, condition]. Retention of juvenile characteristics in the adult.

pedonosology (pē''do-nōs-ōl'ō-jĭ) ["+ *nosos*, disease, + *logos*, study]. The study and classification of children's diseases.

pedophilia (pē''dō-fĭl'ĭ-ă) ["+ *philein*, to love]. 1. Fondness for children. 2. In psychology, an unnatural desire for sexual relations with children.

peduncle (pē-dun'kl) [L. *pedunculus*, a little foot.]. 1. A stem or stalk. SYN: *pedicle.* 2. A brachium of the brain; a band connecting parts of the brain. SYN: *pedunculus.* SEE: *cimbia; crus; sessile.*

    p., cerebellar, inferior. A band of fibers running along lateral border of 4th ventricle connecting spinal cord and medulla with the cerebellum. SYN: *restiform body.*

    p., cerebellar, middle. A band of fibers connecting cerebellum with basilar portion of the pons. SYN: *brachium pontis.*

    p., cerebellar, superior. A band of fibers connecting cerebellum with midbrain. SYN: *brachium conjunctivum.*

    p., cerebral. A pair of white bundles from upper part of the pons to the cerebrum. It constitutes the ventral portion of the midbrain. SYN: *crus cerebri.*

    p. of flocculus. A band of fibers connecting flocculus of cerebellum with vermis.

    p., mammillary. A band of fibers extending from tegmentum of midbrain to mammillary body.

p., pineal. A band from either side of the pineal gland to the anterior pillars of the fornix.

p. of superior olive. A slender band of fibers extending from superior olivary nucleus in medulla to nucleus of abducens nerve.

p., thalamic. One of four groups of fibers known as thalamic radiations which connect thalamus with cerebral cortex. SEE: *radiation, thalamic.*

peduncular (pĕ-dŭn'kū-lar) [L. *pedunculus,* a little foot]. Concerning a peduncle.

pedunculate, pedunculated (pĕ-dŭn'kū-lāt, -ed). Possessing a stalk or peduncle. SYN: *pediculate.*

peeling [ME. *pelen,* to peel]. Shedding of surface layer of skin; desquamation.

peer (pēr). 1. [ME.] One who has an equal standing with another in age, class, or rank. 2. To observe closely.

peinotherapy (pī-nō-thĕr'ă-pī) [Gr. *peina,* hunger, + *therapeia,* treatment]. Treating disease by fasting. SYN: *pinotherapy.*

pejorative (pĭ-jŏr'ă-tĭv, pē'jă-rā'tĭv) [L. *pejor,* worse]. Tending to become or make worse.

pelada (pē-lā'dă). Alopecia areata or loss of body hair in patchy areas.

pelage (pĕl'ĭj) [Fr.]. The collective hair of the body.

Pel-Ebstein's fever. [Pieter K. Pel, Dutch physician, 1852-1919; Wilhelm Ebstein, Ger. physicist, 1836-1912]. Cyclic fever occurring in Hodgkin's disease in which periods of fever lasting from 3 to 10 days are separated by an afebrile period of about the same length.

Pelger-Huët anomaly. [Karel Pelger, Dutch physician, 1885-1931; G.J. Huet, contemporary Dutch physician] Granulocytes of the blood with rodlike, dumbbell, peanut-shaped, and spectacle-like nuclei. The chromatin of the nuclei is unusually coarse. The condition is inherited as a non-sex-linked dominant. The cells function in a normal manner and carriers have no demonstrably lowered resistance to infection.

pelioma (pē-lĭ-ō'mă) [Gr.]. A livid cutaneous patch. SYN: *ecchymosis.*

peliosis (pĕlĭ-ō'sĭs) [Gr.]. A disease marked by purple patches on the mucous membranes and skin. SYN: *purpura.*

p. rheumatica. An acute affection characterized by inflammation of the joints. A form of rheumatism. SYN: *purpura rheumatica; Schonlein's disease.*

SYM: Sore throat, urticaria, moderate fever, purpuric spots over extremities or trunk. Tenderness, swelling, and pain in joints.

pellagra (pĕl-ă'gră, pē-lăg'ră) [L. *pellis,* skin, + Gr. *agra,* seizure]. A deficiency disease or syndrome endemic in certain parts of the world, characterized by cutaneous, gastrointestinal, mucosal, neurologic, and mental symptoms.

ETIOL: Due to deficiency in diet or failure of body to absorb niacin (nicotinic acid) or its amide (niacinamide, nicotinamide). Usually associated with a deficiency of tryptophane-containing proteins such as occurs in a high corn diet. P. may occur secondary to gastrointestinal diseases and alcoholism.

SYM: In advanced cases, scarlet stomatitis and glossitis, diarrhea, dermatitis, and mental symptoms. Cutaneous lesions include erythema followed by vesiculation, crusting, and desquamation. Skin may become dry, scaly, and atrophic. The mucous membranes of mouth, esophagus, and vagina may undergo atrophy; ulcers and cysts may develop. Anemia is common. Nausea, vomiting, and diarrhea occur, the latter being characteristic. Involvement of the central nervous system is first manifested by neurasthenia, followed by organic psychosis characterized by disorientation, impairment of memory, and confusion. Later delirium and clouding of consciousness may occur.

TREATMENT: A diet adequate in all vitamins, minerals, and amino acids supplemented by 500 to 1000 mg. of niacinamide given orally three times daily. If there is any doubt about the ability of the intestinal tract to absorb vitamins, they should be given parenterally.

p. sine pellagra. Pellagra in which the characteristic erythematous rash is absent.

pellagrazein (pĕl-ă-grā'zē-ĭn). Poisonous substance in decomposed cornmeal. At one time was regarded erroneously as the cause of pellagra. SYN: *pellagracein.*

pellagrin (pĕ-lā'grĭn, -lăg'rĭn) [L. *pellis,* skin, + Gr. *agra,* seizure]. A person afflicted with pellagra.

pellagrous (pĕ-lā'grŭs, -lăg'rŭs). Concerning or affected with pellagra.

pellet (pĕl'ĕt) [Fr. *pelote,* a ball]. A tiny pill or small ball of medicine or food.

pellicle (pĕl'ĭ-kl) [L. *pellicula,* a little skin]. 1. A thin piece of cuticle or skin. 2. Film or surface on a liquid. 3. A thin nonliving sheath forming the surface layer of certain one-celled animals. SYN: *scum.*

pellotine (pĕl'ō-tēn). A white, crystalline alkaloid used as a hypnotic.

pellucid (pĕl-lū'sĭd) [L. *pellucidus*]. Translucent; transparent.

p. zone. Clear layer covering the oocyte. SYN: *zona pellucida.*

pelvic (pĕl'vĭk) [L. *pelvis*, basin]. Pert. to a pelvis, usually the bony pelvis.

    p. girdle. Arch made by the innominate bones.

    p. inlet. Upper pelvic entrance, the brim of the pelvis forming its boundary.

    p. outlet. Lower pelvic opening.

pelvilithotomy (pĕl''vĭ-lĭ-thŏt'ŏ-mĭ) ["+ Gr. *lithos*, stone, + *tomē*, a cutting]. Removal of a stone from the renal pelvis. SYN: *nephrolithotomy; pelviolithotomy; pyelolithotomy.*

pelvimeter (pĕl-vĭm'ē-tĕr) ["+ Gr. *metron*, measure]. Device for measuring the pelvis.

pelvimetry (pĕl-vĭm'ĕt-rĭ). Measurement of the pelvic dimensions or proportions. Helps determine whether or not it will be possible to deliver a fetus through the normal route. Done by manual or x-ray methods or both. SEE: *pelvis.*

    p., x-ray. Use of X ray for measurement of the pelvis.

pelviolithotomy (pĕl''vĭ-ō-lĭ-thŏt'ŏ-mĭ) [L. *pelvis*, basin, + Gr. *lithos*, stone, + *tomē*, a cutting]. Incision of the renal pelvis to remove a calculus.

pelvioplasty (pĕl'vĭ-ō-plăs''tĭ) ["+ Gr. *plassein*, to form]. Enlargement of the outlet of the pelvis. SYN: *hebotomy; symphyseotomy.*

pelvioscopy (pĕl''vĭ-ŏs'kō-pĭ) [L. *pelvis*, basin, + Gr. *skopein*, to examine]. Inspection of the pelvis.

pelviotomy (pĕl-vĭ-ŏt'ŏ-mĭ) ["+ Gr. *tomē*, a cutting]. 1. Incision of the pelvic bones, esp. in case of difficult labor. 2. Incision into the renal pelvis.

pelviperitonitis (pĕl''vĭ-pĕr-ĭ-tō-nĭ'tĭs) ["+ Gr. *peritonaion*, peritoneum, + *-itis*, inflammation]. Inflammation of the peritoneum lining the pelvic cavity.

pelvis (pĕl'vĭs) [L., basin]. (pl. *pelves)* [NA] Any basin-shaped structure or cavity. 2. The bony structure formed by the innominate bones, the sacrum, the coccyx, and the

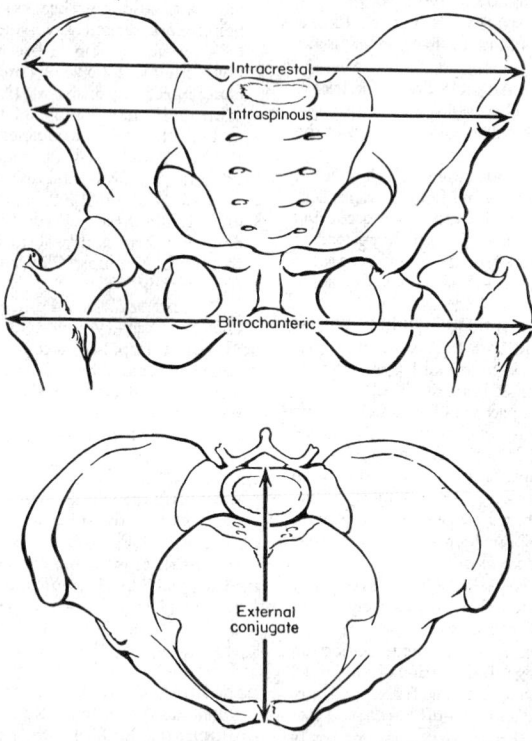

EXTERNAL PELVIMETRY

ligaments uniting them. The structure serves as a support for the vertebral column and for articulation with the lower limbs. 3. The cavity included within these bones.

It is separated into a *false*, or superior p., and a *true*, or inferior one, by the iliopectineal line and the upper margin of the symphysis pubis. The circumference of this area constitutes the *inlet* of the true pelvis. Lower border of true pelvis is formed by the coccyx, the protuberances of the ischia, the ascending rami of the ischia, and the descending rami of the ossa pubis and the sacrosciatic ligaments, and is termed the *outlet.*

The floor of the pelvis is formed by the perineal fascia, levator ani, and the coccygeus muscles.

DIAMETERS: All diameters normally are larger in the female than in the male.

EXTERNAL: *Interspinous:* Distance between outer edges of the anterior superior iliac spines, diameter normally measuring 26 cm. (10 1/4 in.). *Intercristal:* Distance between outer edges of the most prominent portion of the iliac crests, diameter normally being 28 cm. (11 in.). *Intertrochanteric:* Distance between most prominent points of the femoral trochanters, 32 cm. (12 1/2 in.). *Oblique* (right and left): Distance from one posterior superior iliac spine to the opposite anterior superior iliac spine, 22 cm. (8 1/2 in.), right being slightly greater than the left. *External conjugate;* Distance from the undersurface of the spinous process of last lumbar vertebra to the upper margin of anterior surface of the symphysis pubis, 20 cm. (7 7/8 in.). SYN: *Baudelocque's diameter.*

INTERNAL: *True conjugate:* Anteroposterior diameter of the pelvic inlet, 11 cm. (4 1/4 in.), the most important single diameter of the pelvis. *Diagonal conjugate:* Distance between the promontory of the sacrum to undersurface of symphysis pubis, 13 cm. (5 1/8 in.), 2 cm. (3/4 in.) being deducted for the height and inclination of symphysis to obtain diameter of conjugate. *Transverse:* Distance between ischial tuberosities, 11 cm. (4 1/4 in.). *Anteroposterior* (of outlet): Distance between the lower border of symphysis and tip of sacrum, 11 cm. (4 1/4 in.). *Anterior sagittal:* Distance from undersurface of symphysis to center of line between the ischial tuberosities, 7 cm. (2 3/4 in.). *Posterior sagittal:* Distance from the center of line between ischial tuberosities to the tip of the sacrum, 10 cm. (4 in.).

RS: acanthopelvis; brim; cavity, pelvic; Claudius' fossa; diameter; endopelvic; pelvimetry; pelviotomy.

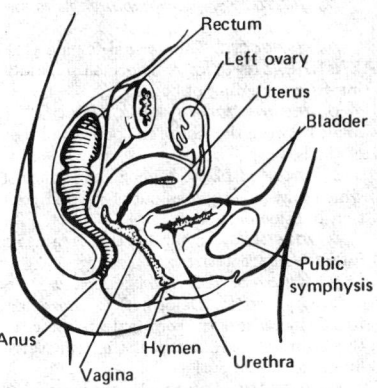

FEMALE PELVIC VISCERA

p. aequabiliter justo major. P. symmetrically larger than standard in all its dimensions.

p. aequabiliter justo minor. P. with all dimensions equally smaller than standard.

p., android. A female p. which resembles that of a male.

p., anthropoid. A female p. resembling that of the great apes in being long and narrow.

p., beaked. P. with the pelvic bones laterally compressed and pushed forward so that outlet is narrow and long.

p., brim of. SEE: inlet of pelvis.

p., contracted. P. in which one or more of the principal diameters is reduced to a degree that parturition is impeded.

p., cordate. P. possessing a heart-shaped inlet.

p., coxalgic. One deformed subsequent to hip joint disease.

p., dwarf. An aequabiliter justo minor pelvis. One reduced in all its diameters and resembling an infantile pelvis. Bones usually united by cartilage. SYN: *p. nana.*

p., elastic. An osteomalacic pelvis.

p., false. Portion above the iliopectineal line.

p. fissa. A split p., q.v.

p., fissured. A rachitic pelvis with ilia pushed forward so as to be almost parallel.

p., flat. One in which anteroposterior diameters are shortened.

p., funnel-shaped. P. in which the outlet is considerably contracted, but the inlet dimensions are normal.

p., giant. SEE: *p. aequabiliter justo major.*

p., gynecoid. The normal female p.

p., halisteretic. A deformed p. resulting from softening of bones.

p., inclination of, obliquity of. The angle between the axis of the pelvis and that of the body.

p., India rubber. A pelvis, the bones of which may be stretched out of normal position in osteomalacia.

p., infantile. An adult p. that retains its infantile characteristics.

p., Kilian's. SEE: *osteomalacic p.*

p., kyphotic. Deformed p. characterized by increase of the conjugate diameter at the brim with reduction of the transverse diameter at the outlet.

p., lordotic. Deformed p. in which the spinal column has an anterior curvature in the lumbar region.

p., major. [NA]. The false pelvis, q.v.

p., malacosteon. SEE: *rachitic p.*

p. masculine. P. of a female resembling that of a male, esp. in being narrower, more conical, heavier boned, and with heart-shaped inlet. SYN: *android pelvis.*

p., Naegele. An obliquely contracted p. in which conjugate diameter assumes an oblique direction.

p. nana. A dwarf p., q.v.

p., osteomalacic. P. distorted as a consequence of osteomalacia.

p., pseudo-osteomalacic. A rickety p. similar to that of a person affected with osteomalacia.

p., rachitic. P. deformed from rickets.

p., reduced. SEE: *aequabiliter justo minor.*

p., renal. [NA]. The expanded proximal end of the ureter. It lies within renal sinus of kidney and receives the urine through the major calyces. SYN: *pelvis renalis.*

p., reniform. P. shaped like a kidney.

p., Robert's. One with an embryonic sacrum and narrowing of the transverse and oblique diameters.

p., rostrate. SEE: *beaked p.*

p., rotunda. A tympanic depression in the inner wall, at the bottom of which is the fenestra rotunda.

p., round. P. with a circular inlet.

p., rubber. An osteomalacic p., q.v.

p., scoliotic. Deformed p. due to spinal curvature.

p., simple flat. P. with a shortened anteroposterior diameter.

p. spinosa. A rachitic pelvis with a pointed crest of the pubis.

p., split. P. with a congenital division at the symphysis pubis.

p., spondylolisthetic. A pelvis in which the last lumbar vertebra is dislocated in front of the sacrum causing occlusion of the brim.

p., triangular. P. whose inlet is triangular.

p., triradiate. SEE: *p., beaked.*

p., true. The part of the p. below the iliopectineal line.

pelvitherm (pĕl′vĭ-thurm) [L. *pelvis,* basin, + Gr. *thermē,* heat]. Device for applying heat to the pelvis.

pelvoscopy (pĕl-vŏs′kō-pĭ) ["+ Gr. *skopein,* to examine]. Inspection of a pelvis.

pemphigoid (pĕm′fĭ-goyd) [Gr. *pemphigōdēs,* breaking out in blisters]. Similar to pemphigus.

pemphigus (pĕm′fĭ-gŭs) [Gr. *pemphix,* a blister]. An acute or chronic disease of adults characterized by occurence of successive crops of bullae which appear suddenly on apparently normal skin and disappear leaving pigmented spots. It may be attended by itching and burning and constitutional disturbance. ETIOL: Unknown.

TREATMENT: Care of general health. In severe and extensive cases patient to be kept on air or water mattress, and given meticulous care of the skin.

p. acutus. Constitutional symptoms severe and outcome often fatal. Bullae 1-10 cm. in diameter often containing blood and serum. If coalescing, denuded areas are formed.

p. circinatus. P. with circular eruptions.

p. foliaceus. Rare type. Large flaccid bullae that develop rapidly, rupture soon, and leave a moist, raw surface covered with seropurulent fluid. Bullous contents are purulent from beginning with sickening odor. Chronic course.

p. vegetans, Hallopeau type. A form of p. vulgaris characterized by pustules instead of bullae. Pustules are followed by warty vegetations. Prognosis, even prior to corticosteroids, was good.

p. vegetans, Neumann type. Variant of p. vulgaris. Initial stage similar, but the lesions persist instead of drying up, resulting in papillary excrescences with no tendency to heal, secreting foul-smelling seropurulent fluid and sodden decomposing masses of epidermis. Prior to the use of corticosteroids most patients with this form of pemphigus died.

p. vulgaris. Uncomplicated form in which replacement of epidermis follows. Lesions develop suddenly and are round or oval, thin walled, tense, and translucent with contents bilateral in distribution. The lesions have little tendency to heal and bleed easily when they burst. Prior to the use of corticosteroids, the outcome was fatal. With the use of corticosteroids, the mortality rate is 40%.

penalge'sia. A reduction in number of touch and pain spots in skin in cases of trigeminal neuralgia.

pendular (pĕn'dū-lĕr) [L. *pendulus*]. Hanging so as to swing by an attached part; oscillating like a pendulum.

pendulous (pĕn'dū-lŭs). Swinging freely like a pendulum; hanging.

penetrate (pĕn'e-trāt) [L. *penetrāre*]. To enter or force into the interior; pierce.

penetrating (pĕn'ĕ-trāt-ĭng). Entering beyond the exterior.

p. power. Penetrating capacity of a lens.

p. wound. Wound entering the interior of an organ or cavity.

penetration (pĕn''ĕ-trā'shŭn) [L. *penetrāre*, to go within]. 1. Process of entering within a part. 2. Capacity to enter within a part. 3. Power of a lens to give a clear focus at varying depths.

penetrometer (pĕn-ĕ-trŏm'ĕ-tĕr) ["+ Gr. *metron*, measure]. An instrument that compares roughly the comparative absorption of roentgen rays in various metals, esp. silver. lead, and aluminum; hence, it gives a rough estimation of the ability of X rays to penetrate tissues. SYN: *penetrameter; qualimeter.*

penicillin (pen-ĭ-sĭl'ĭn). One of a group of antibiotics biosynthesized by several species of molds, esp. Penicillium notatum and P. chrysogenum. P. is bacteriostatic, inhibiting the growth of most Gram-positive bacteria and certain Gram-negative forms. It is effective also against certain molds, spirochetes, and rickettsias. There are many different penicillins, including synthetic ones, and their effectiveness varies for different organisms.

penicillinase (pĕn-ĭ-sĭl'ĭ-nās). A bacterial substance which inactivates most but not all penicillins. Is used to treat allergic reaction to penicillin.

penicilliosis (pĕn''ĭ-sĭl-ĭ-ō'sĭs) [L. *penicillum*, pencil]. Infection with the fungi of the genus Penicillium.

Penicillium (pĕn''ĭ-sĭl'ĭ-ŭm) [L. *penicillum*, pencil, brush]. A genus of molds belonging to the Ascomycetes (Sac fungi). They form the blue molds which grow on fruits, bread, cheese, etc. A number of species (P. chrysogenum, P. notatum, and others) are the source of penicillin. Occasionally in man they produce infections of the external ear, skin, or respiratory passageways. They are common allergens.

penicillus (pĕn''ĭ-sĭl'ŭs) [L., paint brush]. (pl. *penicil'li*) [NA] A group of the branches of arteries in the spleen which are arranged like the bristles of a brush. Each consists of successive portions: the pulp arteries, sheathed arteries, and terminal arteries.

penile (pē'nĭl, -nīl) [L. *penis*, penis]. Pert. to the penis.

p. reflex. 1. Sudden downward movement of penis when the prepuce or gland of a completely relaxed penis is pulled upward. 2. Contraction of bulbocavernous muscle on percussing dorsum of penis. 3. Contraction of bulbocavernous muscle resulting from compression of glans penis.

penis (pē'nĭs) [L.]. (pl. *penes*) [NA] The male organ of copulation and in mammals contains the passage for urine. It is a cylindrical, pendulous organ suspended from the front and sides of the pubic arch. It is composed of three columns of cavernous tissue, the whole being covered with skin, the two lateral columns being known as the corpora cavernosa penis. The third or median column contains the urethra, known as the corpus cavernosum urethrae.

The head of the penis is known as the *glans penis* in which the urethral orifice is situated; it is covered with a movable hood known as the *foreskin* or *prepuce*, under which is secreted a lubricating substance called *smegma*. Hyperemia of the genitals fills the corpora cavernosa with blood as the result of sexual excitement or stimulation, thus causing an *erection*. The hyperemia is lowered following ejaculation of the seminal fluid and the organ returns to its normal condition.

Contrary to popular myths, the size of the penis has no bearing on the male's or female's enjoyment of sexual intercourse. SEE: *urethra* for illustration.

p. captivus. One which is held within the vagina during copulation as a result of vaginismus and contraction of the perineal muscles.

p. clubbed. A condition in which the penis is curved during erection.

p. lunatus. Painful curved erection in gonorrhea. SYN: *chordee*, q.v.

p. muliebris. Clitoris, q.v.; the erectile organ of the female.

p. palmatus. P. enclosed by the scrotum.

p. webbed. P. palmatus.

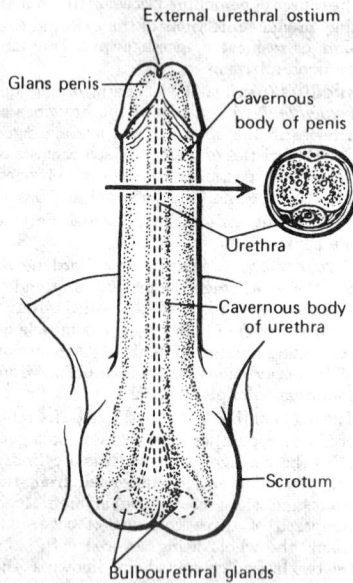

External urethral ostium

Glans penis

Cavernous body of penis

Urethra

Cavernous body of urethra

Scrotum

Bulbourethral glands

**PENIS AND MALE
EXTERNAL GENITALIA**

penis, words pert. to: balanitis; cavernitis; cavernosum; chordee; circumcision; condyloma; cord, spermatic; corpus cavernosum; Cowper's glands; ductus deferens; epispadias; erection; foreskin; frenulum preputii; genitalia, male; hypospadias; words beginning with "mentula-"; nervus erigens; peotomy; prepuce; prostate; scrotum; seminal vesicle; smegma; testes; Tyson's glands; urethra; vas deferens; words beginning with "balano" and "phall."

penischisis (pē-nĭs'kĭ-sĭs) [L. *penis,* penis, + Gr. *schisis,* splitting]. Epispadias, hypospadias, paraspadias, or any fissured condition of the penis.

penitis (pē-nī'tĭs) ["+ Gr. *-itis,* inflammation]. Inflammation of the penis.

penniform (pĕn'ĭ-form) [L. *penna,* feather, + *forma,* shape]. Feather-shaped.

pennyroyal (pĕn'ĭ-roi'ăl). Name for various plants, esp. Hedeoma and Mentha, which yield commercial oil used as carminative and stimulant.

pennyweight (pĕn'ĭ-wāt). Troy weight containing 24 grains or 1/20 of a troy ounce. Equal to 1.555 grams.

pension neurosis. A condition that develops subsequent to an injury in the belief that compensation can be obtained or will be continued by being ill. SEE: *neurosis, compensation.*

pent-, Penta- [Gr.]. Combining form meaning five.

pentad (pĕn'tăd) [Gr. *pente,* five]. 1. A radical or element with a valence of five. 2. Group of five.

pentamethylenediamine (pĕn"tă-mĕth'ĭ-lĕn-dī'ă-mēn). A nontoxic ptomaine occurring in tissue decomposition. SYN: *cadaverine.*

pentane (pĕn'tān). C_5H_{12}. One of the hydrocarbons of the methane series. A product of petroleum distillation.

pentavalent (pĕn"tă-vā'lĕnt, -tăv'ă-lent) [Gr. *pente,* five, + L. *valens,* having power]. Having a chemical valence of 5. SYN: *quinquivalent.*

pentobarbital sodium (pĕn"tō-bar'bĭ-tăl sō'dĭ-ŭm). A barbituric acid derivative used as an oral or intravenous hypnotic agent in preanesthetic medication. Used in labor with or without scopolamine. SYN: *nembutal.*

pentosazon (pĕn"tō-să'zŏn). Abnormal substance in urine which is incapable of fermentation.

pentose (pĕn'tōs) [Gr. *pente,* five]. $C_5H_{10}O_5$. A simple sugar with five atoms of carbon in the molecule.

pentosemia (pĕn"to-sē'mĭ-ă). Pentose in the blood.

pentoside (pĕn'tō-sīd). Pentose combined with some other substance.

pentosuria (pĕn"tō-sū'rĭ-ă). A condition in which pentose is found in the urine.

pentothal sodium (pĕn'tō-thăl so'dĭ-ŭm). Proprietary name for sodium thiopental (USP), an ultra-short-acting anesthetic used intravenously.

peonin (pē'ō-nĭn). A dye used as a hydrogen ion concentration test.

peotillomania (pē"ō-tĭl"ō-mă'nĭ-ă) [Gr. *peos,* penis, + *tillein,* to pull, + *mania,* madness]. A tic resulting in constant pulling at the penis. SYN: *pseudomasturbation.*

peotomy (pē-ŏt'ō-mĭ) ["+ *tomē,* incision]. Surgical removal of the penis.

pepo (pē'pō) [L., pumpkin]. Pumpkin seed which is used as an agent to remove tapeworms.

pepper (pĕp'ĕr) [ME. *peper*]. A spice that is used as a condiment, stimulant, carminative, and counterirritant.

Food value of 100 gm. (sweet green): Cal. 22; protein 1.2 gm.; trace of fat; carbohydrate 4.8 gm.; calcium 9 mg.; vitamin A, 420 I.U.; ascorbic acid 128 mg.

peppermint (pĕp'pĕr-mĭnt). USP. The leaves and tops of the plant Mentha piperita from which oil of peppermint is derived.

USES: Aromatic stimulant, carminative, and flavoring agent.

pepsic (pĕp'sĭk) [Gr. *peptein*, to digest]. Peptic, q.v.

pepsin (pĕp'sĭn) [Gr. *pepsis*, digestion]. The chief enzme of gastric juice which converts proteins into proteoses and peptones. It is formed by the chief cells of gastric glands and produces its maximum activity at a pH of 1.5 to 2. It is obtainable in granular form and in the presence of HCl, will digest proteins in vitro.

pepsinogen (pĕp-sĭn'ō-jĕn) ["+ *gennan*, to produce]. The zymogen or antecedent of pepsin existing in the form of granules in the chief cells of gastric glands.

peptic (pĕp'tĭk) [Gr. *peptikos*]. 1. Concerning digestion. 2. Concerning pepsin.

p. ulcer. An ulcer occurring in lower end of esophagus, in stomach usually along lesser curvature, in duodenum, or on jejunal side of a gastrojejunostomy.

SYM: Pain is the most characteristic symptom, tending to be of uniform quality and usually described as "gnawing." It is localized in the epigastrium and exhibits a rhythmicity and periodicity usually appearing one to three hours after a meal. It is absent before breakfast but may occur during the night. It is relieved by foods and alkalies; it is aggravated by alcohol and condiments. Often periods of remission occur in which pain is absent.

Other symptoms include dyspepsia, heartburn, acid eructations, nausea, vomiting, and anorexia. Diarrhea may occur with loss of weight. In some cases, physical signs may be absent, the first indication of the condition being hemorrhage or perforation. Gastric juice always exhibits hyperacidity.

PROG: Guardedly favorable. Hemorrhage or perforation may occur without warning and relapses from new ulcers not uncommon.

NP: Medicine to reduce acid secretion of stomach. Bed rest initially in calm, quiet atmosphere. Daily bath and oral hygiene. Watch for complications of hemmorrhage and perforation. Examine vomitus and stools for blood. No food or fluid by mouth. No movement; report pain immediately as it is first sign of perforation.

TREATMENT: Symptoms may disappear and the ulcers heal without benefit of any medical therapy, and symptoms may sub-

side without evidence of healing by x-ray evaluation. Therapy includes combinations of the following.

General: Bedrest is indicated if pain is severe, if patient has lost considerable blood, or if he is heavily sedated. Otherwise it is optional according to the physician's instructions. Sedatives probably will be helpful if the patient is under severe and chronic emotional stress.

Diet: The Sippy diet, q.v., is used in the acute phase of the disease. In general however, diet has probably been overemphasized as a means of treating peptic ulcer. Frequent small feedings are usually more effective in relieving pain than three widely-spaced meals. Alcoholic beverages usually are not allowed, but some patients will be greatly relaxed by their use. If alcohol is allowed, be certain it is consumed well diluted and not taken on an empty stomach. This will help to counteract its ability to stimulate gastric acid secretion. The patient may be aware of specific foods which aggravate his symptoms. These should, of course, be avoided. Spices except for black pepper are not harmful. Smoking, being generally detrimental to health, should be discontinued.

Antacids: Excess gastric acid secretion usually is important in causing peptic ulcer, and antacids usually provide prompt relief of pain. Antacids leave the stomach quite rapidly if taken on an empty stomach; therefore they should be given frequently and with small feedings about an hour after the usual meal when the acid secretion is at its peak. Antacids commonly used include calcium carbonate, aluminum hydroxide, aluminum carbonate, magnesium carbonate, magnesium trisilicate, and sodium bicarbonate. The latter should not be used because of its several disadvantages, including gastric distention and the potential for causing edema in those who retain sodium.

Anticholinergics: Used to reduce secretion of acid following food intake. These act synergistically with antacids by causing gastric retention and thus allowing greater time for the antacids to be effective. They are also useful when given at night to help prevent excess acid secretion during sleep. Anticholinergics are increased in dose until blurring of vision and dryness of mouth occur. *CAUTION:* Anticholinergics should not be used in patients who have glaucoma, gastric retention, pyloric obstruction, prostatic hypertrophy, or other conditions which cause retention of urine.

Psychotherapy: Some patients will need extensive psychotherapy in order to change life styles or situations from those which are stressful to those more compatible with them and their stomachs.

peptidase. An enzyme which converts peptides to amino acids.

peptide (pĕp'tĭd) [Gr. *peptein*, to digest]. Compound formed by hydrolytic cleavage of peptones and containing two or more amino acids. A class of substances prepared by synthesis from amino acids and intermediate in molecular weight and chemical properties between the amino acids, which may be made artificially, and the proteins, which may not.
RS: dipeptide; polypeptide; tripeptide.

peptidolytic (pĕp''tĭ-dō-lĭt'ĭk) ["+ *lytikos*, dissolving]. Causing the splitting up or digestion of peptides.

peptinotoxin (pĕp''tĭn-ō-tŏk'sĭn) ["+ *toxikon*, poison]. Poisonous ptomaine found in the body as a result of disordered or defective digestion.

peptization (pĕp''tĭ-zā'shŭn) [Gr. *peptein*, to digest]. In the chemistry of colloids, the process of making a colloidal solution more stable; conversion of a gel to a sol.

peptogenic, peptogenous (pĕp-tō-jĕn'ĭk, -tŏj'ĕn-ŭs) ["+ *gennan*, to produce]. 1. Producing peptones and pepsin. 2. Promoting digestion

peptoid (pĕp'toyd) ["+ *eidos*, resemblance]. A product of protein digestion which does not give the biuret reaction.

peptolysis (pĕp-tŏl'ĭ-sĭs) [Gr. *peptein*, to digest, + *lysis*, dissolution]. The splitting up or hydrolysis of peptones.

peptolytic (pĕp-tō-lĭt'ĭk). Pert. to the splitting up of peptone.

peptone (pĕp'tōn) [Gr. *pepton*, digesting]. A secondary protein formed by the action of proteolytic enzymes, acids, or alkalies on certain proteins. P.'s are nitrogenous compounds soluble in water; they are not coagulated by boiling.

peptonemia (pĕp''tō-nē'mĭ-ă) ["+ *haima*, blood]. Peptones in the blood.

peptonization (pĕp''tō-nĭ-zā'shŭn) [Gr. *peptōn*, digesting]. Process of changing protein substance into peptones by action of proteolytic enzymes.

peptonize. To convert into peptones; to predigest with pepsin.

pep''tonol'ysis. The breakdown of peptones into simpler products, (peptides or amino acids). SYN: *peptolysis*.

peptonuria (pĕp''tō-nū'rĭ-ă) ["+ *ouron*, urine]. Excretion of peptones in the urine.

per, per- [L.]. 1. A word used as a prefix or by itself meaning through, by, by means of. 2.

In chemistry, the highest valence of an element.

peracidity (pŭr''ă-sĭd'ĭt-ĭ) [L. *per*, throughout, + *acidus*, sour]. Abnormal acidity.

peracute (pŭr-ă-kūt') ["+ *acutus*, keen]. Very acute or violent.

per anum (pŭr ā'nŭm) [L.]. Through or by way of the anus.

peratodyn'ia [Gr. *peran*, to pierce, + *odynē*, pain]. Heartburn; pain in region of cardia of stomach.

per cent, percent. Per hundred. For or out of each hundred. Its symbol, %, is used to indicate that the preceding number is a percentage.

p. c. of a solution. Term which designates the number of grams of solute per 100 ml. of solvent or the number of cc. of a liquid dissolved in 100 ml. of another.

percentile (pŭr-sĕn'tĭl). One of 100 equal divisions of a series of items or data. Thus if a value, such as a test score, is higher than 92% of all the other test scores, that result is the 92nd percentile of the range of scores.

perception (pŭr-sĕp'shŭn) [L. *perceptiō*, perceive]. 1. Process of being aware of objects; consciousness. 2. The process of receiving sensory impressions. 3. The elaboration of a sensory impression; the ideational association modifying, defining, and usually completing the primary impression or stimulus. Vague or inadequate association occurs in confused and depressed states.

p., depth. Term used in evaluating visual function. The ability to recognize that an object has depth as well as height and width. It is generally believed that it is essential that both eyes be functioning normally for a person to have normal ability to perceive depth. Sometimes this is true, but most persons with the use of only one eye learn to judge depth quite accurately.

p., extrasensory. Perception not through the recognized senses. SYN: *paranormal perception*.

p., stereognostic. Recognition of objects by touch.

perceptivity (pŭr-sĕp-tĭv'ĭ-tĭ). Power to receive sense impressions.

perclu'sion. Inability to perform a movement.

percolate (pŭr'kō-lāt) [L. *percolare*, to strain through]. 1. To seep through a powdered substance. 2. Any fluid that has been filtered or percolated. 3. To strain a fluid through powdered substances in order to impregnate it with soluble principles of such substances.

percolation (pŭr'kō-lā'shŭn) [L. *percolatiō*]. 1. Filtration. 2. Process of extracting soluble portions of a drug of powdered composition by filtering a liquid solvent through it.

percolator (pŭr′kō-lā″tŭr). Apparatus used for extraction of a drug with a liquid solvent.

per contiguum (pŭr kŏn-tĭg′ū-ŭm) [L.]. Touching, as in the spread of an inflammation from one part to an adjacent structure.

per continuum (pŭr kŏn-tĭn′ū-ŭm) [L.]. Continuous, as the spread of an inflammation from part to part.

percuss (pŭr-kŭs′) [L. *percutere*]. To tap parts of the body to aid diagnosis by sound emitted.

percussion (pŭr-kŭsh′ŭn) [L. *percussio,* a striking]. Tapping the body lightly but sharply to determine position, size, and consistency of an underlying structure and the presence of fluid or pus in a cavity. These conditions are established by resonance and pitch of the sound emitted, vibration elicited, or resistance encountered.

RS: abdomen; bladder; boxnote; chest; heart; intestines; kidney; liver; ovary; palpation; spleen; uterus.

p., auscultatory. P. combined with auscultation.

p., direct. P., immediate, q.v.

p., finger. Striking of the finger resting upon the body with a finger of the other hand.

p., hammer. A hammer with a rubber head used for percussion. SYN: *plexor.*

p., immediate. Performed by striking the surface directly with the fingers.

p., indirect. P., mediate, q.v.

p., mediate. Performed by using fingers of one hand as a plexor and those of the opposite hand as a pleximeter.

p. test. P. along the course of a peripheral nerve to test for its having been interrupted or for its regeneration.

percussor (pŭr-kŭs′or) [L., striker]. Device used for diagnosis by percussion, consisting of hammer with rubber or metal head.

percutaneous (pŭr″kū-tā′nē-ŭs) [L. *per,* through, + *cutis,* skin]. Effected through the skin. Applying a medicated ointment by friction, or removal or injection by needle.

pereirine (pĕ-rā′rēn). [Jonathan Pereira, Eng. pharmacologist, 1804-1853]. An alkaloid obtained from pereira bark which is used as a quinine substitute in treatment of fevers.

perflation (pŭr-flā′shŭn) [L. *perflatio*]. The process of blowing air into a cavity to expand its walls or to force out secretions or other matter.

perforans (pŭr′fō-rǎns) [L.]. Perforating or penetrating, as a nerve or muscle.

perforate (pŭr′fō-rāt) [L. *perforatus,* pierced with holes]. 1. To puncture or to make holes. 2. Pierced with holes.

perforation (pŭr″fō-rā′shŭn). 1. The act or process of making a hole, such as that caused by ulceration. 2. Hole made through substance or part.

p. of stomach or intestine. SYM: Abdominal crisis due to escape of contents of the perforated viscus into the peritoneal cavity. Peritonitis certain unless operated upon in time. Onset is accompanied by acute pain over perforated area spreading all over the abdomen which is rigid. Face is anxious with beads of perspiration on it. Nausea and vomiting will occur. Pulse rapid and feeble, respiration rapid and shallow. Temperature drops, but rises as peritonitis sets in, and pulse becomes fuller.

TREATMENT: Surgical. Pending operation give no fluids. Complete rest. No talking. Apply warmth. SEE: *peritonitis.*

perforator (pŭr′fō-rā-tor) [L., a piercing device]. Instrument for piercing the skull and other bones.

p., tympanum. Instrument for perforating the tympanum.

perfrication (pŭr-frĭ-kā′shŭn) [L. *perfricāre,* to rub]. Thorough rubbing with an ointment or embrocation. SYN: *inunction*

perfusion (pŭr-fū′zhŭn) [L. *perfundere,* to pour through]. 1. Passing of a fluid through spaces. 2. The pouring of a fluid. 3. Supplying an organ or tissue with nutrients and oxygen by injecting blood or a suitable fluid into an artery.

perhydrocyclopentanophenanthrene (pĕr-hī″drō-sī″klō-pĕn-tăn″ō-phĕn-ăn′thrēn). Name of the ring structure of the chemical nucleus of the steroids.

PERHYDROCYCLOPENTANOPHENANTHRENE

peri- [Gr.]. Prefix meaning around or about.

periacinal, periacinous (pĕr'ĭ-ăs'ĭ-năl, -ŭs) [Gr. *peri*, around, + L. *acinus*, grape]. Placed around a saclike dilation.

periadenitis (pĕr'ĭ-ă"dē-nī'tĭs) ["+ *adēn*, gland, + -*itis*, inflammation]. Inflamed condition of tissues surrounding a gland.

perialienitis (pĕr'ĭ-ā"lĭ-ĕn-ī'tĭs) ["+ L. *alienus*, foreign, + Gr. -*itis*, inflammation]. Noninfectious inflammation around a foreign body. SYN: *perixenitis.*

periamygdalitis (pĕr'ĭ-ăm-ĭg"dăl-ī'tĭs) [Gr. *peri*, around + *amygdalē*, tonsil, + -*itis*, inflammation]. Inflammation of connective tissue around the tonsil. SYN: *peritonsillitis.*

periangiitis (pĕr'ĭ-ăn"jĭ-ī'tĭs) ["+ *angeion*, vessel, + -*itis*, inflammation]. Inflamed condition of tissue around a blood or lymphatic vessel.

periangiocholitis (pĕr'ĭ-ăn"jĭ-ō-kō-lī'tĭs) ["+ "+ *cholē*, bile, + -*itis*, inflammation]. Inflamed condition of tissues around the bile ducts.

periaortitis (pĕr'ĭ-ā-or-tī'tĭs) ["+ *aortē*, aorta, + -*itis*, inflammation]. Inflamed condition of adventitia and tissues around the aorta.

periapical (pĕr'ĭ-ăp'ĭ-kăl) [Gr. *peri*, around, + L. *apex*, tip]. Around the apex of the root of a tooth.

periappendicitis (pĕr'ĭ-ă-pĕn"dĭ-sī'tĭs) ["+ L. *appendix*, appendage, + Gr. -*itis*, inflammation]. Inflamed condition of appendix and its surrounding tissues.

    p. decidualis. Decidual cells in the peritoneum of the appendix vermiformis in cases of tubal pregnancy due to adhesions between fallopian tubes and the appendix.

periarterial (pĕr'ĭ-ar-tē'rĭ-ăl) ["+ *artēria*, artery]. Placed around an artery.

periarteritis (pĕr'ĭ-ar-tĕr-ī'tĭs) ["+ "+ -*itis*, inflammation]. Inflammation of external coat of an artery.

    p. gummosa. Gummas in the blood vessels in syphilis.

    p. nodosa. Widespread focal areas of damage due to inflammation of arteries, esp. small and medium-sized ones. Function of organs involved is impaired. When the disease begins, its manifestations are extremely variable. Sym. of a moderate febrile disease are quite common. SYN: *polyarteritis nodosa.*

periarthric (pĕr'ĭ-ar'thrĭk) [Gr. *peri*, around, + *arthron*, joint]. Surrounding a joint. SYN: *circumarticular*

periarthritis (pĕr'ĭ-ar-thrī'tĭs) ["+ "+ -*itis*, inflammation]. Inflammation of area around a joint.

periarticular (pĕr'ĭ-ar-tĭk'ū-lăr) [Gr. *peri*, around, + L. *articulus*, a joint]. Surrounding a joint. SYN: *circumarticular.*

periaxial (pĕr-ĭ-ăk'sĭ-ăl) ["+ *axōn*, axis]. Located around an axis.

periaxillary (pĕr'ĭ-ăk'sĭl-ĕ-rī) [Gr. *peri*, around, + L. *axilla*, armpit.]. Occurring around the axilla.

peribronchiolitis (pĕr'ĭ-brŏng"kĭ-ō-lī'tĭs) ["+ L. *bronchiolus*, bronchiole, + -*itis*, inflammation]. Inflammation of area around the bronchioles.

peribronchitis (pĕr'ĭ-brŏng-kī'tĭs) ["+ *bronkhos*, windpipe, + -*itis*, inflammation]. Inflammation of all tissues surrounding the bronchi or bronchial tubes.

pericardiac, pericardial (pĕr-ĭ-kar'dĭ-ăk, -ăl) [Gr. *peri*, around, + *kardia*, heart]. Concerning the pericardium.

pericardicentesis (pĕr'ĭ-kar"dĭ-sĕn-tē'sĭs) ["+ "+ *kentēsis*, puncture]. Surgical piercing of the pericardium.

pericardiectomy (pĕr'ĭ-kar-dĭ-ĕk'tō-mĭ) ["+ "+ *ektomē*, excision]. Excision of part or all of the pericardium.

pericardiocentesis (pĕr'ĭ-kar"dĭ-ō-sĕn-tē'sĭs) [Gr. *peri*, around, + *kardia*, heart, + *kentēsis*, puncture]. Surgical perforation of the pericardium. SYN: *pericardicentesis.*

pericardiolysis (pĕr'ĭ-kar"dĭ-ŏl'ĭ-sĭs) ["+ "+ *lysis*, dissolution]. Separation of adhesions between the visceral and parietal pericardium.

pericardiomediastinitis (pĕr'ĭ-kar"dĭ-ō-mē-dĭ-ăs"tĭ-nī'tĭs) ["+ "+ L. *mediastinum*, + Gr. -*itis*, inflammation]. Inflamed condition of the pericardium and mediastinum.

pericardiopexy ["+ "+ *pexis*, putting together]. Surgical procedure designed to increase the blood supply to the heart by joining the pericardium to an adjacent tissue.

pericardiophrenic (pĕr-ĭ-kar"dĭ-ō-frĕn'ĭk) [Gr. *peri*, around, + *kardia*, heart, + *phrēn*, diaphragm]. Concerning the pericardium and diaphragm.

pericardiopleural (pĕr'ĭ-kar"dĭ-ō-plŭ'răl) ["+ "+ *pleura*, rib]. Concerning the pericardium and pleura.

pericardiorrhaphy (pĕr'ĭ-kar"dĭ-or'ă-fĭ) ["+ "+ *rhaphē*, a sewing]. Suture of a wound in the pericardium.

pericardiostomy (pĕr'ĭ-kar"dĭ-ŏs'tō-mĭ) [Gr. *peri*, around, + *kardia*, heart, + *stoma*, opening]. Formation of an opening into the pericardium for drainage.

pericardiosymphysis (pĕr'ĭ-kar"dĭ-ō-sĭm'-fĭ-sĭs) ["+ "+ *symphysis*, a joining]. Adhesion between the layers of the pericardium.

pericardiotomy (pĕr′ĭ-kar-dĭ-ŏt′ō-mĭ) ["+ "+ *tomē*, a cutting]. Incision of pericardial sac around heart.

pericarditic (pĕr-ĭ-kar-dĭt′ĭk). Concerning the pericardium.

pericarditis (pĕr-ĭ-kar-dĭ′tĭs) [Gr. *peri*, around, + *kardia*, heart, + *-itis*, inflammation]. Inflammation of pericardium.

ETIOL: Tuberculosis, mycoses, infection by pyogenic organisms, collagen disease, uremia, myocardial infarction, neoplasms, trauma.

SYM: Moderate fever, precordial pain and tenderness, dry cough, dyspnea, and palpitation. Pulse, first rapid, forcible, then weak and irregular.

First stage: Auscultation reveals to and fro friction sound heard over 4th left intercostal space near sternum. Inspection and palpation sometimes reveal a diffuse apex beat. Friction rub may sometimes be palpated.

Second stage: Serofibrinous effusion. Bulging of precordium. Increased area of dullness, triangular in shape, base down. Heart sounds muffled, distant, feeble. Purulent effusion yields similar signs, but in addition high, irregular fever; sweats; chills, and progressive pallor; sometimes edema over the precordium. In doubtful cases the aspirating needle reveals pus.

PROG: Fair in early stages. In purulent and fibrinous, extremely grave.

TREATMENT: *General:* Absolute bed rest, light diet. For relief of pain apply ice bag over precordium or administer pain-relieving drugs, depending on its intensity. *Specific:* Appropriate antibiotic for specific organisms involved. If purulent effusion occurs, aspiration or surgical drainage. If gallop rhythm or signs of heart failure occur, restrict fluids and salt. For chronic constrictive pericarditis, resection of pericardium.

p., acute fibrinous. P. characterized by fibrinous exudation.

p., acute nonspecific. A disease of unknown etiology usually following respiratory infections.

p. adhesiva. Form in which the layers of pericardium adhere.

p., constrictive. P. in which adhesions form between visceral and parietal layers of the peritoneum.

p. externa. Inflammation of exterior surface of the pericardium.

p., fibrinous. Membrane is covered with butterlike exudate which organizes and unites the pericardial surfaces.

SYM: Precordial bulging, a weak apex beat with loud sounds, a systolic retraction at apex and over large part of precordium, peculiar diastolic collapse of jugular veins, feeble apex beat with a forcible impulse over body of heart. Signs of heart failure, as dyspnea, dropsy, cyanosis.

p., hemorrhagic. P. in which the exudate contains blood.

p., idiopathic. SEE: *p., acute nonspecific.*

p., ischemic. P. resulting from myocardial infarction.

p., neoplastic. P. due to invasion of pericardium by malignant tumors of adjoining structures.

p. obliterans. Pericardial inflammation causing adhesions and obliteration of the pericardial cavity.

p., serofibrinous. P. in which there is a considerable quantity of serous exudate but little fibrin.

p., uremic. P. resulting from uremia.

p., viral. SEE: *p., acute nonspecific.*

pericardium (pĕr′ĭ-kar′dĭ-ŭm) [Gr. *peri*, around, + *kardia*, heart]. [NA]. The double, membranous, fibroserous sac enclosing the heart and the origins of the great blood vessels. It is composed of an inner serous layer (visceral pericardium or epicardium) and an outer fibrous layer (parietal pericardium). The space between the two constitutes the pericardial cavity which is normally filled with a small amount of serous fluid. Its base is attached to the diaphragm, its apex extending upward as far as the first subdivision of the great blood vessels. It is attached in front to the sternum, laterally to the mediastinal pleura, and posteriorly to the esophagus, trachea, and principal bronchi. Normally, p. contains a thin serous fluid.

p., adherent. Condition in which fibrous bands form between the two layers obliterating pericardial cavity. SEE: *pericarditis, constrictive.*

p., bread and butter. Condition seen in fibrinous pericarditis in which pericardium has a peculiar appearance due to fibrinous deposits on the two opposing surfaces.

p. externum. The outer fibrous layer of the pericardium.

p. internum. Serous inner layer of the pericardium.

p., parietal. The outer fibrous layer of the pericardium.

p., shaggy. Condition occurring in fibrinous pericarditis in which loose shaggy deposits of fibrin are seen on surfaces of pericardium.

p., visceral. Serous inner layer of the pericardium.

pericecal (pĕr″ĭ-sē′kăl) [Gr. *peri*, around, + L. *caecum*, blind]. Situated around the cecum.

pericecitis (pĕr-ĭ-sē-sī′tĭs) [" "+ Gr. *-itis*, inflammation]. Inflamed condition of area around the cecum. SYN: *perityphlitis.*

pericementitis (pĕr″ĭ-sē-mĕn-tī′tĭs) [Gr. *peri*, around, + L. *caementum*, cement, + Gr. *-itis*, inflammation]. Progressive neocrosis of the alveoli of the teeth. SYN: *periodontitis.*

pericementoclasia (pĕr″ĭ-sē-mĕn″tō-klā′zĭ-ă) [" "+ Gr. *klasis*, a breaking]. Dissolution of the pericementum with alveolar absorption. SYN: *pyorrhea alveolaris.*

pericementum (pĕr″ĭ-sē-mĕn′tŭm). Fibrous tissue covering the root of a tooth.

perichareia (per″ĭ-kă-rī′ă) [Gr.]. Excessive or abnormal rejoicing, seen in certain psychoses.

pericholangitis (pĕr″ĭ-kō-lăn-jī′tĭs) [Gr. *peri*, around, + *cholē*, bile, + *angeion*, vessel, + *-itis*, inflammation]. Inflammation of tissues surrounding a bile duct. SYN: *periangiocholitis.*

pericholecystitis (pĕr″ĭ-kō-lē-sĭs-tī′tĭs) ["+ "+ *kystis*, a sac, + *-itis*, inflammation]. Inflammation of tissues situated around the gallbladder.

perichondral, perichondrial (pĕr-ĭ-kon′drăl, -drĭ-ăl) [Gr. *peri*, around, + *chondros*, cartilage]. Concerning the membrane that covers cartilage.

perichondritis (pĕr-ĭ-kŏn-drī′tĭs) [" "+ *-itis*, inflammation]. Inflamed condition of perichondrium.

perichondrium (pĕr-ĭ-kŏn′drĭ-ŭm) [Gr. *peri*, around, + *chondros*, cartilage]. [NA]. Membrane of fibrous connective tissue around surface of cartilage.

perichondroma (pĕr″ĭ-kŏn-drō′mă) [" "+ *-ōma*, tumor]. A tumor arising from fibrous tissue which covers cartilage.

perichordal (pĕr-ĭ-kor′dăl) [Gr. *peri*, around, + *chordē*, cord]. Placed around the notochord.

perichorioidal, perichoroidal (pĕr″ĭ-kō-rĭ-oy′dăl, -roy′dăl) [Gr. *peri*, around, + *chorioeidēs*, skinlike]. Situated around the choroid coat.

perichrome (pĕr″ĭ-krōm) [" + *chrōma*, color]. A nerve cell in which the tigroid mass is arranged in rows throughout the protoplasm.

pericolic (pĕr-ĭ-kō′lĭk) [Gr. *peri*, around, + *kōlon*, colon]. Around or encircling the colon.

pericolitis (pĕr″ĭ-kō-lī′tĭs) ["+ "+ *-itis*, inflammation]. Inflammation of area around the colon.

pericolonitis (pĕr″ĭ-kō-lŏn-ī′tĭs). Inflamed condition of region around the colon.

pericolpitis (pĕr″ĭ-kŏl-pī′tĭs) [Gr. *peri*, around, + *kolpos*, vagina, + *-itis*, inflammation]. Inflammation of connective tissues surrounding the vagina.

periconchal (pĕr-ĭ-kŏng′kăl) ["+ *konchē*, concha]. Around the concha of the ear.

p. sulcus. Groove on posterior surface of the auricle.

periconchitis (pĕr″ĭ-kŏng-kī′tĭs) ["+ "+ *-itis*, inflammation]. Inflamed condition of the lining of the orbit.

pericorneal (pĕr″ĭ-kor′nē-ăl) [Gr. *peri*, around, + L. *cornu*, horn]. Placed around the cornea.

pericranitis (pĕr″ĭ-krā-nī′tĭs) [Gr. *peri*, around, + *kranion*, skull, + *-itis*, inflammation]. Inflamed condition of pericranium.

pericranium (pĕr″ĭ-krā′nĭ-ŭm). [NA]. Fibrous membrane surrounding the cranium; periosteum of the skull.

p. internum. Lining surface of the cranium. SYN: *endocranium.*

pericystitis (pĕr″ĭ-sĭs-tī′tĭs) [Gr. *peri*, around, + *kystis*, a bladder, + *-itis*, inflammation]. Inflamed condition of tissues about the bladder.

pericytial (pĕr-ĭ-sĭsh′ăl) ["+ *kytos*, cell]. Placed around a cell.

peridendritic (pĕr″ĭ-dĕn-drĭt′ĭk) ["+ *dendron*, a tree]. Surrounding a dendrite of a nerve cell.

peridental (pĕr″ĭ-dĕn′tăl) [Gr. *peri*, around, + L. *dens, dent-*, tooth]. Surrounding a tooth or part of one. SYN: *periodontal.*

peridenti′tis [" "+ *-itis*, inflammation]. Inflammation of tissues surrounding a tooth; periodontoclasia.

per′iderm [" + *derma*, skin]. Thin layer of flattened cells forming a transient layer of embryonic epidermis. SYN: epitrichial layer; epitrichium.

peridesmitis (pĕr″ĭ-dĕz-mī′tĭs) [Gr. *peri*, around, + *desmion*, band, + *-itis*, inflammation]. Inflammation of the areolar tissue around a ligament.

peridesmium (pĕr″ĭ-dĕz′mĭ-ŭm). The connective tissue membrane sheathing a ligament.

peridiverticulitis (pĕr″ĭ-dī″vĕr-tĭk″ū-lī′tĭs) [Gr. *peri*, around, + L. *diverticulāre*, to turn aside, + Gr. *-itis*, inflammation]. Inflammation of tissues situated around an intestinal diverticulum.

periductal (pĕr-ĭ-dŭk′tăl) [" + L. *ductus*, a passage]. Situated around a duct.

periduodenitis (pĕr'ĭ-dū"ō-dē-nĭ'tĭs) ["+ L. *duodeni,* twelve, + Gr. *-itis,* inflammation]. Inflammation around the duodenum often causing adhesions attaching it to the peritoneum.

periencephalitis (pĕr'ĭ-ĕn-sĕf'ă-lĭ'tĭs) [Gr. *peri,* around, + *enkephalos,* brain, + *-itis,* inflammation]. Inflamed condition of the surface of the brain.

periencephalomeningitis (pĕr'ĭ-ĕn-sĕf'ă-lō-mĕn"ĭn-jĭ'tĭs) ["+ "+ *mēninx,* membrane, + *-itis,* inflammation]. Inflamed condition of cerebral cortex and the meninges.

periendothelioma (pĕr'ĭ-ĕn"dō-thē"lĭ-ō'mă) ["+ *endon,* within, + *thēlē,* nipple, + *-ōma,* tumor]. A tumor arising from the endothelium of the lymphatics and the perithelium of blood vessels.

perienteritis (pĕr'ĭ-ĕn"tĕr-ĭ'tĭs) [Gr. *peri,* around, + *enteron,* intestines, + *-itis,* inflammation]. Inflamed condition of peritoneal lining of intestines.

periesophagitis (pĕr'ĭ-ē-sŏf'ă-jĭ'tĭs) ["+ *oisophagos,* esophagus, + *-itis,* inflammation]. Inflamed condition of tissues around the esophagus.

perifistular (pĕr-ĭ-fĭs'tū-ler) ["+ L. *fistula,* pipe]. Located around a fistula.

perifolliculitis (pĕr'ĭ-fō-lĭk"ū-lĭ'tĭs) [Gr. *peri,* around, + L. *folliculus,* a little sac, + *-itis,* inflammation]. Inflamed condition of area around the hair follicles.

perigangliitis (pĕr'ĭ-găng"lĭ-ĭ'tĭs) ["+ *ganglion,* knot, + *-itis,* inflammation]. Inflamed condition of region around a ganglion.

perigastritis (pĕr'ĭ-găs-trĭ'tĭs) ["+ *gastēr,* belly, + *-itis,* inflammation]. Inflammation of peritoneal covering of stomach.

perihepatitis (pĕr'ĭ-hĕp-ă-tĭ'tĭs) [Gr. *peri,* around, + *he'par, hēpat-,* liver, + *-itis,* inflammation]. Inflammation of peritoneal covering of the liver, usually occurring in circumscribed areas.

perijejunitis (pĕr'ĭ-jĕj-ū-nĭ'tĭs) ["+ L. *jejunum,* empty, + Gr. *-itis,* inflammation]. Inflamed condition of tissues around the jejunum.

perikaryon (pĕr'ĭ-kăr'ĭ-ŏn) [Gr. *peri,* around, + *karyon,* nucleus]. The cell body of a neuron.

perikeratic (pĕr'ĭ-kĕr-ă'tĭk) ["+ *keras, kerat-,* horn]. About the cornea. SYN: pericorneal.

perilabyrinthitis (pĕr'ĭ-lăb'ĭr-ĭn-thĭ'tĭs) ["+ *labyrinthos,* a maze of canals, + *-itis,* inflammation]. Inflammation of tissues around the labyrinth.

perilaryngitis (pĕr'ĭ-lăr'ĭn-jĭ'tĭs) [Gr. *peri,* around, + *larynx,* larynx, + *-itis,* inflammation]. Inflamed condition of tissues around the larynx.

perilymph (pĕr'ĭ-lĭmf) ["+ L. *lympha,* serum]. The pale, limpid fluid contained in the space between the membranous and bony labyrinth of the internal ear.

perilymphangitis (pĕr'ĭ-lĭmf-ăn-jĭ'tĭs) ["+ "+ *angeion,* vessel, + *-itis,* inflammation]. Inflammation of tissues around a lymphatic vessel.

perimeningitis (pĕr'ĭ-mĕn'ĭn-jĭ'tĭs) [Gr. *peri,* around, + *mēninx,* membrane, + *-itis,* inflammation]. Inflamed condition of the dura mater. SYN: *pachymeningitis.*

perimeter (pĕr-ĭm'ĕt-ĕr) ["+ *metron,* measure]. 1. The outer edge or periphery of a body or measure of the same. 2. Device for determining the extent of the field of vision.

perimetritis (pĕr'ĭ-mē-trĭ'tĭs) ["+ *mētra,* uterus, + *-itis,* inflammation]. Inflammation of the peritoneal covering of the uterus. May be associated with parametritis.

perimetrium (pĕr-ĭ-mē'trĭ-ŭm). [NA]. Serous coat of the uterus.

perimetry (pĕr-ĭm'ē-trĭ) [Gr. *peri,* around, + *metron,* measure]. 1. Circumference, edge, border of a body. 2. Measurement of the scope of the field of vision with a perimeter.

perimolysis. Disappearance of tooth substance with gross loss of enamel. May be due to persistent vomiting with continual exposure of the teeth to the acid from gastric fluid.

perimyelitis (pĕr'ĭ-mĭ"ē-lĭ'tĭs) ["+ *myelos,* marrow, + *-itis,* inflammation]. 1. Inflammation of the pia mater and arachnoid of the brain or spinal cord. SYN: *leptomeningitis.* 2. Inflammation of the endosteum or membrane around medullary cavity of a bone.

perimyelography (pĕr'ĭ-mĭ"ē-lŏg'ră-fĭ) ["+ "+ *graphein,* to write]. X-ray examination of the area around the spinal cord.

perimyoendocarditis (pĕr'ĭ-mĭ"ō-ĕn"dō-kar-dĭ'tĭs) [Gr. *peri,* around, + *mys, my-,* muscle, + *endon,* within, + *kardia,* heart, + *-itis,* inflammation]. Inflammation of the muscular wall of the heart, its endothelial lining, and the pericardium.

perimysial (pĕr-ĭ-mĭs'ĭ-ăl). Concerning, or of the nature of, the fibrous sheath of a muscle.

perimysiitis (pĕr'ĭ-mĭs'ĭ-ĭ'tĭs) [Gr. *peri,* around, + *mys,* muscle, + *-itis,* inflammation]. Inflamed condition of the perimysium, the sheath surrounding a muscle.

perimysium (pĕr'ĭ-mĭs'ĭ-ŭm). (pl. *perimys'ia*) [NA] Connective tissue sheath that envelops each primary bundle of muscle fibers. Sometimes called p. internum.

p. *externum.* The epimysium, q.v.

perinatal (pĕr'ĭ-nā'tal) [Gr. *peri,* around, + L. *nātālis,* birth]. Occurring in the period preceding, during, or after birth.

perineal (pĕr'ĭ-nē'ăl) [Gr. *perinaion,* perineum]. Concerning, or situated on, the perineum.

    p. body. Mass of tissue composed of skin, muscle, and fascia between vagina and rectum in the female, and the urethra and rectum in the male.

    p. fascia. Three layers of tissue between muscles of perineum.

    p. hernia. Hernia perforating the perineum. SYN: *perineocele.*

    p. section. Surgical incision through perineum. SYN: *perineotomy.*

perineo- [Gr. *perinaion*]. Combining form pert. to the perineum.

perineocele (pĕr'ĭ-nē'ō-sēl) [Gr. *perinaion,* perineum, + *kēlē,* hernia]. Hernia in the region of the perineum, between the rectum and vagina or between the rectum and prostate.

perineocolporectomyomectomy (pĕr'ĭ-nē-ō-kŏl"pō-rĕk"tō-mī"ō-mĕk'tō-mĭ) [" + *kolpos,* vagina, + L. *rectus,* straight, + Gr. *mys, myo-,* muscle, + *-ōma,* tumor, + *ektomē,* excision]. Excision of a myoma by incising the perineum, vagina, and rectum.

perineometer (per'ĭ-nē-ŏm'ĕ-ter) [Gr. *perinaion,* perineum, + *metron,* measure]. Apparatus for measuring pressure or force which is produced in the vagina when pubococcygeus and levator ani muscles are contracted voluntarily.

perineoplasty (pĕr'ĭ-nē'ō-plăs"tĭ) [" + *plassein,* to form]. Reparative surgery on the perineum.

perineorrhaphy (pĕr'ĭ-nē-ŏr'ă-fĭ) [" + *rhaphē,* a sewing]. Suture of the perineum to repair a laceration, usually following labor.

    NP: Give external irrigation to perineum following each use of bedpan as sepsis must be avoided. Keep stitches dry and sterile dressing secured with a T-bandage which is changed frequently, at least twice daily. Swab with antiseptic, dry, and put on fresh dressing. Warm glycerin packs are sometimes ordered to relieve pain and reduce edema. Light treatments are ordered by some doctors.

    It is difficult for patient to assume a comfortable position in which to lie. Prop up first on one and then the other side. Encourage the patient to move about. Diet as desired. Prevent hard bowel movements by giving substances to soften feces. Be certain patient is voiding freely.

    p., anterior. Surgical repair of anterior perineum and vaginal wall to correct a cystocele.

    p., colpo-. Removal of part of posterior vaginal wall and suturing of torn perineal body.

    p., posterior. Removal and repair of rectocele.

perineosynthesis (pĕr'ĭ-nē"ō-sĭn'thĕ-sĭs) [Gr. *perinaion,* perineum, + *synthesis,* placing together]. Plastic operation for repair of a lacerated perineum.

perineotomy (pĕr'ĭ-nē-ŏt'ō-mĭ) [" + *tomē,* a cutting]. Surgical incision into the perineum.

perineovaginal (pĕr'ĭ-nē"ō-văj'ĭn-ăl) [" + L. *vagina,* sheath]. Concerning the perineum and vagina.

perinephric (pĕr'ĭ-nĕf'rĭk) [Gr. *peri,* around, + *nephros,* kidney]. Located or occurring around the kidney.

    p. abscess. Abscess formation in peritoneal membrane surrounding the kidney.

perinephritis (pĕr'ĭ-nē-frī'tĭs) [" + " + *-itis,* inflammation]. Inflammation of peritoneal tissues around the kidney. SYN: *paranephritis.*

perinephrium (pĕr'ĭ-nĕf'rĭ-ŭm). The connective and fatty tissue surrounding the kidney.

perineum (pĕr'ĭ-nē'ŭm) [Gr. *perineos*]. 1. [NA]. The structures occupying the pelvic outlet and comprising the pelvic floor. 2. The external region between the vulva and anus in a female or between the scrotum and anus in a male.

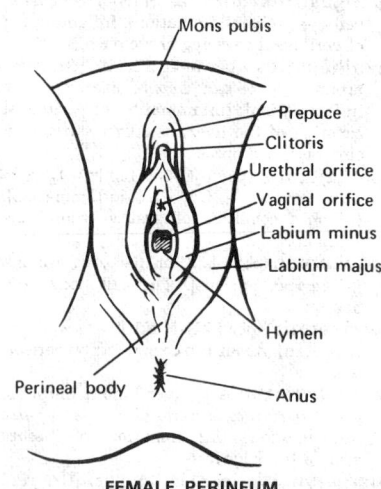

Mons pubis

Prepuce

Clitoris

Urethral orifice

Vaginal orifice

Labium minus

Labium majus

Hymen

Perineal body

Anus

FEMALE PERINEUM, LITHOTOMY POSITION

It is made up of skin, muscle, and fasciae. The muscles of the perineum are the anterior portion of the intact levator ani muscle, the transverse perineal muscle, and the sphincter muscles of the vagina.

RS: bodies, perineal; words beginning with "perine."

p., tears of the. There are three degrees of severity caused by overstretching of vagina and perineum in delivery. Fetal malposition increases the chance of tears occurring.

COMPLICATIONS: Hemorrhage, infection, cystocele, rectocele, descent of uterus, perhaps loss of bowel control.

TREATMENT: Surgery.

p., watering-pot. One riddled with fistulas from urethral stricture.

perineurial (pĕr'ĭ-nū'rī-ăl) [Gr. *peri*, around, + *neuron*, sinew]. Concerning the perineurium, the sheath around a bundle of nerve fibers.

perineuritis (pĕr'ĭ-nū-rī'tĭs) ["+ "+ *-itis*, inflammation]. Inflammation of the sheath enveloping nerve fibers.

perineurium (pĕr'ĭ-nū'rī-ŭm) [Gr. *peri*, around, + *neuron*, sinew]. A connective tissue sheath investing a fasciculus or bundle of nerve fibers. SYN: *perifascicular sheath.*

periocular (pĕr'ĭ-ŏk'ū-ler) ["+ L. *oculus*, eye]. Located around the eye. SYN: *circumocular.*

period (pēr'ĭ-ŏd) [L. *periodus*]. 1. The interval of time between two successive occurrences of any regularly recurring phenomenon or event; a cycle. 2. The menses. 3. Time occupied by a disease in running its course, or by a stage of a disease, such as an incubation p.

p., childbearing. The p. in the female during which she is capable of procreation; puberty to the menopause.

p. of development. SEE: *embryo, development of.*

p., gestation. P. of pregnancy; time from conception to parturition. Average length is 10 lunar months or 280 days measured from onset of last menstrual period. Length varies from 250 to 310 days. SEE: *gestation; pregnancy table.*

p., incubation. Time from moment of infection until appearance of first symptom.

p.'s of an infectious disease. 1. P. of incubation. 2. P. of prodromal symptoms. 3. P. of invasion. 4. Fastigium or acme. 5. P. of decline or defervescence. SEE: *infection.*

p., latent. The time between stimulation and the resulting response.

p., menstrual. Menstruation.

p., neonatal. The first 30 days of infant life.

p., patent. The time in a parasitic disease during which organisms are demonstrable in the body.

p., puerperal. Interval of time from birth of a child to approximately six weeks later, at which time complete involution of the uterus has occurred.

periodic (pēr-ĭ-ŏd'ĭk) [Gr. *periodikos*]. Recurring after definite intervals.

p. law. That which states that the chemical and physical properties of the chemical elements are periodic functions of their atomic weights.

periodicity (pēr'ĭ-ō-dĭs'ĭ-tĭ). 1. State of being regularly recurrent. 2. The rate of rise and fall or interruption of a unidirectional current in physical therapy. 3. Recurrence of the menses.

periodontal (pĕr'ĭ-ō-dŏn'tăl) [Gr. *peri*, around, + *odous, odont-*, tooth]. Located around a tooth.

periodontitis (pĕr'ĭ-ō-dŏn-tī'tis) ["+ "+ *-itis*, inflammation]. Inflammation or degeneration, or both, of the dental periosteum, alveolar bone, cementum, and adjacent gingiva. Suppuration usually occurs, supporting bone is resorbed, teeth become loose, and recession of gingivae occurs. Usually follows chronic gingivitis, Vincent's infection, or poor dental hygiene. Systemic factors may predispose. SYN: *pyorrhea alveolaris; Rigg's disease.*

p., apical. P. of periapical region usually leading to formation of periapical abscess.

periodontium (pĕr-ĭ-ō-dŏn'shĭ-ŭm). [NA]. The tissues surrounding and supporting a tooth. They include periodontal membrane, alveolar bone, and gingiva.

periodontoclasia (pĕr'ĭ-ō-dŏn"tō-klā'zĭ- ă) [Gr. *peri*, around, + *odous, odont-*, tooth, + *klasis*, breaking]. Condition characterized by inflammation accompanied by degenerative and retrogressive changes in the periodontium.

periodontology (pĕr'ĭ-ō-dŏn-tŏl'ō-jĭ) ["+ "+ *logos*, study of]. Field of dentistry dealing with treatment of diseases of the tissues around the teeth.

periodoscope (pĕr'ĭ-ŏd'ō-skōp) [LL. *periodus*, interval of time, + *skopein*, to examine]. Table or dial for calculation of expected date of confinement.

periomphalic (pĕr'ĭ-ŏm-făl'ĭk) [Gr. *peri*, around, + *omphalos*, navel]. Located around or near the umbilicus.

periontogenic ["+ *on*, existing, + *gennan*, to produce]. Diseases caused by the environment.

perionychia (pĕr''ĭ-ō-nĭk'ĭ-ă) ["+ *onyx, onych-*, nails]. Inflammation around a nail.

perionychium (pĕr''ĭ-ō-nĭk'ĭ-ŭm). The epidermis surrounding a nail.

perionyxis (pĕr''ĭ-ō-nĭk'sĭs). Inflammation of epidermis surrounding a nail.

perioophoritis (pĕr''ĭ-ō-ŏf''ō-rī'tĭs) [Gr. *peri*, around, + *oophoron*, ovary, + *-itis*, inflammation]. Inflammation of the surface membrane of the ovary. SYN: *perioothecitis.*

perioophorosalpingitis (pĕr''ĭ-ō-ŏf''ō-rō-sal''pĭn-jī'tĭs) ["+ "+ *salpinx*, tube, + *-itis*, inflammation]. Inflamed condition of tissues around an ovary and oviduct.

perioothecitis (pĕr''ĭ-ō''ō-thē-sī'tĭs) [Gr. *peri*, around, + *ōon*, egg, + *thécē*, box, + *-itis*, inflammation]. Inflammation of the tissues around the ovary. SYN: *perioophoritis.*

perioothecosalpingitis (pĕr''ĭ-ō''ō-thē''kō-săl-pĭn-jī'tĭs) ["+ "+ "+ *salpinx*, tube, + *-itis*, inflammation]. Inflammation of peritoneal membrane around the ovary and oviduct. SYN: *perioophorosalpingitis; perisalpingoovaritis.*

perioptometry (pĕr''ĭ-ŏp-tŏm'ĕ-trĭ) [Gr. *peri*, around, + *optos*, visible, + *metron*, a measure]. Measurement of the visual field.

perioral (pĕr''ĭ-ō'ral) ["+ L. *oralis*, mouth]. Surrounding the mouth. SYN: *circumoral.*

periorbita (pĕr''ĭ-or'bĭ-tă) [Gr. *peri*, around, + L. *orbita*, orbit]. [NA]. Connective tissue covering the socket of the eye.

periorbital (pĕr''ĭ-or'bĭ-tăl). Surrounding the socket of the eye. SYN: *circumorbital.*

periorbititis (pĕr''ĭ-or''bĭ-tī'tĭs) [Gr. *peri*, around, + L. *orbita*, orbit, Gr. *-itis*, inflammation]. Inflamed condition of the periorbita.

periorchitis (pĕr''ĭ-or-kī'tĭs) ["+ *orchis*, testicle, + *-itis*, inflammation]. Inflamed condition of the tissues investing a testicle.

　　p. hemorrhagica. Chronic hematocele of the tunica vaginalis coat of the testis.

periosteal (pĕr-ĭ-ŏs'tĭ-ăl) ["+ *osteon*, bone]. Concerning the periosteum.

periosteitis (pĕr''ĭ-ŏs''tē-ī'tĭs) ["+ "+ *-itis*, inflammation]. Inflammation of membrane investing a bone, the periosteum. SYN: *periostitis.*

periosteoedema (pĕr''ĭ-os''tē-ō-ē-dē'mă) [Gr. *peri*, around, + *osteon*, bone, + *oidema*, swelling]. Edema of the periosteum, the membrane surrounding a bone.

periosteoma (pĕr''ĭ-ŏs-tē-ō'mă) ["+ "+ *-ōma*, tumor]. 1. An abnormal growth surrounding a bone. 2. Tumor of the periosteum, the tissue surrounding a bone.

periosteomyelitis (pĕr''ĭ-ŏs''tē-ō-mī'ĕ-lī'tĭs) ["+ "+ *myelos*, marrow, + *-itis*, inflammation]. Inflammation of bone, including the periosteum and marrow.

periosteophyte (pĕr''ĭ-ŏs'tē-ō-fīt) [Gr. *peri*, around, + *osteon*, bone, + *phyton*, growth]. Abnormal bony growth on periosteum, or arising from it.

periosteorrhaphy (pĕr''ĭ-ŏs''tē-or'ă-fĭ) ["+ *rhaphē*, a sewing]. Joining by suture the margins of a severed periosteum.

periosteotome (pĕr''ĭ-ŏs'tē-ō-tōm) [Gr. *peri*, around, + *osteon*, bone, + *tomē, a cutting*]. Instrument for cutting the periosteum or removing it from the bone.

periosteotomy (pĕr''ĭ-ŏs-tē-ŏt'ō-mĭ). Incision into the periosteum.

periosteous (pĕr''ĭ-ŏs'tē-ŭs) [Gr. *peri*, around, + *osteon*, bone]. Concerning, or of the nature of, periosteum. SYN: *periosteal.*

periosteum (pĕr-ĭ-ŏs'tē-ŭm) [Gr. *periosteon*]. [NA]. The fibrous membrane which forms the investing covering of bones except at their articular surfaces. Consists of a dense *external* layer containing numerous blood vessels and an *inner* layer of connective tissue cells which, when the bone is injured, function as osteoblasts and participate in new bone formation. P. serves as a supporting structure for blood vessels nourishing bone and for attachment of muscles, tendons, and ligaments. It extends over the whole surface except at the cartilaginous articulations.

　　p. externum. P. covering external surfaces of bones.

　　p. internum. Interior p. lining the medullary canal of a bone.

periostitis (pĕr''ĭ-ŏs-tī'tĭs) ["+ *-itis*, inflammation]. Inflamed condition of periosteum, the membrane investing a bone.

　　ETIOL: Infection following infectious diseases, esp. syphilis; also trauma.

　　SYM: Pain over part, esp. under pressure, fever, sweats, leukocytosis, skin inflamed, rigidity of overlying muscles.

　　p., albuminous. P. with albuminous serous fluid exudate beneath the membrane affected.

　　p., alveolar. Inflammation of the peridental membrane. SYN: *periodontitis.*

　　p., dental. P. of a tooth sheath.

　　p., diffuse. P. of the long bones.

　　p., hemorrhagic. P. with extravasation of blood under the periosteum.

periostoma (pĕr''ĭ-ŏs-tō'mă) [Gr. *peri*, around, + *osteon*, bone, + *-ōma*, tumor]. A bony neoplasm around a bone or arising from its membranous sheath.

periostomedullitis (pĕr″ĭ-ŏs″tō-mĕd-ū-lī′tĭs) ["+ "+ L. *medulla*, marrow, + Gr. *-itis*, inflammation]. Inflammation of the marrow or sheath of a bone. SYN: *periosteomedullitis; periosteomyelitis.*

periostosis (pĕr″ĭ-ŏs-tō′sĭs) ["+ "+ *-ōsis*, condition]. A bony neoplasm around a bone or arising from it.

periostotomy (pĕr″ĭ-ŏs-tŏt′ō-mĭ) ["+ "+ *tomē*, incision]. Incision of the periosteum, the sheath covering a bone. SYN: *periosteotomy.*

periotic (pĕr-ĭ-ŏ′tĭk) [Gr. *peri*, around, + *ous, ot-*, ear]. Situated around the ear, esp. the internal ear.

p. bone. The mastoid and petrous portions of the temporal bone.

peripachymeningitis (pĕr″ĭ-pak″ĭ-mĕn-ĭn-jī′tĭs) ["+ *pachys*, thick, + *mēninx*, membrane, + *-itis*, inflammation]. Inflamed condition of connective tissue between the dura mater and the bone.

peripancreatitis (pĕr″ĭ-păn″krē-ă-tī′tĭs) [Gr. *peri*, around, + *pankreas*, pancreas, + *-itis*, inflammation]. Inflammation of tissues about or around the pancreas.

peripatetic (pĕr″ĭ-pă-tĕt′ĭk) [L. *peripateticus*, to walk about while teaching]. Moving from place to place.

periphacitis (pĕr-ĭ-fă-sī′tĭs) [Gr. *peri*, around, + *phakos*, lens, + *-itis*, inflammation]. Inflamed condition of the capsule of the crystalline lens of the eye.

periphakus (pĕr″ĭ-fā′kŭs). The elastic capsule surrounding the crystalline lens.

peripherad (pĕr-ĭf′ĕr-ăd) [Gr. *peri*, around, + *pherein*, to bear, + L. *ad*, to]. In the direction of the periphery.

peripheral (pĕr-ĭf′ĕr-ăl). Located at, or pert. to, the periphery.

peripheraphose (pĕr″ĭf′ĕr-ă-fōs). Subjective sensation of darkness or shadow which originates in peripheral optic structures (optic nerve or eyeball).

peripherophose (per-ĭf′er-ō-fōs). A subjective sensation of light or color which originates in peripheral optic structure (optic nerve or eyeball).

periphery (pĕr-ĭf′-ē-rĭ) [Gr. *periphereia*]. Outer part or surface of a body; part away from the center.

periphlebitis (pĕr″ĭ-flē-bī′tĭs) [Gr. *peri*, around, + *phleps*, vein, + *-itis*, inflammation]. Inflamed condition of external coat of a vein or tissues around it.

periphoria (pĕr-ĭ-fō′rĭ-ă) ["+ *phoros*, bearing]. Tendency of the axis of the eye to deviate from the normal. SYN: *cyclophoria.*

periphrastic (pĕr″ĭ-frăs′tĭk) [Gr. *periphrastikos*]. Rel. to the use of superfluous words in expressing a thought.

periphrenitis (pĕr″ĭ-frē-nī′tĭs) [Gr. *peri*, around, + *phrēn*, diaphragm, + *-itis*, inflammation]. Inflamed condition of the structures around the diaphragm.

Periplaneta (per″ĭ-plă-nē′tă). A genus of cockroaches belonging to the order Orthoptera. Roaches contaminate food by mechanically transporting disease-producing bacteria, ova, and protozoa to the food.

P. americana. The American cockroach.

P. australasiae. The Australian cockroach.

periplast (pĕr′ĭ-plăst) [Gr. *peri*, around, + *plassein*, to form]. 1. Peripheral protoplasm of a cell exclusive of the nucleus. 2. Matrix of a part or organ. 3. A cell wall.

peripleural (pĕr″ĭ-plū′răl) ["+ *pleura*, rib]. Encircling the pleura.

peripleuritis (pĕr-ĭ-plū-rī′tĭs) ["+ "+ *-itis*, inflammation]. Inflamed condition of the connective tissues between the pleura and wall of the chest.

periproctitis (pĕr″ĭ-prŏk-tī′tĭs) [Gr. *peri*, around, + *prōktos*, anus, + *-itis*, inflammation]. Inflammation of areolar tissues in region of the rectum and anus. SYN: *perirectitis.*

periprostatic (pĕr″ĭ-prŏs-tăt′ĭk) ["+ *prostatēs*, prostate]. Surrounding or occurring about the prostate.

periprostatitis (pĕr″ĭ-prŏs-tă-tī′tĭs) ["+ "+ *-itis*, inflammation]. Inflamed condition of tissues surrounding the prostate.

peripylephlebitis (pĕr″ĭ-pī″lĕ-flĕ-bī′tĭs) ["+ *pylē*, gate, + *phleps, phleb-*, vein, + *-itis*, inflammation]. Inflamed condition of tissues about the portal vein.

peripyloric (pĕr″ĭ-pī-lor′ĭk) [Gr. *peri*, around, + *pylōros*, pylorus]. Extending around the pylorus.

perirectal (pĕr″ĭ-rĕk′tăl) ["+ L. *rectus*, straight]. Extending around the rectum.

perirectitis (pĕr″ĭ-rĕk-tī′tĭs) ["+ "+ Gr. *-itis*, inflammation]. Inflamed condition of tissues about rectum and anus. SYN: *periproctitis.*

perirenal (pĕr″ĭ-rē′năl) [Gr. *peri*, around, + L. *ren*, kidney]. Extending around the kidney. SYN: *circumrenal; perinephric.*

perirhinal (pĕr″ĭ-rī′năl) ["+ *rhis, rhin-*, nose]. Located about the nose or nasal fossae.

perirhizoclasia (pĕr″ĭ-rī″zō-klā′zĭ-ă) [Gr. *peri*, around, + *rhiza*, root, + *klasis*, destruction]. Inflammation and destruction of tissues extending around the roots of a tooth.

perisalpingitis (pĕr″ĭ-săl″pĭn-jī′tĭs) ["+ *salpinx, salping-*, tube, + *-itis*, inflammation]. Inflamed condition of peritoneal coat about the oviduct.

perisalpingoovaritis (pĕr″ĭ-săl-pĭn″gō-ō″văr-ī′tĭs) ["+ "+ L. *ovarium*, ovary, + Gr. *-itis*, inflammation]. Inflammation of peritoneal tissues surrounding the fallopian tubes and ovaries. SYN: *perioophorosalpingitis; perioothecosalpingitis.*

periscle′rium [Gr. *peri*, around, + *skléros*, hard]. Fibrous tissue encircling ossifying cartilage.

periscopic (pĕr″ĭ-skŏp′ĭk) ["+ *skopein*, to examine]. Viewing on all sides.

perish (pĕr′ĭsh) [ME. *perisshen*]. To disintegrate or die, esp. by other than natural causes.

perisigmoiditis (pĕr″ĭ-sĭg″moy-dī′tĭs) [Gr. *peri*, around, + *sigma*, Gr. letter S, + *eidos*, like, + *-itis*, inflammation]. Inflamed condition of peritoneal tissues around sigmoid flexure of the colon.

perisinusitis (pĕr″ĭ-sī″nū-sī′tĭs) ["+ L. *sinus*, cavity, + Gr. *-itis*, inflammation]. Inflammation of membranes about a sinus, esp. a venous sinus of the dura mater. SYN: *perisinuitis.*

perispermatitis (pĕr″ĭ-spĕr″mă-tī′tĭs) ["+ *sperma*, seed, + *-itis*, inflammation]. Inflamed condition of tissues about spermatic cord.

    p. serosa. Hydrocele of spermatic cord.

perisplanchnic (pĕr″ĭ-splank′nĭk) [Gr. *peri*, around, + *splanchnon*, viscus]. Extending around a viscus or the viscera.

perisplanchnitis (pĕr″ĭ-splănk-nī′tĭs) ["+ "+ *-itis*, inflammation]. Inflamed condition of the tissues around the viscera. SYN: *perivisceritis.*

perisplenitis (pĕr″ĭ-splē-nī′tĭs) ["+ *splēn*, spleen, + *-itis*, inflammation]. Inflammation of peritoneal coat of the spleen, the splenic capsule.

    p. cartilaginea. Inflammation of capsule of the spleen resulting in thickening and hardening. SYN: *hyalin capsulitis.*

perispondylitis (pĕr″ĭ-spŏn-dĭl-ī′tĭs) [Gr. *peri*, around, + *spondylos*, vertebra, + *-itis*, inflammation]. Inflamed condition of the parts around a vertebra.

perissad (pĕr-ĭs′ăd) [Gr. *perissos*, odd]. 1. Radical or element of odd valence. 2. Having odd valence.

perissodactylous (pĕr-ĭs″sō-dăk′tĭ-lŭs) ["+ *daktylos*, digit]. Having an odd number of fingers or toes.

peristalsis (pĕr-ĭ-stăl′sĭs) [Gr. *peri*, around, + *stalsis*, contraction]. A progressive, wavelike movement that occurs involuntarily in

hollow tubes of the body, esp. the alimentary canal. It is characteristic of tubes possessing longitudinal and circular layers of smooth muscle fibers.

P. is induced reflexly by distention of the walls of the tube. The wave consists of contraction of the circular muscle above the distention with relaxation of the region immediately distal to the distended portion. The simultaneous contraction and relaxation progresses slowly for a short distance as a wave that causes the contents of the tube to be forced onward.

    p., mass. Forced peristaltic movements of short duration, moving contents from one section of the colon to another, occurring three or four times daily.

    p., reverse. In a direction opposite to the normal direction. SYN: *antiperistalsis.*

peristaltic (pĕr″ĭ-stăl′tĭk). Concerning, or of the nature of, peristalsis.

    p. rush. A rapidly moving peristaltic wave that occurs from time to time in the small intestine moving all of the contents before it.

    p. unrest. Increased peristalsis or abnormal motility of the intestinal tract.

    p. wave. The wavelike movement occurring during peristalsis.

peristaphyline (pĕr″ĭ-stăf′ĭ-lĭn) [Gr. *peri*, around, + *staphylē*, uvula]. About the uvula.

peristome (pĕr′ĭ-stōm) ["+ *stoma*, mouth]. Channel leading to the cytosome or mouth in certain types of protozoa.

peristrumitis (pĕr″ĭ-strū-mī′tĭs) ["+ L. *struma*, goiter, + *-itis*, inflammation]. Inflamed condition of tissues around a goiter. SYN: *perithyroiditis.*

perisynovial (pĕr″ĭ-sĭ-nō′vĭ-ăl) [Gr. *peri*, around, + *syn*, with, + *ōon*, egg]. Extending around a synovial structure.

perisystole (pĕr″ĭ-sĭs′tō-lē) ["+ *systolē*, contraction]. The period preceding the systole in the cardiac rhythm. SYN: *presystole.*

peritectomy (pĕr″ĭ-tĕk′tō-mī) [Gr. *peri*, around, + *ektomē*, excision]. Surgical removal of a ring of conjunctiva around the cornea.

peritendineum (pĕr″ĭ-tĕn-dĭn′ē-ŭm) ["+ L. *tendō*, tendon]. [NA]. A sheath of fibrous connective tissue investing a fiber bundle of a tendon.

peritendinitis (pĕr″ĭ-tĕn″dĭ-nī′tĭs) ["+ "+ Gr. *-itis*, inflammation]. Inflamed condition of the sheath of a tendon. SYN: *peritenonitis.*

    p. calcarea. The deposition of calcareous material in tendons and associated regions, characterized by pain, tenderness, and limitation of motion.

peritenonitis (pĕr″ĭ-tĕn″o-nī′tĭs). Inflammation of sheath investing a tendon. SYN: *peritendinitis.*

perithelioma (pĕr″ĭ-thē-lĭ-ō′mä) [Gr. *peri,* around, + *thēlē,* nipple, + *-ōma,* tumor]. A tumor derived from the perithelial layer of the blood vessels.

perithelium (pĕr″ĭ-thē′lĭ-ŭm). Fibrous outer layer of the smaller blood vessels and capillaries.

perithyroiditis (pĕr″ĭ-thī-roy-dī′tĭs) [Gr. *peri,* around, + *thyreos,* shield, + *eidos,* form, + *-ītis,* inflammation]. Inflammation of capsule or tissues sheathing the thyroid gland. SYN: *peristrumitis.*

peritomy (pĕr-ĭt′ō-mĭ) [″+ *tomē,* incision]. 1. Excision of narrow strip of conjunctiva around the cornea in treatment of pannus. 2. Circumcision.

peritoneal (pĕr″ĭ-tō-nē′ăl) [Gr. *peritonaion,* peritoneum]. Concerning the peritoneum.

p. cavity. Region bordered by parietal layer of the peritoneum containing all the abdominal organs exclusive of the kidney. SEE: *cholascos.*

p. dialysis. Removal of toxic substances from the body by perfusing specific warm, sterile chemical solutions through the peritoneal cavity. Used in treating renal failure or in certain poisonings. Some of the drugs and chemicals which may be so removed are salicylates, barbiturates, meprobamate, amphetamines, bromide, methanol, boric acid, sulfonamide, and various antibiotics.

P. dialysis may be dangerous and cause death if not done with adequate supervision of body fluid and electrolyte balance.

p. sac, lesser. The omental bursa or cavity of the great omentum.

peritonealgia (pĕr″ĭ-tō″nē-ăl′jĭ-ă) [″+ *algos,* pain]. Pain of the peritoneum.

peritonealize. During abdominal surgery, to cover a tissue with peritoneum.

peritoneocentesis (pĕr″ĭ-tō″nē-ō-sĕn-tē′sĭs) [Gr. *peritonaion,* peritoneum, + *kentēsis,* puncture]. Piercing of the peritoneal cavity to obtain fluid. SEE: *paracentesis.*

peritoneoclysis (pĕr″ĭ-tō″nē-ō-klī′sĭs) [″+ *klysis,* a washing out]. Introduction of fluid into the peritoneal cavity.

peritoneopathy (pĕr″ĭ-tō-nē-ŏp′ăth-ĭ) [″+ *pathos,* disease]. Any disordered condition of the peritoneum.

peritoneopexy (pĕr″ĭ-tō′nē-ō-pĕks″ĭ) [Gr. *peritonaion,* peritoneum, + *pēxis,* fixation]. Fixation of the uterus by way of the vagina.

peritoneoplasty (pĕr″ĭ-tō′nē-ō-plăs″tĭ) [″+ *plassein,* to form]. Reparative surgery to prevent reformation of loosened adhesions.

peritoneoscope (pĕr″ĭ-tō′nē-ō-skōp) [Gr. *peritonaion,* peritoneum, + *skopein,* to examine]. Long, slender periscope or telescope device with a light at one end and an eye piece at the other. Used to inspect the peritoneal and abdominal cavities through a small incision in the abdominal wall.

peritoneoscopy (pĕr″ĭ-tō″nē-ŏs′kō-pĭ). Examination of peritoneal cavity with the peritoneoscope.

peritoneotomy (pĕr″ĭ-tō″nē-ŏt′ō-mĭ). Process of incising the peritoneum.

peritoneum (pĕr″ĭ-tō-nē′ŭm) [LL.]. [NA]. The serous membrane reflected over the viscera and lining the abdominal cavity.

PALPATION: If palmar surface of hand is applied to side of abdomen at level of the liquid in ascites and light percussion is performed on the opposite side, a sense of fluctuation will be communicated to the hand.

p., parietal. P. lining abdominal and pelvic walls and undersurface of diaphragm.

p., visceral. The p. that invests the abdominal organs. The p. holds the viscera in position by its folds.

peritonitic (pĕr″ĭ-tō-nĭt′ĭk) [″+ *-ītis,* inflammation]. Affected with or concerning peritonitis.

peritonitis (pĕr″ĭ-tō-nī′tĭs) [Gr. *peritonaion,* peritoneum, + *-ītis,* inflammation]. Inflammation of the peritoneum, the membranous coat lining the abdominal cavity and investing the viscera.

ETIOL: Infectious organisms that gain access by way of (1) rupture or perforation of viscus or associated structures, (2) female genital tract, (3) piercing of abdominal wall, (4) blood stream or lymphatic vessels, (5) operative incisions and failure to practice aseptic techniques. Prophylactic measures to prevent development of peritonitis is of utmost importance in the care of all patients.

TREATMENT: Antibiotic therapy.

p., acute diffuse. Generalized p. of a large area.

ETIOL: Rupture of an intra-abdominal viscus, as the appendix or stomach. Infection may take place directly from an adjacent organ which is inflamed or from the blood stream in patients with septicemia.

SYM: Chill; fever, 102°-103° F. (38.9°-39.4° C.) rapid pulse rate; abdominal pain and tenderness so intense abdominal respiration and bodily movement inhibited; patient on back, thighs flexed; features pinched and anxious; vomiting persistent; bowels usually constipated; hiccough; abdominal distention.

PROG: Guarded.

TREATMENT: Surgical intervention. Absolute bed rest; sips of water by mouth; saline or glucose solution, blood, or plasma parenterally; analgesics for pain; suction to gastrointestinal tract; antibiotic therapy.

p., adhesive. P. in which the visceral and parietal layers stick together by means of adhesions.

p., aseptic. P. due to causes other than bacterial infection, such as trauma, presence of chemicals produced naturally or introduced from without, irradiation.

p., chronic. Usually tuberculous, cancerous, or syphilitic; occurs in chronic alcoholism.

SYM: Fever slight or absent. Pain not severe; paroxysms; usually diffuse tenderness; anemia and emaciation may be marked.

PROG: Guarded.

TREATMENT: Rest; light diet; paracentesis. Laparotomy.

p., circumscribed. Localized p.

p., deformans. Chronic p. with thickened membrane and adhesions contracting and causing retraction of the intestines.

p., diffuse. P. which is widespread involving most of the peritoneum. SYN: *generalized peritonitis.*

p., localized. P. in which only a small area is involved.

p., meconium. P. in the newborn due to perforation of the gastrointestinal tract in utero. Neonatal intestinal obstruction may be present. In males a soft hydrocele or scrotal mass may be found.

p., pelvic. P. involving peritoneum of the pelvic region, usually the sequela of uterine tube infection in female.

p., primary. P. resulting from infectious organisms transmitted through blood or lymph.

p., puerperal. P. that develops following childbirth.

p., secondary. P. resulting from extension of infection from adjoining structures, rupture of a viscus, abscess, or trauma.

p., septic. P. caused by a pyogenic bacterium.

p., serous. P. in which there is copious liquid exudation.

p., traumatic. Acute p. due to injury or wound infection.

p., tuberculous. P. caused by numerous tubercle bacilli on the peritoneum.

peritonsillar (pĕr″ĭ-tŏn'sĭ-lăr) [Gr. *peri,* around, + L. *tonsilla,* tonsil]. Extending around a tonsil.

peritonsillitis (pĕr″ĭ-tŏn″sĭ-lī'tĭs) ["+ "+ Gr. *-itis,* inflammation]. Inflamed condition of tissues around the tonsils.

Peritricha (pĕr-īt'rĭ-kă) [Gr. *peri,* around, + *thrix,* hair]. A group of bacteria having flagella over the entire surface.

peritrichous (pĕ-rit'rĭk-ŭs) ["+ *thrix, trich-,* hair]. Indicating microorganisms that have cilia or flagella covering the entire surface.

perityphlitis (pĕr″ĭ-tĭf-lī'tĭs) ["+ *typhlon,* cecum, + *-itis,* inflammation]. Inflamed condition of tissues around the cecum and appendix. SYN: *appendicitis.*

periureteritis (pĕr″ĭ-ū-rē-tĕr-ī'tĭs) [Gr. *peri,* around, + *ourētēr,* ureter, + *-itis,* inflammation]. Inflamed condition of parts about the ureter.

periurethral (pĕr″ĭ-ū-rē'thrăl). Located about the urethra.

periuterine (pĕr″ĭ-ū'tĕr-ĭn) [Gr. *peri,* around, + L. *uterus,* womb]. Located about the uterus. SYN: *perimetric.*

perivaginitis (per″ĭ-vaj″ĭ-nī'tĭs) ["+ L. *vagina,* sheath, + Gr. *-itis,* inflammation]. Inflammation of region around the vagina. SYN: *pericolpitis.*

perivascular (pĕr″ĭ-văs'kū-ler) ["+ L. *vasculus,* a little vessel]. Located around a vessel, esp. a blood vessel.

perivasculitis (pĕr″ĭ-văs″kū-lī'tĭs) ["+ "+ Gr. *-itis,* inflammation]. Inflamed condition of tissues surrounding a blood vessel. SYN: *periangiitis.*

perivisceritis (pĕr″ĭ-vĭs″ĕr-ī'tĭs) ["+ L. *viscera,* internal organs, + Gr. *-itis,* inflammation]. Inflamed condition of the tissues surrounding the viscera.

perixenitis (pĕr″ĭ-zĕ-nī'tĭs) ["+ *xenos,* strange, + *-ītis,* inflammation]. Inflammation occurring around a foreign body in a tissue or organ.

perle (purl) [Fr., pearl]. A soft capsule containing medicine.

perlèche (pĕr-lĕsh') [Fr.]. Disorder marked by fissures and epithelial desquamation at corners of the mouth, esp. seen in children. May be due to oral moniliasis or a symptom of dietary deficiency, esp. riboflavin deficiency.

perlingual (pĕr-ling'gwal) [L. *per,* through, + *lingua,* tongue]. By way of the tongue; method of administering medicines.

permanent (per'mă-nĕnt) ["+ *manere,* to remain]. Enduring; without change.

p. teeth. Teeth developing at the second dentition. SEE: *dens permanens.*

permanganate (pĕr-man'gă-nāt). Any one of the salts of permanganic acid.

permeability (per″mē-ă-bĭl'ĭ-tĭ) [LL. *permeābilis*]. The quality of being permeable.

   p., capillary. The condition of capillary wall that enables substances in the blood to diffuse into tissue spaces or into cells, or vice versa.

permeable (per′mē-ă-bl). Capable of allowing the passage of fluids or substances in solution.

permeation (pĕr″mē-ā'shŭn) [L. *permeāre*, permeate]. Penetration of, and spreading throughout, an organ, tissue, or space.

permutation (pĕr″mū-tā'shŭn) [L. *per*, completely, + *mūtāre*, to change]. Transformation; complete change; act of altering objects in a group.

pernicious (pĕr-nĭsh'ŭs) [L. *perniciōsus*, destructive]. Destructive; fatal; harmful.

   p. anemia. Severe form of blood disease marked by progressive decrease in red blood corpuscles, muscular weakness, and gastrointestinal and neural disturbances. May be fatal if not treated with vitamin B₁₂, iron, and diet. SEE: *anemia, pernicious.*

   p. trend. A psychological term indicating an abnormal departure from conventional ideas and social interests.

pernio (per′nĭ-o) [L.]. Chilblain. Congestion and swelling of the skin due to cold.

   SYM: Attended with severe burning or itching; ulceration may result from vesicles and bullae that sometimes form.

perniosis (per″nĭ-ō'sĭs) ["+ Gr. *ōsis*, condition]. A skin disorder caused by cold. SEE: *chilblain; pernio.*

pero- [Gr. *pēros*, maimed]. Combining form meaning deformed.

perobrachius (pē″rō-brā'kē-ŭs) ["+ *brachiōn*, arm]. Condition in which forearms and hands are deformed.

perocephalus (pē″rō-sĕf'ă-lŭs) ["+ *kephalē*, head]. An individual with a congenitally defective head.

perodactylia (pē″rō-dăk-tĭl'ĭ-ă) ["+ *daktylos*, finger]. Congenital absence of one or more fingers.

peromelia (pē″rō-mē'lĭ-ă) ["+ *melos*, limb]. Congenital absence or deformity of the terminal part of a limb or limbs.

peromelus (pē-rŏm'ĕ-lŭs) [Gr. *peros*, maimed, + *melos*, limb]. An individual with malformation of extremities, including absence of hand or foot.

peroneal (pĕr″ō-nē'ăl) [Gr. *peronē*, pin]. Concerning the fibula.

peroneo- [Gr.]. Combining form pert. to the fibula.

peroneus (pĕr″ō-nē'ŭs) [Gr. *peronē*, pin]. One of several muscles of the leg causing motion in the foot.

peronia (pē-rō'nĭ-ă) [Gr. *pēros*, maimed]. Malformation.

peroral (pĕr-ōr'ăl) [L. *per*, through, + *os, or-,* mouth]. Administered through the mouth.

per os [L.]. By mouth.

peroxidase (per-ŏk'sĭ-dās) [L. *per*, through, + *oxys*, acid, + *ase*, enzyme]. An enzyme that hastens the transfer of oxygen from peroxide to a tissue that requires oxygen. This process is essential to intracellular respiration.

peroxide (per-ok'sīd). In chemistry, a compound containing more oxygen than the other oxides of the element in question. Ex: peroxides of hydrogen, H_2O_2; sodium, Na_2O_2; magnesium, MgO_2; and nitrogen, NO_2.

perplication (per-plĭ-kā'shŭn) [Gr. *per*, through, + *plicāre*, to fold]. Inserting the cut end of an artery through an incision in its own wall to arrest bleeding.

per primam, per primam intentionem (per prī'măm ĭn-tĕn-tĭ-ō'nĕm) [L.]. By first intention. SEE: *healing, first intention.*

per rectum (per rĕk'tŭm) [L.]. By the rectum; through the rectum.

persalt (per'sawlt). In chemistry, a salt containing largest possible amount of an acid radical.

per secundam (per sē-kŭn'dăm) [L.]. By second intention. SEE: *healing.*

perseveration (per-sĕv″ĕr-ā'shŭn) [L. *perseverāre*, to persist]. Continued repetition of a meaningless word or phrase, or repetition of answers which are not related to successive questions asked.

persimmon (per-sĭm'ĕn) [AmerInd.]. Food value of 100 gm. (raw, native to U.S.A.): Cal. 64; protein 0.8 gm.; trace of fat; carbohydrate 20 gm.; calcium 27 mg. (Vitamin A content in the Japanese persimmon is quite high (2710 I.U.), but the value in native persimmon has not been determined.) Vitamin C 66 mg.

persona (pĕr-sō'nă) [L., mask]. The outer attitude or appearance a person presents to others.

personal [L. *persōnalis*]. Characteristic of an individual.

   p. equation. In scientific observation, factors depending on personal qualities of individual observers.

personality (per″son-al'ĭ-tĭ) [LL. *persōnālitās*]. The unique organization of traits, characteristics, and modes of behavior of an individual, setting him apart from other individuals and at the same time determining how others react to him. Personality refers to the mental aspects of an individual in contrast to physique.

RS: consciousness; dissociation; somnambulism; vigilambulism.

p., double. SEE: *p., dual.*

p., dual. Mental dissociation in which one individual shows in alternation two very different personalities. SEE: *dual personality.*

p., extroverted. P. in which activities or libido are directed to other individuals or the environment.

p., introverted. One in which activities or libido are directed to the individual himself.

p., multiple. State in which three or more personalities alternate in the same individual, usually with each personality unaware of the others. SEE: *multiple personality.*

p., neurotic. P. characterized by behavior intermediate between normal and that of a neurotic individual.

p., psychopathic. Individual whose behavior is mostly amoral and antisocial. Actions are impulsive, irresponsible, and serve immediate interests without evidence of guilt or anxiety and without concern for social or legal consequences.

The term is so general that its use is unacceptable; nevertheless it continues to be used.

p., schizoid. P. characterized by shyness, oversensitivity, seclusiveness, dissociation from close interpersonal or competitive relationships, eccentricity, daydreaming, and inability to express hostility and aggression in situations that would call for such reactions.

perspiration (per″spĭr-ā′shŭn) [L. *perspīrāre*, breathe through]. Salty fluid secreted through the skin; sweat. Essentially it is a weak solution of sodium chloride, but it also contains potassium, lactate, and urea.

P. is a means of removing heat from the body. This is best accomplished by sweat evaporating from the skin rather than dripping off. Evaporation of a liter of sweat removes 580 Cal. of heat from the body. Sweat loss will vary from 100 to 1000 ml. per hour but may be many times that in a hot climate.

P. is increased by temperature and humidity of the atmosphere, exercises, pain, nausea, nervousness, mental excitement, dyspnea, diaphoretics, and shock.

P. is decreased by cold, diarrhea, voiding large quantities of urine, and using certain drugs.

p., insensible. Evaporation of water vapor from the body without appearing as moisture.

p., sensible. P. which occurs so as to form drops.

perspiration, words pert. to: adiaphoresis; adiapneustia; anhidrosis; bromohyperhidrosis; bromidrosis; chlorephidrosis; chromidrosis; diaphoresis; meridrosis; panidrosis; polyhidrosis; secretion; sudor; sweat; sweating; transpiration; uridrosis.

perspire (per-spīr′) [L. *perspīrāre*, breathe through]. To excrete fluid through the pores of the skin. SYN: *sweat.*

perstriction (pĕr-strĭk′shŭn) [L. *per*, through, + *strictus*, tighten]. Ligation of a bleeding vessel for the arrest of hemorrhage.

persulfate (per-sul′fāt). One of a series of sulfates containing more sulfuric acid than the others in same series.

per tertiam intentionem (per tĕr′shĭ-ăm ĭn-tĕn-shĭ-ō′nĕm) [L.]. By third intention. SEE: *healing.*

Perthes' disease (pār′tās). [Georg C. Perthes, Ger. surgeon, 1869-1927]. Disease in which changes take place in bone at head of femur with deformity resulting. SYN: *osteochondritis deformans juvenilis.*

SYM: Similar to tuberculous hip joint disease.

per tubam (pĕr tū′băm) [L.]. Through a tube.

perturbation (per″ter-bā′shŭn) [L. *perturbāre*, thoroughly disorder]. State of being greatly disturbed or agitated; uneasiness of mind.

pertussis (pĕr-tŭs′ĭs) [L. *per*, intensive, + *tussis*, cough]. An acute, infectious disease characterized by a catarrhal stage, followed by a peculiar paroxysmal cough, ending in a whooping inspiration. P. may be prevented by immunization of infants beginning at three months of age. SYN: *whooping cough.*

ETIOL: Due to a small, nonmotile, gram-negative bacillus, Bordetella pertussis.

INCUBATION: Seven to 10 days.

SYM: Elevated white blood count with marked lymphocytosis. May be in excess of 30,000 per cubic millimeter.

Often divided into three stages: *Catarrhal.* At this time the symptoms chiefly suggestive of the common cold—slight elevation of fever, sneezing, rhinitis, and dry cough. Irritability and loss of appetite.

Paroxysmal stage sets in after approx. 2 weeks. The cough is more violent and consists of a series of several short coughs, followed by long drawn inspiration during which the typical whoop is heard, this being occasioned by the spasmodic contraction of the glottis. Often with the beginning of each paroxysm, the patient assumes a worried expression, sometimes even one of terror. The face becomes cyanosed, eyes injected, veins distended. With conclusion of the paroxysm, vomiting is common. Also at this time there may be epistaxis, subconjunctival hemorrhages, or hemorrhages in other portions of body. Number of paroxysms in 24 hours may vary from three to four up to 40-50. Cough is precipitated by eating, drinking, or by pressing on the trachea. It is associated often with vomiting.

Decline begins after an indefinite period of several weeks. Paroxysms grow less frequent and less violent. Nutrition of child improves, and after a period which may be prolonged for several months the cough finally ceases.

    p. immune globulin. USP. A sterile solution of globulins derived from the blood of adults who have been immunized with pertussis vaccine. Used to produce passive immunity to pertussis.

    p. vaccine. USP. Sterile bacterial fraction of killed pertussis bacilli. Used for active immunization against pertussis.

pertussoid (pĕr-tŭs'oyd) [L. *per,* intensive, + *tussis,* cough, + Gr. *eidos,* resemblance]. 1. Of the nature of whooping cough. 2. A cough generally similar to that of whooping cough.

perversion (per-ver'zhun) [L. *perversus,* perverted]. Deviation from the normal path, whether it be in the area of one's intellect, emotions, actions, or reactions.

    p., sexual. Maladjustment of sexual life in which satisfaction is sought in ways deviating from the accepted norm. In judging the sexual actions of individuals it is important to remember that what is normal behavior in one society may be regarded as grossly abnormal or perverted in another. Nevertheless, most social groups regard homosexuality, sexual molesting of children, and sexual exhibitionism as abnormal.

pervert [L. *pervetere,* to turn the wrong way]. 1. (per-vert') To turn from the normal; to misuse. 2. (per'vert) One who has turned from the normal or socially acceptable path, esp. sexually.

per vias naturales (per vī'ăs năt''ū-rā'lēz) [L.]. Through natural ways.

pervigilium (pĕr''vī-jĭl'ĭ-ŭm) [L.]. Inability to sleep. SYN: *insomnia; wakefulness.*

pervious (per'vĭ-ŭs) [L. *pervius*]. 1. Capable of being penetrated. SYN: *permeable.* 2. Penetrating.

pes (pĕs) [L.]. (pl. *pedes*) [NA]. The foot or a footlike structure.

    p. anserinus. Three primary branches of the facial nerve after leaving the stylomastoid foramen.

    p. cavus. Abnormal hollowness of the sole of the foot.

    p. contortus. Clubfoot. SYN: *talipes,* q.v.

    p. corvinus. Wrinkles radiating from the outer canthi of the eyes. SYN: *crow's foot.*

    p. equinus. Deformity marked by walking without touching heel to the ground. SYN: *talipes equinus,* q.v.

    p. gigas. An abnormally large foot. SYN: *macropodia.*

    p. hippocampi. [NA]. Lower portion of the hippocampus major.

    p., infraorbital. Terminal radiating branches of the infraorbital nerve after exit from the infraorbital canal.

    p. planus. Flatfoot.

    p. valgoplanus. P. planus, q.v.

    p. valgus. Clubfoot in which sole turns outward. SYN: *talipes valgus.*

    p. varus. Clubfoot in which sole turns inward. SYN: *talipes varus.*

pessary (pes'ă-rī) [L. *pessarium*]. A device inserted into the vagina to function as a supportive structure for the uterus or as a contraceptive device.

    p., cup. One which has a cup-shaped hollow that fits over the os uteri.

    p., diaphragm. Cup-shaped rubber p. used as a contraceptive device.

    p., Gariel's. Inflatable hollow rubber p.

    p., Hodge's. P. used to correct retrodeviations of the uterus.

    p., lever. P. designed according to the principles of a lever.

    p., ring. Round pessary.

    p., stem. P. with stem that fits into the uterine canal.

pes'simism [L. *pessimus,* worst]. Morbid state of mind in which outlook toward life is gloomy or the worst interpretation is applied to events occurring; lacking in hope. Opposed to optimism.

pest (pĕst) [L. *pestis,* plague]. 1. Fatal epidemic disease, esp. plague. 2. A noxious, destructive insect.

pesticide (pĕs'tĭ-sīd') ["+ *cida,* killer]. Any chemical used to kill pests, esp. rodents and insects.

    p. residue. The amount of any pesticide remaining on or in food or beverages intended for human consumption.

pestiferous (pĕs-tĭf'ĕr-ŭs) [L. *pestiferus*]. Producing a pestilence; carrying infection. SYN: *pestilential.*

pestilence (pĕs'tĭl-ēns) [L. *pestilentia*]. 1. An epidemic contagious disease. 2. An epidemic caused by such a disease.

pestilential (pĕs-tĭ-lĕn'shăl). Concerning or causing a pestilence. SYN: *pestiferous.*

pestis (pĕs'tĭs) [L.]. Plague, q.v.

pestle (pĕs'l) [L. *pistillum*]. Device for macerating drugs in a mortar.

petechiae (pē-tē'kĭ-ē) [It. *petecchia*, skin spot]. (sing. *petechia*) 1. Small, purplish, hemorrhagic spots on the skin which appear in certain severe fevers and are indicative of great prostration, as in typhus. May be due to abnormality of blood clotting mechanism. Also applied to similar spots occurring on mucous membranes or serous surfaces. 2. Red spots from bite of a flea.

petechial (pē-tē'kĭ-ăl). Marked by presence of petechiae.

petiole (pĕt'ē-ōl) [LL. *petrolus*]. A slender stalk or stem, as petiole of the epiglottic cartilage.

Petit (pĕt-ē'). [Francois Pourfour du Petit, Fr. anatomist and surgeon, 1664-1741].

   P.'s canal. A space or cleft encircling lens between points of attachment of fibers of suspensory ligament. SYN: *zonular spaces.*

   P.'s sinuses. Hollows in aortic and pulmonary arteries behind semilunar valves.

Petit (pĕt-ē'). [Jean Louis Petit, Fr. surgeon, 1674-1750].

   P.'s triangle. Area on lateral abdominal wall bounded by crest of ilium, posterior margin of exterior oblique, and lateral margin of latissimus dorsi. SYN: *trigonum lumbale.*

petit mal (pĕt-ē' mähl') [Fr., little illness]. Mild form of epileptic attack. Consciousness may be lost, but there is an absence of convulsions. SEE: *epilepsy; pyknolepsy.*

Petri dish (pe'tre). [Julius Petri, Ger. bacteriologist, 1852-1921]. A shallow dish made of plastic or glass with a cover. Used to hold solid media for culturing bacteria.

petrifaction (pĕt-rĭ-făk'shŭn) [L. *petra*, stone, + *facere*, to make]. Process of changing into stone or hard substance.

petrified (pĕt'rĭ-fīd). Changed into stone; rigid.

petrify (pĕt'rĭ-fī). Convert into stone; make rigid.

pétrissage (pä"trē-säzh') [Fr.]. A kneading movement in massage. Performed generally by the tips of the thumbs, with index finger and thumb, or with palm of hand.

   It is used principally on the extremities. The operator picks up a special muscle or tendon and, placing one finger on each side of the part, proceeds in centripetal motion with a firm pressure. SYN: *kneading.*

petro- [L. *petra*, stone]. Combining form meaning stone. Pert. to petrous portion of temporal bone.

petrolatoma (pĕt"rō-lă-tō'mă) [L. *petrolatum*, petroleum]. Tumor or swelling caused by introduction of liquid petrolatum under the skin.

petrolatum (pĕt"rō-lā'tŭm) [L.]. A purified semisolid mixture of hydrocarbons obtained from petroleum. SYN: *petroleum jelly; soft paraffin.*

   ACTION AND USES: As a base for ointments. It is not suitable for use as a vaginal lubricant because it is not miscible in body secretions.

   p., liquid. A mixture of liquid hydrocarbons obtained from petroleum.

   ACTION AND USES: A vehicle for medicinal substances for local applications. Light p. employed as a spray. Heavy p. given internally in treatment of constipation.

   p., white. USP. Purified mixture of semisolid hydrocarbons obtained from petroleum. It is decolorized and may contain a suitable stabilizer.

petroleum (pĕ-trō'lē-ŭm) [L. *petra*, stone, + *oleum*, oil]. An oily inflammable liquid found in the upper strata of the earth; a hydrocarbon mixture.

pet"romas'toid. Pert. to petrous portion of temporal bone and occipital bone.

petrosa (pĕ-trō'să) [L., stony]. The petrous part of the temporal bone.

petrosal (pĕt-rō'săl) [L. *petrōsus*, stony]. Of, pert. to, or situated near the petrous portion of the temporal bone.

petrositis (pĕt"rō-sī'tĭs) ["+ *-ītis*, inflammation]. Inflamed condition of the petrous region of the temporal bone.

petrosphenoid (pĕt"rō-sfē'noyd) ["+ Gr. *sphēn*, wedge, + *eidos*, form]. Pert. to petrous portion of temporal bone and sphenoid bone.

petrosquamous (pĕt"rō-skwă'mŭs) [L. *petrōsus*, stony, + *squamosus*, scaly]. Pert. to petrous and squamous portions of temporal bone.

petrous (pĕt'rŭs) [L. *petrōsus*]. 1. Resembling stone. 2. Rel. to the petrous portion of the temporal bone. SYN: *petrosal.*

   p. ganglion. Inferior ganglion of the glossopharyngeal nerve.

Peutz-Jeghers syndrome. Polyps of the small intestine and melanin pigmentation of the lips, mucosa, fingers, and toes. Anemia due to bleeding from the intestinal polyps is a common finding. It is an inherited disorder.

Peyer's patch (pī'ĕr). [Johann Conrad Peyer, Swiss anatomist, 1653-1712]. An aggregation of solitary nodules or groups of lymph nodules found chiefly in the ileum near its junction with the colon. They are circular or oval, about 1 cm. wide and 2 to 3 cm. long. They lie in the mucosa and submucosa and always occur on side of intestine opposite to attachment of mesentery. In typhoid fever, they undergo hyperplasia and often become ulcerated. Also called aggregated or agminated nodules or follicles.

Peyronie's disease (pā-rō-nē'). [Francois de la Peyronie, Fr. surgeon, 1678-1747]. Hardening of the corpora cavernosa of the penis. This causes distortion or deflection of the penis, esp. when erect.

Pfeiffer's bacillus (fīfer). [Richard F. Pfeiffer, Ger. bacteriologist, 1859 —] Hemophilus influenzae, q.v.

Pfeiffer's phenomenon. A discovery announced in 1894 stating that serum of guinea pigs immunized with cholera vibrios destroyed cholera organisms in peritoneal cavity of immune and nonimmune guinea pigs and that same reaction occurred in vitro. Also that same lytic reaction occurred with typhoid and colon bacteria.

Ph. 1. Abbr. for *Pharmacopoeia.* 2. Chem. symb. for phenyl.

pH. [potential of Hydrogen] In chemistry, the degrees of acidity or alkalinity of a substance are expressed in pH values. The neutral point, where a solution would be neither acid or alkaline, is pH 7. Increasing acidity is expressed as a number less than 7 and increasing alkalinity as a number greater than 7. Maximum acidity is pH 0 and maximum alkalinity is pH 14.

Because each unit on the scale represents a logarithm, there is a tenfold difference between each unit. Ex: pH 5 is 10 times as acid as pH 6 and pH 4 is 100 times as acid as pH 6. Expressed mathematically pH is logarithm of the hydrogen ion concentration

divided into one, i.e.

$$\text{Log}\ \frac{1}{\text{H}^+}.$$

The pH of a solution may be determined electrically by a pH meter or colorometrically by the use of indicators. A list of indicators and the pH range registered by each is given under indicator, q.v. SEE: *pH Table* in *Appendix.*

phacitis (fā-sī'tĭs) [Gr. *phakos,* lens, + *-itis,* inflammation]. Inflamed condition of the crystalline lens. SYN: *phakitis.*

phaco- [Gr. *phakos*]. Prefix pert. to lens of the eye.

phacoanaphylaxis (fāk"ō-ăn"ă-fĭ-lăk'sĭs) ["+ *ana,* excessive, + *phylaxis,* protection]. Hypersensitivity to protein of the crystalline lens.

phacocele (fāk'ō-sēl) ["+ *kēlē,* swelling]. Displacement of the crystalline lens into the interior chamber of the eye.

phacocyst (fāk'ō-sĭst) [Gr. *phakos,* lens, + *kystis,* a sac]. Capsule of the crystalline lens.

phacocystectomy (fāk"ō-sĭs-tĕk'tō-mī) ["+ "+ *ektomē,* excision]. Surgical excision of part of crystalline lens capsule for cataract.

phacocystitis (fāk"ō-sĭs-ti'tĭs) ["+ "+ *-itis,* inflammation]. Inflamed condition of capsule of crystalline lens.

phacoemulsification (fāk"ō-ē-mŭl'sĭ-fĭ-kā"shŭn). A method of treating cataracts of the crystalline lens of the eye.

phacoerysis (fāk"ō-ĕr-ē'sĭs) ["+ *erēsis,* removal]. Removal of crystalline lens by suction method.

phacoglaucoma (fāk"ō-glaw-kō'mă) [Gr. *phakos,* lens, + *glaukos,* green, + *-ōma,* tumor]. Glaucoma and the changes it induces in the crystalline lens. SEE: *glaucoma.*

phacohymenitis (fāk"ō-hī"mĕn-ī'tĭs) ["+ *hymēn,* membrane, + *-itis,* inflammation]. Inflamed condition of capsule of crystalline lens.

phacoid (fāk'oyd) [Gr. *phakos,* lens, + *eidos,* form]. Lentil- or lens-shaped.

phacoidoscope (fā-koyd'ō-skōp) ["+ "+ *skopein,* to examine]. Instrument for observing accommodative changes of the lens. SYN: *phacoscope.*

phacolysis (fāk-ōl'ĭ-sĭs) ["+ *lysis,* dissolution]. 1. Dissection and removal of the lens of the eye in treatment of cataract. 2. Any dissolution or disintegration of the crystalline lens.

phacomalacia (fāk"ō-ma-lā'sĭ-ă) [Gr. *phakos,* lens, + *malakia,* softening]. A softening of the lens usually due to a soft cataract.

Simple Table of pH

Material	pH
Decinormal HCl.	1.0
Gastric juice	1.0 to 5.0
Thousandth-normal HCl	3.0
Pure water (neutral) at 25° C.	7.0
Blood plasma	7.35 to 7.45
Pancreatic juice	8.4 to 8.9
Thousandth-normal NaOH	11.0
Decinormal NaOH	13.0

phacomatosis (fā"kō-mă-tō'sĭs) ["+ -ōma, tumor, + -ōsis, intensive]. One of a group of diseases that are congenital and probably hereditary in origin, manifested by cutaneous and neurological syndromes. They include the following: neurofibromatosis (von Recklinghausen's disease); von Hippel-Lindau disease; Sturge-Weber syndrome; and tuberous sclerosis. SYN: neurodermatoses.

phacometachoresis (fāk"ō-mĕt"ă-kōrē'sĭs) ["+ metachōrēsis, displacement]. Dislocation of the crystalline lens. SYN: phacocele.

phacometer (fāk-ŏm'ē-tĕr) [Gr. phakos, lens, + metron, measure]. Device for ascertaining refractive power of a lens.

phacoplanesis (fāk"ō-plăn-ē'sĭs) ["+ planēsis, wandering]. Abnormal mobility of the crystalline lens.

phacosclerosis (fāk"ō-sklĕr-ō'sĭs) [Gr. phakos, lens, +sklērōsis, a hardening]. Hardening of the crystalline lens of eye.

phacoscope (fāk'ō-skōp) ["+ skopein, to examine]. Instrument for observing change of curvature of crystalline lens during accommodation.

phacoscotasmus (fāk"ō-scō-tăs'mŭs) ["+ skotasmos, clouding]. Clouding of crystalline lens of the eye.

Phaedra complex. [Wife of King Theseus of Athens] The love and attraction between a stepparent and a stepchild. So named because of Phaedra's tragic love for the son (Hippolytus) of her husband by a previous marriage.

phag-, phago- [Gr. phagein, to eat]. Combining form meaning an eater, or pertaining to ingestion, or engulfing.

phage (fāj) [Gr. phagein, to eat]. A particulate, transmissible, ultramicroscopic substance that dissolves or exerts a lytic effect upon bacteria. It is of viral origin. SEE: bacteriophage.

phagedena (fāj-ē-dē'nă) [Gr. phagedaina]. A sloughing ulcer that spreads rapidly.

    p., sloughing. Hospital gangrene; bed sores.

phagedenic (fāj-ē-dĕn'ĭk). Concerning, or of the nature of, phagedena.

phagocyte (făg'ō-sīt) [Gr. phagein, to eat, + kytos, cell]. A cell which has the ability to ingest and destroy particulate substances such as bacteria, protozoa, cells and cell debris, dust particles, and colloids. EX: Cells of the reticuloendothelial system (macrophages or histiocytes, reticular cells of lymph nodes, Kupffer's cells of liver, dust cells of lung) and leukocytes.

    There are two classes: macrophages, large mononucleated cells which ingest dead tissues and cells, and microphages, which ingest bacteria.

    RS: histiocyte; macrophage; reticuloendothelial system.

phagocytic (făg'ō-sĭt'ĭk). Concerning phagocytes or phagocytosis.

    p. index. The average number of bacteria ingested by each leukocyte after incubation of the bacteria in a mixture of serum and bacterial culture. SEE: opsonic index.

phagocytolysis (făg"ō-sī-tŏl'ĭ-sĭs) ["+ "+ lysis, dissolution]. Destruction or disintegration of phagocytes. SYN: phagolysis.

phagocytolytic (făg"ō-sī"tō-lĭt'ĭk). Destroying phagocytes.

phagocytosis (făg"ō-sī-tō'sĭs) [Gr. phagein, to eat, + kytos, cell, + -ōsis, intensive]. Ingestion and digestion of bacteria and particles by phagocytes.

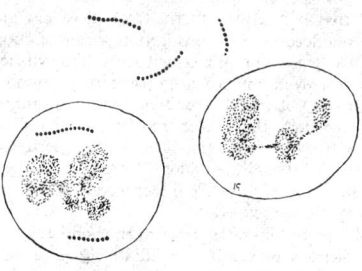

PHAGOCYTOSIS

A small drop of blood was mixed with a drop of a suspension of dead streptococci; the mixture was kept at 37° C. for 20 minutes. A smear under microscopic examination showed (1) polys containing streptococci in their cytoplasm, (2) polys which did not contain streptococci, and (3) a few chains of streptococci which lay free in the medium and must have escaped phagocytosis.

phagodynamometer (fag"ō-dī"nă-mŏm'ē-ter) ["+ dynamis, power, + metron, measure]. Device that measures energy expended in chewing food.

phagokaryosis (făg"ō-kăr"ĭ-ō'sĭs) ["+ karyon, nucleus, + -ōsis, intensive]. Phagocytic action which is performed by a cell nucleus.

phagolysis (făg-ōl'ĭ-sĭs) [Gr. phagein, to eat, + lysis, dissolution]. Disintegration of phagocytes. SYN: phagocytolysis.

phagomania (făg"ō-mā'nĭ-ă) ["+ mania, madness]. Abnormal craving for food.

phagopyrism (făg"ō-pi'rĭzm) ["+ pyr, fever, + ismos, condition]. Hypersensitiveness to certain foods which induce symptoms of poisoning upon ingestion.

phagotherapy (făg″ō-thĕr′ă-pī) ["+ *therapeia*, treatment]. Treatment by feeding or overfeeding.

phakitis (făk-ī′tĭs) [Gr. *phakos*, lens, + *-itis*, inflammation]. Inflamed condition of the crystalline lens. SYN: *phacitis.*

phakolysis (făk-ŏl′ĭs-ĭs) ["+ *lysis*, dissolution]. Disintegration or removal of the crystalline lens. SYN: *phacolysis.*

phalacrosis (făl-ă-krō′sĭs) [Gr. *phalakrōsis*]. Baldness. SYN: *alopecia.*

phalacrotic (făl-ă-krŏt′ĭk). Bald; baldheaded.

phalacrous (făl-ăk′rūs). Bald. SYN: *phalacrotic.*

phalangeal (fă-lăn′jē-ăl) [Gr. *phalanx*, closely-knit row]. Concerning a phalanx.

    p. cells, inner. A row of cells along surface of inner pillar cells in the organ of Corti.

    p. cells, outer. Cells arranged in rows which support the outer hair cells in the organ of Corti. SYN: *cells of Deiters.*

phalangectomy (făl-ăn-jĕk′tō-mī) ["+ *ektomē*, excision]. Excision of one or more phalanges.

phalanges (fă-lăn′jēz). (sing. *phalanx*) [NA] Bones of a finger or toe. SEE: *skeleton.*

phalangitis (fă-lăn-jī′tĭs) [Gr. *phalanx*, closely-knit row, + *-itis*, inflammation]. Inflamed condition of one or more phalanges.

phalanx (fā′lănks) [Gr., closely-knit row]. (pl. *phalanges*) 1. [NA]. Any one of the bones of fingers or toes. 2. One of a set of plates formed of phalangeal cells (inner and outer) forming the reticular membrane of the organ of Corti.

    p., distal. The p. most remote from the metacarpus or metatarsus.

    p., metacarpal; p., metatarsal. SEE: *p., proximal.*

    p., middle. The p. (where there are three) intermediate between distal and proximal phalanges.

    p., proximal. The p. articulating with a metacarpal or metatarsal bone.

    p., terminal; p., ungual; p., unguicular. SEE: *p., distal.*

phalalgia (făl-ăl′jī-ă) [Gr. *phallos*, penis, + *algos*, pain]. Pain in the penis.

phallic (făl′ĭk). Concerning the penis.

phallitis (făl-ī′tĭs) [Gr. *phallos*, penis, + *-itis*, inflammation]. Inflamed condition of the penis.

phallocampsis (făl-ō-kămp′sĭs) ["+ *kampsis*, a bending]. Painful downward curvature of penis when erect.

phallodynia (făl-ō-dĭn′ĭ-ă) ["+ *odynē*, pain]. Pain in the penis. SYN: *phallalgia.*

phalloid (făl′oyd) [Gr. *phallos*, penis, + *eidos*, form]. Similar to a penis.

phalloncus (făl-ŏn′kŭs) ["+ *onkos*, mass]. Tumor or swelling on the penis.

phalloplasty (făl′ō-plăs″tī) ["+ *plassein*, to form]. Reparative or plastic surgery on the penis.

phallorhagia (făl-ō-rā′jī-ă) [Gr. *phallos*, penis, + *rhēgnynai*, to burst forth]. Hemorrhage from the penis.

phallus (făl′ŭs) [Gr. *phallos*, penis]. 1. The penis. 2. An artificial penis, used as a symbol. 3. Embryonic structure developing at tip of genital tubercle which in the male develops into the penis, and in the female, the clitoris.

phanero-, phaner- [Gr. *phaneros*, visible]. Combining forms meaning evident, visible.

phaneromania (făn″ĕr-ō-mā′nĭ-ă) [Gr. *phaneros*, visible, + *mania*, madness]. Abnormal tendency to bite the nails or pick, scratch, or pull a pimple, wart, hair, beard, or mustache.

phaneroscope (făn′ĕr-ō-skōp) ["+ *skopein*, to examine]. Instrument for securing transparency of skin by illumination.

phaneroscopy (făn″ĕr-ŏs′kō-pī). Observation of skin by phaneroscope. Use of a lens to concentrate light in examination of skin lesions.

phanerosis (făn″ĕr-ō′sĭs) [Gr.]. The process of becoming visible.

phanic (făn′ĭk) [Gr. *phainein*, to show]. Manifest; apparent.

phantasia (făn-tā′zĭ-ă) [Gr.]. An appearance that is imaginary.

phantasm (făn′tăzm) [Gr. *phantasma*]. An optical illusion; an apparition, or illusion of something that does not exist.

phantasmatomoria (făn-taz″măt-ō-mo′rĭ-ă) ["+ *mōria*, folly]. Dementia with silly fancies; childishness in the demented.

phantasy (făn′tă-sī) [Gr. *phantasia*, imagination]. A daydream. Phantasy-thinking is a form of wish fulfillment, a disregard for reality which one would escape through revelling in imaginative possibilities.

    RS: delirium; delusion; hallucination; hysteria; illusion; phobia.

phantogeusia (făn-tō-gū′sĭ-ă) ["+ *geusis*, taste]. An intermittent or persistent taste sensation in the mouth not produced by an external stimulus.

phantom (făn′tŭm) [Gr. *phantasma*, an appearance]. 1. An apparition. 2. A model of the body or of one of its parts.

    p. corpuscle. A colorless erythrocyte.

    p. limb. An illusion, following amputation of a limb, that the limb still exists. The sensation that pain exists in the removed part is known as *phantom-limb pain.*

    p. pregnancy. Pseudopregnancy, q.v.

p. tumor. An apparent tumor due to muscular contractions or flatus seen in hysteria.

phantom vision. An experience, usually transient, of visual sensations in an eye which has been surgically removed.

phantosmia (făn-tŏs'mĭ-ă) ["+ osmē, smell]. Intermittent or persistent perception of odor when no odor is inhaled.

pharmacal (făr'măk-ăl) [Gr. pharmakon, drug]. Concerning pharmacy.

pharmaceutical (făr-mă-sū'tĭ-kăl) [Gr. pharmakeutikos]. Concerning drugs or pharmacy.

pharmaceutics (făr-mă-sū'tĭks). Science of dispensing medicines. SYN: pharmacy.

pharmacist (făr'mă-sĭst) [Gr. pharmakon, drug]. A druggist; one licensed to prepare and dispense drugs. SYN: apothecary.

pharmaco- [Gr. pharmakon, drug]. Combining form meaning drug, medicine, poison.

pharmacodiagnosis (făr''mă-kō-dī''ăg-nō'sĭs) [Gr. pharmakon, drug, + dia, through, + gnōsis, knowledge]. Use of drugs in making a diagnosis.

pharmacodynamics (făr''mă-kō-dinām'ĭks) ["+ dynamis, power]. Study of drugs and their actions on living organisms.

pharmacogenetics (far''mă-ko-jĕn-ĕt'ĭks) ["+ genēsis, produce]. Study of the influence of hereditary factors on response of individual organisms to drugs.

pharmacognosy (făr''mă-kŏg'nō-sĭ) [Gr. pharmakon, drug, + gnōsis, knowledge]. The science of crude drugs and their physical, botanical, and chemical properties.

pharmacography (făr''mă-kŏg'ră-fĭ) ["+ graphein, to write]. Treatise on the properties of drugs.

pharmacology (făr''mă-kŏl'ō-jĭ) [Gr. pharmakon, drug, + logos, a study]. The study of drugs and their origin, nature, properties, and effects upon living organisms.

pharmacomania (făr''mă-kō-mā'nĭ-ă) ["+ mania, madness]. Abnormal desire for giving or taking medicines.

pharmacopedia (făr''mă-kō-pē'dĭ-ă) ["+ paideia, education]. Information concerning drugs and their preparation.

pharmacopeia (făr''mă-kō-pē'ă) [Gr. pharmakopoiia, preparation of drugs]. Authorized treatise on drugs and their preparation, esp. a book containing formulas and information which is a standard for preparation and dispensation of drugs.

Pharmacopeia, United States. A pharmacopeia issued every five years, prepared under supervision of a national committee of pharmacists, pharmacologists, physicians, chemists, biologists, and other scientific and allied personnel. The United States Pharmacopeia was adopted as standard in 1906. ABBR: USP; U.S. Phar.

pharmacophobia (făr''mă-kō-fō'bĭ-ă) [Gr. pharmakon, drug, + phobos, fear]. Abnormal fear of taking medicines.

pharmacopsychosis (făr''mă-kō-sī-kō'sĭs) ["+ psychē, soul, + -ōsis, disease]. Addiction to drugs.

pharmacotherapy (făr''mă-kō-thĕr'ă-pĭ) ["+ therapeia, treatment]. Use of medicine in treatment of disease.

pharmacy (făr'mă-sĭ) [Gr. pharmakon, drug]. 1. The practice of compounding and dispensing medicinal preparations. 2. A drugstore.

pharyngalgia (făr-ĭn-găl'jĭ-ă) [Gr. pharynx, pharynx, + algos, pain]. Pain in the pharynx. SYN: pharyngodynia.

pharyngeal (far-ĭn'jē-ăl) [L. pharyngeus]. Concerning the pharynx.

p. bursa. A small, inconstant, blind sac often present in lower portion of pharyngeal tonsil.

p. hypophysis. A small structure anterior to pharyngeal bursa. It is derived from lower portion of Rathke's pouch and occasionally gives rise to a cyst or tumor.

p. reflex. Attempt to swallow following any application of stimulus to pharynx.

p. tonsil. Lymphoid tissue on posterior superior wall of the pharynx. When hypertrophied called adenoids.

pharyngectomy (făr-ĭn-jĕk'tō-mĭ) ["+ ektomē, excision]. Partial excision of the pharynx to remove growths, abscesses, etc.

pharyngemphraxis (făr-ĭn-jĕm-frăk'sĭs) ["+ emphraxis, stoppage]. Pharyngeal obstruction.

pharyngismus (făr''n-jĭz'mŭs) [Gr. pharynx, pharynx, + ismos, condition]. Spasm of the muscles in the pharynx. SYN: pharyngospasm.

pharyngitis (făr'ĭn-jī'tĭs) [Gr. pharynx, pharynx, + -itis, inflammation]. Inflammation of pharynx.

p., acute. SYM: Malaise, fever, dysphagia, pain in throat, postnasal secretion.
TREATMENT: Local: Gargles, lozenges, topical application to oral pharynx. General: Bed rest, adequate fluids, analgesics. Appropriate antibiotic after material has been taken for bacterial study, esp. beta hemolytic streptococci.

p., atrophic. Chronic form with some atrophy of mucous glands and abnormal secretion. SYN: p. sicca.

p., chronic. Associated with pathology in nose and sinuses, mouth breathing, excessive smoking, and chronic tonsillitis.

SYM: Dryness and irritation of throat; cough.

TREATMENT: Intranasal medication and removal of sinus pathology; tonsillectomy.

p., croupous. P. with the false membrane of croup.

p., diphtheritic. Sore throat with general symptoms of diphtheria.

p., follicular. SEE: *p., granular.*

p., gangrenous. Gangrenous inflammation of mucous membrane of pharynx. SYN: *angina maligna.*

p., granular. Chronic p. with granulations seen on the pharynx.

p., hypertrophic. A chronic form with thickened, red mucous membrane on each side with a glazed central portion.

p. sicca. SEE: *p., atrophic*

p. ulcerosa. P. with fever, pain, and the formation of ulcerations.

pharyngo- [Gr. *pharynx*, pharynx]. Combining form pert. to the pharynx.

pharyngoamygdalitis (fă-rĭn″gō-ă-mĭg″dăl-ī′tĭs) [Gr. *pharynx*, pharynx, + *amygdale*, tonsil, + *-itis*, inflammation]. Inflamed condition of the pharynx and tonsil.

pharyngocele (făr-ĭn′gō-sēl) ["+ *kēlē*, hernia]. Hernia through pharyngeal wall.

pharyngodynia (făr-ĭn″gō-dĭn′ī-ă) ["+ *odyne*, pain]. Pain in the pharynx. SYN: *pharyngalgia.*

pharyngokeratosis (făr-ĭn-gō-kĕr″ă-tō′sĭs) [Gr. *pharynx*, pharynx, + *keras*, horn, + *-osis*, condition]. Thickening and hardening of mucous lining of pharynx.

pharyngolaryngitis (făr-ĭn″gō-lăr-ĭn-jī′tĭs) ["+ *larynx*, larynx, + *-itis*, inflammation]. Inflamed condition of pharynx and larynx.

pharyngolith (făr-ĭn′gō-lĭth) ["+ *lithos*, stone]. Concretion in pharyngeal walls.

pharyngology (făr″ĭn-gŏl′ō-jī) [Gr. *pharynx*, pharynx, + *logos*, a study]. Branch of medicine dealing with the pharynx.

pharyngolysis (făr″ĭn-gŏl′ī-sĭs) ["+ *lysis*, dissolution]. Paralysis of the pharynx.

pharyngomycosis (făr-ĭn″gō-mī-kō′sĭs) ["+ *mykēs*, fungus, + *-osis*, disease]. Disease of pharynx due to fungi.

pharyngoparalysis (făr-ĭn″gō-păr-ăl′ī-sĭs) [Gr. *pharynx*, pharynx, + *paralysis*, a loosening at the side]. Paralysis of the muscles of the pharynx. SYN: *pharyngoplegia.*

pharyngopathy (făr″ĭn-gŏp′ă-thī) ["+ *pathos*, disease]. Any disorder of the pharynx.

pharyngoperistole (făr-ĭn″gō-pĕr-ĭs′tō-lē) ["+ *peristolē*, contracture]. Narrowing or stricture of the lumen of the pharynx.

pharyngoplasty (făr-ĭn′gō-plăs″tĭ) ["+ *plassein*, to form]. Reparative surgery of the pharynx.

pharyngoplegia (făr-ĭn″gō-plē′jĭ-ă) [Gr. *pharynx*, pharynx, + *plēgē*, a stroke]. Paralysis of muscles of pharynx. SYN: *pharyngoparalysis.*

pharyngorhinitis (făr-ĭn″gō-rī-nī′tĭs) ["+ *rhis, rhin-*, nose, + *-itis*, inflammation]. Inflamed condition of the nasopharynx.

pharyngorhinoscopy (făr-ĭn″gō-rī-nŏs′kō-pĭ) ["+ "+ *skopein*, to examine]. Inspection of the nasopharynx and posterior nares.

pharyngorrhea (făr″ĭn-gō-rē′ă) ["+ *rhoia*, flow]. Discharge of mucus from the pharynx.

pharyngoscope (făr-ĭn′gō-skōp) [Gr. *pharynx*, pharynx, + *skopein*, to examine]. Instrument for examination of the pharynx.

pharyngoscopy (făr″ĭn-gŏs′kō-pĭ). Examination of the pharynx.

NP: Watch for difficult breathing and cyanosis from edema. Steam inhalations are sometimes ordered.

pharyngospasm (făr-ĭn′gō-spăzm) [Gr. *pharynx*, pharynx, + *spasmos*, a spasm]. Spasmodic contraction of muscles of the pharynx. SYN: *pharyngismus.*

pharyngotherapy (făr-ĭn″gō-thĕr′ă-pĭ) ["+ *therapeia*, treatment]. Treatment of pharyngeal disturbances or diseases.

pharyngotome (făr-ĭn′gō-tōm) ["+ *tomē*, an incision]. Instrument for incision of the pharynx.

pharyngotomy (făr-ĭn-gŏt′ō-mĭ). Incision of the pharynx.

pharynx (făr′inks) [Gr.]. (pl. *pharynges*) [NA]. Serves as passageway for air from nasal cavity to larynx and food from mouth to esophagus. Also acts as a resonating cavity.

A musculomembranous tube extending from base of skull above to level of the 6th vertebra below where it becomes continuous with the esophagus. Upper portion is lined with pseudostratified ciliated epithelium, middle portion with stratified columnar epithelium, and lower portion with stratified squamous epithelium.

Communicates with posterior nares, eustachian tube, mouth, esophagus, and larynx. *Nasopharynx* is section above the palate, *oropharynx* between palate and hyoid bone, and *laryngopharynx* part below the hyoid bone.

The nerves are autonomic, vagus, and glossopharyngeal. Blood vessels branch from the exterior carotid artery. Veins form an extensive pharyngeal plexus and drain into interior jugular vein.

phase (fāz) [Gr. *phasis,* an appearance]. 1. A stage of development. 2. A transitory appearance. 3. The state of a component of a heterogeneous system, as when oil is mixed with water, which is homogeneous throughout itself and bounded by an interface with other phases of the system.

p., continuous. State of substance in a heterogeneous system in which particles are continuous. EX: The water particles in which oil has been dispersed.

p., contraction. SEE: *isometric contraction.*

p., contrast microscope. SEE: *microscope, phase.*

p., disperse. State of a substance in a heterogeneous system in which particles are separated from each other. Also called dis-. continuous phase. EX: Oil particles in water.

phase-shift balloon pumping. A device for aiding circulation of blood. A ballon attached to a catheter is inserted through the femoral artery in the aorta. As the heart rests in diastole, the balloon is quickly filled with helium so that blood is forced on its way peripherally as well as into the coronary arteries. The balloon, which is 15 cm. long, deflates just before systole. This inflation-deflation cycle is timed and activated by the patient's electrocardiogram. This complicated device requires a team of physicians and nurses to work it. It is used as an emergency procedure in patients with shock due to myocardial infarction.

phasic (fā'sĭk). Of, or pertaining to, a phase.

phatne (făt'nē) [Gr., socket]. Socket of a tooth.

phatnoma (făt-nō'mă) ["+ -*ōma,* tumor]. (pl. *phatnomas, phatnomata*) Tumor of a tooth socket.

phatnorrhagia (făt"nō-rā'jĭ-ă) ["+ *rhēgnynai,* to burst forth]. Hemorrhage from the socket of a tooth.

Ph.D. Abbr. for *Doctor of Philosophy.*

phenate (fē'nāt). A salt of phenic acid (phenol).

phengophobia (fĕn"gō-fō'bĭ-ă) [Gr. *phengos,* light, + *phobos,* fear]. Abnormal dread of light. SYN: *photophobia.*

phenic acid (fē'nĭk). Carbolic acid, q.v. SYN: *phenol.*

phenobarbital (fē"nō-bar'bĭ-tăl). USP. Phenylethylbarbituric acid, a white crystalline substance soluble in alcohol.

ACTION AND USES: A hypnotic, long-acting sedative and anticonvulsant. Used, often in combination with diphenylhydantoin sodium, in treatment of epilepsy because it has depressive effect on motor areas of the cerebral cortex.

p., sodium. Soluble phenobarbital. More rapidly absorbed than phenobarbital but has the same uses.

phenol (fē'nōl). USP. C_6H_5OH. 1. A crystalline, colorless or light pink solid, melting at 43° C., obtained from the distillation of coal tar, having a characteristic odor, and dangerous because of its rapid corrosive action on tissues. When used carefully, it is effective as a bacteriostatic agent. SYN: *carbolic acid.* 2. Any of the aromatic derivatives of benzene with one or more hydroxyl groups attached.

POISONING SYM: Strong solutions cause burning, pain, and later anesthesia. The skin and mucous membrane first become pale, then grayish-white, opalescent, and finally brown to black. Even a 1% solution may cause local gangrene. It is absorbed from intact skin wounds and mucous membrane to cause general effects, including collapse and coma. When taken by mouth, it causes whitish discoloration of mucous membranes, intense burning, nausea and rarely vomiting, followed shortly by faintness, weakness, and collapse. Pulse slow and weak and hypothermia with respiratory arrest may be present. Perspiration is increased, and it causes renal damage.

Profound coma may occur within 30 minutes of exposure of skin to phenol.

F. A. TREATMENT: Remove poison from stomach as soon as possible. While waiting to do this administer 5-6 teaspoons (25-30 ml.) of activated charcoal in water. Turn the patient from side to side to insure all portions of the stomach come in contact with the charcoal.

A well-lubricated stomach pump should be used with caution. Give extensive lavage with charcoal. If this isn't available use olive oil, leaving some in the stomach. If olive oil is not available, use cottonseed oil or water. Do not use ethyl alcohol as lavage fluid because it speeds absorption of phenol. Demulcents such as egg whites or milk may be left in the stomach when lavage is finished.

Remove contaminated clothing instantly and wash external burns with large amounts of water or with olive oil. Use external heat, oxygen therapy, and morphine as required. Intravenous sodium bicarbonate may provide symptomatic relief, but its mechanism of action is not understood.

A guarded prognosis should always be given, for although the patient may improve at first, damage to the mucous membrane and absorption of phenol may lead to serious complications later.

p. red. An indicator used in determining hydrogen ion concentration.

phenolphthalein (fē″nŏl-thăl′ē-ĭn, fē″nŏl-thăl′ēn). A white or yellowish crystallized powder, produced by the interaction of phenol and phthalic anhydride.

ACTION AND USES: As a laxative.

phenolsulfonphthalein (fē″nŏl-sŭl″fŏn-thăl′ē-in). Phenol compound used to test renal function and as an indicator of hydrogen ion concentration. SYN: *phenol red.*

phenoluria (fē″nŏl-ū′rĭ-ă). Elimination of phenols in the urine.

phenomenon (fē-nŏm′ē-nŏn) [Gr. *phainomenon,* appearing]. (pl. *phenomena*) A change, perceivable by the senses, that occurs in an organ or vital function; a symptom.

p., Bell's. Rolling of the eyeball upward and outward when an attempt is made to close the eye on the side of the face affected in peripheral facial paralysis.

phenotype (fē′nō-tĭp) [Gr. *phainein,* to show, + *typos,* type]. 1. The physical appearance or makeup of an individual. Some phenotypes, such as the blood groups, are completely determined by heredity, while others, such as hair color, are readily altered by environmental agents. 2. In genetics, a group of individuals who resemble each other in appearance but may differ in genetic makeup. SEE: *genotype.*

phenozygous (fē-nŏz′ĭ-gŭs) ["+ *zygon,* yoke]. Possessing a cranium much narrower than the face.

phenyl (fĕn′ĭl, fē′nĭl). In chemistry, the univalent radical of phenol C_6H_5.

phenylephrine hydrochloride. USP. Adrenergic compound used in a suitably-weak concentration to produce nasal decongestion. May also be used in opthalmic solutions.

phenylhydrazine (fĕn″ĭl-hī′drǎ-zēn). Oily nitrogenous base used as a test for presence of sugar in the urine.

phenylketonuria (fĕn″ĭl-kē″tō-nū′rĭ-ă). 1. Phenylpyruvic acid in the urine. 2. A disease caused by the body's failure to oxidize an amino acid (phenylalanine) to tyrosine, perhaps because of a defective enzyme. Due to a recessive hereditary trait. Brain damage may occur causing severe mental retardation. Test for p. should be made at birth. ABBR: PKU.

SYM: Tremor, spasticity, convulsions, hyperactivity, mental deficiency, eczema, unusual hand posturing, and offensive odor of urine and sweat.

The disease is seen equally in the sexes and in the United States occurs approximately once in each 40,000 births. The incidence in England is 1 in 25,000 births.

TREATMENT: Low phenylalanine diet.

PROGNOSIS: Excellent if treatment is started early postnatal. If started after three years no improvement will occur because of brain damage.

phenylpyruvic acid (fĕn″ĭl-pī-rū′vĭk). A metabolic derivative of phenylalanine.

p. a. amentia. SEE: *p. a. oligophrenia.*

p. a. oligophrenia. A form of inherited mental deficiency resulting from an inborn error of metabolism. Characterized by inability to oxidize phenylpyruvic acid which is excreted in urine. Defect is congenital and familial. SEE: *phenylketonuria.*

phenylthiocarbamide (fĕn″ĭl-thī″ō-car′bă-mĭd). Used in studying medical genetics. About 70% of the population inherit the ability to note the taste of PTC to be extremely bitter. To the remainder of the population, it is tasteless. The inheritance of this trait is due to a single dominant gene pair. ABBR: PTC. SYN: *phenylthiourea.*

pheochromocytoma (fē-o-krō″mō-sī-tō′mă) [Gr. *phaios,* dusky, + *chrōma,* color, + *kytos,* cell, + *-ōma,* tumor]. A chromaffin cell tumor of the sympatho-adrenal system which produces catecholamines, i.e. norepinephrine and epinephrine. Although the tumor usually is benign, it produces hypertension which may be paroxysmal in about half the cases. Patient will complain of attacks of pounding headaches, sweating, palpitation, apprehension, flushing of the face, nausea and vomiting, and tingling of the extremities.

TREATMENT: Surgical removal of the tumor.

pheromone (fĕr′ō-mōn). A substance that provides chemical means of communication between animals and certain insects, usually of the same species. Probably detected by smell. May affect development, reproduction, or behavior of other individuals.

Ph.G. Abbr. for *Graduate in Pharmacy; German Pharmacopeia.*

phial (fī′ăl) [Gr. *phiale,* a bowl]. A small vessel for medicine; a vial.

-philia (fĭl′ĭ-ă) [Gr. *philein,* to love]. Combining form meaning love for, tendency towards, craving for.

philoneism (fĭ-lō′nē-ĭzm) [Gr. *philein,* to love, + *neos,* new]. Excessive love or fondness for newness or change. Opposed to misoneism.

philoprogenitive (fĭ″lō-prō-jĕn′ĭ-tĭv) ["+ *pro,* for, + *gennan,* to produce]. Producing a large number of offspring. SYN: *prolific.*

phil'ter, phil'tre [Gr. *philtron*]. A potion or drug which is supposed to induce love or promote sexual activity.

phil'trum. [NA]. The median groove on external surface of upper lip.

phimosis (fĭ-mō'sĭs) [Gr., a muzzling]. Stenosis or narrowness of preputial orifice so that the foreskin cannot be pushed back over the glans penis.

  TREATMENT: Circumcision.

  p. vaginalis. Narrowness or closure of the vaginal orifice.

pHisoHex (fī'sō-hĕks). Proprietary name for an antibacterial skin cleanser containing hexachlorophene as a main ingredient.

phlebangioma (flĕb''ăn-jĭ-ō'mă) [Gr. *phleps*, vein, + *angeion*, vessel, + *-ōma*, tumor]. An aneurysm occurring in a vein.

phlebarteriectasia (flĕb''ăr-tē''rĭ-ĕk-tā'zĭ-ă) ["+ *artēria*, artery, + *ektasis*, dilatation]. Varicose aneurysms; dilatation of blood vessels.

phlebarteriodialysis (flĕb''ăr-tē''rĭ-ō-dĭ-ăl'ĭ-sĭs) ["+ "+ *dialysis*, separation]. Arteriovenous aneurysm.

phlebectasia, phlebectasis (flĕb-ĕk-tā'zĭ-ă, -ĕk'tă-sĭs) [Gr. *phlebos*, vein, + *ektasis*, dilatation]. Venous dilatation. SYN: *varicosity.*

phlebectomy (flĕb-ĕk'tō-mĭ) ["+ *ektomē*, excision]. Surgical removal of a vein or part of a vein.

phlebectopia (flĕb''ĕk-tō'pĭ-ă) ["+ *ek*, out, + *topos*, place]. Abnormal position of a vein.

phlebemphraxis (flĕb''ĕm-frăk'sĭs) [Gr. *phlebos*, vein + *emphraxis*, stoppage]. Artificial obstruction of a vein.

phlebismus (flĕb-ĭz'mŭs) ["+ *ismos*, condition]. Venous congestion and dilatation.

phlebitis (flĕ-bī'tĭs) [Gr. *phlebos*, vein, + *-itis*, inflammation]. Inflammation of a vein. SYN: *phlegmasia alba dolens; milk leg; thrombophlebitis.*

  ETIOL: Unknown. May occur in acute or chronic infections or following operations or childbirth.

  SYM: Pain and tenderness along course of vein; discoloration of skin; inflammatory swelling, and acute edema below obstruction; rapid pulse; mild elevation of temperature; pain in joints.

  p., adhesive. P. in which vein tends to become obliterated.

  p., migrating. A transitory p. which appears in a portion of a vein, then clears up only to reappear later in another location.

  p. nodularis necrotisans. Circumscribed inflammation of cutaneous veins resulting in nodules that ulcerate.

  p., obliterative. P. in which the lumen of a vein becomes closed. SYN: *obstructive p.; adhesive p.*

  p., plastic. Adhesive phlebitis, q.v.

  p., proliferative. Adhesive phlebitis, q.v.

  p., puerperal. Venous inflammation following childbirth.

  p., sclerosing. P. in which the veins become obstructed and hardened.

  p., sinus. Inflammation of a sinus of the cerebrum.

  p., suppurative. P. characterized by the formation of pus.

phlebo- [Gr. *phleps, phlebos*]. Combining form meaning vein.

phlebocholosis (flĕb''ō-kō-lō'sĭs) ["+ *cholos*, maimed]. Diseased condition of a vein.

phleboclysis (flĕb-ŏk'lĭ-sĭs) ["+ *klysis*, injection]. The introduction of medicinal substances into a vein.

  p., drip. Intravenous injection instilled slowly drop by drop. SEE: *Murphy's drip.*

phlebogram (flĕb'ō-grăm) [Gr. *phlebos*, vein, + *gramma*, mark]. A tracing of the venous pulse.

phlebography (flĕ-bŏg'ră-fĭ) ["+ *graphein*, to write]. A study of the structure and function of the veins.

phleboid (flĕb'oyd) ["+ *eidos*, form]. Pert. to, resembling, or of the nature of a vein; venous.

phlebolite, phlebolith (flĕb'ō-līt, -lĭth) [Gr. *phlebos*, vein, + *lithos*, a stone]. A calcareous concretion in a vein.

phlebolithiasis (flĕb''ō-lĭ-thī'ă-sis) ["+ *lithiasis*, forming stones]. The formation of phleboliths in veins.

phlebology (flĕb-ŏl'ō-jĭ) [Gr. *phlebos*, vein, + *logis*, study]. The science of veins and their diseases.

phlebometritis (flĕb''ō-mē-trī'tĭs) ["+ *mētra*, uterus, + *-itis*, inflammation]. Inflammation of uterine veins.

phlebomyomatosis (flĕb''ō-mī''ō-mă-tō'sĭs) ["+ *mys, my-*, muscle, + *-ōma*, tumor, + *-ōsis*, disease]. Thickening of the tissue of a vein from overgrowth of muscular fibers.

phlebopexy (flĕb'ō-pĕk''sĭ) [Gr. *phlebos*, vein, + *pēksis*, fixation]. Extraserous transplantation of the testes for varicocele, with preservation of venous network.

phleboplasty (flĕb'ō-plăs''tĭ) ["+ *plassein*, to form]. Plastic repair of a wounded vein.

phleborrhagia (flĕb''ō-rā'jĭ-ă) ["+ *rhegnynai*, to burst forth]. Bleeding from a vein.

phleborrhaphy (flĕb-or'ă-fĭ) ["+ *rhaphē*, a sewing]. Suturing of a vein.

phleborrhexis (flĕb''ō-rĕk'sĭs) [Gr. *phlebos*, vein, + *rhēxis*, rupture]. Rupture of a vein.

phlebosclerosis (flĕb″o-sklē-rō′sĭs) ["+ *sklērōsis*, hardening]. Fibrous hardening of a vein's walls.

phlebostasia, phlebostasis (flĕb-ō-stā′zĭ-ă, -ŏs′tă-sĭs) ["+ *stasis*, stoppage]. Compression of veins temporarily removing an amount of blood from the general circulation. SYN: *bloodless phlebotomy.*

phlebothrombosis (flĕb″ō-thrŏm-bō′sĭs) ["+ *thrombos*, a clot]. Clotting in a vein; phlebitis with secondary thrombosis.

phlebotome (flĕb′ō-tŏm) [Gr. *phlebos*, vein, + *tomē*, a cutting]. Lancet used in cutting a vein.

phlebotomize (flĕ-bŏt′ō-mīz). To take blood from a person.

Phlebotomus (flĕ-bŏt′ō-mŭs) [Gr. *phlebos*, vein, + *tomē*, incision]. A genus of insects, the sandflies, belonging to the family Psychodidae, order Diptera. The bloodsucking insects are annoying and transmit various forms of leishmaniasis, sandfly (pappataci) fever, and Oroyo fever.

    P. argentipes. In India, the transmitter of Leishmania donovani, causative agent of kala-azar.

    P. chinensis. Transmitter of kala-azar in China.

    P. papatasii. Transmitter of the causative agent of sandfly fever. The virus is capable of being transmitted through the offspring of flies.

    P. sergenti. Transmitter of kala-azar in Middle East and India.

    P. verrucarum. The transmitter of Bartonella bacilliformis, causative agent of Oroyo fever (Carrion's disease), in S. America.

phlebotomy (flĕ-bŏt′ō-mĭ) [Gr. *phlebos*, vein, + *tomē*, an incision]. Opening a vein. SYN: *venesection*, q.v.

    p., bloodless. Compression of veins of the extremities, cutting off some of the blood from the general circulation. SYN: *phlebostasia.*

phlegm (flĕm) [Gr. *phlegma*]. 1. Thick mucus, esp. that from the respiratory passages. 2. One of the four "humors" of early physiology.

phlegmasia (flĕg-mā′zĭ-ă) [Gr. *phlegmasia*]. Inflammation.

    p. alba dolens. Acute edema, esp. of leg from venous obstruction, usually thrombosis. SYN: *milk leg; white leg.*

    SYM: Usually begins, esp. in women who have recently given birth, with slight fever. Pain in lower part of abdomen follows, extends to hips and back, passes under Poupart's ligament, and thence down the thigh into calf of leg. Sometimes proceeds from calf upwards. Whole extremity becomes excessively swollen, hot and painful but not red, hence the name. Lochia and milk may or may not be suppressed. Constitutional disturbance and fever become greatly increased.

    Tenderness on pressure most marked along course of femoral vein, and veins of the affected region together with associated lymphatics may be felt to be hard and cordlike. Sometimes marked by faint red line. Progress rapid, frequently doubling size of limb in 24 hours or less; parts within pelvis become irritable; often difficulty in evacuating bladder and rectum; glands in groin sometimes swell and suppurate; and abscesses may form in different parts of limb.

    TREATMENT: Elevate limb, protect with a cradle, and apply warm fomentations. Anticoagulants to prevent clot formation. Vasodilator drugs and paracervical block may be used to combat vasospasm. Ligation of main venous channel proximal to thrombus may be done to prevent embolus.

    NP: Complete rest, immobilization of the limb. An elastic bandage, usually cotton, may be ordered by the physician. There is danger of a piece of thrombus becoming detached to form an embolus. No excitement.

    p., cellulitic. Septic inflammation of connective tissue of the leg following childbirth.

    p. malabarica. Inflammation with hypertrophy and induration of the skin. SYN: *elephantiasis.*

    p., thrombotic. SEE: *p. alba dolens.*

phlegmatic (flĕg-măt′ĭk) [Gr. *phlegmatikos*]. Of sluggish or dull temperament. SYN: *apathetic.*

phlegmon (flĕg′mŏn) [Gr. *phlegmonē*, inflammation]. Acute suppurative inflammation of subcutaneous connective tissue, esp. a pyogenic inflammation that spreads along fascial planes or other natural barriers.

    p., bronze. Gaseous p. causing bronze spots near incision.

    p., diffuse. Diffuse inflammation of subcutaneous tissues with sepsis.

    p., gas. Gas gangrene.

    p., Holz. A chronic cellulitis of the deep tissues of the floor of the mouth.

phlegmonous (flĕg′mŏn-ŭs). Pert. to inflammation of subcutaneous tissues.

phlogistic (flō-jĭs′tĭk) [Gr. *phlogistos*]. Pert. to, or inducing, inflammation.

phlogogenic, phlogogenous (flō-gō-jĕn′ĭk, -goj′ĕn-ŭs) [Gr. *phlogosis*, inflamma-

Phobias*

Fear of	Condition
air	aerophobia
aloneness	autophobia, eremophobia, monophobia
animals	zoophobia
anything new	kainophobia, neophobia
bacilli	bacillophobia
bad men	pavor sceleris, scelerophobia
barren space	cenophobia, kenophobia
bearing a deformed child	teratophobia
bees	apiphobia, melissophobia
birds	ornithophobia
blood	hematophobia, hemophobia
blushing	ereuthrophobia, erythrophobia
brain disease	meningitophobia
bridges	gephyrophobia
burglars	scelerophobia
buried alive	taphephobia
cats	ailurophobia, galeophobia, gatophobia
change	kainophobia, kainotophobia, neophobia
childbirth	maieusiophobia
choking	anginophobia, pnigophobia
cold	cheimaphobia, psychrophobia
color	chromatophobia, chromophobia
comet	cometophobia
confinement	claustrophobia
contamination	molysmophobia, mysophobia
corpses	necrophobia
crossing streets	dromophobia
crowds	demophobia, ochlophobia
cumbersome pseudoscientific terms	hellenophobia
dampness	hygrophobia
darkness	nyctophobia, scotophobia
dawn	eosophobia
daylight	phengophobia
death	thanatophobia
defecation	rhypophobia
definite disease	monopathophobia
deformity	dysmorphophobia
demons	demonophobia, demonomania, entheomania
depth	bathophobia
devil	demonophobia, satanophobia
dirt	mysophobia, rupophobia
disease	nosophobia, pathophobia
dogs	cynophobia
dolls	pediophobia
dust	amathophobia
eating	pagophobia
electricity	electrophobia
emptiness	kenophobia
enclosed, being	clithrophobia
everything	panphobia, panophobia, pantophobia
examination	examination phobia
excrement	coprophobia

* Adapted from Hinsie, L. E., and Campbell, R. J.: Psychiatric Dictionary, ed 4. Oxford University Press, Fair Lawn, N.J., 1970.

Phobias (*Continued*)

Fear of	Condition
eyes	ommatophobia
failure	kakorrhaphiophobia
fatigue	kopophobia
fearing	phobophobia
feathers	pteronophobia
female genitals	eurotophobia
fever	fibriphobia, pyrexeophobia
filth	mysophobia, rupophobia
filth, personal	automysophobia
fire	pyrophobia
fish	icthyophobia
floods	antlophobia
fog	homichlophobia
food	cibophobia, sitophobia
forest	hylophobia
frogs	batrachophobia
functioning	ergasiophobia
ghosts	phasmophobia
girls	parthenophobia
glass	crystallophobia, hyelophobia
God	theophobia
gravity	barophobia
hair	trichopathophobia
heat	thermophobia
height	acrophobia, hyposophobia
hell	hadephobia, stygiophobia
heredity	patroiophobia
high objects	batophobia
house	domatophobia, oikophobia
ideas	ideophobia
infinity	apeirophobia
injury	traumatophobia
innovation	neophobia
insanity	lyssophobia, maniaphobia
insects	acarophobia, entomophobia
jealousy	zelophobia
justice	dikephobia
knife	aichmophobia
large objects	megalophobia
left	levophobia
light	photophobia
lightning	astraphobia, astrapophobia, keraunophobia
locked in, being	claustrophobia, clithrophobia
looked at, being	scopophobia
machinery	mechanophobia
man	androphobia
many things	polyphobia
marriage	gamophobia
materialism	hylephobia
medicine	pharmacophobia
metals	metallophobia
meteors	meteorophobia
mind	psychophobia
mirror	eisoptrophobia, spectrophobia
missiles	ballistophobia
moisture	hygrophobia

Phobias (*Continued*)

Fear of	Condition
money	chrematophobia
motion	kinesophobia
mouse	musophobia
myths	mythophobia
naked body	gymnophobia
name	onomatophobia
needles	belonephobia
Negroes	negrophobia
night	noctiphobia, nyctophobia
northern lights	auroraphobia
novelty	kainophobia, kainolophobia
odor	olfactophobia, osmophobia, osphresiophobia
odor, personal	bromidrosiphobia
open space	agoraphobia
pain	algophobia, odynophobia
parasites	parasitophobia
people	anthropophobia
place	topophobia
pleasure	hedonophobia
points	aichmophobia
poison	iophobia, toxicophobia
poverty	peniaphobia
precipices	cremnophobia
punishment	poinephobia
rabies	cynophobia, lyssophobia
railroad or train	siderodromophobia
rain	ombrophobia
rectal excreta	coprophobia
rectum	proctophobia
red	erythrophobia
responsibility	hypengyophobia
ridicule	categelophobia
right	dextrophobia
river	potamophobia
robbers	harpaxophobia
rod	rhabdophobia
ruin	atephobia
sacred things	hierophobia
scabies	scabiophobia
school	school phobia
scratches	amychophobia
sea	thalassophobia
self	autophobia
semen	spermatophobia
sex	genophobia
sexual intercourse	coitophobia
shock	hormephobia
sin	hamartophobia
sinning	peccatiphobia
sitting	thaasophobia
sitting down	kathisophobia
skin disease	dermatosiophobia
skin lesion	dermatophobia
skin of animals	doraphobia
sleep	hypnophobia
small objects	microphobia, microbiophobia

Phobias (Continued)

Fear of	Condition
smothering	pnigerophobia
snake	ophidiophobia
snow	chionphobia
solitude	eremophobia
sounds	acousticophobia
sourness	acerophobia
speaking	laliophobia
speaking aloud	phonophobia
spider	arachneophobia
stairs	climacophobia
standing up	stasiphobia
standing up and walking	stasibasiphobia
stars	siderophobia
stealing	kleptophobia
stillness	eremiophobia
stories	mythophobia
strangers	xenophobia
street	agyiophobia
string	linonophobia
sunlight	heliophobia
symbolism	symbolophobia
syphilis	syphilophobia
talking	laliophobia
tapeworms	taeniophobia
taste	geumaphobia
teeth	odontophobia
thinking	phronemophobia
thunder	astraphobia, brontophobia
time	chronophobia
touched, being	haphephobia
travel	hodophobia
trembling	tremophobia
trichinosis	trichinophobia
tuberculosis	phthisiophobia, tuberculophobia
vaccination	vaccinophobia
vehicle	amaxophobia
venereal disease	cypridophobia, cypriphobia
void	kenophobia
vomiting	emetophobia
walking	basiphobia
water	hydrophobia
weakness	asthenophobia
wind	anemophobia
women	gynophobia, horror feminae
words, hearing certain	onomatophobia
work	ponophobia
writing	graphophobia

tion, + *gennan,* to produce]. Producing or exciting inflammation.

phlogosin (flō-gō'sĭn). Substance isolated from cultures of Staphylococcus aureus, producing suppuration.

phlogosis (flō-gō'sĭs) [Gr., inflammation]. 1. Inflammation. 2. Erysipelas.

phlyctena (flĭk-tē'nă) [Gr. *phlyktaina*]. (pl. *phlyctenae*) A thin ichor- or lymph-containing vesicle, esp. one of many after a first-degree burn.

phlyctenoid (flĭk'tĕ-noyd) ["+ *eidos,* resemblance]. Resembling a blister or pustule.

phlyctenosis (flĭk″tĕ-nō'sĭs) ["+ -ōsis, intensive condition]. Appearance of blisters or pustules.

phlyctenula (flĭk-tĕn'ū-lă) [L.]. (pl. *phlyctenulae*) A tiny vesicle or pustule, esp. that seen on the cornea.

phlyctenular (flĭk-tĕn'ū-lăr). Resembling or pert. to vesicles or pustules.

phlyctenule (flĭk'tĕn-ūl) [Gr. *phlyktaina*, a blister; L. *phlyctaenulaly*]. A small vesicle or blister, as on cornea or conjunctiva.

phlyctenulosis (flĭk-tĕn-ū-lō'sĭs) ["+ -ōsis, intensive]. The formation of many phlyctenules.

phobia (fō'bĭ-ă) [Gr. *phobos*, fear]. Any abnormal fear.

-phobia [Gr.]. Suffix indicating abnormal fear of, or aversion to, a subject.

phobic (fō'bĭk) [Gr. *phobos*, fear]. Concerning a phobia.

  p. desensitization. Method of treating phobias in which the patient is taught to relax while slowly reentering the phobic situation, first in imagination and then in real life. Anxiety and fear are kept to a minimum at all times. SEE: *implosion.*

phobophobia (fō″bō-fō'bĭ-ă) ["+ *phobos*, fear]. Morbid fear of acquiring a phobia.

phocomelia (fō″kō-mē'lĭ-ă) [Gr. *phōkē*, seal, + *melos*, limb]. A congenital malformation wherein the proximal portion of the extremities are poorly developed or absent. Thus the hands and feet are attached to the trunk directly or by means of a poorly formed bone. In some cases this is due to a drug taken during early pregnancy. That drug, a sleeping pill, is no longer sold.

phon-. SEE: *phono-.*

phonacoscope (fō-năk'ō-skōp) [Gr. *phōnē*, voice, + *skopein*, to examine]. A device for increasing the percussion note or voice sounds.

phonacoscopy (fō-nă-kŏs'kō-pĭ). Inspection of the chest with the phonacoscope.

phonal (fō'năl) [Gr. *phōnē*, voice]. Concerning the voice.

phonasthenia (fōn-ăs-thē'nĭ-ă) ["+ *asthenia*, weakness]. Vocal weakness or hoarseness due to straining the voice.

phonation (fō-nā'shŭn). Process of uttering vocal sounds.

phonatory (fō'nă-tō″rĭ) [Gr. *phōnē*, voice]. Concerning utterance of vocal sounds.

phonautograph (fōn-aw'tō-grăf) ["+ *autos*, self, + *graphein*, to write]. Device for registering the voice's vibrations.

phone. An element of speech; a single speech sound.

-phone [Gr. phōnē, voice]. Combining form indicating sound or voice.

phoneme (fō'nēm) [Gr. *phōnēma*, an utterance]. 1. Auditory hallucination of voices and spoken words. May include neologisms, q.v., where patients may repeat a thought or the part of a sentence just read. 2. In linguistics, the smallest unit of speech which distinguishes one utterance or word from another.

phonendoscope (fō-nĕn'dō-skōp) [Gr. *phōnē*, voice, + *endon*, within, + *skopein*, to examine]. A stethoscope that intensifies sounds.

phonendoskiascope (fō-nĕn″dō-skī'ă-skōp) ["+ "+ *skia*, shadow, + *skopein*, to examine]. Device for observing the cardiac movements and for hearing heart sounds.

phonetics (fō-nĕt'ĭks) [Gr. *phōnētikos*, spoken]. Science of speech and pronunciation. SYN: *phonology.*

phoniatrics (fō″nĭ-ăt'rĭks) [Gr. *phōnē*, voice, + *iatrikē*, treatment]. The study of the voice and treatment of its disorders.

phonic (fō'nĭk). Concerning the voice or sound.

phonism (fō'nĭzm) [Gr. *phōnē*, voice, + *-ismos*, condition]. An auditory sensation occurring when another sense is stimulated. SEE: *synesthesia.*

phono- [Gr. phōnē, voice]. Combining form indicating sound, voice.

phonocardiography (fō″nō-kar″dĭ-ŏg'ră-fĭ) ["+ *kardia*, heart, + *graphein*, to write]. Mechanical or electronic registration of heart sounds.

phonogram (fō'nō-grăm) ["+ *gramma*, a mark]. A graphic curve indicating intensity and duration of a sound.

phonograph (fō'nō-grăf) ["+ *graphein*, to write]. Instrument used for reproduction of sounds.

phonology (fō-nŏl'ō-jĭ) [Gr. *phōnē*, voice, + *logos*, a study]. Science of vocal sounds. SYN: *phonetics.*

pho'noma'nia (Gr. *phonos*, murder, + *mania*, madness). Insanity characterized by homicidal tendencies.

phonomassage (fō″nō-mă-săzh') [Gr. *phōnē*, voice, + *massein*, to knead]. Exciting movements of the ossicles of the ear by means of noise or alternating suction and pressure directed through the external auditory meatus.

phonometer (fō-nŏm'ē-tĕr) ["+ *metron*, measure]. Device for determining intensity of vocal sounds.

phonomyoclonus (fō″nō-mī-ŏk'lō-nŭs) [Gr. *phōnē*, voice, + *mys, myo-*, muscle, + *klonos*, a contraction]. Invisible fibrillary muscular contractions revealed by auscultation.

phonomyogram (fō"nō-mī'ō-grăm) ["+ *gramma*, mark]. A recording of sound produced by action of a muscle.

phonomyography (fō"nō-mī-og'ră-fī) ["+ "+ *graphein*, to write]. The recording of sounds made by contracting muscular tissue.

phonopathy (fō-nŏp'ă-thī) [Gr. *phōnē*, voice, + *pathos*, disease]. Any disease of organs affecting speech.

pho"nopho'bia ("+ *phobos*, fear). 1. Morbid fear of sound or noise. 2. Fear of speaking or hearing one's own voice.

phonopsia (fō-nŏp'sī-ă) [Gr. *phōne*, voice, + *opsis*, vision]. The subjective perception of sensations upon hearing certain sounds.

phonoscope (fō'nō-skōp) ["+ *skopein*, to examine]. Device for recording photographs of heart sounds.

phoresis (fō-rē'sīs) [Gr. *phorēsis*, being borne]. In physical therapy, the migration of ions through a membrane by the action of an electric current. The direction of migration is sometimes distinguished by the use of the terms *cataphoresis* and *anaphoresis* for migrations toward cathode and anode, respectively.

-phoria [Gr. *phorēsis*, being borne]. In ophthalmology, a combining form meaning a turning with reference to the visual axis. EX: cyclophoria.

Phormia (for'mī-ă). A genus of blowflies belonging to the family Calliphoridae. Their larvae normally live in decaying flesh of dead animals, but they may infest neglected wounds or sores giving rise to myiasis.

phorology (fō-rŏl'ō-jī) [Gr. *phoros*, carrying, + *logos*, study]. Science dealing with disease carriers.

phorotone (fō'rō-tōn) [Gr. *phora*, motion, + *tonos*, tension]. Device for exercising eye muscles.

phose (fōz) [Gr. *phōs*, light]. A subjective sensation of light or color. SEE: *centraphose; centrophose; chromophose.*

phosgene (fōs'jēn) ["+ *genes*, born]. Carbonyl chloride ($COCl_2$), a poisonous gas causing nausea and suffocation when inhaled. Used in chemical warfare, esp. during World War I; now used in industry in preparation of pharmaceutical and chemical products.

phosphatase (fōs'fă-tās). One of a group of enzymes which catalyzes the hydrolysis of phosphoric acid esters. They are of importance in absorption and metabolism of carbohydrates, nucleotides, and phospholipids and are essential in the calcification of bone.

p., acid. P. whose optimum pH is between 4.0 and 5.4. Present in kidney, semen, serum, and prostate gland.

p., alkaline. P. whose optimum pH is about 9.0. Present in teeth, developing bone, plasma, kidney, and intestine. It is excreted by the liver, hence increases in blood in obstructive jaundice.

phosphate (fōs'fāt) [Gr. *phosphas*]. A salt of phosphoric acid. Phosphates are important in maintenance of acid-base balance of the blood, the principal ones being monosodium and disodium phosphate. The former is acid, the latter alkaline. In the blood, because of their low concentration, they exert a minor buffering action. In the formation of urine, by altering the proportions of acid and alkaline phosphates, an acid urine is formed and the body's fixed base, chiefly Na but also K, Mg, and Ca, is conserved.

Decreased p. excretion in urine occurs when alkaline reserve is high; in nephritis, tetany (hypoparathyroidism), adrenal cortical deficiency, and certain bone diseases.

Increased p. excretion in urine occurs when alkali reserve is low; in starvation, hyperparathyroidism, high protein diet, and extreme muscular exercise.

p., acid. P. in which only one or two of hydrogen atoms of phosphoric acid have been replaced by a metal.

p. -bond-energy. Energy derived from phosphorylated compounds such as adenosine triphosphate (ATP) and creatine phosphate.

p., normal. P. in which all three hydrogen atoms of phosphoric acid have been replaced by metals.

phosphatemia (fōs"fă-tē'mī-ă) [Gr. *phosphas*, phosphate, + *haima*, blood]. Phosphates in the blood.

phosphatide (fōs'fă-tīd). A phospholipid, q.v.

phosphatoptosis (fōs"fă-tŏp-tō'sīs) [Gr. *phosphas*, phosphate, + *ptōsis*, a dropping]. Spontaneous precipitation of phosphates in urine.

phosphaturia (fōs"fă-tū'rī-ă) ["+ *ouron*, urine]. Excessive amount of phosphates in the urine. Often causes renal calculi. SYN: *phosphoruria; phosphuria.*

SYM: Cloudy urine, opaque and pale. Reaction alkaline. Pearly or pinkish white deposits of phosphates in standing urine.

phosphene (fōs'fēn) [Gr. *phōs*, light, + *phainein*, to show]. A subjective sensation of light caused by pressure upon the eyeball.

p., accommodation. P. resulting from contraction of ciliary muscles in accommodation. Seen esp. in the dark.

phosphide (fŏs'fīd) ["+ *pherein*, to carry]. Binary compound of phosphorus with an element or radical.

phosphite (fŏs'fīt). A salt of phosphoric acid.

phosphocreatine (fŏs"fō-krē'ă-tĭn). A compound, found in muscle, of equal parts of phosphoric acid and creatine.

phospholipid (fŏs"fō-lĭp'ĭd) [Gr. *phŏs*, light, + *pherein*, to carry, + *lipos*, fat]. A lipoid substance containing phosphorus, fatty acids, and nitrogenous base, as lecithin. SYN: *phosphatide; phospholipin.*

phospholipin (fŏs"fō-lĭp'ĭn). A lipoid compound containing phosphorus. SYN: *phosphatide; phospholipid.*

phosphonecrosis (fŏs"fō-nē-krō'sĭs) [Gr. *phŏs*, light, + *pherein*, to carry, + *nekros*, dead, + *-ōsis*, disease]. Necrosis of the alveolar process in persons working with phosphorus.

phosphonuclease (fŏs"fō-nū'klē-ās). An enzyme that catalyzes the hydrolysis of nucleotides to nucleosides and phosphoric acid.

phosphopenia (fŏs"fō-pē'nĭ-ă) [Gr. *phŏs*, light, + *phorein*, to carry, + *penia*, lack]. Deficiency of phosphorus in the body.

phosphoprotein (fŏs"fō-prō'tē-ĭn) ["+ "+ *prōtos*, first]. One of a group of proteins in which the protein is combined with phosphorus-containing compound. Ex: caseinogen; vitellin.

Formerly called nucleoalbumin.

phosphorated (fŏs'fō-rā"tĕd) [Gr. *phŏs*, light, + *phorein*, to carry]. Impregnated with phosphorus.

phosphorescence (fŏs-fō-rĕs'ĕns). The induced luminescence that persists after cessation of the irradiation that caused it. The emission of light without appreciable heat.

phosphorhidrosis (fŏs"for-hĭd-rō'sĭs) [Gr. *phŏs*, light, + *phorein*, to carry, + *hidrōsis*, sweating]. Secretion of luminous perspiration. SYN: *phosphoridrosis.*

phosphoribosyltransferase. An important enzyme which catalyzes reconversion to the ribonucleotide stage of the purine bases, hypoxanthine and guanine. A deficiency of the enzyme causes gout. The deficiency is inherited as an X chromosome-linked trait.

phosphoric acid (fŏs-for'ĭk). Orthophosphoric acid, H_3PO_4, a tribasic acid.

phosphoridrosis (fŏs"for-ĭd-rō'sĭs) [Gr. *phŏs*, light, + *phorein*, to carry, + *hidrōsis*, perspiration]. Secretion of perspiration that is luminous. SYN: *phosphorhidrosis.*

phosphorism (fŏs'for-ĭzm) ["+ "+ *ismos*, condition]. Chronic poisoning from phosphorus.

phosphorous acid (fŏs-fō'rŭs) ["+ *phoros*, carrying]. H_3PO_3. Crystalline acid formed when phosphorus is oxidized in moist air.

phosphoruria (fŏs"for-ū'rĭ-ă) [Gr. *phŏs*, light, + *phorein*, to carry, + *ouron*, urine]. Phosphorus in the urine in excess of normal. SYN: *phosphaturia; phosphuria.*

phosphorus (fŏs'fō-rŭs) [Gr. *phŏs*, light, + *phoros*, carrying]. SYMB: *P*. At. wt. 30.9738; at. no. 15. A nonmetallic element not found in a free state but in combination with alkalies.

The adult body contains from 600 to 900 gm. of phosphorus in various forms. 70–80% in bones and teeth, principally combined with calcium, 10% in muscle and 1% in nerve tissue. Minimum daily requirement is approx. 800 mg. Amount should be increased during pregnancy and lactation. Vitamin D is important in the absorption and metabolism of phosphorus. Excesses of phosphorus are excreted by kidney and intestine, about 60% being excreted in urine principally as phosphates.

Phosphorus compounds (adenosine triphosphate and phosphocreatine) are the principal sources of energy in muscle contraction, and phosphorus is essential in the conversion of glycogen to glucose.

P. is found in the protein of food. Ex: Almonds, beans, barley, bran, cheese, cocoa, chocolate, eggs, lentils, liver, milk, oatmeal, peanuts, peas, walnuts, whole wheat, and rye. Good: Asparagus, beef, cabbage, carrots, celery, cauliflower, chard, chicken, clams, corn, cream, cucumbers, egg plant, fish, figs, meat, prunes, pineapples, pumpkin, raisins, and string beans.

DEFICIENCY SYM: Perverted appetite, retarded growth, loss of weight, weakness, rickets, imperfect bone and teeth development.

POISONING: Prior to the introduction of safety matches (which contain no yellow phosphorus) phosphorus poisoning was quite common. However, acute phosphorus poisoning still is seen following ingestion of rat and roach poisons which contain yellow phosphorus.

POISONING SYM: Acute irritation of gastrointestinal tract followed by symptoms resembling acute yellow atrophy of liver and marked blood changes. Bloody vomitus, garlic odor of breath, cramps, headache, liver and kidney damage. Profound weakness, hemorrhage, heart failure. Occasionally nervous symptoms predominate. Metabolism changes.

F.A. TREATMENT: Prolonged gastric lavage, part of which should contain a small amount of cupric sulfate, 0.2%, or potassium permanganate which may aid in oxidizing the phosphorus. This should, of course, be washed out. Protect patient and attendants from vomitus, gastric washings, and feces because the p. in them can burn the skin and eyes. Oils, creams, and fats should be avoided because these promote absorption of phosphorus. Intravenous isotonic sodium chloride and sodium lactate are useful in combating shock, dehydration, and acidosis. Otherwise treat symptomatically. Blood transfusion is helpful. SEE: *Table of Poisons* in *Appendix*.

phosphorylase (fŏs-fŏr'ĭ-lās). An enzyme that catalyzes the formation of glucose-1-phosphate from glycogen.

phosphuria (fŏs-fū'rĭ-ă) [Gr. *phŏs*, light, + *phoros*, a bearer, + *ouron*, urine]. Excess of phosphorus in the urine. SYN: *phosphaturia; phosphoruria*.

phot (fŏt) [Gr. *phŏs, phot-*, light]. The unit of photochemical energy equal to 1 lumen per square centimeter or about 929 foot candles. ABBR: ph.

phot-. SEE: words beginning with *photo-*.

photalgia (fō-tăl'jĭ-ă) [Gr. *phŏs, phot-*, light, + *algos*, pain]. Pain produced by light. SYN: *photodynia; photophobia*.

photaugiophobia (fō-tă-jĭ-ă-fō'bĭ-ă) [Gr. *phōtaugeia*, glare, + *phobos*, fear]. Intolerance of bright light.

photesthesis (fō''tĕs-thē'sĭs) [Gr. *phŏs, phot-*, light, + *aisthesis*, sensation]. Sensitivity to light.

photic (fō'tĭk). Concerning light. In biology, pert. to the production of light by certain organisms.

   p. sneezing. Sneezing initiated or hastened in its onset by light stimulus. Sometimes due to light causing tears which upon draining into the nasal area cause sneezing.

photism (fō'tĭzm) [Gr. *phos, phot-*, light, + *ismos*, condition]. A subjective sensation of color or light produced by a stimulus of another sense, such as smell, hearing, taste, or touch. SEE: *synesthesia*.

photo- [Gr. *phŏtos*]. Combining form indicating light.

photoallergic contact dermatitis. Inflammation of the skin due to substances made allergenic by the effect of ultraviolet or light in the visible spectrum. SEE: *photoallergy*.

photoallergy (fō''tō-ăl'er-jĭ) [Gr. *photos*, light, + *allos*, other, + *ergon*, work]. An immunological reaction produced by interaction of light rays and certain chemicals. It is a form of contact allergic reaction wherein light is necessary to cause the sensitivity reaction. Some of the photocontact allergens are phenothiazine, sulfonamides, hexachlorophene, sunscreen agents, optical bleaches, and topical antihistamines. SEE: *photosensitivity; phototoxic.*

photobiotic (fō''tō-bī-ŏt'ĭk) ["+ *bios*, life]. Capable of living only in the light.

photocauterization (fō''tō-kaw''tĕr-ĭ-zā'shŭn) ["+ *kautērion*, a branding iron]. Cauterization using radioactive means, as X rays.

photoceptor (fō''tō-sĕp'tor) ["+ L. *ceptor*, a receiver]. A nerve ceptor receiving light ray sensations.

photochemistry (fō''tō-kĕm'ĭs-trĭ) [Gr. *photos*, light, *chemeia*, chemistry]. Phase of science dealing with chemical changes produced by light rays.

photochromogen ["+ *chroma*, color, + *gennan*, to produce]. Certain microorganisms in which a pigment develops when it is grown in the presence of light. Ex: Mycobacterium kansasii.

photocoagulation. Alteration of proteins in tissue by the use of light energy in the form of ordinary light rays or a laser beam. Used esp. in treating retinal detachments or bleeding from the retina.

photodermatitis (fō''tō-der-mă-tī'tĭs) ["+ *dermatos*, skin, + *-itis*, inflammation]. Sensitivity of the epithelium to light. May be due to photoallergy, q.v., or to phototoxic, q.v., reaction.

photodromy (fō-tŏd'rō-mĭ) ["+ *dromos*, running]. The condition of particles in suspension wherein they move toward (positive p.) or away from (negative p.) light.

photodynamic (fō''tō-dī-năm'ĭk) [Gr. *photos*, light, + *dynamis*, force]. Pert. to the energy or force effected by light on organisms.

   p. action. Action exerted by certain dyes, such as methylene blue and eosin, on certain biological systems when subjected to light.

photodynia (fō''tō-dīn'ĭ-ă) ["+ *odynē*, pain]. Pain produced by rays of light. SYN: *photalgia*.

photodysphoria (fō''tō-dĭs-fōr'ĭ-ă) ["+ *dysphoria*, distress]. Extreme intolerance of light. SYN: *phengophobia; photophobia*.

photoelectricity (fō''tō-ē-lĕk-trĭ'sĭ-tĭ) [Gr. *photos*, light, + *ēlektron*, amber]. Electricity formed by action of light.

photofluorography (fō''tō-flū''er-ŏg'ră-fĭ). Photographing the images seen during fluoroscopic examination.

photogene (fō'tō-jen) [Gr. *phŏtos*, light, + *gennan*, to produce]. Prolonged retinal image. SYN: *after-image*.

photogenic, photogenous (fō″tō-jĕn′ĭk, -tŏj′ĕn-ŭs). Induced by, or inducing, light.

photograph′ic radiom′eter. An instrument containing a half-tone color index for strips of photographic paper after exposure to roentgen rays and, after development, used to estimate the quantity of roentgen rays.

photohemotachometer (fō″tō-hĕm″ō-tăk-ŏm′ē-tĕr) [Gr. *photos*, light, + *haima*, blood, + *tachys*, swift, + *metron*, measure]. Device for photographing rate of blood flow.

photokinetic (fō″tō-kĭn-ĕt′ĭk) [″+ *kinētikos*, motion]. Reacting with motion to stimulus of light.

photoluminescence (fō″tō-lū-mĭ-nĕs′ĕnts) [″+ L. *lumen*, light]. The power of an object to become luminescent when acted on by light.

photolysis (fō-tŏl′ĭ-sĭs) [″+ *lysis*, dissolution]. Dissolution or disintegration under stimulus of light rays.

photolytic (fō″tō-lĭt′ĭk). Dissolved by stimulus of light rays.

photomania (fō″tō-mā′nĭ-ă) [Gr. *photos*, light, + *mania*, madness]. 1. A psychosis produced by prolonged exposure to intense light. 2. A psychotic desire for light.

photometer (fō-tŏm′ĕt-ĕr) [Gr. *photos*, light, + *metron*, measure]. A device for measuring the intensity of light.

photometry (fō-tŏm′ĕ-trĭ). Measurement of light rays.

photomicrograph (fō″tō-mī′krō-grăf) [Gr. *photos*, light, *mikros*, small, + *graphein*, to write]. Photograph of an object under the microscope.

photom′otor. Pert. to muscular contraction induced by light.

photon (fō′tŏn) [Gr. *photos*, light]. A light quantum or unit of energy of a light ray or other form of radiant energy. Generally considered to be a discrete particle with zero mass, no electric charge, and indefinitely long life.

photonosus (fō-tŏn′ō-sŭs) [″+ *nosos*, disease]. Disease due to prolonged exposure to intense light.

photoperceptive (fō″tō-pĕr-cĕp′tĭv) [″+ *percipere*, to receive]. Capable of perceiving light.

photoperiodism (fō″tō-pĭr′ĭ-ō-dĭzm) [″+ LL. *periodus*, period, + Gr. *ismos*, condition]. The periodic occurrence of biological phenomena in relationship to the presence or absence of light. In most animals, the sleep-wakefulness cycle is a form of periodism.

photophilic (fō-tō-fĭl′ĭk) [Gr. *photos*, light, + *philein*, to love]. Seeking, or fond of, light.

photophobia (fō″tō-fō′bĭ-ă) [″+ *phobos*, fear]. Unusual intolerance of light. Occurs in measles and rubella, meningitis, and inflammation of the eyes. SYN: *phengophobia; photodysphoria.*

photophone (fō′tō-fōn) [″+ *phōnē*, voice]. Device for production of sound by action of light.

photopic (fō-tŏp′ĭk). Pert. to bright light.

    p. vision. Vision in bright light involving the formation of images and discrimination of color. SEE: *scotopic vision.*

photopsia, photopsy (fō-tŏp′sĭ-ă, fō-tŏp′sĭ) [Gr. *photos*, light, + *opsis*, vision]. Subjective sensation of sparks or flashes of light in retinal, optic, or brain diseases.

photoptarmosis (fō″tō-tar-mō′sĭs) [″+ *ptarmōsis*, sneezing]. Sneezing caused by the effect of light.

photoptometer (fō-tŏp-tŏm′ē-tĕr) [″+ *opsis*, vision, + *metron*, measure]. Device for determining the smallest amount of light that will make an object visible.

photoreceptive (fō″tō-rē-sĕp′tĭv) [″+ *receptor*, a receiver]. Capable of perceiving light rays.

photoreceptor (fō″tō-rē-sĕp′tor). Sensory nerve endings or cells which are capable of being stimulated by light. In man, rods and cones of the retina.

pho′toscan. A map of the concentration of a radioisotope outlining an organ in the body. The map is printed on photographic paper.

photoscope (fō′tō-skōp) [Gr. *photos*, light, + *skopein*, to examine]. A variety of fluoroscope used to observe light.

photoscopy (fō-tŏs′kō-pĭ). Examination with a fluorescent screen. SYN: *fluoroscopy; skiascopy.*

photosensitiv′ity [Gr. *photos*, light, + L. *sensitivus*, feeling]. Sensitive to light. SEE: *photoallergy.*

photosensitization (fō″tō-sĕn″sĭ-tĭ-zā′-shŭn). Condition in which the skin reacts abnormally to light, esp. ultraviolet rays or sunlight; due to the presence of drugs, hormones, or heavy metals in the system. SEE: *photoallergy.*

photosensitizer (fō″tō-sĕn″sĭ-tī′zĕr). Substance which, in combination with light, will cause a sensitivity reaction in the substance or organism.

photosynthesis (fō″tō-sĭn′thĕ-sĭs) [Gr. *photos*, light, + *synthesis*, placing together]. The process by which plants are able to manufacture carbohydrates by combining carbon dioxide from the air and water from the soil, utilizing light energy in the presence of chlorophyll.

The basic chemical reaction is as follows:

$$6CO_2 + 6H_2O + energy$$
(4.1 Cal. per gm. of glucose)
$$C_6H_{12}O_6 + 6H_2O.$$

Only plants containing chlorophyll are capable of thus producing sugars. The red and blue waves of the spectrum are absorbed by the chlorophyll, but all other rays are rejected. CO_2 and H_2O are also necessary factors.

When simple sugar is formed, the plant splits up CO_2, uses the carbon by photosynthesis, and liberates the oxygen. The sources of energy for this disruption are the blue and red rays which are absorbed by the plant. To make 1 gm. of natural sugar the plant uses 750 cu. ft. (21,237 liters) of CO_2.

phototaxis (fō″tŏ-tăk′sĭs) [" + *taxis*, arrangement]. The reaction and movement of cells and microorganisms under the stimulus of light.

phototherapy (fō″tŏ-thĕr′ă-pĭ) [" + *therapeia*, treatment]. 1. Exposure to sunlight or artificial light for therapeutic purposes. 2. Reduction of serum bilirubin concentration in the newborn infant by exposure to sunlight or artificial blue light. Infant's eyes must be protected from the light used.

photothermal (fō″tŏ-thĕr′măl) [Gr. *photos*, light, + *thermē*, heat]. Concerning heat produced by light.

   p. radiation. Radiation of heat by a source of light, as that from an electric bulb.

phototopia (fō″tŏ-tō′pĭ-ă). A subjective sensation of light.

phototoxic (fō″tŏ-tŏk′sĭk) [Gr. *photos*, light, + *toxikon*, poison]. Pert. to the harmful reaction produced by light energy, esp. that produced in the skin. Simple sunburn of the skin is an example of phototoxicity.

phototoxis (fō″tŏ-tŏk′sĭs). Disorder produced by effects of overexposure to light or radiation.

phototropism (fō-tŏt′rō-pĭzm) [Gr. *photos*, light, + *tropos*, turning]. A tendency exhibited by green plants and some microorganisms to turn toward or grow toward light.

photuria (fō-tū′rĭ-ă) [" + *ouron*, urine]. Excretion of phosphorescent urine.

phren (frĕn) [Gr.]. 1. The mind. 2. The diaphragm.

phrenalgia (frē-năl′jĭ-ă) [" + *algos*, pain]. 1. Pain of mental origin or caused by a mental process. SYN: *psychalgia.* 2. Pain in the diaphragm.

phrenasthenia (frĕn″ăs-thē′nĭ-ă) [" + *astheneia*, weakness]. Mental deficiency.

phrenemphraxis (frĕn″ĕm-frăk′sĭs) [Gr. *phrēn*, diaphragm, + *emphraxis*, stoppage]. Crushing of the phrenic nerve in order to induce temporary paralysis of the diaphragm; a therapeutic measure which was previously employed in treatment of pulmonary tuberculosis.

phrenetic (frĕn-ĕt′ĭk) [Gr. *phrēn*, mind]. 1. Maniacal; frenzied. 2. A maniac.

-phrenia. Combining form indicating mental disorder.

phrenic (frĕn′ĭk) [Gr. *phrēn*, mind, diaphragm]. 1. Concerning the diaphragm, as the p. nerve. 2. Concerning the mind.

   p. avulsion. Elevation of a side of the diaphragm and semi-collapse of corresponding lung by means of excision of part of the phrenic nerve.

   p. nerve. One arising in the cervical plexus entering the thorax and passing to the diaphragm. A motor nerve to the diaphragm with sensory fibers to the pericardium. SYN: *nervus phrenicus* [NA].

phrenicectomy (frĕn-ĭ-sĕk′tŏ-mĭ) [" + *ektomē*, excision]. Resection of a part of the phrenic nerve. Used to collapse the lung on one side by paralyzing the diaphragm.

phrenicoexairesis. SYN: *phrenicoexeresis*, q.v.

phrenicoexeresis (frĕn″ĭ-kō-ĕk-ser′ĕ′sĭs) [L. *phrenicus*, diaphragm, + Gr. *exairesis*, taking out]. Excision of part of the phrenic nerve.

phrenicotomy (frĕn″ĭ-kŏt′ō-mĭ) [" + *tomē*, a cutting]. Cutting of the phrenic nerve to produce immobilization of a lung by inducing paralysis of one side. This causes the diaphragm to rise; it compresses the lung and diminishes respiratory movement, thus resting the lung on that side.

phrenitis (frē-nī′tĭs) [" + *-itis*, inflammation]. 1. Acute delirium or frenzy. 2. Inflammation of the brain. SYN: *encephalitis.* 3. Inflammation of the diaphragm.

phreno- [Gr.]. Combining form meaning mind or diaphragm.

phrenocardia (frē″nŏ-kar′dĭ-ă) [Gr. *phrēn*, mind, + *kardia*, heart]. Cardiovascular neurasthenia.

   SYM: Cardiac arrhythmia, dyspnea with psychic disturbances, and submammary pain.

phrenocolopexy (frĕn″ŏ-kō′lō-pĕk″sĭ) [Gr. *phrēn*, mind, diaphragm, + *kōlon*, colon, + *pēxis*, fixation]. Suture of the transverse colon to the diaphragm.

phrenodynia (frĕn″ŏ-dĭn′ĭ-ă) [" + *odynē*, pain]. Pain in the diaphragm.

phrenograph (frĕn′ŏ-grăf) [Gr. *phrēn*, diaphragm, mind, + *graphein*, to write]. Device for registering movements of diaphragm.

phrenopathy (frē-nŏp′ă-thĭ) [" + *pathos*, disease]. Any mental disorder.

phrenopericarditis (frē″nō-pĕr-ĭ-kar-dī′tĭs) ["+ *peri*, around, + *kardia*, heart, + *-itis*, inflammation]. Attachment of the heart by adhesions to the diaphragm.

phrenoplegia (frĕn-ō-plē′jĭ-ă) [Gr. *phrēn*, mind, diaphragm, + *plēgē*, stroke]. 1. A sudden psychopathic attack. 2. Paralysis of the diaphragm.

phrenosin (frĕn′ō-sĭn). A cerebroside isolated from brain tissue. SYN: *cerebron.*

phrictopathic (frĭk-tō-păth′ĭk) [Gr. *phriktos*, shuddering, + *pathos*, disease]. Pert. to or having a shuddering sensation; applied to a shuddering sensation due to irritating a hysterical anesthetic area.

phronesis (frō-nē′sĭs) [Gr.]. Soundness of mind.

phrynoderma (frĭn-ō-der′mă) [Gr. *phrynē*, toad, + *derma*, skin]. A form of follicular keratosis of unknown etiology but thought to be related to one of several vitamin deficiencies.

phthalylsulfathiazole (thăl′ĭl-sŭl-fă-thī′ă-zōl). USP. A poorly absorbed sulfonamide used to treat intestinal infections.

phthiriasis (thĭr-ĭ′ă-sĭs) [Gr. *phtheiriasis*]. Condition of being infested with lice. SYN: *pediculosis.*

phthiriophobia (thĭr″ĭ-ō-fō′bĭ-ă) ["+ *phobos*, fear]. Abnormal dread of lice.

Phthirus (thĭr′ŭs) [Gr. *phtheir*, louse]. A genus of sucking lice belonging to the order Anoplura.

    P. pubis. The crab louse. Infests primarily pubic region but also found in armpits, beard, eyebrows, and eyelashes. SEE: *pediculosis pubis.*

phthisic (tĭz′ĭk) [Gr. *phthisikos*]. 1. Affected with pulmonary tuberculosis. 2. Asthma. 3. One afflicted with phthisis or asthma. 4. Wasted away or emaciated.

phthisical (tĭz′ĭ-kăl). Concerning, or afflicted with, phthisis.

phthisicky (tĭz′ĭ-kĭ) Suffering from asthma or phthisis.

phthisis (tĭ′sĭs) [Gr., a wasting]. 1. Pulmonary tuberculosis. 2. Any wasting or atrophic disease.

    p., abdominal. Intestinal tuberculosis.

    p., black. Lung disease from inhaled coal dust. SYN: *anthracosis.*

    p. bulbi. Atrophy of eyeball following intraocular inflammation.

    p., fibroid. 1. Interstitial pneumonia. 2. Pulmonary tuberculosis with dense layers of fibrous tissues surrounding a cavity.

    p., miner's. SEE: *p., black.*

    p., pulmonary. Tuberculosis of the lungs.

    p., stonecutter's. A wasting form of bronchopneumonia due to inhalation of stone dust with consequent irritation.

phycology (fī-kŏl′ō-jĭ) [Gr. *phykos*, seaweed, + *logos*, study]. Study of algae.

Phycomycetes (fī″kō-mī-sē′tēz) ["+ *mykes*, fungus]. An order of fungi rarely pathogenic in man.

phycomycosis (fī″kō-mī-kō′sĭs) ["+ "+ *osis*, condition]. Fungal infection caused by Phycomycetes. The lungs, central nervous system, and other parts of the body may be affected.

phygogalactic (fī″gō-găl-ăk′tĭk) [Gr. *pheugein*, to avoid, + *gala*, milk]. Checking, or that which checks or arrests, milk secretion. SYN: *galactophygous; ischogalactic; lactifuge.*

phylacogogic (fĭ-lăk″ō-gŏj′ĭk) [Gr. *phylakē*, guarding, + *agōgos*, leading]. Stimulating the formation of protective antibodies.

phylactic (fĭ-lăk′tĭk) [Gr. *phylaktikos*, preservative]. Concerning or producing phylaxis.

    p. agent. One with protective power.

    p. power. Power of an organism to ward off infection.

phylaxin (fī-lăk′sĭn) [Gr. *phylaxis*, protection]. Antibody. Protecting and defensive substances produced by the body after exposure to bacterial infection.

phylaxis (fĭ-lăk′sĭs) [Gr., protection]. The active defense of the body against infection.

phyletic (fī-lĕt′ĭk) [Gr. *phyletikos*]. Pert. to a phylum or race. SYN: *phylogenetic.*

phyllo- [Gr. *phyllon*, leaf]. Combining form meaning leaf.

phylogenesis (fī″lō-jĕn′ĕsĭs) [Gr. *phylē*, tribe, + *genesis*, generation]. The evolutionary development of a group, race, or species. SEE: *phylogeny.*

phylogenetic (fī″lō-jĕ-nĕt′ĭk). Concerning the development of a race or group.

phylogeny (fī-lŏj′ē-nĭ). Development and growth of a group or race. SEE: *ontogeny.*

phylum (fī′lŭm) [Gr. *phylon*, tribe]. (pl. *phyla*) One of the primary divisions of the animal or plant kingdom, next higher than a class.

phyma (fī′mă) [Gr., a growth]. (pl. *phymata*) A small, rounded skin tumor.

phymatoid (fī′mă-toyd) ["+ *eidos*, resemblance]. Like a tumor.

phymatorrhysin (fī″mă-to-rī′sĭn). A pigment present in hair and melanotic tumors.

phymatosis (fī-mă-tō′sĭs) ["+ *-ōsis*, disease]. A disease marked by the presence of phymata or small nodules in the skin.

physaliform, physalliform (fī-sal´ī-form) [Gr. *physallis*, bubble, + L. *forma*, shape]. Resembling a bleb or bubble.

Physaloptera (fis´´ă-lŏp´ter-ă) ["+ *pteron*, wing]. A genus of nematode worms belonging to the suborder Spiruata.

   P. caucasica. Species that occurs in and damages the upper gastrointestinal tract.

physiatrics (fĭz´´ī-ăt´rĭks) [Gr. *physis*, nature, + *iatrikē*, surgery, medicine]. The curing of disease by natural methods, esp. physical therapy.

physic (fĭz´ĭk) [Gr. *physikos*, natural]. 1. The art of medicine and healing. 2. A medicine, esp. a cathartic. 3. Drugs in general. 4. To treat with a physic, esp. to purge.

physical (fĭz´ī-kăl). 1. Of or pert. to nature or material things. 2. Concerning or pert. to the body; bodily.

   p. examination. Examination of the body by auscultation, palpation, percussion, inspection, and smelling.

   p. fitness. The ability to carry out daily tasks with vigor and alertness, without undue fatigue, and with ample energy to enjoy leisure-time pursuits and meet unforeseen emergencies. It is the ability to withstand stress and persevere under difficult circumstances where an unfit person would quit. Implied in this is more than lack of illness; it is a positive quality which everyone has to some degree. P. fitness is minimal in the severely ill and maximal in the highly trained athlete.

   p. signs. Disease symptoms revealed by physical examination.

   p. therapist. One skilled in physical therapy.

   p. therapy. The therapeutic use of physical agents other than drugs. It comprises the use of physical, chemical, and other properties of heat, light, water, electricity, massage, exercise, and radiation.

   p. therapy technician or aide. A lay assistant or a nurse trained to apply the physical measures of treatment that have been prescribed by a physician.

   p. unit. SEE: *coulomb, erg, dyne;* and *metric system* and *weights and measures* in Appendix.

physician (fĭ-zĭsh´ŭn) [O. Fr. *physicien*]. A person who has successfully completed the prescribed course of studies in medicine in a medical school officially recognized by the country in which it is located and who has acquired the requisite qualifications for licensing in the practice of medicine.

   p., house. P. who lives in a hospital and is available at all times.

   p., primary. The physician to whom a family or individual goes initially when ill or for a periodic health check.

   p., resident. A physician who lives in a hospital to continue his training after internship. Commonly called resident.

physicist (fĭz´ī-sĭst) [L. *physics*, natural sciences]. A specialist in the science of physics.

physico- [Gr. *physikos*]. Combining form indicating physical or natural.

physics (fĭz´ĭks) [Gr. *physis*, nature]. The study of forces and properties of matter, and of natural phenomena.

physinosis (fĭz´ī-nō´sĭs) ["+ *nosos*, disease]. A disease caused by physical agents.

physio- [Gr. *physis*]. Combining form indicating relationship to nature.

physiocogenic (fĭz´´ī-ō-kō-jĕn´ĭk) [Gr. *physikos*, natural, + *gennan*, to produce.]. Originating from physical causes.

physiocopyrexia (fĭz´´ī-ō-kō´´pī-rĕk´sī-ă) ["+ *pyressein*, feverish]. Fever produced artificially by physical means.

physiognomy (fĭz´´ī-ŏg´nō-mĭ) [Gr. *physis*, nature, + *gnōmōn*, a judge]. 1. The countenance. 2. Assumed ability to see the mental or moral character and qualities by the face.

physiognosis (fĭz´´ī-ŏg-nō´sĭs) ["+ *gnōsis*, knowledge]. Diagnosis determined from one's facial expression and appearance of the eyes.

physiological (fĭz´´ī-ō-lŏj´ī-kăl) [Gr. *physis*, nature, + *logos*, study]. 1. Normal; not diseased. 2. Concerning body function.

   p. chemistry. Chemistry of living organisms. SEE: *biochemistry.*

physiological salt solution. An isotonic sterile solution consisting of 0.85% sodium chloride in distilled water. A teaspoonful of table salt in a pint of water approximates a physiological salt solution.

   Used in irrigating mucuos membranes and raw surfaces, in replenishing of body water in dehydration, and in shock or hemorrhage to restore circulating blood volume.

   ABBR: P.S.S. SYN: *normal salt solution; normal saline.* SEE: *enema, physiological salt solution.*

physiology (fĭz´´ī-ŏl´ō-jī) [Gr. *physis*, nature, + *logos*, study]. The science of the functions of cells, tissues, and organs of the living organism.

physiolysis (fĭz´´ī-ŏl´ī-sĭs) ["+ *lysis*, dissolution]. Natural decay and dissolution of tissue.

physiotherapy (fĭz´´ī-ō-thĕr´ă-pĭ) ["+ *therapeia*, treatment]. Treatment with physical and mechanical means, as massage, electricity, etc. SYN: *physical therapy.*

physique (fĭ-zēk′) [Fr.]. Body build; the structure and organization of the body.

physo- [Gr. *physa*, air]. Combining form indicating air or gas.

physocele (fĭ′sō-sēl) [Gr. *physa*, air, + *kēlē*, tumor]. 1. A tumor filled with gas or circumscribed swelling due to gas. 2. A gas-distended hernial sac.

physohematometra (fĭ″sō-hĕm″ă-tō-mē′tră) [″+ *haima*, blood, + *mētra*, uterus]. Gas and blood distending the uterus.

physohydrometra (fĭ″sō-hī″drō-mē′tră) [″+ *hydōr*, water, + *mētra*, uterus]. Air or gas and serum in the uterus.

physometra (fĭ″sō-mē′tră) [Gr. *physa*, air, + *mētra*, uterus]. Air or gas in the uterine cavity.

physopyosalpinx (fĭ″sō-pī″ō-săl′pĭnks) [″+ *pyon*, pus, + *salpinx*, tube]. Pus and gas in the fallopian tube.

physostigmine salicylate (fĭ″sō-stĭg′mĭn săl-ĭs′ĭl-āt). USP. The salicylate of an alkaloid usually obtained from the dried ripe seed of Physostigma venenosum. SYN: *eserine salicylate.*

ACTION AND USES: Cholinergic. It inactivates cholinesterase, thus prolonging and intensifying the action of acetylcholine. It improves the tone and action of skeletal muscle; through its effects on parasympathetic nervous system, it increases intestinal peristalsis; in the eye, it acts as a miotic. It is used in tetanus and strychnine poisoning and in the treatment of myasthenia gravis.

phytalbumose (fĭ-tăl′bū-mōs) [Gr. *phyton*, plant, + L. *albumen*, white protein]. An albumose found in plants and vegetables.

phytase (fĭ′tās) [″+ *ase*, enzyme]. An enzyme found in grains and present in the kidneys; important in splitting phytin or phytic acid into inositol and phosphoric acid.

phytin (fĭ′tĭn). A calcium or magnesium salt of inositol and hexaphosphoric acid, present in cereals. SEE: *inositol.*

phyto-, phyt- [Gr. *phyton*]. Combining forms indicating a plant or that which grows.

phytobezoar (fĭ″tō-bē′zŏr) [Gr. *phyton*, plant, + Persian *badzahr*, concretion]. A mass composed of vegetable matter found in the stomach. SYN: *food ball.*

phytogenesis (fĭ″tō-jĕn′ĕ-sĭs) [″+ *genesis*, generation]. The origin and development of plants. SYN: *phytogeny.*

phytohemagglutinin (fĭ″tō-hĕm-ă-glū′tĭ-nĭn) [″+ *haima*, blood, + L. *agglutināre*, to glue to]. A substance, which present in plants, agglutinates red blood cells.

phytoid (fĭ′toyd) [″+ *eidos*, like]. Plantlike. 1. Any disease of vegetable parasitic origin. 2. The production of a disease by plant parasites. 3. The presence of plant parasites in an organism.

phytonadione (fĭ″tō-nă-dĭ′ōn). USP. Synthetic vitamin K₁. Used as a prothrombogenic agent.

phytosterol (fĭ″tō-stē′rŏl). Any sterol present in vegetable oil or fat.

phytotoxin (fĭ″tō-tŏk′sĭn) [Gr. *phyton*, plant, + *toxicon*, a poison]. A toxin produced by one of the higher plants. EX: ricin from castor bean.

pia (pī′ă, pē′ă) [L.]. Tender, soft. SEE: *pia mater.*

pia-arachnitis (pē″ă-ăr″ăk-nī′tĭs, pī′ă). Piarachnitis, q.v.

pia-arachnoid. Piarachnoid, q.v.

pial (pī′ăl). Concerning the pia mater.

pia mater (pī′a mā′ter, pē′ă mā′ter) [L. *pia*, soft, + *mater*, mother]. A thin vascular membrane closely investing the brain and spinal cord and proximal portions of the nerves. Innermost of the three meninges.

pian (pē-än′) [Fr.]. Contagious skin disease of the tropics. SYN: *yaws.*

pianists′ cramp (pē′ăn-ĭsts, pē-än′ĭsts). Spasm, or occupational neurosis, of muscles of fingers and forearms from piano playing.

piarachnitis (pī-ăr-ăk-nī′tĭs) [L. *pia*, tender, + Gr. *arachnē*, spider, + *-itis*, inflammation]. Inflammation of the arachnoid and pia mater. SYN: *leptomeningitis.*

piarachnoid (pī″ăr-ăk′noyd) [″+ ″+ *eidos*, like]. The pia mater and arachnoid membranes when regarded as one structure. SYN: *leptomeninges; leptomeninx.*

pica (pī′kă) [L., magpie]. A perversion of appetite with craving for substance not fit for food, as the practice by some women in pregnancy of ingesting starch, clay, ashes, or plaster.

Condition seen in pregnancy, chlorosis, hysteria, helminthiasis, and in certain psychoses. SEE: *appetite; taste.*

piceous (pī′sē-ŭs) [L. *piceus*, pitch]. Like pitch.

Pick's disease. 1. [Arnold Pick, Czechoslovakian physician, 1851-1924]. Presenile dementia; a brain disorder involving atrophy of cerebral cortex. SYM: asthenia, loss of speech, progressive dementia.

2. [Friedel Pick, Czechoslovakian physician, 1867-1926]. Nonrheumatic chronic pericarditis of unknown etiology.

3. [Ludwig Pick, Ger. physician, 1868-1935]. Niemann-Pick disease, q.v.

Pickwickian syndrome. [Pickwick, an obese character in the works of Charles

Dickens] Obesity, decreased pulmonary function, and polycythemia.

picornaviruses (pī-kŏr″nă-vī′rū-sĕs) [It. *pico*, small, + RNA, ribonucleic acid, + L. *virus*, virus]. Very small viruses which are insoluble in a lipid solvent such as ether. Those which affect humans have been classified as Coxsackie virus A (24 species), Coxsackie virus B (6 species), ECHO virus (26 species), poliovirus (3 species), and rhinovirus (approx. 75 species).

picrate (pĭk′rāt). A salt of picric acid.

picro-, picr- [Gr. *pikros*, bitter]. Combining forms meaning bitter.

picrocarmine (pĭk″rō-kar′mĭn). A stain used in microscopy.

picroformal (pĭk″rō-fŏr′măl). Solution of picric acid, formaldehyde, and water used as a fixing agent.

picrol (pĭk′rōl). Antiseptic powder used as a dressing for wounds.

picrotoxin (pĭk″rō-tŏk′sĭn) [Gr. *pikros*, bitter, + *toxikon*, poison]. A powerful stimulant to the central nervous system, obtained from the seed of Anamirta cocculus, a shrub. It is used as a respiratory stimulant.

piebald skin (pī′bald) [ME. *pie*, magpie, + *ballede*, bald]. Skin with spots of pigmentation, or patches with loss of pigment. SEE: *leukoderma; vitiligo.*

piedra (pī-ā′drä) [Sp., stone]. A fungus disease, affecting the hair only, in which hard nodules form on the hair shafts. *Black piedra* is caused by the fungus Piedraia hortae, and *white piedra* by Trichosporon beigelii. Either form of the disease is cured by shaving or cutting the hair.

piesesthesia (pī-ē″zĕs-thē′zĭ-ä) [Gr. *piesis*, pressure, + *aisthēsis*, sensation]. Sensibility to pressure. SYN: *pressure sense.*

piesimeter, piesometer (pī″ē-sĭm′ĕ-tĕr, -sŏm′ĕ-tĕr) ["+ *metron*, measure]. Device for measurement of skin's sensitiveness to pressure.

piezogenic pedal papules (pī-ē′zō-jĕn′ĭk) [Gr. *piezein*, to press, + *gennan*, to produce]. Soft painful skin-colored papules present on the nonweight-bearing portion of the heel. They disappear when weight is taken off the foot and heel. Caused by herniation of fat through connective tissue defects.

pigeon breast (pī′jĕn brĕst). Deformity in which the sternum projects anteriorly. SEE: *breast, chicken.*

pigeon-toed (pī′jĕn-tōd″). Pes varus; walking with feet turned inward.

pigment (pĭg′mĕnt) [L. *pigmentum*, paint]. Any organic coloring matter in the body. SEE: *albino;* words beginning with *chrom-.*

p., bile. P. in bile: bilirubin and bileverdin and their derivatives (e.g., urobilinogen, urobilin, bilicyanin, bilifuscin). SEE: *bile pigments.*

p., biliary. Bilirubin, biliverdin, q.v.

p., blood. P. in blood (hemoglobin) or a derivative of it (hematin, hemin, methemoglobin, hemosiderin).

p., endogenous. P. produced within the body, as melanin.

p., exogenous. P. produced outside the human body.

p., hematogenous. P. from hemoglobin of the erythrocytes.

p., hepatogenous. P. from hemoglobin destruction in the liver. SYN: *bile pigment.*

p., skin. Melanin, melanoid, and carotene, q.v.

p., urinary. Urochrome and sometimes urobilin, q.v.

p., uveal. P. found in cells on inner or posterior surface of the iris, choroid, and ciliary processes.

pigmentary (pĭg′mĕn-tĕr′ĭ) [L. *pigmentum*, paint]. Concerning, or like, a pigment.

pigmentation (pĭg″mĕn-tā′shŭn). Coloration due to deposition of pigments.
RS: albinism; carotenemia; words beginning with "chrom-."

pigmentophage (pĭg-mĕn′tō-fāj) [L. *pigmentum*, paint, + Gr. *phagein*, to eat]. Cell that absorbs pigment.

pigmentum nigrum (pĭg-mĕn″tŭm nĭ′grŭm) [L., black paint]. The black pigment of the lamina vitrea of the choroid of the eye.

piitis (pī-ī′tĭs) [L. *pia*, tender, + Gr. *-ītis*, inflammation]. Inflamed condition of the pia mater.

Pil. Abbr. of L. *pilula*, pill, or *pilulae*, pills.

pila (pī′lä) [L., pillar]. (pl. *pi′lae*) A pillarlike structure in spongy bone.

pilar, pilary (pī′lar, pĭl′ă-rĭ) [L. *pilaris*]. Concerning, or covered with, hair.

pilaster (pī-lăs′ter) [L. *pilastrum*, small pillar]. A prominent ridge sometimes seen on the femur.

pile [L. *pila*, a ball, a pillar]. A single hemorrhoid. SEE: *piles.* 2. The hair. 3. A battery for production of electricity. 4. An apparatus for producing and regulating a nuclear chain-reaction fission process.

pileous (pī′lē-ŭs) [L. *pilus*, hair]. Hairy; hirsute.

piles (pīls) [L. *pila*, a mass]. Dilated blood vessels in the rectal mucosa forming a vascular tumor. SYN: *hemorrhoids,* q.v.

pileus (pī′lē-ŭs) [L., a cap]. 1. A hemisphere of the cerebellum. 2. Membrane which sometimes covers the head of an infant at birth. 3. A nipple shield. 4. Top of the head of a bird. SYN: *pileum*.

pili (pī'lē). Plural of pilus. Hairs.

p. annulata. Condition in which hairs have a ringed appearance; monilethrix.

p. incarnati. Condition of ingrowing hair, esp. in the beard area.

p. tactiles. Sensitive or tactile hairs.

p. torti. Condition in which hairs are broken and twisted.

piliation (pī-lī-ā'shŭn) [L. *pilus*, hair]. Formation and development of hair.

piliform (pĭl'ī-form) ["+ *forma*, shape]. Hairlike.

pilimiction (pī"lĭ-mĭk'shŭn) ["+ *mictio*, micturition]. Passing of urine containing hairlike or filamentous substances.

pill (pĭl) [L. *pilula*, small mass]. 1. Medicine in the form of a tiny mass or pellet to be swallowed or chewed. May be coated. 2. In current usage it also means a contraceptive medicine taken as a pill.

pillar (pĭl'ĕr) [L. *pila*, a column]. An upright support; column, or structure resembling a column.

p. of the abdominal ring. One of the columns on either side of abdominal ring.

p.'s, anterior, of fornix. Two diverging columns extending downward from anterior extremity of body of the fornix.

p. cells. Two groups of cells (inner and outer) resting on basement membrane of organ of Corti in which elongated bodies (pillars) develop. These enclose the inner tunnel (Corti's tunnel).

p.'s of Corti. Two layers resting on membrana basilaris in the ear. SYN: *rods of Corti*.

p.'s of diaphragm. Crura of diaphragm, two bundles of muscle fibers extending from lumbar vertebrae to central tendon and forming sides of hiatus aorticus.

p.'s of the fauces. Folds of mucous membrane, one on each side of the fauces, q.v. and between which is situated the tonsil. SYN: *glossopalatine* and *pharyngopalatine arches*.

p.'s, posterior, of fornix. Two bands forming prolongation of fornix posteriorly.

pilleus, pilleum (pĭl'ē-ŭs, -ŭm) [L., a cap]. A membrane sometimes covering a baby's head at birth. SYN: *caul*.

p. ventriculi. The first portion of the duodenum. SYN: *pyloric cap*.

pillion (pĭl'yŭn) [L. *pellis*, skin]. Temporary form of artificial leg, esp. a peg-leg type of stump.

pilo- [L. *pilus*]. Combining form indicating hair.

pilocarpine hydrochlor'ide (pī"lō-kär'-pīn). USP. $C_{11}H_{16}N_2O_2 \cdot HCl$. Hydrochloride of an alkaloid obtained from leaflets of Pilocarpus jaborandi and P. microphyllus.

ACTION AND USES: Cholinergic. Causes contraction of the pupil. Used topically as a miotic, esp. in glaucoma.

p. ni'trate. USP. Nitrate of the alkaloid obtained from leaves of the jaborandi tree.

ACTION AND USES: Same as pilocarpine hydrochloride.

pilocystic (pī"lō-sĭs'tĭk) [L. *pilus*, hair, + Gr, *kystis*, bladder]. Encysted and containing hair, said of a dermoid cyst.

pilojection ["+ *jacere*, to throw]. Introduction of hairs, by use of a pneumatic gun, into an aneurysm to induce clotting in the aneurysmal sac. Has been used in treating intracranial aneurysms.

pilomatrixoma. Benign calcifying tumor of the skin. It is small and firm with normal skin over it.

pilomotor (pī"lō-mō'tor) [L. *pilus*, hair, + *motor*, mover]. Causing movements of hairs, as the arrectores pilorum, q.v.

p. reflex. Gooseflesh formation when skin is cooled or as a result of emotional reaction.

pilonidal (pī"lō-nī'dăl) ["+ *nidus*, nest]. Containing hairs in a dermoid cyst in nest formation.

p. cyst. A cyst in the saccrococcygeal region, usually at the upper end of the intergluteal cleft. The cyst is due to a developmental defect which permits epithelial tissue to be trapped below the skin. May become symptomatic in early adulthood when an infected draining sinus forms.

p. fistula. Fistula beneath the skin at the lower end of the spinal column resulting from a pilonidal cyst.

p. sinus. P. fistula.

pilose (pī'lōs) [L. *pilosus*]. Hairy, downy.

pilosebaceous (pī"lō-sē-bā'shŭs) [L. *pilus*, hair + *sebaceus*, fatty]. Concerning the hair and sebaceous glands.

pilosis (pi-lō'sĭs) [L. *pilosus*, hairy, + Gr. -*ōsis*, intensive]. Excessive formation of hair.

pilosity (pī-lŏs'ĭ-tĭ). Hairiness.

pilous (pī'lŭs) [L. *pilus*, hair]. Covered with hair; hirsute.

Piltz's reflex (pĭltz). [Jan Piltz, Polish neurologist, 1870-1931]. Change in size of pupil on sudden fixation of attention.

pilula (pĭl'ū-lă) [L., pill]. (pl. *pil'ulae*) A small amount of medicine intended to be swallowed whole and to produce medicinal action. May be ready-prepared pills or may be made by the druggist according to prescription. The former often are coated with sugar, gelatin, chocolate, etc.

pilular (pĭl'ū-lar). Pert. to, or of the nature of, pills.

pilus (pī'lŭs) [L.]. (pl. *pi'li*) [NA]. A hair.

pimel- [Gr. *pimelē*, fat]. Combining form or prefix indicating an association with fat.

pimelitis (pĭm-ĕl-ī'tĭs) [Gr. *pimelē*, fat, + *-itis*, inflammation]. Inflammation of adipose, and of connective tissue in general.

pimeloma (pĭm″ē-lō'mä) [″+ *-ōma*, tumor]. A fatty tumor. SYN: *lipoma.*

pimelopterygium (pĭm″ē-lō-tĕ-rĭj'ĭ-ŭm) [″+ *pterygion*, wing]. A fatty outgrowth of the conjunctiva.

pimelorrhea (pĭm″ĕl-ōr-ē'ä) [Gr. *pimelē*, fat, + *rhoia*, flow]. Discharge of fat in loose stools.

pimelorthopnea (pĭm″ĕl-or″thŏp'nē-ä) [″+ *orthos*, straight, + *pnoia*, breath]. Difficulty in breathing when lying down, resulting from obesity.

pimelosis (pĭm″ē-lō'sĭs) [″+ *-ōsis*, intensive]. 1. Conversion into fat. 2. Fatty degeneration of any tissue. 3. Corpulence; obesity.

pimeluria (pĭm″ĕl-ū'rĭ-ä) [″+ *ouron*, urine]. Excretion of fat or oil in urine. SYN: *lipuria.*

pimple (pĭm'pl) [ME. *pinple*]. Protuberance of the skin, sometimes going on to suppuration.

Often seen in clusters on skin of the adolescent. Patients should be warned not to pick at pimples because infection may take place. SYN: *papule; pustule.*

pincement (păns-mä') [Fr.]. Pinching or nipping of the flesh in massage.

pineal (pĭn'ē-ăl) [Fr., pine cone]. 1. Shaped like a pine cone. 2. The small red gland attached to posterior part of third ventricle of brain. 3. Pert. to the pineal body, q.v.

p. body. A small ovoid body that extends from the roof of posterior extremity of third ventricle of brain. Consists of ependymal cells and neuroglia embedded in connective tissue stroma. Often contains calcareous granules (brain sand). SYN: *epiphysis cerebri.*

pinealectomy (pĭn″ē-ăl-ĕk'tō-mĭ) [L. *pineus*, pineal body, + Gr. *ektomē*, excision]. Removal of the pineal body.

pinealism (pĭn″ē-ăl-ĭzm) [″+ Gr. *ismos*, condition]. Disorder caused by abnormal secretion of the pineal body.

pinealoma (pĭn″ē-ă-lō'mä) [″+ Gr. *-ōma*, tumor]. A tumor of the pineal body, usually encapsulated. Often associated with precocious puberty.

pinealopathy (pĭn″ē-ă-lŏp'ă-thĭ) [″+ Gr. *pathos*, disease]. Any disorder of the pineal gland.

pineapple (pīn'ăp-l) [AS. *pinappel*]. A large fruit of the species Ananas comosus. It often ranges from 3 to 5 pounds (1.361-2.268 kilograms) in weight. COMP: Very rich in cane sugar. Contains bromelin, a proteolytic enzyme.

Food value of 100 gm. (raw): Cal. 52; protein 0.4 gm.; trace of fat; carbohydrate 14 gm.; calcium 17 mg.; 70 I.U. vitamin A; ascorbic acid 17 mg.

pineoblastoma (pĭn″ē-ō-blăs-tō'mä) [L. *pineus*, pineal body, + Gr. *blastos*, germ, + *-oma*, tumor]. A blastoma of the pineal body.

pine tar (pīn'tăr). A product obtained from the distillation of pine wood. Used as an expectorant, and in certain skin preparations.

pinguecula (pĭn-gwĕk'ū-lä) [L. *pinguiculus*, fatty]. Yellowish thickening of bulbar conjunctiva, triangular in shape, on inner and outer margins of the cornea. Base of triangle is toward the limbus. Yellowish color is due to increase in elastic fibers.

pinhole (pĭn'hōl) [AS. *pinn*, pin, + *hol*, hole]. Small perforation made by, or size of that made by, a pin.

p. os. A very small os uteri in young women.

p. pupil. Extreme contraction of the iris. The condition is seen in locomotor ataxia, after use of miotics, in some brain diseases, and in opium poisoning.

piniform (pĭn'ĭ-form) [L. *pineas*, pine cone, + *forma*, shape]. Conical; shaped like a pine cone.

pink-eye (pĭnk'ī) [D. *pinck oog*]. Epidemic form of acute conjunctivitis caused by various organisms. Sporadic noninfectious cases may result from irritation by various agents such as intense light, or they may accompany exanthematous disease such as measles.

pinna (pĭn'ä) [L., wing]. (pl. *pinnae*) The auricle or projected part of the exterior ear. It collects and directs sound waves into the external acoustic meatus and thence to the tympanic membrane.

p. nasi. Protruding cartilaginous extension on each nostril. SYN: *ala nasi.*

pinocytosis (pī″nō-sī-tō'sĭs) [Gr. *pinein*, to drink, + *kytos*, cell, + *-ōsis*, condition]. Term for the absorption of liquids by phagocytic cells.

Pins' sign. [Emil Pins, Aust. physician, 1845-1913]. In pericarditis, the disappearance of symptoms of pleurisy when patient assumes knee-chest position.

pint (pīnt) [ME. *pinte*]. In the U.S.A. a measure of capacity equal to one-half a quart; 16 fluid ounces; 473.2 ml. ABBR: pt. SEE: *Table of Weights and Measures* in *Appendix.*

pinta (pēn'tä) [Sp., paint]. A disease caused by the spirochete Treponema carateum. Manifested by depigmented spots or patches. SYN: *azul; carate; mal del pinto; spotted sickness.*

pinworm (pīn'wurm). A parasitic nematode Enterobius vermicularis, causing enterobiasis, infection of intestines and rectum.

pionemia (pī''ō-nē'mī-ā) [Gr. *pion,* fat, + *haima,* blood]. An abnormally large amount of fat in the blood. SYN: *lipemia.*

piper (pī'pĕr) [L.]. Pepper.

piperazine (pī-pĕr'ā-zēn). A white crystalline powder. Used in the treatment of ascariasis and enterobiasis.

pipet, pipette (pī-pĕt') [Fr. *pipette,* tiny pipe]. Narrow glass tube with both ends open for transferring and measuring liquids by sucking them into the tube.

piptonychia (pīp''tō-nĭk'ĭ-ā) [Gr. *piptein,* to fall, + *onych-,* nails]. The shedding of nails.

Pirogoff's amputation (pīr''ō-gŏf'). [Nicolai I. Pirogoff, Russian surgeon 1810-1881]. Foot amputation at the ankle, removing a portion of the os calcis.

Pirquet's test (pĕr-kā'). [Clemens P. Pirquet, Aust. pediatrician, 1874-1929]. Test for tuberculosis by means of a skin reaction, used esp. in children.

pisiform (pī'sĭ-form) [L. *pisum,* pea, + *forma,* shape]. 1. Name of small pealike sesamoid bone of the wrist. 2. Peashaped. 3. The smallest carpal bone, located in proximal row on ulnar side.

pit (pĭt) [ME. *pitt,* hole]. 1. A tiny hollow or pocket. SYN: *depression; fossa.* 2. To be or become marked with a shallow depression; to cause a depression on pressure in edema.

p., auditory. A pit which develops in auditory placode.

p., gastric. One of many minute depressions (foveolae) in gastric mucosa into which the gastric glands open.

p., nasal. One of two horseshoe-shaped depressions on ventrolateral surface of head bounded by lateral and median nasal processes. It gives rise to nostrils and portion of nasal fossa.

p., olfactory. Nasal pit, q.v.

p., primitive. Minute depression at anterior end of primitive groove or streak and immediately posterior to primitive knot.

p. of the stomach. 1. Depression at end of the ensiform process. 2. The center of the abdominal region above the navel. SYN: *scrobiculus cordis.*

pitch (pĭch) [ME. *picchen,* to fix]. That quality of the sensation of sound that enables one to classify it in a scale from high to low. It is dependent principally on frequency of vibrations.

pithecoid (pĭth'ē-koyd) [Gr. *pithēkos,* ape, + *eidos,* like]. Apelike; resembling an ape.

pithiatic (pĭth-ĭ-at'ĭk) [Gr. *peithein,* to persuade, + *iatrikos,* healing]. Capable of being soothed or relieved by persuasion or by suggestion.

pithiatism (pĭth-ĭ'ă-tĭzm) ["+ *iatos,* curable]. 1. Hysteria induced by suggestion. 2. To cure mental disorder by suggestion.

pithing (pĭth'ĭng) [ME. *pithe*]. Destruction of the central nervous system by the piercing of brain or spinal cord, as in vivisection. Done on experimental animals to render them insensible to pain and to inhibit controlling effects of the central nervous system. SYN: *decerebration.*

pitocin (pī-to'sĭn). Proprietary name for an aqueous solution containing the oxytocic fraction of the posterior pituitary gland. SEE: *oxytocin injection.*

Pitres' sections (pē-trēs'). [Jean A. Pitres, Fr. physician, 1848-1927]. Series of six coronal vertical sections of the brain for study. The sections are prefrontal, pediculofrontal, frontal, parietal, pediculoparietal, and occipital.

pitressin (pĭt-rĕs'ĭn). Proprietary name for vasopressin, a product obtained from the posterior lobe of the pituitary gland containing pressor and antidiuretic principles. SEE: *principle, antidiuretic; vasopressin.*

USES: Increasing blood pressure, increasing the muscular contraction of the intestinal tract, and diminishing urinary output in diabetes insipidus.

pitting (pĭt'ĭng) [ME. *pitt,* hole]. The formation of pits, depressions, or scars, as in smallpox.

pituicyte (pī-tū'ĭ-sĭt) [L. *pituita,* phlegm, + Gr. *kytos,* cell]. A branched, modified, neuroglia cell characteristic of pars nervosa of posterior lobe of pituitary gland. Also present in infundibular stalk.

pituitarism (pĭt-ū'ĭ-tā-rĭzm) ["+ Gr. *ismos,* condition]. Any disorder of the pituitary gland and its function.

pituitarium (pī-tū'ī-tār'ĭ-ŭm) [L.]. Pituitary, q.v.

pituitary (pī-tū'ĭ-tār'ĭ) [L. *pituitārius,* phlegm]. 1. Concerning phlegm. 2. The pituitary body or gland, q.v.; the hypophysis cerebri.

p., anterior. Preparation consisting of dried, defatted, powdered anterior lobe of p. gland of domestic animals.

p. body. SEE: *p. gland.*

p. disorders. Hypersecretion of anterior lobe: gigantism, acromegaly, p. basophilism (Cushing's disease). *Hyposecretion of anterior lobe:* dwarfism, p. cachexia (Simmond's disease), Sheehan's syndrome, acromicria, eunuchoidism or hypogonadism. *Posterior lobe deficiency or hypothalamic lesion:* diabetes insipidus. *Anterior and posterior lobe deficiency and hypothalamic lesion:* Frohlich's syndrome (adiposogenital dystrophy), p. obesity.

p. gland. A small, gray, rounded body attached to the base of the brain by the infundibular stalk, a downward extension of the floor of the third ventricle. It averages 1.3 x 1.0 x 0.5 cm. in size and 0.55 to 0.6 gm. in weight. SYN: *hypophysis cerebri.*

FUNCTIONS: The p. is an endocrine gland secreting a number of hormones which regulate many bodily processes including growth, reproduction, and various metabolic activities. It is often referred to as the master gland of the body.

Evidence indicates that the hormones are secreted by neurosecretory cells of the hypothalamus and pass through fibers of the supraopticohypophyseal tracts in the infundibular stalk to the neurohypophysis where they are stored.

Hormones are secreted in the following lobes: *Intermediate lobe:* In cold-blooded animals, intermedin is secreted, influencing the activity of pigment cells (chromatophores) of fishes, amphibians, and reptiles. In warm-blooded animals no effects are known.

Anterior lobe: somatotrophic, or growth, hormone (STH), which regulates growth; adrenocorticotrophic hormone (ACTH), which regulates functional activity of the adrenal cortex; thyrotrophic hormone (TTH), which regulates functional activity of thyroid gland; gonadotrophic hormones which include follicle-stimulating hormone (FSH) which stimulates development of ovarian follicles and spermatogenesis in the testis, luteinizing hormone (LH), also called interstitial cell stimulating hormone (ICSH), which in conjunction with FSH induces secretion of estrogens, ovulation, and development of corpus luteum, and luteotrophic hormone (LTH), which maintains mature corpora lutea and induces secretion of progesterone. It also induces secretion of milk in a fully developed mammary gland. Because of this action, it is sometimes called the lactogenic hormone.

Posterior lobe: oxytocin, which acts specifically on smooth muscle of uterus increasing tone and contractility; vasopressin, which induces contraction of smooth muscles of the blood vessels. The latter is associated with an antidiuretic principle which prevents excessive loss of water through the kidneys.

p., posterior. Dried, powdered posterior lobe of p. gland of animals used as food by man.

p., whole. Dried, defatted, powdered entire p. gland of domestic animals.

pituitrin (pĭ-tū′ĭ-trĭn). Proprietary name for posterior pituitary extract.

ACTION AND USES: Used to stimulate contraction of blood vessels, peristalsis in intestines, and uterine contractions in labor.

pityriasis (pĭt′ĭ-rī′ă-sĭs) [Gr. *pityron,* bran, + *-iasis,* disease]. A skin disease characterized by branny scales.

p. alba. Superficial eczema of unknown etiology.

p. amiantacea. Sticky scaling of the scalp following infection or trauma. SYN: *tinea amiantacea.*

p. capitis. Dandruff, q.v.

p. lichenoides, acute. A skin disorder characterized by development of an edematous pink papule which undergoes central vesiculation and hemorrhagic necrosis. This may progress to a depressed scar or ulcer.

p. linguae. Transitory benign plaques of the tongue.

p. nigra. Tinea nigra, q.v.

p. rosea. A skin disease characterized by development of distributed patches which are circinate in outline, slightly scaly, a faint red color. SYN: *p. maculata et circinata.*

Acute inflammatory disease marked by a macular eruption on the trunk, obliquely to the ribs. Rose red and somewhat scaly with a clearing in the center, or reddish ring-shaped patches symmetrically distributed over the limbs.

ETIOL: Unknown.

SYM: Macular or circinate lesions; yellowish, salmon or red; rounded, oval or irregular; thinly covered with fine branny scales, increasing in size; when centers clear up, giving rise to slightly elevated reddish rings with fawn-colored centers, coalescence of rings resulting in segmental or gyrate lesions of various sizes. Spontaneous disappearance within three to four weeks but may last several months.

TREATMENT: Locally: antipruritics.

p. rubra pilaris. Persistent general exfoliative dermatitis of unknown etiology.

p. versicolor. A mild, chronic, symptomless fungus infection of the superficial layer of the skin. Characterized by scaly discolored areas. Due to a fungus Malassezia furfur. Treatment is necessary only for cosmetic purposes.

pityroid (pĭt′ĭ-royd) [Gr. *pityron*, bran, + *eidos*, like]. Branny; resembling bran.

pix (piks) [L.]. Pitch.

PK. Abbr. for *psychokinesis.*

PKU. Abbr. for *phenylketonuria.*

placebo (plă-sē′bō) [L., I shall please]. Inactive substance given to satisfy patient's demand for medicine.

Also used in controlled studies of drugs. The placebo is given to a group of patients, and the drug being tested is given to a similar group; then the results obtained in the two groups are compared.

placenta (plă-sĕn′ta) [L., a flat cake]. (pl. *placentae, placentas*) [NA]. The oval or discoid spongy structure in the uterus through which the fetus derives its nourishment.

The placenta consists of a fetal portion, the chorion frondosum, bearing many chorionic villi that interlock with the decidua basalis of the uterus which constitutes the maternal portion. The chorionic villi lie in spaces in the uterine endometrium where they are bathed in maternal blood and lymph. Groups of villi are separated by placental septa forming about twenty distinct lobules called cotyledons.

Attached to the margin of the placenta is a membrane which encloses the embryo. It is a composite of several structures (decidua parietalis, decidua capsularis, chorion laeve, and amnion). At the center of the concave side is attached the umbilical cord through which the umbilical vessels (two arteries and one vein) pass to the fetus. The cord is approx. 50 cm. long at full term.

The mature placenta is 15 to 18 cm. (6 to 7 in.) in diameter and weighs about 450 gm. (1 lb.). When expelled following parturition it is known as the afterbirth.

Maternal blood enters the intervillous spaces of the placenta through spiral arteries, branches of the uterine arteries. It bathes the chorionic villi and flows peripherally to the marginal sinus which leads to uterine veins. Food substances, oxygen, and antibodies pass into fetal blood of the villi; metabolic waste products pass from fetal blood into the mother's blood. In general, there is no admixture of fetal and maternal blood. The placenta also serves as an endocrine organ. It produces chorionic gonadotrophins, the presence of which in urine is the basis of pregnancy tests. Estrogen and progesterone are also secreted by the placenta.

p., abruption of. Premature separation of placenta. SYN: *abruptio placentae,* q.v.

p. accreta. A placenta in which the cotyledons have invaded the uterine musculature and, as a result of this, separation of the placenta is very difficult or even impossible.

p., adherent. P. that remains adherent to the uterine wall after normal period following childbirth.

p., annular. A p. that extends like a belt around the interior of the uterus.

p., battledore. A form of insertion of the umbilical cord into margin of the p. in which it spreads out to resemble a battledore.

p., bipartite. P. that is divided into two separate parts. SYN: *p. bipartita.*

p., circinate. P. that is cup-shaped.

p. cirsoides. P. with appearance of varicose veins.

p., cordiform. P. having a marginal indentation giving it a heart shape.

p., deciduate. A p. of which the maternal part escapes with delivery.

p., discoid. P. which constitutes practically one mass, circumscribed and circular in form.

p., double. A placental mass of the two placentae of a twin gestation.

p. duplex. P. bipartite, q.v.

p., fetal. That part of the p. formed by aggregation of chorionic villi in which the umbilical vein and arteries ramify.

p., fundal. P. attached to the uterine wall within the fundal zone.

p., horseshoe. A formation in which the two placentae of a twin gestation are united.

p., incarcerated. P. retained in the uterus by irregular uterine contractions after delivery.

p., lateral. P. attached to lateral wall of uterus.

p., maternal. Portion of p. that develops from decidua basalis of uterus.

p., membranous. A thinning of the p. from atrophy.

p., nondeciduate. One that does not shed the maternal portion.

p. previa. Placenta which is implanted in the lower uterine segment. There are three types: centralis, lateralis, and marginalis. *Placenta previa centralis* is the condition where the placenta has been implanted in the lower uterine segment and has grown to completely cover the internal cervical os. *Placenta previa lateralis* is the condition when the placenta lies just within the lower uterine segment. *Placenta previa marginalis* is the condition where the placenta partially covers the internal cervical os.

SYM: Slight hemorrhage, recurrent with greater severity, appears 7th or 8th month; gradual anemia, pallor, rapid weak pulse, air hunger, low blood pressure.

DIAG: Painless bleeding during last three months; placenta in lower portion of uterus.

PROG: Depends upon control of hemorrhage and asepsis.

TREATMENT: Conserve blood supply during delivery and before; prevent and control postpartum hemorrhage; combat anemia before and after labor; and prevention of sepsis.

p. reniformis. A kidney-shaped placenta.

p., retained. P. not expelled for two hours after 2nd stage of labor.

p. spuria. An outlying portion of p. which has not maintained its vascular connection with the decidua vera.

p. succenturiata. An accessory p.

p. tripartita. A three-lobed p.

p., triple. A placental mass of three placentae of a triple gestation.

p., velamentous. A p. with the umbilical cord attached to the membrane a short distance from the placenta, the vessels entering the placenta at its margin.

p., zonary. Annular p., q.v.

placental (plă-sĕn'tăl) [L. *placenta,* a flat cake]. Rel. to the placenta.

p. bruit, p. souffle. Sound heard in auscultation over the placenta in pregnancy; due to circulation of the blood.

placentation (plă"sĕn-tā'shŭn). The process of formation and attachment of the placenta.

placentitis (plă"sĕn-tī'tĭs) [L. *placenta,* flat cake, + Gr. *-itis,* inflammation]. Inflamed condition of placenta.

placentography (plă"sĕn-tŏg'ră-fĭ) ["+ Gr. *graphein,* to write]. Examination of the placenta by roentgenography.

placentoid (plă-sĕn'toyd) [L. *placenta,* flat cake, + Gr. *eidos,* like]. Like the placenta.

placentolysin (plă"sĕn-tŏl'ĭ-sĭn) ["+ Gr. *lysis,* dissolution]. A lysin obtained by injecting placental tissue into an animal, the serum thus obtained being destructive to placental cells of the species of animal from which the placenta was originally taken.

placentoma (plă"sĕn-tō'mă) ["+ Gr. *-ōma,* tumor]. A new growth derived from retained placental tissue.

placentotherapy (plă-sĕn"tō-thĕr'ă-pĭ) ["+ Gr. *therapeia,* treatment]. Therapeutic use of placental extract.

Placido's disk (plă-sē'dō). [Antonio Placido, Portuguese ophthalmologist, 1848-1916]. A disk marked with black and white circles used in determining amt. and character of corneal astigmatism.

placode (plăk'ōd) [Gr. *plax,* plate, + *eidos,* form]. In embryology, a platelike thickening of epithelium, usually ectoderm, which serves as the anlage of an organ or structure.

p., auditory. A dorsolateral placode located alongside hindbrain which gives rise to otocyst which in turn develops into internal ear.

p., lens. P. developing in ectoderm directly overlying optic vesicle. Forms lens vesicle which becomes enclosed in optic cup and eventually becomes lens of eye.

p., olfactory. P. which gives rise to olfactory pit and finally major portion of nasal cavity.

pladaroma (plăd-ă-rō'mă) [Gr. *pladaros,* damp, + *-ōma,* tumor]. A soft growth like a wart on the eyelid.

pladarosis (plăd-ă-rō'sĭs) ["+ *-ōsis,* disease]. Pladaroma.

plagiocephalic (plā-jĭ-ō-sĕ-făl'ĭk) [Gr. *plagios,* oblique, + *kephalē,* head]. Marked by or rel. to plagiocephaly.

plagiocephalism (plā"jĭ-ō-sĕf'ă-lĭzm). Plagiocephaly, q.v.

plagiocephaly (plā"jĭ-ō-sĕf'ă-lĭ). Malformation of the skull producing the appearance of a twisted and lopsided head. Due to irregular closure of the cranial sutures.

plague (plāg) [ME., calamity]. 1. A word once used to describe any widespread contagious disease associated with a high death rate. Now applied specifically to disease caused by Pasteurella pestis infection. 2. A highly fatal disease with high fever, restlessness, staggering gait, mental confusion, prostration, delirium, shock, and coma. Exists in several forms: *bubonic* with acutely inflamed lymph nodes (buboes); *septicemic* with absence of buboes; *primary pneumonic* characterized by pulmonary symptoms. The pneumonic form may be spread from man to man by droplets. Streptomycin, tetracyclines, and chloramphenicol are effective in treating plague.

p., ambulatory. Mild but often fatal. SYN: *pestis minor.*

p., black. An epidemic disease with high mortality that swept Europe during the 14th century. So called because of appearance of petechiae or black spots about 3rd day of disease. SYN: *black death.*

p., bubonic. The more common form of plague marked by formation of buboes.

p., murine. Plague infecting rats.

p., pneumonic. A highly virulent form of plague with extensive involvement of the lungs. Occurs as sequela of bubonic plague, or as a primary infection.

p., septicemic. Bubonic plague accompanied by septicemia.

p., sylvatic. Plague infecting various species of rodents.

plane (plān) [L. *planus*]. 1. A flat or relatively smooth surface. SYN: *planum*. 2. A flat surface formed by making a cut, imaginary or real, through the body or a part of it. Planes are used as points of reference by which positions of parts of the body are indicated. In the human subject, all planes are based on body being in an upright, anatomic position, q.v.

p.'s, Addison's. Planes used as landmarks in thoracoabdominal topography.

p., Aeby's. P. perpendicular to the median plane of the cranium through the basion and nasion.

p., alveolocondylar. P. tangent to the alveolar point with most prominent points on lower aspects of condyles of the occipital bone.

p., Baer's. P. through upper border of the zygomatic arches.

p., coccygeal. The fourth parallel plane of the pelvis.

p., coronal. Vertical p. at right angles to a sagittal p. dividing the body into anterior and posterior portions.

p., datum. An assumed horizontal p. from which craniometric measurements are taken.

p., Daubenton's. P. passing through the opisthion and inferior borders of the orbits.

p.'s, focal. Two planes through anterior and posterior principal foci of a dioptric system and perpendicular to the line connecting the two.

p., frontal. A coronal plane, q.v.

p., Hodge's. P. running parallel to the pelvic inlet and passing through the 2nd sacral vertebra and upper border of the os pubis.

p., horizontal. A transverse plane at right angles to the vertical axis of body.

p.'s, inclined, of the pelvis. Anterior and posterior inclined planes of the pelvic cavity, two unequal sections divided by the sciatic spines. In the larger, anterior section, the lateral walls slope toward the symphysis and arch of the pubes; and the posterior walls slope in the direction of the sacrum and coccyx. The anterior inclined planes are the declivities over which rotation of the occiput takes place in the mechanism of normal labor.

p., intertubercular. A horizontal plane passing through tubercles of crests of ilia. Lies approximately at level of 5th lumbar vertebra.

p., Listing's. A transverse vertical p. lying perpendicular to anteroposterior axis of the eye and containing center of motion of the eyes. In it also lie the transverse and vertical axes of voluntary ocular rotation.

p., Mechel's. P. through the auricular and alveolar points.

p., medial; p. median; p. mesial. Anteroposterior p. dividing a body or organ into two equal and symmetrical parts. The median p. of the body is known as the meson.

p., midsagittal. Vertical p. dividing body into symmetrical right and left halves.

p., Morton's. P. passing through the most projecting points of the parietal and occipital protuberances.

p.'s, parallel, of the pelvis. P.'s intersecting the axis of the pelvic canal at right angles. The first plane is that of the superior strait. The second plane is that extending from middle of the sacral verte-

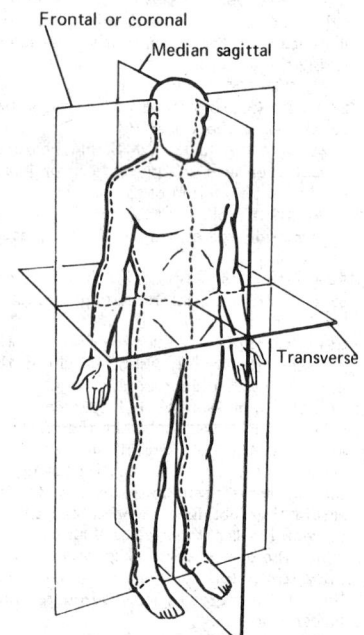

Frontal or coronal

Median sagittal

Transverse

BODY PLANES

bra to the level of the subpubic ligament. The third plane is at the level of spines of the ischia, and the fourth plane is at the outlet.

p.'s of the pelvis. Imaginary ones touching the same parts of the pelvic canal on both sides.

p. of refraction. P. passing through a refracted ray of light and drawn perpendicular to the surface at which refraction takes place.

p. of regard. P. through the fovea of the eye and fixation point.

p., sagittal. Vertical p. parallel to the midsagittal p. One which divides body into right and left portions.

p., subcostal. Horizontal p. passing through lowest points of 10th costal cartilages. Lies approximately at level of 3rd lumbar vertebra.

p., transverse. A horizontal p.

p., visual. P. passing the visual axis of the eye.

planigram (plā'nĭ-grăm) [L. *planus*, plane, + Gr. *gramma*, mark]. An x-ray photograph of a layer or section of the body.

planimeter (plă-nĭm'ĕ-ter) ["+ Gr. *metron*, measure]. Apparatus used to measure the area of a plane figure by passing a tracer around the boundaries.

planoconcave (plā"nō-kŏn'kāv) ["+ *concavus*, hollow]. Flat on one side and concave on the other.

planoconvex (plā"nō-kŏn'vĕks) [L. *planus*, flat, + L. *convexus*, arched]. Flat on one side and convex on the other.

planomania (plā"nō-mā'nĭ-ă) [Gr. *plane*, wandering, + Gr. *mania*, madness]. Morbid desire to wander and to be free of social restraints.

Planorbis (plăn-ōr'bĭs). A genus of freshwater snails serving as intermediate hosts for certain species of blood flukes (Schistosoma).

plant (plănt) [L. *planta*, a sprout]. An organism which contains chlorophyll and manufactures carbohydrates from carbon dioxide and water or, if lacking these characteristics, is similar in structure and life history to those organisms which do possess chlorophyll and manufacture food.

planta (plăn'tă) [L.]. (pl. *plantae*) [NA]. The sole of the foot.

plantar (plăn'tăr). Concerning the sole of the foot.

p. arch. Vascular arch in sole of foot. The union of the plantar and dorsalis pedis arteries in the sole. SYN: *arcus plantaris.*

p. reflex. Contraction of toes upon irritation of the sole.

p. wart. Wart occurring on sole of the foot; usually quite painful. SYN: *verruca plantaris.*

plantarflexion. Extension of the foot so that the forepart is depressed with respect to the position of the ankle. SEE: *dorsiflexion.*

plantaris (plăn-tăr'ĭs) [L.]. [NA]. A long slim muscle of the calf between the gastrocnemius and soleus. It is sometimes double and at other times missing.

plan'tigrade [L. *planta*, sole, + *gradi*, to walk]. Type of foot posture in which entire sole of foot is placed on ground in walking. EX: bear, rabbit, man.

planum (plā'nŭm) [L.]. (pl. *pla'na*) A flat or relatively smooth surface. A plane, q.v.

p. nuchale. Outer surface of occipital bone between foramen magnum and superior nuchal line.

p. occipitale. Outer surface of occipital bone lying above superior nuchal line.

p. orbitale. Portion of maxilla which forms greater part of floor of orbit.

p. popliteum. Smooth triangular area on posterior surface of distal end of femur. Bordered by medial and lateral supracondylar lines and forms floor of popliteal fossa.

p. sternale. Anterior or ventral surface of sternum.

p. temporale. Depressed area on side of skull below inferior temporal line. Underlies the temporal fossa.

planuria (plā-nū'rĭ-ă) [Gr. *plane*, wandering, + *ouron*, urine]. The voiding of urine from an abnormal passage of the body.

plaque (plăk) [Fr., a plate]. 1. A patch on the skin or on a mucous surface. 2. A blood platelet.

p., dental. A gummy mass of microorganisms which grows on the crowns and spreads along the roots of teeth. It usually is too small to be seen and is both colorless and transparent. Dental plaques are the forerunners of dental caries and periodontal disease. They may be prevented by proper daily self-care of the teeth. SEE: *caries; periodontitis; pyorrhea.*

plasma (plăz'mă) [Gr. *plasma*, a thing formed]. 1. The liquid part of the lymph and of the blood. 2. Protoplasm, cell substance outside the nucleus. 3. An ointment base of glycerol and starch.

In the blood, corpuscles and platelets float in p. It consists of serum, q.v., and protein substances in solution.

Blood plasma consists of water in which numerous chemical compounds, both solids and gases, are dissolved. Included are water, electrolytes, sugar, glucose, proteins, nonprotein nitrogenous compounds and fats, bile pigment or bilirubin, gases.

In general, plasma is a medium for circulation of blood cells, carries nutritive substances to various structures, and removes waste products of metabolism from those structures. P. makes possible chemical communication between different portions of the body, carrying minerals, hormones, vitamins, and antibodies.

Different constituents of p. have specific functions within the blood. Proteins, bicarbonates, carbon dioxide, chlorides, phosphates, and ammonia serve to keep the acid-base equilibrium of the blood constant when acid or base substances are added to it. Proteins, esp. albumin, by virtue of their osmotic pressure, tend to prevent undue leakage of fluids out of the capillaries and to maintain a proper exchange of fluid between capillaries and tissues.

Normal plasma is thin and colorless when free from corpuscles, or it has a faint yellow tinge when seen in thick layers.

After clotting of the blood, the liquid squeezed out by the clot is called blood serum. If whole blood is prevented from clotting either by chilling it or by adding anticoagulants, such as sodium citrate, it can be centrifuged. The clear fluid which then occupies the upper half of the centrifuge tube is called plasma. SEE: *blood; coagulation; serum.*

p., blood. Fluid in which cellular elements of the blood are suspended.

p. cell. Cell found in bone marrow and loose connective tissue, probably derived from lymphocytes. SEE: *plasmocyte.*

p. expander. A synthetic solution given intravenously to increase the plasma volume. Used to treat loss of whole blood or plasma. Ex: dextran.

p., lymph. Lymph without its corpuscles.

p., normal human. Sterile pooled plasma obtained from citrated whole blood of eight or more healthy human subjects. It is stored as fluid plasma at 4° C. or as dried plasma prepared by lyophilization technique, i.e., drying in a vacuum at low temperatures. Its usefulness is limited by its ability to cause infectious hepatitis.

plasmacyte (plăz′mă-sĭt) [Gr. *plasma*, a thing formed, + *kytos*, cell]. A plasma cell, one of those found in connective tissue with an eccentrically placed round nucleus and filled with a chromatin mass that stains deeply.

plasmacytoma (plăz″ma-sĭ-tō′mă) ["+ "+ -*ōma*, tumor]. A plasma cell myeloma occur-

ring in bone marrow. SEE: *myeloma, multiple.*

plasmagel (plăz′mă-jĕl″) [Gr. *plasma*, a thing formed, + L. *gelāre*, to congeal]. The peripheral portion of the endoplasm of a cell such as in an ameba. It is immobile and of the nature of a gel.

plasmagene (plăz′mă-jēn″) ["+ *gennan*, to produce]. A cytoplasmic hereditary determiner.

plasmapheresis (plăz″mă-fēr-ē′sĭs) ["+ *aphairesis*, removal]. The removal of blood from the body and centrifuging it. The packed red cells then are suspended in a physiological solution. They may be reinjected into the donor or injected into a patient who requires red cells rather than whole blood.

plasmasome (plăz′mă-sōm) ["+ *sōma*, body]. A leukocyte granule; nucleolar substance (nonchromatin-staining) in the cytoplasm.

plasmatherapy (plăz″mă-thĕr′ă-pī) [Gr. *plasma*, a thing formed, + *therapeia*, service]. The use of blood plasma for therapeutic purposes, as injection in treatment of shock.

plasmatic (plăz-măt′ĭk). 1. Rel. to plasma. 2. Formative or plastic.

p. layer. Blood plasma adjacent to the capillary walls. SYN: *plasmic.*

plasmatorrhexis (plăz″mă-tō-rĕk′sĭs) [Gr. *plasma*, a thing formed, + *rhēxis*, rupture]. Rupture of a cell with loss of its plasma, caused by internal pressure due to swelling.

plasmin (plăz′mĭn). Fibrinolytic enzyme derived from its precursor plasminogen.

plasminogen (plăz-mĭn′ō-jĕn). A protein found in many tissues and body fluids. It is important in preventing fibrin clot formation.

plasmocyte (plăz′mō-sĭt″) [Gr. *plasma*, a thing formed, + *kytos*, cell]. Cells found in bone marrow, connective tissue, and sometimes in blood plasma. Considered by some to be abnormal leukocytes. They are numerous in plasma cell myeloma. SYN: *plasma cell.*

plasmocytoma (plăz″mō-sĭ-tō′mă) ["+ "+ -*ōma*, tumor]. A plasma cell myeloma.

Plasmodium (plăz-mō′dĭ-ŭm). (pl. *plasmodia*). A genus of protozoa belonging to subphylum Sporozoa, class Telosporidea. Includes causative agents of malaria in man and lower animals. SEE: *malaria; mosquito.*

P. falciparum. Causative agent for malignant tertian (estivo-autumnal) malaria.

P. malariae. Causative agent for quartan malaria.

P. ovale. Causative agent for benign tertian or ovale malaria.

P. vivax. Causative agent for benign tertian or vivax malaria.

plasmodium (plăz-mō'dĭ-ŭm) [Gr. *plasma*, a thing formed, + *eidos*, form]. (pl. *plasmodia*). A multinucleate mass of naked protoplasm, occurring commonly among slime molds.

plas"mog'amy ["+ *gamos*, marriage]. The fusion of cells.

plasmogen (plăz'mō-jĕn) ["+ *gennan*, to produce]. Essential part of protoplasm.

plasmology (plăz-mŏl'ō-jĭ) [Gr. *plasma*, a thing formed, + *logos*, a study]. The study of the cells and plasma. SYN: *histology.*

plasmolysis (plăz-mŏl'ĭ-sĭs) ["+ *lysis*, dissolution]. Shrinking of cytoplasm in a living cell due to loss of water by osmosis.

plasmolyze (plăz'mō-līz). To bring about loss of water by osmosis.

plasmorrhexis (plăz"mo-rĕk'sĭs) ["+ *rhēxis*, rupture]. Rupture of a cell with loss of plasma. SYN: *erythrocytorrhexis; erythrorrhexis; plasmatorrhexis.*

plasmoschisis (plăz-mŏs'kĭ-sĭs) [Gr. *plasma*, a thing formed, + *schisis*, a splitting]. The splitting of a cell.

plasmotomy (plăz-mŏt'ō-mĭ) ["+ *tomē*, incision]. Mitosis in which the cytoplasm divides into two or more masses.

plasmotropism (plăz-mŏt'rō-pĭzm) ["+ *tropein*, to turn, + *ismos*, condition]. The action of spleen, liver, and bone marrow, causing the destruction of red blood cells.

plasson (plăs'ŏn) [Gr. *plassōn*, forming]. Primitive protoplasm in cytode or non-nucleated cell stage.

plaster (plăs'tŭr) [Gr. *emplastron*]. External medicinal preparation in which the constituents are formed into a tenacious mass of substance harder than an ointment and spread upon muslin, linen, skin, or paper. Mustard or belladonna may be applied to check secretions, allay pain, or act as a counterirritant.

p., adhesive. Plaster made of a strong cloth coated on one side with an adhesive substance. Used to immobilize a part, to relieve pressure upon sutures, to protect wounds, to secure traction in fractures, to exert pressure, to hold dressings in place, etc. Hair on the area should be removed before applying any plaster. P. should never be applied to abraded or raw surfaces. In reapplying, dead skin should be removed. Surface should be dry and clean. Removal should be made by stripping from both ends up to the wound, first moistening with benzine or ether.

p. bandage. Bandage stiffened with plaster of Paris.

p., blistering. P. made of cantharides.

p. jacket. P. for the trunk made of plaster of Paris.

p., mustard. P. made of powdered mustard paste spread on cloth; used as a rubefacient.

p. of Paris. Gypsum cement, $CaSo_4 \cdot 1/2H_2O$, mixed with water to form a paste which sets rapidly; used to make casts and stiff bandages.

p., porous. Perforated p.; plaster spread on a cloth perforated with holes.

p., resin; p., rosin. P. containing resin, wax, and lead plaster; used as a soothing agent, esp. for children.

p., rubber. SEE: *adhesive p.*

p., warming. P. of cantharides and pitch employed as a counterirritant.

plas'ter cast. Rigid dressing made of gauze impregnated with plaster of Paris, used to immobilize an injured part, esp. in bone fractures.

NP: Patient's position is indicated by fracture. A fracture table should be used when possible and various supplies should be in readiness. Place a plaster bandage, end up, in tepid water. When about saturated, water is gently squeezed by pressing both ends (otherwise the plaster will be forced out through the ends of bandage). As one bandage is passed to the physician, another is placed in water. There should be extra plaster of Paris in perforated cans so it can be shaken on in smoothing the cast.

plastic (plăs'tĭk) [Gr. *plastikos*, fit for molding]. 1. Capable of being molded. 2. Contributing to building tissues.

p. bronchitis. Bronchitis with fibrin exudate adhering in the form of a cast to the bronchial tubes.

p. force. The impetus that builds tissues; generative force.

p. lymph. The exudate covering inflamed serous surfaces, as in wounds.

p. surgery. The restoration and repair of external physical defects by use of grafts of bone or tissues. SEE: *chalinoplasty.*

plasticity (plăs-tĭs'ĭ-tĭ). The ability to be molded.

plastid (plăs'tĭd) [Gr. *plastos*, formed]. A cytoplasmic organoid found in plant cells. Includes *chloroplasts* (which contain chlorophyll), *leukoplasts* (colorless), *chromoplasts* (contain pigment), and *amyloplasts* (store starch). Plastids are centers of chemical activity involved in cell metabolism.

plas'tron [Fr., breastplate]. The sternum and attached cartilages.

plate (plāt) [Gr. *platē*, flat]. 1. A thin flattened part or portion. SYN: *lamina, lamella.* 2. A flattened process of bone. SYN: *lamina, lamella.* 3. An artificial denture or structure for holding false teeth. 4. A shallow covered dish for culturing microorganisms. 5. To inoculate and culture microorganisms in a culture plate.

   p., approximation. A disk of decalcified bone used in intestinal surgery.

   p., auditory. Bony roof of the external auditory meatus.

   p., axial. The primitive streak of the embryo.

   p., blood. Platelet.

   p., bone. Flat, round or oval, decalcified bone or metal disk, employed in pairs, used in approximation.

   p., culture. A small, covered plastic or glass dish containing a bacterial culture medium, such as agar.

   p., dorsal. One of two prominences of the notochord in the embryo.

   p., end. The terminal mass of a nerve fiber ending on a muscle cell.

   p., foot. [NA]. Flat portion of stapes. SYN: *basis stapedis*

   p., medullary. Central portion of the ectoderm in the embryo developing into neural canal.

   p., neural. SEE: *p., medullary.*

   p., palate. Part of the palate bone forming the lateral half of roof of mouth.

   p., tympanic. Bony plate between anterior wall of the external auditory meatus and the tympanum.

platelet (plāt'lĕt) [Gr. *platē*, flat]. A round or oval disk, 2-4 micra (micrometers) in diameter, found in the blood of vertebrates. Platelets number 200,000-350,000/cu. mm. They contain no hemoglobin. SYN: *thromboplastid; thrombocyte.* SEE: *blood.*

   FUNCTIONS: Platelets play an important role in blood coagulation, hemostasis, and blood thrombus formation. When a small vessel is injured, platelets adhere to each other and the edges of the injury and form a plug which covers the area. The plug or blood clot formed soon retracts and stops the loss of blood.

   Thrombocytopenia (reduced platelet count) occurs in acute infections, anaphylactic shock, certain hemorrhagic diseases and anemias. *Thrombocytosis* (increased platelet count) occurs after operations, esp. splenectomy, and following violent exercise and also following tissue injury.

plat'ing. In bacteriology, inoculation of liquefiable, solid media (gelatin or agar) with microorganisms and pouring of medium into a shallow flat dish. SYN: *plating out.*

platinosis. Cutaneous and respiratory allergic reactions to exposure to complex salts of platinum.

platinum (plăt'ĭ-nŭm) [Sp. *platina*]. SYMB: *pt.* At. wt. 195.09; at. no. 78.; sp. gr. 21.45. Heavy silver-white metal.

platy- [Gr. *platys*, broad]. Combining form meaning broad.

platycelous (plăt-ĭ-sē'lŭs) [Gr. *platys*, broad, + *koilos*, hollow]. Concave ventrally and convex dorsally, said of vertebrae.

platycephalic (plăt'ĭ-sĕ-făl'ĭk) ["+ *kephalē*, head]. Having a wide skull with vertical index less than 70.

platycephalous (plăt'ĭ-sĕf'ă-lŭs). Platycephalic, q.v.

platycnemia (plăt-ĭk-nē'mĭ-ă) [Gr. *platys*, broad, + *knēmē*, leg, + *ia*, condition]. 1. Having an unusually broad tibia. 2. Broadlegged.

platycnemic (plăt'ĭk-nē'mĭk). Having unusually broad tibia.

platycnemism (plăt'ĭk'nē-mĭzm). Platycnemia, q.v.

platycoria (plăt'ĭ-kŏr'ĭ-ă) [Gr. *platys*, broad, + *korē*, pupil]. Mydriasis; dilatation of the pupil.

platycoriasis (plăt'ĭ-kŏr'ĭ-ă'sĭs). Platycoria, q.v.

Platyhelminthes (plăt'ĭ-hĕl-mĭn'thēz) [Gr. *platys*, broad, + *helmins, helminth-*, worm]. A phylum of flatworms including the classes Turbellaria, Trematoda (flukes), and Cestoidea (tapeworms). The last two are parasitic and include many species of medical importance. SEE: *Cestoda; Cestoidea; fluke, tapeworm; trematode.*

platyhieric (plă'ĭ-hī-ĕr'ĭk) [Gr. *platys*, broad, + *hieron*, sacrum]. Having a broad sacrum with a sacral index over 100.

platymeric (plăt'ĭ-mē'rĭk) ["+ *mēros*, thigh]. Having an unusually broad femur.

platymorphia (plăt'ĭ-mor'fĭ-ă) ["+ *morphē*, form]. Having an eye with shortened anteroposterior diameter. Results in hyperopia, q.v.

platyopia (plăt'ĭ-ō'pĭ-ă) ["+ *ōps*, face]. Having a very broad face, the nasomalar index being less than 107.5.

platypellic, platypelvic (plăt'ĭ-pĕl'ĭk, -vĭk) [Gr. *platys*, broad, + *pella*, a basin]. Having a broad pelvis.

platypodia (plăt'ĭ-pō'dĭ-ă) ["+ *pous, pod-*, foot]. Condition of being flatfooted.

platyrrhine (plăt'ĭr-ĭn) ["+ *rhis, rhin*, nose]. 1. Having a very wide nose in proportion to length. 2. Pert. to a skull with a nasal index between 51.1 and 58.

platysmal reflex (plă-tĭz″măl rē′flĕks). Dilation of pupil resulting from sharp pinching of platysma myoides.

platysma myoides (plă-tĭz′mă mī-oy′dēz) [Gr. *platysma*, plate, + *mys*, *my-*, muscle, + *eidos*, form]. Broad, thin platelike layer of muscle that extends from the fascia of both sides of the neck to jaw and muscles around the mouth. Acts to wrinkle the skin of the neck and to depress the jaw.

platyspondylisis (plăt″ĭ-spŏn-dĭl′ĭ-sĭs) [Gr. *platys*, flat, + *spondylos*, vertebra]. Flatness of the vertebral bodies.

platystencephaly (plăt″ĭ-stĕn-sĕf′ă-lĭ) ["+ *kephalē*, head]. Having a skull wide at occiput.

plea′sure prin′ciple. In psychology, the avoidance of pain and the seeking of pleasure, indicative of the early stages of man's development. SYN: *hedonism*.

pledget (plĕj′ĕt) [origin uncertain]. Small, flat compress, usually of gauze or absorbent cotton, used to apply or absorb fluid, to protect, to exclude air, etc.

plegaphonia (pleg″a-fō′nĭ-ă) [Gr. *plēgē*, stroke, + *a-*, neg. + *phōnē*, voice]. A sound produced in percussion of the larynx when the glottis is open during auscultation of the chest.

-plegia (plē′jĭ-ă) [Gr. *plēgē*, stroke]. Suffix meaning paralysis or stroke.

pleio-, pleo-, plio- [Gr. *pleiōn, pleōn*, more]. Combining forms meaning more.

pleochroic (plē″ō-krō′ĭk) [Gr. *pleōn*, more, + *chroia*, color]. Pleochromatic, q.v.

pleochromatic (plē″ō-krō-măt′ĭk) ["+ *chroma*, color]. Pert. to the property of crystals and some other bodies in which they show different colors when seen from different axes.

pleocytosis (plē″ō-sī-tō′sĭs) ["+ *kytos*, cell, + *-ōsis*, condition]. Increased number of lymphocytes in the cerebrospinal fluid.

pleomastia, pleomazia (plē″ō-măs′tĭ-ă, -mā′zĭ-ă) [Gr. *pleōn*, more, + *mastos, mazos*, breast]. The state of having more than two mammae. SYN: *polymastia*.

pleomorphic (plē-ō-mor′fĭk) ["+ *morphē*, form]. Having many shapes.

pleomorphism (plē-ō-mor′fĭzm) ["+ "+ *ismos*, condition]. 1. Property of crystallizing into two or more different forms. 2. Occurrence of more than one form in a life cycle.

pleomorphous (plē-ō-mor′fŭs). Having many shapes or crystallizing into several forms.

pleonasm (plē′ō-năzm) [Gr. *pleonasmos*, exaggeration]. 1. State of having more than normal number of organs or parts. 2. The use of more words than necessary to express an idea.

pleonectic (plē″ō-nĕk′tĭk) [Gr. *pleonexia*, greediness]. 1. Being saturated with more than the normal amount of oxygen, said of blood. SEE: *mesectic; mionectic*. 2. Rel. to excessive urge to possess; greedy.

pleonexia (plē″ō-nĕk′sĭ-ă) [Gr.]. Having morbid desire for possession.

pleoptics. A method of eye exercises created to stimulate and train an amblyopic eye.

plerosis (plē-rō′sĭs) [Gr. *plērōsis*, filling up]. Restoration of lost tissue.

plesiomorphous (plē″sĭ-ō-mor′fŭs) [Gr. *plesios*, close, + *morphē*, form]. Of, like, or nearly the same in form.

plesiopia (plē″sĭ-ō′pĭ-ă) [+ *ops*, eye]. Increase in convexity of lens of eye.

plessesthesia (plĕs″ĕs-thē′zĭ-ă) [Gr. *plēssein*, to strike, + *aisthēsis*, sensation]. Palpatory percussion with left middle finger pressed against body and the index finger of right hand percussing in contact with left finger.

plessimeter (plĕs-sĭm′ē-ter) ["+ *metron*, a measure]. A disk which is struck in mediate percussion while being held over the surface of the body. SYN: *pleximeter*.

plessor (plĕs′or) [Gr. *plēssein*, to strike]. A hammer for performing percussion. SYN: *plexor*.

plethora (plĕth′ō-ră) [Gr. *plēthōrē*, fullness]. 1. Overfullness of blood vessels or of the total quantity of any fluid in the body. SEE: *sanguine*. 2. Congestion causing distention of blood vessels.

plethoric (plē-thor′ĭk, plĕth′ō-rĭk). Pert. to or characterized by, plethora; overfull.

plethysmograph (plē-thĭz′mō-grăf) [Gr. *plēthysmos*, increase, + *graphein*, to write]. Device for finding variations in size of a part due to variations in amount of blood passing through or contained in the part.

pleur-, pleuro- [Gr. *pleura*, rib, side]. Prefix indicating relationship to the pleura, the side, or a rib.

pleura (plū′ră) [Gr., side]. (pl. *pleur′ae*) [NA]. Serous membrane that enfolds lungs and is reflected upon the walls of the thorax and diaphragm. There are two pleurae, right and left. They are moistened with a serous secretion which reduces friction during respiratory movements of the lungs. SEE: *mediastinum; thorax*.

    p., costal. P., parietal, q.v.

    p. diaphragmatica. [NA]. Part of p. covering upper surface of diaphragm.

    p., parietal. Extends from roots of the lungs covering the sides of the pericardium to chest wall and backward to the spine. The visceral and costal pleural layers are separated only by a lubricating secretion. These layers may become adherent or separated by fluid or air in diseased conditions. SYN: *parietal layer of pleura.*

p. pericardiaca. Portion covering the pericardium.

p. phrenica. P. diaphragmatica, q.v.

p. pulmonalis. [NA]. The p. investing the lungs and fissures between the lobes.

p., visceral. P. which invests the lungs and enters into and lines the interlobar fissures. It is loose at the base and at sternal and vertebral borders to allow for lung expansion.

pleural (plū′răl) [Gr. *pleura*, a side]. Concerning the pleura.

p. cavity. Space between the parietal and visceral layers of the pleura. SEE: *chylothorax.*

p. fibrosis. Condition occurring in pulmonary tuberculosis in which pleura becomes thickened and pleural cavity often is obliterated.

pleuralgia (plū-răl′jĭ-ă) ["+ *algos*, pain]. Pain in the pleura, or in the side. SYN: *neuralgia, intercostal.*

pleurapophysis (plū-ră-pŏf′ĭ-sĭs) ["+ *apo*, from, + *physis*, a growth]. A rib or a vertebral lateral process.

pleurectomy (plū-rĕk′tō-mĭ) [Gr. *pleura*, a side, + *ektomē*, excision]. Excision of part of the pleura.

pleurisy (plū′rĭs-ĭ) [Gr. *pleuritis*]. Inflammation of pleura. May be primary or secondary; unilateral, bilateral, or local; acute or chronic; fibrinous, serofibrinous, or purulent. SEE: *Andral's decubitus.*

NP: In simple pleurisy, absolute rest is essential with plenty of sunlight and fresh air. Routine nursing is in order, but the patient should not be permitted to exert himself and he should be kept cheerful. Assistance should be given in moving the patient. Increase fluid intake. The doctor may strap the affected side to help immobilize the chest.

p., acute. Chilliness, stabbing pain or stitch in affected side, intensified by coughing or deep breathing. Fever, 101°-103° F.; cough short, dry, partially suppressed; face pale, anxious; patient usually lies on affected side. An effusion of fluid in the pleural space which remains unabsorbed is characteristic of chronic pleurisy.

p., diaphragmatic. Inflammation of diaphragmatic pleura.

SYM: Intense pain under margin of ribs, sometimes referred into abdomen, with tenderness on pressure; thoracic breathing;

tenderness over phrenic nerve referred to supraclavicular region in neck or same side; hiccough; extreme dyspnea.

p., dry. Condition in which the pleural membrane is covered with a fibrinous exudate. It clings together, causing pain during respiration. There is slight pain when apical pleura is inflamed, but there is acute stabbing pain in costal or diaphragmatic pleural inflammation.

p., encysted. P. with effusion limited by adhesions.

p., fibrinous. Pain severe and continuous. Aspiration gives negative results, later much retraction of affected side.

p., hemorrhagic. P. with hemorrhage.

p., interlobar. P. in interlobar spaces.

p., purulent. High, irregular fever; sweats; chills; anemia; sometimes pitting from edema of surface; purulent effusion found on aspiration.

p., secondary. Infectious p. resulting from some specific inflammation.

p., serofibrinous. P. with fibrinous exudate and serous effusion.

p., suppurative. SEE: *p., purulent.*

p., tuberculous. A common cause of pleurisy that is apparently primary in tuberculosis. Effusion apt to be bloody, but presents same symptoms as ordinary serofibrinous pleurisy.

pleuritic (plū-rĭt′ĭk) [Gr. *pleuritis,* pleurisy]. Relating to, or like, pleurisy.

pleuritis (plū-rī′tĭs) [Gr.]. Inflammation of the pleura. SYN: *pleurisy.*

pleurocele (plū′rō-sēl) [Gr. *pleura,* a side, + *kēlē,* a swelling]. 1. Hernia of lungs or of pleura. 2. A serous pleural effusion.

pleurocentesis (plū″rō-sĕn-tē′sĭs) ["+ *kentēsis,* a piercing]. Surgical puncture of the pleural cavity. SYN: *thoracentesis; thoracocentesis.*

pleurocentrum (plū″rō-sĕn′trŭm) ["+ *kentron,* center]. (pl. *pleurocentra*) The lateral half of the centrum of a vertebra.

pleurocholecystitis (plū″rō-kō″lē-sĭst-i′tĭs) [Gr. *pleura,* a side, + *cholē,* bile, + *kystis,* bladder, + *-itis,* inflammation]. Inflamed condition of the pleura and gallbladder.

pleuroclysis (plū-rŏk′lĭ-sĭs) ["+ *klysis,* a washing]. Injection of fluid into the pleural cavity and washing out the cavity.

pleurodynia (plū″rō-dĭn′ĭ-ă) ["+ *odynē,* pain]. Pain of sharp intensity in intercostal muscles due to chronic inflammatory changes in chest fasciae; pain of the pleural nerves.

p., epidemic. Epidemic disease with sudden attack of pain in the region of the attachment of the diaphragm; intermittent

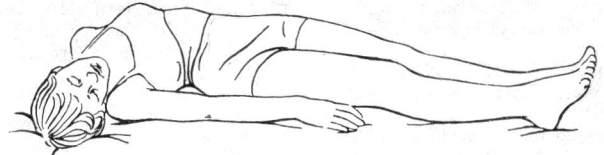

PLEUROTHOTONOS

fever; headache; nausea; malaise. Due to Coxsackie virus, type B1. SYN: *devil's grip*.

pleurogenic (plŭ″rō-jĕn′ĭk) [Gr. *pleura*, a side, + *gennan*, to produce]. Arising in the pleura. SYN: *pleurogenous*.

pleurogenous (plŭ-rŏj′ĕn-ŭs). Having origin in the pleura. SYN: *pleurogenic*.

pleurography (plŭ-rŏg′ră-fĭ) ["+ *graphein*, to write]. X-ray examination of the lungs and pleura.

pleurohepatitis (plŭ″rō-hĕp″ă-tī′tĭs) ["+ *hēpar*, *hēpat-*, liver, + *-itis*, inflammation]. Inflammation of pleura and the liver.

pleurolith (plŭ′rō-lĭth) ["+ *lithos*, stone]. A calculus in the pleura.

pleurolysis (plŭ-rŏl′ĭ-sĭs) [Gr. *pleura*, a side, + *lysis*, a loosening]. Loosening of parietal pleura from intrathoracic fascia to facilitate contraction of the lung or artificial pneumothorax.

pleuroparietopexy (plŭ″rō-păr-ī′ĕt-ō-pĕk″sĭ) ["+ L. *pariēs*, *pariet-*, wall, + Gr. *pēxis*, fixation]. Fastening the lung to the wall of the chest by binding the visceral pleura to the wall of its cavity.

pleuropericarditis (plŭ″rō-pĕr″ĭ-kar-dī′tĭs) ["+ *peri*, around, + *kardia*, heart, + *-itis*, inflammation]. Pleuritis accompanied by pericarditis.

pleuroperitoneal (plŭ″rō-pĕr″ĭ-tō-nē′ăl) ["+ *peritonaion*, peritoneum]. Rel. to the pleura and peritoneum.

    ***p.* cavity.** The body cavity. SYN: *celom*.

pleuropneumonia (plŭ″rō-nū-mō′nĭ-ă) [Gr. *pleura*, a side, + *pneumōn*, lung]. Pleurisy accompanied by pneumonia.

pleuropneumonia-like organisms. The name once given organisms which are now called mycoplasmas, q.v. ABBR: PPLO.

pleuropneumonolysis (plŭ″rō-nū″mōn-ŏl′ĭ-sĭs) [Gr. *pleura*, a side, + *pneumōn*, lung, + *lysis*, a loosening]. Resection of one or more ribs from one side to collapse the lung in unilateral pulmonary tuberculosis.

pleurorrhea (plŭ″rō-rē′ă) ["+ *rhoia*, flow]. Effusion of fluid into the pleura.

pleuroscopy (plŭ-rŏs′kō-pī) ["+ *skopein*, to examine]. Inspection of the pleural cavity through an incision into the thorax.

pleurothotonos (plŭ″rō-thŏt′ō-nŏs) [Gr. *pleurothen*, from the side, + *tonos*, tension]. Tetanic spasm in which the body position is arched to one side.

    RS: emprosthotonos; opisthotonos; orthotonos; position; posture.

pleurotomy (plŭ-rŏt′ō-mĭ) [Gr. *pleura*, a side, + *tomē*, incision]. Incision of the pleura.

pleurotyphoid (plŭ″rō-tī′foyd) ["+ *typhos*, fever, + *eidos*, form]. Typhoid fever with pleural involvement.

pleurovisceral (plŭ″rō-vĭs′ĕr-ăl) ["+ L. *viscus*, *viscer-*, viscera]. Concerning the pleura and the viscera.

plexal (plĕk′săl) [L. *plexus*, a braid]. Pert. to, or of the nature of, a plexus.

plexiform (plĕk′sĭ-form) ["+ *forma*, shape]. Resembling a network or plexus.

pleximeter (plĕks-ĭm′ĕ-tĕr) [Gr. *plēxis*, stroke, + *metron*, measure]. Device for receiving the blow of the percussion hammer.

plexor (plĕks′or). Hammer or other device for striking upon the pleximeter in percussion.

plexus (plĕk′sŭs) [L., a braid]. (pl. *plexus* or *plexuses*) [NA]. A network of nerves or of blood or lymphatic vessels. SEE: *rete; Table of Plexuses* in *Appendix*.

    ***p.,* cavernous.** *Of the nose:* a venous p. in mucosa covering superior and middle conchae. *Of the penis:* nerve p. at root of penis giving rise to large and small cavernous nerves. *Of the clitoris:* nerve p. at base of clitoris formed of fibers from uterovaginal p. *Of the cavernous sinus:* a sympathetic p. supplying fibers to internal carotid artery and its branches within cranium.

    ***p.,* enteric.** One of two p.'s of nerve fibers and ganglion cells which lie in wall of alimentary canal. Include myenteric (Auerbach's) and submucosal (Meissner's) plexus.

    ***p.,* nerve.** SEE: *Table of Plexuses* in *Appendix*.

    ***p.,* pampiniform.** In male, a complicated network of veins lying in spermatic cord and draining the testis; in female, a network of veins lying in mesovarium and draining the ovary.

    ***p.,* prevertebral.** One of three p.'s of autonomic division which lie in body cavities. Includes cardiac, celiac, and hypogastric (pelvic) plexuses. SEE: *Table of Plexuses* in *Appendix.*

pliability (plī″ă-bĭl'ĭ-tĭ) [O. Fr. *pliant,* bend, + L. *ābilis,* able]. Capacity of being bent or twisted easily.

plica (plī'kă) [L.]. (pl. *pli'cae*) [NA]. A fold.

    p. circularis. One of the transverse folds in the intestinal mucosa.

    p. epiglottica. One of three folds of mucosa between the tongue and the epiglottis.

    p. lacrimalis. [NA]. Mucosal fold at the lower orifice of the nasolacrimal duct.

    p. palmatae. [NA]. Radiating fold in the uterine mucosa on anterior and posterior walls of cervical canal.

    p. polonica. Tangled matted hair in which crusts and vermin are embedded.

    p. semilunaris coli. [NA]. Transverse fold of mucosa of large intestine lying between sacculations.

    p. semilunaris conjunctivae. [NA]. Mucosal fold at the inner canthus of the eye.

    p. synovialis. [NA]. A fold of synovial membrane which projects into a joint cavity.

    p. transversalis recti. One of the mucosal folds in the rectum.

plicate (plī'kāt) [L. *plicatus*]. Braided or folded.

plication (plī-kā'shŭn) [L. *plicāre,* to fold]. Stitching folds in an organ's walls to reduce its size.

plicotomy (plī-kŏ'ō-mĭ) ["+ Gr. *tomē,* a cutting]. Section of the posterior fold of the tympanic membrane.

plombage (plŏm-băzh') [Fr. *plomber,* to plug]. A method of collapsing the apex of lung by stripping the parietal pleura from the chest wall at the site of desired collapse and packing the space between the lung and chest wall with an inert substance, such as small balls made of certain plastic materials.

plug (plŭg) [Middle Dutch *plugge*]. A mass obstructing a hole or intended for closing a hole.

    p., vaginal. Closed tube for maintaining patency of vagina following operation for fistula.

plumbic (plŭm'bĭk) [L. *plumbicus,* leaden]. Pert. to, or containing, lead.

plumbism (plŭm'bĭzm) [L. *plumbum,* lead, + Gr. *ismos,* condition]. Poisoning from lead, q.v.

plumbum (plŭm'bŭm) [L.]. Lead; a bluish-white metal.

plumose (plū'mōs) [L. *plumosus*]. Having a delicate, feathery growth.

plumper (plŭm'pĕr) [Middle Low German, *plump,* to fill]. Pad for filling out sunken cheeks, sometimes in form of extended artificial dentures.

pluri- [L. *plus,* more]. Prefix meaning several or more.

pluriceptor (plū″rĭ-sĕp'tor) [L. *plus, plur-,* more, + *ceptor,* a receiver]. A receptor which has more than two groups uniting with the complement.

pluridyscrinia (plū″rĭ-dĭs-krĭn'ĭ-ă) ["+ Gr. *dys,* bad, + *krinein,* to secrete]. Disorder of several endocrine organs at the same time.

pluriglandular (plu″rĭ-glănd'ū-lĕr) ["+ *glandula,* gland]. Pert. to several glands.

plurigravida (plū″rĭ-grăv'ĭ-dă) [L. *plus, plur-,* more, + *gravida,* pregnant]. A pregnant woman who has had two or more pregnancies.

plurilocular (plū″rĭ-lŏk'ū-lăr) ["+ *loculus,* a cell]. Composed of several compartments or cavities. SYN: *multilocular.*

pluripara (plū-rĭp'ă-ră) ["+ *parēre,* to bring forth]. A woman who has given birth to three or more children in at least three pregnancies.

pluriparity (plū″rĭ-păr'ĭ-tĭ). Condition of having borne three or more children.

plutomania (plū″tō-mā'nĭ-ă) [Gr. *ploutos,* wealth, + *mania,* madness]. Delusion that one is very rich.

plutonium (plū-tō'nĭ-ŭm). [Named after the planet *Pluto*] SYMB: *Pu.* At. wt. of the most stable isotope is 244; at. no. 94. A chemical element obtained from neptunium which in turn is obtained from uranium.

Pm. Chem. symb. for promethium.

PMSG. Abbr. for *pregnant mare serum gonadotrophin.* SEE: *gonadotrophin, chorionic.*

pneo- (nē'ō) [Gr. *pnein,* to breathe]. Combining form meaning pert. to breath or breathing. SEE: *pneum-.*

pneocardiac reflex (nē″ō-kar'dĭ-ăk) [Gr. *pnein,* to breathe, + *kardia,* heart]. Change in rate and rhythm of heart when an irritant vapor enters air passages.

pneodynamics (nē″ō-dī-năm'ĭks) ["+ *dynamis,* force]. The mechanism of breathing. SYN: *pneumodynamics.*

pneograph (nē'ō-grăf) ["+ *graphein,* to write]. Apparatus for registering respiratory movements.

pneometer (nē-ŏm'ĕ-tĕr) ["+ *metron,* a measure]. Instrument for measuring lung respiration. SYN: *spirometer, q.v.*

pneophore (nē'ō-for) [Gr. *pnein,* to breathe, + *phoros,* bearing]. Device to aid artificial respiration.

pneopneic reflex (nē-ŏp-nē'ĭk) ["+ *pnein,* to breathe]. Change in respiratory depth and rate, coughing, suffocation and pulmonary edema, when an irritant vapor enters air passages.

pneoscope (nē'ō-skōp) ["+ *skopein,* to examine]. Device for measuring movements of respiration.

pneum-, pneuma-, pneumato- [Gr. *pneuma,* air, breath]. Combining form meaning pert. to air, or gas, or respiration.

pneumarthrosis (nū-mär-thrō'sĭs) [Gr. *pneuma,* air, + *arthron,* joint, + *-ōsis,* intensive]. Accumulation of gas or air in a joint.

pneumascope (nū'mă-skōp) ["+ *skopein,* to examine]. SEE: *pneumatoscope.*

pneumatic (nū-măt'ĭk) [Gr. *pneumatikos,* pert. to air]. 1. Concerning gas or air. 2. Rel. to respiration. 3. Rel. to rarefied or compressed air.

pneumatinuria (nū"măt-ĭn-ū'rĭ-ă) [Gr. *pneuma,* air, + *ouron,* urine]. Excretion of urine containing free gas. SYN: *pneumaturia.*

pneumatocardia (nū"măt-ō-kar'dĭ-ă) ["+ *kardia,* heart]. Air or gas in the heart chambers.

pneumatocele (nū-măt'ō-sēl) ["+ *kēlē,* hernia]. 1. Hernial protuberance of lung tissue. 2. A swelling containing gas or air, esp. a swelling of the scrotum. SYN: *pneumonocele.*

pneumatodyspnea (nū"măt-ō-dĭsp-nē'ă) ["+ *dys,* bad, + *pneia,* breath]. Dyspnea caused by pulmonary emphysema.

pneumatogram (nū-măt'ō-grăm) [Gr. *pneuma,* air, + *gramma,* a mark]. A tracing or record made by a pneumatograph.

pneumatograph (nū-măt'ō-grăf) ["+ *graphein,* to write]. Device for registering respiratory movements. SYN: *pneograph.*

pneumatology (nū"mă-tŏl'ō-jĭ) ["+ *logos,* a study]. Science of gases and air, their chemical properties and use in treatment.

pneumatometer (nū"măt-ŏm'ĕ-tĕr) [Gr. *pneuma,* air, + *metron,* a measure]. Device for measuring quantity of air involved in inspiration and expiration. SYN: *spirometer.*

pneumatometry (nū"măt-ŏm'ĕ-trĭ). Measurement of respiratory force as a means of diagnosis.

pneumatorachis (nū"măt-ōr'ă-kĭs) ["+ *rachis,* spine]. Air in the spinal canal.

pneumatoscope (nū-măt'ō-skōp) ["+ *skopein,* to inspect]. 1. Device for ascertaining presence of foreign bodies in mastoid sinuses. 2. Apparatus used to measure the gas in expired air. 3. Apparatus for internal

thoracic auscultation. 4. Instrument used to measure the respiratory movements. SYN: *pneumascope.*

pneumatosis (nū"mă-tō'sĭs) [Gr. *pneumatōsis*]. Presence of air or gas in an abnormal location in the body.

   p. abdominis. Air in the peritoneal cavity. SYN: *pneumoperitoneum.*

   p. cystoides intestinalis. Presence of thin-walled gas-filled cysts in the intestines.

pneumatotherapy (nū"măt-ō-thĕr'ă-pĭ) [Gr. *pneuma,* air, + *therapeia,* treatment]. 1. Treatment of diseases by use of rarefied or condensed air. 2. Treatment of diseases of the lungs. SYN: *pneumotherapy.*

pneumatothorax (nū"măt-ō-thō'răks) ["+ *thōrax,* chest]. Air or gas accumulation in the pleural cavities. SYN: *pneumothorax, q.v.*

pneumaturia (nū"măt-u'rĭ-ă) ["+ *ouron,* urine]. Excretion of urine containing free gas.

pneumatype (nū'mă-tip) ["+ *typos,* type]. Deposit of moisture on glass from the breath exhaled through the nostrils with the mouth closed for purpose of comparing the airflow through the nostrils.

pneumectomy (nū-mĕk'tō-mĭ) [Gr. *pneumōn,* lung, + *ektomē,* excision]. Excision of all or part of a lung.

pneumo-, pneumono- [Gr. *pneumōn,* lung]. Combining forms meaning air; lung.

pneumocele (nū'mō-sēl). SEE: *pneumatocele.*

pneumocentesis (nū"mō-sĕn-tē'sĭs) [Gr. *pneumōn,* lung, *kentēsis,* a piercing]. Paracentesis, q.v., or surgical puncture of a lung to evacuate a cavity.

pneumocephalus (nū"mō-sĕf'ă-lŭs) ["+ *kephalē,* head]. Gas or air in the cavity of the cranium.

pneumochysis (nū-mōk'ĭs-ĭs) ["+ *chysis,* a pouring]. Edema of the lung.

pneumococcal (nū"mō-kŏk'ăl) [Gr. *pneumōn,* lung, + *kokkos,* berry]. Concerning or caused by pneumococci.

pneumococcemia (nū"mō-kŏk-sē'mĭ-ă). Presence of pneumococci in the blood.

pneumococci (nū"mō-kŏk'sĭ). Plural of pneumococcus, q.v.

pneumococcolysis (nū"mō-kŏk-ŏl'ĭ-sĭs) [Gr. *pneumōn,* lung, + *kokkos,* berry, + *lysis,* destruction]. Destruction or lysis of pneumococci.

pneumococcus (nū"mō-kŏk'ŭs) [Gr. *pneumon,* lung, + *kokkos,* berry]. (pl. *pneumococci*) An oval-shaped, encapsulated, nonspore-forming, gram-positive organism occurring usually in pairs (diplococcus) having lancet-shaped ends. There are more than 75 serological types of pneumococci. In addition to causing pneumonia, pneumococci are also found to be the cause of infections such as otitis media, mastoiditis, meningitis, bronchitis, bloodstream infections, keratitis and conjunctivitis.

Pneumococcal infections are effectively treated with penicillin. Erythromycin may be used if patient is hypersensitive to penicillin.

pneumoconiosis (nū″mō-kō-nĭ-ō′sĭs) [Gr. *pneumōn*, lung, + *konis*, dust, + *-ōsis*, disease]. A condition of the respiratory tract due to inhalation of dust particles. An occupational disorder such as that caused by mining or stonecutting.

RS: anthracosis; chalicosis; coal worker's pneumoconiosis; pneumomelanosis; siderosis; silicosis.

pneumoderma (nū″mō-dĕr′mă) [Gr. *pneumōn*, air, + *derma*, skin]. Emphysema under the skin.

pneumodynamics (nū″mō-dī-năm′ĭks) ["+ *dynamis*, force]. Branch of science dealing with force employed in respiration.

pneumoempyema (nū″mō-ĕm-pī-ē′mă) [Gr. *pneumōn*, lung, + *en*, in, + *pyon*, pus]. Empyema accompanied by an accumulation of gas.

pneumoencephalog′raphy (nū″mō-ĕn-sĕf-ă-lŏg′ră-fĭ) [Gr. *pneumōn*, air, + *graphein*, to write]. Roentgenographic examination of ventricles and subarachnoid spaces of brain following withdrawal of cerebrospinal fluid and injection of air or gas via lumbar puncture.

pneumoenteritis (nū″mō-ĕn-tĕr-ī′tĭs) ["+ *enteron*, intestine, + *-ītis*, inflammation]. Pneumonia and enteritis combined.

pneumoerysipelas (nū″mō-ĕr′ĭ-sip′e-las) [Gr. *pneumōn*, lung, + *erythros*, red, + *pella*, skin]. Erysipelas with pneumonia.

pneumogalactocele (nū″mō-găl-ăk′tō-sēl) [Gr. *pneumōn*, air, + *gala, galakt*, milk, + *kēlē*, hernia]. A breast tumor containing milk and gas.

pneumogastric (nū″mō-găs′trĭk) [Gr. *pneumōn*, lung, + *gastēr*, stomach]. Pert. to the lungs and stomach.

p. nerve. Term formerly used for the vagus nerve.

pneumogram (nū′mō-grăm) ["+ *gramma*, a mark]. 1. A record of respiratory movements. 2. A roentgenogram following injection of air. SYN: *pneumatogram*.

pneumography (nū-mŏg′ră-fĭ) ["+ *graphein*, to write]. 1. Anatomical description or illustration of the lung. 2. Recording of

respiratory movements on a graph. 3. X-ray study of a part or organ after air injection.

p., pelvic. X-ray study of pelvis after CO_2 has been injected into the peritoneal cavity.

pneumohemopericardium (nū″mō-hĕm″ō-pĕr-ĭ-kăr′dĭ-ŭm) [Gr. *pneumōn*, lung, + *haima*, blood, + *peri*, around, + *kardia*, heart]. The accumulation of air and blood in the pericardium.

pneumohemorrhagia (nū″mō-hĕm-ŏr-hā′-jĭ-ă) ["+ "+ *rhēgnynai*, to burst forth]. Hemorrhage into pulmonary air cells; apoplexy of the lungs.

pneumohemothorax (nū″mō-hĕm″ō-thō′-răks) ["+ "+ *thōrax*, chest]. Gas or air and blood collected in the pleural cavity.

pneumohydrometra (nū″mō-hī″drō-mē′tră) [Gr. *pneumōn*, air, + *hydor*, water, + *metra*, uterus]. The accumulation of gas and fluid in the uterus.

pneumohydropericardium (nū″mō-hī″drō-pĕr-ĭ-kăr′dĭ-ŭm) [Gr. *pneumōn*, lung, + *hydōr*, water, + *peri*, around, + *kardia*, heart]. Air and fluid accumulated in the pericardium.

pneumohydrothorax (nū″mō-hī″drō-thō′-răks) ["+ "+ *thōrax*, chest]. Gas or air and fluid in the pleural cavity.

pneumohypoderma (nū″mō-hī″pō-dĕr′mă) [Gr. *pneumōn*, air, + *hypo*, under, + *derma*, skin]. Air in the tissues under the skin.

pneumokidney (nū″mō-kĭd′nĭ) ["+ ME. *kydney*, kidney]. Air in the pelvis of the kidney.

pneumolith (nū′mō-lĭth) [Gr. *pneumōn*, lung, + *lithos*, stone]. A pulmonary calculus.

pneumolithiasis (nū″mō-lĭth-ī′ăs-ĭs) ["+ "+ *-iasis*, condition]. Formation of concretions in the lungs.

pneumology (nū-mŏl′ō-jĭ) ["+ *logos*, a study]. The scientific study of diseases of the lungs and air passages.

pneumolysis (nū-mŏl′ĭs-ĭs) ["+ *lysis*, a loosening]. Separation of an adherent lung from costal pleura.

pneumomalacia (nū″mō-mă-lā′sĭ-ă) ["+ *malakia*, a softening]. Abnormal softening of the lung

pneumomassage (nū″mō-măs-sazh′) [Gr. *pneumōn*, air, + *massein*, to knead]. Massage of the tympanum with air to cause movement of the ossicles.

pneumomelanosis (nū″mō-mĕl-ăn-ō′sĭs) [Gr. *pneumōn*, lung, + *melas, melan-*, black, + *-ōsis*, disease]. Pigmentation of lung seen in pneumoconiosis, q.v.

pneumometer (nū-mŏm′ĕt-ĕr) ["+ *metron*, measure]. Instrument for measuring amount of air inspired and expired in respiration. SYN: *spirometer,* q.v.

pneumomycosis (nū″mō-mī-kō′sĭs) ["+ *mykēs,* fungus, + *-ōsis,* disease]. A fungus pulmonary disease. SYN: *pneumonomycosis.*

pneumomyelography (nū″mō-mī-ĕl-ŏg′rä-fĭ) [Gr. *pneumōn,* air, + *myelos,* marrow, + *graphein,* to write]. X-ray inspection of the spinal canal following injection of air or gas.

pneumonectasia, pneumonectasis (nū″mŏn-ĕk-tā′zĭ-ä, ĕk′tä-sĭs) [Gr. *pneumōn,* lung, + *ektasis,* dilatation]. Distention of lungs with air.

pneumonectomy (nū″mŏn-ĕk′tō-mĭ) ["+ *ektomē,* excision]. Removal of a lung. SYN: *pulmonectomy; pneumectomy.*

pneumonemia (nū″mō-nē′mĭ-ä) ["+ *haima,* blood]. Congestion of the lungs.

pneumonia (nū-mō′nĭ-ä) [Gr. *pneumōn,* lung, + *-ia,* condition]. Inflammation of the lungs caused primarily by bacteria, viruses, chemical irritants, vegetable dusts and allergy. There are more than 50 different causes; the most common ones are listed in the accompanying table.

Pneumonias caused by pneumococci, staphylococci, streptococci, and bacilli often begin suddenly.

SYM: Chills, high fever, pain in chest, cough, sputum purulent and often bloody. Mortality 30 percent unless treated with antibiotics.

NP: Bed rest necessary. For restlessness or pain, drugs or other therapeutic agents should be used as prescribed by the physician. All measures to promote comfort should be taken.

A careful watch over the patient's general condition: his color, his general appearance, and his pulse, temperature, and respiration. Cyanosis or a rising respiratory rate calls for administration of oxygen, or for increase in the amount of oxygen if it is already being given. The nurse must understand how to regulate the flow of oxygen and to adjust the intranasal tube or the temperature in the oxygen tent. High fever demands tepid sponges, rarely the use of antipyretics. Any marked change in the patient's general condition should be reported to the doctor at once.

Measures to prevent and combat abdominal distention. The bowels should act daily; to accomplish this an enema may be given, or the physician may prescribe a laxative. If distention appears, a rectal tube is inserted.

Unless patient is sensitive, penicillin is drug of choice for pneumococcal and streptococcal p.; otherwise sulfadiazine, erythro-

Pneumonias

Specific Microbial Causes	Diseases Accompanied by Pneumonia	Pneumonias Not Caused by Infections
Viruses	Tularemia	Oil aspiration
influenza	Brucellosis	Radiation
adeno-	Rheumatic fever	Chemicals
respiro-	Syphilis	Allergy
syncytial	Typhus	Vegetable dusts
etc.	Rocky Mountain fever	Silo-filler's disease
Mycoplasma pneumoniae	Infectious mono-	
(Primary atypical pneumonia)	nucleosis	
	Trichiniasis	
Cocci		
Pneumococcus		
Staphylococcus		
Hemolytic streptococcus		
Bacilli		
Hemophilus influenzae		
Mycobacterium tuberculosis		
Klebsiella (Friedlander's bacillus)		
Gram-negative bacilli		
Fungi		
Histoplasma capsulatum		
Coccidioides immitis		

mycin, or tetracycline. Special penicillins for penicillin-resistant staphylococci. Tetracycline for p. caused by Mycoplasma pneumoniae; streptomycin for gram-negative bacillary p. Anticipate untoward reactions to antibiotics.

p., acute lobar. P. caused by pneumococci.

p., aspiration. P. after inhaling foreign matter into the lungs.

p., atypical. SEE: *p., primary atypical.*

p., chronic interstitial. Chronic disease of lung with overgrowth of fibrous tissue.

SYM: Moderate dyspnea and chronic cough, expectoration, slight or profuse, fetid, from being retained in bronchiectatic cavities. No fever. May live years.

p., croupous. SEE: *p., acute lobar.*

p., desquamative interstitial. Chronic pulmonary condition of unknown etiology characterized by dyspnea, weight loss, cough, pleural complications, and recurrent pneumothorax. Diagnosis is established by lung biopsy which reveals distal air spaces filled with large alveolar cells.

TREATMENT: Corticosteroid therapy is helpful but symptoms return immediately when it is withdrawn.

p., eosinophilic. Inflammation of the lung characterized by transient or prolonged pulmonary changes. The principal causes are parasites such as roundworms or filaria; fungus infection; drugs or chemicals such as nickel, penicillin, paramonosalicylic acid, nitrofurantoin, and sulfonamides. In most cases, however, the cause is unknown.

p., hypostatic. P. caused by constantly remaining in same position. Gravity causes blood to become congested in one part of the lung. Infection aids development of true p.

NP: Change position of patient frequently and whenever patient is uncomfortable. Have patient breathe deeply several times each hour for full aeration of lungs. Short, shallow breaths predispose to pulmonary complications. Measures to fully expand the lung such as forcibly blowing up a balloon are helpful.

p., lipid. P. after aspiration of oily substances such as oily nose drops or mineral or other bland oil.

p., migratory. P. in which infected area shifts from one part of the lung to another part.

p., primary atypical. A relatively mild p. characterized by cough, fever, pharyngitis and x-ray evidence of lung infiltration out of proportion to the minimal

findings upon examining the lungs. Caused by Mycoplasma pneumoniae.

TREATMENT: Broad spectrum antibiotics; penicillin, sulfonamides and streptomycin are ineffective.

p., terminal. P. occurring secondary to another disease and resulting in death.

p., tuberculous. Condition which simulates p. caused by tubercle bacilli. May result in rapid and widespread inflammatory exudation. If untreated may run a malignant course ending fatally or it may subside and become chronic.

p., tularemic. P. caused by Pasteurella tularensis. May be primary or associated with tularemia, q.v.

p., viral. P., primary atypical, q.v.

pneumonic (nū-mŏn′ĭk) [Gr. *pneumōn*, lung]. Concerning the lungs or pneumonia.

pneumonitis (nū″mō-nī′tĭs) ["+ -*ītis,* inflammation]. Inflammation of the lung. SYN: *pneumonia.*

pneumono- (nū-mŏn-ō) [Gr. *pneumōn,* lung]. Combining form pert. to the lung.

pneumonocele (nū-mŏn′ō-sēl) ["+ *kēlē,* hernia]. A pulmonary hernia. SYN: *pneumocele.*

pneumonocirrhosis (nū″mō-nō-sĭr-ō′sĭs) ["+ *kirros,* orange]. Interstitial pneumonia; cirrhosis of the lung.

pneumonoconiosis (nū″mō-nō-kō-nĭ-ō′sĭs) ["+ *konis,* dust, + -*ōsis,* disease]. Fibrous inflammation or chronic induration of the lungs resulting from inhalation of dust. SYN: *pneumoconiosis,* q.v.

pneumonograph (nū-mō′nō-grăf) [Gr. *pneumōn,* lung, + *graphein,* to write]. X-ray photograph of the lungs.

pneumonography (nū-mō-nŏg′ră-fĭ). The taking and developing of x-ray pictures of the lungs.

pneumonolysis (nū-mō-nŏl′ĭs-ĭs) ["+ *lysis,* loosening]. Loosening of an adherent lung from the chest wall to induce collapse of lung. SYN: *pneumolysis.*

p., extrapleural. Separation of parietal pleura from chest wall. SEE: *apicolysis.*

p., intrapleural. Separation of adhering visceral and parietal layers of pleura.

pneumonomelanosis (nū″mō-nō-mĕl-ăn-ō′-sĭs) ["+ *melas, melan-,* black, + -*ōsis,* disease]. Darkening of the lung tissue as a result of inhalation of black dust particles such as coal dust. SYN: *pneumomelanosis.*

pneumonomycosis (nū-mō″nō-mĭ-kō′sĭs) [Gr. *pneumon,* lung, + *mykēs,* fungus, + -*ōsis,* disease]. Disease of the lungs caused by fungi. SYN: *pneumomycosis.*

pneumonopathy (nū-mō-nŏp′ăth-ĭ) ["+ *pathos,* disease]. Any diseased condition of the lung.

pneumonoperitonitis (nū″mō-nō-pĕr″ĭ-tō-nī′tĭs) ["+ *peritonaion,* peritoneum, + *-itis,* inflammation]. Peritonitis with gas in the peritoneal cavity.

pneumonopexy (nū-mō″nō-pĕk′sĭ) ["+ *pēxis,* fixation]. Surgical attachment of the lung to the chest wall. SYN: *pneumopexy.*

pneumonorrhaphy (nū″mō-nŏr′ă-fĭ) ["+ *raphē,* a sewing]. Suture of a lung.

pneumonosis (nū-mō-nō′sĭs) [Gr. *pneumōn,* lung, + *-ōsis,* disease]. Any noninfective disease or disorder of the lungs, esp. those resulting from degenerative processes.

  p., traumatic. In aviation medicine, a condition resulting from quick deceleration which may result in hemorrhage, emphysema, and other pulmonary changes.

pneumonotherapy. Pneumotherapy, q.v.

pneumonotomy (nū-mō-nŏt′ō-mĭ) ["+ *tomē,* incision]. Incision into the lung. SYN: *pneumotomy.*

pneumono-ultramicroscopicsilicovolcanoconiosis (nu″mō-nō-ŭl″tră-mĭ-krō-skŏp′ĭk-sĭl″ĭ-kō-vŏl-kăn′ō-kō″nĭ-ō′sĭs). Noninfectious form of silicosis, miner's lung disease.

pneumopericardium (nū″mō-pĕr-ĭ-kăr′dĭ-ŭm) [Gr. *pneumōn,* lung, + *peri,* around, + *kardia,* heart]. Air or gas in the pericardial sac.

  ETIOL: Traumatism or communication between the esophagus, stomach, or lungs and the pericardium.

  SYM: Unusual metallic heart sounds, tympany over precordial area.

pneumoperitoneum (nū″mō-pĕr-ĭ-tō-nē′ŭm) ["+ *peritonaion,* peritoneum]. Condition in which air or gas is collected in the peritoneal cavity. May be artificially injected to treat tuberculous peritonitis or where pneumothorax is impossible.

pneumoperitonitis (nū″mō-pĕr-ĭ-tō-nī′tĭs) [Gr. *pneumōn,* lung, + *peritonaion,* peritoneum, + *-itis,* inflammation]. Peritonitis with gas accumulation.

pneumopexy (nū″mō-pĕks′ĭ) ["+ *pēxis,* fixation]. Surgical attachment of a lung to the thoracic wall.

pneumopleuritis (nū″mō-plū-rī′tĭs) ["+ *pleura,* a side, + *-itis,* inflammation]. Inflamed condition of lungs and pleura.

pneumopleuroparietopexy (nū″mō-plū″rō-pă-rī′ĕt-ō-pĕk″sĭ) ["+ "+ L. *pariēs,* wall, + Gr. *pēxis,* fixation]. The operation of attaching the lung with its parietal pleura to the border of a thoracic wound.

pneumopyelography (nū″mō-pī-ĕ-lŏg′ră-fĭ) [Gr. *pneumōn,* lung, + *pyelos,* pelvis, + *graphein,* to write]. X-ray examination of the renal pelvis and ureters after they are injected with oxygen.

pneumopyopericardium (nū″mō-pī″ō-pĕr-ĭ-kar′dĭ-ŭm) ["+ *pyon,* pus, + *peri,* around, + *kardia,* heart]. Air, gas and pus collected in the pericardial sac.

pneumopyothorax (nū″mō-pī″ō-thō′răks) ["+ "+ *thōrax,* chest]. Air and pus collected in the pleural cavity.

pneumoradiography (nū″mō-rā-dī-ŏg′ră-fĭ) ["+ L. *radius,* ray, + Gr. *graphein,* to write]. Injection of air into a part for taking an x-ray picture.

pneumorrachis (nū″mō-rā′kĭs) [Gr. *pneumōn,* lung, + *rhachis,* spine]. Gas accumulation in the spinal canal.

pneumorrhagia (nū″mō-rā′jĭ-ă) ["+ *rhēgnynai,* to burst forth]. Pulmonary hemorrhage. SYN: *hemoptysis.*

pneumoserothorax (nū″mō-sē-rō-thō′răks) [Gr. *pneumōn,* lung, + L. *serum,* whey, + Gr. *thōrax,* chest]. Air or gas and serum collected in the pleural cavity.

pneumotachograph (nū″mō-tăk′ō-grăf) [Gr. *pneuma,* air, + *tachus,* swift, + *graphein,* to write]. Device for registering velocity of inspiration and expiration of air.

pneumotherapy (nū-mō-thĕr′ă-pĭ) [Gr. *pneumōn,* lung, + *therapeia,* treatment]. 1. Treatment of diseases of the lungs. 2. Treatment of diseases by the use of rarefied or condensed gases. SYN: *pneumatotherapy.*

pneumothermomassage (nū″mō-ther″mō-măs-azh′) [Gr. *pneuma,* air, + *thermē,* heat, + *massein,* to knead]. Application to the body of air of varying temperature and pressure.

pneumothorax (nū-mō-thō′răks) ["+ *thōrax,* chest]. A collection of air or gas in the pleural cavity.

  The gas enters as the result of a perforation through the chest wall or the pleura covering the lung (visceral pleura). This perforation may be the result of an injury or the rupture of an emphysematous bleb or superficial lung abscess; the most common latter condition is a tuberculous abscess in the presence of pulmonary tuberculosis.

  SYM: The onset is sudden, usually with a severe sticking pain in the side and marked dyspnea. Fluid very frequently is found, developing within 48 hours (hydropneumothorax). The physical signs are those of a distended unilateral chest, tympanitic resonance, absence of breath sounds, and with fluid, a splash or succussion on shaking patient.

p., artificial. P. induced intentionally by artificial means employed in the treatment of pulmonary tuberculosis or pneumonia.

P. gives the diseased lung temporary rest. The lung collapses when the air enters the pleural space which is not possible if there are adhesions.

Scattered adhesions may afford only a partial collapse. Effusion may occur in about one third of the cases. Hazards are small.

NP: Explain procedure to patient. Instruct not to cough but to warn physician when so impelled. Patient lies on affected side, arm overhead, and held by nurse. Observe color of face, respiration, and pulse. Record intrapleural pressure. Watch for pleural shock and effusion (pain in side, weak pulse, dyspnea, sweating are instances). Physician gives or orders hypodermics or inhalation of oxygen. Complications may be air embolism from puncture of a vein; puncture of lung; surgical emphysema.

Postoperative care: Rest for an hour after. Record temperature every 4 hours for 48 hours. Report dyspnea because it is serious.

p., spontaneous. Spontaneous entrance of air into the pleural cavity.

The pressure may collapse the lung and displace the heart.

SYM: Sudden sharp pain, dyspnea, and cough. Pain may be referred to the shoulder. Majority of cases are mild and require only rest. Rarely shock and collapse occur.

p., valvular. P. characterized by an opening through the pleura which has a slit with a valvelike action allowing the air to pass in but not out. SYN: *tension pneumothorax.*

pneumotomy (nū-mŏt'ō-mĭ) [Gr. *pneumon,* lung, + *tomē,* a cutting]. Incision of the lung.

pneumotoxin (nū"mō-tŏks'ĭn) ["+ *toxikon,* poison]. A toxin produced by pneumococcus.

pneumotyphus (nū"mō-tī'fŭs) ["+ *typhos,* fever]. 1. Typhoid fever with pneumonia at onset. 2. Development of pneumonia during typhoid fever.

pneumouria (nū"mō-ū'rĭ-ă) [Gr. *pneuma,* air, + *ouron,* urine]. Excretion of urine with free gas. SYN: *pneumaturia.*

pneumoventricle (nū"mō-vĕn'trĭ-kl) ["+ L. *ventriculus,* little belly]. Air accumulation in the cerebral ventricles.

pneumoventriculography (nū"mō-vĕn-trĭk"-ū-lŏg'ră-fĭ) ["+ "+ Gr. *graphein,* to write]. Radiography of the lateral ventricles of the brain, after removal of fluid content and injection with air. SYN: *ventriculography.*

pneusis (nū'sĭs) [Gr. *pnein,* to breathe]. 1. Respiration. 2. Panting. SYN: *anhelation.*

pnigophobia (nĭ"gō-fō'bĭ-ă) [Gr. *pnigos,* choking, "+ *phobos,* fear]. Morbid fear of choking; sometimes experienced in angina pectoris.

pock (pŏk) [AS. *poc,* pustule]. A pustule of an eruptive fever, esp. of smallpox.

pocket (pŏk'ĕt) [ME. *poket,* pouch]. A saclike cavity.

pock'eting. Method of treating the pedicle in ovariotomy by enclosing it within the edges of the wound.

pockmarked. Pitted or marked with cicatrices from healed pustules, esp. those due to smallpox.

podagra (pō-dăg'ră) [Gr. *pous, pod-,* foot, + *agra,* seizure]. Gout, esp. of the joints of the foot or of the great toe.

podalgia (pō-dăl'jĭ-ă) ["+ *algos,* pain]. Pain in the feet.

podalic (pō-dăl'ĭk) [Gr. *pous, pod-,* foot]. Pert. to the feet.

p. version. Shifting position of a fetus to bring the feet to the outlet in labor.

podarthritis (pŏd"ar-thrī'tĭs) ["+ *arthron,* joint, + *-itis,* inflammation]. Inflammation of joints of the feet. SYN: *podagra.*

podiatrist (pō-dī'ă-trĭst") [Gr. *pous, pod-,* foot, + *iatreia,* treatment]. One who treats foot disorders; a chiropodist.

podiatry (pō-dī'ă-trĭ'). Treatment of foot disorders. SYN: *chiropody.*

podo-, pod- [Gr. *pous, podos,* foot]. Combining forms indicating relationship to the foot.

podobromidrosis (pŏd"ō-brō"mĭ-drō'sĭs) ["+ *bromos,* stench, + *hidrōs,* perspiration]. Offensive perspiration of the feet.

pododynamometer (pŏd"ō-dī"nă-mŏm'ĕ-tĕr) ["+ *dynamis,* force, + *metron,* measure]. A device for testing strength of the leg and foot muscles.

pododynia (pŏd"ō-dĭn'ĭ-ă) ["+ *odynē,* pain]. Pain in the feet, esp. a neuralgic pain in the heel with swelling and redness.

podogram (pŏd'ō-grăm) ["+ *gramma,* a mark]. An imprint or outline of the sole of the foot.

podology (pŏd-ŏl'ō-jĭ) [Gr. *podos,* foot, + *logos,* a study]. The study of the anatomy and physiology of the foot.

podophyllum (pŏd-ō-fĭl'ŭm) ["+ *phyllon,* leaf]. USP. The dried rhizome and roots of Podophyllum peltatum. Used as a caustic for certain papillomas such as verruca acuminata.

pogoniasis (pō"gō-nī'ă-sĭs) [Gr. *pōgōn,* beard, + *-iasis,* disorder]. 1. Excessive growth of the beard. 2. Growth of a beard in a woman.

pogonion (pō-gō′nĭ-ŏn). The most anterior projecting midpoint of the chin.

-poietic [Gr.]. Suffix meaning making or producing.

poikilocyte (poy′kĭl-ō-sīt) [Gr. *poikilos*, varied, + *kytos*, cell]. A large, irregular, malformed blood corpuscle.

poikilocytosis (poy″kĭl-ō-sī-tō′sĭs) ["+ "+ *-ōsis*, intensive]. Variation in shape of red blood corpuscles; a condition characterized by poikilocytes in the blood.

poikiloderma (poy-kĭl-ō-dĕr′mä) ["+ *derma*, skin]. A skin disorder characterized by pigmentation, telangiectasis, purpura, pruritus, and atrophy.

poikilotherm (poy-kĭl′ō-thĕrm) ["+ *thermē*, heat]. An animal in which the body temperature varies according to that of the environment. Called a cold-blooded animal. Ex: frogs and snakes. Opposed to homoiotherm, q.v.

point (poynt) [O.Fr., a prick, a dot]. 1. The sharp end of any object. 2. Point at which an abscess is about to rupture on a surface. 3. A minute spot. 4. Position in space, time, or degree.

p., anterior focal. Focal p., q.v.

p., anterior nodal. Nodal p., q.v.

p., auricular. Center of external orifice of auditory canal.

p., Boas′. Tender spot in gastric ulcer left of 12th thoracic vertebra.

p., boiling. The temperature at which a liquid will boil.

p., Broca′s. Center of the external auditory meatus; the auricular p.

p.′s, Capuron′s. Four fixed points in pelvic inlet, the two iliopectineal eminences and the two sacroiliac joints.

p.′s, cardinal. 1. Six p.′s determining direction of light rays emerging from and entering the eye. SEE: *p.′s, principal; p.′s, nodal.* 2. P.′s, Capuron′s, q.v.

p.′s, corresponding. P. in the retina of the two eyes which, when stimulated simultaneously, result in a single visual sensation.

p., craniometric. One of the fixed p.′s of the skull used in craniometry.

p., critical, of gases. Temperature at or above which a gas can no longer be liquefied by pressure.

p., critical, of liquids. Temperature above which no pressure may retain a body in a liquid form.

p.′s, deaf, of the ear. Point at lower end of tragus and one where helix intersects line of motion when vibrating tuning fork held in front of ear cannot be heard when started from the lower edge of the zygoma and moved backward toward the occiput.

p., dew. The temperature at which moisture begins to be deposited as dew.

p., disparate. P.′s on the retinae unequally paired.

p., external orbital. The prominent p. at outer edge of orbit above the frontomalar suture.

p., far. The p. (20 ft. or more) at which distinct vision is possible without aid of the muscles of accommodation. It is nearer than 20 ft. according to degree of myopia. There is no far point in the hypermetropic eye.

p., fixation. P. at which the two visual axes converge.

p., focal. The point at which a group of light rays converge.

p., freezing. Temperature at which liquids become solid.

p.′s, hysterogenic. Circumscribed areas of the body which produce symptoms of a hysterical aura, and eventually a hysterical attack when rubbed or pressed.

p.′s, identical retinal. P.′s in the two retinae upon which the images are seen as one.

p., jugal. Posterior border of frontal process of the malar bone where cut by a line tangent to upper border of zygoma.

p., lacrimal. Outlet of lacrimal canaliculus. SYN: *punctum lacrimale* [NA].

p., Lanz′s. P. on line between two anterior superior iliac spines, one third of the distance from right spine, indicating origin of the vermiform appendix.

p., Lian′s. P. at junction of outer and middle thirds of a line from the umbilicus to anterior superior spine of ilium where trocar may be introduced safely for paracentesis.

p., malar. The most prominent p. on external tubercle of the malar bone.

p., McBurney′s. P. 1 1/2 to 2 in. (4.1 to 5.1 cm.) above anterior superior spine of ilium, on line between the ilium and umbilicus, where pressure shows tenderness in acute appendicitis.

p., motor. A p. usually about the middle of a muscle where a motor nerve enters the muscle at which a minimal electrical stimulus to the overlying skin will elicit a visible contraction.

p., Munro′s. P. halfway between left anterior iliac spine and the umbilicus.

p.′s, nasal genital. Point at anterior end of lower turbinated bone, and one at the tuberculum septi, irritation of which, when in a hyperesthetic state, produces pain in the hypogastrium and in sacral region.

p., near. Nearest p. at which the eye can accommodate for distinct vision.

p.'s, nodal. An anterior and posterior cardinal point on the surface of lens of the eye so related that every ray directed toward the anterior point is represented after refraction by a ray emanating from the posterior point.

p.'s, painful. P.'s over which a neuralgic nerve is tender on pressure. SYN: *p.'s, Valleix's.*

p.'s, pressure. 1. P.'s on the skin which, when stimulated, give rise to sensation of pressure. 2. P.'s where arteries come near the surface and at which pressure may be applied to stop arterial bleeding. SEE: *pressure points.*

p.'s, principal. Two p.'s so situated that the optical axis is cut by the two principal planes.

p.'s, Valleix's. Tender spots upon pressure over the course of a nerve in neuralgia. SYN: *points douloureux.*

pointillage (pwähn″tĭ-yahzh′) [Fr.]. Massage with finger tips.

pointing. Reaching a point.

p. of an abscess. An abscess that is about to rupture spontaneously.

p., past. Inability to accurately place finger or some other part of the body on a selected point. Seen in certain neurological disorders.

Poiseuille's law (pwä-zē′ē). [Jean Marie Poiseuille, Fr. physiologist, 1799-1869]. The rapidity of the capillary current is in direct proportion to the square of the diameter of the capillary tube, the pressure on the fluid, and indirectly to the viscosity of the liquid and length of the tube.

Poiseuille's layer or space. The inert capillary current in which leukocytes move slowly, the erythrocytes moving more rapidly in the middle current.

poison (poy′zn) [L. *potio,* a poisonous draft]. Any substance which, taken into the body whether by ingestion, inhalation, injection, absorption, etc., interferes with normal physiological functions. Virtually any substance can be poisonous if consumed in sufficient quantity; therefore the term poison more often implies an excessive degree of dosage rather than any list of substances. Aspirin is not usually thought of as a poison, but overdoses of this drug kill more children accidentally each year than any of the traditional poisons. Since the list of poisonous substances is infinite, it defies classification in any simple way. One of the most widely employed classifications is found in *Standard Nomenclature of Diseases and Operations,* 5th ed., McGraw-Hill Book Co., New York, 1961. For a list of commonly encountered hazardous substances in the home, see *Poisons and Poisoning Table* in *Appendix.*

p., economic. Pesticides. Chemicals whose toxic properties are commercially exploited in agriculture, industry, or commerce to increase quantity, improve quality, or generally to promote consumer acceptability of a variety of products. Common types of economic poisons include insecticides, rodenticides, herbicides, fungicides, insect repellants, molluscicides, and some kinds of food additives. The wide variety of economic poisons that are commonly found in and around the home constitutes an important group in accidental poisonings. SEE: *Table of Poisons and Poisoning* in *Appendix.*

poison control center. A facility meeting the staffing and equipment standards of the American Association of Poison Control Centers and recognized to be able to give information on, or treatment to patients suffering from, poisoning. A poison information center consists only of a reference library and does not have treatment facilities. Over 400 poison centers of these two types are scattered throughout the U. S. Staffed largely by volunteer personnel, they offer service at any time of the day or night. By virtue of their function, they are commonly associated with or are part of large hospitals or medical schools. A government agency—the Poison Control Branch of the Division of Accident Prevention, Public Health Service, Department of Health, Education, and Welfare—is also active in poison control programs and in coordinating the efforts of individual centers. SEE: *Poison Control Centers* in *Appendix.*

poisoning (poy′zn-ing) [L. *potio,* a poisonous draft]. 1. The state produced by introduction of a poison into the body. 2. Administration of a poison. Symptoms of poisoning vary widely with the agent. SEE: *Table of Poisons and Poisoning* in *Appendix.*

F.A.: Avoid becoming excited. Contact a physician or a poison control center immediately and explain the nature of the emergency. Attempt to identify the nature of the poison by looking for the container, questioning the patient, noting burns, stains, odors, or symptoms. Do not discard the poison; keep a sample and the original container, but clean up any spilled material which might be a hazard to another member of the family. If the patient vomits, preserve a sample of the vomitus. Take all specimens and containers to the hospital with the patient.

Dilute the poison at once with large quantities of milk, water, or a slurry of activated charcoal in water. Diluting delays absorption, and it is easier to induce emesis when the stomach is full. Do not attempt to induce emesis in an unconscious or stuporous patient or if strong alkali, mineral acid, or kerosene was ingested.

The primary emphasis should be directed toward getting the patient to a medical facility in the shortest possible time. The following suggestions are to be employed only if they will not delay professional treatment appreciably.

Emesis may be induced by stroking or gently tickling the back of the patient's throat with a finger or the handle of a teaspoon. Sometimes a glass or two of warm water containing either 3 teaspoonsful of table salt or 1 teaspoonful of dry mustard will produce vomiting. If attempts to induce vomiting are successful, readminister large amounts of milk, condensed milk, egg whites, flour and water, or a slurry of activated charcoal in water.

If the patient is unconscious and shows signs of impending vomiting, lay him on his side with his head a few inches below the rest of his body. Watch for difficulty in breathing and be prepared to give artificial respiration if the patient stops spontaneous breathing.

If the patient convulses, do nothing except prevent him from falling or otherwise injuring himself. Blankets, wet compresses, and gentle massage can do no harm and may serve some purpose. Strong black coffee or tea should be given if the patient becomes drowsy.

If material was spilled on the patient's skin, clothing, or splashed in the eyes, discard the garments and flush with running tap water. It may be necessary to hold the victim's eyelids open under water to effect good rinsing. If the material is a gas or a vapor, remove the patient and other persons from the area.

Make notes of all that is said by the patient, but do not repeat any of this to anyone except the physician or a court official.

NOTE: Do not be hasty in concluding that a patient has been poisoned. Many disease states mimic the symptoms of poisoning. Cerebral hemorrhage, epilepsy, overdose of insulin, diabetic coma, meningitis, thrombosis, and uremia may simulate poisoning. Acute indigestion, appendicitis, gastritis, re-nal colic, or peptic ulcer may minic poisoning by corrosive substances.

p., acute. A state of intoxication produced by a single dose administered rapidly. Acute p. does not refer to the rapidity with which symptoms develop after exposure to a toxic agent, although it follows that a large dose of a poison given rapidly usually produces symptoms within a relatively short time.

p., blood. SEE: *bacteremia; pyemia; septicemia; toxemia.*

p., chronic. A state of intoxication produced by multiple small doses given over a period of time, not one dose of which would have produced the full toxic syndrome if given alone.

p., convulsive. SEE: *convulsant poisons.*

p., corrosive. SEE: *corrosive poisons.*

p., cumulative. Chronic poisoning.

p., fish. SEE: *fish poisoning.*

p., food. SEE: *food poisoning.*

p. by unknown substances. In cases where there is no information concerning the nature of the poison taken, and the signs and symptoms are not recognized as being due to any particular substance, it is obvious that specific antidotes cannot be given. There are, however, certain agents which act in a general manner and may be efficacious. One of these is activated charcoal, which is available from many sources. Although a slurry of this in water is messy and offensive to the patient, it is a highly effective adsorbent for certain kinds of poisons.

Another substance is referred to as the universal antidote. It consists of a mixture of 2 parts activated charcoal, 1 part magnesium oxide, and 1 part tannic acid. The universal antidote has been used empirically for a number of years and prepackaged units now are available commercially. It is doubtful if this mixture offers any real advantage over activated charcoal, which has a proven effectiveness against many substances.

Both these materials may be given as a slurry made from several heaping teaspoonsful in a glass of water. Since the ingredients are essentially harmless and since the efficiency is increased by increasing the amount of adsorbent relative to the amount of poison, the dose may be repeated several times.

poison ivy. A climbing vine, Rhus toxicodendron, which on contact produces a severe form of dermatitis. Rhus species contain urushiol, an extremely irritating oily resin.

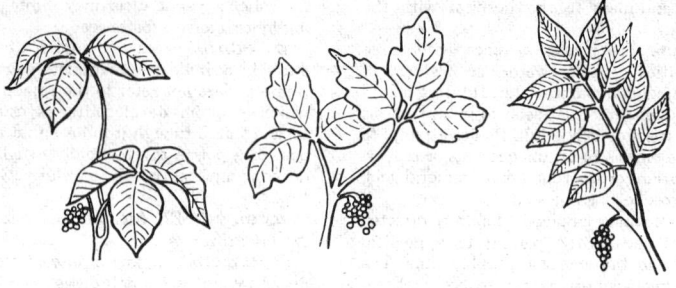

POISON IVY   POISON OAK   POISON SUMAC

Urushiol may also be a potent sensitizer since in many cases subsequent contacts produce increasingly severe reactions.

poison ivy dermatitis. Dermatitis resulting from irritation or sensitization of the skin by the resin of the poison ivy plant. There is no absolute immunity although susceptibility varies greatly even in the same individual.

SYM: Always an interval between time of contact of poison with skin and first appearance of symptoms, varying from a few hours to several days and depending on sensitivity of the patient and possibly condition of skin. Moderate itching or burning sensation soon followed by small blisters; later manifestations vary. Blisters usually rupture and are followed by oozing of serum and subsequent crusting.

FA: Thorough washing of the skin with soap and water and complete change of clothing are advised if there has been known exposure.

TREATMENT: In mild dermatitis, a lotion to relieve itching is usually sufficient. In severe dermatitis, cool wet dressings or compresses, potassium permanganate baths, and perhaps a course of intramuscular or oral corticosteroid therapy are advised. Sedation is also necessary in some cases.

poison oak. A climbing vine, Rhus radicans or R. diversiloba, closely related to poison ivy and containing the same active principle. The symptoms and treatment are identical with those for poison ivy dermatitis, q.v.

poisonous (poy′zn-ŭs) [L. *potio,* a poisonous draft]. Having the properties or qualities of a poison; venomous.

p. plants. Do not eat: castor bean, chinaberry, European bittersweet, wild or black cherry, horse chestnuts, poisonous hemlock, laurel, mushroom or death cup, black nightshade or deadly nightshade, Jimson weed.

Do not touch: poison ivy, poison oak, poison sumac.

poison sumac. A shrublike plant, Rhus vernix, widely distributed in the U.S. as are all Rhus species. Since it contains the same active principle as poison ivy, the symptoms and treatment are the same as in poison ivy dermatitis, q.v.

poker back. Stiffness of the spine. May result from spondylitis, q.v., or rheumatoid arthritis.

pokeroot (pōk′rŭt). The dried root of Veratrum viride used internally as an antihypertensive agent.

p. poisoning. Poisoning resulting from ingestion of pokeroot.

SYM: Nausea, vomiting, drowsiness, vertigo, and possibly convulsions and respiratory paralysis.

TREATMENT: Emetic or lavage.

po′lar [L. *polaris*]. Concerning a pole.

polarimeter (pō″lăr-ĭm′ĕ-tĕr) ["+ Gr. *metron,* a measure]. Instrument for measuring amount of polarization of light, or rotation of polarized light.

polarimetry (pō″lar-ĭm′ĕ-trĭ). Measurement of the amount and rotation of polarized light.

polariscope (pō-lăr′ĭ-skōp) [L. *polaris,* pole, + Gr. *skopein,* to examine]. Apparatus used in measurement of polarized light.

polarity (pō-lăr′ĭ-tĭ). 1. The quality of having poles. 2. The exhibition of opposite effects at the two extremities in physical therapy.

polarization (pō″lăr-ĭ-zā′shŭn) [L. *polaris,* pole]. 1. Condition in a ray of light in which vibrations occur in only one plane or in curves. 2. In a galvanic battery, collection of hydrogen bubbles on negative plate and oxygen on the positive plate, whereby generation of current is impeded. 3. Condition in which ions of opposite charges are separated by a semipermeable membrane such as a cell membrane.

pole (pōl) [L. *polus*]. 1. The extremity of any axis about which forces acting on it are symmetrically disposed. 2. One of two points in a magnet, cell, or battery having opposite physical qualities.

p., animal. P. opposite the yolk in an ovum. At this point, polar bodies are formed and pinched off and protoplasm is concentrated and has greatest activity.

p.'s of the eye. The anterior and posterior extremities of the optic axis.

p., frontal. Most projecting part of the anterior extremity of both cerebral hemispheres.

p., germinal. The p. of an ovum at which the development begins.

p.'s of the kidney. The kidney's upper and lower extremities.

p., occipital. The posterior extremity of the occipital lobe.

p., pelvic. Breech of a fetus.

p., placental, of the chorion. Spot at which the domelike placenta is situated.

p., temporal. The anterior extremity of the temporal lobe.

p.'s of the testicle. The upper and lower extremities of a testicle.

p., vegetal. Part of the egg containing the food yolk. SYN: *vegetative* or *antigerminal pole.*

policlinic (pŏl'ĭ-klĭn'ĭk) [Gr. *polis*, city, + *klinē*, bed]. A city hospital or clinic for outpatients. SEE: *polyclinic.*

pol'io. Acute anterior poliomyelitis, q.v.

polio- [Gr. *polios*, gray]. Combining form indicating relationship to the gray matter of the nervous system.

polioclastic (pōl'ĭ-ō-klăs'tĭk) ["+ *klastos*, breaking]. Destructive to gray matter of the nervous system.

polioencephalitis (pōl'ĭ-ō-ĕn-sĕf'ă-lī'tĭs) [Gr. *polios*, gray, + *enkephalos*, brain, + *-itis*, inflammation]. Condition characterized by inflammatory lesions of the gray matter of the brain.

p., anterior superior. A disease involving necrotic changes in gray matter about 3rd ventricle, anterior portion of 4th ventricle, and aqueduct of Sylvius. Characterized by ocular abnormalities, mental disturbances, and ataxia. Of nutritional origin, probably thiamine (vitamin B₁) deficiency. SYN: *Wernicke's encephalopathy.*

p. hemorrhagica. P. accompanied by hemorrhagic lesions.

p., posterior. P. involving gray matter about 4th ventricle.

polioencephalomeningomyelitis (pōl'ĭ-ō-ĕn-sĕf'ăl-ō-mĕn-ĭn-gō-mī-ĕl-ī'tĭs) ["+ "+ *mēninx*, membrane, + *myelos*, marrow, +

-ītis, inflammation]. Inflammation of the gray matter of the brain and spinal cord and their meninges.

polioencephalomyelitis (pōl'ĭ-ō-ĕn-sĕf'ăl-ō-mĭ-ĕl-ī'tĭs). Inflamed condition of the gray matter of the brain and spinal cord. SYN: *Heine-Medin disease.*

polioencephalopathy (pōl'ĭ-ō-ĕn-sĕf'ăl-ŏp'ă-thĭ) [Gr. *polios*, gray, + *enkephalos*, brain, + *pathos*, disease]. Diseased condition of the gray matter of the brain.

poliomyelencephalitis (pōl'ĭ-ō-mī''ĕl-ĕn-sĕf'ăl-ī'tĭs) ["+ *myelos*, marrow, + *enkephalos*, brain, + *-ītis*, inflammation]. Poliomyelitis with polioencephalitis.

poliomyelitis (pōl'ĭ-ō-mī''ĕl-ī'tĭs) ["+ "+ *-itis*, inflammation]. Inflammation of the gray matter of the spinal cord.

p., abortive. P. in which illness is mild with no involvement of central nervous system.

p., acute anterior. An acute infectious inflammation of the anterior horns of the gray matter of the spinal cord.

This is an acute, systemic, infectious disease in which paralysis may or may not occur. In the majority of patients, the disease is mild, being limited to respiratory and gastrointestinal symptoms, such constituting the minor illness or the abortive type which lasts only a few days. In the major illness, paralysis or weakness of muscles occurs with loss of superficial and deep reflexes. In such cases, characteristic lesions are found in the gray matter of the spinal cord, medulla, motor area of cerebral cortex, and cerebellum.

SYN: *acute lateral paralysis; acute wasting paralysis; epidemic paralysis; Heine-Medin's disease; infantile paralysis; polio; spinal paralytic paralysis.*

ETIOL: Causative agent is a virus consisting of particles from 270 to 300 Angstrom units in diameter. The virus is resistant and stable, remaining viable for months outside the body. Three immunologic types exist.

SYM: Onset often is abrupt, although the ordinary manifestations of a severe cold or some gastrointestinal disturbances may come on gradually, accompanied by slight elevation of temperature, frequently enduring for not more than three days. At the end of this period, paralysis may or may not develop. The extent of any paralysis necessarily depends upon degree of nerve involvement. Consequently, paralysis may be confined to one small group of muscles or affect one or all extremities. In some instances, the respiratory muscles also are involved, and it is in these cases that death is so likely to ensue. In the average paralytic case it is the extensor muscles in particular that are affected.

COMPLICATIONS: Any paralysis occurring in this disease may be regarded as a complication. Atrophy of muscles and ultimate deformities may likewise be classed in a similar way. Aside from bronchopneumonia, which may develop in very severe cases, other complications are surprisingly few.

DIFFERENTIAL DIAG: Among the diseases confused with this infection are the various types of meningitis and rheumatism, traumatic conditions, tuberculosis involving bones or joints, and occasionally scurvy or rickets in infants.

INCIDENCE: Poliomyelitis is endemic throughout the world but occurs in epidemics in certain countries, including the U.S. However, the disease in the U.S. has been brought under almost complete control by vaccination.

Epidemics are seasonal, occurring in summer and fall. Children are more susceptible than adults. Infection is spread by direct contact, the virus probably entering the body via mouth. How it reaches the central nervous system is not known.

INCUBATION PERIOD: From 3 to 21 days, but usually 7 to 12 days.

PROG: Ordinarily the outcome as to life is good. It is only the bulbar and respiratory types in which death is likely to occur. In fact, these two types constitute nearly all of the fatal cases. Even in those cases in which paralysis is present, complete restoration of the parts may finally be brought about. In the more severe types, however, some paralysis may remain.

PROPHYLAXIS: Passive immunization with gamma globulin gives a limited amount of protection. Active immunization with Live Oral Poliovirus Vaccine (USP) has greatly reduced the incidence of paralytic poliomyelitis. The oral vaccine containing all three types of the virus should be given to young infants in three doses 1-2 months apart. Booster doses should be given at 1 1/2 and 5 years of age. Oral poliovirus vaccine and measles vaccine should be given separately at intervals of at least one month.

PREDISPOSING FACTORS: Tonsillectomy and other nose and throat operations, routine immunizations, excessive physical strain and fatigue. Pregnant women are especially susceptible during epidemics.

NP: No known specific drug treatment. Treatment is systematic, aimed at relieving symptoms, preventing deformities, and saving life. In abortive cases, bed rest for 7 to 10 days and light diet are adequate. In severe cases, muscle tenderness and pain are alleviated by proper positioning, gentle passive movement, and by application of hot, moist packs at 20-min. intervals or by hot baths for children. Mild analgesics and sedatives may be used. Fluid and salt balance should be maintained.

Retention of urine and constipation are troublesome complications. The former may be treated by a parasympathetic stimulating drug, the latter by mild laxatives and warm saline enemas.

Respiratory failure may occur in bulbar poliomyelitis. It may result from paralysis of respiratory muscles, failure of respiratory centers in the medulla, obstruction of air passageways resulting from weakness of pharyngeal or laryngeal muscles, or pulmonary edema. Oxygen administration, tracheotomy, or use of respirator may be indicated.

Convalescence of the paralyzed patient necessitates careful attention, often involving physical and occupational therapy and orthopedic treatment as well as an understanding and amelioration of psychological difficulties. Mechanical supports for weakened structures may be necessary.

p., anterior. Inflamed state of the anterior horns of the spinal cord.

p., ascending. P. in which paralysis begins in lower extremities and progresses up legs, thighs, trunk, and finally involves respiratory muscles.

p., bulbar. P. in which gray matter of the medulla oblongata is involved, resulting in paralysis and usually respiratory failure. SYN: *bulbar paralytic poliomyelitis.* SEE: *p., acute anterior.*

p., chronic anterior. Progressive wasting of the muscles. Myelopathic progressive muscular atrophy.

p., epidemic. SEE: *p., acute anterior.*

p., nonparalytic. Pain and stiffness in the muscles of the axial skeleton, esp. of the neck and back; mild fever; increased proteins and leukocytes in the cerebrospinal fluid. Diagnosis depends on the isolation of the virus and serological reactions. SYN: *preparalytic p.*

p., paralytic. Poliomyelitis with a variable combination of signs of damage of the central nervous system. These include weakness, incoordination, muscle tenderness and spasms, flaccid paralysis, and disturbance of consciousness.

p., paralytic, bulbar. SEE: *p., acute anterior.*

p., paralytic, spinal. SEE: *p., acute anterior.*

poliomyelopathy (pŏl″ĭ-ō-mī″ĕl-ŏp′ă-thĭ) [Gr. *polios,* gray, + *myelos,* marrow, + *pathos,* disease]. Any diseased condition of the gray matter of the spinal cord.

polioplasm (pŏl′ĭ-ō-plăzm) ["+ *plasma,* a thing formed]. Granular protoplasm.

poliosis (pŏl′ĭ-ō′sĭs) ["+ *-osis,* condition]. Absence of pigment in the hair. SYN: *canities; grayness.*

politzerization (pŏl″ĭt-sĕr-ĭ-zā′shŭn). The inflation of the middle ear using a Politzer bag, q.v.

Politzer's bag (pŏl′ĭt-zer). [Adam Politzer, Hungarian otologist, 1835-1920]. Soft rubber bag with rubber tip for inflating the middle ear by increasing the pressure in the nasopharynx.

pollakiuria (pŏl-ă-kĭ-ū′rĭ-ă) [Gr. *pollakis,* often, + *ouron,* urine]. Abnormally frequent passage of urine.

pollen (pŏl′ĕn) [L., dust]. The microspores of a seed plant that develop in the anther at tip of stamen. Each pollen grain develops a pollen tube and constitutes the male gametophyte. Within it develops a tube nucleus and two sperm nuclei, the latter constituting the male reproductive elements.

pollenogenic (pŏl″ĕn-ō-jĕn′ĭk) ["+ Gr. *gennan,* to produce]. Caused by the pollen of plants, or producing plant pollen.

pollenosis (pŏl″ĕn-ō′sĭs) ["+ Gr. *-osis,* disease]. Pollinosis, q.v.

pollex (pŏl′ĕks) [L.]. (pl. *pol′lices*) [NA]. The thumb.

p. extensus. Backward deviation of thumb.

p. flexus. Permanent flexion of thumb.

p. pedis. The great toe. SYN: *hallux.*

p. valgus. Abnormal deviation of thumb toward ulnar side.

p. varus. Abnormal deviation of thumb toward radial side.

pollinosis (pŏl-ĭn-ō′sĭs) [L. *pollen,* dust, + Gr. *-osis,* disease]. Nasal congestion of mucous membranes due to contact with pollen. SYN: *hay fever.*

pollution (pŭ-lū′shŭn) [ME. polluten]. 1. State of making impure or defiling. 2. Voluntary or involuntary emission of semen at times other than in coition.

polonium (pō-lō′nĭ-ŭm). [L. Polōnia, Poland, native country of its discoverers, the Curies]. SYMB: *Po.* At. wt. 210; at. no. 84. Radioactive element isolated from pitchblende. SYN: *radium F.*

polus (pō′lŭs) [L.]. (pl. *po′li*) [NA]. Pole; the extremity of an organ.

poly (pŏl′ĭ). Abbr. for *polymorphonuclear leukocyte.*

poly- [Gr. *polys,* many]. Prefix indicating many or much.

polyadenitis (pŏl′ĭ-ad″ē-nī′tĭs) ["+ Gr. *adēn,* gland, + *-itis,* inflammation]. Condition of inflamed lymph nodes, esp. the cervical lymph nodes.

polyadenomatosis (pŏl′ĭ-ăd″ē-nō-mă-tō′sĭs) ["+ "+ *-oma,* tumor, + *-osis,* disease]. Adenomas in many glands.

polyadenous (pŏl′ĭ-ad′ē-nŭs). Involving or rel. to many glands.

polyalgesia (pol′ĭ-ăl-jē′zĭ-ă) [Gr. *polys,* many, + *algēsis,* sensation]. A single stimulus of a part, producing sensation in many parts.

polyandry (pŏl′ĭ-ăn′drĭ) ["+ *aner, andr-,* man]. The practice of having more than one husband at the same time. SEE: *polygamy.*

polyarteritis (pŏl′ĭ-ăr″tĕr-ī′tĭs) ["+ *artēria,* artery, + *-itis,* inflammation]. Inflammation of several arteries at the same time.

p. nodosa. Widespread focal areas of damage due to inflammation of arteries, esp. small and medium-sized ones. Function of organs involved is impaired. When the disease begins, its manifestations are extremely variable. Symptoms of a moderate febrile disease are quite common. SYN: *periarteritis nodosa.*

polyarthric (pŏl′ĭ-ar′thrĭk) [Gr. *polys,* many, + *arthron,* joint]. Affecting or pert. to several joints.

polyarthritis (pol-ĭ-ar-thrī′tis) ["+ "+ *-itis,* inflammation]. Inflammation of a number of joints.

polyarticular (pŏl′ĭ-ăr-tĭk′ū-lăr) [Gr. *polys,* many, + L. *articulus,* a joint]. Affecting many joints. SYN: *multiarticular.*

polyatomic (pŏl′ĭ-ă-tŏm′ĭk) ["+ *atomon,* atom]. 1. Having several atoms. Having more than two replaceable hydrogen atoms.

polyblast (pŏl′ĭ-blăst) ["+ *blastos,* a germ]. Large mononuclear phagocyte present in inflammation derived from an embryonic wandering cell.

polyblennia (pŏl-ĭ-blĕ′nĭ-ă) [Gr. *polys,* many, + *blennos,* mucus]. Secretion of more mucus than normal.

polycholia (pŏl′ĭ-kō′lĭ-ă) ["+ *cholē,* bile]. Abnormal secretion of bile.

polychrest (pŏl′ĭ-krĕst) ["+ *chrēstos,* useful]. A medicine useful in many diseases.

polychromasia (pŏl′ĭ-krō-mā′zĭ-ă) [Gr. *polys,* many, + *chrōma,* color]. Quality of having many colors.

polychromatic (pŏl′ĭ-krō-măt′ĭk). Multicolored.

polychromatophil(e   (pŏl'ĭ-krō-măt'ō-fĭl)
[Gr. *polys,* many, + *chrōma,* color, + *philein,* to love]. A cell, esp. an erythrocyte,
which is stainable with more than one kind
of stain.

polychromatophilia   (pŏl'ĭ-krō-măt"ō-fĭl'ĭ-
ă) ["+ "+ *philein,* to love]. 1. The quality of
being stainable with more than one stain. 2.
Polychromatophil cells in the blood to excess.

polychromemia   (pŏl'ĭ-krō-mē'mĭ-ă) [Gr. *polys,* many, + *chrōma,* color, + *haima,*
blood]. Increase in the hemoglobin of the
blood.

polychylia   (pŏl'ĭ-kī'lĭ-ă) ["+ L. *chylus,* juice].
Excessive secretion of chyle.

polyclinic   (pŏl'ĭ-klĭn'ĭk) ["+ *klinē,* bed]. Hospital or clinic treating many diseases; a
general hospital.

polyclonia   (pŏl'ĭ-klō'nĭ-ă)   ["+ *klonos,* tu-
mult]. A disease characterized by many
clonic spasms, but distinct from chorea or
tic.

polycoria   (pŏl'ĭ-kō'rĭ-ă) ["+ *korē,* pupil]. The
state of having more than one pupil in one
eye.

polycrotic   (pŏl'ĭ-krŏt'ĭk) [Gr. *polys,* many, +
krotos, beat]. Having several pulse waves for
each heart beat.

polycrotism   (pŏl-ĭk'rō-tĭzm) ["+ "+ *ismos,*
condition]. Condition of having several pulse
waves for each heart beat.

polycystic   (pŏl'ĭ-sĭs'tĭk) ["+ *kystis,* cyst].
Composed of many cysts.

polycythemia   (pŏl'ĭ-sī-thē'mĭ-ă) [Gr. *polys,*
many, + *kytos,* cell, + *haima,* blood]. An
excess of red blood cells. SEE: *erythrocytosis.*

*p. megalosplenica; p., myelopath-
ic; p. rubra.* Polycythemia vera, q.v.

p., primary. P. in which there is hyperplasia of blood-forming cells in bone marrow. SYN: *p. vera,* q.v.

p., relative. Relative increase in number of erythrocytes which occurs in hemo-
concentration.

p., secondary. P. resulting from some
physiological condition such as lowered oxygen tension in the blood which stimulates
erythropoiesis. SYN: *erythrocytosis; symptomatic p.*

p., splenomegalic. P. in which enlargement of the spleen occurs. SEE: *p. vera.*

p. vera. A slowly progressive disease
characterized by an increased number of red
blood cells and increase in total blood
volume. SYN: *erythremia; p., primary; p.
rubra; splenomegalic p.; Osler's disease;
Vaquez's disease.*

SYM AND SIGNS: Weakness, fatigue,
vertigo, tinnitus, irritability, enlarged
spleen, flushing of face, redness and pain of
extremities, black and blue spots. Basal
metabolism increased and bone marrow
shows increased cellularity.

ETIOL: Unknown.

TREATMENT: Permanent cure cannot
be achieved today, but remissions of many
months can be produced. Venesection and
radioactive phosphorus (P^{32}) have proved to
be effective.

polydactylism   (pŏl'ĭ-dăk'tĭ-lĭzm) [Gr. *polys,*
many, + *daktylos,* digit, + *-ismos,* condi-
tion]. State of having supernumerary fingers or toes.

polydipsia   (pŏl'ĭ-dĭp'sĭ-ă) ["+ *dipsa,* thirst].
Excessive thirst.

polyemia   (pŏl'ĭ-ē'mĭ-ă)   ["+ *haima,* blood].
Abnormal amount of blood in the system.
SYN: *polycythemia.*

polyesthesia   (pŏl'ĭ-ĕs-thē'zĭ-ă) [Gr. *polys,*
many, + *aisthēsis,* sensation]. Abnormal
sensation of touch in which a single stimulus
is felt at two or more places.

polyesthetic   (pŏl'ĭ-ĕs-thĕt'ĭk). 1. Pert. to
polyesthesia, q.v. 2. Pert. to several senses or
sensations.

polyethylene   (pŏl'ē-ĕth'ĭ-lēn). In chemistry,
a polymerized resin of ethylene. Used to
make a wide variety of products, including
tubing used in medicine.

p. glycol 400. USP. A polymer of ethylene oxide and water. Has formula of
$H(OCH_2CH_2)_nOH$ in which the value of n is
from 8.2 to 9.1. Used as a water-soluble
ointment base.

p. glycol 4000. USP. A polymer of ethylene oxide and water. The formula is
$H(OCH_2CH_2)_nOH$ in which the value of n is
from 68 to 84. Used as a water-soluble
ointment base.

polygalactia   (pŏl'ĭ-gă-lăk'shĭ-ă) [Gr. *polys,*
many, + *galaktos,* milk]. Excessive secretion or flow of milk.

polygamy   (pō-lĭg'ă-mĭ)   ["+ *gamos,* mar-
riage]. Practice of having several wives,
husbands, or mates at the same time, esp.
wives.

polygastria   (pŏl'ĭ-găs'trĭ-ă) ["+ *gastēr,* sto-
mach]. Excessive secretion or flow of gastric
juice.

polygenic.   Pert. to or caused by several
genes.

polyglandular   (pŏl'ĭ-glăn'dū-lăr)   ["+ L.
glandula, a little kernel]. Pert. to or affecting many glands. SYN: *pluriglandular.*

polygram   (pŏl'ĭ-grăm) [Gr. *polys,* many, +
gramma, a mark]. Sphygmographic record

made by polygraph of simultaneous pulse beats.

polygraph (pŏl'ĭ-grăf) ["+ *graphein*, to write]. A device which records simultaneously tracings of several different pulsations, as arterial and venous pulse waves, apex beat of heart, and other pulsations. Has been used as a so-called lie dectector. SYN: *sphygmograph.*

polygyria (pŏl'ĭ-jĭ'rĭ-ă) ["+ *gyros*, circle]. Excess of the normal number of convolutions in the brain.

polyhedral (pŏl'ĭ-hē'drăl) [Gr. *polys*, many, + *hedra*, base]. Having many surfaces.

polyhemia (pŏl'ĭ-hē'mĭ-ă) ["+ *haima*, blood]. Abnormal increase in amount of the blood. SYN: *polyemia.*

polyhidrosis (pŏl'ĭ-hĭ-drō'sĭs) ["+ *hidrōsis,* perspiration]. Excessive perspiration.

polyhistor (pŏl'ē-hĭs'tŭr) ["+ *histōr,* learned]. A scholar or physician who has great and varied abilities and knowledge. Ex: Hippocrates, Galen, Paracelsus, Boerhaave, Richard Mead, and Thomas Jefferson. SYN: *polymath.*

polyhydramnios (pŏl'l-hī-drăm'nĭ-ŏs) ["+ *hydōr,* water, + *amnion,* amnion]. An excess of amniotic fluid in the bag-of-waters in pregnancy. SEE: *amnion.*

polyhydruria (pŏl'ĭ-hĭ-drŭ'rĭ-ă) ["+ "+ *ouron,* urine]. Excessive amt. of water in urine.

polyhypermenorrhea (pŏl'ĭ-hī''pĕr-mĕn''ōrē'ă) [Gr. *polys*, many, + *hyper*, over, + *mēn*, month, + *rhoia*, flow]. Frequent menstruation with excessive discharge.

polyhypomenorrhea (pŏl'ĭ-hī''pō-mĕn''ō-rē'ă) ["+ *hypo*, under, + *mēn*, month, + *rhoia*, flow]. Frequent menstruation with scanty discharge.

Poly I:C. A complex of synthetic polyriboinosinic and polyribocytidylic acids. They are a form of double-stranded ribonucleic acids which may help to induce resistance to virus infection. Poly I:C stimulates production of interferon, q.v.

polyinfection (pŏl'ĭ-ĭn-fĕk'shŭn) ["+ ME. *infecten,* infect]. Infection with two or more microorganisms. SYN: *multiinfection.*

polykaryocyte (pŏl'ĭ-kăr'ĭ-ō-sīt) ["+ *karyon,* nucleus, + *kytos,* cell]. A cell possessing several nuclei.

polyleptic (pŏl'ĭ-lĕp'tĭk) [Gr. *polys*, many, + *lēpsis,* a seizure]. Characterized by numerous remissions and exacerbations, as malaria.

polymastia (pŏl'ĭ-măs'tĭ-ă) ["+ *mastos,* breast]. Condition of having more than two breasts.

polymastigote (pŏl'ĭ-măs'tĭ-gōt) [Gr. *polys*, many, + *mastix, mastig-,* whip]. Possessing several flagella.

polyma'zia ["+ *mastos, mazos,* breast]. Condition of having more than two breasts. SYN: *polymastia.*

polymenia (pŏl'ĭ-mē'nĭ-ă) ["+ *mēn*, month]. Polymenorrhea, q.v.

polymenorrhea (pŏl'ĭ-mĕn-ō-rē'ă) ["+ "+ *rhoia,* a flow]. Menstrual flow occurring too frequently. SYN: *polymenia.*

polymer (pŏl'ĭ-mĕr) [Gr. *polys*, many, + *meros,* a part]. A natural or synthetic substance formed by a combination of two or more molecules (and up to millions) of the same substance. EX: paraformaldehyde (HCHO)₃ formed from three molecules of formaldehyde, HCHO.

  p. fume fever. Condition resulting from breathing fumes produced by certain polymers when they are heated to 300°-700° C. or higher.

  SYM: Tight, gripping sensation of the chest associated with shivering, sore throat, fever, and weakness.

  TREATMENT: Discontinue exposure to fumes.

  SEE: *metal fume fever.*

polymeria (pŏl-ĭ-mē'rĭ-ă). Condition of having supernumerary parts of the body.

polymeric (pŏl''-ĭ-mĕr'ĭk). 1. Having the characteristics of a polymer. 2. Muscles derived from more than one myotome.

polymerism (pŏl'ĭ-mĕr'ĭzm, pō-lĭm'ĕr-ĭzm) [Gr. *polys*, many, + *meros,* part, + *ismos,* condition]. Condition of having more than normal number of parts. SYN: *polymeria.*

polymerization (pŏl'ĭ-mĕr'ĭ-zā'shŭn). Process of changing into another compound having same elements in same proportions, but a higher molecular weight.

polymitus (pō-lĭm'ĭ-tŭs) [Gr. *polys*, many, + *mitos,* thread]. Stage in reproduction of microorganisms in which threads of protoplasm, now being detached, constitute the microgamete.

polymorph (pŏl'ĭ-mŏrf) ["+ *morphē,* form]. A polymorphonuclear leukocyte.

polymor'phic. Occurring in more than one form.

pol''ymor'phism [Gr. *polys*, many, + *morphē*, form, + *-ismos,* condition]. 1. Capacity for appearing in many forms. 2. Existence of several types in the same group or species. SYN: *pleomorphism.*

polymorphocellular (pŏl'ĭ-mŏr-fō-sĕl'ū-lar) ["+ "+ L. *cellula,* a small chamber]. Composed of cells of many forms.

polymorphonuclear (pŏl'ĭ-mor''fō-nū'klē-ăr) ["+ "+ L. *nucleus,* a kernel]. Possessing a nucleus consisting of several parts or lobes connected by fine strands.

p. leukocyte. A white blood cell which possesses a nucleus composed of two or more lobes or parts; a granulocyte (neutrophil, eosinophil, basophil).

polymorphous (pŏl'ĭ-môr'fŭs). Appearing in many forms. SYN: *polymorphic.*

polymyalgia rheumatica. A poorly understood condition characterized by muscle pain in the shoulder and pelvic girdle; a patient almost always over 60 years of age; marked elevation of erythrocyte sedimentation rate; absence of evidence of inflammatory arthritis of any kind; absence of signs of muscle disease such as atrophy, weakness, or fibrillation; and prompt and dramatic response to low doses of corticosteroid therapy.

Corticosteroid relieves symptoms and the sedimentation rate approaches normal. Temporal and cranial arteritis may be associated with this disease.

polymyoclonus (pŏl'ĭ-mī-ōk'lō-nŭs) [Gr. *polys,* many, + *mys, myo-,* muscle, + *klonos,* tumult]. A shocklike muscular contraction, occurring in various parts at the same time. SYN: *myoclonus multiplex; paramyoclonus.*

polymyositis (pŏl'ĭ-mī''ō-sī'tĭs) ["+ "+ -*itis,* inflammation]. Simultaneous inflammation of many muscles.

polymyxin (pŏl'ĭ-mĭks'ĭn). One of several closely related antibiotics isolated from Bacillus polymyxa and designated polymyxins A, B, C, D, and E.

p. B. Least toxic of the antibiotic fractions of polymyxin, and the only one used therapeutically.

polynesic (pŏl'ĭ-nē'sĭk) [Gr. *polys,* many,' + *nēsos,* island]. Appearing in many separate locations or foci.

polyneural (pŏl'ĭ-nū'răl) ["+ *neuron,* sinew]. Pert. to, innervated, or supplied by many nerves.

polyneuralgia (pŏl'ĭ-nū-răl'jĭ-ă) ["+ "+ *algos,* pain]. Neuralgia in several nerves.

polyneuritic (pŏl'ĭ-nū-rĭt'ĭk) ["+ "+ -*itis,* inflammation]. Suffering from inflammation of several nerves at once.

p. psychosis. P. seen in chronic alcoholism with disturbed orientation, polyneuritis, hallucinations, falsification of memory, etc.

polyneuritis (pŏl'ĭ-nū-rī'tĭs) ["+ "+ -*itis,* inflammation]. A neuritis involving two or more nerves, usually a large number.

p., acute idiopathic. A disorder of peripheral nerves characterized by ascending muscular weakness, impairment of reflexes, and sensory disorders. Often follows

a febrile illness. Cause unknown. SYN: *infectious polyneuritis; Landry's paralysis; Guillain-Barrésyndrome.*

p., Jamaica ginger. P. esp. of nerves of extremities following ingestion of Jamaica ginger. SYN: *ginger paralysis.*

p., metabolic. P. resulting from metabolic disorders such as nutritional deficiency, esp. lack of thiamine; gastrointestinal disorders; or pathological conditions such as diabetes, pernicious anemia, toxemias of pregnancy, etc.

p., toxic. P. resulting from poisons such as heavy metals, alcohol, carbon monoxide, various organic compounds, etc.

polyneuropathy (pŏl'ĭ-nū-rŏp'ă-thĭ) ["+ "+ *pathos,* disease]. Term applied to any disorder or affection of peripheral nerves, but preferably restricted to those of a noninflammatory nature. SYN: *polyneuritis; multiple neuritis.*

p., amyloid. P. characterized by deposition of amyloid in nerves.

p., buckthorn. A symmetrical progressive polyneuropathy which starts in the lower limbs and ascends until there is respiratory paralysis when the brain stem becomes affected. If the patient survives, improvement is slow but may progress to almost complete functional recovery. There is no specific therapy.

Disease is due to ingestion of the fruit of poisonous shrub of the buckthorn family. This plant grows in central and northern Mexico and in Texas and New Mexico.

p., erythredema. A condition of unknown etiology occurring in children, and characterized by degenerative changes in peripheral nerves, skin disorders, motor and sensory disturbances. SYN: *acrodynia; Feer's disease; pink disease.*

p., porphyric. P. resulting from acute porphyria, characterized by pains and paresthesias in the extremities and by flaccid paralysis.

p., progressive hypertrophic. A rare familial disease beginning in childhood and characterized by increased size of peripheral nerves due to multiplication and hypertrophy of cells of sheath of Schwann. SYN: *Dejerine-Sottas disease.*

polynuclear (pŏl'ĭ-nū'klē-ăr) [Gr. *polys,* many, + L. *nucleus,* a kernel]. Possessing more than one nucleus; multinuclear.

polynucleotidase (pŏl'ĭ-nū''klē-ō'tĭ-dās). An enzyme present in intestinal mucosa and intestinal juice that catalyzes the breakdown of nucleic acids to nucleotides.

polynucleotide (pŏl″ĭ-nū′klē-ō-tīd). Nucleic acid composed of four nucleotides; a tetranucleotide.

polyodontia (pŏl″ĭ-ō-dŏn′shĭ-ă) [Gr. *polys*, many, + *odous, odont-*, tooth]. State of having supernumerary teeth.

polyopia, polyopsia (pŏl″ĭ-ō′pĭ-ă, -ŏp′sĭ-ă) ["+ *opsis*, vision]. Multiple vision; perception of more than one image of the same object.

polyorchidism (pŏl″ĭ-or′kĭ-dĭzm) ["+ *orchis*, testicle, + *-ismos*, condition]. Condition of having more than two testicles.

polyorchis (pŏl″ĭ-or′kĭs). An individual with more than two testicles.

polyorrhymenitis (pŏl″ĭ-or″hĭ-mĕn-ĭ′tĭs) [Gr. *polys*, many, + *orrhos*, serum, + *hymēn*, membrane, + *-itis*, inflammation]. Malignant inflammation and wasting of serous membranes. SYN: *Concato's disease.*

polyotia (pŏl″ĭ-ō′shĭ-ă) ["+ *ous, ot-*, ear]. State of having more than two ears.

polyp (pŏl′ĭp) [Gr. *polys*, many, + *pous*, foot]. A tumor with a pedicle. Commonly found in vascular organs such as the nose, uterus, and rectum. Polyps bleed easily; if there is a possibility that they will become malignant, they should be removed surgically. SYN: *polypus.*

   p., bleeding. Angioma of nasal mucous membrane.

   p., fibrinous. P. containing fibrin and blood, and located in the uterine cavity.

   p., mucous. A p. of soft or jellylike consistency and exhibiting mucoid degeneration.

   p., vascular. A pedunculated angioma.

polyparesis (pŏl″ĭ-păr′ĕs-ĭs) [Gr. *polys*, many, + *paresis*, relaxation]. General progressive paralysis of paralytic dementia.

polypathia (pŏl″ĭ-păth′ĭ-ă) ["+ *pathos*, disease]. The presence of several diseases at one time, or their frequent recurrence.

polypeptide (pŏl″ĭ-pĕp′tĭd) ["+ *peptein*, to digest]. A union of three or more amino acids. SEE: *peptide.*

polypeptidemia (pŏl″ĭ-pĕp″tĭ-dē′mĭ-ă) ["+ "+ haima, blood]. Polypeptides present in the blood.

polypeptidorrhachia (pŏl″ĭ-pĕp″tĭ-dō-rā′kĭ-ă) ["+ "+ *rhachis*, spine]. Polypeptides in the cerebrospinal fluid.

polyphagia (pŏl″ĭ-fā′jĭ-ă) [Gr. *polys*, many, + *phagein*, to eat]. Eating abnormally large amounts of food at a meal.

   RS: acoria; anorexia; bulimia; parorexia; taste.

polyphalangism (pŏl″ĭ-fă-lăn′jĭzm) ["+ *phalanx*, phalanx, + *ismos*, condition]. An extra number of phalanges on a finger or toe.

polypharmacy (pŏl″ĭ-făr′mă-sĭ) ["+ *pharmakon*, drug]. 1. Excessive use of drugs or overdose of a drug. 2. Prescription of many drugs given at one time.

polyphobia (pŏl″ĭ-fō′bĭ-ă) [Gr. *polys*, many, + *phobos*, fear]. Excessive or abnormal fear of a number of things.

polyphrasia (pŏl″ĭ-frā′zĭ-ă) ["+ *phrasis*, speech]. Excessive talkativeness, a manifestation of insanity. SYN: *verbigeration.*

polyphyletic (pŏl″ĭ-fĭ-lĕt′ĭk) ["+ *phylē*, tribe]. Having more than one origin. Opposed to monophyletic, q.v.

polyplastic (pŏl″ĭ-plăs′tĭk) [Gr. *polys*, many, + *plastos*, formed]. 1. Having had many evolutionary modifications. 2. Having many substances in cellular composition.

polyplastocytosis (pŏl″ĭ-plăs″tō-sĭ-tō′sĭs) ["+ "+ *kytos*, cell, + *-ōsis*, intensive]. Increase of formation of blood platelets.

polyplegia (pŏl″ĭ-plē′jĭ-ă) ["+ *plēgē*, stroke]. Paralysis affecting several muscles.

polyploid (pŏl″ĭ-ployd). 1. Characterized by polyploidy. 2. An individual in which the chromosome number is two or more times the normal haploid number.

polyploidy (pŏl″ĭ-ploy-dĭ). Condition in which the chromosome number is two or more times the normal haploid number found in gametes.

polypnea (pŏl″ĭp-nĭ′ă) [Gr. *polys*, many, + *pnoia*, breath]. Very rapid breathing. SYN: *panting.*

polypodia (pŏl″ĭ-pō′dĭ-ă) ["+ *pous, pod-*, foot]. Possession of more than the normal number of feet.

polypoid (pŏl″ĭ-poyd) ["+ "+ *eidos*, like]. Like a polyp.

polyporous (pŏl-ĭp′ō-rŭs) [Gr. *polys*, many, + *poros*, pore]. Possessing many small openings or pores.

polyposis (pŏl″ĭ-pō′sĭs) ["+ *pous*, foot, + *-ōsis*, intensive]. The presence of numerous polypi.

   p. coli. P. of the large intestine.

   p. ventriculi. Presence of numerous polyps, sometimes involving entire mucosa, accompanied by chronic atrophic gastritis.

polyp′otome ["+ "+ *tomē*, a cutting]. Instrument for excision of polyps.

polypsychotropia (pŏl″ĭ-sī-kō-trō′pĭ-ă). The simultaneous use of two or more psychotropic drugs. SEE: *psychotropic drugs.*

polypus (pŏl′ĭ-pŭs) [L.]. (pl. *pol′ypi*) A polyp, q.v.

   p., bleeding. Angioma of nasal mucous membrane.

   p., cellular. Mucous polypus.

p., cervical. A polyp, either fibrous or mucous, on the cervical mucosa.

p., fibrous. A pedunculated fibroid tumor within the uterine or cervical cavities.

p., fleshy. A submucous myoma in the uterus.

p., placental. A polyp composed of retained placental tissue.

polyradiculitis (pŏl″ĭ-ră-dĭk″ū-lī′tĭs) [Gr. *polys,* many, + L. *radix,* root, + *-itis,* inflammation]. Inflammation of nerve roots, esp. those of spinal nerves.

polyrexia (pŏl″ĭ-rĕks′ĭ-ă). Insatiable appetite, excessive hunger. SYN: *bulimia.*

polyrrhea, polyrrhoea (pŏl″ĭ-rē′ă) [Gr. *polys,* many, + *rhoia,* flow]. Excessive secretion of fluid.

polysaccharide (pŏl″ĭ-săk′ă-rīd) [″ + *sakcharon,* sugar]. One of a group of carbohydrates which upon hydrolysis yield more than two molecules of simple sugars. They are complex carbohydrates of high molecular weight, usually insoluble in water but, when soluble, form colloidal solutions. Their basic formula is $(C_6H_{12}O_6)_x$.

They include two groups: starch group (Ex: starch, inulin, glycogen, dextrin); cellulose group (Ex: cellulose and hemicelluloses). The hemicelluloses include the pentosans (Ex: gum arabic), hexosans (Ex: agar-agar), and hexopentosans (Ex: pectin).

SEE: *carbohydrates; monosaccharide; disaccharide.*

polysaccharose (pŏl″ĭ-săk′ă-rōs). A polysaccharide, q.v.

polysarcia (pŏl″ĭ-săr′sĭ-ă) [″ + *sarx,* flesh]. Fleshiness; obesity.

polysar′cous. Very fleshy; fat.

polyscelia (pŏl″ĭ-sē′lĭ-ă) [Gr. *polys,* many, + *skelos,* leg]. Condition of having more than the normal number of legs.

polyscope (pŏl″ĭ-skōp) [″ + *skopein,* to examine]. Instrument for illumination and examination of cavities. SYN: *diaphanoscope.*

polyserositis (pŏl″ĭ-sē-rō-sī′tĭs) [″ + L. *serum,* whey, + *-itis,* inflammation]. General progressive inflammation, esp. in upper abdominal cavity. SYN: *multiple serositis.*

p., chronic. P. involving fibrous adhesions in pleural and pericardial cavities.

polysinuitis (pŏl″ĭ-sĭn″ū-ī′tĭs). Polysinusitis, q.v.

polysinusitis (pŏl″ĭ-sī″nŭs-ī′tĭs) [Gr. *polys,* many, + L. *sinus,* a hollow, + Gr. *-itis,* inflammation]. Inflammation of several sinuses simultaneously. SYN: *polysinuitis.*

polyspermia (pŏl″ĭ-sper′mĭ-ă) [″ + *sperma,* seed]. 1. Excessive secretion of seminal fluid. 2. Entrance of several spermatozoa into one ovum. SYN: *polyspermism.*

polyspermism (pŏl″ĭ-sperm′ĭzm). Polyspermia, q.v.

polystichia (pŏl″ĭ-stĭk′ĭ-ă) [Gr. *polys,* many, + *stichos,* a row]. Condition in which there are two or more rows of eyelashes.

polystomatous (pŏl″ĭ-stō′mă-tŭs) [″ + *stoma,* mouth]. Possessing many mouths or openings.

polythelia (pŏl″ĭ-thē′lĭ-ă) [″ + *thēlē,* nipple, + *-ismos,* condition]. Presence of more than one nipple on a mamma. SYN: *polythelism.*

polythelism (pŏl″ĭ-thē′lĭzm). Polythelia, q.v.

polytocous (pŏ-lĭt′ō-kŭs) [Gr. *polys,* many, + *tokos,* birth]. Producing several offspring at one time.

polytrichosis (pŏl″ĭ-trĭ-kō′sĭs) [″ + *thrix, trich-,* hair, + *-osis,* intensive]. Excessive growth of hair. SYN: *hypertrichosis.*

polytrophia (pŏl″ĭ-trō′fĭ-ă) [″ + *trophē,* nourishment]. Excessive or abundant nutrition. SYN: *polytrophy.*

polytrophy (pō-lĭt′rō-fĭ). Polytrophia, q.v.

pol″ytrop′ic [Gr. *polys,* many, + *tropē, a turning*]. Affecting more than one type of cell, said of viruses, or affecting more than one type of tissue, said of certain poisons.

polyunsaturated. In chemistry, rel. to long-chain carbon compounds, esp. fats which have many carbon atoms joined by double or triple bonds.

polyuria (pŏl″ĭ-ū′rĭ-ă) [Gr. *polys,* many, + *ouron,* urine]. Excessive secretion and discharge of urine. The urine does not, as a rule, contain abnormal constituents. Several hundred ounces a day may be voided. It is pale in color. Sp. gr. 1.000-1.002, and higher in diabetes.

ETIOL: Occurs in diabetes insipidus; diabetes mellitus; chronic nephritis; nephrosclerosis; following edematous states, esp. those induced by heart failure treated with diuretics; in hyperthyroidism; and following excessive intake of liquids.

polyvalent (pŏl″ĭ-vā′lĕnt, pō-lĭv′ă-lĕnt) [″ + L. *valēre,* to be strong]. Multivalent; having a combining power of more than two atoms of hydrogen.

p. serum. One with antibodies produced by injecting several strains of microorganisms of the same species, or by injecting different species.

p. vaccine. One produced from cultures of a number of strains of the same species.

polyvinylpyrrolidone (pŏl″ĭ-vī″nĭl-pĕr-rŏl′ĭ-dōn). A polymeric substance used to treat conditions associated with decreased blood volume. It is given intravenously. ABBR: PVP.

pomade (pō-mād′) [Fr. *pommade*]. A perfumed ointment, esp. one for the hair. SYN: *pomatum*.

pomatum (pō-mā′tŭm). A perfumed unguent, esp. one used on the hair. SYN: *pomade*.

pompholyx (pŏm′fō-lĭks) [Gr., bubble]. Acute inflammatory condition characterized by bullae limited to hands and feet.

ETIOL: Not known. Occurs in 2nd to 4th decade in coffee and tobacco users and in those with lowered vitality.

SYM: Symmetrical eruptions of crops of deeply seated vesicles and bullae with itching, hyperemia, lasting 4-6 weeks. Secondary infection may occur.

TREATMENT: Hygienic regimen. Locally soothing lotions, potassium permanganate compresses, salicylic acid in alcohol. X-irradiation in resistant cases.

pomphus (pŏm′fŭs) [L.]. (pl. *pomphi*) A blister or a circumscribed elevation on the skin; a wheal.

pomum (pō′mŭm) [L.]. An apple

p. Adami. Prominence in middle line of throat, caused by junction of two lateral wings of the thyroid cartilage. SYN: *Adam's apple.*

ponderal (pŏn′dĕr-ăl) [L. *pondus*, weight]. Rel. to weight.

p. index. The ratio of an individual's height to the cube root of his weight. Expressed as:

$$\frac{\text{height (in inches)}}{\sqrt[3]{\text{weight (in pounds)}}}$$

ponograph (pō′nō-grăf) [Gr. *ponos*, toil and fatigue, + *graphein*, to write]. Device for measuring and registering sensitiveness to pain or fatigue.

ponopalmosis (pŏn″ō-păl-mō′sĭs) ["+ *palmos*, palpitation, + *-ōsis*, intensive]. Palpitation of the heart produced by slight exertion. SYN: *neurocirculatory asthenia.*

ponophobia (pō″nō-fō′bĭ-ă) ["+ *phobos*, fear]. 1. Abnormal distaste for exerting one's self. 2. Dread of pain.

pons (pŏnz) [L., bridge]. (pl. *pontes*) 1. A process of tissue connecting two or more parts. 2. [NA]. Pons varolii, q.v.

p. cerebelli. Pons varolii, q.v.

p. hepatis. Part of liver occasionally extending from quadrate lobe to left lobe across the umbilical fissure.

p. varolii. [Costanzo Varolio, It. anatomist, 1544-1575]. A rounded eminence on ventral surface of the brain stem. It lies between the medulla and cerebral peduncles, and appears externally as a broad band of transverse fibers. It is connected to the cerebellum by the midcerebellar peduncle or brachium pontis. It contains fiber tracts connecting medulla oblongata and cerebellum with upper portions of the brain; the origins of the abducens, facial, trigeminal, and cochlear division of the 8th (vestibulocochlear) nerves are at the borders of the pons. RS: cerebropontile.

pontic (pŏn′tĭk) [L. *pons, pontis*, bridge]. An artifical tooth set in a bridge.

pontile (pŏn′tēl). Pert. to the pons varolii.

p. hemiplegia. One due to lesion of the pons. The arm and leg on one side and face on the other are affected.

p. nuclei. The gray matter in the pons.

pontine (pŏn′tēn). Pert. to the pons varolii.

pon″tobulb′ar. Pert. to the pons and the medulla oblongata.

Pontocaine Hydrochlo′ride (pŏn′tō-kān). A proprietary name for tetracaine hydrochloride. Is available in several forms for use as a topical or spinal anesthetic.

popliteal (pŏp-lĭt-ē′ăl, pŏp-lĭt′ē-al) [L. *poples, poplit-*, ham]. Concerning the posterior surface of the knee.

popliteus (pŏp-lĭt′ē-ŭs, -lĭt-ē′ŭs). Muscle located in hind part of the knee joint which flexes the leg and aids it in rotating. SEE: *Table of Muscles* in *Appendix.*

poppy. Any of the several plants of the genus Papaver. Opium is obtained from the juice of the unripe pods of Papaver somniferum.

population of world. A variable depending upon the rate at which number of people on earth increases. It took approx. three to four million years for the world to attain a population of one billion (1,000,000,000) by 1650. By 1850 the population had grown to two billion; by 1930 it was three billion. It is estimated that there will be four billion people on the earth by 1975.

poradenitis (pōr-ăd-ē-nī′tĭs) [Gr. *poros*, pore, + *adēn*, gland, + *-ītis*, inflammation]. Formation of small abscesses in the iliac glands. SYN: *lymphogranuloma venereum*, q.v.

porcelaneous, porcelanous (pŏr″sĕ-lā′nē-ŭs, -sĕl′ăn-ŭs) [Fr. *porcelaine*]. Translucent or white like porcelain, as the skin.

porcupine disease (pŏr′kū-pīn) [L. *porcus*, swine]. A chronic skin disease with scaly epidermal plates. SYN: *ichthyosis*, q.v.

pore (pōr) [L. *porus*, a pore]. 1. A minute opening, esp. one on an epithelial surface. SYN: *porus* [NA]. 2. Opening of excretory duct of a sweat gland.

RS: skin; stoma; sweat glands.

p., alveolar. A minute opening which is thought to exist between adjacent alveoli of the lung.

p., gustatory. A taste pore, q.v.

p., taste. The external opening of a taste bud. SYN: *gustatory pore.* SEE: *taste.*

porencephalia, porencephaly (pōr″en-sĕf-ā′lĭ-ă, pōr″en-sĕf′ă-lĭ) [L. *pŏrus,* pore, + *enkephalos,* brain]. An anomalous condition in which the ventricles of the brain are connected with the subarachnoid space.

porencephalitis (pōr″en-sĕf′ă-lĭ′tĭs) ["+ "+ -*itis,* inflammation]. Inflammation of the brain with development of cavities communicating with the subarachnoid space.

por″enceph′alous. Pert. to porencephalia, q.v.

po′ri. Pl. of porus, q.v.

por″ioma′nia (Gr. *poreia,* walking, + *mania,* madness). Morbid desire to wander from home.

pork [L. *porcus*]. The meat of hogs.

    Food value of 100 gm. (roasted, medium-fat pork loin): Cal. 373; protein 22.6 gm.; fat 30.6 gm.; calcium 10 mg.; iron 2.3 mg.; thiamine 0.50 mg.

pornography (pōr-nŏg′ră-fĭ) [Gr. *pornē,* prostitute, + *graphein,* to write]. Written or graphic forms of communication which either are intended to, or may, incite sexual interest.

porocephaliasis, porocephalosis (pō″rō-sĕf′ă-lĭ′ă-sĭs, -lō′sĭs) [L. *porus,* pore, + *kephalē,* head]. Infection with a species of Porocephalus.

Porocephalus (pō″rō-sĕf′ă-lŭs). A genus of wormlike arthropods found commonly in snakes. The young sometimes infest mammals, including man.

porokeratosis (pō″rō-kĕr″ă-tō′sĭs) [L. *porus,* pore, + *keras,* a horn, + -*ōsis,* disease]. Skin disease marked by thickening of stratum corneum in linear arrangement, followed by its atrophy. P. appears on smooth areas. It is irregular in form and size with circumscribed outline and affects hands and feet, forearms and legs, the face, neck, and scalp.

poro′ma [Gr.]. Inflammatory hardening or callosity.

poro′sis [L. *porus,* pore]. Bone condition marked by formation of pores or cavities and increased translucency to roentgen rays. SEE: *osteoporosis.*

porosity (pō-rōs′ĭ-tĭ) [L. *porus,* pore]. The state of being porous.

porous (pō′rŭs). Full of pores; able to admit passage of a liquid.

por′phin. The basic ring structure forming the framework of all porphyrins. Consisting of four pyrrole rings united by methene couplings.

porphobilinogen (por″fō-bĭ-lĭn′ō-jĕn). A substance sometimes found in the urine of patients with acute porphyria. The urine

may appear to be normal when fresh, but will change to a Burgundy wine color or even to black when heated with dilute hydrochloric acid to 100° C.

porphyria (por-fĭ′rĭ-ă) [Gr. *porphura,* purple]. Condition of having porphyrin in the blood.

p., acute intermittent. A rare metabolic disorder characterized by excessive excretion of porphyrins, acute abdominal pain, and neurological disturbances, inherited as a mendelian dominant trait. Sometimes precipitated by excessive use of sulfonamides, barbiturates, or other drugs. Sensitivity to light is characteristic.

p., congenital. A rare condition due to an inborn error of metabolism. Inherited as a mendelian recessive trait.

p. cutanea tarda hereditaria. P. inherited as a non-sex-linked mendelian dominant characteristic. Onset of symptoms usually occurs between the ages of 10 and 30.

p. erythropoietica. P. due to a defect in the synthesis of hemoglobin.

p. hepatica. P. due to disturbance in liver metabolism such as occurs following hepatitis, poisoning by heavy metals, certain anemias, and other conditions.

porphyrin (por′fĭ-rĭn) [Gr. *porphura,* purple]. One of a group forming basis of animal and plant respiratory pigments, obtained from hemoglobin and chlorophyll.

porphyrinuria (por″fĭ-rĭ-nū′rĭ-ă) ["+ *ouron,* urine]. The excretion of an increased amount of porphyrin in the urine.

porphyrization (por″fĭr-ĭ-zā′shŭn). Process of pulverizing.

porphyruria (por″fĭr-ū′rĭ-ă) [Gr. *porphura,* purple, + *ouron,* urine]. Excretion of an increased amount of porphyrin in urine.

Porro's operation (por′ō). [Eduardo Porro, It. obstetrician, 1842-1902]. Removal of a pregnant uterus, the ovaries, and tubes through an incision in the abdominal wall; cesarean hysterectomy.

por′ta [L., gate]. (pl. *por′tae*) The point of entry of nerves and vessels into an organ or part.

p. hepatis. [NA]. The fissure of the liver where the portal vein and hepatic artery enter and the hepatic duct leaves.

p. lienis. Hilus of the spleen where vessels enter.

p. pulmonis. Pulmonary hilus for entry and exit of the bronchi, nerves, and vessels.

p. renis. Hilus of the kidney for entry of the vessels.

por′tal [L. *porta,* gate]. 1. An entryway. 2. Concerning a porta or entrance to an organ, esp. that through which the blood is carried to liver.

p. circulation. Blood brought into the liver by the p. vein and out by the hepatic vein.

p. of entry. The avenue by which infectious organisms gain access to the body.

p., intestinal. The opening of the midgut or yolk sac into the foregut or hindgut of an embryo.

p. system. The p. vein and its branches by which blood is collected from abdominal viscera and conveyed to the sinusoids of the liver from which it passes through the hepatic veins to the inferior vena cava.

p. vein. One formed by the veins of the splanchnic area conveying its blood into the liver. It is made of the combined superior and inferior mesenteric, splenic, gastric, and cystic veins.

portio (pŏr'shĭ-ō) [L.]. (pl. *portio'nes*) [NA]. A part. In anatomy, designates a certain portion of a structure or organ.

p. dura. The 7th cranial nerve; the facial nerve.

p. vaginalis. The part of the cervix within the vagina.

port-wine mark or stain. A purplish-red, superficial birthmark. SYN: *nevus*, q.v.

porus (pō'rŭs) [L.]. A meatus or foramen; a tiny aperture in a structure; a pore.

p. acusticus externus. [NA]. The outer opening of the external acoustic meatus.

p. acusticus internus. [NA]. The opening of the internal acoustic meatus into the cranial cavity.

p. lactiferous. Opening of a lactiferous duct on tip of nipple of mammary gland.

p. opticus. Opening in center of optic disk through which retinal vessels (central artery and vein) reach retina through lamina cribrosa of sclera.

p. sudoriferus. [NA]. Opening of a sweat gland.

posiomania (po"sĭ-ō-mā'nĭ-ă) [Gr. *posis*, drinking, + *mania*, madness]. Addiction to alcoholic drinks. SYN: *dipsomania.*

position (pō-zĭsh'ŭn) [L. *positiō*]. 1. Place in which a thing is put. 2. Manner in which a body is arranged, as by the nurse or physician for examination. 3. In obstetrics, the relation of some arbitrarily chosen portion of the child in the pelvis to the right or left side of the mother, the occiput, chin, sacrum, and scapula being the points that are most common.

p., anatomic. P. assumed when a person is standing erect with arms at the sides, palms forward.

Positions of Fetus in Utero

Vertex Presentation (point of designation—occiput):

Left occiput anterior	LOA
Right occiput posterior	ROP
Right occiput anterior	ROA
Left occiput posterior	LOP
Right occiput transverse	ROT
Occiput anterior	OA
Occiput posterior	OP

Breech Presentation (point of designation—sacrum):

Left sacroanterior	LSA
Right sacroposterior	RSP
Right sacroanterior	RSA
Left sacroposterior	LSP
Sacroanterior	SA
Sacroposterior	SP
Left sacrotransverse	LST
Right sacrotransverse	RST

Face Presentation (point of designation—chin [mentum]):

Left mentoanterior	LMA
Right mentoposterior	RMP
Right mentoanterior	RMA
Left mentoposterior	LMP
Mentoposterior	MP
Mentoanterior	MA
Left mentotransverse	LMT
Right mentotransverse	RMT

Transverse Presentation (point of designation—scapula of presenting shoulder):

Left scapuloanterior	LScA
Right scapuloposterior	RScP
Right scapuloanterior	RScA
Left scapuloposterior	LScP

p., dorsal. P. in which patient is on his back. SYN: *supine.*

p., dorsal elevated. On back, with head and shoulders elevated at angle of 30° or more. Employed in digital examination of genitalia and in bimanual examination.

p., dorsal recumbent. On back, extremities moderately flexed and rotated outward. Employed in application of obstetrical forceps, repair of lesions following parturition, vaginal examination, bimanual palpation. SEE: *dorsal recumbent p.* for illustration.

p., dorsosacral. P., lithotomy, q.v.

p., Edebohl's. SYN: *Simon's p.*, q.v.

p., Elliott's. P. in which supports are placed under small of back so that patient resembles a double inclined plane.

p., English. SEE: *p., left lateral recumbent.*

p., erect. Occiput and heels on line; also nose, groins, and great toes in same vertical plane. Employed in practice of ballottement, differentiation of tumors, cystic and solid hernia.

p., Fowler's. P. when the head of the patient's bed is raised above the level about 1 1/2 ft. (46 cm.), and knees are elevated. SEE: *Fowler's p.* for illustration.

p., genucubital. Patient on knees, thighs upright, body resting on elbows, head down on hands. Employed when not possible to use the classic knee-chest p.

p., genupectoral. Patient on knees, thighs upright, head and upper part of chest resting on table, arms crossed above head. Employed in displacement of prolapsed fundus, dislodgment of impacted head of fetus, management of transverse presentation, replacement of retroverted uterus or displaced ovary, flushing of intestinal canal.

p., horizontal. Lying supine, feet extended. Employed in palpation, in auscultation of fetal heart, and in operative procedures. SEE: *horizontal p.* for illustration.

p., horizontal abdominal. Patient flat on abdomen, feet extended. Employed in examination of back and spinal column.

p., jackknife. Patient on back, shoulders elevated, legs flexed on thighs, thighs at right angles to abdomen. Employed when passing urethral sound.

p., knee-chest. SYN: *genupectoral p.,* q.v. SEE: *knee-chest p.* for illustration.

p., knee-elbow. SEE: *p., genucubital.*

p., kneeling-squatting. Patient squatting, knees pressed on abdomen, trunk erect. Employed in childbirth in difficult cases and in underdeveloped nations.

p., lateroprone. Sims' p., q.v.

p., laterosemiprone. Sims' p., q.v.

p., left lateral recumbent. Patient on left side, right knee and thigh drawn up. Employed in childbirth.

p., lithotomy. Patient on back, thighs flexed on abdomen, legs on thighs, thighs abducted. Employed in operation on genital tract, in vaginal hysterectomy, diagnosis and treatment of diseases of urethra and bladder.

p., obstetrical. P., left lateral recumbent, q.v.

p., orthograde. P., anatomic, q.v.

p., prone. P. in which patient is lying face downward.

p., reclining. P., jackknife, q.v.

p., side, semiprone. P., Sims', q.v.

p., Simon's. Exaggerated lithotomy position. Patient flat on back, legs flexed on thighs, thighs on abdomen, hips somewhat elevated, thighs strongly abducted. Employed in operations on vagina.

p., Sims'. Patient on left side, right knee and thigh drawn well up above left, left arm back of patient and hanging over edge of table, chest inclined forward so that patient rests upon it. Employed in curettement of uterus, intrauterine irrigation after labor, tamponade of vagina, rectal exploration, operations on cervix. SEE: *Sims' position* for illustration.

p., Trendelenburg. Dorsal position, body elevated at angle of about 45°, feet and legs hanging over end of table, head down. Employed in abdominal surgery to favor gravitation upward of abdominal viscera.

p., Walcher. Patient with hips on edge of table and lower extremities hanging down.

positioner (pō-zĭsh'ŭn-ĕr). Apparatus for holding or placing the body or part, esp. the head, in a certain position.

positive (pŏz'ĭ-tĭv) [L. *positivus,* ruling]. 1. Definite; affirmative; opposed to negative. 2. Indicating the reaction in laboratory work. 3. Indicating an abnormal condition in examination and diagnosis. 4. Indicates pathological change in postmortem examination. 5. Noting a quantity greater than zero.

Often in laboratory findings and mathematical expressions, p. is indicated by a plus (+) sign.

positron (pŏz'ĭ-trŏn). A particle having the same mass as a negative electron, but possessing a positive charge.

posological (pŏ"sō-lŏj'ĭ-kăl) [Gr. *posos,* how much, + *logos,* a study]. Concerning dosage.

posology (pō-sŏl'ō-jĭ). Branch of scientific study dealing with dosage.

possession (pō-zĕsh'ŭn) [ME. *possessen*]. Psychological state of being dominated by an idea, a passion, or a mental obsession.

p., demoniacal. Belief of being under the influence of an evil spirit or demon.

Possum (pŏs'ŭm). [*p*atient *o*perated *s*elector *m*echanism]. A device that permits a disabled individual to control and operate various machines, such as switches, telephones, and typewriters, by breathing into the master control of the apparatus.

post- [L.]. A prefix meaning behind or after.

postabortal (pōst"ă-bor'tăl) [L. *post,* after, + *abortus,* abortion]. Happening subsequent to abortion.

postaxial (pōst-ăk'sĭ-ăl) ["+ Gr. *axōn,* axis]. Situated or happening behind an axis.

postcapillary (pōst-kăp'ĭl-lā-rĭ). A terminal vessel of a capillary network which leads to a venule. SYN: *venous capillary.*

postcava (pōst-kā'vă) [L. *post*, after, + *cavus*, a hollow]. The ascending or inferior vena cava.

postca'val. Concerning the postcava.

postcentral (pōst-sĕn'trăl) [L. *post*, after, + Gr. *kentron*, center]. 1. Situated or happening behind a center. 2. Located behind the fissure of Rolando.

postcibal (pōst-sī'băl) ["+ *cibum*, food]. Occurring after meals.

postclavicular (pōst"klă-vĭk'ū-lăr) ["+ *clavicula*, a little key]. Located or occurring behind the clavicle.

postclimacteric (pōst"klī-măk-tĕr'ĭk, mak'tĕr-ĭk) [L. *post*, after, + Gr. *kilmaktēr*, rung of a ladder, crisis]. Occurring after the menopause.

postcoital (pōst-kō'ĭt-ăl) ["+ *coitiō*, a coming together]. Subsequent to sexual intercourse.

postconnubial (pōst"kŏn-ū'bĭ-ăl) ["+ *connubium*, marriage]. Occurring after marriage.

postconvulsive (pōst"kŏn-vŭl'sĭv) ["+ *convulsus*, pull violently]. Occurring after a convulsion.

postdiastolic (pōst-dī-ăs-tŏl'ĭk) ["+ *diastolē*, expansion]. Occurring after the cardiac diastole.

postdicrotic (pōst-dī-krŏt'ĭk) [L. *post*, after, + Gr. *dikrotos*, beating double]. Occurring after the dicrotic pulse wave.

   p. wave. A recoil or second wave (not always present) in a sphygmographic tracing.

postdiphtheritic (pōst-dĭf-thĕr-ĭt'ĭk). Following diphtheria.

postencephalitis (pōst"ĕn-sĕf-ă-lī'tĭs) [L. *post*, after, + *enkephalos*, brain, + -*itis*, inflammation]. Occurring after encephalitis. An abnormal state remaining after the acute stage of encephalitis has passed.

postepileptic (pōst"ĕp-ĭ-lĕp'tĭk) ["+ Gr. *epi*, upon, + *lēpsis*, a seizure]. Following an epileptic seizure.

posterior (pŏs-tē'rĭ-ŏr) [L. *posterus*, coming after]. [NA]. 1. Toward the rear or caudal end; opposed to anterior. 2. In man, toward the back; dorsal. 3. Situated behind; coming after.

postero- (pŏs'tĕr-ō) [L.]. Prefix indicating posterior, situated behind, or towards the back.

posteroexternal (pŏs"tĕr-ō-ĕks-tĕr'năl) [L. *posterus*, behind, + *externus*, outer]. Towards the back and outer side.

pos"terointer'nal ["+ *internus*, inner]. Towards the back and inner side.

pos"terolat'eral ["+ *latus, later-*, a side]. Located behind and at the side of a part.

posteromedial (pŏs"tĕr-ō-mē'dĭ-ăl) [L. *posterus*, behind, + *medius*, middle]. Toward the back and toward the median plane.

pos"terome'dian. Situated posteriorly and in the median plane.

posterosuperior (pŏs"tĕr-ō-sū-pē'rĭ-ŏr) [L. *posterus*, behind, + *superior*, upper]. Located behind and above a part.

postesophageal (pōst"ē-sŏf'ă-jē'ăl) [L. *post*, after, + Gr. *oisophagos*, gullet]. Located behind the esophagus.

postethmoid (pōst-ĕth'moyd) ["+ Gr. *ēthmos*, sieve, + *eidos*, form]. Located behind the ethmoid bone.

postfebrile (pōst-fē'brĭl) ["+ *febris*, fever]. Occurring after a fever.

postganglionic (pōst"găn-glĭ-ŏn'ĭk) ["+ Gr. *ganglion*, knot]. Situated posterior or distal to a ganglion.

   p. fiber. The axon of a postganglionic neuron which passes from an autonomic ganglion to a visceral effector.

   p. neuron. The second of a series of efferent neurons that transmit impulses from the central nervous system to a visceral effector. Its cell body lies in one of the autonomic ganglia.

posthetomy (pŏs-thĕt'ō-mī) [Gr. *posthē*, foreskin, + *tomē*, a cutting]. Surgical removal of all or part of the foreskin. SYN: *circumcision*.

posthioplasty (pŏs'thĭ-ō-plas"tĭ) ["+ *plastos*, formed]. Plastic surgery of the prepuce or foreskin.

posthitis (pŏs-thī'tĭs) ["+ -*itis*, inflammation]. Inflamed condition of the foreskin.

posthumous (pŏs'tū-mŭs) [L. *postumus*, last]. 1. Occurring after death. 2. Born after death of father. 3. Said of a child taken by cesarean section after death of mother.

posthypnotic (pōst"hĭp-nŏt'ĭk) [L. *post*, after, + Gr. *hypnos*, sleep]. Occurring or performed subsequent to the hypnotic state.

   p. suggestion. Suggestion given during the hypnotic state influencing a later action when individual returns to normal state.

postictal (pōst-ĭk'tăl) ["+ *ictus*, a blow or stroke]. Following a sudden attack or stroke, as an epileptic seizure or apoplexy.

posticteric (pōst"ĭc-tĕr'ĭc) ["+ Gr. *ikteros*, jaundice]. Following jaundice.

post mor'tem [L.]. After death.

postmor'tem [L.]. Occurring or performed after death.

   p. examination. Dissection of a dead body to ascertain cause of death and the changes wrought by disease. SYN: *autopsy*.

postna'tal [L. *post*, after, + *natus*, birth]. Happening after birth.

postnecrotic (pōst″nē-krŏt′ĭk) ["+ Gr. *nekros*, dead]. After death of a tissue or a part.

postocular (pōst-ŏk′ū-lăr) ["+ *oculus*, eye]. Behind the eye.

    p. neuritis. Inflammation of the optic nerve behind the eyeball.

postolivary (pōst-ŏl′ĭ-vā-rĭ) ["+ *oliva*, olive]. Behind the olivary body; back of the anterior pyramid of the medulla.

postoperative (pōst-ŏp′ĕr-ā-tĭv) [L. *post*, after, + *operatus*, work]. After or following a surgical operation.

    NP (postoperative recovery): When you are called to transfer a patient to the recovery room have essential materials, such as emesis basin and aspiration equipment, at bedside. See that bed is ready and furniture moved so stretcher can be placed beside it. Be careful when handling unconscious patient; he is a dead weight and will not be able to help himself. Get assistance. See that there are no drafts and that room temperature and ventilation are adequate. Do not let direct light shine on patient's face.

    When he vomits keep his head turned to one side and elevate foot of bed so vomitus will not be swallowed or inhaled. Change patient's gown when wet or soiled, rubbing patient dry with bath towel. Watch him carefully when consciousness begins to return, for it is at this time he becomes restless. Note pulse, respiration, blood pressure, and other signs as required by the routine of your hospital. Signs vary with the operation.

postoperculum (pōst-ō-pūr′kū-lŭm) [L. *post*, after, + *operculum*, a cover]. The fold covering the insula that is formed of part of the supertemporal gyrus. SYN: *operculum temporal.*

postoral (pōst-ŏr′ăl) ["+ *os, or-*, mouth]. Behind, or in the posterior part of, the mouth.

postpallium (pōst-păl′ĭ-ŭm) ["+ *pallium*, cloak]. That part of the cerebral cortex behind the fissure of Rolando.

postpaludal (pōst-pal′ū-dăl) ["+ *palus, palud-*, swamp]. After a malarial attack.

postparalytic (pōst″păr-ă-lĭt′ĭk) ["+ *para*, beside, + *lyein*, to loosen]. Subsequent to an attack of paralysis.

post partum (pōst-păr′tŭm) [L. *post*, after, + *partus*, birth]. After childbirth.

postpar′tum. Occurring after childbirth.

    p. hemorrhage. Hemorrhage that occurs after childbirth.

    NP: When hemorrhage occurs despite preventive measures, drastic steps must be employed for its control. An icebag placed on the fundus is used as early routine postpartum measure by some physicians. Massage of uterus with a piece of ice on the abdomen frequently is used when bleeding persists. Packing the lower segment of uterus and vagina is an excellent method of controlling hemorrhage. The large tubular packer is preferred here to a dressing forceps in order to avoid contamination of the packing by contact with the vulva and vaginal tract. Packing the vagina may be done by the nurse, if absolutely necessary, when a physician is not available.

    If the above procedures fail to halt the hemorrhage, the physician may insert one hand into the fundus and at the same time massage the uterus with the other hand on the abdomen. A sterile pair of long gloves should be ready in this case. Keep the patient warm during this time. Elevate the lower extremities as soon as possible. Oxytocic drugs may be ordered intravenously by some physicians. Note the pulse and general condition frequently. Stimulants are given as necessary. Usually blood transfusions are given to maintain and increase the patient's resistance.

    Massage the uterus. The fingertips may be kept lightly on the fundus to discover any relaxation. Give massage only when relaxation occurs.

    Hypodermoclysis and intervenous injections are used if patient is unable to take and retain fluids. Retching may start another hemorrhage; however force fluids as soon as patient's condition warrants. When tolerated, the patient may be given a limited number of oral preparations of ergot, preferably the ones that are not nauseating. These keep the uterus contracted and lessen the chance of infection to which the patient has been predisposed by the loss of blood, lowered resistance, and much manipulation.

    Perfect asepsis must be maintained at all times. Since the patient is predisposed to sepsis, her general resistance must be built up and maintained by plenty of fluids, nourishing foods and, above all, rest.

postpontile (pōst-pŏn′tĭl) [L. *post*, after, + *pons, pont-*, bridge]. Situated behind the pons varolii.

post″prand′ial. Following a meal.

postpubescent (pōst″pū-bĕs′ĕnt) [L. *post*, after, + *pubescens*, becoming hairy]. Following puberty.

postpyramidal (pōst-pĭ-răm′ĭd-ăl). Behind a pyramidal tract.

    p. nucleus. Mass of gray matter in posterior column of the medulla. SYN: *nucleus funiculi gracilis.*

post-transfusion syndrome. Condition of fever, splenomegaly, atypical lymphocytes, abnormal liver function tests, and occasionally a skin rash which develops following blood transfusion or perfusion of an organ during surgery. The syndrome appears three to five weeks after transfusion or perfusion with fresh (less than 24-hour old) blood usually in large quantities. The causative agent is thought to be cytomegalic virus.

postulate (pŏs'chĕ-lāt) [L. *postulāre*, to request]. A supposition or view, usually self-evident, which is assumed without proof. SEE: *Koch's law or postulates*.

postural (pŏs'chū-răl) [L. *postura*, position]. Pert. to or affected by posture.

p. drainage. Drainage of secretions from the bronchi or a cavity in the lung by placing the patient's head lower than the area to be drained. Used in bronchiectasis and before operation for lobectomy, q.v. The position aggravates coughing, resulting in expectoration of much sputum, 5 to 10 oz. (148 to 296 ml.) in severe cases. Five to 10 minutes morning and evening is recommended. High protein diet to replace protein lost.

posture (pŏs'chŭr) [L. *postura*]. Attitude or position of the body.

p., coiled. Body on one side with legs drawn up to meet the trunk. Noted in cerebral diseases and in hepatic, intestinal, or renal colic.

p., dorsal rigid. Patient on back with both legs drawn up. Seen in peritonitis, meningitis, ascites, tympanites. In appendicitis the right leg is drawn up. Also occurs in pelvic inflammation or peritonitis of right side, renal calculus in right ureter, and in psoas abscess.

p., opisthotonos. An uncommon dorsal position in which the body rests upon the head and heels, with the trunk arched upward. It is seen in strychnine poisoning, tetanus, hysteria, epilepsy, the convulsions of rabies, and to a slight extent in meningitis. In the latter case, the neck is rigid and the head retracted, seeming to press into the pillow. SEE: *opisthotonos*.

p., orthopnea. Patient sitting upright, hands or elbows resting upon some support.

Seen in spasmodic asthma, emphysema, dyspnea, ascites, effusions into the pleural and pericardial cavities, and in late stages of diseases of the heart.

p., orthotonos. Neck and trunk extended rigidly in straight line; seen in tetanus, strychnine poisoning, rabies, or meningitis.

p., prone. P. assumed after abdominal colic or because of tuberculosis of spine, eroded vertebrae, abdominal pain, or gastric ulcer.

p., semireclining. Used in diseases of heart and interference with respiration in asthma and pleural effusions.

p., unilateral. Patient on right side in acute pleurisy, lobar pneumonia of right side, and in a greatly enlarged liver; or left side in lobar pneumonia, pleurisy on that side, and in large pericardial effusions.

postuterine (pŏst-ū'tĕr-ĭn) [L. *post*, after, + *uterus*, womb]. Situated behind the uterus.

pot. Slang term for marijuana.

potable (pō'tă-bl) [L. *potabilis*]. Suitable for drinking.

Potain's apparatus (pō-tān'). [Pierre C.E. Potain, Fr. physician, 1825-1901]. A form of aspirator.

Potain's disease. Pulmonary edema.

Potain's sign. Dullness on percussion of the aorta in dilatation, extending from the manubrium sterni toward the third costal cartilage on the right, the base of the sternum in segment of a circle to the right marking the upper limit.

potamophobia (pŏt"ă-mō-fō'bĭ-ă) [Gr. *potamos*, river, + *phobos*, fear]. A morbid fear of large bodies of water.

potash (pŏt'ăsh). Potassium carbonate, q.v.

p. caustic. Potassium hydroxide, q.v.

p., sulfurated. USP. Liver-colored or greenish yellow substance made up of potassium thiosulfate and potassium polysulfides and containing 12.8% sulfur as a sulfide. A principal ingredient of white lotion (USP).

potassemia (pŏt-ă-sē'mĭ-ă) [L. *potassa*, + Gr. *haima*, blood]. Presence of excessive quantity of potassium in the blood.

potassic (pō-tăs'ĭk). Composed of or containing potash.

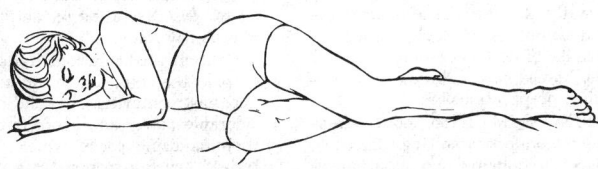

UNILATERAL POSTURE FOR COMFORT

potassium (pō-tăs'ĭ-ŭm) [L. *potassa*, potash]. SYMB: *K*. At. wt. 39.102; at. no. 19; sp. gr. 0.86. Mineral element found in combination with other elements in the body and constituting 0.35% of body weight. SYN: *kalium*.

FUNCTIONS: Potassium is the principal cation in intracellular fluid and is of primary importance in its maintenance. In conjunction with sodium and chloride, it aids in regulation of osmotic pressure and acid-base balance. A proper balance of potassium, calcium, and magnesium ions is essential for normal excitability of muscle tissue, esp. cardiac muscle, and it plays a role in the conduction of nerve impulses.

The usual intake of potassium is 50-150 mEq./day. Intake must be watched carefully to be certain it is adequate in prolonged intravenous feeding, during severe diarrhea or diabetic acidosis, and in patients receiving diuretics. In these conditions an intake of 1-3 mEq./kg./day usually is adequate.

DEFICIENCY SYM: Muscle weakness, dizziness, thirst, mental confusion, and changes in the electrocardiogram.

SOURCES: Found in most foods. Excellent sources are cereals, dried peas and beans, fresh vegetables, fresh or dried fruits, nuts, molasses, cocoa, fresh fish, and fresh poultry.

p. acetate. A white powder or crystalline flakes. CH₃COOK.

ACTION AND USES: Alkaline diuretic.

p. bicarbonate. USP. White crystals or powder. KHCO₃.

ACTION AND USES: To neutralize acid of stomach and to treat acid-base imbalance.

p. bitartrate. Cream of tartar. White powder or crystalline salt. KHC₄H₄O₆.

ACTION AND USES: As a dusting powder, in place of starch, for surgical gloves.

p. bromide. White cubical crystals or powder.

ACTION AND USES: Sedative.

p. carbonate. A white crystalline powder, K₂CO₃, used in pharmaceutical and chemical preparations. SYN: *potash.*

p. chlorate. KClO₃, an explosive white cyrstalline salt soluble in water. Formerly used internally in treatment of pharyngitis and stomatitis but its use has been discontinued because of destructive effect on red blood cells. Its use now is limited to veterinary medical preparations.

POISONING SYM: Large doses cause abdominal discomfort, vomiting, diarrhea, hematuria with nephritis, and disturbances of the blood.

F. A. TREATMENT: Stomach should be washed out. Otherwise treatment must be symptomatic.

p. chloride. USP. KCl, a white cyrstalline salt, soluble in water. One of the three chlorides used in preparation of Ringer's solution. Used in treatment of potassium deficiencies and digitalis intoxication.

p. chromate. Used as dye, furniture stain, in manufacture of batteries, in photography, and in pathology to preserve tissues.

SYM: May be inhaled or may contact the nose from fingers, causing deep, indolent ulcers. When taken by mouth has a disagreeable taste, causes cramping, pain, vomiting, diarrhea, slow respiration; may affect liver and kidneys.

F. A. TREATMENT: Treat as an acid; dilute and give weak alkalies as chalk, baking soda, magnesia, etc., followed by soothing mucilaginous drinks. Treat symptomatically.

p. citrate. Transparent prismatic crystals.

ACTION AND USES: Similar to potassium acetate.

INCOMPATIBILITIES: Caffeine sodium benzoate.

p. cyanide. SEE: *cyanide.*

p. hydroxide. USP. KOH. Grayish-white compound used in preparation of soap. It is used also as a chemical reagent. SYN: *caustic potash.*

POISONING SYM: Nausea; soapy taste; burning pain in mouth which causes bloody, slimy vomitus; abdominal cramping; bloody purging and prostration.

TREATMENT: Dilute with weak, acidulated water such as vinegar, lemon juice, orange juice, grape juice. Household oils likewise reduce the free alkali but more slowly. Follow with olive oil, sweet melted butter, or lard.

p. iodide. USP. Colorless or white crystals having a faint odor of iodine.

ACTION AND USES: Expectorant.

p. permanganate. KMnO₄. Dark purple prisms, odorless, with sweet taste.

ACTION AND USES: As a topical astringent and antiseptic, and as an oxidizing agent. Also useful as an antidote in phosphorus poisoning.

Concentrated solutions irritate and even corrode the skin, and when swallowed induce gastroenteritis. The solutions have considerable power as disinfectants, owing to their oxidizing power which destroys bacteria. They fail to penetrate deeply in an active form and this renders them of less value than many other disinfectants, except for use in very superficial infections.

p. sulfate. Has been used as a laxative, but because of its irritant qualities not to be recommended.

potato (pō-tā'tō) [Sp. *patata*]. The tuber of any of the plants of the genus Solanum. The tuber is widely used as an excellent source of carbohydrate in the diet. Freshly dug potatoes contain about 20 mg. of ascorbic acid in each 100 gm. This value decreases as they are stored so that in 3 months only half this amount of vitamin C remains.

Food value depends on method of preparation, with frying in deep fat (french fries) or mashing with butter greatly increasing Cal. value.

100 gm. (cooked, baked in skin): Cal. 76; protein 2.1 gm.; trace of fat; carbohydrate 17 gm.

potbelly. Selective deposition of adipose tissue in the abdominal subcutaneous tissue. This usually occurs in middle-aged persons who have sedentary occupations. The condition is accentuated by weakening of the anterior abdominal musculature and lumbar lordosis.

TREATMENT: Weight reduction; exercises to strengthen abdominal muscles; and therapy for lordosis.

potency (pō'těn-sĭ) [L. *potentia,* power]. 1. Strength; force; power. 2. Strength of a medicine. 3. Ability of male to perform coitus.

potent (pō'těnt) [L. *potēns,* powerful]. 1. Powerful. 2. Highly effective medicinally. 3. Having power of procreation.

potentia coeundi (pō-těn'shĭ-ă kō-ē-ŭn'dĭ) [L.]. Complete ability to perform sexual intercourse in a normal manner.

poten'tial. 1. Latent; existing in possibility. 2. In electricity, voltage or electrical pressure; a condition in which a state of tension or pressure exists capable of doing work. When two electrically charged bodies of different potentials are brought together, an electric current passes from the body of high potential to that of low.

p., action. The electrical changes that are associated with conduction of a nerve impulse or contraction of a muscle. They may be visualized by use of a cathode-ray oscillograph. ABBR: A.P.

p., after. On an oscillograph, smaller waves following a sharp rising curve of action potential. SEE: *p., spike.*

p., demarcation. The difference in potential between an intact longitudinal surface and the injured end of a muscle or nerve. SYN: *injury potential.*

p., injury. SEE: *p., demarcation.*

p., spike. A change in potential indicated by a sharp spikelike curve indicating a negative deflection.

potentiate (pō-těn'shĭ-āt). To augment or increase the potency or action.

po"tentia'tion. The synergistic action of two substances, e.g., hormones, in which the total effects are greater than the sum of the independent effects of the two substances. SYN: *augmentation.*

potion (pō'shŭn) [L. *potiō,* draft]. A drink or draught; a dose of poison or liquid medicine.

potocytosis (pō"tō-sĭ-tō'sĭs) [Gr. *potos,* drinking, + *kytos,* cell, + *-ōsis,* condition]. The submicroscopic imbibing or taking up of water by cells in contrast to pinocytosis, q.v.

potomania (pō"tō-mā'nĭ-ă) ["+ *mania,* madness]. Delirium tremens, q.v.

Pott's disease. [Percivall Pott, Br. surgeon, 1713-1788]. Caries or osteitis of the vertebrae, usually of tuberculous origin; tubercular inflammation of bodies of the vertebrae. The disease is primarily a disease of children and of adults up to age 40. Destruction and compression of affected vertebrae often results in kyphosis with resulting compression of spinal cord and nerves. Often infection spreads to paravertebral tissues giving rise to paravertebral abscesses.

SYM: Child will complain of pain in region supplied by the nerves arising from affected segment of the cord. (1) If disease is lumbar, pains are abdominal and apt to be associated with vesical irritability; (2) if dorsal, pains are epigastric or intercostal, and respiration sometimes irregular and hurried from failure of respiratory muscles to take the full share in the work; (3) if cervical, neuralgic pain or numbness in hands, a tickling cough and difficult swallowing. Pains apt to be symmetrical.

Increase of pain on jumping or flexing or rotating spine is extremely significant. If child can jump painlessly from chair to floor it is almost certain no inflammation of the body of a vertebra exists. If vertebrae are crowded together by pressure on head or shoulders while patient sits or stands, or while he lies face downward across knees of surgeon, pain much increased.

If stretched, so spine is elongated, relief follows. Involuntary immobilization of spine, as a result of pain on movement, is very characteristic military attitude. If child is asked to look at something behind him, he turns whole trunk. If requested to pick up something from floor, he stoops by bending the thighs upon the trunk and knees upon thighs, never by flexing spinal column in usual way.

In walking, moves as if on ice, sliding or shuffling along so as to avoid jar of successive steps. In standing, he fixes upper portion of column by aid of trapezii and other scapular muscles, action of which at same time raises shoulders and throws arms out from sides. In standing or sitting, there is an involuntary transfer of the weight of head and shoulders and parts above diseased area to the pelvis, by means of the upper extremities. Hands placed upon the hips and arm muscles are tense. In walking about room, lays hold of furniture for aid. Spinal abscess occurs later, location varying with seat of caries. Paralysis may occur, always motor at first, not affecting sensation at all.

TREATMENT: Endeavor to secure resolution of the tuberculous osteitis. Limit destruction of tissue and resulting deformity. Promote ankylosis if indicated. Evacuate pus. Remove a sequestrum or the focus of carious bone. Relieve cord from pressure by pus or bone. Rest in bed in recumbent position. Adequate diet and exercise care to prevent development of decubitous ulcers. Chemotherapy as for pulmonary tuberculosis.

SEE: *gibbosity; kyphosis.*

Pott's fracture. Fracture of lower end of fibula and medial malleolus of the tibia with dislocation of foot outwards and backwards. After reduction, foot and leg are put in plaster in which a walking iron is incorporated. The patient is able to walk, and plaster is removed in about 6 weeks.

pouch (powch) [ME. *pouche*]. Any pocket or sac. SYN: *sacculation.*

    p., branchial. SEE: *p., pharyngeal.*

    p., Broca's. A sac in tissues of the labia majora.

    p. of Douglas. SEE: *p., rectouterine.*

    p., laryngeal. Blind pouch of mucosa entering the ventral portion of the ventricle of the larynx.

    p., Pavlov. A stomach pouch formed surgically for the experimental study of gastric secretion. A section of the stomach is separated from the main stomach left, or attached by only a small pedicle, and fistulized so as to drain to exterior of body.

    p., pharyngeal. One of a series of five pairs of entodermal outpocketings which develop in lateral walls of pharynx of embryo.

    p., Rathke's. An outpocketing of the roof of embryonic stomodeum. Gives rise to anterior lobe of hypophysis cerebri.

    p., rectouterine. Pouch between anterior rectal wall and posterior uterine wall. SYN: *cul-de-sac; excavatio rectouterina* [NA]; *p. of Douglas.*

    p., rectovesical. A fold of peritoneum that in the male extends downward between bladder and rectum.

poudrage (pū-drŏzh') [Fr.]. Application of an irritating, but otherwise nontoxic, powder to the pleural space of the lung in order to produce pleural adhesions.

poultice (pōl'tĭs) [L. *pultēs*, thick paste]. A hot, moist mass of linseed, mustard, or soap and oil between two pieces of muslin applied to the skin to relieve congestion or pain, to stimulate absorption of inflammatory products, and to act as a counterirritant. SEE: *plaster.*

pound (pownd) [L. *pondus*, weight]. SYMB: lb. A measure of weight, 16 ounces. SEE: *Weights and measures* in *Appendix.*

    p., avoirdupois. Sixteen ounces, 7000 gr. and equal to 453.59 gm.

    p., foot-. Power necessary to raise one pound one foot high.

    p., troy. Twelve ounces, 5760 gr. and equal to 373.242 gm.

Poupart's ligament (pū-par'). [Francois Poupart, Fr. anatomist, 1616-1708]. The ligament forming the lower border of aponeurosis of external oblique muscle between anterior superior spine of the ilium and spine of the pubis. SYN: *inguinal ligament.*

powder (pow'dĕr) [ME. *poudre*]. 1. Aggregation of particles. 2. Fine particles of one or more substances that may be passed through fine meshes. 3. A dose of such a powder, contained in a paper.

power (pow'er) [ME. *pouer*]. 1. Rate at which work is done. 2. Capacity for action. 3. In optics, the degree to which a lens or optical instrument magnifies. 4. In microscopy, the number of times the diameter of an object is magnified, indicated by placing an × after the number. Ex: 10×.

pox (pŏks) [ME. *pokkes*, pits]. 1. An eruptive, contagious disease. 2. A papular eruption that becomes pustular. SEE: *chickenpox; smallpox.*

P.P. Abbr. for *punctum proximum,* near point of accommodation (in vision).

P.P.D. Abbr. for *purified protein derivative,* substance used in intradermal test for tuberculosis.

P.P.F. Abbr. for the *pellagra preventive factor* in vitamin B.

PPLO. Abbr. for *pleuropneumonia-like organisms,* now called Mycoplasma. SEE: *Mycoplasmas.*

Ppt. Abbr. for *precipitate; prepared.*

Pr. 1. Abbr. for *presbyopia.* 2. Chem. symb. for praseodymium.

P.R. Abbr. for *punctum remotum,* far point of visual accommodation.

practice (prăk'tĭs) [Gr. *praktikē,* business]. The use, by a physician, of his medical knowledge and skill in diagnosing and treating disease and in preventing illness.

practitioner (prăk-tĭsh'ŭn-ēr). One who has met the medical requirements and is engaged in the profession of medicine.

prae-. SEE: words beginning with *pre-.*

praecox (prē'kŏks) [L.]. Early.

praevia, praevius (prē'vĭ-ă, prē'vĭ-ŭs) [L.]. Going before in time or place.

pragmatagnosia (prăg''măt-ăg-nō'zĭ-ă) [Gr. *pragma,* object, + *agnōsia,* lack of recognition]. Inability to recognize objects once familiar.

pragmatamnesia (prăg''măt-ăm-nē'zĭ-ă) ["+ *amnēsia,* forgetfulness]. Inability to recall the appearance of an object.

p., visual. Name for the mental condition making possible pragmatamnesia.

pragmatic (prăg-măt'ĭk) [Gr. *pragma,* a thing done]. Pert. to, or concerned with, the practical side of anything.

pragmatism (prăg'mă-tĭzm) ["+ *ismos,* condition]. A belief that the practical application of a principle should be the determining factor.

pragmatist (prăg'mă-tĭst). One who believes that practical application should be the determining factor of a principle.

prandial (prăn'dĭ-ăl) [L. *prandium,* breakfast]. Rel. to a meal.

praseodymium (prā''sē-ō-dĭm'ĭ-ŭm). SYMB: *Pr.* At. wt. 140.907; at. no. 59. A metallic element obtained from rare earth.

praxinoscope (prăk-sĭn'ō-skōp) [Gr. *praxis,* action, + *skopein,* to examine]. Contrivance for studying the larynx.

praxiology (prăk''sĭ-ŏl'ō-jĭ) ["+ *logos,* study]. Study of behavior.

Prayer of Maimonides. [Rabbi Moses ben Maimon, Jewish philosopher and physician in Egypt, 1135-1204] A prayer used at graduation ceremonies by some medical schools.

Thy eternal providence has appointed me to watch over the life and health of Thy creatures. May the love for my art actuate me at all times; may neither avarice nor miserliness, nor thirst for glory, or for a great reputation engage my mind; for the enemies of truth and philanthropy could easily deceive me and make me forgetful of my lofty aim of doing good to Thy children.

May I never see in the patient anything but a fellow creature in pain.

Grant me strength, time and opportunity always to correct what I have acquired, always to extend its domain; for knowledge is immense and the spirit of man can extend indefinitely to enrich itself daily with new requirements.

Today he can discover his errors of yesterday and tomorrow he can obtain a new light on what he thinks himself sure of today. Oh, God, Thou has appointed me to watch over the life and death of Thy creatures; here am I ready for my vocation and now I turn unto my calling. SEE: *Declaration of Geneva; Hippocratic oath.*

pre-. [L. *prae,* before]. Prefix indicating before or in front of.

preagonal (prē-ăg'ō-năl) [L. *prae,* before, + Gr. *agōnia,* agony]. Pert. to condition immediately before death agony.

prealbuminuric (prē''ăl-bū''mĭn-ū'rĭk) ["+ *albumen,* white of egg]. Before the appearance of albuminuria.

preanal (prē-ā'năl) ["+ *anus,* anus]. In front of the anus.

preanesthetic (prē''ăn-ĕs-thĕt'ĭk) [L. *prae,* before, + Gr. *anaisthēsia,* lack of sensation]. Preliminary drug given to facilitate induction of general anesthesia.

preantiseptic (prē''ăn''tĭ-sĕp'tĭk) ["+ Gr. *anti,* against, + *sēpsis,* decay]. Before the adoption of antisepsis in surgery.

preaortic (prē''ā-or'tĭk) ["+ Gr. *aortē,* aorta]. Located in front of the aorta.

preataxic (prē-ă-tăk'sĭk) ["+ Gr. *ataxia,* disorder]. Before the onset of ataxia.

preaxial (prē-ăk'sĭ-ăl) [L. *prae,* before, + Gr. *axōn,* axis]. In front of the axis of a limb or of the body.

precancerous (prē-kăn'sēr-ŭs) ["+ *cancer,* crab]. Said of a growth that is not yet, but probably will become, cancerous.

precap'illary [L. *prae,* before, + *capillaris,* hairlike]. An arterial capillary; one which branches from an arteriole or venule. SYN: *metarteriole.*

precava (prē-kā'vă) ["+ *cavus,* hollow]. The descending or superior vena cava.

precentral (prē-sĕn'trăl) ["+ Gr. *kentron,* center]. In front of a center, as the central fissure of the brain.

p. convolution. The ascending frontal convolution.

prechordal (prē-kōr'dăl) ["+ Gr. *chordē,* cord]. In front of the notochord.

precipitant (prē-sĭp'ĭ-tănt) [L. *praecipitāre,* to cast down]. A substance bringing about precipitation.

precipitate (prē-sĭp'ĭ-tāt). 1. A deposit separated from a suspension or solution by precipitation, the reaction of a reagent that causes the deposit to fall to the bottom or float near the top. 2. To separate as a precipitate. 3. Occurring suddenly or unexpectedly.

precipitation (prē-sĭp'ĭ-tā'shŭn) [L. *praecipitatio*]. Process of a substance being separated from a solution by action of a reagent.

    p. test. One in which positive reaction is indicated by formation of a precipitate in the solution being tested.

precipitin (prē-sĭp'ĭ-tĭn). An antibody formed in the blood serum of an animal due to presence of a soluble antigen, usually a protein. When added to a solution of the antigen, it brings about precipitation. The injected protein is called the *antigen* and the antibody produced is the *precipitin*. SEE: *autoprecipitin; precipitinogen.*

    p. reaction. The formation of a precipitate in a solution containing a soluble antigen upon addition of serum containing the specific precipitin. The reaction is very specific. The test is used for identification of unknown proteins; determination of types of pneumococci and meningococci; determination of types of blood stains, whether human or animal; and for diagnosis of plague, anthrax, and echinococcus disease. SYN: *precipitin test.*

precipitinogen (prē-sĭp''ĭ-tĭn'ō-jĕn). Any protein which, acting as an antigen, stimulates the production of a specific precipitin.

precipitinoid (prē-sĭp'ĭt-ĭn-oyd). Precipitin which can no longer cause precipitation when mixed with its antigen, but retains its affinity to the antigen.

precipitophore (prē-sĭp'ĭt-ō-fōr''). Group in a precipitin which produces the actual precipitation. Opposed to haptophore precipitum.

precipitum (prē-sĭp'ĭ-tŭm). The precipitate produced by action of a precipitin.

preclinical (prē-klĭn'ĭ-kăl) [L. *prae,* before, + Gr. *klinikē,* medical treatment in bed]. Occurring before diagnosis of a definite disease is possible.

    p. medicine. Medical training engaged in prior to the actual study of patients, usually constituting the first two years of medical study.

preclival (prē-klī'văl) ["+ *clivus,* slope]. In front of the cerebellar clivus.

precocity (prē-kŏs'ĭ-tĭ) [L. *praecox,* ripening early]. Premature development of physical or mental traits.

    p., sexual. Premature genital maturation; precocious sexual maturity.

precoital (prē-kō'ĭ-tăl) [L. *prae,* before, + *coitiō,* a going together]. Prior to sexual intercourse.

preconscious (prē-kŏn'shŭs) ["+ *conscius,* aware]. Not present in consciousness but able to be recalled as desired.

preconvulsive (prē''kŏn-vŭl'sĭv) ["+ *convulsiō,* pulling together]. Before a convulsion.

precordia (prē-kōr'dĭ-ă) [L. *praecordia*]. The precordium, q.v.

precordial (prē-kōr'dĭ-ăl). Pert. to the precordium or epigastrium.

precordialgia (prē''kōr-dĭ-ăl'jĭ-ă) [L. *praecordia,* precordia, + Gr. *algos,* pain]. Pain in the chest or precordial area.

precordium (prē-kor'dĭ-ŭm). The area on the anterior surface of the body overlying the heart, its great vessels, the pericardium, and whatever pulmonary tissue lies anterior to these structures and the anterior chest wall. SYN: *precordia.*

precornu (prē-kōr'nū) [L. *prae,* before, + *cornu,* horn]. Anterior horn of lateral ventricle of the brain.

precuneus (prē-kū'nē-ŭs) ["+ *cuneus,* wedge]. [NA]. The division of the mesial surface of a cerebral hemisphere between the cuneus and the paracentral lobule.

prediastolic (prē''dī-ă-stŏl'ĭk) ["+ Gr. *diastolē,* expansion]. Before the diastole, or interval in the cardiac cycle that precedes it.

predicrotic (prē''dī-krŏt'ĭk) ["+ Gr. *dikrotos,* beating double]. Preceding the dicrotic wave of the sphygmographic tracing.

predigestion (prē''dī-jĕs'chŭn) [L. *prae,* before, + *digestiō,* carrying apart]. Artificial proteolysis or digestion of proteins and amylolysis of starches before ingestion for use in illness.

predisposing (prē-dĭs-pōz'ĭng) ["+ *disponere,* to dispose]. Indicating a tendency to, or susceptibility to, disease.

predisposition (prē''dĭs-pō-zĭsh'ŭn). A tendency to develop a certain disease, either acquired or hereditary.

    p., acquired. P. to disease not due to innate or inherited factors, such as that resulting from malnutrition, excessive fatigue, etc.

predormition (prē-dŏr-mĭ'shŭn) [L. *prae,* before, + *dormire,* to sleep]. State of unconsciousness immediately preceding actual sleep.

preeclampsia (prē''ē-klămp'sĭ-ă) ["+ Gr. *ek,* out, + *lampein,* to flash]. A toxemia of pregnancy characterized by increasing hypertension, headaches, albuminuria, and edema of the lower extremities. If this condition is neglected or not treated properly, the patient may develop true eclampsia. SEE: *eclampsia*.

prefrontal (pre-fron'tăl) ["+ *frons, front-,* front]. 1. The middle portion of the ethmoid bone. 2. In anterior part of the frontal lobe of the brain.

p. leukotomy. P. lobotomy. SEE: *lobotomy*.

p. lobotomy. SEE: *lobotomy*.

preganglionic (pre"găng-lĭ-ŏn'ĭk) [L. *prae,* before, + Gr. *ganglion,* knot]. Situated in front of or anterior to a ganglion.

p. fiber. The axon of a preganglionic neuron.

p. neuron. The first of a series of two efferent neurons that transmit impulses to visceral effectors. Its cell body lies in the central nervous system. Its axon terminates in an autonomic ganglion.

pregenital (pre-jĕn'ĭ-tăl) ["+ *genitalia,* genitals]. In psychology, rel. to that period when erotic interest in the reproductive organs and functions is not yet organized.

preglobulin (pre-glŏb'ū-lĭn) ["+ *globulus,* a small sphere]. A proteid in cell protoplasm derived from cytoglobulin.

pregnancy (prĕg'năn-sĭ) [L. *praegnans*]. The condition of carrying a developing embryo in the uterus.

SYM AND SIGNS: Amenorrhea, nausea and vomiting, inordinate appetite, pigmentation of the areola of the breasts, the development of Montgomery's tubercles around the nipple, changes in the uterus (softening and progressive enlargement), vaginal discoloration, and frequent urination.

Positive signs are hearing and counting the fetal heart beat, finding x-ray evidence of the fetal skeleton, and detection by the physician of movements of the fetus. There are various biological tests for pregnancy and these are 90-95% accurate.

The duration of pregnancy is approximately 280 days. SEE: *Pregnancy Table.* To estimate the day of delivery, count back 3 months from the day of onset of the last menstrual period and then add 7 days. For example, if the last menstrual period began June (6/10), subtracting 3 months leaves 3/10 and adding 7 days results in 3/17 (that is, the expected day of delivery would be March 17 of the next year). This method assumes all months have the same number of days; thus the date determined will not agree exactly with that found by using the Pregnancy Table.

PHYSICAL CHANGES: *Uterus:* Changes shape, size, and consistency; lining undergoes changes; peritoneal covering enlarges; muscles increase enormously; blood vessels penetrate through uterine muscle.

Vaginal Canal: Elongation caused by rising of uterus in pelvis; mucosa thickens; secretion increased; increased vascularity and elasticity; cervix, vagina, and vulva become softer.

Abdominal Changes: Growing distention and flattened navel; striae gravidarum.

Breasts: Enlarged and painful; skin thin and sensitive; nipples erectile, enlarged, and darker; escape of colostrum; primary and secondary areola; tingling sensation.

Endocrine Glands: Thyroid increases in size and activity; parathyroids enlarge and secretion increases; pituitary increases its activity; placenta gives forth hormones, affecting ovaries and corpus luteum.

Circulatory System: Increased activity; increased blood volume; blood pressure should be normal; varicose veins common; no blood sugar change.

Skeletal Changes: Pelvic joints soften; pelvic joints more movable; bones and teeth affected.

Respiratory Changes: Lungs impeded in late pregnancy; breathing deeper and more frequent.

Digestive Tract: Nausea and vomiting in early pregnancy; appetite affected; loss of weight in early pregnancy with slight anemia; basal metabolism raised in later pregnancy; constipation frequent.

Liver: Enlarged and displaced in late pregnancy.

Skin: Sudoriparous and sebaceous glands very active; deposit of brown pigment (mask of pregnancy); linea nigra.

Weight: Increased.

Posture: Changes, as enlargment of abdomen advances; sacroiliac joints and symphysis pubis more movable; painful locomotion and backache; waddling gait.

Urinary Tract: Increased kidney activity; failure of kidneys produces nephritic toxemia; ureters, esp. right one, dilated; pressure on bladder with increased circulation; frequent urination; bladder lifted into abdomen and pressure diminished. Bladder later pressed upon by presenting part; urinary output varies; presence of albumin abnormal. Sugar found in later part of pregnancy; may be diabetes or glycosuria.

DISORDERS OF: *Nausea and Vomiting:* May be noted when stomach is empty, but may occur at any time. Food may help on arising; four or five small meals per day; psychic causes may be responsible

Constipation and Flatulence: Pressure of uterus on intestines may be a cause; laxative diet and exercise may aid; intestinal stasis may cause flatulence; gas-forming foods should be avoided.

Muscular Cramps: Retention of waste products a cause; poor circulation may cause retention. Applying pressure on foot, extension of leg helps. Rest between periods of standing needed. Tetany may ensue because of deficient calcium supply; calcium and vitamin D indicated.

Pressure Edema: May occur at end of p., better in morning, worse at night. Frequent rest and elevation of limbs indicated. May be due to calcium deficiency. Toxemia must be ruled out by frequent blood pressure and urinalysis.

Headache: Cause may be intestinal intoxication and constipation, eyestrain, temporary hypertrophy of pituitary, sinusitis, or toxemia. Take blood pressure and urinalysis to check latter cause.

Neuralgic Pains: Rest periods and abdominal support indicated; knee-chest position after retiring.

Toothache: May be due to caries induced by deficient calcium. Frequent dental examinations desirable.

Backache: Abnormal balance caused by protruding abdomen; proper shoes indicated. Intra-abdominal pressure may be a cause; flatulence aggravates; enemas may help. Knee-chest position at night is helpful.

Dyspnea: Pressure of uterus upward on transverse colon and stomach; aggravated by flatulence, esp. when lying down. Alkalies may help; pillows under head and shoulder indicated: reexamination of heart indicated.

Vaginal Discharge: Increased blood supply to glands of cervix; cleanliness, but no douches, indicated. Foul, blood-tinged, or profuse discharge should be reported.

Pruritus: Breasts, abdomen, and vulva may be affected; stretching of skin of abdomen a cause in that area. If general, a toxic or nervous origin may be cause. Sugar in urine may cause pruritus of vulva.

Heartburn: Hyperacidity or nervous tension may be responsible. Sedation, frequent small meals, no highly seasoned foods.

Salivation: May be associated with extreme nausea and vomiting; usually an expression of neurosis. Mild astringents may be employed. If due to a toxemia, refer to the physician.

Varicose Veins: Congenitally acquired; aggravated by pregnancy. May occur in pelvis, vulva, and legs; marked on right side.

Avoid round garters, tight clothing, and standing. Rest and supporting stockings indicated; elevation of lower limbs while sleeping; Sims' position, pillow under hips to shift uterus.

Hemorrhoids: Avoid constipation; ointments, wet compresses, suppositories on doctor's orders; carbolized or mentholated petrolatum in absence of doctor's advice; incision by surgeon.

p., abdominal. Implantation of the ovum in the abdominal cavity.

p., ampullar. P. in ampulla of uterine tube.

p., bigeminal. P. with twins in utero.

p., cervical. Implantation of the ovum in the cervical canal.

p., cornual. P. in one of the horns of the bicornuate uterus.

p., ectopic. Extrauterine p., q.v.

p., extrauterine. P. outside the uterine cavity.

p., false. Phantom p., q.v.

p., heterotropic. Combined intrauterine and extrauterine pregnancies.

p., hydatid. P. giving rise to a hydatidiform mole. SEE: *hydated mole.*

p., interstitial. P. occurring in the uterine wall which forms part of the oviduct.

p., intraligamentary. P. occurring within the broad ligament.

p., intramural. P., interstitial, q.v.

p., mask of. Area of brown pigmentation sometimes appearing on the face during p.

p., membranous. P. in which amniotic sac ruptures and fetus comes to lie in direct contact with uterine wall.

p., mesenteric. P., tuboligamentary, q.v.

p., multiple. State of having more than one fetus in the uterus at the same time.

p., ovarian. Implantation of the fertilized ovum in the substance of the ovary.

p., phantom. Enlargement of the abdomen simulating p. SEE: *pseudocyesis.*

p. table. See table accompanying this entry for calculation of expected date of delivery from the first day of the last menstrual period.

p., tuboabdominal. P. in which part of fetus is in uterine tube and part in abdominal cavity.

p., tuboligamentary. P. occuring in uterine tube and extending into broad ligament.

p., tuboovarian. P. in which development of fetus occurs in both uterine tube and ovary.

Pregnancy Table for Expected Date of Delivery

Find the date of the last menstrual period in the top line (light-face type) of the pair of lines. The dark number (bold-face type) in the line below will be the expected day of delivery.

	1	2	3	4	5	6	7	8	9	10	11	12	13	14	15	16	17	18	19	20	21	22	23	24	25	26	27	28	29	30	31	
Jan.	1	2	3	4	5	6	7	8	9	10	11	12	13	14	15	16	17	18	19	20	21	22	23	24	25	26	27	28	29	30	31	
Oct.	8	9	10	11	12	13	14	15	16	17	18	19	20	21	22	23	24	25	26	27	28	29	30	31	1	2	3	4	5	6	7	Nov.
Feb.	1	2	3	4	5	6	7	8	9	10	11	12	13	14	15	16	17	18	19	20	21	22	23	24	25	26	27	28				
Nov.	8	9	10	11	12	13	14	15	16	17	18	19	20	21	22	23	24	25	26	27	28	29	30	1	2	3	4	5				Dec.
Mar.	1	2	3	4	5	6	7	8	9	10	11	12	13	14	15	16	17	18	19	20	21	22	23	24	25	26	27	28	29	30	31	
Dec.	6	7	8	9	10	11	12	13	14	15	16	17	18	19	20	21	22	23	24	25	26	27	28	29	30	31	1	2	3	4	5	Jan.
April	1	2	3	4	5	6	7	8	9	10	11	12	13	14	15	16	17	18	19	20	21	22	23	24	25	26	27	28	29	30		
Jan.	6	7	8	9	10	11	12	13	14	15	16	17	18	19	20	21	22	23	24	25	26	27	28	29	30	31	1	2	3	4		Feb.
May	1	2	3	4	5	6	7	8	9	10	11	12	13	14	15	16	17	18	19	20	21	22	23	24	25	26	27	28	29	30	31	
Feb.	5	6	7	8	9	10	11	12	13	14	15	16	17	18	19	20	21	22	23	24	25	26	27	28	1	2	3	4	5	6	7	Mar.
June	1	2	3	4	5	6	7	8	9	10	11	12	13	14	15	16	17	18	19	20	21	22	23	24	25	26	27	28	29	30		
Mar.	8	9	10	11	12	13	14	15	16	17	18	19	20	21	22	23	24	25	26	27	28	29	30	31	1	2	3	4	5	6		April
July	1	2	3	4	5	6	7	8	9	10	11	12	13	14	15	16	17	18	19	20	21	22	23	24	25	26	27	28	29	30	31	
April	7	8	9	10	11	12	13	14	15	16	17	18	19	20	21	22	23	24	25	26	27	28	29	30	1	2	3	4	5	6	7	May
Aug.	1	2	3	4	5	6	7	8	9	10	11	12	13	14	15	16	17	18	19	20	21	22	23	24	25	26	27	28	29	30	31	
May	8	9	10	11	12	13	14	15	16	17	18	19	20	21	22	23	24	25	26	27	28	29	30	31	1	2	3	4	5	6	7	June
Sept.	1	2	3	4	5	6	7	8	9	10	11	12	13	14	15	16	17	18	19	20	21	22	23	24	25	26	27	28	29	30		
June	8	9	10	11	12	13	14	15	16	17	18	19	20	21	22	23	24	25	26	27	28	29	30	1	2	3	4	5	6	7		July
Oct.	1	2	3	4	5	6	7	8	9	10	11	12	13	14	15	16	17	18	19	20	21	22	23	24	25	26	27	28	29	30	31	
July	8	9	10	11	12	13	14	15	16	17	18	19	20	21	22	23	24	25	26	27	28	29	30	31	1	2	3	4	5	6	7	Aug.
Nov.	1	2	3	4	5	6	7	8	9	10	11	12	13	14	15	16	17	18	19	20	21	22	23	24	25	26	27	28	29	30		
Aug.	8	9	10	11	12	13	14	15	16	17	18	19	20	21	22	23	24	25	26	27	28	29	30	31	1	2	3	4	5	6		Sept.
Dec.	1	2	3	4	5	6	7	8	9	10	11	12	13	14	15	16	17	18	19	20	21	22	23	24	25	26	27	28	29	30	31	
Sept.	7	8	9	10	11	12	13	14	15	16	17	18	19	20	21	22	23	24	25	26	27	28	29	30	1	2	3	4	5	6	7	Oct.

pregnanediol (prĕg-năn'ē-dī-ŏl). $C_{21}H_{36}O_2$. The inactive end product of metabolism of progesterone present in the urine. Amount in urine increases during premenstrual or luteal phase of menstrual cycle and during pregnancy.

pregnant (prĕg'nănt) [L. *praegnans*]. Having conceived; with child. SYN: *gravid*.

pregnenolone (prĕg-nĕn'ō-lōn). A synthetic hormone. A direct oxidation product of cholesterol with a formula closely related to that of cortisone. Used in arthritis.

pregravidic (prē-gră-vĭd'ĭk) [L. *prae*, before, + *gravida*, pregnant]. Before pregnancy.

prehallux (prē-hăl'ŭks) ["+ *hallux*, the great toe]. A supernumerary bone, accessory naviculare pedis, or sometimes a prolongation inward of it on the foot.

prehemiplegic (prē"hĕm-ĭ-plē'jĭk) ["+ Gr. *hemi*, half, + *plēgē*, a stroke]. Occurring before an attack of hemiplegia.

prehensile (prē-hĕn'sĭl) [L. *prehendere*, to seize]. Adapted for grasping or holding, esp. by encircling an object.

prehension (prē-hĕn'shŭn). The act of grasping or seizing.

preimmunization (prē-ĭm"ū-nĭ-zā'shŭn) [L. *prae*, before, + *immunis*, safe]. Immunization produced artificially in very young infants.

Preiser's disease (prī'zĕr). [Georg K.F. Preiser, Ger. orthopedic surgeon, 1879-1913]. A porous condition of bone, osteoporosis, caused by trauma and affecting the carpal scaphoid bone of the wrist.

prelum (prē'lŭm) [L.]. A press.

  p. abdominale. Squeezing of abdominal viscera between the diaphragm and abdominal wall. Occurs in defecation, urination, and parturition.

premature (prē-mă-chūr') [L. *praemātūrus*, ripening early]. Not mature; before term or full development.

  p. beat. A cardiac contraction occurring before the normal one. SYN: *extrasystole*.

  p. infant. One born before term. May be caused by uterine disease, shock, accident, toxemia of pregnancy, syphilis, or any serious organic disease.

  p. labor. Onset of labor before full term.

prematurity. The state of low birth weight of infants.

  The normal gestation period for the human being is forty weeks; infants born prior to the thirty-eighth week of intrauterine life are considered premature. As difficulties are encountered in obtaining accurate and objective data as to the exact length of gestation, a birth weight of 2500 gm. (5 1/2 pounds) or less has been accepted internationally as the clinical criterion of prematurity regardless of the period of gestation. Other measures suggestive of prematurity are crown-heel length (47 cm. or less), crown-rump length (32 cm. or less), occipitofrontal circumference (33 cm. or less), occipitofrontal diameter (11.5 cm. or less), and ratio of the thorax circumference to the head circumference (less than 93%).

  The use of a single criterion measure (birth weight) imposes limitations in accurately identifying those infants born before adequate development of body organs and systems has been achieved; it can easily include mature infants who are of low birth weight for reasons other than a shortened gestation period. The Expert Committee on Prematurity of the World Health Organization (1961) has recommended that the concept of prematurity in the international definition be replaced by that of low birth weight. This term, *low birth weight*, more accurately describes the infant population encompassed by a 2500 gm. birth weight criterion than does the term *prematurity;* the latter should be reserved for those neonates within the low birth weight group that show signs of immaturity.

  During 1962 there were 4,167,362 live births in the United States. Eight per cent of these infants weighed 2500 gm. or less at birth. Chances of survival depend upon degree of maturity achieved, general condition, and quality of care received. See accompanying table.

  Prematurity is the leading cause of death in the neonatal period; mortality among infants weighing less than 2500 gm. at birth is twenty times greater than among infants with birth weight above 2500 gm. Chief causes of mortality are abnormal pulmonary ventilation, infection, intracranial hemorrage, abnormal blood conditions, and congenital anomalies.

  ETIOL: The incidence of neonates of low birth weight is more frequent among the female sex, the nonwhite race, the plural born, and the first and fifth (and over) born infants. Delivery of infants of low birth weight is reported to be more frequent among women who are less than 19 years of age and more than 30, are poorly nourished, have had little or no prenatal care, are unmarried, are cigarette smokers, have bacteriuria that has not been treated, live in urban areas, work during pregnancy, live in high altitude areas, are of lower social classes, and when pregnancies occur within a two-year period or beyond a six-year period of the previous pregnancy.

Factors contributing to prematurity and/ or low birth weight are premature rupture of the membranes, antepartum hemorrhage, toxemia of pregnancy, chronic diseases, acute infections, pelvic abnormalities, physical and emotional trauma, blood incompatibilities, malformation of the fetus, and multiple births. In more than 50% of these deliveries, the cause for low birth weight cannot be stated.

COMPLICATIONS; Frequently premature infants are handicapped by a number of anatomical and physiological limitations. These limitations vary in direct proportion to the degree of immaturity present. Limitations include weakness of the sucking and swallowing reflexes, small capacity of stomach, lowered tolerance of alimentary tract, impairment of renal function, incomplete development of capillaries of medulla and lungs, immature alveoli of the lungs, weakness of the cough and gag reflexes, weakness of the thoracic cage and muscles used in respiration, inadequate regulation of body temperature, incomplete enzyme systems, hepatic immaturity, and deficient placental transfer and antenatal storage of minerals, vitamins, and immune substances.

NP: Care of low birth weight infants should be individualized and reflect the needs of the developing organism in relation to the presence of anatomical and physiological handicaps. Evaluation for degree of immaturity present and the identification of special problems appearing after birth will dictate care required by these infants. In general, care revolves around the prevention of infection, stabilization of body temperature, maintenance of respiration, provision for adequate nutrition and hydration, and conservation of energy.

Aseptic technique is practiced to prevent infection. An incubator or heated bed provides a suitable environment for maintenance of body temperature. A high humidity environment may be of value in respiratory difficulties. Gentle suctioning will aid to keep airways clear. Use of oxygen should be restricted to those minimal amounts required for survival of infant. Because of the danger of retrolental fibroplasia, the oxygen concentration should not exceed 40%.

Depending upon the ability of the infant to suck and swallow, gavage feedings may be necessary. Some of these infants may not be given anything by mouth for as long as 72 hours following birth. Caloric and fluid intakes are gradually increased until 100-120 Cal./kg. and 140-150 ml./kg. in 24 hours are reached. The time required to achieve these intakes depends upon the size and condition of the baby. Small, frequent feedings may be needed to cope with the small capacity of the stomach, to prevent vomiting and distention, and to meet caloric and fluid requirements of the body. Over-feeding should be avoided. During early days of life, clyses sometimes are administered to maintain adequate hydration.

The infant should not be allowed to

Percentage Distribution and Survival of Low Birth Weight Infants

Birth Weight Group	Total Live Births* (per cent)	Low Birth Weight Infants Only* (per cent)	Approximate Survival of Low Birth Weight Infants** (per cent)
Under 1000 grams	0.5	6.25	10
1001–1500 grams	0.7	8.75	50
1501–2000 grams	1.5	18.75	85
2001–2500 grams	5.3	66.25	95
Total 2500 grams or less:	8.0	100.00	85***
Total 2500 grams or over:	92.0		
Total Live Births:	100.0		

* U.S. National Vital Statistics 1962.
** New York City Infant Mortality Rates 1962.
*** Weighted average.

become fatigued either from excessive handling, prolonged feeding procedures, or too much crying. His position should be changed every 2-4 hours. Minimal handling regimen should not be used indiscriminately; gentle handling, rather than minimal handling, should be practiced.

premaxilla (prē''măk-sĭl'ă) [L. *prae*, before, + *maxilla*, upper jaw]. The intermaxillary bone forming median anterior part of superior maxillary bones.

premaxillary (prē-măk'sĭ-lĕr'ĭ). Located before the maxilla.

p. bone. The intermaxillary bone. SYN: *incisive bone.*

premedication (prē''mĕd-ĭ-kā'shŭn) [L. *prae*, before, + *medicari*, to heal]. Induction of unconsciousness by internal drugs prior to administration of inhalation anesthesia. SYN: *prenarcosis.*

premenstrual (prē-mĕn'strū-ăl) ["+ *menstruāre*, to menstruate]. Before menstruation.

premenstruum (prē-mĕn'strū-ŭm) ["+ *menstruum*, monthly fluid]. The period of time prior to menstruation.

premolar (prē-mō'lĕr) [L. *prae*, before, + *moles*, a mass]. 1. A bicuspid tooth. 2. Before a molar tooth.

premonition (prē-mē-nĭsh'ŭn) [L. *praemonēre*, to warn beforehand]. A feeling of an impending event.

premonitory (prē-mŏn'ĭ-tō-rĭ) [LL. *praemonitorius*]. Giving a warning, as an early symptom.

premonocyte (prē-mŏn'ō-sīt) [L. *prae*, before, + Gr. *monos*, alone, + *kytos*, cell]. An embryonic cell transitional in development prior to a monocyte.

premunition (prē''mū-nĭsh'ŭn) ["+ *munitio*, a fortification]. Immunity depending upon existence of a long-continued latent infection.

premyelocyte (prē-mī'ĕl-ō-sīt) ["+ Gr. *myelos*, marrow, + *kytos*, cell]. The cell that is the immediate precursor of a myelocyte.

prenarcosis (prē-năr-kō'sĭs) [L. *prae*, before, + Gr. *narkōsis*, stuporous condition]. Induction of unconsciousness by drugs before administration of a general inhalation anesthetic. SYN: *premedication.*

prenatal (prē-nā'tl) ["+ *natalis*, birth]. Before birth.

p. care. The care of the pregnant woman during the period of gestation. This care consists of periodic examinations for the determination of blood pressure, weight, urinalysis, changes in the size of the uterus, and condition of the fetus as determined by the heart tones and position. By such examinations, changes in the condition of the patient can be noted and toxemias prevented by the institution of treatment as soon as any abnormal signs are present.

preoperative (prē-op'ĕr-ă-tĭv) ["+ *operatus*, work]. Preceding an operation.

NP (preoperative preparation): Prepare area indicated according to technique of your hospital. Warm water and liquid soap for shaving and cleansing the skin; cold liquids on the abdomen give the patient a disagreeable shock. See that patient is attended by his clergyman if this was not arranged prior to admittance. This is absolutely essential in the case of patients who are members of the Roman Catholic Church or the Church of Jesus Christ of Latter Day Saints (Mormon).

Have patient get as much sleep as possible. If he is wakeful and you do not wish to give sedative early, find reading matter for him. Give enemas ordered for the morning as late as you can if he is asleep so as to give him as much rest as possible. Get order for catheterization if you think it will be needed; never send a patient to the operating table with a full bladder. Give preanesthetic medication or basal anesthetic at exactly the time specified.

Place dentures in a glass of water which is marked with the patient's name and room number; remove and identify contact lenses or glasses; remove makeup, nail polish, hair pins, jewelry, etc.; tape wedding ring in place. Dress patient in gown and cap; do not use straight pins. Wrap blankets around neck when he is placed on stretcher. Send patient's chart on stretcher to surgery. Refrain from unnecessary conversation with other nurses and attendants. However, reassure anxious relatives.

preoral (prē-ō'răl) [L. *prae*, before, + *os, or-*, mouth]. In front of the mouth.

prep (prĕp). Abbr. for *prepare; preparation.* Used esp. when referring to preparation for surgery.

preparalytic (prē''păr-ă-lĭt'ĭk) ["+ Gr. *para*, at the side, + *lyein*, to loosen]. Before the appearance of paralysis.

preparation (prĕp-ă-rā'shŭn) [L. *praeparatio*]. 1. The making ready, esp. of a medicine for use. 2. A specimen set up for demonstration in anatomy, pathology, or histology.

p.'s often given rectally.

Chloral hydrate: 0.5 to 1.0 gm. dissolved in 90 ml. of warmed olive oil, or 90 ml. of very warm milk, or 90 ml. of thin, boiled cornstarch water. This makes a good preparation or a base in which to hold the medicine in suspension. The patient's pulse should be taken 5 minutes before and 5 minutes after the administration to determine the heart action. If adverse effects are noticed, action may be taken to prevent further absorption.

Paraldehyde: 1 to 4 ml. may be mixed with water in the proportion of 1:8 and in this ratio it may be mixed with thin starch water for rectal medication. There should be about 90 ml. of starch water.

Sodium bicarbonate: One tablespoonful, or 4 gm. to 500 ml., or 1 pint of water aids in the expulsion of the bowel content. The neutralizing action of the acidity of the bowel content brought about by the sodium bicarbonate solution leaves the bowel soothed.

RS: active principle; alkaline effects of foods; antidotes; dosage; drug action; drugs and their administration; enema; names of individual drugs in alphabetical order; names of poisons; poison; poisoning; prescription writing; proctoclysis.

prepatellar (prē"pă-těl'ar) [L. *prae,* before, + *patella,* pan]. In front of the patella.

p. bursitis. Inflammation of the bursa in front of patella. SYN: *housemaid's knee.* SEE: *bursitis.*

prepat'ent. Before becoming evident or manifest.

p. period. Period between the time of introduction of parasitic organisms into the body and their appearance in the blood or tissues.

prepuce (prē'pūs) [L. *praeputium,* prepuce]. The foreskin or fold of skin over the glans penis in the male. Excision constitutes circumcision, a common religious practice, but also performed in cases of phimosis and for hygienic purposes. A sebaceous secretion under the prepuce is called smegma.

RS: acrobystiolith, acrobystitis, acroposthitis, aposthia, frenulum, penis, phimosis, smegma, urethra (of male).

p. of the clitoris. Fold of the labia minora which covers the clitoris. SEE: *clitoris.*

preputial (prē-pū'shăl). Concerning the prepuce.

p. glands. Small sebaceous glands of the corona of the penis that secrete an odoriferous discharge. SYN: *Tyson's glands.*

preputium (prē-pū'shĭ-ŭm). (pl. *preputia*) [NA]. The fold of skin that covers the glans penis. SYN: *prepuce, q.v.*

p. clitoridis. [NA]. Prepuce of the clitoris, a fold overhanging the glans clitoridis formed by the union of the two labia minora.

p. penis. [NA]. Fold of skin covering the glans penis. SYN: *foreskin.*

prepyloric (prē"pī-lŏr'ĭk). Anterior to, or preceding, the pylorus of the stomach.

presbyacusia, presbyacousia (prĕz"bĭ-ă-kū'sĭ-ă) [Gr. *presbys,* old, + *akousis,* hearing]. Hearing less acutely, due to old age. SYN: *presbycusis.*

presbyatrics, presbyatry (prĕz-bĭ-ăt'rĭks, prĕz'bĭ-ăt-rĭ) ["+ *iatrikos,* healing]. That branch of medicine dealing with the diseases of old age. SYN: *geriatrics.*

presbycardia (prĕz-bĭ-kăr'dĭ-ă) ["+ *kardia,* heart]. Disease or decreased functional capacity of the heart associated with aging.

presbycusis, presbykousis (prĕz-bĭ-kū'sĭs) ["+ *akousis,* hearing]. Impairment of hearing in old age. SYN: *presbyacusia.*

presbyophrenia (prĕz"bĭ-ō-frē'nĭ-ă) [Gr. *presbys,* old, + *phrēn,* mind]. Senile psychotic syndrome involving confabulation and disorientation with preservation of mobility, loquacity, and good spirits. SYN: *Wernicke's syndrome.*

presbyopia (prĕz-bĭ-ō'pĭ-ă) ["+ *ōps,* eye]. Defect of vision in advancing age involving loss of accommodation or recession of near point. Due to loss of elasticity of crystalline lens. The onset usually occurs between 40 and 45 years of age. SYN: *farsightedness.*

presbytiatrics (prĕz"bĭ-tĭ-ăt'rĭks) ["+ *iatrikos,* healing]. Science of old age and its treatment. SYN: *geriatrics; presbyatrics; presbyatry.*

prescription (prē-skrĭp'shŭn) [L. *praescriptiō*]. A written order for dispensing drugs signed by a physician. A prescription consists of four main parts.

Superscription: Represented by the symbol Rx which signifies Recipe, from the Latin *recipere,* meaning to take.

Inscription: Containing the ingredients. This again is generally constructed of four parts: the *basis* or principal drug; the *adjuvant,* which assists the action of the basis; the *corrective,* which diminishes unpleasant taste or pain or griping, etc.; the *vehicle* to hold the drugs either in solution or suspension.

Subscription: Directions to the dispenser as to the manner of preparation of the drugs.

Signature: Directions to the patient with regard to the manner of taking, dosage, etc.; finally the physician's signature, address, telephone number, date, and whether or not the prescription may be refilled. When applicable, the physician's narcotics registry number should be included.

p. carbons. In physical therapy, carbons impregnated with various substances

Terms Used in Prescription Writing*

Abbreviation	Word or Phrase	English Equivalent
āā or a	ana	of each
abs. feb.	absente febre	fever being absent
ad	ad	to, up to
add.	adde	add
ad. feb.	adstante febre	fever being present
adhib.	adhibendus	to be administered
ad. lib.	ad libitum	at pleasure
admov.	admove	apply
ad part. dolent.	ad partes dolentes	to the painful parts
agit.	agita	shake, stir
alb.	albus	white
alter	alter	the other
alt. hor.	alternis horis	every other hour
ante cib. or A. C.	ante cibum	before food
aq. bull.	aqua bulliens	boiling water
aq. dest.	aqua destillata	distilled water
aq. font.	aqua fontis	spring water
aq. pur.	aqua pura	pure water
aut	aut	or
bene	bene	well
b. i. d.	bis in die	twice daily
bib.	bibe	drink
bis	bis	twice
bol.	bolus	a large pill
bull.	bulliat	let (it) boil
c̄	cum	with
cap.	capsula	a capsule
chart. or cht.	chartula	a small medicated paper
coch. mag.	cochleare magnum	a tablespoonful
coch. med	cochleare medium	a dessertspoonful
coch. parv.	cochleare parvum	a teaspoonful
collyr.	collyrium	an eyewash
commisce	commisce	mix together
comp.	compositus	compounded of
cong.	congius	a gallon
cont. rem.	continuantur remedia	continue the medicine
cotula	cotula	a measure
cras mane sum	cras mane sumendus	take tomorrow morning
cuj. lib.	cujus libet	of any you please
d., det.	da, detur	give, let be given
d. d. in d.	de die in diem	from day to day
dec.	decanta	pour off
dent. tal. dos.	dentur tales doses	give of such doses
dexter	dexter	the right
dieb. alt.	diebus alternis	every other day
dieb. tert.	diebus tertiis	every 3rd day
dil.	dilue, dilutus	dilute, diluted
dim.	dimidius	one-half
div.	divide	divide
div. in p. aeq.	dividatur in partes aequales	let it be divided into equal parts
donec alv. sol. ft.	donec alvus soluta fuerit	until bowels are open

*Many of these abbreviations are used rarely if at all. They are recorded for their historical interest.

Terms Used in Prescription Writing (*Continued*)

Abbreviation	Word or Phrase	English Equivalent
dos.	dosis	dose
dur. dolor.	durante dolore	while pain lasts
e.m.p.	ex modo prescripto	as directed
emp.	emplastrum	plaster
emuls.	emulsio	an emulsion
en.	enema	an enema
epistom.	epistomium	a stopper
ext.	extende	spread
febris	febris	fever
ferv.	fervens	boiling
filt.	filtra	filter
ft.	fiat	let be made
garg.	gargarisma	a gargle
grad.	gradatim	by degrees
gr.	granum	a grain
gtt.	gutta, guttae	a drop, drops
guttat.	guttatim	by drops
h.	hora	an hour
haust.	haustus	a draught
hor. decub.	hora decubitus	bedtime
hor. som. or h. s.	hora somni	bedtime
hor. 1 spat.	horae unius spatio	one hour's time
idem	idem	the same
ind.	indies	daily
inf.	infusum	let it infuse
int.	intime	thoroughly
lin.	linimentum	a liniment
liq.	liquor	a solution
lot.	lotio	a lotion
M.	misce	mix
mac.	macera	macerate
man. prim.	mane primo	first thing in the morning
mas.	massa	mass
med.	medicamentum	a medicine
m. et n.	mane et nocte	morning and night
mitt.	mitte	send
mitt. x tal.	mitte decem tales	send 10 like this
mod.	modicus	moderate sized
mod. praesc.	modo praescripto	in the manner written
moll.	mollis	soft
mor. dict.	more dicto	in the manner directed
mor. sol.	more solito	as accustomed
ne tr. s. num.	ne tradas sine nummo	deliver not without the money
no.	numerus	number
noct. maneq.	nocte maneque	night and morning
non. rep., n. r.	non repetatur	let it not be repeated
nunc	nunc	now
o.	octarius	a pint
O.D.	oculus dexter	right eye
O.L.	oculus laevus	left eye
omn. bih.	omni bihoris	every 2nd hour
omn. hor.	omni hora	every hour
om. ¼ h.	omni quadrantae horae	every 15 minutes
om. mane vel. noc.	omni mane vel nocte	every morning or night
part. vic.	partitus vicibus	individual doses

Terms Used in Prescription Writing (*Continued*)

Abbreviation	Word or Phrase	English Equivalent
p. c.	post cibum	after meals
pil.	pilula	a pill
p. p. a.	phiala prius agitata	the bottle being first shaken
p. r. n.	pro re nata	as occasion arises
pro. rat. aet.	pro ratione aetatis	according to patient's age
pulv.	pulvis	powder
q. h.	quaque hora	every hour
q. l.	quantum libet	as much as pleases
q. s.	quantum sufficiat	as much as suffices
quotid.	quotidie	daily
red. in pulv.	redactus in pulverem	reduced to powder
repetat., rep.	repetatur	to be repeated
rub.	ruber	red
sec. a., or s. a.	secundem artem	according to art
semih.	semihora	half an hour
sig.	signa	write
sing.	singulorum	of each
sol.	solutio	solution
s. o. s.	si opus sit	if need exists
solv.	solve	dissolve
ss.	semi or semisse	a half
stat.	statim	immediately
st.	stet or stetem	let it (or them) stand
subind.	subinde	frequently
sum.	sume	take
sum. tal.	sumat talem	take 1 such
suppos.	suppositoria	a suppository
s.v.r.	spiritus vini rectificatus	rectified spirit of wine
tab.	tabella	a tablet
tere	tere	rub
tere bene	tere bene	rub well
t. i. d.	ter in die	three times daily
tinct.	tinctura	a tincture
trit.	tritura	triturate or grind
ult. praes.	ultimus praescriptus	the last ordered
ung.	unguentum	an ointment
ut dict.	ut dictum	as directed
vitel.	vitellus	yolk of an egg

Weights and Measures

♏	Minimum, -i, n., minim, of a fluidram.
Gtt.	Gutta, -ae, f., a drop.
gr.	Granum, -i, n., a grain.
℈	Scrupulus, -i, m., a scruple, 20 grains.
℥	Drachma, -ae, f., a dram, 60 grains.
f℥	Fluidrachma, -ae, f., a fluidram, 60 minims.
℥	Uncia, -ae, f., a troy ounce, 480 grains.
f℥	Fluiduncia, -ae, f., a fluidounce, 8 fluidrams.
lb.	Libra, -ae, f., a pound (troy), 5760 grains.
O.	Octarius, -i, m., a pint, 16 fluidounces.
C.	Congius, -i, m., a gallon, 8 pints.
ss.	Semis, indecl., a half.

Quantities are designated by Roman numerals following the symbol. SEE: *charting*.

for use in treatment of specific conditions.

p. drug. A medicine that can be obtained only when prescribed by a physician.

p., shotgun. Indiscriminate prescription for a large number of drugs in the hope that at least one of them will accomplish the desired effect.

prescription writing. Modern practice is to write prescriptions entirely in the language of the country in which written (as English in the United States) and to use few, if any, abbreviations. All drug quantities should be shown by using the metric system of weights and measures (grams, milligrams, liters, milliliters, etc.).

p.w., Latin used in. (*NOTE:* The following classical presentation of the art of prescription writing is included primarily for its historical interest): An official Latin name is in the nominative case. Drugs are written in the genitive case because the prescription is an order, meaning "take thou." The word "of" is not written in Latin but is indicated by the ending of a word: *quinina* means *quinine,* but changing the termination to "ae" we have *quininae,* meaning *of quinine.*

ALKALOIDS: Written the same as in English, except that the final "e" is changed to "a" to form the nominative case, as *quinina,* for the English quinine. To form the genitive case, the final "e" is changed to "ae," as *quininae.*

ACTIVE PRINCIPLES: These, such as glucosides, resinoids and others, add "um" to the nominative and "i" to the genitive, so that Strophanthin becomes *strophanthinum* to form the Latin nominative, and *strophanthini,* to form the Latin genitive.

ACIDS: The names of these are formed in the same way as those of alkaloids, except that the adjective is formed in the same way and follows the nominative, as *Acidum Hydrochloricum,* or the genitive, *Acidi Hydrochlorici.*

METALS: Latin names of metals, except those of a few known to the ancients, are the same as English forms ending in "um," as in *Sodium,* forming the Latin nominative, but ending in "i" to form the genitive, *Sodii.*

SALTS: Written first with the name of the base in its genitive form, next the acid radical in the nominative, followed by the qualitative adjective in the nominative, as *Ferri Sulfas Exsiccatus,* exsiccated sulfate of iron.

NAMES OF PREPARATIONS: Show the class to which it belongs first, the name of the ingredient next, and the qualifying adjective last, as *Syrupus Scillae Compositus*

(Compound Syrup of Squills). First and last words are in nominative case and middle one in genitive.

DRUGS WITH TWO NAMES: Both should be in the genitive, as *Liquor Potassi Arsenitis.* (-ate endings): The Latin nominative ends in "as," as *sulfas,* for sulfate; and the genitive in "atis," as *sulfatis.* (-ite endings): If the English word ends in "ite," as *sulfite,* the Latin nominative ends in "is," as *sulfis,* and the genitive in "itis," as *sulfitis.* (-ide endings): If an English word has this ending, as "bromide," the Latin nominative ends in "um," dropping the final "e" in the English form, as *Bromidum;* the genitive dropping the "um" to add "i," as *Bromidi.*

(-a, -us, -um endings): English words with these endings are the same in the Latin nominative, but the genitive is formed by changing "a" to "ae," or the "us" or "um" to "i." (-in endings): An English word having this ending adds "um" (usually) to form the Latin nominative as Benzoin and *Benzoinum,* the genitive being formed by merely adding "i," as *Benzoini.* (-ol endings): The Latin nominative is the same as the English, as in Phenol, but "is" is added to form the genitive, as *Phenolis.* (-al endings): To form the Latin nominative, "um" is added, as Chloral and *Chloralum.* To form the genitive, "i" is added to the English form, as *Chlorali.*

There are, of course, exceptions to the foregoing. Many Latin words have the same form as in English. Fortunately, perhaps, most drugs are indicated in prescription by abbreviations which may not discriminate between the Latin nominative and genitive.

RS: active principle; antidotes; dosage; drug action; drugs and their administration; names of individual drugs in alphabetical order; names of poisons; poison; poisoning; preparations, often given rectally.

presentation (prē″zĕn-tā′shŭn) [L. *praesentatio*]. Term applied to the manner of the fetus presenting itself to the examining finger in the vagina or rectum. Thus longitudinal (normal) and transverse (pathological) presentation.

p., breech. When buttocks of fetus present. Breech presentation is of three types: *Complete breech,* when the thighs are flexed on the abdomen and the legs flexed upon the thighs; *frank breech,* when the legs are extended over the anterior surface of the body; and *footling,* when a foot or feet present. Footling can be single, double, or if the leg remains flexed, knee presentation.

p., brow. When the brow presents.

p., cephalic. P. of the head in any position.

p., face. When the head is sharply extended so that the face presents.

p., footling. Presenting feet first.

p., placental. Presentation of the placenta first. SYN: *placenta previa.*

p., sinciput. When the large fontanel presents.

p., transverse. With fetus lying crosswise.

p., vertex. P. of the upper and back part of the head.

preservative (prē-zĕr'vă-tĭv) [L. *prae,* before, + *servāre,* to keep]. A substance added to medicines or foods to prevent them from spoiling. It may act by interfering with certain chemical reactions or with the growth of molds, fungi, bacteria, or parasites. Some common preservatives are sugar, salt, vinegar, ethyl alcohol, sulfur dioxide, and benzoic acid.

presphenoid (prē-sfē'noyd) ["+ Gr. *sphēn,* wedge, + *eidos,* form]. Anterior region of the body of the sphenoid bone.

presphygmic (prē-sfĭg'mĭk) ["+ Gr. *sphygmos,* pulse]. Pert. to period preceding the pulse wave.

prespinal (prē-spī'năl) [L. *prae,* before, + *spina,* thorn]. In front of the spine, or ventral to it.

prespondylolisthesis (prē-spŏn"dĭl-ō-lĭs-thē'sĭs) ["+ Gr. *spondylos,* vertebra, + *olisthanein,* to slip]. A congenital defect of both pedicles of the fifth lumbar vertebra without displacement. This predisposes to spondylolisthesis.

pressinervoscopy (prĕs"ĭ-nĕr-vŏs'kō-pĭ) [L. *pressus,* press, + *nervus,* a nerve, + Gr. *skopein,* to examine]. Diagnosis by pressing upon the parasympathetic and sympathetic nerves.

pressor (prĕs'ŏr) [OF. *presser,* to press]. 1. Stimulating, increasing the activity of a function, esp. of vasomotor activity, as a nerve. 2. Inducing an elevation in blood pressure.

p. base. One of several amines or nitrogenous bases of plant or animal origin that, when injected, have the ability to increase blood pressure. SYN: *p. amine.*

p. nerves. Nerves which when stimulated bring about an increase in blood pressure.

p. reflex. Any reflex in which the response to stimulation is increased by blood pressure.

pressoreceptor (prĕs"ō-rē-sĕp'tŏr). Sensory nerve ending, such as those in the aorta and carotid sinus, that are stimulated by changes in blood pressure.

pressure (prĕsh'ŭr) [L. *pressura*]. 1. A compression. 2. Stress or force exerted on a body, as by tension, weight, pulling, etc. 3. In psychology, quality of sensation aroused by moderate compression of the skin. 4. In physics, the quotient obtained by dividing a force by the area of the surface on which it acts.

RS: atmosphere; blood; hypertonic; isotonic.

p., after-. A feeling of p. which remains for a few seconds after removal of a weight or other pressure.

p., arterial. P. of blood in the arteries. For a normal young man at physical and mental rest and in sitting position, systolic blood pressure averages about 120 mm. Hg; diastolic pressure about 80 mm. Hg. There is a wide range of normal variation due to constitutional, physical, and psychic factors. For women the figures are lower. For older people they are higher. There is little difference in the b.p. of the two arms.

p., atmospheric. P. of weight of atmosphere; at sea level it averages about 760 mm. of mercury.

p., back. P. resulting from interference in flow of blood from the ventricles, such as occurs in valvular disorders. Results in reduced venous return to the heart and consequent venous engorgement.

p., blood. P. exerted by blood against the walls of blood vessels. SEE: *blood pressure.*

p., diastolic. Arterial pressure during diastole or dilatation of heart chambers.

p., endocardiac. Blood pressure within the heart. SYN: *intracardiac p.*

p., hydrostatic. P. exerted by a fluid within a closed system.

p., intra-abdominal. P. within the abdominal cavity, such as that caused by descent of the diaphragm.

p., intracranial. P. of the cerebrospinal fluid in the subarachnoid space between the skull and the brain. The pressure is normally the same as that found during lumbar puncture.

p., intraocular. Normal tension within the eyeball, equal to approximately 12-20 mm. of mercury.

p., intrathoracic. P. within the thorax but outside of the lungs. In quiet expiration it is about –4.5 mm., in forced inspiration as high as –30 mm., but in quiet inspiration –7.5 mm.

p., intraventricular. P. within the ventricles of the heart during different phases of diastole and systole.

p., oncotic. Osmotic pressure, q.v.

p., osmotic. The force with which a solvent, usually water, passes through a semipermeable membrane separating solutions of different concentrations. It is measured by determining the hydrostatic (mechanical) pressure which must be opposed to the osmotic force to bring the passage to a standstill. The osmotic pressure of blood serum and of solutions isotonic with it is 6.7 atmospheres. SYN: *oncotic p.*

p. palsy. Temporary paralysis due to p. on a nerve trunk.

p. paralysis. Paralysis due to p. on the spinal cord.

ETIOL: Injury, tumor, gummata.

p. points. Areas for exerting p. to control bleeding. For control of hemorrhage, p. above bleeding point when an artery passes over a bone may be sufficient. Principal pressure points follow.

Common carotid artery, two inches above clavicle, press backwards against spine. *Temporal artery,* at side of face in front of ear. *Occipital artery,* behind mastoid process. *Subclavian artery* behind clavicle, pressing down onto first rib. *Axillary artery,* by compression in axilla. *Brachial artery,* compressed by pressure at inner edge of biceps muscle halfway down arm and also above bend of elbow before artery divides into radial and ulnar arteries. *Radial artery,* press on thumb side of wrist against radius. *Ulnar artery,* press on little finger side of wrist against ulna. *Deep palmar arch,* in thumb opposite root of abducted thumb. *Abdominal artery,* may be compressed against lumbar vertebrae to left of middle line when patient lies on his back. *Femoral artery,* by abduction and external rotation of thigh, bringing head of femur forward into groin and compressing artery against it. *Popliteal artery,* in popliteal space over artery. *Anterior tibial artery,* at front of bend of ankle. *Posterior tibial artery,* behind internal malleolus as it passes into foot.

p., pulse. The difference between systolic and diastolic pressures.

p. sore. A sore caused by p. as from a splint or other appliance, or from the body itself when it has remained immobile in bed for extended periods of time. SYN: *bed sore; decubitus ulcer.*

p., systolic. Arterial p. at time of the contraction of the ventricles, or the ventricular systole.

p., venous. P. of the blood within the veins. It is highest near the periphery, diminishing progressively from capillaries to the heart. Near the heart the p. may be below zero (negative pressure) due to negative intrathoracic pressure.

presternum (prē-ster'nŭm) [L. *prae,* before, + Gr. *sternon,* chest]. The upper part of the sternum. SYN: *manubrium sterni* [NA].

presuppurative (prē-sŭp'ū-rā''tĭv) ["+ *sub,* under, + *puris,* pus]. Rel. to period of inflammation before suppuration.

presylvian fissure (prē-sĭl'vĭ-ăn). The anterior division of the sylvian fissure.

presystole (prē-sĭs'tō-lē) [L. *prae,* before, + Gr. *systolē,* contraction]. The period in the heart's cycle just before the systole.

presystolic (prē-sĭs-tŏl'ĭk). Before the systole of the heart.

pretarsal (prē-tar'săl) [L. *prae,* before, + Gr. *tarsos,* tarsus]. In front of the tarsus.

pretibial (prē-tĭb'ĭ-ăl) ["+ *tibia,* shin]. In front of the tibia.

p. fever. A viral disease characterized by fever, rash on legs, prostration, splenomegaly, and respiratory disturbances. SYN: *Fort Bragg fever.*

preurethritis (prē''ū-rē-thrī'tĭs) ["+ Gr. *ourēthra,* urethra, + *-itis,* inflammation]. Inflammation around the urethral orifice of the vaginal vestibule.

prev'alence [L. *praevalens,* prevail]. The number of cases of a disease present in a specified population at a given time.

preventive (prē-vĕn'tĭv) [ME. *preventen,* to anticipate]. Hindering the occurrence of something, esp. disease. SYN: *prophylactic.*

p. medicine. The branch of medicine concerned with preventing the occurrence of both mental and physical illness and disease. There are three levels of preventive effort.

Primary p. is concerned with preventing the development of disease in a susceptible or potentially susceptible population. These efforts include general promotion of health and specific protection such as immunization. *Secondary p.* involves early diagnosis and prompt therapy to shorten duration of illness, reduce the severity of disease, reduce possibility of contagion, and limit sequellae. *Tertiary p.* is important in limiting degree of disability and promoting rehabilitation in chronic and irreversible diseases.

prevertebral (prē-ver'tē-brăl) [L. *prae,* before, + *vertebra,* vertebra]. In front of a vertebra.

prevertiginous (prē-ver-tĭj'ĭ-nŭs) ["+ *vertigo,* dizziness]. Having a tendency to fall forward. SYN: *dizzy.*

prevesical (prē-vĕs'ĭ-kl) ["+ *vesica,* bladder]. Located in front of the bladder.

pre'via, prae'via [L.]. Appearing before or in front of.

prezon'ular. Pert. to the posterior chamber of the eye, the space between iris and ciliary zonule (suspensory ligament).

priapism (prī'ă-pĭzm) [L. *priapismus*]. Abnormal, painful, and continued erection of the penis due to disease, usually without sexual desire.

ETIOL: May be due to lesions of the cord above the lumbar region, or turgescence of corpora cavernosa without erection may exist. It may be reflex from peripheral sensory irritants, from organic irritation of nerve tracts or nerve centers when libido may be lacking. Is sometimes seen in patients with acute leukemia.

RS: erection; gonorrhea; satyriasis.

priapitis (prī-ă-pī'tĭs) [" + -*itis*, inflammation]. Inflammation of the penis.

priapus (prī'ă-pŭs). The penis.

prickle cell (prĭk'l). A cell with rod-shaped processes, intercellular bridges connecting with similar adjoining cells.

p. c. layer. The innermost layer of the epidermis. SYN: *stratum germinativum; stratum spinosum; malpighian layer.*

prickly heat (prĭk'lĭ hēt). Noncontagious cutaneous eruption of red pimples, with itching and tingling of the affected parts, seen usually in hot weather.

ETIOL: Inflammation of skin around sweat glands. SYN: *lichen tropicus; miliaria.*

Priessnitz compress (prēs'nĭtz). [Vincent Priessnitz, Silesian farmer, 1799-1852]. A cold wet compress. SEE: *Neptune girdle.*

primae viae (prī'mē vī'ē) [L., first passages]. The alimentary canal; the secondary ones consisting of the lacteals.

primary (prī'mă-rĭ) [L. *primarius*, principal]. First in time or order. SYN: *principal.*

p. amputation. One before inflammation has set in.

p. bubo. A simple adenitis of an inguinal gland. SYN: *bubon d'emblée.*

p. cell. In physical therapy, a device consisting of a container, two solid conducting elements, and an electrolyte for the production of electric current by chemical energy.

p. hemorrhage. Bleeding at time of an injury.

p. lesion. 1. An original lesion from which a second one originates. 2. Lesion of syphilis, a chancre, q.v.

p. physician. The physician to whom a family or individual goes intially for check-up or when ill.

p. sore. The initial sore or hard chancre of syphilis.

primate (prī'māt) [L. *primus*, first]. A member of the order Primates.

Primates (prī-mā'tēz). An order of vertebrates belonging to the class Mammalia, subclass Theria. Includes the lemurs, tarsiers, monkeys, apes, and man. This order is most highly developed with respect to the brain and nervous system.

prime (prim) [L. *primus*, first]. Period of greatest health and strength.

p. mover. The muscle primarily responsible for a specific action. SYN: *agonist; protagonist.*

primigravida (prī-mĭ-grăv'ĭ-dă) [" + *gravida*, pregnant]. A woman during her first pregnancy.

primipara (prī-mĭp'ă-ră) [" + *parēre*, to bear offspring]. A woman who has had or who is giving birth to her first child.

primipar'ity. Condition of having given birth to only one child.

primip'arous. Pert. to a primipara, a woman giving birth to, or having had, her first child.

primitiae (prī-mĭsh'ĭ-ē) [L. *primus*, first]. Liquor amnii appearing before the fetus at birth. SEE: *amnion; bag of waters; liquor amnii; labor.*

primitive (prĭm'ĭ-tīv) [L. *primitivus*]. Original; early in point of time; embryonic.

p. groove. The longitudinal depression in the dorsum of the embryonic area.

p. streak. A dark, thickened longitudinal band that forms at caudal end of the embryonic disk, consisting of a surface layer of ectoderm overlying a thickened mass of mesoderm cells. It marks the future longitudinal axis of the embryo.

primordial (prī-mōr'dĭ-ăl) [L. *primordialis*]. 1. Existing first. 2. Existing in an undeveloped, primitive, or early form.

primor'dium [L., origin]. (pl. *primor'dia*) In embryology, the beginnings of a future organ or part. SYN: *anlage.*

primum non nocere (prī'mŭm nŏn nō'sĕ-ră) [L.]. "First do no harm." An adage which all individuals working in the healing arts should remember constantly.

princeps (prĭn'sĕps) [L., chief]. 1. Original; first. 2. The name of certain arteries. EX: princeps cervicis.

principal (prĭn'sĭ-păl). 1. Chief. 2. Outstanding.

principle (prĭn'sĭ-pl) [L. *principium*, foundation]. 1. A constituent of a compound representing its essential properties. 2. A fundamental truth. 3. An established rule of action.

p., antianemic. Antianemic factor. SEE: *factor, antianemic.*

p., antidiuretic. The antidiuretic hormone (ADH) present in extracts of the posterior lobe of hypophysis.

p.'s gastrointestinal. Substances, secreted by mucosa of stomach and intestine, which are absorbed by the blood and act as hormones. SEE: *cholecystokinin; gastrin; secretin.*

p., oxytocic. A hormone in extracts of posterior lobe of hypophysis which stimulates contraction of uterine muscle.

p., proximate. A substance that may be extracted from its complex form without destroying or altering its chemical properties.

prism (prĭzm) [Gr. *prisma*]. A solid with sides that are parallelograms whose bases are similar plane figures.

p., enamel. A minute rod of calcareous material deposited at the end of an ameloblast in the formation of the enamel of a tooth.

prismoptometer (prĭz-mŏp-tŏm'ĕ-tĕr) ["+ *opsis*, vision, + *metron*, measure.]. Device for estimating abnormal refraction of the eye by using prisms.

privates (prī'vĕts) [L. *privatus*, peculiar to an individual]. The external genitalia of the male or female.

privileged communication. Confidential information furnished (in order to facilitate diagnosis and treatment) by patient to a professional authorized by law to care for him. In some states the person who has received this communication may not be made to divulge it. When this is the case, communication between the patient and the recipient is classed as privileged.

p.r.n. Abbr. for L. *pro re nata,* as circumstance may require. Sometimes used in prescription writing.

pro- [L., Gr. *pro,* before]. Prefix indicating for, in front of, before, from, in behalf of, on account of, etc.

proaccelerin. The fifth factor (Factor V) in blood coagulation. Present in normal plasma but deteriorates rapidly at room temperature. Its function in blood coagulation is unclear. SYN: *thrombogen.*

proactinomycin (prō-ăk"tĭ-nō-mī'sĭn). An antibiotic obtained from Nocardia gardneri. Effective against gram-positive bacteria.

proagglutinoid (prō"ă-glū'tĭ-noyd). An agglutinoid having a greater affinity for the agglutinogen than that possessed by the agglutinin.

proamnion (prō-ăm'nĭ-ŏn) [Gr. *pro,* before, + *amnion,* amnion]. A region anterior to the head in a vertebrate embryo in which mesoderm is lacking.

proantithrombin (prō"ăn-tĭ-thrŏm'bĭn). A substance present in blood plasma or serum which, through the action of heparin, is converted into antithrombin.

pro'band. The original individual who, because of his mental or physical disorder, causes a study of his hereditary and genetic factors in order to determine if other members of the family have had the same disease or carry it. SYN: *propositus.*

probationary (prō-bā'shŭn-ăr-ĭ) [L. *probātiō,* probation]. One who is in a trial period waiting, as for admission or for a test.

probationer (prō-bā'shŭn-ĕr). A person working during a trial period, as a student nurse just after entering training.

probe (prōb) [L. *probare,* to test]. An instrument, usually flexible, for exploring the depth and direction of a wound or sinus.

probenicid. A benzoic acid derivative useful in treating gout. In large doses it prevents reabsorption of uric acid by the kidney.

procaine hydrochlor'ide (prō'kān). USP. White, colorless, crystalline compound.

ACTION AND USES: A safe, local anesthetic, less toxic than cocaine. Used in infiltration anesthesia, nerve block, and spinal anesthesia. Its effect is prolonged by simultaneous injection of epinephrine.

procatarctic (prō"kă-tark'tĭk) [Gr. *pro,* before, + *katarchein,* to begin]. Predisposing or inciting, as the cause of a disease.

procatarxis (prō"kă-tark'sĭs). Inception of a disease through a predisposing cause.

procedure (prō-sē'dūr) [L. *procedere,* to proceed.]. A particular way of accomplishing a desired result.

procelous (prō-sē'lŭs) [Gr. *pro,* before, + *koilos,* hollow]. Concave anteriorly.

procephalic (prō"sē-făl'ĭk) ["+ *kephalē,* a head]. Of, or relating to, the anterior part of the head.

procercoid (prō-sĕr'koyd). The first larval stage in the development of certain cestodes belonging to order Pseudophillidea. It is an elongated structure which develops in crustaceans.

process (prŏs'ĕs) [L. *processus,* going before]. 1. A method of action. 2. State of progress of a disease. 3. A projection or outgrowth of bone or tissue.

p., acromion. The acromion, q.v.

p., alar. A process of cribiform plate of ethmoid bone which articulates with frontal bone.

p., alveolar. 1. The inferior border of the maxilla containing sockets for upper teeth. 2. The superior border of body of mandible containing sockets for lower teeth.

p., articular, of vertebra. One of four processes (two superior and two inferior) by which vertebrae articulate with each other.

p., basilar. Narrow part of the base of occipital bone, in front of foramen magnum, articulating with the sphenoid bone. SYN: *pars basilaris.*

p., caudate. P. of caudate lobe of liver extending under right lobe.

p., ciliary. One of about 70 prominent meridional ridges projecting from corona ciliaris of choroid coat of eye to which suspensory ligament of lens is attached.

p., condyloid. Posterior process on superior border of ramus of mandible which articulates with temporal bone.

p., coracoid. A beak-shaped process extending upward and laterally from neck of scapula.

p., coronoid. 1. P. extending upward from anterior portion of ramus of mandible. 2. Sharp projection forming anterior and lower border of semilunar notch of ulna.

p., ensiform. The xiphoid process of the sternum.

p., ethmoidal. Small p. on superior border of inferior concha which articulates with uncinate process of ethmoid.

p., falciform. An extension of posterior edge of sacrotuberous ligament to ramus of ischium.

p., frontal. Upward projection of maxilla which articulates with frontal bone. Forms part of orbit and nasal fossa.

p., frontosphenoidal. Upward projecting process of zygomatic bone.

p., head. An axial strand of cells in vertebrate embryos extending forward from primitive knot. Forms primitive axis about which embryo differentiates. SYN: *notochordal plate.*

p., infraorbital. Medially projecting process of zygomatic bone which articulates with maxilla. Forms inferior lateral margin of orbit.

p., jugular. P. of occipital bone lying lateral to occipital condyle.

p., lacrimal. A short process of inferior concha which articulates with lacrimal bone.

p., lenticular. A knob on the malleus in the ear which articulates with the stapes.

p., lyophile. Lyophilization, q.v.

p., mandibular. Posterior portion of first branchial arch from which lower jaw develops.

p., mastoid. Projection of mastoid portion of the temporal bone.

p., maxillary. 1. Anterior portion of first branchial arch which, with medial

nasal processes, forms upper jaw. 2. P. of inferior nasal concha extending laterally and covering orifice of antrum. 3. P. on anterior border of perpendicular portion of palatine bone.

p., odontoid. Toothlike process extending upward from axis about which the axis rotates. SYN: *dens.*

p., olecranon. The olecranon, an extension at proximal end of ulna.

p., orbital. 1. P. at tip of perpendicular portion of palatine bone directed upward and backward. 2. P. of zygomatic bone which forms anterior boundary of temporal fossa.

p., palatine. P. extending transversely from medial surface of maxilla. With corresponding process from other side, it forms major portion of hard palate.

p., postglenoid. P. of temporal bone separating mandibular fossa from external acoustic meatus.

p., pterygoid. P. of sphenoid bone extending downward from junction of the body and great wing. Consists of the lateral and medial pterygoid plates.

p., styloid. Styloid process, q.v.

p., transverse. P. extending laterally and dorsally from the arch of a vertebra.

p., vermiform. Vermiform appendix, q.v.

p., vocal. P. of arytenoid cartilage which serves for attachment of vocal ligament.

p., xiphoid. Thin, elongated process extending caudally from body of sternum. SYN: *ensiforme p.*

processus (prō-sĕs′ŭs) [L.]. (pl. proces′sus) [NA]. Process or processes.

    p. cochleariformis. [NA]. Curved portion of a thin plate of bone separating eustachian tube from canal for tensor tympani muscle over which tendon of muscle passes before insertion into manubrium of malleus.

    p. retromandibularis. Wedge-shaped portion of parotid gland which projects medially toward the pharynx.

    p. uncinatus. [NA]. 1. Curved process of ethmoid labyrinth projecting from lateral wall of middle meatus which forms inferior border of hiatus semilunaris. 2. A hooklike portion of the head of pancreas which curves around the superior mesenteric vessels. SYN: *pancreas of Winslow.*

procheilon (prō-ki′lŏn) [Gr. *pro,* before, + *cheilon,* lip]. Prominence in central portion of the upper lip.

prochondral (prō-kŏn′drăl) ["+ *chondral,* cartilage]. Preceding the formation of cartilage.

prochoresis (prō″kō-rē′sĭs) [Gr. *prochōresis*, advancement]. Movement of partially digested food through the pyloric canal.

prochromosome (prō-krō′mō-sōm) [Gr. *pro*, before, + *chroma*, color, + *sōma*, body]. Chromocenter; false or chromatin nucleolus; karyosome, q.v.

procidentia (prō″sĭ-dĕn′shĭ-ă) [L.]. A complete prolapse, esp. of the uterus to such an extent that the uterus lies outside of the vulva with everted vaginal walls.

ETIOL: Generally due to injury of pelvic floor. SEE: *descensus uteri*.

pro′create [L. prōcreāre]. To beget; to bring forth young.

procreation (prō″krē-ā′shŭn). The act or state of bringing forth young. SYN: *reproduction*.

proctagra (prŏk-tăg′rä) [Gr. *prōktos*, anus, + *agra*, seizure]. Sudden rectal pain.

proctalgia (prŏk-tăl′jī-ă) [" + *algos*, pain]. Pain in or about the anus and rectum.

p. fugax. Rectal pain due to an unknown cause. May occur following sexual excitement and is sometimes relieved by defecation.

proctatresia (prŏk″tă-trē′zĭ-ă) [" + *atresis*, imperforation]. Imperforation of the anus.

proctectasia (prŏk″tĕk-tā′sĭ-ă) [Gr. *prōktos*, anus, + *ektasis*, dilatation]. Dilatation of the anus or rectum.

proctectomy (prŏk-tĕk′tō-mĭ) [" + *ektomē*, excision]. Excision of the rectum or anus.

proctenclisis (prŏk″tĕn-klĭ′sĭs) [" + *enkleiein*, to shut in]. Stricture of the anus or rectum.

procteurynter (prŏk″tū-rĭn″tĕr) [Gr. *prōktos*, anus, + *eurynein*, to widen]. Instrument for dilation of the anus or rectum.

procti′tis [" + *-itis*, inflammation]. Inflammation of rectum and anus. SEE: *rectitis*.

ETIOL: Infectious organisms; trauma; radiation injury; drugs, esp. broad-spectrum antibiotics; allergy.

p., acute or chronic. Rectal discomfort; repeated urge to evacuate rectum accompanied by inability to pass feces; presence of mucus, blood, or pus in stools; tenesmus.

p., diphtheritic. Diphtheritic and albuminous membrane forms over surface of mucous membrane: headache, with roaring in ears; constipation, gas, bloating; neurasthenia.

p., dysenteric. May result from ordinary diarrhea, affects upper part the most. May have ulcers, afterwards cicatricial scars.

p., gonorrheal. Gonorrheal infection.

p., traumatic. Pain, pressure as if bowels were going to move; irritable; mucous membrane red, eroded. Surface tissues sensitive to touch. Chronic constipation.

procto-, proct- [Gr. *prōktos*, anus]. Combining forms indicating relationship to the anus and rectum.

proctocele (prŏk′tō-sēl) [" + *kēlē*, hernia]. A protrusion of the rectal mucosa.

p., vaginal. Hernia of the rectum into the vagina. SYN: *rectocele*

proctoclysis (prŏk-tŏk′lĭ-sĭs) [" + *klysis*, a washing out]. A continuous infusion into the rectum and colon in which the solution is introduced drop by drop. SYN: *Murphy drip*. SEE: *enteroclysis*.

THERAPEUTIC PURPOSES: To supply fluid in postoperative cases when fluids cannot be taken otherwise; to supply the body with fluid as in hemorrhage, vomiting, or diarrhea; to relieve thirst as in persistent vomiting; to lower body temperature by giving ice water enemas.

SOLUTIONS USED: The solution usually consists of a normal saline solution, a sodium bicarbonate solution, or plain tap water at body temperature. Normal salt solution half strength frequently is used. This need not be a sterile solution unless so ordered. Sodium bicarbonate of 2%-5% strength. A glucose solution of 2%-5%, but no stronger. A combination of these may also be ordered: as a normal saline with glucose and sodium bicarbonate, 5% and 2%, respectively, or other combinations may be given as an order.

NP: Usually a cleansing enema is given; then the fluid at body temperature introduced through a lubricated rectal catheter inserted to approx. 4 inches (10 cm.). The liquid is given at a rate of 40-60 drops/min. If given faster, the bowel will be stimulated. Do not give more than 6 ounces (180 ml.) in a single continuous proctoclysis. Turn the patient frequently during the treatment. If rectal gas needs to be passed, clamp the tube temporarily. Discontinue if pain or distention develops.

proctococcypexia, proctococcypexy (prŏk″tō-kŏk-sĭ-pĕk′sĭ-ă, -kŏk′sĭ-pĕk″sĭ) [Gr. *prōktos*, anus, + *kokkyx*, coccyx, + *pēxis*, fixation]. Suture of rectum to the coccyx.

proctocolitis (prŏk″tō-kō-lī′tĭs) [" + *kolon*, colon, + *-itis*, inflammation]. Inflamed condition of colon and rectum.

proctocolonoscopy (prŏk″tō-kō′lŏn-ŏs′kō-pĭ) [" + " + *skopein*, to examine]. Examination of interior of rectum and lower colon.

proctocystotomy (prŏk″tō-sĭs-tŏt′ō-mĭ) [Gr. *prōktos*, anus, + *kystis*, bladder, + *tomē*, a cutting]. Incision into the bladder through the rectum.

proctodeum (prŏk-tō-dē'ŭm) ["+ *hodaios*, a way]. An ectodermal depression located caudally which, upon rupture of the cloacal membrane, forms the anal canal.

proctodynia (prŏk″tō-dĭn'ĭ-ă) ["+ *odynē*, pain]. Pain in the rectum or about the anus.

proctologist (prŏk-tŏl'ō-jĭst) [Gr. *prōktos*, anus, + *logos*, study]. One who specializes in diseases of the colon, rectum, and anus.

proctology (prŏk-tŏl'ō-jĭ). Phase of medicine dealing with treatment of diseases of colon, rectum, and anus.

proctoparalysis (prŏk″tō-păr-ăl'ĭ-sĭs) [Gr. *prōktos*, anus, + *para*, at the side, + *lyein*, to loosen]. Paralysis of the anal sphincter muscle.

proctopexia, proctopexy (prŏk-tō-pěk'sĭ-ă, prŏk'tō-pěk″sĭ) ["+ *pēxis*, fixation]. Suture of the rectum to some other part.

proctophobia (prŏk″tō-fō'bĭ-ă) ["+ *phobos*, fear]. Abnormal apprehension in those suffering from rectal disease.

proctoplasty (prŏk'tō-plăs″tĭ) [Gr. *prōktos*, anus, + *plastos*, formed]. Plastic surgery of the anus or rectum.

proctoplegia (prŏk″tō-plē'jĭ-ă) ["+ *plēgē*, a stroke]. Paralysis of the anal sphincter. SYN: *proctoparalysis*.

proc″topto'sis ["+ *ptōsis*, a dropping]. Prolapse of the anus and rectum. SEE: *procidentia*.

proctorrhagia (prŏk″tō-rā'jĭ-ă) [Gr. *prōktos*, anus, + *rhēgnynai*, to burst forth]. Bleeding from the rectum.

proctorrhaphy (prŏk-tŏr'ă-fĭ) ["+ *rhaphē*, a sewing]. Suturing of rectum or anus.

proctorrhea (prŏk-tō-rē'ă) ["+ *rhoia*, flow]. Mucous discharge from the anus.

proc'toscope [Gr. *prōktos*, anus, + *skopein*, to examine]. Instrument for inspection of the rectum.

proctoscopy (prŏk-tŏs'kō-pĭ). Instrumental inspection of the rectum.

proctosigmoiditis (prŏk″tō-sĭg″moyd-ī'tĭs) [Gr. *prōktos*, anus, + *sigma*, letter S, + *eidos*, form, + *-ītis*, inflammation]. Inflamed condition of the rectum and sigmoid.

proc'tospasm ["+ *spasmos*, a contracting]. Rectal spasm.

proctostasis (prŏk″tō-stā'sĭs) ["+ *stasis*, stoppage]. Constipation resulting from failure of rectum to respond to defecation stimulus.

proctostenosis (prŏk″tō-stěn-ō'sĭs) [Gr. *prōktos*, anus, + *stēnōsis*, narrowing]. Stricture of the anus or rectum.

proctostomy (prŏk-tŏs'tō-mĭ) ["+ *stoma*, mouth]. Surgical creation of a permanent opening into the rectum.

proc'totome ["+ *tomē*, a cutting]. Knife for incision into rectum.

proctotomy (prŏk-tŏt'ō-mĭ). Incision of the rectum or anus.

NP: Patient in Simon's position, q.v. Dress incision with iodoform gauze and T-bandage.

proctotoreusis (prŏk″tō-tō-rū'sĭs) [Gr. *prōktos*, anus, + *toreusis*, boring]. The making of an opening in an imperforate anus.

proctovalvotomy (prŏk″tō-văl-vŏt'ō-mĭ) ["+ L. *valva*, valve, + Gr. *tomē*, a cutting]. Incision of the rectal valves.

procum'bent [L. *prōcumbens*, lying down]. Lying face down. SYN: *prone*.

procursive (prō-kŭr'sĭv) [L. *procursivus*]. Having an involuntary tendency to run forward.

prodromal (prō-drō'măl) [Gr. *prodromos*, running before]. Pert. to the initial stage of a disease; the interval between the earliest symptoms and the appearance of the rash or fever.

 p. rash. One that precedes the true rash of an infectious disease.

pro'drome. (pl. *prodromes, prodromata*) A symptom indicative of an approaching disease.

product (prŏd'ŭkt) [L. *prōductum*]. Anything which is made naturally or artificially. SEE: *catabolite.*

production (prō-dŭk'shŭn). Development or formation of a substance.

productive (prō-dŭk'tĭv). Forming, esp. new tissue.

 p. inflammation. Inflammation producing new tissue with or without an exudate.

proenzyme (prō-ĕn'zīm) [Gr. *prō*, before, + *en*, in, + *zymē*, a leaven]. The inactive form of an enzyme found within a cell which, upon leaving the cell, is converted into the active form. EX: pepsinogen. SYN: *zymogen.*

proerythroblast (prō″ē-rĭth'rō-blăst) ["+ *erythros*, red, + *blastos*, germ]. The earliest cells which show differentiation in the direction of erythrocyte formation. SYN: *basophilic erythroblast.*

proestrus (prō-ĕs'trŭs). The period preceding estrus in females, characterized by development of ovarian follicles and uterine endometrium.

profer'ment [Gr. *pro*, before, + L. *fermentum*, leaven]. An inactive precursor of a ferment. Zymogen.

professional (prō-fĕsh'ŭn-ăl) [ME. *profession*, sacred vow]. 1. Pert. to a profession. 2.

Caused by the practice of a profession, as writer's cramp.

profluvium (prō-flū'vĭ-ŭm) [L.]. An excessive flow or discharge; a flux.

p. lactis. Excessive flow of milk.

p. seminis. Flow of semen from the vagina deposited during coition.

profondometer (prō"fŏn-dŏm'ĕ-tĕr) [L. *profundus*, deep, + Gr. *metron*, a measure]. Device for locating a foreign body with the fluoroscope.

profun'da [L.]. Deep seated; term applied to certain deeply located blood vessels.

progenitor (prō-jĕn'ĭ-tor) [L.]. An ancestor.

progeny (prŏj'ĕ-nĭ) [ME. *progenie*]. Offspring.

progeria (prō-jē'rĭ-ă) [Gr. *pro*, before, + *gēras*, old age]. Premature senility occurring in childhood.

ETIOL: Unknown.

SYM AND SIGNS: Small stature, face looks old and wizened, skin is dry and thin, hair is scanty, and sex organs are infantile.

progesterone (prō-jĕs'tĕr-ōn). $C_{21}H_{30}O_2$, a steroid hormone obtained from the corpus luteum, adrenals, or placenta. It is responsible for changes in uterine endometrium in second half of menstrual cycle preparatory for implantation of blastocyst; development of maternal placenta after implantation; development of mammary glands.

USES: In treatment of menstrual disorders (amenorrhea, dysmenorrhea) and threatened abortion.

progestin (prō-jĕs"tĭn). A corpus luteum hormone which prepares the endometrium for the fertilized ovum. This word is now used to cover a large group of synthetic drugs which have a progesteronelike effect on the uterus. SYN: *progesterone*.

proglossis (prō-glŏs'ĭs) [Gr.]. Tip of the tongue.

proglot'tid. Proglottis, q.v.

proglot'tis [Gr. *pro*, before, + *glōssa*, tongue]. (pl. *proglot'tides*) A segment of a tapeworm, containing both male and female reproductive organs. SEE: *Cestoda; tapeworm.*

prognathism (prŏg'nă-thĭzm) ["+ *gnathos*, jaw, + *ismos*, condition]. Projection of jaws beyond projection of forehead.

prog'nathous. Having jaws projecting forward beyond rest of the face.

prognosis (prŏg-nō'sĭs) [Gr., foreknowledge]. Prediction of course and end of disease, and outlook based on it.

p. anceps. Doubtful prognosis.

p. fausta. Favorable prognosis.

p. infausta. Unfavorable prognosis.

prognos'tic. Rel. to prediction of outcome of a disease.

prognosticate (prŏg-nŏs'tĭ-kāt) [Gr. *prognōstikon*, knowing before]. To make a statement on the probable outcome of an illness.

progonoma (prō"gō-nō'mă) [Gr. *pro*, before, + *gonos*, sperm, + -*oma*, tumor]. A tumor, such as a hairy mole, which develops from displacement of embryonic cells.

progranulocyte (prō-grăn'ŭ-lō-sīt) ["+ L. *granula*, granule, + Gr. *kytos*, hollow vessel]. A promyelocyte, q.v.

prograv'id ["+ L. *gravidus*, pregnant]. Before or preceding pregnancy.

p. phase. The secretory phase of the menstrual cycle, q.v.

progression (prō-grĕsh'ŭn) [L. *prōgressus*]. Advancing or moving forward.

p., backward. Walking backward; a sym. seen in certain nervous disorders. SYN: *retropulsion.*

progressive (prō-grĕs'ĭv). Advancing, as a disease from bad to worse.

p. muscular atrophy. Gradual advancing atrophy of groups of muscles due to spinal cord degeneration. SEE: *atrophy.*

p. ossifying myositis. Tendency to bony deposits in the muscles with chronic inflammation.

proinsulin. A precursor of insulin produced in the beta cells of the pancreas.

proiosystole (prō-ĭ-ō-sĭs'tō-lĭ) [Gr. *prōi*, early, + *systolē*, contraction]. A cardiac contraction occuring before its normal time.

proiosystolia (prō"ĭ-ō-sĭs-tō'lĭ-ă). A condition marked by occurrence of systoles before the normal time.

proiotia (prō"ĭ-ō'shĭ-ă) [Gr. *prōiotēs*, early]. Genital precocity.

projectile vomiting. Vomiting in which the stomach contents are forcibly ejected, but not preceded by nausea.

projection (prō-jĕk'shŭn) [Gr. *pro*, before, + *jacere*, to throw]. 1. The act of throwing forward. 2. A part extending beyond the level of its surroundings. 3. The mental process by which sensations are referred to the sense organs or receptors stimulated, or outside the body to the object which is the stimulus. 4. Distortion of a perception as a result of its repression, resulting in such a phenomenon as hating without cause one who has been dearly loved, or attributing to others one's own undesirable traits. Characteristic of the paranoid reaction.

prolabium (prō-lā'bĭ-ŭm) ["+ *labium*, lip]. The entire central portion of the upper lip.

prolac'tin ["+ *lac*, milk]. Hormone produced by the anterior lobe of the pituitary gland.

It is capable of initiating and sustaining lactation, but only when other essential hormones such as estrogen, progesterone, and oxytocin are present. P. has other metabolic functions which are not completely understood.

prolamin(e (prō-lăm'ĭn, prō'lă-mĭn). Any one of a class of proteins found in seeds, soluble in 70%-80% alcohol, and insoluble in water alone or in absolute alcohol. SYN: *gliadin.*

prolan (prō'lan). A hormone principle formerly believed to be from the anterior pituitary body, but now known to be chorionic gonadotrophins. SEE: *gonadotrophin, chorionic.*

prolapse (prō-lăps') [L. *prolapsus*]. A falling or dropping down of an organ or internal part, such as the uterus or rectum. SYN: *ptosis; procidentia.*

     p. of anus. Prolapsus ani; p. of rectum, q.v.

     p. of the cord. Expulsion of umbilical cord prematurely. SEE: *labor.*

     p. of iris. Protrusion of iris through an injury in the cornea.

     p. of rectum. Protrusion of rectal mucosa through the anus.

     p. of uterus. Prolapsus uteri, q.v.

prolap'sus. A falling or downward displacement of some part of the body, as the uterus.

     p. ani. Protrusion of lower portion of digestive tract through external sphincter of anus. SEE: *prolapse of rectum.*

     p. uteri. Downward displacement of uterus, the cervix sometimes protruding from the vaginal orifice. SYN: *descensus uteri.*

prolep'sis [Gr. *pro*, before, + *lēpsis*, a seizure]. Return of paroxysmal attacks at successively shorter intervals.

prolep'tic. Recurrring before the time expected, said of paroxysms.

proleukocyte (prō-lū'kō-sīt) [Gr. *pro*, before, + *leukos*, white, + *kytos*, cell]. An undeveloped leukocyte. SYN: *leukoblast.*

proliferate (prō-lĭf'ĕr-āt) [L. *proles*, offspring, + *ferre*, to bear]. To increase by reproduction of similar forms.

proliferation (prō-lĭf'ĕr-ā'shŭn). 1. Reproduction rapidly and repeatedly of new parts, as by cell division. SEE: *auxesis.* 2. Process or result of rapid reproduction.

prolif'erous. 1. Multiplying, as by formation of new tissue cells. 2. Bearing offspring.

     p. cyst. One with epithelial lining, proliferating and projecting from inner surface of the cyst.

prolif'ic [L. *prōlificus*]. Fruitful; reproductive. SYN: *fertile.*

proligerous (prō-lĭj'ĕr-ŭs) [L. *proles*, offspring, + *gerere*, to bear]. Producing offspring. SYN: *germinating.*

pro'linase. An enzyme found in animal tissues and yeast which hydrolyzes proline peptids to simpler peptids and proline.

proline (prō'lēn). An important amino acid formed by protein decomposition, having the formula $C_4H_8N \cdot COOH$.

prolymphocyte (prō''lĭmf'ō-sīt) [Gr. *pro*, before, + L. *lympha*, water, + Gr. *kytos*, cell]. A cell intermediate between a lymphoblast and lymphocyte.

promegakaryocyte (prō-mĕg''ă-kăr'ĭ-ō-sīt) ["+ *megas*, big, + *karyon*, nucleus, + *kytos*, cell]. Cell from which a megakaryocyte develops.

promegaloblast (prō-mĕg'ă-lō-blast'') ["+ "+ *blastos*, germ]. A cell of the erythrocyte series preceding the megaloblast.

promethium (prō-mē'thĭ-ŭm). SYMB: *Pm.* At. wt. 147; at. no. 61. A radioactive element of the rare earth series.

promine. A tissue extract which promotes growth of certain tumors in mice.

prominence (prŏm'ĭ-nĕns) [L. *prōminēns*, project]. A projection or protrusion. SEE: *prominentia* [NA].

prominentia (prŏm''ĭ-nĕn'shĭ-ă) [L.]. (pl. *prominen'tiae*) [NA]. A projection.

     p. laryngea. [NA] The laryngeal prominence; Adam's apple. SYN: *pomum adami.*

     p. spiralis. [NA] A small ridge extending entire length of cochlea located on inner surface of spiral ligament. It projects slightly into cochlear canal and contains blood vessels including the vas prominens. SYN: *spiral prominence.*

promontory (prŏm'ŭn-tōr''ĭ) [L. *promontorium*]. A projecting process or part.

     p. of sacrum. The anterior projecting portion of the pelvic surface of base of the sacrum. With the 5th lumbar vertebra, it forms the sacrovertebral angle.

     p. of tympanic cavity. Projection on medial wall of tympanic cavity produced by first turn of the cochlea.

promyelocyte (prō-mī'ĕl-ō-sīt) [Gr. *pro*, before, + *myelos*, marrow, + *kytos*, cell]. 1. A large mononuclear myeloid cell seen in the blood in leukemia. 2. Cell development between myeloblast and a myelocyte, resembling a myeloblast.

pronation (prō-nā'shŭn) [L. *prōnus*, prone]. 1. The act of lying prone or face downward. 2. The act of turning hand so that palm faces downward or backward.

pronator. A muscle that pronates. SEE: *Table of Muscles* in *Appendix.*

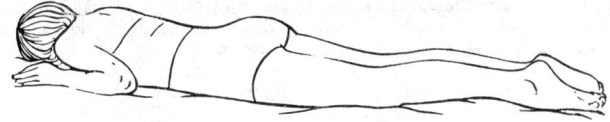

PRONE POSITION

pronaus, pronaeus (prō-nā'ŭs) [Gr. *pro*, before, + *naos*, temple]. The vagina or vestibule of the vagina.

prone (prōn) [ME.]. 1. Lying horizontal with face downward. 2. Denoting the hand with the palms turned downward. Opposed to supine, q.v.

pronephric (prō-nĕf'rĭk) [Gr. *pro*, before, + *nephros*, kidney]. Pert. to the pronephron, q.v.

p. duct. Duct that connects posteriorly to cloaca and to which pronephric tubules are connected.

p. tubules. Several pairs of segmentally arranged tubules which open into cranial portion of pronephric duct. They communicate with coelom through a ciliated funnel-shaped nephrostome. They are vestigial in higher vertebrates.

pronephron, pronephros (prō-nĕf'rŏn, -rŏs). The earliest and simplest type of excretory organ of vertebrates, functional in simpler forms (cyclostomes) and serving as a provisional kidney in some fishes and amphibians. In reptiles, birds, and mammals, it appears in the embryo as a temporary, functionless structure.

pronograde (prō'nō-grād) [L. *prōnus*, prone, + *gradus*, a step]. Walking on hands and feet or resting with the body in a horizontal position. Opposed to orthograde, q.v.

pronometer (prō-nŏm'ĕ-tĕr) ["+ Gr. *metron*, a measure]. Device for showing amount of pronation or supination of forearm.

pronucleus (prō-nū'klē-ŭs) [Gr. *pro*, before, + *nucleus*, little kernel]. Nucleus of the ovum (the female p.) or of the spermatozoon (the male p.) after fertilization of the ovum.

prootic (prō-ŏt'ĭk, -ō'tĭk) ["+ *ous, ot-*, ear]. In front of the ear.

propagation (prŏp-ă-gā'shŭn) [L.]. Act of reproducing or giving birth. SYN: *generation; reproduction.*

prop'aga"tive. Pert. to or taking part in reproduction.

propalinal (prō-pāl'ĭ-năl) [Gr. *pro*, before, + *palin*, back]. Applied to a backward and forward movement, as of the jaws.

propanolol. A drug used in treating cardiac arrhythmias, particularly supraventricular tachycardia. The drug should be used with digitalis.

propep'tone ["+ *peptein*, to digest]. An intermediate product in the digestive conversion of protein into peptone. SYN: *hemialbumose.*

propeptonuria (prō"pĕp-tō-nū'rĭ-ă) ["+ "+ *ouron*, urine]. Excretion of propeptone in the urine. SYN: *hemialbumosuria.*

properdin (prō-pĕrd'ĭn). A serum protein which, in the presence of magnesium ions and complement, has the ability to help destroy gram-negative bacteria and viruses. The exact method of action is not fully understood.

prophase (prō'fāz) [Gr. *pro*, before, + *phasis*, phase of the moon]. First stage of indirect cell division. SEE: *centriole; metaphase; mitosis.*

prophylactic (prō-fĭ-lăk'tĭk) [Gr. *prophylaktikos*, guarding]. 1. Warding off disease. 2. Agent which wards off disease. 3. A chemical substance or physical device used to prevent venereal disease. Usually used during or following sexual intercourse.

prophylaxis (prō-fĭ-lăk'sĭs, prō-fĭl-ăks'ĭs) [Gr. *prophylassein*, to guard against]. 1. Observance of rules necessary to prevent disease. 2. In dentistry, cleaning the teeth's surface, esp. the scales that develop at the gingival margins.

propositus (prō-pŏz'ĭ-tŭs) [L. *proponere*, to put on view]. The initial individual whose condition led to investigation of an hereditary disorder. SYN: *proband.*

proprietary medicine (prō-prī'ĕ-tar'ĭ) [L. *proprietarius*, pert. to property]. Any chemical, drug or similar preparation used in the treatment of diseases, if such article is protected against free competition as to name, product, composition or process of manufacture by secrecy, patent or copyright, or by another means. SEE: *patent medicine.*

proprioception (prō"prī-ō-sĕp'shŭn) [L. *proprius*, one's own, + *capio*, to take]. The awareness of posture, movement, and changes in equilibrium and the knowledge of position, weight, and resistance of objects in relation to the body.

proprioceptive (prō"prī-ō-sĕp'tĭv). Pert. to proprioception.

p. impulses. Afferent impulses arising in proprioceptors, q.v.

p. sense. Muscle sense; kinesthetic sense.

proprioceptor (prō″prī-ō-sĕp′tor) [L. *proprius,* one's own, + *ceptor,* a receiver]. A receptor that responds to stimuli originating within the body itself, esp. those responding to pressure, position, or stretch. EX: muscle spindles, Golgi tendon organs, pacinian corpuscles, and labyrinthine receptors.

proptometer (prŏp-tŏm′ĕ-tĕr) [Gr. *proptōsis,* protrusion, + *metron,* a measure]. An instrument for measuring extent of exophthalmos.

proptosis (prŏp-tō′sĭs). A downward displacement, as of the uterus or of the eyeball in exophthalmic goiter, or in inflammatory conditions of the orbit.

propulsion (prō-pŭl′shŭn) [L. *prōpulsus,* driven forward]. 1. A tendency to push or fall forward in walking. 2. A condition seen in paralysis agitans. SEE: *festination.*

propylthiouracil (prō″pĭl-thī″ō-ū′ră-sĭl). USP. Antithyroid drug used in treatment of hyperthyroidism, thyroiditis, and thyrotoxicosis. Also employed for preoperative therapy and in cases where surgery is contraindicated.

pro re nata (prō rā nă′tă) [L.]. According to the circumstances. ABBR: p.r.n.

prorennin (prō-rĕn′ĭn). The preliminary material which is converted into rennin. SYN: *prorenninogen.*

prorrhaphy (prō′ră-fī) [Gr. *pro,* before, + *rhaphē,* suture]. Surgical movement of a muscle or tendon insertion to a point farther away. Done to change the action of a muscle. SYN: *advancement.*

prosecretin (prō″sē-krē′tĭn) ["+ *secretiō,* a secretion]. Substance present in the duodenal mucosa which, when acted on by hydrochloric acid in chyme, is converted into secretin. SEE: *secretin.*

prosector (prō-sĕk′tor) [L.]. One who prepares cadavers for dissection or dissects for demonstration.

prosencephalon (prŏs″ĕn-sĕf′ă-lŏn) [Gr. *prosō,* before, + *enkephalos,* brain]. The embryonic forebrain which gives rise to the telencephalon and diencephalon, q.v.

proso- [Gr. *prosō,* forward]. Combining form indicating forward or anterior.

prosodemic (prŏs″ō-dĕm′ĭk) [Gr. *prosō,* forward, + *dēmos,* people]. Spread by individual contact; said of a disease. Opposed to epidemic.

prosopagnosia (prŏs″ō-păg-nō′sĭ-ă) ["+ *a,* not, + *gnōsis,* recognition]. Inability to recognize faces, even one's own face.

prosopalgia (prŏs″ō-păl′jĭ-ă) [Gr. *prosōpon,* face, + *algos,* pain]. Neuralgic pain in the trigeminal nerve and its branches. SYN: *prosopodynia; tic douloureux.*

prosopectasia (prŏs″ō-pĕk-tā′zĭ-ă) ["+ *ektasis,* dilatation]. Enlarged size of the face.

prosopic (prō″sŏp′ĭk). Pert. to face or facial skeleton that is convex anteriorly.

prosopoanoschisis (prŏs″ō-pō″ă-nŏs′kĭ-sĭs) [Gr. *prosōpon,* face, + *ana,* up, + *schisis,* cleft]. Oblique facial cleft, a slanting furrow extending from mouth to eye.

prosopodiplegia (prŏs″ō-pō-dī-plē′jĭ-ă) ["+ *dis,* double, + *plēgē,* a stroke]. Paralysis on both sides of the face.

prosopodynia (prŏs″ō-pō-dĭn′ĭ-ă) ["+ *odynē,* pain]. Pain in the face. SYN: *tic douloureux.*

prosoponeuralgia (prŏs″ō-pō-nū-răl′jĭ-ă) ["+ *neuron,* sinew, + *algos,* pain]. Facial neuralgia. SYN: *prosopalgia.*

prosopoplegia (prŏs″ō-pō-plē′jĭ-ă) [Gr. *prosōpon,* face, + *plēgē,* stroke]. Paralysis of the face.

prosopoplegic (prŏs″ō-pō-plē′jĭk). Rel. to, or afflicted with, facial paralysis.

prosoposchisis (prŏs-ō-pŏs′kĭ-sĭs) [Gr. *prosōpon,* face, + *schisis,* a cleft]. Congenital cleft of the face.

prosopospasm (prŏs′ō-pō-spăzm) ["+ *spasmos,* a spasm]. Facial spasm.

prosopotocia (prŏs″ō-pō-tō′shĭ-ă) ["+ *tokos,* birth]. Presentation of the face in parturition.

pros′opus va′rus [Gr. *prosōpon,* face, + L. *varus,* crooked]. Congential obliquity of the face due to atrophy of one side of the head.

pros′taglandins. A group of fatty acid derivatives present in many tissues including prostate gland, menstrual fluid, brain, lung, kidney, thymus, seminal fluid, and pancreas. There are more than a dozen prostaglandins. They are extremely active biological substances which affect the cardiovascular system, smooth muscle, and stimulate the uterus to contract.

prostatalgia (prŏs-tă-tăl′jĭ-ă) [Gr. *prostatēs,* prostate, + *algos,* pain]. Pain of the prostate gland.

prostate (prŏs′tāt) [Gr. *prostatēs*]. A gland which surrounds the neck of the bladder and the urethra in the male. It is partly glandular, with ducts opening into the prostatic portion of the urethra, and partly muscular. Consists of a median lobe and two lateral lobes.

About 2 × 4 × 3 cm., and weighing about 20 gm., it is enclosed in a fibrous capsule containing smooth muscle fibers in its inner layer. Muscle fibers also separate the glandular tissue and encircle the urethra.

The gland secretes a thin, opalescent, slightly alkaline fluid which forms part of semen.

PATHOLOGY: Inflammation of the prostate may occur, often the result of gonorrheal urethritis. Enlargement of the prostate is common, esp. after middle age. This results in urethral obstruction, impeding urination and sometimes leading to retention. Benign and malignant tumors, calculi, and nodular hyperplasia are common, particularly in men past 60.

prostatectomy (prŏs″tă-tĕk′tō-mĭ) ["+ *ektomē*, excision]. Excision of part or all of the prostate gland. Operation may be performed with an incision in the perineum (perineal p.), into the bladder (suprapubic p.), or through the urethra (transurethral p.).

After prostatectomy, the patient is unable to ejaculate but his libido is unaffected.

COMPLICATIONS: Retention of urine, hematuria, cystitis, infection of kidney, pyelitis, infective nephritis, renal failure.

prostathelcosis (prŏs″tă-thĕl-kō′sĭs) ["+ *helkosis*, ulceration]. Ulceration of prostate gland.

prostatic (prŏs-tăt′ĭk) [Gr. *prostatēs*, prostate]. Concerning the prostate gland.

p. calculus. A stone in the prostate.

p. plexus. 1. Veins around the base and neck of the bladder and prostate gland. 2. Nerves from the pelvic plexus to the prostate gland, erectile tissue of the penis, and to the seminal vesicles.

p. syncope. Fainting during examination of the prostate. This is a rare occurrence which can be avoided by examining the patient in the left lateral recumbent position.

p. urethra. Part of the urethra surrounded by the prostate gland.

prostatism (prŏs′tă-tĭzm) ["+ *-ismos*, condition]. Any condition with obstruction of the prostate gland, resulting in retention of urine in the bladder.

ETIOL: Benign hypertrophy, carcinoma, prostatitis, nodular hyperplasia.

SYM: Frequent, uncomfortable urination, nocturia. Retention of urine may occur with development of uremia.

prostatitis (prŏs″tă-tī′tĭs) ["+ *-itis*, inflammation]. Inflamed condition of the prostate gland. May be a complication of gonorrheal infection.

p., acute. Discomfort and pain in perineal area. Frequent urination; later, retention of urine. If severe, marked malaise, rise of temperature, constipation, chills, and vomiting.

p., chronic. Dull, aching pain in perineal region. Discharge from the penis.

prostatocystitis (prŏs″tă-tō-sĭs-tī′tĭs) [Gr. *prostatēs*, prostate, + *kystis*, bladder, + *-itis*, inflammation]. Inflammation of the prostatic urethra involving the bladder.

prostatocystotomy (prŏs″tă-tō-sĭs-tŏt′ō-mĭ) ["+ "+ *tomē*, a cutting]. Surgical incision of the prostate and bladder.

prostatodynia (prŏs″tă-tō-dĭn′ĭ-ă) ["+ *odynē*, pain]. Pain in the prostate gland. SYN: *prostatalgia.*

pros″tat′olith [Gr. *prostatēs*, prostate, + *lithos*, stone]. A calculus of the prostate gland.

prostatomegaly (prŏs″tă-tō-mĕg′ă-lĭ) ["+ *megas, megal-*, large]. Enlargement of the prostate gland.

pros″tatom′eter ["+ *metron*, a measure]. Device for measuring enlargement of the prostate.

prostatomy (prŏs-tăt′ō-mĭ) [Gr. *prostatēs*, prostate, + *tomē*, a cutting]. Incision into the prostate.

prostatomyomectomy (prŏs″tă-tō-mĭ″ō-mĕk′tō-mĭ) ["+ *mys, my-*, muscle, + *ektomē*, excision]. Surgical excision of a prostatic myoma.

prostatorrhea (prŏs″tă-tō-rē′ă) ["+ *rhoia*, flow]. Abnormal discharge from the prostate gland.

prostatotomy (prŏs″tă-tŏt′ō-mĭ) ["+ *tomē*, a cutting]. Incision into prostate gland.

prostatovesiculectomy (prŏs″tă-tō-vē-sĭk″ū-lĕk′tō-mĭ) [Gr. *prostatēs*, prostate, + L. *vesiculus*, a little sac, + Gr. *ektomē*, excision]. Removal of the prostate gland and seminal vesicles.

prostatovesiculitis (prŏs″tă-tō-vē-sĭk″ū-lī′tĭs) ["+ "+ Gr. *-itis*, inflammation]. Inflammation of the seminal vesicles and prostate gland.

prosternation (prō″stĕr-nā′shŭn) [Gr. *pro*, before, + *sternon*, chest]. Habitual flexion of the trunk forward. SYN: *camptocormia.*

prostheon (prŏs′thē-ŏn) [Gr. *prosthios*, foremost]. The alveolar point; midpoint of lower border of upper alveolar arch.

prosthesis (prŏs′thē-sĭs) [Gr., an addition]. (pl. *prosthe′ses*) 1. Replacement of a missing part by an artificial substitute. 2. An artificial organ or part. 3. Device to augment performance of a natural function. Ex: hearing aid.

p., dental. Replacement of a tooth or of a section of teeth by partial or full dentures.

p., maxillofacial. Repair and artificial replacement of face and jaw missing because of disease or injury.

prosthetic group (prŏs-thĕt'ĭc). In chemistry, the linking of a protein to another compound by some means other than through an amino acid.

prosthetics (prŏs-thĕt'ĭks). The branch of surgery dealing with replacement of missing parts.

prosthetist (prŏs'thē-tĭst). 1. Specialist in artificial dentures. 2. Maker of artificial limbs.

prosthetosclerokeratoplasty. Surgical procedure for replacement of diseased scleral and corneal tissue with a transparent prosthesis.

pros"thodon'tics [Gr. *prosthesis*, an addition, + *odous, odont-*, tooth]. Branch of dentistry dealing with construction of artificial appliances for the mouth.

pros"thodon'tist. A dentist who specializes in the mechanics of making and fitting artificial teeth.

prosthokeratoplasty (prŏs"thō-kĕr'ă-tō-plăs"tĭ) ["+ *keras*, horn, + *plassein*, to form]. Surgical replacement of diseased or scarred corneal tissue with a transparent prosthesis.

prostigmin (prō-stĭg'mĭn). Registered trademark for a brand of neostigmine, q.v.

prostitute (prŏs'tĭ-tūt) [L. *prostituere*, to prostitute]. 1. A woman or, less frequently, a man who solicits or accepts payment for sexual relations. 2. To sell one's self basely, such as to prostitute one's talents.

prostitution (prŏs"tĭ-tū'shŭn). Act or practice of prostituting. Prostitution is a major cause of the spread of venereal disease.

prostrate (prŏs'trāt) [Gr. *pro*, before, + L. *sternere*, stretch out]. 1. Lying with body extended. 2. To deprive of strength or to exhaust.

pros"tra'ted. Depleted of strength; exhausted.

prostration (prŏs-trā'shŭn). Absolute exhaustion.

    p., heat. Exhaustion resulting from exposure to excessive heat.

    p., nervous. General physical and nervous exhaustion. SYN: *neurasthenia.*

protactinium (prō"tăk-tĭn'ĭ-ŭm). SYMB: *Pa*. At. wt. 231; at. no. 91. A radioactive element.

protal (prō'tăl) [Gr. *prōtos*, first]. Existing from time of birth or before. Hereditary.

protamine (prō'tă-mĭn). 1. One of a class of simple proteins which are strongly basic, noncoagulable in heat, and yield diamino acids when hydrolyzed. 2. An amine, $C_{16}H_{32}O_2N_9$, isolated from spermatozoa and spawn of fish.

    Found in fish sperm and named from the fish from which it is derived. SEE: *salmine; sturine.*

p. insulin, p. zinc insulin. Preparations of insulin which are more slowly dissolved and absorbed by body tissues than ordinary insulin. Act longer and keep the blood sugar normal for 20-24 hr. One injection is sufficient for this period.

protanopia (prō-tăn-ō'pĭ-ă) [Gr. *prōtos*, first, + *an-*, negative, + *opsis*, vision]. Defect in color vision characterized by red blindness.

protean (prō'tē-ăn). 1. [Gr. *Proteus*, a god who changed shapes at will]. Having ability to change form, as the ameba. Variable. 2. [Gr. *prōtos*, first]. One of the primary derivatives of protein resulting from action of water, enzymes, or dilute acids.

protease (prō'tē-ās) [Gr. *prōtos*, first, + *ase*, enzyme]. A protein-splitting enzyme.

protective (prō-tĕk'tĭv) [L. *protectus*, shielding]. 1. Covering, preventing infection, providing immunity. 2. An agent that will mechanically protect the part to which applied. Ex: collodion, plaster. SYN: *dressing.*

proteidogenous (prō"tē-ĭd-ōj'ĕn-ŭs). Producing proteins.

protein (prō'tē-ĭn, prō-tēn) [Gr. *prōtos*, first]. One of a class of complex nitrogenous compounds which occur naturally in plants and animals, give amino acids when hydrolyzed, and are essential for the growth and repair of animal tissue. In mammals there is a strict order of priority of the use the body makes of available protein. First priority goes to the manufacture of hemoglobin; second to making blood plasma proteins; and finally when those requirements are made, protein is used in the repair of tissue.

    CLASSIFICATION: Proteins have been classified in three groups: simple, conjugated, and derived proteins, q.v.

    COMPOSITION: Proteins are composed of carbon, hydrogen, oxygen, nitrogen, phosphorus, sulfur, and iron which make up the greater part of plant and animal tissue. Amino acids represent the basic structure of proteins. Some foods containing p. consist of different numbers and kinds of amino acids. A *complete p.* is one that contains all the essential amino acids (tryptophane, lysine, methionine, valine, leucine, isoleucine, phenylalanine, threonine, arginine, and histidine). These are necessary for growth and maintenance of body weight.

    FUNCTIONS: Proteins are a source of heat and energy to the body. They are essential for growth, the building of new tissue, and the repair of injured or broken-down tissue. They form an integral part of the protoplasm of every cell. They are oxidized in the body, thus liberating heat. One gm. supplies 4 Cal. of heat.

Children require from 2-3 gm. per kilogram of body weight per day. This should be calculated on the basis of ideal, rather than actual, weight of the child. Age also is a factor in determining p. requirements, the amount decreasing with age. Physical work, menstruation, lactation, and convalescence demand increased p. requirement. Excess p. in the diet results in increased nitrogen excretion in the urine.

SOURCES: Milk, eggs, cheese, meat, fish, and some vegetables, such as soy beans, are the best sources. Proteins are found in both vegetable and animal forms. *Principal animal proteins* are ovalbumin in eggs; lactalbumin in milk; serumalbumin in serum; myogen or myosinogen in striated muscle tissue; crystallins found in the lens of the eye; fibrinogen in blood; ovoglobulin in eggs; lactoglobulin in milk; serum globulin in serum; myosin in striated muscle tissue; thyroglobulin in thyroid; globin in blood; thymus histones in thymus; collagen and gelatin in connective tissue; elastin; and keratin. Nucleoprotein is found in the thymus, pancreas, liver, animal cells, and glands; chondroprotein is found in tendons and cartilage; mucin and mucoids are found in various secreting glands and animal mucilaginous substances; caseinogen in milk; vitellin in egg yolk; hemoglobin in blood; and lecithoprotein in blood, brain, and bile.

p. balance. Equilibrium between protein intake and anabolism, and protein catabolism and elimination of nitrogenous products. SEE: *nitrogen equilibrium.*

p., Bence Jones. P. that occurs in urine. Its presence is symptomatic of certain pathologic conditions: multiple myeloma, lymphosarcoma, leukemia, or Hodgkin's disease.

p., biological value of. The proportion of absorbed nitrogen retained in the body when a protein is ingested.

p.'s, blood. P.'s present in blood. Include *hemoglobin* in red blood cells and *plasma p.'s.* Normal values are hemoglobin, 13-16 gm./100 ml. in men, and 12-14 gm./100 ml. in women; albumin, 4-5 gm./100 ml. of serum; globulin, 2-3 gm./100 ml. of serum; fibrinogen, 0.15-0.30 gm./100 ml. of plasma. The amount of albumin in relation to the amount of globulin is referred to as the albumin-globulin (A/G) ratio, which is normally 1.5 to 2.5 : 1.

p.- calorie malnutrition. Malnutrition in persons, usually infants and young children, whose diets are deficient in proteins and calories. Clinically the condition

may be precipitated by other factors such as infections or intestinal parasites.

p., complete. P. containing all the essential amino acids.

p., conjugated. P.'s containing the p. molecule with some other molecule or molecules. *Chromoproteins:* Ex: hemoglobin. *Glycoproteins:* Ex: mucin. *Lecithoproteins:* Compounds of lecithins or similar substances with the protein molecule. *Nucleoproteins. Phosphoproteins:* Ex: casein.

p., denatured. P. whose amino acid composition and stereochemical structure has been altered by physical or chemical means.

p., derived. P.'s not occurring naturally but derived through the action of heat, reagents, enzymes, etc.

p.-high diet. 1.5-2 gm. protein per kg. ideal body weight per day in adults.

p., incomplete. P. lacking one or more of the essential amino acids.

p., native. A p. in its natural state; one which has not been denatured.

p.'s, plasma. P.'s present in blood plasma, i.e., albumins, globulins, fibrinogen.

p. sensitization. Condition in which patient is hypersensitive to foreign proteins, so that severe reaction occurs upon their administration.

p., serum. P.'s present in blood serum, i.e., albumins and globulins.

p., simple. Those which produce alpha amino acids on hydrolysis. *Albumins:* Soluble in water and coagulated by heat. Ex: egg albumin. *Globulins:* Insoluble in water, soluble in salt solutions, coagulated by heat. Ex: edestin from hemp seed. *Glutelins, Prolamines:* alcohol-soluble proteins. Ex: gliadin from wheat. *Albuminoids:* Ex: keratin from corn. *Histones, Protamines:* Ex: salmon from the ripe sperm of salmon.

p. sparer. A substance in the diet (carbohydrates or fat) that relieves the body tissues of the necessity of giving up p. for energy.

p., tissue. P. within the solid tissues of the body in contrast to those in circulating blood.

proteinase (prō'tē-ĭn-ās) [Gr. *protos,* first, + *ase,* enzyme]. A proteolytic enzyme; an enzyme that acts on native proteins.

proteinic (prō''tē-ĭn'ĭk). Rel. to protein.

proteinivorus (prō''tē-ĭn-ĭv'ō-rŭs) ["+ L. *vorāre,* to devour]. Living on protein.

proteinogenous (prō''tē-ĭn-ŏj'ĕn-ŭs) [Gr. *protos,* first, + *gennan,* to produce]. Developing from a protein.

proteinophobia (prō″tē-ĭn-ō-fō′bĭ-ă) ["+ *phobos*, fear]. Aversion to foods containing protein.

proteinosis (prō″tē-ĭn-ō′sĭs) ["+ *-osis*, condition]. Accumulation of proteins in the tissues.

   p., lipid. A rare condition resulting from an undefined metabolic defect. Yellow deposits of a mixture of protein and lipoid occur, esp. on the mucous surface of the mouth and tongue. Nodules may appear on the face, extremities, and on the epiglottis and vocal cords. This latter abnormality produces hoarseness. SYN: *hyalinosis cutis et mucosae.*

proteinuria (prō″tē-ĭn-ū′rĭ-ă) [Gr. *prōtos*, first, + *ouron*, urine]. Protein, usually albumin, in the urine.

proteogens (prō′tē-ō-jĕns) ["+ *gennan*, to produce]. Preparations of plant proteins for injection hypodermically.

proteolysin (prō″tē-ōl′ĭ-sĭn) [Gr. *prōtos*, first, + *lysis*, dissolution]. A specific substance causing decomposition of proteins.

proteolysis (prō″tē-ōl′ĭ-sĭs). The hydrolysis of proteins, usually by enzyme action, into simpler substances.

proteolytic (prō″tē-ō-lĭt′ĭk). Hastening the hydrolysis of proteins.

proteometabolism (prō″tē-ō-mē-tăb′ō-lĭzm) [Gr. *prōtos*, first, + *metabolē*, change, + *ismos*, condition]. Digestion, absorption, and assimilation of proteins.

proteopeptic (prō″tē-ō-pĕp′tĭk) ["+ *peptein*, to digest]. Pert. to the digestion of protein.

proteopexic (prō-tē-ō-pĕks′ĭk) ["+ *pēxis*, fixation]. Pert. to fixation of proteins within the organism.

proteopexy (prō″tē-ō-pĕks′ĭ). The fixation of proteins within the body.

proteose (prō′tē-ōs) [Gr. *prōtos*, first]. One of the class of intermediate products of proteolysis between protein and peptone.

   p., primary. First formed products during proteolysis of proteins.

   p., secondary. P. resulting from further hydrolysis of primary proteoses.

proteosuria (prō″tē-ōs-ū′rĭ-ă) ["+ *ouron*, urine]. Proteose in urine. SYN: *albumosuria.*

proteuria (prō″tē-ū′rĭ-ă). Proteins in the urine. SYN: *proteinuria.*

Proteus (prō′tē-ŭs) [Gr., a god who could change his form]. A genus of enteric bacilli, found in intestines and decaying material, causing protein decomposition.

   P. morganii. May cause urinary tract infections and acute enteritis.

   P. vulgaris. An essentially saprophytic form, but may produce urinary tract infections.

prothesis (prŏth′ē-sĭs) [Gr. *protithenai*, to add to]. Replacement by an artificial part. SYN: *prosthesis.*

prothrombase (prō-thrŏm′bās) [Gr. *pro*, before, + *thrombos*, a clot]. A substance which becomes a fibrin ferment when activated by thrombokinase. SYN: *prothrombin; thrombogen.*

prothrom′bin. A chem. substance existing in circulating blood, and which, through the medium of thrombokinase, interacts with calcium salts to produce thrombin. SYN: *thrombogen.*

prothrom″bine′mia. Presence of prothrombin in the blood.

prothrombinopenia (prō-thrŏm″bĭ-nō-pē′nĭ-ă). Deficiency of prothrombin in the blood. SYN: *hypoprothrombinemia.*

Protis′ta [L., simplest organisms]. Term applied to kingdom of organisms including the simpler animals and plants characterized by being acellular or unicellular. Includes bacteria, some algae, spirochetes, protozoa, and other forms not easily classified as being either plants or animals.

protistologist (prō-tĭs-tŏl′ō-jĭst) ["+ *logos*, study]. One who studies the Protista, the unicellular organisms.

protistology (prō-tĭs-tŏl′ō-jĭ). The science of Protista or unicellular plants and microorganisms. SYN: *microbiology.*

proto- [Gr. *prōtos*, first]. 1. Prefix signifying first. 2. The lowest of a series of compounds having the same elements.

protobiology (prō″tō-bĭ-ŏl′ō-jĭ) ["+ *bios*, life, + *logos*, study]. The phase of science dealing with forms more minute than bacteria, i.e., the ultraviruses and bacteriophages.

protoblast (prō′tō-blăst) ["+ *blastos*, a germ]. 1. A naked cell with no cell wall yet formed. 2. Blastomere of segmenting ovum which is parent cell of a part or organ.

protoblastic (prō″tō-blăs′tĭk). Pert. to a protoblast.

protocol (prō′tō-kŏl) [Gr. *prōtokollon*, first notes glued to manuscript]. 1. A clinical report from first notes taken. 2. Minutes of a meeting. 3. Description of steps taken in an experiment.

protodiastole (prō″tō-dī-ăs′tō-lĭ) [Gr. *prōtos*, first, + *diastolē*, expansion]. The first of four phases of ventricular diastole characterized by drop in intraventricular pressure and closure of semilunar valves. Occurs immediately after second heart sound.

protogala (prō-tŏg′ă-lă) ["+ *gala*, milk]. A mother's first milk after birth of a child. SYN: *colostrum*.

protogaster (prō″tō-găs′ter) ["+ *gastēr*, belly]. The archenteron or gastrocele; the cavity in a gastrula or developing embryo from which the digestive tract develops.

protoleukocyte (prō″tō-lū′kō-sīt) [Gr. *prōtos*, first, + *leukos*, white, + *kytos*, cell]. A minute lymphoid cell in red bone marrow and in the spleen.

Protomastigida (prō″tō-măst-ij′ĭ-dă) ["+ *mastix*, whip, + *eidos*, form]. An order of flagellate protozoa. It contains several pathogenic forms including Leishmania and Trypanosoma.

proton (prō′tŏn) [Gr., first]. A positively charged particle forming the nucleus of hydrogen and present in the nuclei of all elements, the atomic number of the element indicating the number of protons present. Its mass is 1836 times that of an electron. SEE: *atom; atomic theory; electron; element*.

pro″topath′ic ["+ *pathos*, suffering]. Primitive, undiscriminating. SEE: *sensibility*.

protoplasia (prō-tō-plā′zĭ-ă) ["+ *plassein*, to form]. The primary formation of tissue.

protoplasm (prō′tō-plăzm) [Gr. *prōtos*, first, + *plasma*, a thing formed]. A thick, viscous colloidal substance which constitutes the physical basis of all living activities, exhibiting the properties of assimilation, growth, motility, secretion, irritability, and reproduction. It is a complex mixture of heterogeneous substances surrounded by an invisible membrane that regulates the interchange of substances with the surrounding medium. It possesses the physical properties of a colloidal mass, the medium of dispersion being water.

It consists of inorganic substances (water, mineral compounds) and organic substances (proteins, carbohydrates, and lipids). The principal elements present are oxygen, carbon, hydrogen, nitrogen, calcium, and phosphorus which comprise about 99% of protoplasm. Others present in small amounts are potassium, sulfur, chlorine, sodium, magnesium, iron together with trace elements (copper, cobalt, manganese, zinc, and others).

RS: cell; cytoplasm; nucleus.

protoplasmic (prō-tō-plăz′mĭk). Pert. to protoplasm, or composed of it.

protoplast (prō′tō-plăst) [Gr. *prōtos*, first, + *plassein*, to form]. 1. A cell. 2. A mass of protoplasm. SYN: *protoplasm*.

protoporphyrin (prō″tō-pŏr′fĭ-rĭn). $C_{34}H_{34}$-N_4O_4, a derivative of hemoglobin containing four pyrrole nuclei. Formed from heme (ferriprotoporphyrin) by deletion of an atom of iron. Occurs naturally.

protoproteose (prō″tō-prō′tē-ōz). A primary proteose which, upon further digestion, is converted to deuteroproteose.

protospasm (prō′tō-spăzm) [Gr. *prōtos*, first, + *spasmos*, a spasm]. A spasm beginning in one area and extending to other parts.

prototoxin (prō″tō-tŏks′ĭn) ["+ *toxikon*, poison]. Dissociation product of a toxin having greatest affinity for the antitoxin.

prototrophic (prō″tō-trō′fĭk) ["+ *trophē*, nourishment]. Requiring simple inorganic elements as food.

protovertebra (prō″tō-vĕr′tē-bră) [Gr. *prōtos*, first, + L. *vertebra*, vertebra]. Primitive vertebra in the notochord. SYN: *metamere; somite*.

Protozo′a ["+ *zōon*, animal]. The phylum of the animal kingdom which includes the simplest animals. Most are unicellular, although some are colonial. Reproduction usually asexual by fission, although conjugation and sexual reproduction occur.

protozoacide (prō-tō-zō′ă-sĭd) [Gr. *prōtos*, first, + *zōon*, animal, + L. *cidus*, kill]. Destructive to, or that which kills, protozoa.

protozoal (prō″tō-zō′ăl). Pert. to protozoa, unicellular organisms.

p. diseases. Those produced by single-celled organisms. Ex: amebic dysentery, sleeping sickness, and malaria.

protozoology (prō″tō-zō-ŏl′ō-jĭ) [Gr. *prōtos*, first, + *zōon*, animal, + *logos*, study]. Phase of science dealing with study of protozoa.

pro″tozo′on. (pl. *protozoa*) Unicellular organism. SEE: *protozoa*.

protozoophage (prō″tō-zō′ō-fāj) [Gr. *prōtos*, first, + *zōon*, animal, + *phagein*, to eat]. A phagocyte which ingests protozoa.

protractor (prō-trăk′tŏr) [L. *prōtractus*, dragged out]. 1. Instrument for removing foreign bodies from wounds. 2. A muscle that draws a part forward. Opposed to retractor.

protrude [L. *prōtrūdere*]. To project; to extend beyond a border or limit.

protrusion (prō-trū′zhŭn). State or condition of being thrust forward or projecting.

protuberance (prō-tū′bĕr-ans) [Gr. *pro*, before, + L. *tuber*, bulge]. A part that is prominent beyond a surface, like a knob.

proud flesh. A mass of excessive granulation formed when a wound shows no other sign of healing or tendency to cicatrization.

provisional (prō-vĭzh′ŭn-ăl) [L. *prōvīsiō*, provision]. Serving a temporary use pending

Table of Pathogenic Protozoa

Subphylum	Genus and Species	Disease Caused
Mastigophora	*Borrelia recurrentis*	Relapsing fever
Locomotion by flagella	*Borrelia duttonii*	Relapsing fever
	Borrelia bronchialis	Bronchial infection
	Borrelia vincentii	Vincent's disease
	Leptospira icterohaemorrhagiae	Weil's disease
	Leishmania donovani	Kala-azar
	Leishmania braziliensis	American leishmaniasis
	Leishmania tropica	Oriental sore
	Giardia lamblia	Intestinal disturbances
	Trypanosoma gambiense	Sleeping sickness
	Trypanosoma rhodesiense	Sleeping sickness
	Trypanosoma cruzi	Chagas' disease
Sarcodina	*Entamoeba histolytica*	Amebic dysentery
Locomotion by pseudopodia	*Dientamoeba fragilis*	Diarrhea, fever
Sporozoa	*Plasmodium malariae*	Quartan malaria
No locomotion in adult stage	*Plasmodium falciparum*	Malignant tertian malaria
	Plasmodium vivax	Benign tertian malaria
	Plasmodium ovale	Ovale malaria
Ciliophora Possess cilia in some stage of life cycle	*Balantidium coli*	Balantidiasis

permanent arrangements.

provitamin (prō-vī′tă-mĭn) [L. *pro*, before, + *vita*, life, + *amine*]. An inactive substance that can be transformed in the body to a corresponding active vitamin and thus function as a vitamin.

    p. A. Carotene, the precursor of vitamin A.

proximad (prŏk′sĭm-ăd) [L. *proximus*, next, + *ad*, toward]. Toward the proximal or central point.

proximal (prŏk′sĭm-ăl). Nearest the point of attachment, center of the body, or point of reference. Opposed to distal.

proximate (prŏk′sĭm-āt). Closely related with respect to space, time, or sequence. Next to, or nearest.

proximoataxia (prŏk″sĭ-mō-ă-tak′sĭ-ă) [L. *proximus*, nearest, + Gr. *ataxia*, lack of order]. Lack of coordination in muscles of the proximal area of an extremity, as the arm, forearm, thigh, or leg.

pro′zone. That portion of the low dilution range of a homologous serum that fails to agglutinate bacteria that are agglutinated by the same serum in a higher dilution.

prozymogen (prō-zī′mō-jĕn) [Gr. *pro*, before, + *zymē*, leaven, + *gennan*, to produce]. An intranuclear substance that becomes zymogen. SYN: *prezymogen*.

prune (prūn) [L. *pruna*]. A dried plum, rich in carbohydrate. Contains a substance which is useful in stimulating the bowel, esp. for those who suffer from chronic constipation. The ability of prunes and prune juice to exert a laxative effect is due to the presence of dihydroxyphenyl isatin.

    Food value of 100 gm. (cooked, unsweetened): Cal. 119; protein 0.8 gm.; fat 0.3 gm.; carbohydrate 31 gm.; calcium 24 mg.; vitamin A, 750 I.U.

prune-belly defect. A nonstandard, but descriptive, term for children with congenital absence of abdominal muscles.

pruriginous (prū-rĭj′ĭ-nŭs) [L. *prurigō*, itch]. Pert. to, or of the nature of, prurigo.

prurigo (prū-rī′gō) [L., the itch]. This term is used by dermatologists throughout the world, but it has not received a universally-acceptable definition. P. is a chronic skin disease marked by constantly-recurring, discrete, pale, deep-seated, intensely-itchy papules on extensor surfaces of limbs. Superimposed exanthematous manifestations may mask the true nature.

ETIOL: Exciting cause unknown. Hygienic factors are supplementary.

PROG: Guarded. P. begins in childhood and may last a lifetime.

TREATMENT: Constitutional and local. Hygienic regimen. Antipruritics locally.

p. estivalis. A form of polymorphic light eruption characterized by prurigo and photodermatitis. Recurring every summer and continuing during hot weather.

p. nodularis. Eruption in skin of hard nodules with great itching. Occurs most commonly in middle-aged women.

ETIOL: Unknown.

p., pregnancy. A form which usually has its onset in the middle trimester of pregnancy or later. The lesions occur on the proximal portion of the limbs and upper part of the trunk. The skin lesions usually improve spontaneously before term or rapidly after delivery.

p., simple acute. Simple form of p. with recurring tendency. Thought to be caused by reaction to bites in sensitive subjects.

pruritus (prū-rī'tŭs) [L., itching]. Severe itching. May be symptomatic, or occur idiopathically as a neurosis without structural change.

ETIOL: Predisposing factor is cutaneous hyperesthesia. Localized causes are present in pruritus ani, pruritus vulvae, focal infection, intestinal parasites (pinworms), mycotic infection, bath itch, etc.

TREATMENT: Exciting or contributory cause located and removed. Hygienic regimen. Pilocarpine, phenacetin, bromide. In anal and vulvar pruritus, examination by competent gynecologist or proctologist before cutaneous therapy is instituted. In bath avoid too sudden changes of temperature. For dry skins, avoid frequent soap and water bathing. Soft, nonirritating underclothing, soothing lotions, oil rubs, antipruritics.

p. ani. Itching about the anus. May be due to pinworms, fistula in anus, hemorrhoids, contact with soap or detergents that remain in underclothing following improper washing, or irritation.

p., essential. P. without apparent skin lesion.

p. estivalis. P. with prickly heat occurring in hot weather. SYN: *summer itch.*

p. hiemalis. Winter itch. Occurs in cold weather and is provoked by cooling of the skin.

p. senilis. P. in aged with degenerative skin changes.

p., symptomatic. P. as a symptom of some other disorder.

p. vulvae. Disorder marked by severe itching of external female genitalia. Often an early sign of diabetes mellitus. May be sign of vaginitis.

Prussak's space (prŭ'săk). [Alexander Prussak, Russ. otologist, 1839-1897]. Tiny space in middle ear between Shrapnell's membrane laterally and neck of malleus medially.

prussic acid (prŭs'ĭk). A violent and rapid poison. SYN: *acid, hydrocyanic,* q.v.

psalterium (săl-tē'rĭ-ŭm) [Gr. *psaltērion,* harp]. A transverse band of fibers that connect the crura of the fornix immediately posterior to the body of the fornix. SYN: *hippocampal fissure; lyre.*

psammoma (săm-ō'mă) [Gr. *psammos,* sand, + *-ōma,* tumor]. A small tumor of the brain, the choroid plexus, and other areas, containing calcareous particles.

p. bodies. Laminated concretions often found in the pineal body. SYN: *brain sand; corpora arenacea.*

psammosarcoma (săm"ō-sar-kō'mă) ["+ *sarx,* flesh, + *-ōma,* tumor]. A sarcoma in which psammoma bodies are present.

psammotherapy (săm"ō-thĕr'ă-pī) ["+ *therapeia,* treatment]. The application of sand baths in treatment.

psammous (săm'ŭs). Sandy, gritty.

pselaphesia, pselaphesis (sĕl-ă-fē'zĭ-ă, -sĭs) [Gr. *pselaphēsis,* touch]. 1. Sense of touch. 2. Plucking at bedclothes with the fingers, a sign observed in delirium. SYN: *carphology.*

psellism, psellismus (sĕl'ĭzm, sĕl-ĭz'mŭs) [Gr. *psellisma,* stammer]. Defective pronunciation, stuttering, or stammering.

p. mercurialis. Jerking, hurried, unintelligible speech in mercurial tremor.

pseudacousma (sū"dă-kūz'mă) [Gr. *pseudēs,* false, + *akousma,* a thing heard]. Condition in which all sounds are heard falsely, seeming to be altered in quality of pitch, or imaginary sounds are heard.

pseudacusis (sū"dă-kū'sĭs). State in which sounds are heard falsely or imagined. SYN: *pseudacousma.*

pseudagraphia (sū"dă-grăf'ĭ-ă) ["+ *graphein,* to write]. A form of agraphia in which a person is unable to write independently, but is able to copy words or letters. SYN: *pseudoagraphia.*

pseudaphia (sū-dā'fī-ă) [Gr. *pseudēs*, false, + *haphē*, touch]. A false or defective perception of touch. SEE: *paraphia; pseudesthesia.*

pseudarthritis (sū"dăr-thrī'tĭs) ["+ *arthron*, joint, + *-ītis*, inflammation]. Hysterical disease of the joints.

pseudarthrosis (sū"dăr-thrō'sĭs) ["+ "+ *-ōsis*, disease]. A false joint developing after a fracture that has not united.

pseudesthesia (sū"dĕs-thē'zĭ-ă) ["+ *aisthēsis*, sensation]. 1. An imaginary or false sensation, as that after amputation felt in the lost part. 2. Sense of feeling not caused by external stimulation. SEE: *paraphia; pseudaphia.*

pseudo- (sū'dō) [Gr. *pseudēs*, false]. A prefix meaning false.

pseudoagglutination (sū"dō-ă-glū"tĭ-nā'shŭn). The clumping together of red blood cells as in the formation of rouleaux, but differing from true agglutination in that they can be dispersed by shaking.

pseudoagraphia. Pseudagraphia, q.v.

pseudoalbinism (sū"dō-ăl'bĭ-nizm) [Gr. *pseudēs*, false, + L. *albus*, white, + Gr. *-ismos*, condition]. Loss of pigment of the skin as occurs in leukopathia or vitiligo.

pseudoanemia (sū"dō-ă-nē'mĭ-ă) ["+ *an-*, negative, + *haima*, blood]. Pallor of mucous membranes and skin without other signs of true anemia.

pseudoangina (sū"dō-ăn'jĭ-na, -ăn-jī'nă) ["+ L. *angina*, a choking]. False symptoms of nervous origin, resembling angina pectoris.

SYM: Functional attacks in cardiac region but not associated with any disease of the heart or its vessels.

pseudoapoplexy (sū"dō-ăp'ō-plĕk"sī). Condition simulating apoplexy, but not accompanied by cerebral hemorrhage.

pseudoataxia (sū"dō-ă-tăk'sĭ-ă) [Gr. *pseudēs*, false, + *ataxia*, lack of order]. Condition resembling ataxia, but not due to tabes dorsalis. SEE: *pseudotabes.*

pseudobacterium (sū"dō-băk-tē'rĭ-ŭm) ["+ *baktērion*, a little rod]. Any microscopic cell similar to a bacterium.

pseudoblepsia, pseudoblepsis (sū"dō-blĕp'sĭ-ă, -sĭs) ["+ *blepsis*, sight]. False or imaginary vision. SYN: *parablepsia; pseudopsia.*

pseudobulbar paralysis (sū"dō-bŭl'bĕr) ["+ *bolbos*, a swollen end]. Paralysis resembling bulbar paralysis, but due to lesion of cortical centers.

pseudocartilaginous (sū"dō-kăr"tĭ-lăj'ĭ-nŭs) [Gr. *pseudēs*, false, + L. *cartilāgō*, gristle]. Pert. to, or formed of, a substance resembling cartilage.

pseudocast (sū'dō-kăst) ["+ ME. *casten*, a throwing off]. A sediment in urine resembling a true cast; a false cast.

pseudocele (sū'dō-sēl) ["+ *koilos*, hollow]. The cavity of the septum pellucidum, the so-called 5th ventricle. SYN: *cavum sept. pellucidi* [NA]; *pseudocoele.*

pseudocholinesterase (sū"dō-kō"lĭn-ĕs'tĕr-ās). A nonspecific cholinesterase that hydrolyzes noncholine esters as well as acetylcholine. Found in blood serum and pancreatic tissue.

pseudochorea (sū"dō-kō-rē'ă) [Gr. *pseudēs*, false, + *choreia*, a dance]. Hysterical state resembling chorea. SYN: *spurious chorea.*

pseudochromesthesia (sū"dō-krō"mĕs-thē'zĭ-ă) ["+ *chrōma*, color, + *aisthēsis*, sensation]. A condition in which sounds, esp. of the vowels, seem to induce a sensation of a distinct visual color. SEE: *phonism; photism.*

pseudochromidrosis (sū"dō-krō"mĭd-rō'sĭs) ["+ "+ *hidrōs*, perspiration, + *-ōsis*, condition]. Appearance of colored sweat in which the sweat acquires its color after it is excreted.

pseudocirrhosis (sū"dō-sĭr-ō'sĭs) [Gr. *pseudēs*, false, + *kirros*, orange yellow, + *-ōsis*, disease]. A condition with symptoms of cirrhosis of liver, due usually to pericarditis.
SYM: Cyanosis, ascites, dyspnea.

pseudocoele (sū'dō-sēl) ["+ *koilos*, hollow]. The 5th ventricle of brain. SYN: *pseudocele.*

pseudocoloboma (sū"dō-kŏl-ō-bō'mă) ["+ *kolōboma*, imperfection]. A scarcely noticeable scar on the iris from an embryonic fissure.

pseudocrisis (sū-dō-krī'sĭs) [Gr. *pseudēs*, false, + *krisis*, crisis.]. A false crisis; a temporary fall of body temperature which may be followed by a rise.

pseudocroup (sū-dō-krūp'). False croup. SYN: *laryngismus stridulus.*

pseudocyesis (sū"dō-sī-ē'sĭs) [Gr. *pseudēs*, false, + *kyēsis*, pregnancy]. A condition in which a patient has nearly all of the usual signs and symptoms of pregnancy such as enlargement of abdomen, weight gain, cessation of menses, and morning sickness, but is not pregnant.

Usually seen in women who either are very desirous of having children or wish to avoid pregnancy. When the patient is under anesthesia or hypnosis or is asleep, the abdominal enlargement disappears.

Treatment usually is done by psychiatric means. P. also has been reported as occurring in men. SYN: *phantom pregnancy.*

pseudocyst (sū'dō-sĭst) ["+ *kystis*, bladder]. A dilatation resembling a cyst.

seudodementia (sū″dō-dē-měn′shǐ-ă) ["+ L. *de-*, negative, + *mens, ment-*, mind]. Exaggerated indifference to environment without impairment of mental capacity.

seudodiphtheria (sū″dō-dǐf-thē′rǐ-ă) ["+ *diphthera*, membrane]. A condition resembling diphtheria, but not due to Corynebacterium diphtheriae.

seudoedema (sū″dō-ē-dē′mă) [Gr. *pseudēs*, false, + *oidēma*, a swelling]. A puffy condition of the skin simulating edema.

seudoemphysema (sū″dō-ěm-fǐ-zē′mă) ["+ *emphysēma*, an inflation]. A bronchial condition simulating emphysema, due to temporary blockage of the bronchi.

seudoencephalitis (sū″dō-ěn-sěf″ă-lǐ′tǐs) ["+ *enkephalos*, brain, + *-itis*, inflammation]. A false encephalitis due to profuse diarrhea.

pseudoerysipelas (sū″dō-ěr-ǐ-sǐp′ě-lăs) [Gr. *pseudēs*, false, + *erythros*, red, + *pella*, skin]. An inflammation of subcutaneous cellular tissue simulating erysipelas.

pseudoesthesia (sū″dō-ěs-thē′zǐ-ă) ["+ *aisthēsis*, sensation]. An imaginary sensation or a false one. SYN: *pseudesthesia*.

pseudofracture (sū″dō-frăk′chŭr). A ribbonlike zone of decalcification seen in certain types of osteomalacia.

pseudoganglion (sū″dō-găn′glǐ-ŏn) [Gr. *pseudēs*, false, + *gagglion*, knot]. A slight thickening of a nerve, resembling a ganglion.

pseudogeusesthesia (sū″dō-gūs″ěs-thē′zǐ-ă) ["+ *geusis*, taste, + *aisthēsis*, sensation]. A sense of taste stimulated by one of the other senses.

pseudogeusia (sū″dō-gū′sǐ-ă). A subjective sensation of taste not produced by external stimulus.

pseudoglioma (sū″dō-glǐ-ō′mă) [Gr. *pseudēs*, false, + *glia*, glue, + *-ōma*, tumor]. Inflammatory changes occurring in the vitreous body which simulate glioma of retina, but due to iridochoroiditis.

pseudoglobulin (sū″dō-glŏb′ū-lǐn) ["+ L. *globulus*, little globe]. One of a class of globulins characterized by being soluble in salt-free water. SEE: *euglobulin*.

pseudoglottis (sū″dō-glŏt′ǐs) ["+ *glōttis*, glottis]. Area between false vocal cords.

pseudogout (sū′dō-gout″). Recurrent acute attacks of chronic arthritis which resembles gout. It is due to deposition of crystals of calcium pyrophosphate dihydrate in the joint space.

TREATMENT: Aspiration of affected joint and phenylbutazone therapy if salicylates do not control the pain. SYN: *chondrocalcinosis*.

pseudohemoptysis (sū″dō-hē-mŏp′tǐ-sǐs) [Gr. *pseudēs*, false, + *haima*, blood, + *ptyein*, to spit]. Spitting of blood which does not arise from the bronchi or the lungs.

pseudohermaphroditism (sū″dō-hěr-măf′rō-dǐt″ǐzm) ["+ *Hermaphroditos*, mythical two-sexed god]. A congenital abnormality of the external genitalia and of the body in which one resembles the other sex. SEE: *intersex*.

p., female. Condition in a female marked by a large clitoris, resembling the penis, and hypertrophied labia majora, resembling the scrotum, thus resembling a male. Can be caused by disease of the adrenal gland.

p., male. Condition in a male marked by a small penis, perineal hypospadias, and scrotum without testes, thereby resembling the vulva. Can be due to disease of the adrenal or condition of feminizing testis.

pseudohypertrophic (sū″dō-hī-pěr-trō′fǐk) [Gr. *pseudēs*, false, + *hyper*, above, + *trophē*, nourishment]. Pert. to a false hypertrophy.

p. paralysis. Paralysis with enlargement and loss of motion of muscles.

pseudohypertrophy (sū″dō-hī-pěr′trō-fǐ). Increase in size of an organ or structure due to hypertrophy or hyperplasia of tissue other than parenchyma. Often accompanied by diminution of function.

pseudohypoparathyroidism. Hereditary disease resembling hypoparathyroidism but caused by an inadequate response to parathyroid hormone rather than a deficiency of the hormone. Some, but not all, of the patients will be obese with short, stocky build and moonfaced. Mental deficiency may be present along with cataracts, strabismus, tetany, stridor, convulsions, and muscular cramps.

pseudoisochromatic (sū″dō-ī″sō-kro-măt′ǐk) [Gr. *pseudēs*, false, + *isos*, equal, + *chroma*, color]. Seemingly of the same color; colors used in charts testing for color blindness.

pseudologia (sū-dō-lō′jǐ-ă) [Gr. *pseudēs*, false, + *logos*, a study]. Falsification in writing or in speech, a form of pathological lying.

p. fantastica. Pathological lying; one of the forms of the psychopathic state.

pseudomania (sū-dō-mā′nǐ-ă) ["+ *mania*, madness]. 1. A psychosis in which the patient falsely accuses himself of crimes which he thinks he has committed. 2. Pathological lying.

pseudomasturbation (sū″dō-măs-tŭr-bā′shŭn) ["+ L. *manus*, hand, + *stuprare*, to rape]. A nervous habit of pulling at the penis. SYN: *peotillomania*.

pseudomelanosis (sū″dō-měl-ā-nō′sĭs) [Gr. *pseudēs*, false, + *melas, melan-*, black, + *-ōsis*, disease]. Discoloration of tissues after death.

pseudomembrane (sū″dō-měm′brān) ["+ L. *membrana*, membrane]. A false membrane, as in diphtheria.

pseudomembranous (sū″dō-měm′brā-nŭs). Pert. to, or marked by, false membranes.

pseudomeningitis (sū″dō-měn-ĭn-jī′tĭs) [Gr. *pseudēs*, false, + *mēninx*, membrane, + *-itis*, inflammation]. A condition resembling symptoms of meningitis without lesions of meningeal inflammation.

pseudomenstruation (sū″dō-měn″strū-ā′shŭn) ["+ L. *menstruare*, menstruate]. Bleeding from the uterus not accompanied by the usual changes in the endometrium.

pseudomnesia (sū″dōm-nē′zĭ-ă) ["+ *mnēsis*, memory]. A memory perversion in which patient remembers that which never occurred.

Pseudomonas (sū-dō-mō′năs) [Gr. *pseudēs*, false, + *monas*, single]. A genus of small, motile, gram-negative bacilli with polar flagella. Most are saprophytic living in soil and decomposing organic matter. Some produce blue and yellow pigments.

   P. aeruginosa. A species which is sometimes pathogenic for man. May cause urinary tract infections or otitis externa.

pseudomucin (sū-dō-mū′sĭn) [Gr. *pseudēs*, false, + L. *mucus*, mucus]. A variety of mucin found in ovarian cysts.

pseudomyxoma (sū″dō-mĭk-sō′mă) ["+ *myxa*, mucus, + *-ōma*, tumor]. A peritoneal tumor resembling a myxoma and containing a thick viscid fluid.

   p. peritonei. A type of tumor developing in peritoneum from implantation metastases resulting from rupture of ovarian cystadenoma or cells escaping during surgical removal. Numerous papillomas develop attached to abdominal wall and intestine, and peritoneal cavity becomes filled with mucuslike fluid.

pseudoneoplasm (sū-dō-nē′ō-plăsm) ["+ *neos*, new, + *plasm*, something formed]. A false or phantom tumor. A temporary swelling that simulates a tumor, usually of an inflammatory nature.

pseudoneuroma (sū″dō-nū-rō′mă) [Gr. *pseudēs*, false, + *neuron*, sinew, + *-ōma*, tumor]. A mass of interlacing, coiled nerve fibers, cells of Schwann, and fibrous tissue forming a mass at end of amputation stump. Also called amputation or traumatic neuroma. It is not a true neuroma. SYN: *neurofibroma*.

pseudonuclein (sū″dō-nū′klē-ĭn) ["+ L. *nucleus*, a nut]. A combination of albumin with metaphosphoric acid. SYN: *paranuclein*.

pseudonucleolus (sū″dō-nū-klē-ōl′ŭs). The false nucleolus or karyosome.

pseudoparalysis (sū″dō-pă-răl′ĭ-sĭs) [Gr. *pseudēs*, false, + *para*, at the side, + *lyein*, to loosen]. A loss of muscular power not due to lesion of the nervous system.

pseudoparaplegia (sū″dō-păr-ă-plē′jĭ-ă) ["+ "+ *plēgē*, a stroke]. Seeming paralysis of the lower extremities without impairment of the reflexes.

pseudoparasite (sū″dō-păr′ă-sīt) ["+ "+ *sitos*, food]. 1. Anything resembling a parasite. 2. Organism that can live as a parasite, although it is normally not one. SEE: *parasite, facultative*.

pseudoparesis (sū″dō-păr-ē′sĭs, -păr′ĕ-sĭs) ["+ *paresis*, relaxation]. A condition simulating paresis, but unlike the ordinary forms, and due to hysteria.

Pseudophyllidea (sū″dō-fĭ-lĭd′ē-ă). An order belonging to the class Cestoidea, subclass Cestoda. Includes tapeworms with scolex bearing two lateral (or one terminal) sucking grooves (bothria). Includes Diphyllobothrium, the fish tapeworm of man.

pseudoplegia (sū″dō-plē′jĭ-ă) [Gr. *pseudēs*, false, + *plēgē*, a stroke]. Paralysis of hysterical origin. SYN: *pseudoparalysis*.

pseudopod (sū′dō-pŏd) ["+ *pous, pod-*, foot]. Temporary protruding protoplasmic process in protozoa for the purpose of taking up food and aiding in locomotion. SYN: *pseudopodium*.

pseudopodium (sū″dō-pō′dĭ-ŭm). (pl. *pseudopodia*) 1. A temporary protruding process of a protozoan or an ameboid cell, such as a leukocyte, that aids in locomotion and the engulfing of food particles or foreign substances, as in phagocytosis. SYN: *pseudopod*, 2. An irregular projection at the edge of a wheal.

pseudopregnancy (sū″dō-prěg′năn-sī) [Gr. *pseudēs*, false, + L. *praegnans*, with child]. 1. Condition occurring in lower animals following sterile matings in which anatomical and physiological changes occur similar to those of pregnancy. 2. Phantom pregnancy, q.v. SEE: *pseudocyesis*.

pseudopsia (sū-dŏp′sĭ-ă) ["+ *opsis*, vision]. Visual hallucinations or false perceptions. SYN: *pseudoblepsis*.

pseudoptosis (sū-dō-tō′sĭs) ["+ *ptōsis*, fall]. Apparent ptosis of the eyelid, resulting from fold of skin or fat projecting below edge of eyelid.

pseudorabies (sū″dō-rā′bēz, -rā′bĭ-ēz) [Gr. *pseudēs*, false, + L. *rabere*, to rage]. A condition resembling rabies. SYN: *lyssophobia*.

pseudoreaction (sū″dō-rē-ăk′shŭn). A false reaction. A response to injection of a test substance into the tissues, due to presence of an allergen other than one for which test is made.

pseudorubella (sū″dō-rū-bĕl′ă). Roseola infantum, q.v.

pseudoscarlatina (sū″dō-skăr-lă-tē′nă). A septic febrile condition with rash resembling scarlatina.

pseudosclerosis (sū″dō-sklē-rō′sĭs) [Gr. *pseudēs*, false, + *sklērōsis*, a hardening]. A condition with the symptoms, but without the lesions, of multiple sclerosis of the nervous system.

pseudosmia (sū-dŏz′mĭ-ă) [″+ *osmē*, smell]. An olfactory hallucination or perversion of the sense of smell.

pseudostoma (sū-dŏs′tō-mă) [″+ *stoma*, a mouth]. An apparent aperture between endothelial cells that have been stained.

pseudostratified (sū-dō-străt′ĭ-fīd) [Gr. *pseudēs*, false, + L. *strata*, sheets]. Apparently composed of layers.

   p. epithelium. E. in which basal ends of all cells rest on basement membrane but distal ends may or may not reach the surface. Their nuclei lie at different levels, giving the appearance of being stratified.

pseudosyphilis (sū″dō-sĭf′ĭ-lĭs). A nonspecific condition resembling syphilis.

pseudotabes (sū″dō-tā′bēz) [Gr. *pseudēs*, false, + L. *tabēs*, a wasting]. A neural disease simulating tabes dorsalis.

pseudotetanus (sū″dō-tĕt′ă-nŭs) [″+ *tetanos*, tension]. Persistent muscular contractions resembling tetanus.

pseudotuberculosis (sū″dō-tū-ber″kū-lō′sĭs) [″+ L. *tuberculus*, tubercle, + G. *-ōsis*, disease]. Disease resembling tuberculosis, but caused by Pasteurella pseudotuberculosis. The multiple necrotic lesions resemble tubercles grossly but not histologically. Has been erroneously used to indicate infections caused by unclassified or atypical mycobacteria.

pseudotumor cerebri (sū″dō-tū′mŏr sĕr″ĕ-brī). Condition which produces general signs and sym. of brain tumor even though a tumor is not present. SYN: *benign intracranial hypertension.*

pseudotympany (sū″dō-tĭm′pă-nĭ) [Gr. *pseudēs*, false, + *tympanon*, drum]. Flattening of arch of diaphragm and swelling of abdomen with increased respiration. It disappears under anesthesia and is of purely nervous origin. SYN: *accordion abdomen.*

pseudotyphoid (sū″dō-tī′foyd) [″+ *typhos*, fever, + *eidos*, resemblance]. Condition resembling typhoid fever, but not caused by the typhoid bacillus.

pseudoxanthoma (sū″dō-zăn-thō′mă) [″+ *xanthos*, yellow, + *-ōma*, tumor]. Condition resembling xanthoma.

   p. elasticum. Chronic, degenerative cutaneous disease marked by yellow patches and stretching of skin. Associated with hypertension and degeneration of elastic coat of arteries. Angioid streaks in retina common.

psilosis (sī-lō′sĭs) [Gr. *psilōsis*, a stripping]. 1. Falling out or removal of hair. 2. Tropical diarrhea of severe, often fatal form. SYN: *sprue.*

   ETIOL: Disease of pancreas, invasion by bacteria, or sensitivity to gluten in diet.

   SYM: Diarrhea; large, lightly-colored, acid stools containing fat. No pain or tenesmus. Inflamed, eroded, and cracked tongue and mouth.

psittacosis (sĭt-ă-kō′sĭs) [Gr. *psittakos*, parrot, + *-ōsis*, disease]. An infectious disease of parrots and other birds that may be transmitted to man. Tetracyclines, erythromycin, or penicillin are effective in treatment. SYN: *ornithosis.* SEE: *chlamdia.*

   SYM AND SIGNS (in man): Headache, epistaxis, nausea, chill followed by fever, constipation, sometimes pulmonary disorders.

psoas (sō′ăs) [Gr. *psoa*]. One of two muscles of the loins. SEE: *Table of Muscles* in *Appendix.*

   p. abscess. A cold abscess in sheath of the psoas major muscle. It follows the sheath of this muscle until it reaches the surface and points. Generally it occurs above Poupart's ligament in the iliac fossa, or near the attachment of the psoas muscle to the femur.

   ETIOL: Usually tuberculous disease of vertebrae accompanied by pus.

psoitis (sō-ī′tĭs) [Gr. *psoa*, muscle of the loin, + *-itis*, inflammation]. Inflammation of the psoas muscles or of the area of the loins.

psora (sō′ră) [Gr., itch]. 1. An itching disease of the skin; scabies. 2. Psoriasis, an erythematous, scaling, cutaneous eruption.

psorelcosis (sō″rĕl-kō′sĭs) [″+ *helkōsis*, ulceration]. Ulceration occurring as a result of scabies.

psoriasis (sō-rī′ă-sĭs) [Gr. *psōriasis*, an itching]. A common, genetically-determined dermatitis consisting of discrete pink or

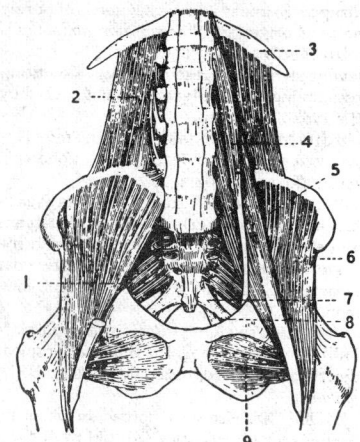

PSOAS, ILIACUS, AND
QUADRATUS LUMBORUM
1, Pyriformis. 2, Quadratus lumborum. 3,
Twelfth rib. 4, Psoas minor. 5, Psoas major. 6,
Iliacus. 7, Sarcospinous ligament. 8, Sarco-
tuberous ligament. 9, Obturator externus.

dull-red lesions surmounted by characteristic silvery scaling. Lesions may become
confluent. Although they come and go, they
usually are chronic. A specific type of arthritis frequently is associated with the disease.

ETIOL: Unknown.

SYM: May begin at any age as flat-topped
papule covered with thin, grayish-white
scale spreading peripherally; lesions coalescing; centers regressing, forming circinate lesions. Under the dry scales are red
bleeding points (papillae).

TREATMENT: General and nonspecific
measures are utilized to give comfort to the
patient as well as to help control the disease.
There is no cure for the disease.

p., elephantine. A rare, but persistent,
p. which occurs on the back, thighs, and hips
in thick scaling plaques.

p., guttate. Characterized by small, distinct lesions that generally occur over the
body. Appear particularly in the young
following acute streptococcal infections.

p., nummular. The most common form
of p. with discs and plaques of varying sizes
on the extremities and trunk. There may be
a great number of lesions, or a solitary
lesion.

p., rupioid. P. with hyperkeratotic lesions on the feet.

psorophthalmia (sō″rŏf-thăl′mĭ-ă) [Gr.].
Marginal inflammation of the eyelids with
ulceration.

psorous (sō′rŭs) [Gr. *psōros*]. Rel. to, or affected with, itch.

P.S.P. Abbr. for *phenolsulfonphthalein;* a
substance used to test kidney function.

psychagogy (sī″kă-gō′jē) [Gr. *psyche*, soul,
mind, + *agein*, to lead]. A psychotherapeutic, reeducational procedure which stresses
proper social adjustment of the individual.

psychalgia (sī-kăl′jĭ-ă) ["+ *algos*, pain]. 1.
Mental distress or pain, esp. in melancholia.
2. Pain of hysterical origin.

psychanalysis (sī-kăn-ăl′ĭ-sĭs) ["+ *analysis*,
breaking apart]. Discovery of the pathogenic
links between the objective and subjective
consciousness by a system of recall. SYN:
psychoanalysis, q.v.

psychanopsia (sī-kăn-ŏp′sĭ-ă) ["+ *an-*, not,
+ *opsis*, vision]. Sight with failure to recognize anything seen, due to brain lesion.
SYN: *psychic blindness*.

psychataxia (sī″kă-tăk′sĭ-ă) [Gr. *psyche*,
soul, + *ataxia*, lack of order]. Disordered
power of concentration.

psychauditory (sĭk-ŏ′dĭ-tor-ĭ) ["+ L.
auditorius, hearing]. Pert. to the perception
and interpretation of sounds.

psyche (sī′kē) [Gr. *psyche*, soul, mind]. All
that constitutes the mind and its processes.

psychedelic (sī″kĕ-dĕl′ĭk) ["+ *delos*, mani-
fest]. Originally used in 1963 to mean mind-
manifesting. Now used by lay persons to
describe some of the subjective aspects of
intoxication, particularly with a drug such
as lysergic acid diethylamide (LSD), or other
psychotogenic medicines.

psychiatric (sī-kĭ-ă′trĭk) ["+ *iatrikos*, heal-
ing]. Pert. to psychiatry, the science concerned with the study, diagnosis, and
prevention of mental illness.

psychiatrist (sī-kī′ă-trĭst). A physician who
specializes in study, treatment, and prevention of mental disorders.

psychiatry (sī-kī′ă-trĭ). The branch of medicine which deals with diagnosis, treatment,
and prevention of mental illness.

psychiatry, words pert. to: abalienatio
mentis; abalienation; aberration; abnormality; abreaction; abulia; acatalepsia; acatamathesia; acataphasia; acousma; acous-
matagnosis; acousmatamnesia; acrasia;
affect; agnosia; agraphia; agrypnia;
ahypnia; akathisia; akinesia; alcoholism;
alexia; algesia; algolagnia; algopsychalia;
alienation; alienism; alienist; alliteration;
allophasis; allopsychic; allotropic; Alzheimer's disease; ambitendency; ambivalence;
amentia; amimia; amnesia; amnestic; amok;

amoralia; amusia; anaclitic choice; anacroasia; anal erotism; ananabasia; ananastasia; anandria; anergastic reaction; anhedonia; anoesia; anoia; anomia; anorexia; apandria; apanthropia; apastia; apathy; aphasia; aphemesthesia; aphemia; aphonia; aphrasia; aphrenia; aphronesia; aphthenxia; apodemialgia; apraxia; aprosexia; apsithyria; apsychosis; asemia; asitia; association; assonance; astereognosis; asyllabia; asymbolia; asynesia; atactilia; atavism; ataxaphasia; ataxia, intrapsychic; ataxophemia; ateliosis; athymia; attitude; autism; autistic child; autoanalysis; automatism; autoecholalia; autophagia; autophilia; autophobia; autoplastic; autopsychosis; autosuggestion; autosynnoia; avulsion; behaviorism; blocking; bradylalia; bradylexia; brain storm; catatonia; catharsis; cenesthesia; censor; chorea; claustrophilia; claustrophobia; complex; compulsion; conation; condensation; confabulation; conflict; constellation; coprolagnia; coprolalia; coprophilia; cretinism; cryptesthesia; cycloid; cyclothymia; deafness; delire de toucher; delirium; delusion; dementia; depersonalization; depression; dereistic; determinism; disorientation; displacement; dissociation; distractibility; divagation; dysbulia; dyschiria; dyscinesia; dysmnesia; dysphrenia; dysthymia; echolalia; echomimia; ego; egocentric; ekphorize; emotion; emotivity; empathy; eremophobia; erethism; ergasiomania; ergasiophobia; erotism; erotomania; erythrophobia; eschrolalia; eviration; exhibitionism; extrovert; fabrication; fastidium; fear; feeblemindedness; fixation; folie; free association; fugue; furor amatorius; Ganser's syndrome; geophagia; graphorrhea; hallucination; hallucinosis; haphalgesia; hebephrenia; heterolalia; holergastic; hyperhedonia; hyperprosexia; hypersthenia; hyperthymia; hypnagogic; hypnoidal; hypnosis; hypnotic; hypnotism; hypochondria; hypochondriac; hypochondriasis; hypophrenia; hysteria; idea; idiocy; idiot; idiotropic type; illusion; image; imago; imbecile; imperious acts; impulsion; incoherence; incompetent; infantilism; inhibition; insanity; instinct; integration; intelligence; intrapsychic; introjection; introversion; introvert; katatonia; kinesthesia; Korsakoff's psychosis; latent content; lethargy; lethologica; logamnesia; logopathia; logorrhea; malingerer; masochism; melancholia; mesmerism; mind; misocainea; misologia; misopedia; moramentia; moria; moron; morosis; narcissism; narcotism; necrophilaus; necrophilism; negativism; neologism; neurosis; noctambulism; non compos

mentis; nookleptia; nunnation; object choice; obsession; oligergasia; oligopnea; omnipotence of thought; oneiric; oneirism; oneirodynia; organic psychoses; orthopsychiatry; overdetermination; overtone; paragraphia; paralexia; paralogia; paramimia; paramnesia; paranoia; paranomia; parapathia; paraphasia; paraphonia; parapraxis; parent fixation; paresis; pathergasia; pavor nocturnus; pedophilia; periphrastic; perseveration; personality; phantasia; phantasm; phantasmatomoria; phantasy; phantom; phoneme; pica; pithiatism; pleasure principle; pragmatism; pragmatagnosia; preconscious; rationalization; reaction; reality principle; recapitulation theory; repression; resistance; restraint; retardation; rut formation; safety symbolism; satyriasis; schizoid; schizophrenia; scotomization; sexual bondage; shell shock; stereotypy; stupor; subconscious; subjective; sublimation; subliminal; suggestion; surrogate; sycophancy; symbiosis; symbol; symbolism; syntonic; threshold of consciousness; transfer; transvestism; trend; twilight state; tyrannism; unconscious; verbigeration; vesanic; vigil; vigilambulism; vision; voice; word blindness; word salad; words beginning with "psych."

psychic (sī′kĭk) [Gr. *psychikos*]. 1. Concerning the mind or psyche. 2. One said to be endowed with semisupernatural powers, such as the ability to read the minds of others, or to foresee coming events; one apparently sensitive to nonphysical forces.

    p. blindness. Sight without recognition of that which is seen.

    p. contagion. Communication of another's nervous disorder by imitation, as a tic.

    p. deafness. Inability to recognize sounds heard.

    p. determinism. The theory that mental processes are determined by conscious or unconscious motives, and are never irrelevant.

    p. force. Force generated apart from physical energy.

psychinosis (sī-kĭ-nō′sĭs) [Gr. *psychē*, mind, + *nosos*, disease]. Any functional disease affecting the mind.

psycho-, psych- [Gr. *psychē*, mind]. Combining form indicating relationship to the mind or mental processes.

psychoanalysis (sī″kō-ă-năl′ĭ-sĭs) ["+ *analysis,* a loosening apart]. Method of obtaining a detailed account of past and present mental and emotional experiences and repressions in order to determine the source and to eliminate or diminish the undesirable effects of unconscious conflicts by making the patient aware of their existence, origin, and inappropriate expression in emotions and behavior.

Largely a system that is the creation of Sigmund Freud, q.v., and was originally the outgrowth of his observations of neurotics. Frequently the term is used synonymously with freudianism, but more commonly it is used for a more extensive system of psychological fact and theory applying both to normal and abnormal groups.

In addition to freudian method, other schools of thought or disciplines utilized in analysis of the psyche include *analytical psychology* (Jung), *psychobiology* (Meyer), and *individual psychology* (Adler).

P. is based upon the theory that abnormal phenomena are caused by repression of painful or undesirable past experiences which, although totally forgotten, later manifest themselves in various abnormal ways. P. includes a study of the ego in relationship to reality, and more particularly the herd and the conflicting goals so created. This conflict is solved by repressing one component. This repressed or censored emotion-laden complex of ideas exists in the subconscious, manifesting itself in the hidden content of dreams, in neuroses, and tension states. Anger outbursts, rationalization of unfair attitudes, slips of the tongue, etc., occur because the patient is unaware of the influence of the subconscious.

Repressed material is largely sexual, and the peculiar conditioning of the patient is chiefly determined by emotional experiences of earlier years. Reactions of inferiority may result in a compensatory reaction of goodness, ambition, etc. Sublimation is the escape of creative interest on levels not socially taboo.

Therefore p. makes an effort to bring forgotten memories into the conscious mind. The patient thus is enabled to view the occurrence in its true perspective, and so loses its harmful effect.

psychoanalyst (sī″kō-ăn′ă-līst) [Gr. *psychē*, mind, + *analysis*, breaking apart]. One who practices psychoanalysis.

psychobiology (sī″kō-bī-ŏl′ō-jī) [Gr. *psychē*, soul, + *bios*, life, + *logos*, a study]. 1. The study of the biology of the psyche, including the anatomy, physiology, and pathology of the mind. SYN: *biopsychology*. 2. A method of psychoanalysis employing distributive analysis, which includes a study of all mental and physical factors involved in the growth and development of an individual.

p., objective. P. in which special emphasis is placed on the relationship of the individual to his environment.

psychocardiac reflex (sī″kō-kăr′dī-ăk). Change in circulatory rate and consciousness of heart thumping, resulting from memory of, or subconscious dream state recollection of, an emotional impression or experience.

psychocatharsis (sī″kō-kă-thăr′sĭs) [Gr. *psychē*, mind, + *katharsis*, purging]. The bringing of so-called traumatic experiences and their affective associations into consciousness by interview, hypnosis, or by use of drugs such as sodium amytal.

psychochrome (sī″kō-krōm) ["+ *chrōma*, color]. Color impression resulting from sensory stimulation of a part other than the visual organ.

psychochromesthesia (sī″kō-krōm″ĕs-thē′zī-ă) ["+ "+ *aisthēsis*, sensation]. Color sensation produced by the stimulus of a sense organ other than that of vision. SEE: *pseudochromesthesia.*

psychocoma (sī″kō-kō′mă) [Gr. *psychē*, mind, + *kōma*, stupor]. Condition of mental stupor.

psychocortical (sī″kō-kor′tĭ-kăl) ["+ L. *cortex,* rind]. Pert. to the cerebral cortex as the seat of sensory, motor, and psychic functions.

psychodiagnostics (sī″kō-dī″ăg-nŏs′tĭks). The use of psychological testing as an aid in diagnosing mental disorders.

Psychodidae (sī″kŏd′ī-dē). A family of the order Diptera, characterized by minute size, long legs, and hairy bodies and wings. Includes moth flies, owl midges, and sand flies. SEE: *Phlebotomus.*

psychodometry (sī″kō-dŏm′ĕ-trī) [Gr. *psychē*, mind, + *hodos*, way, + *metron*, measure]. Measurement of rate of mental activity.

psychodrama (sī″kō-dram′ă) ["+ L. *drama*, drama]. A form of group psychotherapy. Patients act out assigned roles and, in so doing, are able to gain insight into their own mental disturbances.

psychodynamics (sī″kō-dī-năm′īks) ["+ *dynamis*, power]. The scientific study of mental action or force.

psychoepilepsy (sī″kō-ĕp′ī-lĕp′sī) ["+ *epilēpsia*, seizure]. A form of hysterical neurosis accompanied by movements resembling those of epilepsy.

psychogenesis (sī″kō-jĕn′ĕ-sĭs) [Gr. *psychē*, mind, + *genesis*, formation]. 1. The origin and development of mind; the formation of mental traits. 2. Origination within the mind or psyche.

psychogenetic (sī″kō-jĕn-ĕt′ĭk). 1. Originating in the mind, as a disease. 2. Concerning formation of mental traits.

psychogenic (sī-kō-jĕn′ĭk) [Gr. *psyche*, mind, + *gennan*, to produce]. 1. Of mental origin. 2. Concerning the development of the mind. SYN: *psychogenetic.*

psychogeusic (sī″kō-gū′sĭk) ["+ *geusis*, taste]. Pert. to perception of taste.

psychogram (sī′kō-grăm) ["+ *gramma*, a writing]. A subjective visualization of a mental concept.

psychograph (sī′kō-grăf) ["+ *graphein*, to write]. 1. A chart showing personality traits. 2. A history of the personality of an individual.

psychokinesia (sī″kō-kĭ-nē′zĭ-ă) [Gr. *psyche*, mind, + *kinesis*, motion]. Explosive or impulsive maniacal action caused by defective inhibition. SYN: *psycheclampsia.*

psychokinesis (sī″kō-kĭ-nē′sĭs). Influence exerted on a physical object by a subject without any intermediate physical energy or instrumentation.

psycholagny (sī″kō-lăg′nĭ) [Gr. *psyche*, mind, + *lagneia*, lust]. Sexual excitation brought about by mental imagery; psychic or mental masturbation.

psycholepsy (sī″kō-lĕp′sĭ) ["+ *lepsis*, a seizure]. Sudden alteration of moods in which mental inertia and hopelessness are manifested.

psycholeptic (sī″kō-lĕp′tĭk). Concerning sudden shifting of moods, particularly to one marked by hopelessness and mental inertia.

psychological (sī″kō-lŏj′ĭ-kăl) [Gr. *psyche*, mind, + *logos*, a study]. Pert. to study of the mind in all of its relationships, normal and abnormal.

psychologist (sī-kŏl′ō-jĭst). One who is trained in methods of psychological analysis, therapy, and research.

psychology (sī-kŏl′ō-jĭ) [Gr. *psyche*, soul, mind, + *logos*, a study]. The science dealing with mental processes, both normal and abnormal, and their effects upon behavior. There are two main approaches to the study: introspective, i.e., looking inward or self-examination of one's own mental processes; objective, i.e., studying the minds of others. SEE: words beginning with *psych.*

    p., abnormal. The study of deviational behavior and the mental phenomena associated with such.

    p., analytic. Psychoanalysis based on the concepts of Carl Jung, de-emphasizing sexual factors in motivation and emphasizing the "collective unconscious" and "psychological types" (introvert and extrovert).

    p., animal. The study of animal behavior.

    p., applied. The application of the principles of p. to special fields, i.e., clinical, industrial, educational, nursing, or pastoral.

    p., dynamic. The p. of motivation; that which seeks the causes of mental phenomena.

    p., experimental. Study of mental acts by tests and experiments.

    p., Gestalt. That which emphasizes the wholeness of psychological processes and behavior, maintaining that such cannot be adequately explained by breaking down into constituent parts.

    p., individual. A system of psychological thinking developed by Alfred Adler in which an individual is regarded as having three life goals; physical security, sexual satisfaction, and social integration. Self-evaluations lead to feelings of inferiority and inadequacy which often lead to overcompensation or a striving for superiority.

    p., physiologic. That which deals with the structure and function of the nervous system and other bodily organs and their relationship to behavior.

psychometry (sī-kŏm′ĕ-trĭ) [Gr. *psyche*, mind, + *metron*, a measure]. The measurement of psychological variables, such as intelligence, aptitude, behavior, and emotional reactions.

psychomotor (sī″kō-mō′tor) ["+ L. *motor,* a mover]. Concerning or causing physical activity associated with mental processes.

psychoneurosis (sī″kō-nū-rō′sĭs) [Gr. *psyche*, mind, + *neuron*, sinew, + *-osis*, condition]. Emotional maladaptation due to unresolved unconscious conflicts. This leads to disturbances in thought, feelings, attitudes, and behavior. There is little, if any, loss of contact with reality, but the patient's effectiveness in performing his or her usual responsibilities is handicapped.

    Psychoneurosis is a major category in classifying mental illness. The patient usually recognizes that the altered thoughts and feelings are abnormal and indeed unwelcome. This is in contrast to the patient with a psychosis or character disorder.

    Neuroses are classified according to the symptoms which predominate.

    p., anxiety reaction. Anxiety with apprehension out of proportion to any obvious external cause.

    p., conversion reaction. P. wherein unacceptable unconscious impulses are converted into hysterical somatic symptoms. Although the symptoms have a specific symbolic meaning to the patient, their interpretation is different in each individual.

p., depressive reaction. P. marked by depression out of proportion to any obvious cause.

p., dissociated reaction. Characterized by dissociated behavior, such as amnesia, fugue, sleepwalking, and dream states. Important to differentiate from schizophrenia, q.v.

p., obsessive-compulsive reaction Persistent, repetitive impulses to perform certain acts or rituals, such as handwashing, touching something, or counting.

p., phobic reaction. Irrational fear of any of a variety of situations, persons, or objects.

psychoneurotic (sī″kō-nū-rŏt′ĭk) [Gr. *psychē*, mind, + *neuron*, sinew]. 1. Pert. to a functional disorder of mental origin. 2. A person suffering from a psychoneurosis.

psychonomy (sī-kŏn′ō-mī) ["+ *nomos*, law]. The science of the laws of the mind and its functions.

psychoparesis (sī″kō-pă-rē′sĭs, -păr′ē-sĭs) ["+ *paresis*, relaxation]. Weakness or enfeeblement of the mind.

psychopath (sī′kō-păth) [Gr. *psychē*, mind, + *pathos*, disease]. Individual with a psychopathic personality. SEE: *personality, psychopathic.*

psychopath′ia. Psychopathy, q.v.

psychopathic (sī″kō-păth′ĭk). 1. Concerning or characterized by a mental disorder. 2. Concerning treatment of mental disorders. 3. Abnormal.

p. personality. SEE: *personality, psychopathic.*

psychopathology (sī″kō-păth-ŏl′ō-jī) [Gr. *psychē*, mind, + *pathos*, disease, + *logos*, a study]. The study of the causes and nature of mental disease or abnormal behavior.

psychopathy (sī-kŏp′ă-thī). Any mental disease, esp. one characterized by defective character or personality.

psychopharmacology (sī″kō-făr″mă-kŏl′ō-jī). The science of drugs having an effect on psychomotor behavior and emotional states.

psychophonasthenia (sī″kō-fō″năs-thē′nĭ-ă) [Gr. *psychē*, mind, + *phōnē*, voice, + *astheneia*, weakness]. A speech defect of mental origin.

psychophysical (sī″kō-fĭz′ĭ-kăl) ["+ *physikos*, natural]. Concerning the relationship of the physical and the mental. RS: childbirth, psychophysical preparation for.

p. law. Intensity of sensation increases as the logarithms of the stimuli.

psychophysics (sī″kō-fĭz′ĭks). 1. The study of mental processes in relationship to physi-

cal processes. 2. The study of stimuli in relationship to the effects they produce.

psychophysiologic (sī″kō-fĭz-ĭ-ōlō′jĭk). Pert. to psychophysiology, q.v.

p. autonomic and visceral disorders. Term applied to a large number of disorders of organs and viscera innervated by the autonomic nervous system in which emotional factors are a primary causative factor. Formerly called psychosomatic disease or disorder.

psychophysiology (sī″kō-fĭz″ĭ-ŏl′ō-jī). Physiology of the mind; science of the correlation of body and mind.

psychoplegic (sī″kō-plē′jĭk) [Gr. *psychē*, mind, + *plēgē*, a stroke]. An agent reducing excitability of the mental processes.

psychoprophylactic childbirth. Mental and physical training of the mother in preparation for delivery. The goals of the preparation are the dispelling of the fear of pain and the delivery of a healthy child.

psychorhythmia (sī″kō-rĭth′mĭ-ă) ["+ *rhythmos*, rhythm]. Mental condition in which involuntary repetition of previous voluntary actions occurs.

psychorrhea (sī″kō-rē-ă) ["+ *rhoia*, flow]. A mental condition characterized by an incoherent stream of thought resulting in vague and often bizarre theories and ideas.

psychosensory (sī″kō-sĕn′so-rī) ["+ L. *sensorius*, sensation]. 1. Understanding and interpreting sensory stimuli. 2. Concerning perceptions not arising in sensory organs, as hallucinations.

psychosexual (sī″kō-sĕks′ū-ăl) [Gr. *psychē*, soul, mind, + L. *sexus*, sex.]. Concerning the emotional components of sexual instinct.

p. development. Evolution of personality through infantile and pregenital periods to sexual maturity.

psychosin (sī-kō′sĭn). A cerebroside occurring in brain tissue.

psychosis (sī-kō′sĭs) [Gr. *psychē*, mind, soul, + *-osis*, condition]. (pl. *psychoses*) A term formerly applied to any mental disorder, but now generally restricted to those disturbances of such magnitude that there is personality disintegration and loss of contact with reality. The disturbances are of psychogenic origin, or without clearly defined physical cause or structural change in the brain. They usually are characterized by delusions and hallucination, and hospitalization generally is required.

A condition manifested in the behavior, emotional reaction, and ideation of the patient. He fails to mirror reality as it is, reacts erroneously to it, and builds up false concepts regarding it. His behavior responses are peculiar, abnormal, inefficient, or definitely antisocial.

All this does not include amentia because defective intelligence merely lessens comprehension of reality but does not distort it. The psychopathic personality reacts badly because of intrinsic emotional differences playing upon an undistorted world of reality.

p., depressive. P. characterized by extreme depression, melancholia, and feelings of unworthiness. SYN: *psychotic depressive reaction.*

p., involutional. P. occurring during involutional period of bodily and intellectual decline. In women from ages 40-55; in men from 50-65.

p., manic-depressive. Ordinarily a series of periods of psychotic depression or excessive well-being, appearing in any sequence and alternating with longer periods of relative normalcy.

Though intensity may vary greatly, the manic shows an elated though unstable mood, a flight of ideas, and great physical activity. The case of primary depression finds all exertion exhausting; there is difficulty in thinking or acting and victim is very unhappy.

p., organic. The result of a pathological condition of the central nervous system, such as paresis.

p., postinfectious. P. following an infectious disease such as meningitis, pneumonia, typhoid fever.

p., postpartum. Occurring in the period following childbirth.

p., senile. Due to old age.

p., toxic. P. resulting from toxic agents.

p., traumatic. P. resulting from head injuries and belonging to the organic group.

psychosomat'ic (sī''kō-sō-măt'ĭk) [Gr. *psychē*, mind, + *sōma*, body]. 1. Pert. to the mind and body. 2. Indicating illnesses in which some portion of the etiology is related to emotional factors.

When so used the impression is created that the mind and body are separate entities and that a disease may be purely somatic in its effect or entirely emotional. This partitioning of the human being is not possible; thus no disease is limited to only the mind or the body. A complex interaction is always present even though in specific instances a disease might on superficial examination appear to involve only the body or the mind.

p. disorder. A disease thought to be etiologically related to emotional factors. SEE: *psychophysiologic autonomic and visceral disorders.*

p. medicine. Branch of medicine which recognizes the importance of mind-body interrelationship in all illnesses and in which therapy and management are based on this fact.

psychosurgery (sī''kō-sūr'jer-ĭ) ["+ L. *chirurgia*, surgery]. Brain surgery for mental illness. The term includes such procedures as lobotomy, topectomy, and thalamotomy.

psychotechnics (sī''kō-tĕk'nĭks) ["+ *technē*, art]. Application of psychological methods in the study of economic and social problems.

psychotherapeutic drugs. Drugs which are used because of the effects they have in ameliorating the principal symptoms which occur in mentally disturbed persons, i.e. anxiety, depression, and psychosis.

psychotherapy (sī-kō-thĕr'ă-pĭ) [Gr. *psychē*, mind, + *therapeia*, treatment]. A method of treating disease, esp. nervous disorders, by mental means rather than physical. EX: suggestion, hypnotism, psychoanalytic therapy.

psychotogenic (sī-kŏt''ō-jĕn'ĭk) ["+ *gennan*, to produce]. Producing a psychosis, usually temporary and due to certain powerful drugs.

psychotomimetic (sī-kŏt''ō-mĭ-mĕ'tĭk) ["+ *mimetikos*, imitative]. A hallucinogen producing weird illusions and phantasms.

psychotropic drugs ["+ *tropē*, a turning]. Drugs which affect psychic function, behavior, or experience. Many drugs can be classed as being intentionally psychotropic, but many other drugs may occasionally produce undesired psychotropic side effects also.

psychroalgia (sī-krō-ăl'jĭ-ă) [Gr. *psychros*, cold, + *algos*, pain]. Painful sensation of cold.

psychroesthesia (sī''krō-ĕs-thē'zĭ-ă) ["+ *aisthēsis*, sensation]. A sensation of cold in a part of the body, although it is warm.

psychrometer (sī-krŏm'ĕ-tĕr) ["+ *metron*, measure]. Device for measuring relative humidity of the atmosphere. Calculations are made utilizing the readings of two thermometers, one with a dry bulb and one with a wet bulb.

psychrophilic (sī-krō-fĭl'ĭk) [Gr. *psychros*, cold, "+ *philein*, to love]. Preferring cold, as bacteria which thrive best at low temperatures between 0° and 30° C. (32° and 86° F.).

psychrophobia (sī-krō-fō'bĭ-ă) ["+ *phobos*, fear]. Abnormal aversion or sensitiveness to cold.

psychrophore (sī'krō-fōr) [Gr. *psychros*, cold, + *phorein*, to carry]. Apparatus for

Psychotherapeutic Drugs*

Indication	Drugs	Clinical Use	Note
Antianxiety	Barbiturates Meprobamate Tybamate Chlordiazepoxide Diazepam Oxazepam	Anxiety Nervousness Psychoneuroses Insomnia	Patients may become tolerant to the drug, or abuse the drug and become addicted. Use may delay definitive therapy.
Antidepressants	Tricyclic compounds or Dibenzazepines (imipramine, desipramine, amitryptyline, nortriptyline) Lithium Carbonate (used experimentally)	Depression	Uncertain response. Use may delay electroconvulsive therapy or psychotherapy.
Antipsychotics	Phenothiazines (chlorpromazine, thioridazine, trifluoperazine) Thioxanthenes Butyrophenones Reserpine	Schizophrenic reactions Excitement Chronic brain syndromes Mental retardation	May have long-term undesired side effects; autonomic nervous system effects; extrapyramidal tract effects.

* Adapted from Hollister, L. E.: Clinical Use of Psychotherapeutic Drugs. Postgraduate Medicine, January 1970.

applying cold to the urethra, or any canal.

psychrotherapy (sĭ″krō-thĕr′ă-pĭ) ["+ *therapeia,* treatment]. Treatment of disease by administration of cold.

psyllium seed (sĭl′ĭ-ŭm). The dried, ripe seed of a plant grown in France, Spain, and India. Used as a mild laxative.

ptarmic (tăr′mĭk) [Gr. *ptarmikos,* causing to sneeze]. 1. Causing sneezing. 2. Agent that causes sneezing. SYN: *sternutatory.*

ptarmus (tăr′mŭs). Spasmodic sneezing.

pterion (tē′rĭ-ŏn) [Gr. *pteron,* wing]. Point of suture of frontal, parietal, temporal, and sphenoid bones.

pteroylglutamic acid. SEE: *folic acid.*

pterygium (tĕr-ĭj′ĭ-ŭm) [Gr. *pterygion,* wing]. Triangular thickening of bulbar conjunctiva extending from inner canthus to border of the cornea with apex toward pupil.

p., progressive. Stage in which the growth extends toward center of cornea.

p., stationary. Stage in which the head of pterygium remains permanently attached to same point on the cornea.

TREATMENT: Surgical.

pterygoid (tĕr′ĭ-goyd) [Gr. *pterygōdēs*]. Wing-shaped. SYN: *alate.*

p. process. One of two large processes of sphenoid bone extending downward from junction of body and great wings, each consisting of lateral and medial pterygoid plates.

pterygomaxillary (tĕr′ĭ-gō-măk′sĭ-lĕr′ĭ) ["+ L. *maxillaris,* upper jaw]. Concerning the pterygoid process and the upper jaw.

pterygopalatine (tĕr′ĭ-gō-păl′ă-tīn) ["+ L. *palatinus,* palate]. Rel. to the pterygoid process and the palate bone.

PTH. Abbr. for *parathyroid hormone.*

ptilosis (tĭ-lō′sĭs) [Gr.]. Loss of eyelashes.

ptomaine (tō′mān) [Gr. *ptōma,* dead body]. One of a class of nitrogenous organic bases formed in the action of putrefactive bacteria on proteins and amino acids. Ex: cadaverine, $NH_2(CH_2)_5NH_2$.

ptomainuria (tō-mā′ĭ-nū′rĭ-ă) ["+ *ouron,* urine]. Presence of ptomaines in urine.

ptosis (tō′sĭs) [Gr. *ptōsis,* a dropping]. Dropping or drooping of an organ or part, as the upper eyelid from paralysis, or the visceral organs from weakness of the abdominal muscles.

p., abdominal. Sagging of transverse colon, sometimes almost to the pelvic floor.

ETIOL: Obesity or lack of abdominal muscle tone.

TREATMENT: A properly adjusted abdominal belt may help. This is contraindicated if the patient shows dependence upon belt rather than on exercising and developing abdominal muscles.

ptyalagogue (tĭ-ăl′ă-gŏg) [Gr. *ptyalon,* saliva, + *agōgos,* leading]. Causing, or that which causes, a flow of saliva. SYN: *sialogogue.*

ptyalin (tĭ′ă-lĭn). A salivary amylolytic enzyme converting starch into maltose and dextrin. SEE: *enzyme; ptyalism; saliva.*

ptyalism (tĭ′ă-lĭzm) [Gr. *ptyalon,* saliva, + *-ismos,* condition]. Excessive secretion of saliva.

ETIOL: May be due to pregnancy, stomatitis, rabies, exophthalmic goiter, menstruation, epilepsy, hysteria, nervous conditions, and gastrointestinal disorders. May be induced by mercury, iodides, pilocarpine, and other drugs. SYN: *salivation.* SEE: *xerostomia.*

ptyalith (tĭ′ă-lĭth) ["+ *lithos,* stone]. A calculus in a salivary gland.

ptyalocele (tĭ-ăl′ō-sēl) ["+ *kēlē,* hernia]. A salivary cystic tumor or cystic dilatation of a salivary duct.

p., sublingual. SEE: *ranula.*

ptyalogenic (tĭ″ăl-ō-jĕn′ĭk) [Gr. *ptyalon,* saliva, + *gennan,* to produce]. Of salivary origin.

ptyalogogue (tĭ″ăl′ō-gŏg) ["+ *agōgos,* leading]. An agent that causes the flow of saliva. SYN: *sialogogue, q.v.*

ptyalogram (tĭ-ăl′ō-grăm) [Gr. *ptyalon,* saliva, + *gramma,* a writing]. An x-ray film of the salivary glands.

ptyalography (tĭ″ăl-ŏg′ră-fĭ) ["+ *graphein,* to write]. X-ray inspection of the salivary glands and ducts. SYN: *sialography.*

ptyalolith (tĭ′ă-lō-lĭth) ["+ *lithos,* stone]. A salivary concretion.

ptyalolithiasis (tĭ″ă-lō-lĭ-thī′ă-sĭs). Presence of a concretion in a salivary gland or duct.

ptyalolithotomy (tĭ″ăl-ō-lĭ-thŏt′ō-mĭ) [Gr. *ptyalon,* saliva, + *lithos,* stone, + *tomē,* a cutting]. Surgical removal of a concretion from a salivary duct or gland.

ptyalorrhea (tĭ″ă-lō-rē′ă) ["+ *rhoia,* flow]. An excessive flow of saliva.

ptysis (tĭ′sĭs) [Gr.]. Spitting; the ejection of saliva from the mouth.

ptysmagogue (tĭz′mă-gŏg) ["+ *agōgos,* leading]. An agent that induces the flow of saliva.

pubarche (pū-băr′kē) [L. *puber,* grown up, + Gr. *arkhē,* beginning]. 1. The beginning of puberty. 2. Beginning development of pubic hair.

puber (pū′bŭr) [L., grown up]. One at onset of puberty.

puberal (pū′bĕr-ăl) [L. *pubertas,* puberty]. Concerning puberty.

pubertal. Pert. to puberty.

pubertas (pū′ber-tăs) [L.]. Puberty.

p. plena. Complete puberty.

p. praecox. Precocious puberty or puberty at an early age.

puberty (pū′bĕr-tĭ). Period in life at which one of either sex becomes functionally capable of reproduction. A period of rapid change in boys and girls. It occurs between the ages of 13 and 15 in boys, and from 9 to 16 in girls, and ends in the attainment of sexual maturity.

RS: hebephrenia; hebetic; interstitial; latent period; menacme; nubility.

p., timing of. Boys: Between the ages of 13 and 15 there is a relatively rapid increase in height and weight with broadening of the shoulders and increase in size of the penis and testicles. Pubic hair and the beard begin to grow. Endocrine and sebaceous gland activity is increased. Nocturnal emissions occur.

Young boys should be assured that the size of the penis is not related to the degree of masculinity and is not an important factor in experiencing or providing sexual gratification.

Girls: Between the ages of 9 and 16 a marked increase in growth rate is accompanied by breast enlargement and appearance of pubic hair. Within one to two years after these changes, underarm hair grows and the normal whitish vaginal secretion (physiological leukorrhea) characteristic of the adult female is noticed. Several months later the first menstrual period (menarche) occurs. Each individual will vary somewhat from this schedule.

The young girl should be told prior to puberty about menstruation and the technique of menstrual protection through use of perineal pads or tampons. In addition, she should be told that a certain amount of vaginal discharge is normal but if the secretion is malodorous or causes irritation of the vulva a physician should be consulted. SEE: *menstruation.*

pubes (pū′bēz) [L., grown up]. (sing. pubis) 1. Anterior part of innominate bone; os pubis. 2. The pubic region. 3. [NA] Hair of the pubic region.

pubescence (pū-bĕs′ĕns) [L. *pubescens,* becoming hairy]. 1. Puberty or its approach. 2.

Covering of fine, soft hairs on the body. SYN: *lanugo*.

pubescent (pū-bĕs'ĕnt). 1. Reaching puberty. 2. Covered with downy hair.

pubetrotomy (pū"bĕ-trŏt'ō-mĭ) [L. *pubes*, grown up, + Gr. *ētron*, belly, + *tomē*, a cutting]. Section through the os pubis and lower abdominal wall.

pubic (pū'bĭk) [L. *pubes*, grown up]. Concerning the pubes.

 p. bone. The lower anterior part of the innominate bone. SYN: *os pubis*.

 p. hair. Hair over the pubes which appears at onset of sexual maturity. The distribution is somewhat different in men as compared to women.

pubio-, pubo- [L. *pubes*, grown up]. Combining form meaning the pubic hair of the pubic bone or region.

pubiotomy (pū-bĭ-ŏt'ō-mĭ) ["+ *tomē*, a cutting]. Incision across the pubis in order to enlarge the pelvic passage, facilitating the delivery of the fetus when pelvis is malformed.

pubis (pū'bĭs) [L., grown up]. (pl. *pubes*) Pubic bone; os pubis.

pubofemoral (pū"bō-fĕm'ōr-ăl) ["+ *femur*, *femor-*, thigh bone]. Pert. to the os pubis and the femur.

puboprostatic (pū"bō-prŏs-tăt'ĭk) ["+ Gr. *prostatēs*, prostate]. Rel. to the os pubis and prostate gland.

pubovaginal device. Apparatus which is fitted for use in the vagina to help prevent urinary incontinence.

pubovesical (pū"bō-vĕs'ĭ-kl) ["+ *vesiculus*, a little sac]. Pert. to the os pubis and bladder.

pudenda (pū-dĕn'dă) [L.]. (sing. *pudendum*) The external genitalia, esp. of the female. SYN: *vulva*.

pudendagra (pū"dĕn-dăg'ră) ["+ Gr. *agra*, seizure]. Pain in the external genitals.

pudendal (pū-dĕn'dăl) [L. *pudenda*, external genitals]. Rel. to the external genitals of female.

pudendum (pū-dĕn'dŭm) [L.]. (pl. *pudenda*) The external genitals, esp. those of the female; the vulva.

 p. muliebre. External genitals of the female.

pudic (pū'dĭk) [L. *pudicus*, modest]. Concerning external female genitalia. SYN: *pudendal*.

Puente's disease (pū-ĕn'tă). Simple glandular cheilitis.

puericulture (pū-er'ĭ-kŭl"chŭr) [L. *puer*, child, + *cultura*, culture]. Science concerned with prenatal care of unborn children, and the art of raising and training children.

puerile (pū'ē-rĭl) [L. *puerilis*]. Concerning a child; childlike.

 p. respiration. That heard in auscultation of healthy children.

puerilism (pū'ĕr-ĭl-ĭzm) ["+ Gr. *-ismos*, condition]. Childishness; second childhood.

puerpera (pū-ĕr'pĕr-ă) [L. *puer*, child, + *parēre*, to bear]. Woman during the period following the 3rd stage of labor, i.e., delivery of the placenta, lasting until there is complete involution of the uterus.

puerperal (pū-ĕr'pĕr-ăl) [L. *puerperalis*]. Concerning puerperium.

 p. eclampsia. Convulsions during puerperium.

 p. fever. Septicemia following childbirth. SYN: *childbed fever*.

 p. period. Period immediately following childbirth.

 p. sepsis. A toxemia of puerperium accompanied by a rise in temperature during the first 21 days after childbirth. Prior to effective antibiotic therapy this was the greatest single cause of death due to childbirth.

 CHARACTERISTICS: Lowered resistance a danger; toxemia, anemia, exhaustion in labor, abrasions and lacerations, loss of blood predisposing factors. May be autogenous or heterogeneous. Other foci aside from genitals may be responsible for invasion; infection may remain localized or it may spread; infected thrombi from veins of placental site may enter blood stream; metastatic areas of infection may be caused by infected blood. Spreading along mucous membranes, the infection may reach the tubes, ovaries, and peritoneum. Thrombophlebitis in pelvic veins may lead to thrombophlebitis in veins of the leg.

 Localized infections indicated by fever, rapid pulse, pain, and pelvic tenderness; fever about 3rd day, 103° F. to 104° F. (39.4° to 40° C.). In endometritis, tenderness confined to uterus. Lochia may be scant without odor; lochia profuse and foul if any membranes are retained. Parametritis in more severe infections; swelling due to inflammatory exudate, giving place to suppuration after a few days, accompanied by chill and rise in temperature. Peritonitis possible, esp. if gonococcus is present. Spread of disease indicated by rise in temperature, and perhaps chills. Drainage may be necessary. Permanent sterility possible.

 PREVENTION: Aseptic technique in all obstetric cases; masking of those who come in contact with patient. Complete bacteriological survey following any infection to determine possible source and exclusion of all positive carriers from attendence upon maternity cases. Better intrapartum care of patient in long labor, use of least traumatizing type of delivery, avoidance of blood loss, and wider use of blood transfusions.

TREATMENT: Active surgical intervention during infection seldom indicated. Good nursing care, high caloric and vitamin diet, and restriction of visitors. All manipulative procedures kept at a minimum. Excellent results have been obtained from use of broad-spectrum antibiotics.

puerperalism (pū-ĕr′pĕr-ăl-ĭzm) [L. *puer,* child, + *parēre,* to bear, + Gr. *ismos,* condition]. Pathological conditions accompanying childbirth.

p., infantile. Any pathogenic condition of the newborn.

p., infectious. Puerperal disease caused by infection.

puerperant (pū-ĕr′pĕr-ănt). A woman in labor, or one who recently has been delivered.

puerperium (pū″ĕr-pē′rī-ŭm) [L.]. Period following the 3rd stage of labor, lasting until involution of pelvic organs takes place; usually 3-6 weeks.

RS: sepsis, puerperal.

puerperous (pū-ĕr′pĕr-ŭs) [L. *puer,* child, + *parēre,* to bear]. In the period following childbirth. SYN: *puerperal.*

Pu′lex (pū′lĕks) [L., flea]. A genus of fleas belonging to the order Siphonaptera.

P. irritans. The human flea, which also infests dogs, hogs, and other mammals. May serve as intermediate host of the tapeworms Dipylidium caninum and Hymenolepsis diminuta.

pulicaris (pū″lī-kā′rĭs). Marked by spots resembling flea bites.

pulicatio (pū″lĭ-kā′tī-ō). Infested with fleas.

Pulicidae (pū-lĭs′ī-dē). A family of fleas belonging to the order Siphonaptera, which includes the genera Pulex, Echidnophaga, Ctenocephalides, and Xenopsylla. SEE: *flea.*

pulicide (pū′lĭ-sīd) [L. *pulex,* flea, + *caedere,* to kill]. An agent that kills fleas.

pullulate (pŭl′ū-lāt) [L. *pullulare,* to sprout]. To bud or germinate.

pullulation (pŭl″ū-lā′shŭn). The act of budding or germinating, as seen in yeast plant.

pulmo- [L.]. Combining form meaning lung.

pulmoaortic (pŭl″mō-ā-or′tĭk) [″+ Gr. *aortē,* aorta]. 1. Concerning the lungs and the aorta. 2. Rel. to the pulmonary artery and aorta.

pulmometer (pŭl-mŏm′ĕ-tĕr) [″+ Gr. *metron,* measure]. Device for measuring lung capacity. SYN: *spirometer.*

pulmometry (pŭl-mŏm′ĕ-trī). Determination of capacity of the lungs.

pulmonary (pŭl′mō-nĕ-rī) [L. *pulmonarius*]. Concerning or involving the lungs.

p. arterial webs. Weblike deformities seen in pulmonary angiograms at the site of previous pulmonary thromboembolism.

p. circulation. Passage of blood from heart to lungs and back again for purification. The blood flows from the right cardiac ventricle through the lungs, there to be oxygenated; then back to the left cardiac atrium. SEE: *circulation* for illustration.

p. incompetence, p. insufficiency. Failure of the pulmonary valve to close properly.

p. stenosis. Narrowing of opening into the pulmonary artery from right cardiac ventricle.

pulmonary surfactant. A phospholipid substance important in controlling the surface tension of the air-liquid emulsion which is present in the lungs. Abnormalities in this surfactant have been noted in prematurity, hyaline membrane disease, and pulmonary edema.

pulmonectomy (pŭl″mō-nĕk′tō-mī) [L. *pulmo, pulmon-,* lung, + Gr. *ektomē,* excision]. Removal of part or all of a lung's tissue. SYN: *pneumonectomy.*

pulmonitis (pŭl-mō-nī′tĭs) [″+ Gr. *-ītis,* inflammation]. Inflamed condition of the lung. SYN: *pneumonia.*

pulmotor (pŭl′mō-tor) [″+ *motor,* mover]. Apparatus for inducing artificial respiration by forcing oxygen into the lungs and drawing out carbon dioxide.

pulp [L. *pulpa,* flesh]. 1. The soft part of fruit. 2. The soft part of an organ. 3. Mass of partly digested food passed from stomach to duodenum. SYN: *chyme.* 4. In dentistry, the soft vascular portion of the center of a tooth.

p. cavity. Hollow space within a tooth containing dental p.

p. cells. Those in the p. cavity of any organ.

p. cords. Anastomosing cords of red p. of the spleen traversed by venous sinuses. SYN: *cords of Billroth.*

p., digital. Elastic, soft prominence on the palmar or plantar surface of the last phalanx of a finger or toe.

p., enamel. Cells forming a stellate reticulum lying between outer and inner layers of the enamel organ of a tooth.

p., red. The portion of splenic p. consisting of venous sinuses plus p. cords.

p., splenic. Soft, spongelike tissue-forming substance of the spleen.

p., white. Portion of splenic p. consisting of a compact type of lymphatic tissue which forms a sheath about certain arteries.

pulpal (pŭl'păl). Rel. to pulp.

pulpefaction (pŭl-pĭ-făk'shŭn) [L. *pulpa*, pulp, + *facere*, to make]. Conversion into pulpy substance.

pulpitis (pŭl-pī'tĭs) ["+ *-itis*, inflammation]. (pl. *pulpit'ides*) Inflammation of the pulp of a tooth.

pulpy (pŭl'pĭ). Resembling pulp; flabby. SYN: *pultaceous.*

pulsate (pŭl'sāt) [L. *pulsāre*]. To throb or beat in rhythm.

pulsatile (pŭl'să-tĭl). Pulsating; characterized by a rhythmic beat. SYN: *throbbing.*

pulsation (pŭl-sā'shŭn) [L. *pulsatio*, a beating]. The rhythmic beat, as of the heart and blood vessels; a throbbing. SEE: *pulse.*

ABNORMAL CENTERS OF PULSATION: *Epigastric p.:* May result from excited action of heart from any cause; enlargement of right ventricle; pulsating aorta noted in certain nervous and anemic patients; aortic aneurysm; tumors of left lobe of liver resting on the aorta. *P. in left axillary region:* May result from enlargement of heart; a tense purulent effusion in left pleural sac (pulsating empyema); aneurysm; chronic disease of left lung and pleura associated with retraction.

Unnatural p. in carotids: May result from excitement of heart from any cause; exophthalmic goiter; anemia; valvular disease, esp. aortic regurgitation; aneurysm or dilatation of the vessels; unnatural elasticity of the vessels noted in certain nervous and anemic patients. *Jugular p.:* The jugular vein often becomes distended in forced expiration and coughing. Sometimes distention noted in adherent pericardium. A true rhythmical venous pulsation usually results from tricuspid regurgitation. A pulsation may be transmitted to the jugular vein from the underlying carotid, but this false pulsation will continue when light pressure is made on root of neck, while the true venous pulse will cease.

pulse (pŭls) [L. *pulsus*, beating]. 1. Rate, rhythm, condition of arterial walls, compressibility and tension, and size and shape of the wave. 2. Rhythmical throbbing. 3. Throbbing caused by the regular contraction and alternate expansion of an artery; the periodic thrust felt over arteries in time with the heartbeat.

Normal pulse rate of adult is 70-72 in men and 78-82 in women, and is usually felt in radial artery of the wrist.

POINTS TO BE OBSERVED: Hour, frequency, pressure, regularity, force. Temperature and respiration are of clinical importance to the physician. Right and left radial arteries are usually tested and differences, if any or absent, should be noted. Pressure should not be too great on artery. Thumb should not be used because examiner may be counting pulse in own thumb rather than patient's. Count for at least one-half minute.

A tracing of this is called a sphygmogram and consists of a series of waves in which the upstroke is called the *anacrotic* limb, and the downstroke (on which is normally seen the dicrotic notch), the *catacrotic.*

p., accelerated. A common symptom in all fevers. The pulse of the adult rarely exceeds 150 beats per minute even in acute inflammatory infections; when it exceeds 170 it may portend a fatal issue.

A pulse of 170 is known as *tachycardia,* and in some diseases it is a common symptom. If such an acceleration does not diminish within a short time it is esp. unfavorable. A rate of 150 is not necessarily fatal. When quick and bounding it indicates acute fever or inflammation, or may result from a toxic goiter; organic heart disease; pressure at the base of the brain sufficient to paralyze the pneumogastric nerve, as in clot, tumor, and advanced meningitis; shock; reflex irritation, as in ovarian or uterine disease; rheumatoid arthritis; independent paroxysmal neurosis, or the use of certain drugs such as belladonna, nitrites, or alcohol.

p., alternating. P. with alternating weak and strong pulsations.

p., anacrotic. P. showing a secondary wave on ascending limb of the main wave.

p., angry. A tense p. SYN: *wiry p.*

p., asymmetrical radial. P. in which beats vary in force. SYN: *unequal p.*

p., bigeminal. Two regular beats followed by a longer pause. It has the same significance as an irregular p.

p., bounding. P. which reaches a higher level than normal, then disappears quickly. Best detected when arm is held aloft. Due to shortened ventricular systole and reduced peripheral pressure. SYN: *collapsing p.*

p., capillary. Alternating redness and pallor of capillary region, as in the matrices beneath the nails, occuring chiefly where an excessive cardiac impulse coincides with general arterial narrowing.

p., catacrotic. P. showing one or more secondary waves on descending limb of the main wave.

p., central. P. recorded near the origin of the carotid or subclavian arteries.

p., collapsing. P. feebly striking the finger, then subsiding abruptly and completely. SYN: *p., bounding*, q.v.

p., Corrigan's. One of aortic insufficiency. SEE: *p., waterhammer.*

p., decurtate. P. which gradually decreases in force. SYN: *myurous p.*

p., deficit. The number of p. beats counted at the wrist is less than those counted in the same period of time at the heart. Seen in auricular fibrillation.

p., dicrotic. A double beat, one heartbeat for two arterial pulsations, or a seeming weak wave between the usual heartbeats. This weak wave should not be counted as a regular beat. It is indicative of low arterial tension and is noted in fevers, in low states of the nervous system, and sometimes in typhoid fever.

p., entopic. Intermittent subjective sensations of light which accompany the heartbeat.

p., febrile. A full, bounding p. at onset of fever, becoming feeble and weak when fever subsides or on prostration.

p., female. More frequent than male p. by 8-10 beats. There is an important correlation between the pulse, respiration, and temperature which must be considered in most disease states.

p., filiform. Thready p., q.v.

p., formicant. A small, feeble p.

p. frequency. Depends upon sex, age, exertion, position of body, and health. It is higher in children and increases with very old age. It is slower in tall persons than it is in short persons. It is 10-12 beats more frequent in standing than sitting. Physical exertion will increase it normally to as much as 200 beats per minute in young healthy persons. Eating and drinking likewise increase heart action. It is less frequent when sleeping or lying down.

p., full. A distended one in an artery giving a tense feeling; observed in sthenic inflammation.

p., gaseous. A soft, full p.

p., hard. One with sensation of hardness due to changes in the arterial wall or to vascular distention.

p., hepatic. P. due to expansion of veins of the liver at each ventricular contraction.

p., high-tension. P. in which force of beat is relatively increased and which may be roughly estimated by noting the amount of pressure of the fingers that is required to arrest the beat. It is observed in many conditions: cardiac diseases, such as hyper-

trophy; chronic nephritis; cerebral affections; irritation of the vasomotor center as in apoplexy, tumors, and beginning meningitis; after the use of certain drugs such as digitalis, ergot, and alcoholic stimulants; chills; angina pectoris; epileptic and hysterical seizures; gout; and uremia.

p., incident. P. with 2nd beat weaker than 1st, the 3rd weaker than the 4th, followed by a stroke as strong as the 1st.

p., infrequent. Observed in organic heart disease, esp. fatty degeneration and fibroid induration; jaundice; pressure at base of brain sufficient to irritate the vagus, as in beginning meningitis; and at the close of febrile diseases, as in typhoid fever, and pneumonia. May follow the use of certain drugs such as digitalis, aconite, and opium. Physiological slowness is noted in repose, during fasting, in the puerperium, and old age; it is habitual in certain people (40-60 beats per minute).

p., intermediate. That recorded in proximal portions of carotid, femoral, and brachial arteries.

p., intermittent. P. in which occasional beats are skipped. Caused by an apparent drop of a heartbeat. It is not inconsistent with health; yet it is commonly an indication of disease, frequently from gastric, hepatic, uterine, and renal causes. It is common in fatty degeneration of the heart and is habitual in certain people after exercise, eating, or excitement.

p., irregular. P. with a variation in force and frequency. Has same significance as intermittent p. Common in myocarditis and valvular diseases, esp. in mitral regurgitation. Heart trouble may be noted by long continued irregular pulse.

p., jerky. That of aortic regurgitation, because from a state of emptiness the artery is suddenly filled with blood.

p., jugular. Venous p. felt in jugular vein.

p., long. P. in which duration of the systolic wave is comparatively long.

p., low-tension. P. with sudden onset, short duration, and rapid decline, esp. noted in degeneration of the heart, collapse, debility, fevers, and low states of the nervous system.

p., male. From 70 to 72 beats per minute, but not an invariable rule, as some are healthy with a pulse rate of 50 or even 90.

p., monocrotous. P. with a sphygmogram showing a simple ascending and descending, uninterrupted line and no dicrotism; indicative of a grave condition of the circulation and of impending death.

p., myurous. P. which decreases in force. SYN: *decurtate p.*

p., paradoxical. P. which is more or less suppressed at close of each full inspiration. Thought to be due to compression of the great vessels by inflammatory adhesions, the latter being stretched during act of inspiration. Frequently noted in adherent pericardium.

p., peripheral. P. recorded in arteries (radial or pedal) in distal portion of limbs.

p., pistol-shot. P. resulting from rapid distention and collapse of an artery as occurs in aortic regurgitation.

p., plateau. P. that slowly rises but is maintained.

p. pressure. The difference between the systolic and the diastolic pressure.

This is really expressive of the tone of the arterial walls. Ex:

120 is systolic pressure
<u>100</u> is diastolic pressure
20 is the pulse pressure

130 is the systolic pressure
<u>90</u> is the diastolic pressure
40 is the pulse pressure

Normal pulse pressure: The systolic pressure is normally about 40 points greater than the diastolic. *Abnormal pulse pressure:* A pulse pressure over 50 points or under 30 points is considered abnormal.

p., quick, full, bounding. Indicates inflammation or fever of acute inflammatory character.

p., quick, hard. Characteristic of diphtheria and scarlatina. It also indicates inflammation or fever of acute inflammatory nature.

p., Quincke's. P., capillary, q.v.

p., rapid. P., accelerated, q.v.

p. rate. The average normal beats per minute are as follows:

Pulse of embryo	150
At birth	140–130
During 1st year	130–115
During 2nd year	115–100
During 3rd year	100– 90
About 7th year	90– 85
About 14th year	85– 80
In middle life	75– 70
Old age	65– 50

p., regular. When the force and frequency are the same, i.e., when the length of beat and number of beats per minute and the strength are the same.

p., respiratory. Alternate dilatation and contraction of the large veins of the neck occurring simultaneously with inspiration and expiration following rapid exercise.

p., running. A weak, rapid p. with one wave continuing into the next.

p., senile. That of the aged. The sphygmogram shows a high position of the secondary waves in descent with great size of the 1st secondary wave as compared with the 2nd.

p., short. P. with a short, quick systolic wave.

p., shuttle. P. that feels as though it is floating something solid as well as fluid.

p., slow. A very slow pulse, fully accentuated, often found among the aged. It is a habitual rate among those inclined to be slow and easy in their actions. Such a pulse rate ranges between 40-60 beats per minute.

p., sluggish, full. Common in diseases attended with coma resulting from concussion or compression of brain and chronic softening.

p., small and rapid. Seen in great prostration from wasting diseases or hemorrhage.

p., soft. P. which may be stopped by digital compression.

p., thready. A fine, scarcely perceptible pulse.

p., tremulous. P. in which a series of oscillations is felt with each beat.

p., trigeminal. Three regular beats followed by a pause. SEE: *p., irregular.*

p., undulating. P. that seems to have several successive waves.

p., unequal. P. in which beats vary in force.

p., vagus. A slow p. resulting from vagus inhibition of the heart.

p., venous. P. in a vein, esp. one of the large veins near the heart, such as the internal and external jugular. Normally is undulating and scarcely palpable. In conditions such as tricuspid regurgitation, it is pronounced.

p., vermicular. A small, frequent p. with a wormlike feeling.

p., waterhammer. Characterized by a short, powerful, jerky beat which suddenly collapses. The peculiar pulsation may be distinctly visible, not only in the carotids, but throughout the brachial artery. It is diagnostic of aortic regurgitation during the period of compensation, and its force is due to excessive ventricular hypertrophy and to the large amount of blood expelled with each systole; its sudden recession is due to the incompetent valves failing to support the column of blood. SYN: *Corrigan's p.*

p. wave. A wave in the blood column and the arterial walls which is initiated by the ejection of blood from the left ventricle into the aorta. It travels at a rate of 7-9 meters per sec.

p., wiry. A tense p. that feels like a wire or firm cord. SYN: *angry p.*

pulse, words pert. to: acrotic; acrotism; Adams-Stokes syndrome; anacrotic; anadicrotic; anadicrotism; anatricrotic pulse; arrhythmia; artery; asphyctic; auricular; bisferious; bradycrotic; bradydiastole; bradysphygmia; cardiopuncture; catacrotism; catadicrotic; catadicrotism; centesis; Corrigan's p.; diastasis; diastole; diastolic pressure; dicrotic; heart; hemisystole; infant; intercadence; intercalary; phlebogram; pulsate; pulsation; pulsus; respiration; sphygmoid; sphygmogram; sphygmomanometer; spinal; systaltic; systole; systolic pressure; thermometry; vein.

pulsimeter (pŭl-sĭm'ĕt-ẽr) [L. *pulsus,* a beat, + Gr. *metron,* measure]. Contrivance for measuring frequency and force of the pulse. SYN: *sphygmometer.*

pulsion (pŭl'shŭn). Driving or propelling in any direction.

p., lateral. Movement, particularly walking as if pulled to one side.

pulsus (pŭl'sŭs) [L.]. Pulse.

p. alternans. A succession of strong and weak beats alternating.

p. bigeminus. Paired beats.

p. celer. Fast pulse, particularly that associated with high pulse pressure in aortic regurgitation.

p. paradoxus. One in which the pulse becomes weaker during inspiration.

p. tardus. Slow pulse, esp. that felt in aortic stenosis.

pultaceous (pŭl-tā'shŭs) [L. *pultaceus*]. Resembling a poultice. SYN: *pulpy.*

pulv. [L.]. Abbr. for *pulvis,* powder.

pulverization (pŭl-vẽr-ĭ-zā'shŭn) [L. *pulvis,* powder]. The crushing of any substance to powder or tiny particles.

pulverulent (pŭl-vẽr'ū-lĕnt). Of the nature of, or resembling, powder. SYN: *powdery.*

pulvinar (pŭl-vī'nẽr) [L., cushioned seat]. [NA] Part of the thalamus comprising a portion of the posterior nuclei. Projects posteriorly and medially partially overlying midbrain.

pulvinate (pŭl'vĭ-nāt) [L. *pulvinus,* cushion]. Very convex; shaped like a cushion.

pul'vis [L.]. Powder.

pump [ME. *pumpe*]. 1. Apparatus that transfers fluids or gases by pressure or suction. 2. To force air or fluid into a cavity, as heart pumps blood.

p., air. Device for forcing air in or out of a chamber.

p., breast. Apparatus for removing milk from the breasts.

p., dental. Apparatus for removing saliva from the mouth during operation on teeth or jaws.

p., stomach. Apparatus for removing contents of stomach.

pumpkin (pŭmp'kĭn) [Gr. *pepōn,* ripe]. A trailing vine with large, pulpy, round fruit. Edible when cooked.

Food value of 100 gm. (canned): Cal. 33; protein 1.0 gm.; fat 0.3 gm.; carbohydrate 8.0 gm.; calcium 86 mg.; 6400 I.U. vitamin A.

punch drunk. An imprecise term used to indicate disordered brain function due to multiple concussions. Characterized by slow body movement and impairment of intellect. Seen in boxers, particularly those who began boxing before the calvarium and supportive structures of the brain were fully developed.

punched out. Appears as if holes have been made; used to describe appearance of bones (as seen on x-ray film) in certain pathological states.

puncta (pŭnk'tă) [L.]. (sing. *punctum*) Points.

p. dolorosa. Painful points in course of, or at exit of, nerves affected by neuralgia.

p. lacrimalia. Orifices of lacrimal ducts situated at tip of lacrimal papillae located on inner margins of eyelids about 6 mm. from medial canthus.

p. vasculosa. Minute red areas which mark the cut surface of white central substance of the brain, caused by blood escaping from divided blood vessels.

punctate (pŭnk'tāt) [L. *punctum,* point]. Having pinpoint punctures or depressions on the surface; marked with dots.

p. keratoses. Discrete yellow-to-brown firm keratotic papules of the palms and soles. Most probably due to the performing of manual labor.

p. pits. Depressed areas of the skin, esp. of the palmar creases of the hands and soles.

p. rash. One with minute red points.

punctiform (pŭnk'tĭ-form) ["+ *forma,* shape]. 1. Formed like a point. 2. In bacteriology, referring to pinpoint colonies of less than 1 mm. in diameter.

punctograph (pŭnk'tō-grăf) ["+ Gr. *graphein,* to write]. Device employing radiography for localization of foreign bodies in the tissues.

punctum (pŭnk'tŭm) [L.]. (pl. *puncta*) Point.

p. caecum. Spot in fundus of the eyeball where the optic nerve enters. SYN: *blind spot.*

p. lacrimale. [NA] Outlet of lacrimal canaliculus.

p. nasale inferius. Lower portion of suture joining the nasal bones. SYN: *rhinion.*

p. proximum. Visual accomodation near point. ABBR: P.P.

p. remotum. Visual accommodation far point. ABBR: P.R.

p. saliens. First trace of the embryonic heart.

puncture (pŭnk'chŭr) [L. *punctura,* a point]. 1. A hole or wound made by a sharp pointed instrument. 2. To make a hole with such an instrument.

p., diabetic. P. in floor of 4th ventricle which results in glycosuria. SYN: *Bernard's puncture.*

p., exploratory. Piercing of a cavity or cyst for purpose of examining fluid or pus removed.

p., lumbar. P. of the lumbar spinal membranes to relieve dropsy or for examination of spinal fluid. SEE: *cisternal puncture; lumbar puncture; cerebrospinal fluid.*

p., ventricular. P. of a ventricle of the brain for purpose of withdrawing fluid or introducing air for ventriculography.

p. wound. A wound made by piercing with a sharp instrument. SEE: *wound, puncture.*

pungency (pŭn'jĕn-sĭ) [L. *pungēns,* prick]. Quality of being sharp, strong or bitter, as an odor or taste.

pungent (pŭn'jĕnt). Acrid, sharp, as applied to an odor or taste.

P. U. O. Abbr. for *pyrexia of unknown origin.*

pupa (pū'pă) [L., girl]. Stage, in complete metamorphosis of an insect, that follows the larva and precedes the adult or imago. Insect does not feed in this stage and usually is inactive.

pupil (pū'pĭl) [L. *pupilla*]. The contractile opening at the center of the iris of the eye. It contracts when exposed to strong light, and when the focus is on a near object. It dilates in the dark, and when the focus is on a distant object. Average diameter is 4 to 5 mm. Both pupils should be equal.

CONSTRICTION OF: Occurs in old age and photophobia; induced by morphine, pilocarpine, physostigmine, eserine, and other miotic drugs.

DILATION OF: May occur in blindness or deficient sight from any cause; from distress or strong emotion; in fevers and comatose states, oculomotor nerve paralysis, glaucoma. May be induced by belladonna (atropine), cocaine, eucatropine, homatropine,

hyoscine (scopolamine), and other mydriatic drugs.

RS: accommodation; adaptation; anisocoria; ciliospinal center; corectasia; corenclesis; eye; hippus; iridoplegia; isocoria; miosis; miotic; mydriasis; mydriatic; myosis; myotic; reflex; seclusio pupillae.

p., Argyll Robertson. P. which reacts to accommodation, but not to light. Seen in tabes dorsalis and occasionally in other diseases affecting midbrain.

p., artificial. P. made by iridectomy when normal pupil is occluded.

p., bounding. Rapid dilatation of pupil alternating with contraction.

p., cat's-eye. One narrow and slitlike.

p., occlusion of. P. with opaque membrane shutting off the pupillary area.

p., pinhole. P. of minute size; one excessively constricted. Seen after use of miotics, in opium poisoning, and in certain brain disorders.

p., tonic. P. which reacts slowly in accommodation-convergence reflexes.

pupillary (pū'pĭ-lĕr-ĭ) [L. *pupilla,* pupil]. Concerning the pupil.

p. reflex. 1. Constriction of pupil upon stimulation of retina by light. 2. Constriction of pupil upon accommodation for near vision, and dilatation upon accommodation for far vision. SYN: *accommodation reflex.* 3. Constriction of pupil of one eye in response to stimulation of the other by light. SYN: *commensal light reflex.* 4. Constriction of pupil upon attempted closure of eyelids which are held apart. SYN: *Westphal's pupillary reflex, lid or orbicularis reflex.* SEE: *ciliospinal reflex; hippus.*

pupillometer (pū-pĭl-ŏm'ĕ-tĕr) [L. *pupilla,* pupil, + Gr. *metron,* measure]. Device for measurement of diameter of a pupil.

pupilloscopy (pū-pĭl-os'kō-pĭ) ["+ Gr. *skopein,* to examine]. 1. Measurement of eye refraction by effect of light and shadow on the retina. SYN: *skiascopy.* 2. Examination of the pupil.

pupillostatometer (pū"pĭl-ō-stă-tŏm'ĕ-tĕr) ["+ Gr. *statos,* placed, + *metron,* measure]. Device for measuring distance between centers of the pupils.

pure (pyūr) [ME.]. 1. Free from pollution; uncontaminated. 2. Chaste.

p. line. 1. The progeny of a single homozygous individual obtained by self-fertilization. 2. The progeny of an individual reproducing asexually by simple fission, or by buds, runners, stolons, etc. 3. The progeny of two homozygous individuals reproducing sexually.

purgation (pŭr-gā'shŭn) [L. *purgatio*]. 1. Cleansing. 2. Evacuation of the bowels caused by action of a purgative medicine. SYN: *catharsis*.

purgative (pŭr'gă-tĭv) [L. *purgativus*]. 1. Cleansing. 2. An agent that will cause watery evacuation of the intestinal contents. Ex: castor oil; magnesium sulfate. SEE: *catharsis; cathartic.*

   p., cholagogue. Stimulates flow of bile, producing green stools.

   p., drastic. Produces violent action of bowels with cramps and griping.

   p. enema. A strong, high colonic one that produces evacuation when other enemas fail. SEE: *enema.*

   p., saline. Produces copious watery discharges.

   p., simple. Produces free discharge from bowels with some griping.

purge (pŭrj) [L. *purgare*, to cleanse]. 1. To evacuate the bowels by means of a cathartic. 2. A drug that causes evacuation of the bowels.

puriform (pū'rĭ-form) [L. *pus, pur-*, pus, + *forma*, shape]. Resembling pus.

purine (pū'rēn) [L. *purum*, pure, + *uricus*, uric acid]. Parent of a group of heterocyclic nitrogen compounds including purine itself, $C_5H_4N_4$; caffeine, adenine, guanine, xanthine, and uric acid. Purines are the end products of nucleoprotein digestion and may be synthesized in the body. They break down to form uric acid. SEE: *meat.*

   p. body. P. or any base derived from it. Included are adenine, guanine, xanthine, and hypoxanthine. SYN: *p. base.*

   p., endogenous. P. originating from nucleoproteins within the tissues.

   p., exogenous. P. present in, or derived from, foods.

   p. -free diet. Diet which excludes the following: meat, esp. sweetbreads, liver, kidney; poultry; fish; condiments; alcohol; and foods that are difficult to digest such as concentrated sweets, rich pastries, and fried foods.

   p. -low diet. Excludes foods such as meat, fish, fowl, spinach, lentils, mushrooms, peas, asparagus.

Purkinje (pŭr-kĭn'jĕ). [Johannes E. von Purkinje, Hungarian physiologist, 1787-1869].

   P. cells. Large neutrons which have dendrites extending to the molecular layer of the cerebellar cortex and into the white matter of the cerebellum.

   P. fibers. Atypical muscle fibers lying beneath endocardium constituting the impulse-conducting system of the heart.

   P. figures. Dark lines produced by the vessels of the retina.

   P. network. Fibrous network of large muscle cells found in cardiac muscle beneath the endocardium.

   P. phenomenon, pupillomotor. When the eye adapts from light to dark conditions, the maximum pupillary movement is caused by green instead of yellow light.

   P. vesicle. The nuclear portion of an ovum. SYN: *germinal vesicle.*

Purkinje-Sanson's images (pŭr-kĭn'jĕ-sŏ-sō'). [J. E. Purkinje; Louis J. Sanson, Fr. physician, 1790-1841] Three images of one object seen in the pupil of the eye.

purohepatitis (pū'rō-hĕp''ă-tī'tĭs) [L. *pus, pur-*, pus, + Gr. *hepar, hepat-*, liver, + *-itis*,

Purines in Food

Group A: High concentrations (150 to 1000 mg. per 100 grams)	
Liver	Sardines (in oil)
Kidney	Meat extracts
Sweetbreads	Consomme
Brains	Gravies
Heart	Fish roes
Anchovies	Herring

Group B: Moderate amounts (50 to 150 mg. per 100 grams)	
Meat, game and fish other than those mentioned in Group A	
Fowl	Asparagus
Lentils	Cauliflower
Whole grain cereals	Mushrooms
Beans	Spinach
Peas	

Group C: Very small amounts. Need not be restricted in diet of persons with gout.	
Vegetables other than those mentioned above	
Fruits of all kinds	Coffee
Milk	Tea
Cheese	Chocolate
Eggs	Carbonated beverages
Refined cereals, spaghetti & macaroni	
Butter, fats, nuts & peanut butter*	
Sugars and sweets	Tapioca
Vegetable soups	Yeast

*Fats interfere with the urinary excretion of urates and thus should be limited when attempting to control the excretion of uric acid.

inflammation]. Purulent inflammation of the liver.

puromucous (pū"rō-mū'kŭs) ["+ *mucus,* phlegm]. Mucopurulent, containing both mucus and pus.

purpura (pūr'pū-ră) [L., purple]. An affection with various manifestations and diverse causes, characterized by hemorrhages into the skin, mucous membranes, internal organs, and other tissues. Hemorrhage into the skin shows red, darkening into purple, then brownish-yellow and finally disappearing in 2-3 weeks. Areas of discoloration do not disappear under pressure.

   p., allergic. A group of purpuras due to a variety of agents including bacteria, drugs, and food.

   p. annularis telangiectodes. Eruption of ring-shaped spots on lower limbs with pronounced telangiectasia. SYN: *Majocchi's disease.*

   p., fibrinolytic. P. resulting from excess fibrinolytic activity of blood.

   p. fulminans. A rapidly progressing form occurring principally in children; of short duration and frequently fatal.

   p., hemorrhagic. Idiopathic thrombocytopenic p., q.v.

   p., idiopathic thrombocytopenic. A hemorrhagic disorder in which there is a pronounced reduction in circulating blood platelets, due to presence in blood plasma of a substance which agglutinates platelets. Primary cause unknown. ABBR: ITP. SYN: *purpura hemorrhagica; Werlhof's disease.*

   SYM: Bleeding from mouth and skin upon slight injury. Bleeding may also occur from mucous membranes, in serous membranes, and sometimes into brain. Increased bleeding time and reduced platelet count. Clot is nonretractile, but the coagulation time is normal.

   p., nonthrombocytopenic. Allergic p., q.v.

   p., senile. P. occurring in debilitated and aged persons; ecchymoses and petechiae on legs.

   p., thrombocytopenic. Idiopathic thrombocytopenic p., q.v.

purpuric (pūr-pū'rĭk) [L. *purpura,* purple]. Pert. to, resembling, or suffering from purpura.

purpurin (pūr'pū-rĭn). 1. An acid dye used to stain nuclei. 2. Uroerythrin, a red pigment sometimes present in urine.

purpurinuria (pūr"pū-rĭn-ū'rĭ-ă) [L. *purpura,* purple, + Gr. *ouron,* urine]. Purpurin in urine.

purring thrill. Thrill or vibration, like a cat's purring, due to mitral stenosis, aneurysm,

or valvular erosion of the heart; felt by palpation over the precordium.

purulence (pūr'ū-lĕns) [L. *purulentia*]. The state of containing pus. SYN: *suppuration.*

purulency (pūr'ū-lĕn"sĭ). Purulence.

purulent (pūr'ū-lĕnt) [L. pūrulentus]. Suppurative; forming or containing pus. SEE: *sputum.*

puruloid (pūr-ū'loyd) [L. *pus, pur-,* pus, + Gr. *eidos,* form]. Like pus. SYN: *puriform.*

pus (pŭs) [L.]. Liquid product of inflammation composed of albuminous substances, a thin fluid, and leukocytes or their remains; generally yellow in color. If red it suggests rupture of small vessels. If blue or green it indicates presence of Pseudomonas aeruginosa.

   ETIOL: Streptococci, staphylococci, gonococci, pneumococci, and other species of bacteria.

   p. cells. Leukocytes, generally dead and showing degenerative changes. Found in suppurative inflammation.

   p., cheesy. Very thick pus.

   p., concrete. Fibropurulent coagula seen in infective endocarditis.

   p., ichorous. P. that is thin with shreds of sloughing tissue. It may have a fetid odor.

   p., sanious. Ichorous p. colored by blood.

   p., serous. P. mostly of thin serum containing flakes.

   p. in urine. Condition when there are more than the normal number of pus or white blood cells in the urine. It may be due to cystitis, pyelitis, urethritis, tuberculosis of the kidney, infection of the genitourinary tract, or trauma. SYN: *pyuria.*

   Freshly passed urine may be cloudy due to presence of phosphates or pus. If the former, the addition of acid will cause it to clear; if pus is present it will not clear but may become gelatinous.

pus, words pert. to: apyetous; apyous; archepyon; burrowing; cell; empyema; empyesis; pyemia; resorption; saprogenic; suppurate; suppuration; words beginning with "pyo."

pustulant (pŭs'tū-lănt) [L. *pustula,* blister]. 1. Causing pustules. 2. Agent that produces the formation of pustules.

pustular (pŭs'tū-lĕr). Pert. to, or characterized by, pustules.

pustulation (pŭs"tū-lā'shŭn). The development of pustules.

pustule (pŭs'tūl) [L. *pustula,* blister]. Small elevation of skin filled with lymph or pus. Pustules may be circumscribed, flat, rounded, or umbilicated. They occur in eczema pustulosum, acne vulgaris, dermatitis herpetiformis, impetigo simplex, ecthyma, varicella, syphilis, or in smallpox. SEE: *pus; pustulant.*

p., malignant. Severe infectious disease with formation of hard pustule and symptoms of collapse. SYN: *anthrax,* q.v.

pustulocrustaceous (pŭs″tū-lō-krŭs-tā′shŭs) [L. *pustula,* blister, + *crusta,* shell]. Characterized by formation of pustules and crusts.

pustulosis (pŭs″tū-lō′sĭs) ["+ Gr. *-ōsis,* disease]. A generalized eruption of pustules.

putamen (pū-tā′mĕn) [L., shell]. [NA]. The darker, outer layer of the lenticular nucleus.

putrefaction (pū″trĕ-făk′shŭn) [L. *putrefactio*]. Decomposition of animal matter, esp. protein associated with malodorous and poisonous products such as the ptomaines, mercaptans, and hydrogen sulfide, caused by certain kinds of bacteria and fungi. Decomposition occurring spontaneously in sterile tissue after death is called autolysis. SEE: *intestinal putrefaction; sepsis.*

putrefactive (pū″trĕ-făk′tĭv) [L. *putrefacēre,* to putrefy]. 1. Causing, or pert. to, putrefaction. 2. Agent promoting putrefaction.

putrefy (pū′trĕ-fī) [L. *putrefacere,* to putrefy]. To undergo putrefaction.

putrescence (pū-trĕs′ĕns) [L. *putrēscens,* grow rotten]. Decay; rottenness.

putrid (pū′trĭd) [L. *putridus*]. Decayed; rotten; foul.

putrilage (pū′trĭl-ĕj) [L. *putrilago*]. Product of putrefaction.

pyarthrosis (pī″ăr-thrō′sĭs) [Gr. *pyon,* pus, + *arthron,* joint, + *-ōsis,* condition]. Pus in the cavity of a joint.

pycnemia (pĭk-nē′mĭ-ă) [Gr. *pyknos,* thick, + *haima,* blood]. Thickening of the blood. SYN: *pyknemia.*

pycno- (pĭk′nō) [Gr. *pyknos,* thick]. Combining form meaning dense, thick. SEE: words beginning with *pykno-.*

pyecchysis (pī-ĕk′ĭ-sĭs) [Gr. *pyon,* pus, + *ek,* out, + *chein,* to pour]. An effusion of pus.

pyelectasia, pyelectasis (pī″ĕ-lĕk-tā′zĭ-ā, -ĕk′tăs-ĭs) [Gr. *pyelos,* pelvis, + *ektasis,* dilatation]. Dilatation of the renal pelvis.

pyelitic (pī″ĕ-lĭt′ĭk). Rel. to, or affected with, pyelitis.

pyelitis (pī″ĕ-lī′tĭs) [Gr. *pyelos,* pelvis, + *-itis,* inflammation]. Inflammation of the kidney pelvis and its calices.

p., calculous. P. resulting from a calculus.

pyelo- [Gr. *pyelos,* pelvis]. Combining form meaning the pelvis.

pyelocystitis (pī′ĕ-lō-sĭs-tī′tĭs) ["+ *kystis,* bladder, + *-itis,* inflammation]. Inflamed condition of the kidney, pelvis, and bladder.

pyelocystostomosis (pī′ĕ-lō-sĭs″tō-sto-mō′sĭs) ["+ "+ *stoma,* mouth, + *-ōsis,* condition]. Establishment of surgical communication between the kidney and the bladder.

pyelogram, pyelograph (pī′ĕ-lō-grăm, -grăf) [Gr. *pyelos,* pelvis, + *gramma,* a mark]. A roentgen picture of the ureter and renal pelvis.

pyelography (pī″ĕ-lŏg′ră-fī) ["+ *graphein,* to write]. X-ray examination of a renal pelvis and ureter.

pyelolithotomy (pī″ĕ-lō-lĭth-ŏt′ŏ-mī) ["+ *lithos,* stone, + *tome,* incision]. Removal of calculus from the pelvis of a kidney through an incision.

pyelometer (pī″ĕ-lŏm′ĕ-ter) [Gr. *pyelos,* pelvis, + *metron,* measure]. Device to measure the pelvic diameters. SYN: *pelvimeter.*

pyelometry (pī″ĕ-lŏm′ĕ-trī). 1. Measurement of the kidney's pelvis. 2. Measurement of the diameters of the pelvis. SYN: *pelvimetry.*

pyelonephritis (pī″ĕ-lō-nĕ-frī′tĭs) [Gr. *pyelos,* pelvis, + *nephros,* kidney, + *-itis,* inflammation]. Inflammation of kidney substance and pelvis.

ETIOL: Bacterial, metastatic, or urogenous (ascending from bladder).

SYM: Sudden onset of chilliness and fever with dull pain in the flank over either or both kidneys. There is tenderness when the kidney is palpated. Usually there are signs of cystitis, i.e., urgency with burning and frequency of urination. White blood cells will be present in the urinary sediment.

PROG: Depends upon character and virulence of infection, accessory etiological factors, drainage of kidney, presence or absence of complications, and general physical condition.

TREATMENT: Recognition and removal of cause (focal infection, etc.); measures to increase resistance of patient; bed rest. Avoidance of drugs irritating to kidney, condiments, and alcohol. Hot water bag, antipyretic drugs, and antibiotics. Surgery if necessary (nephrotomy, nephrectomy, pyelotomy).

pyelonephrosis (pī″ĕ-lō-nĕ-frō′sĭs) [Gr. *pyelos,* pelvis, + *nephros,* kidney, + *-ōsis,* disease]. Disease of the pelvis of the kidney.

pyelopathy (pī″ĕ-lŏp′ăth-ī) ["+ *pathos,* disease]. Any disease of the pelvis of the kidney. SYN: *pyelonephrosis.*

pyeloplasty (pī′ĕ-lō-plăs″tī) ["+ *plastos,* formed]. Reparative operation on the kidney pelvis.

pyeloplication (pī''ĕ-lō-plī-kā'shŭn) [Gr. *pyelos*, pelvis, + L. *plicāre*, to fold]. Shortening of the wall of a dilated renal pelvis by taking tucks in it.

pyeloscopy (pī''ĕlŏs'kō-pī) ["+ *skopein*, to examine]. Examination of the pelvis of the kidney using fluoroscopy.

pyelostomy (pī''ĕ-lŏs'tō-mī) ["+ *stoma*, mouth]. Creation of an opening into the renal pelvis.

pyelotomy (pī''ĕ-lŏt'ō-mī) [Gr. *pyelos*, pelvis, + *tomē*, incision]. Incision of renal pelvis.

NP: Keep patient dry, watch skin for decubitus. If retention catheter present, keep draining at all times. Accurate record of intake and output of urine.

pyelovenous backflow (pī''ĕ-lō-vē'nŭs) ["+ L. *vena*, vein]. Drainage from the renal pelvis into the venous system because of back pressure.

pyemesis (pī-ĕm'ī-sīs) [Gr. *pyon*, pus, + *emesis*, vomiting]. Vomiting of pus.

pyemia (pī-ē'mī-ă) ["+ *haima*, blood]. A form of septicemia due to presence of pus-forming organisms in the blood, manifested by formation of multiple abscesses of a metastatic nature.

SYM: High intermittent temperature with recurrent chills; metastatic processes in various parts of the body, esp. in lungs; septic pneumonia, empyema. Results may be fatal.

TREATMENT: Antibiotics. Prophylactic treatment consists in prevention of suppuration.

p., arterial. P. resulting from dissemination of emboli from a thrombus in cardiac vessels.

p., cryptogenic. P., the focus of which is hidden in the deeper tissues.

p., metastatic. Multiple abscess resulting from infected pyemic thrombi.

p., portal. Suppurative inflammation of portal vein.

pyemic (pī-ē'mīk) [Gr. *pyon*, pus, + *haima*, blood]. Rel. to, or affected with, blood poisoning.

pyencephalus (pī''ĕn-sĕf'ă-lŭs) ["+ *enkephalos*, brain]. A brain abscess with suppuration within the cranium. SYN: *pyocephalus.*

pyesis (pī-ē'sīs). Formation of pus. SYN: *suppuration.*

pygal (pī'găl) [Gr. *pygē*, rump]. Concerning the buttocks.

pygalgia (pī-găl'jī-ă) ["+ *algos*, pain]. Pain in the rump or buttocks.

pygmalionism (pĭg-mā'lī-ŏn-ĭzm). [Pygmalion, a sculptor and king in Gr. mythology, who fell in love with a figure he had carved].

Psychopathic condition in which a person is in love with a creation of his own.

pygo- [Gr. *pygē*, rump]. Combining form meaning the rump.

pyin (pī'īn) [Gr. *pyon*, pus]. A substance of albuminous nature sometimes present in pus.

pyknic type (pīk'nīk) [Gr. *pyknos*, thick]. A body type characterized by broad head, thick shoulders, large chest, short neck, and stocky body.

Individuals of this type often are happy, carefree persons whose emotional reactions are obvious. They are interested in others apart from themselves. They are extroverts. SEE: *asthenic body type.*

pykno- [Gr. *pyknos*, thick]. Combining form meaning thick, compact, dense, frequent. SEE; words beginning with *pycno.*

pyknocardia (pīk-nō-kär'dī-ă) ["+ *kardia*, heart]. Rapid pulse. SYN: *tachycardia.*

pyknohemia (pīk''nō-hē'mī-ă) ["+ *haima*, blood]. Thickening of the blood. SYN: *pyknemia.*

pyknolepsy (pīk''nō-lĕp'sī) [Gr. *pyknos*, thick, + *lēpsis*, seizure]. Attacks similar to petit mal or minor epileptic seizures, usually occurring in childhood.

pyknometer (pīk-nŏm'ĕ-tĕr) ["+ *metron*, measure]. Device for determining specific gravity of liquids.

pyknomorphous (pīk''nō-mōrf'ŭs) ["+ *morphē*, form]. Characterized by compact arrangement of the stainable portions, said esp. of certain nerve cells.

pyknophrasia (pīk''nō-frā'zī-ă) [Gr. *pyknos*, thick, + *phrasis*, speech]. Thickness of words uttered in speech.

pyknosis (pīk-nō'sīs) ["+ *-ōsis*, intensive]. Inspissation; thickness, esp. shrinking of cells through degeneration.

pyle- [Gr. *pylē*, gate]. Combining form meaning orifice, esp. that of the portal vein.

pylemphraxis (pī''lĕm-fräk'sīs) ["+ *emphraxis*, stoppage]. Occlusion of the portal vein.

pylephlebectasia, pylephlebectasis (pī''lē-flē-bĕk-tā'zī-ă, -bĕk'tă-sīs) ["+ *phleps*, *phleb-*, vein, + *ektasis*, dilatation]. Distention of the portal vein.

pylephlebitis (pī''lē-flē-bī'tīs) ["+ "+ *-ītis*, inflammation]. Inflamed condition of the portal vein, generally suppurative.

p., adhesive. Thrombosis of the portal vein.

p. obturans. P. with obstructed flow in the portal vein.

pylethrombosis (pī''lē-thrŏm-bō'sīs) [Gr. *pylē*, gate, + *thrombos*, a clot, + *-ōsis*, intensive]. Occlusion of portal vein by a thrombus.

pylometer (pī-lŏm'ĕ-tĕr) ["+ *metron*, measure]. Device for measuring obstructions at vesical opening.

pyloralgia (pī'lō-răl'jĭ-ă) [Gr. *pyloros*, gatekeeper, + *algos*, pain]. Pain around the pylorus, distal aperture of the stomach.

pylorectomy (pī'lō-rĕk'tō-mī) ["+ *ektomē*, excision]. Surgical removal of the pylorus.

pyloric (pī-lor'ĭk) [Gr. *pyloros*, gatekeeper]. Pert. to the opening between the stomach and duodenum.

   p. antrum. The first part of the pyloric portion of the stomach; portion leading to pyloric canal. SYN: *p. vestibule; p. sinus.*

   p. canal. The narrow constricted region of pyloric portion of stomach that opens through pylorus into duodenum.

   p. gland. A gland of the stomach near the pylorus.

   p. obstruction and dilatation. P. obstruction increases the resistance offered to the expulsion of food. In its efforts to overcome this the stomach first becomes hypertrophied, then dilated. Causes of dilatation are pyloric obstruction, laxness of walls from simple atony, excessive ingestion of food or drink.

   SYM: The general symptoms of dyspepsia with the following symptoms relating to vomit. Vomiting occurs long after eating, sometimes several hours or days. Amount often excessive, sometimes several quarts; is sour and fermented, and on standing separates into a sediment of undigested food and a turbid, frothy liquid. Ejected fluid rich in torulae and sarcinae, forms of bacteria. Obstinate constipation.

   SIGNS: Bulging over epigastrium; in thin subjects the outline of stomach may be visible. Palpation gives a splashing fremitus. In percussion there is an increased area of gastric tympany. In auscultation, splashing sounds often are audible at some distance. Ordinarily an esophageal sound may be inserted a distance of 60 cm. from the teeth. In dilatation may be inserted 65-70 cm.

   PROG: Guarded. More favorable in dilatation without obstruction.

   TREATMENT: Diet light, nutritious, not bulky, and should be given in small amounts at frequent intervals. An abdominal support often relieves some of distressing symptoms.

   p. orifice. Opening or passage between the stomach and duodenum.

   p. stenosis. Narrowing of the p. orifice. Also due to excessive thickening of circular muscle of pylorus (hypertrophic pyloric

stenosis), or hypertrophy and hyperplasia of mucosa and submucosa.

pyloristenosis (pī-lōr-ĭ-stĕn-ō'sĭs) [Gr. *pyloros*, gatekeeper, + *stenōsis*, a narrowing]. Constriction of the pylorus.

pyloritis (pī-lō-rī'tĭs) ["+ -*itis*, inflammation]. Inflamed condition of the pylorus.

pyloro- [Gr. *pyloros*, gatekeeper]. Combining form meaning gatekeeper; applied to the pylorus.

pyloroduodenitis (pī-lōr"ō-dū"ō-dē-nī'tĭs) ["+ L. *duodeni*, twelve, + Gr. -*itis*, inflammation]. Inflammation of the mucosa of the pylorus and duodenum.

pylorogastrectomy (pī-lōr"ō-găs-trĕk'tō-mī) ["+ *gastēr*, belly, + *ektomē*, excision]. Excision of pyloric portion of the stomach.

pyloromyotomy (pī-lōr"ō-mī-ŏt'ō-mī) [Gr. *pyloros*, gatekeeper, + *mys, my-*, muscle, + *tomē*, a cutting]. Incision and suture of the pyloric sphincter.

pyloroplasty (pī-lōr'ō-plăs"tĭ) ["+ *plassein*, to form]. Operation to repair the pylorus, esp. one to increase the caliber of the pyloric opening by stretching.

pyloroptosia, pyloroptosis (pī-lō"rŏp-tō'sĭ-ă, -rŏp'tō-sĭs) ["+ *ptōsis*, a dropping]. Displacement downward of the pyloric end of the stomach.

pyloroschesis (pī'lōr-ō-shē'sĭs). Obstruction of pyloric orifice.

pyloroscopy (pī-lō-rŏs'kō-pī) [Gr. *pyloros*, gatekeeper, + *skopein*, to examine]. Fluoroscopic examination of the pylorus.

pylorospasm (pī-lōr'ō-spăzm) ["+ *spasmos*, a spasm]. Spasmodic contraction of the pyloric orifice. Usually due to a disturbance in motor mechanism of pylorus. May occur secondary to lesions of stomach and duodenum near to pylorus.

pylorostenosis (pī-lōr"ō-stĕn-ō'sĭs) ["+ *stenosis*, narrowing]. Abnormal narrowing or stricture of the pyloric orifice. SEE: *pyloric stenosis.*

pylorostomy (pī-lōr-ŏs'tō-mī) [Gr. *pyloros*, gatekeeper, + *stoma*, opening]. Formation of an opening through the abdominal wall into the pylorus.

pylorotomy (pī-lōr-ŏt'ō-mī) ["+ *tomē*, a cutting]. Incision of the pyloric submucosa to relieve hypertrophic stenosis.

pylorus (pī-lōr'ŭs) [Gr. *pyloros*, gatekeeper]. The lower orifice of the stomach opening into the duodenum. The pylorus is closed most of the time but opens at intervals permitting acid chyme to enter duodenum. The primary factor in the opening of pylorus is elevation of gastric pressure over duodenal pressure.

   p., spasm of. Pylorospasm, q.v.

pyo-, py- [Gr. *pyon*, pus]. Combining forms meaning pus.

pyocele (pī'ō-sēl) [Gr. *pyon*, pus, + *kēlē*, hernia]. A hernia or distended cavity containing pus.

pyocelia (pī''ō-sē'lī-ā) [" + *koilia*, cavity]. Pus formation in the abdominal cavity.

pyocephalus (pī''ō-sēf'ā-lŭs) [" + *kephalē*, head]. Effusion of purulent nature within the cranium.

> **p., circumscribed.** Abscess of the brain.
>
> **p., external.** Suppuration of the meninges.
>
> **p., internal.** Pus in the cerebrospinal fluid.

pyochezia (pī''ō-kē'zī-ā) [Gr. *pyon*, pus, + *chezein*, to defecate]. Pus in the feces.

pyococcus (pī''ō-kŏk'ŭs) [" + *kokkos*, berry]. A micrococcus which causes suppuration, as the Streptococcus pyogenes.

pyocolpocele (pī''ō-kŏl'pō-sēl) [" + *kolpos*, vagina, + *kēlē*, mass]. A vaginal tumor containing pus. SEE: *pyocolpos*.

pyocolpos (pī''ō-kŏl'pŏs). Accumulation of pus in the vagina.

pyoculture (pī'ō-kŭl''chŭr) [Gr. *pyon*, pus, + L. *cultura*, growth]. Comparative tests for cultivation of pus from a wound, a portion being left in the collecting tube and a portion being cultivated on artificial media.

pyocyanase (pī''ō-sī'ā-nāz). An antibiotic obtained from Psuedomonas aeruginosa. Active principally against gram-positive organisms on which it has a lytic action.

pyocyanic (pī''ō-sī-ăn'ĭk) [Gr. *pyon*, pus, + *kyanos*, dark blue]. Pert. to pyocyanin or blue pus.

pyocyanin (pī''ō-sī'ā-nĭn). An antibiotic obtained from Pseudomonas aeruginosa, effective principally against gram-positive organisms.

pyocyst (pī'ō-sĭst) [Gr. *pyon*, pus, + *kystis*, sac]. A cyst containing pus.

pyoderma (pī-ō-dŭr'mă) [" + *derma*, skin]. Any acute inflammatory, destructive skin disease of unknown origin. Bacteria may be cultured from the lesions, but they are the normal resident flora.

> **p. gangrenosum.** P. usually associated with ulcerative colitis or rheumatoid arthritis. Occurs principally on the trunk.

pyodermatitis (pī''ō-dŭr''mă-tī'tĭs) [" + " + *-itis*, inflammation]. Pyogenic infection of the skin causing a dermatitis.

pyodermatosis (pī''ō-dŭr''mă-tō'sĭs) [" + " + *-osis*, condition]. Any skin condition of pyogenic origin. SYN: *pyodermia*.

pyodermia (pī''ō-dŭr'mī-ā). Any suppurative skin disease.

pyofecia (pī''ō-fē'sī-ā) [Gr. *pyon*, pus, + L. *faeces*, feces]. Pus in the stools.

pyogenesis (pī''ō-jĕn'ĕ-sĭs) [" + *genesis*, formation]. The formation of pus.

pyogenic (pī-ō-jĕn'ĭk) [" + *gennan*, to produce]. Producing pus.

> **p. microorganisms.** M. forming pus. The principal ones are Staphylococcus aureus, S. albus, Streptococcus hemolyticus, Bacillus anthracis, B. subtilis, Clostridium perfringens, Pseudomonas aeruginosa, and Neisseria gonorrhoeae.

pyohemothorax (pī''ō-hē''mō-thō'răks) [Gr. *pyon*, pus, + *haima*, blood, + *thōrax*, chest]. Pus and blood in the pleural cavity.

pyoid (pī'oyd) [" + *eidos*, like]. Resembling pus.

pyolabrinthitis (pī''ō-lăb''ĭ-rĭn-thī'tĭs) [" + *labyrinthos*, a maze, + *-itis*, inflammation]. Inflammation with suppuration of the labyrinth of the ear.

pyometra (pī''ō-mē'trā) [Gr. *pyon*, pus, + *mētra*, uterus]. Retained pus accumulation in the uterine cavity.

pyometritis (pī''ō-mē-trī'tĭs) [" + " + *-itis*, inflammation]. Purulent inflammation of the uterus.

pyonephritis (pī''ō-nef-rī'tĭs) [Gr. *pyon*, pus, + *nephros*, kidney, + *-itis*, inflammation]. Inflammation of the kidney, suppurative in character.

pyonephrolithiasis (pī''ō-nĕf''rō-lĭth-ī'ā-sĭs) [" + " + *lithos*, stone]. Pus and calculi in the kidney.

pyonephrosis (pī''ō-nĕf-rō'sĭs) [" + " + *-osis*, condition]. Pus accumulation in the pelvis of kidney.

pyoovarium (pī''ō-ō-vā'rī-ŭm) [Gr. *pyon*, pus, + L. *ovarium*, ovary]. Abscess formation in an ovary.

pyopericarditis (pī''ō-pĕr''ĭ-kăr-dī'tĭs) [" + *peri*, around, + *kardia*, heart, + *-itis*, inflammation]. Pericarditis with suppuration.

pyopericardium (pī''ō-pĕr''ĭ-kăr'dī-ŭm) ["]. Pus formation in the pericardium.

pyoperitoneum (pī''ō-pĕr''ĭ-tō-nē'ŭm) [Gr. *pyon*, pus, + *peritonaion*, peritoneum]. Pus formation in the peritoneal cavity.

pyoperitonitis (pī''ō-pĕr''ĭ-tō-nī'tĭs) [" + " + *-itis*, inflammation]. Purulent inflammation of the lining of peritoneum.

pyophagia (pī''ō-fā'jĭ-ā) [" + *phagein*, to eat]. Swallowing of purulent substance.

pyophthalmia, pyophthalmitis (pī''ōf-thăl'mĭ-ā, -thăl-mī'tĭs) [Gr. *pyon*, pus, + *ophthalmos*, eye, + *-itis*, inflammation]. Suppurative inflamed condition of the eye.

pyophylactic (pī''ō-fī-lăk'tĭk) [" + *phylaxis*, protection]. Guarding against formation of pus.

p. membrane. Lining membrane of an abscess cavity separating it from healthy tissue.

pyophysometra (pī″ō-fī″sō-mē′tră) ["+ *physa*, air, + *mētra*, uterus]. Pus and gas accumulation in the uterus.

pyoplania (pī″ō-plā′nĭ-ă) ["+ *planos*, wandering]. Spreading of pus by infiltration into other tissue.

pyopneumocholecystitis (pī″ō-nū″mō-kō-lē-sĭs-tī′tĭs) [Gr. *pyon*, pus, + *cholē*, bile, + *kystis*, sac, + *-itis*, inflammation]. Distention of the gallbladder with air and pus.

pyopneumocyst (pī″ō-nū″mō-sĭst) ["+ "+ *kystis*, bladder]. A cyst enclosing pus and gas.

pyopneumopericardium (pī″ō-nū″mō-pĕr″ĭ-kăr′dĭ-ŭm) ["+ "+ *peri*, around, + *kardia*, heart]. Pus and air or gas in pericardium.

pyopneumoperitonitis (pī″ō-nū″mō-pĕr″ĭ-tō-nī′tĭs) ["+ "+ *peritonaion*, peritoneum]. Pus and air in the peritoneal cavity complicating peritonitis.

pyopoiesis (pī″ō-poy-ē′sĭs) [Gr. *pyon*, pus, + *poiein*, to make]. Formation of pus. SYN: *pyogenesis; suppuration.*

pyopoietic (pī″ō-poy-ĕt′ĭk). Pert. to formation of pus. SYN: *suppurative.*

pyoptysis (pī-ŏp′tĭ-sĭs) [Gr. *pyon*, pus, + *ptysis*, spitting]. Spitting of pus.

pyorrhagia (pī-ōr-ă′jĭ-ă) ["+ *rhēgnynai*, to burst forth]. Profuse flow of pus, as when an abscess ruptures.

pyorrhea (pī″ō-rē′ă) ["+ *rhoia*, flow]. A discharge of purulent matter.

p. alveolaris. A periodontal disease characterized by inflammatory or degenerative changes of the periosteum, alveolar bone, and tooth cementum. Resorption of alveolar bone occurs, resulting in loosening of teeth and recession of gums. SYN: *periodontitis; periodontoclasia; Riggs' disease.*

pyosalpingitis (pī″ō-săl″pĭn-jī′tĭs) [Gr. *pyon*, pus, + *salpinx*, tube, + *-itis*, inflammation]. Retained pus in the oviduct with inflammation.

pyosalpingo-oophoritis (pī″ō-săl-pĭn″gō-ō″ŏf-ō-rī′tĭs) ["+ "+ *ōon*, ovum, + *phoros*, a bearer, + *-itis*, inflammation]. Inflammation of ovary and oviduct with suppuration.

pyosalpinx (pī″ō-săl′pĭnks). Pus in the fallopian tube. SEE: *pyosalpingitis.*

pyosis (pī-ō′sĭs) [Gr.]. Formation of pus. SYN: *suppuration.*

pyospermia (pī″ō-spŭr′mĭ-ă) [Gr. *pyon*, pus, + *sperma*, seed]. Pus in the semen.

pyostatic (pī″ō-stăt′ĭk) ["+ *statikos*, halting]. 1. Preventing pus formation. 2. Agent checking the development of pus.

pyotherapy (pī″ō-thĕr′ă-pī) ["+ *therapeia*, treatment]. Treatment of disease with pus.

pyothorax (pī″ō-thō′răks) [Gr. *pyon*, pus, + *thōrax*, chest]. Pus in the pleural cavity. SYN: *empyema.*

pyotorrhea (pī″ō-tōr-ē′ă) ["+ *ous, ot-*, ear, + *rhoia*, flow]. Purulent discharge from the ear.

pyotoxinemia (pī″ō-tōk″sĭ-nē′mĭ-ă) ["+ *toxikon*, poison, + *haima*, blood]. Infection from toxic products of pus organisms in the blood.

pyoturia (pī″ō-tū′rĭ-ă) [Gr. *pyon*, pus, + *ouron*, urine]. Pus cells in the urine. SYN: *pyuria.*

pyourachus (pī″ō-ū′ră-kŭs) ["+ *ourachos*, fetal urinary canal]. Accumulation of pus in the urachus.

pyoureter (pī″ō-ū-rē′tĕr) ["+ *ourēter*, ureter]. Pus collection in the ureter.

pyovesiculosis (pī″ō-vĕ-sĭk″ū-lō′sĭs) [Gr. *pyon*, pus, + L. *vesiculus*, a small vessel, + Gr. *-ōsis*, condition]. Pus collection in the seminal vesicles.

pyoxanthin (pī″ō-zăn′thĭn) ["+ *xanthos*, yellow]. A yellow pigment resulting from oxidation of pyocyanin. Sometimes present in pus.

pyramid (pĭr′ă-mĭd) [Gr. *pyramis*, a pyramid]. 1. A solid on the base with three or more sides, the triangular planes of which meet at an apex. 2. Any part of the body resembling a pyramid. 3. A compact bundle of nerve fibers in the medulla oblongata. 4. Petrous portion of temporal bone.

p. of cerebellum. A median ventral projection of vermis of cerebellum lying between tuber and uvula.

p., malpighian. Renal pyramid, q.v.

p. of the medulla. A pair of elongated tapering prominences on anterior surface of medulla oblongata, composed of descending corticospinal fibers.

p., renal. One of a number of cone-shaped structures comprising medulla of the kidney along with renal columns. Each p. has an external base in the kidney's boundary with an apex that projects as a renal papilla into the renal sinus. P.'s converge. SYN: *p. of Malpighi; malpighian p.*

p. of temporal bone. The pyramis or petrous portion of the temporal bone.

p. of the thyroid. A conical process sometimes present, extending cephalad from the isthmus of the thyroid gland. SYN: *pyramidal or median lobe.*

p. of the tympanum. A hollow projection on inner wall of the tympanum through which passes the stapedius muscle. SYN: *pyramidal eminence.*

pyramidal (pĭ-răm'ĭ-dăl). In the shape of a pyramid.

   p. cell. Pyramid-shaped cell of cerebral cortex.

   p. tract. One of three descending tracts (lateral, ventral, ventrolateral) of the spinal cord. Consists of fibers arising from giant pyramidal cells of Betz present in motor area of cerebral cortex SYN: *cortispinal tract.*

pyramidalis (pĭ-răm''ĭ-dal'ĭs) [L.]. The muscle which arises from the crest of the pubis and is inserted into the linea alba upward about half way to the naval.

   p. auriculae. Small muscle inserted into auricle of ear. Often absent.

   p. nasi. Small muscle overlying nasal bone. Inserted into skin at root of nose. SYN: *procerus muscle.*

pyrenemia (pī''rĕ-nē'mĭ-ă) [Gr. *pyrēn,* fruit stone, + *haima,* blood]. Condition in which there are nucleated red cells in the blood.

pyrenin (pī'rĕ-nĭn). The oxyphilic substance found in the nucleolus.

pyrenoid (pī'rĕ-noyd) [Gr. *pyrēn,* fruit stone, + *eidos,* like]. A colorless, highly refractive body in certain protozoan chromatophores.

pyretherapy (pī''rĕ-thĕr'ă-pī) [Gr. *pyr,* fever, + *therapeia,* treatment]. Artificial fever treatment.

pyrethrins (pī-rē'thrĭnz). General name of substances derived from pyrethrum flowers (chrysanthemums). Used as insecticides.

pyretic (pī-rĕt'ĭk) [Gr. *pyretos,* fever.]. Concerning fever.

   p. therapy. Treatment of disease by artificial induction of fever, either by heat or the inoculation of malarial organisms.

pyreticosis (pī-rĕt''ĭ-kō'sĭs) [" + -*ōsis,* intensive]. Feverishness.

pyreto- (pī-rĕt'ō) [Gr. *pyretos,* fever.]. Prefix meaning fever.

pyretogen (pī-rĕt'ō-jĕn) [" + *gennan,* to produce]. A substance producing fever.

pyretogenesia, pyretogenesis (pī''rĕ-tō-jĕn-ē'zĭ-ă, -jĕn'ĕ-sĭs) [" + *genesis,* production]. Origin and production of fever.

pyretogenic (pī''rĕt-ō-jĕn'ĭk). Producing or causing fever.

   p. bacteria. Pathogenic bacteria causing fever.

   p. stage. Period in a fever when it is rising slowly.

pyretogenous (pī''rĕ-tŏj'ĕn-ŭs). 1. Producing or causing fever. 2. Caused by fever.

pyretography (pī''rĕ-tŏg'ră-fī) [Gr. *pyretos,* fever, + *graphein,* to write]. A treatise on fever.

pyretology (pī''rĕ-tŏl'ō-jĭ) [" + *logos,* a study]. Science of fevers and their characteristics.

pyretolysis (pī''rĕ-tŏl'ĭ-sĭs) [" + *lysis,* dissolution]. 1. Reduction of fever. 2. Lysis of symptoms of disease process which is accelerated by fever.

pyretotherapy (pī''rĕ-tō-thĕr'ă-pī) [" + *therapeia,* treatment]. 1. Treatment by artificially raising the patient's temperature. 2. Treatment of fever.

pyretotyphosis (pī''rĕ-tō-tī-fō'sĭs) [" + *typhōsis,* delirium]. The delirious or stuporous characteristic of fever.

pyrexia (pī-rĕk'sĭ-ă) [Gr. *pyressein,* to be feverish]. Condition in which the temperature is above normal. SYN: *fever.*

   Some classify it as:

Low	99°–101° F.
Moderate	101°–103° F.
High	103°–105° F.

   p., local. Acute inflammation of a part.

pyrexial (pī-rĕk'sĭ-ăl). Concerning fever.

pyrexin (pī'rĕks'ĭn). A substance extracted from inflammatory exudates which induces fever.

pyridoxal 5-phosphate. A derivative of pyridoxine, which serves as a coenzyme of certain amino-acid decarboxylases in bacteria, and in animal tissues of 3,4-Dihydroxyphenyalanine (dopa) decarboxylase.

pyridoxamine (pĭr''ĭ-dŏks'ă-mĭn). One of the vitamin B_6 group; a 4-aminoethyl analog of pyridoxine.

4-pyridoxic acid (pĭr''ĭ-dŏks'ĭk). The principal end product of pyridoxine metabolism excreted in human urine.

pyridoxine (pī-rĭ-dŏks'ēn). One of a group of substances, including pyridoxal and pyridoxamine, which make up vitamin B_6. SEE: *vitamin B_6.*

pyriform (pĭr'ĭ-form) [L. *pīrum,* pear, + *forma,* shape]. Shaped like a pear.

pyrimidine (pī-rĭm'ĭd-īn). The parent of a group of heterocyclic nitrogen compounds, $C_4H_4N_2$, including uracil, cytosine, and thymine, some of which are components of nucleic acid.

pyrithiamine (pĭr''ĭ-thī'ă-mĭn). A synthetic analog of thiamine which acts as an antithiamine substance. When administered, it produces many of the sym. of thiamine deficiency.

pyro- (pī'rō) [Gr. *pyr,* fire]. Prefix meaning heat or fire.

pyrogen (pī''rō-jĕn) [Gr. *pyr,* fire, + *gennan,* to produce]. Any substance which produces fever.

   NP: Do not give fluids intravenously which have been opened previously and allowed to stand, even though the top may have been closed tightly.

p., leukocytic. A substance found in blood during fever which acts upon the thermoregulatory centers of the hypothalamus.

p., reaction. A febrile reaction seen within the first few minutes of a blood transfusion or intravenous solution which contains a pyrogen. Seldom seen now that pyrogen-free water and plastic disposable containers and administration sets are used.

pyrogenic (pī"rō-jěn'ĭk) [Gr. *pyr,* fire, + *gennan,* to produce]. Producing fever.

py"rolag'nia ("+ *lagneia,* lust). Insane desire to see or produce fires; accompanied by sexual gratification.

pyrollic amino acids. Proline and oxyproline.

pyrolysis (pī-rŏl'ĭ-sĭs) ["+ *lysis,* dissolution]. Decomposition of organic matter when there is a rise in temperature.

pyromania (pī"rō-mā'nĭ-ă) ["+ *mania,* madness]. Fire madness; mania for setting fires or seeing them.

pyrometer (pī-rŏm'ē-tĕr) [Gr. *pyr,* fire, + *metron,* measure]. Device for measuring extreme degrees of heat.

pyronyxis (pī"rō-nĭk'sĭs) ["+ *nyxis,* a piercing]. Treatment or cauterization by puncturing a part with hot needles. SYN: *ignipuncture.*

pyrophobia (pī"rō-fō'bĭ-ă) ["+ *phobos,* fear]. Abnormal fear of fire.

pyroptothymia (pī"rŏp-tō-thī'mĭ-ă) [Gr. *pyr,* fire, + *ptoein,* to scare, + *thymos,* mind]. A psychosis in which one imagines himself surrounded by flames.

pyropuncture (pī"rō-pŭnk'chŭr) ["+ L. *punctura,* piercing]. Treatment by puncture

of a part with hot needles. SYN: *pyronyxis.* SEE: *counterirritation.*

pyrosis (pī-rō'sĭs) [Gr. *pyrōsis,* burning]. A burning sensation in the epigastric and sternal region, with raising of acid liquid from stomach. SYN: *heartburn; waterbrash.*

    NP: Note whether it occurs before or after food is taken, the time and duration, and whether different foods give rise to it. SEE: *taste.*

pyrotic (pī-rŏt'ĭk) [Gr. *pyrōtikos*]. 1. Caustic; burning. 2. Pert. to pyrosis.

pyrotoxin (pī"rō-tŏk'sĭn) [Gr. *pyr,* fire, + *toxikon,* poison]. A toxin generated by a febrile process.

pyroxylin (pī-rŏk'sĭ-lĭn) ["+ *xylon,* wood]. A product obtained by the action of a mixture of nitric and sulfuric acids on cellulose.

    USES: In the preparation of collodion.

    INCOMPATIBILITIES: Sulfides, alkalies.

pyrrol cells. Cells of the reticuloendothelial system so called because of their ability to ingest colloidal dyes (pyrrol blue). SYN: *histiocytes.*

pyruvate (pī'rū-vāt). A salt or ester of pyruvic acid.

pyruvic acid (pī-rū'vĭk). $CH_3CO\cdot COOH$, an organic acid which plays an important role in Krebs cycle, it being an intermediate product in the metabolism of carbohydrates, fats, and amino acids. It increases in quantity in the blood and tissues in thiamine deficiency, thiamine being essential for its oxidation.

pyuria (pī-ū'rĭ-ă) [Gr. *pyon,* pus, + *ouron,* urine]. Pus in the urine; evidence of renal disease.

    ETIOL: Lesion of urethra, ureters, bladder, kidneys, infection.

    RS: cystitis; kidney; pyelitis, ureteritis; urethritis.

PZI. Abbr. for *protamine zinc insulin.*

Q

Q. 1. Abbr. for *electric quantity; quart.* 2. Symb. for *coulomb.*

Q$_{co2}$. Number of microliters of CO_2 given off per milligram of dry weight of tissue per hour.

Q$_{o2}$. Number of microliters of O_2 taken up per milligram of dry weight of tissue per hour.

q. d. Abbr. for L. *quaque die,* every day.

Q disk. A dark, doubly refractile, anisotropic band of a striated muscle myofibril. SYN: *Q band; Q stripe, A disk.*

Q fever [Q is for "query" because its etiology was unknown]. An acute infectious disease characterized by headache, fever, malaise, myalgia, and anorexia. Caused by the rickettsial organism, Coxiella burnetii. Contracted by inhaling infected dusts, drinking unpasteurized milk from infected animals, or by handling infected animals such as goats, cows, or sheep. Spread by human contact is rare but has occurred. An effective vaccine is available for prevention of infection in persons who have a good chance of being exposed to the disease. Tetracyclines are effective in treating Q fever. SYN: *ninemile fever; quadrilateral fever.*

q. h. Abbr. for L. *quaque hora,* every hour.

q. i. d. Abbr. for L. *quater in die,* four times a day.

q. l. Abbr. for L. *quantum libet,* as much as one pleases.

Q law. As temperature decreases, chemical activity decreases. A principle used in treatment of gastric ulcers by using cold therapy to arrest hemorrhage and acid secretion.

q. m. Abbr. for L. *quaque matin,* every morning.

q. n. Abbr. for L. *quaque nox,* every night.

QRS complex. The Q, R, and S waves or deflections of an electrocardiogram produced during the transmission of the excitation wave through the conductile tissue of the heart. Normal duration is 0.06-0.08 sec.

QRST complex. The Q, R, S, and T waves of an electrocardiogram. Duration is approx. same as that of mechanical systole. SYN: *ventricular complex.*

q. s. Abbr. for *quantum sufficit,* as much as necessary.

qt. Abbr. for *quart.*

quack (kwăk) [Dutch *kwaksalven,* to peddle salve]. One who pretends to have knowledge or skill in medicine. SYN: *charlatan.*

quackery (kwăk'ĕr-ĭ). The practice or misrepresentation by a quack. SYN: *charlatanry.*

quadrangular (kwŏd-răng'ū-lĕr) [L. *quadri,* four, + *angulus,* angle]. Having four angles and four sides.

 q. lobe. A region forming superior portion of each cerebellar hemisphere.

 q. membrane. The upper portion of the elastic membrane of the larynx. Extends from aryepiglottic folds above the level of ventricular folds below.

quadrant (kwŏd'rănt) [L. *quadrans,* a fourth]. 1. The 4th of a circle. 2. One of four corresponding regions, as of the abdomen, divided for descriptive and diagnostic purposes.

quadrantanopsia (kwŏd"rănt-ăn-ŏp'sĭ-ă) ["+ Gr. *an-,* negative, + *opsis,* vision]. Loss of sight in approximately one fourth of the visual field.

quadrate (kwŏd'rāt) [L. *quadratus,* squared]. Square, or having four equal sides.

 q. lobe. A small lobe of liver located on visceral surface and lying in contact with pylorus and duodenum.

 q. lobule. The square lobule of the upper surface of the cerebellum.

quadri-, quadr- [L. *quattuor,* four]. Combining forms meaning having four or consisting of four.

quadriceps (kwŏd'rĭ-sĕps) [L. *quattuor,* four, + *ceps,* head]. Four-headed, as a quadriceps muscle.

 q. femoris. A large muscle on anterior surface of thigh composed of four muscles, rectus femoris, vastus lateralis, vastus medialis, and vastus intermedius. These muscles are inserted by a common tendon on tuberosity of tibia. Q. femoris is an extensor of the leg. SEE: *Table of Muscles* in *Appendix.*

 q. reflex. Extension of the leg following contraction of the quadriceps muscle resulting from a quick tap of the patellar tendon. SYN: *knee jerk; patellar reflex.*

quadrigemina (kwŏd"rĭ-jĕm'ĭn-ă) ["+ *geminus,* twin]. The corpora quadrigemina. SEE: *colliculus inferior; colliculus superior.*

quadrigeminal (kwŏd"rĭ-jĕm'ĭn-ăl). Fourfold; having four symmetrical parts. Pert. to corpora quadrigemina.

quadrilateral (kwŏd"rĭ-lăt'ĕr-ăl) [L. *quattuor,* four, + *latus, later-,* side]. Having four sides.

quadripara (kwŏd-rĭp'ă-ră) ["+ *parere,* to bear]. A woman in her fourth confinement or who has had four children.

quadripartite (kwŏd"rĭ-păr'tĭt) ["+ *partīre,* to divide]. Divided into four parts.

quadriplegia (kwŏd″rĭ-plē′jĭ-ă) [L. *quattuor,* four, + Gr. *plēgē,* stroke]. Paralysis affecting all four limbs.

quadrisect (kwŏd′rĭ-sĕkt) ["+ *sectiō,* a cutting]. To divide into four parts.

quadritubercular (kwŏd″rĭ-tū-bŭr′kŭ-lĕr) ["+ *tuberculum,* a tubercle]. Having four tubercles or cusps.

quadrivalent (kwŏd″rĭ-vā′lĕnt) ["+ *valens,* powerful]. Having ability to replace four atoms of hydrogen in a compound.

quadroon (kwŏd-rūn′) [Sp. *cuarterón*]. The offspring of a white person and a mulatto; a person having one quarter Negro blood.

quadruped (kwŏd″rū-pĕd) [L. *quattuor,* four, + *pes,* foot]. 1. Four-footed animal. 2. Assuming a position with hands and feet on floor.

quadrupedal reflex (kwŏd-rūp′ĕd-ăl). Extension of flexed arm on assuming quadrupedal posture.

quadruplet (kwŏd′rū-plĕt, kwŏ-drū′plĕt) [L. *quadruplus,* fourfold]. One of four children born of the same mother at same labor. SEE: *Hellin's law.*

quale (kwā′lē) [L. *quālis,* of what kind]. The quality of anything, esp. of a sensation.

qualimeter (kwŏl-ĭm′ĕt-ĕr) ["+ Gr. *metron,* measure]. Device to determine hardness of the roentgen rays. SEE: *penetrometer.*

qualitative (kwŏl′ĭ-tā″tĭv) [L. *qualitativus*]. Referring to the quality of anything.

   q. analysis. In chemistry, an analysis that determines the nature of the elements of a compound, or the identity of the components of a mixture. SEE: *quantitative.*

quality (kwŏl′ĭ-tĭ) [L. *qualitās,* quality]. That which constitutes or characterizes a thing; the natural character.

quanta (kwŏn′tă) [L.]. Pl. of quantum, q.v.

quantimeter (kwŏn-tĭm′ĕt-ĕr) [L. *quantus,* how great, + Gr. *metron,* measure]. Colorimetric standard for measuring quantity of roentgen rays to which a subject is exposed.

quanti-Pirquet (kwŏn″tĭ-pēr-kā′). [Clemens Pirquet, Aust. physician, 1874-1929] Quantitative cutaneous test of amount of sensitiveness to tuberculin by use of graduated dilutions.

quantitative (kwŏn″tĭ-tā′tĭv) [LL. *quantitativus*]. Concerning quantity.

   q. analysis. Analysis that determines the proportionate parts of elements in a compound, or the percentage of components of a mixture. SEE: *qualitative.*

quantity (kwŏn′tĭ-tĭ) [L. *quantitās,* quantity]. Amount; portion.

   q., unit of. Coulomb, the measure of amount of electric current passing a given point in a conductor in a given time.

quantum (kwŏn′tŭm) [L., how much]. (pl. *quan′ta*) 1. A definite amount. 2. A unit of radiant energy.

   q. theory. Radiation is an intermittent, not continuous, emission of energy in varying multiples of quanta action.

quantum libet (kwŏn′tŭm lĭ′bĕt) [L.]. As much as desired.

quantum sufficit (kwŏn′tŭm sŭf′fĭ-sĭt) [L.]. As much as needed. ABBR: q.s.

quarantine (kwŏr′ăn-tēn″) [It. *quarantina,* 40 days]. 1. The period of debarring from entrance to a country, or the isolation of persons exposed to infectious diseases—formerly 40 days. 2. Period of isolation from public communication following onset of a contagious disease.

   Complete q. is limitation of freedom of movement of such well persons or domestic animals as have been exposed to a communicable disease, for a period of time equal to the longest incubation period of the disease, in such a manner as to prevent effective contact with those not so exposed.

   SEE: *contagious; isolation.*

quart (kwŏrt) [L. *quartus,* a fourth]. A unit of fluid or dry measure; one fourth part of a gallon or two pints; one eighth part of a peck. ABBR: qt.

quartan (kwŏr′tăn) [L. *quārtāna,* of the fourth]. 1. Occurring every 4th day. 2. Malarial fever with a paroxysm every 4th day, figuring from and including the 1st day of paroxysm. SEE: *fever; malaria.*

   q., double. Malaria in which there are two concurrent cycles resulting in fever occurring on two successive days.

   q., triple. Malaria in which there are three concurrent cycles resulting in fever occurring every day.

quartile (kwŏr′tĭl) [L. *quartus,* a fourth]. One of the two middle values of each half of a series of variables.

quartipara (kwŏr-tĭp′ă-ră) ["+ *parēre,* to bear]. A woman who has borne her fourth child. SYN: *quadripara.*

quartiparous (kwŏr-tĭp′ă-rŭs). Having given birth to four children or having been in labor four times.

quartz (kwărts) [Ger. *quarz*]. Silicon dioxide, the principal ingredient of sandstone (crystallized silica; rock crystal). When crystal is clear and colorless it permits the passage of ultraviolet radiations in large proportions.

   q. applicator. Quartz rod of various shapes and angles to conduct, by total internal reflection, ultraviolet radiation from a water-cooled mercury arc quartz lamp.

   q. glass. Crystalline quartz is used for prisms and lenses; fused quartz for windows, etc., through which ultraviolet radiations are freely transmitted.

quassation (kwă-sā'shŭn) [L. *quassatio*]. A beating, a shaking; breaking up of crude materials into small pieces.

quassia (kwŏsh'ă, kwŏsh'ĭ-ă) [*Quassi*, Surinam inhabitant who discovered its medicinal value]. The wood of a tree, quassia amara, grown in tropical America.

USES: Once considered valuable as a bitter tonic, and as an injection for certain intestinal parasites.

quassin (kwŏs'ĭn). $C_{22}H_{30}O_6$, a bitter principle extracted from the wood of quassia.

quater in die (kwŏ'tĕr ĭn dĭ-ă) [L.]. Four times a day. ABBR: q.i.d.

quaternary (kwŏ-tĕr'nă-rĭ) [L. *quarternarius*, of four]. 1. The 4th in order. 2. Composed of four elements.

Queckenstedt's sign (kwĕk'ĕn-stĕt). [Hans Queckenstedt, Ger. physician, 1887-1918] Upon compression of the veins of the neck, unilaterally or bilaterally, cerebrospinal fluid pressure rises rapidly in healthy persons; this disappears when pressure is released. In vertebral canal block, the pressure is scarcely affected by this procedure.

querulent (kwĕr'ū-lĕnt) [L. *querulus*, complaining]. 1. Complaining; fretful. 2. One who is dissatisfied, complaining, and suspicious.

quick (kwĭk) [ME. *quicke*, alive]. 1. A part susceptible to keen feeling, esp. part of a finger or toe to which nail is attached. 2. Pregnant with fetal movements.

quickening (kwĭk'ĕn-ĭng). First movements of the fetus felt in utero. Occurs from 18th to 20th week of pregnancy. Movements have been felt as early as the tenth week and rarely are not felt during the entire pregnancy.

quicklime. CaO. Calcium oxide, unslaked lime. Forms calcium hydroxide when water is added to it.

quicksilver (kwĭk'sĭl-vĕr) [ME. *quicke*, alive, + *silver*, silver]. The metal mercury.

quillaja (kĕl-yŏ'hŏ) [Sp.]. The inner bark of a tree grown in South America.

USES: As an emulsifying agent. It has been used unwisely in the production of foam on nonalcoholic beverages. Has no authorized use in modern medicine.

quinacrine hydrochloride. USP. An agent used in the treatment of malaria. Also used in infestations of Giardia lamblia, a parasite. SYN: *atabrine*, q.v.

quince (kwĭns) [ME. *quynce*]. Applelike fruit of a tree native to western Asia. Contains 3 times as much cellulose as cherries. Also contains tannin.

Food value of 100 gm. (raw): Cal. 57; protein 0.4 gm.; fat 0.1 gm.; carbohydrate 15.3 gm.; vitamin C, 15 mg.

Quincke (kwĭnk'ē). [Heinrich I. Quincke, Ger. physician, 1842-1922].

Q.'s disease. Angioneurotic edema of skin; urticaria; giant hives.

Q.'s pulse. Capillary pulse. Seen under fingernails and indicated by alternate reddening and blanching; a sign of aortic insufficiency.

Q.'s puncture. Lumbar p. to determine tension of spinal fluid, or to remove some of spinal fluid.

quinidine sulfate (kwĭn'ĭ-dēn). USP. The sulfate of an alkaloid obtained from cinchona bark; a white, crystalline substance with a bitter taste.

ACTION AND USES: To regulate heart rhythm, esp. to prevent fibrillation.

quinine (kwĭ'nĭn", kwĭ-nēn') [Sp. *quina*]. Bitter, white crystalline alkaloid derived from cinchona bark.

USES: Analgesic, antipyretic, antimalarial. Usually administered in the form of its salts.

q. bisulfate. The acid sulfate of quinine.

ACTION AND USES: Same as quinine sulfate, but having greater solubility.

q. dihydrochloride. The dihydrochloride of quinine, freely soluble in water, 1 gm. dissolving in 0.6 cc. of water. Suitable for intravenous injection.

q. hydrochloride. The hydrochloride of quinine. Used in treatment of malaria.

q. sulfate. USP. The sulfate of an alkaloid obtained from cinchona.

ACTION AND USES: Antipyretic and specific in malaria.

q. tannate. A nearly tasteless and odorless compound of quinine and tannic acid. A means of administering quinine to young children.

q. and urea hydrochloride. USP. In dilute solutions, used as a sclerosing agent for injection treatment of hemorrhoids and varicose veins.

quininism (kwĭ'nĭn-ĭzm, kwĭ-nēn'ĭzm) [Sp. *quina*, + Gr. *-ismos*, condition]. Poisoning by cinchona or its alkaloids. SYN: *cinchonism*.

quinoline (kwĭn'ō-lēn"). C_9H_7N, a tertiary amine derived from coal tar. It is a solvent and antiseptic and many of its salts are used medicinally as antipyretics, analgesics, and in the treatment of amebic dysentery and other infections.

quinone (kwĭn'ōn). 1. Yellow, crystalline oxidation product of quinic acid. 2. Class of organic compounds in which two atoms of hydrogen are replaced by two oxygen atoms.

quinoxyl (kwĭn-ōk'sĭl). Chiniofon.

quinqu- [L.]. Combining form meaning five.

Quinquaud's disease (kăn-kō'). [Charles E. Quinquaud, Fr. physician, 1841-1894] Purulent inflammation of scalp's hair follicles resulting in bald patches.

quinquina (kwĭn-kwī'nă, kĭn-kē'nă). Cinchona, q.v.

quinsy (kwĭn'zē) [ME. *quinesye*, sore throat]. Peritonsillar abscess due to bacterial inflammation of the tonsillar area. Abscess may rupture spontaneously; if not, surgical incision may be required.

quintan (kwĭn'tăn) [L. *quintanus*, of a fifth]. 1. Occurring every fifth day. 2. Intermittent fever, the paroxysms occurring every 5th day with intermission of three days.

quinti- [L. *quintus*, fifth]. Combining form meaning fifth.

quintipara (kwĭn-tĭp'ă-ră) ["+ *parēre*, to bear]. A woman in her 5th pregnancy, or one who has had five children.

quintuplet (kwĭn'tū-plĕt, -tŭp'lĕt) [LL. *quintuplex*, fivefold]. One of five children born of one mother during the same confinement. SEE: *Hellin's law; twin.*

quotidian (kwō-tĭd'ĭ-ăn) [L. *quotidianus,* daily]. Occurring daily.

   q. fever. A malarial fever characterized by daily paroxysms.

quotient (kwō'shĕnt) [L. *quotiens,* how many times]. Number of times one number is contained in another.

   q., caloric. Result obtained by dividing heat (in cal.) by the oxygen consumed (in mg.) in metabolism.

   q., intelligence. Division of the patient's mental age by his actual age.

   q., respiratory. The result of dividing amount of carbon dioxide in expired air by the oxygen inhaled, normally 0.9.

q. v. Abbr. for *quantum vis,* as much as you like; *quod vide,* which see.

Q wave. A downward or negative wave of an electrocardiogram following the P wave. It is usually not prominent and may be absent without significance.

R

R. 1. Abbr. for *roentgen; respiration; right.* 2. In chem., a radical.

R—. Abbr. used in organic chemistry to indicate part of a molecule.

–R. Rinne negative. SEE: *Rinne's test.*

+R. Rinne positive. SEE: *Rinne's test.*

℞. Symb. for L. *recipe,* to take.

RA. Abbr. for *rheumatoid arthritis.*

Ra. Chem. symb. for radium.

rabbetting (răb'ĕt-ĭng) [Fr. *raboter,* to plane]. Interlocking of the jagged edges of a fractured bone.

rabbit fever. Tularemia, q.v.

rabiate (rā'bē-āt) [L. *rabiēs,* rage]. Suffering from rabies. SYN: *rabid.*

rabic (răb'ĭk). Concerning rabies.

rabicidal (răb-ĭ-sī'dăl) ["+ *cidus,* kill]. Destructive to causative virus of rabies.

rabid (răb'ĭd). Pert. to, or affected with, rabies. SYN: *rabiate.*

rabies (rā'bēz) [L. *rabiēs,* rage]. An acute infectious disease of mammals, esp. carnivores. Dogs, cats, and cattle are the domestic animals particularly susceptible. Characterized by involvement of central nervous system, resulting in paralysis and finally death. May be communicated to man through the bite of a rabid animal, usually a dog. SYN: *hydrophobia.*

PERIOD OF INCUBATION: Usually 4-6 weeks, but may be as short as 6 days or as long as a year, depending on deepness of laceration and site of wound.

ETIOL: A neurotropic filtrable virus present in saliva of rabid animals.

PREVENTION: Thoroughly clean all bites or scratches made by any animal with strong (20%) medicinal soap solution. Deep puncture wounds should be opened to permit access of solution.

TREATMENT: If animal is caught, confine and observe for 10 days. Give vaccine to exposed person at first sign of physical or laboratory evidence of rabies in the observed animal. If animal is not caught and rabies is known to be present in the area, start vaccination immediately. In severe bites, rabies hyperimmune serum may be used in addition to the vaccine. SEE: *dog bite.*

SYM: General malaise, depression of spirits or intense excitement and aggressiveness, respiratory problems, swelling of lymphatics near wound, tetanic spasms, fever. Usually vomiting, unusual saliva, and albuminuria.

race (rās) [Fr.]. 1. A class of individuals with common interests, characteristics, appearance, habits, etc., as if derived from a common ancestor. 2. Division of mankind with traits sufficient to mark it as a distinct human type.

racemose (răs'ē-mōs) [L. *racēmōsus,* full of clusters]. Resembling a clustered bunch of grapes, as a gland, divided and subdivided, ending in a bunch of follicles.

rachi-, rachio- [Gr. *rhachis,* spine]. Combining forms indicating spine.

rachialbuminimeter (rā"kĭ-ăl-bū"mĭn-ĭm'ĕt-ĕr) ["+ L. *albumen,* white protein, + Gr. *metron,* measure]. Device for determining the amount of albumin in the cerebrospinal fluid.

rachialbuminimetry (rā"kĭ-ăl-bū"mĭn-ĭm'ĕt-rĭ). Determining the amount of albumin in the cerebrospinal fluid.

rachialgia (rā-kĭ-ăl'jĭ-ă) [Gr. *rhachis,* spine, + *algos,* pain]. Pain in the spine.

rachianalgesia (rā"kĭ-ăn-ăl-jē'zĭ-ă) ["+ *analgesia,* lack of pain]. Spinal anesthesia. SYN: *rachianesthesia.*

rachianesthesia (rā"kĭ-ăn-ĕs-thē'zĭ-ă) ["+ *an-,* negative, + *aisthēsis,* sensation]. Spinal anesthesia.

rachicele (rā'kĭ-sēl) [Gr. *rhachis,* spine, + *kēlē,* hernia]. Protrusion of contents of spinal canal in spina bifida.

rachicentesis (rā"kĭ-sĕn-tē'sĭs) ["+ *kentēsis,* puncture]. Puncture into the spinal canal.

rachidian (rā-kĭd'ĭ-ăn). Rel. to the spinal column.

rachigraph (rā'kĭ-grăf) [Gr. *rhachis,* spine, + *graphein,* to write]. Device for outlining the curves of the spine.

rachilysis (rā-kĭl'ĭ-sĭs) ["+ *lysis,* dissolution]. Mechanical treatment of lateral curvature of the spine through traction and pressure.

rachiocampsis (rā-kĭ-ō-kamp'sĭs) ["+ *kampsis,* a bending]. Curvature of spine.

rachiochysis (rā-kĭ-ok'ĭ-sĭs) [Gr. *rhachis,* spine, + *chysis,* a pouring]. Accumulation of fluid within the spinal canal.

rachiodynia (rā-kĭ-ō-dĭn'ĭ-ă) ["+ *odynē,* pain]. Painful condition of spinal column. SYN: *rachialgia.*

rachiometer (rā-kĭ-ŏm'ē-tĕr) ["+ *metron,* measure]. Instrument for measuring a curvature of the spine.

rachiopagus (rā"kĭ-ŏp'ă-gŭs) [Gr. *rhachis,* spine, + *pagos,* something fixed]. Twins united back to back, but involving only the spinal column.

rachioplegia (rā-kĭ-ō-plē′jĭ-ă) ["+ *plēgē*, a stroke]. Paralysis of spine.

rachioscoliosis (rā″kĭ-ō-skō″lĭ-ō′sĭs) ["+ *skoliōsis*, bending]. Lateral curvature of the spine.

rachiotome (rā″kĭ-ō-tōm″) [Gr. *rhachis*, spine, + *tomē*, a cutting]. Instrument for dividing the vertebrae.

rachiotomy (rā″kĭ-ŏt′ō-mĭ). Surgical cutting of the vertebral column.

rachis (rā′kĭs) [Gr. *rhachis*]. (pl. *rachises*) The spinal column.

rachischisis (rā-kĭs′kĭ-sĭs) ["+ *schisis*, cleft]. Congenital spinal column fissure. SYN: *spina bifida; cleft spine.*

rachitic (rā-kĭt′ĭk). Pert. to, or affected with, rickets.

   r. beads. Rachitic rosary, q.v.

   r. flat pelvis. Pelvic deformity due to having had rickets in childhood.

   r. rosary. Beadlike prominences at junction of the ribs with their cartilages.

rachitis (rā-kī′tĭs) [Gr. *rhachis*, spine, + *-itis*, inflammatory]. 1. Inflammation of the spine, commonly rickets. 2. Rickets, q.v. SEE: *rachitic beads.*

   r. fetalis annularis. Congenital enlargement of epiphyses of long bones.

   r. fetalis micromelica. Congenital shortness of the bones.

rachitism (răk′ĭ-tĭsm). Tendency to rickets.

rachitogenic (rā-kĭt″ō-jĕn′ĭk) [Gr. *rhachis*, spine, + *genesis*, production]. Causing or inducing development of rickets.

rachitome (răk′ĭ-tōm″) ["+ *tomē*, a cutting]. Instrument employed for opening spinal canal.

raclage (ră-klŏzh′) [Fr.]. Destruction and removal of a soft growth by scraping or rubbing. SYN: *raclement.*

rad. Abbr. for *radiation absorbed dose.*

radectomy (ră-dĕk′tō-mĭ) [L. *radix*, root, + Gr. *ektomē*, excision]. Surgical removal of a tooth or part of one.

radiability (rā″dĭ-ă-bĭl′ĭ-tĭ) [L. *radius*, ray, + *habilitās*, able]. Capability of being penetrated readily by roentgen ray.

radiad (rā′dĭ-ăd) [L. *radialis*, radial, + *ad*, toward]. In direction of the radial side.

radial (rā′dĭ-ăl). 1. Radiating out from a given center. 2. Pert. to the radius.

   r. reflex. Flexion of forearm resulting when lower end of radius is percussed.

radiant (rā′dĭ-ănt) [L. *radians*]. 1. Emitting beams of light. 2. Transmitted by radiation. 3. Emanating from a common center.
   RS: energy; flux; heat.

radiate (rā′dĭ-āt) [L. *radiatus*]. To spread from a common center.

radiation (rā-dĭ-ā′shŭn) [L. *radiatio*]. 1. Process by which energy is propagated through space or matter. 2. Emission of rays in all directions from a common center. 3. Treatment with a radioactive substance. 4. In neurology, a group of fibers which diverge from a common origin.

A general term for any form of radiant energy emission or divergence, as of energy in all directions from luminous bodies, roentgen ray tubes, radioactive elements, and fluorescent substances.

   r. absorbed dose. Unit indicating absorbed dose of ionizing radiation.

   r., acoustic. Auditory r., q.v.

   r., auditory. A band of fibers that connects auditory areas of cerebral cortex with medial geniculate body of thalamus. SYN: *acoustic r.; thalamotemporal r.*

   r. of corpus callosum. Total of fibers radiating from corpus callosum into each cerebral hemisphere.

   r. exposure limit. Recommended limit of accumulated exposure of an individual to ionizing radiation to prevent excess exposure.

The National Council on Radiation and Protection and Measurements recommends that radiation exposure to the whole body, active blood-forming organs, gonads, or ocular lens accumulated at any age shall not exceed 5 rems multiplied by the number of years beyond age 18 and that exposure in any 13 consecutive weeks shall not exceed 3 rems. This can be expressed by the formula: MPL = 5 (N-18) rems. MPL is the maximum permissive accumulated exposure in dose equivalents (rems) and N is the individual's age in years. These limits apply to persons who are designated radiation workers. Members of the general population should be allowed only 10% of these limits.

Both patients and those who work where they may be exposed to ionizing radiation should be prevented from excess exposure. Nurses caring for patients treated with radioisotopes are exposed to the radiation given off by the isotope present in the patient's body and in the patient's excreta and bandages. Hospital personnel working with radioisotopes should wear a device for monitoring their exposure to radiation.

   r., heterogeneous. R. containing waves of various wave lengths.

   r., homogeneous. R. containing waves of only one wave length.

r., infrared. Near or short infrared extends 7200 A. U.-14,000 A. U.; far or long infrared 15,000-120,000.

r. injury, ionizing. Injury to cell life because of therapeutic r.

Ionizing r. has the ability to penetrate cells and deposit energy within them in a random fashion, unaffected by the usual cellular barriers. This form of energy, when sufficiently intense, kills cells by inhibiting their division. The sensitivity of cells to ionizing r. varies considerably in different stages of cell life. Because of this effect of ionizing r., the amount of exposure to all forms of it, including X rays, radioisotopes, and other radioactive sources, is limited to a certain amount each year and to a specific total life-time dose.

RS: radiation accident cases, emergency handling of.

r., interstitial. R. accomplished by insertion of radium or radon directly into tissues.

r., ionizing. R. which either directly or indirectly induces ionization of radiation-absorbing material.

r., irritative. Overdosage of ultraviolet irradiation resulting in erythema, and, in exceptional cases, blister formation.

r., mitogenetic. Hypothetical radiations given off by cells during mitosis which induce mitosis. SYN: *Gurvich r.*

r., occipitothalamic. Optic r., q.v.

r., optic. A system of fibers extending from lateral geniculate body of thalamus through sublenticular portion of internal capsule to the calcarine occipital cortex (striate area). SYN: *geniculocalcarine tract.*

r., photochemical. From a therapeutic standpoint the electromagnetic spectrum divided into photothermal and photochemical radiations. Photochemical r.'s penetrate only to fractions of mm., are absorbed by protoplasm, and cause physical and biological changes.

r., photothermal. Photothermal radiations penetrate subcutaneous tissues, heat the blood, accelerate vital reactions, and act instantaneously. SEE: *r., photochemical.*

r. sickness. R. syndrome, q.v.

r., solar. Radiations of the sun, 60% in infrared region and 40% visible and ultraviolet, shortest wave length.

r., striomesencephalic. Fibers originating in corpus striatum and terminating principally in substantia nigra of midbrain.

r., striosubthalamic. A system of fibers consisting of three groups emerging from medial aspect of lentiform nucleus and entering subthalamic region, most terminating there but some continuing into the midbrain. SYN: *ansa lenticularis.*

r., striothalamic. Groups of fibers connecting the corpus striatum with thalamus and subthalamus.

r. syndrome. 1. Illness resulting from exposure of body tissue to ionizing radiations from radioactive substances (radium, radon) or roentgen rays. Mild acute illness is manifested by anorexia, headache, nausea, vomiting, and diarrhea. Delayed effects resulting from repeated or prolonged exposure may result in amenorrhea, sterility, disturbances in blood cell formation, cataract formation, carcinogenesis, and leukemia.

2. Illness resulting from effects of explosion of an atomic bomb. Effects include destruction of lymphatic tissue, extensive hemorrhages, aplastic bone marrow, prolonged clotting and bleeding times, loss of hair and teeth, and possible genetic changes. In massive exposure to radiation such as would occur in persons close to the center of the atomic bomb explosion, death may occur within several weeks if the individual is not fortunate enough to die immediately from the physical effects of the explosion.

SYN: *r. sickness.*

r., thalamic. Groups of fibers that connect thalamus with cerebral hemispheres. Include frontal, centroparietal occipital, and optic radiations. SYN: *thalamic peduncles or stalks.*

r., ultraviolet. Radiant energy extending from 3900 to 200 A. U. Divided into *near ultraviolet,* extending from 3900 to 2900 A. U., and *far ultraviolet,* from 2900 to 200 A. U.

r., unit. SEE: *angstrom unit; maché unit.*

r., visible. Visible spectrum may be broken up into different wave lengths representing different colors:

Violet, 4000-4500 A. U.
Blue, 4500-4900 A. U.
Green, 4900-5500 A. U.
Yellow, 5500-5900 A. U.
Orange, 5900-6300 A. U.
Red, 6300-7800 A. U.
SEE: *spectrum.*
RS: heliotherapy; helium.

radiation accident cases, emergency handling of. As the field of nuclear energy expands in industry, medicine, and university studies it is to be expected that there will be a rise in contamination accidents. The following has been prepared by the U.S. Atomic Energy Commission in cooperation with A.M.A., 1969, and is used with permission of *Industrial Medicine and Surgery,* 39:(No. 1) 87, 1970.

Emergency Handling of Radiation Exposure or Radioactive Contamination Cases should not be feared. The handling of these cases is a matter involving common sense, cleanliness and good housekeeping.

Radiation can be detected and measured by a simple instrument—a survey meter. Radiation accident problems have parallels in other conditions handled frequently by Emergency Rooms and Rescue Squads without concern and following simple rules. Your group, your hospital can be involved. There are a few things you should know.

There are four types of radiation accident patients. The individual who has received whole or partial body external radiation may have received a lethal dose of radiation but he is no hazard to attendants, other patients or the environment. He is no different than the radiation therapy or diagnostic x-ray patient.

Another type is the individual who has received internal contamination by inhalation or ingestion. He also is no hazard to attendants, other patients or the environment. Following cleansing of minor amounts of contaminated material deposited on the body surface during airborne exposure, he is similar to the chemical poisoning case such as lead. His body wastes should be collected and saved for measurements of the amount of nuclides to assist in determination of appropriate therapy.

External contamination of body surface and/or clothing by liquids or by dirt particles presents a third type, with problems similar to vermin infestation. Surgical isolation technique to protect attendants and cleansing to protect other patients and the hospital environment must take place to confine and remove a potential hazard.

When external contamination is complicated by a wound, care must be taken not to cross-contaminate surrounding surfaces from the wound and vice versa. The wound and surrounding surfaces are cleansed separately and sealed off when clean. When crushed dirty tissue is involved, early preliminary wet debridement following wound irrigation may be indicated. Further debridement and more definitive therapy can await sophisticated measurement and consultant guidance.

STANDING ORDERS FOR EMERGENCY HANDLING: If the ambulance or Rescue Squad that picks up the radiation accident case has a radio or telephone, the Emergency Room should be alerted to expect a patient who may have had radiation exposure or radioactive contamination.

It is the responsibility of the senior Hospital Emergency Room person on duty, nurse or physician, on receipt of notification of the momentary arrival of a case involving radiation exposure or contamination, to:

1. Notify responsible staff physician or nurse and aides (trained health physicists or trained technicians from x-ray or nuclear medicine departments, if the hospital has such persons on its staff).

2. Get appropriate survey meter, if one is on hand in the hospital. If hospital has no meter, notify *hospital administrator* or responsible hospital official so he may obtain survey meter and other pertinent equipment by calling the Police Department.

3. Notify the hospital administrator so he may *seek expert professional consultation* for technical management of the case.

4. If contamination is suspected, prepare separate space, using either isolation room or cubicle if available. Some hospitals use the morgue, since the autopsy table lends itself to washing with water. The morgue entrance would then be used rather than the Emergency Room. When morgue is used the patient and his family must be reassured of why that space is used. If no separate space is available, cover a floor area immediately adjacent to the entrance way to the Emergency Room with absorbent paper...the area to be adequate for stretcher-cart, disposal hampers, and working space for professional attendants. Mark and close off this area. If dust is involved be prepared to shut off air-circulation system to prevent spread of contamination.

On Ambulance Arrival, the responsible physician or nurse in the Emergency Room should:

1. Check patient on stretcher for contamination (preferably as stretcher is removed from the ambulance) by use of a survey meter.

2. If seriously injured, give emergency lifesaving assistance immediately.

3. Handle contaminated patient and wound as one would a surgical procedure, i.e., gown, gloves, cap, mask, etc.

4. If possible external contamination is involved save all clothing and bedding from ambulance, blood, urine, stool, vomitus, and all metal objects (e.g., jewelry, belt buckles, dental plates, etc.). Label with name, body location, time and date. Save each in appropriate containers; mark containers clearly, "Radioactive—Do not Discard."

5. Decontamination should start, if medical status permits, with cleansing and scrubbing the area of highest contamination first.

If an extremity alone is involved, clothing may serve as an effective barrier and the affected limb alone may be scrubbed and cleansed. Initial cleansing should be done with soap and warm water. If the body as a whole is involved or clothing generally permeated by contaminated material showering and scrubbing will be necessary. Pay special attention to hair parts, body orifices and body folds areas. Remeasure and record measurement after each washing or showering.

If a wound is involved, prepare and cover the wound with self-adhering disposable surgical drape. Cleanse neighboring surfaces of skin. Seal off cleansed areas with self-adhering disposable surgical drapes. Remove wound covering and irrigate wound with sterile water, catching the irrigating fluid in a basin or can to be marked and handled as described in rule 4 above. Each step in the decontamination should be preceded and followed by monitoring and recording of the location and extent of contamination.

6. Save physicians', nurses and attendants scrub or protective clothing, as described for patients. Doctors, nurses and attendants must follow the same monitoring and decontamination routine as the patients.

7. The physician in attendance in the Emergency Room, if confronted with a grossly contaminated wound with dirt particles and crushed tissue, should be prepared to do a preliminary simple wet debridement. Further measurements may necessitate sophis-ticated wound counting detection instruments supplied by the consultant who will advise if further definitive debridement is necessary.

When the accident has occurred at a plant, university or medical group regularly working with nuclear material, the health physicist, supervisor, co-worker and the patient should be able to inform the rescue squad of the nature of the accident, type of radiation exposure or radioactive contamination involved and possible body areas that may be affected.

REGIONAL COORDINATING OFFICES FOR RADIOLOGICAL EMERGENCY ASSISTANCE: The U.S. Atomic Energy Commission has regional offices for information and assistance on radiological emergencies. Contacts may be made in person or by phone.

radiator (rā'dĭ-ā"tor) [L. *radiatus*, radiate]. Device for radiating heat or light.

   r., infrared. Device for transmitting infrared rays.

radical (răd'ĭ-kăl) [L. *radicalis*]. 1. A group of atoms acting as a single unit, passing without change from one compound to another, but not able to exist in a free state. 2. Anything that reaches the root or origin; original. 3. A foundation or principle.

   r. treatment. A treatment that seeks an absolute cure, as r. surgery; not palliative. Opposed to conservative treatment.

radicle (răd'ĭ-kl) [L. *radicula*, little root]. 1. A structure resembling a rootlet, as a r. of a nerve or vein. 2. Group of elements unaffected by chemical change, unable to exist in the free state.

U.S. Atomic Energy Commission's Regional Coordinating Offices for Radiological Emergency Assistance

CALIFORNIA: Berkeley 94704
2111 Bancroft Way
Phone: 415-841-5121 (ext. 664 duty hrs.; 415-841-9244 off hrs.)
(Includes Hawaii)

IDAHO: Idaho Falls 83401
P.O. Box 2108
Phone: 208-526-0111, ext. 1515

ILLINOIS: Argonne 60439
9800 S. Cass Avenue
Phone: 312-739-7711 (ext. 2111 duty hrs.; ext. 4451 off hrs.)

NEW MEXICO: Albuquerque 87115
P.O. Box 5400
Phone: 505-264-4667
(Includes Canal Zone)

NEW YORK: Uptown, Long Island 11973
Phone: 516-924-6262

SOUTH CAROLINA: Aiken 29801
P.O. Box A
Phone: 803-824-6331, ext. 3333
(Includes Puerto Rico and the Virgin Islands)

TENNESSEE: Oak Ridge 37830
P.O. Box E
Phone: 615-483-8611, ext. 3-4510

WASHINGTON: Richland 99352
P.O. Box 550
Phone: 509-942-7381
(Includes Alaska)

radicotomy (răd''ĭ-kŏt'ō-mĭ) [L. *radix, radic-*, root, + Gr. *tomē*, a cutting]. Section of spinal nerve roots. SYN: *rhizotomy*. SEE: *radiculectomy*.

radiculalgia (ră-dĭ-kū-lăl'jĭ-ă) ["+ Gr. *algos*, pain]. Neuralgia of roots of nerves.

radicular (ră-dĭk'ū-lăr) [L. *radix, radic-*, root]. Concerning a root or radicle.

radiculectomy (ră-dĭk''ū-lĕk'tō-mĭ) ["+ Gr. *ektomē*, excision]. 1. Excision of a spinal nerve root. 2. Resection of posterior spinal nerve root. SEE: *radicotomy*.

radiculitis (ră-dĭk''ū-lī'tĭs) [L. *radicula*, radicle, + Gr. *-itis*, inflammation]. Inflammation of spinal nerve roots, accompanied by pain and hyperesthesia.

radiculomeningomyelitis (ră-dĭk''ū-lō-mē-nĭn''gō-mĭ-ĕl-ī'tĭs) ["+ Gr. *mēninx*, membrane, + *myelos*, marrow, + *-itis*, inflammation]. Inflamed condition of nerve roots, meninges, and spinal cord. SYN: *rhizomeningomyelitis*.

radiculomyelopathy (ră-dĭk''ū-lō-mī''ĕ-lŏp'ă-thĭ) ["+ Gr. *myelos*, marrow, + *pathos*, disease]. Any diseased condition involving spinal cord and roots of spinal nerves.

radiculoneuritis (ră-dĭk''ū-lō''nū-rī'tĭs) [L. *radicula*, radicle, + Gr. *neuron*, sinew, + *-itis*, inflammation]. Inflammation of roots of spinal nerves.

radiculopathy (ră-dĭk''ū-lŏp'ă-thĭ) ["+ Gr. *pathos*, disease]. Any diseased condition of roots of spinal nerves.

radio- [L. *radius*, ray]. 1. Combining form indicating relationship to radiant energy or radioactive substances. 2. As a prefix to a chemical element indicating a radioactive isotope.

radioactinium (rā''dĭ-ō-ăk-tĭn'ĭ-ŭm). A radioactive product formed from disintegration of the element actinium.

radioactive (rā''dĭ-ō-ăk'tĭv) [L. *radius*, ray, + *activus*, acting]. Capable of emitting radiant energy.

    r. decay. The decrease with passage of time in the number of radioactive atoms in a radioactive substance. This occurs when the nuclei disintegrate spontaneously by emitting radiant energy.

radioactive patient. An individual who originally was treated or accidentally contaminated with radioactive materials and who continues to be radioactive. If he is still emitting radiation when discharged from the hospital, he should be told how long to avoid close contact with children.

    RS: radiation accident cases, emergency handling of.

radioactivity (rā''dĭ-ō-ăk''tĭv'ĭ-tĭ). The ability of a substance to emit rays or particles (alpha, beta, gamma) from its nucleus.

    r., artificial. R. resulting from bombardment of a substance with high-energy particles in a cyclotron, betatron, or other apparatus.

    r., induced. Temporary r. of a substance which has been within the sphere of influence of a radioactive element.

    r., natural. R. possessed by a number of elements which are continuously disintegrating and emitting alpha particles (helium nuclei) or beta particles (electrons) atom by atom. Ex: radium.

radioautograph (rā''dĭ-ō-ŏ'tō-grăf) [L. *radius*, ray, + Gr. *autos*, self, + *graphein*, to write]. A photograph of a histologic section of a tissue showing the distribution of radioactive substances in the tissue. SYN: *autoradiogram*.

radiobe (rā'dĭ-ōb'') ["+ Gr. *bios*, life]. A peculiar structure formed in sterilized bouillon as a result of radium radiation. It resembles bacteria in appearance.

radiobiology (rā''dĭ-ō-bī-ŏl'ō-jĭ). Branch of biology which deals with the effects of radiations on living organisms.

radiocarpal (rā''dĭ-ō-kar'păl) [L. *radius*, ray, + Gr. *karpos*, wrist]. Concerning the radius and carpus.

radiochemistry (rā''dĭ-ō-kĕm'ĭs-trĭ) ["+ Gr. *chemeia*, chemistry]. The phase of chemistry dealing with radioactive phenomena.

radiochroism (rā''dĭ-ō-krō'ĭzm) ["+ Gr. *chroa*, color]. The ability of a substance to absorb radioactive rays.

radiochrometer (rā''dĭ-ō-krŏm'ē-tĕr) ["+ Gr. *chrōma*, color, + *metron*, measure]. Device for measuring penetrating powers of X rays and the character of roentgen tubes. SEE: *penetrometer*.

radiocystitis (rā''dĭ-ō-sĭs-tī'tĭs) [L. *radius*, ray, + Gr. *kystis*, bladder, + *-itis*, inflammation]. Inflammation of the bladder following treatment by radium or roentgen rays.

radiode (rā'dĭ-ōd) ["+ Gr. *hodos*, way]. Metal container for radium used in therapeutic application.

radiodermatitis (rā''dĭ-ō-dŭr''mă-tī'tĭs) ["+ Gr. *derma*, skin, + *-ōsis*, condition]. Inflammation of the skin caused by exposure to roentgen rays or radioactive elements.

radiodiagnosis (rā''dĭ-ō-dī''ăg-nō'sĭs) [L. *radius*, ray, + Gr. *dia*, through, + *gnōsis*, knowledge]. Diagnosis by means of roentgen rays.

radiodontia (rā''dĭ-ō-dŏn'shĭ-ă) ["+ Gr. *odous, odont-*, teeth]. Roentgenography of the teeth.

radioelectrocardiography (rā″dĭ-ō-ē-lĕk″trō-kär″dĭ-ŏg′ră-fĭ) [L. *radius*, ray, + Gr. *ēlektron*, amber, + *kardia*, heart, + *graphein*, to write]. Recording of changes in heart beats by radio wave from subject to receiver without direct attachment of apparatus, thus allowing recordings to be made during normal life activities of the patient.

radioelectrophysiolography (rā″dĭ-ō-ē-lĕk″trō-fĭs″ĭ-ō-lŏg′ră-fĭ) [″+ ″+ *physis*, nature, + *graphein*, to write]. Recording of changes in electrical tension or pressure of the brain by radio transmission to an electroencephalogram at some other site. SEE: *radioelectrocardiography.*

radioelement (rā″dĭ-ō-ĕl′e-mĕnt) [″+ *elementum*, element]. Any of the elements possessing power of radioactivity.

radioepidermitis (rā″dĭ-ō-ĕp″ĭ-dŭr-mī′tĭs) [L. *radius*, ray, + Gr. *epi*, upon, + *derma*, skin, + *-itis*, inflammation]. Destructive changes in the skin caused by radioactive rays.

radioepithelitis (rā″dĭ-ō-ĕp″ĭ-thē-lī′tĭs) [″+ ″+ *thēlē*, nipple, + *-itis*, inflammation]. Disintegration of epithelium due to exposure to irradiation.

radiofrequency electrophrenic respiration. Method of stimulating respiration in cases of respiratory paralysis from injury of the spinal cord at the cervical level.

Electrical stimuli to the phrenic nerves are supplied by a radiofrequency transmitter implanted subcutaneously. The diaphragmatic muscles contract in response to intermittent electrical stimuli.

radiogenic (rā″dĭ-ō-jĕn′ĭk) [″+ *gennan*, to produce]. Caused by radioactivity.

radiogram (rā′dĭ-ō-grăm) [L. *radius*, ray, + Gr. *gramma*, a writing]. X-ray picture, esp. of internal organs. SYN: *actinogram; skiagram; roentgenogram.*

radiograph (rā′dĭ-ō-grăf) [″+ Gr. *graphein*, to write]. 1. A record produced on a photographic plate, film, or paper by the action of roentgen rays or radium; specifically an x-ray photograph. SEE: *skiagraph,* 2. To make a radiograph of.

radiographer (rā″dĭ-ŏg′ră-fŭr). A person skilled in making roentgenograms or radiographs.

radiography (rā-dĭ-ŏg′ră-fĭ). The making of x-ray pictures. SYN: *roentgenography; skiagraphy.*

radiohumeral (rā″dĭ-ō-hū′mĕr-ăl) [L. *radius*, ray, + *humerus*, humerus]. Concerning the radius and humerus.

radioimmunoassay. A very sensitive method of determining the concentration of substances, particularly the proteins in hormones, in blood plasma. The procedure is based on the competitive inhibition of binding of radioactively-labeled hormones to a specific antibody. Concentrations of protein in the picogram (10^{-12} gm.) range can be measured by using this technique.

radioiodine (rā″dĭ-ō-ī′ō-dĭn). A radioactive isotope of iodine. Used in the diagnosis and treatment of thyroid disorders. The most commonly used isotope is I^{131}.

radioisotopes (rā″dĭ-ō-ī′sō-tōps). Radioactive forms of chemicals.

radiologist (rā-dĭ-ŏl′ō-jĭst) [L. *radius*, ray, + Gr. *logos*, study]. One who practices diagnosis and treatment by radiant energy.

radiology (rā-dĭ-ŏl′ō-jĭ). The branch of science which deals with roentgen rays, radium rays, and other radiations and their curative properties.

radiolucency (rā″dĭ-ō-lū′sĕn-sĭ) [L. *radius*, ray, + *lucere*, to shine]. Property of being partly or wholly permeable to radiant energy.

radiolus (rā-dĭ′ō-lŭs) [L., a little ray]. A sound or probe.

radiometer (rā-dĭ-ŏm′ē-ter) [L. *radius*, ray, + Gr. *metron*, measure]. Instrument for measuring intensity of radiation.

radiomimetic (rā″dĭ-ō-mĭm-ĕt′ĭk) [″+ Gr. *mimētikos*, imitation]. Imitating the biological effects of radiation.

radion (rā′dĭ-ōn) [″+ Gr. *ōn*, being]. One of the particles of the alpha, beta rays or cathode rays given off by radioactive matter.

radionecrosis (rā″dĭ-ō-nĕ-krō′sĭs) [L. *radius*, ray, + Gr. *nekrōsis*, death]. Disintegration of tissue by exposure to radiant energy.

radioneuritis (rā″dĭ-ō-nū-rī′tĭs) [″+ Gr. *neuron*, sinew, + *-itis*, inflammation]. Neuritis caused by exposure to radioactive substance.

radionuclides. Atoms that disintegrate by emission of electromagnetic radiation.

radiopaque (rā-dĭ-ō-pāk′) [″+ *opacus*, dark]. Impenetrable to the X ray or other forms of radiation.

radioparent (rā″dĭ-ō-par′ĕnt) [″+ *parere*, to appear]. Penetrable by radioactive rays.

radiopathology (rā″dĭ-ō-pă-thŏl′ō-gĭ) [L. *radius*, ray, + Gr. *pathos*, disease, + *logos*, study]. Study of pathological changes induced by radiation.

radiopelvimetry (rā″dĭ-ō-pĕl-vĭm′ĕt-rĭ) [″+ *pelvis*, basin, + Gr. *metron*, measure]. Measurement of the pelvis by roentgen ray.

radiopharmaceuticals. Radioactive chemicals either in the form of individual elements or elements attached to other substances called carriers. They are used in testing the location, size, outline, or function

Clinical Uses of Radiopharmaceuticals*

Use	Isotope	Half-Life		Carrier
Thyroid Studies	^{131}I	8.08	days	sodium iodide, thyroxine, liothyronine
Kidney Studies	^{131}I	8.08	days	iodohippurate sodium
	^{197}Hg	65	hours	chlormerodrin
	^{203}Hg	46	days	chlormerodrin
Liver Studies	^{131}I	8.08	days	rose bengal sodium
	^{198}Au	64.8	hours	gold colloid
Gastrointestinal Tract Studies	^{131}I	8.08	days	triolein, oleic acid, tolpovidone
	^{57}Co	270	days	vitamin B_{12}
	^{51}Cr	27.8	days	sodium chromate
Blood Studies	^{131}I	8.08	days	serum albumin
	^{51}Cr	27.8	days	sodium chromate
	^{59}Fe	44.5	days	ferric chloride, ferrous citrate, ferrous sulfate
Brain Studies	^{131}I	8.08	days	serum albumin
	^{74}As	17.9	days	sodium aresenate
	^{197}Hg	65	hours	chlormerodrin
	^{99m}Tc	6	hours	pertechnetate
Eye Studies	^{32}P	14.3	days	sodium phosphate
Electrolyte Studies	^{22}Na	2.58	years	sodium chloride
	^{42}K	12.5	hours	potassium chloride
	^{45}Ca	165	days	calcium chloride
	^{47}Ca	4.56	days	calcium chloride
Cancer Therapy	^{131}I	8.08	days	sodium iodide
	^{131}I	8.08	days	ethiodized oil
	^{198}Au	64.8	hours	gold colloid
	^{32}P	14.3	days	chromic phosphate
Thyroid Therapy	^{131}I	8.08	days	sodium iodide
Blood Disease Therapy	^{32}P	14.3	days	sodium phosphate

*Adapted from Radioisotopes in Medicine. Abbott Laboratories/Radiopharmaceutical Products Division, N. Chicago, Ill. 1970.

of tissues, organs, vessels, or body fluids. The presence and location of radiopharmaceutical substances in the body is detected by special methods or apparatus which record or take an x-ray picture of the radioactivity produced. These compounds may also be used to treat certain diseases.

CAUTION: Radiopharmaceuticals must be handled in accordance with prescribed methods in order to prevent the patient or those treating the patient from being exposed to unnecessary ionizing radiation.

radiopraxis (rā″dĭ-ō-prăk′sĭs) [″ + Gr. *praxis,* practice]. Diagnosis or treatment by use of some radioactive substance.

radioprotective drugs. Drugs which protect man against the damaging or lethal effects of ionizing radiation.

ra″dioresis′tant. Resistant to the action of radiation, esp. of a tumor which cannot be destroyed by treatment with radiation.

radioscopy (rā-dǐ-ŏs'kō-pǐ) [L. *radius,* ray, + Gr. *skopein,* to examine]. Inspection and examination of the inner structures of the body by means of roentgen rays. SYN: *fluoroscopy.*

radiosensibility. Quality of sensitivity to radioactive substances.

radiosensitive. Capable of being destroyed by radiation, as a tumor by x-ray treatment.

radiosurgery (rā"dǐ-ō-sūr'jěr-ǐ) [L. *radius,* ray, + Gr. *cheirurgia,* handwork]. The use of high-energy protons and alpha particles in the form of beams as an "atomic knife" in treating diseases such as cancer or in selectively destroying an overactive endocrine gland.

radiotelemetry (rā"dǐ-ō-těl-ěm'ě-trǐ) [L. *radius,* ray, + Gr. *tēle,* at a distance, + *metron,* measure]. Transmission of data, including biological data, via radio. Developed in order to be able to monitor heart rate, ECG, and body temperature data from astronauts. Now used also in hospitals.

radiotherapist (rā"dǐ-ō-thěr'ǎ-pǐst) ["+ Gr. *therapeia,* treatment]. One trained in use of radiant energy for therapeutic purposes.

radiotherapy (rā"dǐ-ō-thěr'ǎ-pǐ). The treatment of disease by application of roentgen rays, radium, ultraviolet, and other radiations.

radiothermy (rā"dǐ-ō-thěr'mǐ) [L. *radius,* ray, + Gr. *thermē,* heat]. 1. Use of radiant heat or heat from radioactive substances for therapeutic purposes. 2. Short-wave diathermy.

radiotoxemia (rā"dǐ-ō-tŏk-sē'mǐ-ǎ) ["+ Gr. *toxikon,* poison, + *haima,* blood]. Toxemia produced by exposure to radioactive substance. SYN: *actinotoxemia.*

radiotransparent (rā"dǐ-ō-trǎns-par'ěnt) ["+ *trans,* across, + *parere,* to appear]. Penetrable by radiation.

ra"diotrop'ic [L. *radius,* ray, + Gr. *tropos,* turning]. Affected by radiation.

radioulnar (rā"dǐ-ō-ŭl'nǎr) ["+ *ulna,* arm]. Concerning the radius and ulna.

radish (rǎd'ǐsh) [L. *radix,* root]. Pungent root high in oxalic acid. Of little food value, but desirable for its minerals.

　　Food Value of 100 gm. (raw): Cal. 17; protein 1.0 gm.; trace of fat; carbohydrate 3.6 gm.; calcium 30 mg.

radium (rā'dǐ-ŭm) [L. *radius,* ray]. SYMB: *Ra.* There are more than a dozen isotopes, but radium with a half-life of 1622 years and an atomic weight of 226 is the most common. At. no. 88. A metallic element found in very small quantities in pitchblende. It is radioactive and fluorescent.

　　Radiation is of three kinds: alpha (α-rays), beta (β-rays), and gamma (γ-rays) which are analogous to X rays. SEE: words beginning with *actin-.*

　　r. intratumoral application. Implanting r. into tumors for therapeutic purposes.

　　r. needles. Slender containers for r. These are inserted into tissue in order to kill malignant cells.

radiumization (rā"dǐ-ŭm-ǐ-zā'shŭn). Exposure to action of radium rays.

radiumology (rā"dǐ-ŭm-ŏl'ō-jǐ) [L. *radius,* ray, + Gr. *logos,* study]. The science of radium therapy.

radium therapy ["+ Gr. *therapeia,* treatment]. The treatment of disease by means of radium or radon, its emanation, or its active deposit.

ra'dius [L. *radius,* ray]. (pl. *ra'dii*) 1. A line extending from a circle's center point to its circumference. 2. [NA] The outer and shorter bone of the arm which revolves partially about the ulna. Its head articulates with the capitulum of the humerus. Its lower extremity articulates by the ulnar notch with the ulna, and by another articulation with the navicular and lunate bones of the wrist.

　　r., fracture of. Colles' fracture. A fracture and dislocation of lower end of radius, generally caused by falling on the outstretched hand.

radix (rā'dǐks) [L., root]. (pl. *radi'ces*) [NA] 1. The root portion of a cranial or spinal nerve. 2. The root of a plant.

radon (rā'dŏn) [L. *radius,* ray]. SYMB: *Rn.* At. wt. 222; at. no. 86. A radioactive, gaseous element resulting from disintegration of radium.

rage. [ME.]. Violent anger.

ragsorters' disease. A febrile pulmonary disease arising in persons who sort paper and rags, due to inhalation of bacillus causing anthrax, q.v.

ragweed. One of several species of the genus Ambrosia whose pollen is an important allergen. Pollen-producing period of grasses is, in temperate zones, from middle of August to the first hard frost, usually the middle of October.

Raillietina (rǐ"lē-ě-tǐ'nǎ). A genus of cyclophyllidean tapeworms belonging to family Davaineidae.

　　R. demerariensis. A species that infests humans, reported from several S. American countries, esp. Ecuador. SYN: R. *quitensis.*

railway sickness. Motion sickness resulting from movement of a train.

raised (rāzd) [ME. *reisen,* to rise]. In bacteriology, having a thick, elevated growth with terraced edges.

raisin [ME]. A sweet grape, dried either in the sun or artificially.

Food value of 100 gm. (dried): Cal. 289; protein 2.5 gm.; trace of fat; carbohydrate 77.4 gm.; calcium 62 mg.

rale (rŏl) [Fr., rattle]. An abnormal sound heard on auscultation of the chest, produced by passage of air through bronchi which contain secretion or exudate or which are constricted by spasm or a thickening of their walls. May be heard on either inspiration or expiration.

CLASS: There is no general agreement as to classification of the sounds. They are designated moist and dry. Moist rales are also called crackling and these in turn, coarse, medium, or dry. If loud and sharp, they are consonating. Dry rales are sometimes designated musical and may be tinkling, sonorous, snoring, or low pitched, or they may be whistling, piping, and high pitched.

r., atelectatic. Crepitant r., q.v.

r., bronchiectatic. Heard over bronchiectatic cavities filled with accumulated secretion. Disappears with expectoration.

r., bubbling medium. Heard in inspiration and expiration, produced by passage of air through mucus in the larger tubes. Larger than the small bubbling moist r. Heard in capillary bronchitis, esp. in children.

r., cavernous. Heard in inspiration and expiration, produced by passage of air through a small cavity with flaccid walls that collapse with expiration. Hollow and metallic.

r., clicking. Heard in inspiration only, produced by passage of air through softening material in smaller bronchi. Small, sticky. Heard in pulmonary tuberculosis, early stage.

r., coarse. Originates in the larger bronchi.

r., consonating. A loud, sharp rale sounding as though close to the ear. Usually associated with consolidation of tissues about bronchial tubes.

r., crackling, medium. Heard chiefly in inspiration, produced by fluid in the finer bronchi. Larger than the small r., crackling, dry. Heard in softening of the tubercular deposit or pneumonic exudation.

r., crepitant. Heard at end of inspiration, produced by passage of air into collapsed vesicles containing fibrinous exudation, usually at base of lungs. Small,

like rubbing hair between the fingers. Heard in pneumonia, in early stage edema of lungs, hypostatic pneumonia. It is localized in pulmonary tuberculosis.

r., dry. Heard in inspiration and expiration, produced by narrowing of the bronchial tubes from thickening of their mucous lining, from spasmodic contraction of the muscular coat, viscid mucus within or pressure from without. Large and sonorous, small, hissing or whistling. Heard in bronchitis, asthma, and localized in beginning pulmonary tuberculosis.

r., gurgling. Heard in inspiration and expiration, produced by passage of air through fluid in cavities of large bubbles. Heard in pulmonary tuberculosis after formation of cavities.

r., moist. Produced by passage of air through bronchi containing fluid.

r. redux, r. de retour. Heard in inspiration and expiration, produced by passage of air through fluid in bronchial tubes. Crackling, unequal. Heard in pneumonia, in the stage of resolution.

r., sibilant. High pitched, whistling, and frequent at end of inspiration.

r., sonorous. Low snoring, greater in volume, continuing during inspiration.

r., subcrepitant. Heard in inspiration and expiration, produced by passage of air through mucus in the capillary bronchial tubes. Small, moist. Heard in capillary bronchitis.

r., submucous. Higher pitched and more numerous than large mucous rale. Heard in interscapular and supramammary regions and indicating involvement of many tubes of small caliber.

r., vesicular. Crepitant r., q.v.

rami (rā'mī) [L.]. Pl. of ramus, q.v.

ramification (răm'ĭ-fĭ-kā'shŭn) [L. *rāmificāre,* to make branches]. 1. Process of branching. 2. A branch. 3. Arrangement in branches.

ramify (răm'ĭ-fī). To branch; to spread out in different directions.

ramisection (răm'ĭ-sĕk"shŭn) [L. *ramus,* branch, + *sectio,* a cutting]. Surgical division of a ramus communicans between a spinal nerve and a ganglion of the sympathetic trunk.

ramisectomy (răm-ĭs-ĕk'tō-mĭ) ["+ Gr. *ektomē,* excision]. Excision of a ramus, specifically ramus communicans. SEE: *ramisection.*

ramollissement (rŏ"mŏl-ēs-mŏ') [Fr.]. Morbid softening of some organ or tissue, esp. of brain.

ra'mose [L. *ramus*, branch]. Branching; having many branches.

ram'ulus [L.]. (pl. *ram'uli*) A small branch or ramus.

ramus (rā'mŭs) [L., branch]. (pl. *ra'mi*) [NA] 1. A branch of one of the divisions of a forked structure. 2. Posterior portion of lower jawbone. 3. Primary division of a blood vessel or nerve.

r., anterior. A primary division of a spinal nerve which supplies the lateral and ventral portions of body wall, the limbs, and perineum. SYN: *ventral r.*

r., bronchial. Collateral branches of each primary bronchus.

r. communicans. [NA] One of the primary branches of a spinal nerve which connects with a sympathetic ganglion. Each consists of a *gray* portion (gray ramus communicans) of myelinated preganglionic sympathetic fibers, and a *white* portion (white ramus communicans) composed of unmyelinated postganglionic fibers.

r., meningeal. One of the primary branches of a spinal nerve which reenters vertebral foramen and supplies meninges and vertebral column. SYN: *recurrent branch.*

r., posterior. One of the primary branches of a spinal nerve which supplies muscles and skin of the back. SYN: *dorsal r.*

rancid (rǎn'sĭd) [L. *rancidus*]. Offensive; having a sour smell or taste from partial decomposition, as a fat.

range [ME., series]. The difference between the highest and lowest in a set of variables or in a series of values or observations.

r. of accommodation. Difference between least and greatest distance of distinct vision. SEE: *accommodation.*

ranine (rā'nīn) [L. *rana,* a frog]. 1. Pert. to a ranula, or to the region beneath the tip of the tongue. 2. Branch of the lingual artery supplying that area. 3. Pert. to frogs.

ranula (rǎn'ū-lǎ) [L., little frog]. A large cystic tumor seen on underside of tongue on either side of the frenum; a retention cyst of the submaxillary or sublingual ducts. The swelling may be small or as large as an egg.

SYM: Semitranslucent; soft, large, dilated veins coursing over it. Fullness and discomfort. Usually no pain. Contains clear, glairy fluid, due to dilatation of ducts of salivary glands and to obstruction of those of sublingual mucous glands.

TREATMENT: Periodic emptying of sac by careful needle aspiration will provide temporary relief. Surgical intervention is required to completely remove.

r., pancreatic. Cystic disease of pancreas due to obstruction of its ducts.

Ranvier's nodes (rŏn-vē-āz'). [Louis A. Ranvier, Fr. pathologist, 1835-1922]. Constrictions in the medullary substance of a nerve fiber at more or less regular intervals. SEE: *nerve fiber.*

rape (rāp) [L. *rapere,* to snatch]. Coitus with a female without her consent, or when she is too young or without sufficient intelligence to give legal consent. It is a crime punishable by death in some states. It is very difficult legally to prove rape. Rape of a vigorous girl by an unassisted male is considered almost impossible if the victim is conscious and free to defend herself.

RS: age of consent; coitus; sexual intercourse; virginity.

raphania (rō-fā'nī-ă) [Gr. *rhaphanos,* radish]. A spasmodic disease caused by eating seeds of the wild radish; allied to ergotism, q.v. SYN: *rhaphania.*

raphe (rā'fē) [Gr. *rhaphē*]. [NA] A crease, ridge, or seam noting union of the halves of a part.

r., buccal. R. on cheek indicating line of fusion of maxillary and mandibular processes.

r., palatine. A line or ridge in median line of palate.

r. of penis. [NA] A median ridge on posterior surface of penis, a continuation of raphe of scrotum.

r., perineal. A line or ridge in midline of perineum.

r. of scrotum. A ridge in midline of scrotum.

r. of tongue. A median groove on dorsum of tongue.

rapport (rǎ-pōr') [Fr. *rapporter,* to bring back]. A relationship of mutual sympathy and understanding, esp. between patient and physician.

raptus (rǎp'tŭs) [L.]. A sudden seizure or attack; rape.

r. hemorrhagicus. A sudden, massive hemorrhage.

r. maniacus. A sudden maniacal attack.

r. melancholicus. A sudden attack of agitation occurring during melancholia.

r. nervorum. A sudden attack of extreme nervousness; a cramp or spasm.

rarefaction (rar''ē-fǎk'shŭn) [L. *rarefacere,* to make thin]. Process of decreasing density and weight, as of air. The farther from the surface of the earth, the less dense the atmosphere becomes.

r. of bone. The process of making bone more porous because of absorption of mineral substances.

ETIOL: Disturbed calcium-phosphorus metabolism possibly resulting from excess parathyroid hormone. SEE: *osteoporosis; parathyroid.*

rarefy (răr'ĕ-fī). To make less dense, or to increase porosity of.

rarefying osteitis. Chronic bone inflammation marked by development of granulation tissue in marrow spaces with absorption of surrounding hard bone. SEE: *osteitis.*

rash (răsh) [O. Fr. *rasche*]. General term applied to any eruption of the skin, esp. those associated with communicable diseases. Usually temporary. The r. usually is a shade of red, which varies with disease. SYN: *exanthema.* SEE: *eruption; lesion; roseola.*

NP: Observe the following: Extent, whether localized, discrete, diffuse, or confluent; character, whether consisting of macules, papules, wheals, vesicles, pustules, bullae, or petechia; course, whether onset is gradual or sudden. Note changes in character.

r., cable. An acneiform eruption caused by contact with chlorinated waxes.

r., diaper. Inflammation of skin of infants in the diaper area due to one or more diverse primary irritants. Improperly processed diapers and metabolic by-products of wastes are probable irritant sources.

r., drug. One caused by use of certain drugs, such as bromide or iodine. SYN: *dermatitis medicamentosa,* q.v. SEE: *idiosyncrasy; drug rashes.*

r., ecchymotic. A hemorrhagic rash, q.v.

r., enema. R. caused by soap in an enema.

r., gum. A red, papular eruption of the chin and anterior chest area of children seen during teething. A form of miliaria due to excess saliva coming in contact with the skin. SYN: *strophulus.*

r., heat. Miliaria, q.v.

r., hemorrhagic. A r. consisting chiefly of hemorrhages or ecchymoses.

r., mulberry. R. seen in typhus fever; dusky in color.

r., nettle. Smooth, elevated, itchy, white patches. SYN: *hives; urticaria.*

r., red. Gum r., q.v.

r., rose. Any rose-colored r. SYN: *roseola.*

r., serum. R. accompanying serum sickness resulting from injection of a foreign serum. SEE: *serum sickness.*

r., tooth. Gum r., q.v.

r., vaccination. R. that sometimes follows vaccination.

r., wandering. SEE: *geographic tongue.*

raspatory (răs'pă-tō"rĭ) [L. *raspatorium*]. File used in surgery, esp. for trimming surfaces of bone. SYN: *xyster.*

raspberry (răz'bĕr'ĭ). Edible berries consisting of a mass of small, fleshy drupelets. Contains three times as much cellulose and less ash than strawberry.

Food value of 100 gm. (red, raw): Cal. 57; protein 1.2 gm.; fat 0.5 gm.; carbohydrate 13.6 gm.; calcium 22 mg.; iron 0.9 mg.; vitamin A 130 I.U.; ascorbic acid 25 mg.

rasura, rasure (rō-sū'ră, rā'zhūr) [L. *rasura,* a scraping]. 1. Process of scraping or shaving. 2. Scrapings or filings.

rat [ME]. A rodent, rattus, found in and around human habitations. In addition to causing enormous economic loss, rats are of primary importance in the spread of human and animal diseases in that they serve as hosts of various protozoans, flukes, tapeworms, and threadworms; reservoirs of amebiasis, murine and scrub typhus, plague (bubonic, septicemic, pneumonic). The plagues are transmitted to man principally through arthropods (rat flea). Rats also transmit ratbite fever, q.v. SEE: *flea.*

ratbite fever. Either of two infectious diseases contractible from the bite of a rat. They are caused by Streptobacillus moniliformis, characterized by skin inflammation, headache, vomiting, and back and joint pain; or Spirillum minus, with ulceration, rash, and recurrent fever. The latter disease is rare in the U.S.A.

rate (rāt) [L. *rata,* calculated]. The speed or frequency of occurrence of an event. Usually expressed with respect to time or some other known standard.

r., case fatality. The number of deaths per 100 cases of a specific disease.

r., morbidity. The number of cases per year of a certain disease in relation to the population in which they occur.

r., mortality. The frequency of all deaths over a period of time in relation to the population (sick and well) in which the deaths occur. SYN: *death rate; mortality.*

ratio (rā'shĭ-ō) [L., computation]. Relationship in degree or number between two things.

r., A-G. Albumin-globulin r., q.v.

r., albumin-globulin. Ratio of albumin to globulin in blood plasma or serum. Normally 1.3:1 to 3.0:1. Values less than one (1) are indicative of pathologic conditions.

r., body-weight. Body weight in gm. divided by body height in cm.

r., curative. Therapeutic r., q.v.

r., dextrose-nitrogen. Ratio of dextrose to nitrogen in urine.

r., mendelian. A r. obtained between groups of offspring of parents which differ in certain unit characters. Ratios will vary depending on degree of dominance of one character over the other, whether parents are homozygous, etc.

r., sex. R. of males to females in a given population. Usually expressed as number of males per 100 females.

r., therapeutic. R. obtained by dividing effective therapeutic dose by minimum lethal dose.

ration (rā'shŭn). Fixed allowance of food and drink for a certain period.

rational (răsh'ŭn-ăl) [L. *rationalis,* reasoning]. 1. Of sound mind. SYN: *sane.* 2. Reasonable or logical. 3. Employing treatments based on reasoning or general principles, opposed to empiric.

rationalization (răsh"ŭn-ăl-ĭ-zā'shŭn). In psychology, rational or plausible explanation to justify behavior or belief actually determined by some process other than reason.

rattle (răt'l) [Me. *ratelen*]. A sound or rale heard on auscultation.

r., death. A gurgling sound or subcrepitant rale heard in the trachea of the dying.

raucous (rŏ'kŭs) [L. *raucus*]. Hoarse, harsh, as the sound of a voice.

rauwolfia (rŏ-wolf'ĭ-ă). [Leonhard Rauwolf, Ger. botanist, — 1596]. The dried roots of Rauwolfia serpentina. Extracts are potent hypotensive agents and sedatives with low toxicity. Derivatives are serpentine, serpentinine, and reserpine, q.v.

rave (rāv) [ME. *raven,* to be delirious]. To talk irrationally, as in delirium.

rav'ing. 1. Irrational utterance. 2. Talking irrationally.

ray (rā) [L. *radius,* ray]. 1. One of a number of lines diverging from a common center. 2. Line of propagation of any form of radiant energy, esp. light or heat; loosely, any narrow beam of light.

RS: energy; energy, radiant; fluorescence; heat; radiation; words beginning with "roentgen;" spectrum; X ray.

r., actinic. A solar r. of the spectrum, capable of producing chemical changes.

r., alpha. R. composed of positively charged particles of helium derived from atomic disintegration of radioactive elements. Velocity one tenth that of light. Alpha r.'s are completely absorbed by a thin sheet of paper and possess powerful fluorescent, photographic, and ionizing properties. They are less penetrative than beta rays.

r., antirachitic. Ultraviolet r. from 2700 to 3020 A. U.

r., bactericidal. R. between 1850 and 2600 A. U. which is strongly bactericidal.

r.'s, Becquerel's. Those from radium, uranium, and other radioactive substances.

r.'s, beta. Negatively charged electrons expelled from atoms of disintegrating radioactive elements.

r.'s, border; r.'s, borderline; r.'s, Bucky. SEE: *grenz rays.*

r.'s, canal. Positive rays in a vacuum tube going from anode toward cathode. Old name for positive r.

r.'s, cathode. Negatively charged electrons discharged by the cathode through a vacuum, moving in a straight line and, upon hitting solid matter, producing roentgen rays.

r., characteristic. Secondary roentgen rays, the wavelengths of which are determined by the chemical constitution of the object that emits, transmits, or scatters them.

r., chemical. Actinic r., q.v.

r., cosmic. Electromagnetic waves (radiation) coming from sources in outer space. Cosmic rays have a short wavelength and exceptionally high velocity and penetrative power. SYN: *Millikan rays.*

r.'s, delta. Highly penetrative ether waves given off by radioactive substances.

r.'s, dynamic. Rays which are physically or therapeutically active.

r., erythema-producing. R. between 1800 and 4000 A. U., which produces erythema, with those around 2540 and between 2050 and 3100 A. U. being most effective.

r., Finsen; light. Ultraviolet radiation from the Finsen lamp.

r.'s, fluorescent roentgen. Secondary rays whose wavelengths are characteristic of the substance which emits them.

r. fungus. Genus of parasitic fungi with radiating formation.

r., gamma. Heterogeneous vibrations caused by electronic disturbance in atoms of radioactive elements during their disintegration. They appear identical with roentgen rays except that the wavelengths range from about 1.4 to 0.01 angstroms. They have high velocity and penetrative power. They lie between ultraviolet and roentgen rays.

r., grenz. Soft roentgen r. with an average wave length of 2 angstroms (range from 1 to 3 angstroms); obtained with peak voltage of less than 10 kilo-volts.

r.'s, hard. X-rays of short wave-length and great penetration.

r.'s, heat. Visible rays from 4000 to 7000 A. U. and infrared rays from 6000 to 14,000 A. U. The heating effect of visible rays on deeper tissue is proportionately stronger than that of infrared rays, because the visible rays have greater penetrating power. SEE: *heat.*

r.'s, Hertzian. Electromagnetic waves of great wavelength. Used in radio communication.

r.'s, infrared. Radiations just beyond the red end of the spectrum. Their wavelengths range between 7700 and 500,000 angstroms. The therapeutic range extends from about 7700 to about 14,000 angstroms.

r's, lenard's. Cathode rays that have passed outside the discharge tube. SEE: *cathode ray.*

r., luminous. Visible r.

r., medullary. One of many slender processes composed of straight tubules which project into the cortex from the bases of renal pyramids. SYN: *pars radiata; processes of rays of Ferrein.*

r.'s, Millikan. Cosmic rays, q.v.

r.'s, monochromatic. Rays characterized by a definite wavelength, as secondary rays.

r.'s, pigment-producing. Rays at 2500 and 3000 A. U. are most effective in causing pigmentation, a local response to irritation of cutaneous prickle-cells.

r., positive. R. of positively charged ions which, in a discharge tube, go from the anode toward the cathode.

r., primary. R. discharged directly from a radioactive substance, as the alpha, beta, and gamma rays.

r., roentgen. X rays discovered by Wilhelm Konrad Roentgen. They have a penetrative power through opaque substances; used for photographing internal organs and parts, and for diagnostic and therapeutic purposes.

r.'s, scattered. Roentgen rays or gamma rays which, in their passage through a substance, have deviated in direction and also may have been changed by an increase in wavelength.

r.'s, Schumann. Rays in the region bounded between 1220 and 1850 angstroms.

r.'s, secondary. Roentgen rays emitted in all directions by any matter irradiated with roentgen rays.

r.'s, ultraviolet. Invisible rays of the spectrum which are beyond the violet rays, and of varying wavelengths. Of luminous ether which may be refracted, reflected, and polarized, but which will not traverse many substances impervious to the rays of the visible spectrum. They do not affect the retina, but rapidly destroy the vitality of bacteria. They produce photochemical and photographic effects.

r.'s, X. SEE: *roentgen rays.*

Raynaud's disease or syndrome (ra-nō'). [Maurice Raynaud, Fr. physician, 1834-1881]. A condition caused by an abnormal degree of spasm of the blood vessels of the extremities, esp. in response to cold temperature which would not affect a normal person. Emotional stress may cause the symptoms. Heat relieves the symptoms. The disease is rare in males.

SYM: Appears in two forms. (1) A part, usually a finger or toe, becomes pale, cold, anesthetic. After a time these phenomena disappear and are followed by redness, heat, and tingling. Attacks may be excited by cold and come and go without damaging the part. (2) Affected part becomes swollen, dark, red, painful; if attack persists, bullae may appear and gangrene develop. Gangrenous areas often symmetrical, involving a finger on each hand, toe on each foot, or both ears.

PROG: Attacks persist, but life not endangered. In rare instances, extensive gangrene develops and death follows. Gangrene may be absent in mild forms.

TREATMENT: Mild cases may be treated merely by protecting the patient from the cold by wearing warmer clothes or moving to a warmer climate. Psychotherapy and reassurance are helpful. In severe cases sympathectomy is indicated.

Rb. Chem. symb. for rubidium.

RBC, rbc. Abbr. for *red blood count.*

R.C.D. Abbr. for *relative cardiac dullness.*

R.C.P. Abbr. for Royal College of Physicians.

R.C.S. Abbr. for Royal College of Surgeons.

R.D.A. Abbr. for *right dorsoanterior,* presentation position of the fetus.

R.D.P. Abbr. for *right dorsoposterior,* presentation position of the fetus.

R. E. Abbr. for *radium emanation; right eye; reticuloendothelium.*

Re. Chem. symb. for rhenium.

re- [L.]. Prefix meaning back or again.

reaction (rē-ăk'shŭn) [LL. *reactus,* reacted]. 1. Response of an organism, or part of it, to a stimulus. 2. In chem., a chemical process or change; the result of a test to determine the pH (hydrogen-ion concentration) of a solution and designated acid, neutral, or alkaline. 3. An opposing or counteraction. 4. Emotional and mental state created by a situation.

There are two forms of r. *Anesthesia dolorosa:* pain associated with anesthesia of a part, as in thalamic lesions. *Subjective sensations:* these may include causalgia; paresthesia; pseudomyelia paresthetica, a false sensation, as of movement in a paralyzed limb or part, or sensation of lack of movement in a moving limb.

SEE: *method; reflex; response; test.*

r., affective. SEE: *affective psychosis; psychosis, manic-depressive.*

r., alarm. The first stage in the general adaptation syndrome (G-A-S) which includes changes occurring in the body when subjected to stressful stimuli. Physiological changes which occur are direct results of damage and/or shock, or reactions of the body to defend itself against shock.

r., allergic. A reaction resulting from hypersensitivity to an antigen.

r., anamnestic. The reappearance of antibodies which may occur when an antigen is injected a considerable time after the first injection.

r., anaphylactic. R. which follows injection or administration of a foreign substance to an animal which has been sensitized to it. The principal manifestation of the antigen-antibody r., q.v. SYN: *anaphylaxis.*

r., anaphylactoid. R. similar to an anaphylactic r. but not as severe. Induced by introducing into subject a substance to which he has not become hypersensitive.

r., antigen-antibody. The combination of molecules of an antigen with one or more molecules of its specific antibody.

r., atopic. Atopic sensitivity.

r., complement fixation. A test based on the principle that the complement enters into combinations formed between soluble or particulate antigens and antibody. Used for diagnosis of certain diseases, esp. syphilis. SEE: *complement.*

r., consensual. 1. An involuntary action. 2. A crossed reflex.

r., cross. A r. between an antibody and an antigen which is not specific for the antibody but closely allied to the one which is.

r. of degeneration. The change in muscle reactivity to electricity, seen in lower motor neuron paralysis.

r., delayed. R. occurring a considerable time after a stimulus, esp. a reaction such as inflammation of the skin occurring hours or days after exposure to the allergen.

r., false-positive. A positive r. in a test, esp. test for syphilis, which is due to faulty technique or to presence of another disease.

r. formation. The checking of infantile impulses and tendencies that might become those of an antisocial nature later, or which might hold the individual upon an infantile level, and the attributes developed from such partial repressions as modesty, shame, or disgust.

r., immune. A r. which demonstrates the presence of antibodies in the blood. Indicative of a high degree of immunity.

r., inflammatory. SEE: *inflammation.*

r., local. R. occurring at point of stimulation or injection of exciting substances.

r., myasthenic. Gradual decrease and eventual cessation of muscle contractions when a muscle is stimulated repeatedly by direct current.

r., neutral. In chemistry, a reaction indicating absence of acid or alkaline properties. Expressed as pH 7.0.

r., ophthalmic. Local r. of conjunctiva to introduction of toxins of tuberculosis and typhoid fever; more severe in those having the diseases.

r., quellung. The swelling of capsules of bacteria when mixed with their specific immune serum. SYN: *Neufeld's reaction.*

r., time. Time elapsing between application of a stimulus and the response to it.

r., transfusion. R. following transfusion of incompatible blood resulting from agglutination and hemolysis of red blood cells.

reac'tivate. To make active again, esp. the process of reactivating immune serum that has lost its potency by the addition of fresh normal serum, thus restoring the complement which had become inactive through age, heat, or other factors.

reactive depression. In psychology, a psychosis resulting from bereavement, sadness, or a situation causing such emotions, lasting longer and more marked than the normal reaction.

reading. The comprehending of written or printed material.

r. disorders. Conditions which interfere with or prevent comprehension of written or printed material. A term used esp. in reference to children. The condition seen in some adults may have developed due to injury to the brain or may have persisted from infancy. SEE: *dyslexia.*

r., lip. Interpretation of what is being spoken by watching movements of the speaker's lips.

reagent (rē-ā′jĕnt) [L. *reagere,* to react]. 1. A substance involved in a chemical reaction. 2. A substance used to detect the presence of another substance. 3. Subject of a psychological experiment, esp. one reacting to a stimulus.

reagin (rē-ō′jĭn). 1. An antibody associated with atopic hypersensitivity; one associated with manifestations of hay fever, asthma, urticaria, angioedema, and infantile eczema. 2. A substance present in serum and cerebrospinal fluid that induces flocculation in complement fixation and similar tests.

   r., atopic. Antibodies, present in naturally hypersensitive persons, which will produce passive hypersensitivity when injected into a normal subject.

reality principle (rē-ăl′ĭ-tĭ). Awareness of external demands and adjustment in a manner that meets these demands, yet assures a continued self-gratification.

re″amina′tion. The restoration of an amino group to a compound from which an amino group had previously been removed.

rean′imate [ME. *re,* again, + L. *animāre,* fill with life]. To reactivate, restore to life, revive, resuscitate.

reapers′ keratitis (rēp′ĕrs kĕr-ă-tī′tĭs). Keratitis caused by dust from grain.

rebound [ME. *rebounden,* to leap back]. Response seen in reflexes in which sudden withdrawal of stimulus is followed by fresh activity, such as a strong contraction following a moderate one, marked relaxation following moderate relaxation, or contraction replacing inhibition.

   r. phenomenon. When a limb or a part is acting against a resistance and the resistance is suddenly removed, the limb will move forcibly in direction toward which effort was being directed.

recalcification (rē″kăl-sĭ-fĭ-kā′shŭn) [ME. *re,* again, + L. *calx,* lime, + *facere,* to make]. The restoration of mineral salts to tissues from which they have been withdrawn.

recall′ ["+ AS. *ceallian,* to call]. Act of bringing back to mind that which has been previously learned or experienced.

recapitulation theory (rē″kă-pĭt-ū-lā′shŭn) ["+ *capitulum,* a section]. The theory that an individual in its development from the ovum to maturity passes through successive stages which approximate the series of adult ancestors from which that organism has descended. Summarized in the statement, "Ontogeny recapitulates phylogeny."

receiver (rē-sēv′er) [ME. *re,* again, + *capere,* to take]. 1. Container for holding a gas or a distillate. 2. Apparatus for receiving electrical waves or current, i.e., a radio receiver.

receptaculum (rē″sĕp-tăk′ū-lŭm) [L.]. (pl. *receptac′ula*) A vessel or cavity in which a fluid is contained.

   r. chyli. Inferior, pear-shaped, expanded portion of the lower end of the thoracic duct, near 1st and 2nd lumbar vertebrae, into which the right and left lumbar trunks, an intestinal trunk, and some thoracic vessels empty.

receptor (rē-sĕp′tōr) [L., a receiver]. 1. Molecular group in cells which have a special affinity for toxins, amboceptors, etc. SEE: *Ehrlich's side-chain theory.* 2. Group of cells functioning in reception of stimuli; a sense organ; endings of afferent (sensory) nerves.

   r., auditory. The hair cells in the organ of Corti in cochlea of ear.

   r., contact. A r. that gives rise to a sensation such as touch, temperature, pain which can be localized in or on surface of body.

   r., cutaneous. R. which is located in the skin.

   r., distance. A r. that responds to stimuli originating at a distance from the body. Includes visual, auditory, and olfactory sense organs. SYN: *telereptor.*

   r., gravity. Macula hair cells of utricle and saccule which respond to changes in position of the head and linear acceleration.

   r., olfactory. The olfactory cells, bipolar nerve cells, found in olfactory epithelium, whose axons form fibers of olfactory nerve.

   r., optic. The rods and cones of the retina.

   r., proprioceptive. Muscle and tendon spindles, the receptors of the muscle or kinesthetic sense.

   r., rotary. The hair cells in the cristae of the ampulla of semicircular ducts, which are stimulated by angular acceleration or rotation.

   r., sensory. A sensory nerve-ending, a cell or group of cells, or a sense organ which, when stimulated, gives rise to an afferent or sensory impulse.

   CLASSIFICATION: *Exteroreceptors:* those located on or near surface and respond to stimuli of outside world; include eye and ear (distance receptors) and touch, temperature, and pain receptors (contact receptors). *Interoceptors:* those in mucous linings of alimentary and digestive tracts which respond to internal stimuli; also called visceroceptors. *Proprioceptors:* those responding to stimuli arising within body tissues.

Receptors also are classified on the basis of nature of stimuli to which they respond: *chemoreceptors,* those that respond to chemical substances (taste buds, olfactory cells, receptors in aortic and carotid bodies); *pressoreceptors,* those that respond to pressure (receptors in aortic arch and carotid sinus); *photoreceptors,* those that respond to light (rods and cones); *tangoreceptors,* those that respond to touch (Meissner's corpuscle).

r., stretch. Neuromuscular and neurotendinar spindles and organs of Golgi which are stimulated by stretch. SEE: *proprioceptor.*

r., taste. The gustatory cells of the taste buds.

r., temperature. Krause's end-bulbs (receptors of cold) and Ruffini's corpuscles (receptors for warmth).

r., touch. Merkel's disks, Meissner's corpuscles, and nerve plexus about the roots of hairs.

re'cess [L. *recessus,* receded]. A small indentation, depression, or cavity. SEE: *recessus.*

r., cochlear. A small concavity lying between the two limbs of the vestibular crest in vestibule of ear which lodges the beginning of the cochlear duct.

r., elliptical. A small concavity lying superiorly and posteriorly on medial wall of vestibule that lodges the utricle.

r., epitympanic. That portion of the tympanic cavity that lies above the level of tympanic membrane. It contains the head of the malleus and short limb of incus. SYN: *attic.*

r., infundibular. A small projection of third ventricle which extends into infundibular stalk of hypophysis.

r., lateral, of fourth ventricle. One of two lateral extensions of the 4th ventricle, forming narrow pockets on each side and around upper portions of the restiform bodies.

r., lineal. R., omental, q.v.

r., nasopalatine. A small depression on floor of nasal cavity near nasal septum. Lies immediately over incisive foramen.

r., omental. One of three pocketlike extensions of the omental bursa. The *superior r.* extends upward behind caudate lobe of liver, the *inferior r.* extends downward into great omentum, and the *lienal r.* extends laterally to hilus of spleen.

r., optic. A pocket of the 3rd ventricle lying anterior to infundibular r. It is bound inferiorly by optic chiasma.

r., pharyngeal. R. in lateral wall of nasal pharynx lying above and behind opening to auditory tube. SYN: *fossa of Rosenmüller.*

r., pineal. A r. of roof of 3rd ventricle extending into stalk of pineal body.

r., pyiform. A deep depression in wall of laryngeal pharynx lying lateral to orifice of larynx. It is bounded laterally by thyroid cartilage and medially by cricoid and arytenoid cartilages. It is a common site for lodgement of foreign objects.

r., sphenoethmoidal. Small space in nasal fossa lying above superior concha. Lies between ethmoid bone and anterior surface of body of sphenoid bone and posteriorly receives opening of sphenoidal sinus.

r., spherical. R. on medial wall of vestibule of inner ear which accommodates the saccule.

r., suprapineal. A posterior extension of roof of 3rd ventricle forming a small cavity above pineal body.

r., tympanic membrane. One of two pouches of tympanic mucous membrane (anterior and posterior) lying between tympanic membrane and anterior and posterior malleolar folds.

r., umbilical. A dilatation on left main branch of portal vein which marks position where umbilical vein was originally attached.

recession (rē-sĕsh'ŭn) [L. *recessus,* recess]. The withdrawal of a part from its normal position.

r. of gums. Shrinkage of gums away from necks of teeth. SYN: *ulatrophia.*

recess'ive. Tending to recede or go back; lacking control; not dominant.

r. character. A mendelian character which does not express itself in the offspring unless it is transmitted by both genes. SEE: *gene; factor; heredity.*

r. gene. A gene which, in the presence of its dominant allelomorph, does not express itself.

recessus (rē-sĕs'ŭs) [L.]. A small hollow or recess.

recidivation (rē-cĭd''ĭ-vā'shŭn) [L. *recidivus,* falling back]. 1. The relapse of a disease. 2. The relapsing into crime.

recid'ivism. Habitual criminality; repetition of antisocial acts.

recid'ivist. 1. A confirmed criminal. 2. A patient, esp. one with mental illness who has repeated relapses, esp. a mentally ill patient who relapses into behavior marked by antisocial acts.

recidiv'ity. Tendency to relapse, or to return to a former condition.

recipe (rĕs'ĭ-pē) [L., take]. 1. Take, indicated by the sign ℞. 2. A prescription or formula for a medicine. SEE: *prescription*.

recipient (rē-sĭp'ĭ-ĕnt) [L. *recipiēns*, receiving]. One who receives anything, esp. those who receive blood, tissues, or organs provided by a donor, as in a blood transfusion or kidney transplant. SEE: *donor*.

reciprocal (rē-sĭp'rō-kăl) [L. *reciprocus*, alternate]. Interchangeable in character.

   r. reception. Articulation with convex surface in one direction and concave surface in another.

Recklinghausen (rĕk'lĭng-how"zĕn). [Friedrich D. von Recklinghausen, Ger. pathologist, 1833-1910].

   R.'s canals. Rootlets of the lymphatics, minute spaces in connective tissue.

   R.'s disease or syndrome. Pigmentation of skin, multiple small fibrous tumors on same with tenderness along nerves, pain in joints, sluggishness, multiple neurofibromatosis.

   R.'s tumor. An adenoleiomyofibroma on wall of the fallopian tube, or posterior uterine wall.

reclination (rĕk"lĭ-nā'shŭn) [L. *reclinatio*, lean back]. The turning of the eye lens covered with a cataract over into the vitreous to remove it from line of vision. SYN: *couching*.

recline (rē-klīn') [L. *reclīnāre*]. To be in recumbent position; to lie down.

Reclus' disease (rā-klū'). [Paul Reclus, Fr. surgeon, 1847-1914] Multiple, benign, cystic growths in the mammary gland.

recomposition [L. *re*, again, + *composer*, to place together]. The recombining of constituents or parts.

recompres'sion ["+ LL. *compressāre*, press together]. Resubjecting a person to increased atmospheric pressure, a procedure used in the treatment of caisson disease (bends).

reconstituent (rē"kŏn-stĭt'ū-ĕnt) [L. *re*, again, + *constituens*, constituting]. An agent that improves or strengthens one or more parts or functions of the body by replacing lost material. Ex: calcium; iron; phosphorus. SYN: *tonic*.

reconstitution (rē"kŏn-stĭ-tū'shŭn). A substance, previously altered for preservation and storage, returned to its original state. Ex: dried blood plasma.

recover (rē-kŭv'ŭr) [O. Fr. *recoverer*]. To regain health after illness; to regain a former state of health. To regain a normal state as to *recover* from fright.

recovery (rē-kŭv'ŭr-ĭ). The process or act of recovering.

   r. room. Area provided with equipment and nurses needed to care for patients who have just come from surgery. Patients remain there until they regain consciousness and are no longer drowsy and stuporous from the effects of anesthesia.
   RS: postoperative.

recrement (rĕk'rē-mĕnt) [L. *recrēmentum*, sifted again]. Secretion which, after having performed its function as the saliva or part of the bile, is reabsorbed into the blood.

recrementitious (rĕk"rē-mĕn-tĭsh'ŭs). Of the nature of a secretion which, having performed its function, is reabsorbed into the blood.

recrudescence (rē"krū-dĕs'ĕns) [L. *recrudescere*, to get worse]. Return of symptoms. SYN: *relapse*.

recrudescent (rē"krū-dĕs'ĕnt). Assuming renewed activity after dormant or inactive period.

recruitment (rē-krūt'mĕnt) [O. Fr. *recrute*, new growth]. Condition in which response in a reflex action increases to a maximum when a stimulus is prolonged, even though strength of stimulus is unchanged; due to activation of increasingly greater numbers of motor neurons. Ex: If, while testing the patellar reflex, the normal patient clasps his hands together and attempts to pull them apart, the intensity of the reflex response will be increased.

   r. of end organs. Increase in discharge from sensory end organs, resulting from increase of stimulus accounted for by increase in number of end organs discharging and increase in frequency in discharge from each.

rectal (rĕk'tăl) [L. *rectus*, straight]. Pert. to the rectum.

   r. alimentation. Rectal feeding, q.v.

   r. anesthesia. Introduction of anesthetic into rectum for local desensitization, used esp. in labor. SEE: *anesthesia, labor*.

   r. crisis. Tenesmus and rectal pain in locomotor ataxia.

   r. feeding. The introduction of nutrients in fluid form into the colon through the rectum. SYN: *nutrient enema*. SEE: *enema, nutrient*.

   r. reflex. The normal desire to evacuate feces present in rectum.

rectalgia (rĕk-tăl'jĭ-ă) [L. *rectus*, straight, + Gr. *algos*, pain]. Pain in rectum.

rectectomy (rĕk-tĕk'tō-mĭ) ["+ Gr. *ektomē*, excision]. Excision of the rectum or anus. SYN: *proctectomy*.

rectification (rĕk"tĭ-fĭ-kā'shŭn) ["+ *facere*, to make]. 1. The process of refining or purifying a substance. 2. Act of straightening or correcting.

rectified (rĕk'tĭ-fīd). Made pure or straight. Set right.

    r. spirit. One resulting from fractional or repeated distillation of alcohol, as whiskey.

rectifier (rĕk'tĭ-fī"ẽr) [L. *rectum*, straight, + *-ficāre*, to make]. In electricity, a device for transforming an alternating current into a direct one.

rectitis (rĕk-tī'tĭs) ["+ Gr. *-itis*, inflammation]. Inflamed condition of the rectum. SYN: *proctitis.*

recto- [L. *rectum*, straight]. Combining form meaning straight or the rectum.

rectocele (rĕk'tō-sēl) ["+ Gr. *kēlē*, hernia]. Protrusion or herniation of posterior vaginal wall with anterior wall of rectum through the vagina. SEE: *cystocele.*

rectoclysis (rĕk-tŏk'lĭ-sĭs) ["+ Gr. *klysis*, a washing out]. Slow introduction of fluid into rectum. SYN: *Murphy drip; proctoclysis.*

rectococcypexia (rĕk"tō-kŏk-sĭ-pĕks'sĭ-ă) [L. *rectum*, straight, + Gr. *kokkyx*, coccyx, + *pēxis*, fixation]. Fixation of rectum by suturing it to coccyx.

rectocolitis (rĕk"tō-kō-lī'tĭs) ["+ Gr. *kolon*, colon, + *-itis*, inflammation]. Inflamed condition of rectum and colon. SYN: *proctocolitis.*

rectocystotomy (rĕk"tō-sĭs-tŏt'ō-mĭ) ["+ Gr. *kystis*, bladder, + *tomē*, a cutting]. Incision of the bladder through rectum, usually to remove a calculus.

rectopexy (rĕk'tō-pĕk-sĭ) [L. *rectum*, straight, + Gr. *pēxis*, fixation]. Fixation of rectum by suturing to another part. SYN: *proctopexy.*

rectophobia (rĕk"tō-fō'bĭ-ă) ["+ Gr. *phobos*, fear]. Morbid fear in those patients with rectal disease.

rectoplasty (rĕk'tō-plăs"tĭ) ["+ Gr. *plassein*, to form]. Plastic operation on the anus and rectum. SYN: *proctoplasty.*

rectorrhaphy (rĕk-tor'ă-fĭ) [L. *rectum*, straight, + Gr. *rhaphē*, a sewing]. Suture of rectum and anus. SYN: *proctorrhaphy.*

rectoscope (rĕk'tō-skōp) ["+ Gr. *skopein*, to examine]. A speculum to examine the rectum.

rectosigmoid (rĕk"tō-sĭg'moyd) ["+ Gr. *sigma*, letter S, + *eidos*, form]. Upper part of rectum and adjoining portion of the sigmoid colon.

rectostenosis (rĕk"tō-stĕn-ō'sĭs) [L. *rectum*, straight, + Gr. *stenōsis*, a narrowing]. Stricture of the rectum.

rectostomy (rĕk-tŏs'tō-mĭ) ["+ Gr. *stoma*, a mouth]. Creation of an artificial opening into the rectum to relieve stricture. SYN: *proctostomy,* q.v.

rectotomy (rĕk-tŏt'ō-mĭ) ["+ Gr. *tomē*, an incision]. Incision for stricture of the rectum or other purposes. SYN: *proctotomy,* q.v.

rectourethral (rĕk"tō-ū-rē'thrăl) [L. *rectum*, straight, + Gr. *ourēthra*, urethra]. Concerning the rectum and urethra.

rectouterine (rĕk"tō-ū'tĕr-ĭn) ["+ *uterus*, womb]. Concerning the rectum and uterus.

rectovaginal (rĕk"tō-văj'ĭ-năl) ["+ *vagina*, sheath]. Concerning the rectum and vagina.

rectovesical (rĕk"tō-vĕs'ĭ-kăl) ["+ *vesica*, a small vessel]. Concerning the rectum and bladder.

rectum (rĕk'tŭm) [L., straight]. Lower part of large intestine, about 5 in. (12.7 cm.) long, between sigmoid flexure and the anal canal. The centers for the defecation reflex are located in the medulla and 2nd, 3rd, and 4th sacral segments.

PREPARATIONS SOMETIMES GIVEN BY RECTUM: *Chloral Hydrate:* Prescribed dose dissolved in 3 oz. (90 ml.) of warm olive oil, 3 oz. (90 ml.) of very warm milk, or 3 oz. (90 ml.) of thin, boiled cornstarch water. This makes a good preparation or base in which to hold the medicine in suspension. The patient's pulse should be taken 5 minutes before and at 5-minute intervals for one-half hour after the administration, to observe the heart action. If adverse effects are noticed, action should be taken to prevent further absorption.

Paraldehyde: Prescribed dose may be mixed with water in the proportion of 1:8, and in this ratio it may be mixed with thin starch water for rectal medication. There should be about 3 oz. (90 ml.) of starch water.

Sodium Bicarbonate: One teaspoonful, or 4 gm. to 500 cc., or 1 pint, of water aids in the expulsion of the bowel content. The neutralizing action on the acidity of the bowel content brought about by the sodium bicarbonate solution leaves the bowel soothed and with a bland reaction.

    RS: anorectal; anus; archocele; archoptosis; archorrhagia; archostenosis; cloaca; colon; enema; feeding; hemorrhoid; sigmoid; words beginning with "proct-" or "rect-."

rectus (rĕk'tŭs) [L.]. 1. Straight; not crooked. 2. Any straight muscle.

    r. muscles. 1. Two external abdominal muscles, one on each side, from pubic bone to the ensiform cartilage and 5th, 6th, and 7th ribs. 2. Four short muscles of the eye-exterior, interior, superior, and inferior.

recumbency (rē-kŭm'bĕn-sĭ) [L. *recumbēns*, lying down]. State of leaning or reclining.

recumbent. 1. Lying down. SEE: *left lateral recumbent position; prone.* 2. Inactive, idle.

recuperation (rē-kū″pŭr-ā′shŭn) [L. *recuperāre,* to recover]. Restoration to normal health.

recurrence (rē-kŭr′ĕns) [L. *re,* again, + *currere,* to run]. Return of symptoms after a period of quiescence, as in recurrent fever and in yellow fever. SYN: *relapse.*

recurrent (rē-kŭr′ĕnt) [L. *recurrens,* returning]. Returning at intervals, as a fever.

    r. fever. Relapsing fever, q.v.

recurvation (rē″kŭr-vā′shŭn) [L. *recurvus,* bent back]. The act of bending backwards.

recurve (rē-kŭrv′). Bend backward.

red (rĕd) [AS. *rēad*]. A primary color of the spectrum.

    r. blindness. Inability to see red hues. The most frequent color blindness.

    r. blood cell. Blood corpuscle containing hemoglobin. SYN: *erythrocyte,* q.v.

    r. lead. Lead tetroxide, Pb_3O_4; minium.

    r. nucleus. Gray matter in the tegmentum of midbrain. SYN: *nucleus ruber.*

    r. precipitate. Red mercuric oxide. POISONING SYM: Similar to mercuric chloride, q.v.

    r. softening. Hemorrhagic softening of the brain and cord.

red. in pulv. Abbr. for *reductus in pulverum,* reduced to powder.

redia (rē′dĭ-ă). [Francesco Redi, It. naturalist, 1626-1698]. (pl. *re′diae*) Stage in life cycle of a trematode following the sporocyst. The organisms are sac-like structures, possessing an oral sucker and a blind gut. They arise parthenogenetically from germ masses within the sporocyst and in turn give rise to 2nd or 3rd generation rediae or to cercaria.

redintegration (rĕd-ĭn″tĕ-grā′shŭn) [L. *redintegratio*]. 1. Restitution of a part. 2. Restoration to health. 3. Recall by mental association.

red-out (rĕd′out). A term used in aerospace medicine to describe what happens to the vision and central nervous system, i.e., seeing red and perhaps experiencing unconsciousness, when the aircraft is doing part or all of an outside loop at high speed, or any other maneuver that causes the pilot to experience negative G. The condition is due to engorgement of the vessels of the head including those of the retina.

redox. Abbr. for *oxidation-reduction.*

redressment (rē-drĕs-man′) [Fr.]. 1. Correction of a deformity. 2. Dressing of a wound more than once.

reduce (rē-dūs′) [L. *re,* again, + *ducere,* to lead]. 1. To restore to usual relationship, as the ends of a fractured bone. 2. To weaken,

as a solution. 3. To diminish, as in bulk or weight.

reducible (rē-dūs′ĭ-bl). Capable of being replaced in a normal position, as a dislocated bone, a hernia, etc.

reducing agent. A substance that loses electrons easily, hence causes other substances to be reduced. Ex: hydrogen sulfide; sulfur dioxide.

reductase (rē-dūk′tās) [L. *re,* again, + *ducere,* to lead, + *ase,* enzyme]. An enzyme accelerating process of reduction of chemical compounds.

reduction (rē-dūk′shŭn) [L. *reductiō,* leading back]. 1. Restoration to normal position, as a fractured bone or a hernia. 2. In chemistry, a type of reaction in which hydrogen is taken up by the given compound, or oxygen is removed, or the valence of the metallic element is lowered. SEE: *oxidation.*

    r. diet. One which reduces the caloric content sufficently to cause loss of weight. Normal metabolism must be preserved. Bulk, mineral, protein, vitamin, and water requirements must be maintained. Energy value should be 600 to 1500 Cal. below maintenance requirements. For a person of average size, this could be accomplished by a diet containing the following amounts of nutrients: protein 60 gm.; carbohydrate 50 gm.; fat 45 gm.

    r. division. Division occurring in gametogenesis following synapsis in which diploid number of chromosomes is reduced to the haploid number (one half the diploid number). SYN: *meiosis; miosis.*

redundant (rē-dŭn′dĕnt) [L. *redundāre,* to overflow]. More than necessary.

reduplicated (rē-dū′plĭ-kā″tĕd) [L. *re,* again, + *duplicāre,* to double]. 1. Doubled. 2. Bent backward upon itself, as a fold.

reduplication (rē-dū″plĭ-kā′shŭn). 1. A doubling, as of the heart sounds in some morbid conditions. 2. A fold.

Reduviidae (rē″dū-vī′ĭ-dī). A family of the order Hemiptera, including the assassin bugs.

Reduvius (rē-dū′vĭ-ŭs). A genus of true bugs belonging to the family Reduviidae.

    R. personatus. A species which normally feeds on other insects, but sometimes attacks man, inflicting painful bites about the face. In some individuals, these bugs may cause severe allergic symptoms. SYN: *kissing bug; masked hunter.*

re-education (rē″ĕd-ū-kā′shŭn) [L. *re,* again, + *educāre,* to educate]. 1. Training to partially restore lost competence to a disabled or mentally disordered person. 2. Physical means for restoring muscular tone and activity.

refection (rē-fĕk'shŭn) [L. *reficere*]. 1. Act of restoring after fatigue or exhaustion. 2. Recovery from symptoms of vitamin B-complex deficiency on a diet deficient in vitamin B. Thought to be due to bacterial synthesis of vitamins by intestinal bacteria.

reference man. Concept used in nutritional investigation and surveys. A man 22 years of age, weight 70 kg., living in an environment with a mean temperature of 20° C., wearing clothing compatible with thermal comfort, engaged in light physical activity, and with an estimated calorie allowance of 2800 kcal.

reference woman. A woman used in nutritional references, described the same as reference man except in weight (58 kg.) and calorie allowance (2000 kcal.). SEE: *reference man.*

referred pain (rē-fūrd'pān). Pain felt in a part removed from its point of origin. SYN: *synalgia.*

refine (rē-fīn) [L. *re*, again, + ME. *fin*, finished]. To purify or render free from foreign material.

reflection (rē-flĕk'shŭn) [L. *reflexio*, a bending back]. 1. Condition of being turned back upon itself, as when the peritoneum passes from wall of a body cavity to and around an organ and back to the body wall. 2. The throwing back of a ray of radiant energy from a surface not penetrated. 3. Mental consideration of some subject matter.

reflector (rē-flĕk'tŏr) [L. *re*, again, + *flectere*, to bend]. Device or surface which reflects waves of radiant energy or sound.

reflex (rē'flĕks) [L. *reflexus*, bent back]. An involuntary response to a stimulus; a reflex action. Reflexes are specific and predictable and are usually purposeful and adaptive. Reflexes depend upon an intact neural pathway between point of stimulation and responding organ (muscle or gland). This pathway is called r. arc. In a simple r. this includes a sensory receptor, afferent or sensory neuron, r. center in brain or spinal cord, one or more efferent neurons, and an effector organ (muscle or gland). Most reflexes, however, are more complicated and include internuncial or associative neurons intercalated between afferent and efferent neurons.

RS: Achilles jerk; areflexia; chemoreflex; chin jerk; conditioned r.; consensual; intestinal; jerk; reaction; reinforcement; Setschenow's inhibitory center; and reflexes under their individual names.

  •*r.,* **abdominocardiac.** A change in heart rate, usually a slowing, resulting from mechanical stimulation of abdominal viscera.

r., **acquired.** A conditioned r., q.v.

r. **action.** An involuntary response to a stimulus, a reflex.

r., **after-discharge of.** R. activity which persists for a time after cessation of the stimulus.

r's. **allied.** Reflexes initiated by several stimuli originating in widely separated receptors whose impulses follow the final common path to effector organ and reinforce one another.

r's, **antagonistic.** Two or more reflexes initiated simultaneously in different receptors which involve the same motor center but produce opposite effects. The most important or adaptive response takes place.

r. **arc.** The neural pathway or circuit between point of stimulation and responding organ in a r. action. SEE: *reflex.*

r., **autonomic.** Any r. involving the response of a visceral effector (cardiac muscle, smooth muscle, glands). Such reflexes always involve two efferent neurons (a preganglionic and postganglionic).

r., **autonomic, true.** A visceral response in which afferent impulses do not pass through central nervous system, but instead enter prevertebral ganglia where connections are made with efferent neurons.

r., **axon.** A r. which does not involve a complete r. arc, hence is not a true r. The afferent and efferent limbs of the r. are branches of a single nerve fiber, the axon (axonlike dendrite) of a sensory neuron. Ex: vasodilation resulting from stimulation of skin.

r., **biceps.** Flexion of forearm upon percussion of tendon of biceps brachii.

r. **center.** A region, usually in brain or spinal cord, where impulses from an afferent limb of a r. arc initiate impulses in the efferent limb.

r., **conditioned.** A r. acquired as a result of training in which the cerebral cortex is an essential part of the neural mechanism. Any r. not inborn or inherited.

r., **consensual.** R., crossed, q.v.

r., **convulsive.** Condition in which a weak stimulus will induce a convulsion resulting in widespread uncoordinated and purposeless actions. Seen in strychnine poisoning.

r., **cranial.** Any r. whose center lies in the brain.

r., **crossed.** R. in which stimulation of one side of body results in response on opposite side.

r., deep. R. caused by stimulation of parts beneath skin, like tendons or bones, as the jaw, elbow, wrist, triceps, knee, and ankle jerk reflexes.

r., delayed. R. not taking place until some seconds after application of stimulus.

r., elbow. Triceps r., q.v.

r., elementary. A typical r. common to all vertebrates. Includes postural, flexion, stretch, and extensor thrust reflexes.

r., extensor thrust. A quick and brief extension of a limb upon application of pressure to plantar surface.

r., inborn. An unconditioned r.; an innate or inherited r.

r., indirect. A crossed r. SEE: *crossed reflexes.*

r.'s, inhibition of. The stoppage or prevention of a r. action, as inhibiting a sneeze by pressure on facial nerve just under upper lip or through action of higher cerebral centers.

r., intersegmental. R. in which several segments of spinal cord are involved.

r., intestinal. R., myenteric, q.v.

r., intrasegmental. R. that involves only a single segment of the spinal cord.

r.'s, irradiation of. The spreading of reflexes through the central nervous system whereby impulses entering the cord in one segment activate motor neurons located in many segments.

r., kinetic. R., labyrinthine, q.v.

r., knee-jerk. Extension of the leg resulting from percussion of patellar tendon. This is an example of a myotactic or stretch r. of importance in the maintenance of posture. The r. is diminished or abolished in lesions of the nerve supplying the muscle and tendon, lesions of posterior roots involving sensory pathway as in tabes dorsalis, lesions of anterior root involving motor pathways, or lesions of lower motor neurons in anterior horns of gray matter of spinal cord, as in poliomyelitis. If, however, the upper motor neuron is destroyed, muscle tone and the motor response are greatly increased. So-called pathologic reflexes under these conditions may appear. Reflexes are also modified by higher centers, e.g., emotional tension increases the knee jerk (and muscle tension generally). SEE: *Babinski's sign.*

r., labyrinthine. A r., esp. a postural r., resulting from stimulation of receptors in semicircular ducts, utricle, and saccule of inner ear. SYN: *accelerator r; kinetic r.*

r., local. R. which does not involve the central nervous system. Ex: the myenteric r.

which occurs even though extrinsic nerves to intestine have been cut.

r., long. R. involving many segments of the spinal cord.

r., mass. Condition following a section of spinal cord in which a weak stimulus through irradiation brings about widespread responses due to release from inhibition of higher cortical centers.

r., monosynaptic. R. involving only two neurons, an afferent and efferent.

r., myenteric. R. caused by distention of intestine resulting in contraction above point of stimulation, and relaxation below it. SYN: *intestinal reflex.*

r., myotatic. A stretch r., q.v.

r., near. Accommodation r., q.v.

r., nociceptive. A r. initiated by a painful stimulus.

r., palm-chin. Vigorous stroking or scratching of the thenar eminence, producing contraction of the skin and lower lip muscles on the same side.

r., patellar. SEE: *knee-jerk r.; r., knee-jerk.*

r., pathologic. Abnormal r. due to disease and seen as one of its symptoms.

r., postural. Any r. that is concerned with maintenance of posture.

r., pressor. A r. that results in elevation of blood pressure brought about by constriction of arterioles.

r., pupillary. When a beam of light strikes the retina it normally causes the pupil to contract (protective against excessive stimulation). The same effect results with accommodation to near objects.

r., righting. Any of the many reflexes that enable an animal to maintain the body in a definite relationship to the head and thus maintain its body right side up.

r., sexual. Reflexes concerned with sexual activities, esp. erection and ejaculation.

r., short. R. involving one, or a few, segments of spinal cord.

r., somatic. R. induced by stimulation of somatic sensory nerve endings.

r., spinal. A r. whose center is in the spinal cord.

r., static. R. concerned with establishment and maintenance of posture when body is at rest.

r., statokinetic. Reflexes occurring when body is moving, i.e., walking or running.

r., stretch. Contraction of a muscle as a result of stretching the same muscle. SYN: *myotatic reflex.*

r., superficial. Cutaneous r. caused by irritation of the skin or areas depending upon the spinal cord as a motor center, such as the scapular, epigastric, abdominal, cremasteric, gluteal, and plantar reflexes; or upon centers in the medulla, as conjunctival, pupillary, and palatal reflexes.

r., tendon. Deep r. obtained by tapping skin over tendon of a muscle sharply. It is exaggerated in disease of an upper neuron and diminished or lost in disease of lower neuron.

r., triceps. Sharp extension of forearm resulting from tapping of triceps tendon while arm is held loosely in bent position.

r., unconditioned. A natural or inherited r. action; one not acquired.

r., vascular. R., vasomotor, q.v.

r., vasomotor. Constriction or dilatation of a blood vessel in response to a stimulus, i.e., becoming pale from fright.

r., visceral. Any r. induced by stimulation of visceral nerves.

r., visceromotor. Contraction or tenseness of skeletal muscles resulting from painful stimuli originating in visceral organs.

reflexogenic (rē-flĕks″ō-jĕn′ĭk) [L. *reflexus,* bent back, + Gr. *gennan,* to produce]. Causing a reflex action.

reflexograph (rē-flĕks′ō-grăf) [″+ Gr. *graphein,* to write]. Device for charting a reflex.

reflexometer (rē″flĕks-ŏm′ĕ-tĕr) [″+ Gr. *metron,* measure]. Instrument for measuring force of the tap required to produce a reflex.

reflexophil (rē-flĕks′ō-fĭl) [L. *reflexus,* reflex, + Gr. *philein,* to love]. Characterized by activity of, or exaggerated, reflexes.

reflexotherapy (rē-flĕks″ō-thĕr′ă-pī) [″+ Gr. *therapeia,* treatment]. Treatment by manipulation, anesthetizing, or cauterizing an area distant from seat of the disorder. SEE: *spondylotherapy; therapy, zone.*

reflux (rē′flŭks) [L. *re,* back, + *fluxus,* flow]. A return or backward flow. SEE: *regurgitation.*

refract (rē-frăkt′) [L. *refractus,* broken away]. 1. To turn back. 2. To deflect a light ray. 3. To detect errors of refraction in the eyes and to correct them.

refracta dosi (rē-frak′tă dō′sī) [L.]. In divided doses, denoting a definite amount of a drug taken within a given time in a number of fractional equal parts.

refraction (rē-frăk′shŭn) [L. *refractio,* break back]. 1. Deflection from a straight path, as of light rays as they pass through media of different densities; the change of direction of a ray when it passes from one medium to another of a different density. 2. Determination of amount of ocular refractive errors and their correction.

RS: ametropia; anisometropia; astigmatism; emmetropia; hypermetropia; myopia; presbyopia.

r., angle of. The angle formed by a refracted ray of light with a line perpendicular to surface at point of r.

r., coefficient of. The quotient or sine of angle of incidence divided by sine of angle of r.

r., double. Birefringence, or possessing more than one refractive index.

r., dynamic. Static refraction of the eye plus that accomplished by accommodation; the reciprocal of the near-point distance.

r., errors of. Condition in which parallel rays of light are not brought to a focus upon the retina because of a defect in shape of eyeball or in refracting media of the eye. SYN: *ametropia.*

r., index of. 1. Ratio of angle made by incident ray with the perpendicular (angle of incidence) to that made by emergent ray (angle of refraction). 2. The ratio of speed of light in air to its speed in another substance. The refractive index of water is 1.33; of crystalline lens, 1.413.

r., ocular. R. of the eye, q.v.

r. of the eye. Ocular r. brought about by refractive media of the eye (cornea, aqueous humor, crystalline lens, vitreous body).

r., static. R. of the eye when accommodation is at rest or paralyzed.

refractionist (rē-frăk′shŭn-ĭst) [L. *refractio,* break back]. One skilled in determining and correcting ocular refractive errors by means of glasses.

refractive (rē-frăk′tĭv) [L. *refractus*]. Concerning refraction.

r. index. SEE: *refraction, index of.*

r. power. The degree to which a transparent body deflects a ray of light from a straight path. SEE: *diopter.*

refractometer (rē-frăk-tŏm′ĕt-ĕr) [″+ Gr. *metron,* measure]. Device for measuring refractive power, as of the eye.

refractory (rē-frăk′tō-rī) [L. *refractarius*]. 1. Obstinate, stubborn. 2. Resistant to ordinary treatment. 3. Resistant to stimulation, said of muscle or nerve.

r. period, relative. Period of relaxation of a muscle during which excitability is depressed. If stimulated it will respond, but a stronger stimulus is required and response is less.

refracture (rē-frăk′chūr) [L. *refractus,* broken away]. 1. To break again, as a bone set wrongly. 2. Rebreaking of a fracture united in the wrong position.

refrangible (rē-frăn'jĭ-bl) [L. *re*, again, + ME. *frangible*, breakable]. Capable of refraction.

refresh (rē-frĕsh') [O.Fr. *refreschir*, to renew]. 1. To restore strength; to relieve from fatigue; to renew; to revive. 2. To scrape epithelial covering from two opposing surfaces of a wound to cause them to unite.

refrigerant (rē-frĭj'ĕr-ănt) [L. *refrigerans*, to make cold]. 1. Allaying heat or fever; cooling. 2. Medicine or agent that relieves thirst, is cooling, or reduces a fever. SEE: *algefacient.*

    r. gases. A number of these gases are used in ordinary household refrigerators; poisoning due to leaks, faulty connections or breakage, and gas dissipated into atmosphere may occur.

refrigeration (rē-frĭj''ĕr-ā'shŭn) [L. *refrigeratio*]. Cooling; reduction of heat.

    r. anesthesia. Anesthesia resulting from cold, such as that produced in a limb by immersion in cold water.

    r. therapy. Use of low temperatures as a therapeutic procedure. SYN: *cryotherapy.* SEE: *hypothermia.*

refrin'gent. Refractive, q.v.

refusion (rē-fū'zhŭn) [L. *refusus*, poured back]. The return of blood into the same circulatory system from which it was removed.

regeneration (rē-jĕn''ĕr-ā'shŭn) [L. *re*, again, + *generare*, to produce]. Repair, regrowth, or restoration of a part, as tissues. Opposed to degeneration, q.v.

regimen (rĕj'ĭ-mĕn) [L., rule]. 1. Regulation of diet, sleep, exercise, and manner of living to improve or maintain health. 2. Hygiene.

region (rē'jŭn) [L. *regiō*, boundary line]. A portion of the body with natural or arbitrary boundaries. SEE: *abdomen.*

    RS: epigastrium; inguinal; Kiesselbach's area; temple.

regional (rē'jŭn-ăl). Concerning a region.

register [LL. *registra*, list]. 1. An official recording of names, facts, etc. 2. The compass or range of a voice. 3. A series of tones of like quality or character, as low or high register, chest or head register, etc.

registrant (rĕj'ĭs-trănt) [L. *registrāns*, registering]. A nurse who is named on the books of a registry as being "on call" or available to be called for duty.

registrar (rĕj'ĭs-trar) [O.Fr. *registreur*]. The official manager of a registry.

registra'tion [L. *registratiō*]. The act of recording, such as births, deaths, etc.

registry (rĕj'ĭs-trĭ) [LL. *registra*, list]. An office or book where a list of nurses ready for duty is kept; a placement bureau for nurses.

regression (rē-grĕsh'ŭn) [L. *regressiō*, a going back]. 1. A turning back or return to a former state. 2. A return of symptoms. 3. Retrogression. 4. In psychology an abnormal return to earlier reaction, characterized by mental state and behavior inappropriate to the situation. R. may occur as a result of frustration or in states of fatigue, dreams, hypnosis, intoxication, illness, and in certain psychoses (schizophrenia).

    r., filial. In biology, tendency of offspring to deviate less from the average of a population than their parents.

regressive (rē-grĕs'ĭv). Concerning or marked by regression.

regular (rĕg'ū-lar) [L. *rēgula*, rule]. 1. Conforming to rule or custom. 2. Methodical, steady in course, as pulse. SYN: *normal; typical.*

regula'tion. 1. State of being controlled or directed. 2. The ability of an individual, such as a developing embryo, to develop normally in spite of experimental modifications.

    r. development. In embryology, condition in which a single blastomere, or a portion of an embryo, can give rise to a whole embryo. Opposed to mosaic development, q.v.

regula'tive. Pert. to regulation.

regulator. A device for adjusting or controlling the rate of flow or administration of fluids, oxygen, blood, etc.

regurgitant (rē-gŭr'jĭ-tănt) [L. *re*, again, + *gurgitāre*, to flood]. Throwing back or flowing in a direction opposite to the normal.

regurgitation (rē-gŭr''jĭ-tā'shŭn). 1. Return of solids or fluids to the mouth from the stomach. R. may be a complication of diphtheria. It occurs in paralysis of the soft palate and in some digestive disorders. SEE: *taste.* 2. Return of blood backward through a defective heart valve.

    r., aortic. Backflow of blood into left ventricle as a result of incompetetent aortic valves.

    r., cardiac. Backward flow of blood through the aortic, mitral, or tricuspid valves due to incomplete closure.

    r., duodenal. Return flow of chyme from duodenum to stomach.

    r., functional. R. not due to valvular disorder but to dilatation of ventricles, the great vessels, or valve rings.

    r., mitral. Backflow of blood from left ventrical into left atrium resulting from imperfect closure of mitral or bicuspid valve.

r., pulmonic. Backflow of blood from pulmonary artery into the right ventricle.

r., tricuspid. Backflow of blood from the right ventricle into the right atrium.

rehabilitation (rē″hā-bĭl′ĭ-tā′shŭn) [L. *rehabilitāre*]. Process of restoring to useful life a person who has been ill or who is handicapped. This is accomplished through education and therapy.

rehalation (rē″hă-lā′shŭn) [L. *re*, again, + *halāre*, to breathe]. Rebreathing process occasionally employed in anesthesia.

Reichert's cartilage (rī′kĕrts). [Karl B. Reichert, Ger. anatomist, 1811-1884]. The second branchial arch of the embryo which gives rise to stapes, styloid process, stylohyoid ligament, and lesser cornua of hyoid bone.

Reichmann's disease (rīk′man). [Nikolas Reichmann, Pol. physician, 1851-1918]. Excessive gastric secretion without intermission. SYN: *gastrochronorrhea; gastrorrhea; gastrosuccorrhea.*

Reid's base line (rēd). [Robert W. Reid, Scottish anatomist, 1851-1938]. Line extending from lower edge of the orbit to center of aperture of external auditory canal backward to center of occipital bone.

Reil's island (rīl). [Johann C. Reil, Ger. anatomist, 1759-1813] Three or more small convolutions at bottom of fissure of Sylvius. SYN: *insula* [NA]; *island of Reil*, q.v.

reimplantation (rē″ĭm-plăn-tā′shŭn) [L. *re*, again, + *in*, into, + *plantāre*, to set]. Replacement of a part from where it has been taken out, as a tooth.

reinfection (rē″ĭn-fĕk′shŭn) ["+ *infectus*, infect]. A second infection with the same organism.

reinforcement (rē″ĭn-fors′mĕnt) [L. *re*, again, + *inforce*, enforce]. Strengthening; augmentation of force.

r. of reflex. Strengthening of the response to one stimulus by concurrent action of another; the exaggeration of a reflex by nervous activity elsewhere. Thus, during the raising of a heavy weight the knee jerk is stronger.

reinfusion (rē″ĭn-fū′shŭn) ["+ *infusio*, to pour in]. The reinjection of blood serum or cerebrospinal fluid.

reinnervation (rē″ĭn-ŭr-vā′shŭn) ["+ *in*, into, + *nervus*, nerve]. 1. Anastomosis of a paralyzed part with a living nerve. 2. Grafting of a fresh nerve for restoration of function in a paralyzed muscle.

reinoculation (rē″ĭn-ŏk″ū-lā′shŭn) [L. *re*, again, + *in*, into, + *oculus*, bud]. A second inoculation with the same virus or organism. SEE: *reinfection.*

re″integra′tion. In psychology, the resumption of normal behavior and mental functioning following disintegration of personality in mental illness.

reinversion (rē″ĭn-vŭr′shŭn) [L. *re*, again, + *in*, into, + *versiō*, turning]. Correction of an inverted organ, as of an inverted uterus by pressure on the fundus.

Reissner's membrane (rīs′nĕr). [Ernest Reissner, Ger. anatomist, 1824-1878]. Delicate membrane separating the cochlear canal from scala vestibuli. SYN: *membrana vestibularis.*

Reiter's syndrome (rī′ter). [Hans Reiter, Ger. bacteriologist, 1881 —] A group of symptoms which appears as a complication of nonspecific urethritis. Symptoms include urethritis, arthritis, and conjunctivitis. The oral mucosa and skin may be involved also.

   ETIOL: Unknown, but a virus seems to be related to the cause of some, if not all, of the cases.

   PROG: Generally good; however recurrences are common.

   TREATMENT: There is no specific therapy. Broad spectrum antibiotics are used for urethritis. Symptomatic therapy for pain.

rejection [L. *rejicere*, to throw back]. 1. Refusal to accept or to show affection for. In lower animals the young may be ignored or driven away by their mother. 2. In transplantation of tissues and organs, destruction of transplanted material at the cellular level by the host's immune mechanism.

r., acute. Very early destruction of grafted or transplanted material. May be reversed by increased use of immunosuppressive agents.

r., chronic. Slow destruction of grafted or transplanted material. This may occur over a period of months or years.

r., hyperacute. Immediate, intense, and irreversible destruction of grafted material.

rejuvenation (rē-jū″vĕ-nā′shŭn) [L. *re*, again, + *juvenis*, young]. A return to youthful conditions or to the normal.

rejuvenescence (rē-jū″vĕ-nĕs′ĕns) ["+ *juvenescere*, to become young]. The renewal of youth or return to earlier stage of existence.

relapse (rē-lăps′) [L. *relapsus*]. Recurrence of a disease or symptoms after apparent recovery.

relaps′ing. Recurring after apparent recovery.

r. fever. An infectious disease marked by intermittent attacks of high fever.

   ETIOL: Several species of spirochetes belonging to genus Borrelia and transmitted by head lice, body lice, and ticks of the genus Ornithodorus.

TREATMENT: Symptomatic treatment with bed rest. Penicillin and broadspectrum antibiotics have replaced the use of arsenicals except in cases where spirochetes are resistant. The use of antipyretics and antinauseants may be indicated, and dehydration and electrolyte imbalance should be combatted by parenteral injections.

relax [L. *relaxāre*, to loosen]. To decrease tension or intensity, or to be rid of strain, anxiety, and nervousness.

relaxant (rē-lăk'sănt) [to loosen]. 1. Rel. to or producing relaxation. 2. A drug which reduces tension. 3. A laxative.

   r., muscle. A drug or therapeutic treatment that specifically relieves muscular tension.

relaxation (rē-lăk-sā'shŭn). 1. A lessening of tension or activity in a part. 2. Phase or period in a single muscle-twitch following contraction in which tension decreases, fibers lengthen, and muscle returns to resting position.

   r., general. R. of the entire body.

   r., heat of. That portion of initial heat, about 35%, in muscle activity during r.

   r., local. R. limited to a particular muscle group, or to a certain part.

relaxed movement. Form of bodily movement which the operator carries through without the assistance or resistance of the patient. SYN: *passive exercise.*

relaxin (rē-lăk'sĭn). A polypeptide hormone secreted in the corpus luteum during pregnancy. Obtained commercially from ovaries of pregnant sows. It has been used as a uterine relaxant and to soften the cervix. Has no estrogenic or progestational effect.

relief (rē-lēf') [ME.]. Alleviation or removal of a distressing or painful symptom.

relieve [L. *relever*]. To provide relief.

R.E.M. Abbr. for *rapid eye movement.* Movement of the closed eyes observed or recorded during sleep. Movements occur while the subject is dreaming.

rem. Abbr. for *roentgen equivalent* (in) *man.*

Remak (rā'măk). [Robert Remak, Ger. neurologist, 1815-1865].

   R.'s axis cylinder. The conducting part of a nerve.

   R.'s band. The axis cylinder of a neuron.

   R.'s fibers. The nonmedullated nerve fibers.

   R.'s ganglion. A group of nerve cells in coronary sinus near its entry into right atrium.

Remak's sign or symptom. [Ernest Julius Remak, Ger. neurologist, 1849-1911]. 1. Polyesthesia. A single stimulus is perceived as if it were several stimuli applied in separate locations. 2. Delay in perception of stimuli. Both are seen in tabes dorsalis.

remedial (rē-mē'dĭ-ăl) [L. *remedialis*]. Curative; intended for a remedy.

remedy (rĕm'ĕd-ĭ) [L. *remedium,* medicine]. 1. Anything that relieves or cures a disease. 2. To cure or relieve a disease.

   r., local. Agent to relieve a local condition, as a sore.

   r., systemic. Agent to relieve or cure a disease affecting the entire organism.

remission (rē-mĭsh'ŭn) [L. *remissiō,* remit]. 1. Lessening of severity, or abatement of symptoms. 2. The period during which symptoms abate.

remittent (rē-mĭt'ĕnt) [L. *remittere,* to send back]. Alternately abating and returning at certain intervals. SEE: *fever.*

   r. fever. A fever alternately abating and returning, without intervals of afebrility. SEE: *fever* for illustration; *malaria.*

ren (rĕn) [L.]. (pl. *renes*) [NA]. The kidney.

   r. amyloidens. Amyloid degeneration of the kidneys.

   r. mobilis. Movable kidney.

   r. unguliformis. Horseshoe kidney.

renal (rē'nal) [LL. *rēnālis*]. 1. Pert. to the kidney. SEE: *urinary tract* for illustration. 2. Shaped like a kidney.

   r. failure, acute. Acute failure of the kidney to perform its essential functions. May be due to trauma; any condition which impairs the flow of blood to the kidneys; certain toxic substances such as mercury, carbon tetrachloride, or ethylene glycol; bacterial toxins; glomerulonephritis; acute obstruction of the urinary tract.

   TREATMENT: Specific therapy for primary disease; either peritoneal dialysis or hemodialysis.

   r. insufficiency. The reduced capacity of the kidney to perform its functions.

   r. papillary necrosis. Destruction of the papillae of the kidney. May be caused by a variety of conditions including diabetes mellitus, acute pyelonephritis, urinary obstruction, sickle cell trait, and repeated use of phenacetin. Management consists of ureteral catheter irrigation of r. pelvis to remove obstruction; appropriate antibiotics; and adequate hydration.

   r. scanning. Method of determining r. function and shape of the kidney. A radioactive substance which concentrates in the kidney is given intravenously. The irradiation emitted from the substance as it accumulates in the kidneys is recorded on a suitable photographic film.

r. transplantation. Surgical implantation of a donor kidney to replace one removed from a patient. The procedure has been successful technically, but the problem of testing for rejection has not been resolved.

r. tubule. A nephron, q.v.

renal clearance test. A kidney function test based on the ability of the kidney to eliminate a given substance in a standard time. Urea, phenolsulfonphthalein (PSP), Diodrast, and other substances are employed. Normal urea clearance is 75, i.e., the quantity of urea removed from circulation in one minute equals that contained in 75 ml. of blood. Diodrast clearance is 500-700 ml./min. in females and 560-830 in men.

renifleur (rǎ-nǐ-flūr') [Fr.]. One stimulated sexually by certain odors, esp. by the urine of others.

reniform (rěn'ǐ-form) [L. *rēn*, kidney, + *forma*, shape]. Shaped like a kidney.

ren'in. A protein formed in an ischemic kidney; acts as an enzyme converting an alpha-2-globulin of the blood into angiotensin I which is rapidly transformed into angiotensin II, a powerful vasoconstrictor.

r. substrate. Alpha-2-globulin of the plasma. SYN: *hypertensinogen.*

renipuncture (rěn'ǐ-pŭnk'chūr) [L. *rēn*, kidney, + *punctūra*, a piercing]. Surgical puncture of capsule of kidney.

rennet (rěn'ĕt) [ME.]. 1. An infusion of inner coat of calf's stomach. 2. A fluid containing rennin, a coagulating enzyme, used for making junket or cheese.

rennin (rěn'ǐn). A coagulating enzyme found in the stomach of ruminants, which curdles milk. It is the active principle of rennet. It acts on caseinogen in the presence of calcium ions converting it to insoluble casein.

renninogen, rennogen (rěn-ǐn'ō-jěn, rěn'ō-jěn) [ME. *rennet*, rennet, + Gr. *gennan*, to produce]. Antecedent or zymogen from which rennin is formed. The inactive form of rennin.

renogastric (rē'nō-gǎs'trǐk) [L. *rēn*, kidney, + Gr. *gastēr*, belly]. Concerning the kidney and stomach.

renogram (rē'nō-grǎm) ["+ Gr. *gramma*, a mark]. 1. List of results of a group of kidney function tests. 2. Record of rate of removal from the blood by the kidneys of an intravenously injected dose of radioactive iodine (I^{131}).

renography (rē-nǒg'rǎ-fǐ) ["+ Gr. *graphein*, to write]. Study of the kidney by means of an x-ray picture.

renointestinal (rē'nō-ǐn-těs'tǐn-ǎl) [L. *rēn*, kidney, + *intestinum*, intestine]. Concerning the kidney and the intestine.

renopathy (rē-nop'ǎ-thǐ) ["+ Gr. *pathos*, disease]. Any pathological condition of the kidneys.

renotrophic (rē'nō-trǒf'ǐk) ["+ Gr. *trophē*, nourishment]. Having the ability to induce hypertrophy of the kidney.

Renshaw cells (rěn'shǒ). Small cells with short axons which serve to connect motor nerve axons with each other. The process functions to inhibit motor neurons.

reovirus (rē'ō-vī'rŭs). [Acronym for *r*espiratory *e*nteric *o*rphan *virus*] Viruses found in the respiratory and digestive tracts of apparently healthy persons. Their exact importance in producing disease is not known. This group of viruses was formerly classed as Echo virus, type 10.

repair (rē-pār') [L. *reparāre*, to prepare again]. To remedy, replace, or heal, as a wound or a lost part.

r. solution. Any solution given intravenously to treat an electrolyte or metabolic disturbance.

repell'ance [L. *repellere*, drive back]. Condition in which certain individuals are relatively immune to bites of arthropods.

repell'ent. 1. An agent which repels noxious organisms such as insects, ticks, and mites. Repellents may be applied to surface of body as a liquid, spray, or dust, or they may be used to impregnate clothing. 2. Reducing a swelling. 3. Agent which lessens a swelling.

repercolation (rē'pŭr-kō-lā'shŭn) [L. *re*, again, + *percolāre*, to filter]. Repeated percolation using same materials.

repercussion (rē-pŭr-kŭsh'ŭn) [L. *repercussiō*, rebound]. 1. Reciprocal action. 2. Action involved in causing subsidence of a swelling, tumor, or eruption. 3. In obstetrics, diagnosis of pregnancy by insertion of a finger into the vagina to push the uterus, causing embryo to rise and fall. SYN: *ballottement.*

re"percuss'ive. 1. Causing repercussion. 2. An agent which repels; a repellent.

replacement. The act of replacing.

r. bone. Bone which is formed in cartilage preceding the definitive bone. SYN: *cartilage bone; endochondral bone; substitution bone.*

replanta'tion [L. *re*, again, + *planto*, to plant]. Planting again.

r. of a tooth. Replacement of a tooth which has been removed from its socket.

repletion (rē-plē'shŭn) [L. *replētio*, a filling up]. 1. Condition of being full or satisfied. 2. Fullness of blood. SYN: *plethora.*

re"polariza'tion. Reestablishment of a polarized state in a muscle or nerve fiber following contraction or conduction of a nerve impulse.

reportable diseases. Diseases which must be reported by the physician to the health authorities. There are six diseases which, by international sanitary regulations, are required universally to be reported. They are cholera, plague, louse-borne relapsing fever, smallpox, louse-borne typhus fever, and yellow fever.

reposition (rē"pō-zīsh'ŭn) [L. *repositio,* a replacing]. Restoration of an organ or tissue to its correct or original position.

repos'itor. Instrument for restoring a tissue or an organ to its normal position.

r., inversion. Instrument for replacement of an inverted uterus.

r., uterine. A lever for replacement of the uterus when out of normal position.

repression (rē-prĕsh'ŭn) [L. *repressus,* press back]. In psychology, refusal to entertain distressing or painful ideas, thus submerging them in the unconscious where they continue to exert their influence upon the individual. Psychoanalysis seeks to discover and to release these repressions.

reproduction (rē-prō-dŭk'shŭn) [L. *re,* again, + *productio,* production]. 1. Process by which plants and animals give rise to offspring. 2. The creation of a similar structure or situation; the act of duplicating.

r., asexual. R. in which sex cells are not involved, as by fission or budding.

r., sexual. R. by means of sexual or germ cells. Usually a male cell (spermatozoon) fuses with a female cell egg or ovum. Sometimes ova may develop without fertilization. SYN: *syngamy.* SEE: *parthenogenesis.*

reproductive (rē"prō-dŭk'tĭv). Concerning, or employed in, reproduction.

repulsion (rē-pŭl'shŭn) [L. *repulsio,* a thrusting back]. 1. Act of driving back. 2. The force exerted by one body on another to cause separation. Opposed to attraction.

RES. Abbr. for *reticuloendothelial system.*

research (rĭ-sŭrch', rē'sŭrch) [O. Fr. *recerche,* research]. Scientific and diligent study, investigation, or experimentation in order to establish facts and analyze their significance.

r., clinical. R. based mainly on bedside observation of the patient, rather than through laboratory work.

r., laboratory. R. done principally in the laboratory.

r., medical. R. concerned with any phase of medical science.

resect (rē-sēkt') [L. *resectus,* cut off]. To cut off, or to cut out, a portion of a structure or organ, as to cut off the end of a bone or to remove a segment of the intestine.

resectable (rē-sēk'tā-bl). Able to be removed, esp. by surgical means. Usually used in reference to malignant growths which can be removed completely by use of surgery.

resection (rē-sēk'shŭn) [L. *resectio,* a cutting off]. Partial excision of a bone or other structure.

r., window. R. of a portion of the nasal septum after reflection of a flap of mucous membrane. SYN: *submucous resection.*

resectoscope (rē-sēk'tō-skōp) [L. *resectus,* cut off, + Gr. *skopein,* to examine]. An instrument for resection of prostate gland through the urethra.

resectoscopy (rē"sēk-tōs'kō-pī). Resection of the prostate through the urethra.

reserpine (rē-sŭr'pīn). USP. A chemically pure derivative of Rauwolfia serpentina. An old snakeroot remedy used in India for centuries for snake bite, mental illness, anxiety states. It lowers blood pressure and acts as a tranquilizer.

reserve (rē-zerv') [L. *reservāre,* to keep back]. 1. That which is held back for future use. 2. Self control of one's feelings and thoughts.

r. air. Additional amount of air that can be expelled from the lungs over the normal quantity, 1200-1600 cc.

r., alkali. Alkali content of body available for neutralization of acid. SEE: *alkaline reserve.*

r., cardiac. The ability of the heart to increase cardiac output to meet the needs of the body.

reservoir (rēz'ŭr-vwŏr) [Fr.]. A place or cavity for storage of fluids.

reservoir of infection. A source of supply of an infectious agent or disease. These may be man, animals, plants, or organic matter which will allow an infectious agent to live. For example, the reservoir for tuberculosis usually is man, but may be in other animals such as the milk from tubercular cows.

res'ident. A physician who continues to further his clinical training after his internship. Usually this is done as a member of the house staff of a hospital.

r. physician. A resident.

residual (rē-zĭd'ū-ăl) [L. *residuum,* remaining]. 1. Rel. to that which is left as a residue. 2. In psychology, any internal aftereffect of experience influencing later behavior.

r. air. Air remaining in the lungs after the strongest possible (forced) expiration.

r. urine. Urine left in bladder after urination; occurring in cases of enlarged prostate.

residue (rĕz'ĭ-dū). The remainder of something after a part is removed.

r. free diet. Diet without cellulose or roughage. Purées, semisolids, and bland foods are included.

r., high, diet. A diet with increased amounts of cellulose (fiber), water, mineral salts, and vitamins (esp. vitamin B).

r., low, diet (solid). An inadequate diet including solid food in which r. is reduced to a minimum. SEE: *nonlaxative diet.*

residuum (rĕ-zĭd'ū-ŭm) [L.]. (pl. *resid'ua*) Residue; the remainder.

resilience (rē-zĭl'ĭ-ĕns) [L. *resiliens,* leaping back]. The quality of coming back to normal after straining, as a stretched rubber band when released. SYN: *elasticity.*

resilient (rē-zĭl'ĭ-ĕnt). Elastic.

resin (rĕz'ĭn) [L. *resina*]. 1. An amorphous, nonvolatile solid or soft solid substance, a natural exudation from plants. It is practically insoluble in water, but soluble in alcohol. Ex: guaiac, rosin. 2. Any of a large group of polymerized synthetic or chemically modified natural resins. Included are polyvinyl, polyethylene, and polystyrene. These are combined with chemicals such as epoxies, plasticizers, pigments, fillers, and stabilizers to form plastics.

r., ion-exchange. Ionizable synthetic substances, which may be acid or basic, used accordingly to remove either acid or basic ions from solutions. Thus *anionic-exchange resins* may be used to absorb acid in the stomach. *Cationic-exchange resins* have the ability to remove basic (alkaline) ions from solutions.

resinous (rĕz'ĭ-nŭs). Of the nature of, or pert. to, resin.

resistance (rē-zĭs'tăns) [L. *resistens,* standing back]. Opposition to, or the ability to oppose, anything. Ex: power of a fluid to retard that which is passing through it; of the air; or opposition of the body to passage of an electric current. 2. The sum total of body mechanisms which interpose barriers to the progress of invasion, multiplication of infectious agents, or damage by their toxic products. *Immunity* is r. associated with the presence of antibodies having a specific action on infectious microorganisms. *Inherent r.* is the ability to resist disease independently of antibodies. 3. The force exerted to penetrate the unconscious or to submerge memories in the unconscious. 4. In psychoanalysis, condition in which ego avoids bringing into consciousness conflicts and unpleasant events responsible for neurosis; reluctance of subject to give up old patterns of thought and behavior.

r. transfer factor. A genetic factor in bacteria which controls r. to certain antibiotic drugs. The factor is spread by bacteria to bacteria. This makes it possible for nonpathogenic bacteria to become resistant to antibiotics and to transfer that r. to pathogens, thereby establishing a potential source for an epidemic.

resolution (rĕz-ō-lū'shŭn) [L. *resolūtio,* a relaxing]. 1. Decomposition; absorption or breaking down of the products of inflammation. 2. Cessation of inflammation without suppuration. The return to normal. 3. The ability of the eye or series of lenses to distinguish fine detail.

resolve (rē-zŏlv') [L. *resolvere,* to release]. 1. To return to normal as after a pathological process. 2. To separate into component parts.

resolvent (rē-zŏl'vĕnt) [ME. *resolven,* releasing]. 1. Promoting disappearance of inflammation. 2. That which reduces inflammation or swelling.

resonance (rĕz'ō-nǎns) [L. *resonantia,* resound]. 1. Quality or act of resounding. 2. Quality of the sound heard on percussion of a hollow structure such as chest or abdomen. Absence of resonance is termed *flatness;* diminished resonance, *dullness.* 3. In physics, modification of sound due to vibrations of a body which are set up by waves of another vibrating body. 4. In electricity, state in which two electrical circuits are in tune with each other.

r., amphoric. Sound, as that when blowing across mouth of an empty bottle.

r., bandbox. R., tympanitic, q.v.

r., bell-metal. Sound heard in pneumothorax in auscultation when coin is held against chest wall and it is struck by another coin.

r., cracked-pot. A sound having a peculiar clinking quality sometimes heard on percussion of chest in cases of advanced tuberculosis when cavities are present.

r., normal. Normal pulmonary r.

r., skodaic. Increased percussion sound over upper lung when there is pleural effusion in lower part.

r., tympanitic. R. obtained by percussion of a hollow structure, such as the stomach or colon, when moderately distended with air.

r., vesicular. Normal pulmonary r.

r., vocal. The vibrations of the voice transmitted to the ear, normally more marked over the right apex.

Abnormally increased in pneumonic consolidation, lungs infiltrated with tuberculosis, or cavities that freely communicate with a bronchus.

Vocal r. is diminished or absent in pleural effusion (air, pus, serum, lymph, or blood); emphysema; pulmonary collapse; pulmonary edema; egophony, a modified bronchophony characterized by a trembling, bleating sound usually heard above the upper border of dullness of pleural effusions and occasionally heard in beginning pneumonia.

r., whispering. Auscultation sound heard when patient whispers.

resonat'ing [L. *resonantia,* resound]. Vibrating sympathetically with a source of sound or electrical oscillations.

r. cavities. The resonator of the human voice. Includes upper portion of larynx, pharynx, nasal cavity, paranasal sinuses, and mouth cavity.

resonator (rĕz'ō-nā"tür). 1. A structure that is capable of being set into sympathetic vibration when sound waves of the same frequency from another vibrating body strike it. 2. In electricity, an apparatus consisting of an electrical circuit in which oscillations of a certain frequency are set up by oscillations of the same frequency in another circuit. When this occurs, the circuits are said to be in syntony.

resorbent (rē-sōr'bĕnt) [L. *resorbens,* sucking in]. An agent that promotes the absorption of abnormal matter, as exudates or blood clots. Ex: potassium iodide, ammonium chloride.

resorption (rē-sōrp'shŭn) [L. *resorbēre,* to suck in]. 1. Act of removal by absorption, as resorption of an exudate or pus. 2. Removal of hard parts of a tooth as a result of lysis and phagocytic action.

respirable (rē-spīr'ă-bl, rĕs'pŭr-ă-bl) [L. *respīrāre,* breathe again]. Fit or adapted for respiration.

respiration (rĕs"pĭr-ā'shŭn) [L. *respiratio,* breathing]. 1. The interchange of gases between an organism and the medium in which it lives. More specifically the taking in of oxygen, its utilization in the tissues, and the giving off of carbon dioxide. 2. The act of breathing.

ADVENTITIOUS SOUNDS: *Friction sounds:* Sounds produced by the rubbing together of roughened pleural surfaces; may be heard both in inspiration and expiration. Often resemble subcrepitant rales, but are more superficial and localized than the latter, and are not modified by cough or deep inspiration.

Metallic tinkling: Silvery bell-like sounds heard at intervals over a pneumohydrothorax or large cavity. Speaking, coughing, and deep breathing usually induce them. Must not be confounded with similar sound produced by liquids in the stomach.

Rales: Abnormal bubbling sounds heard in air cells or bronchial tubes, q.v.

Succussion-splash or hippocratic succussion: A splashing sound produced by the presence of air and liquid in the chest, may be elicited by gently shaking the patient while auscultating. Nearly always indicates either a hydro- or a pyopneumothorax, although it has been detected over very large cavities. Air and liquid in stomach produce similar sounds.

AUSCULTATION OF RESPIRATORY ORGANS: Normal respiration. Vesicular breathing is heard over the body of the lungs and is characterized by a soft, breezy inspiration, and a short, low-pitched expiration. Normally, expiration is not more than one half as long as inspiration. Auscultation over trachea or main bronchi in the interscapula space yields bronchial breathing.

MODIFICATION OF THE RESPIRATORY MURMUR: Amphoric and cavernous breathing. These two are almost identical. Sounds loud, expiration prolonged and hollow. Pitch of amphoric breathing a little higher than cavernous. May be imitated by blowing over the mouth of an empty jar. Heard in phthisical or bronchiectatic cavities, pneumothorax when the opening to the lung is patulous, area of consolidation near a large bronchus, sometimes over lung compressed by a moderate effusion.

Respiration, Pulse and Temperature Ratio

Respiration	Pulse	Temperature	
18	80	99° F.	(37.2° C.)
19	88	100	(37.8)
21	96	101	(38.3)
23	104	102	(38.9)
25	112	103	(39.4)
27	120	104	(40)
28	128	105	(40.6)
30	136	106	(41.1)

r., abdominal. R. where chiefly the diaphragm exerts itself, while walls of chest are nearly at rest. Utilized in normal, quiet breathing, esp. by males, and in pathological conditions as in pleurisy, pericarditis, and fracture of ribs. SYN: *diaphragmatic breathing.*

r., absent. R. in which respiratory sounds are suppressed.

r., accelerated. Considered accelerated when more than 25/minute after 15 years of age. Increased frequency may result from exercise, physical exertion, or mental disturbances.

Frequently occurs in disease. In disease it may be preternaturally frequent or slow, rising to 60 or 80 or falling to 8 to 10/minute. It is present in many disorders of the lungs, i.e., pneumonia, bronchiectasis, advanced pulmonary tuberculosis, consolidation or compression of a lobe or of entire lung, congestion, asthma, emphysema, abscess, tumors, aneurysms, diseases of the chest wall, hernia of the diaphragm, and partial obstruction to the entrance of air into the lungs. It may be seen in diseases of the blood, such as the anemias; in kidney troubles; febrile disease; diseases of the heart; and as a result of drugs or nervous conditions.

r., aerobic. R. in which air or free oxygen is utilized.

r., amphoric. R. having amphoric resonance. SEE: *resonance, amphoric.*

r., anaerobic. R. in which oxygen is obtained from chemical reactions not involving the liberation of free oxygen.

r., apneustic. Breathing characterized by prolonged inspiration unrelieved by attempts to expire. Seen in patients who have had the upper part of the pons of the brain removed or damaged.

r., artificial. Artificial methods to restore r. in cases of suspended breathing. SEE: *artificial r.*

r., Biot's. Breathing with irregularly alternating periods of apnea and hyperpnea. Occurs in meningitis and disorders of the brain which cause increased intracranial pressure.

r., cell. The combination of oxygen with various substances within cells resulting in formation of CO_2 and H_2O and release of energy. There are many intermediary reactions in which substances other than oxygen act as oxidizing agents, i.e., hydrogen or electron acceptors. Reactions are catalyzed by respiratory enzymes which include the flavoproteins, cytochromes, and other enzymes. Certain vitamins (nicotinamide, riboflavin, thiamine, pyridoxine, and pantothenic acid) are essential in the formation of components of various enzyme systems.

r., Cheyne-Stokes. Breathing in which respirations gradually increase in rapidity and volume until they reach climax, then gradually subside and cease entirely for 5-50 seconds when they begin again.

Due to some disturbance of respiratory center, exact nature of which is as yet undetermined. Usually forerunner of death, but may last several months, or few days, and disappear.

This type of r. is not necessarily associated with disease. It is observed in normal persons during sleeping, esp. the aged, or during visits to moderately high altitude.

r., cogwheel. R., interrupted, q.v.

r., costal. Costal breathing. R. in which chest cavity is enlarged by raising the ribs.

r., decreased. It occurs in uremia, diabetic coma, affections of the brain, shock, hysteria, stenosis of the larynx, chronic fibroid phthisis, poisoning with opium or its derivatives, and approaching death.

r., diaphragmatic. R., abdominal, q.v.

r., difficult. Dyspnea, q.v.

r., direct. R. in which an organism, such as a one-celled ameba, secures its oxygen and gives up carbon dioxide directly to the surrounding medium.

r., external. The processes involved in ventilating the lungs (breathing) and the exchange of gases (O_2 and CO_2) between the air in lungs and the blood within capillaries in the walls of alveoli. SYN: *pulmonary respiration.* SEE: *air; spirometer.*

Inspiration or drawing in of air is accomplished by enlargement of the thoracic cavity. This is brought about by contraction of the diaphragm and raising the ribs and sternum. *Expiration* or the expulsion of air may be active or passive. In ordinary breathing it is passive, no muscular effort being needed to bring chest wall back to normal position. In forced or labored respiration, muscular effort is involved.

If the aspiration of air is accomplished chiefly by contraction of the diaphragm, the abdomen will bulge with each inspiration because the diaphragm, forming at once the floor of the thorax and the roof of the abdominal cavity, is dome-shaped with its concavity downward. In contracting, it pushes the abdominal viscera down. This type of r. is called diaphragmatic or abdominal. Its opposite is the thoracic type in which the ribs and sternum must be raised and which is seen when the abdomen is confined by tight clothing.

RS: air; breathing; diaphragm; expiration; inspiration; spirometer.

r., fetal. Exchange of gases in the placenta between blood of fetus and maternal blood.

r., forced. Voluntary hyperpnea (increase in rate and depth of breathing).

r., forms of. Jerking, spasmodic, stertorous, stridulous, whistling, wavy, lack of evenness, abdominal, or thoracic.

r., frequent. Common in all febrile and inflammatory diseases, esp. in children. As a rule, rapid breathing is a sign of thoracic disease. In hysteria patient often breathes 60-70 times/minute. Frequent r. may occur in acute respiratory affections, lesions of medulla; or it may be induced by atropine, carbon dioxide, or cocaine.

r., internal. The passage of oxygen from the blood into the cells, its utilization by the cells, and the passage of carbon dioxide from cells into the blood.

Oxygen is carried in combination with hemoglobin. Oxyhemoglobin gives arterial blood its red color; reduced hemoglobin gives venous blood its blue color. Carbon dioxide is carried in combination with metallic elements in the blood as bicarbonates and also as carbonic acid. Normally the partial pressure of oxygen in the blood is 75-100 mm. of mercury, depending upon age; and for CO_2 it is 35-45 mm.

r., interrupted. R. in which inspiration or expiration sounds are not continuous.

r., intrauterine. R. by fetus before birth. SEE: *r., fetal.*

r., Kussmaul's. Deep, gasping r. SEE: air hunger.

r., labored. Dyspnea or difficult breathing; r. which involves active participation of accessory inspiratory and expiratory muscles.

r., method of counting. With the hand in the same position as when taking the pulse, watch the patient's chest, without his knowledge if possible, because breathing is controlled by both the voluntary and involuntary muscles. Count each inspiration and expiration as one breath. Observe for one full minute by watching rise and fall of chest or upper abdomen. When the movements are scarcely perceptible, place the hand gently but firmly on the chest or back and count in this manner. Note hour, frequency, and any abnormal condition, such as pain associated with breathing.

TOTAL LUNG CAPACITY (T.L.C.): In normal adult males, depending upon their size, T.L.C. range is 3.6-9.4 liters. In females, 2.5-6.9 liters.

r., muscles of. *Inspiration:* diaphragm and external intercostals. *Forced inspira-*

tion: (assist in elevating ribs and sternum) scaleni, levatores costorum, sternocleidomastoideus, pectoralis major, platysma myoides, and serratus posterior superior. *Expiration:* (voluntary deep breathing or forced expiration) rectus abdominis, external and internal oblique, transverse abdominis.

The following accessory muscles may assist in depressing the ribs: internal intercostals, serratus posterior inferior, quadratus lumborum. SEE: *diaphragm; expiration; inspiration.*

r., paradoxical. 1. R. occurring in open pneumothorax in which lung fills on expiration and is deflated on inspiration. 2. Condition seen in paralysis of diaphragm in which diaphragm ascends during inspiration.

r., periodic. Breathing of uneven rhythm as in Cheyne-Stokes r., q.v.

r. pigment. A pigment which carries oxygen. Ex: hemoglobin and hemocyanin.

r., placental. R., fetal, q.v.

r. quotient. SEE: *quotient, respiratory.*

r., radiofrequency electrophrenic. Method used in cases of r. paralysis in spinal cord injury. SEE: *radiofrequency electrophrenic r.*

r., rate of. Depends on several factors including age, altitude, and whether subject is exercising or at rest.

Rate of Respiration

Premature infant	40–90/min
Newborn	30–80/min
1st year	20–40/min
2nd year	20–30/min
5th year	20–25/min
15th year	15–20/min
Adult	15–20/min

r., slow. Breathing in which there are less than 12 respirations/minute. Generally result of some structural or functional derangement of the nervous system. Observed in apoplexy, effusion of serum within cranium, softening of the brain, brain compressions and hemorrhage, uremia, and in most of the circumstances that occasion coma. It may be induced by carbon monoxide and opium or its derivatives.

r., stertorous. Rattling or bubbling sounds which obscure normal respiratory sounds. Usually caused by breathing with mouth open with resultant vibration of soft palate.

r., stridulous. A high-pitched, crowing or barking sound heard during inspiration caused by an obstruction in vicinity of glottis or in respiratory passageway.

r. system. The lungs and the respiratory passages. The latter include nasal cavities, pharynx, mouth (if open), larynx, trachea, bronchi, and bronchioles.

r., thoracic. R. performed entirely by expansion of the chest when abdomen does not move. Observed when peritoneum or diaphragm is inflamed, when abdominal cavity is physically restricted by tight bandages or clothes, or during abdominal surgery.

respiration, words pert. to: air, complemental; a., minimal; a., reserve; a., residual; a., supplemental; a., tidal; anapnea; apnea; asphyxia; Biot's breathing; blowing; Bouchut's respiration; chest; Cheyne-Stokes respiration; diaphragmatic; dyspnea; eupnea; hyperpnea; hypopnea; infant; inspiration; oligopnea; orthopnea; polypnea; respirator; respiratory; stridor; stridulus; tachypnea; thermometry.

respirator (rĕs″pĭ-rā″tor) [L. *respirāre*, to breathe]. 1. A machine for prolonged artificial respiration. SEE: *Drinker respirator.* 2. A device by which inspired air is purified, warmed, or medicated when passing through it.

respiratory (rē-spir′ă-tō-rĭ, rĕs′pĭ-ră-tō″rĭ). Pert. to respiration.

r. center. A region in the medulla oblongata which regulates movements of respiration. Consists of an inspiratory center, located in rostral half of reticular formation overlying olivary nuclei, and an expiratory center, located dorsal to inspiratory center. A pneumotaxic center, located in the pons, also is concerned with respiratory movements.

r. failure, acute. Acute failure of the lungs to perform their ventilatory function. This may be due to impairment of gas exchange in the lung or obstruction to the free flow of air in and out of the lungs.

TREATMENT: If due to obstruction, remove the cause. If due to impaired gas exchange, positive pressure ventilation is indicated.

r. minute volume. The amount of air breathed in one minute. ABBR: RMV.

r. syncytial virus. A virus which induces formation of syncytial masses in infected cell cultures. It is an important cause of acute respiratory disease in children.

r. system. The lungs, pleura, bronchi, pharynx, larynx, tonsils, and the nose.

respiratory distress syndrome. A condition, formerly known as hyaline membrane disease, accounting for more than 25,000

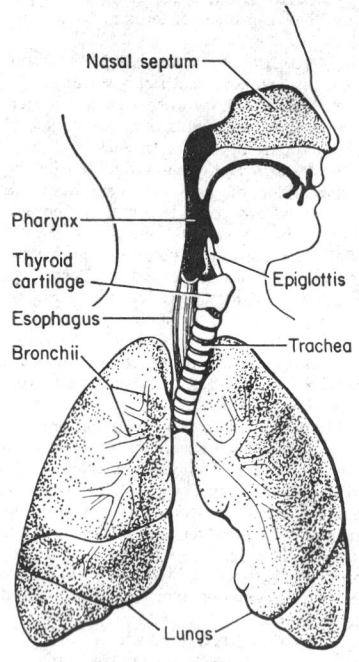

Nasal septum

Pharynx

Thyroid cartilage

Esophagus

Bronchii

Epiglottis

Trachea

Lungs

RESPIRATORY SYSTEM

infant deaths per year in the USA. Clinical signs, including delayed onset of respiration and low Apgar Score, are usually present at birth. Etiol. is unknown but prematurity, maternal diabetes, and antepartum maternal hemorrhage are predisposing factors.

SYM: Dyspnea, rapid breathing, expiratory grunt, cyanosis, limpness, cardiac failure, respiratory disease, and cardiac arrest.

TREATMENT: No specific therapy. Supportive measures include oxygen, correction of dehydration and acid-base imbalance, control of humidity and temperature of environment. Use digitalis for heart failure.

PROG: Good if the arterial blood oxygen content increases when the patient breathes 100% oxygen. If death occurs, it is almost always within the first three days.

respirometer (rĕs″pĭr-ŏm′ĕt-ĕr) [L. *respirāre*, to breathe, + Gr. *metron*, a measure]. Instrument to ascertain character of respirations.

response [L. *respondere*, reply]. 1. A reaction, such as contraction of a muscle or secretion of a gland, resulting from a stimulus. SEE: *reaction.* 2. The sum total of reactions of an individual to specific conditions, i.e., the response (favorable or unfavorable) of a patient to a certain treatment.

   r., inverse. The acquisition of a refractoriness to repeated injections of a hormone. May be due to antibody reaction to the injected hormone.

   r., triple. Three phases of vasomotor reactions occurring when a pointed instrument is drawn across the skin. Includes red reaction, flare or spreading flush, and wheal.

rest (rĕst) [AS. *raest*]. 1. Repose of body due to sleep. 2. Freedom from activity, as of mind or body. 3. To lie down; to cease from motion. 4. A remnant of embryonic tissue that persists in the adult. SYN: *epithelial* or *fetal rest.*

restiform (rĕs'tĭ-form) [L. *restis*, rope, + *forma*, shape]. Ropelike; rope-shaped.

resting. Inactive, motionless, at rest.

   r. body. Inferior cerebellar peduncle SYN: *corpus restiforme.*

   r. cell. 1. A cell not in the process of dividing. 2. A cell which is not performing its normal function, i.e., a nerve cell that is not conducting an impulse or a muscle cell that is not contracting.

   r. potential. The potential difference that exists across a cell membrane between the outside and the inside of a resting cell.

restitutio integrum [L.]. Complete restoration to health.

restitution (rĕs″tĭ-tū'shŭn) [L. *restitutio*]. 1. A return to a former status. 2. The act of making amends. 3. The turning of a fetal head to the right or left after it has completely emerged through the vagina.

restless legs. A condition of unknown etiology characterized by an intolerable creeping and internal-itching sensation occurring in the lower extremities. Symptoms are worse at the end of the day when either seated or in bed. Patient is compelled to move legs and this brings relief.

restorative (rē-stōr'ă-tiv) [L. *restaurāre*, to fix]. 1. Pert. to restoration. 2. An agent that is effective in the regaining of health and strength.

restraint (rē-strānt') [O.Fr. *restrainte*]. 1. The process of confining from any action, mental or physical. 2. State of being hindered. 3. That which hinders or restricts; device or method used to keep a patient from injuring himself. Various states have laws concerning methods to be used in restraining patients.

   r. in bed. Move bed against wall, place straight backed chairs along open side of bed. Tie them into place by interlacing with rope and then tying to foot and head of bed, or place a wide board the length of bed on either side and fasten through three or four holes bored near ends of the boards. Fold sheet lengthwise to width of one foot. Place under patient's back and cross in front below armpits. At sides secure hem ends to side bar or springs of bed. This allows some freedom for turning from side to side. The hands and feet may be restrained by a clove hitch of wide bandage around wrists and ankles and tied to side or foot of bed.

   r. (of the) lower extremities. Tie a sheet across knees and tie feet together with a figure-of-eight bandage. Start loop under ankles, cross between feet, bring ends around feet, and tie on top.

   r., mechanical. R. by physical devices, esp. r. of insane.

   r., medicinal. R. of violent mentally ill patients through use of narcotics or sedatives.

resuscitation (rē-sŭs″ĭ-tā'shŭn) [L. *resuscitātio*]. Act of bringing one back to full consciousness. SEE: *artificial respiration.*

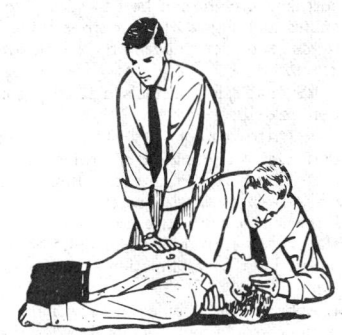

RESUSCITATION
Note correct position of patient's head and neck.

   r., heart-lung. The American Heart Association recommends the following:

   IF UNCONSCIOUS: Be certain there is an adequate airway. Elevate head and push jaw up. Then clear vomitus, false teeth, or other matter from mouth and pharynx.

   IF NOT BREATHING: SEE: *r., oral.*

   IF PULSE IS ABSENT: If the pupils are dilated and there is a deathlike appearance, massage the heart by using the following *closed chest* (i.e., not surgical method) *compression method:* Press on the sternum with sufficient force to depress it 1 1/2 to 2 inches (3.8 to 5.1 cm.). Do this once per second. At the same time continue mouth-to-mouth r.

Continue both mouth-to-mouth r. and intermittent chest compression until spontaneous pulse and respiration return. If one person is doing the resuscitation, alternate two quick inflations with 15 chest compressions. If there are two operators, do these maneuvers at the rate of one inflation for every fifth chest compression.

r., oral. Wipe any foreign matters from mouth and pharynx. Bend head back, chin pointing up. Pull or push jaw outward, moving tongue from back of throat. Open mouth wide and place your mouth tightly over victim's mouth. Close patient's nostrils by pinching them together with the fingers. Blow into victim's mouth. If mouth has been damaged hold mouth and lips shut and blow into patient's nose. In small children place mouth over child's nostrils and mouth, and blow into both. Remove your mouth, turn head to side and listen for return rush of air. Repeat blowing. Blow vigorously at rate of 12 breaths a minute; for a child, about 20 shallow breaths a minute. If initial failure to get air exchange, recheck head and jaw position. A child can be up-ended holding ankles and slapped two or three times between shoulder blades. SYN: *mouth-to-mouth r.*

RS: anabiosis; anastasis; artifical respiration; revivification.

resuscitator (rē-sŭs'ĭ-tā"tor) [L. *resuscitare,* to revive]. An automatic breathing machine that forces oxygen into the lungs under pressure of 4 oz. per square inch (1.4 mm. Hg) when back pressure of 3 oz. (about 1 mm. Hg) trips the machine for exhalation. May be used for several patients at the same time.

ret. Abbr. for *roentgen equivalent therapy.* It is analogous to rem, q.v., used in describing radiation protection or exposure.

retardation (rē"tŏr-dā'shŭn) [L. *retardāre,* to delay]. 1. A holding back or slowing down; delay. 2. Delayed mental or physical response due to pathological conditions. SEE: *mental deficiency.*

retarded depression. The depressed state of manic-depressive psychosis.

retch (rĕch) [AS. *hraecan,* to cough up phlegm]. Involuntary attempt to vomit, q.v.

retching (rĕch'ĭng). Attempting to vomit.

rete (rē'tē) [L.]. (pl. *retia*) [NA]. A network. A plexus of nerves or blood vessels.

r., articular. R. about a joint, esp. a deep anastomosis at knee joint.

r., cutaneum. A network of blood vessels at junction of the corium and superficial fascia.

r. mirabile. [NA]. A plexus formed by sudden division of a vessel into small twigs which unite again to form one vessel, as in the glomeruli of the kidneys.

r. olecrani. A network of vessels at back of elbow formed by divisions of the recurrent ulnar arteries.

r. ovarii. A group of rudimentary cellcords lying in broad ligament and mesovarium of ovary. They are homologous to rete testes in male.

r. patellae. [NA]. A superficial network of vessels lying about the patella. Formed by branches of genicular arteries.

r. subpapillare. A network of vessels between papillary and reticular layers of the dermis.

r. testis. [NA]. A network of tubules in mediastinum testis which receives sperm through the tubuli recti from the seminiferous tubules. From the rete testis, efferent ducts convey sperm to the epididymis.

r., vertebral. SEE: *retia, venous, of the vertebra.*

retention (rē-tĕn'shŭn) [L. *retentio,* a holding back]. Retaining in the body that which does not belong there, or which should be excreted, as urine, feces, or perspiration.

r. cyst. One caused by retention of a secretion in a gland, due to closure of the gland's duct.

r. defect. Inability to recall a name, number, or fact shortly after the subject was requested to remember it.

r. enema. Enema to be retained to provide nourishment, medicate the mucosa, or act as anesthetic. SEE: *enema, retention.*

r. of urine. Inability to empty bladder. This may be due to a number of causes, such as loss of muscle tone of the bladder from anemia, old age, exposure to cold, prolonged operation, or a greatly distended bladder without voiding for a considerable length of time; lesions involving nervous pathways to and from the bladder; lesions involving reflex centers in brain and spinal cord; obstruction of the urethra which may result from inflammation, stricture, stones, diverticula, cysts, tumors, or pressure from the outside as in cases of hypertrophy of the prostate; psychogenic factors; medication such as morphine or certain antihistamines.

r. with overflow. Spasm of sphincter, causing failure to empty the bladder at one voiding; with only overflow dribbling away; due to same causes as urine retention.

retia. Pl. of rete.

r., venous, of the vertebrae. Two plexuses within vertebral canal extending from foramen magnum to coccyx. They lie posteriorly and laterally to dura and between dura and arches of vertebrae.

reticula (rē-tĭk'ū-lō) [L.]. Pl. of reticulum.

reticular (rē-tĭk'ū-lăr) [L. *reticula*, net]. Meshed, or in the form of a network.

   r. activating system. The alerting system of the brain consisting of the reticular formation, subthalamus, hypothalamus, and medial thalamus. It extends from central core of the brain stem to all parts of the cerebral cortex. This system is essential in initiating and maintaining wakefulness and introspection, and in directing attention. Some of the tranquilizing drugs act on this system.

   r. apparatus of Golgi. SEE: *Golgi apparatus.*

   r. cells. 1. Phagocytic cells present in lymphatic and myeloid tissues. 2. The cells of r. connective tissue. SEE: *r. tissue.*

   r. fibers. Extremely fine argyrophilic (i.e., silver-staining) fibers found in r. tissue, q.v.

   r. formation. Groups of cells and fibers arranged in a diffuse network throughout the brain stem. These both fill the spaces and connect the tracts which ascend and descend through the area. They are important in controlling or influencing alertness, waking, sleeping, and various reflexes.

   r. layer. Layer of connective tissue forming deeper portion of dermis. Lies beneath papillary layer.

   r. membrane. Membrane formed by cuticular plates of distal ends of supporting cells in the organ of Corti.

   r. tissue. A form of connective tissue consisting of a network of r. fibers and cells. Cells are stellate with protoplasmic processes anastomosing with adjacent cells. Protoplasm also encloses and extends along the fibers. Found principally in bone marrow and lymphatic organs (lymph nodes). Also found in various organs (liver, kidney), in tissue underlying mucous membranes, and in walls of blood vessels.

retic'ulate. Of the nature of a network.

   r. substance. Reticular formation, q.v.

reticulated (rē-tĭk'ū-lā″tĕd) [L. *reticula*, net]. Netlike; pert. to a reticulum. SYN: *reticular.*

reticulation (rē-tĭk″ū-lā'shŭn). The formation of a network mass.

reticulin (rē-tĭk'ū-lĭn) [L. *reticula*, net]. An albuminoid or scleroprotein substance in the connective tissue framework of lymphatic tissues.

reticulocyte (rē-tĭk'ū-lō-sīt) ["+ Gr. *kytos*, cell]. A red blood cell containing a network of granules or filaments representing an immature stage in development. Normally comprise about 1% of circulating red blood cells.

reticulocytopenia (rē-tĭk″ū-lō-sī″tō-pē'nĭ-ă) ["+ "+ *penia*, poverty]. Lowering of the number of the reticulocytes of the blood.

reticulocytosis (rē-tĭk″ū-lō-sī-tō'sĭs) ["+ "+ -ōsis, intensive]. Increase in number of reticulocytes in circulating blood. Indicative of active erythropoiesis in red bone marrow. Occurs after hemorrhage, in high altitudes, and following treatment for pernicious anemia. SYN: *reticulosis.*

reticuloendothelial (rē-tĭk″ū-lō-ĕn″dō-thē'-lĭ-ăl) [L. *reticula*, net, + Gr. *endon*, within, + *thēlē*, nipple]. Pert. to the r. system, q.v.

   r. cell. A phagocytic cell of the r. system, q.v. SYN: *histiocyte; macrophage.*

   r. system. Term applied to those cells scattered throughout the body which have the power to ingest (phagocytose) particulate matter (bacteria, colloidal particles). Includes macrophages (histiocytes, clasmatocytes, or resting wandering cells) of loose connective tissue; reticular cells of lymphatic organs and myeloid tissues; Kupffer cells of the liver; cells lining blood sinuses of spleen, bone marrow, adrenal cortex, and hypophysis; microglia of central nervous system; adventitial cells about blood vessels; and dust cells of the lungs.

   The above types are called fixed R.E. cells. Under certain conditions, esp. inflammatory stimuli, fixed cells may become wandering R.E. cells, i.e., they become actively motile. Monocytes of the blood also are included in this group. R.E. cells function in elimination of worn out cells, esp. red blood cells; in repair of injured tissue; and in defense mechanisms, both local and general, of the body.

   Diseases of the RES include lymphosarcoma, reticulum cell sarcoma, Hodgkin's disease, follicular lymphoma, mycosis, fungoides, Gaucher's disease, and Niemann-Pick's disease. ABBR: RES.

reticuloendotheliosis (rē-tĭk″ū-lō-ĕn″dō-thē-lĭ-ō'sĭs) [L. *reticula*, net, + Gr. *endon*, within, + *thēlē*, nipple, + *ōsis*, intensive]. Hyperplasia of reticuloendothelium.

reticuloendothelium (rē-tĭk″ū-lō-ĕn″dō-thē'lĭ-ŭm). Tissue of the reticuloendothelial system, q.v. ABBR: R.E.

reticulosis (rē-tĭk-ū-lō'-sĭs) [L. *reticula*, net, + Gr. -ōsis, intensive]. Reticulocytosis, q.v.

reticulum (rē-tĭk'ū-lŭm) [L., a little net]. (pl. *reticula*) A network.

   r. of nucleus. A fine network of linin threads on which are arranged masses of chromatin.

r. stellate. The enamel pulp consisting of stellate cells lying between inner and outer epithelial layers of enamel organ of developing tooth.

retiform (rĕt'ĭ-form) [L. *rēte*, net, + *forma*, shape]. Resembling a network. SYN: *reticular.*

retina (rĕt'ĭ-nă) [L.]. (pl. *retinae*) [NA]. Innermost or 3rd tunic of the eye which receives image formed by the lens and is immediate instrument of vision.

The r. is a light-sensitive structure upon which light rays come to a focus. It extends from the point of entrance of the optic nerve anteriorly to the margin of the pupil, completely lining the interior of the eye. It consists of three parts: *pars optica,* the nervous or sensory portion extending from optic disc forward to ora serata, a wavy line immediately behind ciliary process; *pars ciliaris,* part lining inner surface of ciliary process; and *pars iridica,* part forming posterior surface of iris. Slightly lateral to posterior pole of the eye is a small, oval, yellowish spot, the macula lutea, in center of which is a depression, the fovea centralis. This region contains only cones and is the region of most acute vision. About 3.5 mm. nasally from the fovea is the optic papilla (optic disk), point at which nerve fibers from retina make their exit and form optic nerve. This region is devoid of rods and cones and is insensitive to light, hence named the *blind spot.*

The layers of the retina from without inward are layer of pigment epithelium, layer of rods and cones, external limiting membrane, external nuclear layer, external plexiform layer, internal nuclear layer, internal plexiform layer, layer of ganglion cells, layer of nerve fibers, and internal limiting membrane.

COLOR: Normally a purplish-red tint, varying with complexion. It is colorless in severe anemia or in ischemia. It is reddened in hyperemia.

VESSELS: The arteries shown are branches of a single central artery, a branch of the ophthalmic artery. The central artery enters at the center of the optic papilla, and it supplies the inner layers of retina. The outer layers, including rods and cones, are nourished by capillaries of the choroid layer. The veins lack muscular coats. They parallel the arteries, blood leaving by a central vein which leads to the superior ophthalmic vein.

r., coarctate. Condition in which there is an effusion of fluid between retina and choroid, giving retina a funnel shape.

r., detachment of. Complete or partial separation of retina from the choroid.

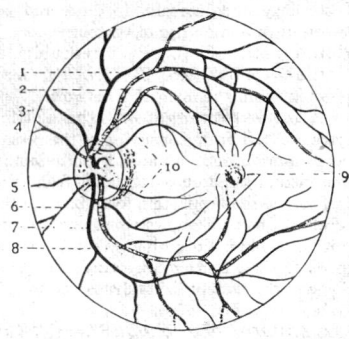

DIAGRAM OF RETINAL VESSELS

1, Superior temporal artery. 2, Superior temporal vein. 3, Superior nasal vein. 4, Superior nasal artery. 5, Inferior nasal vein. 6, Inferior nasal artery. 7, Inferior temporal vein. 8, Inferior temporal artery. 9, Macula lutea. 10, Macular veins.

May follow trauma, choroidal hemorrhages, or tumors.

r., shot-silk. R. having an opalescent appearance, sometimes seen in young persons. SYN: *watered-silk r.*

r., tigroid. R. having a spotted or striped appearance seen in retinitis pigmentosa.

retinaculum (rĕt'ĭ-năk'ū-lŭm) [L., halter]. (pl. *retinac'ula*) [NA]. A band or membrane holding any organ or part in its place. Thickenings of the deep fascia in distal portions of limbs which hold tendons in position when muscles contract, called r. tendinum.

r. cutis. [NA]. A fibrous band connecting the corium with underlying fascia.

r., extensor, of ankle. 1. The superior extensor retinaculum, a band which crosses the extensor tendons of foot and is attached to lower portion of tibia and fibula. 2. The inferior extensor retinaculum, a band located on dorsum of foot. Consists of two limbs having common origin or lateral surface of calcaneum. The upper limb is attached to medial malleolus; lower limb curves around instep and is attached to fascia of abductor hallucis on medial side of foot.

r., extensor, of wrist. An oblique band attached medially to styloid process of ulna, hammate bone, and medial ligament of wrist joint. Laterally it is attached to anterior border of radius. Contains six separate compartments for passage of extensor tendons to hand.

r., flexor, of ankle. R. extending from medial malleolus to medial tubercle of calcaneum.

r., flexor, of wrist. R. extending from trapezium and scaphoid bones laterally to hammate and pisiform bones medially.

r. of hip joint. Any one of three flat bands lying along neck of femur and continuous with capsule of hip joint. SYN: *cervical ligaments.*

r. mammae. Strands of connective tissue in mammary gland extending from glandular tissue through fat towards the skin where they are attached to deep fascia. Over cephalic portion of mammae they are well developed and called suspensory ligaments of Cooper.

r., patellar. Two fibrous bands (medial and lateral r.) lying on either side of knee joint and forming part of joint capsule. They are extensions of the insertions of the medial and lateral vastus muscles.

r., peroneal. Two fibrous bands on lateral side of foot which contain tendons of peroneus longus and brevis muscles. The superior peroneal r. extends from lateral malleolus to lateral surface of calcaneum; the inferior peroneal r. is attached below to calcaneum, above to lower border of inferior extensor retinaculum.

r. tendinum. SEE: *retinaculum.*

retinal (rĕt'ĭ-năl) [L.]. Concerning the retina.

r. breaks. A break in the continuity of the retina. Usually caused by trauma to the eye. Detachment of the retina may follow appearance of break.

r. correspondence. Condition in which simultaneous stimulation of points in the retinas of two eyes results in formation of a single visual sensation. Such points are called corresponding points. These lie in the foveas of the two retinas, or in the nasal half of one retina and the temporal half of the other. Abnormal correspondence results in double vision (diplopia) and usually is the result of inequality of ocular muscles. SEE: *strabismus.*

r. detachment. Separation of the inner sensory layer of the retina from the outer pigment epithelium, leading to loss of retinal function. Usually caused by a hole or break in the inner sensory layer which permits fluid to accumulate between the two layers.

r. purple. Rhodopsin or visual purple, q.v.

retine. A tissue extract which inhibits growth of certain tumors in mice.

retinene (rĕt'ĭ-nēn). An orange-yellow carotenoid pigment formed in retina as a result of the action of light on rhodopsin; an aldehyde of vitamin A. In dark adaptation, rhodopsin is regenerated from retinene. SYN: *visual yellow; xanthopsin.*

retinitis (rĕt-ĭ-nī'tĭs) [L. *retina*, retina, + Gr. *-itis*, inflammation]. Inflamed condition of the retina.

SYM: Diminished vision, contractions of fields or scotomata, alteration in size of objects, photophobia.

TREATMENT: Absolute rest of eyes, protection from light, treat underlying cause.

r., actinic. R. due to exposure to intense light or other forms of radiant energy.

r. albuminurica. R. associated with chronic kidney disease and malignant hypertension. Shows general signs of retinitis and is distinguished by white patches in the fundus, esp. surrounding the papilla and in the macular region.

r., apoplectic. R. associated with hemorrhaging of retinal vessels.

r. circinata. R. in which there is a circle of white spots about the macula.

r. circumpapillaris. R. in which there is a proliferation of outer layers of retina about optic disk.

r., diabetic. R. occurring in diabetics, esp. that of long duration. Characterized by aneurysmal dilatation of blood vessels, hemorrhages, and waxy and cotton-wool exudates.

r. disciformis. R. accompanied by degeneration of retina in region of macula.

r., exogenous purulent. R. following introduction of infectious organisms into eye as a result of perforating wound or ulcer.

r., external exudative. Condition in which large masses of white and yellow crystals occur beneath retina as a result of organization of hemorrhages. SYN: *external hemorrhagic r.; Coats' disease.*

r., metastatic. Acute purulent retinitis resulting from lodgement of infective emboli in retinal vessels.

r. pigmentosa. A chronic progressive disease characterized by degeneration of retinal neuroepithelium, esp. rods; atrophy of optic nerve; and widespread pigmentary changes in retina. A degenerative condition without inflammation.

ETIOL: Unknown but a hereditary tendency is manifested. Usually appears in childhood. SYN: *primary pigmentary degeneration of retina.*

r. proliferans. Vascularized masses of connective tissue which project from retina into the vitreous. End result of recurrent hemorrhage from retina into the vitreous.

r. punctata albescens. A non-progressive degenerative, familial disease characterized by presence of innumerable minute white spots scattered over entire retina, and without pigmentary changes. Usually starts early in life. SYN: *degeneratio punctata albescens.*

r., punctate, central. R. characterized by numerous white or yellow spots in fundus of eye.

r. septica. A mild benign condition occurring in patients with systemic infections. Characterized by white spots, usually surrounded by hemorrhagic areas, and seen near the optic disk. These are called Roth's spots. SYN: *r. of Roth.*

r., solar. R. resulting from exposure of retina to rays of sun.

r., stellate. R. characterized by presence of exudates, hemorrhages, blurring of optic disk, and formation of a star-shaped figure about macula. SYN: *pseudonephritic r.; toxic exudative r.*

r., syphilitic. R. resulting from, or associated with, syphilis. May involve not only retina but also optic nerve (syphilitic neuroretinitis).

retinoblastoma (rĕt′ĭ-nō-blăs-tō′mă) [L. *retina,* retina, + Gr. *blastos,* germs, + *-ōma,* tumor]. A malignant glioma of the retina. Occurs in young children and shows a hereditary pattern. Usually unilateral.

retinochoroiditis (rĕt′ĭ-nō-kō-royd-ī′tĭs) ["+ Gr. *chorioeidēs,* skinlike, + *-itis,* inflammation]. Inflamed condition of retina and choroid.

retinocystoma (rĕt′ĭ-nō-sĭs-tō′mă) ["+ Gr. *kystis,* sac, + *-ōma,* tumor]. Glioma of the retina.

retinoid (rĕt′ĭ-noyd). 1. [L. *retina,* retina, + Gr. *eidos,* resemblance]. Like the retina. 2. [Gr. *rhētinē,* resin, + *eidos,* resemblance]. Resembling a resin; resinous.

retinopapillitis (rĕt′ĭ-nō-pă″pĭl-ī′tĭs) [L. *retina,* retina, + *papilla,* nipple, + Gr. *-itis,* inflammation]. Inflamed condition of retina and optic papilla. SYN: *papilloretinitis.*

ret″inop′athy ["+ Gr. *pathos,* disease]. Any disorder of the retina.

r., arteriosclerotic. R. accompanying generalized arteriosclerosis and moderate hypertension.

r., diabetic. R. occurring in diabetics.

r., hypertensive. R. associated with hypertension, toxemia of pregnancy, glomerulonephritis.

r., solar. Pathological changes in the r. after looking directly at the sun. Seen frequently following an eclipse of the sun. SYN: *eclipse blindness.*

r., syphilitic. R. occurring in later stages of syphilis.

retinoscope (rĕt′ĭ-nō-skōp) ["+ Gr. *skopein,* to examine]. An instrument used in performing retinoscopy.

retinos′copy. Objective method of determining refractive errors of the eye. The examiner projects light into eyes and judges error of refraction by movement of reflected light rays. SYN: *skiascopy.*

retisolution (rĕt′ĭ-sō-lū′shŭn) [L. *rēte,* net, + *solutio,* dissolution]. Dissolution of the Golgi structures.

retispersion (rĕt′ĭ-spŭr′zhŭn) ["+ *spersio,* a scattering]. Transference of Golgi structures to periphery of the cell.

retort (rē-tort′) [L. *retortus,* bent back]. A flasklike, long-necked vessel used in distillation.

retothelium (rē″tō-thē′lĭ-ŭm) [L. *rēte,* net, + Gr. *thēlē,* nipple]. Cellular layers covering reticular tissue. SYN: *reticuloendothelium; reticulothelium.*

re″tract′ [L. *retractus*]. To draw back.

retractile (rē-trăkt′ĭl) [L. *retractilis*]. Capable of being drawn back or in.

retraction (rē-trăk′shŭn). A shortening; the act of drawing backward or state of being drawn back.

r. ring. A ridge sometimes felt on uterus above the pubes, marking line of separation between upper contractile and lower dilatable segments of the uterus. Seen in prolonged or obstructed labor. SYN: *Bandl's ring.*

r., uterine. The process by which muscular fibers of the uterus remain permanently shortened to a small degree following each contraction or labor pain.

retrac′tor. 1. Instrument for holding back the margins of a wound. 2. Muscle which draws in any organ or part.

retreat (rē″trēt′) [ME. *retret,* draw back]. Act of retiring or withdrawing from difficult life situations. May be direct, as in physical flight, or indirect, as in malingering, illness, abnormal preoccupation, and self-deception.

retrench′ment [Fr. *retrenchier,* to cut back]. Procedure used in plastic surgery to remove excess tissue.

retro- [L.]. Prefix meaning backward.

retroaction (rĕt″rō-ăk′shŭn). Action in a reverse direction.

retroauricular (rĕt″rō-ŏ-rĭk′ū-lar) [L. *retrō,* backward, + *auricula,* ear]. Behind the auricle or ear.

retrobuccal (rĕt′rō-bŭk′ăl) ["+ *bucca,* cheek]. Concerning the back part of the mouth or area behind the mouth.

retrobulbar (rĕt″rō-bŭl′bar) ["+ Gr. *bulbus*, bulb]. 1. Behind the eyeball. 2. Posterior to the medulla oblongata.

retrocedent (rĕt″rō-sē′dĕnt) [L. *retrocedere*]. 1. Going backward; returning. 2. A condition affecting some interior organ and disappearing from the surface.

retrocervical (rĕt″rō-sĕr′vĭ-kăl) [L. *retrō*, backward, + *cervix*, neck]. Back of the cervix uteri.

retrocession (rĕt″rō-sĕsh′ŭn) [L. *retrocessio*, going back]. 1. A going back; a relapse. 2. Metastasis of a condition from the surface to an internal organ. 3. An abnormal position of the uterus; backward displacement.

retrocolic (rĕt″rō-kŏl′ĭk) [L. *retrō*, backward, + Gr. *kōlon*, colon]. Back of the colon.

retrocollic (rĕt″rō-kŏl′ĭk) ["+ *collum*, neck]. Concerning the back of the neck.

    r. spasm. Wryneck with spasms affecting posterior muscles of neck.

retrocollis (rĕt″rō-kŏl′ĭs). Spasm of posterior muscles of the neck with drawing of the head backward. SYN: *torticollis*.

retrocursive (rĕt″rō-kŭr′sĭv) [L. *retrō*, backward, + *curro*, to run]. Stepping or turning backward.

retrodeviation (rē″trō-dē″vĭ-ā′shŭn) ["+ *deviāre*, to turn aside]. Backward displacement, as of an organ.

retrodisplacement (rē″trō-dĭs-plās′mĕnt) ["+ Fr. *desplacer*, displace]. Displacement backwards of a part.

retroesophageal (rĕt″rō-ē-sŏf″ă-jē′ăl) [L. *retro*, backward, + Gr. *oisophagos*, gullet]. Located behind the esophagus.

retroflexed (rĕt′rō-flĕkst″) ["+ *flexus*, bent]. Bent backward.

retroflexion (rĕt″rō-flĕk′shŭn). A bending or flexing backward.

    r. of uterus. A condition of the womb in which its body is bent backward at an angle with the cervix whose position usually remains unchanged.

retrogasserian (rĕt″rō-găs-sē′rĭ-ăn). Referring to the posterior root of the gasserian ganglion.

retrograde (rĕt′rō-grād, rē′trō-grād) [L. *retrō*, backward, + *gradi*, to step]. Moving backward; degenerating from better to worse state.

    r. amnesia. Loss of memory for events and situations just preceding time of patient's illness.

    r. flow. The flow of fluid in a direction opposite to that which is considered normal.

retrography (rē-trŏg′ră-fĭ) [L. *retrō*, backward, + Gr. *graphein*, to write]. Mirror writing, a symptom of certain brain diseases.

retrogression (rĕt″rō-grĕsh′ŭn) [L. *retrō-gressus*, go backward]. 1. A going backward as in the involution, degeneration, or atrophy of a tissue or structure. 2. Passing from a more complex to a simpler type of structure in the development of an organ, an individual, or a race. 3. The return of symptoms in recovery from a disease.

ret″rogres′sive changes. Changes to lower type of organization, such as in atrophy, degeneration, necrosis, hypertrophy, etc.

retroinfection (rē″trō-ĭn-fĕk′shŭn) [L. *retrō*, backward, + *infectiō*, infection]. Infection communicated by the fetus in utero to the mother.

retroinsular (rĕt″rō-ĭn′sū-lar) ["+ *insula*, island]. Situated behind the island of Reil in the brain.

retrojection (rĕt″rō-jĕk′shŭn) ["+ *jacio*, to throw]. Washing out a cavity from within by injection of a fluid.

retrolabyrinthine (rē″trō-lăb″ĭ-rĭn′thĭn) [L. *retrō*, backward, + Gr. *labyrinthos*, a maze]. Situated behind the labyrinth of the ear.

retrolent′al. Behind the crystalline lens.

    r. fibroplasia. Condition in which an opaque fibrous membrane develops on posterior surface of the lens. Occurs chiefly in premature infants weighing less than 2000 gm., esp. those subjected to high oxygen concentrations while in an incubator for a considerable period of time. ABBR: RLF.

retrolingual (rĕt″rō-lĭng′gwal) [L. *retrō*, backward, + *lingua*, tongue]. Behind the tongue.

retromammary (rĕt″rō-măm′mă-rĭ) ["+ *mamma*, breast]. Located behind the mammary gland.

retromandibular (rē″trō-măn-dĭb′ū-lar) ["+ *mandibulum*, jaw]. Located behind the lower jaw.

retromastoid (rē″trō-măs′toyd) [L. *retrō*, backward, + Gr. *mastos*, breast, + *eidos*, like]. Situated behind the mastoid process.

retromorphosis (rē″trō-mōr′fō-sĭs) ["+ Gr. *morphē*, form, + *-ōsis*, intensive]. 1. Change in shape accompanying a transition from a higher to a lower type of structure. 2. Retrogressive changes within cells or tissues; catabolism, q.v.

retronasal (rĕt″rō-nā′zăl) ["+ *nasus*, nose]. Rel. to, or situated at, the back part of the nose.

retroocular (rĕt″rō-ŏk′ū-lar) [L. *retrō*, backward, + *oculus*, eye]. Located behind the eye.

retroperitoneal (rē″trō-pĕr-ĭ-tō-nē′ăl) ["+ Gr. *peritonaion*, peritoneum]. Located behind the peritoneum.

retroperitoneum (rē″trō-pĕr-ĭ-tō-nē′ŭm). The space behind the peritoneum.

retroperitonitis (rē″trō-pĕr″ĭ-tō-nī′tĭs). Inflammation behind the peritoneum.

retropharyngeal (rē″trō-făr-ĭn′jē-ăl) [L. *retrō*, backward, + Gr. *pharynx*, pharynx]. Behind the pharynx.

retropharyngitis (rē″trō-făr″ĭn-jī′tĭs) [″+ ″+ -*itis*, inflammation]. Inflammation of the retropharyngeal tissue.

retroplacental (rē″trō-plă-sĕn′tăl) [″+ *placenta*, a flat cake]. Behind the placenta, or behind both the placenta and the uterine wall.

retroplasia (rē″trō-plā′zĭ-ă) [L. *retrō*, backward, + Gr. *plassein*, to form]. Degenerative change of a cell or tissue into a more primitive form.

retroposed (rĕ-trō-posd′) [″+ *positus*, placed]. Displaced backward.

retropulsion (rē″trō-pŭl′shŭn) [″+ *pulsiō*, a thrusting]. 1. Pushing back of any part, as of the fetal head in labor. 2. A walking or running backward involuntarily, seen in some nervous disorders.

re″troster′nal [″+ Gr. *sternon*, chest]. Behind the sternum.

   r. pulse. Venous pulse felt over suprasternal notch.

retrotarsal (rē″trō-tar′săl) [″+ Gr. *tarsos*, edge of eyelid]. Located behind the tarsus of the eye.

retrouterine (rē″trō-ū″tĕr-ĭn) [L. *retrō*, backward, + *uterus*, womb]. Located behind the uterus.

retrovaccina′tion. Vaccination with virus obtained from a calf inoculated with smallpox virus obtained from a human.

retroversion (rĕt″rō-vŭr′shŭn, rē″trō-vŭr′shŭn) [L. *retrō*, backward, + *versio*, turning]. A turning, or state of being turned back, esp. an entire organ being tipped.

   r. of uterus. Displacement of the uterus backward with cervix pointing forward toward symphysis pubis. Normally, the cervix points toward the lower end of the sacrum with the fundus toward the suprapubic region.

re″trude′ [L. *rē*, back, + *trudere*, to shove]. To force inward or backward.

retrusion (rē-trū′shŭn). 1. Process of forcing backward, esp. with reference to teeth. 2. Condition in which teeth are retroposed.

Retzius (rĕt′zĭ-ŭs). [Anders Adolf Retzius, Swedish anatomist, 1796-1860].

   R., space of. Space in lower portion of abdomen between bladder and pubic bones and bounded superiorly by peritoneum. Contains areolar tissue, fat, and a plexus of veins. SYN: *cavum Retzii; prevesical space; retropubic space.*

   R., veins of. Veins forming communications between the mesenteric veins and inferior vena cava. SYN: *retroperitoneal veins.*

Retzius, lines of (rĕt′zĭ-ŭs). [Magnus Gustav Retzius, Swedish anatomist, 1842-1919]. Brownish, concentric lines in the enamel of a tooth.

Reuss′ test (roys). [August R. von Reuss, Austrian ophthalmologist, 1841-1924]. Test for atropine, employing sulfuric acid and an oxidizing agent.

revellent (rē-vĕl′ĕnt) [L. *re*, back, + *vellere*, to draw]. 1. Producing revulsion, the diversion of disease or blood from one part of the body to another. 2. Agent producing revulsion.

re″verbera′tion [L. *reverberāre*, to cause to rebound]. Process by which closed chains of neurons, when excited by a single impulse, will continue to discharge impulses from collaterals of their cells.

reversal (rē-vŭr′săl) [L. *reversus*, revert]. 1. A change, or turning in the opposite direction. 2. In psychology, a change in an instinct to its opposite, as from love to hate.

reversion (rē-vŭr′zhŭn). 1. Return to a previously existing condition. 2. In genetics, the appearance of traits possessed by a remote ancestor. SEE: *atavism*.

revivification (rē-vĭv″ĭ-fĭ-kā′shŭn) [L. *re*, again, + *vivere*, to live, + *facere*, to make]. 1. Attempt to restore life to those apparently dead; restoration to life or consciousness. Also restoring life in local parts, as a limb after freezing. 2. Paring of surfaces to facilitate healing, as in a wound.

revulsant (rē-vŭl′sănt) [L. *revulsio*, pulling back]. 1. Causing transfer of disease or blood from one part of the body to another. 2. Drug which draws blood to an inflamed part.

revulsion (rē-vŭl′shŭn). 1. Act of driving backward, as diverting disease from one part to another by a quick withdrawal of the blood from that part. 2. In physical therapy, circulatory changes obtained by sudden and intense reactions to heat and cold. The Scotch douche is a powerful revulsive measure. SEE: *counterirritation*.

revulsive (rē-vŭl′sĭv). 1. Causing revulsion. 2. A counterirritant.

RF. Abbr. for *rheumatoid factor*, q.v.

R. factor. Resistance transfer factor, q.v.

Rh. 1. Chem. symbol for rhodium. 2. Abbr. for *rhesus*, a monkey (Macaca rhesus) in which the Rh factor was first identified.

Rh antiserum. Human serum which contains Rh antibodies. SYN: *anti-Rh-serum.*

Rh blood factor. A factor discovered in erythrocytes of the rhesus monkey and present in about 85% of human population, such individuals being designated Rh+ (Rh positive). In the remaining 15% (Rh−, or Rh negative) it causes, when injected, the formation of anti-Rh agglutinin. Subsequent transfusions of Rh+ blood may result in serious transfusion reactions (agglutination and hemolysis of red blood cells). A pregnant woman may become sensitized by blood of an Rh+ fetus. In subsequent pregnancies, if the fetus is Rh+, Rh antibodies produced in maternal blood may cross the placenta and destroy fetal cells giving rise to erythroblastosis fetalis, q.v.

Rh genes. A series of eight allelic genes which are responsible for the various Rh blood types and designated by Wiener as R^1, R^2, R^0, R^z, r, r′, r″, and r_y. Genes represented by small r's are responsible for Rh− persons; those by large R's for Rh+ persons.

Rh-Hr agglutinogens (antigens). Substances present in red blood cells which stimulate antibody formation.

Rh immune globulin. A solution of gamma globulin containing anti-Rh. Given within 72 hours after delivery of an Rh positive infant to an Rh negative mother. It acts to prevent and suppress the Rh immune response. Also indicated in abortion done on an Rh negative mother.

Rhabditis (răb-dĭ'tĭs) [Gr. *rhabdos*, rod]. A genus of small nematode worms, some of which are parasitic.

rhabdo- [Gr. *rhabdos*, rod]. Combining form meaning rod.

rhabdomyoma (răb″dō-mī-ō'mă) ["+ *mys*, my-, muscle, + -*ōma*, tumor]. A striated muscular tissue tumor.

rhabdophobia (răb-dō-fō'bĭ-ă) ["+ *phobos*, fear]. Abnormal fear of being hit or beaten with a stick or rod.

rhachialgia (ră″kĭ-ăl'jĭ-ă) [Gr. *rhachis*, spine, + *algos*, pain]. Pain in the spine.

rhachiocampsis (ră″kĭ-ō-kămp'sĭs) ["+ *kampsis*, a bending]. Curvature of spine.

rhachioplegia (ră″kĭ-ō-plē'jĭ-ă) ["+ *plēgē*, a stroke]. Spinal paralysis.

rhachioscoliosis (ră″kĭ-ō-skō-lĭ-ō'sĭs) ["+ *skoliōsis*, bending]. Curvature of the spine laterally.

rhachis (ră'kĭs) [Gr.]. Spinal column.

rhachischisis (ră-kĭs'kĭ-sĭs) ["+ *schisis*, fissure]. A congenital cleft in the spinal column.

rhachitis (ră-kī'tĭs) ["+ -*itis*, inflammation]. Constitutional disease of infancy marked by faulty nutrition and bone deformity. SYN: *rachitis, rickets*, q.v.

rhacoma (ră-kō'mă) [Gr. *rhakōma*, rags]. 1. Ragged, irregular abrasion, usually of the skin. 2. Relaxation of integument of scrotum.

rhagades (răg'ă-dēz) [Gr., tears]. Linear fissures appearing in skin, esp. at the corner of the mouth or anus, causing pain. If due to syphilis, they form a radiating scar on healing.

rhagadiform (ră-găd'ĭ-form) [Gr. *rhagas*, tear, + L. *forma*, shape]. Fissured; having cracks.

-rhage, -rhagia [Gr. *rhēgnynai*, to burst forth]. Suffix meaning bleeding, profuse discharge.

rhaphania (ră-fā'nĭ-ă) [Gr. *raphanos*, radish]. Spasmodic disease caused by eating wild radish. SYN: *raphania*.

rhaphe (ră'fē) [Gr.]. A seam or ridge. SYN: *raphe*.

-rhaphy [Gr. *rhaphē*]. Suffix meaning joining in a seam, or suturation.

-rhea [Gr. *rhoia*, flow]. Suffix meaning to flow.

rhegma (rĕg'mă) [Gr. *rhēgma*, a tear]. Rupture, fracture, or rent. Ex: vessel walls, a bone, or an abscess.

rhembasmus (rĕm-băs'mŭs) [Gr. *rhembasmos*]. Wandering of mind; indecision.

rhenium (rē'nĭ-ŭm). SYMB: *Re*. At. wt. 186.2; at. no. 75. A metallic element similar to manganese.

rheo- [Gr. *rheos*, current]. Combining form indicating current, stream, or to flow.

rheobase (rē'ō-bās) ["+ *basis*, step]. In unipolar testing with the galvanic current using negative as active pole, the minimal voltage required to produce a stimulated response. This is the rheobase, or threshold of excitation. SEE: *chronaxie*.

rheochord (rē'ō-kord) ["+ *chordē*, cord]. Type of rheostat used for measuring resistance of an electric current. SEE: *rheostat*.

rheometer (rē-ŏm'ĕt-ĕr) [Gr. *rheos*, current, + *metron*, measure]. 1. Instrument for qualitative determination of presence of an electric current. SYN: *galvanometer*. 2. Device for measuring rapidity of the blood current.

rheonome (rē'ō-nōm) ["+ *nemein*, to distribute]. Device for ascertaining the effect of irritation on a nerve.

rheophore (rē'ō-fōr) ["+ *phoros*, bearing]. A cord conducting an electrical current, as one between patient and electrical apparatus. SYN: *electrode*.

rheoscope (rē'ō-skōp) [Gr. *rheos*, current, + *skopein*, to examine]. Device indicating the existence of an electric current. SYN: *galvanoscope*.

rheostat (rē′ō-stăt) ["+ *statos*, standing]. A device maintaining fixed or variable resistance for controlling the amount of current entering a circuit.

rheostosis (rē-ŏs-tō′sĭs) ["+ *osteon*, bone]. A hypertrophying and condensing osteitis occurring in streaks, involving long bones.

rheotachygraphy (rē″ō-tă-kĭg′ră-fĭ) [Gr. *rheos*, current, + *tachys*, swift, + *graphein*, to write]. Graphic recording of variation of electromotive force in a muscle.

rheotaxis (rē″ō-tăk′sĭs) ["+ *taxis*, arrangement]. Reaction to a current of fluid, causing the part acted upon to move against the current.

rheotome (rē′ō-tōm) ["+ *tomē*, a cutting]. A device for interrupting electrical current at required intervals.

rheotrope (rē′ō-trōp) ["+ *tropos*, a turning]. An instrument for automatically reversing a current of electricity.

rhestocythemia (rĕs″tō-sī-thē′mĭ-ă) [Gr. *rhaistos*, destroyed, + *kytos*, cell, + *haima*, blood]. Condition of degenerated red blood cells in the peripheral circulation.

rheum, rheuma (rūm, rūm′ă) [Gr. *rheuma*, discharge]. Any catarrhal or watery discharge.

   r., salt. Various skin eruptions; chronic eczema.

rheumatic (rū-măt′ĭk) [Gr. *rheumatikos*]. Pert. to rheumatism.

   r. chorea. SEE: *chorea, Sydenham's.*

   r. fever. A systemic, febrile disease; inflammatory and nonsuppurative in nature; variable in severity, duration, and sequelae. It is frequently followed by serious heart or kidney disease.

   ETIOL: Unknown, but its onset follows a preceding infection with a strain of group A beta hemolytic streptococci. Attacks usually occur in childhood; an individual is esp. susceptible to subsequent attacks.

   SYM: Sometime following a streptococcal infection the patient will experience the sudden occurrence of fever and joint pain; this is the most common type of onset. Other sym. include fever, migratory polyarthritis, pain upon motion, abdominal pain, chorea, cardiac involvement (pericarditis, myocarditis, and endocarditis).

   Later gives rise to precordial discomfort and development of heart murmurs. Skin manifestations include erythema marginatum or circinatum, and development of subcutaneous nodules. Epistaxis is common.

   R. fever may occur without any sign or sym. of joint involvement.

   TREATMENT: Enforced bed rest until signs of active rheumatic fever have disappeared. Salicylates for symptomatic relief. Penicillin administered to eradicate streptococci. Complications, esp. those involving heart, require special treatment.

   PROPHYLAXIS: Prompt and adequate treatment of streptococcal infections with penicillin preferably, or erythromycin in appropriate dose, for a minimum of 10 days. Following an attack of rheumatic fever, individuals should receive continuous prophylaxis with penicillin or sulfonamide for an indefinite period.

rheumatism (rū′mŏ-tizm) [Gr. *rheumatismos*]. A general term for acute and chronic conditions characterized by soreness and stiffness of muscles, and pain in joints and associated structures. It includes arthritis (infectious, rheumatoid, gouty); arthritis due to rheumatic fever or trauma; degenerative joint disease; neurogenic arthropathy; hydroarthrosis; myositis; bursitis; fibromyositis; and many other conditions. SEE: *arthritis; rheumatic fever.*

   r., acute articular. SEE: *rheumatic fever.*

   r., chronic. R. associated with a joint disorder, such as rheumatoid arthritis, gout, or degenerative joint disease, usually resulting in deformity of the joint.

   r., gonorrheal. Arthritis resulting from gonorrheal infection. SEE: *gonorrhea.*

   r., muscular. Term applied to a number of muscular conditions characterized by tenderness, soreness, pain, and local spasm. Includes such conditions as fibromyositis, myositis, myalgia, and torticollis, q.v.

   r., psychogenic. R. of psychic origin, esp. that occurring under emotional stress.

   r., soft tissue (non-articular). General term for a variety of localized and generalized conditions which cause pain around joints but which are not related to or caused by joint disease. Included in this general classification are bursitis, tennis elbow, tendinitis, perichondritis, stiff man syndrome, and Tietze's disease.

rheumatoid (rū′mă-toyd) [Gr. *rheuma*, discharge, + *eidos*, like]. Of the nature of rheumatism; resembling rheumatism.

   r. arthritis. Form of arthritis with inflammation of the joints, stiffness, swelling, cartilaginous hypertrophy, and pain. SEE: *arthritis.*

   r. factor. An immunoglobulin present in serum of 50-95% of adults with r. arthritis. This factor, though not specific for r. arthritis, is quite helpful in diagnosing and investigating the disease.

rhexis (rĕk′sĭs) [Gr., rupture]. Rupture of any organ, blood vessel, or tissue.

rhicnosis (rĭk-nō'sĭs) [Gr. *rhytis*, wrinkle, + *-ōsis*, condition]. Wrinkling of the skin due principally to atrophy of subcutaneous tissue, esp. elastic fibers.

rhigosis (rĭ-gō'sĭs) [Gr. *rhigōsis*, shivering]. Perception of cold.

rhinal (rī'năl) [Gr. *rhis, rhin-*, nose]. Concerning the nose. SYN: *nasal.*

rhinalgia (rĭ-năl'jĭ-ă) ["+ *algos*, pain]. Pain in nose; nasal neuralgia.

rhinencephalon (rĭ-nĕn-sĕf'ă-lŏn) ["+ *enkephalos*, brain]. Portion of brain concerned with reception and integration of olfactory impulses. Includes olfactory bulb, olfactory tract and striae, intermediate olfactory area, pyriform area, paraterminal area, hippocampal formation, and fornix. It constitutes the paleopallium and archipallium.

rhinesthesia (rĭ-nĕs-thē'zĭ-ă) ["+ *aisthēsis*, sensation]. The sense of smell.

rhineurynter (rĭn"ū-rĭn'ter) ["+ *eurynein*, to dilate]. Elastic bag used for dilating the nostrils.

rhinion (rĭn'ĭ-ŏn) [Gr.]. Lower end of the suture between nasal bones; a craniometric point. SYN: *punctum nasale inferius.*

rhinitis (rī-nī'tĭs) [Gr. *rhis, rhin-*, nose, + *-itis*, inflammation]. Inflammation of the nasal mucosa. SEE: *endorhinitis; ozena.*

   r., acute. Acute congested condition of nose with increased secretion of mucus. SYN: *common head cold; coryza.*

   TREATMENT: No specific treatment is known. General measures include rest, adequate fluids, well-balanced diet. Analgesics and antipyretics may be used to make patient comfortable. Sulfonamides and antibiotics are of no value and should not be administered. Antihistamines may relieve early symptoms but do not abort or alter course. Vasoconstrictors in form of inhalants, nasal sprays, or drops may give temporary relief. Their use helps prevent the development of middle ear infections by helping to maintain the patency of the eustachian tubes.

   r., allergic. R. due to sensitivity of nasal mucosa to an allergen. SYN: *atopic r.; hay fever; vasomotor r.*

   r., atrophic. Chronic inflammation with marked atrophy of mucous membrane and with considerable dry crusting and disturbance in the sense of smell. Usually accompanied by ozena. The throat is dry and, as a rule, contains crusts. A husky voice or hoarseness often is common.

   SYM: Fetid odor from nose and throat with considerable crusting.

   TREATMENT: Irrigation of nose with warm alkalinized saline solution twice daily.

General hygienic measures. Correction of any associated disorders. Surgical treatment seldom helpful.

   r. caseosa. Characterized by accumulation of offensive cheeselike masses in nose and sinuses and accompanied by a seropurulent discharge.

   r., chronic hyperplastic. Chronic inflammation of mucous membrane accompanied by polypoid formation and underlying sinus pathology. SEE: *sinus.*

   r., chronic hypertrophic. Inflammation of the mucous membrane of the nose characterized by hypertrophy of the mucous membrane of the turbinates and the septum.

   SYM: Those of nasal obstruction, postnasal discharge, and recurrent head colds.

   TREATMENT: Consists in surgical removal of hypertrophic or mulberry ends of inferior turbinates and cauterization of mucosa of inferior turbinates and septum.

   r., fibrinous. R. characterized by formation of a false membrane in nasal cavities.

   r., perennial. R. which is nonseasonal, but continues indefinitely with variations in severity.

   r., periodic. R., allergic, q.v.

   r., pseudomembranous. R., fibrinous, q.v.

   r., vasomotor. R. with rhinorrhea due to increased secretion of mucus from the nasal mucosa. May be caused by allergy or neurovascular imbalance.

rhino- [Gr. *rhis*]. Combining form indicating the nose.

rhinoantritis (rī"nō-ăn-trī'tĭs) ["+ *antron*, cavity, + *-itis*, inflammation]. Inflamed condition of the nasal cavities and one or both maxillary antra.

rhinobyon (rī-nō'bĭ-ŏn) ["+ *byein*, to plug]. A tampon or plug for the nose.

rhinocanthectomy (rī"nō-kăn-thĕk'tō-mĭ) [Gr. *rhis, rhin-*, nose, + *kanthos*, canthus, + *ektomē*, excision]. Excision of inner corner of the eye. SYN: *rhinommectomy.*

rhinocele (rī'nō-sēl) ["+ *koilia*, hollow]. The ventricle or hollow of the olfactory lobe or rhinoencephalon.

rhinocheiloplasty (rī"nō-kī'lō-plăs-tĭ) ["+ *cheilos*, lip, + *plastos*, formed]. Plastic surgery of the nose and upper lip.

rhinocleisis (rī-nō-klī'sĭs) [Gr. *rhis, rhin-*, nose, + *kleisis*, closure]. Nasal obstruction.

rhinodacryolith (rī"nō-dăk'rĭ-ō-lĭth) ["+ *dakryon*, tear, + *lithos*, stone.]. A nasal calculus.

rhinodynia (rī"nō-dĭn'ĭ-ă) ["+ *odynē*, pain]. Nasal pain. SYN: *rhinalgia.*

Rhinoestrus (rī-nĕs'trŭs). A genus of flies belonging to family Oestridae. Larvae may be deposited in eye, nasal, or buccal cavities of mammals.

R. purpureus. Russian gadfly, whose larvae sometimes cause nasomyiasis and ophthalmomyiasis in man.

rhinogenous (ri-nŏj'ĕn-ŭs) [Gr. *rhis, rhin-,* nose, + *gennan,* to produce]. Originating in the nose.

rhinokyphosis (rī"nō-ki-fō'sīs) ["+ *kyphos,* hump, + *-osis,* intensive]. A deformity of the bridge of the nose.

rhinolalia (rī"nō-lā'lĭ-ă) ["+ *lalia,* speech]. Nasal quality of voice.

r. aperta. R. caused by undue patency of posterior nares.

r. clausa. R. caused by closure of nasal passages.

rhinolaryngitis (rī"nō-lăr"ĭn-jī'tĭs) [Gr. *rhis, rhin-,* nose, + *larynx,* larynx, + *-itis,* inflammation]. Simultaneous inflammation of mucosa of nose and larynx.

rhinolith (rī'nō-līth) ["+ *lithos,* stone]. Nasal concretion.

rhinolithiasis (rī"nō-līth-ī'ă-sīs) ["+ "+ *-iasis,* condition]. The formation of nasal calculi.

rhinologist (ri-nŏl'ō-jĭst) [Gr. *rhis, rhin-,* nose, + *logos,* study]. A specialist in diseases of the nose.

rhinology (ri-nŏl'ō-jĭ). Science of the nose and its diseases.

rhinomanometer (rī"nō-măn-ŏm"ĕt-ĕr) [Gr. *rhis, rhin-,* nose, + *manos,* thin, + *metron,* a measure]. A device for measuring the amount of nasal obstruction.

rhinometer (ri-nŏm'ĕt-ĕr). Device for measurement of the nose or its cavities.

rhinomiosis (rī"nō-mī-ō'sīs) [Gr. *rhis, rhin-,* nose, + *meiōsis,* a lessening]. Surgical reduction in size of the nose. SYN: *rhinomeiosis.*

rhinommectomy (rī"nŏm-mĕk'tō-mĭ) ["+ *omma,* eye, + *ektomē,* excision]. Surgical excision of the inner canthus.

rhinomycosis (rī"nō-mĭ-kō'sīs) ["+ *mykēs,* fungus, + *-ōsis,* condition]. Fungi in mucous membranes and secretions of the nose.

rhinonecrosis (rī"nō-nē-krō'sīs) [Gr. *rhis, rhin-,* nose, + *nekrōsis,* death]. Necrosis of the nasal bones.

rhinopathy (ri-nŏp'ă-thĭ) ["+ *pathos,* disease]. Any nasal disease.

rhinopharyngitis (rī"nō-făr-ĭn-jī'tĭs) ["+ *pharynx,* pharynx, + *-itis,* inflammation]. Inflamed condition of the nasopharynx.

rhinopharyngocele (rī"nō-făr-ĭn'gō-sēl) [Gr. *rhis, rhin-,* nose, + *pharynx,* pharynx, + *kēlē,* mass]. A nasopharyngeal tumor.

rhinopharyngolith (rī"nō-făr-ĭn'gō-lĭth) ["+ "+ *lithos,* stone]. Concretion in the nasal pharynx.

rhinopharynx (rī"nō-făr'ĭnks). Upper portion of pharynx continuous with the nasal passages. SYN: *nasopharynx.*

rhinophonia (rī"nō-fō'nĭ-ă) [Gr. *rhis, rhin-,* nose, + *phōnē,* voice]. A nasal tone in speaking.

rhinophyma (rī-nō-fī'mă) ["+ *phyma,* growth]. Lobular hypertrophy of nose, with red coloration, congestion, and retention of sebum. SYM: *acne rosacea.*

rhinoplasty (rī'nō-plăs-tĭ) ["+ *plastos,* formed]. Plastic surgery of the nose.

rhinopolypus (rī"nō-pŏl'ĭ-pŭs) [Gr. *rhis, rhin-,* nose, + *polys,* many, + *pous,* foot]. Polypus of the nose.

rhinorrhagia (rī"nō-rā'jĭ-ă) ["+ *rhēgnynai,* to burst forth]. Profuse hemorrhage from nose. SYN: *epistaxis; nosebleed.*

rhinorrhea (rī"nō-rē'ă) ["+ *rhoia,* a flow]. Thin, watery discharge from nose.

r., cerebrospinal. Discharge of spinal fluid from nose due to defect in cribriform plate.

r., gustatory. Flow of a thin watery material from the nose while eating.

rhinosalpingitis (rī"nō-săl"pĭn-jī'tĭs) [Gr. *rhis, rhin-,* nose, + *salpinx,* tube, + *-itis,* inflammation]. Inflammation of the mucosa of the nose and eustachian tube.

rhinoscleroma (rī"no'-sklĕ-rō'mă) ["+ *sklēros,* hard, + *-ōma,* tumor]. A chronic, infectious disease involving nose and upper portions of respiratory tract in which growths of almost stony hardness develop, sometimes leading to marked deformity.

ETIOL: Klebsiella rhinoscleromatis, a gram-negative encapsulated bacillus.

SYM: The disease presents a hard, nodular growth, which usually begins at anterior end of nose and spreads to the lower respiratory tract. There usually is no pain and no tendency to ulceration.

TREATMENT: Surgical, in combination with streptomycin.

rhinoscope (rī'nō-skōp) ["+ *skopein,* to examine]. Instrument for examination of the nose.

rhinoscopy (ri-nŏs'kō-pĭ). Examination of nasal passages.

r., anterior. Examination through anterior nares.

r., posterior. Examination through posterior nares, usually with small mirror in nasopharynx.

rhinosporidiosis (rī"nō-spō-rīd"ĭ-ō'sīs) [Gr. *rhis, rhin-,* nose, + *sparidion,* little seed, + *-ōsis,* condition]. Condition caused by a fungus, Rhinosporidium seeberi, characterized by development of pedunculated polyps on mucous membranes of nose, larynx, eyes, penis, vagina, and sometimes skin of various parts of body. Disease is contracted from cattle. Found in India, Ceylon, and other parts of the world.

Rhinosporidium (rī″nō-spō-rĭd′ĭ-ŭm). A genus of fungi which is pathogenic to man.

   R. seeberi. Causative agent of rhinosporidiosis, q.v.

rhinostenosis (rī″nō-stĕn-ō′sĭs) [Gr. *rhis, rhin-*, nose, + *stenōsis*, a narrowing]. Obstruction of the nasal passages. SYN: *rhinocleisis.*

rhinotomy (rī-nŏt′ō-mĭ) [″+ *tomē*, incision]. Incision of the nose for drainage purposes.

rhinovaccination (rī″nō-văk-sĭn-ā′shŭn) [″+ L. *vaccinus*, pert. to a cow]. Vaccine applied to the mucosa of the nose.

Rhipicephalus (rī″pĭ-sĕf′ă-lŭs) [Gr. *rhipis*, fan, + *kephalē*, head]. A genus of ticks belonging to the family Ixodidae. Several species, esp. R. sanguineus, serve as vectors for the organisms of spotted fever, boutonneuse fever, and other rickettsial diseases.

rhitidectomy (rĭt″ĭ-dĕk′tō-mĭ) [Gr. *rhytis*, wrinkle, + *ektomē*, excision]. Removal of wrinkles by operation. SYN: *rhytidectomy.*

rhitidosis (rĭt-ĭ-dō′sĭs) [Gr. *rhytidōsis*]. 1. Wrinkling of face without corresponding signs of age. 2. Wrinkling of the cornea, indicating its disintegration. One of the signs of approaching death. SYN: *rhytidosis.*

rhizo- [Gr. *rhiza*]. Combining form meaning root.

rhizodontropy (rī″zō-dŏn′trō-pĭ) [Gr. *rhiza*, root, + *odous, odont-*, tooth, + *tropē*, a turning]. Process of pivoting an artificial crown upon the root of a tooth.

rhizodontrypy (rī″zō-dŏn′trī-pĭ) [″+ ″+ *trypē*, a hole]. Puncture of root of a tooth.

rhizoid (rī′zoyd) [″+ *eidos*, form]. 1. Rootlike. 2. A rootlike structure, usually one-celled, occurring in lower forms of plant life. 3. In bacteriology, term applied to a colony showing an irregular rootlike system of branching.

rhizome (rī′zōm) [Gr. *rhizōma*, mass of roots]. A rootlike stem growing horizontal along or below the ground and sending out roots and shoots. SYN: *rootstalk; rootstock.*

rhizomelic (rī-zō-mĕl′ĭk) [Gr. *rhiza*, root, + *melos*, limb]. Concerning the hip joint and shoulder joint.

Rhizopoda (rī-zŏp′ō-dă) [″+ *pous, pod-*, foot]. A subclass of the class Sarcodina, phylum Protozoa, characterized by possession of lobose pseudopodia and lacking a central

filament. Includes the amebae and foraminifera.

rhizotomy (rī-zŏt′ō-mĭ) [″+ *tomē*, a cutting]. Section of a root, as of a nerve or tooth.

   r., anterior. Section of ventral root of spinal nerve.

   r., posterior. Section of dorsal root of spinal nerve for the relief of pain.

rhodium (rō′dĭ-ŭm). SYMB: Rh. At. wt. 102.905; at. no. 45. A rare metallic element.

rhodo- (rō′dō) [Gr. *rhodon*, rose]. Combining form meaning red.

rhodogenesis (rō″dō-jĕn′ĕ-sĭs) [Gr. *rhodon*, rose, + *genesis*, formation]. Regeneration of visual purple that has been bleached by light.

rhodophane (rō′dō-fān) [″+ *phainein*, to show]. A red pigment found in retinal cones of birds and fishes.

rhodophylaxis (rō″dō-fĭ-lăk′sĭs) [″+ *phylaxis*, protection]. Ability of the retinal epithelium to regenerate visual purple which has been bleached by light.

rhodopsin (rō-dŏp′sĭn) [″+ *opsis*, vision]. Visual purple, a pigment in outer segment of retinal rods.

rhombencephalon (rŏm″bĕn-sĕf′ă-lŏn) [Gr. *rhombos*, rhomb, + *enkephalos*, brain]. [NA] A primary division of the embryonic brain which gives rise to metencephalon and myelencephalon. Includes the pons, cerebellum, and medulla oblongata. SYN: *hindbrain.*

rhombocele (rŏm′bō-sēl) [″+ *koilos*, a hollow]. The cavity of the rhombencephalon.

rhomboid (rŏm′boyd) [″+ *eidos*, shape]. An oblique parallelogram.

   r. fossa, r. sinus. The 4th ventricle of the brain.

rhomboideus (rŏm-bō-ĭd′ĭ-ŭs) [L.]. One of two muscles beneath the trapezius muscle. SEE: *Table of Muscles* in *Appendix; muscles* for illustration.

rhoncal, rhonchial (rŏng′kăl, rŏng′kĭ-ăl) [Gr. *rhonchos*, a snore]. Pert. to, or produced by, a rattle in the throat.

rhonchus (rŏng′kŭs). A rale or rattling in the throat, esp. when it resembles snoring.

rhotacism (rō′tō-sĭzm) [Gr. *rhōtakizein*, to overuse letter "r"]. Overuse or improper utterance of "r" sounds, with too much emphasis upon this letter.

rhubarb (rū′barb) [ME. *rubarbe*]. Extract made from roots and rhizome of Rheum officinale, R. palmatum, and other species. Used as a cathartic and astringent. High in oxalic acid. Of little food value, but desirable for its mineral content.

Food value of 100 gm. (cooked, sugar added): Cal. 141; protein 0.5 gm.; trace of fat; carbohydrate 36 gm; calcium 78 mg.

Rhus (rūs) [L. *rhosis*]. A genus of trees and shrubs, some of which are poisonous, i.e., poison ivy (R. toxicodendron) or poison sumac (R. venenala), and which produce a severe dermatitis.

rhyostomaturia (rī″ō-sto″mă-tū′rĭ-ă) [Gr *rhyas*, fluid, + *stoma*, mouth, + *ouron*, urine]. The elimination of urinary elements by the salivary glands.

rhyparia (rĭ-pā′rĭ-ă) [Gr., filth]. 1. Foul substance which collects in mouth in low fevers. SYN: *sordes*. 2. Filth.

rhypophagy (rĭ-pŏf′ă-jĭ) [Gr. *rhypos*, filth, + *phagein*, to eat]. The eating of filth. SYN: *scatophagy*.

rhypophobia (rī″pō-fō′bĭ-ă) ["+ *phobos*, fear]. Abnormal disgust at the act of defecation, feces, or filth.

rhythm (rĭth′ŭm) [Gr. *rhythmos*, measured motion]. 1. A measured time or movement; regularity of occurrence of action or function. 2. Marking the intermenstrual periods of fertility and sterility in the female. SEE: *cacorhythmic*.

r., alpha. In electroencephalography, rhythmical oscillations in electric potential occurring at a rate of 8 1/2 to 12 per second. SYN: *alpha wave.*

r., atrioventricular nodal. Rhythmic discharge of impulses from atrioventricular (A-V) node which occurs when activity of S-A node is depressed or abolished. If impulses arise in upper or atrial portion of node, the atria are activated slightly before ventricles (*upper nodal rhythm*); if in middle portion, atria and ventricles contract simultaneously (*middle nodal rhythm*); if in lower or ventricular portion, atria are activated slightly before ventricles (*lower nodal rhythm*). SYN: *A-V nodal rhythm.*

r., beta. In electroencephalography, waves ranging in frequency from 15-30/sec. and of lower voltage than alpha waves. More pronounced in frontomotor leads. SYN: *beta waves.*

r., bigeminus. The coupling of extrasystoles with previously normal beats.

r., cantering. Gallop rhythm, q.v.

r., coupled. R. in which every other heartbeat produces no pulse at the wrist.

r., delta. In electroencephalography, slow waves with a frequency of 1/2-3/sec. and of relatively high voltage (20-200 microvolts). May be found over the area of a gross lesion such as a tumor or hemorrhage. SYN: *delta waves.*

r., ectopic. A cardiac r. originating outside S-A node. May be homotropic or heterotropic.

r., gallop. Abnormal heart r. with three sounds in each cycle, resembling gallop of a horse.

r., idioventricular. R. of ventricles occurring in heart block resulting from establishment of a new center of rhythmicity in ventricular myocardium usually in bundle of His.

r. method. A means of preventing conception by avoiding coitus on the days immediately preceding and following expected time of ovulation.

r., nodal. R., atrioventricular nodal, q.v.

r., pendulum. R. with the two heart sounds alike, similar to the sound of a ticking clock.

r., sinus. Normal cardiac r. proceeding from the sinoatrial node.

r., tic-tac. A state of cardiac distress in which the first and second heart sounds are the same quality. SYN: *embryocardia.*

r., ventricular. Very slow ventricular contractions in heart block.

rhyth′mic [Gr. *rhythmos*]. Rhythmical; pert. to, or marked by, rhythm.

rhythmicity (rĭth-mĭs′ĭ-tĭ). Characterized by rhythmic activity.

rhytidectomy (rĭt′ĭ-dek′tō-mĭ) [Gr. *rhytis*, wrinkle, + *ektomē*, excision]. Excision of wrinkles by plastic surgery.

rhytidosis (rĭt′ĭ-do′sĭs) ["+ *-ōsis*, condition]. 1. Wrinkling of the skin. 2. Wrinkling of cornea. Occurs in cases of great diminution in tension of eyeball, particularly after the escape of aqueous or vitreous humor, usually near death. SYN: *rhitidosis.*

rib (rĭb) [AS. *ribb*]. One of a series of 12 pairs of narrow, curved bones extending laterally and anteriorly from sides of thoracic vertebrae and forming a part of the skeletal thorax. With the exception of the floating ribs, they are connected to the sternum by means of costal cartilages.

r., asternal. R., false, q.v.

r., bicipital. Irregular condition resulting from fusion of two ribs, usually involving the first rib.

r., cervical. A supernumerary rib sometimes developing in connection with a cervical vertebra, usually the lowest.

r.'s, false. Five ribs on each side which are not directly attached to the sternum.

r.'s, floating. Two lower ribs not attached to the sternum.

r., lumbar. A rudimentary r. which develops in relation to a lumbar vertebra.

r., sternal. A true rib.

r.'s, true. The upper seven ribs on each side which join the sternum by separate cartilages.

riboflavin (rī″bō-flā′vĭn). USP. A water-soluble vitamin of the B complex group. It is an orange-yellow crystalline powder ($C_{17}H_{20}N_4O_6$), comparatively stable to heat and air but unstable in light. SYN: *lactoflavin; vitamin B_2; vitamin G.*

SOURCES: Milk and milk products, leafy green vegetables, liver, beef, fish, dry yeast. Also synthesized by bacteria in body.

DAILY REQUIREMENT: Adults: 0.55 mg./1000 Cal. of food intake. Infants, children, pregnant and lactating women: require increased amounts.

EFFECTS OF DEFICIENCY: Eye disorders, cheilosis, glossitis, seborrheic dermatitis, esp. of face and scalp.

FUNCTIONS: It is a constituent of certain flavoproteins which function as coenzymes in cellular oxidations. Essential for tissue repair.

ribonuclease (rī″bō-nū′klē-ās). An enzyme which catalyzes the depolymerization of ribonucleic acid (RNA) with formation of mononucleotides. ABBR: RNA-ase.

ribonucleic acid (rī″bō-nū′klē-ĭk). A nucleic acid found principally in the nucleolus, microsomes, and mitochondria of cells. It appears to play an important role in synthetic reactions within cells. ABBR: RNA.

ribose (rī′bōs). $C_5H_{10}O_5$, a pentose sugar present in ribonucleic acids, riboflavin, and some nucleotides.

rice (rīs) [Gr. *oryza*]. 1. A cereal grass (Oryza sativa) raised extensively in warm climates for its seed or grain. 2. The seeds of rice plant widely used as a food.

COMP: Poor in nitrogen and fats, high in carbohydrates. Cellulose is higher than in bread, and residue greater. During cooking, the starch is partly converted into dextrin. Food value of 100 gm. (cooked, parboiled): Cal. 106; protein 2.1 gm; fat 0.1 gm.; carbohydrate 23 gm.; calcium 19 mg.

r., polished. R. which has been milled to produce the white product commercially available in Western countries. This treatment removes the hull which contains the majority of the vitamin B_1.

r. water stools. Those of cholera, resembling water in which rice has been boiled.

ricin (rī″sĭn). A white, amorphous, highly toxic protein (albumin) present in the seed of the castor bean, Ricinus communis.

ricinine (rĭs′ĭn-ēn, -ĭn). A poisonous alkaloid present in the leaves and seeds of castor bean plant, Ricinus communis.

ricinoleic acid. 12-hydroxy-9-octadecenoic acid. An unsaturated hydroxy acid comprising about 80% of fatty acids in the glycerides of castor oil. Has a strong laxative action.

rickets (rĭk′ĕts). A form of osteomalacia in children. Results from deficient deposition of lime salts in developing cartilage and newly formed bone, causing abnormalities in shape and structure of bones. SYN: *avitaminosis D; rachitis.*

ETIOL: Due primarily to vitamin D deficiency which affects the absorption of calcium and phosphorus from the intestine and the reabsorption of phosphorus by the renal tubules. May also result from inadequate intake or excessive loss of calcium.

SYM: Restlessness and slight fever at night (101-102° F. or 38.3-38.9° C.); free perspiration about head; diffuse soreness and tenderness of body; pallor; slight diarrhea; enlargement of liver and spleen; delayed dentition and eruption of badly formed teeth; head large and more or less square in outline; craniotabes or skull bones often so thin they crackle like parchment.

Sides of thorax flattened; sternum prominent; nodules can be felt at sternal end of ribs, forming rachitic rosary. Deformity may be kyphosis, lordosis, or scoliosis. Liver and spleen may be considerably enlarged; long bones are curved and prominent at their extremities.

PROG: Serum phosphatase studies are helpful in making diagnosis and prognosis. Usually favorable. Deformity disappears in 90% of cases.

PROPHYLAXIS AND TREATMENT: *Prevention:* Exposure to ultraviolet light (sunlight or artificial light) and administration of vitamin D in quantities to provide 400 I.U. of vitamin D activity per day.

Active rickets: Careful regulation of diet to meet nutritive requirements of the child, plus administration of 2200 I.U. of vitamin D per day usually is effective. Some bone deformities may require surgery.

CAUTION: Excessive use of vitamin D (in infants, over 20,000 I.U. daily; in adults over 100,000 I.U. daily) is to be avoided because of danger of hypervitaminosis D.

r., renal. A disturbance in epiphyseal growth during childhood due to severe chronic renal insufficiency resulting in persistent acidosis. Dwarfism and failure of gonadal development result. Prognosis is poor. SYN: *renal osteitis fibrosa generalisata.*

TREATMENT: Diet low in meat, milk, cheese, and egg yolk. Administration of calcium lactate or calcium gluconate in large doses.

Rickettsia (rĭ-kĕt′sĭ-ă). [Howard T. Ricketts, Amer. pathologist, 1871-1910]. Generic name applied to a group of microorganisms, family Rickettsiaceae, order Rickettsiales, which occupy a position intermediate between viruses and bacteria. They differ from bacteria in that they are obligate parasites requiring living cells for growth, and differ from viruses in that they are retained by the Berkefeld filter. They are the causative agents of many diseases, and are usually transmitted by arthropods (lice, fleas, ticks, mites) which serve as vectors. SEE: *rickettsial disease, rickettsiosis.*

rickettsia (rĭ-kĕt′sĭ-ă). (pl. *rickett′siae*) Term applied to any of the microorganisms belonging to the genus Rickettsia, q.v.

rickettsial disease. A disease caused by an organism of the genus Rickettsia. The most common types are spotted-fever group (Rocky Mt. spotted fever, rickettsialpox); epidemic typhus, endemic typhus, Brill's disease; Q fever; scrub typhus; trench fever.

rickettsialpox (rĭ-ket′sĭ-ăl-pŏks″). An acute, febrile, self-limited disease caused by Rickettsia akari. It is transmitted from mouse to man by a small colorless mite, Allodermaanyssus sanguineus.

rickettsiosis (rĭ-kĕt″sĭ-ō′sĭs). Infection with rickettsiae.

riders′ bone (rī′derz). Bony formation in adductor muscle of leg. Seen in those who ride horses extensively. SYN: *cavalry bone.*

riders′ leg, riders′ sprain. Sprain of adductor muscles of the thigh.

ridge (rĭj) [ME. *rigge*]. An elongated projecting structure or crest.

   r., carotid. A sharp ridge between carotid canal and jugular fossa.

   r., epicondylic. One of two ridges for muscular attachments on the humerus.

   r., gastrocnemial. A ridge on posterior femoral surface for attachment of gastrocnemius muscles.

   r., genital. R. which develops on ventromedian surface of urogenital r. and gives rise to gonads.

   r., gluteal. A r. extending obliquely downward from great trochanter of femur for the attachment of the gluteus maximus muscle.

   r., interosseous. A r. on the fibula for attachment of the interosseous membrane.

   r., mesonephric. R. which develops on lateral surface of urogenital r. and gives rise to mesonephros.

   r., pronator. Oblique r. on the anterior surface of ulna, giving attachment to the pronator quadratus.

   r., pterygoid. R. at angle of junction of temporal and infratemporal surface of great wing of the sphenoid bone.

   r., superciliary, r., supraorbital. Curved r. of the frontal bone over supraorbital arch.

   r., supracondylar. One of two ridges (lateral and medial) on distal end of humerus extending upward from lateral to medial epicondyles.

   r., tentorial. R. on upper inner surface of the cranium to which is attached the tentorium.

   r., trapezoid. An oblique r. on the upper surface of the clavicle giving attachment to the trapezoid ligament.

   r., urogenital. R. on dorsal wall of coelom which gives rise to genital and mesonephric ridges, q.v. SYN: *urogenital fold; wolffian ridge.*

   r., wolffian. R., mesonephric, q.v.

ridgel, ridgil, ridgeling, ridgling (rĭj′ĕl, -ĭl, -ĭng). A male human being or animal with only one testicle, or only one descended testicle.

Riedel's lobe (rē′dĕl). [Bernhard M.C.L. Riedel, Ger. surgeon, 1846-1916] A tongue-shaped process of liver, frequently found protruding over gallbladder in cases of chronic cholecystitis.

rifampin. An antibiotic synthesized from natural rifamycin which in turn is produced by fermentation of Streptomyces mediterranei. It is used in treating Mycobacterium tuberculosis and carriers of Neisseria meningitidis.

Riga-Fede's disease (rē′gă, fā′dā). [Antonio Riga, It. physician, 1832-1919; Francesco Fede, It. physician, 1832-1913] Ulceration of frenum of the tongue with membrane formation. Occurs after abrasion by the lower central incisors.

right (rīt) [AS. *riht*]. Dexter. Pert. to the side of the body in which the liver normally is located. ABBR: R; rt.

right-handed. Voluntary preference for use of the right hand.

rigid (rĭj′ĭd) [L. *rigidus*]. Stiff, hard, unyielding.

rigidity (rĭ-jĭd′ĭ-tĭ). 1. Tenseness; immovability; stiffness; inability to bend or be bent. 2. In psychiatry, refers to one who is excessively resistant to change.

   r., cadaveric. Rigor mortis.

   r., cerebellar. Stiffness of body and extremities resulting from lesion of middle lobe of cerebellum.

r., cogwheel. Condition noted upon passively stretching a hypertonic muscle in which resistance is jerky.

r., decerebrate. Sustained contraction of extensor muscles of limbs resulting from a lesion in the brain stem between superior colliculi and vestibular nuclei.

rigor (rĭg'ŭr) [L. *rigor*, stiffness]. 1. A sudden, paroxysmal chill with high temperature, called the cold stage, followed by a sense of heat and profuse perspiration, called the hot stage. 2. A state of hardness and stiffness, as in a muscle. Rigor chills may be coarse, fine, diffuse, trembling.

r. mortis. The stiffness seen in corpses. SEE: *dead; Nysten's law.*

rima (rī'mă) [L., a slit]. (pl. *rimae*) [NA] A slit, fissure, or crack.

r. cornea'lis. Groove in the sclera holding edge of the cornea. SYN: *corneal cleft.*

r. glottidis. [NA] An elongated slit between the vocal folds.

r. oris. [NA] Aperture of the mouth.

r. palpebrarum. [NA] Slit between the eyelids.

r. pudendi. [NA] Space between the labia majora through which uretha and vagina open. SYN: *pudendal slit; urogenital cleft; vulval slit.*

r. respiratoria. Space behind the arytenoid cartilages.

r. vestibuli. [NA] Space between the false vocal cords. SYN: *glottis spuria.*

r. vocalis. R. glottidis, q.v.

rimose (rī'mōs, rī-mōs') [L. *rimōsus*]. Fissured or marked by cracks.

rimous (rī'mŭs). Filled with cracks or fissures. SYN: *rimose.*

rimula (rĭm'ū-lă) [L.]. (pl. *rim'ulae*) A minute fissure or slit, esp. of the spinal cord or brain.

rind (rĭnd) [AS.]. A thick or firm outer coating of an organ, plant, animal, etc.

r. tumor. Neoplasm arising from lining membrane tissue of the embryo. SYN: *lepidoma.*

ring (rĭng) [AS. *hring*]. 1. Any round organ or band around a circular opening. SEE: *annulus.* 2. In bacteriology, a growth like a ring around upper margin of a liquid culture, adhering to the glass more or less closely.

r, abdominal. SEE: *abdominal rings.*

r., ciliary. Portion of ciliary body consisting of a bandlike zone lying directly anterior to ora serrata. SYN: *orbicularis ciliaris.*

r., femoral. The superior aperture of femoral canal.

r., inguinal, abdominal. The abdominal opening of the inguinal canal. SYN: *internal abdominal ring.*

r., inguinal, subcutaneous. The external opening of inguinal canal. SYN: *external abdominal ring.*

r., removal of, from swollen finger Technique for removal of ring from an injured or swollen finger. Pass one end of a length of string under the ring. Push the ring as far away from the swollen area toward the hand as is possible; wrap the string on the side of the swollen area around the finger for a dozen turns or so. Grasp the end of the string which extends under the ring and while holding it firmly unwind the string from the hand side of the ring. This will move the ring toward the free end of the finger. Continue this until the ring is free.

r., tympanic. A r. of bone formed by three elements (squamous, petromastoid, and tympanic); develops into tympanic plate.

Ringer's solution (rĭng'er). [Sydney Ringer, Eng. physiologist, 1835-1910] USP. An aqueous solution containing 8.6 gm. sodium chloride, 0.3 gm. potassium chloride, 0.33 gm. calcium chloride per liter.

ringworm (rĭng'wŭrm). A dermatomycosis due to various species of fungi belonging to the genera Microsporum and Trichophyton.

Ringworm of the scalp is called tinea capitis; of the body, tinea corporis; of the beard, tinea barbae; of the nails, tinea unguium. SEE: *tinea.*

SYM: Red-ringed patch of vesicles, itching, pain, scaling.

TREATMENT: Griseofulvin may be helpful in certain types. At the same time,

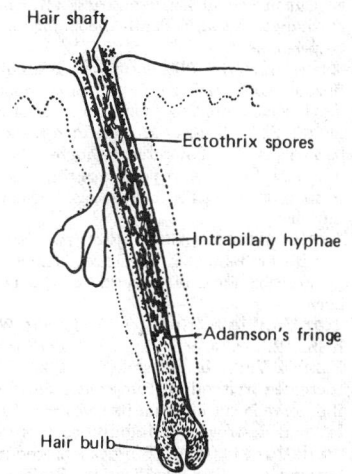

Hair shaft

Ectothrix spores

Intrapilary hyphae

Adamson's fringe

Hair bulb

RINGWORM OF HAIR

treatment with topical fungistatic preparations is important.

r., crusted. SYN: *favus; tinea favosa,* q.v.

r., honeycomb. SEE: *tinea favosa.*

Rinne's test (rĭn'nĕh). [Heinrich A. Rinne, Ger. otologist, 1819-68] Use of tuning fork to compare bone conduction hearing with air conduction. The vibrating fork is held by its stem on the mastoid process of the ear until it is no longer heard by the patient. Then it is held close to the external auditory meatus. If the subject still hears the vibrations this is called a *positive Rinne test.*

If the fork is not heard by air conduction the test is repeated; but first air conduction is tested until the sound is no longer heard, then the stem of the fork is placed on the mastoid process of the ear. If the sound is still heard, this is called a *negative Rinne test.*

Riolan (rē"ō-lahn'). [Jean Riolan, Fr. anatomist, 1580-1657].

R.'s arch. Arch formed by the mesentery of the transverse colon.

R.'s bouquet. Two ligaments and three muscles attached to styloid process of temporal bone.

R.'s muscle. Ciliary portion of orbicularis oculi. SYN: *musculus ciliaris.*

ripa (rī'pă) [L., bank]. Any line of reflection of the ependyma of the brain from the ventricular wall to the choroid plexus.

Ripault's sign (rē-pō'). [Louis H.A. Ripault, Fr. physician, 1807-56] Change in shape of pupil produced by unilateral (external) pressure upon eyeball. During life it is a transitory change, but after death the change may be permanent.

risorius (rī-sŏ'rĭ-ŭs) [L., laughing]. Muscular fibrous band arising over masseter muscle and inserted into tissues at the corner of the mouth. SEE: *Table of Muscles* in *Appendix.*

risus (rī'sŭs) [L.]. Laughter; a laugh.

r. sardonicus. A peculiar grin, as seen in tetanus, caused by acute spasm of facial muscles.

Ritter's disease (rĭt'ĕr). [Gottfried Ritter von Rittershain, Ger. physician, 1820-83] A generalized form of impetigo of the newborn.

Ritter-Valli law (rĭt"ĕr, văl'ī). [Johann Wilhelm Ritter, Ger. physicist, 1776-1810; Eusebio Valli, It. physiologist, 1726-1810] Increased irritability from center outward, if a nerve is cut off from its center or if the latter is destroyed. Irritability soon is lost.

ritualistic surgery. Surgical procedures without scientific justification. Performed in primitive societies without direction toward treatment or prevention of disease. Included in this are alterations of the skin, ears, lips, teeth, genitalia, and head.

In some cases, even in nonprimitive societies, surgical procedures without rational justification are considered to be ritualistic.

ri'valry strife. Alternate sensations of color and shape when the fields of vision of the two eyes cannot combine in one visual image.

Rivinus canals or ducts (rē-vē'nŭs). [August Quirinus Rivinus, Ger. anatomist, 1652-1723] Ducts of sublingual gland.

Rivinus' glands. Sublingual glands.

Rivinus' ligament. Small portion of the drum membrane in notch of Rivinus. SYN: *Shrapnell's membrane.*

riziform (rĭz'ĭ-form) [Fr. *riz,* rice, + *forma,* form]. Resembling rice grains.

RLF. Abbr. for *retrolental fibroplasia,* q.v.

RLQ. Abbr. for *right lower quadrant* (of abdomen).

R. M. A. Abbr. for *right mentoanterior presentation* (of the fetal face).

R. M. P. Abbr. for *right mentoposterior presentation* (of the fetal face).

R. N. Abbr. for *registered nurse.*

RNA. Abbr. for *ribonucleic acid,* q.v.

RNA, messenger. Ribonucleic acid which carries information from the nucleus to cytoplasmic sites.

RNA, transfer. Ribonucleic acid which reacts with and carries an activated amino acid to participate in the manufacture of a protein molecule.

Robertson's pupil. Argyll Robertson pupil, q.v.

roborant (rŏb'ō-rănt) [L. *roborans,* strengthening]. 1. A tonic. 2. Strengthening.

Rochelle salt (rō-shĕl'). Potassium sodium tartrate; a colorless, transparent powder having a cooling and saline taste.

ACTION AND USES: Saline cathartic.

Rocky Mountain spotted fever. An infectious disease caused by a parasite, Rickettsia rickettsii, and transmitted by a wood tick; marked by fever, pains in bones and muscles, and profuse reddish eruption. Occurs in the Rocky Mountains and on the Pacific Coast. Mortality is no longer high because of prompt diagnosis and treatment. SEE: *spotted fever; tick fever.*

rod (rŏd) [AS. *rodd,* club]. 1. Slender, straight bar. 2. One of the slender, long sensory bodies in retina responding to faint light. 3. Bacterium shaped like a rod.

r.'s and cones. The light-sensitive portions of rod and cone visual cells of the retina. They form the 2nd layer lying between external limiting membrane and pigment epithelium. The rods contain visual purple (rhodopsin), essential for vision in dim light.

r.'s, enamel. Minute calcareous rods or prisms laid down by ameloblasts and forming enamel of a tooth.

rodenticide (rō-děn'tĭ-sīd) [L. *rōdens*, gnawing, + *caedere*, to kill]. An agent which kills rodents.

rodent ulcer (rō'děnt) ["+ *ulcus*, ulcer]. A slowly-growing, gnawing cancer which slowly destroys soft tissues and bones, causing great destruction. Usual sites are on outer angle of the eye, near side and on tip of nose, and on edges of the scalp. SEE: *ulcer, rodent.*

rodonalgia (rō-dō-năl'jĭ-ă) [Gr. *rhodon,* rose, + *algos*, pain]. Vasomotor condition marked by redness and neuralgic pain of the extremities, swelling, and fever. SYN: *erythromelalgia.*

Roentgen (rěnt'gĕn). [Wilhelm Konrad Roentgen, Ger. physicist, 1845-1923]. Discovered roentgen rays in 1895, won the Nobel prize in physics in 1901.

roentgen (rěnt'gĕn). An obsolete unit of roentgen radiation.

roentgenogram (rěnt-gĕn'ō-grăm). Film produced by roentgenography.

roentgenography (rěnt'gĕn-ŏg'rä-fĭ) [roentgen, + Gr. *graphein*, to write]. The process of obtaining pictures by use of roentgen rays.

roentgenologist (rěnt''gĕn-ōl'ō-jĭst) ["+ Gr. *logos,* study]. A physician skilled in roentgen diagnosis, roentgen therapy, or both.

roentgenology (rěnt''gĕn-ōl'ō-jĭ). The science of applying roentgen rays for diagnostic and therapeutic purposes.

roentgenotherapy, roentgentherapy (rěnt''gĕn-ō-thĕr'ăp-ĭ, rěnt''gĕn-thĕr'ä-pĭ) [roentgen, + Gr. *therapeia,* treatment]. The treatment of disease by exposure of the patient to roentgen rays.

roentography (rěn-tŏg'rä-fĭ) ["+ Gr. *graphein,* to write]. The making of x-ray pictures. SYN: *roentgenography, skiagraphy.*

roeteln, roetheln (rět'ĕln) [Ger.]. German measles, q.v. SYN: *rubella.*

Rokitansky's disease (rō''kĭ-tăn'skĭ). [Karl Freiherr von Rokitansky, Austrian pathologist, 1804-1878]. Acute yellow atrophy of the liver.

Rolan'do's area. [Luigi Rolando, It. anatomist, 1773-1831]. Motor area in the cerebral cortex.

Rolando's fissure. Fissure between parietal and frontal lobes. SYN: *sulcus centralis.*

role (rōl) [O. Fr. *rolle,* roll of paper on which a part is written]. The characteristic and expected social behavior of an individual in relationship to the group.

r. playing. Using drama as a therapeutic means of understanding and treating emotional conflicts.

roller (rōl'er) [O. Fr., roll]. 1. Strip of muslin on other cloth rolled up in cylinder form for surgeon's use. 2. A roller bandage. SEE: *bandage.*

romaine (rō-mān') [Fr., Roman]. A leafy vegetable in the lettuce family. SYN: *cos; cos lettuce.*

    Food value of 100 gm.; Cal. 18; protein 1.3 gm.; calcium 68 mg.; potassium 264 mg.; vitamin A, 1900 I.U.

Roman numerals. Those used by the Romans in contradistinction to the Arabic numerals which we now use. In Roman notations values are increased either by adding one or more symbols to the initial symbol, as III for 3, or by subtracting a symbol from one or more to the right of it, as IV for 4, IX for 9, etc. SEE: *Roman numerals* in *Appendix.*

romanopexy (rō-măn'ō-pěk''sĭ) [L. *romanum,* the sigmoid, + Gr. *pēxis,* fixation]. Fixation of the sigmoid flexure for prolapse of the rectum. SYN: *sigmoidopexy.*

romanoscope (rō-măn'ō-skōp) ["+ Gr. *skopein,* to examine]. Instrument for examining the sigmoid flexure.

Romberg's sign (rŏm'bŭrg). [Maritz Heinrich Romberg, Ger. physician, 1795-1873]. Inability to maintain the body balance when the eyes are shut and the feet close together. Seen in tabes dorsalis, severe alcoholic neuritis, etc.

rongeur (rŏ-zhŭr') [Fr., to gnaw]. A gouge forceps, an instrument for removing tiny fragments of bone.

roof nucleus. Small mass of gray matter in white substance of vermis of the cerebellum. SYN: *nucleus fastigii* [NA].

rooming-in. The placing of infants in the same hospital room as their mothers, beginning immediately following birth.

room, clean. A room, particularly one housing delicate electronic medical instruments, which is constructed so as to be isolated from the free entry of air. Air entering is filtered, and personnel wear special clothing to prevent particles from their body becoming freely dispersed in the room.

room, dustfree. A type of room designed to eliminate or reduce particulate matter, including airborne microorganisms, from circulating. This kind of room is useful in housing burn patients, removing allergens from the air, in transplantation surgery, and in preparing drugs and solutions for intravenous use.

root (rŭt) [AS. *rōt*]. 1. The underground part of a plant. Ex: Stillingia; glycyrrhiza; belladonna. 2. Proximal end of a nerve. 3. Portion of an organ implanted in tissues.

   r., anterior. One of two roots by which a spinal nerve is attached to spinal cord. Contains efferent nerve fibers. SYN: *motor root; ventral root.*

   r. arteries. Arteries accompanying nerve roots into the spinal cord. SYN: *radicular vessels.*

   r. canal. Pulp cavity of root of tooth.

   r., posterior. One of two roots by which a spinal nerve is attached to spinal cord. Contains afferent nerve fibers. SYN: *dorsal root; sensory root.*

   r. resorption of teeth. Condition of the roots of teeth caused by endocrine imbalance or excessive pressure of orthodontic appliances. X-ray photographs demonstrate roots which appear to be sawed off or shortened. SYN: *blunting of the roots.*

   r. sheath. Epithelium covering the hair follicle.

   r. zone. Burdach's column of the spinal cord. Outer tract of posterior funiculus or white column of the cord. SYN: *fasciculus cuneatus.*

R. O. P. Abbr. for *right occipitoposterior* presentation, i.e., the occiput of fetus being in relationship to the right sacroiliac joint of the mother.

rosa (rō'ză) [L.]. Rose.

   r. asturica. Deficiency disease due to lack of vitamin B_2. SYN: *pellagra,* q.v.

rosacea (rō-zā'sĭ-ă) [L. *rosaceus,* rosy]. A syndrome of unknown cause associated with varying degrees of papules, pustules, and hyperplasia of the sebaceous glands. Predominantly on the nose, face, and chin. The onset is usually between 30 and 50 years of age but may be as early as 10 or occur first in old age. In adults it occurs three times as often in females as in males.

   TREATMENT: Symptomatic. Tetracyclines in small doses may help. If sunlight makes the disease worse, chloroquine for six weeks should be tried. Firm massage, using a bland oil as a lubricant, repeatedly moving the fingers from the nose to the edge of the face for five to ten minutes each evening, is the single most effective measure.

rose cold. Summer or June cold; hay fever of early summer attributed to inhaling rose pollen. SYN: *rose fever.* SEE: *hay fever.*

Rosenbach's sign (rō'zĕn-bŏk). [Ottomar Rosenbach, Ger. physician, 1851-1907]. Absence of abdominal skin reflex in intestinal inflammation.

Rosenmüller's body (rō'zĕn-mĭl''ĕr). [Johann Christian Rosenmüller, Ger. anatomist, 1771-1820]. Rudimentary tubule in the mesosalpinx between the fallopian tube and ovary. SYN: *epoophoron; parovarium.*

Rosenmüller's cavity, Rosenmüller's fossa. Slitlike depression in the pharyngeal wall behind opening of the eustachian tube.

roseo- [L. *roseus,* rosy]. 1. Combining form meaning rose-colored. 2. A prefix in chemical terms.

roseola (rō-zē'ō-lă) [L. *roseus,* rosy]. 1. Skin condition marked by maculae or red spots of varying sizes on the skin; a rose-colored rash. 2. Measles or German measles. SYN: *rose rash.*

   r. idiopathica. Macular eruptions not associated with any well-defined symptoms.

   r. infantum. A noninfectious roseola occurring in infants. Characterized by high fever, splenomegaly, and a rash which appears just as the fever subsides. SYN: *exanthem subitum.*

   r. symptomatica. Macular eruption occurring in well-defined diseases.

roseolous (rō-zē'ō-lŭs) [L. *roseus,* rosy]. Resembling or pert. to roseola.

rose rash. Any red-colored eruption. SYN: *roseola.*

rosette [Fr., small rose]. 1. Something that resembles a rose. 2. A spherical group of fine red vacuoles surrounding cytocentrum of a monocyte.

rose water. Saturated aqueous solution of the oil of rose. Used to impart agreeable odor to lotions, etc.

rosin (rŏz'ĭn) [L. *resina*]. Substance distilled from oil of turpentine and used as adhesive and stimulant on plasters.

Rossbach's disease (rŏs'bŏk). [Michael Josef Rossback, Ger. physician, 1842-1899]. Excessive secretion of gastric acid. SYN: *gastroxynsis; hyperchlorhydria.*

Ross' bodies. [Edward Halford Ross, Eng. pathologist]. Copper-colored, round bodies showing dark granules. Found in blood and tissue fluids in syphilis. Sometimes they exhibit ameboid movements.

Rossolimo's reflex (rŏs''ō-lē'mō). [Gregorij I. Rossolimo, Russian neurologist, 1860-1928]. Plantar flexion of 2nd to 5th toes in response to percussion of plantar surface of the toes.

rostellum (rŏs-tĕl'lŭm) [L., little beak]. (pl. *rostel'la*) A fleshy protrusion on anterior end of scolex of tapeworms bearing one or more rows of spines or hooks.

rostral (rŏs'trăl) [L. *rostralis*]. 1. Resembling a beak. 2. Toward the front or cephalic end of the body.

rostrate (rŏs'trāt) [L. *rostratus*, beaked]. Having a beak or hook formation.

rostrum (rŏs'trŭm) [L., beak]. (pl. *ros'trums, ros'tra*) Any hooked or beaked structure.

rosulate (rŏs'ū-lāt) [L. *rosulatus*, like a rose]. Shaped like a rosette.

rot (rŏt) [ME. *roten*]. To decay or decompose.

   r., jungle. Common term for certain fungus diseases of the skin which occur in the tropics.

rotate (rō'tāt) [L. *rotāre*, to turn]. To twist or revolve.

rotation (rō-tā'shŭn) [L. *rotatio*, a turning]. Process of turning on an axis.

   r., fetal. Twisting of the fetal head as it follows the curves of the birth canal downward.

rotator (rō-tā'tōr). (pl. *rotatores*) A muscle revolving a part on its axis.

röteln, rötheln (rĕt'ĕln) [Ger. *rot*, red]. German measles. SYN: *roeteln; rubella.*

Rouget's cells (rū-zhā'). [Charles M.B. Rouget, Fr. physiologist, 1824-1904]. Contractile cells which surround the capillaries, observed in frogs and salamanders.

roughage (rŭf'ĭj) [AS. *rūh*, rough]. Indigestible fiber of fruits, vegetables, and cereals which acts as a stimulant to aid intestinal peristalsis. Plenty of water should be added to consumption of roughage. Should not be used in colitis or in intestinal irritation. SEE: *cellulose.*

   r. diet. Diet with large amounts of cellulose, water, mineral salts, and vitamins. SYN: *high residue diet.*

rouleau (rū-lō') [Fr., roll]. (pl. *rouleaux*) A group of red blood corpuscles arranged like a roll of coins.

round (rownd) [O. Fr. *ronde*]. 1. Circular in shape. 2. Spherical, globular.

   r. ligament. 1. Curved fibrous cord attached to center of articular surface of head of femur. 2. Two round cordlike structures passing from front of the body of the uterus in anterior wall of broad ligament, below the fallopian tubes, outward through the inguinal canals to soft tissues of the labia majora. 3. Fibrous cord which is the remnant of umbilical vein.

roundworm. Any member of the phylum Nemathelminthes (Aschelminthes), esp. one belonging to the class Nematoda, q.v. SYN: *threadworm.*

Routes of medication. SEE: *medication routes.*

RPF. Abbr. for *renal plasma flow.*

rpm. Abbr. for *revolutions per minute.*

RPS. Abbr. for *renal pressor substance.* SEE: *renin.*

R. Q. Abbr. for *respiratory quotient.*

-rrhagia (rā'jĭ-ā) [Gr. *rhēgnynai*, to burst forth]. Combining form indicating abnormal discharge, hemorrhage.

R.S.A. Abbr. for *right sacroanterior* position of fetus.

R.S.P. Abbr. for *right sacroposterior* presentation of fetus.

R.T. Abbr. for *reading test; registered technician.*

R.U. Abbr. for *rat unit.*

Ru. Chem. symbol for ruthenium.

rubber-dam. Thin rubber tissue used by dentists to seal off the tooth during dental treatment from saliva in the mouth.

rubedo (rū-bē'dō) [L.]. Temporary redness of the skin. SYN: *blushing.*

rubefacient (rū'bŭ-fā'shĕnt) [L. *rubefaciēns*, making red]. 1. Causing redness, as of the skin. 2. Agent which reddens the skin producing a local congestion, the vessels becoming dilated and the supply of blood increased. Rubefacients include mustard, turpentine, capsicum, flaxseed, arnica, and liniments.

rubella (rū-bĕl'lă) [L. *rubellus*, reddish]. Acute infectious disease resembling both scarlet fever and measles, but differing from these in its short course, slight fever, and freedom from sequelae. SYN: *German measles; röteln; three-day measles.*

   INCUBATION: 14-21 days. R. produces a maculopapular rash that vanishes by slight desquamation in from two to three days.

   SYM: Prodromes, slight or altogether absent. Drowsiness, slight fever, sore throat. Eruption 1st or 2nd day. In some cases rash composed of pale red, scarcely elevated papules, more or less discrete rubella morbilliforme; in others rash is bright red and diffuse like that of scarlet fever, rubella scarlatiniforme. Rash begins on face, spreads rapidly over whole body, but fades so rapidly that face may be clear before extremities are affected. Slight desquamation frequently present, though not always. Superficial cervical and posterior auricular glands more swollen than in measles. Duration, 3 to 5 days.

   COMPLICATIONS: R. in pregnant women, esp. in first two or three months of gestation, is serious in that it may give rise to fetal anomalies, esp. congenital cataract.

   PROG: Good.

   TREATMENT: Nonspecific. Local antipruritics for itching; rest; liquid diet; sponging with tepid water.

rubeola (rū-bē'ō-lă) [L., reddish]. 1. Acute, contagious disease, marked by fever, catarrhal symptoms, and a typical cutaneous eruption. SYN: *measles*. 2. Term occasionally applied to acute infectious disease with mild symptoms and rose-colored macular eruption. SYN: *rubella*, q.v.

rubeosis iridis. Vascularization of the iris associated with vascular disease which affects the retinal vein of the eye. Leads to painful, hemorrhagic glaucoma.

rubescent (rū-bĕs'ĕnt) [L. *rubescere*, to grow red]. Growing red; flushing.

rubidium (rū-bĭd'ĭ-ŭm) [L. *rubidus*, red]. SYMB: *Rb*. At. wt. 85.47; at. no. 37. A soft, silvery metal which decomposes water with violence and bursts into flame spontaneously in air. Its salts are used medicinally.

rubiginous (rū-bĭj'ĭ-nŭs) [L. *rubīginōsus*]. Rusty or rust-colored.

rubigo (rū-bī'gō) [L. rust]. Rust; mildew.

Rubin's test (rū'bĭn). [Isidor Clinton Rubin, Amer. physician, 1883-1958]. Transuterine insufflation with carbon dioxide of the fallopian tubes to test their patency. SEE: *sterility*.

rubor (rū'bōr) [L.]. Discoloration or redness caused by inflammation. One of the classical symptoms of inflammation. RS: calor; dolor; tumor.

rubrospinal (rū"brō-spī'năl) [L. *ruber*, red, + *spina*, thorn]. A descending tract consisting of a small bundle of nerve fibers in lateral funiculus of spinal cord. Fibers arise in cells of the red nucleus of midbrain and terminate in ventral horn of gray matter.

rubrum (rū'brŭm) [L., red]. Reddish nucleus of gray matter in crus cerebri near optic thalamus.

    r. scarlatinum. Scarlet red, a substance used as a healing agent and stain.

ructus (rŭk'tŭs) [L.]. Belching of air from stomach. SYN: *eructation.*

rudiment (rū'dĭ-mĕnt [L. *rudimentum*, beginning]. 1. That which is undeveloped. 2. In biology, a part just beginning to develop. 3. An organ arrested in an early stage of development. 4. Remains of a part functional only at an earlier stage of an individual or in his ancestors.

rudimentary (rū"dĭ-mĕn'tă-rĭ). 1. Elementary. 2. Undeveloped; not fully formed; remaining from an earlier stage. SYN: *vestigial.*

Ruffini's corpuscles (rū-fē'nē). [Angelo Ruffini, It. anatomist, 1864-1929]. Encapsulated sensory nerve endings found in subcutaneous tissue, thought to mediate sense of warmth.

rufous (rū'fŭs) [L. *rufus,* red]. Ruddy; having a ruddy complexion and reddish hair.

ruga (rū'gă) [L.]. (pl. *ru'gae*) A fold or crease, esp. one of the folds of mucous membrane seen on internal surface of stomach.

    r. of the vagina. Small ridges on inner surface of vagina extending laterally and upward from the columna rugarum (long ridges on anterior and posterior walls). SYN: *rugae vaginales* [NA].

Ruggeri's reflex. Increase in pulse rate when eyes are strongly converged on a near object.

rugose, rugous (rū'gōs, -gŭs) [L. *rūgōsus*, wrinkled]. Having many wrinkles or creases. SYN: *corrugated.*

rugosity (rū-gŏs'ĭ-tĭ) [L. *rūgōsitas*]. 1. Condition of being folded or wrinkled. 2. A ridge or wrinkle.

R.U.L. Abbr. for *right upper lobe* of lung.

rule (rūl) [ME. *riule*]. A guide or principle based on experience or observation.

rumination (rū"mĭ-nā'shŭn) [L. *rūminatiō*]. 1. Regurgitation, esp. with rechewing, of previously swallowed food. 2. In psychiatry, obsessional preoccupation of mind by a single idea or a set of thoughts, and inability to dismiss or dislodge them.

rump (rŭmp) [ME. *rumpe*]. Posterior end of the back, the gluteal region or buttocks.

Rumpf's symptom (rŭmpf). [Heinrich Theodor Rumpf, Ger. physician, 1851–]. 1. In neurasthenia, quickening of the pulse when pressure is exerted over a painful spot. 2. Twitching after strong faradization, in traumatic neuroses.

run [AS. *rinnan*, run]. To exude pus or mucus.

runaround, runround. Superficial infection encircling the fingernail. SYN: *felon; paronychia; whitlow.*

rupia (rū'pĭ-ă) [Gr. *rhypos*, filth]. A cutaneous eruption, usually of tertiary syphilis, which manifests itself at first by large elevations of the epidermis filled with a clear or blood-stained serum, soon becoming turbid and purulent. The bulla bursts and allows some fluid to escape. As it desiccates it is covered with a crust which dries, accumulates new layers, and becomes covered with greenish-brown scales, sometimes to depth of 1/2 in. (13 mm.). Thickest of all syphilides and presents most extensive ulcerations.

    TREATMENT: Constitutional, antisyphilitics.

rupophobia (rū"pō-fō'bĭ-ă) ["+ *phobos,* fear]. Abnormal dislike for dirt or filth. SYN: *rhypophobia.*

rupture (rŭp'chŭr) [L. *ruptūra*, breaking]. 1. A breaking apart of an organ or tissue. 2. Hernia, q.v.

r. of membranes. R. of amniotic sac as normal result of dilation of the cervix uteri in labor.

r. of perineum. R. of perineum in labor, a condition the obstetrician seeks to avoid. More frequent in primiparae.

r. of tubes. R. of a fallopian tube, a serious event in extrauterine pregnancy. May occur without the woman's knowledge of her pregnancy.

r. of uterus. Rare r., and due to unrelieved obstructed labor.

RUQ. Abbr. for *right upper quadrant* of abdomen.

Russell's bodies (rŭs'ĕl). [William Russell, Eng. physician, 1852-1940]. Hyaline, small, spherical bodies in cancerous and simple inflammatory growths.

Russian bath. Hot vapor bath followed by friction and plunge in cold water.

rusts. Members of an order of parasitic fungi (Uredinales), all of which are parasitic on plants. Many are allergens.

Rust's disease (rŭst). [Johann N. Rust, Ger. surgeon, 1775-1840]. Tuberculosis of cervical vertebrae and their articulations.

rusty (rŭst'ĭ) [AS. *rustig*]. Reddish in color. Resembling, or containing, rust. SYN: *rubiginous.*

r. sputum. Reddish sputum expectorated in pneumonia.

rut (rŭt) [O. Fr. *ruit,* roaring of deer]. Seasonal period of sexual excitement in lower animals during which ovulation and mating usually take place. SYN: *estrus; heat.*

rutabaga (rū"tā-bā'gă) [Swedish *rotabagge*]. A large variety of turnip.

Food value of 100 gm. (cooked, boiled): Cal. 35; protein 0.9 gm.; trace of fat; carbohydrate 8.2 gm.

rut-formation. Loss of interest in environment, fixation upon a single object, and concentration of emotional or other interests in a groove or rut.

ruthenium (rū-thē'nĭ-ŭm). SYMB: *Ru.* At. wt. 101.07; at. no. 44. A hard, brittle, metallic element of platinum group.

ruth'erford. [Ernest Rutherford, British physicist, 1871-1937]. A unit of radioactivity representing 10^6 disintegrations per second. ABBR: rd.

rutidosus (rū-tĭ-dō'sŭs) [Gr. *rhytis,* wrinkle]. Contraction or puckering of cornea just before death.

rutilizm (rū'tĭl-ĭzm) [L. *rutilis,* red, + Gr. *-ismos,* condition]. Having red or auburn-colored hair.

rutin (rū'tĭn). A crystalline glucoside of quercetin, closely related to hesperidin.

Derived from buckwheat but present in many plants.

Rx. Symb. for *recipe; take.* SEE: *prescription.*

rye (rī) [AS. *ryge*]. A cereal grass which produces a grain used in food and beverage production. When rye grain is infected with a certain fungus, ergot is produced.

Food value of 100 gm. (medium flour): Cal. 350; protein 11.4 gm.; fat 1.7 gm.; carbohydrate 68 gm.

rytidosis (rĭt'ĭ-dō'sĭs) [Gr. *rhytis,* a wrinkle, + *ōsis,* condition]. Wrinkling or contraction of cornea preceding death. SYN: *rutidosis.*

S

S. Abbr. for *signa*, mark, or let it be written, term used in prescription writing; *smooth*, description of bacterial colonies; *spherical* or *spherical lens; subject* (pl. Ss), participant in an experiment.

S. Chem. symb. for sulfur.

s. Abbr. for *semis*, half; *sinister*, left.

s̄, s̥. Symb. for (L.) *sine*, without; used in charts.

S 1, S2, etc. Abbr. for *first sacral nerve, second sacral nerve*, etc.

S 1. Abbr. for *first heart sound*.

S2. Abbr. for *second heart sound*.

saber shin. Anterior border of the tibia marked with sharp convexity, found in hereditary syphilis.

sabulous (săb'ū-lŭs) [L. *sabulosus*, sand]. Gritty; sandy.

saburra (să-bŭr'ră) [L., sand]. Foulness of stomach or mouth due to decayed food. SYN: *sordes*.

saburral (să-bŭr'ăl). 1. Pert. to foulness of mouth or stomach due to accumulation of decayed food. 2. Pert. to sand, as in application of a hot sand bath for relief from pain, as in muscular rheumatism.

sac (săk) [L. *saccus*, pouch]. A baglike part of an organ, a cavity or pouch, sometimes containing fluid. SEE: *cyst*.

s., air. An alveolar cell in the lung.

s., allantoic. The expanded end of the allantois, well developed in birds and reptiles. SYN: *allantoic vesicle*.

s., alveolar. The terminal portion of an air passageway within the lung. Its wall contains pocketlike structures (alveoli) and each alveolar sac is connected to a respiratory bronchiole by an alveolar duct. SYN: *air sac*.

s., amniotic. A thin membrane, containing a serous fluid, enclosing the embryo. SYN: *amnion*.

s., chorionic. Saclike structure, consisting of chorion, which encloses the developing embryo. SYN: *chorionic vesicle*.

s., conjunctival. The cavity, lined with conjunctiva, which lies between the eyelids and anterior surface of the eye.

s., dental. The mesenchymal tissue surrounding a developing tooth.

s., endolymphatic. The expanded distal end of the endolymph duct.

s., hernial. A saclike protrusion of the peritoneum containing a herniated organ. SEE: *hernia; hernial sac*.

s., lacrimal. Upper dilated portion of the nasolacrimal duct.

s., lesser peritoneal. A large sacculation developing from an invagination of the dorsal mesogastrium which gives rise to the great omentum. It communicates with greater peritoneal cavity through the epiploic foramen. SYN: *omental bursa*.

s., vitelline. The yoke sac, q.v.

s., yolk. An extra-embryonic membrane that encloses the yolk in reptiles, birds, and monotremes. It is formed of an inner layer of entoderm invested by splanchnic mesoderm. In marsupials and placental mammals which lack a yolk mass, the yolk sac is a rudimentary vesicle lying within the chorionic sac.

saccadic (să-kăd'ĭk) [Fr. *saccade*, jerk]. Pert. to rapid intermittent movements, esp. of the eye. This type of eye movement is important when the fovea follows a moving target. SEE: *vergence*.

saccate (săk'ăt) [L. *saccatus*, baglike]. 1. Pert. to, like, or enclosed in a sac. SYN: *encysted*. 2. In bacteriology, marking a sac-shaped form, as in a type of liquefaction.

saccharase (săk'ă-rās) [Sanskrit *śarkarā*, sugar]. An enzyme which catalyzes the breakdown of disaccharides to monosaccharides, esp. the hydrolysis of sucrose to dextrose. Ex: sucrase; invertase.

saccharide (săk'ă-rid). A group of carbohydrates including sugars. The group is divided into the following classifications: monosaccharides, disaccharides, trisaccharides, and polysaccharides.

sacchariferous (săk''ă-rĭf'ĕr-ŭs) [Sanskrit *śarkarā*, sugar, + L. *ferre*, to carry]. Producing or containing sugar.

saccharin (săk'ă-rĭn). USP. ($C_7H_5NO_3S$) A sweet, white, powdered, synthetic product derived from coal tar, 300-500 times as sweet as sugar. Used as an artificial sweetener.

saccharine (săk'ă-rĭn, -rīn) [L. *saccharinus*]. Of the nature of, or having the quality of, sugar. SYN: *sweet*.

saccharo- [Sanskrit *śarkarā*, sugar]. Combining form meaning sugar.

saccharogalactorrhea (săk''ă-rō-gă-lăk''tō-rē'ă) ["+ Gr. *gala, galakt-*, milk, + *rhoia*, flow]. Excessive lactose secreted in milk.

saccharolytic (săk''ă-rō-lĭt'ĭk) ["+ Gr. *lysis*, dissolution]. Able to split up sugar.

Saccharomyces (săk''ă-rō-mī'sēz) [Sanskrit *śarkarā*, sugar, + *mykēs*, fungus]. (pl. sac-

charomycetes) A genus of fungi, reproducing by budding. SYN: *yeasts.*

saccharomycosis (săk″ă-rō-mī-kō′sĭs) ["+ "+ -ōsis, condition]. Any disease or pathological condition due to yeasts or Saccharomycetes.

saccharorrhea (săk″ă-rō-rē′ă) [Sanskrit *śarkarā*, sugar, + *rhoia*, flow]. Presence of sugar in the body fluids, as in urine or perspiration. SEE: *diabetes mellitus; glycosuria.*

saccharose (săk′ă-rōs). 1. Sucrose; cane, beet, or maple sugar. 2. One of the group of carbohydrates having the same chemical formula, $C_{12}H_{22}O_{11}$.

saccharosuria (săk″ă-rō-sū′rĭ-ă) [Sanskrit *śarkarā*, sugar, + *ouron*, urine]. Saccharose in the urine.

saccharum (săk′ă-rŭm) [L., sugar]. Sugar.

    s. album. Pure or white crystallized sugar.

    s. canadense. Maple sugar.

    s. candidum. Rock candy.

    s. lactis. Sugar of milk. SYN: *lactose.*

    s. purificatum. Pure white sugar.

    s. ustum. Burnt sugar; caramel.

saccharuria (săk″ă-rū′rĭ-ă) [Sanskrit *śarkarā*, sugar, + *ouron*, urine]. Sugar in the urine.

sacciform (săk′sĭ-form) [L. *saccus*, pouch, + *forma*, shape]. Bag-shaped or like a sac. SYN: *saccate.*

sacculated (săk′ū-lāt″ĕd) [L. *sacculātus*, baglike]. Consisting of small sacs or saccules.

sacculation (săk″ū-lā′shŭn). 1. Formation into a sac or sacs. 2. Group of sacs, collectively.

saccule (săk′ūl) [L. *sacculus*, a little bag]. 1. A small sac. 2. The smaller of two sacs comprising the portion of the membranous labyrinth occupying the vestibule of inner ear. It communicates with the utricle, cochlear duct, and endolymphatic duct, all of which are filled with endolymph. In its wall is the macula sacculi, a sensory area.

    s. of the larynx. A small diverticulum extending ventrally from the laryngeal ventricle lying between ventricular fold and thyroarytenoid muscle. SYN: *ventricular appendix.*

    s., vestibular. SEE: *saccule.*

sacculus (săk′ū-lŭs) [L., a small bag]. (pl. *sacculi*) A saccule or little sac.

saccus (săk′ŭs) [L., a bag]. (pl. *sacci*) [NA]. A sac or pouch.

    s. endolymphaticus. [NA]. Dilated, blind end of the ductus endolymphaticus.

    s. lacrimalis. [NA]. The lacrimal sac, into which empty the two lacrimal ducts.

sacrad (sā′krăd) [L. *sacrum*, sacred, + *ad*, toward]. In the direction of the sacrum.

sacral (sā′krăl) [L. *sacralis*]. Rel. to the sacrum.

    s. bone. A triangular bone made up of five fused vertebrae just above the coccyx.

    s. canal. Continuation of the vertebral canal in the sacrum.

    s. flexure. Rectal curve in front of the sacrum.

    s. index. S. breadth multiplied by 100 and divided by s. length.

    s. nerves. Five pairs of spinal nerves, the upper four of which emerge through the posterior sacral foramina, the 5th pair through the sacral hiatus (termination of sacral canal). All are mixed nerves (motor and sensory).

    s. plexus. Plexus of s. nerves from which sciatic nerve originates. It is a part of the lumbosacral plexus.

    s. vertebra. Fused segments forming the sacrum.

sacralgia (sā-krăl′jĭ-ă) [L. *sacrum*, sacred, + Gr. *algos*, pain]. Pain in the sacrum. SYN: *hieralgia.*

sacralization (sā″krăl-ĭ-zā′shŭn). Union of the sacrum and the 5th lumbar vertebra.

sacra media (sā′kră mē′dĭ-ă) [L.]. Middle sacral artery.

sacrectomy (sā-krĕk′tō-mī) [L. *sacrum*, sacred, + Gr. *ektomē*, excision]. Excision of part of sacrum.

sacro- (sā′krō) [L. *sacrum*, sacred]. Prefix indicating relationship to the sacrum.

sacroanterior (sā″krō-ăn-tē′rĭ-ōr) ["+ *anterior*, before]. Denoting intrauterine fetal position in which the fetal sacrum is directed anteriorly.

sacrococainization (sā″krō-kō-kăn″ĭ-zā′-shŭn). Injection of cocaine through the sacrolumbar space into the spinal cord.

sacrococcygeal (sā″krō-kŏk-sĭj′ē-ăl) [L. *sacrum*, sacred, + Gr. *kokkyx*, coccyx]. Concerning the sacrum and coccyx.

sacrococcygeus (săk″rō-kŏk-sĭj′ē-ŭs). One of two small muscles (anterior and posterior) extending from sacrum to coccyx.

sacrocoxalgia (sā″krō-kŏks-ăl′jĭ-ă) [L. *sacrum*, sacred, + *coxa*, hip, + Gr. *algos*, pain]. Pain in sacroiliac joint, usually due to inflammation. SEE: *sacrocoxitis.*

sacrocoxitis (sā″krō-kŏks-i′tĭs) ["+ "+ Gr. *-itis*, inflammation]. Inflammation of the sacroiliac joint, frequently tuberculous.

sacrodynia (sā″krō-dĭn′ĭ-ă) [L. *sacrum*, sacred, + *odynē*, pain]. Pain in the region of the sacrum.

sacroiliac (sā″krō-ĭl′ĭ-ăk) ["+ *iliacus*, hipbone]. Of, or pert. to, the sacrum and ilium.

s. disease. Tuberculous disease of the sacroiliac joint.

s. joint. The articulation between the hipbone and sacrum. It is a diarthrodial joint, a narrow joint cavity being present. However, joint movement is limited because of interlocking of articular surfaces.

sacrolumbar (sā″krō-lŭm′băr) ["+ *lumbus*, loin]. Of, or concerning, the sacrum and loins.

s. angle. Angle formed by articulation of the last lumbar vertebra and the sacrum.

sacroposterior (sā″krō-pŏs-tē′rĭ-ōr) [L. *sacrum*, sacred, + *posterior*, coming after]. Denoting intrauterine fetal position in which the fetal sacrum is directed posteriorly.

sacrosciatic (sā″krō-sī-ăt′ĭk) ["+ *sciaticus*, hipjoint]. Concerning the sacrum and ischium.

sacrospinalis ["+ *spina*, spine]. A large muscle lying on either side of vertebral column extending from sacrum to head. Its two chief components are the iliocostalis and longissimus muscles. SEE: *Table of Muscles* in *Appendix*.

sacrotomy (sā-krŏt′ō-mĭ) [L. *sacrum*, sacred, + Gr., a cutting]. Surgical excision of the lower part of the sacrum.

sacrouterine (sā″krō-ū′tĕr-ĭn) ["+ *uterus*, womb]. Concerning the sacrum and uterus.

sacrovertebral (sā″krō-vŭr′te-brăl) ["+ *vertebra*, vertebra]. Concerning the sacrum and the vertebrae.

s. angle. Angle formed by base of sacrum and 5th lumbar vertebra.

sacrum (sā′krŭm) [L., sacred]. The triangular bone situated dorsal and caudal from the two ilia between the 5th lumbar vertebra and the coccyx. It is formed of five united vertebrae and is wedged between the two innominate bones, its articulations forming the sacroiliac joints. It forms the base of the vertebral column and, with the coccyx, forms the posterior boundary of the true pelvis. The sacrum in a male is narrower and more curved than in a female.

sactosalpinx (săk″tō-săl′pĭnks) [Gr. *saktos*, stuffed, + *salpinx*, tube]. Dilated fallopian tube due to retention of secretions, as in pyosalpinx or hydrosalpinx.

saddle joint. Joint with articulating surfaces convex in one direction and concave in the other. Ex: carpometacarpal joint of the thumb.

saddle nose. A nose with a depressed bridge.

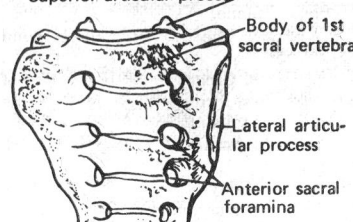

SACRUM

sadism (sā′dĭzm, săd′ĭzm). [Comte Donatien Alphonse Francois de Sade, Marquis de Sade, 1740-1814]. Conscious or unconscious sexual pleasure derived from inflicting mental or physical pain on others. SEE: *algolagnia; masochism.*

sadist (sā′dĭst, săd′ĭst). One who practices sadism.

sadness. A normal emotional feeling of dejection or melancholy. A result of an unhappy event or situation which warrants a change in the emotional state. Not to be confused with depression in which the person is melancholy for no apparent reason.

sadomasochism (sā″dō-măs′ĕ-kĭzm, săd″ō-măs′ĕ-kĭzm). Sexual pleasure related to both sadism and masochism.

Saemisch's ulcer (sā′mĭsh). [Edwin Theodor Saemisch, Ger. ophthalmologist, 1833-1909]. Serpiginous, infectious ulcer of the cornea.

Saenger's operation (zĕng′ŭr). [Max Saenger, Austrian gynecologist, 1853-1903]. A form of cesarean section by which the uterus is taken out before the fetus.

safety symbolism. Engagements to marry, the engagement ring, the wedding, the wedding ring, marriage itself, the public announcement of wedding anniversaries, the advent of children, are all symbols which announce to the world that a man or a woman is the possession of one or the other; a warning, as it were, to protect the other partner from the attentions of one of the opposite sex.

sagittal (săj′ĭ-tăl) [L. *sagittalis*]. Arrowlike; in an anteroposterior direction.

s. plane. A vertical plane through the longitudinal axis of the trunk dividing the body into right and left portions. If it is through the midaxis dividing body into right and left halves, it is called a median or midsagittal plane.

   s. sinus. The superior longitudinal sinus.

   s. sulcus. Groove on inner surface of parietal bones, forming a channel for the superior sagittal sinus.

   s. suture. Suture between the two parietal bones.

sago (sā′gō) [Malay *sagu*]. A substance prepared from various palms, consisting principally of starches. Used as a demulcent and as a food with little residue.

   ACTION: Easy to digest. Fattening. Leaves little residue. Indicated in convalescence, emaciated conditions, and when little residue is desired. SEE: *carbohydrates; starch.*

Saint Anthony's fire. Any of certain inflammations or gangrenous skin conditions, esp. erysipelas, hospital gangrene, and ergotism, q.v.

Saint Vitus' dance. Nervous disease with involuntary, jerking motions. SYN: *chorea.*

sal (săl) [L.]. Salt; or a substance resembling salt.

   s. ammoniac. Chloride of ammonia.

salaam convulsion (sŭ-lŏm) [Arabic *salām*, peace]. Clonic muscular spasm of the trunk resulting in a bowing movement. SYN: *nodding spasm.*

salacious (sĕ-lā′shŭs) [L. *salāx, salāc-*, lustful]. Lustful or inciting to lust.

salicylate (săl′ĭ-sĭl′āt, săl-ĭs′ĭl-āt). Any salt of salicylic acid.

   s., methyl. The principal constituent of oil of wintergreen. It is applied externally as a counterirritant.

   s., sodium. White crystalline substance with disagreeable taste, in some cases even nauseating. Used to reduce pain and temperature. SEE: *aspirin.*

salicylated (sălĭs′ĭl-āt-ĕd). Impregnated with salicylic acid.

salicylic acid (săl′ĭ-sĭl′ĭk). USP. ($C_7H_6O_3$) A white crystalline acid derived from phenol.

   USES: In making aspirin, as a preservative and flavoring agent, and in external treatment of certain skin conditions.

salicylism (săl′ĭ-sĭl′ĭzm). Toxic condition caused by an overdose of salicylic acid or its derivatives.

salicylsulfonic acid test. Test for albumin in urine. SEE: *albumin.*

salicyluric acid (săl′ĭ-sĭ-lū′rĭk). Acid in urine after taking salicylic acid or its derivatives.

salifiable (săl′ĭ-fī′ăbl) [L. *sal*, salt, + *fieri*, to be made]. Capable of forming a salt by combining with an acid.

salimeter (sŏ-lĭm′ĕ-ter) ["+ Gr. *metron*, a measure]. Device for testing strength of saline solutions.

saline (sā′lĭn) [L. *salinus*, of salt]. 1. Containing or pert. to salt; salty. 2. A mineral salt that produces evacuation of the intestinal contents. Ex: magnesium sulfate, sodium sulfate, and potassium citrate.

   s. enema. Enema used to excite peristalsis and evacuation. Magnesium sulfate, 1 oz. (28.35 gm.) in 2 oz. (59.15 ml.) of very warm water (115° F. or 46.1° C.), given with a small bore tube. SEE: *enema, physiological salt solution.*

   s. purgative. Any salt producing evacuation, as Epsom salts.

   s. solution. A solution of sodium chloride and distilled water; a 0.9% solution of sodium chloride is an isotonic solution.

   A normal s. solution consists of 0.85% salt solution, which is necessary to maintain osmotic pressure and the stimulation and regulation of muscular activity. SYN: *physiological salt solution,* q.v.

saliva (să-lī′vă) [L.]. Salivary gland and oral mucous gland fluid, the secretion which begins the process of digesting food. SYN: *spittle.*

   CHARACTER: It is tasteless, clear, odorless, viscid, and weakly alkaline, being neutralized after being acted upon by the gastric juice in the stomach. Sp. gr. 1.002-1.006. Amount secreted in 24 hr., 1000-1500 cc.

   CONSTITUENTS: *Inorganic substances* include water, 99.5% salts (chlorides, carbonates, phosphates, sulfates); gasses in solution; and sometimes abnormal substances being excreted from body, i.e., acetone. *Organic substances* include enzymes (ptyalin, maltase, lysozyme); proteins (serum albumin and globulin, mucin); and small amounts of urea, uric acid, creatine, and amino acids. *Cellular elements* include epithelial cells and leukocytes.

   FUNCTION: To moisten food, facilitating mastication and deglutition; to moisten and lubricate mouth parts; to act as a solvent; for excretion of waste products; to initiate digestion of starches; to assist in regulation of water balance.

   RS: angiosialitis; aptyalia; aptyalism; asialia; glycosialia; insalivation; parotid; ptyalin; ptyalism; salivary digestion; s. glands; sialagogue.

   s., artificial. A solution which is useful in treating excessive dryness of the mouth (xerostomia). The formula is 20 ml. of a 4%

solution of methylcellulose, 10 ml. of glycerin, add sufficient normal saline to make 90 ml., and one drop of lemon oil.

salivary (săl'ĭ-vĕr-ĭ) [L. *salivarius*]. Pert. to, producing, or formed from saliva.

   s. amylase. Ptyalin, q.v. SEE: *s. digestion.*

   s. calculus. Concretion in a salivary duct.

   s. corpuscles. Nucleated, spherical bodies in saliva thought to be modified leukocytes from lymphatic tissue.

   s. digestion. That occurring in the mouth resulting from action of salivary enzymes. Ptyalin, a salivary amylase, acts on boiled starch, converting it successively by hydrolysis to erythrodextrin, achrodextrin, maltose, and isomaltose. Small quantities of maltose may be converted to glucose by action of maltase in saliva. Oral digestion is limited because of the short time food remains in the mouth, but digestion continues in the stomach until food becomes acidified by gastric juice. Ptyalin is active at a pH of 6.7-6.8, but inactivated by a pH below 6.

   s. glands. Parotid glands, one on each side of the face below the ear; *submaxillary* glands, principally in the floor of mouth; *sublingual* glands, principally in floor of mouth; *buccal* glands, scattered beneath the mucous membrane of lips and cheeks. They form saliva.

   S. secretion is under nervous control, being reflexly initiated by mechanical, chemical, or radiant stimuli acting on taste buds (gustatory receptors) in the mouth, olfactory receptors, visual receptors (eyes), or other sense organs. Secretion may also occur as a result of conditioned reflexes, as when one thinks about food or hears a dinner bell.

   NERVES: Facial and glossopharyngeal, also the autonomic system.

   BLOOD SUPPLY: Branches from the external carotid artery. SEE: *saliva; salivary digestion.*

salivation (săl'ĭ-vā'shŭn) [L. *salivātio*]. 1. The act of secreting saliva. 2. Excessive secretion of saliva. SYN: *ptyalism.*

salivatory (săl'ĭ-vă-tōr'ĭ). Producing secretion of saliva.

Salk vaccine (sŏlk). [Jonas E. Salk, Amer. microbiologist, 1914 —]. First successful poliomyelitis vaccine. A vaccine that contains three types of poliomyelitis viruses and induces immunity against the disease.

sallow (săl'ō) [AS. *salo*]. Of a pale, sickly, yellowish color, usually said of complexion or skin.

sallowness (săl'ō-nĕs). A sickly, yellowish tint, often helpful in diagnosing diseases. SEE: *face; skin.*

salmin(e (săl'mēn, -mĭn) [L. *salmō*, salmon]. $C_{30}H_{57}N_{14}O_6$. A toxic protamine obtained from spermatozoa of salmon. SEE: *protamine, protein.*

salmon (săm'ŭn). (pl. *salmon, -ons*) Various large food and game fish of northern waters having a delicate pinkish flesh.

   Food value of 100 gm. (canned, pink liquid and solid): Cal. 203; protein 21.7 gm.; fat 12.2 gm.

salmon patch. Salmon-colored area of the cornea in syphilitic keratitis. SYN: *Hutchinson's patch.*

Salmonella (săl'mō-nĕl'ă) [L.]. [Daniel E. Salmon, Amer. pathologist, 1850-1914]. A genus of bacteria belonging to the family Enterobacteriaceae. S. are gram-negative, usually motile rods. Several species are pathogenic, some producing mild gastroenteritis, others producing a severe and often fatal food poisoning. SEE: *salmonellosis.*

   S., choleraesuis. A species often found to be the cause of septicemia.

   S. enteritidis. Cause of Salmonella gastroenteritis and Salmonella food poisoning in man.

   S. schottmülleri. Species causing paratyphoid fever, Type B.

   S. typhimurium. A species frequently isolated from persons having acute gastroenteritis.

   S. typhosa. The causative agent of typhoid fever.

salmonellosis (săl-mō-nĕ-lō'sĭs). Infestation with bacteria of genus Salmonella. There are three forms of salmonella infection which occur in man: *enteric fever* (Ex: typhoid fever); *septicemia* which usually is caused by Salmonella choleraesuis; *acute gastroenteritis* which can be caused by a variety of species of salmonella.

salpingectomy (săl''pĭn-jĕk'tō-mĭ) [Gr. *salpinx, salping-*, tube, + *ektomē*, excision]. Surgical removal of the fallopian tube.

salpingemphraxis (săl''pĭn-jĕm-frăk'sĭs) ["+ Gr. *emphraxis*, a stoppage]. 1. Obstruction of the eustachian tube causing deafness. 2. Obstruction of a fallopian tube.

salpingian (săl-pĭn'jĭ-ăn). Concerning the eustachian tube or fallopian tube.

salpingion (săl-pĭn'jĭ-ōn). A point at inferior surface of the apex of the petrous portion of temporal bone.

salpingitis (săl''pĭn-jī'tĭs) [Gr. *salpinx, salping-*, tube, + *-itis*, inflammation]. Inflammation of the fallopian tube or, less commonly, of the eustachian tube.

ETIOL: The condition may be acute, suba-cute, or chronic. The organisms most often associated with salpingitis are the gonococ-cus, staphylococcus, streptococcus, colon bacillus, and tubercle bacillus.

s., eustachian. Inflammation of the eustachian tube. SYN: *eustachitis.*

salpingo- [Gr. *salpinx*, tube]. Combining form indicating eustachian or fallopian tube.

salpingocatheterism (săl-pĭng″gō-kăth′ĕt-ĕr-ĭzm) ["+ *kathetēr*, catheter, + *-ismos*, process]. Catheterization of the eustachian tube.

salpingocele (săl-ping′gō-sēl) ["+ *kēlē*, hernia]. Hernial protrusion of a fallopian tube.

salpingocyesis (săl-pĭng″ō-sī-ē′sĭs) [Gr. *sal-pinx*, tube, + *kyēsis*, pregnancy]. Pregnancy in which fetus begins to develop in a fallopi-an tube; tubal pregnancy.

salpingo-oophorectomy (săl-pĭng″gō-ō″ŏf-ō-rĕk′tō-mĭ) ["+ *ōōn*, egg, + *phoros*, a bear-er, + *ektomē*, excision]. Excision of an ovary and fallopian tube.

OPER. NP: Needle layout, sutures, and operating procedure identical to those for hysterectomy. In the operation for a rup-tured ectopic pregnancy it is well to have three times the usual number of laparotomy pads and packs ready, as well as an extra amount of very warm saline solution for flushing out the abdominal cavity. This is because there may be a great quantity of both fresh and clotted blood to be removed. POSITION: Horizontal.

salpingo-oophoritis (săl-pĭng″ō-ō″ŏf-ō-rī′tĭs) ["+ "+ "+ *-ĭtis*, inflammation]. In-flammation of the tube and ovary. SYN: *salpingo-oothecitis.*

salpingo-oophorocele (săl-pĭng″gō-ō-ŏf′ōr-ō-sēl) [Gr. *salpinx*, tube, + *ōōn*, egg, + *phoros*, a bearer, + *kēlē*, hernia]. Hernia enclosing the ovary and fallopian tube.

salpingo-oothecitis (săl-pĭng″gō-ō″ō-thē-sī′tĭs) ["+ "+ *thēkē*, box, + *-ĭtis*, inflamma-tion]. Inflammation of a fallopian tube and ovary. SYN: *salpingo-oophoritis.*

salpingo-oothecocele (săl-pĭng″gō-ō″ō-thē′kō-sēl) ["+ "+ "+ *kēlē*, hernia]. Hernia of ovary and fallopian tube.

salpingo-ovariectomy (săl-pĭng″gō-ō″vār-ĭ-ĕk′tō-mĭ) [Gr. *salpinx*, tube, + L. *ovarium*, ovary, + Gr. *ektomē*, excision]. Surgical removal of an ovary and fallopian tube. SYN: *salpingo-oophorectomy.*

salpingopexy (săl-pĭng′ō-pĕk″sĭ) ["+ *pēxis*, fixation]. Fixation of a fallopian tube.

salpingopharyngeus (săl-pĭng″gō-făr-ĭn′jē-ŭs) ["+ *pharynx, pharyng-*, pharynx].

The muscle arising near opening of the eustachian tube. Raises nasopharynx.

salpingorrhaphy (săl″pĭng-gŏr′ă-fĭ) [Gr. *sal-pinx*, tube, + *rhaphē*, a seam]. Suture of a fallopian tube.

salpingosalpingostomy (săl-pĭng′gō-săl″pĭng-gŏs′tō-mĭ) ["+ *salpinx*, tube, + *stoma*, a mouth]. The operation of attaching one fallopian tube to the other.

salpingoscope (săl-pĭng′gō-skōp″) ["+ *sko-pein*, to see]. Device for examining the nasopharynx and eustachian tube.

salpingostenochoria (săl-pĭng′gō-stĕn″ō-kŏr′ĭ-ă) [Gr. *salpinx*, tube, *stenōsis*, stenosis, + *choreia*, dance]. Stenosis or stricture of eustachian tube.

salpingostomatomy (săl-pĭng′gō-stō-măt′ō-mĭ) ["+ *stoma*, a mouth, + *tomē*, a cutting]. Creation of an artificial opening in a fallopian tube after it has been occluded as a result of inflammation and scarring.

salpingostomy (săl-pĭng-ŏs′tō-mĭ). Surgical opening of a fallopian tube which has been occluded, or for drainage purposes.

salpingotomy (săl-pĭng-ŏt′ō-mĭ) [Gr. *sal-pinx*, tube, + *tomē*, a cutting]. Incision of a fallopian tube.

salpingo-ureterostomy (săl-pĭng″gō-ūr-ēt″ĕr-ŏs′tō-mĭ) ["+ *ourēter*, ureter, + *stoma*, opening]. Surgical connection of the ureter and the fallopian tube.

salpingysterocyesis (săl″pĭng-jĭs″tĕr-ō-sī-ē′sĭs) ["+ *hystera*, uterus, + *kyēsis*, preg-nancy]. Pregnancy in which the embryo is located at the entrance of the fallopian tube into the uterus; ectopic pregnancy.

salpinx (săl′pĭnks) [Gr., tube]. (pl. *salpinges*) The fallopian or eustachian tube.

salsify (săl′sĭ-fĭ″) [It. *salsífica*]. A plant, native to Europe which has a root that is eaten as a vegetable. Has an oysterlike flavor and sometimes is called oyster plant.

Food value of 100 gm. (cooked): Cal. (value may be as low as 13 Cal. in the fresh product, or as high as 82 Cal. in that which has been stored); protein 2.6 gm.; fat 0.6 gm.; carbohy-drate 15.1 gm.

salt [AS. *sealt*]. 1. White crystalline com-pound occurring in nature, known chemical-ly as sodium chloride, $NaCl$. 2. Containing, tasting of, or treated with salt. 3. To treat with salt. 4. In the plural, any mineral salt or saline mixture used as an aperient or cathartic, esp. Epsom salts or Glauber's salt. 5. In chemistry, a compound consisting of a positive ion other than hydrogen, and a negative ion other than hydroxyl. 6. A chemical compound, usually crystalline, re-sulting from the interaction of an acid and a base.

Salts and water are the inorganic or mineral constituents of the body. They play specific roles in the functions of cells and are indispensable for life. The principal salts are chlorides, carbonates, bicarbonates, sulfates, and phosphates which are compounds of sodium, potassium, calcium, magnesium, and iron with chlorine, CO_2, sulfur, and phosphorus.

In general, salts serve the following roles in the body: maintenance of proper osmotic conditions; maintenance of water balance and regulation of blood volume; maintenance of proper acid-base balance; provision for essential constituents of tissue, esp. bones and teeth; maintenance of normal irritability of muscle and nerve cells; maintenance of condition for coagulation of the blood; provision for essential components of certain enzyme systems, respiratory pigments, and hormones; regulation of cell membrane and capillary permeability.

RS: chlorite; low-salt diet; normal; rheum; sal; saline; salt-free diet; salt glow; secretion; "sial-" words.

s., buffer. A s. in the blood, which fixes excess amounts of acid or alkali without a change in hydrogen-ion concentration.

s., Epsom. Magnesium sulfate.

s., Glauber's. Sodium sulfate.

s., iodized. S. containing 1 part sodium or potassium iodide to 10,000 parts of sodium chloride. An important source of iodine in the diet. The use of this form of s. will prevent goiter. S. which has not been iodized should not be used in the diet.

s., Rochelle. Sodium and potassium tartrate.

s., rock. Native sodium chloride.

s. solution, normal. S. solution, physiological, q.v.

s. solution, physiological. A sterile solution containing 0.85% of sodium chloride in chemically pure distilled water (8.5 gm. sodium chloride in 1000 ml. or one liter of distilled water).

NP: When salt solution is given intravenously or hypodermically, rigid aseptic precautions must be observed. Usually injected in front of thighs or under breasts, as loose tissue is found in these areas. The temperature of the solution is about 100° F., so that when the blood is reached solution will be at body temperature. If speed is not necessary, administration via the rectum is the least risky, as it is not painful and there is no risk of infection. The patient placed on left side, hips are elevated by a pillow, and the solution, by means of a rectal tube, is instilled into the rectum. The solution is allowed to run in at the rate of about 1 quart per hour.

saltation (săl-tā'shŭn) [L. saltātiō, leaping]. 1. Act of leaping or dancing, as in chorea. 2. Abrupt variation in character of a species. SYN: mutation.

saltatory (săl'tă-tō''rĭ). Marked by dancing or leaping.

s. conduction. Skipping from node to node, said of movement of the potential along myelinated neurons.

s. spasm. Tic of muscles of lower extremity, causing convulsive leaping upon attempt to stand. SEE: palmus.

salt-free diet. It is impractical to attempt to maintain a diet absolutely free of sodium chloride. Thus salt-free means a low sodium diet. A diet which allows 500 mg. (0.5 gm.) of salt per day. On this diet, table salt should not be added to the food. Also, it is important to know the amount of salt in the drinking water, because some areas have water containing a large amount of sodium. Some medicines (for example, sodium salicylate) are quite high in sodium content. Exclusion of sodium-containing medicines is important in attempting to regulate the amount of sodium consumed.

RS: salt; sodium chloride.

salt glow. Name given to a rub of the entire body with moist salt for stimulation.

salting out. A method of separating a specific protein from a mixture of proteins by the addition of a salt, i.e., ammonium sulfate.

saltpeter, saltpetre (sawlt'pē'ter) [L. sal, salt, + petra, rock]. A common name for potassium nitrate.

s., Chile. A common name for sodium nitrate, $NaNO_3$. Crystalline powder, saline in taste and soluble in water.

salt-poor diet. All food prepared and served without the addition of salt, including salt-free bread and butter. Milk intake is limited.

salts. Pl. of salt, q.v.

salubrious (să-lū'brĭ-ŭs) [L. salubris]. Promoting or favorable to health. SYN: wholesome.

salutary (săl'ū-tā''rĭ) [L. salutaris]. Healthful; promoting health; curative.

salvarsan (săl'văr-săn) [L. salvus, safe, + Gr. arsen, arsenic]. An arsenical, yellowish powder preparation developed by Ehrlich for treatment of syphilis. Since the development of penicillin, there has been little need for salvarsan in the treatment of syphilis. RS: arsphenamine.

salve (săv) [AS. sealf]. 1. An ointment applied to wounds. 2. In pharmacology, any ointment or cerate made with a base of a fat, oil, petrolatum, resin, etc.

samarium (sŏ-mā'rĭ-ŭm). SYMB: *Sm.* or *Sa.* At. wt. 150.35; at. no. 62; sp. gr. approx. 7.50.

sanative (săn'ă-tĭv) [L. *sanāre,* to heal]. Of a healing nature. SYN: *curative.*

sanatorium (săn"ă-tō'rĭ-ŭm) [L. *sanatōrius,* healing]. An establishment for preservation of health, or for the treatment of the chronically sick. SYN: *sanitarium.*

sanatory (săn'ă-tō"rĭ). Curative; conducive to health.

sand (sănd) [AS.]. Fine grains of disintegrated rock.

   s., auditory. Calcareous concretion in labyrinth of the ear. SYN: *otolith.*

   s. bath. Therapeutic covering of the body with hot s.

   s., brain. Concretion of matter near base of the pineal gland. SYN: *acervulus cerebri.*

   s. tumor. Tumor made up of calcareous particles and located in membrane of the brain, choroid plexus, other areas. SYN: *psammoma.*

sandflies. Flies of the order Diptera belonging to the genus Phlebotomus. They transmit sandfly fever, Oroya fever, and various types of leishmaniasis.

sandfly fever. A mild virus disease which clinically resembles influenza, except for absence of respiratory symptoms. The causative organism, any one of three species of arboviruses, is transmitted by the common sandfly Phlebotomus papatasii, a small hairy blood-sucking midge which bites at night and has a limited flight range. The disease occurs in tropical and subtropical areas which experience long periods of hot, dry weather. SYN: pappataci fever, phlebotomus fever, three-day fever.

Sandwith's bald tongue (sănd'wĭth). [Fleming M. Sandwith, Br. physician, 1777-1843]. Abnormally clean tongue seen in late stages of pellagra.

sane (sān) [L. *sanus*]. Sound of mind; mentally normal.

sanguicolous (săng-gwĭk'ō-lŭs) [L. *sanguis,* blood, + *colere,* to dwell]. Inhabiting the blood, as a parasite.

sanguifacient (săng-gwĭ-fā'shĕnt) ["+ *facere,* to make]. Making blood.

sanguiferous (săng-gwĭf'ĕr-ŭs) ["+ *ferre,* to carry]. Conducting or containing blood, as the circulatory organs.

sanguification (săng-gwĭ-fĭ-kā'shŭn) ["+ *facere,* to make]. Conversion into, or formation of, blood. SYN: *hematopoiesis.*

sanguimotor, sanguimotory (săng'gwĭ-mō'tor, -tō-rĭ) [L. *sanguis,* blood, + *motor,* a mover]. Pert. to blood circulation.

sanguine (săng'gwĭn) [L. *sanguineus,* bloody]. 1. Optimistic; cheerful. 2. Plethoric,

bloody; marked by abundant and active blood circulation, particularly a ruddy complexion. 3. Pert. to, or consisting of, blood.

sanguineous (săng-gwĭn'ē-ŭs) [L.]. 1. Bloody; rel. to blood. 2. Having an abundance of blood. SYN: *plethoric.*

sanguinolent (săng-gwĭn'ō-lĕnt) [L. *sanguinolentus*]. Containing, or tinged with, blood.

sanguinopoietic (săng"gwĭn-ō-poy-ĕt'ĭk) [L. *sanguis,* blood, + *poiein,* to form]. Forming or making blood. SYN: *hematopoietic; sanguifacient.*

sanguirenal (săng"gwĭ-rē'năl) ["+ *rēn,* kidney]. Pert. to the blood supply of the kidneys.

sanguis (săng'gwĭs) [L.]. [NA]. Blood.

sanguisuga (săng-gwĭ-sū'gă) ["+ *sugere,* to suck]. A leech or bloodsucker. SEE: *Hirudo.*

sanies (sā'nĭ-ēz) [L.]. A thin, fetid, greenish discharge from a wound or ulcer, presenting appearance of pus tinged with blood.

saniopurulent (sā"nĭ-ō-pū'rū-lĕnt) [L. *sanies,* diseased blood, + *purulentus,* full of pus.]. Having characteristics of sanies and pus; pert. to a fetid, serous, blood-tinged discharge containing pus.

sanioserous (sā"nĭ-ō-sē'rŭs) ["+ *serum,* whey]. Composed of sanies and serum.

sanious (sā'nĭ-ŭs) [L. *saniosus*]. Of the nature of fetid, purulent fluid from an ulcer; sanies.

sanitarium (săn-ĭ-tā"rĭ-ŭm) [L. *sanatōrius,* healing]. Institution for treatment and recuperation of persons having physical or mental disorders; occasionally limited to place where conditions are prophylactic rather than therapeutic. SYN: *sanatorium.*

sanitary (săn'ĭ-tā"rĭ) [L. *sanitarius*]. Promoting, or pert. to, conditions improving health.

   s. napkin. Perineal pad, esp. one used during menstruation.

   s. towel. Perineal pad used during menstruation.

sanitation (săn"ĭ-tā'shŭn) [L. *sanitas,* health]. The formulation and application of measures to promote and establish conditions favorable to health, esp. public health. SEE: *assanation; hygiene.*

sanity (săn'ĭ-tĭ). Soundness of health or mind; normal mentality. SEE: *sane.*

santonin (săn'tō-nĭn). A colorless, crystalline substance obtained from the unexpanded flower heads of species of the plant Artemisia cina.

   ACTION AND USES: A vermifuge against the roundworm. Because of its toxicity it is not the drug of choice.

sap (săp) [AS. *saep*]. 1. Any fluid essential to life and vitality of a living structure. 2. To cause gradual exhaustion or weakness, as to sap one's strength.

s., cell. Hyaloplasm, q.v.

s., nuclear. Liquid portion of a cell nucleus. SYN: *karyolymph.*

saphena (să-fē'nă) [Gr. *saphēnēs,* manifest]. (pl. *saphenae*) Name given to two large veins of the leg.

saphenous (să-fē'nŭs). Pert. to, or associated with, a saphenous vein or nerve in the leg. Superficial, manifest.

    s. nerve. A deep branch of the femoral nerve. In lower leg, it follows the long saphenous vein supplying medial side of leg, ankle, and foot.

    s. opening. An aperture in the fascia, oval in shape, in inner and upper part of thigh transmitting the saphenous vein below Poupart's ligament. SYN: *fossa ovalis.*

    s. veins. Two veins, long and short, passing up the leg — the long from the foot to the saphenous opening, the short one behind outer malleolus up back of leg joining the popliteal. SEE: *vein.*

sapid (săp'ĭd) [L. *sapidus,* tasty]. Savory; tasty; opposed to insipid.

sapo (sā'pō) [L.]. Soap prepared from pure olive oil and sodium hydroxide.

saponaceous (să"pō-nā'shŭs) [L. *saponaceus,* soapy]. Soapy; resembling soap in feel or quality.

saponatus (să"pō-nā'tŭs) [L.]. Mixed with soap.

saponification (să-pŏn"ĭ-fĭ-kā'shŭn) [L. *sapo,* soap, + *-ficāre,* to make]. 1. Conversion into soap; chemically, the hydrolysis or the splitting of fat by an alkali yielding glycerol and three molecules of alkali salt of the fatty acid, the soap. 2. In chemistry, hydrolysis of an ester into corresponding alcohol and acid (free or in form of a salt).

    s. number. In analysis of fats, the number of mg. of potassium hydroxide needed to neutralize the fatty acids in 1 gm. of oil or fat. SYN: *saponification value.*

saponify (să-pŏn'ĭ-fī). To convert into a soap, as when fats are treated with an alkali to produce a free alcohol plus the salt of the fatty acid.

    Thus, stearin, saponified with sodium hydroxide, yields the alcohol glycerol plus the soap sodium stearate.

saponin (săp'ō-nĭn) [Fr. *saponine,* soap]. Unabsorbable glucoside contained in the roots of some plants forming a lather in an aqueous solution. Saponins cause hemolysis of red blood cells even in high dilutions. When taken orally, can produce diarrhea and vomiting.

saporific (săp"ō-rĭf'ĭk) [L. *saporificus,* producing taste]. Imparting a taste or flavor.

sapphism (săf'ĭzm) [Gr. *Sapphō,* Gr. poetess, 7th century B.C.]. Female homosexuality.

    Sappho was the reputed instigator of lesbianism.

sapremia (să-prē'mĭ-ă) [Gr. *sapros,* rotten, + *haima,* blood]. A toxic condition caused by the absorption into the blood of toxins or poisons produced by saprophytes or putrefactive bacteria. SEE: *septicemia.*

sapro- [Gr. *sapros,* rotten]. Combining form meaning putrid or rotten.

saprodontia (săp"rō-dŏn'shĭ-ă) ["+ *odous, odont-,* tooth]. Caries of the teeth; tooth decay.

saprogen (săp'rō-jĕn) ["+ *gennan,* to produce]. Any microorganism causing or produced by putrefaction.

saprogenic (săp"rō-jĕn'ĭk). Causing putrefaction, or resulting from it.

saprophilous (săp-rŏf'ĭl-ŭs) [Gr. *sapros,* rotten, + *philein,* to love]. Living on decaying or dead substances, as a microorganism. SYN: *saprophytic.*

saprophyte (săp'rō-fīt) ["+ *phyton,* plant]. Any organism living on decaying or dead organic matter. Most of the higher fungi are saprophytes. SEE: *parasite.*

saprophytic (săp"rō-fīt'ĭk). Living or growing in decaying or dead matter; characteristic of a saprophyte.

saprozoic (săp"rō-zō'ĭk) [Gr. *sapros,* rotten, + *zōon,* animal]. Living on decaying or dead organic matter.

sarapus (săr'ă-pŭs) [Gr. *sarapous*]. A person having flat feet.

sarcitis (săr-sī'tĭs) [Gr. *sarx, sarkos,* flesh, + *-ītis,* inflammation]. Inflammation of muscle tissue. SYN: *myositis.*

sarco- [Gr. *sarx, sarkos,* flesh]. Combining form indicating flesh.

sarcoadenoma (săr"kō-ăd"en-ō'mă) ["+ *adēn,* gland, + *-ōma,* tumor]. A fleshy tumor of a gland. SYN: *adenosarcoma.*

sarcobiont (săr"kō-bī'ŏnt) ["+ *bioun,* to live]. A microorganism that lives on flesh.

sarcoblast (săr'kō-blăst) [Gr. *sarkos,* flesh, + *blastos,* a germ]. Embryonic cell which develops into a muscle cell. SYN: *myoblast.*

sarcocarcinoma (săr"kō-kăr-sĭn-ō'mă) ["+ *karkinos,* crab cancer, + *-ōma,* tumor]. A tumor of malignant growth of sarcomatous and carcinomatous types.

sarcocele (săr'kō-sēl) ["+ *kēlē,* a mass]. A fleshy tumor of the testicle.

Sarcocystis (săr"kō-sĭs'tĭs) [Gr. *sarkos,* flesh, + *kystis,* bladder]. A genus of sporozoons found in the muscles of higher vertebrates (reptiles, birds, and mammals).

    S. lindemanni. A species infesting muscles of man.

Sarcodina (săr-kō-dī′nă) ["+ *eidos,* form]. A class of Protozoa characterized by absence of a thick pellicle and movement by pseudopodia. S. are typically holozoic and reproduce principally by asexual methods. Includes the families Amoebidae and Endamoebidae, the latter including many forms parasitic and pathogenic in man.

sarcogenic (săr″kō-jĕn′ĭk) [Gr. *sarkos,* flesh, + *gennan,* to produce]. Producing flesh or muscle.

sarcoid (săr′koyd) ["+ *eidos,* form]. 1. Resembling flesh. 2. A small epithelioid tubercle-like lesion characteristic of sarcoidosis, q.v.

sarcoidosis (săr″koyd-ō′sĭs) ["+ "+ -*ōsis,* condition]. A chronic granulomatous disease of unknown etiology characterized by the formation of tubercle-like lesions in the organs most generally affected. These are the skin, lymph nodes, lungs, and bone marrow. The term now includes a number of diseases previously considered as separate entities (Boeck's sarcoid; Schaumann's disease).

sarcolemma (săr″kō-lĕm′ă) ["+ *lemma,* a rind]. A delicate membrane surrounding each striated muscle fiber.

sarcology (săr-kŏl′ō-jī) [Gr. *sarkos,* flesh, + *logos,* a study]. Branch of medicine dealing with study of the soft tissues of the body.

sarcolysis (săr-kŏl′ĭ-sĭs) ["+ *lysis,* a dissolution]. Decomposition of the soft tissues or flesh.

sarcolytic (săr″kō-lĭt′ĭk). Decomposing flesh.

sarco′ma [Gr. *sarx,* flesh, + -*ōma,* tumor]. (pl. *sarcomas, -mata*) Cancer arising from underlying tissue: muscle, bone, and other connective tissue. May affect the bones, bladder, kidneys, liver, lungs, parotids, and spleen.

   s., botryoid. S. of uterus composed of polypoid mass of soft edematous tissues.

   s., chondro-. S. composed of masses of cartilage.

   s., Ewing's. A diffuse endothelioma or endothelial myeloma forming a fusiform swelling on a long bone.

   s., fibro-. A malignant tumor with fibrous tissue, many spindle cells, and dilated vessels.

   s., giant cell. S. from cancellous bone tissue with large cells with many nuclei. A special type called an epulis is seen in the jaw. SYN: *osteoclastoma.*

   s., lipo-. A rare tumor of bone containing cells of various types with small vacuoles of fat.

   s., lymphangio-. S. arising from endothelium of lymph vessels in a lymph gland.

   s., myeloid. S., giant cell, q.v.

   s., myxo-. A benign tumor of mucoid tissue, such as that of the umbilical cord. SYN: *myxoma.*

   s., osteogenic. S. composed of osseous tissue containing variously shaped cells.

   s., reticulum cell. A variety of malignant lymphoma involving the lymph nodes and other lymphatic tissue. SYN: *Hodgkin's sarcoma.*

   s., rhabdomyo-. An embryonal tumor of striated muscle containing multinucleated cells with a striated cytoplasm.

   s., spindle cell. S. consisting of small and large spindle-shaped cells.

sarcomatoid (săr-kō′mă-toyd) [Gr. *sarx,* flesh, + -*ōma,* tumor, + *eidos,* form]. Resembling a sarcoma.

sarcomatosis (săr″kō-mă-tō′sĭs) ["+ "+ -*ōsis,* condition]. Condition marked by presence and spread of a sarcoma; sarcomatous degeneration.

sarcomatous (săr-kō′mă-tŭs, săr-kō′mătŭs). Of the nature of, or like, a sarcoma.

sarcomere (săr′kō-mēr) [Gr. *sarx, sarkos,* flesh, + *meros,* a part]. The portion of a striated muscle fibril lying between two adjacent dark lines (Krause's membranes).

sarcomphalocele (săr″kŏm-fāl′ō-sēl) ["+ *omphalos,* umbilicus, + *kēlē,* mass]. Fleshy tumor at the umbilicus.

sarcomyces (săr″kō-mī′sēz) ["+ *mykēs,* fungus]. A fleshy growth having the appearance of a fungus.

Sarcophagidae (săr″kō-fāj′ĭ-dē) [Gr. *sarkos,* flesh, + *phagein,* to eat]. The family of the order Diptera which includes the flesh flies. Females deposit their eggs or larvae on decaying flesh of dead animals. Larvae of two genera, Sarcophaga and Wohlfahrtia, frequently infest open sores and wounds of man giving rise to cutaneous myiasis.

sarcophagy (săr-kŏf′ă-jī). Practice of eating flesh.

sarcoplasm (săr′kō-plăzm) [Gr. *sarkos,* flesh, + *plasma,* a thing formed]. Semifluid interfibrillary substance of striated muscle cells. The cytoplasm of muscle cells.

sarcopoietic (săr″kō-poy-ĕt′ĭk) ["+ *poiein,* to form]. Forming muscle or flesh.

Sarcoptidae (sar″kŏp′tĭ-dē). A family of mites of the order Acarina, class Arachnida, which includes Sarcoptes scabiei, the causative agent of scabies or itch in man and mange and scab in other animals.

sarcosis (săr-kō′sĭs) [Gr. *sarkos,* flesh, + *ōsis,* condition]. 1. The development of multiple fleshy tumors. 2. Abnormal formation of flesh.

sarcosome (săr'kō-sōm) ["+ *sōma,* body]. Term previously used for mitochondria, particularly of muscle cells.

Sarcosporidia (săr''kō-spō-rĭd'ĭ-ă) ["+ *sporos,* a seed]. An order of protozoa belonging to the class Sporozoa which are parasitic in the muscles of higher vertebrates. Includes the genus Sarcocystis.

sarcosporidiosis (săr''kō-spō-rĭd-ĭ-ō'sĭs) ["+ "+ *-ōsis,* condition]. Infestation with Sarcosporidia or condition produced by them.

sarcostosis (săr-kŏs-tō'sĭs) [Gr. *sarkos,* flesh, + *osteon,* bone, + *ōsis,* condition]. Ossification of fleshy or muscular tissue.

sarcostyle (săr'kō-stīl) ["+ *stylos,* a column]. Any one of the fine longitudinal fibrillae of a striated muscle fiber.

sarcotic (săr-kŏt'ĭk) [Gr. *sarx, sarkos,* flesh]. 1. Producing or pert. to flesh formation. 2. Agent producing growth of flesh.

sarcous (sar'kŭs). Concerning flesh or muscle.

    s. substance. Substance of a sarcous element.

sardine (săr-dēn') [L. *sardina*]. Any of numerous small silvery fish.

    Food value of 100 gm. (canned in oil: solids and liquids): Cal. 311; protein 20.6 gm.; carbohydrate 0.6 gm.; fat 24.4 gm.; calcium 354 mg.; vitamin A, 180 I.U.

sardon'ic laugh. Old term for a spasmodic affection of facial muscles, giving an appearance of laughter. SYN: *risus sardonicus.*

sartorius (săr-tō'rĭ-ŭs) [L. *sartor,* tailor]. A long, ribbon-shaped muscle of the thigh. The longest muscle in the body, it aids in flexing the knee. So called from its use in crossing the legs, as tailors do. SEE: *Table of Muscles* in *Appendix.*

SAT. 1. Abbr. for *satellite.* 2. Abbr. for (L.) *sine acido thymonucleinico,* without thymonucleic acid.

sat. Abbr. for *saturated.*

SAT-chromosome. Chromosome possessing a satellite, q.v.

satellite (săt'l-īt) [L. *satelles,* attendant]. A small structure attached to a larger one, esp. a minute body attached to a chromosome by a slender chromatic filament.

    s., bacterial. A bacterial colony that grows best when close to a colony of another microorganism.

    s. cells. 1. Flat epithelium-like cells forming the inner portion of a double-layered capsule which covers a neuron. 2. Neuroglial cells enclosing the cell bodies of neurons in spinal ganglia.

satellitosis (săt''l-ĭ-tō'sĭs) [L. *satelles,* companion, + *-ōsis,* condition]. The accumulation of satellite cells about neurons of the central nervous system, seen in certain degenerative and inflammatory conditions.

satiety (sa-tī'ĕt-ĭ) [L. *satietās,* sufficiency]. Being full to satisfaction, esp. with food.

saturated (săt'ū-rā''tĕd) [L. *saturatio*]. 1. Holding all that can be absorbed, received, combined, etc. 2. Term applied to a solution in which no more of a substance can be dissolved. 3. Term applied to carbon compounds in which all the atoms are linked by single bonds.

    s. compound. A compound incapable of additional products, as any in the methane series. SEE: *unsaturated compound.*

    s. solution. Solution containing as much of the solid drug as can be dissolved.

    s. time. Time required for peripheral blood of a person inhaling pure oxygen to become saturated.

saturation (săt'ū-rā'shŭn). The holding in solution of all of a solid that can be dissolved therein.

Saturday night paralysis. A musculospiral paralysis, occurring often in alcoholics, from lying immobile with arm pressed against a projecting surface. SYN: *Sunday morning paralysis.*

saturnine (săt'ŭr-nīn) [L. *saturnus,* lead]. Concerning or produced by lead.

    s. breath. Sweet breath produced by lead poisoning.

    s. gout. Goutlike symptoms produced by lead poisoning.

saturnism (săt'ŭr-nĭzm) ["+ Gr. *ismos,* condition]. Lead poisoning, q.v. SYN: *plumbism.*

satyriasis (săt-ĭ-rī'ă-sĭs) [LL.]. Excessive, and often uncontrollable, sex drive in men.

Sauerbruch's cabinet (sow'ĕr-brook). [Ferdinand Sauerbruch, Ger. surgeon, 1875-1951]. An airtight cabinet for operation on the chest under negative pressure. The patient's head is outside the cabinet and his body and the surgeon's are within it.

sauerkraut (sowr'krowt) [Ger. *sauer,* sour, + *kraut,* cabbage]. Shredded cabbage that is salted and fermented in its own juice.

    Food value of 100 gm. (solid and liquids): Cal. 18; protein 1.0 gm.; fat 0.2 gm.; carbohydrate 4.0 gm.; vitamin A, 50 I.U.; vitamin C, 14 mg.

sausage (sŏ'sĭj) [ME. *sausige*]. Chopped and seasoned meat, esp. pork, stuffed into a casing and cooked or cured.

    Food value of 100 gm. (pork, cooked): Cal. 476; protein 18.1 gm.; fat 44.2; trace of carbohydrate.

savory (sā'vō-rĭ) [O.Fr. *savouré,* tasty]. Having a pleasant or appetizing taste or odor.

saw (sŏ) [AS. *sagu*]. A cutting instrument with an edge of sharp toothlike projections; used esp. for cutting bone in surgery.

saxifragant (săks-ĭf'rā-gănt) [L. *saxum*, rock, + *frangere*, to break]. Dissolving or breaking calculi, esp. in the bladder.

Sayre's jacket (sār). [Lewis Albert Sayre, Amer. surgeon, 1820-1900] A jacket of plaster of Paris worn to support the spine in vertebral diseases.

Sb. Symb. for antimony.

SbCl₃. Antimony trichloride.

Sb₂O₅. Antimonic oxide; antimony pentoxide.

Sb₄O₆. Antimonious oxide.

Sc. Chem. symbol for scandium.

s.c. Abbr. for *subcutaneously*.

scab (skăb) [ME. *scabbe*]. 1. Crust of a cutaneous sore, wound, ulcer, or pustule formed by drying up of the discharge. 2. To become covered with a crust.

scabicide (skā'bĭ-sīd). An agent which kills mites, esp. the causative agent of scabies, q.v.

scabies (skā'bĭ-ēz, -bēz) [L. *scabiēs*, itch]. A highly communicable skin disease caused by an arachnid, Sarcoptes scabiei, the itch mite. SYN: *itch; seven-year itch.*

SYM: Papules, vesicles, pustules, burrows, and intense itching resulting in eczema. The impregnated females live in burrows which appear as slightly discolored lines several mm. to several cm. in length. Eggs deposited within the tunnel hatch within 4-8 days.

Parts most commonly affected are hands; between the fingers; wrists; axillae; genitalia; beneath the mammae; and inner aspect of the thighs.

PROG: Favorable.

TREATMENT: Benzyl benzoate 25% solution applied to the entire body, except the eyes, nose, and mouth, after the patient has taken a prolonged hot bath or shower. The affected areas are scrubbed thoroughly and then the medicine is applied. A second application is made the following morning.

scabiphobia (skā'bĭ-fō'bĭ-ă) [L. *scabies*, itch, + *phobos*, fear]. Morbid fear of acquiring scabies. SYN: *acarophobia.*

scabrities (skā-brĭsh'ĭ-ēz) [L. *scaber*, rough]. 1. Scaly, roughened condition of the skin. 2. A morbid roughness of inner surface of eyelids causing sensation as if sand were in eyes.

s. unguium. Morbid degeneration of the nails making them rough, thick, distorted, and separated from the flesh at the root. Symptomatic of syphilis and leprosy.

scala (skā'lā) [L. *scālae*, stairs]. Any one of the three spiral passages of the cochlea. SEE: *cochlea.*

s. media. The cochlear duct which lies between the s. tympani and s. vestibuli. Its floor contains the spiral organ of Corti. It extends from saccule to tip of cochlea and is filled with endolymph.

s. tympani. Canal filled with perilymph lying below spiral lamina of cochlea. Extends from tip of cochlea to round cochlear window.

s. vestibuli. A canal forming the upper portion of the osseous canal of the cochlea. It lies above the spiral lamina and extends from floor of vestibule to tip of cochlea where it communicates with scala tympani through an aperture, the helicotrema.

scald (skŏld) [LL. *excaldāre*, wash in hot water]. 1. Burn to skin or flesh caused by moist heat and hot vapors, as steam. 2. To cause a burn with hot liquid or steam. 3. Cutaneous disease marked by scab formation on the head.

A scald is deeper than a burn from dry heat, and should be treated as a burn, q.v. Healing is slower and scar formation greater.

Emergency treatment of a scalded area should be the immediate application of cold in the most readily available form, i.e., ice packs or very cold water. This should be continued for at least an hour.

scalded skin syndrome. Necrosis of the epidermal layer of the skin with very little damage to underlying dermis. As much as 80% of the skin may be affected.

ETIOL: Staphylococcal infections, drug reactions, or unknown causes.

TREATMENT: Appropriate antibiotic if caused by staphylococcal infection. Adrenal cortical hormones if caused by drugs.

scale (skāl). 1. [O.Fr. *escale*, husk]. A small, thin, dry exfoliation shed from upper layers of skin. 2. Film of tartar encrusting the teeth. 3. To remove a film of tartar from the teeth. 4. To form a scale on. 5. To shed scales. 6. [ME. *scole*, balance] An instrument for weighing. 7. [L. *scāla*, ladder] A graduated or proportioned measure, a series of tests, or an instrument for measuring quantities or for rating, i.e., individual intelligence.

Shedding of scales from skin in small amounts is normal. More shedding is seen in cutaneous disorders such as squamous eczema, seborrhea sicca, psoriasis, ichthyosis, syphilis, lupus erythematosus, pityriasis rosea, and tinea tonsurans. SEE: *macule; rash.*

s., absolute. A s. used for indicating low temperatures based on absolute zero. SEE: *absolute temperature; absolute zero.*

s., centigrade. Thermometric scale running from 0°, the melting point of ice, to 100°, the boiling point of water. SYN: *Celsius scale.* SEE: *centigrade; thermometer* for table.

s., Fahrenheit. S. in which the freezing point of water is 32° and the boiling point is 212°. SEE: *Fahrenheit; thermometer* for table.

scalene (skā-lēn′) [Gr. *skalēnos,* uneven]. 1. Having unequal sides and angles, said of a triangle. 2. Designating a scalenus muscle.

s. tubercle. Tubercle on upper surface of 1st rib, the insertion of the scalenus anticus muscle. SYN: *tubercle, Lisfranc's.*

scaleniotomy (skā-lēn′ĭ-ŏt′ō-mĭ) ["+ *tomē,* a cutting]. Incision of scalenus muscles near their insertion to check expansive movements in tuberculosis of the apex of the lung.

scalenus (skā-lē′nŭs) [L.]. One of three deeply situated muscles on each side of the neck, extending from the tubercles of the transverse processes of 3rd through 6th cervical vertebrae to the 1st or 2nd rib. Known as scalenus anterior, medius, and posterior. SEE: *Table of Muscles* in *Appendix.*

s. anticus syndrome, s. syndrome. A symptom complex characterized by brachial neuritis with or without vascular or vasomotor disturbance in the upper extremities.

SYM: Not clearly defined, but pain, tingling, and numbness may occur anywhere from shoulder to fingers. Atrophy of small muscles of the hand or even the deltoid or other muscles of arm.

TREATMENT: Correction of posture, avoidance of fatigue, and sometimes immobilization of arm and shoulder. When relief is not obtained, surgical correction may be required.

scall (skŏl) [Norse *skalli,* baldhead]. Dermatitis of the scalp producing a crusted, scabby eruption.

scalp (skălp) [ME.]. The hairy integument of the head. In anatomy, includes skin, dense subcutaneous tissue, occipitofrontalis muscle with the galea aponeurotica, loose subaponeurotic tissue, and the cranial periosteum.

scalpel (skăl′pĕl) [L. *scalpellum,* little knife]. A small, straight surgical knife with a convex edge and thin, keen blade.

scalpriform (skăl′prĭ-form) [L. *scalper,* knife, + *forma,* shape]. Shaped like a chisel.

scalprum (skăl′prŭm) [L.]. (pl. *scalpra*) 1. A toothed instrument for removal of carious bone or for trephining. 2. A large scalpel. 3. Cutting edge of an incisor tooth.

scaly (skā′lĭ) [O.Fr. *escale,* husk]. Resembling or characterized by scales.

scandium (L. *Scandia,* Scandinavia). SYMB: *Sc.* At. wt. 44.956; at. no. 21. A rare metal belonging to the aluminum group.

scanning. Recording, on a photographic plate, the emission of radioactive waves from a specific substance injected into the body. The radioactive agent selected is one that is concentrated in a specific tissue such as thyroid, brain, or liver.

scan'ning speech. Pronunciation of words in syllables, or slowly and hesitatingly; a symptom of disseminated sclerosis, q.v. SEE: *speech.*

scanty (skăn′tĭ) [ME. *skant,* short]. Not abundant; insufficient, as a secretion.

scapha (skā′fă) [L., skiff]. [NA]. Elongated depression of the ear between the helix and anthelix. SYN: *scaphoid fossa.*

scapho- [Gr. *skaphē,* skiff]. Combining form meaning boat.

scaphocephalic, scaphocephalous (skăf′ō-sĕf-ăl′ĭk, -sĕf′ăl-ŭs) ["+ *kephalē,* head]. Having a deformed head, projecting like a boat's keel.

scaphocephalism (skăf′ō-sĕf′ăl-ĭzm) ["+ "+ *-ismos,* condition]. Condition of having a deformed head, projecting like the keel of a boat.

scaphoid (skăf′oyd) [Gr. *skaphē,* skiff, + *eidos,* resemblance]. 1. Boat-shaped, navicular, hollowed. 2. A proximal, boat-shaped bone of the carpus on radial side. SYN: *navicular bone; os scaphoideum.* 3. A boat-shaped bone on inner side of the tarsus between the talus and three cuneiform bones. SYN: *navicular bone.*

s. abdomen. Abdomen with hollowed anterior wall.

s. bone. Navicular bone. SEE: *scaphoid.*

scaphoiditis (skăf′oyd-ī′tĭs) ["+ "+ *-itis,* inflammation]. Inflamed condition of the scaphoid bone.

scapula (L.). (pl. *scapulae*) [NA]. The large, flat, triangular bone of the shoulder. It articulates with the clavicle and the humerus. SYN: *shoulder blade.* SEE: *triceps.*

s., winged. Condition in which medial border of scapula is prominent, usually the result of paralysis of serratus anterior or trapezius muscles. SYN: *scapula alata.*

RS: acromial; acromial angle; acromioclavicular joint; acromiocoracoid; acromion; angel's wing; glenoid cavity.

scapulalgia (skăp-ū-lăl′jĭ-ă) [L. *scapula,* shoulder blade, + Gr. *algos,* pain]. Pain in the region of the shoulder blade.

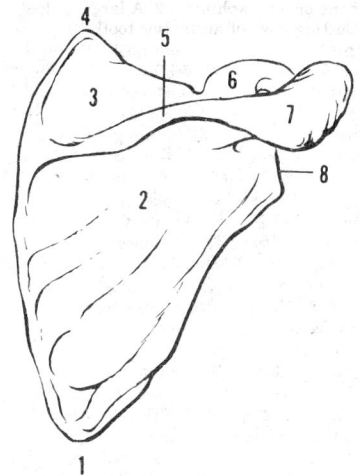

SCAPULA
1, Inferior angle. 2, Infraspinatous fossa. 3,
Supraspinatous fossa. 4, Superior angle. 5,
Spine. 6, Coracoid process. 7, Acromion process.
8, Anterior angle.

scapular (skăp'ū-lăr). Of, or pert. to, the
shoulder blade.
    s. reflex. Scapular muscular contrac-
tion following percussion or stimulus between the scapulae.

scapulary (skăp'ū-lā-rĭ). A shoulder bandage
for keeping a body bandage in place. A broad
roller bandage is split in half. The undivided
section of the roller bandage is fastened in
front with the two ends passing over the
shoulders and attached to the back of the
body bandage.

scapulectomy (skăp''ū-lĕk'tō-mĭ) [L. *scapula,* shoulder blade, + Gr. *ektomē,* excision].
Surgical excision of the scapula.

scapulo- [L. *scapula,* shoulder blade]. Combining form meaning shoulder.

scapuloclavicular (skăp''ū-lō-klă-vĭk'ū-lăr)
["+ *clavicula,* a little key]. Concerning the
scapula and the clavicle.

scapulodynia (skăp''ū-lō-dĭn'ĭ-ă) ["+ *odynē,*
pain]. Inflammation and pain in the shoulder muscles.

scapulohumeral (skăp''ū-lō-hū'mĕr-ăl) [L.
scapula, shoulder blade, + *humerus,* shoul-
der]. Concerning the scapula and the humerus.
    s. reflex. When vertebral border of
scapula is percussed, upper arm is adducted
and rotated outwards.

scapulopexy (skăp''ū-lō-pĕk'sĭ) ["+ Gr.
pēxis, fixation]. Fixation of the scapula to
the ribs.

scapulothoracic (skăp''ū-lō-thō-răs'ĭk) ["+
Gr. *thōrax,* chest]. Concerning the scapula
and the thorax.

scapus (skā'pŭs) [L. *scapus,* stalk]. (pl. *sca'pi*)
A shaft or stem.
    s. penis. Shaft of penis.
    s. pili. [NA]. Major portion of a hair, esp.
that section that extends beyond the outer
scalp. SYN: *hair shaft.*

scar (skăr) [Gr. *eskhara,* scab caused by a
burn]. Mark left in skin or internal organ by
healing of a wound, sore, or injury because
of replacement by connective tissue of the
injured tissue. Scars may result from
wounds that have healed, lesions of diseases,
or surgical operations.
    When first developed it is red or purple,
later whitish and glistening. When on the
head scars may be the result of wounds
which have healed or of skin disease. On the
skin they may be the result of trauma or
surgery. SYN: *cicatrix.* SEE: *cicatricotomy;
keloid.*
    s., cicatricial. A scar or cicatrix with
considerable contraction. It may be necessary to divide the scar and graft on new skin,
as in burns.
    s., keloid. A red, raised, smooth scar
containing blood vessels, often irritable.
    s., painful. S. which is painful because
of involvement of a nerve during healing.
The end of the nerve may become bulbous.
    TREATMENT: Dissection of scar or exci-
sion of nerve.

scar"abi'asis [L. *scarabaeus,* scarab, + Gr.
-iosis, condition]. Condition in which intestine is invaded by the dung beetle. Occurs
principally in children. SYN: *beetle disease.*

scarf'skin [O.Fr. *escarpe,* scarf, + O. Norse
skinn, skin]. Epidermis or outermost layer of
skin, esp. the cuticle.

scarification (skăr'ĭ-fĭ-kă'shŭn) [Gr. *skari-
phismos,* scratching up]. Making of numerous superficial incisions in the skin.

scar'ifica"tor. Instrument for making small
incisions in the skin. SYN: *scarifier.*

scarlatina (skăr''lă-tē'nă) [L.]. Scarlet fever,
q.v.
    s. simplex. Mild type of scarlet fever.

scarlatinal (skăr''lă-tē'năl). Concerning or
due to scarlatina.

scarlatinella (skăr-lăt''ĭ-nĕl'ă) [L.]. A mild
disease resembling measles and scarlet fever. SYN: *fourth disease.*

scarlatiniform, scarlatinoid (skăr-lă-
tĭn'ĭ-form, -lăt'ĭ-noyd) [L. *scarlatina,* scar-

latina, + *forma,* shape, + Gr. *eidos,* form].
Resembling scarlatina or its rash.

scarlet fever (skăr'lĕt) [L. *scarlatum,* red].
An acute contagious disease characterized
by sore throat, strawberry tongue, fever,
punctiform scarlet rash, and rapid pulse.
SYN: *scarlatina.*

ETIOL: Many strains (over 40) of Type A
hemolytic, toxin-producing streptococci
have been recovered from scarlet fever patients. The erythema-producing toxin was
discovered by Dick and Dick (1924-25). SEE:
Dick method.

INCUBATION: Probably never less than
24 hr. May be 1-3 days, rarely longer.

SYM: Onset sudden, rarely with a chill,
but sometimes with a convulsion in very
young children. As a rule, begins with sore
throat, temperature from 101° to 105° F.
(38.3° to 40.6° C.), frequent vomiting; followed within 12-36 hr. by a rash, first on
neck and chest, rapidly extending over body,
finally involving the extremities. Face
flushed and may be characterized by the
well-known circumoral pallor, the punctiform rash on the remainder of the body,
seldom seen on face.

With first eruption, throat is markedly
injected, tonsils are swollen, tongue heavily
coated, and the papillae are enlarged, projecting through it; the tongue properly described as a strawberry tongue. In mild or
average case, duration of rash is 2-3 days. By
end of 3rd day, the coating has disappeared
from tongue though the papillae are still
enlarged, the remainder of tongue presenting a deep red appearance. In this stage, the
tongue may be referred to as the raspberry
tongue.

With disappearance of rash in an uncomplicated case, the temperature closely approaches normal and recovery is uneventful.
Extremely mild cases occur in which the
rash is very faint and of very short duration,
possibly not exceeding 24 hr. Scarlet fever
may actually occur without any rash what-
soever. In any form, a leukocytosis is to be
expected in the average case. Number of
leukocytes may range from 10,000 to 20,000
with 75-90% neutrophils.

SPECIFIC TREATMENT: Penicillin is
the agent of choice although other antibiotics may be used to combat the septic factor
in the disease; however, these have little
effect on toxic manifestations.

Penicillin should be given for a minimum
of 10 days no matter how mild the infection
in order to prevent the subsequent development of complications such as rheumatic
fever and acute glomerulonephritis. Im-

mune serum and antitoxin are effective
against toxic manifestations but exert little
effect against the streptococcal organisms.
Serum therapy has largely been abondoned
because of dangers of serum sickness. It is
reserved for rare cases in which toxic manifestations suggest a possibly fatal outcome.

GENERAL TREATMENT: Isolation, rest,
and diet are of utmost importance. Patient
with uncomplicated scarlet fever should be
kept in bed during acute phase of the illness.

s. f., afebrile. S. f. without fever.

s. f., anginal. S. f. with severe throat
symptoms.

s. f., hemorrhagic. S. f. with blood extravasated into mucous membranes and the
skin.

s. f., latent. S. f. without rash but complicated by nephritis.

s. f., malignant. S. f. with great prostration and severe symptoms.

s. f., rheumatic. S. f. with joint pain.

s. f. without angina. S. f. without sore
throat.

scarlet rash. A rose-colored rash, specifically that of German measles, q.v.

scar'let red. An azo dye, of the color its
name suggests.

USES: To stimulate healing of indolent
ulcers, burns, wounds, etc. In histology, as a
stain.

SYN: *rubrum scarlatinum.*

Scarpa (skär'pä). [Antonio Scarpa, It. anatomist, 1747-1832].

S.'s fascia. Deep layer of superficial abdominal fascia around edge of the subcutaneous inguinal ring.

S.'s fluid. Fluid in membranous labyrinth of the ear. SYN: *endolymph.*

S.'s foramina. Bony passages opening
into the incisor canal for passage of the
nasopalatine nerves.

S.'s ganglion. The vestibular ganglion.
SEE: *ganglion, vestibular.*

S.'s liquor. S.'s fluid, q.v.

S.'s membrane. Membrane that closes
the fenestra rotunda of the tympanic cavity.

S.'s triangle. Triangular space bounded laterally by inner edge of sartorius, above
by Poupart's ligament, and medially by the
adductor longus.

scatacratia (skăt'ă-krā'shĭ-ă) [Gr. *skatos,*
dung, + *akratia,* lack of control]. Fecal
incontinence.

scatemia (skă-tē'mĭ-ă) ["+ *haima,* blood]. Intestinal toxemia from retained fecal matter.

scato- [Gr. *skōr, skatos,* dung]. Combining
form denoting relationship to dung or fecal
matter.

scatology (skă-tŏl′ō-jĭ) ["+ *logos,* study]. 1. Scientific study and analysis of the feces. SYN: *coprology.* 2. Interest in obscene things, esp. literature.

scatoma (skă-tō′mă) ["+ *-ōma,* tumor]. Mass of inspissated feces in colon or rectum resembling an abdominal tumor. SYN: *coproma; fecaloma; stercoroma.*

scatophagy (skă-tŏf′ă-jĭ) [Gr. *skatos,* dung, + *phagein,* to eat]. The eating of excrement. SYN: *coprophagy.*

scatoscopy (skă-tŏs′kō-pĭ) ["+ *skopein,* to examine]. Examination of excreta for diagnostic purposes.

scavenger cell (skăv′ĕn-jer) [ME. *skawager,* toll collector]. A phagocytic cell, such as a macrophage or a neutrophil leukocyte, which functions in the removal of disintegrating tissues.

S.C.C.M. Abbr. for *Society of Critical Care Medicine.*

Schafer's method of artificial respiration (shā′fer). [Sir Edward A. Sharpey-Schafer, Eng. physiologist, 1850-1935] A method of artificial respiration in which the subject lies prone with both arms extended forward, with one flexed so that hand rests under cheek and mouth. Operator kneels astride one or both thighs and places palms of hands on back over lower ribs. Operator rhythmically applies pressure with his hands on the patient's back at a rate of 12 times per minute.

This method formerly was widely used, but has been replaced by mouth-to-mouth breathing technique. SEE: *artificial respiration; resuscitation.*

Schäffer's reflex (shā′fer). [Max Schäffer, Ger. neurologist, 1852-1923]. Dorsal flexion of toes and flexion of foot resulting when middle portion of tendo achillis is pinched.

schematic (skē-măt′ĭk) [L. *schematicus,* planned]. Pert. to a diagram or model; showing part for part in a diagram.

scheroma (shē-rō′mă). A condition caused by lack of lacrimal fluid. SYN: *xerophthalmia.*

Schick test (shĭk). [Béla Schick, Amer. pediatrician, 1877-1967] Injection intradermally of 0.1 ml. of dilute diphtheria toxin, 1/50 MLD. (MLD: *minimum lethal dose,* the amount of diphtheria toxin which would kill a small guinea pig in four days.)

Results 3-4 days later. Susceptibility (*positive test*) is indicated by the development of a red, inflamed area at point of injection, which slowly disappears after a few days. A *negative test* (little or no reaction) indicates the presence of antibodies sufficient to neutralize the toxin, hence the person is immune. SEE: *diphtheria.*

Schilder's disease. [Paul Ferdinand Schilder, Austrian-Amer. neurologist, 1886-1940]. A rare, but invariably fatal, disease of the central nervous system. It probably is a special form of multiple sclerosis.

Schiller's test (shĭl′er). [Walter Schiller, Austrian-Amer. pathologist, 1887 —]. Test for superficial cancer, esp. of the cervix uteri. Paint tissue with solution of iodine. Cancer cells not containing glycogen fail to stain, thus revealing their presence.

Schilling's classification. [Victor Schilling, Ger. hematologist, 1883-1960] Method of classifying polymorphonuclear neutrophils into four categories according to number and arrangement of the nuclei in the cells. SYN: *Schilling blood count.*

Schilling test. [Robert F. Schilling, Amer. hematologist, 1919 —]. A test, utilizing radioactive vitamin B_{12}, for gastrointestinal absorption of vitamin B_{12}. For diagnosis of primary pernicious anemia.

schindylesis (skĭn″dĭ-lē′sĭs) [Gr. *schindylēsis,* a splintering]. A form of wedge and groove suture in which a crest of one bone fits into a groove of another.

schisto- (skĭs′to) [Gr. *schistos,* split]. Combining form meaning split or cleft.

schistocelia (skĭs″tō-sē′lĭ-ă) ["+ *koilia,* belly]. Congenital abdominal fissure.

schistocyte (skĭs′tō-sĭt) ["+ *kytos,* a cell]. A fragmented segment of a red blood cell. Seen in patients with hemolytic anemia.

schistocytosis (skĭs″tō-sī-tō′sĭs) ["+ "+ *-ōsis,* condition]. Schistocytes in the blood.

schistoglossia (skĭs″tō-glos′ĭ-ă) [Gr. *schistos,* split, + *glōssa,* tongue]. A cleft tongue.

schistoprosopia (skĭs″tō-prō-sō′pĭ-ă) ["+ *prosōpon,* face]. Congenital fissure of the face.

schistorrhachis (skĭs-tōr′ă-kĭs) ["+ *rhachis,* spine]. Protrusion of membranes through a congenital cleft in lower vertebral column. SYN: *spina bifida.*

Schistosoma (skĭs′tō-sō′mă) [Gr. *schistos,* a cleft, + *sōma,* body]. A genus of blood flukes belonging to the family Schistosomatidae, class Trematoda. Adults live in blood vessels of visceral organs. Eggs make their way into bladder or intestine and are discharged in urine or feces. Eggs hatch into miracidia which enter snails and transform into sporocysts. These develop daughter sporocysts which give rise to fork-tailed cercaria. These leave snail and enter final host directly through skin or through mucus membrane.

S. haematobium. A species common in Africa and southwestern Asia. Adults infest pelvic veins of vesicle plexus. Eggs work their way through bladder wall and are discharged through urine. Cause of urinary schistosomiasis.

S. japonicum. A species common in many parts of Orient. Adults live principally in branches of superior mesenteric vein. Eggs work their way through intestinal wall into lumen and are discharged with feces. Cause of Oriental schistosomiasis.

S. mansoni. A species occurring in many parts of Africa and tropical America (W. Indies, northern part of S.A.). Adults live in branches of inferior mesenteric veins. Eggs discharged through either intestine or bladder. Cause of bilharzial dysentery or Manson's intestinal schistosomiasis.

schistosome dermatitis (skĭs'tō-sōm). Dermatitis resulting from penetration of skin of humans by cercariae of non-human blood flukes. Common in lake region of northern U.S. It is not associated with visceral schistosomiasis. SYN: *swimmer's itch.*

schistosomiasis (skĭs''tō-sō-mī'ăs-ĭs) [Gr. *schistos,* a cleft, + *sōma,* body, + *-iasis,* infection]. A parasitic disease due to infestation with blood flukes belonging to the genus Schistosoma, q.v. The disease is widespread throughout Asia, Africa, and tropical America. Man becomes infested by wading or bathing in water containing cercaria which have issued from snails. SYN: *bilharziasis.*

schistothorax (skĭs''tō-thō'răks) ["+ *thōrax,* chest]. Fissure of the thorax.

schizamnion (skĭz-ăm'nĭ-ŏn) ["+ *amnion,* lamb]. An amnion formed by development of a cavity in the inner cell mass.

schizaxon (skĭs-ăk'sŏn) ["+ *axōn,* axle]. An axon that divides in two equal, or nearly equal, branches.

schizo- (skĭz'ō) [Gr. *schizein,* to divide]. Combining form indicating division.

schizoblepharia (skĭz-ō-blĕf'ă-rĭ-ă) ["+ *blepharon,* eyelid]. Fissure of an eyelid.

schizocytosis (skĭz''ō-sī-tō'sĭs) ["+ *kytos,* cell, + *-ōsis,* condition]. SYN: *schistocytosis.*

schizogenesis (skĭz''ō-jĕn'ĕs-ĭs) [Gr. *schizein,* to divide, + *genesis,* production]. Reproduction by fission.

schizogony (skĭz-ŏg'ō-nĭ) ["+ *gonē,* seed]. Reproduction by multiple asexual fission characteristic of sporozoans, esp. the life-cycle of the malarial parasite.

schizogyria (skĭz''ō-jĭ'rĭ-ă) ["+ *gyros,* a circle]. A break or cleft in the cerebral convolutions.

schizoid (skĭz'oyd) [Gr. *schizein,* to split, + *eidos,* resemblance]. Resembling schizophrenia.

    s. personality. The type of person characterized by seclusiveness, inability to devel-

op close emotional attachments to others, reduced initiative, morbid introspection, and oftentimes queer behavior. The so-called shut-in type.

Schizomycetes (skĭz''ō-mī-sē'tēz) ["+ *mykēs,* fungus]. Class of plant microorganisms or fungi which multiplies by fission. Includes the bacteria.

schizont (skĭz'ŏnt) ["+ *ontos,* being]. 1. A stage appearing in the life cycle of a sporozoan protozoon resulting from multiple division or schizogony. 2. Stage in asexual phase of life cycle of Plasmodium found in red blood cells. By schizogony, each gives rise to 12-24 or more merozoites. An early schizont is called a presegmenter; a mature schizont is called a rosette or segmenter. SEE: *malaria* for illustration.

schizonychia (skĭz''ō-nĭk'ĭ-ă) [Gr. *schizein,* to split, + *onyx, onych-,* nail]. Split condition of the nails.

schizophasia (skĭz''ō-fā'zĭ-ă) ["+ *phasis,* speech]. Muttered and incomprehensible speech of the schizophrenic.

schizophrenia (skĭz''ō-frē'nĭ-ă) [Gr. *schizein,* to split, + *phrēn,* mind]. A group of mental disorders characterized by disturbances of thinking, mood, and behavior. There is an altered concept of reality, and in some cases delusions and hallucinations. Mood changes include inappropriate emotional responses and loss of empathy. Withdrawn, regressive, and bizarre behavior may be noted.

    This term includes all cases of dementia precox of the older writers. It may also apply to numerous borderline cases which would not have been included in dementia precox.

    Usually four types of schizophrenic reactions are differentiated, although the dominant reaction in any patient may vary from time to time. The types are simple, paranoid, catatonic, and hebephrenic. In the *simple* type, the patient becomes dull emotionally, loses ambition, and tends to withdraw; however, there is no serious intellectual impairment. The *paranoid* type develops extensive delusions of persecution. The *catatonic* may show stereotyped excitement or simulate a stupor, though lucid and clearly recalling the episode if recovery occurs. A vague sense of being two personalities and of having changed occurs in all types. The *hebephrenic* shows silly mannerisms, speech anomalies, hysteroid symptoms, delusions, hallucinations, and often childish behavior and mannerisms. It is important to note that a person who has made a fairly successful adjustment in one society might appear to be markedly abnormal by observers from a society with a different set of mores.

ETIOL: Unknown.

PROG: Always guarded.

NP: Expert and careful nursing care is required during the hospital stay.

TREATMENT: Hospitalization is essential in most cases. Psychotherapy is used. Drug therapy involving use of tranquilizing agents such as chlorpromazine or reserpine is effective in certain cases.

schizophrenic (skĭz″ō-frĕn′ĭk) [Gr. *schizein,* to split, + *phrēn,* mind]. Afflicted with, or person afflicted with schizophrenia.

schizoprosopia (skĭz″ō-prō-sō′pĭ-ă) ["+ *prosōpon,* face]. Fissure of the face, i.e., harelip or cleft palate.

schizotrichia (skĭz″ō-trĭk′ĭ-ă) ["+ *thrix, trich-,* hair]. Splitting of the tips of the hair.

Schlemm's canal (shlĕm). [Friedrich S. Schlemm, Ger. anatomist, 1795-1858]. Irregular space or spaces in the sclerocorneal region of the eye. It receives the aqueous humor from the anterior chamber of the eye. SYN: *sinus venosus sclera.*

Schmorl's disease. [Christian G. Schmorl, Ger. pathologist, 1861-1932] Herniation of the nucleus pulposus.

schneiderian membrane (shnī-dē′rĭ-ăn). [Conrad Victor Schneider, Ger. physician, 1610-1680]. The nasal mucosa.

Schönlein's disease (shän′lĭn). [Johann Lukas Schönlein, Ger. physician, 1793-1864] An allergic or anaphylactic purpura occurring in individuals, esp. children, with drug sensitivities, serum sickness, and other allergic disorders. It is usually accompanied by pains in joints and abdomen. SYN: *purpura hemorrhagica; Schönlein-Henoch purpura.*

Schultze's bundle (shūltz). [Max Johann Schultze, Ger. biologist, 1825-1874]. Longitudinal mass of descending fibers, shaped like a comma, in the fasciculus cuneatus of spinal cord.

Schultze's cells. Olfactory cells.

Schultze's granule masses. Fine, granular masses formed by breaking up of plaques in the blood.

Schwabach test (shvŏ′băk). [Dagobert Schwabach, Ger. otologist, 1846-1920]. A test for hearing by use of 5 tuning forks, each of a different tone. SEE: *test.*

Schwann's cells (shvŏn). [Theodor Schwann, Ger. anatomist, 1810-1882]. Cells of ectodermal origin which comprise the neurilemma.

Schwann's sheath. The neurilemma of a nerve fiber. SYN: *neurilemma.*

Schwann's white substance. Myelin of a medullated nerve fiber.

sciage (sē-azh′) [Fr., a sawing]. A movement in massage resembling that in sawing.

sciatic (sī-ăt′ĭk) [L. *sciaticus*]. 1. Pert to the hip or ischium. 2. Pert. to, due to, or afflicted with sciatica, q.v.

s. nerve. Largest nerve in the body arising from sacral plexus on either side, passing from pelvis through greater sciatic foramen, down back of thigh, where it divides into tibial and peroneal nerves. Lesions cause paralysis of flexion and of adduction of toes, abduction and adduction of toes, rotation inward and adduction of foot; of plantar flexion and lowering of ball of foot; anesthesia in cutaneous distribution (external popliteal nerve); paralysis of dorsal flexion and adduction of foot; of rotation of ball of foot outward and of raising external border of foot and of extension of toes; also anesthesia in cutaneous distribution. SYN: *great sciatic nerve; nervus ischiadicus* [NA]. SEE: *Table of Nerves* in *Appendix.*

s. nerve, small. The posterior femoral cutaneous nerve, a cutaneous nerve supplying skin of buttocks, perineum, popliteal region, and back of thigh and leg.

sciatica (sī-ăt′ĭ-kă) [L.]. Severe pain in the leg along the course of the sciatic nerve felt at back of thigh running down the inside of the leg. SEE: *meralgia; sciatic nerve.*

ETIOL: 1. Compression or trauma of the sciatic nerve or its roots, esp. that resulting from ruptured intervertebral disk or osteoarthrosis of lumbosacral vertebrae. 2. Inflammation of sciatic nerve resulting from metabolic, toxic, or infectious disorders. 3. Pain referred to sciatic nerve from other parts of body.

SYM: May begin abruptly or gradually and is characterized by a sharp, shooting pain running down back of thigh. Movement of limb generally intensifies the suffering. Pain may be uniformly distributed along the limb, but not infrequently there are certain spots where it is more intense; numbness, tingling; nerve may be extremely sensitive to touch. Sym. grow worse at night and on approach of stormy weather. Duration of attack varies from few days to several months. In long-standing cases, muscles grow atrophied and rigid.

PROG: Recovery follows in majority of cases when treatment is instituted early and is carried out persistently.

TREATMENT: Surgical intervention if due to ruptured intervertebral disk. In acute stage, rest is essential. Hot fomentations. Morphine or Demerol may be required to control pain, but the danger of habituation must be kept in mind. In rheumatic patients, full doses of salicylate or sodium are useful. In chronically ill patients, prolonged rest. Improve general health; good, nourishing diet; hot applications often help to provide relief. Some patients are relieved by the spraying of ethyl chloride over course of nerve. Nerve stretching by pulling affected leg. Lift in shoe of affected limb.

scieropia (sī-ĕr-ō′pĭ-ă) [Gr. *skieros*, shadow, + *opsis*, vision]. Abnormal vision in which things appear to be in shadow.

scintillascope (sĭn-tĭl′ă-skōp) [L. *scintilla*, spark, + Gr. *skopein*, to examine]. Device for viewing the effect of ionizing radiation, alpha particles, on a fluorescent screen.

scintillation (sĭn″tĭ-lā′shŭn) [L. *scintillatio*]. 1. Sparkling; a subjective sensation, as of seeing sparks. 2. The emissions which come from radioactive substances.

scintiphotography. Photographing the scintillations emitted by radioactive substances injected into the body. Used to determine the outline and function of organs and tissues in which the radioactive substance collects or is secreted.

scintiscan. Use of scintillation scanning to produce a map of scintillations produced when a radioactive substance is introduced into the body. The intensity of the record indicates the differential accumulation of the substance in the various parts of the body.

scirrho- [Gr. *skirrhos*, hard]. Combining form meaning hard, or indicating relationship to a hard tumor or scirrhus.

scirrhoid (skĭr′oyd) [″+ *eidos*, form]. Pert. to, or like, a hard carcinoma or scirrhus.

scirrhoma (skĭr-ō′mă) [″+ *-ōma*, tumor]. A hard carcinoma or scirrhus.

scirrhosarca (skĭr″ō-săr′kă) [″+ *sarx, sark-*, flesh]. Hardening of the flesh, esp. of the newly born. SYN: *sclerema neonatorum; scleroderma.*

scirrhous (skĭr′rŭs) [L. *skirrhosus*]. Hard, like a scirrhus.

scirrhus (skĭr′ŭs) [Gr. *skirrhos*]. A hard, cancerous tumor due to overgrowth of fibrous tissue. A hard form of cancer.

scissor leg (sĭz′ōr lĕg). Abnormal tendency of the legs to cross due to contraction of thigh adductor muscles.

scissor gait. Crossing the legs in walking. SEE: *gait.*

scissors (sĭz′ōrs) [LL. *cisōrium*]. A cutting instrument composed of two opposed cutting blades with handles, held together by a central pin. This allows the cutting edge to be opened and closed. SYN: *pair of scissors.*

scissura (sĭ-sū′ră) [L.]. (pl. *scissu′rae*) A fissure or cleft; a splitting.

sclera (sklē′ră) [Gr. *sklēros*, hard]. (pl. *sclerae*) [NA]. A tough white fibrous tissue which covers the so-called white of the eye. It extends from optic nerve to cornea. SYN: *sclerotica.*

scleradenitis (sklē″rad-ĕn-ī′tĭs) [″+ *adēn*, gland, + *-ītis*, inflammation]. Inflammation and induration of a gland.

scleral (sklē′răl) [Gr. *sklēros*, hard]. Concerning the sclera.

sclerectasia (sklē″rĕk-tā′zĭ-ă) [″+ *extasis*, dilatation]. Protrusion of the sclera.

sclerectoiridectomy (sklĕ-rĕk″tō-ĭr′ĭ-dĕk′tō-mĭ) [″+ *iris, irid-*, iris, + *ektomē*, excision]. Formation of a filtering cicatrix in glaucoma by combined sclerectomy and iridectomy.

sclerectoiridodialysis (sklĕ-rĕk″tō-ĭr″ĭd-ō-dī-ăl′ĭ-sĭs) [″+ ″+ *dialysis*, a loosening]. Sclerectomy and iridodialysis for relief of glaucoma.

sclerectomy (sklē-rĕk′tō-mĭ) [Gr. *sklēros*, hard, + *ektomē*, excision]. 1. Excision of a portion of the sclera. 2. Removal of adhesions in chronic otitis media.

scleredema (sklē″rĕ-dē′mă) [″+ *oidēma*, a swelling]. A condition usually following an acute infection characterized by edema and induration of the skin. It is a benign, self-limited disease occurring more frequently in females than males. It is often confused with scleroderma, q.v. SYN: *scleredema adultorum of Buschke; scleriasis.*

sclerema (sklē-rē′mă) [Gr. *sklēros*, hard]. Hardening of the skin. SYN: *scleroderma.*

   s. adiposum. S. neonatorum, q.v.

   s. adultorum. Scleroderma, q.v.

   s. neonatorum. Progressive hardening of the skin in the newborn; usually fatal.

sclerencephalia (sklē″rĕn-sĕ-fā′lĭ-ă) [Gr. *sclēros*, hard, + *enkephalos*, brain]. Sclerosis of the brain.

scleriasis (sklē-rī′a-sĭs) [Gr. *sklēriasis*]. 1. Progressive hardening of the skin. SYN: *scleroderma.* 2. Hardening of the eyelid.

scleriritomy (sklē″rĭ-rĭt′ō-mĭ) [″+ *iris*, iris, + *tomē*, a cutting]. Incision of iris and sclera.

scleritis (sklē-rī′tĭs) [″+ *-ītis*, inflammation]. Superficial and deep inflammation of the sclera. SEE: *episcleritis.*

   s., annular. Inflammation limited to the area surrounding the limbus of the cornea. A complete ring is formed.

scleroblastema (sklē″rō-blăs-tē′mă) [Gr. *sklēros*, hard, + *blastēma*, a sprout]. The embryonic tissue from which formation of bone takes place.

scleroblastemic (sklē″rō-blăs-tĕm′ĭk). Rel. to or derived from scleroblastema.

sclerocataracta (sklē″rō-kăt-ă-rak′tă) [Gr. *sklēros*, hard, + *katarraktēs*, a pouring down]. A hard cataract.

sclerochoroiditis (sklē″rō-kō″roid-i′tĭs) ["+ *chorioeidēs*, skinlike, + *-itis*, inflammation]. Inflammation of the sclera and choroid coat of the eye.

   s., posterior. Myopic choroiditis, posterior staphyloma.

scleroconjunctival (sklē″rō-kon″jŭnk-tī′văl) ["+ L. *conjunctivus*, to bind together]. Pertaining to the sclera and conjunctiva.

sclerocornea (sklē″rō-kor′nē-ă) ["+ L. *cornu*, a horn]. The sclera and cornea together considered as one coat.

sclerodactylia (sklē″rō-dăk-tĭl′ĭ-ă) ["+ *daktylos*, a finger]. Induration of the skin of the digits.

scleroderma (sklē-rō-der′mă) [Gr. *sklēros*, hard, + *derma*, skin]. A progressive disease of the skin involving collagen tissue resulting in diffuse leathery induration of the skin frequently followed by atrophy and pigmentation. The localized form is known as morphea. Involvement of internal organs is to be expected. SYN: *progressive systemic sclerosis.*

   ETIOL: Unknown.

   SYM: Smooth, waxy, edematous skin; later becomes hard, yellowish, and adherent to underlying tissue, causing masklike expression (face) or clawlike appearance of hands (sclerodactylia). When chest is involved respiration may be interfered with. Renal and cardiac involvement produce the usual signs of impaired function of these organs.

   PROG: Better in circumscribed form than in extensive scleroderma, but the disease is usually slow to progress.

   TREATMENT: Physiotherapy for comfort and prevention of fixation where applicable; frequent small feedings for dysphagia. Adrenal steroids do not cure this disease but are of considerable help in controlling the swelling and inflammation. This therapy may be required for months or years. When these are used be alert for systemic bacterial infections; if these occur they are treated with appropriate antibiotic drugs.

   s., circumscribed. Skin disease with pink, firm patches which atrophy, leaving scars. SYN: *morphea.*

   s. neonatorum. Hardness and tightness of the skin in early infancy. SYN: *sclerema adiposum.*

sclerodermatitis (sklē″rō-der-mă-tī′tĭs) ["+ "+ *itis*, inflammation]. Inflammation of the skin accompanied by thickening and hardening.

sclerogenous (sklē-rŏj′ē-nŭs) ["+ *gennan*, to produce]. Causing sclerosis or hardening of tissue.

scleroid (sklē′rŏyd) ["+ *eidos*, form]. Having a hard or firm texture.

scleroiritis (sklē″rō-ī-rī′tĭs) [Gr. *sklēros*, hard, + *iris*, iris, + *-itis*, inflammation]. Inflammation of both sclera and iris.

sclerokeratitis (sklē″rō-ker-ă-tī′tĭs) ["+ *keras, kerat-*, horn, + *-itis*, inflammation]. Cellular infiltration with inflammation of the sclera and cornea.

sclerokeratoiritis (sklē″rō-ker″ă-tō-ī-rī′tĭs) ["+ "+ *iris*, iris, + *-itis*, inflammation]. Inflamed condition of the sclera, cornea, and iris.

scleroma (sklē-rō′mă) [Gr. *sklērōma*, induration]. Indurated, circumscribed area of granulation tissue in mucous membrane or skin. SEE: *sclerosis.*

scleromalacia (sklē″rō-mă-lā′sĭ-ă) ["+ *malakia*, a softening]. Softening of the sclera.

   s. perforans. Scleromalacia accompanied by perforation.

scleromere (sklē′rō-mēr) [Gr. *sklēros*, hard, + *meros*, a part]. 1. Any segment or metamere of the skeleton. 2. The caudal half of a sclerotome, q.v.

scleronychia (sklē″rō-nĭk′ĭ-ă) ["+ *onyx*, nail]. Thickening and hardening of the nails.

scleronyxis (sklē-rō-nĭk′sĭs) [Gr. *sklēros*, hard, + *nyxis*, a piercing]. Surgical puncture of the sclera.

sclero-oophoritis (sklē″rō-ō-ŏf″ō-rī′tĭs) ["+ *ōon*, egg, + *phoros*, a bearer, + *-itis*, inflammation]. Induration and inflammation of the ovary.

sclerophthalmia (sklē″rŏf-thăl′mĭ-ă) ["+ *ophthalmos*, eye]. Congenital condition in which opacity of the sclera advances over the cornea.

scleroplasty (sklē′rō-plăs″tĭ) ["+ *plassein*, to form]. Plastic surgery of the sclera.

scleroprotein (sklē″rō-prō′tē-ĭn) ["+ *prōtos*, first]. A group of proteins noted for their insolubility in most chemicals. Found in skeletal tissue, cartilage, hair, nails, and in animal claws and horns. SYN: *albuminoid.*

sclerosed (sklē-rōsd′, sklē′rōsd) [Gr. *sklēros*, hard]. Having sclerosis; hardened. SYN: *indurated.*

sclerosing (sklē-rōs′ĭng). Causing or developing sclerosis.

sclerosis (sklē-rō′sĭs) [Gr. *sklērosis*, a hardening]. 1. A hardening or induration of an organ or tissue, esp. that due to excessive growth of fibrous tissue. 2. Hardening within nervous system, esp. brain and spinal cord resulting from degeneration of nervous elements, as the myelin sheath. 3. Thickening and hardening of the layers in wall of an artery. SEE: *atherosclerosis; arteriosclerosis.*

RS: cerebrosclerosis; Charcot-Marie-Tooth disease; scleritis.

s., Alzheimer's. Hyaline degeneration affecting the small blood vessels of brain.

s., amyotropic lateral. Progressive muscular atrophy resulting from disease conditions, degenerative in nature, involving anterior horn cells and the pyramidal tracts. It is rapidly progressive, usually ending in bulbar paralysis.

s., annular. S. in which sclerosed substance forms a band about spinal cord.

s., arterial. Hardening of the coats of the arteries. SYN: *arteriosclerosis.*

s., arteriolar. S. of arterioles.

s., diffuse. S. affecting large areas of the brain and spinal cord.

s., disseminated. S., multiple, q.v.

s., hyperplastic. S., medial, q.v.

s., insular. S., multiple, q.v.

s., intimal. Atherosclerosis, q.v.

s., lateral. S. of the lateral column of the spinal cord. SEE: *s., amyotropic lateral.*

s., lobar. Sclerosis of cerebrum resulting in mental disturbances.

s., medial. S. involving the tunica media of arteries, usually the result of involutional changes accompanying aging. SYN: *Mönckeberg's sclerosis.*

s., multiple. A chronic, slowly progressive disease of the central nervous system characterized by development of disseminated demyelinated glial patches called plaques. Symptoms and signs are numerous, but in later stages those of Charcot's triad (nystagmus, scanning speech, and intention tremor) are common. Occurs in the form of many clinical syndromes, the most common being the cerebral, brainstem-cerebellar, and spinal. A history of remissions and exacerbations is diagnostic. Etiology is unknown and there is no specific therapy.

s., neural. S. with chronic inflammation of a nerve trunk with branches.

s., posterior spinal. SEE: *tabes dorsalis.*

s., renal. Nephrosclerosis, q.v.

s., vascular. S. of the walls of blood vessels; arterial and venous s.

s., venous. Phlebosclerosis, q.v.

scleroskeleton (sklē″rō-skĕl′ē-tŏn) [Gr. *sklēros,* hard, + *skeleton,* skeleton]. Skeletal parts resulting from ossification of fibrous structures, such as ligaments, fasciae, and tendons.

sclerostenosis (sklē″rō-stĕ-no′sĭs) ["+ *stenōsis,* a narrowing]. Contraction and induration of tissues, esp. those about an orifice.

s. cutanea. Induration of the skin. SYN: *scleroderma.*

sclerostomy (sklē-rŏs′tō-mĭ) ["+ *stoma,* an opening]. Surgical formation of an opening in the sclera.

sclerothrix (sklē′rō-thrĭks) ["+ *thrix,* hair]. Brittleness of the hair.

sclerotic (sklē-rŏt′ĭk) [L. *scleroticus,* hard]. Pert. to or affected with sclerosis.

s. acid. An amorphous, brown powder from ergot. A hemostatic and oxytocic.

s. coat. The membrane forming the exterior coat of the eye. SYN: *sclera, sclerotica.*

s. teeth. Hard, yellowish teeth almost immune to caries.

sclerotica (sklē-rŏt′ĭ-kă) [L. *scleroticus,* hard]. The exterior white coat of the eye. SYN: *sclera; sclerotic coat.*

scleroticectomy (sklē-rŏt′ĭ-sĕk′tō-mĭ) ["+ Gr. *ektomē,* excision]. Excision of a part of the sclera. SYN: *sclerectomy.*

scleroticochoroiditis (sklē-rŏt″ĭ-kō-kō″-roy-dī′tĭs) ["+ Gr. *chorioeidēs,* skinlike, + *-ītis,* inflammation]. Inflammation of sclerotic and choroid coats of the eye. SYN: *sclerochoroiditis.*

scleroticonyxis (sklē-rŏt″ĭ-kō-nĭk′sĭs) ["+ Gr. *nyxis,* a piercing]. Surgical puncture of the sclera. SYN: *scleronyxis.*

scleroticopuncture (sklē-rŏt″ĭ-kō-punk′-tūr) ["+ *punctūra,* a piercing]. Surgical puncture of the sclera. SYN: *scleronyxis; scleroticonyxis.*

scleroticotomy (sklē-rŏt′ĭ-kŏt′ō-mĭ) ["+ Gr. *tomē,* a cutting]. Incision of the sclerotic coat of the eye. SYN: *sclerotomy.*

sclerotitis (sklē-rō-tī′tĭs) [Gr. *sklēros,* hard, "+ *-ītis,* inflammation]. Inflammation of the sclera. SYN: *scleritis.*

sclerotium (sklē-rō′shĭ-ŭm). Hardened "fruit-body" of certain fungi. That formed by ergot is the only one of medical importance.

sclerotome (sklē′rō-tōm) [Gr. *sklēros,* hard, + *tomē,* a cutting]. 1. Knife used in incision of the sclera. 2. One of a series of segmentally arranged masses of mesenchymal tissue lying on either side of the notochord. They give rise to the vertebrae and ribs.

sclerotomy (sklē-rŏt′ō-mĭ). Surgical incision of sclera.

s., anterior. Incision at angle of anterior chamber in glaucoma.

s., posterior. Opening through sclera into the vitreous for detached retina, removal of foreign body, etc.

sclerotrichia (sklē-rō-trĭk'ĭ-ă) [Gr. *sclerosis,* hard, + *thrix,* hair]. Hardness and brittleness of the hair.

sclerous (sklē'rŏs). Hard; indurated.

scobinate (skō'bĭn-āt) [L. *skobina,* rasp]. Having a rough, uneven, nodular surface.

scolex (skō'lĕks) [Gr. *skōlēx,* worm]. (pl. *sco´lices*) The portion of a tapeworm, the so-called head, by which it attaches itself to the wall of the intestine. Scolices usually possess hold-fast organs such as hooks, suckers, or grooves (bothria).

scoliometer (skō''lĭ-ŏm'ĕt-ĕr) [Gr. *skolios,* twisted, + *metron,* measure]. Device for measuring curves, esp. lateral ones of the spine.

scoliorachitic (skō''lĭ-ō-rǎ-kĭt'ĭk) ["+ *rhachis,* spine]. Pert. to, or afflicted with, spinal curvature from rickets.

scoliosiometry (skō''lĭ-ō-sē-ŏm'ĕ-trĭ) ["+ *metron,* a measure]. Measurement of degree of spinal curvature.

scoliosis (skō''lĭ-ō'sĭs) [Gr. *skoliōsis,* curvature]. Lateral curvature of the spine. Usually consists of two curves, the original one and a compensatory curve in the opposite direction.

   s., cicatricial. S. due to cicatricial contraction resulting from necrosis.

   s., congenital. S. present at birth, usually the result of defective development of the spine.

   s., coxitic. S. in the lumbar spine due to tilting of the pelvis in hip disease.

   s., empyematic. S. following empyema and retraction of one side of the chest.

   s., habit. S. due to habitually assumed improper position.

   s., inflammatory. S. due to disease of the vertebrae.

   s., ischiatic. S. due to hip disease.

   s., myopathic. Weakening of spinal muscles causing a lateral curvature.

   s., ocular, s., ophthalmic. S. from tilting of the head due to visual defects or extraocular muscle imbalance.

   s., osteopathic. S., myopathic, q.v.

   s., paralytic. Lateral curvature of the spine due to paralysis of the muscles.

   s., rachitic. S. due to rickets.

   s., rheumatic. S. due to rheumatism of dorsal muscles.

   s., sciatic. Lateral curvature in sciatica.

   s., static. That due to difference in length of legs.

scoliosometry (skō''lĭ-ō-sŏm'ĕt-rĭ) [Gr. *skoliōsis,* curvature, + *metron,* measure]. Determination of degree of spinal curvature. SYN: *scoliosiometry.*

scoliotic (skō-lĭ-ŏt'ĭk). Suffering from, or related to, scoliosis.

scoliotone (skō'lĭ-ō-tōn) [Gr. *skolios,* twisted, + *tonos,* tension]. An apparatus for correcting the curve in scoliosis by stretching the spine.

scoop (skūp) [ME., a ladle]. Surgical spoon-shaped instrument.

   s., bone. Instrument for scraping or removing necrosed bone or contents of suppurative tracts. Ex: Volkmann's; Schede's; Von Brun's; Hebra's; Treve's.

   s., bullet. Instrument for dislodging bullets.

   s., cataract. Instrument for removing fluids, foreign growths; for exerting pressure or center pressure.

   s., ear. Instrument for removing middle ear granulations.

   s., lithotomy. Instrument for dislodging encysted calculi or removing stones, debris, etc.

   s., mastoid. Instrument used in mastoid operations.

   s., renal. Instrument to dislodge or remove small stones from pelvis of kidney.

-scope [Gr. *skopein,* to examine]. Combining form meaning an instrument or device for viewing or examining.

scopolamine hydrobromide (skō-pŏl'ă-mēn hī''drō-brō'mĭd). USP. The hydrobromide of alkaloids obtained from plants of the nightshade family.

   ACTION AND USES: As a sedative; locally as a mydriatic; and with morphine and pentobarbital in labor to produce "twilight" sleep. SYN: *hyoscine hydrobromide.*

scopophobia (skō''pō-fō'bĭ-ă) [Gr. *skopos,* a watcher, + *phobos,* fear]. Abnormal fear of being seen.

scopophobiac (skō''pō-fō'bĭ-ăk). One who is afraid of being seen.

scoptophilia (skŏp''tō-fĭl'ĭ-ă) [Gr. *skopos,* a watcher, + *philein,* to love]. Sexual pleasure derived from visual sources such as nudity and obscene pictures. SYN: *scopophilia.*

scoptophobia (skŏp''tō-fō'bĭ-ă) ["+ *phobos,* fear]. Aversion to being seen.

scoptophobiac (skŏp''tō-fō'bĭ-ăk). One who dreads being seen.

-scopy [Gr. *skopein,* to examine]. Combining form meaning examination.

scoracratia (skōr''ă-krā'shĭ-ă) [Gr. *skōr,* dung, + *akratia,* lack of control]. Inability to retain the feces. SYN: *scatacratia.*

scorbutic (skōr-bū'tĭk) [L. *scorbuticus*]. Concerning or affected with scurvy.

scorbutus (skōr-bū'tŭs) [L., scurvy]. A deficiency disease due to lack of vitamin C in fresh vegetables and fruits. SYN: *scurvy*, q.v. SEE: *deficiency disease; vitamin.*

scordinema (skōr-dĭ-nē'mă) [Gr. *skordinēma*, yawning]. Yawning and stretching with fatigue and heaviness of the head, a prodromal sym. of an infectious disease.

scoretemia (skōr-ĕ-tē'mĭ-ă) [Gr. *skōr*, dung, + *haima*, blood]. Autointoxication resulting from absorption of feces in the intestine or absorption of substances from feces retained in the intestine.

scorp'ion [Gr. *skorpios*]. An arachnid belonging to the order Scorpionida confined principally to warm countries. Scorpions are capable of inflicting a dangerous, and sometimes fatal, sting by means of an erectile tail equipped with a stinger. The venom contains neurotoxins, hemolysins, cardiac toxins, and agglutinins.

s., sting. Sym. resemble those of black widow spider bite or of strychnine poisoning. Severity of sym. depends on age of victim. Stings often are fatal to children under 3 years of age; adults usually recover.

TREATMENT: Same as a black widow spider bite. Apply tourniquet with caution. Apply ice, or freeze with ethyl chloride to slow dissemination of venom. Specific antivenin should be administered if available. In Southwest U.S. it can be secured from Poisonous Animals Research Laboratory, Arizona State College, Tempe, Arizona.

SEE: *spider, black widow.*

scotodinia (skō''tō-dĭn'ĭ-ă) [Gr. *skotos*, darkness, + *dinos*, whirl]. Vertigo with black spots before the eyes and faintness.

scotoma (skō-tō'mă) [Gr. *skotōma*, darkness]. (pl. *scotomata*) Islandlike blind gap in the visual field.

s., absolute. An area in the visual field in which there is absolute blindness.

s., annular. A scotomatous zone which encircles the point of fixation like a ring, not always completely closed, but leaving the fixation point intact.

s., central. An area of depressed vision involving the point of fixation, seen in lesions of the macula.

s., color. Color blindness in a limited portion of visual field.

s., eclipse. An area of blindness in the visual field due to having looked directly at the sun during an eclipse.

s., flittering. S., scintillating, q.v.

s., negative. S. not perceptible by the patient.

s., physiological. Blind spot due to absence of rods and cones where optic nerve enters retina.

s., positive. Area which patient perceives in his visual field as a dark spot.

s., relative. S. in which perception of the object is impaired, but not completely lost.

s., scintillating. An irregular outline around a luminous patch in the visual field following mental or physical labor, eyestrain, or in migraine. SYN: *teichopsia.*

scotomata (skō-tō'mă-tă) [Gr.]. Pl. of scotoma.

scotomatous (skō-tŏm'ă-tŭs) [Gr. *skotōma*, darkness]. Rel. to, of the nature of, or afflicted with scotoma.

scotometer (skō-tŏm'ĕt-ĕr) ["+ *metron*, a measure]. Device for detecting and measuring scotomata in visual field.

scotometry (skō-tŏm'ĕ-trĭ). The locating and measurement of scotomata.

scotomization (skō''tō-mĭ-zā'shŭn) [Gr. *skotōma*, darkness]. Development of blind spots, particularly mental ones wherein the patient denies, or fails to be aware of, that which his ego finds unpleasant.

scotophilia (skō''tō-fĭl'ĭ-ă) [Gr. *skotos*, darkness, + *philein*, to love]. Preference for darkness or for the night. SYN: *nyctophilia.*

scotophobia (skō''tō-fō'bĭ-ă) ["+ *phobos*, fear]. Abnormal dread of darkness.

scotopia (skō-tō'pĭ-ă) ["+ *ōps*, eye]. The adjustment of vision for darkness.

scotopic (skō-tŏp'ĭk). Pert. to scotopia.

s. vision. Dark adaptation; the adjustment of the eyes for vision in dark or dim light.

scotoscopy (skō-tŏs'kō-pĭ) [Gr. *skotos*, darkness, + *skopein*, to examine]. Examination of internal organs by use of the fluoroscope. SYN: *skiascopy.*

scratch (skrăch) [ME. *cracchen*]. 1. A mark or superficial injury produced by scraping with the nails or a rough surface. 2. To make a thin, shallow cut with a sharp instrument. 3. To rub the skin, esp. with fingernails, to relieve itching.

screatus (skrē-ā'tŭs) [L. *screātus*, a hawking]. A neurosis characterized by paroxysmal fits of hawking or snorting.

screen [O.Fr. *escren*]. 1. A flat area upon which movies or slides are viewed, or suitable for visualizing x-ray pictures. 2. To make a fluoroscopic examination. 3. To examine systematically in order to determine suitability. 4. A structure used to protect, guard, or shield from a damaging influence such as X rays.

s., intensifying. An apparatus for intensifying the image produced by x-ray pictures.

screen'ing. Testing or examining an individual or large groups of people by utilizing only a portion of the usual examining procedures. Ex: chest x-rays are used in screening for presence of pulmonary or cardiac diseases, urinalysis is used for detection of diabetes, and determination of intraocular pressure is used for diagnosing glaucoma.

scrivener's palsy (skrīv'ner) [O.Fr. *escrevein*, scribe]. Occupational neurosis caused by excessive use of the hand in writing. SYN: *writer's cramp.*

scrobiculate (skrō-bĭk'ū-lāt) [L. *scrobiculatus*]. Having shallow depressions; pitted.

scrobiculus (skrō-bĭk'ū-lŭs) [L., a little pit]. A small groove or pit.

    s. cordis. Pit of the stomach; precordial or epigastric depression.

scrofula (skrŏf'ū-lǎ) [L., a breeding sow]. A variety of tuberculous adenitis that is most frequently encountered. It is thought to be a secondary involvement of cervical lymph nodes as a result of a localized hematogenous spread from a pulmonary lesion. Most common in childhood.

    TREATMENT: Responds to specific antituberculosis chemotherapy.

scrof'ulid(e). Scrofuloderma.

scrofuloderma (skrŏf'ū-lō-der'mǎ) [L. *scrofula,* a breeding sow, + Gr. *derma,* skin]. A skin manifestation of tuberculous origin, usually secondary to scrofula. Marked by ulcers usually resulting from a tuberculous sinus. Occurs most commonly on chest, neck, and in the axillae and groins, esp. in children and adolescents. Now very rare. SYN: *tuberculosis cutis colliquativa.*

    TREATMENT: Responds to ultraviolet light treatments and specific chemotherapy for tuberculosis.

scrof"ulo'sis. Scrofula, q.v.

scrofulous (skrŏf'ū-lŭs) [L. *scrofula,* a breeding sow]. Of the nature of, or afflicted with, scrofula.

scrotal (skrō'tǎl) [L. *scrotum,* a bag]. Concerning the scrotum.

    s. reflex. Slow vermicular contraction of s. muscle when perineum is stroked or cold applied.

    s. tongue. A furrowed tongue.

scrotectomy (skrō-tĕk'tō-mĭ) ["+ Gr. *ektomē,* excision]. Excision of part of the scrotum.

scroti'tis ["+ Gr. *-ītis,* inflammation]. Inflamed condition of the scrotum.

scrotocele (skrō'tō-sēl) [L. *scrotum,* a bag, + Gr. *kēlē,* hernia]. Hernia in the scrotum.

scrotum (skrō'tŭm) [L., a bag]. (pl. *scro'ta, -ums*) [NA]. The double pouch containing the testicles and part of the spermatic cord, found in most mammals. Constituent parts of the s. are skin; a network of nonstriated muscular fibers called dartos; cremasteric, spermatic, and infundibuliform fasciae; cremasteric muscle; and tunica vaginalis.

    RS: chimney-sweeps' cancer; chyloderma; dartos; oscheal; oscheitis; oscheoncus; rhacoma; urocele.

scrub'bing [M.D. *schrubben*]. Term applied to washing the hands, fingernails, and lower arms in preparation for performing surgery. The precise procedure to follow usually is posted in a special area where the washing is done.

    METHOD: Scrubbing with soap and water and a nail brush, immersion in a mild germicidal solution and the wearing of sterilized rubber gloves, cap, gown, and mask. SEE: *sterilization.*

scrub nurse. Term applied to operating room nurse who hands instruments to the surgeon, and who has previously sterilized her hands and wears sterile rubber gloves.

scrub typhus. An acute febrile illness caused by Rickettsia tsutsugamushi transmitted by several species of mites, including Trombicula akamushi and T. deliensis. Common in the Asiatic-Pacific area. If untreated, fever lasts for about 14 days. Fatality rate varies in untreated cases from 1-4%. SYN: *mite-borne typhus; tsutsugamushi disease.*

    TREATMENT: Tetracycline or chloramphenicol.

scruple (skrū'pl) [L. *scrupulus,* a small stone]. SYMB: ℈. Twenty grains in apothecaries' weight; 1.296 gm. ABBR: scr.

Scultetus' bandage (skŭl-tē'tŭs). [Johann Schultes (Scultetus), Ger. surgeon, 1595-1645] A many-tailed bandage applied, usually around the abdomen, so the ends overlap each other as if they were roof shingles.

Scultetus' position. Position in which head is low and the body on an inclined plane.

scum (skŭm) [ME. *scume*]. Slimy floating islands of bacteria or impurities on the surface of a culture; an interrupted pellicle of bacterial growth.

scurf (skŭrf) [AS. *scurf*]. A branny desquamation of the epidermis, esp. on the scalp. SEE: *dandruff.*

scurvy (skŭr'vĭ) [L. *scorbūtus*]. A deficiency disease characterized by hemorrhagic manifestations and abnormal formation of bones and teeth.

    ETIOL: Deficiency of vitamin C usually resulting from lack of fresh fruits and vegetables in diet.

SYM: Preceded by period of ill health; sallow; loss of energy; pains in legs, limbs, and joints. Anemic; great weakness; spongy, bleeding gums; fetor of breath; loosening of teeth; subcutaneous hemorrhages and hemorrhages from mucus membranes; painful, brawny indurations of muscles.

PROG: Favorable in early stages.

TREATMENT: For infants, 300 mg. of vitamin C (ascorbic acid) daily for one week, then 150 mg. daily for one month, or 4-8 oz. (52-104 ml.) of orange juice or 12-24 oz. (155-311 ml.) of tomato juice daily. For adults, 300 to 500 mg. of ascorbic acid daily until symptoms have disappeared.

s., infantile. A form of s. which sometimes follows the prolonged use of condensed milk, sterilized milk, or proprietary foods. SYN: *Barlow's disease.*

SYM: Anemia, immobility of legs, pseudoparalysis, extreme tenderness, swelling without pitting, thickening of bones from subperiosteal hemorrhage, ecchymoses and tendency to epiphyseal fractures of epiphyses of bones.

scute (skūt) [L. *scūtum,* shield]. 1. A thin plate or scale, esp. the horny plates found on the carapace of turtles. 2. Term formerly applied to the tegmen tympani, q.v.

scutiform (skū'tĭ-form) ["+ *forma,* a shield]. Shield-shaped.

scutulum (skū'tū-lŭm) [L., a little shield]. (pl. *scutula*) Lesion of the scalp caused by the fungus Trichophyton schoenleini. A yellow cup-shaped crust consisting of a dense mass of mycelia and epithelial debris. The cup faces up and its center is pierced by the hair around which it has developed. SEE: *favus.*

scutum (skū'tŭm) [L., shield]. Plate of bone resembling a shield.

scybalous (sĭb'ă-lŭs) [Gr. *skybalon,* dung]. Of the nature of hard fecal matter.

scybalum (sĭb'ă-lŭm) (pl. *scybala*) A hard, rounded mass of fecal matter.

scypho- [Gr. *skyphos,* cup]. Combining form meaning cup.

scyphoid (sī'foyd) ["+ *eidos,* like]. Cup-shaped.

Se. Chem. symbol for selenium.

seabather's eruption. Itching red papules which may appear on the skin within a few hours of swimming in the sea. The lesions progress to form crusted papules and disappear spontaneously in 7 to 10 days. Treatment is symptomatic. Cause is unknown. SEE: *swimmer's itch.*

searcher (sŭrch'ĕr) [ME. *serchen*]. Instrument for locating opening of ureter previous to inserting catheter, exploring sinuses, and

esp. for detecting stones in the bladder. SYN: *sound.*

seasickness (sē'sĭk-nĕs) [AS. *sae,* sea, + *sēocness,* illness]. Disorder due to motion of a vessel at sea, or riding in cars, trains, and elevators. A similar condition affects some air travelers. SYN: *motion sickness.*

ETIOL: Motion affects the middle ear, and the vomiting center in the brain stem is stimulated. There is wide individual variation in susceptibility.

SYM: Giddiness, vomiting, headache, nausea, and often extreme drowsiness, retching, prostration.

PREVENTION: Select position in craft where up-and-down motion is least; avoid dietary and alcoholic excesses; avoid reading or unusual visual stimuli; assume a supine or recumbent position.

TREATMENT: Specific antinausea and antimotion sickness medicine. These include several forms of antihistamines. Sedatives and supportive therapy, such as intravenous fluids, may be required in severe and prolonged cases.

Generally, antinausea pills should not be given to pregnant women during early pregnancy.

RS: motion sickness; nausea.

seatworm (sēt'wŭrm). A species of nematode worms, Enterobius vermicularis, which occurs commonly in man. Adult worms inhabit large intestine in region of cecum and appendix. Gravid females migrate nightly to anus where they deposit eggs in perianal region. Movement of the worms about anus causes intense itching. SYN: *pinworm.*

sebaceous (sē-bā'shŭs) [L., fatty]. Containing, or pert. to, sebum, an oily, fatty matter secreted by the s. glands.

s. cyst. A cyst filled with s. material from a distended s. gland. These cysts are sometimes known as wens. They frequently form on the scalp and consist of a small sac, containing sebaceous matter, which may grow to a large size. They may result from impairment of localized circulation and closure of sebaceous glands or ducts. Drainage does not remove them permanently because they will recur unless entirely extirpated. Extirpation, q.v., should be done with an electric current or cutting knife. One should never attempt to drain such a cyst without taking every precaution against infection.

s. gland. Oil-secreting gland of the skin. The glands are simple or branched alveolar glands, most of which open into hair follicles. They are holocrine glands, their secretion, sebum, arising from disintegration of

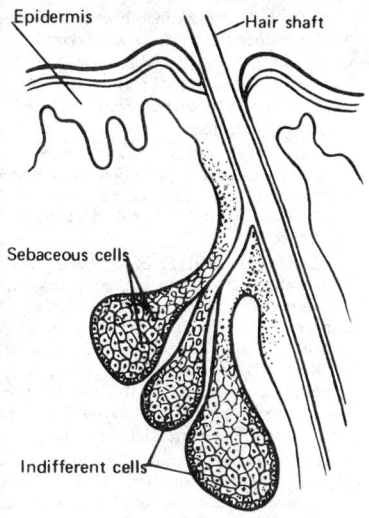

SEBACEOUS GLAND

cells filling the alveoli. Most, but not all, s. glands have a hair follicle associated with them.

sebastomania (sĕ-băs″tō-mā′nĭ-ă) [Gr. *sebastos*, reverend, + *mania*, madness]. Religious insanity.

sebiagogic (sĕb-ĭ-ă-gōj′ĭk) [L. *sebum*, tallow, + Gr. *agōgos*, leading]. Forming fat or sebaceous matter. SYN: *sebiferous; sebiparous.*

sebiferous (sē-bĭf′ĕr-ŭs) [″ + *ferre*, to carry]. Producing fatty or sebaceous matter. SYN: *sebiagogic; sebiparous.*

sebip′arous [″ + *parēre*, to produce]. Producing sebum or sebaceous matter. SYN: *sebiagogic; sebiferous.*

sebolite, sebolith (sĕb′ō-līt, -lĭth) [L. *sebum*, tallow, + Gr. *lithos*, a stone]. Concretion in a sebaceous gland.

seborrhagia (sĕb″ō-rā′jĭ-ă) [″ + Gr. *rhēgnynai*, to burst forth]. Excessive secretion of sebaceous glands. SYN: *seborrhea.*

seborrhea (sĕb-or-ē′ă) [L. *sebum*, tallow, + Gr. *rhoia*, to flow]. Functional disease of the sebaceous glands marked by increase in the amount, and often alteration of the quality, of the sebaceous secretion.

    RS: dermatitis seborrheica; sebaceous; sebum.

    s. capiti. S. of the scalp.

    s. congestiva. Facial form with elevated patches with red borders and covered

with crusts and scars. SYN: *lupus erythematosus.*

    s. corporis. S. of the trunk.

    s. faciei. S. of the face.

    s. furfuracea. Seborrheic dermatitis, q.v.

    s. nigra, s. nigricans. Dark-colored crusts in seborrhea.

    s. oleosa. S. in which fat elements predominate. Shows shiny skin with widely dilated follicular orifices, many of which contain comedones.

    s. sicca. S. with grayish-brown or yellow scale and crust formation in addition to abnormal oiliness. Differentiation from seborrheic dermatitis is difficult. This form most frequently observed on scalp and constitutes what is popularly called dandruff.

    Examination reveals an encrustation composed of thin, yellowish-gray scales. In uncomplicated cases the skin is pale, but often becomes hyperemic or inflamed from irritation. When allowed to continue, nutrition of hair is interfered with, and baldness results.

    On the body, s. sicca appears as yellowish-gray, slightly elevated patches covered with greasy scales. Outlets of follicles are often dilated. There is generally more or less redness of the skin from hyperemia (seborrheal eczema).

seborrheic (sĕb″ō-rē′ĭk) [L. *sebum*, tallow, + Gr. *rhoia,* flow). Afflicted with or like seborrhea.

    s. dermatitis. SYN: *dermatitis seborrheica; seborrhea furfuracea.*

seborrhoic (sĕb″ō-rō′ĭk). Suffering from or like seborrhea, q.v. SYN: *seborrheic.*

sebum (sē′bŭm) [L., tallow]. A fatty secretion of the sebaceous glands of the skin. It varies in different parts of the body. S. from the ears is called cerumen, q.v.; that from the foreskin is called smegma, q.v.

    RS: sebaceous; seborrhea; smegma.

secernent (sē-sĕr′nĕnt) [L. *secernens,* secreting]. 1. Secreting. 2. A secreting organ.

seclusio pupillae [L.]. Shutting off of the pupil due to adherence of iris to the lenticular capsule. SYN: *annular posterior synechia.*

seclusio pupillae siderosis bulbi. Deposit of iron pigment within the eyeball. Seen in cases of iron foreign bodies retained in the eye.

seconal (sē′kōn-ăl). A proprietary barbituric acid derivative.

    USES: Same as the barbiturates.

secondary. 1. Next to or following; second in order. SYN: *subordinate.* 2. Produced by a primary cause.

s. areola. Pigmentation around the nipples during pregnancy. SEE: *areola.*

s. disease. Disease following a previouse disease.

s. hemorrhage. 1. Hemorrhage appearing more than 24 hrs. after an injury or operation and which is due to sepsis and septic ulceration into a blood vessel. 2. Uterine bleeding due to septic infection or from infant's umbilicus due to same cause. SEE: *hemorrhage.*

second cranial nerve. A sensory nerve which conveys visual impulses from eye to thalamus. The two optic nerves undergo partial decussation at the optic chiasma. SEE: *Table of Nerves* in *Appendix.*

second intention. Healing by granulation or indirect union. Granulation tissue is formed to fill the gap between the edges of the wound with a thin layer of fibrinous exudate. It bars bacteria and aids in checking bleeding by the coagulation of the blood. Connective tissue cells support the new capillaries. This form of healing is slower than that by first intention and its grayish-red surface may become pale and flabby if the healing is too long delayed. If the granulations show above the surface they may have to be removed with caustics. If the granulations first form at the top instead of the bottom of the wound, it may have to be kept open with drainage.

RS: healing; intention; resolution.

second sight. Alteration in refractive powers of the lens so that reading is possible again without glasses in incipient cataract. SYN: *gerontopia.*

second stage of labor. Period between complete dilation of cervix and delivery of the child. During this stage involuntary pains become quite strong. This stage normally lasts 2-4 hr. in primiparae and up to 1 hr. in multiparae. SEE: *labor.*

second wind. Condition occuring following strenuous exercise in which the feeling of breathlessness subsides subjectively.

secreta (sē-krē'tă) [L.]. The products of secretion.

secretagogue (sē-krē'tă-gŏg) [L. *secretum*, secretion, + Gr. *agōgos*, leading]. 1. That which stimulates secreting organs. 2. An agent that causes secretion.

secrete' [L. *sēcrētiō*, separation]. To separate from the blood, living organism, or gland; more specifically to form a secretion, q.v.

secretin (sē-krē'tĭn). A hormone formed in the mucous membrane of the duodenum through the influence of acid contents from the stomach whose function is to stimulate the secretion of pancreatic juice and bile.

SEE: *cholecystokinin; digestion, duodenal and intestinal; gastrin; pancreozymin.*

secre'tion [L. *sēcrētiō*, separation]. 1. The process whereby cells of glandular organs produce certain materials from the blood. 2. Substance secreted.

If the useful material flows out through a duct (e.g., saliva) it is called an *external secretion;* if it is returned to the blood or lymph (i.e., insulin) it is called an *internal secretion.*

FLUIDS OF BODY: *Blood:* Composed of 79% water, 21% solids, including the cellular elements of blood. *Bile:* Emulsifies fats and precipitates soluble peptones, 20-24 oz. (259-311 ml.). Sp. gr. 1.026-1.032. Reaction alkaline. *Chyle:* Absorbed by lacteals, the lymphatics of the small intestines. Contains fat absorbed from food. *Chyme:* Food that has undergone gastric digestion only.

Gastric juice: Clear, acid, watery s. of the glands of the stomach. Principal ingredients are hydrochloric acid, mucus, pepsin, and rennin. *Intestinal juice:* Has combined action of saliva and gastric and pancreatic juices. Starch and complex sugars are converted into monosaccharides. Reaction alkaline. *Lymph:* Characteristics vary with site of origin. If derived from a limb, it may be clear and have less than 1 gm. of protein/ 100 ml. If derived from gut, protein is increased and fluid may have milky appearance. *Menstrual:* Menstrual flow. Average 60 ml. during each period. *Pancreatic juice:* Contains enzymes which act on fats, proteins or products of protein digestion, and carbohydrates. Approx. 2000 ml. of a fluid of pH 7.5-8.0 secreted daily. *Perspiration:* The s. of sweat glands. From 100-1000 ml./day under normal conditions. May be many times that amount in extremely hot and dry conditions.

Saliva: Composition varies with particular glands, being watery if from parotid and viscous from submandibular glands. Approx. 1500 ml. secreted/day. Serves to lubricate food and break down starch and glycogen. *Urine:* 1000-2500 ml./24 hours but highly variable. Sp. gr. 1.003-1.025. *Acid:* Contains 50-70 gm. of solids, 20-40 gm. of urea, and 10-15 gm. of chlorides a day. SEE *urine.*

s., apocrine. S. in which the apical end of a secreting cell is broken off and its contents extruded, as in the mammary gland.

s., external. A s. which passes through duct and is discharged upon an epithelial surface, either internal or external.

s., holocrine. S. in which the entire cell and its contents are extruded as a part of the secretory product, as in sebaceous glands.

s., internal. S. imparted to the blood instead of being eliminated by a duct.

s., merocrine. S. in which the product is elaborated within cells and discharged through the cell membrane, the cell itself remaining intact.

s., paralytic. Continuous abundant watery s. from a gland after section of its secretory nerves.

secretion, words pert. to: acrinia; amyxia; anorrhorrhea; apolepsis; asteatosis; athyreosis; athyroidism; cerumen; ceruminal; ceruminosis; ceruminous; choleresis; chromocrinia; crinogenic; diacrisis, errhine; exsiccant; hormone; interstitial; saliva; sebum; secretagogue; secrete; secretin; semen; smegma; succorrhea.

secretogogue (sē-krē'tō-gŏg) [L. *sēcrētiō*, separation, + Gr. *agōgos*, leading]. 1. Causing secretion. 2. That which stimulates secretion. SYN: *secretagogue*.

secretory (sē-krē'tō-rĭ, sē'krē-tō-rĭ). Pert. to or promoting secretion; secreting.

s. capillaries. Very small canaliculi receiving secretion discharged from gland cells.

s. fibers. Centrifugal nerve fibers which excite secretion.

s. granules. SEE: *granule, zymogen*.

sectarian (sĕk-tā'rĭ-ăn) [L. *sectus*, having cut]. A medical man who follows a dogma, tenet, or principle based on some unscientific belief to the exclusion of scientific demonstration.

sectile (sĕk'tĭl) [L. *sectilis*]. Capable of being cut.

section [L. *sectio*, a cutting]. 1. Process of cutting. 2. A division or segment of a part. 3. A surface made by cutting.

s., abdominal. Any abdominal operation. SYN: *laparotomy*, q.v.

s., cesarean. Incision of uterus for delivery of a fetus through abdominal wall or through the vagina. SEE: *cesarean section*.

s., coronal. S., frontal, q.v.

s., frontal. S. dividing the body into two parts, dorsal and ventral.

s., frozen. A thin s. of the body, an organ, or a piece of tissue which has been frozen before being sectioned and then studied microscopically.

s., midsagittal. S. which divides the body into right and left halves.

s., paraffin. A s. of a tissue which has been infiltrated with paraffin.

s., perineal. External incision into urethra to relieve stricture.

s., Pitres'. One of the series of sections made through the brain for postmortem examination.

s., sagittal. A s. cut parallel to the median plane of the body.

s., serial. Microscopic sections made and arranged in consecutive order.

s., vaginal. Incision into the abdominal cavity through the vagina.

sectioning [L. *sectio*, a cutting]. The slicing of thin sections of tissue for examination under the microscope.

RS: microtome.

s., ultrathin. The cutting of sections extraordinarily thin (less than 1 micron in thickness), esp. for use in electron microscopy.

sector (sĕk'tor) [L., cutter]. The area of a circle included between two radii and an arc.

sectorial (sĕk-tō'rĭ-ăl). Having cutting edges, as teeth.

secundigravida (sē-kŭn"dĭ-grăv'ĭd-ă) [L. *secundus*, second, + *gravida*, pregnant]. A woman in her 2nd pregnancy.

secundines (sĕk'ŭn-dĭnz, sĭ-kŭn'dĭnz) [LL. *secundinae*]. The placenta, umbilical cord, and fetal membranes expelled during the 3rd stage of labor. SYN: *afterbirth*.

secundipara (sē"kŭn-dĭp'ă-ră) [L. *secundus*, second, + *parēre*, to give birth]. A woman who has borne two children in separate labors.

secundiparity (sē-kŭn"dĭ-păr'ĭ-tĭ). The condition of being a secundipara.

secundum artem (sē-kŭn'dŭm ăr'tĕm) [L.]. In an approved manner; according to rule or science.

S.E.D. Abbr. for *skin erythema dose*.

Sed [L.]. Abbr. of *sedes*, stool.

sedation (sē-dā'shŭn) [L. *sedatio*, from *sedāre*, to calm]. 1. Process of allaying nervous excitement. 2. State of being calmed.

Usually effected by means of a drug.

sedative (sĕd'ă-tĭv) [L. *sedativus*, calming]. 1. Quieting. 2. An agent which exerts a soothing or tranquilizing effect. They may be general, local, nervous, or vascular.

s., cardiac. S. that decreases the heart's force.

s. enema. Retention enema given for its soothing action and to allay irritability.

s., nervous. S. affecting nervous system.

sedentary (sĕd'ĕn-tā'rĭ) [L. *sedentarius*]. 1. Sitting. 2. Pert. to an occupation or mode of living requiring minimal physical exercise.

sediment (sĕd'ĭ-mĕnt) [L. *sedimentum,* a settling]. The substance settling at bottom of a liquid. SYN: *hypostasis.* SEE: *precipitate.*

sedimentation (sĕd''ĭ-mĕn-tā'shŭn). Formation or depositing of sediment.

s. rate. Laboratory test of speed at which erythrocytes settle when an anticoagulant is added to blood. In this test, blood to which an anticoagulant has been added is placed in a long, narrow tube, and the speed at which the red cells settle is observed.

Various methods of determining the rate have been devised. Some pathologists determine the time required for the cells to settle a certain distance (s. time), while others determine the distance the cells settle in a given time (s. rate), both normally about 5 min./mm. The speed at which the cells settle depends upon the size of the clumps into which the red cells aggregate, and the size of the clumps appears to depend upon the amount of fibrinogen in the blood. The speed of settling is increased in a variety of infections, in cancer, and in pregnancy, and may be decreased in liver disease.

sedimentator (sĕd-ĭ-mĕn-tā'tor). A centrifuge for separating urinary sediment.

seed (sēd) [AS. *saed*]. 1. The ripened ovule of a spermatophyte plant usually consisting of the embryo (germ), and a supply of nutrient material enclosed within the seed coats. It is a resting sporophyte. 2. Sperm; semen. 3. Capsule containing radon, radium, etc., for use in treatment of cancer. 4. Offspring. 5. To introduce microorganisms into a culture medium.

segment (sĕg'mĕnt) [L. *segmentum,* a portion]. 1. A part or section, esp. a natural one, of an organ or body. 2. One of the serial divisions of an animal.

s., body. In the embryo, a somite; in the adult, a portion derived from a somite. SYN: *metamere; somite.*

s., interannular. Portion of a neuron between two nodes of Ranvier.

s., mesodermal. A somite.

segmental (sĕg-mĕn'tăl). Pert. to, resembling, or composed of segments.

s. reflex. A reflex action in which afferent impulses enter the cord in the same segment or segments from which the efferent impulses emerge.

s. static reactions. Postural reflexes in which movements of one extremity result in a movement in an opposite extremity.

segmentation (sĕg''mĕn-tā'shŭn) [L. *segmentum,* a portion]. 1. Division into similar parts. 2. The division of a fertilized egg into many smaller cells or blastomeres. SYN: *cleavage.* SEE: *blastomere; cleavage; embryo.*

s. cavity. Central space in blastula stage of s. of an ovum.

s., rhythmic. Division of the intestine and the chyme within it into segments by contraction of circular muscle fibers. SYN: *segmenting contractions.*

segmenter. Stage in development of the malarial organism (Plasmodium) in which the organism is undergoing schizogony. SYN: *mature schizont; rosette.*

segrega'tion [L. *sēgregāre,* to separate]. 1. Setting apart, separating. 2. In genetics, the process which takes place in the formation of germ cells (gametogenesis) in which each gamete (egg or sperm) receives only one of each pair of genes.

seg'rega"tor. Instrument composed of two catheters for securing urine from each kidney separately. The procedure was done by dividing the bladder into hypothetical halves, and urine was collected from each side. Method has been replaced by the procedure in which a ureteral catheter is placed in each ureter while it is viewed through a cystoscope.

Séguin's signal symptom (sā-găn'). Involuntary contractions of muscles just before an epileptic attack.

Seidlitz powder (sĕd'lĭts, sĭd'lĭtz). [Seidlitz, village in Bohemia]. Effervescent cathartic composed of tartaric acid, sodium bicarbonate, and sodium and potassium tartrate.

seisesthesia (sīz''ĕs-thē'zĭ-ă) [Gr. *seisis,* concussion, + *aisthēsis,* sensation]. Perception of a concussion.

seismesthesia (sīz''mĕs-thē'zĭ-ă) [Gr. *seismos,* earthquake, + *aisthēsis,* sensation]. Perception of vibrations.

seismotherapy (sīz''mō-thĕr'ă-pĭ) ["+ *therapeia,* treatment]. Treatment of disease by vibratory massage. SYN: *sismotherapy.*

seizure (sē'zhŭr) [O.Fr. *seisir,* to take possession of]. A sudden attack of pain, of a disease, or of certain symptoms.

s., convulsive. 1. A convulsion, q.v. 2. An attack of epilepsy.

s., larval. A s. indicated by abnormal brain waves in an electroencephalogram but not evidenced by clinical symptons.

Seldinger technique. Method for introducing a catheter into a vein or artery. The vessel is located with a special needle which contains a wire; the needle is removed. The catheter is threaded into the vein while being guided by the wire over which it is moving. The wire is then removed from the catheter.

selec'tion [L. *sēlectus,* having chosen]. 1. Choice; the process of choosing or selecting. 2. In biology, any process by which a group of individuals, such as a species, is enabled to survive or to avoid extermination.

s., artificial. Process by which man selects individuals possessing desirable characteristics and endeavors to produce through selective breeding a race or strain homozygous for these characteristics.

s., natural. 1. Process by which individuals possessing characteristics which adapt them to their environment survive, whereas those lacking these characteristics die or fail to leave progeny. 2. Darwin's theory of evolution or origin of species. SEE: *natural selection.*

s., sexual. A theory originated to account for differences in secondary sex characteristics between males and females. It assumes that individuals preferentially select for mating individuals of the opposite sex who possess these characteristics.

selenium (sē-lē'nĭ-ŭm) [Gr. *selēnē,* moon]. SYMB: *Se.* At. wt. 78.96; at. no. 34. A chem. element resembling sulfur. It is poisonous to certain animals which feed on plants grown on soil which contains an excess of selenium.

self-digestion. Destruction or disintegration of a cell or tissue by its own juice, as that of the walls of the stomach by the gastric juice occurring in certain diseases of that organ. SYN: *autodigestion.*

self-limited disease. Disease that, without treatment, runs a definite course within a limited time.

sella turcica (sĕl'ă tŭr'sĭ-kă) [L., Turkish saddle]. [NA]. A concavity on superior surface of body of sphenoid bone which houses the hypophysis cerebri (pituitary gland). SYN: *hypophyseal fossa; pituitary fossa.*

semeiology (sē″mī-ŏl'ō-jĭ) [Gr. *sēmeion,* sign, + *logos,* study]. The branch of medicine dealing with the study of symptoms. SYN: *symptomatology.*

semeiosis (sē″mī-ō'sĭs) ["+ *-ōsis,* intensive]. Study of disease by symptoms.

semeiotic (sē″mī-ŏt'ĭk) [Gr. *sēmeiōtikos*]. Of or pert. to symptoms. SYN: *symptomatic.*

semeiotics (sē″mī-ŏt'ĭks). 1. Branch of medical science concerning symptoms. SYN: *semiotics; symptomatology.* 2. Symptoms of a disease in a particular case considered as a whole.

semelincident (sĕm″ĕl-ĭn'sĭ-dĕnt) [L. *semel,* once, + *incidens,* falling upon]. Occurring only once in a person.

semen (sē'mĕn) [L., seed]. (pl. *semina*) A thick, opalescent, viscid secretion discharged from the urethra of the male at the climax of sexual excitement (orgasm). Contains the spermatozoa. S. is the mixed product of various glands (prostate and bulbourethral) plus the spermatozoa which, having been produced in the testicles, are stored in the seminal vesicles.

Normal values for the seminal fluid ejaculate: volume, 2-5 ml.; pH, 7.2-8.0; leukocytes, absent or only an occasional one seen per high power field; sperm count, 60-150 million/ml.; motility, 80% or more should be motile; morphology, 80-90% should be normal.

RS: aspermatic; aspermatism; aspermous; azoospermia; bradyspermatism; coition; coitus; coitus interruptus; copulation; ejaculation; emissio seminis; emission; erection; excitation; fertilization; insemination; libido; orgasm; penis; prostate; sexual intercourse; sperm; sperma; spermatemphraxis; spermatic; spermatorrhea; spermatozoon; vesicle, seminal.

s., frozen. S. stored in a bank for future use in insemination. Offers supply of donors in small communities where it would be impossible to keep anonymity of local donors. However, number of successful pregnancies is lower with frozen semen than fresh semen in therapeutic insemination.

semenuria (sē″mĕn-ū'rĭ-ă) [L. *sēmen,* seed, + Gr. *ouron,* urine]. Excretion of semen in the urine. SYN: *seminuria; spermaturia.*

semi- [L. *semis,* half]. Prefix meaning half.

semicanal (sĕm″ĭ-kăn-ăl') ["+ *canalis,* passage]. A duct open on one side.

semicircular (sĕm″ĭ-sĭr'kū-lăr) ["+ *circulus,* a ring]. In the form of a half circle.

s. canals. Superior, posterior, and inferior passages forming part of inner ear.

semicoma (sĕm″ĭ-kō'mă) ["+ Gr. *kōma,* lethargy]. Mild degree of coma from which it is possible to arouse the patient.

semicomatose (sĕm″ĭ-kō'măt-ōs). In a condition of unconsciousness from which patient may be aroused.

semilunar (sĕm″ĭ-lū'năr) [L. *semis,* half, + *luna,* moon]. Shaped like a crescent.

s. bone. Halfmoon-shaped bone of carpus.

s. cartilages. Two crescentic cartilages (medial and lateral) in the knee joint between the femur and tibia.

s. ganglions. Two small nervous ganglions of the abdominal cavity, supplying solar plexus. The gasserian ganglion.

s. lobe. Lobe on upper surface of the cerebellum.

s. notch. A notch at proximal end of ulna for articulation with trochlea of humerus.

s. valves. Valves of aorta and pulmonary artery. SEE: *Arantius' body.*

semimembranosus (sĕm″ĭ-mĕm″brăn-ō′sŭs) [L.]. Large muscle of inner and back part of thigh. SEE: *Table of Muscles* in *Appendix.*

seminal (sĕm′ĭ-năl) [L. *seminalis*]. Concerning the semen or seed.

s. duct. Any duct which conveys sperm, esp. the ductus deferens and the ejaculatory duct. SYN: *spermatic duct.*

s. emission. Discharge of semen. SEE: *nocturnal emission.*

s. filament. Male seed. SYN: *spermatozoon.*

s. fluid. Semen, male fertilizing fluid.

s. vesicle. One of two saclike structures in the male, lying behind the bladder and connected to the ductus deferens on each side. They secrete a thick viscous fluid which forms a part of the semen.

semination (sĕm-ĭ-nā′shŭn) [L. *seminatio,* a begetting]. Introduction of semen into the female genital tract. Occurs during sexual intercourse or may be introduced artifically. SYN: *insemination.*

s., artificial. Introduction of semen into the vagina or uterus by artificial means. SYN: *artificial insemination.*

seminiferous (sĕm-ĭn-ĭf′ĕr-ŭs) [L. *sēmen,* seed, + *ferre,* to produce]. Producing or conducting semen, as the tubules of the testes.

seminoma (sĕm′ĭ-nō′mă) [″+ Gr. *-ōma,* tumor]. A tumor of the testis.

seminormal (sĕm′ĭ-nŏr′măl) [L. *semis,* half, + *norma,* rule]. One half the normal standard.

s. solution. One having half the quantity of the substance in the normal solution. Indicated thus: 0.5 N or N/2.

seminuria (sē″mĭn-ū′rĭ-ă) [L. *sēmen,* seed, + Gr. *ouron,* urine]. Semen in the urine. SYN: *semenuria; spermaturia.*

semiology (sē″mĭ-ŏl′ō-jĭ) [Gr. *sēmeion,* sign, + *logos,* a study]. Phase of medicine dealing with study of symptoms. SYN: *semeiology; symptomatology.*

semiotic (sē″mĭ-ŏt′ĭk) [Gr. *sēmeiōtikos*]. Like or pert. to symptoms of disease. SYN: *semeiotic; symptomatic.*

semiotics (sē″mĭ-ŏt′ĭks). Scientific study of symptoms as a whole, or in one particular case. SYN: *semeiotics; symptomatology.*

semipermeable (sĕm′ĭ-per′mē-ă-bl) [L. *semis,* half, + *per,* through, + *meāre,* to pass]. Half permeable; said of a membrane which will allow fluids but not the dissolved substance to pass through it. SEE: *membrane; osmosis.*

semiprone (sĕm-ĭ-prōn′) [″+ *pronus,* prone]. In a position on left side and chest, with both thighs flexed on abdomen, the right higher than the left, and left arm back. SYN: *Sims' position.* SEE: *position, Sims'; Sims' position* for illustration.

semirecumbent (sĕm′ĭ-rē-kŭm′bĕnt) [″+ *recumbere,* to lie down]. Reclining, but not fully recumbent.

semis (sē′mĭs) [L.]. Half. ABBR: ss.

semisideratio, semisideration (sĕm′ĭ-sĭd-ĕr-ā′shĭ-ō, -ā′shŭn) [L. *semis,* half, + *sideratio,* a blight]. Paralysis on one side of the body. SYN: *hemiplegia.*

semisopor (sĕm′ĭ-sō′por) [″+ *sopor,* deep sleep]. Light coma from which patient can be roused. SYN: *semicoma.*

semispinalis (sĕm″ĭ-spĭ-năl′ĭs) [L.]. Deep layer of muscle of back on either side of spinal column, divided into three parts. SEE: *Table of Muscles* in *Appendix.*

semisupination (sĕm″ĭ-sū-pĭn-ā′shŭn) [L. *semis,* half, + *supinus,* bent back]. A position halfway between supination and pronation.

semitendinosus (sĕm″ĭ-tĕn″dĭn-ō′sŭs) [L.]. Fusiform muscle of posterior and inner part of thigh. SEE: *Table of Muscles* in *Appendix.*

semper- [L. *semper,* always]. Combining form meaning always.

senescence (sĭ-nĕs′ens) [L. *senēscēns,* growing old]. 1. The process of growing old. 2. The period of old age.

senile (sē′nĭl, sĕn′ĭl) [L. *senilis,* old]. Pert. to growing old or to the aged.

senilism (sē′nĭl-ĭzm, -nĭl-ĭzm) [″+ Gr. *-ismos,* condition]. Old age, particularly when premature. SEE: *progeria.*

senility (sē-nĭl′ĭ-tĭ) [L. *senilis,* old]. 1. The stage of being old. 2. The weakness of old age, mental or physical.

s., premature. Onset of characteristics before the normal time, as early as 40 years.

s., psychosis of. Mental disorder in old age.

senium (sē′nĭ-ŭm) [L.]. Old age, esp. its debility.

senna (sĕn′a) [Arabic *sanā*]. The dried leaves of the plant Cassia acutifolia and C. angustifolia.

ACTION AND USES: As a purgative acting on the large intestine.

senopia (sĕn-ō′pĭ-ă, sē-no′-) [L. *senilis,* old, + Gr. *ōps,* eye]. Improvement in visual power of old people. SYN: *gerontopia.*

sensation (sĕn-sā′shŭn) [L. *sēnsātiō*]. A feeling or awareness of conditions within or without the body resulting from the stimulation of sensory receptors.

s., common. The sum total of all bodily sensations.

s., cutaneous. S. through medium of the skin.

s., delayed. S. not experienced immediately following a stimulus.

s., epigastric. A sinking feeling in the stomach.

s., external. Effect upon the mind of stimuli produced from a source outside the body.

s., girdle. A painful s., as a bandage tightened about a limb or the trunk as in spinal disease. SYN: *zonesthesia.*

s., internal. S., subjective, q.v.

s., palmesthetic. S. felt in the skin from vibration.

s., referred or reflex. S. which seems to arise from a source other than the actual one.

s., subjective. S. not resulting from any external stimulus and perceptible only by the subject.

s., tactile. S. produced through the sense of touch.

sense (sĕns) [L. *sensus,* a feeling]. 1. To perceive through a sense organ. 2. The general faculty by which conditions outside or inside the body are perceived. 3. Any special faculty of sensation connected with a particular organ. 4. Normal power of understanding.

The most important of the senses are sight; hearing; smell; taste; touch and pressure; temperature; weight, resistance, and tension (muscle sense); pain; visceral and sexual sensations; equilibrium; hunger and thirst.

s., color. The perception of various colors.

s., cutaneous. Sensation felt through the skin.

s., genesic. The sexual instinct.

s., kinesthetic. S., muscular, q.v.

s., light. Perception of degree of light.

s., muscle, muscular. Consciousness of muscular movement required in a given act.

s., posture. Ability through muscle sense to differentiate positions of the body or its structures.

s., pressure. Faculty of feeling various degrees of pressure on the body surface.

s., seventh. Subjective sensations of internal organs. Term is obsolete.

s., sixth. General feeling of normal functioning of the bodily organs. SYN: *cenesthesia.*

s., space. That s. by which we recognize objects in space, their relationship, and dimensions.

s.'s, special. Sight, hearing, smell, touch, and taste.

s., stereognostic. Ability to judge consistency and shape of objects held in the fingers.

s., temperature. Ability to detect differences of temperature.

s., time. Ability to detect differences in time intervals, as in sound.

s., tone. Ability to distinguish between different tones.

s., visceral. Perception of the sensations of the internal organs.

sensibilin (sĕn″sĭ-bĭl′ĭn) [L. *sēnsibilis,* a feeling]. A specific antibody formed in the body at first injection of a foreign protein. SYN: *anaphylactic reaction body.*

sensibility (sĕn″sĭ-bĭl′ĭ-tĭ) [L. *sēnsibilitās*]. Capacity to receive and respond to stimuli.

s., deep. 1. The s. existing after an area of the skin is made anesthetic. 2. Sensation by which the position of a limb and estimation of difference in weight and tension are apparent.

s., mesoblastic. S., deep, q.v.

s., palmesthetic. The s. existing in the skin to vibration.

sensibilization (sĕn″sĭ-bĭl-ĭz-ā′shŭn). 1. The process of making sensitive; sensitization. 2. Production of hypersusceptibility to a foreign substance by injecting it into the body. SYN: *anaphylaxis; sensitization.*

sensibilizer (sĕn′sĭ-bĭl-ī″zer). Substance in blood serum produced during the process of immunization or infection. SYN: *amboceptor.*

sensible (sĕn′sĭ-bl) [L. *sēnsibilis,* feeling]. 1. Capable of being perceived by the senses; perceptible. 2. Capable of receiving sensations. SYN: *sensitive.* 3. Having reason. SYN: *intelligent.* 4. Conscious, as opposed to insensible.

sensiferous (sĕn-sĭf′ĕr-ŭs) [L. *sensus,* a feeling, + *ferre,* to bear]. Causing, conducting, or transmitting sensations.

sensigenous (sĕn-sĭj′ĕn-ŭs) ["+ Gr. *gennan,* to produce]. Causing or starting a sensory impulse.

sensimeter (sĕn-sĭm′ĕ-tĕr) ["+ Gr. *metron,* measure]. Machine for recording the degree of sensitiveness of various areas of the body.

sensitinogen (sĕn″sĭ-tĭn′ō-jen) ["+ Gr. *gennan,* to produce]. The collective antigens which sensitize the body.

sensitive (sĕn′sĭ-tĭv) [L. *sensitivus*]. 1. Capable of transmitting a sensation. 2. Able to feel a sensation. 3. Subject to destructive action of a complement. 4. Susceptible to suggestions, as a hypnotic. 5. Abnormally susceptible to a substance, as a drug or foreign protein. SEE: *allergic.*

sensitivity tests, antimicrobial. Laboratory method of determining the susceptibility of the patient's bacterial infection to antibiotics or antibacterials.

The specimen obtained from the patient is cultured in various liquid dilutions of the drugs or on solid media containing various concentrations of the drugs in disks placed on the surface of the media. The disk-type test is not completely reliable.

sensitivity training. A form of group therapy wherein individuals are given the opportunity to relate verbally and physically with complete candor and honesty with other members of the group. The goals of therapy are to increase self-awareness, learn constructive ways of dealing with conflicts, establish a better sense of inner direction, and relate to persons with warmth and affection.

sensitization (sĕn″sĭ-tĭ-zā′shŭn). 1. A condition of being made sensitive to specific stimulus. 2. Rendering of a cell sensitive to the action of a complement by uniting it with a specific amboceptor. 3. Process of making a person susceptible to a substance by repeated injections of it, as a serum. SYN: *anaphylaxis.*

sensitized (sĕn′sĭ-tīzd). Made susceptible to a specific substance.

   s. vaccine. A live culture which has been mixed with its antiserum before introduction.

sensitizer (sĕn′sĭ-tī″zer) [L. *sensitivus,* feeling]. An antibody producing susceptibility to cytolysis. SYN: *amboceptor.*

sensitometer (sĕn″sĭ-tŏm′ĕt-ēr) ["+ Gr. *metron,* a measure]. Device for determining the penetrating power of light.

sensorial (sĕn-sō′rĭ-ăl) [L. *sensorialis*]. Pert. to the sensorium, the seat of sensation.

sensorimotor (sĕn-sō-rĭ-mō′tor) [L. *sēnsus,* sense, + *motor,* motion]. Both sensory and motor. SYN: *sensomotor.*

sensorium (sĕn-sō′rĭ-ŭm) [L. *sensōrium,* sensation]. (pl. *sensoriums, sensoria*) 1. That portion of the brain which functions as a center of sensations. 2. The sensory apparatus of the body taken as a whole.

   s. area. The precentral and postcentral areas of the cerebral cortex taken as a whole.

sensory (sĕn′sō-rĭ) [L. *sensorius*]. 1. Conveying impulses from sense organs to the reflex or higher centers. SYN: *afferent,* q.v. 2. Pert. to sensation.

   s. amusia. Musical deafness; inability to comprehend music or musical sounds.

   s. aphasia. Inability to understand written or spoken words. SYN: *perceptive aphasia.*

   s. area. Any area of the cerebral cortex in which sensations are perceived.

   s. area, somesthetic. Area occupying postcentral gyrus of cerebral cortex and extending into adjacent areas in which sensations of general somatic sensibility are perceived.

   s. decussation. The superior pyramidal decussation.

   s. ending. A termination of an afferent nerve fiber which upon stimulation gives rise to a sensation. SYN: *receptor; sensory end-organ.*

   s. epilepsy. Disturbances of sensation that replace epileptic convulsions.

   s. nerve. An afferent nerve conveying sensory impulses to the sensorium, or one composed of sensory fibers.

   s. unit. A single sensory nerve fiber with all its branches and their terminal nerve endings.

sensual (sĕn′shū-ăl) [L. *sensus,* sense]. Concerning or consisting in the gratification of the senses; indulgence of the appetites; not spiritual or intellectual; carnal, worldly.

sensualism (sĕn′sū-al-ĭzm). State or condition of being sensual; condition in which one's actions are dominated by emotions.

sensuous (sĕn′shū-ŭs) [L. *sensus,* sense]. Pert. to or affecting the senses; susceptible to influence through the senses.

sentient (sĕn′shĭ-ĕnt) [L. *sentiens,* perceive]. Capable of perceiving sensation. SYN: *sensitive.*

sentiment (sĕn′tĭ-mĕnt) [L. *sentio,* to feel]. Feeling, sensibility, esp. susceptibility to tender feelings; an emotional attitude toward an object or a group of objects.

separation. The process of disconnecting, disuniting, or severing.

   s., epiphyseal. S. of the epiphysis from the diaphysis or shaft of a bone.

separator [L. *separator*]. 1. Anything which prevents two substances from mingling. 2. Any device or instrument used for bringing about a separation of two substances such as cream from milk.

separatorium (sĕp″a-rā-tō′rĭ-ŭm) [L. *separatorium*]. Instrument for separating pericranium from skull.

sepsis (sĕp′sĭs) [Gr. *sēpsis,* putrefaction]. Pathologic state usually febrile, resulting from the presence of microorganisms or their poisonous products in the blood stream. May be manifested as cellulitis (local dissemination of infection), lymphangitis or lymphadenitis (dispersion along lymphatic channels) or bacteremia (widespread dissemination by way of blood stream). The latter is commonly called blood poisoning. SYN: *bacteremia; septicemia.*

s., gas. That resulting from infection by gas gangrene bacilli (Clostridium perfringens) and others.

s., puerperal. Infection of the genital tract following childbirth. SYN: *childbed fever; puerperal infection.*

The infection may be brought about by exogenous or endogenous means. The organisms most commonly associated with this type of infection are streptococcus, staphylococcus, Escherichia coli.

PATH: In minor cases of ulceration, the vaginal tract is covered by a dirty membrane. In streptococci infection the endometrium is smooth, and the lymphatics are congested with the invading organism. As a rule, the uterine cavity is filled with very little lochia. The saprophytic type shows an endometrial cavity filled with greenish, purulent, foul-smelling shreds. Microscopically, there is a thick layer of leukocytes under the necrotic layer. The uterus shows poor involution. In the event that the infection extends further than the uterus, the parametrium or cellular tissues show edema, inflammation and in some cases purulent infiltration. Extension of the process to the veins produces infectious thrombi which in turn produce localized abscesses in other parts of the body.

SYM: Onset may be gradual or sudden. Patient begins to have general malaise, headache, chilly sensations or shaking chills and rise in temperature. The uterus is tender, there is some abdominal distention, and the lochia in the saprophytic type is profuse and foul-smelling, while in the streptococcic type it is decreased in amount and of a serous character.

COURSE: Early diagnosis and appropriate therapy will effectively control the course of the disease in most cases.

TREATMENT: General measures include absolute bed rest, light or liquid diet, maintenance of fluid balance by parenteral injections if necessary, blood transfusion if required, analgesics for pain.

sepsometer (sep-som'e-ter) [Gr. *sepsis*, decay, + *metron*, measure]. Device for determining bacterial contamination of air.

septal (sĕp'tăl) [L. *saeptum*, a partition]. Concerning a septum.

septan (sĕp'tăn) [L. *septem*, seven]. Recurring every 7th day, as the paroxysms of malarial fever.

septate (sĕp'tāt) [L. *saeptum*, a partition]. Having a dividing wall.

septectomy (sĕp-tĕk'tō-mĭ) ["+ Gr. *ektomē*, excision]. Excision of a septum, esp. the nasal septum or a part of it.

septemia (sĕp-tē'mĭ-ă) [Gr. *sēptos*, putrid, + *haima*, blood]. Invasion of the blood by pathogenic bacteria or their toxins. SYN: *septicemia.*

septic (sĕp'tĭk) [Gr. *sēptikos*, putrefying]. 1. Pert. to sepsis. 2. Pert. to pathogenic organisms or their toxins.

s. fever, s. infection. Fever or infection due to presence of pathogenic organisms or their products in the blood. SYN: *septicemia.*

s. sore throat. Streptococcic inflammation of throat with fever and marked prostration.

septicemia (sĕp-tĭ-sē'mĭ-ă) ["+ *haima*, blood]. Morbid condition from absorption of septic products into blood and tissues or of pathogenic bacteria which may rapidly multiply there. SYN: *blood poisoning.*

Symptoms and signs usually include chills and fever, petechiae, purpuric pustules, and abscesses.

s., bronchopulmonary. S. following entry, usually by aspiration, of infected material into the bronchi.

s., cryptogenic. S. in which no primary focus of infection can be found.

s., fungal. Presence of pathogenic fungi in the blood. May be seen as a complication of parenteral hyperalimentation. SYN: *fungemia.*

s., puerperal. S. occurring following prolonged and difficult labor or incomplete abortion. SYN: *postabortal sepsis; puerperal infection; septic abortion.*

septicemic (sĕp-tĭ-sē'mĭk). Relating to, resulting from, or of the nature of septicemia.

septicophlebitis (sĕp"tĭ-kō-flē-bī'tĭs) [Gr. *sēptikos*, putrefying, + *phleps*, vein, + *-itis*, inflammation]. Septic inflammation of a vein.

septicopyemia (sĕp"tĭ-kō-pī-ē'mĭ-ă) ["+ *pyon*, pus, + *haima*, blood]. Septicemia and pyemia together.

septigravida (sep"tĭ-grav'ĭ-da) [L. *septem*, seven, + *gravida*, pregnant]. A woman pregnant for the 7th time.

septimetritis (sĕp"tĭ-mē-trī'tĭs) [Gr. *sēptos*, putrid, + *mētra*, uterus, + *-itis*, inflammation]. Inflammation of uterus due to sepsis.

septipara (sĕp-tĭp'ă-ră) [L. *septem*, seven, + *parēre*, to bring forth]. A woman who has borne 7 children separately.

septivalent (sĕp-tĭ-vā'lĕnt, -tĭv'ă-lĕnt) ["+ *valēre*, to be strong]. Having a valency of 7 or combining with or replacing 7 hydrogen atoms.

septomarginal (sep″to-mar′ji-nal). Pert. to the margin or the border of a septum.

septometer (sĕp-tŏm′e-ter). 1. [L. *saeptum*, a partition, + *metrum*, measure]. Calipers for measuring width of nasal septum. 2. [Gr. *sepsis*, putrefaction, + *metron*, a measure]. Device for determining bacterial contamination of air. SYN: *sepsometer*.

septotome (sĕp′tō-tōm) [L. *saeptum*, a partition, + Gr. *tomē*, a cutting]. An instrument for cutting or removing a section of the nasal septum.

septotomy (sĕp-tŏt′ō-mĭ) [″ + Gr. *tomē*, a cutting]. Incision of a septum, esp. the nasal septum.

septu′la [L.]. Pl. of septulum, q.v.

    s. testis. [NA]. Thin partition extending inward from mediastinum testis and separating testis into the lobuli testis.

septulum (sep′tu-lum) [L.]. (pl. *septula*) A small partition or septum.

septum (sĕp′tŭm) [L. *saeptum*, a partition]. (pl. *septa*) A membranous wall dividing two cavities.

    s., atrial. A wall between the atria of the heart.

    s. atriorum cordis, s. auricularum. A wall between the atria of the heart.

    s., crural. S., femoral, q.v.

    s., femoral. Connective tissue which closes the femoral ring.

    s., interatrial. S., atrial, q.v.

    s., intermuscular. 1. A connective tissue septum which separates two muscles, esp. one from which muscles may take their origin. 2. One of two connective tissue septa which separate the muscles of the leg into anterior, posterior, and lateral groups.

    s., interventricular. S., ventricular, q.v.

    s., lingual. A sheet of connective tissue separating the halves of the tongue.

    s. lucidum. 1. A translucent s., the interior boundary of lateral ventricles of the brain. SYN: *septum pellucidum*. 2. The stratum corneum layer of the epidermis.

    s., mediastinal. SEE: *mediastinum*.

    s., nasal. The partition which divides the nasal cavity into two nasal fossae. Bony portion formed by the perpendicular plate of ethmoid and the vomer bone; cartilaginous portion formed by septal and vomeronasal cartilages and medial crura of greater alar cartilages.

    s., orbital. A fibrous sheet extending partially across the anterior opening of the orbit partially closing it.

    s. pectiniforme. Comblike partition that separates the corpora cavernosa.

    s. pellucidum. [NA] A thin triangular sheet of nervous tissue consisting of two lamina attached to corpus callosum above and the fornix below. It forms the medial wall of the lateral ventricles.

    s., rectovaginal. Partition between the rectum and the vagina.

    s. scroti. [NA] Partition dividing the chambers of the scrotum. SYN: *s. of scrotum*.

    s., ventricular. Partition between the ventricles of the heart.

septuplet (sĕp′tŭ-plĕt) [L. *septuplum*, a group of seven]. One of 7 children born from the same gestation.

sequela (sē-kwē′lă) [L. *sequēla*, sequel]. (pl. *sequelae*) A condition following and resulting from a disease.

sequence [L.]. The order or occurrence of a series of phenomena as symptoms.

sequester (sē-kwĕs′tĕr) [L. *sequestrāre*, to separate]. 1. To isolate. 2. A piece of necrosed bone separated from surrounding tissue. SYN: *sequestrum*.

sequestration (sē″kwĕs-tra′shŭn) [L. *sequestrātio*, a separation]. 1. The formation of sequestrum. 2. Isolation of a patient for treatment or quarantine. 3. Reduction of hemorrhage of head or trunk by temporarily stopping the return of blood from the extremities by applying tourniquets to the thighs and arms.

sequestrectomy (sē″kwĕs-trĕk′tō-mĭ) [″ + Gr. *ektomē*, excision]. Excision of a necrosed piece of bone.

sequestrotomy (sē″kwĕs-trŏt′ō-mĭ) [″ + Gr. *tomē*, a cutting]. Operation for removal of a sequestrum, a fragment of necrosed bone. SYN: *sequestrectomy*.

sequestrum (sē-kwĕs′trŭm) [L. *sequestrum*, something set aside]. (pl. *sequestra*) Fragment of a necrosed bone that has become separated from surrounding tissue. Designated primary if piece is entirely detached, secondary if still loosely attached, and tertiary if it is partially detached but still remaining in place.

sera (sē′ră) [L.]. Pl. of serum, q.v.

seralbumin (sēr-ăl-bū′mĭn) [L. *serum*, whey, + *albumen*, white of egg]. Albumin of the blood.

serendipity (sĕr″ĕn-dĭp′ĭ-tĭ). The gift of finding, by chance and wisdom, valuable or agreeable things not sought for. In medical research an unexpected reaction or result may produce new insights into some area totally unrelated to that which prompted the investigation.

serial (sē'rĭ-ăl) [L. *series,* a succession]. In numerical order, in continuity or sequence, as in a series.

sericeps (sēr'ĭ-sĕps) [L. *sericus,* silken, + *caput,* head]. Silk sac used in making traction on fetal head.

series (sēr'ēz) [L. *series,* a succession]. 1. Arrangement of objects in succession or in order. 2. In electricity, batteries or mode of arranging the parts of a circuit by connecting them successively end to end to form a single path for the current. The parts so arranged are said to be "in series."

serin. α-Amino-β-hydroxypropionic acid; an amino acid present in many proteins including casein, vitellin, and others. Found in the urine of normal human beings.

seriscission (sĕr-ĭ-sĭsh'ŭn) [L. *sericum,* silk, + *scindere,* to cut]. Division of soft tissues, as a pedicle, by tying a silk ligature around it.

sero- [L.]. Combining form pert. to serum.

seroalbuminuria (sē"rō-ăl-bū-mĭn-ū'rĭ-ă) [L. *serum,* whey, + *albumen,* white of egg, + Gr. *ouron,* urine]. Serum albumin in the urine.

serochrome (sē'rō-krōm) ["+ Gr. *chrōma,* color]. The pigment of normal serum.

serocolitis (sē"rō-kō-lī'tĭs) ["+ Gr. *kōlon,* colon, + *-itis,* inflammation]. Inflammation of serous coat of the colon. SYN: *pericolitis.*

seroculture (sē'rō-kŭl-chūr) [L. *serum,* whey, + *cultura,* cultivation]. A bacterial culture on blood serum.

serocystic (sē"rō-sĭs'tĭk) ["+ Gr. *kystis,* a cyst]. Composed of cysts containing serous fluid.

serodermatosis (sē"rō-der-mă-tō'sĭs) ["+ Gr. *derma,* skin, + *-ōsis,* condition]. Skin disease with serous effusion into tissues of the epidermis.

serodiagnosis (sē"rō-dī-ăg-nō'sĭs) [L. *serum,* whey, + Gr. *dia,* through, + *gnōsis,* knowledge]. Diagnosis by observing the reactions of blood serum.

seroenteritis (sē"rō-ĕn-ter-ī'tĭs) ["+ Gr. *enteron,* intestine, + *-itis,* inflammation]. Inflammation of serous covering of the intestine.

serofibrinous (sē"rō-fĭb'rĭn-ŭs) ["+ *fibra,* fiber]. 1. Composed of both serum and fibrin. 2. Denoting a serofibrinous exudate.

serohepatitis (sē"rō-hĕp-ă-tī'tĭs) [L. *serum,* whey, + Gr. *hēpar, hepat-,* liver, + *-itis,* inflammation]. Inflammation of the peritoneal covering of the liver.

serolipase (sē"rō-lĭp'ās) [Gr. *lipos,* fat, + *ase,* enzyme]. Lipase found in blood serum.

serologic, serological (sē-rō-lŏj'ĭk, -ăl) ["+ Gr. *logos,* a study]. Pert. to or the study of sera.

serologist (sē-rŏl'ō-jĭst) ["+ Gr. *logos,* a study]. One who has special knowledge and ability in serology.

serology (sē-rŏl'ō-jĭ) [L. *serum,* whey, + Gr. *logos,* a study]. The scientific study of serum.

serolysin (sē-rŏl'ĭs-ĭn) ["+ Gr. *lysis,* dissolution]. A bactericidal substance or lysin found in the blood serum.

seromembranous (sē"rō-mĕm'brăn-ŭs) ["+ *membrana,* membrane]. Both serous and membranous; rel. to a serous membrane.

seromucous (sē"rō-mū'kŭs) [L. *serum,* whey, + *mucus,* mucus]. Pert. to or composed of both serum and mucus.

seronegative (sē"rō-nĕg'ătĭv). Producing a negative reaction to serological tests.

seroperitoneum (sē"rō-pĕr"ĭ-tō-nē'ŭm) [L. *serum,* whey, + Gr. *peritonaion,* peritoneum]. Fluid in the peritoneum. SYN: *ascites, hydroperitoneum.*

seropositive (sē"rō-pŏz'ĭ-tiv). Producing a positive reaction to serological tests.

seroprognosis (sē"rō-prŏg-nō'sĭs) [L. *serum,* whey, + Gr. *prō,* before, + *gnōsis,* knowledge]. Prognosis of disease determined by seroreactions.

seroprophylaxis (sē"rō-prō-fĭ-lăks'ĭs) ["+ Gr. *prō,* before, + *phylaxis,* protection]. Prevention of a disease by injection of serum. SYN: *seroprevention.*

seropurulent (sē"rō-pū-rū-lĕnt) ["+ *purulentus,* full of pus]. Composed of serum and pus, as an exudate.

seroreaction (sē"rō-rē-ăk'shŭn) ["+ *re,* back, + *actio,* action]. 1. Any reaction taking place in or involving serum. SEE: *deviation; fixation, complement.* 2. Reaction to an injection of serum marked by rash, fever, pain, etc. SYN: *serum sickness.*

seroresistance (sē"rō-rē-zĭs'tăns). Failure of a serum reaction to become negative or be reduced in titer following treatment.

serosa (sē-rō'să) [L. *serum,* whey]. A serous membrane, q.v. Examples are peritoneum, pleura, and pericardium. SYN: *tunica serosa.*

serosamucin (sē-rō"să-mū'sĭn) [L. *serosus,* serous, + *mucus,* mucus]. A mucinlike substance in ascitic fluid from inflamed sites.

serosanguineous (sē"rō-săn-gwĭn'ē-ŭs) [L. *serum,* whey, + *sanguineus,* bloody]. Containing or of the nature of serum and blood.

seroscopy (sē-rŏs'kō-pĭ) ["+ Gr. *skopein,* to examine]. Examination of serum for diagnostic purposes.

seroserous (sē″rō-sē′rŭs) [L. *serosus*, serous, + *serum*, whey]. Pert. to two serous surfaces.

serositis (sē″rō-sī′tĭs) ["+ Gr. *-ītis*, inflammation]. (pl. *serositides*) Inflamed condition of a serous membrane.

serosity (sē-rŏs′ĭ-tĭ) [Fr. *sérosité*]. The quality of being serous.

serosynovitis (sē″rō-sĭn″ō-vī′tĭs) [L. *serum*, whey, + Gr. *syn*, with, + *ōon*, egg, + *-ītis*, inflammation]. Synovitis with increase of synovial fluid.

serotherapy (sē″rō-thĕr′ă-pī) ["+ Gr. *therapeia*, treatment]. The treatment of disease by the injection of blood serum, either human or animal, containing antibodies. Concerned with producing temporary artificial immunity in a person by injecting the blood serum of an animal which has acquired active immunity to the disease in question.

serotonin (sĕr″ō-tōn′ĭn). A chemical, 5-hydroxytryptamine (5-HT), present in platelets, gastrointestinal mucosa, mast cells, and in carcinoid tumors. Serotonin is quite similar in its action to epinephrine.

serotype (se′ro-tīp). A microorganism determined by the kinds and combinations of constituent antigens present in the cells.

serous (sĭr′ŭs) [L. *serosus*]. 1. Having the nature of serum. 2. Producing a serous secretion, or containing serum or a serumlike substance.

   s. cavity. A cavity lined by a s. membrane, specifically the pleural, peritoneal, and pericardial cavities.

   s. cell. A cell which secretes a thin, watery, albuminous secretion.

   s. effusion. Escape of serum.

   s. exudate. Exudate consisting mostly of serum.

   s. fluids. Liquids of the body, similar to blood serum, which are in part secreted by s. membranes.

   s. glands. A gland secreting a watery, albuminous fluid. Ex: parotid gland.

   s. inflammation. Inflammation of a part with s. exudate, or inflammation of a s. membrane.

   s. membrane. A membrane lining a s. cavity.

   RS: membrane, serous.

serovaccination. A process with combined injection of serum, to secure immediate passive immunity, and bacterial vaccine, to acquire subsequent active immunity.

serozymogenic (sē″rō-zī″mō-jĕn′ĭk) [L. *serum*, whey, + Gr. *zymē*, ferment, + *gennan*, to produce.]. Pert. to a serous fluid and enzymes.

   s. cell. A cell which produces a serous secretion containing an enzyme.

serpiginous (sĕr-pĭj′ĭ-nŭs) [L. *serpere*, to creep]. Creeping from one part to another.

   s. ulcer. Ulcer, extending in one direction while healing in another direction.

serpigo (sĕr-pī′gō) [ME.]. Any creeping eruption, esp. ringworm, herpes, or tinea.

serrate (sĕr′āt) [L. *serrātus*, toothed]. Notched; toothed. SYN: *dentate*.

Serratia (sĕr-ā′shĭ-ă). [Serafino Serrati, It. physicist, 18th century]. A genus of bacteria of the family Enterobacteriaceae.

   S. marcescens. Formerly called Chromobacterium prodigiosum, and erroneously believed to be nonpathogenic to man.

serration (sĕr-ā′shŭn) [L. *serratio*, a notching]. 1. Formation with sharp projections like the teeth of a saw. 2. A single tooth or notch in a serrated edge.

serra′tus muscle. Any of several muscles arising from the ribs or vertebrae by separate slips. SEE: *Table of Muscles* in *Appendix*.

serrefine (săr-fēn′) [Fr.]. A small, wire, spring forceps for compressing bleeding vessels.

serrenoeud (săr-nŭd) [Fr. *serrer*, to squeeze, + *noeud*, knot]. Device for tightening ligatures, esp. those placed on vessels in a deep cavity out of reach of fingers.

Sertoli′s cells (sĕr-tō′lē). [Enrico Sertoli, It. histologist, 1842-1910]. Supporting, elongated cells of seminiferous tubules which nourish spermatids.

serum (sē′rŭm) [L., whey]. (pl. *serums, sera*) 1. Any serous fluid, esp. the fluid which moistens the surfaces of serous membranes. 2. The watery portion of the blood after coagulation; a fluid found when clotted blood is left standing long enough for the clot to shrink. 3. Serum from an animal rendered immune against a pathogenic organism, to be injected into a patient with the disease resulting from the same organism. It consists of plasma minus fibrinogen.

   s. albumin. A protein found in blood s. SEE: *blood; protein, simple*.

   s., anticrotalus. S. to overcome the effect of rattlesnake poison.

   s., antidiphtheritic. S. used to counteract the effects of diphtheria.

   s., antimeningococcus. S. antagonistic to meningococcus infection.

   s., antipneumococcus. S. for pneumococcus infection.

   s., antitetanic. S. given to counteract tetanus toxin.

s., antitoxic. S. containing the antitoxin of the microorganism against which it is supposed to be protective.

s., antityphoid. S. containing antibodies of the typhoid bacillus.

s., bactericidal. S. having no effect on toxins but destructive to bacteria.

s., bacteriolytic. A s. containing a lysin that destroys certain bacteria.

s., blood. The liquid clear portion of blood without its fibrin and corpuscles.

s., convalescent. Blood s. from a person convalescing from an infection, the s. to be used on others having the same disease.

s., foreign. S. from one animal injected into another animal of another species, or into man.

s. globulin. A protein found in blood s. SEE: *globulin, serum.*

s., immune. A s. containing antibodies for specific antigens.

s., polyvalent. S. containing antibodies to several types of the same bacterial species.

s., pooled. Mixed blood s. from several persons.

s., pregnancy. Blood s. from pregnant women given to premature infants in food.

s., pregnant mare's. A source of hormones, esp. chorionic gonadotrophin. ABBR: pms.

s. protein. Any protein in blood s. S. protein forms weak acids mixed with alkali salts; this increases the buffer effects of the blood but to a lesser extent than cell protein.

s. rash. Rash first seen at site of an injection of serum. It remains thickest there, but it may invade other parts of the body. It resembles a combination of urticarial, morbilliform, and scarlatiniform rashes.

SYM: Severe irritation; marked swelling of skin, esp. of the face; malaise; and constitutional symptoms.

s. sickness. A condition which may occur from several days to 2-3 weeks after administration of antisera or following certain drug therapy.

SYM: Fever, enlarged lymph nodes and spleen, skin rash, and painful joints.

TREATMENT: Symptomatic and adrenal cortical hormones if needed.

serum, words pert. to: agglutinin; agglutinogen; antigen; antitropin; antivenin; autoserodiagnosis; autoserotherapy; autoserous; autoserum; chromodiagnosis; complement; icteric index; isohemagglutinin; opsonic index; opsonin; orrhorrhea; serology; serous; words beginning with *lymph.*

serumal (sē-rū'măl) [L. *serum*, whey]. Rel. to serum.

s. calculus. Calculus formed about the teeth from serous exudate.

serum-fast. Resistant to the action of serum.

servomechanism (sŭr''vō-měk'ă-nĭzm). In biology and physiology, the feedback mechanism which controls the constancy of supply or activity of a function. For example, when in the normal person the blood glucose level rises, the pancreas responds by releasing insulin which enables the glucose to be metabolized. The level of hormones is regulated by this same mechanism when the anterior pituitary responds to either falling or rising levels of hormones by either increasing or decreasing the production of the appropriate substance which causes a gland to produce hormones.

SES. Abbr. for *socioeconomic status.*

sesamoid (sěs'a-moyd) [L. *sesamoides*]. Resembling a grain of sesame in size or shape.

s. bone. An oval nodule of bone or fibrocartilage in a tendon playing over a bony surface. The patella is the largest one.

s. cartilage. One or more small cartilage plates present in fibrous tissue between lateral nasal and greater alar cartilages of the nose.

sesqui- [L.]. Prefix meaning one and a half.

sesquihora (sěs''kwĭ-hō'ră) [L.]. Every hour and a half.

sessile (sěs'ĭl) [L. *sessilis*, low]. Having no peduncle, but attached directly by a broad base.

set. 1. To fix firmly in place, as to set a bone in reduction of a fracture. 2. To allow an amalgam or plaster to harden. 3. In psychology, a group of conditions or attitudes which favor the occurrence of a certain response.

setaceous (sē-tā'shŭs) [L. *setaceus*]. Bristly, hairy; resembling a bristle.

seton (sē'tŏn) [L. *seta*, a thread]. 1. A thread or threads drawn through a fold of skin to act as a counterirritant. 2. A fistulous tract so produced.

se'tose. Having bristlelike appendages.

Setschenow's inhibitory centers (sě'tchn-ŏf). [Ivan M. Setschenow, Russian neurologist, 1829-1903]. Centers in the spinal cord and oblongata for inhibiting reflex movement.

seven basic foods. 1. Leafy green and yellow vegetables. 2. Citrus fruit, tomatoes, raw cabbage. 3. Potatoes and other vegetables and fruits. 4. Milk or milk products. 5. Meat, poultry, fish, eggs. 6. Bread; flour; cereals, whole-grain, enriched, or restored. 7. Butter and fortified margarine.

seven-year itch. Scabies, q.v.

seventh cranial nerve. Facial nerve; nervus facialis.

sevum (sē'vŭm) [L.]. Tallow or suet.

sewer gas. Foul air of a sewer. SEE: *carbon monoxide*.

sex [L. *sexus*]. 1. The distinctive quality which differentiates between male and female. 2. Males or females collectively. 3. The sexual instinct as it manifests itself in behavior.

   s. chromatin. Cells which contain a dark-staining chromatin mass at the periphery of the nuclei when stained with basic dye. They are derived from female subjects and are not present in male cells. The material is thought to be the X chromosome pair present in females. SYN: *Barr bodies*.

   s. chromosomes. The chromosomes in a cell which determine sex.

   s., nuclear. The genetic sex of an individual determined by the absence or presence of sex chromatin in the body cells, particularly blood cells.

   s. ratio. Ratio of females to males. Used in defining proportion of births of the two sexes or in the representation by sexual distribution in certain diseases.

sexdigital (sĕks-dĭj'ĭ-tăl) [L. *sex*, six, + *digitus*, digit]. Having six fingers and toes.

sexivalent (sĕks'ĭ-vā'lĕnt, -ĭv'ăl-ĕnt) ["+ *valēre*, to be strong]. Capable of combining with six atoms of hydrogen.

sex-limited. Expression of a genetic character or trait in one sex only.

sex-linked. A character which is controlled by genes in the sex chromosomes.

sexology [L. *sexus*, sex, + Gr. *logos*, study]. Scientific study of sexuality.

sextan (sĕks'tăn) [L. *sextanus*, of the sixth]. Occurring every 6th day.

sextigravida (sĕks'tĭ-grăv'ĭd-ă) [L. *sextus*, six, + *gravida*, a pregnant woman]. A woman pregnant for the 6th time.

sextipara (sĕks-tĭp'ă-ră) ["+ *parēre*, to bear a child]. A woman who has had six pregnancies resulting in viable offspring.

sextuplet (sĕks'tū-plĕt) [L. *sextus*, six]. One of six children born of a single gestation.

sexual (sĕks'ū-ăl) [L. *sexuālis*]. 1. Pert. to sex. 2. Having sex.

   s. bondage. An abnormal, but not perverse, phenomenon of dependence of one person upon another of the opposite sex, one dominating the other.

   s. intercourse. Sexual union between a male and a female. SYN: *coition; coitus; copulation*.

   RS: clitoris; coitus interruptus; dyspareunia; ejaculation; emission; excitation; penis; semen; telegony; vagina.

   s. inversion. Homosexuality.

   s. involution. The menopause.

   s. metamorphosis. A form of s. aberration in which one adopts the habits and dress of the opposite sex.

   s. psychopathy. A term for the group in which exist perversions of sex. SEE: *bestiality; coprolagnism; exhibitionism; fetishism; frottage; homosexuality; lesbianism; masochism; masturbation; onanism; pedophilia; renifleur; sadism; sodomy; transvestism; voyeur*.

   s. reassignment. Legal, surgical, or social action or decision to assign the appropriate sexuality to an individual who has been considered previously to be of the opposite sex.

   s. reflex. Erection and ejaculation resulting from direct genital stimulation or indirectly from emotion, whether asleep or awake.

sexuality (sĕks-ū-ăl'ĭ-tĭ) [L. *sexus*, sex]. 1. State of having sex; the collective characteristics which mark the differences between the male and the female. 2. Constitution and life of individual as related to sex; all the dispositions related to the love life whether associated with the sex organs or not.

SGOT. Abbr. for *serum glutamic-oxalacetic transaminase*. SEE: *transaminase*.

shad (shăd) [AS. *sceadd*]. A herringlike food fish having a comparatively deep body.

   Food value of 100 gm. (baked): Cal. 201; protein 23.3 gm.; fat 11.3 gm.; vitamin A, 30 I.U.; niacin 8.6 mg.

shad'ow [AS. *sceaduwe*]. A hemolyzed erythrocyte. SYN: *ghost cell; phantom cell*.

shadowgram, shadowgraph ["+ Gr. *graphein*, to write]. A print on a photographic plate exposed to X rays. SYN: *skiagraph*.

shaft [AS. *sceaft*]. 1. The principal portion of any cylindrical body. 2. The diaphysis of a long bone. SEE: *diaphysis*.

   s., hair. The keratinized portion of a hair which extends from a hair follicle beyond the surface of the epidermis.

shakes (shāks) [AS. *sceacen*]. 1. Shivering caused by a chill, esp. in intermittent fever. 2. State of tremulousness and extreme irritability often seen in chronic alcoholics. SYN: *jitters*.

shak'ing. A passive movement in Swedish massage.

shaking palsy. A basal ganglion disease with progressive rigid tremulousness, peculiar gait, muscular contraction, and weakness. SYN: *paralysis agitans; Parkinson's disease*.

shaman (shā'mŭn, shŏ-) [Russ., ascetic]. One who heals or attempts to heal by the use of magic; one acting as both priest and doctor. SYN: *medicine man.* SEE: *shamanism.*

shamanism (shā'mŭn-ĭsm, shŏ'-). 1. Primitive religion of certain peoples of northern Asia who believe good and evil spirits pervade the world and can be influenced only by shamans acting as mediums. 2. Any similar form of primitive spiritualism, such as practiced among American Indian tribes.

shank (shăngk) [AS. *sceanca*]. The tibia or portion of leg from knee to ankle. SYN: *shin.*

shape (shāp) [AS. *sceapan*]. 1. To mold to a particular form. 2. Outward form; contour.

RS: aliform; arcate; arciform; arcuation; arenoid; asbestiform; asteroid; bacciform; belemnoid; bilateralism; bosselated; bosselation; bulbiform; calculus; carinate; caudate; circle; circumvallate.

sharkskin. Condition seen in pellagra (nicotinic acid deficiency) in which openings of sebaceous glands become plugged with a dry, yellowish material.

Sharpey's intercrossing fibers (shär'pē). [William Sharpey, Scot. physiologist, 1802-1880] Fibers forming the lamellae constituting the walls of the haversian canals in bone.

Sharpey's perforating fibers. 1. Fibers extending from the periosteum into the lamellae of bone. 2. F. extending from peridontal membrane into cementum of a tooth.

sheath (shēth) [AS. *sceath*]. A covering structure of connective tissue, usually of an elongated part, such as the membrane covering a muscle.

s., arachnoid or arachnoidean. Delicate partition between pial s. and dural s. of the optic nerve.

s., axon. The myelin s. and/or neurilemma.

s., carotid. Portion of cervical or pretracheal fascia enclosing carotid artery, interior jugular vein, and vagus nerve.

s., crural. Fascial covering of femoral vessels.

s., dentinal. S. lining the dental canals.

s., dural. A fibrous membrane or external investment of the optic nerve.

s., femoral. The fascial covering of femoral vessels.

s. of Henle. S. of Key and Retzius, q.v.

s. of Key and Retzius, connective tissue. Delicate reticular fibrils around individual nerve fibers.

s., lamellar. Connective tissue s. covering bundle of nerve fibers. SYN: *perineurium.*

s., myelin. Layers of lipid and protein substances which form a semifluid covering of nerves. The layers are an extension of the plasma membrane of the Schwann cell. The s. is relatively insensitive to the action of temperature and electrolytes. SEE: *nerve fiber; neuron.*

s., nerve. S., lamellar, q.v.

s. of Neumann. A layer of dentine which lies adjacent to a dentinal tubule.

s., pial. Extension of the pia, closely investing surface of the optic nerve.

s., root. The layers of a hair follicle derived from the epidermis. Includes the *outer root s.* which is a continuation of the stratum germinativum, and the *inner root s.* which consists of three layers of cells closely investing the root of the hair. SEE: *hair.*

s. of Schwann. Membranous covering of myelin s. of a nerve fiber. SYN: *neurilemmal s.*

s. of Schweigger-Seidel. The thickened wall of a sheathed artery of the spleen.

s., synovial. A double-walled tubelike bursa which encloses a tendon. Consists of an inner visceral layer lying upon and adhering to a tendon and an outer parietal layer, the two being separated by a space filled with synovial fluid. Found esp. in the hands and feet where tendons are confined to osteofibrous canals or pass over bony surfaces.

s., tendon. A dense fibrous s. which confines a tendon to an osseous groove converting it into an osteofibrous canal. Found principally in the wrist and ankle. SEE: *s., synovial.*

shedd'ing [ME. *sheden*, shed]. 1. The loss of deciduous teeth. 2. Casting off of surface layer of the epidermis.

sheet (shēt) [AS. *sciete*, cloth]. Linen or cotton bedcovering next to the sleeper.

s., draw. A sheet folded under a patient so it may be withdrawn without lifting the patient. This is accomplished by turning the patient to the side of the bed to allow one side of the sheet to be removed and replaced with a clean one. The patient is then turned to the other side of the bed. The soiled sheet is removed and placement of the clean one is completed. SEE: *draw sheet.*

shell shock. An obsolete term used during World War I to designate a wide variety of psychotic and neurotic disorders associated with the stress of combat. SEE: *hysteria.*

shield (shēld) [AS. *scild*, shield]. 1. Any protecting device. 2. In biology, a protective plate or hard outer covering.

s. bone. The scapula.

s., Buller's. A watch glass to be worn over the eye to protect it from gonorrheal or ophthalmic infection.

s., embryonic. The two-layered blastoderm or blastodisk from which a mammalian embryo develops. SYN: *embryonic disk.* SEE: *disk, embryonic.*

s., nipple. A cover to protect sore nipples during nursing.

s., phallic. An antiseptic covering for the male genitals during operations.

shift [AS. *sciftan,* to arrange]. A change in position or direction.

s., chloride. The shift of chloride ions from the plasma into red blood cells upon the addition of carbon dioxide from the tissues and the reverse movement when carbon dioxide is released in the lungs. It is a mechanism for maintaining constant pH of the blood.

s. to the left. An increase in the number of young polymorphonuclear leukocytes in the blood. SEE: *Arneth's classification of neutrophils.*

s. to the right. An increase in the number of older polymorphonuclear leukocytes in the blood. SEE: *Arneth's classification of neutrophils.*

Shiga's bacillus (shē'gä). [Kiyoshi Shiga, Japanese physician, 1870-1957]. The bacillus causing a form of dysentery. SYN: *Shigella dysenteriae.*

Shigella (shǐ-gel'lä). [Kiyoshi Shiga] A genus of nonlactose-fermenting, nonmotile, gramnegative rods belonging to the family Enterobacteriaceae. It contains a number of species which cause digestive disturbance ranging from mild diarrhea to a severe and often fatal dysentery.

S. dysenteriae. The Shiga bacillus, a virulent form isolated during a severe epidemic of dysentery in Japan in 1896.

shin (shǐn) [AS. *scinu,* shin]. Anterior edge of tibia, portion of leg between the ankle and knee. SYN: *shank.*

s., saber. Condition seen in congenital syphilis in which anterior edge of tibia is extremely sharp.

s. spots. Hyperpigmented and retracted scars of the skin on the anterior lower legs. Condition is usually, but not always, associated with diabetes.

shingles (shǐng'lz) [L. *cingulus,* a girdle]. Eruption of acute, inflammatory, herpetic vesicles on the trunk of the body along a peripheral nerve; occasionally elsewhere. SYN: *herpes zoster,* q.v.

ship fever. A fever due to unhygienic conditons aboard ship, usually typhus fever and occasionally yellow fever.

shiver (shǐv'ēr) [ME. *chiveren*]. 1. A slight tremor of the skin, as from cold or fear. 2. To tremble or shake.

shock (shŏk) [ME. *schokke*]. Term used to designate a clinical syndrome with varying degrees of disturbances of oxygen supply to the tissues and return of blood to the heart. Shock may be caused by a variety of conditions including hemorrhage, infection, drug reaction, trauma, poisoning, myocardial infarction and dehydration. To the lay person "shock" may mean cerebral vascular accident.

Every injury is accompanied by some degree of shock and so should be treated promptly. Syncope is caused by insufficient blood supply to the brain in certain persons and the clinical picture resembles shock.

RS: catalepsy; insulin.

SYM: The most outstanding symptoms are: marked paleness of the skin; a bluish or grayish discoloration (cyanosis of the lips, nails, tips of the fingers and lobes of the ears); the face is pinched and without expression; there may be a staring of the eyes which often lose their characteristic luster and the pupils may be dilated; the pulse is weak and rapid; the breathing rate is increased and is shallow; the blood pressure is decreased and may be unobtainable; there may be urinary retention and incontinence of feces; occasionally there is an unusual restlessness or excitement; and very often the patient expresses an extreme thirst. If conscious the patient seems quite disinterested in the surroundings and complains little of pain even though he may be groaning.

TREATMENT: Keep patient lying down with head lower than body. The lower extremities can be slightly elevated by placing the lower half of the body on pillows, or by elevating the foot of the bed.

Patient should be kept comfortably warm, but application of external heat is not advisable. Avoid unnecessary questions and noises. Do not move patient unnecessarily.

Even though thirst is present, give fluids by mouth sparingly in order to reduce the possibility of vomiting and aspirating vomitus. If bleeding is present it should be controlled. If internal hemorrhage is suspected or presence of head injuries, no stimulants are permissible.

A physician should be called promptly. The use of hypodermics and intramuscular and intravenous injections, such as epinephrine, ephedrine, caffeine, strychnine, etc., may be recommended by the doctor. Oxygen may be necessary. Blood transfusion or even artificial respiration may be required, depending on the seriousness of the condition.

Relieve pain by splints, posture, supporting bandages and drugs. Morphine is valuable. Maintain circulation by posture, have patient lying down with head and shoulders lower than the body. Blood transfusions may be lifesaving. If blood is not available, artificial substances for increasing plasma volume may be used.

Respiration may be aided by administration of oxygen preferably mixed with 4 to 10% carbon dioxide as a respiratory stimulant. Constant, kindly, tactful encouragement and extreme gentleness in all procedures are of importance.

F. A. TREATMENT: Depends on accuracy of diagnosis. In general, treat specific etiological factor; maintain body heat by warm but not hot blankets, water bottles, etc. Stimulants used generously except in presence of suspected bleeding or head injury.

s., anaphylactic. Reaction from injection of protein substance to which patient is sensitized.

s., anesthesia. This is not surgical shock, but is due to an overdose of anesthesia and calls for the immediate cessation of anesthesia.

Artificial respiration and appropriate stimulants should be given at once. The condition is manifested by a weak, rapid pulse, a fall or drop in blood pressure, cold, clammy skin, and shallow respirations.

s. from burns. SEE: *burn, treatment.*

s., deferred or delayed. Late manifestation following injury or burns. May appear in 3 to 30 hours and may be due to transportation, emotional stress, hemorrhage, dehydration, acidosis, or toxemia.

s., electric. The result of passage of electric current through any part of the body. SEE: *electric shock.*

s., epigastric. Result of a blow or other trauma (surgery) in upper abdomen.

s., hypoglycemic. SEE: *insulin shock.*

s., insulin. Condition resulting from overdosages of insulin.

F. A. TREATMENT: Give orange juice, glucose, candy, lump of sugar, etc. If unconscious, inject glucose intravenously. SEE: *insulin.*

s., mental. Due to emotional stress or seeing injury, accidents, etc. SEE: *s., psychic.*

s., peptone or protein. Reaction resulting from parenteral administration of a protein.

s., psychic. S. due to excessive fear, joy, anger, grief.

s., secondary. S., deferred, q.v.

s., serum. One occurring as part of reaction to injection of serum.

s., shell. Obsolete term. SEE: *shell shock.*

s., surgical. Following operations and including traumatic shock. S., traumatic, q.v.

s. therapy. Form of treatment in mental illness. Two types are used: *Electric shock therapy* in which convulsions are induced by passage of electric current through the brain, used chiefly in depression. *Insulin shock therapy* in which hypoglycemia and coma are induced by injection of insulin, used chiefly in depression.

s., traumatic. Shock due to injury or surgery.

May occur as result of abdominal injury from any cause. Shock is proportional to extent of injury. Esp. severe in upper abdomen and more marked when viscera are damaged. If prolonged, indicates hemorrhage or peritonitis or both.

Cerebral injury: Concussion of brain or skull fracture. May come on immediately or later from edema or intracranial hemorrhage.

Chemical injury: S. due to pain from the effect of chemicals, esp. corrosives.

Crushing injury: The greater the extent of injury the more severe the degree of shock.

Fracture: Esp. in compound fracture. Often extensive blood loss into tissues and hence body is not able to maintain circulation.

Heart damage: As in angina pectoris, myocardial infarctions, pericarditis or myocarditis.

Inflammation: As acute general peritonitis or fulminating sepsis anywhere in the body.

Intestinal obstruction: Shock is present when obstruction is acute.

Nerve injury: Contusion of highly sensitive parts, as testicle, solar plexus, eye, urethra, etc.

Operations: May occur even after minor operations, as paracentesis and catheterization.

Perforation or rupture of viscera: As in acute pneumothorax, ruptured aneurysm, perforated peptic ulcer, perforation in appendicitis, ectopic pregnancy.

Strangulation: As in hernia, intussusception, volvulus.

Thermal injury: As burns, frostbite, heat exhaustion.

Torsion of viscera: As of an ovary, testicle.

s., wound. S., traumatic, q.v.

shoe'makers' cramp or spasm. Spasm of muscles of hand and arm occurring in shoemakers.

shortsightedness (short-sīt'ĕd-nĕs). A condition of not being able to see very far. Due to light rays coming to a focus in front of the retina. SYN: *myopia; nearsightedness.*

short stature. Condition of being of less height than that considered to be within the limits of normal variation when compared with individuals of the same chronological age and of similar racial background. In most cases this condition is determined genetically.

shot'gun prescrip'tion. One containing many drugs given with hope that one of them may prove effective. Not a recommended approach to the treatment of disease.

shoulder (shōl'dĕr) [AS. *sculdor*]. The junction of the clavicle and scapula where the arm meets the trunk.

RS: omalgia; omarthritis; omitis; scapula.

s. blade. The scapula.

s., dislocation of. Displacement of shoulder joint. Very frequently accompanied by a fracture. It is believed by all surgeons that it is wiser to have an x-ray examination of the affected bones because fractures are often present. Attempts to reduce dislocations without knowledge of fractures is very dangerous, sometimes resulting in serious paralysis of the entire upper extremity or grave damage to the large blood vessels in the armpit.

CAUSES: The causes of a shoulder dislocation are usually from falling on an outstretched arm or a blow to the arm in some unusual position. It is very common among athletes, esp. football and basketball players. A patient with a dislocated shoulder usually has a hollow in place of the normal bulge of the shoulder. There seems to be a slight depression at the outer end of the clavicle, and the patient cannot place his hand at his opposite shoulder while his elbow is on his chest. Always compare both sides.

TREATMENT: Send for a doctor as soon as possible. Lay the patient on the back, with a pillow (or folded pad) between the shoulders. Place a large, soft pad under the elbow on the affected side, then bind the forearm horizontally across the chest using an open sling which is reinforced by a broad cravat; bandage and apply cold applications to the affected shoulder. Treat for shock.

s. girdle. The two scapulae and two clavicles attaching the bones of the upper extremities to the axial skeleton.

s. joint. Formed by humerus and glenoid cavity of scapula.

show (shō) [AS. *scēawian*, to look at]. The sanguinoserous discharge from the vagina during the first stage of labor or just preceding menstruation.

Shrapnell's membrane (shrăp'nĕl). [Henry J. Shrapnell, English anatomist, 1761-1841]. A small triangular portion of the tympanic membrane lying above the malleolar folds. It is thin and lax and attached directly to the petrous bone at the tympanic notch (notch of Rivinus). SYN: *pars flaccida membranae tympani* [NA].

shred'ded wheat. Food value of 100 gm. (without salt or other added nutrients): Cal. 354; protein 9.9 gm.; carbohydrate 79.9 gm.; fat 2.0 gm.; iron 3.5 mg.; sodium 3.0 mg.; calcium 43 mg.

shreds [AS. *scrēade*]. Slender strands of mucus seen in urine indicative of inflammation of urinary tract or associated organs.

shrimp (shrĭmp) [ME. *shrimpe*]. Any of various small, long-tailed crustaceans, many varieties of which are used for food.

Food value of 100 gm. (raw): Cal. 91; protein 18.1 gm.; carbohydrate 1.5 gm.; fat 0.8 gm.; calcium 63 mg.; sodium 140 mg.

shud'der [ME. *shuddren*]. A temporary convulsive tremor resulting from fright, horror, or aversion.

shunt (shŭnt) [ME. *shunten*, to avoid]. 1. To turn away from; to divert. 2. Anomalous passage or one artificially constructed to divert flow from one main route to another. 3. Electric conductor connecting two points in a circuit to form a parallel circuit through which a portion of the current may pass.

s., right-to-left. Passage of blood from the right side of the heart to the left side through some abnormal opening such as a septal defect. The shunted blood has no opportunity to become oxygenated because of having failed to pass through the lungs.

Si. Chem. symb. for silicon.

siagonantritis (sī''ăg-ŏn-ăn-trī'tĭs) [Gr. *siagōn*, jawbone, + *antron*, cavity, + *-itis*, inflammation]. Inflammation of the maxillary sinus.

sialaden (sī-ăl'ă-dĕn) [Gr. *sialon*, saliva, + *adēn*, gland]. A salivary gland.

sialadenitis (sī''al-ad''ĕ-nī'tis) ["+ "+ *-itis*, inflammation]. Inflamed condition of a salivary gland.

sialadenoncus (sī''ăl-ăd''ĕ-nŏng'kŭs) ["+ "+ *onkos*, tumor]. Tumor of salivary gland.

sialagogue (sī-ăl'ă-gŏg) [Gr. *sialon*, saliva, + *agōgos*, leading]. Agent increasing flow of saliva. Also spelled sialogogue.

sialaporia (sī″ăl-ă-pō′rĭ-ă) ["+ *aporia*, lack]. Deficiency in secretion of saliva.

sialemesis (sī″ăl-ĕm′ĕs-ĭs) ["+ *emesis*, vomiting]. Vomiting of saliva or vomiting caused by an excessive secretion of saliva.

sialine (sī′ă-lĭn) [Gr. *sialon*, saliva]. Concerning the saliva.

sialism, sialismus (sī′ăl-ĭzm, sī-ăl-ĭz′mŭs) ["+ *-ismos*, condition]. An excessive secretion of saliva. SYN: *ptyalism; salivation*.

sialoadenitis (sī″ă-lō-ad″ĕ-nī′tĭs) ["+ *adēn*, gland, + *-itis*, inflammation]. Inflammation of a salivary gland. SYN: *sialadenitis*.

sialoaerophagy (sī″ă-lō-ā″ĕr-of′ă-jī) ["+ *aēr*, air, + *phagein*, to eat]. Constant swallowing, thus taking saliva and air into the stomach.

sialoangitis (sī″ă-lō-ăn-jī′tĭs) [Gr. *sialon*, saliva, + *aggeion*, vessel, + *-itis*, inflammation]. Inflamed condition of the salivary ducts.

sialocele (si′ă-lo-sēl) ["+ Gr. *kēlē*, tumor]. Cyst or tumor of a salivary gland.

sialodochitis (sī″ă-lō-dō-kī′tĭs) ["+ *dochē*, receptacle, + *-itis*, inflammation]. Inflamed condition of salivary ducts.

   s. fibrinosa. S. with duct obstructed by a fibrinous exudate.

sialoductitis (sī″ă-lō-dŭk-tī′tĭs) ["+ L. *ductus*, duct, + Gr. *-itis*, inflammation]. Inflamed condition of Stensen's duct.

sialogenous (sī″ă-lōj′e-nŭs) [Gr. *sialon*, saliva, + *gennan*, to produce]. Forming saliva.

sialogogic (sī″ă-lō-gŏj′ĭk). Producing or promoting a secretion of saliva.

sialogogue (sī-ăl′ō-gŏg) [Gr. *sialon*, saliva, + *agōgos*, leading]. 1. An agent that stimulates the secretion of saliva. 2. Producing or promoting the secretion of saliva. SYN: *sialagogue*.

sialography (sī″ă-lŏg′ră-fĭ) ["+ *graphein*, to write]. Examination of salivary ducts and glands with x-rays. SYN: *ptyalography*.

sialolith (sī-ăl′ō-lĭth) ["+ *lithos*, a stone]. A salivary concretion of calculus.

sialolithiasis (sī″ă-lō-lĭ-thī′a-sĭs) ["+ "+ *-iasis*, condition]. Presence of salivary calculi.

sialolithotomy (sī″ă-lō-lĭ-thot′ō-mĭ) ["+ "+ *tomē*, a cutting]. Removal of a calculus from a salivary gland or duct.

sialoncus (sī″ă-lŏng′kŭs) ["+ *ogkos*, tumour]. A tumor under the tongue caused by obstruction of a salivary gland or duct.

sialoporia (sī″ă-lō-pō′rĭ-ă) [Gr. *sialon*, saliva, + *aporia*, lack]. Deficient secretion of saliva.

sialorrhea (sī″ă-lo-rē′a) ["+ *rhoia*, a flow]. Excessive flow of saliva. SYN: *sialism*.

sialoschesis (sī″ă-lŏs′kĕ-sĭs) ["+ *schesis*, suppression]. Suppression or retention of saliva.

sialosemeiology (sī″ă-lō-sē″mĭ-ŏl′o-jī) ["+ *semeion*, sign, + *logos*, a study]. Diagnosis based upon examination of the saliva.

sialosis (sī-ă-lō′sĭs) [Gr. *sialon*, saliva, + *-ōsis*, condition]. The flow of saliva.

sialostenosis (sī″ă-lō-stĕ-nō′sĭs) ["+ *stenō-sis*, a narrowing]. Closure of a salivary duct.

sialosyrinx (sī″ă-lō-sī′rĭnks) ["+ *syrigx*, a pipe]. 1. Fistula into the salivary gland. 2. A syringe for washing out salivary ducts. 3. Drainage tube for a salivary duct.

sialotic (sī″ă-lŏt′ĭk) [Gr. *sialon*, saliva]. Concerning the flow of saliva.

sialozemia (sī″ă-lō-zē′mĭ-ă) ["+ *zemia*, loss]. Involuntary loss of saliva. SYN: *salivation*.

Siamese twins (sī-ă-mēz′). [After Chang and Eng (1811-1874), joined Chinese twins born in Siam] Congenitally united twins, usually at the hips or buttocks, the members being capable of activity.

sib [AS. *sibb*, kin]. A brother or sister. SYN: *sibling*.

sibilant (sĭb′ĭ-lănt) [L. *sibilans*, hissing]. Hissing or whistling, as a sound heard in a certain rale, q.v.

sibila′tion. Pronunciation in which the hissing sound is predominant.

sibilis′mus. A hissing sound.

   s. aurium. Tinnitus, q.v.

sibilus (sĭb′ĭ-lŭs) [L. *sibilans*, hissing]. A hissing rale.

sibling (sĭb′lĭng) [AS. *sibb*, kin, + *-ling*, having the quality of]. One of two or more children of same parents; a brother or sister.

sibship. Brothers and sisters of a single family.

siccant (sĭk′ănt) [L. *siccus*, dry]. Drying.

siccative (sĭk′ă-tĭv) [L. *siccātivus*, drying]. Drying or that which dries. SYN: *siccant*.

sicchasia (sĭ-kā′shĭ-ă) [Gr. *sikchasia*, loathing]. Nausea.

siccus (sĭk′ŭs) [L.]. Dry.

sick (sĭk) [AS. *seōc*, ill]. 1. Not well. SYN: *ill*. 2. Mentally ill or disturbed. 3. Nauseated or "sick at the stomach." 4. Menstruating.

   s. headache. One with nausea, vomiting, anorexia, etc. SYN: *migraine*, q.v.

   s. at the stomach. Inclined to vomit. SYN: *nauseated*.

sick′le cell. Abnormal red blood corpuscle of crescent shape.

   s. c. anemia. A form of anemia in which abnormal sickle or crescent-shaped erythrocytes are present. Due to the presence of abnormal type of hemoglobin in the red blood cells. SEE: *anemia*.

sicklemia (sĭk-lē′mĭ-ă) [AS. *sicol*, sickle, + Gr. *haima*, blood]. Sickle cells in the blood.

sickling. Tendency of red blood cells to be sickle shaped. SEE: *sickle cell anemia*.

sick′ness [AS. *seóc*, ill]. State of being unwell. SYN: *illness*.

   s., bleeding. Abnormal tendency to bleed. SYN: *hemophilia*.

   s., car. Nausea and malaise from riding in vehicles such as trains or automobiles. SYN: *motion sickness*.

   s., falling. Epilepsy.

   s., green. Form of anemia with greenish pallor. SYN: *chlorosis*.

   s., monthly. Menstruation.

   s., morning. Nausea of early pregnancy.

   s., motion. Nausea and vomiting caused by a variety of motions, such as those experienced on boats, airplanes, trains, automobiles, or rides in amusement parks.

   s., mountain. Nausea and dyspnea caused by insufficient oxygen at high altitudes.

   s., sea. S. caused by motion of a vessel while at sea.

   s., serum. S. following injection of serum.

   s., sleeping. 1. Infection with genus of Trypanosomes with involvement of central nervous system and ultimately continuous sleeping. SYN: *trypanosomiasis*. 2. Acute infectious disease with increasing lethargy. SYN: *lethargic encephalitis*.

side (sīd) [AS. *sīde*]. 1. Left or right part of trunk of the body. 2. An outer portion considered as facing in a particular direction.

   s. effect. The action or effect, usually of a drug, other than that desired. Commonly this is an undesirable effect such as an allergic reaction to penicillin.

   s. position. Lying on one side, thighs flexed, with underarm behind back. SYN: *Sims' position*, q.v.

sideration (sĭd-ĕr-ā′shŭn) [L. *siderāri*, to be struck by a planet]. 1. Therapeutic application of electric sparks. 2. A sudden stroke of disease, as in apoplexy. 3. Lightning stroke.

siderism, siderismus (sĭd′ĕr-ĭzm, -ĭz′mŭs) [Gr. *sidēros*, iron, + *-ismos*, condition]. Therapeutic application of metals to the skin. SYN: *metallotherapy*.

sidero- (sĭd′er-o) [Gr. *sidēros*, iron]. Combining form meaning iron or steel.

siderocyte (sĭd′er-ō-sīt) [″+ *kytos*, cell]. A red blood cell containing iron in a form other than hematin.

sideroderma (sĭd′′ĕr-ō-der′mă) [Gr. *sidēros*, iron, + *derma*, skin]. Bronzed coloration of the skin from disordered hemoglobin disintegration.

siderodromophobia (sīd′′ĕr-ō-drō′′mō-fō′bĭ-ă) [″+ *dromos*, a way, + *phobos*, fear]. Morbid fear of railway travel.

siderofibrosis (sīd′′ĕr-ō-fī-brō′sĭs) [″+ L. *fibra*, fiber, + Gr. *-ōsis*, condition]. Fibrosis associated with deposits of iron.

siderogenous (sĭd′′ĕr-ōj′ĕ-nŭs) [″+ *gennan*, to produce]. Producing or forming iron.

sideropenia (sĭd′′er-o-pe′ne-a) [Gr. *sidēros*, iron, + *penia*, poverty]. Iron deficiency; deficiency of iron in the blood.

sideropenic (sĭd′′er-o-pe′nik). Characterized by deficiency of iron in the blood.

siderophilous (sīd′′ĕr-of′ĭ-lŭs) [Gr. *sidēros*, iron, + *philein*, to love]. Having a tendency to absorb iron, as the red blood corpuscles.

sideroscope (sīd′ĕr-ō-skōp) [″+ *skopein*, to examine]. Instrument for finding particles of iron in the eye.

siderosis (sĭd′′er-ō′sĭs) [Gr. *sidēros*, iron, + *-ōsis*, condition]. A form of pneumoconiosis resulting from inhalation of dust or fumes containing iron particles. It is benign and constitutes no serious health hazard. SYN: *arc-welder's disease*.

Sigault's operation (sē-go′). [Jean René Sigault, Fr. obstetrician, 1740 —] Division of the symphysis pubis to aid obstetrician. SYN: *symphyseotomy*.

sigh [AS. *sican*]. A deep inspiration followed by a slow audible expiration. SYN: *suspirium*.

sight (sīt) [AS. *sihth*]. 1. Power or faculty of seeing. 2. Range of sight. 3. A thing or view seen. SYN: *vision*.

   s., day. Night blindness. SYN: *nyctalopia*.

   s., far-. Rays of light focusing behind the retina. SYN: *hypermetropia; hyperopia*.

   s. meter. Device for measuring intensity of light in foot candles.

   s., near-. Rays of light focusing before the retina. SYN: *myopia*.

   s., night. Day blindness. SYN: *hemeralopia*.

   s., old. Loss of accommodation of near point. SYN: *presbyopia*.

   s., second. Alteration in refractive powers of the lens of the eye so that reading is again possible without glasses. May be caused by incipient cataract.

sight, words pert. to: achromatopsia; afterimage; alexia; amaurosis; amblyopia; ametropia; aniseikonia; anisocoria; anisoiconia; anisometropia; anorthopia; aprosexia; asthenopia; astigmatism; blindness; brachymetropia; hemeralopia; hypermetropia; hyperopia; myopia; nyctalopia; photophobia; presbyopia; squint.

sigmatism (sĭg'mă-tĭzm) [Gr. *sigma,* letter S, + *-ismos,* condition]. Excessive or defective use of "s" sounds in speech.

sigmoid (sĭg'moyd) [Gr. *sigmoeides*]. 1. Shaped like the Greek letter sigma. 2. Pert. to the sigmoid flexure of the colon.

s. flexure. The lower part of descending colon, between iliac crest and the rectum, shaped like the letter S.
RS: cecosigmoidostomy; colon.

sigmoidectomy (sĭg''moyd-ĕk'tō-mĭ) [" + *ektomē,* excision]. Removal of all or part of the sigmoid flexure.

sigmoiditis (sĭg''moid-ī'tĭs) [" + *-itis,* inflammation]. Inflammation of the sigmoid flexure of the colon.

sigmoidopexy (sĭg-moy'dō-pĕk''sĭ) [" + *pēxis,* fixation]. Fixation of the sigmoid to an abdominal incision for prolapse of the rectum.

sigmoidoproctostomy (sĭg-moy''dō-prok-tos'tō-mĭ) [Gr. *sigmoeidēs,* + *prōktos,* rectum, + *stoma,* passage]. Establishment of artificial passage by anastomosis of the sigmoid flexure with the rectum.

sigmoidorectostomy (sĭg-moy''dō-rĕk-tōs'tō-mĭ) [" + L. *rectus,* straight, + Gr. *stoma,* passage]. Anastomosis of sigmoid flexure with the rectum to establish an artificial passage. SYN: *sigmoidoproctostomy.*

sigmoidoscope (sĭg-moy'dō-skōp) [" + *skopein,* to examine]. Tubular speculum for examination of sigmoid flexure.

sigmoidostomy (sĭg-moyd-ŏs'tō-mĭ) [Gr. *sigmoeidēs,* + *stoma,* passage]. Creation of an artificial anus in the sigmoid flexure.

sigmoidotomy (sĭg-moyd-ŏt'ō-mĭ) [" + *tome,* incision]. Surgical incision of the sigmoid.

sign (sīn) [L. *signum*]. 1. Symbol or abbreviation, esp. one used in pharmacy. 2. Any objective evidence or manifestation of an illness or disordered function of the body. They are more or less definitive and obvious, and apart from the patient's impressions, in contrast to symptoms which are subjective. SEE: *symptom.*

s., objective. One recognized by an observer. SYN: *physical s.*

s., physical. One revealed by auscultation, percussion, inspection, etc.

signa (sĭg'nă) [L. *signa*]. A term used in writing prescriptions, q.v., meaning mark. ABBR: S or sig.

signature (sĭg'nă-tūr) [L. *signatura*]. The part of a prescription, q.v., giving instructions to the patient.

silastic. A silicone material which because of its inertness and compatibility with biologi-

cal tissues is used in plastic surgery to help form body structures.

silent. Free from noise; mute; still.

s. disease. A disease which produces no clinically obvious symptoms or signs.

s. period. Period in a tendon reflex that immediately follows the contraction of the responding muscles during which the motor neurons do not respond to afferent impulses entering the reflex center.

silica (sĭl'ĭ-kă) [L. *silex,* flint]. Silicon dioxide, SiO_2.

silicate (sĭl'ĭ-kāt) [L. *silicus,* flintlike]. A salt of silicic acid.

silicic (sĭl-ĭs'ĭk). Pert. to silica or silicon.

s. acid. One of a number of colloid acids.

silicon (sĭl'ĭ-kon) [L. *silex,* flint]. SYMB: *Si.* At. wt. 28.086; at. no. 14; sp. gr. 2.33. A nonmetallic element found in the soil. Silicon comprises approximately 25% of the earth's crust being exceeded only by oxygen. It occurs in traces in skeletal structures (bones and teeth). silicon is commonly combined with oxygen to form silicon dioxide, SiO_2, which occurs in many forms, both crystalline and amorphous. In a pure state it forms quartz or rock crystal. It is present in many abrasive materials and is the principal constituent of glass.

silicone (sĭl'ĭ-kōn) Any of a group of polymeric organic silicon compounds. Used in adhesives, lubricants, synthetic rubber, and prostheses.

s., injectable. Medical grade silicone compounds suitable for implantation in the body. Used in plastic surgery. Use of nonmedical grade silicone for cosmetic breast augmentation has produced unfortunate results.

silicosis (sĭl-ĭ-kō'sĭs) [L. *silex,* flint, + Gr. *-ōsis,* condition]. A form of pneumoconiosis resulting from inhalation of silica (quartz) dust, characterized by formation of small discrete nodules. In advanced cases, a dense fibrosis and emphysema with impairment of respiratory function may develop.

silicotic (sĭl-ĭ-kŏt'ĭk). 1. Relating to silicosis. 2. One affected with silicosis.

silicotuberculosis (sĭl''ĭ-kō-tū-bĕr-kū-lō'sĭs) [L. *silex,* flint, + *tuberculus,* a tubercle, + Gr. *-ōsis,* condition]. Silicosis associated with pulmonary tuberculosis.

siliquose (sĭl'ĭ-kwōs) [L.*siliqua,* pod]. Resembling a two-valve capsule.

s. cataract. Cataract with a dry, wrinkled capsule.

s. desquamation. Shedding of dried vesicles from the skin.

silver (sĭl'ver) [AS. *siolfor*]. SYMB: *Ag.* At. wt. 107.870; at. no. 47; sp. gr. 10.5. A white soft ductile malleable metal, its salts being widely used in medicine for their caustic, astringent, and antiseptic effects.

s. arsphenamine. A brownish-black arsphenamine derivative, containing 19% arsenic and 14% silver.

USES: Same as those of arsphenamine.

s. nitrate. USP. AgNO₃. A toxic preparation made from silver. Most of its former uses have passed out of vogue, but it remains important as a germicide and local astringent.

INCOMPATIBILITIES: Aspirin, sodium chloride.

POISONING: When taken by mouth, causes a grayish discoloration of mucus membranes.

SYM: Burning in throat and stomach; rather prompt vomiting. When small amounts of silver are taken over a long period, as in nose or eye drops, patient develops argyria, a peculiar bluish discoloration of all the exposed tissues of body.

F. A. TREATMENT: Large volumes of ordinary table salt in water precipitate the silver as a slightly soluble chloride; follow with egg whites, oils, and other demulcents.

s. picrate. A compound of silver and picric acid, containing 30% silver. Useful as an antiseptic, similar to other preparations of silver.

s. protein. A combination of silver and protein, containing from 7 to 19% silver.

sil'ver-fork deformity or fracture. Deformity in Colles' fracture of wrist and hand resembling curve on back of a fork.

Silves'ter's method. [Henry Robert Silvester, Eng. physician, 1829-1908] A method of artificial respiration in which the patient lies on his back, his arms are raised to sides of his head, held there temporarily, then brought down and pressed against his chest. Movement repeated 16 times per minute. This method is no longer the preferred or effective method of producing artificial respiration. SEE: *artificial respiration; resuscitation.*

simesthesia (sĭm-ĕs-thē'zĭ-ä) [Gr. *aisthēsis,*

sensation]. Sensibility felt in a bone.

simian crease. A crease on palm of hand, so termed because of its similarity to the transverse flexion crease found in some monkeys.

Normally the palm of the hand at birth contains several flexion creases, two of which are separate and approx. transverse. When these two appear to fuse and thus form a single transverse crease, it is termed simian crease. The crease may be present in a variety of developmental abnormalities including Down's syndrome, rubella syndrome, and Turner's syndrome; and in Klinefelter's syndrome, q.v., pseudohypoparathyroidism, q.v., and gonadal dysgenesis, q.v. SYN: *simian line.*

similia similibus curantur (sĭ-mĭl'ĭ-ä sĭ-mĭl'ĭ-bŭs kū-rahn'tŭr) [L., likes are cured by likes]. The homeopathic doctrine that a drug producing pathological symptoms in those who are well will cure such symptoms in disease states.

Simmonds' disease or syndrome (sĭm'-monds). [Morris Simmonds, Hamburg physician, 1855-1925] Condition in which complete atrophy of the pituitary body causes premature senility and psychic symptoms. SYN: *cachexia, pituitary,* q.v.

Simon's position (zē'mŏn). [Gustav Simon, Ger. surgeon, 1824-1876] An exaggerated lithotomy position in which the hips are somewhat elevated with thighs strongly abducted. Employed in operations on the vagina. SYN: *Odebohls' position.*

simple (sĭm'pl) [L. *simplex*]. 1. Not complex; not compound. 2. Deficient in intellect. 3. A medicinal plant.

s. fracture. Fracture without rupture of ligaments and skin.

s. inflammation. Inflammation without pus or other inflammatory exudates.

s. reflex. A reflex in which only two or possibly three neurons are interposed between receptor and effector organs.

Sims' position (sĭmz). [J. Marion Sims, Am. gynecologist, 1813-1883] A semiprone position. Patient on left side, right knee and thigh drawn well up, left arm along back of

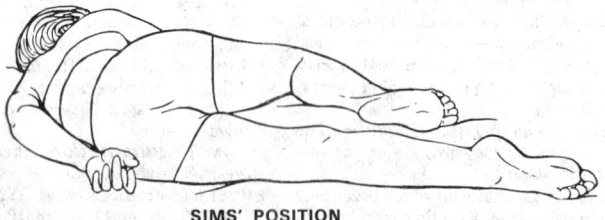

SIMS' POSITION

patient, chest inclined forward so patient rests upon it. Employed in curettement of uterus, intrauterine irrigation after labor, tamponade of vagina, rectal exploration, and operations on cervix.

simul (sī'mŭl) [L.]. At once or at the same time; term used in signature of prescription.

simulation (sĭm-ū-lā'shŭn) [L. *simulātio,* imitation]. Pretense of having a disease; feigning of illness. Imitation of symptoms of one disease by another. SEE: *malingerer.*

Simulium. A genus of insects of the order Diptera which includes the black flies (buffalo gnats) which are important annoyers of domestic animals and man. The females are vicious blood suckers.

    S. damnosum. Species which serves as intermediate host of a filarial worm Onchocerca volvulus.

    S. venustum. A very annoying species common in North America.

Sinapis (sī-na'pĭs) [Gr. *sinapi,* mustard]. A genus of plants, the mustard plant.

sinapiscopy (sĭn-ă-pĭs'kō-pī) ["+ *skopein,* to examine]. Use of mustard in testing for sensory disturbance.

sinapism (sĭn'ă-pĭzm) ["+ *-ismos,* process]. A mustard plaster. Used to produce counter irritation.

    PROPORTIONS: Enough water is added to flour to make a paste. *Adult:* 3-4 parts wheat flour to 1 of mustard flour. *Child:* 8-10 parts wheat flour to 1 of mustard flour. *Infant:* 10-12 parts wheat flour to 1 of mustard flour.

sinapized (sĭn'ă-pīzd) [Gr. *sinapi,* mustard]. Containing mustard.

sincipital (sĭn-sĭp'ĭ-tăl) [L. *sinciput,* half a head]. Concerning the sinciput.

sinciput (sĭn'sĭp-ŭt) [L. *sinciput,* half a head]. [NA]. 1. Fore and upper part of the cranium. 2. Upper half of the skull. SYN: *calvaria.*

sinew (sĭn'ū) [AS. *sinu*]. A tendon.

sing. Abbr. of L. *singulorum,* of each.

singer's node or nodule (sĭn'gerz nōd, nōd'ūl). A swelling between the arytenoid cartilages of singers. SYN: *chorditis nodosa.*

singultus (sĭng-gŭl'tŭs) [L.]. Hiccup, q.v.

sinistrad (sĭn'ĭs-trăd) [L. *sinister,* left, + *ad,* toward]. Toward the left.

sinistral (sĭn'ĭs-trăl) [L.]. 1. Pert. to or showing preference for the left hand, eye, or foot in certain actions. 2. On the left side.

sinistrality (sĭn'ĭs-trăl'ĭ-tī). Left-handedness.

sinistraural (sĭn-ĭs-traw'răl) [L. *sinister,* left, + *auris,* ear]. Having better hearing with the left ear.

sinistro- (sĭn'ĭs-trō) [L.]. Combining form meaning *left.*

sinistrocardia (sĭn-ĭs-trō-kar'dĭ-ă) [L. *sinister,* left, + Gr. *kardia,* heart.]. Displacement of the heart to left of the medial line; opposed to dextrocardia.

sinistrocerebral (sĭn-ĭs-trō-sĕr'ĕ-brăl) ["+ *cerebrum,* brain]. Located in the left cerebral hemisphere.

sinistrocular (sĭn-ĭs-trok'ū-lar) ["+ *oculus,* eye]. Having stronger vision in the left eye.

sinistrocularity (sĭn-ĭs-trŏk-ū-lăr'ĭ-tī). Condition of having better vision in the left eye.

sinistrogyration (sĭn-ĭs-trō-jī-rā'shŭn) [L. *sinister,* left, + Gr. *gyros,* a circle]. Inclination to the left.

sinistromanual (sĭn-ĭs-trō-măn'ū-ăl) ["+ *manus,* hand]. Left-handed.

sinistropedal (sĭn-ĭs-trŏp'ĕd-ăl) ["+ *pes, ped-,* foot]. Left-footed.

sinistrosis (sĭn-ĭs-trō'sĭs) [L. *sinister,* left, unlucky, + Gr. *-ōsis,* condition]. Shell shock, q.v.

sinistrotorsion (sĭn-ĭs-trō-tor'shŭn) ["+ *torsio,* a turning]. A twisting or turning toward the left.

sin'istrous. Awkward, clumsy, unskilled, the opposite to dextrous.

sinoatrial (sin"ō-ā'trĭ-ăl). Pertaining to the sinus venosus and the atrium. SYN: *sinoauricular.*

    s. node. Node at junction of superior vena cava with right cardiac atrium, regarded as starting point of the heartbeat. SYN: *S-A node.*

sinoauricular. Sinoatrial, q.v.

sinogram. X-ray study of a sinus injected with a radiopaque dye to determine the range and course of the sinus.

sinuitis (sī-nū-ī'tĭs) [L. *sinus,* a curve, + Gr. *-ītis,* inflammation]. Inflammation of a sinus. SYN: *sinusitis.*

sinuotomy (sĭn-ū-ŏt'ō-mī) ["+ Gr. *tomē,* a cutting]. Surgical incision into a sinus. SYN: *sinusotomy.*

sinuous (sĭn'ū-ŭs) [L. *sinuōsus,* winding]. Winding; wavy; tortuous.

sinus (sī'nŭs) [L. *sinus,* a curve, hollow]. (pl. *sinuses, sinus*) 1. A canal or passage leading to an abscess. 2. A cavity within a bone. 3. Dilated channel for venous blood. 4. Any cavity having a relatively narrow opening.

    RS: antritis; antronasal; antrotympanic; antrum; cephalhematocele; lateral sinus; sinusitis; transillumination.

    s.'s, accessory nasal. The paranasal sinuses; frontal, maxillary, ethmoidal, and sphenoidal. Anterior group: Frontal, maxillary and anterior ethmoids. Posterior group: Posterior ethmoids and sphenoid.

    Sinuses develop embryologically from nasal cavities, are lined with same type of epithelium, are filled with air, and communicate with nasal cavities through their various ostia. Function of sinuses not definitely known. Various theories give them the same function as nasal cavities, namely, warming, moistening and filtering the air.

s., aortic. Saclike dilatation of the aorta.

s. arrhythmia. Irregularity of heartbeat due to interference with impulses from the sinoatrial node.

s., basilar. S., transverse, q.v.

s., cavernous. A large s. from sphenoidal fissure to apex of petrous portion of temporal bone.

s., circular. A venous s. around the pituitary body, communicating on each side with the cavernous s.

s., coronary, of the heart. A vein in transverse groove between left cardiac auricle and ventricle.

s.'s, cranial. Venous canals between folds of the dura.

s.'s, ethmoidal. Air cavities in the ethmoid bone.

s., frontal. An irregular cavity in frontal bone on each side of midline above the nasal bridge. One may be larger than the other. A duct carries secretions to upper part of nostrils.

s., genitourinary. S., urogenital, q.v.

s., inferior longitudinal. A venous s. along posterior half of lower border of the falx cerebri.

s., inferior petrosal. A large venous s. from cavernous s., running along lower margin of the petrous portion of the temporal bone.

s.'s, intercavernous. The anterior and posterior halves of the circular s.

s., lateral. One of two large venous s.'s in inner side of skull passing near the mastoid antrum, emtying into the jugular vein.

s.'s, lymph. Small spaces throughout the parenchyma of a lymphatic gland.

s., maxillary. A cavity in the maxillary bone opening at upper part of antrum into the nose. SYN: *antrum of Highmore.*

s., occipital. A small venous s. in attached margin of the falx cerebelli extending to margin of the foramen magnum.

s.'s, paranasal. Accessory nasal sinuses. SEE: *paranasal sinuses.*

s.'s, pleural. Spaces in pleural sac along the lower and inferior portions of lung which the lung does not occupy.

s. pocularis. Lacuna in prostatic part of the urethra.

s. prostaticus. S. pocularis, q.v.

s., rhomboid. The fourth cranial ventricle.

s. rhythm. Normal cardiac rhythm commencing at the sinoatrial node.

s.'s, sphenoidal. Air s.'s which occupy the body of sphenoid bone and connect with nasal cavity.

s., sphenoparietal. 1. A venous sinus uniting the cavernous sinus and a meningeal vein. 2. The portion of the cavernous sinus below the ensiform process.

s., straight. One which is continuous with the inferior longitudinal s. and running along the junction of the falx cerebri and tentorium.

s., superior longitudinal. A triangular one along upper edge of the falx cerebri.

s., superior petrosal. A venous canal running in a groove in the petrous portion of the temporal bone.

s., terminal. A vein encircling the vascular area of the blastoderm.

s., transverse. 1. S. that unites the two inferior petrosal sinuses. 2. Venous network in the dura over basilar process of occipital bone.

s., urinogenital or urogenital. 1. Duct into which, in the embryo, the wolffian ducts and bladder empty and which opens into the cloaca. 2. The common receptacle of genital and urinary ducts.

s.'s, uteroplacental. Slanting venous channels from the placenta serving to convey the maternal blood from the intervillous lacunae back into the uterine veins.

s. of Valsalva. A dilatation of the aorta or pulmonary artery opposite the segment of the semilunar valve. SYN: *aortic s.*

s., venous. One conveying venous blood.

s.'s, vertebral. Veins within the vertebrae.

sinusitis (sĭ-nus-ĭ'tĭs) [L. *sinus,* a curve, a hollow, + Gr. *-itis,* inflammation]. Inflammation of a sinus, esp. a paranasal sinus.

ETIOL: A number of causative agents including viruses, bacteria, or allergy.

PREDISPOSING FACTORS: Inadequate drainage which may result from presence of polyps, enlarged turbinates, deviated septum, etc.; chronic rhinitis, general debility, or dental abscess in maxillary bone.

s., acute catarrhal. Inflammation accompanying a similar process in the nose.

s., acute suppurative. Purulent inflammation with symptoms of pain over the sinus, fever, chills, headache, etc.

TREATMENT: Conservative, shrinkage in the nasal mucosa to facilitate ventilation, and drainage of the sinus. Rest in bed, force fluids, anodynes for pain.

s., chronic hyperplastic. Polyps present in sinuses and nose and underlying osteitis of sinus walls.

TREATMENT: *Surgical:* Conservative, removal of polyps and intranasal opening into sinuses for adequate ventilation and drainage. *Radical:* Complete removal of sinus mucosa either through external or intranasal route.

s., chronic hypertrophic. Inflammation found in conjunction with chronic hypertrophic rhinitis. Living in a climate where the temperature fluctuations are not extreme may be beneficial.

sinusoid (sī'nŭs-oyd) [L. *sinus,* a hollow, a curve, + Gr. *eidos,* like]. 1. Resembling a sinus. 2. A minute blood vessel found in such organs as the liver, spleen, adrenal glands, and bone marrow. It is slightly larger than a capillary and has a lining of reticuloendothelium.

sinusoidal (sī-nŭs-oyd'ăl). Pert. to a sinusoid.

s. current. Alternating induced electric current, the two strokes of which are equal.

sinusoidalization (sī''nŭ-soy''dăl-ī-zā'shŭn) [L. *sinus,* a hollow, a curve, + Gr. *eidos,* like]. Use of a sinusoidal current.

sinusotomy (sī-nū-sŏt'ō-mĭ) ["+ Gr. *tomē,* a cutting]. The operation of incising a sinus.

SiO₂. Silicon dioxide.

siphon (sī'fŏn) [Gr. *siphōn,* tube]. A tube bent at an angle to form two unequal lengths for removing liquids by atmospheric pressure.

Siphonaptera (sī''fō-năp'ter-ă) ["+ *apteros,* wingless]. An order of insects commonly called fleas. They are wingless, undergo complete metamorphosis, and have piercing and sucking mouth parts, their food being the blood of birds and mammals. The body is compressed laterally and their legs are adapted for leaping. In addition to being annoying pests, they transmit the causative organisms of several diseases (bubonic plague, endemic or murine typhus, and among rodents, tularemia). They also serve as intermediate hosts of certain tapeworms. SEE: *flea.*

siphonoma (sī-fon-ō'mă) ["+ *-ōma,* tumor]. A tumor made up of fine tubes.

Sippy diet (sĭp'ē). [Bertram W. Sippy, American physician, 1866-1924] Treatment of gastric ulcer by diet, checking acidity of gastric juice. Small amounts of milk and cream every hour and alkaline powders every half hour.

Average mixture: 1 1/2 oz. (44.36 ml.) each of cream and milk given once each hour for a total of 13 feedings during the day. For the next 3 to 4 days continue these feedings but substitute an egg and fine cereal for one feeding in the morning and one at night. The next day, 3 oz. (85.05 gm.) soft cereal added to afternoon feeding; another egg the next day; and finally 3 servings of cereal and 3 eggs per day added to the milk and cream. Purée, custards, and toast added the next week. Decreased feedings as amount of each feeding is increased until 6 feedings are given per day. Each feeding replaces the scheduled milk and cream.

This schedule is monotonous, deficient in vitamins, and provides no feeding at night. It is usually modified to compensate for these deficiencies.

siriasis (sī-rī'ă-sĭs) [Gr. *seirian,* to be hot]. Sunstroke, q.v.

sismotherapy (sĭs''mō-ther'ă-pĭ) [Gr. *seismos,* a shake, + *therapeia,* treatment]. Therapeutic employment of vibration. SYN: *seismotherapy; vibrotherapeutics.*

sister. A term used by the British for nurse, esp. a senior or head nurse.

site. Position or location.

sitieirgia (sĭt-ĭ-ĭr'jĭ-ă) [Gr. *sition,* food, + *eirgein,* to bar out]. Hysterical refusal to take food.

sitio-, sito- [Gr.]. Combining forms meaning bread or made from grain; food, as sitomania.

sitiology (sĭt-ĭ-ŏl'ō-jĭ) [Gr. *sition,* food, + *logos,* a study]. Science of nutrition. SYN: *sitology.*

sitiomania (sĭt-ĭ-ō-mā'nĭ-ă) ["+ *mania,* madness]. Periodic abnormal appetite or craving for food. SYN: *sitomania.*

sitology (sī-tŏl'ō-jĭ) [Gr. *sitos,* food, + *logos,* a study]. Science of nutrition and food. SYN: *sitiology.*

sitomania (sī''tō-mā'nĭ-ă) ["+ *mania,* madness]. 1. Periodic abnormal craving for food. 2. Periodic abnormality of appetite. SYN: *sitiomania.*

sitophobia (sī''tō-fō'bĭ-ă) ["+ *phobos,* fear]. Psychoneurotic abhorrence of food, or morbid dread of, or repugnance to food, whether generally or only to specific dishes.

sitotherapy (sī''tō-ther'ă-pĭ) ["+ *therapeia,* treatment]. The therapeutic use of food.

sitotoxism (sī''tō-tŏks'ĭzm) [Gr. *sitos,* food, + *toxikon,* poison, + *ismos,* condition]. Poisoning by vegetable foods infested with molds or bacteria.

sitotropism (sī-tŏt'rō-pĭzm) ["+ *tropos,* a turning, + *-ismos,* condition]. Response of cells to the attraction or repulsion of food elements.

situs (sī'tŭs) [L.]. A position.

s. inversus viscerum. Abnormal displacement of viscera to opposite side of the body.

s. perversus. Malposition of any visceral structure.

sitz bath (sĭtz bath). Bath to sit in with water above and covering the hips. The tub or fixture is usually shaped to allow the legs to be out of the water. SYN: *hip bath.* SEE: *bath, sitz.*

sixth cranial nerve. Abducens nerve which supplies the external rectus of the eye. SEE: *cranial nerves.*

skatol(e (skăt'ōl) [Gr. *skōr, skat-,* dung]. Betamethyl indole, C_9H_9N, a malodorous, solid, heterocyclic nitrogen compound found in feces, formed by protein decomposition in the intestines and giving them their odor.

skelalgia (skĕ-lăl'jĭ-ă) [Gr. *skelis,* leg, + *algos,* pain]. Pain in the leg.

skeletal (skĕl'ĕ-tăl) [Gr. *skeleton*]. Pert. to the skeleton.

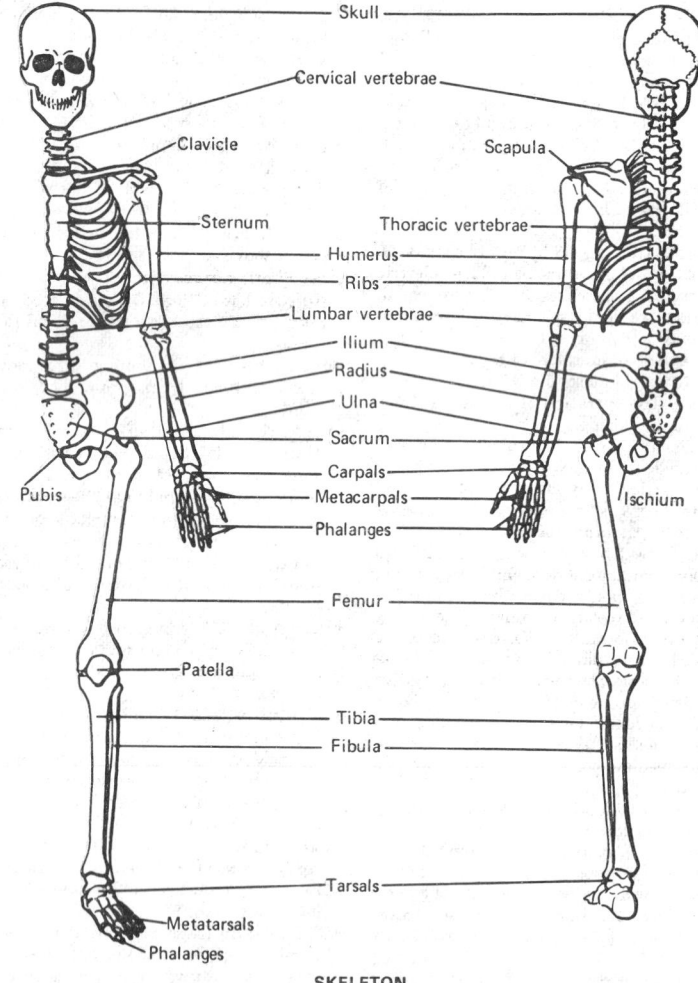

Skull — Cervical vertebrae — Clavicle — Scapula — Sternum — Thoracic vertebrae — Humerus — Ribs — Lumbar vertebrae — Ilium — Radius — Ulna — Sacrum — Carpals — Pubis — Metacarpals — Ischium — Phalanges — Femur — Patella — Tibia — Fibula — Tarsals — Metatarsals — Phalanges

SKELETON

LEFT ANTERIOR   **LEFT POSTERIOR**

s. muscle. Muscle fibers which with few exceptions are attached to parts of the skeleton and involved primarily in movements of the parts of the body. SYN: *striated muscle; voluntary muscle.*

s. traction. Traction exerted directly on long bones.

skeletization (skĕl-ĕt-ĭ-zā'shŭn). 1. Excessive emaciation. 2. Removal of soft parts of the body leaving only the skeleton.

skeleto- (Gr.). Combining form meaning skeleton.

skeletogenous (skĕl-ĕ-tŏj'ĕ-nŭs) [Gr. *skeleton*, skeleton, + *gennan*, to produce]. Forming skeletal structures or tissues.

skeleton (skĕl'ĕt-ŏn) [Gr. *skeletos*, dried up]. The bony framework of the body, consisting of 206 bones —80 axial or trunk and 126 of the limbs. This number does not include teeth. The various bones follow.

AXIAL (80 Bones)
  Head (29 Bones)
    Cerebral cranials (8)
      frontal—1
      parietal—2
      occipital—1
      temporal—2
      sphenoid—1
      ethmoid—1
    Visceral cranials (facial) (14)
      maxilla—2
      mandible—1
      zygoma—2
      lacrimal—2
      nasal—2
      turbinate—2
      vomer—1
      palate—2
    Hyoid (1)
    Auditory ossicles (6)
      malleus—2
      incus—2
      stapes—2
  Trunk (51 Bones)
    Vertebrae (26)
      cervical—7
      dorsal—12
      lumbar—5
      sacrum—1
      coccyx—1
    Ribs (24)
      true rib—14
      false rib—6
      floating rib—4
    Sternum (1)

LIMBS (126 Bones)
  Upper extremities (64 Bones)
    Arms and Shoulders (10)
      clavicle—2

      shoulder blade—2
      humerus—2
      radius—2
      ulna—2
    Wrist (16)
      scaphoid—2
      semilunar—2
      cuneiform—2
      pisiform—2
      trapezium—2
      trapezoid—2
      capitate—2
      hamate—2
    Hands (38)
      metacarpal—10
      phalanx (finger bones)—28
  Lower extremities (62 Bones)
    Legs and Hips (10)
      hip bone—2
      femur—2
      tibīa—2
      fibula—2
      patella (knee cap)—2
    Ankles (14)
      astragaloid—2
      heel bone—2
      scaphoid—2
      cuboid—2
      cuneiform, internal—2
      cuneiform, middle—2
      cuneiform, external—2
    Feet (38)
      metatarsal—10
      phalanx (toe bones)—28

s., axial. Bones of the head and trunk.

s., cartilaginous. Structure from which the bones have been formed through ossification.

Skene's glands (skēn). [Alexander J. C. Skene, American gynecologist, 1838-1900] Glands lying just inside of and on the posterior of the urethra in the female. If the margins of the urethra are drawn apart and the mucus membrane gently everted, the two small openings of Skene's tubules or glands, one on each side of the floor of the urethra, become visible. Trauma frequently causes a gaping of the urethra and ectropion of the mucus membrane. In acute gonorrhea these glands are almost always infected. SYN: *paraurethral glands.*

skenitis (skē-nī'tĭs) [Gr. *-itis*, inflammation]. Inflamed condition of Skene's glands.

skeocytosis (skē-ō-sī-tō'sĭs) [Gr. *skaios*, left, + *kytos*, cell, + *-ōsis*, condition]. Immature white corpuscles in the peripheral blood; also called deviation to the left.

skew (skyōō) [ME. *skewen*, to escape]. Turned to one side; asymmetrical.

s. deviation. Condition in which one eyeball is directed upward and outward, the other inward and downward.

skiagram (skī'ă-grăm) [Gr. *skia*, shadow, + *gramma*, a mark]. An x-ray picture. SEE: *roentgenogram.*

skiagraph (skī'ă-grăf) ["+ *graphein*, to write]. An x-ray picture. SYN: *roentgenograph.*

skiagraphy (skī-ăg'ră-fī). Process of taking pictures with roentgen rays. SYN: *radiography, roentgenography.*

skiameter (skī-ăm'ĕt-ĕr) [Gr. *skia*, shadow, + *metron*, a measure]. Device for determining differences in density and penetration of X rays.

skiascope (skī'ă-skōp) ["+ *skopein*, to examine]. 1. Device for examination by the fluoroscope. 2. Examination of the eye employing movement of shadow and light.

skiascopy (skī-ăs'kō-pī). 1. Retinoscopy or shadow test used in determining the refractive error of an eye. 2. Fluoroscopic inspection of the body.

skin (skĭn) [Old Norse *skinn*]. The integument or external covering of the body.

The skin consists essentially of two layers, the epidermis and the corium. The epidermis (cuticle, scarf skin) is composed of four main layers of stratified epithelium. The outermost, the stratum corneum, is formed of several layers of flattened cells which have become horny and lost their nuclei and which contain keratin. They form a protective covering for the body surfaces. Underneath this layer is the stratum lucidum, which is formed of translucent flattened cells. The 3rd layer, the stratum granulosum, consists of two or three layers of flattened cells containing granules of eleidin, the precursor of keratin. The 4th and last layer is the stratum germinativum (stratum mucosum, stratum Malpighi). The cells in upper portion of this layer are cuboidal; those nearest the corium are columnar. Cells of this layer possess well-defined intercellular bridges which appear as spines projecting from the surface; hence these cells are often called prickle cells and the entire layer, stratum spinosum. These cells contain peculiar fibrils, tonofibrils, which pass through the intercellular bridges. The color of the skin is due principally to the presence of a pigment, melanin, present as granules in stratum germinatum.

The corium (cutis, dermis, derma, true skin) is formed of connective tissue containing lymphatics, nerves and nerve endings, blood vessels, sebaceous and sweat glands, and elastic fibers. It is divided into two layers, a superficial papillary layer and a deep reticular layer. The papillary layer contains conical protuberances, the papillae, which fit into corresponding depressions in the epidermis. Within each papilla is a capillary loop which furnishes the epidermis with a blood supply. The reticular layer is made up in the main of white fibrous tissue supporting the blood vessels and other structures in it. It rests on the subcutaneous connective tissue.

Appendages of the skin are the hair, q.v., and nails, q.v.

FUNCTION: Protection against injuries and parasitic invasion; regulation of body temperature; aids in elimination; prevention of dehydration; reservoir for food and water; sense organ for the cutaneous senses; source of antirachitic vitamin (vitamin D).

DIAGNOSIS: *Abnormal dryness:* May indicate abnormal deficiency of thyroid function, diabetes and other causes. *Ashy:* Malignant diseases, severe anemia, cancer, scrofula, chronic interstitial nephritis. *Bronzing:* Addison's disease, dyes or metals, early stages of pellagra.

Brownish-yellow Spots (liver spots): Noted in pregnancy (chloasma uterinum), in exophthalmic goiter, and uterine and liver malignancies; also freckles, sunburn, cosmetics, mustard, turpentine, and other irritants.

Cherry Red: Carbon monoxide poisoning. *Cold Sweats:* Indicate great prostration, fear or depression of spirits.

Cyanosis: May be congenital; if acquired may be due to asthma, pulmonary tuberculosis, whooping cough, advanced emphysema, croup, tracheal obstruction, aneurysm, goiter, flushing (hyperemia), emotion, febrile disorders, pulmonary tuberculosis, convulsions, large ovarian tumor, plethora, polycythemia. *Cyanosis Alternating with Pallor:* Cerebrospinal diseases, typhoid, vasomotor disturbances, menopause, Gray's argyria, silver salts. May be noted in lips, mucus membranes, fingertips and external ear. If extreme, entire body shows dusky, leaden tint. Indicates lack of oxygen and excess of carbon dioxide in blood. May be due to inflammation of pharynx and larynx, abscess of same, angina Ludovici, croup and disorders affecting respiration. Also to overdose of drugs and asphyxiation by gas.

Discolorations: Seen in icterus, chlorosis, leprosy, administration of silver nitrate, malignant diseases, and asphyxia from gas. *Edema:* Seen in anemia, hydremia, obstruction, inflammation, cardiac, circulatory and renal decompensation. If local, may be due to obstruction of return circulation or heart failure, in which case it will be evident in ankles and often legs, esp. at night. May also be due to renal diseases. *Emphysema:* Due to air or gas in cellular tissue. *Hot and Dry:* Indicates fever, mental excitement, or excessive use of salted provisions. *Moist:* Increased perspiration (hyperhidrosis) may be due to malarial fever; rheumatic, relapsing and septic fever; pneumonic crisis; pulmonary tuberculosis; Graves' disease; neuralgia; migraine; drugs; hot drinks; exercise. Lack of noted in ichthyosis.

Paleness: Nervous prostration, dropsy, paralysis, malnutrition. *Pallor:* Occurs in those living an indoor life, esp. in prisoners and night workers. May be due to lowered circulation, decrease of red blood corpuscles, nonfilling capillaries. Occurs in all anemias. Temporary pallor occurs in syncope, chills, shock, rigors and some vasomotor spasms. If sudden and persistent may be sign of internal hemorrhage. Also seen in lead poisoning and toxic febrile affections. If it gradually becomes permanent may indicate chronic febrile disease, chronic gastrointestinal dis-

ease, cancer, arsenical poisoning, chronic suppuration, chronic mercurial poisoning, hemorrhages, leukemia, cachexia, nephrosis, nephritis, syphilis, parasitic diseases, tuberculosis, malaria. *Purplish:* Interference of circulation common in asthma and typhus.

Rashes: SEE: rash. *Temperature:* Usually correlates with internal temperature, unless raised by local applications of heat or exposure to cold. If generally cold, may be due to poor circulation or obstruction of same, vasomotor spasms, venous or arterial thrombosis, exposure to cold. General abnormal heat seen in febrile disorders, although in some of them a cold and clammy skin is present. *Redness:* Local redness seen in inflammation, skin diseases, chronic alcoholism, vasomotor disturbances, and pyrexia. Local redness with pain indicates inflammation. Sunburn (actinic dermatitis). *Sallowness:* Cachexia, syphilis, chronic gallbladder disease, arthritis deformans, constipation, some anemias, gastric, pancreatic, enteric, or hepatic disorders.

Wrinkling: If permanent may be due to aging; temporary due to prolonged immersion in water or dehydration.

Yellow: Jaundice, liver derangements. If jaundiced, plethoric, hyperemic, or pigmented, it should be noted in any examination. Rashes, scars, and their cause are also diagnostic. Texture and temperature of skin are important signs. Undue moisture, cold or hot spots on body, dryness of skin are other points to look for in diagnosis. SEE: *anemia, pernicious; biliousness; endocarditis, bacterial; face; liver.*

s., alligator. Severe scaling of the skin with formation of thick plates resembling hide of an alligator.

s. cancer. Cancer that may arise on surface of body as a small ulcer, pimple or mole. May be red, brown, black, or white, according to type. May be single or in a group, open or ulcerated. May be localized or invade blood vessels, lymph glands and connecting ducts.

s., deciduous. Shedding of the epidermis. SYN: *keratolysis.*

s., elastic. Skin which has property of great elasticity.

s., fish. SEE: *ichthyosis.*

s., glossy. Shining atrophy of the skin.

s. graft, cadaver. Use of skin obtained from a person shortly after death for grafting on a living patient.

s. grafting. Grafting of skin from another part of body to repair a defect or trauma. SEE: *Thiersch's graft.*

Duct of sweat gland

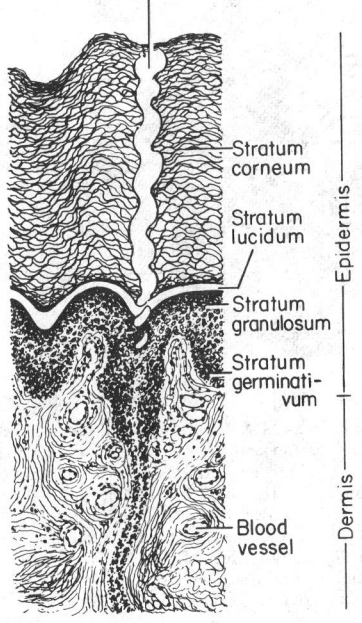

Stratum corneum

Stratum lucidum

Stratum granulosum

Stratum germinativum

Epidermis

Blood vessel

Dermis

LAYERS OF SKIN

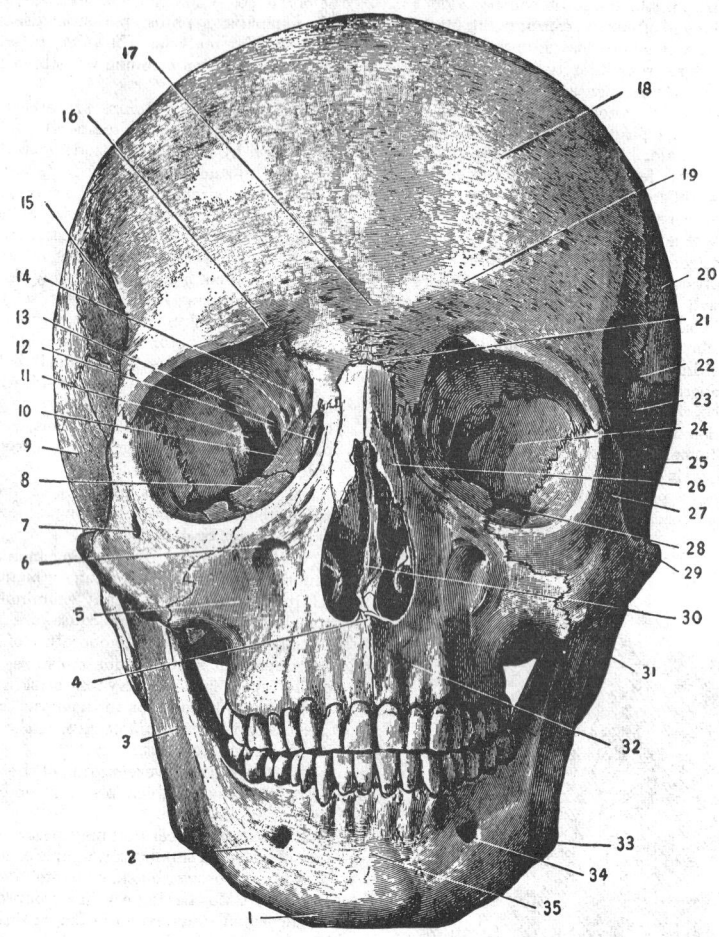

SKULL—FRONT VIEW

1, Mental tubercle. 2, Body of mandible. 3, Ramus of mandible. 4, Anterior nasal spine. 5, Canine fossa. 6, Infraorbital foramen. 7, Zygomaticofacial foramen. 8, Orbital surface of maxilla. 9, Squamous temporal. 10, Lateral surface of ethmoid. 11, Superior orbital fissure. 12, Lacrimal bone and groove. 13, Optic foramen. 14, Ethmoidal foramina. 15, Temporal line. 16, Supraorbital notch. 17, Glabella. 18, Frontal eminence. 19, Superciliary arch. 20, Parietal bone. 21, Nasofrontal suture. 22, Pterion. 23, Great wing of sphenoid. 24, Orbital surface of great wing. 25, Squamous part of temporal. 26, Left nasal bone. 27, Zygomatic bone. 28, Inferior orbital fissure. 29, Zygomatic arch. 30, Apertura piriformis. 31, Mastoid process. 32, Incisive fossa. 33, Angle of mandible. 34, Mental foramen. 35, Symphysis menti.—Robinson (ed.): Cunningham's Textbook of Anatomy, ed. 6., Oxford University Press, New York City.

ONP: Position of patient indicated by location of graft. The appropriate areas of both donor and recipient are prepared in the usual manner for surgical procedure. Patient is draped with sterile sheets and towels so that both areas are exposed. A dressing is applied to area from which the skin is removed. The area receiving skin is covered with a paraffin-coated mesh.

s., hidebound. Scleroderma, q.v.

s., loose. Hypertrophy of the skin.

s., parchment. Atrophy of the skin with stretching.

s., piebald. SEE: vitiligo.

s. rashes. They may cover one small area or most of the body surface if they represent blood cell tumors. Sometimes the patches tend to bleed. They look more like chickenpox than skin cancers. They may not be of leukemic origin.

s., scarf, s., scurf. Cuticle, epidermis, the outer layer of the skin.

s., true. Corium or inner layer of the skin, q.v.

skinfold thickness. Measurement with calibrated calipers of thickness of a fold of skin at a selected body site. The sites usually are upper arm or triceps, subscapular region, and upper abdomen. The measurements are used in evaluating nutritional status.

skin-marking. Application of nontoxic paints or dyes to the skin to provide landmarks during plastic surgery or to permit accurate alignment of the wound edges at the time the skin is closed.

skleriasis (sklē-rī'ăs-ĭs) [Gr. sklēros, hard, "+ -iasis, condition]. Progressive hardening of the skin in patches. SYN: scleroderma.

sklero- [Gr.]. See words beginning with sclero-.

Skoda's rales (skō'dă). [Josef Skoda, Austrian physician, 1805-1881]. Bronchial rales heard through consolidated tissue of the lungs in pneumonia.

Skoda's resonance. Tympanic resonance above the line of fluid in pleuritic effusion, or above consolidation in pneumonia. SYN: Skoda's sign; S.'s tympany.

skull (skŭl) [ME. skulle, bowl]. The bony framework of the head, composed of 8 cranial bones, the 14 bones of the face, and the teeth. SYN: calvaria, cranium. SEE: skeleton.

s. cap. Upper round portion of skull covering the brain.

s., fractured. Fractures of the skull can be classified according to whether the fracture is in the vault or the base, but from the point of view of treatment a more useful classification is as follows:

Simple Uncomplicated Fractures: Not common.

Compound Fractures: If in vault of skull, the bone is depressed and driven inwards with possible damage to brain. Treatment is operative.

slave. A device which allows the body movements to be transferred to a machine either directly or by remote control. Ex: Apparatus for lifting, squeezing, and turning laboratory equipment containing radioactive materials. The remote "hands" are controlled by the operator from sufficient distance to prevent exposure to radiation. Artificial arms and legs equipped to respond to physical or electrical stimulation have been developed.

sleep (slēp) [AS. slǣep]. A condition characterized by more or less periodic loss of consciousness accompanied by reduced cortical and physical activities. It is easily differentiated from the lessened consciousness of stupor in that normal awareness can completely reassert itself when danger threatens and ordinarily continues until sleep can again be resumed.

Emotionalism and anxiety (e.g., fear) are the great enemies of sleep and the most common cause of insomnia. Hypersomnia may be a symptom of hypopituitarism.

s., crescendo. Normal sleep with increased movement during the night.

s. drunkenness. The stupor of sleep in drunkenness. SYN: somnolentia.

s. epilepsy. Uncontrollable desire to sleep at periodic intervals. SYN: narcolepsy.

s., hypnotic. S. induced by hypnotic suggestion.

s. paralysis. Temporary paralysis of a part due to pressure during sleep.

s., paroxysmal. S. epilepsy, q.v.

s., pathological. A term used in encephalitis lethargica (sleeping sickness); here sleep reasserts itself excessively and under conditions not to the best interests of the patient.

s., physiological standards of. Metabolic rate reduced 10-15% below basal level. Systolic pressure falls 10 to 30 mm. of mercury. Pulse rate slows from 10 to 30 beats. Respiration slowed and typically irregular. Temperature drops sharply; lowest about the middle hours of sleep. Muscles relax. Pupils constricted, eyeballs turned upward and outward. Increased sweating. Lacrimal, salivary secretions and volume of urine reduced. Specific gravity raised. Newborn sleeps 18-20 hrs. a day; growing child

12-14 hrs., adult 7-9 hrs. Older persons 5-7 hrs. but it is not necessarily true that older persons require much less sleep than they did when they were young. Women require more sleep than men. Depth of sleep varies from hour to hour. Lessens from the second hour.

s., R.E.M. Abbr. for *sleep* during which *rapid eye movements* are noted. These eye movements are related to dreams.

s., twilight. A procedure of injection of scopolamine and morphine to abolish the subsequent memory of pain felt during childbirth, but it does not completely abolish pain at the time. The patient is delivered in delirium-like state.

s. walking. Walking in one's sleep. SYN: *somnambulism.*

sleep, words pert. to: agrypnia; ahypnia; antilethargic; carotic; dreams; hallucination; hypnagogic; hypnogenic zones; hypnoidal; hypnosis; hypnotic; hypnotism; incubus; insomnia; narcohypnia; narcolepsy; nightmare; noctambulism; oneirodynia; somnambulism; somnifacient; somniloquy; somnolence; somnolent; sopor; soporific; twilight sleep.

sleeping pills. Various medicines including several forms of barbituric acids. Barbiturates may be habit forming or may be taken in excess resulting in acute poisoning. Habitual use may result in psychiatric disorders, especially psychoneuroses, liver and kidney disorders. The drugs most commonly involved are Nembutal, Seconal, Amytal, phenobarbital, and barbital. The action of Seconal is quick but brief. Nembutal has a slower but longer action. The effect is cumulative, so repeated doses may be fatal. In nonfatal cases of overdose, respiratory disorders (atelectasis and bronchopneumonia) are common. Alcohol should not be taken with them. Sudden withdrawal of drugs from a person taking 0.8 gm. or more daily may result in marked withdrawal symptoms (abstinence syndrome).

sleep'ing sick'ness. 1. Acute, infectious disease marked by increasing lethargy, drowsiness, muscular weakness and cerebral symptoms. SYN: *encephalitis lethargica,* q.v. 2. African trypanosomiasis caused by a protozoon introduced into the blood and cerebrospinal fluid by the bite of a tsetse fly; characterized by fever, protracted lethargy, weakness, tremors, and wasting.

slimy (slī'mĭ) [AS. *slim,* smooth]. Resembling slime or a viscid substance; of a growth, adhering to needle so it can be drawn out as a long thread.

sling (slĭng) [AS. *slingan,* to wind]. A support for an injured upper extremity. SEE: *bandage.*

s., clove hitch. Make clove hitch in center of roller bandage. Fit to hand and carry ends over shoulder. Tie beside neck with square knot, making longer ends. They may be carried over and behind the shoulders, brought under each axilla and tied over chest.

s., cravat. The center of cravat is placed under wrist or forearm and ends tied around neck.

s., folded cravat. (lesser arm sling). Place broad fold in position on chest with one end over affected shoulder and other hanging down in front of chest. Flex arm as desired across sling. Bring lower end up over sound shoulder. Knot with other end on affected shoulder.

s., open. The point of the triangle is placed at tip of elbow. The ends are brought around at back of neck and tied. The point should be brought forward and pinned or tied in a single knot, forming a cup to prevent elbow from slipping out.

s., simple figure-of-eight roller arm. Flex arm on chest in desired position, then fix bandage with single turn toward uninjured side around arm and chest, crossing elbow just above external epicondyle of humerus. Make 2nd turn overlapping 2/3 of 1st and bring bandage forward under tip of elbow, then upward along flexed forearm to root of neck of sound side. Then bring downward over scapula and cross chest and arm horizontally, overlapping, turn above and continue as in progressive figure-of-eight.

s., St. John's. Apply triangle with point downwards under elbow, upper end over sound shoulder. Flex arm acutely on chest. Bring lower end under affected arm and around back to knot with upper end on sound shoulder. Bring point up over elbow and fasten to base. Support is wholly for injured shoulder.

s., swathe arm or cravat. (Use wide cravat or folded muslin band.) Place center under acutely flexed elbow, carry front and upwards across the forearm and over affected shoulder. Proceed obliquely across back to sound axilla. Bring other end around front of arm and across body to sound axilla, where it is pinned to other end, continuing around back to part of sling surrounding affected elbow and pinned again.

s., triangular. With suspension from uninjured side (brachioscapular sling). Place triangle on chest with one end over sound shoulder, the point under affected extremity, fold the base. Flex injured arm outside of triangle. Carry lower end upward under axilla of injured side, back of shoulder and tie with upper end behind back. Bring point of triangle anteriorly and medially around back of elbow and fasten to body of bandage. (This bandage changes point of carrying and also relieves the clavicle on injured side of the load.)

   s., triangular, reversed. (reversed brachiocervical sling). Apply with one end over injured shoulder, point toward the sound side, base vertical under injured elbow. Flex arm acutely over triangle. Lower end is brought upwards over front of arm and over sound shoulder. Pull ends taut and tie over sound shoulder. The point is pulled taut over forearm and fixed to anterior and posterior layers between forearm and arm. (Holds elbow more acutely flexed—the weight is supported by the elbow.)

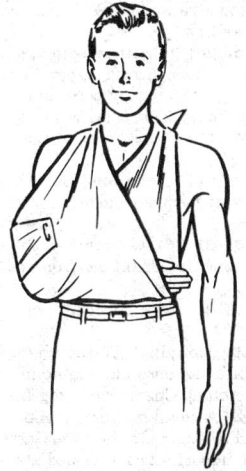

TRIANGULAR BANDAGE SLING

slit [ME. *slitte*]. A narrow opening.

   s., vestibular. The opening between left and right ventricular folds of the larynx.

slough (slŭf) [ME. *slughe*, a skin]. 1. Dead matter or necrosed tissue separated from living tissue or an ulceration. 2. To separate in the form of dead or necrosed parts from living tissue. 3. To cast off, as dead tissue. SEE: *eschar*.

sloughing (slŭf'ĭng). The formation of a slough; separation of dead from living tissue.

   s. phagedena. Hospital gangrene.

slow (slō) [AS. *slāw*, dull]. 1. Mentally dull. 2. Exhibiting retarded speed, as the pulse. 3. Of a morbid condition, or fever, not acute. SEE: words beginning with *brady*.

slows (slōz). An infectious disease of cattle transmitted to man through milk or butter, marked by severe neural symptoms, constipation, vomiting; frequently fatal. SYN: *milk sickness, trembles.*

slow virus infection. Viruses which remain dormant in the body for a prolonged period prior to causing signs and symptoms of illness. They may require from five to ten years to incubate prior to causing such diseases as scrapie in sheep or kuru in man. The disease, subacute sclerosing panencephalitis, may be caused by a slow-acting virus.

sludge (slujh). The semisolid matter deposited in sewage.

   s., activated. Sludge from well-aerated sewage, exposed to oxidizing bacteria, supplying oxidizing organisms sufficient to activate another supply of sewage.

   s., dewatered. Sludge that has been dried.

sludged blood. Condition of the blood in certain abnormal states such as tissue injury or shock in which volume of plasma is reduced and the cells show a pronounced tendency to agglutinate and form large clumps or masses which move slowly through the vessels and sometimes clog the smaller vessels.

slurry (slur'ĭ) [ME. *slory*]. A thin watery mixture.

Sm. Chem. symb. for samarium.

smallpox (smawl'pŏks) [AS. *smael*, tiny, + *poc*, pustule]. An acute, contagious, febrile disease, the constitutional symptoms of which are followed by the appearance of an eruption. SYN: *variola*, q.v.

smear (smēr) [AS. *smerian*, to anoint]. 1. In bacteriology, material spread on a surface, as a microscopic slide or a culture medium. 2. One obtained from infected matter spread over solid culture media. SYN: *s. culture*.

   s., blood. A thin film of blood on a glass slide. Blood is prepared in this manner for staining and microscopic examination.

smegma (smĕg'mă) [Gr. *smēgma*, soap]. Secretion of sebaceous glands, specifically, the thick, cheesy, ill-smelling secretion found under the labia minora about the glans clitoridis and under the male prepuce from Tyson's glands. SYN: *sebum*.

   s. clitoridis. Odoriferous secretion of the glands of the clitoris.

   s. embryonum. Vernix caseosa.

   s. praeputii. Cheesy odoriferous substance collecting under prepuce in the male.

Differential Diagnosis of Smallpox and Chickenpox

	Smallpox	Chickenpox
General symptoms	May be severe, with pyrexia, backache, prostration, etc., for 3 to 4 days before appearance of eruption	Mild Appear at same time as rash
Eruption Type	About 4th day of illness Papules before vesicles; deep, often "shotty"	First day Maculopapular for few hours, then vesicular
Appearance	All spots at same stage of development Pustules appear on the 8th day	Successive crops; therefore, all stages present at the same time Pustules on 3rd or 4th day
Distribution	Maximum on distal parts, not in axillae or groins	Maximum on trunk, present in axillae

smegmatic (smĕg-măt′ĭk). Pert. to or made up of smegma.

smegmolith (smĕg′mō-lĭth) [Gr. *smēgma*, soap, + *lithos,* a stone]. Calcareous mass in the smegma.

smell (smĕl) [ME. *smellen,* to reek]. 1. To perceive by stimulation of the olfactory nerves. 2. To emit an odor, pleasant or offensive. 3. A chemical sense dependent upon end organs on the surface of the upper part of the nasal septum and the superior nasal conch. 4. Property of a thing affecting the olfactory organs, pleasant or unpleasant. SYN: *odor, scent, stench.*

The sense of smell may be affected by many conditions, some of which are the following:

Anosmia: A loss of the sense of smell. It may be a local and a temporary condition resulting from acute and chronic rhinitis, mouth breathing, nasal polyps, dryness of the nasal mucus membrane, pollens, or very offensive odors. It may also result from disease or injury of the olfactory tract, bone disease near the olfactory nerve, disease of the nasal accessory sinuses, basal meningitis, or tumors or gumma affecting the olfactory nerve. It is sometimes found in locomotor ataxia, and frequently in hysteria and neurasthenia. Disease of one cranial hemisphere or of one nasal chamber may account for anosmia. SYN: *anodmia; anosphrasia.*

Hyperosmia: An increased sensitivity to odors.

Kakosmia: The perception of bad odors where none exist; it may be due to head injuries or occur in hallucinations in certain psychoses. SYN: *cacosmia; parosmia.*

Parosmia: A perverted sense of smell.

Odors that are considered agreeable are assumed to be offensive and disagreeable odors may be found pleasant to those suffering from certain functional derangements and in some catarrhs. SYN: *parosphresia.* SEE: *kakosmia.*

smell, words pert. to: anodmia; anosmatic; anosmia; anosphrasia; aroma; aromatic; cacosmia; dysosmia; hyperosmia; jumentous; kakosmia; odor; odoriferous; olfaction; olfactory; osmethesia; osphresis; oxyosphresia.

smog [Blend of smoke and fog]. Dense fog combined with smoke and other forms of air pollution.

smok′er′s can′cer. Cancer of the lip, throat or lung due to irritation from excessive smoking.

SMON. Abbr. for *subacute myelo-optic neuropathy.*

smudging (smŭj′ĭng). A speech defect in which difficult consonants are omitted.

Sn [L. *stannum*]. Chem. symb. for *tin.*

snail [ME.]. A small mollusk having a spiral shell and belonging to the class Gastropoda. They are important as intermediate hosts of many species of parasitic flukes.

snake [ME.]. A creeping reptile possessing scales and lacking limbs, external ears, and functional eyelids. SYN: *serpent.*

s. -bite. Bite of a snake. All snakes should be considered poisonous, although there are only a few that secrete an amount of venom sufficient to inoculate poison deeply into the tissues.

F. A. TREATMENT: Apply tourniquet tight enough to stop venous return of blood, but it should not be tight enough to prevent arterial circulation. Then incise, and induce bleeding. Immobilize patient immediately in order to delay spread of venom. If swelling persists, incise again. This may need to be done frequently. Inject antivenin. If the type of snake cannot be determined, use mixed antivenin. Release tourniquet cautiously for 90 seconds every 10 minutes and observe effect. At the same time, cooling of the entire limb or area is effective in preventing transfer of the venom from the area to the general circulation.

A tourniquet should not be applied too tight or remain on too long. Alcoholic stimulants must not be taken and nothing should be done to increase circulation. Do not cauterize with strong acids or depend upon home remedies. Antibiotics and tetanus prophylaxis are essential.

s., poisonous. A venom-producing snake. Venom is produced in a poison gland which is connected by a tube or groove to a poison fang, one of two sharp, elongated teeth present in upper jaw. The following are poisonous snakes of the U.S.: coral snake, copperhead, water moccasin (cottonmouth), and rattlesnake, of which there are 15 species. All except the coral snake belong to a group known as pit vipers because of presence of a distinct pit between eye and nostril. SEE: *venom, snake.*

A polyvalent antivenin serum for bites by pit vipers is prepared by Wyeth Lab. Inc., Philadelphia, Pa. Antivenin for coral snake bite is available from the Florida State Dept. of Health, Jacksonville, Fla.

Information concerning the nearest source of antivenin may be obtained from the National Institutes of Health, Bethesda, Md.; the Reptile Institute, Silver Springs, Fla.; or from large zoos.

RS: antivenene; antivenom; antivenomous; ophidiophobia; ophidism; ophiotoxemia; venenation; venene; veneniferous; venom.

snapping finger. A snapping sound or feeling produced by bending the finger. In adults it is usually caused by tenosynovitis; in children by the sliding of tendons out of a cramped space when the finger is extended.

snap'ping hip. Slipping of the hip joint with a snap due to displacement over the great trochanter of a tendinous band.

snare (snār) [AS. *sneare,* noose]. Device for excision of polyps, tumors, etc., by tightening wire loops around them.

sneeze (snēz) [AS. *fnēosan,* to pant]. 1. To expel air forcibly through the nose and mouth by spasmodic contraction of muscles of expiration due to irritation of nasal mucosa. The sneeze reflex may be produced by a great number of stimuli. Placing a foot on a cold surface will provoke a sneeze in some

people, while looking at a bright light or sunlight will cause it in others. Firm pressure applied to the middle of the upper lip and just under the nose will sometimes prevent a sneeze which is about to occur. SEE: *photic sneezing.* 2. The act of sneezing.

RS: sternutation, sternutator, sternutatory.

Snellen's chart (snĕl'ĕn). [Herman Snellen, Dutch opthalmologist, 1834-1908]. One used for testing visual acuity.

Snellen's reflex. Congestion of ear on same side resulting when distal end of the divided auriculotemporal nerve is stimulated.

snore (snōr) [AS. *snora*]. 1. To breathe noisily during sleep, due to vibration of the uvula and soft palate. 2. Noisy breathing in sleep or coma. SYN: *rhonchus; stertor.*

snoring rale (snōr'ing rahl). A sonorous rale, low in pitch, resembling a snore.

snow blind'ness. Irritation of the conjunctiva caused by reflection of the sun on the snow.

SYM: Photophobia, blepharospasm, burning pain in the eyes, hyperemia or temporary blindness. SYN: *chionablepsia; niphablepsia; niphotyphlosis.*

snuffles (snŭf'ls) [D. *snuffelen,* to snuff]. Obstructed nasal breathing with discharge from the nasal mucosa, esp. in infants, chiefly in congenital syphilis.

soap (sōp) [AS. *sāpe*]. A cleansing chemical compound formed by an alkali acting on a fatty acid; example: sodium stearate, $NaC_{18}H_{35}O_2$. SEE: *saponification.*

Castile soap is made by saponifying olive oil with sodium hydroxide, and contains mainly sodium oleate, $NaC_{18}H_{33}O_2$.

s., green. S., soft medicinal, q.v.

s. liniment. Liquid opodeldoc. A solution of soap and camphor in alcohol and water.

ACTION AND USES: Stimulant and rubefacient.

s., soft medicinal. A liquid soap made by saponification of vegetable oils excluding coconut oil and palm kernel oil and without removal of glycerin. Used in the treatment of skin diseases. SYN: *green soap.*

s.- suds enema. One given so that the irritating action of the soap will stimulate the bowel. Less harsh forms of enema are preferred. SEE: *enema.*

sob [ME. *sobben,* to catch breath]. 1. To weep with convulsive movements of the chest. 2. A cry or wail resulting from a sudden convulsive inspiration accompanied by spasmodic closure of glottis.

sociology (sō-sĭ-ōl'ō-jĭ) [L. *socius,* companion, + Gr. *logos,* a study]. Study of human social behavior, and the origins, institutions and functions of human groups and societies.

sociomedical. Pert. to sociology and medicine, esp. the interrelationships between the two.

socket (sŏk'ĕt) [ME. *soket*, a spearhead]. A hollow in a joint or part for another corresponding organ, as a bone socket or an eye socket.

s., dry. Alveolitis following tooth extraction characterized by extreme pain but without suppuration.

s., tooth. A dental alveolus of the maxilla or mandible; a cavity which contains the root of a tooth.

soda (sō'dä) [ML. *soda*, headache]. 1. Term loosely applied to various salts of sodium, esp. to caustic soda (sodium hydroxide) and baking soda (sodium bicarbonate). SEE: *sodium.* 2. Short for soda water, which is water charged with carbon dioxide.

s. ash. Commercial sodium carbonate.

s., baking. Sodium bicarbonate.

s., caustic. Sodium hydroxide.

s. lime. USP. A white granular substance consisting of a mixture of calcium hydroxide and sodium hydroxide or potassium hydroxide or both. Used to absorb carbon dioxide.

s., lye. Sodium hydroxide.

s., niter. Nitrate of soda.

s., washing. Sal soda, sodium carbonate.

s. water. A solution of carbon dioxide under pressure; carbonic acid.

sodic (sō'dĭk). Relating to or containing soda or sodium.

sodio-. Combining form denoting a compound containing sodium.

sodium (sō'dĭ-ŭm) [ML. *soda*, headache]. SYMB: *Na.* At. wt. 22.9898; at. no. 11; sp. gr. 0.971. Sodium constitutes approximately 0.15% of elements of the body. Sodium (Na^+), K^+, Ca^{++}, and Mg^{++} constitute the principal cations of the body, their relative concentration determining the integrity of cell membranes and the bioelectric potentials of tissues. Na^+ is the principal cation found in extracellular fluids.

FUNCTIONS: Sodium salts are found in the fluids of the body, serum, blood, and lymph, and in the tissues, the concentration being lower in the tissues. They are necessary to preserve a balance between calcium and potassium to maintain normal heart action and the equilibrium of the body. They regulate osmotic pressure in the cells and fluids, act as an ion balance in tissues, produce a buffer action in the blood, and

guard against an excessive loss of water from the tissues.

DEFICIENCY SYM: Weakness, nerve disorders, loss of weight, "salt hunger," miner's cramps, disturbed digestion.

s. acetate. $NaC_2H_3O_2$. Colorless, odorless, translucent crystals, saline in taste and soluble in water.

ACTION AND USES: Diuretic and laxative.

s. amytal. The monosodium salt of isoamylethylbarbituric acid.

ACTION AND USES: Sedative and hypnotic in control of insomnia; preliminary to surgical anesthesia and in labor.

s. benzoate. USP. A white, odorless powder with sweet taste.

ACTION AND USES: A food preservative.

s. bicarbonate. USP. White, odorless powder with saline taste. $NaHCO_3$.

ACTION AND USES: Orally, as an antacid. Effectiveness for this purpose is questionable. Externally, mild alkaline wash.

INCOMPATIBILITIES: Acids, acid salts, ammonium chloride, lime water, ephedrine hydrochloride, iron chloride.

s. bisulfite. USP. Granular or crystalline powder, sulfurous taste and odor, soluble in water.

ACTION AND USES: As an antioxidant in industry.

s. borate. USP. Borax.

ACTION AND USES: As an ingredient of certain pharmaceutical preparations for external use.

s. carbonate. USP. Na_2CO_3. White crystalline powder (washing soda).

ACTION AND USES: An alkali employed chiefly in alkaline baths.

s. chloride. USP. NaCl. Common salt.

ACTION AND USES: In preparation of normal saline solution, emetic and to add flavor to foods.

INCOMPATIBILITIES: Silver nitrate.

s. citrate. USP. White granular powder, saline in taste and soluble in water.

ACTION AND USES: As an anticoagulant for blood in transfusion.

s. fluoride. USP. NaF. White crystalline powder, saline in taste, soluble in 25 parts of water.

ACTION AND USES: In drinking water and in solution for local application to teeth for prevention of dental caries. Commercially, in etching glassware, for eradication of rats, insects, ants, and other pests.

POISONING: SYM: Optical: conjunctivitis; oral: retching, vomiting, nausea, later cardiac weakness, kidney disturbances, and interference with coagulation of blood.

F.A. TREATMENT: In addition to washing affected areas, precipitate by addition of soluble calcium salts, as lime water, calcium gluconate, calcium lactate. Give emetics and soothing drinks, as milk, cream, egg whites, etc.

s. hydroxide. USP. NaOH. A whitish solid; soluble in water, making a clear solution.

USES: Antacid and caustic. In the laundry and in commercial compounds, in cleaning sink traps, toilets, etc., and in the preparation of soap. *CAUTION:* Use great care in handling it as it rapidly destroys organic tissues. If splashed in eye, may cause blindness.

POISONING: SEE: *potassium hydroxide.*

s. hyposulfite. S. thiosulfate.

s. iodide. USP. NaI. A salt resembling in appearance and action potassium iodide.

s. morrhuate injection. USP. The sodium salt of the fatty acids, found in cod-liver oil.

USES: As a sclerosing agent for the obliteration of varicose veins.

s. nitrite. USP. NaNO₂. White crystalline powder. Antidote for cyanide poisoning.

s. salicylate. USP. C₇H₅NaO₃. White powder or scales with sweet saline taste.

ACTION AND USES: As an analgesic and antipyretic.

INCOMPATIBILITIES: Caffeine citrate, caffeine sodium benzoate.

s. thiosulfate. USP. White crystalline substance, having a cooling taste.

ACTION AND USES: Externally, to remove stains of iodine. Intravenously, as an antidote for cyanide poisoning.

sodokosis (sŏd-ō-kō'sĭs) [Japanese, rat poison]. Infectious febrile disease caused by infection from bite of a rat. SYN: *ratbite fever; sodoku.*

sodoku (sō-do'koo). Infectious febrile disease due to rat bite. SYN: *ratbite fever; sodokosis.*

sodomy (sŏd'ō-mĭ) [LL. *Sodoma,* Sodom]. Anal coitus, usually between males; bestiality, q.v. (concubitus cum bestia), and pederasty, q.v. (concubitus cum persona ejusdem sexus).

Soemmering's bone. [Samuel T. von Soemmering, German anatomist, 1755-1830]. Marginal process of malar (zygomatic) bone.

Soemmering's foramen. The fovea centralis, q.v.

Soemmering's ring. Annular swelling of the periphery of the lens capsule.

Soemmering's spot. The macula lutea of the retina.

soft (sŏft) [AS. *sōfte*]. Not hard, firm or solid.

s. palate. The soft posterior part of the palate. SYN: *palatum molle; velum pendulum palati.*

s. sore. A venereal sore, not due to syphilis, caused by Ducrey's bacillus. SYN: *chancroid.*

soft or convalescent diet. Fish, egg and cheese dishes, chicken, cereals, bread, toast, butter, nothing not soft, semi-solid or liquid. No red meats, vegetables or fruits having seeds or thick skins. No cellulose, raw fruits, or salads.

s. diet, cold. Suitable for tonsillectomies. All forms of milk and cream, iced cocoa, iced coffee and tea, gelatin, junket, custard, strained cereals and fruits if not seeded, such as berries. No fruit juices unless ordered.

s. d., light. Medical liquids, strained cream soups, toast, cream, poached or coddled eggs, mashed potatoes, carrots, peas, and spinach purées, gelatins, junkets, custards, stewed fruits, souffles, jellies, gruels, cereals if strained, ice cream, sherbets.

s. d., l., surgical. Fluids plus thick water gruels, toast, stewed fruits if strained but no seeded fruits.

s. d., modified. Small meals, frequent feedings, gradual additions to full liquid diet—crackers, baked potato, soft cooked egg, cream of wheat, farina, strained oatmeal, applesauce, puréed pears, jelly, simple desserts; later, cottage cheese, puréed vegetables, minced tender meat.

softening (sŏf'ĕn-ĭng) [AS.]. Process of becoming soft. SYN: *malacia, mollities.* RS: words ending in *-malacia.*

s., anemic. White softening of the brain from lack of blood.

s. of bones. Osteomalacia.

s. of brain. Paresis with progressive dementia. SYN: *encephalomalacia.*

s. colliquative. The liquefying of tissues.

s., gray. S. of the brain with absorption of fat following yellow s.

s. of heart. Myomalacia cordis.

s., hemorrhagic. S., red, q.v.

s., mucoid. Myxomatous degeneration.

s., red. S. of the brain with bleeding into necrosed portions.

s. of stomach. Gastromalacia.

s., white. S., anemic, q.v.

s., yellow. S. of brain in a late stage with deposit of changing pigment and fatty degeneration of cells.

soft tissue (non-articular) rheumatism. SEE: *rheumatism, soft tissue (non-articular).*

sol (sŏl, sōl) [Gr. *sole*, salt water]. 1. Abbr. for *solution*. 2. State of a colloid system in which the dispersion medium or solvent forms a continuous phase in which the particles of the solute are dispersed forming a fluid mass. It is called a hydrosol if dispersion medium is a liquid, aerosol if a gas.

solanine (sō'lăn-ĭn). A poisonous narcotic alkaloid obtained from potato sprouts and tomatoes.

solar (sō'lar) [L. *sōlāris*]. Pert. to the sun or its rays.

    s. plexus. The celiac plexus behind the stomach and between the suprarenal glands, and consisting of two large ganglia, the celiac and superior mesenteric ganglia, from which sympathetic fibers pass to visceral organs.

    s. therapy. Treatment with the sun's rays. SYN: *heliotherapy.*

solargentum (sol-ar-jĕn'tŭm). A brand of mild silver protein, containing 19-23% colloidal silver.

solarium (sō-lā'rĭ-ŭm) [L. *solarium*, terrace]. 1. A room or porch exposed to the sun. 2. A room designed for heliotheraphy or for the application of artificial light.

solation (sō-lā'shŭn). In colloidal chemistry, the transformation of a gel into a sol.

soldier's heart. SEE: *asthenia, neurocirculatory.*

sole (sōl) [AS. *sole*]. 1. Underpart of the foot. SYN: *planta.* 2. The portion of a motor end plate at termination of a motor nerve fiber which is directly adjacent to the contractile substance of a muscle fiber. A large number of muscle nuclei are usually aggregated here. SEE: *antithenar; thenar.*

    s. reflex. Contraction of muscles when tickling the sole. SYN: *plantar reflex.*

soleus (sō'lē-ŭs) [L. *solea*, sole of foot]. A flat, broad muscle of calf of leg. SEE: *Table of Muscles* in *Appendix.*

solid (sŏl'ĭd) [L. *solidus*]. 1. Not gaseous, hollow, or liquid. 2. A substance not gaseous, liquid, or hollow.

    s. carbon dioxide therapy. Therapeutic application of solid carbon dioxide. SEE: *refrigeration.*

solipsism (sol'ip-sizm) [L. *solus*, alone, + *ipse,* self]. The theory that the self may know only its own feelings and changes and there is then only subjective reality.

solitary (sŏl'ĭ-tăr-ĭ) [L. *solitarius*]. Alone; single or existing separately.

    s. lymph nodules or follicles. Small spherical lymphatic nodules found in lamina propria of small and large intestine.

solubility (sŏl''ū-bĭl'ĭ-tĭ) [L. *solubilis*, dissolve]. Capability of being dissolved.

soluble (sŏl'ū-bl). Able to be dissolved.

solum tympani. The floor of the tympanic cavity.

solute (sŏl'ūt) [L. *solutus*, dissolved]. The substance that is dissolved in a solution.

solution (sō-lū'shŭn) [L. *solutus*]. 1. Liquid containing dissolved substance. 2. Process by which a solid is homogeneously mixed with a fluid or a solid or gas so that the dissolved substances cannot be distinguished from the resultant fluid. 3. Mixture so formed. 4. Termination of a disease.

    The liquid in which the substances are dissolved is called the *solvent,* q.v., and the substance dissolved, the *solute,* q.v. The strength represents the amt. of substance dissolved by ratio, percentage, or grains to the ounce.

    s., buffer. A solution of a weak acid and its salt (e.g., carbonic acid, sodium bicarbonate) of importance in maintaining a constant pH, esp. of the blood.

    s., colloidal. That in which the solute is suspended and not dissolved, such as gelatin, albumin.

    s., hypertonic. A solution having a greater osmotic pressure than that of cells or body fluids; a solution which draws water out of cells thus inducing plasmolysis. Ex: A concentrated solution of sodium chloride.

    s., hypotonic. A solution having an osmotic pressure less than that of cells or body fluids; a solution which will cause water to enter cells thus inducing turgor and possibly hemolysis. Ex: A sodium chloride solution containing less than 0.9 gm. of NaCl in each 100 ml. of water.

    s., isohydric. A solution having the same hydrogen ion concentration or pH as another.

    s., isosmotic. An isotonic solution, q.v.

    s., isotonic. One which has the same osmotic pressure as that of body cells or fluids. Ex: A sodium chloride solution containing 0.9 gm. of NaCl in each 100 ml. of water.

    s., Locke-Ringer's. A buffered isotonic solution containing sodium chloride 9.0 gm., potassium chloride 0.42 gm., calcium chloride 0.24 gm., sodium bicarbonate 0.5 gm., magnesium chloride 0.2 gm., dextrose 0.5 gm., distilled water, to make 1000 ml.

    s., molar. Solution containing a gram molecular weight or mole of the reagent dissolved in one liter (1000 ml.) of solution. Designated 1M.

    s., normal. Solution containing one gram equivalent weight of reagent in one liter (1000 ml.) of solution. Designated 1N.

s., normal saline. An isotonic saline solution. SEE: *s., isotonic.*

s., physiological saline. An isotonic solution of sodium chloride. SEE: *solution, isotonic.*

s., repair. Any solution given intravenously to treat an electrolyte or metabolic disturbance.

s., Ringer's. A solution containing chlorides of sodium, calcium, and potassium in most favorable concentration. For mammals it contains sodium chloride 8.6 gm., calcium chloride 0.33 gm., potassium chloride 0.3 gm., distilled water to make one liter (1000 ml.). SYN: *Ringer's injection* (USP).

s., saline. A solution of a salt, usually sodium chloride. SEE: *s., isotonic; s., normal saline; s., physiological saline.*

s., saturated. A solution that contains all the solute it can dissolve. This limit is called the saturation point.

s., seminormal. A solution containing one-half of a gram equivalent weight of reagent in one liter (1000 ml.) of solution. ABBR: 0.5N or N/2.

s., standard. A solution containing a definite amount of a substance as a normal solution.

s., supersaturation. Solution in which the saturation point is reached, but when heated it is possible to dissolve more of the solute.

s., test. A reagent solution; one used in performing a particular test. ABBR: T.S.

s., Tyrode's. A modified Ringer's solution containing, in addition, a small amount of magnesium chloride and acid and sodium phosphates.

s., volumetric. A standard solution containing a definite amount (1/2, 1/10, etc.) gram equivalent of a substance in one liter (1000 ml.) of solution. Used in volumetric analysis. ABBR: V.S.

solv. Abbr. of L. *solve, dissolve.*

solvate (sŏl'vāt). A compound formed by reaction between solvent and solute.

solvation (sŏl-vā'shŭn). The formation of a solvate.

solvent (sŏl'vĕnt) [L. *solvens*]. 1. Producing a solution; dissolving. 2. A liquid holding another substance in solution. 3. A liquid which reacts with a solvent bringing it into solution.

soma (sō'mă) [Gr. *sōma*, body]. 1. The body as distinct from the mind. 2. All of the body cells except the germ cells. 3. The body exclusive of the extremities.

somasthenia (sōm"as-the'nĭ-a) [Gr. *sōma*, body, + *astheneia*, weakness]. A condition of chronic bodily weakness. SYN: *somatasthenia.*

somatasthenia (sō-măt-ăs-the'nĭ-ă) ["+ *astheneia*, weakness]. Chronic bodily weakness usually with low blood pressure, but *not* neurasthenia. SYN: *somasthenia.*

somatalgia (sō"mă-tăl'jĭ-ă) ["+ *algos*, pain]. Pain in the body.

somatesthesia (sō-măt-ĕs-the'zĭ-ă) ["+ *aisthēsis*, sensation]. The consciousness of the body; bodily sensation.

somatic (sō-măt'ĭk) [Gr. *sōma*, body]. 1. Pertaining to nonreproductive cells or tissues. 2. Pert. to the body. 3. Pert. to structures of the body wall, e.g., skeletal muscles (somatic musculature) in contrast to structures associated with the viscera, e.g., visceral muscles (splanchnic musculature).

somatoceptors (sō-măt-ō-sĕp'tors). Term applied to proprioceptors and exteroceptors collectively.

somatology (sō-mă-tol'ō-jĭ) [Gr. *sōma*, body, + *logos*, a study]. Comparative study of structure, functions and development of the human body.

somatopathic (sō-mă-tō-păth'ĭk) ["+ *pathos*, disease]. Organically ill, as distinguished from neuropathic or psychopathic diseases.

somatoplasm (sō-măt'ō-plăzm) [Gr. *sōma*, body, + *plasma*, a thing formed]. The protoplasm of all the body cells as distinguished from that of the germ plasm; the soma.

somatopleure (sō-măt'ō-plūr) ["+ *pleura*, a side]. The lateral and ventral body wall of an embryo consisting of the outer ectoderm and a layer of somatic mesoderm underlying it. It continues beyond the embryo as the amnion and chorion.

somatopsychic (sō-măt-ō-sī'kĭk) ["+ *psyche*, mind]. Pert. to both body and mind.

somatopsychosis (sō"mă-tō-si-kō'sĭs) ["+ "+ *-ōsis*, condition]. Any mental disorder which is a symptom of a bodily disease.

somatoscopy (sō-mă-tŏs'kō-pĭ) [Gr. *sōma*, body, + *skopein*, to examine]. Physical examination of the body.

somatotrophic (sō"mă-tō-trŏf'ĭk) ["+ *tropos*, a turning]. 1. Having selective attraction for or influence on body cells. 2. Stimulating growth.

somatotype (sō-măt'ō-tip). A particular build or type of body.

s. theory. A theory that certain body types (endomorphy, mesomorphy, actomorphy) are associated with certain personality types.

somatropin (sō-măt'rō-pĭn) [Gr. *sōma*, body, + *tropos*, a turning]. The anterior pituitary lobe's growth-stimulating principle. In the human, this is called human growth hormone (HGH).

somesthesia (som-es-the'sĭ-ă) [Gr. *sōma*, body, + *aisthēsis*, sensation]. Awareness of bodily sensations. SYN: *somatesthesia.*

somesthetic (sō-měs-thět'ĭk). Pert. to sensations and sensory structures of the body.

s. area. The region in the cortex in which lie the terminations of the axons of general sensory conduction paths.

s. path. General sensory conduction path leading to the cortex.

somite (sō'mĭt) [Gr. *sōma*, body]. 1. Embryonic blocklike segment formed on either side of the neural tube and its underlying notochord. 2. Any one of the embryonic segments.

Each somite gives rise to a muscle mass supplied by a spinal nerve and each pair gives rise to a vertebra.

somnambulism (som-năm'bū-lĭzm) [L. *somnus*, sleep, + *ambulāre*, to walk]. 1. A form of hysteria in which behavior and purposeful actions are not subsequently remembered. 2. Sleepwalking, an affection that prompts the sleeping person to perform, unconsciously, acts that naturally belong to the waking state. SYN: *noctambulism*, q.v.

The term has a more comprehensive meaning in psychiatry than that of noctambulism.

somnambulist (som-năm'bū-lĭst). One who is subject to sleepwalking.

somnarium (som-nā'rĭ-ŭm) [L. *somnus*, sleep]. A sanitarium in which sleep therapy is employed in the treatment of neuroses.

somnifacient (som-nĭ-fā'shĕnt) ["+ *facere*, to make]. 1. Producing sleep. SYN: *hypnotic.* 2. A medicine producing sleep. SYN: *soporific*, q.v.

somniferous (som-nĭf'ĕr-ŭs) ["+ *ferre*, to bear]. Sleep-producing; pert. to that which promotes sleep.

somnific (som-nĭf'ĭk). Producing sleep.

somniloquist (som-nĭl'ō-kwĭst) [L. *somnus*, sleep, + *loqui*, to speak]. One who talks in his sleep.

somniloquy (som-nĭl'ō-kwĭ) ["+ *loqui*, to speak]. Act of talking during sleep or in a hypnotic condition.

somnipathy (som-nĭp'ă-thĭ) ["+ Gr. *pathos*, disease]. 1. Any disorder of sleep. 2. Hypnotism.

somnocinematograph (som-nō-sĭn-ĕ-măt'ō-grăf) ["+ Gr. *kinema*, motion, + *graphein*, to write]. Device for recording motions of those who are asleep.

somnolence (som'nō-lĕns) [L. *somnolentia*, sleepiness]. Prolonged drowsiness or a condi-

tion resembling trance which may continue for a number of days; sleepiness.

somnolent (som'nō-lĕnt) [L. *somnolentus*]. Sleepy; drowsy.

somnolentia (som-nō-lĕn'shĭ-ă) [L.]. 1. Drowsiness. 2. The sleep of drunkenness in which the faculties are only partially in repose.

sone. A unit of loudness; the loudness of a pure tone of 1000 cycles per second, 40 decibels above the listener's threshold of audibility.

sonic boom (son'ĭk) [L. *sonus*, sound]. Noise caused by shock waves from an airborne object traveling at a speed in excess of the speed of sound. When the waves hit the ground they may break windows and affect the hearing.

sonitus (son'ĭ-tŭs) [L.]. Subjective noises in the ear. SYN: *tinnitus aurium*, q.v.

sonometer (sō-nŏm'ĕtĕr) [L. *sonus*, sound, + Gr. *metron*, a measure]. 1. Device for testing the hearing. 2. Device to cause sound for production of anesthesia; used by dentists.

sonorous (sō-nō'rŭs) [L.]. Giving forth a loud and rounded sound.

s. rale. A dry or low pitched rale often caused by vibration of mucuous secretion in a bronchus.

sophistication (sō-fĭs-tĭ-kā'shŭn) [Gr. *sophistikos*, deceitful]. Adulteration of any substances.

sopor (sō'por) [L. *sopor*, deep sleep]. Deep, lethargic sleep. SYN: *stupor.*

soporific (sō-po-rĭf'ĭk) ["+ *facere*, to make]. 1. Inducing sleep. 2. Narcotic; a drug producing sleep.

soporose, soporous (sō'por-ōs, -ŭs) [L.]. Marked by or resembling sound sleep or coma.

sorbefacient (sor"bē-fā'shĕnt) [L. *sorbere*, to suck, + *facere*, to make]. Causing or that which causes or promotes absorption.

sordes (sor'dēz) [L. *sordere*, to be dirty]. 1. Foul, brown crusts or accumulations on the teeth and about the lips from foul stomach or secretions of the mouth in low forms of fever. 2. Filth.

NP: A solution of half glycerin or mineral oil and half lemon juice carefully applied with applicators will remove the condition and help to prevent further accumulation.

sore (sōr) [AS. *sār*, sore]. 1. Tender; painful. 2. A tender or painful ulcer or lesion of the skin.

s., bed-. Gangrene of skin due to pressure. SYN: *decubitus*, q.v., *pressure sore.*

s., canker. A small lesion of the mucous membrane of the mouth. They often accompany a number of systemic conditions. Cause unknown. SYN: *aphthous stomatitis; aphthous ulcer.*

   s., cold. Blister on the lips. SYN: *herpes simplex.*

   s., hard. Syphilitic chancre, q.v., primary lesion of syphilis.

   s., Oriental. Cutaneous leishmaniasis. SYN: *Delhi boil; tropical sore.*

   s., pressure. A bedsore, q.v.

   s., soft venereal. Soft, nonsyphilitic, venereal sore occurring on the genitalia. SYN: *chancroid,* q.v.

   s. throat. Any inflammation of the tonsils, pharynx or larynx.

   s. throat, diphtheritic. Croupous tonsillitis.

   s. throat, quinsy. Peritonsillar abscess. SEE: *quinsy.*

   s. throat, septic. Severe, epidemic, pseudomembranous inflammation of fauces and tonsils caused by the hemolytic streptococcus.

   s., tropical. S., Oriental, q.v.

   s., venereal. S., soft venereal, q.v.

soroche (sō-rō'kā, or skā) [Sp.]. Mountain sickness, esp. that occurring in the Andes.

sororiation (so-ror-ī-ā'shŭn) [L. *sororiäre,* to increase together]. Growth of the breasts at puberty.

s.o.s. Abbr. for L. *si opus sit,* if necessary or required.

souffle (soof'fl) [Fr. *souffler,* to puff]. A soft blowing sound heard in auscultation; a bruit; an auscultatory murmur.

   s., cardiac. Heart murmur.

   s., fetal. The soft blowing sound heard over the location of the umbilical cord of the fetus in utero and synchronous with the fetal heartbeat during late pregnancy.

   s., funic, s., funicular, s., umbilical. S., fetal, q.v.

   s., splenic. Sound heard over spleen in malaria.

   s., uterine. Sound caused by blood entering dilated arteries of uterus in last months of pregnancy; synchronous with maternal pulse. It is more frequent than the fetal souffle and is heard as a loud blowing murmur along left side of uterus, and frequently all over it. An enlarged uterus may cause it. That of pregnancy is variable, whereas other forms are constant.

sound (sownd) [L. *sonus,* sound]. 1. Auditory sensations produced by vibrations; noise. It is measured in decibels, which is the logarithm of the intensity of sound; thus 20 d. represents not twice 10 d., but ten times as much. Conversation represents 90 d's. Exposure to excessively loud noises esp. in certain frequencies if repeated will cause perma-

nent injury to the hearing. SEE: *decibel, noise, sonic boom.* 2. A form of vibrational energy that gives rise to auditory sensations. SEE: *cochlea, ear, organ of Corti, sonic boom.* 3. Healthy, not diseased. 4. Heart sounds. SEE: *diastole, systole.* 5. [Fr. *sonder,* to probe]. Instrument for introduction into a cavity or canal for diagnosis or treatment.

   s., anasarcous. Moist sound heard on auscultation when skin is edematous.

   s., blowing. Organic murmur as of air from an aperture expelled with moderate force.

   s., bottle. Noise as of fluid in a bottle. SYN: *amphoric,* q.v., *murmur.*

   s.'s, breath. Respiratory sounds heard on auscultation of the chest. In a normal chest they are classified as vesicular, tracheal, and bronchovesicular.

   s., bronchial. Sound not heard in normal lung but occurring in pulmonary disease indicating infiltration and solidification of lung.

   s.'s, bronchovesicular. A mixture of bronchial and vesicular sounds.

   s., cracked-pot. A tympanic resonance heard over pulmonary cavities.

   s., fetal heart. Sound made by the fetal heart.

   s., friction. Sound produced by the rubbing together of two inflamed mucous surfaces.

   s.'s, heart. The two sounds "lubb" and "dupp" resulting from closure of atrioventricular and semilunar valves. SEE: *heart, auscultation of.*

   s., to and fro. Rasping friction sounds of pericarditis.

   s., tracheal. That normally heard over the trachea or larynx.

   s., tubular. Sound heard over the trachea or large bronchi.

   s., vesicular. Sound heard over entire lung during inspiration resulting from distention of alveoli with air.

sound, words pert. to: amphoric; anacamptics; aphthongia; aspirate; auscultation; bell-metal resonance; bourdonnement; capotement; clang; clapotage; clapotement; heart; hyperacusis; murmur; rale; resonance; souffle; stridulous; succussion; uterus.

soybean (soi'bēn) [Hind. *soyā,* fennel]. The seed of several varieties of glycine. Contains proteins and a fixed oil (soya oil) and very little starch.

   Food value of 100 gm. (cooked): Cal. 118; protein 9.8 gm.; fat 5.1 gm.; carbohydrates 10.1 gm.; calcium 60 mg.; vitamin A 660 I.U.

sp. Abbr. for L. *spiritus,* spirit; *Species.*

spa. A mineral spring, esp. one having healing properties.

space (spās) [L. *spatium*, space]. An area, region, or segment. RS: chondroporosis, circumscribed.

s., axillary. The axilla or s. beneath the arm.

s., circumlental. S. between equator of lens and ciliary body.

s., epidural. S. between the dura mater and vertebral periosteum, or between the bones of the cranium and the dura mater, assumed to be lymph spaces.

s.'s of Fontana. S. in scleral meshwork in angle of iris through which aqueous humor passes from anterior chamber to canal of Schlemm.

s., interfascial. S., Tenon's, q.v.

s., intervillous. S. in placenta which develops from early chorionic trophoblast. It forms a blood sinus in which chorionic villi of fetus are bathed in maternal blood received from uterine vessels.

s., Nuel's. S. between outer hair cells and rods in the organ of Corti.

s., perforated. S. pierced by blood vessels at base of brain. SYN: *substantia perforata.*

s.'s, perivascular. S. within adventitia of larger blood vessels of the brain. They communicate with subarachnoid space. SYN: *Spaces of Virchow-Robin.*

s., plantar. S. (1 of 4) between fascial layers of the foot. When the foot is infected, pus may be found here.

s., popliteal. S. back of knee joint containing the popliteal artery and vein and small sciatic and popliteal nerves.

s., prezonular. The anterior portion of the posterior chamber of the eye.

s., Pruzzak's. S. in tympanum behind Shrapnell's membrane.

s., retropharyngeal. S. behind pharynx separating prevertebral from visceral fascia. SYN: *retropharyngeal fascial cleft.*

s.'s, subarachnoid. S. between the pia mater and arachnoid containing the cerebrospinal fluid. The spaces, esp. in the cranium, are traversed by numerous trabeculae. SYN: *intraleptomeningeal spaces.*

s., subdural. Narrow s. between dura and the arachnoid.

s., suprasternal. Triangular s. immediately above sternum between layers of deep cervical fascia. SYN: *space of Burns.*

s., Tenon's. Lymph s. between the sclera and Tenon's capsule.

s., thenar. A deep fascial s. in the hand lying anterior to adductor pollicis muscle. SYN: *lateral palmar space.*

s., tissue. Any s. within tissues not lined with epithelium and containing tissue fluid.

s.'s, zonular. S. within zonule (suspensory ligament of lens).

spaghetti (spă-gĕt'ĭ) [It. *spaghetto*, little cord]. Food value of 100 gm. (enriched: cooked, firm stage, "al dente"): Cal. 148; protein 5.0 gm.; fat 0.5 gm.; carbohydrates 30.1 gm.; calcium 11 mg.

Spanish fly (spăn'ĭsh flī). A strong rubefacient and blistering agent produced from these beetles. SYN: *cantharides.*

spanogyny (spăn'o-jĭn'ĭ) [Gr. *spanos*, scarce, + *gynē*, a woman]. More males than females; decrease in female births.

sparer (spăr'er) [AS. *sparian*, to refrain]. A substance destroyed by catabolism, but which, nevertheless, lessens catabolic action upon other substances.

s., protein. Carbohydrates and fats, so designated because their presence in diet prevents tissue proteins from being utilized as a source of energy.

sparganosis (spar-gă-nō'sĭs). Infestation with a variety of Sparganum.

Sparganum (spar'gă-num) [Gr. *sparganon*, swathing band]. (pl. *spargana*) The plerocercoid larva of tapeworms, esp. those of the genus Dibothriocephalus.

S. mansoni. An elongated plerocercoid, 3-14 inches in length found in muscles and connective tissue, esp. that around the eye. Common in Far East.

S. mansonoides. Species occasionally occurring in U.S. The adult form is unknown.

S. proliferum. Minute form infesting man and producing acne-like nodules. It is thought to proliferate by means of budlike outgrowths.

spargosis (spar-gō'sĭs) [Gr. *spargōsis*, swelling]. 1. Distention of the female breasts with milk. 2. Swelling or thickening of the skin. SYN: *elephantiasis.*

spark coil. Coil consisting of primary and secondary coils with an interrupted current passing through them. SYN: *induction coil.*

spark gaps. 1. Arrangement of opposed points or surfaces between which an electric spark may jump. 2. An adjustable gap between needle points or between spheres used to measure high potentials.

s. g., quenched. A multiple spark gap with numerous electrodes about 0.3 mm. apart and equipped with a copper air-cooling device.

sparteine sulfate (spar'tēn) [L. *spartium*, broom]. The salt of an alkaloid obtained from Scoparius.

USES: Once regarded as of value in cardiac diseases and as a diuretic. Also has limited usefulness in obstetrics to stimulate the uterus to contract.

spasm (spăzm) [Gr. *spasmos*, a convulsion]. An involuntary, sudden movement or convulsive muscular contraction. Spasms may be clonic (characterized by alternate contraction and relaxation) or tonic (sustained). They may involve either visceral (smooth) muscle or skeletal (striated) muscle. When contractions are strong and painful, they are called cramps.

The effect depends upon the part affected. Asthma is assumed to be due to spasm of muscular coats of smaller bronchi; renal colic, to spasm of muscular coat of the ureter.

TREATMENT: General measures to reduce tension, induce muscle relaxation and improve circulation. Specific measures include analgesics for relief of pain, physiotherapy (heat, diathermy, electrical therapy). Special orthopedic supports or braces are sometimes effective. For vascular spasm, chemical sympathectomy may give relief.

　s., Bell's. Convulsive tic of the face.

　s. center. Point in the oblongata where it meets the pons.

　s., choreiform. Spasmodic movements resembling chorea.

　s., clonic. Intermittent contractions and relaxation of muscles.

　s. of esophagus. Paroxysmal dysphagia (inability to swallow), often associated with a sense of constriction in the chest.

　Characterized by intense dyspnea and occurs in spasmodic croup, true croup, ulceration of larynx, laryngismus stridulus, whooping cough, tetany, hysteria, hydrophobia, laryngeal crises of locomotor ataxia, when foreign bodies have lodged in larynx, and when aneurysms or mediastinal tumors press on recurrent laryngeal nerve and irritate it.

　PROG: Indefinite regarding duration, not threatening to life.

　TREATMENT: Search for exciting cause and remove. Treatment largely dietetic, hygienic and psychologic. Dilation by passage of a bougie may be of great value.

　s., habit. Spasms due to habit.

　s., nodding. A psychogenic condition in adults, causing nodding of the head from clonic spasms of the sternomastoid muscles.

A similar nodding in babies with head turning from side to side.

　s., saltatory. Term employed to designate a condition allied to hysteria in which a violent spasm seizes the muscles of the leg as soon as the feet touch the ground, and as a result patient is thrown violently in the air.

　s., tetanic. S. in which contractions continue for a time without interruption.

　s., tonic. Continued involuntary contractions.

　s., torsion. Spasm characterized by a turning of a part, esp. the turning of the body at the pelvis.

　s., toxic. S. due to poison.

　s., winking. Spasmus nictitans, q.v.

spasm, words pert. to: campospasm, cardiospasm, carpopedal, child crowing, chirospasm, Chvostek's sign, clonic, clonospasm, clonus, facial, habit, hypertonus, mobile, Raynaud's disease, spasticity, tetanus, tetany, tic douloureux, tonic spasm, trismus.

spasmatic,　spasmodic (spăz-măt'ĭk, -mŏd'ĭk) [Gr. *spasmos*, a convulsion]. Pert. to, like, or marked by, spasm. SEE: *cholepathia spastica.*

　s. asthma. A. caused by spasm of the bronchioles.

　s. croup. Laryngismus stridulus.

　s. stricture. Temporary narrowing of any canal, as the urethra, due to localized spasmodic muscular contraction of its coat.

spasmology (spăz-mŏl'ō-jĭ) [" + *logos*, a study]. The study of spasms, their nature and cause.

spasmolygmus (spăz-mō-lĭg'mŭs) [" + *lygmos*, a sob]. 1. Spasmodic hiccup. 2. Spasmodic sobbing.

spasmolytic (spăz-mō-lĭt'ĭk) [" + *lysis*, dissolution]. Arresting spasms or that which acts as an antispasmodic.

spasmomyxorrhea (spăz"mō-mĭks-or-re'ă) [" + *myxa*, mucus, + *rhoia*, flow]. Excessive secretion of intestinal mucus. SYN: *myxorrhea intestinalis.*

spasmophemia (spăz-mō-fē'mĭ-ă) [Gr. *spasmos*, convulsion, + *phēmē*, speech]. A spasmodic disorder of speech. SYN: *stuttering.*

spasmophilia (spăz-mō-fĭl'ĭ-ă) [" + *philein*, to love]. A tendency to tetany and convulsions; almost always associated with rickets.

spasmous (spăz'mŭs) [Gr. *spasmos*, convulsion]. Of the nature of a spasm.

spasmus (spăz'mŭs) [Gr. *spasmos*, convulsion]. A spasm.

　s. agitans. Paralysis agitans, q.v.

　s. bronchialis. Bronchial asthma.

　s. caninus. Spasm of face causing a constant grin. SYN: *risus sardonicus.*

s. coordinatus. Imitative or compulsive movements, as mimic tics or festination.

s. cynicus. Spasmodic contraction of muscles on both sides of the mouth.

s. Dubini. Rhythmic contractions, in rapid succession, of a group or groups of muscles, starting at an extremity or half of the face, and covering a large part or all of the body. SYN: *electric chorea.*
PROG: Usually fatal.

s. glottidis. Spasm of larynx. SYN: *laryngismus stridulus.*

s. intestinorum. Pain in intestines. SYN: *enteralgia.*

s. nictitans. A winking movement of the eyelid.

s. nutans. Nodding spasm.

spastic (spăs'tĭk) [Gr. *spastikos,* convulsive]. 1. Resembling or of the nature of spasms or convulsions. 2. Produced by spasms. 3. One afflicted with spasms.

s. gait. A stiff movement with toes seeming to catch together and to drag.

s. hemiplegia. Partial hemiplegia with spasmodic muscular contractions.

s. paralysis. Muscular rigidity accompanying partial paralysis. Usually due to a lesion involving upper motor neurons.

s. paraplegia. Paraplegia due to transverse lesions of the cord or sclerosis.

spasticity (spăs-tĭs'ĭ-tĭ). Hypertension of muscles causing stiff and awkward movements: the result of upper motor neuron lesion.

spatial (spā'shăl). Pertaining to space.

s. discrimination. Ability to perceive as separate points of contact the two blunt points of a compass when applied to the skin. SYN: *two-point discrimination.*

spatula (spăt'ū-lă) [L. *spatula,* blade]. Instrument for spreading or mixing semisolids. It is usually flat, thin, somewhat flexible and shaped like a knife.

s., eye. Blades for separating lips of corneal wounds, arresting hemorrhage or for making pressure; sheet metal or rubber.

s., nasal. Device for holding mucous flaps in place or to guard against burning from cautery.

spay (spā) [Gael. *spoth,* castrate]. Surgical removal of ovaries, usually said of animals. SEE: *castration.*

specialist (spĕsh'ăl-ĭst) [L. *specialis*]. A physician who has had postgraduate training in and practices a particular branch of medicine such as surgery, internal medicine, pediatrics, and obstetrics.

species (spē'shēz) [L. *species,* a kind]. In biology, a category of classification for living organisms. This group is just below genus and is usually capable of interbreeding.

specific (spē-sĭf'ĭk) [L. *specificus,* pert. to a kind]. 1. A remedy having a curative effect on a particular disease or symptom. 2. Pert. to a species. 3. A disease always caused by the same organism. 4. Restricted, explicit; not generalized.

s. dynamic action. The increase in metabolic rate resulting from absorption of food. For protein it amounts to about 30%, for carbohydrates, 7%, and for fats, 4%. After a general meal the increase would be 10 to 15%. This effect lasts for 4 to 6 hours. ABBR: SDA.

s. gravity. Weight of a substance compared with an equal volume of water. Water is represented by 1.000.

specificity (spē-sĭ-fĭs'ĭ-tĭ). State of being specific; having a relation to a definite result or to a particular cause.

specillum (spē-sĭl'lŭm) [L. *specere,* to look]. (pl. *specilla*) 1. Lens. 2. Button-shaped silver probe.

specimen (spĕs'ĭ-mĕn) [L. *specere,* to look]. A part of a thing intended to show kind and quality of the whole, as a specimen of urine.

spectacles (spĕk'tăk-lz) [L. *spectāre,* to see]. Two lenses supported by a nose bridge and side pieces passing over the ears. Used to aid vision or protect the eyes. SYN: *eyeglasses; glasses.*

spectro- [L.]. Combining form meaning appearance, image, form, spectrum.

spectrocolorimeter (spĕk-trō-kŭl-or-ĭm'ĕ-tĕr) [L. *spectrum,* image, + *color,* color, + Gr. *metron,* measure]. Device for detecting color blindness by isolating a single spectral color.

spectrograph (spĕk'trō-grăf) ["+ Gr. *graphein,* to write]. An instrument designed to photograph spectra on a sensitive photographic plate.

spectrometer (spĕk-trŏm'ĕt-ĕr) ["+ Gr. *metron,* a measure]. A spectroscope so constructed that angular deviation of a ray of light produced by a prism or by a diffraction grating thus indicates the wavelength.

spectrophotometer (spĕk"trō-fō-tŏm'ĕt-ĕr) ["+ Gr. *photos,* light, + *metron,* a measure]. Device for measuring amt. of color in a solution by comparison with the spectrum.

spectrophotometry (spĕk"trō-fō-tŏm'ĕt-rī) ["+ "+ *metron,* a measure]. Estimation of coloring matter in a solution by use of the spectroscope or spectrophotometer.

spectropyrheliometer (spĕk"trō-pĭr-hē-lĭ-ŏm'ĕ-tĕr) [L. *spectrum,* image, + Gr. *pyr,* fire, + *hēlios,* sun, + *metron,* a measure]. Instrument to measure solar radiation.

spectroscope (spĕk'tro-skōp) ["+ Gr. *skopein*, to examine]. An instrument for separating radiant energy into its component frequencies or wavelengths by means of a prism or grating to form a correct spectrum for inspection.

spectroscopy (spĕk-trŏs'ko-pĭ). The branch of physical science that treats of the phenomena observed with the spectroscope, or those principles on which its action is based; also, the art of using the spectroscope.

spectrum (spĕk'trŭm) [L. image]. (pl. *spectra*) Charted band of wave lengths of electromagnetic vibrations obtained by refraction and diffraction of ray of white light.

   s., invisible. Spectral portion either below the red (infrared) or above the violet (ultraviolet), which is invisible to the eye, the waves being too long or too short to affect the retina.

   The invisible spectrum includes rays less than 3900 A.U. in length (ultraviolet, roentgen or X, gamma, and cosmic rays) and those exceeding 7700 A.U. in length (infrared, high frequency oscillations used in short and long wave diathermy, radio, hertzian, and very long waves). These range in length from 7700 A.U. to 5,000,000 meters.

   s., visible. Portion of spectrum which is visible; consists of wavelengths between 3900 A.U. and 7000 A.U.

   The visible spectrum consists of the colors from red to violet with wavelengths of 3900 A.U. to 7700 A.U. When white light is passed through a prism, the various colors, because of different wavelengths, are refracted to various degrees giving rise to the diverse colors of the rainbow. These are violet, indigo, blue, green, yellow, orange, and red.

speculum (spĕk'ū-lŭm) [L. a mirror]. (pl. *specula*) 1. Instrument for examination of canals. 2. Membrane separating anterior cornua of lateral ventricles of brain. SYN: *septum pellucidum.*

   s., ear. Short, funnel-shaped tubes, tubular or bivalve; former preferable.

   s., eye. Device for separating eyelids. Plated steel wire, plain, Von Graefe's, Steven's or Luer's are most common.

speech [AS. *spaec*]. 1. Verbal expression of one's thought. 2. The act of uttering articulate words or sounds. 3. Words that are spoken.

   Primitively, certain crude sounds served as warnings or threats in much the same way as did facial and bodily expressions. As sounds became highly differentiated, each became associated, and gradually identified with a certain idea. These word-symbols are a most valuable tool in ideation, and thinking is very largely dependent on this internal speech. Further identifications have made possible visual symbols (written language); though primitive written language was entirely unrelated— a series of pictures and crude representations.

   External speech requires the coordination of larynx, mouth, lips, chest, and abdominal muscles. These have no special inervation for speech but the upper neurons respond to complex motor pattern fields which convert the idea into suitable motor stimuli.

   s. abnormalities. Speech failure results in motor aphasia in which the patient is speechless but there is no paralysis of muscles of articulation. Although unable to express his thoughts in words, the patient can still understand what he hears and reads.

   Labialism is the excessive use of labial sounds.

   Absence of speech or hoarseness may be part of a hysteria. Aphasias are also described as sensory.

   When a word is heard, but the patient has no idea of its meaning, we speak of word-deafness. Similarly, word-blindness means that the written symbol might as well be a foreign word. This is sometimes called alexia, q.v. Aphasia, q.v., in right-handed patients is classically referable to left-handed brain lesions, but the concept of centers for internal speech esp. is rather misleading. It is probably a diffuse cortical activity and countless minor distortions occur in addition to those mentioned. Chief of those not enumerated is the slurring speech of paresis, q.v., where letters and syllables are omitted without recognition of defect, and this further identifies the abnormality. Dysarthria, q.v., describes any defect of articulation; muscular tone disturbances as seen in cerebellar disease, chorea, paralysis agitans, lenticular degeneration, multiple sclerosis producing jerky, monotonous or scanning speech.

   Paralysis due to bilateral medullary pathology results in indistinct enunciation (mouthful speech) often entirely unintelligible. Pseudobulbar palsy (as in cases of double hemiplegia) adds a slow spastic characteristic. Peripheral nerve lesions, cleft palate, adenoids, myasthenia gravis, merely suggest the many possible modifications.

   Stammering and stuttering are usually psychogenic.

   Emotional values may be added to speech qualities; tremulousness and tension may render the voice high-pitched, irritating, or unsustained and broken. Emotional flattening may occur in the neuroses and psychoses. In the latter, diagnostic changes may occur in the stream of talk.

Slowing is common in all depressed states. When complete (mutism) it suggests the negativism esp. likely to occur in schizophrenia. Aphonic-like aphasia patients will find some means of communication.

Excessive talk flow is generally seen in mania and excited states. When merely voluble but relevant, it constitutes circumstantiality. If the goal ideal is lost, irrelevancy is associated with a "flight of ideas"—in extreme form a "word salad." The manner of speech often mirrors the mood.

Neologisms are words created by the patient, often of no apparent significance.

Stereotyped speech is constant repetition of a word or phrase. It should be distinguished from perseveration in which the repetition is against the intention or wishes of the patient.

Amentia,q.v., invariably delays speech appearance and its faulty development is of diagnostic value. Its delayed or non-appearance may be referable to deafness (deaf-mutism). Childish indistinctness (e.g., r's replaced by w's) may persist in feebleminded adults (lalling-smudging).

    s., aphonic. Whispering.

    s., ataxic. Defective speech resulting from muscular incoordination usually the result of cerebellar disorder.

    s., clipped. S., scamping, q.v.

    s., echo. Parrotlike repetition of words spoken by others. SYN: *echolalia.*

    s., interjectional. Speech characterized by inarticulate sounds.

    s., mirror. Reversing the order of syllables of a word.

    s., scamping. Omission of consonants or syllables when unable to pronounce them.

    s., scanning. A staccato-like speech with pauses between syllables.

    s., slurring. Slovenly articulation of letters difficult to pronounce.

    s., staccato. Slow and laborious speech with each syllable pronounced separately, as in multiple sclerosis.

speech, words pert. to: acataphasia; alliteration; allolalia; alogia; anarthria literalis; anchone; angophrasia; aphasia; aphemia; aphonia; aphrasia; aphthenxia; aphthongia; area, Broca's; articulation; asaphia; ataxophemia; baryglossia; barylalia; baryphonia; betacism; bradyarthria; bradylalia; bradyphrasia; bradyphrenia; bredouillement; cataphasia; deaf mute; divagation; dyslalia; dyslexia; dysphasia; dysphemia; dysphonia; egophony; hyperplasia; labialism; lallation; lalopathy; laloplegia; monophasia; mute; mutism; nyctophonia; onomatomania; onomatopoiesis; oxylalia; palilalia; palinphrasia; perseveration; scanning speech; stammering; stutter; tachyphasia; Wernicke's syndrome.

sperm (spĕrm) [Gr. *sperma,* seed]. 1. The ejaculate from the male; contains spermatozoa. SYN: *semen,* q.v. 2. Spermatozoa, q.v.

    s. cell. A spermatozoon or spermatid.

    s. center. The spermatozoon's centrosome during fertilization.

    s. nucleus. The head of a spermatozoon.

sperma (spĕr'mă) [Gr.]. 1. Testicular secretion containing the male reproductive cells, spermatozoa. SYN: *semen.* 2. Individual male germ cell. 3. Also used as a combining form.

spermacrasia (spĕr"măk-rā'zĭ-ă) [Gr. *sperma,* seed, + *akrasia,* bad mixture]. Lack of spermatozoa in the semen.

spermatemphraxis (sper-măt-ĕm-frăk'sĭs) ["+ *emphraxis,* stoppage]. An obstruction to emission of semen.

spermatic (sper-măt'ĭk) [Gr. *sperma,* seed]. Pert. to semen or sperm.

    s. arteries. Two long, slender vessels, branches of the abdominal aorta, following each spermatic cord to the testes.

    s. cord. The cord suspending the testis composed of veins, arteries, lymphatics, nerves, and the ductus deferens. SEE: *cord, infundibuloform, varicocele.*

    s. duct. Canal for passage of semen, esp. the ductus deferens and the ejaculatory duct.

    s. vein. One of two veins draining the testes. The right one empties into the inferior vena cava, the left into the left renal vein. In the spermatic cord, each forms a dilated pampiniform plexus.

spermaticidal (spĕrm"ăt-ĭ-sīd'ăl). Destructive to or causing the death of spermatozoa.

spermatid (sper'mă-tĭd). A cell arising by division of the secondary spermatocyte to become a spermatozoon.

spermatin (sperm'ă-tĭn). A mucilaginous substance in the semen.

spermatism (sper'mă-tĭzm) [Gr. *sperma,* seed, + *-ismos,* condition]. Ejaculation of semen, voluntarily or otherwise.

spermatitis (sper"mă-tī'tĭs) ["+ *-itis,* inflammation]. Inflammation of the spermatic cord or of the ductus deferens. SYN: *deferentitis, funiculitis.*

spermato- [Gr. *sperma, spermatos,* seed]. Combining form meaning sperm, to sow seed.

spermatoblast (sper-măt′ō-blăst) [Gr. *spermatos,* seed, + *blastos,* germ]. The rudimentary spermatozoon. SYN: *spermatid.*

spermatocele (sper-măt′ō-sēl) ["+ *kēlē,* mass]. A cystic tumor of the epididymis containing spermatozoa.

spermatocidal (sper″mă-tō-sī′dăl) ["+ L. *cidus,* kill]. Destroying spermatozoa.

spermatocyst (sper-măt′ō-sĭst) [Gr. *spermatos,* seed, + *kystis,* a sac]. 1. A seminal vesicle. 2. Tumor of epididymis containing semen. SYN: *spermatocele.*

spermatocystectomy (sper″măt-ō-sĭs-tĕk′-tō-mĭ) ["+ "+ *ektomē,* excision]. Removal of the seminal vesicles.

spermatocystitis (sper″măt-ō-sĭs-tī′tĭs) ["+ "+ *-itis,* inflammation]. Inflammation of a seminal vesicle. SYN: *seminal vesiculitis.*

spermatocystotomy (sper″măt-ō-sĭs-tŏt′ō-mĭ) ["+ "+ *tomē,* a cutting]. Incision into a seminal vesicle for drainage.

spermatocyte (sper-măt′ō-sīt) [Gr. *spermatos,* seed, + *kytos,* cell]. A cell originating from a spermatogonium which forms by division the spermatids which give rise to spermatozoa.

    s., primary. Cell arising by growth and development from a spermatogonium.

    s., secondary. Cell arising from primary spermatocyte by a miotic division. It undergoes a second miotic division, giving rise to two spermatids with haploid, q.v., number of chromosomes.

spermatogenesis (sper-măt-ō-jĕn′ē-sĭs) ["+ *genesis,* produce]. The formation of mature functional spermatozoa. In the process, undifferentiated spermatogonia become primary spermatocytes each of which divides to form two secondary spermatocytes. Each of these divide to form two spermatids which transform into functional motile spermatozoa. In the process the chromosome number is reduced from the diploid to the haploid number. SEE: *gametogenesis; maturation; miosis.*

spermatogonium (sper-măt-ō-gō′nĭ-ŭm) ["+ *gonē,* generation]. (pl. *spermatogonia*) A large unspecialized germ cell which in spermatogenesis gives rise to a primary spermatocyte. SEE: *spermatogenesis.*

spermatoid (sper′mă-toyd) ["+ *eidos,* form]. Resembling a spermatozoon.

spermatology (sper-mă-tŏl′ō-jĭ) [Gr. *spermatos,* seed, + *logos,* a study]. The study of the seminal fluid.

spermatolysin (sper-măt-ōl′ĭ-sĭn) ["+ *lysis,* dissolution]. A lysin destroying spermatozoa.

spermatolysis (sper-măt-ōl′ĭ-sĭs) ["+ *lysis,* dissolution]. Dissolution or destruction of spermatozoa.

spermatolytic (sper-măt-ō-lĭt′ĭk). Destroying spermatozoa.

spermatopathia,   **spermatopathy** (sper″mă-tō-păth′ĭ-ă, spĕr-mă-tŏp′ă-thĭ) [Gr. *spermatos,* seed, + *pathos,* disease]. Disease of sperm cells or their secreting glands or ducts.

spermatophobia (spĕr-mă-tō-fō′bĭ-ă) ["+ *phobos,* fear]. Abnormal fear of being afflicted with spermatorrhea, involuntary loss of semen.

spermatopoietic (spĕr″măt-ō-poy-ĕt′ĭk) ["+ *poiein,* to make]. Promoting the formation and secretion of semen.

spermatorrhea (spĕr″mă-tō-rē′ă) [Gr. *spermatos,* seed, + *rhoia,* flow]. Abnormally frequent, involuntary loss of semen without orgasm.

spermatoschesis (sper″măt-ŏs′kē-sĭs) ["+ *schesis,* checking]. Suppression of the semen.

spermatospore (sper-mat′ō-spōr) ["+ *sporos,* a seed]. A primitive cell from which spermatozoa arise. SYN: *spermatogonium.*

spermatotoxin (spĕr″mă-tō-tŏk′sĭn) [Gr. *spermatos,* seed, + *toxikon,* poison]. A toxin which destroys spermatozoa. SYN: *spermatoxin.*

spermatovum (spĕr″măt-ō′vŭm) ["+ L. *ovum,* egg]. A fecundated or impregnated ovum.

spermatoxin (sper-mă-tŏks′ĭn) [Gr. *spermatos,* seed, + *toxikon,* poison]. A toxin which causes destruction of spermatozoa. It is formed by injecting spermatozoa from an animal of another species.

spermatozoa (spĕr″măt-ō-zō′ă). Pl. of spermatozoon.

spermatozoon (spĕr″măt-ō-zō′ŏn) [Gr. *sperma,* seed, + *zōon,* life]. (pl. *spermatozoa*) The mature male sex or germ cell formed within the seminiferous tubules of the testes. The s. has a broad, oval, flattened head with a nucleus and a protoplasmic neck or middle piece and tail. It is about 1/500 in. (51 microns or micrometers) in length and resembles a tadpole.

    It has the power of self-propulsion by means of a flagellum. Develops after puberty from the spermatids in the testes in enormous quantities. The head pierces the envelope of the ovum and loses its tail when fusion of the two cells takes place. This process is called fertilization.

RS: acrosome; fertilization; gamete; ovum; semen; sperm; zygote.

spermaturia (spĕr″mă-tū′rĭ-ă) [Gr. *sperma*, seed, + *ouron*, urine]. Semen discharged with the urine.

spermectomy (spĕr-mĕk′tŏ-mĭ) [″ + *ektomē*, excision]. Resection of a portion of the spermatic cord and duct.

spermic (spĕr′mĭk). Concerning sperm, male reproductive cells.

spermicidal (spĕr′mĭ-sĭ′dăl) [Gr. *sperma*, seed, + L. *cidus*, kill]. Killing spermatozoa.

spermicide (spĕr′mĭ-sĭd′). An agent which kills spermatozoa.

spermidine. A protein isolated from spermatozoa.

spermiduct (spĕr′mĭ-dŭkt) [Gr. *sperma*, seed, + L. *ductus*, a duct]. The ejaculatory duct and ductus deferens considered as one.

spermine. A protein isolated from spermatozoa.

spermiogenesis. The processes involved in the transformation of a spermatid to a functional spermatozoon.

spermium. A spermatozoon, q.v.

spermoblast (spĕr′mŏ-blăst) [Gr. *sperma*, seed, + *blastos*, a germ]. A cell developing into a spermatozoon. SYN: *spermatid; spermatoblast.*

spermolith (spĕr′mŏ-lĭth) [″ + *lithos*, stone]. A calculus in the seminal vesicle or spermatic duct.

spermolysin (spĕr-mol′ĭ-sĭn). A cytolysin formed following the inoculation of spermatozoa.

spermolytic (spĕr-mŏ-lĭt′ĭk) [″ + *lysis*, dissolution]. Causing the destruction of spermatozoa.

spermoneuralgia (spĕr″mŏ-nū-răl′jĭ-ă) [Gr. *sperma*, seed, + *neuron*, nerve, + *algos*, pain]. Neuralgic pain in the testicles and spermatic cord.

spermophlebectasia (spĕr″mŏ-flē″bĕk-tā′-zĭ-ă) [″+ *phleps*, vein, + *ektasis*, dilatation]. Varicosity of the spermatic veins.

spermoplasm (spĕr′mŏ-plăzm) [″ + *plasma*, a thing formed]. The protoplasm of a male germ cell.

spermosphere (spĕr′mŏ-sfēr) [Gr. *sperma*, seed, + *sphaira*, a circle]. Mass of spermatoblasts derived from spermatogonia.

spermospore (spĕr′mŏ-spōr) [″ + *sporos*, seed]. A primitive cell from which spermatozoa originate. SYN: *spermatogonium; spermatospore.*

spes phthisica (spēz′ tĭz′ĭ-kă) [L. *spēs*, hope, + *phthisis*, consumption]. A sense of well-being, happiness, and hopefulness in patients ill with tuberculosis. The cause may be an underlying fear from which the pa-tient tries to escape, and accomplishes it by repression, which manifests itself by characteristic behavior of the opposite extreme.

sp. gr. Abbr. for *specific gravity.*

sphacelate (sfăs′ĕl-āt) [Gr. *sphakelos*, gangrene]. 1. To affect with gangrene. 2. Gangrenous. SYN: *mortified; necrosed.*

sphacelation (sfăs″ĕl-ā′shŭn). Mortification; formation of a mass of gangrenous tissue. SYN: *gangrene; necrosis.*

sphacelism (sfăs′ĕl-ĭzm) [Gr. *sphakelos*, gangrene, + *-ismos*, condition]. Condition of being affected with sphacelus or gangrene. SYN: *necrosis.*

sphaceloderma (sfăs″ĕl-ō-dĕr′mă) [″+ *derma*, skin]. Gangrene of the skin, esp. when symmetrical. SEE: *Raynaud's disease.*

sphacelotoxin (sfăs″ĕl-ō-tŏk′sĭn) [″+ *toxikon*, poison]. Poisonous principle obtained from ergot used to produce abortion. SYN: *spasmotin.*

sphacelous (sfăs′ĕl-ŭs) [Gr. *sphakelos*, gangrene]. Pert. to a slough or patch of gangrene. SYN: *gangrenous; necrosed; necrotic.*

sphacelus (sfăs′ĕl-ŭs). 1. A necrosed mass of tissue. SYN: *slough.* 2. Process of becoming gangrenous. SYN: *gangrene; mortification; necrosis.*

sphagiasmus (sfă″jē-ăz′mŭs) [Gr. *sphagiasmos*, a slaying]. Spasm of neck muscles occurring in an epileptic seizure.

sphagitis (sfă-jī′tĭs) [Gr. *sphagē*, throat, + *-itis*, inflammation]. Inflammation of the throat.

sphenion (sfē′nĭ-ŏn) [Gr. *sphēn*, wedge]. (pl. *sphe′nia*) Point at apex of the sphenoidal angle of the parietal bone.

spheno- [Gr. *sphēn*, wedge]. Combining form meaning a wedge, the sphenoid bone.

sphenoethmoid (sfē″nŏ-ĕth′moyd) [″ + *ēthmos*, sieve, + *eidos*, form]. Pert. to the sphenoid and the ethmoid bones.

    s. recess. Groove back and above the superior concha, or turbinate bone.

sphenoid (sfē′noyd) [Gr. *sphēn*, wedge, + *eidos*, form]. Cuneiform or wedge-shaped.

    s. bone. Large bone at base of skull between occipital and ethmoid in front, and the parietal and temporal bones at the side.

    s. fissure. Fissure in s. and frontal bones for nerves and blood vessels.

sphenoiditis (sfē″noy-dī′tĭs) [″ + ″ + *-itis*, inflammation]. 1. Inflammation of the sphenoidal sinus. 2. Necrosis of the sphenoid bone.

sphenoidotomy (″+ ″+ *tomē*, incision]. Incision into sphenoid bone.

sphenomaxillary (sfē″nŏ-măk′sĭ-lā-rĭ) [Gr. *sphēn*, wedge, + L. *maxilla*, jaw]. Concerning the sphenoid and the maxilla.

sphenopalatine (sfē″nō-păl′ă-tēn) ["+ L. *palatum*, palate]. Concerning the sphenoid and palatine bones.

spheno′sis [Gr., wedging]. Condition in which fetus becomes wedged in pelvis.

sphenotresia (sfē″nō-trē′zĭ-ă) [Gr. *sphēn*, wedge, + *trēsis*, boring]. Perforating of the basal part of the fetal skull in craniotomy.

sphenotribe (sfē′nō-trĭb) ["+ *tribein*, to crush]. Instrument for breaking up basal part of fetal cranium.

sphere (sfēr) [Gr. *sphaira*, a globe]. 1. A ball or globelike structure. 2. The environment which one controls or in which one lives and works.

  s., attraction. A clear region in cytoplasm close to nucleus and usually containing a centriole or diplosome (a divided centricle). SYN: *cell center.*

spheresthesia (sfēr″ēs-thē′zĭ-ă) ["+ *aisthēsis*, sensation]. A morbid sensation, as of being in contact with a ball.

spherical (sfēr′ĭ-kăl) [Gr. *sphairikos*]. Having the form of, or pert. to, a sphere. SYN: *globular.*

spherocyte (sfē′rō-sĭt) [Gr. *sphaira*, globe, + *kytos*, cell]. An erythrocyte which assumes a spheroid shape.

spherocytosis (sfē″rō-sī-tō′sĭs) ["+ "+ *-ōsis*, condition]. Condition in which erythrocytes assume a spheroid shape. Occurs in certain hemolytic anemias.

spheroid (sfē′royd) ["+ *eidos*, form]. 1. A body shaped like a sphere. 2. Sphere-shaped.

spherolith (sfē′rō-lĭth) [Gr. *sphaira*, globe, + *lithos*, stone]. A minute concretion in the kidney of the newborn.

spheroma (sfē-rō′mă) ["+ *-ōma*, tumor]. A tumor of spherical form.

spherometer (sfē-rŏm′ĕt-ĕr) ["+ *metron*, measure]. Device to ascertain curvature of a surface.

spherospermia (sfē″rō-spĕr′mĭ-ă) [Gr. *sphaira*, globe, + *sperma*, seed]. Round spermatozoa without tails.

spherule (sfēr′ūl) [LL. *sphaerula*, little globe]. 1. A very small sphere. 2. A minute granule found in center of a centromere of a chromosome.

sphincter (sfĭnk′tĕr) [Gr. *sphinktēr*, a binder]. Circular muscle constricting an orifice. In normal contraction it closes the orifice.

  s. ampullae. Delicate network of fibers about papilla of Vater, occasionally present in adults, a part of s. of Oddi.

  s. ani. S. that closes the anus, the external one being of striated muscle, the internal one, of plain muscle.

  s., bladder. Plain muscle about opening of bladder into the urethra.

  s., cardiac. Plain muscle about the esophagus at cardiac opening into the stomach.

  s. choledochus. Smooth muscle investing common bile duct just before its junction with pancreatic duct; a part of s. of Oddi.

  s., ileocecal. Plain muscle about the ileum at its opening into the cecum.

  s. of Oddi. Contracted region in common bile duct at papilla of Vater.

  s. pancreaticus. Smooth muscle encircling pancreatic duct just before it joins ampulla.

  s., pyloric. A thickening of the muscular wall around the pyloric orifice.

sphincteralgia (sfĭnk″tĕr-ăl′jĭ-ă) [Gr. *sphinkter*, a binder, + *algos*, pain]. Pain in the sphincter ani muscles.

sphincterectomy (sfĭnk″tĕr-ĕk′tō-mĭ) ["+ *ektomē*, excision]. 1. Excision of any sphincter muscle. 2. Excision of part of the iris′ pupillary border. SYN: *oblique blepharotomy.*

sphincterismus (sfĭnk″tĕr-ĭz′mŭs) ["+ *-ismos*, condition]. Spasm of sphincter ani muscles.

sphincteritis (sfĭnk″tĕr-ī′tĭs) [Gr. *sphinktēr*, a binder, + *-ītis*, inflammation]. Inflammation of any sphincter muscle.

sphincterolysis (sfĭnk″tĕr-ŏl′ĭ-sĭs) ["+ *lysis*, dissolution]. Freeing of the iris from the cornea in anterior synechia affecting only the pupillary border.

sphincteroplasty (sfĭnk′tĕr-ō-plăs″tĭ) ["+ *plassein*, to form]. Plastic operation upon any sphincter muscle.

sphincteroscope (sfĭnk′tĕr-o-skōp″) [Gr. *sphinktēr*, a binder, + *skopein*, to examine]. Instrument for inspection of the anal sphincter.

sphincteroscopy (sfĭnk″tĕr-ŏs′kō-pĭ). Inspection of the internal anal sphincter.

sphincterotomy (sfĭnk″tĕr-ŏt′ō-mĭ) [Gr. *sphinktēr*, a binder, + *tomē*, a cutting]. Cutting of a sphincter muscle.

sphygmic (sfĭg′mĭk) [Gr. *sphygmikos*]. Rel. to the pulse.

sphygmo- [Gr. *sphygmos*, pulse]. Combining form indicating pulse.

sphygmobolometer (sfĭg″mō-bō-lŏm′ē-tĕr) ["+ *bōlos*, mass, + *metron*, a measure]. Device to measure force of the pulse rather than the blood pressure.

sphygmocardiogram (sfĭg″mō-kar′dĭ-ō-grăm) ["+ *kardia*, heart, + *gramma*, mark]. A tracing made by a sphygmocardiograph of the heartbeat and radial pulse.

sphygmocardiograph (sfĭg″mō-kăr′dĭ-ō-grăf) ["+ "+ *graphein*, to write]. Device for simultaneous recording of the radial pulse and the heartbeat.

sphygmocardioscope (sfĭg″mō-kăr′dĭ-ō-skōp) ["+ "+ *skopein*, to examine]. Device for recording the action of the pulse and heart. SYN: *sphygmocardiograph.*

sphygmochronograph (sfĭg″mō-krō′nō-grăf) [Gr. *sphygmos*, pulse, + *chronos*, time, + *graphein*, to write]. A sphygmograph recording graphically time between the heartbeat and the pulse.

sphygmogram (sfĭg′mō-grăm) ["+ *gramma*, mark]. A tracing of the pulse made by using the sphygmograph.

sphygmograph (sfĭg′mō-grăf) ["+ *graphein*, to write]. Instrument for recording the shape and force of the pulse wave.

sphygmoid (sfĭg′moyd) [Gr. *sphygmos*, pulse, + *eidos*, form]. Resembling the pulse.

sphygmology (sfĭg-mŏl′ō-jĭ) ["+ *logos*, a study]. Scientific study of the pulse.

sphygmomanometer (sfĭg″mō-măn-ŏm′ĕt-ĕr) ["+ *manos*, thin, + *metron*, measure]. Instrument for determining arterial blood pressure indirectly.

　　s., random-zero. A special type of s. which allows the blood pressure to be taken without the observer knowing where zero pressure is on the device. After the pressure is obtained the mercury comes to rest at a point. The observed pressure is then corrected by subtracting the at-rest value on the device from the pressure obtained. Used to prevent subjective bias in determining blood pressure.

sphygmometer (sfĭg-mŏm′ĕt-ĕr) ["+ *metron*, measure]. Instrument for measuring the pulse. SYN: *sphygmograph.*

sphygmophone (sfĭg′mō-fōn) [Gr. *sphigmos*, pulse, + *phōnē*, voice]. Instrument for hearing the pulse beat.

sphygmoplethysmograph (sfĭg″mō-plĕth-ĭz′mō-grăf) ["+ *plethysmos*, increase, + *graphein*, to write.]. Device which traces the pulse with its curve of fluctuation in volume.

sphygmoscope (sfĭg′mō-skop) ["+ *skopein*, to examine]. Instrument for showing the heart's movements or pulsations of arteries and veins.

sphygmosystole (sfĭg″mō-sĭs′tō-lē) [Gr. *sphigmos*, pulse, + *systolē*, contraction]. The segment of the sphygmogram that corresponds to the heart's systole.

sphygmotonograph (sfĭg″mō-tō′nō-grăf) ["+ *tonos*, tension, + *graphein*, to write) An instrument for simultaneous recording and timing of arterial blood pressure, jugular or carotid pulse, and the brachial pulse.

sphygmotonometer (sfĭg″mō-tō-nŏm′ĕt-ĕr) ["+ "+ *metron*, measure]. Instrument for ascertaining elasticity of walls of an artery.

sphygmus (sfĭg′mŭs) [Gr. *sphygmos*]. A pulse or pulsation.

sphyrectomy (sfĭ-rĕk′tō-mĭ) [Gr. *sphyra*, malleus, + *ektomē*, excision]. Surgical excision of the malleus.

sphyrotomy (sfĭ-rŏt′ō-mĭ) ["+ *tomē*, a cutting]. Surgical excision of a portion of the malleus.

spica (spi′kă) [L., ear of grain]. A reverse spiral bandage, the turn of which crosses like letter V. SEE: *bandage.*

spicular (spĭk′ū-lăr) [L. *spiculum*, a dart]. Pert. to or resembling a spicule; dartlike.

spicule (spĭk′ūl). A small, needle-shaped body.

　　s., bony. A needle-shaped fragment of bone.

spiculum (spĭk′ū-lŭm) [L., a dart]. (pl. *spicula*) A sharp, small spike. SYN: *spicule.*

spider (spi′dĕr). An insect, belonging to the order Araneae, subclass Arachnida, class Arachnoidea, phylum Arthropoda. Body is divided into cephalothorax and abdomen joined by narrow waist. A s. usually possesses four pairs of legs, poison fangs; it breathes by both lungs and trachea and often possesses spinnerets.

　　s. bites or poisoning. Not all spider bites are dangerous.

　　SYM: In general the victim is bitten about the genitalia. Local symptoms are slight burning followed in about half an hour by severe radiating pains, often extending long distances from puncture. Sloughing at site and along lymphatics may occur. Collapse, unconsciousness, convulsions, and death sometimes follow.

　　s., black widow. The female of Latrodectus mactans. It is glossy black in color with a brilliant red or yellow spot, usually shaped like an hourglass or two triangles, on under surface of the abdomen. Its bite causes excruciating pain and may prove fatal.

　　SYM: Initially the sensation resembles the prick of a pin. This pain usually lasts for a short period of time, subsides, and later the abdominal muscles become rigid. Within a half hour severe abdominal cramps begin. The venom which is neurotoxic causes an ascending motor paralysis. Because of the extreme abdominal pain the patient may be suspected of having an acute condition requiring abdominal surgery.

　　TREATMENT: Avoid all stimulants. Suction is of little value as the toxin is rapidly absorbed. Calcium gluconate intravenously often gives relief from pain. Large doses of morphine, repeated when necessary, given slowly by vein, also control pain. Heat, a hot tub, and forcing fluids also recommended. Specific antivenin is available from Merck, Sharp and Dohme, West Point, Pa. This horse serum-containing preparation should be given intramuscularly as soon as the diagnosis is made provided the patient is not sensitive to horse serum. SEE: *bites.*

s., brown recluse. Loxosceles reclusa, a small three-eighth in. (10 mm.) long spider native to North America. Its venom is quite toxic and is capable of causing death. The venom produces a large area of necrosis at the site of the bite. Treatment is symptomatic.

s. cells. Branching cells in neuroglia. SEE: *Deiters' cells; neuroglia cell.*

s. fingers. Abnormally long phalanges of the hands. SYN: *arachnodactyly.*

s. nevus. A branched growth of dilated capillaries on the skin resembling a s. SYN: *nevus araneus; vascular s.*

spigelian line (spī-jē'lī-ăn). [Adrian van der Spiegel, Flemish anatomist, 1578-1625]. Line on abdomen lying parallel to median line and marking edge of rectus abdominis muscle. SYN: *linea semilunaris; semilunar line.*

spigelian lobe. A small lobe behind right lobe of liver. SYN: *lobus caudatus of liver.*

spill (spĭl) [AS. *spillan*, to squander]. An overflow.

s., cellular. Dissemination of cells through lymph or the blood resulting in metastasis.

spiloma, spilus (spī-lō'mă, spī'lŭs) [Gr. *spilōma, spilos*, spot]. A mole or discoloration of skin. SYN: *nevus.*

spiloplania (spī''lō-plā'nī-ă) ["+ *plane*, a wandering about]. Transient and wandering erythema of the skin.

spiloplaxia (spī''lō-plăk'sī-ă) ["+ *plax*, plate]. A red spot appearing in leprosy.

spina (spī'-nă) [L., thorn]. (pl. *spi'nae*) [NA] 1. Any spinelike protuberance. 2. The spine.

s. bifida. Congenital defect in walls of spinal canal caused by lack of union between the laminae of the vertebrae. Lumbar portion is section chiefly affected.

SYM: As result of this deficiency the membranes of the cord are pushed through the opening, forming a tumor known as spina bifida, on account of condition of spine which gives rise to the deformity, and hydrorrhachis due to the fluid contained in the tumor.

s. bifida occulta. Failure of vertebrae to close but lacking hernial protrusion.

spinach (spĭn'ĭch) [Sp. *espinaca*]. A widely cultivated plant having edible leaves eaten as a vegetable. Rich in oxalates. SEE: *atriplicism.*

Food value of 100 gm. (cooked, boiled, drained): Cal. 23; protein 3.0 gm.; fat 0.3 gm.; carbohydrate 4.3 gm.; calcium 93 mg.; vitamin A, 8100 I.U.; ascorbic acid 28 mg.

spinal (spī'năl) [L. *spinalis*]. Pert. to the spine or spinal cord.

s. anesthesia. Anesthesia produced by an anesthetic injected into the spinal canal.

RS: anesthesia; cisternal puncture; lumbar puncture; spinal puncture.

s. canal. Canal of the vertebral column. RS: intrathecal; spina bifida; spinal puncture.

s. column. The vertebral column enclosing spinal cord consisting of 34 bones: 7 cervical, 12 dorsal or thoracic, 5 lumbar, 5 sacral vertebrae forming 1 bone and 4 coccygeal vertebrae fused into 1 bone.

s. cord. An ovoid column of nervous tissue about 44 cm. long, flattened anteroposteriorly, extending from the medulla to the 2nd lumbar vertebra in the spinal canal. All nerves to the trunk and limbs are issued from the spinal cord, and it is the center of reflex action containing the conducting paths to and from the brain.

In cross section, it does not fill the vertebral space, being surrounded by the pia mater, the cerebrospinal fluid, the arachnoid, and the dura mater, which fuses with the periosteum of the inner surfaces of the vertebrae.

The gray substance approximates the shape of an "H," there being a posterior and anterior horn in either half. The anterior horn is composed of motor cells from which the fibers making up the motor portions of the peripheral nerves arise. Sensory neurons enter posteriorly.

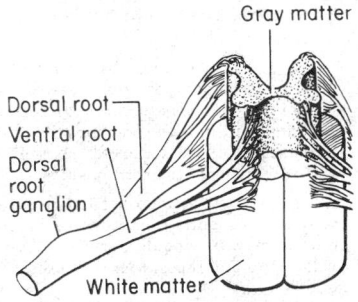

Gray matter

Dorsal root

Ventral root

Dorsal root ganglion

White matter

SPINAL CORD—CROSS SECTION

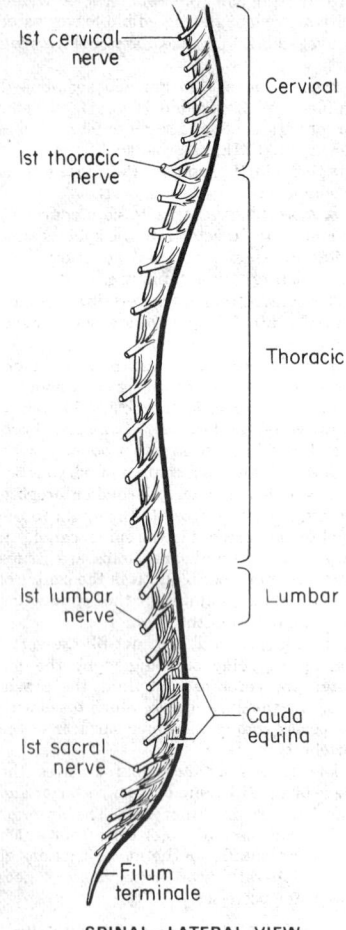

Ist cervical nerve

Cervical

Ist thoracic nerve

Thoracic

Ist lumbar nerve

Lumbar

Cauda equina

Ist sacral nerve

Filum terminale

SPINAL—LATERAL VIEW

The "H" also divides the surrounding white matter into posterior, lateral and anterior bundles. These serve to connect brain and cord in both directions (i.e., with efferent and afferent nerves) as well as various portions of the cord itself.

s. curvature. Abnormal curvature of the spine, frequently constitutional in children. It may be angular (caries), lateral (scoliosis), or anteroposterior (kyphosis, q.v., lordosis, q.v.).

s. curvature, angular. Caries of the spine. SYN: *Pott's disease,* q.v.

s. curvature, lateral. Deviation of spine to one side or the other causing a twist of the spine.

s. fluid. Cerebrospinal fluid, q.v. When normal, it contains 55 to 75 mg. of sugar per 100 cc. The sugar content is lower than that in the blood.

DIAG: *Cell count:* If normal, 0-10 cells per ml. in adults and 0-20 in children. Increased in all diseased states, several hundred or thousands in meningitis, when fluid becomes opaque. *Lymphocytes:* Found in encephalitis and tuberculous meningitis; polymorphonuclears predominate in septic meningitis and epidemic meningitis. *Bloody fluid:* Brain hemorrhages due to arteriosclerosis, high blood pressure, tumors and other causes. Spinal fluid may contain blood due to needle having punctured a small blood vessel. *Encephalitis:* Sugar content is increased, fluid clear, cell count 100 plus. *Globulin:* Negative in health, positive in disease.

Microorganisms: Meningococci, streptococci, pneumococci, tubercle bacilli, and influenza bacilli may be present, any of which may be indicative of meningitis. Epidemic meningitis indicated by gram-negative, intracellular diplococcus, biscuit-shaped microorganisms. Typhoid bacilli may produce meningeal symptoms in typhoid fever. Streptococci enter the meninges through the ear; the invading point of pneumococci, influenza bacilli, and pneumobacilli is the lungs. All these may be found in smears though sometimes missed and found in cultures. *Meningitis:* Lower spinal fluid sugar than sugar content of blood; 25 to 15 mg. If suppurative m., spinal fluid is puslike and turbid, but it is clear in tuberculous m., encephalitis and poliomyelitis. *Poliomyelitis:* Same as encephalitis, q.v.

RS: anhydromyelia; calcinorrhachia; cerebrospinal fluid; meningitis; poliomyelitis.

s. fusion. After removal of herniated disks, the adjacent vertebrae are immobilized by surgical procedure. SEE: *spondylosyndesis.*

s. ganglion. Enlargement on dorsal or posterior root of a spinal nerve composed principally of cell bodies of somatic and visceral afferent neurons.

s. nerves. Nerves arising from the spinal cord: 31 pairs, consisting of 8 cervical, 12 thoracic, 5 lumbar, 5 sacral, and 1 coccygeal, corresponding with the spinal vertebrae. SEE: *skeleton.*

Each spinal nerve is attached to the spinal cord by two roots: a dorsal or posterior sensory root and a ventral or anterior root. The former consists of afferent fibers conveying impulses to the cord; the latter of efferent fibers conveying impulses from the cord. A typical spinal nerve, on passing through the intervertebral foramen, divides into four branches, a recurrent branch, a dorsal ramus or posterior primary division, a ventral ramus, or anterior primary division, and two rami communicantes (white and gray) which pass to ganglia of the sympathetic trunk.

s. puncture. Puncture of the s. cavity with a needle to extract the s. fluid for diagnostic purposes, to introduce anesthetic agents into the s. canal, or to remove fluid so other fluids such as radio-opaque substances may be injected. SYN: *spinal tap.*

SITE OF PUNCTURE: To prevent injury of the nerve fibers, the puncture is usually made at the juncture between the 3rd and 4th lumbar vertebrae. A line drawn posteriorly from the crest of one ilium over the crest of the other will usually pass over the tip of the spinous process of the 4th lumbar vertebra. The point for the needle injection is directly above this line (i.e., toward the head).

NP: Drape a small table with a sterile sheet. Doctor's gown and gloves, flat gauze and iodine sponges are placed on the table. Sterile sponges and adhesive plaster should be in readiness. Patient may be placed sitting with feet over side of table, arms crossed with elbows on knees and head well forward; or in a lateral recumbent "curled-up" position with head and legs flexed. This allows maximum separation of the vertebrae.

If s. puncture is done in order to administer s. anesthesia, position of the patient is quite important. Anesthetic materials which are heavier than the spinal fluid will flow "down-hill" and those which are of less specific gravity than the s. fluid will flow "up-hill." Failure to be aware of this could lead to inadvertent paralysis of the vital centers of the brain. Thus the position of the patient must be specified by the anesthetist and changed only under his direction. *CAUTION:* If the cerebrospinal fluid pressure is elevated it may be dangerous to perform spinal puncture.

s. reflex. Any reflex centering in the s. cord.

s. shock. Effects resulting from transverse section of s. cord and which occur in segments below level of section. Principal effects are anesthesia, paralysis, loss of muscle tone, and suppression of reflexes, both visceral and somatic.

spinalgia (spī-năl′jĭ-ă) [L. *spina,* thorn, + Gr. *algos,* pain]. Pain in a vertebra under pressure.

spinalis (spī-nā′lĭs) [L.]. A muscle attached to the spinal process of a vertebra. SEE: *Table of Muscles* in *Appendix.*

spinant (spī′nănt) [L. *spinatus,* having thorns]. Any agent that increases spinal cord excitability.

spinate (spī′nāt). Having spines or shaped like a thorn.

spindle (spĭn′dl) [AS. *spinel*]. 1. A fusiform-shaped body. 2. The portion of the achromatic apparatus seen in mitosis consisting of a bundle of delicate fibrils which connect the two centrosomes or asters. The chromosomes arrange themselves on the spindle in an equatorial plate.

s., aortic. A dilatation of the aorta following the aortic isthmus.

s. cells. Fusiform cells.

s. legged. Having long, thin legs.

s., neuromuscular. A complex sensory nerve ending consisting of muscle fibers enclosed within a capsule and supplied by an afferent nerve fiber. It mediates proprioceptive sensations and reflexes.

s., neurotendinous. A proprioceptive nerve ending found in a tendon, in muscle septa or sheaths, in a muscle tissue, or at junction of a muscle or tendon. SYN: *Golgi tendon organ.*

spine (spīn). 1. A sharp process of bone. 2. The spinal column, consisting of 33 vertebrae: cervical 7, thoracic 12, lumbar 5, sacral 5, coccygeal 4. The bones of the sacrum and coccyx are ankylosed in adult life and counted as one each. SYN: *backbone.*

RS: cephalorhachidian; cord, spinal; cramp; curvature; rachialgia; rachilysis, "rach-" words; scoliosis.

s., alar, s., angular. Spinous process of the sphenoid bone. SYN: *spina angularis.*

s., anterior nasal. Projection formed by anterior prolongation of inferior border of nasal notch of maxilla.

s., bifid. SEE: *spina bifida.*

s., fracture of. A fractured s. often is treated in a plaster jacket with the spine hyperextended to reduce the fracture. A window is cut over the abdomen. If the fracture is high the neck is included in the jacket which must be short enough to allow flexion of the thighs. The patient is allowed to walk in the jacket which is left on for 3 or 4 months. A vest is put on under this plaster, and the prominences are padded with felt.

The muscles of the back are exercised by carrying weight on the head.

If the fracture involves the cord with paralysis below the injury, a plaster bed lined with felt is made. Bedsores and cystitis must be prevented. An enema is given when needed. Traction to the legs to take the weight off the sacrum and prevent bedsores may be employed.

s., frontal. Sharp-pointed medial process extending downward from nasal process of frontal bone. SYN: *nasal s.*

s., hemal. That part of the hemal arch of a typical vertebra that closes it in.

s., Henle's. S., suprameatal, q.v.

s., iliac. One of four spines of the ilium, namely the anterior and posterior inferior spines and the anterior and posterior superior spines.

s., ischial. S. of the ischium, a pointed eminence on its posterior border.

s., mental. Small process on inner surface of mandible at back of symphysis formed of one or more small projections (genial tubercles).

s., nasal. A sharp process descending in middle line from inferior surface of frontal bone between the superior maxillae.

s., neural. Spinous process of a vertebra. The posterior projection of the neural arch.

s., pharyngeal. Ridge under basilar process of the occipital bone.

s., posterior nasal. S. formed by medial ends of horizontal processes of palatine bones.

s. of the pubes. A prominent tubercle on upper border of the pubis.

s. of the scapula. An osseous plate projecting from the posterior surface of the scapula.

s., sciatic. Same as ischial.

s. of the sphenoid. Spinous process of greater sphenoid wing.

s., suprameatal. A small s. at junction of superior and posterior walls of the external auditory meatus. SYN: *Henle's s.*

s., typhoid. Acute arthritis due to infection causing spinal ankylosis during or following typhoid fever.

spinifugal (spī-nǐf'ū-gǎl) [L. *spina*, thorn, + *fugāre*, to flee]. Moving away from the spinal cord.

spinnbarkheit (spǐn'bǒr-kǐt) [Ger.]. The elasticity of cervical mucus discharge at ovulation. Useful in choosing a day for therapeutic insemination.

The cervical secretion is aspirated and placed on a slide. Spinnbarkheit is measured by pulling upward on the secretion with a forceps. Before ovulation there is no elastici-

ty. On the day of ovulation there is good elasticity, measuring 12-24 cm. or more. The day after ovulation elasticity diminishes.

Not all women have SBK changes that are clear-cut. Therefore this test is used in conjunction with other signs of ovulation. ABBR: SBK. SEE: *fern pattern; mittelschmerz; mucorrhea.*

spinobulbar (spī''nō-bŭl'bǎr) ["+ Gr. *bulbos*, a bulb]. Concerning the spinal cord and medulla oblongata.

spinocellular (spī''nō-sěl'ū-lǎr) ["+ *cellula*, a little chamber]. Pert. to or like prickle cells.

spinocerebellar (spī''nō-sěr-ĕ-běl'ǎr) [L. *spina*, thorn, + *cerebellum*, little brain]. Concerning spinal cord and cerebellum.

spinocortical (spī''nō-kōr'tǐ-kǎl) ["+ *cortex*, rind]. Pert. to the spinal cord and cerebral cortex. SYN: *corticospinal.*

spinoglenoid (spī''nō-glěn'oyd) ["+ Gr. *glēnē*, cavity, + *eidos*, form]. Rel. to the spine of scapula and glenoid cavity.

s. ligament. Ligament joining spine of the scapula to the border of the glenoid cavity.

spinotectal (spī''nō-těk'tǎl) [L. *tectum*, roof]. Pert. to the spinal cord and the tectum, the dorsal portion (corpora quadrigemina) of the midbrain.

spinous (spī'nǔs) [L. *spina*, thorn]. Pert. to or resembling a spine.

s. point. Spot over a spinous process very sensitive to pressure.

s. process. Prominence at posterior part of each vertebra.

spintherism (spǐn'thěr-ǐzm) [Gr. *spinthērizein*, to emit sparks]. Sensation of sparks before the eyes.

spintheropia (spǐn''thěr-ō'pǐ-ǎ) [Gr. *spinthēr*, spark, + *ōps*, eye]. Subjective sensation of sparks before the eyes.

spiradenitis (spī''rǎd-ĕn-ī'tǐs) [Gr. *speira*, coil, + *adēn*, gland, + *-itis*, inflammation]. A funiculus beginning in coil of a sweat gland. SYN: *hidrosadenitis phlegmonous.*

spiradenoma (spī''rǎd-ĕn-ō'mǎ) ["+ "+ *-ōma*, tumor]. Tumor of the sweat glands.

spiral (spī'rǎl) [L. *spiralis*]. Coiling around a center like the thread of a screw.

s. bandage. Roller bandage to be applied spirally.

s. canal of the cochlea. The bony cochlea enclosing the scala tympani, scala vestibuli, and cochlear duct.

s. canal of modiolus. Canal that runs spirally around the modiolus and contains spiral ganglion.

s. lamina. A thin, bony plate projecting from the modiolus into the cochlear canal dividing it into two portions, the upper scala vestibuli and lower scala tympani. SYN: *lamina spiralis.*

s. organ of Corti. Structure in floor of cochlear duct resting on basilar membrane. It contains hair cells, the receptors of stimuli produced by sound. SEE: *Corti, organ of.*

spirilla (spī-rĭl′ă) [L.]. Pl. of spirillum, q.v.

spirillicidal (spī-rĭl′′ĭ-sĭd′ăl) [L. *spirillum,* coil, + *cidus,* kill]. Destroying spirochetes or spirilla.

spirillicide (spī-rĭl′ĭ-sĭd). Destructive to spirilla.

spirillolysis (spī′′rĭ-lŏl′ĭ-sĭs) [L. *spirillum,* coil, + Gr. *lysis,* dissolution]. The destruction of spirilla.

spirillo′sis ["+ Gr. *-ōsis,* condition]. A disease caused by presence of spirilla in the blood.

spirillotropic (spī′′rĭ-lō-trŏp′ĭk) ["+ Gr. *tropē,* a turning]. Having an attraction to spirilla.

spirillotropism (spī′′rĭ-lŏt′rō-pĭzm) ["+ "+ *ismos,* condition]. The ability to attract spirilla.

Spirillum (spī-rĭl′ŭm) [L., coil]. (pl. *Spiril′la*) A genus of spiral-shaped motile microorganisms belonging to the family Pseudomonadaceae, tribe Spirilleae. Found in fresh and salt water.

S. minus. Found in the blood of rats and mice. The causative agent of one form of ratbite fever.

spirillum. (pl. *spiril′la*) A flagellated aerobic bacterium with an elongated spiral shape, of the genus Spirillum.

spirit (spĭr′ĭt) [L. *spiritus,* breath]. 1. A solution of essential or volatile liquid. 2. Any distilled or volatile liquid. 3. Alcoholic beverage.

s. of ammonia. A mixture of ammonia, alcohol, various flavoring oils, and distilled water, employed as a stimulant for persons who feel faint. A pledget of cotton moistened with the s. is held to the nose. SYN: *aromatic s. of ammonia.*

s. of bitter almond. A mixture of oil of bitter almond, almond, and distilled water, employed as flavoring agent.

s. of camphor. A mixture of camphor and alcohol, employed locally as a counterirritant.

s. of glyceryl trinitrate. An alcoholic solution of glyceryl trinitrate employed in angina pectoris, asthma, and as a relaxant in arterial spasm.

s. of juniper. A mixture of oil of juniper and alcohol.

s. of lavender. A mixture of oil of lavender flowers and alcohol, employed as a flavoring agent.

s. of mustard. A solution of volatile oil of mustard in alcohol, employed as a counterirritant.

s. of peppermint. A mixture of oil of peppermint, peppermint and alcohol, employed as a carminative.

spir′itual ther′apy [L. *spiritus,* breath, + Gr. *therapeia,* treatment]. The application of spiritual knowledge in the treatment of all mental and physical disorders. Based upon the assumption that man is a spiritual being living in a spiritual universe, that in proportion to his acceptance of this idea and in proportion to his success in demonstrating it, he may control the body and the material elements in harmony with a Divine plan.

spirituous (spĭr′ĭt-ū-ŭs′) [L. *spiritus,* breath]. 1. Pert. to alcohol. 2. An alcoholic.

spiritus (spĭr′ĭ-tŭs) [L., breath]. Alcoholic solution of a volatile substance. Usually, 5-10% strength. SYN: *spirit.*

s. frumenti. Whiskey.

s. juniperi. Gin.

s. myrciae. Bay rum.

s. vini gallici. Brandy.

Spirochaeta (spī′′rō-kē′tă) [Gr. *speira,* coil, + *chaitē,* hair]. A genus of slender, spiral, motile microorganisms belonging to the family Spirochaetaceae, order Spirochaetales.

S. icterohaemorrhagiae. Species found in Weil's disease or acute febrile jaundice. SYN: *Leptospira icterohemorrhagiae.*

S. nodosa. Assumed pathogenic organism of Weil's disease, q.v. SYN: *Spirillum minus,* q.v.

S. pallida. Treponema pallidum, the microorganism which causes syphilis.

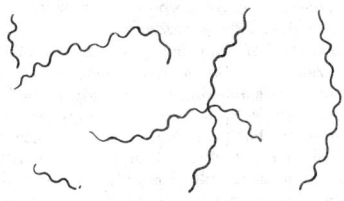

SPIROCHAETA PALLIDA

Spirochaetales (spī′′rō-kē-tā′lēs). An order of slender, flexuous spiral organisms belonging to the class Schizomycetes. It includes the families Spirochaetaceae and Treponemataceae.

spirochetal (spī"rō-kē'tăl) [Gr. *speira*, coil, + *chaitē*, hair]. Pert. to spirochetes, esp. infections caused by them.

spirochetalytic (spī"rō-kē"tă-lĭt'ĭk) ["+ "+ *lysis*, dissolution]. Destructive of spirochetes.

spirochete (spī"rō-kēt). Any member of the order Spirochaetales.

spirochetemia (spī"rō-kē-tē'mĭ-ă) [Gr. *speira*, coil, + *chaitē*, hair, + *haima*, blood]. Spirochetes in the blood.

spirocheticidal (spī"rō-kē"tĭ-sī'dăl) ["+ "+ L. *cidus*, kill]. Destructive to spirochetes.

spirocheticide (spī"rō-kē'tĭ-sīd). Anything that destroys spirochetes.

spirochetolysis (spī"rō-kē-tŏl'ĭ-sĭs) [Gr. *speira*, coil, + *chaitē*, hair, + *lysis*, dissolution]. The destruction of spirochetes by specific antibodies, chemotherapy, or lysins.

spirochetosis (spī"rō-kē-tō'sĭs) ["+ "+ *-osis*, condition]. Any infection caused by spirochetes.

spirochetotic (spī"rō-kē-tŏt'ĭk). Pert. to or marked by spirochetosis.

spirocheturia (spī"rō-kē-tū'rĭ-ă) [Gr. *speira*, coil, + *chaitē*, hair, "+ "+ *ouron*, urine]. Spirochetes in the urine.

spirogram (spī'rō-grăm") [L. *spirāre*, to breathe, + Gr. *gramma*, a mark]. A tracing made by a spirograph indicating respiratory movements.

spirograph (spī'rō-grăf) ["+ Gr. *graphein*, to write.]. Device for recording graphically respiratory movements.

spiroid (spī'royd) [Gr. *speira*, coil, + *eidos*, form]. Resembling a spiral.

spirokinesis (spī"rō-kĭn-ē'sĭs) ["+ *kinesis*, motion]. The tendency of motile organisms, including man, to veer or move in a spiral direction when deprived of external reference points.

spiroma (spī-rō'mă) ["+ *-ōma*, tumor]. Multiple, benign, cystic epithelioma of the sweat glands. SYN: *spiradenoma*.

spirometer (spī-rŏm'ĕt-ĕr) [L. *spirāre*, to breathe, + Gr. *metron*, measure]. An apparatus consisting of a cylindrical bell immersed in water and so equipped with outlets that gases can be exhaled into it or inhaled out of it while measurements of volume are made. The following are typical measurements made on normal men by using the spirometer:

Complemental air (Inspiratory reserve volume): 1600 cc., the amount which a subject can still inhale by special effort after a normal inspiration.

Dead space air: 150 cc., the air inhaled through the nose, which gets only as far as nasopharynx or trachea and does not reach the lungs.

Functional residual air (Functional residual capacity): About 2600 cc., the sum of the supplemental and residual air.

Minimal air: Less than 1000 cc., that which remains in the lungs after complete collapse as in pneumothorax.

Reserve air: Supplemental air, q.v.

Residual air (Residual volume): 1000 cc. that are left in the lungs after a complete expiration.

Supplemental air (Expiratory reserve volume): 1600 cc. which can still be exhaled after a normal exhalation.

Tidal volume: 500 cc., the amount exhaled or inhaled during normal respiration.

spirometry (spī-rŏm'ē-trī) [L. *spirāre*, to breathe, + Gr. *metron*, measure]. Measurement of air capacity of the lungs.

spirophore (spī'rō-fōr) ["+ Gr. *phoros*, a bearer]. A cabinet device used for artificial respiration. SYN: *iron lung*.

spiroscope (spī'rō-skōp) ["+ Gr. *skopein*, to examine]. Device for measuring air capacity of the lungs.

spiroscopy (spī-rŏs'kō-pī). The use of the spiroscope to measure respiratory capacity of the lungs.

spissated (spĭs'ăt-ēd) [L. *spissatus*]. Thickened. SYN: *inspissated*.

spissitude (spĭs'ĭ-tūd) [L. *spissitudo*]. Condition of being inspissated, as a fluid thickened by evaporation almost to a solid; thickness.

spit (spĭt) [AS. *spittan*]. 1. Saliva. SYN: *expectoration; spittle; sputum*. 2. To expectorate spittle.

spit'tle [AS. *spātl*]. The digestive fluid of the mouth. SYN: *saliva*.

splanchna (splăngk'nă) [Gr.]. The intestines or the viscera.

splanchnapophysis (splăngk"nă-pŏf'ĭ-sĭs) [Gr. *splanchnos*, viscus, + *apophysis*, offshoot]. 1. Any skeletal element connected with the alimentary canal, as the lower jaw. 2. Outgrowth of a vertebra on opposite side of a vertebral axis, enclosing some viscus.

splanchnectopia (splăngk"něk-tō'pī-ă) ["+ *ektopos*, out of place]. Dislocation of a viscus or of the viscera.

splanchnemphrasix (splăngk"něm-frăk'-sĭs) ["+ *emphraxis*, stoppage]. Obstruction of any internal organ, particularly of the intestine.

splanchnesthesia (splăngk"něs-thē'zĭ-ă) [Gr. *splanchnos*, viscus, + *aisthēsis*, sensation]. Visceral sensation.

splanchnesthetic (splăngk"něs-thět'ĭk). Rel. to visceral consciousness or sensation.

splanchnic (splăngk'nĭk) [Gr. *splanchnikos*]. Pert. to the viscera.

s. nerves. Three nerves from the thoracic sympathetic ganglia distributed to the viscera.

splanchnicotomy (splăngk"nĭ-kŏt'ō-mĭ) ["+ *tomē*, a cutting]. Section of a splanchnic nerve.

splanchnoblast (splăngk'nō-blăst) [Gr. *splanchnos*, viscus, + *blastos*, germ]. Incipient rudiment of a viscus. SEE *anlage; proton.*

splanchnocele (splăngk'nō-sēl). 1. ["+ *koilos*, a hollow]. That part of the coelom persisting in the adult, giving rise to the visceral cavities. SYN: *splanchnocoele.* 2. ["+ *kēlē*, hernia]. Protrusion of any abdominal viscus.

splanchnocoele (splăngk'nō-sēl) [Gr. *splanchnos*, viscus, + *koilos*, a hollow]. Rudimentary embryonic cavity from which the visceral cavities arise.

splanchnocranium (splănk"nō-krā'nĭ-ŭm) ["+ *kranion*, upper part of head]. The portion of the skull derived from the visceral or branchial skeleton.

splanchnodiastasis (splăngk"nō-dĭ-ăs'tă-sĭs) ["+ *diastasis*, separation]. Displacement or separation of any viscus.

splanchnodynia (splăngk-nō-dĭn'ĭ-ă) [Gr. *splanchnos*, viscus, + *odynē*, pain]. Pain in the abdominal region.

splanchnography (splăngk-nŏg'ră-fĭ) ["+ *graphein*, to write]. Descriptive treatise on anatomy of the viscera.

splanchnolith (splăngk'nō-lĭth) ["+ *lithos*, stone]. An intestinal calculus.

splanchnology (splăngk-nŏl'ō-jĭ) [Gr. *splanchnos*, viscus, + *logos*, a study]. The study of the viscera.

splanchnopathia (splăngk"nō-păth'ĭ-ă) ["+ *pathos*, disease]. Pathological conditions of the viscera.

splanchnopleure (splăngk'nō-plūr) ["+ *pleura*, side]. The embryonic layer formed by the union of the visceral layer of the mesoderm with the entoderm. SEE: *somatopleure.*

splanchnoptosia, splanchnoptosis (splăngk"nō-tō'sĭ-ă, -sĭs) [Gr. *splanchnos*, viscus, + *ptōsis*, a dropping]. Prolapse of the viscera. SYN: *abdominal ptosis; enteroptosia; visceroptosia.*

splanchnosclerosis (splăngk"nō-sklēr-ō'sĭs) ["+ *sklerōsis*, a hardening]. Hardening of any of the viscera through overgrowth of connective tissue.

splanchnoscopy (splăngk-nŏs'kō-pĭ) ["+ *skopein*, to examine]. Examination of the viscera with aid of roentgen rays or transillumination.

splanchnoskeleton (splăngk"nō-skĕl'ē-tŏn) [Gr. *splanchnos*, viscus, + *skeleton*, skeleton]. 1. In primitive vertebrates such as fishes, the cartilaginous or bony arches (branchial) which encircle pharyngeal portion of digestive tract. 2. In higher vertebrates, the bones derived from the branchial arches which include the maxilla, mandible, maleus, incus, stapes, hyoid bone, and cartilages of the larynx. SYN: *branchial skeleton; visceral skeleton.*

splanchnotomy (splăngk-nŏt'ō-mĭ) ["+ *tomē*, a cutting]. Dissection of the viscera.

splanchnotribe (splăngk'nō-trib) ["+ *tribein*, to crush]. A crushing instrument for temporarily closing the lumen of the intestine prior to resection.

splay'foot [ME. *splayen*, to spread out, + AS. *fōt*, foot]. A flatfoot or the deformity flatfoot. SYN: *pes planus; talipes valgus.*

spleen (splēn) [Gr. *splēn*]. The largest collection of reticuloendothelial cells in the body; an elongated, dark red, ovoid body lying in upper left quadrant of abdomen posterior and inferior to the stomach. It is composed of spongelike tissue (splenic pulp) consisting of lymphatic tissue differentiated into white pulp and pulp infiltrated with red blood cells (red pulp). It is enclosed by a dense capsule from which trabeculae extend into substance of spleen. On one side is the hilus through which enter splenic vessels and nerves. SYN: *lien.*

FUNCTIONS: *Blood formation:* In the embryo all types of blood cells are formed but in the adult only lymphocytes and monocytes. *Blood storage:* Smooth muscle and elastic tissue fibers in capsule and trabeculae enable spleen to contract and discharge blood cells into circulation. *Blood filtration:* By which bacteria and particulate matter, esp. worn-out red blood cells, are removed from circulation.

DISORDERS: Acute and chronic infections and certain infectionlike states, hypersplenism, primary splenic thrombocytopenia, primary splenic neutropenia, Felty's syndrome, Banti's disease, congestive splenomegaly, tumors, etc. SEE: *thrombosis.*

s., accessory. Splenic tissue nodules near the spleen.

s., floating or wandering. An enlarged, movable s. which is not protected by the ribs.

s., lardaceous. Enlargement of s. from lardaceous matter. SEE: *degeneration, amyloid.*

s. pulp. The spleen's soft parenchyma.

s., sago. S. having appearance of grains of sago, q.v.

splenadenoma (splēn'ăd-ē-no'mă) [Gr. *splēn*, spleen, + *adēn*, gland, + *-ōma*, tumor]. Enlargement of the spleen caused by hyperplasia of its pulp.

splenalgia (splē-năl'jĭ-ă) ["+ *algos*, pain]. Neuralgic pain in the spleen. SYN: *splenodynia.*

splenceratosis (splēn''sēr-ă-tō'sĭs) ["+ *keras, kerat-*, horn, + *-ōsis*, condition]. Induration of the spleen.

splenectasia (splē''něk-tā'zĭ-ă) [Gr. *splēn*, spleen, + *ektasis*, dilatation]. Enlargement of the spleen.

splenectasis (splē-něk'tă-sĭs). Enlargement of the spleen. SYN: *splenectasia.*

splenectomy (splē-něk'tō-mĭ) [Gr. *splēn*, spleen, + *ektomē*, excision]. Surgical excision of the spleen.

splenectopia, splenectopy (splē''něk-tō'pĭ-ă-něk'tō-pĭ) ["+ *ektopos*, out of place]. Displacement or mobility of the spleen. SYN: *floating spleen.*

splenelcosis (splē''něl-kō'sĭs) ["+ *helkōsis*, ulceration]. Ulceration or abscess of the spleen.

splenemia (splē-nē'mĭ-ă) [Gr. *splēn*, spleen, + *haima*, blood]. 1. Splenic congestion. 2. Leukemia with splenic hypertrophy.

splenemphraxis (splē''něm-frăk'sĭs) ["+ *emphraxis*, stoppage]. Congested condition of the spleen.

splenepatitis (splē''něp-ă-tī'tĭs) ["+ *hēpar, hēpat-*, liver, + *-itis*, inflammation]. Inflammation of both spleen and liver.

splenetic, splenic (splē-nět'ĭk, splēn'ĭk) [Gr. *splēnikos*]. 1. Pert. to the spleen. 2. Suffering with chronic disease of the spleen. 3. Surly, fretful, impatient.

s. cords. Poorly defined cords of red pulp of the spleen. SYN: *cords of Billroth.*

s. flexure. Junction of transverse and descending colon, making a bend on the left side near the spleen.

s. nodule. A concentrated mass of white pulp in the spleen. SYN: *malpighian body*, q.v.; *splenic corpuscle.*

s. sinus. One of a series of wide channels with thin walls forming an anastomosing plexus throughout red pulp of spleen. SYN: *cavernous veins; terminal veins.*

s. vein. Vein carrying blood from spleen to the portal vein.

splenicterus (splē-nĭk'tĕr-ūs) [Gr. *splēn*, spleen, + *ikteros*, jaundice]. Inflammation of spleen associated with jaundice.

splenification (splē''nĭ-fĭkā'shŭn) ["+ L. *facere*, to make]. Change in a structure whereby it resembles splenic tissue. SYN: *splenization.*

splenitis (splē-nī'tĭs) ["+ *-itis*, inflammation]. Inflamed condition of the spleen. Comprises acute and chronic hypertrophy, proliferative splenitis, and suppurative inflammation, the result of acute infectious disease.

SYM: Indefinite or absent. Usually little pain or tenderness unless perisplenitis exists. Considerable enlargement may be attended by sense of weight, tension, or distress in left hypochondrium, accompanied perhaps by slight dyspnea, sudden pain appearing in gastric region followed by vomiting of pus and blood in course of infectious disease, which may be due to abscess of spleen.

PROG: Depends upon systemic condition.

splenium (splē'nī-ŭm) [Gr. *splēnion*, bandage]. 1. A compress or bandage. 2. A structure resembling a bandaged part.

s. corporis callosi. [NA] The thickened posterior end of the corpus callosum.

splenius (splē'nī-ŭs). A flat muscle on either side of back of neck and upper thoracic area. SEE: *muscles* for illustration; *Table of Muscles* in *Appendix.*

splenization (splē''nīzā'shŭn). The change in a tissue, as of the lung, when it resembles splenic tissue.

splenocele (splē'nō-sēl) [Gr. *splēn*, spleen, + *kēlē*, hernia]. 1. A hernia of the spleen. 2. A splenic tumor.

splenoceratosis (splē''nō-sēr''ă-tō'sĭs) ["+ *keras, kerat-*, horn, + *-ōsis*, condition]. Induration of the spleen.

splenocleisis (splē''nō-klī'sĭs) ["+ *kleisis*, closure]. Friction on the surface of the spleen or wrapping with gauze in order to induce the formation of fibrous tissue.

splenocolic (splē''nō-kōl'ĭk) [Gr. *splēn*, spleen, + *kōlon*, colon]. Pert. to the spleen and colon or reference to a fold of peritoneum between the two viscera.

splenocyte (splē'nō-sīt) ["+ *kytos*, cell]. A unicellular leukocyte or lymphocyte of the spleen. It probably orginates elsewhere in the body.

splenodynia (splē''nō-dĭn'ĭ-ă) ["+ *odynē*, pain]. Pain in the spleen. SYN: *splenalgia.*

splenogenic, splenogenous (splē''nō-jěn'ĭk, splē-nŏj'ěn-ūs) [Gr. *splēn*, spleen, + *gennan*, to produce]. Originating in the spleen.

splenography (splē-nŏg'ră-fĭ) ["+ *graphein*, to write]. A treatise on, or a description of, the spleen.

splenohemia (splē″nō-hē′mĭ-ă) ["+ *haima*, blood]. Congestion of the spleen. SYN: *splenemia*.

splenohepatomegaly (splē″nō-hĕp″ă-tō-mĕg′ă-lĭ) [Gr. *splēn*, spleen, + *hēpar, hēpat-*, liver, + *megas*, large]. Enlargement of spleen and liver.

splenoid (splē″noyd) ["+ *eidos*, resemblance]. Resembling the spleen.

splenokeratosis (splē″nō-kĕr″ă-tō′sĭs) ["+ *keras*, horn, + *-ōsis*, condition]. Induration of the spleen.

splenology (splē-nol′ō-jĭ) [Gr. *splēn*, spleen, + *logos*, study]. The study of functions and diseases of the spleen.

splenolysin (splē-nŏl′ĭ-sĭn) ["+ *lysis*, dissolution]. An antibody which destroys splenic tissue.

splenolysis (splē-nŏl′ĭ-sĭs). Destruction of splenic tissue.

splenoma (splē-nō′mă) [Gr. *splēn*, spleen, + *-ōma*, tumor]. (pl. *splenomas, -mata*) A tumor of the spleen. SYN: *splenocele*.

splenomalacia (splē″nō-mă-lā′shĭ-ă) ["+ *malakia*, softening]. Softening of the spleen.

splenomegalia, splenomegaly (splē″nō-mē-gā′lĭ-ă, -mĕg′ă-lĭ) ["+ *megas*, large]. Enlargement of the spleen.

splenomyelomalacia (splē″nō-mī″ĕl-ō-mălā′shĭ-ă) [Gr. *splēn*, spleen, + *myelos*, marrow, + *malakia*, softening]. Abnormal softening of the spleen and bone marrow.

splenonephric (splē″nō-nĕf′rĭk) ["+ *nephros*, kidney]. Rel. to the spleen and the kidney. SYN: *lienorenal*.

splenonephroptosis (splē″nō-nĕf′rŏp-tō′sĭs) ["+ "+ *ptōsis*, a dropping]. Downward displacement of the spleen and kidney.

splenopancreatic (splē″nō-păn″krē-ăt′ĭk) [Gr. *splēn*, spleen, + *pankreas*, pancreas]. Rel. to the spleen and pancreas.

splenopathy (splē-nŏp′ă-thĭ) ["+ *pathos*, disease]. Any disorder of the spleen.

splenopexy (splē′nō-pĕk-sĭ) ["+ *pēxis*, fixation]. Artificial fixation of a movable spleen.

splenopneumonia (splē″nō-nū-mō′nĭ-ă) [Gr. *splēn*, spleen, + *pneumōnia*, inflammation of lung]. Pneumonia with splenization, q.v., of the lung.

splenoptosis (splē″nŏp-tō′sĭs) ["+ *ptosis*, a dropping]. Downward displacement of the spleen.

splenorenal (splēn″ō-rē′năl). Pert. to the spleen and kidney.

    s. shunt. Anastomosis of splenic vein to renal vein to enable blood from portal system to enter general venous circulation. Performed in cases of portal hypertension.

splenorrhagia (splē″nō-rā′jĭ-ă) [Gr. *splēn*, spleen, + *rhēgnynai*, to burst forth]. Hemorrhage from a ruptured spleen.

splenorrhaphy (splē-nōr′ă-fĭ) ["+ *rhaphē*, suture]. Suture of wound of the spleen.

splenotomy (splē-nŏt′ō-mĭ) [Gr. *splēn*, spleen, + *tomē*, a cutting]. Incision of spleen.

splenotoxin ["+ *toxikon*, poison]. Cytotoxin having specific action on splenic cells. SYN: *lienotoxin*.

splenulus (splĕn′ū-lŭs) [L., a little spleen]. A rudimentary or accessory spleen.

splint (splĭnt) [Middle D. *splinte*, a wedge]. An appliance made of bone, wood, metal, and/or plaster of Paris, used for the fixation, union, or protection of an injured part of the body. It may be movable or immovable.

    s., Agnew's. A s. used in fractures of the patella and metacarpus.

    s., airplane. An appliance usually used on ambulatory patients in the treatment of fractures of the humerus, and it takes its name from the elevated (abducted) position in which it holds the arm suspended in air.

    s., anchor. A s. for fracture of the jaw, with metal loops fitting over the teeth and held together by a rod.

    s., Ashhurst's. A bracketed s. of wire with a footpiece to cover the thigh and leg after excision of the knee joint.

    s., Balkan. S. for continuous extension in fracture of the femur.

    s., banjo traction. S. made out of a steel rod bent to resemble the shape of a banjo. Used for the treatment of contractures and fractures of the fingers.

    s., Bavarian. An immovable dressing in which the plaster is applied between two layers of flannel.

    s., Bond's. A s. for fracture of the lower end of the radius.

    s., Bowlby's. A s. for fracture of shaft of humerus.

    s., bracketed. A s. composed of two pieces of metal or wood united by brackets.

    s., Cabot's. A s. composed of a metal structure placed posterior to thigh and leg.

    s., Carter's intranasal. A steel bridge with wings connected by a hinge. Used for operation of depressed nasal bridge.

    s., coaptation. Small s. adjusted about a fractured part to prevent overriding of the fragments of bones. Usually covered by a longer s. for fixation of entire section.

    s., Dupuytren's. A s. to prevent eversion in Pott's fracture, q.v.

    s., Fox's. A s. for fractured clavicle.

    s., Gibson walking. Modification of Thomas' splint.

s., Gordon's. A side s. for the arm and hand in Colles' fracture, q.v.

s., inflatable. Inflatable device for immobilizing part or all of an extremity. The hollow tubular device is placed around the part and then inflated.

CAUTION: Do not inflate tightly enough to prevent flow of blood to and from the extremity. If the patient is to be transported by air, inflatable s. should not be used without carefully monitoring the pressure.

s., Jones' nasal. A s. for fracture of nasal bones.

s., Kanavel. S. for stiffened hands.

s., Levis'. A s. of perforated metal extending from below the elbow to the end of the palm; shaped to fit the arm and hand.

s., McIntire's. A s. shaped like a double inclined plane, used as a posterior s. for leg and thigh.

s., Sayre's. One of three varieties of s.: ankle, knee, and hip joint disease.

s., Stromeyer's. A s. with two hinged sections which can be set at any angle, used esp. for knee.

s. technology. The scientific study of splints.

s., Thomas' knee. A rigid metal used to remove pressure of body weight from weak knee joint by transferring weight to the ischium and perineum.

s., Thomas' posterior. A s. used in hip joint disease.

s., Volkmann's. S. for fracture of lower extremity, consisting of a footpiece and two lateral supports.

splinter (splin'tĕr) [Middle D. *splinte,* a wedge]. 1. A fragment from a fractured bone. 2. A slender, sharp piece of material piercing or imbedded in the skin.

s. hemorrhage. Small linear hemorrhage under the finger- or toenails. May be due to subacute bacterial endocarditis.

splint'ing. Fixation of a dislocation or fracture with a splint.

split (split) [D. *splitten,* to divide]. 1. A longitudinal fissure. 2. Characterized by a deep fissure.

s. foot. Congenital deformity, the division of the toes extending into the metatarsal region.

s. hand. Congenital deformity, the division between the fingers extending into the metacarpal region. SYN: *cleft hand.*

s. pelvis. Congenital failure of pubic bones to form a union at the symphysis.

s. tongue. A cleft or bifid tongue resulting from developmental arrest.

splitting (split'ing) [D. *splitten,* to divide]. In chemistry the breaking up of complex molecules into two or more simpler compounds.

spodogenous (spō-dŏj'ĕn-ŭs) [Gr. *spodos,* ashes, + *gennan,* to produce]. Caused by waste material.

s. splenomegaly. Enlargement of the spleen due to degenerated red blood cells.

spodogram (spŏd'ō-grăm) ["+ *gramma,* mark]. The pattern formed of the ash on microincineration of tissue or other matter.

spodophagous (spō-dŏf'ă-gŭs) ["+ *phagein,* to eat]. Destroying the waste matters in the body; said of scavenger cells.

spondylalgia (spŏn"dĭl-ăl'jī-ă) [Gr. *spondylos,* vertebra, + *algos,* pain]. Painful condition of a vertebra.

spondylarthritis (spŏn"dĭl-ăr-thrī'tĭs) ["+ *arthron,* joint, + *-itis,* inflammation]. Inflammation of a vertebra; arthritis of the spine.

spondylarthrocace (spŏn"dĭl-ăr-thrŏk'ă-sē) ["+ "+ *kakē,* badness]. Tuberculous condition of the vertebrae.

spondyl(e (spŏn'dĭl) [Gr. *spondylos*]. A vertebra.

spondylexarthrosis (spŏn"dĭl-ĕks"ăr-thrō'sĭs) ["+ *exarthrōsis,* dislocation]. Dislocation of a vertebra.

spondylitis (spŏn-dĭl-ī'tĭs) ["+ *-itis,* inflammation]. Inflammation of one or more vertebrae; esp. tuberculous disease of the vertebrae, Pott's disease, q.v.

s. ankylosing. S., rheumatoid, q.v.

s. deformans. Inflammation of the vertebral joints resulting in the outgrowth of bonylike deposits on the vertebrae which may fuse and cause rigid and distorted spine.

s., hypertrophic. Condition occurring in most people over 50 in which bodies of vertebrae hypertrophy. Bony changes such as slipping at bases, development of bony outgrowths on articular processes, etc., occur.

s., Kummell's. Traumatic s. in which symptoms do not appear until some time after the injury.

s., Marie-Strumpell. Ankylosing or rheumatoid spondylitis. SEE: *s., rheumatoid.*

s., rheumatoid. A chronic progressive disease involving the joints between articular processes, costovertebral joints, and sacroiliac joints. Bilateral sclerosis of sacroiliac joints is a diagnostic sign. Changes occurring in joints are similar to those seen in rheumatoid arthritis. Ankylosis may occur giving rise to stiff back (poker spine).

s. rhizomelica. Progressive rigidity of the spine caused by ankylosis of the vertebrae from below upward.

s. tuberculosa. Tuberculosis of the vertebral joints. SYN: *vertebral caries; Pott's disease,* q.v.

spondylizema (spŏn″dĭl-ĭ-zē′mă) [Gr. *spondylos,* vertebrae, + *izēma,* depression]. Downward settlement of a vertebra caused by the disintegration of the one below it.

spondylo- [Gr. *spondylos,* vertebra]. Combining form meaning a vertebra.

spondylocace (spŏn″dĭ-lŏk′ă-sē) [″+ *kakē,* badness]. Tuberculosis of the vertebrae. SYN: *spondylarthrocace.*

spondylodiagnosis (spŏn″dĭ-lō-dī″ăg-nō′sĭs) [″+ *dia,* through, + *gnōsis,* knowledge]. Diagnosis by means of visceral reflexes obtained by percussion over the vertebrae.

spondylodynia (spŏn″dĭ-lō-dĭn′ĭ-ă) [Gr. *spondylos,* vertebra, + *odynē,* pain]. Pain in a vertebra.

spondylolisthesis (spŏn″dĭ-lō-lĭs″thē′sĭs) [″+ *olisthēsis,* a slipping]. Forward subluxation of the lower lumbar vertebrae on the sacrum.

spondylolysis (spŏn″dĭ-lŏl′ĭ-sĭs) [″+ *lysis,* a dissolution]. The breaking down of a vertebral structure.

spondylopathy (spŏn″dĭl-ŏp′ă-thĭ) [Gr. *spondylos,* vertebra, + *pathos,* disease]. Any disorder of the vertebrae.

spondylopyosis (spŏn″dĭ-lō″pī-ō′sĭs) [″+ *pyōsis,* suppuration]. Suppuration with inflammation of a vertebra.

spondyloschisis (spŏn″dĭ-lŏs′kĭ-sĭs) [″+ *schisis,* cleft]. Congenital fissure of one or more of the vertebral arches. SYN: *rhachioschisis.*

spondylosis (spŏn″dĭ-lō′sĭs) [Gr. *spondylos,* vertebra, + *-ōsis,* condition]. Vertebral ankylosis.

s., rhizomelic. Ankylosis interfering with movements of hips and shoulders.

spondylosyndesis (spŏn″dĭ-lō-sĭn′dĕ-sĭs) [″+ *syndesis,* a binding together]. Surgical formation of an ankylosis between vertebrae.

spondylotherapy (spŏn″dĭl-ō-thĕr′ă-pĭ) [″+ *therapeia,* treatment]. Spinal therapeutics; spinal manipulation in the treatment of disease.

spondylotomy (spŏn″dĭl-ŏt′ō-mĭ) [″+ *tomē,* a cutting]. Removal of part of the vertebral column to correct a deformity or facilitate delivery of a fetus. SYN: *rachitomy.*

sponge (spŭnj) [Gr. *sphongos,* sponge]. 1. Elastic, porous mass forming internal skeleton of certain marine animals, or rubber or synthetic substance having absorbent qualities. Used in bathing or to mop up fluids in surgery. 2. An absorbent pad made of gauze and cotton. 3. Short for s. bath. 4. To moisten, clean, or wipe with a s.

s., abdominal. Flat sponges from 1/2 to 1 in. (1.27-2.54 cm.) thick, 3-6 in. (7.62-15.24 cm.) in diameter, used as packing, to prevent closing or obstruction by intrusion of viscera, as covering to prevent tissue injury, and as absorbents.

s., artificial. Constructed of antiseptic gauze.

s. bath. Bathing of the body with a wet s. or wash cloth.

s., gelatin. Spongy substance prepared from gelatin. It is a nonantigenic, readily absorbable material and used esp. to stop internal bleeding. Sold under trade name of Gelfoam.

s. graft. S. placed in an ulcer to cause granulation.

s. tent. S. impregnated with mucilage of acacia, dried in desired shape, to dilate the os uteri or sinuses by absorbing moisture and expanding.

spongiform (spŭn′jĭ-form) [Gr. *sphongos,* sponge, + L. *forma,* shape]. Having the appearance or quality of a sponge.

spongioblast (spun′jĭ-ō-blăst) [″+ *blastos,* germ]. Cell which develops from embryonic neural tube and serves as forerunner of ependymal cells and astrocytes.

spongioid (spŭn′jĭ-oyd) [″+ *eidos,* resemblance]. Resembling a sponge. SYN: *spongiform.*

spongioplasm (spŭnjĭ-ō-plăzm) [Gr. *sphongos,* sponge, + *plasma,* a thing formed]. Fibrillar network supporting protoplasm. SYN: *cytoreticulum.*

spongy (spŭn′jĭ). Resembling a sponge in texture.

spontaneous (spŏn-tā′nē-ŭs) [L. *spontāneus*]. Occurring unaided or without apparent cause; voluntary.

s. fracture. Fracture caused by the state of the bone and causing little or no injury.

ETIOL: Fragilitas ossium; nerve conditions, i.e., tabes; secondary malignant growths; atrophy in bones of the aged.

s. version. The unaided conversion of a transverse presentation of a fetus into a vertex or breech presentation.

spoon [AS. *spōn,* a chip]. Instrument consisting of a small bowl on a handle, used in scooping out tissues, tumors, etc., or in measuring quantities.

s. nail. A nail having a concave outer surface.

sporadic (spō-răd′ĭk) [Gr. *sporadikos*]. Occurring occasionally or in scattered instances, as a disease.

RS: endemic; epidemic; pandemic.

sporangiophore (spō-răn′jĭ-ŏ-fōr) [Gr. *sporos*, seed, + *angeion*, vessel, + *phoros*, a bearer]. In bacteriology, the supporting stalk for a spore sac of certain fungi.

sporangium (spō-răn′jĭ-ŭm). A sac enclosing spores, seen in certain fungi.

spore (spōr) [Gr. *sporos*, seed]. 1. A reproductive cell, usually unicellular, produced by plants and some protozoons. Usually spores are asexual, but certain fungi form sexual spores (oospores, zygospores, or ascospores). Spores usually possess a thick wall enabling the cell to withstand unfavorable environmental conditions.

Sporing is an asexual method of reproduction in many unicellular animals and plants. Certain bacteria also form spores, but more in the nature of a defensive mechanism than for reproduction. The spores of bacteria are difficult to destroy because they are very resistant to heat and require prolonged exposure to high temperatures to destroy them.

RS: apospory; asporogenic; asporous.

sporicidal (spōr-ĭ-sī′dăl) [Gr. *sporos*, seed, + L. *cidus*, kill]. Destructive to spores.

sporicide (spōr′ĭ-sīd). An agent which destroys spores.

sporiferous (spōr-ĭf′ĕr-ŭs) [Gr. *sporos*, seed, + L. *ferre*, to bear]. Producing spores.

sporoblast (spōr′ŏ-blăst) ["+ *blastos*, germ]. Structure within the oocyst of certain parasitic protozoons (Eimeria and Isospora) which gives rise to a sporocyst and eventually a spore.

sporocyst (spōr′ŏ-sĭst) ["+ *kystis*, sac]. 1. Any sac containing spores or reproductive cells. 2. Sac secreted around a sporoblast by certain protozoons prior to spore production. 3. Stage in life cycle of a trematode worm usually found in tissues of 1st intermediate host, a mollusk. It develops from a miracidium and is essentially a germinal sac containing germ cells. It gives rise to daughter sporocysts or redia.

sporogenesis (spōr″ŏ-jĕn′ĕ-sĭs) [Gr. *sporos*, seed, + *genesis*, production]. The production or formation of spores.

sporogenic (spōr″ŏ-jĕn′ĭk) ["+ *gennan*, to produce]. Having the ability of developing into spores.

sporogony (spōr-ŏg′ŏ-nĭ) ["+ *goneia*, generation]. Reproducing by development of spores. SYN: *sporogenesis*.

sporophyte (spōr′ŏ-fīt) [Gr. *sporos*, seed, + *phyton*, plant]. The spore-bearing stage of a plant exhibiting alternation of generation.

sporotrichin (spōr-ŏ′trī-kĭn). Antigenic substance derived from Sporotrichum and used for diagnostic purposes.

sporotrichosis (spōr″ŏ-trĭ-kō′sĭs) [Gr. *sporos*, seed, + *thrix*, hair, + *-ōsis*, condition]. A chronic granulomatous infection usually involving the skin and superficial lymph nodes characterized by formation of abscesses, nodules, and ulcers. It is caused by a fungus Sporotrichum schenckii, q.v.

Sporotrichum (spō-rŏt′rĭ-kŭm). (pl. *Sporotricha*) A yeastlike genus of microorganisms, one of which is the causative agent of sporotrichosis, q.v.

   S. schenckii. The causative agent of sporotrichosis.

Sporozoa (spŏr″ŏ-zō′ă) [Gr. *sporos*, seed, + *zōon*, animal]. A subphylum of the phylum Protozoa which includes a miscellaneous assortment of organisms which are parasitic, usually with complicated life-cycles including sexual and asexual forms and lacking locomotor organs in the adult forms. The medically important genera are Isospora, Plasmodium, and Toxoplasma.

sporozo′an. 1. Pert. to the sporozoa. 2. Sporozoon.

sporozoite (spŏr″ŏ-zō′ĭt) [Gr. *sporos*, seed, + *zōon*, animal]. 1. An animal spore. 2. An elongated sickle-shaped cell which develops from a sporoblast within the oocyst in the life cycle of the malaria organism. Upon bursting of oocyst, sporozoites are released into body cavity and make their way to salivary gland. They are introduced into human blood by a mosquito and almost immediately enter tissue cells. Here they go through two schizogonic divisions and then reenter blood stream and infect erythrocytes.

sporozo′on. (pl. *sporozo′a*) A protozoon belonging to the subphylum Sporozoa.

sport (spōrt) [ME. *sporten*, to divert]. An individual organism which differs spontaneously from the accepted limits of normal variation. SYN: *mutation, q.v.*

sporulation (spōr-ū-lā′shŭn) [L. *sporula*, little spore]. Production of spores, a method of reproduction of unicellular organisms.

spot (spŏt) [Middle D. *spotte*]. A small area of surface differing from surrounding parts in appearance. SYN: *loculus; macula; papule; pustule.*

   s., blind. The optic disk where optic nerve enters the retina.

   s., blue. S., Mongolian, q.v.

   s., cherry-red. Red spot occurring on retina in cases of amaurotic familial idiocy.

s., cold. An area on surface of skin which, when stimulated, gives rise to sensation of coldness.

s., corneal. An opaque area on the cornea. SYN: *leukoma.*

s.'s, Filatow's; s.'s, Flindt's. S.'s, Koplik's.

s., genital. Area on nasal mucosa which tends to bleed during menstruation SEE: *menstruation, vicarious.*

s., germinal. Old term for nucleolus of ovum.

s., hot. S., warm, q.v.

s., hypnogenic. A point which, when pressed, will throw a susceptible person into hypnosis or sleep.

s., hysterogenic. A point which, upon pressure, will induce in a susceptible subject an attack of hysteroepilepsy.

s.'s, Koplik's. Minute white or bluish-white spots on mucous membrane of mouth before appearance of the rash of measles.

s., liver. Chloasma, q.v.

s., milk. 1. A thickened and opaque area seen on epicardium in postmortems. 2. A dense area of macrophages in the omentum.

s., Mongolian. Bluish or mulberry-colored spots usually located in sacral region.

s.'s, rose. Rose-colored maculae occurring on abdomen or loins in eruption of typhoid fever.

s., ruby. A senile angioma. SEE: *angioma.*

s., temperature. A cutaneous area which responds to temperature changes. SEE: *s., cold; s., warm.*

s., warm. Areas on surface of skin which, when stimulated, give rise to sensation of warmth.

s., white. Light-colored, elevated areas of various sizes occurring on ventricular surface of anterior leaflet of mitral valve.

s., yellow. Area surrounding and including the fovea centralis in the retina. SYN: *macula lutea.*

spotted fever. Popular name for various eruptive fevers: typhus; tick fever; cerebrospinal meningitis.

s. f., Rocky Mountain. A febrile disease occurring in eastern and northwestern United States caused by Rickettsia rickettsii, transmitted by dog and wood ticks. SYN: *tick fever.*

s. f., South American. A febrile disease occurring in South America, esp. Brazil. It is caused by Rickettsia pijperi transmitted by the dog tick. SYN: *Sao Paulo* or *Colombian fever.*

spotting. Appearance of blood-tinged discharge from the vagina, usually between menstrual periods or at onset of labor.

sprain (sprān) [O.Fr. *espraindre,* to wring]. Trauma to a joint which causes pain and disability depending upon degree of injury to ligaments. In severe sprain, ligaments may be completely torn. The ankle joint is most often sprained. SEE: *fracture; strain.*

SYM: The signs of a sprain are rapid swelling, heat, and disability; often discoloration and limitation of function.

TREATMENT: Hot or cold compresses and bandaging; elevate the joint. If recovery proves slow, immobilization of the joint is indicated followed by careful massage. Very cold water helps to alleviate the pain and acts to prevent further swelling.

s. of back. Overstretching of muscles, ligaments, or other structures of spinal mechanism, often associated with small fractures.

SYM: Pain, esp. on extreme movements; tenderness; muscle spasm.

F. A. TREATMENT: Have patient lie down on rigid support, do not allow to sit up or walk until fracture is ruled out; intermittent heat, rest, with adhesive strapping, brace, etc.

s. of foot. Tearing of the ligaments of the foot or ankle.

SYM: Pain, tenderness, swelling, discoloration.

TREATMENT: Sprain is best treated as a fracture by complete immobilization until proven otherwise by x-ray examination.

s. fracture. The separation of a tendon or ligament from its insertion taking with it a piece of the bone.

s., riders'. Sprain of the adductor longus muscles of the thigh, resulting from strain in riding horseback.

spray (sprā) [Middle D. *spraeyen,* to sprinkle]. 1. A jet of fine medicated vapor applied to a diseased part or discharged into the air. 2. A pressurized container. SYN: *atomizer.* 3. To discharge fluid in a fine stream.

s. tube. Device for converting liquid into a spray.

spreading (sprĕd'ĭng) [AS. *sprǣdan,* to strew]. Indicating a growth on a bacterial culture, extending much (several mm. or more) beyond the site of inoculation.

s. factor. A substance produced by staphylococci which increases the permeability of connective tissue. SYN: *Duran-Reynal's factor; hyaluronidase.*

spring [AS. *springan,* a rising]. 1. The season of the year which comes after winter and before summer. SYN: *vernal season.* 2. A flying back of a body to its original position through its elasticity.

s. conjunctivitis. A form recurring each year in the spring but disappearing with the first frost. SYN: *vernal catarrh.* Arrested movement of a finger in flexion or extension followed by a jerk. SYN: *trigger finger.*

s. ligament. Interior calcaneoscaphoid ligament of the sole of the foot. It joins the os calcis to the scaphoid bone.

sprue (sprū) [D. *sprouwe*]. A disease endemic in many tropical regions and occurring sporadically in temperate countries, characterized by weakness, loss of weight, steatorrhea, and various digestive disorders, esp. impaired absorption of glucose, fats, and vitamins. It occurs in two forms, tropical and idiopathic or non-tropical sprue. Its cause is unknown.

spud (spŭd) [ME. *spudde,* short knife]. Short, flattened, spadelike blade to dislodge a foreign substance.

spur (spŭr) [AS. *spura,* a pointed instrument]. 1. A sharp or pointed projection. 2. A sharp horny outgrowth of the skin.

s., calcaneal. An exostosis of the heel, often painful and resulting in disability.

s., femoral. Spur sometimes present on medial and underside of neck of femur.

s., scleral. A pointed portion of sclera which projects into the deeper part of cornea immediately behind canal of Schlemm at angle of iris.

spurious (spūrĭ-ŭs) [L. *spurius*]. Not true or genuine; adulterated; false.

sputum (spū'tŭm) [L.]. (pl. *sputa*) Substance expelled by coughing or clearing the throat. It contains a variety of material from the respiratory tract including cellular debris,

Varieties of Sputum*
The Character and Diseases in Which They Occur

Variety of Sputum	Character of Sputum	Diseases in Which the Various Types Occur
Mucoid	Clear, thin, may be somewhat viscid	Early stages of bronchitis
Mucopurulent	Thick, viscid, greenish color, inoffensive, frothy, may have sweetish odor	Later stages of bronchitis, phthisis, pneumonia
Purulent	Thick, viscid yellow; often offensive	Abscess of lung, empyema, advanced phthisis, bronchiectasis
Nummular	Mucopurulent, with small, round, semisolid masses which sink in water	Advanced tuberculosis
Rusty	Mucopurulent, very viscid and gelatinous; rusty tinge	Pneumonia
Prune juice	Dark brown, offensive, often semisolid	Later stages of pneumonia, gangrene of lung, new growth in lung
Red currant jelly	Blood clots resembling currant jelly	New growth in lung
Blood (hemoptysis)	Bright red, frothy, with air bubbles; blood may be in streaks or mixed with sputum, fluid or clotted, or sputum may consist of pure blood	Tuberculosis (ulceration of a vessel in a cavity; other diseases of the lung (pneumonia, new growth, gangrene, abscess, bronchiectasis); mitral stenosis; aneurysm rupturing into the bronchial tubes

* Faber's *Nurses' Pocket Encyclopedia.*

mucus, blood, pus, caseous material, and microorganisms.

Its appearance depends upon the underlying condition as follows: *Amount:* Copious; seen in chronic inflammations of bronchial and pulmonary systems. Scanty; in all pulmonary bronchial acute inflammations and the early stages of lobar pneumonia and beginning bronchopneumonia.

Color: This depends upon its origin, cause, and amount of decomposition.

Conditions: Anthracosis (coal dust): sputum is black. Bronchiectasis: sputum is mucopurulent and foul if expectoration is infrequent. Bronchial asthma: scanty sputum and frothy, later becoming purulent and grayish, containing eosinophils. Bronchitis: sputum is mucous, later purulent, and in chronic cases, greenish-yellow and thick. Bronchopneumonia: frothy, mucoid, thin, mucopurulent, copious often with blood, or prune juice in color. Calcinosis: shows a sputum containing particles of lime or chalky deposits such as plaster of Paris. Empyema: if accompanied by perforations the sputum resembles that of pulmonary abscess. Gangrene of lung and putrid bronchitis: sputum has an obnoxious odor and is purulent, separates on standing into three layers containing pus cells, hematoidin crystals, and leukocytes. Lobar pneumonia: scanty and viscid, yellowish, and somewhat mucopurulent during early stages; in later stages, rusty, bloody, tenacious and viscid, esp. near or soon after crisis. Pulmonary abscess: usually purulent and fetid with many pus cells and pieces of lung tissue. Pulmonary tuberculosis: in early stages, scanty, whitish, or grayish-yellow, frothy, and expectorated in small quantities during coughing; later when consolidation takes place it becomes more copious, tenacious, and yellowish-gray; and in the late stages it becomes mucopurulent, musty and fetid, containing fibers and tubercle bacilli, sometimes blood-tinged or mixed with blood. Pneumonoconiosis: depends upon character of inhaled dust that produced the disease. Siderosis: contains particles of iron or other metals and resembles s. of chronic bronchitis. It also contains alveolar cells. Silicosis: produces s. containing particles of silica or other stone dusts.

RS: albuminoptysis; albuminoreaction; Charcot-Leyden crystals.

NP: Instruct patients to cover mouth and nose while coughing and to avoid exposing other persons to their cough. S. should be collected in covered disposable containers that may easily be burned. It may be disin-fected with 5% phenol or 5% formalin by one hour's exposure. Paper s. cups should be disposed of if there is any evidence of dried s. on them.

Handkerchiefs and gauze should not be used unless disposed of immediately after using. A paper bag should be attached to the bed or the bedside table. Paper wipes, squares of cloth, or soft tissues may be used for wiping away the discharge and disposing of it in the bag. The bag may be made of newspaper in a conical shape and pinned on the sheet; as the deposit accumulates, it is removed and another bag replaced. The patient should be instructed to keep the material deposited well covered. When removed, the paper should be folded over and placed in the waste can or burned at once.

s., bloody. This occurs in hemorrhages. If the blood is mixed with the s., the hemorrhage is in the finer bronchioles. Large quantities of blood indicate rupture of larger vessel.

s., currant jelly or raspberry. Indicates tumor of lung. If of a fetid odor, bronchitis.

s., fruity. Type of s. preceding rupture of an echinococcus cyst. S. may be bloody, mucoid, mucopurulent, purulent, serous, frothy, in plugs; or it may contain elastic fibers, fibrinous bronchial casts, bacteria, tubercles, pneumococci, influenza bacteria, diphtheria bacteria, staphylococci, streptococci, and pneumococci.

s., nummular. Round, coin-shaped, flat forms which sink in water; seen in bronchiectasis and advanced pulmonary tuberculosis.

s., prune juice. Thin, reddish, bloody s. in gangrene, cancer of the lung, and certain pneumonias.

s., rusty. S. seen in lobar pneumonia.

s., septicemia. S. acquired from inoculation with organisms in saliva or s.

squama (skwā′mŭ) [L.]. (pl. squa′mae) 1. A thin plate of bone. 2. A scale from the epidermis.

squamocellular (skwā″mō-sĕl′ū-lār) [L. *squama,* scale, + *cellula,* cell]. Rel. to or having squamous cells.

squamoparietal (skwā″mō-pō-rī′ĕ-tăl) ["+ *paries,* wall]. Rel. to the squamous and parietal bones.

squamosa (skwā-mō′sā) [L., scaly]. The squamous part of temporal bone.

squamous (skwā′mŭs) [L. *squamosus*]. Scale-like.

s. bone. Upper anterior portion of temporal bone.

s. cell. Flat, scaly, epithelial cell.

s. epithelium. Flat form of epithelial cells.

s. suture. Line uniting squamosa and parietal bone.

square knot. Double knot in which ends and standing parts are together and parallel to each other. This knot is used universally because it holds well. It is quite easy to tie but may be very difficult to untie.

Hold one end in each hand, carry right end over left end and make a simple knot. Now reverse by carrying left end over right end and again tying, thus forming a simple symmetrical knot. If this is not done correctly a false or granny knot results, a type of knot which usually slips. To untie, steady the knot, take one end and draw it over knot, and then continue pulling in this direction until knot slips or jumps and forms two half hitches which may be slipped off.

square lobe. 1. The quadrate lobe of the liver. SYN: *lobus quadratus* [NA]. 2. A lobe on upper surface of the cerebellum.

squarrose, squarrous (skwăr'ŏs, -ŭs) [L. *squarrōsus*]. Scurfy or scaly; full of scabs or scales.

squash (skwŏsh) [Amerind. *askootasquash*]. Any of various plants having fleshy edible fruit with many seeds and a hard rind. Several kinds of squash are available and they vary considerably in nutrient value.

Food value of 100 gm. (yellow cooked, drained): Cal. 15; protein 1.0 gm.; fat 0.2 gm.; carbohydrate 3.1 gm.; calcium 25 mg.; vitamin A, 440 I.U.; ascorbic acid 11 mg.

squat'ting position. Position in which person crouches with legs drawn up closely in front of, or beneath, body; sitting on one's haunches and heels. SYN: *kneeling-squatting position.*

squeeze-bottle. Bottle made of a flexible, semirigid material which can be deformed by applying hand pressure to it. Used to contain irrigating solutions, esp. those required in ophthalmology.

squill (skwĭl) [Gr. *skilla*]. A drug once popular as an expectorant and diuretic.

squint (skwĭnt) [ME. *asquint,* sidelong glance]. 1. Abnormality in which both the visual axes do not bear toward an objective point simultaneously. SYN: *strabismus.* 2. To close the eyes partly as in excess light. 3. To be unable to direct both eyes simultaneously toward a point.

s., convergent. Condition existing when eyes are turned toward the medial line. SYN: *esotropia.*

s., divergent. Condition existing when eyes are turned outwards. SYN: *exotropia.*

s., external. S., divergent.

s., internal. S., convergent.

SR. Abbr. for *sedimentation rate.*

Sr. Chem. symb. for strontium.

SS. Abbr. for *saliva sample; sterile solution.*

Ss. Abbr. for *subjects,* as in Ss of an experiment or clinical study.

ss. Abbr. for *semis,* half.

sse. Abbr. for *soapsuds enema.*

s. s. & p. enema. A mixture of one dram of peppermint in soapsuds solution, given to relieve flatulence. SEE: *enema.*

SSS. Abbr. for *sterile saline soak.*

s. s. & t. enema. Compound cleaning enema using a mixture of thick liquid soap and turpentine. SEE: *enema.*

ST. Abbr. for *sedimentation time.*

S.T. 37. Proprietary germicide and disinfectant. SYN: *hexylresorcinol,* q.v.

stab (stăb) [ME. *stob,* stick]. 1. To pierce with a knife. 2. Inoculum plunged deeply into a solid culture medium with a wire or needle. 3. The culture so produced.

s. culture. Bacterial culture in which organism is introduced into a solid gelatin medium with a wire or needle.

stabile (stā'bĭl) [L. *stabilis,* stable]. Not moving; fixed.

s. current. An electric current generated by holding stationary electrodes in a fixed position.

stable (stā'bl). Firm; steady.

staccato speech, utterance (stă-kä'tō) [It. *staccare,* to detach]. Jerky pronunciation with words and syllables separated by pauses. SYN: *scanning speech.* SEE: *speech.*

stactometer (stăk-tŏm'ĕt-ĕr) [Gr. *staktos,* dropping, + *metron,* measure]. Instrument for measuring fluid in drops.

stadium (stā'dĭ-ŭm) [Gr. *stadion,* alteration]. A stage or period in the progress of a disease.

s. acmes. The height of a disease.

s. augmenti. Period of rising temperature or other symptoms.

s. caloris. The hot stage in a fever or disease.

s. decrementi. Period of defervescence or decrease of symptoms.

s. florescentiae. Stage of eruption in an exanthematous disease.

s. frigoris. Cold, shivering stage in intermittent fevers, as malaria.

s. incrementi. Period of increase of fever or symptoms.

s. invasionis. Incubation period of an infectious disease.

s. sudoris. Sweating stage of a paroxysm of malaria.

s. vitimum. Last stage of a febrile disease.

staff (stăf) [AS. *staef,* a stick]. 1. An instrument to be introduced into the urethra and bladder as a guide to a surgical knife. 2. The medical personnel attached to a hospital.

s., attending. The group of physicians and surgeons who are in regular attendance at a hospital.

s., consulting. Physicians and surgeons attached to a hospital who may be consulted by members of the attending staff.

s. of Wrisberg. Prominence of the cuneiform cartilage seen in the normal larynx during examination.

stage (stāj) [O.Fr. *estage*]. 1. A period in the course of a disease or in the life history of an organism. SYN: *stadium.* 2. The platform of a microscope on which the slide is placed.

s., algid. Period of chilliness at the beginning of a fever.

s., amphibolic. S. which intervenes between acme of a disease and its outcome, at a time when the outcome is unknown.

s., asphyxial. Preliminary s. of Asiatic cholera.

s., cold. Chill or rigor of a malarial paroxysm.

s., defervescent. Period in which temperature is declining.

s., eruptive. Period in which an exanthem appears.

s., expulsive. S. of dilatation of the cervix uteri during which the child is expelled from uterus; second s. of labor.

s., first. Period when the fetal head is molded and the cervix dilated.

s., hot. Febrile s. in a malarial paroxysm.

s. of invasion. Period in which a morbific influence precedes the onset of a disease.

s. of latency. The incubation period of an infectious disorder.

s., placental. Period of labor during which placenta and fetal membranes are discharged; third s. of labor.

s., preeruptive. S. following infection and before appearance of eruption.

s., pyrogenetic. S. of onset in a febrile disease.

s. resting. A s. of relative inactivity between periods of activity as in a cell between mitotic divisions; a dormant s.

s., second. S., expulsive, q.v.

s., sweating. The 3rd or terminal s. of malaria during which sweating occurs.

s., third. S., placental, q.v.

staging. Process of classifying tumors, esp. malignant tumors, with respect to their degree of differentiation, to their potential for responding to therapy, and to the patient's prognosis.

stagnation (stăg-nā'shŭn) [L. *stagnāns,* stagnant]. 1. Cessation of motion. 2. In pathology, a stoppage of motion of any fluid in the body, as blood. SYN: *stasis.*

stain (stān) [O.Fr. *desteindre,* deprive of color]. 1. Any discoloration. 2. A pigment or dye used in coloring microscopic objects and tissues. 3. To apply pigment to a tissue or microscopic object.

s., acid. S. in which the color-bearing ion (chromatophore) is the anion. Ex: eosin, commonly used for staining the cytoplasmic or basic elements of cells.

s., acid-fast. A s. used in bacteriology, esp. for staining tuberculosis bacteria. A special solution of carbolfuchsin is used, which the organism retains in spite of washing with acid alcohol; a decolorizing agent. SYN: *Ziehl-Neelsen s.*

s., basic. One in which the color-bearing ion is the cation. Ex: methylene blue, commonly used to stain the nucleic or acidic elements of cells.

s., Commission Certified. A s. that has been certified by the Biological Stain Commission.

s., contrast. S. used to color one part of a tissue or cell unaffected when another part is stained by another color.

s., counter. A s., usually a contrast s., which is used following the staining of specific elements of a tissue.

s., differential. In bacteriology, a s. such as Gram's s. which enables one to differentiate between different types of bacteria.

s., double. A mixture of two contrasting dyes, usually an acid and a basic s.

s., Gram's. Gram's method, q.v.

s., intravital. A nontoxic dye which when introduced into an organism selectively stains certain cells or tissues. SYN: *vital s.*

s., inversion. A basic s. which when under the influence of a mordant, acts as an acid s.

s., metachromatic. A s. which stains the constituents of cells or tissues a color different from the s. itself.

s., neutral. A combination of an acid and a basic s.

s., nuclear. A basic s. affecting nuclei.

s.'s, removal from linen. SEE: *antistain formulary.*

s., substantive. A s. which is directly absorbed by the tissues when they are immersed in the staining solution.

s., supravital. A s. which will color living cells or tissues which have been removed from the body.

s., vital. S., intravital, q.v.

s., Wright's. A polychrome stain used for staining blood smears. SEE: *Wright's technique for blood smears.*

staining (stān'ĭng) [O.Fr. *desteindre*]. Process of impregnating a substance, esp. a tissue, with pigments so that its component parts may be visible under a microscope. SEE: *Wright's technique for blood smears.*

staircase phenomenon. The effect exhibited by skeletal and heart muscle when subjected to rapidly repeated maximal stimuli following a period of rest. In the resulting series of contractions each is greater than the preceding one until a state of maximum contraction is reached. SYN: *staircase effect; treppe.*

stalagmometer (stă-lăg-mŏm'ĕ-tĕr) [Gr. *stalagmos,* dropping, + *metron,* a measure]. Instrument for measuring number of drops in a given amount of fluid.

stalk (stawk) [ME.]. An elongated structure usually serving to attach or support an organ or structure.

s., belly. Structure in embryo which develops into umbilical cord.

s., body. A bridge of mesoderm which connects the caudal end of embryo with chorion. Into it grow the allantois and embryonic blood vessels, the latter forming the umbilical arteries and vein which connect the embryo with the placenta.

s., cerebellar. One of the cerebellar peduncles which connect the cerebellum with brain stem.

s., infundibular. Stalk which connects diencephalon with neural lobe of hypophysis. SYN: *infundibulum.*

s., optic. Structure which connects optic vesicle or cup to the forebrain.

s., yolk. The narrow constricted portion by which the yolk sac is connected to midgut of embryo. SYN: *vitelline duct.*

stamina (stăm'ĭ-nă) [L., thread of the warp, thread of human life]. Inherent force; constitutional energy; strength; endurance.

stammering (stăm'er-ĭng) [AS. *stamerian*]. Hesitant or faltering speech disorder. May be due to hesitation; mispronunciation; transposing the letters l, r, or s; or repetition. SEE: *speech.*

RS: lalling; mytacism.

s. of bladder. Interrupted and irregular flow of urine, the muscles which control micturition acting spasmodically.

standard (stăn'dard) [O.Fr. *estandard,* marking rallying place]. That which is estab-

lished by custom or authority as a model, criterion, or rule for comparison of measurement.

s. deviation. SYMB: σ. In statistics, commonly used measure of dispersion or variability in a distribution. The square root of the variance, q.v. ABBR: S.D.

s. error. A measure of variability which could be expected of a statistical constant following the taking of random samples of a given size in a particular set of observations. An important S.E. is that of the difference between the means of two samples. ABBR: S.E.

standardization. The process of standardizing, esp. that of determining the strength or scale value of a substance or device by comparing with some standard, as standardization of solutions or thermometers.

s., biological. The standardization of drugs or biological products (vitamins, hormones, antibiotics) by testing their effects upon animals. Utilized when chemical analysis is impossible or impracticable.

standing orders. Orders, rules, regulations, or procedures prepared by the professional staff of a hospital or clinic.

Used as guide lines in preparation for and carrying out medical and surgical procedures. Standing orders serve to assure that such procedures are carried out correctly without being dependent upon an individual's fallible memory.

stand'still. A cessation of activity.

s., atrial. Cessation of atrial contractions. SYN: *auricular standstill.*

s., cardiac. Cessation of contractions of heart.

s., inspiratory. Temporary cessation of inspiration normally following each inspiration resulting from stimulation of proprioceptors in alveoli of lungs. SEE: *Hering-Breuer reflex.*

s., respiratory. Cessation of respiratory movements.

s., ventricular. Cessation of ventricular contractions.

stapedectomy (stā"pē-dĕk'tō-mĭ) [L. *stapes,* stirrup, + Gr. *ektomē,* excision]. Excision of the stapes in the ear.

During the first 24 hours following surgery the patient remains flat in bed, head movements are kept to a minimum, and he is instructed to refrain from blowing his nose or sneezing (if possible). In the second 24 hours the patient moves or raises only if assisted. The patient should not allow the ear to get wet for at least ten days postoperatively. For 30 days following surgery he should not fly, climb to high altitudes, or be exposed to loud sounds such as jet airplanes; and sudden movements, even in elevators, should be avoided.

stape'dial. Rel. to the stapes.

stapediotenotomy (stā-pē″dĭ-ō-tĕn-ŏt′ō-mĭ) [L. *stapes*, stirrup, + Gr. *tenōn*, tendon, + *tomē*, a cutting]. Division of the tendon of the stapedius muscle.

stapediovestibular (stā-pē″dĭ-ō-vĕs-tĭb′ū-lar) ["+ *vestibulum*, an antechamber]. Rel. to the stapes and vestibule of the ear.

stapedius (stā-pē′dĭ-ŭs) [L. *stapes*, stirrup]. A small muscle of the middle ear inserted in the stapes. SEE: *Table of Muscles* in *Appendix*.

stapes (stā′pēz) [L., stirrup]. [NA] Ossicle in middle ear which articulates with the incus. Commonly called stirrup. The footplate of the stapes fits into oval window. SEE: *ear*.

staphyle (stăf′ĭ-lē) [Gr. *staphylē*, bunch of grapes]. Pendulous, fleshy mass hanging from the soft palate. SYN: *uvula*, q.v.

staphylectomy (stăf′ĭ-lĕk′tō-mĭ) ["+ *ektomē*, excision]. Amputation of the uvula. SYN: *staphylotomy; uvulotomy.*

staphyledema (stăf′ĭ-ē-dē′mä) ["+ *oidēma*, swelling]. Swelling of the uvula.

staphyline (stăf′ĭ-lin) [Gr. *staphylē*, a bunch of grapes]. 1. Resembling a bunch of grapes. SYN: *botryoid*. 2. Rel. to the uvula. SYN: *uvular.*

staphylinopharyngeus (stăf′ĭl-ĭn″ō-făr-ĭn′-jē-ŭs) ["+ *pharynx*, pharynx]. Muscle in undersurface of soft palate which contracts the fauces and elevates back of the tongue. SEE: *Table of Muscles* in *Appendix*.

staphylinus (stăf′ĭ-lī′nŭs) [Gr. *staphylē*, a bunch of grapes]. One of two muscles which elevate the soft palate and make it tense. SEE: *Table of Muscles* in *Appendix*.

staphylion (stăf-ĭl′ĭ-ŏn) [Gr., little grape]. 1. Craniometric point at median line of posterior border of hard palate. 2. Uvula. 3. A nipple or teat.

staphylitis (stăf′ĭl-ī′tĭs) [Gr. *staphylē*, a bunch of grapes, + -*itis*, inflammation]. Inflammation of uvula.

staphylo- [Gr. *staphylē*, a bunch of grapes]. Combining form indicating the uvula; pert. to or resembling a bunch of grapes; or pert. to Staphylococcus.

staphyloangina (stăf′ĭl-ō-ăn′jĭ-nä) ["+ L. *angina*, sore throat]. Sore throat due to staphylococcus.

staphylococcal (stăf′ĭl-ō-kŏk′ăl) ["+ *kokkos*, berry]. Pert. to or caused by staphylococci.

   s. actinophytosis. Botryomycosis, a condition characterized by granulomatous lesions resembling those of actinomycoses;

however, when organisms recovered from the lesions are cultured, they grow as staphylococci.

   s. food poisoning. Poisoning by food containing a heat-stable enterotoxin produced by certain strains of staphylococci. When ingested the toxin causes nausea, vomiting, diarrhea, intestinal cramps, and in severe cases prostration and shock. Attack usually lasts three to six hours. Fatalities are rare.

staphylococcemia (stăf′ĭl-ō-kŏk-sē′mĭ-ä) ["+ "+ *haima*, blood]. The presence of staphylococcus in the blood. SEE: *staphylomycosis*.

staphylococci (stăf′ĭl-ō-kŏk′sī). Pl. of staphylococcus.

Staphylococcus (stăf′ĭl-ō-kŏk′ŭs) [Gr. *staphylē*, bunch of grapes, + *kokkos*, berry]. A genus of micrococci belonging to the family Micrococcaceae, order Eubacteriales. They are gram positive and on agar produce white, yellow, or orange colored colonies. Some species are pathogenic causing suppurative conditions and elaborating endotoxins destructive to tissue cells. Some produce enterotoxins and are the cause of a common type of food poisoning. SYN: *Micrococcus*.

   S. albus. A form of low pathogenicity characterized by formation of white colonies. SYN: *Micrococcus pyogenes albus.*

   S. aureus. A species commonly present on skin and mucous membranes, esp. those of nose and mouth, characterized by production of a golden-yellow pigment. A cause of suppurative conditions such as boils, carbuncles, and internal abscesses in man. SYN: *Micrococcus pyogenes aurens.*

   S. cereus aureus. Species found in nasal mucus in coryza.

   S. cereus flavus. Species found in pus causing yellow color.

   S. citreus. A form producing pale yellow colonies. Mildly pathogenic. SYN: *Micrococcus citreus.*

   S. pyogenes albus. Form causing suppuration.

   S. pyogenes aureus. A pus-producing form.

   S. viridis flavescens. Species found in lesions of varicella, causing greenish-yellow color.

staphylococcus (stăf′ĭl-ō-kŏk′ŭs). (pl. *staphylococ′ci*) Term applied loosely to any pathogenic micrococci, esp. Micrococci pyogenes, var. albus and aureus. SEE: *Staphylococcus*.

staphylodermatitis (stăf′ĭl-ō-dĕrm″ă-tī′tĭs) [Gr. *staphylē*, bunch of grapes, + *derma*, skin, + -*itis*, inflammation]. A dermatitis caused by staphylococci.

staphylodialysis (stăf'ĭ-lō-dī-ăl'ĭ-sĭs) ["+ *dialysis*, a loosening]. Relaxed and elongated condition of the uvula.

staphylohemia (stăf'ĭ-lō-hē'mĭ-ă) ["+ *haima*, blood]. Staphylococci in the blood. SYN: *staphylococcemia.*

staphylolysin (stăf'ĭ-lŏl'ĭ-sĭn) ["+ *lysis*, dissolution]. A hemolysin produced by staphylococci.

staphyloma (stăf'ĭl-ō'mă) [Gr.]. A protrusion of the cornea or sclera of the eye.

   s., anterior. Globular enlargement of anterior part of the eye. SYN: *keratoglobus.*

   s., ciliary. S. in region of ciliary body.

   s., corneae. Thinning and bulging of the cornea.

   s., equatorial. S. in equatorial region of the eye.

   s., intercalary. S. in the region of union of sclera with periphery of iris.

   s., partial. Extends in one direction displacing the pupil; the remainder of the cornea is clear.

   s., posterior, s. posticum. Bulging of sclera backward.

   s., total. Opaque, protuberant cicatrix found in place of cornea.

   ETIOL: Perforation of cornea resulting in poor vision, increased tension, rupture of thin scar.

   TREATMENT: Prophylaxis, incision, excision, ablation.

   s. uveale. Protrusion of any portion of the uvea through the sclera.

staphyloncus (stăf'ĭ-lŏng'kŭs) [Gr. *staphylē*, a bunch of grapes, + *onkos*, tumor]. A tumor or enlargement of the uvula.

staphylopharyngeus (stăf'ĭ-lō-făr-ĭn'jē-ŭs) ["+ *pharynx*, pharynx]. Muscle of soft palate narrowing fauces and occluding nasopharynx. SYN: *palatopharyngeus; pharyngopalitinus.*

staphyloplasty (stăf'ĭ-lō-plăs''tĭ) ["+ *plassein*, to form]. Plastic surgery of the uvula or soft palate.

staphyloptosia, staphyloptosis (stăf'ĭ-lŏp-tō'sĭ-ă, -sĭs) ["+ *ptōsis*, a dropping]. Relaxation or elongation of the uvula. SYN: *staphylodialysis.*

staphylorrhaphy (stăf'ĭl-ōr'ă-fĭ) [Gr. *staphylē*, a bunch of grapes, + *rhaphē*, suture]. Suture of a cleft palate.

staphyloschisis (stăf'ĭ-lŏs'kĭ-sĭs) ["+ *schisis*, a fissure]. Fissure of the uvula. SYN: *cleft palate.*

staphylotomy (stăf'ĭ-lŏt'ō-mĭ) ["+ *tomē*, a cutting]. Amputation of the uvula.

staphylotoxin (stăf'ĭ-lō-tŏk'sĭn) [Gr. *staphylē*, a bunch of grapes, + L. *toxicum*, poison]. A toxin elaborated by one of the staphylococci. Among some of the toxins produced are an *enterotoxin*, a cause of food poisoning, and *exotoxins*, including a hematoxin which lyses red blood cells, a lethal toxin, a dermonecrotic toxin, and leukocidins.

staple food. Any food which supplies a substantial part, at least 25-35%, of the caloric requirement and is regularly consumed by a given people or country.

stapling. In surgery, a means of fastening tissues together by using special staples compatible with tissues. The staples are U-shaped lengths of wire which are pushed through the tissues. The ends are then bent over on an anvil.

star [AS. *steorra*]. Any structure resembling a star. SYN: *aster.*

   s., lens. A starlike structure developing in lens of eye as a result of unequal growth of lens fibers.

   s.'s of Verheyen. Star-shaped masses of veins in renal cortex. SYN: *venae stellatae.*

starch [AS. *stercan*]. Noncrystalline carbohydrate of the polysaccharose group found in plants. The polysaccharoses include vegetable starches, animal starch (glycogen), celluloses, pectins, dextrins, and gums, among which it is difficult to make distinctions. All of them are rather easily decomposed, have high molecular weights, and yield monosaccharoses on complete hydrolysis.

   Those which the body is able to hydrolyze into hexoses are useful as concentrated energy-giving foods. They all must be reduced to simple sugars, except cellulose, before they may be absorbed. What is not needed is stored in the liver as glycogen. They are an excellent source of energy. In some fruits the s. is changed to sugar when they ripen, while some vegetables (peas and corn) change sugar into s. as their seeds develop.

   The amylases of saliva and pancreatic juice hydrolyze starches to dextrins and maltose. These in turn are hydrolyzed to glucose, which is absorbed into the blood stream. Glucose not immediately needed for energy is converted into glycogen, a form of s. which is stored in the liver or in muscle tissue.

   Pure starches, having the formula $(C_6H_{10}O_5)_n$, if normally metabolized, leave no residue and give rise only to carbon dioxide and water. Starches yield an acid ash.

   s., animal. Glycogen.

Classification of Starches

Groups

I.	Potato Group	(a) Canna	(b) Potato	(c) Arrowroot
II.	Leguminous Group	(a) Beans	(b) Peas	(c) Lentils
III.	Wheat Group	(a) Wheat	(b) Barley	(c) Rye
IV.	Sago Group	(a) Sago	(b) Cassava	(c) Arum
V.	Rice Group	(a) Rice	(b) Maize	(c) Oats

Starches

Name	From
1. Cornflour	Maize or corn
2. Arrowroot	Maranta
3. Cassava	Brazilian arrowroot
4. Curcuma	East Indian arrowroot
5. Arum	Portland arrowroot
6. Tous-les-mois	Canna (West India)
7. Sago	Palm (East India)
8. Inulin	Dahlia tubers
9. Lichen	Iceland moss
10. Glycogen	Animal livers

NOTE: Starch is soluble at 150° F. (65.6° C.) Only slightly so in cold water.

IODINE acting on starch paste gives a deep blue.

BROMINE acting on starch paste gives an orange-yellow.

The Percentage of Starch in Various Foods

Article	Per cent	Article	Per cent
Arrowroot	23	Oatmeal	68
Bananas	22	Peanuts	18
Barley	79	Peas, dried	60
Beans	61	Peas, green	14
Beans, green	26	Potatoes	17
Bread fruit	7	Potatoes, sweet	26
Buckwheat flour	73	Rice, uncooked	80
Chestnuts, dried	78	Rye flour	73
Lentils	60	Wheat flour	74

s., corn. S. obtained from ordinary corn or maize (Zea mays). It is used as a dusting powder and an absorbent and is a constituent in many pastes and ointments. It is widely used in industry and as a food.

stare (stār) [AS. *starian*]. To gaze fixedly at anyone or anything.

Starling's law of heart. The force of the heartbeat is determined primarily by the length of the fibers comprising its muscular wall, i.e., an increase in diastolic filling increases force of heartbeat.

Starling's law of intestine. [Ernest Henry Starling, Eng. physiologist, 1866-1927] A stimulus within the intestine, i.e., the presence of food, initiating a band of constriction on proximal side and relaxation on distal side. This results in a peristaltic wave.

start'er. A pure culture of bacteria or other microorganism used to initiate a particular fermentation as in the making of cheese.

starva'tion [AS. *steorfan*, to die]. 1. The condition of being without food for a long period of time. When everything but air and water is withheld, the sequence of events is as follows: (1) Hunger, beginning about four hours after the last meal, accompanied by special activity of the stomach and general restlessness, becoming more acute periodically, esp. at times when meals were customarily taken; (2) loss of weight; (3) utilization of glycogen stored in liver and muscles; (4) utilization of stored fat; (5) spells of nausea and diminishing acuteness of the sensation of hunger; (6) destruction of body protein. The greatest loss of weight is in the fatty tissues, spleen, and liver. The nervous system loses little and the heart least of all. 2. Condition in which the supply of a specific food is below minimum bodily requirements. Ex: protein starvation. 3. Condition resulting from failure of the body to digest and absorb essential foodstuffs. SEE: *deficiency disease; diet; dietetics.*

stasibasiphobia (stā″sĭ-bā″sĭ-fō′bĭ-ă) [Gr. *stasis*, a standing, + *basis*, step, + *phobos*, fear]. Delusion of one's inability to stand or walk, or fear to make the attempt.

stasiphobia (stā′sĭ-fō′bĭ-ă) ["+ *phobos*, fear]. Delusion of one's inability to stand erect or hesitation to make the attempt.

stasis (stā′sĭs) [Gr. *stasis*, standing still]. Stagnation of normal flow of fluids, as of the blood, urine, or of the intestinal mechanism.

   s., diffusion. S. with diffusion of lymph or serum.

   s., intestinal. Condition in which peristaltic movements fail to move food along the intestine.

   s., venous. S. of blood caused by venous congestion.

stat [L.]. Abbr. of *statim*, immediately.

state [L. *status*, condition]. 1. A condition. 2. A mode or condition of being.

   s., anxiety. A condition characterized by more or less continuous anxiety and apprehension. SEE: *anxiety neurosis.*

   s., central excitatory. A condition of increased excitability in the central nervous system, esp. in the spinal cord, following an excitatory stimulus. ABBR: c.e.s.

   s., central inhibitory. A condition of decreased excitability in the central nervous system, esp. in the spinal cord, resulting from an inhibitory stimulus. ABBR: c.i.s.

   s., fatigue. Neurasthenia, q.v.

static (stăt′ĭk) [Gr. *statikos*, standing]. At rest; in equilibrium; not in motion.

   s. electricity. Electricity produced by friction.

   s. equilibrium. Equilibrium concerned with recognition of position of head in relation to gravity. Opposed to dynamic equilibrium.

   s. reflex. A reflex action having to do with maintenance of posture or maintenance of muscle tone.

statics (stăt′ĭks). Study of matter at rest and forces bringing about equilibrium. SEE: *dynamics.*

statim (stăt′ĭm) [L.]. Immediately; at once. ABBR: stat.

station (stā′shŭn) [L. *statio*, standing]. 1. The manner of standing. 2. A stopping place.

   s., aid. Site in the army for collecting the wounded in battle.

   s., dressing. A temporary s. for wounded soldiers in the field.

   s., rest. A temporary relief s. for the sick on a military road or railway.

stationary (stā′shŭn-ĕr-ĭ) [L. *stationarius*, belonging to a station]. Remaining in a fixed condition.

statis′tical. Pert. to statistics.

statis′tics [LL. *statisticus*]. The systematic collection, organization, and interpretation of numerical data pert. to any subject.

   s., medical. S. pert. to medical sciences, esp. data pert. to human disease.

   s., morbidity. S. pert. to sickness.

   s., vital. S. dealing with births, deaths, marriages, etc.

statokinetic (stăt″ō-kĭn-ĕt′ĭk) [Gr. *statos*, placed, + *kinētikos*, moving]. Pert. to reactions of the body produced by movement.

   s. reflexes. Reactions which are the result of movement of the body (positive or negative acceleration) or movements of the head. SYN: *kinetic* or *accelerator reflexes.*

statometer (stā-tŏm′ĕt-ĕr) [Gr. *statos*, standing, + *metron*, a measure]. Instrument for measuring amount of abnormal protrusion of eyeball.

stature (stăt′ūr) [L. *statūra*]. Height of the body in a standing position.

status (stā′tŭs) [L.]. (pl. *statuses*) A state or condition.

   s. anginosus. A sustained attack of angina pectoris.

   s. arthriticus. Predisposition to having attacks of gout.

   s. asthmaticus. Persistent and intractable asthma.

   s. dysraphicus. Condition resulting from imperfect closure of neural tube of embryo.

   s. dysmyelinisatus of Vogt. Condition marked by demyelination of the globus pallidus, and various nuclei of the brain, esp. the hypothalamic nuclei and dentate nucleus of cerebellum.

   s. epilepticus. Rapid succession of epileptic attacks without regaining consciousness during the intervals.

   s. lymphaticus. A hyperplastic condition of all lymphatic tissue, the spleen, bone marrow, and thymus. Previously thought to be related to sudden unexpected death of infants. The thymus enlarges together with lymph glands and lymphoid tissue elsewhere in the body.

People with this condition have a delicate framework, slight musculature, delicate cardiovascular system, low blood pressure, low blood sugar, and lymphocytosis. They are particularly susceptible to shock and infection. SYN: *lymphatism*.

s. parathyreoprivus. Condition resulting from loss of parathyroid tissue.

s. praesens. The state of a patient at time observed.

s. raptus. A state of ecstacy.

s. thymicolymphaticus. Condition resembling s. lymphaticus but with enlarged thymus as primary factor.

s. thymicus. S. thymicolymphaticus, q.v.

s. typhosus. Condition in wasting fevers in which symptoms are stupor; great prostration; coma; vigil or muttering delirium; feeble, frequent pulse; involuntary discharge of urine and feces; sordes, and dry, brownish tongue. SYN: *typhoid s.*

s. vertiginosus. Persistent condition of vertigo, q.v.

staunch (stŏnch) [O.Fr. *estanche,* firm]. To stop the flow of blood from a wound.

staurion (stŏ'rĭ-ŏn) [Gr. *stauros,* little cross]. Craniometric point where transverse palatine suture crosses the median one.

stauroplegia (stŏ"rō-plē'jĭ-ă) ["+ *plēgē,* a stroke]. Hemiplegia of a part on one side of the body and another part on the other side. SYN: *crossed hemiplegia.*

S.T.D. Abbr. for *skin test dose.* SEE: *Dick test.*

steam (stēm) [AS. *stēam,* vapor]. 1. Invisible vapor into which water is converted at boiling point by heat. 2. Mist formed by condensation of water vapor. 3. Any vaporous exhalation.

s. tent. A device for inhalation of vapors. If no tent is available a makeshift tent may be improvised in various ways. It is important that the method does not burn the patient.

(1) Tie an old umbrella to the head of the bed; place a pitcher of boiling water in a box beside the patient. Vapors tend to fill the umbrella. Solution may be kept hot by placing in a double boiler or wrapping pitcher in an old woolen cloth or newspapers.

(2) Window screens may be used by fastening them about head of bed and then covering with a blanket or sheet lined with newspapers. Solution may be used as above, or a steaming teakettle placed alongside of bed with the spout directed under tent.

(3) A rod or rope fastened across head of bed and down to foot of bed. Place a blanket across rod to cover patient. Use inhalation as above.

(4) Fasten ropes to all four corners of bed, covering with blankets, etc., forming enclosure for patient. Numerous variations will quickly suggest themselves.

SOLUTIONS: Approx. a quart (a liter) of boiling water to which is added a teaspoonful (5 ml.) of compound tincture of benzoin or a teaspoonful (5 ml.) of tincture benzoin (this does not contain aloe), a few crystals of menthol or camphor, or a few drops of methyl salicylate. These ingredients are pleasant but have relatively little therapeutic effect. Most of the value is in the water vapor. SEE: *croup.*

steapsin (stē-ăp'sĭn) [Gr. *stear,* fat, + *pepsis* digestion]. A lipolytic enzyme present in pancreatic juice that hydrolyzes fats to fatty acid and glycerine. The bile salts prepare the fats for the action of steapsin by emulsifying them. SYN: *pancreatic lipase.* SEE: *enzyme; pancreas.*

stearate (stē'ă-rāt). An ester or salt of stearic acid.

stearic acid (stē-ăr'ĭk) [Gr. *stear,* fat]. A white, fatty acid found in solid animal fats and a few vegetable fats.

steariform (stē-ăr'ĭ-form) ["+ L. *forma,* shape]. Resembling fat.

stearin (stē'ă-rĭn) [Gr. *stear,* fat]. $C_3H_5(C_{18}H_{35}O_2)_3$. A white, crystalline solid in animal and vegetable fats; any of the esters of glycerol and stearic acid, specifically glyceryl tristearate. One of the commonest fats in the body, esp. the solid ones. It breaks down into stearic acid and glycerol.

stearodermia (stē"ă-rō-dĕr'mĭ-ă) ["+ *derma,* skin]. Disease of the sebaceous glands of the skin.

stearoptene (stē"ă-rŏp'tēn) ["+ *ptēnos,* volatile]. The more solid portion of a volatile oil as distinguished from the more fluid portion or eleoptene. Ex: menthol, thymol.

stearrhea (stē"ă-rē'ă) [Gr. *stear,* fat, + *rhoia,* flow]. Excessive secretion of sebum or fat. SYN: *seborrhea oleosa.*

s. flavescens. S. with yellow sebaceous matter deposited on the skin.

s. nigricans. S. with black sweat due to presence of indican. SEE: *chromidrosis; chromodermatosis.*

s. simplex. Excessive discharge of sebum.

steatadenoma (stē-ăt"ăd-ē-nō'mă) [Gr. *steatos,* fat, + *adēn,* gland, + *-ōma,* tumor]. Tumor of the sebaceous glands.

steatitis (stē"ă-tī'tĭs) ["+ *-itis,* inflammation]. Inflammation of adipose tissue.

steato- [Gr. *steatos*, fat]. Prefix meaning fatty.

steatocele (stē-ăt′ō-sēl, stē′ăt-ō-sēl) ["+ *kēlē*, tumor]. Fatty tumor within the scrotum.

steatocryptosis (stē″ă-tō-krĭp-tō′sĭs) ["+ *kryptē*, a sac, + *-ōsis*, disorder]. Any disease of sebaceous glands. SEE: *steatodermia*.

steatocysto′ma multiplex. A skin disorder characterized by development of many sebaceous cysts. SYN: *steatomatosis*.

steatogenous (stē″ă-tŏj′ĕn-ŭs) [Gr. *steatos*, fat, + *gennan*, to produce]. 1. Causing fatty degeneration. 2. Producing any sebaceous gland disease.

steatolysis (stē″ă-tŏl′ĭ-sĭs) ["+ *lysis*, dissolution]. 1. The process by which fats are first emulsified and then hydrolyzed to fatty acids and glycerine preparatory to absorption. 2. The decomposition of fat. SYN: *lipolysis*.

steatolytic (stē″ă-tō-lĭt′ĭk). Concerning steatolysis.

steatoma (stē″ă-tō′mă) [Gr. *steatos*, fat, + *-ōma*, tumor]. 1. Sebaceous cyst. SYN: *wen*. 2. Benign tumor composed of fat cells. SYN: *lipoma*.

S. is called a chalazion when on eyelid and meibomian gland. Smooth, shiny, globular, cutaneous or subcutaneous tumor from pea to orange size arising from sebaceous glands, single or multiple, usually on neck, scalp, back, or scrotum.

ETIOL: Duct occlusion is causative in some.

PROG: Prolonged irritation may cause suppuration.

TREATMENT: Surgical excision by dissection without perforating sac. Packing in suppurative cases.

steatonecrosis (stē″ă-tō-nē-krō′sĭs) [Gr. *steatos*, fat, + *nekros*, dead, + *-ōsis*, condition]. Necrosis of fatty tissue in small patches.

steatopathy (stē-ă-tŏp′ă-thĭ) ["+ *pathos*, disease]. Disease of the sebaceous glands of the skin.

steatopygia (stē″ă-tō-pĭj′ĭ-ă) ["+ *pygē*, buttock]. Abnormal fatness of the buttocks. Seen to an extreme degree in certain parts of Africa. Location of this excess fat accumulation in the buttocks represents adaptation to a very hot climate. If this fat were generally spread throughout the subcutaneous tissue, normal cooling of the skin would be severely limited.

steatorrhea (stē″ă-tō-rē′ă) [Gr. *steatos*, fat, + *rhoia*, flow]. 1. Increased secretion of sebaceous glands. SYN: *seborrhea*, q.v. 2. Fatty stools, as seen in pancreatic diseases.

s., idiopathic. Term applied to gastrointestinal disorders characterized by impaired absorption. SYN: *secondary sprue*.

s. simplex. Excessive secretion of sebaceous glands of the face.

ste″ato′sis ["+ *-ōsis*, condition]. 1. Fatty degeneration. 2. Disease of the sebaceous glands.

steclin (stĕk′lĭn). A proprietary name for tetracycline.

stegnosis (stĕg-nō′sĭs) [Gr. *stegnōsis*, obstruction]. 1. Checking of a secretion or discharge. 2. Closing of a passage. SYN: *stenosis*. 3. Constipation. SYN: *costiveness*.

stegnotic (stĕg-nŏt′ĭk). Bringing about stegnosis. SYN: *astringent; constipating*.

Stegomyia (stĕg″ō-mī′ĭ-ă). A subgenus of mosquito of the genus Aedes, family Culicidae, suspected of transmitting the causative organism of yellow fever.

Steinert's disease (stīn′ŭrt). [Hans Steinert, Ger. physician, 19th century] Myotonia dystrophica, q.v.

stel′la [L.]. (pl. *stel′lae*) Star.

s. lentis hyaloidea. Posterior pole of crystalline lens of eye.

s. lentis iridica. Anterior pole of crystalline lens of eye.

stell′ate [L. *stellātus*]. Star-shaped; arranged with parts radiating from a center.

s. bandage. Bandage wound on the back, crossways.

s. cell. Any cell that appears star-shaped. Ex: neurons of molecular layer of cerebellum, Kupffer's cells of the liver sinusoids, astrocytes.

s. fracture. Fracture with numerous fissures radiating from central point of injury.

s. ganglion. A sympathetic ganglion formed by the fusion of inferior cervical and first thoracic ganglions. SYN: *cervicothoracic ganglion*.

s. ligament. One of the anterior costovertebral ligaments. SYN: *radiate ligament*.

s. veins. Venous plexuses beneath the kidney's capsule. SYN: *stars of Verheyen*.

Stellwag's sign (stĕl′văg). [Carl Stellwag von Carion, Austrian oculist, 1823-1904] Widening of palpebral aperture with absence or lessened frequency of winking, seen in Graves' disease.

stem. 1. [AS. *stemn*, tree trunk] Any stalklike structure. 2. Offspring. 3. To derive from or originate in. 4. [ME. *stemmen*] To check, stop, or hold back.

s., brain. The lower portion of the brain excluding the cerebrum and cerebellum.

Includes the medulla oblongata, pons, midbrain, and diencephalon.

s. cell. A cell which gives rise to a specific type of cell as in hematopoiesis.

stenion (stĕn′ĭ-ŏn) [Gr. *stenos*, narrow]. Craniometric point at extremities of the smallest transverse diameter in the temporal region.

steno- [Gr. *stenos*, narrow]. Combining form meaning narrow or short.

stenocardia (stĕn″ō-kar′dĭ-ă) ["+ *kardia*, heart]. Angina pectoris, q.v.

stenocephaly (stĕn″ō-sĕf′ă-lĭ) ["+ *kephalē*, head]. Narrowness of the cranium in one or more diameters.

stenochoria (stĕn″ō-kō′rĭ-ă) [Gr. *stenos*, narrow, + *chōros*, space]. Partial constriction, esp. of the lacrimal duct. SYN: *stenosis*.

stenocompressor (stĕn″ō-kŏm-prĕs′or) ["+ L. *compressor*, that which presses together]. An instrument for compressing Stensen's ducts to stop the flow of saliva.

stenocoriasis (stĕn″ō-kō-rĭ′ă-sĭs) ["+ *korē*, pupil]. Narrowing of pupil of the eye.

stenopaic, stenopeic (stĕn-ō-pā′ĭk, -pē′ĭk) [Gr. *stenos*, narrow, + *opē*, opening]. Provided with a narrow opening or slit, esp. denoting optical devices to protect against snow blindness.

stenosed (stē-nōst′, stĕn′ōzd). Characterized by stenosis; constricted.

stenosis (stĭ-nō′sĭs) [Gr.]. Constriction or narrowing of a passage or orifice. SYN: *stricture*.

ETIOL: May result from embryonic maldevelopment, hypertrophy and thickening of a sphincter muscle, inflammatory disorders, or excessive development of fibrous tissue. It may involve almost any tube or duct.

s., aortic. Constriction of the aortic orifice at cardiac base, or narrowing of the aorta.

s., cardiac. A narrowing or constriction of any of the orifices leading into or from the heart or between chambers of the heart.

s., cicatricial. S. resulting from any contracted cicatrix.

s., mitral. S. of mitral valve or orifice of heart, or of both. Usually the result of rheumatic heart disease.

s., pyloric. Obstruction caused by hypertrophy of walls of the pyloric orifice.

s., subaortic. Congenital constriction of aortic tract below aortic valves.

stenostomia (stĕn″ō-stō′mĭ-ă) [Gr. *stenos*, narrow, + *stoma*, mouth]. Narrowing of the mouth.

stenother′mal ["+ *thermē*, heat]. Resisting only a small change of temperature. SYN: *stenothermic.*

stenothorax (stĕn″ō-thō′răks) ["+ *thōrax*, chest]. An unusually narrow thorax.

stenot′ic [Gr. *stenōsis*, a narrowing]. Produced by or characterized by stenosis.

Stensen's duct (stĕn′sĕn). [Niels Stensen, Danish anatomist, 1638-1686]. The excretory duct of parotid gland.

Stensen's foramina. Incisive foramina of superior maxillary bone transmitting anterior branches of descending palatine vessels.

stent. [Charles R. Stent, 11th century Eng. dentist] 1. Originally a compound used in making dental molds. 2. Any material used to hold tissue in place or to provide a support for a graft or anastomosis while healing is taking place.

stentorophonic (stĕn″tō-rō-fŏn′ĭk). [Stentor, loud-voiced herald in the *Iliad*] Speaking or sounding very loud. SYN: *stentorian; stentorophonous.*

stephanion (stē-fā′nĭ-ŏn) [Gr. *stephanos*, crown]. Point at intersection of superior temporal ridge and coronal suture.

step′page gait. The high-stepping gait seen in diabetic neuritis of the peroneal nerve and in tabes dorsalis. Patient lifts the foot very high in walking to raise the drooping toes from the ground or floor.

sterco- [L. *stercus*, dung]. Combining form indicating a relationship to feces.

stercobilin (stĕr″kō-bī′lĭn) ["+ *bilis*, bile]. A brown pigment derived from the bile giving the characteristic color to feces. SEE: *urobilin.*

stercobilinogen (stĕr″kō-bī-lĭn′ō-jĕn). A colorless substance derived from stercobilin. It is present in the feces and turns brown on oxidation. SYN: *urobilinogen.*

stercoraceous (stĕr″kō-rā′shŭs) [L. *stercoraceus*]. Having the nature of, pert. to, or containing feces.

stercoral (stĕr′kō-răl) [L. *stercus*, dung]. Pert. to feces. SYN: *stercoraceous.*

stercorolith (stĕr′kō-rō-lĭth) ["+ Gr. *lithos*, stone]. A fecal concretion. SYN: *coprolith; fecalith.*

stercoroma (stĕr″kō-rō′mă) ["+ Gr. *-ōma*, tumor]. A fecal tumorlike mass in the rectum. SYN: *coproma; fecaloma; scatoma.*

stercorous (stĕr′kō-rŭs) [L. *stercorosus*]. Resembling excrement. SYN: *stercoral; stercoraceous.*

stercus (stĕr′kŭs) [L.]. (pl. *ster′cora*) Feces. SYN: *excreta; excrement.*

stere (ster, star) [Gr. *stereos*, solid]. A measure of volume equal to one cubic meter.

stereo- [Gr. *stereos*, solid]. Combining form meaning solid or indicating three-dimensional.

stereoanesthesia (stĕr″ē-ō-ăn″ĕs-thē′zĭ-ă) ["+ *an-*, negative, + *aisthesis*, sensation]. Inability to recognize objects by feeling their form.

stereoarthrolysis (stĕr″ē-ō-ăr-thrŏl′ĭ-sĭs) ["+ *arthron*, joint, + *lysis*, dissolution]. Surgical formation of a movable new joint in bony ankylosis.

stereochemical (stĕr″ē-ō-kĕm′ĭ-kăl) [Gr. *stereos*, solid, + *chēmeia*, chemistry]. Concerning stereochemistry.

stereochemistry (stĕr″ē-ō-kĕm′ĭs-trĭ). That branch of chemistry dealing with atoms in their space relationship.

stereocilia (stĕr″ē-ō-sĭl′ĭ-ă). Nonmotile protoplasmic projections from free surfaces of cells of ductus epididymis and ductus deferens.

stereognosis (stĕr″ē-ŏg-nō′sĭs) [Gr. *stereos*, solid, + *gnōsis*, knowledge]. Ability to recognize form of solid objects by touch.

stereoisomerism (stĕr″ē-ō-ĭ-sō′mĕr-ĭsm). Condition in which two or more substances may have the same empirical formula, but a different structural formula, structural formulas being mirror images of each other.

Ex: dextrose and levulose. Such differ in optical activity with regard to their effect on a plane of polarized light.

stereometry (stē″rē-ŏm′ē-trĭ) [Gr. *stereos*, solid, + *metron*, a measure]. The measurement of a solid body or the cubic contents of a hollow body.

stereoorthopter (stĕr″ē-ō-ōr-thŏp′tĕr) ["+ *orthos*, straight, + *opsis*, vision]. A mirror-reflecting device for treatment of strabismus.

stereophantoscope (stĕr″ē-ō-făn′tō-skōp) [Gr. *stereos*, solid, + *phantos*, visible, + *skopein*, to examine]. A stereoscopic device with rotating disks for testing vision.

stereophorometer (stĕr″ē-ō-fōr-ŏm′ē-ter) ["+ *phoros*, a bearer, + *metron*, a measure]. A prism-refracting device for use in correcting defective vision.

stereophotography (stĕr″ē-ō-fō-tŏg′ră-fĭ) ["+ *phōs, phot-*, light, + *graphein*, to write]. Photography which produces effect of solidity or depth in the pictures.

stereophotomicrograph (stĕr″ē-ō-fō″tō-mĭ′krō-grăf) ["+ "+ *mikros*, tiny, + *graphein*, to write]. A photograph showing solidity or depth of a microscopic subject.

stereoscope (stĕr′ē-ō-skōp) [Gr. *stereos*, solid, + *skopein*, to see]. Instrument which creates an impression of solidity or depth of objects seen by combining images of two pictures.

stereoscop′ic, stereoscop′ical. Pert. to the stereoscope or its use.

s. vision. Vision in which things have the appearance of solidity and relief as though seen in three dimensions. Binocular vision produces this effect.

stereotaxis [Gr. *stereos*, solid, + *taxis*, arrangement]. A method of precisely locating areas in the brain; use of this technique is essential in certain neurosurgical procedures.

stereotropism (stĕr″ē-ŏt′rō-pĭzm) ["+ *tropos*, a turning]. A response toward (positive s.) or away from (negative s.) a solid object. SYN: *thigmotropism*.

stereotypy (stĕr-ē-ō-tī′pĭ) ["+ *typos*, type]. Persistent repetition of words, posture, or movement without meaning; seen in catatonic partial stupors.

sterile (stĕr′ĭl) [L. *sterilis*, barren]. 1. Free from living microorganisms. SYN: *aseptic*. 2. Not fertile; unable to reproduce young. SYN: *barren*.

sterility (stĕr-ĭl′ĭ-tĭ) [L. *sterilitās*, barrenness]. 1. Condition of being free from living microorganisms. 2. Inability to produce offspring.

Investigation into the cause of s. includes investigation of both husband and wife. A routine examination for s. includes a study of the vaginal secretions, a bimanual examination, visualization of the cervix, and in some cases a test for patency of the tubes.

A history of pelvic disorder is of great importance, and any information as to the use of strong chemical douches for the purpose of contraception may be vital.

TREATMENT: Treatment of s. depends upon the finding and correction of any or all causes of the condition. A high percentage of couples who have an infertility problem in the first year of marriage will have produced an offspring within two to three years even without treatment.

s., absolute. Complete and incurable inability to produce offspring as a result of anatomical or physiological factors which prevent production of functional germ cells, conception, or normal development of a zygote.

s., acquired. The failure of further conception after once having given birth to a child. SYN: *secondary s.*

s., facultative. Voluntary sterility; that resulting from contraceptive practices.

s., female. Inability to conceive.

ETIOL: *Congenital abnormalities:* Absence or maldevelopment of the uterus tubes, or ovaries; infantile uterus.

Acquired local conditions: Vagina: Inflammation. *Cervix:* Narrowing of the internal os; acute and chronic endocervicitis; polyps occluding the cervical canal; cervical mucus which, due to either its chemical or physical qualities, is hostile to sperm. *Body of the uterus:* Fibroids of the uterus which block the canal; diseased endometrium, particularly endometritis. *Fallopian tube:* Chronic salpingo-oophoritis with closure of the tubal ostium and where the ovary is embedded in adhesions. *Ovarian dysfunction:* Congenital conditions, or secondary to endocrine disorders, infections, trauma, neoplasms, x-ray or surgical castration, or effects of toxic agents.

Psychological and emotional disturbances. Coital difficulties. Dietary deficiencies.

s., male. Inability of a male to bring about conception.

ETIOL: May result from congenital factors such as cryptorchidism or maldevelopment of testicular ducts or testis; acquired factors; or lack of libido or impotence. SEE: *s., female.*

s., one-child. S. in a woman following the birth of one child.

s., primary. S. resulting from failure of testis or ovary to produce functional germ cells.

s., relative. S. due to causes other than defect of sex organs.

sterilization (ster′ĭl-ĭ-zā′shŭn) [L. *sterilis*, barren]. 1. Process of destruction of all microorganisms on a substance by exposure to chemical or physical agents, exposure to ionizing radiation, or by filtering gas or liquids through porous materials which remove microorganisms. 2. Process of rendering barren. Can be accomplished by surgical removal of testis or ovary (castration) or inactivation by irradiation, or by tying off or removal of a portion of reproductive ducts (ductus deferens or uterine tubes). SEE: *vasectomy; salpingectomy.*

s., dryheat. S. of microorganisms accomplished by subjection to high heat (165°-170° C.) for two to three hours in ovens.

s., fractional. S. of microorganisms in which heating is done at separated intervals, so that spores can develop into bacteria and be destroyed. Usually accomplished by subjecting organisms to free-flowing steam for 15 min. for three or four successive days. SYN: *intermittent sterilization; tyndalization.*

s., gas. Exposure to gases which destroy microorganisms. Ex: formaldehyde, ethylene oxide.

s., intermittent. S., fractional, q.v.

s., steam, by flowing. Exposure of microorganisms at 212° F. (100° C.) to steam in an unsealed receptacle.

s., steam, under pressure. Exposure of microorganisms to steam in an autoclave.

sterilize (ster′ĭ-līz) [L. *sterilis*, barren]. 1. To free from microorganisms. 2. To make incapable of reproduction.

sterilizer (ster′ĭ-lī″zer). Oven or appliance for sterilizing.

s., Arnold steam. A s. using live or streaming steam at atmospheric pressure.

s., steam. An autoclave or steam-pressure cooker which sterilizes by steam under pressure at temperatures above 100° C.

ster′nal [Gr. *sternalis*]. Rel. to the sternum or breastbone.

sternalgia (ster-năl′jĭ-ă) [Gr. *sternon*, sternum, + *algos*, pain]. Pain in the sternum. SYN: *sternodynia.*

sternebra (ster′nē-bră) [″+ L. *vertebra*, vertebra]. Parts of the sternum prior to fusion.

sterno- [Gr.]. Combining form meaning sternum.

sternoclavicular (ster″nō-klă-vĭk′ū-lăr) [Gr. *sternon*, sternum, + L. *clavicula*, a little key]. Concerning the sternum and clavicle.

sternocleidomastoid (ster″nō-klī″dō-măs′-toyd) [″+ *kleis*, clavicle, + *mastos*, breast, + *eidos*, like]. One of two muscles arising from sternum and inner part of clavicle. SEE: *Table of Muscles* in *Appendix.*

sternocostal (ster″nō-kŏs′tăl) [″+ L. *costa*, rib]. Rel. to sternum and ribs.

sternodynia (ster″nō-dĭn′ĭ-ă) [Gr. *sternon*, sternum, + *odynē*, pain]. Pain in the sternum. SYN: *sternalgia.*

sternohyoid (ster′nō-hī′oyd) [″+ *hyoeidēs*, U-shaped]. Muscle from medial end of clavicle and sternum to hyoid bone. SEE: *Table of Muscles* in *Appendix.*

sternoid (ster′noyd) [″+ *eidos*, resemblance]. Resembling the breastbone.

sternomastoid (ster″nō-măs′toyd) [Gr. *sternon*, sternum, + *mastos*, breast, + *eidos*, form]. Pert. to the sternum and mastoid process of temporal bone.

s. region. Wide area on lateral region of neck covered by sternocleidomastoid muscle. SYN: *carotid region.*

sternopericardial (ster″nō-per′ĭ-kăr′dĭ-ăl) [″+ *peri*, around, + *kardia*, heart]. Concerning the sternum and pericardium.

sternoschisis (ster-nŏs′kĭ-sĭs) [″+ *schisis*, cleft]. A cleft or fissured sternum.

sternothyroid (stĕr″nō-thī′royd) [Gr. *sternon*, breast, + *thyreos*, shield, + *eidos*, like]. Muscle extending beneath the sternohyoid which depresses thyroid cartilage. SEE: *Table of Muscles* in *Appendix*.

sternotomy (stĕr-nŏt′ō-mĭ) ["+ *tomē*, a cutting]. The operation of cutting through the sternum.

sternotrypesis (stĕr″nō-trī-pē′sĭs) ["+ *trypēsis*, a boring]. Surgical perforation of the sternum.

sternum (stĕr′nŭm) [L.]. [NA]. The narrow, flat bone in the median line of the thorax in front. It consists of three portions, distinguished as the manubrium, the gladiolus, and the ensiform or xiphoid process. SYN: *breastbone*.

RS: chicken breast; chondrosternal; chondroxiphoid; cleft; ensiform; gladiolus; manubrium; xiphoid process.

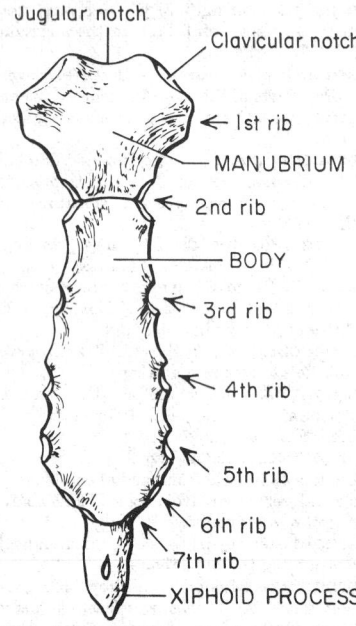

Jugular notch — Clavicular notch — 1st rib — MANUBRIUM — 2nd rib — BODY — 3rd rib — 4th rib — 5th rib — 6th rib — 7th rib — XIPHOID PROCESS

STERNUM—POSTERIOR VIEW

s., cleft. Congenital fissure of the s.

sternutament (stĕr-nū′tăm-ĕnt) [L. *sternutāre*, to sneeze]. A substance causing sneezing.

sternutatio (stĕr-nū-tā′shē-ō) [L.]. Sneezing.

s. convulsiva. Paroxysmal sneezing as in hay fever.

sternutation (stĕr-nū-tā′shŭn). Act of sneezing.

s., convulsive. Spasmodic or paroxysmal sneezing with profusion of watery secretion from the nose.

sternutator (stĕr′nū-tā″tor) [L. *sternutatorius,* causing sneezing]. An agent, such as a war gas, which induces sneezing.

sternutatory (stĕr-nū′tă-tō″rĭ). Causing sneezing.

steroid (stĕr′oid). 1. An organic compound containing in its chemical nucleus the perhydrocyclopentanophenanthrene ring. SEE: *perhydrocyclopentanophenanthrene.* 2. Term applied to any one of a large group of substances chemically related to sterols. Includes sterols, D vitamins, bile acids, certain hormones, saponins, glucosides of digitalis, and certain carcinogenic substances.

s. hormones. The sex hormones and hormones of the adrenal cortex.

steroid hormone therapy. Treatment with various steroid hormones, esp. those from the adrenal cortex. If therapy is continued for longer than a few days, the following general precautions should be observed: low salt diet; restricted fluid intake; high protein diet; control gastric acidity; adequate potassium intake; determine need for covering antibiotic such as isoniazid in sarcoidosis or in those who have a positive tuberculin test; nitrogen balance (androgen or estrogen therapy may be needed); observe for osteoporosis, particularly in postmenopausal women.

sterol (stĕr′ōl, stĕr′ōl) [Gr. *stereos,* solid, + L. *oleum,* oil]. One of a group of substances related to fats and belonging to the lipoids. They are alcohols with a cyclic nucleus (cyclopentanoperhydrophenanthrene) and are found free or esterified with fatty acids (cholesterides). They are found in animals (zoosterols) or in plants (phytosterols).

Generally colorless, crystalline compounds, nonsaponifiable and soluble in certain organic solvents. Ex: cholesterol.

stertor (stĕr′tōr) [L. *stertor*]. Snoring or laborious breathing due to obstruction of air passages in the head, seen in certain diseases as apoplexy.

stertorous (stĕr′tō-rŭs). Pert. to laborious breathing provoking a snoring sound.

stetho- [Gr. *stēthos*, chest]. Combining form indicating the *chest*.

stethogoniometer (stĕth″ō-gō″nĭ-ŏm′ĕt-ĕr) ["+ *gōnia*, angle, + *metron*, measure]. Device for measuring the curvature of the chest.

stethograph S-104 stilet, stilette

stethograph (stĕth'ō-grăf) ["+ *graphein,* to write]. Device to record chest movements in respiration.

stethokyrtograph (stĕth"ō-kir'tō-grăf) [Gr. *stēthos,* chest, + *kyrtos,* bent, + *graphein,* to write]. Device for measuring and recording the dimensions and amount of curves of the chest.

stethometer (stĕth-ŏm'ĕt-ĕr) ["+ *metron,* measure]. Device for measuring the chest's expansion during respiration.

stethophonometer (stĕth"ō-fō-nŏm'ĕt-ĕr) ["+ *phōnē,* voice, + *metron,* measure]. Instrument for determining intensity of sound emitted in auscultation.

stethoscope (stĕth'ō-skōp) [Gr. *stēthos,* chest, + *skopein,* to examine]. Instrument used to mediate sounds produced in the body. Ordinarily consists of rubber tubing in a Y-shape.

   s., binaural. S. designed for use with both ears.

   s., compound. More than one set attached to the same fork and chest piece.

   s., double. S. with two earpieces and tubes.

   s., percussion. Solid cylinder of wood, one end wedge-shaped, the other enlarged into an earpiece adapted for intercostal use.

   s., single. For one ear only; rigid or flexible. SYN: *monaural s.*

stethoscopy (stĕth-ŏs'kō-pī) [Gr. *stēthos,* chest, + *skopein,* to see]. Examination by means of the stethoscope.

stethospasm (stĕth'ō-spăzm) ["+ *spasmos,* spasm]. Spasm of the pectoral or chest muscles.

STH. Abbr. for *somatotrophin,* the growth hormone.

sthenia (sthē'nĭ-ă) [Gr. *sthenos,* strength]. Normal or unusual strength. Opposed to asthenia.

sthenic (sthĕn'ĭk). Active; strong.

sthenometer (sthĕn-ŏm'ĕ-tĕr) [Gr. *sthenos,* strength, + *metron,* measure]. Device for measuring muscular strength.

sthenometry (sthĕn-ŏm'ĕ-trī). Determination of bodily strength.

stibialism (stĭb'ĭ-ăl-ĭzm) [L. *stibium,* antimony, + Gr. *-ismos,* condition]. Antimonial poisoning.

stibium (stĭb'ĭ-ŭm) [L.]. Antimony.

stichochrome (stĭk'ō-krōm) [Gr. *stichos,* row, + *chrōma,* color]. A nerve cell in which the stainable bodies (tigroid mass) are arranged in parallel rows.

stiff [AS. *stif*]. Rigid, firm, inflexible

   s. joint. Joint with reduced mobility.

   s. neck. Rigidity of neck resulting from spasm of neck muscles. It is a symptom of

many disorders. SYN: *torticollis; wryneck.*

   s. -neck fever. 1. Dengue. 2. Cerebrospinal meningitis.

stiff man syndrome. Intermittent aching, tightness, and stiffness of the muscles which progresses to permanent stiffness to the extent of limiting voluntary movement. Disease is not limited to men but only 30% of cases occur in women.

   Etiol. unknown. Dramatic improvement with diazepam has been reported.

stigma (stĭg'mă) [Gr., mark]. (pl. *stigmata, -mas*) 1. A mark or spot on the skin. 2. Spot on ovarian surface where rupture of a graafian follicle will occur. 3. Red spot due to extravasation of blood produced by nervous influence. 4. Mental or physical mark characterizing a specific disease.

   s. of degeneration. Any of the bodily variations from the normal. Formerly thought to be associated with mental degeneracy.

   DEGENERATIVE CHANGES: *Face:* May be unusually hairy in the female and abnormally smooth in the male. *Fingers and toes:* May be an extra one, or adherent or webbed. *Forehead:* May be sloping and very low. *Eyes:* May be different in color or set at different levels. *Ears:* Unusual in many ways. *Jaws:* Either one may project unusually. *Head:* May be unusually large or small. *Teeth:* May be irregular or project. *Roof of mouth:* May be high and pointed or unusually narrow. Only several of these irregularities may be considered as indicative of defective mentality.

   s., hysterical. Any of the peculiar marks or symptoms of hysteria such as spots on the skin, impairment of sensory functions.

   s., psychic. Mental state characterized by susceptibility to suggestion.

stigmatic (stĭg-măt'ĭk) [Gr. *stigma,* mark]. Pert. to or marked with a stigma.

stigmatism. 1. Condition characterized by possession of stigmata. 2. Condition in which the rays of light are accurately focused on retina. SEE: *astigmatism.*

stigmatization (stĭg"mă-tĭ-zā'shŭn). The formation of stigmata, esp. hysterical stigmata on the skin.

stigmatometer (stĭg'mă-tŏm'ĕ-tĕr) [Gr. *stigma,* mark, + *metron,* measure]. Device for testing eye refraction. SYN: *astigmatometer.*

stilbestrol (stĭl-bĕs'trŏl). Diethylstilbestrol, q.v.

stilet, stilette (stĭ-lĕt) [Fr. *stilette*]. 1. Small, sharp-pointed instrument for probing. 2.

Wire used to pass through or stiffen a flexible catheter.

stillbirth (stĭl′bĕrth) [AS. *stille,* quiet, + ME. *burth,* birth]. Birth of a dead fetus.

stillborn (stĭl′bŏrn) [" + *boren,* to bring forth]. Dead at birth.

stillicidium (stĭl′ĭ-sĭd′ĭ-ŭm) [L. *stilla,* drop, + *cadere,* to fall]. A dribbling or flowing, drop by drop.

    s. lacrimarum. Watering of the eye. SYN: *epiphora.*

    s. narium. Watery mucus discharged at onset of coryza.

    s. urinae. Urinary incontinence from a distended bladder. SYN: *strangury.*

stimulant (stĭm′ū-lănt) [L. *stimulāns,* goading]. Any agent temporarily increasing functional activity. Stimulants may be classified according to the organ upon which they act as follows: cardiac, bronchial, gastric, cerebral, intestinal, nervous, motor, vasomotor, respiratory, and secretory.

stimulate (stĭm′ū-lāt) [L. *stimulāre,* to goad on]. To increase functional activity of an organ or structure.

stimulation (stĭm″ū-lā′shŭn). 1. Process of being stimulated. 2. Irritating action of agents on muscles, nerves, or sensory end organs by which activity in a part is evoked.

stimulus (stĭm′ū-lŭs) [L., a goad]. (pl. *stim′uli*) 1. Any agent or factor able to influence living protoplasm directly, as one capable of causing muscular contraction or secretion in a gland, or of initiating an impulse in a nerve. 2. A change of environment of sufficient intensity to evoke a response in an organism. 3. An excitant or irritant.

    s., adequate. 1. Any stimulus capable of evoking a response, i.e., an environmental change possessing a certain intensity, acting for a certain length of time and occurring at a certain rate. 2. A stimulus capable of initiating a nerve impulse in a specific type of receptor.

    s., chemical. A chemical substance (liquid, gaseous, or solid) which is capable of evoking a response.

    s., conditioned. A s. that gives rise to a conditioned response. SEE: *reflex, conditioned.*

    s., electric. A s. resulting from the initiation of, or cessation of, a flow of electrons as from a battery, induction coil, or generator.

    s., homologous. A s. which acts only on specific sensory end organs.

    s., iatrotropic. The s. or event which makes a person seek or receive medical attention; also called the sick person's chief complaint. However there are many reasons

why medical care is voluntarily sought by apparently-healthy people, i.e., an Armed Forces draft examination, preemployment or premarital examination, or in a health screening survey. Thus it is possible for disease to be discovered prior to the time when the disease would make itself known to the individual. This is called lanthanic disease, q.v.

    s., liminal. S., threshold, q.v.

    s., mechanical. A s. produced by a physical change such as contact with objects, changes in pressure, etc. SYN: *physical s.*

    s., minimal. S., threshold, q.v.

    s., nociceptive. A painful and usually injurious s.

    s., subliminal. Less than a threshold s.

    s., thermal. S. produced by a change in temperature of the skin, a rise giving sensations of warmth; a fall giving sensations of coldness.

    s., threshold. The least or weakest stimulus that is capable of initiating a response or giving rise to a sensation. SYN: *liminal s.; minimal s.*

sting [AS. *stingan*]. 1. Sharp, smarting sensation, as of a wound or astringent. 2. A sharp offensive weapon of an insect such as a bee or wasp. 3. A wound made by a sting.

stingray. A group of rays of the family Dasayatidae. A number of species are found in the coastal waters of the United States. It is flat with wide pectoral fins which resemble wings. A venomous spine runs along the top of its whip-like tail, with which it can inflict severe injuries.

    TREATMENT: Pain relievers, debridement of wound, irrigation with removal of foreign material and stinger if it is present, and injection of site with local anesthetic. Soak area in hot water (45-60° C.) 30-60 minutes to inactivate venom.

S-T interval. The interval in an electrocardiogram which represents the initial and final ventricular complexes.

stippling (stĭp′lĭng) [Dutch *stippelen,* to spot]. A spotted condition, as in retina in certain ocular diseases or in basophilic red corpuscles.

stirrup, stirrup bone (stĭr′ŭp) [AS. *stigrāp,* a stirrup]. Stapes of the ears.

stitch (stĭch) [AS. *stice,* a pricking]. 1. A local, sharp, lancinating, or spasmodic pain. 2. A single loop of suture material passed through skin or flesh by a needle, to facilitate healing of a wound. 3. To unite skin or flesh with a needle and suture material. Some stitches are removed after a few days

and other types are absorbed by the body.
SYN: *suture.*

   s. abscess. Abscess developing in a suture; due to infection.

stochastic model (stō-kăs'tĭk) [Gr. *stokastikos,* skillful in guessing]. A statistical model which attempts to reproduce that sequence of events which would be expected to occur in a real-life situation. This technique has some usefulness in predicting the importance and extent of disease in a specified population.

stock (stŏk) [AS. *stocc,* tree trunk]. The original individual, race, or tribe from which others have descended.

   s. culture. Permanent culture of a microorganism reinforced from time to time by fresh media.

Stokes-Adams syndrome (stōks-ād'ăms). [William Stokes, Irish physician, 1804-1878; Robert Adams, Irish physician, 1791-1875]. A series of symptoms in those suffering from heart block. Onset is sudden, resembling epilepsy, for which it is sometimes mistaken. SYN: *Adams-Stokes syndrome.*

   ETIOL: Due to complete heart block with consequent decrease in blood flow to the brain.

   TREATMENT: Intracardiac epinephrine, a sharp blow to the precordium or use of an external electric pacemaker.

Stokes' law (stōks). A muscle is frequently a seat of paralysis if lying above an inflamed serous or mucous membrane.

Stokes' lens. [George G. Stokes, Eng. physicist, 1819-1903]. Device used to diagnose astigmatism.

stoma (stō'mă) [Gr. *stoma,* mouth]. (pl. *stomata, -mas*) 1. A mouth, small opening, or a pore. 2. Artificially created opening between two passages or body cavities or between a cavity or passage and the body's surface. 3. A minute opening between cells of certain epithelial membranes, esp. peritoneum and pleura.

stomach (stŭm'ăk) [Gr. *stomachos,* stomach]. A dilated, saclike, distensible portion of the alimentary canal below the esophagus and below the diaphragm to right of spleen, partly under the liver. It is composed of a *fundus,* or round part; a *body,* or middle portion; and *pyloric portion* which is the small end.

   It has two openings; the upper cardiac orifice opens into the esophagus, and the lower pyloric orifice opens into the duodenum. The stomach is composed of four layers; the outer serous coat covers almost all of the organ. The muscular layer just beneath is formed of three layers of smooth

muscle fibers: an outer longitudinal layer, a medial circular layer, and an inner oblique layer. Submucous layer is a connecting medium between the muscular and mucous layer, the inner lining of the stomach.

   The cardiac, fundic (parietal or oxyntic), and pyloric glands of the stomach are composed of columnar and tubular cells which secrete gastric juice containing hydrochloric acid, pepsin, etc.

   FUNCTIONS: The s. secretes gastric juice and converts proteins into peptones. In addition to its basic function of serving as an organ of digestion, the stomach also serves in the following ways: it regulates the admission of food to the remainder of the gut, acting as a reservoir; its acid kills a large proportion of the microbes present in most food; it has some power to absorb; it is important in the acid-base equilibrium of the body, particularly when electrolytes are removed from the body during vomiting; it can excrete some drugs, administered parenterally, into the gastric juice; it acts as a kind of receptor for chemical and nervous mechanisms by which secretion and movement are stimulated in lower parts of the gastrointestinal tract; it forms a hematinic principle (antianemic factor), effective in prevention of pernicious anemia, by the action of an intrinsic factor (present in gastric juice) on an extrinsic factor (vitamin B_{12}) present in foods.

   DIET IN SOME DISORDERS: *Atony and Hypomotility:* Food is retained longer than normal and decomposition may occur if hydrochloric acid is deficient. Liquids are retained longer than solids. Therefore diet

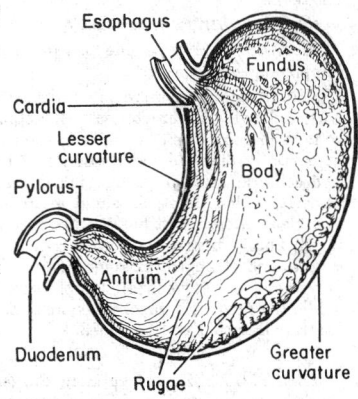

THE STOMACH

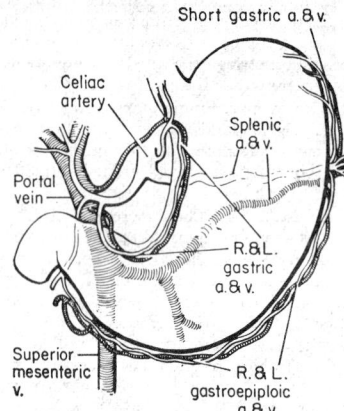

Short gastric a. & v.

Celiac artery

Splenic a. & v.

Portal vein

R. & L. gastric a. & v.

Superior mesenteric v.

R. & L. gastroepiploic a. & v.

THE STOMACH—ANTERIOR VIEW

should consist of quickly and easily digested foods—cream, butter, soft-cooked vegetables, chicken, fish, strained beef, and moderate amount of milk. Avoid liquids, pastries, and rich gravies. *Hypermotility:* The stomach empties too rapidly; therefore, diet should be liquid, soft, in small amounts, and in frequent feedings. Fats delay the emptying of the stomach. *Hyperacidity:* Give protein to combine with acid, thus inhibiting its secretion by moderate amount of fat. Avoid stimulating secretion of acid. Five small meals or three meals and two lunches.

s. ache. Pain in the stomach. SYN: *gastralgia; gastrodynia; stomachalgia; stomachodynia.*

s., bilocular. S., hourglass, q.v.

s. cancer. May be due to carcinoma, lymphoma, sarcoma, etc.

SYM: General symptoms of dyspepsia with following characteristic symptoms: continued pain, often tenderness; vomiting of partially digested food; absence of free hydrochloric acid in gastric juice; hematemesis or blood in stools, slight in amount and blood-altered so it has a coffee-grounds appearance; presence of tumor; loss of weight and strength; extreme anemia; involvement of superficial lymph glands. When the pylorus is involved, symptoms of gastric dilatation will be added.

PROG: Very poor.

TREATMENT: Early treatment. Surgery; liquid or semiliquid diet; rest; constitutional treatment as indicated.

s., cardiac. Fundus of the stomach.

s., cascade. A form of hourglass stomach in which there is a constriction between cardiac and pyloric portions. Cardiac portion fills first and then contents cascade into pyloric portion. SYN: *cup-and-spill stomach.*

s., cow horn. A high, transversely placed stomach. SYN: *steer horn s.*

s., foreign bodies in. In the average case there is no concern. Foreign bodies usually pass through the alimentary tract without disturbance. However, these patients should be under a doctor's care. Usually symptoms are absent, but the patient may be alarmed. Give nothing by mouth. Under no circumstances should salts, cathartics, and enemas be used inasmuch as they can only make the condition worse.

s., hourglass. S. resembling an hourglass, caused by constriction from a band of fibrous exudate.

s. intubation. Passage of a tube into the stomach to obtain gastric contents for examination, for prophylaxis and treatment of ileus, or to remove ingested poisons.

s., leather-bottle. S. caused by hypertrophy of the s. walls or their infiltration with malignant tissue.

s. pump. Device for removing contents of the stomach through a tube inserted through the mouth.

s., thoracic. Condition in which stomach lies above diaphragm. May result from embryonic anomaly in which stomach fails to descend, or from hernia of diaphragm. Latter results in so-called upside-down stomach.

s. tooth. A lower canine tooth during first dentition.

s. tube. Tube used to wash out or feed the stomach.

s., water-trap. S. with the pylorus situated unusually high, causing slow emptying.

stomach, words pert. to: abdominal cavity; absorption; achylia gastrica; acidity; anachlorhydria; anadenia; anticardium; atony; atretogastria; capotement; cardialgia; cardiopyloric; cardiospasm; catastalsis; chlorhydria; cholangiogastrostomy; clapotement; clapotage; digestion; ectasia; endogastritis; feeding, artificial; gastric juice; gastric lavage; "gastr-" words; gavage; hourglass stomach; hunger; lavage; linitis; myxorrhea gastrica; pneumatosis; pneumogastric; pylorus; reflex, gastrocolic; saburra; secretagogue; ulcer; ventriculus.

stomachal (stŭm'ă-kăl) [Gr. *stomachos,* stomach]. 1. Rel. to the stomach. 2. A gastric tonic.

stomachal'gia ["+ *algos,* pain]. Pain in the stomach.

stomachic (stō-măk'ĭk). 1. Concerning the stomach. 2. Medicine exciting action of the stomach. SYN: *stomachal.*

stomachos'copy [Gr. *stomachos,* stomach, + *skopein,* to inspect]. Examination of the stomach. SYN: *gastroscopy.*

sto'mata. Pl. of stoma, q.v.

stomatalgia (stō"mă-tăl'jĭ-ă) [Gr. *stoma, stomat-,* mouth, + *algos,* pain]. Pain in the mouth. SYN: *stomatodynia.*

stomat'ic. Pert. to or rel. to the mouth.

stomatitis (stō"mă-tī'tĭs) [Gr. *stoma, stomat-,* mouth, + *-itis,* inflammation]. Inflammation of the mouth.

SYM: Heat, pain, increased flow of saliva, fetor of breath, restlessness, languor, disinclination to nurse in infants, sometimes fever.

ETIOL: S. may be caused by many factors or conditions. Among them are pathogenic organisms, including bacteria and viruses; mechanical trauma; irritants such as alcohol, tobacco, hot foods, spices; sensitization to chemical substances in tooth pastes, mouthwashes, etc.; nutritional deficiencies, esp. avitaminoses; blood disorders; poisoning by drugs, esp. heavy metals; certain skin disorders; systemic infections such as measles, scarlet fever, syphilis. There are also several forms with unknown etiology.

RS: gangrene; noma, thrush.

s., aphthous. Formation of tiny ulcers (canker sores) on mucosa of the mouth.

SYM: General symptoms of stomatitis and on inspection numerous small, round vesicles on cheeks, lips, and tongue, which soon break and leave little shallow ulcers with red areola.

PROG: Good.

TREATMENT: For infants, sterilize milk. Nurse at regular intervals. Wash mouth with clean linen cloth. In adults, correct gastric disturbance or other cause.

s., catarrhal. Simple s.

SYM: General symptoms of s. with diffuse red swelling of mucous membrane.

TREATMENT: Good hygienic conditions; cleanse mouth with weak solution of boric acid or chlorate of potassium as a wash.

s., corrosive. S. resulting from intentional or accidental exposure to corrosive substances.

s., diphtheritic. Diphtheria of mucous membranes of the gums or cheeks. SYN: *buccal diphtheria.*

s., follicular. S., aphthous, q.v.

s., gangrenous. This form seen in debilitated children from 2 to 6 years; usual-ly follows one of the specific fevers, esp. measles and whooping cough. SYN: *cancrum oris; noma.*

SYM: General. An inspection shows cheek is affected—externally, swollen, hard, red and glazed; internally, irregular, sloughing ulcer.

COMPLICATIONS: Perforation, septicemia, lobular pneumonia from aspirated sloughs, and diarrhea from swallowing fetid material.

PROG: Grave. Death common from exhaustion or complications. Recovery often attended with deformity.

TREATMENT: Excision with electrocautery knife early. Nutritious food, good hygiene.

s., herpetic. S. characterized by cold sores (fever blisters).

s., membranous. S. accompanied by the formation of a false or adventitious membrane.

s., mercurial. This form is seen in artisans who work with mercury; after the administration of very large doses of mercurials, and after small doses where there has been unnatural susceptibility.

PREMONITORY SYM: Tenderness of gums, redness near insertion of teeth, metallic taste, increase of saliva.

LATER SYM: Profuse salivation, fetor of breath; redness, swelling, and tenderness of gums. Tongue may be similarly affected and protrude from mouth. In severe cases ulceration of mucous membrane, loss of teeth, and necrosis of jaw result.

TREATMENT: If due to acute poisoning, early administration of British antilewisite will be helpful. If chronic, remove patient from source of poison and treat symptomatically. SEE: *ptyalism.*

s., myotic. Thrush, q.v.

s., parasitica. S. caused by a yeastlike fungus, Candida albicans. SYN: *thrush.*

SYM: Of general s. with milk-white elevations on tongue and mouth which on removal leave a raw surface. Disease may extend to pharynx, esophagus, and larynx. Microscopic examination reveals fungus.

PROG: Good.

TREATMENT: Correct hygiene. Treat any gastric disturbance; locally, mild alkaline mouthwash. Diluted gentian violet mouthwash is effective also. Topical application of diluted nystatin solution may be necessary.

s., simple. Erythematous inflammation of the mouth occurring in patches on the mucous membranes.

s., traumatic. S. resulting from mechanical injury as from ill-fitting dentures, sharp jagged teeth, biting cheek, etc.

s., ulcerative. Thought by some to be an infectious disease, as it often occurs in epidemics and attacks both children and adults when congregated and subjected to bad hygienic conditions. SYN: *trench mouth.*

SYM: Of the general form. Gums of lower jaw chiefly affected, are swollen, red, and spongy. Linear ulcers soon form and may extend to cheek; gland under jaw swollen. In severe cases loosening of teeth and necrosis of jaw may form.

PROG: Guardedly favorable.

TREATMENT: Correct hygiene; antiseptic mouthwashes such as hydrogen peroxide; no smoking.

s., vesicular. S., aphthous, q.v.

s., Vincent's. Ulcerative s.

stomato- [Gr.]. Combining form indicating mouth.

stomatodynia (stō''mă-tō-dĭn'ĭ-ă) [Gr. *stoma, stomat-,* mouth, + *odynē,* pain]. Pain in the mouth. SYN: *stomatalgia.*

stomatodysodia (stō''mă-tō-dĭs-ō'dĭ-ă) ["+ *dysōdia,* stench]. Foul odor from the mouth.

stomatogastric (stō''mă-tō-găs'trĭk) ["+ *gastēr,* belly]. Concerning the stomach and mouth.

stomatography (stō''mă-tŏg'ră-fĭ) [Gr. *stoma, stomat-,* mouth, + *graphein,* to write]. A treatise on the mouth.

stomatologist (stō''mă-tŏl'ō-jĭst) ["+ *logos,* a study]. Specialist in treatment of diseases of the mouth.

stomatology (stō''mă-tŏl'ō-jĭ). Science of the mouth and teeth and their diseases.

stomatomalacia (stō''mă-tō-mă-lā'shĭ-ă) [Gr. *stoma, stomat-,* mouth, "+ *malakia,* softening]. Pathological softening of any structures of the mouth.

stomat'omy ["+ *tomē,* a cutting]. Surgical nicking of the edges of the os uteri to facilitate delivery.

stomatomycosis (stō''mă-tō-mī-kō'sĭs) ["+ *mykēs,* fungus, + *-ōsis,* condition]. Any mouth disease resulting from fungi.

stomatonecrosis, stomatonoma (stō''mă-tō-nē-krō'sĭs, -nō'mă) ["+ *nekrosis,* death, + *nomē,* a spreading]. Gangrenous, ulcerative inflammation of the mouth. SYN: *cancrum oris; gangrenous stomatitis; noma.*

stomatopathy (stō''mă-tŏp'ă-thĭ) [Gr. *stomatos,* mouth, + *pathos,* disease]. Any mouth disease.

stomatoplasty (stō''mă-tō-plăs'tĭ) ["+ *plassein,* to form]. Plastic surgery or repair of the mouth.

stomatorrhagia (stō''mă-tō-rā'jĭ-ă) ["+ *rhēgnynai,* to burst forth]. Hemorrhage from the mouth or gums.

stomat'oscope [Gr. *stomatos,* mouth, + *skopein,* to examine]. Instrument for examining the mouth.

stomato'sis ["+ *-osis,* condition]. Any disease of the mouth.

stomodeum (stō''mō-dē'ŭm) ["+ *hodaios,* a way]. An external depression lined with ectoderm and bounded by frontonasal, mandibular, and maxillary processes of the embryo. It forms anterior portion of oral cavity. Its floor, the pharyngeal membrane, separates s. from the foregut.

stone [AS. *stān*]. Hardened mineral matter, as a gallstone, q.v. SYN: *calculus,* q.v.

stool (stūl) [AS. *stōl,* a seat]. 1. Evacuation of the bowels. 2. Waste matter discharged from the bowels. SYN: *feces,* q.v.

COLOR: Iron and bismuth turn the stool black, and certain vegetables and berries darken it or produce a distinct color. Pathological stools are usually grayish or a whitish glistening color, and tarry in hemorrhage or show fresh blood.

CHARACTER OR NATURE OF STOOLS: *Fatty stools:* These are observed in obstructive jaundice, cancer of the pancreas, pancreatic calculi, and in indigestion or overfeeding in infants.

Frothy, poorly formed stools: They may indicate a spastic colon, the presence of gas, or intestinal inflammation.

Lienteric stools: These contain much undigested food and are noted in inflammatory conditions of the stomach and upper bowel.

Tarry stools: They may indicate gastric hemorrhage, swallowed blood from the nose or lungs, bleeding ulcers of the gastrointestinal tract, hepatic cirrhosis, or cancer.

Membranous shreds: They may exist in cancer of the colon, dysentery, relapsing fever, acute proctitis, and in sloughing of intestinal mucosa.

Mucus stools: Exist in catarrhal or inflamed conditions of the intestines or rectum, in dysentery, enterocolitis, proctitis, impaction, and ulcerative colitis.

SHAPE OF: *Cylindrical:* If of small caliber, they may be indicative of prolapsus ani, annular rectal stricture, or intestinal spasms.

Ribbon-shaped: Indicative of stricture or cancer of the rectum; possibly enlargement of the prostate in males, hemorrhoids, spasm of the lower bowel and anus, prostatic abscess, and prolapse of the uterus.

Scybala: Rounded masses or balls of fecal matter or hardened feces, the result of habitual constipation, atony or sacculation (diverticulum) of the colon, gastric ulcer, dilation, rectal cancer, or dysentery.

s., bilious. Yellowish or yellowish-brown discharges in diarrhea becoming darker on exposure.

s., fatty. Fat in the feces, as in pancreatic disease.

s., pea soup. Liquid stools of typhoid.

s., rice water. Watery serum stools with detached epithelium, as in cholera.

s. softeners. Substances which act as wetting agents and thus promote soft malleable bowel movements. They are not laxatives and therefore are not indicated for constipation caused by decreased or absent peristaltic activity. Dioctyl sodium sulfosuccinate or dioctyl calcium sulfosuccinate is used to soften stools.

stop needle. One with eye at tip and a disk to prevent penetration deeper than desired.

stoppage (stŏp′ăj) [AS. *stoppian*]. Obstruction of an organ. SEE: *cholestasia*.

storm [AS.]. A sudden outburst or exacerbation of symptoms of a disease.

s., renal. A sudden attack of renal symptoms accompanying a neurosis sometimes occurring in patients suffering from aortic regurgitation.

stout (stowt) [O.Fr. *estout*, bold]. Having a bulky body. SYN: *corpulent.*

STP. Abbr. for *standard temperature and pressure.*

STPD. Abbr. for *standard temperature, and pressure, dry.* Gas volume at 0° C. 760 mm. of mercury total pressure and partial pressure of water of 0° C.

Str. Abbr. for *Streptococcus.*

strabismic (stră-bĭz′mĭk) [Gr. *strabismos,* a squint]. Pert. to or afflicted with strabismus.

strabismometer (stră-bĭz-mŏm′ĕt-ĕr) ["+ *metron,* a measure]. Instrument for determining amount of strabismus.

strabismus (stră-bĭz′mŭs) [Gr. *strabismos,* a squinting]. Disorder of eye in which optic axes cannot be directed to same object, due to lack of muscular coordination. The squinting eye always deviates to the same extent when the eyes are carried in different directions: *unilateral* when same eye always deviates; *alternating* when either deviates, the other being fixed; *constant* when the squint remains permanent; *periodic* when eyes are occasionally free from it. Muscles may lead to squint, but prime factor is found in errors of refraction, in hypermetropia or in myopia with or without astigmatism. SYN: *heterotropia; squint.* SEE: *microstrabismus.*

s., accommodative. S. due to disorder of ocular accommodation.

s., alternating. S. affecting either eye alternately.

s., bilateral. S., accommodative, q.v.

s., concomitant. Form in which both eyes move freely, but retain false relationship to each other.

s., convergent. The deviating eye turns inward. SYN: *internal squint.*

s. deorsum vergens. Vertical s., the deviating eye turning downward. SYN: *hypotropia.*

s., divergent. Deviating eye turns outward.

s., intermittent. S. recurring at intervals.

s., monocular. S. in which the same eye habitually deviates.

s., monolateral. S. with the squinting eye always the same.

s., paralytic. S. which is due to paralysis of a muscle. The deviation is present only in the sphere of action of the paralyzed muscle. In paralytic squint the secondary deviation is greater than the primary. This condition is due to paralysis of one or more ocular muscles and may point to grave cerebral disease or to presence of some constitutional disease.

This form of s. is recognized by the fact that if a candle or the finger of the surgeon is carried from right to left before the face of the patient, the deviating eye fails to follow to its proper limit and leads the physician to look for lesions of the 6th nerve in failure of external rectus, of 3rd nerve in failure of internal rectus of either side, of 4th nerve in impairment of superior oblique muscles. In adults this usually is due to syphilitic disease involving the nerve centers or trunks, or to rheumatism.

PROG: In general, guarded.

TREATMENT: Directed to the cause. Eyeglasses.

s., spastic. S. due to contraction of an ocular muscle.

s. sursum vergens. Vertical squint upward. SYN: *hypertropia.*

ETIOL: Defects of fusion faculty, errors of refraction, poor vision in one eye, anisometropia.

TREATMENT: Refraction with prescribing of glasses, orthoptic training (training of fusion), operative.

s., vertical. Eye turns upward. The vision is double (diplopia) unless there is unconscious suppression of the image in squinting eye. Expression of face is bizarre and sometimes malign. Vertical s. usually is the result of ametropia in childhood, or of central nervous system disease in adult life.

strabometer (strä-bŏm′ĕt-ẽr) [Gr. *strabos,* squinting, + *metron,* a measure]. Instrument to ascertain the degree of strabismus.

strabotomy (strä-bŏt′ō-mĭ) ["+ *tomē,* a cutting]. Operation for strabismus.

strain (strān). 1. [AS. *strēon,* offspring]. A stock, said of bacteria or protozoa from a specific source and maintained in successive cultures or animal inoculation. 2. Hereditary streak or tendency. 3. [O.Fr. *estreindere,* to draw tight]. To pass through, as a filter. 4. To injure by making too strong an effort or by excessive use. 5. Excessive use of a part of the body so that it is injured. 6. Trauma to the muscle or the musculotendinous unit from violent contraction or excessive forcible stretch. May be associated with failure of synergistic action of muscles. SEE: *sprain.*

F. A. TREATMENT: Apply cold applications and a firm dressing. Immobilize for some time. Adhesive strapping helpful. Operative repair sometimes necessary.

s. x-ray. X-ray picture taken with the part, usually a bone or joint, under static force or tension. Used to better demonstrate the pathological change which might be inapparent if this technique were not employed.

strainer (strān′ẽr). Device used for retaining solid pieces while liquid passes through. SYN: *filter.*

strait (strāt) [O.Fr. *estreit,* narrow]. A constricted or narrow passage.

s., inferior. The lower outlet of the pelvic canal.

s. -jacket. Shirt with long sleeves laced on patient and fastened to restrain the arms. SYN: *camisole.*

s.'s of the pelvis. The inferior and superior openings of the true pelvis.

s., superior. The upper opening or inlet of the pelvic canal.

stramonium (strä-mō′nĭ-ŭm) [L.]. Jamestown weed, Jimson weed. The dried leaves of Datura stramonium.

USES: An ingredient in asthma powder for its antispasmodic effect. Local anodyne.

POISONING: Related to atropine. SEE: *atropine sulfate.*

strangalesthesia (strang′′gäl-ĕs-thē′zĭ-ä) [Gr. *strangalizein,* to choke, + *aisthēsis,* sensation]. A girdlelike sensation of constriction. SYN: *zonesthesia.*

strangle (strang′gl) [L. *strangulāre*]. To choke or suffocate or be choked from compression of the trachea.

strangulated (străng′ū-lā″tĕd). Constricted so that air or blood supply is cut off, as a s. hernia.

strangulation (străng′′ū-lā′shŭn) [L. *strangulāre*]. Compression or constriction of a part, as the bowel or throat, such as causes suspension of breathing or of passage of contents; congestion accompanies condition.

s., internal. Slipping of a coil of the intestine through the diaphragm or an abnormal opening.

strangury (străng′ū-rĭ) [Gr. *stranx,* a drop, + *ouron,* urine]. Painful and interrupted urination in drops produced by spasmodic muscular contraction of urethra and bladder.

strap (străp) [Gr. *strophos,* a cord]. 1. A band, as one of adhesive plaster, used to hold dressings in place or to approximate surfaces of a wound. 2. To bind with strips of adhesive plaster.

strapping (străp′ĭng). 1. Adhesive plaster or other substance used to bind surfaces together or hold dressings in place. 2. Application of adhesive plaster strips on a part so as to give it support or compress it.

stratified (străt′ĭ-fīd) [L. *stratificāre,* to arrange in layers]. In strata or in the form of layers.

s. epithelium. Epithelium in superimposed layers with differently shaped cells in the various layers.

stratiform (străt′ĭ-form) [L. *stratum,* layer, + *forma,* shape]. Arranged in layers, as manner of liquefaction of gelatin stab culture, in which there is liquefaction to the walls of the tube at the top and then downward horizontally.

stratum (strā′tŭm, străt′ŭm) [L.]. (pl. *stra′ta*) A layer.

s. basale. The innermost or deepest layer of the endometrium of uterus.

s. compactum. The superficial or outermost layer of the endometrium.

s. corneum. Outermost horny layer of the epidermis.

s. disjunction. The outermost layer of the stratum corneum which is being shed constantly.

s. germinativum. Innermost layer of epidermis. A row of columnar cells which divide to replace rest of the epidermis as it wears away. SEE: *prickle cell.*

s. granulosum. A layer of cells containing deeply staining granules of keratohyalin found in epidermis of skin and lying between s. germinativum and s. lucidum.

s. lucidum. A translucent layer of the epidermis lying between s. corneum and s. granulosum. Frequently it is absent.

s. malpighii. Inner layer of the epidermis. SYN: *rete mucosum; s. germinativum.*

s mucosum. S. malpighii, q.v.

s. papillare. The papillary of the corium lying adjacent to the epidermis.

s. reticulare. The recticular layer of the corium lying just beneath the papillary layer.

s. spinosum. S. malpighii, q.v.

s. spongiosum. Middle layer of decidua.

s. submucosum. Layer of smooth muscle fibers of the myometrium lying contiguous with endometrium.

s. subserosum. Layer of smooth muscle fibers of myometrium which lies immediately under serous coat.

s. supravasculare. A layer of circular and longitudinal muscle fibers lying between s. subserosum and s. vasculare.

s. vasculare. A layer of smooth muscles in myometrium lying between s. submucosum and s. supravasculare.

strawberry (strŏ'bĕr'ĭ) [AS. *strēawberige*]. Various low-growing plants producing red, fleshy, edible fruit.

    COMP: Contain little cellulose. Sugar is low. They contain much lime and a salicylic element. ACTION: The salicylic element is irritating to many and may result in a skin rash.

    Food value of 100 gm. (frozen, sliced, sweetened): Cal. 109; protein 0.5 gm.; fat 0.2 gm.; calcium 14 mg.; carbohydrate 27.8 gm.; vitamin C, 53 mg.

strawberry mark. A soft, nodular, vascular nevus usually present on face or neck, occurring at birth or shortly afterwards. Usually disappears without treatment. SYN: *cavernous angioma; simplex hemangioma.*

strawberry tongue. The peculiar red, papillated tongue of scarlatina, q.v. SEE: *tongue.*

straw itch. A skin condition accompanied by itching due to working in straw or sleeping on a straw mattress.

streak (strēk) [AS. *strica*]. A line or stripe. SYN: *stria.*

s., angioid. A dark s. seen in retina in individuals with pseudoxanthoma elasticum.

s. culture. A bacterial culture in streaks.

s., medullary. Deep longitudinal groove on dorsal surface of the embryo which becomes the medullary tube. SYN: *dorsal groove.*

s., meningitic. A red line across the skin formed by drawing a pointed article

across it; seen in meningitis and nerve center affections. SYN: *tache cérébrale.*

s. reflex. A white, shining s. along center of retinal vessels.

strephosymbolia (strĕf'ō-sĭm-bō'lĭ-ă) [Gr. *strephein*, to twist, + *symbolon*, symbol]. 1. Difficulty in distinguishing between letters which are similar but face in opposite directions. Ex: p-q, b-d. 2. Perception of objects reversed as in a mirror.

strephotome (strĕf'ō-tōm) ["+ *tomē*, a cutting]. Instrument for invagination of a hernial sac.

strep'itus [L.]. A sound or noise, as that heard on auscultation.

strepticemia (strĕp"tĭ-sē'mĭ-ă) [Gr. *streptos*, twisted, + *haima*, blood]. Streptococci present in the blood stream, causing infection. SYN: *streptococcemia.*

strepto- [Gr. *streptos*, twisted]. Combining form meaning twisted.

streptoangina (strĕp"tō-ăn-jī'nă) ["+ L. *angina*, a choking]. Sore throat with membranous formation due to streptococci.

streptobacillus (strĕp"tō-bă-sĭl'ŭs). A bacillus in which individual bacilli form a chain-like colony.

streptococcal (strĕp"tō-kŏk'ăl) [Gr. *streptos*, twisted, + *kokkos*, berry]. Caused by or pert. to streptococci.

streptococcemia (strĕp"tō-kŏk-sē'mĭ-ă) ["+ "+ *haima*, blood]. Presence of streptococci in the blood causing infection.

streptococcic (strĕp"tō-kŏk'sĭk) [Gr. *streptos*, twisted, + *kokkos*, berry]. Resembling, produced by, or pert. to streptococci.

s. sore throat. Severe epidemic form with membranous formation caused by beta hemolytic streptococci.

streptococcicosis (strĕp"tō-kŏk"sĭ-kō'sĭs) ["+ "+ -ōsis, condition]. Any streptococcal infection.

streptococcolysin (strĕp"tō-kŏk-kŏl'ĭ-sĭn) ["+ "+ *lysis*, dissolution]. A lysin produced by streptococci.

Streptococcus (strĕp"tō-kŏk'ŭs) [Gr. *streptos*, twisted, + *kokkos*, berry]. (pl. *Streptococci*) A genus of bacteria belonging to the family Lactobacillaceae, tribe Streptococceae. They are gram-positive cocci occurring in chains.

    Most species are harmless saprophytes, but some are among the most common and dangerous pathogens of man. They are differentiated on the basis of their reactions on blood-agar plates into three types: alpha (α), beta (β), and gamma (γ). Those of the alpha type (Streptococcus viridans) form a greenish coloration about colonies and partially hemolyze blood; those of the beta or hemo-

lytic type form clear zones about colonies
and completely hemolyze blood (Ex: Str.
pyogenes); those of the gamma type are
nonhemolytic and produce a grayish coloration about colonies (Ex: Str. anhemolyticus).

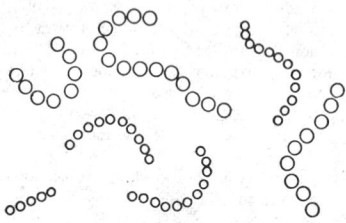

STREPTOCOCCUS
Cocci of varying size in chains.

Str. anhemolyticus. A species of low
pathogenicity often found as secondary invaders.

Str. equinus. Variety found in intestines of horses, and in bovine and in human
feces.

Str. pyogenes. Any of the hemolytic
streptococci causing suppurative processes.
The causative agent of scarlet fever, erysipelas, septic sore throat, puerperal sepsis, and
various pyogenic infections.

Str. salivarius. α-hemolytic species of
the Viridans group. Normally present in the
nose, mouth, and throat of human beings.

Str. thermophilus. An organism
found in dairy products.

Str. viridans. A group of α-hemolytic
streptococci which are normally present in
the upper respiratory tract. Minor trauma
such as vigorous chewing may result in their
being admitted to the blood stream. Thus
when heart valves are damaged these organisms are the ones which most frequently
colonize on them. When this occurs, subacute bacterial endocarditis has an excellent
chance of developing.

streptocolysin (strĕp"tō-kŏl'ĭ-sĭn)   [Gr.
streptos, twisted, + *lysis,* dissolution]. A
hemolysin produced by streptococci. SYN:
streptococcolysin; streptolysin.

streptodermatitis (strĕp"tō-dĕr"mă-tī'tĭs)
["+ *derma,* skin, + *-itis,* inflammation].
Inflammation of the skin caused by streptococci.

streptodornase (strĕp"tō-dōr'nās). One of
the enzymes (streptokinase is another)
elaborated by certain strains of hemolytic
streptococci, and capable of liquefying fibrinous and purulent exudates. Useful in
pneumococcic and tuberculous empyema.

streptokinase (strĕp"tō-kī'nās). SEE: *streptodornase.*

streptoleukocidin   (strĕp"tō-lū"kō-sī'dĭn)
[Gr. *streptos,* twisted, + *leukos,* white, + L.
cidus, to kill]. A toxin produced by streptococci, destructive to leukocytes.

streptolysin (strĕp-tŏl'ĭ-sĭn). A hemolysin
excreted by a streptococcus. SYN: *streptococcolysin; streptocolysin.*

s. O. A s. resistant to heat and acid but
sensitive to oxygen.

s. S. A s. insensitive to oxygen but rapidly destroyed by heat and acid.

streptomycin (strĕp"tō-mī'sĭn). An antibiotic derived from a soil microbe, Streptomyces
griseus.

streptomycosis (strĕp"tō-mī-kō'sĭs) [Gr.
streptos, twisted, + *mykēs,* fungus, + *-ōsis,*
condition]. Infection caused by microorganisms of the genus Streptomyces.

streptosepticemia (strĕp"tō-sĕp"tĭ-sē'mĭ-ă)
["+ *sēptikos,* putrid, + *haima,* blood]. Septicemia resulting from streptococcus infection. SYN: *streptococcemia; streptomycosis.*

streptothricin (strĕp-tō-thrī'sĭn). An antibiotic biosynthesized by Streptomyces laven-
dulae. It is effective against both
gram-negative and gram-positive bacteria
and some fungi. It is more toxic than streptomycin.

streptothricosis (strĕp"tō-thrī-kō'sĭs) [Gr.
streptos, twisted, + *thrix,* hair, + *-ōsis,*
condition]. Infection caused by a species of
Streptothrix.

SYM: Chronic suppurative inflammation.

Streptothrix (strĕp'tō-thrĭks). A genus of
Chlamydobacteriaceae, of which one form is
the cause of actinomycosis and another is
assumed to be cause of ratbite fever.

stress (strĕs) [O.Fr. *estresse,* narrowness]. In
medicine, the result produced when a structure, system, or organism is acted upon by a
stressor. It is generally believed that biological organisms require a certain amount of s.
in order to maintain their well-being. However when s. occurs in quantities that the
system cannot handle it produces pathological changes.

This biological concept of s. was developed
by Hans Selye who intended originally for s.
to indicate cause rather than effect. But
through a linguistic error, he gave the term
s. to effect and then later had to create the
word *stressor* for the cause.

s. ulcer. Peptic ulcer caused by acute or
chronic stress such as cerebral trauma,
burns, surgery, acute infection.

stress'or. An agent or condition capable of
producing stress. SEE: *stress.*

s., systemic. S. which produces generalized systemic responses.

s., topical. S. which causes mild inflammation or local damage.

stretch (strĕch) [AS. *streccan*, extend]. To draw out or extend to full length.

s. receptor. A proprioceptor located in a muscle or tendon which is stimulated by a stretch or pull.

s. reflex. The contraction of a muscle as a result of a pull exerted upon the tendon of the responding muscle. S. reflexes are of primary importance in maintenance of posture. SYN: *myotactic reflex.*

stretcher (strĕch'ĕr). A litter for carrying the sick, injured, or dead.

stretching of contractures. Process performed to loosen contracted ligaments, muscles, and adhesions in stiff joints. There should be a slow, steady, and gradually increasing pull by the operator or with gradually increasing weights.

stria (strī'ă) [L., a channel]. (pl. *stri'ae*) [NA] A line or band elevated above or depressed below surrounding tissue, or differing in color and texture.

s. acusticae. Horizontal white stripes on floor of the 4th ventricle of the brain. SYN: *striae medullares.*

s. atrophica. A fine pinkish-white or gray line, usually 14 cm. in length, seen in parts of body where skin has been stretched. Commonly seen on thighs, abdomen, and breasts of women who are or have been pregnant; in persons whose skin has been stretched by obesity, tumor, or dropsy; or in persons who have taken adrenocortical hormones for a prolonged period.

s. cerebellares. S. medullares; s. acusticae, q.v.

s. distensae. S. atrophica, q.v.

s. gravidarum. S. atrophica, q.v.

s. longitudinalis lateralis. One of the longitudinal bands of gray matter, slightly elevated on upper part of the corpus callosum.

s. medullares. S. acusticae, q.v.

s. terminalis. A band of fibers in roof of inferior horn running to floor of body of the lateral ventricle.

striate, striated (strī'āt, strī'ā-tĕd) [L. *striatus*]. Striped; marked by streaks or striae.

s. arteries. Branches of the middle cerebral artery which supply basal nuclei of brain.

s. body. Mass of gray and white bands in each cerebral hemisphere. SYN: *corpus striatum.*

s. muscle. Skeletal muscle, consisting of fibers marked by cross striations. SEE: *muscle.*

s. veins, inferior. Branches of basal vein which drain corpus striatum.

striation (strī-ā'shŭn) [L. *striatus*, striped]. 1. State of being striped or streaked. 2. One of a series of streaks. SYN: *stria.*

striatum (strī-ā'tŭm) [L., grooved]. The caudate and lentiform nuclei of the brain considered as one. SYN: *corpus striatum.*

stricture (strĭk'chŭr) [L. *strictūra*, contraction]. A narrowing or constricture of the lumen of a tube, duct, or hollow organ such as the esophagus, ureter, or urethra. Strictures may be congenital or acquired. Acquired strictures may result from infection, trauma, fibrosis resulting from mechanical or chemical irritation, muscular spasm, or pressure from outside from adjacent structures or tumors. They may be temporary or permanent, depending on cause.

s., annular. Ringlike obstruction of an organ involving entire circumference of structure.

s., anorectal. Fibrotic narrowing of the anorectal canal.

s., bridle. S. caused by a band of membrane stretched across a tube, partially occluding it.

s., cicatricial. S. resulting from a scar or wound.

s., functional. S. due to muscular spasm.

s., impermeable. S. closing the lumen of a tube or canal so that an instrument cannot pass through it.

s., irritable. S. causing pain when an instrument is passed.

s., spasmodic. S., functional, q.v.

s. of urethra. Most common in men. May be partial or complete.

SYM: Straining to pass urine, esp. at commencement of urination.

ETIOL: Spasm of urethral muscle, congestion of urethra and fibrous formation.

stricturotome (strĭk'chŭr-ō-tōm) [L. *strictūra*, contraction, + Gr. *tomē*, a cutting]. Instrument for cutting strictures.

stricturotomy (strĭk"chŭr-ŏt'ō-mĭ). Operation of cutting strictures.

stridor (strī'dŏr) [L., a harsh sound]. Harsh sound during respiration; high pitched and like the blowing of the wind due to obstruction of air passages.

s., congenital, laryngeal. Inspiration at birth or during first three weeks giving forth a crowing sound.

s., dentium. Noise from grinding of the teeth.

s. serraticus. Sound of respiration like that of sawing, produced by patient's tracheotomy tubes.

stridulous (strĭd'ū-lŭs) [L. *stridulus*]. Making a shrill, grating sound.

string-of-pearls deformity. Fusiform enlargement of proximal and middle phalanges seen in rickets.

string sign. A greatly narrowed terminal ileum seen in roentgenological examination of abdomen in regional enteritis.

strip (strĭp) [AS. *striepan*, to plunder]. To remove all contents from, esp. by gentle pressure, as to strip the seminal vesicles.

strobila (strō-bī'lă) [Gr. *strobilos*, pine cone]. The adult form of a tapeworm.

stroke (strōk) [ME.]. 1. A sudden, severe attack of affliction, as apoplexy; a sharp blow. 2. To rub gently in one direction, as in massage. 3. Gentle movement of the hand across a surface.

   s., apoplectic. Sudden loss of consciousness resulting from intracranial hemorrhage, thrombosis, or embolism. SEE: *apoplexy.*

   s., back. Ventricular recoil of the heart during systole. SYN: *basculation*, q.v.

   s., heat. SEE: *heatstroke.*

   s., paralytic. Sudden onset of paralysis resulting from injury to brain or spinal cord.

   s. volume. The amount of blood ejected by the left ventricle at each beat. Amount varies with age, sex, and exercise. SYN: *systolic discharge.*

stroma (strō'mă) [Gr., mattress]. (pl. *stromata*) [NA] 1. Foundation supporting tissues of an organ. Opposed to parenchyma. 2. Spongy, colorless framework of an erythrocyte.

stromal, stromatic (strō'măl, strō-măt'ĭk). Concerning or resembling the stroma of an organ.

Stromeyer's splint (strō'mĭ-ur). [Georg F. L. Stromeyer, Ger. surgeon, 1804-76]. A hinged splint for a joint, which can be fixed at an angle.

stromuhr (strō'moor) [Ger. *strom*, stream, + *uhr*, clock]. Device for measuring velocity of blood flow. SYN: *rheometer.*

Strongylata (strŏn"jĭ-lō'tă) [Gr., compactly formed]. A suborder of nematode worms which includes the hookworms, strongyles, gapeworms, and lungworms.

strongyle (strŏn'jĭl). A nematode belonging to the suborder Strongylata, often parasitic in gastrointestinal tract of animals.

Strongyloides (strŏn"jĭ-loy'dēz). A genus of roundworms frequently found in the intestines.

   S. intestinalis. An intestinal roundworm.

   S. stercoralis. An intestinal parasite of man similar to the hookworm both in distribution and life cycle. SYN: *S. intestinalis.*

strongyloidosis (strŏn"jĭ-loy-dō'sĭs) [Gr. *strongylos,* compactly formed, + *-osis*, condition]. Infestation with Strongyloides.

strongylosis (strŏn"jĭ-lō'sĭs). Infestation with Strongylus.

Strongylus (strŏn'jĭ-lŭs). A genus of parasitic nematodes.

strontium (strŏn'shĭ-ŭm). [Strontian, mining village in Scotland]. SYMB: *Sr.* At. wt. 87.62; at. no. 38; sp. gr. 2.6. A dark yellowish metal. Medically it is of interest because its radioactive isotope ^{90}Sr constitutes a radioactive hazard in fallout from atom bombs. The isotope has a half-life of 28 years and is stored in bone when ingested.

Strophanthus (strō-făn'thŭs) [Gr. *strophos*, twisted cord, + *anthos*, flower]. Plant yielding a poisonous, white, crystalline glucoside; used chiefly in the form of alkaloid; strophanthin.

   ACTION AND USES: Heart stimulant.

strophulus (strŏf'ū-lŭs) [L.]. An obsolete term used to describe a variety of skin eruptions including milium, prickly heat, and papular urticaria. SYN: *gum rash; red rash; tooth rash.*

   s. albidus. Small, white nodule below the epidermis. SYN: *milium.*

   s. infantum. Urticaria in infants.

   s. pruriginosus. A form with itching papules.

structural (strŭk'tū-răl) [L. *structūra*, structure]. Pert. to organic structure.

   s. disease. A disease effecting changes in any structure.

struma (strū'mă) [L., a mass]. An imprecise term having several meanings, including enlargement of the thyroid gland. SYN: *goiter.*

   s. aberranta. S. of the accessory thyroid glands.

   s., cast iron. Chronic thyroiditis accompanied by extreme development of fibrous tissue.

   s. congenita. Goiter present at birth.

   s. lingualis. Presence of thyroid tissue in tongue in region of foramen cecum.

   s. lymphomatosa. Rare form involving a diffuse and extensive infiltration of the entire gland. SYN: *Hashimoto's s.*

   s. maligna. Carcinoma of the thyroid gland.

   s. ovarii. A form of ovarian teratoma in which mass is composed of typical thyroid follicles filled with colloid.

s., Riedel's. A form of chronic thyroiditis in which gland becomes enlarged, hard, and adherent to adjacent tissues. Follicles become atrophic and fibrosis occurs.

strumiprivous (strū"mĭ-prĭ'vŭs) [L. *struma,* a mass, + *privus,* deprived]. Rel. to or caused by removal of the thyroid gland. SEE: *cachexia.*

strumitis (strū-mī'tĭs) ["+ Gr. *-itis,* inflammation]. Inflammation of a thyroid gland with goiter. SYN: *thyroiditis.*

strumous (strū'mŭs) [L. *strumosus*]. 1. Affected with scrofula. SYN: *scrofulous.* 2. Affected with goiter.

Strümpell's sign (strĭm'pĕl). [Adolf von Strümpell, Ger. physician, 1853-1925]. Dorsiflexion of foot when thigh is flexed on abdomen.

Strümpell-Marie disease. [A.S.; Pierre Marie, Fr. neurologist, 1853-1940] Ankylosing or rheumatoid spondylitis.

strychnine (strĭk'nĭn, -nēn, -nĭn) [Gr. *strychnos,* nightshade]. A poisonous alkaloid obtained from plants, as nux vomica. It has no therapeutic usefulness but has been used as an experimental tool in neuropharmacology.
POISONING TREATMENT: SEE: *Table of Poisons* in *Appendix.*

strychninism (strĭk'nĭn-ĭzm) ["+ *-ismos,* condition]. Chronic strychnine poisoning. SYN: *strychnism.*

strychnism (strĭk'nĭzm). Poisoning from use of strychnine. SYN: *strychninism.*

STS. Abbr. for *serological test for syphilis.*

STU. Abbr. for *skin test unit.*

Stuart factor. The 10th factor (Factor X) in blood coagulation. It is present in plasma and serum and is essential for blood coagulation. SYN: *thrombokinase.*

stump (stŭmp) [ME. *stumpe*]. End of limb left after amputation.
s. hallucination. Sensation of still possessing a limb or arm after its amputation. SYN: *phantom limb.*

stun (stŭn) [O.Fr. *estoner,* a blow]. To render unconscious or stupified by a blow.

stupe (stūp) [L. *stupa,* tow]. Cloth of flannel wrung out of hot water for a fomentation, often saturated with turpentine to produce counterirritation. SEE: *fomentation.*
s., turpentine. S. with 4-8 ml. of turpentine sprinkled evenly over the dry flannel before water is poured on.

stupefacient (stū"pē-fā'shĕnt) [L. *stupefaciens,* stupefying]. Causing or that which causes stupor. SYN: *narcotic; soporific.*

stupemania (stū"pē-mā'nĭ-ă) [L. *stupor,* numbness, + Gr. *mania,* madness]. Insanity with symptoms of numbness.

stupor (stū'pōr) [L.]. 1. Condition of unconsciousness, torpor, or lethargy with suppression of sense or feeling. 2. In psychiatry, a state of lessened responsiveness.
S. occurs in visceral and infectious diseases, melancholia, catatonia, epilepsy, paresis, poisonings, and hysteria. A benign form is seen in manic-depressive psychosis.
RS: carotic; catatonia; collapse; coma; lethargy; narcoma; narcose; syncope; unconsciousness.
s., anergic. S. accompanied with immobility seen in certain psychoses.
s., delusional. S. accompanied by delusions.
s., epileptic. S. sometimes following an attack of epilepsy.
s., lethargic. S. accompanied by lethargy. SEE: *trance.*
s. melancholicus. S. associated with mental depression.
s. vigilans. Catalepsy, q.v.

stu'porous. Affected with stupor.
s. depression. An extremely depressed phase of manic-depressive psychosis characterized by extreme psychomotor retardation and unresponsiveness to surrounding conditions.

stupration, stuprum (stū-prā'shŭn, stū'prŭm) [L. *stuprum,* defilement]. Sexual intercourse with a woman without her consent and by overpowering force or intimidation. SYN: *rape.*

sturine (stū'rĭn) [L. *sturio,* sturgeon]. Protamine obtained from sperm of sturgeon.

stutter (stŭt'er) [ME. *stutten,* to stutter]. To hesitate and repeat or stumble spasmodically in speaking, due to difficulty in pronouncing initial consonants caused by spasm of lingual and palatal muscles.

stuttering (stŭt'er-ĭng). Defect in speech in which there is stumbling and spasmodic repetition of same syllable.
RS: battarism; mogilalia.
s., urinary. Irregular, spasmodic urination. SYN: *stammering of the bladder,* q.v.

sty(e (stī) [AS. *stigan,* to rise). (pl. *styes; sties*). Acute localized bacterial infection of one of several sebaceous glands of the eyelid. In external styes, the glands of Zeiss or Moll at the edge of the lid are inflamed. Internal styes concern the meibomian or tarsal glands under the eyelid. SYN: *hordeolum.*
SYM: General edema of lid, pain, localized conjunctivitis.
TREATMENT: Hot fomentations. When suppuration has taken place, free incision and pressure to evacuate sac. Local and systemic antibiotics will hasten resolution and healing in severe cases. When a succes-

sion of styes occurs, Staphylococcus toxoid or vaccine, or an autogenous vaccine, may be helpful.

s., meibomian. Inflammation of a meibomian gland.

s., Zeisian. Inflammation of one of Zeiss' glands.

styles, stylet (stiles, stī'lĕt) [Gr. *stylos*, pillar]. 1. A slender, solid or hollow, plug of metal for making permanent a canal after operation or for stiffening or clearing a cannula or catheter. 2. A thin probe.

styliscus (stī-lĭs'kŭs) [Gr. *styliskos*, pillar]. A slender, cylindrical plug for dilating a channel or for keeping a wound open.

styloglossus (stī-lō-glŏs'ŭs) [Gr. *stylos*, pillar, + *glōssa*, tongue]. A muscle connecting the tongue and styloid process which raises and retracts the tongue. SEE: *Table of Muscles* in *Appendix.*

stylohyoid (stī-lō-hī'oyd) ["+ *hyoeides*, hyoid]. Pert. to the styloid process of the temporal and hyoid bones.

stylohyoideus (stī''lō-hī-oyd'ē-ŭs). A muscle having its origin on styloid process and insertion on hyoid bone. It draws the hyoid bone upward and backward. SEE: *Table of Muscles* in *Appendix.*

styloid (stī'loyd) [Gr. *stylos*, pillar, + *eidos*, form]. Resembling a stylus or pointed instrument.

s. process. 1. A pointed process of the temporal bone, projecting downward, and to which some of the muscles of the tongue are attached. 2. A pointed projection behind the head of the fibula. 3. A protuberance on distal end of radius' outer portion. 4. An ulnar projection on inner side of the distal end.

styloiditis (stī''loyd-ī'tĭs) ["+ "+ *-itis*, inflammation]. Inflammation of a styloid process.

stylomandibular (stī''lō-măn-dī'bū-lăr) ["+ L. *mandibula*, lower jaw]. Concerning the styloid process of the temporal bone and the mandible.

stylomastoid (stī''lō-măs'toyd) [Gr. *stylos*, pillar, + *mastos*, breast, + *eidos*, form]. Concerning the styloid and mastoid processes of the temporal bone.

stylomaxillary (stī''lō-măks'ĭ-lă-rĭ) ["+ L. *maxilla*, jaw]. Concerning the styloid process of the temporal bone and the mandible.

stylopharyngeus (stī''lō-făr-ĭn'jē-ŭs) ["+ *pharynx*, pharynx]. Muscle connecting the styloid process and pharynx which elevates and dilates the pharynx. SEE: *Table of Muscles* in *Appendix.*

stylus (stī'lŭs) [Gr. *stylos*, a pillar]. 1. A probe or slender wire for stiffening or clearing a canal or catheter. 2. Pointed medicinal

preparation in stick form for external application.

stype (stīp) [Gr. *stypē*, tow]. A pledget or tampon of cotton or other material.

stypsis (stĭp'sĭs) [Gr., contraction]. Astringency or the use of an astringent.

styptic (stĭp'tĭk) [Gr. *styptikos*, contracting]. 1. Contracting a blood vessel; stopping a hemorrhage by astringent action. 2. Anything that stops a hemorrhage. SYN: *astringent; hemostat.*

Ex: alum, ferrous sulfate, tannic acid.

sub- [L. *sub*, under]. Combining form meaning under, beneath, in small quantity, less normal. SYN: [Gr.] *hypo-.*

subabdominal (sŭb''ăb-dŏm'ĭ-năl) [L. *sub*, beneath, + *abdōmen*, abdomen]. Below the abdomen.

subacetate (sŭb-ăs'ē-tāt) ["+ *acetum*, vinegar]. A basic acetate.

subacromial (sŭb-ă-krō'mĭ-ăl) ["+ Gr. *akron*, point, + *omos*, shoulder]. Under the acromion process.

subacute (sŭb''ă-kūt') [L. *sub*, under, + *acutus*, sharp]. Between acute and chronic, but with some acute features, said of the course of a disease.

subacute myelo-optic neuropathy. Neurological disease which usually begins with abdominal pain or diarrhea followed by sensory and motor disturbances in the lower limbs, ataxia, impaired vision, and convulsions or coma. Reported mostly in Japan and Australia. Most patients survive but neurological disability remains.

Many of those who have the disease have a history of taking drugs of the halogenated oxyquinoline group, but a cause-and-effect relationship has not been established. ABBR: SMON.

subacute sclerosing panencephalitis. Encephalitis which occurs in the first two decades of life. Characterized by a progressive course with intellectual deterioration, behavior disorders, and involuntary muscular disorders. Probably due to a viral infection. It is generally agreed that SSPE is the same disease as those previously termed subacute inclusion-body encephalitis and subacute sclerosing leukoencephalitis. ABBR: SSPE.

subalimentation (sŭb-ăl-ĭ-mĕn-tā'shŭn) ["+ *alimentum*, food]. A state of insufficient nourishment.

subanconeus (sŭb''ăn-kŏ'nē-ŭs) ["+ Gr. *ankon*, elbow]. 1. Below the elbow. 2. Muscle beneath the elbow which contracts its posterior ligament. SEE: *Table of Muscles* in *Appendix.*

subaponeurotic (sŭb″ăp-ō-nū-rŏt′ĭk) ["+ Gr. *apo*, from, + *neuron*, tendon]. Below an aponeurosis.

subarachnoid (sŭb″ă-răk′noyd) [L. *sub*, under, + Gr. *arachnē*, spider, + *eidos*, form]. Below the arachnoid membrane.

  s. cisternae. Spaces at the base of the brain where the arachnoid becomes widely separated from the pia giving rise to large cavities.

  s. space. Space between the pia proper and arachnoid containing the cerebrospinal fluid.

subarcuate (sŭb-ăr′kū-āt) ["+ *arcuatus*, arched]. Slightly arched.

  s. fossa. Depression which extends backward as a blind tunnel under the superior semicircular canal of the temporal bone.

subastragalar (sŭb-ăs-trăg′ă-lar) ["+ Gr. *astragalos*, ball of the ankle joint]. Beneath the astragalus.

subastringent (sŭb″ăs-trĭn′jĕnt) [L. *sub*, under, + *astringere*, to contract]. Mildly astringent.

subaural (sŭb-aw′răl) ["+ *auris*, ear]. Below the ear.

subcapsular (sŭb-kăp′sū-lăr) ["+ *capsula*, a little box]. Below any capsule, esp. the capsule of the brain, or a capsular ligament.

subcarbonate (sŭb-kăr′bō-nāt) ["+ *carbo*, coal]. A basic carbonate; one having proportion of carbonic acid radical less than the normal carbonate.

subcartilaginous (sŭb″kăr-tĭ-lăj′ĭn-ŭs) [L. *sub*, beneath, + *cartilāgo*, cartilage]. 1. Located beneath a cartilage. 2. Cartilaginous in part.

subchronic (sŭb-krŏn′ĭk) ["+ Gr. *chronos*, time]. Noting a condition between subacute and chronic; almost chronic.

subclavian (sŭb-klā′vĭ-ăn) ["+ *clavis*, a key]. Under the clavicle or collarbone. SYN: *subclavicular.*

  s. artery. Large artery at base of neck which supplies blood to arm. The right subclavian artery branches from the innominate artery; the left subclavian artery branches from aortic arch.

  s. triangle. Triangle-shaped part of the neck formed by the clavicle and the omohyoid and sternomastoid muscles.

  s. vein. Large vein draining arm. It unites with interior jugular to form the innominate vein.

subclavian steal syndrome. Shunting of blood, which was destined for the brain, away from the cerebral circulation. This occurs in this particular case when the subclavian artery is occluded. Blood then flows from the opposite vertebral artery across to and down the vertebral artery on the side of the occlusion.

  SYM: Signs of insufficient blood flow to the brain. Symptoms are transient and are aggravated by exercise. Usually the blood pressure in the arm on the affected side will be significantly lower than in the other arm.

subclavicular (sŭb″klă-vĭk′ū-lăr) [L. *sub*, under, + *clavicula*, a little key]. Beneath the clavicle. SYN: *subclavian.*

subclavius (sŭb-klā′vĭ-ŭs) ["+ *clavis*, a key]. A tiny muscle from the 1st rib to the undersurface of the clavicle. SEE: *Table of Muscles* in *Appendix.*

subclinical (sŭb-klĭn′ĭ-kal) ["+ Gr. *klinikos*, pert. to a bed]. Pert. to a period before appearance of typical symptoms of a disease.

subcollateral (sŭb-kō-lăt′ĕr-ăl) [L. *sub*, under, + *con*, with, + *latus*, *later-*, side]. Below the collateral fissure, indicating a cerebral convolution.

subconjunctival (sŭb″kŏn-jŭnk-tī′văl) ["+ *conjunctiva*, a joining]. Beneath the conjunctiva.

subconscious (sŭb-kŏn′shŭs) ["+ *conscious*, aware]. Not clearly conscious; pert. to activities of which the mind is not aware or to that which is not cognizable through the physical senses; below the threshold of objective consciousness; that which is activated by involuntary processes; intuitional. Now almost obsolete.

  s. mind. A hypothetical mind acting below the threshold of objective consciousness.

subconsciousness (sŭb-kŏn′shŭs-nĕs). 1. The state of being partially unconscious. 2. Noting of impressions and ideas without conscious knowledge of them.

subcontinuous (sŭb″kŏn-tĭn′ū-ŭs) [L. *sub*, under, + *continuus*, holding together]. Almost continuous; with periods of abatement, but no interruptions to continuity.

  s. fever. Fever with periods of remission and exacerbation. SYN: *remittent fever.*

subcoracoid (sŭb-kōr′ă-koyd) ["+ Gr. *korakoeidēs*, crowlike]. Beneath the coracoid process.

subcortex (sŭb-kōr′tĕks) ["+ *cortex*, rind]. White substance of the brain underlying the cortex.

subcortical (sŭb-kōr′tĭ-kăl). Pert. to the region beneath the cerebral cortex.

subcostal (sŭb-kŏs′tăl) [L. *sub*, under, + *costa*, rib]. Beneath the ribs.

subcostalgia (sŭb″kŏs-tăl′jĭ-ă) ["+ "+ Gr. *algos*, pain]. Pain in region over the subcostal nerve.

subcranial (sŭb-krā′nĭ-ăl) ["+ Gr. *kranion*, skull]. Beneath or below the cranium.

subcrepitant (sŭb-krĕp'ĭ-tănt) [L. *sub*, under, + *crepitāre*, to rattle]. Partially crepitant or crackling in character; noting a rale.

subcrureus (sŭb-krū-rē'ŭs) ["+ *crus, crur-*, leg]. Small muscle between anterior surface of femoral shaft and synovial membrane of knee joint. SEE: *Table of Muscles* in *Appendix.*

subculture (sŭb-kŭl'chŭr) ["+ *cultūra*, cultivation]. To make a culture of bacteria with material derived from another culture.

subcutaneous (sŭb"kū-tā'nē-ŭs) [L. *sub*, under, + *cutis*, skin]. Beneath or to be introduced beneath the skin. SYN: *hypodermic.*

    s. surgery. Operation performed through a small opening in the skin.

    s. wound. A wound with only a small opening through the skin.

subcuticular (sŭb"kū-tĭk'ū-lăr) ["+ *cuticula*, little skin]. Beneath the cuticle or epidermis. SYN: *subepidermal.*

subcu'tis. The layer of connective tissue beneath the skin.

subdelirium (sŭb"dē-lĭr'ĭ-ŭm) [L. *sub*, under, + *dē*, away from, + *lira*, track]. A mild or partial state of delirium.

subder'mal ["+ Gr. *derma*, skin]. Below the skin.

subdiaphragmatic (sŭb"dī-ă-frăg-măt'ĭk) ["+ Gr. *dia*, across, + *phragma*, wall]. Beneath the diaphragm. SYN: *subphrenic.*

subdural (sŭb-dū'răl) [L. *sub*, under, + *durus*, hard]. Beneath the dura mater.

    s. space. Space between the arachnoid and dura mater.

subendocardial (sŭb"ĕn-dō-kăr'dĭ-ăl) ["+ Gr. *endon*, within, + *kardia*, heart]. Below the endocardium.

subendothelial (sŭb"ĕn-dō-thē'lĭ-ăl) ["+ Gr. *endon*, within, + *thēlē*, nipple]. Beneath the endothelium.

subepidermal (sŭb"ĕp-ĭ-dĕr'măl) [L. *sub*, under, + Gr. *epi*, upon, + *derma*, skin]. Beneath the epidermis. SYN: *subcuticular.*

subepithelial (sŭb"ĕp-ĭ-thē'lĭ-ăl) ["+ "+ *thēlē*, nipple]. Beneath the epithelium.

subfascial (sŭb-făsh'ĭ-ăl) ["+ *fascia*, band]. Beneath a fascia.

subfebrile (sŭb-fē'brĭl) [L. *sub*, under, + *febris*, fever]. Mild fever, usually considered to be less than 101° F. (38.3° C.).

subflavous (sŭb-flā'vŭs) ["+ *flavus*, yellow]. Yellowish.

    s. ligament. Yellowish ligament connecting the laminae of the vertebrae. SYN: *ligamentum subflavum.*

subfrontal (sŭb-frŏn'tăl) ["+ *frons, front-*, forehead]. Below a frontal convolution or lobe of the brain.

subglenoid (sŭb-glē'noyd) [L. *sub*, under, + Gr. *glēnē*, cavity, + *eidos*, form]. Below the glenoid fossa or glenoid cavity.

subglossal (sŭb-glŏs'ăl) ["+ Gr. *glōssa*, tongue]. Under the tongue. SYN: *hypoglossal; sublingual.*

subglossitis (sŭb-glŏs-sī'tĭs) ["+ "+ *-ītis*, inflammation]. Inflammation of the undersurface or tissues of the tongue.

subgrondation, subgrundation (sŭb-grŏn-dā'shŭn, -grŭn-dā'shŭn) [Fr.]. Depression of one fragment of a broken bone beneath the other, as of the cranium.

subhyoid (sŭb-hī'oyd) [L. *sub*, beneath, + Gr. *hyoeidēs*, U-shaped]. Beneath the hyoid bone.

subiliac (sŭb-ĭl'ĭ-ăk) ["+ *iliacus*, pert. to the hip]. 1. Below the ilium. 2. Pert. to the subilium.

subilium (sŭb-ĭl'ĭ-ŭm). The lowest part of the ilium.

subincision. Production of a fistula of the penile urethra. May interfere with conception. Used by some primitives, esp. Australian aborigines.

subinfection (sŭb"ĭn-fĕk'shŭn) [L. *sub*, under, + *infectio*, a putting into]. Mild infection with minimal clinical signs or symptoms.

subinflamma'tion ["+ *inflammatio*, a setting on fire]. Very mild inflammation. SYN: *irritation.*

subinflammatory (sŭb"ĭn-flăm'ă-tō-rī). Very mildly inflammatory.

subin'timal [L. *sub*, under, + *intima*, innermost]. Beneath the intima.

subintrant (sŭb-ĭn'trănt) [L. *subintrans*, stealing into]. Having cycles or paroxysms in such rapid succession that they intermingle and thus overlap.

    s. fever. Intermittent fever in which the paroxysms occurs so rapidly that one comes on before the previous one has disappeared.

subinvolution (sŭb"ĭn-vō-lū'shŭn) [L. *sub*, beneath, + *involutio*, a turning into]. Imperfect involution; incomplete return of a part to normal dimensions after physiological hypertrophy, as when the uterus fails to reduce to normal size following childbirth. SEE: *uterus.*

subja'cent ["+ *jacere*, to lie]. Lying underneath.

subject (sŭb'jĕkt) [L. *subjectus*, brought under]. 1. A patient undergoing treatment, observation, or investigation. 2. A body used for dissection. 3. To have a liability to develop attacks of a particular disease. 4. To submit to a procedure or to the action of another.

subjec'tive [L. *subjectivus*]. Arising from or concerned with the individual; not perceptible to an observer. Opposed to objective.

s. sensation. A sensation occurring when stimuli due to internal causes excite the nervous system; one not of objective origin.

s. symptoms. Those which are of internal origin and evident only to the patient.

subjugal (sŭb-jū'găl) [L. *sub*, beneath, + *jugum*, yoke]. Below the malar bone or os zygomaticum.

sublatio (sŭb-lā'shĭ-ō) [L.]. Removal, elevation, or detachment of a part.

s. retinae. Detachment of the retina.

sublethal (sŭb-lē'thăl) [L. *sub*, under, + Gr. *lēthē*, oblivion]. A little less than lethal; almost fatal.

s. dose. Dose containing not quite enough of a toxin or noxious substance to cause death.

sublimate (sŭb'lĭ-māt) [L. *sublimāre*, to elevate]. 1. A substance obtained or prepared by sublimation. 2. To cause a solid or gas to change state without becoming a liquid during transition. Ex: Ice may evaporate without first becoming a liquid. 3. To overcome the libido by diverting it into nonsexual or other socially accepted activities.

sublimation (sŭb''lĭ-mā'shŭn) [L. *sublimatio*]. 1. Altering the state of a gas or solid without first changing it into a liquid. 2. Conversion of the libido into nonsexual channels. A Freudian term pert. to unconscious mental processes whereby the sex instinct finds an outlet through creative mental work.

sublime (sŭb-līm') [L. *sublimis*, to the limit]. To evaporate a substance directly from the solid into the vapor state and condense it again. Thus metallic iodine on heating does not liquefy, but forms directly a violet gas.

subliminal (sŭb-lĭm'ĭn-ăl). 1. Below the threshold of sensation; too weak to arouse sensation or muscular contraction. 2. Below the normal consciousness.

s. self. In psychiatry, part of the normal individual's personality in which his mental processes function without consciousness under normal waking conditions.

sublingual (sŭb-lĭng'gwăl) [L. *sub*, under, + *lingua*, tongue]. Beneath or concerning the area beneath the tongue.

s. gland. The smallest of the salivary glands, located between side of tongue and the mandible, one on each side. It has about 20 ducts, most of which open directly above the gland.

sublinguitis (sŭb''lĭng-gwī'tĭs) ["+ "+ Gr. *-itis*, inflammation]. Inflammation of the sublingual gland.

sublobular (sŭb-lŏb'ū-lăr) [L. *sub*, under, + *lobulus*, a lobule]. Beneath a lobule.

sublumbar (sŭb-lŭm'băr) ["+ *lumbus*, loin]. Below the lumbar region.

subluxation (sŭb''lŭks-ā'shŭn) ["+ *luxatio*, dislocation]. A partial or incomplete dislocation.

submammary (sŭb-măm'ă-rī) [L. *sub*, under, + *mamma*, breast]. Below the mammary gland.

sub''mandib'ular ["+ *mandibula*, lower jaw bone]. Beneath the mandible or lower jaw.

s. gland. The submaxillary gland, q.v.

submarginal (sŭb-măr'jĭn-ăl) ["+ *marginalis*, margin]. Close to or next to a margin or border of a part.

submaxilla (sŭb''măk-sĭl'ă) [L. *sub*, under, + *maxilla*, jaw]. The lower jaw or mandible. SYN: *inferior maxilla*.

submaxillaritis (sŭb-măk''sĭl-ăr-ī't ĭs) ["+ "+ Gr. *-itis*, inflammation]. Inflammation of the submaxillary gland.

submaxillary (sŭb-măk'sĭl-ă-rī). Beneath the lower jaw or inferior maxilla.

s. gland. One of the salivary glands, a mixed tubuloalveolar gland about the size of a walnut which lies in digastric triangle beneath the mandible. Its main duct (Wharton's duct) opens at side of the frenulum linguae. SYN: *submandibular gland.*

submaxillitis (sŭb''măk-sĭl-ī'tĭs) [L. *sub*, under, + *maxilla*, jaw, + Gr. *-itis*, inflammation]. Inflammation of, or mumps affecting, the submaxillary gland.

submen'tal ["+ *mentum*, chin]. Under the chin.

submerge (sŭb-mŭrj) ["+ *mergere*, to immerse]. To place under water.

submi'cron [L. *sub*, under, + Gr. *mikros*, tiny]. A tiny particle invisible except with the ultramicroscope. SYN: *ultramicron.*

sub''microscop'ical ["+ "+ Gr. *skopein*, to examine]. Too minute to be visible under the microscope.

submorphous (sŭb-mŏr'fŭs) ["+ Gr. *morphē*, form]. Neither completely amorphous nor crystalline, as some calculi.

submucosa (sŭb''mū-kō'să) [L. *sub*, under, + *mucosus*, mucous]. The layer of areolar connective tissue under a mucous membrane.

submucous (sŭb-mū'kŭs) ["+ *mucus*, mucus]. Beneath a mucous membrane.

subnarcotic (sŭb-năr-kŏt'ĭk) ["+ Gr. *narkōtikos*, numb]. Mildly narcotic.

subna′sal [L. *sub*, under, + *nasus*, nose]. Under the nose.

s. point. Craniometric point at base of nasal spine.

subneural (sŭb-nū′răl) ["+ Gr. *neuron*, nerve]. Beneath the neural axis or the central nervous system.

subnormal (sŭb-nŏr′măl) ["+ *norma*, rule]. Less than normal or average.

subnucleus (sŭb-nū′klē-ŭs) [L. *sub*, under, + *nucleus*, a nut]. One of the secondary nuclei into which a nucleus of the central nervous system may be divided.

suboccipital (sŭb″ŏk-sĭp′ĭ-tăl) ["+ *occiput*, back of head]. Situated below the occiput or occipital bone.

suboperculum (sŭb″ō-pĕr′kū-lŭm) ["+ *operculum*, covering]. Portion of occipital convolution overlapping the insula. SEE: *operculum*.

suborbital (sŭb-ōr′bĭ-tăl) [L. *sub*, under, + *orbita*, track]. Beneath the orbit.

subpapular (sŭb-păp′ū-lăr) ["+ *papula*, pimple]. Very slightly papular, as papules elevated being scarcely more than macules.

subpatellar (sŭb″pă-tĕl′ar) ["+ *patella*, a pan]. Beneath the patella.

subpeduncular (sŭb″pē-dŭn′kū-lăr) [L. *sub*, under, + *pedunculus*, a stem]. Below a peduncle

s. lobe. Tiny lobe on undersurface of either cerebellar hemisphere. SYN: *flocculus*.

subpericardial (sŭb″pĕr-ĭ-kăr′dĭ-ăl) ["+ Gr. *peri*, around, + *kardia*, heart]. Beneath the pericardium.

subperiosteal (sŭb″pĕr-ĭ-ŏs′tĭ-ăl) ["+ "+ *osteon*, bone]. Beneath the periosteum.

s. operation. Bone surgery without removal of the periosteum.

subperitoneal (sŭb″pĕr-ĭ-tō-nē′ăl) [L. *sub*, under, + Gr. *peritonaion*, peritoneum]. Beneath the peritoneum.

subpharyngeal (sŭb″făr-ĭn′jē-ăl) ["+ Gr. *pharynx*, pharynx]. Beneath the pharynx.

subphrenic (sŭb-frĕn′ĭk) ["+ Gr. *phrēn*, diaphragm]. Beneath the diaphragm. SYN: *subdiaphragmatic*.

s. abscess. Collection of pus beneath the diaphragm.

subplacenta (sŭb″plă-sĕn′tă) ["+ *placenta*, a flat cake]. Part of the decidua directly lining the uterus. SYN: *decidua parietalis* [NA]; *decidua vera*.

subpleural (sŭb-plū′răl) [L. *sub*, under, + Gr. *pleura*, a side]. Beneath the pleura.

subpontine (sŭb-pŏn′tĭn, -tīn) ["+ *pons*, pont-, bridge]. Below the pons.

subpreputial (sŭb″prē-pū′shăl) ["+ *praeputium*, prepuce]. Under the prepuce.

subpubic (sŭb-pū′bĭk) [L. *sub*, under, + *pubes*, pubis]. Beneath the pubic arch, as a ligament, or performed beneath the pubic arch.

subpulmonary (sŭb-pŭl′mō-nă-rĭ) ["+ *pulmōn*, lung]. Below the lung.

subretinal (sŭb-rĕt′ĭ-năl) ["+ *rētē*, a net]. Beneath the retina.

subscapular (sŭb-skăp′ū-lăr) ["+ *scapula*, shoulder]. Below the scapula.

subscription (sŭb-skrĭp′shŭn) [L. *subscriptas*, written under]. That part of a prescription which contains directions for compounding ingredients.

subserous (sŭb-sē′rŭs) [L. *sub*, under, + *serum*, whey]. Beneath a serous membrane.

subsib′ilant ["+ *sibilans*, hissing]. Having the sound of a muffled whistle.

subsidence (sŭb-sīd′ĕnts) [L. *subsīdere*, to sink down]. The gradual disappearance of symptoms or manifestations of a disease.

subspinous (sŭb-spī′nŭs) [L. *sub*, under, + *spina*, thorn]. 1. Beneath any spinous process. 2. Anterior to or beneath the spinal column.

s. dislocation. Dislocation with head of the humerus resting below spine of the scapula.

substage (sŭb′stāj) ["+ O.Fr. *estage*, position]. That part of the microscope below the stage by which attachments are held in place.

substance (sŭb′stăns) [L. *substantia*]. That of which any material thing is composed; matter.

s., anterior perforated. Portion of rhinencephalon lying immediately anterior to optic chiasma. It is perforated by numerous small arteries.

s., anterior pituitary-like. Chorionic gonadotrophin. SYN: *APL substance*. SEE: *gonadotrophin*.

s., chromophilic. Substance found in the cytoplasm of certain cells which stains similar to chromatin with basic dyes. Includes Nissl bodies of neurons and granules in serozymogenic cells. SYN: *basophilic, chromophil*, or *chromidial substance*.

s., colloid. Jellylike s. in colloid degeneration.

s., depressor. Any substance whose action is that of reducing arterial blood pressure. SEE: *vasopressin*.

s., gray. Gray matter of the brain and spinal cord.

s., ground. The matrix or intercellular substance in which the cells of an organ or tissue are embedded.

s., intercellular. The s. occupying the spaces between cells.

s., ketogenic. A s. which, in its metabolism, gives rise to ketone bodies.

s., Nissl. Chromatophilic substance of nerve cells. SEE: *Nissl's bodies.*

s., posterior perforated. A triangular area forming floor of the interpenduncular fossa. It lies immediately behind the corpora mammillaria and contains numerous openings for blood vessels.

s., pressor. A substance which elevates arterial blood pressure.

s., reticular. SEE: *formation, reticular.*

s., specific soluble. A polysaccharide hapten obtained from the capsules of pneumococci. ABBR: SSS.

s., threshold, high. A s. such as glucose or sodium chloride present in the blood and excreted by the kidney only when its concentration exceeds a certain optimum value.

s., threshold, low. A s. such as urea or uric acid which is excreted from the blood almost in its entirety. It occurs in the urine in high concentrations.

s., white. White matter of brain and spinal cord.

s., w., of Schwann. A nerve fiber's medullary sheath.

sub"stan'dard. Failing to meet the usual or accepted standard.

substantia (sŭb-stăn'shĭ-ă) [L.]. [NA]. Substance in general.

s. alba. [NA]. White substance of the brain.

s. cinerea. Gray substance of brain and spinal cord.

s. ferruginea. [NA]. Elongated mass of pigmented cells in the locus ceruleus.

s. gelatinosa. [NA]. Gray matter of the cord surrounding central canal and capping head of posterior horns of spinal cord.

s. grisea. [NA]. Gray matter of the spinal cord.

s. nigra. [NA]. Black substance in a section of the crus cerebri. SYN: *locus niger.*

s. propria membranae tympani. Fibrous middle layer of drum membrane.

substernal (sŭb-stĕr'năl) [L. *sub*, beneath, + Gr. *sternon*, chest]. Situated beneath the sternum.

substitution (sŭb-stĭ-tū'shŭn) [L. *substitutio*, replacing]. 1. Displacing an atom (or more than one) of an element in a compound by atoms of another element, equivalently. 2. In psychiatry, the turning from an obstructed desire to one whose gratification is socially acceptable. 3. The turning from an obstructed form of behavior to a more primitive one, as a s. neurosis. 4. The replacement of a substance by another. 5. In pharmacy,

the replacement of one drug by another drug in dispensing.

s. products. Compounds formed by an element or a radical replacing another element or radical in a compound.

s. therapy. The use in treatment of a substance such as a product of glandular secretion (hormone or enzyme) to replace natural substance in body. This method is employed when glands fail to secrete properly or substance secreted is unavailable to tissues.

substitutive (sŭb'stĭ-tū"tĭv) [L. *substitutivus*]. Causing a change or substitution of characteristics.

s. therapy. Treatment to overcome an inflammation of a specific character by exciting an acute nonspecific inflammation.

substrate, substratum (sŭb'strāt, sŭb-strā'tŭm) [L. *substratum*, to lie under]. 1. An underlying layer or foundation. 2. A base, as of a pigment. 3. The substance acted upon, as by an enzyme. SYN: *zymolyte.* SEE: *enzyme.*

subsultus (sŭb-sŭl'tŭs) [L. *subsultus*, springing up]. Any morbid tremor or twitching, as of the tendons; a grave symptom in certain fevers.

s. clonus, s. tendinum. Involuntary twitchings of muscles, esp. of arms and feet, causing movement of tendons. Observed in certain febrile conditions.

subsylvian (sŭb-sĭl'vĭ-ăn). Below the fissure of Sylvius.

subtarsal (sŭb-tăr'săl) [L. *sub*, under, + Gr. *tarsos*, tarsus]. Below the tarsus.

subtentorial. Located beneath the tentorium.

subthalamic (sŭb"thă-lăm'ĭk) ["+ Gr. *thalamos*, chamber]. Located below the thalamus.

s. nucleus. An elliptical mass of gray matter lying in the ventral thalamus above cerebral peduncle and rostral to substantia nigra. It receives fibers from the globus pallidus. SYN: *body of Luys.*

subthal'amus. Portion of the diencephalon lying below the thalamus and above the hypothalamus. SYN: *ventral thalamus.*

subtile, subtle (sŭb'tĭl, sŭt'l) [L. *subtilis*, fine]. 1. Very fine or delicate. 2. Very acute. 3. Mentally acute or crafty or piercing, as sharp. 4. Operating without attracting attention, as subtle poisons.

subtilin (sŭb'tĭl-ĭn). An antibiotic biosynthesized by Bacillus subtilis. It is of low toxicity and effective against gram-positive organisms.

subtotal (sŭb-tō'tăl) [L. *sub*, under, + *totus*, whole]. Less than total, as subtotal removal of a gland. SYN: *incomplete.*

subtrochanteric (sŭb″trō-kăn-tĕr′ĭk) ["+ Gr. *trochantēr*, a runner]. Below a trochanter.

subtuberal (sŭb-tū′bĕr-ăl) ["+ *tuber*, a knot]. Located under a tuber.

subtympanic (sŭb-tĭm-păn′ĭk) [L. *sub*, under, + Gr. *tympanon*, drum]. Below the tympanum.

sububeres (sŭb-ū′bĕr-ēz) ["+ *ubera*, breast]. Suckling children.

subumbilical (sŭb″ŭm-bĭl′ĭ-kăl) ["+ *umbilicus*, navel]. Below the umbilicus.

s. space. Space within the body cavity below the navel resembling a triangle in shape.

subungual, subunguial (sŭb-ŭng′gwăl, -gwĭ-ăl) ["+ *unguis*, nail]. Situated beneath nail of a finger or toe. SEE: *hyponychium*.

s. hematoma. Collection of blood under the nail as a result of trauma. Condition may be treated by heating the end of a paper clip and then placing its point against the nail. This permits a small hole to be melted in the nail through which the blood escapes.

suburethral (sŭb″ū-rē′thrăl) [L. *sub*, under, + Gr. *ourēthra*, urethra]. Below the urethra.

subvaginal (sŭb-văj′ĭn-ăl) ["+ *vagina*, sheath]. 1. Below the vagina. 2. On inner side of any tubular sheathing membrane.

subvertebral (sŭb-vĕr′tĕ-brăl) ["+ *vertebra*, vertebral]. Beneath or on ventral side of the vertebral column or of a vertebra. SYN: *subspinal*.

subvirile (sŭb-vĭr′ĭl, -vĭ′rĭl) [L. *sub*, under, + *virilis*, male]. Deficient in, or lacking, virility.

subvitrinal (sŭb-vĭt′rĭn-ăl) ["+ *vitrina*, vitreous body]. Located beneath the vitreous body.

subvolution (sŭb″vō-lū′shŭn) ["+ *volutus*, turning]. Method of turning over a flap surgically to prevent adhesions.

succagogue (sŭk′ă-gŏg) [L. *succus*, juice, + Gr. *agōgos*, leading]. 1. To stimulate glandular secretion. 2. A substance which stimulates glandular secretion.

succedaneous (sŭk″sē-dā′nē-ŭs) [L. *succedaneus*, substituting]. Acting as a substitute or relating to one.

succharase. Sucrase, q.v.

succi. Pl. of succus.

succinylsulfathiazole. USP. 2-(N₄-succinylsulfanilamido) thiazole. Member of the sulfonamide family valuable as an antibacterial agent for use in the intestinal tract. Less than 5% is absorbed from the gastrointestinal tract. White crystalline powder sparingly soluble in alcohol, ace-

tone, and water; readily soluble in aqueous bases, as sodium bicarbonate solution.

succorrhea (sŭk-kō-rē′ă) [L. *succus*, juice, + Gr. *rhoia*, flow]. Unnatural increase in secretion of any juice, esp. of a digestive fluid.

succus (sŭk′kŭs) [L. *succus*, juice]. (pl. *suc′ci*) A juice or fluid secretion.

s. entericus. The intestinal juice of the body. It is alkaline. Sp. gr. 1.010. The secretion of the minute glands lining the small intestine.

s. gastricus. The gastric juice.

s. pyloricus. An alkaline secretion by the pyloric end of the stomach.

succussion (sŭ-kŭsh′ŭn) [L. *succussio*, a shaking]. Shaking of a person to detect the presence of fluid in the bodily cavity by listening for a splashing sound, esp. in the thorax.

suck [AS. *sūcan*, to suck]. 1. To draw fluid into the mouth, as from the breast. 2. To exhaust air from a tube and thus siphon fluid from a container. 3. That which is drawn into the mouth by sucking.

sucking pad. Mass of fat in cheeks, esp. well developed in an infant, aiding it to suck. SEE: *myzesis*.

suckle. To nurse at the breast.

sucrase (sū′krās) [Fr. *sucre*, sugar]. An enzyme in the intestinal juice which splits cane sugar into glucose and fructose, the two being absorbed into the portal circulation. SYN: *invertase; saccharase*.

sucroclastic (sū″krō-klăs′tĭk) ["+ Gr. *klastos*, destroyed]. Splitting up or hydrolyzing a sugar.

sucrose (sū′krōs) [Fr. *sucre*, sugar]. USP. A saccharose, $C_{12}H_{22}O_{11}$, obtained from sugar cane, sugar beet, and other sources. It is hydrolyzed in the intestine to glucose and fructose by sucrase present in intestinal juice.

ACTION: Only a little is retained by the stomach, and it is all absorbed in the intestines. The lack of residue tends to cause constipation. S. is stored by the hepatic cells of the liver in the form of glycogen for future use. No chemical changes take place with the simple sugars, as they are directly absorbed.

RS: carbohydrates; disaccharose; fructose; galactose; glucose; lactose; levulose; maltose.

suction [LL. *sūctiō*, sucking]. The act of, or capacity for, sucking up by reduction of air pressure over part of the surface of a substance.

s. abortion. Removing the products of conception from the uterus by using a device which sucks the tissues away from the lining of the uterus.

s. biopsy. Obtaining tissue by use of a device which applies s. to the area from which tissue is desired. This technique is used in obtaining tissue from the mucosa of the stomach and intestines.

s., post-tussive. S. sound over a lung cavity heard on auscultation after a cough.

sudamen (sū-dā'měn) [L., sweat]. (pl. *sudamina*) Noninflammatory eruption from sweat glands characterized by whitish vesicles caused by the retention of sweat in corneous layer of the skin, appearing after profuse sweating or in certain febrile diseases, disappearing by absorption.

sudamina (sū-dăm'ĭn-ă). Pl. of sudamen, q.v.

Sudan (sū-dăn'). One of a number of related biological stains which have a special affinity for fats. Includes Sudan II, Sudan III (G), Sudan IV, and Sudan R.

sudanophil (sū-dăn'ō-fĭl) [*sudan, + Gr. philein,* to love]. A leukocyte which stains readily with Sudan III, indicative of fatty degeneration.

sudanophilia (sū-dăn"ō-fĭl'ĭ-ă). A condition in which minute fat droplets contained in the leukocytes take a brilliant red stain, probably indicative of suppuration.

sudation (sū-dā'shŭn) [L. *sudatio*]. 1. The act of sweating. 2. Excessive perspiration.

sudatoria (sū"dă-tō'rĭ-ă) [L.]. (sing. *sudatorium)* Excessive sweating. SYN: *ephidrosis; hyperidrosis.*

sudatorium (sū"dă-tō'rĭ-ŭm) [L., a sweating room]. (pl. *sudatoria)* 1. A hot air bath or any bath to induce perspiration. 2. A room used to induce sweat baths.

sudden infant death syndrome. Unexplained death of infants, usually during sleep. A variety of explanations have been suggested but none is completely satisfactory.

More cases occur in winter than summer and boys seem to be more susceptible than girls. It is estimated 10,000 children die of this condition each year in the U.S. In England the syndrome is called crib or cot death. ABBR: SIDS.

sudokeratosis (sū"dō-kěr"ă-tō'sĭs) [L. *sudor,* sweat, + Gr. *keras, kerat-,* horn, + *-ōsis,* condition]. Circumscribed, horny overgrowths obstructing the sweat ducts.

sudomotor (sū"dō-mō'tōr) ["+ *motor,* a mover]. Pert. to stimulating the secretion of sweat; noting certain nerves.

sudor (sū'dōr) [L.]. Secretion from the sweat glands. SYN: *perspiration; sweat.*

RS: anhidrosis; bromidrosis; chromidrosis; hydrosis; hematidrosis; perspiration; pore; skin; sweat; sudorific; uridrosis.

s. cruentus. Blood-tinged sweat. SYN: *hematidrosis.*

sudoral (sū'dōr-ăl). Pert. to, caused by, or marked by perspiration.

sudoresis (sū"dō-rē'sĭs) [L.]. Profuse sweating. SYN: *diaphoresis.*

sudoriferous (sū-dōr-ĭf'ĕr-ŭs) [L. *sudor,* sweat, + *ferre,* to bear]. Conveying or producing sweat.

s. glands. Sweat-secreting glands of the skin.

sudorific (sū"dōr-ĭf'ĭk) [L. *sudorificus*]. 1. Secreting or promoting the secretion of sweat. 2. Agent which produces sweating. SYN: *diaphoretic.*

sudoriparous (sū"dōr-ĭp'ă-rŭs) [L. *sudor,* sweat, + *parēre,* to produce]. Secreting sweat. SYN: *sudoriferous.*

suet (sū'ĕt) [Fr. *sewet,* suet]. Hard fat from the ox or sheep's kidneys and loins. Used as the base of certain ointments and as an emollient.

suffocate (sŭf'ō-kāt) [L. *suffocāre*]. To impair respiration; to smother, asphyxiate.

suffocation (sŭf"ō-kā'shŭn). 1. State of being choked by obstruction of air passages by drowning, smothering, throttling, or inhalation of noxious gases. SYN: *asphyxia,* q.v. 2. Act of obstructing the air passages.

SYM: Insensibility, breathing slight, face purple and swollen, livid lips. Sym. not always present.

TREATMENT: Dash cold water in face. Slap chest. Apply ammonia to nostrils. Artificial respiration. Tracheotomy may be required. RS: resuscitation; unconsciousness.

suffusion (sŭ-fū'zhŭn) [L. *suffusio,* a pouring over]. 1. Spreading of a bodily fluid into surrounding tissues. SYN: *extravasation.* 2. Pouring of a fluid over the body as treatment.

sugar (shŭ'găr) [O.Fr. *zuchre*]. A sweet-tasting carbohydrate belonging to the monosaccharose and disaccharose groups. Crystalline carbohydrates of comparatively low molecular weight and generally having a sweet taste.

CLASSIFICATION: First, as to the number of atoms of simple sugars yielded on hydrolysis by a molecule of the given sugar and, secondly, as to the number of carbon atoms in the molecules of the simple sugars so obtained. Thus, dextrose, q.v., is a monosaccharide because it cannot be hydrolyzed to a simpler sugar; it is a hexose because it contains six carbon atoms per molecule.

Sucrose is a disaccharide because on hydrolysis it yields two molecules, one of dextrose and one of levulose.

s., beet. Sucrose obtained from sugar beets.

s., blood. The carbohydrate present in the blood; principally glucose.

s., brain. Galactose.

s., cane. Sucrose obtained from sugar cane.

s., diabetic. Glucose in the urine of diabetics.

s., fruit. Levulose or fructose.

s., grape. Glucose.

s., invert. Consisting of one molecule of glucose and one of fructose resulting from the hydrolysis of sucrose.

s., liver. Glycogen.

s., malt. Maltose.

s., milk. Lactose.

s., muscle. Inositol; it is not a true sugar. SEE: *inositol.*

sugar, words pert. to: aglycosuric; blood; carbohydrate; dextrose; disaccharide; disaccharose; fructose; fruit s.; galactose; glucide; hypoglycemia; invert; invertase; lactose; levulose; melitemia; monosaccharide; monosaccharose; pentose; pentosuria; polysaccharide; polysaccharose; sucrose; xylose; words beginning with "gluco-," "glyco-," and "sacchar-."

suggestibility (sŭg-jĕs″tĭ-bĭl′ĭ-tĭ) [L. *suggestus,* suggested]. A condition in which a person responds readily to suggestions or opinions of another.

suggestible (sŭg-jĕs′tĭ-bl). Very susceptible to the opinions or suggestions of others.

suggestion (sŭg-jĕs′chŭn) [L. *suggestio*]. 1. Imparting an idea indirectly; to imply. 2. The idea so conveyed. 3. The psychological process of having an individual adopt or accept an idea without argument or persuasion.

s., auto-. Self-suggestion as distinguished from that coming from another person, esp. in hypnotic state.

s., posthypnotic. S. made to a subject while under hypnosis. After emerging from the hypnotic state the person performs the suggested act.

suggestive (sŭg-jĕs′tĭv). Stimulating or pert. to suggestion.

s. medicine. Therapy by suggestion either during consciousness or hypnosis.

s. therapeutics. The practice of treating disease by suggestion or hypnotism.

suggillation (sŭg-jĭl-ā′shŭn) [L. *sugillatio*]. A bruise or black and blue mark. SYN: *ecchymosis.*

suicide (sū′ĭ-sĭd) [L. *sui,* of oneself + *caedere,* to kill]. 1. Act or instance of taking one's own life voluntarily. 2. One who attempts or commits self-murder. These individuals often have attacks of temporary insanity or mental depression which may lead to suicide. SEE: *hysteria.*

MENTAL STATES CONDUCIVE TO: Those with sudden impulses; the depressed; those with delusions of persecution, of being ruined, of voices suggesting, of incurable disease. In melancholia; schizophrenia; epilepsy; confusional states; alcoholism. Through accidents causing acute delirium, mania, general paralysis.

METHODS RESORTED TO: Hanging; drowning in tub or otherwise; poisoning; cutting an artery; burning; jumping from window; overdose of various medications; bombs; deliberately crashing vehicles or airplanes. Instruments used may be harmless articles converted into dangerous tools, i.e., matches, knives and spoons, glass, cord, rope, suspenders, bedclothing, nail files. All must be removed if patient is inclined to harm self or others.

NP: In addition to the usual F.A. Treatment for injuries, kindly interrogation and soothing, tranquil conversation are invaluable. In their after-care, such patients should be watched and kept free from needless questioning or emotional display. Sedatives are useful. Persons who have attempted suicide should be observed carefully because of the danger of their attempting to commit suicide again.

sulcal (sŭl′kăl) [L.]. Pert. to a sulcus.

s. artery. A tiny branch of anterior spinal artery.

sulcate, sulcated (sŭl′kāt, -ĕd) [L. *sulcatus*]. Furrowed or grooved.

sulcus (sŭl′kŭs) [L., groove]. (pl. *sul′ci*) A furrow, groove, slight depression, or fissure, esp. of the brain.

s. centralis. Fissure dividing the frontal and parietal lobes of each cerebral hemisphere. SYN: *fissure of Rolando.*

s., intraparietal. Groove that separates the inferior from the superior parietal bones and lobes.

s. precentralis. [NA]. An interrupted s. generally parallel with the fissure of Rolando and anterior to it.

s. pulmonalis. [NA]. Depression on either side of the vertebral column.

s. spiralis cochleae. Groove between the labium tympanicum and labium vestibulare.

sulf-, sulfo- [L. *sulfur*]. Prefix showing that a compound with this prefix contains sulfurous anhydride or the group SO.

sulfacetamide (sŭl″fă-sĕt′ă-mĭd). An antibacterial sulfonamide that is highly soluble. It is particularly useful for topical application to the eye.

sulfadiazine (sŭl″fă-dī′ă-zēn). USP. One of a group of diazine derivatives of sulfanilamide. Because it readily penetrates the blood-brain barrier it has been used extensively in treating meningococcal meningitis. Some strains of meningococci have become resistant to sulfadiazine.

sulfa drugs. Drugs of the sulfonamide group possessing bacteriostatic properties. SEE: *sulfonamides*.

sulfamerazine (sŭl″fă-mĕr′ă-zēn). USP. An antibacterial sulfonamide which is more readily absorbed than sulfadiazine from which it is derived. SEE: *sulfadiazine*.

sulfamethazine (sŭl″fă-mĕth′ă-zēn). USP. An antibacterial sulfonamide similar to sulfadiazine.

sulfanilamide (sŭl″făn-ĭl′ă-mĭd). Para-aminobenzenesulfonamide. white, slightly bitter, crystalline substance from coal tar, the parent of the azo dyes. Formerly it was widely used in the treatment of a number of infections, but because of its toxic reactions it has been superseded by more effective and less toxic sulfonamides.

sulfapyridine (sŭl″fă-pĭr′ĭ-dēn). USP. A sulfonamide, one of the first drugs to have a curative effect upon pneumonia. Formerly used extensively in the treatment of streptococcal, gonococcal, and staphylococcal infections, but its use has been supplanted by other sulfonamides which are less toxic and more effective.

sulfapyr′idine so′dium monohy′drate. A soluble salt of sulfapyridine for intravenous use only.

sulfarsphenamine (sŭlf′ăr-sfĕn′ă-mēn). An arsenic compound; 19% arsenic.
USES: Effective in treating syphilis.

sulfasuxidine (sŭl″fă-sŭks′ĭ-din). Proprietary name for succinylsulfathiazole, a bacteriostatic for infections of the gastrointestinal tract; very poorly absorbed from the gastrointestinal tract.

sulfate (sŭl′fāt) [L. *sulphas*]. A salt or ester of sulfuric acid.

s., iron. Green vitriol; copperas. Fatal in large dosage.
POISONING: Magnesia and diluents.

s., magnesium. Magnesium sulfate, q.v.

sulfathiazole (sŭl″fă-thī′ă-zōl). A rapidly absorbed and excreted sulfanilamide com-

pound; largely replaced by less toxic sulfonamides.

sulfhemoglobin (sŭlf′hēm-ō-glō′bĭn). Substance formed by action of hydrogen sulfide on blood. SYN: *sulfmethemoglobin*.

sulfhemoglobinemia (sŭlf′hēm-ō-glō′bĭn-ē′mĭ-ă). Persistent cyanotic condition due to sulfhemoglobin in blood.

sulfhydryl (sŭlf-hī′drĭl). The univalent radical, SH, of sulfur and hydrogen. SYN: *SH group*.

sulfmethemoglobin (sŭlf′mĕt-hē″mō-glō′-bĭn). The greenish hemoglobin compound formed when hemoglobin and hydrogen sulfide are combined. SYN: *sulfhemoglobin*.

sulfo-. A combining form usually indicating the presence of divalent sulfur or of the sulfo- group, -SO₂OH.

sulfonamides. A group of compounds consisting of amides of sulfanilic acid derived from their parent compound sulfanilamide. They are bacteriostatic, their action on bacteria resulting from interference with functioning of enzyme systems necessary for normal metabolism, growth, and multiplication.

sulfonethylmethane (sŭl″fōn-ĕth′ĭl-mĕth′ān). Trional. White powder or crystalline substance with a bitter taste.
ACTION AND USES: As a hypnotic.

sulfourea (sŭl″fō-ū-rē′ă). Urea with oxygen replaced by sulfur. SYN: *thiourea*.

sulfur (sŭl′fŭr) [L.]. SYMB: *S*. At. wt. 32.06, at. no. 16; sp. gr. 2.07. A pale yellow, crystalline element which burns with a blue flame producing sulfur dioxide.

The amount of sulfur excreted in urine varies with amount of protein in diet but more or less parallels the amount of nitrogen excreted, as both are derived from protein catabolism. The S:N ration is approx. 1:14, i.e., for each gm. of sulfur excreted 14 gm. of nitrogen are excreted. The amount of sulfur excreted daily is about 1 gm. It is oxidized to sulfate and required for the synthesis of body proteins as cystine, cysteine, or their combination.

DEFICIENCY SYM: Dermatitis, imperfect development of hair and nails. Deficiency of cystine or cysteine proteins in diet restricts growth and may be fatal. Tissue oxidation of cystine forms inorganic sulfate if the protein intake is sufficient.

s. dioxide. SO₂. An irritating gas used in industry to manufacture acids. Also used in electrical refrigerators. A bactericide and important disinfectant.
POISONING SYM: Suffocation from a highly irritating gas which forms sulfuric acid when in contact with moisture of the

mouth, eyes, and respiratory passages with resultant pain, swelling, burning, etc.

TREATMENT: Remove patient from the vitiated atmosphere. Oxygen by intermittent positive pressure breathing apparatus or artificial respiration may be necessary. Give heart and respiratory stimulants as needed. Wash affected areas with large amounts of water and weak alkalies, as chalk magnesia, lime water, soapsuds. Follow by bland diet.

sulfurated, sulfureted (sŭl'fū-rā"ted, -rĕt"ĕd). Combined or impregnated with sulfur.

s. hydrogen. H₂S, a colorless, inflammable gas of disagreeable odor resulting from decomposition of organic matter containing sulfur; used as a chemical reagent. SYN: *hydrogen sulfide.*

sulfuric acid (sŭl-fū'rĭk). A colorless, odorless, liquid of heavy, oily consistency. It is extremely caustic and corrosive. It is widely used in manufacturing. SYN: *oil of vitriol.*

POISONING: Sometimes accidentally taken by mouth, as it resembles syrup or glycerin.

SYM: Local effects. Burning, with destruction of skin. If it strikes eye it may result in blindness. If taken by mouth, intense pain extending from mouth to esophagus and down to stomach, causing marked, excruciating pain; swelling of affected tissues; salivation; painful swallowing; often gasping for breath, and hoarse voice. Mucous membrane has a grayish-white coating. There is persistent, painful vomiting. Patient quickly goes into shock.

TREATMENT: Dilute acid with large volumes of water. Neutralize acid with milk of magnesia, baking soda, or other well-diluted alkalies. Follow by soothing substances, as raw eggs.

s. a., dilute. An aqueous 10% solution of H₂SO₄. Used as an astringent and for gastric hypoacidity.

summation (sŭm-ā'shŭn) [L. *summatio,* adding]. Cumulative action or effect, as of stimuli. Thus an organ reacts to two or more weak stimuli as if they were a single strong one.

summer (sŭm'ĕr) [AS. *sumer*]. The warmest season of the year, occurring between spring and autumn.

sunburn (sŭn'bŭrn) [AS. *sunne,* sun, + *bernan,* to burn]. Dermatitis due to excessive exposure to the actinic rays of the sun. SEE: *burn.*

Sunday morning paralysis. Radial nerve palsy, sometimes the indirect result of acute alcoholism resulting from stuporous patient lying immobile with arm pressed over a projecting surface. SYN: *Saturday night paralysis.*

sunflower eyes. Slang term for the appearance of the eyes of patients with Wilson's disease. Deposits of copper around the edge of the cornea (Kayser-Fleischer rings) cause this condition.

sunscreen. Substance used to protect the skin from ultraviolet rays of the sun. Usually applied as an ointment or cream.

sunstroke (sŭn'strōk) [AS. *sunne,* sun, + *strāke,* a blow]. An affection from undue exposure to rays of the sun or excessive heat.

SYM: Extreme prostration; high fever; other symptoms of heatstroke; delirium; collapse; loss of mind; or death. SEE: *heatstroke.*

super- [L.]. Combining form meaning above, beyond, superior.

superalimentation (sūp"ĕr-ăl"ĭ-měn-tā'shŭn) [L. *super,* above, + *alimentum,* food]. Therapeutic administration of food in excess of body needs or appetite. SYN: *hyperalimentation.*

superalkalinity (sūp"ĕr-ăl"kă-lĭn'ĭ-t ĭ) ["+ *alkalinus,* alkaline]. Excessive alkalinity.

superciliary (sū"pĕr-sĭl'ĭ-ă-rĭ) [L. *supercilium,* eyebrow]. Pert. to or in the region of an eyebrow.

supercilium (sū"pĕr-sĭl'ĭ-ŭm) [L.]. (pl. *supercil'ia*) 1. [NA]. Eyebrow. 2. A hair of the eyebrow.

superego (sū"pĕr-ē'gō) [L. *super,* above, + *egō,* I]. In psychoanalytical theory, the portion of the personality associated with ethics, self-criticism, and the moral standard of the community. It is formed in infancy by the individual's adopting as his personal standards the values of the significant persons with whom he identifies. This serves to help form the *conscience.* The superego functions to protect and to reward when the ego-ideal of behavior or thought is satisfied; and to criticize, punish, and evoke a sense of guilt when the reverse is true. In neuroses, symptoms develop when instinctual drives conflict with those dictated by the superego. SEE: *ego.*

superfecundation (sū"pĕr-fē"kŭn-dā'-shŭn) ["+ *fecundāre,* to fertilize]. Successive fertilization by more than one coitus of two or more ova formed during the same menstrual cycle. Fertilization may be by the same or two different males.

super female. A female having three X chromosomes.

superfetation (sū"pĕr-fē-tā'shŭn) [L. *super,* above, + *fetus,* fetus]. Fertilization of two ova in the same uterus at different menstrual periods within a short interval.

superficial (sū″pĕr-físh'ăl) [L. *superficialis*].
1. Confined to the surface. 2. Not thorough;
cursory.

s. reflex. Reflex induced by very light
stimulus, such as stroking skin lightly with
soft cotton wad.

superficialis (sū″pĕr-físh-ĭ-ā'lĭs) [L.]. Superficial; noting a superficial artery, vein, or
nerve, or structure near the surface.

superimpregnation (sū″pĕr-ĭm″prĕg-
nā'shŭn) [L. *super*, over, + *impregnatio*,
impregnation]. Conception during pregnancy; fertilization from two different ovula-
tions. SYN: *superfecundation;
superfetation.*

superinduce (sū″pĕr-ĭn-dūs') ["+ *in*, into, +
ducere, to lead]. To bring on over or above an
already existing condition or situation.

superinfection (sū″pĕr-ĭn-fĕk'shŭn) ["+ *infectio*, a putting into]. A new infection by an
organism different from that which caused
the initial infection.

superinvolution (sū″pĕr-ĭn-vō-lū'shŭn) ["+
involutus, a turning]. Excessive reduction of
the uterus to less than its normal size
following childbirth. SYN: *hyperinvolution.*

superior (sū-pē'rĭ-ŏr) [L. *superus*, upper]. 1.
Higher than; situated above something else.
2. Better than. 3. One in charge of others.

superior'ity com'plex. An exaggerated
conviction of one's own superiority; a pretense of superiority in order to compensate
for supposed inferiority.

superlactation (sū″pĕr-lăk-tā'shŭn) [L. *super*, above, + *lactāre*, to suckle]. Oversecretion of milk, or continuance of lactation
beyond normal time.

superlethal (sū″pĕr-lē'thăl) ["+ *lethum*,
death]. A dose of a drug, or exposure to
trauma, greater than that required to produce death.

supermoron (sū″pĕr-mō'rŏn) ["+ Gr. *mōros*,
stupid]. One slightly subnormal, but above a
moron mentally.

supermotility (sū″pĕr-mō-tĭl'ĭ-tĭ) [L. *super*,
above, + *motilis*, able to move]. Excessive
motility in any part. SYN: *hyperkinesia.*

supernatant (sū″pĕr-nā'tănt) ["+ *natāre*, to
float]. 1. Floating on surface, as oil on water.
2. The clear liquid remaining at the top after
a precipitate settles.

supernate (sū′pĕr-nāt). A supernatant fluid.

supernumerary (sū″pĕr-nū'mĕr-ăr'ĭ) [L.
supernumerarius]. Exceeding the regular
number.

supernutrition (sū″pĕr-nū-trĭ'shŭn) [L. *super*, above, + *nutritio*, nourishment]. More
than normal nutrition.

supersat'urated solution. Solution containing more salt or other substance than it
can dissolve at normal temperature.

superscription (sū″pĕr-skrĭp'shŭn) [L. *super*, above, + *scriptio*, a writing]. The beginning of a prescription noted by the sign Rx,
signifying (L.) *recipe*, take.

supersecretion (sū″pĕr-sē-krē'shŭn) ["+ *secretio*, a separating]. An excess of any secretion.

su″persen'sitive″ness ["+ *sensitivus*,
sensitive]. Excessive susceptibility to a foreign protein or other antigenic substance.
SYN: *hypersensitiveness.*

supersoft (sū″pĕr-sŏft') [L. *super*, above, +
AS. *sōfte*, soft]. Exceptionally soft; noting
roentgen rays of extremely long wave length
and low penetrating power.

supersonic ["+ *sonus*, sound]. 1. Pert. to vibrations of sound space waves of frequencies
above 20,000 cycles which are inaudible to
the human ear. SYN: *ultrasonic.* 2. Used to
describe speeds greater than that of sound.
At sea level, in air at 0° C. the speed of sound
is about 331 meters, or 1087 feet/second (741
miles/hour).

supertension (sū′pĕr-tĕn'shŭn) ["+ *tensio*, a
stretching]. Extremely high tension.

supervenos'ity. Incomplete oxidation of the
blood; a condition of excessive venosity.

supervention (sū″pĕr-vĕn'shŭn) [L. *super-
ventio*, a coming over]. Additional condition
developing, as a complication to an existing
disease.

supervirulent (sū″pĕr-vĭr'ū-lĕnt) [L. *super*,
above, + *virulentus*, poisonous]. More virulent than usual.

supervisor. A person, usually a nurse, who is
responsible for a certain department, ward,
or activity in a hospital or nursing school.

supervitaminosis. Excess accumulation of
vitamins due to administration of an excess
dose. SYN: *hypervitaminosis.*

supinate (sū′pĭ-nāt) [L. *supinatus*, bent back-
wards]. 1. To turn the forearm or hand so
that the palm faces upward. 2. To rotate the
foot and leg outward. 3. To cause to assume,
or to assume, a position of supination.

supination (sū″pĭn-ā'shŭn) [L. *supinatio*]. 1.
Turning of the palm or foot upward. 2. Act
of lying flat upon the back. 3. Condition of
being on the back or having the foot or palm
facing upward.

supinator (sū″pĭn-ā'tŏr) [L.]. A muscle producing the motion of supination of the
forearm. SEE: *Table of Muscles* in *Appendix.*

s. longus reflex. Flexion of the forearm caused by tapping of the tendon of the
supinator longus.

supine (sū-pīn') [L. *supinus*, lying on the back]. 1. Of position, lying on the back or with the face upward. 2. Of the hand or foot, noting position with the palm or foot facing upward. Opposed to prone. SEE: *position*.

supplemental (sŭp″lĕ-mĕn'tăl) [L. *supplementum*, an addition]. Referring to something added to supply a need or to reinforce.

  s. air. The air which by the most forcible effort can be expelled after an ordinary expiration which has followed a normal inspiration. In adult males it averages about 1500 cc. SYN: *reserve air.*

suppository (sŭ-pŏz'ĭ-tō-rī) [L. *suppositorium*, something placed underneath]. (pl. *suppositories*) A semisolid substance for introduction into the rectum, vagina, or urethra where it dissolves. It often serves as a vehicle for medicines to be absorbed. Commonly shaped like cylinder or cone and made of soap, glycerinated gelatin, or cocoa butter (oil of theobroma).

  s., rectal, anodyne. For local or general effects to reduce pain.

  s., rectal, astringent. To contract blood vessels and tissues.

  s., rectal, evacuant. To cause evacuation.

suppression (sŭ-prĕsh'ŭn) [L. *suppressio*, a pressing under]. 1. Repression of the external manifestation of a morbid condition. 2. Complete failure of natural production of a secretion or excretion, as distinguished from retention in which normal secretion occurs but the discharge is retained within the organ or body. 3. In psychoanalysis, conscious inhibition of an idea or desire, as distinguished from repression which is considered an unconscious process.

  s. of menses. 1. Amenorrhea in which menstruation ceases after once being established and from some cause other than pregnancy or the climacteric. 2. Any suppression of the menses.

  s. of urine. Suppression of urine resulting from renal conditions.

suppurant (sŭp'ū-rănt) [L. *suppurans*]. 1. Producing, tending to produce, or characterized by pus formation. 2. Agent causing pus formation. SYN: *suppurative.*

suppurate (sŭp'ū-rāt) [L. *suppurāre*]. To form or generate pus.

suppuration (sŭp-ū-rā'shŭn) [L. *suppurātio*]. 1. The process of pus formation. 2. The discharge produced by suppuration. SYN: *pus.*

  Condition produced by inflammation due to the presence of certain microorganisms called pyogenic (pus-forming) bacteria. Suppuration does not always develop even though microorganisms are present in the affected part, as may be the case in erysipelas and acute joint affections where exudate is serous.

  Liquefaction of tissues and formation of pus will continue so long as the microorganisms are alive. They cause the death of the leukocytes (white cells) and the cells of the part, liquefying the tissue so that the area becomes filled with a liquid containing the dead and dying cells. This fluid is called pus. An abscess may form by the accumulation of this liquid. The abscess is indicated by redness, swelling, heat, and pain. It will show fluctuation which may be felt by palpating it with two fingers. When the abscess reaches the surface it will burst and discharge its contents. In most cases it is wise to surgically incise the abscess rather than to wait for it to burst spontaneously.

  RS: abscess; gangrene; infection; inflammation; purulent; pus; pustulant; pustule; pyogenic.

suppurative (sŭp'ū-rā″tĭv, -ră-tĭv) [L. *suppuratus*]. 1. Producing or associated with generation of pus. 2. Agent producing pus formation.

  s. fever. Pus in the blood causing fever; a form of septicemia. SYN: *pyemia.*

supra- [L.]. Combining form meaning above.

supra-acromial (sū″prǎ-ă-krō'mĭ-ăl) [L. *supra*, above, + Gr. *akron*, point, + *ōmos*, shoulder]. Located above the acromion.

supra-auricular (sū″prǎ-ŏ-rĭk'ū-lăr) ["+ *auricula*, ear]. Located above the auricle.

supracerebellar (sū″prǎ-sĕr″ē-bĕl'ăr) ["+ *cerebellum*, little brain]. On or above the upper surface of the cerebellum.

suprachoroid (sū″prǎ-kō'royd) [L. *supra*, above, + Gr. *chorioeidēs*, skinlike]. 1. Situated upon or above the choroid layer of the eyeball. 2. The s. lamina, q.v. SYN: *epichoroid; lamina suprachoroidea.*

  s. lamina. The superficial layer of the choroid consisting of thin transparent layers, the outermost adhering to the sclera. SYN: *epichoroid lamina suprachoroidea.*

suprachoroidea (sū″prǎ-kō-roy'dē-ă). Outermost layer of the choroid. SYN: *suprachoroid lamina.*

supraclavicular (sū″prǎ-klǎ-vĭk'ū-lăr) [L. *supra*, above, + *clavicula*, a little key]. Located above the clavicle.

  s. fossa. Depression on either side of neck reaching down behind the clavicle.

  s. point. A stimulation point over the clavicle at which contraction of arm muscles may be produced.

supracondylar (sū″prǎ-kŏn'dĭ-lǎr) ["+ Gr. *kondylos*, knuckle]. Above a condyle.

supracotyloid (sū″prä-kŏt′ĭ-loyd) ["+ Gr. *kotyloeidēs*, cup-shaped]. Above the acetabulum.

supradiaphragmatic (sū″prä-dī″ä-frăg-măt′ĭk) [L. *supra*, above, + Gr. *dia*, across, + *phragma*, wall]. Above the diaphragm.

supraglenoid (sū″prä-glē′noyd) ["+ Gr. *glēnē*, cavity, + *eidos*, form]. Above the glenoid cavity or fossa.

s. tuberosity. A rough surface of the scapula above glenoid cavity to which is attached the long head of biceps muscle.

suprahyoid (sū″prä-hī′oyd) ["+ *hyoeidēs*, U-shaped]. Located above the hyoid bone; denoting accessory thyroid glands within the geniohyoid muscle.

s. muscles. The digastric, geniohyoid, mylohyoid, and stylohyoid muscles.

suprainguinal (sū″prä-ĭn′gwĭn-äl) ["+ *inguinalis*, pert. to the groin]. Above the groin.

supraliminal (sū″prä-lĭm′ĭ-näl) [L. *supra*, above, + *limen, limin-*, threshold]. 1. Above the threshold of consciousness; conscious. 2. Exceeding the stimulus threshold. SEE: *subliminal*.

supralumbar (sū″prä-lŭm′bär) ["+ *lumbus*, loin]. Above the lumbar region.

supramalleolar (sū″prä-mŏ-lē′ŏ-lär) ["+ *malleolus*, little hammer]. Located above either malleolus.

supramarginal (sū″prä-măr′jĭn-äl) [L. *supra*, above, + *margo, margin-*, margin]. Above any border.

s. convolution, s. gyrus. A cerebral convolution on lateral surface of the parietal lobe above posterior part of sylvian fissure.

supramastoid (sū″prä-măs′toyd) ["+ *mastos*, breast, + *eidos*, like]. Above the mastoid process of the temporal bone.

s. crest. A ridge on the temporal bone. SYN: *temporal line*.

supramaxilla (sū″prä-măk-sĭl′ä) ["+ *maxilla*, jaw]. The upper jawbone. SYN: *maxilla*.

supramaxillary (sū″prä-măk′sĭ-lĕr-ĭ). 1. Rel. to the upper jaw. 2. Located above the upper jaw.

suprameatal (sū″prä-mē-ā′tăl) [L. *supra*, above, + *meatus*, passage]. Above a meatus, esp. the exterior auditory meatus, noting the spine of Henle, a small, bony projection at posterior superior margin of external auditory meatus.

s. spine. Small bony projection at posterior superior margin of external auditory meatus marking the anterior superior apex of the suprameatal triangle, q.v. SYN: *spine of Henle*.

s. triangle. Triangular space bordered by upper half of posterior wall of external auditory meatus, and the supramastoid crest used to locate the mastoid antrum.

supraoccipital (sū″prä-ŏk-sĭp′ĭ-tăl) [L. *supra*, above, + *occiput*, back of head]. Lying above or in upper portion of the occiput.

s. portion of occipital bone. Portion lying immediately above the foramen magnum and forming lower part of squamous portion of occipital bone.

supraorbital (sū″prä-ŏr′bĭ-tăl) ["+ *orbita*, circuit]. Located above the orbit.

s. neuralgia. Neuralgia of the s. nerve. SYN: *hemicrania*.

s. notch. A notch in superior margin arch of orbit for transmitting supraorbital vessels and nerve.

s. reflex. Contraction of orbicularis oculi muscle with closure of lids resulting from percussion above s. nerve.

suprapelvic (sū″prä-pĕl′vĭk) ["+ *pelvis*, basis]. Located above the pelvis.

suprapontine (sū″prä-pŏn′tĭn) [L. *supra*, above, + *pons, pont-*, bridge]. Located above the pons Varolii.

suprapubic (sū″prä-pū′bĭk) ["+ *pubis*, pubis]. Above the pubic arch.

s. aspiration of urine. Use of a sterile needle and syringe to obtain urine from the bladder.

TECHNIQUE: Patient is instructed to drink fluids and not to urinate. When the bladder is palpable the s. area is cleaned with alcohol and a 21 gauge sterile needle is inserted through the skin into the bladder. Urine is then aspirated. Local anesthetic is not required.

CAUTION: The needle may pierce a loop of bowel which is lying over the anterior surface of the bladder.

s. cystotomy. Surgical opening of the bladder from just above the symphysis pubis.

s. reflex. Deflection of linea alba toward stroked side when abdomen is stroked above Poupart's ligament.

suprarenal (sū″prä-rē′näl) [L. *supra*, above, + *rēn*, kidney]. 1. Above the kidney. 2. Tiny gland above each kidney. SYN: *adrenal; s. body; s. capsule; s. gland*. 3. Pert. to the s. gland.

s. gland. An endocrine gland lying cephalad and mediad to each kidney. SYN: *adrenal gland; glandula suprarenalis*. SEE: *ACTH; adrenal; adrenalin; endocrine gland; epinephrine; corticosterone; cortisone*.

suprarenalopathy (sū″prä-rē-năl-ŏp′ä-thĭ) ["+ " + Gr. *pathos*, disease]. A disorder due to abnormal functioning of the suprarenal glands.

suprarenopathy (sū"prā-rē-nŏp'ă-thĭ). Any disorder of the suprarenal glands.

suprascapular (sū"prā-skăp'ū-lăr) [L. *supra*, above, + *scapula*, shoulder]. Located above the scapula.

suprasegmen'tal ["+ *segmentum*, segment]. Above the segmented portion.

   s. brain. The cerebrum, midbrain, and cerebellum as distinguished from the segmental portion (pons and medulla oblongata).

suprasellar (sū"prā-sĕl'ăr) ["+ *sella*, saddle]. Above or over the sella turcica.

suprasonic (sū"prā-sŏn'ĭk) [L. *supra*, above, + *sonus*, sound]. Noting sound with frequencies of vibration above 20,000 per second. SEE: *supersonic*.

supraspinal (sū"prā-spī'năl) ["+ *spina*, a thorn]. Above a spine.

supraspi'nous. Above any spinous process.

   s. fossa. A groove above the spine of the scapula.

suprasternal (sū"prā-stĕr'năl) [L. *supra*, above, + Gr. *sternon*, chest]. Above the sternum. SYN: *episternal*.

supra"ster'ol. Substance produced by overirradiation of vitamin D.

supratentorial. Located above the tentorium.

supratrochlear (sū"prā-trŏk'lē-ar) [L. *supra*, above, + *trochlea*, pulley]. Above a trochlea, esp. that of the humerus.

supravaginal (sū"prā-văj'ĭ-năl) ["+ *vagina*, sheath]. Above the vagina or any sheathing membrane.

supravergence (sū"prā-vĕr'jĕns) ["+ *vergere*, to be inclined]. Condition in which one eye moves upward in the vertical plane while the other does not.

sura (sū'rā) [L.]. [NA]. Calf of the leg; muscular posterior portion of lower leg.

sural (sū'răl). Rel. to the calf of the leg.

suralimentation (sūr"ăl-ĭm-ĕn-tā'shŭn) [Fr. *sur*, above, + L. *alimentum*, nourishment]. Treatment by overfeeding. SYN: *gavage; superalimentation*.

surdity (sūr'dĭ-tĭ) [L. *surditās*, deafness]. Inability to hear. SYN: *deafness*.

surdomute (sūr'dō-mūt") [L. *surdus*, deaf, + *mutus*, dumb]. 1. A deaf-mute. 2. Deaf and dumb.

surface (sūr'fĕs) [Fr. *sur*, above, over, + *faciēs*, face]. 1. The exterior boundary of a solid object. 2. The external or internal exposed portions of a hollow structure, as the outer or inner surfaces of the cranium or stomach. 3. The face or faces of a body such as a bone.

   s. tension. Condition at the surface of a liquid in contact with a gas or another liquid which causes its surface to act as a stretched rubber membrane. It is the result of mutual attraction of the molecules to each other, thus producing a cohesive state which causes liquids to assume a shape presenting the smallest surface area to the surrounding medium. This accounts for the spherical shape assumed by fluids, such as drops of oil or water. ABBR: S.T.

surfac'tant. An agent that lowers surface tension. Ex: oils and various forms of detergents.

   s., pulmonary. A phospholipid substance important in controlling the surface tension of air-liquid emulsion which is present in the lungs. Abnormalities in this surfactant have been noted in prematurity, hyaline membrane disease, and pulmonary edema.

surfer's knots. Nodular swelling and possibly bone changes of area of lower leg and foot exposed to pressure and trauma while on a surfboard. Nodules may be painful.

surgeon (sūr'jŭn) [O.Fr. *serurgien*]. A medical practitioner who specializes in surgery.

   s., dental. A dentist authorized to operate on the mouth and teeth. SYN: *stomatologist*.

   s., house. A s. in training who works under the supervision of the attending s.

surgery (sūr'jŭr-ĭ) [O.Fr. *serurgerie*]. 1. Branch of medicine dealing with manual and operative procedures for correction of deformities and defects, repair of injuries, diagnosis and cure of diseases, relief of suffering, and prolongation of life. SYN: *chirurgery, chirurgia*. 2. Surgeon's operating room.

   s., aseptic. Operative procedures carried on under aseptic conditions or in the absence of pathogenic organisms.

   s., aural. That pert. to the ear.

   s., conservative. That in which as much as possible of a part or structure is retained.

   s., major. Important and serious operations involving risk to life.

   s., minor. Simple, less serious operations.

   s., oral. That pert. to the mouth and associated structures, esp. the teeth and jaws.

   s., orificial. S. of the orifices of the body such as the mouth, anus, vagina, etc.

   s., orthopedic. S. for correction of deformities.

   s., plastic. S. concerned with the repair or restoration of defective or missing structures, frequently involving the transference of tissue from a part or person to another part or person.

surgical (sŭr'jĭ-kăl). Of the nature of or pert. to surgery.

s. diathermy. The use of high-frequency electrical oscillations in such a way that animal tissues are destroyed.

s. dressing. Sterile protective covering of gauze or other substance applied to an operative wound. SEE: *chemise.*

s. fever. Fever following an operation or injury.

s. neck. Constricted part of shaft of humerus below the tuberosities; commonly the seat of fracture.

surrogate (sŭr'ō-gāt) [L. *surrogatus,* substituted]. 1. Something or someone replacing another; a substitute, esp. an emotional substitute for another. 2. In psychoanalysis, the representation of one whose identity is concealed from conscious recognition as in a dream; a figure of importance may represent one's loved one.

sursumduction (sŭr″sŭm-dŭk'shŭn) [L. *sursum,* upward, + *ducere,* to lead]. Elevation, as the power or act of turning an eye upward independently of the other one.

sursumvergence (sŭr″sŭm-vĕr'jĕns) [" + *vergere,* to turn]. An upward turning, as of the eyeballs.

sursumversion (sŭr″sŭm-vĕr'zhŭn) [" + *versio,* turning]. Process of turning upward; simultaneous movement of both eyes upward.

susceptible (sŭ-sĕp'tĭ-bl) [L. *susceptibilis,* capable of receiving]. 1. Having little resistance to a disease or foreign protein. 2. An individual with little resistance to an infectious disease or who is not known to have become immune to one. 3. Easily impressed or influenced.

suscitate (sŭs'ĭ-tāt) [L. *suscitāre,* to rouse]. To arouse to increased activity; to stimulate.

suscitation (sŭs″ĭ-tā'shŭn) [L. *suscitatio,* arousal]. Act of stimulating to greater activity. SYN: *excitation.*

suspended (sŭs-pĕnd'ĕd) [L. *suspendēre,* to hang up]. 1. Hanging. 2. Temporarily inactive.

s. animation. A cessation of the vital functions temporarily.

suspension (sŭs-pĕn'shŭn) [L. *suspensio,* a hanging]. 1. A condition of temporary cessation, as of any vital process. 2. Treatment by immobilization of a part or whole of a patient by hanging in desired position. 3. State of a solid when its particles are mixed with, but not dissolved in, a fluid or another solid; also a substance in this state.

s., cephalic. Supported suspension of a patient by the head to extend the vertebral column.

s., colloidal. A colloidal solution in which particles of the dispersed phase are relatively large.

s., stability. Degree of speed with which erythrocytes sink to bottom in a mass of citrated blood. SYN: *sedimentation rate.*

s., tendon. Tenodesis; fixation of a tendon.

s. of the uterus. The operation of attaching the uterus to the abdominal wall.

suspensoid (sŭs-pĕn'soyd) [" + Gr. *eidos,* form]. A colloid solution in which the dispersed particles are solid, as distinguished from emulsoid. SYN: *suspension, colloidal.*

suspensory (sŭs-pĕn'sō-rĭ) [L. *suspensorius,* hanging]. 1. Supporting a part, as a muscle, ligament, or bone. 2. A structure of the body which supports a part. 3. Bandage or sac for supporting or compressing a part, esp. the scrotum.

s. bandage. A sling for support of the testicles.

s. ligament. Any one of a number of ligaments which support a specific organ or structure. SEE: *ligament, suspensory.*

suspiration (sŭs″pĭr-ā'shŭn) [L. *suspiratio*]. A sigh or the act of sighing.

suspirious (sŭs-pĭ'rĭ-ŭs) [L. *suspirāre,* to sign]. Breathing with apparent effort; sighing.

sustentacular (sŭs″tĕn-tăk'ū-lŭr) [L. *sustentaculum,* support]. Supporting; upholding.

s. cell. A supporting cell such as those found in the acoustic macula, organ of Corti, olfactory epithelium, taste buds, or testes. SEE: *Sertoli's cells.*

s. fibers of Müller. Fibers forming the supporting framework of the retina.

sustentaculum (sŭs″tĕn-tăk'ū-lŭm) [L.]. (pl. *sustentac'ula*) A supporting structure.

s. hepatis. A fold of peritoneum upon which rests the right margin of the liver.

s. lienis. Phrenocolic ligament which apparently supports the spleen.

s. tali. [NA]. A process of the calcaneum which supports part of the astragalus.

susurrus (sū-sŭr'ŭs) [L., a whisper]. A murmur.

sutura (sū-tū'rä) [L., a seam]. (pl. *suturae*) 1. [NA]. A kind of fibrous union found only in the skull; one in which bony surfaces are closely united by a thin fibrous membrane, the membrane disappearing eventually. 2. Suture of any kind.

s. denta'ta. S. with interlocking of bony processes resembling the teeth of a saw.

s. harmo'nia. Simple apposition of two contiguous bones.

s. limbosa. Beveled suture in which opposing margins fit in parallel ridges as between parietal and frontal bones.

s. no'tha. A false suture with ill-defined projections.

s. serra'ta. [NA]. S. with deeper and more irregular indentations than a dental s.

s. squamosa. [NA]. S. formed by overlapping of contiguous bones by broad beveled edges as in suture between squamous portion of temporal and parietal bones.

s. vera. A true suture in which no movement of united bones can occur.

sutural (sū'tū-răl) [L. *sutura*, a seam]. Rel. to a suture.

s. joint. Articulation between two bones.

s. ligament. Fibers uniting opposed bones forming a cranial suture.

suturation (sū"tū-rā'shŭn). Application of sutures; stitching.

suture (sū'chŭr) [L. *sutura*, a seam]. 1. Line of union in an immovable articulation, as those between the skull bones; also such an articulation itself. SYN: *sutura; synarthrosis.* 2. Operation of uniting parts by stitching them together. 3. The thread or wire or other material used in the operation of stitching parts of the body together. 4. The seam or line of union formed by surgical stitches. 5. To unite by stitching. SEE: *raphe.*

s., absorbable. S. which is gradually dissolved by body tissues and cells. Suture material made of gut tissue is the best example.

s., basilar. The one between the occipital bone and sphenoid bone.

s., bifrontal. Junction of the frontal and parietal bones.

s., biparietal. Suture between the two parietal bones.

s.'s, buried. Those completely covered by skin and not involving that structure at all.

s., button. One in which the threads are passed through buttons on the surface and tied to prevent the thread from cutting into the skin.

s., catgut. Material used in suturing, made from a portion of the small intestine of sheep. It can be sterilized. Eventually it is absorbed by body fluids.

s., coaptation. Superficial s. for cutaneous wounds.

s., cobbler's. A s. in which the thread has a needle at each end.

s., continuous. The closure of a wound by means of one continuous thread, usually by transfixing first one lip and then the other alternately from within outward.

s., coronal. The junction of the frontal and parietal bones.

s.'s, cranial. Those S.'s between the bones of the skull.

s., dentate. An articulation of long and toothlike processes.

s., ethmoidofrontal. S. between the ethmoid and frontal bones.

s., ethmoidolacrimal. S. between the ethmoid and lacrimal bones.

s., ethmosphenoid. S. between the ethmoid and sphenoid bones.

s., false. Any form of s. in which one surface is smooth.

s., figure-of-eight. S. which has shape of the figure eight.

s., frontal. An occasional s. in the frontal bone from the sagittal s. to root of nose.

s., frontolacrimal. S. between the frontal and lacrimal bones.

s., frontomalar. S. between the frontal and malar bones.

s., frontomaxillary. S. between the frontal bone and superior maxilla.

s., frontonasal. The one between the frontal bone and the alae of the sphenoid bone.

s., frontoparietal. S., coronal, q.v.

s., frontotemporal. S. between the frontal and temporal bones.

s., glover's. A continuous s. in which the needle is passed through the loop of the preceding stitch.

s., harmonic. S. in which there is simple apposition of bone.

s., horsehair. S. adapted for light, superficial sutures, alternated with heavier ones and for exposed places like the face, where scar tissue is to be avoided.

s., implanted. A s. formed by placing pins opposite each other on the two sides of a wound, and approximating the lips by winding thread or other similar material about the pins.

s., intermaxillary. S. between the superior maxillae.

s., internasal. S. between the nasal bones.

s., interparietal. S. sagittal, q.v.

s., interrupted. A s. formed by single stitches inserted separately, the needle usually being passed through one lip from without inward, and through the other from within outward.

s., lambdoid. S. between the parietal bones and the two superior borders of the occipital bone.

s., longitudinal. S. sagittal, q.v.

s., mattress. A continuous s. in which a stitch is taken with a needle, the thread tied, and then needle inserted upon the same side as that from which it emerged, and passed in opposite direction through both lips of the wound, the direction of the needle being reversed at each stitch.

s., maxillolacrimal. S. between the maxilla and lacrimal bone.

s., mediofrontal. S., frontal, q.v.

s., metopic. S., frontal, q.v.

s., nasomaxillary. S. between the nasal bone and superior maxilla.

s., nonabsorbable. Silk, silkworm gut, horsehair, and wire; materials which are not absorbed by the body.

s., occipital. S., lambdoid, q.v.

s., occipitomastoid. S. between the occipital bone and mastoid portion of temporal bone.

s., occipitoparietal. S., lambdoid, q.v.

s., palatine. S. between the palatine bones.

s., palatine transverse. S. between the palatine processes and superior maxilla.

s., parietal. S., sagittal, q.v.

s., parietomastoid. S. between parietal bone and mastoid portion of the temporal bone.

s., petrooccipital. S. between the petrous portion of the temporal bone and occipital bone.

s., petrosphenoidal. S. between petrous portion of the temporal bone and ala magna of sphenoid bone.

s., purse-string. S. going in and out around a circular opening, closing when the two are drawn taut.

s., quilled, s., quill. An interrupted s. in which a double thread is passed deep into the tissues below the bottom of the wound, needle being so withdrawn as to leave a loop hanging from one lip and the two free ends of the thread from the other. A quill, or more commonly a piece of bougie, is passed through the loops, which are tightened upon it, and the free ends of each separate thread are tied together over a second quill. Purpose of quill s. is prevention of tearing when tension becomes greater.

s., relaxation. A s. that may be loosened to relieve excessive tension.

s., relief. A row of supplementary S.'s including the tissues to the extent of 1 or 1 1/2 in. on each side of a fistula or a deep wound, for the purpose of lessening the strain on the coaptation S. 's.

s., right-angled. A s. used in sewing intestine. The needle is passed in the same direction as the long axis of the incision and the process repeated on the opposite side of the incision, the suture being continuous.

s., sagittal. S. between the two parietal bones.

s., serrated. An articulation by s. in which there is an interlocking of bones by small, fine, and delicate projections and indentations.

s., shotted. A s. in which both ends of a wire or silkworm gut are passed through a perforated shot that is then compressed tightly over them.

s., silk. Type of s. which does not produce suppuration if sterilized. Twisted, braided, and floss.

s., silkworm gut. Type of s. which causes little friction, is pliable, does not curl or twist, and is less liable to produce irritation.

s., sphenoparietal. S. between the parietal bone and ala magna of the sphenoid bone.

s., sphenosquamous. Articulation of the great wing of the sphenoid with squamous portion of the temporal bone.

s., sphenotemporal. S. between the sphenoid and temporal bones.

s., squamoparietal, s., squamosal. S. between the parietal and squamous portion of the temporal bone.

s., squamosphenoidal. S. between the squamous portion of the temporal bone and great wing of sphenoid.

s., subcuticular. A buried continuous s. in which the needle is passed horizontally under the epidermis into the cutis vera, emerging at the edge of the wound but beneath the skin, then in a similar manner passed through cutis vera of opposite side of the wound, and so on until the other angle of the wound is reached.

s., temporooccipital. S., occipitomastoid, q.v.

s., temporoparietal. S. between the temporal and parietal bones.

s., twisted. A s. in which pins are passed through the opposite lips of a wound, at right angles to direction of wound, and material is wound about the pins, crossing them first at one end and then at the other in a figure-of-eight fashion, thus holding the lips of the wound firmly together.

s., uninterrupted. S., continuous, q.v.

s., wire. Type of s. adapted for cases where there is tension, resection, ends of bones, etc. Usually silver wire.

swab (swŏb) [Dutch *swabbe*, mop]. 1. Cotton or gauze on end of slender stick used for cleansing cavities, applying remedies, or for obtaining a piece of tissue or secretion for bacteriological examination. 2. To wipe with a swab.

s., test tube. S. for cleansing tubes, etc.

s., urethral. Slender rod for holding cotton, used in examinations with speculum, in treating ulcers, removing secretions, etc.

s., urethral, male. Rod about 7 in. long.

s., uterine. Slender, flattened wire, plain rod, or one with coarse thread on distal end for absorbing or wiping away discharges.

swaddling. Restraining an infant by wrapping with strips of cloth. An historic practice which has been used experimentally in modern times.

swallow (swŏ'lō) [AS. *swelgan*]. To cause or enable the passage of something from the mouth through the throat and esophagus into the stomach by muscular action. SYN: *ingest*.

swallowing (swŏ'lō-ĭng). A complicated act usually initiated voluntarily but always completed reflexively, whereby food is moved from the mouth through the pharynx and esophagus to the stomach. It occurs in three stages as follows:

In the first stage, food is placed on surface of tongue. Tip of tongue is placed against hard palate; then elevation of larynx and backward movement of tongue forces food through isthmus of fauces into pharynx.

In the second stage, the food passes through the pharynx. This involves constriction of the walls of the pharynx, backward bending of the epiglottis, and an upward and forward movement of the larynx and trachea. This may be observed externally with the bobbing of the Adam's apple. Food is kept from entering nasal cavity by elevation of soft palate and from entering larynx by closure of the glottis and backward inclination of epiglottis. During this stage, respiratory movements are inhibited by reflex.

In the third stage, food moves down the esophagus and into the stomach. This movement is accomplished by momentum from the second stage, peristaltic contractions, and gravity. With the body in upright position, liquids pass rapidly and do not require assistance from the esophagus. However, second stage momentum and peristaltic contractions are sufficient to allow liquids to be drunk even when the head is lower than the stomach.

Difficulty in swallowing is called dysphagia, q.v. It may be caused by congenital defects such as cleft palate or esophageal obstruction; neural and psychogenic disturbances; muscular dysfunction; or local conditions such as presence of tumors, abscesses, and inflammation. SYN: *deglutition*.

RS: acataposis; aglutition; aphagia; choking; deglutition; dysphagia.

s., air. Swallowing of air. SYN: *aerophagia*.

s. reflex. S. induced by stimulation of soft palate.

s., tongue. Condition in which the tongue has a tendency to fall backward obstructing openings to larynx and esophagus. The tongue is not actually swallowed and the term is inaccurate; nevertheless it is commonly used. The condition is due to excessive flaccidity of tongue during unconsciousness. This requires forceful elevation of the chin and extension of the head during artificial respiration in order to help provide an airway.

swallow's nest. Cerebral depression between the uvula and the posterior velum. SYN: *nidus hirundinis*.

sweat (swĕt) [AS. *sweatan*]. 1. The secretion of the sudoriparous glands of the skin. SYN: *perspiration; sudor*. SEE: *glands, Moll's.* 2. Condition of perspiring or of being made to perspire freely, as to order a sweat for a patient. 3. To emit moisture through the skin's pores. SYN: *perspire.* 4. To cause to emit moisture through the pores.

Perspiration is a colorless, slightly turbid, salty, aqueous fluid, although that from the sweat glands in the axillae, around the anus, and of the ceruminous glands has an oily consistency. It contains urea, fatty substances, and sodium chloride. This salty, watery fluid is difficult to collect without contamination with sebum, q.v.

FUNCTION: To cool the body by evaporation and to rid it of what waste may be expressed through the pores of the skin. The amount per day is about a liter; this figure is subject to extreme variation according to muscular activity and atmospheric conditions, and in extreme conditions may be as much as 10 to 15 liters in 24 hours.

PHYS: Perspiration is controlled by the sympathetic nervous system through true secretory fibers supplying the sweat glands. SEE: *perspiration*.

s., bloody. S. tinged with blood. SYN: *hematidrosis*.

s. centers. Principal centers controlling perspiration located in the hypothalamus; secondary centers are present in the spinal cord.

s., colliquative. Profuse s. of a clammy nature.

s., colored. S. tinged with a pigment. SYN: *chromidrosis*.

s., fetid. S. with foul odor. SYN: *bromidrosis*.

s. glands. Simple, coiled, tubular glands found on all body surfaces except margin of lips, glans penis, and inner surface of prepuce. The coiled secreting portion lies in the corium or subcutaneous portion of skin; the excretory duct follows a straight or oblique course through the dermis, but becomes spiral in passing through the epidermis to its opening, a sweat pore.

Most s. glands are merocrine; those of the axilla, areola, mammary gland, labia majora, and circumanal region are apocrine. S. glands are most numerous on the palms of the hands and soles of the feet.

s., night. Sweating during the night; may be a symptom of pulmonary tuberculosis.

s., profuse. Excessive perspiration. SYN: *hyperhidrosis.*

s., scanty. Abnormally small amount or lack of s. SYN: *anhidrosis.*

sweat, words pert. to: anaphoresis; antisudoral; antisudorin; bromidrosis; chromidrosis; chylidrosis; diaphoresis; diaphoretic; dyshidria; dysidrosis; ephidrosis; hemathidrosis; hidradenitis; hidrorrhea; hidrosis; hydradenitis; hydradenoma; hyperhidrosis, hyphidrosis; ischidrosis; melanidrosis; perspiration; phosphorhidrosis; sudor; sudorific; sudoriparous; uridrosis.

sweating (swĕt'ĭng) [AS. *swāt*, sweat]. 1. Act of exuding sweat. 2. Emitting sweat. 3. Causing profuse s.

To induce s., paint 2 in. square of skin under each axilla with mixture of equal parts of olive oil and guaiacol solution. Cover with several layers of gauze, then flannel, and hold with adhesive tape. Wrap patient in warm blankets.

s., deficiency of. Seen in profuse diarrhea, polyuria, vomiting, hemorrhage, diabetes insipidus, myxedema, general anasarca, ichthyosis, and in high temperature. SYN: *anhidrosis.*

s., excessive. Seen in rheumatic, malarial and relapsing fever, septic fevers, pneumonia at crisis, pulmonary tuberculosis, hyperthyroidism, migraine, neuralgia. Locally of hands and feet in hysteria, neurasthenia, vagotonia, nervous irritability, exophthalmic goiter, fright, and other emotions. SYN: *hyperhidrosis.*

s. sickness. Miliary fever, q.v.

s., urinous. Often found in uremia. SYN: *uridrosis.*

RS: anhidrosis; bromidrosis; chromidrosis; hidrosis; perspiration; pores; skin; sudor; sudorific; sweat; uridrosis.

Swedish gymnastics. System of active and passive exercise of the various muscles and joints of the body without using apparatus.

TYPES: *Active:* Taken by the patient with the assistance or resistance of the operator. *Duplicated active:* Performed by the patient with the operator's assistance. *General active:* Performed by the patient exclusively. *Passive:* All given to the patient by the operator. *General passive:* May be performed while the patient is dressed.

PRINCIPAL MOVEMENTS: *Bending; depression* and *elevation; flexion* and *extension; pressing* and *shaking.* In pressing, the operator uses the tips of his fingers in vertical motion over the principal nerves. In shaking the arm, the operator grasps the hand and shoulder, keeping the arm in an extended position, and shakes as quickly as possible. In shaking the leg, he grasps the foot with one hand and the thigh as high as possible with the other and shakes quickly. These movements are always passive.

Pulling; raising; rotation. This is a rotary movement by which the different joints are brought into motion within their natural limits. Rotation is to lengthen and shorten the veins so as to produce a sucking of their contents, thus stimulating the circulation and assisting the heart in its action.

Separating and *closing; turning.*

POSITIONS: Movements may be performed in five different positions—kneeling, lying, sitting, standing, or suspending. These are called ground positions and have many subdivisions. There are 47 derivative positions—about 800 movements in all. SYN: *Swedish movements.*

Swedish massage. Massage combined with Swedish gymnastics, q.v.

sweet [AS. *swēte*, sweet]. 1. Pleasing to the taste or smell. SEE: *taste.* 2. Containing or derived from sugar. 3. Free from excess of acid, sulfur, or corrosive salts.

s. oil. Olive oil.

sweetbread. The thymus and pancreas glands, esp. of the calf, used as food.

COMP: Nuclein and purines are high.

Food value of 100 gm. (cooked, braised, calf): Cal. 168; protein 32.6 gm.; fat 3.2 gm.

swelling (swĕl'ĭng) [AS. *swellan*, swollen]. An abnormal enlargement, esp. one appearing on the surface of the body.

TREATMENT: Ice water with salt applied to area reduces swelling rapidly.

RS: detumescence; node; nodule; turgescence; turgid.

s., albuminous. S., cloudy, q.v.

s., Calabar. S. occurring in infestations by the nematode, Loa loa. Temporary and painless, the swellings are thought to be the result of temporary sensitization.

s., cloudy. Degeneration of tissues marked by cloudy appearance, swelling, and appearance of tiny albuminoid granules in the cells as observed with the microscope.

s., fugitive. Temporary swellings such as those occurring in infestations of Loa loa which appear at one place, persist for two or three days, then disappear, possibly to recur at another position.

s., glassy. S. occurring in amyloid degeneration of tissues. SYN: *amyloid degeneration; erythredema; pink disease; polyneuropathy.*

s., white. S. seen in tuberculous arthritis, esp. of the knee.

swimmer's ear. A type of external otitis seen in persons who swim for a considerable period of time or fail to completely dry their ear canals after swimming. If excess cerumen is not present, the condition can be prevented by placing a few drops of 70% alcohol in the ear canals at the end of each swimming session.

swimmer's itch. Appearance of papules resembling insect bites on the skin of persons who swim in water containing the cercariae of certain schistosomes. Usually present only on exposed surfaces of the skin. The papules appear from 4-13 days after exposure. Disease is self-limited, thus treatment is symptomatic. SYN: *cercarial dermatitis.* SEE: *seabather's eruption.*

Swiss chard. A variety of beet having large, succulent leaves which are eaten.

Food value of 100 gm. (cooked): Cal. 18; protein 1.8 gm.; fat 0.2 gm.; carbohydrate 3.3 mg.; vitamin A, 5400 I.U.; vitamin C, 16 mg.

switch (swĭch) [Middle Dutch *swijch,* bough]. In physical therapy, device used to break or open an electrical circuit or to divert current from one conductor to another.

s., foot. A s. whereby the operator, using both his hands in application of surgical high-frequency currents, may use his foot to start or break the current.

s., pole-changing. A s. by which the polarity of a circuit may be reversed.

swoon [AS. *swōgan,* to suffocate]. 1. A fainting spell. 2. To faint.

sycoma (sī-kō'mă) [Gr. *sykōma*]. A large, soft wart. SYN: *condyloma.*

sycophancy (sīk'ō-făn-sī) [Gr. *sykophantēs,* informer]. In psychology, the practice or characteristics of one who is intelligently mature. However, he has not developed a sense of responsibility and is more or less dependent upon others.

sycophant (sīk'ō-fănt). One who seeks to incur favor or advance himself by flattery and praise of persons of influence.

sycosiform (sī-kō'sī-form) [Gr. *sykōsis,* figlike disease, + L. *forma,* shape]. Resembling sycosis.

sycosis (sī-kō'sĭs) [Gr. *sykōsis,* figlike disease]. Chronic inflammation of hair follicles.

ETIOL: Staphylococcus aureus and albus entering through hair follicles. Trauma and disability are predisposing factors.

SYM: Inflammation of hairy areas of the body characterized by an aggregation of papules and pustules, each of which is pierced by a hair. Pustules show no disposition to rupture but dry to yellow-brown crusts. Itching and burning. If disease persists may lead to extreme destruction of hair follicles and permanent alopecia.

PROG: Disease is curable under prolonged treatment; relapses occur.

TREATMENT: Local treatment includes topical use of antibiotics. Organism should be cultured and tested to determine antibiotic of choice.

s. barbae. S. of the beard marked by papules and pustules perforated by hairs and surrounded by infiltrated skin. SYN: *folliculitis barbae.*

s., hypogenic. Tinea barbae, q.v.; barber's itch, usually due to species of Trichophyton.

s. tinea. A form due to infection with ringworm commonly affecting the beard.

s. vulgaris. SYN: *barber's itch; folliculitis barbae.* SEE: *s., barbae; tinea barbae.*

Sydenham's chorea (sĭd'ĕn-hăm). [Thomas Sydenham, English physician, 1624-89]. Simple chorea with irregular involuntary movements of the face and extremities.

syllabic utterance (sĭ-lăb'ĭk) [Gr. *syllabikos*]. A staccato accentuation of syllables, slowly but separately, observed in multiple sclerosis. SYN: *scanning speech.*

syllable stumbling (sĭl'ă-bl) [Gr. *syllabē,* syllable]. Hesitating utterance (dysphasia) with difficulty in pronouncing certain syllables.

syllabus (sĭl'ă-bŭs) [Gr. *syllabos,* table of contents]. Abstract of a lecture or outline of a course of study or of a book.

syllepsiology (sĭl'ĕp-sī-ŏl'ō-jī) [Gr. *syllēpsis,* conception, + *logos,* study]. The study of conception and pregnancy.

syllepsis (sĭl-ĕp'sĭs) [Gr. *syllēpsis,* conception]. Conception, impregnation, or pregnancy.

sylvat'ic plague. Bubonic plague which is enzootic among wild rodents, esp. in western

U.S. The causative organism is transmitted by fleas. SEE: *plague*.

sylvian aqueduct (sĭl'vĭ-ăn). [Jacobus Sylvius, Fr. anatomist, 1478-1555]. A narrow canal from 3rd to 4th ventricle. SYN: *aqueduct of Sylvius*.

sylvian artery. [Francois Sylvius, Fr. anatomist, 1614-1672]. Middle cerebral artery in the fissure of Sylvius.

sylvian fissure. The fissure separating the temporal lobe from the frontal and parietal lobes.

sylvian line. One on exterior of cranium, marking direction of the sylvian fissure.

sym- [Gr. *syn*, together]. Combining form meaning with, along, together with, beside.

symbion, symbiont (sĭm'bĭ-ŏn, -ŏnt) [Gr. *syn*, together, + *bios*, life]. An organism which lives with another in a state of symbiosis. SYN: *commensal*.

symbiosis (sĭm''bĭ-ō'sĭs) [Gr.]. The living together in close association of two organisms of different species. If neither organism is harmed, such is referred to as *commensalism;* if the association is beneficial to both, it is *mutualism;* if one is harmed and the other benefited, it constitutes *parasitism*.

symblepharon (sĭm-blĕf'ă-rŏn) [Gr. *syn*, together, + *blepharon*, eyelid]. Adhesion between conjunctivae of lid and eyeball due to injuries, esp. burns from lime, acids, etc. Also seen in trachoma, pemphigus, and following operations.

SYM: Interference with movement of eyeball, conjunctival irritation.

TREATMENT: Division of cicatricial bands and keeping raw surfaces separated. Mucous membrane grafts.

symbol (sĭm'bŏl) [Gr. *symbolon*, a sign]. 1. An object or sign that represents an idea or quality by association, resemblance, or convention. SEE: *prescription writing* for table; *Table of Symbols* in *Appendix*. 2. In psychology, an object used as an unconscious substitute which is not connected consciously with the libido, but into which the libido is concentrated. 3. A mark or letter representing an atom or an element in chemistry. SEE: *Table of Physical Constants of Elements* in *Appendix*.

　　s., phallic. An object which bears some resemblance to the penis.

symbo'lia. Ability to identify or recognize an object by the sense of touch.

symbolism (sĭm'bŏl-ĭzm) [Gr. *symbolon*, a sign, + *-ismos*, condition]. 1. Unconscious substitutive expression of subconscious thoughts of sexual significance in terms recognized by the objective consciousness. 2. An abnormal condition in which everything

that occurs is interpreted as a symbol of the patient's own thoughts.

symboliza'tion. An unconscious process by which an object or idea comes to represent another object or idea on the basis of similarity or association.

symbolophobia (sĭm''bŏl-ō-fō'bĭ-ă) [Gr. *symbolon*, a sign, + *phobos*, fear]. Hesitancy in expressing one's self in words or action for fear that it may be interpreted as possessing a symbolic meaning.

Syme's operation (sīm). [James Syme, Scottish surgeon, 1799-1870]. 1. Amputation of the foot at the ankle joint with removal of the malleoli. 2. Excision of the tongue. 3. External urethrotomy.

symmelia (sĭm-mē'lĭ-ă) [Gr. *syn*, together, + *melos*, limb]. Fusion of limbs.

symmetric, symmetrical (sĭm-ĕt'rĭk, -rĭkl) [Gr. *symmetrikos*, symmetry]. 1. Exhibiting correspondence in size and shape of parts. 2. Denoting an atomic arrangement in a molecule at equal relative intervals.

　　s. gangrene. Gangrene affecting corresponding parts simultaneously and similarly. SYN: *Raynaud's disease*, q.v.

symmetromania (sĭm''ĕ-trō-mā'nĭ-ă) [Gr. *symmetria*, symmetry, + *mania*, madness]. An abnormal impulse to make symmetrical motions, i.e., with both arms instead of one.

symmetry (sĭm'ĕt-rĭ). Correspondence in shape, size, and relative position of parts on opposite sides of a body.

　　s., bilateral. S. of an organism whose right and left halves are mirror images of each other or in which a median longitudinal section divides the organism into equivalent right and left halves.

　　s., radial. S. of an organism whose parts radiate from a central axis.

sympathectomy (sĭm''pă-thĕk'tō-mĭ) [Gr. *sympathētikos*, sympathy, + *ektomē*, excision]. Excision of a portion of the sympathetic division of the autonomic nervous system. It may include a nerve, plexus, ganglion, or a series of ganglia of the sympathetic trunk.

　　s., chemical. The use of chemicals to destroy or temporarily inactivate part of the sympathetic nerve.

　　s., periarterial. Removal of sheath of an artery in which sympathetic nerve fibers are located; used in trophic disturbances.

sympatheoneuritis (sĭm-păth''ē-ō-nū-rī'tĭs) [Gr. *sympathētikos*, sympathy, + *neuron*, nerve, + *-itis*, inflammation]. Inflammation of the sympathetic nerve.

sympathetic (sĭm''pă-thĕt'ĭk). 1. Pert. to sympathetic nervous system, q.v. 2. Caused by or pert. to sympathy.

s. irritation. Irritation of one structure caused by irritation of another related structure.

s. nervous system. A division of the autonomic nervous system.

RS: nervous system; parasympathetic nervous system.

s. ophthalmia. Inflammation of the uveal tract in one eye due to similar inflammation in the other eye.

s. plexuses. Plexuses formed at intervals by the s. nerves and ganglia.

sympatheticalgia (sĭm″pă-thĕt′ĭ-kăl′jĭ-ă) [Gr. *sympathētikos,* sympathy, + *algos,* pain]. Pain in the cervical sympathetic ganglion.

sympatheticless (sĭm″pă-thĕt′ĭk-lĕs) [″+ AS. *laēs,* without]. Indicates absence of the abdominal sympathetic chain.

sympatheticoparalytic (sĭm″pă-thĕt′ĭ-kō-păr″ă-lĭt′ĭk) [″+ *paralysis,* a loosening at the sides]. Resulting from paralysis of the sympathetic nervous system.

sympatheticopathy (sĭm″pă-thĕt′ĭ-kŏp′ă-thĭ) [Gr. *sympathetikos,* sympathy, + *pathos,* disease]. Any condition resulting from disorder of the sympathetic nervous system.

sympatheticotonia (sĭm″pă-thĕt′ĭ-kō-tō′nĭ-ă) [″+ *tonos,* tension]. Condition characterized by excessive tone of the sympathetic nervous system with unusually high blood pressure and tendency to vascular spasm. SYN: *sympathicotonia.*

sympatheticotonic (sĭm″pă-thĕt′ĭ-kō-tŏn′ĭk). Marked by increased arterial tone or vasoconstriction due to overaction of the sympathetic nervous system.

sympathicectomy (sĭm-păth′ĭ-sĕk′tō-mĭ) [Gr. *sympathetikos,* sympathy, + *ektome,* excision]. Excision of part of the sympathetic nervous pathways. SYN: *sympathectomy.*

sympathicoblast (sĭm-păth′ĭ-kō-blăst) [″+ *blastos,* a germ]. A primitive sympathetic nerve cell. SEE: *sympathoblast.*

sympathicoblastoma (sĭm-păth′ĭ-kō-blăs-tō′mă) [″+ ″+ *-ōma,* tumor]. A tumor made up of sympathicoblasts.

sympathicolytic (sĭm-păth′ĭ-kō-lĭt′ĭk) [″+ *lytikos,* dissolving]. Interfering with, opposing, inhibiting, or destroying impulses from the sympathetic nervous system. SYN: *sympatholytic.*

sympathicomimetic (sĭm-păth′ĭ-kō-mĭm-ĕt′ĭk) [Gr. *sympathētikos,* sympathy, + *mimētikos,* imitating]. Producing effects resembling those resulting from stimulation of the sympathetic nervous system, such as effects following the injection of epinephrine.

sympathiconeuritis (sĭm-păth′ĭ-kō-nū-rī′tĭs) [″+ *neuron,* nerve, + *-itis,* inflammation]. Inflammation of the sympathetic nerves.

sympathicotonia (sĭm-păth′ĭ-kō-tō′nĭ-ă) [″+ *tonos,* tension]. Increased tonus of the sympathetic system with marked tendency to vascular spasm and heightened blood pressure. Opposed to vagotonia, q.v.

sympathicotripsy (sĭm-păth′ĭ-kō-trĭp′sĭ) [Gr. *sympathētikos,* sympathy, + *tripsis,* a crushing]. Crushing of the superior cervical ganglion in treatment of mental diseases. SYN: *sympatheticotripsy.*

sympathicotropic (sĭm-păth′ĭ-kō-trŏp′ĭk) [″+ *tropos,* a turning]. Having a special affinity for the sympathetic nerve.

sympathicus (sĭm-păth′ĭ-kŭs). The sympathetic nervous system. SYN: *systema nervorum sympathicum.*

sympathism (sĭm′pă-thĭzm) [Gr. *sympathētikos,* sympathy, + *-ismos,* condition]. Condition of susceptibility to suggest. SYN: *suggestibility.*

sympathoblast (sĭm-păth′ō-blăst) [″+ *blastos,* germ]. A primitive cell from which arises a sympathetic ganglion cell.

sympathoblastoma (sĭm″păth-ō-blăs-tō′mă) [″+ ″+ *-ōma,* tumor]. A malignant tumor made up of sympathetic nerve cells.

sympathoglioblastoma (sĭm″păth-ō-glī″ō-blăs-tō′mă) [Gr. *sympathētikos,* sympathy, + *glia,* glue, + *blastos,* germ, + *-ōma,* tumor]. A tumor made up primarily of sympathoblasts with scattered neuroblasts and spongioblasts.

sympathogonia (sĭm″păth-ō-gō′nĭ-ă) [″+ *gonē,* seed]. Primitive cells from which sympathetic cells are derived.

sympathogonioma (sĭm″pă-thō-gō″nĭ-ō′mă) [″+ *-ōma,* tumor]. A tumor containing sympathogonia.

sympatho′ma [Gr. *sympathētikos,* sympathy, + *-ōma,* tumor]. A tumor composed of tissue similar to that of the sympathetic nervous system.

sympathomimetic (sĭm″pă-thō-mĭm-ĕt′ĭk) [″+ *mimētikos,* imitating]. SYN: *sympathicomimetic,* q.v.

sympathy (sĭm′pă-thĭ) [Gr. *sympatheia*]. 1. Relationship between two organs or parts through which one unaffected part is affected or becomes disordered from disease in the other part without actual transmission of morbific cause. 2. An affective reaction to, and like that of, another person. It may be *imitative s.* in which the reaction is like that of another person as perceived or thought (i.e., weeping because another person is weeping), or *reflective s.* in which the reaction is like that of another person as his situation is understood. 3. Feeling as another feels. SEE: *empathy.*

sympexion (sĭm-pĕks'ĭ-ŏn) [Gr. *sympēxis,* concretion]. A concretion in certain sites such as the prostate or seminal vesicles.

sympexis (sĭm-pĕks'ĭs). Arrangement of red blood cells due to the effect of surface tension.

symphalangism (sĭm-făl'ăn-jĭzm) [Gr. *syn,* together, + *phalanx,* phalanx]. 1. Ankylosis of joints of the fingers or toes. 2. Web-fingered or web-toed condition.

symphyseal (sĭm-fĭz'ē-ăl) [Gr. *symphysis,* growing together]. Pert. to symphysis.

symphyseotomy (sĭm-fĭz"ē-ŏt'ō-mĭ) ["+ *tomē,* incision]. Section of symphysis pubis to enlarge the pelvic diameters during delivery.

symphysiectomy (sĭm-fĭz"ĭ-ĕk'tō-mĭ) ["+ *ektomē,* excision]. Resection of the symphysis pubis to facilitate delivery.

symphysion (sĭm-fĭz'ĭ-ŏn) [Gr. *symphysis,* growing together]. Most anterior point of the alveolar process of the lower jaw.

symphysiotomy (sĭm-fĭz"ĭ-ŏt'ō-mĭ) ["+ *tomē,* a cutting]. Section of the symphysis pubis to facilitate childbirth by enlarging the pelvic outlet.

symphysis (sĭm'fĭ-sĭs) [Gr., growing together]. (pl. *sym'physes*) 1. A line of fusion between two bones which are separate in early development, as s. of mandible. 2. [NA] A form of synchrondrosis in which the bones are separated by a disk of fibrocartilage, as in joints between bodies of vertebrae or between pubic bones. SEE: *intervertebral disk.*

   s. cartilaginosum. A synchondrosis.

   s. of jaw. An anterior, median, vertical ridge upon outer surface of lower jaw representing line of union of its halves.

   s. ligamentosa. Syndesmosis, q.v.

   s. mandibulae. S. menti, q.v.

   s. menti. The s. of the chin or the ridge marking line of union of the two halves of the mandible. SYN: *symphisis mandibulae.*

   s. pubis. The junction of the pubic bones on midline in front; bony eminence under the pubic hair. SEE: *disk, interpubic.*

sympodia (sĭm-pō'dĭ-ă) [Gr. *syn,* together, + *pous, pod-,* foot]. Condition in which lower extremities are united.

symptom (sĭm'tŭm, sĭmp-) [Gr. *symptōma,* occurrence]. Any perceptible change in the body or its functions that indicates disease or the kind or phases of disease.

They may be classified as objective, subjective, cardinal, and sometimes as constitutional. Another classification considers all symptoms as being subjective, objective indications being called signs, q.v. Some of the symptoms affecting different parts follow.

ABDOMEN: May be distended, rigid, flat, flabby, adipose, tympanitic, shiny, enlarged, or bulging in certain areas, certain discolorations, stripings, or markings. Muscles may be tensed and little affected by pressure. May be cold areas. Various sounds may be heard such as splashings, roarings, and rumblings (borborygmus, also known as intestinal flatus).

Closely associated with abdominal symptoms is pain. Locate exact area affected and note nature, time of duration, time when it arises, and any causes that might be responsible.

Emesis is another condition associated with symptoms pert. to the abdominal region. Emesis may be watery, clear, or contain mucus or undigested food; may be stertorous, bilious, frothy, profuse, purulent, colored from food or medication, and contain blood (hematemesis). If blood is present in large quantity and has been acted on by gastric juices it may resemble coffee grounds. Emesis may be sour, have odor of feces or garlic, may be ammoniacal, or have odor characteristic of some food or drug.

The patient may complain of abdominal distention, gas, and pain caused by gas, crowding in the region of the heart, and interference with respiration. Heartburn may be present, or gastritis and regurgitation. Pain may be felt when food enters the stomach, or relieved by eating or shortly after eating, or by changing body position. Distention after eating should be noted, or desire to eructate or to expel flatus from the stomach. Colicky pains in the abdomen may be accompanied by pain in the shoulder. Pain at pit of stomach and in lower right quadrant may be indicative of appendicitis. When over lower right ribs or little below, the gallbladder may be suspected. SEE: *abdomen; emesis.*

BACK: The dorsal side of the body may reveal edema, deformities, irregularities of the spine, discolorations, eruptions, impaired motion, decubitus, or any condition affecting the skin. SEE: *backache.*

BREATH: May have a fecal odor, a sweet (acetone) odor, one of wet hay, an odor of fish, ammonia, urine, blood, or pus. Respiration may be abdominal or thoracic, and show dyspnea, orthopnea, apnea, or it may be normal (eupnea). SEE: *apnea; breath; dyspnea; orthopnea.*

CHEST: The chest may show abnormalities and deformities. Coughing may be whooping, hacking, crowing, hoarse, dry, rasping, or hysterical. There may or may not be expectoration. A cough may be spasmodic or occur on awakening; during deep sleep it may awaken patient; it may occur when swallowing food, when in a horizontal position, or when subjected to change of temperatures. If hiccupping is present, note when it occurs. Sputum may be mucoid, yellowish, thick, tenacious, ropy, gelatinous, dark green, offensive in odor, copious, streaked with bright (brick red) or dark blood (hemoptysis), or it may resemble cheesy lumps. It may be clear and watery, scanty, or profuse.

Frequency of coughing and clearing throat should be noted. Patient's respirations may be shallow; dyspnea may be present, or inability to expand the lungs, complaints of irritation, sticking pains, or catchy pains on inspiration. There may be an accumulation of phlegm in the air passages or a tickling in throat. Patient may not be able to take deep inspirations or may be constantly yawning. There may be migrating, knifelike pains in region of heart or throughout chest. Heart-consciousness may be present, or a fluttering feeling about the heart, or cardiac pain. Queer sensations, the loud beating of the heart, and heaviness in cardiac region are other symptoms. SEE: *apnea; chest; dyspnea; cough; hiccough; sputum.*

DEFECATION: Symptoms to observe are the frequency of defecation; the presence of constipation; hemorrhoids; the nature of the feces, such as formation, i.e., ribbon-shaped, soft, semiformed, hard or scybala, cylindrical, and whether watery, liquid, or semiliquid; the color, whether dark brown, light brown, clay-colored, green, yellowish, black, bloody; and whether lienteric, serous, mucous, purulent, tarry, or containing membranous shreds, calculi, or foreign substances. The amount should be noted, as small, medium, large, or copious. The odor may be characteristic of various conditions: sour, putrid, offensive, or fetid. The nature of the evacuation should be noted, as natural, difficult, involuntary, or painful. SEE: *feces; stool.*

DENTITION: Teeth may be irregular, missing, misshapen, or affected by caries. There may be a partial or complete denture. Dental hygiene may be good or poor. There may be a loosening of teeth, a film over them, or they may show the presence of sordes.

EARS: Tinnitus aurium, q.v., i.e., ringing in the ears, occurs in certain diseases. Pain in or about ears, or swelling under either or both should be noted. Impacted cerumen, foreign bodies, or insects may be present in auditory canals. SEE: *ear.*

EYES: May be staring, have an excited look, or expressionless. Nystagmus, strabismus, and coma vigil may be indicated. Pupils may be contracted or dilated, or one pupil affected. Patient may keep eyes closed constantly, or keep one open and the other closed. Eyes may be sunken or protruding. Lacrimation may be present. Eyelids may be edematous, and eyeball soft to the touch. Accommodation may be faulty. Nictating, squinting, or tremor of the eyelids should always be recorded. Blurring of vision usually is associated with other symptoms. Patient may complain of specks dancing before the eyes (muscae volitantes). These may be colorless or colored. SEE: *eye.*

GAIT: May be faltering, scissors, festinating, unsteady, staggering, weakened, swaying, or movements may be stiff, awkward, or unusual. May be total disability or immobility. SEE: *gait.*

GENERAL APPEARANCE: The face may show an expression of anxiety, have a pinched look or a drawn expression. Patient may have air of apathy, a distorted or a blank look, an emotional expression, a risus sardonicus, or sudden lack of all expression (masklike).

GENERAL SYMPTOMS: Burning sensations may be complained of in various parts of the body, as in the head, throat, arms, chest, or abdomen. They may or may not be accompanied by tenderness. The complaint may be of feeling too hot or too cold without apparent cause, or of having a general feeling of distress.

Anorexia and nausea upon taking food, at the thought of food, or with no reference to food are significant and should be noted; also when nausea obtains: on awakening, when taking fluids, after eating, when changing a position, when taking medication, or in the presence of odors. There always should be an explanation for nausea, either somatic or psychiatric.

Fear of death (angor animi), anxiety, agitation, or panic may be present.

LIMBS: The symptoms pert. to the skin, of course, apply to skin of the limbs. Note if there are deformities, abnormalities, impaired motion, discolorations, sensitivity, varicosities.

LIPS: May be pale, dry, cyanotic, edematous, drawn, deformed, out of proportion, motionless and expressionless, flushed, fissured, or show other lesions or growths. SEE: *lip.*

MOUTH AND GUMS: May be pale or ulcerated, highly inflamed and red, infected, discolored, edematous, or abnormally shaped. Pyorrhea or edema may be present. Patient may complain of certain tastes such as bitter, sweet, salty, sour, fishy, or flat tastes, or an absence of taste. Medication may have much to do with temporary disorders of taste. SEE: *gum; mouth.*

NOSE: May appear deformed, discolored, edematous, or enlarged. Nostrils may discharge or show obstruction. May be inability to breathe through one or both nostrils. Patient may complain of odors not usually manifested as objective symptoms, or for which there is no known cause. SEE: *nose.*

PAIN: The exact area affected must be ascertained, and the wording of the patient's complaint of pain must be charted or reported. Note if pain is in nature of a cramp or spasm, if it is dull, superficial, deep, remittent, shifting, shooting, lancinating, gnawing, fixed, sharp, inflammatory; or if there is an absence of pain, esp. in conditions in which pain usually occurs. Note whether pain is relieved or increased by pressure, heat, cold, change of body position or environment, or other causes. When is pain experienced, how often does the same type of pain recur, and does it awaken the patient from sleep, esp. at night? Observe the facial expression during an attack of pain and listen carefully to the patient's description.

The patient may locate a headache around the eyes and nose, in the center of the forehead, above the nose, in one or both temples accompanied by throbbing, at the top of the head, or at the base of the brain. It may be felt as a tight, bandlike sensation around the head above the eyes. It may be in the center of the forehead above the eyebrow line, in the upper region of the center forehead, all over the top of the head, over one or both ears, or back of both ears. Pain may be sharp, dull, or shifting. It may accompany head noises, or a roaring in the head may be experienced without pain. Vertigo may be present or a sensation of fainting. Pulsations may be felt in the occiput or in the temporal region. A patient may be very sensitive to light and sound, and headaches may be accompanied by nausea, vomiting, the sensation of flashing lights, and chills. Tenderness or soreness may be associated with rigidity. SEE: *headache; pain.*

POSITIONS AND POSTURES: An inability to lie down; to arise; or to lie on one side,

on the back, or in any special position reveals much to the doctor. Whether lying on the affected or unaffected side is also important to observe. The left leg may be flexed or the right one, or both, or there may be an inclination to lie with the arms above the head. SEE: *posture.*

SKIN: May appear pale, flushed all over or in spots; may be cyanotic, jaundiced, shiny, erupted, burned, blistered, sunburned, wrinkled, lacerated, nodular, bruised; or exhibit dermographia, lesions, growth, or deformities; or be puffy and edematous, ashy, gray, wet with perspiration, or discolored. SEE: *skin.*

THROAT: May show abnormalities, discoloration, inflammation, diseased tonsils and presence of adenoids. Dysphagia and hoarseness or aphonia and other conditions affecting the voice may be present. A lump in the throat (globus hystericus), or a dry, scratchy irritation or fullness or pulsations may be present.

TONGUE: May be coated, clean, smooth, atrophic, shiny, dry on top and moist on the sides or dry all over; may look like raw beef or appear furry, glossy, tremulous, or sharp pointed. It may be edematous or abnormal in size; there may be fissures; the papillae may have disappeared; there may be a strawberry-tongue, or it may have various colors. SEE: *tongue.*

URINE: It may be blue, milky, pale, lemon, smoky, brick-colored, clear, amber, straw-colored, orange, or almost any other color. Hematuria may be present. Polyuria or oliguria may be indicated, or there may be frequent urination of small amounts. The odors may be ammoniacal, aromatic, stercorous, or like that of new-mown hay, ripe apples, or violets. There may be retention, suppression, or dribbling, and urination may be painful. SEE: *urine.*

s., accessory. A minor symptom, or one not pathognomonic.

s., accidental. S. occurring incidentally during course of a disease, but having no relationship to the disease.

s., assident. S., accessory, q.v.

s.'s, cardinal. Those pert. to pulse, respiration, and temperature.

s. complex. The entire group of symptoms presenting a clear picture of a disease. SYN: *syndrome,* q.v.

s., concomitant. S. occurring along with the essential symptoms of a disease.

s., constitutional, s., general. S. caused by or indicating disease of the whole body.

s., delayed. S. appearing sometime after precipitating cause.

s., direct. S. resulting from direct effects of disease.

s., dissociation. Anesthesia to heat, cold, and pain without loss of tactile sensibility. Seen in syringomyelia.

s., equivocal. 1. S. that may occur in several diseases, hence of doubtful significance. 2. S. of such degree as to cause doubt of its presence.

s., focal. S. at a specific location.

s., general. S., constitutional, q.v.

s., indirect. S. occurring secondarily as a result of a disease.

s., labyrinthine. A group of symptoms, such as tinnitus, vertigo, or nausea, indicating a disease or lesion of the inner ear.

s., local. S. indicating specifically the seat of the disease or morbid process.

s., negative pathognomonic. S. which never occurs in a certain disease or condition; hence its occurrence rules out the existence of that disease.

s., objective. S. apparent to the observer. SYN: *sign.*

s., passive. S., static, q.v.

s., pathognomonic. S. which unmistakably points out presence of a particular disease.

s.'s, prodromal. S.'s which indicate an approaching disease. SYN: *prodrome,* q.v.

s., rational. S. apparent only to patient. SYN: *subjective s.*

s., signal. A s. which is premonitory of an impending condition such as the aura which precedes an attack of epilepsy or migraine.

s. static. S. pert. to the condition of a single organ or structure without reference to remainder of body.

s., subjective. S. apparent only to the patient.

s., sympathetic. A s. for which there is no specific inciting cause and usually occurring at a point more or less remote from the point of disturbance.

s.'s, withdrawal. Those s.'s following sudden withdrawal of a stimulant from an addict. Generally excitement and collapse.

symptomatic (sĭmp″tō-măt′ĭk) [Gr. *symptōmatikos*]. Of the nature of or concerning a symptom.

symptomatology (sĭmp″tō-mă-tŏl′ō-jĭ) [Gr. *symptōma,* symptom, + *logos,* a study]. 1. Science of symptoms and indications. SYN: *semeiology.* 2. All of the symptoms of a given disease as a whole.

symptomatolytic (sĭmp″tō-măt″ō-lĭt′ĭk) [″+ *lysis,* destruction]. Causing the removal of symptoms.

symptom complex. A group of symptoms which occur together and thus characterize a specific disease. SYN: *syndrome.*

symptomolytic (sĭmp″tō-mō-lĭt′ĭk) [Gr. *symptōma,* symptom, + *lysis,* destruction]. Pert. to the removal of symptoms. SYN: *symptomatolytic.*

symptosis (sĭmp-tō′sĭs) [Gr. *syn,* together, + *ptōsis,* fall]. Emaciation; wasting away of the body or an organ.

syn- [Gr., together]. Prefix meaning joined, together. SEE: words beginning with *con-.*

syn″acto′sis [Gr. *syn,* together, + L. *actio,* function, + Gr. *-ōsis,* condition]. Malformation resulting from the abnormal fusion of parts.

synalgia (sĭn-ăl′jĭ-ă) [″+ *algos,* pain]. Referred or reflex pain felt in a part distant from the site of its origin.

synal′gic. Pert. to or characterized by referred pain.

synanastomosis (sĭn″ăn-ăs″tō-mō′sĭs) [Gr. *syn,* together, + *anastomōsis,* a connecting mouth]. The connection of several vessels.

synanche (sĭn-ăn′kē) [″+ anchein, to choke]. Severe throat infection with impending airway obstruction. SYN: *cynanche.*

synanthema (sĭn″ăn-thē′mă) [″+ *anthein,* to bloom]. Exanthem made up of several different forms of eruption.

synapse (sĭn′ăps) [Gr. *synapsis,* point of contact]. The point of junction between two neurons in a neural pathway, where the termination of the axon of one neuron comes into close proximity with the cell body or dendrites of another. At this point, where the relationship of the two neurons is one of contact only, the impulse traveling in the first neuron initiates an impulse in the second neuron. Synapses are polarized, i.e., the impulses pass in one direction only. They are susceptible to fatigue, offer a resistance to the passage of impulses, and are markedly susceptible to the effects of oxygen deficiency, anesthetics, and other agents, including therapeutic drugs and toxic chemicals.

synapsis (sĭn-ăp′sĭs) [Gr., point of contact]. 1. Synapse, q.v. 2. The process of first maturation division in gametogenesis in which there is conjugation of pairs of homologous chromosomes forming double or bivalent chromosomes. In the resulting miotic division, the chromosome number is reduced from the diploid to the haploid number. It is at this stage that crossing over occurs.

RS: crossing over; miosis; oogenesis; spermatogenesis.

synap'tic. Pert. to a synapse or synapsis.

s. field. A field in cerebral cortex, cerebellar cortex, and retina where large numbers of contacts between neurons can take place.

synaptolemma (sĭn-ăp''tō-lĕm'ă). The membrane at a synapse separating two neurons.

synarthrodia (sĭn''ăr-thrō'dĭ-ă) [Gr. *syn,* together, + *arthron,* joint, + *eidos,* form]. Type of immovable cartilaginous joint without a joint cavity in which bones are separated by only a connective tissue membrane; a fixed articulation. SYN: *synarthrosis.* SEE: *joint.*

synarthro'dial. Pert. to an immovable articulation between bones.

synarthrophysis (sĭn''ăr-thrō-fī'sĭs) [Gr. *syn,* together, + *arthron,* joint, + *physis,* growth]. Progressive ankylosis of joints.

synarthro'sis ["+ *arthrōsis,* joint]. (pl. *synarthroses*) A type of joint in which the skeletal elements are united by a continuous intervening substance (cartilage, fibrous tissue, or bone). Movement is absent or limited and a joint cavity is lacking. It includes the synchondrosis, suture, and syndesmosis types of joints.

syncanthus (sĭn-kăn'thŭs) [Gr. *syn,* together, + *kanthos,* angle]. Adhesion of eyeball to the structures of the orbit.

synchilia (sĭn-kī'lĭ-ă) ["+ *cheilos,* lip]. Congenital adhesions of the lips or atresia of the mouth.

synchiria (sĭn-kī'rī-ă) ["+ *cheir,* hand]. Disorder of sensibility in which stimulus applied to one side of the body is felt on both sides. SYN: *allochiria.*

RS: achiria; dyschiria.

synchondroseotomy (sĭn''kŏn-drō''sē-ŏt'ō-mĭ) [Gr. *syn,* together, + *chondros,* cartilage, + *tomē,* a cutting]. An operation of cutting through the sacroiliac ligaments and closing the arch of the pubes in congenital absence of the anterior wall of the bladder (exstrophy).

synchondrosis (sĭn''kŏn-drō'sĭs) ["+ "+ *-ōsis,* condition]. An immovable joint having surfaces between the bones connected by cartilages. This may be temporary, in which case the cartilage eventually becomes ossified, or permanent.

synchondrotomy (sĭn-kŏn-drŏt'ō-mĭ) ["+ "+ *tomē,* a cutting]. 1. Division of articulating cartilage. 2. Section of the symphysis pubis to facilitate childbirth. SEE: *symphyseotomy.*

synchronism (sĭn'krō-nĭzm) [Gr. *syn,* together, + *chronos,* time, + *-ismos,* condition]. Simultaneous occurrence of acts or events.

synchronous (sĭn'krō-nŭs). Occurring simultaneously.

synchysis (sĭn'kĭs-ĭs) [Gr., confound]. Fluid state of vitreous of the eye.

s. scintillans. Bright flashes of light resulting from presence of crystals of cholesterol or fat substances in vitreous body.

syncinesis (sĭn''sĭn-ē'sĭs) [Gr. *syn,* together, + *kinēsis,* motion]. An involuntary movement produced in association with a voluntary one. SYN: *synkinesis,* q.v.

s., imitative. Involuntary movement occurring on sound side when movement is attempted on paralyzed side.

s., spasmodic. S. occurring on hemiplegic side when muscles of opposed side are voluntarily moved.

synciput (sĭn'sĭ-pŭt). Anterior upper half of the cranium. SYN: *sinciput.*

synclitism (sĭn'klĭt-ĭzm) [Gr. *synklinein,* to lean together]. Parallelism between the planes of the fetal head and those of the maternal pelvis.

synclonus (sĭn'klō-nŭs) [Gr. *syn,* together, + *klonos,* turmoil]. 1. Clonic contraction of several muscles together. 2. A disease marked by muscular spasms.

s. ballismus. Paralysis agitans, q.v.

s. tremens. Generalized tremor.

syncopal (sĭn'kō-păl) [Gr. *synkopē,* fainting]. Rel. to or marked by syncope.

syncope (sĭn'kŭ-pē) [Gr. *synkopē,* fainting]. A transient loss of consciousness due to inadequate blood flow to the brain. SYN: *fainting; swoon.*

ETIOL: Syncope or fainting may be due to deficient blood flow resulting from peripheral circulatory failure, cerebral vascular accident (stroke), cardiac arrhythmia or transient cardiac standstill in Stokes-Adams syndrome, q.v., altered quality of the blood as in hyperventilation or hypoglycemia. Predisposing factors include fatigue, prolonged standing, nausea, pain, emotional disturbances, anemia, dehydration, poor ventilation, and many others.

TREATMENT: Stimulate the heart action, fresh air, treat underlying cause. If patient is seated, depress head between knees, compressing abdominal viscera. Remove tight clothing. Apply sudden dash of cold water, or cold towel which should be removed immediately. Aromatic spirits of ammonia inhalations for only a moment or two. Test to see it is not too strong. When recovered give strong coffee or tea. Keep lying down. Ten to 20 drops of ammonia by mouth in half a glass of water. Call a physician if recovery is not prompt. SEE: *unconsciousness.*

s. anginosa. Syncope occurring with anginal pain.

s., cardiac. Syncope of cardiac origin as in Stokes-Adams syndrome, aortic stenosis, tachycardia, bradycardia, myocardial infarction, etc.

s., carotid sinus. S. resulting from pressure on, or hypersensitivity of, carotid sinus. May result from turning head to one side or from too tight a collar.

s. cough. S. which occurs during a coughing spell. SYN: *tussive s.*

s., hysterical. S. resulting from purely psychological mechanisms.

s., laryngeal. Brief unconsciousness following coughing and tickling in the throat. SYN: *laryngeal vertigo.*

s., local. Numbness of a part with sudden blanching, as of the fingers; a symptom of Raynaud's disease or of local asphyxia.

s., vasovagal. S. resulting from fall in blood pressure due to failure of peripheral resistance with concomitant, reduced venous return, or due to slowing of the heart. May be caused by psychogenic faint, pain, acute loss of blood, fear, or by assuming an upright position after having been in bed for a prolonged period. SYN: *carotid sinus s.; vasodepressor s.*

syncytial (sĭn-sī'shăl). Of the nature of a syncytium.

s. trophoblast. Syntrophoblast, q.v.

syncytiolysin (sĭn''sĭt-ĭ-ŏl'ĭ-sĭn) [Gr. *syn,* together, + *kytos,* cell, + *lysis,* destruction]. A cytolysin that is formed from injections of emulsions of placental tissue.

syncytioma (sĭn''sĭt-ĭ-ō'mă) ["+ "+ *-ōma,* tumor]. A tumor of the chorion. SYN: *chorioma; deciduoma.*

s. benignum. A mole.

s. malignum. A tumor formed of cells from the syncytium and chorion, occurring frequently after abortion or during puerperium at site of placenta.

syncytium (sĭn-sĭt'ĭ-ŭm) [Gr. *syn,* together, + *kytos,* cell]. 1. A multinucleated mass of protoplasm. Ex: a striated muscle fiber. 2. A group of cells in which the protoplasm of one cell is continuous with that of adjoining cells. Ex: mesenchyme cells of the embryo. SYN: *coenocyte.*

syndactylism (sĭn-dăk'tĭl-ĭzm) ["+ *daktylos,* digit, + *ismos,* condition]. A fusion of two or more toes or fingers.

syndectomy (sĭn-dĕk'tō-mĭ) ["+ *dēin,* to bind, + *ektomē,* excision]. Excision of a circular strip of the conjunctiva around cornea to relieve pannus. SYN: *peritomy.*

syndesis (sĭn-dē'sĭs) [Gr. *syn,* together, + *desis,* binding]. 1. Condition of being bound together. 2. Surgical fixation or ankylosis of a joint.

syndesmectomy (sĭn''dĕs-mĕk'tō-mĭ) [Gr. *syndesmos,* ligament, + *ektomē,* excision]. Excision of a section of a ligament.

syndesmectopia (sĭn''dĕs-mĕk-tō'pĭ-ă) ["+ *ektopos,* out of place]. Abnormal position of a ligament.

syndesmitis (sĭn''dĕs-mī'tĭs) ["+ *-ītis,* inflammation]. 1. Inflammation of a ligament or ligaments. 2. Inflammation of the conjunctiva.

syndesmochorial (sĭn''dĕs''mō-kōr'ĭ-ăl). Pert. to a type of placenta found in ungulates (Ex: sheep and goats) in which there is destruction of surface layer of uterine mucosa, thus allowing chorionic villi to come into direct contact with maternal blood vessels.

syndesmography (sĭn-dĕs-mŏg'ră-fĭ) [Gr. *syndesmos,* ligament, + *graphein,* to write]. Treatise on the ligaments.

syndesmology (sĭn''dĕs-mŏl'ō-jĭ) ["+ *logos,* a study]. Study of the ligaments and their disorders.

syndesmoma (sĭn''dĕs-mō'mă) ["+ *-ōma,* tumor]. A connective tissue tumor.

syndesmopexy (sĭn-dĕs'mō-pĕk''sĭ) [Gr. *syndesmos,* ligament, + *pēxis,* fixation]. Joining of two ligaments or fixation of a ligament in a new place, used in correction of a dislocation.

syndesmoplasty (sĭn-dĕs'mō-plăs''tĭ) ["+ *plassein,* to form]. Plastic surgery on a ligament.

syndesmorrhaphy (sĭn''dĕs-mōr'ă-fĭ) ["+ *rhaphē,* suture]. Repair or suture of a ligament.

syndesmosis (sĭn''dĕs-mō'sĭs) [Gr. *syndesmos,* ligament, + *-ōsis,* condition]. (pl. *syndesmoses*) [NA] Articulation in which the bones are united by ligaments. Ex: the distal tibiofibular articulation.

syndesmotomy (sĭn''dĕs-mŏt'ō-mĭ) ["+ *tomē,* a cutting]. Surgical section of ligaments.

syndrome (sĭn'drōm) [Gr., a running together]. A group of signs and symptoms that collectively characterize or indicate a particular disease or abnormal condition; the sum of signs associated with any pathological process. For syndromes not listed here, see the adjectives.

s., Adair-Dighton. A familial condition characterized by fragility of bones, deafness, and blue sclerae.

s., adiposogenital. S., Fröhlich's, q.v.

s., adrenogenital. S. characterized by pubertas praecox in children, overmasculin-

s., Angelucci's. Palpitation, excitable temperament, and vasomotor disturbance in some of those who experience spring conjunctivitis.

s., dumping. Symptom complex which may follow partial or complete gastrectomy. Appears to be related to rapid emptying of gastric pouch. Occurs immediately after eating. Consists of weakness, varying degrees of syncope, nausea, sweating, and palpitation, and sometimes diarrhea and sensation of warmth. Usually lying down affords some relief.

s., Fröhlich's. Increase in fat, atrophy of the genitals, transition to feminine type due to lesions of the hypophysis.

s., Gradenigo's. Paralysis of external rectus muscle with severe tempoparietal pain and suppurative otitis media on affected side. Caused by infection in petrous portion of temporal bone involving 6th nerve.

s., Horner's. Contracted pupil, ptosis, enophthalmos, and dry, cool face on affected side produced by paralysis of sympathetics.

ETIOL: Tumors in neck, trauma, apical tuberculosis, tabes, syringomyelia, and neuritis of cervical plexus.

s., Korsakoff's. A psychosis, ordinarily due to chronic alcoholism, with polyneuritis, disorientation, insomnia, muttering delirium, hallucinations, and a bilateral wrist or foot drop.

s., Marfan's. A hereditary condition of connective tissue, bones, eyes, muscles, ligaments, and skeletal structures. SYM: Irregular, unsteady gait; lean and tall with stooping shoulders.

s., skin-eye. Deposits on the anterior surface of the lens and posterior cornea, and skin pigmentation. Due to extensive medication with some of the phenothiazine type tranquilizers.

s., Stokes-Adams. Bradycardia and intermittent convulsive seizures with loss of consciousness due to complete heart block.

s., Weber's. Paralysis of hypoglossal nerve on one side and of oculomotor nerve on other with paralysis of limbs due to lesion of a cerebral peduncle.

syndromic (sĭn-drŏm'ĭk) [Gr. *syndromē,* a running together]. Pert. to or occurring as a syndrome.

synechia (sĭn-ĕk'ē-ŭ) [Gr. *synecheia,* continuity]. (pl. *synech'iae*) Adhesion of parts, esp. adhesion of iris to lens and cornea.

s., annular. Adhesion of the iris to the lens throughout its entire pupillary margin.

s., anterior. Adhesion of iris to cornea.

s., posterior. Adhesion of iris to capsule of lens.

s., total. Adhesion of entire surface of iris to lens.

synechotomy (sĭn"ĕk-ŏt'ō-mĭ) [Gr. *synecheia,* continuity, + *tomē,* a cutting]. Division of a synechia or adhesion.

synecology (sĭn"ē-kŏl'ō-jĭ) [Gr. *syn,* together, + *oikos,* house, + *logos,* a study]. The study of organisms in relationship to their environment in group form.

syneresis (sĭn-ĕr'ē-sĭs) [Gr. *synairesis,* drawing together]. Contraction of a gel resulting in its separation from the liquid, as a shrinkage of fibrin when blood clots.

synergetic (sĭn"ĕr-jĕt'ĭk) [Gr. *syn,* together, + *ergon,* work]. Exhibiting cooperative action, said of certain muscles; working together. SYN: *synergic.*

synergia (sĭn-ĕr'jĭ-ă). The association and correlation of the activity of synergetic muscle groups.

synergic (sĭn-ĕr'jĭk) [Gr. *syn,* together, + *ergon,* work]. Rel. to or exhibiting cooperation, as certain muscles.

synergism (sĭn'ĕr-jĭzm) ["+ "+ *-ismos,* condition]. The harmonious action of two agents, such as drugs, or organs, such as muscles, producing an effect which neither could produce alone or an effect which is greater than the total effects of each agent operating by itself.

synergist (sĭn'ĕr-jĭst). 1. A remedy that stimulates the action of another. SYN: *adjuvant.* 2. A muscle or organ functioning in cooperation with another, as the flexor muscles.

synergy (sĭn'ĕr-jĭ) [Gr. *synergia*]. Action of two or more agents or organs working with each other; cooperation. Combined action; coordinated action.

synesthesia (sĭn"ĕs-thē'zĭ-ă) [Gr. *syn,* together, + *aisthēsis,* sensation]. 1. A sensation in one area from a stimulus applied to another part. 2. A subjective sensation of another sense than the one being stimulated. Hearing a sound may also produce the sensation of smell. SEE: *chromatism; phonism.*

s. algica. Painful synesthesia.

synesthesialgia (sĭn"ĕs-thē-zĭ-ăl'jĭ-ă) ["+ "+ *algos,* pain]. A painful sensation giving rise to a subjective one of different character. SEE: *synesthesia.*

synezesis (sĭn"ē-zē'sĭs) [Gr. *synizēsis,* a sitting together]. Closure of the pupil.

Syngamus (sĭn'gă-mŭs). A genus of nematode worms parasitic in respiratory tract of birds and mammals.

    S. laryngeus. Species normally parasitic in ruminants, but sometimes accidentally infesting man.

syngamy (sĭn'gă-mĭ) [Gr. *syn*, together, + *gamos*, marriage]. 1. Sexual reproduction. 2. Cell union as of gametes in fertilization.

syngenesious (sĭn″jĕ-nē'shŭs) [″+ *genesis*, origin]. Derived from an individual of the same species, said of tissue transplants.

syngignocism (sĭn-jĭg′nō-sĭzm) [″+ *gignō-skein*, to know]. Hypnotism and its results.

synhidrosis (sĭn″hĭ-drō'sĭs) [Gr. *syn*, together, + *hidrōsis*, a sweating]. Sweating, esp. excessive sweating associated with another condition.

synizesis (sĭn″ĭ-zē'sĭs) [Gr. *synizēsis*]. An occlusion, or shutting.

    s. pupillae. Closure of the pupil of the eye with loss of vision.

synkaryon (sĭn-kăr'ĭ-ŏn) [Gr. *syn*, together, + *karyon*, kernel]. A nucleus resulting from fusion of two pronuclei.

synkinesis (sĭn″kĭ-nē'sĭs) [″+ *kinēsis*, motion]. 1. An involuntary movement of one part occurring simultaneously with reflex or voluntary movement of another part. 2. An involuntary movement in a healthy or normal muscle accompanying an attempted movement of a paralyzed muscle on the opposite side. Called imitative s.

synonym (sĭn'ō-nĭm) [Gr. *synōnymon*]. A word which has the same or very similar meaning; an additional or substitute name for the same disease, sign, symptom, or anatomical structure. ABBR: Syn.

synophrys (sĭn-ŏf'rĭs) [Gr. *syn*, together, + *ophrys*, eyebrow]. Condition in which the two eyebrows grow together.

synopsia (sĭn-ŏp-sĭ-ā) [″+ *opsis*, vision]. Condition in which there is congenital fusion of the eyes.

synopsis (sĭn-ŏp'sĭs) [Gr.]. A summary; a general review of the whole.

synoptophore (sĭn-ŏp'tō-fōr) [Gr. *syn*, together, + *ops*, sight, + *phoros*, bearing]. Apparatus for diagnosing and treating strabismus.

synoptoscope (sĭn-ŏp'tō-skōp) [″+ ″+ *skopein*, to examine]. An instrument for diagnosis and treatment of strabismus. SYN: *synoptophore.*

synorchidism, synorchism (sĭn-ŏr'kĭd-ĭzm, -kĭzm) [″+ *orchis*, testicle, + *-ismos*, condition]. Union or partial fusion of the testicles.

synosteo'sis. SEE: *synostosis.*

synosteotomy (sĭn″ŏs-tē-ŏt'ō-mĭ) [Gr. *syn*, together, + *osteon*, bone, + *tomē*, a cutting]. Dissection of joints.

synostosis (sĭn″ŏs-tō'sĭs) [″+ ″+ *-ōsis*, condition]. (pl. *synosto'ses*) [NA] 1. Articulation by osseous tissue of adjacent bones. 2. Union of separate bones by osseous tissue.

synotia (sĭn-ō'shĭ-ā) [″+ *ous*, ear]. The union of, or approximation of, the ears occurring in embryonic development, usually associated with absence of, or incomplete development of, the lower jaw.

synovectomy (sĭn″ō-věk'tō-mĭ) [Gr. *syn*, together, + L. *ovum*, egg, + Gr. *ektomē*, excision]. Excision of synovial membrane.

synovia (sĭn-ō'vĭ-ā) [L.]. [NA]. A colorless, viscid, lubricating fluid of joints, bursae, and tendon sheaths secreted within synovial membranes. It contains mucin, albumin, fat, and mineral salts. SYN: *synovial fluid.* SEE: *asynovia.*

synovial (sĭn-ō'vĭ-ăl). Pert. to synovia, the lubricating fluid of the joints.

    s. bursa. A cleft in connective tissue between muscles, tendons, ligaments, and bones lined by a s. membrane and containing synovia. SYN: *bursa mucosa.* SEE: *bursa.*

    s. crypt. Diverticulum of a s. membrane of a joint.

    s. cyst. Accumulation of synovia in a bursa, s. crypt, or sac of a synovial hernia, causing a tumor.

    s. fluid. Clear lubricating fluid secreted by the s. membrane of a joint. SYN: *synovia.*

    s. folds. Smooth folds of synovial membrane on inner surface of joint capsule. SYN: *plicae synoviales* [NA].

    s. hernia. Protrusion of a portion of s. membrane through a tear in the stratum fibrosum of a joint capsule.

    s. membrane. Membrane lining the capsule of a joint.

    s. tendon sheaths. Sheaths which develop in osteofibrous canals through which tendons pass. Each is a double layered tube, the space between the two layers being occupied by s. fluid. SYN: *vaginae mucosae.*

    s. villi. Slender avascular processes on the free surface of a s. membrane projecting into the joint cavity. SYN: *haversian fringes.*

synovioma (sĭn″ō-vĭ-ō'mă) [Gr. *syn*, together, + L. *ovum*, + Gr. *-ōma*, tumor]. A tumor arising from a s. membrane.

synovitis (sĭn″ō-vī'tĭs) [″+ ″+ Gr. *-itis*, inflammation]. Inflammation of a synovial membrane.

    ETIOL: Simple inflammation may be the result of an aseptic wound, a subcutaneous injury (contusion or sprain), irritation produced by floating cartilage, or exposure to cold and dampness.

SYM: Joint painful, severely so on motion, esp. at night. Swollen, tense; may be fluctuating. In s. of the knee, patella is floated up from condyles, can be readily depressed, to rise again when pressure is taken off. The part is never in full extension, as this increases the pain. Skin, which is very sensitive to pressure only at certain points, is neither thickened nor reddened. After a few days, when pain lessens and swelling diminishes as the effusion and extravasated blood are absorbed, the limb takes its natural position and recovery follows.

s., chronic. Condition in which active congestion disappears, but an undue amount of fluid remains in the cavity and the membrane itself is edematous. Later if disease does not subside, membrane and articular structures become irregularly thickened by plastic exudation and formation of fibrous tissue. Joint is weak but not esp. painful, except on pressure and sometimes not even then. Movements, esp. in extension, are restricted, and generally attended by some grating or creaking. Symptoms are well marked when there is great accumulation of liquid. Fluid, which is straw-colored, somewhat viscid, sometimes flocculent, and more or less blood stained, may be drawn off with the hypodermic needle.

s., dendritic. S. with villous growths developing in the sac.

s., dry. S. with little or no effusion.

s., purulent. S. with purulent effusion within the sac.

s., serous. S. with nonpurulent, copious effusion.

s., sicca. S., dry, q.v.

s., simple. S. with effusion only slightly turbid, if not clear.

s., tendinous. Inflammation of a tendon sheath. SEE: *synovial tendon sheaths.*

s., vaginal. S., tendinous, q.v.

s., vibration. S. resulting from a wound near a joint.

synovium (sĭn-ō′vĭ-ŭm) [Gr. *syn*, together, + L. *ovum*, egg]. A synovial membrane.

synpneumonic (sĭn-nū-mŏn′ĭk) [Gr. *syn*, together, + *pneumonia*, pneumonia]. Concurrent with pneumonia; complicating pneumonia.

syntasis ["+ *teinein*, to stretch]. Stretching.

syntaxis (sĭn-tăk′sĭs) ["+ *taxis*, arrangement]. A junction between two bones. SYN: *articulation.*

syntexis (sĭn-tĕk′sĭs) [Gr.]. Wasting or cachexia.

synthermal (sĭn-thĕr′măl) [Gr. *syn*, together, + *thermē*, heat]. Having the same temperature.

synthesis (sĭn′thĕs-ĭs) [Gr.]. In chemistry, the union of elements to produce compounds; the process of building up. Opposed to analysis and decomposition. In general, the process or processes involved in the formation of a complex substance from simpler elements or compounds, as the s. of proteins from amino acids.

synthetic (sĭn-thĕt′ĭk) [Gr. *synthetikos*]. Rel. to or made by synthesis; artificially prepared.

syntone (sĭn′tōn) [Gr. *syn*, together, + *tonos*, tension]. An individual whose personality indicates a stable responsiveness to his environment and its social demands. SEE: *syntonic.*

syntonic (sĭn-tŏn′ĭk). Pert. to a personality characterized by an even temperament, a normal emotional responsiveness to life situations. Opposed to schizoid. S. type is exaggerated in manic states or in depression.

syntonin (sĭn′tō-nĭn). An acid albumin; esp. one formed by the action of dilute hydrochloric acid on muscle during gastric digestion.

syntoxoid (sĭn-tŏk′soyd) [Gr. *syn*, together, + *toxikon*, poison, + *eidos*, form]. A toxoid having the same degree of affinity for an antitoxin as that possessed by the toxin.

syntripsis (sĭn-trĭp′sĭs) [Gr., destruction]. A comminuted fracture or act causing it.

syntrophoblast (sĭn-trŏf′ō-blăst) [Gr. *syn*, together, + *trophē*, nourishment, + *blastos*, germ]. The outer syncytial layer of the trophoblast. SEE: *trophoblast.*

synulotic (sĭn″ū-lŏt′ĭk) ["+ *oulē*, scar]. 1. Promoting cicatrization. 2. An agent stimulating cicatrization.

syphilelcosis (sĭf-ĭl-ĕl-kō′sĭs) [*syphilis* + Gr. *helkōsis*, ulceration]. Syphilitic ulceration.

syphilelcus (sĭf′ĭl-ĕl′kŭs) ["+ Gr. *helkos*, ulcer]. A syphilitic ulcer or chancre.

syphilid(e (sĭf′ĭl-ĭd) [Fr.]. (pl. *syphil'ides*) Skin eruption caused by syphilis.

syphilionthus (sĭf′ĭl-ĭ-ŏn′thŭs) [*syphilis* + Gr. *ionthos*, eruption]. A copper-colored, branny-scaled syphilide.

syphiliphobia (sĭf′ĭl-ĭ-fō′bĭ-ă) ["+ Gr. *phobos*, fear]. Morbid fear of syphilis. SYN: *syphilophobia.*

syphilis (sĭf′ĭ-lĭs). [perhaps *Syphilis*, shepherd having the disease in a Latin poem] An infectious, chronic, venereal disease characterized by lesions which may involve any organ or tissue. It usually exhibits cutaneous manifestations, relapses are frequent, and it may exist without symptoms for years. SYN: *lues venerea.*

ETIOL: Treponema pallidum, a spirochete which is transmitted by direct contact between humans, contact with freshly contaminated material, transfusion of infected blood or plasma, or in utero by passage of organism from mother to fetus. The organism may enter through any broken place in skin or mucous membrane.

PRIMARY STAGE SYM: Initial lesion appears 2-4 weeks after inoculation, changing from a small red papule to a small ulcer to a hard chancre. Usually upon prepuce or vulva. Lymph nodes enlarge about two weeks after appearance of lesion. Signs which are almost positive are inflammation at mouth of Stensen's duct and enlargement of epitrochlear lymph nodes.

SECONDARY STAGE SYM: Symptoms appear about 6 weeks after appearance of primary lesion, principally in the form of lesions of the skin and mucus membranes. The character of the skin lesions is protean, syphilis often being called the "Great Imitator." Systemic symptoms such as headache, fever, and malaise are common but may be absent. Enlargement and induration of regional lymph nodes occurs. Eruptions of skin, maculae (roseola), syphilide, reddish-brown coppery spots continuing for a week or two and possibly recurring later.

TERTIARY STAGE SYM: The heart and blood vessels (cardiovascular syphilis) and the central nervous system (neurosyphilis) are frequently involved. Tabes dorsalis, paresis (general paralysis of the insane), and various types of psychoses may result.

DIAG: Laboratory tests for syphilis are based on three procedures: *microscopic:* darkfield demonstration of spirochetes in material taken from a chancre or other early lesion; *biopsy:* examination of cerebrospinal fluid; *serologic tests for syphilis* (S.T.S.) done on blood and spinal fluid. These include flocculation tests (Kahn, Eagle, Mazzini, Kline, Hinton), complement-fixation techniques (Wassermann test and its modifications). The VDRL (Venereal Disease Research Laboratory), treponema pallidum immobilization (TPI), and fluorescent treponemal antibody (FTA) tests also are useful in diagnosing syphilis and distinguishing it from biological false positive serologic reactions.

CAUTION: A person who contracts gonorrhea also may have been exposed to syphilis at the same time. Because the clinical signs and symptoms of gonorrhea develop several weeks prior to those of syphilis, the patient may be treated for that disease. The treatment for gonorrhea may be sufficient to mask or delay the signs of syphilis, but insufficient to rid the patient of the spirochetes. When this occurs syphilis will develop and may be unnoticed by the patient. It is therefore of vital importance either to treat each case of gonorrhea as if syphilis had also been contracted, or to test the patient for serologic evidence of syphilis each month for at least four months following the treatment for gonorrhea.

TREATMENT: Penicillin is the treatment of choice for all types and stages. Should allergic reactions occur, other antibiotics (oxytetracycline, chlortetracycline, or erythromycin) may be substituted. The use of arsenicals, bismuth, and mercurials has been almost completely supplanted by antibiotics.

s., cardiovascular. S. involving the heart and great blood vessels, esp. the aorta. Saccular aneurysms of the aorta and aortic insufficiency frequently result.

s., congenital. S. present at birth.

s., extragenital. S. in which the primary chancre is located elsewhere than on genital organs.

s. innocentium, s. insontium. S. not contracted through coition.

s., latent. Phase in which symptoms are absent, and the disease can be diagnosed only by serological tests.

s., marital. S. acquired from a spouse.

s., meningovascular. A form of neurosyphilis in which the meninges and vascular structures of the brain and spinal cord are involved. May be localized or general.

s., neuro-. Involvement of the nervous system by s.

s., prenatal. S. transmitted from mother to child; congenital s.

s., venereal. S. acquired through illicit sexual relations.

s., visceral. S. in which visceral organs are involved.

syphilitic (sĭf'ĭ-lĭt'ĭk) [L. *syphiliticus*]. Rel. to, caused by, or affected with syphilis.

s. fever. Rise in temperature in early stage of secondary syphilis.

s. macules. Small red eruptions manifested in secondary syphilis, often covering the entire body.

SYM: Associated with chancre or scar, alopecia, pain in bones, swollen glands, and sore throat.

syphiloderm, syphiloderma (sĭf′ĭl-ō-dŭrm″, sĭf′ĭl-ō-dŭr′mă) [*syphilis* + Gr. *derma*, skin]. A syphilitic cutaneous disorder.

syphilogenesis (sĭf′ĭl-ō-jĕn′ĕ-sĭs) [″+ Gr. *genesis*, production]. The development or origin of syphilis. SYN: *syphilogeny.*

syphilogeny (sĭf′ĭl-ŏj′ĕn-ĭ) [″+ Gr. *gennan*, to produce]. The development or origin of syphilis. SYN: *syphilogenesis.*

syphilographer (sĭf′ĭl-ŏg′ră-fĕr) [*syphilis* + Gr. *graphein*, to write]. One who writes about syphilis.

syphilography (sĭf′ĭl-ŏg′ră-fĭ). A treatise on syphilis.

syphiloid (sĭf′ĭ-loyd) [*syphilis* + Gr. *eidos*, form]. 1. Resembling syphilis. 2. A disease akin to syphilis.

syphilogy (sĭf′ĭl-ŏl′ō-jĭ). The study of syphilis and its treatment.

syphilologist (sĭf′ĭl-ŏl′ō-jĭst) [″+ Gr. *logos*, a study]. A specialist in diagnosis and treatment of syphilis.

syphilo′ma [*syphilis* + Gr. *ōma*, tumor]. A syphilitic tumor; a gumma.

syphiloma′nia [″+ Gr. *mania*, madness]. Morbid fear of syphilis or inference that one is suffering with it. SYN: *syphilophobia.*

syphilopathy (sĭf′ĭ-lŏp′ă-thĭ) [″+ Gr. *pathos*, disease]. Any syphilitic disorder.

syphilophobia (sĭf′ĭl-ō-fō′bĭ-ă) [*syphilis* + Gr. *phobos*, fear]. 1. Morbid fear of syphilis. 2. Delusion of having syphilis.

syphilophobic (sĭf′ĭl-ō-fō′bĭk). Pert. to or affected with syphilophobia.

syphilophyma (sĭf′ĭl-ō-fĭ′mă) [*syphilis* + Gr. *phyma*, a growth]. 1. Any growth or excrescence due to syphilis. 2. Syphiloma of the epidermis.

syphilopsychosis (sĭf′ĭl-ō-sī-kō′sĭs) [″+ Gr. *psychē*, soul, + *-ōsis*, condition]. Any mental disease caused by syphilis.

syphilosis (sĭf′ĭ-lō′sĭs) [″+ Gr. *-ōsis*, disease]. Generalized syphilitic disease.

syphilotherapy (sĭf′ĭl-ō-thĕr′ă-pĭ) [*syphilis* + Gr. *therapeia*, treatment]. Treatment of syphilis.

syphilotropic (sĭf′ĭl-ō-trŏp′ĭk) [″+ Gr. *tropos*, a turning]. Esp. susceptible to syphilis.

syphilous (sĭf′ĭl-ūs). Of the nature of or pert. to syphilis. SYN: *syphilitic.*

syphionthus (sĭf′ĭ-ŏn′thŭs) [*syphilis* + Gr. *ionthos*, eruption]. Copper-colored patches seen in syphilis.

syr. Abbr. for *syrupus*, syrup.

syrigmophonia (sĭr′ĭg-mō-fō′nĭ-ă) [Gr. *syrigmos*, a whistle, + *phōnē*, voice]. 1. A sibilant rale. 2. A whistling sound in pronunciation of "s" due to a denture peculiarity.

syrig′mus. A subjective sound such as a hissing or ringing heard in the ears.

syringadenoma (sĭr-ĭng″ă-dē-nō′mă) [Gr. *syrinx*, pipe, + *adēn*, gland, + *-ōma*, tumor]. Tumor of a sweat gland.

syringe (sĭr-ĭnj′, sĭr′ĭnj) [Gr. *syrinx*, pipe]. 1. Instrument for injecting fluids into cavities or vessels. 2. To wash out or introduce fluid with a syringe.

syringectomy (sĭr′ĭn-jĕk′tō-mĭ) [″+ *ektomē*, excision]. Removal of the walls of a fistula.

syringitis (sĭr′ĭn-jī′tĭs) [″+ *-ītis*, inflammation]. Inflammation of eustachian tube.

syringobulbia (sĭr-ĭn″gō-bŭl′bĭ-ă) [Gr. *syrinx*, pipe, + *bulbos*, a bulb]. A chronic progressive disease characterized by development of cavities in the medulla oblongata. SEE: *syringomyelia.*

syringocele (sĭr-ĭn′gō-sēl) [″+ *koilia*, a hollow]. 1. The central canal of the myelon or spinal cord. 2. A form of meningomyelocele which contains a cavity in the ectopic spinal cord.

syringocystadenoma (sĭr-ĭn″gō-sĭs″tă-dē-nō′mă) [″+ *kystis*, a bladder, + *adēn*, gland, + *-ōma*, tumor]. Adenoma of sweat glands characterized by tiny, hard, papular formations.

syringocystoma (sĭr-ĭn″gō-sĭs-tō′mă) [″+ ″+ *-ōma*, tumor]. Cystic tumor having its origin in ducts of the sweat gland.

syringoid (sĭr-ĭn′goyd) [Gr. *syrinx*, pipe, + *eidos*, form]. Resembling a tube; fistulous.

syringoma (sĭr′ĭn-gō′mă) [Gr. *syrinx*, pipe, + *-ōma*, tumor]. Tumor of the sweat glands.

syringomeningocele (sĭr-ĭn″gō-men-ĭn′gō-sēl) [″+ *mēninx*, membrane, + *kēlē*, hernia]. Meningocele which is similar to a syringomyelocele.

syringomyelia (sĭr-ĭn″gō-mī-ē′lĭ-ă) [″+ *myelos*, marrow]. A chronic progressive disease of the spinal cord characterized by the development of cavities and gliosis of surrounding tissue. Usually begins before age of 30 and is more common among males. Its cause is unknown.

SYM: Cavitation occurs in cervical and lumbar regions and soon involves pathways of the cord that carry impulses of pain and temperature sensations, resulting in dissociated sensory loss. Destruction of lateral and anterior gray matter causes muscular atrophy, weakness, and autonomic anomalies.

TREATMENT: There is no satisfactory treatment. Sudden enlargement of cavity may warrant surgical intervention with decompression of cavity. Persistent pain may necessitate chordotomy or medullary tractotomy for relief.

syringomyelitis (sĭr-ĭn″gō-mī″ĕ-lī′tĭs) [Gr. *syrinx*, pipe, + *myelos*, marrow, + *-itis*, inflammation]. Inflammation coincident with abnormal dilation of the central canal of spinal cord.

syringomyelocele (sĭr-ĭn″gō-mī′ĕl-ō-sēl) ["+ "+ *kēlē*, tumor]. A form of spina bifida in which the cavity of the projecting portion communicates with the central canal of the spinal cord.

syringomyelus (sĭr-ĭn″gō-mī′ĕl-ŭs). Abnormal dilatation of central canal of spinal cord.

syringopontia (sĭr-ĭn″gō-pŏn′shĭ-ă) [Gr. *syrinx*, pipe, + L. *pons, pont-*, bridge]. Cavities in the pons Varolii similar to syringomyelia.

syringosystrophy (sĭr-ĭn″gō-sĭs′trō-fĭ) ["+ *systrophē*, a twist]. Twisting of the oviduct.

syringotome (sĭr-ĭn′gō-tōm) ["+ *tomē*, a cutting]. Instrument for incision of a fistula.

syringotomy (sĭr′ĭn-gŏt′ō-mĭ). Operation for cure of fistula by cutting.

syrinx (sĭr′ĭnks) [Gr., pipe]. 1. The eustachian tube. 2. Pathological cavity in the spinal cord or brain. 3. A fistula.

syrup (sĭr′ŭp) [L. *syrupus*]. USP. Concentrated solution of sugar in water. Usually specific medicinal substances are added. S. usually does not represent a very high percentage of the active drug. Some syrups are used principally to give a pleasant odor and taste to solutions. ABBR: syr.

syssarcosis (sĭs″ăr-kō′sĭs) [Gr. *syn*, together, + *sarkōsis*, fleshy growth]. The union of bones by means of muscles; muscular articulation, as of the hyoid and patella.

systaltic (sĭs-tăl′tĭk) [Gr. *systaltikos*, contracting]. Contracting and dilating alternately; having a systole. SYN: *pulsating*.

system (sĭs′tĕm) [Gr. *systēma*, a composite whole]. 1. An organized grouping of related structures. 2. A group of structures or organs related to each other and functioning together in the performance of certain functions. Ex: digestive system. 3. A group of cells or aggregations of cells which perform a particular function. Ex: reticuloendothelial system.

s., autonomic nervous. That portion of the peripheral nervous s. which innervates all smooth muscle, cardiac muscle, and glands, the activities of which are involuntary. It includes the craniosacral (parasympathetic) and thoracolumbar (sympathetic) divisions, each of which provides fibers for most of the visceral structures or organs. SEE: *autonomic nervous s.*

s.'s of body. Circulatory, digestive, endocrine, hematopoietic, integumentary, lymphatic, muscular, nervous, reproductive, respiratory, skeletal, urinary.

s., cardiovascular. The heart and blood vessels (aorta, arteries, arterioles, capillaries, venules, veins, venae cavae).

s., centimeter-gram-second. A system of measurement in units of length, mass, and time. ABBR: CGS; cgs. SYN: *metric s.*

s., central nervous. That portion of nervous s. consisting of the brain and spinal cord. SEE: *central nervous system.*

s., chromaffin. SEE: *chromaffin system.*

s., circulatory. S. concerned with circulation of body fluids. It includes the cardiovascular and lymphatic systems. SYN: *vascular system.*

s., cytochrome. Cytochrome oxidase and three hemochromogen-like pigments (cytochromes a, b, and c) which make molecular oxygen available for the oxidation of hydrogen liberated from cellular metabolites.

s., digestive. The alimentary canal (mouth, teeth, tongue, pharynx, esophagus, stomach, small and large intestines) and accessory glands (salivary glands, liver, pancreas). SEE: *digestion; digestive system* for illustration.

s., endocrine. The ductless glands or the glands of internal secretion.

s., enzyme. A group of enzymes essential for the completion of a series of metabolic and other reactions.

s., extrapyramidal motor. S. including all descending fibers arising in cortical and subcortical motor centers which reach the medulla and spinal cord by pathways other than recognized pyramidal tracts. S. is important in maintenance of equilibrium and muscle tone.

s., genital. S., reproductive, q.v. SEE: *genitourinary system* for illustration.

s., genitourinary. Genitals and urinary organs. SEE: *genitourinary system* for illustration.

s., haversian. The structural unit of bone. SEE: *haversian system.*

s., hematopoietic. The blood-forming tissues and organs of the body. Includes the bone marrow, spleen, and lymphatic tissue.

s., impulse-conducting. A s. of atypical muscle fibers (Purkinje fibers) within the heart which conducts impulses regulating contractions of the atria and ventricles. Includes S-A and A-V nodes and bundle of His.

s., integumentary. The skin and its derivatives (hair, nails, etc.).

s., lymphatic. That concerned with the circulation of lymph. Includes lymph vessels and ducts and lymphatic organs (lymph nodes, tonsils, thymus, spleen). SEE: *lymphatic*.

s., muscular. S. which includes all the muscles (smooth, cardiac, striated, or skeletal). As generally used, the term refers to the skeletal muscles. SEE: *muscle*.

s., nervous. S. which includes the brain, spinal cord, ganglia, and nerves. SEE: *nervous system*.

s., osseous. The bony structures of the body; the skeleton. SEE *skeleton*.

s., portal. The hepatic portal vein and all of its branches. SEE: *portal system*.

s., reproductive. The gonads and their associated structures and ducts. SYN: *genital s.* SEE: *genitourinary system* for illustration.

s., reproductive, female. The ovaries, uterine tubes (oviducts), uterus, vagina, and vulva. SEE: *genitourinary system* for illustration.

s., reproductive, male. The testes, efferent ducts, epididymis, ductus deferens, ejaculatory duct, and urethra with the accessory glands (bulbourethral, prostate, seminal vesicles) and penis. SEE: *genitourinary system* for illustration.

s., respiratory. The air passageways and organs (nasal cavities, oral cavity, pharynx, larynx, trachea, and lungs, including bronchi, bronchioles, alveolar ducts, and alveoli). SEE: *respiratory system* for illustration.

s., reticuloendothelial. Collectively, all the phagocytic cells of the body excepting the leukocytes. Includes macrophages, histiocytes, Kupffer's cells of the liver, reticular cells of lymphatic organs, microglia of the brain, and many others. ABBR: RES. SEE: *reticuloendothelial system*.

s., sympathetic nervous. The thoracolumbar or sympathetic division of the autonomic nervous s.

s., urinary. The kidneys, ureters, bladder, and urethra.

s., urogenital. The urinary and reproductive systems combined. SEE: *genitourinary system* for illustration.

s., vascular. Vessels of the body (heart, blood vessels, and lymphatics).

s., vegetative nervous. The autonomic nervous system, q.v.

s., visceral efferent. S. which includes all efferent nerve fibers conveying impulses to the visceral organs; the autonomic nervous system, q.v.

systema (sĭs-tē'mă) [Gr. *systēma*, a composite whole]. System, q.v.

systemic (sĭs-tĕm'ĭk). Pert. to a whole body rather than to one of its parts; somatic.

s. circulation. The blood flow from the left ventricle through the aorta and all its branches (arteries) to the capillaries of the tissues and its return to the heart through veins and the venae cavae which empty into the right atrium.

s. remedies. Remedies which will act on the body as a whole.

systemoid (sĭs'tĕ-moyd) [Gr. *systēma*, a composite whole, + *eidos*, form]. 1. Resembling a system. 2. Pert. to tumors made up of several types of tissues.

systole (sĭs'tō-lē) [Gr., contraction]. That part of the heart cycle in which the heart is in contraction, i.e., the myocardial fibers are tightening and shortening. Occurs in the interval between first and second heart sound during which blood is surged through the aorta and pulmonary artery.

RS: diastole; murmur; presystole.

s., aborted. A premature cardiac s. Arterial pressure is increased little if at all because of inadequate filling of ventricles due to shortening of preceding diastole.

s., anticipated. S. that is aborted because it occurs before the ventricle is filled.

s., arterial. The rebound or recoil of the stretched elastic walls of the arteries following ventricular s.

s., atrial. The contraction of the atria. Precedes the ventricular s.

s., electrical. The total duration of the QRS-T complex in an electrocardiogram. Approximately the same as that of the mechanical systole.

s., extra-. A premature s. occurring in addition to the fundamental rhythm.

s., premature. S. slightly preceding a normal s. SYN: *extrasystole*.

s., ventricular. Ventricular contraction.

systolic (sĭs-tŏl'ĭk) [Gr. *systolē*, contraction]. Pert. to the systole.

s. discharge. The amount of blood ejected by the heart at each systole.

s. murmur. A cardiac murmur during systole.

s. pressure. Blood pressure is expressed in terms of the s. pressure; the greatest force exerted by the heart and the highest degree of resistance put forth by the arterial walls.

RS: blood pressure; diastolic pressure pulse; pulse pressure; systole.

systolometer (sĭs″tō-lŏm′ĕt-ĕr) [Gr. *systole*, contraction, + *metron*, measure]. Device for determining quality and character of cardiac murmurs.

systremma (sĭs-trĕm′ă) [Gr. *systremma*, anything twisted together]. Cramp in calf of the leg, the muscles assuming form of a hard knot.

syzygial (sĭ-zĭj′ĭ-ăl) [Gr. *syzygia*, conjunction]. Pert. to a syzygium.

syzygiology (sĭ-zĭj″ĭ-ŏl′ō-jĭ) [" + *logos*, a study]. Study of interdependence or interrelationship of the whole as opposed to that of isolated functions or separate parts.

syzygium (sĭ-zĭj′ĭ-ŭm) [Gr. *syzygia*, conjunction]. Fusion of two parts or structures without loss of identity of the parts.

syzygy (sĭz′ĭ-jĭ). Fusion of organs, each remaining distinct.

T

T. Abbr. for *temperature; time; intraocular tension.*

t. Abbr. for *temporal;* L. *ter,* three times.

T₁T₂. First thoracic vertebra, second thoracic vertebra, etc.

T-bandage. Bandage resembling the letter T. SEE: *bandage.*

T-wave. One of the waves or elevations in an electrocardiogram due to ventricular activity.

T.A. Abbr. for *toxin-antitoxin.*

Ta. Chem. symbol for tantalum.

tabacism (tăb'ă-sĭzm) [L. *tabacum,* tobacco, + Gr. *-ismos,* condition]. Chronic tobacco poisoning. SYN: *tabacosis.*

tabacosis (tăb"ă-kō'sĭs) [" + Gr. *-ōsis,* condition]. Chronic tobacco poisoning, esp. from inhaling tobacco dust.

tabacum (tă-bā'kum, tăb'ă-kum) [L.]. Tobacco.

tabagism (tăb'ă-jĭzm) [" + Gr. *-ismos,* condition]. Tobacco poisoning. SYN: *tabacosis.*

Tabanidae (tŭ-băn'ĭ-dē) [L. *tabānus,* horsefly]. A family of insects belonging to the order Diptera. It includes horseflies, gadflies, deer flies, and mango flies, all bloodsucking insects which attack man and other warm-blooded animals. T. is of medical importance in that flies serve in the transmission of the filaria worm, Loa loa, tularemia, anthrax, and other diseases. Their bites are extremely painful and heal with difficulty.

tabardillo (tăb'är-dē'lyō) [Sp.]. Mexican typhus. SEE: *typhus.*

tabatière anatomique (tŏ-bŏ''tē-ăr'ŏ-nä''tō-mēk') [Fr., anatomical snuffbox]. Depression at base of thumb in back when thumb is extended.

tabella (tă-bĕl'ă) [L., tablet]. (pl. *tabel'lae*) A medicated mass of material formed into a small disk.
RS: disk; lozenge; tablet; troche.

tabes (tā'bēz) [L., wasting away]. 1. A gradual, progressive wasting in any chronic disease. 2. Tabes dorsalis, q.v.

SYM: Postural instability, esp. when eyes are closed, and a staggering, wide-base gait are characteristic; hence the name locomotor ataxia. Pains and paresthesias are common, esp. lightning pains, described as sharp, stabbing, and paroxysmal. Ankle and knee reflexes are diminished or lost. Many symptoms characteristic of syphilis such as pupillary changes; optic atrophy; bladder disturbances; development of trophic ulcers, esp. on feet, make diagnosis certain.

TREATMENT: Antiluetic treatment as in syphilis. Special measures should be taken to relieve pains which are most troublesome. Rehabilitation measures are often essential for those with disturbed gait. SEE: *syphilis.*

t., cerebral. Chronic degenerative brain disease with physical and mental deterioration. SYN: *general paresis.*

t., cervical. T. first affecting the upper extremities.

t., diabetic. Peripheral neuritis affecting diabetics. May affect spinal cord and simulate t. dorsalis.

t. dorsalis. A form of neurosyphilis characterized by chronic and usually progressive degeneration of ascending fibers of sensory neurons in posterior columns of spinal cord and usually also involving dorsal roots and ganglia of spinal nerves. SYN: *locomotor ataxia; tabetic neurosyphilis.*

t. ergotica. T. resulting from the use of ergot.

t., marantic. T. with great emaciation.

t. mesenterica. Emaciation and general disorder of the functions of nutrition due to engorgement and tubercular degeneration of the mesenteric glands.

tabetic (tă-bĕt'ĭk) [L. *tabes,* wasting away]. Pert. to or afflicted with tabes or tabes dorsalis.

t. ataxia. Occurs when there are lesions of first order of sensory neurons.

t. crises. Paroxysms of pain or other acute manifestations of episodic character in tabes dorsalis.

t. foot. Twisted foot in locomotor ataxia.

tabetiform (tă-bĕt'ĭ-fōrm) [" + *forma,* shape]. Resembling or characteristic of tabes.

table (tā'bl) [L. *tabula,* a board]. 1. A flat-topped structure, as an operating table. 2. A thin, flat plate, as of bone.

t.'s of skull. Inner and outer condensed layers of the cranial bone separated by diploe (cancellous bony tissue).

t., vitreous. The inner cranial t.

t.'s of weights and measures. SEE: *Table of weights and measures* in *Appendix.*

tablespoon (tā'bl-spūn). A rough measure utilizing a household spoon. When instructed to administer a tablespoon of medicine, give 15 ml. of the substance. ABBR: tbsp.

tablet (tăb'lĕt) [O.Fr. *tablete,* a small table]. A small, disklike mass of medicinal powder.

t., coated. Usually made by coating compressed tablets with sugar, chocolate, etc.

t., compressed. Made by forcibly compressing the powdered substances into the desired shape; usually made to contain from 65 to 650 mg. of the active drug. Frequently they are very hard and not readily soluble.

t., dispensing. T.'s that contain a comparatively large amount of the active drug, as 1 gr. of strychnine sulfate. Used by pharmacists and dispensing physicians to avoid the necessity of weighing small amounts of a potent drug in filling prescriptions.

t., hypodermic. T.'s which frequently contain in addition to the active drug, some agents that produce chemical action when water is added, thus causing a rapid disintegration of the mass. Ex: t. triturates, q.v. Used to form injectable solutions.

t., sublingual. A small, flat, oval t. placed beneath the tongue to permit direct absorption of the active substance.

t. triturates. T.'s made by moistening the powder with a volatile liquid, as alcohol, and then molding into shape and allowing the liquid to evaporate. They seldom contain more than 65 mg. of the active agent. They usually disintegrate readily and are a very desirable form for administering certain drugs.

tablier (tă-blyā′) [Fr., apron]. Pudendal apron. Enlarged vulvae.

taboo [Polynesian *tabu, tapu,* inviolable]. An act, object, or social custom separated or set aside as being sacred or profane, thus forbidden for general use. SYN: *banned; prohibited.*

taboparalysis (tā″bō-păr-ăl′ĭ-sĭs) [L. *tabes,* a wasting, + *paralysis,* a loosening at the sides]. Tabes associated concurrently with general paralysis.

taboparesis (ta″bō-păr-ē′sĭs, -păr′ē-sĭs) [″+ Gr. *paresis,* relaxation]. General paralysis in combination with tabes. SYN: *taboparalysis.*

tabophobia (tā″bō-fō′bĭ-ă) [″+ Gr. *phobos,* fear]. A morbid fear of being afflicted with tabes, a common symptom of neurasthenia.

tabular (tăb′ū-lăr) [L. *tabula,* a table]. 1. Resembling a table. 2. Set up in columns, as a tabulation.

t. bone. A flat bone, or one with two compact bonelike parts with cancellous tissue between them.

tache (tŏsh) [Fr., spot]. A colored spot or macule on the skin, as a freckle.

t. blanche. A white spot on liver in some infectious diseases.

t. bleuatre. A blue spot on skin, usually due to bite of cutaneous parasites. SYN: *macula caerulea.*

t. cérébrale. The red line that occurs in meningitis and other nervous disorders, when the fingernail is drawn across the skin. q.v.

t. motrice. The motor end plate of a striated muscle fiber.

t. noir. A small round or oval ulcer covered by a black scab; the primary lesion of boutonneuse fever and rickettsialpox.

tachetic (tăk-ĕt′ĭk) [Fr. *tache,* spot]. Marked by purple or reddish blue patches (taches).

tachogram (tăk′ō-grăm) [Gr. *tachos,* speed, + *gramma,* mark]. A graphic tracing of rate of flow of blood.

tachography (tăk-ŏg′ră-fĭ) [″+ *graphein,* to write]. The recording of the speed of the blood circulation.

tachy- [Gr. *tachys,* swift]. Combining form meaning swift.

tachyarrhythmia (tăk″ĭ-ă-rĭth′mĭ-ă) [″+ *a,* not, + *rhythmos,* rhythm]. Irregularity of heart beat combined with rapid rate.

tachyauxesis (tăk″ĭ-ŏk-sē′sĭs) [″+ *auxesis,* increase]. Condition in which a part of an organism grows more rapidly than the whole.

tachycardia (tăk″ĭ-kăr′dĭ-ă) [″+ *kardia,* heart]. Abnormal rapidity of heart action.

t., atrial. SEE: *auricular fibrillation.*

t., atrioventricular. T. arising from stimuli in the A-V node characterized by sudden onset and cessation.

t., essential. Rapid, persistent heart action due to functional disturbance.

t., extrinsic. T. caused by factors outside the heart, as increased metabolism or instability of the nervous system.

t., intrinsic. T. caused by infection, as from rheumatism.

t., nodal. T. resulting from an increase in rhythmicity of A-V node over the S-A node. May be the result of digitalis therapy.

t., paroxysmal. Sudden and abrupt acceleration of cardiac rate, ceasing abruptly. Due to stimulus of cardiac contraction having its origin at an abnormal point. May go as high as 250 beats/minute. SEE: *arrhythmia; bradycardia.*

t., paroxysmal atrial. Paraoxysmal t. originating in an ectopic or abnormal focus in the atria. Occurs commonly in early childhood or early adulthood and usually in the absence of heart disease. Its cause is unknown.

t., paroxysmal ventricular. Paroxysmal t. originating in an ectopic or abnormal focus in the ventricles.

t., reflex. T. resulting from stimuli outside the heart, reflexly accelerating heart rate or depressing vagal tone.

t., sinus. Uncomplicated t. when sinus rhythm is faster than 100 beats/minute, as that due to exercise. Causes other than exercise include hyperthermia, thyrotoxicosis, hemorrhage, anoxia, infections, cardiac failure, and certain drugs such as atropine, epinephrine, and nicotine.

TREATMENT: T. sometimes ceases following procedures which cause vagal stimulation. Among these are pressure on one or both carotid sinuses, pressure on eyeballs, induction of gagging or vomiting, attempted expiration with glottis closed, lying down with feet in air, and bending over. If above procedures when employed singly are unsuccessful, two or more combined may produce desirable results. If these general measures are ineffective, specific therapy based on etiological factors will be required.

t. strumosa exophthalmica. T. occurring as a symptom of exophthalmic goiter.

t., ventricular. Rapid contractions of the ventricle, the atrial rhythm remaining unchanged.

tachycardiac (tăk″ĭ-kar′dĭ-ăk) [Gr. *tachys,* swift, + *kardia,* heart]. Pert. to or afflicted with tachycardia.

tachylalia (tăk″ĭ-lā′lĭ-ă) ["+ *lalein,* to speak]. Rapid speech.

tachymeter (tăk-ĭm′ĕ-tĕr) ["+ *metron,* measure]. Instrument for estimating the rapidity of any body in motion.

tachyphagia (tăk″ĭ-fā′jĭ-ă) [Gr. *tachys,* swift, + *phagein,* to eat]. Rapid eating.

tachyphasia (tăk″ĭ-fā′zĭ-ă) ["+ *phasis,* speech]. Very rapid or voluble speech. SYN: *tachyphrasia.*

tachyphrasia (tăk″ĭ-frā′zĭ-ă) ["+ *phrasis,* speech]. Excessive volubility or rapidity of speech, as seen in mental disorders. SYN: *tachyphasia.*

tachyphrenia (tăk″ĭ-frē′nĭ-ă) [Gr. *tachys,* swift, + *phrēn,* mind]. Abnormally rapid mental activity.

tachyphylaxis (tăk″ĭ-fĭ-lăk′sĭs) ["+ *phylaxis,* protection]. Rapid immunization to a toxic dose of a substance by previously injecting tiny doses of the same substance.

tachypnea (tăk″ĭp-nē′ă) ["+ *pnoia,* breath]. Abnormal rapidity of respiration.

t., nervous. Breathing with forty or more respirations per minute. It occurs in hysteria, neurasthenia, etc. If prolonged, this will cause excess loss of CO_2 and the hyperventilation syndrome will develop. SEE: *alkalosis, respiratory; hyperventilation.*

tachypsychia (tăk″ĭ-sī′kĭ-ă) [Gr. *tachys,* swift, + *psychē,* soul]. Rapid action of psychic processes.

tachyrhythmia (tăk″ĭ-rĭth′mĭ-ă) ["+ *rhythmos,* rhythm]. 1. Rapid heart action. SYN: *tachycardia.* 2. Increase in frequency of brain waves in electroencephalography up to 12-50/sec.

tachysterol (tă-kĭs′tĕ-rŏl). One of the isomers of ergosterol, q.v., obtained by irradiation.

tachysystole (tăk″ĭ-sĭs′tō-lē) [Gr. *tachys,* swift, + *systolē,* contraction]. Abnormally rapid systole. SEE: *extrasystole.*

tachytrophism (tăk″ĭ-trō′fĭzm) ["+ *trophē,* nourishment, + *-ismos,* condition]. Accelerated metabolism.

tactile (tăk′tĭl) [L. *tactilis*]. Perceptible to the touch.

t. corpuscles. Minute elongated bodies enclosing the endings of several afferent nerve fibers and serving as the receptor for slight pressure or touch. They are located in dermal papillae just beneath the epidermis and are most numerous on finger tips, toes, soles, palms, lips, nipples, and tip of tongue. SYN: *Meissner's corpuscle.*

t. disk. Tiny expanded end of a sensory nerve fiber found in epidermis and in epithelial root sheath of a hair. SYN: Merkel's disk.

t. system. That portion of the nervous system concerned with the sensation of touch. Includes sensory nerve endings (Meissner's corpuscles, Merkel's tactile disks, hair-root endings), afferent nerve fibers, conducting pathways in the cord and brain, and sensory (somesthetic) area of cerebral cortex.

tactometer (tăk-tŏm′ĕt-ĕr) [L. *tactus,* touch, + Gr. *metron,* measure]. Instrument for determining acuity of tactile sensitiveness.

tactual (tăk′tū-ăl) [L. *tactus,* touch]. Rel. to the sense of touch. SYN: *tactile.*

tactus (tăk′tŭs) [L.]. Touch.

t. eruditus, t. expertus. Sensitiveness of touch acquired by long practice, as by a diagnostician or surgeon.

taedium vitae (tē′dĭ-ŭm-wē′tē) [L.]. Weariness of life with suicidal inclination.

Taenia (tē′nĭ-ă) [L., tape]. A genus of parasitic flatworms belonging to the class Cestoda, phylum Platyhelminthes. They are elongated, ribbonlike worms consisting of a scolex, usually armed, and a chain of segments (proglottids). Adults live as intestinal parasites of vertebrates; larvae parasitize both vertebrates and invertebrates which serve as intermediate hosts. SEE: *taeniasis; tapeworm.*

T. rata. Diphyllobothrium latum. Causes vitamin B$_{12}$ deficiency in the host. SYN: *fish tapeworm.*

T. saginata. Tapeworm whose larval stages live in cattle, the adult living in the intestine of man. Humans acquire it by eating insufficiently cooked beef infested with the encysted larval form (cysticercus or bladder worm). Adult worms may reach a length of 15 to 20 ft. (4.6 to 6.1 meters) or longer. SYN: *beef tapeworm.*

T. solium. Tapeworm whose larval stages live in hogs, the adult living in the intestine of man. Humans acquire it by eating insufficiently cooked pork infested with larval form. Infected pork containing the bladder worm (Cysticercus cellulosae) is called measly pork. The cysticerci may also develop in humans, infection occurring from self-infection with eggs from contaminated hands or by hatching of eggs liberated in the intestine. SYN: *pork tapeworm.*

taenia (tē'nĭ-ă) [L., tape]. 1. Any bandlike structure. SYN: *tenia* [NA]. 2. A tapeworm.

t. coli. One of three bands of the large intestines into which muscular fibers are collected, i.e., t. mesocolica (mesenteric insertion), t. libera (opposite mesocolic band), and t. omentalis (at place of adhesion of omentum to transverse colon).

t. of the fimbriae. The folded or recurved lateral edge of the fimbria to which the epithelium covering the choroid plexus of the inferior horn of the lateral ventricle is attached.

t. pontis. One or two small transverse bands of fiber at rostral border of the pons. SYN: *fila lateralia.*

t. semicircularis. Stria terminalis, q.v.

t. thalami. Structure separating superior surface from lateral surface of thalamus, its lateral portion containing the stria medullaris.

t. ventriculi quarti. The thickened line of attachment of the arachnoid to lateral surface of the medulla. SYN: *ligula.*

t. ventriculi tertii. The taenia of the third ventricle. SYN: *stria medullaris thalami.*

taeniacide (tē'nĭ-ă-sīd) [L. *taenia,* tapeworm, + *cidus,* kill]. An agent that kills tapeworms.

taeniasis (tē-nĭ'ă-sĭs) ["+ Gr. *-iasis,* condition]. Condition of being infested with tapeworms of the genus Taenia, q.v. SEE: *tapeworm.*

taeniform (tē'nĭ-form) ["+ *forma,* shape]. Having the structure of, or resembling, a tapeworm.

taenifuge (tē'nĭ-fūj) [L. *taenia,* tapeworm, + *fuga,* flight]. An agent which expels tapeworms.

taeniophobia (tē"nĭ-ō-fō'bĭ-ă) ["+ Gr. *phobos,* fear]. Morbid fear of becoming infested with tapeworms.

tagging. Making a chemical or organic material easily measured or detected by using isotopes of the substance or by introducing radioactive elements into the formula. This technique is used to follow the metabolic path of substances as they travel through the body.

tagliacotian operation (tŏ-lē-ŏ-kŏ'shĭ-ăn). [Gasparo Tagliacozzi, It. surgeon, 1546-99]. Plastic operation on the nose in which skin is used from another part of the body. SYN: *rhinoplasty.*

tagma (tăg'mă) [Gr., a thing arranged]. (pl. *tagmas, tagmata*) An aggregate of molecules; protoplasm.

tail (tāl) [AS. *taegel*]. Posterior, long, flexible terminus, as the extremity of the spinal column. SEE: *cauda* [NA].

t. bone. Bone at caudal end of spine. SYN: *coccyx.*

tailor's cramp or spasm (tā'lor). An occupational neurosis characterized by spasm of the muscles of the arms and hands.

Tait's law (tāt). [Lawson Tait, Eng. gynecologist, 1849-1899]. A code that exploratory laparotomy should be made in every case of obscure abdominal or pelvic disease which is a threat to health or life.

Tait's operation. Repair of a torn perineum. SYN: *perineorrhaphy.*

take. A non-medical term used to indicate satisfactory response to smallpox vaccination or skin graft.

talalgia (tăl-ăl'jĭ-ă) [L. *talus,* heel, + Gr. *algos,* pain]. Pain in the heel or ankle. SYN: *pternalgia.*

talar (tā'lăr) [L. *tālāris,* of the ankle]. Pert. to the talus, the ankle.

talc (tălk) [Persian *talk*]. USP. Powdered soapstone; a soft, soapy powder; native hydrous magnesium silicate used as a dusting powder.

talcum (tălk'ŭm) [L.]. SEE: *talc.*

talipes (tăl'ĭ-pēz) [L. *talus,* ankle, + *pēs,* foot]. Any of a number of deformities of the foot, esp. those occurring congenitally; a nontraumatic deviation of the foot in the direction of one or the other of the four lines of movement, or of two of these combined.

t. arcuatus. Exaggerated normal arch of the foot. SYN: *t. cavus.*

t. calcaneus. Flexion of foot; condition in which the heel alone touches the ground, causing the patient to walk on inner side of heel. Often follows infantile paralysis of muscle of tendo Achillis.

t. cavus. T. arcuatus, q.v.

t. equinus. Extension of foot; form in which the person walks on the toes.

t. percavus. Excessive plantar curvature.

t. valgus. Abduction of foot; form with everted foot.

t. varus. Adduction of foot; condition in which foot is inverted.

talipomanus (tăl″ĭp-ŏm′ăn-ŭs) [L. *talus*, ankle, + *pēs*, foot, + *manus*, hand]. Deformity of the hand in which it is twisted out of shape. SYN: *clubhand.*

talocalcaneal (tā″lō-kăl-kā′nē-ăl) [″ + *calcaneum,* heel bone]. Pert. to the talus and calcaneus, bones of the tarsus.

talocrural (tā″lō-krū′răl) [″ + *crus,* leg]. Pert. to the talus and leg bones.

t. articulation. The ankle joint, a ginglymus or hinge joint.

talonid (tăl′ō-nĭd) [ME. *talon,* heel]. The crushing region, the posterior or heel part, of a lower molar tooth.

talus (tā′lŭs) [L., ankle]. (pl. *ta′li*) [NA] The ankle bone articulating with the tibia, fibula, calcaneus, and navicular bone. SYN: *astragalus.*

tambour (tŏm-būr′) [Fr., drum]. A shallow, drum-shaped appliance used in transmitting and registering arterial pulsations, blood pressure, respiratory movements, peristaltic contractions, and other slight movements.

Tamm-Horsfall urinary mucoprotein. The matrix of all casts in the urine. It is virtually invisible in ordinary bright-field microscopy but is readily seen using phase-contrast microscopy.

tampol. A medicated tampon.

tampon (tăm′pŏn) [Fr., plug]. A roll or pack made of various absorbent substances, cotton, rayon, wool, gauze, used to arrest hemorrhage or absorb secretions from a wound or body cavity.

t., menstrual. An absorbent material suitably shaped and prepared to provide a hygienic means of absorbing menstrual fluid in the vagina. A cord is attached and this remains outside the vagina to facilitate removal. These tampons are made for self-insertion. This is facilitated by the use of disposable hygienic paper container applicator tubes.

t., Mikulicz's. A large scale capillary drain. It consists of a square piece of iodoform gauze of requisite size, placed in a cavity and filled with narrow strips of plain gauze until the necessary degree of compres-

sion is secured. Used where there is parenchymatous oozing. Serves as a t. to arrest bleeding and also acts as a capillary drain.

t., nasal. Soft rubber bulb dilated with compressed air, used in plugging nostrils to stop hemorrhage from the nose.

t., rectal. T. made of piece of rubber tubing size of thumb, 12 in. (31 cm.) in length, covered with iodoform gauze. Into this tube is inserted a glass cylinder 3 in. (7.6 cm.) in length, over which the rubber tubing should extend 2 in. (5.1 cm.). An umbrella of iodoform gauze, 12x12 in. (31x31 cm.), is fastened to the tube by tying a silk ligature over it at a point corresponding with the glass cylinder. Strips of sterilized gauze are used in packing the space between the tube and umbrella or mantle of gauze after the tube has been inserted into rectum.

tamponade, tamponage (tăm″pŏn-ād′, tăm′pŏn-ōj) [Fr., plug]. To use or make use of a tampon.

t., balloon. Producing pressure against some object by use of a catheter surrounded by a balloon. Often used in the esophagus to arrest bleeding from varices. The catheter is placed in the esophagus and the balloon is inflated to approx. 35-44 mm. of mercury pressure.

NP: Patient's vital signs must be monitored carefully if balloon t. is used for esophageal t. When the balloon is in place the patient cannot swallow, thus appropriate oral intake orders will be followed. In addition patient will be instructed to expectorate saliva instead of swallowing it. If patient is unconscious, continuous drainage of the esophagus above the balloon will be required.

t., cardiac. Condition resulting from accumulation of excess fluid in the pericardium. May result from pericarditis or injuries to the heart or great blood vessels, with accumulation of blood.

tannin (tăn′ĭn) [Fr. *tanin*]. 1. Acid substance found in bark of certain plants and trees or their products, usually from nutgall. Found in coffee and to a greater extent in tea. 2. Any of several substances containing tannin.

ACTION AND USES: Astringent, antidote for various poisons, for burns, and as a hemostatic. It is constipating. It is partly eliminated in the urine as gallic acid.

tantalum (tăn′tă-lŭm). SYMB: *Ta.* At. wt. 180.947; at. no. 73. A metallic element derived from tantalite. Because it is noncorrosive and malleable, it has been used to repair cranial defects and as a wire suture.

tap (tăp). 1. [AS. *taeppa*]. To puncture or to empty of fluid by paracentesis. 2. [O.Fr. *taper*]. A slight blow.

tape (tāp) [AS. *taeppe*]. 1. A long, flexible, narrow strip of linen, cotton, paper, plastic, etc., such as adhesive t. 2. To wrap a part with a long bandage made of adhesive or other type of material.

tapetum (tă-pē'tŭm) [LL., a carpet]. A layer of fibers from the corpus callosum forming roof and lateral walls of inferior and posterior horns of lateral ventricles of the brain. Fibers pass to temporal and occipital lobes.

tapeworm (tāp'wŭrm) [AS. *taeppe*, a narrow band, + *wyrm*, worm]. Any of the species of parasitic worms belonging to the class Cestoda, phylum Platyhelminthes. A typical tapeworm consists of a scolex with hooks and suckers for attachment, and a series of segments or proglottids which vary in number from a few to several thousand. New proglottids are budded off of the scolex, so that a worm is actually a linear colony consisting of immature, mature, and ripe or gravid proglottids.

Adults live as endoparasites in the intestine. The terminal ripe proglottids containing the ova break off and pass out with the feces. Upon disintegration eggs develop into minute six-hooked oncospheres which when ingested by proper intermediate host, usually another vertebrate, develop in muscle tissues into an encysted larva known as a cysticercus or bladder worm. Infestation occurs when uncooked meat containing bladder worms is eaten. These develop into the mature adult in the primary host.

Species of medical importance are: Diphyllobothrium latum, Echinococcus granulosus, Hymenolepis nana, H. diminuta, Taenia saginata, and T. solium. q.v. SEE: *cysticercosis; cysticercus; hydatid; parganum; taeniasis.*

SYM: Often absent. If numerous, may cause intestinal obstruction. Occasionally mild systemic symptoms may occur from absorption of metabolic wastes. Sometimes there are dyspeptic symptoms.

t., armed. Taenia solium, the pork tapeworm, whose scolex possesses a row of hooks about the rostellum.

t., beef. Taenia saginata, q.v.

t., dog. Dipylidium caninum, q.v.

t., dwarf. Hymenolepis nana, q.v.

t., fish. Diphyllobothrium latum, q.v.

t., mouse. Hymenolepis diminuta.

t., pork. Taenia solium, q.v.

t., rat. Hymenolepis diminuta.

taphephobia, taphophobia (tăf'ē-fō'bĭ-ă, -ō-fō'bĭ-ă) [Gr. *taphos*, grave, + *phobos*, fear]. Abnormal fear of being buried alive.

tapinocephalic (tăp'ĭn-ō-sĕf-ăl'ĭk) [Gr. *tapeinos*, lying low, + *kephalē*, head]. Pert. to flatness of top of cranium.

tapinocephaly (tăp'ĭn-ō-sĕf'ă-lĭ). Flatness of top of the skull.

tapioca (tăp'ĭ-ō'kă) [AmerInd. *tipioca*]. The starchy substance of the cassava plant; a strictly carbohydrate food.

Food value of 100 gm. (cooked cream pudding): Cal. 134; protein 5.0 gm.; fat 5.1 gm.; carbohydrate 17.1 gm.; calcium 105 mg.

tapiroid (tā'pĭr-oyd) [Amerind. *tapira*, tapir, + Gr. *eidos*, form]. Resembling a tapir's snout; said of an elongated cervix uteri.

tapotement (tă-pōt-mā') [Fr.]. Percussion in massage. It is divided into *beating* with the clenched hand, used for sciatica and muscular atrophy; *clapping* performed with the palm of the hand, used to reach superficial nerves; *hacking* with the ulnar border of the hand, used principally around a nerve center and upon the muscles; *punctuation* with the tips of the fingers, used principally around the heart and upon the head.

The strength of the manipulations is a principal point in the massage treatment, and care must be taken not to bruise the patient. As a rule, begin with moderate pressure, ascertaining from the patient his sensation. White petrolatum or some other oleaginous substance should be used to avoid abrading the skin. SEE: *massage.*

tapping (tăp'ĭng). 1. [O.Fr. *taper*, of imitative origin]. Percussion in massage. SYN: *tapotement.* 2. [AS. *taeppa*, tap]. Removal of fluid from a cavity. SYN: *paracentesis.* SEE: *thoracentesis.*

tarantism (tăr'ăn-tĭzm) [It. *taranto*, tarantula, + Gr. *-ismos*, condition]. A nervous affection marked by stupor, melancholy and uncontrollable dancing mania. Popularly attributed to bite of tarantula.

tarantula (tă-răn'tū-lă). A large venomous spider much feared by many people; however, its bite is relatively harmless. SEE: *spider bites.*

tarassis (tă-ras'is) [Gr. *taraxis*, disturbance]. Hysteria in the male.

Tardieu's ecchymoses or spots (tăr-dyū'). [Auguste A. Tardieu, Fr. physician, 1818-79]. Subpleural spots of ecchymosis following death by strangulation.

tardive (tăr'dĭv) [Fr.]. Descriptive of a disease wherein the characteristic sign or symptom appears late in the course of the disease.

target (tăr'gĕt) [O.Fr. *targette*, light shield]. 1. The electrode on which cathode rays within an x-ray tube are focused and from which roentgen rays are emitted; usually of a heavy metal such as tungsten. 2. A tiny figure on an ophthalmometer's arm whose image is used to determine the amount of corneal astigmatism. SYN: *mire,* q.v.

t. cell. An abnormal erythrocyte with rounded central area which stains deeply, surrounded by a lightly staining area which in turn is surrounded by denser cytoplasm at the periphery of the cell, the whole somewhat resembling a target with a bull's eye; found in certain types of anemia and after splenectomy.

t. cell anemia. Thalassemia, q.v.

t. organ. The organ or structure toward which the effects of a drug, hormone, or therapeutic agent are primarily directed.

Tarnier's sign (tŏr-nē-ā′). [Etienne Stéphene Tarnier, French obstetrician, 1828-1897] A sign of impending abortion; the disappearance of angle between upper and lower uterine segments in pregnancy.

tarsadenitis (tăr-săd″ĕn-ī′tĭs) [Gr. *tarsos,* flat surface, + *adēn,* gland, + *-itis,* inflammation]. Inflamation of the tarsal or meibomian glands of eyelid.

tarsal (tăr′săl) [Gr. *tarsalis*]. 1. Pert. to the tarsus or supporting plate of the eyelid. 2. Pert. to the ankle or tarsus.

t. arches. Two branches, superior and inferior of the median palpebral artery supplying the eyelid.

t. bones. The seven bones of the ankle.

t. cartilage. The dense connective tissue of the tarsus of the eyelid. It is not cartilage. SYN: *palpebral cartilage.*

t. glands. Branched alveolar, sebaceous glands embedded in tarsus and opening on margin of eyelid. SYN: *meibomian glands.*

t. lacrimal glands. Accessory lacrimal glands located on inner surface of eyelids, esp. upper lid.

tarsalgia (tăr-săl′jĭ-ă) [Gr. *tarsos,* flat of the foot, + *algos,* pain]. Pain in tarsus or ankle. May be due to flatfoot, shortening of Achilles tendon, or other causes.

tarsalia (tar-sā′lĭ-ă) [L.]. (sing. *tarsale*) The tarsal bones.

tarsalis (tăr-sā′lĭs) [L.]. One of the tarsal muscles. SEE: *Table of Muscles* in *Appendix.*

tarsectomy (tăr-sĕk′tō-mĭ) [Gr. *tarsos,* flat of the foot, edge of eyelid, + *ektomē,* excision]. 1. Excision of tarsus or a tarsal bone. 2. Removal of tarsal plate of an eyelid.

tarsi. Pl. of tarsus, q.v.

tarsitis (tăr-sī′tĭs) [″ + *-itis,* inflammation]. 1. Inflammation of tarsus of the foot. 2. Inflammation of eyelid's border. SYN: *blepharitis.*

tarso- [Gr. *tarsos,* a broad flat surface]. Combining form meaning the flat of the foot, edge of the eyelid.

tarsocheiloplasty (tar″sō-kī′lō-plăs″tĭ) [Gr. *tarsos,* edge of eyelid, flat of the foot, + *cheilos,* lip, + *plassein,* to form]. Plastic surgery of borders of the eyelid.

tarsoclasia, tarsoclasis (tar″sō-klā′sĭ-ă, tar-sŏk′lās-ĭs) [″+ *klasis,* a breaking]. Surgical fracture of the tarsus for correction of clubfoot.

tarsomalacia (tar″sō-mă-lā′sĭ-ă) [″ + *malakia,* a softening]. Softening of the tarsal cartilages of the eyes.

tarsometatarsal (tar″sō-mĕt″ă-tar′săl) [″+ *meta,* between, + *tarsos,* flat of the foot]. Pert. to the tarsus and the metatarsus.

tarsophyma (tar″sō-fī′mă) [″+ *phyma,* a growth]. Any tarsal tumor of the eyelid. SYN: *hordeolum, sty.*

tarsoplasia, tarsoplasty (tar″sō-plā′zĭ-ă, tar′sō-plăs′tĭ) [Gr. *tarsos,* edge of eyelid, flat of the foot, + *plassein,* to form]. Plastic surgery of margin of the eyelid. SYN: *blepharoplasty.*

tarsoptosis (tars″ŏp-tō′sĭs) [″+ *ptōsis,* a dropping]. Falling of the tarsus. SYN: *flatfoot.*

tarsorrhaphy (tar-sor′ă-fĭ) [Gr. *tarsos,* edge of eyelid, flat of the foot, + *rhaphē,* a seam]. The operation of uniting the edges of the lids at the outer commissure for the purpose of reducing the width of the palpebral fissure.

tarsotomy (tar-sŏt′ō-mĭ) [″ + *tomē,* a cutting]. 1. Incision of tarsal cartilage of an eyelid. 2. Any surgical incision of the tarsus of the foot.

tarsus (tar′sus) [Gr. *tarsos,* a flat surface]. (pl. *tarsi*) 1. The ankle, with its seven bones located between bones of lower leg and metatarsus. It forms the proximal portion of the foot. It consists of the following bones: *calcaneus* (os calcis), *talus* (astragalus), *cuboid* (os cuboideum), *navicular* (scaphoid), and *first, second,* and *third cuneiform* bones. The talus articulates with the tibia and fibula; the cuboid and cuneiform bones with the metatarsals. SEE: *foot; skeleton; names of individual bones.*

2. A curved plate of dense white fibrous tissue forming supporting structure of eyelid. SYN: *tarsal plates.*

tartar (tar′tĕr) [Gr. *tartaron,* dregs]. Calcareous matter deposited upon the teeth. SYN: *calculus* or *dental calculus.*

t., cream of. Potassium bitartrate.

tartaric acid (tar-tăr′ĭk). Any one of four isomers of an organic compound, $C_4H_6O_6$. Used in making potassium acid tartrate which is cream of tartar.

tart cells. Certain cells containing altered nuclear material appearing along with L.E. cells in suspensions of leukocytes or bone marrow cells.

tar'trate. A salt of tartaric acid.

taste (tāst) [OFr. *taster*, to feel, to taste]. 1. To attempt to determine the flavor of a substance by touching it with the mouth. 2. A chemical sense dependent upon sense organs on the surface of the tongue. These organs, called taste buds, when appropriately stimulated, produce one or a combination of the four fundamental taste sensations: sweet, bitter, sour, and salt. The nervous impulses are carried to the brain by the lingual (from the anterior two-thirds of the surface) and the glossopharyngeal (from the posterior third) nerves.

Loss of taste may be due to bilateral disease of chorda tympani nerve and of gustatory fibers of the glossopharyngeal nerve.

RS: ageusia; agnosia; alliaceous; allotriogeustia; amblygeustia; appetite; degustation; dysgeusia; gustation; gustatory; hypergeusesthesia; hypogeusia; oxygeusia; parageusia; pseudogeusia.

t., after. The persistence of a taste sensation after removal of original stimulus.

t. area. Area in cerebral cortex at lower end of somesthetic area.

t. blindness. Inability to taste certain substances such as phenylthiocarbamide (PTC). May be due to a hereditary factor which is transmitted as a mendelian recessive trait.

t. buds. Sensory end organs which mediate the sensation of taste. They are oval structures located on surface of tongue, esp. sides of circumvallate papillae, on soft palate, epiglottis, and portions of pharynx. Each contains sensory, gustatory (taste) cells and supporting (sustentacular) cells. When stimulated by chemical stimuli, they give rise to sense of taste. SEE: *taste cells*.

t. cells. Neuroepithelial cells within a taste bud which serve as receptors for the sense of taste. Each possesses on the free surface a short taste hair which projects through the inner taste pore. SYN: *gustatory cells*.

T.A.T. Abbr. for *toxin-antitoxin* or *tetanus antitoxin*.

tattooing. Indelible marking of the skin produced by introducing minute amounts of pigments into the skin. Tattooing is usually done to produce a certain design, picture, or name dear to the recipient. When done commercially, sterile procedures are rarely used and infectious hepatitis virus may be transmitted to the customer. Technic may also be used to conceal a corneal leucoma, to mask pigmented areas of skin or to color skin to look like areola in mammoplasty.

taurocholemia (taw″rō-kō-lē′mĭ-ă) [Gr. *tauros*, a bull, + *cholē*, bile, + *haima*, blood]. Taurocholic acid in the blood.

tauto- [Gr.]. Prefix meaning the same.

tautomeral, tautomeric (taw-tŏm′ĕr-ăl, -tō-mĕr′ĭk) [Gr. *tauto*, the same, + *meros*, a part]. Noting certain neurons which send processes to the white matter on the same side of the spinal cord.

tautomerism (taw-tŏm′ĕr-ĭzm) [″ + ″ + -*ismos*, condition]. Phenomenon in which two formulae are possible and exist in dynamic equilibrium so that as the amount of one substance is altered the second is changed into the other form in order to maintain the equilibrium.

tautorotation (taw″tō-rō-tā′shŭn) [″ + L. *rotāre*, to turn round]. A change in specific rotation which occurs when a solution of certain sugars stands a while.

taxis (tăk′sĭs) [Gr. *taxis*, arrangement]. 1. Manual replacement or reduction of a hernia or dislocation. 2. The response of an organism to its environment; a turning toward (positive taxis) or away from (negative taxis) a particular stimulus, e.g. *chemotaxis*, q.v.

t., bipolar. Replacing of a retroverted uterus by drawing down the cervix in the vagina and pressing upward through the rectum.

taxonomy (tăks-ŏn′ō-mĭ) [″ + *nomos*, law]. Laws and principles of classification of animals and plants.

Tay-Sachs disease. [Warren Tay, English physician, 1843-1927; Bernard Sachs, American neurologist, 1858-1944]. The infantile form of amaurotic family idiocy characterized by a cherry-red macula lutea seen in ophthalmoscopic examination. It is a disorder of lipid metabolism. SEE: *amaurotic familial idiocy, infantile*.

Tb. Abbr. for *terbium*.

T.b. Abbr. for *tubercle bacillus; tuberculosis*.

TBP. Abbr. for *thyroxine-binding protein*.

tbsp. Abbr. for *tablespoon*.

Tc. Symb. for *technetium*.

t.d.s. Abbr. for L. *ter die sumendum*, to be taken three times a day.

Te. 1. Chem. symb. for tellurium. 2. Abbr. for *tetanus*.

tea (tē) 1. An infusion of a medicinal plant. 2. Leaves of plant Thea chinensis, from which a beverage is made.

COMP: The principal ingredients are caffeine and tannin but also contains dextrin, gum, nitrogenous extracts, oxalates, and traces of theobromine and theophylline.

t., black. Tea made from leaves which have been fermented before they are dried.

t., green. Tea prepared by heating leaves in open trays.

t., Paraguay copper. A tea made from the leaves and stems of the Ilex paraguayensis. It is a stimulating drink and contains volatile oil, tannin, and caffeine.

TEAB. Abbr. for *tetraethylammonium bromide.*

TEAC. Abbr. for *tetraethylammonium chloride,* q.v.

tear (tār). To separate or pull apart by force.

tear gas. SEE: *gas, tear.*

tears (tērz) [AS. *tēar*]. 1. The watery saline solution secreted by the lacrimal glands, q.v. They lubricate the surfaces between the eyeball and eyelids, i.e. the conjunctiva. 2. Hardened lumps or tearlike drops of any gummy or resinous material.

tease (tēz) [AS. *taesan,* to pluck]. To separate a tissue into minute parts with a needle to prepare it for the microscope.

teaspoon (tē'spōōn). A spoon holding approximately five ml. Teaspoons used in the home vary from three to six ml. When a teaspoon dose is prescribed or ordered, give five ml. of the substance. ABBR: tsp.

teat (tēt) [M.E. *tete,* from AS. *tit,* teat]. 1. The nipple of the mammary gland. SYN: *papilla mammilla.* 2. Any protuberance resembling a nipple.

teatulation (tēt"ū-lā'shŭn) [AS. *tit,* teat]. The development of a nipplelike elevation.

technetium (tĕk-nē'shĭ-ŭm). SYMB: *Tc.* At. wt. 99; at. no. 43. A metallic chemical element.

technetium⁹⁹ᵐ dioxide. A radioactive compound used in determining blood flow to certain organs by use of scanning technique. It has a half-life of six hours.

technic (tĕk'nĭk) [Gr. *technē,* art]. SEE: *technique.*

technical (tĕk'nĭ-kăl) [Gr. *tekhnikos,* skilled]. Requiring technic or special skill.

technician (tĕk-nĭsh'ăn) [Gr. *technē,* art]. One skilled in a special technique.

t., medical laboratory. A person who has received special training in medical laboratory procedures.

technique (tek-nēk') [Gr. *tekhnikos*]. 1. Systematic procedure or methods by which an involved or scientific task is completed. 2. The skill in performing details of a procedure or operation.

techno- [Gr.]. Combining form meaning art, skill.

technologist (tĕk"nŏl'ō-jĭst). A technician, esp. one who is highly trained.

t., medical. One who is certified by the Registry of Medical Technologists of the American Society of Clinical Pathologists.

tecno- [Gr.]. Combining form meaning child.

tectocephaly (tĕk-tō-sĕf'ăl-ĭ) [L. *tectum,* roof, + Gr. *kephalē,* head]. Possession of a boat-shaped cranium. SYN: *scaphocephalism.*

tectonic (tĕk-tŏn'ĭk) [Gr. *tektōn,* a builder]. Relating to plastic surgery or to surgery for the restoration of lost parts.

tectorial (tĕk-tō'rĭ-ăl) [L. *tectum,* roof]. Pert. to a roof or covering. SYN: *tegmental.*

tectorium (tĕk-tō'rĭ-ŭm) [L. *tectorium,* a covering]. 1. Any rooflike structure. 2. Corti's membrane. SYN: *membrana tectoria.*

tectospinal (tĕk"tō-spī'năl) [L. *tectum,* roof, + *spina,* thorn]. From the tectum mesencephali to the spinal cord.

t. tract. A tract of white fibers of the spinal cord passing from the tectum of midbrain and going down through the medulla to the spinal cord. It begins on one side and crosses to the other.

tectum (tĕk'tŭm) [L., roof]. 1. Any structure serving as, or resembling, a roof. 2. The dorsal portion of the midbrain consisting of the superior and inferior colliculi (corpora quadrigemina).

t. mesencephali. Roof of the midbrain including the corpora quadrigemina.

teenage. Pert. to those who are thirteen to nineteen years of age. SYN: *adolescent.*

teeth (tēth) [AS. *tōth,* tooth]. (sing. *tooth*) Hard, bony projections in jaws serving as organs of mastication, there being 32 permanent teeth, 16 in each jaw. They include the following types: incisors, canines, (cuspids), premolars (bicuspids), and molars. An average child should have 6 teeth at 1 year, 12 at 18 months, 16 at 2 years, and 20 at 2 1/2

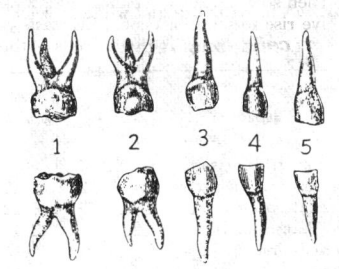

DECIDUOUS TEETH
1, Second molar. 2, First molar. 3, Canine. 4, Second incisor. 5, First incisor.

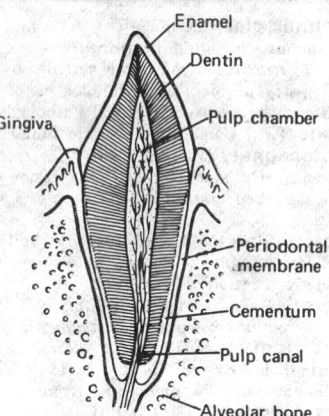

STRUCTURE OF TOOTH AND
RELATED TISSUES

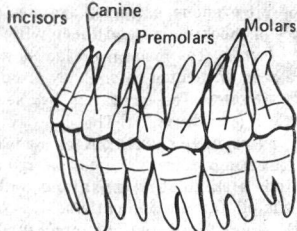

ADULT TEETH—LEFT SIDE

years. A child may be born with teeth, and in other cases the teeth may not appear until 16 months.

t., anterior. Two canine and four incisors in each jaw.

t., auditory. Minute toothlike projections along the free margin of the labium vestibulare of the cochlea. SYN: *Huschke's a. teeth.*

t., back. All posterior teeth (to the canines) of the molar series.

t., deciduous. Temporary or milk teeth; those comprising the first set, which are shed.

t., Hutchinson's. Lateral incisors of upper jaw when pegged and central incisors of same jaw having convex sides and crescentic notches on their cutting edges; noted only on permanent teeth, indicating hereditary syphilis.

t., malacot'ic. Those which are apt to decay, soft in structure and white in color.

t., milk. The first set of teeth. SYN: *deciduous teeth.*

t., permanent. Those of the second dentition, replacing the deciduous teeth.

t., sclerotic. Yellowish teeth that are naturally hard and not subject to ready decay.

t., secondary. The permanent teeth erupting about the 6th year and being complete about the 15th year.

t., temporary. Those of the first dentition; the milk or deciduous teeth.

teething (tēth'ĭng) [AS. *tŏth*, tooth]. Eruption of the teeth. SYN: *dentition.*

tegmen (tĕg'mĕn) [L. *tegmen*, covering]. (pl. *tegmina*) A structure that covers a part.

t. mastoidem. Bony roof of mastoid cells.

t. tympani. Roof of tympanum separating middle ear from cranial cavity.

t. ventriculi quarti. The roof of the fourth ventricle.

tegmental (tĕg-mĕn'tăl) [L. *tegmentum*, covering]. Relating to a tegument or tegmentum; covering.

t. nuclei. Several masses of gray matter lying in tegmentum of midbrain and upper portion of the pons. Include the dorsal, pedunculopontile, reticular, and ventral nuclei.

Deciduous Teeth	
Name	**Erupt (months)**
Lower central incisors	5–9
Upper central incisors	8–12
Upper lateral incisors	10–12
Lower lateral incisors	12–15
Anterior (first) molars	12–15
Canines	18–24
Posterior (second) molars	24–30

Permanent Teeth	
Name	**Erupt (years)**
First molars	6–7
Central incisors	7–8
Lateral incisors	7–8
First premolars	9–10
Second premolars	9–10
Canines	12–14
Second molars	12–15
Third molars	17–25

tegmentum (tĕg-mĕn'tŭm) [L., covering]. 1. A roof or covering. 2. The dorsal portion of cruri cerebri of the midbrain. It contains the red nucleus and nuclei and roots of the oculomotor nerve.

tegument (tĕg'ū-mĕnt). 1. The skin; the covering of the body. SYN: *integument.* 2. A covering structure.

tegumental, tegumentary (tĕg"ū-mĕn'tăl, -tă-rĭ). Concerning the skin or tegument; covering.

teichopsia (tĭ-kŏp'sĭ-ä) [Gr. *teichos,* wall, + *opsis,* vision]. Zigzag lines bounding a luminous area appearing in the visual field causing a temporary blindness in that portion of the eye, sometimes accompanying migraine headaches and mental or physical strain. SYN: *scotoma, scintillating; scotoma, fortification spectra.*

teinodynia (tī"nō-dĭn'ĭ-ä) [Gr. *tenōn,* tendon, + *odynē,* pain]. Pain in the tendons. SYN: *tenodynia.*

tela (tē'lä) [L. *tēla,* web]. (Pl. *telae*) Any weblike structure.

    t. choroi'dea. Part of the pia mater covering roof of the 3rd and 4th cerebral ventricles.

    t. subcutanea. Subcutaneous connective tissue; superficial fascia.

    t. submucosa. The submucosa of the intestine.

telalgia (tĕl-ăl'jĭ-ä) [Gr. *tēle,* far away, + *algos,* pain]. Pain felt at a distance from its stimulus. SYN: *pain, referred.*

telangiectasia, telangiectasis (tel-ăn"jĭ-ĕk-tā'zhĭ-ä, -ĕk'tă-sĭs) [Gr. *telos,* end, + *angeion,* vessel, + *ektasis,* dilatation]. Dilatation of capillaries and sometimes of terminal arteries producing an angioma of macular appearance, or hyperemic spot.

    It may be as a birthmark, or become apparent in young children. May occur anywhere in the skin but is seen most frequently on the face and thighs.

    t. faciei. Acne rosacea, q.v.

    t., hereditary hemorrhagic. A hereditary disease characterized by thinness of walls of blood vessels of nose, skin, and digestive tract and tendency to hemorrhage. SYN: *Osler-Weber-Rendu disease.*

    t. lymphat'ica. Tumor composed of dilated lymph vessels.

    t., spider. A stellate angioma (nevus araneus).

telangiectoma (tĕl-ăn-jĭ-ĕk-tō'mä) ["+ "+ "+ -ōma, tumor]. Angioma from dilatation of capillaries or arterioles. SYN: *telangioma.*

telangiitis (tĕl-ăn-jĭ-ī'tĭs) ["+ "+ -ītis, inflammation]. Inflammation of the capillaries.

telangioma (tĕl-lăn"jĭ-ōmä) [Gr. *tele,* far off, + *angeion,* vessel, + *-ōma,* tumor]. A tumor made up of dilated capillaries or arterioles.

telangiosis (tĕl"ăn-jĭ-ō'sĭs) ["+ "+ -ōsis, condition]. Disease of capillary vessels.

tele-, tel- [Gr.]. Combining forms meaning at a distance, far off.

telecardiogram (tel"ĕ-kar'dĭ-ō-grăm) [Gr. *tele,* distant, + *kardia,* heart, + *gramma,* a writing]. A cardiogram which records at a distance from the patient. SYN: *telelectrocardiogram.*

telecardiography (tĕl"ĕ-kar"dĭ-og'ră-fĭ) ["+ "+ *graphein,* to write]. Process of taking telecardiograms.

telecardiophone (tĕl"ĕ-kar'dĭ-ō-fōn) ["+ "+ *phōnē,* voice]. A stethoscope which will magnify heart sounds so that they may be heard at a distance from patient.

teleceptive (tĕl-ĕ-sĕp'tĭv) ["+ L. *-ceptivus,* take]. Relating to a teleceptor.

teleceptor (tĕl'ĕ-sĕp-tor) [Gr. *tele,* distant, + L. *ceptor,* a receiver]. A distance receptor; a sense organ that responds to stimuli arising some distance from the body. Ex: eye, ear, nose. SYN: *teloceptor.*

telecinesia (tĕl"ĕ-sĭn-ē'zĭ-ä) ["+ *kinēsis,* movement]. Apparent automatic movement of an object produced without contact with any stimulus or power. SYN: *telekinesia.*

telecurietherapy (tĕl-ĕ-kū-rĭ-thĕr'ă-pĭ) [Gr. *tele,* distant, + *curie* + Gr. *therapeia,* treatment]. Application of radium rays from a distance from a patient.

teledendrite, teledendron (tĕl-ĕ-dĕn'drĭt, -dĕn'drŏn) ["+ *dendron,* a tree]. The terminal processes of an axon. SYN: *telodendron.*

telediastolic (tĕl"ĕ-dī-ă-stŏl'ĭk) [Gr. *telos,* end, + *diastolē,* a dilatation]. Concerning the last phase of the diastole.

telegony (tĕl-ĕg'ō-nĭ) [Gr. *tēle,* distant, + *gonē,* offspring]. An alleged theory that the male sperm from a dam's first sexual contact modifies the blood of the female, thus influencing the offspring resulting from mating with another sire.

telelectrocardiogram (tĕl"ĕ-lĕk"trō-kar'dĭ-ō-grăm) ["+ *elektron,* amber (electricity), + *kardia,* heart, + *gramma,* a writing]. One taken with a galvanometer attached to the patient by a wire some distance from the instrument. SYN: *telecardiogram.*

telemeter (tĕl-ĕ-mē'tĕr) ["+ *metron,* measure]. To transmit information to a distant point by using electronic devices.

telencephalic (těl-ěn-sěf-al'ĭk) ["+ *enkephalos*, brain]. Pert. to the endbrain (telencephalon).

telencephalon (těl-ěn-sěf'ă-lŏn) [Gr. *telos*, end, + *enkephalos*, brain]. The embryonic endbrain or anterior division of the prosencephalon from which the cerebral hemispheres, corpora striata, and rhinencephalon develop.

teleo- [Gr.]. Combining form meaning perfect, complete.

teleology (těl-ē-ŏl'ō-jĭ) [Gr. *telos*, end, + *logos*, a study]. The belief that everything is directed toward some final purpose. The doctrine of final causes.

teleoperator. Device used to extend and amplify man's muscular dexterity. Usually used as a mechanical extension of the hands and arms into areas where it would be impossible for a man to work. Ex: a hot oven; into a laboratory containing radioactive isotopes.

teleopsia (těl-ē-ŏp'sĭ-ă) ["+ *ops*, eye]. A visual disorder in which objects perceived in space have excessive depth or close objects appear far away.

teleorganic (těl''ē-or-găn'ĭk) ["+ *organon*, organ]. Necessary to organic life. SYN: *vital*.

teleotherapeutics (těl''ē-ō-ther-ă-pū'tĭks) [Gr. *tēle*, far off, + *therapeutikē*, treatment]. The use of hypnotic suggestion in the treatment of disease. SYN: *suggestive therapeutics*.

telepathist (tě-lěp'ă-thĭst) [Gr. *tēle*, distant, + *pathos*, feeling]. One who claims the ability to read the mind of others.

telepathy (tě-lěp'ă-thĭ) ["+ *pathos*, feeling]. Supposed communication of one mind with another at a distance without any means known to physical or psychological science.

teleradiography (těl''ē-rā-dĭ-og'ră-fĭ) [Gr. *tēle*, distant, + L. *radius*, ray, + Gr. *graphein*, to write]. Radiography with the tube about two meters (6 1/2 ft.) from the body. Done to minimize distortion by having rays virtually parallel at that distance. SYN: *teleroentgenography*.

telergy (těl'ěr-jĭ) ["+ *ergon*, work]. 1. Action without conscious exercise of the will. SYN: *automatism*. 2. Hypothetical action of one individual's thoughts upon brain of another by transmission of some unknown form of energy.

teleroentgenography (těl''ē-rěnt'gěn-ŏg'ră-fĭ) ["+ *roentgen*+ Gr. *graphein*, to write]. Radiography in which the tube is about two meters (6 1/2 ft.) from the body. SYN: *teleradiography*.

telesthesia (těl-ěs-thē'zĭ-ă) ["+ *aisthēsis*, sensation]. 1. An impression received at a distance without normal operation of organs of sense. 2. Distance perception. SYN: *telepathy*.

telesystolic (těl''ē-sis-tol'ĭk) [Gr. *telos*, end + *systolē*, contraction]. Pert. to the termination of the cardiac systole.

teletactor (tel''ē-tăk'tŏr) ["+ L. *tactus*, touch]. A device used by the deaf to receive vibrations through the skin.

teletherapy (těl-ē-thěr'ă-pĭ) [Gr. *tēle*, distant, + *therapeia*, treatment]. Absent treatment; treatment of disease by telepathy, q.v.; method of mental healers.

telluric (tě-lūr'ĭk) [L. *tellūs*, earth]. Of or rel. to the earth.

tellurium (těl-ū'rĭ-ŭm) [L. *tellus*, earth]. SYMB: *Te*. At. wt. 127.60; at. no. 52; sp. gr. 6.24. A nonmetallic element used as an electric rectifier and in coloring glass.

POISONING SYM: Garlic odor of all secretions and excretions. A disagreeable odor to the breath with suppression of perspiration and saliva, resulting in dry skin and mouth. Anorexia, nausea, drowsiness, and weakness.

F.A. TREATMENT: Give saline cathartics; increase fluid intake; induce perspiration; otherwise treatment is symptomatic.

teloceptor. Teleceptor, q.v.

telodendron (těl-ō-děn'drŏn) [Gr. *telos*, end, + *dendron*, a tree]. The more or less diffuse arborizations at the end of an axon or its collaterals.

telolecithal (těl-ō-lěs'ĭ-thăl) ["+ *lekithos*, yolk]. Term applied to an ovum in which the yolk is concentrated at one end.

telolemma (těl''ō-lěm'mă) ["+ *lemma*, rind]. The membrane covering motor end plate in a striated muscle fiber.

telophase (těl'ō-fāz) [Gr. *telos*, end, + *phasis*, a phase]. The final phase or stage of mitosis (karyokinesis) during which reconstruction of the daughter nuclei takes place and the cytoplasm of the cell divides giving rise to two daughter cells.

telosynapsis (těl''ō-sĭ-năp'sĭs) ["+ *synapsis*, conjunction]. End-to-end union of pairs of homologous chromosomes during gametogenesis.

telotism (těl'ō-tĭzm) ["+ *-ismos*, process]. The entire performance of a function, as that of one of the senses.

TEM. Abbr. for *triethylene melamine.* SEE: *nitrogen mustard.*

tempeh. A wheat-soy bean food developed as an excellent source of protein for children in economically depressed countries. Quality of protein is almost equal to casein.

temperament (těm'per-ă-měnt) [L. *temperamentum*, mixture]. The combination of intellectual, emotional, ethical, and physical characteristics of a specific individual.

t., bilious. Temperament characterized by olive or dark skin, brunet hair, well-developed physique, a hot or quick temper.

t., choleric. Same as bilious t.

t., melancholic. Temperament characterized by a state of depression; melancholia.

t., sanguine. Temperament marked by a ruddy complexion, fair hair, light-colored eyes, active blood circulation, and a generally optimistic mental outlook.

temperate (tĕm′per-ĭt). Moderate; not excessive.

temperature (tĕm′per-ă-tūr) [L. *temperatura,* proportion]. 1. Degree of heat of a living body; loosely, body heat above normal. 2. Degree of hotness or coldness of a substance.

Body t. varies with different organs' areas and with the time of day. The t. in the liver may by 105° F. (40.6° C.), while that under the tongue is 98.6° F. (37° C.); the t. under the arm at 2 P.M. may be 99.0° F. (37.2° C.) and at 2 A.M. 96.7° F. (35.9° C.); the rectal temperature is likely to be 0.5-1.0° F. (.28°-.56° C.) above the oral.

One of the mechanisms for raising t. is muscular work (as in shivering); one for lowering it is sweating. The interplay of such processes keeps the body t. constant.

Body t. may be measured by a clinical thermometer placed in the mouth, rectum, or under the arm. Rectal t. usually is from 0.5-1.0° F. (.28°-.50° C.) higher than by mouth; axillary t. about 0.5° F. (.28° C.) lower than by mouth. Oral t. may be inaccurate if taken just after the patient has eaten or drunk cold substances.

Body t. is the result of the balance between heat production and heat loss. 85% of body heat is lost through the skin, the remainder via lungs and through digestive and urinary excretions. Regulation of body t. is accomplished principally through thermoregulatory centers located in the hypothalamus. Elevation of t. above normal is designated fever (pyrexia), subnormal t. is hypothermia.

t., absolute. T. measured from absolute zero, which is –273° C.

t., axillary. Thermometer is placed in apex of axilla with arm pressed closely to side of body. Temperature obtained by this method is usually 0.5 to 1.0° F. (.28°-.56° C.) lower than oral.

t., body. The t. of the body.

t., critical. The t. below which a gas may be converted to liquid form by pressure.

t. curve. Line indicating the fluctuations of t. for a given period.

t. equivalents. SEE: *Fahrenheit scale.* To convert Fahrenheit t. to Centigrade use this formula:

$$°C. = \frac{(F. - 32)}{9} \times 5.$$

To convert Centigrade t. to Fahrenheit use this formula:

$$°F. = \frac{9}{5} C. + 32.$$

t., inverse. Condition in which body temperature is higher in the morning than in the evening.

t., maximum. T. above which bacterial growth will not take place.

t., mean. The average t. for a stated period in a given locality.

t., minimum. T. below which bacterial growth will not take place.

t., normal. T. of the body, taken orally, in a healthy individual; 98.6° F. (37° C.) in man.

t., optimum. T. at which an operation is best carried out, as the culture of a given organism or the action of a new enzyme.

t., oral. Thermometer is held for three minutes under patient's tongue with lips closed. It should not be taken for at least 10 min. after ingestion of hot or cold liquids. It is not advisable for infants, mouth-breathers, comatose patients, or those extremely ill.

t., rectal. The thermometer should be inserted at least 1 1/2 in. (3.8 cm.) and allowed to remain 3-5 minutes. Do not take following a rectal operation or if rectum is diseased. Rectal t. is more accurate than either oral or axillary temperatures. It averages about 1° F. (.56° C.) higher than by mouth.

t., room. T. between 65-80° F. (18.3° to 26.7° C.).

t. scale. Graduated device marked at regular intervals on a thermometer to register temperature.

RS: thermometer scale.

t. scale, absolute. One in which absolute zero (–273° C. or –459.4° F.) is taken as zero. This is the point at which molecular motion has ceased, and there is complete absence of heat.

t. senses. The sensations of warmth resulting from raising the temperature of the skin and that of cold aroused by lowering it. The sensation of warmth is mediated by Ruffini's corpuscles, that of cold by end-bulbs of Krause. These receptors are distribut̃ed so as to form cold and warm spots on the skin. Afferent impulses from receptors, on reaching the thalamus, may give rise to crude uncritical temperature sensations; on being relayed to the somesthetic area of the cortex they result in discrete and fairly well localized sensations of heat and cold. Adaptation is rapid.

t., subnormal. T. below the normal of 98.6° F. (37° C.).

temperature, words pert. to: algid; a. stage; algogenic; chauffage; cold; frigid; frigidity; frigorific; hardening; heat; infant; myothermic; pseudocrisis; respiration; temperature scale; "therm-" words.

template (těm-plāt). A pattern, mold, or form used as a guide in duplicating a shape, structure, or device.

temple (těm'pl) [O.Fr. from L. *tempora,* pl. of *tempus,* temple]. The region of head in front of ear and over the zygomatic arch.

tempolabile (těm″pō-lā'bl) [L. *tempus,* time, + *labilis,* unstable]. Becoming altered spontaneously within a definite time.

temporal (těm'por-ăl) [L. *temporalis,* pert. to time; pert. to temples]. 1. Pert. to or limited in time. 2. Relating to the temples.

t. bone. A bone on both sides of the skull at its base. Composed of squamous, mastoid, and petrous portions, the latter enclosing the organ of hearing. SYN: *os temporale.* SEE: *Arnold's canal; mastoid; petrosa; petrosal; squamous; styloid process.*

t. line. One of two lines on lateral surface of frontal and parietal bones which mark upper limit of temporal fossa.

t. lobe. Lobe of cerebrum located laterally and below frontal and occipital lobes. Contains auditory receptive areas.

temporalis (těm″pō-rā'lĭs) [L.]. Muscle in temporal fossa which elevates the mandible. SEE: *Table of Muscles* in *Appendix.*

temporo- [L.]. Combining form meaning temples of the head.

temporomaxillary (těm″pō-rō-măk'sĭ-lěr-ĭ) [L. *tempus, tempor-,* temple]. Pert. to the temporal and maxillary bones.

temporo-occipital (těm″pō-rō-ŏk-sĭp'ĭ-tăl) ["+ *occipitalis,* pert. to the occiput]. Pert. to the temporal and occipital bones or their regions.

temporosphenoid (těm″pō-rō-sfē'noyd) ["+ Gr. *sphēn,* wedge, + *eidos,* form]. Pert. to the temporal and sphenoid bones.

temulence (těm'ū-lěns) [L. *temulentia,* intoxication]. Drunkenness; intoxication.

tenacious (tě-nā'shŭs) [L. *tenax*]. Adhering to; adhesive; retentive.

tenacity (tě-năs'ĭ-tĭ). The condition of being tough, stubborn, obstinate.

tenaculum (těn-ăk'ū-lŭm) [L. a holder]. Sharp, hooklike, pointed instrument with slender shank for grasping and holding a part, as an artery.

t., abdominal. Longer than others with smaller hook. Ex: Sim's, Emmet's, Kelly's.

t., uterine. Heavier and shorter hook used for manipulating uterus.

tenalgia (těn-ăl'jĭ-ă) [Gr. *tenōn,* tendon, + *algos,* pain]. Pain in a tendon. SYN: *tenodynia.*

t. crepitans. Inflammation of a tendon sheath which on movement results in a crackling sound. SYN: *tendosynovitis crepitans.*

tenderizers. Preparations, containing proteolytic enzymes such as papain or bromelin, used to make meat more tender.

tenderness (těn'dẽr-něs). Sensitiveness to pain upon pressure.

t., rebound. Production of or intensification of pain when pressure is released.

tendinitis (těn″dĭn-i'tĭs) [L. *tendo,* tendon, + Gr. *-itis,* inflammation]. Inflammation of a tendon. SYN: *tenonitis; tenontitis.*

tendinoplasty (těn'dĭ-nō-plăs″tĭ) ["+ Gr. *plassein,* to form]. Plastic surgery of tendons. SYN: *tenontoplasty; tenoplasty.*

tendinosuture (těn″dĭn-ō-sū'chŭr) ["+ *sutura,* sewing]. The suturing of a divided tendon. SYN: *tenorrhaphy.*

tendinous (těn'dĭ-nŭs) [L. *tendinōsus*]. Pert. to, composed of, or resembling tendons.

t. synovitis. Inflammation of a tendon's synovial sheath.

ten'do [L.]. (pl. *tendines*) [NA] A tendon.

t. Achillis. The tendon of the soleus and gastrocnemius muscles inserted into the tuberosity of the os calcis.

t. calca'neus. [NA] T. Achillis, q.v.

tendolysis (těn-dŏl'ĭ-sĭs) [L. *tendo,* tendon, + Gr. *lysis,* a loosening]. The process of freeing a tendon from adhesions.

tendon (těn'dŭn) [L. *tendo,* tendon]. Fibrous connective tissue serving for the attachment of muscles to bones and other parts. SYN: *sinew.*

RS: Achilles jerk; achillobursitis; achillotomy; aponeurotomy; "teno-" words.

t., Achilles. The large tendon at lower end of gastrocnemius muscle, inserted into the os calcis. It is the strongest and thickest t. in the body.

t., calcaneous. T., Achilles, q.v.

t., cells. Fibroblasts of white fibrous connective tissue of tendons arranged in parallel rows.

t., central. The central portion of the diaphragm consisting of a flat aponeurosis in which fibers of the diaphragm are inserted.

t. reflex. Reflex act in which a muscle contracts when its t. is percussed.

t. r., patellar. Slight extension of the leg when t. of quadriceps muscle is tapped immediately below the patella. Tested with the leg slightly bent at the knee if patient is in bed. May be tested while leg hangs free when patient is sitting on edge of bed. SYN: *knee jerk; patellar reflex.*

t. spindle. Fusiform nerve ending in a t.

t., superior, of Lockwood. Portion of fibrous ring from which superior oblique muscle of eye originates.

t. of Zinn. Portion of the fibrous ring (annulus tendineus communis) from which inferior rectus muscle of eye originates.

tendonitis [L. *tendo,* tendon, + Gr. *itis,* inflammation]. Inflammation of a tendon.

tendoplasty (těn′dō-plăs″tĭ) [L. *tendo,* tendon, + Gr. *plassein,* to mold]. Reparative surgery of an injured tendon. SYN: *tenoplasty; tenontoplasty.*

tendosynovitis (těn″dō-sĭn″ō-vī′tĭs) ["+ *syn,* with, + *ovum,* egg, + Gr. *-itis,* inflammation]. Inflammation of a sheath of a tendon or the tendon. SYN: *tendovaginitis, tenosynovitis.*

t. crepitans. T. accompanied by a crackling sound on movement.

tendotome (těn′dō-tōm) ["+ Gr. *tomē,* cutting]. Instrument for severing a tendon. SYN: *tenotome.*

tendotomy (těn-dŏt′ō-mĭ). Division of a tendon. SYN: *tenotomy.*

tendovaginal (těn″dō-văj′ĭ-năl) [L. *tendo,* tendon, + *vagina,* sheath]. Rel. to a tendon and its sheath.

tendovaginitis (těn″dō-văj′ĭn-ī′tĭs) ["+ "+ Gr. *-itis,* inflammation]. Inflamed condition of a tendon and its sheath. SYN: *tenosynovitis.*

Tenebrio (tě-něb′rĭ-ō). A genus of beetles including the species of T. molitor which serves as intermediate host for the tapeworm Hymenolepis diminuta.

tenec′tomy [Gr. *tenōn,* tendon, + *ektomē,* excision]. Excision of a lesion of a tendon or tendon sheath; removal of a ganglion or xanthoma.

tenesmic (těn-ěz′mĭk) [Gr. *teinesmos,* a stretching]. Pert. to or like tenesmus.

tenesmus (tě-něz′mŭs). Spasmodic contraction of anal or vesical sphincter with pain and persistent desire to empty the bowel or bladder, with involuntary, ineffectual straining efforts.

teni-. SEE: words beginning with *taeni.*

teniasis (tē-nī′ă-sĭs) [L. *taenia,* tapeworm, + Gr. *-iasis,* a condition]. Presence of tapeworms in the body.

tenifuge (těn′ĭ-fūj) ["+ *fuga,* flight]. Causing or that which causes explusion of tapeworms. SYN: *teanifuge.*

ten′nis el′bow. An obscure, insidious, distressing complaint after playing tennis following a period of muscular inactivity of the arm or following a long duration of play.

SYM: Pain over lateral epicondyle of humerus radiating to outer side of arm and forearm and aggravated by dorsiflexion and supination of wrist. Weakness of wrist and difficulty in grasping objects.

TREATMENT: In mild cases, immobilization by a splint or adhesive strapping, supplemented by heat or diathermy. In long continued cases, surgical intervention may be indicated.

teno- [Gr. *tenōn*]. Combining form indicating tendon.

tenodesis (těn-ŏd′ě-sĭs) [Gr. *tenōn,* tendon, + *desis,* a binding]. Suturing of the end of a tendon to a point of attachment.

tenodynia (těn″ō-dĭn′ĭ-ă) ["+ *odynē,* pain]. Pain in a tendon. SYN: *tenalgia.*

tenomyoplasty (těn′ō-mī′ō-plăs″tĭ) ["+ *mys,* muscle, + *plassein,* to form]. Reparative operation upon a tendon and muscle. SYN: *tenontomyoplasty.*

tenomyotomy (těn″ō-mī-ŏt′ō-mĭ) ["+ "+ *tomē,* a cutting]. Excision of lateral portion of a tendon or muscle.

tenonec′tomy [Gr. *tenōn,* tendon, + *ektomē,* excision]. Excision of a portion of a tendon.

tenonitis (těn″ō-nī′tĭs). 1. [Gr. *tenōn,* tendon, + *-itis,* inflammation]. Inflammation of a tendon. SYN: *tenontitis.* 2. [*tenon* + Gr. *-itis,* inflammation]. Inflammation of Tenon's capsule, q.v.

tenonometer (těn″ō-nŏm′ě-těr) [Gr. *teinein,* to stretch, + *metron,* measure]. Device for measuring amount of intraocular tension.

Tenon's capsule (tě-nŏn′). [Jacques R. Tenon, Fr. surgeon, 1724-1816]. A thin connective tissue envelope of the eyeball behind the conjunctiva.

Tenon's space. Space between the post. surface of the eyeball and Tenon's capsule.

tenontitis (těn″ŏn-tī′tĭs) [Gr. *tenōn,* tendon, + *-itis,* inflammation]. Inflammation of a tendon. SYN: *tendinitis; tenositis.*

tenontodynia (těn″ŏn-tō-dĭn′ĭ-ă) ["+ *odynē,* pain]. Pain in a tendon. SYN: *tenalgia; tenodynia.*

tenontography (těn″ŏn-tŏg′ră-fĭ) ["+ *graphein,* to write]. A treatise on the tendons.

tenontology (tĕn″ŏn-tŏl′ō-jĭ) [Gr. *tenōn*, tendon, + *logos*, a study]. The study of the tendons.

tenontomyoplasty (tĕn-ŏn″tō-mĭ′ō-plăs″tĭ) ["+ *mys*, muscle, + *plassein*, to form]. Plastic surgery, including muscle and tendon repair, in treatment of hernia. SYN: *tenomyoplasty.*

tenontomyotomy (tĕn-ŏn″tō-mĭ-ŏt′ō-mĭ) ["+ "+ *tomē*, a cutting]. Cutting of the principal tendon of a muscle with excision of the muscle in part or in whole. SYN: *myotenotomy.*

tenontoplasty (tĕn-ŏn′tō-plăs″tĭ) [Gr. *tenōn*, tendon, + *plassein*, to form]. Plastic surgery of defective or injured tendons. SYN: *tenoplasty.*

tenontothecitis (tĕn-ŏn″tō-thē-sī′tĭs) ["+ *thēkē*, sheath, + *-itis*, inflammation]. Inflammation of a tendon and its sheath. SYN: *tendosynovitis; tendovaginitis; tenosynovitis.*

    t. stenosans. A chronic form of t. with narrowing of the sheath.

tenophyte (tĕn′ō-fīt) ["+ *phyton*, a growth]. A cartilaginous or osseous growth on a tendon.

tenoplasty (tĕn′ō-plăs″tĭ) [Gr. *tenōn*, tendon, + *plassein*, to form]. Reparative surgery of tendons. SYN: *tenontoplasty.*

tenorrhaphy (tĕn-ōr′ă-fĭ) ["+ *rhaphē*, suture]. Suturing of a tendon.

tenositis (tĕn″ō-sī′tĭs) ["+ *-itis*, inflammation]. Inflammation of a tendon. SYN: *tenontitis.*

tenostosis (tĕn″ŏs-tō′sĭs) [Gr. *tenōn*, tendon, + *osteon*, bone, + *-ōsis*, condition]. Conversion of a tendon into bony tissue.

tenosuspension (tĕn″ō-sŭs-pĕn′shŭn) ["+ L. *suspensiō*, a hanging under]. Suspension of the humerus by a layer of a tendon to the acromion process.

tenosuture (tĕn″ō-sū′chŭr) ["+ L. *sutura*, sewing]. Reunion of a divided tendon. SYN: *tenorrhaphy.*

tenosynovectomy (tĕn″ō-sĭn″ō-vĕk′tō-mĭ) ["+ *syn*, with, + L. *ovum*, egg, + Gr. *ektomē*, excision]. Excision of a tendon sheath.

tenosynovitis (tĕn″ō-sĭn″ō-vī′tĭs) ["+ "+ "+ Gr. *-itis*, inflammation]. Inflammation of a tendon sheath.

    t. crepitans. Inflammation of a tendon sheath in which a cracking sound is heard on motion. Most commonly affects flexor tendons.

    ETIOL: May follow puncture wounds, contusions, and lacerations, or be caused by lymphatic extension from an abrasion.

    SYM: Pain, finger rigid, excessive tenderness.

    TREATMENT: Early drainage, rest.

    t. hyperplastica. Painless swelling of extensor tendons over the wrist joint.

tenotome (tĕn′ō-tōm) ["+ *tomē*, cutting]. Instrument for section of a tendon.

tenotomist (tĕn-ŏt′ō-mĭst). Specialist in tenotomy.

tenotomy (tĕn-ŏt′ō-mĭ). Surgical section of a tendon.

tenovaginitis (tĕn″ō-văj″ĭn-ī′tĭs) [Gr. *tenōn*, tendon, + L. *vagina*, sheath, + Gr. *-itis*, inflammation]. Inflammation of a tendon sheath. SYN: *tenontothecitis.*

tension (tĕn′shŭn) [L. *tensio*, a stretching]. 1. Process or act of stretching; state of being strained or stretched. 2. Pressure, as arterial tension. 3. Expansive force of a gas or vapor.

    t., arterial. Tension resulting from the force exerted by the blood on the walls of arteries. SYN: *arterial blood pressure.*

    t. of gases. Gas pressure measured in millimeters of mercury (mm. Hg).

    When in solution, gases are measured by gas pressure in surrounding medium sufficient to prevent gas from escaping from the solution.

    t. headache. Headache caused by sustained tension of muscles of the face, neck, and scalp.

    t., intraocular. Internal pressure of liquid within eyeball.

    t., intravenous. Force exerted by the blood on the walls of a vein.

    t., muscular. That condition of a muscle in which fibers tend to shorten and thus perform work, or liberate heat.

    t., premenstrual. Condition occurring periodically usually a week or ten days before menstruation characterized by extreme nervousness and irritability, emotional instability, headaches, and sometimes depression. Usually disappears a short time after onset of menstrual flow.

    t., surface. Molecular property of film on surface of a liquid to resist rupture, the particles tending to pull inward.

    t. suture. One used to reduce pull of the edges of a wound.

tensiophone (tĕn′sĭ-ō-fōn) [L. *tensio*, tension, + Gr. *phōnē*, sound]. Device for obtaining blood pressure readings by auscultation and palpation.

tensor (tĕn′sor) [L. *tensor*, a stretcher]. A muscle making a part tense. SEE: *Table of Muscles* in *Appendix.*

tent (tĕnt) [O.Fr. *tente*, from L. *tenta*, stretched out]. 1. To keep open with a tent.

2. A portable covering or shelter composed of fabric.

t., oxygen. A tent which can be placed over a bed for the administration of oxygen.

tentative (tĕn′tă-tĭv) [L. *tentativus*]. Noting a diagnosis subject to change because of insufficient data; experimental.

tenth cranial nerve. Nerve supplying most of the abdominal viscera, the heart, lungs, and esophagus. SYN: *vagus nerve.* SEE: *cranial nerves* in *Appendix; vagus.*

tentigo (tĕn-tī′gō) [L.]. Abnormal sexual desire. SYN: *lasciviousness; lust; nymphomania; satyriasis.*

tentorial (tĕn-tō′rĭ-ăl). Pertaining to a tentorium.

    t. notch. An arched cavity formed by the anterior and inner border of the tentorium cerebelli. SYN: *foramen ovale of Pacchioni.*

    t. pressure cone. Projection of a portion of temporal lobe of cerebrum through the incisure of the tentorium due to increased intracranial pressure.

tentorium (tĕn-tō′rĭ-ŭm) [L. *tentōrium*, tent]. A tentlike structure or part.

    t. cerebelli. [NA]. The process of the dura mater between the cerebrum and cerebellum supporting the occipital lobes.

tentum (tĕn′tŭm) [L. *tenta*, from *tendere*, to stretch]. The penis.

tenuate (tĕn′ū-āt). To make thin.

tenuity (tĕn-ū′ĭ-tĭ) [L. *tenuitās*, from *tenuis*, thin]. The state or condition of being thin.

tenuous (tĕn′ū-ŭs). Thin, slender, minute.

tephromalacia (tĕf′rō-măl-ā′sĭ-ă) [Gr. *tephros*, gray, + *malakia*, softening]. Softening of the gray substance of brain or spinal cord.

tephromyelitis (tĕf′rō-mī″ĕl-ī′tĭs) [″ + *myelos*, marrow, + *-itis*, inflammation]. Inflammation of the gray matter of the spinal cord. SYN: *poliomyelitis.*

tephrosis (tĕf-rō′sĭs) [″ + *-ōsis*, condition]. Incineration; cremation.

tephrylometer (tĕf″rĭ-lom′ĕ-tĕr) [″ + *ylē,* matter, + *metron,* measure]. Device for measuring the thickness of the cerebral cortex, the gray matter of brain.

tepid (tĕp′ĭd) [L. *tepidus,* lukewarm]. Slightly warm; lukewarm.

    t. bath. One about 86° F. (30° C.).

tepidarium (tĕp″ĭd-ā′rĭ-ŭm) [L.]. A place for a warm bath.

TEPP. Abbr. for *tetraethylpyrophosphate.*

ter- [L.]. Combining form meaning thrice.

teramorphous (tĕr-ă-mŏr′fŭs) [Gr. *teras,* monster, + *morphē,* form]. Similar to, or of the nature of, a congenitally deformed fetus, infant, or child.

teras (tĕr′ăs) [L., Gr.]. (pl. *ter′ata*) A severely deformed fetus.

teratic (tĕr-ăt′ĭk) [Gr. *teratikos,* monstrous]. Pert. to a severely malformed fetus.

teratism (tĕr′ă-tĭzm) [Gr. *teratisma*]. An anomaly or structural abnormality either inherited or acquired.

    t., acquired. Abnormality resulting from a prenatal environmental influence.

    t., atresic. T. in which natural openings such as the mouth or anus fail to form.

    t., casemic. T. in which a normal union of parts fails to occur.

    t., ectogenic. Condition in which parts are absent or defective.

    t., ectopic. Abnormality in which a part becomes displaced.

    t., hypergenetic. T. in which a part is exceptionally large.

    t., symphysic. T. in which parts which are normally separate are fused.

terato- [Gr. *teratos,* monster]. Combining form indicating a severely malformed fetus.

teratoblastoma (tĕr″ă-tō-blăs-tō′mă) [″ + *-blastos,* germ, + *-ōma,* tumor]. A tumor containing embryonic material but which is not representative of all three germinal layers. SEE: *teratoma.*

teratogenesis (tĕr″ă-tō-gĕn′ĕ-sĭs) [″ + *genesis,* production]. The development of abnormal structures in an embryo; the development of a severely deformed fetus.

teratoid (tĕr′ă-toyd) [Gr. *teratos,* monster, + *eidos,* form]. Resembling a severely malformed fetus.

    t. tumor. Tumor of embryonic remains from all of the germinal layers. SYN: *teratoma.*

teratology (tĕr-ă-tŏl′ō-jĭ) [″ + *logos,* a study]. Branch of science dealing with the study of congenitally deformed fetuses.

teratoma (tĕr-ă-tō′mă) [″ + *-ōma,* tumor]. Congenital tumor containing embryonic elements of all three primary germ layers, as hair, teeth, etc. SYN: *dermoid.*

teratomatous (ter″ă-tō′mă-tŭs). Pert. to or resembling a teratoma.

teratophobia (tĕr″ă-tō-fō′bĭ-ă) [Gr. *teratos,* monster, + *phobos,* fear]. Abnormal fear of giving birth to a malformed fetus or of being in contact with one.

teratosis (tĕr″ă-tō′sĭs) [″ + *-ōsis,* condition]. A deformed fetus.

ter′bium. SYMB: *Tb.* At. wt. 158.9254; at. no. 65; sp. gr. 8.272. A metal of the rare earths.

tere (tē′rē) [L.]. Rub.

terebinthinate (tĕr″ē-bĭn′thĭ-nāt) [L. *terebinthus,* turpentine]. Containing turpentine.

terebrant, terebrating (tĕr'ē-brănt, -brăt''ing) [L. *terebrans*, boring]. Boring or piercing, said of pain.

terebration (tĕr''ē-brā'shŭn) [L. *terebratio*]. 1. The act of boring. SYN: *trephining.* 2. A boring pain.

teres (tē'rēz) [L., round]. 1. Round and smooth; cylindrical. 2. A cylindrical muscle.

    t. major. A muscle that draws the arm down and back.

    t. minor. A muscle inserted in the great tuberosity of the humerus, which rotates the humerus outward and abducts it.

tereti- [L.]. Combining form meaning round.

tergo- [L.]. Combining form indicating the back.

tergum (tĕr'gŭm) [L.]. The back.

ter in die (tĕr-ĭn-dē'ā) [L.]. Three times a day. ABBR: t.i.d.

term (term) [L. *terminus*, a boundary]. 1. A limit or boundary. 2. A definite period. 3. The normal period of pregnancy, approx. nine calendar months.

    t. birth. Birth occurring at expected time of delivery; one not premature.

terminal (tĕr'mĭ-năl) [L. *terminalis*]. Pert. to or placed at the end.

    t. arteriole. Arteriole with no branches, but which splits into capillaries.

    t. bars. Minute bars of dense intercellular cement which occupy and close spaces between epithelial cells and bind them together.

    t. ganglia. Those of the parasympathetic division of the autonomic nervous system that are located in or close to walls or visceral structures such as heart, intestines. SYN: *peripheral ganglia.*

    t. illness. An illness which because of its nature can be expected to cause the patient to die. Usually an unrelenting chronic disease for which there is no known cure.

    t. infection. Infection appearing in the late stage of another disease; often fatal.

    t. veins. One of two veins (anterior and posterior) draining portions of the brain and emptying into interior cerebral veins.

termination [L. *terminatio*, limiting]. 1. The distal end of a part. 2. The cessation of anything.

terminology (tĕr-mĭ-nŏl'ō-jĭ) [L. *terminus*, term, + Gr. *logos*, word]. The vocabulary of scientific and technical terms used in specific arts, trades, or professions. SYN: *nomenclature.*

ternary (tĕr'nă-rĭ) [L. *ternarius*, triple]. 1. Threefold; triple; third. 2. Composed of three elements.

    t. acid. An inorganic acid containing hydrogen and two other elements.

teropterin (tĕr-ŏp'tĕr-ĭn). Trade name for sodium pteroyl triglutamate solution. Used for palliation of certain symptoms of malignancy in treatment adjunctive to x-ray, radium, and surgical treatment.

ter'pin hy'drate. White crystalline substance with a turpentine taste; made by the interaction of rectified spirits of turpentine, alcohol, and nitric acid.

    ACTION AND USES: As an expectorant.

terra (tĕr'ā) [L.]. Earth; soil.

    t. alba. White clay.

    t. fullonica. Fuller's earth.

terracing (tĕr'ăs-ĭng) [O.Fr. *terrasse*]. Suturing in several rows through thick tissues in closing a wound.

terramycin (tĕr''ă-mī'cĭn). A proprietary name for the oxy derivative of tetracycline. An antibiotic biosynthesized by Streptomyces rimosus. It is a broad spectrum antibiotic effective against both gram-negative and gram-positive bacteria, rickettsias, and some viruses. SEE: *oxytetracycline; tetracycline.*

terror (tĕr'ŏr) [L.]. Very great fear.

    t., night. Nightmare, esp. of children.

tertian (tĕr'shŭn) [L. *tertianus*, the third]. Occurring every 3rd day.

    t. fever. A malarial fever with paroxysms every other day.

    t. malaria. Caused by Plasmodium vivax, q.v. SEE: *malaria.*

tertiary (tĕr'shĭ-ār-ĭ) [L. *tertiarius*]. Third in order or stage.

    t. alcohol. Alcohol containing the trivalent group COH.

    t. syphilis. Third and most advanced stage of syphilis.

tertipara (tĕr-tĭp'ă-ră) [L. *tertius*, third, + *parēre*, to bring forth]. A woman who has given birth to three children.

tessellated (tĕs'ē-la''tĕd) [L. *tessella*, a square]. Composed of little squares.

test (test) [L. *testum*, earthen vessel]. 1. An examination. 2. Method to determine the presence or nature of a substance or the presence of a disease. 3. A chemical reaction. 4. A reagent or substance used in making a t.

    t., acetone. T. for presence of acetone in the urine; made by adding a few drops of sodium nitroprusside to the urine along with strong ammonia water. Presence of acetone causes formation of a magenta ring at outline of contacts.

    t., Allen-Doisy. T. to determine amount of estrogen content in female blood serum by its reaction on secretions of mice.

t., Aschheim-Zondek. T. for pregnancy by injecting the patient's urine subcutaneously into immature female mice.

t., Binet-Simon. Method of ascertaining the mental capacity of children by asking a series of suitable questions.

t., biuret. T. for the presence of proteins or urea.

t., Friedman. T. for pregnancy by injecting urine of the patient into unmated mature female rabbits, a positive reaction being indicated by formation of corpora lutea and corpora haemorrhagica.

t., Gelle's. T. for ear lesions by employing rubber tubing and a tuning fork.

t., Huhner. Aspiration of vagina within an hour after coitus, to investigate sperm activity.

t., Kahn. Precipitation t. for syphilis.

t. paper. Paper used in making tests, as litmus paper.

t., pregnancy. T. to determine pregnancy.

t., Rubin. T. for patency of the fallopian tubes by insufflation with carbon dioxide; used in determining cause of sterility.

t., Schiller's. T. for cancer of the cervix by painting with iodine solution; areas which contain glycogen are stained by the iodine. Those sites which do not stain, but become white or yellow, are assumed to be malignant. Tissue is taken from those areas for microscopic examination.

t., Schneider's. A pregnancy t. using female rabbits.

t., Schwabach. T. for hearing using tuning forks.

t. solution. A standard solution used in making a t.

t. tube. A plain tube of thin glass, closed at one end, used for simple tests.

t., urea balance. T. of the kidney function by measuring intake and output of urea.

t., Wassermann. Diagnostic t. for syphilis based on principle of fixation of complement.

testectomy (těs-těk'tō-mǐ) [L. *testis*, testicle, + Gr. *ektomē*, excision]. 1. Removal of a testicle. SYN: *castration.* 2. Removal of a corpus quadrigeminum.

testes (těs'tēs) [L.]. Pl. of testis, q.v.

testicle (těs'ti-kl) [L. *testiculus*, a little *testis*]. A testis, q.v.

testicular (těs-tǐk'ū-lǎr). Rel. to a testicle.

testis (těs'tǐs) [L.]. (pl. *tes'tes*) [NA] The male gonad. One of two reproductive glands located in the scrotum which produce the male reproductive cells or spermatozoa and the male hormone, testosterone. SYN: testicle.

Each is an ovoid body about 4.0 cm. long and 2-2.5 cm. in width and thickness enclosed within a dense inelastic fibrous tunica albuginea. The testis is divided into numerous lobules separated by septa, each lobule containing one to three seminiferous tubules within which the spermatozoa arise. The lobules lead to straight ducts which join a plexus, the rete testis, from which 15-20 efferent ducts lead to the epididymis. The epididymis leads to the ductus deferens through which sperm are conveyed to the urethra.

Between the seminiferous tubules are located the interstitial cells (cells of Leydig) which are considered to be the source of the male hormone(s).

The testes are suspended from the body by the spermatic cord, a structure extending

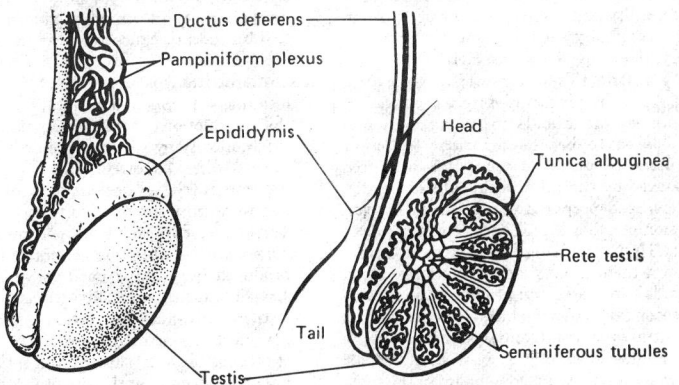

TESTIS AND RELATED STRUCTURES

from inguinal ring to testis. It contains the ductus deferens, testicular vessels (spermatic artery, vein, lymph vessels) and nerves.

Hyperfunction (hypergonadism) may cause early maturity such as dentition, large sexual organs with early functional activity, and growth of hair.

Hypofunction (hypogonadism) is indicated by undeveloped testes, absence of body hair, high-pitched voice, sterility, smooth skin, loss of sex desire, low metabolism, and eunuchoid or eunuch type.

t., abdominal. An undescended t. which remains within body cavity.

t. compression reflex. Contraction of abdominal muscles following moderate compression of t.

t., descent of. Change in position of the testis from abdominal cavity to scrotum during fetal life.

t., displaced. A t. located abnormally within the inguinal canal or pelvis.

t., femoral. An inguinal t. which is near or over the femoral ring.

t., inverted. A t. reversed in the scrotum so that the epididymis attaches to the anterior instead of posterior part of gland.

t., perineal. T. which is located in the perineal region outside the scrotum.

t., puboscrotal. T. located over pubic tubercle.

t., undescended. T. remaining in the inguinal canal or abdominal cavity at birth.

testitis (tĕs-tī'tĭs) [L. *testis*, testicle, + Gr. *-itis*, inflammation]. Inflammation of a testis. SYN: *orchitis.*

testitoxicosis (tĕs"tĭ-tŏk-sĭ-kō'sĭs) ["+ Gr. *toxikon*, poison, + *-ōsis*, condition]. A toxic state sometimes following ligation of the ductus deferens.

test meal. A meal usually small and of definite quality and composition, given to aid in chemical analysis of the stomach contents or x-ray diagnosis of the stomach.

testosterone (tĕs-tŏs'tĕr-ōn) [L. *testis*, testicle]. An androgen isolated from the testes of a number of animals including man and considered to be the principal testicular hormone produced in man. It is a steroid produced by the interstitial cells of Leydig. It has been prepared synthetically by conversion of other sterols, esp. cholesterol.

ACTION: It accelerates growth in tissues upon which it acts and stimulates blood flow. It stimulates and promotes the growth of secondary sexual characteristics and is essential for normal sexual behavior and the occurrence of erections. It is essential for normal growth and development of the male accessory sexual organs. It is responsible for deepening of the male voice at puberty, greater muscular development in men, development of beard and pubic hair, and distribution of fat in adult men. It also affects many metabolic activities.

tetanic (tē-tăn'ĭk) [Gr. *tetanikos*]. 1. Pert. to or producing tetanus. 2. Any agent producing tetanic spasms.

t. convulsion. A tonic one with constant muscular contraction.

tetaniform (tē-tăn'ĭ-form) [Gr. *tetanos*, tetanus, + L. *forma*, shape]. Resembling tetanus.

tetanigenous (tĕt"ă-nĭj'ĕ-nŭs) ["+ *gennan*, to produce]. Causing tetanus or tetanic spasms.

tetanilla (tĕt"ă-nĭl'ă) [L.]. 1. Mild form of tetany, q.v., without rigidity. 2. Twitchings of a limited group of muscular fibers with clonic paroxysmal contractions.

tetanism (tĕt'ă-nĭzm) [Gr. *tetanos*, tetanus, + *-ismos*, condition]. Persistent muscular hypertonicity resembling tetanus, esp. in infants.

tetanization (tĕt"ă-nī-zā'shŭn) [Gr. *tetanos*, tetanus]. 1. Production of tetanus or tetanic spasms by induction of the disease. 2. Induction of tetanic contractions in a muscle by electrical stimuli.

tetanize (tĕt'ă-nīz). To induce tonic muscular spasms.

tetanode (tĕt'ă-nōd) [Gr. *tetanos*, tetanus, + *eidos*, form]. 1. Resembling tetanus. SYN: *tetanoid.* 2. Noting interval between recurrent tonic spasms in tetany.

tetanoid (tĕt'ă-noyd) ["+ *eidos*, form]. Resembling tetanus. SYN: *tetaniform.*

t. paraplegia. Paralysis of lower extremities due to lateral sclerosis of spinal cord. SYN: *spastic paraplegia.*

tetanolysin (tĕt"ă-nŏl'ĭ-sĭn). A hemolytic component of the toxin produced by Clostridium tetani, causative organism of tetanus.

tetanomotor (tĕt"ăn-ō-mō'tor) [Gr. *tetanos*, tetanus, + L. *motor*, a mover]. Appliance for the production of tetanic motor spasms mechanically by shocking a nerve.

tetanophil, tetanophilic (tĕt"ăn-ō-fĭl, tĕt"ăn-ō-fĭl'ĭk) ["+ *philein*, to love]. Possessing an affinity for tetanus toxin.

tetanospasmin (tĕt"ă-nō-spăs'mĭn) ["+ L. *spasmus*, spasm]. A component of the toxin produced by tetanus bacillus which is responsible for tetanic convulsions.

tetanus (tĕt'ă-nŭs) [Gr. *tetanos*, tetanus]. 1. An infectious, acute disease due to the toxin of tetanus bacillus, Clostridium tetani growing anaerobically at the site of injury. There is a state of more or less persistent, painful tonic spasm of some of the voluntary muscles. 2. A state of sustained contraction of a muscle, esp. that induced experimentally.

T. usually begins gradually but may begin suddenly, may be of brief duration or last some weeks. The first sign is stiffness of the jaw, esophageal muscles, and some of the muscles of the neck. Soon the jaws become rigidly fixed (trismus or lockjaw), the voice is altered, and muscles of the face contract producing a wild, excited expression, a compound of bitter laughter and crying (risus sardonicus). The muscles of back, extremities, and penis become tetanic.

If the patient is bent back in a bow, the condition is termed opisthotonos; if he is bent to the side, pleurothotonos; if he is bent forward, emprosthotonos.

The paroxysms are reflex and are excited by noises, currents of air, and irritation of bedclothes. The temperature usually rises and may become extremely high. The pain is great, patient also suffering from hunger, thirst, and want of sleep. The mind is clear. This disease is usually, but not always, fatal, the patient expiring from asphyxia or exhaustion.

RS: emprosthotonos; lockjaw; opisthotonos; pleurothotonos; posture; risus sardonicus.

t., anticus. Form in which the body is bowed forward.

t. antitoxin. An antibody which develops in the blood of man or other animals (horse) as a result of infection by the t. organism (Clostridium tetani) or inoculation with t. toxin or toxoid. 2. An antitoxin derived from the blood of horses or cattle immunized against t. toxin. It is used to produce passive immunity to prevent the development of t. and in the treatment of active t. Prophylactic dose is 1500 units injected subcutaneously; for active tetanus, 5000 to 20,000 units injected intravenously or subcutaneously.

t., artificial. Form produced by a drug like strychnine or by mechanical appliance.

t., ascending. T. in which muscle spasms occur first in lower part of body and then spread upward, finally involving muscles of head and neck.

t., cephalic. Form due to a wound of the head, esp. one near the eyebrow. It is marked by trismus, facial paralysis on one side, and pronounced dysphagia; resembles rabies; often fatal.

t., cerebral. A form produced by inoculating the brain of animals with t. antitoxin. marked by epileptiform convulsions and excitement.

t., chronic. 1. A latent infection in a healed wound, reactivated upon opening the wound. 2. A form of t. in which onset and progress of the disease is slower and more prolonged and symptoms less severe. SYN: *delayed t.*

t., descending. T. in which muscle spasms occur first in head and neck and later are manifested in other muscles of the body.

t. dorsalis. T. in which the body is bent backward.

t., extensor. T. which affects the extensors especially.

t., hydrophobic. T., cephalic, q.v.

t., idiopathic. T. which occurs without any visible lesion.

t., imitative. Hysteria which simulates t.

t. infantum. T. of young infants due to infection of umbilicus.

t., intermittent. SYN: tetany, q.v.

t. lateralis. Form in which the body is bent sideways.

t., local. T. characterized by spasticity of a group of muscles near the wound. Trismus contraction of jaw muscles usually is absent.

t. neonatorum. T. of very young infants, usually due to infection of navel.

t. paradoxus. Cephalic t. in which condition is combined with paralysis of the facial or other cranial nerve.

t., postoperative. T. which follows an operation.

t., puerperal. T. which occurs following childbirth.

t., rheumatic. Form due to exposure to cold and wet.

t., Ritter's. Tetanic contractions at opening of a constant current which has been passing along a nerve for some time; seen in tetany.

t., toxic. Produced by overdose of nux vomica or strychnine.

t. toxoid. T. toxin modified by treatment with formaldehyde so that its toxicity is greatly reduced but its capacity to promote active immunity has been retained.

t., traumatic. T. following a wound.

tetany (tĕt′ă-nĭ) [Gr. *tetanos,* tetanus]. A nervous affection characterized by intermittent tonic spasms which are usually paroxysmal and involve the extremities; most frequent in the young; frequently associated with pregnancy or lactation.

ETIOL: Tetany is induced by changes in pH and extracellular calcium which increase nervous and muscular excitability. Causative factors are parathyroid deficiency or inadvertent operative removal of parathyroids during thyroidectomy, alkalosis, or vitamin-D deficiency.

SYM: Characterized by nervousness, irritability and apprehension, numbness and tingling of the extremities, cramps of the various muscles, particularly those of the hands, producing a typical accoucheur type of hand and extreme extension of the feet. Bilateral tonic spasms in arms and legs, jaws rarely involved. Contractions usually paroxysmal and are attended with pain. Electrocontractility of muscles greatly exaggerated. May be slight edema. Sensation not disturbed; mind clear; fever slight or absent.

SIGNS: Characteristic diagnostic signs are Trousseau's sign, Chvostek's sign, and the peroneal sign. Prolongation of the isoelectric phase of the ST segment of the ECG usually is indicative of low calcium. SEE: *Chvostek's sign; Trousseau's sign.*

PROG: Usually favorable. Attacks following thyroidectomy sometimes fatal.

t., alkalotic. That resulting from respiratory alkalosis, as in hyperventilation, or from metabolic alkalosis induced by excessive intake of sodium bicarbonate or excessive loss of chlorides by vomiting, gastric lavage, or suction.

t., duration. Continuous contraction, esp. in degenerated muscles, in response to a continuous electric current.

t., epidemic. A form of t. occurring in Europe, esp. in the winter season. It is of short duration and seldom fatal. SEE: *rheumatic t.*

t., gastric. Severe t. from stomach disorders accompanied by tonic, painful spasms of extremities.

t., gutturotetany. Stammering resulting from tetanoid laryngeal spasm.

t., hyperventilation. T. caused by continued forced respiration.

t., hypocalcemic. T. due to low serum calcium and high serum phosphate levels. May be due to lack of vitamin D, factors which interfere with calcium absorption such as steatorrhea or infantile diarrhea, or defective renal excretion of phosphorus.

t., latent. T. which requires mechanical or electrical stimulation of nerves to show characteristic signs of excitability.

t., manifest. T. in which the characteristic symptoms such as carpopedal spasm, laryngospasm, and convulsions are present. Opposed to latent t.

t., parathyroid. T. resulting from excision of the parathyroid gland or from hyposecretion of the parathyroid gland as a result of disease or disorders of the gland. SYN: *hypoparathyroidism.*

t., rachitic. T. due to hypocalcemia accompanying vitamin D deficiency.

t., thyreoprival. T. resulting from removal of thyroid gland accompanied by removal of parathryoid glands.

tetarcone (tĕt′ăr-kōn) [Gr. *tetartos,* fourth, + *konos,* cone]. Fourth or distolingual cusp of an upper molar tooth. SYN: *tetartocone.*

tetartanopia, tetartanopsia (tĕt″ăr-tăn-ō′pĭ-ă, -ŏp′sĭ-ă) [″+ *opsis,* vision]. Symmetrical blindness in the same quadrant of each visual field. SYN: *quadrantanopia.*

tetartocone (tĕt-ăr′tō-kōn). The distolingual cusp of an upper molar tooth. SYN: *tetartocone.*

tetra-, tetr- [Gr. *tetras,* four]. Combining forms meaning four.

tetrabasic (tĕt″ră-bā′sĭk) [Gr. *tetras,* four, + *basis,* base]. Having four replaceable hydrogen atoms, said of an acid or acid salt.

tetrablastic (tĕt″ră-blăs′tĭk) [″+ *blastos,* germ]. Having four germinal layers: the ectoderm, endoderm, and two mesodermic layers.

tetrabromofluorescein (tĕt″ră-brŏm″ō-flū-or-ĕs′ĭn, -ē-ĭn). A dye, $C_{20}H_8Br_4O_5$, obtained from action of bromine on fluorescein, used as a stain in microscopy. SYN: *eosin.*

tetracaine hydrochloride. USP. A surface, infiltration, and intraspinal anesthetic.

tetrachlorethylene (tĕt″ră-klōr-ĕth′ĭ-lēn) USP. A clear, colorless liquid with a characteristic odor. An anthelmintic.

tetracid (tĕ-trăs′ĭd) [Gr. *tetra,* + L. *acidus,* sour]. 1. Able to react with four molecules of a monoacid or two of a diacid to form a salt or ester, said of a base or alcohol; term disapproved by some authorities. 2. Having four hydrogen atoms replaceable by basic atoms or radicals, said of acids.

Tetracoccus (tĕt″ră-kŏk′ŭs) [″+ *kokkos,* berry]. Genus of micrococcus arranged in groups of four by division into two planes.

tetracrotic (tĕt″ră-krŏt′ĭk) [″+ *krotos,* beat]. Noting a pulse or pulse tracing with four upward strokes in the descending limb of the wave. SYN: *catatricrotic.*

tetracycline (tĕt″ră-sī′klēn). USP. A member of the tetracycline group of broad-spectrum antibiotics having similar pharmacological activity (i.e., tetracycline, chlortetracycline, oxytetracycline). Esp. effective in treatment of Q fever, typhus fever, psittacosis, acute brucellosis, granuloma inguinale.

tetrad (tĕt′răd) [Gr. *tetras, tetrad-,* four]. 1. A group of four things with something in common. 2. An element having a valence or combining power of four. 3. A group of four similar bodies. 4. A group of four parts, said of cells produced by division in two planes, or of a chromosome in four parts in preparation for two mitotic divisions in maturation.

tetraethylammonium chloride (tĕt-rā-ĕth-ĭl-ăm-ō'nĭ-ŭm-klō'rĭd). A quaternary ammonium compound used as a ganglionic blocking agent in diagnosis and treatment of circulatory diseases. ABBR: TEAC.

tetraethylpyrophosphate (tĕt-rā-ĕth'ĭl-pī-rō-fŏs'fāt). A powerful cholinesterase inhibitor used as an insecticide; poisonous to man. Has had some use in treatment of myasthenia gravis. ABBR: TEPP.

tetragenous (tĕt-răj'ĕn-ŭs) [Gr. *tetras,* four, + *gennan,* to produce]. Pert. to organisms, esp. bacteria, which divide into groups of four.

tetralogy of Fallot. An anomaly of the heart consisting of pulmonary stenosis, interventricular septal defect, dextroposed aorta which receives blood from both ventricles, and hypertrophy of the right ventricle.

tetramastia (tĕt"rā-măs'tĭ-ă) [Gr. *tetras,* four, + *mastos,* breast]. Condition characterized by presence of four breasts. SYN: *tetramazia.*

tetramazia (tĕt"rā-mā'zĭ-ă) ["+ *mazos,* breast]. Condition of having four breasts. SYN: *tetramastia.*

tetrameric, tetramerous (tĕt"rā-mĕr'ĭk, tĕt-răm'ĕr-ŭs) ["+ *meros,* a part]. Having four parts.

tetranopsia (tĕt"rā-nŏp'sĭ-ă) [Gr. *tetras,* four, + *an,* no, + *opsis,* vision]. Obliteration of one quarter of the visual field.

tetraplegia (tĕt"rā-plē'jĭ-ă) ["+ *plēgē,* a stroke]. Paralysis of both arms and legs.

tetrasomic (tĕt-rā-sō'mĭk) ["+ *sōma,* body]. Possessing four instead of the usual two of a pair of chromosomes, that is, having a chromosome number of 2n + 2.

tetraster (tĕt-răs'tĕr) [Gr. *tetras,* four, + *astēr,* star]. A mitotic figure in which there are four asters instead of more commonly two; occurring abnormally in mitosis.

tetravalent (tĕt"rā-vā'lĕnt). Having a valence or combining power of four. SYN: *quadrivalent.*

tetrodotoxin (tĕt"rō-dō-tŏks'ĭn). A powerful nerve poison found in the eggs of the California newt and in certain fish in Japan. In concentrated form is more toxic than cyanide.

tetter (tĕt'ĕr) [AS. *teter*]. 1. Obsolete term for various vesicular cutaneous diseases as herpes, ringworm, or eczema. 2. A pimple or blister.

textiform (tĕks'tĭ-form) [L. *textum,* something woven, + *forma,* shape]. Resembling a network, web, or mesh.

textoblastic (tĕks"tō-blăs'tĭk) [L. *textus,* tissue, + Gr. *blastos,* germ]. Forming adult tissue; regenerative; noting cells.

textural (tĕks'tū-răl) [L. *textura,* weaving]. Concerning the texture or constitution of a tissue.

T fracture. Fracture in which bone splits both longitudinally and transversely.

T-groups. Groups of individuals who meet in sensitivity training sessions in order to become more sensitive to themselves and others.

Th. Chem. symbol for thorium.

thalamic (thăl-ăm'ĭk) [Gr. *thalamos,* inner chamber]. Pert. to the thalamus.

    t. syndrome. Vascular lesions of the thalamus causing disturbances of sensation and partial or complete paralysis of one side of the body. An extremely severe, sharp, boring-type pain may occur spontaneously. There also is a tendency to overrespond to a sensory stimulus and awareness of the stimulus long after it has ceased. SYN: *Dejevine-Roussy syndrome.*

    ETIOL: Optic thalamus lesion.

thalamo- [Gr.]. 1. Combining form meaning chamber, part of brain at which a nerve originates. 2. Pert. to the thalamus.

thalamocele, thalamocoele (thăl'ăm-ō-sēl) [Gr. *thalamos,* chamber, + *koilia,* a hollow]. The 3rd ventricle of the brain.

thalamocortical (thăl"ăm-ō-kŏr'tĭ-kăl) ["+ L. *cortex, cortic-,* rind]. Pert. to the optic thalamus and the cerebral cortex.

thalamolenticular (thăl"ăm-ō-lĕn-tĭk'ū-lăr) ["+ L. *lenticula,* a small lentil]. Concerning the optic thalamus and the lenticular nucleus.

thalamotomy (thăl-ă-mŏt'ō-mī) [Gr. *thalamos,* chamber, + *tomē,* incision]. Destruction by one of several methods of a portion of the thalamus in order to treat psychosis or intractable pain.

thalamus (thăl'ă-mŭs) [L.]. (pl. *thal'ami*) [NA]. The largest subdivision of the diencephalon on either side, consisting chiefly of an ovoid, gray nuclear mass in the lateral wall of the 3rd ventricle. Each consists of a number of nuclei (anterior, medial, lateral, and ventral), the medial and lateral geniculate bodies, and the pulvinar.

    FUNCTIONS: All sensory stimuli, with the exception of olfactory, are received by the thalamus. These are associated, synthesized, and then relayed through thalamocortical radiations to specific cortical areas. Impulses are also received from the cortex, hypothalamus, and corpus striatum and relayed to visceral and somatic effectors. The t. is also the center for appreciation of primitive, uncritical sensations of pain, crude touch, and temperature.

t. opticus. SYN: *thalamus.*

thalassemia (thăl-ă-sē'mĭ-ă) [Gr. *thalassa,* sea, + *haima,* blood]. An hereditary anemia, due to genetically-transmitted abnormalities, with familial or racial incidence. The disorder is in the synthesis of hemoglobins. There are two chief forms of the disease and no specific therapy.

t. major. The homozygous type, most severe form of the disease. It is found in children. Characterized by mongoloid facies, fatigue, splenomegaly, severe anemia, enlargement of heart, and slight jaundice. Prognosis varies; however, the younger the child when the disease appears, the more unfavorable the outcome.

SYN: *Cooley's anemia; erythroblastic anemia; hereditary leptocytosis; Mediterranean disease.*

t. minor. The heterozygous form, a mild disease which is difficult to detect. Usually revealed by chance or as a result of study of the family of an individual having t. major. Prognosis is excellent.

thalassophobia (thăl-ăs''ō-fō'bĭ-ă) [Gr. *thalassa,* sea, + *phobos,* fear]. Abnormal fear of the sea.

thalassotherapy (thăl-ăs''sō-ther'ă-pĭ) ["+ *therapeia,* treatment]. Treatment of disease by living at the seaside, by sea bathing, sea voyages, or sea air.

thalidomide (thă-lid'ō-mĭd). A chemical substance, *a* (N-phthalimido) glutarimide, used extensively as a sedative and sleeping pill in Europe in the early 1960's. Its use was discontinued when it was discovered to cause severe malformation in limbs of developing fetuses exposed to the drug in their very early intrauterine life.

thallinization (thăl'ĭn-ĭ-zā'shŭn). Treatment with doses of thalline or its salts.

thallitoxicosis (thăl'ĭ-tŏks'ĭ-kō'sĭs). Poisoning by accidental ingestion of thallium-sulfate-containing pesticides. SEE: *Table of Poisons and Poisoning* in *Appendix.*

thallium (thăl'ĭ-ŭm) [L., a young shoot]. SYMB: *Tl.* At. wt. 204.37; at. no. 81; sp. gr. 11.85. A metallic element. Its salts are active poisons.

thamuria (thă-mū'rĭ-ă) [Gr. *thamys,* often, + *ouron,* urine]. Abnormally frequent urination.

thanato- [Gr. *thanatos,* death]. Combining form meaning death.

thanatobiological (thăn''ă-tō-bī-ō-lŏj'ĭ-kăl) [Gr. *thanatos,* death, + *bios,* life, + *logos,* study]. Rel. to the processes of life and death.

thanatognomonic (thăn''ăt-ŏg-nō-mŏn'ĭk) ["+ *gnōmonikos,* knowing]. Indicative of the approach of death.

thanatoid (thăn'ă-toyd) ["+ *eidos,* form]. Resembling death.

thanatology (thăn''ă-tŏl'ō-jĭ) [Gr. *thanatos,* death, + *logos,* science]. The science of death.

thanatomania (thăn''ă-tō-mā'nĭ-ă) ["+ *mania,* madness]. Condition of homicidal or suicidal mania.

thanatometer (thăn''ă-tŏm'ĕt-ĕr) ["+ *metron,* measure]. Instrument for determining occurrence of death by internal temperature.

thanatophobia (thăn''ă-tō-fō'bĭ-ă) [Gr. *thanatos,* death, + *phobos,* fear]. Morbid fear of death.

thanatophoric dwarfism. Dwarfism caused by generalized failure of endochondral bone formation. Characterized by large head, prominent forehead, hypertelorism, saddle nose, and short limbs extending straight out from the trunk. Most of these infants die soon after birth.

thanatopsia, thanatopsy (thăn''ă-tŏp'sĭ-ă, thăn'ă-tŏp'sĭ) ["+ *opsis,* view]. Examination of a dead body to determine cause of death. SYN: *autopsy; necropsy.*

thanatos (thăn'ă-tŏs) [Gr., death]. The death instinct. In psychoanalysis, all the instinctive tendencies leading to senescence and death.

thaumato- [Gr. *thauma,* wonder]. Combining form meaning wonder, marvel.

Thayer-Martin medium. A special medium used for growing the causative organism of gonorrhea, Neisseria gonorrhoeae.

theaism (thē'ă-ĭzm) [L. *thea,* tea, + Gr. *-ismos,* condition]. Chronic poisoning from excess of tea drinking. SYN: *theinism; themism.*

thebaism (thē'bă-ĭzm) [Gr. *Thebai,* opium of Thebes]. Condition produced by opium.

Thebesian foramina (thē-bē'zĭ-ăn). [Adam Christian Thebesius, Ger. physician, 1686-1732]. Orifices of the Thebesian veins, opening into the right auricle of the heart.

Thebesian valve. An endocardial fold at entrance of the coronary sinus into right auricle.

Thebesian veins. Venules conveying blood from the myocardium to the auricles or ventricles.

theca (thē'kă) [Gr. *thēkē,* sheath]. (pl. *the'cae*) A sheath of investing membrane.

t. cell tumor. Thecoma, q.v.

t. cordis. Pericardium which sheathes the heart.

t. folliculi.[NA]. Outer wall of a graafian follicle, consisting of an inner vascular layer (theca interna) and outer fibrous layer (theca externa).

thecal (thē′kăl) [Gr. *thēkē,* sheath]. Pert. to a sheath.

thecitis (thē-sī′tĭs) ["+ -*itis,* inflammation]. Inflammation of the sheath of a tendon.

theco- [Gr. *thēkē,* sheath]. Combining form meaning sheath, case, receptacle.

thecodont (thē′kō-dŏnt) [Gr. *thēkē,* sheath, + *odous, odont-,* tooth]. Having teeth which are inserted in sockets.

thecoma (thē-cō′mă) ["+ -*ōma,* tumor]. A tumor of the ovary usually occurring during or following the menopause. Only rarely is it malignant. SYN: *theca cell tumor; thecalutein-cell tumor.*

thecostegnosia, thecostegnosis (thē′′kō-stĕg-nō′sĭ-â, -nō′sĭs) ["+ *stegnōsis,* a narrowing]. Constriction of a tendon sheath.

theine (thē′ēn). Caffeine, q.v.

thelalgia (thē-lăl′jĭ-ă) [Gr. *thēlē,* nipple, + *algos,* pain]. Pain in the nipples.

thelarche (thē-lăr′kē) ["+ *archē,* beginning]. The beginning of breast development at puberty.

thelasis (thē-lăs′ĭs) ["+ -*asis,* condition]. The act of sucking.

Thelazia (thē-lā′zĭ-ă) [Gr. *thēlazō,* to suck]. A genus of nematodes that inhabits the conjunctival sac and lacrimal ducts of various species of vertebrates. Occasionally T. are found in man.

thelaziasis (thē′′lā-zī′ă-sĭs) ["+ -*iasis,* condition]. Condition of being infested by worms of the genus Thelazia.

theleplasty (thē′lĕ-plăs′′tī) [Gr. *thēlē,* nipple, + *plassein,* to form]. Plastic surgery of the nipple.

thelerethism (thĕl-ĕr′ĕ-thĭzm) ["+ *erethisma,* stimulation]. Erection of the nipple.

thelitis (thē-lī′tĭs) ["+ -*itis,* inflammation]. Inflammation of the nipples.

thelium (thē′lĭ-ŭm) [L.]. (pl. *the′lia*) 1. A papilla. 2. A nipple. 3. A cellular layer.

thelon′cus [Gr. *thēlē,* nipple, + *onkos,* mass]. A tumor of a nipple.

thelophlebostemma (thē′′lō-flĕb′′ō-stĕm′mă) ["+ *phleps,* vein, + *stemma,* wreath]. A dark or venous circle of veins about the nipple.

thelorrhagia (thē′′lo-rā′gĭ-ă) [Gr. *thēlē,* nipple, + *rhēgnynai,* to burst forth]. Hemorrhage from a nipple.

thelothism (thē′lō-thĭzm) ["+ *erethisma,* stimulation]. Erection of a nipple brought about by contraction of smooth muscle fibers. SEE: *thelerethism.*

thenad (thē′năd) [Gr. *thenar,* palm, + L. *ad,* toward]. Toward the palm or thenar eminence.

thenal (thē′năl) [Gr. *thenar,* palm]. Pert. to the palm or thenar prominence.

t. aspect. Outer side of the palm.

t. eminence. Ball of the thumb. SYN: *thenar.*

thenar (thē′nar) [Gr. *thenar,* palm]. 1. Palm of hand or sole of foot. 2. Fleshy eminence at base of thumb. 3. Concerning the palm.

t. cleft. A fascial cleft of the palm overlying volar surface of adductor pollicis muscle. SYN: *thenar space.*

t. eminence. One at the base of the thumb.

t. fascia. A thin membrane covering the short muscles of the thumb.

t. muscles. Abductor and flexor muscles of the thumb.

theobromine (thē-ō-brō′mēn) [Gr. *theos,* god, + *brōma,* food]. A white powder obtained from Theobroma cacao.

ACTION AND USES: Dilates blood vessels in the heart and peripherally. Used as a mild stimulant and as a diuretic.

theomania (thē-ō-mā′nĭ-ă) [Gr. *theos,* god, + *mania,* madness]. Religious insanity; esp. that in which patient thinks he is the Deity or has Divine inspiration.

theophobia (thē′′ō-fō′bĭ-ă) ["+ *phobos,* fear]. Abnormal fear of the wrath of God.

theophylline (thē′′ō-fĭl′ēn, -ĭn) [L. *thea,* tea, + Gr. *phyllon,* plant]. A white crystalline powder with action resembling caffeine and theobromine.

theory (thē′ō-rē) [Gr. *theōria,* speculation as opposed to practice]. A supposition or an assumption based on certain evidence or observations but lacking scientific proof. When a theory becomes generally accepted and firmly established, it then becomes a doctrine or principle.

theotherapy (thē′′ō-thĕr′ă-pī) [Gr. *theos,* god, + *therapeia,* treatment]. Treatment of disease by spiritual and religious methods.

therapeutic (thĕr-ă-pū′tĭk) [Gr. *therapeutikos,* treating]. 1. Pert. to results obtained from treatment. 2. Having medicinal or healing properties. 3. A healing agent.

t. exercise. Scientific supervision of exercise for the purpose of preventing muscular atrophy, restoring joint and muscle function, increasing muscular strength, and improve efficiency of cardiovascular and pulmonary function. SEE: *exercise.*

therapeutics (thĕr′′ă-pū′tĭks) [Gr. *therapeutikē,* treatment]. That branch of medicine concerned with the application of remedies and the treatment of disease. SYN: *therapy,* q.v.

t., suggestive. Treatment of a condition by using hypnotic suggestion.

therapeutist (thĕr-ă-pū'tĭst) [Gr. *therapeuein,* to treat medically]. One who practices therapeutics.

therapia sterilisans magna (thĕr"ă-pē'ästē-rĭl'ĭ-säns măg'nă) [L.]. Ehrlich's method of administering chemical agent which will destroy in one large does all the parasites in the body of a patient without causing serious injury to the patient.

therapy (thĕr'ă-pĭ) [Gr. *therapeia,* treatment]. Treatment of a disease or pathological condition.

t., inhalation. Administration of medicines, water vapor, gases (such as oxygen, carbon dioxide, or helium), or anesthetics by inhalation. The medicines usually are nebulized by using an aerosol or spray apparatus. SEE: *intermittent positive pressure breathing.*

t., light. Treatment with radiation from the visible spectrum.

t., maggot. Use of maggots in suppurating wounds of bones and soft tissues to remove necrotic areas.

t., mental. The use of suggestion in the treatment of disease.

t., nonspecific. Use of injections of foreign proteins, bacterial vaccines, etc., in treatment of infection to stimulate general cellular activity. SEE: *therapy, specific.*

t., opsonic. Use of bacterial vaccines to elevate the opsonic index of the blood.

t., physical. Use of physical agents in the treatment of disease, as massage, heat, hydrotherapy, radiation, electricity, and exercise.

t., serum. Use of injections of blood serum from immunized animals or persons in the treatment of disease. SYN: *serotherapy.*

t., specific. Administration of a remedy acting directly against the cause of a disease, as arsphenamine or mercury for syphilis, or quinine for malaria.

t., spiritual. The application of spiritual knowledge in the treatment of disease. SEE: *spiritual therapy.*

t., substitution. Administration of a substance which the body normally produces, i.e., a hormone.

t., vaccine. Injection of bacteria or their products to produce active immunization against a disease. SYN: *opsonic therapy.*

t., zone. Mechanical manipulation or stimulation of an area in the same longitudinal zone as disorder causing distress.

therm (therm) [Gr. *thermē,* heat]. Term used to indicate a variety of quantities of heat.

thermacogenesis (thĕr"mă-kō-jĕn'ĕs-ĭs) [Gr. *thermē,* heat, + *genesis,* production]. Production of an increase of body temperature by drug therapy.

thermaerotherapy (thĕr-mā"er-ō-ther'ă-pĭ) ["+ *aēr,* air, + *therapeia,* treatment]. Therapeutic application of hot air.

thermal (ther'măl) [Gr. *thermē,* heat]. Pert. to heat.

t. capacity. Heat necessary to raise any body from 0° to 1° C.

t. death point. Degree of heat that will kill a fluid culture in 10 minutes.

t. radiation. Heat radiation.

t. sense. Capacity for recognition of heat. SYN: *thermesthesia.*

thermalgia (thĕr-măl'jĭ-ă) ["+ *algos,* pain]. Neuralgia accompanied by intense burning sensation, pain, redness, and sweating of the area involved. SYN: *causalgia.*

thermanalgesia (thĕrm"ăn-ăl-jē'zĭ-ă) ["+ *an-,* not, + *algēsis,* pain]. Inability to experience reaction to heat because of cerebral lesion.

thermanesthesia (thĕrm"ăn-ĕs-thē'zĭ-ă) ["+ *an-,* not, + *aisthēsis,* sensation]. Inability to recognize sensations of heat and cold; insensibility to heat changes. It sometimes occurs in syringomyelia. SYN: *thermoanesthesia.*

thermatology (thĕr-mă-tŏl'ō-jĭ) [Gr. *thermē,* heat, + *logos,* science]. The study of heat in treatment of disease.

thermelometer (thĕr-mĕl-ŏm'ĕ-tĕr) ["+ *ēlektron,* amber, + Gr. *metron,* a measure]. An electric thermometer used to indicate temperature changes too slight to be measured on an ordinary thermometer.

thermesthesia (thĕr-mĕs-thē'zĭ-ă) ["+ *aisthēsis,* sensation]. Capability of perceiving heat and cold; temperature sense. SYN: *thermoesthesia.*

thermesthesiometer (thĕrm"ĕs-thē-zĭ-ŏm'ĕt-ĕr) [Gr. *thermē,* heat, + *aisthēsis,* sensation, + *metron,* a measure]. Device for determining sensibility to heat.

thermhypesthesia (thĕrm-hĭ-pĕs-thē'zĭ-ă) ["+ *hypo,* under, + *aisthēsis,* sensation]. Lessened sensibility of the temperature sense. SYN: *thermohypesthesia.*

thermic (thĕr'mĭk) [Gr. *thermē,* heat]. Pert. to heat.

t. sense. The temperature sense; ability to react to heat stimuli.

thermo- [Gr. *thermē*, heat]. Combining form indicating hot, heat.

thermoalgesia (thĕr″mō-ăl-jē'zĭ-ă) [Gr. *thermē*, heat, + *algēsis*, pain]. Condition in which pain is caused by application of moderate heat. SYN: *thermalgesia*.

thermoanalgesia (thĕr″mō-ăn″ăl-jē'zĭ-ă) ["+ *an-*, not, + *algēsis*, pain]. Loss of heat sensation. SYN: *thermanalgesia*.

thermoanesthesia (thĕr″mō-ăn″ĕs-thē'zĭ-ă) ["+ "+ *aisthēsis*, sensation]. 1. Inability to distinguish between heat and cold. 2. Insensibility to heat or temperature changes.

thermobiosis (thĕr″mō-bī-ō'sĭs) [Gr. *thermē*, heat, + *biōsis*, way of life]. Ability to withstand high temperature.

thermobiotic (thĕr″mō-bī-o'ĭk) ["+ *bios*, life]. Able to exist at high temperature.

thermocauterectomy (thĕr″mō-kō-tĕr-ĕk'tō-mī) ["+ *kautērion*, branding iron, + *ektomē*, excision]. Excision by thermocautery.

thermocautery (thĕr″mō-kō'tĕr-ĭ). 1. Cautery by application of heat. 2. Cauterizing iron. SEE: *actual cautery*.

thermocoagulation (thĕr″mō-kō-ăg-ū-lā'shŭn) [Gr. *thermē*, heat, + L. *coagulāre*, to clot]. The use of high frequency currents to produce coagulation to destroy tissue.

thermocouple (thĕr'mō-kŭ″pl) ["+ L. *copula*, a bond]. Device for measuring slight temperature changes. SYN: *thermopile*.

thermode. A device for heating or cooling a part of the body. T.'s have been used in studying the effect on body function when temperature of some organ or tissue is changed.

thermoduric (thĕr″mō-dū'rĭk) ["+ L. *durus*, resistant]. Able to live in high temperatures. SEE: *thermophylic*.

thermoesthesia (thĕr″mō-ĕs-thē'zĭ-ă) [Gr. *thermē*, heat, + *aisthēsis*, sensation]. Ability to recognize temperature differences. SYN: *thermesthesia*.

thermoexcitory (thĕr″mō-ĕk-sī'tōr-ĭ) ["+ L. *excitāre*, to irritate]. Stimulating the production of heat in the body.

thermogenesis (thĕr″mō-jĕn'ē-sĭs) ["+ *genesis*, production]. The production of heat, esp. in the body.

thermograph (thĕr'mō-grăf) [Gr. *thermē*, heat, + *graphein*, to write]. Device for registering variations of heat.

thermog'raphy. In medicine, the use of a device which detects and records the heat present in very small areas of the part being studied. When these multiple readings are accumulated the relatively hot and cold spots on the body surface are revealed. The

technique has been used to study blood flow to limbs and to detect cancer of the breast.

thermohyperalgesia (thĕr″mō-hī″pĕr-ăl-gē'zĭ-ă) ["+ *hyper*, above, + *algesis*, pain]. Unbearable pain upon the application of heat.

thermohyperesthesia (thĕr″mō-hī″pĕr-ĕs-thē'zĭ-ă) [Gr. *thermē*, heat, + *hyper*, above, + *aisthēsis*, sensation]. Exceptional sensitiveness to heat.

thermohypesthesia (thĕr″mō-hī″pĕs-thē'-zĭ-ă) ["+ *hypo*, under, + *aisthēsis*, sensation]. Diminished perception of heat.

thermoinhibitory (thĕr″mō-ĭn-hĭb'ĭ-tōr'ĭ) ["+ L. *inhibere*, to restrain]. Arresting or impeding the generation of body heat.

thermolabile (thĕr″mō-lā'bĭl) [Gr. *thermē*, heat, + *labilis*, unstable]. Destroyed or changed easily by heat; unstable. SEE: *heat; heat, latent*.

thermolysis (thĕr-mŏl'ĭ-sĭs) ["+ *lysis*, dissolution]. 1. Loss of heat from the body, as by evaporation. 2. Chemical decomposition by heat.

thermometer (thĕr-mŏm'ĕ-tĕr) [Gr. *thermē*, heat, + *metron*, measure]. An instrument for indicating the degree of heat or cold. First mention of a t. in diagnosis of disease was given by It. physician, Sanctorius, in 1626. The instrument he used is little different from that used today.

    t., air or gas. T. filled with air or gas, the expansion of which registers high tem-

Comparative Thermometric Scale

	Centigrade	Fahrenheit*
Boiling point		
of water	100°	212°
	90°	194°
	80°	176°
	70°	158°
	60°	140°
	50°	122°
	40°	104°
	30°	86°
	20°	68°
	10°	50°
Freezing point		
of water	0°	32°
	−10°	14°
	−20°	−4°

CONVERSION: *F. to Centigrade:* Subtract 32 and multiply by 5/9. *C. to Fahrenheit:* Multiply by 9/5 and add 32.

* Also called *Celsius*.

peratures.

t., alcohol. T. containing alcohol.

t., Celsius. Centigrade t.

t., centigrade. T. generally used in Latin America and in Europe, and in scientific work. Temperature of boiling water at sea level 100° and freezing point 0°, with 100° between.

t., clinical. T. for measuring temperature of body; one in which the mercury remains stationary at registration point until shaken down.

t., differential. T. recording slight variations.

t. disinfection. Disinfection with a substance that is able to kill ordinary bacteria and Mycobacterium tuberculosis as well as viruses. A variety of chemical solutions are used but the effectiveness of these agents can be greatly diminished if the thermometer is not washed thoroughly prior to being disinfected.

t., Fahrenheit. T. used in English-speaking countries and in Holland. Boiling point 212°, freezing point 32°.

t., mercury. T. containing mercury.

t. scale. Graduated device on a t. to indicate a temperature.

t., self-registering. T. recording variations of temperature.

t., spirit. T. filled with alcohol instead of mercury for registering low temperatures.

t., surface. T. for indicating temperature of the body's surface.

t., wet and dry bulb. A device for determining relative humidity consisting of two thermometers, the bulb of one being kept saturated with water vapor. The difference in temperatures between the two is dependent upon relative humidity.

thermometric (thĕr″mō-mĕt′rĭk) [Gr. *thermē*, heat, + *metron*, measure]. Pert. to heat measurement or a thermometer.

thermometry (thĕr-mŏm′ĕ-trĭ). Measurement of temperature.

t., clinical. Oral temperature of healthy body ranges between 96.6° and 100° F. (35.9°-37.8° C.). During a 24 hr. period, a person's body temperature may vary 0.5°-2.0° F. (.28°-1.1° C.). It is highest in late afternoon, lowest during sleep in early hours of the morning. Slightly increased by eating, exercising, and

Thermometric Equivalents

C	F	C	F	C	F	C	F
0	32	27	80.6	54	129.2	81	177.8
1	33.8	28	82.4	55	131	82	179.6
2	35.6	29	84.2	56	132.8	83	181.4
3	37.4	30	86.0	57	134.6	84	183.2
4	39.2	31	87.8	58	136.4	85	185
5	41	32	89.6	59	138.2	86	186.8
6	42.8	33	91.4	60	140	87	188.6
7	44.6	34	93.2	61	141.8	88	190.4
8	46.4	35	95	62	143.6	89	192.2
9	48.2	36	96.8	63	145.4	90	194
10	50	37	98.6	64	147.2	91	195.8
11	51.8	38	100.4	65	149	92	197.6
12	53.6	39	102.2	66	150.8	93	199.4
13	55.4	40	104	67	152.6	94	201.2
14	57.2	41	105.8	68	154.4	95	203
15	59	42	107.6	69	156.2	96	204.8
16	60.8	43	109.4	70	158	97	206.6
17	62.6	44	111.2	71	159.8	98	208.4
18	64.4	45	113	72	161.6	99	210.2
19	66.2	46	114.8	73	163.4	100	212
20	68	47	116.6	74	165.2		
21	69.8	48	118.4	75	167		
22	71.6	49	120.2	76	168.8		
23	73.4	50	122	77	170.6		
24	75.2	51	123.8	78	172.4		
25	77	52	125.6	79	174.2		
26	78.8	53	127.4	80	176		

external heat; reduced about 1.5° F. (.80° C.) during sleep. In disease the temperature of body deviates several degrees above and below the average of health.

In facial erysipelas, acute meningitis, pneumonia, scarlatina, typhus, smallpox, and intermittent fever it sometimes rises as high as 106°-107° F. (41.1°-41.7° C.). In other febrile diseases it rarely reaches 104° F. (40° C.). However, temperature may reach as high as 110 ° F. (43.3° C.) as in sunstroke, with patient recovering. The lowest extreme of temperature is found sometimes in cold stage of cholera when temperature may be very low (90°-85° F. or 32.2°-29.4° C.) for several days.

Subnormal temperatures, below 98° F. (36.7° C.) are observed in the following conditions: during convalescence from certain febrile conditions, after pneumonia and typhoid fever; in collapse resulting from shock, hemorrhage, or rupture of a viscus, as the bowel in typhoid, the lung in phthisis, or stomach in perforating ulcer.

In general, for every degree of fever the pulse rises 10 beats per minute, but rise of temperature to 99.5° F. (37.5° C.) gives more evidence of disease than rising of pulse from 70-90 beats per minute. If temperature remains above normal after general symptoms denote convalescence, patient is in danger of a relapse or the supervention of some other disease. The range of the increase of heat in different febrile diseases extends to 110° F. (43.3° C.) and as a rule the amount of increase is a criterion of the intensity of the disease.

Artificial fever induced through diathermy, continuous hot bath, or malarial injections was formerly utilized in some diseases, but is seldom used in modern medicine.

thermoneurosis (thĕr″mō-nū-rō′sĭs) [Gr. *thermē*, heat, + *neuron*, nerve, + *-ōsis*, condition]. Elevation of body temperature in hysteria and other nervous conditions.

thermopenetration (thĕr″mō-pĕn-ĕ-trā′shŭn) ["+ L. *penetrāre*, to penetrate]. Application of heat to the deeper tissues of the body by diathermy.

thermoperiodicity (thĕr″mō-pĕr-ĭ-ō-dĭs′ĭ-tĭ). Condition in which an organism grows better when exposed to alternating high and low temperatures.

thermophagy (thĕr-mŏf′ă-gĭ) [Gr. *thermē*, heat, + *phagein*, to eat]. Swallowing extremely hot foods.

thermophilic (thĕr″mō-fĭl′ĭk) ["+ *philein*, to love]. Preferring or thriving best at high temperatures, said of bacteria which thrive best at temperatures between 40°-70° C. (104° and 158° F.).

thermophobia (thĕr″mō-fō′bĭ-ă) ["+ *phobos*, fear]. Abnormal dread of heat.

thermophore (thĕr′mō-fōr) [Gr. *thermē*, heat, + *phoros*, a bearer]. Apparatus for applying heat to a part, consisting of water heater and tubes conveying water to a coil and returning to heater, or salts which produce heat when moistened.

thermophylic (thĕr″mō-fī′lĭk) ["+ *phylakē*, guard]. Resistant to destruction by heat, characteristic of certain bacteria.

thermopile (thĕr′mō-pīl) ["+ L. *pila*, pile]. In physical therapy, thermoelectric battery used in measuring small variations in the degree of heat. It consists of a number of dissimilar metallic plates connected together. Under the influence of heat, these produce an electric current.

thermoplegia (thĕr″mō-plē′jĭ-ă) [Gr. *thermē*, heat, + *plēgē*, a stroke]. Heatstroke; sunstroke.

thermopolypnea (thĕr″mō-pŏl-ĭp-nē′ă) ["+ *polys*, many, + *pnoia*, breath]. Quickened breathing caused by high fever or great heat.

thermoradiotherapy (thĕr″mō-rā″dĭ-ō-thĕr′ă-pī) ["+ L. *radius*, ray, + Gr. *therapeia*, treatment]. Application of heat to deep tissues by diathermy. SYN: *thermopenetration*.

thermoreceptor (thĕr″mō-rē-sĕp′tor) [Gr. *thermē*, heat, + L. *receptor*, receiver]. A sensory receptor which is stimulated by a rise of body temperature.

thermoregulatory (thĕr″mō-rĕg′ū-lă-tōr-ĭ). Pert. to the regulation of temperature, esp. body temperature.

   t. centers. Centers in the hypothalamus which regulate heat production and heat loss, esp. the latter, so that a normal body temperature is maintained. They are influenced by nervous impulses from cutaneous receptors and by the temperature of the blood flowing through them.

thermoresistant (thĕr″mō-rē-zĭs′tănt) [Gr. *thermē*, heat, + L. *resistentia*, resistance]. Ability to survive in relatively high temperature. Characteristic of some types of bacteria.

thermostabile (thĕr″mō-stā′bl) ["+ L. *stabilis*, stationary]. Not changed or destroyed by heat.

thermostat (thĕr′mō-stăt) [Gr. *thermē*, heat, + *statos*, standing]. An automatic device for regulating the temperature.

thermosteresis (thĕr″mō-stĕ-rē′sĭs) ["+ *sterēsis*, deprivation]. The deprivation or loss of heat.

thermosterilization. 1. Bacterial sterilization by use of heat. 2. Sexual sterilization, usually temporary, by application of heat to the testicular area.

thermosystaltic (thĕr″mō-sĭs-tăl′tĭk) ["+ systellein, to contract]. Pert. to contraction of the muscles under stimulus of heat.

thermotactic, thermotaxic (thĕr″mō-tăk′tĭk, -tăks′ĭk) ["+ taktikos, regulating]. Rel. to regulation of the body temperature.

thermotaxis (thĕr″mō-tăks′ĭs) [Gr. thermē, heat, + taxis, arrangement]. 1. Regulation of bodily temperature. 2. Reaction of organisms or of protoplasm in the living body to heat. 3. The movement of certain organisms or cells toward (positive thermotaxis) or away from (negative thermotaxis) heat. SYN: thermometropism.

thermotherapeutics (thĕr″mō-thĕr-ă-pū′tĭks) ["+ therapeutikē, treatment]. Use of heat in treatment of disease. SYN: thermotherapy.

thermotherapy (thĕr″mō-thĕr′ă-pĭ) ["+ therapeia, treatment]. The therapeutic application of heat. Heat may be applied locally by radiant heating devices which give off infrared rays and by conductive heating which utilizes hot water bottles, paraffin baths, hot packs, etc. The temperature of the body may be increased by artificial fever, by raising environmental temperature, or by preventing heat loss from the body. SEE: heat; hyperthermia.

thermotolerant (thĕr″mō-tŏl′ĕr-ănt) [Gr. thermē, heat, + L. tolerāre, to tolerate]. Able to live normally in high temperature.

thermotoxin (thĕr″mō-tŏks′ĭn) ["+ toxikon, poison]. A poison formed in the tissues by excessive heat.

thermotropism (thĕr-mŏt′rō-pĭzm) ["+ tropē, turning]. Thermotaxis, q.v.

thesaurismosis (thē-sö″rĭs-mō′sĭs) [Gr. thesaurosis, treasure, + -osis, condition]. Abnormal or excessive storage of substances in certain cells. Usually due to a metabolic disease such as lipoidosis.

thesis (thē′sĭs) [LL., affirmation]. An essay on a given subject offered by a candidate for a collegiate degree.

thi′amin(e). A white crystalline compound ($O_{12}H_{17}N_4OS$) occurring naturally and produced synthetically. It is widely distributed in various animal and plant foods, dry yeast and wheat germ being the richest natural resources. It occurs in the outer layers of seeds and in nuts, legumes, most vegetables, and in some meats (pork, muscle, liver, heart, and kidneys). SYN: vitamin B_1.

FUNCTION: It is essential for the normal metabolism of carbohydrates and fats. It acts as a coenzyme of carboxylases in the carboxylation of pyruvic acid, hence is essential for the liberation of energy and disposal of pyruvic acid.

EFFECTS OF DEFICIENCY: Moderate deficiency results in impaired functioning of nervous, circulatory, digestive, and endocrine systems. Neurasthenia, neurological disorders, and cardiac and gastrointestinal symptoms may result. Loss of appetite, fatigue, muscle tenderness, and increased irritability are symptoms. Severe and prolonged deficiency result in beriberi, q.v.

DAILY REQUIREMENTS: For children and adults 0.5 mg./1000 Cal. of food intake.

Thiersch's graft, method (tērsh). [Karl Thiersch, Ger. surgeon, 1822-1895]. A method of skin grafting using epidermis and a portion of the dermis.

thigh (thī) [AS. theoh]. The proximal portion of the lower extremity; the portion lying between the hip joint and the knee. SEE: hip; pectineus; sartorius.

    t. bone. The femur.

    t. joint. The hip joint. SYN: articulatio coxae.

thigmesthesia (thĭg″mĕs-thē′zĭ-ă) [Gr. thigma, touch, + aisthēsis, sensation]. Sensitive to touch.

thigmotaxis (thĭg″mō-tăks′ĭs) ["+ taxis, arrangement]. The negative or positive response of certain motile cells to touch.

thigmotropism (thĭg-mŏt′rō-pĭzm) ["+ tropos, a turning, + -ismos, condition]. The response of certain motile cells to move toward something which touches them.

thio- [Gr. theion, sulfur]. Prefix denoting presence of sulfur replacing oxygen.

thiogenic (thī″ō-jĕn′ĭk) [Gr. theion, sulfur, + gennan, to produce]. Able to convert hydrogen sulfide into higher sulfur compounds, said of bacteria in the water of some mineral springs.

thioneine (thī′ō-nēn) ["+ neos, new]. Thiol-histidine-betaine, compound containing crystalline sulfur, found in ergot and red blood cells. SYN: ergthioneine.

thiopectic, thiopexic (thī-ō-pĕk′tĭk, -pĕks′ĭk) ["+ pexis, fixation]. Pert. to the fixation of sulfur.

thiopexy (thī′ō-pĕks′ĭ). The fixation of sulfur.

thiophil, thiophilic (thī′ō-fĭl, thī″ō-fĭl′ĭk) [Gr. theion, sulfur, + philein, to love]. Thriving in the presence of sulfur or its compounds, as some bacteria.

thiouracil (thī″ō-ū′ră-sĭl). An antithyroid drug which is little used now. SEE: propylthiouracil.

thiourea (thī″ō-ūr-ē′ă) [Gr. theion, sulfur, + ouron, urine]. Colorless crystalline compound of urea in which sulfur replaces the oxygen.

third cranial nerve. Oculomotor nerve. SEE: *Table of Cranial Nerves* in *Appendix.*

third intention. Healing of a wound by filling with granulations. SEE: *resolution.*

third ventricle. Third ventricle of the brain, a narrow cavity between the two optic thalami. It communicates anteriorly with the lateral ventricles and posteriorly, via the cerebral aqueduct of Silvius, with the 4th ventricle. SYN: *ventriculus tertius.*

thirst [AS. *thurst*]. 1. Desire for fluid, esp. for water. This may occur in fevers and certain other maladies, or it may be entirely lacking in some conditions. The nurse should note whether the intake of fluids allays the patient's thirst. 2. The sensation resulting from the lack of or the need of water. Thirst may result from drying of mucous membranes, esp. those of the pharynx, or from reduced salivary secretion. It also results from general dehydration as may occur following hemorrhage, profuse sweating, vomiting, or excessive loss of urine as in diabetes mellitus or insipidus.

RS: adipsia; anadipsia; aposia; taste.

t., absence of. Adipsia, aposia.

t., excessive. Polydipsia.

t., false. Pseudodipsia; not sated by drinking water.

t., morbid. Dipsosis.

Thiry's fistula (tē′rē). [Ludwig Thiry, Austrian physiologist, 1817-1897]. An artificial fistula placed in a dog's intestines for obtaining intestinal juices for experimental purposes.

Thomsen's disease (tŏm′sĕn). [Asmus Julius Thomsen, Danish physician, 1815-1896]. Myotonia congenita, q.v.

thoracalgia (thō″răk-ăl′jĭ-ă) [Gr. *thōakos*, chest, + *algos*, pain]. Pain in the chest wall. SYN: *pleurodynia.*

thoracectomy (thō″ră-sĕk′tō-mĭ) [″+ *ektomē*, excision]. Incision of the chest wall with resection of a portion of rib.

thoracentesis (thō″rā-sĕn-tē′sĭs) [″+ *kentēsis*, a puncture]. Surgical puncture of the chest wall for removal of fluids. Usually done by using a large-bore needle. SYN: *pleurocentesis*, q.v.

NP: Have patient well supported. Watch for signs of collapse during and following treatment.

thoracic (thō-răs′ĭk) [Gr. *thōrax*, chest]. Pert. to the chest or thorax.

t. cavity. The space lying above the diaphragm and enclosed within the walls of the thorax; the space occupied by the t. viscera. It includes the pleural cavities occupied by the lungs and the mediastinum, the space between the lungs occupied by the heart lying within the pericardium, the thoracic aorta, pulmonary artery and veins, vena cava, thymus gland, lymph nodes, trachea, bronchi, esophagus, and thoracic duct. It is separated from the abdominal cavity by the diaphragm.

RS: chyle; cisterna chyli; lacteal; lymphatic, lymphatic system.

t. duct. The main lymph duct of the body having its origin at the cisterna chyli on the abdomen. It passes upward through the diaphragm into the thorax, continuing upward alongside aorta and esophagus to the neck where it turns to the left and enters the left subclavian vein near its junction with the left internal jugular vein. It receives lymph from all parts of the body except right side of head, neck, and thorax and right upper extremity.

t. limbs. Upper extremities.

t. squeeze. A rare occurrence in divers who are skilled enough to go approx. 80-100 feet (24.4-30.5 meters) deep while holding their breath. The lungs become compressed sufficiently to cause rupture of alveolar capillaries.

TREATMENT: Immediate removal from the water; artificial respiration preferably with an apparatus which will deliver increased oxygen concentration rather than air.

thoraco- [Gr. *thōrax, thōrakos*, chest]. Combining form meaning chest or chest wall.

thoracobronchotomy (thō″răk-ō-brŏn-kŏt′-ō-mĭ) [″+ *bronchos*, windpipe, + *tomē*, a cutting]. Incision through the thoracic wall into the bronchus.

thoracocautery (thō″răk-ō-kŏ′tĕr-ĭ) [″+ *kautērion*, branding iron]. The use of cautery in breaking up pulmonary adhesions to collapse the lung.

thoracoceloschisis (thō″răk-ō-sĕ-lŏs′kĭ-sĭs) [Gr. *thōrakos*, chest, + *koilia*, belly, + *schisis*, a fissure]. Congenital fissure of the thoracic and abdominal cavities.

thoracocentesis (thō″răk-ō-sĕn-tē′sĭs) [″+ *kentēsis*, a puncture]. Surgical entry into the thoracic cavity in order to remove fluid. Usually done by using a needle. SYN: *thoracentesis.*

thoracocyllosis (thō″răk-ō-sĭl-ō′sĭs) [″+ *kyllōsis*, crippling]. Deformity of the chest.

thoracocyrtosis (thō″răk-ō-sĭr-tō′sĭs) [Gr. *thōrakos*, chest, + *kyrtōsis*, curvature]. Excessive curvature of the chest.

thoracodynia (thō″răk-ō-dĭn′ĭ-ă) [″+ *odynē*, pain]. Pain in the thorax.

thoracogastroschisis (thō″răk-ō-găs-trŏs′kĭ-sĭs) [″+ *gastēr*, belly, + *schisis*, a fissure]. Congenital fissure of abdomen and thorax.

thoracolumbar (thō″răk-ō-lŭm′băr) [Gr. *thōrakos*, chest, + L. *lumbus*, loin]. Pert. to the thoracic and lumbar parts of the spine; noting their ganglia and the fibers of the sympathetic nervous system.

thoracolysis (thō″răk-ŏl′ĭ-sĭs) [″+ *lysis*, dissolution]. The freeing of a lung which is attached to the chest wall. SYN: *pneumonolysis.*

thoracometry (thō″ră-kŏm′ĕt-rĭ) [″+ *metron*, measure]. The measurement of the thorax.

thoracomyodynia (thō″ră-kō-mī″ō-dĭn′ĭ-ă) [Gr. *thōrakos*, chest, + *mys*, *my-*, muscle, + *odynē*, pain]. Pain in chest muscles.

thoracopagus (thō″ră-kŏp′ă-gŭs) [″+ *pagos*, fixed]. Two malformed fetuses joined at the thorax.

thoracopathy (thō″răk-ŏp′ă-thĭ) [″+ *pathos*, disease]. Any disease of the thorax, thoracic organs, or tissues.

thoracoplasty (thō″ră-kŏ-plăs″tĭ, thō-rā′kō-plăs″tĭ) [Gr. *thōrakos*, chest, + *plassein*, to form]. A plastic operation upon the thorax; removal of portions of the ribs in stages to collapse diseased areas of the lung. SEE: *empyema.*

thoracopneumoplasty (thō″ră-kō-nū′mō-plăs-tĭ) [″+ *pneumon*, lung, + *plassein*, to form]. Plastic surgery involving the chest and lung.

thoracoschisis (thō″ră-kŏs′kĭ-sĭs) [″+ *schisis*, fissure]. Congenital fissure of the chest wall.

thoracoscope (thō-rā′kō-skōp, -răk′ō-skōp) [Gr. *thōrakos*, chest, + *skopein*, to examine]. 1. Instrument for inspection of the thoracic cavity. It has an electric light and is inserted through an intercostal space. 2. An instrument used in auscultation to convey the sounds of the chest to the ear. SYN: *stethoscope.*

thoracoscopy (thō″ră-kŏs′kō-pĭ). Diagnostic examination of the pleural cavity with an endoscope.

thoracostenosis (thō″ră-kō-stĕn-ō′sĭs) [Gr. *thōrakos*, chest, + *stenōsis*, a contraction]. Narrowness of the thorax. SYN: *waspwaist.*

thoracostomy (thō″răk-ŏs′tō-mĭ) [″+ *stoma*, mouth]. Resection of chest wall to allow room for enlarged heart or for drainage.

thoracotomy (thō″răk-ŏt′ō-mĭ) [″+ *tomē*, a cutting]. Surgical incision of the chest wall.

thorax (thō′răks) [Gr.]. (pl. *thoraces, thoraxes*) [NA] That part of the body between the base of the neck superiorly and the diaphragm inferiorly.

The surface of the thorax is divided into regions as follows: *Anterior surface:* supraclavicular, above the clavicles; suprasternal, above the sternum; clavicular, over the clavicles; sternal, over the sternum; mammary, the space between the 3rd and 6th ribs on either side; inframammary, below the

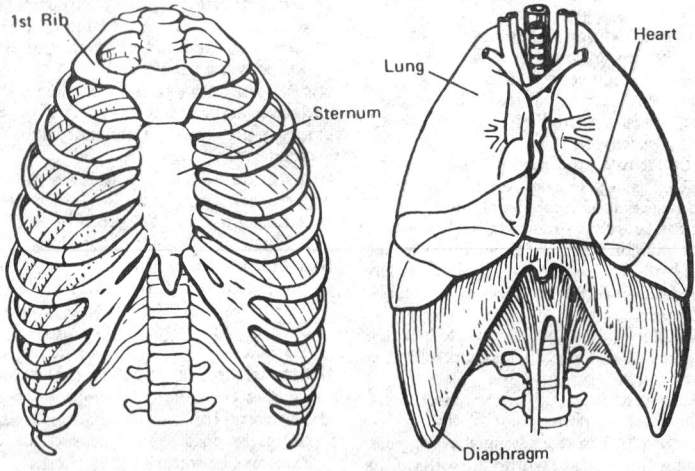

THORAX
Left, bony thorax; Right, visceral thorax.

mamma and above the lower border of the 12th rib on either side. *Posterior surface:* scapular, over the scapulae; interscapular, between the scapulae; infrascapular, below the scapulae. *On sides:* axillary, above the 6th rib. SYN: *chest.*
RS: acromiothoracic; cholohemothorax; "thorac-" words.

t., Amazon. A chest with only one breast.

t., barrel-shaped. A malformed chest rounded like a barrel seen in pulmonary emphysema.

t., fusiform. A chest deformed by long continued tight lacing.

t. paralyticus. The long, flat chest of patients with constitutional visceroptosis.

t., Peyrot's. A chest that has an obliquely oval, deformed shape, seen in large pleural effusions.

thorazine (thōr-ā′zēn). A proprietary name for chlorpromazine hydrochloride. It is a central nervous system depressant and employed as a sedative and antiemetic. It potentiates the effects of sedatives and general anesthetics and is of value in quieting severely excited psychiatric patients.

thorium (thō′rǐ-ŭm). SYMB: *Th.* At. wt. 232.038; at. no. 90. A metallic element occurring in combination. It is radioactive. At one time it was used to outline blood vessels.

thoron (thō′rŏn). SYMB: *Tn.* At. wt. 220; at. no. 86. A radioactive isotope of radon. It has a half-life of 51.5 seconds.

thread′worm. Common name applied to the pinworm, Enterobius vermicularis.

three-day fever. A viral disease transmitted by the sandfly, Phlebotomus papatasii. The disease resembles dengue but is less severe. SYN: *pappataci fever; sandfly fever.*

thremmatology (thrĕm″ă-tŏl′ō-jĭ) [Gr. *thremma,* nursling, + *logos,* science]. Scientific breeding of plants and animals.

threonine (thrē′ō-nǐn). Alpha-amino beta-hydroxy butyric acid. One of the essential amino acids.

threpsology (thrĕp-sŏl′ō-jĭ) [Gr. *threpsis,* nutrition, + *logos,* study]. Science of nutrition.

threshold (thresh′ōld) [AS. *therscold*]. 1. Point at which a psychological or physiological effect begins to be produced. 2. A measure of the sensitivity of an organ or function which is obtained by finding the lowest value of the appropriate stimulus that will give the response.

t., absolute. The stimulus of least intensity that will give rise to a sensation or a response.

t., auditory. Minimum audible sound.

t. of consciousness. In psychoanalysis, point at which a stimulus is just barely perceived.

t., differential. The lowest limit at which two stimuli can be differentiated from each other.

t., erythema. Stage in which erythema of the skin due to radiation just begins.

t., ketosis. The lower limit at which ketone bodies (acetoacetic acid, hydroxybutyric acid, and acetone), upon their accumulation in the blood, are excreted by the kidney. At that point ketone bodies are being produced faster by the liver than the body can oxidize them.

t. limit value. The concentration in air of a substance to which workers can be exposed without affecting their health or well-being.

t., renal. The concentration at which a substance in the blood normally not excreted by the kidney begins to appear in the urine. The renal threshold for glucose is 160-180 mg./100 ml.

t., sensory. The minimal stimulus for any sensory receptor which will give rise to a sensation.

t., stimulus. The least or minimal stimulus that will give rise to a sensation or bring about a response such as a muscle contraction. SYN: *liminal stimulus; rheobase.*

t. substance. A substance present in the blood which on being filtered through glomeruli of the kidney is reabsorbed by the tubules up to a certain limit, that being the upper limit of the concentration of the substance in normal plasma. *High-threshold* substances are those which are entirely or almost entirely reabsorbed. Ex: chlorides; glucose. *Low-threshold* substances are those which are reabsorbed in limited quantities. Ex: phosphates; urea. *No-threshold* substances are those excreted in their entirety. Ex: creatinine sulfate.

thrill (thrĭl) [ME. *thrillen,* to pierce]. 1. Abnormal tremor accompanying a vascular or cardiac murmur felt on palpation. SYN: *fremitus.* 2. A tingling or shivering sensation of tremulous excitement as from pain, pleasure, or horror.

t., aneurysmal. T. felt on palpation of an aneurysm.

t., aortic. T. heard over aortic aperture on lesions of valves.

t., arterial. T. heard over an artery.

t., diastolic. T. felt over the heart during diastole of the ventricle.

t., hydatid. Peculiar tremor felt on palpation of a hydatid cyst.

t., presystolic. T. sometimes felt over apex of the heart preceding ventricular contraction.

throat (thrōt) [AS. *throte*]. 1. The pharynx and the fauces. 2. Cavity from arch of palate to glottis and superior opening of the esophagus. 3. The front of the neck. 4. Any narrow orifice.

t., foreign bodies in. Symptoms depend somewhat on the location and size of the foreign body, and vary from simple discomfort to distressing coughing, difficulty in breathing, retching and cyanosis, and, if not relieved, suffocation resulting in unconsciousness.

TREATMENT: If not causing serious distress, the patient should lie down with the head lower than the body. The common practice of a sudden slap on the back often helps to dislodge bodies in the trachea or throat, and in youngsters is esp. efficacious when the child is inverted. If this does not succeed, it is possible to introduce a finger through the mouth into the throat, possibly to the larynx, and so dislodge the foreign body. It has been possible in this way to dislodge a bean from the larynx of an unconscious child.

Summon a physician immediately. Make sure to tell him the nature of the case so that he may bring the proper instruments as it may be necessary for him to open the trachea. Folk remedies such as cathartics, enemas, and eating coarse food such as corn bread are of no value whatever, and may be dangerous. SEE: *symptom, throat.*

t., sore. Inflammation of tonsils, larynx, or pharynx. SYN: *pharyngitis; tonsillitis.*

throb (thrŏb) [ME. *throbben*, of imitative orgin]. 1. A beat or pulsation, as of the heart. 2. To pulsate.

throbbing (thrŏb'ĭng). Pulsation; a beating; rhythmic movement.

Throckmorton's reflex (thrŏk'mōr"tŭn). [Thomas Bentley Throckmorton, Amer. neurologist, 1885 —]. Extension of great toe and flexion of others when dorsum of foot is percussed in metatarsophalangeal region.

throe (thrō) [AS. *thruve*, paroxysm]. A severe spasm of pain, esp. one in childbirth.

thrombasthenia (thrŏm"băs-thē'nĭ-ă) [Gr. *thrombos*, clot, + *astheneia*, weakness]. 1. Deficiency or abnormality of the blood platelets. 2. A congenital bleeding disorder characterized by a normal platelet count, prolonged bleeding time, and defective clot retraction.

thrombectomy (thrŏm-bĕk'tō-mĭ) [Gr. *thrombos*, clot, + *ektomē*, excision]. Excision of a thrombus.

thrombi (thrŏm'bī). Pl. of thrombus.

thrombin (thrŏm'bĭn) [Gr. *thrombos*, clot]. 1. An enzyme formed in shed-blood from prothrombin which reacts with soluble fibrinogen converting it to fibrin which forms the basis of a blood clot. SEE: *coagulation.*

thrombinogen (throm-bin'o-jen). An obsolete term for prothrombin.

thrombo- [Gr.]. Combining form meaning clot of blood; a thrombus.

thromboangiitis (thrŏm"bō-ăn"jĭ-ī'tĭs) [Gr. *thrombos*, clot, + *angeion*, vessel, + *-itis*, inflammation]. Inflammation of inner coat of a blood vessel with clot formation. SEE: *thrombosis.*

t. oblit'erans. Chronic recurring inflammatory occlusive disease, chiefly of the peripheral arteries and veins, with an extraordinary affinity for young men. SYN: *Buerger's disease.*

SYM: Occlusion; thrombosis; excruciating pain in leg or foot, worse at night; cyanotic, clammy cold extremity; diminished sense of heat and cold; gangrene of toes or foot may set in.

thromboarteritis (thrŏm"bō-ar-tĕ-rī'tĭs) ["+ *artēria*, artery, + *-itis*, inflammation]. Inflammation of an artery in connection with thrombosis.

thromboclasis (thrŏm-bŏk'lă-sĭs) ["+ *klasis*, a breaking]. The breaking up or lysis of a thrombus. SYM: *thrombolysis.*

thromboclastic (thrŏm-bō-klăs'tĭk). Pert. to or producing the dissolution of a thrombus. SYM: *thrombolytic.*

thrombocyst, thrombocystis (thrŏm'bō-sĭst, -sĭs'tĭs) [Gr. *thrombos*, clot, + *kystis*, a sac]. A membranous sac enveloping a thrombus.

thrombocyte (thrŏm'bō-sīt) [Gr. *thrombos*, a clot, + *kytos*, cell]. An old term for blood platelets, q.v.

thrombocytocrit (thrŏm'bō-sī'tō-krĭt) ["+ *kytos*, cell, + *krinein*, to separate]. Device for estimating the platelet content of the blood.

thrombocytolysis (thrŏm"bō-sī-tŏl'ĭ-sĭs) ["+ "+ *lysis*, dissolution]. Dissolution of thrombocytes.

thrombocytopenia (thrŏm"bō-sī"tō-pē'nĭ-ă) ["+ "+ *penia*, lack]. Abnormal decrease in number of the blood platelets. SYN: *thrombopenia.*

thrombocytopoiesis (thrŏm"bō-sī"tō-poy-ē'sĭs) ["+ "+ *poiēsis*, production]. The formation of blood platelets.

thrombocytosis (thrŏm"bō-sī-tō'sĭs) [Gr. *thrombos*, clot, + *kytos*, hollow vessel]. Increase in number of thrombocytes.

thromboembolism (thrŏm″bō-ĕm′bō-lĭsm) [Gr. *thrombos*, clot, + L. *embolismus*, obstruction]. An embolism; the blocking of a blood vessel by a thrombus which has become detached from its site of formation.

thromboendocarditis (thrŏm″bō-ĕn″dō-kär-dī′tĭs) [Gr. *thrombos*, clot, + *endon*, within, + *kardia*, heart, + *-itis*, inflammation]. Formation of a clot on inflamed surface of a heart valve.

thrombogen (thrŏm′bō-jĕn) [Gr. *thrombos*, clot, + *gennan*, to produce]. A synonym for the fifth factor (*Factor V*) in blood coagulation. SYN: *proaccelerin*, q.v.

thrombogenesis (thrŏm″bō-jĕn′ĕ-sĭs) [Gr. *thrombos*, a clot, + *genesis*, production]. The formation of a blood clot.

thrombogenic (thrŏm″bō-jĕn′ĭk) [″+ *gennan*, to produce]. Producing or tending to produce a clot.

thromboid (thrŏm′boyd) [″+ *eidos*, form]. Resembling a thrombus or clot.

thrombokinase (thrŏm″bō-kĭn′ās) [Gr. *thrombos*, a clot, + *kinēsis*, motion]. A synonym for the tenth blood coagulation factor (Factor X) or Stuart factor, q.v.

thrombokinesis (thrŏm″bō-kĭ-nē′sĭs) [Gr. *thrombos*, a clot, + *kinēsis*, motion]. The coagulation of the blood.

thrombolymphangitis (thrŏm″bō-lĭm″făn-jī′tĭs) [″+ L. *lympha*, lymph, + Gr. *angeion*, vessel, + *-itis*, inflammation]. Inflammation of a lymphatic vessel due to obstruction by thrombus formation.

thrombolysis (thrŏm-bŏl′ĭ-sĭs) [″+ *lysis*, destruction]. The breaking up of a thrombus. SYN: *thromboclasis*.

thrombolytic (thrŏm″bō-lĭt′ĭk). Pert. to or causing the breaking up of a thrombus.

thrombopathy (thrŏm-bŏp′ă-thī) [″+ *pathos*, disease]. A defect in the coagulation apparatus of the blood. SYN: *hemophilia*, q.v.

thrombopenia (thrŏm-bō-pē′nĭ-ă) [Gr. *thrombos*, a clot, + *penia*, lack]. Lessening of the number of blood platelets.

thrombophilia (thrŏm-bō-fĭl′ĭ-ă) [Gr. *thrombos*, a clot, + *philein*, to love]. A tendency to the occurrence of clot formation.

thrombophlebitis (thrŏm″bō-flē-bī′tĭs) [Gr. *thrombos*, a clot, + *phleps*, *phleb-*, vein, + *-itis*, inflammation]. Inflammation of a vein developing before the formation of a thrombus. SYN: *alba dolens; milk leg; phlebitis, phlegmasia*.

NP: Immobilize the affected limb, elevate it and support with a pillow. The weight of bedclothes should be removed by supporting them on a cradle. Application of local heat by continuous use of moist, hot packs.

TREATMENT: Absolute rest to avoid the greatest danger, which is an embolus. Leg elevated so hip and knee are in flexion and heat is applied. Patient must not get up until the temperature has been normal for at least a week; if there have been infarcts, for about 2 weeks. Anticoagulants and ligation of large vein proximal to the thrombus are often used. Elastic stockings, not roller bandages should be placed on unaffected leg; and on both legs as soon as the acute phase has subsided.

thromboplastic (thrŏm″bō-plăs′tĭk) [″+ *plassein*, to form]. Pert. to or causing acceleration of clot formation in the blood.

thromboplastin (thrŏm″bō-plăs′tĭn) [″+ *plassein*, to form]. The third blood coagulation factor (Factor III). A substance found in both blood and tissues. Tissue thromboplastin is found in most parts of the body as an intracellular substance. A substance with thromboplastic activity is also present in red blood cells. Even though these two substances are separate and act in different manners, both are able to accelerate the clotting of blood.

thrombopoiesis (thrŏm″bō-poy-ē′sĭs) [″+ *poiēsis*, production]. The formation of blood platelets.

thrombosed (thrŏm′bōzd) [Gr. *thrombos*, a clot]. 1. Coagulated; clotted. 2. Denoting a vessel containing a thrombus.

thrombosin (thrŏm-bō′sĭn) [Gr. *thrombos*, clot]. An obsolete term for thrombin.

thrombosinusitis (thrŏm″bō-sī-nŭs-ī′tĭs) [″+ L. *sinus*, cavity, + Gr. *-itis*, inflammation]. Thrombus formation of a dural sinus.

thrombosis (thrŏm-bō′sĭs) [Gr. *thrombos*, clot, + *-ōsis*, condition]. The formation or development of a blood clot or thrombus.

It is a solid aggregation formed in circulating blood and such changes constitute thrombosis. When a thrombus is detached from its original site and found in another part, it is called a thrombotic embolus.

ETIOL: Trauma, esp. following an operation and parturition; cardiac and vascular disorders, obesity, heredity, increasing age, an excess of erythrocytes and of platelets, an overproduction of fibrinogen, and sepsis are predisposing causes.

SYM: *Lungs:* Obstruction of smaller vessels in the lungs causes an infarct manifested by sudden pain in the side of the chest, similar to pleurisy; also the spitting of blood, a pleural friction rub, and signs of consolidation. *Kidneys:* Blood appears in the urine, and small hemorrhagic spots in the skin. *Spleen:* Pain is felt in the left upper abdomen. *Extremities:* If a large artery in one of the extremities, such as the brachial, is suddenly obstructed, the part becomes cold, pale, bluish, and the pulse disappears below the obstructed site. Gangrene of the digits or of the whole limb may ensue. Same symptoms may apply to embolisms, q.v.

NP: In thrombosis of a limb rest in bed is essential. Patient must not be permitted to move himself; not even the upper portion of his body. Elevate the affected limb on a pillow and steady it with sandbags. Cotton or wool may be lightly wrapped about the limb to protect it.

If limb is badly swollen watch for pressure sores. Guard against burning with hot water bottle or electric pad. From six days to several weeks bedrest may be necessary depending on condition of patient.

Anticoagulant therapy necessary. When a thrombus or embolus is large, surgical removal may be necessary.

RS: embolus, "thromb-" words, angina pectoris.

t., atrophic. T. resulting from malnutrition.

t., cardiac. T. of an artery supplying the heart muscle (myocardium).

t., coagulation. T. due to coagulation of fibrin in a blood vessel.

t., compression. T. due to compression between a thrombus and the heart.

t., coronary. T. of the coronary arteries. A common cause of myocardial infarction.

SYM: Sudden onset of severe and prolonged substernal oppression and pain, the pain arising over the precordium and being referred to the upper and middle sternum and often radiating to the left and sometimes right arm and into the neck or back. Blood pressure usually falls, pulse becomes rapid, fever and leukocytosis usually observed within 24 hours. Erythrocyte sedimentation rate becomes elevated and electrocardiographic changes occur.

TREATMENT: Complete physical and mental rest for a variable length of time depending upon severity. This is sometimes best accomplished by allowing the patient to rest in a reclining chair rather than a bed; and to use a bedside toilet instead of having to strain to use a bedpan. Special nursing care is desirable. Prompt and complete relief from pain by use of morphine sulfate; oxygen administration sometimes necessary. Vasopressor drugs to elevate blood pressure; digitalis when there is evidence of congestive heart failure; treatment of cardiac arrhythmias, esp. tachycardia; anticoagulants. Treatment in coronary care unit is highly desirable.

DIET: Low protein and carbohydrate intake of approx. 1000 cal. Fluids to produce urinary output of 1500 ml. daily. Restrict salt intake.

POSSIBLE COMPLICATIONS: Shock; acute pulmonary edema; paroxysmal ventricular tachycardia; congestive heart failure; aneurysm of the ventricle.

t., dilatation. T. due to dilatation of a vein.

t., embolic. T. due to an embolus obstructing a vessel.

t., infective. T. due to bacterial infection.

t., marasmic. T. due to wasting diseases of infancy and old age.

t., placental. Thrombi in the placenta and veins of the uterus.

t., plate. Thrombus formed from an accumulation of blood platelets.

t., puerperal. Coagulation in veins following labor.

t., sinus. T. of the venous sinus.

Lateral: ETIOL: Associated with middle ear disease. SYM: Sudden rise of temperature with remission, chills, prostration, sweats, headache, mental symptoms, dullness or delirium, high leukocyte count.

Cavernous: Sinus structures involved, edema and venous stasis in and about the eye.

t., traumatic. T. due to a wound or injury of a part.

t., venous. T. of a vein.

thrombostasis (thrŏm-bŏs'tă-sĭs) [Gr. *thrombos,* clot, + *stasis,* a standing still]. Stasis of blood in a part causing or due to formation of thrombus.

thrombotic (thrŏm-bŏt'ĭk) [Gr. *thrombos,* clot]. Related to, caused by, or of the nature of, a thrombus.

thrombus (thrŏm'bŭs) [Gr. *thrombos*]. A blood clot obstructing a blood vessel or a cavity of the heart.

Anticoagulants are being used in prevention and treatment of this condition.

t., annular. One whose circumference is attached to the walls of a vessel, an opening still remaining in the center.

t., antemortem. A clot formed before death in heart or large vessels.

t., ball. A round clot in the heart, esp. in the auricles.

t., hyaline. One having a glassy appearance usually occurring in smaller blood vessels.

t., Laennec's. A globular thrombus which forms in the heart, usually in cases of fatty degeneration.

t., lateral. A mural one, q.v.

t., milk. A curdled milk tumor in the female breast due to obstruction in a lactiferous duct.

t., mural. One attached to the wall of a vessel or the heart. SYN: *lateral t., parietal t.*

t., obstructing. One completely occluding the lumen of a vessel.

t., progressive. One which increases in size.

t., stratified. One composed of layers. SYN: *fibrolaminar.*

t., white. SYN: *antemortem thrombus,* q.v.

through drainage. Drainage by passing a perforated tube into cavity to be drained and flushing cavity by injection of fluids.

through illumination. Passage of light through the walls of an organ or cavity for medical examination. SYN: *transillumination.*

thrush (thrŭsh) [D. *tröske,* rotten wood]. Fungus infection of mouth or throat, esp. in infants and young children, characterized by formation of white patches and ulcers, frequently fever and gastrointestinal inflammation. SYN: *aphtha; sprue; stomatitis,* q.v.

    ETIOL: Candida (Monilia) albicans.

thrypsis (thrĭp'sĭs) [Gr., breaking in pieces]. A fracture in which the bone is splintered or crushed.

thulium (thū'lĭ-ŭm). SYMB: *Tm.* At. wt. 168.934; at. no. 69. A rare metallic element found in combination with minerals.

thumb (thŭm) [AS. *thūma,* thumb]. The short, thick, first finger on radial side of the hand, having but two phalanges and greater freedom of movement than other fingers. SYN: *pollex.*

t. sign. Protrusion of the thumb across the palm and beyond the clenched fist. Seen in children with Marfan's syndrome.

t. sucking. The habit of sucking one's own thumb. Intermittent thumb sucking is not abnormal, but prolonged and intensive thumb sucking past the time the first permanent teeth erupt at five or six years of age can lead to misshaped mouths and displaced teeth. If the habit persists, combined dental and psychological therapy should be instituted.

thus (thŭs) [L.]. Frankincense, the oleoresin obtained as an exudate from trees of the Pinus species. Genuine frankincense is obtained from the bark of Boswellia carterii.

thylacitis (thī''lă-sī'tĭs) [Gr. *thylax,* pouch, + *-itis,* inflammation]. Inflammation of the sebaceous glands of the skin.

thymectomy (thī-měk'tō-mĭ) [Gr. *thymos,* thymus, + *ektomē,* excision]. Surgical removal of the thymus gland.

thymelcosis (thī''měl-kō'sĭs) ["+ *helkōsis,* ulceration]. Ulceration of the thymus gland.

thymic (thī'mĭk) [L. *thymicus*]. Rel. to the thymus gland.

thymicolymphatic (thī''mĭ-kō-lĭm-făt'ĭk). Rel. to the thymus and lymph glands.

thymion (thĭm'ĭ-ŏn) [Gr.]. A wart.

thymitis (thī-mī'tĭs) [Gr. *thymos,* thymus, + *-itis,* inflammation]. Inflammation of the thymus gland.

thymo-. 1. [Gr. *thymos,* thymus]. Combining form indicating relationship to the thymus. 2. [Gr. *thymos,* mind, spirit]. Combining form indicating relationship with the soul or emotions.

thymokesis (thī''mō-kē'sĭs) [Gr. *thymos,* thymus]. Abnormal enlargement and persistence of the thymus in the adult.

thymol (thī'mŏl) ["+ L. *oleum,* oil]. White crystals obtained from oil of thyme. Formerly used in treatment of hookworm.

thymolysis (thī-mŏl'ĭ-sĭs) ["+ *lysis,* dissolution]. Dissolution of thymus tissue.

thymolytic (thī''mō-lĭt'ĭk). Destructive to thymus tissue.

thymoma (thī-mō'mă) [Gr. *thymos,* thymus, + *-ōma,* tumor]. A tumor originating in epithelial tissues of the thymus gland.

thymopexy (thī''mō-pěks'ĭ) ["+ *pēxis,* fixation]. Fixation of an enlarged thymus in a new position.

thymotoxic (thī''mō-tŏks'ĭk) ["+ *toxikon,* poison]. Poisonous to thymus tissue.

thymus (thī'mŭs) [Gr. *thymos*]. An unpaired organ located in the mediastinal cavity anterior to and above the heart. It consists of two flattened symmetrical lobes each enclosed in a capsule, from which trabeculae extend into the gland dividing each lobe into many lobules, each consisting of a cortex and medulla. The cortex is composed of dense lymphoid tissue containing many cells (thymocytes) closely packed together. The medulla also contains thymocytes but they are less numerous. It also contains characteristic thymic (Hassall's) corpuscles.

    At birth the average weight of the thymus is 13 grams. Growth is rapid during the first two years, then slow, attaining a weight of about 30 gm. at puberty, after which it begins to undergo involution and the thymic tissue is replaced with adipose and connective tissue.

    FUNCTIONS: Important in development of immune response in newborn. Its removal during early childhood has been associated with an increased susceptibility to acute infectious diseases at a later time.

PATH: Sometimes it is much larger than it should be and is then known as enlarged or persistent thymus. Children having these enlarged structures should be carefully followed. The practice of routinely treating the enlarged thymus with x-irradiation is not advisable. Children who have been treated frequently develop thyroid cancer.

SEE: *status thymicolymphaticus; thymic asthma.*

t., accessory. A lobule isolated from the mass of the thymus gland.

t. persistens hyperplastica. A thymus persisting into adulthood, sometimes hypertrophying.

thymusectomy (thī″mŭs-ĕk′tō-mĭ) [Gr. *thymos,* thymus, + *ektomē,* excision]. Surgical excision of the thymus.

thyreo-, thyro- [Gr.]. Combining forms meaning oblong, shield, thyroid.

thyreoplasia. Defective functioning of the thyroid gland due to abnormal development.

thyroadenitis (thī″rō-ăd-e-nī′tĭs) [Gr. *thyreos,* shield, + *adēn,* gland, + *-itis,* inflammation]. Inflammation of thyroid gland.

thyroaplasia (thī″rō-ă-plă′zĭ-ă) [″+ *a-,* not, + *plasis,* a molding]. Imperfect development of the thyroid gland.

thyroarytenoid (thī″rō-ă-rīt′en-oyd) [″+ *arytaina,* ladle, + *eidos,* form]. Rel. to the thyroid and arytenoid cartilages.

thyrocardiac (thī″rō-kar′dĭ-ăk) [Gr. *thyreos,* shield, + *kardia,* heart]. 1. Pert to the heart and thyroid gland. 2. A person suffering from thyroid disease complicated by heart disorder.

thyrocele (thī′rō-sēl) [″+ *kēlē,* mass]. Enlarged condition of the thyroid gland. SYN: *goiter.*

thyrochondrotomy (thī″rō-kŏn-drŏt′ō-mĭ) [″+ *chondros,* cartilage, + *tomē,* a cutting]. Surgical incision of thyroid cartilage. SYN: *laryngotomy.*

thyrocricotomy (thī″rō-krī-kŏt′ō-mĭ) [Gr. *thyreos,* shield, + *krikos,* ring, + *tomē,* a cutting]. Tracheotomy; division of the cricothyroid membrane.

thyroepiglottic (thī″rō-ĕp″ĭ-glŏt′ĭk) [″+ *epi,* upon, + *glōttis,* glottis]. Rel. to the thyroid and epiglottis.

t. muscle. Muscle arising on inner surface of thyroid cartilage. It extends upward and backward and is inserted on epiglottis. It depresses the epiglottis.

thyroepiglottideus (thī″rō-ĕp″ĭ-glŏt-ĭd′ē-us). Muscle in the thyroid cartilage that depresses the epiglottis.

thyroglobulin (thī″rō-glŏb′ū-lĭn) [Gr. *thyreos,* shield, + L. *globulus,* a tiny sphere]. An iodine-containing protein secreted by the thyroid gland and stored within its colloid substance. SYN: *iodothyroglobulin.*

thyroglos′sal. Pert. to the thyroid gland and the tongue.

t. duct. A duct which in the embryo connects the thyroid diverticulum with the tongue. It eventually disappears, its point of origin being indicated as a pit, the foramen cecum. It sometimes persists as an anomaly.

thyrohyoid (thī″rō-hī′oyd) [″+ *hyoeidēs,* U-shaped]. Rel. to thyroid cartilage and hyoid bone. SYN: *hyothyroid.*

thyroid (thī′royd) [Gr. *thyreos,* shield, + *eidos,* form]. 1. Thyroid extract, q.v. 2. A gland of internal secretion in the neck, anterior to and partially surrounding the thyroid cartilage and upper rings of the trachea. SEE: *t. gland.*

t. cachexia. Exophthalmic goiter.

t. cartilage. The principal cartilage of the larynx consisting of two broad lamina united anteriorly to form a V-shaped structure. It forms a subcutaneous projection, the laryngeal prominence or Adam's apple.

t. crisis. thyroid storm, q.v.

t. extract. USP. The dried thyroid glands of the ox or sheep.

ACTION AND USES: Used in cases of deficient action of the gland, i.e., hypothyroidism.

ADMINISTRATION: Tablet form by mouth. The maximum effect will not be obtained for at least 7 to 10 days. It is advisable to start with a small dose and increase it gradually until the proper dose is established. Because the patient may take thyroid extract for all of his life, the least expensive form of therapy, Thyroid (USP), should be used.

t. function tests. Tests for evidence of increased or decreased t. function including clinical physical examination, which is usually reliable, and a variety of reliable laboratory tests. Some of the more common tests are based on direct or indirect determination of the two t. hormones, thyroxine (T-4) and triiodothyronine (T-4). Also frequently used are tests on radioactive iodine uptake by the t. and direct measurement of free thyroxine in the serum.

Most t. function tests are unreliable in certain circumstances. They may be influenced by the patient's having been exposed to organic or inorganic iodides or to drugs that interfere with the binding capacity of serum proteins.

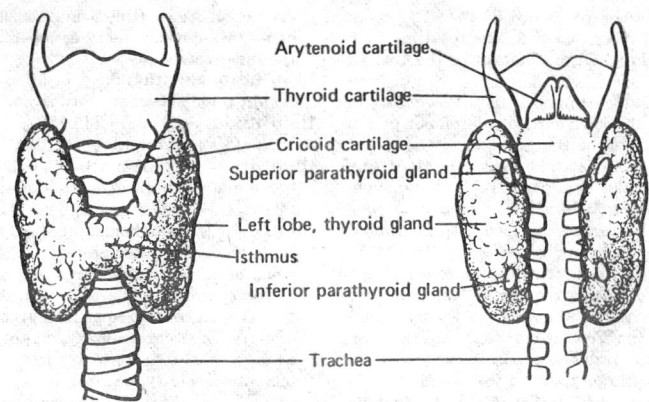

THYROID
Left, anterior aspect with related structures; right, posterior aspect.

t. gland. A gland of internal secretion located in the base of the neck on both sides of the lower part of the larynx and upper part of trachea.

It consists of two lateral lobes connected by an isthmus. Sometimes a third medial or pyramidal lobe extends upward from the isthmus. Histologically it consists of a large number of closed vesicles called follicles which contain a homogeneous substance called colloid which contain the thyroglobulin which in turn contains various active substances such as thyroxine. Enlarged in goiter. It may pulsate.

RS: endocrine gland; hormone hyperthyroidism, hypothyroidism; iodine; struma; thyrotropic hormone; thyroxine.

t. storm. A complication of thyrotoxicosis which if untreated is almost uniformly fatal. Consists of abrupt onset of fever, sweating, tachycardia, pulmonary edema or congestive heart failure, tremulousness, and restlessness. Occurs in a patient in whom existing thyrotoxicosis has been treated poorly or not at all. It usually is precipitated by infection, trauma, or a surgical emergency. SYN: *thyroid crisis.*

TREATMENT: Catecholamine inhibitors. Both guanethedine and propanol have been reported to be quite effective.

t. therapy. Thyroid extract treatment.

thyroidectomized (thī″roy-dĕk′tō-mīzd) [Gr. *thyreos,* shield, + *eidos,* form, + *-ektomē,* excision]. With the thyroid gland removed.

thyroidectomy (thī″royd-ĕk′tō-mĭ) ["+ "+ *ektomē,* excision]. Excision of the thyroid gland.

POSTOPERATIVE CARE: Patient in sitting position as soon as recovered from anesthesia, head and arms well supported. Watch for edema or swelling due to bleeding into the wound. Also observe for hoarseness and evidence of injury to parathyroid glands. The early signs of decreased parathyroid gland function are tingling and tightness of the fingers, anxiety and mental depression.

thyroiditis (thī″royd-ī′tĭs) [Gr. *thyreos,* shield, + *eidos,* form, + *-itis,* inflammation]. Inflammation of the thyroid gland. SEE: *Riedel's struma.*

t., giant cell. Thyroiditis characterized by presence of giant cells, round-cell infiltration, fibrosis, and destruction of follicles.

thyroidization (thī″royd-ĭ-zā′shŭn) [Gr. *thyreos,* shield, + *eidos,* form]. Thyroid extract therapy.

thyroidotomy (thī″royd-ŏt′ō-mĭ) ["+ "+ *tomē,* a cutting]. Incision of thyroid gland.

thyroidotoxin (thī″royd-ō-tŏk′sĭn). A substance which is toxic for cells of the thyroid gland.

thyrolytic (thī″rō-lĭt′ĭk) [Gr. *thyreos,* shield, + *lysis,* dissolution]. Causing destruction of thyroid tissue.

thyroparathyroidectomy (thī″rō-păr″ă-thī″royd-ĕk′tō-mĭ) ["+ *para,* beside, + *thyreos,* shield, + *eidos,* form, + *ektomē,* excision]. Surgical removal of the thyroid and parathyroid glands.

thyropenia (thī″rō-pē′nĭ-ă) ["+ *penia,* lack]. Defective thyroid secretion.

thyroprival (thī″rō-prī′văl) ["+ L. *privus*, lacking]. Pert. to a condition resulting from loss of function or removal of the thyroid gland.

thyroptosis (thī″rŏp-tō′sĭs) ["+ *ptōsis*, a dropping]. Downward displacement of the thyroid into the thorax.

thyrosis (thī-rō′sĭs) ["+ -*ōsis*, condition]. Any condition due to abnormal thyroid function.

thyrotherapy (thī″rō-ther′ă-pī) [Gr. *thyreos*, shield, + *therapeia*, treatment]. Treatment with thyroid gland extracts.

thyrotome (thī′rō-tōm) ["+ *tomē*, a cutting]. Knife for cutting the thyroid cartilage.

thyrotomy (thī-rŏt′ō-mī) ["+ "]. 1. The splitting of the thyroid cartilage anteriorly in midline in order to expose laryngeal structures. 2. Surgery on the thyroid gland.

thyrotoxic (thī″rō-tŏks′ĭk) [Gr. *thyreos*, shield, + *toxikon*, poison]. Pert. to, affected by, or marked by toxic activity of the thyroid gland.

thyrotoxicosis (thī″rō-tŏks″ĭ-kō′sĭs) ["+ "+ -*ōsis*, condition]. Toxic condition due to hyperactivity of the thyroid gland. SYN: *exophthalmic goiter*, q.v.

SYM: Rapid heart action; tremors; elevated basal metabolism; enlarged gland; exophthalmos; nervous symptoms; and loss of weight.

thyrotropic (thī″rō-trŏp′ĭk) [Gr. *thyreos*, shield, + *tropē*, a turning]. That which has an affinity for or stimulates the thyroid gland.

   t. hormone. The thyroid-stimulating hormone secreted by the anterior lobe of hypophysis. ABBR: TSH. SYN: *thyroid-stimulating hormone.*

thyrotropin (thī-rŏt′rō-pĭn). The thyrotropic hormone, q.v.

thyroxine (thī-rŏks′ēn) [Gr. *thyreos*, shield]. 3,5,3′,5′-Tetraiodothyronine, an amino acid obtained from the thyroid gland considered to be the principal thyroid hormone. Used in the treatment of hypothyroidism.

   t. -binding protein. The globin protein responsible for binding the greater part of thyroxine in the plasma. ABBR: TBP.

Ti. Chem. symb. for titanium.

tibia (tĭb′ĭ-ă) [L., shinbone]. The inner and larger bone of the leg between the knee and ankle articulating with the femur above and with the talus below. Also called shin bone.

   t., Lannelongue′s. A syphilitic tibia.

   t., saber-shaped. A deformity of the tibia due to gummatous periostitis (syphilitic) in which it curves outward.

tibialis (tĭb″ĭ-ā′lĭs) [L.]. Tibia; shin bone.

tibioadductor reflex (tĭb″ĭ-ō-ăd-dŭk′tor) [L. *tibia*, shinbone, + *adducere*, to lead to].

Adduction of either the stimulated leg or the opposite one when the tibia is percussed on the inner side.

tibiofemoral (tĭb′ĭ-ō-fem′ōr-ăl) ["+ L. *femur*, thigh]. Rel. to the tibia and femur.

tibiofibular (tĭb″ĭ-ō-fĭb′ū-lăr) ["+ L. *fibula*, buckle]. Rel. to the tibia and fibula.

tibiotarsal (tĭb″ĭ-ō-tăr′săl) ["+ Gr. *tarsos*, broad flat surface]. Rel. to the tibia and tarsus.

tic (tĭk) [Fr.]. A spasmodic muscular contraction, most commonly involving the face, head, neck, or shoulder muscles.

The spasms may be tonic, q.v. or clonic, q.v. The movement appears purposeful, is often repeated, involuntary, can be inhibited for a short time, only to burst forth with increased severity. SYN: *habit spasm.*

ETIOL: Certain of these cases are due to structure changes, many psychogenic; the expression of frustration; and its correlated muscular tension. The former group most commonly encountered in patients who have suffered from lethargic encephalitis. SEE: *tiqueur.*

   t., convulsive. Facial muscle spasm.

   t. douloureux. Degeneration of or pressure on the trigeminal nerve, resulting in neuralgia of that nerve. The pain comes on in severe lightning-like stabs and radiates from angle of the jaw along one of the involved branches. If the first branch, a shocklike pain is felt along the eye and back over the forehead. If it is the middle fiber, the upper lip, nose, and cheek under the eye are affected. If it is the third branch, pain is in the lower lip and outer border of tongue on affected side. Pain is momentary but may occur repetitively for as long as 20 seconds. Paroxysms may last for hours and then subside for weeks or months. SYN: *trigeminal neuralgia.*

TREAT: Injection of the nerve with alcohol. Other measures as anticonvulsants may be helpful to shorten attacks or cause remission. Surgical therapy may be required.

RS: neuralgia.

   t., facial. SEE: *convulsive tic.*

   t., habit. Habitual repetition of a grimace or muscular action.

   t. rotatoire. Spasmodic torticollis in which head and neck are forcibly rotated or turned from one side to the other.

   t., spasmodic. Tonic contractions and paralysis of muscles of one or both sides of the face.

tick (tĭk) [ME. *tyke*]. Any of the numerous bloodsucking arachnids of the order Acarida. Ixodidae is the hard tick family and

Argasidae the soft. They transmit specific diseases to man and lower animals.

t. fever. A general term used to indicate a variety of tick-borne rickettsial diseases similar to Rocky Mountain spotted fever. It is caused by a rickettsial organism (Rickettsia rickettsii) transmitted by a tick.

SYM: Incubation period: From the bite to the first symptom, 5-7 days. Onset may be gradual or sudden, but generally for a period of 1 or more days; if so, it is preceded by weakness, chilly sensations and then a definite chill.

Other symptoms are nausea and vomiting; headache in front and back of head, or both; more or less bloodshot eyes with sensitivity to light; eyeballs sore to touch; deep, dusky flush on face; pain in muscles, bones, and joints; backache, esp. in lower portion; bronchial cough; nosebleed; constipation, and marked weakness. The skin becomes spotted between the 3rd and 5th day after onset. The spots resemble those of measles but differ in distribution. In Rocky Mountain spotted fever spots are apt to be concentrated on the wrist, ankles, and feet, instep, soles, and then spread to the trunk. The spots appear to disappear on pressure but later become hemorrhagic, changing to a rust color due to disintegration. Relative bradycardia may be present during fever. Development of hypotension is a grave prognostic sign.

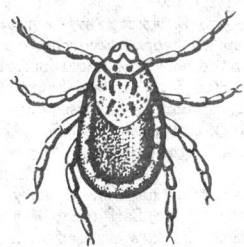

FEMALE ROCKY MOUNTAIN WOOD TICK
Enlarged view of tick .635 cm. in length.

tickle (tĭk'l) [ME. *tikelen*]. 1. Peculiar sensation caused by titillation or touching, esp. in certain regions, resulting in reflex muscular movements, laughter, or hysteria. 2. To arouse such a sensation by touching a surface lightly.

tickling (tĭk'lĭng). Gentle stimulation of a sensitive surface and its reflex effect, such as involuntary laughter, etc. SYN: *titillation.*

tictology (tĭk-tŏl'ō-jĭ) [Gr. *tiktein*, to give birth, + *logos*, science]. Obstetrics.

t. i. d [L. *ter in die*]. Abbr. for L. *ter in die,* three times a day.

tidal (tī'dăl). Periodically rising and falling, increasing and decreasing.

t. air. That which is inhaled and exhaled during normal quiet breathing. SEE: *air; respiration.*

t. drainage. The drainage of a paralyzed bladder by use of an automatic irrigation apparatus.

tide [AS. *tīd*, time]. Alternate rise and fall; a space of time.

t., acid. A temporary increase in acidity of urine due to increased secretion of alkaline substances into the duodenum or after fasting.

t., alkaline. Temporary decrease in acidity of urine following awakening and after meals. The former results from hyperpnea in which excess CO_2 is eliminated; the latter results from increase of base in the blood following the secretion of HCl into gastric juice.

Tietze's disease or syndrome (tēt'sēz). [Alexander Tietze, Ger. surgeon, 1864-1927]. Inflammation of the costochondral cartilage. A self-limiting disease of unknown etiology. Pain may be confused with that of myocardial infarction. There is no specific therapy.

tigering [Gr. *tigris*, tiger]. Tiger-like striped appearance of heart muscle due to irregular areas of fatty degeneration. Seen in conditions which cause severe anoxemia such as anemia. SYN: *tiger-heart, tiger-lily heart.*

tigretier (tē-grĕt″ē-ā′) [Fr.]. A dancing mania or form of tarantism due to bite of a poisonous spider, occurring in Tigré, Abyssinia.

tigroid (tī'groyd) [Gr. *tigroeidēs*, tiger-spotted]. Striped, spotted, or marked like a tiger.

t. bodies. Masses of chromophil substance present in the cell bodies of neurons. SYN: *Nissl bodies.*

tigrolysis (tĭg″rol'ĭ-sĭs). Dissolution and disappearance of chromophil substance of a nerve cell. May occur following injury to an axon (retrograde degeneration) or subsequent to direct injury to a nerve cell. SYN: *chromatolysis.*

tilmus (tĭl'mŭs) [Gr. *tilmos*, a plucking]. Delirious picking at the bedclothes by the patient. SYN: *carphology; floccillation.*

tiltometer (tĭl-tŏm'ĕ-tĕr). A device for measuring the degree of tilt of a bed or operating table. Used when spinal anesthesia has been given in order to know which end of the spinal canal is lower.

timbre (tĭm'ber, tahn'br) [Fr., a bell to be struck with a hammer]. Resonance quality of a sound by which it is distinguished, other than pitch or intensity, depending upon the number and character of vibrating body's overtones.

time (tim) [AS. *tima,* time]. Interval between beginning and ending; measured duration. Age.

    t., bleeding. Time required for bleeding from a small wound to cease. Usually tested by puncturing lobe of ear. Normal time, 1-3 min.

    t., clot retraction. Time required following withdrawal of blood for a clot to completely contract and express the serum entrapped within the fibrin net. Normal time, about 1 hour. Clot retraction is dependent upon number of platelets.

    t., coagulation. Time required for clotting to occur in whole blood which has been placed in tubes coated with silicone. Time required is somewhat different for each laboratory but will usually vary from 20 to 60 minutes.

    t., prothrombin. That needed for oxalated plasma to clot, measured in seconds, after adding thromboplastin and recalcifying.

    t., reaction. Period between application of a stimulus and the response.

    t., thermal death. Time required to kill a bacterium at a certain temperature.

timer (tim'ẽr). A device for measuring, signaling, recording, or regulating time. Various forms of timers are used in x-ray, surgical, and laboratory work.

tin (tĭn) [AS. *tin*]. SYMB: Sn. At. wt. 118.69; at. no. 50. A metallic element, used in medicine.

    POISONING: Tin in tinned or soldered containers in the past has occasionally been responsible for poisoning. This is exceedingly rare and for practical purposes need not be considered.

    SYM: Metallic taste, gastrointestinal irritation, nausea, vomiting, cramping, and diarrhea.

    F. A. TREATMENT: Wash out stomach and administer bland or soothing drinks.

tinctorial (tĭnk-tō'rĭ-al) [L. *tinctōrius,* dyeing]. Rel. to staining or color.

tinctura (tĭnk-tū'rä) [L., a dyeing]. (pl. *tincturae*) Tincture, q.v.

tincture (tĭngk'chŭr). Diluted alcoholic solutions of nonvolatile substances, 10% being standard strength for powerful drugs and 20% for weaker ones. Simple alcoholic solutions of pure substances such as iodine and quinine are no longer called tinctures.

The name of any fluid contained in the tincture other than alcohol is added to the name of the tincture.

This class of preparations usually contain tannic acid, so, in most instances, cannot be employed with agents that are incompatible with that drug. Those tinctures that contain much resinous matter or oils will precipitate with water. Some examples are tinctures of ginger, benzoin, guaiac. Tinctures of the most potent drugs usually represent 10% of the crude drug, as tinctures of opium, digitalis. Where more than a teaspoon of a 10% tincture would have to be taken to get a dose of the drug, the tincture is usually made to represent 20%, or more, of the agent.

    t. iodine. Obsolete term for simple alcoholic solution of iodine. POISONING: This commonly used antiseptic is sometimes taken by mouth either accidentally or for the purpose of suicide.

    SYM: Very strong irritation of mouth, esophagus, and stomach. Stains membranes dark brown or black. Pain intense, and leads to early vomiting and purging; extreme thirst, often collapse.

    TREATMENT: Give large amounts of water, milk and starchy paste; gruels, as boiled rice or cream of wheat. Gastric lavage with either one to 10% starch solution, or sodium thiosulfite or protein solution such as egg white or milk. Control pain, circulatory collapse and fluid and electrolyte balance with appropriate therapy. Tracheotomy may be required.

tinea (tĭn'ē-ä) [L., worm]. Any fungus skin disease, esp. ringworm, occurring on various parts of the body, the name indicating the part affected. Ex: t. barbae (beard), t. corporis (body). A dermatomycosis, q.v.

    SYM: Of two types. *Superficial* is marked by scaling; slight itching; reddish or grayish patches; dry, brittle hair which is easily extracted with hair shaft. *Deep type* is characterized by flat, reddish, kerionlike tumors, the surface studded with dead or broken hairs or by gaping follicular orifices; nodules may be broken down in center, discharging pus, etc., through dilated follicular openings.

    TREATMENT: Griseofulvin, q.v., given orally for all types of true trichophyton infections. Local treatment alone is of little benefit in ringworm of the scalp, nails, and in most cases the feet.

    After the 5th day of treatment with griseofulvin, scrubbing with soap and water is advisable. Topical preparations containing fungicidal agents are useful in treatment of t. cruris and t. pedis.

Personal hygiene is important in controlling these two common diseases. The use of antiseptic foot baths to control t. pedis does not prevent spread of the infection from person to person. Persons affected should not allow their personal items, such as clothes, towels, and sports equipment, to be used by others.

Ringworm of the scalp, t. capitis, is particularly resistant if due to Microsporum audouini. Do not treat topically. Griseofulvin is quite effective.

t. barbae. A fungus skin disease of the bearded portions of neck and face. SYN: *barber's itch; t. sycosis.*

t. capitis. A fungus skin disease of the scalp; ringworm of the scalp. May be due to one of several types of Microsporum.

t. corporis. T. of the body. Begins with red, slightly elevated scaly patches which on examination reveal minute vesicles or papules. New patches spring from the periphery while central portion clears up. Often considerable itching. SYN: *t. circinata.*

t. cruris. A fungus skin disease of surfaces of contact in the scrotal, crural, anal, and genital areas. SYN: *dhobie itch; jock itch.*

t. nigra. An asymptomatic superficial fungal infection which affects the skin of the palms. Characterized by deeply-pigmented macular, non-scaly patches.
ETIOL: Cladosporium werneckii or C. mansonii.

t. nodosa. Sheathlike, nodular masses in hair of beard and mustache from growth of either Piedraia hortai, which causes black piedra, or Trichosporon bigelii, which causes white piedra. The masses surround the hairs which become brittle; hairs may be penetrated by fungus and thus split. SYN: *piedra.*

t. pedis. A fungus skin disease of the foot; ringworm of the foot. SYN: *dermatophytosis; athlete's foot.*

t. sycosis. Rare type of t. barbae, q.v.

t. versicolor. Fungus infection of skin producing branny patches which are yellow or fawn-colored. SYN: *pityriasis versicolor.*

Tinel's sign. [Jules Tinel, Fr. neurologist, 1879-1952] Cutaneous tingling sensation produced by pressing on or tapping the nerve trunk which has been damaged or is healing following trauma.

tine test. A skin test for tuberculosis. The tuberculin is on metal tines which are pressed into the skin. The test is read in 48 and 72 hours. The unit is sterile and disposable and therefore is very useful in mass surveys.

tingle (tĭng′gl). A prickling or stinging sensation. May be caused by cold or nerve injury.

tinnitus (tĭn′ĭ-tŭs, tĭn-ī′tŭs) [L. *tinnitus,* a jingling]. A subjective ringing or tinkling sound in the ear.

t. aurium. Ringing, tinkling, buzzing, or other sounds in the ear.
Found in certain diseases of exterior, middle, or inner ear.
ETIOL: Impacted cerumen; myringitis; otitis media; labyrinthitis; Ménière's symptom complex; otosclerosis; hysteria; etc. Also follows overdosage of drugs such as quinine.

tintometer (tĭn-tŏm′ĕ-ter) [L. *tinctus,* a dyeing, + Gr. *metron,* a measure]. A scale of different shades of color to determine by comparison the intensity of color of the blood or other fluid.

tintometric (tĭn″tō-mĕt′rĭk). Rel. to tintometry.

tintometry (tĭn-tŏm′ĕ-trĭ). Estimation of a color by comparison with a scale of colors.

tip (tĭp). A point or apex of a part.

tiqueur (tĭ-kŭr′) [Fr.]. One afflicted with a tic.

tire (tīr) [AS. *tēorian,* to tire]. 1. Exhaustion; fatigue. 2. To exhaust or fatigue. 3. To become fatigued.

tirefond (tēr-fon′) [Fr.]. Appliance like a corkscrew for raising depressed portions of bone or for removing foreign bodies.

tires (tīrz). Condition marked by constipation, vomiting, muscular tremors, and pain. SYN: *trembles.*

tissue (tĭsh′ū) [O. Fr. *tissu,* from L. *texere,* to weave]. A group or collection of similar cells and their intercellular substance which act together in the performance of a particular function. The primary tissues are (a) epithelial, (b) connective, (c) muscular, and (d) nervous.

t., adipose. Areolar tissue containing aggregations of densely packed fat cells. SYN: *fat.*

t., areolar. A form of loose connective tissue consisting of interlacing collagenous and elastic fibers embedded in a semifluid matrix together with fibroblasts, histiocytes, mast cells, plasma cells, and other cellular elements. It is widely distributed forming the interstitial tissue of most organs, the membranes surrounding blood vessels and nerves, and constituting the principal portion of fascia.

t., cartilage. SEE: *cartilage.*

t., chondroid. Embryonic cartilage.

t., chromaffin. Tissues containing cells which give the chromaffin reaction. Found in the adrenal medulla and ganglia of the parasympathetic nervous system. SEE: *chromaffin system.*

t., chromophil. Those tissues which give a chromophil reaction; found in the medulla and sympathetic ganglia.

t., connective. T. which supports and connects other tissues and parts. The cells of connective tissue are comparatively few in number, the bulk of the tissue consisting of intercellular substance or matrix, the nature of which gives each type of connective tissue its particular properties. Connective tissues are highly vascular with the exception of cartilage. Connective tissue proper includes the following types: mucous, fibrous (areolar, white fibrous, yellow fibrous, or elastic), reticular, and adipose. Dense connective tissue includes cartilage and bone (osseous tissue).

t., elastic. A form of connective tissue in which yellow elastic fibers predominate. Found in certain ligaments, and the walls of blood vessels, esp. the larger arteries.

t., embryonic. T., mucous, q.v.

t., epithelial. A form of tissue composed of cells arranged in a continuous sheet consisting of one or several layers. It forms epidermis of skin, covers surfaces of organs, lines cavities and canals, forms tubes and ducts and secreting portions of glands. SYN: *epithelium.*

t., erectile. Spongy tissue, the spaces of which fill with blood, causing it to harden and expand. Found in the penis, clitoris, and nipples.

t., fibrous. Connective tissue consisting principally of fibers. Includes three types: areolar or loose connective, white fibrous, and yellow fibrous or elastic.

t., interstitial. Connective t. forming a network with the cellular elements of an organ.

t., mucous. Jelly-like tissue from which connective tissue is derived.

t., muscular. *Voluntary:* Striped or striated tissue principally connected with the bony framework. In animals it is known as lean meat or flesh. It is a cross-striped, muscular tissue, the fibers like a long cylinder with flattened sides and conical ends, enveloped in a delicate sheath, the sarcolemma. *Involuntary:* Smooth or unstriped, or nonstriated, not under control of the will. Principally found in walls of hollow organs, tubes, arteries, and veins.

t., osseous or bone. Connective tissue with intercellular substance impregnated with phosphate and carbonate of calcium, the mineral substances being 2/3 of the bone's dry weight.

t., reticular or retiform. A type of connective tissue consisting of delicate fibers forming interlacing networks. Fibers stain selectively with silver stains and are called argyrophil fibers. It supports lymph nodes and is found in muscular tissue and in bone marrow, the spleen, liver, lungs, kidneys, and mucous membranes of the gastrointestinal tract.

t., subcutaneous. Areolar tissue under and becoming part of the corium.

t., subcutaneous, adipose. Adipose tissue within subcutaneous tissue.

t. typing. Techniques utilized in determining the histocompatibility of tissues to be used in grafts and transplants with the recipient's tissues and cells. SEE: *transplantation.*

t., white fibrous. Connective t. with white, inelastic fibers, forming tendons, ligaments, and resistant membranes.

t., w. nervous. Nervous tissue of medullated nerve fibers.

t., yellow elastic. T., elastic, q.v.

titanium (tī-tā′nĭ-ŭm) [L. *titan,* the sun]. SYMB: *Ti.* At. wt. 47.90; at. no. 22; sp. gr. 4.54. A metallic element found in combination in minerals.

titer (ti′ter) [Fr. *titre,* standard]. Standard of strength per volume of volumetric test solution.

t., agglutination. The highest dilution of a serum which will cause clumping or agglutination of the bacteria being tested.

t. of a serum. Amount of specific antibody in an antiserum, or strength of a serum.

titillation (tĭt″ĭl-ā′shŭn) [L. *titillatio,* a tickling]. 1. Act of tickling, as in the throat. 2. State of being tickled. 3. Sensation produced by tickling.

titration (tĭ-trā′shŭn) [Fr. *titre,* a standard]. 1. Estimation of the concentration of a chemical solution by adding known amounts of standard reagents until alteration in color or electrical state occurs. 2. Determination of quantity of antibody in an antiserum.

titre. SEE: *titer.*

titrimetric (tĭt″trĭ-mĕt′rĭk) [Fr. *titre,* a standard, + Gr. *metron,* a measure]. Employing the process of titration.

titubation (tĭt″ū-bā′shŭn) [L. *titubatio,* a staggering]. A staggering gait, seen in diseases of the cerebellum.

t., lingual. Stuttering, stammering.

Tl. Chem. symb. for thallium.

TLC. Abbr. for *tender loving care,* a concept embodying one of the most basic and important therapeutic procedures. Administration of TLC is of particular importance in a hospital setting where the patient may feel human beings have deserted him because he is left to the impersonal care of a machine.

Tm. 1. Chem. symb. for thulium. 2. Symb. for maximal tubular excretory capacity of the kidneys.

Tn. Symb. for normal intraocular tension.

TNM classification. Method of classifying malignant tumors with respect to primary tumor, involvement of regional lymph nodes, and presence or absence of metastases.

TO. Abbr. for *original; old tuberculin* (also abbr. OT).

toadskin (tōd'skĭn). Condition characterized by excessive dryness, wrinkling, and scaling of skin sometimes seen in vitamin deficiencies. SEE: *phrynoderma.*

toadstool (tōd'stool). Any of various fungi with an umbrella-shaped cap; popularly a poisonous mushroom.

POISONING SYM: Usually come on from a few minutes to 15 hours after ingestion, characterized by marked abdominal pain, vomiting and intense diarrhea associated with blood and mucus. Profound weakness comes early and remains. Sometimes perspiration and lacrimation present and occasionally convulsions or coma.

F.A. TREATMENT: Absolute bed rest. Empty stomach and bowels promptly and completely with gastric lavage and quick-acting cathartic and enemata. Atropine is especially helpful and may be given by any route. Fluid, and sodium chloride and carbohydrate intake should be maintained intravenously if required. Coffee, tea, and milk are helpful. Charcoal may be given early if available. Treat for shock.

NOTE: Call nearest Poison Control Center for availability and advisability of using thioctic acid in emergency treatment. SEE: *Poison Control Centers* in *Appendix.*

tobacco (tō-băk'ō) [Sp. *tabaco*]. Dried leaves of Nicotiana tabacum and other species. It contains nicotine, pyridine, picoline, and collidin. Widely used in forms of cigars, cigarettes, pipe tobacco, snuff, and chewing. During its combustion, various products are given off, the most important being nicotine, q.v., and certain compounds which have an adverse effect on the lungs. For this reason, the use of tobacco products may be injurious to health.

t., Indian. Lobelia.

tocodynamometer (tō"kō-dī"năm-ŏm'ē-ter) [Gr. *tokos*, birth, + *dynamis*, power, + *metron*, a measure]. Device for estimating expulsive force of uterine contractions in childbirth.

tocogony (tō-kŏg'ō-nĭ) ["+ *gonos*, seed]. Parental generation as opposed to abiogenesis.

tocograph (tŏk'ō-grăf) ["+ *graphein*, to write]. A device for estimating and recording the force of uterine contractions.

tocology (tō-kŏl'ō-jĭ) ["+ *logos*, science]. Science of parturition and obstetrics.

tocomania (tō"kō-mā'nĭ-ă) [Gr. *tokos*, birth, + *mania, madness*]. Puerperal insanity.

tocometer (tō-kŏm'ĕt-ĕr) ["+ *metron*, a measure]. Device for estimating expulsive force of the uterus in labor. SYN: *tocodynamometer.*

tocopherol (tō-kŏph'ĕr-ōl) ["+ *pherein*, to carry, + L. *oleum*, oil]. One of three substances collectively referred to as vitamin E, q.v.

tocophobia (tō"kō-fō'bĭ-ă) ["+ *phobos*, fear]. Abnormal fear of childbirth.

tocus (tō'kŭs) [L.]. Parturition; childbirth.

toe (tō) [AS. tā]. A digit of the foot.

RS: acroataxia; acrodynia; bunion; camptodactylia; clavus; dactyl; dactylus; digit; gout; hallux; metatarsus.

t., claw. Hammer toe, q.v.

t. clonus. Contraction of the big toe in sudden extension of the first phalanx.

t., dislocations of. These are treated essentially same as dislocations of the fingers. SEE: *finger, dislocation of.*

t. drop. Inability to lift the toes.

t.'s. fanning of. Spreading of toes, esp. when sole is stroked.

t., hammer. SEE: *hammer toe.*

t., Morton's. Metatarsalgia, q.v.

t., pigeon. Walking with the toes turned inward.

t. reflex. When great toe is strongly flexed all muscles below knee become tense.

toilet (toy'lĕt) [Fr. *toilette*, a little cloth.]. 1. Cleansing of a wound after operation or of an obstetrical patient. 2. An apparatus for use during defecation and urination to collect these waste products. The disposal may be immediate by flushing with water or by chemical digestion.

toko- [Gr.]. Combining form meaning birth. SEE: words beginning *toco-.*

tolerance (tŏl'ĕr-ăns) [L. *tolerantia*, tolerance]. Capacity for enduring climatic conditions, a poison, or a food or drug which may be harmful if taken in excess; power of resistance to such, or point at which such resistance ends; amount of a drug or food which may be so tolerated.

t., exercise. The amount of physical activity which can be done safely.

t., glucose. The ability of the body to absorb and utilize glucose. SEE: *glucose tolerance test.*

t., heat. Ability of a person or animal to withstand a hot environment.

t. levels. The limits of amounts of a food additive permissible. Amounts are specified for each food additive by the U.S. Food and Drug Administration. Specified levels are below those which would be harmful. SEE: *food additives.*

tol′erant. Capable of enduring or withstanding drugs without experiencing ill-effects.

toma′to. A plant with edible, fleshy fruit which may be eaten raw or cooked.

Food value of 100 gm. (raw): Cal. 22; protein 1.1 gm.; fat 0.2 gm.; carbohydrate 4.7 gm.; vitamin A, 900 I.U.; ascorbic acid 23 mg. (During certain growing periods, the ascorbic acid content may be less than 23 mg.)

-tome [Gr.]. Combining form meaning a cutting, a cutting instrument.

tomograph (tō′mō-gräf). A special type of x-ray apparatus which demonstrates the organ or tissue at a particular depth.

tomography (tō-mŏg′rä-fī) [" + *graphein*, to write]. Any of several special techniques of roentgenography designed to show detailed images of structures in a selected plane of tissue by blurring images of structures in all other planes. SYN: *analytical roentgenography; laminagraphy; planigraphy; sectional roentgenography; stratigraphy.*

tomomania (tō″mō-mā′nĭ-ă) [Gr. *tomē,* a cutting, + *mania,* madness]. 1. Tendency of a surgeon to resort to unnecessary surgical operations. 2. Abnormal desire to be operated upon.

tomotocia (tō″mō-tō′sĭ-ă) [" + *tokos,* birth]. Delivery of the fetus by cesarean section.

tonaphasia (tō″nă-fā′sĭ-ă) [L. *tonus,* a stretching, + *a-,* not, + *phasis,* speech]. Inability to remember a tune due to cerebral lesion. SYN: *amusia, vocal.*

tone (tōn) [L. *tonus,* a stretching]. 1. That state of a body or any of its organs or parts in which the functions are healthy and normal. In a more restricted sense, the resistance of muscles to passive elongation or stretch. 2. Normal tension or responsiveness to stimuli, as of arteries or muscles, seen particularly in involuntary muscle (such as the sphincter of the urinary bladder). 3. A musical or vocal sound.

t. deafness. Inability to detect differences in musical sounds. SYN: *amusia.*

t., muscular. Condition in which a muscle is in a steady state of contraction; the ability of a muscle to resist a force for a considerable period of time without change in length.

tongue (tŭng) [AS. *tunge*]. A freely-movable muscular organ lying partly in the floor of the mouth and partly in the pharynx. Its function is manipulation of food in mastication and deglutition; speech production; and taste. Its surface is covered with mucous membrane.

ANAT: It consists of a body and root and is attached by muscles to the hyoid bone below, the mandible in front, the styloid process behind, and the palate above, and by mucous membrane to the floor of the mouth, the lateral walls of the pharynx, and the epiglottis. A median fold, the frenulum linguae, connects the tongue to the floor of the mouth. The surface of the tongue bears numerous papillae of three types, filiform, fungiform, and vallate. Taste buds are present on the surfaces of many of the papillae, esp. the vallate papillae. Mucous and serous glands (lingual glands) are present, their ducts opening on the surface. Lymphoid tissue comprising the lingual tonsils is present in the posterior third of the tongue. A median fibrous septum extends the entire length of the tongue.

Arteries: Lingual, exterior maxillary, and ascending pharyngeal. *Muscles:* Extrinsic muscles include genioglossus, hypoglossus, and styloglossus. Intrinsic muscles consist of four groups: superior, inferior, transverse, and vertical lingualis muscles. *Nerves:* Lingual nerve (containing fibers from trigeminal and facial nerves); glossopharyngeal; vagus; and hypoglossal.

CONDITIONS: *Pain:* Occurs in local lesions; fissures; glossitis; malignancies; and pernicious anemia. *Protrusion and Movement:* This occurs with very sick patients, as in advanced typhoid fever and toxemia. The tongue is tremulous in early typhoid and in meningitis. In chorea it is thrust out suddenly and at once withdrawn. If it is protruded very slowly or if left exposed after being shown, it is a sign of great exhaustion, vascular congestion or disorder of the nerve supply. If the tongue when protruded points to the right or left involuntarily then a central or peripheral lesion of the nerve supply is present. Some persons have the ability to curl the tongue along its long axis. This ability is genetically determined.

Scars: These may be the result of injury or bulbar palsy causing ulceration and resulting in scars. *Sharp-pointed:* Observed in irritation and inflammation of the brain, smoker's tongue, leukoplakia. *Spasm:* Occurs in multiple sclerosis; general paresis; melancholia; and in stuttering. *Tremors:* Noted in asthenia; alcoholism; bulbar palsy; Graves' disorder; and in hemiplegia it is turned toward the paralyzed side if face is affected. If turned toward the unaffected side, it denotes lesion of the medulla. *Tremulous:* In all acute diseases but no particular significance in chronic nervous disorders.

Colored: The tongue may be temporarily discolored by a variety of colored medicines, foods, and liquids. *Black coating:* Glossophytia; may be due to stain or presence of microphytes. In dysentery, indicates exhaustion; mortification; death. In jaundice, denotes organic disease of liver. Onset of jaundice is usually first detectable in the yellowish discoloration of the area seen under the tongue when its tip is placed against the roof of the mouth.

Bluish: Denotes impaired circulation; interference with respiration; heart disease; asthma; cyanosis. *Dark brown:* Addison's disease. *Pale:* Indicates severe anemia; the tongue appears smaller than normal. *Red:* An early sign in typhoid fever. *Bright red:* Indicates inflammation of gastric or intestinal mucous membrane; glossitis; stomatitis. *Clean red:* With papillae prominent, or a white-coated tongue with papillae projecting through the fur, indicates scarlatina.

Red tip and edges, or having red, dry streak in center typical of typhoid. *Strawberry:* White fur through which project bright red and prominent papillae. Seen in early stage of scarlet fever. *Yellow:* With thick fur covering the tongue, indicates jaundice.

Macroglossia: large tongue, generally congenital, or may result from inflammation; Ludwig's angina; glossitis; actinomycosis; acromegaly; myxedema. If localized, may be due to gumma; carcinoma; or local trauma. *Microglossia:* small tongue, observed in anemia; emaciation; convalescence from typhoid. These conditions are temporary. *Thrust to one side:* Indicates hemiplegia if continually held in this position.

t., bifid. One with a cleft at its anterior end; a forked tongue.

t., black, hairy. Condition in which tongue possesses a brown, furlike area on its dorsum. The area is composed of hypertrophied filiform papillae pigment, and possibly microorganisms. Sometimes results from excessive use of oxygen-liberating mouthwashes or antibiotic therapy. SYN: *hyperkeratosis linguae; lingua nigra; lingua villosa nigra.*

t., burning. SEE: *Glossopyrosis.*

t., cleft. A bifid or trifid tongue, q.v.

t., coated. One covered with layer of whitish or yellowish material consisting of desquamated epithelium; bacteria; food de-

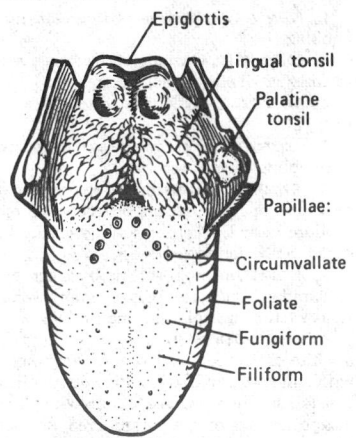

TONGUE—SUPERIOR VIEW

bris, etc. Significance is difficult to interpret. May mean only that patient slept with mouth open or has not eaten because of loss of appetite. If darkly coated, it may indicate a fungus infection.

t., deviation of. Marked turning of tongue from the midline when protruded. Indicative of lesions of the hypoglossal nerve.

t., dry. One that is dry and shriveled, usually indicative of a dehydration. May also be the result of mouth breathing.

t., fern-leaf. One possessing a prominent central furrow and lateral branches.

t., filmy. One possessing symmetrical whitish patches.

t., fissured. One bearing deep furrows in its epithelium. May be normal. Causes obscure. If deep and inflamed, may be due to syphilitic infection, or dissecting glossitis; a broken tooth; chronic dysentery; hepatic disease; or diabetes mellitus. SYN: *furrowed tongue; lingua plicata.*

t., forked. T., bifid, q.v.

t., furred. Coated tongue on which surface epithelium appears as a coat of white fur. Seen in nearly all fevers.

Unilateral furring may result from disturbed innervation, as in condition affecting the 2nd and 3rd branches of the 5th nerve. Has been noted in neuralgia of those branches and in fractures of the skull involving the foramen rotundum.

Yellow fur indicates jaundice.

t., geographic. One possessing white, raised areas resembling mountain ranges on a relief map. Areas consist of heaped-up epithelium surrounding areas of atrophy.

t., hairy. One possessing fine elongated papillae.

t., magenta. One magenta-colored seen in cases of riboflavin deficiency.

t., parrot. A dry shriveled tongue, seen in typhus.

t., scrotal. Furrowed and fissured. Resembling skin of scrotum.

t., smoker's. Condition characterized by white, opaque patches of thickened epithelium later thickening and becoming fissured. SYN: *leukoplakia.*

t., smooth. One resulting from atrophy of papillae. Characteristic of many conditions such as anemia and malnutrition.

t., strawberry. Tongue which first has a white coat except at tip and along edges, with enlarged papillae standing out distinctly against white surface. Later white coat disappears leaving a bright red surface. Characteristic of scarlet fever.

t., tremulous. Due to hyperthyroidism.

t., trifid. One in which anterior end is divided into three parts. SEE: *symptoms, throat.*

tongue, words pert. to: circumvallate papillae; cleft; frenulum; "gloss-" words; hypoglossal; lingua; macroglossia; microglossia; lingual; ranula; strawberry; sublingual; s. gland.

tongue-swallowing. The tendency, in an unconscious person lying on the back, for the relaxed tongue to slip back into the pharynx. This blocks the airway and seriously interferes with respiration. To correct, elevate the shoulders and extend the head; this maneuver will open the airway. Also a mechanical airway device may be used to hold or push the tongue forward. Unless this is done, attempts to apply artificial respiration to an unconscious person may be in vain.

tongue-tie. This is a congenital shortening of the frenum.

SYM: Interference in sucking and in articulation.

TREATMENT: Surgical.

tonic (tŏn'ĭk) [Gr. *tonikos,* pert. to tone]. 1. Pert. to or characterized by tension or contraction, esp. muscular tension. 2. Restoring tone. 3. A medicine that increases strength and tone. They are subdivided according to action, as cardiac; general, etc. Ex: iron; digitalis.

t. spasm. A persistent, involuntary, firm or violent muscular contraction. See: *clonic.*

tonicity (tō'-nĭs'ĭ-tĭ) [Gr. *tonos,* tone]. 1. Property of possessing tone, esp. muscular tone. 2. State of normal tension or partial contrac-

tion of muscle fibers while at rest. SYN: *tone.*

tonoclonic (tŏn''o-klŏn'ĭk) ["+ *klonos,* tumult]. Both tonic and clonic, said of muscular spasms.

tonograph (tŏn'ō-grăf) ["+ *graphein,* to write]. Device for recording blood pressure.

tonometer (tŏn-ŏm'ĕ-tĕr) ["+ *metron,* a measure]. Instrument for measuring tension or pressure, esp. intraocular pressure.

tonometry (tŏn-ŏm'ĕ-trĭ). The measurement of tension of a part, as intraocular tension. This test is extremely useful in detecting glaucoma, q.v.

tonophant (tŏn'ō-fănt) [Gr. *tonos,* tone, + *phainein,* to show]. Device for making acoustic or sound energy visible.

tonsil (tŏn'sĭl) [L. *tonsilla,* almond]. 1. A mass of lymphatic tissue located in depressions of the mucous membrane of fauces and pharynx. SEE: *lingual, palatine; pharyngeal tonsil.* 2. A rounded mass on inferior surface of cerebellum lying lateral to the uvula.

FUNCTION: Acts as filter to protect body from invasion of bacteria, and aids in the formation of white cells.

t., cerebellar. One of a pair of cerebellar lobules on either side of the uvula, q.v., projecting from inferior surface of cerebellum.

t., faucial. SEE: *tonsil* (def. 1).

t., lingual. A mass of lymphoid tissue located in root of tongue.

t., Luschka's. T., pharyngeal, q.v.

t., nasal. Lymphoid tissue on the nasal septum.

t., palatine. A mass of lymphoid tissue which lies in tonsillar fossa on each side of oral pharynx between glossopalatine and pharyngopalatine arches. The free surface of each tonsil is covered with stratified squamous epithelium which forms deep indentations or crypts extending into substance of tonsil. The lateral surface of each tonsil is covered with a firm fibrous capsule. Efferent lymph vessels convey lymph from the tonsil. No afferent vessels are present.

t., pharyngeal. Lymphoid tissue on posterior superior wall of pharynx. SEE: *adenoid.*

t., tubal. Lymphatic tissue present in mucous membrane of auditory tube near its opening into pharynx.

tonsillar (tŏn'sĭ-lăr). Pert. to a tonsil, esp. the faucial or palatine t.

t. area. Area composed of the palatine arch, tonsillar fossa, glossopalatine sulcus, and posterior faucial pillar.

t. crypt. A deep indentation into pharyngeal surface of a tonsil. It is lined with stratified epithelium.

t. fossa. A depression between the glossopalatine and pharyngopalatine arches in which the palatine tonsil is situated.

t. ring. The almost complete ring of tonsilar tissue encircling the pharynx. Includes the palatine, lingual and pharyngeal tonsils. SYN: *Waldeyer's ring.*

t. sinus. Space lying between plica triangularis and anterior surface of palatine tonsil.

tonsillectomy (tŏn-sĭl-ĕk'tō-mĭ) [L. *tonsilla,* almond, + Gr. *ektomē,* excision]. Surgical removal of the tonsils.

OPER. NP: Patient is placed in dorsal position with head extended and covered with a sterile sheet up to neck in usual manner; over sterile sheet, at neck, place a sterile towel.

Immediately following operation patient is turned on side or face down, so that vomitus or blood is not inhaled, and ice compress is placed around throat. Pulse rate should be taken frequently and any marked increase that might indicate a possible hemorrhage should be reported to the doctor immediately. It is important for nurse to test suction apparatus before operation. Cold water should be flushed through the suction tip into bottle after operation to prevent stoppage through clotting of blood.

tonsillitis (tŏn-sĭl-i'tĭs) [L. *tonsilla,* almond, + Gr. *-itis,* inflammation]. Inflammation of a tonsil, esp. the faucial tonsil.

t., acute. Inflammation of the lymphatic tissue of the pharynx, esp. the palatine or faucial tonsils. May occur sporadically or in epidemic form. SYN: *scarlatina; scarlet fever; epidemic sore throat; septic sore throat.*

ETIOL: May be caused by a variety of organisms. If due to group A hemolytic streptococci, its clinical importance because of possible sequelae must be considered.

SYM: Onset is sudden, usually accompanied by chills. Temperature may reach 105° F. (40.6° C.). Malaise; headache; pains and aches in back and extremities; pain in tonsils, esp. when swallowing may be present. Tonsils appear enlarged, red; and yellowish exudate projects from crypts.

PROG: Usually self-limited but serious complications may occur such as sinusitis; otitis media; mastoiditis; or peritonsillar abscess.

TREATMENT: *General:* Bedrest; liquid diet; antipyretics; hot saline or 30% glucose gargles or throat irrigations. *Specific:* Procaine penicillin or tetracycline drugs.

If the disease is thought to be due to group A hemolytic streptococci, the throat should be cultured and then penicillin therapy instituted for a full ten-day course. If in the meantime the report on the culture is negative for these organisms, the penicillin therapy may be discontinued when clinical signs of infection have subsided.

If throat culture technique is not available and infection with group A hemolytic streptococci is suspected, then a full ten-day course of penicillin should be given. This regimen will prevent the streptococci from elaborating the toxic substances which cause rheumatic fever, rheumatic heart disease, and certain kidney diseases. Administration of penicillin for less than ten days when tonsillitis is due to group A hemolytic streptococci is not advisable, even though clinical signs of infection may disappear within the first several days of treatment.

tonsillolith (tŏn'sĭl-ō-lĭth) [L. *tonsilla,* almond, + Gr. *lithos,* stone]. A concretion within a tonsil. SYN: *amygdalolith.*

tonsilloscopy (tŏn"sĭl-los'kō-pĭ) [" + Gr. *skopein,* to examine]. Inspection of the tonsils.

tonsillotomy (tŏn"sĭl-ŏt'ō-mĭ) [" + Gr. *tomē,* a cutting]. Incision of the tonsils.

tonus (tō'nŭs) [L., tone]. That partial, steady contraction of muscle which determines tonicity or firmness. SYN: *tone; tonicity.*

tooth (tooth) [AS. *tŏth*]. (pl. *teeth*) One of the conical hard structures in the upper and lower jaws used for mastication.

A tooth consists of a crown or portion above gum, a root, portion embedded in socket (alveolus) of jaw bones, and neck or cervix, constricted region between crown and root which is covered by the gum or gingiva. The major portion of a tooth consists of dentin, an ivorylike substance harder than bone, which surrounds the pulp cavity. A layer of enamel covers the crown and cementum covers the dentin of the root. A periodontal membrane surrounds the root and holds the tooth firmly in its socket. The pulp cavity contains dental pulp which consists of connective tissue, capillaries, lymph vessels and nerve endings. SEE: *dentition, teeth,* words beginning with *odonto-.*

toothache. Pain in a tooth or the region about a tooth. SYN: *odontalgia, odontodynia.*

topagnosis (tŏp"ăg-nō'sĭs) [Gr. *topos,* place, + *a,* not, + *gnōsis,* recognition]. Loss of ability to localize site of origin of tactile sensations.

topectomy (tō-pĕkt'ō-mĭ) [" + *ektomē,* excision]. A modified form of frontal lobotomy in which small incisions are made through the thalamofrontal tracts. A psychosurgical procedure used in the treatment of certain mental diseases.

topesthesia (top″es-the′zĭ-ă) [″+ *aisthēsis*, sensation]. Ability through tactile sense to determine any part that is touched.

tophaceous (tō-fā′shŭs) [L. *tophaceus*, sandy]. 1. Relating to a tophus. 2. Sandy, gritty.

tophus (tō′fŭs) [L. *tophus*, porous stone]. (pl. *tophi*) 1. Deposit of sodium biurate in tissues near a joint in gout. 2. A salivary calculus. 3. Tartar on the teeth.

tophyperidrosis (tŏf′ĭ-pĕr″ĭ-drō′sĭs) [Gr. *topos*, place, + *hyper*, above, + *hidrōs*, perspiration]. Excessive sweating in local areas.

top′ical [Gr. *topos*, place]. Pert. to a definite area; local.

topoalgia (tō″pō-ăl′jĭ-ă) [″+ *algos*, pain]. Localized pain; common in neurasthenia following emotional upsets.

topoanesthesia (tō″pō-ăn″ĕs-the′zĭ-ă) [″+ *an-*, not, + *aisthēsis*, sensation]. Loss of ability to recognize the location of a tactile sensation.

topognosia, topognosis (tō″pŏg-nō′sĭ-ă, -sĭs) [″+ *gnōsis*, knowledge]. Recognition of the location of a tactile sensation. SYN: *topesthesia.*

topographic (top″ō-grăf′ĭk) [″+ *graphein*, to write]. Pert. to description of special regions.

    t. anatomy. A study of all the structures and their relationships in a given region, for example, the axilla. SYN: *regional anatomy.*

topography (tō-pŏg′ră-fī). Description of a part of the body.

toponarcosis (tō″pō-năr-kō′sĭs) [Gr. *topos*, place, + *narkōsis*, stupor]. Local anesthesia.

toponeurosis (tō″pō-nū-rō′sĭs) [″+ *neuron*, nerve, + *-ōsis*, condition]. Neurosis of a limited area.

topophobia (tō″pō-fō′bĭ-ă) [″+ *phobos*, fear]. A fear of psychoneurotic origin in relation to a particular locality.

topothermesthesiometer (top″ō-ther″mĕs-the-zhĭ-ŏm′ĕ-ter) [″+ *thermē*, heat, + *aisthēsis*, sensation, + *metron*, measure]. Device for measuring local temperature sense.

TOPS. Acronym for an organization which assists obese persons to *T*ake *O*ff *P*ounds *S*ensibly.

tormen (tor′mĕn) [L. *tormen*, a twisting]. (pl. *tormina*) Acute griping pain in the intestinal tract.

tormina (tor′mĭn-ă) [L. twistings]. (sing. *tormen*) Intestinal colic with griping pains.

torose, torous (tō′rōs, -rŭs) [L. *torosus*, full of muscle]. Knobby or bulging; tubercular.

torpent (tor′pĕnt) [L. *torpens*, numbing]. 1. Medicine which modifies irritation. 2. Not capable of fu.nctioning; dormant, apathetic, torpid.

torpid (tor′pĭd) [L. *torpidus*, numb]. Not acting vigorously; sluggish.

torpidity (tor-pĭd′ĭ-tĭ). Sluggishness; inactivity.

torpor (tor′por) [L. *torpor*, numbness]. Abnormal inactivity; dormancy; numbness; apathy.

    t. intestino′rum. Constipation.

    t. peristal′ticus. Atonic constipation.

    t. retinae. Reduced sensitivity of retina to light stimuli.

torsion (tor′shŭn) [L. *torsio*, a twisting]. 1. Act of twisting or condition of being twisted. 2. Rotation of the vertical meridians of the eye.

torsive (tor′sĭv). Twisted, as in a spiral.

torso (tor′sō) [It.]. The trunk of the body.

torsoclusion (tor″sōk-lū′zhun) [″+ L. *occlusio*, a shutting out]. 1. Acupressure in combination with torsion to stop a bleeding vessel. 2. Malocclusion characterized by rotation of a tooth on its long axis.

torticollis (tor″tĭ-kŏl′ĭs) [L. *tortus*, twisted, + *collum*, neck]. Stiff neck caused by spasmodic contraction of neck muscles drawing the head to one side with chin pointing to the other side. Congenital or acquired. SYN: *wryneck.*

    ETIOL: Result of scars; disease of cervical vertebrae; adenitis; tonsillitis; rheumatism; enlarged cervical glands; retropharyngeal abscess; cerebellar tumors. It may be spasmodic (clonic) or permanent (tonic). The latter type may be due to Pott's disease (tuberculosis of the spine).

    The muscles affected are principally those supplied by the spinal accessory nerve.

    t., fixed. Abnormal position of head due to organic shortening of the muscles.

    t., intermittent. T., spasmodic, q.v.

    t., ocular. T. from inequality in sight of the two eyes.

    t., rheumatic. T., symptomatic, q.v.

    t., spasmodic. T. with recurrent but transient contractions of muscles of neck and esp. of the sternocleidomastoid.

    t., spurious. T. from caries of the cervical vertebrae.

    t., symptomatic. Rheumatic stiff neck.

tortipelvis (tor″tĭ-pĕl′vĭs) [L. *tortus*, twisted, + *pēlvis*, basin]. Muscular spasms in children distorting the spine and hip. SYN: *dystonia musculorum deformans.*

Torula (tor′ū-lă). Former name of a genus of yeastlike organism, now called Cryptococcus.

toruloid (tor′ū-loyd) [L. *torulus,* a little bulge, + Gr. *eidos,* form]. Beaded; noting an aggregate of colonies like those seen in the budding of yeast.

Torulopsis glabrata. A yeast of the family Cryptococcaceae. It is closely related to the Candida species. Usually nonpathogenic for man but may cause serious illness in patients receiving immunosuppressive drugs, antibiotics, or corticosteroids.

torulosis (tor-ū-lō′sĭs). Infestation with Torula or yeast cells. SYN: *cryptococcosis* which is the preferable term.

torulus (tor′ū-lŭs) [L. *torulus,* a little elevation]. A very small elevation. SYN: *papilla.*

   t. tac′tilis. A tactile cutaneous elevation on palms and soles.

torus [L., swelling]. A rounded elevation or swelling.

total hip replacement. Surgical procedure used in treating severe arthritis of the hip.

   Both the head of the femur and the acetabulum are replaced with metal components. The acetabulum replacement is covered with a plastic material so that there is metal-to-plastic contact rather than metal-to-metal. In general the operation has not been done on persons of less than 50 years of age. SYN: *total hip arthroplasty.*

totipotent [L. *totus,* all, + *potentia,* power]. A cell capable of differentiating into a large variety of cells. The fertilized ovum has this ability.

touch (tŭtsh) [O.Fr. *tochier*]. 1. To perceive by the tactile sense; to feel with the hands, to palpate. 2. The sense by which pressure on the skin or mucosa is perceived; the tactile sense. 3. Examination with the hand. SYN: *palpation.*

   Various disorders may disturb or impair the tactile sense or the ability to feel normally. There are a number of words pert. to sensation and its modifications, a few of the more important ones being listed as follows: algesia; -algia; anesthesia; dysesthesia, -dynia; esthesia; esthesioneurosis; hyperesthesia; paresthesia; synesthesia.

   t., abdominal. Palpation of the abdomen.

   t., after. Persistence of the sensation of touch after contact with stimulus has ceased.

   t., double. Vaginal and rectal examination made at same time.

   t., rectal. Digital examination of the rectum.

   t., vaginal. Digital examination of the vagina.

   t., vesical. Digital examination of the bladder.

touch, words pert. to: amblyaphia; anaphia; anaptic; astereognosis; atopognosis; delire de toucher; dysaphia; hallucinations; haphephobia; haptic; polyesthesia; stereognosis; tactile.

tour de maitre (tūr″deh mā-tr′) [Fr., the master's turn]. A method of introducing a catheter or sound into the male bladder or into the uterus.

Tournay's sign (tūr-nā′). Dilatation of the pupil of the eye on unusually strong lateral fixation.

tourniquet (tūr′nĭ-kĕt) [Fr., a turning instrument]. Any constrictor used on an extremity to make pressure over an artery and thereby control bleeding; also used to distend veins to facilitate venipuncture or intravenous injections.

   Tourniquets are made more effective by placing a firm object such as a padded stone or a padded piece of wood over an artery to concentrate pressure at that point.

   Tourniquet should never be left in place too long. Ordinarily, it should be released from 12 to 18 minutes after application to determine whether bleeding has ceased. If it has, leave tourniquet loosely in place so that it may be retightened if necessary. If not retighten at once.

   In general, a tourniquet should not be used if steady, firm pressure over the bleeding site will stop the flow.

   Arterial hemorrhage: Apply between the wound and the heart, close to the wound, placing a hard pad over point of pressure. Should be discontinued as soon as possible and a tight bandage substituted under the loosened tourniquet.

   Venous hemorrhage: Place below bleeding point, but close to the wound. The tourniquet should remain in place with periodic momentary loosening until released by a physician.

   t. paralysis. Injury to a nerve due to a tourniquet's having been applied for too long a period or too tightly.

   t. test. Test for determining the ability of capillaries to withstand increased pressure.

Touton cells (toot′ōn). [Karl Touton, Ger. dermatologist, born 1858] Giant multinucleated cells found in lesions of xanthomatosis.

tow (tō) [AS. *tow,* a weaving]. Coarse fibers of flax, used for surgical dressings.

towelette (tow′ĕl-ĕt′) [ME. *towelle*, towel]. A small towel for surgical or obstetrical use.

toweling, towelling (tow′ĕl-ĭng). Friction with a coarse towel.

toxalbumin (tŏks′′ăl-bū′mĭn) [L. *toxicum*, poison, + *albumen*, white of egg]. A poisonous albumin or protein.

toxalbumose (tŏks-ăl′bŭ-mōs). A poisonous albumose.

toxanemia (tŏks′′ă-nē′mĭ-ă) [L. *toxium*, poison, + Gr. *an-*, not, + *haima*, blood]. Anemia due to a hemolytic toxin.

toxemia (tŏks-ē′mĭ-ă) [L. *toxicum*, poison, + Gr. *haima*, blood]. Distribution throughout body of poisonous products of bacteria growing in a focal or local site, thus producing generalized symptoms.

SYM: Fever; diarrhea; vomiting; pulse and respiration quickened or depressed; shock.

In tetanus, the nervous system is esp. affected; in diptheria, nerves and muscles.

    t., eclamptogenic. Toxemia of pregnancy, q.v. SEE: *eclampsia.*

    t. of pregnancy. Various conditions affecting women in pregnancy.

    ETIOL: Unknown.

    FORMS: Simple vomiting; pernicious vomiting (hyperemesis gravidarum); acute yellow atrophy of the liver; renal failure; preeclampsia; and eclampsia.

toxenzyme (tŏks-ĕn′zīm) ["+ Gr. *en*, in, + *zymē*, leaven]. A poisonous enzyme.

toxic (tŏks′ĭk) [L. *toxicum*, poison]. Pert. to, resembling or caused by poison. SYM: *poisonous.*

    t. erythema. Redness of skin or a rash resulting from toxic agents such as drugs.

toxicant (tŏks′ĭ-kănt) [L. *toxicans*, poisoning]. Poisonous; toxic. 2. Any poison.

toxicide (tŏks′ĭ-sīd) [L. *toxicum*, poison, + *cidus*, from *caedere*, to kill]. 1. Destructive to toxins. 2. A chemical antidote for poisons.

toxicity (tŏks-ĭs′ĭ-tĭ). The extent, quality, or degree of being poisonous.

toxico- [Gr. *toxikon*, poison]. Combining form meaning poisonous.

toxicoderma (tŏks′′ĭ-kō-der′mă) [Gr. *toxikon*, poison, + *derma*, skin]. Any skin disease resulting from a poison.

toxicodermatitis (tŏks′′ĭ-kō-derm-ă-tī′tĭs) ["+ "+ *-itis*, inflammation]. Inflammation of the skin due to a poison.

toxicodermatosis (tŏks′′ĭ-kō-derm-ă-tō′sĭs) ["+ "+ *-osis*, condition]. Toxicoderma, q.v.

toxicogenic (tŏks′′ĭ-kō-jĕn′ĭk) [Gr. *toxikon*, poison, + *gennan*, to produce]. Caused by, or producing, a poison.

toxicoid (tŏks′ĭ-koyd) ["+ *eidos*, resemblance]. Of the nature of a poison.

toxicologist (tŏks′′ĭ-kŏl′ō-jĭst) ["+ *logos*, study]. A specialist in the field of poisons or toxins.

toxicology (tŏks′′ĭ-kŏl′ō-jĭ). The science of poisons, their nature, effects, and antidotes.

toxicomania (tŏks′′ĭ-kō-mā′nĭ-ă) [Gr. *toxikon*, poison, + *mania*, madness]. Abnormal craving for narcotics, intoxicants, or poisons.

toxicopathic (tŏks′′ĭ-kō-păth′ĭk) ["+ *pathos*, disease]. Pert. to any condition caused by a poison.

toxicopathy (tŏks′′ĭ-kop′ă-thĭ) [Gr. *toxikon*, poison, + *pathos*, disease]. Any disease caused by a poison.

toxicophobia (tŏks′′ĭ-kō-fō′bĭ-ă) ["+ *phobos*, fear]. Abnormal fear of being poisoned by any medium: food, gas, water, drugs, etc.

toxicosis (tŏks′′ĭ-kō′sĭs) ["+ *-osis*, condition]. A diseased condition resulting from poisoning. SYN: *toxicopathy.*

    t., endogen′ic. Disease due to poisons generated within the body. SYN: *autointoxication.*

    t., exogen′ic. Any disease resulting from a poison not generated in the body.

    t., retention. T. from retained products which normally are excreted as formed.

toxidermitis (tŏks′′ĭ-der-mī′tĭs) [Gr. *toxikon*, poison, + *derma*, skin, + *-itis*, inflammation]. Any inflammatory skin disease due to poisoning. SYN: *toxicodermatitis.*

toxiferous (tŏks-ĭf′ĕr-ŭs) ["+ L. *ferre*, to carry]. Containing a poison. SYN: *poisonous.*

toxigenic (tŏks′′ĭ-jĕn′ĭk) ["+ *gennan*, to produce]. Producing toxins or poisons.

toxigenicity (tŏks′′ĭ-jĕn-ĭs′ĭ-tĭ). The virulence of a toxin-producing pathogenic organism.

toxignomic (tŏks′′ĭg-nŏm′ĭk) [Gr. *toxikon*, poison, + *gnomikos*, knowing]. Having the toxic action peculiar to a poison.

toxin (tŏks′ĭn) [L. *toxicum*, poison]. A poisonous substance of animal or plant origin.

    RS: antibody; antitoxin; bacteria; phytotoxin; toxoid.

    t., bacterial. T. produced by bacteria. Includes *exotoxins* which diffuse from bacterial cells into surrounding medium, and *endotoxins* which are liberated only when the bacterial cell is destroyed. SEE: *bacteria.*

    t., extracellular. SEE: *exotoxin.*

    t., intracellular. SEE: *endotoxin.*

toxin-antitoxin (tŏks′ĭn-ăn′′tĭ-tŏks′ĭn) [L. *toxicum* poison, + Gr. *anti*, against, + L. *toxicum*]. Diptheria toxin with its antitoxin in a nearly neutral mixture, the diptheria toxin being about 85% neutralized.

    Used for immunization against diptheria. SYN: *T. A. T. mixture.*

toxinemia (tŏks″ĭn-ē′mĭ-ă) ["+ Gr. *haima,* blood]. Blood poisoning. SYN: *toxemia.*

toxinfection (tŏks″ĭn-fĕk′shŭn) ["+ *infectio,* a putting into]. Infection caused by toxins or other poisons.

toxinicide (tŏks-ĭn′ĭs-ĭd) ["+ *cidus,* kill]. That which is destructive to toxins.

toxinosis (tŏks″ĭn-ō′sĭs) ["+ Gr. *-ōsis,* condition]. Disease due to a toxin.

toxipathy (tŏks-ĭp′ă-thĭ) [L. *toxicum,* poison, + Gr. *pathos,* disease]. Any disease due to poison.

toxiphobia (tŏks″ĭ-fō′bĭ-ă) ["+ Gr. *phobos,* fear]. Abnormal fear of being poisoned.

toxitabellae (tŏks″ĭ-tăb-ĕl′ē) ["+ *tabella,* tablet]. Poisonous tablets. Usually designated by having an angular shape or by having the word "poison" or the "skull and crossbones design" stamped upon them.

toxitherapy (tŏks″ĭ-thĕr′ă-pĭ) ["+ Gr. *therapeia,* treatment]. Use of toxins in treatment of disease.

toxituberculid (tŏks″ĭ-tū-bĕr′kū-lĭd). A skin lesion resulting from action of toxin of tuberculosis organism.

toxogenin (tŏks-ŏj′ĕn-ĭn) [Gr. *toxikon,* poison, + *gennan,* to produce]. Hypothetical substance in the blood caused by injection of antigens, innocuous in itself, but causing anaphylaxis upon addition of fresh antigen.

toxoalexin (tŏks″ō-ăl-ĕks′ĭn) ["+ *alexein,* to ward off]. An alexin which counteracts bacterial toxins.

toxocariasis (tŏks″ō-kăr-ĭ′ă-sĭs). Disease due to infection with nematode worms, Toxocara canis or T. cati.

In man, the eggs penetrate the bowel wall and enter the circulation. Larvae may be carried to any part of the body where the blood vessel is large enough to accomodate them. They may end up in the brain, retinal vessels, liver, lung, or heart. The larvae cause hemorrhage, inflammation, and necrosis in these tissues. Thus the patient may have myocarditis, endophthalmitis, epilepsy, or encephalitis.

Diagnosis is made by immunological tests. It is important that t. be considered in cases diagnosed as retinoblastoma.

toxoid (tŏks′oyd) ["+ *eidos,* form]. A toxin treated so as to destroy its toxicity, but still capable of inducing formation of antibodies on injection.

　　t., alum-precipitated. T. of diphtheria or tetanus precipitated with potash-alum.

　　t., diphtheria. Diphtheria toxin detoxified by formaldehyde treatment.

toxolecithin (tŏks″ō-lĕs′ĭ-thĭn) [Gr. *toxikon,* poison, + *lekithos,* yolk of egg]. A compound of lecithin with a toxin such as certain snake venoms.

toxolysin (tŏks-ŏl′ĭ-sĭn) ["+ *lysis,* dissolution]. Substance destroying toxins. SYN: *antitoxin, toxicide.*

toxomucin (tŏks″ō-mū′sĭn) ["+ L. *mucus,* mucus]. Specific toxic albuminoid from cultures of tubercle bacilli.

toxon, toxone (tŏks′ŏn, -ōn) [Gr. *toxikon,* poison]. A bacterial toxin with lessened activity, producing paralysis and delayed death.

toxonoid (tŏks′ō-noyd) ["+ *eidos,* form]. A nontoxic substance with a weak affinity for antitoxin.

toxonosis (tŏks″ō-nō′sĭs) ["+ *-ōsis,* condition]. A disease caused by poisoning. SYN: *toxicosis, toxinosis.*

toxopeptone (tŏks″ō-pĕp′tŏn) ["+ *pepton,* digesting]. A protein derivative produced by action of a toxin on peptones.

toxophil(e) (tŏks′ō-fĭl, -fĭl) ["+ *philein,* to love]. Having a special affinity for toxins.

toxophore (tŏks′ō-fōr) [Gr. *toxikon,* poison, + *phoros,* a bearer]. That portion of a toxin which gives to a toxin its poisonous qualities.

toxophore group (tŏks′ō-fōr). Poison-bearing group of a toxin.

toxophylaxin (tŏks″ō-fĭ-lăks′ĭn) [Gr. *toxikon,* poison, + *phylax,* guard]. A substance which neutralizes bacterial toxins. SYN: *toxicophylaxin.*

Toxoplasma (tŏks″ō-plăs′mă). A genus of protozoa.

　　T. gondii. The causative agent of toxoplasmosis, q.v.

toxoplasmosis (tŏks-ō-plăs-mō′sĭs). A disease due to infection with the protozoa, Toxoplasma gondii. The organism is found in many mammals and birds. Symptoms may be so mild as to be barely noticeable or may be more severe with lymphadenopathy, malaise, muscle pain, and little if any fever. In the severe disseminated form there are pneumonitis, hepatitis, and encephalitis. In the congenital form, destructive lesions of the central nervous system, jaundice, anemia, and generalized lymphadenopathy usually are present.

　　DIAG: By identification or culture of the organism and by serologic test.

　　TREATMENT: Even though treatment is not entirely satisfactory, pyrimethamine with sulfonamides is indicated.

toxosozin (tŏks″ō-sō′zĭn) [Gr. *toxikon,* poison, + *sōzein,* to save]. A protein substance, normally present in the blood, which neutralizes bacterial toxins.

T.P.I. test. Abbr. for *Treponema pallidum immobilizing test* (for syphilis).

TPN. Abbr. for *triphosphopyridine nucleotide.*

t.p.r. Abbr. for *temperature, pulse, respiration.*

tr. Abbr. for L. *tinctura,* tincture.

trabecula (tră-bĕk'ū-lă) [L. *trabecula,* a little beam]. (pl. *trabeculae*) [NA]. Fibrous cord of connective tissue, serving as supporting fiber by forming septum extending into an organ from its wall or capsule.

trabeculae carneae. [NA]. Thick muscular tissue bands attached to inner walls of the ventricles of the heart.

trabs, trabs cerebri (trăbz ser'ĕ-brī) [L. *trabs,* a beam]. Arched band of white fibers connecting the cerebral hemispheres. SYN: *corpus callosum.*

trace (trās) [O.Fr. *tracier,* from L. *tractus,* a dragging]. 1. A very small quantity. 2. A mark.

t. elements. Organic elements normally found in minute traces in foods and tissues, such as aluminum; bromine; cobalt; copper; fluorine; manganese; nickel; silicon; zinc; and other physiologically rare minerals.

t., primitive. Pale white streak in germinal area indicating beginning of development of the blastoderm. SYN: *primitive streak.*

tracer. A radioactive isotope, capable of being incorporated into compounds, which when introduced into the body "tags" a specific portion of the molecule so that its course may be traced. Used in absorption and excretion studies, for identifying intermediary products of metabolism, and determination of distribution of various substances in the body. Radioactive carbon (C^{14}), calcium (Ca^{42}) and iodine (I^{131}) are examples of tracers commonly used.

trachea (trā'kē-ă) [Gr. *tracheia,* rough]. (pl. *tracheae*) [NA] A cylindrical cartilaginous tube, 4 1/2 inches (11.3 cm.) long, from the larynx to the bronchial tubes.

It extends from the sixth cervical to the fifth dorsal vertebra. Here it divides into two bronchi, one for each lung. It is lined with mucous membrane. Its inner surface is lined with ciliated epithelium. SYN: *windpipe.*

tracheaectasy (trā'kē-ă-ĕk'tă-sī) [Gr. *tracheia,* rough, + *ektasis,* dilatation]. Dilatation of the trachea.

tracheal (trā'kē-ăl). Pertaining to the trachea.

t. tugging. Pulsation of the larynx or downward pull of the trachea, symptomatic of thoracic aneurysm.

trachealgia (trā'kē-ăl'jī-ă) [*+ algos,* pain]. Pain in the trachea.

trachealis (trā-kē-ā'lĭs) [L.]. A muscle composed of smooth muscle fibers which extends between the ends of the tracheal rings. Its contraction reduces the size of the' lumen.

tracheitis (trā"kē-ī'tĭs) [Gr. *tracheia,* rough, + *-itis,* inflammation]. An inflammation of the trachea.

It may be acute or chronic and may be associated with bronchitis and laryngitis.

NP: It is necessary to keep patient in bed, as the condition may spread and give rise to bronchial complications. Pulse and temperature must be carefully checked and recorded. Camphorated oil may be rubbed on the chest, which is then covered with warm wool. Lemonade should be within reach of the patient as constant small sips will help relieve irritation from coughing.

trachelagra (trā"kĕl-ăg'ră) [Gr. *trachelos,* neck, + *agra,* seizure]. Rheumatism or gout of neck muscles resulting in torticollis.

trachelectomopexy (trā"kĕ-lĕk'tom-o-pek"sī) ["+ *ektomē,* a cutting out, + *pēxis,* fixation]. Fixation of uterine neck with partial excision.

trachelectomy (trā"kĕl-ĕk'tō-mī) [Gr. *trachēlos,* neck, + *ektomē,* excision]. Amputation of the cervix uteri.

trachelematoma (trā"kĕl-ē-mă-tō'mă) ["+ *haima,* blood, + *-ōma,* tumor]. A hematoma situated on the neck.

trachelism, trachelismus (trā'ke-lĭzm, trā-ke-lĭz'mŭs) ["+ *-ismos,* condition]. Backward spasm of the neck, sometimes preceding an epileptic attack.

trachelitis (trā-kĕ-lī'tĭs) ["+ *-itis,* inflammation]. Inflammation of mucous membrane of the cervix uteri. SYN: *cervicitis.*

trachelo- [Gr.]. Combining form, meaning neck.

trachelobregmatic (trā'kĕ-lō-brĕg-măt'ĭk) [Gr. *trachēlos,* neck, + *bregma,* front of the head]. Pert. to the neck and the bregma.

trachelocystitis (trā"kĕl-ō-sĭs-tī'tĭs) ["+ *kystis,* bladder, + *-itis,* inflammation]. Inflammation of neck of bladder.

trachelodynia (trā"kĕ-lō-dĭn'ĭ-ă) ["+ *odynē,* pain]. Pain in the neck.

trachelokyphosis (trā-kĕl-ō-kī-fō'sĭs) ["+ *kyphōsis,* humpback]. Excessive anterior curvature of cervical portion of spine.

trachelology (trā"ke-lŏl'ō-jī) ["+ *logos,* study]. Scientific study of the neck, its diseases and injuries.

trachelomastoid (trā"kē-lō-măs'toyd) [Gr. *trachēlos,* neck, + *mastos,* breast, + *eidos,* form]. A muscle of the neck. SYN: *longissimus capitus.* SEE: *Table of Muscles* in *Appendix.*

trachelomyitis (trā″ke-lō-mī-i′tĭs) ["+ *mys*, muscle, + *-itis*, inflammation]. Inflammation of muscles of neck.

trachelopexy (trā′kel-ō-pĕks″ĭ) ["+ *pēxis*, fixation]. Surgical fixation of the cervix uteri to an adjacent part.

tracheloplasty (trā′kel-ō-plas″tĭ) [Gr. *trachēlos*, neck, + *plassein*, to form]. Either surgical repair or plastic surgery of the neck of the uterus.

trachelorrhaphy (trā″kel-or′ă-fĭ) ["+ *rhaphē*, seam]. Suturing of a torn cervix uteri.

trachelotomy (trā″kel-ŏt′ō-mĭ) ["+ *tomē*, a cutting]. Incision of the cervix of the uterus.

tracheo- [Gr.]. Combining form meaning trachea, windpipe.

tracheoaerocele (trā″ke-ō-ā′ēr-ō-sēl) [Gr. *tracheia*, trachea, + *aēr*, air, + *kēlē*, hernia]. Hernia or cyst of trachea containing air.

tracheobronchoscopy (trā″ke-ō-brŏng-kŏs′kō-pĭ) ["+ *bronchos*, windpipe, + *skopeō*, to examine]. Inspection of the trachea and bronchi through a bronchoscope.

tracheocele (trā′ke-ō-sēl) ["+ *kēlē*, hernia]. Protrusion of mucous membrane through the wall of the trachea.

tracheoesophageal (trā″ke-ō-ē-sō-făj′ī-al) ["+ *oisophagos*, esophagus]. Pert. to the trachea and esophagus.

tracheolaryngotomy (trā″ke-ō-lăr-ĭn-gŏt′ō-mĭ) ["+ *larynx*, larynx, + *tomē*, a cutting]. Incision into larynx and trachea.

tracheopathia, tracheopathy (trā″ke-ō-păth′ĭ-ă, -ŏp′ă-thĭ) [Gr. *tracheia*, trachea, + *pathos*, disease]. Diseased condition of the trachea.

tracheopharyngeal (trā″ke-ō-far-in′je-ăl) ["+ *pharynx*, pharynx]. Pert. to both the trachea and pharynx.

tracheophonesia (trā″ke-ō-fōn-ē′zhĭ-ă) ["+ *phōnēsis*, a sounding]. Cardiac auscultation at the sternal notch.

tracheophony (trā″ke-ŏf′ō-nĭ) [Gr. *tracheia*, trachea, + *phōnē*, a sound]. Sound heard over the trachea in auscultation.

tracheoplasty (trā″ke-ō-plăs″tĭ) ["+ *plassein*, to form]. Plastic operation on the trachea.

tracheopyosis (trā″ke-ō-pī-ō′sĭs) ["+ *pyon*, pus, + *-ōsis*, condition]. Tracheitis with suppuration.

tracheorrhagia (trā″ke-or-ā′jĭ-ă) [Gr. *tracheia*, trachea, + *rhēgnynai*, to burst forth]. Tracheal hemorrhage.

tracheoschisis (trā″ke-ŏs′kĭs-ĭs) ["+ *schisis*, a cleft]. Fissure of the trachea.

tracheoscopy (trā″ke-ŏs′kō-pĭ) ["+ *skopein*, to examine]. Inspection of interior of trachea, by means of reflected light.

tracheostenosis (trā″ke-ō-sten-ō′sĭs) ["+ *stenōsis*, a narrowing]. Contraction or narrowing of lumen of the trachea.

tracheostomy (tra″ke-os′to-mĭ). SEE: *tracheotomy*.

tracheotome (trā″ke-ō-tōm) [Gr. *tracheia*, trachea, + *tomē*, a cutting]. Instrument used in opening of trachea.

tracheotomy (trā″ke-ŏt′ō-mĭ). Operation of cutting into the trachea usually for insertion of tube to overcome tracheal obstruction. SYN: *tracheostomy*.

NP: Temperature of tracheotomy room must not be less than 80° F. and atmosphere should be saturated with steam. The outer tube should not be removed by nurse, but inner one should be removed every hour or oftener if so directed by physician. It is held in place by a tape connected to each side and joined at the back of the patient's neck. This prevents the tube's being coughed out. The movable or inner tube should be washed, rinsed, and dried thoroughly. Usually there are two or more inner tubes available. Thus each can be sterilized and ready for replacement when a soiled one is removed. Before replacing inner tube, the tube remaining in trachea should also be cleaned to remove mucus that collects in and around tube. The patient will require almost continual observation during the acute phase of the condition which necessitated the tracheotomy. The nurse must check the suctioning apparatus and be familiar with its operation. SEE: *diphtheria*.

t. tube. T. to insert into opening made in tracheotomy.

trachitis (tră-kī′tĭs) [Gr. *tracheia*, trachea, + *-itis*, inflammation]. Inflammation of the trachea. SYN: *tracheitis*.

trachoma (tră-kō′mă) [Gr. *trachōma*, roughness]. A chronic contagious form of conjunctivitis, noted by hypertrophy of conjunctiva, formation of follicles with subsequent cicatricial changes. The disease affects 400,000,-000 people, mostly in Asia and Africa; but is also seen in the southwestern part of the United States. Approximately 20,000,000 persons have been blinded by this disease. SYN: *conjunctivitis, granular; ophthalmia, Egyptian*.

ETIOL: A virus which is readily transmitted especially in early stages of disease. Transmission is by direct contact with trachomatous material or indirectly through contaminated articles such as towels, handkerchiefs, etc.

COMPLICATIONS: Pannus, ptosis, corneal ulcers.

SEQUELAE: Blindness; corneal opacities; ectropion; entropion; staphyloma; symblepharon; trichiasis.

TREATMENT: Either tetracyclines or sulfonimides given orally are effective. Surgery may be necessary when lid deformities occur. It is possible that a vaccine for trachoma will be available.

t., brawny. T. with general lymphoid infiltration without granulation of the conjunctiva.

t. deformans. Vulvitis with cicatricial contractions.

t., diffuse. T. with large granulations.

trachychromatic (trä″kĭ-krō-mat′ĭk) [Gr. *trachys,* rough, + *chrōma,* color]. Pert. to a nucleus with very deeply staining chromatin.

trachyphonia (trä″kĭ-fō′nĭ-ä) ["+ *phōnē,* voice]. Roughness of the voice.

tract (träkt) [L. *tractus,* extent]. 1. A course or pathway. 2. A group or bundle of nerve fibers within the spinal cord or brain which constitutes an anatomical and functional unit. SEE: *fasciculus.* 3. A group of organs or parts forming a continuous pathway.

t., afferent. An ascending tract, q.v.

t., alimentary. The canal or passage from the mouth to the anus.

t., ascending. Afferent white fibers in spinal cord.

t., descending. Efferent fibers in the spinal cord.

t., digestive. SEE: *alimentary tract.*

t., genitourinary. The genital and urinary pathways.

t., motor. Descending pathway conveying motor impulses from brain to lower portions of spinal cord.

t., olfactory. A narrow white band extending from olfactory bulb to anterior perforated substance of brain.

t., optic. A band of fibers extending from optic chiasma to lateral geniculate body of thalamus. Some fibers of the tract continue on to midbrain and hypothalamus.

t., pyramidal. Any of columns of motor fibers in the spinal cord which are continuations of pyramids in the medulla.

t., respiratory. The respiratory organs in continuity.

t., rubrospinal. A descending tract of fibers arising from cell bodies located in red nucleus of midbrain. Fibers terminate in gray matter of spinal cord.

t., sensory. Any tract of fibers conducting sensation to the brain.

t., supraopticohypophyseal. A tract consisting of fibers arising from cell bodies located in supraoptic and paraventricular nuclei of hypothalamus and terminating in post. lobe of hypophysis.

t., urinary. The urinary passageway from kidney to the outside. Includes the pelvis of kidney, ureter, bladder, and urethra.

traction (träk′shŭn) [L. *tractio*]. Process of drawing or pulling.

t., axis. Traction in line with the long axis of a course through which a body (fetus) is to be drawn.

t., elastic. Traction exerted by elastic devices such as rubber bands.

t., head. Traction applied to the head as in the treatment of injuries to cervical vertebrae.

t., weight. Traction exerted by means of weights.

tractotomy (träk-tŏt′ō-mĭ). Surgical section of a fiber tract of the central nervous system. Sometimes resorted to for relief of intractable pain.

tractus (träk′tŭs) [L.]. (pl. *tractus*) A tract or path.

tragacanth (trag′ă-kănth) [Gr. *tragakantha,* a goat thorn]. The dried gummy exudation from a plant (Astragalus gummifer) and related species, grown in Asia, used in the form of mucilage as a greaseless lubricant, and as an application for chapped skin.

tragal (trä′găl) [Gr. *tragos,* goat]. Relating to the tragus.

tragi. Pl. of tragus, q.v.

t., lamina. The cartilage of the tragus.

tragicus (trăj′ĭk-ŭs) [L.]. Muscle on the outer surface of the tragus. SEE: *Table of Muscles* in *Appendix.*

tragomaschalia (trag″ō-măs-kāl′ĭ-ä) [Gr. *tragos,* goat, + *maschalē,* the armpit]. Odorous perspiration (bromidrosis) of the axilla.

tragophonia, tragophony (trăg″ō-fō′nĭ-ä, -of′ō-nĭ) ["+ *phōnē,* voice]. A bleating sound heard in auscultation at level of fluid in hydrothorax. SYN: *egophony.*

tragopodia (trăg″ō-pō′dĭ-ä) ["+ *pous, pod-,* foot]. Knock-knee.

tragus (trä′gŭs) [Gr. *tragos,* goat]. [NA]. 1. Cartilaginous tonguelike projection in front of the exterior meatus of the ear. 2. One of the hairs at the entrance of the exterior auditory meatus.

train (trān). To participate in a special program of instruction in order to attain competence in a certain occupation or profession.

trait (trāt). A distinguishing feature; a characteristic or property of an individual.

t., acquired. One that is not inherited; one resulting from effects of environment.

t., inherited. One due to hereditary determiners or genes transmitted through germ cells.

trajector (tră-jĕk'tor) [L. *trajectus*, thrown across]. Device for determining approximate location of a bullet in a wound.

trance (trăns) [L. *transitus*, a passing over]. A sleeplike state, as in deep hypnosis, appearing also in hysteria and in some spiritualistic mediums, with limited sensory and motor contact with the ordinary surroundings, and with subsequent amnesia of what has occurred during the state.

t., death. Trance simulating death.

t., induced. Trance caused by some external event such as hypnosis.

tranquilizer (tran"kwĭ-liz'er) [L. *tranquillus*, calm, + *-ize*, to make, + *-er*, agent]. A drug which acts to reduce mental tension and anxiety without interfering with normal mental activity. This ideal state of tranquilization is difficult to attain. Thus patients taking these medicines may find that their reactions are slowed. The use of tranquilizers has facilitated the treatment of severely disturbed psychiatric patients. Among the drugs in use are chlorpromazine (Thorazine); meprobamate (Miltown, Equanil); promazine (Sparine); reserpine (Serpasil).

Side effects, particularly from chlorpromazine and reserpine, have included jaundice; nausea; rashes; and in some surprising instances severe mental depression. The U. S. Public Health Service has warned of "a significant incidence of severe depression, with suicidal tendencies in some instances," in persons under heavy reserpine dosage.

trans- [L.]. Prefix meaning across, over, beyond, through.

transamidination. The transfer of an amidine group from one amino acid to another.

transaminase. An enzyme that catalyzes transamination.

t., glutamic-oxalacetic. ABBR: GOT or SGOT for serum GOT.

t., glutamic-pyruvic. Enzymes present in many tissues; the highest concentrations are found in the liver and cardiac muscle. Injury of either of those tissues liberates the enzymes into the bloodstream. Thus measurement of their levels in the serum (SGOT or SGPT) provides a valuable test for hepatic cell or myocardial injury. ABBR: GPT or SGPT for serum GPT.

transamination (trăns"ăm-ĭ-nā'shŭn). The transfer of an amino group from one compound to another or the transposition of an amino group within a single compound.

transanimation (trans"ăn-ĭ-mā'shŭn) [L. *trans*, across, + *anima*, breath]. Resuscitation of a stillborn infant.

transaudient (trăns"aw'dĭ-ent) ["+ *audire*, to hear]. Permeable to sound waves.

transcalent (trăns-kā'lĕnt) ["+ *calere*, to be hot]. Permeable by heat rays. SYN: *diathermanous.*

transcapillary (trăns"kăp'ĭl-lă-rĭ) ["+ *capillaris*, relating to hair]. Across the endothelial wall of a capillary.

t. exchange. The passage of substances between blood and tissue (interstitial) fluid.

transducer (trăns-dū'sĕr) [L. *trans*, across, + *ducere*, to lead]. A device which converts one form of energy to another. Used in medical electronics to receive the energy produced by sound or pressure and relay it as an electrical impulse to another transducer which can either convert the energy back into its original form or make a record of it on a recording device. The telephone is an example of this.

transduction (trăns-dŭk'shŭn). A phenomenon causing genetic change in bacteria in which DNA is carried from one bacterium to another by bacteriophage. SEE: *transformation.*

transection (trăn-sĕk'shŭn) [L. *trans*, across, + *sectio*, a cutting]. A cutting made across a long axis; a cross section.

transfer, transference (trans'fer, transfer'ĕns) ["+ *ferre*, to bear]. 1. The mental process whereby a person transfers patterns of feelings and behavior which had previously been experienced with important figures such as parents or siblings to another person. Quite often these feelings are shifted to the psychiatrist. 2. State in which the symptoms of one area are transmitted to a similar area on the other side, as in hysteria.

t. neuroses. Compulsion neuroses and hysteria.

t. situation. The emotional state of a patient existing between him and his physician during psychoanalysis.

Either affection or distrust is transferred by the patient to the physician, although such feelings are not related to reality.

t., thought. Transference of one's thoughts to another. SYN: *telepathy.*

transferase (trăns'fĕr-ās). An enzyme which catalyzes the transfer of atoms or groups of atoms from one chemical compound to another.

transfix (trăns-fĭks') [L. *trans*, across, + *figere*, to fix]. To pierce through or impale with a sharp instrument.

transfixion (trăns-fĭk′shŭn). Maneuver in performing an amputation in which a knife is passed into the soft parts and cutting is from within outward.

transforation (trăns″for-ā′shŭn) [L. *trans,* across, + *forāre,* to pierce]. The perforation of the fetal skull at the base in craniotomy.

transforator (trăns′fo-rā″tor). Instrument for perforating fetal skull.

transformation (trăns″for-mā′shŭn) [L. *trans,* across, + *formatio,* a forming]. 1. Change of shape or form. SYN: *metamorphosis.* 2. Change of one tissue into another. 3. Degeneration. 4. A type of mutation occurring in bacteria. It results from DNA of a bacterial cell penetrating the host cell and becoming incorporated into the genotype of host.

transformer (trăns-form′er) [″+ *formāre,* to form]. A stationary induction apparatus to change electrical energy at one voltage and current to electrical energy at another voltage and current through the medium of magnetic energy, without mechanical motion.

transfusion (trăns-fū′zhŭn) [″+ *fusio,* a pouring]. 1. Injection of the blood of one person into the blood vessels of another. SEE: *blood transfusion, donor.*

2. Injection of saline or other solutions into a vein for a therapeutic purpose.

    t., cadaver blood. T. using blood obtained from a cadaver within a short time after death.

    t., direct. Transfer of blood directly from one person to another.

    t., exchange. Method for reducing the risk of death or injury in infants born with hemolytic disease. The sensitized red blood cells are removed from an artery at the same time compatible Rh negative blood is given intravenously. It is not advisable to give more blood than is removed.

    t., indirect. T. of blood from a donor to a suitable storage container and then to the patient.

    t., replacement. Procedure in treatment of erythroblastosis fetalis of the newborn in which major portion of total blood volume is withdrawn in small amounts at a time and replaced with Rh-negative blood.

    t., single unit. Administration of a single unit of blood.

    In general it is believed that this is not indicated. However, attempts to regulate transfusion resulted in administration of two units, an amount not always necessary. Therefore the committee on Blood of A.M.A. proposed that the appropriate amount of blood always be administered.

    t., subcutaneous. Infusion of saline solution or other fluid beneath the skin.

    t. syndrome, multiple. Development of hemorrhagic tendency caused by multiple transfusions with blood low in platelets and by increased fibrinolytic activity in the blood. TREATMENT: Transfuse with blood which is only a few hours old and give fibrinogen. SEE: *post-transfusion syndrome.*

transgrow. A special medium for culturing Neisseria gonorrhoeae. The specimen may be placed in the medium and then shipped to the laboratory. The bacteria will remain viable even though they were not incubated while being transported.

transiliac (trăns-ĭl′ī-ăk) [″+ *iliacus,* pert. to a haunch bone]. Extending between the two ilia.

transillumination (trăns″ĭl-lū″mĭ-nā′shŭn) [L. *trans,* across, + *illūmināre,* to enlighten]. Inspection of a cavity or organ by passing a light through its walls.

    When pus or lesion or degeneration is present, the reflection of light is diminished or absent.

transition (trănz-ĭ′shŭn) [L. *transitio,* a going across]. Passage from one state or position to another, or from one part to another part. SEE: *transitional.*

transitional (trănz-ĭsh′ŭn-ăl). Marked by or relating to a transition.

translucent (trăns-lū′sĕnt) [L. *trans,* across, + *lucens,* shining]. Not transparent but permitting passage of light.

transmethylation (trans″meth-ĭ-lā′shŭn). Process in the metabolism of amino acids in which a methyl group is transferred from one compound to another; for example, the conversion in the body of homocysteine to methionine. In this case the methyl group is furnished by choline or betaine.

transmigration (trăns″mī-grā′shŭn) [L. *trans,* across, + *migratio,* migration]. Wandering across or through, especially the passage of white blood cells through capillary membranes into the tissues.

    t., external. Transfer of an ovum from an ovary to an opposite tube through the pelvic cavity.

    t., internal. Transfer of an ovum through the uterus to the opposite oviduct.

transmissible (trăns-mĭs′ĭ-bl) [L. *transmissio,* a sending across]. Capable of being carried from one person to another, as an infectious disease.

transmission (trăns-mĭsh′ŭn). Transfer of anything, as a disease or hereditary characteristics.

    t., biological. Condition in which organism transmitting causative agent of disease plays an essential role in the life history of a parasite or germ.

t., duplex. Passage of impulses through a nerve trunk in both directions.

t., mechanical. The passive transfer of causative agents of disease, esp. by arthropods. May be indirect, as when flies pick up organisms from excreta of a man or animals and deposit them on food, or direct, as when they pick up organisms from body of a diseased individual and directly inoculate them into body of another individual by bites or through open sores.

t., neuromyal. The transmission of excitation from a motor neuron to a muscle fiber at a neuromyal (myoneural) junction.

t., placental. The transmission of substances in the mother's blood to the blood of the fetus by way of the placenta.

t., synaptic. The mechanism by which an impulse in one neuron gives rise to an impulse in another neuron.

t., transovarial. The transmission of causative agents of disease to offspring following invasion of ovary and infection of eggs. Occurs in ticks and mites.

transmutation   (trăns″mū-tā′shŭn)   [L. *transmutātio,* a changing across]. A transformation or change, as of one species into another.

transonance (trăns′ō-nǎns) [L. *trans,* across, + . *sonaus,* sounding]. Transmission of sounds through an organ, as heart sounds through the lungs and chest wall.

transparent (trăns-pǎr′ěnt) [″+ *parere,* to appear]. 1. Transmitting light rays so that objects are visible through the substance. 2. Pervious to radiant energy. SEE: *clearing agent.*

transpirable (trăns-pī′rā-bl) [″+ *spirāre,* to exhale]. Permitting excretion through the skin or membranes, as perspiration.

transpiration (trăns″pī-rā′shŭn) [″+ *spiratio,* exhalation]. 1. Act of exhaling water, gas, or vapor through the skin or a membrane. SEE: *perspiration.* 2. Substance exhaled.

t., cutaneous. Giving off sweat from pores of the skin. SYN: *perspiration.*

t., pulmonary. Escape of watery vapor from the blood to the air in the lungs.

transplantation (trăns″plăn-tā′shŭn) [″+ *plantāre,* to plant]. The taking of a portion of living tissue from its normal position in the body or from the body of another person and uniting it with like tissue in another place, to lessen defect or remedy deformity or injury. SEE: *autotransplantation, graft.*

t., autoplastic. Transplantation of tissue from one part to another part of the same body.

t., hetero. The transplantation of an organ or tissue from one individual to another of a different species.

t., heteroplastic. The transplantation of a part from one individual to another individual of the same or a closely related species.

t., heterotopic. One in which transplant is placed in a different location in host than it had in donor.

t., homo-. Transplantation of tissue from one individual of the same species to another.

t., homoplastic. An autoplastic transplant, q.v.

t., homotopic. One in which transplant occupies same location in host that it had in donor.

t. of cornea. Keratoplasty, q.v.

t., tenoplastic. Transplantation of tissue between individuals belonging to different genera.

transport. Movement or transfer of substances including electrolytes, nutrients, and liquids across cell membranes. T. may occur actively, passively, or with the assistance of a carrier.

t., active. Transfer of a substance across a membrane even though its concentration may be higher on the side toward which the movement is taking place.

transportation of the injured. *Carrying in arms:* Patient is picked up in both arms as a child.

One-arm assist: Patient's arm is placed about neck of bearer and bearer's arms are placed about waist, thus assisting patient to walk.

Chair carry, chair stretcher: (Method I): Any ordinary firm chair may be used. Patient is placed seated upon it tilted back. One bearer grasps back of the chair and the other the legs of the chair (either the front or rear, depending on the construction of the chair). Both bearers face in the same direction. Patient's head rests either on chest or back of the head bearer. (Method II): Turn two chairs to the ground; overlap the backs and tie or wire them together, using the legs as handles.

Double loop: A sheet is rolled on its long axis, tied and placed over the shoulder of both bearers. Patient sits on the long loop and rests his back against a short upper loop with the bearers supporting him. The weight is thus distributed on shoulders of both bearers.

Fireman's drag: Patient's wrists are crossed and tied with tie, belt, etc. Bearer kneels astride patient, places his head under patient's wrists, and walks on all fours dragging patient beneath him.

Fireman's lift: Bearer grasps patient's left wrist with right arm; places patient's head under left armpit drawing patient's body over his left shoulder. Left arm should encircle both thighs, then lift patient. Patient's wrist is transferred to bearer's left hand, thus leaving one hand free to remove obstacles or to open doors, etc.

Four-handed basket seat: Each of two bearers grasps his own wrist and then grasps partner's free wrist. Patient sits upon this support.

Pack-strap carry: Patient lies on bearer's back. Patient's right arm is brought over bearer's right shoulder and held by his left hand. Left arm is brought over left shoulder and held by his right hand. Patient is thus carried on the back with arms resembling pack straps.

Pickaback carry: This is the pack strap carry only bearer supports patient's knees in flexed position. This leaves patient practically in a sitting position astride bearer's back with his arms around the bearer's neck or trunk.

Saddle-back carry: Bearer places arm under patient's armpit around his back and grasps it around armpit. Patient's body is across bearer's back. Rescuer's free arm grasps both thighs, allowing patient to rest across the bearer's back.

Shirt-tail Carry: Bearer grasps patient's coat, blouse, or shirt tail, twists it to make a handle and brings it over his shoulder thus carrying patient back to back.

Six- or eight-man carry: This is done as the three-man carry except three or four bearers are on each side of patient, thus dividing weight more uniformly.

Three-handed basket seat: Bearer grasps his own wrist, partner grasps the other wrist and leaves one arm free for supporting patient.

Three- or four-man carry: The litter-type carry used by emergency squads. Three men kneel on one side of patient, place their hands under him and lift him up. The head bearer supports head and shoulders, center bearer lifts waist and hips, and third bearer lifts both lower extremities. If a fourth man is available, he should help steady patient while he is being lifted.

Triangular or greater arm sling, or branchiocervical sling: Place triangle on chest with one end over the sound shoulder, the point at elbow of affected side. Fold the base. Flex injured arm outside of triangle above the horizontal. Carry other end upward outside of arm back over shoulder of affected side. Tie to side of neck with square knot. Bring point anteriorly around back of elbow and fasten to ascending base or tie forming a cup at elbow. (In this bandage the weight is taken from entire length of forearm.)

Two-handed seat: Bearers kneel on either side of patient. Each passes one arm around back (under armpits) and other arm under knees and lifts him carefully. Patient is in a sitting position.

Wheel chair, improvised: Fastening casters to ordinary chair: Tie on a broom handle or similar stick for footrest by placing chair legs on parallel boards and fastening roller skates, wheels, etc.

Fastening as rocker to roller skates: Remove legs from an old chair and fasten to frame of a baby carriage, or play wagon.

t. by vehicle. Ambulances are desirable if available and usually contain appropriate stretchers. When not obtainable, stretchers may be made with poles, chairs or ladders. When entering or leaving an airplane one must remember to tie the patient to the stretcher. SEE: *stretcher.*

t. by automobile. This is difficult except in a station wagon or similar vehicle. One bearer should be in the car and one or two outside to assist patient. A small chair stretcher can sometimes be used with advantage. A door or ladder slung across the open windows or from front to rear seats may be used.

transposition (trăns″pō-zĭ′shŭn) [L. *trans,* across, + *positio,* a placing]. 1. A transfer of position from one spot to another. SEE: *metathesis.* 2. Displacement of an organ, esp. a viscus, to the opposite side. 3. Transplantation of a flap of tissue without severing it entirely from its original position until it has united in the new position.

transsegmental (trăns″sĕg-mĕn′tăl) ["+ *segmentum,* a cutting]. Extending across or beyond a segment, as of a limb.

transseptal (trăns-sĕp′tăl) ["+ *saeptum,* partition]. Across a septum.

transsexual (trăns-sĕks′shū-ăl) [L. *trans,* across, + *sexus,* sex]. 1. An individual who has an overwhelming desire to be the opposite sex. 2. An individual who has had his external sex changed by surgery.

t., female-to-male. A person who has all the anatomical and chromosomal features of a female but feels she is a male and attempts to live in this cross-gender role.

Etiological factors of this condition unknown.

t., male-to-female. A person who has all the anatomical and chromosomal features of a male but feels he is a female and attempts to live in this cross-gender role. Etiological factors unknown.

t. surgery. Surgical therapy for alteration of the anatomical sex of an individual whose psychological gender is not consistent with the anatomical sexual characteristics.

transtemporal (trăns-tĕm'pō-răl) ["+ temporalis, pert. to a temple]. Crossing the temporal or the cerebrum.

transthalamic (trăns''thăl-ăm'ĭk) ["+ Gr. thalamos, chamber]. Passing across the optic thalamus.

transthermia (trăns-thĕr'mĭ-ă) [L. trans, across, + Gr. thermē, heat]. Production of heat in the deep tissues by electric currents. SYN: diathermy, thermopenetration.

transthoracic (trăns''thō-răs'ĭk) ["+ Gr. thōrax, chest]. Across the thorax.

transthoracotomy (trăns''thō-ră-kŏt'ō-mĭ) [L. trans, across, + Gr. thōrax, chest, + tomē, a cutting]. The operation of incising across the thorax.

transubstantiation (trăn''sŭb-stăn''shĭ-ă'shŭn) ["+ substantia, substance]. The process of replacing one tissue by another.

transudate (trăns'ū-dāt) ["+ sudare, to sweat]. The fluid which passes through the pores of a membrane, esp. that which passes through capillary walls. Compared to an exudate, q.v., a transudate has fewer cellular elements and would be of a lower specific gravity.

transudation (trăns-ū-dā'shŭn). Oozing of a fluid through pores or interstices, as of a membrane.

transurethral (trăns''ū-rē'thrăl) [L. trans, across, + Gr. ourēthra, urethra]. Pert. to an operation performed through the urethra.

transvaginal (trăns-văj'ĭn-ăl) ["+ vagina, sheath]. Through the vagina or across its wall as in a surgical procedure.

transversalis (trans''vĕr-sā'lĭs) ["+ vertere, to turn]. Transverse to or at right angles to the long axis of the body.

t. fascia. A thin membrane forming the peritoneal surface of the transversus muscle and its aponeurosis.

transverse (trăns-vĕrs') [L. transversus]. Lying across; crosswise.

t. fora'men. Canal in each transverse process of a cervical vertebra for the arteries and veins.

transversectomy (trăns''vĕr-sĕk'tō-mĭ) ["+ Gr. ektomē, excision]. Excision of a transverse vertebral process.

transversospinalis (trăns-vĕr''sō-spī-nā'lĭs) [L. transversus, turned across, + spina, thorn]. Semispinalis capitus, s. cervicis. SEE: Table of Muscles in Appendix.

transversus (trăns-vĕr'sŭs) [L.]. 1. Any of several small muscles. SEE: Table of Muscles in Appendix. 2. Lying across the long axis of a part or organ.

transvestism, transvestitism (trăns-vĕst'ĭzm, -ĭ-tĭzm) [L. trans, across, + vestitus, clothed, + Gr. -ismos, condition]. The abnormal desire to dress in the clothes of and be accepted as a member of the opposite sex. Sexual pleasure is derived from this activity. SYN: eonism, q.v.

trapezium (tră-pē'zĭ-ŭm) [Gr. trapezion, a little table]. The first bone in the distal row of carpal bones. It lies between navicular and first metacarpal bones. SYN: greater multangular bone; os trapezium.

trapezius (tră-pē'zĭ-ŭs). A flat, triangular muscle covering posterior surface of neck and shoulder. SEE: Table of Muscles in Appendix.

trapezoid (trăp'ē-zoyd) [Gr. trapezoeidēs, table-shaped]. A plane four-sided figure having two sides parallel.

t. body. A bundle of transverse fibers in the ventral portion of tegmentum of pons. SYN: corpus trapezoideum.

t. bone. The second bone in the distal row of carpal bones. It lies between the greater multangular and capitate. SYN: lesser multangular bone.

t. ligament. The lateral portion of the coraco-clavicular ligament.

trauma (traw'mă) [Gr. trauma, wound]. (pl. traumata or traumas) An injury or a wound.

t., psychic. A painful, emotional experience, which may cause a neurosis.

traumatic (traw-măt'ĭk) [Gr. traumatikos]. Caused by or relating to an injury.

t. fever. One following an injury.

t. psychosis. One resulting from physical injuries or emotional shock.

traumatism (traw'mă-tĭzm) [Gr. traumatismos]. 1. Morbid condition of system due to an injury or wound. 2. Incorrectly, a trauma.

traumatology (traw-mă-tŏl'ō-jĭ) [Gr. trauma, wound, + togos, science]. The branch of surgery dealing with wounds and their care.

traumatopnea (traw''mă-tŏp-nē'ă) ["+ pnoia, breath]. Passage of air in and out of a wound in the chest wall.

treatment (trēt'ment) [ME. treten, to handle]. 1. Medical, surgical or psychiatric management of a patient. 2. Any specific procedure used for the cure or the amelioration of a disease or pathological condition. SEE: *therapy.*

t., active. Treatment directed specifically toward cure of a disease.

t., after. That employed during convalescence following an operation or an illness.

t., causal. Treatment directed toward removal of the cause of the disease.

t., conservative. 1. The withholding of administration of medicine or utilization of operative procedures until such procedures are clearly indicated. 2. In surgical cases, the preservation of the organ or part if at all possible with the least possible mutilation.

t., dietetic. Treatment based on regulation of diet.

t., electric shock. Electroshock therapy, shock therapy, q.v.

t., empiric. One based on observation and experience rather than having a scientific basis.

t., expectant. Relief of symptoms as they arise, i.e., not directed at the specific cause.

t., hypoglycemic shock. Insulin shock therapy, shock therapy, q.v.

t., palliative. One designed for the relief of symptoms of the disease rather than curing the disease.

t. paralysis. A serious and sometimes fatal complication following the administration of antirabic vaccine.

t., preventive, prophylactic. T. directed to prevention of disease.

t., rational. One based on scientific principles.

t., shock. Shock therapy, q.v.

t., specific. T. directed to the cause of a disease.

t., starvation. Treatment employed in which food is withheld as in cases of bacillary dysentery, following hemorrhage, etc. 2. The treatment of diabetes in which there are days of fasting followed by a restricted and carefully controlled diet.

t., supportive. Special measures employed to supplement specific therapy.

t., surgical. T. by means of operation.

t., symptomatic. Treatment directed toward constitutional symptoms such as pyrexia, shock, and pain.

tree. In anatomy, a treelike structure.

t., bronchial. The right or left bronchus with its branches and their terminal arborizations.

Trematoda (trem″ă-tō′dă) [Gr. *trēmatōdēs,* pierced]. A class of flatworms commonly called flukes belonging to the phylum Platyhelminthes. It includes two orders:

Monogenea, which are external or semi-external parasites having direct development with no asexual multiplication, and Digenea, internal parasites with asexual generation in their life cycle. The Digenea usually require two or more hosts, the hosts alternating. SEE: *fluke.*

trematode (trĕm′ă-tōd). A fluke, a parasitic flatworm belonging to the class Trematoda. SEE: *cercaria; fluke.*

trematodiasis (trĕm″ă-tō-dī′ă-sīs). Infestation with a trematode.

tremble (trem′bl) [O. Fr. *trembler*]. 1. An involuntary quivering or shaking. 2. To shiver, quiver, or shake.

trembles (trĕm′blz). A condition resulting from ingestion of plants such as snakeroot (Eupatorium urticaefolium) or jimmey weed (Aploppus heterophyllus). Common in domestic animals and may occur in humans as a result of ingesting the plants or more commonly from drinking milk or eating the meat of poisoned animals. Symptoms are weakness; anorexia; nausea and vomiting; prostration, and possibly death. SYN: *milk sickness.*

tremetol (trĕm′ĕ-tōl). A poisonous substance occurring in snakeroot, rayless goldenrod, and other plants which may cause trembles in animal or man. SEE: *trembles.*

tremogram (trĕm′ō-grăm) [L. *tremere,* to shake, + Gr. *gramma,* a mark]. Graphic representation made by a tremograph.

tremograph (trĕm′ō-grăf) [″ + Gr. *graphein,* to write]. Device for recording tremors.

tremolabile (trē″mō-lā′bl) [″ + *labilis,* unsteady]. Easily destroyed or inactivated by shaking; said of a ferment.

tremophobia (trē″mō-fō′bĭ-ă) [″ + Gr. *phobos,* fear]. Abnormal fear of trembling.

tremor (trĕm′or, trē′mor) [L. *tremor,* a shaking]. 1. A quivering, esp. continuous quivering of a convulsive nature. 2. An involuntary movement of a part or parts of the body resulting from alternate contractions of opposing muscles.

Tremors may be classified as involuntary; static; dynamic; kinetic; hereditary; and hysteric. Pathologic tremors are independent of the will. The trembling may be fine or coarse, rapid or slow, may appear on movement (intention tremor) or improve when the part is employed. Often due to organic disease; trembling may express an emotion (e.g., fear).

TREATMENT: Varies with underlying cause. SEE: *subsultus.*

t., alcoholic. The visible t. exhibited by alcoholics.

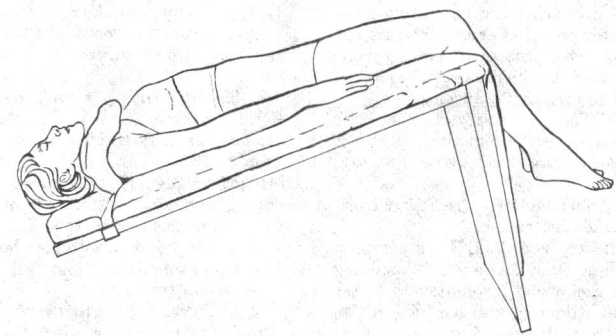

TRENDELENBURG POSITION
Shoulder braces on table prevent patient from slipping.

t., coarse. One in which oscillations are relatively slow.

t., continuous. One that resembles tremors of paralysis agitans.

t., fibrillary. One caused by consecutive contractions of separate muscular fibrillae, rather than of a muscle or muscles.

t., fine. A rapid tremor.

t., flapping. Coarse tremor of a muscle group. The supported part momentarily loses its support and there is an attempt to regain the support. When seen in the outstretched arm and hand the part flaps like a wing. Seen in hepatic coma and other diseases which cause encephalopathy. SYN: *asterixis.*

t., forced. T. continuing after voluntary motion has ceased.

t., hysterical. A fine tremor occurring in hysteria. May be limited to one extremity or generalized.

t., intention. T. when voluntary motion is attempted.

t., intermittent. One common to paralyzed muscles in hemiplegia when attempting voluntary movement.

t., muscular. Slight oscillating muscular contractions in rhythmical order.

t., physiologic. A transient tremor occurring in normal individuals, resulting from excessive physical exertion; excitement; hunger; fatigue; or other causes.

t., rest. One present when the involved part is at rest but absent or diminished when active movements are attempted.

t., senile. A tremor occurring in old age.

t., static. One present when muscles involved are at rest. SYN: *rest tremor.*

t., volitional. Trembling of limbs or of body when making a voluntary effort. Seen in multiple sclerosis and other nervous diseases. SEE: *intention tremor.*

tremulous (trĕm'ū-lŭs) [L. *tremere,* to shake]. Trembling or shaking.

trench foot. A condition resembling frostbite affecting feet of soldiers who are obliged to stand in cold water for long periods of time.

trench mouth. Painful pseudomembranous ulceration of the mucous membranes of the mouth and pharynx. SYN: *Vincent's angina,* q.v. SEE: *mouth, trench.*

trend [ME. *trenden,* to revolve]. The inclination to proceed in a certain direction or at a certain rate. Used to describe the prognosis or course of a symptom or disease.

Trendelenburg position (trĕn-dĕl'ĕn-bŭrg). [Friedrich Trendelenburg, Ger. surgeon, 1844-1925] The bed or table is raised from the foot, greatly elevating the knees, the legs projecting on an extended leg rest.

In this position the abdominal organs are pushed up toward the chest by gravity. The legs are elevated at an angle of 45°. The head is lower than the hips and legs. The foot of the bed may be elevated by resting on blocks or pins.

This position is sometimes used in abdominal surgery, in case of shock, or low blood pressure.

trepan (trē-păn') [Gr. *trypanon,* a borer]. 1. To perforate the skull with a trepan to relieve brain from pressure. 2. An instrument resembling a carpenter's bit for incision of the skull. SYN: *trephine.*

trephination (trĕf'ĭn-ā'shŭn) [Fr. *tréphine,* a bore]. Process of cutting out a piece of bone with the trephine.

trephine (trĕ-fīn'). 1. To perforate with a trephine. 2. A cylindrical saw for cutting circular piece of bone out of skull. SYN: *trepan.*

trephin'ing. The process of cutting bone with a trephine. 2. The removal of a piece of cornea for the relief of glaucoma.

trephone (trĕf'ōn) [Gr. *trephein*, to nourish]. Hypothetical growth-promoting substance in the blood serum, used by cells as food material.

trepidant (trĕp'ĭ-dănt) [L. *trepidans*, trembling]. Marked by tremor.

trepidation (trĕp'ĭ-dā'shŭn) [L. *trepidatio*, a trembling]. 1. Fear, anxiety. 2. Trembling movement, esp. when involuntary.

Treponema (trĕp''ō-nē'mă) [Gr. *trepein*, to turn, + *nēma*, thread]. A genus of spirochetes, parasitic in man, with undulating or rigid bodies. They belong to the family Treponemataceae.

    T. carateum. The causative agent of pinta, an infectious disease of the skin.

    T. pallidum. Causative organism of syphilis. SYN: *Spirochaeta pallida.*

    T. pertenue. Causative organisms of yaws (frambesia).

Treponemataceae (trĕp''ō-nē''mă-tā'sĭ-ē). A family of spiral organisms belonging to the order Spirochaetales. Includes the genera Borrelia; Leptospira; and Treponema.

treponemiasis (trĕp''ō-nē-mī'ă-sĭs) [Gr. *trepein*, to turn, + *nēma*, thread, + *iasis*, condition]. Infestation with Treponema.

treponemicidal (trĕp''ō-nē''mĭ-sī'dăl) ["+ "+ L. *cidus*, from *caedere*, to kill]. Destructive to Treponema.

trepopnea (trĕp-ŏp'nē-ă) ["+ *pnoia*, breath]. Condition of being able to breathe with less difficulty when in a certain position.

treppe (trĕp'eh) [Ger. *treppe*, staircase]. Increase in height of contractions when the heart or a muscle is stimulated rapidly at regular intervals. SYN: *staircase phenomenon,* q.v.

tresis (trē'sĭs) [Gr. *trēsis*, perforation]. Perforation.

tri- [Gr. *treis*, three]. Combining form meaning three.

triad (trī'ăd) [Gr. *trias*, group of three]. 1. Any three things having something in common. 2. A trivalent element. 3. Trivalent.

    t., Hutchinson's. Notched teeth, interstitial keratitis, and eighth-nerve deafness due to meningeal involvement; a syndrome characteristic of prenatal syphilis.

triage (trē-ahzh') [Fr. *trier*, sort out]. The classification of sick, wounded or injured persons in order to ensure the efficient use of medical and nursing manpower, equipment, and facilities. Classification is concerned

with the casualties who would live without therapy of any kind, those who would die no matter what treatment is provided, and those who would survive if given adequate care.

triakaidekaphobia (trī''ă-kī''dĕk-ă-fō'bĭ-ă) [Gr. *treis*, three, + *kai*, and, + *deka*, ten, + *phobos*, fear]. Superstition regarding the number 13.

triangle (trī'ăng-l) [L. *tres*, three, + *angulus*, angle; *triangulum*]. A figure or area formed by three angles and three sides.

    t., anal. Triangle with base between the two ischial tuberosities and apex at coccyx. SYN: *rectal triangle.*

    t., anterior, of the neck. The space bounded by the middle line of the neck, the anterior border of the sternocleidomastoid, and a line running along the lower border of the mandible and continued to the mastoid process of the occipital bone.

    t., carotid, inferior. The space bounded by the middle line of the neck, the sternomastoid and the anterior belly of the omohyoid muscle.

    t., carotid, superior. The space bounded by the anterior belly of the omohyoid muscle, the posterior belly of the digastricus and the sternomastoid.

    t., cephalic. A t. on the anteroposterior plane of the skull formed by lines joining the occiput and forehead and chin, and one uniting the two latter.

    t., facial. A t. bounded by lines uniting the basion and the alveolar and nasal points and one uniting the two latter.

    t., femoral. T. on the inner part of the thigh, bounded by the sartorius and adductor longus muscle, and above by inguinal ligament.

    t., frontal. A t. bounded by the maximum frontal diameter and lines joining its extremities and the glabella.

    t., Hesselbach's. The interval in the groin bounded by Pouparts's ligament, edge of rectus muscle, and deep epigastric artery.

    t., inferior occipital. Area having the bimastoid diameter for its base and the inion for its apex.

    t., inguinal. T., femoral, q.v.

    t., Lesser's. Space bounded below by anterior and posterior bellies of the digastri muscle and above by the hypogastric nerve

    t., lumbocostoabdominal. Th space bounded in front by the obliquu abdominis externus, above by the lowe border of the serratus posticus inferior an the point of the 12th rib, behind by the oute edge of the erector spinae, and below by th obliquus abdominis internus.

t., muscular. T., carotid, inferior, q.v.

t., mylohyoid. The triangular space formed by the mylohyoid muscle and the two bellies of the digastric muscle.

t., occipital, of the neck. The space bounded by the sternocleidomastoid, the trapezius, and the omohyoid.

t., omoclavicular. T., subclavian, q.v.

t., omohyoid. T., carotid, superior, q.v.

t. of Petit. The space above the hipbone, between the exterior oblique muscle, the latissimus dorsi, and interior oblique muscle.

t., posterior cervical; t., posterior, of the neck. The space bounded by the upper border of the clavicle, the posterior border of the sternocleidomastoid muscle,

and the anterior border of the trapezius muscle.

t., pubourethral. A triangular space in the perineum, bounded externally by the ischiocavernous muscle, internally by the bulbocavernous muscle, and posteriorly by the transversus perinei muscle.

t., Scarpa's. T., femoral, q.v.

t., subclavian. A space bounded by the posterior belly of the omohyoid, the upper border of the clavicle, and the posterior margin of the sternocleidomastoid.

t., submaxillary. The space between the lower border of the inferior maxilla, the parotid gland, and the mastoid process of the temporal bone above, the posterior belly of the digastric and the stylohyoid below, and

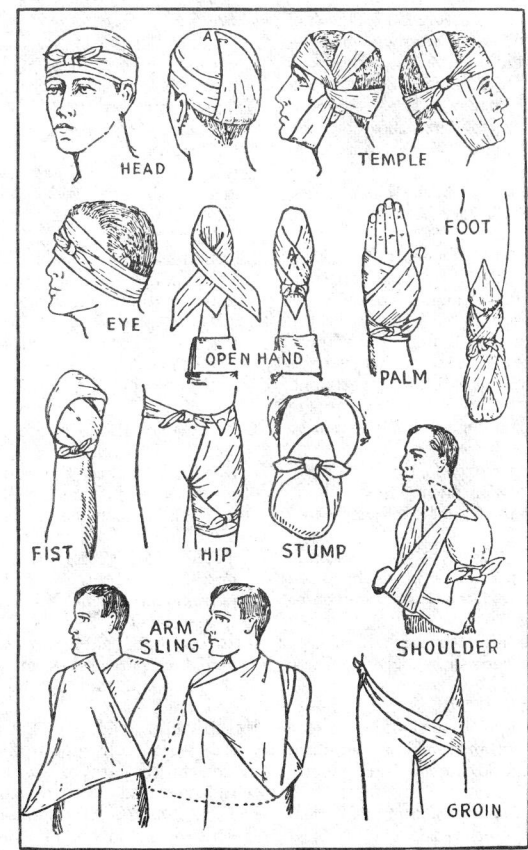

TRIANGULAR BANDAGES

the middle line of the neck in front.

t., supraclavicular. T., subclavian.

t., suprameatal. Triangle slightly above and behind exterior auditory meatus. It is bounded above by root of zygoma and anteriorly by posterior wall of exterior auditory meatus.

t., urogenital. Triangle with base formed by line between the two ischial tuberosities and its apex just below symphysis pubis.

t., vesical. The trigone, q.v.

triang'ular. Having three sides; shaped like a triangle.

t. ligament. One of two ligaments, right and left, connecting posterior portions of right and left lobes of liver with corresponding portions of diaphragm.

t. nucleus (of Schwalbe). The chief or dorsal nucleus of the vestibular division of the eighth cranial nerve. Located in pons occupying most of area acoustica of rhomboid fossa. SYN: *medial nucleus.*

triangular bandage. One folded diagonally. When folded, the several thicknesses afford support.

triangularis (trī-ăng″gū-lā′rĭs) [L.]. A muscle of the chin. SEE: *Table of Muscles* in *Appendix.*

Triatoma (trī-ăt′ō-mă). A genus of bloodsucking bugs belonging to the order Hemiptera, family Reduviidae. Commonly called conenosed bugs or assassin bugs. It includes the species T. braziliensis; T. dimidiata; T. infestans; T. protracta; T. recurva; T. rubida and others. They are house-infesting pests and some species especially T. infestans serve to transmit Trypanosoma cruzi, causative agent of Chagas' disease.

tribade (trĭb′ăd) [Gr. *tribein,* to rub]. A woman, usually one with an enlarged clitoris, who plays the part of a male in homosexual practices.

tribadism (trĭb′ăd-ĭzm) ["+ *-ismos,* condition]. A form of perversion in which women attempt to imitate heterosexual intercourse with each other.

tribasilar (trī-băs′ĭl-ăr) [Gr. *treis,* three, + L. *basilaris,* from *basis,* base]. Having three bases.

t. synostosis. Condition resulting from premature fusion of three skull bones—the occipital, sphenoid, and temporal. Results in arrested cerebral development and mental deficiency.

tribe (trīb) [L. *tribus,* division of the Roman people]. In biology, an occasional subdivision of a family; often equal to or below subfamily.

triboluminescence (trī′bō-lū″mĭ-něs′ĕns) [Gr. *tribein,* to rub, + L. *lūmen,* light, + O.Fr. *escence,* continuing]. Luminescence or sparks produced by friction or mechanical force applied to certain chemicals. Has been observed when wintergreen mints are broken by the teeth in the dark.

tribromide (trī-brō′mĭd) [Gr. *treis,* three, + *brōmos,* stench]. A compound having three atoms of bromine in the molecule.

tribromoethanol (trī-brō″mō-eth′ăn-ŏl). A white crystalline substance which is used in anesthesia.

tricephalus (trī-sĕf′ă-lŭs) [Gr. *treis,* three, + *kephalē,* head]. A fetal monster having three heads.

triceps (trī′sĕps) ["+ L. *caput,* head]. A muscle arising by three heads with a single insertion. SEE: *Table of Muscles* in *Appendix.*

t. reflex. Sharp extension of forearm resulting from tapping of triceps tendon while arm is held loosely in bent position.

Tricercomonas (trī″sĕr-cŏm-ō′năs). SEE *Enteromonas hominis.*

trichangiectasia, trichangiectasis (trik″ăn-jī-ĕk-tā′zī-ă, -ĕk′tă-sĭs) [Gr. *thrix, trich-,* hair, + *angeion,* vessel, + *ektasis,* dilatation]. Dilatation of capillaries. SYN *telangiectasia.*

trichatrophia (trĭk″ă-trō′fĭ-ă) [Gr. *thrix* hair, + *atrophia,* atrophy]. Brittleness of hair resulting from atrophy of root of hair.

trichauxe, trichauxis (trĭk-awk′sē, -sĭs) ["+ *auxē,* increase]. Excessive growth of hair. SYN: *hypertrichosis.*

trichi-, tricho- [Gr.]. Combining forms meaning hair.

trichiasis (trĭk-ī′ăs-ĭs) [Gr. *trichiasis,* hair condition]. Inversion of eyelashes so that they rub against the cornea, causing a continual irritation of the eyeball.

SYM: Photophobia, lacrimation, and feeling of foreign body in eye.

TREATMENT: Epilation, electrolysis and operation, such as correcting the underlying entropion with which this condition is usually associated.

Trichina (trĭk-ī′nă) [Gr. *trichinos,* of hair]. A nematoid, parasitic worm usually found in the intestinal tract of certain lower animals and man.

Trichinella (trĭk″ī-něl′lă). A genus of nematode worms belonging to the suborder Trichurata. They are parasitic in humans, hogs, rats, and many other mammals.

T. spiralis. The species of Trichinella which commonly infests man causing trichinosis. Infection occurs when raw or improperly cooked meat, particularly pork containing cysts is eaten. Larvae encyst in the duodenum and invade mucosa of small intestine becoming adults in five to seven days. After fertilization, each female deposits 1000 to 2000 living larvae which enter blood or lymph vessels and are circulated to various parts of the body where they encyst in striated muscle. SEE: *trichinosis.*

trichinelliasis (trĭk″ĭ-nĕl-lī′ă-sĭs). SEE: *trichinosis.*

trichinellosis (trĭk″ĭ-nĕl-lō′sĭs) [Gr. *trichinos,* of hair, + *-ōsis,* condition]. Disease caused by Trichinella spiralis. SYN: *trichinosis,* q.v.

trichinization (trĭk″ĭn-ĭ-zā′shŭn). Infestation with trichinae.

trichinophobia (trĭk″ĭn-ō-fō′bĭ-ă) [Gr. *trichinos,* of hair, + *phobos,* fear]. Abnormal fear of developing trichinosis.

trichinosis (trĭk″ĭn-ō′sĭs) [″ + *-ōsis,* condition]. Disease caused by the ingestion of Trichina spiralis into the system through eating raw or insufficiently cooked pork.

SYM: Sometimes lacking. When large numbers have been ingested, gastrointestinal symptoms develop in a few days. These are pain, nausea, vomiting and serous diarrhea.

In from one to two weeks muscular symptoms develop, muscles become swollen, firm, extremely painful; movement is inhibited, and dyspnea results from involvement of respiratory muscles. Edema, esp. of face, is a prominent symptom. Profuse sweating sometimes observed and high fever commonly present. Blood shows an eosinophilia.

PROG: Depends on number of worms ingested. Majority recover.

TREATMENT: For acute stage thiabendazole may be helpful. In later stages after worms have involved muscles, muscle pains should be relieved by analgesics. Treatment is in general symptomatic and supportive to enable patient to survive the acute toxemia following invasion of muscles. After encystment the only symptom is vague muscular pains which may persist for weeks.

trichinous (trĭk′ĭn-ŭs) [Gr. *trichinos,* of hair]. Infested with trichinae.

trichitis (trĭk-ī′tĭs) [Gr. *thrix,* hair, + *-itis,* inflammation]. Inflammation of hair bulbs.

trichloroethylene (trī″klor-ō-ĕth′ĭl-ēn) A colorless, clear, volatile liquid with a specific gravity of 1.47 at 59° F. (15° C.). Used as an analgesic and anesthetic agent. It is a halogenated hydrocarbon having the chemical formula $CCl_2{:}CHCl$. Marketed under the trade names Trilene and Trimar. It should not be used with epinephrine.

tricho- [Gr. *thrix, trichos,* hair]. A prefix denoting a relationship to hair.

trichobacteria (trĭk″ō-băk-tē′rĭ-ă) [Gr. *trichos,* hair, + *baktērion,* rod]. 1. Filamentous bacteria. 2. Bacteria possessing flagella.

trichobezoar (trĭk″ō-bē′zō-ar) [″+ Persian *pad-zahr,* antidote]. A hair ball or concretion in the intestine or stomach.

trichocardia (trĭk-ō-kar′dĭ-ă) [″+ *kardia,* heart]. Pericardial inflammation with elevations resembling hair. SYN: *cor hirsutum; hairy heart; shaggy pericardium.*

trichoclasia, trichoclasis (trĭk″ō-klā′zĭ-ă, -ok′lăs-ĭs) [″+ *klasis,* a breaking]. Brittleness of the hair. SYN: *trichorrhexis.*

trichocryptosis (trĭk″ō-krĭp-tō′sĭs) [″+ *kryptos,* concealed]. Any disease of the hair follicles.

trichoepithelioma (trĭk″ō-ĕp″ĭ-thē-lĭ-ō′mă) [Gr. *trichos,* hair, + *epi,* upon, + *thēlē,* nipple, + *-ōma,* tumor]. A benign skin tumor originating in the hair follicles.

trichoesthesia (trĭk″ō-ĕs-thē′zĭ-ă) [″+ *aisthēsis,* sensation]. 1. Sensation felt when a hair is touched. 2. A paresthesia causing a sensation of the presence of a hair on a mucous membrane or on the skin.

trichoesthesiometer (trĭk″ō-ĕs-thē″zĭ-ŏm′ĕ-ter) [″ + ″+ *metron,* a measure]. Device for testing sensibility of the scalp by means of the hair.

trichogen (trĭk′ō-jĕn) [″+ *gennan,* to produce]. An agent stimulating growth of hair.

trichogenous (trĭk-ŏj′ĕn-ŭs). Promoting hair growth.

trichoglossia (trĭk″ō-glŏs′sĭ-ă) [Gr. *trichos,* hair, + *glōssa,* tongue]. Hairy condition of the tongue.

trichoid (trĭk′oyd) [″+ *eidos,* resemblance]. Hairlike.

trichokryptomania (trĭk″ō-krĭp″tō-mā′nĭ-ă) [″+ *kryptos,* hidden, + *mania,* madness]. Abnormal desire to break off the hair or beard with the fingernail. SYN: *trichorrhexomania.*

trichology (trĭk-ŏl′ō-jĭ) [″+ *logos,* a study]. Study of the hair and its care and treatment.

trichoma (trĭk-ō′mă) [Gr. *trichōma,* hairiness]. 1. Inversion of one or more eyelashes. SYN: *entropion.* 2. Matted, verminous, encrusted state of the hair. SYN: *plica polonica.*

trichomatosis (trĭk″ō-mă-tō′sĭs) [″+ *-ōsis,* condition]. Entangled, matted hair due to fungus disease of scalp and want of cleanliness. SYN: *plica polonica.*

trichomatous (tri-kŏm′ă-tŭs). Of the nature of, or affected with trichoma.

Trichomonas (trĭk-ŏm'ō-năs) [Gr. *trichos,* hair, + *monas,* unit]. Genus of flagellate parasitic protozoa.

 T. hom'inis. Species in human intestines sometimes causing diarrhea and bacillary dysentery.

 T. vaginalis. Vaginitis caused by a species of T. in secretions of the vagina. A fairly common condition in women, esp. during pregnancy or following vaginal surgery. It is sometimes found in the male urethra and is communicated through intercourse.

 SYM: Persistent burning and itching of the vulvar tissue, associated with a profuse white frothy discharge. Occasionally T. vaginalis is present but asymptomatic.

 TREATMENT: Metromidazole taken orally by the female and her sex partner.

trichomoniasis (trĭk"ō-mō-nī'ăs-ĭs) ["+ "+ *-iasis,* infection]. Infestation with a parasite of genus Trichomonas.

trichomycosis (trĭk"ō-mī-kō'sĭs) ["+ *mykēs,* fungus, + *-ōsis,* condition]. Any disease of the hair due to a fungus.

 t. axillaris. An affection of the axillary region and sometimes pubic hairs caused by Nocardia tenuis. SYM: *trichomycosis nodosa,* q.v.

 t. nodosa. Disease marked by nodule formations on the hair shafts. SYM: *piedra.*

trichonosis, trichonosus (trĭk-ō-nō'sĭs, -ŏn'ō-sŭs) [Gr. *trichos,* hair, + *nosos,* disease]. Any diseased condition of the hair.

trichopathophobia (trĭk"ō-păth"ō-fō'bĭ-ă) ["+ *pathos,* disease, + *phobos,* fear]. Morbid fear of hair on the face experienced by women, or any abnormal anxiety regarding hair.

trichopathy (trĭk-ŏp'ă-th-ĭ) ["+ *pathos,* disease]. Any disease of the hair.

trichophagia, trichophagy (trĭk-ō-fā'jĭ-ă, -of'ă-jĭ) ["+ *phagein,* to eat]. The habit of swallowing hair.

trichophobia (trĭk"ō-fō'bĭ-ă) [Gr. *trichos,* hair, + *phobos,* fear]. Abnormal dread of hair or of touching it.

trichophytic (trĭk"ō-fĭt'ĭk) ["+ *phyton,* plant]. 1. Relating to Trichophyton. 2. Promoting hair growth.

trichophytid (trĭ-kŏf'ĭ-tĭd). A skin disorder considered to be an allergic reaction to fungi of the genus Trichophyton.

trichophytin (trĭ-kŏf'ĭ-tĭn). An extract prepared from cultures of the fungi of the genus Trichophyton. Used as an antigen for skin tests and for the treatment of certain trichophytid infections.

trichophytobezoar (trĭk-ō-fī"tō-bē'zŏr) [Gr. *trichos,* hair, + *phyton,* plant, + Persian *pād-zahr,* antidote]. A hair ball found in stomach or intestine composed of hair, vegetable fibers, and miscellaneous debris.

Trichophyton (trĭk-ŏf'ĭt-ŏn). A genus of parasitic fungi which lives in or on the skin or its appendages (hair and nails) and is the cause of various dermatomycoses and ringworm infections. Species which produce spores arranged in rows on the outside of the hair are designated ectothrix; if spores are within the hair, endothrix.

 T. schoenleinii. Causative agent of favus of the scalp.

 T. tonsurans. The most frequent cause of ringworm of the scalp. SEE: *tinea capitis.*

 T. violaceum. Causative agent of some forms of ringworm of the scalp, beard or nails.

trichophytosis (trĭk"ō-fī-tō'sĭs) [Gr. *trichos,* hair, + *phyton,* plant, + *-ōsis,* condition]. Infestation with trichophyton fungi.

trichoptilosis (trĭk"ŏp-tĭl-ō'sĭs) ["+ *ptilon,* feather, + *-ōsis,* condition]. 1. The splitting of hairs at their ends, giving them a featherlike appearance. 2. Disease of hair marked by development of nodules along the hair shaft at which point it splits off. SYN: *trichorrhexis nodosa.*

trichorrhea (trĭk-or-ē'ă) ["+ *rhoia,* a flow]. Rapid loss of hair.

trichorrhexis (trĭk"ō-rĕks'ĭs) [Gr. *trichos,* hair, + *rhēxis,* a breaking]. Condition in which the hair splits. SYN: *fragilitas orinium; trichoschisis.*

 t. nodo'sa. Longitudinal splitting of hair at nodules formed on the shaft. SYN: *clastothrix; trichoclasia.*

trichorrhexomania (trĭk"ō-rĕks"ō-mā'nĭ-ă) ["+ "+ *mania,* madness]. The abnormal habit of breaking off the hair with the fingernails.

trichoschisis (trĭ-kos'kis-ĭs) ["+ *schisis,* a fissure]. Splitting of the hairs.

trichoscopy (trĭk-ŏs'kō-pĭ) [Gr. *trichos,* hair, + *skopein,* to examine]. Inspection of the hair.

trichosis (trĭ-kō'sĭs) ["+ *-ōsis,* condition]. Any disease of the hair or its abnormal growth or development in an abnormal place.

 t. dec'olor. Any abnormal coloring or lack of coloring of the hair. SYN: *canities.*

 t. seto'sa. Coarse hair.

Trichosporon (trĭ-kŏs'pō-rŏn) [Gr. *trichos,* hair, + *sporos,* a seed]. A genus of fungi which grows on hair causing piedra.

 T. beigelii. The causative agent of white piedra, q.v.

trichosporosis (trĭk"ō-spō-rō'sĭs) ["+ "+ *-ōsis,* condition]. Infestation of the hair with Trichosporon.

trichostrongyliasis (trĭk″ō-strŏn-jĭ-lĭ′ă-sĭs). Infestation with the intestinal parasite Trichostrongylus. A rare disease in the U.S.A.

Trichothecium (trĭk″ō-thē′sĭ-ŭm) ["+ thēkē, a box]. A genus of mold fungi causing disease of the hair.

T. ro′seum. A species of mold fungus found in certain cases of inflammation of the eardrum (mycomyringitis).

trichotillomania (trĭk″ō-tĭl″ō-mā′nĭ-ă) ["+ tillein, to pull, + mania, madness]. The unnatural impulse to pull out one's own hair.

trichotomy (trĭ-kŏt′ō-mĭ) [Gr. tricha, three-fold, + tomē, a cutting]. Division into three parts.

trichotoxin (trĭk″ō-tŏks′ĭn) [Gr. trichos, hair, + toxikon, poison]. An antibody or cytotoxin which destroys ciliated epithelial cells.

trichotrophy (trĭ-kŏt′rō-fĭ) ["+ trophē, nourishment]. Nutrition of the hair.

trichroic (trĭ-krō′ĭk) [Gr. treis, three, + chroa, color]. Presenting three different colors when viewed along each of three different axes.

trichroism (trĭ′krō-ĭzm) ["+ "+ -ismos, condition]. Quality of showing a different color when viewed along each of three axes.

trichromatic (trĭ″krō-măt′ĭk) ["+ chrōma, color]. Rel. to or able to see the three primary colors; denoting normal color vision.

trichromic (trĭ-krō′mĭk). Pert. to normal color vision or ability to see the three primary colors. SYN: trichromatic.

trichuriasis (trĭk″ū-rĭ′ă-sĭs) [Gr. trichos, hair, + oura, tail]. Presence of worms of genus Trichuris in the colon, or in the ileum.

Trichuris (trĭ-kū′rĭs). A genus of Trematoda.

T. trichiur′ia. The whipworm.

tricipital (trĭ-sĭp′ĭ-tăl) [Gr. treis, three, + L. caput, head]. Three-headed, as the triceps muscle.

tricornic, tricornute (trĭ-kor′nĭk, -nūt) ["+ L. cornu, horn]. Having three horns or cornua.

tricrotic (trĭ-krŏt′ĭk) [Gr. trikrotos, rowed with a triple stroke]. Condition in which three accentuated waves or notches occur on a sphygmograph tracing from one beat of the pulse.

tricrotism (trĭ′krŏt-ĭzm) ["+ -ismos, condition]. Condition of being tricrotic.

tricuspid (trĭ-kŭs′pĭd) [Gr. treis, three, + L. cuspis, a point]. 1. Pert. to the tricuspid valve. 2. Having three points or cusps. 3. A tooth having three cusps.

t. area. Lower portion of body of sternum where sounds of right atrioventricular orifice are best heard.

t. atresia. Stenosis of the tricuspid valve. A fairly uncommon congenital malformation which causes cyanosis and clubbing.

SYM: Paroxysmal dyspnea. Difficulty in feeding.

t. murmur. One caused by stenosis of the tricuspid valve or by its incompetency.

t. orifice. Right atrioventricular cardiac aperture.

t. tooth. One with a crown having three cusps.

t. valve. Right atrioventricular valve. SYN: valvula tricuspidalis.

trident, tridentate (trī′dĕnt, trī-dĕn′tāt) [L. trēs, tria, three, + dens, dent-, tooth]. Having three prongs.

tridermic (trī-der′mĭk) [Gr. treis, three, + derma, skin]. Developed from the ectoderm, endoderm, and mesoderm.

tridermoma (trī″dĕr-mō′mă) ["+ "+ -ōma, tumor]. A teratoid growth containing all three germ layers.

trielcon (trī-ĕl′kŏn) ["+ helkein, to draw]. Instrument with three branches for removing bullets or other foreign substances from wounds.

triethylenemelamine (trī-ĕth′ĭ-lēn-mĕl′ă-mēn). One of the nitrogen mustard compounds. ABBR: TEM. SEE: nitrogen mustards.

trifacial (trī-fā′shăl) [L. trifacialis]. Pert. to the 5th pair of cranial nerves. SYN: trigeminal.

t. neuralgia. Neuralgia of one of the branches of the 5th cranial nerve; often severe. SYN: tic douloureux.

trifid (trī′fĭd) [L. trifidus, split thrice]. Split into three; having three clefts.

trigastric (trī-găs′trĭk) [Gr. treis, three, + gastēr, belly]. Having three bellies, as certain muscles.

trigeminal (trī-jĕm′ĭn-ăl) [L. trēs, tria, three, + geminus, twin]. Pert. to the trigeminus or 5th cranial nerve.

t. cough. A reflex cough from irritation of the trigeminal terminations in respiratory upper passages.

t. nerve. The 5th cranial nerve, a large mixed nerve arising superficially from the side of the pons near its superior border. It is attached to the brain stem by two roots: a large sensory root and a small motor root. The sensory root bears an enlargement, the semilunar Gasserian ganglion, from which three large branches arise. These are ophthalmic, purely sensory, from skin of upper part of head, mucous membranes of nasal cavity and sinuses, cornea and conjunctiva; *maxillary,* purely sensory, from dura mater, gums and teeth of upper jaw, upper lip, and orbit; *mandibular,* the largest division, containing sensory fibers from tongue, gums and teeth of lower jaw, skin of cheek, lower jaw and lip, and motor fibers supplying principally muscles of mastication. SYN: *nervus trigeminus.*

   t. neuralgia. Facial neuralgia. SYN: *tic douloureux.*

   t. pulse. One with longer or shorter interval after each three beats because the 3rd beat is an extrasystole. SYN: *pulsus trigeminus.*

trigeminus (trī-jĕm'ĭ-nŭs). The 5th cranial nerve. SYN: *trigeminal nerve,* q.v. SEE: *Table of Cranial Nerves* in *Appendix.*

trigeminy (trī-jĕm'ĭ-nĭ). Occurring in threes, especially three pulse beats in rapid succession.

trigenic (trī-jĕn'ĭk) [Gr. *treis,* three, + *gennan,* to produce]. In genetics, condition in which three instead of two alleles are present at any particular locus on the chromosome.

trigger (trĭg'er) [D. *trekker,* something pulled]. To initiate or start with suddenness.

   t. action. A physiologic process or a pathologic change initiated by a sudden stimulus.

   t. finger. State in which flexion or extension is arrested temporarily, but finally completed with a jerk.

   t. material. T. substance, q.v.

   t. substance. A chemical substance which initiates a function or action.

   t. zone. 1. An area which when stimulated will initiate an attack of neuralgia. 2. An area of cerebral cortex which when stimulated produces abnormal reactions similar to those in acquired epilepsy. SEE: *epileptogenic zone.*

triglyceride (trī-glĭs'ĕr-īd). Combination of glycerol with the three fatty acids—stearic, oleic, palmitic. Most animal and vegetable fats are triglycerides.

trigonal (trĭg'ō-năl) [Gr. *trigōnon,* a three-cornered figure]. Triangular; pert. to a trigone.

trigone (trī'gŏn). A triangular space, esp. one at the base of the bladder. SYN: *trigonum.*

trigonid (trī-gō'nĭd). The first three cusps of a lower molar tooth.

trigonitis (trĭg"ō-nī'tĭs) [Gr. *trigōnon,* a three-cornered figure + *-itis,* inflammation]. Inflammation of trigone of bladder confined to its mucous membrane.

trigonocephalic (trī"gō-nō-se-fāl'ĭk) ["+ *kephalē,* head]. Having a head shaped like a triangle.

trigonum (trī-gō'nŭm) [L.]. Any triangular area. SYN: *trigone.*

trihybrid (trī-hī'brĭd) [Gr. *treis,* three + L. *hybrida,* mongrel]. In genetics, the offspring of a cross between two individuals differing in three unit characters.

trilabe (trī'lāb) ["+ *labē,* a handle]. Three-pronged forceps for removing foreign substances from the bladder. SEE: *lithotrite.*

trill (trĭl) [It. *trillare,* probably imitative]. A tremulous sound, esp. in vocal music.

trilocular (trī-lok'ū-lăr) [Gr. *treis,* three + L. *loculus,* cell]. Having three compartments.

trimanual (trī-măn'ū-ăl) [Gr. *treis,* three, + *manualis,* by hand]. Performed with three hands, as an obstetrical maneuver.

trimensual (trī-mĕn'shū-ăl) ["+ *mensualis,* monthly]. Occurring quarterly or every three months.

trimorphous (trī-mor'fŭs) [Gr. *treis,* three, + *morphē,* form]. 1. Having three different forms as the larva, pupa, and adult of certain insects. 2. Having three different forms of crystals.

trinitrophenol (trī"nĭ-trō-fē'nŏl). Picric acid, a yellow crystalline powder, explosive when heated. Used as a dye and as a reagent.

triorchid, triorchis (trī-or'kĭd, -kĭs) [Gr. *treis,* three, + *orchis,* testicle]. One having three testicles.

triorchidism (trī-or'kĭd-ĭzm) ["+ "+ *-ismos,* condition]. The condition of having three testicles.

triose (trī'ōs). A monosaccharide having three carbon atoms in its molecule.

trip. A slang term used to refer to hallucinations produced by various drugs including LSD, mescaline, and some narcotics.

tripara (trĭp'ă-ră) [L. *trēs, tria,* three, + *parĕre,* to bear]. A woman who has had three children in separate pregnancies. Designated Para III. SYN: *tertipara.*

tripeptide (trī-pĕp'tĭd) [Gr. *treis,* three, + *peptōn,* digested]. Product of combination of three amino acids formed during proteolytic digestion.

triphalangia (trī"fă-lan'jĭ-ă) ["+ *phalanx,* phalanx]. Deformity marked by presence of three phalanges in a thumb or great toe.

triphasic (trī-fā'sĭk) ["+ *phasis,* phase]. Consisting of three phases or stages, said of electric currents.

Tripier's amputation (trĭp-ē-ā'). [Léon Tripier, French surgeon, 1842-1891]. Amputation of a foot with part of the calcaneus removed.

triple [L. *triplus*, threefold]. Consisting of three; threefold; treble.

   t. response. The three reactions of the skin to injury: a red reaction along line of injury; a red area (flare or erythema) about injury; and an elevated area (welt or wheal) resulting from localized edema.

triplegia (trī-plē'jī-ă) [Gr. *treis*, three, + *plēgē*, stroke]. Hemiplegia with paralysis of one limb on the other side of the body.

triplet (trĭp'lĕt) [L. *triplus*, threefold]. 1. One of three children born at one birth. SEE: *Hellin's law.* 2. A combination of three of a kind.

triplex (trī'plĕks, trĭp'lĕks) [Gr. *triploos*, triple]. Triple; threefold.

triploblastic (trĭp''lō-blăst'ĭk) ["+ *blastos*, germ]. Consisting of three germ layers: ectoderm, entoderm, and mesoderm.

triplokoria (trĭp''lō-kor'ī-ă) ["+ *korē*, pupil]. Possessing three pupillary openings in one eye.

triplopia (trĭp-lō'pī-ă) [Gr. *triploos*, triple, + *ōpē*, vision]. Condition in which three images of the same object are seen.

triquetral (trī-kwēt'răl) [L. *triquetrous*]. Triangular; the triquetral bone, q.v.

   t. bone. 1. The third carpal bone in the proximal row, enumerated from radial side. 2. Any wormian bone. SYN: *cuneiform bone, os triquetrum.*

triquetrous (trī-kwē'trŭs) [L. *triquetrus*, triangular]. Triangular.

   t. bone. 1. A wormian bone. 2. The cuneiform bone of the carpus.

trisaccharide (trī-săk'ă-rīd). A carbohydrate which upon hydrolysis yields three molecules of simple sugars (monosaccharides).

trismoid (trĭz'moyd) [Gr. *trismos*, trismus, + *eidos*, form]. 1. Of the nature of trismus. 2. A form of trismus nascentium; once thought to be due to pressure on occiput during delivery.

trismus (trĭz'mŭs) [Gr. *trismos*, grating]. 1. Tonic contraction of the muscles of mastication. May occur in mouth infections, encephalitis, inflammation of salivary glands, and tetanus. 2. Old term for tetanus (lockjaw).

trisomic (trī-sōm'ĭk). In genetics, an individual possessing 2n + 1 chromosomes, that is, one with three chromosomes of a given kind with two only of each of the remaining chromosomes of the haploid set.

trisomy (trī'sō-mī). In genetics, having three of a specific numbered chromosomes per cell instead of a pair.

   t. 13-15. Severe congenital deformation and mental retardation. These children, who usually do not survive past the first

year of life, have a large broad nose, widely-spaced small eyes (hypertelorism), low set ears, and poorly formed lower jaw. SYN: *D trisomy.*

   t. 17-18. Severe deformity and mental retardation. These children usually do not survive beyond the first year of life. Characterized by prominent occiput, overlapping of index finger over third finger, frequent facial abnormalities, straight nose coming off sharply from the forehead, low set ears, and cleft palate and lip. SYN: *E trisomy.*

   t. 21. Down's syndrome (mongolism), q.v.

trisplanchnic (trī-splănk'nĭk) [Gr. *treis*, three, + *splanchna*, viscera]. Pert. to the three large body cavities: the skull, thorax, and abdomen.

   t. nervous system. Sympathetic nervous system.

tristichia (trī-stĭk'ī-ă) ["+ *stichos*, row]. The presence of three rows of eyelashes.

tristimania (trĭs''tĭ-mā'nĭ-ă) [L. *tristis*, sad, + Gr. *mania*, madness]. Melancholia.

trisulcate (trī-sŭl'kāt) [L. *trēs, tria*, three, + *sulcus*, groove]. Having three grooves or furrows.

TRIT. Abbr. for *triiodothyronine*.

tritanopia (trī''tă-nō'pī-ă) [Gr. *tritos*, third, + *an-*, not, + *ōpē*, vision]. Color blindness in which blue and yellow appear gray.

tritiate (trĭt'ī-āt). To treat with tritium.

triticeous (trĭt-ĭsh'ŭs) [L. *triticeus*, of wheat]. Shaped like a grain of wheat.

   t. cartilage, t. nodule. A cartilaginous nodule in the thyrohyoid ligament.

tritium (trĭt'ī-um) [Gr. *tritos*, third]. The mass three isotope of hydrogen; triple-weight hydrogen.

triturable (trĭt'ū-ră-bl) [L. *tritūrāre*, to pulverize]. Capable of being powdered.

triturate (trĭt'ū-rāt). 1. To reduce to a fine powder by rubbing. 2. A finely divided substance made by rubbing.

trituration (trĭt-ū-rā'shŭn) [LL. *tritūrāre*, to pulverize]. 1. The act of reducing to a powder. 2. A finely ground and easily mixed powder.

trivalent (trī-vā'lĕnt, trĭv'ăl-ĕnt) [Gr. *treis*, three, + L. *valens*, powerful]. Combining with or replacing three hydrogen atoms.

trocar (trō'kăr) [Fr. *trois quarts*, three quarters]. A sharply pointed surgical instrument contained in a metal cannula. Used for aspiration or removal of fluids from cavities.

troch. Abbr. for *trochiscus*. SEE: *troche.*

trochanter (trō-kăn'ter) [Gr. *trokhantēr*, a runner]. Either of the two bony processes below the neck of the femur.

   t., greater. T. major, q.v.

   t., lesser. T. minor, q.v.

t. major. [NA]. A thick process at upper end of the femur projecting upward externally to union of neck and shaft.

t. minor. [NA]. A conical tuberosity upon inner and posterior surface of upper end of femur, at junction of shaft and neck.

t. tertius. [NA]. The gluteal ridge of the femur when it is unusually prominent.

t., third. T. tertius, q.v.

trochanterian, trochanteric (trō″kăn-tē′rĭ-ăn, trō-kăn-ter′ĭk). Rel. to a trochanter.

troche (trō′kē) [Gr. *trokhiskos*, a small wheel]. Solid, discoid, or cylindrical mass consisting chiefly of medicinal powder, sugar, and mucilage.

They are intended to be used by placing them in the mouth and allowing them to remain until, through slow solution or disintegration, their purpose of mild medication is effected. SYN: *lozenge; trochiscus.*

trochlea (trok′lē-ă) [Gr. *trokhileia*, system of pulleys]. (pl. *trochleae*) 1. A structure having the function of a pulley; a ring or hook through which a tendon or muscle projects. 2. The articular smooth surface of a bone upon which glides another bone.

trochlear (trok′lē-ăr). 1. Of the nature of a pulley. 2. Pert. to a trochlea.

t. fovea. A depression on orbital plate of frontal bone for attachment of cartilaginous pulley of superior oblique muscle.

t. nerve. A small mixed nerve making its exit from dorsal surface of midbrain. It contains efferent motor fibers to superior oblique muscle of eye and afferent sensory fibers conveying proprioceptive impulses from the same muscle. SYN: *nerve trochlearis; 4th cranial nerve.* SEE: *Table of Cranial Nerves* in *Appendix.*

trochlearis (trok′lē-ă′rĭs) [L.]. Superior oblique muscle of the eye. SEE: *Table of Muscles* in *Appendix.*

trochocardia (trō″kō-kar′dĭ-ă) [Gr. *trokhos*, a wheel, + *kardia*, heart]. Rotary displacement of the heart on its axis.

trochocephalia, trochocephaly (trō″kō-se-fā′lĭ-a, -sĕf′ă-lĭ) ["+ *kephalē*, head]. Roundheadedness, a deformity due to premature union of frontal and parietal bones.

trochoid (trō′koyd) [Gr. *trokhos*, a wheel, + *eidos*, form]. Rotating or revolving, noting an articulation resembling a pivot or pulley.

t. joint. A pivot joint. SEE: *joint, pivot.*

trochoides (trō-koy′dēz). A pivot or rotary joint.

Troglotrematidae (trŏg′lō-trē-măt′ĭ-dē). A family of flukes which includes Paragonimus (human lung fluke) and Troglotrema

Nanophyetus, the fluke associated with salmon poisoning in dogs.

Trombicula (trŏm-bĭk′ū-lă). A genus of mites belonging to the Trombiculidae. The larvae called redbugs or chiggers are annoying pests causing an irritating dermatitis and rash. They may serve as vectors of various diseases.

T. akamushi. Species of mite transmitting causative agent of scrub typhus.

trombidiiasis, trombidiosis (trŏm-bĭ″dĭ-ī′ă-sĭs, -bĭd′ĭ-ō′sĭs). Infestation with the Trombidium irritans.

tromomania (trŏm″ō-mā′nĭ-ă) [Gr. *tromos*, a trembling, + *mania*, madness]. Delirium tremens.

troph-, tropho- [Gr.]. Combining forms meaning nourishment.

trophedema, trophoedema (trŏf′ē-dē′mă) [Gr. *trophē*, nourishment, + *oidēma*, a swelling]. Localized edema due to congenital hypoplasia of lymphatic vessels or resulting secondarily from obstruction to lymph flow by external pressure or to repeated low grade infection. SYN: *hereditary trophedema* or *Milroy's disease.*

trophic (trŏf′ĭk) [Gr. *trophikos*]. Concerned with nourishment.

Applied particularly to a type of efferent nerves believed to control the growth and nourishment of the parts they innervate. SEE: *autotrophic.*

trophoblast (trŏf′ō-blăst) [Gr. *trophē*, nourishment, + *blastos*, germ]. The outermost layer of the developing blastocyst (blastodermic vesicle) of a mammal. It differentiates into two layers, the cytotrophoblast and syntrophoblast, the latter coming into intimate relationship with the uterine endometrium with which it establishes nutrient relationships. SYN: *trophectoderm.*

trophoblastoma (trŏf′ō-blăs-tō′mă) ["+ "+ -*ōma*, tumor]. A neoplasm due to excessive proliferation of chorionic epithelium. SYN: *chorioepithelioma.*

trophoderm (trŏf′ō-derm) [Gr. *trophē*, nourishment, + *derma*, skin]. Term applied to the trophoblast and its underlying layer of mesoderm. It is homologous to the serosa of birds, reptiles, and lower mammals.

trophology (trō-fŏl′ō-jĭ) ["+ *logos*, a science]. The science of nutrition.

trophoneurosis (trŏf″ō-nū-rō′sĭs) ["+ *neuron*, nerve, + -*ōsis*, condition]. Any trophic disorder due to defective function of the nerves concerned with nutrition of the part.

t., disseminated. Thickening and hardening of the skin. SYN: *sclerema, scleroderma.*

t., facial. Progressive facial atrophy.

t., muscular. Muscular changes in connection with nervous disorders.

trophoneurotic (trŏf′ō-nū-rŏt′ĭk). Rel. to a trophoneurosis.

trophonosis (trŏf′ō-nō′sĭs) ["+ *nosos,* disease]. Any disease due to a nutritional defect.

trophonucleus (trŏf′ō-nū′klē-ŭs) [Gr. *trophē,* nourishment, + L. *nucleus,* kernel]. Protozoan nucleus concerned with vegetative functions in metabolism and not reproduction. SYN: *macronucleus.*

trophopathia, trophopathy (trŏf′ō-path′ĭ-ā, trof-op′ă-thĭ) ["+ *pathos,* disease]. 1. Any disorder of the nutrition. 2. A trophic disease.

trophotaxis (trŏf′ō-tăks′ĭs) ["+ *taxis,* arrangement]. The movement of cells away from or toward nutrients. SYN: *trophotropism.*

trophotherapy (trŏf′ō-thĕr′ă-pĭ) ["+ *therapeia,* service]. The therapeutic use of foods. SYN: *dietotherapy.*

trophotonos (trŏf-ŏt′ŏn-ŏs) ["+ *tonos,* tension]. A rigid state of contractile tissue resulting from trophic disorder.

trophotropism (trŏf-ot′rō-pĭzm) [Gr. *trophē,* nourishment, + *tropos,* a turning, + *-ismos,* condition]. Attraction and repulsion of cells to nutritive substances; positive and negative trophotropism respectively. SYN: *trophotaxis.*

trophozoite (trŏf′ō-zō′ĭt) ["+ *zōon,* animal]. A sporozoan nourished by its hosts during its growth stage.

tropia (trō′pĭ-ā) [Gr. *trope,* turn]. Deviation of the eye or eyes away from the visual axis. Observed with the eyes open and uncovered. Esotropia indicates inward or nasal deviation; exotropia, outward; hypertropia, upward; hypotropia, downward. SYN: *manifest squint; strabismus.*

tropical (trŏp′ĭ-kăl) [Gr. *tropikos,* turning]. Pert. to the tropics.

    t. immersion foot. Syndrome with severe wrinkling and maceration of the soles of the feet and marked lowering of the threshold of pain. Due to prolonged exposure of the feet to warm water as would occur in the tropics. May be prevented by allowing feet to dry thoroughly each night and by protecting the feet with silicone grease.

    t. lichen. Prickly heat, acute inflammation of the sweat glands.

tropin (trō′pĭn). A substance present in blood serum which stimulates the engulfment of bacteria by phagocytic cells. SEE: *bacteriotropin.*

-tropin [Gr. *tropos,* a turn]. Suffix indicating the stimulating effect of a substance, esp. a hormone, on its target organ.

tropism (trō′pĭsm) [Gr. *tropē,* a turn, + *-ismos,* condition]. 1. Reaction of living organisms involuntarily toward or away from light, darkness, heat, cold, or other stimuli. 2. The involuntary response of an organism as a bending, turning, or movement toward (positive tropism) or away from (negative tropism) an external stimulus. SYN: *taxis.* SEE: *chemotropism; galvanotropism; phototropism.*

-tropism. Combining form meaning a response to or a turning towards or away from an external stimulus.

tropometer (trŏp-om′ē-ter) [Gr. *tropē,* a turn, + *metron,* a measure]. 1. Device for measuring the rotation of the eyeballs. 2. Instrument for measuring torsion in long bones.

Trousseau's sign (trū-sō′). [Armand Trousseau, French physician, 1801-1867]. Muscular spasm resulting from pressure applied to nerves and vessels of the upper arm. It is indicative of latent tetany. Also occurs is osteomalacia.

Trousseau's spots. Streaking of the skin with the fingernail, seen in meningitis and other cerebral diseases. SYN: *meningitic streak.*

Trousseau's symptom. Spasmodic muscular contractions produced by pressing the principal vessel and nerve of the limb. Presence of this symptom is a sign of tetany.

troy weight. A system of weighing gold, silver, precious metals, and jewels. 5.760 grains equal 1 lb. SEE: *Appendix* for apothecaries, avoirdupois, household weights and measures; metric system.

TRU. Abbr. for *turbidity reducing unit.*

true (trū) [AS. *trēowe,* faithful]. Not false; real; genuine.

    t. pelvis. Portion below the iliopectineal line.

    t. ribs. The seven upper ones on each side with cartilages articulating directly with the sternum. SYN: *costa vera.* SEE: *rib.*

truncal (trŭng′kăl) [L. *truncus,* trunk]. Rel. to the trunk.

truncate (trŭng′kāt) [L. *truncāre,* to cut off]. 1. Having a square end as if it were cut off; lacking an apex. 2. To shorten by cutting off the end; to amputate.

truncus (trŭng′kŭs). Trunk.

trunk (trŭnk) [L. *truncus,* trunk]. 1. The body exclusive of the head and limbs. SYN: *torso.* 2. Main stem of a lympathic vessel, nerve, or blood vessel.

truss (trŭs) [ME. *trusse*, a bundle]. Device for holding a hernia in its place.

truth serum. One of several hypnotic drugs supposedly having the effect of causing a person upon questioning to talk freely and without inhibition.

trypanocide, trypanocidal (trĭp-ăn'ō-sĭd, trĭp"ăn-ō-si'dăl) [Gr. *trypanon*, a borer, + L. *caedere*, to kill]. 1. Destructive to trypanosomes. 2. An agent which kills trypanosomes. SYN: *trypanosomicide.*

trypanolysis (trĭp-an-ŏl'ĭ-sĭs) ["+ *lysis*, dissolution]. The dissolution of trypanosomes.

Trypanoplasma (tri"păn-ō-plăz'mă) ["+ *plasma*, a thing formed]. A genus of protozoan parasites resembling trypanosomes.

Trypanosoma (trī"păn-ō-sō'mă) [Gr. *trypanon*, a borer, + *sōma*, a body]. A genus of parasitic, flagellate protozoa found in the blood of many vertebrates including man. They are transmitted by insect vectors.

    T. brucei. The causative agent of trypanosomiasis in horses and other domestic animals. Nonpathogenic in man.

    T. cruzi. The causative agent of American trypanosomiasis in many animals and specifically Chagas' disease in humans. It is transmitted by blood-sucking insects (triatomids) belonging to the family Reduviidae.

    T. gambiense. The causative agent of African sleeping sickness. It is transmitted by the tsetse fly.

    T. rhodesiense. An organism parasitic in wild game and domestic animals of portions of Africa. May cause East African sleeping sickness in humans.

trypanosomal (tri-păn-ō-sō'măl). Pert. to trypanosomata.

trypanosome (tri'păn-ō-sōm). Any protozoan belonging to the genus Trypanosoma.

    t. fever. Sleeping sickness.

trypanosomiasis (tri-păn"ō-sō-mī'ă-sĭs) [Gr. *trypanon*, a borer, + *sōma*, body, + -*iasis*, infection]. Any of the several diseases occurring in man and domestic animals caused by a species of Trypanosoma. SEE: *sleeping sickness.*

    t., African. African sleeping sickness, caused by Trypanosoma gambiense, q.v.

    t., American. Trypanosomiasis in the western hemisphere. In man, Chagas' disease is caused by Trypanosoma cruzi transmitted by blood-sucking triatomids.

trypanosomid (tri-pan'ō-sō-mĭd). A skin eruption in any disease caused by a trypanosome.

tryparsamide (trĭp"ars'ă-mĭd, -mĭd). An arsenic compound containing about 25% arsenic.

USES: Chiefly in neurosyphilis and sleeping sickness.

trypesis (trĭp-ē'sĭs) [Gr. *trypēsis*, a boring]. An incision of the skull to reduce pressure by removing a disk of bone. SYN: *trephining.*

trypsin (trĭp'sĭn) [Gr. *tripsis*, a rubbing]. A proteolytic enzyme formed in the intestine from the action of enterokinase of the intestinal juice (succus entericus) on trypsinogen secreted by the pancreas and present in pancreatic juice. It catalyzes the hydrolysis of peptide bonds in partly digested proteins and some native proteins, the final products being amino acids and various polypeptides. SEE: *chymotrypsin; digestion; enzyme; pancreas.*

trypsinized (trĭp'sī-nīzd). Subjected to action of trypsin, thus having antitryptic power abolished.

trypsinogen (trĭp-sĭn'ō-jĕn) [Gr. *trypsis*, a rubbing, + *gennan*, to produce]. The proenzyme, or inactive form of trypsin found in pancreatic juice. Activated when mixed in the intestine with the enterokinase of the succus entericus.

tryptic (trĭp'tĭk). Rel. to trypsin.

tryptolysis (trĭp-tŏl'ĭ-sĭs) [Gr. *tripsis*, a rubbing, + *lysis*, dissolution]. The hydrolysis of proteins or their derivatives by trypsin.

tryptonemia (trĭp"tō-nē'mĭ-ă) ["+ *haima*, blood]. Tryptones in the blood.

tryptophan (trĭp'tō-făn). An amino acid produced by digestion of proteins. It is an essential amino acid and is required for normal growth and development.

tryptophanuria (trĭp"tō-fă-nū'rĭ-ă) [*tryptophan*, + Gr. *ouron*, urine]. Tryptophan in the urine.

T/S. Abbr. for *thyroid:serum* (thyroid to serum iodine ratio).

T.S. Abbr. for *test solution; triple strength.*

TSD. Abbr. for *target skin distance.*

tsetse fly (tsĕt'sē) [S. African]. One of several species of blood-sucking flies belonging to the genus Glossina, order Diptera, confined to Africa south of the Sahara Desert. It is an important transmitter of trypanosomes, the causative agents of African sleeping sicknesses in man, and nagana and other diseases of cattle and game animals. SEE: *Trypanosoma, trypanosomiasis.*

TSH. Abbr. for *thyroid-stimulating hormone.*

tsp. Abbr. for *teaspoon.*

tsutsugamushi disease (soot"soo-gă-moo-sh'ĭ) [Japanese, dangerous bug]. Scrub typhus, q.v.

TT. Abbr. for *transit time* of blood through heart and lungs.

T.U. Abbr. for *toxic unit; transmission unit.*

tub (tŭb) [ME. *tubbe*]. 1. A receptacle for bathing. 2. The use of the cold bath. 3. To treat by using a cold bath.

tubal (tū′băl) [L. *tuba*, tube]. Pert. to a tube, esp. the fallopian tube.

    t. nephritis. Inflammation of kidney tubules.

    t. pregnancy. Pregnancy in one of the oviducts.

tubatorsion (tū″bă-tor′shŭn) ["+ *torsio*, a twisting]. The twisting of an oviduct.

tube (tūb) [L. *tuba*, a tube]. A long, hollow, cylindrical structure.

    t., Cantor. SEE: *t., intestinal decompression.*

    t., cathode-ray. A vacuum t. with a thin window at the end opposite the cathode to allow the cathode rays to pass outside. More generally, any discharge t. in which the vacuum is fairly high.

    t., Coolidge. A kind of hot cathode tube, which is so highly exhausted that the residual gas plays no part in the production of the cathode stream, and which is regulated by variable heating of the cathode filament.

    t., Crookes'. T. with an exhausted vacuum, used in producing roentgen rays.

    t., drainage. A glass or rubber t. which, when inserted into a cavity, drains away its fluid contents.

    t., esophageal. T., stomach, q.v.

    t., eustachian. The t. passing from the throat to the middle ear.

    t., fallopian. One of two oviducts.

    t., hot-cathode. A vacuum t. in which the cathode is electrically heated to incandescence and in which the supply of electrons depends on the temperature of the cathode.

    t., h.c. roentgen-ray. A vacuum roentgen-ray t. in which the electron stream is supplied by a heated cathode. The cathode stream may be regulated by varying the current through the cathode filament.

    t., intestinal decompression. A t. placed in the intestinal tract, usually via the nose and esophagus, in order to relieve gas pressure produced when paralytic ileus or intestinal obstruction is present. T.'s may be plain, made of rubber, plastic, or silicone; or they may be equipped with a mercury-filled tip to facilitate passage into the intestinal tract. The latter is called a Cantor t. The t.'s are impregnated with a radio-opaque substance in order to allow x-ray visualization of their location.

    t., intubation. A tube for passing into the larynx to facilitate breathing.

    t., oscillator vacuum. Method of producing alternating current. Current pro-

duced by this is a continuous sine wave current in contradistinction to the damped harmonic wave of spark gap diathermy machine.

    t., Southey's. Very small tube pushed into tissue to help drain edema fluid. Used in severe congestive heart failure to relieve edema of the legs.

    t., stomach. A rubber tube for introducing food into the stomach or for washing out the stomach.

    t., tracheotomy. A tube for inserting into the trachea.

tuber (tū′ber) [L. *tuber*, a swelling]. (pl. *tubers, tubera*) A swelling or enlargement.

tubercle (tū′ber-kl) [L. *tuberculum*, a little swelling]. 1. A small rounded elevation or eminence on a bone. 2. A small nodule, esp. a circumscribed solid elevation of the skin or mucous membrane. 3. The characteristic lesion resulting from infection by tubercle bacilli. It consists typically of three parts: a central giant cell, a midzone of epithelioid cells, and a peripheral zone of nonspecific structure. SEE: *tuberculosis.*

    t., adductor. That part of femur to which is attached the tendon of the adductor magnus.

    t. bacillus. Organism causing tuberculosis.

    t., deltoid. T. in clavicle for attachment of deltoid muscle.

    t., genial. T. on either side of lower jawbone.

    t., genital. The embryonic structure that becomes the clitoris, or the penis.

    t., lacrimal. T. on upper jawbone.

    t., laminated. The cerebellar nodule.

    t., Lisfranc's. T. for scalenus anticus muscle on the 1st rib.

    t., miliary. A small tubercle resembling a millet seed; the lesion of tuberculosis.

    t., zygomatic. T. on the zygoma at junction of anterior root.

tubercular (tū-ber′kū-lar) [L. *tuberculum*, a little swelling]. 1. Relating to or marked by nodules. 2. Person with tuberculosis. SEE: *torose.*

tuberculate, tuberculated (tū-ber′kū-lăt, -lāt″ed) [L. *tuberculum*, a small swelling]. Covered with nodules. SYN: *tubercular.*

tuberculation (tū-ber″kū-lā′shŭn). The formation of tubercles.

tuberculid(e (tū-ber′kū-lĭd, -līd) [L. *tuberculum*, a little swelling]. A tuberculous cutaneous eruption due to toxins of tuberculosis.

    t., follicular. That characterized by presence of groups of follicular lesions, esp. on trunk.

t., papulonecrotic. Form characterized by symmetrically distributed bluish papules, esp. on extremities. These undergo central necrosis and, on healing, leave deep scars.

tuberculigenous (tū-ber-kū-lĭj'ĕn-ŭs) ["+ Gr. *gennan,* to produce]. Causing or predisposing to tuberculosis.

tuberculin (tū-bĕr'kū-lĭn) [L. *tuberculum,* a little swelling]. A soluble cell substance prepared from the tubercle bacillus, usually the human type, which is used to determine the presence of a tuberculosis infection. Among the types of tuberculin used are Koch's original or old tuberculin (ABBR: OT or TO) and tuberculin purified protein derivative (ABBR: PPD).

   t. test. A test to determine the presence of a tuberculous infection based on positive reaction of subject to tuberculin. Tests commonly used are *Mantoux test,* injection intradermally of tuberculin; *von Pirquet test,* rubbing tuberculin on scarified skin; and *Vollmer patch test,* the application to skin of a piece of gauze impregnated with dried tuberculin. In all three tests a local inflammatory reaction is observed in infected persons after 48-96 hours. Tests do not reveal whether infection is active or inactive. SEE: *tine test.*

   t. tine test. Tuberculin test performed by using a special disposable instrument which contains multiple sharp points or prongs for piercing the skin. These tines penetrate the skin and introduce the tuberculin which has been applied to them. The test is read in 48 and 72 hours.

tuberculoderma (tū-ber"kū-lō-der'mă) ["+ Gr. *derma,* skin]. A tuberculous lesion of the skin. SYN: *tuberculide.*

tuberculofibroid (tū-ber'kū-lō-fī'broyd) [L. *tuberculum,* a little swelling, + *fibra,* fiber, + Gr. *eidos,* form]. Denoting fibroid degeneration of tubercles.

tuberculofibrosis (tū-ber"kū-lō-fĭ-brō'sĭs) ["+ "+ Gr. *-ōsis,* condition]. 1. Chronic pulmonary inflammation with formation of fibrous tissue. 2. Interstitial pneumonia.

tuberculoid (tū-ber'kū-loyd) [L. *tuberculum,* a little swelling, + Gr. *eidos,* resemblance]. Resembling tuberculosis or a tubercle.

tuberculoma (tū-ber-kū-lō'mă) ["+ Gr. *-ōma,* tumor]. 1. A tuberculous abscess. 2. Any tuberculous neoplasm.

tuberculophobia (tū-ber"kū-lō-fō'bĭ-ă) [L. *tuberculum,* a little swelling, + Gr. *phobos,* fear]. An abnormal fear of being infected with tuberculosis.

tuberculoprotein (tū-bĕr"cū-lō-prō'tē-ĭn). A protein derived from tubercle bacilli.

tuberculosis (tū-bĕr"kū-lō'sĭs) [L. *tuberculum,* a little swelling, + Gr. *-ōsis,* disease]. An infectious disease caused by the tubercle bacillus, Mycobacterium tuberculosis, and characterized pathologically by inflammatory infiltrations, formation of tubercles, caseation, necrosis, abscesses, fibrosis, and calcification.

   It most commonly affects the respiratory system but other parts of the body such as gastrointestinal and genito-urinary tracts, bones, joints, nervous system, lymph nodes, and skin may become infected. Fish, amphibians, birds, and mammals (cattle) are subject to the disease. Three types of the tubercle bacillus exist, namely human, bovine and avian. Man may become infected by any of the three types but in the U. S. the human type predominates. Infection usually is acquired from contact with an infected person or an infected cow or through drinking contaminated milk.

   T. may occur in an acute generalized form (miliary tuberculosis) or in a chronic localized form. In man, the primary infection usually consists of a localized lesion and regional adenitis, these constituting the primary complex. From this state, lesions may heal by fibrosis and calcification and the disease exist in an arrested or inactive stage. Reactivation or exacerbation of the disease or reinfection gives rise to the chronic progressive form.

   NOTE: Many varieties of Mycobacteria which previously were thought to be nonpathogenic for man have been found to cause chronic progressive pulmonary disease closely resembling pulmonary t. These organisms have been termed anonymous or atypical Mycobacteria. They have been classified into four groups: photochromogens, scotochromogens, nonphotochromogens and rapid growers.

   TREATMENT: Sanitorium care is recommended for active cases; however, recent developments in chemotherapy have greatly altered time-honored views. In advanced cases, bed rest, adequate well-balanced diet, relief from emotional tension, collapse therapy (pneumoperitoneum, pneumothorax, phrenemphraxis) and, in some cases, surgery (thoracoplasty) may be required. Among chemotherapeutic drugs, three are widely used: streptomycin, para-amino-salicylic acid (PAS), and isoniazid. Kanamycin and ethionamide are useful in cases where the tubercle bacillus has become resistant to the usual drugs. Symptomatic treatment is necessary for cough, hemoptysis, chest pain, and other symptoms. RS: myobacterium;

tubercle; tubercle bacillus; tuberculin; tuberculin test.

tuberculostatic (tū-bĕr″cū-lō-stăt′ĭk). Arresting the growth of tubercle bacillus.

tuberculous (tū-ber′kū-lŭs) [L. *tuberculum*, a little swelling]. Relating to or affected with tuberculosis, or conditions marked by infiltration of a specific tubercle, as opposed to the term tubercular, referring to nonspecific tubercle.

tuberculum (tū-ber′kū-lŭm) [L. a little swelling]. (pl. *tubercula*) A small knot or nodule; a tubercle.

     t. acus′ticum. Dorsal nucleus of the cochlear nerve.

     t. majus humeri. [NA]. Larger tuberosity of the humerus at upper end of its lateral surface giving attachment to infraspinatus, supraspinatus, and teres minor muscles.

     t. minus humeri. The projection at proximal end of anterior humerus providing attachment to subscapularis muscle.

tuberin (tu′ber-ĭn) [L. *tuber*, a swelling]. A simple protein; a globulin in pototoes.

tuberositas (tū-ber-ŏs′ĭt-ăs) [L.]. (pl. *tuberosita′tes*) A projection, nodule, or prominence.

tuberosity (tū-ber-ŏs′ĭ-tĭ) [L. *tuberositas*, tuberosity]. 1. An elevated round process of a bone. 2. A tubercle or nodule.

tuberous (tū′bĕr-ŭs). Pert. to or having tubers.

tuberous sclerosis. A syndrome manifested by convulsive seizures, progressive mental disorder, adenoma sebaceum, and tumors of the kidneys and brain with projections into the cerebral ventricles.

tubo- [L.]. Combining form meaning tube.

tuboabdominal (tū″bō-ăb-dŏm′ĭn-ăl) [L. *tubus*, tube, + *abdominalis*, pert. to the abdomen]. Pert. to the fallopian tubes and the abdomen.

     t. pregnancy. Ectopic gestation with embryo partly in tube and partly in the abdominal cavity.

Tubocurarine chloride (tū″bō-cū-ră′rin-klō-rĭd). USP. Drug used to produce skeletal muscle relaxation during anesthesia and convulsive states, and in treating poisoning due to black widow spider bites. Tubocurarine was originally obtained from the Indian arrow poison, curare. SEE: *curare.*

     CAUTION: Tubocurarine should be administered only by those who are fully capable of providing artificial ventilation, tracheal intubation, appropriate antidotes, and additional therapy in case of overdose.

tuboligamentous (tū″bō-lĭg-ă-mĕn′tŭs) [L. *tubus*, tube, + *ligamentum*, a band]. Pert. to

the fallopian tube and broad ligament of the uterus.

tuboovarian (tū″bō-ō-vā′rĭ-ăn) ["+ *ovarium*, egg holder]. Pert. to the fallopian tube and the ovary.

tuboovariotomy (tū″bō-ō-vā-rĭ-ŏt′ō-mĭ) [L. *tubus*, tube, + *ovarium*, egg holder, + Gr. *tomē*, a cutting]. Excision of ovaries and oviducts. SYN: *salpingo-oothecotomy.*

tuboperitoneal (tū″bō-pĕr-ĭ-tō-nē′ăl) ["+ Gr. *peritonaion*, peritoneum]. Rel. to the oviduct and peritoneum.

tuborrhea (tū-bor-rē′ă) ["+ Gr. *rhoia*, a flow]. Discharge from the eustachian tube.

tubotympanal (tū″bō-tĭm′pă-năl) ["+ Gr. *tympanon*, a drum]. Rel. to the tympanum of the ear and the eustachian tube.

tubouterine (tū″bō-ū′tĕr-ĭn) ["+ *uterinus*, pert. to the uterus]. Rel. to the oviduct and the uterus.

tubular (tū′bū-lar) [L. *tubularis*, like a tube]. Rel. to or having the form of a tube or tubule.

     t. excretory capacity, maximum. Abbr. Tm. The difference between the amount of a substance that is filtered and that appearing in urine per minute. Tm. gives valuable information concerning glomerular and tubular activity.

tubule (tū′būl) [L. *tubulus*, a tubule]. A small tube or canal.

     t., collecting. T. in renal medulla which is part of the discharging tubule.

     t., excretory. The uriniferous tubules in medullary portion of kidneys.

     t., junctional. Short part of a uriniferous t. connecting with a collecting t.

     t's., seminiferous. Very small channels of the testes in which spermatozoa develop and through which they leave the testes.

     t., uriniferous. Minute canals forming the glandular substance of the kidney, originating in Bowman's capsules and emptying into pelvis of kidney.

tubuloalveolar. Consisting of tubes and alveoli.

     t. gland. Branched, compound glands in which some of the terminal secreting portions are tubular, others alveolar (acinar), i.e., salivary glands. SYN: *tubuloacinar gland.*

tubulodermoid (tū″bū-lō-der′moyd) [L. *tubulus*, tubule, + Gr. *derma*, skin, + *eidos*, form]. A dermoid tumor due to the persistent embryonic tubular structure.

tubulus (tū′bū-lŭs) [L.]. (pl. *tubuli*) [NA]. A tubule; a small tube.

tuft. A small clump, cluster, or coiled mass.

t., enamel. Abnormal structure formed in development of enamel consisting of poorly calcified twisted rods.

tug'ging. A dragging or pulling.

t., tracheal. An indication of thoracic aneurysm.

SYM: A sense of downward pulling of larynx with cardiac systole when thyroid cartilage is gently raised between the finger and thumb.

tularemia (tū-lär-ē'mĭ-ă) [*Tulare,* part of California where disease was first discovered]. An acute plague-like infectious disease caused by Pasteurella tularensis. Transmitted to man by the bite of an infected tick or other blood-sucking insect; direct contact with infected animals; by eating inadequately cooked meat or drinking water containing the organism.

TREATMENT: Streptomycin and tetracyclines are effective.

SYM: From one to 10 days but averaging three days after infection, headache, chilliness, vomiting, aching pains, and fever develop. Site of infection develops into an ulcer. Glands at elbow or in armpit become enlarged, tender, and painful; later may develop into an abscess. Sweating, loss of weight, and debility.

tumbu fly. Species of fly belonging to the genus Cordylobia in Africa and the genus Dermatobia in tropical America. Their larvae develop in the skin of wild and domesticated animals, and man is frequently attacked.

tumefacient (tū-mĕ-fā'shĕnt) [L. *tumefaciens,* producing swelling]. Producing or tending to produce swelling; swollen.

tumefaction (tū''mĕ-făk'shŭn) [L. *tumefactio,* a swelling]. 1. A swelling. 2. Act of swelling or the state of being swollen.

tumentia (tū-mĕn'shĭ-ă) [L.]. Swelling.

t., vasomotor. Irregular swellings in lower extremities associated with vasomotor disturbances.

tumescence (tū-mĕs'ĕns). 1. Condition of being swollen or tumid. 2. A swelling.

tumid (tū'mĭd) [L. tumidus]. Swollen.

tumor (tū'mor) [L. *tumor,* a swelling]. 1. A swelling or enlargement. 2. A spontaneous new growth of tissue forming an abnormal mass which performs no physiologic function. It is with few exceptions of unknown cause, noninflammatory, and develops independent of, and unrestrained by normal laws of growth and morphogenesis. SYN: *neoplasm.* SEE: *cancer.*

TYPES OF TUMORS: *Myeloid Sarcomata, Giant Celled S:* Consist of elements formed chiefly of protoplasm containing two or more nuclei, up to 20 or even 50; with a varying number of round, spindle, or mixed cells. Vary in consistency from that of jelly to that of muscle. More frequently occurs on lower jaw, femur, and tibia. *Round Celled Sarcomata:* Usually soft, vascular, rapidly growing, become large, and early give rise to metastatic deposits in distant parts and in viscera. Occur in periosteum, bone, lymphatic glands, subcutaneous tissue, testicle, eye, ovary, uterus, lung, kidneys; though may occur wherever fibrous tissue exists. *Glioma:* Grows from the connective tissue of nerve centers and its basic substance resembles that structure. Occurs in retina and brain.

Melanotic Sarcoma: In cells may be of either round or spindle variety. Is the most malignant form. *Spindle-cell Sarcoma:* Cells vary much in size, from small oat-shaped cells to greatly elongated bodies with long, fine, tapering extremities. Chiefly in bones. *Endotheliomata:* Attack, in different forms, the testicle, pia mater, pleura, and peritoneum. *Acinous or Spheroidal-celled Carcinoma:* Hard, spheroidal-celled (scirrhus or chronic c.). Soft, spheriodal-celled (encephaloid, or acute c.); resembles brain tissue in appearance and consistency. Occurs in testicle, liver, bladder, kidney, ovary, fundus oculi, more rarely in the breast. SEE: *scirrhus.*

Colloid Carcinoma: Really one of preceding varieties which has undergone mucoid degeneration, and so distended the alveoli they may be seen by naked eye. Occurs in stomach, intestine, omentum, ovary. *Epithelial Carcinoma:* (1) The squamous-celled epitheliomata which always spring from skin or mucous membranes, or their glands, esp. at junctions of mucous and cutaneous surfaces. Are not encapsulated. Commence as wart-like growth, flattened tubercle, or fissure, ulceration in all these forms setting in early. (2) Cylindrical or columnar-celled. Less common form of carcinoma. Originates from either the cylindrical surface epithelium of a mucous membrane, or of its glands, closely imitating these structures in microscopic appearance. These growths form indurated, infiltrating masses in the walls of organs attacked, producing considerable stenosis of lumen, of hollow viscera; as rectum and small intestinal obstruction. Occur in uterus and intestinal tract.

Warty or Villous Growth (Papillomata): Resemble in their structure hypertrophied papillae of skin—or mucous membrane. These include condylomata and mucous tubercles. Occur about anus and genitals, or in mouth and throat. Warts and warty growths on skin of hands and genitalia, and mucous surface of larynx. Villous growths, bladder, rectum, and larynx. *Teratoma:* Tumors containing bone, hair, teeth, etc., usually situated in ovaries or testicles but may also be present in other tissues.

tumoraffin (tū'mor-ăf-ĭn) [L. *tumor,* a swelling, + *affinis,* related]. Having an affinity for tumor cells. SYN: *oncotropic.*

tumor angiogenesis factor. A protein present in animal and human cancer tissue which in experimental studies appears to be essential to growth of the cancer. The substance is thought to act by stimulating the growth of new blood capillaries for supplying the tumor with nutrients and removing waste products. ABBR: T.A.F.

tumultus (tū-mŭl'tŭs) [L.]. Excessive or agitated activity.

　　t. cordis. Irregular heart action with palpitation.

　　t. sermo'nis. Extreme stuttering due to pathologic cause.

tuna fish (tū'nă). Any of various, often large marine and food fishes, several of which are commercially important sources of canned fish.

　　Food value of 100 gm. (canned in oil, solids and liquids): Cal. 288; protein 24 gm.; fat 20 gm.; calcium 6 mg.

Tunga (tŭng'ă). A genus of fleas commonly called chiggers. It belongs to the family Tungidae, order Siphonaptera.

　　T. penetrans. SYN: *chigger, chigoe, jigger, sand flea.* A small flea common in tropical regions which infests man, cats, dogs, rats, pigs, and other animals. They produce a severe local inflammation frequently liable to secondary infection.

tungsten (tŭng'stĕn). SYMB: *W* (for wolfram). At. wt. 183.85; at. no. 74. A metallic element.

tunic (tū'nĭk) [L. *tunica,* a sheath]. An investing membrane.

tunica (tū'nĭ-kă) [L. *tunica,* a sheath]. (pl. *tunicae*) An enveloping or covering membrane.

　　t. adventitia. [NA] Outer coat of an artery or any tubular structure.

　　t. albuginea. The white fibrous coat of the eye, testicle, ovary, or spleen.

　　t. externa. Outer coat of an artery.

　　t. interna. T. intima, q.v.

　　t. intima. Lining coat of an artery.

　　t. media. Middle muscular coat of an artery.

　　t. propria. Deep portion of the corium containing blood vessels, nerves, glands, and hair follicles.

　　t. vaginalis. Serous membrane surrounding the front and sides of the testicle.

tunnel (tŭn'ĕl). A narrow channel or passageway.

　　t. disease. Caisson disease, q.v.

　　t., inner. Triangular canal lying between the inner and outer pillars of Corti in the organ of Corti of inner ear. SYN: *tunnel of Corti.*

tunnel vision. 1. A condition seen in hysteria wherein the field of vision is the same regardless of distance from the visual screen. SYN: *tubular vision.* 2. Severe constriction of the visual field due to advanced chronic glaucoma. 3. An expression used to indicate a lack of ability to visualize the broad or long-range aspects of a problem or situation. When used this way the term has no reference to actual visual difficulty.

turbid (tŭr'bĭd) [L. *turba,* a tumult]. Cloudy; not clear. SEE: *turbidity.*

turbidimeter (tŭr-bĭ-dĭm'ĕ-ter) [L. *turbidus,* disturbed, + Gr. *metron,* a measure]. Device for estimating degree of turbidity of a fluid.

turbidimetry (tŭr-bĭ-dĭm'ĕ-trĭ) ["+ Gr. *metron,* a measure]. Estimation of the turbidity of a liquid.

turbidity (tŭr-bĭd'ĭ-tĭ) [L. *turbiditas,* turbidity]. 1. Quality of not having translucent appearance of liquid due to growth of microorganisms. 2. Having flaky or granular particles suspended in a clear liquid giving it a cloudy appearance. SEE: *clarificant.*

turbinate(d (tur'bĭ-nā"tĕd) [L. *turbo, turbin-,* a whirl]. Top- or cone-shaped.

　　t. bones. SYN: *conchae.* SEE: *conchae, nasal.*

turbinectomy (tŭr-bĭn-ĕk'tō-mĭ) ["+ Gr. *ektomē, excision*]. Excision of a turbinated bone.

turbinotome (tŭr-bĭn'ō-tōm) ["+ Gr. *tomē,* a cutting]. Instrument for excision of a turbinated bone.

turbinotomy (tŭr-bĭn-ŏt'ō-mĭ) ["+ Gr. *tomē,* incision]. Surgical incision of a turbinated bone.

turgescence (tur-jĕs'ĕns) [L. *turgescens,* swelling]. Swelling or enlargement of a part.

turgescent (tur-jĕs'ĕnt) [L. *turgescens,* swelling]. Swelling; inflated.

turgid (tur'jĭd) [L. *turgidus,* swollen]. Swollen; bloated.

turgor (tur'gor) [L. *turgor,* a swelling]. 1. Normal tension in a cell. 2. Distention, swelling.

　　t. vita'lis. Normal fullness of the capillaries and blood vessels.

turkey (tŭr'kĭ). A large North American bird that is widely domesticated for food.

Food value of 100 gm. (cooked, roasted light meat): Cal. 176; protein 33 gm.; fat 4 gm.

Dark meat has 10 per cent more calories than white meat.

turning (turn'ĭng) [AS. *turnian,* to turn]. Process of manually changing position of fetus in utero to permit normal delivery. SYN: *version.*

turnip (tŭr'nĭp). A widely cultivated plant having a large yellow or white root. This root is eaten as a vegetable.

Food value of 100 gm. (cooked): Cal. 23; protein 0.8 gm.; fat 0.2 gm.; carbohydrate 5.0 gm.; calcium 35 mg.; vitamin C 22 mg.

turnip greens (tŭr'nĭp grēnz). The leaves of young turnips sometimes eaten as food.

Food value of 100 gm. (boiled, and drained after cooking in a large amt. of water for a long time): Cal. 20; protein 2.2 gm.; fat 0.2 gm.; carbohydrate 3.3 gm.; vitamin A, 5700 I.U.; vitamin C, 47 mg.; calcium 174 mg.

Cooking in a small amt. of water for a short length of time allows less of the vitamin C to be lost.

turpentine (tur'pĕn-tin) [Gr. *terebinthos,* turpentine tree]. Oleoresin obtained from various species of pine trees. A mixture of terpenes and other hydrocarbons obtained from pine trees used externally in liniments and counterirritants. The source of oil of turpentine or spirits of turpentine.

POISONING: May occur from inhalation.

SYM: Warm or burning sensation in the gullet and stomach, followed by cramping, vomiting, and diarrhea. Pulse and respiration become weak, slow, and irregular; irritation of urinary tract and central nervous system resembling alcoholic intoxication.

F. A. TREATMENT: Gastric lavage, soothing drinks, and stimulants. Increase fluid intake.

turunda (tu-run'dă) [L.]. 1. A surgical tent, drain, or tampon. 2. A suppository.

tussal (tŭs'ăl) [L. *tussis,* cough]. Rel. to a cough. SYN: *tussive.*

tussis (tŭs'ĭs) [L. *tussis,* a cough]. A cough, as bronchial tussis, senile tussis, etc.

t. convulsi'va. Pertussis or whooping cough, q.v.

t. stomacha'lis. Reflex cough from irritation of the mucosa of the stomach.

tussive (tŭs'ĭv) [L. *tussis,* cough]. Relating to a cough. SYN: *tussal.*

twelfth cranial nerve. One of a pair of cranial nerves distributing to the base of the tongue. SEE: *hypoglossal nerve; Table of Nerves* in *Appendix.*

twilight sleep (twī'lĭt slēp). A state of partial anesthesia and hypoconsciousness in

which pain sense has been greatly reduced by the injection of morphine and scopolamine. Patient responds to pain, but afterward memory of pain is dulled or effaced. SEE: *labor.*

twilight state. One in which consciousness is disordered, making possible actions subsequently forgotten. Evidenced in hysteria, epilepsy, and dementia precox.

twin (twĭn) [AS. *twinn*]. One of two children developed within the uterus at the same time from the same impregnation. SEE: *Hellin's law.*

RS: enzygotic; fetus papyraceus.

t's., biovular. Dizygotic twins, q.v.

t's., conjoined. Twins which are united. SEE: *Siamese twins.*

t's., dizygotic. Those from two separate ova fertilized at the same time.

t's., fraternal. Dizygotic twins, q.v.

t's., identical. Twins which develop from a single fertilized ovum. Twins of this type have the same genetic makeup, consequently are of the same sex and resemble each other strikingly in physical, physiological, and mental traits. They develop within a common chorionic sac and have a common placenta. Each usually develops its own amnion and umbilical cord. Such twins may result from development of two inner cell masses within a blastocyst, development of two embryonic axes on a single blastoderm, or the division of a single embryonic axis into two centers.

t's., interlocked. Twins in which the neck of one becomes interlocked with the head of the other making vaginal delivery impossible.

t's., monozygotic. Those developing from a single fertilized ovum. These give rise to identical twins, q.v. Also called monochorionic, uniovular, or similar twins.

t., parasitic. The smaller of a pair of conjoined twins, when there is a marked disparity in size.

t's., Siamese. Symmetrical conjoined twins. SEE: *Siamese twins.*

t's., true. Monozygotic twins.

t's., uniovular. Those developing from a single ovum.

twinge (twĭnj) [AS. *twengan,* to pinch]. A sudden, keen pain.

twitch (twĭch) [ME. *twicchen*]. 1. A simple, quick, spasmodic contraction of a muscle. 2. To jerk convulsively. SEE: *myokymia, myopalmus.*

tylion (tĭl'ĭ-ŏn) [Gr. *tyleion,* knot]. Point at middle of anterior edge of the optic groove.

tyloma (tĭ-lō'mă) [Gr. *tylos,* knot, + *-ōma,* tumor]. A callosity.

tylosis (tī-lō'sĭs) ["+ *-ōsis,* condition]. 1. A callosity. SYN: *tyloma.* 2. Formation of a callus.

tympanal (tĭm'păn-ăl) [Gr. *tympanon* drum]. Rel. to the tympanum. SYN: *tympanic.*

tympanectomy (tĭm″păn-ĕk'tō-mĭ) ["+ *ektomē,* excision]. Excision of the tympanic membrane.

tympanic (tĭm-păn'ĭk) [Gr. *tympanon,* drum]. 1. Pert. to the tympanum. 2. Resonant.

   t. membrane. Membrane serving as the lateral wall of the tympanic cavity and separating it from the external acoustic meatus. SYN: *drum membrane; eardrum.* SEE: *tympanum.*

tympanism (tĭm'păn-ĭzm) [Gr. *tympanon,* drum, + *-ismos,* condition]. Abdominal inflation from gas. SYN: *tympanites.*

tympanites (tĭm-păn-ī'tēz). Abdominal distention due to intestinal gas.

tympanitic (tĭm-păn-ĭt'ĭk) [Gr. *tympanitēs,* distention]. 1. Pert. to or characterized by tympanites. 2. Resonant. SYN: *tympanic.*

   t. resonance. A sound produced by percussion over an air- or gas-filled cavity.

tympanitis (tĭm-păn-ī'tĭs) [Gr. *tympanon,* drum, + *-itis,* inflammation]. Inflammation of the middle ear. SYN: *otitis media.*

tympano- [Gr.]. Combining form meaning eardrum, tympanum of the ear.

tympanomastoiditis (tĭm″păn-ō-măs-toy-dī'tĭs) ["+ *mastos,* breast, + *eidos,* form, + *-itis,* inflammation]. Inflammation of the tympanum and mastoid cells.

tympanoplasty (tĭm″păn-ō-plăs'tĭ) [Gr. *tympanon,* drum, + *plassein,* to form]. Any one of several surgical procedures designed to either cure a chronic inflammatory process in the middle ear or to restore function to the sound-transmitting mechanism of the middle ear.

tympanosis (tĭm-pă-nō'sĭs) ["+ *-osis,* condition]. Tympanites, q.v.

tympanotomy (tĭm″păn-ŏt'ō-mĭ) ["+ *tomē,* a cutting]. Incision of the membrana tympani. SYN: *myringotomy.*

tympanous (tĭm'păn-ŭs) [Gr. *tympanon,* a drum]. Marked by abdominal distention with gas.

tympanum (tĭm'păn-ŭm) [Gr. *tympanon*]. The middle ear or tympanic cavity. SYN: *cavum tympani, eardrum.* SEE: *ear, middle.*

   t. antrum. The space by which the epitympanic recess of the tympanic cavity proper communicates with the mastoid cells.

   t. cavity. The cavity of the middle ear. SEE: *tympanum.*

tympany (tĭm'pă-nĭ). 1. Abdominal distention with gas. 2. Tympanic resonance on percussion. It is a clear hollow note like that of a drum having no vesicular quality. It indicates a pathological condition of the lung or of a cavity.

type (tīp) [Gr. *typos,* mark]. The general character of a person, a disease, or substance.

   RS: Aztec; koinotropic; sexual psychopathy; syntonic.

   t., asthenic. One who is slender with a long chest that is flat and who has poor muscular development.

   t., pyknic. One with a rounded body, thick shoulders, large chest, short neck, and broad head.

   t., vagotonic. One with deficient adrenal gland secretion, with slow pulse, low blood pressure, and high sugar tolerance.

typhlatonia, typhlatony (tĭf-lă-tō'nĭ-ă, -lăt'ō-nĭ) [Gr. *typhlon,* cecum, + *tonos,* tone]. Deficient motor activity of the cecum.

typhlectasis (tĭf-lĕk'tă-sĭs) ["+ *ektasis,* dilatation]. Cecal distention.

typhlectomy (tĭf-lĕk'tō-mĭ) ["+ *ektomē,* excision]. Excision of the cecum. SYN: *cecectomy.*

typhlenteritis (tĭf-lĕn-ter-ī'tĭs) [Gr. *typhlon,* cecum, + *enteron,* intestine, + *-itis,* inflammation]. Inflammation of the cecum. SYN: *typhlitis.*

typhlitis (tĭf-lī'tĭs) ["+ *-itis,* inflammation]. Inflammation of the cecum.

typhlodicliditis (tĭf'lō-dĭk-lĭ-dī'tĭs) ["+ *diklis,* door, + *-itis,* inflammation]. Inflammation of the ileocecal valve.

typhloempyema (tĭf'lō-ĕm-pī-ē'mă) ["+ *en,* in, + *pyon,* pus, + *haima,* blood]. An abdominal abscess following appendicitis.

typhloenteritis (tĭf'lō-ĕn-ter-ī'tĭs) [Gr. *typhlon,* cecum, + *enteron,* intestine, + *-itis,* inflammation]. Inflammation of the cecum. SYN: *typhlenteritis, typhlitis.*

typhlolexia (tĭf'lō-lĕks'ĭ-ă) [Gr. *typhlos,* blind, + *lexis,* speech]. Inability to recognize written or spoken words. SYN: *word blindness.*

typhlolithiasis (tĭf'lō-lĭ-thī'ă-sĭs) [Gr. *typhlon,* cecum, + *lithos,* stone, + *-iasis,* condition]. Formation of a concretion in the cecum.

typhlology (tĭf-lŏl'ō-jĭ) [Gr. *typhlos,* blind, + *logos,* study]. Study of blindness, its causes and effects.

typhlopexy (tĭf'lo-pĕks'ĭ) [Gr. *typhlon,* cecum, + *pexis,* fixation]. Suturing of a movable cecum to the abdominal wall.

typhlosis (tĭf-lō'sĭs) [Gr. *typhlos,* blind, + *-ōsis,* condition]. Blindness.

typhlospasm (tĭf'lō-spăsm). Spasm of the cecum.

typhlostenosis (tĭf-lō-stĕn-ō'sĭs) [Gr. *typh-lon*, cecum, + *stenōsis*, a narrowing]. Stenosis or stricture of the cecum.

typhlostomy (tĭf-lŏs'tō-mĭ) ["+ *stoma*, opening]. Establishment of a permanent cecal fistula.

typhlotomy (tĭf-lŏt'ō-mĭ) [Gr. *typhlon*, cecum, + *tomē*, a cutting]. Incision of the cecum.

typhloureterostomy (tĭf'lō-ū-rē''ter-ŏs'tō-mĭ) ["+ *ourētēr*, ureter, + *stoma*, opening]. Implantation of a ureter in the cecum.

typho- [Gr.]. Combining form pert. to fever, typhoid.

typhobacillosis (tī''fō-băs-ĭl-ō'sĭs) [Gr. *ty-phos*, stupor, + L. *bacillus*, little stick, + Gr. *-ōsis*, condition]. Poisoning due to toxins produced by the typhoid bacillus.

typhohemia (tī''fō-hē'mĭ-ă) ["+ *haima*, blood]. Degeneration of the blood due to presence of bacilli.

typhoid (tī'foyd) [Gr. *typhos*, stupor, + *eidos*, form]. Resembling typhus.

    t. fever. An acute, infectious disease characterized by definite lesions in Peyer's patches, mesenteric glands, and spleen accompanied by fever, headache, and abdominal symptoms.

    ETIOL: Causative organism Salmonella typhosa (Eberthella typhi, a gram-negative, motile bacillus. Common in early adult life and esp. prevalent during fall and early winter. It may be transmitted by infected water or milk supplies. Well water in country districts sometimes contaminated through the soil from outhouses. Human carriers, particularly when food handlers may be responsible for spread of infection. Body discharges from active or convalescent cases may be the means of infecting others.

    INCUBATION: Average, two weeks; varies from one to three weeks.

    SYM: Early symptoms are: Headache, general weakness, indefinite pains, nosebleed; constipation may occur. Within a few days to a week the temperature may reach a maximum of 104°-105° F. (40°-40.6° C.) and during this time, or up to the 10th day, rose spots can usually be seen, particularly on the abdomen, though they may be observed on the chest and back. They usually come out in crops during a period of several days and disappear upon pressure. Abdominal tenderness develops and with it, generally, distention. Splenomegaly will be found in more than half of the cases by the end of the first week.

    During following weeks fever is characterized by marked daily remissions, evening temperature being from 1°-3° F. (.56°-1.7° C.)

higher than the morning. In the young, the temperature often rises very abruptly. When the diurnal remissions are slight, a protracted case is forecast. As defervescence advances, the temperature becomes more irregular. Remissions are more decided and not infrequently a higher temperature is recorded in the morning. Hurried respiration, slight cough, and bronchial rales are common. Pulse is usually slow in comparison with the temperature rise, and is dicrotic. Heart sounds often feeble, expression dull and heavy, cheeks somewhat flushed, conjunctivae clear, pupils dilated.

    Tongue tremulous; at first red at tip and edges, and covered posteriorly with a whitish fur. In severe cases, tongue becomes dry, brown and fissured, and sordes collect on teeth. Gastric symptoms not common, but obstinate. Vomiting sometimes develops and becomes a serious complication. Abdomen tympanitic, tenderness on palpation, esp. in iliac fossa. Diarrhea generally present, though not a constant symptom. Discharges vary from three to six or more a day; thin, offensive, yellowish. Stupor, muttering, delirium, twitching of the tendons, carphologia, and coma vigil may be present. Urine usually shows albumin. Retention common.

    White blood count demonstrates a leukopenia. Convalescence marked by anemia, falling of hair, often desquamation. The patient gives evidence of having suffered from a protracted illness that has produced general enfeeblement of mind and body.

    VARIETIES: *Abortive:* Abrupt onset with severe symptoms, but convalescence follows within a few days. Often seen in children. *Mild form:* Moderate fever with marked remissions, diarrhea slight, nervous symptoms often absent, rash usually present and often abundant. *Ambulatory type* (walking typhoid): Symptoms mild and often disregarded by patient, who refuses to go to bed. However, grave symptoms may suddenly develop and even death from intestinal perforation may follow. *Typhoid of children:* Rash often absent, fever rises abruptly, cerebral symptoms may be sufficiently marked to suggest meningitis.

    RELAPSES: These are common in typhoid. There may be a complete repetition of all symptoms experienced during primary attack, but they are usually of shorter duration.

    RECRUDESCENCE: This is a sudden, temporary elevation of temperature occurring during convalescence, and is not associated with a return of other symptoms. It may be due to constipation, excitement, or irritating food.

COMPLICATIONS: These occur in approximately 25% of cases and account for the majority of the deaths. The most frequent and dangerous complications are intestinal hemorrhage and intestinal perforation. An abrupt fall of several degrees in temperature is suggestive of intestinal hemorrhage or perforation. Usually occurs during 3rd or 4th week.

DIFFERENTIAL DIAG: Paratyphoid, pneumonia, dysentery, meningitis, smallpox, appendicitis. Diagnostic points of value will be the presence of rose spots, splenomegaly, leukopenia, the Widal serological test, blood culture and examination of feces for presence of causative organism.

PROG: Should always be guarded, no matter how mild the case appears to be. Fatality rate varies in different epidemics. Hemorrhages in any form, together with excessive diarrhea, are unfavorable signs.

PROPHYLAXIS: Safeguards adopted for the supply of drinking water in large cities and the more or less general pasteurization of milk are probably chief factors in the great reduction of typhoid fever in well-governed communities. Active immunization is a factor in reduction of mortality. Individual immunity can ordinarily be established by administerng two injections of high-antigenicity vaccine spaced by several weeks. SEE: *typhoid vaccine.*

TREATMENT OF THE ACTIVE CASE: General care, isolation of patient, and disinfection of all discharges are of primary importance. Those caring for the typhoid patient should be immunized against the disease. All precautions applicable to such infections must be adopted. Articles in contact with the patient must be sterilized or disinfected before being handled by persons other than the immediate attendant. It is necessary to guard against development of bedsores. Since delirium is not infrequent, patient may require constant watching to prevent his leaving the bed, which might result in fatal consequences. The mouth should be kept as clean as possible to prevent development of sordes.

Ampicillin is the drug of choice, but chloramphenicol may be required in severe cases.

DIET: A bland or liquid diet of 3000 Cal. should be given until the patient improves, then frequent relatively high-calorie feedings. If intestinal symptoms prevent oral feedings intravenous fluids and feedings will be required. The starvation diet, once so common in treatment of typhoid fever, is seldom followed in the present day.

Ice bags and cold sponging are little used at the present time. On the other hand, sponging with tepid water, or with alcohol, is sometimes used when the temperature has reached unusual heights. Surgical intervention will be necessary if antibiotics and bowel decompression fail to control severe hemorrhage or intestinal perforation.

NP: The objectives are to support the patient's strength, to lessen toxemia, and to prevent complications and the spread of the disease. Strict isolation technique should be followed.

Quiet is essential; visitors, excitement, and noise are not conducive to quiet or peace of mind. Bright lights, heavy bedclothing, and everything that might irritate the patient should be avoided. An airy, well-ventilated room is essential. The bed must be comfortable and protection provided in case of incontinence. If the patient becomes emaciated an air bed may be necessary.

Position of patient: Usually he lies on one side with knees drawn up. If sores are apt to develop, the knees should be wrapped in wool to prevent chafing when together. Extra pillows are permissible if desired by the patient. The patient should make no muscular effort while the bed is being made.

Care of the mouth: Frequent soft swabs and bland lotions should be used, as sordes gather on the teeth and the mouth is dry, brown, and fissured. Keeping the mouth moist cannot be overemphasized.

Care of the skin: A morning and night cleansing bath should be given. In the meantime, tepid sponging will remove perspiration and help maintain the function of the skin and also assist in elimination. Because the secretion of the skin carries infection, water used for bathing should be disposed of and the basin disinfected. The patient's hands should be kept scrupulously clean to prevent them from being contaminated with excreta. Ointment should be used to protect the skin in cases of incontinence.

Headache and backache: A severe frontal headache may last from 10-14 days from inception of the fever. The light should be shaded and cold compresses applied. The legs and back should be suppported with pillows.

Restlessness: This may induce sleeplessness. A change of position, a sponge bath, taking off a cover if the patient is hot or adding one if cold, and washing the face and brushing the hair will do much to rest the patient.

Urine: This should be measured and tested daily for albumin. Watch for sign of retention due to atony of the bladder's muscular wall in the latter weeks of illness.

Stools: Inspection for presence of undigested food, blood, and flatus is very important. Frequency should be noted. Four or five movements per day is normal in diarrhea, but 8-12 indicate complications. Constipation is not unusual with these patients; nevertheless, laxatives and enemas should not be used. Stool softeners may be used. When complicated by hemorrhages, and frequent stools, the patient may be too exhausted to use a bedpan, in which case the excreta should be received on pads.

Abdominal distention: This may become a dangerous complication; in any event it is distressing. Decompression by gastric or intestinal drainage may be used, but this is hazardous because of the danger of causing perforation or hemorrhage.

Bathing: Baths, their nature and frequency should be left to the discretion of the physician; otherwise routine care such as cleansing and sponge baths may be used unless contraindicated.

Delirium: This is usually of the low muttering type, and the patient stares with a fixed gaze upon the ceiling and plucks on the bedclothing. Utensils and other articles should not be left within his reach and he must not be left alone.

Charting: A four-hour chart should be kept of temperature, pulse, and respiration, although the pulse should be taken much more frequently than this. In the 3rd week, the temperature should be taken every two hours. A sudden drop in temperature indicates hemorrhage.

Disinfection: The usual methods of disinfection should be observed in handling all excreta and secretions, linens, and utensils. Disinfection for the nurse is also very important.

t. state. Condition in many diseases marked by profound prostration and other symptoms like those of typhus or typhoid fever.

t. vaccine. A vaccine containing killed typhoid bacilli. Even though its effectiveness in preventing typhoid fever is debatable, its use is advisable in persons who will be exposed to typhoid bacilli.

t., walking. T. fever with mild general constitutional symptoms, the patient being able to be up and to walk. SYN: *ambulatory typhoid.*

typhoidal (tĭ-foy'dăl) [Gr. *typhos,* stupor, + *eidos,* resemblance]. Resembling typhoid.

typholysin (tĭ-fŏl'ĭ-sĭn) ["+ *lysis,* dissolution]. A lysin destructive to typhoid bacilli.

typhomalarial (tĭ''fō-mă-lā'rĭ-ăl) [Gr. *typhos,* stupor, + Italian *malaria,* bad air]. Having symptoms of both typhoid and malarial fever.

typhomania (tĭ-fō-mā'nĭ-ă) [Gr. *typhos,* stupor, + *mania,* madness]. Muttering delirium characteristic of typhoid fever and typhus.

typhopneumonia (tĭ''fō-nū-mō'nĭ-ă) ["+ *pneumōnia,* inflammation of lungs]. 1. Pneumonia occurring in typhoid fever. 2. Pneumonia with typhoid symptoms.

typhous (tĭ'fŭs) [Gr. *typhos,* stupor]. Pert. to typhus fever.

typhus, typhus fever (tĭ'fŭs) [Gr. *typhos,* stupor]. One of a group of acute, infectious diseases characterized by great prostration, severe headache, generalized maculopapular rash, sustained high fever, and usually progressive neurologic involvement, ending in a crisis in 10 to 14 days.

Three diseases are included in the group: epidemic (louse-borne) typhus, Brill-Zinsser disease (recrudescent typhus), and murine (flea-borne) typhus. Although clinically and pathologically similar, they differ in intensity of symptoms, severity, and mortality rate.

Epidemic typhus is particularly prevalent amid unsanitary conditions. It often develops on shipboard, in army camps, and where living conditions are unfavorable and congestion is marked. The disease is rare in the U.S., infection being found principally at the seaboard as a result of imported cases.

INCUBATION: Six to 14 days.

SYM: Onset sudden. Severe headache, pain in back and limbs, extreme prostration. Fever rises rapidly, often reaching 104° to 105° F. (40°-40.6° C.) in from two to three days. Remains high for about 10 days, when

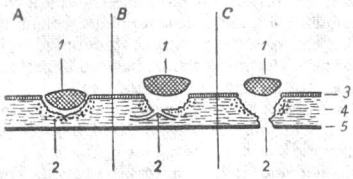

TYPHOID ULCERS
A, In Peyer's patch: 1, slough in ulcer; 2, lymphoid tissue. B, Erosion of blood vessel with separation of slough, causing hemorrhage: 1, slough separated; 2, eroded artery. C, Perforation of ulcer through peritoneum: 1, slough separated; 2, peritoneal perforation; 3, mucous membrane; 4, muscle layer; 5, peritoneum.

it falls by crisis. Pulse rapid, weak, often dicrotic. Tongue tremulous, may be covered with whitish fur; in severe cases becomes black and rolled up like a ball in back of mouth. Face dusky, conjunctivae injected, pupil contracted, headache, stupor, delirium, muscle twitching, picking at the bedclothes (carphologia).

From 4th to 5th day, bluish spots appear over body, esp. on abdomen. These are petechial in character and do not disappear on pressure. The extent of eruption is indicative of severity of attack. Sometimes there is a diffuse, dark red, subcuticular mottling. Bowels are constipated, urine is scanty, high-colored and often albuminous.

COMPLICATIONS: Bronchopneumonia more frequent than lobar, hypostatic congestion of lungs, nephritis, and parotid abscess.

DIFFERENTIAL DIAG: Typhoid fever, hemorrhagic smallpox, Henoch's purpura, epidemic meningitis of fulminating type, and ulcerative endocarditis may have to be considered.

PROG: Variable. Mortality may be quite high in epidemic typhus and almost nonexistent in murine typhus. Broad-spectrum antibiotics will be life saving if given early enough.

TREATMENT: *Preventive:* Absolute cleanliness, sterilization of clothing, and the use of apparel to prevent infestation of the body louse. The delousing camps, so common during the late war, were examples of the precautions necessary to prevent its spread. Patient must be isolated. Absolute rest necessary, and a liquid diet. *Specific:* Broad-spectrum antibiotics, such as the tetracyclines and chloramphenicol, give excellent results. PABA (para-aminobenzoic acid) is also useful.

t., classic. T., epidemic, q.v.

t., endemic. T., murine, q.v.

t., epidemic. An infectious disease caused by Rickettsia prowazekii and transmitted by the human body louse (Pediculus humanus corporis). SYN: *louse-borne t.*

t., flea-borne. T., murine, q.v.

t., Mexican. A louse-borne epidemic typhus present in certain portions of Mexico. SYN: *tabardillo.*

t., mite-borne. Tsutsugamushi disease or scrub typhus.

t., murine. A disease caused by Rickettsia mooseri and occurring in nature as a mild infection of rats and transmitted from rat to rat by the rat-louse or flea. Humans may acquire it by being bitten by infected rat-fleas or ingesting food contaminated by rat-urine or flea-feces. SYN: *flea-borne t.*

t., rat. T., murine, q.v.

t., recrudescent. A recurrence or recrudescence of a preceding attack of epidemic typhus after initial attack. SYN: *Brill's disease; Brill-Zinsser disease.*

t., rural. T., scrub, q.v.

t., scrub. A self-limited febrile disease of two weeks duration caused by Rickettsia tsutsugamushi and transmitted by two species of mites (chiggers) of the genus Thrombicula. Occurs principally in Pacific-Asiatic area. SYN: *mite-borne* or *rural typhus; Japanese river fever; Tsutsugamushi disease.*

t., shop. T., murine, q.v.

t., urban. T., epidemic, q.v.

typical (tĭp'ĭ-kăl) [Gr. *typikos,* pert. to type]. Having the characteristics of, pert. to, or conforming to, a type or condition or group.

typing (tĭp'ĭng). The determination of the specific blood group to which an individual belongs or testing of tissue. Also the determination of the specific type or subdivision of a species to which certain bacteria (e.g., Salmonella or Diplococcus pneumoniae) belong. SEE: *blood transfusion.*

t., tissue. Techniques utilized in determining the histocompatibility of tissues to be used in grafts and transplants with the recipient's tissues and cells. SEE: *transplantation.*

typo- [Gr.]. Combining form meaning a type.

typoscope (tĭ'pō-skōp) ["+ *skopein,* to examine]. Device to aid patients with amblyopia and cataract in reading.

tyramine (tī'rä-mēn). Intermediate product in the conversion of tyrosine to epinephrine.

T. is found in some ripened, aged cheese; and in beer, broad bean pods, yeast, wine, and chicken liver. When persons taking certain types of antidepressant monoamine oxidase inhibitors also eat this type of cheese they may experience severe hypertension, headache, palpitation, neck pain, and perhaps intracranial hemorrhage. This is due to the tyramine's not being inactivated by monoamine oxidation. This has been called the "cheese reaction."

tyrannism (tĭr'ăn-ĭzm) [Gr. *tyrannos,* tyrant, + *-ismos,* condition]. Abnormal tendency to exercise cruelty. SYN: *sadism,* q.v.

tyremesis (tī-rĕm'ĕ-sĭs) [Gr. *tyros,* cheese, + *emesis,* vomiting]. Infant vomiting of curdy or cheesy substances.

tyrogenous (tī-rŏj'ĕn-ŭs) ["+ *gennan,* to produce]. Having origin in cheese or produced by it.

Tyroglyphus (tī-rŏg'lĭ-fūs) [Gr. *tyros,* cheese, + *glyphein,* to carve]. A genus of sarcoptoid mites commonly known as cheese mites. They infest cheese and dried vegetable food products and occassionally infest man causing a pruritus. Contains species causing grocer's itch, vanillism and copra itch.

tyroid (tī'royd) ["+ *eidos,* form]. Caseous; cheesy.

tyromatosis (tī-rŏ-mă-tō'sĭs) ["+ "+ *-osis,* condition]. Cheesy degeneration. SYN: *caseation.*

tyrosinase (tī-rō'sĭn-ās) [Gr. *tyros,* cheese]. An enzyme which acts on tyrosine to produce melanin.

tyrosine (tī'rō-sĭn). An amino acid present in many proteins, esp. casein. It serves as a precursor of epinephrine, thyroxine, and melanin. Two vitamins, ascorbic acid and folic acid, are essential for its metabolism.

tyrosinosis (tī-rō-sĭn-ō'sĭs) [Gr. *tyros,* cheese, + *-osis,* condition]. Condition resulting from faulty metabolism of tyrosine, whereby its oxidation products appear in the urine.

tyrosinuria (tī-rō-sĭn-ū'rĭ-ă) ["+ *ouron,* urine]. Tyrosine in the urine.

tyrosis (tī-rō'sĭs) [Gr. *tyros,* cheese, + *-osis,* condition]. 1. Curdling of milk. 2. Vomiting of cheesy substance by infants. SYN: *tyremesis,* q.v. 3. Cheesy degeneration. SYN: *tyromatosis.*

tyrotoxism (tī-rō-tŏks'ĭzm) ["+ "+ *-ismos,* condition]. Poisoning produced by a milk product or by cheese.

Tyrrell's fascia (tĭr-rĕlz). [Frederick Tyrrell, Eng. anatomist, 1797-1843] An ill-defined fibromuscular layer from the middle aponeurosis of the perineum, behind the prostate gland. SYN: *rectovesical fascia.*

Tyson's glands (tī-sŭnz). [Edward Tyson, Eng. physician and anatomist, 1649-1708] Modified sebaceous glands located on neck of penis and inner surface of prepuce. Their secretion is one of the components of smegma. SYN: *preputial glands.*

Tzank test. [Arnault Tzank, Russ. dermatologist in Paris, 1886-1954] Test of cells obtained from floor of pemphigus bulla to substantiate the diagnosis.

U

U. 1. Chem. symbol of uranium. 2. Abbr. for *unit.*

uarthritis (ū″ar-thrī′tĭs) [Gr. *arthron*, joint, + *-itis*, inflammation]. Gout supposed to result from excess of uric acid. SYN: *arthritis urica.*

uberous (ū′bĕr-ŭs) [L. *uber*, udder]. Prolific; fruitful; fertile.

uberty (ū′bĕr-tĭ) [L. *uber*, udder]. Fruitfulness; fertility.

UBI. Abbr. for *ultraviolet blood irradiation.*

Uffelmann's test (oof′ĕl-mahn). [Jules Uffelmann, Ger. physician, 1837-1894]. Test for determination of lactic acid in gastric juice.

Uhthoff's sign (ūt′hŏf). [Wilhelm Uhthoff, Ger. ophthalmologist, 1853-1927]. The nystagmus which occurs in multiple disseminated sclerosis.

ulaganactesis (ū-lăg″ă-năk′tĕ-sĭs) [Gr. *oulon*, gum, + *aganektesis*, irritation]. Disagreeable sensations or irritation in or about the gums.

ulalgia (ū-lăl′jĭ-ă) [Gr. *oulon*, gum, + *algos*, pain]. Pain in the gums.

ulatrophia (ū-lă-trō′fĭ-ă) [Gr. *oulon*, gum, + *atrophos*, ill-nourished]. Shrinking of gums; recession of the gums.

ulcer (ŭl′ser) [L. *ulcus, ulcer-*, ulcer]. An open sore or lesion of the skin or mucous membrane of the body, with loss of substance, sometimes accompanied by formation of pus.

Simple ulcers may result from trauma, caustics, or intense heat or cold. They may occur as a complication of varicose veins.

In syphilis, they are deep seated, having an offensive secretion; in epithelioma, they have a single center and a thickened, infiltrated edge with a scanty, bloody secretion; in lupus vulgaris, they are superficial.

RS: abscission; anabrosis; anthracosis; aphtha; argema; carcinelcosis; carcinomelcosis; chalarosis; dieresis; duodenal u.; peptic; phagedena; rodent u.; slough; stomach.

u., amputating. U. which destroys tissue to the bone by encircling the part.

u., atonic. A chronic ulcer.

u., callous. A chronic u. with indurated, elevated edges and no granulations, which does not heal.

u., Curling's. Peptic ulcer which sometimes occurs following a severe burn.

u., decubitus. A bedsore; a pressure sore. SEE: *bed, air; bed, float.*

u., duodenal. An u. on the mucosa of the duodenum, due to the action of the gastric juice.

u., erethistic. U. with an inflamed, red, painful surface.

u., follicular. A tiny u. having its origin in a lymph follicle and affecting a mucous membrane.

u., fungus. U. in which the granulations protrude above edges of wound and bleed easily.

u., gastric. U., peptic, q.v.

u., healthy. An u. which tends toward healing, its surface being soft and smooth with tiny red granulations.

u., indolent. Nearly painless u. usually found on leg, characterized by indurated and elevated edge, and nongranulating base.

u., peptic. An u. of the mucosa of the duodenum or stomach.

u., perforating. An u. which permeates the entire thickness of the part, as the foot or intestine.

u., phagedenic. An u. which sloughs particles, spreading rapidly and disintegrating the tissues.

u., rodent. A deeply infiltrating u. which slowly destroys bones and soft tissues; commonly affects the upper part of the face.

u., round. U., peptic, q.v.

u., serpiginous. A creeping u. which heals in one part and extends to another.

u., simple. A local u. with no severe inflammation or pain.

u., specific. An u. caused by a specific disease, as syphilis or lupus.

u., stercoral. 1. U. caused by pressure from impacted feces. 2. U. through which feces escape.

u., stress. Peptic u. due to acute or chronic stress such as may be present with cerebral trauma, burns, surgery, acute infection, prolonged adrenal corticosteroid therapy, or central nervous system disease.

ulcera. Pl. of ulcus, q.v.

ulcerate (ŭl′sĕr-āt) [L. *ulcerāre*, to ulcerate]. To produce or become affected with an ulcer.

ulcerated (ŭl′sĕr-ā″tĕd). Of the nature of an ulcer or affected with one.

u. sore throat. Putrid sore throat, a gangrenous inflammation.

u. tooth. Suppuration of the alveolar periosteum with ulceration of gum surrounding the decaying root of a tooth.

ulceration (ŭl″sĕr-ā′shŭn). Suppuration taking place on a free surface, as on the skin or on a mucous membrane.

A termination of inflammation.

ulcerative (ŭl′sĕr-ā-tĭv) [L. *ulcerāre*, to form ulcers]. Pert. to or causing ulceration.

   u. scrofuloderma. Tubercular scrofuloderma.

ulcerogenic drugs. Medicines which, because of their systemic rather than local effects, may cause peptic ulcers.

ulceromembranous (ŭl″sĕr-ō-mĕm′brăn-ŭs) ["+ *membrana*, membrane]. Pert. to ulceration and formation of a fibrous pseudomembrane.

   u. tonsillitis. Tonsillitis that ulcerates and develops a membranous film.

ulcerous (ŭl′sĕr-ŭs). Pert. to or affected with an ulcer.

ulcus (ŭl′kŭs) [L.]. (pl. *ulcera*) Ulcer.

   u. cancro′sum. Cancerous ulcer which eats away the tissues. SYN: *rodent ulcer.*

   u. cruris. Indolent ulcer of the leg.

   u. durum. Lesion of syphilis. A hard ulcer. SYN: *chancre.*

   u. induratum. A chancre, q.v.

   u. molle. Chancroid or soft chancre, q.v.

   u. tuberculo′sum. Tuberculosis of the skin. SYN: *lupus.*

ulectomy (ū-lĕk′tō-mĭ). 1. [Gr. *oulē*, scar, + *ektomē*, excision]. Excision of scar tissue, esp. in secondary iridectomy. 2. [Gr. *oulon*, gum, + *ektomē*, excision]. Removal of gum tissue, as in pyorrhea alveolaris. SYN: *gingivectomy.*

ulegyria (ū″lē-jĭ′rĭ-ă) [Gr. *oulē*, scar, + *gyros*, ring]. Condition in which gyri of the cerebral cortex are abnormal due to scar tissue from injuries usually occurring in early development.

ulemorrhagia (ū″lĕm-ō-rā′jĭ-ă) [Gr. *oulon*, gum, + *rhēgnynai*, to burst forth]. Bleeding from the gums.

ulerythema (ū-lĕr-ĭ-thē′mă) [Gr. *oulē*, scar, + *erythēma*, redness]. An erythematous disorder with atrophic scar formation. SEE: *lupus erythematosus.*

   u. centrifugum. Lupus erythematosus.

   u. ophryog′enes. Folliculitis of eyebrows.

   SYM: Falling out of hair and scarring.

   u. sycosiforme. Inflammation of the hair follicles of the beard with alopecia in the affected area. SYN: *lupoid sycosis.*

uletic (ū-lĕt′ĭk) [Gr. *oulon*, gum]. Pert. to the gums.

uletomy (ū-lĕt′ō-mĭ) [Gr. *oulē*, scar, + *tomē*, a cutting]. Incision of a scar to relieve tension. SYN: *cicatricotomy.*

uliginous (ū-lĭj′ĭ-nŭs) [L. *uliginosus*, wet]. Muddy; slimy.

ulitis (ū-lī′tĭs) [Gr. *oulon*, gum, + *-ītis*, inflammation]. Inflammation of the gums.

   u., interstitial. Inflammation of connective tissue of gums about the necks of the teeth.

ulna (ŭl′nă) [L. *ulna*, elbow]. The inner and larger bone of the forearm, between the wrist and the elbow, on the side opposite that of the thumb.

   It articulates with the head of the radius and humerus above and with the radius below.

   RS: coronoid process; cubital; cubitus; olecranon; skeleton.

ulnad (ŭl′năd) ["+ *ad*, toward]. In the direction of the ulna.

ulnar (ŭl′nar) [L. *ulna*, elbow]. 1. Rel. to the ulna, or to nerve or artery named from it. 2. Cuneiform carpal bone. SYN: *ulnare.*

ulnocarpal (ŭl″nō-kar′păl) [L. *ulna*, elbow, + Gr. *karpos*, wrist]. Relating to the carpus and ulna, or to the ulnar side of the wrist.

ulnoradial (ŭl″nō-rā′dĭ-ăl) ["+ *radius*, spoke of a wheel]. Rel. to the ulna and radius, as their ligaments and articulations.

ulocace (ū-lŏk′ā-sē) [Gr. *oulon*, gum, + *kakē*, badness]. Ulcerative inflammation of the gums.

ulocarcinoma (ū″lō-kar-sĭn-ō′mă) ["+ *karkinos*, cancer, + *-ōma*, tumor]. Carcinoma of the gums.

ulodermatitis (ū″lō-derm-ă-tī′tĭs) [Gr. *oulē*, scar, + *derma*, skin, + *-ītis*, inflammation]. Dermatitis with scar tissue formation.

uloglossitis (ū″lō-glos-ī′tĭs) ["+ *glossa*, tongue, + *-ītis*, inflammation]. Inflammation of the gums and tongue.

uloid (ū′loyd) [Gr. *oulē*, scar, + *eidos*, resemblance]. 1. Scarlike. 2. A scarlike lesion caused by subcutaneous degeneration. SYN: *u. cicatrix.*

   u. cicatrix. A scarlike lesion caused by subcutaneous degeneration.

uloncus (ū-lŏn′kŭs) [Gr. *oulon*, gum, + *onkos*, mass]. Swelling or tumor of the gums. SEE: *epulis.*

ulorrhagia (ū-lor-ā′jĭ-ă) [Gr. *oulon*, gum, + *rhēgnynai*, to burst forth]. Bleeding from the gums.

ulorrhea (ū″lor-rē′ă) ["+ *rhoia*, a flow]. Slow bleeding from the gums.

ulosis (ū-lō′sĭs) [Gr. *oulē*, scar, + *-ōsis*, condition]. Formation of scar tissue. SYN: *cicatrization.*

ulotic (ū-lŏt′ĭk) [Gr. *oulē*, scar]. Causing cicatrization. SYN: *cicatricial.*

ulotomy (ū-lŏt′ō-mĭ). 1. [Gr. *oulē*, scar, + *tomē*, a cutting]. The cutting of scar tissue to relieve deformity or tension. 2. [Gr. *oulon,* gum, + *tomē,* a cutting]. Incision of the gums.

ulotrichous (ū-lŏt'rĭk-ŭs) [Gr. *oulos,* woolly, + *thrix, trich-,* hair]. Having short, woolly hair, characteristic of some races.

ulotripsis (u"lo-trip'sĭs) [Gr. *oulon,* gum, + *tripsis,* massage]. Stimulation of the gums by massage.

ultex (ŭl'tĕks). A bifocal glass in which the near section is ground integral with the spherical curve.

ultimate (ŭl'tĭm-āt) [L. *ultimus,* last]. Final or last.

ultimobranchial bodies (ŭl-tĭ-mō-brăng'kĭ-ăl). Two embryonic pharyngeal pouches usually considered as rudimentary fifth pouches. They become separated from the pharynx and incorporated into substance of the thyroid gland where they lose their identity. SYN: *postbranchial bodies.*

ultra- [L.]. Prefix meaning beyond, excess.

ultrabrachycephalic (ŭl"trä-brăk"ĭ-sē-făl'-ĭk) [L. *ultra,* beyond, + Gr. *brachys,* short, + *kephalē,* head]. Having a cephalic index of 90 or over.

ultracentrifuge (ŭl-trä-sĕn'trĭ-fūj) [L. *ultra,* beyond, + *centrum,* center, + *fugere,* to flee]. A high speed centrifuge capable of producing centrifugal forces more than 100,-000 times gravity. Used in the study of proteins, viruses, etc.

ultrafilter (ŭl-trä-fĭl'tĕr). A filter by which colloidal particles may be separated from their dispersion medium or from crystalloids.

ultrafiltration (ŭl"trä-fĭl-trä'shŭn) ["+ *filtrum,* a filter]. Filtration of a colloidal substance in which the dispersed particles, but not the liquid, are held back.

ultraligation (ŭl"trä-lĭ-gā'shŭn) [L. *ultra,* beyond, + *ligāre,* to bind]. Ligation of a blood vessel beyond the origin of a branch.

ultramicrobe (ŭl"trä-mī'krōb) ["+ Gr. *mikros,* tiny, + *bios,* life]. A microorganism too small to be visible by the ordinary microscope.

ultramicroscope (ŭl"trä-mī'krō-skōp) ["+ "+ *skopein,* to examine]. Microscope by which objects invisible through an ordinary microscope may be seen by means of powerful side illumination.

ultramicroscopy (ŭl"trä-mī-krŏs'kō-pī). The use of the ultramicroscope.

ultrasonic (ŭl-trä-sŏn'ĭk) [L. *ultra,* beyond, + *sonus,* sound]. Pertaining to sounds of frequencies above 16,000 cycles per second. They are inaudible to the human ear. SEE: *ultrasound.*

ultrasonics (ŭl-trä-sŏn'ĭks). Inaudible sounds with frequencies greater than 16,000 cycles per sec. Biological effects may result depending on itensity of beams. Heating effects are produced by beams of low intensity, paralytic effects by those of moderate intensity, and lethal effects by those of high intensity. The lethal action of ultrasonics is primarily the result, either directly or indirectly, of cavitation. Ultrasonics are utilized clinically for therapeutic and diagnostic purposes. SEE: *ultrasound.*

ultrasonography. Use of ultrasound to produce an image or photograph of an organ or tissue. Ultrasonic echoes are recorded as they strike tissues of different densities.

ultrasound. Inaudible sound in the frequency range of 16,000 to 10,000,000,000 cycles/second. U. has different velocities in tissues which differ in density and elasticity from others. This property permits the use of u. in outlining the shape of various tissues and organs in the body. Use of u. for diagnostic and therapeutic purposes requires special equipment. SEE: *ultrasonography.*

ultraviolet (ŭl"trä-vī'ō-lĕt) ["+ *violet*]. Beyond the visible spectrum at its violet end, said of rays. SEE: *infrared rays.*

   u. rays. Invisible rays emitted by very hot bodies and ionized gases with wave lengths between 3900 and 1800 angstroms. From a therapeutic standpoint, physiological effects include erythema production, pigmentation of skin, antirachitic effect through production of vitamin D, bactericidal effects, and various effects on metabolism. In clinical practice, dosage is measured in terms of minimum erythema dose (M.E.D.).

   u. therapy. Treatment with ultraviolet radiation. SEE: *heliotheraphy; light therapy.*

ultravirus (ŭl"trä-vī'rŭs) ["+ *virus,* poison]. A virus which is filtrable but which can be demonstrated by inoculation test. SEE: *virus, filtrable.*

umbilical (ŭm-bĭl'ĭkăl) [L. *umbilicus,* navel]. Pert. to the umbilicus.

   u. artery catheter. Catheter placed in the u. artery of the infant in order to facilitate administration of medicines parenterally or to do an exchange transfusion.

   u. cord. The attachment connecting the fetus with the placenta, surgically severed at birth of the child.

   It leaves a depression on the abdomen of the child called the navel or umbilicus, where the cord was attached to the fetus. It contains two arteries and one vein surrounded by a gelatinous substance, Wharton's jelly. The embryo receives nourishment from the blood. This is supplied by the arteries of the umbilical cord which go from the placenta to the fetus.

Cord should not be cut or tied until umbilical vessels have ceased pulsating. This gives the infant a better blood supply. SEE: *Wharton's jelly.*

u. fissure. Portion of hepatic longitudinal fissure in which the umbilical vein is lodged.

u. hernia. A hernia in the region of the umbilicus.

u. souffle. A hissing sound said to arise from the u. cord.

u. vesicle. That part of the embryonic yolk sac leading from the umbilicus.

umbilicate (ŭm-bĭl'ĭ-kāt) [L. *umbilicātus,* dimpled]. Pert. to or shaped like the navel, noting a bacterial colony with a central depression resembling an umbilicus.

umbilication (ŭm-bĭl-ĭ-kā'shŭn) [L. *umbilicātus,* dimpled]. 1. A depression resembling a navel. 2. Formation at apex of a pustule or vesicle of a pit or depression.

umbilicus (ŭm-bĭ-lī'kŭs, -bĭl'ĭ-kŭs) [L., a pit]. (pl. *umbilici*). A depressed point in the middle of the abdomen; the scar which marks the former attachment of the umbilical cord to the fetus.

RS: angiolysis; funic; f. souffle; funiculus; funis; hydromphalus; mesogastrium; navel; "omphal-" words; umbilical cord; varicocomphalus; Wharton's jelly.

umbo (ŭm'bō) [L., boss]. Projecting center of a round surface.

u. of tympanic membrane. The central depressed portion of concavity on lateral surface of tympanic membrane. It marks the point where the handle (manubrium of malleus) is attached to inner surface.

umbrascopy (ŭm-brăs'kō-pĭ) [L. *umbra,* shadow, + Gr. *skopein,* to view]. Use of shadows in refraction of the eye or use of roentgen rays. SYN: *skiascopy.*

umbrella filter. Filter placed in a blood vessel in order to prevent emboli from passing that point. Has been used in the vena cava to prevent emboli in the veins from reaching the lungs.

umbrella pack. SEE: *pack, umbrella.*

un- [AS. *un-,* against]. Prefix meaning back, reversal, annulment of, not.

unciform (ŭn'sĭ-form) [L. *uncus,* hook, + *forma,* shape]. Hook-shaped.

u. bone. Hook-shaped bone on ulnar side of distal row of the carpus. SYN: *os hamatum.*

u. fascioulus. Bundle of fibers connecting frontal cerebral lobes with the temporosphenoid ones.

u. process. 1. Long, thin lamina of bone from orbital plate of the ethmoid articulating with the inferior turbinate. 2. Hook at anterior end of hippocampal gyrus. 3. Hooked end of unciform bone.

uncinate (ŭn'sĭn-āt) [L. *uncinātus,* hooked]. Hook-shaped; hooked.

u. bundle of Russell. Fibers arising in fastigial superior cerebellar peduncle and pass inferiorly to vestibular nuclei and reticular formation by which impulses are carried to muscles, esp. those of neck and body. SYN: *fastigiobulbar tract.*

u. convolution. U. gyrus, q.v.

u. epilepsy. Form of e. occurring in disease of uncinate area of the temporal lobe.

u. fasciculus. Bundle of fibers connecting orbital gyri of frontal lobe with rostral portion of temporal lobe. They curve sharply as they pass over lateral fissure of cerebrum.

u. fits. Episodic attacks characterized by olfactory and gustatory hallucinations, usually disagreeable, a sense of unreality, and sometimes convulsions and temporary loss of senses of taste and smell. Associated with lesions of uncinate gyrus.

u. gyrus. A gyrus of the temporal lobe consisting of recurved rostral portion of hippocampal gyrus. SYN: *uncinate convolution; uncus.*

unconditioned reflex. An inborn or natural reflex; one not dependent upon previous experience or training.

unconscious (ŭn-kŏn'shŭs) [AS. *un,* not, + L. *conscius,* aware]. 1. Insensible; lacking in awareness of the environment. 2. State in which a person experiences no sensory impressions and has no subjective experiences. SEE: *unconsciousness.* 3. In psychiatry, that part of our personality consisting of a complex of feelings and drives of which we are unaware and which are not available to our consciousness.

unconsciousness (ŭn-kŏn'shŭs-nĕs) [AS. *un,* not, + L. *conscius,* aware]. State of being insensible or without conscious experiences. Unconsciousness physiologically occurs in sleep; pathologically it may occur temporarily as in syncope (fainting) or be prolonged and vary in depth from stupor (semiconsciousness) to coma (profound unconsciousness).

CAUSES: Anoxia; alcohol, barbiturate and bromide intoxication; brain tumor; cerebral accident (hemorrhage, thrombosis, embolism), concussion; cardiac decompensation; carbon monoxide poisoning; diabetes; epilepsy; eclampsia; fear; fracture of skull; fright; heat stroke; hemorrhage (especially subarachnoid); hypertensive encephalopathy; meningitis; neurosyphilis; opium poisoning; pneumonia; subdural hematoma; severe infections; uremia.

SYM: Patient unable to swallow; eyes do not react, insensible to surroundings.

If face is flushed or if hemorrhage is present or suspected, do not lower head and do not give stimulants. In all other instances, it is desirable to lower head and shoulders, loosen clothing, and keep patient comfortably warm but not hot. Turn head to one side to prevent vomit, if any, from being drawn into lungs. Fresh air and, if necessary, artificial respiration. Look for fractures, paralysis. Test pulse, respiration, odor of breath, condition of skin and pupils of eyes. Make a diagnosis prior to further treatment.

MOVING UNCONSCIOUS PATIENT, STRETCHER TO BED: *Method I:* Fold draw sheet in half lengthwise and place it across center of stretcher, pleating the excess and tucking the ends under for about six in. before patient is put on stretcher. (When patient is on stretcher this sheet should be under the buttocks). Place stretcher parallel with bed and as close as you can get it. Get three other people to help you. Have one person at patient's head, one at feet, one at side, and one at far side of bed. The people at the sides take firm hold of the ends of the draw sheet and all four lift together, the person at the far side pulling the draw sheet toward her.

Method II: This movement requires three people. Place stretcher at right angles to the foot of the bed with patient's head at end nearest bed. Standing side by side the three people put their arms under patient, lift him, and swing him around onto the bed.

unconsciousness, words pert. to: aochlesia; aphrenia; aphronia; apoplexy; apopsychia; asphyctic; asphyxial; asphyxiation; catalepsy; collapse; coma; fainting; gas; shock; sleep; stupor; syncope; trance; twilight sleep.

unction (ŭnk'shŭn) [L. *unctio*, ointment]. 1. The applicaton of an ointment. 2. Substance used for anointing. SYN: *unguent.*

unctuous (ŭnk'chū-ŭs) [L. *unctus,* an ointment]. Oily; greasy.

uncus (ŭn'kŭs) [L. *uncus,* hook]. 1. Any structure that is hook-shaped. 2. Hooked anterior end of hippocampal gyrus.

undernutrition (ŭn"dĕr-nū-trĭsh'ŭn) [AS. *under,* beneath, + LL. *nūtrĭtiō,* nourish]. Inadequate nutrition from any cause.

SYM: Loss of body weight representing at first mostly loss of body fat; then loss of

protein manifested by atrophy of muscles, weakness, edema.

undertoe (ŭn'dĕr-tō) ["+ *tā,* toe]. Condition of displacement of the great toe underneath the others.

underweight (ŭn'dĕr-wāt). Condition in which body weight is at least 10% less than what would be considered within normal limits for a particular individual. It is an imprecise term.

undifferentiation (ŭn-dĭf-ĕr-ĕn-shĭ-ā'shŭn) [AS. *un,* not, + L. *differens,* bearing apart]. Alteration in cell character to a more embryonic type or toward a malignant state. SYN: *anaplasia.*

undine (ŭn'dĭn) [L. *unda,* wave]. A small glass flask used for irrigating the eye.

undinism (ŭn'dĭn-ĭzm). Awakening of the libido by running water, as by urination or at sight of urine.

undulant (ŭn'dū-lănt) [L. *undulatio,* wavy]. Rising and falling like waves, or moving like them.

  u. fever. An infectious disease characterized by fever which rises to 104° or 105° F. (40°-40.6° C.) in the evening and drops gradually to normal in the morning. Other symptoms are weakness, sweats, chills, anorexia, general malaise, and nervous symptoms. Caused by one of three species of Brucella affecting animals: Br. abortus (cattle, hogs), Br. suis (hogs), and Br. melitensis (goats). SYN: *brucellosis; Malta fever.*

undulate (ŭn'dū-lāt) [L. *undulatio,* wavy]. Wavy; having a wavy border with shallow sinuses, said of bacterial colonies.

undulation (ŭn-dū-lā'shŭn). A continuous wavelike motion or pulsation.

  u., jugular. A venous pulse.

  u., respiratory. Fluctuations in blood pressure due to respiratory movements.

ung [L.]. Abbr. of *unguentum,* ointment.

ungual (ŭng'gwăl) [L. *unguis,* nail]. Pert. to or resembling the nails. SYN: *unguinal.*

  u. phalanx. Terminal phalanx of each finger and toe.

  u. tuberosity. Spatula-shaped extremity of the terminal phalanx which supports the nails of fingers and toes.

unguent (ŭng'gwĕnt) [L. *unguentum,* ointment]. A lubricant or salve for sores, burns, etc. SYN: *ointment.*

unguentum (ŭn-gwĕn'tŭm). 1. Fatty, soft, solid preparation intended to be applied to the skin by inunction. 2. Simple ointment. SYN: *ointment,* q.v.

unguis (ŭng'gwĭs) [L. *unguis,* nail]. (pl. *ungues*) 1. A fingernail or toenail. SYN: *onyx.* 2. The lacrimal bone. 3. A white prominence on floor of the lateral ventricle's posterior horn. SYN: *hippocampus minor.*

u. incarnatus. An ingrowing nail, esp. a toenail.

ungula (ŭn'gū-lä) [L. *ungula,* claw]. Instrument for removal of dead fetus from the uterus.

uni- [L.]. Combining form meaning one.

uniarticular (u''nī-ar-tik'u-lar) [L. *unus,* one, + *articulus,* joint]. Pertaining to a single joint. SYN: *monoarticular.*

unicellular (ū''nī-sĕl'ū-lar) ["+ *cellula,* a little box]. Having only one cell.

uniceps (u'nī-seps) [L. *unus,* one, + *caput,* head]. Having a single head or origin, as in muscles.

unicorn (ū'nī-korn) ["+ *cornū,* horn]. Having a single cornu or horn.

u. uterus. A uterus with but one horn perfectly formed.

unicornous (ū-nī-kor'nŭs). Having but one horn or cornu.

unigravida (ū''nī-grăv'ĭ-dä) [L. *unus,* one, + *gravida,* pregnant]. Woman who is pregnant for the first time.

unilateral (ū''nī-lăt'ĕr-al) ["+ *latus, later-,* side]. Affecting or occurring on only one side. SEE: *ipsilateral; homolateral; contralateral.*

unilocular (ū''nī-lŏk'ū-lar) [L. *unus,* one, + *loculus,* a little place]. Having but one cavity.

uninuclear, uninucleate(d (ū''nī-nū'klē-ar, -ăt, -ā-tĕd) ["+ *nucleus,* a kernel]. Having only one nucleus.

uniocular (ū''nī-ok'ū-lar) [L. *unus,* one, + *oculus,* eye]. Pert. to or having only one eye.

union (ūn'yŭn) [L. *unio,* oneness, union]. 1. Act of joining two or more things into one part, or state of being so united. 2. Growing together of severed or broken parts, as of bones or lips of a wound. SEE: *healing.*

u., non-. Failure to unite, as a fractured bone.

u., secondary. A healing by second intention with adhesion of granulating surfaces.

u., vicious. Union of ends of a broken bone in such a way as to cause deformity.

unioval (ū''nī-ō'văl) [L. *unus,* one, + *ovum,* egg]. Developed from one ovum, as identical twins.

unipara (ū-nĭp'ă-rä) ["+ *parere,* to bring forth]. A woman who has had only one child.

uniparous (ū-nĭp'ă-rŭs) [L. *unus,* one, + *parere,* to bring forth]. 1. Having produced but one child. 2. Giving birth to one offspring at a time.

unipolar (ū''nī-pō'lar) ["+ *polus,* pole]. 1. Having or pert. to one pole. 2. Having a single process as a unipolar neuron.

unit (ū'nĭt) [L. *unus,* one]. 1. One of anything. 2. A determined amount adopted as a standard of measurement.

u., Allen-Doisy. SEE: *unit, mouse; unit, rat.*

u., amboceptor. The smallest amount of amboceptor required in the presence of which a given quantity of red blood corpuscles will be hemolyzed by an excess of complement.

u., Angström. An internationally adopted unit of measurement of wave length, 1/10,000,000 of a millimeter, or 1/254,000,000 of an inch. ABBR: Å or A.U.

u., antigen. Smallest quantity of antigen required to fix one unit of complement, preventing hemolysis.

u., antitoxic. A unit for expressing the strength of an antitoxin. Originally the various units were defined biologically but now are compared to a weighed standard specified by the U. S. Public Health Service and the World Health Organization.

u., British thermal. The amt. of heat necessary to raise one pound of water at 39° F. one degree. Equivalent to about 252 Calories.

u. of capacity. Capacity of a condenser which gives a difference of potential of one volt when charged with one coulomb. SYN: *curie; farad.*

u., cat. The amount of drug per kg. of weight of animal just sufficient to kill a cat when injected intravenously slowly and continuously.

u., complement. Smallest quantity of complement required for hemolysis of a given amount of red blood corpuscles with one amboceptor unit present.

u. dose medication. The technique of dispensing medicines so that each dose is contained in an individual package. Each package is labeled to identify the medicine, dose, control number, and expiration date if applicable. All forms of medicine may be dispensed in this manner.

u., electrical. SEE: *ampere; ohm; volt; watt.*

u., hemolytic. The amount of inactivated immune serum which causes complete hemolysis of 1 ml. of a 5% emulsion of washed red blood corpuscles, in the presence of complement.

u., immunizing. Antitoxic u., q.v.

u., international. One defined and adopted by the International Conference for Unification of Formulae.

u., i., of vitamin A. The vitamin activity of 0.0006 mg. of the international standard carotene.

u., i., of vitamin B. The vitamin activity of 10 mg. of the international standard absorption product.

u., i., of vitamin C. The vitamin activity of 0.05 mg. of the international standard levo-ascorbic acid.

u., i., of vitamin D. The vitamin activity of 1 mg. of the international standard solution of irradiated ergosterol.

u., light. A foot-candle, or the amount of light one ft. from a standard candle.

u., Mache. Unit of measurement of radium emanation. ABBR: M.U.

u., mouse. Least amount of estrus-producing hormone which induces, in a spayed mouse, a characteristic desquamation of the vaginal epithelium.

u., physical. SEE: *Units of Measurement* in Appendix.

u., radiation. SEE: *u., Mache.*

u., rat. Greatest dilution of an estrus-producing hormone which will cause desquamation and cornification of vaginal epithelium during 1st day, if given to a mature spayed rat in three injections, every four hours.

unitarian (ū-nĭ-tā′rĭ-an) [L. *unitarius*]. Composed of a single unit.

unitary (ū′nĭ-tā-rĭ). Rel. to a single unit.

uniterminal (ū″nĭ-ter′mĭn-ăl) [L. *unus*, one, + *terminus*, end]. Having only one terminal. SEE: *monoterminal.*

univalent (ū″nĭ-vā′lĕnt, ū-nĭv′ă-lĕnt) [″+ *valens*, to be powerful]. 1. Possessing the power of combining or replacing one atom of hydrogen. 2. Single, noting a chromosome which lacks or fails to unite with a synaptic mate.

universal (ū″nĭ-ver′săl) [L. *universalis*, combined into one whole]. General.

u. antidote. Two parts activated charcoal; one part tannic acid; one part magnesium oxide. Give orally a paste of five heaping teaspoonsful of the mixture dissolved in a glass of water. After the patient has swallowed the antidote, the stomach contents should then be removed by gastric lavage. Use in cases of poisoning where specific antidote is unknown or not available.

u. donor. A person belonging to blood group O whose blood as a rule may be transfused without danger of untoward reactions into persons belonging to any of the other blood groups.

NOTE: Because there are multiple blood type factors in addition to those of ABO, it would be dangerous to assume that group O blood could, without further tests of compat-

ibility, be given to persons of different blood type.

u. recipient. A person belonging to blood group AB, whose serum will not agglutinate the cells of any blood group.

unofficial (ŭn-of-ĭsh′ăl) [AS. *un*, not, + L. *officialis*, doing work]. Indicates a drug not listed by the pharmacopeia or National Formulary.

unorganized (ŭn-or′găn-īzd) [″+ L. *organizāre*, to form a structure]. 1. Not organized into an organic structure. 2. Without the characteristics of a living organism; inorganic.

unphysiological (ŭn-fĭz-ē-ō-loj′ĭk-ăl). Contrary to physiological principles.

unrest. Turbulence, instability, or irregularity.

unsaturated (ŭn-săt′ū-rāt″ĕd) [AS. *un*, not, + L. *saturāre*, to sate]. 1. Capable of dissolving or absorbing to a greater degree. 2. Not combined to the greatest possible extent.

u. compound. An organic compound having double or triple bonds between the carbon atoms.

unsex (ŭn-sĕks′) [″+ L. *sexus*, sex]. 1. To castrate; to spay or excise the ovaries. 2. To deprive of sexual character.

unstriated (ŭn-strī′āt-ĕd) [AS. *un-*, not, + *striātus*, striped]. Unstriped, as smooth muscle fiber.

unwell (ŭn-wĕl′) [″+ *wel*, well]. 1. Sick; ill; indisposed. 2. Menstruating.

upsiloid (ŭp′sĭ-loyd) [Gr. *upsilon*, letter U, + *eidos*, form]. Shaped like the letter U or V.

urachal (ū′ră-kăl) [Gr. *ourachos*, fetal urinary canal]. Rel. to the urachus.

urachus (ū′ră-kus) [Gr. *ourachos*, fetal urinary canal]. An epithelioid cord surrounded by fibrous tissue extending from apex of bladder to umbilicus. In the embryo it is continuous with the allantoic stalk; postnatally it forms the middle umbilical ligament of the bladder.

u., patent. Condition in which urachus remains as a hollow tube connecting vertex of bladder with umbilicus resulting in an umbilical urinary fistula.

uracil (u′ră-sil). A pyrimidine base, $C_4H_4N_2O_2$, found in ribonucleic acids.

uracrasia (ū-ră-krā′sĭ-ă) [Gr. *ouron*, urine, + *akrasia*, bad mixture]. 1. A disordered condition of urine. 2. Inability to retain the urine. SYN: *urinary incontinence.*

uracratia (ū-ră-krā′shĭ-ă) [″+ *akratia*, incontinence]. Incontinence of the urine.

uragogue (ū′ră-gog) [″+ *agogos*, leading]. Increasing the secretion of urine. SYN: *diuretic.*

uranisconitis (ū-răn-ĭs″kon-ī′tĭs) [Gr. *ouraniskos*, palate, + *-itis*, inflammation]. Inflammation of the palate.

uraniscoplasty (ū-răn-ĭs′kō-plăs″tĭ) ["+ *plassein*, to form]. Operation for repair of cleft palate. SYN: *uranoplasty, uranorrhaphy.*

uraniscorrhaphy (ū-răn-ĭs-kor′ră-fĭ) ["+ *rhaphē*, a seam]. Operation for suturing of a cleft palate. SYN: *uraniscoplasty.*

uraniscus (ū-răn-ĭs′kŭs) [Gr. *ouraniskos*, palate]. Palate, or roof of mouth.

uranism (ū′răn-ĭzm) [Gr. *ouranos*, heaven, + *-ismos*, condition]. Homosexuality.

uranist (ū′răn-ĭst). A homosexual.

uranium (ū-rā′nĭ-ŭm) [Gr. *ouranos*, sky]. SYMB: *U.* At. wt. 238.029; at. no. 92. Primary radioactive element, the parent of radium and other radioelements.

uranoplasty (ū′răn-ō-plăs″tĭ) [Gr. *ouranos*, palate, + *plassein*, to form]. Operation for cleft palate. SYN: *uraniscoplasty.*

uranoplegia (ū″ră-nō-plē′jĭ-ă) ["+ *plēgē*, stroke]. Paralysis of muscles of the soft palate.

uranorrhaphy (ū-răn-or′ră-fĭ) ["+ *rhaphē*, a seam]. Operation for suture of a cleft palate. SYN: *uraniscorrhaphy.*

uranoschisis (ū-răn-ŏs′kĭs-ĭs) [Gr. *ouranos*, sky, + *schisis*, a fissure]. Cleft palate.

uranostaphyloplasty (ū″răn-ō-stăf′ĭl-ō-plăs″tĭ) ["+ *staphylē*, uvula, + *plassein*, to form]. Operation for correction of a defect of the soft and hard palates.

uranostaphylorrhaphy (ū″răn-ō-stăf-ĭl-or′ă-fĭ) ["+ "+ *rhaphē*, a seam]. Operation for repair of cleft of hard and soft palates.

urapostema (u-ră-pos-te′mă) [Gr. *ouron*, urine, + *apostema*, abscess]. An abscess containing urine.

uraroma (ū-ră-rō′mă) ["+ *aroma*, spice]. Aromatic, spicy odor of the urine.

urase (ū′rās). Urease, q.v.

urate (ū′rāt) [Gr. *ouron*, urine]. Combination of uric acid with a base; a salt of uric acid.
Urates are normally present in urine.

uratemia (ū″ră-tē′mĭ-ă) ["+ *haima*, blood]. Urates, esp. sodium urate, in the blood.

uraturia (ū″ră-tū′rĭ-ă) [Gr. *ouron*, urine]. Excess of urates in the urine. SYN: *lithuria.*

urceiform (ŭr-se′ĭ-form) [L. *urceus*, pitcher, + *forma*, shape]. Pitcher shaped.

urea (ū-rē′ă) [Gr. *ouron*, urine]. The diamide of carbonic acid, a crystalline solid having the formula $CO(NH_2)_2$; found in blood, lymph, and urine. It is formed in the liver from ammonia derived from amino acids by deamination. It may also be formed directly from arginine.

U. is the chief nitrogenous constituent of urine and final product of protein metabolism in the body. In normal conditions, urea represents 80-90% of the total urinary nitrogen.

It is without odor and is colorless, appearing as white prismatic crystals, and forming salts with acids. Its excess is one of the causes of uremia, q.v. The amount of u. excreted varies directly with the amount of protein in the diet. Excretion is increased in fever, diabetes, or increased activity of the adrenal gland.

USES: As a diuretic.

u. frost. White flaky deposits of urea seen on skin in patients with advanced uremia.

u. nitrogen. The nitrogen of urea as distinguished from nitrogen in blood proteins. ABBR: BUN.

ureagenetic (ū-rē″ă-jĕn-ĕt′ĭk) [Gr. *ouron*, urine, + *genesis*, production]. Pert. to or producing urea.

ureal (ū-rē′ăl). Rel. to or containing urea.

ureameter (ū-rē-ăm′et-er) [Gr. *ouron*, urine, + *metron*, a measure]. Device for determining amount of urea in urine. SYN: *ureometer.*

ureametry (ū-rē-ăm′ĕt-rĭ). Determination of amt. of urea in urine.

urease (ū′rē-ās) [Gr. *ouron*, urine]. An enzyme which accelerates hydrolysis of urea into ammonium carbonate and hippuric acid into glycocoll and benzoic acid.

It is found in alkaline fermentation of urine, is produced by many microorganisms, and is also found in jack beans and soybeans.

It is used in determining the amount of urea in blood or in urine.

urecchysis (ū-rĕk′ĭs-ĭs) ["+ *ekchysis*, a pouring out]. Effusion of urine into areolar tissue.

uredema (ū-re-dē′mă) ["+ *oidēma*, a swelling]. Urine in the subcutaneous tissues distending them.

uredo (ū-rē′dō) [L. *uredo*, a blight]. 1. Burning sensation in the skin. 2. Skin disorder marked by smooth, white elevations which itch severely. SYN: *hives; urticaria*, q.v.

ureide (ū′rē-īd) [Gr. *ouron*, urine]. Any compound of urea in which acid radicals have taken the place of one or more of its hydrogen atoms.

urelcosis (ū-rĕl-kō′sĭs) ["+ *helkōsis*, ulceration]. Ulceration of the urinary tract.

uremia (ū-rē′mĭ-ă) [Gr. *ouron*, urine, + *haima*, blood]. Toxic condition associated with renal insufficiency and the retention in the blood of nitrogenous substances normally excreted by the kidney.

ETIOL: Result of disturbed kidney function seen in nephritis and due to suppression or deficient secretion of urine from any cause.

SYM: Nausea, vomiting, headache, dizziness, dimness of vision, coma or convulsions, urinous odor of breath, and perspiration. Stupor, stertorous respiration. No change in pupillary reaction; dry skin; hard, rapid pulse; elevated blood pressure; scanty urine containing casts and albumin. There is a reduction of urea, and presence of tube casts in uremic coma. Urea retention 150 to 500 mg. or more per 100 ml. SEE: *azotemia; coma, uremic.*

u., extrarenal. Uremia, prerenal, q.v.

u., prerenal. Uremia occurring not as a result of primary renal disease but due to other conditions such as disturbances in circulation, fluid balance, or metabolism arising in other parts of the body. Also called prerenal azotemia.

uremic (ū-rē′mĭk). Pert. to or caused by uremia.

uremide (ū′re-mĭd) [Gr. *ouron*, urine, + *haima*, blood]. The skin lesions of uric acid poisoning.

uremigenic (u-rē-mĭ-jĕn′ĭk) ["+ "+ *gennan*, to produce]. Caused by uremia or producing it.

ureogenesis. Formation of urea.

ureometer (ū″rē-ŏm′ĕt-ĕr) [Gr. *ouron*, urine, + *metron*, a measure]. Appliance used to determine the amt. of urea in urine. SYN: *ureameter.*

ureometry (ū-rē-ŏm′ĕt-rĭ). Estimation of amt. of urea in urine.

uresiesthesia, uresiesthesis (ū-rē″sĭ-ĕs-thē′-zĭ-ă, -sĭs) [Gr. *ouresis*, urination, + *aisthēsis*, sensation]. The normal inclination to void urine.

uresis (ū-rē′sĭs). The passage of urine. SYN: *urination.*

ureter (ū′rĕ-ter, ū-rē′tĕr) [Gr. *ourētēr*, ureter]. One of two tubes carrying urine from the kidneys to the bladder, beginning with the pelvis of the kidney, and emptying into the base of the bladder.

The ureters are from 28 to 34 cm. long with the right being slightly shorter than the left. They vary in diameter from 1 mm. to 1 cm. Its wall consists of three layers: the mucosal, muscular, and fibrous coats.

RS: autonephrectomy; kidney; urelcosis; "uret-" words.

ureteralgia (ū-rē-ter-ăl′jĭ-ă) ["+ *algos*, pain]. Pain in the ureter.

uretercystoscope (ū-rē″tĕr-sĭs′tō-skōp) ["+ *kystis*, bladder, + *skopein*, to examine]. A cystoscope combined with a ureteral catheter.

ureterectasis (ū-rē″tĕr-ĕk′tă′sĭs) [Gr. *ourētēr*, ureter, + *ektasis*, dilatation]. Dilatation of the ureter.

ureterectomy (ū-rē″tĕr-ĕk′tō-mĭ) ["+ *ektomē*, excision]. Excision of a ureter.

ureteritis (ū-rē″tĕr-ī′tĭs) ["+ *-itis*, inflammation]. Inflammation of the ureters.

ureterocele (ū-rē′tĕr-ō-sēl) [Gr. *ourētēr*, ureter, + *kēlē*, hernia]. Cystlike dilatation of ureter near its opening into the bladder usually due to congenital stenosis of ureteral orifice.

ureterocolostomy (ū-rē″tĕr-ō-kō-lŏs′tō-mĭ) ["+ *kōlon*, colon, + *stoma*, passage]. The implantation of the ureter into the colon.

ureterocystoneostomy (ū-rē″tĕr-ō-sĭst″ō-nē-ŏs′tō-mĭ) [Gr. *ourētēr*, ureter, + *kystis*, bladder, + *neos*, new, + *stoma*, passage]. Ureteroneocystostomy, q.v.

ureterocystostomy (ū-rē″tĕr-ō-sĭs-tŏs′tō-mĭ) ["+ "+ *stoma*, passage]. Ureteroneocystostomy, q.v.

ureterodialysis (ū-rē″tĕr-ō-dī-ăl′ĭ-sĭs) ["+ *dialysis*, a separation]. Rupture of a ureter. SYN: *ureterolysis.*

ureteroenterostomy (ū-rē″tĕr-ō-ĕn-ter-ŏs′tō-mĭ) [Gr. *ourētēr*, ureter, + *enteron*, intestine, + *stoma*, passage]. Formation of a passage between a ureter and the intestine.

ureterography (ū-rē″tĕr-ŏg′ră-fĭ) ["+ *graphein*, to write]. X-ray photography of the ureter after injection of a radiopaque substance into it.

ureterohydronephrosis (ū-rē″tĕr-ō-hī″drō-nē-frō′sĭs) [Gr. *ourētēr*, ureter, + *hydōr*, water, + *nephros*, kidney, + *ōsis*, condition]. Dilatation of ureter and pelvis of kidney resulting from an obstruction, either mechanical or of an inflammatory nature, in the urinary tract.

ureterolith (ū-rē′ter-ō-lĭth) [Gr. *ourētēr*, ureter, + *lithos*, stone]. A stone or calculus in the ureter.

ureterolithiasis (ū-rē″ter-ō-lĭth-ī′ăs-ĭs) ["+ "+ *-iasis*, condition]. Development of a calculus in the ureter.

ureterolithotomy (ū-rē″ter-ō-lĭth-ŏt′ō-mĭ) ["+ "+ *tomē*, a cutting]. Surgical incision for removal of a calculus from ureter.

ureterolysis (ū-rē″ter-ŏl′ĭ-sĭs) [Gr. *ourētēr*, ureter, + *lysis*, loosening]. 1. Rupture of the ureter. SYN: *ureterodialysis.* 2. Paralysis of the ureter. 3. The process of loosening adhesions around the ureter.

ureteroneocystostomy (ū-rē″ter-ō-nē″ō-sĭs-tŏs′tō-mĭ) ["+ *neos*, new, + *kystis*, bladder, + *stoma*, passage]. Surgical formation of a new passage between a ureter and the bladder. SYN: *ureterocystoneostomy; ureterocystostomy.*

ureteroneopyelostomy (ū-rē″ter-ō-nē″ō-pī-ĕ-lŏs′tō-mĭ) ["+ "+ *pyelos,* pelvis, + *stoma,* passage]. Excision of a portion of the ureter with attachment of the severed end of the lower portion to a new aperture in the renal pelvis. SYN: *ureteropyeloneostomy.*

ureteronephrectomy (ū-rē″ter-o-nef-rĕk′-tō-mĭ) [Gr. *ourētēr,* ureter, + *nephros,* kidney, + *ektomē,* excision]. Removal of a kidney and its ureter.

ureteropathy (ū-rē-ter-ŏp′ă-thĭ) ["+ *pathos,* disease]. Any diseased condition of the ureter.

ureterophlegma (ū-rē″ter-ō-flĕg′mă) ["+ *phlegma,* phlegm]. Mucus accumulation in the ureter.

ureteroplasty (ū-rē′ter-ō-plăs″tĭ) [Gr. *ourētēr,* ureter, + *plassein,* to form]. Plastic surgery of the ureter.

ureteroproctostomy (ū-rē″ter-ō-prŏk-tŏs′-tō-mĭ) ["+ *prōktos,* anus, + *stoma,* passage]. Formation of a passage from the ureter to the lower rectum.

ureteropyelitis (ū-rē″ter-ō-pī-ĕl-ī′tĭs) ["+ *pyelos,* pelvis, + *-itis,* inflammation]. Inflammation of the pelvis of the kidney and a ureter.

ureteropyeloneostomy (ū-rē″ter-ō-pī″ĕl-ō-nē-ŏs′tō-mĭ) ["+ "+ *neos,* new, + *stoma,* passage]. Ureteroneopyelostomy, q.v.

ureteropyelonephritis (ū-rē″ter-ō-pī″ĕl-ō-nef-rī′tĭs) ["+ "+ *nephros,* kidney, + *-itis,* inflammation]. Inflammation of the renal pelvis and the ureter.

ureteropyeloplasty (ū-rē″ter-ō-pī″ĕl-o-plăs″tĭ) ["+ "+ *plassein,* to mold]. Plastic surgery of the ureter and renal pelvis.

ureteropyosis (ū-rē″tĕr-ō-pī-ō′sĭs) [Gr. *ourētēr,* ureter, + *pyon,* pus, + *-ōsis,* condition]. Suppurative inflammation within a ureter.

ureterorrhagia (ū-rē″ter-or-rā′jĭ-ă) ["+ *rhēgnynai,* to burst forth]. Hemorrhage from the ureter.

ureterorrhaphy (ū-rē″ter-or′ră-fĭ) [Gr. *ourētēr,* ureter, + *rhaphē,* a seam]. Suture of the ureter, as for fistula.

ureterosigmoidostomy (ū-rē″ter-ō-sĭg-moyd-ŏs′tō-mĭ) [Gr. *ourētēr,* ureter, + *sigma,* letter S, + *eidos,* shape, + *stoma,* passage]. Surgical implantation of the ureter into the sigmoid flexure.

ureterostenosis (ū-rē″ter-ō-stĕn-ō′sĭs) ["+ *stenōsis,* a narrowing]. Stricture of a ureter.

ureterostomy (ū-rē″ter-ŏs′tō-mĭ) ["+ *stoma,* passage]. Formation of a permanent fistula for drainage of a ureter.

ureterotomy (ū-rē″ter-ŏt′ō-mĭ) ["+ *tomē,* a cutting]. Incision or surgery of the ureter.

ureteroureterostomy (ū-rē″ter-ō-ū-rē″ter-ŏs′tō-mĭ) [Gr. *ourētēr,* ureter, + *ourētēr,* ureter, + *stoma,* passage]. 1. Formation of a connection from one ureter to the other. 2. Reestablishment of a passage bet. the ends of a divided ureter.

ureterovaginal (ū-rē″ter-ō-văj′ĭ-năl) ["+ L. *vagina,* sheath]. Relating to a ureter and the vagina, noting a fistula connecting them.

ureterovesical (ū-rē″ter-ō-vĕs′ĭ-kăl) ["+ L. *vesica,* bladder]. Pert. to a connection bet. the ureter and the bladder.

ureterovesicostomy (ū-rē″ter-ō-vĕs″ĭ-kŏs′tō-mĭ) ["+ "+ Gr. *stoma,* passage]. Reimplantation of a ureter into the bladder.

urethra (ū-rē′thră) [Gr. *ourēthra,* urethra]. A canal for the discharge of urine extending from the bladder to the outside. In the female its orifice lies in the vestibule between vagina and clitoris; in the male, the urethra transverses the penis opening at the tip of the glans penis. In the male it serves as the passage for semen as well as urine.

Its inner lining, the mucosa, is thrown into folds and contains openings of lacunae into which glands of Littre open. Surrounding the mucosa is a lamina propria containing many elastic fibers and blood vessels, outside of which is an indefinite muscular layer. SEE: *penis.*

    u. mulie′bris. The female urethra. SYN: *u. femina* [NA].

    u. viri′lis. The male urethra. SYN: *u. masculina* [NA].

urethra, words pert. to: aerourethros-

MALE REPRODUCTIVE TRACT

copy; anaspadias; ankylurethria; atreturethria; bulb; bulbourethral glands; corpus spongiosum; gleet; habenula urethralis; hypospadias; meatus urinarius; Skene's glands; urelcosis; "urethr-" words.

urethral (ū-rē′thrăl) [Gr. *ourēthra*, urethral]. Relating to the urethra.

urethralgia (ū-rē-thrăl′jĭ-ă) ["+ *algos*, pain]. Urethral pain; pain in the urethra.

urethratresia (ū-rē-thră-trē′zĭ-ă) ["+ *atrēsis*, imperforation]. Occlusion, or imperforation of the urethra.

urethrectomy (ū-rē-thrĕk′tō-mĭ) [Gr. *ourēthra*, urethra, + *ektomē*, excision]. Surgical excision of the urethra or part of it.

urethremphraxis (ū-rē-thrĕm-frăk′sĭs) ["+ *emphraxis*, obstruction]. Urethral obstruction. SYN: *urethrophraxis*.

urethreurynter (ū-rē-thrū-rĭn′ter) [Gr. *ourētēr*, ureter, + *eurynein*, to dilate]. Appliance for dilating the urethra.

urethrism, urethrismus (ū′rē-thrĭzm, ū′′rē-thrĭz′mŭs) ["+ *-ismos*, condition]. Irritability or spasm of the urethra.

urethritis (ū-rē-thrī′tĭs) [Gr. *ourēthra*, urethra, + *-itis*, inflammation]. Inflammation of the urethra.

u., anterior. Inflammation of that portion of the urethra ant. to the ant. layer of the triangular ligament.

u., gonococcal. U. caused by gonococcus.

u., nonspecific. Inflammation and irritation of the urethra but not known to be caused by a specific organism. It is usually transmitted by sexual intercourse. Treatment is not always successful. Both tetracyclines and sulfonamides are used.

u., posterior. Inflammation of membranous and prostatic portions of the urethra.

u., specific. Urethritis due to a specific organism, usually gonococcus.

urethro- [Gr.]. Combining form meaning urethra.

urethrocele (ū-rē′thrō-sēl) [Gr. *ourēthra*, urethra, + *kēlē*, hernia]. 1. Pouchlike protrusion of the urethral wall in the female. 2. Thickening of connective tissue around the urethra in the female.

urethrocystitis (ū-rē′′thrō-sĭs-tī′tĭs) ["+ *kystis*, bladder, + *-itis*, inflammation]. Inflammation of urethra and bladder.

urethrography (ū-rē-thrŏg′ră-fĭ) ["+ *graphein*, to write]. X-ray photography of the urethra, after the injection of a radiopaque substance into it.

urethrolysis. Surgical lysis or excision of constricting elastic tissue surrounding the distal third of the urethra in girls.

urethrometer (ū-rē-thrŏm′et-er) [Gr. *ourēthra*, urethra, + *metron*, a measure]. Instrument for measuring diameter of urethra or lumen of a stricture.

urethropenile (ū-rē′′thrō-pē′nĭl) ["+ L. *penis*, penis]. Relating to the urethra and penis.

urethroperineal (ū-rē′′thrō-pĕr-ĭ-nē′ăl) [Gr. *ourēthra*, urethra, + LL. *perinaion*, perineum]. Rel. to the urethra and perineum.

urethroperineoscrotal (ū-rē′′thrō-pĕr-ĭ-nē′′-ō-skrō′tăl) ["+ "+ L. *scrotum*, pouch]. Relating to the urethra, perineum, and scrotum.

urethropexy (u-rēth′ro-pex-ĭ) ["+ Gr. *pexis*, fixation]. Surgical fixation of the urethra.

urethrophraxis (ū-rē-thrō-frăks′ĭs) [Gr. *ourēthra*, urethra, + *phrassein*, to obstruct]. Urethral obstruction. SYN: *urethremphraxis*.

urethrophyma (ū-rē-thrō-fī′mă) ["+ *phyma*, growth]. A neoplasm in the urethra.

urethroplasty (ū-rē′thrō-plăs′′tĭ) ["+ *plassein*, to mold]. Reparative surgery of the urethra.

urethrorectal (ū-rē′′thrō-rĕk′tăl) [Gr. *ourēthra*, urethra, + L. *rectus*, straight]. Rel. to the urethra and the rectum.

urethrorrhagia (ū-rē′′thror-ā′jĭ-ă) ["+ *rhēgnynai*, to burst forth]. Hemorrhage from urethra.

urethrorrhaphy (ū-rē-thror′ăf-ĭ) ["+ *rhaphē*, a seam]. Suture of the urethra, as a urethral fistula.

urethrorrhea (ū-rē′′thror-ē′ă) [Gr. *ourēthra*, urethra, + *rhoia*, a flow]. Abnormal discharge from the urethra.

u. ex libidine. The discharge of normal glandular secretions resulting from sexual stimulation, esp. that preceding sexual intercourse.

urethroscope (ū-rē′thrō-skōp) ["+ *skopein*, to examine]. Device for examining interior of urethra.

urethroscopic (ū-rē′′thrō-skŏp′ĭk) ["+ *skopein*, to examine]. Relating to the urethroscope or urethroscopy.

urethroscopy (ū-rē-thrŏs′kō-pĭ). An examination of the mucous membrane of the urethra with a urethroscope.

urethrospasm (ū-rē′thrō-spăzm) [Gr. *ourēthra*, urethra, + *spasmos*, a spasm]. Spasmodic stricture of the urethra.

urethrostaxis (ū-rē′′thrō-staks′ĭs) ["+ *staxis*, a dropping]. Oozing of blood from the urethral mucous membrane.

urethrostenosis (ū-rē′′thrō-sten-ō′sĭs) ["+ *stenōsis*, a narrowing]. Stricture of the urethra.

urethrostomy (ū-rē-thrŏs'tō-mǐ) ["+ *stoma,* opening]. Formation of a permanent fistula opening into the urethra by perineal section and fixation of membranous urethra in perineum.

urethrotome (ū-rē'thrō-tōm) [Gr. *ourēthra,* urethra, + *tomē,* a cutting]. An instrument for incision of urethral stricture.

urethrotomy (ū-rē-thrŏt-ō-mǐ). Incision of a urethral stricture.

urethrovaginal (ū-rē"thrō-văj'ǐ-năl) [Gr. *ourēthra,* urethra, + L. *vagina,* sheath]. Pert. to the urethra and vagina.

urhydrosis (ūr-hǐ-drō-sǐs) [Gr. *ouron,* urine, + *hidrōs,* sweat]. Excretion of urea in sweat.

uric (ū'rǐk) [Gr. *ourikos,* urine]. Of or pert. to urine.

   u. acid. $C_5H_4N_4O_2$, a crystalline acid, occurring as an end-product of purine metabolism. It is formed from purine bases derived from nucleoproteins. It is a common constituent of urinary and renal calculi, and gouty concretions.

   OUTPUT: Between 0.5 and 1 gm./day on ordinary mixed diet. Uric acid must be excreted, as it cannot be destroyed within the body.

   Increased Elimination: Observed in ingestion of proteins, gout, leukemia, acute articular rheumatism, after exercise, and the ingestion of nitrogenous foods. Decreased Elimination: Observed in nephritis, chlorosis, lead poisoning, and protein-free diet.

   u. a., endogenous. U. acid derived from purines undergoing metabolism from the nucleoprotein of body tissues.

   u. a., exogenous. U. acid derived from those purines from food made up of free purines and nucleoproteins. SEE: *urate; uraturia.*

uricacidemia (ū"rǐk-ăs-ǐd-ē'mǐ-ă) [Gr. *ourikos,* urine, + L. *acidus,* sour, + Gr. *haima,* blood]. Excess uric acid in the blood.

uricaciduria (ū"rǐk-ăs-ǐd-ū'rǐ-ă) ["+ "+ Gr. *ouron,* urine]. Excessive amount of uric acid in the urine.

uricase (ū'rǐ-kāz) [Gr. *ourikos,* urine, + *ase,* enzyme]. An enzyme present in the liver and kidneys of most mammals, but not man. This enzyme is capable of oxidizing uric acid into allantoin and carbon dioxide.

uricemia (ū-rǐ-sē'mǐ-ă) [Gr. *ourikos,* urine, + *haima,* blood]. Excess uric acid in the blood. SYN: *uricacidemia.*

uricocholia (ū"rǐ-kō-kō'-lǐ-ă) ["+ *cholē,* bile]. Uric acid in the bile.

uricolysis (ū-rǐ-kŏl-ǐ-sǐs) ["+ *lysis,* dissolution]. The decomposition of uric acid.

uricolytic (ū"rǐ-kō-lǐt'ǐk). Decomposing uric acid.

uricometer (ū-rǐk-ŏm'ě-těr) [Gr. *ourikos,* urine, + *metron,* a measure]. Apparatus for quantitative estimation of uric acid in the urine.

uricopoiesis (ū-rǐ-kō-poy-ē-sǐs) ["+ *poiēsis,* formation]. Producing uric acid.

uricosuria (ū-rǐ-kō-sū'rǐ-ă) ["+ *ourikos,* urine]. The excessive excretion of uric acid in the urine.

uricosuric (ū'rǐ-kō-sū'rǐk). Potentiating the excretion of uric acid in the urine.

   u. agent. A drug (such as probenecid) that increases the urinary excretion of uric acid, thereby reducing the concentration of uric acid in the blood. Used in treatment of gout.

uricoxydase (ū"rǐk-oks'ǐ-dās) [Gr. *ourikos,* urine, + *oxys,* sharp, + *ase,* enzyme]. An enzyme capable of oxidizing uric acid.

uridrosis (ū-rǐ-drō-sǐs) ["+ *hidrōsis,* a sweating]. The presence of urea in the sweat. Evaporation may show white scales, the crystals of urea.

   u. crystalli'na. White powder of uric acid deposited on the skin. SYN: *urea frost.*

uriesthesis (ū-re-ěs-thē'sǐs) ["+ *aisthēsis,* sensation]. Normal desire to void urine.

urina (ū-rī'nă) [L.]. Urine.

   u. cibi. Urine voided after a full meal.

   u. galactodes. Urine of a milky color.

   u. hysterica. Watery, pale urine following hysteria.

   u. jumentosa. Cloudy urine.

   u. potus. U. voided after drinking.

urinal (ū'rǐn-ăl) [L. *urina,* urine]. 1. A vessel for the urine. 2. A toilet for the male consisting of a vessel attached to a wall.

urinalysis (ū-rǐ-năl-ǐ-sǐs) ["+ Gr. *ana,* apart, + *lysis,* a loosening]. Analysis of the urine.

urinary (ū'rǐ-năr"ǐ) [L. *urina,* urine]. Pert. to, secreting, or containing urine.

   u. bladder. Receptacle for urine before it is voided. SEE: *bladder.*

   u. calculi. Concretions formed in the urinary passages. They vary in composition but may contain urates, calcium, oxalate, calcium carbonate, phosphates, and cystine.

   u. casts. Casts of kidney tubules passed in the urine.

   u. organs. The structures concerned with the secretion and excretion of urinary products, consisting of the two kidneys, two ureters, the bladder, and the urethra.

   u. pigments. Urochrome, urobilin, uroerythrin, and hematoporphyrin.

   u. reflex. Desire to void resulting from accumulation of urine in bladder.

   u. sediments. Substances found in standing urine, i.e., bacteria, mucus, phosphates, uric acid, calcium oxalate, calcium carbonate, calcium phosphate, magnesium and ammonium phosphate; more rarely, cystine, tyrosine, xanthine, hippuric acid, hematoidin.

u. stammering. Temporary interruptions in voiding urine.

u. stuttering. Same as u. stammering.

u. system. Kidneys, ureters, bladder, and urethra.

u. tract. Organs and ducts participating in secretion and elimination of urine.

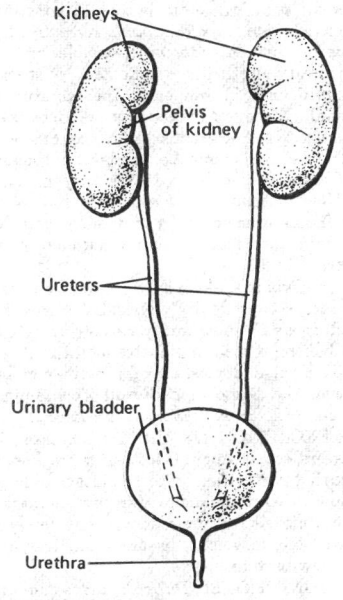

Kidneys

Pelvis of kidney

Ureters

Urinary bladder

Urethra

URINARY TRACT

urinate (ū′rĭ-nāt) [L. *urināre*, to discharge urine]. To pass the urine from the bladder. SYN: *micturate.*

urination (ū-rĭ-nā-shŭn) [L. *urinātio*, a discharging of urine]. The act of voiding urine. SYN: *micturition.*

Although this act is somewhat under voluntary control, it is accomplished chiefly by the action of involuntary muscles. The musculus sphincter vesicae relaxes, while the general musculature of the wall of the urinary bladder contracts to force out its contents.

INCREASED FREQUENCY: Seen in polyuria; nervous excitement; irritation of bladder, urethra, or urinary meatus; disease of spinal cord; enlarged prostate in male;

pregnancy in female; beer drinking; interstitial nephritis; diabetes; phimosis.

DECREASED FREQUENCY: After sweating, diarrhea, or bleeding; in anuria, oliguria, uremia, brain disease, drug poisoning, coma, and parenchymatous nephritis. SEE: *urine.*

urination, words pert. to: anisuria; bacilluria; bladder; bradyuria; catheterization; diuresis; diuretic; dysuria; enuresis; kidney; melanuria; micturate; micturition; nocturia; nycturia; oliguria; polyuria; strangury; uracratia; urea; "uret-" words; uric acid; "urin-" words; void.

urine (ū′rĭn) [L. *urina*, from Gr. *ouron,* urine]. The fluid secreted from the blood by the kidneys, stored in the bladder, and discharged, usually voluntarily, through the urethra. It is conveyed to the bladder by two ureters from the kidneys.

In health, urine is of amber color, slightly acid reaction, and it has a peculiar odor with a bitter, saline taste, frequently depositing a precipitate of phosphates when fresh, but esp. on standing, and having a specific gravity that varies from 1.005 to 1.030.

The greater the amt. excreted, the lower is the specific gravity. The normal amt. of nonprotein nitrogen is from 25-35 mg./100 cc. of blood. The amt. of this substance present in the blood is related to how well the kidneys are functioning.

The daily output is equally variable, being adapted to the amt. of water taken in, and to the amt. lost by evaporation from the respiratory and cutaneous surfaces.

CONSTITUENCY: Urine consists of water (95%) and solids (5%). Solids amount to 30-70 gm./liter and include the following (figures are in grams/24 hours unless otherwise noted): *Organic substances:* urea, uric acid (0.5 to 0.8), creatine (60 to 150 mgm.), creatinine (1.0 to 1.8), ammonia (0.3 to 1.0). *Inorganic substances:* sodium chloride (9 to 16), potassium chloride (2.5), calcium (0.1 to 0.2), magnesium (0.05 to 0.2), phosphorus (2.0 to 2.5).

In addition to the above, many other substances may be present depending on diet and state of health of the individual. Among substances indicating pathological states are albumin, glucose, ketone bodies, blood, pus, casts, and bacteria.

DIAGNOSIS: *Normal urine:* amber color. Its color is imparted by urobilin, q.v., a pigment mainly derived from bilirubin, q.v., in the bile. This pigment is found in more than normal quantities in fever and it may be indicative of blood destruction. The effect of food and medication must be considered before concluding that the color of the urine reflects a pathological condition.

Black: Melanuria; malignant pigmented tumor; melanotic cancer or carbolic acid poisoning. *Bile-colored:* Seen in jaundice. *Blue:* May result from methylene blue or the presence of indigo. *Colorless:* This is known as achromaturia. *Milky:* May be due to chyluria, lipuria, or pus. *Orange-red:* May indicate the presence of pyridine dyes. *Pale:* Indicates an excess of water, it is found in conditions causing polyuria. *Red or reddish color:* May be due to the presence of blood in the urine, hematuria, or to senna or rhubarb which may color the urine either brown or orange.

Acid u.: May be found in acidosis and pyelonephritis. *Alkaline urine:* Shows a white sediment. *Bacteria in u.:* Appears cloudy. *Bloody urine:* It shows a smoky sediment, and is reddish-brown. *Pus:* This is mucoid and shows a white sediment; it is found in bacterial infections of the urinary tract.

Ammoniacal odor: May result from decomposition products. *Aromatic:* This is the odor of a normal urine. *Fecal odor:* Due to fistulous communication between the intestinal and urinary tracts. *Fishy:* Cystitis. *New-mown hay odor:* Indicative of diabetes. *Overripe apple:* Indicative of acetonuria or the presence of acetone bodies in the urine. *Violet:* May be caused by turpentine.

URINARY PRODUCTS IN DISEASE: *Albumin:* Due to nephritis and inflammation of mucous membrane of any portion of the urinary apparatus. *Acetone:* Represents the by-products of excessive fat metabolism excreted by the kidneys and known as ketonuria. *Animal parasites:* Rare, found as result of contamination. *Bacteria:* Usually regarded as being of little importance if fewer than 100,000 can be cultured from each ml. of urine. *Bile:* Bile in the urine indicates abnormal retention of bile. *Blood:* Indicates hemorrhagic nephritis, calculi, congestion of a kidney, renal carcinoma, tuberculosis of kidney, chronic infections. *Casts:* These indicate renal disease. A few hyaline casts in the aged denote slight damage to the kidneys. Casts are found in large numbers in nephritis. The less acute the disease, the finer are the granular casts. *Crystals:* Acid urine produces crystals, calcium oxalate, and urates; alkaline urine, ammonium biurate and phosphates. Crystals have little significance, excepting leucine and tyrosine crystals which may indicate liver disease.

Cylindroids: No special significance. *Diacetic acid:* Deficient carbohydrate metabolism of an advanced stage; it is preceded by the presence of acetone. *Epithelial cells* (squamous): If in large numbers from urinary bladder and ureters they indicate inflammation of these parts; renal epithelial cells of kidney indicate serious damage to the same.

Fat droplets: Fatty degeneration of kidneys and lipemia. *Froth:* Around standing urine indicates presence of bile. *Indican:* Small significance but is seen in intestinal putrefaction. *Lipoids, double refractile:* Epstein's lipoidal *Mucus:* If visible and in quantity, urethritis is indicated. No special significance in women if the quantity is small. *Mucous threads:* Mucoid, ribbonlike structures of no great significance. *Pus cells:* Their presence may be normal if not many; if accompanied by red cells they indicate inflammation. *Red blood cells:* Stones or inflammation of kidney or urinary tract. No significance if due to contamination by menstrual fluid.

Sediment: Pinkish due to excess of urates; white, caused by phosphates. *Sugar* (glucose): Denotes faulty carbohydrate metabolism as seen in diabetes mellitus. *Urea:* Principal end product of protein metabolism. *Yeasts and molds:* Result of contamination. SEE: *urea; urinary conditions.*

EXCRETION OF URINE: Increased in fevers, esp. if weight is lost, after pregnancy, during parturition, after the intake of large quantities of liquid and after protein intake. Diminished in pregnancy, convalescence with gain in weight, disease of the liver, and in low protein intake.

CONDITIONS: *Difficult urination* (dysuria): Found in urethral stricture, enlarged prostate, atony and impairment of the bladder's muscular power, and in gonorrhea and other inflammatory conditions involving the urethra, bladder, or lower ureter. *Diminished* (oliguria): Cardiac failure; scanty in all fevers. Accompanies acute, chronic, and parenchymatous nephritis; obstruction of return venous circulation of kidney; thrombosis of renal vein or inferior vena cava; loss of fluids through hemorrhages, vomiting, or diarrhea; obstruction or pressure upon ureter; lead poisoning.

Incontinence (enuresis, q.v.): Inability to retain urine because of paralysis or relaxation of sphincters or contraction of longitudinal muscular layer of bladder; incontinence and dribbling are results. All forms of coma, shock, sunstroke and some forms of insanity, typhoid, typhus. Injuries

Significance of Changes in Urine
Quantity

Normal	Abnormal	Significance
1000–1500 ml. (96% H_2O)		Depends upon water and fluid foods consumed, exercise, temperature, kidney function, etc.
	High (polyuria)	Diabetes mellitus, diabetes insipidus, nervous diseases, certain types of chronic nephritis (kidney disorder), diuretics (drugs as caffeine, calomel, digitalis, causing increased urinary excretion)
	Low (oliguria)	Acute nephritis, heart disease, fevers, eclampsia, diarrhea, vomiting
	None (anuria)	Uremia (urinary substances in blood), acute nephritis, metal poisoning, e.g., due to bichloride of mercury

Color

Normal	Abnormal	Significance
Yellow to amber		Depends upon concentration of pigment (urochrome)
	Pale	Diabetes insipidus, granular kidney, due to a very dilute urine
	Milky	Fat globules, pus corpuscles in genitourinary infections
	Reddish	Blood pigments, drugs, or food pigments
	Greenish	Bile pigment, associated with jaundice
	Brown-black	Poisoning (mercury, lead, phenol), hemorrhages

Transparency

Normal	Abnormal	Significance
Clear		No significance
Cloudy on standing		Precipitation of mucin from urinary tract; not pathological
Turbid		Precipitation of calcium phosphate; not pathological
	Milky	Presence of fat globules; pathological
	Turbid	Presence of pus as result of inflammation of urinary tract; pathological

Significance of Changes in Urine (*Continued*)
Odor

Normal	Abnormal	Significance
Faintly aromatic		No significance
	Pleasant (sweet)	Acetone, associated with diabetes mellitus
	Unpleasant	Decomposition or ingestion of certain drugs or foods

Specific Gravity

Normal	Abnormal	Significance
1.015 to 1.025 sp. gr.		Ordinarily, sp. gr. inversely proportional to volume
	Low	Dilution if volume is large; otherwise nephritis
	High	Acute nephritis; concentrated if volume is small; otherwise if volume is large and light colored, diabetes mellitus

Acidity

Normal	Abnormal	Significance
Acid (slight)		Diet of acid-forming foods (meats, eggs, prunes, wheat, etc.) overbalancing the base-forming foods (vegetables and fruits)
	High acidity	Acidosis, diabetes mellitus, many pathological disorders (fevers, starvation)
	Alkaline	Putrefying bacteria change urea into ammonium carbonate; infection or ingestion of alkaline compounds

to spinal cord and tumors of same and lesions; transverse myelitis, spinal meningitis, locomotor ataxia, paralysis. Reflex excitability of nervous system. Local irritation. Cystitis, phimosis, vesical calculus, meatus contracted, ascarides, diabetic or too concentrated urine. Relaxation of vesical sphincters. Hydrocyanic acid poisoning.

Increased (polyuria): May be indicative of chronic interstitial nephritis; diabetes (mellitus or insipidus); amyloid disease of kidney; reabsorption of effusions; functional disease of nervous system as hysteria, neurasthenia, migraine, etc. Persistent in bulbar, cerebellar, and spinal tumors, locomotor ataxia, and meningitis. *Obstructive:* Result of occlusion of one or both ureters. *Painful:* Dysuria, q.v., vesical tenesmus; there is a persistent desire to urinate. *Residual:* That remaining in bladder after urination; usually indicative of a pathological condition such as prostatic disease, cystocele.

Retention (ischuria): Inability to urinate; almost same diseases and injuries of cord producing incontinence. All forms of coma; typhoid; peritonitis; hysteria; atony; prostatic enlargement; urethral stricture; urethritis, cystitis, or tumors of bladder; calculus in urethra. *Strangury:* Painful and spasmodic. May be indicative of cystitis; neuralgia; acute nephritis; tuberculosis; cancer or ulceration of bladder; urethritis; urethral stricture; hypertrophied, cancerous, or inflamed prostate; prolapsus uteri; pelvic peritonitis and abscess; metritis; cancer of cervix; dysmenorrhea; vesical tenesmus.

Pain and burning often caused by concentrated or acid urine. *Suppression:* Failure of kidneys to secrete urine. May be complete (anuria) or partial (oliguria). Failure of kidneys to secrete the urine or failure to reach the bladder if secreted may be found in acute nephritis or congestion, renal abscess, last stages of chronic nephritis. Renal damage caused by patient's having received a blood transfusion with incompatible blood.

SEDIMENT, HOW TO OBTAIN: The examination should be made quickly after urine is voided by centrifuging for three minutes.

urine, words pert. to: acathectic; acetone; a. bodies; a., tests for; acetonuria; achromaturia; acidaminuria; acromaturia; adrenaluria; albiduria; albinuria; albuminaturia; albuminorrhea; albuminuria; albumosuria; alkalinuria; alkaluretic; alkaptone; alkaptonuria; allantoinuria; allotriuria; alloxuria; aminosuria; ammoniuria; amylosuria; amyluria; anisuria; antidiuresis; antidiuretic; anuresis; anuria; arabinosuria; azoturia; baruria; Bence-Jones protein; Benedict's test; bilirubinuria; bladder, urinary; bladder stammering; bladder percussion; blennuria; blood, test for; brick dust; calcariuria; carbohydraturia; carboluria; carbonuria; cast; ceramuria cerebrosuria; chlorides, test for; chloriduria; chloruremia; chloruria; choleuria; choluria; chondroituria; chromaturia; chyluria; diacetic acid test; enuresis; epithelium; erythruria; galactosuria; galacturia; glucose; glycosuria; Heller's test; hemoglobinuria; hippuria; hyaline casts; hydruria; incontinence; ischuria; ketonuria; ketosis; kidney; lactosuria; lipuria; lithuria; litmus; melanuria; mucus; myosinuria; nocturia; oliguresis; oxaluria; pentosuria; pus; pyuria; residual; residuum; retention; secretion; tyrosinuria; uraturia; urea; urechysis; uredema; uremia; ureter; uric acid; urinalysis; "uro-" words.

urinemia (ū″rĭ-nē′mĭ-ă) [L. *urina,* urine, + Gr. *haima,* blood]. Accumulation in the blood of substances such as urea, which are normally excreted in the urine. SYN: *uremia,* q.v.

uriniferous (ū-rĭ-nĭf′ĕr-ŭs) ["+ *ferre,* to bear]. Carrying urine.

uriniparous (ū-rĭ-nĭp-ă-rŭs) ["+ *parere,* to bear]. Producing or secreting urine.

urinogenital (ū-rĭ-nō-jĕn-ĭ-tăl) ["+ *genitalia,* genitals]. Pert. to the genital and urinary organs. SYN: *urogenital.*

urinogenous (ū-rĭ-nŏj-ĭ-nŭs) [Gr. *ouron,* urine, + *gennan,* to produce]. 1. Producing urine. 2. Originating in urine. SYN: *urogenous.*

urinology (ū-rĭ-nŏl-ō-jĭ) ["+ Gr. *logos,* study]. Scientific study of the urine and the urinary tract. SYN: *urology.*

urinoma (ū″rĭ-nō′mă) [L. *urina,* urine, + Gr. *-ōmo,* mass]. A cyst containing urine.

urinometer (ū″rĭ-nŏm′ĕ-tĕr) ["+ Gr. *metron,* a measure]. Device for determining urine's specific gravity.

urinometry (ū″rĭ-nŏm′ĕt-rĭ) ["+ Gr. *metron,* a measure]. Determination of specific gravity of the urine.

urinophil (ū′rĭ-nō-fīl) [Gr. *ouron,* urine, + *philein,* to love]. Capable of existing in the urine, as bacteria which grow best in urine.

urinoscopy (ū-rĭ-nŏs′kō-pĭ) ["+ Gr. *skopein,* to examine]. Examination of the urine.

urinose, urinous (ū′rĭ-nōs, ū′rĭ-nŭs) [L. *urina,* urine]. Having the characteristics of, or containing urine.

urisolvent (ū″rĭ-sŏl′vĕnt) ["+ *solvens,* dissolving]. Dissolving uric acid or causing it to be dissolved.

urningism, urnism (oorn′ĭng-ĭzm, oorn′-ĭzm) [Ger.]. Condition in which sexual desire is only for one of the same sex. SYN: *amor lesbicus; homosexuality; lesbianism; sapphism; tribadism,* q.v.

uro- [Gr.]. Combining form meaning pert. to urine.

uroacidimeter (ū″rō-ăs-ĭ-dĭm′ĕ-tĕr) [Gr. *ouron,* urine, + L. *acidus,* sour, + Gr. *metron,* a measure]. An apparatus for measuring the degree of acidity of the urine.

urobilin (ū″rō-bī′lĭn) [Gr. *ouron,* urine, + L. *bilis,* bile]. A brown pigment formed by the oxidation of urobilinogen, a decomposition product of bilirubin. Urobilin may be formed in stools or in urine after exposure to air.

urobilinemia (ū″rō-bī″lĭn-ē′mĭ-ă) ["+ "+ Gr. *haima,* blood]. Urobilin in blood.

urobilinicterus (ū″rō-bī-lĭn-ĭk′tĕr-ŭs) [Gr. *ouron,* urine, + L. *bilis,* bile, + Gr. *ikteros,* jaundice]. Jaundice resulting from urobilinemia.

urobilinogen (ū-rō-bĭ-lĭn′ō-jĕn) ["+ "+ Gr. *gennan,* to produce]. A colorless derivative of bilirubin from which it is formed by the action of intestinal bacteria. SYN: *stercobilinogen.*

urobilinogenemia (ū″rō-bī″lĭn-ō-jĕn-ē′mĭ-ă) [Gr. *ouron,* urine, + L. *bilis,* bile, + Gr. *gennan,* to produce, + *haima,* blood]. Urobilinogen in the blood.

urobilinuria (ū″rō-bī″lĭn-ū′rĭ-ă) ["+ "+ Gr. *ouron,* urine]. Excess of urobilin in the urine.

urocele (ū′rō-sēl) [Gr. *ouron,* urine, + *kēlē,* hernia]. Escape of urine into the scrotum.

urocheras (ū-rŏk'ĕr-ăs) [Gr. *ouron*, urine, + *cheras*, gravel]. Gravel or calcareous sediment in the urine. SYN: *uropsammus.*

urochesia (ū-rō-kē'zǐ-ă) [Gr. *ouron*, urine, + *chezein*, to defecate]. A discharge of urine in the feces.

urochrome (ū'rō-krōm) ["+ *chrōma*, color]. The substance which gives urine its characteristic color. It is derived from urobilin.

uroclepsia (ū-rō-klĕp'sǐ-ă) ["+ *kleptein*, judge]. Involuntary urination without being aware of it.

urocrisis (ū-rŏk'rǐ-sǐs) ["+ *krisis*, crisis]. 1. Change (generally favorable) which supervenes in the crisis of a disease accompanied by copious urination. 2. A crisis marked by excessive urination. 3. Pain in bladder in locomotor ataxia.

urocyanogen (ū″rō-sī-ăn'ō-jĕn) [Gr. *ouron*, urine, + *kyanos*, blue, + *gennan*, to produce]. A blue pigment in urine, esp. in cholera patients.

urocyanosis (ū″rō-sī-ăn-ō'sǐs) [Gr. *ouron*, urine, + *kyanos*, blue, + *-ōsis*, condition]. Blue discoloration of the urine. May be due to presence of indigo blue from oxidation of indican, or from ingestion of drugs such as methylene blue. SYN: *indicanuria.*

uroedema (ū″rō-ē-dē'mă) ["+ *oidēma*, a swelling]. Extravasation of urine distending the tissues. SYN: *uredema.*

uroerythrin (ū″rō-er'ǐth-rǐn) ["+ *erythros*, red]. A reddish pigment sometimes present in urine. SYN: *urerythrin.*

urofuscin (ū″rō-fūs'ǐn) [Gr. *ouron*, urine, + L. *fuscus*, tawny]. A reddish-brown pigment sometimes found in samples of urine, esp. in cases of porphyrinuria.

urofuscohematin (ū″rō-fūs″kō-hĕm'ăt-ǐn) ["+ L. *fuscus*, tawny, + Gr. *haima*, blood]. A red-brown pigment in urine in some diseases.

urogastrone (ū″rō-găs'trōn) [Gr. *ouron*, urine, + *gastĕr*, belly]. A hormone-like substance present in urine which has an inhibitory effect on gastric secretion.

urogenital (ū″rō-jĕn'ǐ-tăl) ["+ L. *genitalia*, genitals]. Pert. to the urinary and reproductive organs. SYN: *urinogenital.*

urogenous (ū-rŏj'ĕn-ŭs) ["+ *gennan*, to produce]. 1. Producing urine. 2. Originating in urine. SYN: *urinogenous.*

urogram (ū'rō-grăm) [Gr. *ouron*, urine, + *gramma*, a mark]. An x-ray photograph of any part of the urinary tract.

urography (ū-rŏg'ră-fǐ) [Gr. *ouron*, urine, + *graphein*, to write]. Roentgenography of any part of the urinary tract, after introduction of a radiopaque substance.

urohematin (ū″rō-hĕm'ăt-ǐn) ["+ *haima*, *haimat-*, blood]. Pigment in urine, considered as identical with hematin, q.v. which alters color of urine in proportion to degree of oxidation.

urohematonephrosis (ū-rō-hĕm″ă-tō-nē-frō'sǐs) [Gr. *ouron*, urine, + *haima*, blood, + *nephros*, kidney]. Pathological condition of kidney in which pelvis is distended with blood and urine.

urohematoporphyrin (ū″rō-hĕm″ă-tō-por ′-fīr-ǐn) ["+ "+ *porphyra*, purple]. Iron-free hematin in urine when hemolysis occurs.

urokinase (u-ro-ki'nās). An enzyme obtained from human urine. Used experimentally for dissolving intravascular clots. It is administered intravenously.

urokinetic (ū-rō-kǐ-nĕt'ǐk) [Gr. *ouron*, urine, + *kinēsis*, movement]. Resulting reflexly from stimulation of the urinary organs.

urolagnia (ū-rō-lăg'nǐ-ă) [Gr. *ouron*, urine, + *lagneia*, lust]. Sexual excitation associated with urine or urination.

urolith (ū'rō-lǐth) ["+ *lithos*, stone]. A concretion in the urine.

urolithiasis (ū-rō-lǐ-thǐ-ă-sǐs) [Gr. *ouron*, urine, + *lithos*, stone, + *iasis*, condition]. Formation of urinary calculi and the illness associated with the presence of calculi in the urinary tract. SEE: *calculus, renal.*

urolithology (ū-rō-lǐ-thŏl'ō-jǐ) ["+ "+ *logos*, a study]. Science dealing with urinary calculi.

urologic (ū-rō-lŏj'ǐk) [Gr. *ouron*, urine, + *logos*, study]. Pert. to urology.

urologist (ū-rŏl'ō-jǐst) ["+ *logos*, a study]. One who specializes in the practice of urology.

urology (ū-rŏl'ō-jǐ) [Gr. *ouron*, urine, + *logos*, a study]. The branch of medicine concerned with the urinary tract in both sexes and the genital tract in the male.

urolutein (ū″rō-lū'tē-ǐn) ["+ L. *luteus*, yellow]. A yellow pigment seen in the urine.

uromancy (ūr'ō-măn″sǐ) ["+ *manteia*, a divination]. Use of urinalysis for diagnosis of disease.

uromelanin (ū-rō-mĕl'ăn-ǐn) [Gr. *ouron*, urine, + *melas*, black]. A black pigment occurring in urine resulting from the decomposition of urochrome.

urometer (ū-rŏm'ĕt-ĕr) ["+ *metron*, a measure]. Instrument for determining specific gravity of urine. SYN: *urinometer.*

uroncus (ū-rŏn'kŭs) [Gr. *ouron*, urine, + *onkos*, a mass]. A swelling or cyst containing urine.

uronephrosis (ū″rō-nĕf-rō'sǐs) [Gr. *ouron*, urine, + *nephros*, kidney, + *-ōsis*, condition]. Dilatation of renal structures from

obstruction of urinary flow. Distention of renal pelvis and tubules with urine. SYN: *hydronephrosis*.

uronology (ū-rō-nŏl'ō-jī) ["+ *logos*, a study]. The science of urine and genitourinary diseases. SYN: *urology*.

uronophile (ū-rŏn'ō-fil) ["+ *philein*, to love]. Developing best in a culture containing urine, noting a microorganism.

uropathy (ū-rŏp'ă-thī) ["+ *pathos*, disease]. Any disease affecting the urinary tract.

 u., obstructive. Any disease resulting from obstruction of the urinary tract.

uropenia (ū-rō-pē'nī-ă) [Gr. *ouron*, urine, + *penia*, a lack]. Lack of urinary secretion.

urophan (ū'rō-făn) [Gr. *ouron*, urine, + *phainein*, to appear]. A substance which when taken into the body appears unchanged in the urine.

urophanic (ū-rō-făn'ĭk). Appearing in the urine.

urophein, urophaein (ū"rō-fē'ĭn) [Gr. *ouron*, urine, + *phaios*, gray]. Gray pigment in urine said to cause its characteristic odor.

urophosphometer (ū"rō-fŏs-fŏm'ē-tĕr) ["+ L. *phosphas*, phosphorus]. Device for estimating amt. of phosphorus in the urine.

uroplania (ū"rō-plā'nī-ă) ["+ *planē*, a wandering]. Condition in which urine is present or discharged from parts other than the urinary organs.

uropoiesis (ū"rō-poy-ē'sĭs) ["+ *poiēsis*, production]. Formation of urine by the kidneys.

uropoietic (ū"rō-poy-ĕt-ĭk) [Gr. *ouron*, urine, + *poiein*, to form]. Concerned in the formation of urine, or uropoiesis.

uroporphyrin (ū-rō-por'fī-rin). A reddish pigment present in the urine and feces in cases of porphyria. May also be present in the urine of persons taking certain drugs.

uropsammus (ū"rō-săm'ŭs) [Gr. *ouron*, urine, + *psammos*, sand]. Gravel or calcareous sediment in the urine. SYN: *urocheras*.

uropyonephrosis (ū"rō-pī-ō-nĕf-rō'sĭs) ["+ *pyon*, pus, + *nephros*, kidney, + -*ōsis*, condition]. Urine and pus in the renal pelvis.

uropyoureter (ū"rō-pī"ō-ū-rē'tĕr) ["+ "+ *ourētēr*, ureter]. Accumulation of urine and pus in the ureter.

urorosein (ū"rō-rō'zē-ĭn) ["+ L. *roseus*, rosy]. A rose-colored pigment in urine, which is increased in certain diseases. SYN: *urorrhodin*.

urorrhagia (ū-rō-ră'jī-ă) ["+ *rhēgnynai*, to burst forth]. Excessive secretion of urine. SYN: *polyuria*.

urorrhea (ū-rō-rē'ă) ["+ *rhoia*, a flow]. Involuntary flow of urine. SYN: *enuresis*.

urorrhodin (ū-rō-rō'dĭn) ["+ *rhodon*, rose]. A rose-colored pigment in the urine. SYN: *urorosein*, q.v.

urorrhodinogen (ū-rō-rō-dĭn'ō-jĕn) [Gr. *ouron*, urine, + *rhodon*, rose, + *gennan*, to produce]. A chromogen of the urine which, when decomposed, forms urorrhodin.

urorubin (ū-rō-rū'bĭn) ["+ L. *ruber*, red]. A red pigment obtained from urine by treatment with hydrochloric acid.

urorubrohematin (ū"rō-rū"brō-hĕm'ă-tĭn) ["+ "+ Gr. *haima, haimat-*, blood]. A reddish pigment occasionally found in the urine in some chronic diseases.

urosacin (ū-rō'să-sĭn) [Gr. *ouron*, urine]. A red pigment in the urine. SYN: *urorrhodin*.

uroscheocele (ū-rŏs'kē-ō-sēl) ["+ *oscheon*, scrotum, + *kēlē*, mass]. Swelling of scrotum from extravasation of urine into scrotal sac. SYN: *urocele*.

uroschesis (ū-rŏs'kĕs-ĭs) ["+ *schesis*, a holding]. 1. Suppression of urine. 2. Retention of the urine.

uroscopy (ū-rŏs'kō-pī) [Gr. *ouron*, urine, + *skopein*, to examine]. 1. Examination of the urine. 2. Diagnosis by examination of the urine.

urosemiology (ū"rō-sē-mī-ŏl'ō-jī) ["+ *sēmeion*, sign, + *logos*, study]. Examination of the urine as an aid to diagnosis.

urosepsin (ū-rō-sĕp'sĭn) ["+ *sēpsis*, putrefaction]. A toxic substance formed from decomposition of urine in the tissues.

urosepsis (ū-rō-sĕp'sĭs). Septic poisoning due to retention and absorption of urinary products in the tissues.

urospectrin (ū-rō-spĕk'trĭn) [Gr. *ouron*, urine, + L. *spectrum*, image]. A pigment derived from normal urine seen when shaken with acetic ether.

urostealith (ū"rō-stē'ă-lĭth) ["+ *stear*, fat, + *lithos*, stone]. A fatty substance in some urinary calculi.

urotoxicity (ū"rō-tŏks-ĭs'ĭ-tī) ["+ *toxikon*, poison]. The toxic character of the urine.

uroureter (ū"rō-u'rē-tĕr, -ū-rē'tĕr) ["+ *ourētēr*, ureter]. Distention of the ureter with urine, due to stricture or obstruction.

urous (ū'rŭs) [Gr. *ouron*, urine]. Having the nature of urine.

uroxanthin (ū"rō-zăn'thĭn) ["+ *xanthos*, yellow]. Yellow coloring matter of the urine; an indigo-forming substance.

uroxin (ū-rŏk'sĭn) ["+ *oxys*, sharp]. A derivative of alloxan, q.v.

urtica (ŭr'tĭk-ă, ŭr-tī'kă) [L., a stinging nettle]. (pl. *urti'cae*) A wheal.

urticae. Pl. of urtica, q.v.

urticaria (ŭr-tĭ-kā'rī-ă) [L. *urtica*, nettle]. A vascular reaction of the skin characterized by the eruption of pale, evanescent wheals, which are associated with severe itching. SYN: *hives; nettle rash.* SEE: *allergy; angioneurotic edema (giant hives).*

ETIOL: Contact with an external irritant as the nettle rash, physical agents, foods, insect bites, serum sickness, pollens, drugs, neurogenic factors.

SYM: Sudden general eruption of papules or wheals associated with intense itching.

TREATMENT: *General measures.* Because the skin manifestation is an allergic reaction, identify and remove the antigenic offender if possible. Check diet for common offenders such as wheat, milk, eggs, chocolate, and other food allergens. Avoid unnecessary medication as drugs are often causative factors. *Specific measures.* Antihistaminic drugs often give quick relief. Injection of epinephrine (subcutaneous). Ephedrine may be used. In severe cases ACTH or cortisone used with caution has proved effective. Locally, antipruritic lotions and baths are frequently beneficial.

u., aquagenic. U. caused by exposure of the skin to ordinary water.

u. bullo′sa. Eruption of temporary vesicles with infusion of fluid under the epidermis.

u. facti′tia. Wheals following slight irritation of the skin. SYN: *dermatographia.*

u. haemorrhagica. U. with lesions infiltrated with blood.

u. maculo′sa. A chronic form of u. with red-colored lesions.

u. mariti′ma. U. due to salt water bathing.

u. medicamento′sa. U. due to certain drugs.

u. papulosa. In this form the wheal is followed by a lingering papule which is attended by considerable itching. Most commonly observed in debilitated children. SYN: *lichen urticatus; prurigo simplex.*

u. solaris. Urticaria occurring in certain individuals following exposure to sunlight.

u. vesiculo′sa. U. bullosa, q.v.

urticarial, urticarious (ŭr″tĭ-kā′rĭ-ăl, ŭr″tĭ-kā′rĭ-ŭs) [L. *urtica,* a nettle]. Pert. to urticaria.

urtication (ŭr-tĭ-kā′shŭn). 1. Flogging of a part with nettles to induce counterirritation. 2. Burning or itching sensation. 3. Eruption of itching wheals. SYN: *urticaria.*

urushiol (ū′rū-shĭ-ol″) [Jap. *urushi,* lac, + L. *oleum,* oil]. The principal toxic irritant substance of plants such as poison ivy which produce severe dermatitis upon contact.

U. S. A. N. Abbr. for *United States Adopted Name.* A non-proprietary name for a drug.

U. S. P., U. S. Phar. Abbr. for *United States Pharmacopeia.*

U. S. P. H. S. Abbr. for *United States Public Health Service.*

ustilaginism (ŭs-tĭl-ăj′ĭn-ĭzm) [L. *ustulatus,* scorched]. Poisoning resulting from eating corn infected with smut fungus, Ustilago maydis.

Ustilago (us-tĭl-ā′gō). A moldlike fungus, Ustilago maydis, commonly called smut.

ustion (ŭs′chŭn) [L. *ustio,* a burning]. 1. Cauterization with actual cautery. 2. Incineration.

ustulation (ŭs-tū-lā′shŭn) [L. *ustulāre,* to scorch]. Roasting, parching, or drying of a moist substance.

ustus (ŭs′tŭs) [L.]. Burned. SEE: *calcination.*

uta (ū′tă). American leishmaniasis. SEE: *leishmaniasis, American.*

ut dict. Abbr. for L. *ut dictum,* as directed.

utend. Abbr. for L. *utendus,* to be used.

uter-, utero [L. *uterus,* womb]. Combining forms, denoting relationship to the uterus.

uteralgia (ū-tĕr-ăl′jĭ-ă) [L. *uterus,* womb, + Gr. *algos,* pain]. Uterine pain.

uterectomy (ū-tĕr-ĕk′tō-mĭ) ["+ Gr. *ektomē,* excision]. Removal of uterus through the abdomen or vagina. SYN: *hysterectomy,* q.v.

uterine (ū′tĕr-ĭn, -īn) [L. *uterinus*]. Pert. to the uterus.

u. bleeding. Bleeding from the uterus. Physiologic bleeding via the vagina occurs in normal menstruation. Abnormal forms include excessive menstrual flow (hypermenorrhea, menorrhagia) or too frequent menstruation (polymenorrhea). Nonmenstrual bleeding is called metrorrhagia. Pseudomenstrual or withdrawal bleeding may occur following estrogenic therapy. Breakthrough bleeding is the term used for intermenstrual bleeding which sometimes occurs in women who take progestational agents.

SEE: *menstruation; napkin, sanitary; pad, perineal; tampon, vaginal.*

u. cake. The placenta.

u. glands. The tubular glands in the endometrium.

u. milk. A milky, white substance between the gravid uterus and the placental villi.

u. souffle. Vascular sound in the pregnant uterus heard with stethoscope.

u. subinvolution. Failure of the uterus to return to normal size after childbirth. A uterus which weighs more than 100 gm. is considered to be enlarged.

u. tubes. Small tubes attached to either side of the uterus, and leading from the region of the ovary. SYN: *fallopian tubes.*

uterismus (ū″tĕr-ĭs′mŭs). Painful contractions of the uterus.

uteritis (ū-tĕr-ī′tĭs) [L. *uterus,* womb, + Gr. *-itis,* inflammation]. Inflammation of the uterus. SYN: *metritis.*

uteroabdominal (ū″tĕr-ō-ăb-dŏm-ĭ-năl) ["+ *abdominalis,* pert. to abdomen]. Pert. to both the uterus and abdomen.

uterocele (ū-tĕr′ō-sēl) ["+ Gr. *kēlē,* hernia]. Hernia containing the uterus.

uterocervical (ū″tĕr-ō-sĕr′vĭ-kăl) [L. *uterus,* womb, + *cervix,* neck]. Rel. to the uterus and the cervix.

uterocystostomy (ū″tĕr-ō-sĭs-tŏs′tō-mĭ) ["+ Gr. *kystis,* bladder, + *stoma,* mouth]. Formation of a passage between the uterine cervix and the bladder.

uterofixation (ū″tĕr-ō-fĭks-ā′shŭn) ["+ *fixātio,* a fixing]. Fixation of a displaced uterus. SYN: *hysteropexy.*

uterogestation (ū-tĕr-ō-jĕs-tā′shŭn) [L. *uterus,* womb, + *gestātio,* a carrying]. Pregnancy in the uterus; normal pregnancy.

uterography (ū″tĕr-ŏg′ră-fĭ) ["+ Gr. *graphein,* to write]. Roentgenography of the uterus.

uterolith (ū′tĕr-ō-lĭth) [L. *uterus,* womb, + Gr. *lithos,* stone]. A uterine concretion.

uterometer (ū″tĕr-ŏm′ĕt-ĕr) ["+ Gr. *metron,* measure]. Device for measuring the uterus and for determining its position.

uteroovarian (ū″tĕr-ō-ō-vā′rĭ-ăn) [L. *uterus,* womb, + *ovarium,* ovary]. Rel. to the uterus and ovary.

uteropexia, uteropexy (ū″tĕr-ō-pĕks′ĭ-ă, ū′tĕr-ō-pĕks-ĭ) ["+ Gr. *pexis,* fixation]. Fixation of the uterus to the abdominal wall. SYN: *hysteropexy.*

uteroplacental (ū″tĕr-ō-plă-sen′tăl) [L. *uterus,* womb, + *placenta,* a flat cake]. Rel. to the placenta and uterus.

uteroplasty (ū″tĕr-ō-plăs′tĭ) ["+ Gr. *plassein,* to form]. Plastic surgery of the uterus.

uterosacral (ū″tĕr-ō-sā′krăl) ["+ *sacralis,* pert. to the sacrum]. Rel. to the uterus and sacrum.

uterosalpingography (ū″tĕr-ō-săl-pĭng-ŏg′ră-fĭ) [L. *uterus,* womb, + Gr. *salpinx,* tube, + *graphein,* to write]. Visualization of the interior of the uterus and fallopian tubes by X ray.

uteroscope (ū′tĕr-ō-skōp) ["+ Gr. *skopein,* to examine]. Device for viewing the uterine cavity.

uterotome (ū′tĕr-ō-tōm) ["+ Gr. *tomē,* a cutting]. An instrument used for uterotomy. SYN: *hysterotome.*

uterotomy (ū-tĕr-ŏt′ō-mĭ) ["+ Gr. *tomē,* a cutting]. Incision of the uterus.

uterotonic (ū″tĕr-ō-tŏn′ĭk) [L. *uterus,* womb, + Gr. *tonos,* tone]. Giving muscular tone to the uterus.

uterotractor (ū″tĕr-ō-trăk′tor) ["+ *tractor,* a drawer]. An instrument for applying traction to the cervix uteri.

uterotubal (ū″tĕr-ō-tū′băl) ["+ *tuba,* tube]. Relating to the uterus and the oviducts.

uterovaginal (ū″tĕr-ō-văj′ĭ-năl) [L. *uterus,* womb, + *vagina,* sheath]. Rel. to the uterus and vagina.

uterovesical (ū″tĕr-ō-vĕs′ĭ-kăl) ["+ *vesica,* bladder]. Rel. to the uterus and bladder.

uterus (ū′tĕr-ŭs) [L. *uterus,* womb]. An organ of the female for containing and nourishing the embryo and fetus from the time the fertilized egg is implanted to the time of birth of the fetus. SYN: *womb.*

ANAT: A muscular, hollow, pear-shaped structure of the female. It is partly covered by peritoneum, the cavity lined by mucous membrane which is the endometrium.

The uterus consists of three areas: the body or expanded upper portion, the isthmus or constricted central area, and the cervix, the lowermost cylindrical portion at the upper end of the vagina. The rounded portion of the body lying above the openings of the two uterine tubes is the fundus. It is supported in this position by the pelvic diaphragm, supplemented by two broad ligaments, two round ligaments, and two uterosacral ligaments, as well as other lesser ligaments.

The upper part of the body is called the fundus and the ends of the fundus to which the tubes are attached are called the cornual ends. The cavity of the uterus is triangular in shape, with the base of the triangle in the fundal portion. The canal of the cervix is long and narrow and is constricted at the upper end by the internal os and at the lower end by the external os.

The largest portion of the uterus is made up of musculature which is longitudinal and circular. The outer covering of the uterus is peritoneum, with the exception of that part upon which the bladder rests and the vaginal portion of the cervix. The inner lining of the body of the uterus varies in form and histological structure with the period of life in which it is studied, the prepuberty stage, the actively menstruating stage, and the menopausal stage each having its own characteristics.

The uterus is situated in the mid-pelvis approximately halfway between the sacrum and the symphysis pubis. It is supported in this position by the two broad ligaments, the round ligaments, the uterosacral ligaments, and the ligaments attached to bladder. The uterus is normally anteflexed. The blood supply of the uterus is derived from the uterine and ovarian arteries.

POSITIONS: Anteflexion: Bending forward. Anteversion: Forward displacement of fundus towards pubis, while cervix is tilted up towards sacrum. Retroflexion: Bending backward, at junction of body and cervix. Retroversion: Inclination backward with retention of normal curve; opposed to anteversion.

AUSCULTATION: After the 4th month of gestation if uterus contains a living fetus three distinct sounds may be heard. *Fetal heart sounds:* Consist of a succession of short, rapid, double pulsations varying in frequency from 120 to 140 per minute. First sound is short, feeble, and obscure, while the 2nd, the one usually heard, is loud and distinct; sounds like ticking of a watch wrapped in a napkin. Sound is usually transmitted over space of three or four inches square. Location is determined by position of fetus. Generally, when maximum intensity is on level of or above umbilicus a breech presentation; when low down in front on left side, 1st position; low in front on right side, in 2nd position. During labor, examinations, if made, should be between uterine contractions. In protracted labors the fetal heart sound is of value in indicating the time for manual or instrumental interference to save life of child.

Sounds: Irregularity and feebleness of sound are the most threatening to the life of the child.

Funic souffle: A sound usually heard at a point quite remote from the uterine bruit. It is short, blowing in character, and corresponds in pregnancy with the fetal pulsation. Supposed to depend upon obstruction to the transmission of blood through the umbilical arteries, as from twirling or knotting of the umbilical cord or from external pressure. Is not a constant or even frequent sound, the conditions of production being rarely met with.

Uterine bruit: This sound is single, intermittent in character, and a combination of blowing and hissing sounds. Increases in intensity up to the period of labor. Believed to depend upon rapid passage of blood from the arteries into the distended venous sinuses of the uterus. Synchronous with maternal pulse, subject to same variations, and is always heard before the pulsations of the fetal heart; area over which is audible

varies, greatest point of intensity in median line a little above pubes.

PALPATION: During pregnancy in 3rd month, if walls of abdomen are not too thick, palpate by placing patient upon her back with head raised and thighs flexed, and pressing points of fingers gently downward and backward above the pubes. A hard, round mass will be found on the median line, rising out of the pelvis. Two or four weeks later the increase is much more strongly marked. As pregnancy advances, the mass loses more and more of its hardness, and becomes more elastic, like a cyst filled with water. In doubtful cases where decided enlargement of abdomen is present, exploration per vaginum becomes of great importance.

By vaginal examination one may be able to diagnose the stage of gestation, stage of parturition, or whether the woman is in that state, the progress of labor, the presentation and position of the child, and the position of uterus. May be practiced with the woman standing, lying on either side, or back. The sensation of the tip of cervix of unimpregnated uterus to the touch is like that imparted to the finger by touching the tip of the nose, firm and cartilaginous; of the impregnated, like that of touching the lips. Feels soft like velvet, but deeper, beyond the softness, is a hardness, as of board.

PERCUSSION: Unimpregnated uterus is inaccessible to touch externally, or to percussion. In pregnancy at end of 2nd month a dull sound on percussion just above pubes indicates the enlarging uterus; later, as uterus increases in volume and rises into abdomen, one is able, by oval tumor felt in hypogastrium and by circumscribed area of dullness corresponding to situation of the tumor, to establish strong presumptive evidence of pregnancy. This presumption becomes strengthened if the area of dullness increases with the regularity proper to gestation. Palpation and percussion, however, are not sufficient to determine whether the enlargement is due to pregnancy or to some other form of new growth. After the 5th month both these methods are inferior to auscultation.

SUBINVOLUTION: The lack of involution of the uterus following childbirth. It is manifested by a large uterus and a continuation of lochia rubra beyond the usual time. The factors in its causation are usually puerperal infection, multiparity, overdistention of the uterus by multiple pregnancy or polyhydramnios, lack of lactation, malposition of the uterus, and retained secundines.

Involution is aided by being certain that the placenta is intact at the time of delivery, and the use of ecbolics to cause contraction of the uterus.

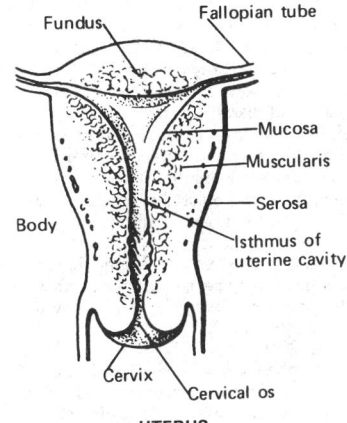

UTERUS

u. acollis. Uterus without a cervix.

u. arcuatus. Uterus with a depressed arched fundus.

u. bicornis. Uterus in which the fundus is divided into two parts.

u. biforis. Uterus in which the external os is divided into two parts by a septum.

u. bilocularis. Uterus in which the cavity is divided into two parts by a partition.

u., bipartite. Uterus in which body is partially divided by a median septum.

u., cancer of. Malignant neoplasm of the uterus. Detected by size, intermittent bleeding, purulent discharge, vaginal or Papanicolau smear, or cervical or endometrial biopsy. May produce sterility, abortion, hemorrhage, sepsis. Extremely rare in pregnancy; however, growth will increase with pregnancy.

u. cordiformis. A heart-shaped uterus.

u. didelphys. Double uterus.

u. duplex. A double uterus resulting from failure of union of mullerian ducts.

u., fetal. One which is retarded in development and possessing an extremely long cervical canal.

u. gravid. Pregnant uterus.

u. masculinus. The prostatic utricle. SEE: *utricle, masculinus.*

u. parvicollis. Normal uterus with disproportionately small vaginal portion.

u., prolapse of. Downward displacement of uterus, the cervix sometimes pro-

truding from the vaginal orifice. SEE: *descensus uteri.*

u., pubescent. An adult uterus which resembles a uterus of a prepuberal female.

u., rupture of, in pregnancy. Rare but serious. May be spontaneous or traumatic. Child and amniotic sac may be expelled into peritoneal cavity. Active movements of child with death ensuing.

ETIOL: Obstruction, weakness of uterine wall. Scars may cause weakness.

SYMP. AND SIGNS: Obstruction usually precedes symptoms. Abdominal pains, shock, hemorrhage. Child easily palpated. However, spontaneous rupture may occur without warning.

TREATMENT: Combat shock and hemorrhage.

u. septus. U. bilocularis, q.v.

u., tumors of. May cause sterility, abortion, or obstruct labor; may become infected or twisted on their attachments. Myomata possible, but not common in young women; fibroids common beyond 30 and in negro race. Subserous tumors do not affect pregnancy; may bar labor; may disappear following labor. Interstitial and submucous type may interfere with pregnancy and produce abortion.

EFFECTS UPON LABOR: Usually have no effect. If low, may cause malpresentation or impossible labor; labor pains may be weak and inefficient. Often severe pains and rupture of uterus. Submucous tumors may protrude before or after birth. Placenta may be retained. Tumor may be infected postpartum. Knee-chest position helps patient if tumor is in pelvis. If in fundus, delivery is through vagina; if not, cesarean section may be needed. Control hemorrhage by packing.

u. unicornis. Uterus which possesses only one lateral half and usually having only one uterine tube.

utricle (ū'trĭk-l) [L. *utriculus,* a little bag]. 1. One of two sacs of the membranous labyrinth in the bony vestibule of the inner ear. The utricle communicates with the semicircular ducts by five openings on posterior wall and with the sacculus and endolymphatic duct by an opening on anterior wall. On its inner surface is an area of sensory epithelium, the macula utriculi containing cells which respond to movement of otoliths due to changes in position. 2. Any small sac.

u., prostatic. A small blind pouch of the urethra extending into substance of prostate gland. It is a remnant of the embryonic mullerian duct. SYN: *uterus masculinus.*

u. of the urethra. The prostatic vesicle of the male.

u. of vestibule. Vestibular cavity connecting with the semicircular canals.

utricular (ū-trĭk'ū-lar) [L. *utriculus,* a little bag]. 1. Pert. to the utricle. 2. Like a bladder.

utriculitis (ū-trĭk-ū-lī'tĭs) ["+ Gr. *-itis,* inflammation]. Inflammation of the utricle, either that of the vestibule or the prostatic utricle.

utriculoplasty (ū-trĭk'ū-lō-plăs''tĭ) ["+ Gr. *plassein,* to form]. Reduction of the uterus by excision of a longitudinal, wedge-shaped section.

utriculosaccular (ū-trĭk''ū-lō-săk'ū-lar) ["+ *sacculus,* a small cavity]. Pert. to the utricle and saccule of the labyrinth.

u. duct. A duct uniting the utricle and saccule.

utriculus (ū-trĭk'ū-lŭs) [L. *utriculus,* a little bag]. A utricle, q.v.

u. masculin'us. SEE: *utricle, prostatic.*

u. prostaticus. SEE: *utricle, prostatic.*

utriform (ū'trĭ-form) [L. *uter, utri-,* a skin bag, + *forma,* shape]. Having a shape like a bottle.

Utus paste. Soap medicated with iodine, potassium iodide, thymol, and astringents. Has been used to induce abortions by placing it in the uterus.

uvea (ū'vē-ă) [L. *uva,* grape]. The 2nd or vascular coat of the eye lying immediately beneath the sclera. It consists of iris, ciliary body and choroid, forming pigmented layer.

uveal (ū'vē-ăl). Pert. to the middle coat of the eye, or uvea.

uveitic (ū-vē-ĭt'ĭk) ["+ Gr. *-itis,* inflammation]. Marked by or pert. to uveitis.

uveitis (ū-vē-ī'tĭs). Inflammation of the iris, ciliary body, and choroid, or the entire uvea.

uveoparotitis (ū''vē-ō-păr-ō-tī'tĭs) [L. *uva,* grape, + Gr. *para,* near, + *ous, ot-,* ear, + *-itis,* inflammation]. Inflammation of parotid gland and uveitis.

uveoplasty (ū'vē-ō-plăs''tĭ) ["+ Gr. *plassein,* to form]. Reparative operation of the uvea.

uviofast (ū'vĭ-ō-făst). Unaffected by ultraviolet radiation.

uviol (ū'vĭ-ōl). Glass which is unusually transparent to ultraviolet rays.

u. lamp. Electric l. with uviol glass globe.

uviolize (ū'vē-ō-līz). To use ultraviolet rays therapeutically.

uvioresistant (ū''vĭ-ō-rē-zĭs'tănt). Resistant to effects of ultraviolet rays. SYN: *uviofast.*

uviosensitive (ū''vĭ-ō-sĕn'sĭ-tĭv). Sensitive to effects of ultraviolet rays.

uvula (ū'vū-lă) [L. *uvula,* a little grape]. Small, soft structure hanging from free edge of soft palate in midline above the root of the tongue. It is composed of muscle, connective tissue and mucous membrane.

RS: cion; staphyle.

u. of cerebellum. A small lobule of the cerebellum lying on inferior surface of inferior vermis, anterior to the pyramis.

u. fissa. A cleft uvula.

u. palatine. SEE: *uvula.*

u. vesicae. A median projection of mucous membrane of urinary bladder located immediately anterior to orifice of urethra.

uvulaptosis (ū''vū-lăp-tō'sĭs) [L. *uvula,* little grape, + Gr. *ptōsis,* a dropping]. A relaxed condition of the uvula. SYN: *uvuloptosis.*

uvular (ū'vū-lar) [L. *uvula,* little grape]. Pert. to the uvula.

uvularis (ū-vū-lā'rĭs) [L.]. The azygos uvulae muscle. SEE: *Table of Muscles* in *Appendix.*

uvulatome (ū'vū-lă-tōm) [L. *uvula,* little grape, + Gr. *tomē,* a cutting]. Instrument for removal of uvula.

uvulatomy (ū-vū-lăt'ō-mĭ). Excision of the uvula.

uvulitis (ū''vū-lī'tĭs) [L. *uvula,* little grape, + Gr. *-itis,* inflammation]. Inflammation of the uvula.

uvuloptosis (ū-vū-lŏp-tō'sĭs) ["+ Gr. *ptōsis,* a dropping]. Relaxed condition of the palate.

uvulotome (ū'vū-lō-tōm) [L. *uvula,* little grape, + Gr. *tomē,* a cutting]. Instrument for performing uvulotomy. SYN: *uvulatome.*

uvulotomy (ū-vū-lŏt'ō-mĭ). Amputation of the uvula.

V

V. 1. Abbr. for *Vibrio; vision; visual acuity.* 2. Chem. symb. for vanadium.

v. Abbr. for L. *vena,* vein; *volt.*

vaccigenous (văk-sĭj'ĕn-ŭs) [L. *vaccīnus,* pert. to cows, + Gr. *gennan,* to produce]. Producing vaccine. SYN: *vaccinogenous.*

vaccinal (văk'sĭn-ăl). Rel. to vaccine or to vaccination.

    v. fever. A mild fever that may follow vaccination.

vaccinate (văk'sĭn-āt) [L. *vaccinus,* pert. to cows]. 1. To inoculate with cowpox vaccine to prevent or mitigate an attack of smallpox. 2. To inoculate with any vaccine to produce immunity against disease.

vaccination (văk″sĭ-nā'shŭn) [L. *vaccinus,* pert. to cows]. 1. Inoculation with a vaccine to prevent smallpox. 2. Inoculation with any vaccine to establish resistance to a specific infectious disease. 3. A scar left on the skin by inoculation of a vaccine.

    Smallpox v. should be given in the 2nd year of life in smallpox-free countries and as soon after birth as possible in countries where smallpox is endemic and in countries adjacent to endemic areas. In endemic areas v. should be repeated at one year with revaccination every 3-5 years thereafter. Evidence of revaccination within three years is required in international travelers. Persons whose work indicates contact with international travelers, or hospital employees and morticians in endemic areas, should be revaccinated annually.

    The use of a fully-potent vaccine at the time of inoculation is of the utmost importance. To retain its potency vaccine may be freeze-dried; this is esp. useful in the tropics. Glycerinated vaccine will maintain its potency for at least 6 months if it is kept below freezing constantly until the time of use. If stored below 10° C. (50° F.) it should maintain its potency for at least 14 days.

    Preferred site of v. is the upper, outer portion of the arm. Do not cleanse the skin unless it is obviously dirty. If it needs cleansing wipe the area gently with clean cloth or cotton and water and allow the spot to dry.

    There are two techniques for applying vaccine. The *multiple pressure* technique involves applying pressure with a sharp needle held perpendicular to the skin over the site where a small drop of vaccine has been placed. Usually 6-10 strokes are required for primary v. and 30 for revaccina-

tion. The appearance of several minute drops of blood is evidence that the correct amount of pressure was applied. The *jet injection* technique involves a device which deposits about 0.1 ml. of a special, less-potent vaccine intradermally through use of a jet of air.

    A major reaction is one in which a vesicular or pustular lesion with a scab or ulcer develops one week after v. Any other reaction is classed as equivocal and indicates the need for revaccination. No bandage should be placed on the v. unless there is oozing later. Then a loose nonocclusive dressing may be used.

    CONTRAINDICATION: In endemic areas serious acute illness is the only contraindication to v. In smallpox-free countries the following are contraindications: eczema or other chronic dermatitis; leukemia, lymphoma, and other reticuloendothelial malignancies; dysgammaglobulinemia; therapy with immunosuppresive drugs or ionizing radiation; and pregnancy. If a person with one of these contraindications has had a possible exposure to smallpox, he should be given vaccinia immune globulin (VIG) 0.3 ml./kg. at time of v. In the United Kingdom VIG is called human antivaccinal immunoglobulin.

vaccine (văk'sēn) [L. *vaccinus,* pert. to cows]. A suspension of infectious agents or some part of them, given for the purpose of establishing resistance to an infectious disease.

    Vaccines are of four general classes: those containing living attenuated infectious organisms; those containing infectious agents killed by physical or chemical means; those containing soluble toxins of microorganisms, sometimes used as such, but generally forming toxoids; and substances extracted from infectious agents.

    Examples of the 1st class are the BCG vaccine for tuberculosis and vaccines for smallpox and yellow fever.

    Examples of the 2nd class are vaccines used to protect human beings against typhoid fever, rabies, and whooping cough. Vaccines of this class have been prepared for use in preventing several other diseases including cholera, dysentery, undulant fever, and plague, but they are less reliable as preventives against these.

    An example of the 3rd class is toxoid used in the prevention of diphtheria and tetanus.

Examples of the 4th class are capsular polysaccharides extracted from pneumococci.

FUNCTION: To stimulate the development of specific defensive mechanisms in the body which result in more or less permanent protection against a disease. An attack of smallpox or diphtheria, for example, usually leaves the recovered patient permanently immune to those diseases. As a result of infection, the body succeeds in building up its own defenses, so that a new infection causes no illness. A successful vaccine does the same thing without risk of illness.

v., aqueous. V. employing physiological salt solution as the vehicle.

v., autogenous. Bacterial v. taken from the individual to be inoculated.

v., bacterial. Any substance for preventive inoculation, esp. a suspension of bacteria, killed or attenuated, in saline solution. Used for injection into body to induce development of active immunity to the same organism.

v., BCG. (Calmette-Guerin bacillus). Substance used in prophylactic vaccination of infants against tuberculosis. Virulence of the bacillus has been reduced by repeated cultures on glycerinated ox bile.

v., cholera. V. made from killed Vibrio cholerae. It is effective for only a few months.

v., epidemic typhus fever. V. made of killed Rickettsia prowazekii for treating epidemic typhus fever.

v., heterologous. V. prepared from organisms obtained from a source other than the person to be inoculated.

v., homologous. An autogenous v., q.v.

v., humanized. V. obtained from vaccinia vesicles in human beings.

v., influenza. A polyvalent v. containing antigenic variants of the influenza virus available for use in areas which can be expected to have epidemics. Its use is particularly helpful to the aged and chronically ill.

v., killed. V. consisting of killed infectious agents.

v., live, attenuated, measles virus V. for immunization against measles. This type of measles v. is the preferred form except in patients who have one of the following: lymphoma, leukemia, or other generalized malignancy; radiation therapy; pregnancy; active tuberculosis; egg sensitivity; prolonged treatment with drugs which suppress the immune response; administration of gamma globulin, blood, or plasma.

v., measles virus inactivated. V. for immunization against measles. Protection provided is short-lived. This preparation should be used only when there are contraindications to the use of live, attenuated measles vaccine, q.v.

v., mixed. V. prepared from more than one infectious agent.

v., multivalent. V., polyvalent, q.v.

v., mumps. A live, attenuated vaccine used to prevent mumps. Its use should be governed by the same restrictions listed for live attenuated measles virus v., q.v.

v., plague. V. made from a crude fraction of plague bacilli for immunizing against plague.

v. point. A needle or quill coated with v. lymph at its tip.

v., polyvalent. V. made from several strains of the same species of bacterium or virus.

v., rabies. V. prepared from fixed virus of rabies, used prophylactically following bite by a rabid animal. SEE: *rabies.*

v., Sabin. Oral poliomyelitis v. SEE: *poliomyelitis.*

v., sensitized. V. made more active by treatment of the bacteria with their specific immune serum.

v., smallpox. V. made from lymph of cowpox vesicles obtained from healthy vaccinated bovine animals.

v., TAB. A mixture of typhoid, paratyphoid A, and paratyphoid B vaccines.

v. therapy. Treatment of a disease by inoculation with a v. specific for that disease.

v., triple. TAB vaccine for typhoid.

v., typhoid. V. made of killed Salmonella typhosa organisms for immunizing against typhoid. May not be effective if person receives unusually large doses of the live organism at time of exposure.

v., yellow fever. V. made from attenuated strain of yellow fever virus.

vaccinia (văk-sĭn′ĭ-ă) [L. *vaccinus,* pert. to cows]. A contagious disease resulting from inoculation with cowpox virus. Papules form about 3rd day after vaccination, changing to umbilicated vesicles about the 5th day, and at end of 1st week becoming umbilicated pustules surrounded by a red areola. They dry and form scabs which fall off about the 2nd week, leaving a white, pitted depression. Inoculation of humans with this virus confers immunity against smallpox. SYN: *cowpox.*

RS: vaccination; varicella; variola.

v. immune globulin. Hyperimmune gamma globulin. The therapeutic agent of choice for dermal complications of vaccination for smallpox, i.e., eczema vaccinatum and progressive vaccinia. May be obtained commercially or by contacting one of the designated consultants listed by the Regional Blood Centers of the American Red Cross.

v. necrosum. Spreading necrosis at the site of smallpox vaccination. May be accompanied by similar necrotic areas elsewhere on the body.

vacciniform (văk-sĭn′ĭ-form) [L. *vaccinus,* pert. to cows, + *forma,* shape]. Of the nature of vaccinia or cowpox.

vacciniola (văk″sĭn-ĭ-ō′lă) [L., little cows]. Secondary general eruption after local eruption from vaccine.

vaccinogenous (văk″sĭn-ŏj′ĕn-ŭs) [L. *vaccinus,* pert. to cows, + Gr. *gennan,* to produce]. Producing vaccine or pert. to its production.

vaccinoid (văk′sĭn-oyd) [″ + Gr. *eidos,* form]. 1. Resembling vaccinia. 2. Modified or spurious vaccinia.

vaccinotherapeu′tics, vaccinother′apy. Treatment by injection of bacterial vaccines.

vacuolar (văk′ū-ō-lär) [L. *vacuum,* vacuum]. Pert. to or possessing vacuoles.

v. degeneration. Swelling of cells with increase in number and size of vacuoles. Also called parenchymous, albuminous, or hydropic degeneration; or cloudy swelling.

vac′uolat″ed. Possessing or containing vacuoles.

vacuolation (văk″ū-ō-lā′shŭn). Formation of vacuoles. SYN: *vacuolization.*

vacuole (văk′ū-ōl) [L. *vacuum,* vacuum]. A clear space in cell protoplasm filled with fluid or air.

v. autophagic. A v. that contains recognizable fragments of the cells own cytoplasm.

v. heterophagous. A v. that contains substances which come from outside the cell.

v., plasmocrin. A v. present in cytoplasm of secretory cell which is filled with crystalloid material.

v., rhagiocrin. A v. present in cytoplasm of secretory cell which is filled with colloid material.

vacuolization (văk″ū-ō-lĭ-zā′shŭn) [L. *vacuum,* vacuum]. Vacuolation, q.v.

vacuum (văk′ū-ŭm) [L., empty]. A space exhausted of its air content.

v. extractor. Device, using a suction cup attached to the fetal head, for applying traction to the fetus during delivery. Its use may be hazardous except in the hands of experts.

v. treatment. Insertion of a limb in a partial v.

v. tube. A vessel of insulating material (usually glass) which is sealed and has a vacuum sufficiently high to permit the free flow of electrons between the electrodes which extend into the tube from the outside. In England it is called a v. valve.

vade mecum (vā″dē-mē′kŭm) [L., go with me]. A useful object which a person has available with him at all times. A dictionary or handbook.

vag′abond′s disease. Discoloration of skin caused by exposure and scratching due to presence of lice. SEE: *pediculosis corporis.*

vagal (vā′găl) [L. *vagus,* wandering]. Pert. to the vagus nerve.

v. attack. A condition of dyspnea with cardiac distress and a fear of impending death. A sinking sensation assumed to be the result of vasomotor spasm.

v. escape. Condition in which one or more beats of the heart occurs even though the vagus nerve is being continuously stimulated. Stimulation of the vagus normally inhibits heart beat.

v. substance. Substance liberated at termination of vagus nerve fibers in the heart. SEE: *acetylcholine.*

v. tone. Condition in which impulses over the vagus nerve exert a continuous inhibitory effect upon the heart.

vagi (vā′gī). Pl. of vagus.

vagina (vă-jī′nă) [L., sheath]. (pl. *vaginae, vaginas*) 1. A sheathlike part. 2. [NA] A musculomembranous tube which forms the passageway between the uterus and the entrance to the vagina between the vulvae.

ANAT: In the uppermost part, the cervix divides the vagina into four fornices, the two lateral, the anterior, and the posterior.

The bladder is situated adjacent to the anterior wall of the v. and the rectum is behind the posterior wall. The v. represents a potential space, the walls of which are in contact with each other. Close to the cervix uteri the walls form a horizontal crescent shape, at the midpoint an H shape, and close to the vulva the shape of a vertical slit. The vagina is lined by mucous membrane made up of squamous epithelium. It is surrounded by fascias which allow for easy distensibility. The blood supply of the vagina is furnished from the inferior vesical, inferior hemorrhoidal, and uterine arteries.

FUNCTION: A passage for the intromission of the penis, the reception of the semen, and for the discharge of the menstrual flow; also as the passageway through which the fetus is delivered.

SEE: *puberty, timing of.*

v., bulb of. Small erectile body on each side of the vaginal vestibule. SYN: *Bartholin's glands; bulbi vestibuli.*

v. fibrosa tendinis. A fibrous sheath surrounding a tendon which usually confines it to an osseous groove.

v. masculinus. The prostatic utricle, q.v.

v. mucosa tendinis. A synovial sheath which develops about a tendon.

v., septate. Congenital condition in which the v. is divided longitudinally into two parts. Division may be partial or complete.

vagina, words pert. to: bulb of the vestibule; coitus; "colp-" words; cystocele; "elytr-" words; endocolpitis; enterocele; fistula; fornix; fourchette; gynatresia; hematocolpometra; hydrocolpos; hymen; leukorrhea; lochiocolpos; paravaginal; pronaus; rectocele; supravaginal; transvaginal; "vagin-" words.

vaginal (văj'ĭn-ăl) [L. *vagina,* sheath]. Pert. to the vagina or to any enveloping sheath.

v. hysterectomy. Surgical removal of uterus through vagina.

vaginalectomy (văj'ĭn-ăl-ĕk'tō-mĭ) ["+ Gr. *ektomē,* excision]. Excision of the tunica vaginalis. SYN: *vaginectomy.*

vaginalitis (văj-ĭn-ăl-ī'tĭs) ["+ Gr. *-itis,* inflammation]. Inflammation of tunica vaginalis testis.

vaginapexy (văj'ĭn-ă-pĕk'sĭ) [L. *vagina,* sheath, + Gr. *pēxis,* fixation]. Repair of a relaxed and prolapsed vagina. SYN: *colpopexy; vaginofixation.*

vaginate (văj'ĭn-āt) [L. *vaginatus*]. Forming or enclosed in a sheath.

vaginectomy (văj-ĭn-ĕk'tō-mĭ) [L. *vagina,* sheath, + Gr. *ektomē,* excision]. 1. Resection of tunica vaginalis. 2. Excision of the vagina or a part of it.

vaginismus (văj'ĭn-ĭz'mŭs) [L.]. Painful spasm of vagina from contraction of the muscles surrounding the vagina. May interfere with coitus. V. may indicate neurotic aversion to coitus. Extraordinary hyperesthesia of nerve supply to mucous membrane of vagina at or near site of the hymen, resulting in spasmodic constriction of sphincter vaginae muscle, preventing coitus. May also be due to local trauma, ulceration, lack of physiological lubrication, vaginitis, menopausal involution, or congenital malformation.

SYM: Extreme sensitiveness. Spasmodic closure of vaginal orifice on slightest touch.

TREATMENT: Psychotherapy; correction of primary causative factors; education correcting misinformation and fear.

v., deep. V. caused by spasm of the levator ani muscle.

v., hysterical. V. associated with hysteria.

v., mental. V. resulting from aversion to sexual intercourse. SYN: *psychogenic vaginismus.*

v., posterior. V. due to contraction of the levator ani muscle.

vaginitis (văj-ĭn-ī'tĭs) [L. *vagina,* sheath, + Gr. *-itis,* inflammation]. 1. Inflammation of a sheath. 2. Inflammation of the female vagina.

ETIOL: May be caused by microorganisms, e.g., gonococci, staphylococci, streptococci, spirochetes; chemical irritation, e.g., use of too strong chemicals in douching; fungus infection (moniliasis) caused by Candida albicans; protozoan infection (Trichomonas vaginalis); irritation from foreign bodies (pessaries, etc.); vitamin deficiency as in pellagra; conditions involving vulva and surrounding areas, as uncleanliness, intestinal worms.

SYM: Free, purulent vaginal discharge, sometimes offensive and occasionally stained with blood. There is irritation and itching of the vulvae and perineum, frequently of micturition, and smarting pain on the passage of urine. The vaginal mucous membrane is reddened and there may be superficial ulceration.

TREATMENT: Specific therapy as indicated. Improve perineal hygiene by instructing in proper method of cleaning anus after a bowel movement, proper use of menstrual protection materials, and necessity of drying vulvae following urination. Douching is not essential to the maintenance of vaginal health or cleanliness.

v. adhaesiva. Inflammation of the vagina causing adhesions between its walls.

v., atrophic. V. following the menopause, whether natural or artificial. SYN: *postmenopausal v.; senile v.*

v., diphtheritic. V. with membranous exudate caused by infection with Corynebacterium diphtheriae.

v., emphysematous. V. with gas-bubble formation in connective tissues.

v., granular. V. with cellular infiltration and enlargement of papillae.

v., postmenopausal. Atrophic v., q.v. Usually due to insufficient estrogens.

v., senile. V., atrophic, q.v.

v. testis. Inflammation of the tunica vaginalis of the testis.

v., Trichomonas vaginalis. V. associated with, or caused by, infection by Trichomonas vaginalis, a flagellate protozoon. T. vaginalis may be present in the vagina without causing disease in the host. Because the causative organism may be spread by direct contact during sexual intercourse, T. vaginalis v. is classified as a venereal disease.

vaginoabdominal (văj′ĭn-ō-ăb-dŏm′ĭn-ăl) [L. *vagina*, sheath, + *abdominalis*, abdominal]. Rel. to the vagina and abdomen.

vaginocele (văj′ĭn-ō-sēl) [″+ Gr. *kēlē*, hernia]. Vaginal hernia. SYN: *colpocele*.

vaginodynia (văj′ĭn-ō-dĭn′ĭ-ă) [″+ Gr. *odynē*, pain]. Pain in the vagina.

vaginofixation (văj′ĭn-ō-fĭks-ā′shŭn) [L. *vagina*, sheath, + *fixātio*, a fixing]. 1. Process of rendering the vagina immovable. 2. Attachment of uterus to vaginal peritoneum.

vaginogenic (văj′ĭn-ō-jĕn′ĭk) [″+ Gr. *gennan*, to produce]. Developed from or originating in the vagina.

vaginography (văj-ĭn-ŏg′ră-fĭ) [″+ Gr. *graphein*, to write]. The taking of x-ray pictures of the vagina.

vaginolabial (văj′ĭn-ō-lā′bĭ-ăl) [L. *vagina*, sheath, + *labium*, lip]. Rel. to the vagina and the labia. SYN: *vaginovulvar; vulvovaginal*.

vaginometer (văj-ĭn-ŏm′ĕ-tĕr) [L. *vagina*, sheath, + Gr. *metron*, measure]. Device for measuring the length and expansion of the vagina.

vaginomycosis (văj′ĭn-ō-mī-kō′sĭs) [″+ Gr. *mykēs*, fungus, + *-ōsis*, disease]. A fungus infection (mycosis) of the vagina.

vaginoperineal (văj′ĭn-ō-pĕr-ĭ-nē′ăl) [L. *vagina*, sheath, + Gr. *perinaion*, perineum]. Rel. to the vagina and perineum.

vaginoperineorrhaphy (văj′ĭn-ō-pĕr′ĭ-nē-or′ăf-ĭ) [″+ ″+ *rhaphē*, a sewing]. Repair of a laceration involving both the perineum and vagina. SYN: *colpoperineorrhaphy.*

vaginoperineotomy (văj′ĭn-ō-pĕr′ĭn-ē-ŏt′ō-mĭ) [″+ ″+ *tomē*, a cutting]. Surgical incision of the vagina and perineum. Usually done in order to facilitate childbirth.

vaginoperitoneal (văj′ĭn-ō-pĕr′ĭ-tō-nē′ăl). Rel. to the vagina and peritoneum.

vaginopexy (vă-jĭ′nō-pĕk″sĭ) [L. *vagina*, sheath, + Gr. *pēxis*, fixation]. Fixation of the vagina. SYN: *colpopexy.*

vaginoplasty (vă-jĭ′nō-plăs″tĭ) [″+ Gr. *plassein*, to form]. Plastic surgery on the vagina.

vaginoscope (văj′ĭn-ō-skōp) [″+ Gr. *skopein*, to examine]. Instrument for inspection of the vagina. May be a speculum or an optical instrument.

vaginoscopy (vă″jĭn-ŏs′kō-pĭ). Visual examination of the vagina.

vaginotome (văj-ĭ′nō-tōm) [L. *vagina*, sheath, + Gr. *tomē*, a cutting]. An instrument for making an incision in the vaginal walls.

vaginotomy (văj′ĭ-nŏt′ō-mĭ) [″+ Gr. *tomē*, a cutting]. Incision of vagina.

vaginovesical (văj′ĭ-nō-vĕs′ĭ-kăl) [″+ *vesica*, bladder]. Rel. to the vagina and bladder. SYN: *vesicovaginal.*

vaginovulvar (văj′ĭn-ō-vŭl′văr) [L. *vagina*, sheath, + *vulva*, a covering]. Pert. to the vulva and vagina.

vagitis (vă-jī′tĭs) [L. *vagus*, wandering, + *-itis*, inflammation]. Inflammation of the vagal nerve.

vagitus (vă-jī′tŭs) [L. *vagire*, to squall]. First cry of newly-born infant.

v. uterinus. Crying of the fetus before birth while still in the uterus.

v. vaginalis. Cry of an infant with head still in the vagina.

vagomimetic (vă″gō-mī-mĕt′ĭk) [L. *vagus*, wandering, + Gr. *mimetikos*, imitating]. Resembling action caused by stimulation of the vagus nerve.

vagosympathetic (vă″gō-sĭm-pă-thĕt′ĭk) [″+ Gr. *sympathētikos*, suffering with]. The cervical sympathetic and the vagus nerves considered together.

vagotomy (vă-gŏt′ō-mĭ) [″+ Gr. *tomē*, a cutting]. Section of the vagus nerve.

vagotonia (vă″gō-tō′nĭ-ă) [L. *vagus*, wandering, + Gr. *tonos*, tension]. Hyperirritability of the parasympathetic nervous system. SYN: *vasomotor instability.* SEE: *sympatheticotonia.*

vagotonic (vă″gō-tŏn′ĭk). Pert. to vagotonia.

vagotropic (vă″gō-trŏp′ĭk) [L. *vagus*, wandering, + Gr. *tropos*, a turning]. Acting upon the vagus nerve.

vagotropism (vă-gŏt′rō-pĭzm) [″+ ″+ *-ismos*, condition]. Affinity for the vagus nerve, as a drug.

vagrant (vă′grănt) [L. *vagrans*]. 1. Wandering from place to place. 2. A vagabond.

v's. disease. Cutaneous discoloration and irritation caused by filth and body lice. SYN: *vagabond's disease.*

vagus (vă′gŭs) [L., wandering]. (pl. *va′gi*) The pneumogastric or 10th cranial nerve. It is a mixed nerve, having motor and sensory functions and a wider distribution than any of the cranial nerves.

v. pulse. Decreased heart rate due to the slowing action of stimuli from the vagus nerve. SEE: *vagotomy; vagotonia.*

valence, valency (vă′lĕns, -lĕn-sĭ) [L. *valens*, powerful]. 1. Property of an atom or group of atoms causing them to combine in definite proportion with other atoms or groups of atoms. Valency may be as high as 8. 2. Degree of the combining power or replacing power of an atom or group of atoms, the hydrogen atom being unit of comparison. The number indicates how many atoms of hydrogen can unite with one atom of another element.

v., antibody. In immunology the number of reactive sites of an antibody molecule which can be bound by an appropriate antigen. SEE: *ligand.*

Valentin's ganglion (văl'ĕn-tĕn). [Gabriel Gustav Valentin, Ger. physician, 1810-1883]. A small ganglion at junction of middle and posterior branches of the superior dental plexus.

valetudinarian (văl-ĕ-tū-dĭn-ā'rĭ-ăn) [L. *valetudinarius*]. Chronically ill; an invalid.

valgus (văl'gŭs) [L. *valgus*, bowlegged]. A term denoting position, meaning bent outward or twisted, applied esp. to deformities in which a part is bent outward and away from the midline of the body, as talipes valgus, q.v., hallux valgus, q.v.

valine (văl'ĕn, vā'lĕn). $C_5H_{11}NO_2$, an amino acid derived from digestion of proteins. It is essential for normal growth in infants and for nitrogen balance in adults.

vallate (văl'āt) [L. *vallātus*, walled]. Having a rim around a depression.

v. papilla. A circumvallate papilla; one of a group of papillae forming a V-shaped row on posterior dorsal surface of tongue.

vallecula (văl-lĕk'ū-lă) [L., a depression]. [NA]. A depression or crevice.

v. cerebel'li. [NA]. A deep fissure on inferior surface of the cerebellum.

v. epiglottica. [NA]. Depression lying lateral to the median epiglottic fold and separating it from the pharyngoepiglottic fold.

v. ova'ta. A depression in the liver in which rests the gallbladder.

v. syl'vii. A depression marking beginning of the fissure of Sylvius.

v. un'guis. Fold of skin in which the proximal and lateral edges of the nails are embedded.

valley of the cerebellum. Hollow on inferior surface of cerebellum. SYN: *vallecula cerebelli* [NA].

vallum unguis (văl'um ŭng'gwĭs). [NA]. Fold of skin overlapping the nail.

Valsalva's maneuver, experiment (văl-săl'vă). [Antonio Maria Valsalva, It. anatomist, 1666-1723] Attempt to forcibly exhale with the glottis, nose, and mouth closed. If the eustachian tubes are not obstructed the pressure on the tympanic membranes will be increased. Maneuver can also be done with just the glottis closed, but only intrathoracic pressure will be increased. This causes increased intrathoracic pressure, slowing of the pulse, decreased return of blood to the heart, and increased venous pressure.

Valsalva's sinuses. Three dilatations in wall of the aorta behind the flaps of the three aortic semilunar valves.

valvate (văl'vāt) [L. *valva*, valve]. Pert. to or provided with valves. SYN: *valvular.*

valve (vălv) [L. *valva*, a fold]. Any one of various structures for temporarily closing an orifice or passage, or for allowing movement of fluid in one direction only.

v., aortic. The semilunar v. preventing regurgitation at the entrance of the aorta to the heart, composed of three segments.

v., bicuspid. V. closing orifice between left cardiac atrium and left ventricle.

v., Houston's. Mucosal folds of the rectum. SYN: *plicae transversales recti.*

v., ileocecal. Valve between ileum and large intestine to prevent regurgitation of intestinal contents; composed of two membranous folds.

v., mitral. V., bicuspid, q.v.

v., pulmonary. V. composed of three cusps separating pulmonary artery and right ventricle.

v., pyloric. Prominent circular membranous fold at pyloric orifice of the stomach.

v., semilunar. Valve between heart and the aorta and valve between the heart and the pulmonary artery.

v., tricuspid. Valve between the right cardiac atrium and right ventricle.

v., vacuum. The name of a vacuum tube in England.

v. of Varolius. V., ileocecal, q.v.

valvotomy [L. *valva*, a fold, + Gr. *tomē*, a cutting]. Incision into a valve, esp. Houston's valves of the rectum. SYN: *diclidotomy.*

valvula (văl'vū-lă) [L., a tiny fold]. [NA]. A valve, specifically a small valve.

v. bicuspidalis. Valve between left cardiac atrium and left ventricle.

v. coli. Valve between ileum and large intestine. SYN: *ileocecal valve.*

v. pylori. Prominent mucosal fold at pyloric entrance of the stomach.

v. semilunaris. [NA]. Valve separating heart and aorta and heart and pulmonary artery.

v. tricuspidalis. Valve between the right atrium and right ventricle of the heart.

valvulae (văl'vū-lē). Pl. of valvula.

v. conniventes. Circular membranous folds projecting into lumen of small intestine; they do not disappear on distention of bowel, and act by retarding passage of the food along the bowel; they also provide a greater absorbing area. SYN: *plica circularis.*

valvular (văl'vū-lăr) [L. *valvula,* a small fold]. Rel. to or having a valve. SYN: *valvate.*

valvulitis (văl″vū-lī'tĭs) [″ + Gr. *-itis,* inflammation]. Inflammation of a valve, esp. a cardiac valve. SYN: *dicliditis.*

valvulotome (văl'vū-lō-tōm) [″ + Gr. *tomē,* a cutting]. An instrument for incising a valve.

valvulotomy (văl″vū-lŏt'ō-mī). Process of cutting through a valve, as a rectal fold which is too rigid. SYN: *valvotomy.*

vanadium (vă-nā'dī-ŭm). SYMB: *V.* At. wt. 50.941; at. no. 23. A light gray metallic element.

van Buren's disease (văn bū'rĕn). [William Holme van Buren, Amer. surgeon, 1819-1883]. Induration of the corpora cavernosa.

van den Bergh's test (văn-dĕn-bŭrg'). [A. A. Hysman van den Bergh, Dutch physician, 1869-1943]. A test to detect the presence of bilirubin in blood serum.

vanilla (vŭ-nĭl'ŭ) [Sp. *vainilla,* little sheath]. Any one of a group of tropical orchids. The cured fruits of V. planifolia contains an aromatic substance, vanillin, which is used as a flavoring substance.

vanil'lin. USP. A flavoring substance used in foods and drugs. SEE: *vanilla.*

vanillism (vă-nĭl'lĭzm). Irritation of the skin, mucous membranes, and conjunctiva sometimes experienced by workers handling vanilla. It is caused by a mite.

vanillylmandelic acid. 4-Hydroxy-3-methoxymandelic acid. Approx. 90% of the catecholamines epinephrine and norepinephrine are metabolized to VMA and are secreted in the urine.

Persons with pheochromocytoma produce excess amounts of catecholamines; thus VMA is present in their urine in increased amount. ABBR: VMA.

vapor (vā'pŏr) [L., steam]. 1. Gaseous state of any substance. 2. Medicinal substance for administration in form of inhaled vapor.

v. bath. Exposure of body to hot v.

v. cabinet. Cabinet in which vapor baths are given.

vaporium (vă-pō'rĭ-ŭm) [L.]. Apparatus for applying hot, cold, or medicated vapors.

vaporization (vā″pŏr-ĭ-zā'shŭn) [L. *vapor,* steam]. 1. The conversion of a liquid or solid into vapor. 2. Therapeutic use of a vapor. SYN: *nebulization.*

vaporizer (vā'pŏr-ĭ-zĕr). Device for converting liquids into a vapor spray.

vaporous (vā'pŏr-ŭs) [L. *vapor,* steam]. Consisting of, pert. to, or producing vapors.

Vaquez's disease (vă-kā'). [Louis Henri Vaguez, Fr. physician, 1860-1936]. Polycythemia vera, q.v.

variance. In statistics, the mean of the squares of the variations from the mean of a frequency distribution.

varicella (văr′ĭ-sĕl'ă) [L., a tiny spot]. An acute, highly contagious viral disease characterized by an eruption that makes its appearance in successive crops, and passes through stages of macules, papules, vesicles, and crusts. SYN: *chickenpox.*

ETIOL: Varicella-zoster virus which also is the causative agent of herpes zoster. May occur at any age, though far less common in adults than in children. Epidemics most frequent in winter and spring; in temperate zones. Approx. 3/4 of children will have had chickenpox by age 15.

INCUBATION: From 2-3 weeks; usually 13-17 days.

SYM: There may be but slight elevation of temperature at onset, followed within 24 hours by appearance of the eruption, after which time temperature usually rises still further. Eruption first appears on back and chest, crops continuing to make their appearance for a period of from 2-3 days on an average.

Each crop requires about 36 hours to pass through the several stages. Because of this, macules, papules, vesicles and crusts may be found side by side in the same general locality. Lesions are superficial and rupture very easily.

They have a tendency to be ovoid. On the chest their distribution is often particularly marked along the course of the intercostal nerves. Some, though possibly few, scars nearly always remain as evidence of a chickenpox attack. The extremities are relatively free as compared with the trunk.

COMPLICATIONS: Secondary infections due to scratching, which may result in abscess formation; at times development of erysipelas or even septicemia. Occasionally lesions in the vicinity of the larynx may cause edema of the glottis and threaten the life of the patient. Encephalitis is a rare complication. Chickenpox is a severe disease in children taking adrenal cortical steroids.

DIFFERENTIAL DIAG: Confusion between this disease and smallpox is responsible for the chief importance given chickenpox. Impetigo, dermatitis herpetiformis, herpes zoster, and furunculosis may require consideration.

PROG: Always favorable except in a very severe type which is described as varicella gangrenosa. In this variety, gangrene may develop about the site of the lesions.

TREATMENT: Isolation. Restrain the hands in the case of infants or young children in order that the lesions may not be scratched. Use of calamine lotion locally may alleviate irritation. Keep the skin, bedclothes, and sheets clean to help prevent skin infections. Also keep patient's fingernails well trimmed. The usual duration of the disease is from 2-3 weeks. Cases usually classed as contagious from five days prior to the skin eruption until not more than 6 days after the first crop of vesicles.

v. gangrenosa. V. in which necrosis occurs around the vesicles resulting in gangrenous ulceration.

varices (văr′ĭ-sēz) [L.]. Pl. of varix, q.v.

variciform (văr-ĭs′ĭ-fôrm) [L. *varix*, a twisted vein, + *forma*, shape]. Resembling a varix. SYN: *varicose.*

varicoblepharon (văr′ĭ-kō-blĕf′ă-ron) ["+ Gr. *blepharon*, eyelid]. Varicose tumor of the eyelid.

varicocele (văr′ĭ-kō-sēl) ["+ Gr. *kēlē*, hernia]. Enlargement of the veins of the spermatic cord (pampiniform plexus), commonly occurring on the left side in adolescent males; these seldom require treatment.

SYM: Vessels on affected side of scrotum are full, feeling like a bundle of worms, sometimes purplish in color. Dull ache along the cord. Slight dragging sensation in groin.

TREATMENT: Dragging sensation from exceptionally large varicocele may be relieved by a suspensory. Surgery is required for persistent symptomatic varicocele.

v., ovarian. Varicosity of veins of the ovarian or pampiniform plexus of the broad ligament.

v., utero-ovarian. Varicosity of the veins of the ovarian (pampiniform) plexus and uterine plexus of the broad ligament.

varicocelectomy (văr′ĭ-kō-sē-lĕk′tō-mĭ) [L. *varix*, twisted vein, + Gr. *kēlē*, hernia, + *ektomē*, excision]. Excision of portion of scrotal sac with ligation of the dilated veins to relieve varicocele.

varicography (văr′ĭ-kŏg′ră-fĭ) ["+ Gr. *graphein*, to write]. X-ray photography of varicose veins.

varicomphalus (văr′ĭ-kŏm′fă-lŭs) ["+ Gr. *omphalos*, navel]. Varicose tumor of the navel.

varicophlebitis (văr′ĭ-kō-flē-bī′tĭs) [L. *varix*, twisted vein, + Gr. *phleps, phleb-*, vein, +

-itis, inflammation]. Phlebitis combined with varicose veins.

varicose (văr′ĭ-kōs) [L. *varicosus*]. Pert. to varices; distended, swollen, knotted veins.

v. veins. Enlarged twisted veins. May occur in almost any part of the body but are most commonly observed in the lower extremity.

ETIOL: Congenitally defective venous valves, pregnancy, occupations requiring standing positions, and obesity.

SYM: Pain in feet and ankles, swelling, ulcers on skin. Severe bleeding if a vein is injured.

F. A. TREATMENT: For hemorrhage elevation of extremity and gentle, but firm, pressure over wound will stop bleeding. The use of a tourniquet is undesirable. Sterile dressing should be held in place with a firm bandage. Patient should not be permitted to walk for some time.

In general treatment consists of rest, elevation of extremity, and use of an external support. The use of elastic stockings is much preferred to elastic bandages. Unna's paste boots recommended for elderly or debilitated persons. Injection of sclerosing solutions may be utilized for small varicosities. High ligation and removal of vein by stripping may be necessary for major varicosities.

RS: cirsenchysis, cirsodesis, cirsomphalos, cirsotomy.

varicosity (văr′ĭ-kŏs′ĭ-tĭ) [L. *varix*, twisted vein]. 1. Condition of being varicose. 2. A swollen, twisted vein. SYN: *varix.*

varicotomy (văr′ĭ-kŏt′ō-mĭ) ["+ Gr. *tomē*, a cutting]. Excision of a varicose vein.

varicula (văr-ĭk′ū-lă) [L., a tiny dilated vein]. A small varix, esp. of the conjunctiva.

vari'ety [L. *varietās*, variety]. A term used in classifying individuals in a subpopulation of a species.

variola (vă-rī′ō-lă) [L., pustule]. An acute, contagious, systemic, viral disease characterized by a prodromal stage during which the constitutional symptoms usually are severe, followed by an eruption which passes through the successive stages of macules, papules, vesicles, pustules, and crusts. SYN: *smallpox.*

ETIOL: Causative agent is variola virus. More common during colder seasons; no age exempt; may occur in utero; no preference as to sex. Acquired chiefly by direct contact with patient. May also be spread through the handling of articles contaminated by the patient. Susceptibility practically universal in those unprotected by proper vaccination, or before a first attack of smallpox, although second attacks have been reported.

INCUBATION: Eight to 17 days; usually 10-12 days to onset of illness and 2-4 more days to onset of rash.

SYM: True variola or variola major, which occurs in those who have not been vaccinated against smallpox, characterized by abrupt onset with chills. Headache usually frontal, intense lumbar pains, elevation of temperature which may rise to 104° F. (40° C.) or higher, nausea, or more frequently, vomiting. Fever remains high until evening of 3rd or morning or 4th day, when it falls sharply, often to normal.

With drop in temperature, the eruption makes its appearance, normally coming out first about the face and soon afterward on extremities and to lesser extent on trunk. Eruption is of same character in any one general location, in this respect differing markedly from eruption of chickenpox.

About 2nd day of eruption, the macules become papular, and from 3rd to 5th day these papules become vesicles. The vesicles increase in size and from 7th to 8th day, well developed pustules are present. Finally scabs form. These fall off at the end of 3rd to 4th week.

The lesions of smallpox, being deepseated, do not rupture easily, for two reasons. First, the smallpox lesion is not single celled, but multilocular. Second, intramuscularly, of the deeper invasion, there is a thicker protective covering. It is because of the first of these reasons that 213/245-8411.) smallpox lesion does not collapse when pricked by a needle.

Variola minor or alastrim is characterized by the same signs and symptoms as true variola, but it is milder and complications are less frequent.

COMPLICATIONS: Abscesses, iritis, conjunctivitis, cervical adenitis, nephritis, and pneumonia are among the more common ones.

PROG: In true variola, recovery is doubtful, but in variola minor recovery is to be expected.

TREATMENT: *Prophylactic:* Successful vaccination against smallpox is an absolute preventive. However, this should always be repeated during an epidemic or when individual has been exposed to smallpox.

General: Absolute isolation of patient in a screened, but well ventilated, room. This is continued until all scabs and crusts have disappeared. If there are many lesions on mucous membranes a liquid diet may be essential. In the discrete type, patient need

not be limited as to diet, unless there is some contraindication. Plenty of water, fruit juices, and vegetables should be given. Milk is often soothing as well as nourishing in those cases in which the throat symptoms are severe.

Closest attention should be given to the eyes. They may be irrigated several times each day with 2% sodium bicarbonate solution. It is not advisable to use ointments on the skin before desiccation is complete, as such treatment only blocks the surface and increases likelihood of abscess formation.

Itching is not a common complaint; when present, calamine lotion may be applied. In the confluent type, weak iodine baths, or weak permanganate tubbings are often necessary, not merely for cleansing skin but for purpose of acting as a deodorant.

TREATMENT OF EXPOSED SUSCEPTIBLES: Vaccinia immune globulin (human), VIG, will, if given within 24 hours of exposure, modify or prevent smallpox. This is given intramuscularly, not intravenously. (In the U.S.A. VIG may be obtained from Hyland Laboratories, 4501 Colorado Boulevard, Los Angeles, Calif., 90039. Phone 213/245-8411.)

variolar (văr-ĭ'ō-lăr) [L. *variola,* pustule]. Pert. to smallpox.

variolate (văr'ĭ-ō-lāt). 1. To vaccinate with smallpox virus. 2. Having lesions like those of smallpox.

variolation, variolization (văr'ĭ-ō-lā'shŭn, văr'ĭ-ō-lĭ-zā'shŭn) [L. *variola,* pustule]. Inoculation with smallpox.

varioloid (văr'ĭ-ō-loyd) ["+ Gr. *eidos,* form]. 1. Resembling smallpox. 2. Pert. to varioloid. 3. A mild but contagious type of smallpox in those who have had smallpox or have been vaccinated.

variolous (vă-rĭ'ō-lŭs). Rel. to smallpox.

varix (vă'rĭks) [L., a twisted vein]. (pl. *var'ices*) 1. A tortuous dilatation of a vein. SEE: *varicose veins.* 2. Less commonly, dilatation of an artery or lymph vessel.

   v., aneurysmal. A direct communication between an artery and a varicose vein without an intervening sac.

   v., chyle. A v. of a lymphatic vessel which conveys chyle.

   v. lymphaticus. Dilatation of lymphatic vessel.

   v., turbinal. Permanent dilatation of veins of turbinate bodies.

varolian (vă-rō'lĭ-ăn). [Costanzo Varolio, It. surgeon, 1543-1575]. Rel. to the pons Varolii.

varolian bend. Anterior extension of hindgut on its ventral surface in the fetus.

varus (vā'rŭs) [L.]. 1. Turned inward; bow-legged. 2. A condition in which a clubfooted person walks on outer border of the foot. SYN: *talipes varus.* SEE: *valgus.*

vas (văs) [L. *vas,* vessel]. (pl. vasa) [NA]. A vessel or duct.

　　v. aberrans. 1. A narrow tube varying in length from 1 1/2 to 14 inches, occasionally found connected with the lower part of the canal of the epididymis or with the commencement of the vas deferens. 2. Vestige of the biliary ducts sometimes found in the liver.

　　v. afferens. [NA]. An afferent vessel of a lymph node.

　　v. afferens glomeruli renis. [NA]. The afferent arteriole which conveys blood to the glomerulus of a renal corpuscle.

　　v. capillare. [NA]. A capillary blood vessel.

　　v. deferens. The excretory duct of the testis, the continuation of the canal of the epidymis. This slim muscular tube approximately 18 inches (45.7 cm.) in length transports the sperm from each testis to the prostatic urethra. SYN: *ductus deferens* [NA].
　　RS: ampullitis; cord; deferentitis; spermatic.

　　v. lymphaticum. [NA]. One of the vessels carrying the lymph.

　　v. prominens. [NA]. Blood vessel on the cochlea's accessory spiral ligament.

　　v. spirale. A large blood vessel beneath the tunnel of Corti in the basilar membrane.

vasa (vā'să) [L. *vas,* vessel]. Pl. of vas.

　　v. afferen'tia. [NA]. The lymphatic vessels entering a lymph node.

　　v. bre'via. Branches of the splenic artery going to greater curvature of the stomach.

　　v. efferen'tia. 1. Lymphatics which leave a lymph node. 2. Excretory ducts of the testis to the head of the epididymis.

　　v. prae'via. The blood vessels of the umbilical cord presenting before the fetus.

　　v. rec'ta. 1. Tubules which become straight prior to entering the mediastinum testis. 2. Straight collecting tubules of the kidney.

　　v. vaso'rum. [NA]. Tiny blood vessels which are distributed to walls of larger veins and arteries.

　　v. vortico'sa. Stellate veins of the choroid, carrying blood to the superior ophthalmic vein. SYN: *venae choroideae oculi* [NA].

vasal (vā'săl) [L. *vas,* vessel]. Rel. to a vas or vessel.

vasalgia (vă-sal'jĭ-ă). Pain in a vessel of any kind.

vascular (văs'kū-lăr) [L. *vasculum,* a small vessel]. Pert. to or composed of blood vessels.

　　v. reflex. Constriction or dilation of vascular trunk or area resulting from mental or physical irritation.

　　v. system. The heart, blood vessels, lymphatics and their parts considered collectively.
　　It includes the pulmonary and portal systems.

　　v. tuft. One of the vascular processes on the chorion in the fetus at an early stage of development. SYN: *chorionic; villi.*

　　v. tumor. One containing dilated blood vessels. SYN: *angioma, telangioma.*

vascularization (văs"kū-lăr-ĭ-zā'shŭn) [L. *vasculum,* a tiny vessel]. Development of new blood vessels in a structure.

vascularize (văs'kū-lăr"īz) [L. *vasculum,* a tiny vessel]. To become vascular by development of new blood vessels.

vasculature. The arrangement of veins in the body or any part of it, including their relationship and functions.

vasculitis (văs"kū-li'tīs) [L. *vasculum,* a small vessel, + *-itis,* inflammation]. Inflammation of a vessel. SYN: *angiitis.*

vasculum (văs'kū-lŭm) [L.]. A tiny vessel.

vasectomy (văs-ĕk'tō-mĭ) [L. *vas,* vessel, + Gr. *ektomē,* excision]. Removal of all or a segment of the vas deferens. Usually done bilaterally to produce sterility in the male.
　　NOTE: Persons who have had this surgical procedure ejaculate in a normal manner but the ejaculate does not contain sperm. There are no anatomical or physiological reasons for sterilization by this method to alter the sex drive or libido.

vasifactive (văs"ĭ-făk'tĭv) ["+ *facere,* to make]. Forming new vessels. SYN: *vasofactive; vasoformative.*

vasiform (văs'ĭ-form) ["+ *forma,* shape]. Resembling a tubular structure or vas.

vaso- [L.]. Combining form meaning a vessel, as a blood vessel.

vasoactive (văs"ō-ak'tiv). Affecting blood vessels.

vasoconstrictive (văs"ō-kŏn-strĭk'tĭv) [L. *vas,* vessel, + *constrictus,* bound]. Causing constriction of the blood vessels.

vasoconstrictor (văs"ō-kŏn-strĭk'tor) ["+ *constrictor,* a binder]. 1. Causing constriction of blood vessels. 2. That which constricts or narrows the caliber of blood vessels, as a drug or a nerve.

vasodentin (văs"ō-dĕn'tin) ["+ *dentīnus,* pert. to a tooth]. Modified dentine provided with blood capillaries.

vasodepression (văs″ō-dē-prĕsh′ŭn) ["+ *depressio*, a pushing down]. Vasomotor depression or collapse.

vasodepressor (văs″ō-dē-prĕs′or) [L. *vas*, vessel, + *depressor*, that which pushes down]. 1. Having a depressing influence on the circulation, lowering blood pressure by dilatation of blood vessels. 2. An agent which depresses circulation.

vasodilatation (văs″ō-dĭl-ă-tā′shŭn) ["+ *dilatāre*, to widen]. Dilatation of blood vessels, esp. small arteries and arterioles.

   v., antidromic. Vasodilatation resulting from stimulation of dorsal root of a spinal nerve.

   v., reflex. Blood vessel dilation due to stimulation of its dilator nerves or inhibition of its constrictor substance or nerves. This can be done by stimulating the sensory reflex arc.

vasodilator (văs″ō-dī-lā′tor) ["+ *dilatāre*, to widen]. 1. Causing relaxation of the blood vessels. 2. A nerve or drug which dilates the blood vessels.

vasoepididymostomy (văs″ō-ĕp″ĭ-dĭd-ĭ-mŏs′tō-mī) ["+ Gr. *epi*, upon, + *didymos*, testicle, + *stoma*, passage]. Formation of a passage between the vas deferens and the epididymis.

vasofactive (văs″ō-făk′tĭv) [L. *vas*, vessel, + *facere*, to make]. Forming new blood vessels. SYN: *vasifactive; vasoformative.*

vasoformative (văs″ō-for′mă-tĭv) ["+ *formāre*, to form]. Forming new blood vessels. SYN: *vasifactive; vasofactive.*

vasography (văs-ŏg′ră-fī) ["+ Gr. *graphein*, to write]. X-ray photography of the blood vessels.

vasohypertonic (văs″ō-hī″pĕr-tŏn′ĭk) ["+ Gr. *hyper*, over, + *tonikos*, pert. to tension]. Causing or that which causes constriction of blood vessels. SYN: *vasoconstrictor.*

vasohypotonic (văs″ō-hī″pō-tŏn′ĭk) [L. *vas*, vessel, + Gr. *hypo*, under, + *tonikos*, pert. to tension]. Relaxing or that which relaxes blood vessels. SYN: *vasodilator.*

vasoinhibitor (văs″ō-ĭn-hĭb′ĭ-tor) ["+ *inhibere*, to restrain]. An agent that depresses vasomotor nerves.

vasoinhibitory (văs″ō-ĭn-hĭb′ĭ-tor-ī). Restricting vasomotor activity.

vasoligation (văs″ō-lĭ-gā′shŭn) [L. *vas*, vessel, + *ligāre*, to bind]. Ligation of a vessel, specifically the vas deferens.

vasomotion (văs″ō-mō′shŭn) ["+ *motio*, movement]. Change in caliber of a blood vessel.

vasomotor (văs″ō-mō′tor) [L. "+ *motor*, a mover]. Pert. to the nerves having muscular control of the blood vessel walls.

The circularly arranged fibers of the muscles of arteries and veins can contract or relax; the affected region is accordingly either blanched or flushed. The former effect can commonly be produced by stimulating sympathetic fibers, and is consequently called vasoconstrictor; certain other nerves on stimulation cause vasodilation, examples being the nervus chorda tympani and the nervi erigentes.

A vasomotor reflex is one in which the stimulus, e.g., a horrifying sight, results in a change in vasomotor tone, e.g., pallor. SEE: *vasoconstrictor; vasodilator.*

   v. epilepsy. E. with vasomotor changes in the skin.

   v. nerves. Those which cause either contraction or dilation of blood vessels.

   v. spasm. Spasm of smaller arteries.

vasomotory (văs″ō-mō′tor-ī). Controlling changes in the size of the blood vessels. SYN: *vasomotor.*

vasoneurosis (văs″ō-nū-rō′sĭs) [L. *vas*, vessel, + Gr. *neuron*, nerve, + *-ōsis*, condition]. A neurosis affecting blood vessels; a disorder of the vasomotor system. SEE: *angioneurosis.*

vaso-orchidostomy (văs″ō-or′kĭd-ŏs′tō-mī) ["+ Gr. *orchis*, orchid-, testicle, + *stoma*, mouth]. Surgical connection of the epididymis to the severed end of the vas deferens.

vasoparesis (văs″ō-păr-ē′sĭs) ["+ Gr. *paresis*, relaxation]. Partial paralysis or weakness of the vasomotor nerves.

vasopressin (văs″ō-prĕs′ĭn) ["+ *press*, stem of *premere*, to press]. A hormone formed in supraoptic and paraventricular nuclei of hypothalamus and transported to posterior lobe of hypophysis through the hypothalamo-hypophyseal tract. It has an antidiuretic and a pressor effect elevating blood pressure. SYN: *antidiuretic hormone* (ABBR: ADH.); *pitressin.* SEE: *oxytocin.*

vasopuncture (văs′ō-pŭnk″chŭr) [L. *vas*, vessel, + *punctura*, a piercing]. Puncture of the vas deferens.

vasorelaxation (văs″ō-rē-lăk-sā′shŭn) ["+ *relaxāre*, to loosen]. Lessening of vascular pressure.

vasorrhaphy (văs-or′ă-fī) ["+ Gr. *rhaphē*, a seam]. Surgical suture of the vas deferens.

vasosection (văs″ō-sĕk′shŭn) ["+ *sectio*, a cutting]. Surgical division of the vasa deferentia.

vasosensory (văs″ō-sĕn′sō-rī) [L. *vas*, vessel, + *sensōrius*, pert. to sensation]. Rel. to sensation in the blood vessels.

vasospasm (văs′ō-spăzm) ["+ Gr. *spasmos*, a spasm]. Spasm of any vessel, esp. of a blood vessel. SYN: *angiospasm; vasoconstriction.*

vasostimulant (văs″ō-stĭm′ū-lănt) ["+ *stimulāre*, to goad]. Exciting vasomotor action.

vasostomy (va-zos′to-mĭ) [L. *vas*, vessel, + Gr. *stoma*, mouth]. Surgical procedure of making an opening into the vas deferens.

vasotomy (văs-ŏt′ō-mĭ) ["+ Gr. *tomē*, a cutting]. Incision of the vas deferens.

vasotonic (văs″ō-tŏn′ĭk) ["+ Gr. *tonikos*, pert. to tone]. 1. Pert. to the tone of a vessel. 2. Causing vasotonia.

vasotribe (văs′ō-trĭb) [L. *vas*, vessel, + Gr. *tribein*, to crush]. Pressure forceps used for controlling hemorrhages. SYN: *angiotribe*.

vasotripsy (văs′ō-trĭp-sĭ) ["+ Gr. *tripsis*, a crushing]. Arrest of hemorrhages with a strong forceps by crushing an artery. SYN: *angiotripsy.*

vasotrophic (văs″ō-trŏf′ĭk) [L. *vas*, vessel, + Gr. *trophē*, nourishment]. Concerned with the nutrition of blood vessels.

vasovastomy (văs″ō-văs-ŏt′ō-mĭ). Surgical anastomosis of the two cut ends of the vas deferens.

vasovesiculectomy (văs″ō-vē-sĭk″ū-lĕk′tō-mĭ) ["+ *vesicula*, tiny sac, + Gr. *ektomē*, excision]. Excision of the vas deferens and seminal vesicles.

vasovesiculitis (văs″ō-vē-sĭk″ū-lī′tis) ["+ *vesicula*, tiny sac, + Gr. *-itis*, inflammation]. Inflammation of the vas deferens and seminal vesicles.

vastus (văs′tŭs) [L., vast]. 1. Great, large, extensive. 2. One of three muscles of the thigh. SEE: *Table of Muscles* in *Appendix.*

Vater (fŏ′ter). [Abraham Vater, Ger. anatomist, 1684-1751].

    V., ampulla of. Former name for papilla of Vater, q.v.

    V.'s corpuscles. Ovoid end organs of nerves supplying the skin. SYN: *Vater-Pacini corpuscles.*

    V., papilla of. The duodenal end of the drainage systems of the pancreatic and common bile ducts. Formerly called ampulla of Vater. SYN: *vaterian segment.*

V.D. Abbr. for *venereal disease.*

V.D.G. Abbr. for *venereal disease—gonorrhea.*

V.D.H. Abbr. for *valvular disease of the heart.*

VDRL. Abbr. for *Venereal Disease Research Laboratories.*

veal (vēl) [ME. *veel*]. The meat of a calf. To be distinguished from beef which is the meat of a full-grown cow or bull.

    Food value of 100 gm. (broiled loin, medium-fat class, 77% lean, 23% fat): Cal. 234; protein 29 gm.; fat 13 gm.; niacin 5 mg.

vectis (vĕk′tĭs) [L., pole]. A curved lever for making traction on the presenting part of the fetus.

vector (vĕk′tor) [L., a carrier]. An animal, usually an arthropod (insect or tick) which transmits the causative organisms of disease from infected to noninfected individuals, esp. one in which the organism goes through one or more stages in its life cycle.

    v., biological. An animal vector wherein the disease-causing organism multiplies or develops prior to becoming infective for a susceptible individual.

    v., cardiac. SEE: *vectorcardiogram.*

    v., mechanical. A vector in or upon which growth and development of the infective agent does not occur.

vectorcardiogram (vĕk″tor-kăr′dē-ō-gram). At any moment the electrical activity of the heart can be represented as an electrical vector with a specific direction and magnitude. This is called the instantaneous cardiac vector. These vectors may be established for the entire cardiac cycle. By joining the tips of these vectors with a continuous line, the vectorcardiogram loop is formed. The configuration so obtained may be projected on the frontal plane or viewed as a three-dimensional loop.

    Three vectorcardiogram loops are formed during each cardiac cycle: one for the electrical activity of the auricle; one for ventricular depolarization; one for ventricular repolarization. Analysis of the configuration of these loops permits certain statements to be made about the state of health or disease of the myocardium.

vectorial (vĕk-tō′rĭ-ăl) [L. *vector,* a carrier]. Rel. to a vector.

vegan (vĕj′ăn). An extreme vegetarian who omits all animal protein from the diet.

vegetable (vĕj′ĕ-tă-bl) [O.Fr.]. 1. Pert. to, of the nature of, or derived from plants. 2. A herbaceous plant, esp. one cultivated for food. 3. The edible part or parts of plants which are used as food, including the leaves, stems, seeds and seed pods, flowers, roots, tubers, and fruits.

    Vegetables play an important dietary role as they are important sources of minerals and vitamins, provide bulk which stimulates intestinal motility, and are sources of energy. Caloric value is indirectly proportional to water content.

    Vegetables in general are valuable for their mineral content and for their cellulose. Copper is estimated at 1.2 milligrams per kg. for leafy vegetables, and 0.7 milligram per kg. for nonleafy ones. They are deficient in fat, which can be corrected by adding milk, cream, butter in their preparation. SEE: *names of minerals.*

All starches in vegetables must be changed to sugars before they can be absorbed in the system. Dry heat changes starch to dextrin; heat and acid or a ferment change dextrin to dextrose; in germinating grain, starch is changed to dextrin and dextrose. Dextrose in fermentation turns to alcohol and carbon dioxide. SEE: *sugar.*

vegetal (vĕj′ĕ-tăl). 1. Pertaining to plants. 2. Tropic or nutritional, esp. with reference to that part of an ovum which contains the yolk. SEE: *pole, vegetal.*

vegetarian (vĕj-ĕ-tā′rĭ-ăn) [from *vegetable,* coined 1847 by Vegetarian Society]. One who eats no animal products, but who lives on vegetables.

vegetarianism (vĕj-ĕ-tā′rĭ-ăn-ĭzm) ["+ Gr. *-ismos,* condition]. The belief and practice of eating vegetables and fruits only.

vegetate (vĕj′ĕ-tāt) [LL. *vegetāre,* to grow]. 1. To grow luxuriantly with the production of fleshy or warty outgrowths such as a polyp. 2. To lead a passive existence either mentally or physically; to do little more than eat and maintain unconscious body functions.

vegetation (vĕj-ĕ-tā′shŭn). A morbid luxurious outgrowth on any part, esp. wartlike projections made up of collections of fibrin in which are enmeshed white and red blood cells; sometimes seen on denuded areas of the endocardium covering the valves of the heart.

 v., adenoid. Fungus-like masses of lymphoid tissue in nasopharynx.

vegetative (vĕj′ĕ-tā″tĭv). 1. Having the power to grow, as plants. 2. Functioning involuntarily. 3. Quiescent, passive, noting a stage of development.

 v. nervous system. The sympathetic nervous system, q.v.

 v. pole. Area at end of ovum containing nutritive matter.

vehicle (vē′ĭ-kl) [L. *vehiculum,* that which carries]. A substance, usually inactive therapeutically, used in a medicinal preparation as the agent for carrying the active ingredient, for example, a syrup in liquid preparations.

veil (vāl) [L. *velum,* a covering]. 1. Any veil-like structure. 2. A piece of the amniotic sac occasionally covering the face of a newborn infant. SYN: *caul.* 3. Slight alteration in the voice in order to disguise it.

 v., acquired. Slight imperfection of the voice due to strain or exposure.

 v., Hottentot. Elongated labia present in Hottentot women. SYN: *Hottentot apron.*

 v., uterine. Device for covering the cervix uteri to prevent impregnation.

vein (vān) [L. *vena,* vein]. Vessel carrying dark red (unaerated) blood to the heart, except for pulmonary vein, which carries oxygenated blood.

Veins have three coats: inner, middle, and outer. They differ from arteries in their larger capacity and greater number; also in their thinner walls, larger and more frequent anastomoses and presence of valves which prevent backward circulation. They consist of two sets, superficial or subcutaneous and the deep veins with frequent communications. The former do not usually accompany an artery, as do the latter. The systemic veins consist of three groups: Those entering the heart through the superior vena cava, those through the inferior vena cava, and those through the coronary sinus. Blood from the capillary plexuses enters the right auricle of the heart. SEE: *circulation; Table of Veins* in *Appendix.*

vein, words pert. to: basilic; cava; innominate; intravenous; jugular; phlebectomy; phlebitis; phlebogram; phlebotomy; phlegmasia alba dolens; portal; thrombophlebitis; thrombus; "varic-" words; varix; vascular; vasoconstrictor; vasodilator; vasomotor; vasoparesis; vena; vena cava; venesection; venosity; venotomy; venous; venule.

velamen (vĕ-lā′mĕn) [L. *velamen,* veil]. (pl. *velamina*) Any covering membrane.

 v. nativum. The skin covering the body.

 v. vul′vae. Abnormal elongation of the nymphae. SYN: *Hottentot apron* or *veil.*

velamentous (vĕl″ā-mĕn′tŭs). Expanding like a veil, or sheet.

velamentum (vĕl″ā-mĕn′tŭm) [L. *velamentum,* a cover]. (pl. *velamenta*) A membranous covering.

velar (vē′lar) [L. *velum,* a veil]. Pert. to a veil or veil-like structure.

vellication (vĕl-ĭk-ā′shŭn) [L. *vellicāre,* to twitch]. Spasmodic twitching of muscular fibers.

velosynthesis (vĕl″o-sĭn′thĕs-ĭs) [L. *velum,* veil, + Gr. *synthesis,* a placing together]. Suture of a cleft palate, particularly the soft palate. SYN: *staphylorrhaphy.*

Velpeau′s bandage (vĕl-pō). [Alfred Velpeau, Fr. surgeon, 1795-1867] A bandage for the shoulder. SEE: *bandage.*

Velpeau′s deformity. D. seen in Colles′ fracture, q.v., in which lower fragment is displaced backward.

velum (vē′lŭm) [L. *velum,* veil]. [NA] Any veil-like structure.

 v. palati′num. [NA]. The soft palate.

vena (vē′nă) [L.]. (pl. *venae*) A vein. SEE: *Table of Veins* in *Appendix.*

v. cava inferior. [NA] The principal vein draining lower portion of the body. It is formed by junction of the two common iliac veins and terminates in right atrium of the heart. SEE: *heart.*

v. cava superior. [NA] The principal vein draining the upper portion of the body. It is formed by the junction of the right and left innominate veins and empties into right atrium of the heart. SEE: *heart.*

venae comitantes [L.]. Two or more veins accompanying an artery. They are usually present with the deep arteries of the extremities.

vena'tion. The distribution of veins to an organ or structure.

venenation (věn″ē-nā'shŭn) [L. *venenum,* poison]. 1. Condition of being poisoned. 2. Act of poisoning.

venene (vē-nēn'). A mixture of venoms from poisonous snakes.

veneniferous (věn″ē-nĭf'ĕr-ŭs) [L. *venenum,* poison, + *ferre,* to carry]. Transmitting or carrying poison.

venenific (věn″ē-nĭf'ĭk) ["+ *facere,* to make]. Producing poison.

venenous (věn'ĕn-ŭs) [L. *venenum,* poison]. Poisonous.

venepuncture (věn'ē-pŭnk″chŭr) [L. *vena,* vein, + *punctura,* a piercing]. Venipuncture, q.v.

venereal (vē-nē'rē-ăl) [L. *venereus*]. Pert. to or resulting from sexual intercourse.

v. bubo. Enlarged lymph node in the groin, the result of a venereal disease.

v. collar. Mottled condition of the neck seen occasionally in syphilis.

v. disease. One acquired ordinarily as a result of sexual intercourse with an individual who is afflicted. The diseases are gonorrhea, syphilis and chancroid. Trichomonas vaginalis vaginitis can be, but is not always, contracted through sexual intercourse.

v. sore, v. ulcer. Chancroid.

v. urethritis. Urethritis occurring in gonorrhea.

v. wart. Moist reddish elevation on genitals and anus. SYN: *condyloma; verruca acuminata.*

venereologist (vē-nēr″ē-ŏl'ō-jĭst) ["+ Gr. *logos,* a study]. A doctor who specializes in the treatment of venereal diseases.

venereology (vē-nēr″ē-ŏl'ō-jĭ). The scientific study and treatment of venereal diseases.

venereophobia (vē-nēr″ē-ō-fō'bĭ-ă) ["+ Gr. *phobos,* fear]. Abnormal fear of venereal disease. SYN: *cypridophobia.*

venesection, venisection (věn″-ĕ-sĕk'shŭn) [L. *vena,* vein, + *sectio,* a cutting].

Surgical opening of a vein for withdrawal of blood. SYN: *phlebotomy.*

venin(e (věn'ĭn) [L. *venenum,* poison]. Toxic substance in snake venom. SYN: *venene.*

venin-antivenin (věn″ĭn-ăn″tĭ-věn'ĭn). Vaccine to counteract snake poison.

veniplex (věn'ĭ-plĕks) [L. *vena,* vein, + *plexus,* a braid]. A plexus of veins.

venipuncture (věn'ĭ-pŭnk″chŭr) ["+ *punctura,* a piercing]. Puncture of a vein for any purpose.

venisuture (věn'ĭ-sū″chŭr) ["+ *sutura,* a stitch]. Suture of a vein. SYN: *phleborrhaphy.*

venoatrial (venoauricular) (vē″nō-āt'rī-ăl, -aw-rĭk'ū-lăr) [L. *vena,* vein, + *atrium,* corridor]. Rel. to the vena cava and the atrium.

venoclysis (vē-nŏk'lĭ-sĭs) ["+ Gr. *klysis,* injection]. The continuous injection of medicinal or nutrient fluid intravenously. SYN: *phleboclysis.*

venogram (vē'nō-grăm) ["+ Gr. *gramma,* a writing]. 1. A roentgenogram of the veins. SYN: *phlebogram.* 2. A tracing of the venous pulse.

venography (vē-nŏg'ră-fĭ) ["+ Gr. *graphein,* to write]. 1. Roentgenography of veins. 2. The making of a tracing of the venous pulse.

venom (věn'ŏm) [L. *venenum,* poison]. A poison excreted by some animals, such as insects or snakes, and transmitted by bites or stings.

v., snake. The poisonous secretion of the labial glands of certain snakes. Venoms contain proteins, chiefly toxins and enzymes, which are responsible for their toxicity. They are classified as neurocytolysins, hemolysins, hemocoagulins, proteolysins, and cytolysins on the basis of the effects produced.

venomotor (vē″nō-mō'tor) [L. *vena,* vein, + *motus,* moving]. Pert. to constriction or dilatation of veins.

venomous (věn'ō-mŭs) [L. *venenum,* poison]. Poisonous.

v. snake. In the USA, the coral snakes and pit vipers (copperhead, cottonmouth moccasin, and rattlesnake). SEE: *snake, poisonous.*

venoperitoneostomy (vē″nō-pĕr″ĭ-tō″nē-ŏs'tō-mĭ) [L. *vena,* vein, + Gr. *peritonaion,* peritoneum, + *stoma,* passage]. Surgically inserting the cut end of the saphenous vein into the cavity of the peritoneum. This is done to allow ascitic fluid from the peritoneal cavity to drain into the vein.

venopressor (vē″nō-prěs″or) ["+ *pressor,* that which squeezes.]. Pert. to venous blood pressure.

venosclerosis (vē″nō-sklĕ-rō'sĭs) ["+ Gr. *sklērōsis*, a hardening]. Sclerosis of veins. SYN: *phlebosclerosis*.

venosity (vē-nŏs'ĭ-tĭ) [L. *vena*, vein]. 1. Condition in which there is an excess of venous blood in a part causing venous congestion. 2. Deficient aeration of venous blood.

venospasm (vē'nō-spăzm) ["+ Gr. *spasmos*, a convulsion]. Contraction of a vein. May follow infusion of cold or irritating substance into the vein.

venostasis (vē″nō-stā'sĭs) ["+ Gr. *stasis*, a standing]. The trapping of blood in an extremity by compression of veins, a method sometimes employed for reducing the amount of blood in circulation.

venostat (vē'nō-stăt) [L. *vena*, vein, + Gr. *statikos*, standing]. Appliance for performing venous compression.

venothrombotic (vē-nō-thrŏm-bŏt'ĭk). Having the property of inducing the formation of thrombi in veins.

venotomy (vē-nŏt'ō-mĭ) [L. *vena*, vein, + Gr. *tomē*, a cutting]. Incision of a vein.

venous (vē'nŭs) [L. *vena*, vein]. Pert to the veins or blood passing through them.

 v. blood. The dark blood in the veins.

 v. hum. Murmur heard upon auscultation over larger veins of the neck.

 v. hypere'mia. Excess of venous blood in a part. SYN: *venosity*.

 v. return. The amount of blood returning to the atria of the heart.

 v. sinus. A channel which carries venous blood. Important venous sinuses are those of the dura mater draining the brain and those of the spleen.

 v. sinus of sclera. The canal of Schlemm. SEE: *canal, Schlemm's*.

venovenostomy (vē″nō-vē-nŏs'tō-mĭ) [L. *vena*, vein, + *vena*, vein, + Gr. *stoma*, mouth]. Formation of an anastomosis of a vein into a vein.

vent (vĕnt) [O.Fr. *fente*, slit]. An opening in any cavity, esp. one for excretion.

 v., alveolar. An opening between adjacent alveoli of the lung.

venter (vĕn'ter) [L. *venter*, belly]. 1. A belly-shaped part. 2. The cavity of the abdomen. 3. [NA] The wide swelling part or belly of a muscle.

ventilation (vĕn″tĭ-lā'shŭn) [L. *ventilāre*, to air]. 1. Circulation of air or amt. of fresh air in a room and withdrawal of foul air. 2. Oxygenation of blood. 3. In physiology, the amt. of air inhaled per day. This can be estimated by spirometry, multiplying the tidal air by the number of respirations per day. An average figure is 10,000 liters. This must not be confused with the total amt. of oxygen consumed, which is on the average only 360 liters/day.

 v. coefficient. The amount of air that must be respired for each liter of oxygen absorbed.

 v., continuous positive pressure. Method of mechanically assisting pulmonary v. A device administers air or mixture of gases to the lungs under continuously positive pressure. The pressure in the airway fluctuates in order to allow air to flow in and out of the lungs, but the pressure never returns to zero.

 v., intermittent positive pressure. Mechanical method for assisting pulmonary ventilation employing a device which administers air or a mixture of gases to the lungs under positive pressure intermittently at a rate approx. equal to the normal respiratory rate.

 v., pulmonary. The inspiration and expiration of air from the lungs.

 v. rate. The amount of air breathed in one minute. ABBR: VR. SYN: *respiratory minute volume (RMV).*

ventrad (vĕn'trăd) [L. *venter*, belly, + *ad*, toward]. Toward the ventral aspect. Opposed to *dorsad.*

ventral (vĕn'trăl) [L. *ventralis*, pert. to the belly]. Pert. to the belly, hence, in quadrupeds, pertaining to the lower or underneath side of the body; in man, pertaining to the anterior portion or the front side of the body.

 v. hernia. Hernia through the abdominal wall, esp. at points other than the umbilicus and groin.

ventricle (vĕn'trĭk-l) [L. *ventriculus*, a little belly]. 1. A small cavity. 2. Either of two lower chambers of the heart which when filled with blood contract to propel it into the arteries. The right v. forces blood into the pulmonary artery and thence into the lungs; the left, through the aorta. 3. One of the cavities of the brain.

 RS: Arantius' body; aula; aulatela; carneous; heart.

 v., aortic. Left v. of the heart.

 v. of the larynx. The space between the true and false vocal cords.

ventricornu (vĕn″trĭ-kor'nū) [L. *venter*, belly, + *cornu*, horn]. The anterior ventral horn of gray matter of the spinal cord.

ventricose (vĕn'trĭ-kōs) [L. *ventricōsus*, big-bellied]. 1. Inflated or distended. 2. Corpulent.

ventricular (vĕn-trĭk'ū-lar) [L. *ventriculus*, a little belly]. Pert. to a ventricle.

v. folds. The false vocal cords or folds of mucous membrane parallel or above the true vocal cords.

v. ligament. A narrow band of fibrous tissue lying within each ventricular fold.

v. tertius. Third ventricle of the brain.

ventriculography (věn-trǐk″ū-lǒg′rǎ-fǐ) ["+ Gr. *graphein*, to write]. An x-ray process used for visualizing the size and shape of the cerebral ventricles by injecting air to displace the cerebrospinal fluid which normally fills these cavities.

ventriculometry (věn-trǐk″ū-lǒm′ě-trǐ) ["+ Gr. *metron*, a measure]. The measurement of the intraventricular cerebral pressure.

ventriculonector (věn-trǐk″ū-lō-něk′tor) [L. *ventriculus*, a little belly, + *nector*, a joiner]. The atrioventricular bundle.

ventriculoscopy (věn-trǐk″ū-lǒs′kō-pī) ["+ Gr. *skopein*, to examine]. Examination of the ventricles of the brain with an endoscope.

ventriculus (věn-trǐk′ū-lǔs) [L. a little belly]. [NA] 1. Ventricle. 2. The stomach. 3. A ventricle of the brain or heart.

ventricumbent (věn″trǐ-kǔm′běnt) [L. *venter*, belly, + *cumbere*, to lie]. Lying on the belly. SYN: *prone*.

ventriduct (věn′trǐ-dǔkt) ["+ *ductus*, leading]. To draw toward the abdomen.

ventrimeson (věn″trǐ-měs′ǒn) ["+ Gr. *mesos*, middle]. The median line on the ventral surface of the body.

ventripyramid (věn″trǐ-pir′ǎ-mǐd) [L. *venter*, belly, + Gr. *pyramis*, pyramid]. An anterior pyramid of the medulla oblongata.

ventro- [L. *venter*, belly]. Combining form denoting the abdomen or ventral (anterior) surface of the body.

ventrocystorrhaphy (věn″trō-sǐs-tor′ǎ-fǐ) ["+ Gr. *kystis*, sac, + *rhaphē*, a seam]. Suture of a cyst or the bladder to the abdominal wall.

ventrofixation (věn″trō-fǐks-ā′shǔn) ["+ *fixāre*, to fix]. The suture of a displaced viscus to the abdominal wall.

ventrohysteropexy (věn″trō-hǐs′těr-ō-pěks′ǐ) ["+ Gr. *hystera*, uterus, + *pēxis*, fixation]. Attachment of the uterus to the abdominal wall.

ventroscopy (věn-trǒs′kō-pī) [L. *venter*, belly, + Gr. *skopein*, to examine]. Examination of the abdominal cavity by illumination. SYN: *celioscopy*.

ventrose (věn′trōs). Having a belly or swelling like one.

ventrosity (věn-trǒs′ǐ-tǐ). Having an enlarged belly; corpulence.

ventrosuspension (věn″trō-sǔs-pěn′shǔn) [L. *venter*, belly, + *suspensio*, a hanging].

Fixation of displaced uterus to abdominal wall.

ventrotomy (věn-trǒt′ō-mǐ) ["+ Gr. *tomē*, a cutting]. Incision into abdominal cavity. SYN: *celiotomy; laparotomy*, q.v.

ventrovesicofixation (věn″trō-věs″ǐ-kō-fǐks-ā′shǔn) ["+ *vesica*, bladder, + *fixāre*, to fix]. Suture of uterus to abdominal wall and bladder. SYN: *hysterocystopexy*.

venturimeter (ven″tūr-im′ē-ter). [Giovanni Battista Venturi, It. physicist, 1746-1822] Device for measuring flow of fluids through vessels.

venula (věn′ū-lǎ) [L., little vein]. Venule.

venule (věn′ūl) [L. *venula*, little vein]. A tiny vein continuous with a capillary.

Venus (vē′nŭs). The Roman goddess of love.

V.'s collar. Pigmentation around the neck in eruption due to syphilis.

V., crown of. An eruption around the hairline caused by syphilis.

V., mount of. The mons pubis (mons veneris), q.v.

verbigeration (věr-bǐj″ěr-ā′shŭn) [L. *verbigerāre*, to chatter]. Repetition of words which are either meaningless or have no significance.

verbomania (věr″bō-mā′nǐ-ǎ) [L. *verba*, word, + Gr. *mania*, madness]. The flow of talk in some forms of psychosis.

verdigris (věr′dǐ-grǐs) [O.Fr. *vert de Grece*, green of Greece]. 1. Mixture of basic copper acetates. 2. Deposit of copper carbonate upon copper and bronze vessels. These are of a greenish gray color.

   POISONING TREATMENT: Same as for copper sulfate.

verdohemoglobin (věr″dō-hēm′ō-glōb-ǐn). A greenish pigment occurring as an intermediate product in the formation of bilirubin from hemoglobin.

Verga's ventricle (věr′gǎ). [Andrea Verga, It. neurologist, 1811-1895] Cleftlike space between the corpus callosum and the body of the fornix of the brain.

vergence (věr′jěns) [L. *vergere*, to bend]. A turning of one eye with reference to the other. May be horizontal (convergence or divergence) or vertical (infravergence or supravergence).

Verheyen's stars (fěr-hī′ěn). [Philippe Verheyen, Flemish anatomist, 1648-1710] Starlike venous plexuses on surface of the kidney below its capsule.

vermicidal (věr″mǐ-sī′dǎl) [L. *vermis*, worm, + *cidus*, kill]. Destroying worms parasitic in the intestines.

vermicide (věr′mǐ-sīd). 1. Destroying worms. 2. An agent that will kill intestinal worms.

vermicular (vĕr-mĭk′ū-lăr) [L. *vermicularis*]. Resembling a worm.

v. movements. The wormlike movements of peristalsis.

v. pulse. Small, rapid pulse resulting in wormlike feeling in the fingers.

vermiculation (vĕr-mĭk″ū-lā′shŭn) [L. *vermiculāre*, to wriggle]. A wormlike motion, as in the intestines. SEE: *peristalsis.*

vermiculose, vermiculous (vĕr-mĭk′ū-lōs, vĕr-mĭk′ū-lŭs) [L. *vermicularis*, wormlike]. 1. Infested with worms or larvae. 2. Wormlike.

vermiform (vĕr′mĭ-form) [L. *vermis*, worm, + *forma*, shape]. Contoured like a worm.

v. appendix. A long, narrow, worm-shaped tube connected to the cecum. It varies in length from less than 1 to more than 8 in. (2.5 to 20.3 cm.) with an average of about 3 in. (7.6 cm.). Its distal end is closed. It is lined with mucosa similar to that of the large intestine. Inflammation of it is called appendicitis, q.v.

vermifugal (vĕr-mĭf′ū-găl) [″+ *fugāre*, to put to flight]. Expelling worms from the intestines.

vermifuge (vĕr′mĭ-fūj). Agent for expelling intestinal worms. SEE: *anthelmintic; vermicide.*

vermilion border. The junction of the pinkish red area of the lips with the surrounding skin.

vermin (vĕr′mĭn) [L. *vermis*, worm]. Small insects and animals, such as mice, lice, bedbugs which are annoying or cause destruction or disease.

vermination (vĕr″mĭn-ā′shŭn). Vermin or worm infestation.

verminosis (vĕr″mĭn-ō′sĭs) [L. *vermis*, worm, + Gr. *-ōsis*, condition]. Infestation with vermin.

verminous (vĕr′mĭn-ŭs). Pert. to or infested with worms.

vermiphobia (vĕr″mĭ-fō′bĭ-ă) [L. *vermis*, worm, + Gr. *phobos*, fear]. An abnormal fear of being infested with worms.

vermis (vĕr′mĭs) [L. *vermis*, worm]. 1. A worm. 2. Median connecting lobe of the cerebellum.

v. cerebel′li. [NA] Same as vermis, 2.

v., inferior. The anterior inferior portion of the vermis of the cerebellum. Includes the nodule, uvula, pyramis, and tuber.

v., superior. The posterior, dorsal portion of the vermis. Includes the folium, declive, culmen, and central lobule.

vernal (vĕr′năl) [L. *vernalis*, pert. to spring]. Occurring in or pert. to the spring.

vernix (vĕr′nĭks) [L.]. Varnish.

v. caseo′sa. A sebaceous deposit covering the fetus due to secretion of skin glands. Most abundant in creases and flexor surfaces. Consists of exfoliations of outer skin layer, lanugo, and secretions of sebaceous glands. It is not necessary to remove this after the fetus is delivered. SEE: *sebum.*

verruca (vĕr-rū′kă) [L. *verruca*, wart]. (pl. *verrucae*) Tumor of the epidermis of the skin. Produces a circumscribed elevated area of hypertrophy of the papillae. SYN: *wart.*

ETIOLOGY: Caused by a virus.

PROGNOSIS: Essentially benign and may disappear spontaneously, particularly in children and young adults. In elderly with longstanding dry seborrhea, lesions may have potential malignancy.

TREATMENT: Removal with sharp spoon curet under local anesthesia. If elevated, clip off with sharp scissors and touch with iodine. Freezing with carbon dioxide snow or fulguration.

v. acuminata. A pointed reddish moist wart about the genitals and the anus.

Develops near mucocutaneous junctures, forming pointed, tufted, or pedunculated, pinkish or purplish projections of varying lengths and consistence.

Venereal warts should be treated with applications of podophyllum resin followed by removal of the resin by washing with soap and water about six hours after application. SYN: *venereal wart.*

v. digitata. Form seen on face and scalp, possibly serving as starting point of cutaneous horns, forming several filiform projections with horny caps closely grouped on a comparatively narrow base which in turn may be separated from skin surface by slightly contracted neck.

v. filiformis. Small threadlike growths on neck and eyelids covered with smooth and apparently normal epidermis.

v. gyri hippocampi. One of the small wartlike protuberances on the convex surface of the gyrus hippocampi.

v. plantaris. Warts on the soles of the feet. SYN: *plantar wart.*

v. vulgaris. Common warts, usually on backs of hands and fingers but may occur anywhere on the skin.

verruciform (vĕ-rū′sĭ-form) [L. *verruca*, wart, + *forma*, shape]. Wartlike.

verrucose, verrucous (vĕr′rū-kōs, vĕr-rū′kŭs) [L. *verrucosus*, wartlike]. Wartlike, with raised portions.

verruga peruana (vĕ-rū′gă pĕr-wăn′ă) [Sp. Peruvian wart]. The eruptive second clinical stage of bartonellosis, q.v. Oroya fever is the first or febrile stage. SYN: *Verruca peruana; verruca peruviana.*

versicolor (vĕr'sĭ-kŭl"er) [L. *versicolor,* of changing colors]. 1. Having many shades or colors. 2. Changeable in color. SEE: *tinea versicolor.*

version (ver'zhŭn) [L. *versio,* a turning]. 1. Altering the position of the fetus in the uterus. Done in order to facilitate delivery. 2. Deflection of an organ such as the uterus from its normal position.

v., cephalic. Turning of fetus so that the head presents.

v., combined. Done by combined internal and external manipulation.

v., external. Manipulation of the fetus through the abdominal wall.

v., internal. Manipulation of the fetus by the hand placed inside the uterus.

v., pelvic. Manipulation of a cross presentation until it is changed to a pelvic presentation.

v., podalic. Manipulation of fetus by the feet so that the breech presents.

v., spontaneous. V. of fetus by uterine muscular contraction without artificial assistance.

vertebra (ver'tĕ-brä) [L.]. (pl. *vertebrae*) [NA] Any one of the 33 bony segments of the spinal column.

The vertebrae are comprised of 7 cervical, 12 thoracic (dorsal), 5 lumbar, 5 sacral, and 4 coccygeal. In adults, the five sacral vertebrae fuse to form a single bone, the sacrum, and the four rudimentary coccygeal vertebrae fuse to form the coccyx.

A typical vertebra consists of a ventral body and a dorsal or neural arch. In the thoracic region the body bears on each side two costal pits for reception of the head of a rib. The arch which encloses the vertebral foramen is formed of two roots or pedicles and two lamina. The arch bears seven processes: a dorsal spinous process, two lateral transverse processes, and four articular processes (two superior and two inferior). A deep concavity, inferior vertebral notch, on the inferior border of the arch provides a passageway for a spinal nerve. The successive vertebral foramina surround the spinal cord.

The bodies of successive vertebrae articulate with one another and are separated by intervertebral disks, disks of fibrous cartilage enclosing a central mass, the nucleus pulposus. The inferior articular processes articulate with the superior articular processes of the next succeeding vertebra in the caudal direction. Several ligaments (supraspinous, interspinous, anterior and posterior

longitudinal, and the ligamenta flava) hold the vertebrae in position yet permit a limited degree of movement.

SEE: *sacrum* for illustration. RS: acantha; anapophysis; anticlinal; atlas; axis; cervical v.; lamina; spondyle; spondylitis; spondylotherapy.

v., basilar. The lowest of the lumbar vertebrae.

v., cervical. The 7 vertebrae of the neck.

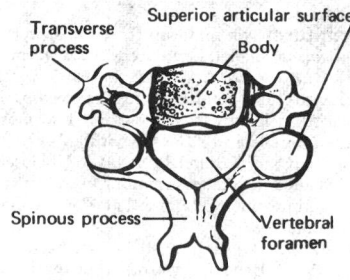

CERVICAL VERTEBRA

v., coccygeal. The rudimentary vertebrae of the coccyx.

v. dentata. The second cervical vertebra. SYN: *axis.*

v., false. One of the segments of the sacrum and the coccyx.

v., fixed. False vertebrae, q.v.

v., flexion. All except the atlas and axis.

v., lumbar. The five vertebrae between the dorsal vertebrae and the sacrum.

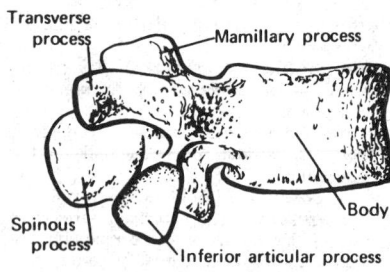

LUMBAR VERTEBRA

v. magnum. The sacrum.

v., odontoid. Same as v. dentata.

v. prominens. [NA] The seventh cervical vertebra.

v., rotation. The first two cervical vertebrae, the atlas and axis.

v., sacral. The five fused segments forming the sacrum. SEE: *sacrum* for illustration.

v., sternal. The segments of the sternum.

v., thoracic. The 12 vertebrae which connect the ribs and form part of the posterior wall of the thorax. SYN: *dorsal v.*

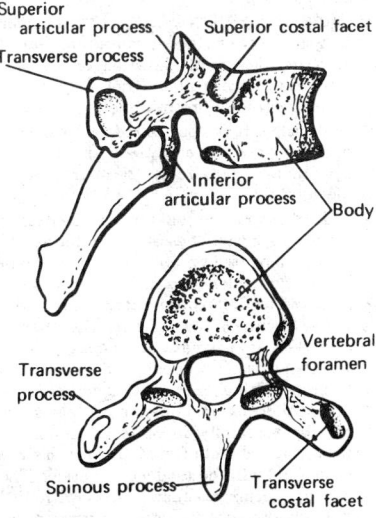

THORACIC VERTEBRAE

v., true. The vertebrae which remain unfused through life.

vertebral (ver'tĕ-brăl) [L. *vertebra,* vertebra]. Pertaining to a vertebra or the vertebral column.

v. arch. The thoracic portion of a vertebra which encloses a vertebral foramen.

v. canal. Cavity of the spinal (vertebral) column which contains the spinal cord.

v. column. Spinal column.

v. foramen. 1. The hollow space enclosed by a vertebral arch. 2. A vertebrarterial foramen.

v. groove. Groove lying on either side of the spinous processes of the vertebrae.

v. notch. Notch on inferior surface of vertebral arch for transmission of a spinal nerve.

v. ribs. The lower two, or floating, ribs.

Vertebrata (vĕr″tĕ-brāt'ă). A subphylum of the phylum Chordata characterized by possession of segmented backbone or spinal column. They possess an axial notochord at some period of their existence. Includes the following classes: Agnatha (cyclostomes); Chondrichthyes (cartilaginous fishes); Osteichthyes (bony fishes); Amphybia; Reptilia; Aves; and Mammalia.

vertebrate, vertebrated (ver'tĕ-brāt, ver'-tĕ-brā-tĕd) [L. *vertebra*]. Having or resembling a vertebral column.

vertebrectomy (ver″tĕ-brĕk'tō-mĭ) ["+ Gr. *ektomē,* excision]. Excision of a vertebra or part of one.

vertebrochondral (ver″tĕ-brō-kŏn'drăl) ["+ Gr. *chondros,* cartilage]. Denoting the false ribs (8th, 9th, 10th) connected with a vertebra at one end and the costal cartilages at the other.

vertebrocostal (ver″tĕ-brō-kŏs'tăl) [L. *vertebra + costa,* rib]. Pert. to a vertebra and a rib. SYN: *costovertebral.*

vertebromammary (ver″tĕ-brō-măm'mă-rĭ) ["+ *mammarius,* pert. to a breast]. Pert. to the vertebral and mammary area.

v. diameter. The anteroposterior diameter of the thorax.

vertebrosternal (ver″tĕ-brō-ster'năl) ["+ Gr. *sternon,* chest]. Pert. to a vertebra and the sternum.

vertex (ver'tĕks) [L. *vertex,* summit]. [NA]. The top of the head. SYN: *crown.*

v. cordis. Apex of the heart.

v. presentation. Presentation in labor of vertex of the fetal skull.

vertical (ver'tĭ-kăl) [L. *vertex, vertic-,* summit]. 1. Pert. to or situated at the vertex. 2. Perpendicular to the plane of the horizon of the earth; upright.

verticillate (ver-tĭs'ĭl-āt, -tĭs-ĭl'āt) [L. *verticillus,* a little whirl]. Arranged like the spokes of a wheel or a whorl.

vertiginous (ver-tĭj'ĭ-nŭs) [L. *vertigo, vertigin-,* a turning round]. Pert. to or afflicted with vertigo.

vertigo (ver'tĭ-gō, ver-tī'gō) [L. *vertigo,* a turning round]. True vertigo is the sensation either of moving around in space or of having objects move about the person. The subject has difficulty maintaining equilibrium. This is due to a disturbance of the sense of balance. Vertigo is not faintness, lightheadedness, or dizziness.

ETIOL: May be caused by a variety of entities including middle ear disease; toxic conditions such as those caused by salicylates; alcohol; streptomycin; sunstroke; postural hypotension; toxemia due to food poisoning or infectious diseases.

v., auditory, v., aural. V. due to disease of the ear.

v., cerebral. V. due to brain disease.

v., epileptic. V. attending an epileptic attack or following it.

v., essential. V. from an unknown cause.

v., gastric. V. from gastric disturbance.

v., hysterical. V. accompanying hysteria.

v., labyrinthine. V. due to disease of labyrinth of the ear. SYN: *Ménière's disease.*

v., laryngeal. V. accompanying laryngeal spasm.

v., objective. V. when objects seen appear to be moving when stationary.

v., ocular. V. caused by disease of the eye.

v., organic. V. from a brain lesion.

v., peripheral. V. from disturbance distant from the brain.

v., subjective. V. in which patient seems to be turning or rotating.

v., toxic. V. from presence of a toxin in the body.

verumontanitis (ver″ū-mŏn″tăn-i′tĭs) [L. *verumontānum,* mountainous ridge, + Gr. *-itis,* inflammation]. Inflammation of the verumontanum. SYN: *colliculitis.*

verumontanum (ver″ū-mŏn-tā′nŭm) [L. *verumontānum,* mountainous ridge]. An elevation on the floor of the prostatic portion of the urethra where the seminal ducts enter.

vesalianum (vĕs-a-lĭ-ā′nŭm). [Andreas Vesolius, Flemish anatomist and physician, 1514-1564] One of the sesamoid bones in the tendon of origin of the gastrocnemius muscle, and another on outer border of foot in the angle between the cuboid and fifth metatarsal.

Vesalius, foramen of (vĕs-ā′lĭ-ŭs). Opening in base of the skull transmitting an emissary vein.

Vesalius, vein of. Small emissary vein from cavernous sinus passing through foramen of Vesalius and conveying blood to the pterygoid plexus.

vesanic (vĕs-ăn′ĭk) [L. *vesania,* insanity]. Pertaining to insanity.

vesica (vĕ-sī′kă) [L. *vesica,* a bladder]. [NA] A bladder.

v. fellea. [NA]. The gallbladder.

v. prostat'ica. A minute pouch in the prostatic urethra, remnant of müllerian duct. SYN: *utriculus prostaticus.*

v. urinaria. [NA]. The urinary bladder.

vesical (vĕs′ĭ-kăl). Pert. to or shaped like a bladder.

v. reflex. Inclination to urinate caused by moderate bladder distention.

vesicant (vĕs′ĭ-kănt) [L. *vesicāre,* to blister]. 1. Blistering; causing or forming blisters. 2. Agent used to produce blisters. It is much less severe in its effects than escharotics. 3. A blistering gas used in chemical warfare.

vesication (vĕs′ĭ-kā′shŭn). 1. Process of blistering. 2. A blister.

vesicatory (vĕs′ĭ-kă-tor′ĭ). 1. Causing or pert. to blisters. 2. Agent causing blisters. SYN: *vesicant.*

vesicle (vĕs′ĭ-kl) [L. *vesicula,* a little bladder]. 1. A small sac or bladder containing fluid. 2. A blisterlike small elevation on the skin containing serous fluid. They may vary in diameter from a few millimeters to a cm.

Vesicles may be round, transparent, opaque, or dark elevations of the skin, sometimes containing seropurulent or bloody fluid.

They are seen in sudamina as the result of sweat which cannot escape from the skin; in herpes, mounted on an inflammatory base, having no tendency to rupture but associated with burning pain. In herpes zoster they follow the line of the nerve trunks. They are also seen in dermatitis venenata, as the result of poison ivy or oak, and accompanied by great itching, in dermatitis herpetiformis or multiformis, in impetigo contagiosa, occurring especially in children in discrete form, flat and umbilicated, filled with straw-color fluid with no tendency to break. They dry up, forming yellow crusts with little itching; also seen in vesicular eczema, miliaria (prickly heat or heat rash), in chickenpox, smallpox, and in scabies.

RS: chiropompholyx; herpes; miliaria.

v., auditory. That portion of the cerebral v. from which the exterior ear is formed.

v., blastodermic. Sac developed from the blastoderm.

v., cerebral. Expansion of neural embryonic canal from which the brain develops.

v., seminal. One of the two membranous, sacculated tubes situated at the base of the bladder, between it and the rectum, serving as a reservoir for the semen and having a secretion of its own.

v., umbilical. Portion of embryonic yolk sac outside the body cavity.

vesico- (ves′ĭ-ko) [L.]. Combining form meaning bladder.

vesicocele (ves′ĭ-kō-sēl) [L. *vesica,* bladder, + Gr. *kēlē,* hernia]. Hernia of bladder. SYN: *cystocele.*

vesicocervical (vĕs″ĭ-kō-ser′vĭ-kăl) ["+ *cervix*, neck]. Rel. to the urinary bladder and cervix uteri.

vesicoclysis (vĕs-ĭ-kŏk′lĭ-sĭs) ["+ Gr. *klysis*, a washing out]. Injection of fluid into the bladder.

vesicofixation (ves″ĭ-kō-fĭks-ā′shŭn) [L. *vesica*, bladder, + *fixātio*, a fixing]. Attachment of the uterus to the bladder or the bladder to the abdominal wall.

vesicoprostatic (vĕs″ĭ-kō-prŏs-tăt′ĭk) ["+ Gr. *prostatēs*, prostate]. Relating to the bladder and prostate.

vesicopubic (vĕs″ĭ-kō-pū′bĭk) ["+ *pubis*, pubis]. Pert. to the bladder and the os pubis.

vesicospinal (vĕs″ĭ-kō-spī′năl) ["+ *spina*, a thorn]. Relating to the urinary bladder and spinal cord.

vesicotomy (vĕs″ĭ-kŏt′ō-mĭ) [L. *vesica*, a bladder, + Gr. *tomē, a cutting*]. Incision of the bladder.

vesicouterine (ves″ĭ-kō-ū′ter-ĭn) ["+ *uterinus*, pert. to the womb]. Pert. to the urinary bladder and the uterus.

    v. pouch. Downward extension of the peritoneal cavity located between bladder and uterus. SYN: *uterovesical pouch.*

vesicovaginal (vĕs″ĭ-kō-văj′ĭ-năl) ["+ *vagina*, a sheath]. Pert. to the urinary bladder and vagina.

vesicula (vĕ-sĭk′ū-lă) [L. *vesicula*, a tiny bladder]. (pl. *vesiculae)* [NA] A small bladder, or vesicle.

    v. seminalis. [NA]. Tiny reservoir of semen at base of the bladder. SYN: *seminal,* q.v.; *vesicle.*

vesicular (vĕ-sĭk′ū-lar). Pert. to vesicles or small blisters.

    v. breathing. Murmur heard in normal breathing.

    v. eczema. E. accompanied by formation of vesicles.

    v. murmur. The normal sound of respiration heard on auscultation. Same as v. breathing.

    v. rale. The crepitant rale, a crackling sound heard at end of inspiration.

    v. resonance. Percussion sound heard over the normal lung.

vesiculase (vĕ-sĭk′ū-lās). An enzyme in prostatic fluid said to coagulate semen.

vesiculation (vĕ-sĭk″ū-lā′shŭn) [L. *vesicula*, a tiny bladder]. Formation of vesicles or state of having or forming them.

vesiculectomy (vĕ-sĭk″ū-lĕk′tō-mĭ) ["+ Gr. *ektomē*, excision]. Partial or complete excision of a vesicle, particularly a seminal vesicle.

vesiculiform (vĕ-sĭk″ū-lĭ-form) ["+ *forma*, shape]. Having the shape of a vesicle.

vesiculitis (vĕ-sĭk″ū-lī′tis) [L. *vesicula*, a tiny bladder, + Gr. *-ītis*, inflammation]. Inflammation of a vesicle, particularly the seminal vesicle.

vesiculocavernous (vĕ-sĭk″ū-lō-kăv′ĕr-nŭs) ["+ *cavernōsis*, hollow]. Vesicular and cavernous.

vesiculogram (vĕ-sĭk′ū-lō-grăm) ["+ Gr. *gramma*, a mark]. An x-ray picture of the seminal vesicles.

vesiculography (vĕ-sĭk″ū-lŏg′ră-fĭ) [L. *vesicula*, a tiny bladder, + Gr. *graphein*, to write]. X-ray photography of the seminal vesicles.

vesiculopapular (vĕ-sĭk″ū-lō-păp′ū-lăr) ["+ *papula*, a pimple]. Composed of vesicles and papules.

vesiculopustular (vĕ-sĭk″ū-lō-pŭs′tū-lăr) ["+ *pustula*, pustule]. Having both vesicles and pustules.

vesiculotomy (vĕ-sĭk″ū-lŏt′ō-mĭ) [L. *vesicula*, a tiny bladder, + Gr. *tomē*, a cutting]. Surgical incision into a vesicle, as a seminal vesicle.

vesiculotympanic (vĕ-sĭk″ū-lō-tĭm-păn′ĭk) ["+ Gr. *tympanon*, drum]. Having both vesicular and tympanic qualities.

vespajus (vĕs-pā′jŭs). Follicular, suppurative inflammation of the hairy part of the scalp.

vessel (vĕs′ĕl) [O. Fr. from L. *vascellum*, a little vessel]. A tube, duct, or canal to convey the fluids of the body. SYN: *vas.*

    RS: anastomose; anastomosis; angiitis; angiodystrophia; arrosion; atresic; endothelial; intima; rhegma; vas; vascular.

    v.'s, absorbent. The lacteals, lymphatics and capillaries of the intestines.

    v.'s, blood. Arteries, veins, and capillaries.

    v.'s, chyliferous. V.'s arising in the villi of the intestinal walls carrying chyle and terminating in the thoracic duct.

    v.'s, lymphatic. V.'s conveying lymph.

    v.'s, nutrient. Those supplying interior of the bones.

    v., radicular. Branch of a vertebral artery supplying cerebral nerve root.

vestibular (vĕs-tĭb′ū-lăr) [L. *vestibulum*, vestibule]. Pert. to a vestibule.

    v. bulbs. Two sacculated collections of veins, lying on either side of the vagina beneath the bulbocavernosus muscle, connected anteriorly by the pars intermedia, and through this strip of cavernous tissue communicating with the erectile tissue of the clitoris.

    Injury during labor may give rise to troublesome bleeding. The vestibular bulbs are the homologues of the male corpus spongiosum. SEE: *Bartholin's glands; vagina; vestibule.*

v. nerve. A main division of the auditory nerve. Arises in vestibular ganglion. Is concerned with equilibrium.

vestibule (věs'tĭ-būl). A small space or cavity at the beginning of a canal, such as the aortic v.

v. of ear. The middle part of the inner ear, behind the cochlea, and in front of the semicircular canals; it contains the utriculus and sacculus.

v. of larynx. The portion of the larynx above the vocal cords.

v. of nose. The anterior part of the nostrils containing the vibrissae.

v. of vagina. An almond-shaped space between the lines of attachment of the labia minora. At the anterior angle the clitoris is situated; the posterior boundary is the fourchette. The vestibule appears approximately four or five cm. long and two cm. in greatest width when the labia minora are separated. Four major structures open into vestibule: The urethra anteriorly, the vagina posteriorly, and the two excretory ducts of the glands of Bartholin, laterally. The covering membranes are pink in color and constructed of delicate stratified squamous epithelium. Collections of cavernous tissue are disposed beneath the integument. SEE: *Bartholin's glands; vagina; vestibular bulbs.*

vestibulitis (věs-tĭb-ū-lī'tĭs) [L. *vestibulum,* vestibule, + *ītis,* inflammation]. A dermatitis of the nasal vestibule; common in diabetics.

vestibulocochlear nerve (věs-tĭb''ū-lō-kŏk'lĭ-ăr) ["+ *cochlea,* snail shell]. The 8th cranial nerve which emerges from the brain behind the facial nerve, between the pons and medulla oblongata. SYN: *acoustic nerve.*

vestibulotomy (věs-tĭb''ū-lŏt'ō-mĭ) ["+ Gr. *tomē,* a cutting]. Surgical incision into the vestibule of the inner ear.

vestibulourethral (věs-tĭb''ū-lō-ū-rē'thrăl) ["+ Gr. *ourēthra,* urethra]. Rel. to the vestibule of vagina and urethra.

vestibulum (věs-tĭb'ū-lŭm) [L. *vestibulum,* vestibule]. (pl. *vestibula*) Vestibule.

vestige (věs'tĭj) [L. *vestigium,* footstep]. A small degenerate or incompletely developed structure which has been more fully developed in the embryo or in a previous stage of species.

vestigial (věs-tĭj'ĭ-ăl). Of the nature of a vestige. SYN: *rudimentary.*

vestigium (věs-tĭj'ĭ-ŭm) [L. a footstep]. (pl. *vestigia*) Vestige.

veta (vā'ta) [Sp.]. Mountain sickness, esp. that which occurs in Andean rail travelers.

veterinarian (vĕt''ĕr-ĭ-nār'-ĭ-ăn). One who practices veterinary medicine.

veterinary (vĕt'ĕr-ĭ-nār'ĭ). Pert. to the diseases of animals and their treatment. 2. A veterinarian.

v. medicine. That which deals with diseases of animals and their treatment.

V.H. Abbr. for *viral hepatitis.*

via (vī'ă) [L. way]. (pl. *viae*) Any passage in the body such as nasal, intestinal, or vaginal.

viability (vī''ă-bĭl'ĭ-tĭ) [L. *vita,* life, + *habilis,* fit]. Ability to live, grow and develop.

viable (vī'ă-bl) [L. *vita,* life, + *habilis,* fit]. Capable of living, as a newborn or a fetus which has reached a stage, usually 28 weeks or older, which will permit it to live outside the uterus.

vial (vī'ăl) [Gr. *phialē,* a drinking cup]. A small glass bottle for medicines or chemicals.

vibex (vī'beks) [L. *vibix,* mark of a blow]. (pl. *vibices*) Narrow linear mark, as a line of blood in subcutaneous tissue.

vibrapuncture. Medical use of tattoo technique to introduce medicine into skin lesions. Multiple punctures are made into the skin by a needle which has passed through a small amount of the solution of medicine placed on the site.

vibratile (vī'bră-tĭl) [L. *vibrāre,* to shake]. Adapted to or used in vibratory motion; moving to and fro. SEE: *vibratory.*

vibration (vī-brā'shŭn). 1. A to and fro movement. SYN: *oscillation.* 2. Therapeutic shaking of the body, a form of massage.

Consists of a quick motion of the fingers or the hand vertical to the body or use of a mechanical vibrator.

vibrator (vī'bră-tor) [L. *vibrator,* a shaker]. Device for causing artificial vibration of body or its parts.

v., mechanical. Machine driven by hand or motor to give general shake-up of part desired.

vibratory (vī'bră-tō''rĭ) [L. *vibrator,* a shaker]. Having a vibrating or oscillatory movement.

v. sense. The ability to perceive vibrations transmitted through the skin to deep tissues. Usually tested by placing a vibrating tuning fork over bony prominences.

Vibrio (vib'rĭ-ō) [L. from *vibrāre,* to shake]. A genus of curved, motile, gram-negative bacilli. The only one pathogenic for man is V. cholerae. It is, in fresh culture, shaped like a comma.

V. cholerae. The etiological agent of cholera.

vibrissae (vī-brĭs'ē) [L. *vibrissa*, that which shakes]. (sing. *vibrissa*) Stiff hairs within the nostrils at the anterior nares.

vibromassage (vī"brŏ-mă-sŏzh'). Massage given by a mechanical vibrator.

vibromasseur (vī"bro-mă-sūr'). Instrument used to produce vibratory massage of the ear.

vibrometer (vī-brŏm'ĕt-ĕr) [L. *vibrāre*, to shake, + Gr. *metron*, a measure]. Device which produces rapid vibrations of the membrana tympani. A form of massage treatment for deafness.

vibrotherapeutics (vī"brŏ-thĕr"ă-pū'tĭks) ["+ Gr. *therapeutikē*, treatment]. The therapeutic application of vibration.

vicarious (vī-kā'rĭ-ŭs) [L. *vicarius*, substitute]. Acting as a substitute; pert. to assumption of the function of one organ by another.

   v. menstruation. Blood loss during menstruation at some site other than the vagina, as hemorrhage from the nose, from the breast, or eyes.

   v. respiration. Increased r. in one lung when respiration in the other is lessened or abolished.

Vicq d'Azyr's tract (vĭk da-zēr'). [Félix Vicq d'Azyr, Fr. anatomist, 1748-1794] A large myelinated bundle arising in mammillary nuclei and terminating in anterior thalamic nuclei. SYN: *mammallothalamic tract.*

vidian artery (vĭd'ĭ-ăn). [Guido Guidi (L. *Vidius*), Italian physician, 1500-1569]. Branch of int. maxillary artery passing through the vidian canal.

   v. canal. A canal in medial pterygoid plate of the sphenoid bone for transmission of pterygoid (vidian) vessels and nerve. SYN: *pterygoid canal.*

   v. nerve. A branch from the sphenopalatine ganglion. SEE: *Table of Nerves* in *Appendix.*

vigil (vĭj'ĭl) [L. awake]. Insomnia, wakefulness.

   v., coma. Condition of muttering delirium in which patient is partially conscious and not completely comatose. SEE: *vigilambulism.*

vigilambulism (vĭj"ĭl-ăm'bū-lĭzm) [L. *vigil*, awake, + *ambulāre*, to walk, + Gr. *-ismos*, condition]. Automatism which occurs while the person is awake. Resembles somnambulism.

vigintinormal (vī-jĭn"tĭ-nor'măl) [L. *viginti*, twenty, + *norma*, rule). Consisting of one-twentieth of what is normal, as a solution.

vigor (vig'or) [L.]. Active force or strength of body or mind.

villi (vĭl'ī). Pl. of L. *villus*, tuft of hair.

   v., chorionic. Tiny branching processes of surface of chorion which become vascular and help to form the placenta.

villiferous (vĭl-ĭf'ĕr-ŭs) ["+ *ferre*, to bear]. Having villi, or tufts of hair.

villoma (vī-lo'mă) [L. *villus*, tuft of hair + Gr. *-ōma*, tumor]. A villous tumor.

villose, villous (vĭl'ōs, vĭl'ŭs) [L. *villus*, tuft of hair]. Pert. to or furnished with villi or with fine hairlike extensions.

villositis (vĭl-ōs-ī'tĭs) ["+ Gr. *-itis*, inflammation]. Inflammation of the placental villi.

villus (vĭl'ŭs) [L. *villus*, tuft of hair]. (pl. *villi*) The short filamentous processes found on certain membranous surfaces.

   v., chorionic. Tiny vascular projections on the chorionic surface which help to form the placenta. SEE: *chorion.*

Vincent's angina (vĭn'sĕnts ăn-jī'nă). [Henri Vincent, Fr. physician, 1862-1950]. Painful pseudomembranous ulceration of the gums, oral mucous membranes, pharynx and tonsils. SYN: *necrotizing ulcerative gingivostomatitis; trench mouth,* q.v. SEE: *Borrelia vincentii.*

   Bacteroides fusiformis and Borrelia vincentii. Poor oral hygiene, mental and physical stress, nutritional deficiencies. Absorption of heavy metals, such as mercury and bismuth, predisposes to development of the disease. Not considered to be a contagious disease.

   SYM: Painful swelling of lymphatic nodes, inflammation of tonsils extending to floor of mouth. Pseudomembranous exudate, later ulceration; fever.

vinculum (vĭn'kū-lŭm) [L. *vinculum,* a band]. (pl. *vincula*) A uniting band or bundle. SYN: *frenulum, frenum, ligament.*

   v. ten'dinum. 1. Tendinous, slender filaments connecting the phalanges with the flexor tendons. 2. The ringlike ligament of the ankle or wrist.

vinegar (vĭn'ē-găr) [ME. *vinegre,* from Fr. *vin,* wine, + *aigre,* sour]. The product of the oxidation of fermented alcoholic solutions such as beer or wine. A weak and impure solution of acetic acid. Usually contains 4 to 6% acetic acid. SEE: *condiment.*

vinous (vī'nŭs) [L. *vinum,* wine]. Containing or of the nature of wine.

vinum (vī'nŭm) [L. *vinum,* wine]. Wine.

   The medicated wines are solutions of medicinal substances in wine. They are not often prescribed. None are official.

vioform (vī'ō-form). A proprietary product (iodochlorhydroxyquin) containing 41% iodine and having antibacterial and antifungal action.

violate [L. *violāre*, to injure]. To harm or injure a person, especially to rape a female.

violence (vī′ō-lĕnts) [L. *violentia*]. The use of force or physical compulsion. It may be expected in acute delirious mania. After epileptic furor, patients have no memory of their violent attacks. Many attacks of violence may be averted by recognizing warning signs and by knowing the patient.

violet (vī′ō-lĕt) [ME. *violett*, from L. *viola*, violet]. One of the colors of the spectrum resembling purple.

    v. blindness. Inability to see violet tints. SYN: *amianthinopsy.*

viomycin (vī-ō-mī′sĭn). An antibiotic produced by strains of streptomyces griseus.

viosterol (vī-ŏs′tĕr-ōl). A solution of irradiated ergosterol in vegetable oil. SYN: *calciferol.*

    USES: Same as cod liver oil.

viraginity (vĭr″ă-jĭn′ĭ-tĭ) [L. *virāgo*, an amazon or manlike woman]. Presence in a woman of masculine qualities and sexual tendencies.

viral. Pert. to or caused by a virus.

    v. disease. One which is caused by a virus. SEE: *virus diseases.*

viremia (vī″rēm′ĭ-ă). Presence of viruses in the blood.

vires. Pl. of vis, q.v.

virgin (vĭr′jĭn) [L. *virgo*, a maiden]. 1. A woman (or man) who has not had sexual intercourse. 2. Uncontaminated; fresh; new.

virginal (vĭr′jĭn-ăl) [L. *virgo*, a maid.]. Relating to a virgin or to virginity.

    v. membrane. The tissue surrounding the entrance to the vagina. Its absence cannot be regarded as proof that the individual has had sexual intercourse. SYN: *hymen.*

virginity (vĭr-jĭn′ĭt-ĭ) [L. *virginitas*, maidenhood]. The state of being a virgin; not having experienced sexual intercourse.

viricidal (vī-rĭ-sī′dăl) [L. *virus*, poison, + *cidus*, from caedere, to kill]. Destructive to or inhibiting a virus. SYN: *virucidal.*

virile (vĭr′ĭl) [L. *virilis*, masculine]. Having characteristics of a mature male. SYN: *masculine.*

    v. reflex. 1. Sudden downward movement of penis when the prepuce or gland of a completely relaxed penis is pulled upward. SYN: *bulbocavernous reflex.* 2. Contraction of bulbocavernous muscle on percussing dorsum of penis. 3. Contraction of bulbocavernous muscle resulting from compression of glans penis.

virilescence (vĭr-ĭl-ĕs′ĕns) [L. *virilis*, masculine]. The acquisition of masculine characteristics in the female.

virilia (vĭr-ĭl′ĭ-ă) [L. *virilia*, male genitalia]. The male sexual organs.

virilism (vĭr′ĭl-ĭzm) [L. *virilis*, masculine, + Gr. *-ismos*, condition]. Presence or development of male secondary characteristics in a woman.

virility (vĭr-ĭl′ĭ-tĭ) [L. *virilitas*, masculinity]. 1. The state of possessing masculine qualities. 2. Sexual potency in the male.

virion. A complete virus particle; a unit of genetic material surrounded by a protective coat which serves as a vehicle for its transmission from one cell to another.

viripotent (vĭr-ĭp′ō-tĕnt) [L. *vir*, man, + *potens*, able]. 1. Sexually mature, said of male. 2. Marriageable, applied only to a female. SYN: *nubile.*

virology (vĭr-ŏl′ō-jĭ) [L. *virus*, poison, + Gr. *logos*, study]. The study of viruses and viral diseases.

virose, virous (vī′rōs, vī′rŭs) [L. *virus*, poison]. Having poisonous qualities or effects. SYN: *poisonous.*

virtual (vĭr′tū-ăl) [L. *virtus*, capacity]. Appearing to exist but not in actual fact or form.

virucidal (vĭ-rū-sī′dăl) [L. *virus*, poison, + *cidus*, from caedere, to kill]. Destructive of a virus.

virulence (vĭr′ū-lĕns) [L. *virulentia*, a stench]. 1. Relative power and degree of pathogenicity possessed by organisms to produce disease. 2. Property of being virulent; venomousness, as of a disease. SEE: *attenuation; avirulent.*

virulent (vĭr′ū-lĕnt) [L. *virulentus*, full of poison]. 1. Very poisonous. 2. Infectious; able to overcome the host's defensive mechanism.

viruliferous (vĭr-ū-lĭf′ĕr-ŭs) [L. *virus*, poison, + *ferre*, to bear]. Conveying or producing a virus.

virus (vī′rŭs) [L. *virus*, poison]. 1. Originally this word meant any organism capable of causing an infection, but this usage is obsolete. 2. Minute organisms not visible with ordinary light microscopy. They are parasitic and depend on nutrients inside cells for their metabolic and reproductive needs.

    Some bacteria share these properties but not the distinctive features of viruses such as their simple organization and composition and their mechanism of replication.

    Viruses cause a variety of diseases.

    A virus was synthesized in the laboratory for the first time in 1967. This was done by using natural virus DNA (deoxyribonucleic acid) as a template for forming the synthetic virus DNA.

    v., attenuated. A virus so treated that its pathogenicity is decreased.

v., cytomegalic. SEE: *cytomegalic virus.*

v. dehumanized. Vaccine obtained by the inoculation of a heifer with virus from a human being.

v. diseases. Smallpox, chickenpox, measles, mumps, the common cold, poliomyelitis, rabies, epidemic encephalitis, and v. pneumonia are only a few of the virus diseases of man.

v., filtrable. A virus causing infectious disease, the essential elements of which are so tiny that they retain infectivity after passing through a filter of the Berkefeld type. SEE: *filter, Berkefeld.*

v., neurotropic. Those which reproduce in nervous tissue.

v., parainfluenza. One of a group of viruses which affect infants and young children. Causes respiratory infections which may be mild or may progress to pneumonia. Most infections are so mild as to be clinically inapparent.

virusemia (vi″rus-ēm′ĭ-ā) ["+ Gr. *haima,* blood]. Virus in the blood. SYN: *viremia.*

virustatic (vīr″ū-stăt′ĭk) [L. *virus,* poison, + Gr. *statikos,* bringing to a standstill]. Stopping the growth of viruses.

vis (vĭs) [L. *vis,* force]. (pl. *vires*) Force, strength, energy, power.

v. afron′te. Force that attracts.

v. formati′va. Energy resulting in development of new tissue.

v. medica′trix natu′rae. The healing power of nature.

viscera (vĭs′ĕr-ā) [L. *viscus, viscer-,* body organ]. Pl. of viscus, q.v. Internal organs, esp. the abdominal.

RS: celosomia; evisceration; splanchnic.

viscerad (vĭs′ĕr-ăd) ["+ *ad,* toward]. Toward the viscera.

visceral (vĭs′sĕr-ăl) [L. *viscus, viscer-,* body organ]. 1. Pert. to viscera. 2. Pert. to or derived from the gill arches of vertebrates.

v. arches. Branchial arches, q.v.

v. cavity. Body cavity containing the viscera.

v. clefts. The fissures separating the visceral arches.

v. skeleton. The pelvis, ribs and sternum enclosing the viscera.

visceralgia (vĭs″ĕr-ăl′jĭ-ā) ["+ Gr. *algos,* pain]. Neuralgia of any of the viscera.

viscero- (vĭs′ĕr-o). Combining form meaning pertaining to the viscera.

viscerogenic (vĭs″ĕr-ō-jĕn′ĭk) [L. *viscus, viscer-,* body organ, + Gr. *gennan,* to produce]. Originating in the viscera.

visceroinhibitory (vĭs″ĕr-ō-ĭn-hĭb′ĭ-tō-rĭ) ["+ *inhibere,* to restrain]. Checking the action of the viscera.

visceromegaly (vĭs″ĕr-ō-mĕg′ă-lĭ) ["+ Gr. *megal,* great]. Generalized enlargement of the abdominal visceral organs.

visceromotor (vĭs″ĕr-ō-mō′tor) [L. *viscus, viscer-,* body organ, + *motor,* a mover]. Conveying motor impulses to the viscera. SYN: *viscerimotor.*

v. reflex. Increase in tonus of abdominal muscles resulting from painful stimuli originating in a viscus.

visceroparietal (vĭs″ĕr-ō-pă-rī′ĕ-tăl) ["+ *paries, pariet-,* wall]. Rel. to the viscera and the abdominal wall.

visceroperitoneal (vĭs″ĕr-ō-pĕr′ĭ-tō-nē′ăl) ["+ Gr. *peritonaion,* peritoneum]. Rel. to the abdominal viscera and peritoneum.

visceropleural (vĭs″ĕr-ō-plū′răl) [L. *viscus, viscer-,* body organ, + Gr. *pleura,* a side]. Rel. to the thoracic viscera and the pleura. SYN: *pleurovisceral.*

visceroptosis (vĭs″ĕr-ŏp-tō′sĭs) ["+ Gr. *ptōsis,* fall]. Downward displacement of a viscus.

visceroreceptors (vĭs″ĕr-ō-rĭ-sĕp′tŏrz). A group of receptors which includes those located in visceral organs. Their stimulation gives rise to poorly localized and ill-defined sensations. In hollow visceral organs they are stimulated principally by excessive contraction or by distention.

viscerosensory (vĭs″ĕr-ō-sĕn′sō-rĭ) [L. *viscus, viscer-,* body organ, + *sensorius,* sensory]. Pert. to sensations aroused by stimulation of visceroreceptors.

v. reflex. Pain or tenderness elicited in somatic structures (skin and muscle) due to visceral disorder. SEE: *referred pain.*

visceroskeletal (vĭs″ĕr-ō-skĕl′ĕt-ăl) ["+ Gr. *skeleton,* skeleton]. Rel. to the visceral skeleton.

viscerosomatic (vĭs″ĕr-ō-sō-măt′ĭk) ["+ Gr. *sōma,* body]. Rel. to the viscera and the body.

v. reaction. A reaction occurring in muscles of the body-wall as a result of stimulation of visceroreceptors.

viscerotonia (vĭs″ĕr-ō-tōn′ĭ-ā) [L. *viscus, viscer-,* body organ, + LL. *-tonia,* suffix denoting tonicity, from Gr. *tonos,* tension.]. A personality type typical of the endomorphic, characterized by predominance of social over intellectual and physical traits. Individual is sociable, convivial, and exhibits gluttony for food, company, affection, and social support.

viscerotrophic (vĭs″ĕr-ō-trŏf′ĭk) ["+ Gr. *trophē,* nourishment]. Pertaining to trophic conditions related to or associated with visceral conditions.

viscerotropic (vĭs″ĕr-ō-trŏp′ĭk) ["+ Gr. *tropos*, a turn]. Primarily affecting the viscera.

viscerovisceral reaction (vĭs″ĕr-ō-vĭs′ĕr-ăl). A reaction taking place in the viscera as a result of stimulation of visceral receptors. Such reactions are usually below the level of consciousness.

viscid (vĭs′ĭd) [L. *viscidus*, sticky]. Adhering, glutinous, sticky.

In bacteriology, said of a colony which strings out by clinging to a needle when it is touched to the culture and withdrawn. The sediment rises in a coherent whirl when the liquid culture is shaken.

viscidity (vĭs-ĭd′ĭ-tĭ). The property of being viscid or sticky. SYN: *viscosity*.

viscosimeter (vĭs″kŏs-ĭm′ĕ-tĕr) [L. *viscōsus*, sticky, + Gr. *metron*, a measurer]. Device for estimating the viscosity of a fluid, esp. of blood.

viscosity (vĭs″kŏs′ĭ-tĭ) [L. *viscōsus*, sticky]. 1. State of being sticky or gummy. 2. Resistance offered by a fluid to change of form or relative position of its particles due to attraction of molecules to each other.

v., specific. The internal friction of a fluid, measured by comparing the rate of flow of the liquid through a tube with that of some standard liquid, or by measuring the resistance to rotating paddles.

viscous (vĭs′kŭs). Sticky, gummy, gelatinous.

viscus (vĭs′kŭs) [L. *viscus*, body organ]. (pl. *viscera*) Any internal organ enclosed within a cavity, such as the thorax or abdomen. SEE: *viscera*.

visibility. Quality of being visible.

visible. Capable of being seen.

visile (vĭz′ĭl) [L. *visum*, seeing]. 1. Pert. to vision. 2. Readily recalling what is seen, more than that which is audible or motile.

vision (vĭzh′ŭn) [L. *visio*, a seeing]. 1. Act of viewing external objects. SYN: *sight*. 2. Sense by which light and color are apprehended. 3. An imaginary sight.

v., achromatic. Complete color blindness.

v., artificial. A technique, still in experimental stage, designed to make it possible for some blind persons to see.

v., binocular. Visual sensation which is produced when the images perceived by each eye are fused to appear as one.

v., central, v., direct. Vision with the fovea centralis.

v., day. Condition in which patient sees better during the day than at night, found in

peripheral lesions of the retina, such as retinitis pigmentosa.

v., double. Seeing of one object as two. SYN: *diplopia*.

v., field of. The space within which an object can be seen while the eye remains fixed on some one point.

v., half. Blindness in one or both eyes for half of the visual field. SYN: *hemianopia*.

v., indirect, v., peripheral. Vision with the retina outside of the macular field.

v., monocular. Utilizing only one eye.

v., multiple. Seeing of one object as two or more. SYN: *polyopia*.

v., night. Ability to see when illumination is reduced.

v., phantom. An experience of visual sensations in an eye which has been surgically removed. Usually a transient condition.

vision, words pert. to: aberration; accommodation; aftercataract; afterimage; ambiopia; amblyopia; ametropia; amphodiplopia; anianthinopsy; anopsia; anotropia; asthenope; asthenopic; astigmatic; astigmatism; autophony; bifocal; blind; chloropia; chloropsia; chromatic; chromatopsia; chromopsia; convergence; cyanopia; cyclophoria; diplopia; emmetropia; erythropsia; farpoint; farsightedness; field; fogging; gerontopia; glare; halation; hypermetropia; hypometropia; ianthinopsia; image; macropsia; metamorphosis; micropsia; monoblepsia; muscae volitantes; myope; myopia; night blindness; nyctalopia; nyctamblyopia; nyctotyphlosis; ocular; oculist; orthophrenia; oxyblepsia; polyopia; scintillation; scotoma; second sight; spintherism; strabismus; vergence; visile; visual; xanthopsia; words ending in "-phoria."

visual (vĭzh′ū-ăl) [L. *visio*, a seeing]. 1. Pert. to vision. 2. One whose learning and memorizing processes are largely of a visual nature.

v. acuity. A measure of the resolving power of the eye. Usually determined by having the subject read letters of various sizes at a standard distance from the test chart. The result is expressed as a fraction. For example, 20/20 is normal vision. This means the subject's eyes have the ability to see from a distance of 20 feet (6.1 meters) what the normal eye would see at that distance. 20/40 means that a person sees at 20 feet (6.1 meters) what the normal eye could see at 40 feet (12.2 meters), etc.

v. angle. Angle between line of sight and the extremities of object seen.

v. axis. The line of vision, from object seen through the pupil's center to macula lutea.

v. cone. The cone whose vertex is at the eye and whose generating lines touch the boundary of a visible object.

v. field. The area within which objects may be seen when the eye is fixed.

v. line. The visual axis.

v. plane. The plane in which both optic axes lie.

v. point. Center of vision.

v. purple. A purple pigment in retinal rods. SYN: *rhodopsin.*

visuoauditory (vĭzh″ū-ō-aw′dĭ-tor′ĭ) [L. *visio,* a seeing, + *auditōrius,* pert. to hearing]. Rel. to sight and hearing, as connecting nerve fibers between auditory and visual centers.

visuognosis (vĭzh″ū-ŏg-nō′sĭs) ["+ Gr. *gnōsis,* knowledge]. The recognition and appreciation of what is seen.

visuopsychic (vĭzh″ū-ō-sī′kĭk) ["+ Gr. *psychē,* soul]. Both visual and psychic, applied to cerebral area involved in apprehension of visual sensations.

visuosensory (vĭzh″ū-ō-sĕn′sō-rĭ) [L. *visio,* a seeing, + *sensorius,* sensory]. Rel. to the recognition of visual impressions.

vitaglass (vī′tă-glăs) [L. *vita,* life + glass]. Window glass containing quartz for transmitting the ultraviolet rays of sunlight.

vital (vī′tăl) [L. *vitalis,* pert. to life]. 1. Pert. to or characteristic of life. 2. Contributing to or essential for life.

v. capacity. Volume of air that can be expelled following full inspiration.

v. center. Respiratory center in medulla.

v. signs. Respiration, pulse, and temperature.

v. statistics. A record of births, marriages, disease, and deaths in an area.

vitalism (vī′tăl-ĭzm) ["+ Gr. *-ismos,* condition]. The opinion that a vital force neither chemical nor mechanical is responsible for the phenomenon of life.

vitalist (vī′tăl-ĭst) [L. *vitalis,* pert. to life]. One who believes in vitalism.

vitalistic (vī-tăl-ĭs′tĭk). Relating to vitalism.

vitality (vī-tăl′ĭ-tĭ). 1. That which distinguishes living things from the nonliving. 2. Animation, action. SYN: *strength.* 3. State of being alive.

vitals (vī′tălz) [L. *vita,* life]. Organs of the body, esp. the heart, liver, lungs, and brain, essential to life.

vitamer (vī′tă-mĕr). Any one of a number of compounds which differ in structure from vitamins but which exert vitaminlike function.

vitamin (vī′tă-mĭn) [L. *vita,* life, + amine]. Any of a group of organic substances other than proteins, carbohydrates, fats, minerals, and organic salts which are essential for normal metabolism, growth, and development of the body.

Vitamins are not sources of energy nor do they contribute significantly to the substance of the body, but they are indispensable for normal functions and the maintenance of health. They are effective in minute quantities. They act principally as regulators of metabolic processes and play a role in energy transformations, usually acting as coenzymes in enzymatic systems.

Vitamins are extremely complex chemical substances, but the nature, chemical structure, and composition of most of them are known. Most have been isolated and some have been synthesized. In general, none of the vitamins can be formed in the body but must be obtained preformed from animal or plant sources. Exceptions to the above are the formation of vitamin A from its precursor, carotene; the formation of vitamin D by the action of ultraviolet light on the skin; and the formation of vitamin K by symbiotic bacteria of the intestines.

Vitamins are unstable, being readily destroyed by oxidation; by heat, esp. in an alkaline medium; strong acids, light, and aging. SEE: *Table of Vitamins* in *Appendix.*

RS: avitaminosis; deficiency disease.

v., antiberiberi. Thiamine (vitamin B₁). SEE: *thiamine.*

v., antidermatitis. Vitamin B₆.

v., antihemorrhagic. Vitamin K.

v., anti-infective. Vitamin A.

v., antineuritic. Thiamine (B₁), q.v.

v., antipellagra. Nicotinamide (pellagra-preventing factor).

v., antirachitic. The vitamin D group.

v., antiscorbutic. Vitamin C.

v., antixerophthalmic. Vitamin A.

v., coagulation. Vitamin K.

vitamin A. A fat-soluble vitamin formed in the body from precursors, yellow pigments of plants (alpha, beta, and gamma carotene). It is essential for normal growth and development, the integrity of epithelial tissues, and for normal teeth and bone development. It is stored in the liver. SYN: *vitamin, anti-infective; v., antixerophthalmic. SEE: Table of Vitamins* in *Appendix.*

ACTION: Essential to the normal function of epithelial cells and visual purple.

STABILITY: Resists boiling for some time if not exposed to oxidation. Quite stable to heat but not to continued high temperatures (above 100° C.). Vit. A is present in most canned fruits and vegetables.

VITAMIN A DEFICIENCY DISORDERS: Interference with growth, reduced resistance to infections, interference with nutrition of cornea, conjunctiva, trachea, hair follicles, renal pelvis. Thus these tissues have an increased susceptibility to infections. Interference with ability of eyes to adapt to darkness (night blindness). Visual acuity will also be impaired. Children will experience impaired growth and development.

SOURCES OF VITAMIN A: Butter, butter fat in milk, egg yolks, and cod liver oil are rich sources. Green leafy and yellow vegetables and some fruits; prunes, pineapples, oranges, limes, cantaloupes, liver.

vitamin A₁. Form found in fish liver oils.

vitamin A₂. A compound found in the livers of fresh-water fish. Similar in properties to vitamin A but with different absorption spectrum in the ultraviolet.

vitamin B complex. A large number of water-soluble vitamins isolated from liver, yeast, and other sources. Among vitamins included are: thiamine (B₁), riboflavin (B₂), niacin (nicotinic acid), pyridoxine (B₆), biotin, inositol, p-aminobenzoic acid (PABA), cyanocobalamine (B₁₂), and folic acid.

ACTION: Affects growth, appetite, lactation, gastrointestinal, nervous, and endocrine systems; aids in marasmus and lymphocytosis; stimulates appetite; reduces sugar content in diabetes; stimulates biliary action; aids in treating tuberculosis; and is necessary for carbohydrate metabolism.

Only grain-made yeast that is dried at once preserves its potency.

B₁, thiamine, for growth and nutrition and carbohydrate metabolism. B₂, riboflavin, for growth and cellular metabolism. Nicotinic acid prevents pellagra.

Although not destroyed by ordinary cooking, it may be destroyed by excessive heating for 2-4 hours. Soda in cooking aids destruction. Riboflavin and nicotinic acid, more stable than thiamine, are not destroyed by heat or oxidation.

VITAMIN B DEFICIENCY DISORDERS: Beriberi, pellagra, digestive disturbances, enlargement of liver, reduction of pancreas, affects the thyroid, causes degeneration of sex glands, reduces catalysis of tissues, affects the nervous system, deranges the endocrines; induces edema, affects the heart, liver, spleen and kidneys, enlarges the adrenals and deranges function of the pituitary and salivary glands, and cause of some disorders in diabetes.

Polyneuritis, gastrointestinal disorders, achlorhydria, anorexia, and failure of lactation have been attributed to deficiency of B₁.

SOURCES OF VITAMIN B: *Thiamine:* Whole grains, wheat embryo, brewer's yeast, legumes, nuts, egg yolk, fruits and vegetables.

Riboflavin: Brewer's yeast, liver, meat, esp. pork and fish, poultry, eggs, milk, and green vegetables.

Nicotinic Acid: Brewer's yeast, liver, meat, poultry, and green vegetables.

Pyridoxine: Rice, bran, yeast.

Folic Acid: Leafy, green vegetables, organ meats, lean beef and veal, wheat cereals.

STABILITY: Long-continued cooking or high temperature destroys and soda in cooking aids its destruction. Not destroyed by ordinary cooking or heat.

vitamin B₁. Thiamine, or thiamine hydrochloride. Recommended daily allowance: 0.5 mg./1000 Cal. SEE: *Table of Vitamins* in *Appendix.*

vitamin B₂. Riboflavin, q.v. SEE: *Table of Vitamins* in *Appendix.*

vitamin B₆. Pyridoxine. Found in rice, bran, and yeast. SEE: *Table of Vitamins* in *Appendix.*

vitamin B₁₂. A red, crystalline substance extracted from liver which is essential for the formation of red blood cells. Its deficiency results in pernicious anemia. It is used for prophylaxis and treatment of these and other diseases in which there is defective red cell formation. Recommended daily requirement: 5 micrograms per day for adults. SYN: *antipernicious anemia principle; cyanocobalamin.*

vitamin C. Ascorbic acid, a factor necessary for formation of intercellular substance of connective tissue and essential in maintenance of integrity of intercellular cement in many tissues, especially capillary walls. Deficiency leads to scurvy. SYN: *ascorbic acid.* SEE: *Table of Vitamins* in *Appendix.* *NOTE:* Large daily doses of vitamin C have been recommended for prevention and treatment of the common cold. The effectiveness of vitamin C for this purpose has not been established.

STABILITY: Destroyed easily by heat in the presence of oxygen, as in open-kettle boiling. Less affected by heat in an acid medium; otherwise stable.

VITAMIN C DEFICIENCY DISORDERS: Scurvy, imperfect prenatal skeletal formation, defective teeth, pyorrhea, anorexia, anemia, undernutrition, injury to bone, cells and blood vessels.

SOURCES OF VITAMIN C: Raw cabbage, young carrots, orange juice, lettuce, celery, onions, tomatoes, radishes and green peppers. Citrus fruits are especially rich in this vitamin. Strawberries are about as rich a source as tomatoes, apples, pears, apricots, plums, peaches, and pineapples. Rutabagas are also rich in this vitamin.

vitamin D. One of several vitamins having antirachitic activity. The vitamin D group includes D_2 (calciferol), D_3 (irradiated 7-dehydrocholesterol), D_4 (irradiated 22-dihydroergosterol) and D_5 (irradiated dehydrositosterol). It is essential in calcium and phosphorus metabolism; consequently it is essential for normal development of bones and teeth. SEE: *Table of Vitamins* in *Appendix.*

ACTION: Related to utilization of calcium and phosphorus in blood and bone building. It is called the antirachitic vitamin because deficiency of it interferes with calcium and phosphorus utilization, which in turn causes rickets, q.v. Exposure to the sun or ultraviolet ray synthesizes this vitamin in the body. Necessary for most efficient absorption of calcium and phosphorus. A specific in treatment of infantile rickets, spasmophilia (infantile tetany), and softening of bone; valuable also in prevention. Important in normal growth and mineralization of skeleton and teeth.

VITAMIN D DEFICIENCY DISORDERS: Imperfect skeletal formation; bone diseases; rickets; caries.

SOURCES OF VITAMIN D: Milk; cod liver oil; salmon and cod livers; egg yolk; butter fat. Ergosterol activated by sunlight or the ultraviolet ray possesses vitamin D potency.

STABILITY: Not affected by oxidation or by heat unless over 100° C. (212° F.) or long-continued cooking.

vitamin E. An essential nutrient for man, although the exact biochemical mechanism whereby vitamin E functions in the body is unknown. Because of the amount of vitamin E present in foods, deficiency of this vitamin is absent in the general population. SYN: *alpha tocopherol.*

vitamin K. An antihemorrhagic factor whose activity is associated with compounds derived from naphthoquinone. Vitamin K is from alfalfa; vitamin K_2 from fishmeal; vitamin K_3 is synthesized as menadione sodium bisulfite USP. Vitamin K aids blood coagulation, and is necessary for formation of prothrombin. Its deficiency prolongs blood-clotting time and causes hemorrhages.

ACTION: Helps to eliminate prolonged bleeding in operations and in biliary tract of jaundiced patients. Bile salts necessary for its absorption.

SOURCES OF VITAMIN K: Found in fats, fishmeal, oats, wheat, rye and alfalfa.

vitamin loss. Commercial canning destroys from 50 to 85% of vitamin C in peas, lima beans, spinach, and asparagus. The wheat embryo is removed from wheat flour in milling. As the wheat embryo is rich in vitamin B_1, this vitamin is lost in milling. Apple pie and freshly prepared applesauce retain only from 20 to 30% of the vitamin C value of the apple. Pickling, salting, curing, or fermenting usually causes complete loss of vitamin C. Pasteurization, unless special precautions are observed, causes a loss of from 30 to 60% of vitamin C.

vitaminoid (vī'tăm-ĭn-oyd) [L. *vita,* life, + amine, + Gr. *eidos,* resemblance]. Of the nature of vitamin.

vitellary (vĭt'ĕl-ă-rĭ) [L. *vitellus,* yolk of an egg]. Pert. to the vitellus. SYN: *vitelline.*

vitellin (vī-tĕl'ĭn). A protein which can be extracted from egg yolk and contains lecithin. SEE: *nucleoprotein; ovovitellin.*

vitelline (vī-tĕl'ēn). Pert. to the yolk of an egg or the ovum.

v. circulation. The embryonic circulation of blood to the yolk sac via vitelline arteries and its return to general circulation through the vitelline veins.

v. duct. The narrow duct connecting the yolk sac with the embryonic gut.

v. membrane. 1. The membrane forming the surface layer of an ovum. 2. In a chicken egg, the membrane forming the surface layer of the vitellus or yolk.

v. veins. Two veins conveying blood from the yolk sac. SYN: *omphalomesenteric veins.*

vitellus (vī-tĕl'ŭs) [L. *vitellus,* yolk of egg]. The yolk of an ovum, esp. the yolk of a hen's egg.

vitiation (vĭsh'ĭ-ā'shŭn) [L. *vitiāre,* to corrupt]. Injury, contamination, impairment of use or efficiency.

vitiligo (vĭt-ĭl-ĭ'gō) [L.]. An acquired cutaneous affection characterized by milk-white patches, surrounded by areas of normal pigmentation. More common in tropics and in Negroes. Cause unknown. SYN: *leukoderma, piebald skin.*

v. capitis. Vitiligo of the scalp with depigmentation of the hairs of the affected area.

v. perinevoid. Vitiligo surrounding a nevus.

vitiligoidea (vĭt'ĭl-ĭg-oyd'ē-ă) [L. *vitilīgō,* tetter, + Gr. *eidos,* appearance]. Disease marked by formation of tiny yellow patches or nodules on the skin, as on the eyelids. SYN: *xanthoma.*

vitium (vĭsh′ĭ-ŭm) [L. *vitium,* fault]. (pl. *vitia*) A fault, defect, or vice.

v. cordis. An organic heart lesion.

vitreocapsulitis (vĭt″rē-ō-kăp″sū-lī′tĭs) [L. *vitreus,* glassy, + *capsula,* capsule, + Gr. *-itis,* inflammation]. Inflammation of the vitreous humor. SYN: *hyalitis.*

vitreous (vĭt′rē-ŭs) [L. *vitreus,* glassy]. 1. Glassy. 2. Pertaining to the vitreous body of the eye. 3. The vitreous body, q.v.

v. body. A transparent jellylike mass that fills the cavity of the eyeball, enclosed by the hyaloid membrane.

v. chamber. The portion of the cavity of the eyeball behind the lens.

v. degeneration. Retrogressive change of a part into a translucent shining substance, esp. of a blood vessel wall. SYN: *hyaline degeneration.*

v. humor. The clear, watery fluid filling the interstices of the stroma of the vitreous body.

v. membrane. 1. Inner one of the choroid. 2. The innermost layer of the connective tissue sheath surrounding a hair follicle. SYN: *hyaline layer.*

v. table. The inner layer of compact tissue characteristic of most of the bones of the cranium.

vitrescence (vĭ-trĕs′ĕns). Becoming hard and transparent like glass.

vitriol (vĭt′rē-ol) [L. *vitriolum,* from *vitrium,* glass (from glassy appearance of sulfates)]. A sulfate of any of various metals.

v., blue. Copper sulfate, q.v.

v., green. Ferrous sulfate, q.v.

v., oil of. Sulfuric acid, q.v.

v., white. Zinc sulfate, q.v.

vitro, in. SEE: *in vitro.*

vitropression (vĭt″rō-prĕsh′ŭn) [L. *vitrum,* glass, + *pressio,* a squeezing]. Method of temporarily eliminating redness of the skin caused by hyperemia by pressure with a glass slide on the skin for purpose of studying any lesions or discolorations.

Vitus′ dance, St. (vī′tŭs). A functional nervous disorder causing muscular spasms. SYN: *chorea,* q.v.

vivi- (vĭv′ĭ) [L.]. Combining form meaning alive.

vividiffusion (vĭv-ĭ-dĭf-ū′zhŭn) [L. *vivus,* alive, + *diffusio,* a pouring apart]. The process of removing diffusible substances from blood of a living animal by allowing it to flow through dialyzing membranes immersed in saline solution.

vivification (vĭv-ĭ-fĭ-kā′shŭn) [″+ *facere,* to make]. 1. Trimming of the surface layer of a wound to aid union of tissues. 2. Transformation of protein food through assimilation into the living matter of cellular organisms.

viviparous (vĭv-ĭp′ăr-ŭs) [″+ *parere,* to bear young]. Developing young within the body, the young being expelled and born alive, the opposite of oviparous.

vivisect (vĭv′ĭ-sĕkt) [L. *vivus,* alive, + *sectio,* a cutting]. To dissect a living animal for experimental purposes.

vivisection (vĭv′ĭ-sĕk′shŭn) [″+ *sectio,* a cutting]. Cutting of or operation upon a living animal for physiological investigation and the study of disease. The operations are usually performed upon an anesthetized animal under conditions similar to those encountered in an operating room of a hospital.

vivisectionist (vĭv′ĭ-sĕk′shŭn-ĭst). One who practices or believes in vivisection. SEE: *antivivisectionist.*

vivisector (vĭv-ĭs-ĕk′tor) [L. *vivus,* alive, + *sector,* a cutting]. One who practices vivisection.

vivo, in. SEE: *in vivo.*

Vleminckx′s solution (flĕm′ĭnks). [Jean François Vleminckx, Belgian physician, 1800-1876] A solution of sulfurated lime.

USES: In various skin diseases.

VMA. Vanillylmandelic acid, q.v.

vocal (vō′căl) [L. *vox, voc-,* voice]. Pert. to the voice.

v. cords, false. The ventricular folds, q.v.

v. cords, true. The vocal cords, q.v.

v. folds. The thin edges of the vocal lips, each of which encloses the vocal ligament. They form the edges of the rima glottidis, and are concerned with the production of sound.

v. frem′itus. Chest-wall vibration felt on palpation while patient is speaking.

v. ligament. A strong band of elastic tissue lying within vocal fold.

v. lips. Two shelflike projections of lateral walls of the larynx. Their edges bear the vocal folds, q.v.

v. muscle. The inner portion of the thyroarytenoid muscle which lies in vocal lip lateral to and in contact with the vocal ligament.

v. process. That of the arytenoid cartilage to which are attached the vocal cords.

v. res′onance. Sound heard in auscultation of lung while patient is speaking.

v. signs. Indication of disease by changes in the voice.

voice (voys). Sound uttered by human beings, produced by vibration of the vocal cords.

voice, words pert. to: amphoricity; amphoriloquy; amphorophony; anepia; apsithyria; arytenoid; heterophonia; hoarseness; mogiphonia; paraphonia; phonation; resonance; rhinolalia; rhinophonia; trachyphonia.

voiceprint. Technique for depicting graphically the characteristics of an individual's speech pattern. Because voiceprints, like fingerprints, can be used to distinguish one person from another, the technique is useful in medicine and in identifying the voices of criminal suspects.

voices (voys'ĕs). In psychiatry, verbal, auditory hallucinations expressed as being heard by the patient.

void (voyd) [O. Fr. *voider*, to empty]. To evacuate the bowels or bladder.

vol. Abbr. for *volume*.

vol%. Abbr. for *volume per cent*.

vola (vō'lä) [L.]. The sole of foot or palm of the hand.

    v. manus. Palm of hand.

    v. pedis. Sole of foot.

volar (vō'lär) [L. *vola*, palm, sole]. Relating to the palm, or sole of foot.

volatile (vol'ă-tĭl) [L. *volatilis*, from *volāre*, to fly]. Easily vaporized or evaporated.

    Examples of volatile liquids are ether (boiling point, 34.5° C.) and ethyl chloride (b. p. 12.2° C.).

volatilization (vŏl"ă-tĭl-ĭ-zā'shŭn). Conversion of a solid or liquid into a vapor.

volition (vō-lĭsh'ŭn) [L. *volitio*, will]. The act or power of willing or choosing.

Volkmann's contracture (fŏlk'mahn). [Richard von Volkmann, Ger. surgeon, 1830-1899]. Degeneration, contracture, fibrosis, and atrophy of a muscle resulting from injury to its blood supply. Usually seen in the hand.

volley (vŏl'ĕ) [L. *volāre*, to fly]. The simultaneous or nearly simultaneous discharge of a number of nerve impulses from a center within the brain or spinal cord.

volsella (vŏl-sĕl'ä) [L. *volsella*, a tweezer]. Forceps with sharp pointed hooks at end of each blade.

volt (vŏlt). An electrical unit of pressure, the electromotive force required to produce one ampere of current through a resistance of one ohm.

voltage (vōl'tĭj). Electromotive force or difference in potential expressed in volts.

volubility (vŏl"u-bĭl'ĭ-tĭ) [L. *volubilitas*, flow of discourse]. Excessive speech.

volume (vol'ūm). The space occupied by a substance. Usually expressed in cubic units.

    v. index. The mean volume of an average erythrocyte compared with the mean volume of the normal erythrocyte. Varies from 0.9 to 1.10. Indices below this indicate abnormally small red cells; above, abnormally large ones. The volume index is found by dividing the percentage of red cells into the hematocrit (q.v.) percentage. ABBR: V.I. SEE: *color index*.

    v., mean corpuscular. The mean volume of an average erythrocyte. Normal values range from 82 to 92 cubic microns. ABBR: M.C.V.

    v., minute. The amount of blood discharged from one ventricle in one minute.

    v., packed cell. The volume of packed erythrocytes in a sample of centrifuged blood. Average volume equals 47% of blood volume in men, 42% in women. SYN: *hematocrit*.

    v. per cent. The number of cubic centimeters (milliliters) of a substance (usually O_2 or CO_2) contained in 100 cc. (or ml.) of another substance, e.g., blood. ABBR: vol.%.

    v., stroke. The amount of blood discharged by a ventricle in one contraction. Determined by dividing the minute volume by the number of heartbeats occurring in one minute.

volumetric (vŏl"ū-mĕt'rĭk) [L. *volūmen*, a volume, + Gr. *metron*, a measure]. Pert. to measurement of volume.

voluntary (vŏl'ŭn-tĕr'ĭ) [L. *voluntas*, will]. Pert. to or under control of the will.

    v. muscles. Voluntary muscles are generally attached to the skeleton, are innervated by myelinated nerves coming directly from the brain or spinal cord, and under the microscope are seen to consist of long cylindrical fibers bearing crosswise striations.

    Voluntary, striped, striated, cross striated, and skeletal are practically synonymous when applied to muscle.

voluptuous (vō-lŭp'tū-ŭs) [L. *voluptas*, pleasure]. 1. Pert. to, arising from, or provoking consciously or otherwise, sensual desire, usually applied to the female sex. 2. Given to sensualism.

volupty (vŏl'ŭp-tĭ) [O. Fr. *volupté*, pleasure]. Sexual pleasure.

volute (vō-lūt') [L. *volutus*, rolled]. Spiral, rolled up. SYN: *convoluted*.

volvulus (vŏl'vū-lŭs) [L. *volvere*, to roll]. A twisting of the bowel upon itself causing obstruction. Prolapsed mesentery predisposing cause. Usually occurs at sigmoid and ileocecal areas of intestines.

vomer (vō'mer) [L. *vomer*, plowshare]. The plow-shaped bone which forms the lower and posterior portion of the nasal septum, articulating with the ethmoid, sphenoid, the two palate bones, and two superior maxillary bones.

vomerine (vō'mĕr-ĭn). Pert. to the vomer.

vomeronasal (vō"mĕr-ō-nā'săl). Pert. to the vomer and the nasal bones.

    v. cartilages. Two narrow strips of cartilage lying along anterior portion of inferior border of septal cartilage of nose.

    v. organ (of Jacobson). A small tubular epithelial sac lying on anterior inferior surface of nasal septum. Rudimentary in man.

vomica (vŏm'ĭ-kă) [L. *vomica*, ulcer]. (pl. *vomicae*) 1. A cavity in the lungs, as from suppuration. 2. Sudden and profuse expectoration of putrid, purulent matter.

vomicose (vŏm'ĭ-kōs). Marked by many ulcers; ulcerous; purulent.

vomit (vŏm'ĭt) [L. *vomere*, to vomit]. 1. That which is ejected from the stomach through the mouth. 2. To eject stomach contents through the mouth.

    PHYS: The act is usually reflex involving coordinated activity of both voluntary and involuntary muscles. A certain position is assumed, the glottis is closed, the diaphragm and abdominal muscles contract, and the cardiac sphincter of the stomach relaxes while antiperistaltic waves course over the duodenum, stomach and esophagus.

    RS: melena; nausea; vomiting.

    v., bilious. Bile forced back into the stomach and ejected with vomited matter.

    v., black. Vomit containing blood acted on by the gastric juice. Seen in worst form of yellow fever.

    v., coffee-ground. V. having the appearance and consistency of coffee grounds because of blood mixed with gastric contents. Occurs in conditions such as cancer of stomach.

vomiting (vŏm'ĭt-ing) [L. *vomere*, to vomit]. Ejection through the mouth of the gastric contents.

    Vomiting may result from toxins from ptomaines, drugs, uremia, and specific fevers; cerebral tumors and meningitis (often unaccompanied by nausea and does not relieve associated headache); diseases of the stomach such as ulcer, cancer, dilatation, dyspepsia; reflex from pregnancy, uterine, or ovarian disease, irritation of the fauces, worms, biliary colic; intestinal obstruction; motion sickness; nervous affections as hysteria and migraine. Periodic vomiting may be in itself a neurosis or associated with the gastric crises of locomotor ataxia; esophageal vomiting results from obstruction, and the vomitus (q.v.) is alkaline in reaction. SYN: *emesis.*

TREATMENT: Antinausea medicines by mouth if possible, otherwise intramuscularly or intravenously. Fluids may be given by mouth if patient will accept them. If vomiting continues, fluids and electrolytes intravenously will be required to replace those lost in the vomitus.

    In pregnancy (hyperemesis gravidarum, q.v.): Fluid intake by mouth should be restricted but maintained by intravenous route. Frequent small feedings of more or less dry foods are advisable. Sedatives and antiemetics are useful. *CAUTION:* Give only those medicines which do not interfere with normal fetal development.

POSTOPERATIVE NP: Position patient to help prevent aspiration of vomitus, i.e. elevate foot of bed and turn head to one side. Suction apparatus should be available and used to keep vomited material out of airway. At first sign restrict fluids for 1/2 hour, then resume in gradually increasing amts. In certain cases (gastric) record time, color, amt., whether regurgitant or projectile. Save specimen for examination. Wash mouth frequently. Take specimen of urine if vomiting is persistent. (May be due to acidosis. If so, alkalies and glucose may be given.) Odor, ammoniacal, fecal, garlic, etc., should be charted. Fecal v. indicates intestinal obstruction. SEE: *hematemesis.*

POISONS: Vomiting may result from taking arsenic, aconite, antimony, barium, colchicum, cantharides, copper, corrosive alkalis, acids, digitalis, iodine, mercury, phenol, phosphorus, veratrum, wood alcohol, foot poisons, and zinc.

    RS: anacatharsis; antiemetic; cyclic v.; emesis; emetic; hyperemesis; tyremesis; vomit; vomitus.

    v., cyclic. Recurring paroxysms of vomiting.

    v., dry. Nausea without vomitus.

    v., epidemic. Sudden, unexplained attacks of gastroenteritis characterized by nausea, vomiting, and sometimes diarrhea. Though not proven, the symptoms are believed to be due to a virus. Treatment is symptomatic.

    v., incoercible. Uncontrollable vomiting.

    v., pernicious. Severe vomiting of pregnancy.

    v. of pregnancy. That of morning sickness.

    v., projectile. Ejection of vomitus with great force.

    v., stercoraceous. Vomiting of fecal matter.

vomitory (vŏm′ĭ-tō-rĭ) [L. *vomitōrius*, pert. to vomit]. 1. Causing vomiting. 2. An agent inducing emesis. 3. A vessel to receive ejecta.

vomiturition (vŏm″ĭ-tū-rĭsh′ŭn) [L. *vomitus*, vomit]. Repeated ineffective efforts to vomit. SYN: *retching.*

vomitus (vŏm′ĭ-tŭs). 1. Act of ejecting matter from the stomach through the mouth. 2. Material ejected from the stomach by vomiting.

NATURE OF VOMITUS: *Ammoniacal odor:* Indicates uremia.

Bilious: Green or greenish-yellow, containing bile, appears after frequent and violent vomiting; if early in the act of vomiting, it may be grass-green; a symptom of peritonitis which also precedes fecal vomiting in intestinal obstruction.

Fecal: This is indicative of intestinal obstruction, general peritonitis, and abnormal communication between the intestines and stomach.

Garlic odor: Denotes phosphorus poisoning.

Hematemesis: The vomiting of blood. If bright and fluid it has not been long in the stomach; otherwise, it has the appearance of coffee grounds, reddish-brown, or it forms in clots. This may indicate, also, rupture of aneurysms into the stomach or esophagus, or rupture of esophageal varicose veins; gastric ulcer, cirrhosis of liver, enlarged spleen, carcinoma of the stomach. It is not necessarily fatal.

It may result from swallowed blood. It may occur in vicarious menstruation, gastritis, corrosive poisoning, in the presence of strong alkalies or acids, or it may result from anemia, leukemia, Hodgkin's disease and it is sometimes present in chronic nephritis, scurvy, purpura hemorrhagica, acute yellow atrophy of the liver, and in malaria.

Profuse: The ejection of large quantities of frothy fermented material is highly significant of gastric dilatation.

Purulent: This may result from the rupture of an abscess into the esophagus or stomach.

Without nausea, distress, or other phenomena: This may occur in certain neuroses of the stomach, in hysteria, uremia, brain disease, as from a tumor, or as a precursor of apoplexy. The vomitus may be colored by certain fruits, by wine, coffee, cocoa, soups and bile. SEE: *blennemesis; cholemesis.*

v., coffee-ground. Vomitus of dark red or black granular material (resembling coffee grounds) which is blood. The blood has been in the stomach or intestinal tract long enough to be changed from red to black by the action of gastric and intestinal juices.

v. cruentus. Bloody vomit.

v. mari′nus. Seasickness.

v. matutinus. The vomiting of morning sickness.

von Gierke's disease (fŏn gēr′kĕ). [Edgar von Gierke, Ger. pathologist, 1877 —]. Condition in which excessive amounts of glycogen are stored in tissues and body is unable to use it. Results in excessive production of ketones. SYN: *glycogen storage disease; glycogenosis.*

von Graefe's sign (fŏn gra′fĕ). [Albrecht von Graefe, Ger. ophthalmologist, 1828-1870]. Failure of lid to move downward promptly with eyeball, the lid moving tardily and jerkily; seen in exophthalmic goiter.

von Pirquet's test (fŏn pēr′kā). [Clemens Freiherr von Pirquet, Austrian pediatrician, 1874-1929]. A diagnostic test for tuberculosis, in which a little tuberculin is applied to a scarified area of the skin of the arm.

A positive reaction is seen if a red papillar eruption appears at the site of inoculation.

von Recklinghausen's disease (fŏn rĕk′lĭng-how″zĕn). [Friedrich D. von Recklinghausen, Ger. pathologist, 1833-1910] 1. Multiple neurofibromata of nerve sheaths. They occur along peripheral nerves, where they are quite obvious, and on spinal and cranial nerve roots. Extremely variable in size, number, and shape. Area over tumor may be hyperpigmented. Symptoms may be completely absent or may be those of pain due to pressure on spinal cord or on the brain.

TREATMENT: Surgical as required to relieve symptoms.

Voorhees' bag (voor′ĕz). [James Ditmors Voorhees, Amer. obstetrician, 1869-1929]. An inflatable rubber bag for dilating the cervix uteri to induce labor.

voracious (vō-rā′shŭs) [L. *vorāre*, to devour]. Having an insatiable or ravenous appetite.

vortex (vor′tĕks) [L. *vortex*, a whirlpool]. (pl. *vortices*) A structure having a spiral or whorled appearance.

v., coccygeal. The region over coccyx where lanugo hairs of embryo come to a point. SYN: *vortex coccygeus.*

v. lentis. Spiral patterns on the surface of the lens due to concentric pattern of fiber growth.

v. of the heart. Region at apex of heart where muscle fibers of the ventricles make a tight spiral and turn inward.

vortices. Pl. of vortex.

v. pilorum. Hair whorls as in arrangement of hairs on the scalp.

vorticose (vor'tĭk-ōs) [L. *vortex, vortic-*, a whirlpool]. Whirling or having a whorled arrangement.

v. veins. Four veins (two superior and two inferior) which receive blood from all parts of the choroid of the eye. They empty into posterior ciliary and superior ophthalmic veins.

vox (vŏks) [L. *vox*]. (pl. *voces*) Voice.

v. abscissa. Loss of voice.

v. capitus. Falsetto voice or a voice in the upper register.

v. choler'ica. The suppressed voice of last stages of cholera.

v. rauca. A hoarse voice.

voyeur (vwŏ-yūr') [Fr., one who sees]. One who derives sexual pleasure from observing the sexual activity of others.

V.R. Abbr. for *right vision; ventilation rate; vocal resonance.*

V.S. Abbr. for *vesicular sound; vital sign; volumetric solution.*

vuerometer (vū''ĕr-ŏm'ĕ-tĕr) [Fr. *vue*, sight, + Gr. *metron*, a measure]. Apparatus for measuring interpupillary distance of the eyes.

vulgaris (vŭl-gā'rĭs) [L. *vulgaris*, common]. Ordinary, common.

vulnerable (vŭl'nĕr-ă-bl) [L. *vulnerāre*, to wound]. Easily injured or wounded.

vulnerary (vŭl'nĕr-ār-ĭ). 1. Pert. to wounds. 2. An agent used to assist wound healing.

vulnerate (vŭl'nĕr-āt). To wound.

vulnus (vŭl'nŭs) [L. *vulnus*, wound]. (pl. *vulnera*) A wound or injury.

Vulpian-Heidenhain-Sherrington phenomenon. Contraction of denervated skeletal muscle by stimulating autonomic cholinergic fibers innervating its blood vessels. SYN: *pseudomotor phenomenon.*

vulsella, vulsellum (vŭl-sĕl'ă, vŭl-sĕl'ŭm) [L. *vulsella*, tweezers]. A forceps with a hook on each blade. SYN: *volsella.*

vulva (vŭl'vă) [L., a covering]. (pl. *vulvae*) That portion of the female genitalia lying beneath the mons veneris consisting of the labia majora, labia minora, clitoris, vestibule of the vagina, and bulbs of the vestibule. SYN: *pudendum femininum* [NA].

v. connivens. Vulva in which the labia majora are in apposition.

v. hians. Vulva in which labia majora are gaping.

v., velamen. Abnormally elongated clitoris. SYN: *Hottentot apron.*

vul'val, vul'var [L. *vulva*, covering]. Relating to the vulva.

v. leukoplakia. Condition characterized by diffuse or focal, translucent thickening of the vulva. Often gives rise to carcinoma.

vulvectomy (vŭl-vĕk'tō-mĭ) ["+ Gr. *ektomē*, excision]. Excision of the vulva.

vulvismus (vŭl-vĭz'mŭs) ["+ Gr. *-ismos*, condition]. Painful spasm of the vagina. SYN: *vaginismus.*

vulvitis (vŭl-vī'tĭs) [L. *vulva*, covering, + Gr. *-itis*, inflammation]. Inflammation of the vulva.

v., acute nongonorrheal. V. resulting from chafing of opposed lips of vulva or from accumulated sebaceous material around the clitoris.

v., follicular. Inflammation of hair follicles of vulva.

v., gangrenous. Necrosis and sloughing of areas of vulva, often a complication of infectious diseases such as diphtheria, scarlatina, typhoid fever.

v., leukoplakic. A chronic atrophic vulvitis. SEE: *kraurosis vulvae.*

v., mycotic. V. caused by various fungi, most commonly by *Candida albicans.*

v., salivary. Inflammation of the vulval area caused by oral-genital contact to such extent as to traumatize the area.

vulvo- [L.]. Combining form meaning a covering, the vulva.

vulvocrural (vŭl''vō-krū'răl) [L. *vulva*, covering, + *cruralis*, pert. to the leg]. Rel. to the vulva and the thigh.

vulvopathy (vŭl-vŏp'ă-thĭ) [L. *vulva*, covering, + Gr. *pathos*, disease]. Any disorder of the vulva.

vulvouterine (vŭl''vō-ū'tĕr-in) ["+ *uterinus*, pert. to the uterus]. Rel. to the vulva and uterus.

vulvovaginal (vŭl''vō-văj'ĭ-năl) ["+ *vagina*, a sheath]. Pert. to the vulva and vagina.

v. glands. Small glands on either side of the vulvar orifice. SEE: *Bartholin's glands.*

vulvovaginitis (vŭl''vō-văj''ĭ-nī'tĭs) ["+ "+ Gr. *-itis*, inflammation]. Inflammation of both the vulva and vagina at the same time, or of the vulvovaginal glands.

v., diabetic. Mycotic vulvar infection commonly occurring with diabetes.

vv. Abbr. for *veins.*

W

W. Chem. symbol for tungsten.

w. Abbr. for *watt,* a unit of electric energy; *week; wife; with.*

Wachendorf's membrane (vŏk'ĕn-dôrf). [Eberhard J. Wachendorf, Ger. anatomist, 18th century]. 1. A thin membrane occluding the pupil of the embryo. SYN: *membrana pupillaris.* 2. The outer membrane ensheathing a cell.

wafer (wā'fēr) [Ger. wāfel]. 1. A thin sheet of flour paste used to enclose a medicinal dose of powder. 2. A flat vaginal suppository.

Wagstaffe's fracture (wăg'stăf). [William Warwick Wagstaffe, Eng. surgeon, 1843-1910]. Fracture with separation of the internal malleolus of the ankle.

waist (wāst) [ME. *wast,* growth]. Small part of the human trunk between thorax and hips. SEE: *cincture sensation.*

wakeful (wāk'fŭl) [AS. *wacian,* to be awake, + *full,* complete]. Not able to sleep; sleepless.

Walcher's position (vŏl'kĕr). [Gustav Adolf Walcher, Ger. gynecologist, 1856-1935]. Position in which the patient assumes dorsal recumbent posture with hips at the edge of the bed and legs hanging down.

Wald cycle. The transformations involved in the breakdown of resynthesis of rhodopsin.

Waldeyer's neuron (vŏl'dī-ēr). [Wilhelm von Waldeyer, Ger. anatomist, 1836-1921]. The nerve cell and its processes.

Waldeyer's ring. The ring of tonsillar (lymphatic) tissue which encircles the naso- and oropharynx. Consists of the two palatine tonsils, lingual and pharyngeal tonsils.

walker. A mobile device used to assist a person in walking. A stable platform, made of tubing, that the patient grasps while taking a step. The w. is then moved forward and another step is taken. SEE: *crutch.*

walking [AS. *wealcan,* to roll]. Act of moving on foot; advancing by steps.

RS: abasia; akathisia; astasia; atremia; basophobia; claudication; dysbasia; gait.

w. cast. A cast which allows the patient to be ambulatory.

w., sleep. Somnambulism, q.v.

w. typhoid. Typhoid fever in which the symptoms are mild so that the patient is ambulatory.

wall [AS. *weall*]. The limiting or surrounding substance or material of a cell, vessel, or cavity such as an artery, vein, chest, or bladder.

Wallenberg's syndrome (vŏl'ĕn-bĕrg). [Adolf Wallenberg,.Ger. physician, 1862-1949]. A complex of symptoms resulting from occlusion of the posterior inferior cerebellar artery or one of its branches supplying lower portion of brain stem. Dysphagia, muscular weakness or paralysis, impairment of pain and temperature senses, and cerebellar dysfunction are characteristic.

wallerian degeneration (wŏl-ē'rī-ăn). [Augustus Volney Waller, Eng. physician, 1816-1870]. Degeneration of a nerve fiber (axon) which has been severed from its cell body. The myelin sheath also degenerates and is transformed into a chain of lipoid droplets which stains by the Marchi method, a method utilized in tracing the course of injured nerve fibers. The neurilemma does not degenerate but forms a tube which directs the growth of the regenerating axon.

walleye [ME. *wawil-eghed*]. 1. Eye in which iris is light-colored or white. 2. Leukoma or dense opacity of cornea. 3. Squint in which both visual axes diverge. SYN: *divergent strabismus.*

wal'nut [AS. *wealhhnutu,* a foreign nut]. A tree of the genus Juglans, and its fruit. Occurs in two forms, black and English.

Food value of 100 gm. (English, raw): Cal. 651; protein 14.8 gm.; fat 64 gm.; carbohydrate 15.8 gm.

wan'dering [AS. *wandrian*]. Moving about; not fixed.

w. abscess. Abscess that burrows and comes to the surface at a point distant from its origin.

w. kidney, w. spleen. Dislocated floating kidney or spleen.

w. mind. Daydream or reverie.

Wangensteen's method (wăn'gĕn-stēn). [Owen H. Wangensteen, Am. surgeon, 1898 —] Technique for relieving postoperative abdominal distention, nausea, vomiting, and certain cases of mechanical bowel obstruction. It involves use of an intranasal catheter in combination with a suction siphonage apparatus. SEE: *decompression; distention.*

Warburg apparatus. [Otto H. Warburg, Ger. biochemist, 1883 —] A capillary manometer used for determining oxygen consumption and CO_2 production of small bits of cellular tissue. Widely used in metabolism studies.

ward [AS. *weard,* watching over]. A large room or hall in a hospital for the care of several patients.

w., accident. W. reserved for accident cases.

w., isolation. W. for isolation of those having or suspected of having a contagious disease.

w., probationary. W. for temporary detention of patients suspected of having a communicable disease.

w., psychopathic. W. in a general hospital for mentally ill patients.

Wardrop's disease (war'drŏp). [James Wardrop, Eng. surgeon, 1782-1869]. Acute inflammation of matrix of the nail in scrofulous children. SYN: *onychia maligna.*

Wardrop's operation. Ligation of an artery for aneurysm at a distance beyond the sac.

warehousemen's itch. Eczema of hands from touching irritating substances.

war gases. Any chemical substances, whether solid, liquid, or vapor, used to produce poisonous or irritant effects. SEE: *gases, war.*

wart (wŏrt) [AS. *wearte*]. A circumscribed cutaneous elevation resulting from hypertrophy of the papillae and epidermis. It is caused by a virus. SYN: *verruca.*

RS: condyloma; keratosis, seborrheic; sycoma; venereal; verrucose.

w., fig. A growth of filiform projections usually occurring on genitalia. Frequently they are covered with a foul-smelling secretion. SYN: *condyloma acuminatum; venereal wart; verruca acuminata.*

w., plantar. W. on pressure-bearing areas, esp. sole of foot.

w., seborrheic. Patch of corneous hypertrophy on face of the aged.

w., senile. W., seborrheic, q.v.

w.'s, venereal. Vegetating growths upon skin, esp. on the mucocutaneous juncture of the genitals, having an offensive discharge. SYN: *verruca acuminata.*

wash. 1. Act of cleaning, esp. a part or all of the body. 2. A medicinal preparation used in washing or coating.

w., eye. A lotion for the eyes. SYN: *collyrium.*

washerwoman's itch. Eczema of the hands of laundry workers.

wasp [AS. *waesp*]. Term sometimes applied to all insects belonging to the suborder Apocrita, order Hymenoptera (except the Formicidae or ants), but more generally restricted to the superfamilies Scolioidea, Vespoidea, and Specoidea. Members have base of abdomen constricted and females have a piercing ovipositor which in many species is modified into a sting. Many are social, living in large colonies. Common representatives are yellow jackets and hornets.

w. sting. The injection of wasp venom into the skin resulting in a painful wound and sometimes a mild systemic reaction. Multiple stings may be dangerous, esp. to sensitized individuals.

TREATMENT: Apply bicarbonate of soda paste, strong Epsom salt, or household ammonia solution locally. If pain is severe, infiltrate area with 2% procaine solution. Severe allergic reaction may require injection of epinephrine and cortisone. Application of cold to a large area around bite will slow absorption of the venom.

w. waist. Condition seen in some cases of muscular dystrophy in which atrophy of trunk muscles is pronounced.

Wassermann-fast (wăs'ĕr-măn). [August Paul von Wassermann, Ger. bacteriologist, 1866-1925]. Indicating a positive reaction shown by a Wassermann test which continues after adequate antisyphilitic medication.

Wassermann reaction. Serum complement fixation test as a diagnosis of syphilis. A general term loosely applied to almost any serological test for syphilis.

The results are designated as 1, 2, 3, and 4 plus, the intensity of the reaction usually corresponding to the severity of the infection. The disease may still exist with a negative reaction. Several such reactions would indicate its absence. Several years should pass after treatment and after last negative test before cure is definitely accepted.

waste (wāst) [L. *vāstus*, empty]. 1. To shrink in physical bulk or strength, as from disease. SYN: *cachexia.* 2. Loss by breaking down of bodily tissue. 3. Refuse material no longer useful to an organism.

w. products. Carbon dioxide, organic and inorganic salts, urine, dead skin, hair, nails, undigested foods.

w. products, metabolic. Soluble salts in the form of nitrogenous salts (urea) and inorganic salts (sodium chloride); gas in form of carbon dioxide, and liquid in the form of water. They are excreta, removed by the process of elimination, q.v.

wasting (wāst'ĭng) [L. *vāstāre*, to devastate]. Enfeebling; causing loss of strength or size; emaciating. SEE: *marasmus.*

w. palsy or paralysis. Chronic disease marked by gradual atrophy of muscular tissue with paralysis. SYN: *progressive muscular atrophy.*

water (wŏ-tĕr) [AS. *waeter*]. 1. H_2O, hydrogen and oxygen, a tasteless, clear, odorless fluid.

2. The urine. 3. A solution in water of a volatile substance. W. freezes at 32° F. (0° C.) and boils at 212° F. (100° C.). It is the principal chemical constituent of the body, comprising approx. 75%. It is distributed within the intracellular fluid and outside of the cells in the extracellular fluid. W. is indispensable for metabolic activities within cells as it is the medium in which chemical reactions can take place. Outside of cells, w. is the principal transporting agent of the body. The following are properties of w. which are of importance to living organisms: It is almost a universal solvent; it is a medium in which acids, bases, and salts ionize, and the concentrations of these substances (electrolytes) must be and are normally regulated quite precisely by the body; it possesses a high specific heat and a high latent heat of vaporization, of importance in regulation and maintenance of a constant body temperature; it possesses a high surface tension; it is an important reacting agent and essential in all hydrolytic reactions.

W. is the principal constituent of all body fluids (blood, lymph, tissue fluid), of all secretions (salivary juice, gastric juice, bile, sweat, etc.), and all excretory fluids (urine). Intake of w. is determined principally by the sense of thirst. Excessive intake may lead to water intoxication; excessive loss to dehydration.

w. balance. Condition in which intake of w. equals output.

w.- bed. A rubber mattress partially filled with warm w. (temp. 100° F. or 37.8° C.); must not be too full or it will be hard. Has been used in treating and preventing bed sores.

w., bound. W. which in protoplasm is attached to organic substances. It is not available for metabolic processes.

w. on brain. Disease marked by abnormal increase in cerebral spinal fluid. SYN: *hydrocephalus.*

w. brash. Gastric burning pain with eructations. SYN: *heartburn.*

w.- cure. Use of w. in treatment. SYN: *hydrotherapy.*

w., deionized. W. that has been passed through a substance which removes cations and anions present as contaminants.

w., distilled. W. which has been purified by distillation, q.v. Used for pharmaceutical purposes.

w., emergency preparation of safe drinking. W. must be purified when only unclean w. is available or if there is reason to believe that available drinking w. has become contaminated. One of the following methods may be used: (1) Strain w. through a clean cloth and boil w. vigorously for one minute. (2) Add three drops of alcoholic solution of iodine to each quart (approx. 1 liter) of w. Mix well and let it stand for 30 minutes prior to using. (3) Add either 10 drops of 1% chlorine bleach, or 2 drops of 4-6% chlorine bleach, or 1 drop of 7-10% chlorine bleach to each quart (liter) of w. Mix well and let stand for 30 minutes. If w. is cloudy to begin with, use double the amount of chlorine.

w.- hammer pulse. Pulse marked by quick, powerful beat, collapsing suddenly. SYN: *Corrigan's pulse,* q.v. SEE: *pulse.*

w., hard. W. which contains dissolved salts of magnesium or calcium.

w., heavy. (D_2O) An isotopic variety of w., esp. deuterium oxide, in which hydrogen has been displaced by its isotope, deuterium. Its properties differ from ordinary w. in that heavy w. has a higher freezing and boiling point and in the fact that it is incapable of supporting life.

w. (for) injection. W. for parenteral use that has been distilled and sterilized within 24 hours or w. that has been distilled (sometimes redistilled), sterilized, and placed in sealed containers so that it remains free of pyrogens. SEE: *w., pyrogen-free.*

w. intoxication. Intoxication resulting from ingestion of large quantities of w. or in cases of kidney disorder when urinary secretion is reduced. Death may occur.

SYM: headache, dizziness, vomiting, convulsions, and coma.

w. itch. Schistosome dermatitis, q.v.

w., purified. W. which is mineral free. Obtained by distillation, q.v., or deionization, q.v.

w., pyrogen-free. W. that has been rendered free of fever-producing proteins (bacteria and their metabolic products). SEE: *water (for) injection.*

w., soft. W. which contains very little, if any, dissolved salts of magnesium or calcium.

watercress. A plant with green leaves and white flowers; usually grows in fresh running water. The leaves and stems are used in salads.

Food value of 100 gm. (raw): Cal. 19; protein 2.2 gm.; fat 0.3 gm.; carbohydrate 3.0 gm.; vitamin A, 4900 I.U.; vitamin C, 79 mg.

watermelon. The large, round or oblong fruit of a vine of the same name. Its red, sweet, juicy center is eaten.

Food value of 100 gm. (raw): Cal. 26; protein 0.5 gm.; fat 0.2 gm.; carbohydrate 6.4 gm.; vitamin C, 13 mg.

waters. Common term for the amniotic fluid surrounding the fetus.

w., bag of. Sac enclosing liquor amnii surrounding the fetus. SYN: *amniotic sac.*

wave (wāv) [ME. *wave*]. 1. A disturbance, usually orderly and predictable, observed as a moving ridge on the surface of a liquid. 2. An undulating or vibrating motion. 3. An oscillation seen in the recording of an electrocardiogram, electroencephalogram, or other graphic record of physiological activity.

w., excitation. The excitatory impulse(s) which originate in the sinuatrial node of the heart and sweep through the musculature of the atria stimulating the atrioventricular node and then continuing through the conductile tissue of the ventricles. They bring about the contraction of the chambers of the heart.

w., hertzian. Electromagnetic radiations used in radio and wireless transmission.

w., pulse. The pressure w. originated by the systolic discharge of blood into the aorta. It is not due to the passage of the ejected blood but is the result of the impact being transmitted through the arterial walls. Its speed of transmission varies with nature of the arterial wall increasing with age as the arteries become less resilient. Thus in arteriosclerosis, the velocity is increased over normal.

w.'s, sound. Vibrations of a vibrating medium which, upon stimulating sensory receptors of the cochlea, are capable of giving rise to sensations of sound. Velocity: In dry air 1087 ft. (331.6 meters)/sec. at 0° C.; in water, approx. 4 times faster than in air.

wax [AS. *weax*]. 1. Beeswax, secreted by bees; a substance that is solid at room temperature. In medicine, a purified form, white wax (USP), is used in making ointments and to stop bleeding from bones during surgery. 2. Any substance with the consistency of beeswax. 3. Earwax. SYN: *cerumen.* SEE: *ceroplasty.*

waxy (wāks'ĭ) [AS. *weax*, wax]. Resembling or pert. to wax.

w. cast. Dense, highly refractile urinary cast. Such casts have clean-cut contours, sometimes irregular curves and notches. Occurs in severe chronic renal disease.

w. degeneration. Amyloid degeneration seen in wasting diseases.

W.B.C. Abbr. for *white blood count; white blood cells.*

weak (wēk) [Old Norse *veikr,* flexible]. Lacking physical strength or vigor; infirm.

RS: asthenia; atony; cardiasthenia; enervation; ergasthenia; fatigue; lassitude.

wean (wēn) [AS. *wenian*]. To accustom an infant to discontinuation of breast milk by substitution of other nourishment.

wean'ling. A young child or infant recently changed from breast to formula feeding.

w. diarrhea. Severe gastroenteritis which sometimes occurs in infants who recently have been weaned.

webbed (wĕbd) [AS. *webb,* a fabric]. Having a membrane or tissue connecting adjacent structures, as the duck's feet.

w. fingers, w. toes. Two or more toes or fingers connected by a membrane.

Weber-Christian disease (wĕb'ĕr-krĭs'-chĕn). [Friedrich Weber, Eng. physician, 1863-1962; Henry A. Christian, Amer. physician, 1876-1951] Relapsing, febrile, nodular, nonsuppurative panniculitis, a generalized disorder of fat metabolism characterized by recurring episodes of fever and development of crops of subcutaneous fatty nodules.

Weber's paralysis (wĕb'ĕr). [Sir Hermann David Weber, Eng. physician, 1824-1918]. Paralysis of oculomotor nerve on one side with contralateral spastic hemiplegia. SYN: *Weber's syndrome.*

ETIOL: Lesion of the crus cerebri.

weep'ing [AS. *wēpan*, to lament]. 1. Shedding tears. 2. Moist, dripping.

w. eczema. Dermatitis with eruption of vesicles exuding serum.

w. sinew. Circumscribed cystic swelling of a tendon sheath.

Weidel's reaction (vī'dĕl). [Hugo Weidel, Austrian chemist, 1849-99]. Test for presence of xanthine bodies or uric acid.

Weigert's law (vī'gĕrt). [Karl Weigert, Ger. pathologist, 1843-1904]. An observation which states that loss or destruction of tissue results in an excess of new tissue during repair.

weight (wāt) [AS. *gewiht*]. The measure of heaviness or the mass of something.

W. of the body increases in pathological obesity and decreases in Addison's disease, cancer, chronic diarrhea, chronic suppurations, diabetes, hysteria, anorexia, fevers, lactation when prolonged, marasmus, obstruction of pylorus or thoracic duct, tuberculosis, ulcer of stomach.

Normal w. depends upon the frame of the individual. Determination of one's own frame is difficult.

w., atomic. W. of an atom of an element compared with that of oxygen which is taken as 16; the mean value of the isotopic weights of an element.

w., molecular. The sum of all the atomic weights of all the elements in one molecule of a compound. ABBR: M.

weight'lessness. Condition of not being acted upon by the force of gravity. This is present when astronauts travel in areas so distant from the earth, moon, or planets that the force of gravity is virtually absent.

weights and measures. SEE: *Table of Weights and Measures* in *Appendix.*

Weil-Felix reaction (vil-fā′lĭk). [Edmund Veil, Ger. physician, 1880-1922; Arthur Felix, Ger. bacteriologist, 1887-1956]. The agglutination of certain Proteus organisms due to the development of Proteus antibodies in certain rickettsial diseases. SYN: *Weil-Felix test.*

Weil's disease (vil). [Adolf Weil, Ger. physician, 1848-1916]. Any one of several sero-types of Leptospira such as L. icterohemorrhagica, L. pomona, L. canicola, or L. autumnalis.

ETIOL: An organism found in rat urine and feces, and acquired by man through contaminated food or water or by contact of broken skin with an infected rat or its feces or urine.

It is a specific infection accompanied by muscular pains, fever, jaundice, and enlargement of liver and spleen.

TREATMENT: Largely symptomatic because there is no specific therapeutic agent. Penicillin may shorten the course of the disease.

Weir Mitchell's treatment (wēr-mĭt′-chĕl). [S. Weir Mitchell, Amer. neurologist, 1829-1914]. Treatment for hysteria and neurasthenia which consists of rest in bed, massage, nourishing diet, and isolation.

Welch's bacillus (wĕlsh). [William Henry Welch, Amer. pathologist, 1850-1934]. Clostridium perfringens, the causative organism of gas gangrene. SEE: *Clostridium perfringens; gangrene, gas.*

welt [ME. *welte*]. An elevation on the skin produced by a lash, blow, or allergic stimulus. The skin is unbroken and the mark is reversible.

wen (wĕn) [AS.]. A cyst resulting from the retention of secretion in a sebaceous gland. SYN: *steatoma.*

SYM: One or more rounded or oval elevations, varying in size from peas to large walnuts, slowly appear on scalp, face, or back; painless, rather soft, containing a yellowish-white caseous mass.

Desirable Weights for Men and Women of 25 and Over*

	Women				Men		
Height (with shoes on) 2-inch heels	Weight (in pounds fully clothed)			Height (with shoes on) 1-inch heels	Weight (in pounds fully clothed)		
Ft. In.	Small Frame	Medium Frame	Large Frame	Ft. In.	Small Frame	Medium Frame	Large Frame
4 10	92–98	96–107	104–119	5 2	112–120	118–129	126–141
4 11	94–101	98–110	106–122	5 3	115–123	121–133	129–144
5 0	96–104	101–113	109–125	5 4	118–126	124–136	132–148
5 1	99–107	104–116	112–128	5 5	121–129	127–139	135–152
5 2	102–110	107–119	115–131	5 6	124–133	130–143	138–156
5 3	105–113	110–122	118–134	5 7	128–137	134–147	142–161
5 4	108–116	113–126	121–138	5 8	132–141	138–152	147–166
5 5	111–119	116–130	125–142	5 9	136–145	142–156	151–170
5 6	114–123	120–135	129–146	5 10	140–150	146–160	155–174
5 7	118–127	124–139	133–150	5 11	144–154	150–165	159–179
5 8	122–131	128–143	137–154	6 0	148–158	154–170	164–184
5 9	126–135	132–147	141–158	6 1	152–162	158–175	168–189
5 10	130–140	136–151	145–163	6 2	156–167	162–180	173–194
5 11	134–144	140–155	149–168	6 3	160–171	167–185	178–199
6 0	138–148	144–159	153–173	6 4	164–175	172–190	182–204

*Courtesy of Metropolitan Life Insurance Company.

TREATMENT: Sac and contents should be carefully dissected in order to prevent its recurrence. SEE: *sebaceous gland.*

Werdnig-Hoffmann's disease (vĕrd'nĭg-hŏf'man). [Guido Werdnig, Austrian neurologist, 19th century; Johann Hoffmann, Ger. neurologist, 1857-1919] Infantile muscular atrophy, considered by some to be identical with amyotonia congenita.

Werlhof's disease (vĕrl'hŏf). [Paul G. Werlhof, Ger. physician, 1699-1767]. Form of progressive purpura marked by hemorrhages from the mucous membranes and severe prostration. SYN: *idiopathic thrombocytopenic; purpura.*

SYM: Large reduction of blood platelets, spontaneous hemorrhages into and from tissues, enlargement of spleen.

Wernicke's syndrome (ver'nĭk-ē). [Karl Wernicke, Ger. neurologist, 1848-1905]. Frequent condition of old age marked by loss of memory and disorientation with confabulation. SYN: *presbyophrenia,* q.v.

Westphal-Edinger nucleus. [Karl Westphal, Ger. neurologist, 1833-1890; Ludwig Edinger, Ger. neurologist, 1855-1918]. Small group of nerve cells in rostral portion of nucleus of oculomotor nerve. Efferent fibers pass to ciliary ganglion conveying impulses destined for intrinsic muscles of the eye.

wet (wĕt) [AS. *wāēt*]. Soaked with moisture.

w. brain. Increased amt. of cerebrospinal fluid with edema of the meninges, due to alcoholism.

w. cup. A cupping glass used after scarification.

w. dream. Nocturnal seminal emission.

w.- nurse. A woman who breast-feeds another's child.

w. pack. A form of bath, given by wrapping patient in hot or cold wet sheets, covered with a blanket, used esp. to reduce fever.

WEUP. Abbr. for *willful exposure to unwanted pregnancy.*

Wharton's duct (hwăr'tŏn). [Thomas Wharton, Eng. anatomist, 1614-73]. Duct of the submandibular salivary gland opening into the mouth at side of the frenum linguae.

Wharton's jelly. A gelatinous intercellular substance consisting of primitive connective tissue of the umbilical cord. It is rich in hyaluronic acid.

wheal (hwēl) [AS. *hwēle*]. More or less round and evanescent elevation of the skin, white in center with pale red periphery, accompanied by itching. Seen in urticaria, insect bites, anaphylaxis, angioneurotic edema. SYN: *pomphus.*

wheat (hwēt) [AS. *hwāēte*]. Any of various cereal grasses, widely cultivated for its important edible grain used in making flour. Boiled whole wheat is an excellent food. SEE: *bread.*

Food value of 100 gm. (flour from hard wheat): Cal. 333; protein 13.3 gm.; fat 2.0 gm.; carbohydrate 71 gm.; iron 33 mg.; calcium 41 mg.; phosphorus 372 mg.; niacin 4.3 mg.

STRUCTURE OF A GRAIN OF WHEAT: Husk or outer coat, removed before grinding; bran coats, removed in making white flour and containing the mineral substances; gluten, contains the fat and protein; starch, center of the kernel.

WHEAT PREPARATIONS AND PASTAS: Macaroni, vermicelli, noodles, etc., are made from flour and water, molded, dried, and slightly baked. They are easy to digest and not over 10% of nitrogen content is lost.

wheeze (hwēz) [ME. *whesen*]. A whistling or sighing sound resulting from narrowing of the lumen of a respiratory passageway. Often only noted by use of stethoscope. Occurs in asthma, croup, hay fever, mitral stenosis, and pleural effusion. May result from presence of tumors, foreign obstructions, bronchial spasm, tuberculosis, obstructive emphysema, or edema.

wheez'ing. Production of whistling sounds during difficult breathing such as occurs in asthma, coryza, croup, and other respiratory disorders. SEE: *wheeze.*

whelk (hwĕlk) [AS. *hwylca*]. A wheal; a protuberance on the face as a nodule or tubercle.

whey (hwā) [AS. *hwaeg*]. The liquid left after milk has been coagulated by the aid of rennet. SEE: *buttermilk; milk.*

Food value of 100 gm. (liquid): Cal. 26; protein 0.9 gm.; fat 0.3 gm.; carbohydrate 5.1 gm.; calcium 51 mg.

whiff. 1. A slight gust or puff of air, esp. one conveying an odor. 2. A quick inhalation or exhalation, as of tobacco smoke.

whinolallia. Hypernasality and distortion of speech. Occurs in incompetent palatal syndrome.

whiplash injury. Imprecise term for injury to the cervical vertebrae and adjacent soft tissues. Produced by a sudden jerking or relative backward or forward acceleration of the head with respect to the vertebral column. Injury may occur to those in a vehicle which is suddenly and forcibly struck from the rear.

Whipple's disease (hwĭp'ĕl). [George Hoyt Whipple, Amer. pathologist, 1878 –]. Intestinal lipodystrophy, characterized by fatty stools, loss of weight and strength, chronic arthritis, a distinctive lesion of the mucosa of the jejunum and ileum, and other signs of a malabsorption syndrome. This rare disease resembles idiopathic steatorrhea.

TREATMENT: Tetracycline.

whipworm. A roundworm often parasitic in the human intestines. SYN: *Trichuris trichiura.*

whirl (hwûrl) [Old Norse *hvirfla*]. 1. To revolve rapidly. 2. To feel giddiness.

whirl'bone. 1. The kneecap. SYN: *patella.* 2. The head of the femur.

whisky, whiskey (hwĭs'kē). A distilled alcoholic liquor made from grain. The alcohol present is ethyl alcohol. *CAUTION:* Wood or methyl alcohol should never be used in alcoholic beverages intended for human consumption. It is extremely toxic and may cause death. In those who survive, blindness is a common occurrence. SYN: *spiritus frumenti.*

whisper (hwĭs'per) [AS. *hwisprian*]. 1. Speech without voice; a low, sibilant sound. 2. To utter in a low, nonvocal sound.

    w., cavernous. Direct transmission of a whisper through a cavity in auscultation.

white (hwĭt) [AS. *hwīt*]. 1. The achromatic color of maximum lightness. 2. Of the color of milk.

    w. cell, w. corpuscle. The leukocyte. SEE: *blood; corpuscle.*

    w. of egg. The albumin of an egg.

    w. of eye. Conjunctiva, q.v.

    w. gangrene. Gangrene due to local anemia.

    w. leg. Phlebitis of femoral vein marked by w. swelling of the leg. SYN: *phlegmasia alba dolens, q.v.*

    w. line. W. tendinous attachment of abdominal oblique and transverse muscles. Visible in the midline of the skin covering the anterior wall of the abdomen. SYN: *linea alba.*

    w. matter, w. substance. Any nervous structure composed of w. medulated nerve fibers.

    w. precipitate. A w. amorphous powder used principally in ointments for external treatment of some skin diseases. SYN: *ammoniated mercury.*

    w. softening. Stage of softening of any substance in which the affected area has become w. and anemic.

white'fish. North American freshwater fish of a silvery color.

    Food value of 100 gm. (smoked): Cal. 155; protein 20.9 gm.; fat 7.3 gm.; no carbohydrate.

whites. A medical colloquialism for a thick, whitish vaginal discharge. SYN: *leukorrhea,* q.v.

whitlow (hwĭt'lō) [ME. *whitflawe,* white flow]. Suppurative inflammation at the end of a finger or toe. It may be deep seated, involving the bone and its periosteum, or superficial, affecting parts of the nail. SYN: *felon; panaris; paronychia,* q.v.

whoop (hūp) [AS. *hwōpan,* to threaten]. The sonorous and convulsive inspiratory crow following a paroxysm of whooping cough.

whooping cough. An acute infectious disease with recurrent spasms of coughing ending in a whooping inspiration. SYN: *pertussis,* q.v.

whorl (hwûrl) [ME. *whorle*]. 1. Spiral arrangement of cardiac muscular fibers. SYN: *vortex.* 2. A type of fingerprint in which the central papillary ridges turn through at least one complete circle.

whortleberry (hwûr'tl-bĕr'ĭ). A sweet European blueberry. SEE: *blueberry* for food value.

Widal's reaction or test (vē-dŏl'). [Fernand Widal, Fr. physician, 1862-1929]. An agglutination test for typhoid fever.

wild cherry. USP. The dried bark of prunus virginiana, used principally in the form of syrup as a flavored vehicle for cough medicine.

will [AS.]. 1. The mental faculty used in choosing or deciding upon an act or thought. 2. Power of controlling one's actions or emotions.

    RS: acrasia; bulesis; volition; voluntary.

Willis' circle. An intercommunicating set of arteries which encircles optic chiasma and hypophysis from which the principal arteries supplying the brain are derived. It receives blood from the two internal carotid arteries and the basilar artery formed by union of the two vertebrals.

Willis' cords (wĭl'ĭs). [Thomas Willis, Eng. anatomist, 1621-1675]. Cords crossing the superior longitudinal sinus transversely.

Wilson's disease (wĭl'sŭn). A rare disease of degeneration of corpus striatum and cirrhosis of the liver characterized by tremulous distortion of the muscles (increased by activity), dysarthria, dysphagia, and emotionalism. It is thought to be the result of abnormal copper metabolism.

Winckel's disease (vĭng'kĕl). [Franz von Winckel, Ger. gynecologist, 1837-1911]. A fatal disease of the newborn characterized by profuse hemorrhages, hematuria, jaundice, enlarged spleen, collapse, and convulsions.

windchill. The cooling effect wind has on exposed human skin.

w. factor. Loss of heat from exposure of skin to wind. Heat loss is proportional to the speed of the wind. Thus skin exposed to a wind velocity of 20 miles/hour when the temperature is 0° F. (–17.8° C.) will be cooled at the same rate it would be in still air at –46° F. (–43.3° C.) Similarly when the temperature is 20° F. (–6.7° C.) and the wind is 10, 20, or 35 MPH (16.1, 32.2, or 56.3 kilometers per hour), the equivalent skin temperature would be –4°, –18°, or –28° F. (–20°, –27.8°, or –33.3° C.) respectively.

W. factor is calculated for dry skin. Skin, wet from any cause and exposed to wind, will lose heat at a much higher rate than dry skin. W. blowing over wet skin can cause frostbite, even on a comfortably warm day as judged by the thermometer.

w. index. A table listing the w. factor for various combinations of temperature and wind velocity. SEE: *w. factor.*

winding sheet. A sheet used to wrap a dead body. SYN: *shroud.*

window [Old Norse *vindauga*]. 1. An aperture for the admission of light or air or both. 2. A small aperture into a cavity, esp. that of inner ear. SEE: *fenestra.*

w., cochlear. The fenestra rotunda, q.v. SYN: *fenestra cochlea; round window.*

w., oval. The fenestra ovalis, q.v. SYN: *fenestra vestibuli.*

w., round. The fenestra rotunda, q.v. SYN: *fenestra cochlea.*

w., vestibular. The oval window. SYN: *fenestra ovalis,* q.v.

wind'pipe. Air passage from the larynx to the lungs. SYN: *trachea,* q.v.

wine (wīn) [L. *vīnum,* wine]. 1. Fermented juice of any fruit, usually made from grapes and contains 10-15% alcohol. 2. Solution of a medicinal substance in wine. SYN: *vinum.*

Food value of 100 gm. (table wine, about 12% alcohol by volume, slightly more than 3 fluid ounces): Cal. 85; protein 0.1 gm.; no fat; carbohydrate 4.2 gm.; calcium 9.0 mg.

w. glass. A fluid measure of approx. two fluid ounces (60 ml.).

w. sores. Slang term for superficial infected areas of the skin seen in alcoholics with poor personal hygiene. Erroneously thought to be due to specific action of the wine.

wing [Old Norse *vaengi*]. A structure resembling the wing of a bird, esp. the great and small wings of the sphenoid bone, q.v. SEE: *ala.*

winged scapula. SEE: *scapula, winged.*

wink [AS. *wincian*]. 1. To close and open the eyelids quickly. 2. Act of closing and opening the eyelids quickly. SEE: *nictation.*

Winslow, foramen of (wĭnz'lō). [Jacob B. Winslow, Fr. anatomist, 1669-1760] The epiploic foramen.

Winslow, ligament of. The oblique popliteal ligament located at back of knee.

Winslow, pancreas of. The processus uncinatus of the pancreas.

win'ter itch. Itching occurring only in cold weather. Probably due to drying of skin which is deficient in natural lubrication. SYN: *pruritus hiemalis.*

Wirsung, duct of (vēr'sūng). [Johann Georg Wirsung, Ger. physician, 1600-43]. Excretory duct of the pancreas. SYN: *pancreatic duct.*

wisdom tooth (wĭz'dŏm). The last molar tooth on each side of the jaw. These four molars may appear as late as the 25th year.

witches' milk. Milk secreted by the newly born infant's breast, stimulated by the lactating hormone circulating in the mother.

withdrawal. Cessation of administration of a drug, esp. a narcotic, to which the individual has become either physiologically or psychologically addicted. W. symptoms vary with the type of drug used. SEE: *drug addiction.*

Wohlfahrtia (vōl-fär'tĭ-ā). A genus of flies parasitic in animal tissue, belonging to the family Sarcophagidae, order Diptera.

W. magnifica. Species found in southeast Europe. The larvae may occur in human and animal wounds.

W. opaca. Species occurring in Canada, a common parasite of wild animals. Human babies may become infested.

W. vigil. Species found in Canada and north United States.

wolffian body (wŭl'fĭ-ăn). [Kaspar Friedrich Wolff, Ger. anatomist, 1733-94]. An embryonic organ on each side of the vertebral column. SYN: *mesonephros.* SEE: *archinephron; embryo; paroophoron; parovarium.*

wolffian cyst. One of the broad ligaments of the uterus.

wolffian duct. Duct in embryo leading from mesonephros to cloaca. From it develop the ductus epididymis, ductus deferens, seminal vesicle, ejaculatory duct, ureter and pelvis of kidney. SYN: *mesonephric duct.*

wolffian tubules. One of 30 to 34 tubules which develop within the mesonephros and empty into mesonephric duct. Most are transitional persisting for only a short time. Some persist in adult males as the efferent ductules of the testis, others persist only as vestigial structures. SYN: *mesonephric tubules.* SEE: *epoophoron; paradidymis; paroophoron.*

Wolhynian fever. Trench fever.

womb (wūm) [AS. *wamb*]. Female organ for protection and nourishment of the fetus. SYN: *uterus*, q.v.

wood alcohol. (CH₃OH) Alcohol obtained by distillation from wood. It is a poisonous substance and frequently causes loss of sight. SEE: *methyl alcohol; whiskey.*

Wood's rays. [Robert Williams Wood, Amer. physicist, 1868 —]. Ultraviolet rays. Used to detect fluorescent materials in the skin and hair in certain disease states such as tinea capitis. The terms Wood's light and Wood's lamp have become synonymous for Wood's rays, even though these are misnomers.

wood tick. Dermacentor andersoni, an important N. Amer. species of tick which causes tick paralysis and transmits causative organisms of Rocky Mountain spotted fever and tularemia.

wool fat. Anhydrous lanolin, a fatty substance obtained from sheep's wool. Used as a base for ointments.

wool'sorter's disease. A pulmonary form of anthrax which develops in those who handle wool contaminated with Bacillus anthracis.

word blindness. Inability to comprehend written words; a form of aphasia, q.v. SYN: *alexia.*

word salad. The use of words with no apparent meaning attached to them or to their relationship with one another. Usually found in schizophrenia.

work (wûrk) [Ger. *wirken*]. Mental or physical effort made in order to accomplish or produce something. SEE: *calorie; erg; unit.*

worm (wûrm) [AS. *wyrm*]. 1. An elongated invertebrate belonging to one of the following phyla: Platyhelminthes (flatworms); Nemathelminthes or Aschelminthes, round- or threadworms; Acanthocephala, spinyheaded worms; and Annelida (Annulata), segmented worms. SYN: *helminth.* SEE: individual worms by name. 2. Any small, limbless, creeping animal. 3. Median portion of the cerebellum. 4. Any wormlike structure.

wormian bones (wûr'mĭ-ăn). [Olaus Worm, Dan. anatomist, 1588-1654]. Small, irregular bones in the course of the cranial sutures.

wound (woond) [AS. *wund*]. Break in the continuity of soft parts of body structures caused by violence or trauma to tissues. In treating any wound, the patient should be given a tetanus toxoid booster injection if he

has been immunized previously. If not, he must be given human tetanus antitoxin. If human tetanus antitoxin is not available, the equine form may be used but the patient must be tested for hypersensitivity prior to administering the full dose.

w., abdominal. Frequently sustained; ordinarily involves structure of abdominal wall. In such instances, the w. may be treated as ordinary wounds. Where a cavity has been opened, and esp. if viscera have been exposed, the area should be kept sterile and moist with a sterile normal salt solution prepared by dissolving a teaspoonful of salt in pint of warm water, or use the clearest water at hand, because allowing viscera to dry encourages the development of gangrene.

w., bullet. A puncture w. from a bullet. Usually there is a small point of entrance; if the bullet left the body, a larger point of exit; it is associated with injuries of bone, tendon, blood vessels, etc.

SYM: Depend on site, speed, and character of bullet.

F.A. TREATMENT: Antitetanic serum. Antiseptic to wound and dressing. Treat complications and shock.

w., cellulitis of. Local inflammation of a w., occurring when w. has been closed without drainage, esp. in appendicitis.

SYM: Elevation of temperature from 4th to 7th day with accompanying tenderness. Inspect dressing and chart findings.

TREATMENT: Evacuation of the abscess; hot wet dressings; antibiotics.

w., contused. A bruise. It may be caused by a blunt instrument. The skin need not be broken. However, injury of the tissues under skin, leaving skin unbroken, traumitizes the soft tissue. The blood vessels ruptured underneath the skin cause discoloration. If extravasated blood becomes encapsulated it is termed hematoma; if it is diffused, an ecchymosis. SEE: *ecchymosis; hematoma.*

TREATMENT: Cold compresses, pressure, and rest. Elevation of injured area will help prevent or reduce swelling. When acute stage is over (24-48 hours), continued rest, heat, and elevation are prescribed. Aseptic drainage may be indicated.

w., crushing. If bleeding, apply cold cloths; if not, apply dressing and treat as an ordinary wound until patient can be given definitive surgical treatment. If bone is fractured, apply splint.

w., fishhook. Embedded fishhooks are difficult to remove. Push the hook through, then cut off barb with an instrument, and pull the remainder of the fishhook out by the route it entered. Antitetanus treatment as indicated. Frequently these injuries become infected, so carefully saturate with an antiseptic, cover with a dressing, and observe for several days.

w., gunshot. Penetrating or perforating w. which may contain a foreign body as a bullet.

F.A. TREATMENT: Should be conservative. Apply antiseptic, sterile dressing; treat hemorrhage. Antitetanus therapy if indicated. Do not probe the w.

w., incised. A clean-cut w. Caused by a keen cutting instrument, and so there are no jagged edges. Any sharp cut in which the tissues are not severed is an incised w. It may be either an aseptic or infected w., depending on circumstances which caused it.

An aseptic w., one occurring under surgical conditions, should heal if conditions are favorable and no contaminations due to pathogenic organisms or foreign material enter into it. During healing process, area of the w. must be kept aseptic. The skin must be cleansed with plain soap and water, rinsed thoroughly, and covered securely with sterile dressings to keep the w. clean. A clean w. should be left alone. The dressings should be changed only often enough to keep w. clean. There should be no squeezing or pulling of its edges.

w., lacerated. A torn w., a type which provides many avenues for infection. It is not a clean wound; the edges are ragged. May be caused by many kinds of implements, and the implement may be covered with any kind of pathogenic bacteria. Thus a variety of types of w. infections may be expected. Antitetanus and gas gangrene prophylaxis may be needed.

TREATMENT: The w. should be cleansed with mild soap and water and rinsed thoroughly. If w. edges are ragged, they will need to be trimmed and dead tissue removed. The patient should be given tetanus antitoxin. The w. should never be sealed. It is well to hold it open with some form of drain.

w., nonpenetrating. W. in which the surface of skin remains intact.

w., open. Contusion where skin is also broken, such as a gunshot w., incised w., or lacerated w.

w., penetrating. W. in which the skin is broken and the agent causing the wound enters subcutaneous tissue or a deep-lying structure or cavity.

w., perforating. W. in which the object which caused the w. entered the body and emerged, i.e., a bullet, projectile, or knife.

w., poisoned. This may be classed as a lacerated w. or a puncture w., depending on tearing of tissue. The poisoned w. may be caused by a diseased animal, a snake or dog, or some of the wild animals, such as a coon or squirrel.

TREATMENT: A poisoned w. should be treated the same as a puncture w. If possible, the animal should be put under observation for rabies, q.v.

w., puncture. W. made by a sharp-pointed instrument, such as a dagger, ice pick, or needle. The chief danger is from thrombosis and possible release of emboli. A puncture w. usually is collapsed. This provides ideal conditions for infection. Placement of a drain, antitetanus therapy, and gas gangrene prophylaxis may be required. This will depend on the nature of the instrument which caused the injury.

w., subcutaneous. All wounds which are unaccompanied by break in skin, i.e., contusions.

w., tunnel. W. having a small entrance and exit and of uniform diameter.

W.R. Abbr. for *Wassermann reaction,* q.v.

Wright's stain. [James H. Wright, Amer. pathologist, 1871-1928]. A combination of eosin and methylene blue used in studying blood corpuscles and revealing malarial parasites. SEE: *Wright's technique for blood smears.*

Wright's technique for blood smears. Cover the dried blood smear with 5 to 10 drops of Wright's stain. Let stand one minute. Add an equal amount of neutral distilled water to the stain. Let diluted stain stand for 3-10 minutes. A metallic sheen should appear. Remove stain by gently washing with distilled water. Stand slide on end and allow to dry. Mount in balsam or methacrylate. If staining results are good, red cells will have a pinkish or copper color; white cells will have densely stained blue nuclei, and the cytoplasmic granules will stain variously in the different types of leukocytes. SEE: *leukocytes.*

wrinkle (rĭng'kl) [AS. *gewrinclian,* to wind]. 1. A crevice, furrow, or ridge in the skin. 2. To make creases or furrows as in the skin by habitual frowning.

Wrisberg's cardiac ganglion (rĭs'bŭrg). [Heinrich August Wrisberg, Ger. anatomist, 1739-1808]. A small ganglion sometimes found in cardiac plexus to the right of the ligamentum arteriosus.

Wrisberg's cartilages. The cuneiform cartilages of the larynx.

Wrisberg's nerve. 1. The medial brachial cutaneous nerve, a branch of the medial cord of the brachial plexus. 2. The nervus intermedius (pars intermedia), a branch of the facial nerve lying between the motor root and the acoustic nerve.

wrist (rĭst) [AS.]. The joint, or region, lying between the hand and the forearm.

   w. bones. The carpus consisting of eight bones. SEE: *skeleton.*

   w. drop. Condition in which hand is flexed at wrist and cannot be extended; due to injury of radial nerve or paralysis of extensor muscles of wrist and hand.

writer's cramp. A cramp affecting muscles of the thumb and two adjacent fingers after prolonged writing.

writing. The act of placing characters, letters, or words on a surface, usually paper, for the purpose of communicating ideas.

   w., defects of. SEE: *agraphia.*

   w., dextrad. W. that progresses from left to right.

   w., mirror. W. so that letters and words are reversed and appear as in a mirror.

writing hand. Position seen in paralysis agitans marked by contraction of muscle of the hand. The fingers assume the position similar to holding a pen.

wryneck (rĭ'nĕk). Contracted state of one or more muscles of the neck, producing an abnormal position of the head. SYN: *torticollis.*

   Occasionally it is acute, due to cold or trauma; more commonly it is chronic, spastic in character, and dependent upon nerve irritation. Has been produced by habitual malposition of the head assumed because of existing ocular defect. May be congential.

   When acute, generally passes away under influence of rest, heat, and time. Chronic may require surgical therapy.

w.s. Abbr. for *water soluble.*

wt. Abbr. for *weight.*

Wuchereria (vū″kĕr-ē'rĭ-ă). [Otto Wucherer, Ger. physician, 1820-73]. A genus of filarial worms belonging to the superfamily Filarioidea, class Nematoda. Common in warm regions of the world.

   W. bancrofti. The causative agent of elephantiasis. Adults of the species live in lymph nodes and ducts of man. Females give birth to sheathed microfilariae which remain in internal organs during the day but at night are in circulating blood where they are sucked up by night-biting mosquitoes in which they continue their development, becoming infective larvae in about two weeks. They are then passed on to the human when the mosquito bites. SYN: *Filaria bancrofti.*

   W. malayi. Species occurring in Southeast Asia and largely responsible for lympyangitis and elephantiasis in that region. Closely resembles W. bancrofti.

wuchereriasis (vū″kĕr-ē-rī'ă-sĭs). Infestation with filaria worms of the genus Wuchereria. SYN: *elephantiasis,* q.v.; *filariasis.*

w/v. Abbr. for *weight in volume.* It indicates the amount by weight of a solid substance dissolved in a measured quantity of liquid. Per cent w/v expresses number of grams of an ingredient in 100 ml. of solution.

w/w. Abbr. for *weight in weight.* It indicates the amount by weight of a solid substance dissolved in a known amount (by weight) of liquid. Per cent w/w expresses the number of grams of one ingredient in 100 grams of solution.

X

X. Roman numeral 10.

xanthelasma (zăn″thĕl-ăz′mă) [Gr. *xanthos,* yellow, + *elasma,* plate]. 1. Yellow. 2. Flat or slightly-raised yellowish tumor occurring in elderly persons, found most frequently on the upper and lower lids, esp. near the inner canthus. SYN: *xanthoma.*

xanthelasmoidea (zăn″thĕl-ăz-moy′dē-ă) [″+ ″+ *eidos,* resemblance]. Chronic disease of childhood marked by wheals and followed by brownish-yellow patches. SYN: *urticaria pigmentosa.*

xanthemia (zăn-thē′mĭ-ă) [″+ *haima,* blood]. Yellow pigment in the blood. SYN: *carotenemia.*

xanthic (zăn′thĭk) [Gr. *xanthos,* yellow]. 1. Yellow. 2. Pert. to xanthine.

   x. calculus. A urinary concretion containing xanthine.

xanthine (zăn′thĭn, -thēn). A nitrogenous extractive contained in muscle tissue, liver, spleen, pancreas, and other organs, and in the urine, formed during the metabolism of nucleoproteins.

   x. bases. Nitrogenous substances resulting from splitting up of nucleins.

xanthinuria (zăn″thĭn-ū′rĭ-ă) [Gr. *xanthos,* yellow, + *ouron,* urine]. Excretion of large amounts of xanthine in the urine.

xanthochroia (zăn″thō-krō′ĭ-ă) [″+ *chroia,* skin]. Yellowish discoloration of the skin.

xanthochromia (zăn″thō-krō′mĭ-ă) [″+ *chrōma,* color]. Yellow discoloration, as of the skin in patches or of the cerebrospinal fluid, resembling jaundice.

xanthochroous (zăn-thŏk′rō-ŭs) [Gr. *xanthochroos*]. Having a yellowish or light complexion.

xanthocyanopia, xanthocyanopsia (zăn″thō-sī-ăn-ō′pĭ-ă, -ŏp′sī-ă) [Gr. *xanthos,* yellow, + *kyanos,* blue, + *opsis,* sight]. A form of color blindness in which yellow and blue are distinguishable, but not red and green.

xanthocyte (zăn″thō′sīt) [″+ *kytos,* cell]. A cell containing yellow pigment.

xanthoderma (zăn″thō-dĕr′mă) [″+ *derma,* skin]. Yellowness of the skin.

xanthodont, xanthodontous (zăn′thō-dŏnt, zăn″thō-dŏn′tŭs) [Gr. *xanthos,* yellow, + *odous, odont-,* tooth]. Having yellow teeth.

xanthogranuloma (zăn″thō-grăn″u-lō′mă) [″+ L. *granulum,* grain, + *-ōma,* tumor]. A tumor having characteristics of both an infectious granuloma and an xanthoma.

xanthokyanopy (zăn″thō-kī-ăn′ō-pī) [″+ *kyanos,* blue, + *opsis,* sight]. Partial blindness for color, only yellow and blue being discerned. SYN: *xanthocyanopia.*

xanthoma (zăn-thō′mă) [Gr. *xanthos,* yellow, + *-ōma,* tumor]. Flat, slightly elevated, soft, rounded plaque or nodule, usually on the eyelids. May occur in patches of yellowish macule on orbital regions, confined to middle life or later, and to the female sex, consisting of a degenerative process involving fibers of the orbicularis muscle.

   x. diabeticorum. Cutaneous disease associated with diabetes mellitus.

   x. disseminatum. Condition characterized by presence of x. throughout body, esp. on face, in tendon sheaths, and in mucous membranes.

   x. multiplex. Xanthomas all over the body.

   x. palpebrarum. X. affecting the eyelids.

   x. tuberosum. A form which may appear on the neck, shoulders, trunk, or extremities, consisting of small, elastic, and yellowish-colored nodules.

xanthomatosis (zăn″thō-mă-tō′sĭs) [Gr. *xanthos,* yellow, + *ōma,* tumor]. Condition in which there is a deposition of lipid in tissues usually accompanied by hyperlipemia. Cholesterol may accumulate in tumor nodules (xanthoma) or in individual cells, esp. histiocytes and reticuloendothelial cells.

xanthoproteic (zăn″thō-prō-te′ĭk) [″+ *prōtos,* first]. Derived from or pert. to xanthoprotein.

xanthoprotein (zăn″thō-prō′tē-ĭn). Yellowish substance produced by heating proteins with nitric acid.

xanthopsia (zăn-thŏp′sĭ-ă) [Gr. *xanthos,* yellow, + *opsis,* sight]. Condition in which objects appear to be yellow.

xanthopsin (zăn-thŏp′sĭn). Visual yellow, the visual purple produced by light acting on rhodopsin.

xanthopsis (zăn-thŏp′sĭs). Yellow pigmentation seen in certain cancers and degenerating tissue.

xanthorrhea (zăn″thō-rē′ă) [Gr. *xanthos,* yellow, + *rhoia,* to flow]. Discharge of a yellow, purulent substance from the vagina.

xanthosis (zăn-thō′sĭs) [″+ *ōsis,* condition]. A yellowing of the skin seen in carotenemia resulting from ingestion of excessive quantities of carrots, squash, egg yolk, and other foods containing carotenoids. Condition usually harmless but it may indicate increase of lipochromes in blood due to other conditions such as hypothyroidism or diabetes.

xanthous (zăn′thŭs) [Gr. *xanthos*, yellow]. Yellow.

xanthuria (zăn-thū′rĭ-ă) [″+ *ouron*, urine]. Excretion of an excess of xanthine in the urine. SYN: *xanthinuria*.

X chromosome. The chromosome that determines that female sex characteristics will develop in an individual. In the normal female there are two X chromosomes and in the male only one. SEE: *chromosome, X.*

Xe. Chem. symbol for xenon.

xeno- [Gr. *xenos*, guest]. Combining form indicating strange or a foreign material.

xenogenous (zĕn-ŏj′ĕn-ŭs) [Gr. *xenos*, strange, + *gennan*, to produce]. 1. Caused by a foreign body. 2. Originating in the host, as a toxin resulting from stimuli applied to cells of the host.

xenology (zĕn-ŏl′ŏ-gĭ) [″+ *logos*, study]. The study of parasites and their hosts and their relationships to one another.

xenomenia (zĕn-ō-mē′nĭ-ă) [″+ *mēniaia*, menses]. Menstruation from a part of the body other than the normal one. SYN: *vicarious menstruation*.

xenon (zē′nŏn) [Gr. *xenos*, strange]. SYMB: *Xe.* At. wt. 131.30; at. no. 54. A gaseous element in the atmosphere.

xenon[133]. A radioactive isotope of xenon used in photoscanning studies of the lung.

xenophobia (zĕn″ō-fō′bĭ-ă) [Gr. *xenos*, strange, + *phobos*, fear]. Abnormal dread of strangers.

xenophonia (zĕn″ō-fō′nĭ-ă) [″+ *phōnē*, voice]. Alteration in accent and intonation of a person's voice due to defect of speech.

xenophthalmia (zĕn″ŏf-thăl′mĭ-ă) [″+ *ophthalmia*, eye inflammation]. Inflammation of the eye caused by a foreign body.

Xenopsylla (zĕn″ŏp-sĭl′ă) [Gr. *xenos*, strange, + *psylla*, flea]. A genus of fleas belonging to the family Pulicidae, order Siphonaptera.

    X. cheopis. The rat flea, but other hosts include man and various animals. It is a vector and transmitter of a number of pathogens including Hymenolepis nana, the dwarf tapeworm, Salmonella, and causative organisms of bubonic and sylvatic plague, and endemic typhus.

xenorexia (zĕn″ō-rĕk′sĭ-ă) [″+ *orexis*, appetite]. An abnormality of appetite marked by persistent swallowing of foreign objects.

xeransis (zē-răn′sĭs) [Gr., drying up]. Loss of moisture in tissues or drugs brought about gradually. SYN: *siccation*.

xerantic (zē-răn′tĭk). Causing dryness. SYN: *siccant; siccative*.

xerasia (zē-rā′sĭ-ă) [Gr. *xēros*, dry]. Disease of the hair in which there is abnormal dryness, brittleness, and eventual loss of hair.

xero- [Gr. *xēros*]. Prefix meaning dry.

xerocheilia (zē″rō-kī′lĭ-ă) [Gr. *xeros*, dry, + *cheilos*, lip]. Dryness of the lips; a type of cheilitis.

xeroderma (zē″rō-dĕr′mă) [″+ *derma*, skin]. Roughness and dryness of the skin; mild ichthyosis.

    x. pigmentosum. A rare disease of the skin starting in childhood marked by disseminated pigment discolorations, ulcers, cutaneous and muscular atrophy, and death. SYN: *Kaposi's disease*.

xeroma (zē-rō′mă) [Gr. *xēros*, dry, + *ōma*, mass]. An abnormally dry state of the conjunctiva. SYN: *xerophthalmia*.

xeromenia (zē″rō-mē′nĭ-ă) [″+ *mēniaia*, menses]. The occurrence of the usual physical disturbances during menses without menstrual flow.

xeromycteria (zē″rō-mĭk-tē′rĭ-ă) [″+ *myktēr*, nose]. Dryness of the nasal passages.

xeronosus (zē-rŏn′ō-sŭs) [Gr. *xēros*, dry, + *nosos*, disease]. Dryness of the skin.

xerophagia (zē″rō-fā′jĭ-ă) [″+ *phagein*, to eat]. The eating of dry food only.

xerophthalmia (zē-rŏf-thăl′mĭ-ă) [″+ *ophthalmos*, eye]. Conjunctival dryness with keratinization of epithelium following chronic conjunctivitis and in disease due to deficiency of vitamin A.

xerosis (zē-rō′sĭs) [Gr.]. 1. Abnormal dryness of skin, mucous membranes, or of the conjunctiva. 2. Normal sclerosis of tissues in the aged. SYN: *asteatosis*.

xerostomia (zē″rō-stō′mĭ-ă) [Gr. *xēros*, dry, + *stoma*, mouth]. Dryness of the mouth caused by the arresting of normal salivary secretion. It occurs in diabetes, hysteria, paralysis of facial nerve involving chorda tympani, acute infections, some types of neuroses, and is induced by certain drugs such as nicotine and atropine. SEE: *ptyalism*.

xerotes (zē′rō-tēz) [Gr. *xērotēs*, dryness]. Dryness of the body; dryness.

xerotic (zē-rŏt′ĭk) [Gr. *xēros*, dry]. Dry; characterized by dryness.

xerotocia (zē″rō-tō′sĭ-ă) [″+ *tokos*, birth]. Dry labor due to diminished amount of amniotic fluid.

xerotripsis (zē″rō-trĭp′sĭs) [″+ *tripsis*, rubbing]. Dry friction.

xiphi-, xipho- [Gr. *xiphos*, sword]. Prefixes pert. to the xiphoid cartilage.

xiphisternum (zĭf'ĭ-stĕr'nŭm) [Gr. *xiphos*, sword, + *sternon*, chest]. The pointed process of the lower end of the sternum. SYN: *xiphoid cartilage*.

xiphocostal (zĭf'ō-kŏs'tăl) ["+ L. *costa*, rib]. Rel. to the xiphoid cartilage and the ribs.

    x. ligament. Ligament connecting the xiphoid cartilage to the cartilage of the 8th rib.

xiphodynia (zĭf'ō-dĭn'ĭ-ă) ["+ *odynē*, pain]. Pain in the ensiform cartilage.

xiphoid (zĭf'oyd) [Gr. *xiphos*, sword, + *eidos*, process]. Sword-shaped, ensiform.

    x. process. The lowest portion of the sternum, a sword-shaped cartilaginous process supported by bone. It has no ribs attached to it, but some of the abdominal muscles are attached to it. It ossifies in the aged.

xiphoiditis (zĭf'oyd-ī'tĭs) ["+ "+ *-itis*, inflammation]. Inflammation of the ensiform or xiphoid cartilage.

X ray. A high energy electromagnetic wave varying in length from .05-100 Angstrom units. X rays are produced by bombarding a target in a vacuum tube with high velocity electrons. Because of their ability to penetrate solid matter and to act on photographic film they are used both in diagnosis and therapy. SYN: *roentgen ray*.

x-ray. A photograph obtained by use of X rays.

    x., bite-wing. X-ray picture taken with the film holder held between the teeth and the film parallel to the teeth. This technique permits film to be taken of several upper and lower teeth at the same time.

    x. dermatitis. Cutaneous inflammation due to exposure to X rays.

    x. strain. X-ray taken with the part, usually a bone or joint, under static force or tension. Used to better demonstrate the pathological change which might be inapparent if this technique were not employed.

xylenin (zī'lē-nĭn) [Gr. *xylon*, wood]. A toxic substance extracted by xylene from tubercle bacilli.

xylo- [Gr. *xylon*, wood]. Prefix pert. to wood.

xylose (zī'lōs) [Gr. *xylon*, wood]. Wood sugar, a crystalline, nonfermentable pentose.

xyrospasm (zī'rō-spăzm) [Gr. *xyron*, razor, + *spasmos*, spasm]. Occupational neurosis of the fingers seen in barbers.

xysma (zĭz'mă) [Gr. *zysma*, filings]. Shreds of tissue sometimes seen in diarrhea stools.

xyster (zĭs'tĕr) [Gr., scraper]. File or rasp used in surgery.

Y

Y. Chem. symb. for yttrium.

yard [AS. *gerd,* a rod]. A measure of 3 feet or 36 inches. Equal to 0.9144 meter. SEE: *Table of Measures* in *Appendix.*

yaw (yŏ). The primary lesion of yaws, q.v.

y., mother. The primary lesion of yaws occurring at site of inoculation 3-4 weeks after infection.

yawn (yŏn) [AS. *geonian*]. 1. To open the mouth involuntarily as in drowsiness or fatigue. 2. Involuntary act of gaping, accompanied by attempts at inspiration, excited by drowsiness.

yawning (yŏn'ĭng). Deep inspiration with mouth wide open; induced by drowsiness or fatigue. SYN: *oscitation.* SEE: *pandiculation.*

yaws (yŏz) [Cariban]. An infectious tropical disease caused by a spirochete, Treponema pertenue. SYN: *frambesia.*

SYM: Febrile disturbances, rheumatism, eruption of tubercles with a caseous crust on hands, feet, face, and external genitals.

TREATMENT: Penicillin.

Yb. Chem. symb. for ytterbium.

Y car'tilage. The cartilage uniting the three pelvic bones at bottom of the acetabulum early in life.

Y chromosome. One of a pair of sex chromosomes (X and Y) which is present in fetuses which have male sexual characteristics. SEE: *chromosome, Y.*

yeast (yēst) [AS. *gist*]. 1. Any of several unicellular fungi of the genus Saccharomyces which reproduce by budding. They are capable of fermenting carbohydrates. 2. A commercial product composed of meal impregnated with living yeast.

y., brewer's. Y. obtained during the brewing of beer. May be used in the dried form as a good source of vitamin B.

yelk (yĕlk). Variant of yolk.

yellow (yĕl'ō) [AS. *geolu*]. 1. One of the primary colors resembling that of a ripe lemon. 2. Colored yellow as the skin in disease.

y. body. The corpus luteum, q.v.

y. enzyme. SEE: *enzyme, yellow.*

y. fever. An acute infectious disease characterized by jaundice, epigastric tenderness, vomiting, hemorrhages, and a febrile course consisting of two paroxysms.

ETIOL: A filtrable virus transmitted by the bite of a female mosquito, Aedes segypti, with a 3-6 day incubation period.

TREATMENT: Water and electrolyte balance should be carefully watched. Parenteral fluids containing dextrose and saline should be given in cases of persistent vomiting.

PROPHYLAXIS: Preventive measures include mosquito control by screening, spraying with nontoxic insecticides, and destruction of breeding areas. Preventive vaccines are available for those who plan to travel or live in areas where the disease is endemic.

SYM: *First Stage:* Disease begins with sudden onset of fever, sometimes accompanied by a chill, followed by pain in head, back, and limbs. Temperature rises rapidly till it reaches its maximum 103°-105° F. (39.4°-40.6° C.). Face flushed, conjunctivae injected, pupils small, gastroenteritis, urine scanty and albuminous. This stage lasts from a few hours to several days. It is followed by a marked fall in temperature and an improvement in general symptoms. At this time convalescence may begin or patient may pass into second febrile paroxysm. Jaundice rarely appears before the third day.

Second Stage, Period of Intoxication: Three to nine days. Fever rises to its original height, skin becomes yellow, vomiting persistent; vomitus may contain dark blood. Sometimes hemorrhages occur from other mucous membranes. Pulse rapid but not proportionate to the fever. Urine becomes very scanty and contains albumin and casts. Death frequently results from exhaustion or uremia, though recovery may follow the gravest symptoms.

PROG: Always grave. Mortality 5% for natives of an area where the disease is endemic.

TREATMENT: There is no specific therapy. Absolute rest; cool, well-ventilated room; liquid diet, Vitamin K and calcium gluconate for hemorrhagic tendency. Dehydration and electrolyte balance must be controlled by appropriate fluid replacement therapy. Transfusion may be required. Control fever by cool applications. Analgesics for pain.

y. softening. A stage of softening of the brain marked by fatty degeneration and yellow discoloration.

y. spot. 1. Yellowish nodule of anterior end of vocal cord. SYN: *macula flava.* 2. Center of the retina, the point of clearest vision. SYN: *macula lutea.*

y. vision. Condition in which objects seem yellow in color. SYN: *xanthopsia.*

yerba (yĕr′bă) [Sp.]. An herb.

   y. maté. Paraguayan tea.

Yersin's serum (yĕr′sĭn). [Alexandre J. E. Yersin, Swiss bacteriologist, 1863-1943] An antitoxic serum for the plague.

yoga [Sanskrit, union]. A system of beliefs and practices the goal of which is to attain a union of the individual self with Supreme Reality or the Universal Self.

   The term yoga as used in the Western world has been associated almost exclusively with physical postures and regulation of breathing. These are yoga exercises but not yoga in the spiritual sense.

-yl [Gr. *hylē*, matter, substance]. Suffix signifying a radical in chemistry.

-ylene. Suffix denoting a bivalent hydrocarbon radical in chemistry.

Y ligament. A y-shaped band covering the upper and front portions of the hip joint. SYN: *iliofemoral, q.v.; ligament.*

yogurt, yoghurt (yōg′hĕrt) [Turkish]. A form of curdled milk, curdling caused by action of Lactobacillus bulgaricus. Extensive claims have been made concerning the therapeutic value of yoghurt for various ailments. These have not been substantiated. SEE: *milk.*

yolk (yōk) [AS. *geolca*]. The contents of the ovum; sometimes only the nutritive portion. SYN: *vitellus*, q.v. SEE: *zona pellucida.*

   y. sac. Membranous sac surrounding food yolk in the embryo.

   y. stalk. The umbilical duct connecting the yolk sac with the embryo.

Young-Helmholtz theory (yŭng-hĕlm′hōlts). [Thomas Young, Eng. physician, 1773-1829; H. L. F. Helmholtz, Ger. physician, 1821-94] Belief that color vision depends on three different sets of retinal fibers responsible for perception of red, green, and violet. The loss of either red, green, or violet as color perceptive elements in the retina causes an inability to perceive a primary color or any color of which it forms a part.

Young's rule (yŭng). A rule for calculating the dose of medicine a child should receive. Divide the age by the age plus 12. The result represents the fraction of the adult dose suitable for the child. Ex: a child of 4 years of age requires

$$\frac{4}{4+12} = \frac{1}{4}$$

of the adult dose.

youth (yūth) [AS. *geoguth*]. Period between childhood and maturity.

ypsiliform (ĭp-sĭl′ĭ-form). Y-shaped.

y.s. Abbr. for *yellow spot* of the retina.

ytterbium (ĭ-tŭr′bĭ-ŭm). SYMB: *Yb.* At. wt. 173.04; at. no. 70. A rare metallic element.

yttrium (ĭt′rĭ-ŭm). SYMB: *Y.* At. wt. 88.905; at. no. 39. A metallic element.

Z

Z. 1. Abbr. for Ger. *Zuckung,* contraction. 2. Symb. for atomic number.

z. Abbr. for *zero; zone.*

Zaglas' ligament (zā'glŭs). The part of the posterior sacroiliac ligament from posterior superior spinous process of ilium to side of sacrum.

Zahn's lines, ribs (zŏn). [Frederick W. Zahn, Ger. pathologist, 1845-1904] Transverse whitish marks on the free surface of a thrombus made by the edges of the lamellae of blood platelets.

Zang's space (zang). [Christoph B. Zang, Ger. surgeon, 1772-1835] Space between the two lower tendons of the sternomastoid muscle in the supraclavicular fossa.

zein (zē'ĭn) [Gr. *zeia,* a kind of grain]. A protein obtained from maize. It is deficient in tryptophan and lysine.

Zeiss' gland (zīs). [Carl Zeiss, Ger. optician, 1816-1888] One of the sebaceous glands at free edges of eyelids.

zelotypia (zē'lŏ-tĭp'ĭ-ă) [Gr. *zēlos,* zeal, + *typtein,* to strike]. 1. Morbid or monomaniacal zeal in the interest of any project or cause. 2. Insane jealousy.

Zenker's degeneration, zenkerism (zĕng'kĕr, -ĭzm). [Friedrich A. Zenker, Ger. pathologist, 1825-1898]. A glassy or waxy, hyaline degeneration of skeletal muscles in acute infectious diseases, esp. in typhoid.

zephiran (zĕf'ĭ-răn). Proprietary name for refined benzalkonium chloride.

zero (zē'rō) [It.]. 1. Corresponding to nothing. SYMB: 0. SYN: *cipher.* 2. The point from which the graduation of a scale commences.

On the centigrade scale zero (0°) is the temperature of melting ice, equivalent to 32° on the Fahrenheit scale. To obtain this fixed point the thermometer is immersed in melting ice, and when the mercury column ceases to fall, the level at which it remains is fixed as 0° on the C. and as 32° on the F. scale. SEE: *thermometer.*

z., absolute. The temperature at which all atoms and molecules cease movement, or at which all gases liquify; -273.15°C. or -459.67°F.

z. gravity. Absence of effect of gravity. Condition exists in space travel.

z., limes. The greatest amount of toxin which, when mixed with one unit of antitoxin and injected into a guinea pig weighing 250 gm., will cause no local edema. SYMB: L0.

zero population growth. The dermographic condition when in a given period of time the population neither increases nor decreases. ABBR: ZPG.

zestocausis (zĕs'tō-kŏw'sĭs) [Gr. *zestos,* boiling hot, + *kausis,* burning]. Cauterization with a tube containing heated steam.

Ziehl-Neelsen method (zēl-nēl'sĕn). [Franz Ziehl, Ger. bacteriologist, 1857-1926; Friederich K. A. Neelsen, 1854-1894] Method for staining Mycobacterium tuberculosis.

zinc (zĭnk) [L. *zincum*]. SYMB: *Zn.* At. wt. 65.37; at. no. 30; sp. gr. 7.13. A bluish-white, crystalline metallic element which boils at 906°C. It is found as a carbonate and silicate, known as calamine, and as a sulfide (blende).

z. acetate. White, pearly crystals.
ACTION AND USES: Astringent and antiseptic. Used chiefly in eye solutions, in a 1/10 to 5/10% solution.

z. chloride. USP. White granular powder.
ACTION AND USES: Antiseptic.

z. ointment. An ointment consisting of 20% of zinc oxide mixed with petrolatum and white ointment, used in treating skin diseases.

z. oxide. USP. Very fine white powder.
ACTION AND USES: Slightly antiseptic and astringent. Used chiefly in the form of ointment, 20%.

z. salts. A bluish-white metal used to make various containers and also to galvanize iron to prevent rust. The most commonly used compounds are zinc oxide as a pigment for paints, in ointments, and in chloride and sulfate which resemble Epsom salts and have been administered accidentally. The salts also are used as a wood preservative, in soldering, and in medicine to neutralize tissue, and in dilute solutions as an astringent and emetic.
POISONING SYM: Metallic taste with prompt burning of mouth, throat, esophagus, and stomach; violent vomiting, often bloody; increased salivation; painful diarrhea; coma. If patient recovers, nervous complications are frequent.
F. A. TREATMENT: Wash out stomach and treat as for sulfuric acid.

z. stearate. Very fine, smooth powder.
USES: A nonirritating antiseptic and astringent for burns, scalds, abrasions

z. sul'fate. White, transparent crystals.
ACTION AND USES: Externally, astringent and styptic. Internally, as an emetic.

Z-1

Zinn's ligament (zĭn). [Johann G. Zinn, Ger. anatomist, 1727-1759] Connective tissue giving attachment to the rectus muscles of the eyeball. SEE: *zonule of Zinn.*

zirconium (zĭr-kō'nĭ-ŭm). SYMB: *Zr.* At. wt. 91.22; at. no. 40. A metallic element found only in combination.

Zn. Chem. symb. for zinc.

zoanthropy (zō-ăn'thrō-pĭ) [Gr. *zōon,* animal, + *anthropos,* man]. Delusion that one is an animal.

zoetic (zō-ĕt'ĭk) [Gr. *zōē,* life]. Pert. to life. SYN: *vital.*

Zollinger-Ellison syndrome. [R.M. Zollinger and E.M. Ellison, contemporary American surgeons] Condition caused by noninsulin-secreting tumors of the pancreas which secrete excess amounts of gastrin. This stimulates the stomach to secrete great amounts of hydrochloric acid and pepsin which in turn leads to peptic ulceration of the stomach and small intestines. About 60% of the tumors are malignant.

TREATMENT: Total gastrectomy and local excision of pancreatic tumor if metastases have not appeared.

zona (zō'nă) [L., a girdle]. (pl. *zo'nae*) 1. A band or girdle. 2. An acute inflammatory disease, characterized by groups of small vesicles mounted on inflammatory bases, associated with neuralgic pain and following the distribution of certain nerve trunks. SYN: *herpes zoster.*

    z. ciliaris. Ciliary processes taken together. SYN: *corona ciliaris.*

    z. facialis. Herpes zoster of the face.

    z. pellucida. Inner, solid, thick, membranous envelope of the ovum. It is pierced by many radiating canals, giving it a striated appearance.

    z. radiata. Z. pellucida, q.v.

zonae. Pl. of zona, q.v.

zonal (zō'năl) [L. *zonalis*]. Pert. to a zone.

zonary (zō'năr-ĭ) [L. *zona,* a girdle]. Pert. to or shaped like a zone.

    z. placenta. Placenta arranged in the form of a broad ring around the chorion.

Zondek-Aschheim test (zŏn'dĕk-ash'hīm). [Berhardt Zondek, Ger. gynecologist, 1891 —; Selmar Aschheim, Ger. gynecologist, 1878 —]. A test for pregnancy. SEE: *test, Aschheim-Zondek.*

zone (zōn) [L. *zona,* a girdle]. A small zone or belt.

    z's., erogenous, erotogenic. Areas of the body which may produce erotic desires when stimulated. These areas include the breasts, lips, genital and anal regions, buttocks, and sometimes the special senses

which cause sexual excitation, such as certain odors.

zonesthesia (zōn"ĕs-thē'zĭ-ă) [Gr. *zōnē,* girdle, + *aisthēsis,* sensation]. A sensation, as a cord constricting the body. SYN: *cincture sensation.*

zonifugal (zō-nĭf'ū-găl) [L. *zona,* zone, + *fugere,* to flee]. Passing outward from within any zone or area.

zoning. The occurrence of a stronger fixation of complement in a lesser amount of suspected serum; a phenomenon occasionally observed in diagnosing syphilis by complement fixation method.

zonipetal (zō-nĭp'ĕt-ăl) [L. *zona,* zone, + *petere,* to seek]. Passing from without into a zone or area of the body.

zonula (zōn'ū-lă) [L.]. A small zone. SYN: *zonule.*

    z. ciliaris. [NA] Suspensory ligament of the crystalline lens.

zonular (zōn'ū-lăr). Pert. to a zonula.

    z. cataract. Cataract with opacity limited to certain layers of the lens.

    z. fibers. Interlacing fibers of the zonula ciliaris.

    z. spaces. Spaces between fibers of ligaments of the lens.

zonule (zōn'ūl) [L. *zonula,* small zone]. A small band or area. SYN: *zonula.*

    z. of Zinn. Suspensory ligament of the crystalline lens. SYN: *zonula ciliaris.*

zonulitis (zōn-ū-lī'tĭs) ["+ Gr. *-itis,* inflammation]. Inflammation of Zinn's zonule.

zoodermic (zō"ō-dĕr'mĭk) [Gr. *zōon,* animal, + *derma,* skin]. Performed with the skin of an animal, said of a method of skin grafting.

zoogenous (zō-ōj'ĕn-ŭs) ["+ *gennan,* to produce]. Derived or acquired from animals.

zooglea (zō"ō-glē'ă) ["+ *gloios,* sticky]. A stage in development of certain organisms in which colonies of microbes are embedded in a gelatinous matrix.

zoograft (zō'ō-grăft) [Gr. *zōon,* animal, + L. *graphium,* a grafting knife]. A graft of tissue obtained from an animal.

zoografting (zō'ō-grăft'ĭng) Use of animal tissue in grafting on a human body.

zooid (zō'oyd) [Gr. *zōon,* animal, + *eidos,* resemblance]. 1. Resembling an animal. 2. A form resembling an animal; an organism produced by fission. 3. An animal cell which can move or exist independently.

zoolagnia (zō"ō-lăg'nĭ-ă) ["+ *lagneia,* lust]. Sexual desire for animals.

zoologist (zō-ōl'ō-jĭst) ["+ *logos,* a study]. A person who specializes in the study of animal life.

zoology (zō-ōl'ō-jĭ). The science of animal life.

zoomania (zō″ō-mā′nĭ-ă) [Gr. *zōon*, animal, + *mania*, madness]. A morbid and excessive affection for animals.

zoonoses (zo-o-no′sēz) ["+ *nosos*, disease]. Diseases communicable from animals to man under natural conditions.

zooparasite (zō″ō-păr′ă-sīt) ["+ *parasitos*, parasite]. An animal parasite.

zoopathology (zō″ō-păth-ŏl′ō-jĭ) [Gr. *zōon*, animal, + *pathos*, disease, + *logos*, a study]. Science of the diseases of animals.

zoophagous (zō-ŏf′ă-gŭs) ["+ *phagein*, to eat]. Living upon animal food.

zoophilism (zō-ŏf′ĭl-ĭzm) ["+ *philein*, to love, + *-ismos*, condition]. Abnormal love of animals.

zoophobia (zō″ō-fō′bĭ-ă) [Gr. *zōon*, animal, + *phobos*, fear]. Abnormal fear of animals.

zoophyte (zō′ō-fīt) ["+ *phyton*, plant]. A plantlike animal; any of numerous invertebrate animals resembling plants in appearance or mode of growth.

zooplasty (zō′ō-plăs-tĭ) ["+ *plassein*, to form]. Transplantation of animal tissue to man.

zoopsia (zō-ŏp′sĭ-ă) [Gr. *zōon*, animal, + *opsis*, vision]. Hallucinations involving animals.

zoosmosis (zō″ōs-mō′sĭs) [Gr. *zōē*, life, + *ōsmos*, impulsion]. Process of passage of living protoplasm into the tissues from blood vessels.

zoospore (zō′ō-spōr) ["+ *sporos*, seed]. A motile asexual spore which moves by means of one or more flagella.

zootoxin (zō″ō-tŏks′ĭn) [Gr. *zōon*, animal, + *toxikon*, poison]. Any toxin or poison produced by an animal, as snake venom.

zoster (zŏs′tĕr) [Gr. *zōstēr*, girdle]. Acute inflammatory disease with vesicles grouped in the course of cutaneous nerves. SYN: *herpes zoster; zona.*

   z. auricularis. Herpes zoster of the ear.

   z. opthalmicus. Herpes affecting the opthalmic nerve.

zosteriform (zŏs-tĕr′ĭ-fōrm) ["+ L. *forma*, shape]. Resembling herpes zoster. SYN: *zosteroid.*

zosteroid (zŏs′tĕr-oyd) ["+ *eidos*, form]. Resembling herpes zoster. SYN: *zosteriform.*

ZPG. Zero population growth, q.v.

Z-plasty. A technique with a Z-shaped incision used in plastic surgery to relieve tension in scar tissue. The area under tension is lengthened at the expense of the surrounding elastic tissue.

Zr. Chem. symb. for zirconium.

zwieback (zwī′bŏk) [Ger., twice baked]. A kind of bread, baked, then sliced and toasted.

Food value of 109 gm.: Cal. 423; protein 10.7 gm.; fat 8.8 gm.; carbohydrate 74.3 gm.; vitamin A, 40 I.U.

zygapophysis (zī″gŏ-pŏf′ĭ-sĭs) [Gr. *zygon*, yoke, + *apo*, from, + *physis*, growth]. One of the articular processes of the neural arch of a vertebra.

zygion (zĭj′ĭ-ŏn) [Gr. *zygon*, yoke]. (pl. *zygia*) Craniometrical point on the zygoma at either end of bizygomatic diameter.

zygodactyly (zī″gō-dăk′tĭl-ĭ) ["+ *daktylos*, digit]. Fusion of two or more fingers or toes. SYN: *syndactylism.*

zygoma (zĭ-gō′mă) [Gr., cheekbone]. 1. The long arch that joins zygomatic processes of the temporal and malar bones on the sides of the skull. SYN: *arcus zygomaticus* [NA]. 2. The malar bone. SYN: *os zygomaticum* [NA].

zygomatic (zī″gō-măt′ĭk). Pert. to the zygoma.

   z. arch. The formation on each side of the cheeks of the zygomatic process of each malar bone articulating with the zygomatic process of the temporal bone. SYN: *arcus zygomaticus* [NA].

   z. bone. Bone on either side of the face below the eye. SYN: *malar bone; os zygomaticum* [NA].

   z. process. 1. A thin projection from the temporal bone bounding its squamous portion. 2. A part of the malar bone helping to form the zygoma.

   z. reflex. Movement of lower jaw toward percussed side when zygoma is percussed.

zygomaticoauricularis (zī″gō-măt″ĭ-kō-ă-rĭk″ū-lā′rĭs) [L.]. Muscle which draws the pinna of the ear forward. SEE: *Table of Muscles* in *Appendix.*

zygomaticum (zī″gō-măt′ĭ-kŭm) [L.]. The zygomatic bone.

zygomaticus (zī″gō-mat′ĭk-ŭs) [L.]. A muscle which draws the upper lip upward and outward. SEE: *Table of Muscles* in *Appendix.*

zygomaxillary (zī″gō-măks′ĭl-ār-ĭ) [Gr. *zygoma*, cheekbone, + L. *maxilla*, jaw]. Pert. to the cheekbone and upper jaw.

   z. point. A craniometrical point marked at the lower end of the zygomatic suture.

zygote (zī′gŏt) [Gr. *zygōtos*, yoked]. Cell produced by union of two gametes. The fertilized ovum. SYN: *zygocyte.*

zymase (zī′mās) [Gr. *zymē*, leaven, + *ase*, enzyme]. Any of a group of enzymes which, in the presence of oxygen, convert certain carbohydrates into carbon dioxide and water or, in absence of oxygen, into alcohol and carbon dioxide or lactic acid. It is found in yeast, bacteria, and higher plants and animals. SEE: *enzymes; ferment.*

zyme (zīm) [Gr., leaven]. 1. An enzyme or ferment. 2. An agent that produces an infectious disease.

zymogen (zī′mō-jĕn) [Gr. *zymē,* leaven, + *gennan,* to produce]. A substance that develops into a chemical ferment or enzyme. It exists in an inactive form antecedent to the active enzyme. SYN: *proenzyme.* SEE: *pepsinogen; trypsinogen.*

zymogene (zī′mō-gēn). Microbe causing fermentation.

zymogenic (zī″mō-jĕn′ĭk). 1. Causing a fermentation. 2. Pert. to or producing a zymogen.

zymohydrolysis (zī″mō-hī-drŏl′ĭ-sĭs) [Gr. *zymē,* leaven, + *hydor,* water, + *lysis,* dissolution]. Decomposition brought about by a ferment. SYN: *zymosis,* q.v.

zymologic (zī″mō-lŏ′jĭk) [″ + *logos,* a study]. Rel. to zymology.

zymologist (zī-mŏl′ō-jĭst). One who specializes in study of ferments.

zymology (zī-mŏl′ō-jī). The science of fermentation.

zymolysis (zī-mŏl′ĭ-sĭs) [Gr. *zymē,* leaven, + *lysis,* a dissolution]. Changes produced by an enzyme; action of enzymes. SYN: *fermentation; zymosis,* q.v.

zymolyte (zī′mō-līt′). Substance upon which a ferment acts. SYN: *substrate.*

zymolytic (zī″mō-lĭt′ĭk) [Gr. *zymē,* leaven, + *lytikos,* dissolved]. Causing fermentation; fermentative.

zymometer (zī-mŏm′ĕ-tĕr) [″ + *metron,* measure]. Device for measuring fermentation. SYN: *zymosimeter.*

Zymonema (zī″mō-nē′mă) [″ + *nēma,* thread]. A genus of fungi.

zymonematosis (zī″mō-nē″măt-ō′sĭs) [″ + ″ + *-ōsis,* condition]. Infestation with Zymonema.

zymophore (zī′mō-fōr) [Gr. *zymē,* leaven, + *phoros,* a bearer]. Noting the atomic group bearing the ferment.

zymophoric, zymophorous (zī″mō-for′ĭk, zī-mŏf′ōr-ŭs). Having fermentative properties.

zymophyte (zī′mō-fīt) [Gr. *zymē,* leaven, + *phyton,* growth]. A microorganism causing fermentation.

zymoplastic (zī″mō-plăs′tĭk) [″ + *plassein,* to form]. Producing a ferment.

zymoscope (zī′mō-skōp) [″ + *skopein,* to examine]. Device for determining zymotic power of yeast.

zymose (zī′mōs) [Gr. *zymē,* leaven, + *ose,* sugar]. An enzyme that changes a disaccharide into a monosaccharide, such as cane sugar into invert sugar. SYN: *invertin.*

zymosimeter (zī″mō-sĭm′ĕ-tĕr) [″ + *metron,* measure]. Device for determining amount of fermentation.

zymosis (zī-mō′sĭs) [Gr. *zymōsis,* fermentation]. 1. Fermentation. 2. Process by which an infectious disease is supposed to develop. 3. An infectious disease.

    z. gas′trica. Organic acid in the stomach due to action of yeasts.

zymosthenic (zī-mōs-thĕn′ĭk) [Gr. *zymē,* leaven, + *sthenos,* strength]. Increasing the power and activity of an enzyme.

zymotic (zī-mŏt′ĭk). Rel. to or produced by fermentation.

Z.Z.'Z.". Symb. for increasing strengths of contraction.

Appendix

Index to Appendix

Units of Measurement

Metric System

Weights

Scale	Table		Grams		Grains
Kilo	1 Kilogram	=	1000.0	=	15,432.35
Hecto	1 Hectogram	=	100.0	=	1,543.23
Deca	1 Decagram	=	10.0	=	154.323
Unit	1 Gram	=	1.0	=	15.432
Deci	1 Decigram	=	0.1	=	1.5432
Centi	1 Centigram	=	0.01	=	0.15432
Milli	1 Milligram	=	0.001	=	0.01543
Micro	1 Microgram	=	10^{-6}	=	15.432×10^{-6}
Nano	1 Nanogram	=	10^{-9}	=	15.432×10^{-9}
Pico	1 Picogram	=	10^{-12}	=	15.432×10^{-12}

Arabic numbers are used with weights and measures, as 10 gm., or 3 ml., etc. Portions of weights and measures are usually expressed decimally. 10^{-1} indicates 0.1; $10^{-6} = 0.000006$; etc.

Rules for Converting One System to Another

To Convert Grains, Drams, and Ounces into Grams or Milliliters

Divide the number of grains by 15.
Multiply the number of drams by 4.
Multiply the number of ounces by 30.
The result = the number of grams or milliliters.

To Convert from the Metric System

Milligrams to grains: Multiply by 0.0154.
Grams to grains: Multiply by 15.
Grams to drams: Multiply by 0.257.
Grams to ounces: Multiply by 0.0311.

To Convert into Metric Fluid Measures

Minims to cubic millimeters: Multiply by 63.
Minims to milliliters: Multiply by 0.06.

To Convert Metric Fluid Measures

Cubic millimeters to minims: Divide by 63 (or multiply by 0.016).
Milliliters to minims: Multiply by 16.7.
Milliliters to fluid ounces: Divide by 30 (or multiply by 0.033).
Liters to pints (U.S.): Multiply by 2.1.
Liters to pints (Imperial): Multiply by 1.76.

To Convert Centigrade or Celsius Degrees to Fahrenheit Degrees

Multiply the number of Centigrade degrees by 9/5 and add 32 to the result.
Example: 55° C. $\times$ 9/5 = 99 + 32 = 131° F.

To convert Fahrenheit degrees to Centigrade degrees: Subtract 32 from the number of Fahrenheit degrees and multiply the difference by 5/9.
Example: 243° F. − 32 = 211 $\times$ 5/9 = 117.2° C.

Tables of Data

Arabic numbers are used with weights and measures, as 10 gm., or 3 ml., etc. Portions of weights and measures are usually expressed decimally. For practical purposes, one cc. is equivalent to one milliliter and one drop (gtt) of water is equivalent to a minim (m).

Units of Length

	Millimeters	Centimeters	Inches	Feet	Yards	Meters
1 mm. = 1.00	0.100	0.03937	0.00328	0.0011	0.0010
1 cm. = 10.0	1.00	0.3937	0.03281	0.0109	0.0100
1 in. = 25.4	2.54	1.00	0.0833	0.0278	0.0254
1 ft. = 304.8	30.48	12.00	1.00	0.333	0.305
1 yd. = 914.0	91.4	36.0	3.00	1.000	0.914
1 m. = 1000.0	100.0	39.37	3.2808	1.094	1.00

1 μ = 1 mu = 1 micron* = 0.001 millimeter. One mm. = 1000 μ.
1 km. = 1 kilometer = 1000 meters = 0.6215 mile.
1 mile = 5280 feet = 1.609 kilometers.
*Micron is also called micrometer. μm = 10^{-6}.

Units of Volume

	Cubic Centimeters	U.S. Fluid Drams	Cubic Inches	U.S. Fluid Ounces	Quarts (U.S. Fluid)	Liters
1 cc. = 1.00	0.270	0.0610	0.03381	0.00106	0.00100
1 fl. ʒ = 3.70	1.000	0.226	0.1250	0.00391	0.00370
1 cu. in. = 16.38706	4.43	1.000	0.554	0.0173	0.01639
1 fl. ℥ = 29.574	8.00	1.805	1.000	0.03125	0.0296
1 qt. = 946.35	256.0	57.75	32.00	1.000	0.946
1 L. = 1000.0	270.52	61.03	33.81	1.0567	1.000

1 cubic millimeter = 0.001 cubic centimeter; 1 cc. = 1000 cu. mm.
1 gallon = 4 quarts = 8 pints = 3.785 liters.
1 pint = 473.16 ml.

Units of Weight

	Grains	Grams	Apothecary Ounces	Avoirdupois Pounds	Kilograms
1 gr. = 1.000	0.0648	0.00208	0.0001429	0.000065
1 gm. = 15.43	1.000	0.03215	0.002205	0.001000
1 ℥ = 480.0	31.1	1.000	0.06855	0.0311
1 lb. = 7000.0	453.6	14.58	1.000	0.4536
1 kg. = 15432.0	1000.0	32.15	2.205	1.000

1 γ = 1 gamma = 1 microgram = 0.001 milligram; 1000 γ = 1 mg.
1 mg. = 1 milligram = 0.001 gm.; 1000 mg. = 1 gm.
1 grain = 64.8 mg.; 1 mg. = 0.0154 grain.

Weights* and Measures

APOTHECARIES' WEIGHT

20 grains = 1 scruple   3 scruples = 1 dram
8 drams = 1 ounce   12 ounces = 1 pound
The ounce and pound in this are the same as in Troy Weight.

AVOIRDUPOIS WEIGHT

$27^{11}/_{32}$ grains = 1 dram   16 drams = 1 ounce
16 ounces = 1 pound   100 pounds = 1 hundredweight
2000 pounds = 1 short ton   2240 pounds = 1 long ton
1 oz. Troy = 480 grains   1 oz. Avoirdupois = $437^1/_2$ grains
1 lb. Troy = 5760 grains   1 lb. Avoirdupois = 7000 grains

CIRCULAR MEASURE

60 seconds = 1 minute   60 minutes = 1 degree
90 degrees = 1 quadrant   4 quadrants = 360 degrees = circle

CUBIC MEASURE

1728 cubic inches = 1 cubic foot   27 cubic feet = 1 cubic yard
2150.42 cubic inches = 1 standard bushel   268.8 cubic inches = 1 dry (U.S.) gallon
1 cubic foot = about four-fifths of a bushel   128 cubic feet = 1 cord (wood)

DRY MEASURE

2 pints = 1 quart   8 quarts = 1 peck   4 pecks = 1 bushel

LIQUID MEASURE

16 ounces = 1 pint   4 quarts = 1 gallon   2 barrels = 1 hogshead
1000 milliliters = 1 liter $31^1/_2$ gallons = 1 barrel   1 quart = 0.946 liters
4 gills = 1 pint   2 pints = 1 quart

Barrels and hogsheads vary in size. A gallon (U.S.) is equal to 0.8327 British gallon; therefore
a British gallon is equal to 1.201 U.S. gallons.
1 liter is equal to 1.0567 quarts.

LINEAR MEASURE

1 inch = 2.54 centimeters   40 rods = 1 furlong   8 furlongs = 1 statute mile
12 inches = 1 foot   3 feet = 1 yard $5^1/_2$ yards = 1 rod
3 miles = 1 league

TROY WEIGHT

24 grains = 1 pennyweight   20 pennyweights = 1 ounce   12 ounces = 1 pound
Used for weighing gold, silver, and jewels.

*For abbreviations and symbols of these weights, see *Symbols* in *Appendix*.

HOUSEHOLD MEASURES AND WEIGHTS

Approximate Equivalents: 60 gtt. = 1 teaspoonful = 4 cc. or
ml. = 60 minims = 60 grains = 1 dram = $1/_8$ ounce.

	Equivalents
1 teaspoon*	$1/_8$ fl. oz.; 1 dram
4 teaspoons	1 tablespoon
1 tablespoon	$1/_2$ fl. oz.; 4 drams
16 tablespoons (liquid)	1 cup
12 tablespoons (dry)	1 cup
1 cup	8 fl. oz.
1 tumbler or glass	8 fl. oz.; $1/_2$ pint

*Some household teaspoons will hold 5 ml. of liquid substances.

Miscellaneous

UNITS OF TIME

1 millisecond = one thousandth (0.001) of a second   1 minute = 1/60 of an hour
1 second = 1/60 of a minute   1 hour = 1/24 of a day

UNITS OF TEMPERATURE

Given a temperature on the Fahrenheit scale; to convert it to Centigrade, subtract 32 and multiply by 5/9. Given a temperature on the Centigrade scale; to convert it to Fahrenheit, multiply by 9/5 and add 32. Celsius degrees are equivalent to Centigrade degrees.

UNITS OF ENERGY

1 gram-centimeter = 980.665 dynes-centimeter
1 foot-pound = 13,600,000 ergs = 13,825.5 gram-centimeters
1 Joule = .2389 Calorie
1 Calorie = 4.26649×10^7 gram-centimeters = 3085.46 foot-pounds
1 kilocalorie = 1000 calories = 4.1855 Joules
A large Calorie, or kilocalorie, is always written with a capital C.

pH TABLE

In trying to understand the following pH table, there is no need to be concerned about the intricate mathematical theory implied in the symbol "pH." The facts are simple and suffice. Imagine three beakers containing a weak acid solution, purified (distilled) water, and a weak alkaline solution. If a fourth, unknown, solution is tested with litmus paper, phenolphthalein, and other indicators, it is possible to place the unknown in one of four plaes in the series, thus:

(1) Un Ac   W   —   Al   (3)   Ac   —   W   Un   Al
(2)   Ac   Un   W   —   Al   (4)   Ac   —   W   —   Al   Un

Its position will depend on whether it is of strong or weak acidity or strong or weak alkalinity.

The pH scale is simply a series of numbers stating where a given solution would stand in a series of solutions arranged according to acidity or alkalinity. At one extreme (i.e., high pH) lies an alkaline solution made by dissolving 4 gm. of sodium hydroxide in water to make a liter of solution; at the other is a solution containing 3.65 gm. of hydrogen chloride per liter. Halfway between lies purified water, which is neutral. All other solutions can be arranged on this scale, and their acidity or alkalinity can be stated by giving the numbers that indicate their relative positions.

Tenth-normal HCl	1.00	Litmus is red in
Gastric juice	*1.4	this acid range.
Urine	*6.0	
Water	7.00-Neutral	
Blood	7.45	
Bile	7.5	Litmus is blue in
Pancreatic juice	8.5	this alkaline range.
Tenth-normal NaOH	13.00	

If one is told that the pH of a certain solution is 5.3, one knows at once that it falls between gastric juice and urine on the above scale, is moderately acid, and will turn litmus red.
* These body fluids vary rather widely in pH; typical figures have been used for simplicity. Urine samples obtained from normal people may have pH's anywhere between 4.7 and 8.0.

PREPARATION OF PERCENTAGE SOLUTIONS

When the metric system is used, the preparation of percentage solutions is simple: a 1% solution contains 1 gm. in 100 ml.; a 0.1% solution contains 0.1 gm. (or 100 milligrams) per 100 ml.

When the apothecaries' system is used the following are helpful: 4.55 grains to the ounce, or 2.5 drams to 32 ounces; or 3.25 drams to 40 ounces, all make a 1% solution.

To Prepare a Dilute Solution From One Which Is Stronger:

For example, to make 80% alcohol from 95%: Dilute 80 ml. of the 95% alcohol to 95 ml. with distilled water.

Rule: Dilute a volume equal to the percent desired to a volume equal to the percent used.
SEE: *Dosage*.

Table of Physical Constants of the Elements

Element*	Symbol	Valence	Atomic Number	Atomic Weight†	Density (g/ml)	Melting Point °C	Boiling Point °C
Actinium	AC	3	89	(227)		1050.0	
Aluminum	Al	3	13	26.9815	2.70	660.0	2450.0
Americium	Am	3, 4, 5, 6	95	(243)	11.7		
Antimony	Sb	3, 5	51	121.75	6.62	630.5	1380.0
Argon	Ar	0	18	39.948	1.40	−189.4	−185.8
Arsenic	As	3, 5	33	74.9216	5.72	817.0	613.0‡
Astatine	At	1, 3, 5, 7	85	(210)		(302)	
Barium	Ba	2	56	137.34	3.5	714.0	1640.0
Berkelium	Bk	3, 4	97	(247)			
Beryllium	Be	2	4	9.01218	1.85	1277.0	2770.0
Bismuth	Bi	3, 5	83	208.9806	9.8	271.3	1560.0
Boron	B	3	5	10.80	2.34	(2030)	
Bromine	Br	1, 3, 5, 7	35	79.904	3.12	−7.2	58.0
Cadmium	Cd	2	48	112.40	8.65	320.9	765.0
Calcium	Ca	2	20	40.08	1.55	838.0	1440.0
Californium	Cf	3	98	(251)			
Carbon	C	2, 4	6	12.011	2.26	3727.0‡	4830.0
Cerium	Ce	3, 4	58	140.12	6.67	795.0	3468.0
Cesium	Cs	1	55	132.9055	1.90	28.7	690.0
Chlorine	Cl	1, 3, 5, 7	17	35.453	1.56	−101.0	−34.7
Chromium	Cr	2, 3, 6	24	51.996	7.19	1875.0	2665.0
Cobalt	Co	2, 3	27	58.9332	8.9	1495.0	2900.0
Columbium	SEE:	*Niobium*					
Copper	Cu	1, 2	29	63.546	8.96	1083.0	2595.0
Curium	Cm	3	96	(247)			
Dysprosium	Dy	3	66	162.50	8.54	1407.0	2600.0
Einsteinium	Es		99	(254)			
Erbium	Er	3	68	167.26	9.05	1497.0	2900.0
Europium	Eu	2, 3	63	151.96	5.26	826.0	1439.0
Fermium	Fm		100	(253)			
Fluorine	F	1	9	18.9984	1.11	−219.6	−188.2
Francium	Fr	1	87	(223)		(27)	
Gadolinium	Gd	3	64	157.25	7.87	1312.0	3000.0
Gallium	Ga	2, 3	31	69.72	5.91	29.8	2237.0
Germanium	Ge	4	32	72.59	5.32	937.4	2830.0
Glucinum	SEE:	*Beryllium*					
Gold	Au	1, 3	79	196.9665	19.3	1063.0	2970.0
Hafnium	Hf	4	72	178.49	13.1	2222.0	5400.0
Helium	He	0	2	4.0026	0.126	−269.7	−268.9
Holmium	Ho	3	67	164.9303	8.80	1461.0	2600.0
Hydrogen	H	1	1	1.008	0.071	−259.2	−252.7
Indium	In	3	49	114.82	7.31	156.2	2000.0
Iodine	I	1, 3, 5, 7	53	126.9045	4.94	113.7	183.0
Iridium	Ir	3, 4	77	192.22	22.5	2454.0	5300.0
Iron	Fe	2, 3	26	55.847	7.86	1536.0	3000.0
Krypton	Kr	0	36	83.80	2.6	−157.3	−152.0
Lanthanum	La	3	57	138.9055	6.17	920.0	3470.0
Lawrencium	Lw		103	(257)			
Lead	Pb	2, 4	82	207.2	11.4	327.4	1725.0
Lithium	Li	1	3	6.941	0.53	108.5	1330.0
Lutecium	Lu	3	71	174.97	9.85	1652.0	3327.0
Magnesium	Mg	2	12	24.305	1.74	650.0	1107.0
Manganese	Mn	2, 3, 4, 6, 7	25	54.938	7.43	1245.0	2150.0
Mendelevium	Md		101	(256)			
Mercury	Hg	1, 2	80	200.59	13.6	−38.4	357.0
Molybdenum	Mo	3, 4, 6	42	95.94	10.2	2610.0	5560.0

*The 103 chemical elements known at the present time are included in this table. Some of those recently discovered have been obtained only as unstable isotopes.

†Based on Carbon-12. Figures enclosed in parentheses represent the mass number of the most stable isotope.

‡Element sublimes unless under pressure.

Table of Physical Constants of the Elements (*Continued*)

Element*	Symbol	Valence	Atomic Number	Atomic Weight†	Density (g/ml)	Melting Point °C	Boiling Point °C
Neodymium	Nd	3	60	144.24	7.00	1024.0	3027.0
Neon	Ne	0	10	20.179	1.20	−248.6	−246.0
Neptunium	Np	4, 5, 6	93	237.0482	19.5	637.0	
Nickel	Ni	2, 3	28	58.71	8.9	1453.0	2730.0
Niobium	Nb	3, 5	41	92.9064	8.4	2415.0	3300.0
Nitrogen	N	3, 5	7	14.0067	0.81	−210.0	−195.8
Nobelium	No		102	(254)			
Osmium	Os	2, 3, 4, 8	76	190.2	22.6	2700.0	5500.0
Oxygen	O	2	8	15.9994	1.14	−218.8	−183.0
Palladium	Pd	2, 4, 6	46	106.4	12.0	1552.0	3980.0
Phosphorus	P	3, 5	15	30.9738	1.82	44.2	280.0
Platinum	Pt	2, 4	78	195.09	21.4	1769.0	4530.0
Plutonium	Pu	3, 4, 5, 6	94	(242)		640.0	3235.0
Polonium	Po	2, 4	84	(209)	(9.2)	254.0	
Potassium	K	1	19	39.102	0.86	63.7	760.0
Praseodymium . . .	Pr	3	59	140.9077	6.67	935.0	3127.0
Promethium	Pm	3	61	(145)		(1027)	
Protactinium	Pa		91	(231)	15.4	(1230)	
Radium	Ra	2	88	(226)	5.0	700.0	
Radon	Rn	0	86	(222)		(−71)	(−61.8)
Rhenium	Re		75	186.2	21.0	3180.0	5900.0
Rhodium	Rh	3	45	102.9055	12.4	1966.0	4500.0
Rubidium	Rb	1	37	85.4678	1.53	38.9	688.0
Ruthenium	Ru	3, 4, 6, 8	44	101.07	12.2	2500.0	4900.0
Samarium	Sm	2, 3	62	150.4	7.54	1072.0	1900.0
Scandium	Sc	3	21	44.9559	3.0	1539.0	2730.0
Selenium	Se	2, 4, 6	34	78.96	4.79	217.0	685.0
Silicon	Si	4	14	28.086	2.33	1410.0	2680.0
Silver	Ag	1	47	107.868	10.5	960.8	2210.0
Sodium	Na	1	11	22.9898	0.97	97.8	892.0
Strontium	Sr	2	38	87.62	2.6	768.0	1380.0
Sulfur	S	2, 4, 6	16	32.06	2.07	119.0	444.6
Tantalum	Ta	5	73	180.9479	16.6	2996.0	5425.0
Technetium	Tc	6, 7	43	98.9062	11.5	2200.0	
Tellurium	Te	2, 4, 6	52	127.60	6.24	449.5	989.8
Terbium	Tb	3	65	158.9254	8.27	1356.0	2800.0
Thallium	Tl	1, 3	81	204.37	11.85	303.0	1457.0
Thorium	Th	4	90	232.0381	11.7	1750.0	3850.0
Thulium	Tm	3	69	168.9342	9.33	1545.0	1727.0
Tin	Sn	2, 4	50	118.69	7.30	231.9	2270.0
Titanium	Ti	3, 4	22	47.90	4.51	1668.0	3260.0
Tungsten	W	6	74	183.85	19.3	3410.0	5930.0
Uranium	U	4, 6	92	238.029	19.07	1132.0	3818.0
Vanadium	V	3, 5	23	50.9414	6.1	1900.0	3450.0
Xenon	Xe	0	54	131.30	3.06	−111.9	−108.0
Ytterbium	Yb	2, 3	70	173.04	6.98	824.0	1427.0
Yttrium	Y	3	39	88.9059	4.47	1509.0	3030.0
Zinc	Zn	2	30	65.37	7.14	419.5	906.0
Zirconium	Zr	4	40	91.22	6.49	1852.0	3580.0

* The 103 chemical elements known at the present time are included in this table. Some of those recently discovered have been obtained only as unstable isotopes.

† Based on Carbon-12. Figures enclosed in parentheses represent the mass number of the most stable isotope.

Physiological Standards, Average Normal

Blood

(Expressed per 100 ml. of whole blood unless otherwise stated)

Albumin (serum)	4–5 gm.
Ammonia (blood)	40–70 micrograms
Amylase	4–25 Russell units
Ascorbic acid	0.4–1.5 mg.
Bilirubin, total (indirect)	0.3 mg.
Bleeding time	1–5 min.
Calcium, total (serum)	8.5–10.5 mg.
Carbon dioxide content (serum)	26–28 mEq./L.
Chlorides (as chloride) (serum)	100–106 mEq./L.
Cholesterol, total (serum)	150–280 mg.
Clotting time (Lee-White method)	Below 20 min. 4th tube
Creatinine	0.7–1.5 mg.
Fibrinogen (plasma)	0.15–0.30 gm.
Glucose, fasting level	100 mg.
Hematocrit	42–50 mm. (males)
	40–48 mm. (females)
Hemoglobin	13–16 gm. (males)
	12–14 gm. (females)
Iodine, protein bound (serum)	3.5–8.0 micrograms
Iron, inorganic (plasma)	50–150 micrograms
Lactic acid	6–16 mg.
Lipids, total fatty acids	190–420 mg.
Magnesium (serum)	1.5–2.5 mEq./L.
Oxygen partial pressure	75–100 mm. of mercury
pH (serum)	7.35–7.45
Phosphorus, inorganic (serum)	3.0–4.5 mg.
Platelets	200,000–350,000/cu.mm.
Potassium (serum)	3.5–5.0 mEq./L.
Red Blood cells (Erythrocytes)	4,000,000–5,000,000/cu.mm.
Diameter	5.5–8.8 microns
Reticulocytes	0.5–1.5% of red cells
Sodium (serum)	136–145 mEq./L.
Sulfates, inorganic (serum)	0.5–1.5 mg.
Urea nitrogen (BUN)	8–25 mg.
Uric acid	3–7 mg.
Water	78%
White blood cells (Leukocytes)	5000–10,000/cu.mm.
Neutrophils (segmented)	54–62%
Lymphocytes	25–33%
Monocytes	3–7%
Eosinophils	1–3%
Basophils	0–0.75%

Cerebrospinal Fluid

Character	Clear; colorless; no coagulum
Pressure	70–180 mm. of water
Specific gravity	1.006–1.008
Total protein (Lumbar)	15–45 mg./100 ml.
Glucose	50–75 mg./100 ml.
Nonprotein nitrogen	12–30 mg./100 ml.
Chlorides	120–130 mEq./L.
Cells	0–5 mononuclear cells/cu.mm.
Colloidal gold reaction	Negative

Symbols

♏	Minim.	μ	Micron.*
Ɖ	Scruple.	μμ	Micromicron.
℥	Dram.	+	Plus; excess; acid reaction; positive.
f℥	Fluid dram.	−	Minus; deficiency; alkaline reaction; negative.
℥	Ounce.	±	Plus or minus; either positive or negative; indefinite.
f℥	Fluid ounce.	#	Number; following a number; pounds.
O	Pint.	÷	Divided by.
℔	Pound.	×	Multiplied by; magnification.
℞	Recipe; take.	=	Equals.
M	Misce; mix.	>	Greater than; from which is derived.
āā, āa	Of each.	<	Less than; derived from.
A, Å	Angstrom unit.	≮	Not less than.
C′	Complement.	≯	Not greater than.
c, c̄	[L. *cum*.]. With.	≦	Equal to or less than.
E_0	Electroaffinity.	≧	Equal to or greater than.
F_1	First filial generation.	≠	Not equal to.
F_2	Second filial generation.	√	Root; square root; radical.
mμ	Millimicron, micromillimeter.	²√	Square root.
μg	Microgram.	³√	Cube root.
mEq	Milliequivalent.	∞	Infinity.
mg	Milligram.	:	Ratio; "is to."
mg. %	Milligrams percent; milligrams per 100 ml.	::	Equality between ratios; "as."
Q_{O_2}	Oxygen consumption.	∴	Therefore.
m-	Meta-.	°	Degree.
o-	Ortho-.	%	Percent.
p-	Para-.	π	3.1416—ratio of circumference of a circle to its diameter.
s̄s̄, ss	[L. *semis*]. One-half.	☐, ♂	Male.
′	Foot; minute; primary accent; univalent.	○, ♀	Female.
″	Inch; second; secondary accent; bivalent.	⇌	Denotes a reversible reaction.
μm	Micrometer.		

* Common term for micrometer.

Abbreviations, Prefixes, Suffixes, Latin and Greek Nomenclature

Principal Medical Abbreviations

Abbreviation	Latin (unless indicated)	English Definition
a or āā	ana (Greek)	of each
a. c.	ante cibos	before meals
ad.	ad	to; up to
ad lib.	ad libitum	as desired
alt. dieb.	alternis diebus	every other day
alt. hor.	alternis horis	every other hour
alt. noc.	alternis noctus	every other night
aq..	aqua	water
aq. com.	aqua communis	common water
aq. dest.	aqua destillata	distilled water
aq. tep.	aqua tepida	tepid water
arg.	argentum	silver
av.	(French)	avoirdupois
bib.	bibe	drink
b. i. d.	bis in die	twice a day
b. i. n.	bis in noctus	twice a night
C.	Centigradus	centigrade
C.	congius	gallon
c̄	cum	with
cap.	capsula	capsule
cc.	(French)	cubic centimeter
cg.	(French)	centigram
cm.	(French)	centimeter
comp.	compositus	compound
cong.	congius	gallon
def.	defaecatio	defecation
Dil., dil.	dilue	dilute
dr.	drachma	dram or drams
elix.	(Arabic)	elixir
emp.	emplastrum	a plaster
et	et	and
ext.	extractum	extract
F.	(proper name)	Fahrenheit
Fld.	fluidus	fluid
fl. dr.	fluidrachma	fluid dram
fl. oz.	fluidus uncia	fluid ounce
Ft., ft.	fiat	let there be made
Gm.; gm.	gramme (French)	gram
gr.	granum	grain
Gtt., gtt.	guttae	drops
H.	hora	hour
h.n.	hac nocte	tonight
hor. interm.	horis intermediis	at intermediate hours
h.s.	hora somni	at bedtime or hour of sleep
hypo	(Greek)	hypodermically
inf.	infusum	infusion
L.		liter
lb.	libra	pound
liq.	liquor	liquid; fluid
M.	(French)	meter
m.	minimum	minim

Principal Medical Abbreviations (*Continued*)

Abbreviation	Latin (unless indicated)	English Definition
mEq.		milliequivalent
mg.		milligram
mist.	mistura	mixture
ml.		milliliter
mm.	(French)	millimeter
n.b.	nota bene	note well
no.	numero	number
non rep.	non repetatur	don't repeat
noxt.	nocte; noxte	at night
O.	octarius	pint
ol.	oleum	oil
omn. hor.	omni hora	every hour
omn. noct.	omni nocte	every night
os.	os; ora	mouth
oz.	uncia	ounce
p.c.	post cibum	after food; after meals
per.		through or by
pil.	pilula	pill
p.o.	per os	by mouth
p.r.n.	pro re nata	as needed; as desired
pt.	pinte (French)	pint
pulv.	pulvis	powder
Q.h.	quaque hora	every hour
Q. 2h.		every two hours
Q. 3h.		every three hours
q.i.d.	quater in die	four times a day
Q.s.	quantum sufficiat	a sufficient quantity
qt.	quartina	quart
quotid.	quotidie	every day
Q.v.	quantum vis	as much as you will
R	recipe	take
rep.	repetatur	let it be repeated
S.	signa	mark
s	sans	without
S.c.	sub cutis	subcutaneously
Sig.	signetur	let it be marked
Sol.	solutio	solution
solv.	solve	dissolve
s.o.s.	si opus sit	if occasion requires; if necessary
sp. gr.	gravitus	specific gravity
spt.	spiritus	spirit
ss.	semis	half
stat.	statim	immediately
syr.	syrupus	syrup
T.	temperatura	temperature
tab.	tabella	tablet
t.i.d.	ter in die	three times a day
t.i.n.	ter in nocte	three times a night
tr., tinct.	tinctura	tincture
ung.	unguentum	ointment
Ur.	urina	urine
vin	vinum	wine
vol. %		volume per cent
Wt.	wiht (Old English)	weight
w/v.		weight by volume

SEE: *Symbols* in *Appendix.*

A Glossary of Latin Medical Words

Latin words which have become a part of the general medical vocabulary
are listed in alphabetical order in the text.

abacus, -ī. *m.* Shelf.

abdōminālis, -e. Abdominal.

abdūcēns, -ntis. Leading or drawing from (the median line); applied also to 6th pair of cranial nerves.

aberrāns, -ntis. Wandering.

abstractum, -ī. *n.* Abstract.

accessōrius, -a, -um. Accessory.

accidō, -ere, -cidī. Occur; happen.

ācer, ācris, ācre. Sharp; severe.

acervulus, -ī. *m.* (Lit., little heap), acervulus.

acētābulum, -ī. *n.* (Lit., vinegar cup), the bony cuplike cavity of the hip joint; acetabulum.

acetās, -ātis. *m.* Acetate.

acētum, -ī. *n.* Vinegar.

acidum, -ī. *n.* Acid.

acinus, -ī. *m.* A terminal compartment or secreting portion of a gland; acinus.

acusticus, -a, -um. Auditory.

acūtus, -a, -um. Acute.

adeps, adipis. *m.* and *f.* Fat; lard.

adjūtor, -ōris. *m.* Helper; assistant.

adjuvō, -āre, -jūvī, -jūtus. Aid; assist.

adsum, -esse, -fuī. Be present.

aeger, -gra, -grum. Sick.

aegrōtus, -a, -um. Sick.

āēr, āēris. *m.* Air.

aeternus, -a, -um. Eternal.

aether, -is. *m.* Ether.

āla, -ae. *f.* Wing.

ālāris, -e. Winglike; alar.

albicāns, -ntis. Whitening; white.

albūgineus, -a, -um. White.

albulus, -a, -um. Whitish.

albus, -a, -um. White.

alcoholicus, -a, -um. Alcoholic.

aliquandō. Sometimes.

alius, -a, -ud. Other.

aloina, -ae. *f.* Aloin.

alter, -tera, -terum. Other.

altus, -a, -um. High.

alūmen, -inis. *n.* Alum.

alvus, -ī. *f.* Belly, or its contents.

amārus, -a, -um. Bitter.

amīcus, -ī. *m.* Friend.

āmissiō, -ōnis. *f.* Loss.

āmissus, -ūs. *m.* Loss.

ammōnium, -ī. *n.* Ammonium.

amygdala, -ae. *f.* Almond.

anaestheticus, -a, -um. Producing insensibility; anesthetic.

anastomoticus, -a, -um. Anastomosing.

ānellus, -ī. *m.* Ring.

angulus, -ī. *m.* Angle.

anima, -ae. *f.* Breath; life.

anīsum, -ī. *n.* Anise.

ānnulāris, -e. Ringlike; annular.

ānnulus, -ī. *m.* Ring.

anterius, -a, -um. Anterior.

antīcus, -a, -um. Foremost.

antidōtum, -ī. *n.* Antidote.

antimōniālis, -e. Of antimony; antimonial.

antimōnium, -ī. *n.* Antimony.

antipyreticus, -a, -um. Reducing the temperature; antipyretic.

antisepticus, -a, -um. Destroying germ life; antiseptic.

antitrāgus, -ī. *m.* A conical eminence opposite the tragus, q.v.; antitragus.

antīquus, -a, -um. Ancient.

aperiēns, -ntis. Laying open; laxative; aperient.

appellō, -āre, -āvī, -ātus. Call.

aptē. Aptly.

apud. Near.

aqua, -ae. *f.* Water.

aqueductus, -ūs. *m.* A canal; aqueduct.

aquōsus, -a, -um. Watery.

arbor, -oris. *f.* Tree.

arceō, -ēre, -uī, -tus. Ward off.

arcuātus, -a, -um. Curved like a bow.

arcus, -ūs. *m.* A bow; arch.

āreola, -ae. *f.* Small area, especially around the nipple.

argentum, -ī. *n.* Silver.

arōmaticus, -a, -um. Aromatic.

arsenicum, -ī. *n.* Arsenic.

arsenis, -itis. *m.* Arsenite.

artēria, -ae. *f.* Artery.

articulāris, -e. Articular.

articulō, -āre, -āvī, -ātus. Articulate.

artus, -ūs. *m.* Joint.

ascendēns, -ntis. Ascending.

asepticus, -a, -um. Free from putrefactive matter; aseptic.

asper, -a, -um. Rough.

astrictus, -a, -um. Bound up.

astūtus, -a, -um. Shrewd; artful.

atropīna, -ae. *f.* Active principle of belladonna; atropine.

attollēns, -ntis. Raising up; elevating.

attrāhēns, -ntis. Drawing to or towards.

audītōrius, -a, -um. Auditory.

aurantium, -ī. *n.* Orange.

auricula, -ae. *f.* Auricle.

auris, -is. *f.* Ear.

axis, -is. *m.* (Lit., that about which a body turns), 2nd cervical vertebra; axis.

azygos. (Gr.) Without a fellow.

Latin Medical Words (*Continued*)

balneum, -ī. *n.* Bath.
basīlāris, -e. Basilar.
basis, -is. *f.* Base.
bene. Well.
benignus, -a, -um. Mild; benign; not malignant.
berberis, -idis. *f.* Barberry.
bibō, -ere, bibī. Drink.
bicarbonās, -ātis. *m.* Bicarbonate.
biceps, -cipitis. Two-headed.
bifidus, -a, -um. Cleft.
biliaris, -e. Pert. to or conveying bile; bilary.
bīnī, -ae, -a. Two each.
bismuthum, -ī. *n.* Bismuth.
bitartrās, -ātis. *m.* Bitartrate.
bonus, -a, -um. Good.
borās, -ātis. *m.* Borate.
brachiālis, -e. Of the arm; brachial.
brāchium, -ī. *n.* Arm.
brevis, -e. Short.
brōmidum, -ī. *n.* Bromide.
būbula, -ae. *f.* Beef.
būccinātor, -ōris. *m.* The trumpeter muscle; buccinator.
bulbus, -ī. *m.* Bulb.
caecus, -a, -um. Blind.
calamus, -ī. *m.* Reed.
calcaneum, -ī. *n.* The heelbone (os calcis).
calcium, -ī. *n.* Calcium.
calidus, -a, -um. Hot.
callōsus, -a, -um. Hard, tough.
calor, -ōris. *m.* Heat.
calumba, -ae. *f.* Calumba.
calvārium, -ī. *n.* The skullcap.
calx, -cis. *f.* Lime.
calyx, -icis. *f.* Cup; calyx.
camphora, -ae. *f.* Camphor.
camphorātus, -a, -um. Camphorated.
canāliculus, -ī. *m.* Small duct or canal.
canālis, -is. *m.* Canal.
canīnus, -a, -um. Of a dog, canine.
canis, -is. *m.* and *f.* Dog.
cānitiēs, -ēī. *f.* A gray color, hoariness.
cannabis, -is. *f.* Hemp.
cantharis, -idis. *f.* Spanish fly.
canthus, -ī. *m.* The corner or angle of the eye.
capiō, -ere, cēpī, captus. Take.
capitulum, -ī. *n.* A knob or protuberance of bone received into a concavity of another bone.
capsicum, -ī. *n.* Cayenne pepper; capsicum.
capsula, -ae. *f.* A small box; capsule.
carbō, -ōnis. *m.* Carbon; coal; charcoal.
carbolicus, -a, -um. Carbolic.
carbonās, -ātis. *m.* Carbonate.
cardamōmum, -ī. *n.* Cardamom.
careō, -ēre, -uī, -itus. Need; want.
carneus, -a, -um. Fleshy.
carpus, -ī. *m.* Wrist.
cartilāginōsus, -a, -um. Cartilaginous.
cartilāgo, -inis. *f.* Cartilage.

caruncula, -ae. *f.* A little piece of flesh; caruncle.
cataplasma, -atis. *n.* Poultice; cataplasm.
catharticus, -a, -um. Cathartic.
cauda, -ae. *f.* Tail.
caudātus, -a, -um. Having a tail; caudate.
causa, -ae. *f.* Cause.
causō, -āre, -āvī, -ātus. Cause.
cavernōsus, -a, -um. Hollow; cavernous.
cavitās, -ātis. *f.* Cavity.
cavus, -a, -um. Hollow.
celeriter. Quickly.
centrālis, -e. Central.
centrum, -ī. *n.* Center.
cephalalgia, -ae. *f.* Headache.
cērātum, -ī. *n.* Waxed dressing; cerate.
cerātus, -a, -um. Waxed.
cerevisa, -ae. *f.* Beer.
certus, -a, -um. Sure; certain.
cēterus, -a, -um. Other.
charta, -ae. *f.* Medicated paper.
chartula, -ae. *f.* Small paper (powder).
chirāta, -ae. *f.* Chirata.
chīrurgia, -ae. *f.* Surgery.
chīrurgus, -ī. *m.* Surgeon.
chlōral. *n.* Chloral.
chlōrās, -ātis. *m.* Chlorate.
chlōridum, -ī. *n.* Chloride.
chlōrōformum, -ī. *n.* Chloroform.
choledochus, -ī. *m.* Holding or receiving bile.
chorda, -ae. *f.* Cord.
chronicus, -a, -um. Chronic.
chylum, -ī. *n.* Chyle.
cibus, -ī. *m.* Food.
cicātrōsus, -a, -um. Full of scars, scarred.
ciliāris, -e. Ciliary.
cinchōna, -ae. *f.* Cinchona.
cinchonīna, -ae. *f.* Cinchonine.
cinereus, -a, -um. Ash-colored.
cinnamōmum, -ī. *n.* Cinnamon.
circulāris, -e. Circular.
circulatiō, -ōnis. *f.* Circulation.
circulus, -ī. *m.* Circle.
circum. Around.
circumdō, -dare, -dedī, -datus. Surround.
citō. Promptly; quickly.
citrās, -ātis. *m.* Citrate.
clārus, -a, -um. Clear, distinguished.
claudus, -a, -um. Lame.
clāvus, -ī. *m.* A corn, usually on the toes.
cludō, -ere, -sī, -sus. Shut; close.
cochlea, -ae. *f.* (Lit., snail shell), spiral cavity of the internal ear; cochlea.
cochleāre, -is. *n.* Spoon.
codeina, -ae. *f.* An alkaloid of opium; codeine.
coeliacus, -a, -um. Relating to the stomach; celiac.
colicus, -a, -um. Of or pert. to the colon.
collateriālis, -e. Collateral.

Latin Medical Words (*Continued*)

collum, -ī. *n.* Neck.

colocynthis, -idis. *f.* Colocynth.

color, -ōris. *m.* Color.

cōlum, -ī. *n.* Large intestine; colon.

columna, -ae. *f.* Column.

comes, -itis. *m.* Companion.

commissūra, -as. *f.* A joining; commissure.

communicāns, -ntis. Communicating.

commūnis, -e. Common.

compōnō, -ere, -posuī, -positus. Compound.

conarium, -ī. *n.* A synonym for the pineal gland; conarium.

concha, -ae. *f.* (Lit., a shell), hollow part of the external ear; concha.

confectiō, -ōnis. *f.* Confection.

conium, -ī. *n.* Poison, hemlock; conium.

conīveō, -āre, -nīvī. Blink; half close.

conjectūra, -ae. *f.* Guess.

contineō, -ēre, -tinuī, -tentus. Contain.

contrāhō, -ere, -xī, -ctus. Draw together; contract.

contusiō, -ōnis. *f.* Bruise.

cōnus, -ūs. *m.* Cone.

convalescō, -ere, -valuī. Regain health.

cor, cordis. *n.* Heart.

cornicula, -ae. *f.* Little horn.

cornu, -ūs. *n.* Horn; horn-shaped process.

corōna, -ae. *f.* Crown.

coronārius, -a, -um. Encircling like a crown; coronary.

corpus, -oris. *n.* Body.

corrōsīvus, -a, -um. Corrosive.

corrugātor, -ōris. *m.* A muscle which wrinkles; corrugator.

cortex, -icis. *m.* and *f.* Bark; rind; external layer; cortex.

costa, -ae. *f.* Rib.

craniālis, -e. Cranial.

crās. Tomorrow.

crassus, -a, -um. Gross; large.

creasōtum, -ī. *n.* Creasote.

crēber, -bra, -brum. Frequent.

crēdō, -ere, -credidī, -creditus. Trust; believe.

crēta, -ae. *f.* Chalk.

cribriformis, -e. Sievelike; cribriform.

cribrōsus, -a, -um. Having holes like a sieve.

crista, -ae. *f.* Crest; comb of a cock (gallus).

crūrālis, -e. Of the leg; crural.

crūreus, -a, -um. Of the leg.

crūs, crūris. *n.* The leg.

crusta, -ae. *f.* Crust.

cubēba, -ae. *f.* Cubeb.

cubitum, -ī. *n.* Elbow.

cuboideus, -a, -um. Cubelike; cuboid.

cum. With.

cuneiformis, -e. Wedge-shaped; cuneiform.

cūra, -ae. *f.* Care.

cūrō, -āre, -āvī, -ātus. Treat; cure.

cutis, -is. *f.* Skin.

decem. Ten.

deciduus, -a, -um. That which falls off.

decoctum, -ī. *n.* Decoction.

deferēns, -ntis. Bearing away.

defessus, -a, -um. Tired; wearied.

deformāns, -ntis. Deforming.

deformitās, -ātis. *f.* Deformity.

demonstrō, -āre, -āvī, -ātus. Show; prove.

dēns, dentis. *m.* Tooth.

dentātus, -a, -um. Toothed; dentate.

depressor, -ōris. *m.* That which depresses; depressor.

descendēns, -ntis. Descending.

dexter, -tra, -trum. Right.

diabeticus, -a, -um. Diabetic; one having diabetes.

diabolus, -ī. *m.* Devil.

dīcō, -ere, -dixī, dictus. Say.

diēs, -ēī. *m.* Day.

difficilis, -e. Difficult.

digitus, -ī. *m.* Finger (digitus pedis, a toe).

dilātor, -ōris. *m.* That which dilates; dilator.

dilūtus, -a, -um. Dilute.

dimidius, -a, -um. Half.

discipulus, -ī. *m.* A learner; pupil; student.

diū. For a long time.

diureticus, -a, -um. Diuretic.

dividō, -ere, -vīsī, -vīsus. Divide.

dō, dare, dedī, datus. Give.

doctus, -a, -um. Learned.

dolōr, -ōris. *m.* Pain.

dolōrōsus, -a, -um. Painful.

domicilium, -ī. *n.* Abode.

dorsālis, -e. Of the back; dorsal.

dorsum, -ī. *n.* Back.

dosis, -is. *f.* Dose.

drachma, -ae. *f.* Dram.

dustus, -ūs. *m.* Duct.

dulcis, -e. Sweet.

duo, duae, du. Two.

dūrus, -a, -um. Hard.

dyspepticus, -a, -um. Dyspeptic; a dyspeptic.

edō, -ere, -ēdi, -ēsus. Eat.

efferēns, -ntis. Bearing out or away; efferent.

effervescēns, -ntis. Boiling up.

elegāns, -ntis. Elegant.

ēluviēs, -ēī. *f.* Discharge.

emeticus, -a, -um. Causing vomiting; emetic.

ēminentia, -ae. *f.* Eminence.

emō, -ere, -ēmī, emptus. Buy.

empiricus, -ī. *n.* Quack; empiric.

emplastrum, -ī. *n.* Plaster.

ensiformis, -e. Sword-shaped; ensiform.

eō, īre, īvī, itus. Go.

epilepsia, -ae. *f.* Epilepsy.

epiploicus, -a, -um. Relating to the epiploön (omentum).

equīnus, -a, -um. Of a horse; equine.

ergota, -ae. *f.* Ergot.

Latin Medical Words (*Continued*)

errō, -āre, -āvī, -ātus. Wander; err.

ērudītus, -a, -um. Learned; educated; erudite.

et. And.

et-et. Both - and.

ethmoidālis, -e. Ethmoid.

etiam. Even.

euonymus, -ī. *m.* Wahoo; Euonymus.

eupatōrium, -ī. *n.* Boneset; eupatorium.

excessus, -ūs. *m.* Departure.

excīdō, -ere, -īdī, -īsus. Cut out; excise.

excitō, -āre, -āvī, -ātus. Excite.

expectatiō, -ōnis. *f.* Expectation.

experimentum, -ī. *n.* Experiment.

expressiō, -ōnis. *f.* Expression.

exsiccātus, -a, -um. Dried out.

exsudō, -āre, -āvī, -ātus. Sweat out; exude.

externus, -a, -um. External.

extractum, -ī. *n.* Extract.

faciēs, -ēī. *f.* Face; countenance.

faciō, -ere, fēcī, factus. Make.

falx, -cis. *f.* Sickle (a sickle-shaped process).

familia, -ae (or -as). *f.* Family.

fasciculus, -ī. *m.* A small bundle of fibers.

febrifuga, -ae. *f.* Agent that reduces fever; febrifuge.

febris, -is. *f.* Fever.

fēmina, -ae. *f.* Woman.

femorālis, -e. Of the thigh; femoral.

fenestra, -ae. *f.* Window; an opening in the wall of the tympanum.

ferē. Almost.

ferrum, -ī. *n.* Iron.

fibrilla, -ae. *f.* Filament; fibril.

fibrōsus, -a, -um. Fibrous.

fides, -eī. *f.* Faith; trustworthiness.

fīdus, -a, -um. Faithful; trustworthy.

filia, -ae. *f.* Daughter.

filius, -ī. *m.* Son.

filix, -icis. *f.* Fern.

fimbria, -ae. *f.* Fringe.

fimbriātus, -a, -um. Fringed; fimbriated.

finiō, -īre, -īvī, -ītus. End; finish.

fiō, fierī, factus. Be made.

fissūra, -ae. *f.* Cleft; fissure.

flavus, -a, -um. Yellow.

flexilis, -e. Flexible.

flōs, flōris. *m.* Flower.

fluidus, -a, -um. Fluid.

flūmen, -inis. *n.* River.

fluō, -ere, fluxī, fluxus. Flow.

fluor, -ōris. *m.* Flux; flow.

foetidus, -a, -um. Offensive, fetid.

folium, -ī. *n.* Leaf.

folliculus, -ī. *m.* A small secretory sac; follicle.

fons, -ntis. *m.* Fountain; spring.

formō, -āre, -āvī, -ātus. Form.

fornicātus, -a, -um. Arched.

fornix, -icis. *m.* Arch; vault; fornix.

fortis, -e. Strong; brave.

fossa, -ae. *f.* Ditch; depression; fossa.

fovea, -ae. *f.* Small pit; depression.

fractus, -a, -um. Broken.

fragilitās, -ātis. *f.* Brittleness.

frēnum, -ī. *n.* A bridle; a membranous fold; frenum.

frigidus, -a, -um. Cold.

fructus, -ūs. *m.* Fruit.

frumentum, -ī. *n.* Corn; grain.

frustum, -ī. *n.* Piece; bit.

functiō, -ōnis. *f.* Execution; normal action; function.

fuscus, -a, -um. Brown.

fūsiformis, -e. Spindle-shaped; fusiform.

gallus, -ī. *m.* Cock.

ganglioniformis, -e. Ganglionlike.

gelsemium, -ī. *n.* Gelsemium; yellow jasmine (root).

gemellus, -a, -um. Paired; twin.

gena, -ae. *f.* The cheek.

geniōhyoglossus, -ī. *m.* Muscle attached to chin, hyoid bone and tongue.

gentiāna, -ae. *f.* Gentian.

genu, -ūs. *n.* Knee.

genus, generis. *n.* Kind.

germinātīvus, -a, -um. Germinative; germinal.

glabrus, -a, -um. Smooth.

glaciēs, -ēī. *f.* Ice.

globus, -ī. *m.* Globe.

glomerulus, -ī. *m.* Small ball or tuft of vessels; glomerule.

glūteus, -a, -um. Of the buttock; gluteal.

glycerīnum, -ī. *n.* Glycerin.

glycerītum, -ī. *m.* Glycerite.

glycyrrhiza, -ae. *f.* Licorice.

gracilis, -e. Slender; graceful.

granulōsus, -a, -um. Granular.

granum, -ī. *n.* Grain.

gratus, -a, -um. Agreeable; pleasing.

gubernāculum, -ī. *n.* (Lit., a helm), applied to fetal cord directing descent of testes; gubernaculum.

gummi. Gum.

gustō, -āre, -āvī, -ātus. Taste.

gutta, -ae. *f.* Drop.

gyrus, -ī. *m.* Circle; ring; convolution (of the brain).

habeō, -ēre, -uī, -itus. Have.

habitō, -āre, -āvī, -ātus. Inhabit.

hallex, -icis, or hallux, -ucis. *f.* The great toe.

harmonia, -ae. *f.* Harmony, "suture of harmony."

helix, -icis. *f.* Outer ring of the external ear; helix.

hemisphericus, -a, -um. Hemispherical.

hēpar, hepatis. *n.* Liver.

herba, -ae. *f.* Herb.

herī. Yesterday.

hiātus, -ūs. *m.* Opening; aperture.

hīc, haec, hoc. This.

hilāris, -e. Cheerful.

Latin Medical Words (*Continued*)

hīlus, -ī. *m.* Small fissure or depression.

hippocampus, -ī. *m.* (Lit., sea horse), applied to two convolutions of brain (major and minor); hippocampus.

homo, -inis. *m.* Man.

horribilis, -e. Horrible.

humānus, -a, -um. Human.

hūmor, -ōris. *m.* Fluid; humor.

hydrargyrum, -ī. *n.* Mercury.

hydrastis, -is. *f.* Golden seal (root); hydrastis.

hyoideus, -a, -um. Hyoid.

Hyoscyamus, -ī. *m.* Henbane; Hyoscyamus.

īdem, eadem, idem. Same.

ignārus, -a, -um. Ignorant.

iliacus, -a, -um. Of or pert. to the flanks or ilium; iliac.

ille, illa, illud. He; she; it.

immōbilis, -e. Immovable.

immōbilitas, -ātis. *f.* Immobility.

impar, -is. Without a mate or fellow.

impediō, -īre, -īvī, -ītus. Hinder; check; prevent.

imperītus, -a, -um. Unskilled.

impūrus, -a, -um. Impure.

īmus, -a, -um. Lowest.

incisūra, -ae. *f.* Groove or notch.

Indicus, -a, -um. Indian.

infans, -ntis. *m.* and *f.* Infant.

inflammatiō, -ōnis. *f.* Inflammation.

infraspinātus, -a, -um. Beneath the spine (of the scapula); infraspinate.

infūsum, -ī. *m.* Infusion.

ingressus, -ūs. *m.* Entrance.

innominātus, -a, -um. Unnamed; innominate.

intermittō, -ere, -mīsī, -missus. Intermit.

internōdium, -ī. *n.* Space between two joints; internode.

internus, -a, -um. Inner.

interpositus, -a, -um. Placed between.

intertragicus, -a, -um. Between the tragus, q.v., and antitragus.

intestīnum, -ī. *n.* Intestine.

intumescentia, -ae. *f.* An enlargement; intumescence.

inveniō, -īre, -vēnī, -ventus. Find; discover.

inversiō, -ōnis. *f.* Inversion.

iodidum, -ī. *n.* Iodide.

ipecacuanha, -ae. *f.* Ipecac.

ipse, ipsa, ipsum. Himself; herself; itself.

iris, iridis. *f.* Iris.

is, ea, id. He; she; it.

iter, itineris. *n.* Way; passageway.

jecur, jecinoris. *n.* Liver.

jūcundē. Happily; pleasantly.

jūglans, juglandis. *f.* Walnut.

jugulāris, -e. Jugular.

jūniperus, -ī. *f.* Juniper tree.

juvenis. *m.* and *f.*, *adj.*, and *subst.* Young; a youth.

labium, -ī. *n.* Lip.

lacer, -a, -um. Lacerated; mutilated.

lacrima, -ae. *f.* Tear.

lacrimālis, -e. Pert. to tears; lacrimal.

lactās, -ātis. *m.* A salt of lactic acid; lactate.

lactiferus, -a, -um. Milk-bearing; lactiferous.

lacus, -ūs. *m.* Lake; basin; reservoir.

lamella, -ae. *f.* Layer.

lamina, -ae. *f.* Thin plate; layer.

lāna, -ae. *f.* Wool.

lassus, -a, -um. Weary.

laterālis, -e. Lateral.

lātus, -a, -um. Broad.

laudō, -āre, -āvī, -ātus. Praise.

lavandula, -ae. *f.* Lavender.

lavō, -āre, -āvī, -ātus or lavi, lautus. Wash.

laxātor, -ōris. *m.* A muscle that loosens; relaxer.

legō, -ere, -lēgī, lectus. Bring together; collect.

leniō, -īre, -īvī, -ītus. Calm; soothe; assuage.

lenticulāris, -e. Lentil-shaped (double-convex); lenticular.

lentus, -a, -um. Sticky.

letifer, -a, -um. Deadly.

levis, -e. Light.

lienālis, -e. Of the spleen.

ligamentōsus, -a, -um. Ligamentous.

ligamentum, -ī. *n.* Ligament.

lignum, -ī. *n.* Wood.

limbus, -ī. *n.* Border; band; fringe.

līmitāns, -ntis. Limiting.

limon, -ōnis. *f.* Lemon.

linea, -ae. *f.* Line.

lingua, -ae. *f.* Tongue.

linguālis, -e. Of the tongue; lingual.

linimentum, -ī. *n.* Liniment.

linum, -ī. *n.* Flax.

liquidus, -a, -um. Liquid.

lobulus, -ī. *m.* Lobule.

lobus, -ī. *m.* Lobe.

longitudinālis, -e. Longitudinal.

longus, -a, -um. Long.

lotiō, -ōnis. *f.* Wash; lotion.

lucidus, -a, -um. Clear; transparent.

lumbālis, -e. Of the loins; lumbar.

lumbus, -ī. *m.* Loin.

lūnula, -ae. *f.* Small crescent; lunula.

lupulīna, -ae. *f.* Yellow powder from the scales of the hop; lupulin.

luteus, -a, -um. Yellow.

luxātiō, -ōnis. *f.* Dislocation.

lympha, -ae. *f.* Chyle; lymph.

mācerō, -āre, -āvī, ātus. Soak; macerate.

magister, -trī. *m.* Teacher; master.

magnus, -a, -um. Large; great.

māla, -ae. *f.* The cheekbone.

malignus, -a, -um. Malignant.

malus, -a, -um. Bad.

mandibulum, -ī. *n.* A jaw.

māne. *n.* Morning.

manūbrium, -ī. *n.* (Lit., a handle, hilt), upper part of sternum; manubrium.

manus, -ūs. *f.* Hand.

Latin Medical Words (Continued)

massa, -ae. *f.* Mass.

masticō, -āre, -āvī, -ātus. Chew.

mastoideus, -a, -um. Nipplelike: mastoid.

mater, -tris. *f.* Mother.

māteria, -ae. *f.* Materials.

māternus, -a, -um. Maternal.

matrix, -īcis. *f.* Source; origin.

maxilla, -ae. *f.* Jawbone; jaw.

meātus, -ūs. *m.* Opening; passage.

mediānus, -a, -um. Middle; median.

medicāmen, -inis. *n.* Drug.

medicāmentārius, -a, -um. Medicated.

medicāmentum, -ī. *n.* Drug.

medicātus, -a, -um. Medicated.

medicīna, -ae. *f.* Medicine.

medicus, -ī. *m.* Physician; doctor.

medius, -a, -um. Middle.

membrāna, -ae. *f.* Membrane.

membrum, -ī. *n.* Member.

memoria. -ae. *f.* Memory.

mentha, -ae. *f.* Mint.

mentum, -ī. *n.* Chin.

mesentericus, -a, -um. Of the mesentery; mesenteric.

metus, -ūs. *m.* Fear.

mīles, -itis. *m.* Soldier.

minerālis, -e. Mineral.

misceō, -ēre, miscuī, mixtus. Mix.

miser, -a, -um. Poor; wretched.

mistūra, -ae. *f.* Mixture.

mītis, -e. Mild.

mitto, -ere, mīsī, missus. Send.

mobilis, -e. Movable.

mobilitās, -ātis. *f.* Mobility.

modiolus, -ī. *m.* (Lit., a small measure), hollow cone in the cochlea of the ear, modiolus.

molāris, -e (mola, mill). The grinder teeth; molar.

molliō, -īre, -īvī, -ītus. Soften; mitigate.

mollis, -e. Soft.

mollitīes, -ēī. *f.* Softness.

mons, -ntis. *m.* Mountain.

montānus, -a, -um. Of a mountain; mountain.

monticulus, -ī. *m.* Small eminence.

morbus, -ī. *m.* Disease.

mordeō, -ēre, momordī, morsus. Bite.

moritūrus, -a, -um. About to die.

morphīna, -ae. *f.* Morphine.

morrhua, -ae. *f.* A genus of fishes, including the cod; cod.

mors, mortis. *f.* Death.

morsus, -ūs. *m.* Bite.

mortarium, -ī. *n.* Mortar.

mōtor, -ōris. *m.* That which moves; mover.

moveō, -ēre, mōvī, mōtus. Move.

mox. Presently; soon; directly.

mucilāgō, -inis. *f.* Mucilage.

mucōsus, -a, -um. Mucous.

mulceō, -ere, mulsi, mulsus. Soothe; allay.

multifidus, -a, -um. Many-clefted.

multus, -a, -um. Much; many.

muriāticus, -a, -um. Muriatic.

musculus, -ī. *m.* Muscle.

mūtātiō, -ōnis. *f.* Change.

myristica, -ae. *f.* Nutmeg.

myrtiformis, -e. Shaped like the myrtle leaf or berry; myrtiform.

nāris, -is. *f.* Nostril.

nāsus, -ī. *m.* Nose.

natō, -āre, -āvī, -ātus. Swim; float.

natūra, -ae. *f.* Nature.

nauta, -ae. *m.* Sailor.

naviculāris, -e. Boat-shaped; navicular.

neglectus, -a, -um. Neglected.

nemō, -inis. *m.* and *f.* No one.

nervus, -ī. *m.* Nerve.

nescio, -īre, -īvi, -ītus. Not know; be ignorant of.

neurilemma, -atis. *n.* Nerve sheath.

nictitāns, -ntis. Winking.

nil. Nothing.

nimium. Too often.

nisi. Unless.

nitrās, -ātis. *m.* Nitrate.

nitricus, -a, -um. Nitric.

nitrōsus, -a, -um. Nitrous.

nōmen, -inis. *m.* Name.

nōminō, -āre, -āvī, -ātus. Name.

nōn. Not.

nondum. Not yet.

nōnus, -a, -um. Ninth.

nosco, -ere, nōvī, nōtus. Learn; know.

novem. Nine.

novus, -a, -um. New.

nox, noctis. *f.* Night.

nucha, -ae. *f.* Nape of neck.

nullus, -a, -um. No; none.

numerus, -ī. *m.* Number.

nunc. Now.

oblīquus, -a, -um. Oblique.

oblongātus, -a, -um. Oblong.

octō. Eight.

oculus, -ī. *m.* Eye.

officīna, -ae. *f.* Office.

officinālis, -e. Officinal.

oleorēsīna, -ae. *f.* Oleoresin.

oleum, -ī. *n.* Oil.

olfactōrius, -a, -um. Olfactory.

omentum, -ī. *n.* Epiploon; omentum.

omnis, -e. Every; all.

operculum, -ī. *n.* (Lit., a cover or lid), applied to a group of convolutions in the cerebrum, between the two divisions of the fissure of Sylvius.

ophthalmicus, -a, -um. Of the eye; ophthalmic.

oppōnēns, -ntis. Opposing.

opticus, -a, -um. Optic.

opus, operis. *n.* Work.

orbita, -ae. *f.* The cavity which lodges the eye; orbit.

Latin Medical Words (Continued)

ordō, -inis. *m.* Row.

orificium, -ī. *n.* Opening.

orior, -īrī, ortus. Arise.

ōs, ōris. *n.* Mouth.

os, ossis. *n.* Bone.

ossiculum, -ī. *n.* Small bone.

ostium, -ī. *n.* An opening.

ovālis, -e. Egg-shaped; oval.

oxalās, -ātis. *m.* A salt of oxalic acid, oxalate.

oxidum, -ī. *n.* Oxide.

palātum, -ī. *n.* Palate.

palpēbra, -ae. *f.* Eyelid.

pālus, -ūdis. *f.* Marsh; swamp.

pancreāticus, -a, -um. Pancreatic.

papillāris, -e. Resembling or covered with papillae; papillary.

pār, paris. *n.* A pair.

parasiticus, -a, -um. Parasitic.

paries, -iētis. *m.* Wall.

parō, -āre, -āvī, -ātus. Prepare.

pars, partis. *f.* Part.

partus, -ūs. *m.* Parturition; childbirth.

parvus, -a, -um. Small.

pater, -tris. *m.* Father.

patheticus, -a, -um. That which moves the passions; a name given to the 4th pair of nerves.

patria, -as. *f.* Fatherland; country.

paucus, -a, -um. Few.

pectinātus, -a, -um. Resembling the teeth of a comb; pectinate.

pectineus, -a, -um. Comblike.

pectiniformis, -e. Comblike.

pectus, pectoris. *n.* Breast; bosom.

pellūcidus, -a, -um. Transparent.

pensō, -āre, -āvī, -ātus. Weigh.

pepsīnum, -ī. *n.* Pepsin.

percolō, -āre, -āvī, -ātus. Filter; strain.

perforō, -āre, -āvī, -ātus. Bore through; perforate.

periculōsus, -a, -um. Dangerous.

perītus, -a, -um. Skilled.

peronēus, -a, -um. Relating to the fibula; peroneal.

persōna, -ae. *f.* Person.

perspiratōrius, -a, -um. Relating to perspiration; perspiratory.

pēs, pedis. *m.* Foot.

petō, -ere, -īvī, -ītus. Seek.

petrolātum, -ī. *n.* Petrolatum; vaseline.

petrōsus, -a, -um. Rocklike; petrous.

pharmacopoeia, -a. *f.* Pharmacopoeia.

phiala, -ae. *f.* Vial.

philosophus, -ī. *m.* Philosopher.

phosphās, -ātis. *m.* A salt of phosphoric acid; phosphate.

phrenicus, -a, -um. Of the diaphragm; phrenic.

physostigma, -atis. *n.* Calabar bean; physostigma.

piger, -gra, -grum. Lazy.

pigmentum, -ī. *n.* Pigment.

pilula, -ae. *f.* Pill.

pilus, -ī. *m.* Hair.

pineālis, -e. Resembling a pine cone; pineal.

pinna, -ae. *f.* (Lit., feather), pavillion of the ear; pinna.

piper, piperis. *n.* Pepper.

piperītus, -a, -um. Pepper, peppery.

pistillum, -ī. *n.* Pestle.

pituitārius, -a, -um. (pituita, phlegm or mucus), pituitary (applied to a reddish-gray body occuping the sella Turcica of the sphenoid bone from a former erroneous belief that it discharged mucus into the nostrils).

pius, -a, -um. Tender.

pix, picis. *f.* Pitch.

plantāris, -e. Relating to the sole of the foot; plantar.

plānus, -a, -um. Flat; level; smooth.

plexus, -a, -um. Network; plexus.

plica, -ae. *f.* Fold.

plumbum, -ī. *n.* Lead.

poculum, -ī. *n.* Cup.

pollex, -icis. *f.* The thumb.

pomum, -ī. *n.* Apple.

pons, pontis. *m.* Bridge.

poples, poplitis. *m.* Ham of the knee; popliteal space.

poplitēus, -a, -um. Relating to the ham; popliteal.

populus, -ī. *m.* People.

portō, -āre, -āvī, -ātus. Carry.

portiō, -ōnis. *f.* Portion.

porus, -ī. *m.* Channel; canal.

post. Behind; after.

posteā. Afterward.

posticus, -a, -um. Hindmost.

potēns, -ntis. Powerful.

potiō, -ōnis. A drink; draught.

potō, -āre, -āvī, -ātus. Drink.

potus, -ūs. *m.* Drink.

praeparō, -āre, -āvī, -ātus. Prepare.

praeparatiō, -ōnis. *f.* Preparation.

praeputium, -ī. *n.* Foreskin; prepuce.

praescrībō, -ere, -scrīpsī, -scrīptus. Prescribe.

praescriptum, -ī. *n.* Prescription.

praesēns, -ntis. Present.

praestāns, -ntis. Excellent.

pressiō, -ōnis. *f.* Pressure.

primus, -a, -um. First.

princeps, -ipis. The first; chief; principal.

privō, -āre, -āvī, -ātus. Deprive.

prō. For; in behalf of.

processus, -ūs. *m.* A prominence; process.

profundus, -a, -um. Deep.

pronātor, -ōris. *m.* A muscle which turns the palm of the hand downward; pronator.

properō, -āre, -āvī, -ātus. Hasten.

proprius, -a, -um. One's own; special; proper.

prudēns, -ntis. Prudent.

Latin Medical Words (Continued)

pterygium, -ī, *n.* An eye disease; pterygium.
publicus, -a, -um. Public.
puella, -ae. *f.* Girl.
pugnō, -āre, -āvī, -ātus. Fight.
pulcher, -chra, -chrum. Beautiful.
pulmo, -ōnis. *m.* Lung.
pulmonālis, -e. Of the lungs; pulmonary.
pulverō, -āre, -āvī, -ātus. Powder; pulverize.
pulvis, pulveris. *m.* Powder.
punctum, -ī. *n.* Point.
puniō, -īre, -īvī, -ītus. Punish.
pūpilla, -ae. *f.* Pupil (of eye).
pupillāris, -e. Pupillary; applied to a delicate membrane which covers the pupil of the eye in the fetus.
purgātīvus, -a, -um. Purgative.
purificātus, -a, -um. Purified.
pūrus, -a, -um. Pure.
pyramidālis, -e. Pyramidal.
pyramis, -idis. *f.* Pyramid.
pyriformis, -e. Pear-shaped; pyriform.
quadrātus, -a, -um. Four-sided; square.
quadriceps, -cipitis. Four-headed.
quadrigeminus, -a, -um. Fourfold; four.
quaestiō, -ōnis. *f.* Question.
quam. Than.
quartus, -a, -um. Fourth.
quatuor. Four.
quatuordecim. Fourteen.
que. And.
quinīna, -ae. *f.* Quinine.
quis, quae, quid. Who; which; what.
quondam. Formerly.
quoque. Also.
quot. How many.
radiālis, -e. Of the radius; radial.
radiātus, -a, -um. Radiated.
rādix, -īcis. *f.* Root.
ramus, -ī. *m.* Branch.
rārō. Rarely.
rārus, -a, -um. Rare.
recens. Recently.
recipiō, -ere, -cēpī, -ceptus. Take.
recreō, -āre, -āvī, -ātus. Refresh.
rectus, -a, -um. Straight.
reductio, -ōnis. *f.* A bringing back.
reflexus, -a, -um. Turned back; reflected.
relevō, -āre, -āvī, -ātus. Relieve.
remedium, -ī. *n.* Remedy.
remittō, -ēre, -mīsī, -missus. Send back; remit.
removeō, -ēre, -mōvī, -mōtus. Remove.
rēn, rēnis. *m.* (usually pl.), kidney.
rēnalis, -e. Of the kidney; renal.
reperiō, -īre, -perī, -pertus. Find.
reprimō, -ēre, -pressī, -pressus. Check; repress.
requiesco, -ēre, -ēvī, -ētus. Rest.
rēs, reī. *f.* Thing.
rēsīna, -ae. *f.* Resin.
rēspīrātiō, -ōnis. *f.* Respiration.
rēte, -is. *n.* Net.

reticulāris, -e. Like a net; reticular.
retrāhēns, -ntis. Drawing back; retracting.
rheumatismus, -ī. *m.* Rheumatism.
ricinus, -ī. *m.* (Lit., a tick, which the seeds resemble), the castor oil plant (Ricinus communis).
rima, -ae. *f.* Slit; cleft.
rogō, -āre, -āvī, -ātus. Ask.
rosa, -ae. *f.* Rose.
rostrum, -ī. *n.* Beak.
rotundus, -a, -um. Round.
ruber, -bra, -brum. Red.
rubor, -ōris. *m.* Redness.
rūga, -ae. *f.* A wrinkle; fold.
rumex, -icis. *m.* and *f.* Sorrel.
sabulum, -ī. *n.* Sand.
saccharātus, -a, -um. Saccharated.
saccharum, -ī. *n.* Sugar.
sacciformis, -e. Saclike.
saccus, -ī. *m.* A sack or bag.
saepe. Often.
sal, -is. *m.* and *f.* Salt.
salicīnum, -ī. *n.* Salicin.
salicylās, -ātis. *m.* Salicylate.
salix, -īcis. *f.* Willow.
sānābilis, -e. Curable.
sanguis, -guinis. *m.* Blood.
sānitās, -ātis. *f.* Healing.
sānō, -āre, -āvī, -ātus. Heal; cure.
sapientia, -ae. *f.* Wisdom.
sapō, -ōnis. *m.* Soap.
sartōrius, -ī. *m.* The tailor's muscle; sartorius.
scāla, -ae. *f.* Ladder.
scalēnus, -a, -um. Of unequal sides.
scaphoideus, -a, -um. Boat-shaped; scaphoid.
schola, -ae. *f.* (Lit., leisure given to learning), school.
scientia, -ae. *f.* Knowledge; science.
scilla, -ae. *f.* Squill.
sciō, -īre, -īvī, -ītus. Know.
scrībō, -ēre, scripsī, scrīptus. Write.
scriptōrius, -a, -um. Of a writer; writer's.
secundus, -a, -um. Second.
sed. But.
sedes, -is. *f.* Seat.
segmentum, -ī. *n.* Segment.
sella, -ae. *f.* Saddle.
sēmicirculāris, -e. Semicircular.
sēmiellipticus, -a, -um. Semielliptical.
sēmilunāris, -e. Semilunar.
sēmimembranōsus, -a, -um. Semimembranous.
sēminālis, -e. Seminal.
sēmis, sēmissis. *m.* Half.
sēmitendinōsus, -a, -um. Semitendinous.
senectus, -tūtis. *f.* Old age.
senex, senis. *m.* Old man.
senilitās, -ātis. The feebleness of old age; senility.
sentiō, -īre, -sī, -sus. Feel.
septem. Seven.

Latin Medical Words (*Continued*)

sequestrum, -ī. *n.* A portion of dead bone; sequestrum.

sermō, -ōnis. *m.* Conversation.

serrātus, -a, -um. Notched like a saw; serrated.

servus, -ī. *m.* Servant; assistant.

sesamoideus, -a, -um. Like a sesame seed; sesamoid (applied to a bone developed in a tendon).

seu. Whether.

signō, -āre, -āvī, -ātus. Write; direct.

similō, -āre, -āvī, -ātus. Simulate.

simplex, -icis. Simple.

sināpis, -is. *f.* Mustard.

sitis, -is. *f.* Thirst.

solitārius, -a, -um. Solitary.

somnificus, -a, -um. Sleep-producing.

somnus, -ī. *m.* Sleep.

sopor, -ōris. *m.* Deep sleep.

spectrum, -ī. *n.* Image.

spēs, speī. *f.* Hope.

sphenoideus, -a, -um. Wedge-shaped; sphenoid.

spīna, -ae. *f.* (A thorn), a process on the surface of a bone; the backbone.

spinālis, -e. Spinal.

spinōsus, -a, -um. Spiny.

spirālis, -e. Spiral.

spiritus, -ūs. *m.* Spirit.

splēnius, -a, -um. Resembling the spleen; applied to a muscle of the back and neck.

spongiōsus, -a, -um. Spongy.

squamōsus, -a, -um. Scaly; squamous.

stapēdius, -ī. *m.* A muscle acting upon the stapes; stapedius.

stertor, -ōris. *m.* Snoring.

stomachālis, -e. Stomachic.

stomachus, -ī. *m.* Stomach.

stramōnium, -ī. *n.* Jamestown weed; stramonium.

stria, -ae. *f.* Stripe; stria.

striātus, -a, -um. Striped; striated.

struō, -ēre, -xī, -ctus. Arrange.

strychnīna, -ae. *f.* Strychnine.

subacetās, -ātis. *m.* Subacetate.

subanconeus, -a, -um. Under the elbow.

subitō. Suddenly.

subitus, -a, -um. Sudden.

sublīmis, -e. Deep.

submuriās, -ātis. *m.* Submuriate.

subnitras, -ātis. *m.* Subnitrate.

subscapulāris, -e. Under the scapula; subscapular.

substantia, -ae. *f.* Substance.

subsultus, -ūs. *m.* A jumping; a twitching.

succus, -ī. *m.* Juice.

sudor, -ōris. *m.* Sweat.

sulcus, -ī. *m.* Furrow.

sulphās, -ātis. *m.* Sulfate.

sulphonal. Sulfonal.

sulphuricus, -a, -um. Sulfuric.

sum, esse, fui. Be.

sūmō, -ēre, -psi, -ptus. Take.

supercilium, -ī. *n.* Eyebrow.

superficialis, -e. Superficial.

superficiēs, -ēī. *f.* Surface.

suppositōrium, -ī. *n.* Suppository.

supraspinātus, -a, -um. Above the spine (of scapula); supraspinate.

suspensōrium, -ī. *n.* That which suspends.

suspensōrius, -a, -um. Suspensory.

sustentaculum, -ī. *n.* A prop; support.

sutūra, -ae. *f.* Seam; suture.

sympatheticus, -a, -um. Sympathetic.

symptōma, -atis. *n.* Symptom.

synoviālis, -e. Synovial.

tabacum, -ī. *n.* Tobacco.

taenia, -ae. *f.* A band. (t. semicirculāris, a layer in the cerebrum; also a genus of intestinal worms, the tapeworm).

talus, -ī. *m.* The heel.

tam. So.

tapētum, -ī. *n.* (tapēte, carpet, tapestry), a lining membrane; also, the radiating fibers of the corpus callōsum.

taraxacum, -ī. *n.* Dandelion root; taraxacum.

tarsus, -ī. *m.* Ankle.

tartaricus, -a, -um. Tartaric.

tartrās, -ātis. *m.* Tartrate.

tectōrium, -ī. *n.* A covering.

tectōrius, -a, -um. Protecting; covering.

tegō, -ēre, -xī, -ctum. Cover; protect.

temporālis, -e. Temporal.

tempus, -oris. *n.* Time.

tenax, -ācis. Holding fast; tenacious.

tendineus, -a, -um. Tendinous.

tendō, -ēre, tetendī, tentus. Stretch; reach.

tendō, -dinis. *m.* Tendon.

teneō, -ēre, -uī, -tus. Keep; hold.

tener, -a, -um. Delicate; tender.

tensor, -ōris. *m.* Stretcher; tensor.

tentō, -āre, -āvī, -ātus. Test, try.

tentōrium, -ī. *n.* A tent; covering.

tenuis, -e. Thin; small.

tepidus, -a, -um. Lukewarm.

terebinthina, -ae. *f.* Turpentine.

teres, -etis. Rounded; smooth.

tergum, -ī. *n.* Back.

terminus, -ī. *m.* End.

tertius, -a, -um. Third.

theobrōma, -ātis. *n.* Cacao (food of the gods).

thoracicus, -a, -um. Thoracic.

thyroideus, -a, -um. Having the shape of an oblong shield; thyroid.

tiglium, -ī. *n.* The specific name of the croton oil plant.

tinctūra, -ae. *f.* Tincture.

tonicus, -a, -um. Tonic.

tonsilla, -ae. *f.* Tonsil.

torcular, -āris. *n.* A wine press.

tracheālis, -e. Tracheal.

tractō, -āre, -āvī, -ātus. Handle.

Latin Medical Words (*Continued*)

tragus, -ī. *m.* Small nipple in front of external auditory meatus, so called because sometimes covered with hair; tragus.

transversālis, -e. Transverse.

transversus, -a, -um. Transverse.

trapezoideus, -a, -um. Like a trapezium; trapezoid.

trauma, -atis. *n.* Injury; wound.

trēs, tria. Three.

triangulāris, -e. Triangular.

triceps, -ipitis. Three-headed.

trigeminus, -a, -um. Three-fold.

trīgīnta. Thirty.

trigōnum, -ī. *n.* Triangle.

triquetrus, -a, -um. Three-cornered; triangular.

trochiscus, -ī. *m.* Troche.

tuba, -ae. *f.* (Trumpet), tube.

tuber, -eris. *n.* Swelling, protuberance.

tuberculum, -ī. *n.* A protuberance; tubercle.

tubulus, -ī. *m.* Small tube.

tubus, -ī. *m.* Tube.

tunica, -ae. *f.* Coat; covering.

tussiō, -īre, -īvī, -ītus. Cough.

tūtāmen, -minis. *n.* Means of defense; a protection.

tūtō. Safely.

tympanicus, -a, -um. Of the tympanum; tympanic.

ubi. Where.

ulna, -ae. *f.* Larger bone of forearm; ulna.

ulnāris, -e. Of the ulna; ulnar.

uncia, -ae. *f.* Ounce.

unciformis, -e. Hooked.

uncinātus, -a, -um. Hooked; uncinate.

unguentum, -ī. *n.* Ointment.

unguis, -is. *m.* Nail.

ūnus, -a, -um. One.

urbānus, -a, -um. Of the city; urbane.

urīna, -ae. *f.* Urine.

uriniferus, -a, -um. Urine-bearing; uriniferous.

usque. Continuously; constantly.

uterīnus, -a, -um. Of the uterus; uterine.

ūtilis, -e. Useful.

uvula, -ae. *f.* A small appendix or tubercle; uvula.

uxor, -ōris. *f.* Wife.

vaginālis, -e. Sheathlike; vaginal.

valeriānās, -ātis. *m.* Valerianate.

valetūdō, -inis. *f.* Health.

validus, -a, -um. Strong; sturdy; healthy.

valvula, -ae. *f.* Valve.

vās, vāsis. *n.* Vessel.

vasculōsus, -a, -um. Vascular.

vasculum, -ī. *n.* Small vessel.

vastus, -a, -um. Extensive; large.

vegetābilis, -e. Vegetable.

vehiculum, -ī. *n.* Vehicle.

vel. Either.

vēlum, -ī. *n.* Veil.

vēna, -ae. *f.* Vein.

vendō, -ēre, vendidī. Sell.

veneficus, -ī. *m.* Poisoner.

venēnum, -ī. *n.* Poison.

venōsus, -a, -um. Venous.

venter, -tris. *m.* Belly.

ventriculus, -ī. *m.* Ventricle.

vērātrum, -ī. *n.* Hellebore; veratrum.

vermiformis, -e. Wormlike.

veru, -ūs. *n.* A spit (for roasting upon); used only in **verumontanum,** a longitudinal ridge in the floor of the male urethra.

verus, -a, -um. True.

vesica, -ae. *f.* Urinary bladder.

vesicatōrium, -ī. *n.* Blister.

vesicula, -ae. *f.* Vesicle.

vesiculāris, -e. Full of vesicles or cells; vesicular.

vestibulāris, -e. Relating to the vestibule of the ear; vestibular.

vetus, veteris. Old.

vigilō, -āre, -āvī, -ātus. Watch.

vīgintī. Twenty.

villus, -ī. *m.* Tuft of hair; villus.

vinculum, -ī. *n.* Link; chain.

vinum, -ī. *n.* Wine.

vir, virī. *m.* Man.

viridis, -e. Green.

vīs, vīs, pl. vīres, -ium. *f.* Force; power.

viscus, -eris. *n.* Any internal organ of the body.

visiō, -ōnis. *f.* Vision.

vīsus, -ūs. *m.* Vision.

vīta, -ae. *f.* Life.

vitellus, -ī. *m.* Yolk.

vitreus, -a, -um. Resembling glass; vitreous.

vocālis, -e. Vocal.

vocō, -āre, -āvī, -ātus. Call.

vola, -ae. *f.* Palm of the hand (sole of the foot).

vorticōsus, -a, -um. Resembling an eddy or whirlpool.

vulnerō, -āre, -āvī, -ātus. Wound.

vulnus, vulneris. *n.* A wound.

vultus, -ūs. *m.* Countenance.

zincum, -ī. *n.* Zinc.

zingiber, -eris. *n.* Ginger.

zōna, -ae. *f.* Zone; belt.

zōnula, -ae. *f.* Little zone, or belt; zonule.

SEE: *prescription writing.*

English with Latin and Greek Equivalents

acid. Acidum.
ague. Febris.
and. Et.
arm. Brachium. Gr., brachion.
artery. Arteria.
attachment. Adhesio.
back. Tergum; dorsum.
backbone. Spina.
backward. Retro.
bath. Balneum.
beef. Bubula.
belly. Venter; abdomen.
bend. Flexus.
bile. Bilis. Gr., chole.
bladder. Vesica.
bleed. Fluere.
blind. Obscurus.
blister. Pustulo; vesicatorium.
bloat. Tumeo.
blood. Sanguis. Gr., haima.
blood vessel. Vena.
body. Corpus. Gr., soma.
boiling up. Effervescens.
bone. Os. Gr., osteon.
bony. Osseus.
bowels. Intestina; viscera.
bowlegged. Valgus.
brain. Cerebrum. Gr., enkephalos.
breach. Ruptura.
breast. Mamma. Gr., mastos.
breath. Halitus.
bubble. Pustula.
bulb. Bulbus.
buttock. Clunis. Gr., gloutos.
calcareous. Calci similis.
canal. Canalis.
cartilage. Cartilago. Gr., chondros.
catarrh. Coryza.
cavity. Caverna.
change. Mutatio.
chest. Thorax. Gr., thorax.
chin. Mentum. Gr., geneion.
choke. Strangulo.
clavicle. Clavicula.
confinement. Puerperium.
congestion. Conglobatio.
consumption. Phthisis, pulmonaria.
convulsion. Convulsio.
cord. Corda.
corn. Callus-clavus.
cornea. Cornu. Gr., keras.
costive. Astrictus.
cough. Tussio.
countenance. Vultus.
cramp. Spasmus.
crisis. Dies crisimus.
cup. Poculum.
cure. Sano.
curvature. Curvatura.

cuticle. Cuticula.
daily. Diurnus.
dandruff. Furfures capitas.
day. Dies.
dead. Mortuus; defunctus.
deadly. Lethalis.
deafness. Surditas.
decompose. Dissolvo.
dental. Dentalis.
depression. Depressio.
digestive. Digestorius; pepticus.
dilute. Dilutus.
discharge. Eluvies; effluens.
disease. Morbus.
dorsal. Dorsalis.
dose. Potio.
dram. Drachma.
drink. Bibo; potis.
dropsy. Hydrops; opis.
drug. Medicamentum.
duct. Ductus.
dysentery. Dysenteria.
ear. Auris. Gr., ous.
eat. Edo.
egg. Ovum.
elbow. Cubitum. Gr., ankon.
embryo. Partus immaturus.
emission. Emissio.
entrails. Viscera.
epidemic. Epidemus.
epilepsy. Morbus comitalis; epilepsia.
epileptic. Epilepticus.
erection. Erectio.
erotic. Amatorius.
eunuch. Eunuchus.
every. Omnis.
excrement. Excrementum.
excretion. Excrementum; excretio.
exhalation. Exhalatio.
exhale. Exhalo.
expel. Expello.
expire. Expiro.
external. Externus.
extract. Extractum.
eye. Oculus. Gr., ophthalmos.
eyeball. Pupula.
eyebrow. Supercilium.
eyelid. Palpebra.
eyetooth. Dens caninus.
face. Facies.
faculty. Facultas.
faint. Collabor.
fat. Adeps. Gr., lipos.
feature. Lineomentum.
febrile. Febriculosus.
fecundity. Fecunditas.
feel. Tactus.
fever. Febris.
film. Membranula.

English with Latin and Greek Equivalents (*Continued*)

filter. Percolo.
finger. Digitus. Gr., daktylos.
fistula. Fistula putris.
fit. Accessus.
flesh. Carnis. Gr., sarx.
fluid. Fluidus.
food. Cibus.
foot. Pes, pedis. Gr., pous.
forearm. Brachium.
forehead. Frons.
freckle. Lentigo.
gall. Bilis.
gangrene. Gangraena.
gargle. Gargarizo.
gland. Glandula.
gleet. Ichor.
gout. Morbus articularis; (in feet), podagra.
grain. Granum.
gravel. Calculus.
grinder tooth. Dens maxillaris.
gullet. Gula.
gum. Gingiva.
gut. Intestinum.
hair. Capillus. Gr., thrix.
half. Dimidius.
hand. Manus. Gr., cheir.
harelip. Labrum fissum.
haunch. Clunis.
head. Caput. Gr., kephale.
heal. Sano.
healer. Medicus.
healing. Salutaris.
health. Sanitas.
healthful. Salutaris; saluber.
healthy. Sanus.
hear. Audio.
hearing. Auditio; (sense of) auditus.
heart. Cor. Gr., kardia.
heartburn. Redundatio stomachi.
heat. Calor.
hectic. Hecticus.
heel. Calx, talus.
hirsute. Hirsutus.
homeopathic. Homeopathicus.
hysterics. Hysteria.
illness. Morbus.
incisor. Dens acutus.
infant. Infans; puerilis.
infect. Inficio.
infectious. Contagiosus.
infirm. Infirmus; debilis.
inflammation. Inflammatio; (of lungs) inflammatio pulmonaria.
injection. Injectio.
insane. Insanus.
intellect. Intellectus.
intercourse. Congressus.
internal. Intestinus.
intestine. Intestinum. Gr., enteron.
itch. Scabies.

itching. Pruritus.
jaw. Maxilla.
joint. Artus. Gr., arthron.
jugular vein. Vena jugularis.
kidney. Ren. Gr., nephros.
knee. Genu. Gr., gonu.
kneepan. Patella.
knuckle. Condylus.
labor. Partus.
labyrinth. Labyrinthus.
lacerate. Lacero.
larynx. Guttur.
lateral. Lateralis.
leech. Sanguisuga.
leg. Tibia.
leprosy. Leprosus.
ligament. Ligamentum. Gr., syndesmos.
ligature. Ligatura.
limb. Membrum.
lime. Calx.
listen. Ausculto.
liver. Jecur. Gr., hepar.
livid. Lividus.
loin. Lumbus. Gr., lapara.
looseness. Laxitas.
lotion. Lotio.
lukewarm. Tepidus.
lung. Pulmo. Gr., pneumon.
lymph. Lympha.
mad. Insanus.
malady. Morbus.
male. Masculinus.
malignant. Malignus.
maternity. Conditio matris.
medicated. Medicatus.
medicine. (Remedy) Medicamentum.
milk. Lac.
mind. Animus.
mix. Misceo.
mixture. Mistura.
moist. Humidus.
molar. Dens molaris.
month. Mensis.
monthly. Menstruus.
morbid. Morbidus.
mouth. Os. Gr., stoma.
mucous. Mucosus.
muscle. Musculus. Gr., mys.
mustard. Sinapis.
nail. Unguis.
navel. Umbilicus. Gr., omphalos.
neck. Cervix; collum. Gr., trachelos.
nerve. Nervus. Gr., neuron.
nipple. Papilla.
no, none. Nullus.
normal. Normalis.
nose. Nasus. Gr., rhis.
nostril. Naris.
not. Non.
nourish. Nutrio.

nourishment. Alimentus.
now. Nunc.
nudity. Nudatio.
nurse. Nutrix.
obesity. Obesitas.
ocular. Ocularis.
oculist. Ocularis medicus.
oil. Oleum.
ointment. Unguentum.
operator. Manus curatio.
opiate. Medicamentum somnificum.
optics. Optice.
orifice. Foramen.
pain. Dolor.
palate. Palatum.
palm. Palma.
parasite. Parasitus.
part. Pars.
patient. Patiens.
pectoral. Pectoralis.
pedal. Pedale.
phlegm. Pituita.
pill. Pilus.
pimple. Pustula.
plaster. Emplastrum.
poison. Venenum.
poultice. Cataplasma.
powder. Pulvis.
pregnant. Gravida.
prepare. Paro.
prescribe. Praescribo.
prescription. Praescriptum.
puberty. Pubertas.
pubic bone. Os pubis. Gr., pecten.
pulverize. Pulvero.
pupil. Pupilla.
purgative. Purgativus.
putrid. Putridus.
quinsy. Cynanche; angina.
rash. Exanthema.
recover. Convalesco.
recumbent. Recumbens.
recur. Recurro.
redness. Rubor.
remedy. Remedium.
respiration. Respiratio.
rheum. Fluxio.
rib. Costa.
rigid. Rigidus.
ringing. Tinnitus.
rupture. Hernia.
saliva. Sputum.
sallow. Salix.
salt. Sal.
salve. Unguentum.
sane. Sanus.
scab. Scabies.
scalp. Pericranium.
scaly. Squamosus.
scar. Cicatrix.

sciatica. Ischias.
scruple. Scrupulum.
seed. Semen.
senile. Senilis.
serum. Sanguinis pars equosa.
sheath. Vagina.
shin. Tibia.
shock. Concussio; (of electricity), ictus electricus.
short. Brevis.
shoulder. Humerus. Gr., omos.
shoulder blade. Scapula.
shudder. Tremor.
sick. Aegrotus.
side. Latus.
sinew. Nervus.
skeleton. Gr., skeleton.
skin. Cutis. Gr., derma.
skull. Cranium. Gr., kranion.
sleep. Somnus.
smallpox. Variola.
smell. Odoratus.
soap. Sapo.
socket. Cavum.
soft. Mollis.
solid. Solidus.
solution. Dilutum.
soporific. Soporus.
sore. Ulcus.
spasm. Spasmus.
spinal. Dorsalis; spinalis.
spine. Spina.
spirit. Spiritus.
spittle. Sputum.
spleen. Lien.
spoon. Cochleare.
sprain. Luxatio.
stomach. Stomachus. Gr., gaster.
stone. Calculus.
stricture. Strictura.
sugar. Saccharum.
suture. Sutura.
swallow. Glutio.
sweat. Sudor. Gr., hidros.
symptom. Symptoma.
system. Systema.
tail. Cauda.
take. Sumo.
tapeworm. Taenia.
taste. Gustatus.
tear. Lacrima.
teeth. Dentes.
tendon. Tendo. Gr., tenon.
testicle. Testis. Gr., orchis.
thigh. Femur.
throat. Fauces. Gr., pharynx.
throb. Palpito.
thumb. Pollex.
tongue. Lingua. Gr., glossa.
tonsil. Tonsilla.

English with Latin and Greek Equivalents (*Continued*)

tooth. Dens. Gr., odous.
troche. Trochiscus.
tube. Tuba.
twin. Geminus.
twitching. Subsultus.
ulcer. Ulcus.
unless. Nisi.
urine. Urina.
uterine. Uterinus.
vaccine. Vaccinum.
vagina. Vagina. Gr., kolpos.
valve. Valvula.
vein. Vena. Gr., phleps.
vertebra. Vertebra. Gr., spondylos.
vessel. Vas.

wash. Lavo.
water. Aqua.
wax. Cera.
waxed dressing. Ceratum.
weary. Lassus.
wet. Humidus.
windpipe. Arteria aspera.
wine. Vinum.
woman. Femina.
womb. Uterus. Gr., hystera.
worm. Vermis.
wound. Vulnus.
wrist. Carpus. Gr., karpos.
yolk. Luteum.

COLORS

black. Niger; nigra; nigrum.
blue. Caeruleus; cyaneus; lividus.
brown. Fulvus.
crimson. Coccum; coccineus.
gray. Cinereus.
green. Viridis.
lemon. Citreum.
pink. Rosaceus.
purple. Purpura; purpureus.
red. Ruber.
scarlet. Coccineus.
violet. Violaceus.
white. Albus.
yellow. Flavus; luteus; croceus.

QUALITIES

bitter. Acerbus.
chill. Friguscolum.
cold. Frigidus.
dry. Aridus.
dull. Stupidus; hebes.
faintness. Languor.
fat. Obesus; pinguis.
heat. Calor; ardor; fervor.
short. Brevis.
sour. Acidus.
sweet. Dulcis.
tall. Longus; celsus; procerus.
thick. Densus.
heavy. Gravis; ponderosus.
hot. Calidus; fervens; candens.
light. Levis.
liquid. Liquidus.
moist. Humidus; uvidus.
sharp. Acutus.
thin. Tenuis; macer.
warm. Calidus.
warmth. Calor.
weary. Lassus; languidus; fatigatus.
wet. Humidus.

METALS

copper. Cuprum; cuprinus.
gold. Aurum; aureus.
iron. Ferrum; ferreus.

silver. Argentum; argenteus.
tin. Stannum; plumbum album.

TIME

afternoon. Post meridiem.
age. Aetas; maturas; adultus; impubis.
autumn. Autumnus.
birth. Partus; natales.
breakfast. Prandium.
child. Infans; puer; filius.
daily. Diurnus.
date. Status dies.
dawn. Prima lux.
day. Dies.
death. Mors.
dinner. Cena.
evening. Vesper.
hour. Hora.
infant. Infans.
maturity. Maturitas; aetas matura.
meal. Epulae.
midnight. Media nox.
midsummer. Media aestas.
moment. Punctum.
month. Mens.
monthly. Menstruus.
morning. Matutinum.
night. Nox, noctis.
noon. Meridies.
old. Antiquus.
puberty. Pubertas.
second. Secundum.
spring. Ver; veris.
summer. Aestas.
sunrise. Solis ortus.
sunset. Solis occasus.
supper. Cena.
time. Tempus.
winter. Hiems, hiemis.
year. Annus.
young. Parvus; infans.
youth. Adolescentia.

NUMERALS (ROMAN)

SEE: *Latin Numerals* in *Appendix.*

Greek and Latin Singulars and Plurals

Singular	Plural	Singular	Plural
addendum	addenda	focus	foci
aden	adena	fornix	fornices
adenoma	adenomata	fossa	fossae
ala	alae	glans	glandes
albacans	albacantes	gonad	gonades
amygdala	amygdalae	gonococcus	gonococci
antenna	antennae	gyrus	gyri
antiad	antiades	ilium	ilia
antrum	antra	keratosis	keratoses
apertura	aperturae	labium	labia
apex	apices	lamina	laminae
aponeurosis	aponeuroses	loculus	loculi
appendix	appendices	locus	loci
aqua	aquae	medium	media
arcus	arcus	mucosa	mucosae
ascaris	ascarides	naevus	naevi
ascus	asci	nodus	nodi
atrium	atria	nox	noxa
axis	axes	os	ora
bacillus	bacilli	ovum	ova
bacterium	bacteria	papilla	papillae
bronchus	bronchi	pathema	pathemata
bulla	bullae	pes	pedes
bursa	bursae	petechia	petechiae
cactus	cacti	pilula	pilulae
cadaver	cadavera	polypus	polypi
calcaneum	calcanea	ramus	rami
calculus	calculi	septum	septa
calix	calices	sequestrum	sequestra
cantharis	cantharides	serosa	serosae
canthus	canthi	spasmus	spasmi
cornu	cornua	spectrum	spectra
corpus	corpora	speculum	specula
crisis	crises	sperma	spermata
cuniculus	cuniculi	stoma	stomata
dens	dentes	sudamen	sudamina
diagnosis	diagnoses	sulcus	sulci
diaphoreticus	diaphoretici	tarsus	tarsi
diastema	diastemata	tela	telae
digitus	digiti	tinctura	tincturae
dorsum	dorsi	toxicosis	toxicoses
echolatus	echolati	typha	typhae
enema	enemata	ulcus	ulcera
ensis	enses	varix	varices
epididymis	epididymides	vas	vasa
esthesis	estheses	vesicula	vesiculae
fibroma	fibromata	vis	vires
filix	filices	viscus	viscera
filum	fila	vomica	vomicae
flagellum	flagella	zygoma	zygomata

Numerals, Latin

Cardinals		Ordinals	
1	unus	1st	primus
2	duo	2nd	secundus
3	tres	3rd	tertius
4	quattuor	4th	quartus
5	quinque	5th	quintus
6	sex	6th	sextus
7	septem	7th	septimus
8	octō	8th	octāvus
9	novem	9th	nōnus
10	decem	10th	decimus
11	ūndecim	11th	ūndecimus
12	duodecim	12th	duodecimus
13	tredecim	13th	tertius decimus
14	quattuordecim	14th	quartus decimus
15	quīndecim	15th	quīntus decimus
16	sēdecim	16th	septus decimus
17	septendecim	17th	septimus decimus
18	duodēvīgintī	18th	duodēvīcēsimus
19	ūndēvīgintī	19th	ūndēvīcēsimus
20	vīgintī	20th	vīcēsimus
21	vīgintī ūnus, *or* ūnus et vīgintī	21st	vīcēsimus primus, *or* prīmus et vīcēsimus
22	vīgintī duo, *or* duo et vīgintī	22nd	vīcēsimus secundus, *or* duo et vīcēsimus
28	duodētrīgintā	28th	duodētrīcēsimus
29	ūndētrīgintā	29th	ūndētrīcēsimus
30	trīgintā	30th	trīcēsimus
40	quadrāgintā	40th	quadrāgēsimus
50	quīnquāgintā	50th	quīnquāgēsimus
60	sexāgintā	60th	sexāgēsimus
70	septuāgintā	70th	septuāgēsimus
80	octōgintā	80th	octōgēsimus
90	nōnāgintā	90th	nōnāgēsimus
100	centum	100th	centēsimus
101	centum ūnus, *or* centum et ūnus	101st	centēsimus prīmus, centēsimus et prīmus
102	centum duo, *or* centum et duo	102nd	centēsimus secundus, centēsimus et secundus
200	ducentī	200th	ducentēsimus
300	trecentī	300th	trecentēsimus
400	quadringentī	400th	quadringentēsimus
500	quīngentī	500th	quīngentēsimus
600	sēscentī, *or* sexcentī	600th	sēscentēsimus
700	septingentī	700th	septingentēsimus
800	octingentī	800th	octingentēsimus
900	nōngentī	900th	nōngentēsimus
1,000	mīlle	1,000th	mīllēsimus
2,000	duo mīllia	2,000th	bis mīllēsimus
10,000	decem millia	10,000th	decies mīllēsimus
100,000	centum mīllia	100,000th	centiēs mīllēsimus

Numerals, Roman

A line placed over a letter increases its value one thousand times.

1	I	6	VI	11	XI	40	XL	90	XC	5000	$\overline{\text{V}}$
2	II	7	VII	12	XII	50	L	100	C	10,000	$\overline{\text{X}}$
3	III	8	VIII	15	XV	60	LX	500	D	100,000	$\overline{\text{C}}$
4	IV	9	IX	20	XX	70	LXX	1000	M	1,000,000	$\overline{\text{M}}$
5	V	10	X	30	XXX	80	LXXX	2000	MM		

Prefixes and Suffixes

a-, an. Negative.

a-, ab-, abs-. Away from.

ad-, -ad. Toward.

-aemia. Blood.

aer-. Air.

-aesthesia. Sensation.

-algesia, algia. Suffering; pain.

algi-. Pain.

all-. Other.

amb-. Both; on both sides.

amph-. Around; on both sides.

ana-, an-. Up.

angio-. Relating to blood or lymph vessels.

ante-. Before.

anti-. Against.

apo-. From; opposed.

-ase. Enzyme.

aut-, auto-. Self.

bi, bis-. Twice; double.

brachy-. Short.

brady-. Slow.

cac-, caco-. Bad; evil.

cat, cata, cath-. Down.

-cele. A tumor; a cyst; a hernia.

cent-. Hundred.

cephal-. Relating to a head.

chrom-, chromo-. Color.

-cide. Causing death.

circum-. Around.

co, com, con-. Together.

contra-. Against.

cyst-, -cyst. Bag; bladder.

-cyte. A cell.

dacry-. Tears.

dactyl-. Fingers.

de-. From; not.

deca-. Ten.

deci-. Tenth.

demi-. Half.

dent-. Relating to the teeth.

derma-. The skin.

di-. Double; apart from.

dia-. Through; between; asunder.

dipla, diplo-. Double.

dis-. Negative; double; apart; absence of.

-dynia. Pain.

dys-. Difficult; bad.

ec, ecto-. Out; on the outside.

-ectomy. A cutting out.

ef, es, ex, exo-. Out.

-emesis. Vomiting.

-emia. Blood.

en-. In, into.

endo-. Within.

entero-. Relating to the intestine.

ento-. Within.

epi-. Upon.

-esthesia. Sensation.

eu-. Well.

ex-, exo-. Out.

extra-. On the outside; beyond.

fore-. Before; in front of.

-form. Form.

-fuge. To drive away.

galact, galacto-. Milk.

gaster, gastro-. The stomach; the belly.

-gene, -genesis, -genetic, -genic. Production; origin; formation.

glosso-. Relating to the tongue.

-gog, gogue. To make flow.

-gram. A tracing; a mark.

-graphy. A writing; a record.

hem, hemato-. Relating to the blood.

hemi-. Half.

hepa-, hepar-, hepato-. Liver.

hetero-. Other; indicating dissimilarity.

holo-. All.

homo, homeo-. Same; similar.

hydra, hydro-. Relating to water.

hyp, hyph, hypo-. Under.

hyper-. Over; above; beyond.

hypo-. Under.

-iasis. Condition; pathological state.

idio-. Peculiar to the individual or organ.

ileo-. Relating to the ileum.

in-. In; into; not.

infra-. Beneath.

inter-. Between.

intra, intro-. Within.

-ism. Condition; theory.

iso-. Equal.

-itis. Inflammation.

-ize. To treat by special method.

juxta-. Near.

karyo-. Nucleus; nut.

kata-, kath-. Down.

kera-. Horn; indicates hardness.

kinesi-. Movement.

-kinesis. Motion.

lact-. Milk.

laparo-. The loin; relating to the loin or abdomen.

laryng, laryngo-. The larynx.

latero-. Side.

lepto-. Small; soft.

leuko-. White.

-lite, -lith. A stone; a calculus.

lith-. A stone.

-logia, -logy. Science of; study of.

-lysis. Setting free; disintegration.

macro-. Large; long; big.

mal-. Bad; poor; evil.

med-, medi-. Middle.

mega, megal-. Large; great.

-megalia or megaly. Large; great; extreme.

melan-, melano-. Black.

mes-, meso-. Middle.

meta-. Beyond; over; between; change, or transposition.

-meter. Measure.

metra, metro-. The uterus.
micro-. Small.
mio-. Less; smaller.
mono-. Single.
multi-. Many.
my, myo-. Muscle.
myel, myelo-. Marrow.
myxa, myxo-. Mucus.
neo-. New.
nephr, nephra, nephro-. Kidney.
neu, neuro-. Nerve.
niter, nitro-. Nitrogen.
non-, not-. No.
nucleo-. Nucleus.
ob-. Against.
oculo-. The eye.
-ode, oid. Form; shape; resemblance.
odont-. A tooth.
-oid. Form; shape; resemblance.
oligo-. Few.
-oma. A tumor.
omo-. Shoulder.
o-. An egg; ovum.
oophoron-. Ovary.
opisth-. Backward.
orchid-. Testicle.
ortho-. Straight; normal.
os-. A mouth; a bone.
-osis. Condition; disease; intensive.
oste, osteo-. A bone.
-ostomosis, ostomy. To furnish with a mouth or an outlet.
-otomy. Cutting.
oxy-. Sharp; acid.
pachy-. Thick.
pan-. All; entire.
para-. Alongside of.
path-, -path, -pathy. Disease; suffering.
-penia. Lack.
per-. Excessive; through.
peri-. Around.
-phobia. Fear.
-phylaxis. Protection.
-plasm. To mold.
-plastic. Molded; indicates restoration of lost or badly formed features.

-plegia. A stroke.
plur-. More.
pneu-. Relating to the air or lungs.
poly-. Much; many.
post-. After.
pre-. Before.
pro-. Before; in behalf of.
proto-. First.
pseud-, pseudo-. False.
psych-. The soul; the mind.
py-, pyo-. Pus.
re-. Back; again.
retro-. Backward.
-rhage, -rhagia. Hemorrhage; flow.
-rhaphy. A suturing or stitching.
-rhea. To flow; indicates discharge.
sacchar-. Sugar.
sacro-. Sacrum.
salping, salpingo-. A tube; relating to a fallopian tube.
sarco-. Flesh.
sclero-. Hard; relating to the sclera.
-sclerosis. Dryness; hardness.
-scopy. To see.
semi-. Half.
-stomosis, -stomy. To furnish with a mouth or outlet.
sub-. Under.
super, supra-. Above.
syn-. With; together.
tele-. Distant; far.
tetra-. Four.
thio-. Sulfur.
thyro-. Thyroid gland.
-tomy. Cutting.
trans-. Across.
tri-. Three.
-trophic. Relating to nourishment.
tropho-. Relating to nutrition.
uni-. One.
-uria. Relating to the urine.
urino, uro-. Relating to the urine or urinary organs.
vaso-. A vessel.
venter, ventro-. The abdomen.
xanth-. Yellow.

Anatomy and Physiology

Muscles of the Body with Their Action, Origin, Insertion and Innervation

The muscles in the body number over 650, the totals varying according to the authority, as some list as separate muscles what others regard as portions of adjacent muscles. Most of the muscles occur in pairs; five are single muscles.

HEAD AND FACE

attolens aurem (ăt-ōl'ĕnz aw'rĕm). SAME AS: *auricularis superior.*

attrahens aurem (ăt'ră-hĕnz aw'rĕm). SAME AS: *auricularis anterior.*

auricularis anterior (aw-rĭk″ū-lā'rĭs an-tē'rĭ-or). ACTION: Draws pinna of ear forward. ORIGIN: Superficial temporal fascia. INSERTION: Helix of ear anteriorly. INNERVATION: Facial. SYN: *atrahens aurem.*

auricularis posterior (aw-rĭk″ū-lā'rĭs pŏs-tē'rĭ-or). ACTION: Draws pinna of ear backward. ORIGIN: Mastoid process. INSERTION: Root of auricle. INNERVATION: Facial. SYN: *retrahens aurem.*

auricularis superior (aw-rĭk″ū-lā'rĭs sū-pē'rĭ-or). ACTION: Elevates pinna of ear. ORIGIN: Galea aponeurotica. INSERTION: Upper portion of pinna of ear. INNERVATION: Facial. SYN: *attolens aurem.*

buccinator (bŭk″sĭn-ā'tor). ACTION: Compresses cheek, retracts angle of mouth. ORIGIN: Alveolar process of maxilla, pterygomandibular ligament, buccinator ridge of mandible. INSERTION: Orbicularis oris. INNERVATION: Facial.

caninus (kā-nī'nŭs). SAME AS: *levator anguli oris.*

choroideus (kō-roy'dē-ŭs). SAME AS: *ciliaris.*

ciliaris (sĭl-ĭ-ā'rĭs). ACTION: Alters shape of crystalline lens in accommodation. ORIGIN: (1) Meridional: Junction of cornea and sclera. (2) Circular: Fibers forming a circle close to iris. INSERTION: (1) External layers of choroid. (2) Ciliary process. INNERVATION: Short ciliary.

compressor naris (kòm-près'or nā'rĭs). Old term for pars transversa of nasalis muscle.

corrugator supercilii (kor'ū-gā-tor sū-pĕr-sĭl'ĭ-ī). ACTION: Draws eyebrows down and in. ORIGIN: Inner end of superciliary arch. INSERTION: Skin above orbital arch. INNERVATION: Facial.

depressor alae nasi (dē-près'or ā'lē nā'sī). SAME AS: *depressor septi.*

depressor anguli oris (dē-près'or ăng'ū-lī ō'rĭs). ACTION: Depresses angle of mouth. ORIGIN: External oblique line of mandible. INSERTION: Angle of mouth. INNERVATION: Facial. SYN: *triangularis.*

depressor labii inferioris (dē-près'or lā'-bĭ-ī ĭn-fē″rĭ-ō'rĭs). ACTION: Depresses lower lip. ORIGIN: External oblique line of the mandible. INSERTION: Lower lip and orbicularis oris. INNERVATION: Facial. SYN: *quadratus labii inferioris; quadratus menti.*

depressor septi (dē-près'or sĕp'tī). ACTION: Draws outer wall of nostril downward. ORIGIN: Incisive fossa of superior maxillary bone. INSERTION: Septum and ala of nose. INNERVATION: Facial. SYN: *depressor alae nasi.*

dilatator naris anterior (dĭl'ă-tā-tor nā'rĭs ăn-tē'rĭ-or). ACTION: Dilates apertures of nostril. ORIGIN: Cartilage of ala of nose. INSERTION: Border of ala. INNERVATION: Facial.

dilatator naris posterior (dĭl'ă-tā-tor nā'rĭs pŏs-tē'rĭ-or). ACTION: Dilates apertures of nostril. ORIGIN: Nasal notch of superior maxilla and the sesamoid cartilages. INSERTION: Integument of margin of nostril. INNERVATION: Facial.

epicranius (ĕp-ĭ-krā'nĭ-ŭs). Scalp muscles consisting of occipitofrontalis and temporoparietalis connected by galea aponeurotica.

frontalis (frŏn-tā'lĭs). SEE: *occipitofrontalis.*

levator anguli oris (lē-vā'tor ăng'ū-lī ō'rĭs). ACTION: Elevates angle of mouth. ORIGIN: Canine fossa of maxilla. INSERTION: Angle of mouth and orbicularis oris. INNERVATION: Facial. SYN: *caninus.*

levator labii inferioris (lē-vā'tor lā'bĭ-ī ĭn-fē″rĭ-ō'rĭs). SAME AS: *mentalis.*

levator labii superioris (lē-vā'tor lā'bĭ-ī sū-pē″rĭ-ō'rĭs). ACTION: Elevates and extends upper lip. ORIGIN: Lower margin of orbit, malar bone. INSERTION: Upper lip. INNERVATION: Infraorbital branch of facial.

levator labii superioris alaeque nasi (lē-vā'tor lā'bĭ-ī sū-pē″rĭ-ō'rĭs ā-lē'kwĕ nā'sī). ACTION: Elevates upper lip, dilates nostril. ORIGIN:

Muscles of the Body (Continued)

Nasal process of maxilla. INSERTION: Cartilage of ala of nose and upper lip. INNERVATION: Infraorbital branch of facial.

levator menti (lē-vă′tor mĕn′tī). SAME AS: *mentalis.*

levator palpebrae superioris (lē-vă′tor păl′pē-brē sū-pē″rĭ-ō′rĭs). ACTION: Raises upper eyelid. ORIGIN: Lesser wing of the sphenoid bone. INSERTION: Upper tarsal cartilage. INNERVATION: Oculomotor.

masseter (mă-sē′tĕr). ACTION: Mastication. ORIGIN: Zygomatic arch and malar process of superior maxilla. INSERTION: Angle ramus, and coronoid process of mandible. INNERVATION: Mandibular division of trigeminal.

mentalis (mĕn-tā′lĭs). ACTION: Elevates and protrudes lower lip; wrinkles skin of chin. ORIGIN: Incisive fossa of mandible. INSERTION: Integument of chin. INNERVATION: Facial. SYN: *levator labii inferioris; levator menti.*

nasalis (nă-sā′lĭs). Consists of pars transversa and depressor septi.

obliquus oculi inferior (ŏb-lī′kwŭs ŏc′ū-lī ĭn-fē′rĭ-or). ACTION: Rotates eyeball up and out. ORIGIN: Orbital plate of superior maxillary bone. INSERTION: Sclerotic coat at right angles to insertion of rectus externus just below it. INNERVATION: Oculomotor.

obliquus oculi superior (ŏb-lī′kwŭs ŏc′ū-lī sū-pē′rĭ-or). ACTION: Rotates eyeball down and out. ORIGIN: Above optic foramen. INSERTION: By a tendon through trochlea to the sclerotic coat. INNERVATION: Trochlear.

occipitalis (ŏk-sĭp″ĭ-tā′lĭs). SEE: *occipitofrontalis.*

occipitofrontalis (ŏk-sĭp″ĭ-tō-frŏn-tā′lĭs). Consists of (1) occipitalis and (2) frontalis bellies. ACTION: (1) Draws scalp back. (2) Draws scalp forward; raises eyebrows. ORIGIN: (1) Occipital and temporal bones. (2) Procerus, corrugator. and orbicularis oris muscles. INSERTION: Galea aponeurotica. INNERVATION: Facial.

orbicularis oculi (or-bĭk″ū-lā′rĭs ŏk′ū-lī). ACTION: Closes eyelid, wrinkles forehead vertically, compresses lacrimal sac. ORIGIN: (1) (*Pars lacrimalis*) Lacrimal bone. (2) (*Pars orbitalis*) Frontal processes of maxilla and frontal bone. (3) (*Pars palpebralis*) Inner canthus. INSERTION: (1) Joins palpebral portion. (2) Encircles orbit to orbit. (3) Outer canthus. INNERVATION: Facial.

orbicularis oris (or-bĭk″ū-lā′rĭs). ACTION: Closes lips. ORIGIN: Nasal septum and canine fossa of mandible by accessory fibers. INSERTION: Buccinator and adjacent muscles surrounding mouth. INNERVATION: Facial.

orbicularis palpebrarum (or-bĭk″ū-lā′rĭs păl-pē-brā′rŭm). SAME AS: *orbicularis oculi (Pars palpebralis).*

orbitalis (or-bĭ-tā′lĭs). Circular division of ciliaris.

orbitopalpebralis (or″bĭ-tō-păl″pē-brā′lĭs). SAME AS: *levator palpebrae superioris.*

procerus (prō-sē′rŭs). ACTION: Draws skin of forehead down. ORIGIN: Bridge of nose. INSERTION: Skin over root of nose. INNERVATION: Facial. SYN: *pyramidalis nasi.*

pterygoideus lateralis (tĕr-ĭ-goyd′ē-ŭs lăt-ĕr-ăl′ĭs). ACTION: Brings jaw forward; moves jaw from side to side; opens jaws. ORIGIN: (1) Outer plate of pterygoid process. (2) Great wing of sphenoid and infratemporal ridge. INSERTION: Neck of condyle of mandible. INNERVATION: Lateral pterygoid from trigeminal n.

pterygoideus medialis (tĕr-ĭ-goyd′ē-ŭs mē-dĭ-ā′lĭs). ACTION: Closes jaw by raising and advancing it. ORIGIN: Pterygoid fossa of sphenoid bone. INSERTION: Inner surface of angle of mandible. INNERVATION: Medial pterygoid from trigeminal n.

pyramidalis nasi (pī-răm″ĭ-dā′lĭs nā′sī). SAME AS: *procerus.*

quadratus labii inferioris (kwăd-rā′tŭs lā′-bĭ-ī ĭn-fē″rĭ-ō′rĭs). SAME AS: *depressor labii inferioris.*

quadratus labii superioris (kwăd-rā′tŭs lā′bĭ-ī sū-pēr″ĭ-ō′rĭs). Composed of *levator labii superioris alaeque nasi, levator labii superioris, zygomaticus minor.*

quadratus menti (kwăd-rā′tŭs mĕn′tī). SAME AS: *depressor labii inferioris.*

rectus externus or **lateralis** (rĕk′tŭs ĕks-ter′nŭs, lăt-ĕr-ā′lĭs). ACTION: Rotates eyeball outward. ORIGIN: Margin of sphenoidal fissure and outer margin of optic foramen. INSERTION: Sclerotic coat. INNERVATION: Abducent.

rectus inferior (rĕk′tŭs ĭn-fē′rĭ-or). ACTION: Rotates eyeball downward. ORIGIN: Lower margin of optic foramen. INSERTION: Sclerotic coat. INNERVATION: Oculomotor.

rectus internus or **medialis** (rĕk′tŭs ĭntĕr′-nŭs, mē-dĭ-ā′lĭs). ACTION: Rotates eyeball inward. ORIGIN: Lower margin of optic foramen. INSERTION: Sclerotic coat. INNERVATION: Oculomotor.

rectus superior (rĕk′tŭs sū-pē′rĭ-or). ACTION: Rotates eyeball upward. ORIGIN: Upper margin of optic foramen. INSERTION: Sclerotic coat. INNERVATION: Oculomotor.

retrahens aurem (rĕt′ră-hĕns aw′rĕm). SAME AS: *auricularis posterior.*

risorius (rĭ-sō′rĭ-ŭs). ACTION: Draws angle of mouth outward and compresses cheek (laughing muscle). ORIGIN: Fascia over masseter muscle. INSERTION: Angle of mouth. INNERVATION: Facial; buccal branch.

temporalis (tĕm-pō-rā′lĭs). ACTION: Closes jaws. ORIGIN: Temporal fossa and temporal fascia.

Muscles of the Body (*Continued*)

INSERTION: Coronoid process of lower jaw. INNERVATION: Trigeminal; mandibular division. SYN: *temporal*.

tensor tarsi (tĕn'sor tar'sĭ). SAME AS: *Pars lacrimalis of orbicularis oculi muscle.*

triangularis (trī-ăng"gū-lā'rĭs). SAME AS: *depressor anguli oris.*

zygomaticus major (zī-gō-măt'ĭ-kŭs mā'-jor). ACTION: Draws upper lip backward, upward and outward. ORIGIN: Malar bone, zygomatic arch. INSERTION: Angle of mouth. INNERVATION: Facial.

zygomaticus minor (zī-gō-măt'ĭ-kŭs mī'-nor). ACTION: Draws the upper lip up and out. ORIGIN: Malar bone behind the maxillary arch. INSERTION: Angle of mouth, orbicularis oris. INNERVATION: Facial.

EAR

antitragicus (an-tĭ-tră'jĭ-kŭs). ORGIN: Anterior part of antitragus. INSERTION: Opposite side at larger auricular fissure. INNERVATION: Posterior auricular branch of facial.

helicis major and **minor** (hĕl'ĭ-sĭs mā'jŏr, mī'nŏr). ACTION: Tighten the skin of auditory canal. ORIGIN: Tuberosity on helix. INSERTION: Rim of helix. INNERVATION: Auriculotemporal and posterior auricular.

obliquus auriculae (ŏb-lĭ'kwŭs aw-rĭk'ū-lē). ORIGIN: Conch of the ear. INSERTION: Fossa of antihelix. INNERVATION: Posterior auricular branch of facial.

stapedius (stă-pē'dĭ-ŭs). ACTION: Depress base of the stapes. ORIGIN: Interior of pyramid. INSERTION: Neck of stapes. INNERVATION: Tympanic branch of facial.

tensor tympani (tĕn'sor tĭm'păn-ĭ). ACTION: To draw the membrana tympani tense. ORIGIN: Temporal tube, eustachian tube and canal. INSERTION: Handle of malleus. INNERVATION: Branch of mandibular through otic ganglion.

tragicus (tră'jĭ-kŭs). ORIGIN and INSERTION: Outer part of tragus. INNERVATION: Temporal branch of facial.

transversus auriculae (trăns-vĕr'sŭs aw-rĭk'ū-lē). ACTION: Retracts helix. ORIGIN: Cranial surface of pinna. INSERTION: Circumference of pinna. INNERVATION: Posterior auricular branch of facial.

NECK

amygdaloglossus (ăm-ĭg"dă-lō-glŏs'ŭs). ACTION: Lifts edge of tongue. ORIGIN: Pharyngeal aponeurosis over tonsil. INSERTION: Continuous with palatoglossus.

azygos uvulae (ăz'ĭ-gŏs ū'vū-lē). SAME AS: *uvulae.*

cephalopharyngeus (sĕf"ă-lō-făr-ĭn-jē'ŭs). SAME AS: *constrictor pharyngis superior.*

circumflexus palati (sĭr-kŭm-flĕks'ŭs pal-ā'tĭ). SAME AS: *tensor veli palatini.*

constrictor pharyngis inferior (kŏn-strĭk'tor făr-ĭn'gĭs ĭn-fēr'ĭ-ŏr). ACTION: Narrows the pharynx, as in swallowing. ORIGIN: Sides of cricoid and thyroid cartilages. INSERTION: Posterior raphe of pharyngeal wall. INNERVATION: Pharyngeal plexus. SYN: *inferior constrictor; laryngopharyngeus.*

constrictor pharyngis medius (kŏn-strĭk'tor făr-ĭn'gĭs mē'dĭ-ŭs). ACTION: Narrows pharynx, as in swallowing. ORIGIN: Both cornua of hyoid bone and stylohyoid ligament. INSERTION: Middle of posterior pharyngeal wall. INNERVATION: Pharyngeal plexus. SYN: *middle constrictor; hyopharyngeus.*

constrictor pharyngis superior (kŏn-strĭk'tor făr-ĭn'gĭs sū-pēr'ĭ-ŏr). ACTION: Narrows pharynx, as in swallowing. ORIGIN: Internal pterygoid plate, pterygomandibular ligament, jaw, side of tongue. INSERTION: Posterior pharyngeal wall. INNERVATION: Pharyngeal plexus. SYN: *superior constrictor; cephalopharyngeus.*

digastricus (dī-găs'trĭ-kŭs). Consists of (1) anterior and (2) posterior bellies. ACTION: (1) Draws hyoid bone forward. (2) Draws hyoid bone backward. ORIGIN: (1) Lower border of lower jaw. (2) Mastoid groove of temporal bone. INSERTION: Intermediate tendon between both bellies. INNERVATION: (1) Mylohyoid. (2) Facial.

genioglossus (jē-nī"ō-glŏs'ŭs). ACTION: Protrudes and retracts tongue, elevates hyoid. ORIGIN: Mental spine of inferior maxilla. INSERTION: Hyoid and bottom of tongue. INNERVATION: Hypoglossal.

geniohyoglossus (jē-nī"ō-hī"ō-glŏs'ŭs). SAME AS: *genioglossus.*

geniohyoideus (jē-nī"ō-hī-oyd'ē-ŭs). ACTION: Elevates and advances hyoid and helps to depress jaw. ORIGIN: Mental spine of inferior maxilla. INSERTION: Hyoid. INNERVATION: Hypoglossal. SYN: *geniohyoid muscle.*

glossopalatinus (glŏs"ō-păl-ă-tī'nŭs). ACTION: Elevates back of tongue and constricts fauces. TION: Side of tongue. INNERVATION: Pharyngeal plexus. SYN: *palatoglossus.*

hyoglossus (hī"ō-glŏs'ŭs). ACTION: Depresses side of tongue and retracts tongue. ORIGIN: Cornua and body of hyoid. INSERTION: Side of tongue. INNERVATION: Hypoglossal.

hyopharyngeus (hī"ō-făr-ĭn-jē'ŭs). SAME AS: *constrictor pharyngis medius.*

laryngopharyngeus (lăr-ĭn"gō-făr-ĭn-jē'ŭs). SAME AS: *constrictor pharyngis inferior.*

latissimus colli (lăt-ĭs'ĭ-mŭs kŏl'ĭ). SAME AS: *platysma.*

levator palati (lē-vā'tor păl'ă-tĭ). SAME AS: *levator veli palatini.*

levator veli palatini (lē-vā'tor vē'lĭ păl"ă-tī'nĭ). ACTION: Elevates soft palate. ORIGIN: Pet-

Muscles of the Body (*Continued*)

rous portion of temporal bone and cartilaginous eustachian tube. INSERTION: Aponeurosis of soft palate. INNERVATION: Pharyngeal plexus.

lingualis (lĭng-gwā'lĭs). ACTION: Elevates sides and center of tongue. ORIGIN: Undersurface of tongue. INSERTION: Edge of tongue. INNERVATION: Hypoglossal.

longus capitis (lŏng'ŭs kăp'ĭ-tĭs). ACTION: Flexes head. ORIGIN: Transverse processes of 3rd to 6th cervical vertebrae. INSERTION: Occipital bone, basilar process. INNERVATION: Branches of 1st to 3rd cervical nerves. SYN: *rectus capitis anticus major.*

longus cervicis (lŏng'ŭs sĕr'vĭ-sĭs). SAME AS: *longus colli.*

longus colli (lŏng'ŭs kŏl'ī). Consists of three parts: (1) superior oblique, (2) inferior oblique, and (3) vertical. ACTION: Twists and bends neck forward. ORIGIN: (1) Transverse processes of 3rd to 5th cervical vertebrae. (2) Bodies of 1st to 3rd thoracic vertebrae. (3) Bodies of three upper thoracic and three lower cervical vertebrae. INSERTION: (1) Anterior tubercle of atlas. (2) Transverse processes of 5th and 6th cervical vertebrae. (3) Bodies of 2nd to 4th cervical vertebrae. INNERVATION: Branches of 2nd to 7th cervical nerves.

mylohyoideus (mī''lō-hī-oyd'ē-ŭs). ACTION: Elevates floor of mouth and hyoid, depresses jaw. ORIGIN: Mylohyoid line of mandible. INSERTION: Body of hyoid and median raphe. INNERVATION: Mylohyoid. SYN: *mylohyoid muscle.*

omohyoideus (ō''mō-hī-oyd'ē-ŭs). ACTION: Depresses hyoid. ORIGIN: Upper border of scapula. INSERTION: Hyoid bone. INNERVATION: Upper cervical through ansa hypoglossi. SYN: *omohyoid muscle.*

palatoglossus (păl''ă-tō-glŏs'ŭs). SAME AS: *glossopalatinus.*

palatopharyngeus (păl''ă-tō-făr-ĭn'jē-ŭs). SAME AS: *pharyngopalatinus.*

pharyngopalatinus (făr-ĭng''gō-păl-ă-tī'nŭs). ACTION: Narrows fauces and shuts off nasopharynx. ORIGIN: Soft palate. INSERTION: Thyroid cartilage and aponeurosis of the pharynx. INNERVATION: Pharyngeal plexus.

platysma (plă-tĭz'mă). ACTION: Wrinkles skin of neck and chest; depresses jaw and lower lip. ORIGIN: Clavicle, acromion and fascia over deltoid, and pectoralis major. INSERTION: Lower border of mandible, risorius and opposite platysma. INNERVATION: Cervical branch of facial. SYN: *latissimus colli; tetragonus.*

rectus capitis anterior (rĕk'tŭs kăp'ĭ-tĭs ăn-tēr'ĭ-or). ACTION: Turns and inclines the head. ORIGIN: Base of atlas. INSERTION: Occipital bone, basilar process. INNERVATION: Between 1st and 2nd cervical.

rectus capitis anticus major (rĕk'tŭs kăp'ĭ-tĭs ăn-tī'kŭs mā'jor). SAME AS: *longus capitis.*

rectus capitis anticus minor (rĕk'tŭs kăp'ĭ-tĭs ăn-tī'kŭs mī'nor). SAME AS: *rectus capitis anterior.*

rectus capitis lateralis (rĕk'tŭs kăp'ĭ-tĭs lătĕr-ā'lĭs). ACTION: Inclines head laterally and supports it. ORIGIN: Transverse process of atlas. INSERTION: Jugular process of occipital bone. INNERVATION: Between 1st and 2nd cervical nerves.

salpingopharyngeus (săl-pĭn''gō-făr-ĭn'jē-ŭs). ACTION: Elevates nasopharynx. ORIGIN: Eustachian tube close to nasopharynx. INSERTION: Posterior portion of the pharyngopalatinus. INNERVATION: Pharyngeal plexus.

scalenus anterior (skā-lē'nŭs ăn-tē'rī-or). ACTION: Elevates 1st rib and flexes neck. ORIGIN: Transverse processes of 3rd to 6th cervical vertebrae. INSERTION: Tubercle of 1st rib. INNERVATION: Cervical plexus. SYN: *scalenus anticus.*

scalenus medius (skā-lē'nŭs mē'dĭ-ŭs). ACTION: Elevates 1st rib and flexes neck. ORIGIN: Transverse processes of 2nd to 6th cervical vertebrae. INSERTION: First rib. INNERVATION: Cervical plexus.

scalenus posterior (skā-lē'nŭs pŏs-tēr'ī-ōr). ACTION: Elevates 2nd rib and flexes neck. ORIGIN: Transverse processes of 4th to 6th cervical vertebrae. INSERTION: Second rib. INNERVATION: Cervical and brachial plexus. SYN: *scalenus posticus.*

sphenosalpingostaphylinus (sfē''nō-săl-pĭn''gōstăf-ĭ-lī'nŭs). SAME AS: *tensor veli palatini.*

sternocleidomastoideus (stĕr''nō-klī-dō-măstoyd'ē-ŭs). ACTION: Rotates and depresses head. ORIGIN: By two heads, from sternum and clavicle. INSERTION: Mastoid process and outer part of superior curved line of occipital bone. INNERVATION: Spinal accessory. SYN: *sternomastoid muscle.*

sternohyoideus (stĕr''nō-hī-oyd'ē-ŭs). ACTION: Depresses hyoid bone. ORIGIN: Manubrium sterni and 1st costal cartilage. INSERTION: Body of hyoid bone. INNERVATION: Upper cervical through ansa hypoglossi. SYN: *sternohyoid muscle.*

sternothyreoideus (stĕr''nō-thī-rē-oyd'ē-ŭs). ACTION: Depresses thyroid cartilage. ORIGIN: Sternum and 1st costal cartilage. INSERTION: Side of thyroid cartilage. INNERVATION: Upper cervical through ansa hypoglossi. SYN: *sternothyroid muscle.*

styloglossus (stī'lō-glŏs'ŭs). ACTION: Retracts and elevates tongue. ORIGIN: Styloid process. INSERTION: Side of tongue. INNERVATION: Hypoglossal.

stylohyoideus (stī''lō-hī-oyd'ē-ŭs). ACTION: Fixes hyoid, drawing it up and back. ORIGIN:

Muscles of the Body (*Continued*)

Styloid process. INSERTION: Body of hyoid bone. INNERVATION: Facial. SYN: *stylohyoid muscle.*

stylopharyngeus (stī″lŏ-fär-ĭn′jē-ŭs). ACTION: Elevates and dilates pharynx. ORIGIN: Styloid process. INSERTION: Thyroid cartilage and side of pharynx. INNERVATION: Glossopharyngeal.

tensor palati (tĕn′sŏr păl-ă′tī). SAME AS: *tensor veli palatini.*

tensor veli palatini (tĕn′sŏr vē′lī păl″ă-tī′nī). ACTION: Stretches soft palate. ORIGIN: Spine of sphenoid, scaphoid fossa of internal pterygoid process and eustachian tube. INSERTION: Posterior border of hard palate and aponeurosis of soft palate. INNERVATION: Otic ganglion, trigeminal nerve. SYN: *tensor palati; circumflexus palati; sphenosalpingostaphylinus.*

tetragonus (tĕt-ră-gō′nŭs). SAME AS: *platysma.*

thyreohyoideus (thī-rē-ō-hī-oyd′ē-ŭs). ACTION: Depresses hyoid bone; elevates thyroid cartilage if hyoid bone is fixed. ORIGIN: Side of thyroid cartilage. INSERTION: Cornu and body of hyoid bone. INNERVATION: Hypoglossal. SYN: *thyrohyoid muscle.*

uvulae (ū′vū-lē). ACTION: Elevates the uvula. ORIGIN: Posterior nasal spine. INSERTION: Forms large part of uvula. INNERVATION: Pharyngeal plexus.

LARYNX AND EPIGLOTTIS

aryepiglotticus (ăr-ĭ-ĕp-ĭ-glŏt′ĭk-ŭs). ACTION: Closes glottis opening. ORIGIN: Arytenoid cartilage. INSERTION: Epiglottis. INNERVATION: Laryngeal, recurrent.

arytenoideus (ăr-ĭ-tē-noyd′ē-ŭs). Consists of (1) arytenoideus obliquus and (2) arytenoideus transversus. ACTION: Closes glottis opening. ORIGIN: Arytenoid cartilage. INSERTION: (1) Aryepiglottic fold. (2) Crosses between the two cartilages of the obliquus portion. INNERVATION: Laryngeal, recurrent.

cricoarytenoideus lateralis (krī″kŏ-ăr-ĭ-tē-noyd′ē-ŭs lăt-ĕr-ā′lĭs). ACTION: Narrows glottis. ORIGIN: Upper border of arch of cricoid cartilage. INSERTION: Muscular process of arytenoid cartilage. INNERVATION: Laryngeal, recurrent.

cricoarytenoideus posterior (krī″kŏ-ăr-ĭ-tē-noyd′ē-ŭs pŏs-tē′rĭ-or). ACTION: Opens glottis. ORIGIN: Back of cricoid cartilage. INSERTION: Muscular process of arytenoid cartilage. INNERVATION: Laryngeal, recurrent.

cricothyroideus (krī″kŏ-thī-royd′ē-ŭs). ACTION: Tightens vocal cords. ORIGIN: Anterior surface of cricoid cartilage. INSERTION: Thyroid cartilage. INNERVATION: Laryngeal, superior. SYN: *cricothyroid.*

thyreoarytenoideus (thī″rē-ō-ăr-ĭ-tē-noyd′ē-ŭs). ACTION: Relaxes vocal cords. ORIGIN: Thy-

roid cartilage. INSERTION: Arytenoid cartilage. INNERVATION: Laryngeal, recurrent. SYN: *thyroarytenoid.*

thyreoepiglotticus (thī″rē-ō-ĕp-ĭ-glŏt′ĭk-ŭs). ACTION: Depresses epiglottis. ORIGIN: Thyroid cartilage. INSERTION: Epiglottis and sacculus laryngis. INNERVATION: Laryngeal, recurrent. SYN: *thyroepiglotticus.*

BACK

accessorius (ăk″sĕs-sō′rĭ-ŭs). SAME AS: *iliocostalis thoracis.*

biventer cervicis (bī-vĕn′tĕr sĕr′vĭ-sĭs). SAME AS: *spinalis capitis.*

cervicalis ascendens (sĕr-vī-kā′lĭs ă-sĕn′dĕns). SAME AS: *iliocostalis cervicis.*

complexus (kŏm-plĕks′ŭs). SAME AS: *semispinalis capitis.*

erector spinae (ē-rĕk′tor spī′nē). SAME AS: *sacrospinalis.*

iliocostalis cervicis (ĭl″ĭ-ō-kŏs-tā′lĭs sĕr′vĭ-sĭs). ACTION: Extends cervical spine. ORIGIN: Angles of 3rd to 6th ribs. INSERTION: Transverse processes of 4th to 6th cervical vertebrae. INNERVATION: Branches of cervical. SYN: *cervicalis ascendens.*

iliocostalis dorsi (ĭl″ĭ-ō-kŏs-tā′lĭs dor′sī). SAME AS: *iliocostalis thoracis.*

iliocostalis lumborum (ĭl″ĭ-ō-kŏs-tā′lĭs lŭmbō′rŭm). ACTION: Extends lumbar spine. ORIGIN: With sarcospinalis. INSERTION: In angles of 5th to 12th ribs. INNERVATION: Branches of dorsal and lumbar. SYN: *sacrolumbalis.*

iliocostalis thoracis (ĭl″ĭ-ō-kŏs-tā′lĭs thō-răs′ĭs). ACTION: Keeps dorsal spine erect. ORIGIN: Angles of 12th to 7th ribs. INSERTION: Sixth tó 1st ribs and 7th cervical vertebra. INNERVATION: Branches of dorsal. SYN: *iliocostalis dorsi; accessorius.*

interspinales (ĭn″tĕr-spī-nā′lēz). A series. ACTION: Support and extend vertebral column. ORIGIN: Undersurface of spine of one vertebra. INSERTION: Spine of vertebra above. INNERVATION: Branches of spinal.

intertransversales (ĭn-tĕr-trăns-vĕr-sā′lēz). SAME AS: *intertransversarii.*

intertransversarii (ĭn″tĕr-trăns-vĕr-sā′rī-ī). ACTION: Flex vertebral column. ORIGIN: Between transverse processes of contiguous vertebrae. INNERVATION: Branches of ventral and dorsal divisions of spinal. SYN: *intertransversales.*

latissimus dorsi (lăt-ĭs′ĭ-mŭs dŏr′sī). ACTION: Adducts, extends and rotates arm. ORIGIN: Lower thoracic and lumbar vertebrae, sacrum and tip of iliac crest. INSERTION: Intertubercular groove of humerus. INNERVATION: Brachial plexus.

levator scapulae (lē-vā′tor skăp′ū-lē). ACTION: Elevates posterior angle of scapula. ORIGIN:

Muscles of the Body (*Continued*)

Transverse processes of four upper cervical vertebrae. INSERTION: Superior edge of scapula. INNERVATION: Dorsal scapular from 5th cervical, and branches of 3rd and 4th cervical. SYN: *levator anguli scapulae*.

logissimus capitis (lŏn-jĭs'ĭ-mŭs kăp'ĭ-tĭs). ACTION: Keeps head erect, draws it backward or to one side. ORIGIN: Upper thoracic and lower and middle cervical vertebrae. INSERTION: Mastoid process. INNERVATION: Branches of cervical. SYN: *trachelomastoid*.

longissimus cervicis (lŏn-jĭs'ĭ-mŭs sĕr'vĭ-sĭs). ACTION: Extends cervical spine. ORIGIN: Upper thoracic vertebrae. INSERTION: Ribs and upper lumbar and thoracic vertebrae. INNERVATION: Branches of dorsal divisions of spinal. SYN: *transversalis colli*.

longissimus dorsi (lŏn-jĭs'ĭ-mŭs dor'sī). SAME AS: *longissimus thoracis*.

longissimus thoracis (lŏn-jĭs'ĭ-mŭs thŏr-ā'sĭs). ACTION: Extends spinal column. ORIGIN: Transverse processes of lumbar and dorsal vertebrae. INSERTION: Lowest ribs and lumbar and dorsal vertebrae. INNERVATION: Lumbar and dorsal divisions of spinal. SYN: *longissimus dorsi*.

multifidus (mŭl-tĭf'ĭd-ŭs). ACTION: Rotates spinal column. ORIGIN: Sacrum, iliac spine, lumbar, cervical, and dorsal vertebrae. INSERTION: Laminae and spinous processes of next four vertebrae above. INNERVATION: Branches of dorsal divisions of spinal.

multifidus spinae (mŭl-tĭf'ĭd-ŭs spī'nē). SAME AS: *multifidus*.

obliquus capitis inferior (ŏb-lī'kwŭs kăp'ĭ-tĭs ĭn-fēr'ĭ-or). ACTION: Rotates head. ORIGIN: Spine of axis. INSERTION: Transverse process of atlas. INNERVATION: Suboccipital.

obliquus capitis superior (ŏb-lī'kwŭs kăp'ĭ-tĭs sū-pēr'ĭ-or). ACTION: Rotates head. ORIGIN: Transverse process of atlas. INSERTION: Occipital bone. INNERVATION: Suboccipital.

rectus capitis posterior major (rĕk'tŭs kăp'ĭ-tĭs pŏs-tē'rĭ-or mā'jor). ACTION: Rotates and draws head backward. ORIGIN: Spine of axis. INSERTION: Inferior curved line of occipital bone. INNERVATION: Suboccipital. SYN: *rectus capitis posticus major*.

rectus capitis posterior minor (rĕk'tŭs kăp'ĭ-tĭs pŏs-tē'rĭ-or mī'nor). ACTION: Rotates and draws head backward. ORIGIN: Posterior tubercle of atlas. INSERTION: Inferior curved line of occipital bone. INNERVATION: Suboccipital. SYN: *rectus capitis posticus minor*.

rhomboideus major (rŏm-boy'dē-ŭs mā'jor). ACTION: Elevates scapula. ORIGIN: Spinous processes of 2nd to 5th thoracic vertebrae. INSERTION: Vertebral border of scapula below spine. INNERVATION: Dorsal scapular from brachial plexus.

rhomboideus minor (rŏm-boy'dē-ŭs mī'nor).

ACTION: Retracts and elevates scapula. ORIGIN: Spinous processes of 7th cervical vertebra and 1st thoracic vertebra. INSERTION: Border of scapula above spine. INNERVATION: Dorsal scapular from brachial plexus.

rotatores (rō-tā-tō'rēz). ACTION: Extend and rotate the vertebral column. ORIGIN: Transverse processes of 2nd to 12th dorsal vertebrae. INSERTION: Lamina of next vertebra above. INNERVATION: Branches of dorsal divisions of spinal. SYN: *rotatores spinae*.

rotatores spinae (rō-tā-tō'rēz spī'nē). SAME AS: *rotatores*.

sacrolumbalis (sā"krō-lŭm-bā'lĭs). SAME AS: *iliocostalis lumborum*.

sacrospinalis (sā"krō-spī-nā'lĭs). ACTION: Extends vertebral column. ORIGIN: Sacrum, lumbar vertebrae, iliac crest. INSERTION: Iliocostalis and longissimus dorsi. INNERVATION: Posterior branches of spinal.

semispinalis capitis (sĕm"ĭ-spī-nā'lĭs kăp'ĭ-tĭs). ACTION: Rotates and draws head backward. ORIGIN: Transverse processes of upper six or seven thoracic and lower four cervical vertebrae. INSERTION: Occipital bone, between inferior and superior curved line. INNERVATION: Branches of dorsal divisions of cervical. SYN: *complexus*.

semispinalis cervicis (sĕm"ĭ-spī-nā'lĭs sĕr'vĭ-sĭs). ACTION: Erects cervical spine. ORIGIN: Transverse processes of upper five or six thoracic vertebrae. INSERTION: Spines from axis to 5th cervical vertebra. INNERVATION: Branches of dorsal divisions of spinal.

semispinalis colli (sĕm"ĭ-spī-nā'lĭs kŏl'ĭ). SAME AS: *semispinalis cervicis*.

semispinalis dorsi (sĕm"ĭ-spī-nā'lĭs dor'sī). SAME AS: *semispinalis thoracis*.

semispinalis thoracis (sĕm"ĭ-spī-nā'lĭs thō-rā'sĭs). ACTION: Erects vertebral column. ORIGIN: Transverse processes of 6th to 10th thoracic vertebrae. INSERTION: Spines of upper four thoracic and lower two cervical vertebrae. INNERVATION: Branches of dorsal divisions of spinal. SYN: *semispinalis dorsi*.

serratus posterior inferior (sĕr-ā'tŭs pŏs-tē'rĭ-or ĭn-fē'rĭ-or). ACTION: Draws ribs back and downward. ORIGIN: Spines of lower two thoracic and upper two lumbar vertebrae. INSERTION: Lower four ribs. INNERVATION: Branches of ventral divisions of 9th to 12th thoracic. SYN: *serratus posticus inferior*.

serratus posterior superior (sĕr-ā'tŭs pŏs-tē'rĭ-or sū-pē'rĭ-or). ACTION: Elevates the ribs. ORIGIN: Spines of 7th cervical and two upper thoracic vertebrae. INSERTION: Angles of 2nd to 5th ribs. INNERVATION: Branches of ventral divisions of thoracic. SYN: *serratus posticus superior*.

spinalis capitis (spī-nā'lĭs kăp'ĭ-tĭs). ORIGIN: Inconstant; from spines of upper dorsal and

Muscles of the Body (*Continued*)

lower cervical vertebrae. INSERTION: Blends with the semispinalis capitis. SYN: *biventer capitis.*

spinalis cervicis (spĭ-nā′lĭs sĕr′vĭ-sĭs). ACTION: Extends cervical spine. ORIGIN: Spines of 5th, 6th, and 7th cervical vertebrae. INSERTION: Axis and occasionally, the two vertebrae below. INNERVATION: Branches of cervical.

spinalis thoracis (spĭ-nā′lĭs thō-rā′sĭs). ACTION: Erects spinal column. ORIGIN: Spines of first two lumbar and last two thoracic vertebrae. INSERTION: Spines of middle and upper thoracic vertebrae. INNERVATION: Dorsal branches of spinal. SYN: *spinalis dorsi.*

splenius capitis (splē′nĭ-ŭs kăp′ĭ-tĭs). ACTION: Rotates and extends head. ORIGIN: Ligamentum nuchae, 7th cervical and first three thoracic vertebrae. INSERTION: Mastoid process and superior curved line of occiput. INNERVATION: Branches of dorsal divisions of cervical.

splenius cervicis (splē′nĭ-ŭs sĕr′vĭ-sĭs). ACTION: Rotates and flexes head and neck. ORIGIN: Spines of 3rd to 6th thoracic vertebrae. INSERTION: Transverse processes of 1st and 2nd cervical vertebrae. INNERVATION: Branches of dorsal divisions of cervical. SYN: *splenius colli.*

splenius colli (splē′nĭ-ŭs kŏl′ī). SAME AS: *splenius cervicis.*

supraspinatus (sū-pră-spī-nā′tŭs). ACTION: Abducts arm. ORIGIN: Supraspinatous fossa. INSERTION: Greater tuberosity of humerus. INNERVATION: Branches of suprascapular.

suspensorius duodeni (sŭs-pĕn-sō′rĭ-ŭs dū″ō-dē′nĭ). Wide, flat band of unstriped muscle attached to the left crus of diaphragm and continuous with the muscular coat of the duodenum at its line of junction with the jejunum.

trachelomastoid (trā″kē-lō-măs′toyd) SAME AS: *longissimus capitis.*

transversalis colli (trăns″vĕr-sā′lĭs kŏl′ī) SAME AS: *longissimus cervicis.*

trapezius (tră-pē′zĭ-ŭs). ACTION: Draws head back and to the side, rotates scapula. ORIGIN: Superior curved line of occipital, spinous processes of 7th cervical and all thoracic vertebrae. INSERTION: Clavicle, acromion, base of spine of scapula. INNERVATION: Spinal accessory and cervical plexus.

ABDOMEN

cremaster (krē-măs′tĕr). ACTION: Raises testicle. ORIGIN: Midportion of inguinal ligament. INSERTION: Cremasteric fascia and pubic bone. INNERVATION: Genitofemoral.

obliquus externus abdominis (ōb-lī′kwŭs ĕks-tĕr′nŭs ăb-dŏm′ĭ-nĭs). ACTION: Contracts abdomen and viscera. ORIGIN: Lower eight ribs. INSERTION: Iliac crest, Poupart's ligament,

linea alba, pubic crest. INNERVATION: Iliohypogastric, ilioinguinal, and branches of intercostal.

obliquus internus abdominis (ōb-lī′kwŭs intĕr′nŭs ăb-dŏm′ĭ-nĭs). ACTION: Compresses viscera, flexes thorax forward. ORIGIN: Iliac crest, inguinal ligament, lumbar fascia. INSERTION: Few lowest ribs, linea alba, pubic crest. INNERVATION: Iliohypogastric, ilioinguinal, and branches of intercostal.

pyramidalis (pĭ-răm-ĭ-dā′lĭs). ACTION: Tightens linea alba. ORIGIN: Pubic crest. INSERTION: Linea alba. INNERVATION: Branch of 12th thoracic.

quadratus lumborum (kwăd-rā′tŭs lŭm-bō′-rŭm). ACTION: Flexes trunk laterally and forward. ORIGIN: Iliac crest, iliolumbar ligament, lower lumbar vertebrae. INSERTION: Twelfth rib and the upper lumbar vertebrae. INNERVATION: Branches of 1st lumbar and 12th thoracic.

rectus abdominis (rĕk′tŭs ăb-dŏm′ĭ-nĭs). ACTION: Compresses abdomen. ORIGIN: Pubis. INSERTION: Cartilage of 5th to 7th ribs. INNERVATION: Branches of 7th to 12th intercostal.

spincter pylori (sfĭnk′tĕr pī-lō′rī). A thickening of middle circular layer of the gastric musculature surrounding the pylorus.

transversalis abdominis (trăns″vĕr-sā′lĭs ăbdŏm′ĭ-nĭs). SAME AS: *transversus abdominis.*

transversus abdominis (trăns″vĕr′sŭs ăb-dŏm′ĭ-nĭs). ACTION: Compresses abdomen, flexes thorax. ORIGIN: Lumbar fascia, 7th to 12th costal cartilages, inguinal ligament, iliac crest. INSERTION: Xiphoid cartilage, linea alba, pubic crest and iliopectineal line. INNERVATION: Iliohypogastric, ilioinguinal, and branches of intercostal.

PERINEUM

accelerator urinae (ăk-sĕl-ĕ-rā′tŏr ū-rī′nē). SAME AS: *bulbocavernosus.*

bulbocavernosus (bŭl-bō-kă-vĕr-nō′sŭs). ACTION: Constricts bulbous urethra in male; in female constricts urethra. ORIGIN: Central point of perineum and median raphe. INSERTION: Undersurface of bulb, spongy and cavernous part of penis; root of clitoris. INNERVATION: Perineal branch of pudendal.

coccygeus (kŏk-sĭj′ē-ŭs). ACTION: Supports coccyx, closes pelvic outlet. ORIGIN: Ischial spine and sarcospinous ligament. INSERTION: Coccyx and lowest portion of sacrum. INNERVATION: Third and 4th sacral.

compressor urethrae (kŏm-prĕs′ŏr ū-rē′thrē). SAME AS: *sphincter urethrae membranaceae.*

constrictor urethrae (kŏn-strĭk′tŏr ū-rē′thrē). SAME AS: *sphincter urethrae membranaceae.*

corrugator cutis ani (kor-ū-gā′tŏr kū′tĭs ā′nĭ). ACTION: Wrinkles skin of anus. ORIGIN: Submucous tissue, interior of anus. INSERTION: Subcutaneous tissue on opposite side of anus. INNERVATION: Sympathetic.

depressor urethrae (dē-prĕs'ōr ū-rē'thrē). ACTION: Depresses urethra. ORIGIN: Ramus of ischium near the transversus perinei profundus. INSERTION: Fibers of constrictor vaginae.

erector clitoridis (ē-rĕk'tōr klĭ-tōr'ĭ-dĭs). SAME AS: *ischiocavernosus.*

erector penis (ĕ-rĕk'tōr pē'nĭs) SAME AS: *ischiocavernosus.*

ischiocavernosus (ĭs"kĭ-ō-kă-vĕr-nō'sŭs). ACTION: Maintains erection of penis or clitoris. ORIGIN: Tuberosity of ischium and great sacrosciatic ligament. INSERTION: Corpus cavernosum of clitoris or penis. INNERVATION: Perineal branch of pudendal. SYN: *erector clitoridis* (in female); *erector penis* (in male).

ischiococcygeus (ĭs"kĭ-ō-kŏk-sĭj'ē-ŭs). SAME AS: *coccygeus.*

levator ani (lē-vā'tōr ā'nī). ACTION: Supports rectum and pelvic floor, aids in defecation. ORIGIN: Pubis, pelvic fascia, ischial spine. INSERTION: Rectum, coccyx and fibrous raphe of perineum. INNERVATION: Sacral and perineal.

sphincter ani externus (sfĭnk'tĕr ā'nī ĕks-tĕr'nŭs). ACTION: Closes anus. ORIGIN: Ring of fibers surrounding anus. INSERTION: Coccyx and central point of perineum. INNERVATION: Hemorrhoidal branch of pudendal.

sphincter ani internus (sfĭnk'tĕr ā'nī ĭn-tĕr'nŭs). ACTION: Contracts rectum and anus, but not voluntarily. ORGIN: Muscular ring of rectal fibers above canal.

sphincter urethrae membranaceae (sfĭnk'tĕr ū-rē'thrē mĕm-brā-nā'sē-ē). ACTION: Constricts membranous urethra. ORIGIN: Ramus of pubis. INSERTION: Behind and in front of urethra. INNERVATION: Perineal branch of pudendal. SYN: *compressor urethrae; constrictor urethrae.*

sphincter vaginae (sfĭnk'tĕr vă-jī'nē). SAME AS: *bulbocavernosus.*

sphincter vesicae (sfĭnk'tĕr vĕs'ĭ-kē). ACTION: Shuts off internal orifice of urethra. ORIGIN: Near urethra orifice of bladder. INNERVATION: Sacral and hypogastric.

transversus perinei profundus (trăns-vĕr'sŭs pĕr-ĭ-nē'ī prō-fŭn'dŭs). ACTION: Assists compressor urethrae. ORIGIN: Ramus of ischium. INSERTION: Central tendon. INNERVATION: Perineal branch of pudendal.

transversus perinei superficialis (trăns-vĕr'sŭs pĕr-ĭ-nē'ī sū"pĕr-fĭsh-ĭ-ā'lĭs). ACTION: Tenses central tendon. ORIGIN: Ramus of ischium. INSERTION: Central point of perineum. INNERVATION: Perineal branch of pudendal.

THORAX

diaphragma (dī"ă-frăg'mă). ACTION: Increases chest capacity. ORIGIN: Ensiform cartilage, 7th to 12th ribs, arcuate ligaments and lumbar vertebrae. INSERTION: Central tendon. INNERVATION: Phrenic.

infracostales (ĭn"fră-kŏs-tā'lēz). SAME AS: *subcostales.*

intercostales externus (ĭn"tĕr-kŏs-tā'lēz ĕks-tĕr'nŭs). ACTION: Draw ribs together and raise ribs. ORIGIN: Lower border of rib. INSERTION: Upper border of rib below. INNERVATION: Intercostal.

intercostales internus (ĭn"tĕr-kŏs-tā'lēz ĭn-tĕr'nŭs). ACTION: Draw ribs together and lower ribs. ORIGIN: Lower border of rib. INSERTION: Upper border of rib below. INNERVATION: Intercostal.

levatores costarum (lē-vā-tō'rēz kŏs-tā'rŭm). ACTION: Raise ribs; flex vertebral column. ORIGIN: Transverse process of 7th cervical and upper eleven thoracic vertebrae. INSERTION: Rib next below. INNERVATION: Branches of intercostal.

subcostales (sŭb-kŏs-tā'lēz). ACTION: Draw ribs together and lower ribs. ORIGIN: Inconstant; inner surface of the ribs. INSERTION: Inner surface of one of ribs just below. INNERVATION: Intercostal.

transversus thoracis (trăns-vĕr'sŭs thōr-ā'sĭs). ACTION: Narrows the chest. ORIGIN: Xiphoid cartilage and sternum. INSERTION: Costal cartilages, 2nd to 6th ribs. INNERVATION: Branches of intercostal.

triangularis sterni (trī"ăn-gū-lā'rĭs stĕr'nī). SAME AS: *transversus thoracis.*

SHOULDER

deltoideus (dĕl-toy'dē-ŭs). ACTION: Raises arm and rotates it. ORIGIN: Clavicle, acromion process, and spine of scapula. INSERTION: Shaft of humerus. INNERVATION: Axillary (circumflex) from brachial plexus. SYN: *deltoid.*

infraspinatus (ĭn"fră-spī-nā'tŭs). ACTION: Rotates arm back and out. ORIGIN: Infraspinous fossa of scapula. INSERTION: Great tuberosity of humerus. INNERVATION: Suprascapular from brachial plexus.

pectoralis major (pĕk-tō-rā'lĭs mā'jōr). ACTION: Flexes, adducts, and rotates arm. ORIGIN: Sternum, clavicle, and cartilages of 1st to 6th ribs. INSERTION: Bicipital ridge of humerus. INNERVATION: Anterior thoracic from brachial plexus.

pectoralis minor (pĕk-tō-rā'lĭs mī'nōr). ACTION: Draws down scapula and point of shoulder, raises ribs. ORIGIN: Third to 5th ribs. INSERTION: Coracoid process of scapula. INNERVATION: Anterior thoracic from brachial plexus.

Muscles of the Body (*Continued*)

serratus anterior (sĕr-ā′tŭs ăn-tēr′ĭ-ōr). AcTION: Elevates ribs, rotates scapula. ORIGIN: Upper eight or nine ribs. INSERTION: Angles and vertebral border of scapula. INNERVATION: Long thoracic from brachial plexus.

serratus magnus (sĕr-ā′tŭs măg′nŭs). SAME AS: *serratus anterior.*

subclavius (sŭb-klā′vĭ-ŭs). ACTION: Draws clavicle down and forward or elevates the 1st rib. ORIGIN: First rib and its cartilage. INSERTION: Undersurface of clavicle. INNERVATION: Special nerve with fibers from 5th and 6th cervical.

subscapularis (sŭb-skăp-ū-lā′rĭs). ACTION: Rotates humerus inward and lowers it. ORIGIN: Subscapular fossa. INSERTION: Lesser tubercle of humerus. INNERVATION: Subscapular.

supraspinatus (sŭp-ră-spī-nā′tŭs). ACTION: Abducts and raises arm. ORIGIN: Supraspinous fossa of scapula. INSERTION: Greater tubercle of humerus. INNERVATION: Branches of suprascapular.

teres major (tē′rēz mā′jor). ACTION: Rotates arm inward, draws it down and back. ORIGIN: Axillary border of scapula. INSERTION: Lesser tubercle of humerus. INNERVATION: Branch of lower subscapular.

teres minor (tē′rēz mī′nor). ACTION: Rotates arm outward. ORIGIN: Axillary border of scapula. INSERTION: Greater tubercle of humerus. INNERVATION: Branch of axillary (circumflex).

ARM AND FOREARM

abductor pollicis longus (ăb-dŭk′tŏr pŏl′ĭ-sĭs lŏn′gŭs). ACTION: Abducts thumb and wrist. ORIGIN: Dorsal surface of radius, ulna, and interosseous membrane. INSERTION: Base of 1st metacarpal. INNERVATION: Branch of radial. SYN: *extensor ossis metacarpi pollicis.*

anconeus (ăn-kō′nē-ŭs). ACTION: Extends forearm. ORIGIN: Lateral epicondyle of humerus. INSERTION: Olecranon and posterior surface of ulna. INNERVATION: Branch of radial.

biceps brachii (bī′sĕps brā′kĭ-ī). ACTION: Flexes arm and forearm and supinates hand. ORIGIN: (1) Short head from coracoid process. (2) Long head from scapula above glenoid fossa. INSERTION: Bicipital tuberosity of radius. INNERVATION: Musculocutaneous.

brachialis (brā″kĭ-ā′lĭs). ACTION: Flexes forearm. ORIGIN: Lower half of anterior surface of humerus. INSERTION: Coronoid process of ulna. INNERVATION: Musculocutaneous and radial.

brachioradialis (brā″kĭ-ō-rā″dĭ-ā′lĭs). ACTION: Flexes and supinates forearm. ORIGIN: Supracondylar ridge of radius. INSERTION: Styloid process of radius. INNERVATION: Branch of radial. SYN: *supinator longus.*

coracobrachialis (kor-ă-kō-brā″kĭ-ā′lĭs). Ac-

TION: Raises and adducts arm. ORIGIN: Coracoid process of scapula. INSERTION: Middle of inner border of humerus. INNERVATION: Musculocutaneous.

extensor carpi radialis brevis (ĕks-tĕn′sōr kar′pī rā″dĭ-ā′lĭs brĕ′vĭs). ACTION: Extends and abducts wrist. ORIGIN: External condyloid ridge of humerus. INSERTION: Base of 3rd metacarpal. INNERVATION: Branch of radial.

extensor carpi radialis longus (ĕks-tĕn′sōr kar′pī rā″dĭ-ā′lĭs lŏng′gŭs). ACTION: Extends and abducts wrist. ORIGIN: External condyloid ridge of humerus. INSERTION: Base of 2nd metacarpal. INNERVATION: Branch of radial.

extensor carpi ulnaris (ĕks-tĕn′sōr kar′pī ŭlnā′rĭs). ACTION: Extends and abducts wrist. ORIGIN: Lateral epicondyle of humerus. INSERTION: Base of 5th metacarpal. INNERVATION: Branch of radial.

extensor digiti minimi (ĕks-tĕn′sōr dĭj′ĭ-tī mĭn′ĭm-ī). ACTION: Extends little finger. ORIGIN: External epicondyle of humerus. INSERTION: Dorsum of 1st phalanx of little finger. INNERVATION: Branch of radial. SYN: *extensor digiti quinti proprius.*

extensor digiti quinti proprius (ĕks-tĕn′sōr dĭj′ĭ-tī kwĭn′tī prō′prĭ-ŭs). SAME AS: *extensor digiti minimi.*

extensor digitorum communis (ĕks-tĕn′sōr dĭj-ĭ-tō′rŭm kŏm-mū′nĭs). ACTION: Extends fingers and wrist. ORIGIN: External epicondyle of humerus. INSERTION: Second and 3rd phalanges. INNERVATION: Branch of radial.

extensor indicis (ĕks-tĕn′sōr ĭn′dĭ-sĭs). ACTION: Extends index finger. ORIGIN: Dorsal surface of ulna and interosseous membrane. INSERTION: First tendon of extensor digitorum communis. INNERVATION: Branch of radial.

extensor ossis metacarpi pollicis (ĕks-tĕn′sōr ŏs′ĭs mĕt″ă-kar′pī pŏl′ĭ-sĭs). SAME AS: *abductor pollicis longus.*

extensor pollicis brevis (ĕks-tĕn′sōr pŏl′ĭ-sĭs brĕ′vĭs). ACTION: Extends thumb and abducts 1st metacarpal. ORIGIN: Dorsal surface of radius. INSERTION: Base of 1st phalanx of thumb. INNERVATION: Branch of radial.

extensor pollicis longus (ĕks-tĕn′sōr pŏl′ĭ-sĭs lŏng′gŭs). ACTION: Extends terminal phalanx of thumb and abducts hand. ORIGIN: Dorsal surface of ulna. INSERTION: Base of 2nd phalanx of thumb. INNERVATION: Branch of radial.

extensor primi internodii pollicis (ĕks-tĕn′sōr prī′mī ĭn″tĕr-nō′dĭ-ī pŏl′ĭ-sĭs). SAME AS: *extensor pollicis brevis.*

extensor secundi internodii pollicis (ĕks-tĕn′sōr sē-kŭn-dī ĭn″tĕr-nō′dĭ-ī pŏl′ĭ-sĭs). SAME AS: *extensor pollicis longus.*

flexor carpi radialis (flĕks′or kăr′pī rā″dĭ-ā′lĭs). ACTION: Flexes and abducts wrist. ORIGIN: Medial epicondyle of humerus. INSERTION:

Base of 2nd metacarpal. INNERVATION: Branch of median. SYN: *radiocarpus*.

flexor carpi ulnaris (flĕks′or kăr′pī ŭl-nā′rĭs). Consists of (1) humeral head and (2) ulnar head. ACTION: Flexes and adducts wrist. ORIGIN: (1) Medial epicondyle of humerus. (2) Olecranon process and posterior border of ulna. INSERTION: Pisiform bone and 5th metacarpal. INNERVATION: Branch of ulnar.

flexor digitorum profundus (flĕks′or dĭj-ĭ-tō′rŭm prō-fŭn′dŭs). ACTION: Flexes the phalanges. ORIGIN: Upper three fourths of shaft of ulna. INSERTION: Terminal phalanges of fingers. INNERVATION: Branch of ulnar and branch of median.

flexor digitorum sublimis (flĕks′or dĭj-ĭ-tō′rŭm sŭb-lī′mĭs). SAME AS: *flexor digitorum superficialis*.

flexor digitorum superficialis (flĕks′or dĭj-ĭ-tō′rŭm sū″pĕr-fĭsh-ē-ā′lĭs). Consists of three heads: (1) humeral, (2) ulnar and (3) radial. ACTION: Flexes middle phalanges and hand. ORIGIN: (1) Medial epicondyle of humerus. (2) Medial side of coronoid process. (3) Outer border of radius. INSERTION: Second phalanx of each finger. INNERVATION: Branches of median. SYN: *flexor digitorum sublimis*.

flexor pollicis longus (flĕks′or pŏl′ĭ-sĭs long′gŭs). ACTION: Flexes thumb. ORIGIN: Anterior surface of middle 3rd of radius. INSERTION: Terminal phalanx of thumb. INNERVATION: Branch of median.

palmaris longus (păl-mā′rĭs lŏng′gŭs). ACTION: Tightens palmar fascia, flexes wrist. ORIGIN: Medial epicondyle of humerus. INSERTION: Transverse carpal ligament and palmar fascia. INNERVATION: Branch of median.

pronator quadratus (prō-nā′tor kwăd-rā′tŭs). ACTION: Pronates forearm. ORIGIN: Lower 4th of ulna. INSERTION: Lower 4th of radius. INNERVATION: Volar interosseous.

pronator teres (prō-nā′tor tē′rĕz). Consists of (1) humeral head and (2) ulnar head. ACTION: Pronates hand. ORIGIN: (1) Medial epicondyle of humerus. (2) Coronoid process of ulna. INSERTION: Lateral surface of shaft of radius. INNERVATION: Branch of median.

radiocarpus (rā″dĭ-ō-kăr′pŭs). SAME AS: *flexor carpi radialis*.

subanconeus (sŭb-ăn-kō′nē-ŭs). ACTION: Tightens posterior ligament of elbow. ORIGIN: Lower portion of humerus. INSERTION: Posterior ligament of elbow joint. INNERVATION: Radial.

supinator (sū″pĭ-nā′tor). ACTION: Supinates hand. ORIGIN: Lateral epicondyle of humerus; oblique line of ulna; elbow joint. INSERTION: Outer surface of radius. INNERVATION: Branch of radial. SYN: *supinator radii brevis*.

supinator longus (sū″pĭ-nā′tor lŏng′gŭs). SAME AS: *brachioradialis*.

supinator radii brevis (sū″pĭ-nā′tor rā′dĭ-ī brĕ′vĭs). SAME AS: *supinator*.

triceps brachii (trī′sĕps brā′kĭ-ī). Consists of three heads: (1) long, (2) lateral, and (3) medial. ACTION: Extends forearm and arm. ORIGIN: (1) Infraglenoid tubercle of scapula. (2) Posterior surface of humerus below great tubercle. (3) Humerus below radial groove. INSERTION: Olecranon process of ulna. INNERVATION: Branches of radial.

HAND

abductor digiti quinti (ăb-dŭk′tor dĭj′ĭ-tī kwĭn′tī). ACTION: Abducts little finger. ORIGIN: Pisiform bone and ligaments. INSERTION: Inner side of 1st phalanx of little finger. INNERVATION: Ulnar, palmar branch.

abductor minimi digiti (ăb-dŭk′tor mĭn′ĭ-mī dĭj′ĭ-tī). SAME AS: *abductor digiti quinti*.

abductor pollicis brevis (ăb-dŭk′tor pŏl′ĭ-sĭs brĕ′vĭs). ACTION: Abducts thumb. ORIGIN: Ridge of trapezium and transverse carpal ligament. INSERTION: Outer side of 1st phalanx of thumb. INNERVATION: Branch of median.

abductor pollicis longus (ăb-dŭk′tor pŏl′ĭ-sĭs lŏng′gŭs). ACTION: Abducts and assists in extending thumb. ORIGIN: Posterior surfaces of radius and ulna. INSERTION: Outer side of base of 1st metacarpal. INNERVATION: Branch of radial.

adductor pollicis (ăd-dŭk′tor pŏl′ĭ-sĭs). ACTION: Adducts thumb. ORIGIN: Third metacarpal bone. INSERTION: Inner side of base of 1st phalanx of thumb. INNERVATION: Ulnar.

flexor brevis minimi digiti (flĕks′or brĕ′vĭs mĭn′ĭ-mī dĭj′ĭ-tī). SAME AS: *flexor digiti quinti brevis*.

flexor digiti quinti brevis (flĕks′or dĭj′ĭ-tī kwĭn′tī brĕ′vĭs). ACTION: Flexes 1st phalanx of little finger. ORIGIN: Unciform bone. INSERTION: First phalanx of little finger. INNERVATION: Branch of ulnar.

flexor pollicis brevis (flĕks′or pŏl′ĭ-sĭs brĕ′-vĭs). ACTION: Flexes 1st phalanx of thumb. ORIGIN: Transverse carpal ligament, metacarpal bone. INSERTION: Base of 1st phalanx of thumb. INNERVATION: Branch of median and of ulnar.

interossei dorsales manus (ĭn″tĕr-ŏs′ē-ī dōr-sā′lēz mā′nŭs). Four. ACTION: Abduct and adduct fingers. ORIGIN: Sides of metacarpal bones. INSERTION: First phalanges. INNERVATION: Branch of ulnar.

interossei palmares (ĭn″tĕr-ŏs′ē-ī păl-mā′rēz). SAME AS: *interossei volares*.

interossei volares (ĭn″tĕr-ŏs′ē-ī vō-lā′rĕz). Three. ACTION: Adduct index finger, abduct ring and little fingers. ORIGIN: Metacarpal bones laterally. INSERTION: Ulnar side of index finger, and radial sides of ring and little fingers. INNERVATION: Branch of ulnar.

Muscles of the Body (*Continued*)

lumbricales manus (lŭm-brī-kā'lēz mā'nŭs). Four. ACTION: Flex 1st and extend 2nd and 3rd phalanges. ORIGIN: Tendon of flexor digitorum profundus. INSERTION: First phalanx and extensor tendon. INNERVATION: Median and ulnar.

opponens digiti quinti (ŏp-pō'nĕns dĭj'ĭ-tī kwĭn'tī). ACTION: Flexes and adducts little finger. ORIGIN: Unciform bone; transverse carpal ligament. INSERTION: Fifth metacarpal bone. INNERVATION: Branch of ulnar.

opponens minimi digiti (ŏp-pō'nĕns mĭn'ĭ-mī dĭj'ĭ-tī). SAME AS: *opponens digiti quinti.*

opponens pollicis (ŏp-pō'nĕns pŏl'ĭ-sĭs). ACTION: Flexes and adducts thumb. ORIGIN: Trapezium and transverse carpal ligament. INSERTION: First metacarpal bone. INNERVATION: Median.

palmaris brevis (păl-mā'rĭs brē'vĭs). ACTION: Wrinkles skin on inner side of hand. ORIGIN: Central portion of palmar aponeurosis and transverse carpal ligament. INSERTION: Skin of ulnar side of hand. INNERVATION: Branch of ulnar.

HIP, THIGH, LOWER EXTREMITY

adductor brevis (ăd-dŭk'tŏr brē'vĭs). ACTION: Flexes and adducts thigh. ORIGIN: Ramus of pubis. INSERTION: Upper portion of linea aspera of femur. INNERVATION: Branch of obturator.

adductor longus (ăd-dŭk'tŏr lŏng'gŭs). ACTION: Adducts and flexes thigh. ORIGIN: Pubic crest and symphysis. INSERTION: Middle of linea aspera of femur. INNERVATION: Branch of obturator.

adductor magnus (ăd-dŭk'tŏr măg'nŭs). ACTION: Adducts thigh and rotates it outward. ORIGIN: Ramus of ischium and pubis. INSERTION: Linea aspera of femur and medial condyle. INNERVATION: Branch of sciatic and obturator.

articularis genu (ăr-tĭk"ū-lā'rĭs jē'nū). ACTION: Elevates capsule of knee joint. ORIGIN: Lower quarter of anterior surface of femoral shaft. INSERTION: Synovial membrane of knee joint. INNERVATION: Branch of femoral. SYN: *subcrureus.*

biceps femoris (bī'sĕps fĕm'ō-rĭs). ACTION: Flexes knee and rotates it outward. ORIGIN: (1) Short head from linea aspera. (2) Long head from ischial tuberosity. INSERTION: Head of fibula; lateral condyle of tibia. INNERVATION: (1) Peroneal, and (2) tibial portions of sciatic.

crureus (krū'rē-ŭs). SAME AS: *vastus intermedius.*

gemellus inferior (jē-mĕl'ŭs ĭn-fē'rĭ-ōr). ACTION: Rotates thigh outward. ORIGIN: Ischial tuberosity. INSERTION: Greater trochanter. INNERVATION: Sacral.

gemellus superior (jē-mĕl'ŭs sū-pē'rĭ-ōr). ACTION: Rotates thigh outward. ORIGIN: Spine of ischium. INSERTION: Greater trochanter. INNERVATION: Sacral plexus.

gluteus maximus (glū'tē-ŭs măks'ĭ-mŭs). ACTION: Extends and rotates thigh. ORIGIN: Superior curved iliac line and crest, coccyx, and sacrum. INSERTION: Fascia lata and femur below greater trochanter. INNERVATION: Inferior gluteal.

gluteus medius (glū'tē-ŭs mē'dĭ-ŭs). ACTION: Abducts and rotates thigh. ORIGIN: Lateral surface of ilium. INSERTION: Greater trochanter. INNERVATION: Branches of superior gluteal.

gluteus minimus (glū'tē-ŭs mĭn'ĭ-mŭs). ACTION: Abducts and extends thigh. ORIGIN: Lateral surface of ilium. INSERTION: Greater trochanter. INNERVATION: Branch of superior gluteal.

gracilis (grăs'ĭ-lĭs). ACTION: Flexes and adducts leg; adducts thigh. ORIGIN: Symphysis pubis and pubic arch. INSERTION: Medial surface of shaft of tibia. INNERVATION: Branch of obturator.

iliacus (ĭ-lī'ă-kŭs). ACTION: Flexes and rotates thigh. ORIGIN: Margin of iliac fossa. INSERTION: Lesser trochanter. INNERVATION: Branches of femoral.

obturator externus (ŏb-tū-rā'tŏr ĕks-tĕr'nŭs). ACTION: Rotates thigh outward. ORIGIN: Margin of thyroid foramen and obturator membrane. INSERTION: Digital fossa of greater trochanter. INNERVATION: Branch of obturator.

obturator internus (ŏb-tū-rā'tŏr ĭn-tĕr'-nŭs). ACTION: Rotates thigh outward. ORIGIN: Pubes, ischium, obturator foramen. INSERTION: Inner surface of great trochanter. INNERVATION: Sacral plexus.

pectineus (pĕk-tĭn'ē-ŭs). ACTION: Flexes and adducts thigh. ORIGIN: Pubic spine; iliopectineal line. INSERTION: Pectineal line of femur. INNERVATION: Branch of obturator and femoral.

piriformis (pī-rĭ-fŏr'mĭs). ACTION: Abducts and rotates thigh outward. ORIGIN: Margins of anterior sacral foramina and great sacrosciatic notch of ilium. INSERTION: Upper margin of greater trochanter. INNERVATION: Branch of sacral.

psoas major (sō'ăs mā'jor). ACTION: Flexes thigh, adducts and rotates it medially. ORIGIN: Last thoracic and all of the lumbar vertebrae. INSERTION: Lesser trochanter of femur. INNERVATION: Lumbar plexus. SYN: *psoas magnus.*

psoas minor (sō'ăs mī'nor). ACTION: Tenses iliac fascia. ORIGIN: Twelfth thoracic and 1st lumbar vertebrae. INSERTION: Iliac fascia and iliopectineal tuberosity. INNERVATION: Branch of lumbar. SYN: *psoas parvus.*

Muscles of the Body (*Continued*)

pyriformis (pĭ-rĭ-fôr′mĭs). SAME AS: *piriformis*.

quadratus femoris (kwăd-rā′tŭs fĕm′ŏ-rĭs). ACTION: Rotates thigh outward. ORIGIN: Ischial tuberosity. INSERTION: Intertrochanteric ridge. INNERVATION: Sciatic.

quadriceps extensor femoris (kwăd′rĭ-sĕps ĕks-tĕn′sor fĕm′ŏ-rĭs). SAME AS: *quadriceps femoris*.

quadriceps femoris (kwăd′rĭ-sĕps fĕm′ŏ-rĭs). ACTION: Extends leg. ORIGIN: By four heads: rectus femoris, vastus medialis, vastus lateralis and vastus intermedius. INSERTION: Patella and tibial tuberosity. INNERVATION: Branches of femoral.

rectus femoris (rĕk′tŭs fĕm′ŏ-rĭs). ACTION: Extends leg. ORIGIN: Iliac spine, upper margin of acetabulum. INSERTION: Base of patella, INNERVATION: Femoral.

sartorius (săr-tō′rĭ-ŭs). ACTION: Flexes and rotates thigh and leg. ORIGIN: Anterior superior iliac spine. INSERTION: Tibial tuberosity. INNERVATION: Branches of femoral.

semimembranosus (sĕm″ĭ-mĕm-brä-nō′-sŭs). ACTION: Flexes and rotates leg; extends thigh. ORIGIN: Ischial tuberosity. INSERTION: Medial condyle of tibia. INNERVATION: Tibial portion of sciatic.

semitendinosus (sĕm″ĭ-tĕn-dĭ-nō′sŭs). ACTION: Flexes and rotates leg; extends thigh. ORIGIN: Ischial tuberosity. INSERTION: Shaft of tibia below internal tuberosity. INNERVATION: Tibial portion of sciatic.

subcrureus (sŭb-krū′rē-ŭs). SAME AS: *articularis genu.*

tensor fasciae latae (tĕn′sor făs′ĭ-ē lā′tē). ACTION: Flexes and rotates thigh. ORIGIN: Iliac crest, iliac spine, fascia lata. INSERTION: Iliotibial band of fascia lata. INNERVATION: Branch of superior gluteal.

tensor fasciae femoris (tĕn′sor făs′ĭ-ē fĕm′ŏ-rĭs). SAME AS: *tensor fasciae latae.*

vastus lateralis (văs′tŭs lăt-ĕr-ā′lĭs). ACTION: Extends knee. ORIGIN: Linea aspera to greater trochanter. INSERTION: Common tendon of quadriceps femoris. INNERVATION: Branches of femoral. SYN: *vastus externus.*

vastus intermedius (văs′tŭs ĭn″tĕr-mē′dĭ-ŭs). ORIGIN: Upper part of anterior surface of shaft of femur. INSERTION: Common tendon of quadriceps femoris. INNERVATION: Branches of femoral. SYN: *crureus.*

vastus medialis (văs′tŭs mē-dĭ-ā′lĭs). ACTION: Extends leg; draws patella in. ORIGIN: Linea aspera of femur. INSERTION: Common tendon of quadriceps femoris. INNERVATION: Branches of femoral. SYN: *vastus internus.*

LEG

extensor digitorum longus (ĕks-tĕn′sor dĭj-ĭ-tō′rŭm lŏng′gŭs). ACTION: Extends toes, flexes foot. ORIGIN: External tuberosity of tibia; body of fibula. INSERTION: Second and 3rd phalanges of toes. INNERVATION: Branches of peroneal.

extensor hallucis longus (ĕks-tĕn′sor häl-ū′sĭs lŏng′gŭs). ACTION: Extends great toe; flexes foot. ORIGIN: Front of fibula and interosseous membrane. INSERTION: Terminal phalanx of great toe. INNERVATION: Branch of peroneal.

extensor proprius hallucis (ĕks-tĕn′sŏr prŏ′prĭ-ŭs häl-ū′sĭs). SAME AS: *extensor hallucis longus.*

flexor digitorum longus (flĕks′ŏr dĭj-ĭ-tō′rŭm lŏng′gŭs). ACTION: Flexes phalanges and extends toes. ORIGIN: Posterior surface of tibia. INSERTION: Terminal phalanges of four lesser toes. INNERVATION: Branch of tibial.

flexor hallucis longus (flĕks′ŏr häl-ū′sĭs lŏng′gŭs). ACTION: Flexes great toe and extends foot. ORIGIN: Lower portion of shaft of fibula. INSERTION: Distal phalanx of great toe. INNERVATION: Posterior tibial.

gastrocnemius (găs-trŏk-nē′mĭ-ŭs). ACTION: Flexes foot and leg. ORIGIN: External and internal femoral condyles. INSERTION: By tendo calcaneus into os calcis. INNERVATION: Branches of tibial.

peroneus brevis (pĕr-ō-nē′ŭs brē′vĭs). ACTION: Extends and abducts foot. ORIGIN: Midportion of shaft of fibula. INSERTION: Base of 5th metatarsal bone. INNERVATION: Branch of peroneal.

peroneus longus (pĕr-ō-nē′ŭs lŏng′gŭs). ACTION: Extends, abducts, and everts foot. ORIGIN: Upper fibula and external condyle of tibia. INSERTION: By tendon to internal cuneiform and 1st metatarsal bone. INNERVATION: Branch of peroneal.

peroneus tertius (pĕr-ō-nē′ŭs tĕr′shĭ-ŭs). ACTION: Flexes foot. ORIGIN: Lower part of fibula. INSERTION: Fifth metatarsal bone. INNERVATION: Branch of peroneal.

plantaris (plăn-tā′rĭs). ACTION: Extends foot. ORIGIN: External supracondyloid ridge of femur. INSERTION: Inner border of tendo calcaneus. INNERVATION: Branch of tibial.

popliteus (pŏp″lĭ-tē′ŭs). ACTION: Flexes leg and rotates it inward. ORIGIN: External condyle of femur. INSERTION: Posterior surface of tibia. INNERVATION: Branch of tibial.

soleus (sō′lē-ŭs). ACTION: Extends and rotates foot. ORIGIN: Upper shaft of fibula, oblique line of tibia. INSERTION: By tendo calcaneus to os calcis. INNERVATION: Tibial.

tibialis anterior (tĭb-ĭ-ā′lĭs ăn-tē′rĭ-ŏr). ACTION: Elevates and flexes foot. ORIGIN: Upper tibia, interosseous membrane and intermuscular septum. INSERTION: Internal cuneiform and 1st metatarsal. INNERVATION: Branch of peroneal. SYN: *tibialis anticus.*

tibialis posterior (tĭb-ĭ-ā′lĭs pŏs-tē′rĭ-ŏr). ACTION: Extends tarsus and inverts foot. ORIGIN:

Shaft of fibula and tibia. INSERTION: Tuberosity of scaphoid, 2nd to 4th metatarsal, internal cuneiform. INNERVATION: Branch of tibial. SYN: *tibialis posticus.*

FOOT

abductor digiti quinti (ăb-dŭk'tŏr dĭj'ĭ-tī kwĭn'tī). ACTION: Abducts little toe. ORIGIN: Outer tuberosity of calcaneus, plantar fascia, and intermuscular septum. INSERTION: External side of 1st phalanx of little toe. INNERVATION: Lateral plantar.

abductor hallucis (ăb-dŭk'tŏr hăl-ū'sĭs). ACTION: Abducts great toe. ORIGIN: Inner tuberosity of os calcis, plantar fascia. INSERTION: Inner side, 1st phalanx of great toe. INNERVATION: Medial plantar.

abductor minimi digiti (ăb-dŭk'tŏr mĭn'ĭ-mī dĭj'ĭ-tī). SAME AS: *abductor digiti quinti.*

adductor hallucis (ăd-dŭk'tŏr hăl-ū'sĭs). ACTION: Adducts great toe. ORIGIN: Tarsal terminations of middle metatarsal bones. INSERTION: Base of 1st phalanx of great toe. INNERVATION: Branch of lateral plantar.

adductor obliquus hallucis (ăd-dŭk'tŏr ŏb-lī'kwŭs hăl-ū'sĭs). SAME AS: *adductor hallucis.*

adductor transversus hallucis (ăd-dŭk'tŏr trăns-vĕr'sŭs hăl-ū'sĭs). SAME AS: *adductor hallucis.*

extensor digitorum brevis (ĕks-tĕn'sŏr dĭj-ĭ-tō'rŭm brē'vĭs). ACTION: Extends toes. ORIGIN: Dorsal surface of os calcis. INSERTION: To 1st phalanx of great toe and the tendons of extensor digitorum longus. INNERVATION: Branch of peroneal.

flexor accessorius (flĕks'ōr ăk-sĕ-sō'rĭ-ŭs). SAME AS: *quadratus plantae.*

flexor brevis minimi digiti (flĕks'ōr brē'vĭs mĭn'ĭ-mī dĭj'ĭ-tī). SAME AS: *flexor digiti quinti brevis.*

flexor digiti quinti brevis (flĕks'ōr dĭj'ĭ-tī kwĭn'tī brē'vĭs). ACTION: Flexes the little toe. ORIGIN: Base of metatarsal of little toe and sheath of peroneus longus. INSERTION: Outer side of base of 1st phalanx of little toe. INNERVATION: External plantar.

flexor digitorum brevis (flĕks'ōr dĭj'ĭ-tō'rŭm brē'vĭs). ACTION: Flexes toe. ORIGIN: Os calcis and plantar fascia. INSERTION: Second phalanges of lesser toes. INNERVATION: Internal plantar.

flexor hallucis brevis (flĕks'ōr hăl-ū'sĭs brē'vĭs). ACTION: Flexes great toe. ORIGIN: Internal surface of cuboid and middle and external cuneiform bones. INSERTION: Sides of base of 1st phalanx of great toe. INNERVATION: Internal and external plantar.

interosseus dorsalis pedis (ĭn"tĕr-ŏs'ē-ŭs dōr-sā'lĭs pē'dĭs). Four. ACTION: Adduct 2nd toe; abduct 2nd, 3rd, and 4th toe. ORIGIN: Shafts of adjacent metatarsal bones. INSERTION: First phalanges of lesser toes. INNERVATION: External plantar.

interosseus plantaris (ĭn"tĕr-ŏs'ē-ŭs plăn-tā'rĭs). Three. ACTION: Adduct three outer toes. ORIGIN: Third, 4th, and 5th metatarsal bones. INSERTION: First phalanx of corresponding toe. INNERVATION: External plantar.

lumbricalis (lŭm-brĭ-kā'lĭs). Four. ACTION: Flex the 1st and extend the 2nd and 3rd phalanges. ORIGIN: Tendons of flexor digitorum longus. INSERTION: First phalanx and extensor tendon. INNERVATION: External and internal plantar.

pronator pedis (prō-nā'tŏr pē'dĭs). SAME AS: *quadratus plantae.*

quadratus plantae (kwăd-rā'tŭs plăn'tē). ACTION: Assists flexing of toes. ORIGIN: Inferior surface of os calcis by two heads from outer and inner borders. INSERTION: Tendons of flexor digitorum longus. INNERVATION: Branch of lateral plantar. SYN: *flexor accessorius.*

transversus pedis (trăns-vĕr'sŭs pē'dĭs). INSERTION: Transverse head of adductor hallucis.

GENERAL

arrectores pilorum (ăr-rĕk-tō'rēz pī-lō'rŭm). ACTION: Elevates hairs of skin. ORIGIN: Papillary layer of skin. INSERTION: Hair follicles. INNERVATION: Sympathetic.

Principal Joints

Type	Variety	Ligaments
Acromioclavicular	Arthrodial	Capsular; superior and inferior acromio-clavicular; articular disk; coracocla-vicular (trapezoid and conoid)
Ankle	Ginglymus	Capsular; deltoid; anterior and posterior talofibular; calcaneofibular
Atlas	Trochoid; arthrodial	Capsular; anterior and posterior atlanto-axial; transverse
Calcaneocuboid	Arthrodial	Capsular; dorsal calcaneocuboid; bifurcated; long plantar; plantar calcaneocuboid
Carpometacarpal	Arthrodial	Dorsal; volar; interosseous
Elbow	Ginglymus (hinge)	Capsular; ulnar and radial collateral
Hip	Enarthrodial	Capsular; iliofemoral; pubocapsular; ischiofemoral; round ligament of femur; transverse acetabular
Intercarpal Carpal, proximal Carpal, distal Carpal bones, two rows with each other	 Arthrodial Arthrodial	 Dorsal; volar; interosseous Dorsal; volar; interosseous Volar; dorsal; collateral
Intermetacarpal		Dorsal; volar; interosseous; transverse metacarpal
Intermetatarsal	Arthrodial	Dorsal; plantar; interosseous
Interphalangeal	Ginglymus	Collateral; volar in fingers and plantar in toes
Knee	Condyloid and Arthrodial	Capsular; patellar; oblique and arcuate popliteal; tibial and fibular collateral; anterior and posterior cruciate; medial and lateral menisci; transverse; coronary
Mandible (Jaw)	Ginglymus: arthrodial	Capsular; temporomandibular; spheno-mandibular; articular disk; stylomandi-bular
Metacarpophalangeal	Condyloid	Volar; collateral
Metatarsophalangeal	Condyloid	Plantar; collateral
Pubic	Amphiarthrodial	Superior and arcuate pubic; interpubic fibrocartilaginous layer
Radioulnar, distal	Trochoid (pivot)	Ulnar collateral; articular disk

Type	Variety	Ligaments
Radioulnar, middle	Trochoid	Oblique; interosseous
Radioulnar, proximal	Trochoid	Annular
Ribs, heads of	Arthrodial	Capsular; radiate; intra-articular
Ribs, tubercles and necks of	Arthrodial	Capsular; anterior and posterior costo-transverse; neck of rib; tubercle of rib
Sacrococcygeal	Amphiarthrodial	Anterior, posterior, and lateral sacrococcygeal; interposed fibrocartilage; inter-articular
Sacroiliac	Amphiarthrodial	Anterior and posterior sacroiliac; interosseous
Sacrum and ischium		Sacrotuberous; sacrospinous
Shoulder	Enarthrodial (ball-and-socket)	Capsular; coracohumeral; glenohumeral; transverse humeral; glenoid of humerus
Sternoclavicular	Double arthrodial	Capsular; anterior and posterior sternoclavicular; inter- and costoclavicular; articular disk
Sternocostal	Arthrodial	Capsular; radiate and intra-articular sternocostal; costoxiphoid
Subtalar	Arthrodial	Capsular; anterior, posterior, lateral, medial, and interosseous; talocalcaneal
Talo-calcaneonavicular	Arthrodial	Capsular; dorsal talonavicular
Tarsometatarsal	Arthrodial	Dorsal; plantar; interosseous
Tibiofibular	Arthrodial	Capsular; anterior; posterior
Tibiofibular syndesmosis	Arthrodial	Anterior and posterior tibiofibular; inferior transverse; interosseous
Vertebral arches	Arthrodial	Capsular; flaval; supraspinal; nuchal; interspinal; intertransverse
Vertebral bodies	Amphiarthrodial	Anterior and posterior longitudinal; intervertebral fibrocartilages
Vertebral column with cranium	Condyloid	Capsular; anterior and posterior atlanto-occipital membrane; lateral; tectorial membrane; alar; apical odontoid
Wrist	Condyloid	Volar and dorsal radiocarpal; ulnar and radial collateral

Nerves

Name	NA Term	Origin	Function	Distribution
Abducent (6th cranial n.)	N. abducens	Pons	Motor	Lateral rectus muscle of eye.
Accessory (11th cranial n.)	N. accessorius	Medulla oblongata and spinal cord	Motor	Sternomastoid and trapezius muscles.
Auditory (8th cranial n.)	N. vestibulocochlearis	Cochlea	Special sense of hearing	Internal auditory meatus.
Auricular, great	N. auricularis magnus	Second and third cervical through cervical plexus	Sensory	Side of neck; skin of ear and cheek.
Auricular, posterior	N. auricularis posterior	Facial	Motor	Posterior auricular muscle.
Auriculotemporal	N. auriculotemporalis	Mandibular div. of trigeminal	Sensory	Side of scalp.
Buccal	N. buccalis	Mandibular div. of trigeminal	Sensory	Skin and mucous membrane of cheek.
Calcanean, internal		Posterior tibial	Sensory	Sole of foot.
Cervical n., superficial (cutaneous cervical n.; transverse n. of neck)	N. transversus colli	Second and third cervical through cervical plexus	Sensory	Skin of front of neck.
Chorda, tympani		Facial	Motor	Sublingual and submaxillary glands.
Ciliary, long	Nn. ciliares longi	Nasal	Sensory and motor	Cornea, iris, and ciliary body.

App. 46

Ciliary, short	Nn. ciliares breves	Ciliary ganglion	Sensory and motor	Cornea, iris, and ciliary body.
Circumflex (Axillary)	N. axillaris	Posterior cord of brachial plexus	Motor and sensory	Deltoid, teres minor, shoulder joint, and overlying skin.
Coccygeal	N. coccygeus	Spinal cord	Motor and sensory	Coccygeus muscle and skin over coccyx.
Cochlear. SEE: *Vestibulocochlear* n.		Auditory	Special sense of hearing	Cochlea.
Crural, anterior. SEE: *Femoral* n.				
Cutaneous, internal	N. cutaneus antebrachii medialis	Inner cord of brachial plexus	Sensory	Skin of inner aspect of forearm.
Cutaneous, lesser internal	N. cutaneus brachii medialis	Inner cord of brachial plexus	Sensory	Skin of inner aspect of upper arm.
Dental, inferior	N. alveolaris inferior	Mandibular div. of trigeminal	Sensory and motor	Teeth of lower jaw, mylohyoid muscle, and skin of chin.
Dental, superior	Nn. alveolares superiores	Maxillary div. of trigeminal	Sensory	Upper teeth and gums.
Digastric		Facial	Motor	Stylohyoid and posterior belly of digastric muscle.
Facial (7th cranial n.)	N. facialis	Pons	Motor	Muscles of expression.
Femoral (anterior crural n.)	N. femoralis	2nd, 3rd, and 4th lumbar	Motor and sensory	Muscles and skin of thigh.

Nerves (Continued)

Name	NA Equivalents	Origin	Function	Distribution
Frontal	N. frontalis	Ophthalmic div. of trigeminal	Sensory	Skin of forehead.
Genitofemoral (genitocrural n.)	N. genitofemoralis	1st and 2nd lumbar	Sensory and motor	Cremaster muscle and skin of groin and upper part of thigh.
Glossopharyngeal (9th cranial n.)	N. glossopharyngeus	Medulla oblongata	Motor and sensory	Muscles and mucous membrane of pharynx, fauces, and posterior third of tongue.
Gluteal, inferior	N. gluteus inferior	5th lumbar and 1st and 2nd sacral	Motor	Gluteus maximus.
Gluteal, superior	N. gluteus superior	4th and 5th lumbar and 1st sacral	Motor	Gluteus medius and minimus, tensor fasciae femoris.
Hypogastric	N. hypogastricus	Iliohypogastric	Motor and sensory	Muscles and skin of abdominal wall.
Hypoglossal (12th cranial n.)	N. hypoglossus	Hypoglossal nucleus in medulla oblongata	Motor	Intrinsic muscles of tongue.
Iliac	Ramus cutaneus lateralis	Iliohypogastric	Sensory	Skin of gluteal region.
Iliohypogastric	N. iliohypogastricus	1st lumbar	Sensory and motor	Muscles and skin of hypogastrium.
Ilioinguinal	N. ilioinguinalis	1st lumbar	Sensory and motor	Muscles of abdominal wall, skin of upper thigh, skin of root of penis and scrotum (in male),

Infraorbital	N. infraorbitalis	Maxillary div. of trigeminal	Sensory	Skin of cheek and all upper teeth except molars.
Infratrochlear	N. infratrochlearis	Nasociliary	Sensory	Skin of lower eyelid and root of nose, conjunctiva, and lacrimal sac and caruncle.
Intercostal	Nn. intercostales	Thoracic	Sensory and motor	Muscles and skin of back, thorax, and upper abdomen.
Intercostobrachial	Nn. intercosto-brachiales	2nd intercostal	Sensory	Skin of axilla and medial side of arm.
Interosseous anterior (volar interosseous n.)	N. interosseus anterior	Median	Motor	Deep flexor and pronator muscles of forearm.
Interosseous, posterior	N. interosseus posterior	Musculospiral (radial)	Motor and sensory	Muscles and skin of back of forearm and wrist.
Lacrimal	N. lacrimalis	Ophthalmic div. of trigeminal	Sensory	Lacrimal gland, conjunctiva, and skin of upper eyelid.
Laryngeal, inferior	N. laryngeus inferior	Branch of recurrent laryngeal	Motor	Muscles of larynx except crico-thyroid.
Laryngeal, recurrent	N. laryngeus recurrens	Vagus	Motor	Muscles of larynx except crico-thyroid.
Laryngeal, superior	N. laryngeus superior	Vagus	Motor and sensory	Mucous membrane of larynx; arytenoid and cricothyroid muscles.

and skin of mons pubis and labium majus (in female).

Nerves (Continued)

Name	NA Equivalents	Origin	Function	Distribution
Lingual	N. lingualis	Mandibular div. of trigeminal	Sensory	Mucous membrane of anterior two thirds of tongue and floor and outer wall of mouth.
Lumbar	Nn. lumbales	Spinal cord	Motor and sensory	Loins and front of lower abdomen and thigh to help in forming lumbar and sacral plexuses.
Mandibular	N. mandibularis	Trigeminal	Motor and sensory	Teeth, gums, and skin of lower jaw and cheek; muscles of mastication; mucous membrane of anterior two thirds of tongue.
Masseteric	N. massetericus	Mandibular div. of trigeminal	Motor	Masseter muscle.
Maxillary	N. maxillaris	Trigeminal	Sensory	Nasal pharynx, palate, teeth of upper jaw and skin of cheek.
Median	N. medianus	Internal and external cords of brachial plexus	Motor and sensory	Pronators and flexors of forearm, two external lumbricales, thenar muscles, skin of palm of first four fingers.
Mental	N. mentalis	Inferior dental	Sensory	Skin and mucous membrane of lower lip and chin.
Musculocutaneous	N. musculocutaneus	External cord of brachial plexus	Motor and sensory	Flexors of upper arm and skin of external aspect of forearm.

Musculospiral. SEE: *Radial n.*

Mylohyoid	N.mylohyoideus	Inferior dental	Motor	Mylohyoid muscle and anterior belly of digastric muscle.
Nasal (nasociliary n.)	N.nasociliaris	Ophthalmic div. of trigeminal	Sensory	Ciliary ganglion, iris, conjunctiva, ethmoid cells, mucous membrane and skin of nose.
Nasopalatine	N.nasopalatinus	Meckel's ganglion (sphenopalatine ganglion)	Sensory	Mucous membrane of nose and palate.
Obturator	N.obturatorius	2nd, 3rd, and 4th lumbar through lumbar plexus	Motor and sensory	Adductors of thigh, hip and knee joints; skin of inner aspect of thigh.
Occipital, greater	N.occipitalis major	2nd cervical	Motor and sensory	Muscles of back of neck; skin over occiput.
Occipital, lesser	N.occipitalis minor	2nd and 3rd cervical	Sensory	Skin behind ear and on back of scalp.
Occipital, third	N.occipitalis tertius	3rd cervial	Sensory	Skin of back of head and nape of neck.
Oculomotor (3rd cranial n.)	N.oculomotorius	Floor of aqueduct of Sylvius	Motor	All ocular muscles except lateral rectus and superior oblique.
Olfactory (1st cranial n.)	N. olfactorii	Olfactory lobe	Special sense of smell	Nasal mucous membranes in olfactory region.
Ophthalmic	N.ophthalmicus	1st div. of trigeminal	Sensory	Lacrimal gland, conjunctiva, skin of forehead, skin and mucous membrane of nose.

Nerves *(Continued)*

Name	NA Equivalents	Origin	Function	Distribution
Optic (2nd cranial n.)	N. cticus	Corpora quadrigemina	Special sense of sight	Retina.
Palatine, anterior, middle, and posterior	Nn.alatini	Meckel's ganglion	Motor	Mucous membrane of palate.
Perineal	N. prineales	Pudendal	Motor and sensory	Muscles and skin of perineum.
Peroneal, common (lateral popliteal n.)	N. proneus communis	Sciatic	Motor and sensory	Extensor muscles of lower leg and foot and overlying skin.
Phrenic	N. arenicus	3rd, 4th, and 5th cervical	Motor and sensory	Diaphragm.
Pneumogastric. SEE: *Vagus n.*				
Popliteal, deep. SEE: *Tibial n.*				
Popliteal, lateral. SEE *Peroneal n., comon.*				
Pterygoid	N. terygoideus	Mandibular div. of trigeminal	Motor	Lateral and medial pterygoid muscles.
Pterygoid canal, n. of. SEE: *Vidian n.*				
Pudendal	N. adendus	2nd, 3rd, and 4th sacral	Sensory	Skin and muscles of perineum and genitalia.
Radial (musculospiral n.)	N. idialis	Brachial plexus	Motor and sensory	Skin of back of entire arm and hand; extensor muscles of entire arm and hand.

Sacral	Nn. sacrales	Spinal cord	Motor and sensory	Muscles and skin of loins and lower extremities.
Saphenous, external or short. SEE: *Sural n.*				
Saphenous, internal or long	N. saphenus	Femoral	Sensory	Skin of inner aspect of knee, leg, ankle, and dorsum of foot.
Sciatic (great sciatic n.)	N. ischiadicus	Sacral plexus	Motor and sensory	Muscles of calf and back of thigh; skin of lower calf and upper surface of foot.
Sphenopalatine	N. pterygopalatini	Maxillary div. of trigeminal	Sensory	Meckel's ganglion.
Spinal accessory (accessory n.; 11th cranial n.)	N. accessorius	Floor of 4th ventricle and cervical cord	Motor	Sternomastoid and trapezius muscles.
Stapedial	N. stapedius	Facial	Motor	Stapedius muscle.
Stylohyoid		Facial	Motor	Stylohyoid muscle.
Suboccipital	N. suboccipitalis	Posterior div. of 1st cervical	Motor	Complexus oblique and rectus muscles of back of neck.
Subscapular	—	Posterior cord of brachial plexus	Motor	Teres major and subscapularis muscles.
Supraclavicular, intermediate (supraclavicular n, middle; supraclavicular n.)	Nn. supraclaviculares intermedii	3rd and 4th cervical	Sensory	Skin of fossa below collar bone.
Supraclavicular, lateral (supra-clavicular n., posterior; supra-acromial n.)	N. supraclaviculares laterales	3rd and 4th cervical	Sensory	Skin of shoulder.

Nerves (Continued)

Name	NA Equivalents	Origin	Function	Distribution
Supraclavicular, medial (supraclavicular n., anterior; suprasternal n.)	N. supraclaviculares mediales	3rd and 4th cervical	Sensory	Skin over upper part of thorax.
Supraorbital	N. supraorbitalis	Frontal	Sensory	Forehead, upper eyelid, scalp, and frontal sinus.
Suprascapular	N. suprascapularis	5th and 6th cervical	Motor	Supraspinatus and infraspinatus muscles and the shoulder joint.
Supratrochlear	N. supratrochlearis	Frontal	Sensory	Skin of upper eyelid and root of nose.
Sural	N. suralis	Common peroneal and tibial n.'s	Sensory	Skin of calf and medial side of foot to great toe.
Temporal, deep	N. temporalis profundi	Mandibular div. of trigeminal	Motor	Temporal muscle.
Thoracic	Nn. thoracici	Spinal cord	Motor and sensory	Muscles and skin of thorax.
Thoracic, anterior		Brachial plexus	Motor	Pectoralis minor and major muscles.
Thoracic, long (posterior thoracic n.; external respiratory n. of Bell).	N. thoracicus longus	5th, 6th, and 7th cervical	Motor	Serratus anterior muscle.
Tibial	N. tibialis	Sciatic	Motor and sensory	Flexor muscles of back of knee joint and calf; skin of lower leg.

App. 54

Trigeminal (5th cranial n.; tri-facial n.)	N. trigeminus	Midbrain and pons	Motor and sensory	Skin of face, tongue, teeth; muscles of mastication.
Trochlear (4th cranial n.; pathetic n.)	N. trochlearis	Floor of aqueduct of Sylvius	Motor	Superior oblique muscle of eye.
Tympanic (Jacobson's n.)	N. tympanicus	Glossopharyngeal	Sensory	Tympanum, eustachian tube, and structures of middle ear.
Ulnar	N. ulnaris	Medial cord of brachial plexus	Motor and sensory	Muscles and skin of forearm and hand.
Vagus (10th cranial n.; pneumo-gastric n.)	N. vagus	Medulla oblongata	Motor and sensory	Pharynx, larynx, heart, lungs, stomach.
Vestibulocochlear (8th cranial n.; acoustic n.; auditory n.)	N. vestibulocochlearis	Ganglion of Scarpa and ganglion of Corti	Sense of hearing	Internal auditory meatus.
Vidian	N. canalis pterygoidei	Facial	Sensory	Meckel's ganglion (sphenopalatine ganglion).
Zygomatic	N. zygomaticus	Maxillary div. of trigeminal	Sensory	Skin of temple and cheek bone.

Nerve Plexuses of the Sympathetic and Cerebrospinal Systems

aortic (ā-or'tĭk). (*Abdominal*). ORIGIN: Semilunar, lumbar ganglia, renal and solar plexuses. LOCATION: Sides and front of aorta. DISTRIBUTION: Inferior mesenteric, spermatic and hypogastric plexus. Filaments to inferior vena cava. (*Thoracic*). ORIGIN: Thoracic ganglia of sympathetic nerve, cardiac plexus. LOCATION: Surrounding the thoracic aorta. DISTRIBUTION: Solar plexus, aorta.

*brachial (brā'kĭ-ăl). ORIGIN: Anterior branches of 5th, 6th, 7th, 8th, cervical, and greater part of 1st dorsal nerves. LOCATION: Lower part of neck to axilla. DISTRIBUTION: Sixteen branches of suprascapular, subscapular, rhomboid, median, ulnar, musculospiral, posterior thoracic, musculothoracic, circumflex, musculocutaneous nerves.

cardiac (kar'dĭ-ăk). (*Great or Deep*). ORIGIN: Cardiac nerves of cervical ganglion of sympathetic and vagus. LOCATION: In front of bifurcation of trachea. DISTRIBUTION: Pulmonary, coronary and cardiac plexuses. (*Superficial or Anterior*). ORIGIN: Left superior cardiac nerve, branch of vagus and filaments of deep cardiac plexus. LOCATION: Beneath arch of aorta. Front of right pulmonary artery. DISTRIBUTION: Coronary and pulmonary plexuses.

carotid (kăr-ŏt'ĭd). (*External*). ORIGIN: Pharyngeal plexus, superior cardiac nerve, and superior cervical ganglion. LOCATION: Around external carotid artery. DISTRIBUTION: External carotid artery and its branches. (*Internal*). ORIGIN: Asympathetic plexus. LOCATION: Surrounding internal carotid artery. DISTRIBUTION: Tympanic plexus, sphenopalatine ganglion, abducens and oculomotor nerves, the cerebral vessels, and the ciliary ganglion.

cavernous (kăv'ĕr-nŭs). ORIGIN: 3rd to 6th cranial nerves and ophthalmic ganglion. LOCATION: Cavernous sinus. DISTRIBUTION: Wall of internal carotid artery.

celiac (sē'lĭ-ăk). ORIGIN: Solar plexus, branches from lesser splanchnic and vagus nerves. LOCATION: Behind stomach, in front of aorta at level of origin of celiac artery. DISTRIBUTION: Coronary, hepatic, pyloric gastroduodenal, gastroepiploic and splenic plexuses. SYN: *solar plexus.*

*cervical (ser'vĭ-kăl). ORIGIN: Anterior branches of first four cervical nerves. LOCATION: Beneath sternocleidomastoid muscle opposite first four cervical vertebrae. DISTRIBUTION: Cutaneous, muscular, and communicating rami.

*coccygeal (kŏk-sĭj'ē-ăl). ORIGIN: Fourth and 5th sacral and the coccygeal nerves. LOCATION: Dorsal surface of coccyx and caudal end of sacrum. DISTRIBUTION: Anococcygeal nerves.

cystic (sĭs'tĭk). ORIGIN: Hepatic plexus. LOCATION: At gallbladder. DISTRIBUTION: Gallbladder.

esophageal (ē-sō-fāj'ē-ăl). ORIGIN: Vagus nerve, thoracic sympathetic ganglia. LOCATION: Around the esophagus. DISTRIBUTION: Esophagus.

gastric (găs'trĭk). ORIGIN: Celiac plexus and continuations of esophageal plexuses. LOCATION: Gastric artery. DISTRIBUTION: Abdominal viscera.

hemorrhoidal (hĕm″ō-roy'dăl). ORIGIN: Pelvic and inferior mesenteric plexuses. LOCATION: Rectum and sides of rectum. DISTRIBUTION: Rectum.

hepatic (hē-păt'ĭk). ORIGIN: Celiac plexus, left vagus, right phrenic. LOCATION: Accompanies hepatic artery. DISTRIBUTION: Liver.

hypogastric (hī″pō-găs'trĭk). ORIGIN: Aortic plexus and lumbar ganglia. LOCATION: Promontory of sacrum. DISTRIBUTION: Pelvic plexus.

*lumbar (lŭm'bar). ORIGIN: First four lumbar nerves. LOCATION: Psoas muscle. DISTRIBUTION: Iliohypogastric, ilioinguinal, genitocrural, external cutaneous, obturator, accessory, and anterior crural nerves.

Meissner's (mīs'nĕr). ORIGIN: Superior mesenteric plexus (controls secretions of the bowels). LOCATION: Submucous coat of small intestines. DISTRIBUTION: Intestinal walls.

mesenteric (mĕs-ĕn-tĕr'ĭk). ORIGIN: Celiac plexus and left side of aortic plexus. LOCATION: Surrounding the inferior and superior mesenteric arteries. DISTRIBUTION: Descending colon, sigmoid, rectum, intestines.

myenteric (mī-ĕn-tĕr'ĭk). ORIGIN: Sympathetic system (controls peristalsis). LOCATION: Between the circular and longitudinal coats of small intestines. DISTRIBUTION: Intestinal walls.

ophthalmic (ŏf-thăl'mĭk). ORIGIN: Internal carotid plexus. LOCATION: Around

---

* Plexuses of central nervous system.

Nerve Plexuses (*Continued*)

ophthalmic artery and optic nerve. DISTRIBUTION: Optic region.

pancreatic (păn-krē-ăt′ĭk). ORIGIN: Splenic plexus. LOCATION: Near pancreas. DISTRIBUTION: Filaments to pancreas.

pancreaticoduodenal (păn-krē-ăt″ĭ-kō-dū″ō-dē′năl). ORIGIN: Hepatic plexus. LOCATION: Near head of pancreas. DISTRIBUTION: Filaments to pancreas and duodenum.

pelvic (pĕl′vĭk). ORIGIN: Hypogastric plexus, 2nd to 4th sacral nerves, 1st and 2nd sacral ganglia (pelvic brain). LOCATION: Side of rectum and bladder. DISTRIBUTION: Viscera of pelvis, pelvic plexus.

phrenic (frĕn′ĭk). ORIGIN: Solar plexus, semilunar ganglia. LOCATION: Accompanies phrenic artery to diaphragm. DISTRIBUTION: Diaphragm and suprarenal capsules.

prostatic (prŏs-tăt′ĭk). ORIGIN: Hypogastric plexus. LOCATION: Vesical arteries. DISTRIBUTION: Bladder.

pulmonary (pŭl′mō-nā″rĭ). ORIGIN: Anterior and posterior pulmonary branches of vagus and sympathetic nerves. LOCATION: Root of lungs, front and back. DISTRIBUTION: Root of lungs.

pyloric (pī-lor′ĭk). ORIGIN: Hepatic plexus. LOCATION: Near pylorus, DISTRIBUTION: Filaments to pylorus.

renal (rē′năl). ORIGIN: Solar and aortic plexuses and semilunar ganglia. LOCATION: Renal artery. DISTRIBUTION: Kidneys, posterior vena cava, spermatic plexus.

*sacral (sā′krăl). ORIGIN: Anterior branch of 4th and 5th lumbar and 1st, 2nd, 3rd, and 4th sacral nerves. LOCATION: Front of sacrum on piriformis muscle. DISTRIBUTION: Muscular, pudic, superior gluteal, great and small sciatic nerves.

* Plexuses of central nervous system.

solar (sō′lar). (*Epigastric*). ORIGIN: Splanchnics and right vagus. LOCATION: Back of stomach. DISTRIBUTION: Semilunar ganglia, phrenic, suprarenal, renal, spermatic, celiac, superior mesenteric, and aortic plexuses. Called *abdominal brain*. SYN: *celiac plexus.*

spermatic (spĕr-măt′ĭk). (*Ovarian*). ORIGIN: Aortic plexus. LOCATION: Accompanies spermatic vessels to testes or ovaries. DISTRIBUTION: Testes or ovaries.

splenic (splē′nĭk). ORIGIN: Celiac plexus, left semilunar ganglion, right vagus nerve. LOCATION: Accompanies splenic artery. DISTRIBUTION: Spleen, pancreatic plexus, left gastroepiploic plexus.

suprarenal (sū-prä-rē′năl). ORIGIN: Diaphragmatic, solar, and renal plexuses. LOCATION: Around suprarenal capsules. DISTRIBUTION: Filaments to medulla of suprarenal capsules.

thyroid (thī′royd). (*Inferior*). ORIGIN: Middle cervical ganglion. LOCATION: Around external carotid and inferior thyroid arteries. DISTRIBUTION: Larynx, pharynx, thyroid gland. (*Superior*). ORIGIN: Superior laryngeal and cardiac nerves. LOCATION: Around the thyroid gland. DISTRIBUTION: Thyroid region.

uterine (ū′tĕr-ĭn). ORIGIN: Pelvic plexus. LOCATION: Accompanies uterine arteries. DISTRIBUTION: Cervix and lower part of uterus.

vaginal (văj′ĭ-năl). ORIGIN: Pelvic plexus. LOCATION: Vaginal walls. DISTRIBUTION: Vagina.

vertebral (vĕrt′ĕ-brăl). ORIGIN: First part thoracic ganglion, upper cervical nerves. LOCATION: Surrounding basilar and vertebral arteries. DISTRIBUTION: Vertebral and cerebellar regions.

vesical (vĕs′ĭ-kăl). ORIGIN: Pelvic plexus. LOCATION: Accompanies vesical arteries. DISTRIBUTION: Vesicula seminalis, vas deferens.

Cranial Nerves

No.	Name	NA Term	Origin	Function	Distribution
1st	Olfactory	Nn. olfactorii	Olfactory lobe	Smell	Nasal mucous membrane
2nd	Optic	N. opticus	Retina	Sight	Retina
3rd	Oculomotor	N. oculomotorius	Floor of aqueduct of Sylvius	Motor	All ocular muscles except lateral rectus and superior oblique
4th	Trochlear	N. trochlearis	Floor of aqueduct of Sylvius	Motor	Superior oblique muscle of eye
5th	Trigeminal	N. trigeminus	Midbrain and pons	Motor and chief sensory n. of face	Skin of face; tongue; teeth; muscles of mastication
6th	Abducent	N. abducens	Pons	Motor	Lateral rectus muscle of eye
7th	Facial	N. facialis	Pons	Motor	Muscles of expression
8th	Auditory	N. vestibulocochlearis	Brain	Hearing	Internal auditory meatus
9th	Glossopharyngeal	N. glossopharyngeus	Medulla oblongata	Motor and sensory	Sensation of pharynx and posterior third of tongue; parotid gland
10th	Vagus	N. vagus	Medulla oblongata	Motor and sensory	Pharynx; larynx; heart; lungs; esophagus; stomach; abdominal viscera
11th	Accessory	N. accessorius	Medulla oblongata and spinal cord	Motor	Sternomastoid and trapezius muscles
12th	Hypoglossal	N. hypoglossus	Medulla oblongata	Motor	Intrinsic muscles of tongue

Arteries

Name	NA	Origin	Distribution	Branches
Alveolar, inferior	A. alveolaris inferior	Maxillary	Lower anterior skull	Dental; mylohyoid; mental
Angular	A. angularis	Terminal branch of external maxillary	Neck and face	
Aorta SEE: *aorta* in vocabulary				
Arcuate (Metatarsal a.)	A. arcuata	Dorsal a. of foot	Foot and toes	Deep plantar; dorsal metatarsal; dorsal digital
Auditory, internal	A. labyrinthici	Middle of basilar or anterior inferior cerebellar	Internal ear	
Auricular, deep	A. auricularis profunda	Maxillary	Skin of auditory canal, tympanic membrane, and temporomandibular joint	
Auricular, posterior	A. auricularis posterior	External carotid	Middle ear; mastoid cells; auricle; parotid gland	Stylomastoid; auricular; occipital
Axillary	A. axillaris	Subclavian	Forms brachial and seven branches	Superior; thoracic; thoracoacromial; lateral thoracic; subscapular; anterior and posterior humeral; thoracodorsal; brachial
Basilar	A. basilaris	Vertebral	Pons	Posterior cerebral; pontine; internal auditory; anterior inferior cerebellar; superior cerebellar

Arteries (*Continued*)

Name	NA	Origin	Distribution	Branches
Brachial	A. brachialis	Axillary	Upper arm	Deep brachial; nutrient; superior and inferior collateral; muscular
Brachial, deep	A. profunda brachii	Brachial	Accompanies radial nerve	
Brachiocephalic SEE: *Innominate a.*				
Bronchial	Rr. bronchiales	Thoracic aorta	Bronchi; lower trachea; pulmonary vessels; pericardium; part of esophagus	Left and right bronchial
Buccal (Buccinator a.)	A. buccalis	Maxillary	Buccinator muscle; mucous membrane of mouth	
Bulbar SEE: *Medullary a.*				
Capsular, middle SEE: *Suprarenal a., middle.*				
Carotid, common	A. carotis communis	Brachiocephalic trunk (right); aortic arch (left)	Neck and thyroid	External and internal carotid
Carotid, external	A. carotis externa	Common carotid	Neck; face; skull	Superior thyroid; ascending pharyngeal; lingual; facial; occipital; posterior auricular; superficial temporal; maxillary
Carotid, internal	A. carotis interna	Common carotid	Anterior brain; eyes; forehead; nose	Caroticotympanic; Vidian; cavernous; hypophyseal; semilunar; anterior meningeal; ophthalmic; anterior and middle

Artery	Latin	Origin	Distribution	Branches
				cerebral; posterior communicating; choroidal
Celiac	Truncus celiacus	Abdominal aorta	Stomach; liver; pancreas; duodenum; spleen	Left gastric; common hepatic; splenic
Cerebellar, anterior inferior	A. cerebelli inferior anterior	Basilar	Anterior undersurface of cerebellum	
Cerebellar, posterior inferior	A. cerebelli inferior posterior	Vertebral	Cerebellum	
Cerebellar, superior	A. cerebelli superior	Near termination of basilar	Upper cerebellum; midbrain; pineal body	
Cerebral, anterior	A. cerebri anterior	Internal carotid	Cerebrum	Cortical; central; anterior communicating
Cerebral, middle SEE: *Cerebral a., anterior.*				
Cerebral, posterior	A. cerebri posterior	Basilar	Cerebrum	Central; posterior choroidal; cortical temporal; calcarine; parieto-occipital
Cervical, ascending	A. cervicalis ascendens	Inferior thyroid	Muscles of neck and spinal cord	
Cervical, superficial		Thyroid axis	Muscles of shoulder	
Cervical, transverse	A. transversa colli	Thyroid axis	Muscles and glands of neck	Deep and superficial rami
Choroidal, anterior (Choroid)	A. choroidea anterior	Internal carotid	Internal capsule	
Ciliary, anterior	Aa. ciliares anteriores	Ophthalmic and lacrimal	Iris; conjunctiva	

Arteries (Continued)

Name	NA	Origin	Distribution	Branches
Ciliary, long posterior	Aa. ciliares posteriores longae	Ophthalmic	Iris and ciliary process	
Ciliary, short posterior	Aa. ciliares posteriores breves	Ophthalmic	Choroid coat of eye	
Circumflex, anterior humeral	A. circumflexa humeri anterior	Lateral side of axillary	Shoulder joint and upper arm	
Circumflex, posterior humeral	A. circumflexa humeri posterior	Axillary	Deltoid and shoulder joint; upper arm	
Colic, left	A. colica sinistra	Inferior mesenteric	Descending and transverse colon	Ascending and descending colic
Colic, middle	A. colica media	Superior mesenteric	Transverse colon	Right and left colic
Colic, right	A. colica dextra	Superior mesenteric	Ascending colon	Ascending and descending colic
Collateral, inferior ulnar	A. collateralis ulnaris inferior	Brachial	Muscles at back of elbow	
Collateral, superior ulnar	A. collateralis ulnaris superior	Brachial	Elbow joint and triceps muscles	
Communicating, posterior	A. communicans posterior	Internal carotid	Hippocampus; thalamus	
Coronary, left	A. coronaria sinistra	Ascending aorta	Left ventricle and atrium	Anterior descending coronary; circumflex
Coronary, right	A. coronaria dextra	Ascending aorta	Right ventricle and atrium	Posterior descending; marginal

Cystic	A. cystica	Proper hepatic	Gallbladder; liver	
Digital, common palmar	Aa. digitales palmares communes	Palmar arch	Fingers	Proper palmar digital
Digital, proper palmar (Collateral digital a.)	Aa. digitales palmares propriae	Common palmar digital	Fingers	
Dorsal, of foot	A. dorsalis pedis	Continuation of anterior tibial	Foot	Lateral and medial tarsal; deep plantar; arcuate; first dorsal metatarsal
Epigastric, inferior	A. epigastrica inferior	External iliac	Abdominal muscles; peritoneum	Cremasteric
Epigastric, superficial	A. epigastrica superficialis	Femoral	Skin of abdomen; superficial fascia; inguinal lymph nodes	
Epigastric, superior	A. epigastrica superior	Internal thoracic	Abdominal muscles and skin; diaphragm	
Esophageal		In front of aorta	Esophagus	
Ethmoidal, anterior	A. ethmoidalis anterior	Ophthalmic	Ethmoidal cells and frontal sinus; dura mater; nasal cavity	Anterior meningeal
Ethmoidal, posterior	A. ethmoidalis posterior	Ophthalmic	Ethmoidal cells; dura mater; nasal cavity	Posterior meningeal
Facial (External maxillary a.)	A. facialis	Carotid triangle	Face; tonsil; palate; submandibular gland	Ascending palatine; tonsillar; submental; inferior and superior labial; angular; glandular; lateral nasal; muscular

Arteries (*Continued*)

Name	NA	Origin	Distribution	Branches
Facial, transverse	A. transversa faciei	Superficial temporal	Parotid gland; skin of face; masseter muscle	
Femoral	A. femoralis	Continuation of external iliac	Lower abdominal wall; external genitalia; lower extremity	Superficial epigastric; superficial circumflex iliac; external pudendal; deep femoral; descending genicular
Femoral, deep	A. profunda femoris	Femoral	Thigh muscles; hip joint; gluteal muscles; femur	Perforating; medial and lateral circumflex
Femoral, lateral circumflex	A. circumflexa femoris lateralis	Deep femoral a.	Hip joint; thigh muscles	Ascending; descending; transverse
Femoral, medial circumflex	A. circumflexa femoris medialis	Medial aspect of deep femoral a.	Hip joint; thigh muscles	Deep; acetabular; transverse; superficial
Fibular SEE: *Peroneal a.*				
Frontal	A. supratrochlearis	Ophthalmic	Forehead muscles; cranium	
Gastric, left	A. gastrica sinistra	Celiac trunk	Abdominal section of esophagus; stomach; left lobe of liver	Anterior and posterior gastric; cardioesophageal
Gastric, right	A. gastrica dextra	Common hepatic	Lesser curvature of stomach	
Gastric, short	Aa. gastricae breves	End of splenic	Greater curvature of stomach	
Gastroduodenal	A. gastroduodenalis	Common hepatic trunk	Stomach; duodenum;	Superior pancreaticoduodenal;

Gastroepiploic	A. gastroepiploica dextra	Gastroduodenal	pancreas; greater omentum	right gastroepiploic; retroduodenal
Genicular, descending	A. genus descendens	Femoral	Stomach; greater omentum	Pyloric; epiploic; right and left gastroepiploic
Genicular, inferior	A. genus inferior	Popliteal	Knee joint; skin of upper and medial section of leg	Saphenous; musculo-articular
Genicular, middle	A. genus media	Popliteal	Knee joint; skin of upper and middle leg	
Genicular, superior	A. genus superior	On either side of popliteal	Knee joint; ligaments and synovial membrane of knee	
Gluteal, inferior (Sciatic a.)	A. glutea inferior	Internal iliac	Knee joint; femur; patella	
Gluteal, superior	A. glutea superior	Internal iliac	Buttocks and back of thigh	Muscular; coccygeal; anastomotic; articular; cutaneous; comitans nervi; ischiadici
Hemorrhoidal, middle	A. rectalis media	Internal iliac	Gluteal region	Superficial and deep gluteal
Hemorrhoidal, superior	A. rectalis superior	Inferior mesenteric	Rectum; prostate; seminal vesicles	
Hepatic, common	A. hepatica communis	Celiac trunk	Rectum	
			Stomach; pancreas; duodenum; liver; gallbladder; greater omentum	Right gastric; gastroduodenal; proper hepatic

App. 65

Arteries (*Continued*)

Name	NA	Origin	Distribution	Branches
Hepatic, proper	A. hepatica propria	Common hepatic	Liver and gallbladder	Cystic
Hypogastric SEE: *Iliac a., internal.*				
Ileocolic	A. ileocolica	Superior mesenteric	Ileum; cecum; appendix; ascending colon	Superior and inferior ileocolic; appendicular
Iliac, common	A. iliaca communis	End of abdominal aorta	Pelvis; abdominal wall; lower limbs	External and internal iliac
Iliac, deep circumflex	A. circumflexa ilium profunda	External iliac	Muscles of skin and lower abdomen	
Iliac, external	A. iliaca externa	Common iliac	Abdominal wall; external genitalia; lower limb	Inferior epigastric; deep circumflex iliac
Iliac, internal (Hypogastric a.)	A. iliaca interna	Common iliac	Walls and viscera of pelvis, buttocks, reproductive organs; medial side of thighs	Superior, middle, and inferior vesical; middle hemorrhoidal; obturator; internal pudendal; inferior gluteal; uterine; vaginal; iliolumbar; lateral sacral; superior gluteal
Iliac, superficial circumflex	A. circumflexa ilium superficialis	Femoral	Inguinal glands; skin of thigh and abdomen	
Infraorbital	A. infraorbitalis	Maxillary	Maxillary sinus; center face	Anterior superior alveolar; orbital
Innominate	Truncus brachiocephalicus	Arch of aorta	Right side of head, neck, and arm	Right subclavian; right common carotid

Intercostal	Aa. intercostales posteriores	Thoracic aorta	Intercostal spaces; back muscles; vertebral column; thoracic wall	
Interosseous, anterior (Volar interosseous a.)	A. interossea anterior	Common interosseous	Deep structures of anterior forearm	Median; nutrient; muscular
Interosseous, common	A. interossea communis	Ulnar	Deep structure of forearm	Anterior and posterior interosseous
Interosseous, posterior	A. interossea posterior	Common interosseous	Muscles of posterior forearm	Recurrent interosseous
Intestinal		Superior mesenteric	Jejunum and ileum	
Labial, inferior	A. labialis inferior	Near angle of mouth	Lower lip	
Labial, superior	A. labialis superior	Near angle of mouth	Upper lip	
Lacrimal	A. lacrimalis	Ophthalmic	Lacrimal gland; eyelid; conjunctiva	Lateral palpebral; zygomatic; recurrent
Laryngeal, inferior	A. laryngea inferior	Inferior thyroid	Muscles and mucous membrane of trachea and larynx	
Laryngeal, superior	A. laryngea superior	Superior thyroid	Muscles, mucous membrane, and glands of larynx	
Lienal SEE: *Splenic a.*				
Lingual	A. lingualis	External carotid	Undersurface of tongue; tonsil; epiglottis	Suprahyoid; dorsal and deep lingual; sublingual
Lingual, deep	A. profunda linguae	End of lingual	Undersurface of tongue	

Arteries (Continued)

Name	NA	Origin	Distribution	Branches
Lingual, dorsal	R. dorsales linguae	Lingual	Mucous membrane on dorsum of tongue; glossopalatine arch; tonsil; soft palate; epiglottis	
Lumbar	Aa. lumbales	Abdominal aorta	Abdominal wall; vertebrae; lumbar muscles; renal capsule	Posterior lumbar; muscular
Malleolar, lateral anterior	A. malleolaris anterior lateralis	Anterior tibial	Ankle joint	
Malleolar, medial anterior	A. malleolaris anterior medialis	Anterior tibial	Ankle joint	
Malleolar, medial posterior	Rr. malleolares mediales	Peroneal	Tibial malleolus	
Mammary SEE: *Thoracic.*				
Masseteric	A. masseterica	Maxillary	Masseter muscle	
Maxillary (Internal maxillary a.)	A. maxillaris	External carotid	Jaws and teeth; muscles of mastication; ear; meninges; nose; nasal sinus; palate	Anterior tympanic; deep auricular; middle and accessory meningeal; inferior and posterior superior alveolar; deep temporal; pterygoid; masseteric; buccal; infraorbital; greater palatine; pharyngeal; sphenopalatine
Maxillary, external SEE: *Facial a.*				

Mediastinal, anterior	Rr. mediastinales	Internal thoracic	Anterior mediastinal cavity; portion of thymus	
Medullary (Bulbar a.)		Vertebral	Medulla oblongata	
Meningeal, middle	A. meningea media	Maxillary	Dura mater; cranial bones	Superficial; petrosal; superior tympanic; orbital; temporal; and numerous small vessels
Mesenteric, inferior	A. mesenterica inferior	Abdominal aorta	Left half of transverse colon; descending, iliac, and sigmoid colon; part of rectum	Left colic; sigmoid; superior hemorrhoidal
Mesenteric, superior	A. mesenterica superior	Abdominal aorta	Small intestine; cecum; ascending colon; part of transverse colon	Inferior pancreaticoduodenal; jejunal; ileal; ileocolic; right and middle colon
Metacarpal, palmar (Palmar interosseous a.)	Aa. metacarpeae palmares	Deep palmar arch	Interosseous muscles and bones	
Metatarsal SEE: *Arcuate a.*				
Metatarsal, first dorsal		Dorsal a. of foot	Toes	
Musculophrenic	A. musculophrenica	Internal thoracic	Diaphragm; abdominal and thoracic walls	
Nasal	A. dorsalis nasi	Ophthalmic	Lacrimal sac; integuments of nose	Lacrimal
Obturator	A. obturatoria	Internal iliac	Pelvis and thigh	Iliac; vesical; pubic; anterior and posterior obturator

Name	NA	Origin	Distribution	Branches
Occipital	A. occipitalis	Posterior part of external carotid	Muscles of neck and scalp; meninges; mastoid	Muscular; meningeal; sternomastoid; descending occipital; auricular
Ophthalmic	A. ophthalmica	Internal carotid	Eye and adjacent structures of face	Lacrimal; supraorbital; posterior and anterior ethmoidal; medial palpebral; frontal; dorsal nasal; central a. of retina; short posterior, long posterior, and anterior ciliary; muscular
Ovarian	A. ovarica	Abdominal aorta	Ovaries; uterine tubes; ureter	Ureteral
Palatine, ascending	A. palatina ascendens	Facial	Base of skull; palate; auditory tube	
Palatine, greater	A. palatina major	Maxillary	Palate and tonsils	Greater and lesser palatine
Palpebral, medial (Internal palpebral a.)	A. palpebrales mediales	Ophthalmic	Upper and lower eyelids	Superior and inferior palpebral
Pancreaticoduodenal, inferior	Aa. pancreaticoduodenales inferiores	Superior mesenteric	Pancreas; duodenum	
Pancreaticoduodenal, superior	Aa. supraduodenales superiores	Gastroduodenal	Pancreas; duodenum	
Perforating	Aa. perforantes	Deep femoral	Back of thigh	
Pericardiacophrenic	A. pericardiacophrenica	Internal thoracic	Diaphragm; pericardium; pleura	

Peroneal	A. peronea	Posterior tibial	Ankle; deep calf muscles	Perforating; communicating; calcaneal; tibial and fibular nutrient; lateral and medial malleolar
Pharyngeal, ascending	A. pharyngea ascendens	Posterior part of external carotid	Pharynx, soft palate; ear; meninges; cranial nerves; capitis muscles	Pharyngeal; palatine; posterior meningeal; prevertebral; inferior tympanic
Phrenic	Aa. phrenicae	Aorta	Diaphragm; suprarenal glands	Medial, lateral, and superior suprarenal
Plantar, deep	R. plantaris profunda	Dorsal a. of foot	Sole of foot	First plantar metatarsal
Plantar, lateral	A. plantaris lateralis	Posterior tibial	Toes and sole of foot	Plantar arch and plantar metatarsal
Plantar, medial	A. plantaris medialis	Posterior tibial	Muscles and skin of sole of foot and toes	Superficial digital
Popliteal	A. poplitea	Continuation of femoral	Knee and calf	Anterior and posterior tibial; lateral and medial superior genicular; middle, sural, lateral, and medial inferior genicular; genicular articular
Pudendal, external	Aa. pudendae externae	Femoral	External genitalia; medial thigh	
Pudendal, internal	A. pudenda interna	Internal iliac	External genitalia	Posterior scrotal or posterior labial; inferior hemorrhoidal; perineal; urethral; a. of bulb of penis or vestibule; deep a. of penis or clitoris; dorsal a. of penis or clitoris

Arteries (Continued)

Name	NA	Origin	Distribution	Branches
Pulmonary	Truncus pulmonalis	Right ventricle	Lungs	Right and left pulmonary
Pulmonary, left	A. pulmonalis sinistra	Pulmonary trunk	Left lung	Numerous branches
Pulmonary right	A. pulmonalis dextra	Pulmonary trunk	Right lung	Numerous branches
Radial	A. radialis	Brachial	Forearm; wrist; hand	Recurrent radial; muscular; palmar and dorsal carpal; superficial palmar; first dorsal metacarpal; principal a. of thumb; perforating; recurrent; palmar
Radial, of index finger	A. radialis indicis	Principal a. of thumb	Index finger	
Recurrent	A. recurrens tibialis anterior	Anterior tibial	Knee joint	
Recurrent, posterior tibial	A. recurrens tibialis posterior	Anterior tibial	Knee joint	
Recurrent, radial	A. recurrens radialis	Below elbow from radial	Elbow joint; muscles of forearm	
Recurrent, ulnar	A. recurrens ulnaris	Ulnar	Elbow joint; skin and muscles of elbow	Anterior and posterior recurrent
Renal	A. renalis	Abdominal aorta	Kidney; suprarenal gland; ureter	Inferior suprarenal
Retroduodenal		Gastroduodenal	Head of pancreas; duodenum; bile duct	
Sacral, lateral	Aa. sacrales laterales	Internal iliac	Coccyx and sacrum	

Sacral, middle	A. sacralis mediana	Abdominal aorta	Sacrum; coccyx; rectum	Lowest lumbar
Scapular, circumflex	A. circumflexa scapulae	Subscapular	Lateral border of scapula; infraspinous fossa; muscles of upper arm	
Scapular, descending (Dorsal scapular a.)	A. scapularis descendens	Subclavian	Medial border of scapula	
Scapular, transverse SEE: *Suprascapular a.*				
Sciatic SEE: *Gluteal a., inferior.*				
Sigmoid	Aa. sigmoideae	Inferior mesenteric	Iliac, sigmoid, and pelvic colon	
Spermatic, internal SEE: *Testicular a.*				
Sphenopalatine (Nasopalatine a.)	A. sphenopalatina	Maxillary	Nose	Posterior lateral nasal; posterior septal
Spinal, anterior (Ventral spinal a.)	A. spinalis anterior	Vertebral	Anterior spinal cord	
Spinal, posterior (Dorsal spinal a.)	A. spinalis posterior	Vertebral	Posterior spinal cord	
Splenic (Lienal a.)	A. lienalis	Celiac trunk	Pancreas; spleen; stomach; greater omentum	Pancreatic; left gastroepiploic; short gastric; splenic
Sternomastoid	Rr. sternocleidomastoidei	Occipital or external carotid	Sternocleidomastoid muscles	
Stylomastoid	A. stylomastoidea	Posterior auricular	Mastoid; tympanic cavity; stapedius muscle	

App. 73

Arteries (Continued)

Name	NA	Origin	Distribution	Branches
Subclavian	A. subclavia	Innominate (right); arch of aorta (left)	Brain; meninges; spinal cord; neck; thoracic walls; upper limbs	Vertebral; internal thoracic; thyro-cervical; costocervical; transverse cervical
Subcostal	A. subcostalis	Thoracic aorta	Upper abdominal wall	Dorsal and spinal
Sublingual	A. sublingualis	Anterior margin of hypoglossus	Sublingual gland and mucous membrane of mouth and gums	
Submental	A. submentalis	Facial	Mylohyoid muscle; submandibular and sublingual glands; lower lip	
Subscapular	A. subscapularis	Axillary	Shoulder	Scapular circumflex and thoracodorsal
Supraorbital	A. supraorbitalis	Ophthalmic	Forehead; frontal sinus; upper eyelid; upper muscles of orbit	
Suprarenal, middle (Middle capsular a.)	A. suprarenalis media	Abdominal aorta	Suprarenal gland	
Suprascapular (Transverse scapular a.)	A. suprascapularis	Thyroid axis	Scapular; clavicle; shoulder joint	Acromial; suprasternal
Sural	Aa. surales	Popliteal opposite knee joint	Calf	
Tarsal, lateral	A. tarsea lateralis	Dorsal a. of foot	Muscles and joints of tarsus	

Tarsal, medial	Aa. tarseae mediales	Dorsal a. of foot	Middle portion of foot	
Temporal, middle	A. temporalis media	Above zygomatic arch	Temporal muscle	
Temporal, superficial	A. temporalis superficialis	End of external carotid	Parotid gland; auricle; scalp; skin of face; masseter muscle	Transverse facial; middle temporal; anterior auricular; frontal; parietal
Testicular (Internal spermadic a.)		Abdominal aorta	Ureter; epididymis; testes	Ureteral
Thoracic, internal (Internal mammary a.)	A. thoracica interna	Subclavian	Anterior thoracic wall; mediastinal structures; diaphragm	Pericardiacophrenic; anterior mediastinal; pericardial; sternal; intercostal; perforating; musculophrenic; superior epigastric
Thoracic, lateral	A. thoracica lateralis	Axillary	Shoulder muscles and axillary glands	In the female, external mammary
Thoracic, superior	A. thoracica suprema	Thoracoacromial	Muscles of chest	
Thoracoacromial	A. thoracoacromialis	Axillary	Muscles and skin of upper arm, shoulder, and chest	Pectoral; acromial; clavicular; deltoid
Thoracodorsal	A. thoracodorsalis	Subscapular	Posterior portion of axillary	
Thumb, principal a. of	A. princeps pollicis	Radial	Sides and palmar aspect of thumb	Radial a. of index finger
Thyroid, inferior	A. thyroidea inferior	Thyroid axis	Thyroid gland; esophagus	Inferior laryngeal; tracheal; muscular; esophageal; ascending cervical

Arteries *(Continued)*

Name	NA	Origin	Distribution	Branches
Thyroid, superior	A. thyroidea superior	External carotid	Hyoid muscles; larynx; thyroid gland; pharynx	Hyoid; sternomastoid; superior laryngeal; cricothyroid
Tibial, anterior	A. tibialis anterior	Popliteal	Leg; ankle; foot	Anterior and posterior tibial recurrent; fibular; lateral and medial anterior malleolar
Tibial, posterior	A. tibialis posterior	Lower end of popliteal	Leg; foot; heel	Peroneal; lateral and medial posterior malleolar; communicating; plantar; tibial and fibular nutrient
Tympanic, anterior	A. tympanica anterior	Maxillary	Lining of tympanic arch	
Tympanic, inferior	A. tympanica inferior	Ascending pharyngeal	Tympanic cavity	
Ulnar	A. ulnaris	Brachial	Forearm; wrist and hand	Anterior and posterior recurrent; common interosseous; muscular; palmar and dorsal carpal; deep palmar; superficial palmar arch
Uterine	A. uterina	Internal iliac	Uterus; uterine tubes; ovary; vagina	Vaginal; ovarian; tubal
Vaginal	A. vaginalis	Uterine	Vagina; bladder	
Vertebral	A. vertebralis	Subclavian	Muscles of neck; vertebrae; spinal cord; cerebellum; interior of cerebrum	Spinal; muscular; anterior and posterior spinal; posterior inferior cerebellar; medullary
Vesical, inferior	A. vesicalis inferior	Internal iliac	Bladder; prostate; seminal vesicles	

Name	NA	Description	Origin	Distribution
Vesical, middle		Superior vesical	Bladder; seminal vesicles	
Vesical, superior	Aa. vesicales superiores	Internal iliac	Upper part of bladder	A. to the ductus deferens
Vidian (A. of the pterygoid canal)	A. canalis pterygoidei		Roof of pharynx; auditory (eustachian) tube	

Veins

Name	NA	Description	Origin	Distribution
Angular	V. angularis	Short superficial v. in nasal region	Union of supratrochlear and supraorbital veins	Continues inferiorly as facial v.
Antebrachial, median	V. mediana antebrachii	Superficial v. of forearm	Base of dorsum of thumb	Ascends forearm between cephalic and basilic veins to elbow where it joins these veins
Auricular, posterior	V. auricularis posterior	Superficial v. which drains parietal and posterior part of temporal region	Plexus on side of head	From side of head it descends behind the pinna where it unites with retromandibular v. to form the external jugular v.
Axillary	V. axillaris	Portion of venous trunk of upper extremity	Junction of basilic and brachial veins	Lower border of teres major muscles to lateral border of first rib where it becomes the subclavian v.
Azygos	V. azygos	Trunk which connects superior and inferior vena cavae	Arises from ascending lumbar v.	From level of diaphragm up posterior thoracic wall on right of vertebral bodies to superior vena cava

Veins (*Continued*)

Name	NA	Description	Origin	Distribution
Basilic	V. basilica	Superficial v. of hand and forearm	Ulnar side of dorsal rete of hand	Ascends posteriorly on the forearm. Below the elbow it moves to exterior surface where it joins axillary v.
Brachial	Vv. brachiales	Each v. drains an arm	Tributaries from structures in upper arm	Follows course of brachial artery and joins axillary v.
Brachiocephalic (Innominate v.)	Vv. brachiocephalicae (dextra et sinistra)	Paired veins which draw blood from head, neck, and upper extremities. They unite to form superior vena cava	Union of internal jugular and subclavian veins	From sternal end of clavicle it ascends vertically to unite below the cartilage of first rib to form superior vena cava
Bronchial	Vv. bronchiales	Several veins which return blood from larger bronchi and roots of lungs	Capillaries of bronchi and roots of lungs	Empties into azygos v. on the right and into hemiazygos or superior intercostal veins on left
Cardiac	Vv. cordis	Drain blood from tissues of heart	Capillaries of tissues of heart	Circulates throughout heart, usually emptying into coronary sinus
Cardinal		First veins to appear in body of embryo	Each v. receives a v. from caudal and cephalic portions of embryo	Include precardinal and postcardinal veins
Cephalic	V. cephalica	Superficial v. of arm and forearm	Radial border of dorsal rete of hand	Winds anteriorly up arm and empties into axillary v.
Cerebellar, inferior	Vv. cerebelli inferiores	Large veins of undersurface of cerebellum	Undersurface of cerebellum	Empty into transverse, superior, petrosal, and occipital sinuses

Cerebellar, superior	Vv. cerebelli superiores	Veins from upper surface of cerebellum	Upper surface of cerebellum	Empty into straight sinus or transverse sinus
Cerebral, great	V. cerebri magna	Short median trunk	Formed by union of two internal cerebral veins	Curves backward and upward around the splenium of the corpus callosum and continues as a straight sinus
Cerebral, inferior	Vv. cerebri inferiores	Small-sized veins which drain undersurfaces of hemispheres	Tributaries in lobes of cerebrum	From various lobes they empty into cavernous and transverse sinuses
Cerebral, internal	Vv. cerebri internae	Two veins which drain deep parts of hemisphere	Formed near interventricular foramen by union of terminal and choroid veins	Run backward parallel to one another and unite at the splenium of the corpus callosum to form great cerebral v.
Cerebral, superficial middle	V. cerebri media superficialis	Drains lateral surface of cerebral hemisphere	Lateral surface of cerebral hemisphere	Follows lateral cerebral fissure and empties into cavernous sinus
Cerebral, superior	Vv. cerebri superiores	Eight to twelve veins which drain the surface of the cerebral hemisphere	Capillaries of cerebrum	From cerebrum to longitudinal cerebral fissure, opening into superior sagittal sinus
Cervical, deep	V. cervicalis profunda	Deep v. of neck	Plexus in suboccipital triangle	Follows deep cervical artery down neck and empties into vaginal or brachiocephalic v.
Cervical, transverse	Vv. transversae colli	Drain blood from supraspinous region of scapula and neck	Capillaries of supraspinous region of scapula and neck	From supraspinous region of scapula diagonally across shoulder to subclavian or external jugular v.
Cutaneous	SEE: *Superficial v.*			

Veins (Continued)

Name	NA	Description	Origin	Distribution
Cystic	V. cystica	Drains gallbladder	Capillaries of gallbladder	From gallbladder along cystic duct to enter right branch of portal v. just below liver
Deep		Accompany homonymous arteries and usually are enclosed in sheaths with those vessels	Extremities	Throughout the body
Digital, palmar	Vv. digitales palmares	Superficial veins of palmar surface of fingers	Capillaries of superficial tissues of palmar surface of fingers	Along proper and common digital arteries
Digital, plantar	Vv. digitales plantares	Veins of plantar surface of toes	Capillaries of toes	Along plantar surface of toes to foot to form four metatarsal veins
Diploic	Vv. diploicae	Large veins of the skull. Main veins are frontal, anterior and posterior temporal, and occipital	Bony tissue between internal and external skull surface	Connect with meningeal veins, sinuses of the dura mater, and veins of the pericranium
Emissary	Vv. emissariae	One of the small valveless veins which establish communication between sinuses inside the skull and veins external to it	Cerebral sinuses	Pass through foramina of skull
Epigastric, inferior	V. epigastrica inferior	V. of lower anterior abdominal wall	Capillaries of internal surface of lower anterior abdominal walls	Internal surface of abdominal wall diagonally across wall to flow into external iliac v.

Epigastric, superficial	V. epigastrica superficialis	Drains lower and medial portion of abdominal wall	Superficial tissues of lower portion of anterior abdominal wall	Follows superficial epigastric artery and opens into great saphenous v.
Esophageal	Vv. esophageae	One of several small trunks which drain esophagus	Capillaries of esophagus	From esophagus empties into inferior thyroid, hemiazygos, azygos, or left brachiocephalicus v.
Facial	V. facialis	Deep v. of face. Branches drain deep structures of face	Continuation of angular v.	From inner angle of orbit it passes diagonally downward and outward to lower jaw
Femoral	V. femoralis	Large v. of thigh	Continuation of popliteal v.	From posterior region of knee it follows course of femoral artery, becoming external iliac v. at inguinal ligament
Femoral, deep	V. profunda femoris	Deep v. of thigh	Tributaries from posterior region of thigh	Accompanies deep femoral artery to femoral v. in femoral triangle where it joins femoral v.
Fibular SEE: *Peroneal v.*				
Frontal SEE: *Supratrochlear v.*				
Gastric, left	V. gastrica sinistra	Drains both surfaces of stomach	Gastrohepatic omentum	Right to left along lesser curvature of stomach to enter portal v.
Gastric, right (Pyloric)	V. gastrica dextra	Drains upper portion of stomach	Small v. from upper portion of stomach	From upper stomach runs left to right along pyloric portion of lesser curvature of stomach to end in portal v.
Gastric, short	Vv. gastricae breves	Drains wall of stomach	Capillaries of fundus of stomach	From wall of stomach empty into splenic v.

Veins (Continued)

Name	NA	Description	Origin	Distribution
Gastroepiploic, left	V. gastroepiploica sinistra	V. of upper stomach	Branches from stomach and greater omentum	Right to left on greater curvature of stomach to empty into splenic v.
Gastroepiploic, right	V. gastroepiploica dextra	V. of lower stomach	Branches from greater omentum and lower surfaces of stomach	Left to right on greater curvature of stomach to empty into superior mesenteric v.
Gluteal, inferior (Sciatic v.)	Vv. gluteae inferiores	V. of lower region of hip	Capillaries of upper part of back of thigh	Upper back thigh through lower sciatic foramen where they unite into a single v. and empty into internal iliac v.
Gluteal, superior	Vv. gluteae superiores	Drains muscles of buttocks	Capillaries of gluteal and adjacent muscles	From tissues of hip they pass through sciatic foramen to empty into internal iliac v.
Hemiazygos	V. hemiazygos	Single v. of lower left thoracic wall	Left ascending lumbar v.	Lumbar region through diaphragm, crossing in front of spine and emptying into azygos v.
Hemiazygos, accessory	V. hemiazygos accessoria	Drains blood from intercostal spaces above level of sixth to seventh	Capillaries of upper intercostal spaces	From left side of vertebra crosses over spine to enter azygos v.
Hemorrhoidal plexus	Plexus venosus rectalis	Surround the rectum	Muscular wall and submucosa of rectum	Tissues of rectum via hemorrhoidal veins to internal pudendal v. to hypogastric v. to commencement of inferior mesenteric v.
Hepatic	Vv. hepaticae	Drain the liver	Tissues of liver	From liver empty into inferior vena cava

Ileocolic	V. ileocolica	Large tributary of mesenteric v. which drains the ileum, appendix, cecum, and lower part of ascending colon	Capillaries of organs in area of ileum and colon	From lower portion of ascending colon runs parallel with ileocolic artery and empties into superior mesenteric v.
Iliac, common	V. iliaca communis	Large v. which draws blood from pelvis and leg. One on each side meets to form inferior vena cava	Union of internal and external iliac veins	Diagonally across pelvis
Iliac, deep circumflex	V. circumflexa ilium profunda	V. of deep structures of iliac region	Capillaries of deep muscles of upper portion of thigh and lower portion of abdomen	Deep tissues of anterior superior spine along inner surface of pelvic brim to external iliac v.
Iliac, external	V. iliaca externa	Upward continuation of external iliac v.	Begins behind inguinal ligament as continuation of external iliac v.	Behind inguinal ligament to sacroiliac articulation where it unites with internal iliac v. to form common iliac v.
Iliac, internal (Hypogastric v.)	V. iliaca interna	Short v. which draws blood from pelvis	Near upper part of greater sciatic foramen	Upper part of greater sciatic foramen
Innominate SEE: *Brachiocephalic v.*				
Intercostal		One of a number of veins (anterior, posterior, right, left, superior, and highest) which drains blood from intercostal spaces	Tributaries of other veins of intercostal spaces	Intercostal spaces to region of lower ribs

Veins (Continued)

Name	NA	Description	Origin	Distribution
Invertebral	V. invertebralis	One of numerous veins which drain vertebral plexuses and accompany spinal nerves	Vertebral plexuses	Vertebral plexuses through intervertebral foramina where they empty into regional veins
Jugular, anterior	V. jugularis anterior	Superficial v. of anterior region of neck	From veins of region of lower lip	From lower jaw descends neck anteriorly and enters external jugular v.
Jugular, external	V. jugularis externa	A large superficial v. which receives greater part of blood from exterior of cranium and deep parts of face	Formed at parotid gland by union of posterior auricular and retromandibular veins	From parotid gland descends perpendicularly in neck to empty into subclavian, internal jugular, or brachiocephalic v.
Jugular, internal	V. jugularis interna	Largest v. of head and neck. Collects blood from brain, superficial parts of face, and neck	Continuous from transverse sinus at base of skull	Runs vertically in neck and unites with subclavian v. at root of neck to form the brachiocephalic v.
Lingual	V. lingualis	Deep v. of tongue	Capillaries of tongue and sublingual areas	Follows distribution of lingual artery
Lumbar	Vv. lumbales	Four or five veins of abdominal walls	Capillaries of abdominal walls	Abdominal walls to ascending lumbar v., inferior vena cava, and iliolumbar v.
Lumbar, ascending	V. lumbalis ascendens	Longitudinal v. which connects lumbar veins	Lateral sacral veins	Lateral sacral v. along lateral border of spinal column to first lumbar vertebra where it becomes azygos v. on right side and hemiazygos v. on left side
Meningeal	Vv. meningeae	Multiple veins of dura	Meninges of brain	Accompany meningeal arteries

Mesenteric, superior	V. mesenterica superior	Large v. from small intestine	Capillaries of small intestine	From ileum in right iliac fossa it follows distribution of its artery and unites with splenic v. behind pancreas to form portal v.
Mesenteric, inferior	V. mesenterica inferior	Drains blood from rectum and sigmoid and descending parts of colon	Capillaries of colon and rectum	As a continuation of superior rectal v. ascends behind peritoneum and enters splenic v.
Metacarpal, dorsal	Vv. metacarpeae dorsales	Superficial veins of back of hand	Capillaries of hand	From digital venous arches join to form dorsal venous rete of hand
Metacarpal, palmar	Vv. metacarpeae palmares	Deep veins on both sides of hand	Capillaries of palm	Deep tissues of palm along metacarpal bone to deep venous arches
Metatarsal, dorsal	Vv. metatarseae dorsales pedis	Deep veins of back of foot	Dorsal digital veins of toes	Through metatarsal spaces to unite to form dorsal venous arch
Metatarsal, plantar	Vv. metatarseae plantares	Deep veins of solar aspect of foot	Plantar digital veins	From toes to ankles and open into plantar venous arch
Musculophrenic	Vv. musculophrenicae	Drains blood from thoracic surface of diaphragm and from walls of thorax and abdomen	Capillaries of upper abdominal wall, lower intercostal spaces, and diaphragm	Along thoracic surface of diaphragm upward lateral to sternum to unite with superior epigastric v. to form internal thoracic v.
Obturator	Vv. obturatoriae	Drains blood from obturator foramen	Union of tributaries of hip and muscle of upper posterior thigh	From upper portion of adductor region of thigh run through upper part of obturator foramen and run back to empty into internal iliac v.

Veins (*Continued*)

Name	NA	Description	Origin	Distribution
Occipital	V. occipitalis	Superficial v. which drains occipital region	Plexus at back part of vertex of skull	From plexus of occipital region, occasionally following course of occipital artery, extends to internal or external jugular v.
Ophthalmic, inferior	V. ophthalmica inferior	Ophthalmic v. which divides into two terminal branches	Venous network at fore-part of orbit	Runs backward in lower orbit and divides into two branches. One passes through inferior orbital fissure and joins pterygoid venous plexus; the second enters cranium through superior orbital fissure and ends in cavernous sinus
Ophthalmic, superior	V. ophthalmica superior	Paired veins of orbital cavity	Inner angle of orbit	Follows course of ophthalmic artery into cavernous sinus
Ovarian	V. ovarica	Drains ovary	Capillaries of ovaries, uterine tubes, and adjacent structures	Pampiniform plexus of broad ligament into inferior vena cava on right and left renal v. on left
Palatine, external	V. palatina externa	Draws blood from tonsils and soft palate	Capillaries of deep tissues of neck	Palatine regions into facial v.
Pancreatic	Vv. pancreaticae	V. of pancreas	Capillaries of pancreas	From pancreas into splenic and superior mesenteric veins
Parietal	V. emissaria parietalis	Small v. which passes through the parietal foramen of the skull	Upper skull	Connects superior sagittal sinus with extra cranial veins
Parumbilical	Vv. parumbilicales	Small important veins which establish com-	Cutaneous veins in region of umbilicus	From region of umbilicus run backward and upward to left

		munication between portal v. and superior and inferior epigastric veins		portal v.
Penis, dorsal v. of	V. dorsalis penis profunda	Two (deep and superficial) veins of penis	Capillaries of skin or tissue of penis	Runs length of penis between two dorsal arteries
Peroneal (Fibular v.)	Vv. peroneae (fibulares)	Deep v. of leg	Veins of ankle and capillaries of tissues of leg	From venous plexus in region of heel upward along lateral region of deep tissue to flow into posterior tibial v. below knee
Pharyngeal	Vv. pharyngeae	Drain pharyngeal plexus	Pharyngeal plexus	Empty from pharyngeal plexus into internal jugular v.
Phrenic, inferior	Vv. phrenicae inferiores	Drain abdominal surface of diaphragm	Tissues of diaphragm	From diaphragm flow to inferior vena cava on right side and left suprarenal v. on left side
Popliteal	V. poplitea	Large v. in posterior region of knee	Union of tibial veins at lower border of popliteus muscle	From tibial veins upward to adductor hiatus to become femoral v.
Portal	V. portae	Subdivision of systemic venous system. Collects blood from digestive tract and conveys it to the liver	Union of superior mesenteric and splenic veins	Abdominal cavity
Pudendal, external	Vv. pudendae externae	Drain blood from superficial regions of medial aspect of upper thigh and receive subcutaneous dorsal veins of external genitals	Capillaries of superficial tissues of lower abdomen, scrotum or labia	From lower abdomen transversely across upper region of thigh to great saphenous or femoral v.

Veins (Continued)

Name	NA	Description	Origin	Distribution
Pudendal, internal	V. pudenda interna	Drains the perineum and external genitals	Deep veins of penis or clitoris	Follows course of internal pudendal artery and opens into internal iliac v.
Pulmonary	Vv. pulmonales	Four veins which return oxygenated blood from lungs to left atrium of heart	Capillaries upon walls of air sacs of lungs	Lungs to left atrium
Pyloric SEE: *Gastric v., right.*				
Radial	Vv. radiales	Large deep veins on radial side of forearm	Palmar arches of hand	From palmar arches of hand accompany radial artery along lateral side of forearm in deep tissues to unite with ulnar v. to form brachial v.
Rectal, inferior	Vv. rectales inferiores	Drain the rectal plexus	Venous plexus of anal canal	Anal canal to internal pudendal v.
Rectal, middle	Vv. rectales mediae	Drain the rectal plexus	Rectal plexus with tributaries from bladder, prostate, and seminal vesicles	Run laterally from rectal plexus to internal iliac v.
Rectal, superior	V. rectalis superior	Drains upper part of rectal plexus	Capillaries of rectum	Ascends from rectal plexus to brim of pelvis into inferior mesenteric v.
Renal	Vv. renales	Short thick trunks which drain the kidneys. The left is longer than the right	Capillaries of kidneys. The left v. receives the left suprarenal v. and left gonadal v.	From kidneys transversely across posterior abdominal wall to inferior vena cava

Sacral, lateral	Vv. sacrales laterales	Large v. of posterior pelvic wall veins	Tissues of posterior pelvic wall	Posterior pelvic wall upward along sacrum to empty into internal iliac v.
Sacral, middle	V. sacralis mediana	Large v. of posterior pelvic wall	Capillaries of tissues of posterior pelvic wall	From pelvic wall in sacral region follows middle sacral artery to empty into common iliac v.
Saphenous, great	V. saphena magna	Longest v. in body	Medial marginal v. of dorsum of foot	Dorsum of foot to femoral v. just below the inguinal ligament
Saphenous, small	V. saphena parva	Large superficial v. of back of leg	Continuation of marginal v.	From behind malleolus ascends back of leg to knee joint where it opens into popliteal v.
Sciatic SEE: *Gluteal v., inferior.*				
Spermatic	V. testicularis	Receives blood from testis and epididymis	Testicular v. in male and ovarian v. in female	From brim of pelvis upward along posterior abdominal wall to inferior vena cava on right and renal v. on left
Spinal	Vv. spinales	Network of veins drawing blood from spinal cord	Spinal cord and its pia mater	Spinal cord through roots to internal vertebral venous plexuses
Splenic	V. lienalis	Large v. which draws blood from spleen and part of stomach	Union of several small veins at the hilus of the spleen	From spleen transversely across abdomen to head of pancreas where it forms portal v. by joining the superior mesenteric v.
Subcardinal		Paired vessels in embryo which replace post-cardinal veins. SEE: *Cardinal v.*		

Veins (Continued)

Name	NA	Description	Origin	Distribution
Subclavian	V. subclavia	Main venous trunk of upper extremity	Continuation of axillary v.	Outer border of first rib to sternal end of clavicle where it joins the internal jugular v. to form the brachiocephalic v.
Superficial (Cutaneous v.)		Veins located beneath superficial layers of superficial fascia immediately beneath the skin	Capillaries of superficial tissues of body wall	Throughout subcutaneous tissue of body wall
Supraorbital	V. supraorbitalis	Drains upper portion of orbital cavity	Capillaries and superficial tissues of region of eye	From region of eye along lateral wall of orbital cavity to root of nose where it unites with supratrochlear v. to form angular v.
Suprarenal, left	V. suprarenalis sinistra	V. of left adrenal gland	Capillaries of left adrenal gland	Hilum of left suprarenal gland, ascending to left renal v.
Suprarenal, right	V. suprarenalis dextra	V. of right adrenal gland	Capillaries of right adrenal gland	Hilum of right adrenal gland to inferior vena cava
Supratrochlear (Frontal v.)	Vv. supratrochleares	Drain the anterior scalp	Capillaries of anterior region of scalp	From venous plexuses in forehead diagonally to left of root of nose where they unite with supraorbital v. to form angular v.
Temporal, middle	V. temporalis media	Superficial v. of lateral portion of stomach	Substance of temporal muscle	From lateral superficial plexus of skull it passes to zygoma where it joins superficial temporal v. to form retromandibular v.
Temporal, superficial	Vv. temporales superficiales	Veins of superficial tissues of skull	Lateral scalp in parietal and frontal region	Temporal region of scalp diagonally to ear and downward to mandible where they unite with

App. 90

Name	Latin	Description	Origin	Course / Termination
Thoracic, internal	Vv. thoracicae internae	Deep v. of chest draining intercostal spaces	Tributaries from tissues of intercostal spaces	Tributaries form a single trunk which runs up medial side of internal thoracic artery and ends in brachiocephalic v.
Thoracic, lateral (Long thoracic v.)	V. thoracica lateralis	A large tributary v. of the axillary v. which drains the lateral thoracic wall	Capillaries of muscles and glands of anterior chest	Tissues of anterior chest muscles to axillary v.
Thoracoepigastric	Vv. thoracoepigastricae	Superficial v. of trunk which establishes an important communication between the femoral and axillary veins	Region of superficial epigastric v.	Run laterally along trunk from superficial epigastric v. to lateral thoracic v.
Thyroid, inferior	V. thyroidea inferior	Two or more veins which arise in venous plexuses on thyroid gland	Veins from thyroid glands	Downward to brachiocephalic v.
Thyroid, superior		One v. from either side of thyroid	Substance and surface of thyroid gland	Accompanies superior thyroid artery and empties into internal jugular v.
Tibial, anterior	Vv. tibiales anteriores	Deep veins of anterior aspect of leg	Capillaries of leg tissue and dorsal metatarsal v.	Accompany anterior tibial artery, ascending between tibia and fibula and uniting with posterior tibial v. to form popliteal v.
Tibial, posterior	Vv. tibiales posteriores	Deep veins of back of leg	Capillaries of deep tissues of leg	From ankle upward posterior aspect of leg to unite with anterior tibial v. to form popliteal v. just below knee

Veins (Continued)

Name	NA	Description	Origin	Distribution
Ulnar	Vv. ulnares	Large deep veins of medial aspect of forearm	Palmar arches of hand	Palmar arches of hand upward in deep tissues along ulnar side of forearm to form brachial v. with radial v. at elbow
Umbilical	V. umbilicalis sinistra	V. which carries blood from placenta to fetus	Placental tissues	Along umbilical cord through umbilicus to liver upward through inferior vena cava to heart
Uterine	Vv. uterinae	Veins carrying blood from uterus	Tissues of uterus	Uterine plexus through part of the broad ligament to empty into internal iliac v.
Vena cava inferior	V. cava inferior	Returns blood from lower half of body	Right and left iliac veins	From union of iliac veins at level of fifth lumbar vertebra to right atrium of heart
Vena cava superior	V. cava superior	Drains blood from upper half of body	Two innominate veins	From below right costal cartilage to right atrium of heart
Vertebral	V. vertebralis	Drains blood from internal vertebral venous plexuses	Numerous small tributaries in the suboccipital triangle	Base of skull down neck, opening into brachiocephalic v.
Vertebral, anterior	V. vertebralis anterior	Small v.	Plexus around transverse process of upper cervical vertebrae	Descends from region of upper cervical vertebrae with ascending cervical artery and opens into terminal part of vertebral v.

Dietetics

Recommended Daily Dietary Allowances, Revised 1968*

	Age[1] Years from–to	Weight kg	Weight lbs	Height cm	Height in.	Kilogram calorie[†]	Protein gm	Vitamin A Activity I.U.	Vitamin D I.U.	Vitamin E Activity I.U.	Ascorbic Acid mg	Folacin[3] mg	Niacin mg equiv.[4]	Riboflavin mg	Thiamine mg	Vitamin B6 mg	Vitamin B12 µg	Calcium gm	Phosphorus gm	Iodine µg	Iron mg	Magnesium mg
								Fat Soluble Vitamins								Water Soluble Vitamins						
Infants	0–1/6	4	9	55	22	kg x 120	kg x 2.2[2]	1500	400	5	35	0.05	5	0.4	0.2	0.2	1.0	0.4	0.2	25	6	40
	1/6–1/2	7	15	63	25	kg x 110	kg x 2.0[2]	1500	400	5	35	0.05	7	0.5	0.4	0.3	1.5	0.5	0.4	40	10	60
	1/2–1	9	20	72	28	kg x 100	kg x 1.8[2]	1500	400	5	35	0.1	8	0.6	0.5	0.4	2.0	0.6	0.5	45	15	70
Children	1–2	12	26	81	32	1100	25	2000	400	10	40	0.1	8	0.6	0.6	0.5	2.0	0.7	0.7	55	15	100
	2–3	14	31	91	36	1250	25	2000	400	10	40	0.2	8	0.7	0.6	0.6	2.5	0.8	0.8	60	15	150
	3–4	16	35	100	39	1400	30	2500	400	10	40	0.2	9	0.8	0.7	0.7	3	0.8	0.8	70	10	200
	4–6	19	42	110	43	1600	30	2500	400	10	40	0.2	11	0.9	0.8	0.9	4	0.8	0.8	80	10	200
	6–8	23	51	121	48	2000	35	3500	400	15	40	0.2	13	1.1	1.0	1.0	4	0.9	0.9	100	10	250
	8–10	28	62	131	52	2200	40	3500	400	15	40	0.3	15	1.2	1.1	1.2	5	1.0	1.0	110	10	250
Males	10–12	35	77	140	55	2500	45	4500	400	20	40	0.4	17	1.3	1.3	1.4	5	1.2	1.2	125	10	300
	12–14	43	95	151	59	2700	50	5000	400	20	45	0.4	18	1.4	1.4	1.6	5	1.4	1.4	135	18	350
	14–18	59	130	170	67	3000	60	5000	400	25	55	0.4	20	1.5	1.5	1.8	5	1.4	1.4	150	18	400
	18–22	67	147	175	69	2800	60	5000	400	30	60	0.4	18	1.6	1.4	2.0	5	0.8	0.8	140	10	400
	22–35	70	154	175	69	2800	65	5000	—	30	60	0.4	18	1.7	1.4	2.0	5	0.8	0.8	140	10	350
	35–55	70	154	173	68	2600	65	5000	—	30	60	0.4	17	1.7	1.3	2.0	5	0.8	0.8	125	10	350
	55–75+	70	154	171	67	2400	65	5000	—	30	60	0.4	14	1.7	1.2	2.0	6	0.8	0.8	110	10	350
Females	10–12	35	77	142	56	2250	50	4500	400	20	40	0.4	15	1.3	1.1	1.4	5	1.2	1.2	110	18	300
	12–14	44	97	154	61	2300	50	5000	400	20	45	0.4	15	1.4	1.2	1.6	5	1.3	1.3	115	18	350
	14–16	52	114	157	62	2400	55	5000	400	25	50	0.4	16	1.4	1.2	1.8	5	1.3	1.3	120	18	350
	16–18	54	119	160	63	2300	55	5000	400	25	50	0.4	15	1.5	1.2	2.0	5	1.3	1.3	115	18	350
	18–22	58	128	163	64	2000	55	5000	400	25	55	0.4	13	1.5	1.0	2.0	5	0.8	0.8	100	18	350
	22–35	58	128	163	64	2000	55	5000	—	25	55	0.4	13	1.5	1.0	2.0	5	0.8	0.8	100	18	300
	35–55	58	128	160	63	1850	55	5000	—	25	55	0.4	13	1.5	1.0	2.0	5	0.8	0.8	90	18	300
	55–75+	58	128	157	62	1700	55	5000	—	30	60	0.4	12	1.5	1.0	2.0	6	0.8	0.8	80	18	300
Pregnancy						+200	65	6000	400	30	60	0.8	15	1.8	+0.1	2.5	8	+0.4	+0.4	125	18	450
Lactation						+1000	75	8000	400	30	60	0.5	20	2.0	+0.5	2.5	6	+0.5	+0.5	150	18	450

[1] Entries on lines for age range 22–35 years represent the reference man and woman at age 22. All other entries represent allowances for the midpoint of the specific age range.

[2] Assumes protein equivalent to human milk. For proteins not 100% utilized, factors should be increased proportionately.

[3] The folacin allowances refer to dietary sources as determined by Lactobacillus casei assay. Pure forms of folacin may be effective in doses less than ¼ of the RDA.

[4] Niacin equivalents include dietary sources of the vitamin itself plus 1 mg. equivalent for each 60 mg. of dietary tryptophan.

* From Goldsmith, G. A.: The New Total Dietary Allowances. Nutrition Today 3:16–19, Dec., 1968.

† One thousand calories (called a small calorie) equals one kilogram calorie (abbr. kcal. or C.).

Vitamins

(Summary of Vitamins Significant in Human Diet)

Vitamin	Chief Functions	Results of Deficiency	Characteristics	Good Sources	Daily Allowances Recommended
VITAMIN A Provitamin, carotene	Essential for maintaining the integrity of epithelial membranes. Helps maintain resistance to infections. Necessary for the formation of rhodopsin and prevention of night blindness.	*Mild:* Retarded growth. Increased susceptibility to infection. Abnormal function of gastrointestinal, genitourinary and respiratory tracts due to altered epithelial membranes. Skin dries, shrivels, thickens, sometimes pustule formation. Night blindness. *Severe:* Xerophthalmia, a characteristic eye disease, and other local infections.	Fat soluble. Not destroyed by ordinary cooking temperatures. Is destroyed by high temperatures when oxygen is present. Marked capacity for storage in the liver. NOTE: Excessive intake of carotene from which vitamin A is formed may produce yellow discoloration of the skin (carotenemia).	Animal fats butter cheese cream egg yolk whole milk. Fish liver oil. Liver *Vegetable* 1. green leafy, esp. escarole, kale, parsley 2. yellow, esp. carrots. *Artificial:* Concentrates in several forms. Irradiated fish oils.	*Males (Ages 10–75⁺ yrs.):* 4500 to 5000 I.U. *Females (Ages 10–75⁺ yrs.):* 4500 to 5000 I.U. *In pregnancy:* 6000 I.U. *In lactation:* 8000 I.U. *Children:* 2000 to 3500 I.U. *Infants:* 1500 I.U.
THIAMINE Vitamin B₁	Important role in carbohydrate metabolism. Essential for mainte-	*Mild:* Loss of appetite. Impaired digestion of starches and sugars. Colitis, constipation, or	Water soluble. Not readily destroyed by ordinary cooking temperature.	Widely distributed in plant and animal tissues but seldom occurs in high concentration, exception	*Males* (10–75⁺ yrs.): 1.3 to 1.5 mg. *Females*

Vitamin	Function	Deficiency symptoms	Properties	Sources	Requirements
	nance of normal digestion and appetite. Essential for normal functioning of nervous tissue.	diarrhea. Emaciation. *Severe:* Nervous disorders of various types. Loss of coordinating power of muscles. Beriberi Paralysis in man.	Destroyed by exposure to heat, alkali, or sulfites. Is not stored in body.	in brewer's yeast. Other good sources are: Whole grain cereals Peas, Beans Peanuts Oranges Glandular—heart, liver, kidney Many vegetables and fruits Nuts. *Artificial:* Concentrates from yeast. Rice polishings. Wheat germ.	*(10–75+ yrs.):* 1.0 to 1.1 mg. *In pregnancy:* 1.1 to 1.2 mg. *In lactation:* 1.5 to 1.6 mg. *Children:* 0.6 to 1.2 mg. *Infants:* 0.2 to 0.5 mg.
RIBOFLAVIN Vitamin B$_2$	Important in formation of certain enzymes and in cellular oxidation. Normal growth. Prevention of cheilosis and glossitis. Participates in light adaption.	Impaired growth. Lassitude and weakness. Cheilosis. Glossitis. Atrophy of skin. Anemia. Photophobia. Cataracts.	Water soluble. Alcohol soluble. Not destroyed by heat in cooking unless with alkali. Unstable in light, esp. in presence of alkali.	Eggs Green vegetables Liver Kidney Lean meat Milk Wheat germ Yeast, dried Enriched foods.	*Males (10–75+ yrs.):* 1.3–1.7 mg. *Females (10–75+ yrs.):* 1.3–1.5 mg. *In pregnancy:* 1.8 mg. *In lactation:* 2.0 mg. *Children:* 0.6 to 1.2 mg. *Infants:* 0.4 to 0.6 mg.

Vitamins (*Continued*)

Vitamin	Chief Functions	Results of Deficiency	Characteristics	Good Sources	Daily Allowances Recommended
NIACIN Nicotinic acid Nicotinamide Antipellagra vitamin	As the component of two important enzymes, it is important in glycolysis, tissue respiration, and fat synthesis. Nicotinic acid but not nicotinamide causes vasodilation and flushing. Prevents pellagra.	Pellagra. Gastrointestinal disturbances. Mental disturbances.	Soluble in hot water and alcohol. Not destroyed by heat, light, air or alkali. Not destroyed in ordinary cooking.	Yeast Lean meat Fish Legumes Whole grain cereals and peanuts Enriched foods.	*Males (10–75+ yrs.):* 14 to 20 mg. *Females (10–75+ yrs.):* 12 to 16 mg. *In pregnancy:* 15 mg. *In lactation:* 20 mg. *Children:* 8 to 15 mg. *Infants:* 5 to 8 mg.
VITAMIN B$_{12}$ Cyanocobalamin	Produces remission in pernicious anemia. Essential for normal development of red blood cells.	Pernicious anemia.	Soluble in water or alcohol. Unstable in hot alkaline or acid solutions.	Liver Kidney Dairy products. Most of vitamin required by humans is synthesized by intestinal bacteria.	*Males and Females (10–75+ yrs.):* 5 to 6 mcg. *In pregnancy:* 8 mcg. *In lactation:* 6 mcg.

VITAMIN C Ascorbic acid	Essential to formation of intracellular cement substances in a variety of tissues including skin, dentine, cartilage and bone matrix. Important in healing of wounds and fractures of bones. Prevents scurvy. Facilitates absorption of iron.	*Mild:* Lowered resistance to infections. Joint tenderness. Susceptibility to dental caries, pyorrhea, and bleeding gums. *Severe:* Hemorrhage. Anemia. Scurvy.	Soluble in water. Easily destroyed by oxidation; heat hastens the process. Lost in cooking, particularly if water in which food was cooked is discarded. Also loss is greater if cooked in iron or copper utensils. Quick frozen foods lose little of their vitamin C. Stored in the body to a limited extent. Abundant in most fresh fruits and vegetables, esp. citrus fruit and juices, tomato and orange. *Artificial:* Ascorbic acid. Cevitamic acid.	*Children:* 2 to 5 mcg. *Infants:* 1 to 2 mcg. *Males* *(10–75+ yrs.):* 40 to 60 mg. *Females* *(10–75+ yrs.):* 40 to 55 mg. *In pregnancy:* 60 mg. *In lactation:* 60 mg. *Children:* 40 mg. *Infants:* 35 mg. The infant diet is likely to be deficient in vitamin C unless orange or tomato juice or other form is added.

Vitamins (Continued)

Vitamin	Chief Functions	Results of Deficiency	Characteristics	Good Sources	Daily Allowances Recommended
VITAMIN D	Regulates absorption of calcium and phosphorus from the intestinal tract. Antirachitic.	*Mild:* Interferes with utilization of calcium and phosphorus in bone and teeth formation. Irritability. Weakness. *Severe:* Rickets, may be common in young children. Osteomalacia in adults.	Soluble in fats and organic solvents. Relatively stable under refrigeration. Stored in liver. Often associated with vitamin A.	Butter Egg yolk Fish liver oils Fish having fat distributed through the flesh, salmon, tuna fish, herring, sardines Liver Oysters Yeast and foods irradiated with ultraviolet light. Formed in the skin by exposure to sunlight. Artificially prepared forms.	*Males and Females (10–22 yrs.):* 400 I.U. After age 22, none except during pregnancy or lactation. *In pregnancy:* 400 I.U. *In lactation:* 400 I.U. *Children:* 400 I.U. *Infants:* 400 I.U.
VITAMIN E Alpha tocopherol	Normal reproduction in rats. Prevention of muscular dystrophy in rats.	Red blood cell resistance to rupture is decreased.	Fat soluble. Stable to heat in absence of oxygen.	Lettuce and other green, leafy vegetables. Wheat germ oil Margarine Rice.	*Males (10–75+ yrs.):* 20 to 30 I.U. *Females (10–75+ yrs.):* 20 to 25 I.U. *In pregnancy:* 30 I.U. *In lactation:* 30 I.U.

Vitamin	Function	Characteristics	Sources	Recommended Daily Amounts
				Children: 10 to 15 I.U. *Infants:* 5 I.U.
VITAMIN B₆ Pyridoxine	Essential for metabolism of tryptophan. Needed for utilization of certain other amino acids.	Soluble in water and alcohol. Rapidly inactivated in presence of heat, sunlight, or air.	Blackstrap molasses Meat Cereal grains Wheat germ.	*Males and Females* (10–75⁺ yrs.): 1.4 to 2.0 mg. *In pregnancy:* 2.5 mg. *In lactation:* 2.5 mg. *Children:* 0.5 to 1.2 mg. *Infants:* 0.2 to 0.4 mg.
	Dermatitis around eyes and mouth. Neuritis. Anorexia, nausea, and vomiting.			
FOLIC ACID Folacin	Essential for normal functioning of hematopoietic system.	Slightly soluble in water. Easily destroyed by heat in presence of acid. Decreases when food is stored at room temperature. NOTE: A large dose may prevent appearance of anemia in a case of pernicious anemia but still permit neurological symptoms to develop.	Glandular meats Yeast Green, leafy vegetables.	*Males and Females* (10–75⁺ yrs.): 0.4 mg. *In pregnancy:* 0.8 mg. *In lactation:* 0.5 mg. *Children:* 0.1 to 0.3 mg. *Infants:* 0.05 to 0.1 mg.
	Anemia.			

Medical Emergencies

Convulsions

Type	History	Clonic or Tonic	Pulse	Breathing	Color	Muscles	Eyes	Pathology	Treatment
Apoplexy. Intracranial hemorrhage	Usually sequel to cerebral hemorrhage. May be result of vascular disease. Occurs usually after age of 40 years.	Usually tonic. May be limited to different areas, or to one side of the body.	Strong and of a bounding quality.	Respirations are deep and stertorous.	Red. Skin has a florid and flushed appearance.	Spastic in tonic usage with hemiplegia. One side of body shows paralysis; other is normal.	Pupils may be unequal in size.	Arteriosclerosis. Intracranial hemorrhage.	Keep the patient absolutely quiet with an icecap to head. No stimulants. If vomiting, prevent aspiration of vomitus.
Diabetic Convulsions.	Diabetes mellitus, hyperglycemia, acidosis.	Clonic and tonic.	Rapid and weak to irregular.	Deep breathing, rapid with extreme effort.	Dry skin. Very soft, cyanotic in convulsion.	Tonic and clonic.	Eyeballs soft. Cataracts are frequent.	Generalized arteriosclerosis. Kidneys are enlarged. Degeneration in islets of Langerhans.	Use of insulin. Diabetic diet. Care of skin. Bedrest.
Eclampsia.	Occurs in toxemia of pregnancy in antepartum and postpartum stages.	Prolonged tonic convulsions are characteristic with the whole body in a state of rigidity. Both tonic and clonic types may occur.	Rapid, becoming thready.	Respirations are irregular, shallow, and hissing. Breathholding may occur.	Blue. Patient may become very cyanotic.	Rigidity of the body. Extremities are flexed. General tonic spasm of body may be followed by clonic spasm.	Pupils may be dilated and may be of unequal size.	Hypertension. Pathological changes in liver, kidney, brain and adrenals. Rapid gain of weight.	Control convulsions. Give proper antenatal care for toxemia of pregnancy. Control of diet, elimination and prevention of hypertension. Magnesium sulfate intramuscularly.
Epilepsy. Grand mal type.	Previous history of fits. Attack may be preceded	Generalized tonic, clonic type but may be	Rapid.	Respirations are rapid, deep, and stertorous.	Blue. Patient may become very cyanotic.	Rigid in tonic and in clonic origin.	Pupils may be contracted and occasionally of	Abnormal electroencephalographic pattern.	Prevent the patient from injuring himself or from falling.

Condition	Cause / Onset	Type of Convulsions	Pulse	Respirations	Skin	Muscles	Pupils	Remarks / Consciousness	Treatment
	by aura. In some patients convulsions may occur only at night.	focal.					unequal size.		Place on floor with pillow, etc. Use no stimulant. For safety, do not place fingers in mouth but use a suitable padded gag to prevent patient's biting his tongue. Loosen clothing around neck.
Hysteria.	Onset usually is not sudden. Accompanied by laughter and crying. Seizure may be more prolonged than epilepsy.	May be of the stimulation types and take on those of epilepsy. Usually are of the tonic nature.	Shows no definite changes unless slightly rapid due to excitement.	Respirations may become rapid.	No change in color of skin.	Rigidity or relaxed as the victim wishes to demonstrate.	Pupils are normal and react to light. Muscles of eye resist when forced opening is attempted.	Patient seldom loses consciousness. May fall but not in an area where an injury may occur. Highly reactive to suggestion.	Inhalation of aromatic spirit of ammonia. Ice water dashed upon the face. Seizure usually ends when the audience disappears.
Tetanus.	After injury, deep wound, and entrance of tetanus bacillus. Ex: gunshot wound.	Tonic convulsions and tonic spasms of voluntary muscles.	Rapid.	Rapid. Labored to irregular.	Cyanotic in convulsions.	Constant rigidity. Trismus may not appear for 24 hrs. after symptoms.	Normal.	Disease is due to the action of tetanus toxin, which is thought to act centrally rather than on the affected muscles.	Human tetanus immune globulin. Maintain airway. This may require tracheotomy. Oxygen therapy.
Uremic Convulsions.	Condition is usually accompanied by chronic or acute nephritis or chronic cardiac conditions. Marked edema noted.	Clonic (mild) to severe forms of muscle jerking.	Rapid to weak. Muscles are rigid, making it difficult to find pulse.	Respirations are slow and stertorous.	Skin is pale, dry, scaly and has waxy appearance.	Tonic and clonic.	Pupils may be pin points.	Arterial hypertension. Albuminuria. Suppression of urine. Visual disturbance.	Measures to reduce high blood pressure. Treatment by use of artificial kidney may be lifesaving.

Dislocations

Type	History	Pathology	Muscles	Complications	Treatment	Strapping and Support	Differentiation
Ankle.	From violence of undue weight or twisting upon the knee.	Production of scar tissue and contractures, which produce prolonged restriction of motion. Usually a short period of disability and then satisfactory recovery.	Rigid with pain. May include swelling and discoloration (May be delayed).	Fractures—Minor or Major as determined by accident. Temporary or permanent disability.	Continuous application of cold for 24 to 48 hours. Then heat, massage, and passive and active exercise.	Allow no use (fracture may be present). Check x-ray film for fracture. Immobilize the foot and ankle on a pillow or a rigid splint.	Satisfactory reduction is made when the ankle can be dorsiflexed within a right angle.
Back.	Sudden and violent twisting of the back.	Cervical dislocation—Paraplegia may occur. Respiratory failure or dorsal dislocation; urinary infection.	Affected side relaxed; uninjured side spastic. Muscle spasm holds back in rigidity with severe pain when any movement is made.	Damage to cord. Incomplete paraplegia. Failure to replace results in kyphosis deformity. Weakness and arthritis.	Do not allow patient to sit up or to be turned. Prepare patient for cast and brace. Watch for decubitus.	Treat as for fracture. Transport in prone position on rigid stretcher. Keep the body in hyperextension with cast or brace.	Compression fracture of first lumbar vertebrae is the most common injury of the spine. Decided excursion of the ilium (noted when the back is extended or flexed) is corrected. No crepitus. Discoloration, swelling, and persistent pain in muscle.
Clavicle.	May be due to a heavy blow or fall upon the side of the shoulder.	Posterior dislocation causes pressure on structures at base of neck; rupture of sternoclavicular ligament.	Hyperextended. Fatigue results if prolonged.	Increased deformity and insecurity of movement of shoulder. Prolonged disability.	Symptomatic. Slight massage. Adhesive strapping. Sling for four weeks.	In recumbent position with small narrow sand bag between scapulae. Posterior Dislocation—press shoulders backward. Make traction on arm as it is held abducted at right angle—clavicle returns to position.	Complete reduction corrects the deformity at the sternoclavicular joint, no crepitus is present. Stretched ligaments and torn muscles are manifested by swelling, discoloration, and generalized pain. Shoulder has secure movement.

Elbow.	In childhood between ages 8 to 12 years. Child falls upon the outstretched hand. Produces hyperextension of the elbow.	Elbow swollen. Held midway between flexion and extension. Head of radius is felt rotating behind humerus.	Tension in biceps muscle. Muscle ossification at the elbow.	Arthritis in joint. Muscle tissue ossification. Recurrence of dislocation.	Apply splint. Immobilize elbow until replacement can be made. Treat symptomatically.	Supinate the forearm. Make traction forward and downward on the forearm until radius and ulna slip back into position.	The ability to acutely flex the elbow when dislocation is satisfactorily reduced.
Foot.	Force of violent nature upon plantar flexor of foot. Misstepping.	May include a compound dislocation of the ankle. Slight to increased amount of trauma and strain upon all soft tissue of foot.	Tense; marked swelling and discoloration.	Fracture of ankle. Weakness of muscles of plantar arch.	Continuous application of cold for 24 to 48 hours. Then heat, massage, and passive and active exercise.	Pillow splint or rigid splint as for fractures. Watch for swelling and cyanosis in part.	Satisfactory reduction is made when the displaced astragalus (projecting on the back of the foot) has been leveled.
Hand.	Occurs most frequently in thumb due to forced hyperextension of the thumb or finger.	Head of metacarpal bone is wedged between flexor tendons (may necessitate an operation).	Marked tension.	Deformity and permanent disability unless successful reduction is made.	Hyperextend the phalanx or thumb and then flex it. Use adhesive strapping. Cold applications for 24 to 48 hours.	Hyperextension of thumb as local pressure is made—thereby replacement is effected. Very early reduction is necessary.	Displacement of the thumb is the most frequent injury of the hand. Swelling, discoloration, and deformity (without point tenderness) are present.
Hip.	If posterior by indirect violence upon head of femur. If anterior by violent hyperabduction.	Injury to capsular and surrounding tissues of capsule of the acetabulum.	Posterior dislocation—hip is held rigidly flexed. Adduction, inward rotation and flexion of the thigh. Anterior dislocation—hip is immovable in abduction and external rotation. Knee flexed.	Torn tendons and ligaments. Fracture of the neck of femur.	Symptomatic for discomfort. Splinting—since fracture is frequently a sequel. Preparation for reduction of the dislocation.	Board or rigid splint. Keep limb in slight elevation unless fracture is imminent.	Reduction will be complete when flexion with extension and adduction of the thigh are possible.

Type	History	Pathology	Muscles	Complications	Treatment	Strapping and Support	Differentiation
Jaw.	The too-wide opening of the mouth, for example, in yawning, laughing, or eating.	Capsule of Glenoid fossa is too loose. Muscles are soft. Tissues lock in chronic displacement. Jaw becomes locked beneath maxillary prominence.	Muscles spastic. Later become fatigued.	Embarrassment in the unexpected recurrence. Trauma and fatigue in muscles. Predisposes infection.	Symptomatic treatment. Replacement by pressure of operator's thumbs upon molars until normal placement in the mandibular cavity.	Replacement. Jaw bandage (supporting).	Anterior dislocation manifests partly opened and locked jaws with the teeth projecting forward. Complete reduction will restore the jaw for normal occlusion.
Knee.	After violent fall or force upon knee.	Torn ligaments. Traumatized muscles of patellar and popliteal area. Loss of synovial fluid after rupture of bursa.	Rigid with pain. May include slight to marked swelling. Ecchymosis—slight or marked.	Disability and deformity. Permanently stiffened knee when synovial fluid is lost.	Splint as for fracture of femur and lower leg. Symptomatic (to relieve discomfort). Treat for shock.	Board or rigid splint. Keep knee and limb in slight elevation unless fraction is present.	The depression adjacent to the patella is diminished and complete flexion of the knee is restored.
Neck.	Caused by violent twists, fall upon the head, or diving into a pool.	Bilateral dislocation. Severs spinal cord. Death usually follows. Nerve injury caused by tension or displacement. Permanent torticollis and limited neck motion.	Torticollis. Muscles spastic on uninjured side, relaxed on injured side.	Severance of cord. Pressure on cord causing predisposal to recurrence of dislocation, permanent torticollis, paralysis, death.	Keep patient in recumbent position in hyperextension of the neck. Reduction by leverage and not by manual traction. Keep traction by collar or plaster cast.	Reduction done by leverage. Application of plaster collar or rigid collar which must be worn until recovery of the ligaments to prevent recurrence.	Unilateral dislocation produces torticollis with head tilted on side and chin rotated away from displaced vertebrae. Reduction aids in complete disappearance of torticollis.
Shoulder.	ANTERIOR. Force was from behind—head of the humerus lies just below the coracoid process. POSTERIOR. Direct force upon the flexed elbow. Head of humerus is placed in front	Rupture of tendon. Injury to circumflex nerve or brachial plexus. Disability. Injury to axillary vessels. Greater tuberosity (coracoid). Acromion processes fractured.	Muscle tension in the biceps muscle. Triceps muscle immobilized, may be slightly rigid.	Chronic arthritis. Cartilage displacement. Complete loss of function. Recurrences if a repeated injury or improper or inadequate mobilization after the first injury.	Kocher method of Replacement. Kept in sling. 1. Flex elbow to a right angle and place elbow against body. Rotate arm outward until forearm points away from body. 2. Keep elbow and arm (lower arm) flexed on upper. Raise elbow forward until it reaches a right angle position to the long axis (or horizontal) of the body. 3. Arm is directed obliquely inward and hand placed on opposite shoulder so that		Dislocation of shoulder is corrected when the hand (unassisted) can be placed upon the opposite shoulder. Repeated recurrence of dislocation of the shoulder may be common.

and lower than the axilla.

reduction or replacement is complete. Immobilize by sling. X-ray study is necessary.

Type	History	Pathology	Complications	Hemorrhage	Color of Area	Treatment	Transportation
Wrist.	Caused by the hyperextended hand or by severe blows upon the dorsal portion of the wrist.	Dislocation of Semilunar bone. Flexion of the wrist is blocked by displaced bone. Usually results in a permanently weak wrist.	Muscles of back of hand tense. Usually marked swelling in area of the sprain.	Permanent pain, weakness, and limitation of motion. Flexion limited. Displaced bones may have to be removed by surgical methods.	Surgical removal of displaced bone if unable to replace it. Support by splint or strapping. Cold applications for 24 to 48 hours.	Apply traction upon hand. Put firm pressure of the thumb upon the displaced bone.	Flexion of the wrist with slight limitations of motion and manifestation of weakness will indicate satisfactory reduction of the wrist.

Fractures

Type	History	Pathology	Complications	Hemorrhage	Color of Area	Treatment	Transportation
Comminuted	Injury due to crushing blow.	Bone is broken into two or more fragments.	Malunion; unstableness; infection.	Occurs in area of injury.	Discoloration is delayed. Appears in area of deeper bones.	Splint before transportation. Replacement of fracture. Occasionally requires open reduction.	Splint and traction.
Compound	Fall or accident.	Injury where either one or both fragments are through the skin.	Infection; hemorrhage; shock.	May or may not hemorrhage.	Slight to marked increase in ecchymosis.	Immediate debridement in hospital. Further treatment elective.	Cover with sterile dressing. Maintain traction. For leg fracture use Thomas splint.
Greenstick	Fall or accident. (In children)	Fracture is incomplete but there is bowing of the bone.	Complete fracture; deformity.	Probably no hemorrhage will occur.	Discoloration may be slight or it may be marked.	Splint for preparation for transportation. Reduction of the curvature and place in cast.	Splint.
Impacted	Crushing force causing fracture. Fragments telescoped.	One fragment is jammed into another.	Deformity; loss of function; pain; osteomyelitis.	Occurs in area of injury.	Discoloration according to extent of bone injury. It may be delayed.	Traction must be made while reduction and proper cast is fitted to hold extremity in place.	Splint and traction.

Fractures (Continued)

Type	History	Pathology	Complications	Hemorrhage	Color of Area	Treatment	Transportation
Simple	Fall or accident.	A complete fracture with no fragments.	Pressure on the blood supply; malunion; osteomyelitis.	Subcutaneous or capillary.	Slight to marked increase in ecchymosis.	Splint before preparation for transportation. Reduction (depending upon skill of operator).	In splint.
Transverse and Spiral	Sudden twisting violence exerted upon extremity.	Fracture line across the bone. Fracture through the bone or around it.	Malfunction; loss of function; cutting of blood supply; infection of bone.	Frequently occurs around area of fracture.	Same as compound fracture.	Depending on site. Splint and traction.	Traction and immobilization.
Ankle (Potts Fracture)	A sudden or forceful wrenching of the lower end of tibia and fibula.	Fracture of the lower ends of the fibula and tibia. Foot is displaced outward. Impairment of tissues, vessels, etc., from trauma.	Dislocation and sprains may occur simultaneously.	May or may not hemorrhage. Discoloration.	Slight or marked areas of ecchymosis.	Immobilize immediately by pillow splint or rigid splint.	Keep limb well supported with slight elevation.
Back	Occurs after jackknife fall and other accidents.	Usually crushing body of vertebrae.	Paralysis and Shock (depending upon location of the fracture).	None in surrounding tissues.	Usually no change in color of the skin.	Extreme care in preparation and transportation. Rigid support. Place in hyperextension for 8 weeks. Body cast.	Place and secure in prone position. Keep patient in hyperextension. Restrain if necessary. Rigid stretcher or improvision.
Coccyx	Falling into sitting position.	Fracture may be from sacral region or from tip of coccyx.	Constant pain; abscesses; osteomyelitis.	None in surrounding tissues.	No change in color of the skin.	Hot sitz bath after 24–48 hours of cold applications to area. Rest in bed. Perform coccygectomy if not cured.	Carry patient on rigid stretcher. Keep in dorsal recumbent position.
Femur or Thigh	Usually sudden and severe trauma to thigh.	Bone and nerve injury; paralysis and permanent disability.	Deformity and shortening of the limb where an endocrine disturbance is present; severance of nerves and blood vessels.	May or may not hemorrhage. Discoloration may be delayed.	Slight to marked increase in ecchymosis.	Splint to leg and body. Keep patient flat. Provide and retain traction. Watch for shock.	Use rigid stretcher. Keep leg in traction until ready for reduction.

sels; paralysis and gangrene.

Forearm and Colles' Fracture	Result of a twisting force upon the lower arm or wrist, or from violence exerted upon the arm in preventing the body from falling.	Fracture and displacement of the distal end of the radius. Tip of styloid process of ulna broken off. Backward displacement of radius.	Trauma and swelling of tissues. Dislocations and sprains.	Slight. Increased if fracture is not immediately immobilized.	Slight to marked.	Rigid splint, arm support with a sling.	Place in a sling after splinting.
Hip	Usually found in elderly people.	Fracture through neck or through trochanter or both.	Loss of function; deformity and shortening.	Hemorrhage but not in large amounts.	Ecchymosis but it may be delayed.	Traction; Smith-Peterson Nail.	Place in Thomas Splint as improvised.
Humerus	Result of a twisting force or blow upon upper arm.	Injury to the osseous structures. Trauma and lacerations of tissues, muscles, etc., if compound fracture.	Severance of nerves and blood vessels; temporary deformity.	Slight. Increased if compound fracture.	Slight or marked areas of discoloration.	Immobilize immediately by splint or sling (weight of forearm usually provides the necessary traction).	Keep arm in sling or splint.
Neck	Diving into pools; auto wrecks; accidents.	Break extends through body of vertebrae or the laminae.	Paralysis (total or partial). Death.	None noted in the tissues.	No change in color of the skin.	Keep neck in hyperextension. Place rolled blanket under shoulders. Minor fracture needs traction for 5-6 weeks. Major (with cord injury) cast or collar for 10-12 months.	Patient must not move the neck under any circumstances. Keep neck and head hyperextended. Restrain if necessary. Rigid stretcher or improvision for rigidity.
Pelvis	A blow or crushing force.	Bone impairment; involvement of sacral nerves. Paralysis, torn ligaments, and lacerated muscles.	Rupture of bladder and rectum; deformity and shortening of limb; sprain of pelvic joints.	Same as in compound fracture. Discoloration may be delayed.	Same as in compound fracture if compound. Otherwise delayed.	Keep in dorsal recumbent position; after reduction keep prone. Reduction of fragments; symptomatic treatment.	On rigid stretcher in dorsal recumbent position. Keep body extended.

Fractures (Continued)

Type	History	Pathology	Complications	Hemorrhage	Color of Area	Treatment	Transportation
Skull	Fall or blow upon the skull.	In Vault. Little or no intracranial trauma. Linear fracture may be overlooked. In Base. Serious compression in brain. Concussion injury to vital cranial nerves.	Concussion; paralysis of limbs of the body; infection of brain; compression of brain.	Bleeding (bright) from mouth and ears. Clots on the brain. Extent and nature determined by location of injury. Dangers of pressure upon the brain.	Ecchymosis over the mastoid process	Place in dorsal recumbent position. Watch for infection. Allow skull base fractures to bleed. Limit fluids.	Place on rigid stretcher. Keep flat. Keep patient quiet.

Poisons and Poisoning

(Note: See Poison Control Centers, United States and Canada, in Appendix.)

Toxic Substance	History	Probable Lethal Dose for Adult Humans (mg./Kg. body wt.)*	Symptoms of Poisoning	Emergency Measures	Supportive and Follow-up Treatment	Pathology
Acetophenetidin or Acetanilid	50 to 500 mg.		Sweating; nausea; vomiting; chills; ringing in ears; fall in blood pressure; circulatory collapse; cyanosis; coma; convulsions; death from respiratory failure.	Gastric lavage or induce emesis. Instill sodium bicarbonate into stomach. Whole blood or plasma. Artificial respiration or oxygen. Analeptics.	Keep patient warm and quiet. If cyanosis becomes severe, 1-2 mg./kg. of 1% methylene blue.	Methemoglobinemia, CNS stimulation, kidney and liver injury.
Acids (acetic, hydrochloric, nitric, phosphoric, sulfuric,	Variable		Immediate pain and corrosion of mucous membranes of mouth, throat, and esophagus; difficulty in swallowing; stomach pain; nausea; coffee-ground vomitus; thirst, shock syndrome with	Give orally, magnesium oxide, milk of magnesia, lime water, or aluminum hydroxide gel. Avoid carbonates as neutralizers. Give	Correct shock with fluids, plasma, or whole blood. Tracheotomy or gastrectomy may become necessary.	Asphyxia from glottic edema, gastric and pyloric strictures, and stenosis or perforation.

phine for pain.

Name	Amount	Symptoms	Treatment		Pathology
Amanita (phalloides, mushroom)	Variable. May be only one mushroom.	After 6 to 15 hours, abdominal pain, nausea, vomiting, purging, weakness, thirst, shock syndrome, restlessness, delirium, hallucinations, coma, late jaundice, acute renal failure. Death may be from cardiac, kidney, liver, or CNS lesions.	Slurry of activated charcoal as lavage fluid, leaving some in stomach along with saline cathartic. Contact nearest Poison Control Center for availability and advisability of using thioctic acid.	Correct fluid and electrolyte balance. Prepare to treat renal or hepatic failure. Treatment with artificial kidney may be required. Maintain high carbohydrate intake. Give I.V. if necessary.	Acute yellow atrophy of the liver, acute renal failure, cardiac damage.
Aminophylline or Caffeine	50 to 500 mg.	Restlessness; excitement alternating with drowsiness; ringing in ears; fast pulse; nausea; vomiting; fever; diuresis; dehydration; thirst; tremor; delirium; convulsions; coma; death in cardiovascular and respiratory collapse.	Lavage, induce emesis with saline cathartic unless vomiting and purging have already begun. Treat CNS excitation with appropriate barbiturate therapy.	Oxygen and artificial respiration. Maintain high fluid and electrolyte balance.	CNS stimulation and gastric ulceration.
Ammonia	Variable. Even a small amount may kill.	Irritation of eyes and respiratory tract (sometimes pulmonary edema, glottic spasm, or laryngeal edema). Other symptoms are like lye poisoning (SEE: Lye in table).	Give large amounts of diluted vinegar, lemon juice, or orange juice. Demulcents and morphine for pain. Oxygen under pressure to help prevent pulmonary edema.	Treat for shock. Tracheotomy may be needed. NOTE: Do not give drugs such as narcotics which would depress respiration.	Corrosive esophagitis and gastritis, laryngeal edema, pulmonary edema.
d-Amphetamine	5 to 50 mg. but variable	Excitement; talkativeness; restlessness; tremors; dizziness; hyperactive reflexes; dry mouth; nausea; vomiting; diarrhea; palpitations; fever; dehydration; mydriasis; tachycardia; hallucinations; delirium; mania; convulsions; coma; death in circulatory collapse.	Gastric lavage with tap water and activated charcoal, or induce emesis. Treat symptoms of CNS with appropriate barbiturate therapy.	Isolate patient and avoid sensory stimuli. Ice packs and sponge baths for hyperpyrexia. Chlorpromazine, 1-2 mg./kg. I.M., may be required.	CNS and peripheral sympathetic stimulation; petechial hemorrhages in the brain.

* Most of these values from Gleason, M. N., Gosselin, R. E., Hodge, H. C. and Smith, R. P.: Clinical Toxicology of Commercial Products, 3rd ed. The Williams & Wilkins Co., Baltimore, 1969.

Poisons and Poisoning (Continued)

Toxic Substance	Probable Lethal Dose for Adult Humans [mg./kg. body wt.]*	Symptoms of Poisoning	Emergency Measures	Supportive and Follow-up Treatment	Pathology
Aniline	50 to 500 mg.	Intense cyanosis; headache; nausea; dryness in throat; confusion; ataxia; vertigo; weakness; disorientation; drowsiness; death in cardiovascular collapse.	Lavage with 1:5000 potassium permanganate. Instill saline cathartic. Oxygen and artificial respiration. Give 1-2 mg./kg. of body weight of 1% methylene blue.	Whole blood transfusions if needed.	Intense methemoglobinemia; mild liver and kidney injury.
Antabuse (disulfiran)	Unknown	Circulatory collapse.	Oxygen therapy, intravenous 5% glucose in water. Intravenous sodium ascorbate. In severe cases very slow injection of 5 ml. of a 2% solution of saccharated iron oxide may be of benefit.	Complete rest with postural drainage. Continue oxygen inhalation and maintain fluid balance.	Unknown.
Antihistaminics (tripelennamine, diphenhydramine, Chlorpheniramine etc.)	5 to 50 mg.	Drowsiness; lethargy; fatigue; ataxia; dryness of mouth; coma. Sometimes however, only excitement is seen with tremors, anxiety, delirium, convulsions, hyperpyrexia, nausea, vomiting, diarrhea, death in cardiovascular collapse or respiratory arrest.	Lavage or induce emesis. Cautious sedation if excited. Oxygen and artificial respiration.	Ice packs and alcohol sponges for hyperpyrexia.	Mechanism of death not precisely known. Cerebral edema is described.
Arsenic or Antimony	5 to 50 mg.	Symptoms may be delayed several hours. Metallic taste and odor of garlic on breath; burning pain throughout gastrointestinal tract; vomiting and purging; dehydration; shock syndrome;	Gastric lavage with 1% sodium bicarbonate solution. Administer dimercaprol (BAL) in accordance with supplier's dosage schedule.	Maintain fluid and electrolyte balance. Morphine for pain. Treat for shock. Treat anemia and renal failure if either is present.	Shock secondary to hemorrhagic gastroenteritis. Skin eruptions are of no toxicological significance.

coma; convulsions; paralysis; severe diarrhea which becomes bloody. Death may occur.

Atropine	Less than 5 mg.	Dryness of mouth and burning pain in throat; thirst; mydriasis; skin is dry, hot, and flushed; hyperpyrexia; tachycardia; palpitations; restlessness; excitement; confusion; mania; delirium. Death is rare.	Lavage with slurry of activated charcoal or 4% tannic acid. Pilocarpine will make patient more comfortable, but barbiturates must be used to control excitement. Do not use long-acting barbiturates. For depression, use mild stimulants. If severe, use oxygen and artificial respiration.	Oxygen and artificial respiration. Ice packs or alcohol sponges for hyperpyrexia. Catheterize if necessary. Ophthalmic pilocarpine.	Intense CNS excitation and parasympathetic paralysis.
Barbiturates	50 to 500 mg.	Confusion; drowsiness; ataxia; vertigo; slurred speech; headache; stupor; coma; areflexia; cyanosis; hypotension; shallow pulse; cardiovascular collapse; death in respiratory arrest.	Establish airway, gastric lavage, artificial respiration, oxygen with CO_2 inhalation, maintain fluid and electrolyte balance. Use of artificial kidney to remove barbiturate has been helpful.	Record vital signs frequently. Correct airway obstruction. Oxygen and artificial respiration as needed. When vital signs have stabilized and kidney function assured, induce diuresis with urea, and alkalinize urine. Antibiotic therapy if aspiration of vomitus has occurred.	CNS depression with respiratory arrest. Pulmonary edema occurs in prolonged coma.
Barium salts, Chloride, and other soluble salts	Quite variable	Salivation; nausea; vomiting; abdominal cramps; violent and bloody diarrhea; slow and irregular pulse; ringing in ears; dizziness; twitching; convulsions or paralysis; death from respiratory failure and cardiac arrest.	Give sodium magnesium or aluminum sulfate rapidly by mouth. Lavage or induce emesis, then leave more of the above in the stomach. Atropine or morphine may relieve abdominal pain. Quinidine or procainamide to prevent cardiac arrest. Artificial respiration and oxygen.	Intravenous saline for dehydration. Treat for shock.	Violent peristalsis, atrial hypertension, cardiac disturbances, late kidney damage. Barium stimulates contraction of muscles.

Toxic Substance	Probable Lethal Dose for Adult Humans [mg./kg. body wt.]*	Symptoms of Poisoning	Emergency Measures	Supportive and Follow-up Treatment	Pathology
Benzene or Xylene or Toluene	50 to 500 mg.	Burning sensation in mouth and stomach; nausea; vomiting; chest pains; cough; headache; giddiness; vertigo; ataxia; confusion; stupor; restless coma; late severe blood dyscrasias. Death from respiratory failure or ventricular fibrillation.	Lavage with tap water; leave mineral oil and saline cathartic in the stomach.	Oxygen, artificial respiration, parenteral fluids. Avoid fats, oils, alcohol, and epinephrine.	Respiratory failure from CNS depression or ventricular fibrillation. Severe and possibly fatal bone marrow damage.
Benzene hexachloride	50 to 500 mg.	Irritability; vomiting; restlessness; ataxia; spasms; convulsions; coma; respiratory failure.	Lavage with tap water and instill saline cathartic into the stomach. Control convulsions by cautious use of barbiturates.	Rest and quiet. Avoid fats, oils, alcohol and epinephrine.	CNS depression, liver damage, and hyaline changes in the renal tubules.
Boric acid and borate salts	50 to 500 mg.	Headache; nausea; vomiting; diarrhea; stomach pain; weakness and lethargy; restlessness; tremor; convulsions; coma. Distinctive, fine, bright red rash. Shock with death in vascular collapse.	Lavage stomach with 1% sodium bicarbonate solution and instill saline cathartic. Oxygen and plasma or whole blood transfusions as indicated.	Fluids and electrolytes for replacement therapy.	Cause of death not known. Both kidney and liver damage are occasionally reported.
Botulinum toxin	Possibly most poisonous substance known to man. Microgram amounts are lethal.	After 12 to 36 hours but may be as early as three hours: nausea, vomiting, occasionally diarrhea, difficulties in vision and swallowing, weakness and paralysis of respiratory muscles. Profuse sweating, and pulse is rapid and weak.	Lavage with tap water or a slurry of activated charcoal if within a few hours postingestion. Instill saline cathartic. Give specific or polyvalent botulinus antitoxin. NOTE: Call the U.S. National Center for Disease Control,	Oxygen and artificial respiration. Tracheotomy if needed.	Blocks transmission of nerve impulses at motor end plate. Congestion and hemorrhage in all organs, especially the CNS.

			Atlanta, Georgia, telephone (404)633-3311 (day) or (404)634-2561 (night), for the location of nearest supply of antitoxin.	
Bromides (sodium, potassium, ammonium, etc.)	500 to 5000 mg.	Prompt vomiting; drowsiness; irritability; ataxia; vertigo; confusion; mania; hallucinations; coma; skin rashes; neurological signs; sensory disturbances; increased spinal fluid pressure. Death is rare.	Give sodium or ammonium chloride 6-12 gm. daily in divided doses with 4 liters of water. Give saline cathartic. If intoxication is severe enough, use of artificial kidney to hasten removal of bromide may be indicated.	Acne-like skin eruption, inflammation of mucous membranes, CNS depression.
Cadmium salts	Several hundred mg.	Nausea; vomiting; diarrhea; salivation; abdominal cramps; headache; vertigo; exhaustion; collapse; shock and immediate death or delayed death from acute renal failure. Inhaling dusts and fumes very hazardous, producing pulmonary edema.	Demulcents; lavage with milk or water if vomiting is not prompt. Give saline cathartic. If pulmonary edema develops, treat with positive pressure oxygen administration.	Severe gastroenteritis, mild liver damage, and acute renal failure. If inhaled as a dust or fume, produces pulmonary edema.
Camphor	50 to 500 mg.	Nausea; vomiting; feeling of warmth; headache; confusion; vertigo; excitement; restlessness; delirium; hallucinations; tremor; convulsions; depression; coma; death from respiratory failure.	Protect the patient from all possible sensory stimuli. Oxygen and artificial respiration as needed. Avoid fats, oils, alcohol, and opiates. Short-acting intravenous barbiturates to prevent or stop convulsions. Be very careful not to overdose. Gastric lavage with tap water.	Intense CNS excitation.
Carbon disulfide	500 to 5000 mg.	Irritation of skin, eyes, and mucous membranes; headache; nausea; vomiting; diarrhea; weak pulse; palpitations; fatigue; ataxia; vertigo; mania; hallucinations; CNS depression with respiratory paralysis.	Artificial respiration and oxygen. Lavage with tap water. Mild CNS stimulants. Convulsions may be controlled by short-acting intravenous barbiturates.	CNS depression sometimes with permanent neurological sequelae.

Poisons and Poisoning (*Continued*)

Toxic Substance	Probable Lethal Dose for Adult Humans (mg./Kg. body wt.)*	Symptoms of Poisoning	Emergency Measures	Supportive and Follow-up Treatment	Pathology
Carbon monoxide	1.5% concentration in the air causes unconsciousness in a few minutes. Continued exposure will cause death. Young children are more susceptible than adults.	Mild headache; breathlessness on moderate exertion; irritability; fatigue; nausea; vomiting; confusion; ataxia; syncope with periods of convulsions; incontinence of urine and feces; death from respiratory arrest.	Artificial respiration and oxygen. Give 100% oxygen in a pressure chamber if possible. Glucose, 50% solution, I.V. for cerebral edema.	Keep patient warm. Use antibiotics at the first sign of infection. Give whole blood transfusions or washed red blood cells.	High concentrations of carboxyhemoglobin in circulating erythrocytes lead to an asphyxial death.
Carbon tetrachloride	5 to 10 ml. Total dose	Nausea; vomiting; intense abdominal pain; headache; confusion; drowsiness; CNS depression; coma; late kidney and/or liver injury with possible acute renal failure. Death from respiratory arrest, circulatory collapse, or ventricular fibrillation.	If swallowed: Gastric lavage or emetic. If inhaled: Artificial respiration, oxygen, stimulants but avoid alcohol. Remove clothes contaminated with carbon tetrachloride.	No specific therapy but be prepared to treat renal and hepatic failure.	CNS depression, hepatic central lobular necrosis, necrosis of renal tubular epithelium.
Chloral hydrate	50 to 500 mg.	Symptoms much like those seen in barbiturate poisoning except that large doses produce vomiting from hemorrhagic gastritis and enteritis. Combinations of chloral hydrate and alcohol (Mickey Finn) are no longer thought to exhibit more than simple additive depression.	SEE: *Barbiturates* in table.	SEE: *Barbiturates* in table.	CNS depression. May sensitize myocardium to endogenous epinephrine.

Chlorate salts or Bromate salts	50 to 500 mg.	Vomiting; diarrhea; abdominal pain; methemoglobinemia; intravascular hemolysis; delirium; coma; convulsions; cyanosis; icterus; death in acute renal failure.	Gastric lavage. Demulcents and meperidine for pain. Oxygen and whole blood transfusions if needed.	Supportive treatment for acute renal failure.	Methemoglobinemia, intravascular hemolysis, acute renal failure.
Chlordane or Heptachlor	50 to 500 mg.	Irritability; hyperexcitability; convulsions and tremors punctuated by periods of depression; late liver damage.	Gastric lavage with tap water, saline cathartic, ether, or ultrashort-acting barbiturates for convulsions.	Oxygen and artificial respiration. Avoid fats, oils, demulcents, and epinephrine.	CNS excitement and severe gastroenteritis have been described.
Chlorpromazine or other Phenothiazines	50 to 500 mg.	Drowsiness; somnolence; stupor; coma; areflexia; hypotension; tachycardia; hypothermia; restlessness; tremor; spasm; rigidity; convulsions; respiratory or vasomotor collapse.	Lavage with tap water. Levarterol for severe shock.	Fluids and electrolytes. Oxygen or artificial respiration. Blood transfusion may be required.	CNS depression, extra-pyramidal seizures, liver damage.
Copper salts, Sulfate	50 to 500 mg.	Prompt emesis; pain in mouth, esophagus, and stomach; diarrhea with abdominal pain; metallic taste; shock; convulsions; paralysis; coma; death.	Gastric lavage, calcium disodium edetate, penicillamine.	Heat, artificial respiration.	Widespread capillary damage, kidney injury, liver damage.
Cyanide (sodium, potassium, hydrogen, etc.)	Less than 5 mg.	Large doses produce immediate death. In smaller doses, an acrid taste is noted preceding numbness in the throat, anxiety, confusion, vertigo, hyperpnea followed by dyspnea, odor of bitter almonds on breath, unconsciousness followed by convulsions and death from respiratory arrest.	Start artificial respiration immediately, keeping airway clear. Give inhalations from amyl nitrite perles every 2–3 minutes for 15–20 seconds. Inject 10 ml. of freshly prepared 3% sodium nitrite I.V. over a 2- to 4-minute period. Do not remove needle. Urgency may necessitate use of nonsterile solutions. Through the same needle give 50 ml. of 25% sodium thiosulfate over a 10-minute period.	If symptoms recur, repeat injections of half doses at hourly intervals. Positive pressure oxygen. Gastric lavage may now be performed with 1:5000 potassium permanganate.	Cyanide combines with enzymes which are essential in transfer of oxygen to the cells. Death is due to tissue anoxia.

Poisons and Poisoning (Continued)

Toxic Substance	Probable Lethal Dose for Adult Humans (mg./kg. body wt.)*	Symptoms of Poisoning	Emergency Measures	Supportive and Follow-up Treatment	Pathology
DDT	50 to 500 mg.	Vomiting (may be delayed); numbness and tickling of lips, tongue, and face; headache; sore throat; fatigue; tremors; ataxia; confusion; convulsions; coma; death from respiratory failure.	Lavage with tap water and instill saline cathartic. Phenobarbital may be given prophylactically, or parenteral short-acting barbiturates to control convulsions once they have begun. O_2 plus 5% CO_2 inhalation.	Avoid fats, oils, alcohol, epinephrine, sensory stimuli. Calcium gluconate is said to be beneficial in controlling convulsions in addition to barbiturates.	No significant pathological findings in animals except those from convulsions due to CNS excitation.
2,4-Dichlorophenoxyacetic acid (2,4-D)	50 to 500 mg.	Weakness; lethargy; diarrhea; spastic myotonia; ventricular fibrillation and cardiac arrest. Possibly hypermetabolism and hyperpyrexia with convulsions and coma.	Induce emesis or lavage with tap water. Quinidine may be of value for both cardiac symptoms and myotonia.	If fever occurs, treat vigorously with cold packs, alcohol sponges, and other means for promoting heat loss.	Mechanism of death not known; abnormal EEG's have been recorded and severe protracted peripheral neuropathy has occurred.
Dieldrin or Aldrin	5 to 50 mg.	Headache; nausea; vomiting; dizziness; tremors; sudden convulsions alternating with periods of severe CNS depression; death from respiratory arrest.	Lavage with warm water unless convulsions have already begun. Instill saline cathartic. Control convulsions with appropriate barbiturate therapy.	Avoid sensory stimuli. Use oxygen and artificial respiration as needed.	Intense CNS stimulation; mild and transient kidney and liver injury.
Digitalis	50 to 500 mg.	Nausea; salivation; vomiting; headache; fatigue; weakness; drowsiness; confusion; disorientation; delirium; hallucinations; visual disturbances; death from ventricular fibrillation.	Slurry of activated charcoal followed by induced emesis or gastric lavage. Disturbances in cardiac rate and rhythm can be tempo-	Nitroglycerin for anginal pain. Preserve water and electrolyte balance.	Produces cardiac arrhythmia and all grades of impaired conduction. Striking lack of human pathological changes in comparison with those

			rarily influenced by appropriate choices from atropine, potassium or salts, quinidine, procainamide, or sodium EDTA.		seen in experimentally poisoned animals.
2,4 Dinitrophenol	5 to 50 mg.	Fatigue; insatiable thirst; sweating; flushing; nausea; vomiting; abdominal pain; restlessness; excitement; severe hyperpyrexia; tachycardia; hyperpnea; dyspnea; cyanosis; coma; death in respiratory or circulatory collapse.	Lavage with 5% sodium bicarbonate solution and instill saline cathartic. Ice packs, alcohol sponges, or cold water enemas to reduce body temperature.	Appropriate fluid therapy for dehydration or acidosis, mild stimulants, oxygen, artificial respiration.	Tremendously increased BMR through uncoupling of oxidative phosphorylation.
Ergot	5 to 50 mg.	Vomiting; diarrhea; dizziness; weak pulse; thirst; tingling in feet; numbness and coldness of extremities; variable effects on blood pressure; dyspnea; convulsions; loss of consciousness.	Slurry of activated charcoal by mouth followed by emesis or lavage. Instill saline cathartic. Atropine sulfate for pain and spasm, 10% solution of calcium gluconate for myalgia. Artificial respiration and oxygen if necessary.	Keep patient warm and quiet; massage extremities; treat for shock.	Congestion and inflammatory changes in gastrointestinal tract and kidneys. Gangrene of fingers and toes from persistent peripheral vasoconstriction.
Ethyl alcohol	Variable: one pint to more than one quart.	Emotional instability and moods depending on personality, circumstances, and surroundings. Impaired motor coordination; slurred speech; ataxia; peripheral vasodilation with flushing, rapid pulse, and sweating; nausea and vomiting; drowsiness; stupor and coma; peripheral vascular collapse; hypotension; tachycardia; hypothermia; death from respiratory or circulatory failure.	Lavage with tap water or 3% sodium bicarbonate, mild stimulants, oxygen and artificial respiration.	Intravenous saline or lactate for circulatory collapse, dehydration, or acidosis. Mild external heat. Avoid aspiration of vomitus. Hypertonic glucose or urea for cerebral edema. Watch for hypoglycemia in young children.	Irregularly descending CNS depression leading to respiratory or circulatory failure.

Toxic Substance	Probable Lethal Dose for Adult Humans (mg./kg. body wt.)*	Symptoms of Poisoning	Emergency Measures	Supportive and Follow-up Treatment	Pathology
Ethylene glycol	Less than 5 mg.	Transient excitement; nausea; vomiting; abdominal cramps; weakness; muscle cramps; ataxia; vertigo; stupor; coma; death from respiratory paralysis or delayed acute renal failure with uremia.	Gastric lavage with 1:5000 potassium permanganate. Calcium gluconate, 10% I.V. Mild stimulants, oxygen and artificial respiration. Immediate use of artificial kidney.	Supportive measures for acute renal failure.	CNS depression and hydropic degeneration of renal tubular epithelium.
Ferrous or Ferric salts	500 to 5000 mg.	Severe gastroenteritis; abdominal pain; vomiting and diarrhea which eventually becomes bloody; dehydration; pallor; cyanosis; shock leading to death in 3 to 4 hours.	Milk by mouth and induce vomiting if not already spontaneous. Gastric lavage with 5% sodium bicarbonate. The specific antidote desferrioxamine should be given orally and intravenously in appropriate dose.	Intravenous fluids for dehydration and whole blood or plasma for shock.	Shock secondary to local tissue damage, mild hepatic cirrhosis and pyloric stenosis.
Fluoride (salts, sodium)	50 to 500 mg.	Peculiar taste with salivation and thirst; nausea; abdominal pain, vomiting, diarrhea; muscle weakness; tremors; central depression; death in shock.	Give 10 ml. of 10% calcium gluconate I.V. Repeat at signs of tetany. Start drip of glucose in saline. Lavage with solution of lime water or calcium chloride, leaving some solution in the stomach.	Treat shock vigorously by keeping up blood volume and giving norepinephrine. Calcium gluconate I.M. to establish depots.	Hemorrhagic gastroenteritis, inhibition of cellular glycolysis, hypocalcaemia.
Fluoroacetate (salts, sodium)	Less than 5 mg.	Vomiting; paresthesias of face; CNS excitation progressing to	Induced vomiting or lavage. Leave 15-30	Oxygen, artificial respiration, short-acting barbiturates for convulsions.	Cardiac disturbances leading to fatal ven-

Name	Amount	Symptoms	Treatment	Pathology
		convulsions, punctuated by periods of severe CNS depression; disturbances in heartbeat; ventricular fibrillation; death.	gm. sodium or magnesium sulfate in stomach. Most effective antidote appears to be monoacetin (sodium glycerol monoacetate) which is not available in pharmaceutical form. Regardless of sterility, inject this material in doses of 0.5 ml./kg. I.M. every half hour, or dilute 1-5 with sterile saline for I.V. use.	tricular fibrillation.
Formaldehyde	500 to 5000 mg.	Pain in epigastrium; nausea; vomiting; anxiety; weak and rapid pulse; coma; collapse; death in respiratory failure.	Give 30 ml. ammonium acetate solution, 15 ml. of aromatic spirits of ammonia, or 10 to 20 drops of household ammonia diluted with water.	Inflammation and ulceration of gastrointestinal tract, acidosis, kidney damage, circulatory collapse.
Hydrogen sulfide or Alkaline salts	Highly toxic. 0.1 to 0.2% in air usually fatal.	Sudden collapse and unconsciousness in acute poisoning with death from respiratory paralysis. Subacutely, gas is an irritant to eyes, respiratory tract, and skin.	Terminate exposure immediately; artificial respiration; oxygen with 5% CO_2; mild stimulants.	No significant pathological changes except in chronic poisoning in which pulmonary edema may be seen.
Hypochlorite salts or solutions (liquid household bleach)	Variable. Several ounces of usual household bleach (4–6% available chlorine)	Pain and inflammation of mouth, pharynx, esophagus, and stomach; coffee-ground vomitus; circulatory collapse; confusion; delirium; coma; edema of glottis. All systemic symptoms are secondary to local injury and shock.	Milk, egg whites, starch paste, or milk of magnesia. Lavage with tap water or 2% sodium thiosulfate. Morphine for pain. Treat shock with intravenous fluids. Tracheotomy or gastrectomy may be indicated.	Edema of pharynx, glottis, or larynx. Perforation of stomach or esophagus. Fumes may produce pulmonary edema.

Toxic Substance	Probable Lethal Dose for Adult Humans [mg./kg. body wt.]*	Symptoms of Poisoning	Emergency Measures	Supportive and Follow-up Treatment	Pathology
Iodine	5 to 50 mg.	Burning pain in mouth, throat, and stomach; lips and mouth are stained brown; thirst; vomiting (blue vomitus if stomach contained starches); bloody diarrhea; anuria or strangury, urine containing albumin or blood. Death from circulatory collapse, asphyxia from glottic edema or aspiration pneumonia.	Immediately give orally cornstarch or flour solution, 15 gm. in 500 ml. (2 cups) water. Lavage with starch solution or 2% sodium thiosulfate. Morphine for pain and mild stimulants as indicated. Epinephrine, diphenhydramine (Benadryl) or hydrocortisone for anaphylaxis.	Give fluids and electrolytes, supportive therapy for circulatory collapse, antibiotics for secondary infections, prepare for emergency tracheotomy.	Irritation and swelling within throat (glottic edema), esophagus, and stomach. Shock secondary to fluid and electrolyte loss. More rarely, late esophageal stenosis.
Ipecac syrup or fluid-extract	Variable. 1 to 2 ounces of fluid-extract (14 times more concentrated than the syrup).	Nausea; vomiting; diarrhea; albuminuria; abdominal cramps; bloody vomitus and feces; dehydration; myocarditis; myocardial infarction; cardiac arrest or shock secondary to cardiac depression and fluid loss.	Lavage or induce emesis if spontaneous vomiting has not occurred. Do not give additional emetic agents. Saline cathartic if purging has not occurred. Once toxin has been removed vomiting may respond to intravenous chlorpromazine.	General supportive and symptomatic measures for impending shock.	Intractable vomiting and diarrhea due to intense irritation of entire gastrointestinal tract leading to shock. Direct, specific cardiac damage.
Isopropyl alcohol	500 to 5000 mg.	Dizziness, incoordination, headache, confusion, stupor, and coma. Symptoms closely resemble ethyl alcohol intoxication. Death from circulatory collapse or respiratory failure.	Lavage with tap water; oxygen and artificial respiration; mild stimulants.	Intravenous glucose and saline. Anticipate liver or kidney injury.	Acetonuria without glycosuria is pathognomonic. Severe CNS depression. Aspiration pneumonitis.

Poison	Dose	Symptoms	Treatment	Treatment	Pathology
Kerosene (Coal Oil)	500 to 5000 mg. if retained in stomach. If aspirated, a few ml. can be lethal.	Burning sensation in mouth, throat, and stomach; nausea with vomiting and diarrhea; drowsiness; restlessness; disorientation; coma. Signs of pulmonary involvement indicate grave prognosis of impending fulminating hemorrhagic bronchopneumonia.	If risks of lavage are undertaken, an endotracheal tube with inflatable cuff should be employed. Dilute sodium bicarbonate is satisfactory lavage fluid; follow with the instillation of olive oil and saline cathartic.	Antibiotics for secondary infection and positive pressure oxygen. Corticosteroids for pulmonary edema.	Severe chemical pneumonitis.
Lead or its salts	30 gm. (Chronic poisoning is much more common than acute.)	Dryness in mouth; burning pain in stomach and abdomen; constipation followed by diarrhea; muscular weakness; paralysis of extremities; skin cold and cyanotic; delayed severe anemia; death in peripheral vascular collapse or encephalopathy.	Gastric lavage with magnesium or sodium sulfate. Morphine and atropine for pain. Milk or egg white as demulcent. Intravenous calcium salts may relieve colic. Intravenous calcium disodium edetate in accordance with supplier's directions.	Keep patient quiet. Maintain fluid and electrolyte balance. Urea, 4% I.V. for encephalopathy with increased intracranial pressure.	Gastrointestinal inflammation, liver and kidney injury when sufficient lead has been absorbed. Encephalopathy is frequent in children. Precise mechanism of death is not known.
Lye, Sodium and Potassium hydroxides and Carbonates	Total dose of 10 gm. may be fatal.	Severe pain in mouth and difficulty in swallowing; gastrointestinal pain and purging; weak and rapid pulse; death in shock or asphyxia from glottic edema.	Large amounts of water by mouth; diluted vinegar or lemon juice; avoid emetics and lavage. Olive oil by mouth or milk and egg whites. Mild stimulants to prevent shock. Tracheotomy may be required.	Morphine for pain; fluids and electrolytes; cortisone. Use of bougies to prevent esophageal stricture. Broad-spectrum antibiotics.	Laryngeal or glottic edema; corrosion and possible perforation of upper gastrointestinal tract; late esophageal stenosis.
Meprobamate, Equanil, or Miltown	500 to 5000 mg.	Drowsiness; relaxation; stupor; sleep; coma; areflexia; muscular flaccidity; severe and persistent hypotension.	Lavage or induce emesis; plasma or pressor agents for hypotension; mild stimulants. Artificial respiration and oxygen.	Symptomatic and supportive care with frequent recording of vital signs.	No significant pathological changes in tissues.

Poisons and Poisoning (Continued)

Toxic Substance	Probable Lethal Dose for Adult Humans (mg./kg. body wt.)*	Symptoms of Poisoning	Emergency Measures	Supportive and Follow-up Treatment	Pathology
Mercuric chloride or other soluble salts	5 to 50 mg.	Metallic taste and burning in mouth and throat; abdominal pain and cramps with nausea and vomiting; diarrhea and bloody stools; scanty urine containing albumin; collapse in shock with weak, rapid pulse, slow and shallow respirations, and cold and clammy skin. If patient survives acute episode, he may die in renal failure after several days. Chronic mercury poisoning is also common with primarily neurological symptoms.	Egg white, milk, or flour by mouth. Lavage with 3% sodium formaldehyde sulfoxylate; if unavailable, 2–5% sodium bicarbonate solution should be used. Dimercaprol (BAL) I.M. in accordance with supplier's directions. Penicillamine.	Saline cathartic if purging has not already occurred. Demulcents and analgetics. Treat for shock. Prepare for management of acute renal failure.	Ulceration of gums and mouth, loosening of teeth, progressive peripheral neuritis are all seen in chronic poisonings or cases in which death is delayed. In acute cases, usual cause of death due to peripheral vascular collapse secondary to fluid or electrolyte loss, or acute renal failure.
Methyl alcohol	500 to 5000 mg.	Exhilaration accompanied by headache, muscular weakness, nausea, vomiting, and abdominal pain; delirium with visual disturbances which may progress to blindness; weak and rapid pulse; rapid and shallow respirations; cyanosis; coma; death from respiratory failure.	Gastric lavage with 5% sodium bicarbonate, leaving some solution in the stomach. Inject 3% sodium bicarbonate I.V. at the rate of 1000 ml./hour but do not continue after acidosis is corrected. To prevent formation of formic acid, give 10 ml. of ethyl alcohol orally. If poisoning is severe, give ethyl alcohol I.V. in 5% solution in bicarbonate or saline.	Bedrest, treat for shock; mild external heat, stimulants as indicated, protect patient's eyes from light. Oxygen.	Intense metabolic acidosis. Partial to complete blindness due to atrophy of the ganglion cells of the retina if patient survives.
Morphine	5 to 50 mg.	Gross overdosages produce prompt depression, but smaller doses	Gastric lavage, even if several hours after in-	Keep patient awake with mild stimulation. Correct airway obstruction.	Pulmonary congestion. Death is from respira-

		...may cause transient period of excitement before drowsiness. Weariness; loss of pain sensation; nausea; vomiting; pinpoint pupils; coma with muscular relaxation and slowing of respiratory rate; cyanosis; slow pulse; fall in blood pressure; death in respiratory arrest.	...gestion, with 1:10,000 potassium permanganate; saline cathartic left in stomach. Nalorphine is specific antagonist given I.V. in doses of 5-10 mg. Artificial respiration. Inhalation of oxygen with 5% CO_2.	Maintain fluid and electrolyte balance. Keep patient warm. ...tral depression, but circulatory insufficiency may be contributory.
Muscaria mushrooms	Unknown. The ingestion of two or three of Amanita phalloides type may be fatal.	Violent vomiting; diarrhea; apprehension; miosis; severe abdominal pain; irregular and slow pulse; slow and labored respirations; delirium; late stupor; death from cardiac arrest or circulatory collapse.	Slurry of activated charcoal orally. Lavage or induce emesis if not spontaneous. Saline cathartic. Atropine is specific antagonist if the mushrooms contained muscarine. Artificial respiration. Call nearest Poison Control Center for availability of thioctic acid.	Symptoms mimic intense parasympathetic stimulation. Severe hepatic, renal, and central nervous system damage.
Naphthalene (moth balls)	5 to 15 gm.	Abdominal pain; nausea; vomiting; diarrhea; headache; diaphoresis; coma with or without convulsions. Certain individuals exhibit intense intravascular hemolysis accompanied by anemia, hematuria, and renal insufficiency.	Induce emesis or lavage with tap water, saline cathartic, demulcents, and mild stimulants. Sodium bicarbonate every 4 hours to maintain alkaline urine in order to prevent renal blockage with acid hematin crystals.	Various states of central excitement or depression. Rarely, liver necrosis. Acute hemolytic anemia.
Nicotine	Less than 5 mg.	Burning sensation in mouth and throat; salivation; vomiting; diarrhea; headache; sweating; dizziness; weakness; pupils contracted at first then dilated; pulse slow at first then rapid; respirations deep and rapid at first then dyspneic; death from paralysis of respiratory musculature.	Control convulsions with small doses of intravenous barbiturates. Relief for visceral symptoms is obtained with atropine or phenoxybenzamine (Dibenzyline). Slurry of activated charcoal as lavage fluid with additional portion left in stomach. Artificial respiration and oxygen.	Transient stimulation then depression of CNS, all autonomic ganglia and nerve endings in skeletal muscle.

Poisons and Poisoning (Continued)

Toxic Substance	Probable Lethal Dose for Adult Humans (mg./kg. body wt.)*	Symptoms of Poisoning	Emergency Measures	Supportive and Follow-up Treatment	Pathology
Nitroglycerin	Less than 5 mg.	Prompt fall in blood pressure; intense throbbing in head; dizziness; faintness; excessive muscular relaxation; tremors; nausea; vomiting; skin flushed then cold and cyanotic; postural hypotension; paralysis; anoxic convulsions; death.	Gastric lavage or administer mild emetic. Mild stimulants as indicated. Oxygen and artificial respiration.	Keep patient in reclining position and comfortably warm. Transfusions, if needed, with whole blood or plasma.	Anoxia due to methemoglobinemia aggravated by stagnation of blood in capillaries, venules, and veins from peripheral vasodilatation.
Nitrous fumes nitric oxide, nitrogen dioxide, sulfur dioxide, phosgene	Unknown	Only very high concentrations produce immediate pulmonary symptoms. After day or two, fatigue, restlessness, cough and other signs of developing pulmonary edema; increasing difficulty in breathing; cyanosis; coughing with frothy expectoration; lethargy; coma; circulatory collapse; death in asphyxia.	Enforce complete bedrest; positive pressure oxygen as needed. Antibiotics and corticosteroids as indicated. Small doses of morphine.	Remove frothy exudates by suctioning. Good nursing care essential.	Asphyxial death due to blockage of gas exchange in lungs.
Oxalic acid and Oxalate salts	50 to 500 mg.	Severe gastrointestinal irritation and intense pain in upper gastrointestinal tract; vomiting and intense thirst; pulse weak and thready; skin cold and cyanotic; twitching of facial musculature; convulsions; coma; collapse; death.	Immediately give large amounts of calcium lactate, lime water, magnesia, or chalk orally, or lavage cautiously with any of these. Calcium gluconate or chloride I.V.	Keep patient quiet and in recumbent position. Morphine for pain; demulcents.	Severe gastroenteritis and secondary shock, hypocalcemia and kidney injury.
Parathion, and other Organophosphorus insecticides	Less than 5 mg.	Nausea; vomiting; diarrhea; abdominal cramps; salivation; headache; vertigo; runny nose; pinpoint pupils; generalized and	Give atropine 1 to 4 mg. I.V. immediately and repeat every 3-8 minutes until parasym-	Endotracheal intubation or tracheotomy may be necessary. Artificial respiration and oxygen. Keep patient under constant observation.	All signs and symptoms are referable to the inhibition of the enzyme, acetylcholinesterase,

		Symptoms	Treatment	Pathology
(continued from preceding page)		profound muscular weakness; confusion; jerky movements; convulsions; coma; death in respiratory failure.	pathetic symptoms are controlled. Give oxygen and artificial respiration. If available, valuable adjunct is 2-PAM (pyridine aldoxime methiodide) in accordance with manufacturer's directions.	and consequent accumulation of acetylcholine at all nervous junctions where it is the chemical mediator.
Phenol	50 to 500 mg.	Corrosive burns in mouth, esophagus, and stomach; abdominal pain; bloody diarrhea; pallor; sweating; weakness; headache; dizziness; ringing in ears; shock with weak pulse; fall in blood pressure and body temperature; shallow respiration; cyanosis; coma; death from respiratory failure. Skin contact produces pain followed by numbness and corrosive burn.	NOTE: If stomach wall is severely corroded, passage of a tube into it may cause rupture. Cautious lavage with castor or olive oil. Avoid mineral oils and alcohol. As needed demulcents, morphine; mild respiratory stimulants. Wash skin areas with 10% ethyl alcohol or castor oil. Moderate external heat. Treat shock conservatively and watch for signs of renal insufficiency. Systemic acidosis may require therapy with bicarbonate.	Corrosive burns of skin and mucous membranes; gastric perforation. More rarely, esophageal stricture and kidney shutdown.
Phosphorus	Less than 5 mg.	Skin contact produces painful penetrating burns. Ingestion leads to burning pain in throat or abdomen with intense thirst followed by nausea, vomiting, diarrhea, odor of garlic on breath, luminescent vomitus and feces. Patient often appears to recover for several days, then suddenly relapses with severe liver, kidney, and cardiac damage.	Repeated washing of the stomach with 1% copper sulfate followed by 1:10,000 potassium permanganate. Leave mineral oil in stomach. Give morphine for pain, and vitamin K. Intravenous saline and lactate for shock, dehydration, and acidosis. Supportive therapy for delirium, hepatic insufficiency, and renal failure. For several days avoid fats and oils in the diet because they promote absorption of phosphorus.	Fatty degeneration of liver, kidneys, and heart.
Quaternary ammonium germicides	50 to 500 mg.	Burning pain in mouth and throat; restlessness; confusion; muscle weakness; CNS depression; labored breathing; cyanosis; asphyxial death.	Large quantities of milk or egg whites make good lavage. No specific antidotes or antagonists are known. Artificial respiration and oxygen if necessary. If convulsions are persistent (rare), give intravenous short-acting barbiturates.	Nonspecific irritation, visceral congestion, cloudy swelling, mild pulmonary edema.

Poisons and Poisoning (Continued)

Toxic Substance	Probable Lethal Dose for Adult Humans (mg/kg, body wt.)*	Symptoms of Poisoning	Emergency Measures	Supportive and Follow-up Treatment	Pathology
Rotenone	Rotenone: 50 to 500 mg.	Sensation of numbness in mouth; nausea; vomiting; gastrointestinal pain; tremors; convulsions; stupor; respiratory stimulation followed by depression; death from respiratory arrest.	Slurry of activated charcoal by mouth; induce vomiting or lavage with tap water, saline cathartic. Avoid fats and oils.	Support respiration, oxygen, mild sedation (avoid barbiturates), fluids. Glucose may be needed for hypoglycemia.	Severe hypoglycemia may be seen; otherwise the pathological changes largely unknown.
Salicylate (sodium, methyl, acetylsalicylic acid)	50 to 500 mg.	Mild gastrointestinal pain; nausea, vomiting; deep and rapid breathing; headache; dizziness; ringing in ears; dimness of vision; irritability; nervousness; confusion; delirium; mania; convulsions; coma and death from respiratory failure with or without cardiovascular collapse.	Induce vomiting or lavage with 5% bicarbonate solution; saline cathartic.	Determine acid-base status and if acidosis is profound, institute sodium lactate therapy. Correct dehydration and hypoglycemia if present. Barbiturates, vitamin K, dialysis procedures or exchange transfusion as indicated.	Disturbed acid-base balance. Children often exhibit metabolic acidosis while adults more commonly show respiratory alkalosis. Intense CNS stimulation followed by depression.
Silver salts, Nitrate, and other soluble salts	3.5 to 35 gm. total dose.	Intense pain in mouth, throat, and gastrointestinal tract; bloody stools; vertigo; coma; convulsions; death.	Gastric lavage with, or administration of, large quantities of table salt and water. Saline cathartic.	Eggs and milk as demulcents, morphine for pain, stimulants as indicated; treat for shock; maintain fluid and electrolyte balance.	Severe corrosion of gastrointestinal tract. Deposits of metallic silver occur under skin in chronic poisoning, but these are of minor cosmetic concern.
Strychnine	Less than 5 mg.	Apprehension; stiffness of muscles; twitching of face and arms; sudden tetanic convulsions of entire body; cyanosis of face and lips; pulse slow and strong; death in 1–3 hours with	Slurry of activated charcoal by mouth or gastric lavage with dilute permanganate or iodine. Such procedures, however, are usually	Place patient in a quiet, dark room. Avoid drafts. Artificial respiration may be needed. Constant nursing care.	Stimulation of spinal cord leading to contraction of respiratory musculature and death from anoxia.

		face fixed in a grin and body arched in hyperextension.	delayed until convulsions are controlled with chloroform, ether, or I.V. barbiturates. NOTE: Do not give morphine.	
Thallium and salts, sulfate	5 to 50 mg.	Severe abdominal pain; vomiting; diarrhea; tremors; delirium; convulsions; paralysis; coma; death. Loss of hair is peculiar to chronic poisoning or in cases of delayed death.	Induce emesis or lavage with 1% sodium or potassium iodide. Leave activated charcoal in stomach. Give saline cathartic and demulcents. Dimercaprol (BAL) in accordance with supplier's directions.	Hemorrhagic gastroenteritis and encephalopathy.
Thiram or Disulfiram	50 to 500 mg.	Nausea; vomiting; diarrhea; ataxia; hyperexcitability; hypothermia; flaccid paralysis. If patient has also ingested ethyl alcohol in even trivial amounts, symptoms are quite different and include flushing, fall in blood pressure, palpitations, sweating, vertigo, confusion, circulatory collapse, coma, and death.	Lavage with tap water. Strictly prohibit alcohol in all forms. Also avoid fats, oils, and oil solvents. Artificial respiration and oxygen.	Symptomatic and supportive care for gastrointestinal symptoms and neurological complications. In case complicated by alcohol, parenteral glucose, ascorbic acid, ephedrine, and diphenhydramine may be beneficial. Wash skin if contaminated and remove clothing.	Hyperemia, ulceration of gastrointestinal tract, renal and hepatic necrosis, demyelinization of cerebellum and medulla.
Turpentine	500 mg. to 5 gm.	Sensation of warmth or pain in mouth, throat, and stomach followed by abdominal pain, vomiting and diarrhea. Aspiration into lungs may cause pneumonitis. Excitement, ataxia, delirium, and stupor, followed by convulsions, coma, and death from respiratory failure.	Gastric lavage with weak bicarbonate solution, followed by demulcents and saline cathartic.	Morphine sulfate for intense pain and a short-acting barbiturate for excitement. Mild stimulation if indicated, e.g., caffeine sodium benzoate. Force fluids.	Irritation of kidneys; hematuria, albuminuria, and sometimes complete urinary suppression. Kidney symptoms appear to be related to composition of the turpentine, and often never appear.

Poisons and Poisoning (Continued)

Toxic Substance	Probable Lethal Dose for Adult Humans (mg./kg. body wt.)*	Symptoms of Poisoning	Emergency Measures	Supportive and Follow-up Treatment	Pathology
Warfarin	50 to 500 mg.	After few days of repeated ingestions; nosebleed; bleeding gums; pallor; hemorrhagic areas in skin, especially knees and buttocks; blood in urine or feces; death in hemorrhagic shock.	Gastric lavage with tap water in case of large single dose. Vitamin K is specific antidote and should be given until prothrombin levels return to normal. Whole blood transfusions may be necessary.	Replacement iron as ferrous sulfate.	Capillary dilatation and increased fragility with hypoprothrombinemia leading to internal hemorrhage.
Zinc salts, (chloride, sulfate, acetate, etc.)	50 to 500 mg.	Increased salivation; violent vomiting and purging, followed by prostration.	Lavage with milk or lime water. Follow with egg white and other demulcents. Morphine for pain.	Recumbent position, external heat to body, morphine for pain; treat for shock; maintain fluid and electrolyte balances.	Stricture of esophagus, pylorus, and destruction of glandular structure of stomach. Ulceration and/or perforation of the stomach.

* Most of these values from Gleason, M. N., Gosselin, R. E., Hodge, H. C., and Smith, R. P.: Clinical Toxicology of Commercial Products, ed. 3. The Williams & Wilkins Co., Baltimore, 1969.

Dose Equivalent Expressed in Household Measures*

mg./kg.		mg./kg.	
Less than 5	A taste; less than 7 drops	500 to 5000 (5 gm.)	Between one ounce and one pint
5 to 50	Between 7 drops and one teaspoon	5000 to 15,000 (5 to 15 gm.)	Between one pint and one quart
50 to 500	Between one teaspoon and one ounce	Greater than 15,000 mg. (15 gm.)	Greater than one quart

* From Gleason, M. N., Gosselin, R. E., Hodge, H. C., and Smith, R. P.: Clinical Toxicology of Commercial Products, ed. 3. The Williams & Wilkins Co., Baltimore, 1969.

App. 128

Suffocation, Asphyxiation, Drowning

Type	History	Pathology	Symptoms and Color	Pulse	Breathing	Muscles	Pupils	Complications	Treatment
Choking	Edema of larynx; diseases of larynx. Foreign bodies aspirated into the larynx.	Trauma of larynx.	Patient in a state of apprehension. Color is cyanotic.	Rapid due to exertion.	Respirations are very rapid or patient may gasp occasionally.	May be voluntarily contracted.	Dilated.	Pneumonia; sinusitis; complete obstruction of the bronchi; lung abscess.	Manual removal of foreign object or encourage coughing by slap on back. Tracheotomy may be required.
Drowning	Body discovered in water.	Waterlogging of lungs and asphyxia.	Patient is unconcious. Color is gray and changing to blue (cyanosis).	If perceptible, it is rapid and may be shallow.	If respirations are present, the patient may gasp occasionally or very irregularly.	Muscles are relaxed and body is very limp.	May be dilated.	Fracture of neck; heart failure; suffocation, shock, and collapse.	Artificial respiration (mouth to mouth); external cardiac massage if needed; oxygen; treat for shock; heart stimulants.
Gas Poisoning	Victim rescued from room with escaping gas from open jet or victim overcome in closed garage.	Changes in the blood chemistry and then anemia. Respiratory paralysis which leads to death.	Patient unconcious. Color typical cherry red, or pallor and cyanosis, carbon monoxide in poisoning.	Rapid; may be irregular.	Respirations are usually slow but may be rapid and shallow very early after the exposure to gas.	Muscles are relaxed and body is very limp.	Varies with the type of gas poisoning.	Respiratory failure; depletion of O_2 supply in the blood.	Artificial respiration; oxygen; shock treatment.
Strangulation and Hanging	Patient found during or after the act. Very definite signs of violence.	Fracture of cervical vertebrae; suffocation; trauma of medulla by odontoid process of axis.	If living, may be unconscious or in a state of excitement or desperation. Cyanotic if death occurred sometime previous to discovery.	May be perceptible or absent.	No respirations, or respirations are very rapid, or patient may gasp occasionally.	May be voluntarily contracted.	Dilated. Unequal if there is cerebral injury.	Fracture of neck; suffocation; contusions on neck.	Release pull of rope by placing chair under patient's feet and cutting rope. Oxygen therapy; artificial respiration; treat for shock; treat fractures.

Unconsciousness

Type	History	Skin and Color	Pupils	Muscles	Pulse	Breathing	Reflexes	Complications	Treatment
Acid and Alkali Poisoning	Accidental or intentional poisoning.	Clammy skin. Skin pale; face cyanotic.	Dilated. Eyes sunken, staring.	Tense. Patient in convulsion.	Rapid, feeble pulse.	Shallow, rapid, labored, irregular.	Increased.	Corrosion of mucous membranes; ulcers of stomach; gastritis; jaundice.	Acids: Milk of magnesia, egg albumin, lime water, no chalk or alkaline carbonate. Alkalies: Neutralize with acetic acid (vinegar). In both cases careful gastric lavage.
Bleeding	Trauma causing bright red spurting or welling bleeding. Bleeding after an operation.	Skin shows pallor which progresses to a yellow or greenish tinge.	Dilated.	Relaxed.	Rapid, becoming thready.	Respirations are rapid and shallow. Air hunger is evident.	Diminished.	Shock; anemia; heart failure; death.	Digital pressure and tourniquet; pad in joint. Keep patient quiet; treat for shock; transfusion if necessary.
Concussion	Head injury caused by fall or blow upon the head.	Skin pale, cold, and clammy. Varies with degree of pathology.	Dilated. Varies with degree and area of injury.	May be spastic.	Pulse rate usually shows a slight increase. May be weak and rapid.	Respirations are usually deep.	Deep tendon reflexes may be increased.	Shock in severe cases; paralysis of limbs may occur.	Bedrest; keep patient flat and warm.
Drowning	Victim is found unconscious in body of water. May have a fractured neck or skull.	Skin is cold, clammy, and cyanotic.	Dilated.	Relaxed if victim is living. Rigor mortis if dead.	If perceptible, it is rapid and weak, or very irregular.	No respirations. Occasional gasp if living.	None.	Heart failure; shock; pneumonia; aspiration of foreign material	Resuscitation (Mouth-to-mouth is most effective method if a manual positive pressure type of device is not available). Keep body warm but not hot. Stimulating drinks when conscious.

Condition	History	Skin/Color	Pupils	Body	Pulse	Respirations	Reflexes	Complications	Treatment
Drunkenness	Victim is unable to cope with the amount of intoxicants taken.	Color varies. Face may be flushed; skin is moist, relaxed, and cool.	Usually dilated but equal.	Relaxed. Body and limbs are limp.	Strong and slow.	Respirations are slow, deep, stertorous, accompanied by characteristic "lip blowing" and Cheyne-Stokes type of breathing.	Involuntary reflexes usually increased.	Pneumonia.	Keep the body warm. If conscious give emetic. Gastric lavage. Give hot coffee or aromatic spirits of ammonia.
Electric Shock	Victim is found after coming in contact with a live wire.	Skin is pale, cold, and clammy.	Pupils may be unequal.	Tense.	Weak and imperceptible.	Respirations cease suddenly.	Deep tendon reflexes usually are increased.	Low voltage affects heart action, makes resuscitation impossible. High voltage affects the respiratory center in medulla and patient may be resuscitated.	Carefully release the patient from current. Artificial respiration by prone pressure; electrical defibrillation may be required. If heart fails to resume contraction, use of an external cardiac pacemaker is indicated. Each moment of delay increases the chances of death.
Epilepsy	Previous occurrence of fits or spells with or without aura.	Pallor to flush followed by cyanosis—may be slight and gradually increased to marked cyanosis.	Pupils are unequal, eyes rolling.	May be spastic. Tonic type of convulsion is followed by the clonic type.	Usually rapid.	Respirations are deep and stertorous.	May be increased.	Injuries in falling or biting the tongue. Patient may react violently (fighting others).	Bedrest. Prevent falling or biting tongue. Sedative.
Fainting	Fatigue, lightheadedness, shock, or horrifying experience.	Face and lips are blanched. Body is cold and clammy.	Normal.	Completely relaxed.	Rapid and thready.	Respirations are rapid and shallow.	Slightly increased.	Shock usually a serious complication. Body injury and fracture if patient falls.	Apply cold water to face, head, and chest. Place head in low position. Have patient inhale aromatic spirits of ammonia.

Unconsciousness (Continued)

Type	History	Skin and Color	Pupils	Muscles	Pulse	Breathing	Reflexes	Complications	Treatment
Freezing	Exposure to intense cold or prolonged period of exposure to cold.	Frostbite: Skin is cold, pale, and blanched. Frozen: Skin is livid and later cyanotic, then turns to purplish or greenish black.	Dilated.	Tense and becoming very rigid.	Rapid and weak.	Breathing is slower and deeper. Patient falls into very deep slumber.	Not discernible.	Pneumonia; certain damage due to mechanical destruction of the cells' sloughing and gangrene of the part previously frozen.	Gradual warming of the parts; slight massage for better circulation; elevation of parts; treatment of dry gangrene.
Gases	Victim rescued from a mine, burning building, or room with open gas jet. Overcome in garage or car.	In carbon monoxide poisoning, skin is cyanotic and changing to cherry red color.	Eyes fixed. Pupils are usually fully dilated. Varies with type of gas.	Relaxed if victim is living. Rigor mortis if dead.	Weak, slow, and irregular.	Respirations irregular and jerky to only an occasional gasp.	None.	Respiratory failure; asphyxia; collapse.	Place the patient in the open air; give oxygen and resuscitation (mouth-to-mouth). Treat for shock.
Hanging	Victim is found hanging with constriction of the neck.	Skin is pale and face is cyanotic.	Dilated and unequal if cerebral injury.	Relaxed. Varies with the level of tenure.	Pulse is rapid, weak, and irregular if strangulation is incomplete. If complete, pulse is absent.	Respirations have ceased or an occasional gasp is observed.	None	Respiratory and circulatory failure; fracture of neck.	Release the patient and cut the rope. Artificial respiration; treat for shock and possible fracture of neck.
Heat Exhaustion	Victim is overcome by the degree of heat and loss of sodium chloride through perspiration.	Skin may be pale and cool. Temperature is usually normal.	Moderately contracted.	Tense with muscle cramps.	Rapid and may become weak.	Respirations shallow with rigidity of the chest muscles.	Increased.	Shock.	Treat for shock; keep body warm. Give salt by mouth and I.V.
Heat Stroke	Exposure to intense degree, or	Skin is flushed and hot when	Dilated.	Relaxed.	Rapid and weak.	Respirations may be	Increased.	Suppressed sweating for prolonged	Place patient in cool area. Cold appli-

Condition	History	Skin	Pupils	Muscles	Pulse	Respiration		Complications	Treatment
(sun stroke, heat hyperpyrexia)	prolonged period, of heat from environment.	touched. Body temperature may be 106° F. (41° C.) or higher.				shallow and gasping or deep and slow.		period. Paralysis of vasomotor centers within medulla. Paralysis of heart, collapse, and death.	cation to head and body. Rub body with ice or alcohol containing ice. Fan body during procedure to increase rate of cooling. Wrap in cold, wet sheet. Continue to lower body temperature. No stimulants or sedatives unless required to treat convulsions. Judge effectiveness of therapy by continual monitoring of rectal temperature.
Mineral Poisoning	Accidental or suicidal poisoning.	Skin is cold and clammy. Pallor.	Dilated. Eyes fixed, staring.	Tense, convulsive to relaxed when in stupor.	Rapid, feeble to imperceptible.	Respirations are shallow, rapid, labored.	Increased.	Nephritis; liver degeneration; colitis.	Gastric lavage; emetics.
Narcotic Poisoning	History of addiction or allergic reaction to the drug.	Skin is ashen, cyanotic, and cold.	Pupils are contracted to pinpoint if due to opiate derivative.	Relaxed.	Usually slow but varies with type of drug poisoning.	Respirations slow, irregular, stertorous.	Diminished.	Addiction to drug or production of a marked sensitivity to a drug.	Removal of the drug by emetics or lavage; use of antidotes; specific counteractives.
Obstruction in throat	Aspiration of a foreign body or respiratory tract is obstructed by edema or disease.	Skin is cyanotic.	Dilated.	Sternal retraction. Muscles are tense with efforts of trying to breathe and remove obstruction.	Rapid and very weak.	Respirations are deep and labored.	Increased.	Asphyxia; pulmonary infection; shock.	Remove obstruction. Give respiratory stimulant or artificial respiration; treat for shock. Tracheotomy if indicated.

Unconsciousness (Continued)

Type	History	Skin and Color	Pupils	Muscles	Pulse	Breathing	Reflexes	Complications	Treatment
Shock	Result of a blow or damage to the central nervous system.	Cold skin; subnormal temperature. Skin is an ashen to cyanotic color.	Dilated.	Relaxed.	Rapid, becoming thready and feeble.	Respirations are rapid and shallow.	Diminished (not significant).	Respiratory and circulatory embarrassment to collapse and death.	Elevate foot of bed; keep body warm; transfusions usually indicated for depression of vascular system.
Stroke (Apoplectic)	Patient may have history of hypertension and arteriosclerosis. Usually past 40 years of age.	Skin is injected. May be cyanotic or ashen. Hot and dry to touch. Flushed. Elevation of temperature.	Pupils vary. May be dilated, often unequal. Inactive in deep coma.	Muscles of the involved side (hemiplegia) are usually spastic with a facial palsy.	Slow, full with increased tension.	Respirations are slow, loud, usually deep.	Diminished on one side. May be hyperactive on the other side.	Pneumonia; injury from falling.	Rest and absolute quiet with head of bed elevated and feet lowered. Ice cap to head; no stimulants.

Wounds

Type	History	Pathology	Symptoms and Color	Points of Identification	Treatment	Transportation	Complications
Bite (human, animal, or insect).	Bite of a reptile or rabid human or animal. Sting or bite of poisonous insect.	Tissue degeneration at site of wound. Muscular paralysis. Venom has a drastic effect upon respiratory nerve centers.	Type of wound: Snake—two fang wound. Human—shape of denture. Dog—laceration. Patient shows rabid disposition. Insect—elevated wheal with pain and itching or burning sensation,	Shape of wound; odor of colon bacillus about the wound in human bite; presence of stinger.	Dog bite: Observe victim and dog for signs of rabies for two weeks. Pasteur treatment if necessary. Snake bite: Apply tourniquet just tight enough to prevent venous return. Use ice packs to prevent absorp-	Keep patient quiet; avert apprehension; keep muscles of the area elevated and at rest.	Infection introduced by pathogenic organisms. Venom of toxic nature depresses victim. Death if delay in treatment.

Injury	Cause	Description	Symptoms	Treatment	Nursing Care	Complications
	or single or double red dot.			tion of venom. Incision and suction as swelling rises. Sting: Neutralize with alkalies. Treat for shock. Respiratory stimulants for snake or insect venom. Specific antivenins are available for certain snake bites.		
Brush Burns or Abrasions.	Friction of body against rough surface.	Surface effaced with nicks and dotted with small drops of blood.	Surface of the skin is brushed completely away, or remains very lightly attached to the area.	Carefully brush away loose dirt. Cleanse the wound with soap and water. Use antiseptic solutions, ointment, and apply dressings. Tetanus toxoid or antitoxin as required.	Use loose applications of sterile dressings held in place by loose-fitting triangle.	Infection. May retain rough, unsightly scars.
Contusions.	Blow or fall.	A bruise (hematoma) or petechial area with underlying injury.	Skin surface is rough; the area includes a large or small hematoma (depending upon the extent of injury). Skin is not broken. Underlying tissues may be slightly or markedly crushed.	Apply cold to area for 24–48 hours.	Keep part well elevated. If there is additional abrasion, cover with loose-fitting bandage.	Destruction of underlying tissue if hematoma is not aspirated early. Infection if skin is punctured or probed.
Gun Shot.	Accident in care of a gun. Victim of deliberate gunfire.	Wound of single outer puncture site with deep injury consisting of twisting and tearing of tissue. Aperture is small. Powder burns occasionally are found.	Puncture site. Deep wound shows characteristic twisting of the deeper tissues.	Cleanse and irrigate. Debridement when necessary. Wet antiseptic dressings. Tetanus toxoid or antitoxin as required.	Keep patient very quiet; head slightly lower than body. Treat for shock. Watch T.P.R. and blood pressure if blood has been lost or patient is in shock.	Shock; internal hemorrhage; tetanus bacillus infection.

Wounds (Continued)

Type	History	Pathology	Symptoms and Color	Points of Identification	Treatment	Transportation	Complications
Lacerations.	Accident wherein sharp instruments have cut and torn an area of the body.	Jagged or torn and roughened edges of tissues. May include evulsion of certain parts.	Injury has produced area of two raw or bleeding edges of the skin. Blood may be oozing or spurting from the wound.	Wound edges are jagged and irregular. Wound may contain amount of debris or dirt and usually is infected.	Remove the large debris and dirt. Clean the wound by water dripping from sterile cloth, or use soap and warm water; mild antiseptics and sterile dressings.	Edges of wound may be united by flamed strip of adhesive tape. Cover the area with loose dressings held by triangle or cravat bandage. Tetanus toxoid or antitoxin as required.	Infection and septicemia. Wound usually heals with very unsightly scar if not properly sutured.
Puncture.	Accidental or intentional piercing of body with a pointed object.	Tissues are pierced. Small opening through the tissues providing an excellent course or inlet for infection.	Area usually manifests no bleeding. Trauma of tissues usually evident.	Puncture site is very small. Object usually withdrawn with fair amount of ease.	Probe the wound very carefully to enlarge bore for irrigation with antiseptic solutions. Tetanus toxoid or antitoxin as required. Treatment for prevention of gas gangrene may be required.	Cover the area with sterile dressings and triangle or cravat bandage.	Infection of the anaerobic type (Tetanus bacillus) and septicemia.
Stab.	Injury by a blunt or pointed object, incurred during a fight or acquired by a fall or push.	Size of hole in the tissues varies with the size of the instrument. Foreign material and pathogenic bacteria of anaerobic nature are usually introduced.	Evidence of the instrument that was used, such as knife, ice pick, etc. Victim shows pallor, syncope, and later collapse.	Large, very deep puncture site. Instrument may still be in wound. Victim may be pinned to an object by the force of the blow.	Cleanse and irrigate the wound when possible. Irrigation and inclusion of antiseptic drain or wet dressings. Early use of antitetanic sera. Tetanus toxoid or antitoxin as required.	Keep patient very quiet with head and chest slightly elevated. Treat for shock. If chest is involved, watch T.P.R. and blood pressure.	Internal hemorrhage from, or damage to, organs underlying site of wound, such as puncture and collapse of lung, abdominal visceral injury, or severance of a nerve. Pulmonary hemorrhage. Infection of body by anaerobic organisms.

Directory of Poison Control Centers*
United States and Canada

State and province listing of Centers providing information on a 24-hour basis concerning treatment or prevention of accidents involving poisonous substances.

United States and Territories

State	Telephone, Coordinator, and Address
Alabama	(205) 265-2341 Division of Accident Prevention State Department of Public Health Montgomery 36104
Alaska	(907) 586-6311 Child Health State Department of Health and Welfare Juneau 99801
Arizona	(602) 884-0111 Professor of Pharmacology University of Arizona Tucson 85721
Arkansas	(501) 661-2242 Health Educator State Board of Health Little Rock 72201
California	(415) 843-7900 Emergency Health Services Unit Department of Public Health Berkeley 94704
Canal Zone	2-2600 Poison Information Center Gorgas Hospital Balboa Heights
Colorado	(303) 388-6111 Emergency Health Services State Department of Public Health Denver 80220
Connecticut	(203) 566-3456 Technical Director State Department of Health Hartford 06115
Delaware	(302) 655-3389 Poison Information Service 501 W. 14th St. Wilmington 19899
District of Columbia	Poison Control Center Children's Hospital 13th & W Streets, N.W. Washington 20009

* Additional listing may be obtained by writing (in U.S.A.) to Division of Hazardous Substances and Poison Control, Food and Drug Administration, U.S. Department of Health, Education, and Welfare, Washington, D.C. 20204 (telephone (202) 496-7606) or (in Canada) to Food and Drug Directorate, National Health and Welfare Department, Ottawa, Ontario, Canada.

Florida	(904) 354-3961 Emergency Medical Services Program Department of Health and Rehabilitative Services Jacksonville 32201
Georgia	(404) 656-4839 Injury Control, EHS Department of Public Health Atlanta 30334
Guam	42-4158 Department of Public Health and Social Services Agana 96910
Hawaii	(808) 531-7776 Injury Control Branch Department of Health Honolulu 96801
Idaho	(208) 384-2494 Poison Control Coordinator State Department of Health Boise 83701
Illinois	(217) 525-7747 Bureau of Hazardous Substances and Poison Control Department of Public Health Springfield 62706
Indiana	(317) 633-5490 Hazardous Products Section Division of Drug Control State Board of Health Indianapolis 46206
Iowa	(515) 281-5787 Division of Maternal & Child Health Department of Health Des Moines 50319
Kansas	(913) 296-3708 Food and Drug Division State Department of Health Topeka 66612
Kentucky	(502) 564-4830 Division of Health State Department of Health Frankfort 40601
Louisiana	(504) 527-5822 Division of Public Health Education State Department of Health New Orleans 70160
Maine	(207) 623-1511 Commissioner Department of Health & Welfare Augusta 04330
Maryland	(301) 382-2668 Division of Maternal and Child Health State Department of Health Baltimore 21201

Massachusetts	(617) 727-2700 Commissioner of Public Health State Department of Public Health Boston 02133
Michigan	(517) 373-1320 Chief, Developmental Service Department of Public Health Lansing 48914
Minnesota	(612) 378-1150 Poison Information Center State Department of Health Minneapolis 55440
Mississippi	(601) 354-6650 Division of Preventable Disease Control State Board of Health Jackson 39205
Missouri	(314) 635-4111 Accident Prevention Program Missouri Division of Health Jefferson City 65101
Montana	(406) 449-2544 State Department of Health Helena 59601
Nebraska	(402) 477-5211 Division of Laboratories State Department of Health Lincoln 68509
Nevada	(702) 882-7458 Bureau of Preventive Medicine Department of Health & Welfare Carson City 89701
New Hampshire	(603) 225-6611 Division of Maternal & Child Health & Crippled Children's Services Department of Health & Welfare Concord 03301
New Jersey	(609) 292-5616 State Department of Health Trenton 08625
New Mexico	(505) 827-2663 Food Protection Unit, Health and Social Services Department of Public Health Santa Fe 87501
New York	(518) 744-2121 Bureau of Maternal and Child Health State Department of Health Albany 12208
North Carolina	(919) 829-3446 Accident Prevention Section Division of Epidemiology State Board of Health Raleigh 27602

North Dakota	(701) 224-2348 Injury Control Program State Department of Health Bismarck 58501
Ohio	(614) 469-2544 Accident Prevention Unit Department of Health Columbus 43216
Oklahoma	(405) 427-6232 Laboratory Services and Communicable Disease Control State Department of Health Oklahoma City 73111
Oregon	(503) 228-9181 Poison Control Registry Pediatrics Department University of Oregon Medical School Portland 97201
Pennsylvania	(717) 787-6436 Drug Program Consultant Division of Drug Control State Department of Health Harrisburg 17120
Puerto Rico	(809) 765-4800, 765-0615 University of Puerto Rico Rio Piedras 00928
Rhode Island	(401) 521-7100 Division of Public Health, Education & Research State Department of Health Providence 02903
South Carolina	(803) 758-5664 Bureau of Community Health Services State Board of Health Columbia 29201
South Dakota	(605) 224-5911 State Department of Health Pierre 57501
Tennessee	(615) 741-3644 Division of Preventive Health Services State Department of Public Health Nashville 37219
Texas	(512) 453-6631 Industrial Hygiene Program Division of Occupational Health State Department of Health Austin 78756
Utah	(801) 328-6191 Bureau of Disease Prevention State Division of Health Salt Lake City 84113
Vermont	(802) 223-2311 Poison Control Department of Health Montpelier 05602

Directory of Poison Control Centers (*Continued*)

Virgin Islands	(809) 774-1321, ext. 275 Drug and Narcotic Control Department of Health St. Thomas 00801
Virginia	(703) 644-4111 State Department of Health Richmond 23219
Washington	(206) 753-5871 Maternal and Child Health Section State Department of Health Olympia 98502
West Virginia	(304) 348-2971 Administrative Assistant State Department of Health Charleston 25305
Wisconsin	(608) 266-1511 Safety Consultant Department of Health and Social Services Madison 53701
Wyoming	(307) 777-7275 Division of Preventive Medicine State Department of Public Health Cheyenne 82001

Canada

Province	*Telephone and Address*
Alberta	(403) 439-5911 Poison Treatment Centre University Hospital Edmonton
British Columbia	(604) 386-3131 Royal Jubilee Victoria
Manitoba	(204) 775-8311 Winnipeg Children's Hospital Winnipeg
New Brunswick	(506) 475-3351 Victoria Public Hospital Fredericton
Newfoundland (and Labrador)	(709) 722-5100 The Dr. Chas. A. Janeway Child Health Centre St. John's (Newfoundland) (709) 944-2632 Capt. Wm. Jackman Memorial Hospital Labrador City
Nova Scotia	(506) 422-8441 The Izaak Walton Killam Hospital for Children Halifax

Ontario	(705) 461-8272 East General and Orthopaedic Hospital Toronto
Prince Edw. Island	(902) 894-5561 Charlottetown Hospital Charlottetown
Quebec	(418) 529-8711 Hopital de L'Enfant-Jesus Quebec City
Saskatchewan	(306) 522-1811 Regina General Hospital Regina

The Interpreter

Five Language Outline
for
Basic Medical Diagnosis and Treatment
in a
Foreign Language
English, Spanish, Italian, French, German

Table of Contents

Introduction

When attempting to communicate with a person whose language is foreign to you it is important to establish that while you may be able to say a few words in his language you will not be able to understand his replies. He may need to use signs in replying. The following paragraphs are given for your convenience in explaining your language difficulty to the patient.

Hello. I want to help you. I do not speak (English) but will use this book to ask you some questions. I will not be able to understand your spoken answers. Please respond by shaking your head or raising one finger to indicate "no"; nod your head or raise two fingers to indicate "yes."

(Spanish)

(Translation)

Saludos. Quiere ayudarlo. Yo no hablo español, pero voy a usar este libro para hacerle algunas preguntas. No voy a poder entender sus contestas verbalmente. Favor de responder meniando la cabeza o levantando un dedo para contestar -no.- Para indicar -si- menee la cabeza para arriva y para abajo o levante dos dedos.

(Phonetic)

Sah-loo'dohs. Ki-air'oh ah-joo-dar'loh. Joh noh ah'bloh es'panyohl, pair'oh voy ah oo-sawr' es'tay lee'broh pahr'ah ah-sair'lay ahl-goo'nahs pray-goon'tahs. Noh voy ah poh-dair' en-ten-dair' soos kohn-tes'tahs vair-bahl-men'tay. Fah-vohr' day ray-spohn-dair' men-ih-ahn'doh lah kah-bay'thah oh lay-vahn-tahn'doh oon day'doh pahr'ah kohn-tes-tahr' noh. Pahr'ah in'dih-kahr see' men-ay'ay lah kah-bay'thah pahr'ah ahr-ree'vah ee pahr'ah ah-bah'hoh oh lay-vahn'tay dohs day'dos.

(Italian)

(Translation)

Buon giorno. Vi voglio aiutare. Non parlo Italiano ma userò questo libro per chiederui qualche domande. Non potrò comprendere levostre risposte. Per favore rispondete da scuòtere latesta. Alzare un dito per indicare "no"; muovete lavostra testa su e qiu o alzate due diti per indicare "si."

(Phonetic)

Bwon jih-or'noh. Vee vol'yoh ah-yoo-tar'day. Non par'loh ee-towl-ee-ah'noh mah oo-say'roh kwes'toh lee'broh pehr kee-dair'vee kwall-kay' doh-mahn'day. Non poh'throh kohm-prehn'deh-ray lay-vohl'stray reh-spoh'stih. Pehr fah-vohr'ay ray-spohn-day'tay dah shah-oh-tair'ay lah-tes'tah. Ahl-zah'ray oon dee'toh pehr in-dee-kar'ay noh; moo-eh-vay'tay lah-vahs'trah tes'tay soo ay joo ah ahl-zah'tay doo'ay dee'tee pehr in-dee-kar'ay see.

(French)

(Translation)

Bonjour. Je désire vous aider. Je ne parle pas de français, mais j'emploierai ce livre pour vous poser des questions. Je ne pourrai pas comprendre vos réponses parlées. Veuillez répondre en secourant la tête ou en levant un doigt pour indiquer "non"; movez la tête en haut et en bas ou levez deux doigts pour indiquer "oui."

(Phonetic)

Bon-zhoor'. Zheh day-zeer' voo say-day'. Zheh neh parl pah deh frahn-say', may zhahm-ploy-air-ay' seh lee'vrah por voo poh-say' day kehs-tih-on'. Zheh neh poo-ray' pa kahm-prahn'drah voh ray-pahns' par-lay'. Vwee-ay ray-pahn'drah ahn seh-koo-rahnt la teht oo ahn lehv-ahnt un dwoit por ahn-dee-kay' noh; moh-vay la teht ahn hoh eh ahn bah oo leh-vay duh dwoit por ahn-dee-kay' wee.

(German)

(Translation)

Hallo! Ich möchte Ihnen helfen. Ich spreche nicht deutsch aber ich werde dieses Buch benützten um Sie einiges zu fragen. Ich werde ihre Antworten nicht verstehen. Deshalb antworten Sie mir indem Sie ihren Kopf schütteln oder heben Sie ihren Finger um nein auszudrücken; nicken Sie mit dem Kopf oder heben Sie zwei Finger um ja auszudrücken.

(Phonetic)

Ha-loh! Ich möhh'tuh ee'nuhn hel'fuhn. Ich shpre'huh nihht doitsh, ah'buhr ich ver'duh dee'zuhs bookh bā-nüt'zuhn um zee ī'ni-guhs tsoo frah'guhn. Ich ver'duh ee'ruh ant'vor-tuhn nihht fer-shtay'uhn. Dās-halb' ant'vor-tuhn zee meer in-dām' zee ee'ruhn kopf shü'tln ō'der hāb'uhn zee ee'ruhn fing'uhr um nīn ows'tsoo-drük-uhn; nick'uhn zee mit dām kopf ō'der hāb'uhn zee tsvī fing'uhr um ya ows'tsoo-drük-uhn.

The Interpreter in Five Languages

GENERAL

Basic Questions and Replies

English	Spanish	Italian	French	German
Good morning.	Buenos días.	Buon giorno.	Bonjour.	Guten Morgen.
What is your name?	¿Cómo se llama?	Come vi chiamate?	Quel est votre nom?	Wie heissen Sie?
How are you?	¿Cuantos años tiene?	Che età avete?	Quel âge avez-vous?	Wie alt sind Sie?
Do you understand me?	¿Me entiendes?	Mi capisce?	Me comprenez?	Verstehen Sie mich?
Answer only …	No me conteste más que …	Rispondete solamente …	Répondez seul …	Antworten Sie nur …
Yes No	Sí No	Sì No	Oui Non	Ja Nein
What do you say?	¿Qué dice?	Che cosa dite?	Que dites-vous?	Was sagen Sie?
Speak slower.	Hable más despacio.	Parlate più adagio.	Parlez plus lentement.	Sprechen Sie langsamer.
Say it once again.	Repítalo, por favor.	Ditelo ancora una volta.	Dites cela encore une fois.	Sagen Sie das wieder.
Don't be afraid.	No tenga miedo.	Non abbiate paura.	N'ayez pas peur.	Haben Sie keine Angst.
Try to recollect.	Trate de recordarse.	Cercate di ricordarvi.	Cherchez à vous en rappeler.	Versuchen Sie sich zu erinnern.
You cannot remember?	¿No peude recordarse?	Non vi ricordate?	Vous ne vous en souvenez pas?	Können Sie sich nicht erinnern?
Come to my office.	Venga a mi oficina.	Venite al mio ufficio.	Venez à mon bureau.	Kommen Sie in meins Büro.
You will?	¿Ud. quiere?*	Volete?	Vous voulez bien?	Sie wollen?
You will not?	¿No quiere Ud.?	Non volete?	Vous ne voulez pas?	Sie wollen nicht?
You don't know?	¿No sabe?	Non sapete?	Vous ne savez pas?	Wissen Sie nicht?
It is necessary.	Es necesario.	È necessario.	C'est necéssaire.	Es ist durchaus nötig.
Is it impossible?	¿Es imposible?	È impossibile?	C'est impossible?	Ist es unmöglich?
That is right.	Sí.	Va bene.	C'est bien.	Das ist richtig.

App. 146

Show me ...	Déjeme mirar ...	Fatemi vedere i ...	Montrez-moi ...	Lassen Sie mich einsehen ...
Here There	Aquí Allí	Qui Qua	Ici Là	Hier Da
Which side?	¿En qué lado?	Quale lato?	Quel côté?	Auf welcher, Seite?
Since when?	¿Desde cuándo?	Da quando?	Depuis quand?	Seit wann?
Right	Al derecho	A dritta	A droit	Rechts
Left	A la izquierda	A sinistra	A gauche	Links
More or less	Más o menos	Più o meno	Plus ou moins	Mehr oder weniger
How long?	¿Cuánto tiempo?	Da quando tempo?	Combien de temps?	Wie lange?
Not much	No mucho	Non molto	Pas beaucoup	Nicht viel
Try again.	Tratalo otra vez.	Provateci di nuovo.	Essayez encore une fois.	Versuchen Sie es noch einmal.
Never	Nunca	Mai	Jamais	Niemals
Never mind.	Déjelo.	Non importa.	N'importe pas.	Lassen Sie es gut sein.
That will do.	Bastante.	Basta così.	C'est bien.	Das ist genug.
About how much daily?	¿Más o menos que cantidad diaramente?	Circa quanto al giorno?	Combien à peu près par jour?	Ungefähr wie viel täglich?
So much?	¿Tanto?	Tanto?	Autant?	So viel?
You must be very careful	Debe tener mucho cuidado.	Dovete usare molte precauzioni.	Vous devez prendre garde.	Sie müssen sehr vorsichtig sein.

Seasons

In the spring.	En la primavera.	Nella primavera.	Au printemps.	Im Frühjahr.
In summer.	En el verano.	Nell' estate.	En été.	Im Sommer.
In autumn.	En el otoño.	Nell' autunno.	En automne.	Im Herbst.
In winter.	En el invierno.	Nell' inverno.	En hiver.	Im Winter.

*Ud. — Usted.

The Interpreter in Five Languages (Continued)

English	Spanish	Italian	French	German
		Months		
The months	Los meses	I mesi	Les mois	Die Monate
January	enero	gennaio	janvier	Januar
February	febrero	febbraio	février	Februar
March	marzo	marzo	mars	März
April	abril	aprile	avril	April
May	mayo	maggio	mai	Mai
June	junio	giunio	juin	Juni
July	julio	luglio	juillet	Juli
August	agosto	agosto	août	August
September	septiembre	settembre	septembre	September
October	octubre	ottobre	octobre	Oktober
November	noviembre	novembre	novembre	November
December	diciembre	dicembre	decembre	Dezember
		Days of the Week		
Sunday	domingo	domenica	dimanche	Sonntag
Monday	lunes	lunedì	lundi	Montag
Tuesday	martes	martedì	mardi	Dienstag
Wednesday	miércoles	mercoledì	mercredi	Mittwoch
Thursday	jueves	giovedì	jeudi	Donnerstag
Friday	viernes	venerdì	vendredi	Freitag
Saturday	sábado	sabato	samedi	Sonnabend

Numbers and Time of Day
(office hours, age, diagnosis, treatment)

One	Uno	Uno	Un	Eins
Two	Dos	Due	Deux	Zwei
Three	Tres	Tre	Trois	Drei
Four	Cuatro	Quattro	Quatre	Vier
Five	Cinco	Cinque	Cinq	Fünf
Six	Seis	Sei	Six	Sechs
Seven	Siete	Sette	Sept	Sieben
Eight	Ocho	Otto	Huit	Acht
Nine	Nueve	Noue	Neuf	Neun
Ten	Diez	Dieci	Dix	Zehn
Twenty	Veinte	Venti	Vignt	Zwanzig
Thirty	Treinta	Trenta	Trente	Dreissig
Forty	Cuarenta	Quaranta	Quarante	Vierzig
Fifty	Cincuenta	Cinquanta	Cinquante	Fünfzig
Sixty	Sesenta	Sessanta	Soixante	Sechzig
Seventy	Setenta	Settanta	Soixante-dix	Siebzig
At 10:00	A las diez	Alle dieci	A dix heures	Um zehn Uhr
At 2:30	A las dos y media	Alle due e mezzo	A deux heures et demi	Um halb drei
Early in the morning	Temprano por la mañana	Di buon mattino	Le matin de bonne heure	Frühmorgens
In the daytime	Por el día	Nel giorno	Pendant la journée	Bei Tag
At noon	A mediodía	A mezzo giorno	A midi	Mittags
At bedtime	Al acostarse	All' ora di coricarsi	A l'heure de se coucher	Vor dem Schlafegehen
At night	Por la noche	Alla sera	Le soir	Abends
Before meals	Antes de comer	Prima del pasto	Avant les repas	Vor den Mahlzeiten
After meals	Despues de comer	Dopo il pasto	Après les repas	Nach den Mahlzeiten

The Interpreter in Five Languages (Continued)

English	Spanish	Italian	French	German
Today	Hoy	Oggi	Aujourd'hui	Heute
Tomorrow	Mañana	Domani	Demain	Morgen
Every day	Todos los días	Ogni giorno	Chaque jour	Alle Tage
Every hour	Cada hora	Ogni ora	Chaque heure	Jede Stunde
How long have you felt this way?	¿Desde cuando se siente así?	Da quanto tempo vi sentite così?	Depuis quand vous sentez-vous comme ça?	Seit wann fühlen Sie sich so?
It came all of a sudden?	¿Vino de repente?	Venne tutto ad un tratto?	C'est venu tout d'un coup?	Ist es ganz plötzlich gekommen?
For how many days or weeks?	¿Cuántos días o semanas?	Da quanti giorni o settimane?	Depuis combien de jours ou semaines?	Seit wievielen Tagen oder Wochen?
Do they come every day?	¿Los tiene todos los días?	Vi vengono tutti i giorni?	Les avez-vous tous les jours?	Kommt es jeden Tag?
At the same hour?	¿A la misma hora?	Alla stessa ora?	A la même heure?	Zur selben Stunde?
At intervals?	¿De vez en cuando?	Ad intervalli?	De temps à autre?	Dann und wann?
It will be too late.	Será demasiado tarde.	Sarà troppo tardi.	Ce sera trop tard.	Es wird zu spät sein.
Colors				
Black	Negro	Nero	Noir	Schwartz
Blue	Azul	Blu	Bleu	Blau
Green	Verde	Verde	Vert	Grün
Pink	Rosa	Rosa	Rose	Blassrot
Red	Rojo	Rosso	Rouge	Rot
White	Blanco	Blanco	Blanc	Weiss
Yellow	Amarillo	Giallo	Jaune	Gelb
Parts of Body				
In the abdomen?	En el vientre?	Nel ventre?	Dans le ventre?	Im Leib?
The ankle	El tobillo	La caviglia	La cheville	Der Fussknöchel

English	Spanish	Italian	French	German
The arm	El brazo	Il braccio	Le bras	Der Arm
The back	La espalda	Nel dorso	Le dos	Der Rücken
The bones	Los huesos	La ossa	Les os	Die Knochen
The chest	El pecho	Nel petto	La poitrine	Der Brust
The ears	Los oídos	Le orecchie	Les oreilles	Die Ohren
The elbow	El codo	Il gomito	Le coude	Der Ellenbogen
The eye	El ojo	L'occhio	L'oeil	Das Auge
The foot	El pié	Il piede	Le pied	Der Fuss
The gums	Las encias	Le gengive	Les gencives	Das Zahnfleisch
The hand	La mano	La mano	La main	Die Hand
The head	La cabeza	Nella testa	La tête	Der Kopf
The heart	La corazón	Il cuore	Le coeur	Das Herz
The leg	La pierna	La gamba	La jambe	Das Bein
The liver	El hígado	Il fegato	Le foie	Die Leber
The lungs	Los pulmones	I polmoni	Les poumons	Die Lungen
The mouth	La boca	La bocca	La bouche	Der Mund
The muscles	Los musculos	I muscoli	Les muscles	Die Muskeln
The neck	El cuello	Il collo	Le cou	Der Nacken
The nerves	Los nervios	I nervi	Les nerfs	Die Nerven
The nose	La nariz	Il naso	Le nez	Die Nase
The ribs	Las costillas	Le costole	Les côtes	Die Rippen
The shoulder blades	Las hombros	Nelle spalle	Les épaules	Die Schulterblätter
The side	El flanco	Nel fianco	Le côté	Die Seite
The skin	La piel	La pelle	La peau	Die Haut
The skull	El cerebro	El craneo	Le crâne	Der Schädel
The stomach	El estomago	Lo stomaco	L'estomac	Der Magen

The Interpreter in Five Languages (Continued)

English	Spanish	Italian	French	German
The teeth	Las dientes	La identi	Les dents	Die Zähne
The temples	Las sienes	La tempia	Les tempes	Die Schläfen
The thigh	El muslo	La coscia	La hanche	Der Oberschenkel
The throat	La garganta	La gola	La gorge	Der Hals
The thumb	El dedo pulgar	Il police	Le pouce	Der Daum
The tongue	La lengua	La lingua	La langue	Die Zunge
The wrist	La muñeca	Il polso	Le poignet	Das Handgelenk

Occupations

What work do you do?	¿Qué es su ocupación?	Che lavoro fate?	Qu'est-ce que votre travail?	Welche Arbeit tun Sie?
What work have you done?	¿Qué trabajo ha hecho?	Che lavoro avete fatto?	Qu'est ce que vous avez travaille?	Welche Arbeit haben Sie getan?
A baker	Un panadero	Un fornajo	Un boulanger	Ein Bäcker
A butcher	Un carnicero	Un macellajo	Un boucher	Ein Fleischer
A laborer	Un obrero	Un operajo	Un ouvrier	Ein Arbeiter
A mason	Un albañil	Un muratore	Un maçon	Ein Maurer
A miller	Un molinero	Un mugnaio	Un meunier	Ein Müller
A shoemaker	Un zapatero	Un calzolaio	Un cordonnier	Ein Schuhmacher
A tailor	Un sastre	Un sarto	Un tailleur	Ein Schneider

HISTORY
Family

Are you married?	¿Está Ud. casado?	Siete sposato?	Etes-vous marié?	Sind Sie verheiratet?
A widower?	¿Viudo?	Siete vedovo?	Veuf?	Ein Witwer?
A widow?	¿Viuda?	Siete vedova?	Veuve?	Eine Witwe?
Do you have children?	¿Tiene Ud. hijos?	Avete bambini?	Avez-vous des enfants?	Haben Sie Kinder?

English	Spanish	Italian	French	German
Are they still living?	¿Viven todavía?	Vivono ancora?	Vivent-ils encore?	Sind sie noch am Leben?
Do you have any sisters?	¿Tiene hermanas?	Avete sorelle?	Avez-vous des soeurs?	Haben Sie Schwestern?
Do you have any brothers?	¿Tiene hermanos?	Avete fratelli?	Avez-vous des frères?	Haben Sie Brüder?
Of what did your mother die?	¿De qué se murió su madre?	Di che è morta vostra madre?	De quoi est morte votre mère?	Woran ist Ihre Mutter gestorben?
And your father?	¿Y su padre?	E vostro padre?	Et votre père?	Und Ihr Vater?
Your grandfather?	¿Su abuelo?	Il vostro nonno?	Votre grand-père?	Ihr Grossvater?
Your grandmother?	¿Su abuela?	La votra nonna?	Votre grand-mère?	Ihre Grossmutter?

General

English	Spanish	Italian	French	German
Do you have . . . ?	¿Tiene . . . ?	Avete . . . ?	Avez-vous . . . ?	Haben Sie . . . ?
Have you ever had . . . ?	¿Ha tenido . . . ?	Avete mai avuto . . . ?	Avez-vous jamais eu . . . ?	Haben Sie je . . . gehabt?
Chills	Escalofrío	I brividi	Les frissons	Ein Fieberfrösteln
An attack of fever	Un ataque de calentura	Un attacco di febbre	Une attaque de fièvre	Ein Fieberanfall
Toothache	Dolor de dientes	Dolore di denti	Le mal aux dents	Der Zahnschmerz
Hemorrhages	Hemorragias	Emorragias	Des hémorragies	Die Blutergüsse
Nosebleeds	Hemorragia de la nariz	Emorragia nasale	Saignement du nez	Die Nasenbluten
Hoarseness	Ronquera	Raucedine	Enrouement	Die Heiserkeit

Diseases

English	Spanish	Italian	French	German
What diseases have you had?	¿Cuáles enfermedades ha tenido?	Che malattie avete avuto?	Quelles maladies avez-vous eu?	Welche Krankheiten haben Sie gehabt?
Lead poisoning	Envenenamiento por plomo	Avvelenamento da plombo	Empoisonnement causé par le plomb	Die Bleivergiftung
Liver disease	Enfermedad del hígado	Una malattia del fegato	Une maladie de foie	Eine Leberkrankheit
Measles	Sarampion	Morbillo	La rougeole	Die Masern
Pneumonia	Pulmonia	Polmonite	Pneumonie	Die Lungenentzündung
Rheumatism	Reumatismo	Reumatismo	Le rhumatisme	Der Rheumatismus

The Interpreter in Five Languages (Continued)

English	Spanish	Italian	French	German
Scarlet fever	Escarlatina	La febbre scarlattina	La fièvre scarlatine	Das Scharlachfieber
Tuberculosis	Tuberculosis	Tuberculosi	Tuberculose	Die Tuberkulose
Typhoid fever	Tifoidea	La febbre tifoide	La fièvre typhoïde	Der Typhus
A venereal disease	Una enfermidad venerea	Malattie veneree	Une maladie vénérienne	Ein Geschlechtskrankheit

EXAMINATION
General

English	Spanish	Italian	French	German
How do you feel?	¿Cómo está?	Come state?	Comment vous sentez-vous?	Wie geht es Ihnen?
Good	Bien	Bene	Bien	Gut
Bad	Mal	Male	Mal	Schlecht
Let me see ...	Déjeme ver ...	Lasciatemi vedere ...	Permettez-moi de voir ...	Lassen Sie mich sehen ...
Let me feel your pulse.	Déjeme tomar el pulso.	Lasciatemi sentire il pulso.	Permettez-moi de tâter le pulse.	Lassen Sie mich Ihren Puls fühlen.
Whisper: one, two, three.	Cuchichée: uno, dos, tres.	Dite plano: uno, due, tre.	Dites à voix basse: un, deux, trois.	Flüstern Sie: eins, zwei, drei.
Say it out loud.	A voz alta.	Ditelo ad alta voce.	Dites à haute voix.	Sagen Sie es laut.
Sit down.	Siéntese.	Sedetevi.	Asseyez-vous.	Setzen Sie sich.
Stand up.	Levántese.	Alzatevi.	Levez-vous.	Stehen Sie auf.
Can you not rise quicker?	¿No puede levantarse más rápido?	Non vi potete alzare un po' più presto?	Ne pouvez-vous pas se lever plus vite?	Können Sie sich nicht schneller erheben?
Walk a little way.	Ande algunos pasos.	Camminate un pò.	Allez quelques pas.	Gehen Sie einige Schritte.
Return; go backwards.	Vuelva; ande para atrás.	Ritornate; camminate all' indietro.	Revenez; allez en arrière.	Kommen Sie zurück; gehen Sie rückwärts.
Do you feel like falling?	¿Le parece que se va a caer?	Vi sentite come se doveste cadere?	Vous semblez-vous aller à tomber?	Ist es Ihnen als ob Sie fallen müssen?
Do you feel dizzy?	¿Tiene Ud. vertigo?	Avete delle vertigini?	Avez-vous le vertige?	Sind Sie schwindlig?

English	Spanish	Italian	French	German
Are you tired?	¿Está cansado?	Vi sentite molto stanco?	Avez-vous fatigué?	Sind Sie müde?
Have you slept well?	¿Ha dormido bien?	Avete ben dormito?	Avez-vous bien dormi?	Haben Sie gut geschlafen?
Have you any difficulty in breathing?	Tiene dificultad en respirar?	Avete nessuna difficoltà di respirare?	C'est difficile respirer?	Wird Ihnen das Atemholen schwer?
Have you lost weight?	¿Ha perdido el peso?	Siete dimagrito?	Avez-vous maigri?	Haben Sie abgenommen?
Since when have you had this eruption?	¿Desde cuando tiene esta erupción?	Da quanto tempo avete questa eruzione?	Depuis quand avez-vous cette eráption?	Seit wann haben Sie dieser Ausschlag?
Do you sweat much at night?	¿Suda mucho por la noche?	Sudate molto alla notte?	Transpirez-vous beaucoup à la nuit?	Schwitzen Sie viel in der Nacht?
Are you warm?	¿Tiene calor?	Avete caldo?	Avez-vous chaud?	Sind Sie heiss?
Are you cold?	¿Tiene frío?	Avete freddo?	Avez-vous froid?	Sind Sie kalt?
Have you been exposed much to the wet weather?	¿Se ha estado expuesto a la intemperie?	Vi siete mai esposto alla umidità?	Avez-vous été exposé au temps humide?	Sind Sie dem feuchten Wetter ausgesetzt gewesen?
Can you eat?	¿Puede comer?	Potete mangiare?	Pouvez-vous manger?	Können Sie essen?
Have you a good appetite?	¿Tiene Ud. buen apetito?	Avete buon appetito?	Avez-vous un bon appétit?	Haben Sie guten Appetit?
Are you thirsty?	¿Tiene sed?	Avete sete?	Avez-vous soif?	Haben Sie Durst?
Do you still feel very weak?	¿Se siente muy débil todavía?	Vi sentite ancora molto débole?	Vous sentez-vous encore très faible?	Fühlen Sie sich noch sehr schwach?
Had you been drinking?	¿Había tomado algo alcoholado?	Avevate bevuto?	Est-ce que vous-avez bu quelleque chose alcoolique?	Waren Sie angetrunken?
Are you a drinking man?	¿Toma Ud. algo de alcohol de costumbre?	Avete l'abit di bevere?	Buvez-vous des choses alcooliques d'habitude?	Sind Sie Trinker?
Are you nervous?	¿Está Ud. nervioso?	¿Siete nervoso?	Etes-vous nerveux?	Sind Sie nervös?
When were you first taken sick?	¿Cuándo empezó esta enfermedad?	Quando vi siete ammalato la prima volta?	Depuis quand cette maladie a-t-elle commencé?	Wann hat diese Krankheit begonnen?
How did this illness begin?	¿Cómo empezó esta enfermedad?	Come ha incominciato questa malattia?	Comment cette maladie a-t-elle commencé?	Wie hat diese Krankheit begonnen?

The Interpreter in Five Languages (*Continued*)

English	Spanish	Italian	French	German
Did you take anything for it?	¿Tomó algo pare mejorarla?	Avete preso qualche cosa per curarvi?	Avez-vous pris quelque chose pour cela?	Haben Sie etwas dafür genommen?
Have you taken the medicine?	¿Ha tomado Ud. la medicina?	Avete preso la medicina?	Avez-vous pris la médicine?	Haben Sie die Medizin genommen?
A wound	Una herida	Una piaga	Une plaie	Eine Wunde
Are you subject to them?	¿Se le pasa mucho?	Ne siete soggetto?	Etes-vous sujet?	Haben Sie dieselben häufig?
Did a dog bite you?	¿Le mordío un perro?	Vi ha morsicato un cane?	Vous a-t-il mordu un chien?	Hat Sie ein Hund gebissen?
Did a fly sting you?	¿Le picó una mosca?	Vi ha punto una mosca?	Une mouche vous a-t-elle piqué?	Hat Sie eine Fliege gestochen?
Did you prick yourself with a pin?	¿Se ha picado con un alfiler?	Vi siete punto con una spilla?	Vous êtes-vous piqué avec une épingle?	Haben Sie sich mit einer Stecknadel gestochen?
Did you burn yourself?	¿Se quemó?	Vi siete bruciato?	Vous êtes-vous brulé?	Haben Sie sich verbrannt?
Did you sprain your foot?	¿Se torció el pie?	Vi avete dislocato il piede?	Vous êtes-vous foulé le pied?	Haben Sie Ihren Fuss verstaucht?

Pain

English	Spanish	Italian	French	German
Have you any pain?	¿Tiene dolor?	Avete dolori?	Avez-vous des douleurs?	Haben Sie Schmerzen?
Where does it hurt?	¿Dónde le duele?	Dove che te fa mallo?	Où avez-vous mal?	Wo haben Sie Schmerzen?
Do you have pain here?	¿Le duele aquí?	Avete dolori qui?	Avez-vous mal par ici?	Haben Sie Schmerzen hier?
Do you have a pain in your side?	¿Le duele el costado?	Avete dolori al fianco?	Avez-vous mal au côté?	Haben Sie Seitenschmerzen?
Show me where.	Enséñeme donde.	Mostratemi dove.	Montrez-moi où.	Zeigen Sie mir wo.
What did you feel in the beginning?	¿Qué sentía cuando empezo?	Che sentivate prima?	Qu'avez-vous senti au commencement?	Was haben Sie anfangs gespürt?
Shooting pains?	¿Dolores agudos?	Dei dolori acuti?	Des douleurs percantes?	Stechende Schmerzen?
As if one were pricking you with pins?	¿Como si estuvieran picandole con alfileres?	Come se fossero delle spille?	Comme on vous piquâit avec des épingles?	Als ob man Sie mit Stecknadeln stäche?

English	Spanish	Italian	French	German
Did you feel much pain at the time?	¿Le dolía mucho luego?	Avete sentito molto dolore allora?	Avez-vous eu des douleurs alors?	Haben Sie gleich damals arge Schmerzen gespürt?
Is it worse now?	¿Está peor ahora?	È peggio ora?	Est-ce que c'est epire maintenant?	Ist es jetzt schlimmer?
Does it still pain you?	¿Le duele todavía?	Fa male ancora?	Vous fait-elle encore mal?	Schmerzt er doch?
Do you still have that heavy pain?	¿Le duele mucho todavía?	Avete ancora quel dolore pesante?	Avez-vous encore du mal pesante?	Haben Sie noch den drückenden Schmerz?
Does it pain you to breathe?	¿Le duele respirar?	Vi fa male di respirare?	Est-ce qu'il vous fait mal a respire?	Spüren Sie Schmerzen beim Atmen?

Examination of Arms and Hands

English	Spanish	Italian	French	German
Let me see your hand.	Enséñeme la mano.	Fatemi vedere la vostra mano.	Montrez-moi la main.	Zeigen Sie mir Ihre Hand.
Have you no power in it?	¿No tiene fuerza en la mano?	Non avete forza nella mano?	Est-il complètement inerte?	Ist sie ganz kraftlos?
Grasp my hand.	Apriete mi mano.	Stringete la mia mano.	Serrez-moi la main.	Drücken Sie mir die Hand.
Can you not do it better than that?	¿No puede hacerlo más fuerte?	Non potete farlo meglio?	Vous ne pouvez serrer plus fort que cela?	Können Sie nicht fester greifen?
Your arm feels paralysed?	¿Le parece que el brazo está paralizado?	Vi sentite il braccio paralizzato?	Est-ce que le bras il vous paraît être paralysé?	Ihr Arm erscheint Ihnen gelähmt?
Raise your arm.	Levante el brazo.	Alzate il vostro braccio.	Levez le bras.	Heben Sie den Arm.
Raise it more.	Más alto.	Ancora di più.	Plus haut.	Höher.
Now the other.	Ahora el otro.	Adesso l'altro.	Maintenant l'autre.	Jetzt den andern.
Since when is your arm so powerless?	¿Desde cuando no tenía fuerza en el brazo?	Da quando il vostro braccio e senza forza?	Depuis quand votre bras a-t-il perdu la force?	Seit wann ist Ihr Arm so kraftlos?
Had you been sleeping on your arm?	¿Ha dormido encima del brazo?	Avete dormito col braccio sotto la testa?	Vous êtes-vous endormi sur votre bras?	Sind Sie auf Ihrem Arm eingeschlafen?

Examination of Ears

English	Spanish	Italian	French	German
Do you have ringing in the ears?	¿Tiene el campaneo en los oídos?	Vi tentennano le orecchie?	Avez-vous des bourdonnements d'oreilles?	Haben Sie Ohrenbrausen?

The Interpreter in Five Languages (*Continued*)

English	Spanish	Italian	French	German
Do you have discharge from the ears?	¿Le sale cosas de los oídos?	Vi sorte umore dalle orecchie?	La matière vous coule-t-elle des oreilles?	Eitern Ihre Ohren?
The hearing	El oído	L'udito	L'ouie	Das Gehör
Is it affected?	¿Está afectado?	È ammalato?	Est-elle affectée?	Ist es angegriffen?

Examination of Eyes

English	Spanish	Italian	French	German
Look up.	Mire para arriba.	Guardate sù.	Regardez en haut.	Schauen Sie hinauf.
Look down.	Mire para abajo.	Guardate abbasso.	Regardez en bas.	Schauen Sie hinunter.
Look toward your nose.	Mire a la nariz.	Guardatevi il naso.	Regardez au nez.	Schauen Sie auf Ihre Nase.
Look at me.	Míreme.	Guardateveme.	Regardez-moi.	Sehen Sie mich an.
Can you see what is on the wall?	¿Puede ver lo que está en el pared?	Potete vedere che cosa è questo nel muro?	Pouvez-vous voir ce que c'est sur le mur?	Können Sie sehen was hier an der Wand ist?
You cannot?	¿No puede?	Non potete dire?	Vous ne pouvez pas?	Können Sie es nicht erkennen?
Can you see it now?	¿Ya puede verlo?	Potete vederlo adesso?	Le voyez-vous maintenant?	Können Sie es jetzt sehen?
And now?	¿Y ahora?	Ed ora?	Et maintenant?	Und nun?
What is it?	¿Qué es ésto?	Che cosa è?	Qu'est-ce que c'est?	Was ist es?
Tell me what number it is?	Dígame que es el numero.	Ditemi che numero è.	Dites-moi quel est le numéro.	Sagen Sie mir welche Nummer es ist.
Tell me what letter it is.	Dígame que es la letra.	Ditemi che lettra è.	Dites-moi quelle est la lettre.	Nennen Sir mir diesen Buchstaben.
Do you see things through a mist?	¿Ve las cosas por una niebla?	Vedete cose come se fossero fra la nobbia?	Voyez-vous les choses a travers un brouillard?	Sehen Sie Alles durch einen Nebel?
Can you see clearly?	¿Puede ver claramente?	Potete vedere chiaro?	Voyez-vous clarement?	Sehen Sie klar?
Better at a distance?	¿Mejor a la distancia?	Meglio distanza?	Mieux à distance?	Besser aus einer Entfernung?
Do your eyes water a good deal?	¿Le lagrimean mucho los ojos?	Vi lacrimano gli occhi molto?	Pluerent-ils les yeux beaucoup?	Tränen Ihre Augen stark?

App. 158

English	Spanish	Italian	French	German
Can't you open your eye?	¿No puede abrir el ojo?	Non potete aprire il vostro occhio?	Ne pouvez-vous pas ouvrir l'oeil?	Können Sie Ihr Auge nicht öffnen?
Do not try to open it when you awaken.	No trate de abrir los ojos al dispertarse.	Non forzate ad aprirlo nella mattina dopo il sonno.	N'essayez pas de l'ouvrir en se réveillent.	Versuchen Sie nicht, es beim Aufwachen zu öffnen.
Did anything get into your eye?	¿Le entró algo en el ojo?	Vi è entrata qualche cosa nel l'occhio?	Est-ce que quelque chose il vous entré a l'oeil?	Ist Ihnen etwas ins Auge geflogen?
Do you sometimes see things double?	¿Ve las cosas en doble de vez en cuando?	Vedete qualche volta le cose al doppio?	Voyez-vous les choses en double parfois?	Sehen Sie manchmal doppelt?
Does the eyeball feel as if it were swollen?	¿Le parece el ojo hinchado?	Vi pare come se il globo dell'occhio fosse gonfio?	L'oeil vous semble-t-il gonflé?	Fühlt sich das Auge wie angeschwollen?
You must be careful not to go out yet.	Tenga cuidado de no salir todavía.	Dovete aver cura a non andar fuori.	Ayez soin de ne pas sortir.	Sie dürfen durchaus noch nicht ausgehen.
It would harm your eyes.	Le haría daño a los ojos.	Vi farà gran male ai vostri occhi.	Cela nuirait à vos yeux.	Es würde Ihren Augen schaden.
Since when has your eyesight failed you?	¿Desde cuando ha disminuído su vista?	Da quando tempo la vostra vista si è diminuita?	Depuis quand votre vue s'est-elle diminuée?	Seit wann hat Ihre Sehkraft nachgelassen?

Gastrointestinal Study

English	Spanish	Italian	French	German
Do you have stomach cramps?	¿Tiene calambres del estomago?	Avete dolori acuti di stomaco?	Avez-vous des crampes d'estomac?	Haben Sie Magenkrämpfe?
Since when is your tongue that color?	¿Desde cuando tiene la lengua ese color?	Da quando tempo la vostra lingua è di questo colore?	Depuis quand la langue a-t-elle cette couleur?	Seit wann hat Ihre Zunge jene Farbe?
Have you a pain in the pit of your stomach?	¿Tiene dolor en la boca del estomago?	Avete dolore nella bocca dello stomaco?	Avez-vous des douleurs dans le creux de l'estomac?	Haben Sie Schmerzen in der Magengrube?
Nausea	La nausea	La nausea	La nausée	Die Übelkeit
Does eating make you vomit?	¿El comer le hace vomitar?	Mangiare vi fa vomitare?	Rendez-vous ce que vous mangez?	Erbrechen Sie nachdem Sie gegessen haben?
How are your stools?	¿Cómo son las evacuaciónes del cuerpo?	Come andate del corpo?	Comment vont les selles?	Wie ist der Stuhlgang?

The Interpreter in Five Languages (Continued)

English	Spanish	Italian	French	German
Are they regular?	¿Son regulares?	Andate regolarmente?	Allez-vous aux selles regulierment?	Ist er regelmässig?
Have you noticed their color?	¿Se fijó en el color?	Vi siete accorto di che colore?	Avez-vous remarqué la couleur des selles?	Haben Sie auf die Farbe geachtet?
Are you constipated?	¿Está estreñido?	Siete stitico?	Etes-vous constipé?	Haben Sie Verstopfung?
Do you have diarrhea?	¿Tiene diarrea?	Avete diarrea?	Avez-vous la diarrhée	Haben Sie Durchfall?
Do you pass any blood?	¿Pasa sangre?	Fate del sangue?	Y-a-t-il du sange?	Ist Blut im Stuhl?
Have you vomited?	¿Ha vomitado?	Avete vomitato?	Avez-vous vomi?	Haben Sie erbrechen?
Do you still vomit?	¿Vomita todavía?	Vomitate ancora?	Vomissez-vous encore?	Erbrechen Sie noch immer?
Do you vomit blood?	¿Vomita sangre?	Vomitate sangue?	Vomissez-vous du sange?	Erbrechen Sie das Blut?
Is it of a dark or bright red color?	¿Es de color rojo oscuro o claro?	È esso nero o pure rosso?	Cela a-t-elle une couleur fonçée ou claire?	Ist es dunkel oder hellrot?

Examination of Head

English	Spanish	Italian	French	German
How does your head feel?	¿Cómo va la cabeza?	Come vi sentite il capo?	Comment va la tête?	Wie geht es Ihrem Kopf?
Your memory	Su memoria	La vuestra memoria	Votre mémoire	Ihr Gedächnis
Is it good?	¿Está buena?	È essa buona?	Est-elle bonne?	Ist es gut?
Have you any pain in the head?	¿Le duele la cabeza?	Avete dolori di testa?	Avez-vous mal à la tête?	Haben Sie Kopfschmerzen?
Did you fall and how did you fall?	¿Se cayó, y cómo se cayó?	Siete caduto, e come siete caduto?	Etes-vous tombé et comment êtes-vous tombé?	Sind Sie gefallen und wie sind Sie gefallen?
Did you faint?	¿Se desmayó?	Siete svenuto?	Vous êtes-vous évanoui?	Sind Sie ohnmächtig geworden?
Have you ever had fainting spells?	¿Ha tenido los desmayos?	Siete mai svenuto regolarmente?	Avez-vous jamais eu des évanouissments?	Haben Sie je Ohmmachtsanfälle gehabt?

Kidney Study

English	Spanish	Italian	French	German
Have you any difficulty passing water?	¿Tiene dificultad en orinar?	Avete difficoltà nell' urinare?	Avez-vous de la difficulté à uriner?	Haben Sie Schwierigkeiten beim Wasserlassen?
Do you pass water involuntarily?	¿Orina sin querer?	Urinate involontariamente?	Urinez-vous sans le vouloir?	Lassen Sie den Harn ohne es zu wollen?
Are any of your limbs swollen?	¿Tiene algunas partes hinchadas?	Vi sentite gonfio in qualche parte?	Avez-vous des membres gonflés?	Ist irgend eines Ihrer Glieder geschwollen?
How long have they been swollen like this?	¿Desde cuándo estan hinchados asf?	Da quanto tempo che li avete cosi gonfi?	Depuis quand sont-ils gonflés comme ça?	Seit wann sind sie so angeschwollen?
Were they ever swollen before?	¿Habían estado hinchados antes?	Li avete avuto mai gonfi prima?	Ont-ils jamais été gonflés comme ça?	Sind sie je früher so angeschwollen gewesen?

Examination of Throat and Mouth

English	Spanish	Italian	French	German
Cough.	Tosa Ud.	Tossite.	Toussez.	Husten Sie.
Cough again.	Tosa otra vez.	Tossite ancora.	Toussez encore une fois.	Husten Sie noch einmal.
Open your mouth.	Abra la boca.	Aprite la bocca.	Ouvrez la bouche.	Öffnen Sie den Mund.
Does it hurt you to open your mouth?	¿Le duele al abrir la boca?	Vi fa male di aprire la bocca?	Vous fait-il mal ouvrir la bouche?	Spüren Sie Schmerzen wenn Sie den Mund öffnen?
Since when do you cough?	¿Desde cuando tosa Ud?	Da quanto tempo avete la tosse?	Depuis quand avez-vous la toux?	Seit wann husten Sie?
You cough a little?	¿Tose poco?	Tossite solo poco?	Toussez-vous un peu?	Husten Sie ein wenig?
Take a deep breath.	Tome un aliento profundo.	Prendete un gran respiro.	Prenez une respiration profonde.	Atmen Sie tief.
Do you expectorate much?	¿Escupe mucho?	Sputate molto?	Crochez-vous beaucoup?	Spucken Sie viel aus?
What is the color of your expectorations?	¿De qué color es el escupe?	Che colore ha il vostro escupe?	De quelle couleur est-elle votre expectoration?	Welche Farbe hat der Speichel?
Does your tongue feel swollen?	¿Le parece la lengua hinchada?	Ve la sentite gonfia?	Est-ce que la langue vous paraît gonflée?	Fühlt sich Ihre Zunge wie angeschwollen?
Do you have a sore throat?	¿Le duele la garganta?	Avete mal di gola?	Avez-vous mal à la gorge?	Haben Sie Halsschmerzen
Does it hurt to swallow?	¿Le duele cuando traga?	Vi fa male d'ingojare?	Avez-vous mal a avaler?	Spüren Sie Schmerzen beim Schlucken?

The Interpreter in Five Languages (*Continued*)

English	Spanish	Italian	French	German
		TREATMENT **General**		
It is nothing serious.	No es nada grave.	Non è nulla.	Ce n'est rien de grave.	Es ist nichts ernstliches.
You will get better.	Ud. mejorará.	Vi sentirete meglio.	Vous améliorerez.	Es wird besser werden.
Do exactly as I tell you.	Haga exactamente lo que digo.	Fate esattamente ciò che io vi dico.	Faites exactement ce que je vous dis.	Tun Sie genau wie ich Ihnen sage.
Take a bath.	Tome un baño.	Prendete un bagno.	Prenez un bain.	Nehmen Sie ein Bad.
A sponge bath	Un baño con esponja	Un bagno con la spunga	Un bain à l'éponge	Ein Schwamm Bad
A bran bath	Un baño con salvado	Un bagno con crusca	Un bain au son	Ein Kleie Bad
A soda bath	Un baño con soda	Un bagno con soda	Un bain à la soude	Ein Soda Bad
Bathe with hot water.	Báñese con agua caliente.	Bagnate con acqua calda.	Baignez avec de l'eau chaude.	Baden Sie mit heissem Wasser.
Bathe with cold water.	Báñese con agua fría.	Bagnate con acqua fredda.	Baignez avec de l'eau froide.	Baden Sie mit kaltem Wasser.
Bathe with alcohol.	Báñese con alcohol.	Bagnate con lo spirito.	Baignez avec de l'alcohol.	Baden Sie mit Alkohol.
Paint the swelling with this.	Pinte el hinchazón con esto.	Dovete pitturare il gonfiore con questo.	Vous devez peindre l'enflure avec ceci.	Pinseln Sie die Geschwulst damit.
I will use electricity.	Usaré electricidad.	Userò dell'electricità.	Je utiliserai d'electricité.	Ich werde elektrischen Strom anwenden.
Apply bandage to . . .	Ponga un bendaje a . . .	Mettete una fasciatura . . .	Mettez un bandage à . . .	Nehmen Sie Bandagen . . .
Apply ointment	Aplíquese unguento.	Applicate un unguento.	Appliquez un onguent.	Verwenden Sie Salbe.
Keep very quiet.	Estese muy quieto.	State tranquillo.	Restez tranquille.	Verhalten Sie sich sehr ruhig.
You must not speak.	No debe hablar.	Non dovete parlare.	Vous ne devez pas parler.	Sie dürfen nicht sprechen.
Swallow small pieces of ice.	Trague pedacitos de hielo.	Ingoiate dei piccoli pezzettini di ghiaccio	Avalez des petits morceaux de glace.	Schlucken kleine Eisstücke.

Diet

English	Spanish	Italian	French	German
In a few days you may eat food.	Dentro de algunas días se puede comer algo.	In pochi giorni potrete mangiare.	Dedans quelques jours vous pouvez manger.	In einigen Tagen dürfen Sie essen.
And remain on diet.	Y quédese en diéta.	E rimanere a dièta.	Et suivez un régime.	Und Diät halten.
You may eat ...	Se puede comer ...	Potete mangiare ...	Vous pouvez manger ...	Sie dürfen essen ...
Two eggs	Dos huevos	Un paio d'uova	Quelques oeufs	Ein paar Eier
Toast	Pan tostado	Il pane abbrustolito	Du toast	Geröstetes Brot
Bread	Pan	Pane	Du pain	Das Brot
Oysters	Ostras	Delle óstriche	Des huîtres	Die Austern
Chicken	Pollo	Pollame	Du poulet	Das Huhn
You may drink icewater.	Se puede tomar agua con hielo.	Potete bevere acqua ghiacciata.	Vous pouvez boir de l'eau glacée.	Sie dürfen Eiswasser trinken.
Milk	Leche	Latte	Du lait	Das Milch
Tea	Té	Il té	Du thé	Der Tee
Coffee	Café	Il caffè	Du café	Der Kaffee
Chocolate	Chocolate	La cioccolatta	Du chocolat	Die Schokolade
Beef bouillon	Caldo de carne	Brodo	Le bouillon	Die Bouillon

Operation

English	Spanish	Italian	French	German
An operation will be necessary.	Habrá que operarse.	Una operazione è necessaria.	Il faut que opérer.	Eine Operation ist notwendig.
We will operate ...	Operaremos ...	Noe operiamo ...	Nous opererons ...	Wir werden operieren ...

Medication
(use with numbers and time of day)

English	Spanish	Italian	French	German
I will give you something for that.	Le daré algo por éso.	Vi darò qualche cosa per questo.	Je vous donnerai quelque chose pour cela.	Ich werde Ihnen etwas dafür geben.
I will leave a prescription.	Le dejaré una receta.	Lascerò una ricetta.	Je laisserai une ordonnance.	Ich werde Ihnen ein Rezept lassen.

The Interpreter in Five Languages (Continued)

English	Spanish	Italian	French	German
Use it regularly.	Tomele con regularidad.	Usatelo regolarmente.	En prennez régulièrment.	Gebrauchen Sie es regelmässig.
Take one teaspoonfull three times daily (in water).	Tome una cucharita tres veces al día (con agua).	Bevetene un cucciaio tre volte al giorno (nell' acqua).	Prenez-en une cuillerée trois fois par jour (avec de l'eau).	Nehmen Sie einen Teelöffel voll dreimal täglich (im Wasser).
Gargle.	Haga gargaras.	Gargarizzate.	Gargarisez.	Gurgeln Sie.
Use injection	Tomar una inyección.	Injettate.	Injectez-vous.	Injizieren Sie
Take a purgative.	Tome una purga.	Un purgativo	Un purgatif	Nehmen Sie ein Abführmittel.
A pill	Una pildora	Una pinola	Une pilule	Eine Pille
A powder	Un polvo	Una polvere	Une poudre	Ein Pulver
Drop into one eye.	Vierta gotas en un ojo.	Fate sgocciolare nell' occhio	Laissez dégoutter dans un oeil.	Träufeln Sie in das eine Auge.
Drop into each eye.	Vierta gotas en cada ojo.	Fate sgocciolare in ciascun occhio.	Laissez dégoutter dans chaque oeil.	Träufeln Sie in beide Augen.